Optum

ence

DRG Desk Reference

The ultimate resource for improving MS-DRG assignment practices

2024

optumcoding.com

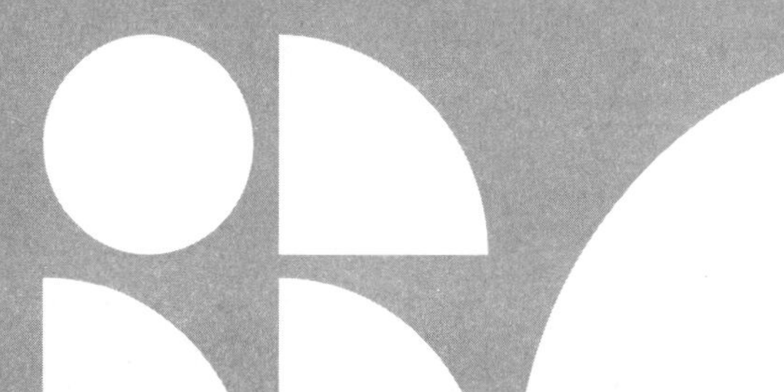

Notice

DRG Desk Reference has been prepared based upon subjective medical judgment and upon the information available as of the date of publication. This publication is designed to provide accurate and authoritative information in regard to the subject covered, and every reasonable effort has been made to ensure the accuracy of the information contained within these pages. *DRG Desk Reference* serves only as a guide. Optum, its employees, agents, and staff make no representation or guarantee that the use of this manual will prevent differences of opinion or disputes with Medicare or other payers as to the amounts that will be paid to providers of services. Optum, its employees, agents, and staff make no representation or guarantee that this manual is free of errors and will bear no responsibility or liability for the results or consequences of its use.

Our Commitment to Accuracy

Optum is committed to producing accurate and reliable materials.

To report corrections, please email customerassistance@optum.com. You can also reach customer service by calling 1.800.464.3649, option 1.

Acknowledgments

Ken Kracker, *Product Manager*
Stacy Perry, *Manager, Desktop Publishing*
Laura M. Anderson, RN, BSN, CCDS, *Subject Matter Expert*
Anita Schmidt, BS, RHIA, AHIMA-approved ICD-10-CM/PCS Trainer, *Subject Matter Expert*
Tracy Betzler, *Senior Desktop Publishing Specialist*
Hope M. Dunn, *Senior Desktop Publishing Specialist*
Katie Russell, *Desktop Publishing Specialist*
Kate Holden, *Editor*

Copyright

Made in the USA

ISBN: 978-1-62254-866-8

About the Subject Matter Experts

Anita Schmidt, BS, RHIA, AHIMA-approved ICD-10-CM/PCS Trainer

Ms. Schmidt has expertise in ICD-10-CM/PCS, DRG, and CPT with more than 15 years' experience in coding in multiple settings, including inpatient, observation, and same-day surgery. Her experience includes analysis of medical record documentation, assignment of ICD-10-CM and PCS codes, and DRG validation. She has conducted training for ICD-10-CM/PCS and electronic health record. She has also collaborated with clinical documentation specialists to identify documentation needs and potential areas for physician education. Most recently she has been developing content for resource and educational products related to ICD-10-CM, ICD-10-PCS, DRG, and CPT. Ms. Schmidt is an AHIMA-approved ICD-10-CM/PCS trainer and is an active member of the American Health Information Management Association (AHIMA) and the Minnesota Health Information Management Association.

Laura M. Anderson, RN, BSN, CCDS

Ms. Anderson is a Registered Nurse and CDI Specialist/Educator with more than 20 years of experience in the healthcare profession. She obtained her BSN at the University of Minnesota and spent most of her bedside nursing career on Medical-Surgical care units. Her clinical documentation experience began in 2007, covering CDI specialist training, education development, and physician engagement. She has served as a CDI Team Lead and consultant, working with senior leadership to incorporate CDI work into documentation compliance and quality metrics. Ms. Anderson also has a BS degree in Biology (Winthrop University), with research experience in liver cancer and radiation-induced leukemia. She has presented at the state and national levels for the Association of Clinical Documentation Integrity Specialists (ACDIS) and serves as a co-lead for the Minnesota state chapter.

Summary of Changes

DRG Desk Reference Website

Optum maintains a website to accompany the *DRG Desk Reference*. Optum will post special reports, CMS information, and updated data files on this website so that the information is available before the next book update. The website address is:

http://www.optumcoding.com/Product/Updates/DRG/

This website is available only to customers who purchase the *DRG Desk Reference*. The following password is needed to access the site: **DRG24**

Summary of Changes for Fiscal 2024

The Centers for Medicare and Medicaid Services (CMS) issued its final rule on changes to the hospital inpatient prospective payment system (IPPS) and fiscal year 2024 rates in the *Federal Register* on August 1, 2023. The Medicare severity diagnosis-related groups (MS-DRGs) are now considered version 41.0 MS-DRGs and are effective for discharges occurring on or after October 1, 2023.

Biannual Code and MS-DRG Updates

The ICD-10-CM and ICD-10-PCS classifications and MS-DRG Grouper and logic will be updated biannually on October 1 and April 1 of each year.

ICD-10-CM/PCS Code Changes

- Added 437 new ICD-10-CM codes (42 effective April 1, 2023)
- Revised 13 ICD-10-CM codes
- Added 112 new ICD-10-PCS codes (34 effective April 1, 2023)
- Revised 14 ICD-10-PCS codes

DRG Grouper Logic Changes

- MDC 02 Diseases and Disorders of the Eye
  - Revised the title of MS-DRG 124 to Other Disorders of the Eye with MCC or Thrombolytic Agent
  - Reassigned eight diagnosis codes describing retinal artery occlusion from MS-DRG 123 to MS-DRGs 124 and 125
  - Added 10 procedure codes describing administration of thrombolytic agent to the list of nonoperating room procedures that affect MS-DRG assignment and assigned these codes to MS-DRG 124
- MDC 04 Diseases and Disorders of the Respiratory System
  - Added new MS-DRG 173 (Ultrasound Accelerated and Other Thrombolysis with Principal Diagnosis Pulmonary Embolism)
  - Revised the logic for MS-DRG 177 to exclude diagnosis codes under the logic list entitled "with Secondary Diagnosis" from acting as an MCC when reported as a secondary diagnosis from the logic list entitled "or Principal Diagnosis"
- MDC 05 Diseases and Disorders of the Circulatory System
  - Added new MS-DRG 212 (Concomitant Aortic and Mitral Valve Procedures)
  - Reassigned procedure code 02HA0RZ for open insertion of short-term external heart assist device as a standalone procedure from MS-DRG 215 to Pre-MDC MS-DRGs 001-002
  - Deleted MS-DRGs 222–223 (Cardiac Defibrillator Implant with Cardiac Catheterization with Acute Myocardial Infarction [AMI], Heart Failure [HF], or Shock with and without MCC)
  - Deleted MS-DRGs 224–225 (Cardiac Defibrillator Implant with Cardiac Catheterization without AMI, HF, or Shock with and without MCC)
  - Deleted MS-DRGs 226–227 (Cardiac Defibrillator Implant without Cardiac Catheterization with and without MCC)
  - Deleted MS-DRGs 246–247 (Percutaneous Cardiovascular Procedures with Drug-Eluting Stent with MCC or 4+ Arteries or Stents and without MCC)
  - Deleted MS-DRG 248–249 (Percutaneous Cardiovascular Procedures with Non-Drug-Eluting Stent with MCC or 4+ Arteries or Stents and without MCC)
  - Revised MS-DRGs 250–251 to Percutaneous Cardiovascular Procedures without Intraluminal Device with and without MCC
  - Added new MS-DRGs 275–277 (Cardiac Defibrillator Implant with Cardiac Catheterization and MCC, with MCC, and without MCC)
  - Added new MS-DRGs 278–279 (Ultrasound Accelerated and Other Thrombolysis of Peripheral Vascular Structures with and without MCC)
  - Added new MS-DRGs 321–322 (Percutaneous Cardiovascular Procedures with Intraluminal Device with MCC or 4+ Arteries/Intraluminal Devices and without MCC)
  - Added new MS-DRGs 323–325 (Coronary Intravascular Lithotripsy with Intraluminal Device with MCC, without MCC, and without Intraluminal Device/MCC)
- MDC 06 Diseases and Disorders of the Digestive System
  - Deleted MS-DRGs 338–340 (Appendectomy with Complicated Principal Diagnosis with MCC, with CC, and without CC/MCC)
  - Deleted MS-DRGs 341–343 (Appendectomy without Complicated Principal Diagnosis with MCC, with CC, and without CC/MCC)
  - Added new MS-DRGs 397–399 (Appendix Procedures with MCC, with CC, and without CC/MCC)
- MDC 16 Diseases and Disorders of Blood, Blood Forming Organs and Immunologic Disorders
  - Revised MS-DRGs 799–801 to Splenic Procedures with MCC, with CC, and without CC/MCC
- Conducted annual review of procedure code assignments grouping to MS-DRGs 981–983 and 987–989
  - Reassigned procedure code 0DTN4ZZ describing percutaneous endoscopic resection of colon to MDC 11 under MS-DRGs 673–675 (Other Kidney and Urinary Tract Procedures with MCC, with CC, and without CC/MCC)
  - Reassigned 28 procedure codes describing open excision of muscle to MDC 05 under MS-DRG 264 (Other Circulatory System O.R. Procedures)
  - Reassigned procedure code 0NR00JZ describing open replacement of skull with synthetic substitute to MDC 09 under MS-DRGs 579–581 (Other Skin, Subcutaneous Tissue and Breast Procedures with MCC, with CC, and without CC/MCC)
  - Reassigned procedure codes 0T768DZ, 0T778DZ, and 0T788DZ describing endoscopic dilation of ureters with intraluminal device to MDC 05 under MS-DRG 264 (Other Circulatory System O.R. Procedures)
  - Reassigned nine procedure codes describing occlusion of splenic artery to MDC 16 under MS-DRGs 799–801 (Splenic Procedures with MCC, with CC, and without CC/MCC)
- Recalibrated the MS-DRG relative weights as required by the Social Security Act
- Revised the list of MCC and CC diagnoses
- Revised the CC Excludes list

Contents

Introduction

The *DRG Desk Reference* is the most comprehensive diagnosis-related group (DRG) resource offering a simplified solution to DRG assignment practices. This portable desk reference is ideal for the coder, DRG/ utilization review coordinators, and compliance auditors to efficiently and effectively manage hospital financial success through easy access to critical coding information. This resource primarily provides:

- Information on the basic characteristics of MS-DRG classification
- Tools to facilitate understanding of MS-DRG grouping and reimbursement methodologies, including optimizing tips for all MDCs.

Basic Steps of Accurate DRG Assignment

There are three basic steps of accurate DRG assignment.

Step 1: assign the working DRG accurately using a DRG guide.

Step 2: assess the working DRG assignment using all the information in the completed medical record to identify any conditions that cause higher facility resource use and, therefore, may qualify for higher reimbursement.

Step 3: determine whether all the required documentation is present to support assignment of the DRG.

The *DRG Desk Reference* primarily provides all the necessary information to complete steps 2 and 3 of the DRG assignment process.

Basic Characteristics of MS-DRG Classification

An MS-DRG is one of 766 groups (version 41.0) that classify patients into clinically cohesive groups that demonstrate similar consumption of hospital resources and length-of-stay patterns.

The MS-DRG system organizes ICD-10-CM/PCS diagnosis and procedure codes into a complex, comprehensive system based on a few simple principles.

Understanding how the MS-DRG system works enables providers to recover the appropriate payment for services rendered, which is consistent with the intent of the federal government when it devised the DRG system. The *DRG Desk Reference* assists providers in understanding MS-DRGs, thus ensuring appropriate payment.

In addition to calculating reimbursement, MS-DRGs have two major functions. The first is to help evaluate the quality of care. Not only are critical pathways designed around MS-DRGs, but benchmarking and outcomes analysis can be launched using the MS-DRG clinical framework, and quality reviews can be performed to assess coding practices and physician documentation. Ongoing education of physicians, coders, clinical documentation specialists, nurses, and utilization review personnel can be guided by the results of MS-DRG analysis.

Second, MS-DRGs assist in evaluating utilization of services. Each MS-DRG represents the average resources needed to treat patients grouped to that MS-DRG relative to the national average of resources used to treat all Medicare patients. The MS-DRG assigned to each hospital inpatient stay also relates to the hospital case mix (i.e., the types of patients the hospital treats). A hospital's Medicare population case complexity is measured by calculation of the case-mix index (CMI), which is an average of all MS-DRG relative weights for the facility during a given period of time. The higher the case-mix index, the more complex the patient population and the higher the required level of resources utilized. Since severity is such an essential component of MS-DRG assignment and case-mix index calculation, documentation and code assignment to the highest degree of accuracy and specificity are of the utmost importance.

Medicare computes the case-mix adjustment for each fiscal year for all hospitals based upon the case-mix data received. This CMI is then used to adjust the hospital base rate, which is a factor in computing the total hospital payment under IPPS. The formula for computing the hospital payment for each MS-DRG is as follows:

DRG Relative Weight x Hospital Base Rate = Hospital Payment

The hospital case-mix complexity includes the following patient attributes:

- Severity of illness—the level of loss of function or mortality associated with disease
- Prognosis—defined as probable outcome of illness
- Treatment difficulty—patient management problems
- Need for intervention—severity of illness that would result due to lack of immediate or continuing care
- Resource intensity—volume and types of services required for patient management

The MS-DRG system was developed to relate case mix to resource utilization. Reimbursement is adjusted to reflect the resource utilization and does not take into consideration severity of illness, prognosis, treatment difficulty, or need for intervention.

Case mix and complexity can be analyzed and monitored in relation to cost and utilization of services. In addition, high-volume conditions and services can be identified and monitored, and MS-DRG trend analysis can aid in forecasting future staff and facility requirements. One important operating parameter is the CMI, which measures the cost of a hospital's Medicare patient mix in relation to the cost of all Medicare patients. A low case mix may indicate unnecessary revenue loss.

MDC and MS-DRG Hierarchies

DRGs divide all possible principal diagnoses into 26 mutually exclusive categories, referred to as major diagnostic categories (MDC). The MDCs were further subdivided into MS-DRGs:

- First—principal diagnosis linked to anatomical system (MDC)
- Second—patient's surgical status
  - principal diagnosis (nonsurgical DRG)
  - extent of surgical procedure (surgical DRG)
- Third—comorbidities, complications, sex, discharge status, and birth weight of neonates

MDC Categories

The diagnoses that define each MDC fall under the umbrella of a single organ system or etiology and are usually grouped by medical specialty, as in MDC 19 Mental Diseases and Disorders, or MDC 14 Pregnancy, Childbirth and the Puerperium. Some cases, such as transplants and tracheostomies, require extremely high resources and may be performed for a variety of different conditions. These cases are assigned to a PRE-MDC DRG, meaning that the Grouper logic's hierarchy for these procedures is higher than that of the principal diagnosis typically used to determine the MS-DRG. Two other MDCs were added to the original list to cover multiple trauma and human immunodeficiency virus (HIV) infections.

MDC Categories

Pre-MDC Heart Transplant or Implant of Heart Assist System (MS-DRGs 001-002)

ECMO or Tracheostomy with Mechanical Ventilation > 96 Hours or PDX Except Face, Mouth & Neck with Major O.R. Procedure (MS-DRG 003)

Tracheostomy with Mechanical Ventilation > 96 Hours or PDX Except Face, Mouth & Neck without Major O.R. Procedure (MS-DRG 004)

Liver Transplant or Intestinal Transplant (MS-DRG 005-006)

Lung Transplant (MS-DRG 007)

Simultaneous Pancreas/Kidney Transplant (MS-DRG 008)

Pancreas Transplant (MS-DRG 010)

Tracheostomy for Face, Mouth & Neck Diagnoses or Laryngectomy (MS-DRGs 011-013)

Allogeneic Bone Marrow Transplant (MS-DRG 014)

Autologous Bone Marrow Transplant (MS-DRGs 016-017)

Chimeric Antigen Receptor (CAR) T-cell and other Immunotherapies (MS-DRG 018)

Simultaneous Pancreas and Kidney Transplant with Hemodialysis (MS-DRG 019)

MDC 1 Diseases and Disorders of the Nervous System (MS-DRGs 020–103)

MDC 2 Diseases and Disorders of the Eye (MS-DRGs 113–125)

MDC 3 Diseases and Disorders of the Ear, Nose, Mouth and Throat (MS-DRGs 135–159)

MDC 4 Diseases and Disorders of the Respiratory System (MS-DRGs 163–208)

MDC 5 Diseases and Disorders of the Circulatory System (MS-DRGs 215–320)

MDC 6 Diseases and Disorders of the Digestive System (MS-DRGs 326–395)

MDC 7 Diseases and Disorders of the Hepatobiliary System and Pancreas (MS-DRGs 405–446)

MDC 8 Diseases and Disorders of the Musculoskeletal System and Connective Tissue (MS-DRGs 453–566)

MDC 9 Diseases and Disorders of the Skin, Subcutaneous Tissue and Breast (MS-DRGs 570–607)

MDC 10 Endocrine, Nutritional and Metabolic Diseases and Disorders (MS-DRGs 614–645)

MDC 11 Diseases and Disorders of the Kidney and Urinary Tract (MS-DRGs 650–700)

MDC 12 Diseases and Disorders of the Male Reproductive System (MS-DRGs 707–730)

MDC 13 Diseases and Disorders of the Female Reproductive System (MS-DRGs 734–761)

MDC 14 Pregnancy, Childbirth and the Puerperium (MS-DRGs 768–788, 796–798, 805–807, 817–819, 831–833, 998)

MDC 15 Newborns and Other Neonates with Conditions Originating in Perinatal Period (MS-DRGs 789–795)

MDC 16 Diseases and Disorders of Blood, Blood Forming Organs and Immunologic Disorders (MS-DRGs 799–804, 808–816)

MDC 17 Myeloproliferative Diseases and Disorders, Poorly Differentiated Neoplasms (MS-DRGs 820–830, 834–849)

MDC 18 Infectious and Parasitic Diseases, Systemic or Unspecified Sites (MS-DRGs 853–872)

MDC 19 Mental Diseases and Disorders (MS-DRGs 876–887)

MDC 20 Alcohol or Drug Use or Induced Organic Mental Disorders (MS-DRGs 894–897)

MDC 21 Injuries, Poisonings and Toxic Effects of Drugs (MS-DRGs 901–923)

MDC 22 Burns (MS-DRGs 927–935)

MDC 23 Factors Influencing Health Status and Other Contacts with Health Services (MS-DRGs 939–951)

MDC 24 Multiple Significant Trauma (MS-DRGs 955–965)

MDC 25 Human Immunodeficiency Virus Infections (MS-DRGs 969–977)

Since the MDCs represent clinically coherent groups based upon diagnosis, cases are defined by the principal diagnosis, the condition established after study to be chiefly responsible for occasioning the admission of the patient to the hospital. Once a patient is assigned to an MDC, the next step is to determine whether the case should be designated as surgical or medical.

Surgical Cases

Cases are considered surgical if there is a valid operating room procedure performed or other non-operating-room procedure that affects DRG assignment. The performance of operating room (OR) procedures brings into play a host of inpatient resources, including anesthesia, nursing care, recovery room, and the operating suite. As a result, DRGs are separated into categories of surgical or medical (nonsurgical) cases.

For one group of DRGs, the Pre-MDC DRGs, the initial step in DRG assignment is based upon the procedure performed, not the principal diagnosis.

Surgical DRGs are chosen based on the ICD-10-PCS procedural code assigned. Keep in mind that a case is first grouped to the MDC according to the principal diagnosis assigned. As an example, in order to be assigned to DRG 405 Pancreas, Liver and Shunt Procedures with MCC, the case must first be assigned a principal diagnosis assigned to MDC 7 Diseases and Disorders of the Hepatobiliary System and Pancreas. In addition the OR procedure performed must be one that is listed under DRG 405. And there must be a condition that is considered a major complication or comorbidity. Other factors that contribute to the DRG assignment process for a case include: complications, comorbidities, sex, discharge status, and birth weight of neonates. For patients undergoing multiple procedures, the most complex applicable DRG in the hierarchy of major surgery, minor surgery, other surgery, and surgery unrelated to principal diagnosis that applies is chosen as driving DRG assignment.

Medical Cases

If no significant procedures were performed, a medical DRG is assigned. Medical diagnoses are divided into categories in the medical DRGs. These categories include neoplasms and symptoms and conditions related to a single anatomical system. The level of service required for medical DRGs is generally less resource-intensive than that for patients who undergo surgery.

Other Factors

The patient's status upon discharge from the hospital is also considered a variable in the definition of an MS-DRG. For example, MS-DRG 280 Acute Myocardial Infarction, Discharged Alive with MCC, requires a patient disposition other than expired on the case. Separate DRGs were designed for patients who leave the hospital against medical advice or expire.

With the implementation of MS-DRGs, effective October 1, 2007, patient age was eliminated as a parameter affecting MS-DRG assignment. All previous MS-DRGs with a reference to "Age 0-17" or "Age greater than 17" were eliminated and collapsed into the corresponding base MS-DRG.

Complications and Comorbidities

Both medical and surgical classes are sometimes further defined by the presence of complications or comorbidities, which are further delineated by being classified as complication/co-morbidity (CC) or major complication/co-morbidity (MCC).

CMS developed lists of MCC and CC conditions for assignment to MS-DRGs. When a CC or MCC is present as a secondary diagnosis, it may affect assignment.

The following are examples of the most commonly missed MCC/CCs:

- Anemia due to blood loss, acute
- Atrial flutter
- Atelectasis
- Cachexia
- Cardiogenic shock
- Cardiomyopathy
- Cellulitis
- Congestive heart failure (CHF) (specific forms)
- Diabetes mellitus with ketoacidosis, hyperosmolarity, other coma
- Hematemesis
- Hyponatremia
- Malnutrition (certain forms)
- Melena
- Pleural effusion
- Pneumothorax
- Renal failure, acute or chronic, Stage IV or V, or ESRD
- Respiratory failure
- Urinary tract infection

The validity of MCC/CCs is dependent on the principal diagnosis. There are some diagnoses that may not function as a CC condition under certain circumstances because they are too closely related to the principal diagnosis. Those CC or MCC conditions that are considered related to other conditions sequenced as principal diagnosis and are excluded as CC/MCC conditions, are referenced as being on the "CC exclusions list." The diagnoses listed under the CC or MCC condition on the exclusions list represent those principal diagnoses for which the diagnosis code in question will not function as a CC or MCC. Note that there is no separate exclusions list for CCs and MCCs. The following parameters are used to determine those secondary diagnoses that are excluded from the CC list:

- Chronic and acute manifestations of the same condition should not be considered MCC/CCs for one another.
- Specific and nonspecific diagnosis codes for a condition should not be considered MCC/CCs for one another.
- Conditions that may not coexist such as partial or total, unilateral or bilateral, obstructed or unobstructed, and benign or malignant should not be considered MCC/CCs for one another.
- The same condition in anatomically proximal sites should not be considered MCC/CCs for one another.
- Closely related conditions should not be considered MCC/CCs for one another.

Principal Diagnosis

To assign a DRG, first determine and code the principal diagnosis, then all secondary diagnoses, and MCC/CCs. With the principal and secondary diagnoses in mind, consult ICD-10-PCS to assign any procedure code(s) that might apply to the patient's case.

Principal Procedure

The *ICD-10-PCS Official Guidelines for Coding and Reporting*, Selection of Principal Procedure provide instructions that should be applied in the selection of the principal procedure and provide clarification on the importance of the principal diagnosis relationship when more than one procedure is performed.

1. Procedure performed for definitive treatment of both principal diagnosis and secondary diagnosis
   a. Sequence procedure performed for definitive treatment most related to principal diagnosis as principal procedure.
2. Procedure performed for definitive treatment and diagnostic procedures performed for both principal diagnosis and secondary diagnosis
   a. Sequence procedure performed for definitive treatment most related to principal diagnosis as principal procedure.
3. A diagnostic procedure was performed for the principal diagnosis and a procedure is performed for definitive treatment of a secondary diagnosis
   a. Sequence diagnostic procedure as principal procedure, since the procedure most related to the principal diagnosis takes precedence.
4. No procedures performed that are related to principal diagnosis; procedures performed for definitive treatment and diagnostic procedures were performed for secondary diagnosis
   a. Sequence procedure performed for definitive treatment of secondary diagnosis as principal procedure, since there are no procedures (definitive or nondefinitive treatment) related to principal diagnosis.

MS-DRG Assignment Process

MS-DRGs are assigned using the principal diagnosis; secondary diagnoses, which include CCs and MCCs; surgical or other invasive procedures; sex of the patient; and discharge status. One MS-DRG is assigned to each inpatient stay.

Diagnoses and procedures are designated by ICD-10-CM and PCS codes.

The following describes the typical decision process used to assign an MS-DRG to a case. A case is assigned to one of 25 major diagnostic categories (MDC), which are mutually exclusive groups based on principal diagnosis. MS-DRG assignment is based upon the following considerations:

- Principal and secondary diagnosis and procedure codes
- Sex of the patient
- Discharge status
- Presence or absence of MCCs and/or presence or absence of CCs
- Birth weight for neonates

Each MDC is organized into one of two sections—surgical or medical. The surgical section classifies all surgical conditions based upon operating room procedures. The medical section classifies all diagnostic conditions based upon diagnosis codes. The majority of MDCs are organized by major body system and are associated with a particular medical specialty.

There are two groups of MS-DRGs that are not assigned to MDCs. First, there is the group that may be associated with all MDCs. This group includes MS-DRGs created specifically to report admissions into a facility that have been assigned principal diagnosis invalid as discharge diagnosis (MS-DRG 998), have O.R. procedures unrelated to a principal diagnosis (MS-DRGs 981–983, and 987–989), or are ungroupable principal diagnoses (MS-DRG 999). Although the scope is too broad for clinical analysis, the MS-DRGs encompass clinically coherent cases.

Another group not assigned to MDCs is called Pre-MDC MS-DRGs which consist of cases that are grouped by surgical procedure rather than principal diagnosis. The Pre-MDC MS-DRG group includes bone marrow and organ transplant cases as well as tracheostomy cases.

Further sorting of medical classifications is performed by principal diagnosis type and/or surgical classifications by type of surgery. Finally the case is analyzed for the presence of MCCs and/or CCs as indicated by ICD-10-CM diagnosis codes, and an MS-DRG is assigned.

Each year, effective October 1, new MS-DRGs are added and/or current MS-DRGs are deleted or revised for the next fiscal year. In addition, MS-DRG assignments are adjusted based on relative weight (RW), arithmetic mean length of stay (AMLOS), and geometric mean length of stay (GMLOS). On April 1, new ICD-10 codes may also be incorporated into the DRG classification.

The information contained in this manual reflects the DRG classification system effective October 1, 2023, Grouper version 41.0. For changes that impact the DRG classification system effective April 1, 2024, please visit our website at: https://www.optum.com/Product/Updates/DRG/.

Grouper Version	Effective Time Period
MS 41.0	10/01/2023 – 03/31/2024
MS 40.1	04/01/2023 – 09/30/2023
MS 40.0	10/01/2022 – 03/31/2023
MS 39.1	04/01/2022 – 09/30/2022
MS 39.0	10/01/2021 – 03/31/2022
MS 38.1	01/01/2021 – 09/30/2021
MS 38.0 R1	10/01/2020 – 12/31/2020
MS 37.2	08/01/2020 – 09/30/2020
MS 37.1 R1	04/01/2020 – 07/31/2020
MS 37.0 R1	10/01/2019 – 03/31/2020
MS 36.0	10/01/2018 – 09/30/2019
MS 35.0	10/01/2017 – 09/30/2018
MS 34.0	10/01/2016 – 09/30/2017
MS 33.0	10/01/2015 – 09/30/2016
MS 32.0	10/01/2014 – 09/30/2015
MS 31.0	10/01/2013 – 09/30/2014
MS 30.0	10/01/2012 – 09/30/2013
MS 29.0	10/01/2011 – 09/30/2012
MS 28.0	10/01/2010 – 09/30/2011
MS 27.0	10/01/2009 – 09/30/2010
MS 26.0	10/01/2008 – 09/30/2009
MS 25.0	10/01/2007 – 09/30/2008
CMS 24.0	10/01/2006 – 09/30/2007
CMS 23.0	10/01/2005 – 09/30/2006
CMS 22.0	10/01/2004 – 09/30/2005
CMS 21.0	10/01/2003 – 09/30/2004
CMS 20.0	10/01/2002 – 09/30/2003
CMS 19.0	10/01/2001 – 09/30/2002
CMS 18.0	10/01/2000 – 09/30/2001
CMS 17.0	10/01/1999 – 09/30/2000
CMS 16.0	10/01/1998 – 09/30/1999
CMS 15.0	10/01/1997 – 09/30/1998
CMS 14.0	10/01/1996 – 09/30/1997
CMS 13.0	10/01/1995 – 09/30/1996
CMS 12.0	10/01/1994 – 09/30/1995
CMS 11.0	10/01/1993 – 09/30/1994
CMS 10.0	10/01/1992 – 09/30/1993
CMS 9.0	10/01/1991 – 09/30/1992
CMS 8.0	10/01/1990 – 09/30/1991
CMS 7.0	10/01/1989 – 09/30/1990
CMS 6.0	10/01/1988 – 09/30/1989
CMS 5.0	10/01/1987 – 09/30/1988
CMS 4.0	10/01/1986 – 09/30/1987
CMS 3.0	05/01/1986 – 09/30/1986
CMS 2.0	10/01/1983 – 04/30/1986

Government Scrutiny

In 1996, the False Claims Act was amended to include claims made to the government in deliberate ignorance or reckless disregard of the truth or falsity of the information. It's not necessary that there be any specific intent to defraud under that provision of the law. A mere pattern or practice of overbilling is sufficient, and that can spell fines of not less than $5,000 and as much as $10,000 per claim, plus treble damages. What's more, government enforcers are using that clause to the maximum effect; numerous settlements have been in the tens and hundreds of millions of dollars.

Federal regulatory agency initiatives to validate documentation and coding as well as proper DRG assignment comes as a result of:

- The shift in responsibility for accuracy of diagnosis and procedure codes from physicians to hospitals
- The internal pressures to increase case mix from one fiscal year to the next
- The fact that the optimization of DRGs has been ingrained into coders since the 1983 inception of the Medicare PPS

It was also expected that there would be increased scrutiny of inpatient coded services due to implementation of MS-DRGs. Because CMS felt strongly that a significant number of hospitals would implement documentation and coding improvement programs that would artificially inflate case mix index values, it included reduction to payments.

CMS also contends that this payment reduction is necessary in order to achieve budget neutrality in the reimbursement of inpatient services. Many of the same high-risk DRG subgroups as those reviewed under the previous CMS DRGs will be scrutinized to ensure appropriate coding and grouping.

Government scrutiny related to DRGs has been focused on the recovery audit contractor (RAC) audits. A demonstration project was completed in early 2008 and the full program was implemented nationwide in 2010. Even after payment of all costs associated with the program were considered, RACs returned $693.6 million to the Medicare Trust Funds through the demonstration project. In the FY 2013 report to Congress, CMS reported:

> "In Fiscal Year (FY) 2013, Recovery Auditors collectively identified and corrected 1,532,249 claims for improper payments, which resulted in $3.75 billion dollars in improper payments being corrected. The total corrections identified include $3.65 billion in overpayments collected and $102.4 million in underpayments repaid to providers and suppliers... After taking into consideration all fees, costs, and first level appeals, the Medicare FFS Recovery Audit Program returned over $3.0 billion to the Medicare Trust Funds…"

A three-year Recovery Audit Prepayment Review Demonstration began on September 1, 2012, in eleven states. These states included seven with high incidences of improper payments and fraud (Florida, California, Michigan, Texas, New York, Louisiana, and Illinois) and four with high claims volumes of short inpatient hospital stays (Pennsylvania, Ohio, North Carolina, and Missouri).

MS-DRGs were selected for review based on Comprehensive Error Rate Testing (CERT) data. Claims in these states containing a selected MS-DRG were flagged for review before the claim was paid.

The following MS-DRGs were under review during the first year of the demonstration:

- MS-DRG 069 Transient Ischemia
- MS-DRG 252 Other Vascular Procedures with MCC
- MS-DRG 253 Other Vascular Procedures with MCC
- MS-DRG 254 Other Vascular Procedures without CC/MCC
- MS-DRG 312 Syncope and Collapse
- MS-DRG 377 GI Hemorrhage with MCC
- MS-DRG 378 GI Hemorrhage with CC
- MS-DRG 379 GI Hemorrhage without CC/MCC
- MS-DRG 391 Esophagitis, Gastroenteritis and Miscellaneous Digestive Disorders with MCC
- MS-DRG 392 Esophagitis, Gastroenteritis and Miscellaneous Digestive Disorders without MCC
- MS-DRG 637 Diabetes with MCC
- MS-DRG 638 Diabetes with CC
- MS-DRG 639 Diabetes without CC/MCC

CMS evaluated the effectiveness of the demonstration.

- The demonstration was successfully implemented and data collected for one year.
- As of September 26, 2013, more than 9,300 Additional Documentation Requests (ADRs) were sent to providers for the selected MS-DRGs as part of the Prepayment Demonstration. Fifty-nine percent of the claims that were reviewed were found to be improper, illustrating the importance of this demonstration.
- The total savings achieved from the first year of the demonstration were $22.3 million.

Both the Recovery Audit Program and the Recovery Audit Prepayment Review Demonstration are of high priority to those involved in coding and reimbursement compliance.

Keys to a Financially Successful DRG Program

Each DRG is assigned a relative weight by CMS based upon charge data for all Medicare inpatient hospital discharges. Each hospital has a customized base rate designed to adjust payment commensurate with the hospital's cost of providing services. The type of hospital and the wage index for the geographic area determines the hospital base rate. DRG relative weights and hospital base rates are adjusted yearly (effective October 1 through September 30) to reflect changes in health care resource consumption as well as economic factors. Payment is determined by multiplying the DRG relative weight by the hospital base rate. The DRG with the highest relative weight is the highest-paying DRG. Regardless of actual costs incurred, the hospital receives only the calculated payment.

The DRG payment system is based on averages. Payment is determined by the resource needs of the average Medicare patient for a given set of diseases or disorders. These resources include the length of stay and the number and intensity of services provided. Therefore, the more efficiently a provider delivers care, the greater its operating margin will be.

The keys to a financially successful DRG program are:

- Decreased length of stay
- Decreased resource utilization (tests or procedures)
- Increased intensity of case management services resulting in optimal length of stay for the patient and facility
- Increased preadmission testing
- Improved medical record documentation, particularly as it relates to specificity of disease processes

The Physician's Role

Proper MS-DRG assignment requires a complete and thorough accounting of the following:

- Principal diagnosis
- Procedures
- Complications
- Comorbidities (all relevant pre-existing conditions)
- Signs and symptoms when diagnoses are not established
- Discharge status

Because MS-DRG assignment is based on documentation in the medical record, the record should:

- Be comprehensive and complete
- Include all diagnoses, procedures, complications, and comorbidities, as well as abnormal test results documented by the physician. It should also include any suspected conditions and what was done to investigate or evaluate them.
- Be timely

All dictation, signatures, etc., should be completed in the medical record as patient care is provided and must be:

- Legible
- Well-documented

The information should be documented properly. With complete information in the medical record, coders can effectively analyze, code, and report the required information. This ensures that proper payment is received. For example, if the physician documents that a patient with a skull fracture was in a coma for less than one hour, MS-DRGs 085–087 may be assigned. If the physician documents that the coma lasted for more than one hour, MS-DRGs 082–084 may be assigned, with a resulting payment difference.

Physicians must be actively involved in the query process. They should respond to queries in a timely fashion and document their responses, as established by the process, to ensure their responses meet regulatory requirements and are maintained, in some form, in the permanent medical record.

ICD-10-CM/PCS Coding Accuracy

Correct ICD-10-CM/PCS coding is essential for correct DRG assignment. Most coding references, whether hard copy or electronic, feature some level of support material to steer the user toward the most specific code selection. For example, the Optum hospital edition of ICD-10-CM features Medicare code edit indicators for codes that affect DRG assignments, including unacceptable principal diagnoses, MCC/CCs, questionable admissions, and sex-specific diagnoses. ICD-10-PCS references also feature indicators for codes that affect DRG assignments, including OR or non-OR procedures or noncovered procedures.

Discharge Status Code Assignment

Required by the Centers for Medicare and Medicaid Services (CMS) and developed and maintained by the National Uniform Billing Committee (NUBC), the discharge status code is a two-digit code entered on the

UB-04 claim that identifies where a patient is going at the conclusion of an inpatient hospital encounter.

The discharge status code is just as important as any other code reported and filed on a claim, and the same processes should be applied for assigning these codes. When two or more discharge status codes may apply, the code reported should be for the highest level of care known. Omitting a code or submitting a claim with an incorrect code is a claim billing error that may result in claim overpayments or underpayments, total recoupment of the original payment, or rejection of the claim entirely. If an inaccurate discharge status code is assigned or the patient does not receive the treatment as planned after discharge, the result may be an unjustified increase or reduction in the transferring hospital's Medicare payment. This is because certain discharge status codes are affected by Medicare's acute care transfer and post-acute care transfer (PACT) provisions. Correct assignment of discharge status codes can avoid these claim billing errors.

In general, a discharge occurs when a Medicare beneficiary does one of the following:

- Leaves a Medicare inpatient prospective payment system (IPPS) acute care hospital after receiving complete acute care treatment
- Dies in the hospital

Medicare makes full MS-DRG payments to IPPS hospitals when the patient is discharged to home or certain types of health care institutions, such as an intermediate care facility (ICF).

Acute Care Transfer

An "acute care transfer" occurs when a Medicare beneficiary in an IPPS hospital (with any MS-DRG) is:

- Transferred to another acute care IPPS hospital or unit for related care
- Leaves against medical advice
- Transferred to a hospital that would ordinarily be paid under prospective payment but is excluded because of participation in a state- or areawide cost control program
- Transferred to a hospital or hospital unit that has not been officially determined to be excluded from PPS, such as:
  - an acute care hospital that would otherwise be eligible to be paid under the IPPS but does not have an agreement to participate in the Medicare program
  - a critical access hospital
- Discharged but then readmitted the same day to another IPPS hospital (unless the readmission is unrelated to the initial discharge). This may occur when a hospital discharges the patient to home and the patient goes to a doctor's appointment the same day and is then admitted to another hospital. If the first hospital was unaware of the planned admission at the second hospital, it is likely the first hospital will have to adjust the previously submitted claim to correct the patient discharge status code to indicate a transfer, reflecting where the patient was later admitted on the same date.

The transferring hospital is paid a per diem payment (when the patient transfers to an IPPS hospital) up to and including the full DRG payment. The transferring hospital may be paid a cost outlier payment. The receiving hospital is paid based on the full prospective payment rate, which may include a cost outlier payment if applicable or be based on the rate of its respective payment system (if not IPPS).

For unrelated admissions, when a transfer case results in treatment in the second hospital under an MS-DRG different from the MS-DRG in the transferring hospital, payment to each hospital is based upon the MS-DRG under which the patient was treated.

For transfers from an IPPS hospital to a hospital or unit excluded from IPPS with an MS-DRG that is not subject to the post-acute care transfer policy, the transferring hospital is paid the full IPPS rate, including an outlier payment, if applicable. The outlier threshold and payment are calculated the same way as any other discharge without a transfer. The payment to the final discharging hospital or unit is made at the rate of its respective payment system.

Post-acute Care Transfer

Effective October 1, 1998, CMS enacted the post-acute care transfer (PACT) policy and payment methodology to reduce hospital payment for certain inpatient stays. This was a result of acute care hospitals' attempts to reduce costs by transferring patients early to post-acute levels of care, such as skilled nursing facilities (SNF) and home health (HH) agencies. CMS determined that Medicare was overpaying for inpatient care of these patients because it was paying the IPPS acute care hospital the full MS-DRG payment and the post-acute provider a separate payment during the same episode of care.

A post-acute care transfer occurs when a Medicare beneficiary in an IPPS hospital stay is grouped to one of the MS-DRGs known as transfer MS-DRGs listed in table 5 of the IPPS final rule and the transfer occurs to:

- A hospital or distinct hospital unit excluded from IPPS:
  - inpatient rehabilitation facilities and distinct units of the hospitals
  - long term care hospitals
  - psychiatric hospitals and distinct units of the hospitals
  - children's hospitals
  - cancer hospitals
- Skilled nursing facilities
- Home, under a written plan of care for home health services that begins within three days of discharge
- Hospice care, home—effective for claims with through date on or after October 1, 2018
- Hospice care, medical facility—effective for claims with through date on or after October 1, 2018

The transferring hospital is paid based upon a per diem rate up to and including the full DRG payment, which may include a cost outlier payment, if applicable. The final discharging hospital is paid based on the full prospective payment rate, which may include a cost outlier payment, if applicable.

Special Payment Post-acute Care Transfer

A special payment post-acute care transfer occurs when a Medicare beneficiary in an IPPS hospital stay is grouped to one of the MS-DRGs listed in table 5 in the column titled, "Special Pay DRG," of the IPPS final rule. For these cases, the transferring hospital is paid 50 percent of the appropriate inpatient prospective payment rate and 50 percent of the appropriate transfer payment.

Planned Acute Care Hospital Inpatient Readmission Discharge Status Codes

Effective October 1, 2013, 15 new discharge status codes were created to capture planned inpatient readmissions to an acute care hospital. All 15 of these readmission status codes apply to the following MS-DRGs only:

280	Acute Myocardial Infarction Discharged Alive with MCC
281	Acute Myocardial Infraction Discharged Alive with CC
282	Acute Myocardial Infarction Discharged Alive without CC/MCC

In addition, readmission status codes 82, 85, and 94 will also apply to MS-DRG 789 Neonates, Died or Transferred to Another Acute Care Facility.

The National Uniform Billing Committee (NUBC) defines a readmission as "an intentional readmission after discharge from an acute care hospital that is a scheduled part of a patient's plan of care." There is no designated timeframe or limitation on when the readmission should occur, and these status codes are unrelated to and in no way affect the Hospital Readmissions Reduction Program.

Accurate assignment of the discharge status codes, especially those that result in post-acute care transfer, is essential to ensuring appropriate payments for both the discharging facility and the transfer facility and avoiding compliance issues. Adding to the complexity, many post-acute care transfer facilities are licensed for multiple levels of care, making it difficult to determine the appropriate discharge status code when the discharging facility's medical record contains no documentation or the documentation does not specify the level of care the transferring facility will provide. Collaboration between hospital staff that facilitate placement of a patient following discharge, that verify appropriate documentation describing the type of placement, or that abstract the actual discharge status code can help mitigate improper assignment of these codes.

Each facility should create an internal action plan to facilitate accurate discharge status code assignment. Hospital staff collaboration would be the primary focus of the action plan and should include the following, when appropriate:

- Case managers
- HIM personnel
- Coding personnel
- CDI personnel
- Discharge planners
- Medicare billers

Policies and procedures should also be developed to clearly define the responsibilities of any hospital staff that document, verify, or code where the patient is going after discharge. The policies should also establish clear lines of reporting and communication. Because the discharge plan can change after discharge, retrospective reviews should be conducted. The facility is responsible for updating and *resubmitting* the discharge disposition when this occurs; these changes can have compliance and financial impacts on the facility.

The following table details the discharge or readmission status codes used on inpatient hospital claims, the definition of the codes, NUBC guidance or instructions, and whether or not a PACT payment applies.

Discharge Status Code	Readmission Status Code[1]	Discharged/Transferred To	Exclusions	PACT[2]
01	81	Home: • On oxygen, if DME only • Any other DME • Home IV services • Under care of home IV provider Self-care Group home Foster care Outpatient programs: • Chemical dependency program • Partial hospitalization Home health services provided by DME supplier Unlicensed residential care facility		No
02	82	Short-term general hospital for inpatient care Nondesignated cancer hospitals Nondesignated children's hospital	Designated children's hospitals and cancer centers—*see* code 05	Yes
03	83	Skilled nursing facility (SNF) in anticipation of skilled care • Medicare certified	Approved swing bed—*see* code 61 Nursing facility without Medicare certification—*see* code 04 Nursing facility with Medicaid certification only—*see* code 64	Yes

[1]Readmission Status Code
Discharge status codes 81–95 are intended for use on the original discharge claim with an intended readmission of the patient as documented in the medical record's discharge plan. Readmission is defined as "an intentional readmission after discharge from an acute care hospital that is a scheduled part of the patient's plan of care."

[2]PACT—Post-Acute Care Transfer Policy
Medicare reimbursement for many MS-DRGs may be reduced when a discharge status code indicates a transfer under the Medicare PACT policy. Discharge status codes with a Yes in the PACT column indicate transfers that may affect reimbursement. Discharge status codes with a No in the PACT column indicate the transfer does not affect reimbursement.

Discharge Status Code	Readmission Status Code[1]	Discharged/Transferred To	Exclusions	PACT[2]
04	84	Facility that provides custodial or supportive care Facility designated at state level: • Intermediate care facilities (ICF) • Medicare-certified for both skilled and intermediate level of care and the patient is transferred to intermediate care Nursing facility: • Without Medicare or Medicaid certification • Medicare-certified but the patient does not qualify for a skilled level of care • Medicare-certified and the patient resides at/there but receives only nonskilled services Assisted living facility (ALF) Convalescent centers	Home care services provided in assisted living facility—*see* code 06 Hospice in nursing facility—*see* code 50	No
05	85	Designated cancer center: • National Cancer Institute list of designated cancer centers can be found at http://www3.cancer.gov/cancercenters/centerslist.html Designated children's hospital	Nondesignated cancer hospital—*see* code 02 Nondesignated children's hospital—*see* code 02	Yes
06	86	Home under care of an organized home health service organization in anticipation of covered skilled care • Admitted to an HHA under a written plan of care and services • Begins within three days after the date of discharge • Includes discharge to assisted living facility when home care services are provided Licensed home health agency (HHA)	Home health services provided by DME supplier—*see* code 01 Home IV provider for home IV services—*see* code 01	Yes
07		Left against medical advice (AMA) Discontinued care	Readmissions to another hospital on the same day the patient leaves AMA, Medicare may retroactively change the code to 02	No
21	87	Court/law enforcement: • Federal or local Jail Prison Other detention or correctional facilities		No
30		Still a patient: • Special circumstances for inpatients that have not been discharged: – for interim billing – leave of absence days		No
43	88	Federal health care facility: • Department of Defense hospital • Veteran's Administration (VA) hospital • VA skilled nursing facility • VA psychiatric unit • Applicable whether or not the patient lives at the facility		No

[1]**Readmission Status Code**

Discharge status codes 81–95 are intended for use on the original discharge claim with an intended readmission of the patient as documented in the medical record's discharge plan. Readmission is defined as "an intentional readmission after discharge from an acute care hospital that is a scheduled part of the patient's plan of care."

[2]**PACT—Post-Acute Care Transfer Policy**

Medicare reimbursement for many MS-DRGs may be reduced when a discharge status code indicates a transfer under the Medicare PACT policy. Discharge status codes with a Yes in the PACT column indicate transfers that may affect reimbursement. Discharge status codes with a No in the PACT column indicate the transfer does not affect reimbursement.

Discharge Status Code	Readmission Status Code[1]	Discharged/Transferred To	Exclusions	PACT[2]
50		Hospice in: • Home • Alternate setting that is considered the patient's home, such as: – nursing facility	Hospice referral but without hospice election or program—*see* code 01	Yes
51		Hospice in: • Qualified inpatient facility with: – inpatient hospice – respite level of care • Qualified nursing home		Yes
61	89	Swing bed: • Medicare certified – SNF level of care – hospital-based		No
62	90	Inpatient rehabilitation facility (IRF): • Independent • Distinct unit of hospital Other rehabilitation facility: • Independent • Distinct unit of hospital		Yes
63	91	Long-term care hospital (LTCH): • Medicare-certified		Yes
64	92	Nursing facility: • Medicaid certified only	Medicare-certified nursing facility—*see* code 03 Nursing facility without Medicare or Medicaid certification—*see* code 04	No
65	93	Psychiatric hospital: • Independent • Distinct unit of hospital	Outpatient psychiatric services—*see* code 01 Psychiatric unit that are not a distinct unit of the hospital (i.e., separate Medicare provider number)—*see* code 02 Psychiatric unit of a federal hospital—*see* code 43	Yes
66	94	Critical access hospital (CAH)	Swing bed in a CAH—*see* code 61	Yes
69		Designated disaster alternative care site: • Armory • Stadium • Other noninstitutional site		No
70	95	Health care institution NEC in the code list Adult treatment unit (ATU) of hospital		No
Status Code		**Expired in**		
20		Hospital		No

[1]Readmission Status Code
Discharge status codes 81–95 are intended for use on the original discharge claim with an intended readmission of the patient as documented in the medical record's discharge plan. Readmission is defined as "an intentional readmission after discharge from an acute care hospital that is a scheduled part of the patient's plan of care."

[2]PACT—Post-Acute Care Transfer Policy
Medicare reimbursement for many MS-DRGs may be reduced when a discharge status code indicates a transfer under the Medicare PACT policy. Discharge status codes with a Yes in the PACT column indicate transfers that may affect reimbursement. Discharge status codes with a No in the PACT column indicate the transfer does not affect reimbursement.

Introduction

Instructions for Using Your *DRG Desk Reference*

Basic Protocols for DRG Assignment

A basic functional understanding of the DRG assignment process is a prerequisite to using this manual. The following are the basic steps for validating DRGs:

Step 1. Identify assigned DRG. Reviewing the complete DRG title is necessary to understand the nature of the cases it comprises.

Step 2. Identify similar DRGs.

Step 3. Compare assigned DRG with similar DRGs. Many diagnoses and procedure codes will group to more than one DRG. Be sure to check every DRG referenced.

The following are key components that provide additional information when determining DRG assignments:

Optimizing Tips

This section lists each MS-DRG, any "Potential DRGs" to which the case may be reassigned, and identifies key elements needed from medical record documentation to group to the "Potential DRG."

ICD-10-CM/PCS Codes by DRG

This section lists each MS-DRG and includes a list of diagnosis and/or procedure codes specific to that MS-DRG.

Appendixes

The resources described below have been included as appendixes for *DRG Desk Reference*.

Appendix A: DRG List

This resource lists all the MS-DRGs in numerical order. Each MS-DRG is listed with its corresponding post-acute or special pay DRG designation (if applicable), the MDC it falls in, the type of DRG (surgical or medical), the DRG title, and the relative weight, arithmetic mean length of stay (AMLOS), and geometric mean length of stay (GMLOS).

Appendix B: Numeric Lists of CCs and MCCs

This resource lists all diagnosis codes designated as CCs or MCCs under the ICD-10 MS-DRGs as provided in the official lists, Table 6I – Complete Major Complication and Comorbidity (MCC) and Table 6J – Complete Complication and Comorbidity (CC) which are posted at https://www.cms.gov/medicare/acute-inpatient-pps/fy-2024-ipps-final-rule-home-page.

Appendix C: Major HIV-Related Conditions (Principal or Secondary Diagnosis)

This resource is the full and complete list of those ICD-10-CM diagnoses that are identified as major related HIV conditions according to the *ICD-10-CM/PCS, MS-DRG v41.0 Definitions Manual*.

Appendix D: Neonate Major Problems (Principal or Secondary Diagnosis)

This resource is the full and complete list of those ICD-10-CM diagnoses that are identified as major problems for neonates per the *ICD-10-CM/PCS, MS-DRG v41.0 Definitions Manual*.

Appendix E: Neonate Other Significant Problems (Principal or Secondary Diagnosis)

This resource is the full and complete list of those diagnoses that are identified as other significant problems for neonates per the *ICD-10-CM/PCS, MS-DRG v41.0 Definitions Manual*.

Appendix F: Root Operation Definitions

This resource is a compilation of all root operations used in section Ø (Medical and Surgical section) and sections 1–9 (Medical and Surgical-related sections) of the ICD-10-PCS code book. It provides a definition and in some cases a more detailed explanation of the root operation, to better reflect the purpose or objective. Examples of related procedure(s) may also be provided.

Appendix G: Body Part Key

Not every anatomical body part has its own body part character in ICD-10-PCS tables. This resource is used to search against anatomical descriptions or sites noted in the documentation to determine the most closely related PCS body part character (character 4) to which that anatomical description or site could be coded.

Appendix H: Device Key and Aggregation Table

The Device Key relates specific devices used in the medical profession, such as stents or bovine pericardial valves, with the appropriate device character (character 6).

The Aggregation Table crosswalks specific device character value definitions for specific root operations in a specific body system to the more general device character value to be used when the root operation covers a wide range of body parts and the device character represents an entire family of devices.

Glossary

This section contains definitions of terms associated with the MS-DRG classification system.

DRG Decision Trees

Optum created DRG decision trees to illustrate the DRG structure for each major diagnostic category (MDC). The decision trees show the surgical and medical partitioning within the MDCs and how they are further divided based on key variables; for example, operating room procedures, combinations of operating room procedures, nonoperating room procedures, complex diagnoses, and complications and/or comorbidities.

Optimizing Tips

Introduction

This section lists each MS-DRG, any "potential DRGs" to which the case may be reassigned, and outlines key elements needed from the medical record documentation in order to group to the potential DRG.

Because of the complexity found in MS-DRG grouper logic, it would not be practical to account for every element needed to optimize a case from a working DRG to a potential DRG. Instead, this resource has simplified the logic, identifying the basic elements typically needed to optimize. Do not assume that an MS-DRG listed as nonoptimized can never be optimized or that the list of potential DRGs is all inclusive. It is entirely possible that a very unusual combination of diagnoses or procedures could legitimately offer optimization potential.

Major Complication/Comorbidity (MCC) and Complication/Comorbidity (CC) Diagnoses

DRG Desk Reference assumes that any MCC or CC condition that is used to group to the working DRG can also be used to group to the potential DRGs.

Example:

In the family of DRGs 011–013, all have relative weights that are more than DRG 146 and, therefore, all could be potential DRGs.

DRG 146	**Ear, Nose, Mouth and Throat Malignancy with MCC**	RW 2.1110
DRG 011	**Tracheostomy for Face, Mouth, and Neck Diagnoses or Laryngectomy with MCC**	RW 5.1563
DRG 012	**Tracheostomy for Face, Mouth, and Neck Diagnoses or Laryngectomy with CC**	RW 4.0049
DRG 013	**Tracheostomy for Face, Mouth, and Neck Diagnoses or Laryngectomy without CC/MCC**	RW 2.6857

However, *DRG Desk Reference* only lists DRG 011 as a potential DRG.

DRG 146 Ear, Nose, Mouth and Throat Malignancy with MCC
Potential DRGs
DRG 011 Tracheostomy for Face, Mouth, and Neck Diagnoses or Laryngectomy with MCC

Because the presence of an MCC did not change, it would not be possible to group to DRGs 012 and 013 as these do not require an MCC.

Resequencing

It is important to understand that resequencing or reassigning codes can also change the MCC and/or CC status for a case.

Example:

DRG 025 Craniotomy and Endovascular Intracranial Procedures with MCC RW 4.4160
Potential DRGs
DRG 020 Intracranial Vascular Procedures with Principal Diagnosis of Hemorrhage with MCC 8.4524

A coder is reviewing a case that has been grouped to the working DRG of 025. After looking at the optimization tips in *DRG Desk Reference*, the coder realizes that by resequencing a cerebral hemorrhage code to PDx, the case can be reassigned to a higher DRG 020. At the working DRG, the cerebral hemorrhage functions as an MCC but after resequencing this code, an MCC is no longer present.

Although the case can still be reassigned to the MS-DRG family of 020–022, optimizing to DRG 020 may not be possible unless another MCC condition is present.

CC Exclusions

CC exclusions are also important factors to consider when grouping a case. There are MCC and CC conditions that when paired with a certain principal diagnosis are excluded from acting as MCCs or CCs. It is entirely possible that when trying to optimize a case, the resequencing or reassignment of the principal diagnosis can then exclude any current condition functioning as an MCC or CC.

Example:

Principal diagnosis	T81.718A	Complication of other artery following a procedure, not elsewhere classified, initial encounter
MCC condition	I26.99	Other pulmonary embolism without acute cor pulmonale

Appendix C of the *ICD-10-CM/PCS, MS-DRG v41.0 Definitions Manual* lists MCC condition I26.99 as being excluded from functioning as an MCC when the principal diagnosis is T81.718A. Instead of this case grouping to DRG 299 Peripheral Vascular Disorders with MCC, it will instead group to 301 Peripheral Vascular Disorders without CC/MCC. Optimization to DRG 300 or DRG 299 will depend on the presence of a CC condition or an additional MCC condition other than I26.99.

Optimizing Tips

Pre MDC

DRG 001 Heart Transplant or Implant of Heart Assist System with MCC — RW 27.0986

No Potential DRGs

DRG 002 Heart Transplant or Implant of Heart Assist System without MCC — RW 12.2441

Potential DRGs

001 Heart Transplant or Implant of Heart Assist System with MCC 27.0986

DRG	PDx/SDx/Procedure	Tips
001	MCC condition	*See* appendix B.

DRG 003 ECMO or Tracheostomy with Mechanical Ventilation > 96 Hours or Principal Diagnosis Except Face, Mouth and Neck with Major O.R. Procedure — RW 21.3203

No Potential DRGs

DRG 004 Tracheostomy with Mechanical Ventilation > 96 Hours or Principal Diagnosis Except Face, Mouth and Neck without Major O.R. Procedure — RW 14.7000

Potential DRGs

003 ECMO or Tracheostomy with Mechanical Ventilation > 96 Hours or Principal Diagnosis Except Face, Mouth and Neck with Major O.R. Procedure 21.3203

DRG	PDx/SDx/Procedure	Tips
003	Extracorporeal membrane oxygenation (ECMO), central or peripheral	Central ECMO provides cardiorespiratory support and involves direct surgical cannulation of the right atrium and aorta via sternotomy. Peripheral (percutaneous) ECMO is a less invasive procedure than central ECMO. Veno-arterial (VA) peripheral ECMO cannulas are inserted percutaneously into both the femoral artery and the femoral vein. This type of ECMO provides both respiratory and circulatory support. Veno-venous (VV) peripheral ECMO may use one or two venous insertions, one in the upper veins and, if used, one in the lower veins, and provides respiratory support only.
	OR	
	Any O.R. procedure not listed under MS-DRGs 987–989	

DRG 005 Liver Transplant with MCC or Intestinal Transplant — RW 10.3500

No Potential DRGs

DRG 006 Liver Transplant without MCC — RW 4.8369

Potential DRGs

005 Liver Transplant with MCC or Intestinal Transplant 10.3500

DRG	PDx/SDx/Procedure	Tips
005	Intestinal transplant	
	OR	
	MCC condition	*See* appendix B.

DRG 007 Lung Transplant — RW 12.2664

Potential DRGs

001 Heart Transplant or Implant of Heart Assist System with MCC 27.0986

DRG	PDx/SDx/Procedure	Tips
001	Heart and lung transplant	
	AND	
	MCC condition	*See* appendix B.

DRG 008 Simultaneous Pancreas and Kidney Transplant — RW 5.2617

Potential DRGs

019 Simultaneous Pancreas and Kidney Transplant with Hemodialysis 7.9935

DRG	PDx/SDx/Procedure	Tips
019	Pancreas and kidney transplant	
	WITH	
	Hemodialysis	Some patients require hemodialysis while waiting for a donor kidney, or after the kidney has been implanted but has not returned to optimal function.

DRG 010 Pancreas Transplant RW 4.8136

Potential DRGs

008	Simultaneous Pancreas and Kidney Transplant	5.2617
019	Simultaneous Pancreas and Kidney Transplant with Hemodialysis	7.9935

DRG	PDx/SDx/Procedure	Tips
008	Pancreas and kidney transplant	
	AND	
	PDx or SDx of diabetes	
	AND	
	PDx or SDx of chronic kidney disease (CKD)	
019	Pancreas and kidney transplant	
	WITH	
	Hemodialysis	Some patients require hemodialysis while waiting for a donor kidney, or after the kidney has been implanted but has not returned to optimal function.
	AND	
	PDx or SDx of diabetes	
	AND	
	PDx or SDx of chronic kidney disease (CKD)	

DRG 011 Tracheostomy for Face, Mouth, and Neck Diagnoses or Laryngectomy with MCC RW 5.1563

Potential DRGs

003	ECMO or Tracheostomy with Mechanical Ventilation > 96 Hours or Principal Diagnosis Except Face, Mouth and Neck with Major O.R. Procedure	21.3203
004	Tracheostomy with Mechanical Ventilation > 96 Hours or Principal Diagnosis Except Face, Mouth and Neck without Major O.R. Procedure	14.7000

DRG	PDx/SDx/Procedure	Tips
003	Extracorporeal membrane oxygenation (ECMO), central or peripheral	Central ECMO provides cardiorespiratory support and involves direct surgical cannulation of the right atrium and aorta via sternotomy. Peripheral (percutaneous) ECMO is a less invasive procedure than central ECMO. Veno-arterial (VA) peripheral ECMO cannulas are inserted percutaneously into both the femoral artery and the femoral vein. This type of ECMO provides both respiratory and circulatory support. Veno-venous (VV) peripheral ECMO may use one or two venous insertions, one in the upper veins and, if used, one in the lower veins, and provides respiratory support only.
	OR	
	Tracheostomy	Tracheostomy carried out elsewhere prior to admission or in an ambulance prior to arrival should not be reported as a current procedure. A tracheostomy procedure may be performed at the bedside and documented in the progress notes or in the operating room and documented in an operative note.
	WITH	
	Mechanical ventilation > 96 hours	Review record documentation for start and stop times. Calculation of mechanical ventilation hours begins when vent is initiated (or time of admission if patient already on a vent) and ends when it is turned off (or the time patient is discharged if still ventilated). The duration includes time spent to wean the patient from the vent. Do not assume that ventilation that spans four calendar days equals > 96 hours; count by the hour not day.
	OR	
	Principal diagnosis not including those related to face, mouth or neck	Any diagnosis not listed under MS-DRG 011.
	WITH	
	Any O.R. procedure not listed under MS-DRGs 987–989	
004	Tracheostomy	*See* DRG 003.
	WITH	
	Mechanical ventilation > 96 hours	*See* DRG 003.
	OR	
	Principal diagnosis not including those related to face, mouth or neck	*See* DRG 003.

DRG 012 Tracheostomy for Face, Mouth, and Neck Diagnoses or Laryngectomy with CC RW 4.0049

Potential DRGs

003	ECMO or Tracheostomy with Mechanical Ventilation > 96 Hours or Principal Diagnosis Except Face, Mouth and Neck with Major O.R. Procedure	21.3203
004	Tracheostomy with Mechanical Ventilation > 96 Hours or Principal Diagnosis Except Face, Mouth and Neck without Major O.R. Procedure	14.7000
011	Tracheostomy for Face, Mouth, and Neck Diagnoses or Laryngectomy with MCC	5.1563

DRG	PDx/SDx/Procedure	Tips
003	Extracorporeal membrane oxygenation (ECMO), central or peripheral	Central ECMO provides cardiorespiratory support and involves direct surgical cannulation of the right atrium and aorta via sternotomy. Peripheral (percutaneous) ECMO is a less invasive procedure than central ECMO. Veno-arterial (VA) peripheral ECMO cannulas are inserted percutaneously into both the femoral artery and the femoral vein. This type of ECMO provides both respiratory and circulatory support. Veno-venous (VV) peripheral ECMO may use one or two venous insertions, one in the upper veins and, if used, one in the lower veins, and provides respiratory support only.
	OR	
	Tracheostomy	Tracheostomy carried out elsewhere prior to admission or in an ambulance prior to arrival should not be reported as a current procedure. A tracheostomy procedure may be performed at the bedside and documented in the progress notes or in the operating room and documented in an operative note.
	WITH	
	Mechanical ventilation > 96 hours	Review record documentation for start and stop times. Calculation of mechanical ventilation hours begins when vent is initiated (or time of admission if patient already on a vent) and ends when it is turned off (or the time patient is discharged if still ventilated). The duration includes time spent to wean the patient from the vent. Do not assume that ventilation that spans four calendar days equals > 96 hours; count by the hour not day.
	OR	
	Principal diagnosis not including those related to face, mouth or neck	Any diagnosis not listed under MS-DRG 011.
	WITH	
	Any O.R. procedure not listed under MS-DRGs 987–989	
004	Tracheostomy	*See* DRG 003.
	WITH	
	Mechanical ventilation > 96 hours	*See* DRG 003.
	OR	
	Principal diagnosis not including those related to face, mouth or neck	*See* DRG 003.
011	MCC condition	*See* appendix B.

DRG 013 Tracheostomy for Face, Mouth, and Neck Diagnoses or Laryngectomy without CC/MCC — RW 2.6857

Potential DRGs

003	ECMO or Tracheostomy with Mechanical Ventilation > 96 Hours or Principal Diagnosis Except Face, Mouth, and Neck with Major O.R. Procedure	21.3203
004	Tracheostomy with Mechanical Ventilation > 96 Hours or Principal Diagnosis Except Face, Mouth and Neck without Major O.R. Procedure	14.7000
011	Tracheostomy for Face, Mouth, and Neck Diagnoses or Laryngectomy with MCC	5.1563
012	Tracheostomy for Face, Mouth, and Neck Diagnoses or Laryngectomy with CC	4.0049

DRG	PDx/SDx/Procedure	Tips
003	Extracorporeal membrane oxygenation (ECMO), central or peripheral	Central ECMO provides cardiorespiratory support and involves direct surgical cannulation of the right atrium and aorta via sternotomy. Peripheral (percutaneous) ECMO is a less invasive procedure than central ECMO. Veno-arterial (VA) peripheral ECMO cannulas are inserted percutaneously into both the femoral artery and the femoral vein. This type of ECMO provides both respiratory and circulatory support. Veno-venous (VV) peripheral ECMO may use one or two venous insertions, one in the upper veins and, if used, one in the lower veins, and provides respiratory support only.
	OR	
	Tracheostomy	Tracheostomy carried out elsewhere prior to admission or in an ambulance prior to arrival should not be reported as a current procedure. A tracheostomy procedure may be performed at the bedside and documented in the progress notes or in the operating room and documented in an operative note.
	WITH	
	Mechanical ventilation > 96 hours	Review record documentation for start and stop times. Calculation of mechanical ventilation hours begins when vent is initiated (or time of admission if patient already on a vent) and ends when it is turned off (or the time patient is discharged if still ventilated). The duration includes time spent to wean the patient from the vent. Do not assume that ventilation that spans four calendar days equals > 96 hours; count by the hour not day.
	OR	
	Principal diagnosis not including those related to face, mouth or neck	Any diagnosis not listed under MS-DRG 011.
	WITH	
	Any O.R. procedure not listed under MS-DRGs 987–989	
004	Tracheostomy	*See* DRG 003.
	WITH	
	Mechanical ventilation > 96 hours	*See* DRG ØØ3.
	OR	
	Principal diagnosis not including those related to face, mouth or neck	*See* DRG ØØ3.
011	MCC condition	*See* appendix B.
012	CC condition	*See* appendix B.

DRG 014 Allogeneic Bone Marrow Transplant — RW 11.4609

No Potential DRG

DRG 016 Autologous Bone Marrow Transplant with CC/MCC — RW 6.1770

Potential DRGs

014	Allogeneic Bone Marrow Transplant	11.4609

DRG	PDx/SDx/Procedure	Tips
014	Allogeneic bone marrow transplant	In allogeneic transplants, the patient receives bone marrow or stem cells from a donor, usually a sibling or parent but an unrelated donor may also be used. In autologous transplants, the patient receives his or her own stem cells.

DRG 017 Autologous Bone Marrow Transplant without CC/MCC — RW 6.1770

Potential DRGs

014	Allogeneic Bone Marrow Transplant	11.4609
016	Autologous Bone Marrow Transplant with CC/MCC	6.1770

DRG	PDx/SDx/Procedure	Tips
014	Allogeneic bone marrow transplant	In allogeneic transplants, the patient receives bone marrow or stem cells from a donor, usually a sibling or parent but an unrelated donor may also be used. In autologous transplants, the patient receives his or her own stem cells.
016	MCC condition	*See* appendix B.
	OR	
	CC condition	*See* appendix B.

DRG 018 Chimeric Antigen Receptor (CAR) T-cell and Other Immunotherapies — RW 36.8427

No Potential DRGs

DRG 019 Simultaneous Pancreas and Kidney Transplant with Hemodialysis — RW 7.9935

No Potential DRGs

MDC 1

Diseases And Disorders Of The Nervous System

DRG 020 Intracranial Vascular Procedures with Principal Diagnosis of Hemorrhage with MCC — RW 8.4524

No Potential DRGs

DRG 021 Intracranial Vascular Procedures with Principal Diagnosis of Hemorrhage with CC — RW 6.1414

Potential DRGs

020 Intracranial Vascular Procedures with Principal Diagnosis of Hemorrhage with MCC 8.4524

DRG	PDx/SDx/Procedure	Tips
020	MCC condition	*See* appendix B.

DRG 022 Intracranial Vascular Procedures with Principal Diagnosis of Hemorrhage without CC/MCC — RW 3.4767

Potential DRGs

020 Intracranial Vascular Procedures with Principal Diagnosis of Hemorrhage with MCC 8.4524
021 Intracranial Vascular Procedures with Principal Diagnosis of Hemorrhage with CC 6.1414

DRG	PDx/SDx/Procedure	Tips
020	MCC condition	*See* appendix B.
021	CC condition	*See* appendix B.

DRG 023 Craniotomy with Major Device Implant/Acute Complex CNS Principal Diagnosis with MCC or Chemotherapy Implant or Epilepsy with Neurostimulator — RW 5.6688

No Potential DRGs

DRG 024 Craniotomy with Major Device Implant/Acute Complex CNS Principal Diagnosis without MCC — RW 3.7888

Potential DRGs

023 Craniotomy with Major Device Implant/Acute Complex CNS Principal Diagnosis with MCC or Chemotherapy Implant or Epilepsy with Neurostimulator 5.6688

DRG	PDx/SDx/Procedure	Tips
023	MCC condition	*See* appendix B.
	OR	
	Chemo Implant	
	OR	
	Epilepsy principal diagnosis	
	WITH	
	Neurostimulator	Insertion of neurostimulator lead in the brain in combination with neurostimulator generator insertion into the skull.

DRG 025 Craniotomy and Endovascular Intracranial Procedures with MCC RW 4.4160

Potential DRGs

020	Intracranial Vascular Procedures with Principal Diagnosis of Hemorrhage with MCC	8.4524
023	Craniotomy with Major Device Implant/Acute Complex CNS Principal Diagnosis with MCC or Chemotherapy Implant or Epilepsy with Neurostimulator	5.6688
955	Craniotomy for Multiple Significant Trauma	6.0902

DRG	PDx/SDx/Procedure	Tips
020	Cerebral hemorrhage	It may be that a cerebral hemorrhage code, that is currently a secondary diagnosis and functioning as the only MCC, can be resequenced as the PDx (when supported by the documentation). Unless another MCC is present, the case may not group to MS-DRG 020 but to one of the other MS-DRGs in this family, MS-DRG 021 or 022, depending on the presence or absence of a CC condition.
	AND	
	Intracranial vascular procedure	
	AND	
	MCC condition	*See* appendix B.
023	Major device implant	Neurostimulator lead insertion in combination with generator insertion.
	OR	
	Acute complex CNS principal diagnoses; meningitis, encephalitis, myelitis, brain abscess, toxic encephalopathy	
	Nontraumatic brain hemorrhage	
	Cerebral infarction	
	AND	
	MCC condition	*See* appendix B.
	OR	
	Chemo Implant	
	OR	
	Epilepsy principal diagnosis	
	WITH	
	Neurostimulator	Insertion of neurostimulator lead in the brain in combination with neurostimulator generator insertion into the skull.
955	Craniotomy for multiple significant trauma; repair, reposition head and facial bones	Craniotomy and PDx of trauma and at least two injuries (assigned as PDx or SDx) that are defined as significant trauma from different body site categories listed under MS-DRG 963.
	Repair traumatic injury to brain, cerebral meninges, dura mater, cerebral ventricle, cerebral hemisphere, basal ganglia, thalamus, hypothalamus, pons, cerebellum, medulla oblongata	

DRG 026 Craniotomy and Endovascular Intracranial Procedures with CC RW 2.9531

Potential DRGs

020	Intracranial Vascular Procedures with Principal Diagnosis of Hemorrhage with MCC	8.4524
021	Intracranial Vascular Procedures with Principal Diagnosis of Hemorrhage with CC	6.1414
023	Craniotomy with Major Device Implant/Acute Complex CNS Principal Diagnosis with MCC or Chemotherapy Implant or Epilepsy with Neurostimulator	5.6688
024	Craniotomy with Major Device Implant/Acute Complex CNS Principal Diagnosis without MCC	3.7888
025	Craniotomy and Endovascular Intracranial Procedures with MCC	4.4160
955	Craniotomy for Multiple Significant Trauma	6.0902

DRG	PDx/SDx/Procedure	Tips
020	Cerebral hemorrhage	It may be that a cerebral hemorrhage code, that is currently a secondary diagnosis and functioning as the only MCC, can be resequenced as the PDx (when supported by the documentation). Unless another MCC is present, the case may not group to MS-DRG 020 but to one of the other MS-DRGs in this family, MS-DRG 021 or 022, depending on the presence or absence of a CC condition.
	AND	
	Intracranial vascular procedure	
	AND	
	MCC condition	*See* appendix B.
021	Cerebral hemorrhage	
	AND	
	Intracranial vascular procedure	
	AND	
	CC condition	*See* appendix B.
023	Major device implant	Neurostimulator lead insertion in combination with generator insertion.
	OR	
	Acute complex CNS principal diagnoses; meningitis, encephalitis, myelitis, brain abscess, toxic encephalopathy	
	Nontraumatic brain hemorrhage	
	Cerebral infarction	
	AND	
	MCC condition	*See* appendix B.
	OR	
	Chemo Implant	
	OR	
	Epilepsy principal diagnosis	
	WITH	
	Neurostimulator	Insertion of neurostimulator lead in the brain in combination with neurostimulator generator insertion into the skull.
024	Major device implant	Neurostimulator lead insertion in combination with generator insertion.
	OR	
	Acute complex CNS principal diagnoses; meningitis, encephalitis, myelitis, brain abscess, toxic encephalopathy	
	Nontraumatic brain hemorrhage	
	Cerebral infarction	
025	MCC condition	*See* appendix B.
955	Craniotomy for multiple significant trauma; repair, reposition head and facial bones	Craniotomy and PDx of trauma and at least two injuries (assigned as PDx or SDx) that are defined as significant trauma from different body site categories listed under MS-DRG 963.
	Repair traumatic injury to brain, cerebral meninges, dura mater, cerebral ventricle, cerebral hemisphere, basal ganglia, thalamus, hypothalamus, pons, cerebellum, medulla oblongata	

DRG 027 Craniotomy and Endovascular Intracranial Procedures without CC/MCC RW 2.4329

Potential DRGs

020	Intracranial Vascular Procedures with Principal Diagnosis of Hemorrhage with MCC	8.4524
021	Intracranial Vascular Procedures with Principal Diagnosis of Hemorrhage with CC	6.1414
022	Intracranial Vascular Procedures with Principal Diagnosis of Hemorrhage without CC/MCC	3.4767
023	Craniotomy with Major Device Implant/Acute Complex CNS Principal Diagnosis with MCC or Chemotherapy Implant or Epilepsy with Neurostimulator	5.6688
024	Craniotomy with Major Device Implant/Acute Complex CNS Principal Diagnosis without MCC	3.7888
025	Craniotomy and Endovascular Intracranial Procedures with MCC	4.4160
026	Craniotomy and Endovascular Intracranial Procedures with CC	2.9531
955	Craniotomy for Multiple Significant Trauma	6.0902

DRG	PDx/SDx/Procedure	Tips
020	Cerebral hemorrhage	It may be that a cerebral hemorrhage code that is currently a secondary diagnosis and functioning as the only MCC can be resequenced as the PDx (when supported by documentation). Unless another MCC is present, the case may not group to MS-DRG 020 but to one of the other MS-DRGs in this family, MS-DRG 021 or 022, depending on the presence or absence of a CC condition.
	AND	
	Intracranial vascular procedure	
	AND	
	MCC condition	*See* appendix B.
021	Cerebral hemorrhage	
	AND	
	Intracranial vascular procedure	
	AND	
	CC condition	*See* appendix B.
022	Cerebral hemorrhage	
	AND	
	Intracranial vascular procedure	
023	Major device implant	Neurostimulator lead insertion in combination with generator insertion.
	OR	
	Acute complex CNS principal diagnoses; meningitis, encephalitis, myelitis, brain abscess, toxic encephalopathy	
	Nontraumatic brain hemorrhage	
	Cerebral infarction	
	AND	
	MCC condition	*See* appendix B.
	OR	
	Chemo Implant	
	OR	
	Epilepsy principal diagnosis	
	WITH	
	Neurostimulator	Insertion of neurostimulator lead in the brain in combination with neurostimulator generator insertion into the skull.
024	Major device implant	Neurostimulator lead insertion in combination with generator insertion.
	OR	
	Acute complex CNS principal diagnoses; meningitis, encephalitis, myelitis, brain abscess, toxic encephalopathy	
	Nontraumatic brain hemorrhage	
	Cerebral infarction	
025	MCC condition	*See* appendix B.
026	CC condition	*See* appendix B.
955	Craniotomy for multiple significant trauma; repair, reposition head and facial bones	Craniotomy and PDx of trauma and at least two injuries (assigned as PDx or SDx) that are defined as significant trauma from different body site categories listed under MS-DRG 963.
	Repair traumatic injury to brain, cerebral meninges, dura mater, cerebral ventricle, cerebral hemisphere, basal ganglia, thalamus, hypothalamus, pons, cerebellum, medulla oblongata	

DRG 028 Spinal Procedures with MCC RW 6.0261

Potential DRGs

456	Spinal Fusion Except Cervical with Spinal Curvature/Malignancy/Infection or Extensive Fusions with MCC	8.4294

DRG	PDx/SDx/Procedure	Tips
456	Noncervical spinal fusion	
	AND	
	PDX of spinal curvature, collapsed vertebra, osteoporosis	Review operative report for scoliosis, kyphosis, lordosis, or malignancy. Review operative report for indication of metastasis.
	Malignancy	Clarify with physician if the pathological fracture is noted, whether possibly due to metastasis when patient has previous history of malignancy.
	Infection	
	OR	
	Secondary diagnosis of spinal curvature	
	OR	
	Extensive fusions	Fusion of eight or more thoracic joints. Fusion of two to seven thoracic joints in combination with fusion of two or more lumbar joints.
	AND	
	MCC condition	*See* appendix B.

DRG 029 Spinal Procedures with CC or Spinal Neurostimulator RW 3.4282

Potential DRGs

028	Spinal Procedures with MCC	6.0261
456	Spinal Fusion Except Cervical with Spinal Curvature/Malignancy/Infection or Extensive Fusions with MCC	8.4294
457	Spinal Fusion Except Cervical with Spinal Curvature/Malignancy/Infection or Extensive Fusions with CC	6.0753

DRG	PDx/SDx/Procedure	Tips
028	MCC condition	*See* appendix B.
456	Noncervical spinal fusion	
	AND	
	PDX of spinal curvature, collapsed vertebra, osteoporosis	Review operative report for scoliosis, kyphosis, lordosis, or malignancy. Review operative report for indication of metastasis.
	Malignancy	Clarify with physician if the pathological fracture is noted, whether possibly due to metastasis when patient has previous history of malignancy.
	Infection	
	OR	
	Secondary diagnosis of spinal curvature	
	OR	
	Extensive fusions	Fusion of eight or more thoracic joints. Fusion of two to seven thoracic joints in combination with fusion of two or more lumbar joints.
	AND	
	MCC condition	*See* appendix B.
457	Noncervical spinal fusion	
	AND	
	PDX of spinal curvature, collapsed vertebra, osteoporosis	Review operative report for scoliosis, kyphosis, lordosis, or malignancy. Review operative report for indication of metastasis.
	Malignancy	Clarify with physician if the pathological fracture is noted, whether possibly due to metastasis when patient has previous history of malignancy.
	Infection	
	OR	
	Secondary diagnosis of spinal curvature	
	OR	
	Extensive fusions	Fusion of eight or more thoracic joints. Fusion of two to seven thoracic joints in combination with fusion of two or more lumbar joints.
	AND	
	CC condition	*See* appendix B.

DRG 030 Spinal Procedures without CC/MCC

RW 2.3190

Potential DRGs

028	Spinal Procedures with MCC	6.0261
029	Spinal Procedures with CC or Spinal Neurostimulator	3.4282
456	Spinal Fusion Except Cervical with Spinal Curvature/Malignancy/Infection or Extensive Fusions with MCC	8.4294
457	Spinal Fusion Except Cervical with Spinal Curvature/Malignancy/Infection or Extensive Fusions with CC	6.0753
458	Spinal Fusion Except Cervical with Spinal Curvature/Malignancy/Infection or Extensive Fusions without CC/MCC	4.5310

DRG	PDx/SDx/Procedure	Tips
028	MCC condition	*See* appendix B.
029	CC condition	*See* appendix B.
	OR	
	Spinal neurostimulator implant	
456	Noncervical spinal fusion	
	AND	
	PDX of spinal curvature, collapsed vertebra, osteoporosis	Review operative report for scoliosis, kyphosis, lordosis, or malignancy. Review operative report for indication of metastasis.
	Malignancy	Clarify with physician if the pathological fracture is noted, whether possibly due to metastasis when patient has previous history of malignancy.
	Infection	
	OR	
	Secondary diagnosis of spinal curvature	
	OR	
	Extensive fusions	Fusion of eight or more thoracic joints. Fusion of two to seven thoracic joints in combination with fusion of two or more lumbar joints.
	AND	
	MCC condition	*See* appendix B.
457	Noncervical spinal fusion	
	AND	
	PDX of spinal curvature, collapsed vertebra, osteoporosis	*See* DRG 456.
	Malignancy	*See* DRG 456.
	Infection	
	OR	
	Secondary diagnosis of spinal curvature	
	OR	
	Extensive fusions	*See* DRG 456.
	AND	
	CC condition	*See* appendix B.
458	Noncervical spinal fusion	
	AND	
	PDX of spinal curvature, collapsed vertebra, osteoporosis	*See* DRG 456.
	Malignancy	*See* DRG 456.
	Infection	
	OR	
	Secondary diagnosis of spinal curvature	
	OR	
	Extensive fusions	*See* DRG 456.

DRG 031 Ventricular Shunt Procedures with MCC RW 4.1166

Potential DRGs

020	Intracranial Vascular Procedures with Principal Diagnosis of Hemorrhage with MCC	8.4524
023	Craniotomy with Major Device Implant/Acute Complex CNS Principal Diagnosis with MCC or Chemotherapy Implant or Epilepsy with Neurostimulator	5.6688
025	Craniotomy and Endovascular Intracranial Procedures with MCC	4.4160

DRG	PDx/SDx/Procedure	Tips
020	Cerebral hemorrhage	
	AND	
	Intracranial vascular procedure	
	AND	
	MCC condition	*See* appendix B.
023	Craniotomy procedure	
	WITH	
	Major device implant	Neurostimulator lead insertion in combination with generator insertion.
	OR	
	Acute complex CNS principal diagnoses; meningitis, encephalitis, myelitis, brain abscess, toxic encephalopathy	
	Nontraumatic brain hemorrhage	
	Cerebral infarction	
	AND	
	MCC condition	*See* appendix B.
	OR	
	Chemo Implant	
	OR	
	Epilepsy principal diagnosis	
	WITH	
	Neurostimulator	Insertion of neurostimulator lead in the brain in combination with neurostimulator generator insertion into the skull.
025	Craniotomy procedure	
	OR	
	Endovascular intracranial procedure	
	AND	
	MCC condition	*See* appendix B.

DRG 032 Ventricular Shunt Procedures with CC

RW 2.1538

Potential DRGs

020	Intracranial Vascular Procedures with Principal Diagnosis of Hemorrhage with MCC	8.4524
021	Intracranial Vascular Procedures with Principal Diagnosis of Hemorrhage with CC	6.1414
023	Craniotomy with Major Device Implant/Acute Complex CNS Principal Diagnosis with MCC or Chemotherapy Implant or Epilepsy with Neurostimulator	5.6688
024	Craniotomy with Major Device Implant/Acute Complex CNS Principal Diagnosis without MCC	3.7888
025	Craniotomy and Endovascular Intracranial Procedures with MCC	4.4160
026	Craniotomy and Endovascular Intracranial Procedures with CC	2.9531
031	Ventricular Shunt Procedures with MCC	4.1166

DRG	PDx/SDx/Procedure	Tips
020	Cerebral hemorrhage	
	AND	
	Intracranial vascular procedure	
	AND	
	MCC condition	*See* appendix B.
021	Cerebral hemorrhage	
	AND	
	Intracranial vascular procedure	
	AND	
	CC condition	*See* appendix B.
023	Craniotomy procedure	
	WITH	
	Major device implant	Neurostimulator lead insertion in combination with generator insertion.
	OR	
	Acute complex CNS principal diagnoses; meningitis, encephalitis, myelitis, brain abscess, toxic encephalopathy	
	Nontraumatic brain hemorrhage	
	Cerebral infarction	
	AND	
	MCC condition	*See* appendix B.
	OR	
	Chemo Implant	
	OR	
	Epilepsy principal diagnosis	
	WITH	
	Neurostimulator	Insertion of neurostimulator lead in the brain in combination with neurostimulator generator insertion into the skull.
024	Craniotomy procedure	
	WITH	
	Major device implant	*See* DRG 023.
	OR	
	Acute complex CNS principal diagnoses; meningitis, encephalitis, myelitis, brain abscess, toxic encephalopathy	
	Nontraumatic brain hemorrhage	
	Cerebral infarction	
	Endovascular intracranial procedure	
025	Craniotomy procedure	
	OR	
	Endovascular intracranial procedure	
	AND	
	MCC condition	*See* appendix B.
026	Craniotomy procedure	
	OR	
	Endovascular intracranial procedure	
	AND	
	CC condition	*See* appendix B.
031	MCC condition	*See* appendix B.

DRG 033 Ventricular Shunt Procedures without CC/MCC RW 1.6229

Potential DRGs

020	Intracranial Vascular Procedures with Principal Diagnosis of Hemorrhage with MCC	8.4524
021	Intracranial Vascular Procedures with Principal Diagnosis of Hemorrhage with CC	6.1414
022	Intracranial Vascular Procedures with Principal Diagnosis of Hemorrhage without CC/MCC	3.4767
023	Craniotomy with Major Device Implant/Acute Complex CNS Principal Diagnosis with MCC or Chemotherapy Implant or Epilepsy with Neurostimulator	5.6688
024	Craniotomy with Major Device Implant/Acute Complex CNS Principal Diagnosis without MCC	3.7888
025	Craniotomy and Endovascular Intracranial Procedures with MCC	4.4160
026	Craniotomy and Endovascular Intracranial Procedures with CC	2.9531
027	Craniotomy and Endovascular Intracranial Procedures without CC/MCC	2.4329
031	Ventricular Shunt Procedures with MCC	4.1166
032	Ventricular Shunt Procedures with CC	2.1538

DRG	PDx/SDx/Procedure	Tips
020	Cerebral hemorrhage	
	AND	
	Intracranial vascular procedure	
	AND	
	MCC condition	*See* appendix B.
021	Cerebral hemorrhage	
	AND	
	Intracranial vascular procedure	
	AND	
	CC condition	*See* appendix B.
022	Cerebral hemorrhage	
	AND	
	Intracranial vascular procedure	
023	Craniotomy procedure	
	WITH	
	Major device implant	Neurostimulator lead insertion in combination with generator insertion.
	OR	
	Acute complex CNS principal diagnoses; meningitis, encephalitis, myelitis, brain abscess, toxic encephalopathy	
	Nontraumatic brain hemorrhage	
	Cerebral infarction	
	AND	
	MCC condition	*See* appendix B.
	OR	
	Chemo Implant	
	OR	
	Epilepsy principal diagnosis	
	WITH	
	Neurostimulator	Insertion of neurostimulator lead in the brain in combination with neurostimulator generator insertion into the skull.
024	Craniotomy procedure	
	WITH	
	Major device implant	Neurostimulator lead insertion in combination with generator insertion.
	OR	
	Acute complex CNS principal diagnoses; meningitis, encephalitis, myelitis, brain abscess, toxic encephalopathy	
	Nontraumatic brain hemorrhage	
	Cerebral infarction	
025	Craniotomy procedure	
	OR	
	Endovascular intracranial procedure	
	AND	
	MCC condition	*See* appendix B.
026	Craniotomy procedure	
	OR	
	Endovascular intracranial procedure	
	AND	
	CC condition	*See* appendix B.
027	Craniotomy procedure	
	OR	
	Endovascular intracranial procedure	
031	MCC condition	*See* appendix B.
032	CC condition	*See* appendix B.

DRG 034 Carotid Artery Stent Procedure with MCC — RW 3.9014

No Potential DRGs

DRG 035 Carotid Artery Stent Procedure with CC — RW 2.2995

Potential DRGs

034	Carotid Artery Stent Procedure with MCC	3.9014

DRG	PDx/SDx/Procedure	Tips
034	MCC condition	*See* appendix B.

DRG 036 Carotid Artery Stent Procedure without CC/MCC — RW 1.8082

Potential DRGs

034	Carotid Artery Stent Procedure with MCC	3.9014
035	Carotid Artery Stent Procedure with CC	2.2995

DRG	PDx/SDx/Procedure	Tips
034	MCC condition	*See* appendix B.
035	CC condition	*See* appendix B.

DRG 037 Extracranial Procedures with MCC — RW 3.3756

Potential DRGs

023	Craniotomy with Major Device Implant/Acute Complex CNS Principal Diagnosis with MCC or Chemotherapy Implant or Epilepsy with Neurostimulator	5.6688
025	Craniotomy and Endovascular Intracranial Procedures with MCC	4.4160
034	Carotid Artery Stent Procedure with MCC	3.9014

DRG	PDx/SDx/Procedure	Tips
023	Craniotomy procedure	
	AND	
	Major device implant	Neurostimulator lead insertion in combination with generator insertion.
	OR	
	Acute complex CNS principal diagnoses; meningitis, encephalitis, myelitis, brain abscess, toxic encephalopathy	
	Nontraumatic brain hemorrhage	
	Cerebral infarction	
	AND	
	MCC condition	*See* appendix B.
	OR	
	Chemo Implant	
	OR	
	Epilepsy principal diagnosis	
	WITH	
	Neurostimulator	Insertion of neurostimulator lead in the brain in combination with neurostimulator generator insertion into the skull.
025	Craniotomy procedure	
	OR	
	Endovascular intracranial procedure	
	AND	
	MCC condition	*See* appendix B.
034	Carotid artery stent placement	Carotid artery stenting only or stenting of vertebral artery or vein, internal or external jugular vein, or right facial vein in combination with stenting of the right common carotid artery.
	AND	
	MCC condition	*See* appendix B.

DRG 038 Extracranial Procedures with CC RW 1.5999

Potential DRGs

023	Craniotomy with Major Device Implant/Acute Complex CNS Principal Diagnosis with MCC or Chemotherapy Implant or Epilepsy with Neurostimulator	5.6688
024	Craniotomy with Major Device Implant/Acute Complex CNS Principal Diagnosis without MCC	3.7888
025	Craniotomy and Endovascular Intracranial Procedures with MCC	4.4160
026	Craniotomy and Endovascular Intracranial Procedures with CC	2.9531
034	Carotid Artery Stent Procedure with MCC	3.9014
035	Carotid Artery Stent Procedure with CC	2.2995
037	Extracranial Procedures with MCC	3.3756

DRG	PDx/SDx/Procedure	Tips
023	Craniotomy procedure	
	AND	
	Major device implant	Neurostimulator lead insertion in combination with generator insertion.
	OR	
	Acute complex CNS principal diagnoses; meningitis, encephalitis, myelitis, brain abscess, toxic encephalopathy	
	Nontraumatic brain hemorrhage	
	Cerebral infarction	
	AND	
	MCC condition	*See* appendix B.
	OR	
	Chemo Implant	
	OR	
	Epilepsy principal diagnosis	
	WITH	
	Neurostimulator	Insertion of neurostimulator lead in the brain in combination with neurostimulator generator insertion into the skull.
024	Craniotomy procedure	
	AND	
	Major device implant	Neurostimulator lead insertion in combination with generator insertion.
	OR	
	Acute complex CNS principal diagnoses; meningitis, encephalitis, myelitis, brain abscess, toxic encephalopathy	
	Nontraumatic brain hemorrhage	
	Cerebral infarction	
025	Craniotomy procedure	
	OR	
	Endovascular intracranial procedure	
	AND	
	MCC condition	*See* appendix B.
026	Craniotomy procedure	
	OR	
	Endovascular intracranial procedure	
	AND	
	CC condition	*See* appendix B.
034	Carotid artery stent placement	Carotid artery stenting only or stenting of vertebral artery or vein, internal or external jugular vein, or right facial vein in combination with stenting of the right common carotid artery.
	AND	
	MCC condition	*See* appendix B.
035	Carotid artery stent placement	*See* DRG 034.
	AND	
	CC condition	*See* appendix B.
037	MCC condition	*See* appendix B.

DRG 039 Extracranial Procedures without CC/MCC RW 1.1410

Potential DRGs

023	Craniotomy with Major Device Implant/Acute Complex CNS Principal Diagnosis with MCC or Chemotherapy Implant or Epilepsy with Neurostimulator	5.6688
024	Craniotomy with Major Device Implant/Acute Complex CNS Principal Diagnosis without MCC	3.7888
025	Craniotomy and Endovascular Intracranial Procedures with MCC	4.4160
026	Craniotomy and Endovascular Intracranial Procedures with CC	2.9531
027	Craniotomy and Endovascular Intracranial Procedures without CC/MCC	2.4329
034	Carotid Artery Stent Procedure with MCC	3.9014
035	Carotid Artery Stent Procedure with CC	2.2995
036	Carotid Artery Stent Procedure without CC/MCC	1.8082
037	Extracranial Procedures with MCC	3.3756
038	Extracranial Procedures with CC	1.5999

DRG	PDx/SDx/Procedure	Tips
023	Craniotomy procedure	
	AND	
	Major device implant	Neurostimulator lead insertion in combination with generator insertion.
	OR	
	Acute complex CNS principal diagnoses; meningitis, encephalitis, myelitis, brain abscess, toxic encephalopathy	
	Nontraumatic brain hemorrhage	
	Cerebral infarction	
	AND	
	MCC condition	*See* appendix B.
	OR	
	Chemo Implant	
	OR	
	Epilepsy principal diagnosis	
	WITH	
	Neurostimulator	Insertion of neurostimulator lead in the brain in combination with neurostimulator generator insertion into the skull.
024	Craniotomy procedure	
	AND	
	Major device implant	Neurostimulator lead insertion in combination with generator insertion.
	OR	
	Acute complex CNS principal diagnoses; meningitis, encephalitis, myelitis, brain abscess, toxic encephalopathy	
	Nontraumatic brain hemorrhage	
	Cerebral infarction	
025	Craniotomy procedure	
	OR	
	Endovascular intracranial procedure	
	AND	
	MCC condition	*See* appendix B.
026	Craniotomy procedure	
	OR	
	Endovascular intracranial procedure	
	AND	
	CC condition	*See* appendix B.
027	Craniotomy procedure	
	OR	
	Endovascular intracranial procedure	
034	Carotid artery stent placement	Carotid artery stenting only or stenting of vertebral artery or vein, internal or external jugular vein, or right facial vein in combination with stenting of the right common carotid artery.
	AND	
	MCC condition	*See* appendix B.
035	Carotid artery stent placement	*See* DRG 034.
	AND	
	CC condition	*See* appendix B.
036	Carotid artery stent placement	*See* DRG 034.
037	MCC condition	*See* appendix B.
038	CC condition	*See* appendix B.

Optimizing Tips

DRG 040 Peripheral/Cranial Nerve and Other Nervous System Procedures with MCC RW 3.8505

Potential DRGs

023	Craniotomy with Major Device Implant/Acute Complex CNS Principal Diagnosis with MCC or Chemotherapy Implant or Epilepsy with Neurostimulator	5.6688
025	Craniotomy and Endovascular Intracranial Procedures with MCC	4.4160
901	Wound Debridements for Injuries with MCC	4.3278

DRG	PDx/SDx/Procedure	Tips
023	Craniotomy procedure	
	AND	
	Major device implant	Neurostimulator lead insertion in combination with generator insertion.
	OR	
	Acute complex CNS principal diagnoses; meningitis, encephalitis, myelitis, brain abscess, toxic encephalopathy	
	Nontraumatic brain hemorrhage	
	Cerebral infarction	
	AND	
	MCC condition	*See* appendix B.
	OR	
	Chemo Implant	
	OR	
	Epilepsy principal diagnosis	
	WITH	
	Neurostimulator	Insertion of neurostimulator lead in the brain in combination with neurostimulator generator insertion into the skull.
025	Craniotomy	
	OR	
	Endovascular intracranial procedure	
	AND	
	MCC condition	*See* appendix B.
901	Principal diagnosis of injury	
	AND	
	Debridement of wound, infection or burn	
	AND	
	MCC condition	*See* appendix B.

DRG 041 Peripheral/Cranial Nerve and Other Nervous System Procedures with CC or Peripheral Neurostimulator

RW 2.2307

Potential DRGs

023	Craniotomy with Major Device Implant/Acute Complex CNS Principal Diagnosis with MCC or Chemotherapy Implant or Epilepsy with Neurostimulator	5.6688
024	Craniotomy with Major Device Implant/Acute Complex CNS Principal Diagnosis without MCC	3.7888
025	Craniotomy and Endovascular Intracranial Procedures with MCC	4.4160
026	Craniotomy and Endovascular Intracranial Procedures with CC	2.9531
040	Peripheral/Cranial Nerve and Other Nervous System Procedures with MCC	3.8505
901	Wound Debridements for Injuries with MCC	4.3278

DRG	PDx/SDx/Procedure	Tips
023	Craniotomy procedure	
	AND	
	Major device implant	Neurostimulator lead insertion in combination with generator insertion.
	OR	
	Acute complex CNS principal diagnoses; meningitis, encephalitis, myelitis, brain abscess, toxic encephalopathy	
	Nontraumatic brain hemorrhage	
	Cerebral infarction	
	AND	
	MCC condition	*See* appendix B.
	OR	
	Chemo Implant	
	OR	
	Epilepsy principal diagnosis	
	WITH	
	Neurostimulator	Insertion of neurostimulator lead in the brain in combination with neurostimulator generator insertion into the skull.
024	Craniotomy procedure	
	AND	
	Major device implant	Neurostimulator lead insertion in combination with generator insertion.
	OR	
	Acute complex CNS principal diagnoses; meningitis, encephalitis, myelitis, brain abscess, toxic encephalopathy	
	Nontraumatic brain hemorrhage	
	Cerebral infarction	
025	Craniotomy	
	OR	
	Endovascular intracranial procedure	
	AND	
	MCC condition	*See* appendix B.
026	Craniotomy	
	OR	
	Endovascular intracranial procedure	
	AND	
	CC condition	*See* appendix B.
040	MCC condition	*See* appendix B.
901	Principal diagnosis of injury	
	AND	
	Debridement of wound, infection or burn	
	AND	
	MCC condition	*See* appendix B.

DRG 042 Peripheral/Cranial Nerve and Other Nervous System Procedures without CC/MCC RW 1.7398

Potential DRGs

023	Craniotomy with Major Device Implant/Acute Complex CNS Principal Diagnosis with MCC or Chemotherapy Implant or Epilepsy with Neurostimulator	5.6688
024	Craniotomy with Major Device Implant/Acute Complex CNS Principal Diagnosis without MCC	3.7888
025	Craniotomy and Endovascular Intracranial Procedures with MCC	4.4160
026	Craniotomy and Endovascular Intracranial Procedures with CC	2.9531
040	Peripheral/Cranial Nerve and Other Nervous System Procedures with MCC	3.8505
041	Peripheral/Cranial Nerve and Other Nervous System Procedures with CC or Peripheral Neurostimulator	2.2307
901	Wound Debridements for Injuries with MCC	4.3278
902	Wound Debridements for Injuries with CC	1.8847

DRG	PDx/SDx/Procedure	Tips
023	Craniotomy procedure	
	AND	
	Major device implant	Neurostimulator lead insertion in combination with generator insertion.
	OR	
	Acute complex CNS principal diagnoses; meningitis, encephalitis, myelitis, brain abscess, toxic encephalopathy	
	Nontraumatic brain hemorrhage	
	Cerebral infarction	
	AND	
	MCC condition	*See* appendix B.
	OR	
	Chemo Implant	
	OR	
	Epilepsy principal diagnosis	
	WITH	
	Neurostimulator	Insertion of neurostimulator lead in the brain in combination with neurostimulator generator insertion into the skull.
024	Craniotomy procedure	
	AND	
	Major device implant	Neurostimulator lead insertion in combination with generator insertion.
	OR	
	Acute complex CNS principal diagnoses; meningitis, encephalitis, myelitis, brain abscess, toxic encephalopathy	
	Nontraumatic brain hemorrhage	
	Cerebral infarction	
025	Craniotomy	
	OR	
	Endovascular intracranial procedure	
	AND	
	MCC condition	*See* appendix B.
026	Craniotomy	
	OR	
	Endovascular intracranial procedure	
	AND	
	CC condition	*See* appendix B.
040	MCC condition	*See* appendix B.
041	CC condition	*See* appendix B.
	OR	
	Peripheral or cranial neurostimulator implant	Neurostimulator lead insertion in combination with generator insertion.
901	Principal diagnosis of injury	
	AND	
	Debridement of wound, infection or burn	
	AND	
	MCC condition	*See* appendix B.
902	Principal diagnosis of injury	
	AND	
	Debridement of wound, infection or burn	
	AND	
	CC condition	*See* appendix B.

DRG 052 Spinal Disorders and Injuries with CC/MCC — RW 1.9445

Potential DRGs

028	Spinal Procedures with MCC	6.0261
029	Spinal Procedures with CC or Spinal Neurostimulator	3.4282
963	Other Multiple Significant Trauma with MCC	2.7343

DRG	PDx/SDx/Procedure	Tips
028	Spinal cord decompression	Includes spinal meninges.
	Spinal fusion or refusion	
	AND	
	MCC condition	*See* appendix B.
029	Spinal cord decompression	*See* DRG 028.
	Spinal fusion or refusion	
	AND	
	CC condition	*See* appendix B.
	OR	
	Spinal neurostimulator implant	Neurostimulator lead insertion in combination with generator insertion.
963	Other multiple significant trauma	Pdx of trauma and at least two significant trauma diagnosis codes from different body site categories. Refer to ED report, interventional radiology reports.
	AND	
	MCC condition	*See* appendix B.

DRG 053 Spinal Disorders and Injuries without CC/MCC — RW 0.9838

Potential DRGs

028	Spinal Procedures with MCC	6.0261
029	Spinal Procedures with CC or Spinal Neurostimulator	3.4282
030	Spinal Procedures without CC/MCC	2.3190
052	Spinal Disorders and Injuries with CC/MCC	1.9445
091	Other Disorders of Nervous System with MCC	1.7892
963	Other Multiple Significant Trauma with MCC	2.7343
964	Other Multiple Significant Trauma with CC	1.5010

DRG	PDx/SDx/Procedure	Tips
028	Spinal cord decompression	Includes spinal meninges.
	Spinal fusion or refusion	
	AND	
	MCC condition	*See* appendix B.
029	Spinal cord decompression	*See* DRG 028.
	Spinal fusion or refusion	
	AND	
	CC condition	*See* appendix B.
	OR	
	Spinal neurostimulator implant	Neurostimulator lead insertion in combination with generator insertion.
030	Spinal cord decompression	*See* DRG 028.
	Spinal fusion or refusion	
052	CC/MCC condition	*See* appendix B.
091	Monoplegia	Review physician documentation, nursing notes, and physical therapy notes to determine functional damage and query physician as necessary to confirm paralysis.
	OR	
	Transient limb paralysis	
	AND	
	MCC condition	*See* appendix B.
963	Other multiple significant trauma	Pdx of trauma and at least two significant trauma diagnosis codes from different body site categories. Refer to ED report, interventional radiology reports.
	AND	
	MCC condition	*See* appendix B.
964	Other multiple significant trauma	*See* DRG 963.
	AND	
	CC condition	*See* appendix B.

DRG 054 Nervous System Neoplasms with MCC — RW 1.4735

Potential DRGs

040	Peripheral/Cranial Nerve and Other Nervous System Procedures with MCC	3.8505

DRG	PDx/SDx/Procedure	Tips
040	Stereotactic radiosurgery	Review interventional radiology notes.
	AND	
	MCC condition	*See* appendix B.

DRG 055 Nervous System Neoplasms without MCC — RW 1.0732

Potential DRGs

040	Peripheral/Cranial Nerve and Other Nervous System Procedures with MCC	3.8505
041	Peripheral/Cranial Nerve and Other Nervous System Procedures with CC or Peripheral Neurostimulator	2.2307
042	Peripheral/Cranial Nerve and Other Nervous System Procedures without CC/MCC	1.7398
054	Nervous System Neoplasms with MCC	1.4735

DRG	PDx/SDx/Procedure	Tips
040	Stereotactic radiosurgery	Review interventional radiology notes.
	AND	
	MCC condition	*See* appendix B.
041	Stereotactic radiosurgery	Review interventional radiology notes.
	AND	
	CC condition	*See* appendix B.
	OR	
	Peripheral or cranial neurostimulator implant	Neurostimulator lead insertion in combination with generator insertion.
042	Stereotactic radiosurgery	Review interventional radiology notes.
054	MCC condition	*See* appendix B.

DRG 056 Degenerative Nervous System Disorders with MCC — RW 2.3940

Potential DRGs

028	Spinal Procedures with MCC	6.0261
040	Peripheral/Cranial Nerve and Other Nervous System Procedures with MCC	3.8505

DRG	PDx/SDx/Procedure	Tips
028	Spinal procedure	
	AND	
	MCC condition	*See* appendix B.
040	Nervous system procedure	
	AND	
	MCC condition	*See* appendix B.

DRG 057 Degenerative Nervous System Disorders without MCC — RW 1.3632

Potential DRGs

028	Spinal Procedures with MCC	6.0261
029	Spinal Procedures with CC or Spinal Neurostimulator	3.4282
030	Spinal Procedures without CC/MCC	2.3190
040	Peripheral/Cranial Nerve and Other Nervous System Procedures with MCC	3.8505
041	Peripheral/Cranial Nerve and Other Nervous System Procedures with CC or Peripheral Neurostimulator	2.2307
042	Peripheral/Cranial Nerve and Other Nervous System Procedures without CC/MCC	1.7398
056	Degenerative Nervous System Disorders with MCC	2.3940

DRG	PDx/SDx/Procedure	Tips
028	Spinal procedure	
	AND	
	MCC condition	*See* appendix B.
029	Spinal procedure	
	AND	
	CC condition	*See* appendix B.
	OR	
	Spinal neurostimulator implant	Neurostimulator lead insertion in combination with generator insertion.
030	Spinal procedure	
040	Nervous system procedure	
	AND	
	MCC condition	*See* appendix B.
041	Nervous system procedure	
	AND	
	CC condition	*See* appendix B.
	OR	
	Peripheral or cranial neurostimulator implant	Neurostimulator lead insertion in combination with generator insertion.
042	Nervous system procedure	
056	MCC condition	*See* appendix B.

DRG 058 Multiple Sclerosis and Cerebellar Ataxia with MCC — RW 1.7279

Potential DRGs

040	Peripheral/Cranial Nerve and Other Nervous System Procedures with MCC	3.8505

DRG	PDx/SDx/Procedure	Tips
040	Insertion of infusion device, monitoring device or other central and peripheral nervous system procedures	
	AND	
	MCC condition	*See* appendix B.

DRG 059 Multiple Sclerosis and Cerebellar Ataxia with CC — RW 1.1872

Potential DRGs

040	Peripheral/Cranial Nerve and Other Nervous System Procedures with MCC	3.8505
041	Peripheral/Cranial Nerve and Other Nervous System Procedures with CC or Peripheral Neurostimulator	2.2307
058	Multiple Sclerosis and Cerebellar Ataxia with MCC	1.7279

DRG	PDx/SDx/Procedure	Tips
040	Insertion of infusion device, monitoring device or other central and peripheral nervous system procedures	
	AND	
	MCC condition	*See* appendix B.
041	Insertion of infusion device, monitoring device or other central and peripheral nervous system procedures	
	AND	
	CC condition	*See* appendix B.
	OR	
	Peripheral or cranial neurostimulator implant	Neurostimulator lead insertion in combination with generator insertion.
058	MCC condition	*See* appendix B.

DRG 060 Multiple Sclerosis and Cerebellar Ataxia without CC/MCC — RW 0.8974

Potential DRGs

040	Peripheral/Cranial Nerve and Other Nervous System Procedures with MCC	3.8505
041	Peripheral/Cranial Nerve and Other Nervous System Procedures with CC or Peripheral Neurostimulator	2.2307
042	Peripheral/Cranial Nerve and Other Nervous System Procedures without CC/MCC	1.7398
058	Multiple Sclerosis and Cerebellar Ataxia with MCC	1.7279
059	Multiple Sclerosis and Cerebellar Ataxia with CC	1.1872

DRG	PDx/SDx/Procedure	Tips
040	Insertion of infusion device, monitoring device or other central and peripheral nervous system procedures	
	AND	
	MCC condition	*See* appendix B.
041	Insertion of infusion device, monitoring device or other central and peripheral nervous system procedures	
	AND	
	CC condition	*See* appendix B.
	OR	
	Peripheral or cranial neurostimulator implant	Neurostimulator lead insertion in combination with generator insertion.
042	Insertion of infusion device, monitoring device or other central and peripheral nervous system procedures	
058	MCC condition	*See* appendix B.
059	CC condition	*See* appendix B.

DRG 061 Ischemic Stroke, Precerebral Occlusion or Transient Ischemia with Thrombolytic Agent with MCC — RW 2.8028

023	Craniotomy with Major Device Implant or Acute Complex CNS PDX with MCC or Chemotherapy Implant or Epilepsy with Neurostimulator	5.6688

DRG	PDx/SDx/Procedure	Tip
023	Craniotomy	
	AND	
	Ischemic stroke	
	AND	
	MCC condition	*See* appendix B.

DRG 062 Ischemic Stroke, Precerebral Occlusion or Transient Ischemia with Thrombolytic Agent with CC — RW 1.8717

Potential DRGs

023	Craniotomy with Major Device Implant or Acute Complex CNS PDX with MCC or Chemotherapy Implant or Epilepsy with Neurostimulator	5.6688
024	Craniotomy with Major Device Implant/Acute Complex Central Nervous System Principal Diagnosis without MCC	3.7888
061	Ischemic Stroke, Precerebral Occlusion or Transient Ischemia with Thrombolytic Agent with MCC	2.8028

DRG	PDx/SDx/Procedure	Tips
023	Craniotomy	
	AND	
	Ischemic stroke	
	AND	
	MCC condition	*See* appendix B.
024	Craniotomy	
	AND	
	Ischemic stroke	
061	MCC condition	*See* appendix B.

DRG 063 Ischemic Stroke, Precerebral Occlusion or Transient Ischemia with Thrombolytic Agent without CC/MCC — RW 1.4868

Potential DRGs

023	Craniotomy with Major Device Implant or Acute Complex CNS PDX with MCC or Chemotherapy Implant or Epilepsy with Neurostimulator	5.6688
024	Craniotomy with Major Device Implant/Acute Complex Central Nervous System Principal Diagnosis without MCC	3.7888
061	Ischemic Stroke, Precerebral Occlusion or Transient Ischemia with Thrombolytic Agent with MCC	2.8028
062	Ischemic Stroke, Precerebral Occlusion or Transient Ischemia with Thrombolytic Agent with CC	1.8717

DRG	PDx/SDx/Procedure	Tips
023	Craniotomy	
	AND	
	Ischemic stroke	
	AND	
	MCC condition	*See* appendix B.
024	Craniotomy	
	AND	
	Ischemic stroke	
061	MCC condition	*See* appendix B.
062	CC condition	*See* appendix B.

DRG 064 Intracranial Hemorrhage or Cerebral Infarction with MCC — RW 2.0030

Potential DRGs

020	Intracranial Vascular Procedures with Principal Diagnosis of Hemorrhage with MCC	8.4524
023	Craniotomy with Major Device Implant or Acute Complex CNS PDX with MCC or Chemotherapy Implant or Epilepsy with Neurostimulator	5.6688
061	Ischemic Stroke, Precerebral Occlusion or Transient Ischemia with Thrombolytic Agent with MCC	2.8028
082	Traumatic Stupor and Coma > 1 Hour with MCC	2.2783
907	Other O.R. Procedures for Injuries with MCC	3.7195

DRG	PDx/SDx/Procedure	Tips
020	Intracranial vascular procedure	
	AND	
	Principal diagnosis of intracranial hemorrhage	Review physician notes for documentation of hemorrhage present on admission, meeting the definition of principal diagnosis.
	AND	
	MCC condition	*See* appendix B.
023	Craniotomy	
	AND	
	Cerebral infarction	
	AND	
	MCC condition	*See* appendix B.
061	Occlusion and stenosis of cerebral or precerebral arteries with cerebral infarction	Review physician notes for documentation of cerebral infarction.
	AND	
	Injection of thrombolytic agent	Review emergency room notes, physician orders, physician progress notes, and medication records for documentation of administration of thrombolytic agent.
	AND	
	MCC condition	*See* appendix B.
082	Principal diagnosis of traumatic stupor and coma > 1 Hr	Physician must document length of time of loss of consciousness. Review ED and other intake reports.
	OR	
	Head trauma diagnosis	
	AND	
	Secondary diagnosis of traumatic stupor and coma > 1 Hr	Physician must document length of time of loss of consciousness. Review ED and other intake reports.
	AND	
	MCC condition	*See* appendix B.
907	Diagnosis of head injury NOS or head/neck vessel injury	
	AND	
	Operations on extracranial, intracranial, or other vessels of head/neck for injuries	
	AND	
	MCC condition	*See* appendix B.

DRG 065 Intracranial Hemorrhage or Cerebral Infarction with CC or tPA in 24 hours — RW 1.0164

Potential DRGs

020	Intracranial Vascular Procedures with Principal Diagnosis of Hemorrhage with MCC	8.4524
021	Intracranial Vascular Procedures with Principal Diagnosis of Hemorrhage with CC	6.1414
023	Craniotomy with Major Device Implant or Acute Complex CNS PDX with MCC or Chemotherapy Implant or Epilepsy with Neurostimulator	5.6688
024	Craniotomy with Major Device Implant/Acute Complex Central Nervous System Principal Diagnosis without MCC	3.7888
061	Ischemic Stroke, Precerebral Occlusion or Transient Ischemia with Thrombolytic Agent with MCC	2.8028
062	Ischemic Stroke, Precerebral Occlusion or Transient Ischemia with Thrombolytic Agent with CC	1.8717
064	Intracranial Hemorrhage or Cerebral Infarction with MCC	2.0030
082	Traumatic Stupor and Coma > 1 Hour with MCC	2.2783
083	Traumatic Stupor and Coma > 1 Hour with CC	1.3564
907	Other O.R. Procedures for Injuries with MCC	3.7195
908	Other O.R. Procedures for Injuries with CC	2.0041

DRG	PDx/SDx/Procedure	Tips
020	Intracranial vascular procedure	
	AND	
	Principal diagnosis of intracranial hemorrhage	Review physician notes for documentation of hemorrhage present on admission, meeting the definition of principal diagnosis.
	AND	
	MCC condition	*See* appendix B.
021	Intracranial vascular procedure	
	AND	
	Principal diagnosis of intracranial hemorrhage	*See* DRG 020.
	AND	
	CC condition	*See* appendix B.
023	Craniotomy	
	AND	
	Cerebral infarction	
	AND	
	MCC condition	*See* appendix B.
024	Craniotomy	
	AND	
	Cerebral infarction	
061	Occlusion and stenosis of cerebral or precerebral arteries with cerebral infarction	Review physician notes for documentation of cerebral infarction.
	AND	
	Injection of thrombolytic agent	Review emergency room notes, physician orders, physician progress notes, and medication records for documentation of administration of thrombolytic agent.
	AND	
	MCC condition	*See* appendix B.
062	Occlusion and stenosis of cerebral or precerebral arteries with cerebral infarction	*See* DRG 061.
	AND	
	Injection of thrombolytic agent	*See* DRG 061.
	AND	
	CC condition	*See* appendix B.
064	MCC condition	*See* appendix B.
082	Principal diagnosis of traumatic stupor and coma > 1 Hr	Physician must document length of time of loss of consciousness. Review ED and other intake reports.
	OR	
	Head trauma diagnosis	
	AND	
	Secondary diagnosis of traumatic stupor and coma > 1 Hr	Physician must document length of time of loss of consciousness. Review ED and other intake reports.
	AND	
	MCC condition	*See* appendix B.
083	Principal diagnosis of traumatic stupor and coma > 1 Hr	*See* DRG 082.
	OR	
	Head trauma diagnosis	
	AND	
	Secondary diagnosis of traumatic stupor and coma > 1 Hr	*See* DRG 082.
	AND	
	CC condition	*See* appendix B.
907	Diagnosis of head injury NOS or head/neck vessel injury	
	AND	
	Operations on extracranial, intracranial, or other vessels of head/neck for injuries	
	AND	
	MCC condition	*See* appendix B.
908	Diagnosis of head injury NOS or head/neck vessel injury	
	AND	
	Operations on extracranial, intracranial, or other vessels of head/neck for injuries	
	AND	
	CC condition	*See* appendix B.

DRG 066 Intracranial Hemorrhage or Cerebral Infarction without CC/MCC RW 0.6875

Potential DRGs

020	Intracranial Vascular Procedures with Principal Diagnosis of Hemorrhage with MCC	8.4524
021	Intracranial Vascular Procedures with Principal Diagnosis of Hemorrhage with CC	6.1414
022	Intracranial Vascular Procedures with Principal Diagnosis of Hemorrhage without CC/MCC	3.4767
023	Craniotomy with Major Device Implant or Acute Complex CNS PDX with MCC or Chemotherapy Implant or Epilepsy with Neurostimulator	5.6688
024	Craniotomy with Major Device Implant/Acute Complex Central Nervous System Principal Diagnosis without MCC	3.7888
061	Ischemic Stroke, Precerebral Occlusion or Transient Ischemia with Thrombolytic Agent with MCC	2.8028
062	Ischemic Stroke, Precerebral Occlusion or Transient Ischemia with Thrombolytic Agent with CC	1.8717
063	Ischemic Stroke, Precerebral Occlusion or Transient Ischemia with Thrombolytic Agent without CC/MCC	1.4868
064	Intracranial Hemorrhage or Cerebral Infarction with MCC	2.0030
065	Intracranial Hemorrhage or Cerebral Infarction with CC or tPA in 24 hours	1.0164
082	Traumatic Stupor and Coma > 1 Hour with MCC	2.2783
083	Traumatic Stupor and Coma > 1 Hour with CC	1.3564
084	Traumatic Stupor and Coma > 1 Hour without CC/MCC	0.9197
907	Other O.R. Procedures for Injuries with MCC	3.7195
908	Other O.R. Procedures for Injuries with CC	2.0041
909	Other O.R. Procedures for Injuries without CC/MCC	1.3563

DRG	PDx/SDx/Procedure	Tips
020	Intracranial vascular procedure	
	AND	
	Principal diagnosis of intracranial hemorrhage	Review physician notes for documentation of hemorrhage present on admission, meeting the definition of principal diagnosis.
	AND	
	MCC condition	*See* appendix B.
021	Intracranial vascular procedure	
	AND	
	Principal diagnosis of intracranial hemorrhage	*See* DRG 020.
	AND	
	CC condition	*See* appendix B.
022	Intracranial vascular procedure	
	AND	
	Principal diagnosis of intracranial hemorrhage	*See* DRG 020.
023	Craniotomy	
	AND	
	Cerebral infarction	
	AND	
	MCC condition	*See* appendix B.
024	Craniotomy	
	AND	
	Cerebral infarction	
061	Occlusion and stenosis of cerebral or precerebral arteries with cerebral infarction	Review physician notes for documentation of cerebral infarction.
	AND	
	Injection of thrombolytic agent	Review emergency room notes, physician orders, physician progress notes, and medication records for documentation of administration of thrombolytic agent.
	AND	
	MCC condition	*See* appendix B.
062	Occlusion and stenosis of cerebral or precerebral arteries with cerebral infarction	*See* DRG 061.
	AND	
	Injection of thrombolytic agent	*See* DRG 061.
	AND	
	CC condition	*See* appendix B.
063	Occlusion and stenosis of cerebral or precerebral arteries with cerebral infarction	*See* DRG 061.
	AND	
	Injection of thrombolytic agent	*See* DRG 061.
064	MCC condition	*See* appendix B.
065	tPA administered within 24 hours	Review emergency room notes, and other intake/transfer reports, as well as physician progress notes, documentation of prior administration of tPA.
	OR	
	CC condition	*See* appendix B.
082	Principal diagnosis of traumatic stupor and coma > 1 Hr	Physician must document length of time of loss of consciousness. Review ED and other intake reports.
	OR	
	Head trauma diagnosis	
	AND	
	Secondary diagnosis of traumatic stupor and coma > 1 Hr	Physician must document length of time of loss of consciousness. Review ED and other intake reports.
	AND	
	MCC condition	*See* appendix B.

DRG 066 (Continued)

DRG	PDx/SDx/Procedure	Tips
083	Principal diagnosis of traumatic stupor and coma > 1 Hr	*See* DRG 082.
	OR	
	Head trauma diagnosis	
	AND	
	Secondary diagnosis of traumatic stupor and coma > 1 Hr	*See* DRG 082.
	AND	
	CC condition	*See* appendix B.
084	Principal diagnosis of traumatic stupor and coma > 1 Hr	*See* DRG 082.
	OR	
	Head trauma diagnosis	
	AND	
	Secondary diagnosis of traumatic stupor and coma > 1 Hr	*See* DRG 082.
907	Diagnosis of head injury NOS or head/neck vessel injury	
	AND	
	Operations on extracranial, intracranial, or other vessels of head/neck for injuries	
	AND	
	MCC condition	*See* appendix B.
908	Diagnosis of head injury NOS or head/neck vessel injury	
	AND	
	Operations on extracranial, intracranial, or other vessels of head/neck for injuries	
	AND	
	CC condition	*See* appendix B.
909	Diagnosis of head injury NOS or head/neck vessel injury	
	AND	
	Operations on extracranial, intracranial, or other vessels of head/neck for injuries	

DRG 067 Nonspecific Cerebrovascular Accident and Precerebral Occlusion without Infarction with MCC

RW 1.4169

Potential DRGs

034	Carotid Artery Stent Procedure with MCC	3.9014
061	Ischemic Stroke, Precerebral Occlusion or Transient Ischemia with Thrombolytic Agent with MCC	2.8028
064	Intracranial Hemorrhage or Cerebral Infarction with MCC	2.0030
070	Nonspecific Cerebrovascular Disorders with MCC	1.7895

DRG	PDx/SDx/Procedure	Tips
034	Carotid artery stent placement	Carotid artery stenting only or stenting of vertebral artery or vein, internal or external jugular vein, or right facial vein in combination with stenting of the right common carotid artery.
	AND	
	MCC condition	*See* appendix B.
061	Occlusion and stenosis of cerebral or precerebral arteries with cerebral infarction	Review physician notes for documentation of cerebral infarction.
	AND	
	Injection of thrombolytic agent	Review emergency room notes, physician orders, physician progress notes, and medication records for documentation of administration of thrombolytic agent.
	AND	
	MCC condition	*See* appendix B.
064	Intracranial hemorrhage or cerebral infarction	Acute disorders only. Code also documented neurologic deficits. Report lacunar infarction here also. Cerebral infarction should be coded only when documented for the current admission, not previous episode of care.
	AND	
	MCC condition	*See* appendix B.
070	Central nervous system disorders	
	Cerebral atherosclerosis	
	Cerebrovascular disease	
	Encephalopathy; metabolic, other or unspecified	Encephalopathy is typically acute (or subacute) in onset and due to a systemic underlying cause that is usually reversible and resolves when the underlying cause is corrected. Common causes of encephalopathy include fever, infection, dehydration, electrolyte imbalance, acidosis, organ failure, sepsis, or hypoxia. Review record documentation carefully for the associated condition or cause. Encephalopathy may be designated as principal diagnosis if it is the condition established after study to be chiefly responsible for the admission.
	AND	
	MCC condition	*See* appendix B.

DRG 068 Nonspecific Cerebrovascular Accident and Precerebral Occlusion without Infarction without MCC RW 0.8710

Potential DRGs

034	Carotid Artery Stent Procedure with MCC	3.9014
035	Carotid Artery Stent Procedure with CC	2.2995
036	Carotid Artery Stent Procedure without CC/MCC	1.8082
061	Ischemic Stroke, Precerebral Occlusion or Transient Ischemia with Thrombolytic Agent with MCC	2.8028
062	Ischemic Stroke, Precerebral Occlusion or Transient Ischemia with Thrombolytic Agent with CC	1.8717
063	Ischemic Stroke, Precerebral Occlusion or Transient Ischemia with Thrombolytic Agent without CC/MCC	1.4868
064	Intracranial Hemorrhage or Cerebral Infarction with MCC	2.0030
065	Intracranial Hemorrhage or Cerebral Infarction with CC or tPA in 24 hours	1.0164
067	Nonspecific Cerebrovascular Accident and Precerebral Occlusion without Infarction with MCC	1.4169
070	Nonspecific Cerebrovascular Disorders with MCC	1.7895
071	Nonspecific Cerebrovascular Disorders with CC	1.0618

DRG	PDx/SDx/Procedure	Tips
034	Carotid artery stent placement	Carotid artery stenting only or stenting of vertebral artery or vein, internal or external jugular vein, or right facial vein in combination with stenting of the right common carotid artery.
	AND	
	MCC condition	*See* appendix B.
035	Carotid artery stent placement	*See* DRG 034.
	AND	
	CC condition	*See* appendix B.
036	Carotid artery stent placement	*See* DRG 034.
061	Occlusion and stenosis of cerebral or precerebral arteries with cerebral infarction	Review physician notes for documentation of cerebral infarction.
	AND	
	Injection of thrombolytic agent	Review emergency room notes, physician orders, physician progress notes, and medication records for documentation of administration of thrombolytic agent.
	AND	
	MCC condition	*See* appendix B.
062	Occlusion and stenosis of cerebral or precerebral arteries with cerebral infarction	Review physician notes for documentation of cerebral infarction.
	AND	
	Injection of thrombolytic agent	*See* DRG 061.
	AND	
	CC condition	*See* appendix B.
063	Occlusion and stenosis of cerebral or precerebral arteries with cerebral infarction	Review physician notes for documentation of cerebral infarction.
	AND	
	Injection of thrombolytic agent	*See* DRG 061.
064	Intracranial hemorrhage or cerebral infarction	Acute disorders only. Code also documented neurologic deficits. Report lacunar infarction here also. Cerebral infarction should be coded only when documented for the current admission, not previous episode of care.
	AND	
	MCC condition	*See* appendix B.
065	Intracranial hemorrhage or cerebral infarction	*See* DRG 064.
	AND	
	tPA administered within 24 hours	Review emergency room notes, and other intake/transfer reports, as well as physician progress notes, documentation of prior administration of tPA.
	OR	
	CC condition	*See* appendix B.
067	MCC condition	*See* appendix B.
070	Central nervous system disorders	
	Cerebral atherosclerosis	
	Cerebrovascular disease	
	Encephalopathy; metabolic, other or unspecified	Encephalopathy is typically acute (or subacute) in onset and due to a systemic underlying cause that is usually reversible and resolves when the underlying cause is corrected. Common causes of encephalopathy include fever, infection, dehydration, electrolyte imbalance, acidosis, organ failure, sepsis, or hypoxia. Review record documentation carefully for the associated condition or cause. Encephalopathy may be designated as principal diagnosis if it is the condition established after study to be chiefly responsible for the admission.
	AND	
	MCC condition	*See* appendix B.
071	Central nervous system disorders	
	Cerebral atherosclerosis	
	Cerebrovascular disease	
	Encephalopathy	*See* DRG 070.
	AND	
	CC condition	*See* appendix B.

DRG 069 Transient Ischemia without Thrombolytic

RW 0.7987

Potential DRGs

020	Intracranial Vascular Procedures with Principal Diagnosis of Hemorrhage with MCC	8.4524
021	Intracranial Vascular Procedures with Principal Diagnosis of Hemorrhage with CC	6.1414
022	Intracranial Vascular Procedures with Principal Diagnosis of Hemorrhage without CC/MCC	3.4767
061	Ischemic Stroke, Precerebral Occlusion or Transient Ischemia with Thrombolytic Agent with MCC	2.8028
062	Ischemic Stroke, Precerebral Occlusion or Transient Ischemia with Thrombolytic Agent with CC	1.8717
063	Ischemic Stroke, Precerebral Occlusion or Transient Ischemia with Thrombolytic Agent without CC/MCC	1.4868
064	Intracranial Hemorrhage or Cerebral Infarction with MCC	2.0030
065	Intracranial Hemorrhage or Cerebral Infarction with CC or tPA in 24 hours	1.0164
067	Nonspecific Cerebrovascular Accident and Precerebral Occlusion without Infarction with MCC	1.4169
068	Nonspecific Cerebrovascular Accident and Precerebral Occlusion without Infarction without MCC	0.8710

DRG	PDx/SDx/Procedure	Tips
020	Intracranial vascular procedure	
	AND	
	Cerebral hemorrhage	
	AND	
	MCC condition	*See* appendix B.
021	Intracranial vascular procedure	
	AND	
	Cerebral hemorrhage	
	AND	
	CC condition	*See* appendix B.
022	Intracranial vascular procedure	
	AND	
	Cerebral hemorrhage	
061	Injection of thrombolytic agent	Review emergency room notes, physician orders, physician progress notes and medication records for documentation of administration of thrombolytic agent.
	AND	
	MCC condition	See appendix B.
062	Injection of thrombolytic agent	*See* DRG 061.
	AND	
	CC condition	See appendix B.
063	Injection of thrombolytic agent	*See* DRG 061.
064	Intracranial hemorrhage or cerebral infarction	Acute disorders only. Code also documented neurologic deficits. Report lacunar infarction here also. Cerebral infarction should be coded only when documented for the current admission, not previous episode of care.
	AND	
	MCC condition	*See* appendix B.
065	Intracranial hemorrhage or cerebral infarction	*See* DRG 064.
	AND	
	tPA administered within 24 hours	Review emergency room notes, and other intake/transfer reports, as well as physician progress notes, documentation of prior administration of tPA.
	OR	
	CC condition	*See* appendix B.
067	Occlusion and stenosis of cerebral and precerebral arteries, without cerebral infarction	
	AND	
	MCC condition	*See* appendix B.
068	Occlusion and stenosis of cerebral and precerebral arteries, without cerebral infarction	

DRG 070 Nonspecific Cerebrovascular Disorders with MCC RW 1.7895

Potential DRGs

020	Intracranial Vascular Procedures with Principal Diagnosis of Hemorrhage with MCC	8.4524
061	Ischemic Stroke, Precerebral Occlusion or Transient Ischemia with Thrombolytic Agent with MCC	2.8028
064	Intracranial Hemorrhage or Cerebral Infarction with MCC	2.0030
100	Seizures with MCC	1.9825

DRG	PDx/SDx/Procedure	Tips
020	Intracranial vascular procedure	
	AND	
	Cerebral hemorrhage	
	AND	
	MCC condition	*See* appendix B.
061	Occlusion and stenosis of cerebral or precerebral arteries with cerebral infarction	Review physician notes for documentation of cerebral infarction.
	AND	
	Injection of thrombolytic agent	Review emergency room notes, physician orders, physician progress notes, and medication records for documentation of administration of thrombolytic agent.
	AND	
	MCC condition	*See* appendix B.
064	Intracranial hemorrhage or cerebral infarction	Acute disorders only. Code also documented neurological deficits. Report lacunar infarction here also. Cerebral infarction should be coded only when documented for the current admission, not previous episode of care.
	AND	
	MCC condition	*See* appendix B.
100	Epilepsy and recurrent seizures	
	OR	
	Convulsions	
	AND	
	MCC condition	*See* appendix B.

DRG 071 Nonspecific Cerebrovascular Disorders with CC RW 1.0618

Potential DRGs

020	Intracranial Vascular Procedures with Principal Diagnosis of Hemorrhage with MCC	8.4524
021	Intracranial Vascular Procedures with Principal Diagnosis of Hemorrhage with CC	6.1414
061	Ischemic Stroke, Precerebral Occlusion or Transient Ischemia with Thrombolytic Agent with MCC	2.8028
062	Ischemic Stroke, Precerebral Occlusion or Transient Ischemia with Thrombolytic Agent with CC	1.8717
064	Intracranial Hemorrhage or Cerebral Infarction with MCC	2.0030
067	Nonspecific Cerebrovascular Accident and Precerebral Occlusion without Infarction with MCC	1.4169
070	Nonspecific Cerebrovascular Disorders with MCC	1.7895
100	Seizures with MCC	1.9825

DRG	PDx/SDx/Procedure	Tips
020	Intracranial vascular procedure	
	AND	
	Cerebral hemorrhage	
	AND	
	MCC condition	*See* appendix B.
021	Intracranial vascular procedure	
	AND	
	Cerebral hemorrhage	
	AND	
	CC condition	*See* appendix B.
061	Occlusion and stenosis of cerebral or precerebral arteries with cerebral infarction	Review physician notes for documentation of cerebral infarction.
	AND	
	Injection of thrombolytic agent	Review emergency room notes, physician orders, physician progress notes, and medication records for documentation of administration of thrombolytic agent.
	AND	
	MCC condition	*See* appendix B.
062	Occlusion and stenosis of cerebral or precerebral arteries with cerebral infarction	Review physician notes for documentation of cerebral infarction.
	AND	
	Injection of thrombolytic agent	*See* DRG 061.
064	Intracranial hemorrhage or cerebral infarction	Acute disorders only. Code also documented neurologic deficits. Report lacunar infarction here also. Cerebral infarction should be coded only when documented for the current admission, not previous episode of care.
	AND	
	MCC condition	*See* appendix B.
067	Occlusion and stenosis of cerebral and precerebral arteries, without cerebral infarction	
	AND	
	MCC condition	*See* appendix B.
070	MCC condition	*See* appendix B.
100	Epilepsy and recurrent seizures	
	OR	
	Convulsions	
	AND	
	MCC condition	*See* appendix B.

DRG 072 Nonspecific Cerebrovascular Disorders without CC/MCC RW 0.7830

Potential DRGs

020	Intracranial Vascular Procedures with Principal Diagnosis of Hemorrhage with MCC	8.4524
021	Intracranial Vascular Procedures with Principal Diagnosis of Hemorrhage with CC	6.1414
022	Intracranial Vascular Procedures with Principal Diagnosis of Hemorrhage without CC/MCC	3.4767
061	Ischemic Stroke, Precerebral Occlusion or Transient Ischemia with Thrombolytic Agent with MCC	2.8028
062	Ischemic Stroke, Precerebral Occlusion or Transient Ischemia with Thrombolytic Agent with CC	1.8717
063	Ischemic Stroke, Precerebral Occlusion or Transient Ischemia with Thrombolytic Agent without CC/MCC	1.4868
064	Intracranial Hemorrhage or Cerebral Infarction with MCC	2.0030
065	Intracranial Hemorrhage or Cerebral Infarction with CC or tPA in 24 hours	1.0164
067	Nonspecific Cerebrovascular Accident and Precerebral Occlusion without Infarction with MCC	1.4169
068	Nonspecific Cerebrovascular Accident and Precerebral Occlusion without Infarction without MCC	0.8710
070	Nonspecific Cerebrovascular Disorders with MCC	1.7895
071	Nonspecific Cerebrovascular Disorders with CC	1.0618
100	Seizures with MCC	1.9825
101	Seizures without MCC	0.9096

DRG	PDx/SDx/Procedure	Tips
020	Intracranial vascular procedure	
	AND	
	Cerebral hemorrhage	
	AND	
	MCC condition	*See* appendix B.
021	Intracranial vascular procedure	
	AND	
	Cerebral hemorrhage	
	AND	
	CC condition	*See* appendix B.
022	Intracranial vascular procedure	
	AND	
	Cerebral hemorrhage	
061	Occlusion and stenosis of cerebral or precerebral arteries with cerebral infarction	Review physician notes for documentation of cerebral infarction.
	AND	
	Injection of thrombolytic agent	Review emergency room notes, physician orders, physician progress notes, and medication records for documentation of administration of thrombolytic agent.
	AND	
	MCC condition	*See* appendix B.
062	Occlusion and stenosis of cerebral or precerebral arteries with cerebral infarction	Review physician notes for documentation of cerebral infarction.
	AND	
	Injection of thrombolytic agent	*See* DRG 061.
	AND	
	CC condition	*See* appendix B.
063	Occlusion and stenosis of cerebral or precerebral arteries with cerebral infarction	Review physician notes for documentation of cerebral infarction.
	AND	
	Injection of thrombolytic agent	*See* DRG 061.
064	Intracranial hemorrhage or cerebral infarction	Acute disorders only. Code also documented neurologic deficits. Report lacunar infarction here also. Cerebral infarction should be coded only when documented for the current admission, not previous episode of care.
	AND	
	MCC condition	*See* appendix B.
065	Intracranial hemorrhage or cerebral infarction	*See* DRG 064.
	AND	
	tPA administered within 24 hours	Review emergency room notes, and other intake/transfer reports, as well as physician progress notes, documentation of prior administration of tPA.
	OR	
	CC condition	*See* appendix B.
067	Occlusion and stenosis of cerebral and precerebral arteries, without cerebral infarction	
	AND	
	MCC condition	*See* appendix B.
068	Occlusion and stenosis of cerebral and precerebral arteries, without cerebral infarction	
070	MCC condition	*See* appendix B.
071	CC condition	*See* appendix B.

DRG 072 (Continued)

DRG	PDx/SDx/Procedure	Tips
100	Epilepsy and recurrent seizures	
	OR	
	Convulsions	
	AND	
	MCC condition	*See* appendix B.
101	Epilepsy and recurrent seizures	
	OR	
	Convulsions	

DRG 073 Cranial and Peripheral Nerve Disorders with MCC — RW 1.5130

Potential DRGs

040 Peripheral/Cranial Nerve and Other Nervous System Procedures with MCC 3.8505

DRG	PDx/SDx/Procedure	Tips
040	Stereotactic radiosurgery	Review interventional radiology notes.
	AND	
	MCC condition	*See* appendix B.

DRG 074 Cranial and Peripheral Nerve Disorders without MCC — RW 1.0262

Potential DRGs

040 Peripheral/Cranial Nerve and Other Nervous System Procedures with MCC 3.8505
041 Peripheral/Cranial Nerve and Other Nervous System Procedures with CC or Peripheral Neurostimulator 2.2307
042 Peripheral/Cranial Nerve and Other Nervous System Procedures without CC/MCC 1.7398
073 Cranial and Peripheral Nerve Disorders with MCC 1.5130

DRG	PDx/SDx/Procedure	Tips
040	Stereotactic radiosurgery	Review interventional radiology notes.
	AND	
	MCC condition	*See* appendix B.
041	Stereotactic radiosurgery	Review interventional radiology notes.
	AND	
	CC condition	*See* appendix B.
	OR	
	Peripheral or cranial neurostimulator implant	Neurostimulator lead insertion in combination with generator insertion.
042	Stereotactic radiosurgery	Review interventional radiology notes.
073	MCC condition	*See* appendix B.

DRG 075 Viral Meningitis with CC/MCC — RW 1.9138

Potential DRGs

094 Bacterial and Tuberculous Infections of Nervous System with MCC 3.6227
095 Bacterial and Tuberculous Infections of Nervous System with CC 2.3842
097 Nonbacterial Infections of Nervous System Except Viral Meningitis with MCC 3.6369
098 Nonbacterial Infections of Nervous System Except Viral Meningitis with CC 2.1545

DRG	PDx/SDx/Procedure	Tips
094	Bacterial infection	Review physician notes for documentation stating due to *H. influenzae*, gram negative anaerobes, *E. coli*, purulent, suppurative, pyogenic, arachnoiditis, meningoencephalitis, meningomyelitis, underlying disease whooping cough.
	AND	
	MCC condition	*See* appendix B.
095	Bacterial infection	*See* DRG 094.
	AND	
	CC condition	*See* appendix B.
097	Meningitis other specified or unspecified cause	Do not assume documentation of clear cerebrospinal fluid excludes a diagnosis of meningitis.
	AND	
	MCC condition	*See* appendix B.
098	Meningitis other specified or unspecified cause	*See* DRG 097.
	AND	
	CC condition	*See* appendix B.

DRG 076 Viral Meningitis without CC/MCC — RW 0.9225

Potential DRGs

075	Viral Meningitis with CC/MCC	1.9138
094	Bacterial and Tuberculous Infections of Nervous System with MCC	3.6227
095	Bacterial and Tuberculous Infections of Nervous System with CC	2.3842
096	Bacterial and Tuberculous Infections of Nervous System without CC/MCC	2.1797
097	Nonbacterial Infections of Nervous System Except Viral Meningitis with MCC	3.6369
098	Nonbacterial Infections of Nervous System Except Viral Meningitis with CC	2.1545
099	Nonbacterial Infections of Nervous System Except Viral Meningitis without CC/MCC	1.3202
177	Respiratory Infections and Inflammations with MCC	1.6964
178	Respiratory Infections and Inflammations with CC	0.9867

DRG	PDx/SDx/Procedure	Tips
075	CC/MCC condition	*See* appendix B.
094	Bacterial infection	Review physician notes for documentation stating due to *H. influenzae*, gram negative anaerobes, *E. coli*, purulent, suppurative, pyogenic, arachnoiditis, meningoencephalitis, meningomyelitis, underlying disease whooping cough.
	AND	
	MCC condition	*See* appendix B.
095	Bacterial infection	*See* DRG 094.
	AND	
	CC condition	*See* appendix B.
096	Bacterial infection	*See* DRG 094.
097	Meningitis other specified or unspecified cause	Do not assume documentation of clear cerebrospinal fluid excludes a diagnosis of meningitis.
	AND	
	MCC condition	*See* appendix B.
098	Meningitis other specified or unspecified cause	*See* DRG 097.
	AND	
	CC condition	*See* appendix B.
099	Meningitis other specified or unspecified cause	*See* DRG 097.
177	Meningitis due to SARS-associated coronavirus (SARS-CoV-2) (COVID-19)	According to ICD-10-CM guidelines when the reason for the encounter/admission is a nonrespiratory manifestation (e.g., viral enteritis) of COVID-19, assign code U07.1 COVID-19, as the principal/first-listed diagnosis and assign code(s) for the manifestation(s) as additional diagnoses.
	AND	
	MCC condition	*See* appendix B.
178	Meningitis due to SARS-associated coronavirus (SARS-CoV-2) (COVID-19)	*See* DRG 177.
	AND	
	CC condition	*See* appendix B.

DRG 077 Hypertensive Encephalopathy with MCC — RW 1.5109

Potential DRGs

020	Intracranial Vascular Procedures with Principal Diagnosis of Hemorrhage with MCC	8.4524
061	Ischemic Stroke, Precerebral Occlusion or Transient Ischemia with Thrombolytic Agent with MCC	2.8028
064	Intracranial Hemorrhage or Cerebral Infarction with MCC	2.0030

DRG	PDx/SDx/Procedure	Tips
020	Intracranial vascular procedure	
	AND	
	Cerebral hemorrhage	
	AND	
	MCC condition	*See* appendix B.
061	Occlusion and stenosis of cerebral or precerebral arteries with cerebral infarction	Review physician notes for documentation of cerebral infarction.
	AND	
	Injection of thrombolytic agent	Review emergency room notes, physician orders, physician progress notes, and medication records for documentation of administration of thrombolytic agent.
	AND	
	MCC condition	*See* appendix B.
064	Intracranial hemorrhage or cerebral infarction	Acute disorders only. Code also documented neurologic deficits. Report lacunar infarction here also. Cerebral infarction should be coded only when documented for the current admission, not previous episode of care.
	AND	
	MCC condition	*See* appendix B.

DRG 078 Hypertensive Encephalopathy with CC

RW 1.0169

Potential DRGs

020	Intracranial Vascular Procedures with Principal Diagnosis of Hemorrhage with MCC	8.4524
021	Intracranial Vascular Procedures with Principal Diagnosis of Hemorrhage with CC	6.1414
061	Ischemic Stroke, Precerebral Occlusion or Transient Ischemia with Thrombolytic Agent with MCC	2.8028
062	Ischemic Stroke, Precerebral Occlusion or Transient Ischemia with Thrombolytic Agent with CC	1.8717
064	Intracranial Hemorrhage or Cerebral Infarction with MCC	2.0030
077	Hypertensive Encephalopathy with MCC	1.5109

DRG	PDx/SDx/Procedure	Tips
020	Intracranial vascular procedure	
	AND	
	Cerebral hemorrhage	
	AND	
	MCC condition	*See* appendix B.
021	Intracranial vascular procedure	
	AND	
	Cerebral hemorrhage	
	AND	
	CC condition	*See* appendix B.
061	Occlusion and stenosis of cerebral or precerebral arteries with cerebral infarction	Review physician notes for documentation of cerebral infarction.
	AND	
	Injection of thrombolytic agent	Review emergency room notes, physician orders, physician progress notes, and medication records for documentation of administration of thrombolytic agent.
	AND	
	MCC condition	*See* appendix B.
062	Occlusion and stenosis of cerebral or precerebral arteries with cerebral infarction	Review physician notes for documentation of cerebral infarction.
	AND	
	Injection of thrombolytic agent	*See* DRG 061.
	AND	
	CC condition	*See* appendix B.
064	Intracranial hemorrhage or cerebral infarction	Acute disorders only. Code also documented neurologic deficits. Report lacunar infarction here also. Cerebral infarction should be coded only when documented for the current admission, not previous episode of care.
	AND	
	MCC condition	*See* appendix B.
077	MCC condition	*See* appendix B.

DRG 079 Hypertensive Encephalopathy without CC/MCC RW 0.7408

Potential DRGs

020	Intracranial Vascular Procedures with Principal Diagnosis of Hemorrhage with MCC	8.4524
021	Intracranial Vascular Procedures with Principal Diagnosis of Hemorrhage with CC	6.1414
022	Intracranial Vascular Procedures with Principal Diagnosis of Hemorrhage without CC/MCC	3.4767
061	Ischemic Stroke, Precerebral Occlusion or Transient Ischemia with Thrombolytic Agent with MCC	2.8028
062	Ischemic Stroke, Precerebral Occlusion or Transient Ischemia with Thrombolytic Agent with CC	1.8717
063	Ischemic Stroke, Precerebral Occlusion or Transient Ischemia with Thrombolytic Agent without CC/MCC	1.4868
064	Intracranial Hemorrhage or Cerebral Infarction with MCC	2.0030
065	Intracranial Hemorrhage or Cerebral Infarction with CC or tPA in 24 hours	1.0164
077	Hypertensive Encephalopathy with MCC	1.5109
078	Hypertensive Encephalopathy with CC	1.0169

DRG	PDx/SDx/Procedure	Tips
020	Intracranial vascular procedure	
	AND	
	Cerebral hemorrhage	
	AND	
	MCC condition	*See* appendix B.
021	Intracranial vascular procedure	
	AND	
	Cerebral hemorrhage	
	AND	
	CC condition	*See* appendix B.
022	Intracranial vascular procedure	
	AND	
	Cerebral hemorrhage	
061	Occlusion and stenosis of cerebral or precerebral arteries with cerebral infarction	Review physician notes for documentation of cerebral infarction.
	AND	
	Injection of thrombolytic agent	Review emergency room notes, physician orders, physician progress notes, and medication records for documentation of administration of thrombolytic agent.
	AND	
	MCC condition	*See* appendix B.
062	Occlusion and stenosis of cerebral or precerebral arteries with cerebral infarction	Review physician notes for documentation of cerebral infarction.
	AND	
	Injection of thrombolytic agent	*See* DRG 061.
	AND	
	CC condition	*See* appendix B.
063	Occlusion and stenosis of cerebral or precerebral arteries with cerebral infarction	Review physician notes for documentation of cerebral infarction.
	AND	
	Injection of thrombolytic agent	*See* DRG 061.
064	Intracranial hemorrhage or cerebral infarction	Acute disorders only. Code also documented neurologic deficits. Report lacunar infarction here also. Cerebral infarction should be coded only when documented for the current admission, not previous episode of care.
	AND	
	MCC condition	*See* appendix B.
065	Intracranial hemorrhage or cerebral infarction	*See* DRG 064.
	AND	
	tPA administered within 24 hours	Review emergency room notes, and other intake/transfer reports, as well as physician progress notes, documentation of prior administration of tPA.
	OR	
	CC condition	*See* appendix B.
077	MCC condition	*See* appendix B.
078	CC condition	*See* appendix B.

DRG 080 Nontraumatic Stupor and Coma with MCC — RW 2.2087

Potential DRGs

020	Intracranial Vascular Procedures with Principal Diagnosis of Hemorrhage with MCC	8.4524
082	Traumatic Stupor and Coma > 1 Hour with MCC	2.2783
085	Traumatic Stupor and Coma < 1 Hour with MCC	2.2728

DRG	PDx/SDx/Procedure	Tips
020	Intracranial vascular procedure	
	AND	
	Cerebral hemorrhage	
	AND	
	MCC condition	*See* appendix B.
082	Principal diagnosis of traumatic stupor and coma > 1 Hr	Physician must document length of time of loss of consciousness. Review ED and other intake reports.
	OR	
	Head trauma diagnosis	
	AND	
	Secondary diagnosis of traumatic stupor and coma > 1 Hr	Physician must document length of time of loss of consciousness. Review ED and other intake reports.
	AND	
	MCC condition	*See* appendix B.
085	Skull fracture or intracranial trauma diagnoses with description of loss of consciousness less than one hour or without loss of consciousness	Mental confusion/disorientation may occur w/o loss of consciousness; physician must document length of time of loss of consciousness.
	AND	
	MCC condition	*See* appendix B.

DRG 081 Nontraumatic Stupor and Coma without MCC — RW 0.9095

Potential DRGs

020	Intracranial Vascular Procedures with Principal Diagnosis of Hemorrhage with MCC	8.4524
021	Intracranial Vascular Procedures with Principal Diagnosis of Hemorrhage with CC	6.1414
022	Intracranial Vascular Procedures with Principal Diagnosis of Hemorrhage without CC/MCC	3.4767
080	Nontraumatic Stupor and Coma with MCC	2.2087
082	Traumatic Stupor and Coma > 1 Hour with MCC	2.2783
083	Traumatic Stupor and Coma > 1 Hour with CC	1.3564
084	Traumatic Stupor and Coma > 1 Hour without CC/MCC	0.9197
085	Traumatic Stupor and Coma < 1 Hour with MCC	2.2728
086	Traumatic Stupor and Coma < 1 Hour with CC	1.3171

DRG	PDx/SDx/Procedure	Tips
020	Intracranial vascular procedure	
	AND	
	Cerebral hemorrhage	
	AND	
	MCC condition	*See* appendix B.
021	Intracranial vascular procedure	
	AND	
	Cerebral hemorrhage	
	AND	
	CC condition	*See* appendix B.
022	Intracranial vascular procedure	
	AND	
	Cerebral hemorrhage	
080	MCC condition	*See* appendix B.
082	Principal diagnosis of traumatic stupor and coma > 1 Hr	Physician must document length of time of loss of consciousness. Review ED and other intake reports.
	OR	
	Head trauma diagnosis	
	AND	
	Secondary diagnosis of traumatic stupor and coma > 1 Hr	Physician must document length of time of loss of consciousness. Review ED and other intake reports.
	AND	
	MCC condition	*See* appendix B.
083	Principal diagnosis of traumatic stupor and coma > 1 Hr	*See* DRG 082.
	OR	
	Head trauma diagnosis	
	AND	
	Secondary diagnosis of traumatic stupor and coma > 1 Hr	*See* DRG 082.
	AND	
	CC condition	*See* appendix B.
084	Principal diagnosis of traumatic stupor and coma > 1 Hr	*See* DRG 082.
	OR	
	Head trauma diagnosis	
	AND	
	Secondary diagnosis of traumatic stupor and coma > 1 Hr	*See* DRG 082.

DRG 081 (Continued)

DRG	PDx/SDx/Procedure	Tips
085	Skull fracture or intracranial trauma diagnoses with description of loss of consciousness less than one hour or without loss of consciousness	Mental confusion/disorientation may occur w/o loss of consciousness; physician must document length of time of loss of consciousness.
	AND	
	MCC condition	*See* appendix B.
086	Skull fracture or intracranial trauma diagnoses with description of loss of consciousness less than one hour or without loss of consciousness	*See* DRG 085.
	AND	
	CC condition	*See* appendix B.

DRG 082 Traumatic Stupor and Coma > 1 Hour with MCC — RW 2.2783

Potential DRGs

003	ECMO or Tracheostomy with Mechanical Ventilation > 96 Hours or Principal Diagnosis Except Face, Mouth and Neck with Major O.R. Procedure	21.3203
004	Tracheostomy with Mechanical Ventilation > 96 Hours or Principal Diagnosis Except Face, Mouth and Neck without Major O.R. Procedure	14.7000
020	Intracranial Vascular Procedures with Principal Diagnosis of Hemorrhage with MCC	8.4524
957	Other O.R. Procedures for Multiple Significant Trauma with MCC	7.2325
963	Other Multiple Significant Trauma with MCC	2.7343

DRG	PDx/SDx/Procedure	Tips
003	Extracorporeal membrane oxygenation (ECMO), central or peripheral	Central ECMO provides cardiorespiratory support and involves direct surgical cannulation of the right atrium and aorta via sternotomy. Peripheral (percutaneous) ECMO is a less invasive procedure than central ECMO. Veno-arterial (VA) peripheral ECMO cannulas are inserted percutaneously into both the femoral artery and the femoral vein. This type of ECMO provides both respiratory and circulatory support. Veno-venous (VV) peripheral ECMO may use one or two venous insertions, one in the upper veins and, if used, one in the lower veins, and provides respiratory support only.
	OR	
	Tracheostomy	Tracheostomy carried out elsewhere prior to admission or in an ambulance prior to arrival should not be reported as a current procedure. A tracheostomy procedure may be performed at the bedside and documented in the progress notes or in the operating room and documented in an operative report. Verify that an actual tracheostomy was performed and not a tube change.
	WITH	
	Mechanical ventilation > 96 hours	Review record documentation for start and stop times. Calculation of mechanical ventilation hours begins when vent is initiated (or time of admission if patient already on a vent) and ends when it is turned off (or the time patient is discharged if still ventilated). The duration includes time spent to wean the patient from the vent. Do not assume that ventilation that spans four calendar days equals > 96 hours; count by the hour not day.
	OR	
	Principal diagnosis not including those related to face, mouth or neck	
	WITH	
	Any O.R. procedure not listed under MS-DRGs 987–989	
004	Tracheostomy	*See* DRG 003.
	AND	
	Mechanical ventilation > 96 hours	*See* DRG 003.
	OR	
	Principal diagnosis not including those related to face, mouth or neck	
020	Intracranial vascular procedure	
	AND	
	Cerebral hemorrhage	
	AND	
	MCC condition	*See* appendix B.
957	Other O.R. procedures for multiple significant trauma	Pdx of trauma and at least two significant trauma diagnosis codes from different body site categories. Refer to ED report, interventional radiology reports.
	AND	
	O.R. procedure other than craniotomy or limb reattachment, hip and femur procedures	
	AND	
	MCC condition	*See* appendix B.
963	Multiple significant trauma	Pdx of trauma and at least two significant trauma diagnosis codes from different body site categories.
	AND	
	MCC condition	*See* appendix B.

DRG 083 Traumatic Stupor and Coma > 1 Hour with CC

RW 1.3564

Potential DRGs

003	ECMO or Tracheostomy with Mechanical Ventilation > 96 Hours or Principal Diagnosis Except Face, Mouth and Neck with Major O.R. Procedure	21.3203
004	Tracheostomy with Mechanical Ventilation > 96 Hours or Principal Diagnosis Except Face, Mouth and Neck without Major O.R. Procedure	14.7000
020	Intracranial Vascular Procedures with Principal Diagnosis of Hemorrhage with MCC	8.4524
021	Intracranial Vascular Procedures with Principal Diagnosis of Hemorrhage with CC	6.1414
080	Nontraumatic Stupor and Coma with MCC	2.2087
082	Traumatic Stupor and Coma > 1 Hour with MCC	2.2783
088	Concussion with MCC	1.5338
957	Other O.R. Procedures for Multiple Significant Trauma with MCC	7.2325
958	Other O.R. Procedures for Multiple Significant Trauma with CC	4.0448
963	Other Multiple Significant Trauma with MCC	2.7343
964	Other Multiple Significant Trauma with CC	1.5010

DRG	PDx/SDx/Procedure	Tips
003	Extracorporeal membrane oxygenation (ECMO), central or peripheral	Central ECMO provides cardiorespiratory support and involves direct surgical cannulation of the right atrium and aorta via sternotomy. Peripheral (percutaneous) ECMO is a less invasive procedure than central ECMO. Veno-arterial (VA) peripheral ECMO cannulas are inserted percutaneously into both the femoral artery and the femoral vein. This type of ECMO provides both respiratory and circulatory support. Veno-venous (VV) peripheral ECMO may use one or two venous insertions, one in the upper veins and, if used, one in the lower veins, and provides respiratory support only.
	OR	
	Tracheostomy	Tracheostomy carried out elsewhere prior to admission or in an ambulance prior to arrival should not be reported as a current procedure. A tracheostomy procedure may be performed at the bedside and documented in the progress notes or in the operating room and documented in an operative report. Verify that an actual tracheostomy was performed and not a tube change.
	WITH	
	Mechanical ventilation > 96 hours	Review record documentation for start and stop times. Calculation of mechanical ventilation hours begins when vent is initiated (or time of admission if patient already on a vent) and ends when it is turned off (or the time patient is discharged if still ventilated). The duration includes time spent to wean the patient from the vent. Do not assume that ventilation that spans four calendar days equals > 96 hours; count by the hour not day.
	OR	
	Principal diagnosis not including those related to face, mouth or neck	
	WITH	
	Any O.R. procedure not listed under MS-DRGs 987–989	
004	Tracheostomy	*See* DRG 003.
	AND	
	Mechanical ventilation > 96 hours	*See* DRG 003.
	OR	
	Principal diagnosis not including those related to face, mouth or neck	
020	Intracranial vascular procedure	
	AND	
	Cerebral hemorrhage	
	OR	
	MCC condition	*See* appendix B.
021	Intracranial vascular procedure	
	AND	
	Cerebral hemorrhage	
	AND	
	CC condition	*See* appendix B.
080	Alteration of consciousness, coma, brain compression, cerebral edema	Review ED and other intake reports for documentation of coma scale. Physician must document length of time of loss of consciousness.
	AND	
	MCC condition	*See* appendix B.
082	MCC condition	*See* appendix B.
088	Concussion	
	AND	
	MCC condition	*See* appendix B.
957	Other O.R. procedures for multiple significant trauma	Pdx of trauma and at least two significant trauma diagnosis codes from different body site categories. Refer to ED report, interventional radiology reports.
	AND	
	O.R. procedure other than craniotomy or limb reattachment, hip and femur procedures	
	AND	
	MCC condition	*See* appendix B.

DRG 083 (Continued)

DRG	PDx/SDx/Procedure	Tips
958	Other O.R. procedures for multiple significant trauma	*See* DRG 957.
	AND	
	O.R. procedure other than craniotomy or limb reattachment, hip and femur procedures	
	AND	
	CC condition	*See* appendix B.
963	Multiple significant trauma	Pdx of trauma and at least two significant trauma diagnosis codes from different body site categories.
	AND	
	MCC condition	*See* appendix B.
964	Multiple significant trauma	*See* DRG 963.
	AND	
	CC condition	*See* appendix B.

DRG 084 Traumatic Stupor and Coma > 1 Hour without CC/MCC

RW 0.9197

Potential DRGs

003	ECMO or Tracheostomy with Mechanical Ventilation > 96 Hours or Principal Diagnosis Except Face, Mouth and Neck with Major O.R. Procedure	21.3203
004	Tracheostomy with Mechanical Ventilation > 96 Hours or Principal Diagnosis Except Face, Mouth and Neck without Major O.R. Procedure	14.7000
020	Intracranial Vascular Procedures with Principal Diagnosis of Hemorrhage with MCC	8.4524
021	Intracranial Vascular Procedures with Principal Diagnosis of Hemorrhage with CC	6.1414
022	Intracranial Vascular Procedures with Principal Diagnosis of Hemorrhage without CC/MCC	3.4767
080	Nontraumatic Stupor and Coma with MCC	2.2087
082	Traumatic Stupor and Coma > 1 Hour with MCC	2.2783
083	Traumatic Stupor and Coma > 1 Hour with CC	1.3564
088	Concussion with MCC	1.5338
089	Concussion with CC	1.1499
957	Other O.R. Procedures for Multiple Significant Trauma with MCC	7.2325
958	Other O.R. Procedures for Multiple Significant Trauma with CC	4.0448
959	Other O.R. Procedures for Multiple Significant Trauma without CC/MCC	2.5324
963	Other Multiple Significant Trauma with MCC	2.7343
964	Other Multiple Significant Trauma with CC	1.5010

DRG	PDx/SDx/Procedure	Tips
003	Extracorporeal membrane oxygenation (ECMO), central or peripheral	Central ECMO provides cardiorespiratory support and involves direct surgical cannulation of the right atrium and aorta via sternotomy. Peripheral (percutaneous) ECMO is a less invasive procedure than central ECMO. Veno-arterial (VA) peripheral ECMO cannulas are inserted percutaneously into both the femoral artery and the femoral vein. This type of ECMO provides both respiratory and circulatory support. Veno-venous (VV) peripheral ECMO may use one or two venous insertions, one in the upper veins and, if used, one in the lower veins, and provides respiratory support only.
	OR	
	Tracheostomy	Tracheostomy carried out elsewhere prior to admission or in an ambulance prior to arrival should not be reported as a current procedure. A tracheostomy procedure may be performed at the bedside and documented in the progress notes or in the operating room and documented in an operative report. Verify that an actual tracheostomy was performed and not a tube change.
	WITH	
	Mechanical ventilation > 96 hours	Review record documentation for start and stop times. Calculation of mechanical ventilation hours begins when vent is initiated (or time of admission if patient already on a vent) and ends when it is turned off (or the time patient is discharged if still ventilated). The duration includes time spent to wean the patient from the vent. Do not assume that ventilation that spans four calendar days equals > 96 hours; count by the hour not day.
	OR	
	Principal diagnosis not including those related to face, mouth or neck	
	WITH	
	Any O.R. procedure not listed under MS-DRGs 987–989	
004	Tracheostomy	*See* DRG 003.
	AND	
	Mechanical ventilation > 96 hours	*See* DRG 003.
	OR	
	Principal diagnosis not including those related to face, mouth or neck	

DRG 084 (Continued)

DRG	PDx/SDx/Procedure	Tips
020	Intracranial vascular procedure	
	AND	
	Cerebral hemorrhage	
	AND	
	MCC condition	*See* appendix B.
021	Intracranial vascular procedure	
	AND	
	Cerebral hemorrhage	
	AND	
	CC condition	*See* appendix B.
022	Intracranial vascular procedure	
	AND	
	Cerebral hemorrhage	
080	Alteration of consciousness, coma, brain compression, cerebral edema	Review ED and other intake reports for documentation of coma scale. Physician must document length of time of loss of consciousness.
	AND	
	MCC condition	*See* appendix B.
082	MCC condition	*See* appendix B.
083	CC condition	*See* appendix B.
088	Concussion	
	AND	
	MCC condition	*See* appendix B.
089	Concussion	
	AND	
	CC condition	*See* appendix B.
957	Other O.R. procedures for multiple significant trauma	Pdx of trauma and at least two significant trauma diagnosis codes from different body site categories. Refer to ED report, interventional radiology reports.
	AND	
	O.R. procedure other than craniotomy or limb reattachment, hip and femur procedures	
	AND	
	MCC condition	*See* appendix B.
958	Other O.R. procedures for multiple significant trauma	*See* DRG 957.
	AND	
	O.R. procedure other than craniotomy or limb reattachment, hip and femur procedures	
	AND	
	CC condition	*See* appendix B.
959	Other O.R. procedures for multiple significant trauma	*See* DRG 957.
	AND	
	O.R. procedure other than craniotomy or limb reattachment, hip and femur procedures	
963	Multiple significant trauma	Pdx of trauma and at least two significant trauma diagnosis codes from different body site categories.
	AND	
	MCC condition	*See* appendix B.
964	Multiple significant trauma	*See* DRG 963.
	AND	
	CC condition	*See* appendix B.

DRG 085 Traumatic Stupor and Coma < 1 Hour with MCC RW 2.2728

Potential DRGs

020	Intracranial Vascular Procedures with Principal Diagnosis of Hemorrhage with MCC	8.4524
957	Other O.R. Procedures for Multiple Significant Trauma with MCC	7.2325
963	Other Multiple Significant Trauma with MCC	2.7343

DRG	PDx/SDx/Procedure	Tips
020	Intracranial vascular procedure	
	AND	
	Cerebral hemorrhage	
	AND	
	MCC condition	*See* appendix B.
957	Other O.R. procedures for multiple significant trauma	Pdx of trauma and at least two significant trauma diagnosis codes from different body site categories. Refer to ED report, interventional radiology reports.
	AND	
	O.R. procedure other than craniotomy or limb reattachment, hip and femur procedures	
	AND	
	MCC condition	*See* appendix B.
963	Multiple significant trauma	Pdx of trauma and at least two significant trauma diagnosis codes from different body site categories.
	AND	
	MCC condition	*See* appendix B.

DRG 086 Traumatic Stupor and Coma < 1 Hour with CC RW 1.3171

Potential DRGs

020	Intracranial Vascular Procedures with Principal Diagnosis of Hemorrhage with MCC	8.4524
021	Intracranial Vascular Procedures with Principal Diagnosis of Hemorrhage with CC	6.1414
080	Nontraumatic Stupor and Coma with MCC	2.2087
082	Traumatic Stupor and Coma > 1 Hour with MCC	2.2783
083	Traumatic Stupor and Coma > 1 Hour with CC	1.3564
085	Traumatic Stupor and Coma < 1 Hour with MCC	2.2728
957	Other O.R. Procedures for Multiple Significant Trauma with MCC	7.2325
958	Other O.R. Procedures for Multiple Significant Trauma with CC	4.0448
963	Other Multiple Significant Trauma with MCC	2.7343
964	Other Multiple Significant Trauma with CC	1.5010

DRG	PDx/SDx/Procedure	Tips
020	Intracranial vascular procedure	
	AND	
	Cerebral hemorrhage	
	AND	
	MCC condition	*See* appendix B.
021	Intracranial vascular procedure	
	AND	
	Cerebral hemorrhage	
	AND	
	CC condition	*See* appendix B.
080	Alteration of consciousness, coma, brain compression, cerebral edema	Review ED and other intake reports for documentation of coma scale. Physician must document length of time of loss of consciousness.
	AND	
	MCC condition	
082	Principal diagnosis of traumatic stupor and coma > 1 Hr	Physician must document length of time of loss of consciousness. Review ED and other intake reports.
	OR	
	Head trauma diagnosis	
	AND	
	Secondary diagnosis of traumatic stupor and coma > 1 Hr	Physician must document length of time of loss of consciousness. Review ED and other intake reports.
	AND	
	MCC condition	*See* appendix B.
083	Principal diagnosis of traumatic stupor and coma > 1 Hr	*See* DRG 082.
	OR	
	Head trauma diagnosis	
	AND	
	Secondary diagnosis of traumatic stupor and coma > 1 Hr	*See* DRG 082.
	AND	
	CC condition	*See* appendix B.
085	MCC condition	*See* appendix B.
957	Other O.R. procedures for multiple significant trauma	Pdx of trauma and at least two significant trauma diagnosis codes from different body site categories. Refer to ED report, interventional radiology reports.
	AND	
	O.R. procedure other than craniotomy or limb reattachment, hip and femur procedures	
	AND	
	MCC condition	*See* appendix B.
958	Other O.R. procedures for multiple significant trauma	*See* DRG 957.
	AND	
	O.R. procedure other than craniotomy or limb reattachment, hip and femur procedures	
	AND	
	CC condition	*See* appendix B.
963	Multiple significant trauma	Pdx of trauma and at least two significant trauma diagnosis codes from different body site categories.
	AND	
	MCC condition	*See* appendix B.
964	Multiple significant trauma	*See* DRG 963.
	AND	
	CC condition	*See* appendix B.

DRG 087 Traumatic Stupor and Coma < 1 Hour without CC/MCC RW 0.8862

Potential DRGs

020	Intracranial Vascular Procedures with Principal Diagnosis of Hemorrhage with MCC	8.4524
021	Intracranial Vascular Procedures with Principal Diagnosis of Hemorrhage with CC	6.1414
022	Intracranial Vascular Procedures with Principal Diagnosis of Hemorrhage without CC/MCC	3.4767
080	Nontraumatic Stupor and Coma with MCC	2.2087
082	Traumatic Stupor and Coma > 1 Hour with MCC	2.2783
083	Traumatic Stupor and Coma > 1 Hour with CC	1.3564
084	Traumatic Stupor and Coma > 1 Hour without CC/MCC	0.9197
085	Traumatic Stupor and Coma < 1 Hour with MCC	2.2728
086	Traumatic Stupor and Coma < 1 Hour with CC	1.3171
957	Other O.R. Procedures for Multiple Significant Trauma with MCC	7.2325
958	Other O.R. Procedures for Multiple Significant Trauma with CC	4.0448
959	Other O.R. Procedures for Multiple Significant Trauma without CC/MCC	2.5324
963	Other Multiple Significant Trauma with MCC	2.7343
964	Other Multiple Significant Trauma with CC	1.5010
965	Other Multiple Significant Trauma without CC/MCC	0.9559

DRG	PDx/SDx/Procedure	Tips
020	Intracranial vascular procedure	
	AND	
	Cerebral hemorrhage	
	AND	
	MCC condition	*See* appendix B.
021	Intracranial vascular procedure	
	AND	
	Cerebral hemorrhage	
	AND	
	CC condition	*See* appendix B.
022	Intracranial vascular procedure	
	AND	
	Cerebral hemorrhage	
080	Alteration of consciousness, coma, brain compression, cerebral edema	Review ED and other intake reports for documentation of coma scale. Physician must document length of time of loss of consciousness.
	AND	
	MCC condition	
082	Principal diagnosis of traumatic stupor and coma > 1 Hr	Physician must document length of time of loss of consciousness. Review ED and other intake reports.
	OR	
	Head trauma diagnosis	
	AND	
	Secondary diagnosis of traumatic stupor and coma > 1 Hr	Physician must document length of time of loss of consciousness. Review ED and other intake reports.
	AND	
	MCC condition	*See* appendix B.
083	Principal diagnosis of traumatic stupor and coma > 1 Hr	*See* DRG 082.
	OR	
	Head trauma diagnosis	
	AND	
	Secondary diagnosis of traumatic stupor and coma > 1 Hr	*See* DRG 082.
	AND	
	CC condition	*See* appendix B.
084	Principal diagnosis of traumatic stupor and coma > 1 Hr	*See* DRG 082.
	OR	
	Head trauma diagnosis	
	AND	
	Secondary diagnosis of traumatic stupor and coma > 1 Hr	*See* DRG 082.
085	MCC condition	*See* appendix B.
086	CC condition	*See* appendix B.
957	Other O.R. procedures for multiple significant trauma	Pdx of trauma and at least two significant trauma diagnosis codes from different body site categories. Refer to ED report, interventional radiology reports.
	AND	
	O.R. procedure other than craniotomy or limb reattachment, hip and femur procedures	
	AND	
	MCC condition	*See* appendix B.
958	Other O.R. procedures for multiple significant trauma	*See* DRG 957.
	AND	
	O.R. procedure other than craniotomy or limb reattachment, hip and femur procedures	
	AND	
	CC condition	*See* appendix B.

DRG 087 (Continued)

DRG	PDx/SDx/Procedure	Tips
959	Other O.R. procedures for multiple significant trauma	*See* DRG 957.
	AND	
	O.R. procedure other than craniotomy or limb reattachment, hip and femur procedures	
963	Multiple significant trauma	Pdx of trauma and at least two significant trauma diagnosis codes from different body site categories.
	AND	
	MCC condition	*See* appendix B.
964	Multiple significant trauma	*See* DRG 963.
	AND	
	CC condition	*See* appendix B.
965	Multiple significant trauma	*See* DRG 963.

DRG 088 Concussion with MCC

RW 1.5338

Potential DRGs

020	Intracranial Vascular Procedures with Principal Diagnosis of Hemorrhage with MCC	8.4524
082	Traumatic Stupor and Coma > 1 Hour with MCC	2.2783
085	Traumatic Stupor and Coma < 1 Hour with MCC	2.2728
957	Other O.R. Procedures for Multiple Significant Trauma with MCC	7.2325
963	Other Multiple Significant Trauma with MCC	2.7343

DRG	PDx/SDx/Procedure	Tips
020	Intracranial vascular procedure	
	AND	
	Cerebral hemorrhage	
	AND	
	MCC condition	*See* appendix B.
082	Principal diagnosis of traumatic stupor and coma > 1 Hr	Physician must document length of time of loss of consciousness. Review ED and other intake reports.
	OR	
	Head trauma diagnosis	
	AND	
	Secondary diagnosis of traumatic stupor and coma > 1 Hr	Physician must document length of time of loss of consciousness. Review ED and other intake reports.
	AND	
	MCC condition	*See* appendix B.
085	Skull fracture or intracranial trauma diagnoses with description of loss of consciousness less than one hour or without loss of consciousness	Mental confusion/disorientation may occur w/o loss of consciousness; physician must document length of time of loss of consciousness.
	AND	
	MCC condition	*See* appendix B.
957	Other O.R. procedures for multiple significant trauma	Pdx of trauma and at least two significant trauma diagnosis codes from different body site categories. Refer to ED report, interventional radiology reports.
	AND	
	O.R. procedure other than craniotomy or limb reattachment, hip and femur procedures	
	AND	
	MCC condition	*See* appendix B.
963	Multiple significant trauma	Pdx of trauma and at least two significant trauma diagnosis codes from different body site categories.
	AND	
	MCC condition	*See* appendix B.

DRG 089 Concussion with CC RW 1.1499

Potential DRGs

020	Intracranial Vascular Procedures with Principal Diagnosis of Hemorrhage with MCC	8.4524
021	Intracranial Vascular Procedures with Principal Diagnosis of Hemorrhage with CC	6.1414
082	Traumatic Stupor and Coma > 1 Hour with MCC	2.2783
083	Traumatic Stupor and Coma > 1 Hour with CC	1.3564
085	Traumatic Stupor and Coma < 1 Hour with MCC	2.2728
086	Traumatic Stupor and Coma < 1 Hour with CC	1.3171
088	Concussion with MCC	1.5338
957	Other O.R. Procedures for Multiple Significant Trauma with MCC	7.2325
958	Other O.R. Procedures for Multiple Significant Trauma with CC	4.0448
963	Other Multiple Significant Trauma with MCC	2.7343
964	Other Multiple Significant Trauma with CC	1.5010

DRG	PDx/SDx/Procedure	Tips
020	Intracranial vascular procedure	
	AND	
	Cerebral hemorrhage	
	AND	
	MCC condition	*See* appendix B.
021	Intracranial vascular procedure	
	AND	
	Cerebral hemorrhage	
	AND	
	CC condition	*See* appendix B.
082	Principal diagnosis of traumatic stupor and coma > 1 Hr	Physician must document length of time of loss of consciousness. Review ED and other intake reports.
	OR	
	Head trauma diagnosis	
	AND	
	Secondary diagnosis of traumatic stupor and coma > 1 Hr	Physician must document length of time of loss of consciousness. Review ED and other intake reports.
	AND	
	MCC condition	*See* appendix B.
083	Principal diagnosis of traumatic stupor and coma > 1 Hr	*See* DRG 082.
	OR	
	Head trauma diagnosis	
	AND	
	Secondary diagnosis of traumatic stupor and coma > 1 Hr	*See* DRG 082.
	AND	
	CC condition	*See* appendix B.
085	Skull fracture or intracranial trauma diagnoses with description of loss of consciousness less than one hour or without loss of consciousness	Mental confusion/disorientation may occur w/o loss of consciousness; physician must document length of time of loss of consciousness.
	AND	
	MCC condition	*See* appendix B.
086	Skull fracture or intracranial trauma diagnoses with description of loss of consciousness less than one hour or without loss of consciousness	*See* DRG 085.
	AND	
	CC condition	*See* appendix B.
088	MCC condition	*See* appendix B.
957	Other O.R. procedures for multiple significant trauma other than craniotomy or limb reattachment, hip and femur procedures	Pdx of trauma and at least two significant trauma diagnosis codes from different body site categories. Refer to ED report, interventional radiology reports.
	AND	
	MCC condition	*See* appendix B.
958	Other O.R. procedures for multiple significant trauma other than craniotomy or limb reattachment, hip and femur procedures	*See* DRG 957.
	AND	
	CC condition	*See* appendix B.
963	Multiple significant trauma	Pdx of trauma and at least two significant trauma diagnosis codes from different body site categories.
	AND	
	MCC condition	*See* appendix B.
964	Multiple significant trauma	*See* DRG 963.
	AND	
	CC condition	*See* appendix B.

DRG 090 Concussion without CC/MCC

RW 0.9348

Potential DRGs

020	Intracranial Vascular Procedures with Principal Diagnosis of Hemorrhage with MCC	8.4524
021	Intracranial Vascular Procedures with Principal Diagnosis of Hemorrhage with CC	6.1414
022	Intracranial Vascular Procedures with Principal Diagnosis of Hemorrhage without CC/MCC	3.4767
082	Traumatic Stupor and Coma > 1 Hour with MCC	2.2783
083	Traumatic Stupor and Coma > 1 Hour with CC	1.3564
085	Traumatic Stupor and Coma < 1 Hour with MCC	2.2728
086	Traumatic Stupor and Coma < 1 Hour with CC	1.3171
088	Concussion with MCC	1.5338
089	Concussion with CC	1.1499
957	Other O.R. Procedures for Multiple Significant Trauma with MCC	7.2325
958	Other O.R. Procedures for Multiple Significant Trauma with CC	4.0448
959	Other O.R. Procedures for Multiple Significant Trauma without CC/MCC	2.5324
963	Other Multiple Significant Trauma with MCC	2.7343
964	Other Multiple Significant Trauma with CC	1.5010
965	Other Multiple Significant Trauma without CC/MCC	0.9559

DRG	PDx/SDx/Procedure	Tips
020	Intracranial vascular procedure	
	AND	
	Cerebral hemorrhage	
	AND	
	MCC condition	*See* appendix B.
021	Intracranial vascular procedure	
	AND	
	Cerebral hemorrhage	
	AND	
	CC condition	*See* appendix B.
022	Intracranial vascular procedure	
	AND	
	Cerebral hemorrhage	
082	Principal diagnosis of traumatic stupor and coma > 1 Hr	Physician must document length of time of loss of consciousness. Review ED and other intake reports.
	OR	
	Head trauma diagnosis	
	AND	
	Secondary diagnosis of traumatic stupor and coma > 1 Hr	Physician must document length of time of loss of consciousness. Review ED and other intake reports.
	AND	
	MCC condition	*See* appendix B.
083	Principal diagnosis of traumatic stupor and coma > 1 Hr	*See* DRG 082.
	OR	
	Head trauma diagnosis	
	AND	
	Secondary diagnosis of traumatic stupor and coma > 1 Hr	*See* DRG 082.
	AND	
	CC condition	*See* appendix B.
085	Skull fracture or intracranial trauma diagnoses with description of loss of consciousness less than one hour or without loss of consciousness	Mental confusion/disorientation may occur w/o loss of consciousness; physician must document length of time of loss of consciousness.
	AND	
	MCC condition	*See* appendix B.
086	Skull fracture or intracranial trauma diagnoses with description of loss of consciousness less than one hour or without loss of consciousness	*See* DRG 085.
	AND	
	CC condition	*See* appendix B.
088	MCC condition	*See* appendix B.
089	CC condition	*See* appendix B.
957	Other O.R. procedures for multiple significant trauma other than craniotomy or limb reattachment, hip and femur procedures	Pdx of trauma and at least two significant trauma diagnosis codes from different body site categories. Refer to ED report, interventional radiology reports.
	AND	
	MCC condition	*See* appendix B.
958	Other O.R. procedures for multiple significant trauma other than craniotomy or limb reattachment, hip and femur procedures	See DRG 957.
	AND	
	CC condition	*See* appendix B.
959	Other O.R. procedures for multiple significant trauma other than craniotomy or limb reattachment, hip and femur procedures	See DRG 957.
963	Multiple significant trauma	Pdx of trauma and at least two significant trauma diagnosis codes from different body site categories.
	AND	
	MCC condition	*See* appendix B.

DRG 090 (Continued)

DRG	PDx/SDx/Procedure	Tips
964	Multiple significant trauma	See DRG 963.
	AND	
	CC condition	*See* appendix B.
965	Multiple significant trauma	See DRG 963.

DRG 091 Other Disorders of Nervous System with MCC

RW 1.7892

Potential DRGs

037	Extracranial Procedures with MCC	3.3756
052	Spinal Disorders and Injuries with CC/MCC	1.9445

DRG	PDx/SDx/Procedure	Tips
037	Suture of vessels, vessel repairs	Review ED reports, interventional radiology reports.
	OR	
	Vein sclerosing agent injection	
	AND	
	MCC condition	*See* appendix B.
052	Late effect of spinal cord injury	
	Unspecified spinal cord injury	
	AND	
	CC/MCC condition	*See* appendix B.

DRG 092 Other Disorders of Nervous System with CC

RW 1.0261

Potential DRGs

037	Extracranial Procedures with MCC	3.3756
038	Extracranial Procedures with CC	1.5999
052	Spinal Disorders and Injuries with CC/MCC	1.9445
091	Other Disorders of Nervous System with MCC	1.7892
102	Headaches with MCC	1.2066

DRG	PDx/SDx/Procedure	Tips
037	Suture of vessels, vessel repairs	Review ED reports, interventional radiology reports.
	OR	
	Vein sclerosing agent injection	
	AND	
	MCC condition	*See* appendix B.
038	Suture of vessels, vessel repairs	*See* DRG 037.
	OR	
	Vein sclerosing agent injection	
	AND	
	CC condition	*See* appendix B.
052	Late effect of spinal cord injury	
	Unspecified spinal cord injury	
	AND	
	CC/MCC condition	*See* appendix B.
091	MCC condition	*See* appendix B.
102	Unspecified headache	
	Headache syndromes	
	Migraine headache	
	Benign intracranial hypertension	
	AND	
	MCC condition	*See* appendix B.

DRG 093 Other Disorders of Nervous System without CC/MCC — RW 0.7744

Potential DRGs

037	Extracranial Procedures with MCC	3.3756
038	Extracranial Procedures with CC	1.5999
039	Extracranial Procedures without CC/MCC	1.1410
052	Spinal Disorders and Injuries with CC/MCC	1.9445
053	Spinal Disorders and Injuries without CC/MCC	0.9838
091	Other Disorders of Nervous System with MCC	1.7892
092	Other Disorders of Nervous System with CC	1.0261
102	Headaches with MCC	1.2066
103	Headaches without MCC	0.8424

DRG	PDx/SDx/Procedure	Tips
037	Suture of vessels, vessel repairs	Review ED reports, interventional radiology reports.
	OR	
	Vein sclerosing agent injection	
	AND	
	MCC condition	*See* appendix B.
038	Suture of vessels, vessel repairs	*See* DRG 037.
	OR	
	Vein sclerosing agent injection	
	AND	
	CC condition	*See* appendix B.
039	Suture of vessels, vessel repairs	*See* DRG 037.
	OR	
	Vein sclerosing agent injection	
052	Late effect of spinal cord injury	
	Unspecified spinal cord injury	
	AND	
	CC/MCC condition	*See* appendix B.
053	Late effect of spinal cord injury	
	Unspecified spinal cord injury	
091	MCC condition	*See* appendix B.
092	CC condition	*See* appendix B.
102	Unspecified headache	
	Headache syndromes	
	Migraine headache	
	Benign intracranial hypertension	
	AND	
	MCC condition	*See* appendix B.
103	Unspecified headache	
	Headache syndromes	
	Migraine headache	
	Benign intracranial hypertension	

DRG 094 Bacterial and Tuberculous Infections of Nervous System with MCC — RW 3.6227

No Potential DRGs

DRG 095 Bacterial and Tuberculous Infections of Nervous System with CC — RW 2.3842

Potential DRGs

094	Bacterial and Tuberculous Infections of Nervous System with MCC	3.6227

DRG	PDx/SDx/Procedure	Tips
094	MCC condition	*See* appendix B.

DRG 096 Bacterial and Tuberculous Infections of Nervous System without CC/MCC — RW 2.1797

Potential DRGs

094	Bacterial and Tuberculous Infections of Nervous System with MCC	3.6227
095	Bacterial and Tuberculous Infections of Nervous System with CC	2.3842
097	Nonbacterial Infections of Nervous System Except Viral Meningitis with MCC	3.6369

DRG	PDx/SDx/Procedure	Tips
094	MCC condition	*See* appendix B.
095	CC condition	*See* appendix B.
097	Meningitis due to other organisms, other specified or unspecified cause	Do not assume documentation of clear cerebrospinal fluid excludes a diagnosis of meningitis.
	AND	
	MCC condition	*See* appendix B.

DRG 097 Nonbacterial Infections of Nervous System Except Viral Meningitis with MCC — RW 3.6369

No Potential DRGs

DRG 098 Nonbacterial Infections of Nervous System Except Viral Meningitis with CC RW 2.1545

Potential DRGs

094	Bacterial and Tuberculous Infections of Nervous System with MCC	3.6227
095	Bacterial and Tuberculous Infections of Nervous System with CC	2.3842
097	Nonbacterial Infections of Nervous System Except Viral Meningitis with MCC	3.6369

DRG	PDx/SDx/Procedure	Tips
094	Bacterial meningitis	Review physician notes for documentation stating due to *H. influenzae*, gram negative anaerobes, *E. coli*, purulent, suppurative, pyogenic, arachnoiditis, meningoencephalitis, meningomyelitis, underlying disease whooping cough.
	AND	
	MCC condition	*See* appendix B.
095	Bacterial meningitis	*See* DRG 094.
	AND	
	CC condition	*See* appendix B.
097	MCC condition	*See* appendix B.

DRG 099 Nonbacterial Infections of Nervous System Except Viral Meningitis without CC/MCC RW 1.3202

Potential DRGs

075	Viral Meningitis with CC/MCC	1.9138
094	Bacterial and Tuberculous Infections of Nervous System with MCC	3.6227
095	Bacterial and Tuberculous Infections of Nervous System with CC	2.3842
096	Bacterial and Tuberculous Infections of Nervous System without CC/MCC	2.1797
097	Nonbacterial Infections of Nervous System Except Viral Meningitis with MCC	3.6369
098	Nonbacterial Infections of Nervous System Except Viral Meningitis with CC	2.1545

DRG	PDx/SDx/Procedure	Tips
075	Viral meningitis	
	Unspecified viral meningitis	
	Herpes zoster with meningitis	
	Mumps meningitis	
	Benign recurrent meningitis [Mollaret]	
	AND	
	CC/MCC condition	*See* appendix B.
094	Bacterial meningitis	Review physician notes for documentation stating due to *H. influenzae*, gram negative anaerobes, *E. coli*, purulent, suppurative, pyogenic, arachnoiditis, meningoencephalitis, meningomyelitis, underlying disease whooping cough.
	AND	
	MCC condition	*See* appendix B.
095	Bacterial meningitis	*See* DRG 094.
	AND	
	CC condition	*See* appendix B.
096	Bacterial meningitis	*See* DRG 094.
097	MCC condition	*See* appendix B.
098	CC condition	*See* appendix B.

DRG 100 Seizures with MCC RW 1.9825

Potential DRGs

061	Ischemic Stroke, Precerebral Occlusion or Transient Ischemia with Thrombolytic Agent with MCC	2.8028
064	Intracranial Hemorrhage or Cerebral Infarction with MCC	2.0030

DRG	PDx/SDx/Procedure	Tips
061	Occlusion and stenosis of cerebral or precerebral arteries with cerebral infarction	Review physician notes for documentation of cerebral infarction.
	AND	
	Injection of thrombolytic agent	Review emergency room notes, physician orders, physician progress notes, and medication records for documentation of administration of thrombolytic agent.
	AND	
	MCC condition	*See* appendix B.
064	Intracranial hemorrhage or cerebral infarction	
	AND	
	MCC condition	*See* appendix B.

DRG 101 Seizures without MCC

RW 0.9096

Potential DRGs

054	Nervous System Neoplasms with MCC	1.4735
055	Nervous System Neoplasms without MCC	1.0732
061	Ischemic Stroke, Precerebral Occlusion or Transient Ischemia with Thrombolytic Agent with MCC	2.8028
062	Ischemic Stroke, Precerebral Occlusion or Transient Ischemia with Thrombolytic Agent with CC	1.8717
063	Ischemic Stroke, Precerebral Occlusion or Transient Ischemia with Thrombolytic Agent without CC/MCC	1.4868
064	Intracranial Hemorrhage or Cerebral Infarction with MCC	2.0030
065	Intracranial Hemorrhage or Cerebral Infarction with CC or tPA in 24 hours	1.0164
070	Nonspecific Cerebrovascular Disorders with MCC	1.7895
071	Nonspecific Cerebrovascular Disorders with CC	1.0618
100	Seizures with MCC	1.9825

DRG	PDx/SDx/Procedure	Tips
054	Nervous system neoplasm, primary or secondary, malignant or benign, uncertain or unspecified behavior	Headache work-up for, or attributed to, nervous system neoplasm.
	AND	
	MCC condition	*See* appendix B.
055	Nervous system neoplasm, primary or secondary, malignant or benign, uncertain or unspecified behavior	*See* DRG 055.
061	Occlusion and stenosis of cerebral or precerebral arteries with cerebral infarction	Review physician notes for documentation of cerebral infarction.
	AND	
	Injection of thrombolytic agent	Review emergency room notes, physician orders, physician progress notes, and medication records for documentation of administration of thrombolytic agent.
	AND	
	MCC condition	*See* appendix B.
062	Occlusion and stenosis of cerebral or precerebral arteries with cerebral infarction	*See* DRG 061.
	AND	
	Injection of thrombolytic agent	*See* DRG 061.
	AND	
	CC condition	*See* appendix B.
063	Occlusion and stenosis of cerebral or precerebral arteries with cerebral infarction	*See* DRG 061.
	AND1.9825	
	Injection of thrombolytic agent	*See* DRG 061.
064	Intracranial hemorrhage or cerebral infarction	Acute disorders only. Report documented neurologic deficits or lacunar infarction. Cerebral infarction should be coded only when documented for the current admission, not previous episode of care.
	AND	
	MCC condition	*See* appendix B.
065	Intracranial hemorrhage or cerebral infarction	*See* DRG 064.
	AND	
	tPA administered within 24 hours	Review emergency room notes, physician progress notes, and other intake/transfer reports for documentation of administration of tPA.
	OR	
	CC condition	*See* appendix B.
070	Encephalopathy; metabolic, other or unspecified	Encephalopathy is typically acute in onset and due to a systemic underlying cause that is usually reversible and resolves when the underlying cause is corrected. Common causes of encephalopathy include fever, infection, dehydration, electrolyte imbalance, acidosis, organ failure, sepsis, or hypoxia. Review documentation carefully for the associated condition or cause. Encephalopathy may be designated as principal diagnosis if it is the condition established after study to be chiefly responsible for the admission.
	Other specified disorders of nervous system, unspecified disorders of nervous system	
	AND	
	MCC condition	*See* appendix B.
071	Encephalopathy	*See* DRG 070.
	Other specified disorders of nervous system, unspecified disorders of nervous system	
	AND	
	CC condition	*See* appendix B.
100	MCC condition	*See* appendix B.

DRG 102 Headaches with MCC — RW 1.2066

Potential DRGs

054	Nervous System Neoplasms with MCC	1.4735
064	Intracranial Hemorrhage or Cerebral Infarction with MCC	2.0030
067	Nonspecific Cerebrovascular Accident and Precerebral Occlusion without Infarction with MCC	1.4169
070	Nonspecific Cerebrovascular Disorders with MCC	1.7895
075	Viral Meningitis with CC/MCC	1.9138
077	Hypertensive Encephalopathy with MCC	1.5109
091	Other Disorders of Nervous System with MCC	1.7892

DRG	PDx/SDx/Procedure	Tips
054	Nervous system neoplasm, primary or secondary, malignant or benign, uncertain or unspecified behavior	Headache work-up for, or attributed to, nervous system neoplasm.
	AND	
	MCC condition	*See* appendix B.
064	Intracranial hemorrhage or cerebral infarction	
	AND	
	MCC condition	*See* appendix B.
067	Occlusion and stenosis of cerebral and precerebral arteries, without cerebral infarction	
	AND	
	MCC condition	*See* appendix B.
070	Encephalopathy; metabolic, other or unspecified	Encephalopathy is typically acute in onset and due to a systemic underlying cause that is usually reversible and resolves when the underlying cause is corrected. Common causes of encephalopathy include fever, infection, dehydration, electrolyte imbalance, acidosis, organ failure, sepsis, or hypoxia. Review documentation carefully for the associated condition or cause. Encephalopathy may be designated as principal diagnosis if it is the condition established after study to be chiefly responsible for the admission.
	Other specified disorders of nervous system, unspecified disorders of nervous system	
	AND	
	MCC condition	*See* appendix B.
075	Viral meningitis	
	Unspecified viral meningitis	
	Herpes zoster with meningitis	
	Mumps meningitis	
	Benign recurrent meningitis [Mollaret]	
	AND	
	CC/MCC condition	*See* appendix B.
077	Hypertensive encephalopathy	Review documentation for hypertensive crisis, diastolic pressure > 140, CSF pressure elevated.
	AND	
	MCC condition	*See* appendix B.
091	Late effect: viral encephalitis, skull/face fracture, intracranial injury	
	Nonruptured cerebral aneurysm	
	AND	
	MCC condition	*See* appendix B.

DRG 103 Headaches without MCC

RW 0.8424

Potential DRGs

054	Nervous System Neoplasms with MCC	1.4735
055	Nervous System Neoplasms without MCC	1.0732
064	Intracranial Hemorrhage or Cerebral Infarction with MCC	2.0030
065	Intracranial Hemorrhage or Cerebral Infarction with CC or tPA in 24 hours	1.0164
067	Nonspecific Cerebrovascular Accident and Precerebral Occlusion without Infarction with MCC	1.4169
068	Nonspecific Cerebrovascular Accident and Precerebral Occlusion without Infarction without MCC	0.8710
070	Nonspecific Cerebrovascular Disorders with MCC	1.7895
071	Nonspecific Cerebrovascular Disorders with CC	1.0618
075	Viral Meningitis with CC/MCC	1.9138
076	Viral Meningitis without CC/MCC	0.9225
077	Hypertensive Encephalopathy with MCC	1.5109
078	Hypertensive Encephalopathy with CC	1.0169
091	Other Disorders of Nervous System with MCC	1.7892
092	Other Disorders of Nervous System with CC	1.0261
102	Headaches with MCC	1.2066

DRG	PDx/SDx/Procedure	Tips
054	Nervous system neoplasm, primary or secondary, malignant or benign, uncertain or unspecified behavior	Headache work-up for, or attributed to, nervous system neoplasm.
	AND	
	MCC condition	*See* appendix B.
055	Nervous system neoplasm, primary or secondary, malignant or benign, uncertain or unspecified behavior	*See* DRG 054.
064	Intracranial hemorrhage or cerebral infarction	Acute disorders only. Report documented neurologic deficits or lacunar infarction. Cerebral infarction should be coded only when documented for the current admission, not previous episode of care.
	AND	
	MCC condition	*See* appendix B.
065	Intracranial hemorrhage or cerebral infarction	*See* DRG 064.
	AND	
	tPA administered within 24 hours	Review emergency room notes, physician progress notes, and other intake/transfer reports for documentation of administration of tPA.
	OR	
	CC condition	*See* appendix B.
067	Occlusion and stenosis of cerebral and precerebral arteries, without cerebral infarction	
	AND	
	MCC condition	*See* appendix B.
068	Occlusion and stenosis of cerebral and precerebral arteries, without cerebral infarction	
070	Encephalopathy; metabolic, other or unspecified	Encephalopathy is typically acute in onset and due to a systemic underlying cause that is usually reversible and resolves when the underlying cause is corrected. Common causes of encephalopathy include fever, infection, dehydration, electrolyte imbalance, acidosis, organ failure, sepsis, or hypoxia. Review documentation carefully for the associated condition or cause. Encephalopathy may be designated as principal diagnosis if it is the condition established after study to be chiefly responsible for the admission.
	Other specified disorders of nervous system, unspecified disorders of nervous system	
	AND	
	MCC condition	*See* appendix B.
071	Encephalopathy; metabolic, other or unspecified	*See* DRG 070.
	Other specified disorders of nervous system	
	Unspecified disorders of nervous system	
	AND	
	CC condition	*See* appendix B.
075	Viral meningitis	
	Unspecified viral meningitis	
	Herpes zoster with meningitis	
	Mumps meningitis	
	Benign recurrent meningitis [Mollaret]	
	AND	
	CC/MCC condition	*See* appendix B.
076	Viral meningitis	
	Unspecified viral meningitis	
	Herpes zoster with meningitis	
	Mumps meningitis	
	Benign recurrent meningitis [Mollaret]	
077	Hypertensive encephalopathy	Review documentation for hypertensive crisis, diastolic pressure > 140, CSF pressure elevated.
	AND	
	MCC condition	*See* appendix B.

DRG 103 (Continued)

DRG	PDx/SDx/Procedure	Tips
078	Hypertensive encephalopathy	*See* DRG 077.
	AND	
	CC condition	*See* appendix B.
091	Late effect: viral encephalitis, skull/face fracture, intracranial injury	
	Nonruptured cerebral aneurysm	
	AND	
	MCC condition	*See* appendix B.
092	Late effect: viral encephalitis, skull/face fracture, intracranial injury	
	Nonruptured cerebral aneurysm	
	AND	
	CC condition	*See* appendix B.
102	MCC condition	*See* appendix B.

Diseases And Disorders Of The Eye

DRG 113 Orbital Procedures with CC/MCC — RW 2.5073

No Potential DRGs

DRG 114 Orbital Procedures without CC/MCC — RW 1.2318

Potential DRGs

113 Orbital Procedures with CC/MCC 2.5073

DRG	PDx/SDx/Procedure	Tips
113	Orbital procedures (involving the eyeball or facial bone)	Principal diagnosis must meet medical necessity for inpatient admission.
	AND	
	CC/MCC condition	*See* appendix B.

DRG 115 Extraocular Procedures Except Orbit — RW 1.5644

Potential DRGs

113 Orbital Procedures with CC/MCC 2.5073

DRG	PDx/SDx/Procedure	Tips
113	Orbital procedures (involving the eyeball or facial bone)	Principal diagnosis must meet medical necessity for inpatient admission.
	AND	
	CC/MCC condition	*See* appendix B.

DRG 116 Intraocular Procedures with CC/MCC — RW 1.8308

No Potential DRGs

DRG 117 Intraocular Procedures without CC/MCC — RW 1.1984

Potential DRGs

115 Extraocular Procedures Except Orbit 1.5644
116 Intraocular Procedures with CC/MCC 1.8308

DRG	PDx/SDx/Procedure	Tips
115	Extraocular procedures such as: excision of lesion of cornea extraocular muscle eyelids conjunctiva lacrimal gland lacrimal duct sclera	Principal diagnosis must meet medical necessity for inpatient admission.
116	CC/MCC condition	*See* appendix B.

DRG 121 Acute Major Eye Infections with CC/MCC — RW 1.2812

Potential DRGs

124 Other Disorders of the Eye with MCC or Thrombolytic Agent 1.3219

DRG	PDx/SDx/Procedure	Tips
124	Herpes virus ophthalmic complications	Principal diagnosis must meet medical necessity for inpatient admission.
		Key terms: chronic infection, uveitis, retinitis, excluding acute endophthalmitis.
	Toxoplasmosis	
	Diabetic retinopathy	
	AND	
	Thrombolytic agent	Applicable codes are found in the Administration section (3EØ) with a seventh-character value of 7 Other thrombolytic, only. Does not include codes with a fourth-character value of 7 Coronary artery.
	OR	
	MCC condition	*See* appendix B.

DRG 122 Acute Major Eye Infections without CC/MCC — RW 0.7445

Potential DRGs

121	Acute Major Eye Infections with CC/MCC	1.2812
124	Other Disorders of the Eye with MCC or Thrombolytic Agent	1.3219
125	Other Disorders of the Eye without MCC	0.7975

DRG	PDx/SDx/Procedure	Tips
121	CC/MCC condition	*See* appendix B.
124	Herpes virus ophthalmic complications	Principal diagnosis must meet medical necessity for inpatient admission. Key terms: chronic infection, uveitis, retinitis, excluding acute endophthalmitis.
	Toxoplasmosis	
	Diabetic retinopathy	
	AND	
	Thrombolytic agent	Applicable codes are found in the Administration section (3E0) with a seventh-character value of 7 Other thrombolytic, only. Does not include codes with a fourth-character value of 7 Coronary artery.
	OR	
	MCC condition	*See* appendix B.
125	Herpes virus ophthalmic complications	*See* DRG 124.
	Toxoplasmosis	
	Diabetic retinopathy	

DRG 123 Neurological Eye Disorders — RW 0.8040

Potential DRGs

091	Other Disorders of Nervous System with MCC	1.7892
092	Other Disorders of Nervous System with CC	1.0261
124	Other Disorders of the Eye with MCC or Thrombolytic Agent	1.3219

DRG	PDx/SDx/Procedure	Tips
091	Disorders of optic chiasm, visual pathways or visual cortex; cortical blindness; internuclear ophthalmoplegia	
	AND	
	MCC condition	*See* appendix B.
092	Disorders of optic chiasm, visual pathways or visual cortex; cortical blindness; internuclear ophthalmoplegia	
	AND	
	CC condition	*See* appendix B.
124	Herpes virus ophthalmic complications	Principal diagnosis must meet medical necessity for inpatient admission. Key terms: chronic infection, uveitis, retinitis, excluding acute endophthalmitis.
	Toxoplasmosis	
	Diabetic retinopathy	
	AND	
	Introduction of thrombolytic agent	Applicable codes are found in the Administration section (3EØ) with a seventh-character value of 7 Other thrombolytic, only. Does not include codes with a fourth-character value of 7 Coronary artery.
	OR	
	MCC condition	*See* appendix B.

DRG 124 Other Disorders of the Eye with MCC — RW 1.3219

Potential DRGs

115	Extraocular Procedures Except Orbit	1.5644
116	Intraocular Procedures with CC/MCC	1.8308

DRG	PDx/SDx/Procedure	Tips
115	Reposition extraocular muscle	Principal diagnosis must meet medical necessity for inpatient admission.
	Transfer extraocular muscle	
116	Glaucoma procedures	Principal diagnosis must meet medical necessity for inpatient admission.
	Lens operations	
	Repair of retinal tear or detachment	
	AND	
	CC/MCC condition	*See* appendix B.

DRG 125 Other Disorders of the Eye without MCC

RW 0.7975

Potential DRGs

115	Extraocular Procedures Except Orbit	1.5644
116	Intraocular Procedures with CC/MCC	1.8308
117	Intraocular Procedures without CC/MCC	1.1984
124	Other Disorders of the Eye with MCC or Thrombolytic Agent	1.3219

DRG	PDx/SDx/Procedure	Tips
115	Reposition extraocular muscle Transfer extraocular muscle	Principal diagnosis must meet medical necessity for inpatient admission.
116	Glaucoma procedures	Principal diagnosis must meet medical necessity for inpatient admission.
	Lens operations	
	Repair of retinal tear or detachment	
	AND	
	CC/MCC condition	*See* appendix B.
117	Glaucoma procedures	*See* DRG 116.
	Lens operations	
	Repair of retinal tear or detachment	
124	Thrombolytic agent	Applicable codes are found in the Administration section (3E0) with a seventh-character value of 7 Other thrombolytic, only. Does not include codes with a fourth-character value of 7 Coronary artery.
	OR	
	MCC condition	*See* appendix B.

Diseases And Disorders Of The Ear, Nose, Mouth And Throat

DRG 135 Sinus and Mastoid Procedures with CC/MCC — RW 2.6521

Potential DRGs

143	Other Ear, Nose, Mouth and Throat O.R. Procedure with MCC	3.3256

DRG	PDx/SDx/Procedure	Tips
143	Drainage mastoid sinus	Diagnostic procedure via open, percutaneous, percutaneous endoscopic approach.
	Excisional biopsy of mastoid sinus	Diagnostic procedure.
	Release of mastoid sinus	
	AND	
	MCC condition	*See* appendix B.

DRG 136 Sinus and Mastoid Procedures without CC/MCC — RW 0.9391

Potential DRGs

135	Sinus and Mastoid Procedures with CC/MCC	2.6521
143	Other Ear, Nose, Mouth and Throat O.R. Procedure with MCC	3.3256
144	Other Ear, Nose, Mouth and Throat O.R. Procedure with CC	1.7305

DRG	PDx/SDx/Procedure	Tips
135	CC/MCC condition	*See* appendix B.
143	Drainage mastoid sinus	Diagnostic procedure via open, percutaneous, percutaneous endoscopic approach.
	Excisional biopsy of mastoid sinus	Diagnostic procedure.
	Release of mastoid sinus	
	AND	
	MCC condition	*See* appendix B.
144	Drainage mastoid sinus	*See* DRG 143.
	Excisional biopsy of mastoid sinus	*See* DRG 143.
	Release of mastoid sinus	
	AND	
	CC condition	*See* appendix B.

DRG 137 Mouth Procedures with CC/MCC — RW 1.5047

Potential DRGs

011	Tracheostomy for Face, Mouth, and Neck Diagnoses or Laryngectomy with MCC	5.1563
012	Tracheostomy for Face, Mouth, and Neck Diagnoses or Laryngectomy with CC	4.0049
140	Major Head and Neck Procedures with MCC	3.7781
141	Major Head and Neck Procedures with CC	2.0717
143	Other Ear, Nose, Mouth and Throat O.R. Procedure with MCC	3.3256
144	Other Ear, Nose, Mouth and Throat O.R. Procedure with CC	1.7305

DRG	PDx/SDx/Procedure	Tips
011	Tracheostomy	Tracheostomy carried out elsewhere before admission or in an ambulance before arrival should not be reported as a current procedure. A tracheostomy procedure may be performed at the bedside and documented in the progress notes or in the operating room and documented in an operative note. Report Bypass, Trachea in Respiratory System (ØB11), with appropriate approach and device characters.
	AND	
	MCC condition	*See* appendix B.
012	Tracheostomy	*See* DRG 011.
	AND	
	CC condition	*See* appendix B.
140	Glossectomy—complete/radical	Resection of tongue/hard palate
	Laryngectomy—partial	Excision of larynx—open, percutaneous endoscopic
	Mandibulectomy—complete, partial	Resection of mandible—open; Excision of mandible—open, percutaneous endoscopic
	AND	
	MCC condition	*See* appendix B.
141	Glossectomy—complete/radical	*See* DRG 140.
	Laryngectomy—partial	*See* DRG 140.
	Mandibulectomy—complete, partial	*See* DRG 140.
	AND	
	CC condition	*See* appendix B.
143	Revision of tracheostomy device	
	Laryngectomy—partial	Excision of larynx—percutaneous, via natural or artificial opening, via natural or artificial opening endoscopic or open as a diagnostic procedure
	AND	
	MCC condition	*See* appendix B.
144	Revision of tracheostomy device	
	Laryngectomy—partial	*See* DRG 144.
	AND	
	CC condition	*See* appendix B.

DRG 138 Mouth Procedures without CC/MCC RW 0.8657

Potential DRGs

011	Tracheostomy for Face, Mouth, and Neck Diagnoses or Laryngectomy with MCC	5.1563
012	Tracheostomy for Face, Mouth, and Neck Diagnoses or Laryngectomy with CC	4.0049
013	Tracheostomy for Face, Mouth, and Neck Diagnoses or Laryngectomy without CC/MCC	2.6857
137	Mouth Procedures with CC/MCC	1.5047
140	Major Head and Neck Procedures with MCC	3.7781
141	Major Head and Neck Procedures with CC	2.0717
142	Major Head and Neck Procedures without CC/MCC	1.5450
143	Other Ear, Nose, Mouth and Throat O.R. Procedure with MCC	3.3256
144	Other Ear, Nose, Mouth and Throat O.R. Procedure with CC	1.7305
145	Other Ear, Nose, Mouth and Throat O.R. Procedure without CC/MCC	1.2211

DRG	PDx/SDx/Procedure	Tips
011	Tracheostomy	Tracheostomy carried out elsewhere before admission or in an ambulance before arrival should not be reported as a current procedure. A tracheostomy procedure may be performed at the bedside and documented in the progress notes or in the operating room and documented in an operative note. Report Bypass, Trachea in Respiratory System (ØB11), with appropriate approach and device characters.
	AND	
	MCC condition	*See* appendix B.
012	Tracheostomy	*See* DRG 011.
	AND	
	CC condition	*See* appendix B.
013	Tracheostomy	*See* DRG 011.
137	CC/MCC condition	*See* appendix B.
140	Glossectomy—complete/radical	Resection of tongue/hard palate
	Laryngectomy—partial	Excision of larynx—open, percutaneous endoscopic
	Mandibulectomy—complete, partial	Resection of mandible—open; Excision of mandible—open, percutaneous endoscopic
	AND	
	MCC condition	*See* appendix B.
141	Glossectomy—complete/radical	*See* DRG 140.
	Laryngectomy—partial	*See* DRG 140.
	Mandibulectomy—complete, partial	*See* DRG 140.
	AND	
	CC condition	*See* appendix B.
142	Glossectomy—complete/radical	*See* DRG 140.
	Laryngectomy—partial	See DRG 140.
	Mandibulectomy—complete, partial	*See* DRG 140.
143	Revision of tracheostomy device	
	Laryngectomy—partial	Excision of larynx—percutaneous, via natural or artificial opening, via natural or artificial opening endoscopic or open as a diagnostic procedure
	AND	
	MCC condition	*See* appendix B.
144	Revision of tracheostomy device	
	Laryngectomy—partial	*See* DRG 144.
	AND	
	CC condition	*See* appendix B.
145	Revision of tracheostomy device	
	Laryngectomy—partial	*See* DRG 144.

DRG 139 Salivary Gland Procedures RW 1.1877

Potential DRGs

011	Tracheostomy for Face, Mouth, and Neck Diagnoses or Laryngectomy with MCC	5.1563
012	Tracheostomy for Face, Mouth, and Neck Diagnoses or Laryngectomy with CC	4.0049
013	Tracheostomy for Face, Mouth, and Neck Diagnoses or Laryngectomy without CC/MCC	2.6857
140	Major Head and Neck Procedures with MCC	3.7781
141	Major Head and Neck Procedures with CC	2.0717
142	Major Head and Neck Procedures without CC/MCC	1.5450

DRG	PDx/SDx/Procedure	Tips
011	Tracheostomy	Tracheostomy carried out elsewhere before admission or in an ambulance before arrival should not be reported as a current procedure. A tracheostomy procedure may be performed at the bedside and documented in the progress notes or in the operating room and documented in an operative note. Report Bypass, Trachea in Respiratory System (ØB11), with appropriate approach and device characters.
	AND	
	MCC condition	*See* appendix B.
012	Tracheostomy	*See* DRG 011.
	AND	
	CC condition	*See* appendix B.
013	Tracheostomy	*See* DRG 011.
140	Neck lymph node dissection—Resection	Lymph node excision implies that only a portion of the node or one node from a group or chain of nodes is removed. Lymph node resection implies that a group or chain of lymph nodes is completely removed. The root operation Excision is "cutting out or off, without replacement, a portion of a body part." Root operation Resection is "cutting out or off, without replacement, all of a body part." It includes all of body part or any subdivision of body part having its own body part value in ICD-10-PCS. Review the description of the procedure for confirmation of removal of the entire group or chain. See appendix G for lymph node/chains included in the Lymphatic, Neck body part. Bilateral removal—report both left and right ICD-10-PCS codes when a bilateral code is not provided.
	Mandibulectomy—complete, partial	Resection of mandible—open; Excision of mandible—open, percutaneous endoscopic
	AND	
	MCC condition	*See* appendix B.
141	Neck lymph node dissection	*See* DRG 140.
	Mandibulectomy—complete, partial	*See* DRG 140.
	AND	
	CC condition	*See* appendix B.
142	Neck lymph node dissection	*See* DRG 140.
	Mandibulectomy—complete, partial	*See* DRG 140.

DRG 140 Major Head and Neck Procedures with MCC RW 3.7781

Potential DRGs

011	Tracheostomy for Face, Mouth and Neck Diagnoses or Laryngectomy with MCC	5.1563
025	Craniotomy and Endovascular Intracranial Procedures with MCC	4.4160

DRG	PDx/SDx/Procedure	Tips
011	Tracheostomy	Tracheostomy carried out elsewhere before admission or in an ambulance before arrival should not be reported as a current procedure. A tracheostomy procedure may be performed at the bedside and documented in the progress notes or in the operating room and documented in an operative note. Report Bypass, Trachea in Respiratory System (ØB11) with appropriate approach and device characters.
	AND	
	MCC condition	*See* appendix B.
025	Craniotomy procedure	
	OR	
	Endovascular intracranial procedure (e.g., embolization)	Occlusion of common carotid artery, right or left (Ø3LH, Ø3LJ) with one of the following devices: Intraluminal Device, Bioactive (coils) (B) or Intraluminal Device (stent) (D).
	AND	
	MCC condition	*See* appendix B.

DRG 141 Major Head and Neck Procedures with CC

RW 2.0717

Potential DRGs

011	Tracheostomy for Face, Mouth and Neck Diagnoses or Laryngectomy with MCC	5.1563
012	Tracheostomy for Face, Mouth and Neck Diagnoses or Laryngectomy with CC	4.0049
025	Craniotomy and Endovascular Intracranial Procedures with MCC	4.4160
026	Craniotomy and Endovascular Intracranial Procedures with CC	2.9531
140	Major Head and Neck Procedures with MCC	3.7781

DRG	PDx/SDx/Procedure	Tips
011	Tracheostomy	Tracheostomy carried out elsewhere before admission or in an ambulance before arrival should not be reported as a current procedure. A tracheostomy procedure may be performed at the bedside and documented in the progress notes or in the operating room and documented in an operative note. Report Bypass, Trachea in Respiratory System (ØB11) with appropriate approach and device characters.
	AND	
	MCC condition	*See* appendix B.
012	Tracheostomy	*See* DRG 011.
	AND	
	CC condition	*See* appendix B.
025	Craniotomy procedure	
	OR	
	Endovascular intracranial procedure (e.g., embolization)	Occlusion of common carotid artery, right or left (Ø3LH, Ø3LJ) with one of the following devices: Intraluminal Device, Bioactive (coils) (B) or Intraluminal Device (stent) (D).
	AND	
	MCC condition	*See* appendix B.
026	Craniotomy procedure	
	OR	
	Endovascular intracranial procedure (e.g., embolization)	*See* DRG 025.
	AND	
	CC condition	*See* appendix B.
140	MCC condition	*See* appendix B.

DRG 142 Major Head and Neck Procedures without CC/MCC

RW 1.5450

Potential DRGs

011	Tracheostomy for Face, Mouth and Neck Diagnoses or Laryngectomy with MCC	5.1563
012	Tracheostomy for Face, Mouth and Neck Diagnoses or Laryngectomy with CC	4.0049
013	Tracheostomy for Face, Mouth and Neck Diagnoses or Laryngectomy without CC/MCC	2.6857
025	Craniotomy and Endovascular Intracranial Procedures with MCC	4.4160
026	Craniotomy and Endovascular Intracranial Procedures with CC	2.9531
027	Craniotomy and Endovascular Intracranial Procedures without CC/MCC	2.4329
140	Major Head and Neck Procedures with MCC	3.7781
141	Major Head and Neck Procedures with CC	2.0717

DRG	PDx/SDx/Procedure	Tips
011	Tracheostomy	Tracheostomy carried out elsewhere before admission or in an ambulance before arrival should not be reported as a current procedure. A tracheostomy procedure may be performed at the bedside and documented in the progress notes or in the operating room and documented in an operative note. Report Bypass, Trachea in Respiratory System (ØB11) with appropriate approach and device characters.
	AND	
	MCC condition	*See* appendix B.
012	Tracheostomy	*See* DRG 011.
	AND	
	CC condition	*See* appendix B.
013	Tracheostomy	*See* DRG 011.
025	Craniotomy procedure	
	OR	
	Endovascular intracranial procedure (e.g., embolization)	Occlusion of common carotid artery, right or left (Ø3LH, Ø3LJ) with one of the following devices: Intraluminal Device, Bioactive (coils) (B) or Intraluminal Device (stent) (D).
	AND	
	MCC condition	*See* appendix B.
026	Craniotomy procedure	
	OR	
	Endovascular intracranial procedure (e.g., embolization)	*See* DRG 025.
	AND	
	CC condition	*See* appendix B.
027	Craniotomy procedure	
	OR	
	Endovascular intracranial procedure (e.g., embolization)	*See* DRG 025.
140	MCC condition	*See* appendix B.
141	CC condition	*See* appendix B.

DRG 143 Other Ear, Nose, Mouth and Throat O.R. Procedures with MCC — RW 3.3256

Potential DRGs

011	Tracheostomy for Face, Mouth and Neck Diagnoses or Laryngectomy with MCC	5.1563
140	Major Head and Neck Procedures with MCC	3.7781

DRG	PDx/SDx/Procedure	Tips
011	Tracheostomy	Tracheostomy carried out elsewhere before admission or in an ambulance before arrival should not be reported as a current procedure. A tracheostomy procedure may be performed at the bedside and documented in the progress notes or in the operating room and documented in an operative note. Report Bypass, Trachea in Respiratory System (ØB11) with appropriate approach and device characters.
	AND	
	MCC condition	*See* appendix B.
140	Revision of tracheostomy device	
	Head/neck lymph node dissection—Resection	Lymph node excision implies that only a portion of the node or one node from a group or chain of nodes is removed. Lymph node resection implies that a group or chain of lymph nodes is completely removed. The root operation Excision is "cutting out or off, without replacement, a portion of a body part." Root operation Resection is "cutting out or off, without replacement, all of a body part." It includes all of body part or any subdivision of body part having its own body part value in ICD-10-PCS. Review the description of the procedure for confirmation of removal of the entire group or chain. See appendix G for lymph node/chains included in the Lymphatic, Neck and Lymphatic, Head body parts. Bilateral removal—report both left and right ICD-10-PCS codes when a bilateral code is not provided.
	Implant of hearing device	Single or Multiple Channel Cochlear device; Hearing device (unspecified) via open approach. Documentation must include all indications for medical necessity. Bilateral implants—report both left and right ICD-10-PCS codes when a bilateral code is not provided.
	Excision (open, percutaneous endoscopic) of:	
	Mandible	
	Larynx	
	AND	
	MCC condition	*See* appendix B.

DRG 144 Other Ear, Nose, Mouth and Throat O.R. Procedures with CC — RW 1.7305

Potential DRGs

011	Tracheostomy for Face, Mouth and Neck Diagnoses or Laryngectomy with MCC	5.1563
012	Tracheostomy for Face, Mouth and Neck Diagnoses or Laryngectomy with CC	4.0049
140	Major Head and Neck Procedures with MCC	3.7781
141	Major Head and Neck Procedures with CC	2.0717
143	Other Ear, Nose, Mouth and Throat O.R. Procedures with MCC	3.3256

DRG	PDx/SDx/Procedure	Tips
011	Tracheostomy	Tracheostomy carried out elsewhere before admission or in an ambulance before arrival should not be reported as a current procedure. A tracheostomy procedure may be performed at the bedside and documented in the progress notes or in the operating room and documented in an operative note. Report Bypass, Trachea in Respiratory System (ØB11) with appropriate approach and device characters.
	AND	
	MCC condition	*See* appendix B.
012	Tracheostomy	*See* DRG 011.
	AND	
	CC condition	*See* appendix B.
140	Revision of tracheostomy device	
	Head/neck lymph node dissection—Resection	Lymph node excision implies that only a portion of the node or one node from a group or chain of nodes is removed. Lymph node resection implies that a group or chain of lymph nodes is completely removed. The root operation Excision is "cutting out or off, without replacement, a portion of a body part." Root operation Resection is "cutting out or off, without replacement, all of a body part." It includes all of body part or any subdivision of body part having its own body part value in ICD-10-PCS. Review the description of the procedure for confirmation of removal of the entire group or chain. See appendix G for lymph node/chains included in the Lymphatic, Neck and Lymphatic, Head body parts. Bilateral removal—report both left and right ICD-10-PCS codes when a bilateral code is not provided.
	Implant of hearing device	Single or Multiple Channel Cochlear device; Hearing device (unspecified) via open approach. Documentation must include all indications for medical necessity. Bilateral implants—report both left and right ICD-10-PCS codes when a bilateral code is not provided.
	AND	
	MCC condition	*See* appendix B.
141	Revision of tracheostomy device	
	Head/neck lymph node dissection (resection)	*See* DRG 140.
	Implant of hearing device	*See* DRG 140.
	AND	
	CC condition	*See* appendix B.
143	MCC condition	*See* appendix B.

DRG 145 Other Ear, Nose, Mouth and Throat O.R. Procedures without CC/MCC RW 1.2211

Potential DRGs

011	Tracheostomy for Face, Mouth and Neck Diagnoses or Laryngectomy with MCC	5.1563
012	Tracheostomy for Face, Mouth and Neck Diagnoses or Laryngectomy with CC	4.0049
013	Tracheostomy for Face, Mouth and Neck Diagnoses or Laryngectomy without CC/MCC	2.6857
140	Major Head and Neck Procedures with MCC	3.7781
141	Major Head and Neck Procedures with CC	2.0717
142	Major Head and Neck Procedures without CC/MCC	1.5450
143	Other Ear, Nose, Mouth and Throat O.R. Procedures with MCC	3.3256
144	Other Ear, Nose, Mouth and Throat O.R. Procedures with CC	1.7305

DRG	PDx/SDx/Procedure	Tips
011	Tracheostomy	Tracheostomy carried out elsewhere before admission or in an ambulance before arrival should not be reported as a current procedure. A tracheostomy procedure may be performed at the bedside and documented in the progress notes or in the operating room and documented in an operative note. Report Bypass, Trachea in Respiratory System (ØB11) with appropriate approach and device characters.
	AND	
	MCC condition	*See* appendix B.
012	Tracheostomy	*See* DRG 011.
	AND	
	CC condition	*See* appendix B.
013	Tracheostomy	*See* DRG 011.
140	Revision of tracheostomy device	
	Head/neck lymph node dissection—Resection	Lymph node excision implies that only a portion of the node or one node from a group or chain of nodes is removed. Lymph node resection implies that a group or chain of lymph nodes is completely removed. The root operation Excision is "cutting out or off, without replacement, a portion of a body part." Root operation Resection is "cutting out or off, without replacement, all of a body part." It includes all of body part or any subdivision of body part having its own body part value in ICD-10-PCS. Review the description of the procedure for confirmation of removal of the entire group or chain. See appendix G for lymph node/chains included in the Lymphatic, Neck and Lymphatic, Head body parts. Bilateral removal—report both left and right ICD-10-PCS codes when a bilateral code is not provided.
	Implant of hearing device	Single or Multiple Channel Cochlear device; Hearing device (unspecified) via open approach. Documentation must include all indications for medical necessity. Bilateral implants—report both left and right ICD-10-PCS codes when a bilateral code is not provided.
	AND	
	MCC condition	*See* appendix B.
141	Revision of tracheostomy device	
	Head/neck lymph node dissection (resection)	*See* DRG 140.
	Implant of hearing device	*See* DRG 140.
	AND	
	CC condition	*See* appendix B.
142	Revision of tracheostomy device	
	Head/neck lymph node dissection (resection)	*See* DRG 140.
	Implant of hearing device	*See* DRG 140.
143	MCC condition	*See* appendix B.
144	CC condition	*See* appendix B.

DRG 146 Ear, Nose, Mouth and Throat Malignancy with MCC RW 2.1110

Potential DRGs

011	Tracheostomy for Face, Mouth and Neck Diagnoses or Laryngectomy with MCC	5.1563
140	Major Head and Neck Procedures with MCC	3.7781

DRG	PDx/SDx/Procedure	Tips
011	Tracheostomy	Tracheostomy carried out elsewhere before admission or in an ambulance before arrival should not be reported as a current procedure. A tracheostomy procedure may be performed at the bedside and documented in the progress notes or in the operating room and documented in an operative note. Report Bypass, Trachea in Respiratory System (ØB11) with appropriate approach and device characters.
	AND	
	MCC condition	*See* appendix B.
140	Revision of tracheostomy device	
	Head/neck lymph node dissection—Resection	Lymph node excision implies that only a portion of the node or one node from a group or chain of nodes is removed. Lymph node resection implies that a group or chain of lymph nodes is completely removed. The root operation Excision is "cutting out or off, without replacement, a portion of a body part." Root operation Resection is "cutting out or off, without replacement, all of a body part." It includes all of body part or any subdivision of body part having its own body part value in ICD-10-PCS. Review the description of the procedure for confirmation of removal of the entire group or chain. See appendix G for lymph node/chains included in the Lymphatic, Neck and Lymphatic, Head body parts. Bilateral removal—report both left and right ICD-10-PCS codes when a bilateral code is not provided.
	AND	
	MCC condition	*See* appendix B.

DRG 147 Ear, Nose, Mouth and Throat Malignancy with CC RW 1.2358

Potential DRGs

011	Tracheostomy for Face, Mouth and Neck Diagnoses or Laryngectomy with MCC	5.1563
012	Tracheostomy for Face, Mouth and Neck Diagnoses or Laryngectomy with CC	4.0049
140	Major Head and Neck Procedures with MCC	3.7781
141	Major Head and Neck Procedures with CC	2.0717
146	Ear, Nose, Mouth and Throat Malignancy with MCC	2.1110

DRG	PDx/SDx/Procedure	Tips
011	Tracheostomy	Tracheostomy carried out elsewhere before admission or in an ambulance before arrival should not be reported as a current procedure. A tracheostomy procedure may be performed at the bedside and documented in the progress notes or in the operating room and documented in an operative note. Report Bypass, Trachea in Respiratory System (ØB11) with appropriate approach and device characters.
	AND	
	MCC condition	*See* appendix B.
012	Tracheostomy	*See* DRG 011.
	AND	
	CC condition	*See* appendix B.
140	Revision of tracheostomy device	
	Head/neck lymph node dissection - Resection	Lymph node excision implies that only a portion of the node or one node from a group or chain of nodes is removed. Lymph node resection implies that a group or chain of lymph nodes is completely removed. The root operation Excision is "cutting out or off, without replacement, a portion of a body part." Root operation Resection is "cutting out or off, without replacement, all of a body part." It includes all of body part or any subdivision of body part having its own body part value in ICD-10-PCS. Review the description of the procedure for confirmation of removal of the entire group or chain. See appendix G for lymph node/chains included in the Lymphatic, Neck and Lymphatic, Head body parts. Bilateral removal – report both left and right ICD-10-PCS codes when a bilateral code is not provided.
	AND	
	MCC condition	*See* appendix B.
141	Revision of tracheostomy device	
	Head/neck lymph node dissection (resection)	*See* DRG 140.
	AND	
	CC condition	*See* appendix B.
146	MCC condition	*See* appendix B.

DRG 148 Ear, Nose, Mouth and Throat Malignancy without CC/MCC — RW 0.8897

Potential DRGs

011	Tracheostomy for Face, Mouth and Neck Diagnoses or Laryngectomy with MCC	5.1563
012	Tracheostomy for Face, Mouth and Neck Diagnoses or Laryngectomy with CC	4.0049
013	Tracheostomy for Face, Mouth and Neck Diagnoses or Laryngectomy without CC/MCC	2.6857
140	Major Head and Neck Procedures with MCC	3.7781
141	Major Head and Neck Procedures with CC	2.0717
142	Major Head and Neck Procedures without CC/MCC	1.5450
146	Ear, Nose, Mouth and Throat Malignancy with MCC	2.1110
147	Ear, Nose, Mouth and Throat Malignancy with CC	1.2358

DRG	PDx/SDx/Procedure	Tips
011	Tracheostomy	Tracheostomy carried out elsewhere before admission or in an ambulance before arrival should not be reported as a current procedure. A tracheostomy procedure may be performed at the bedside and documented in the progress notes or in the operating room and documented in an operative note. Report Bypass, Trachea in Respiratory System (ØB11) with appropriate approach and device characters.
	AND	
	MCC condition	*See* appendix B.
012	Tracheostomy	See DRG 011.
	AND	
	CC condition	*See* appendix B.
013	Tracheostomy	*See* DRG 011.
140	Revision of tracheostomy device	
	Head/neck lymph node dissection—Resection	Lymph node excision implies that only a portion of the node or one node from a group or chain of nodes is removed. Lymph node resection implies that a group or chain of lymph nodes is completely removed. The root operation Excision is "cutting out or off, without replacement, a portion of a body part." Root operation Resection is "cutting out or off, without replacement, all of a body part." It includes all of body part or any subdivision of body part having its own body part value in ICD-10-PCS. Review the description of the procedure for confirmation of removal of the entire group or chain. See appendix G for lymph node/chains included in the Lymphatic, Neck and Lymphatic, Head body parts. Bilateral removal—report both left and right ICD-10-PCS codes when a bilateral code is not provided.
	AND	
	MCC condition	*See* appendix B.
141	Revision of tracheostomy device	
	Head/neck lymph node dissection (resection)	*See* DRG 140.
	AND	
	CC condition	*See* appendix B.
142	Revision of tracheostomy device	
	Head/neck lymph node dissection (resection)	*See* DRG 140.
146	MCC condition	*See* appendix B.
147	CC condition	*See* appendix B.

DRG 149 Dysequilibrium

RW 0.7447

Potential DRGs

073	Cranial and Peripheral Nerve Disorders with MCC	1.5130
074	Cranial and Peripheral Nerve Disorders without MCC	1.0262

DRG	PDx/SDx/Procedure	Tips
073	Zoster encephalitis, Zoster with other nervous system involvement	
	Diabetes mellitus with neurological complications	According to ICD-10-CM guidelines, the classification presumes a causal relationship between diabetes and certain associated manifestations and/or conditions when these terms are linked by the term "with" in the alphabetic index (either under a main term or subterm). These conditions should be coded as related to the diabetes unless the documentation clearly states the conditions are unrelated, in which case they may be coded separately. These conditions do not require provider documentation linking them to diabetes. Review the record and/or query the physician if it is unclear whether a condition is related to diabetes mellitus or the ICD-10-CM classification does not provide instruction.
	Nerve, nerve root and plexus disorders	
	Polyneuropathies and other disorders of the peripheral nervous system	
	Myasthenia gravis and other myoneural disorders	
	Cauda equina syndrome	
	Disorders of autonomic nervous system	
	AND	
	MCC condition	*See* appendix B.
074	Zoster encephalitis, Zoster with other nervous system involvement	
	Diabetes mellitus with neurological complications	*See* DRG 073.
	Nerve, nerve root and plexus disorders	
	Polyneuropathies and other disorders of the peripheral nervous system	
	Myasthenia gravis and other myoneural disorders	
	Cauda equina syndrome	
	Disorders of autonomic nervous system	

DRG 150 Epistaxis with MCC RW 1.3145

Potential DRGs

140	Major Head and Neck Procedures with MCC	3.7781
143	Other Ear, Nose, Mouth and Throat O.R. Procedures with MCC	3.3256
154	Other Ear, Nose, Mouth and Throat Diagnoses with MCC	1.5382
299	Peripheral Vascular Disorders with MCC	1.5762
813	Coagulation Disorders	1.5600
907	Other O.R. Procedures for Injuries with MCC	3.7195

DRG	PDx/SDx/Procedure	Tips
140	Surgical epistaxis control	Report the root operation performed, i.e., Occlusion (ligation) Does not include root operations Control (e.g., cautery or silver nitrate application) or Repair (suture) from the Ear, Nose, Sinus body system (Ø93 and Ø9Q) or root operation Packing from the Placement section (2Y4).
	AND	
	MCC condition	*See* appendix B.
143	Surgical epistaxis control	Report the root operation performed, i.e., Repair (suture) Does not include root operations Control (e.g., cautery or silver nitrate application) from the Ear, Nose, Sinus body system (Ø93) or root operation Packing from the Placement section (2Y4).
	AND	
	MCC condition	*See* appendix B.
154	Benign neoplasm of mouth and pharynx	Key terms: benign neoplasm; sleep apnea (obstructive); congenital malformations; burn/corrosion of mouth/pharynx.
	Benign neoplasm of major salivary glands	
	Benign neoplasm of middle ear, nasal cavity and accessory sinuses	
	Benign neoplasm of larynx	
	Sleep apnea	
	Other congenital malformations of ear, or face and neck, or nose, or larynx, or trachea and bronchus, or salivary glands, or pharynx	
	Burn or corrosion of mouth and pharynx, initial encounter	
	AND	
	MCC condition	*See* appendix B.
299	Epistaxis due to diseases of the capillaries	Hereditary hemorrhagic telangiectasia (HHT) is an autosomal dominant disorder that affects blood vessels throughout the body, resulting in bleeding tendency. Mucocutaneous telangiectases and arteriovenous malformations (AVMs) can affect the nasopharynx. Epistaxis is the most common manifestation. Onset of symptoms may be delayed until age 40 or later. Key term: Osler-Weber-Rendu Syndrome.
	AND	
	MCC condition	*See* appendix B.
813	Hereditary or acquired coagulation, clotting, or factor deficiency	Key terms: Von Willebrand's disease, Hereditary factor XI deficiency, or other clotting factors such as acquired hemophilia or coagulation deficiency, hemorrhagic disorder due to intrinsic or extrinsic circulating anticoagulants, antibodies, or inhibitors, other and unspecified coagulation defects. Do not report a code from D68 series to identify patients on anticoagulant therapy such as Coumadin. It is the intent of this therapy to induce anticoagulation. Review record documentation for indications that the thrust of the treatment is directed towards the coagulation/clotting disorder rather than control of the epistaxis. Treatment could include diagnostic workup, administration of clotting factors, i.e. 4-Factor Prothrombin Complex Concentrate, fibrinogen, Antihemophilic factors, Factor IX, etc.
907	Intraoperative or postoperative hemorrhage, accidental intraoperative laceration	
	WITH	
	O.R. procedure for epistaxis control	Control of epistaxis: report the root operation performed (i.e., Occlusion [ligation], Repair [suture]). Does not include root operation Control (e.g., cautery or silver nitrate application) from the Ear, Nose, Sinus body system (Ø93) or root operation Packing from the Placement section (2Y4).
	OR	
	Laceration or puncture wound, with and without foreign body, bite, or unspecified open wound of nose, unspecified injury of nose	
	WITH	
	Other nasal injury repair or graft	
	AND	
	MCC condition	*See* appendix B.

DRG 151 Epistaxis without MCC

RW 0.7707

Potential DRGs

140	Major Head and Neck Procedures with MCC	3.7781
141	Major Head and Neck Procedures with CC	2.0717
142	Major Head and Neck Procedures without CC/MCC	1.5450
143	Other Ear, Nose, Mouth and Throat O.R. Procedures with MCC	3.3256
144	Other Ear, Nose, Mouth and Throat O.R. Procedures with CC	1.7305
145	Other Ear, Nose, Mouth and Throat O.R. Procedures without CC/MCC	1.2211
150	Epistaxis with MCC	1.3145
154	Other Ear, Nose, Mouth and Throat Diagnoses with MCC	1.5382
155	Other Ear, Nose, Mouth and Throat Diagnoses with CC	0.9466
299	Peripheral Vascular Disorders with MCC	1.5762
300	Peripheral Vascular Disorders with CC	1.0670
813	Coagulation Disorders	1.5600
907	Other O.R. Procedures for Injuries with MCC	3.7195
908	Other O.R. Procedures for Injuries with CC	2.0041
909	Other O.R. Procedures for Injuries without CC/MCC	1.3563

DRG	PDx/SDx/Procedure	Tips
140	Surgical epistaxis control	Report the root operation performed, i.e., Occlusion (ligation) Does not include root operations Control (e.g., cautery or silver nitrate application) or Repair (suture) from the Ear, Nose, Sinus body system (Ø93 and Ø9Q) or root operation Packing from the Placement section (2Y4).
	AND	
	MCC condition	*See* appendix B.
141	Surgical epistaxis control	*See* DRG 140.
	AND	
	CC condition	*See* appendix B.
142	Surgical epistaxis control	*See* DRG 140.
143	Surgical epistaxis control	Report the root operation performed, i.e., Repair (suture) Does not include root operations Control (e.g., cautery or silver nitrate application) from the Ear, Nose, Sinus body system (Ø93) or root operation Packing from the Placement section (2Y4).
	AND	
	MCC condition	*See* appendix B.
144	Surgical epistaxis control	*See* DRG 143.
	AND	
	CC condition	*See* appendix B.
145	Surgical epistaxis control	*See* DRG 143.
150	MCC condition	*See* appendix B.
154	Benign neoplasm of mouth and pharynx	Key terms: benign neoplasm; sleep apnea (obstructive); congenital malformations; burn/corrosion of mouth/pharynx.
	Benign neoplasm of major salivary glands	
	Benign neoplasm of middle ear, nasal cavity and accessory sinuses	
	Benign neoplasm of larynx	
	Sleep apnea	
	Other congenital malformations of ear, or face and neck, or nose, or larynx, or trachea and bronchus, or salivary glands, or pharynx	
	Burn or corrosion of mouth and pharynx, initial encounter	
	AND	
	MCC condition	*See* appendix B.
155	Benign neoplasm of mouth and pharynx	*See* DRG 154.
	Benign neoplasm of major salivary glands	
	Benign neoplasm of middle ear, nasal cavity and accessory sinuses	
	Benign neoplasm of larynx	
	Sleep apnea	
	Other congenital malformations of ear, or face and neck, or nose, or larynx, or trachea and bronchus, or salivary glands, or pharynx	
	Burn or corrosion of mouth and pharynx, initial encounter	
	AND	
	CC condition	*See* appendix B.
299	Epistaxis due to diseases of the capillaries	Hereditary hemorrhagic telangiectasia (HHT) is an autosomal dominant disorder that affects blood vessels throughout the body, resulting in bleeding tendency. Mucocutaneous telangiectases and arteriovenous malformations (AVMs) can affect the nasopharynx. Epistaxis is the most common manifestation. Onset of symptoms may be delayed until age 40 or later. Key term: Osler-Weber-Rendu Syndrome.
	AND	
	MCC condition	*See* appendix B.
300	Epistaxis due to diseases of the capillaries	*See* DRG 299.
	AND	
	CC condition	*See* appendix B.

DRG 151 (Continued)

DRG	PDx/SDx/Procedure	Tips
813	Hereditary or acquired coagulation, clotting, or factor deficiency	Key terms: Von Willebrand's disease, Hereditary factor XI deficiency, or other clotting factors such as acquired hemophilia or coagulation deficiency, hemorrhagic disorder due to intrinsic or extrinsic circulating anticoagulants, antibodies, or inhibitors, other and unspecified coagulation defects. Do not report a code from D68 series to identify patients on anticoagulant therapy such as Coumadin. It is the intent of this therapy to induce anticoagulation. Review record documentation for indications that the thrust of the treatment is directed towards the coagulation/clotting disorder rather than control of the epistaxis. Treatment could include diagnostic workup, administration of clotting factors, i.e. 4-Factor Prothrombin Complex Concentrate, fibrinogen, Antihemophilic factors, Factor IX, etc.
907	Intraoperative or postoperative hemorrhage, accidental intraoperative laceration	
	WITH	
	O.R. procedure for epistaxis control	Does not include root operation Control (e.g., cautery or silver nitrate application) from the Ear, Nose, Sinus body system (Ø93) or root operation Packing from the Placement section (2Y4).
	OR	
	Laceration or puncture wound, with and without foreign body, bite, or unspecified open wound of nose, unspecified injury of nose	
	WITH	
	Other nasal injury repair or graft	
	AND	
	MCC condition	*See* appendix B.
908	Intraoperative or postoperative hemorrhage, accidental intraoperative laceration	
	WITH	
	O.R. procedure for epistaxis control	*See* DRG 907.
	OR	
	Laceration or puncture wound, with and without foreign body, bite, or unspecified open wound of nose, unspecified injury of nose	
	WITH	
	Other nasal injury repair or graft	
	AND	
	CC condition	*See* appendix B.
909	Intraoperative or postoperative hemorrhage, accidental intraoperative laceration	
	WITH	
	O.R. procedure for epistaxis control	*See* DRG 907.
	OR	
	Laceration or puncture wound, with and without foreign body, bite, or unspecified open wound of nose, unspecified injury of nose	
	WITH	
	Other nasal injury repair or graft	

DRG 152 Otitis Media and Upper Respiratory Infection with MCC — RW 1.1882

Potential DRGs

143	Other Ear, Nose, Mouth and Throat O.R. Procedures with MCC	3.3256
177	Respiratory Infections and Inflammations with MCC	1.6964
193	Simple Pneumonia and Pleurisy with MCC	1.3266
865	Viral Illness with MCC	1.6399

DRG	PDx/SDx/Procedure	Tips
143	Myringotomy with intubation	
	Tonsil and/or adenoid procedures	
	AND	
	MCC condition	*See* appendix B.
177	Upper respiratory infection due to SARS-associated coronavirus (SARS-CoV-2) (COVID-19)	According to ICD-10-CM guidelines when the reason for the encounter/admission is a respiratory manifestation of COVID-19, assign code U07.1 COVID-19, as the principal/first-listed diagnosis and assign code(s) for the manifestation(s) as additional diagnoses.
	AND	
	MCC condition	*See* appendix B.
193	Influenza due to other identified or unidentified influenza virus with pneumonia or other respiratory manifestations	Excluding due to COVID-19.
	AND	
	MCC condition	*See* appendix B.
865	Influenza due to other identified or unidentified influenza virus with otitis media	
	AND	
	MCC condition	*See* appendix B.

DRG 153 Otitis Media and Upper Respiratory Infection without MCC — RW 0.7348

Potential DRGs

143	Other Ear, Nose, Mouth and Throat O.R. Procedures with MCC	3.3256
144	Other Ear, Nose, Mouth and Throat O.R. Procedures with CC	1.7305
145	Other Ear, Nose, Mouth and Throat O.R. Procedures without CC/MCC	1.2211
152	Otitis Media and Upper Respiratory Infection with MCC	1.1882
177	Respiratory Infections and Inflammations with MCC	1.6964
178	Respiratory Infections and Inflammations with CC	0.9867
179	Respiratory Infections and Inflammations without CC/MCC	0.7633
193	Simple Pneumonia and Pleurisy with MCC	1.3266
194	Simple Pneumonia and Pleurisy with CC	0.8222
865	Viral Illness with MCC	1.6399
866	Viral Illness without MCC	0.9177

DRG	PDx/SDx/Procedure	Tips
143	Myringotomy with intubation	
	Tonsil and/or adenoid procedures	
	AND	
	MCC condition	*See* appendix B.
144	Myringotomy with intubation	
	Tonsil and/or adenoid procedures	
	AND	
	CC condition	*See* appendix B.
145	Myringotomy with intubation	
	Tonsil and/or adenoid procedures	
152	MCC condition	*See* appendix B.
177	Upper respiratory infection due to SARS-associated coronavirus (SARS-CoV-2) (COVID-19)	According to ICD-10-CM guidelines when the reason for the encounter/admission is a respiratory manifestation of COVID-19, assign code UØ7.1 COVID-19, as the principal/first-listed diagnosis and assign code(s) for the manifestation(s) as additional diagnoses.
	AND	
	MCC condition	*See* appendix B.
178	Upper respiratory infection due to SARS-associated coronavirus (SARS-CoV-2) (COVID-19)	*See* DRG 177.
	AND	
	CC condition	*See* appendix B.
179	Upper respiratory infection due to SARS-associated coronavirus (SARS-CoV-2) (COVID-19)	*See* DRG 177.
193	Influenza due to other identified or unidentified influenza virus with pneumonia or other respiratory manifestations	Excluding due to COVID-19.
	AND	
	MCC condition	*See* appendix B.
194	Influenza due to other identified or unidentified influenza virus with pneumonia or other respiratory manifestations	*See* DRG 193.
	AND	
	CC condition	*See* appendix B.
865	Influenza due to other identified or unidentified influenza virus with otitis media	
	AND	
	MCC condition	*See* appendix B.
866	Influenza due to other identified or unidentified influenza virus with otitis media	

DRG 154 Other Ear, Nose, Mouth and Throat Diagnoses with MCC — RW 1.5382

Potential DRGs

011	Tracheostomy for Face, Mouth, Neck Diagnoses or Laryngectomy with MCC	5.1563
140	Major Head and Neck Procedures with MCC	3.7781
143	Other Ear, Nose, Mouth and Throat O.R. Procedures with MCC	3.3256

DRG	PDx/SDx/Procedure	Tips
011	Tracheostomy	Tracheostomy carried out elsewhere before admission or in an ambulance before arrival should not be reported as a current procedure. A tracheostomy procedure may be performed at the bedside and documented in the progress notes or in the operating room and documented in an operative note. Report Bypass, Trachea in Respiratory System (ØB11) with appropriate approach and device characters.
	AND	
	MCC condition	*See* appendix B.
140	Revision of tracheostomy	
	Nasal fracture reduction, open	Fracture reduction = Reposition.
	AND	
	MCC condition	*See* appendix B.
143	Nasal reconstructive procedures	
	AND	
	MCC condition	*See* appendix B.

DRG 155 Other Ear, Nose, Mouth and Throat Diagnoses with CC RW 0.9466

Potential DRGs

011	Tracheostomy for Face, Mouth, Neck Diagnoses or Laryngectomy with MCC	5.1563
012	Tracheostomy for Face, Mouth, Neck Diagnoses or Laryngectomy with CC	4.0049
140	Major Head and Neck Procedures with MCC	3.7781
141	Major Head and Neck Procedures with CC	2.0717
143	Other Ear, Nose, Mouth and Throat O.R. Procedures with MCC	3.3256
144	Other Ear, Nose, Mouth and Throat O.R. Procedures with CC	1.7305
154	Other Ear, Nose, Mouth and Throat Diagnoses with MCC	1.5382

DRG	PDx/SDx/Procedure	Tips
011	Tracheostomy	Tracheostomy carried out elsewhere before admission or in an ambulance before arrival should not be reported as a current procedure. A tracheostomy procedure may be performed at the bedside and documented in the progress notes or in the operating room and documented in an operative note. Report Bypass, Trachea in Respiratory System (ØB11) with appropriate approach and device characters.
	AND	
	MCC condition	*See* appendix B.
012	Tracheostomy	See DRG 011.
	AND	
	CC condition	*See* appendix B.
140	Revision of tracheostomy	
	Nasal fracture reduction, open	Fracture reduction = Reposition.
	AND	
	MCC condition	*See* appendix B.
141	Revision of tracheostomy	
	Nasal fracture reduction, open	Fracture reduction = Reposition.
	AND	
	CC condition	*See* appendix B.
143	Nasal reconstructive procedures	
	AND	
	MCC condition	*See* appendix B.
144	Nasal reconstructive procedures	
	AND	
	CC condition	*See* appendix B.
154	MCC condition	*See* appendix B.

DRG 156 Other Ear, Nose, Mouth and Throat Diagnoses without CC/MCC — RW 0.6555

Potential DRGs

011	Tracheostomy for Face, Mouth, Neck Diagnoses or Laryngectomy with MCC	5.1563
012	Tracheostomy for Face, Mouth, Neck Diagnoses or Laryngectomy with CC	4.0049
013	Tracheostomy for Face, Mouth, Neck Diagnoses or Laryngectomy without CC/MCC	2.6857
140	Major Head and Neck Procedures with MCC	3.7781
141	Major Head and Neck Procedures with CC	2.0717
142	Major Head and Neck Procedures without CC/MCC	1.5450
143	Other Ear, Nose, Mouth and Throat O.R. Procedures with MCC	3.3256
144	Other Ear, Nose, Mouth and Throat O.R. Procedures with CC	1.7305
145	Other Ear, Nose, Mouth and Throat O.R. Procedures without CC/MCC	1.2211
154	Other Ear, Nose, Mouth and Throat Diagnoses with MCC	1.5382
155	Other Ear, Nose, Mouth and Throat Diagnoses with CC	0.9466

DRG	PDx/SDx/Procedure	Tips
011	Tracheostomy	Tracheostomy carried out elsewhere before admission or in an ambulance before arrival should not be reported as a current procedure. A tracheostomy procedure may be performed at the bedside and documented in the progress notes or in the operating room and documented in an operative note. Report Bypass, Trachea in Respiratory System (ØB11) with appropriate approach and device characters.
	AND	
	MCC condition	*See* appendix B.
012	Tracheostomy	See DRG 011.
	AND	
	CC condition	*See* appendix B.
013	Tracheostomy	*See* appendix B.
140	Revision of tracheostomy	
	Nasal fracture reduction, open	Fracture reduction = Reposition.
	AND	
	MCC condition	*See* appendix B.
141	Revision of tracheostomy	
	Nasal fracture reduction, open	Fracture reduction = Reposition.
	AND	
	CC condition	*See* appendix B.
142	Revision of tracheostomy	
	Nasal fracture reduction, open	Fracture reduction = Reposition.
143	Nasal reconstructive procedures	
	AND	
	MCC condition	*See* appendix B.
144	Nasal reconstructive procedures	
	AND	
	CC condition	*See* appendix B.
145	Nasal reconstructive procedures	
154	MCC condition	*See* appendix B.
155	CC condition	*See* appendix B.

DRG 157 Dental and Oral Diseases with MCC — RW 1.7070

Potential DRGs

140	Major Head and Neck Procedures with MCC	3.7781
143	Other Ear, Nose, Mouth and Throat O.R. Procedures with MCC	3.3256

DRG	PDx/SDx/Procedure	Tips
140	Reduction of facial fractures, open	Fracture/dislocation reduction = Reposition.
	Reduction of TMJ dislocation, open	
	AND	
	MCC condition	*See* appendix B.
143	Fusion of TMJ	
	AND	
	MCC condition	*See* appendix B.

DRG 158 Dental and Oral Diseases with CC RW 0.9385

Potential DRGs

140	Major Head and Neck Procedures with MCC	3.7781
141	Major Head and Neck Procedures with CC	2.0717
143	Other Ear, Nose, Mouth and Throat O.R. Procedures with MCC	3.3256
144	Other Ear, Nose, Mouth and Throat O.R. Procedures with CC	1.7305
157	Dental and Oral Diseases with MCC	1.7070

DRG	PDx/SDx/Procedure	Tips
140	Reduction of facial fractures, open	Fracture/dislocation reduction = Reposition.
	Reduction of TMJ dislocation, open	
	AND	
	MCC condition	*See* appendix B.
141	Reduction of facial fractures, open	Fracture/dislocation reduction = Reposition.
	Reduction of TMJ dislocation, open	
	AND	
	CC condition	*See* appendix B.
143	Fusion of TMJ	
	AND	
	MCC condition	*See* appendix B.
144	Fusion of TMJ	
	AND	
	CC condition	*See* appendix B.
157	MCC condition	*See* appendix B.

DRG 159 Dental and Oral Diseases without CC/MCC RW 0.6752

Potential DRGs

140	Major Head and Neck Procedures with MCC	3.7781
141	Major Head and Neck Procedures with CC	2.0717
142	Major Head and Neck Procedures without CC/MCC	1.5450
143	Other Ear, Nose, Mouth and Throat O.R. Procedures with MCC	3.3256
144	Other Ear, Nose, Mouth and Throat O.R. Procedures with CC	1.7305
145	Other Ear, Nose, Mouth and Throat O.R. Procedures without CC/MCC	1.2211
157	Dental and Oral Diseases with MCC	1.7070
158	Dental and Oral Diseases with CC	0.9385

DRG	PDx/SDx/Procedure	Tips
140	Reduction of facial fractures, open	Fracture/dislocation reduction = Reposition.
	Reduction of TMJ dislocation, open	
	AND	
	MCC condition	*See* appendix B.
141	Reduction of facial fractures, open	Fracture/dislocation reduction = Reposition.
	Reduction of TMJ dislocation, open	
	AND	
	CC condition	*See* appendix B.
142	Reduction of facial fractures, open	Fracture/dislocation reduction = Reposition.
	Reduction of TMJ dislocation, open	
143	Fusion of TMJ	
	AND	
	MCC condition	*See* appendix B.
144	Fusion of TMJ	
	AND	
	CC condition	*See* appendix B.
145	Fusion of TMJ	
157	MCC condition	*See* appendix B.
158	CC condition	*See* appendix B.

Diseases And Disorders Of The Respiratory System

DRG 163 Major Chest Procedures with MCC — RW 4.7136

Potential DRGs

003 ECMO or Tracheostomy with Mechanical Ventilation > 96 Hours or Principal Diagnosis Except Face, Mouth and Neck with Major O.R. Procedure — 21.3203

DRG	PDx/SDx/Procedure	Tips
003	Extracorporeal membrane oxygenation (ECMO), central or peripheral	Central ECMO provides cardiorespiratory support and involves direct surgical cannulation of the right atrium and aorta via sternotomy. Peripheral (percutaneous) ECMO is a less invasive procedure than central ECMO. Veno-arterial (VA) peripheral ECMO cannulas are inserted percutaneously into both the femoral artery and the femoral vein. This type of ECMO provides both respiratory and circulatory support. Veno-venous (VV) peripheral ECMO may use one or two venous insertions, one in the upper veins and, if used, one in the lower veins, and provides respiratory support only.
	OR	
	Tracheostomy	Tracheostomy carried out elsewhere prior to admission or in an ambulance prior to arrival should not be reported as a current procedure. A tracheostomy procedure may be performed at the bedside and documented in the progress notes or in the operating room and documented in an operative note.
	WITH	
	Mechanical ventilation > 96 hours	Review record documentation for start and stop times. Calculation of mechanical ventilation hours begins when vent is initiated (or time of admission if patient already on a vent) and ends when it is turned off (or the time patient is discharged if still ventilated). The duration includes time spent to wean the patient from the vent. Do not assume that ventilation that spans four calendar days equals > 96 hours; count by the hour not day.

DRG 164 Major Chest Procedures with CC — RW 2.5504

Potential DRGs

003 ECMO or Tracheostomy with Mechanical Ventilation > 96 Hours or Principal Diagnosis Except Face, Mouth and Neck with Major O.R. Procedure — 21.3203

163 Major Chest Procedures with MCC — 4.7136

DRG	PDx/SDx/Procedure	Tips
003	Extracorporeal membrane oxygenation (ECMO), central or peripheral	Central ECMO provides cardiorespiratory support and involves direct surgical cannulation of the right atrium and aorta via sternotomy. Peripheral (percutaneous) ECMO is a less invasive procedure than central ECMO. Veno-arterial (VA) peripheral ECMO cannulas are inserted percutaneously into both the femoral artery and the femoral vein. This type of ECMO provides both respiratory and circulatory support. Veno-venous (VV) peripheral ECMO may use one or two venous insertions, one in the upper veins and, if used, one in the lower veins, and provides respiratory support only.
	OR	
	Tracheostomy	Tracheostomy carried out elsewhere prior to admission or in an ambulance prior to arrival should not be reported as a current procedure. A tracheostomy procedure may be performed at the bedside and documented in the progress notes or in the operating room and documented in an operative note.
	WITH	
	Mechanical ventilation > 96 hours	Review record documentation for start and stop times. Calculation of mechanical ventilation hours begins when vent is initiated (or time of admission if patient already on a vent) and ends when it is turned off (or the time patient is discharged if still ventilated). The duration includes time spent to wean the patient from the vent. Do not assume that ventilation that spans four calendar days equals > 96 hours; count by the hour not day.
163	MCC condition	*See* appendix B.

DRG 165 Major Chest Procedures without CC/MCC — RW 1.8764

Potential DRGs

003	ECMO or Tracheostomy with Mechanical Ventilation > 96 Hours or Principal Diagnosis Except Face, Mouth and Neck with Major O.R. Procedure	21.3203
163	Major Chest Procedures with MCC	4.7136
164	Major Chest Procedures with CC	2.5504

DRG	PDx/SDx/Procedure	Tips
003	Extracorporeal membrane oxygenation (ECMO), central or peripheral	Central ECMO provides cardiorespiratory support and involves direct surgical cannulation of the right atrium and aorta via sternotomy. Peripheral (percutaneous) ECMO is a less invasive procedure than central ECMO. Veno-arterial (VA) peripheral ECMO cannulas are inserted percutaneously into both the femoral artery and the femoral vein. This type of ECMO provides both respiratory and circulatory support. Veno-venous (VV) peripheral ECMO may use one or two venous insertions, one in the upper veins and, if used, one in the lower veins, and provides respiratory support only.
	OR	
	Tracheostomy	Tracheostomy carried out elsewhere prior to admission or in an ambulance prior to arrival should not be reported as a current procedure. A tracheostomy procedure may be performed at the bedside and documented in the progress notes or in the operating room and documented in an operative note.
	WITH	
	Mechanical ventilation > 96 hours	Review record documentation for start and stop times. Calculation of mechanical ventilation hours begins when vent is initiated (or time of admission if patient already on a vent) and ends when it is turned off (or the time patient is discharged if still ventilated). The duration includes time spent to wean the patient from the vent. Do not assume that ventilation that spans four calendar days equals > 96 hours; count by the hour not day.
163	MCC condition	*See* appendix B.
164	CC condition	*See* appendix B.

DRG 166 Other Respiratory System O.R. Procedures with MCC RW 4.0578

Potential DRGs

003	ECMO or Tracheostomy with Mechanical Ventilation > 96 Hours or Principal Diagnosis Except Face, Mouth and Neck with Major O.R. Procedure	21.3203
163	Major Chest Procedures with MCC	4.7136
173	Ultrasound Accelerated and Other Thrombolysis with Principal Diagnosis Pulmonary Embolism	3.0750

DRG	PDx/SDx/Procedure	Tips
003	Extracorporeal membrane oxygenation (ECMO), central or peripheral	Central ECMO provides cardiorespiratory support and involves direct surgical cannulation of the right atrium and aorta via sternotomy. Peripheral (percutaneous) ECMO is a less invasive procedure than central ECMO. Veno-arterial (VA) peripheral ECMO cannulas are inserted percutaneously into both the femoral artery and the femoral vein. This type of ECMO provides both respiratory and circulatory support. Veno-venous (VV) peripheral ECMO may use one or two venous insertions, one in the upper veins and, if used, one in the lower veins, and provides respiratory support only.
	OR	
	Tracheostomy	Tracheostomy carried out elsewhere prior to admission or in an ambulance prior to arrival should not be reported as a current procedure. A tracheostomy procedure may be performed at the bedside and documented in the progress notes or in the operating room and documented in an operative note.
	WITH	
	Mechanical ventilation > 96 hours	Review record documentation for start and stop times. Calculation of mechanical ventilation hours begins when vent is initiated (or time of admission if patient already on a vent) and ends when it is turned off (or the time patient is discharged if still ventilated). The duration includes time spent to wean the patient from the vent. Do not assume that ventilation that spans four calendar days equals > 96 hours; count by the hour not day.
163	Open biopsy of bronchus or lung	
	Thoracoscopic or open wedge resection of lung	
	Local excision/destruction of bronchial lesion	
	Destruction of lung lesion or tissue	Review record documentation for use of laser interstitial thermal therapy (LITT) via open or percutaneous endoscopic approach.
	Pulmonary artery embolectomy	The objective of the root operation Extirpation is to remove solid matter from a body part. This may require the solid matter to be broken up (Fragmentation) prior to removal. Only extirpation should be reported when the solid matter is fragmented and removed from the same body part. Percutaneous embolectomy is a minimally invasive option used when thrombolytic therapy fails or is contraindicated. Surgical embolectomy (open approach) is the most invasive treatment and is usually reserved for patients with massive pulmonary embolus and hemodynamic compromise.
	AND	
	MCC condition	*See* appendix B.
173	Principal diagnosis of pulmonary embolism	
	AND	
	Thrombolysis	The objective of the root operation Fragmentation is to break solid matter within a body part into pieces. The pieces are not removed. If the solid matter is fragmented and then removed from the same body part, root operation Extirpation would be reported and the case would group to DRGs 163–165. NOTE: DRG 173 has a lower relative weight than DRG 166; however, based on the surgical hierarchy table, DRG 173 would take precedence over DRG 166.

DRG 167 Other Respiratory System O.R. Procedures with CC RW 1.8198

Potential DRGs

003	ECMO or Tracheostomy with Mechanical Ventilation > 96 Hours or Principal Diagnosis Except Face, Mouth and Neck with Major O.R. Procedure	21.3203
163	Major Chest Procedures with MCC	4.7136
164	Major Chest Procedures with CC	2.5504
166	Other Respiratory System O.R. Procedures with MCC	4.0578
173	Ultrasound Accelerated and Other Thrombolysis with Principal Diagnosis Pulmonary Embolism	3.0750

DRG	PDx/SDx/Procedure	Tips
003	Extracorporeal membrane oxygenation (ECMO), central or peripheral	Central ECMO provides cardiorespiratory support and involves direct surgical cannulation of the right atrium and aorta via sternotomy. Peripheral (percutaneous) ECMO is a less invasive procedure than central ECMO. Veno-arterial (VA) peripheral ECMO cannulas are inserted percutaneously into both the femoral artery and the femoral vein. This type of ECMO provides both respiratory and circulatory support. Veno-venous (VV) peripheral ECMO may use one or two venous insertions, one in the upper veins and, if used, one in the lower veins, and provides respiratory support only.
	OR	
	Tracheostomy	Tracheostomy carried out elsewhere prior to admission or in an ambulance prior to arrival should not be reported as a current procedure. A tracheostomy procedure may be performed at the bedside and documented in the progress notes or in the operating room and documented in an operative note.
	WITH	
	Mechanical ventilation > 96 hours	Review record documentation for start and stop times. Calculation of mechanical ventilation hours begins when vent is initiated (or time of admission if patient already on a vent) and ends when it is turned off (or the time patient is discharged if still ventilated). The duration includes time spent to wean the patient from the vent. Do not assume that ventilation that spans four calendar days equals > 96 hours; count by the hour not day.
163	Open biopsy of bronchus or lung	
	Thoracoscopic or open wedge resection of lung	
	Local excision/destruction of bronchial lesion	
	Destruction of lung lesion or tissue	Review record documentation for use of laser interstitial thermal therapy (LITT) via open or percutaneous endoscopic approach.
	Pulmonary artery embolectomy	The objective of the root operation Extirpation is to remove solid matter from a body part. This may require the solid matter to be broken up (Fragmentation) prior to removal. Only extirpation should be reported when the solid matter is fragmented and removed from the same body part. Percutaneous embolectomy is a minimally invasive option used when thrombolytic therapy fails or is contraindicated. Surgical embolectomy (open approach) is the most invasive treatment and is usually reserved for patients with massive pulmonary embolus and hemodynamic compromise.
	AND	
	MCC condition	*See* appendix B.
164	Open biopsy of bronchus or lung	
	Thoracoscopic or open wedge resection of lung	
	Local excision/destruction of bronchial lesion	
	Destruction of lung lesion or tissue	*See* DRG 163.
	Pulmonary artery embolectomy	*See* DRG 163.
	AND	
	CC condition	*See* appendix B.
166	MCC condition	*See* appendix B.
173	Principal diagnosis of pulmonary embolism	
	AND	
	Thrombolysis	The objective of the root operation Fragmentation is to break solid matter within a body part into pieces. The pieces are not removed. If the solid matter is fragmented and then removed from the same body part, root operation Extirpation would be reported, and the case would group to DRGs 163–165.

Optimizing Tips

DRG 168 Other Respiratory System O.R. Procedures without CC/MCC

RW 1.3557

Potential DRGs

003	ECMO or Tracheostomy with Mechanical Ventilation > 96 Hours or Principal Diagnosis Except Face, Mouth and Neck with Major O.R. Procedure	21.3203
163	Major Chest Procedures with MCC	4.7136
164	Major Chest Procedures with CC	2.5504
165	Major Chest Procedures without CC/MCC	1.8764
166	Other Respiratory System O.R. Procedures with MCC	4.0578
167	Other Respiratory System O.R. Procedures with CC	1.8198
173	Ultrasound Accelerated and Other Thrombolysis with Principal Diagnosis Pulmonary Embolism	3.0750

DRG	PDx/SDx/Procedure	Tips
003	Extracorporeal membrane oxygenation (ECMO), central or peripheral	Central ECMO provides cardiorespiratory support and involves direct surgical cannulation of the right atrium and aorta via sternotomy. Peripheral (percutaneous) ECMO is a less invasive procedure than central ECMO. Veno-arterial (VA) peripheral ECMO cannulas are inserted percutaneously into both the femoral artery and the femoral vein. This type of ECMO provides both respiratory and circulatory support. Veno-venous (VV) peripheral ECMO may use one or two venous insertions, one in the upper veins and, if used, one in the lower veins, and provides respiratory support only.
	OR	
	Tracheostomy	Tracheostomy carried out elsewhere prior to admission or in an ambulance prior to arrival should not be reported as a current procedure. A tracheostomy procedure may be performed at the bedside and documented in the progress notes or in the operating room and documented in an operative note.
	WITH	
	Mechanical ventilation > 96 hours	Review record documentation for start and stop times. Calculation of mechanical ventilation hours begins when vent is initiated (or time of admission if patient already on a vent) and ends when it is turned off (or the time patient is discharged if still ventilated). The duration includes time spent to wean the patient from the vent. Do not assume that ventilation that spans four calendar days equals > 96 hours; count by the hour not day.
163	Open biopsy of bronchus or lung	
	Thoracoscopic or open wedge resection of lung	
	Local excision/destruction of bronchial lesion	
	Destruction of lung lesion or tissue	Review record documentation for use of laser interstitial thermal therapy (LITT) via open or percutaneous endoscopic approach.
	Pulmonary artery embolectomy	The objective of the root operation Extirpation is to remove solid matter from a body part. This may require the solid matter to be broken up (Fragmentation) prior to removal. Only extirpation should be reported when the solid matter is fragmented and removed from the same body part. Percutaneous embolectomy is a minimally invasive option used when thrombolytic therapy fails or is contraindicated. Surgical embolectomy (open approach) is the most invasive treatment and is usually reserved for patients with massive pulmonary embolus and hemodynamic compromise.
	AND	
	MCC condition	*See* appendix B.
164	Open biopsy of bronchus or lung	
	Thoracoscopic or open wedge resection of lung	
	Local excision/destruction of bronchial lesion	
	Destruction of lung lesion or tissue	*See* DRG 163.
	Pulmonary artery embolectomy	*See* DRG 163.
	AND	
	CC condition	*See* appendix B.
165	Open biopsy of bronchus or lung	
	Thoracoscopic or open wedge resection of lung	
	Local excision/destruction of bronchial lesion	
	Destruction of lung lesion or tissue	*See* DRG 163.
	Pulmonary artery embolectomy	*See* DRG 163.
166	MCC condition	*See* appendix B.
167	CC condition	*See* appendix B.
173	Principal diagnosis of pulmonary embolism	
	AND	
	Thrombolysis	The objective of the root operation Fragmentation is to break solid matter within a body part into pieces. The pieces are not removed. If the solid matter is fragmented and then removed from the same body part, root operation Extirpation would be reported, and the case would group to DRGs 163–165.

DRG 173 Ultrasound Accelerated and Other Thrombolysis with Principal Diagnosis Pulmonary Embolism — RW 3.0750

Potential DRGs

163	Major Chest Procedures with MCC	4.7136

DRG	PDx/SDx/Procedure	Tips
163	Pulmonary artery embolectomy	The objective of the root operation Extirpation is to remove solid matter from a body part. This may require the solid matter to be broken up (Fragmentation) prior to removal. Only extirpation should be reported when the solid matter is fragmented and removed from the same body part. Percutaneous embolectomy is a minimally invasive option used when thrombolytic therapy fails or is contraindicated. Surgical embolectomy (open approach) is the most invasive and is usually reserved for patients with massive pulmonary embolus and hemodynamic compromise.
	AND	
	MCC condition	*See* appendix B.

DRG 175 Pulmonary Embolism with MCC or Acute Cor Pulmonale — RW 1.4030

Potential DRGs

003	ECMO or Tracheostomy with Mechanical Ventilation > 96 Hours or Principal Diagnosis Except Face, Mouth and Neck with Major O.R. Procedure	21.3203
004	Tracheostomy with Mechanical Ventilation >96 Hours or Principal Diagnosis Except Face, Mouth and Neck without Major O.R. Procedure	14.7000
163	Major Chest Procedures with MCC	4.7136
166	Other Respiratory System O.R. Procedures with MCC	4.0578
173	Ultrasound Accelerated and Other Thrombolysis with Principal Diagnosis Pulmonary Embolism	3.0750
207	Respiratory System Diagnosis with Ventilator Support > 96 Hours	6.9080
208	Respiratory System Diagnosis with Ventilator Support <= 96 Hours	2.7038
280	Acute Myocardial Infarction, Discharged Alive with MCC	1.5865

DRG	PDx/SDx/Procedure	Tips
003	Extracorporeal membrane oxygenation (ECMO), central or peripheral	Central ECMO provides cardiorespiratory support and involves direct surgical cannulation of the right atrium and aorta via sternotomy. Peripheral (percutaneous) ECMO is a less invasive procedure than central ECMO. Veno-arterial (VA) peripheral ECMO cannulas are inserted percutaneously into both the femoral artery and the femoral vein. This type of ECMO provides both respiratory and circulatory support. Veno-venous (VV) peripheral ECMO may use one or two venous insertions, one in the upper veins and, if used, one in the lower veins, and provides respiratory support only.
	OR	
	Tracheostomy	Tracheostomy carried out elsewhere prior to admission or in an ambulance prior to arrival should not be reported as a current procedure. A tracheostomy procedure may be performed at the bedside and documented in the progress notes or in the operating room and documented in an operative note.
	WITH	
	Mechanical ventilation > 96 hours	Review record documentation for start and stop times. Calculation of mechanical ventilation hours begins when vent is initiated (or time of admission if patient already on a vent) and ends when it is turned off (or the time patient is discharged if still ventilated). The duration includes time spent to wean the patient from the vent. Do not assume that ventilation that spans four calendar days equals > 96 hours; count by the hour not day.
004	Tracheostomy	*See* DRG 003.
	WITH	
	Mechanical ventilation > 96 hours	*See* DRG ØØ3.
163	Pulmonary artery embolectomy	The objective of the root operation Extirpation is to remove solid matter from a body part. This may require the solid matter to be broken up (Fragmentation) prior to removal. Only extirpation should be reported when the solid matter is fragmented and removed from the same body part. Percutaneous embolectomy is a minimally invasive option used when thrombolytic therapy fails or is contraindicated. Surgical embolectomy (open approach) is the most invasive and is usually reserved for patients with massive pulmonary embolus and hemodynamic compromise.
	AND	
	MCC condition	*See* appendix B.

DRG 175 (Continued)

DRG	PDx/SDx/Procedure	Tips
166	Interruption of the vena cava by insertion of implant or sieve (IVC filter)	Root operation Insertion is defined as: "Putting in a non-biological device that monitors, assists, performs, or prevents a physiological function but does not physically take the place of a body part." Root operations Occlusion and Restriction both have the objective of altering the diameter of an orifice or tubular body part. In order to code these root operations correctly, it must be understood whether the objective is to merely narrow or to block the opening or lumen completely.
	Total interruption (Occlusion) of the vena cava	
	Partial interruption (Restriction) of the vena cava	
	AND	
	MCC condition	*See* appendix B.
173	Thrombolysis	The objective of the root operation Fragmentation is to break solid matter within a body part into pieces. The pieces are not removed. If the solid matter is fragmented and then removed from the same body part, root operation Extirpation would be reported, and the case would group to DRGs 163–165.
207	Mechanical ventilation > 96 consecutive hours	Review record documentation for start and stop times. Calculation of mechanical ventilation hours begins when vent is initiated (or time of admission if patient already on a vent) and ends when it is turned off (or the time patient is discharged if still ventilated). The duration includes time spent to wean the patient from the vent. Do not assume that ventilation that spans four calendar days equals > 96 hours; count by the hour not day.
208	Mechanical ventilation for less than or equal to 96 consecutive hours	*See* DRG 207.
280	Acute myocardial infarction, equal to, or less than, four weeks old	
	AND	
	MCC condition	*See* appendix B.

DRG 176 Pulmonary Embolism without MCC RW 0.8156

Potential DRGs

003	ECMO or Tracheostomy with Mechanical Ventilation > 96 Hours or Principal Diagnosis Except Face, Mouth and Neck with Major O.R. Procedure	21.3203
004	Tracheostomy with Mechanical Ventilation >96 Hours or Principal Diagnosis Except Face, Mouth and Neck without Major O.R. Procedure	14.7000
163	Major Chest Procedures with MCC	4.7136
164	Major Chest Procedures with CC	2.5504
165	Major Chest Procedures without CC/MCC	1.8764
166	Other Respiratory System O.R. Procedures with MCC	4.0578
167	Other Respiratory System O.R. Procedures with CC	1.8198
168	Other Respiratory System O.R. Procedures without CC/MCC	1.3557
173	Ultrasound Accelerated and Other Thrombolysis with Principal Diagnosis Pulmonary Embolism	3.0750
175	Pulmonary Embolism with MCC or Acute Cor Pulmonale	1.4030
207	Respiratory System Diagnosis with Ventilator Support > 96 Hours	6.9080
208	Respiratory System Diagnosis with Ventilator Support <= 96 Hours	2.7038
280	Acute Myocardial Infarction, Discharged Alive with MCC	1.5865
281	Acute Myocardial Infarction, Discharged Alive with CC	0.9130

DRG	PDx/SDx/Procedure	Tips
003	Extracorporeal membrane oxygenation (ECMO), central or peripheral	Central ECMO provides cardiorespiratory support and involves direct surgical cannulation of the right atrium and aorta via sternotomy. Peripheral (percutaneous) ECMO is a less invasive procedure than central ECMO. Veno-arterial (VA) peripheral ECMO cannulas are inserted percutaneously into both the femoral artery and the femoral vein. This type of ECMO provides both respiratory and circulatory support. Veno-venous (VV) peripheral ECMO may use one or two venous insertions, one in the upper veins and, if used, one in the lower veins, and provides respiratory support only.
	OR	
	Tracheostomy	Tracheostomy carried out elsewhere prior to admission or in an ambulance prior to arrival should not be reported as a current procedure. A tracheostomy procedure may be performed at the bedside and documented in the progress notes or in the operating room and documented in an operative note.
	WITH	
	Mechanical ventilation > 96 hours	Review record documentation for start and stop times. Calculation of mechanical ventilation hours begins when vent is initiated (or time of admission if patient already on a vent) and ends when it is turned off (or the time patient is discharged if still ventilated). The duration includes time spent to wean the patient from the vent. Do not assume that ventilation that spans four calendar days equals > 96 hours; count by the hour not day.
004	Tracheostomy	*See* DRG 003.
	WITH	
	Mechanical ventilation > 96 hours	*See* DRG ØØ3.

DRG 176 (Continued)

DRG	PDx/SDx/Procedure	Tips
163	Pulmonary artery embolectomy	The objective of the root operation Extirpation is to remove solid matter from a body part. This may require the solid matter to be broken up (Fragmentation) prior to removal. Only extirpation should be reported when the solid matter is fragmented and removed from the same body part. Percutaneous embolectomy is a minimally invasive option used when thrombolytic therapy fails or is contraindicated. Surgical embolectomy (open approach) is the most invasive and is usually reserved for patients with massive pulmonary embolus and hemodynamic compromise.
	AND	
	MCC condition	*See* appendix B.
164	Pulmonary artery embolectomy	*See* DRG 163.
	AND	
	CC condition	*See* appendix B.
165	Pulmonary artery embolectomy (open, percutaneous, percutaneous endoscopic)	*See* DRG 163.
166	Interruption of the vena cava by insertion of implant or sieve (IVC filter)	Root operation Insertion is defined as: "Putting in a non-biological device that monitors, assists, performs, or prevents a physiological function but does not physically take the place of a body part." Root operations Occlusion and Restriction both have the objective of altering the diameter of an orifice or tubular body part. In order to code these root operations correctly, it must be understood whether the objective is to merely narrow or to block the opening or lumen completely.
	Total interruption (Occlusion) of the vena cava	
	Partial interruption (Restriction) of the vena cava	
	AND	
	MCC condition	*See* appendix B.
167	Interruption of the vena cava by insertion of implant or sieve (IVC filter)	*See* DRG 166.
	Total interruption (Occlusion) of the vena cava	
	Partial interruption (Restriction) of the vena cava	
	AND	
	CC condition	*See* appendix B.
168	Interruption of the vena cava by insertion of implant or sieve (IVC filter)	*See* DRG 166.
	Total interruption (Occlusion) of the vena cava	
	Partial interruption (Restriction) of the vena cava	
173	Thrombolysis	The objective of the root operation Fragmentation is to break solid matter within a body part into pieces. The pieces are not removed. If the solid matter is fragmented and then removed from the same body part, root operation Extirpation would be reported, and the case would group to DRGs 163–165.
175	Secondary diagnosis of acute cor pulmonale	
	OR	
	MCC condition	*See* appendix B.
207	Mechanical ventilation > 96 consecutive hours	Review record documentation for start and stop times. Calculation of mechanical ventilation hours begins when vent is initiated (or time of admission if patient already on a vent) and ends when it is turned off (or the time patient is discharged if still ventilated). The duration includes time spent to wean the patient from the vent. Do not assume that ventilation that spans four calendar days equals > 96 hours; count by the hour not day.
208	Mechanical ventilation for less than or equal to 96 consecutive hours	*See* DRG 207.
280	Acute myocardial infarction, equal to, or less than, four weeks old	
	AND	
	MCC condition	*See* appendix B.
281	Acute myocardial infarction, equal to, or less than, four weeks old	
	AND	
	CC condition	*See* appendix B.

DRG 177 Respiratory Infections and Inflammations with MCC — RW 1.6964

Potential DRGs

004	Tracheostomy with Mechanical Ventilation > 96 Hours or Principal Diagnosis Except Face, Mouth and Neck without Major O.R. Procedure	14.7000
207	Respiratory System Diagnosis with Ventilator Support > 96 Hours	6.9080
208	Respiratory System Diagnosis with Ventilator Support <= 96 Hours	2.7038
545	Connective Tissue Disorders with MCC	2.4932
974	HIV with Major Related Condition with MCC	2.9165

DRG	PDx/SDx/Procedure	Tips
004	Tracheostomy	Tracheostomy carried out elsewhere prior to admission or in an ambulance prior to arrival should not be reported as a current procedure. A tracheostomy procedure may be performed at the bedside and documented in the progress notes or in the operating room and documented in an operative note.
	AND	
	Mechanical ventilation > 96 consecutive hours	Review record documentation for start and stop times. Calculation of mechanical ventilation hours begins when vent is initiated (or time of admission if patient already on a vent) and ends when it is turned off (or the time patient is discharged if still ventilated). The duration includes time spent to wean the patient from the vent. Do not assume that ventilation that spans four calendar days equals > 96 hours; count by the hour not day.
207	Mechanical ventilation > 96 consecutive hours	*See* DRG 004.
208	Mechanical ventilation for less than or equal to 96 consecutive hours	*See* DRG 004.
545	Post COVID-19 condition—multisystem inflammatory syndrome (MIS)	Review documentation carefully to determine whether the MIS is a residual effect of a previous COVID-19 infection or an acute manifestation of a current COVID-19 infection. If the MIS is a residual effect, report the code for MIS as principal diagnosis followed by U09.9.
	AND	
	MCC condition	*See* appendix B.
974	Diagnosis of HIV disease	Admission for HIV-related condition: sequence B2Ø first followed by the HIV-related condition code except chapter 15 codes, which take sequencing priority. Any complication of the HIV-related condition would also be coded as a secondary diagnosis. (e.g., acute respiratory failure due to AIDS-related pneumonia).
	AND	
	Opportunistic lung infection	Pneumocystosis candidiasis of lung. See appendix C for the full list of major HIV-related conditions. A diagnosis from this list should not be assumed as HIV-related unless specifically documented as such by the provider.
	AND	
	MCC condition	*See* appendix B.

DRG 178 Respiratory Infections and Inflammations with CC — RW 0.9867

Potential DRGs

004	Tracheostomy with Mechanical Ventilation > 96 Hours or Principal Diagnosis Except Face, Mouth and Neck without Major O.R. Procedure	14.7000
177	Respiratory Infections and Inflammations with MCC	1.6964
193	Simple Pneumonia and Pleurisy with MCC	1.3266
207	Respiratory System Diagnosis with Ventilator Support > 96 Hours	6.9080
208	Respiratory System Diagnosis with Ventilator Support <= 96 Hours	2.7038
545	Connective Tissue Disorders with MCC	2.4932
546	Connective Tissue Disorders with CC	1.1993
974	HIV with Major Related Condition with MCC	2.9165
975	HIV with Major Related Condition with CC	1.3633

DRG	PDx/SDx/Procedure	Tips
004	Tracheostomy	Tracheostomy carried out elsewhere prior to admission or in an ambulance prior to arrival should not be reported as a current procedure. A tracheostomy procedure may be performed at the bedside and documented in the progress notes or in the operating room and documented in an operative note.
	AND	
	Mechanical ventilation > 96 consecutive hours	Review record documentation for start and stop times. Calculation of mechanical ventilation hours begins when vent is initiated (or time of admission if patient already on a vent) and ends when it is turned off (or the time patient is discharged if still ventilated). The duration includes time spent to wean the patient from the vent. Do not assume that ventilation that spans four calendar days equals > 96 hours; count by the hour not day.
177	MCC condition	*See* appendix B.
193	Pneumonia due to Streptococcus	Review lab reports carefully and query the physician if necessary when gram stain reports indicate gram-positive cocci. Both Staphylococcus and Streptococcus are genera of gram-positive cocci. Bacterial pneumonia should be assigned based on physician documentation and not based solely on culture or gram stain reports.
	AND	
	MCC condition	*See* appendix B.
207	Mechanical ventilation > 96 consecutive hours	*See* DRG 004.
208	Mechanical ventilation for less than or equal to 96 consecutive hours	*See* DRG 004.
545	Post COVID-19 condition—multisystem inflammatory syndrome (MIS)	Review documentation carefully to determine whether the MIS is a residual effect of a previous COVID-19 infection or an acute manifestation of a current COVID-19 infection. If the MIS is a residual effect, report the code for MIS as principal diagnosis followed by UØ9.9.
	AND	
	MCC condition	*See* appendix B.
546	Post COVID-19 condition—multisystem inflammatory syndrome (MIS)	*See* DRG 545.
	AND	
	CC condition	*See* appendix B.
974	Diagnosis of HIV disease	Admission for HIV-related condition: sequence B2Ø first followed by the HIV-related condition code except chapter 15 codes, which take sequencing priority. Any complication of the HIV-related condition would also be coded as a secondary diagnosis. (e.g., acute respiratory failure due to AIDS-related pneumonia).
	AND	
	Opportunistic lung infection	Pneumocystosis candidiasis of lung. See appendix C for the full list of major HIV-related conditions. A diagnosis from this list should not be assumed as HIV-related unless specifically documented as such by the provider.
	AND	
	MCC condition	*See* appendix B.
975	Diagnosis of HIV disease	*See* DRG 974.
	AND	
	Opportunistic lung infection	*See* DRG 974.
	AND	
	CC condition	*See* appendix B.

DRG 179 Respiratory Infections and Inflammations without CC/MCC RW 0.7633

Potential DRGs

004	Tracheostomy with Mechanical Ventilation > 96 Hours or Principal Diagnosis Except Face, Mouth and Neck without Major O.R. Procedure	14.7000
177	Respiratory Infections and Inflammations with MCC	1.6964
178	Respiratory Infections and Inflammations with CC	0.9867
193	Simple Pneumonia and Pleurisy with MCC	1.3266
207	Respiratory System Diagnosis with Ventilator Support > 96 Hours	6.9080
208	Respiratory System Diagnosis with Ventilator Support <= 96 Hours	2.7038
545	Connective Tissue Disorders with MCC	2.4932
546	Connective Tissue Disorders with CC	1.1993
974	HIV with Major Related Condition with MCC	2.9165
975	HIV with Major Related Condition with CC	1.3633

DRG	PDx/SDx/Procedure	Tips
004	Tracheostomy	Tracheostomy carried out elsewhere prior to admission or in an ambulance prior to arrival should not be reported as a current procedure. A tracheostomy procedure may be performed at the bedside and documented in the progress notes or in the operating room and documented in an operative note.
	WITH	
	Mechanical ventilation > 96 consecutive hours	
177	MCC condition	*See* appendix B.
178	CC condition	*See* appendix B.
193	Pneumonia due to Streptococcus	Review lab reports carefully and query the physician if necessary when gram stain reports indicate gram-positive cocci. Both Staphylococcus and Streptococcus are genera of gram-positive cocci. Bacterial pneumonia should be assigned based on physician documentation and not based solely on culture or gram stain reports.
	AND	
	MCC condition	*See* appendix B.
207	Mechanical ventilation > 96 consecutive hours	Review record documentation for start and stop times. Calculation of mechanical ventilation hours begins when vent is initiated (or time of admission if patient already on a vent) and ends when it is turned off (or the time patient is discharged if still ventilated). The duration includes time spent to wean the patient from the vent. Do not assume that ventilation that spans four calendar days equals > 96 hours; count by the hour not day.
208	Mechanical ventilation for less than or equal to 96 consecutive hours	*See* DRG 207.
545	Post COVID-19 condition—multisystem inflammatory syndrome (MIS)	Review documentation carefully to determine whether the MIS is a residual effect of a previous COVID-19 infection or an acute manifestation of a current COVID-19 infection. If the MIS is a residual effect, report the code for MIS as principal diagnosis followed by UØ9.9.
	AND	
	MCC condition	*See* appendix B.
546	Post COVID-19 condition—multisystem inflammatory syndrome (MIS)	*See* DRG 545.
	AND	
	CC condition	*See* appendix B.
974	Diagnosis of HIV disease	Admission for HIV-related condition: sequence B2Ø first followed by the HIV-related condition code except chapter 15 codes, which take sequencing priority. Any complication of the HIV-related condition would also be coded as a secondary diagnosis. (e.g., acute respiratory failure due to AIDS-related pneumonia).
	AND	
	Opportunistic lung infection	Pneumocystosis candidiasis of lung. See appendix C for the full list of major HIV-related conditions. A diagnosis from this list should not be assumed as HIV-related unless specifically documented as such by the provider.
	AND	
	MCC condition	*See* appendix B.
975	Diagnosis of HIV disease	*See* DRG 974.
	AND	
	Opportunistic lung infection	*See* DRG 974.
	AND	
	CC condition	*See* appendix B.

DRG 180 Respiratory Neoplasms with MCC RW 1.7382

Potential DRGs

004	Tracheostomy with Mechanical Ventilation > 96 Hours or Principal Diagnosis Except Face, Mouth and Neck without Major O.R. Procedure	14.7000
163	Major Chest Procedures with MCC	4.7136
166	Other Respiratory System O.R. Procedures with MCC	4.0578
207	Respiratory System Diagnosis with Ventilator Support > 96 Hours	6.9080
208	Respiratory System Diagnosis with Ventilator Support <= 96 Hours	2.7038

DRG	PDx/SDx/Procedure	Tips
004	Tracheostomy	Tracheostomy carried out elsewhere prior to admission or in an ambulance prior to arrival should not be reported as a current procedure. A tracheostomy procedure may be performed at the bedside and documented in the progress notes or in the operating room and documented in an operative note.
	WITH	
	Mechanical ventilation > 96 consecutive hours	Review record documentation for start and stop times. Calculation of mechanical ventilation hours begins when vent is initiated (or time of admission if patient already on a vent) and ends when it is turned off (or the time patient is discharged if still ventilated). The duration includes time spent to wean the patient from the vent. Do not assume that ventilation that spans four calendar days equals > 96 hours; count by the hour not day.
163	Thoracoscopic excision of lung lesion or tissue	
	Destruction of lung lesion or tissue	Review record documentation for use of laser interstitial thermal therapy (LITT) via open or percutaneous endoscopic approach.
	AND	
	MCC condition	*See* appendix B.
166	Brachytherapy radioactive implant	
	Destruction of lung lesion or tissue	Review record documentation for use of laser interstitial thermal therapy (LITT) via percutaneous approach.
	Thoracoscopic biopsy of lung	
	AND	
	MCC condition	*See* appendix B.
207	Mechanical ventilation > 96 consecutive hours	*See* DRG 004.
208	Mechanical ventilation for less than or equal to 96 consecutive hours	*See* DRG 004.

DRG 181 Respiratory Neoplasms with CC

RW 1.1011

Potential DRGs

004	Tracheostomy with Mechanical Ventilation > 96 Hours or Principal Diagnosis Except Face, Mouth and Neck without Major O.R. Procedure	14.7000
163	Major Chest Procedures with MCC	4.7136
164	Major Chest Procedures with CC	2.5504
166	Other Respiratory System O.R. Procedures with MCC	4.0578
167	Other Respiratory System O.R. Procedures with CC	1.8198
180	Respiratory Neoplasms with MCC	1.7382
207	Respiratory System Diagnosis with Ventilator Support > 96 Hours	6.9080
208	Respiratory System Diagnosis with Ventilator Support <= 96 Hours	2.7038

DRG	PDx/SDx/Procedure	Tips
004	Tracheostomy	Tracheostomy carried out elsewhere prior to admission or in an ambulance prior to arrival should not be reported as a current procedure. A tracheostomy procedure may be performed at the bedside and documented in the progress notes or in the operating room and documented in an operative note.
	WITH	
	Mechanical ventilation > 96 consecutive hours	Review record documentation for start and stop times. Calculation of mechanical ventilation hours begins when vent is initiated (or time of admission if patient already on a vent) and ends when it is turned off (or the time patient is discharged if still ventilated). The duration includes time spent to wean the patient from the vent. Do not assume that ventilation that spans four calendar days equals > 96 hours; count by the hour not day.
163	Thoracoscopic excision of lung lesion or tissue	
	Destruction of lung lesion or tissue	Review record documentation for use of laser interstitial thermal therapy (LITT) via open or percutaneous endoscopic approach.
	AND	
	MCC condition	*See* appendix B.
164	Thoracoscopic excision of lung lesion or tissue	
	Destruction of lung lesion or tissue	*See* DRG 163.
	AND	
	CC condition	*See* appendix B.
166	Brachytherapy radioactive implant	
	Destruction of lung lesion or tissue	Review record documentation for use of laser interstitial thermal therapy (LITT) via percutaneous approach.
	Thoracoscopic biopsy of lung	
	AND	
	MCC condition	*See* appendix B.
167	Brachytherapy radioactive implant	
	Destruction of lung lesion or tissue	*See* DRG 166.
	Thoracoscopic biopsy of lung	
	AND	
	CC condition	*See* appendix B.
180	MCC condition	*See* appendix B.
207	Mechanical ventilation > 96 consecutive hours	*See* DRG 004.
208	Mechanical ventilation for less than or equal to 96 consecutive hours	*See* DRG 004.

DRG 182 Respiratory Neoplasms without CC/MCC RW 0.7590

Potential DRGs

004	Tracheostomy with Mechanical Ventilation > 96 Hours or Principal Diagnosis Except Face, Mouth and Neck without Major O.R. Procedure	14.7000
163	Major Chest Procedures with MCC	4.7136
164	Major Chest Procedures with CC	2.5504
165	Major Chest Procedures without CC/MCC	1.8764
166	Other Respiratory System O.R. Procedures with MCC	4.0578
167	Other Respiratory System O.R. Procedures with CC	1.8198
168	Other Respiratory System O.R. Procedures without CC/MCC	1.3557
180	Respiratory Neoplasms with MCC	1.7382
181	Respiratory Neoplasms with CC	1.1011
207	Respiratory System Diagnosis with Ventilator Support > 96 Hours	6.9080
208	Respiratory System Diagnosis with Ventilator Support <= 96 Hours	2.7038

DRG	PDx/SDx/Procedure	Tips
004	Tracheostomy	Tracheostomy carried out elsewhere prior to admission or in an ambulance prior to arrival should not be reported as a current procedure. A tracheostomy procedure may be performed at the bedside and documented in the progress notes or in the operating room and documented in an operative note.
	WITH	
	Mechanical ventilation > 96 consecutive hours	Review record documentation for start and stop times. Calculation of mechanical ventilation hours begins when vent is initiated (or time of admission if patient already on a vent) and ends when it is turned off (or the time patient is discharged if still ventilated). The duration includes time spent to wean the patient from the vent. Do not assume that ventilation that spans four calendar days equals > 96 hours; count by the hour not day.
163	Thoracoscopic excision of lung lesion or tissue	
	Destruction of lung lesion or tissue	Review record documentation for use of laser interstitial thermal therapy (LITT) via open or percutaneous endoscopic approach.
	AND	
	MCC condition	*See* appendix B.
164	Thoracoscopic excision of lung lesion or tissue	
	Destruction of lung lesion or tissue	*See* DRG 163.
	AND	
	CC condition	*See* appendix B.
165	Thoracoscopic excision of lung lesion or tissue	
	Destruction of lung lesion or tissue	*See* DRG 163.
166	Brachytherapy radioactive implant	
	Destruction of lung lesion or tissue	Review record documentation for use of laser interstitial thermal therapy (LITT) via percutaneous approach.
	Thoracoscopic biopsy of lung	
	AND	
	MCC condition	*See* appendix B.
167	Brachytherapy radioactive implant	
	Destruction of lung lesion or tissue	*See* DRG 166.
	Thoracoscopic biopsy of lung	
	AND	
	CC condition	*See* appendix B.
168	Brachytherapy radioactive implant	
	Destruction of lung lesion or tissue	*See* DRG 166.
	Thoracoscopic biopsy of lung	
180	MCC condition	*See* appendix B.
181	CC condition	*See* appendix B.
207	Mechanical ventilation > 96 consecutive hours	*See* DRG 004.
208	Mechanical ventilation for less than or equal to 96 consecutive hours	*See* DRG 004.

DRG 183 Major Chest Trauma with MCC — RW 1.5745

Potential DRGs

DRG	Description	RW
004	Tracheostomy with Mechanical Ventilation > 96 Hours or Principal Diagnosis Except Face, Mouth and Neck without Major O.R. Procedure	14.7000
199	Pneumothorax with MCC	1.7741
205	Other Respiratory System Diagnoses with MCC	1.8103
207	Respiratory System Diagnosis with Ventilator Support > 96 Hours	6.9080
208	Respiratory System Diagnosis with Ventilator Support <= 96 Hours	2.7038
963	Other Multiple Significant Trauma with MCC	2.7343

DRG	PDx/SDx/Procedure	Tips
004	Tracheostomy	Tracheostomy carried out elsewhere prior to admission or in an ambulance prior to arrival should not be reported as a current procedure. A tracheostomy procedure may be performed at the bedside and documented in the progress notes or in the operating room and documented in an operative note.
	AND	
	Mechanical ventilation > 96 consecutive hours	Review record documentation for start and stop times. Calculation of mechanical ventilation hours begins when vent is initiated (or time of admission if patient already on a vent) and ends when it is turned off (or the time patient is discharged if still ventilated). The duration includes time spent to wean the patient from the vent. Do not assume that ventilation that spans four calendar days equals > 96 hours; count by the hour not day.
199	Traumatic pneumothorax and hemothorax, initial encounter	
	Traumatic subcutaneous emphysema, initial encounter	
	AND	
	MCC condition	*See* appendix B.
205	Injury of thoracic trachea	Review record documentation for chest trauma with injury specific to the thoracic trachea.
	Foreign body in respiratory tract causing asphyxiation	Review record documentation for chest trauma with respiratory foreign body resulting in asphyxia.
	AND	
	MCC condition	*See* appendix B.
207	Mechanical ventilation > 96 consecutive hours	*See* DRG 004.
208	Mechanical ventilation for less than or equal to 96 consecutive hours	*See* DRG 004.
963	Other multiple significant trauma	PDx of trauma and at least two injuries (assigned as PDx or SDx) that are defined as significant trauma from different body site categories located under MS-DRG 963.
	AND	
	MCC condition	*See* appendix B.

DRG 184 Major Chest Trauma with CC RW 1.0519

Potential DRGs

004	Tracheostomy with Mechanical Ventilation > 96 Hours or Principal Diagnosis Except Face, Mouth and Neck without Major O.R. Procedure	14.7000
183	Major Chest Trauma with MCC	1.5745
189	Pulmonary Edema and Respiratory Failure	1.2320
199	Pneumothorax with MCC	1.7741
200	Pneumothorax with CC	1.0770
205	Other Respiratory System Diagnoses with MCC	1.8103
207	Respiratory System Diagnosis with Ventilator Support > 96 Hours	6.9080
208	Respiratory System Diagnosis with Ventilator Support <= 96 Hours	2.7038
963	Other Multiple Significant Trauma with MCC	2.7343
964	Other Multiple Significant Trauma with CC	1.5010

DRG	PDx/SDx/Procedure	Tips
004	Tracheostomy	Tracheostomy carried out elsewhere prior to admission or in an ambulance prior to arrival should not be reported as a current procedure. A tracheostomy procedure may be performed at the bedside and documented in the progress notes or in the operating room and documented in an operative note.
	AND	
	Mechanical ventilation > 96 consecutive hours	Review record documentation for start and stop times. Calculation of mechanical ventilation hours begins when vent is initiated (or time of admission if patient already on a vent) and ends when it is turned off (or the time patient is discharged if still ventilated). The duration includes time spent to wean the patient from the vent. Do not assume that ventilation that spans four calendar days equals > 96 hours; count by the hour not day.
183	MCC condition	*See* appendix B.
189	Acute respiratory failure	When acute respiratory failure is listed as a secondary diagnosis, review the medical record carefully to determine if ARF meets the criteria for principal diagnosis as determined by the circumstances of the admission, the diagnostic workup, and/or the treatment provided and if appropriate designate as the principal diagnosis.
199	Traumatic pneumothorax and hemothorax, initial encounter	
	Traumatic subcutaneous emphysema, initial encounter	
	AND	
	MCC condition	*See* appendix B.
200	Traumatic pneumothorax and hemothorax, initial encounter	
	Traumatic subcutaneous emphysema, initial encounter	
	AND	
	CC condition	*See* appendix B.
205	Injury of thoracic trachea	Review record documentation for chest trauma with injury specific to the thoracic trachea.
	Foreign body in respiratory tract causing asphyxiation	Review record documentation for chest trauma with respiratory foreign body resulting in asphyxia.
	AND	
	MCC condition	*See* appendix B.
207	Mechanical ventilation > 96 consecutive hours	*See* DRG 004.
208	Mechanical ventilation for less than or equal to 96 consecutive hours	*See* DRG 004.
963	Other multiple significant trauma	PDx of trauma and at least two injuries (assigned as PDx or SDx) that are defined as significant trauma from different body site categories located under MS-DRG 963.
	AND	
	MCC condition	*See* appendix B.
964	Other multiple significant trauma	*See* DRG 963.
	AND	
	CC condition	*See* appendix B.

DRG 185 Major Chest Trauma without CC/MCC

RW 0.7557

Potential DRGs

004	Tracheostomy with Mechanical Ventilation > 96 Hours or Principal Diagnosis Except Face, Mouth and Neck without Major O.R. Procedure	14.7000
183	Major Chest Trauma with MCC	1.5745
184	Major Chest Trauma with CC	1.0519
189	Pulmonary Edema and Respiratory Failure	1.2320
199	Pneumothorax with MCC	1.7741
200	Pneumothorax with CC	1.0770
205	Other Respiratory System Diagnoses with MCC	1.8103
206	Other Respiratory System Diagnoses without MCC	0.9135
207	Respiratory System Diagnosis with Ventilator Support > 96 Hours	6.9080
208	Respiratory System Diagnosis with Ventilator Support <= 96 Hours	2.7038
963	Other Multiple Significant Trauma with MCC	2.7343
964	Other Multiple Significant Trauma with CC	1.5010
965	Other Multiple Significant Trauma without CC/MCC	0.9559

DRG	PDx/SDx/Procedure	Tips
004	Tracheostomy	Tracheostomy carried out elsewhere prior to admission or in an ambulance prior to arrival should not be reported as a current procedure. A tracheostomy procedure may be performed at the bedside and documented in the progress notes or in the operating room and documented in an operative note.
	AND	
	Mechanical ventilation > 96 consecutive hours	Review record documentation for start and stop times. Calculation of mechanical ventilation hours begins when vent is initiated (or time of admission if patient already on a vent) and ends when it is turned off (or the time patient is discharged if still ventilated). The duration includes time spent to wean the patient from the vent. Do not assume that ventilation that spans four calendar days equals > 96 hours; count by the hour not day.
183	MCC condition	*See* appendix B.
184	CC condition	*See* appendix B.
189	Acute respiratory failure	When acute respiratory failure is listed as a secondary diagnosis, review the medical record carefully to determine if ARF meets the criteria for principal diagnosis as determined by the circumstances of the admission, the diagnostic workup, and/or the treatment provided and if appropriate designate as the principal diagnosis.
199	Traumatic pneumothorax and hemothorax, initial encounter	
	Traumatic subcutaneous emphysema, initial encounter	
	AND	
	MCC condition	*See* appendix B.
200	Traumatic pneumothorax and hemothorax, initial encounter	
	Traumatic subcutaneous emphysema, initial encounter	
	AND	
	CC condition	*See* appendix B.
205	Injury of thoracic trachea	Review record documentation for chest trauma with injury specific to the thoracic trachea.
	Foreign body in respiratory tract causing asphyxiation	Review record documentation for chest trauma with respiratory foreign body resulting in asphyxia.
	AND	
	MCC condition	*See* appendix B.
206	Injury of thoracic trachea	*See* DRG 205.
	Foreign body in respiratory tract causing asphyxiation	*See* DRG 205.
207	Mechanical ventilation > 96 consecutive hours	*See* DRG 004.
208	Mechanical ventilation for less than or equal to 96 consecutive hours	*See* DRG 004.
963	Other multiple significant trauma	PDx of trauma and at least two injuries (assigned as PDx or SDx) that are defined as significant trauma from different body site categories located under MS-DRG 963.
	AND	
	MCC condition	*See* appendix B.
964	Other multiple significant trauma	*See* DRG 963.
	AND	
	CC condition	*See* appendix B.
965	Other multiple significant trauma	*See* DRG 963.

DRG 186 Pleural Effusion with MCC RW 1.5521

Potential DRGs

004	Tracheostomy with Mechanical Ventilation > 96 Hours or Principal Diagnosis Except Face, Mouth and Neck without Major O.R. Procedure	14.7000
166	Other Respiratory System O.R. Procedures with MCC	4.0578
180	Respiratory Neoplasms with MCC	1.7382
207	Respiratory System Diagnosis with Ventilator Support > 96 Hours	6.9080
208	Respiratory System Diagnosis with Ventilator Support <= 96 Hours	2.7038

DRG	PDx/SDx/Procedure	Tips
004	Tracheostomy	Tracheostomy carried out elsewhere prior to admission or in an ambulance prior to arrival should not be reported as a current procedure. A tracheostomy procedure may be performed at the bedside and documented in the progress notes or in the operating room and documented in an operative note.
	WITH	
	Mechanical ventilation > 96 consecutive hours	Review record documentation for start and stop times. Calculation of mechanical ventilation hours begins when vent is initiated (or time of admission if patient already on a vent) and ends when it is turned off (or the time patient is discharged if still ventilated). The duration includes time spent to wean the patient from the vent. Do not assume that ventilation that spans four calendar days equals > 96 hours; count by the hour not day.
166	Thoracoscopic pleural cavity drainage	
	Thoracoscopic pleural biopsy	
	AND	
	MCC condition	*See* appendix B.
180	Malignant pleural effusion or underlying pleural or respiratory neoplasm	See "Code first underlying neoplasm" instructional note under code J91.Ø Malignant pleural effusion.
	AND	
	MCC condition	*See* appendix B.
207	Mechanical ventilation > 96 consecutive hours	*See* DRG 004.
208	Mechanical ventilation for less than or equal to 96 consecutive hours	*See* DRG 004.

DRG 187 Pleural Effusion with CC

RW 0.9963

Potential DRGs

004	Tracheostomy with Mechanical Ventilation > 96 Hours or Principal Diagnosis Except Face, Mouth and Neck without Major O.R. Procedure	14.7000
166	Other Respiratory System O.R. Procedures with MCC	4.0578
167	Other Respiratory System O.R. Procedures with CC	1.8198
180	Respiratory Neoplasms with MCC	1.7382
181	Respiratory Neoplasms with CC	1.1011
186	Pleural Effusion with MCC	1.5521
189	Pulmonary Edema and Respiratory Failure	1.2320
207	Respiratory System Diagnosis with Ventilator Support > 96 Hours	6.9080
208	Respiratory System Diagnosis with Ventilator Support <= 96 Hours	2.7038
291	Heart Failure and Shock with MCC	1.2839

DRG	PDx/SDx/Procedure	Tips
004	Tracheostomy	Tracheostomy carried out elsewhere prior to admission or in an ambulance prior to arrival should not be reported as a current procedure. A tracheostomy procedure may be performed at the bedside and documented in the progress notes or in the operating room and documented in an operative note.
	WITH	
	Mechanical ventilation > 96 consecutive hours	Review record documentation for start and stop times. Calculation of mechanical ventilation hours begins when vent is initiated (or time of admission if patient already on a vent) and ends when it is turned off (or the time patient is discharged if still ventilated). The duration includes time spent to wean the patient from the vent. Do not assume that ventilation that spans four calendar days equals > 96 hours; count by the hour not day.
166	Thoracoscopic pleural cavity drainage	
	Thoracoscopic pleural biopsy	
	AND	
	MCC condition	*See* appendix B.
167	Thoracoscopic pleural cavity drainage	
	Thoracoscopic pleural biopsy	
	AND	
	CC condition	*See* appendix B.
180	Malignant pleural effusion or underlying pleural or respiratory neoplasm	See "Code first underlying neoplasm" instructional note under code J91.Ø Malignant pleural effusion.
	AND	
	MCC condition	*See* appendix B.
181	Malignant pleural effusion or underlying pleural or respiratory neoplasm	See "Code first underlying neoplasm" instructional note under code J91.Ø Malignant pleural effusion.
	AND	
	CC condition	*See* appendix B.
186	MCC condition	*See* appendix B.
189	Acute respiratory failure	When acute respiratory failure is listed as a secondary diagnosis, review the medical record carefully to determine if ARF meets the criteria for principal diagnosis as determined by the circumstances of the admission, the diagnostic workup, and/or the treatment provided and if appropriate designate as the principal diagnosis.
207	Mechanical ventilation > 96 consecutive hours	*See* DRG 004.
208	Mechanical ventilation for less than or equal to 96 consecutive hours	*See* DRG 004.
291	Heart failure, all types	Pleural effusion is commonly seen as part of the congestive heart failure process; when evaluated and treated, report as an additional diagnosis.
	Hypertensive heart disease with heart failure	According to the ICD-10-CM guidelines, the classification presumes a causal relationship between hypertension and heart and kidney involvement when these terms are linked by the term "with" in the alphabetic index (either under a main term or subterm). Heart and kidney disease should be coded as related to hypertension unless the documentation clearly states the conditions are unrelated, in which case they may be coded separately. These conditions do not require provider documentation linking them to hypertension.
	Hypertensive heart and kidney disease with heart failure	
	AND	
	MCC condition	*See* appendix B.

DRG 188 Pleural Effusion without CC/MCC RW 0.7465

Potential DRGs

004	Tracheostomy with Mechanical Ventilation > 96 Hours or Principal Diagnosis Except Face, Mouth and Neck without Major O.R. Procedure	14.7000
166	Other Respiratory System O.R. Procedures with MCC	4.0578
167	Other Respiratory System O.R. Procedures with CC	1.8198
168	Other Respiratory System O.R. Procedures without CC/MCC	1.3557
180	Respiratory Neoplasms with MCC	1.7382
181	Respiratory Neoplasms with CC	1.1011
182	Respiratory Neoplasms without CC/MCC	0.7590
186	Pleural Effusion with MCC	1.5521
187	Pleural Effusion with CC	0.9963
189	Pulmonary Edema and Respiratory Failure	1.2320
207	Respiratory System Diagnosis with Ventilator Support > 96 Hours	6.9080
208	Respiratory System Diagnosis with Ventilator Support <= 96 Hours	2.7038
291	Heart Failure and Shock with MCC	1.2839
292	Heart Failure and Shock with CC	0.8565

DRG	PDx/SDx/Procedure	Tips
004	Tracheostomy	Tracheostomy carried out elsewhere prior to admission or in an ambulance prior to arrival should not be reported as a current procedure. A tracheostomy procedure may be performed at the bedside and documented in the progress notes or in the operating room and documented in an operative note.
	WITH	
	Mechanical ventilation > 96 consecutive hours	Review record documentation for start and stop times. Calculation of mechanical ventilation hours begins when vent is initiated (or time of admission if patient already on a vent) and ends when it is turned off (or the time patient is discharged if still ventilated). The duration includes time spent to wean the patient from the vent. Do not assume that ventilation that spans four calendar days equals > 96 hours; count by the hour not day.
166	Thoracoscopic pleural cavity drainage	
	Thoracoscopic pleural biopsy	
	AND	
	MCC condition	*See* appendix B.
167	Thoracoscopic pleural cavity drainage	
	Thoracoscopic pleural biopsy	
	AND	
	CC condition	*See* appendix B.
168	Thoracoscopic pleural cavity drainage	
	Thoracoscopic pleural biopsy	
180	Malignant pleural effusion or underlying pleural or respiratory neoplasm	See "Code first underlying neoplasm" instructional note under code J91.Ø Malignant pleural effusion.
	AND	
	MCC condition	*See* appendix B.
181	Malignant pleural effusion or underlying pleural or respiratory neoplasm	*See* DRG 180.
	AND	
	CC condition	*See* appendix B.
182	Malignant pleural effusion or underlying pleural or respiratory neoplasm	*See* DRG 180.
186	MCC condition	*See* appendix B.
187	CC condition	*See* appendix B.
189	Acute respiratory failure	When acute respiratory failure is listed as a secondary diagnosis, review the medical record carefully to determine if ARF meets the criteria for principal diagnosis as determined by the circumstances of the admission, the diagnostic workup, and/or the treatment provided and if appropriate designate as the principal diagnosis.
207	Mechanical ventilation > 96 consecutive hours	*See* DRG 004.
208	Mechanical ventilation for less than or equal to 96 consecutive hours	*See* DRG 004.
291	Heart failure, all types	Pleural effusion is commonly seen as part of the congestive heart failure process; when evaluated and treated, report as an additional diagnosis.
	Hypertensive heart disease with heart failure	According to the ICD-10-CM guidelines, the classification presumes a causal relationship between hypertension and heart and kidney involvement when these terms are linked by the term "with" in the alphabetic index (either under a main term or subterm). Heart and kidney disease should be coded as related to hypertension unless the documentation clearly states the conditions are unrelated, in which case they may be coded separately. These conditions do not require provider documentation linking them to hypertension.
	Hypertensive heart and kidney disease with heart failure	
	AND	
	MCC condition	*See* appendix B.
292	Heart failure, all types	*See* DRG 291.
	Hypertensive heart disease with heart failure	*See* DRG 291.
	Hypertensive heart and kidney disease with heart failure	
	AND	
	CC condition	*See* appendix B.

DRG 189 Pulmonary Edema and Respiratory Failure — RW 1.2320

Potential DRGs

004	Tracheostomy with Mechanical Ventilation > 96 Hours or Principal Diagnosis Except Face, Mouth and Neck without Major O.R. Procedure	14.7000
183	Major Chest Trauma with MCC	1.5745
186	Pleural Effusion with MCC	1.5521
193	Simple Pneumonia and Pleurisy with MCC	1.3266
196	Interstitial Lung Disease with MCC	1.8954
199	Pneumothorax with MCC	1.7741
205	Other Respiratory System Diagnoses with MCC	1.8103
207	Respiratory System Diagnosis with Ventilator Support > 96 Hours	6.9080
208	Respiratory System Diagnosis with Ventilator Support <= 96 Hours	2.7038
291	Heart Failure and Shock with MCC	1.2839

DRG	PDx/SDx/Procedure	Tips
004	Tracheostomy	Tracheostomy carried out elsewhere prior to admission or in an ambulance prior to arrival should not be reported as a current procedure. A tracheostomy procedure may be performed at the bedside and documented in the progress notes or in the operating room and documented in an operative note.
	WITH	
	Mechanical ventilation > 96 consecutive hours	Review record documentation for start and stop times. Calculation of mechanical ventilation hours begins when vent is initiated (or time of admission if patient already on a vent) and ends when it is turned off (or the time patient is discharged if still ventilated). The duration includes time spent to wean the patient from the vent. Do not assume that ventilation that spans four calendar days equals > 96 hours; count by the hour not day.
183	Principal diagnosis of flail chest (open or closed fracture, initial encounter)	Check physician documentation carefully and query the physician as necessary for underlying cause of pulmonary edema, particularly for trauma patients. Often times pulmonary edema develops rapidly when the chest is crushed and the patient has flail chest.
186	Other specified and unspecified pleural effusion	
	AND	
	MCC condition	*See* appendix B.
193	Simple pneumonia, viral pneumonia, bacterial pneumonia	Excluding pneumonia due to COVID-19.
	AND	
	MCC condition	*See* appendix B.
196	Sarcoidosis	
	Pneumoconiosis and pneumonopathy due to external agents	
	Postinflammatory pulmonary fibrosis, idiopathic interstitial pneumonia	
199	Pneumothorax	
	Interstitial emphysema	
	Traumatic pneumothorax and hemothorax, initial encounter	
	Traumatic subcutaneous emphysema, initial encounter	
	AND	
	MCC condition	*See* appendix B.
205	Respiratory conditions due to chemical fumes, smoke inhalation, vapors, and other/ unspecified external agents	Coding guidelines specify that when a patient is admitted with respiratory failure and another acute condition and they are equally responsible for occasioning the admission to the hospital, either condition may be sequenced as the principal diagnosis. Providing there are no chapter- specific sequencing rules, the circumstances of the admission, diagnostic workup, and treatment provided determines appropriate code sequencing.
	Atelectasis	
	Tracheostomy complications	Review the documentation carefully; code assignment is based on the provider's documentation of a relationship between the condition and the procedure. Unless the classification instructs otherwise, only when there is a clear cause-and-effect relationship between the care provided and the condition and the documentation indicates the condition is a complication, can the condition be coded as such. Query the provider for clarification if the relationship/complication is not clearly documented. See guideline I.B.16.
	Fractured one rib, or rib sprain/strain	
	Contusion of lung, other and unspecified lung injuries	
	Foreign body in trachea, bronchus or lung	
	AND	
	MCC condition	*See* appendix B.
207	Mechanical ventilation > 96 consecutive hours	*See* DRG 004.
208	Mechanical ventilation for less than or equal to 96 consecutive hours	*See* DRG 004.
291	Heart failure, all types	
	Hypertensive heart disease with heart failure	According to the ICD-10-CM guidelines, the classification presumes a causal relationship between hypertension and heart and kidney involvement when these terms are linked by the term "with" in the alphabetic index (either under a main term or subterm). Heart and kidney disease should be coded as related to hypertension unless the documentation clearly states the conditions are unrelated, in which case they may be coded separately. These conditions do not require provider documentation linking them to hypertension.
	Hypertensive heart and kidney disease with heart failure	
	AND	
	MCC condition	*See* appendix B.

DRG 190 Chronic Obstructive Pulmonary Disease with MCC — RW 1.1020

Potential DRGs

004	Tracheostomy with Mechanical Ventilation > 96 Hours or Principal Diagnosis Except Face, Mouth and Neck without Major O.R. Procedure	14.7000
177	Respiratory Infections and Inflammations with MCC	1.6964
189	Pulmonary Edema and Respiratory Failure	1.2320
193	Simple Pneumonia and Pleurisy with MCC	1.3266
207	Respiratory System Diagnosis with Ventilator Support > 96 Hours	6.9080
208	Respiratory System Diagnosis with Ventilator Support <= 96 Hours	2.7038
291	Heart Failure and Shock with MCC	1.2839

DRG	PDx/SDx/Procedure	Tips
004	Tracheostomy	Tracheostomy carried out elsewhere prior to admission or in an ambulance prior to arrival should not be reported as a current procedure. A tracheostomy procedure may be performed at the bedside and documented in the progress notes or in the operating room and documented in an operative note.
	WITH	
	Mechanical ventilation > 96 consecutive hours	Review record documentation for start and stop times. Calculation of mechanical ventilation hours begins when vent is initiated (or time of admission if patient already on a vent) and ends when it is turned off (or the time patient is discharged if still ventilated). The duration includes time spent to wean the patient from the vent. Do not assume that ventilation that spans four calendar days equals > 96 hours; count by the hour not day.
177	Pneumonia with causative organism: Salmonella Klebsiella pneumoniae Pseudomonas Staphylococcus Proteus or other gram-negative organisms	Bacterial pneumonia should be assigned based on physician documentation.
	COVID-19	Sequence UØ7.1 before J12.82 According to the ICD-10-CM guidelines, documentation by the provider that the individual has COVID-19 is sufficient and does not require additional documentation of a positive test result.
	Aspiration pneumonia	If both aspiration pneumonia and bacterial pneumonia or pneumonia due to COVID-19 are documented, code both. Sequencing will depend on the circumstances of admission.
	AND	
	MCC condition	*See* appendix B.
189	Respiratory failure	When acute respiratory failure is listed as a secondary diagnosis, review the medical record carefully to determine if ARF meets the criteria for principal diagnosis as determined by the circumstances of the admission, the diagnostic workup, and/or the treatment provided and if appropriate designate as the principal diagnosis.
	Respiratory failure or pulmonary insufficiency following surgery	
	Pulmonary congestion and hypostasis (pulmonary edema), unspecified acute lung edema	
193	Pneumonia with causative organism of: Viral Pneumococcal/streptococcus H. influenzae Streptococcus Unspecified organism	Excluding pneumonia due to COVID-19.
	AND	
	MCC condition	*See* appendix B.
207	Mechanical ventilation > 96 consecutive hours	*See* DRG 004.
208	Mechanical ventilation for less than or equal to 96 consecutive hours	*See* DRG 004.
291	Heart failure, all types	
	Hypertensive heart disease with heart failure	According to the ICD-10-CM guidelines, the classification presumes a causal relationship between hypertension and heart and kidney involvement when these terms are linked by the term "with" in the alphabetic index (either under a main term or subterm). Heart and kidney disease should be coded as related to hypertension unless the documentation clearly states the conditions are unrelated, in which case they may be coded separately. These conditions do not require provider documentation linking them to hypertension.
	Hypertensive heart and kidney disease with heart failure	
	AND	
	MCC condition	*See* appendix B.

DRG 191 Chronic Obstructive Pulmonary Disease with CC — RW 0.8490

Potential DRGs

004	Tracheostomy with Mechanical Ventilation > 96 Hours or Principal Diagnosis Except Face, Mouth and Neck without Major O.R. Procedure	14.7000
177	Respiratory Infections and Inflammations with MCC	1.6964
178	Respiratory Infections and Inflammations with CC	0.9867
189	Pulmonary Edema and Respiratory Failure	1.2320
190	Chronic Obstructive Pulmonary Disease with MCC	1.1020
193	Simple Pneumonia and Pleurisy with MCC	1.3266
207	Respiratory System Diagnosis with Ventilator Support > 96 Hours	6.9080
208	Respiratory System Diagnosis with Ventilator Support <= 96 Hours	2.7038
291	Heart Failure and Shock with MCC	1.2839

DRG	PDx/SDx/Procedure	Tips
004	Tracheostomy	Tracheostomy carried out elsewhere prior to admission or in an ambulance prior to arrival should not be reported as a current procedure. A tracheostomy procedure may be performed at the bedside and documented in the progress notes or in the operating room and documented in an operative note.
	WITH	
	Mechanical ventilation > 96 consecutive hours	Review record documentation for start and stop times. Calculation of mechanical ventilation hours begins when vent is initiated (or time of admission if patient already on a vent) and ends when it is turned off (or the time patient is discharged if still ventilated). The duration includes time spent to wean the patient from the vent. Do not assume that ventilation that spans four calendar days equals > 96 hours; count by the hour not day.
177	Pneumonia with causative organism: Salmonella Klebsiella pneumoniae Pseudomonas Staphylococcus Proteus or other gram-negative organisms COVID-19	Bacterial pneumonia should be assigned based on physician documentation Sequence U07.1 before J12.82 According to the ICD-10-CM guidelines, documentation by the provider that the individual has COVID-19 is sufficient and does not require additional documentation of a positive test result.
	Aspiration pneumonia	If both aspiration pneumonia and bacterial pneumonia or pneumonia due to COVID-19 are documented, code both. Sequencing will depend on the circumstances of admission.
	AND	
	MCC condition	*See* appendix B.
178	Pneumonia with causative organism: Salmonella Klebsiella pneumoniae Pseudomonas Staphylococcus Proteus or other gram-negative organisms COVID-19	*See* DRG 177.
	Aspiration pneumonia	*See* DRG 177.
	AND	
	CC condition	*See* appendix B.
189	Respiratory failure	When acute respiratory failure is listed as a secondary diagnosis, review the medical record carefully to determine if ARF meets the criteria for principal diagnosis as determined by the circumstances of the admission, the diagnostic workup, and/or the treatment provided and if appropriate designate as the principal diagnosis.
	Respiratory failure or pulmonary insufficiency following surgery	
	Pulmonary congestion and hypostasis (pulmonary edema), unspecified acute lung edema	
190	MCC condition	*See* appendix B.
193	Pneumonia with causative organism of: Viral Pneumococcal/streptococcus pneumoniae H. influenzae Streptococcus Unspecified organism	Excluding pneumonia due to COVID-19.
	AND	
	MCC condition	*See* appendix B.
207	Mechanical ventilation > 96 consecutive hours	*See* DRG 004.
208	Mechanical ventilation for less than or equal to 96 consecutive hours	*See* DRG 004.
291	Heart failure, all types	
	Hypertensive heart disease with heart failure	According to the ICD-10-CM guidelines, the classification presumes a causal relationship between hypertension and heart and kidney involvement when these terms are linked by the term "with" in the alphabetic index (either under a main term or subterm). Heart and kidney disease should be coded as related to hypertension unless the documentation clearly states the conditions are unrelated, in which case they may be coded separately. These conditions do not require provider documentation linking them to hypertension.
	Hypertensive heart and kidney disease with heart failure	
	AND	
	MCC condition	*See* appendix B.

DRG 192 Chronic Obstructive Pulmonary Disease without CC/MCC RW 0.6418

Potential DRGs

004	Tracheostomy with Mechanical Ventilation > 96 Hours or Principal Diagnosis Except Face, Mouth and Neck without Major O.R. Procedure	14.7000
177	Respiratory Infections and Inflammations with MCC	1.6964
178	Respiratory Infections and Inflammations with CC	0.9867
179	Respiratory Infections and Inflammations without CC/MCC	0.7633
189	Pulmonary Edema and Respiratory Failure	1.2320
190	Chronic Obstructive Pulmonary Disease with MCC	1.1020
191	Chronic Obstructive Pulmonary Disease with CC	0.8490
193	Simple Pneumonia and Pleurisy with MCC	1.3266
194	Simple Pneumonia and Pleurisy with CC	0.8222
202	Bronchitis and Asthma with CC/MCC	0.9575
207	Respiratory System Diagnosis with Ventilator Support > 96 Hours	6.9080
208	Respiratory System Diagnosis with Ventilator Support <= 96 Hours	2.7038
291	Heart Failure and Shock with MCC	1.2839
292	Heart Failure and Shock with CC	0.8565

DRG	PDx/SDx/Procedure	Tips
004	Tracheostomy	Tracheostomy carried out elsewhere prior to admission or in an ambulance prior to arrival should not be reported as a current procedure. A tracheostomy procedure may be performed at the bedside and documented in the progress notes or in the operating room and documented in an operative note.
	WITH	
	Mechanical ventilation > 96 consecutive hours	Review record documentation for start and stop times. Calculation of mechanical ventilation hours begins when vent is initiated (or time of admission if patient already on a vent) and ends when it is turned off (or the time patient is discharged if still ventilated). The duration includes time spent to wean the patient from the vent. Do not assume that ventilation that spans four calendar days equals > 96 hours; count by the hour not day.
177	Pneumonia with causative organism: Salmonella Klebsiella pneumoniae Pseudomonas Staphylococcus Proteus or other gram-negative organisms COVID-19	Bacterial pneumonia should be assigned based on physician documentation Sequence U07.1 before J12.82 According to the ICD-10-CM guidelines, documentation by the provider that the individual has COVID-19 is sufficient and does not require additional documentation of a positive test result.
	Aspiration pneumonia	If both aspiration pneumonia and bacterial pneumonia or pneumonia due to COVID-19 are documented, code both. Sequencing will depend on the circumstances of admission.
	AND	
	MCC condition	*See* appendix B.
178	Pneumonia with causative organism: Salmonella Klebsiella pneumoniae Pseudomonas Staphylococcus Proteus or other gram-negative organisms COVID-19	*See* DRG 177.
	Aspiration pneumonia	*See* DRG 177.
	AND	
	CC condition	*See* appendix B.
179	Pneumonia with causative organism: Salmonella Klebsiella pneumoniae Pseudomonas Staphylococcus Proteus or other gram-negative organisms COVID-19	*See* DRG 177.
	Aspiration pneumonia	*See* DRG 177.
189	Respiratory failure	When acute respiratory failure is listed as a secondary diagnosis, review the medical record carefully to determine if ARF meets the criteria for principal diagnosis as determined by the circumstances of the admission, the diagnostic workup, and/or the treatment provided and if appropriate designate as the principal diagnosis.
	Respiratory failure or pulmonary insufficiency following surgery	
	Pulmonary congestion and hypostasis (pulmonary edema), unspecified acute lung edema	

DRG 192 (Continued)

DRG	PDx/SDx/Procedure	Tips
190	MCC condition	*See* appendix B.
191	CC condition	*See* appendix B.
193	Pneumonia with causative organism of: Viral Pneumococcal/streptococcus pneumoniae H. influenzae Streptococcus Unspecified organism	Excluding pneumonia due to COVID-19.
	AND	
	MCC condition	*See* appendix B.
194	Pneumonia with causative organism of: Viral Pneumococcal/streptococcus pneumoniae H. influenzae Streptococcus Unspecified organism	Excluding pneumonia due to COVID-19.
	AND	
	CC condition	*See* appendix B.
202	Acute tracheobronchitis, bronchitis and bronchiolitis	
	Acute bronchospasm	
	AND	
	CC/MCC condition	*See* appendix B.
207	Mechanical ventilation > 96 consecutive hours	*See* DRG 004.
208	Mechanical ventilation for less than or equal to 96 consecutive hours	*See* DRG 004.
291	Heart failure, all types	
	Hypertensive heart disease with heart failure	According to the ICD-10-CM guidelines, the classification presumes a causal relationship between hypertension and heart and kidney involvement when these terms are linked by the term "with" in the alphabetic index (either under a main term or subterm). Heart and kidney disease should be coded as related to hypertension unless the documentation clearly states the conditions are unrelated, in which case they may be coded separately. These conditions do not require provider documentation linking them to hypertension.
	Hypertensive heart and kidney disease with heart failure	
	AND	
	MCC condition	*See* appendix B.
292	Heart failure, all types	
	Hypertensive heart disease with heart failure	*See* DRG 291.
	Hypertensive heart and kidney disease with heart failure	
	AND	
	CC condition	*See* appendix B.

DRG 193 Simple Pneumonia and Pleurisy with MCC — RW 1.3266

Potential DRGs

004	Tracheostomy with Mechanical Ventilation > 96 Hours or Principal Diagnosis Except Face, Mouth and Neck without Major O.R. Procedure	14.7000
177	Respiratory Infections and Inflammations with MCC	1.6964
180	Respiratory Neoplasms with MCC	1.7382
196	Interstitial Lung Disease with MCC	1.8954
207	Respiratory System Diagnosis with Ventilator Support > 96 Hours	6.9080
208	Respiratory System Diagnosis with Ventilator Support <= 96 Hours	2.7038
974	HIV with Major Related Condition with MCC	2.9165

DRG	PDx/SDx/Procedure	Tips
004	Tracheostomy	Tracheostomy carried out elsewhere prior to admission or in an ambulance prior to arrival should not be reported as a current procedure. A tracheostomy procedure may be performed at the bedside and documented in the progress notes or in the operating room and documented in an operative note.
	WITH	
	Mechanical ventilation > 96 consecutive hours	Review record documentation for start and stop times. Calculation of mechanical ventilation hours begins when vent is initiated (or time of admission if patient already on a vent) and ends when it is turned off (or the time patient is discharged if still ventilated). The duration includes time spent to wean the patient from the vent. Do not assume that ventilation that spans four calendar days equals > 96 hours; count by the hour not day.
177	Pneumonia with causative organism: Salmonella Klebsiella pneumoniae Pseudomonas Staphylococcus Proteus or other gram-negative organisms COVID-19	Bacterial pneumonia should be assigned based on physician documentation. Sequence UØ7.1 before J12.82 According to the ICD-10-CM guidelines, documentation by the provider that the individual has COVID-19 is sufficient and does not require additional documentation of a positive test result.
	Aspiration pneumonia	If both aspiration pneumonia and bacterial pneumonia or pneumonia due to COVID-19 are documented, code both. Sequencing will depend on the circumstances of admission.
	AND	
	MCC condition	*See* appendix B.
180	Respiratory neoplasm	
	AND	
	MCC condition	*See* appendix B.
196	Interstitial pneumonia and pneumonitis	
	AND	
	MCC condition	*See* appendix B.
207	Mechanical ventilation > 96 consecutive hours	*See* DRG 004.
208	Mechanical ventilation for less than or equal to 96 consecutive hours	*See* DRG 004.
974	Diagnosis of HIV disease	Admission for HIV-related condition: sequence B2Ø first followed by the HIV-related condition code except chapter 15 codes, which take sequencing priority. Any complication of the HIV-related condition would also be coded as a secondary diagnosis. (e.g., acute respiratory failure due to AIDS-related pneumonia).
	AND	
	Opportunistic lung infection	See appendix C for the full list of major HIV-related conditions. A diagnosis from this list should not be assumed as HIV-related unless specifically documented as such by the provider.
	AND	
	MCC condition	*See* appendix B.

DRG 194 Simple Pneumonia and Pleurisy with CC

RW 0.8222

Potential DRGs

004	Tracheostomy with Mechanical Ventilation > 96 Hours or Principal Diagnosis Except Face, Mouth and Neck without Major O.R. Procedure	14.7000
177	Respiratory Infections and Inflammations with MCC	1.6964
178	Respiratory Infections and Inflammations with CC	0.9867
180	Respiratory Neoplasms with MCC	1.7382
181	Respiratory Neoplasms with CC	1.1011
189	Pulmonary Edema and Respiratory Failure	1.2320
193	Simple Pneumonia and Pleurisy with MCC	1.3266
196	Interstitial Lung Disease with MCC	1.8954
197	Interstitial Lung Disease with CC	0.9975
207	Respiratory System Diagnosis with Ventilator Support > 96 Hours	6.9080
208	Respiratory System Diagnosis with Ventilator Support <= 96 Hours	2.7038
974	HIV with Major Related Condition with MCC	2.9165
975	HIV with Major Related Condition with CC	1.3633

DRG	PDx/SDx/Procedure	Tips
004	Tracheostomy	Tracheostomy carried out elsewhere prior to admission or in an ambulance prior to arrival should not be reported as a current procedure. A tracheostomy procedure may be performed at the bedside and documented in the progress notes or in the operating room and documented in an operative note.
	WITH	
	Mechanical ventilation > 96 consecutive hours	Review record documentation for start and stop times. Calculation of mechanical ventilation hours begins when vent is initiated (or time of admission if patient already on a vent) and ends when it is turned off (or the time patient is discharged if still ventilated). The duration includes time spent to wean the patient from the vent. Do not assume that ventilation that spans four calendar days equals > 96 hours; count by the hour not day.
177	Pneumonia with causative organism: Salmonella Klebsiella pneumoniae Pseudomonas Staphylococcus Proteus or other gram-negative organism COVID-19	Bacterial pneumonia should be assigned based on physician documentation. Sequence UØ7.1 before J12.82 According to the ICD-10-CM guidelines, documentation by the provider that the individual has COVID-19 is sufficient and does not require additional documentation of a positive test result.
	Aspiration pneumonia	If both aspiration pneumonia and bacterial pneumonia or pneumonia due to COVID-19 are documented, code both. Sequencing will depend on the circumstances of admission.
	AND	
	MCC condition	*See* appendix B.
178	Pneumonia with causative organism: Salmonella Klebsiella pneumoniae Pseudomonas Staphylococcus Proteus or other gram-negative organisms COVID-19	*See* DRG 177.
	Aspiration pneumonia	*See* DRG 177.
	AND	
	CC condition	*See* appendix B.
180	Respiratory neoplasm	
	AND	
	MCC condition	*See* appendix B.
181	Respiratory neoplasm	
	AND	
	CC condition	*See* appendix B.
189	Respiratory failure Respiratory failure or pulmonary insufficiency following surgery Pulmonary congestion and hypostasis (pulmonary edema), unspecified acute lung edema	When acute respiratory failure is listed as a secondary diagnosis, review the medical record carefully to determine if ARF meets the criteria for principal diagnosis as determined by the circumstances of the admission, the diagnostic workup, and/or the treatment provided and if appropriate designate as the principal diagnosis.
193	MCC condition	*See* appendix B.
196	Interstitial pneumonia and pneumonitis	
	AND	
	MCC condition	*See* appendix B.
197	Interstitial pneumonia and pneumonitis	
	AND	
	CC condition	*See* appendix B.
207	Mechanical ventilation > 96 consecutive hours	*See* DRG 004.
208	Mechanical ventilation for less than or equal to 96 consecutive hours	*See* DRG 004.

DRG 194 (Continued)

DRG	PDx/SDx/Procedure	Tips
974	Diagnosis of HIV disease	Admission for HIV-related condition: sequence B2Ø first followed by the HIV-related condition code; except Chapter 15 codes which take sequencing priority. Any complication of the HIV-related condition would also be coded as a secondary diagnosis. (i.e., acute respiratory failure due to AIDS-related pneumonia).
	AND	
	Opportunistic lung infection	See appendix C for the full list of major HIV-related conditions. A diagnosis from this list should not be assumed as HIV-related unless specifically documented as such by the provider.
	AND	
	MCC condition	*See* appendix B.
975	Diagnosis of HIV disease	See DRG 974.
	AND	
	Opportunistic lung infection	See DRG 974.
	AND	
	CC condition	*See* appendix B.

DRG 195 Simple Pneumonia and Pleurisy without CC/MCC RW 0.6256

Potential DRGs

004	Tracheostomy with Mechanical Ventilation > 96 Hours or Principal Diagnosis Except Face, Mouth and Neck without Major O.R. Procedure	14.7000
177	Respiratory Infections and Inflammations with MCC	1.6964
178	Respiratory Infections and Inflammations with CC	0.9867
179	Respiratory Infections and Inflammations without CC/MCC	0.7633
180	Respiratory Neoplasms with MCC	1.7382
181	Respiratory Neoplasms with CC	1.1011
182	Respiratory Neoplasms without CC/MCC	0.7590
189	Pulmonary Edema and Respiratory Failure	1.2320
193	Simple Pneumonia and Pleurisy with MCC	1.3266
194	Simple Pneumonia and Pleurisy with CC	0.8222
196	Interstitial Lung Disease with MCC	1.8954
197	Interstitial Lung Disease with CC	0.9975
198	Interstitial Lung Disease without CC/MCC	0.7782
207	Respiratory System Diagnosis with Ventilator Support > 96 Hours	6.9080
208	Respiratory System Diagnosis with Ventilator Support <= 96 Hours	2.7038
974	HIV with Major Related Condition with MCC	2.9165
975	HIV with Major Related Condition with CC	1.3633
976	HIV with Major Related Condition without CC/MCC	0.8453

DRG	PDx/SDx/Procedure	Tips
004	Tracheostomy	Tracheostomy carried out elsewhere prior to admission or in an ambulance prior to arrival should not be reported as a current procedure. A tracheostomy procedure may be performed at the bedside and documented in the progress notes or in the operating room and documented in an operative note.
	WITH	
	Mechanical ventilation > 96 consecutive hours	Review record documentation for start and stop times. Calculation of mechanical ventilation hours begins when vent is initiated (or time of admission if patient already on a vent) and ends when it is turned off (or the time patient is discharged if still ventilated). The duration includes time spent to wean the patient from the vent. Do not assume that ventilation that spans four calendar days equals > 96 hours; count by the hour not day.
177	Pneumonia with causative organism: Salmonella Klebsiella pneumoniae Pseudomonas Staphylococcus Proteus or other gram-negative organisms COVID-19	Bacterial pneumonia should be assigned based on physician documentation. Sequence UØ7.1 before J12.82 According to the ICD-10-CM guidelines, documentation by the provider that the individual has COVID-19 is sufficient and does not require additional documentation of a positive test result.
	Aspiration pneumonia	If both aspiration pneumonia and bacterial pneumonia or pneumonia due to COVID-19 are documented, code both. Sequencing will depend on the circumstances of admission.
	AND	
	MCC condition	*See* appendix B.

DRG 195 (Continued)

DRG	PDx/SDx/Procedure	Tips
178	Pneumonia with causative organism: Salmonella Klebsiella pneumoniae Pseudomonas Staphylococcus Proteus or other gram-negative organisms COVID-19	*See* DRG 177.
	Aspiration pneumonia	*See* DRG 177.
	AND	
	CC condition	*See* appendix B.
179	Pneumonia with causative organism: Salmonella Klebsiella pneumoniae Pseudomonas Staphylococcus Proteus or other gram-negative organisms COVID-19	*See* DRG 177.
	Aspiration pneumonia	*See* DRG 177.
180	Respiratory neoplasm	
	AND	
	MCC condition	*See* appendix B.
181	Respiratory neoplasm	
	AND	
	CC condition	*See* appendix B.
182	Respiratory neoplasm	
189	Respiratory failure Respiratory failure or pulmonary insufficiency following surgery Pulmonary congestion and hypostasis (pulmonary edema), unspecified acute lung edema	When acute respiratory failure is listed as a secondary diagnosis, review the medical record carefully to determine if ARF meets the criteria for principal diagnosis as determined by the circumstances of the admission, the diagnostic workup, and/or the treatment provided and if appropriate designate as the principal diagnosis.
193	MCC condition	*See* appendix B.
194	CC condition	*See* appendix B.
196	Interstitial pneumonia and pneumonitis	
	AND	
	MCC condition	*See* appendix B.
197	Interstitial pneumonia and pneumonitis	
	AND	
	CC condition	*See* appendix B.
198	Interstitial pneumonia and pneumonitis	
207	Mechanical ventilation > 96 consecutive hours	*See* DRG 004.
208	Mechanical ventilation for less than or equal to 96 consecutive hours	*See* DRG 004.
974	Diagnosis of HIV disease	Admission for HIV-related condition: sequence B2Ø first followed by the HIV-related condition code except chapter 15 codes, which take sequencing priority. Admission due to complication of HIV-related condition: sequence B2Ø first followed by the HIV-related condition and the associated manifestation (e.g., acute respiratory failure due to AIDS related pneumonia).
	AND	
	Opportunistic lung infection	See appendix C for the full list of major HIV-related conditions. A diagnosis from this list should not be assumed as HIV-related unless specifically documented as such by the provider.
	AND	
	MCC condition	*See* appendix B.
975	Diagnosis of HIV disease	*See* DRG 974.
	AND	
	Opportunistic lung infection	*See* DRG 974.
	AND	
	CC condition	*See* appendix B.
976	Diagnosis of HIV disease	*See* DRG 974.
	AND	
	Opportunistic lung infection	*See* DRG 974.

DRG 196 Interstitial Lung Disease with MCC — RW 1.8954

Potential DRGs

004	Tracheostomy with Mechanical Ventilation > 96 Hours or Principal Diagnosis Except Face, Mouth and Neck without Major O.R. Procedure	14.7000
163	Major Chest Procedures with MCC	4.7136
166	Other Respiratory System O.R. Procedures with MCC	4.0578
207	Respiratory System Diagnosis with Ventilator Support > 96 Hours	6.9080
208	Respiratory System Diagnosis with Ventilator Support <= 96 Hours	2.7038

DRG	PDx/SDx/Procedure	Tips
004	Tracheostomy	Tracheostomy carried out elsewhere prior to admission or in an ambulance prior to arrival should not be reported as a current procedure. A tracheostomy procedure may be performed at the bedside and documented in the progress notes or in the operating room and documented in an operative note.
	WITH	
	Mechanical ventilation > 96 consecutive hours	Review record documentation for start and stop times. Calculation of mechanical ventilation hours begins when vent is initiated (or time of admission if patient already on a vent) and ends when it is turned off (or the time patient is discharged if still ventilated). The duration includes time spent to wean the patient from the vent. Do not assume that ventilation that spans four calendar days equals > 96 hours; count by the hour not day.
163	Open lung biopsy	
	Lung lesion destruction (open, percutaneous endoscopic, or via natural or artificial opening)	
	AND	
	MCC condition	*See* appendix B.
166	Closed endoscopic lung biopsy	Lung biopsy via percutaneous endoscopic, natural or artificial opening, or natural or artificial opening endoscopic approach.
	Transpleural thoracoscopy	
	AND	
	MCC condition	*See* appendix B.
207	Mechanical ventilation > 96 consecutive hours	*See* DRG 004.
208	Mechanical ventilation for less than or equal to 96 consecutive hours	*See* DRG 004.

DRG 197 Interstitial Lung Disease with CC — RW 0.9975

Potential DRGs

004	Tracheostomy with Mechanical Ventilation > 96 Hours or Principal Diagnosis Except Face, Mouth and Neck without Major O.R. Procedure	14.7000
163	Major Chest Procedures with MCC	4.7136
164	Major Chest Procedures with CC	2.5504
166	Other Respiratory System O.R. Procedures with MCC	4.0578
167	Other Respiratory System O.R. Procedures with CC	1.8198
189	Pulmonary Edema and Respiratory Failure	1.2320
196	Interstitial Lung Disease with MCC	1.8954
207	Respiratory System Diagnosis with Ventilator Support > 96 Hours	6.9080
208	Respiratory System Diagnosis with Ventilator Support <= 96 Hours	2.7038

DRG	PDx/SDx/Procedure	Tips
004	Tracheostomy	Tracheostomy carried out elsewhere prior to admission or in an ambulance prior to arrival should not be reported as a current procedure. A tracheostomy procedure may be performed at the bedside and documented in the progress notes or in the operating room and documented in an operative note.
	WITH	
	Mechanical ventilation > 96 consecutive hours	Review record documentation for start and stop times. Calculation of mechanical ventilation hours begins when vent is initiated (or time of admission if patient already on a vent) and ends when it is turned off (or the time patient is discharged if still ventilated). The duration includes time spent to wean the patient from the vent. Do not assume that ventilation that spans four calendar days equals > 96 hours; count by the hour not day.
163	Open lung biopsy	
	Lung lesion destruction (open, percutaneous endoscopic, or via natural or artificial opening)	
	AND	
	MCC condition	*See* appendix B.
164	Open lung biopsy	
	Lung lesion destruction (open, percutaneous endoscopic, or via natural or artificial opening)	
	AND	
	CC condition	*See* appendix B.
166	Closed endoscopic lung biopsy	Lung biopsy via percutaneous endoscopic, natural or artificial opening, or natural or artificial opening endoscopic approach.
	Transpleural thoracoscopy	
	AND	
	MCC condition	*See* appendix B.
167	Closed endoscopic lung biopsy	*See* DRG 166.
	Transpleural thoracoscopy	
	AND	
	CC condition	*See* appendix B.
189	Respiratory failure	When acute respiratory failure is listed as a secondary diagnosis, review the medical record carefully to determine if ARF meets the criteria for principal diagnosis as determined by the circumstances of the admission, the diagnostic workup, and/or the treatment provided and if appropriate designate as the principal diagnosis.
	Respiratory failure or pulmonary insufficiency following surgery	
	Pulmonary congestion and hypostasis (pulmonary edema), unspecified acute lung edema	
196	MCC condition	*See* appendix B.
207	Mechanical ventilation > 96 consecutive hours	*See* DRG 004.
208	Mechanical ventilation for less than or equal to 96 consecutive hours	*See* DRG 004.

DRG 198 Interstitial Lung Disease without CC/MCC RW 0.7782

Potential DRGs

004	Tracheostomy with Mechanical Ventilation > 96 Hours or Principal Diagnosis Except Face, Mouth and Neck without Major O.R. Procedure	14.7000
163	Major Chest Procedures with MCC	4.7136
164	Major Chest Procedures with CC	2.5504
165	Major Chest Procedures without CC/MCC	1.8764
166	Other Respiratory System O.R. Procedures with MCC	4.0578
167	Other Respiratory System O.R. Procedures with CC	1.8198
168	Other Respiratory System O.R. Procedures without CC/MCC	1.3557
189	Pulmonary Edema and Respiratory Failure	1.2320
196	Interstitial Lung Disease with MCC	1.8954
197	Interstitial Lung Disease with CC	0.9975
207	Respiratory System Diagnosis with Ventilator Support > 96 Hours	6.9080
208	Respiratory System Diagnosis with Ventilator Support <= 96 Hours	2.7038

DRG	PDx/SDx/Procedure	Tips
004	Tracheostomy	Tracheostomy carried out elsewhere prior to admission or in an ambulance prior to arrival should not be reported as a current procedure. A tracheostomy procedure may be performed at the bedside and documented in the progress notes or in the operating room and documented in an operative note.
	WITH	
	Mechanical ventilation > 96 consecutive hours	Review record documentation for start and stop times. Calculation of mechanical ventilation hours begins when vent is initiated (or time of admission if patient already on a vent) and ends when it is turned off (or the time patient is discharged if still ventilated). The duration includes time spent to wean the patient from the vent. Do not assume that ventilation that spans four calendar days equals > 96 hours; count by the hour not day.
163	Open lung biopsy	
	Lung lesion destruction (open, percutaneous endoscopic, or via natural or artificial opening)	
	AND	
	MCC condition	*See* appendix B.
164	Open lung biopsy	
	Lung lesion destruction (open, percutaneous endoscopic, or via natural or artificial opening)	
	AND	
	CC condition	*See* appendix B.
165	Open lung biopsy	
	Lung lesion destruction (open, percutaneous endoscopic, or via natural or artificial opening)	
166	Closed endoscopic lung biopsy	Lung biopsy via percutaneous endoscopic, natural or artificial opening, or natural or artificial opening endoscopic approach.
	Transpleural thoracoscopy	
	AND	
	MCC condition	*See* appendix B.
167	Closed endoscopic lung biopsy	*See* DRG 166.
	Transpleural thoracoscopy	
	AND	
	CC condition	*See* appendix B.
168	Closed endoscopic lung biopsy	*See* DRG 166.
	Transpleural thoracoscopy	
189	Respiratory failure	When acute respiratory failure is listed as a secondary diagnosis, review the medical record carefully to determine if ARF meets the criteria for principal diagnosis as determined by the circumstances of the admission, the diagnostic workup, and/or the treatment provided and if appropriate designate as the principal diagnosis.
	Respiratory failure or pulmonary insufficiency following surgery	
	Pulmonary congestion and hypostasis (pulmonary edema), unspecified acute lung edema	
196	MCC condition	*See* appendix B.
197	CC condition	*See* appendix B.
207	Mechanical ventilation > 96 consecutive hours	*See* DRG 004.
208	Mechanical ventilation for less than or equal to 96 consecutive hours	*See* DRG 004.

DRG 199 Pneumothorax with MCC

RW 1.7741

Potential DRGs

004	Tracheostomy with Mechanical Ventilation > 96 Hours or Principal Diagnosis Except Face, Mouth and Neck without Major O.R. Procedure	14.7000
166	Other Respiratory System O.R. Procedures with MCC	4.0578
207	Respiratory System Diagnosis with Ventilator Support > 96 Hours	6.9080
208	Respiratory System Diagnosis with Ventilator Support <= 96 Hours	2.7038
957	Other O.R. Procedures for Multiple Significant Trauma with MCC	7.2325
963	Other Multiple Significant Trauma with MCC	2.7343

DRG	PDx/SDx/Procedure	Tips
004	Tracheostomy	Tracheostomy carried out elsewhere prior to admission or in an ambulance prior to arrival should not be reported as a current procedure. A tracheostomy procedure may be performed at the bedside and documented in the progress notes or in the operating room and documented in an operative note.
	WITH	
	Mechanical ventilation > 96 consecutive hours	Review record documentation for start and stop times. Calculation of mechanical ventilation hours begins when vent is initiated (or time of admission if patient already on a vent) and ends when it is turned off (or the time patient is discharged if still ventilated). The duration includes time spent to wean the patient from the vent. Do not assume that ventilation that spans four calendar days equals > 96 hours; count by the hour not day.
166	Thoracoscopic pleural cavity drainage	
	AND	
	MCC condition	*See* appendix B.
207	Mechanical ventilation > 96 consecutive hours	*See* DRG 004.
208	Mechanical ventilation for less than or equal to 96 consecutive hours	*See* DRG 004.
957	Other multiple significant trauma (such as traumatic pneumothorax)	PDx of trauma and at least two injuries (assigned as PDx or SDx) that are defined as significant trauma from different body site categories located under MS-DRG 963.
	AND	
	Repair of lung or pleura	Chest tube insertion for multiple significant trauma does not affect MS-DRG assignment and would not move a case from MS-DRG 963 to 957.
	AND	
	MCC condition	*See* appendix B.
963	Other multiple significant trauma (such as traumatic pneumothorax)	*See* DRG 957.
	AND	
	MCC condition	*See* appendix B.

Optimizing Tips

DRG 200 Pneumothorax with CC RW 1.0770

Potential DRGs

004	Tracheostomy with Mechanical Ventilation > 96 Hours or Principal Diagnosis Except Face, Mouth and Neck without Major O.R. Procedure	14.7000
166	Other Respiratory System O.R. Procedures with MCC	4.0578
167	Other Respiratory System O.R. Procedures with CC	1.8198
183	Major Chest Trauma with MCC	1.5745
189	Pulmonary Edema and Respiratory Failure	1.2320
199	Pneumothorax with MCC	1.7741
207	Respiratory System Diagnosis with Ventilator Support > 96 Hours	6.9080
208	Respiratory System Diagnosis with Ventilator Support <= 96 Hours	2.7038
957	Other O.R. Procedures for Multiple Significant Trauma with MCC	7.2325
958	Other O.R. Procedures for Multiple Significant Trauma with CC	4.0448
963	Other Multiple Significant Trauma with MCC	2.7343
964	Other Multiple Significant Trauma with CC	1.5010

DRG	PDx/SDx/Procedure	Tips
004	Tracheostomy	Tracheostomy carried out elsewhere prior to admission or in an ambulance prior to arrival should not be reported as a current procedure. A tracheostomy procedure may be performed at the bedside and documented in the progress notes or in the operating room and documented in an operative note.
	WITH	
	Mechanical ventilation > 96 consecutive hours	Review record documentation for start and stop times. Calculation of mechanical ventilation hours begins when vent is initiated (or time of admission if patient already on a vent) and ends when it is turned off (or the time patient is discharged if still ventilated). The duration includes time spent to wean the patient from the vent. Do not assume that ventilation that spans four calendar days equals > 96 hours; count by the hour not day.
166	Thoracoscopic pleural cavity drainage	
	AND	
	MCC condition	*See* appendix B.
167	Thoracoscopic pleural cavity drainage	
	AND	
	CC condition	*See* appendix B.
183	Open fracture of one rib or multiple rib fractures (open or closed—two or more)	Review record documentation for indications the fractures meet the criteria for principal diagnosis, such as diagnostic workup and therapy provided. According to ICD-10-CM Guidelines, when two or more diagnoses equally meet the criteria for principal diagnosis as determined by the circumstances of admission, diagnostic workup and/or therapy provided, and the Alphabetic Index, Tabular List, or another coding guidelines does not provide sequencing direction, any one of the diagnoses may be sequenced first.
	AND	
	MCC condition	*See* appendix B.
189	Respiratory failure	When acute respiratory failure is listed as a secondary diagnosis, review the medical record carefully to determine if ARF meets the criteria for principal diagnosis as determined by the circumstances of the admission, the diagnostic workup, and/or the treatment provided and if appropriate designate as the principal diagnosis.
	Respiratory failure or pulmonary insufficiency following surgery	
	Pulmonary congestion and hypostasis (pulmonary edema), unspecified acute lung edema	
199	MCC condition	*See* appendix B.
207	Mechanical ventilation > 96 consecutive hours	*See* DRG 004.
208	Mechanical ventilation for less than or equal to 96 consecutive hours	*See* DRG 004.
957	Other multiple significant trauma (such as traumatic pneumothorax)	PDx of trauma and at least two injuries (assigned as PDx or SDx) that are defined as significant trauma from different body site categories located under MS-DRG 963.
	AND	
	Repair of pleura or lung	Chest tube insertion for multiple significant trauma does not affect MS-DRG assignment and would not move a case from MS-DRG 963 to 957.
	AND	
	MCC condition	*See* appendix B.
958	Other multiple significant trauma (such as traumatic pneumothorax)	*See* DRG 957.
	AND	
	Repair of pleura or lung	*See* DRG 957.
	AND	
	CC condition	*See* appendix B.
963	Other multiple significant trauma (such as traumatic pneumothorax)	*See* DRG 957.
	AND	
	MCC condition	*See* appendix B.
964	Other multiple significant trauma (such as traumatic pneumothorax)	*See* DRG 957.
	AND	
	CC condition	*See* appendix B.

DRG 201 Pneumothorax without CC/MCC

RW 0.7061

Potential DRGs

004	Tracheostomy with Mechanical Ventilation > 96 Hours or Principal Diagnosis Except Face, Mouth and Neck without Major O.R. Procedure	14.7000
166	Other Respiratory System O.R. Procedures with MCC	4.0578
167	Other Respiratory System O.R. Procedures with CC	1.8198
168	Other Respiratory System O.R. Procedures without CC/MCC	1.3557
183	Major Chest Trauma with MCC	1.5745
184	Major Chest Trauma with CC	1.0519
185	Major Chest Trauma without CC/MCC	0.7557
189	Pulmonary Edema and Respiratory Failure	1.2320
199	Pneumothorax with MCC	1.7741
200	Pneumothorax with CC	1.0770
207	Respiratory System Diagnosis with Ventilator Support > 96 Hours	6.9080
208	Respiratory System Diagnosis with Ventilator Support <= 96 Hours	2.7038
957	Other O.R. Procedures for Multiple Significant Trauma with MCC	7.2325
958	Other O.R. Procedures for Multiple Significant Trauma with CC	4.0448
959	Other O.R. Procedures for Multiple Significant Trauma without CC/MCC	2.5324
963	Other Multiple Significant Trauma with MCC	2.7343
964	Other Multiple Significant Trauma with CC	1.5010
965	Other Multiple Significant Trauma without CC/MCC	0.9559

DRG	PDx/SDx/Procedure	Tips
004	Tracheostomy	Tracheostomy carried out elsewhere prior to admission or in an ambulance prior to arrival should not be reported as a current procedure. A tracheostomy procedure may be performed at the bedside and documented in the progress notes or in the operating room and documented in an operative note.
	WITH	
	Mechanical ventilation > 96 consecutive hours	Review record documentation for start and stop times. Calculation of mechanical ventilation hours begins when vent is initiated (or time of admission if patient already on a vent) and ends when it is turned off (or the time patient is discharged if still ventilated). The duration includes time spent to wean the patient from the vent. Do not assume that ventilation that spans four calendar days equals > 96 hours; count by the hour not day.
166	Thoracoscopic pleural cavity drainage	
	AND	
	MCC condition	*See* appendix B.
167	Thoracoscopic pleural cavity drainage	
	AND	
	CC condition	*See* appendix B.
168	Thoracoscopic pleural cavity drainage	
183	Open fracture of one rib or multiple rib fractures (open or closed—two or more)	Review record documentation for indications the fractures meet the criteria for principal diagnosis, such as diagnostic workup and therapy provided. According to ICD-10-CM Guidelines, when two or more diagnoses equally meet the criteria for principal diagnosis as determined by the circumstances of admission, diagnostic workup and/or therapy provided, and the Alphabetic Index, Tabular List, or another coding guidelines does not provide sequencing direction, any one of the diagnoses may be sequenced first.
	AND	
	MCC condition	*See* appendix B.
184	Open fracture of one rib or multiple rib fractures (open or closed—two or more)	*See* DRG 183.
	AND	
	CC condition	*See* appendix B.
185	Open fracture of one rib or multiple rib fractures (open or closed—two or more)	*See* DRG 183.
189	Respiratory failure	When acute respiratory failure is listed as a secondary diagnosis, review the medical record carefully to determine if ARF meets the criteria for principal diagnosis as determined by the circumstances of the admission, the diagnostic workup, and/or the treatment provided and if appropriate designate as the principal diagnosis.
	Respiratory failure or pulmonary insufficiency following surgery	
	Pulmonary congestion and hypostasis (pulmonary edema), unspecified acute lung edema	
199	MCC condition	*See* appendix B.
200	CC condition	*See* appendix B.
207	Mechanical ventilation > 96 consecutive hours	*See* DRG 004.
208	Mechanical ventilation for less than or equal to 96 consecutive hours	*See* DRG 004.

DRG 201 (Continued)

DRG	PDx/SDx/Procedure	Tips
957	Other multiple significant trauma (such as traumatic pneumothorax)	PDx of trauma and at least two injuries (assigned as PDx or SDx) that are defined as significant trauma from different body site categories located under MS-DRG 963.
	AND	
	Repair of pleura or lung	Chest tube insertion for multiple significant trauma does not affect MS-DRG assignment and would not move a case from MS-DRG 963 to 957.
	AND	
	MCC condition	*See* appendix B.
958	Other multiple significant trauma (such as traumatic pneumothorax)	*See* DRG 957.
	AND	
	Repair of pleura or lung	*See* DRG 957.
	AND	
	CC condition	*See* appendix B.
959	Other multiple significant trauma (such as traumatic pneumothorax)	*See* DRG 957.
	AND	
	Repair of pleura or lung	*See* DRG 957.
963	Other multiple significant trauma (such as traumatic pneumothorax)	PDx of trauma and at least two injuries (assigned as PDx or SDx) that are defined as significant trauma from different body site categories located under MS-DRG 963.
	AND	
	MCC condition	*See* appendix B.
964	Other multiple significant trauma (such as traumatic pneumothorax)	*See* DRG 963.
	AND	
	CC condition	*See* appendix B.
965	Other multiple significant trauma (such as traumatic pneumothorax)	*See* DRG 963.

DRG 202 Bronchitis and Asthma with CC/MCC

RW 0.9575

Potential DRGs

004	Tracheostomy with Mechanical Ventilation > 96 Hours or Principal Diagnosis Except Face, Mouth and Neck without Major O.R. Procedure	14.7000
177	Respiratory Infections and Inflammations with MCC	1.6964
178	Respiratory Infections and Inflammations with CC	0.9867
189	Pulmonary Edema and Respiratory Failure	1.2320
190	Chronic Obstructive Pulmonary Disease with MCC	1.1020
193	Simple Pneumonia and Pleurisy with MCC	1.3266
207	Respiratory System Diagnosis with Ventilator Support > 96 Hours	6.9080
208	Respiratory System Diagnosis with Ventilator Support <= 96 Hours	2.7038

DRG	PDx/SDx/Procedure	Tips
004	Tracheostomy	Tracheostomy carried out elsewhere prior to admission or in an ambulance prior to arrival should not be reported as a current procedure. A tracheostomy procedure may be performed at the bedside and documented in the progress notes or in the operating room and documented in an operative note.
	WITH	
	Mechanical ventilation > 96 consecutive hours	Review record documentation for start and stop times. Calculation of mechanical ventilation hours begins when vent is initiated (or time of admission if patient already on a vent) and ends when it is turned off (or the time patient is discharged if still ventilated). The duration includes time spent to wean the patient from the vent. Do not assume that ventilation that spans four calendar days equals > 96 hours; count by the hour not day.
177	Pneumonia with causative organism: Salmonella Klebsiella pneumoniae Pseudomonas Staphylococcus Proteus or other gram-negative organisms	Bacterial pneumonia should be assigned based on physician documentation.
	COVID-19	Sequence U07.1 before J12.82 According to the ICD-10-CM guidelines, documentation by the provider that the individual has COVID-19 is sufficient and does not require additional documentation of a positive test result.
	Aspiration pneumonia	If both aspiration pneumonia and bacterial pneumonia or pneumonia due to COVID-19 are documented, code both. Sequencing will depend on the circumstances of admission.
	AND	
	MCC condition	*See* appendix B.
178	Pneumonia with causative organism: Salmonella Klebsiella pneumoniae Pseudomonas Staphylococcus Proteus or other gram-negative organisms	Bacterial pneumonia should be assigned based on physician documentation.
	COVID-19	*See* DRG 177.
	Aspiration pneumonia	*See* DRG 177.
	AND	
	CC condition	*See* appendix B.
189	Respiratory failure	When acute respiratory failure is listed as a secondary diagnosis, review the medical record carefully to determine if ARF meets the criteria for principal diagnosis as determined by the circumstances of the admission, the diagnostic workup, and/or the treatment provided and if appropriate designate as the principal diagnosis.
	Respiratory failure or pulmonary insufficiency following surgery	
	Pulmonary congestion and hypostasis (pulmonary edema), unspecified acute lung edema	
190	Acute exacerbation of chronic bronchitis	
	AND	
	MCC condition	*See* appendix B.
193	Simple pneumonia, viral pneumonia	Excluding pneumonia due to COVID-19.
	AND	
	MCC condition	*See* appendix B.
207	Mechanical ventilation > 96 consecutive hours	*See* DRG 004.
208	Mechanical ventilation for less than or equal to 96 consecutive hours	*See* DRG 004.

DRG 203 Bronchitis and Asthma without CC/MCC RW 0.6949

Potential DRGs

004	Tracheostomy with Mechanical Ventilation > 96 Hours or Principal Diagnosis Except Face, Mouth and Neck without Major O.R. Procedure	14.7000
177	Respiratory Infections and Inflammations with MCC	1.6964
178	Respiratory Infections and Inflammations with CC	0.9867
179	Respiratory Infections and Inflammations without CC/MCC	0.7633
189	Pulmonary Edema and Respiratory Failure	1.2320
190	Chronic Obstructive Pulmonary Disease with MCC	1.1020
191	Chronic Obstructive Pulmonary Disease with CC	0.8490
193	Simple Pneumonia and Pleurisy with MCC	1.3266
194	Simple Pneumonia and Pleurisy with CC	0.8222
202	Bronchitis and Asthma with CC/MCC	0.9575
207	Respiratory System Diagnosis with Ventilator Support > 96 Hours	6.9080
208	Respiratory System Diagnosis with Ventilator Support <= 96 Hours	2.7038

DRG	PDx/SDx/Procedure	Tips
004	Tracheostomy	Tracheostomy carried out elsewhere prior to admission or in an ambulance prior to arrival should not be reported as a current procedure. A tracheostomy procedure may be performed at the bedside and documented in the progress notes or in the operating room and documented in an operative note.
	WITH	
	Mechanical ventilation > 96 consecutive hours	Review record documentation for start and stop times. Calculation of mechanical ventilation hours begins when vent is initiated (or time of admission if patient already on a vent) and ends when it is turned off (or the time patient is discharged if still ventilated). The duration includes time spent to wean the patient from the vent. Do not assume that ventilation that spans four calendar days equals > 96 hours; count by the hour not day.
177	Pneumonia with causative organism: Salmonella Klebsiella pneumoniae Pseudomonas Staphylococcus Proteus or other gram-negative organisms COVID-19	Bacterial pneumonia should be assigned based on physician documentation. Sequence UØ7.1 before J12.82 According to the ICD-10-CM guidelines, documentation by the provider that the individual has COVID-19 is sufficient and does not require additional documentation of a positive test result.
	Aspiration pneumonia	If both aspiration pneumonia and bacterial pneumonia or pneumonia due to COVID-19 are documented, code both. Sequencing will depend on the circumstances of admission.
	AND	
	MCC condition	*See* appendix B.
178	Pneumonia with causative organism: Salmonella Klebsiella pneumoniae Pseudomonas Staphylococcus Proteus or other gram-negative organisms COVID-19	*See* DRG 177.
	Aspiration pneumonia	*See* DRG 177.
	AND	
	CC condition	*See* appendix B.
179	Pneumonia with causative organism: Salmonella Klebsiella pneumoniae Pseudomonas Staphylococcus Proteus or other gram-negative organisms COVID-19	*See* DRG 177.
	Aspiration pneumonia	*See* DRG 177.
189	Respiratory failure	When acute respiratory failure is listed as a secondary diagnosis, review the medical record carefully to determine if ARF meets the criteria for principal diagnosis as determined by the circumstances of the admission, the diagnostic workup, and/or the treatment provided and if appropriate designate as the principal diagnosis.
	Respiratory failure or pulmonary insufficiency following surgery	
	Pulmonary congestion and hypostasis (pulmonary edema), unspecified acute lung edema	
190	Acute exacerbation of chronic bronchitis	
	AND	
	MCC condition	*See* appendix B.
191	Acute exacerbation of chronic bronchitis	
	AND	
	CC condition	*See* appendix B.

DRG 203 (Continued)

DRG	PDx/SDx/Procedure	Tips
193	Simple pneumonia, viral pneumonia	Excluding pneumonia due to COVID-19.
	AND	
	MCC condition	*See* appendix B.
194	Simple pneumonia, viral pneumonia	Excluding pneumonia due to COVID-19.
	AND	
	CC condition	*See* appendix B.
202	CC/MCC condition	*See* appendix B.
207	Mechanical ventilation > 96 consecutive hours	*See* DRG 004.
208	Mechanical ventilation for less than or equal to 96 consecutive hours	*See* DRG 004.

DRG 204 Respiratory Signs and Symptoms

RW 0.8229

Potential DRGs

004	Tracheostomy with Mechanical Ventilation > 96 Hours or Principal Diagnosis Except Face, Mouth and Neck without Major O.R. Procedure	14.7000
189	Pulmonary Edema and Respiratory Failure	1.2320
205	Other Respiratory System Diagnoses with MCC	1.8103
206	Other Respiratory System Diagnoses without MCC	0.9135
207	Respiratory System Diagnosis with Ventilator Support > 96 Hours	6.9080
208	Respiratory System Diagnosis with Ventilator Support <= 96 Hours	2.7038

DRG	PDx/SDx/Procedure	Tips
004	Tracheostomy	Tracheostomy carried out elsewhere prior to admission or in an ambulance prior to arrival should not be reported as a current procedure. A tracheostomy procedure may be performed at the bedside and documented in the progress notes or in the operating room and documented in an operative note.
	WITH	
	Mechanical ventilation > 96 consecutive hours	Review record documentation for start and stop times. Calculation of mechanical ventilation hours begins when vent is initiated (or time of admission if patient already on a vent) and ends when it is turned off (or the time patient is discharged if still ventilated). The duration includes time spent to wean the patient from the vent. Do not assume that ventilation that spans four calendar days equals > 96 hours; count by the hour not day.
189	Respiratory failure	When acute respiratory failure is listed as a secondary diagnosis, review the medical record carefully to determine if ARF meets the criteria for principal diagnosis as determined by the circumstances of the admission, the diagnostic workup, and/or the treatment provided and if appropriate designate as the principal diagnosis.
	Acute respiratory distress syndrome (ARDS)	Acute respiratory distress alone is not synonymous with ARDS; review record documentation carefully and query, if necessary. When acute respiratory failure and ARDS are both documented, only the code for ARDS should be assigned.
	Respiratory failure or pulmonary insufficiency following surgery	
	Pulmonary congestion and hypostasis (pulmonary edema), unspecified acute lung edema	
205	Atelectasis	
	Hypoxemia	
	Fractured one rib, or rib sprain/strain	
	Solitary pulmonary nodule	
	AND	
	MCC condition	*See* appendix B.
206	Atelectasis	
	Hypoxemia	
	Fractured one rib, or rib sprain/strain	
	Solitary pulmonary nodule	
207	Mechanical ventilation > 96 consecutive hours	*See* DRG 004.
208	Mechanical ventilation for less than or equal to 96 consecutive hours	*See* DRG 004.

DRG 205 Other Respiratory System Diagnoses with MCC — RW 1.8103

Potential DRGs

004	Tracheostomy with Mechanical Ventilation > 96 Hours or Principal Diagnosis Except Face, Mouth and Neck without Major O.R. Procedure	14.7000
207	Respiratory System Diagnosis with Ventilator Support > 96 Hours	6.9080
208	Respiratory System Diagnosis with Ventilator Support <= 96 Hours	2.7038
957	Other O.R. Procedures for Multiple Significant Trauma with MCC	7.2325
963	Other Multiple Significant Trauma with MCC	2.7343

DRG	PDx/SDx/Procedure	Tips
004	Tracheostomy	Tracheostomy carried out elsewhere prior to admission or in an ambulance prior to arrival should not be reported as a current procedure. A tracheostomy procedure may be performed at the bedside and documented in the progress notes or in the operating room and documented in an operative note.
	WITH	
	Mechanical ventilation > 96 consecutive hours	Review record documentation for start and stop times. Calculation of mechanical ventilation hours begins when vent is initiated (or time of admission if patient already on a vent) and ends when it is turned off (or the time patient is discharged if still ventilated). The duration includes time spent to wean the patient from the vent. Do not assume that ventilation that spans four calendar days equals > 96 hours; count by the hour not day.
207	Mechanical ventilation > 96 consecutive hours	*See* DRG 004.
208	Mechanical ventilation for less than or equal to 96 consecutive hours	*See* DRG 004.
957	Other multiple significant trauma (such as traumatic pneumothorax)	PDx of trauma and at least two injuries (assigned as PDx or SDx) that are defined as significant trauma from different body site categories located under MS-DRG 963.
	AND	
	Repair of pleura or lung	
	AND	
	MCC condition	*See* appendix B.
963	Other multiple significant trauma (such as traumatic pneumothorax)	*See* DRG 957.
	AND	
	MCC condition	*See* appendix B.

DRG 206 Other Respiratory System Diagnoses without MCC — RW 0.9135

Potential DRGs

004	Tracheostomy with Mechanical Ventilation > 96 Hours or Principal Diagnosis Except Face, Mouth and Neck without Major O.R. Procedure	14.7000
183	Major Chest Trauma with MCC	1.5745
184	Major Chest Trauma with CC	1.0519
189	Pulmonary Edema and Respiratory Failure	1.2320
205	Other Respiratory System Diagnoses with MCC	1.8103
207	Respiratory System Diagnosis with Ventilator Support > 96 Hours	6.9080
208	Respiratory System Diagnosis with Ventilator Support <= 96 Hours	2.7038
957	Other O.R. Procedures for Multiple Significant Trauma with MCC	7.2325
958	Other O.R. Procedures for Multiple Significant Trauma with CC	4.0448
959	Other O.R. Procedures for Multiple Significant Trauma without CC/MCC	2.5324
963	Other Multiple Significant Trauma with MCC	2.7343
964	Other Multiple Significant Trauma with CC	1.5010
965	Other Multiple Significant Trauma without CC/MCC	0.9559

DRG	PDx/SDx/Procedure	Tips
004	Tracheostomy	Tracheostomy carried out elsewhere prior to admission or in an ambulance prior to arrival should not be reported as a current procedure. A tracheostomy procedure may be performed at the bedside and documented in the progress notes or in the operating room and documented in an operative note.
	WITH	
	Mechanical ventilation > 96 consecutive hours	Review record documentation for start and stop times. Calculation of mechanical ventilation hours begins when vent is initiated (or time of admission if patient already on a vent) and ends when it is turned off (or the time patient is discharged if still ventilated). The duration includes time spent to wean the patient from the vent. Do not assume that ventilation that spans four calendar days equals > 96 hours; count by the hour not day.

DRG 206 (Continued)

DRG	PDx/SDx/Procedure	Tips
183	Open fracture of one rib or multiple rib fractures (open or closed—two or more)	Review record documentation for indications the fractures meet the criteria for principal diagnosis, such as diagnostic workup and therapy provided. According to ICD-10-CM Guidelines, when two or more diagnoses equally meet the criteria for principal diagnosis as determined by the circumstances of admission, diagnostic workup and/or therapy provided, and the Alphabetic Index, Tabular List, or another coding guidelines does not provide sequencing direction, any one of the diagnoses may be sequenced first.
	AND	
	MCC condition	*See* appendix B.
184	Open fracture of one rib or multiple rib fractures (open or closed—two or more)	*See* DRG 183.
	AND	
	CC condition	*See* appendix B.
189	Respiratory failure	When acute respiratory failure is listed as a secondary diagnosis, review the medical record carefully to determine if ARF meets the criteria for principal diagnosis as determined by the circumstances of the admission, the diagnostic workup, and/or the treatment provided and if appropriate designate as the principal diagnosis.
	Acute respiratory distress syndrome (ARDS)	Acute respiratory distress alone is not synonymous with ARDS; review record documentation carefully and query, if necessary. When acute respiratory failure and ARDS are both documented, only the code for ARDS should be assigned.
	Respiratory failure or pulmonary insufficiency following surgery,	
	Pulmonary congestion and hypostasis (pulmonary edema), unspecified acute lung edema	
205	MCC condition	*See* appendix B.
207	Mechanical ventilation > 96 consecutive hours	*See* DRG 004.
208	Mechanical ventilation for less than or equal to 96 consecutive hours	*See* DRG 004.
957	Other multiple significant trauma (such as traumatic pneumothorax)	PDx of trauma and at least two injuries (assigned as PDx or SDx) that are defined as significant trauma from different body site categories located under MS-DRG 963.
	AND	
	Repair of pleura or lung	
	AND	
	MCC condition	*See* appendix B.
958	Other multiple significant trauma (such as traumatic pneumothorax)	*See* DRG 957.
	AND	
	Repair of pleura or lung	
	AND	
	CC condition	*See* appendix B.
959	Other multiple significant trauma (such as traumatic pneumothorax)	*See* DRG 957.
	AND	
	Repair of pleura or lung	
963	Other multiple significant trauma	*See* DRG 957.
	AND	
	MCC condition	*See* appendix B.
964	Other multiple significant trauma	*See* DRG 957.
	AND	
	CC condition	*See* appendix B.
965	Other multiple significant trauma	*See* DRG 957.

DRG 207 Respiratory System Diagnosis with Ventilator Support > 96 Hours RW 6.9080

Potential DRGs

004	Tracheostomy with Mechanical Ventilation > 96 Hours or Principal Diagnosis Except Face, Mouth and Neck without Major O.R. Procedure	14.7000

DRG	PDx/SDx/Procedure	Tips
004	Tracheostomy	Tracheostomy carried out elsewhere prior to admission or in an ambulance prior to arrival should not be reported as a current procedure. A tracheostomy procedure may be performed at the bedside and documented in the progress notes or in the operating room and documented in an operative note.
	WITH	
	Mechanical ventilation > 96 consecutive hours	Review record documentation for start and stop times. Calculation of mechanical ventilation hours begins when vent is initiated (or time of admission if patient already on a vent) and ends when it is turned off (or the time patient is discharged if still ventilated). The duration includes time spent to wean the patient from the vent. Do not assume that ventilation that spans four calendar days equals > 96 hours; count by the hour not day.

DRG 208 Respiratory System Diagnosis with Ventilator Support <= 96 Hours RW 2.7038

Potential DRGs

004	Tracheostomy with Mechanical Ventilation > 96 Hours or Principal Diagnosis Except Face, Mouth and Neck without Major O.R. Procedure	14.7000
207	Respiratory System Diagnosis with Ventilator Support > 96 Hours	6.9080

DRG	PDx/SDx/Procedure	Tips
004	Tracheostomy	Tracheostomy carried out elsewhere prior to admission or in an ambulance prior to arrival should not be reported as a current procedure. A tracheostomy procedure may be performed at the bedside and documented in the progress notes or in the operating room and documented in an operative note.
	WITH	
	Mechanical ventilation > 96 consecutive hours	Review record documentation for start and stop times. Calculation of mechanical ventilation hours begins when vent is initiated (or time of admission if patient already on a vent) and ends when it is turned off (or the time patient is discharged if still ventilated). The duration includes time spent to wean the patient from the vent. Do not assume that ventilation that spans four calendar days equals > 96 hours; count by the hour not day.
207	Mechanical ventilation > 96 consecutive hours	*See* DRG 004.

Diseases And Disorders Of The Circulatory System

DRG 212 Concomitant Aortic and Mitral Valve Procedures — RW 10.7707

No Potential DRGs

DRG 215 Other Heart Assist System Implant — RW 10.2148

Potential DRGs

001	Heart Transplant or Implant of Heart Assist System with MCC	27.0986
002	Heart Transplant or Implant of Heart Assist System without MCC	12.2441

DRG	PDx/SDx/Procedure	Tips
001	Insertion of implantable heart assist system or implantation of total internal biventricular heart replacement system	Review operative report carefully to determine extent of all procedures. Implantable ventricular assist devices are mechanical support devices attached to the native heart and can be internal or external. A total artificial heart (TAH) is a surgically implantable biventricular support device that serves as a total replacement for both right and left ventricles of the failing heart. Both ICD-10-PCS procedure codes, Ø2RKØJZ Replacement of right ventricle with synthetic substitute, open approach, and Ø2RLØJZ Replacement of left ventricle with synthetic substitute, open approach, must be reported together to describe a biventricular heart replacement (artificial heart). The excision of the native ventricles is integral to the replacement procedure and is not reported separately.
	OR	
	Insertion of external heart assist system with removal of existing heart assist system (e.g. replacement, exchange)	Review operative report carefully to determine extent of all procedures. External devices (sometimes called percutaneous ventricular assist devices [pVADs]) are generally placed through the femoral artery via catheter. Both insertion and removal must be performed for this DRG.
	OR	
	Removal and revision of heart assist system	Root operation Revision is correcting, to the extent possible, a portion of a malfunctioning device or the position of a displaced device. Removal must be performed in conjunction with revision for this DRG.
	AND	
	MCC condition	*See* appendix B.
002	Insertion of implantable heart assist system or implantation of total internal biventricular heart replacement system	*See* DRG 001.
	OR	
	Insertion of external heart assist system with removal of existing heart assist system (e.g. replacement, exchange)	*See* DRG 001.
	OR	
	Removal and revision of heart assist system	*See* DRG 001.

DRG 216 Cardiac Valve and Other Major Cardiothoracic Procedures with Cardiac Catheterization with MCC — RW 9.7053

Potential DRGs

212	Concomitant Aortic and Mitral Valve Procedures	10.7707

DRG	PDx/SDx/Procedure	Tips
212	Repair or Replacement of aortic valve	Open or percutaneous endoscopic approach.
	AND	
	Repair or Replacement of mitral valve	Open or percutaneous endoscopic approach.
	AND	
	Cardiac catheterization	Measurement of cardiac sampling and pressure (right, left, bilateral) or cardiac rhythm.
	Coronary angiography	

DRG 217 Cardiac Valve and Other Major Cardiothoracic Procedures with Cardiac Catheterization with CC — RW 6.3653

Potential DRGs

212	Concomitant Aortic and Mitral Valve Procedures	10.7707
216	Cardiac Valve and Other Major Cardiothoracic Procedures with Cardiac Catheterization with MCC	9.7053

DRG	PDx/SDx/Procedure	Tips
212	Repair or Replacement of aortic valve	Open or percutaneous endoscopic approach.
	AND	
	Repair or Replacement of mitral valve	Open or percutaneous endoscopic approach.
	AND	
	Cardiac catheterization	Measurement of cardiac sampling and pressure (right, left, bilateral) or cardiac rhythm.
	Coronary angiography	
216	MCC condition	*See* appendix B.

DRG 218 Cardiac Valve and Other Major Cardiothoracic Procedures with Cardiac Catheterization without CC/MCC — RW 5.6967

Potential DRGs

212	Concomitant Aortic and Mitral Valve Procedures	10.7707
216	Cardiac Valve and Other Major Cardiothoracic Procedures with Cardiac Catheterization with MCC	9.7053
217	Cardiac Valve and Other Major Cardiothoracic Procedures with Cardiac Catheterization with CC	6.3653

DRG	PDx/SDx/Procedure	Tips
212	Repair or Replacement of aortic valve	Open or percutaneous endoscopic approach.
	AND	
	Repair or Replacement of mitral valve	Open or percutaneous endoscopic approach.
	AND	
	Cardiac catheterization	Measurement of cardiac sampling and pressure (right, left, bilateral) or rhythm.
	Coronary angiography	
216	MCC condition	*See* appendix B.
217	CC condition	*See* appendix B.

DRG 219 Cardiac Valve and Other Major Cardiothoracic Procedures without Cardiac Catheterization with MCC — RW 7.7112

Potential DRGs

212	Concomitant Aortic and Mitral Valve Procedures	10.7707
216	Cardiac Valve and Other Major Cardiothoracic Procedures with Cardiac Catheterization with MCC	9.7053

DRG	PDx/SDx/Procedure	Tips
212	Repair or Replacement aortic valve	Open or percutaneous endoscopic approach.
	AND	
	Repair or Replacement mitral valve	Open or percutaneous endoscopic approach.
	AND	
	Cardiac catheterization	Measurement of cardiac sampling and pressure (right, left, bilateral) or rhythm.
	Coronary angiography	
216	Cardiac catheterization	Measurement of cardiac sampling and pressure (right, left, bilateral) or cardiac rhythm.
	Coronary angiography	
	AND	
	MCC condition	*See* appendix B.

DRG 220 Cardiac Valve and Other Major Cardiothoracic Procedures without Cardiac Catheterization with CC — RW 5.2446

Potential DRGs

212	Concomitant Aortic and Mitral Valve Procedures	10.7707
216	Cardiac Valve and Other Major Cardiothoracic Procedures with Cardiac Catheterization with MCC	9.7053
217	Cardiac Valve and Other Major Cardiothoracic Procedures with Cardiac Catheterization with CC	6.3653
219	Cardiac Valve and Other Major Cardiothoracic Procedures without Cardiac Catheterization with MCC	7.7112

DRG	PDx/SDx/Procedure	Tips
212	Repair or Replacement aortic valve	Open or percutaneous endoscopic approach.
	AND	
	Repair or Replacement mitral valve	Open or percutaneous endoscopic approach.
	AND	
	Cardiac catheterization	Measurement of cardiac sampling and pressure (right, left, bilateral) or rhythm.
	Coronary angiography	
216	Cardiac catheterization	Measurement of cardiac sampling and pressure (right, left, bilateral) or cardiac rhythm.
	Coronary angiography	
	AND	
	MCC condition	*See* appendix B.
217	Cardiac catheterization	*See* DRG 216.
	Coronary angiography	
	AND	
	CC condition	*See* appendix B.
219	MCC condition	*See* appendix B.

DRG 221 Cardiac Valve and Other Major Cardiothoracic Procedures without Cardiac Catheterization without CC/MCC

RW 4.6486

Potential DRGs

212	Concomitant Aortic and Mitral Valve Procedures	10.7707
216	Cardiac Valve and Other Major Cardiothoracic Procedures with Cardiac Catheterization with MCC	9.7053
217	Cardiac Valve and Other Major Cardiothoracic Procedures with Cardiac Catheterization with CC	6.3653
218	Cardiac Valve and Other Major Cardiothoracic Procedures with Cardiac Catheterization without CC/MCC	5.6967
219	Cardiac Valve and Other Major Cardiothoracic Procedures without Cardiac Catheterization with MCC	7.7112
220	Cardiac Valve and Other Major Cardiothoracic Procedures without Cardiac Catheterization with CC	5.2446

DRG	PDx/SDx/Procedure	Tips
212	Repair or Replacement aortic valve	Open or percutaneous endoscopic approach.
	AND	
	Repair or Replacement mitral valve	Open or percutaneous endoscopic approach.
	AND	
	Cardiac catheterization	Measurement of cardiac sampling and pressure (right, left, bilateral) or rhythm.
	Coronary angiography	
216	Cardiac catheterization	Measurement of cardiac sampling and pressure (right, left, bilateral) or cardiac rhythm.
	Coronary angiography	
	AND	
	MCC condition	*See* appendix B.
217	Cardiac catheterization	*See* DRG 216.
	Coronary angiography	
	AND	
	CC condition	*See* appendix B.
218	Cardiac catheterization	*See* DRG 216.
	Coronary angiography	
219	MCC condition	*See* appendix B.
220	CC condition	*See* appendix B.

DRG 228 Other Cardiothoracic Procedures with MCC

RW 5.0387

Potential DRGs

216	Cardiac Valve and Other Major Cardiothoracic Procedures with Cardiac Catheterization with MCC	9.7053
219	Cardiac Valve and Other Major Cardiothoracic Procedures without Cardiac Catheterization with MCC	7.7112
231	Coronary Bypass with PTCA with MCC	8.1152
233	Coronary Bypass with Cardiac Catheterization or Open Ablation with MCC	7.7996
235	Coronary Bypass without Cardiac Catheterization with MCC	5.8806
266	Endovascular Cardiac Valve Replacement and Supplement Procedures with MCC	6.2461

DRG	PDx/SDx/Procedure	Tips
216	Open valvuloplasty without replacement	Dilation with or without a device, or release. Approach must be open. The objective of root operation Dilation is to enlarge the diameter of a tubular body part or orifice. If a device remains at the end of the procedure to maintain the new diameter, this is an integral part of the procedure and captured with a sixth-character device value. If the sole objective of the procedure is freeing a body part without cutting the body part, the root operation is Release. In the root operation Release, the body part value coded is the body part being freed, not the tissue being manipulated or cut to free the body part.
	OR	
	Cardiac valve replacement, repair, supplement	Open or percutaneous endoscopic approach only.
	AND	
	Cardiac catheterization	Measurement of cardiac sampling and pressure (right, left, bilateral).
	Coronary angiography	
	AND	
	MCC condition	*See* appendix B.
219	Open valvuloplasty without replacement	*See* DRG 216.
	OR	
	Cardiac valve replacement, repair, supplement	*See* DRG 216.
	AND	
	MCC condition	*See* appendix B.

DRG 228 (Continued)

DRG	PDx/SDx/Procedure	Tips
231	Coronary artery bypass procedure with arterial or vein graft	Review operative report carefully to determine the extent of all procedures. DRG 228 includes percutaneous or percutaneous endoscopic in situ coronary venous arterialization, in which the blood flow is rerouted by inserting an intraluminal tubular device similar to a stent, bypassing the coronary artery blockage using a neighboring coronary vein. DRG 231 includes traditional coronary bypass performed with artery or vein grafts using Open or Percutaneous Endoscopic approach.
	AND	
	PTCA—Dilation with or without intraluminal device(s)	Review operative report carefully to determine the extent and intent of all procedures. PTCA with stent for dilation is done for a different indication than in situ coronary venous arterialization.
	AND	
	MCC condition	*See* appendix B.
233	Coronary artery bypass procedure with arterial or vein graft	*See* DRG 231.
	AND	
	Cardiac catheterization	Measurement of cardiac sampling and pressure (right, left, bilateral).
	Coronary angiography	
	OR	
	Open ablation procedures	Review operative report carefully to determine the extent of all procedures. Open ablation procedures in this DRG include destruction of coronary vein, atrial septum, right or left atrium, conduction mechanism, chordae tendineae, right or left pulmonary vein, or left atrial appendage, via an Open approach.
	AND	
	MCC condition	*See* appendix B.
235	Coronary artery bypass procedure with arterial or vein graft	*See* DRG 231.
	AND	
	MCC condition	*See* appendix B.
266	Transapical percutaneous transcatheter aortic, mitral, or pulmonary valve replacement or percutaneous endovascular transcatheter aortic, mitral, or pulmonary valve replacement (TAVR, TAVI)	In transcatheter valve replacements, a bioprosthetic valve made of bovine (cow) pericardium and supported with a metal stent, is inserted via catheter through the femoral artery (percutaneous endovascular approach) or through the apex of the heart by means of a minor thoracotomy incision between the ribs (percutaneous transapical approach). The bioprosthetic valve is placed on the balloon catheter, positioned directly inside the diseased valve, and the balloon is inflated to secure the valve in place. Approach for an aortic, mitral, or pulmonary valve replacement may be percutaneous transapical ***OR*** percutaneous endovascular. Angioplasty is not reported separately.
	OR	
	Transcatheter aortic, mitral, pulmonary, or tricuspid valve supplement	Percutaneous approach.
	AND	
	MCC condition	*See* appendix B.

DRG 229 Other Cardiothoracic Procedures without MCC

RW 3.1796

Potential DRGs

216	Cardiac Valve and Other Major Cardiothoracic Procedures with Cardiac Catheterization with MCC	9.7053
217	Cardiac Valve and Other Major Cardiothoracic Procedures with Cardiac Catheterization with CC	6.3653
218	Cardiac Valve and Other Major Cardiothoracic Procedures with Cardiac Catheterization without CC/MCC	5.6967
219	Cardiac Valve and Other Major Cardiothoracic Procedures without Cardiac Catheterization with MCC	7.7112
220	Cardiac Valve and Other Major Cardiothoracic Procedures without Cardiac Catheterization with CC	5.2446
228	Other Cardiothoracic Procedures with MCC	5.0387
231	Coronary Bypass with PTCA with MCC	8.1152
232	Coronary Bypass with PTCA without MCC	5.9486
233	Coronary Bypass with Cardiac Catheterization or Open Ablation with MCC	7.7996
234	Coronary Bypass with Cardiac Catheterization or Open Ablation without MCC	5.1979
235	Coronary Bypass without Cardiac Catheterization with MCC	5.8806
236	Coronary Bypass without Cardiac Catheterization without MCC	4.0412
266	Endovascular Cardiac Valve Replacement and Supplement Procedures with MCC	6.2461
267	Endovascular Cardiac Valve Replacement and Supplement Procedures without MCC	4.8802

DRG	PDx/SDx/Procedure	Tips
216	Open valvuloplasty without replacement	Dilation with or without a device, or release. Approach must be open. The objective of root operation Dilation is to enlarge the diameter of a tubular body part or orifice. If a device remains at the end of the procedure to maintain the new diameter, this is an integral part of the procedure and captured with a sixth-character device value. If the sole objective of the procedure is freeing a body part without cutting the body part, the root operation is Release. In the root operation Release, the body part value coded is the body part being freed, not the tissue being manipulated or cut to free the body part.
	OR	
	Cardiac valve replacement, repair, supplement	Open or percutaneous endoscopic approach only.
	AND	
	Cardiac catheterization	Measurement of cardiac sampling and pressure (right, left, bilateral).
	Coronary angiography	
	AND	
	MCC condition	*See* appendix B.
217	Open valvuloplasty without replacement	*See* DRG 216.
	OR	
	Cardiac valve replacement, repair, supplement	*See* DRG 216.
	AND	
	Cardiac catheterization	*See* DRG 216.
	Coronary angiography	
	AND	
	CC condition	*See* appendix B.
218	Open valvuloplasty without replacement	*See* DRG 216.
	OR	
	Cardiac valve replacement, repair, supplement	*See* DRG 216.
	AND	
	Cardiac catheterization	*See* DRG 216.
	Coronary angiography	
219	Open valvuloplasty without replacement	*See* DRG 216.
	OR	
	Cardiac valve replacement, repair, supplement	*See* DRG 216.
	AND	
	MCC condition	*See* appendix B.
220	Open valvuloplasty without replacement	*See* DRG 216.
	OR	
	Cardiac valve replacement, repair, supplement	*See* DRG 216.
	AND	
	CC condition	*See* appendix B.
228	MCC condition	*See* appendix B.

DRG 229 (Continued)

DRG	PDx/SDx/Procedure	Tips
231	Coronary artery bypass procedure with arterial or vein graft	Review operative report carefully to determine the extent of all procedures. DRG 228 includes percutaneous or percutaneous endoscopic in situ coronary venous arterialization, in which the blood flow is rerouted by inserting an intraluminal tubular device similar to a stent, bypassing the coronary artery blockage using a neighboring coronary vein. DRG 231 includes traditional coronary bypass performed with artery or vein grafts using Open or Percutaneous Endoscopic approach.
	AND	
	PTCA—Dilation with or without intraluminal device(s)	Review operative report carefully to determine the extent and intent of all procedures. PTCA with stent for dilation is done for a different indication than in situ coronary venous arterialization.
	AND	
	MCC condition	*See* appendix B.
232	Coronary artery bypass procedure with arterial or vein graft	*See* DRG 231.
	AND	
	PTCA—Dilation with or without intraluminal device(s)	*See* DRG 231.
233	Coronary artery bypass procedure with arterial or vein graft	*See* DRG 231.
	AND	
	Cardiac catheterization	Measurement of cardiac sampling and pressure (right, left, bilateral).
	Coronary angiography	
	OR	
	Open ablation procedures	Review operative report carefully to determine the extent of all procedures. Open ablation procedures in this DRG include destruction of coronary vein, atrial septum, right or left atrium, conduction mechanism, chordae tendineae, right or left pulmonary vein, or left atrial appendage, via an Open approach.
	AND	
	MCC condition	*See* appendix B.
234	Coronary artery bypass procedure with arterial or vein graft	*See* DRG 231.
	AND	
	Cardiac catheterization	*See* DRG 233.
	Coronary angiography	
	OR	
	Open ablation procedures	*See* DRG 233.
235	Coronary artery bypass procedure with arterial or vein graft	*See* DRG 231.
	AND	
	MCC condition	*See* appendix B.
236	Coronary artery bypass procedure with arterial or vein graft	*See* DRG 231.
266	Transapical percutaneous transcatheter aortic, mitral, or pulmonary valve replacement or percutaneous endovascular transcatheter aortic, mitral, or pulmonary valve replacement (TAVR, TAVI)	In transcatheter valve replacements, a bioprosthetic valve made of bovine (cow) pericardium and supported with a metal stent, is inserted via catheter through the femoral artery (percutaneous endovascular approach) or through the apex of the heart by means of a minor thoracotomy incision between the ribs (percutaneous transapical approach). The bioprosthetic valve is placed on the balloon catheter, positioned directly inside the diseased valve, and the balloon is inflated to secure the valve in place. Approach for an aortic, mitral, or pulmonary valve replacement may be percutaneous transapical ***OR*** percutaneous endovascular. Angioplasty is not reported separately.
	OR	
	Transcatheter aortic, mitral, pulmonary, or tricuspid valve supplement	Percutaneous approach.
	AND	
	MCC condition	*See* appendix B.
267	Transapical percutaneous transcatheter aortic, mitral, or pulmonary valve replacement or percutaneous endovascular transcatheter aortic, mitral, or pulmonary valve replacement (TAVR, TAVI)	*See* DRG 266.
	OR	
	Transcatheter aortic, mitral, pulmonary, or tricuspid valve supplement	*See* DRG 266.

DRG 231 Coronary Bypass with PTCA with MCC — RW 8.1152

No Potential DRGs

DRG 232 Coronary Bypass with PTCA without MCC — RW 5.9486

Potential DRGs

231 Coronary Bypass with PTCA with MCC 8.1152

DRG	PDx/SDx/Procedure	Tips
231	MCC condition	*See* appendix B.

Optimizing Tips

DRG 233 Coronary Bypass with Cardiac Catheterization or Open Ablation with MCC — RW 7.7996

Potential DRGs

216	Cardiac Valve and Other Major Cardiothoracic Procedures with Cardiac Catheterization with MCC	9.7053
231	Coronary Bypass with PTCA with MCC	8.1152

DRG	PDx/SDx/Procedure	Tips
216	Open valvuloplasty without replacement	Dilation with or without a device, or release. Approach must be open. The objective of root operation Dilation is to enlarge the diameter of a tubular body part or orifice. If a device remains at the end of the procedure to maintain the new diameter, this is an integral part of the procedure and captured with a sixth-character device value. If the sole objective of the procedure is freeing a body part without cutting the body part, the root operation is Release. In the root operation Release, the body part value coded is the body part being freed, not the tissue being manipulated or cut to free the body part.
	OR	
	Cardiac valve replacement, repair, supplement	Open or percutaneous endoscopic approach only.
	AND	
	Cardiac catheterization	Measurement of cardiac sampling and pressure (right, left, bilateral).
	Coronary angiography	
	AND	
	MCC condition	*See* appendix B.
231	PTCA procedure	Dilation with or without intraluminal device(s).
	AND	
	MCC condition	*See* appendix B.

DRG 234 Coronary Bypass with Cardiac Catheterization or Open Ablation without MCC — RW 5.1979

Potential DRGs

216	Cardiac Valve and Other Major Cardiothoracic Procedures with Cardiac Catheterization with MCC	9.7053
217	Cardiac Valve and Other Major Cardiothoracic Procedures with Cardiac Catheterization with CC	6.3653
231	Coronary Bypass with PTCA with MCC	8.1152
232	Coronary Bypass with PTCA without MCC	5.9486
233	Coronary Bypass with Cardiac Catheterization or Open Ablation with MCC	7.7996

DRG	PDx/SDx/Procedure	Tips
216	Open valvuloplasty without replacement	Dilation with or without a device, or release. Approach must be open. The objective of root operation Dilation is to enlarge the diameter of a tubular body part or orifice. If a device remains at the end of the procedure to maintain the new diameter, this is an integral part of the procedure and captured with a sixth-character device value. If the sole objective of the procedure is freeing a body part without cutting the body part, the root operation is Release. In the root operation Release, the body part value coded is the body part being freed, not the tissue being manipulated or cut to free the body part.
	OR	
	Cardiac valve replacement, repair, supplement	Open or percutaneous endoscopic approach only.
	AND	
	Cardiac catheterization	Measurement of cardiac sampling and pressure (right, left, bilateral).
	Coronary angiography	
	AND	
	MCC condition	*See* appendix B.
217	Open valvuloplasty without replacement	*See* DRG 216.
	OR	
	Cardiac valve replacement, repair, supplement	*See* DRG 216.
	AND	
	Cardiac catheterization	*See* DRG 216.
	Coronary angiography	
	AND	
	CC condition	*See* appendix B.
231	PTCA procedure	Dilation with or without intraluminal device(s).
	AND	
	MCC condition	*See* appendix B.
232	PTCA procedure	Dilation with or without intraluminal device(s).
233	MCC condition	*See* appendix B.

DRG 235 Coronary Bypass without Cardiac Catheterization with MCC RW 5.8806

Potential DRGs

216	Cardiac Valve and Other Major Cardiothoracic Procedures with Cardiac Catheterization with MCC	9.7053
219	Cardiac Valve and Other Major Cardiothoracic Procedures without Cardiac Catheterization with MCC	7.7112
231	Coronary Bypass with PTCA with MCC	8.1152
233	Coronary Bypass with Cardiac Catheterization or Open Ablation with MCC	7.7996

DRG	PDx/SDx/Procedure	Tips
216	Open valvuloplasty without replacement	Dilation with or without a device, or release. Approach must be open. The objective of root operation Dilation is to enlarge the diameter of a tubular body part or orifice. If a device remains at the end of the procedure to maintain the new diameter, this is an integral part of the procedure and captured with a sixth-character device value. If the sole objective of the procedure is freeing a body part without cutting the body part, the root operation is Release. In the root operation Release, the body part value coded is the body part being freed, not the tissue being manipulated or cut to free the body part.
	OR	
	Cardiac valve replacement, repair, supplement	Open or percutaneous endoscopic approach only.
	AND	
	Cardiac catheterization	Measurement of cardiac sampling and pressure (right, left, bilateral).
	Coronary angiography	
	AND	
	MCC condition	*See* appendix B.
219	Open valvuloplasty without replacement	*See* DRG 216.
	OR	
	Cardiac valve replacement, repair, supplement	*See* DRG 216.
	AND	
	MCC condition	*See* appendix B.
231	PTCA procedure	Dilation with or without intraluminal device(s).
	AND	
	MCC condition	*See* appendix B.
233	Cardiac catheterization	Measurement of cardiac sampling and pressure (right, left, bilateral).
	Coronary angiography	
	AND	
	MCC condition	*See* appendix B.

DRG 236 Coronary Bypass without Cardiac Catheterization without MCC

RW 4.0412

Potential DRGs

216	Cardiac Valve and Other Major Cardiothoracic Procedures with Cardiac Catheterization with MCC	9.7053
217	Cardiac Valve and Other Major Cardiothoracic Procedures with Cardiac Catheterization with CC	6.3653
218	Cardiac Valve and Other Major Cardiothoracic Procedures with Cardiac Catheterization without CC/MCC	5.6967
219	Cardiac Valve and Other Major Cardiothoracic Procedures without Cardiac Catheterization with MCC	7.7112
220	Cardiac Valve and Other Major Cardiothoracic Procedures without Cardiac Catheterization with CC	5.2446
221	Cardiac Valve and Other Major Cardiothoracic Procedures without Cardiac Catheterization without CC/MCC	4.6486
231	Coronary Bypass with PTCA with MCC	8.1152
232	Coronary Bypass with PTCA without MCC	5.9486
233	Coronary Bypass with Cardiac Catheterization or Open Ablation with MCC	7.7996
234	Coronary Bypass with Cardiac Catheterization or Open Ablation without MCC	5.1979
235	Coronary Bypass without Cardiac Catheterization with MCC	5.8806

DRG	PDx/SDx/Procedure	Tips
216	Open valvuloplasty without replacement	Dilation with or without a device, or release. Approach must be open. The objective of root operation Dilation is to enlarge the diameter of a tubular body part or orifice. If a device remains at the end of the procedure to maintain the new diameter, this is an integral part of the procedure and captured with a sixth-character device value. If the sole objective of the procedure is freeing a body part without cutting the body part, the root operation is Release. In the root operation Release, the body part value coded is the body part being freed, not the tissue being manipulated or cut to free the body part.
	OR	
	Cardiac valve replacement, repair, supplement	Open or percutaneous endoscopic approach only.
	AND	
	Cardiac catheterization	Measurement of cardiac sampling and pressure (right, left, bilateral).
	Coronary angiography	
	AND	
	MCC condition	*See* appendix B.
217	Open valvuloplasty without replacement	*See* DRG 216.
	OR	
	Cardiac valve replacement, repair, supplement	*See* DRG 216.
	AND	
	Cardiac catheterization	*See* DRG 216.
	Coronary angiography	
	AND	
	CC condition	*See* appendix B.
218	Open valvuloplasty without replacement	*See* DRG 216.
	OR	
	Cardiac valve replacement, repair, supplement	*See* DRG 216.
	AND	
	Cardiac catheterization	*See* DRG 216.
	Coronary angiography	
219	Open valvuloplasty without replacement	*See* DRG 216.
	OR	
	Cardiac valve replacement, repair, supplement	*See* DRG 216.
	AND	
	MCC condition	*See* appendix B.
220	Open valvuloplasty without replacement	*See* DRG 216.
	OR	
	Cardiac valve replacement, repair, supplement	*See* DRG 216.
	AND	
	CC condition	*See* appendix B.
221	Open valvuloplasty without replacement	*See* DRG 216.
	OR	
	Cardiac valve replacement, repair, supplement	*See* DRG 216.
231	PTCA procedure	Dilation with or without intraluminal device(s).
	AND	
	MCC condition	*See* appendix B.
232	PTCA procedure	Dilation with or without intraluminal device(s).
233	Cardiac catheterization	Measurement of cardiac sampling and pressure (right, left, bilateral).
	Coronary angiography	
	AND	
	MCC condition	*See* appendix B.
234	Cardiac catheterization	*See* DRG 233.
	Coronary angiography	
235	MCC condition	*See* appendix B.

DRG 239 Amputation for Circulatory System Disorders Except Upper Limb and Toe with MCC — RW 4.8068

No Potential DRGs

DRG 240 Amputation for Circulatory System Disorders Except Upper Limb and Toe with CC — RW 2.8092

Potential DRGs

239	Amputation for Circulatory System Disorders Except Upper Limb and Toe with MCC	4.8068
474	Amputation for Musculoskeletal System and Connective Tissue Disorders with MCC	4.3028
616	Amputation of Lower Limb for Endocrine, Nutritional, and Metabolic Disorders with MCC	3.9577

DRG	PDx/SDx/Procedure	Tips
239	MCC condition	*See* appendix B.
474	Amputation for musculoskeletal system/ connective tissue disorders, such as: Osteomyelitis	Review the medical record carefully for documentation of fever, malaise, localized bone pain, bone penetrated by trauma or surgery, history of diabetes, and previous treatment of surgical debridements. Review laboratory reports for elevated ESR and C-reactive protein. Review radiology reports for CT scans, bone scans, and bone biopsies. Review physician orders and nurse's notes for antibiotic treatment.
	AND	
	MCC condition	*See* appendix B.
616	Diabetes with certain manifestations	Diabetes mellitus with manifestations such as: hyperosmolarity without nonketotic hyperglycemic-hyperosmolar coma (NKHHC), hyperosmolarity with coma, ketoacidosis with/without coma, arthropathy, foot or other skin ulcer, hypoglycemia with/without coma, hyperglycemia, and other specified complications. According to ICD-10-CM guidelines, the classification presumes a causal relationship between diabetes and certain associated manifestations and/or conditions when these terms are linked by the term "with" in the alphabetic index (either under a main term or subterm). These conditions should be coded as related to the diabetes unless the documentation clearly states the conditions are unrelated, in which case they may be coded separately. These conditions do not require provider documentation linking them to diabetes. Review the record and/or query the physician if it is unclear whether a condition is related to diabetes mellitus or the ICD-10-CM classification does not provide instruction.
	AND	
	Lower limb amputation	
	AND	
	MCC condition	*See* appendix B.

DRG 241 Amputation for Circulatory System Disorders Except Upper Limb and Toe without CC/MCC — RW 1.3898

Potential DRGs

239	Amputation for Circulatory System Disorders Except Upper Limb and Toe with MCC	4.8068
240	Amputation for Circulatory System Disorders Except Upper Limb and Toe with CC	2.8092
474	Amputation for Musculoskeletal System and Connective Tissue Disorders with MCC	4.3028
475	Amputation for Musculoskeletal System and Connective Tissue Disorders with CC	2.1447
616	Amputation of Lower Limb for Endocrine, Nutritional, and Metabolic Disorders with MCC	3.9577
617	Amputation of Lower Limb for Endocrine, Nutritional, and Metabolic Disorders with CC	1.9845

DRG	PDx/SDx/Procedure	Tips
239	MCC condition	*See* appendix B.
240	CC condition	*See* appendix B.
474	Amputation for musculoskeletal system/ connective tissue disorders, such as: Osteomyelitis	Review the medical record carefully for documentation of fever, malaise, localized bone pain, bone penetrated by trauma or surgery, history of diabetes, and previous treatment of surgical debridements. Review laboratory reports for elevated ESR and C-reactive protein. Review radiology reports for CT scans, bone scans, and bone biopsies. Review physician orders and nurse's notes for antibiotic treatment.
	AND	
	MCC condition	*See* appendix B.
475	Amputation for musculoskeletal system/ connective tissue disorders, such as: Osteomyelitis	*See* DRG 474.
	AND	
	CC condition	*See* appendix B.
616	Diabetes with certain manifestations	Diabetes mellitus with manifestations such as: hyperosmolarity without nonketotic hyperglycemic-hyperosmolar coma (NKHHC), hyperosmolarity with coma, ketoacidosis with/without coma, arthropathy, foot or other skin ulcer, hypoglycemia with/without coma, hyperglycemia, and other specified complications. According to ICD-10-CM guidelines, the classification presumes a causal relationship between diabetes and certain associated manifestations and/or conditions when these terms are linked by the term "with" in the alphabetic index (either under a main term or subterm). These conditions should be coded as related to the diabetes unless the documentation clearly states the conditions are unrelated, in which case they may be coded separately. These conditions do not require provider documentation linking them to diabetes. Review the record and/or query the physician if it is unclear whether a condition is related to diabetes mellitus or the ICD-10-CM classification does not provide instruction.
	AND	
	Lower limb amputation	
	AND	
	MCC condition	*See* appendix B.
617	Diabetes with certain manifestations	*See* DRG 616.
	AND	
	Lower limb amputation	
	AND	
	CC condition	*See* appendix B.

DRG 242 Permanent Cardiac Pacemaker Implant with MCC — RW 3.4551

Potential DRGs

228	Other Cardiothoracic Procedures with MCC	5.0387
275	Cardiac Defibrillator Implant with Cardiac Catheterization and MCC	7.0358
276	Cardiac Defibrillator Implant with MCC	6.2102

DRG	PDx/SDx/Procedure	Tips
228	Leadless pacemaker insertion	Review the operative report carefully. Leadless or transcatheter pacemakers do not require a subcutaneous pocket or a tunneled lead. The device is placed within the heart chamber (intracardiac), typically the right ventricle via a peripheral vessel.
	AND	
	MCC condition	*See* appendix B.
275	Cardiac defibrillator implant	Two codes must be reported for insertion of the generator and insertion of the lead(s).
	AND	
	Cardiac catheterization	Measurement of cardiac sampling and pressure (right, left, bilateral).
	Coronary angiography	
	AND	
	MCC condition	*See* appendix B.
276	Cardiac defibrillator implant	*See* DRG 275.
	AND	
	MCC condition	*See* appendix B.

DRG 243 Permanent Cardiac Pacemaker Implant with CC RW 2.2776

Potential DRGs

228	Other Cardiothoracic Procedures with MCC	5.0387
229	Other Cardiothoracic Procedures without MCC	3.1796
242	Permanent Cardiac Pacemaker Implant with MCC	3.4551
275	Cardiac Defibrillator Implant with Cardiac Catheterization and MCC	7.0358
276	Cardiac Defibrillator Implant with MCC	6.2102

DRG	PDx/SDx/Procedure	Tips
228	Leadless pacemaker insertion	Review the operative report carefully. Leadless or transcatheter pacemakers do not require a subcutaneous pocket or a tunneled lead. The device is placed within the heart chamber (intracardiac), typically the right ventricle via a peripheral vessel.
	AND	
	MCC condition	*See* appendix B.
229	Leadless pacemaker insertion	*See* DRG 228.
242	MCC condition	*See* appendix B.
275	Cardiac defibrillator implant	Two codes must be reported—insertion of generator and lead(s).
	AND	
	Cardiac catheterization	Measurement of cardiac sampling and pressure (right, left, bilateral).
	Coronary angiography	
	AND	
	MCC condition	*See* appendix B.
276	Cardiac defibrillator implant	*See* DRG 275.
	AND	
	MCC condition	*See* appendix B.

DRG 244 Permanent Cardiac Pacemaker Implant without CC/MCC RW 1.8295

Potential DRGs

228	Other Cardiothoracic Procedures with MCC	5.0387
229	Other Cardiothoracic Procedures without MCC	3.1796
242	Permanent Cardiac Pacemaker Implant with MCC	3.4551
243	Permanent Cardiac Pacemaker Implant with CC	2.2776
275	Cardiac Defibrillator Implant with Cardiac Catheterization and MCC	7.0358
276	Cardiac Defibrillator Implant with MCC	6.2102
277	Cardiac Defibrillator Implant without MCC	4.7824

DRG	PDx/SDx/Procedure	Tips
228	Leadless pacemaker insertion	Review the operative report carefully. Leadless or transcatheter pacemakers do not require a subcutaneous pocket or a tunneled lead. The device is placed within the heart chamber (intracardiac), typically the right ventricle via a peripheral vessel.
	AND	
	MCC condition	*See* appendix B.
229	Leadless pacemaker insertion	*See* DRG 228.
242	MCC condition	*See* appendix B.
243	CC condition	*See* appendix B.
275	Cardiac defibrillator implant	Two codes must be reported—insertion of generator and lead(s).
	AND	
	Cardiac catheterization	Measurement of cardiac sampling and pressure (right, left, bilateral).
	Coronary angiography	
	AND	
	MCC condition	*See* appendix B.
276	Cardiac defibrillator implant	*See* DRG 275.
	AND	
	MCC condition	*See* appendix B.
277	Cardiac defibrillator implant	*See* DRG 275.

DRG 245 AICD Generator Procedures RW 4.5314

Potential DRGs

275	Cardiac Defibrillator Implant with Cardiac Catheterization and MCC	7.0358
276	Cardiac Defibrillator Implant with MCC	6.2102
277	Cardiac Defibrillator Implant without MCC	4.7824

DRG	PDx/SDx/Procedure	Tips
275	Cardiac defibrillator implant	Two codes must be reported—insertion of generator and lead(s).
	AND	
	Cardiac catheterization	Measurement of cardiac sampling and pressure (right, left, bilateral).
	Coronary angiography	
	AND	
	MCC condition	*See* appendix B.
276	Cardiac defibrillator implant	*See* DRG 275.
	AND	
	MCC condition	*See* appendix B.
277	Cardiac defibrillator implant	*See* DRG 275.

DRG 250 Percutaneous Cardiovascular Procedures without Intraluminal Device with MCC RW 2.3508

Potential DRGs

228	Other Cardiothoracic Procedures with MCC	5.0387
231	Coronary Bypass with PTCA with MCC	8.1152
321	Percutaneous Cardiovascular Procedures with Intraluminal Device with MCC or 4+ Arteries/Intraluminal Devices	2.8747
325	Coronary Intravascular Lithotripsy without Intraluminal Device	2.6443

DRG	PDx/SDx/Procedure	Tips
228	Supplement of atrial or ventricular septum	Review interventional radiology reports.
		Code any associated cardiac catheterization, diagnostic ultrasound of heart or esophagoscopy.
	Repair of coronary artery	
	AND	
	MCC condition	*See* appendix B.
231	Coronary artery bypass with arterial or vein graft	Open or percutaneous endoscopic approach.
	AND	
	PTCA	Dilation with or without intraluminal device(s).
	AND	
	MCC condition	*See* appendix B.
321	Insertion of intraluminal device	Device may be drug-eluting or non-drug-eluting.
	AND	
	MCC condition	*See* appendix B.
	OR	
	Procedures on four or more arteries or placement of four or more intraluminal devices	
325	Coronary intravascular lithotripsy	The objective of the root operation Fragmentation is to break solid matter within a body part into pieces. The pieces are not removed.
	AND	
	Dilation of coronary artery	

DRG 251 Percutaneous Cardiovascular Procedures without Intraluminal Device without MCC RW 1.5869

Potential DRGs

228	Other Cardiothoracic Procedures with MCC	5.0387
229	Other Cardiothoracic Procedures without MCC	3.1796
231	Coronary Bypass with PTCA with MCC	8.1152
232	Coronary Bypass with PTCA without MCC	5.9486
250	Percutaneous Cardiovascular Procedures without Intraluminal Device with MCC	2.3508
321	Percutaneous Cardiovascular Procedures with Intraluminal Device with MCC or 4+ Arteries/Intraluminal Devices	2.8747
322	Percutaneous Cardiovascular Procedures with Intraluminal Device without MCC	1.8234
325	Coronary Intravascular Lithotripsy without Intraluminal Device	2.6443

DRG	PDx/SDx/Procedure	Tips
228	Supplement of atrial or ventricular septum	Review interventional radiology reports.
		Code any associated cardiac catheterization, diagnostic ultrasound of heart or esophagoscopy.
	Repair of coronary artery	
	AND	
	MCC condition	*See* appendix B.
229	Supplement of atrial or ventricular septum	*See* DRG 228.
	Repair of coronary artery	
231	Coronary artery bypass with arterial or vein graft	Open or percutaneous endoscopic approach.
	AND	
	PTCA	Dilation with or without intraluminal device(s).
	AND	
	MCC condition	*See* appendix B.
232	Coronary artery bypass with arterial or vein graft	Open or percutaneous endoscopic approach.
	AND	
	PTCA	Dilation with or without intraluminal device(s).
250	MCC condition	*See* appendix B.
321	Insertion of intraluminal device	Device may be drug-eluting or non-drug-eluting.
	AND	
	MCC condition	*See* appendix B.
	OR	
	Procedures on four or more arteries or placement of four or more intraluminal devices	
322	Insertion of intraluminal device	*See* DRG 322.
325	Coronary intravascular lithotripsy	The objective of the root operation Fragmentation is to break solid matter within a body part into pieces. The pieces are not removed.
	AND	
	Dilation of coronary artery	

DRG 252 Other Vascular Procedures with MCC — RW 3.3538

Potential DRGs

268	Aortic and Heart Assist Procedures Except Pulsation Balloon with MCC	6.8547
270	Other Major Cardiovascular Procedures with MCC	5.0569
278	Ultrasound Accelerated and Other Thrombolysis of Peripheral Vascular Structures with MCC	4.4604

DRG	PDx/SDx/Procedure	Tips
268	Endovascular abdominal aortic graft implantation	Endovascular aneurysm repair (EVAR) procedure with insertion of a stent graft into the artery (intraluminal) is reported with root operation Restriction "partially closing an orifice or the lumen of a tubular body part" as the intent is to narrow the artery, not close it completely (Root operation Occlusion "completely closing an orifice or the lumen of a tubular body part"). Endovascular stent grafts are classified as "Intraluminal Devices" in the ICD-10-PCS Definitions of Character 6 – Device and the ICD-10-PCS Device Key. A supplemental procedure to repair an abdominal aortic aneurysm involves placement of a biologic or synthetic graft to physically reinforce and/or augment the weakened and bulging section of the aorta.
	AND	
	MCC condition	*See* appendix B.
270	Embolization or occlusion of head and neck vessels	If the intent of the procedure is to close the vessel completely, report root operation Occlusion "completely closing an orifice or the lumen of a tubular body part."
	AND	
	MCC condition	*See* appendix B.
278	Peripheral intravascular lithotripsy	The objective of the root operation Fragmentation is to break solid matter within a body part into pieces. The pieces are not removed. This procedure may be performed prior to dilation of the vessel. NOTE: When dilation and fragmentation are performed on the same body part, the fragmentation code takes precedence and groups to DRGs 278–279, based on the surgical hierarchy.
	AND	
	MCC condition	*See* appendix B.

DRG 253 Other Vascular Procedures with CC — RW 2.5511

Potential DRGs

252	Other Vascular Procedures with MCC	3.3538
268	Aortic and Heart Assist Procedures Except Pulsation Balloon with MCC	6.8547
269	Aortic and Heart Assist Procedures Except Pulsation Balloon without MCC	4.1586
270	Other Major Cardiovascular Procedures with MCC	5.0569
271	Other Major Cardiovascular Procedures with CC	3.4562
278	Ultrasound Accelerated and Other Thrombolysis of Peripheral Vascular Structures with MCC	4.4604
279	Ultrasound Accelerated and Other Thrombolysis of Peripheral Vascular Structures without MCC	3.2006

DRG	PDx/SDx/Procedure	Tips
252	MCC condition	*See* appendix B.
268	Endovascular abdominal aortic graft implantation	Endovascular aneurysm repair (EVAR) procedure with insertion of a stent graft into the artery (intraluminal) is reported with root operation Restriction "partially closing an orifice or the lumen of a tubular body part" as the intent is to narrow the artery, not close it completely (Root operation Occlusion "completely closing an orifice or the lumen of a tubular body part"). Endovascular stent grafts are classified as "Intraluminal Devices" in the ICD-10-PCS Definitions of Character 6 – Device and the ICD-10-PCS Device Key. A supplemental procedure to repair an abdominal aortic aneurysm involves placement of a biologic or synthetic graft to physically reinforce and/or augment the weakened and bulging section of the aorta.
	AND	
	MCC condition	*See* appendix B.
269	Endovascular abdominal aortic graft implantation	*See* DRG 268.
270	Embolization or occlusion of head and neck vessels	If the intent of the procedure is to close the vessel completely, report root operation Occlusion "completely closing an orifice or the lumen of a tubular body part."
	AND	
	MCC condition	*See* appendix B.

DRG 253 (Continued)

DRG	PDx/SDx/Procedure	Tips
271	Embolization or occlusion of head and neck vessels	*See* DRG 27Ø.
	AND	
	CC condition	*See* appendix B.
278	Peripheral intravascular lithotripsy	The objective of the root operation Fragmentation is to break solid matter within a body part into pieces. The pieces are not removed. This procedure may be performed prior to dilation of the vessel. NOTE: When dilation and fragmentation are performed on the same body part, the fragmentation code takes precedence and groups to DRGs 278–279, based on the surgical hierarchy.
	AND	
	MCC condition	*See* appendix B.
279	Peripheral intravascular lithotripsy	*See* DRG 278.

DRG 254 Other Vascular Procedures without CC/MCC RW 1.7351

Potential DRGs

252	Other Vascular Procedures with MCC	3.3538
253	Other Vascular Procedures with CC	2.5511
268	Aortic and Heart Assist Procedures Except Pulsation Balloon with MCC	6.8547
269	Aortic and Heart Assist Procedures Except Pulsation Balloon without MCC	4.1586
270	Other Major Cardiovascular Procedures with MCC	5.0569
271	Other Major Cardiovascular Procedures with CC	3.4562
272	Other Major Cardiovascular Procedures without CC/MCC	2.4395
278	Ultrasound Accelerated and Other Thrombolysis of Peripheral Vascular Structures with MCC	4.4604
279	Ultrasound Accelerated and Other Thrombolysis of Peripheral Vascular Structures without MCC	3.2006

DRG	PDx/SDx/Procedure	Tips
252	MCC condition	*See* appendix B.
253	CC condition	*See* appendix B.
268	Endovascular abdominal aortic graft implantation	Endovascular aneurysm repair (EVAR) procedure with insertion of a stent graft into the artery (intraluminal) is reported with root operation Restriction "partially closing an orifice or the lumen of a tubular body part" as the intent is to narrow the artery, not close it completely (Root operation Occlusion "completely closing an orifice or the lumen of a tubular body part"). Endovascular stent grafts are classified as "Intraluminal Devices" in the ICD-10-PCS Definitions of Character 6 – Device and the ICD-10-PCS Device Key. A supplemental procedure to repair an abdominal aortic aneurysm involves placement of a biologic or synthetic graft to physically reinforce and/or augment the weakened and bulging section of the aorta.
	AND	
	MCC condition	*See* appendix B.
269	Endovascular abdominal aortic graft implantation	*See* DRG 268.
270	Embolization or occlusion of head and neck vessels	If the intent of the procedure is to close the vessel completely, report root operation Occlusion "completely closing an orifice or the lumen of a tubular body part."
	AND	
	MCC condition	*See* appendix B.
271	Embolization or occlusion of head and neck vessels	*See* DRG 270.
	AND	
	CC condition	*See* appendix B.
272	Embolization or occlusion of head and neck vessels	*See* DRG 270.
278	Peripheral intravascular lithotripsy	The objective of the root operation Fragmentation is to break solid matter within a body part into pieces. The pieces are not removed. This procedure may be performed prior to dilation of the vessel. NOTE: When dilation and fragmentation are performed on the same body part, the fragmentation code takes precedence and groups to DRGs 278–279, based on the surgical hierarchy.
	AND	
	MCC condition	*See* appendix B.
279	Peripheral intravascular lithotripsy	*See* DRG 278.

DRG 255 Upper Limb and Toe Amputation for Circulatory System Disorders with MCC RW 2.7474

Potential DRGs

040	Peripheral/Cranial Nerve and Other Nervous System Procedures with MCC	3.8505
474	Amputation for Musculoskeletal System and Connective Tissue Disorders with MCC	4.3028
616	Amputation of Lower Limb for Endocrine, Nutritional, and Metabolic Disorders with MCC	3.9577
907	Other O.R. Procedures for Injuries with MCC	3.7195

DRG	PDx/SDx/Procedure	Tips
040	Nerve Injury NOS, Malfunctioning or adverse reaction to neuro device/graft, nervous system or CNS complication	Review the documentation carefully; code assignment is based on the provider's documentation of a relationship between the condition and the procedure. Unless the classification instructs otherwise, only when there is a clear cause-and-effect relationship between the care provided and the condition and the documentation indicates the condition is a complication, can the condition be coded as such. Query the provider for clarification if the relationship/complication is not clearly documented. See guideline I.B.16.
	AND	
	Toe amputation	
	AND	
	MCC condition	*See* appendix B.
474	Malignancy of bone, benign neoplasm of bone or soft tissue, arthropathies, osteomyelitis	
	AND	
	Upper limb amputation except finger or thumb	
	AND	
	MCC condition	*See* appendix B.
616	Diabetes with certain manifestations	Diabetes mellitus with manifestations such as: hyperosmolarity without nonketotic hyperglycemic-hyperosmolar coma (NKHHC), hyperosmolarity with coma, ketoacidosis with/without coma, arthropathy, foot or other skin ulcer, hypoglycemia with/without coma, hyperglycemia, and other specified complications. According to ICD-10-CM guidelines, the classification presumes a causal relationship between diabetes and certain associated manifestations and/or conditions when these terms are linked by the term "with" in the alphabetic index (either under a main term or subterm). These conditions should be coded as related to the diabetes unless the documentation clearly states the conditions are unrelated, in which case they may be coded separately. These conditions do not require provider documentation linking them to diabetes. Review the record and/or query the physician if it is unclear whether a condition is related to diabetes mellitus, or the ICD-10-CM classification does not provide instruction.
	AND	
	Lower limb amputation	
	AND	
	MCC condition	*See* appendix B.
907	Traumatic amputation of upper or lower limb, crushing injuries	
	AND	
	Upper limb amputation except finger or thumb	
	OR	
	Lower limb amputation except toes	
	AND	
	MCC condition	*See* appendix B.

DRG 256 Upper Limb and Toe Amputation for Circulatory System Disorders with CC RW 1.6397

Potential DRGs

040	Peripheral/Cranial Nerve and Other Nervous System Procedures with MCC	3.8505
041	Peripheral/Cranial Nerve and Other Nervous System Procedures with CC or Peripheral Neurostimulator	2.2307
255	Upper Limb and Toe Amputation for Circulatory System Disorders with MCC	2.7474
474	Amputation for Musculoskeletal System and Connective Tissue Disorders with MCC	4.3028
475	Amputation for Musculoskeletal System and Connective Tissue Disorders with CC	2.1447
616	Amputation of Lower Limb for Endocrine, Nutritional, and Metabolic Disorders with MCC	3.9577
617	Amputation of Lower Limb for Endocrine, Nutritional, and Metabolic Disorders with CC	1.9845
907	Other O.R. Procedures for Injuries with MCC	3.7195
908	Other O.R. Procedures for Injuries with CC	2.0041

DRG	PDx/SDx/Procedure	Tips
040	Nerve Injury NOS, Malfunctioning or adverse reaction to neuro device/graft, nervous system or CNS complication	Review the documentation carefully; code assignment is based on the provider's documentation of a relationship between the condition and the procedure. Unless the classification instructs otherwise, only when there is a clear cause-and-effect relationship between the care provided and the condition and the documentation indicates the condition is a complication, can the condition be coded as such. Query the provider for clarification if the relationship/complication is not clearly documented. See guideline I.B.16.
	AND	
	Toe amputation	
	AND	
	MCC condition	*See* appendix B.
041	Nerve Injury NOS, Malfunctioning or adverse reaction to neuro device/graft, nervous system or CNS complication	*See* DRG Ø4Ø.
	AND	
	Toe amputation	
	AND	
	CC condition	*See* appendix B.
	OR	
	Peripheral neurostimulator implant	
255	MCC condition	*See* appendix B.
474	Malignancy of bone, benign neoplasm of bone or soft tissue, arthropathies, osteomyelitis	
	AND	
	Upper limb amputation except finger or thumb	
	AND	
	MCC condition	*See* appendix B.
475	Malignancy of bone, benign neoplasm of bone or soft tissue, arthropathies, osteomyelitis	
	AND	
	Upper limb amputation except finger or thumb	
	AND	
	CC condition	*See* appendix B.
616	Diabetes with certain manifestations	Diabetes mellitus with manifestations such as: hyperosmolarity without nonketotic hyperglycemic-hyperosmolar coma (NKHHC), hyperosmolarity with coma, ketoacidosis with/without coma, arthropathy, foot or other skin ulcer, hypoglycemia with/without coma, hyperglycemia, and other specified complications. According to ICD-10-CM guidelines, the classification presumes a causal relationship between diabetes and certain associated manifestations and/or conditions when these terms are linked by the term "with" in the alphabetic index (either under a main term or subterm). These conditions should be coded as related to the diabetes unless the documentation clearly states the conditions are unrelated, in which case they may be coded separately. These conditions do not require provider documentation linking them to diabetes. Review the record and/or query the physician if it is unclear whether a condition is related to diabetes mellitus or the ICD-10-CM classification does not provide instruction.
	AND	
	Lower limb amputation	
	AND	
	MCC condition	*See* appendix B.
617	Diabetes with certain manifestations	*See* DRG 616.
	AND	
	Lower limb amputation	
	AND	
	CC condition	*See* appendix B.
907	Traumatic amputation of upper or lower limb, crushing injuries	
	AND	
	Upper limb amputation except finger or thumb	
	OR	
	Lower limb amputation except toes	
	AND	
	MCC condition	*See* appendix B.

DRG 256 (Continued)

DRG	PDx/SDx/Procedure	Tips
908	Traumatic amputation of upper or lower limb, crushing injuries	
	AND	
	Upper limb amputation except finger or thumb	
	OR	
	Lower limb amputation except toes	
	AND	
	CC condition	*See* appendix B.

DRG 257 Upper Limb and Toe Amputation for Circulatory System Disorders without CC/MCC

RW 0.9910

Potential DRGs

040	Peripheral/Cranial Nerve and Other Nervous System Procedures with MCC	3.8505
041	Peripheral/Cranial Nerve and Other Nervous System Procedures with CC or Peripheral Neurostimulator	2.2307
042	Peripheral/Cranial Nerve and Other Nervous System Procedures without CC/MCC	1.7398
255	Upper Limb and Toe Amputation for Circulatory System Disorders with MCC	2.7474
256	Upper Limb and Toe Amputation for Circulatory System Disorders with CC	1.6397
474	Amputation for Musculoskeletal System and Connective Tissue Disorders with MCC	4.3028
475	Amputation for Musculoskeletal System and Connective Tissue Disorders with CC	2.1447
503	Foot Procedures with MCC	2.6819
504	Foot Procedures with CC	1.7271
505	Foot Procedures without CC/MCC	1.7057
513	Hand or Wrist Procedures, Except Major Thumb or Joint Procedures with CC/MCC	1.6210
616	Amputation of Lower Limb for Endocrine, Nutritional, and Metabolic Disorders with MCC	3.9577
617	Amputation of Lower Limb for Endocrine, Nutritional, and Metabolic Disorders with CC	1.9845
618	Amputation of Lower Limb for Endocrine, Nutritional, and Metabolic Disorders without CC/MCC	1.1615
907	Other O.R. Procedures for Injuries with MCC	3.7195
908	Other O.R. Procedures for Injuries with CC	2.0041
909	Other O.R. Procedures for Injuries without CC/MCC	1.3563

DRG	PDx/SDx/Procedure	Tips
040	Nerve Injury NOS, Malfunctioning or adverse reaction to neuro device/graft, nervous system or CNS complication	Review the documentation carefully; code assignment is based on the provider's documentation of a relationship between the condition and the procedure. Unless the classification instructs otherwise, only when there is a clear cause-and-effect relationship between the care provided and the condition and the documentation indicates the condition is a complication, can the condition be coded as such. Query the provider for clarification if the relationship/complication is not clearly documented. See guideline I.B.16.
	AND	
	Toe amputation	
	AND	
	MCC condition	*See* appendix B.
041	Nerve Injury NOS, Malfunctioning or adverse reaction to neuro device/graft, nervous system or CNS complication	*See* DRG 040.
	AND	
	Toe amputation	
	AND	
	CC condition	*See* appendix B.
	OR	
	Peripheral neurostimulator implant	
042	Nerve Injury NOS, Malfunctioning or adverse reaction to neuro device/graft, nervous system or CNS complication	*See* DRG 040.
	AND	
	Toe amputation	
255	MCC condition	*See* appendix B.
256	CC condition	*See* appendix B.
474	Malignancy of bone, benign neoplasm of bone or soft tissue, arthropathies, osteomyelitis	
	AND	
	Upper limb amputation except finger or thumb	
	AND	
	MCC condition	*See* appendix B.
475	Malignancy of bone, benign neoplasm of bone or soft tissue, arthropathies, osteomyelitis	
	AND	
	Upper limb amputation except finger or thumb	
	AND	
	CC condition	*See* appendix B.
503	Principal diagnosis related to toe disorders and injuries NOT in MDC 5 (Non-circulatory)	
	AND	
	Toe amputation	
	AND	
	MCC condition	*See* appendix B.

DRG 257 (Continued)

DRG	PDx/SDx/Procedure	Tips
504	Principal diagnosis related to toe disorders and injuries NOT in MDC 5 (Non-circulatory)	
	AND	
	Toe amputation	
	AND	
	CC condition	*See* appendix B.
505	Principal diagnosis related to toe disorders and injuries NOT in MDC 5 (Non-circulatory)	
	AND	
	Toe amputation	
513	Diagnosis from MDC8 (Musculoskeletal)	
	AND	
	Amputation and disarticulation of finger or thumb	
	AND	
	CC/MCC condition	*See* appendix B.
616	Diabetes with certain manifestations	Diabetes mellitus with manifestations such as: hyperosmolarity without nonketotic hyperglycemic-hyperosmolar coma (NKHHC), hyperosmolarity with coma, ketoacidosis with/without coma, arthropathy, foot or other skin ulcer, hypoglycemia with/without coma, hyperglycemia, and other specified complications. According to ICD-10-CM guidelines, the classification presumes a causal relationship between diabetes and certain associated manifestations and/or conditions when these terms are linked by the term "with" in the alphabetic index (either under a main term or subterm). These conditions should be coded as related to the diabetes unless the documentation clearly states the conditions are unrelated, in which case they may be coded separately. These conditions do not require provider documentation linking them to diabetes. Review the record and/or query the physician if it is unclear whether a condition is related to diabetes mellitus or the ICD-10-CM classification does not provide instruction.
	AND	
	Lower limb amputation	
	AND	
	MCC condition	*See* appendix B.
617	Diabetes with certain manifestations	*See* DRG 616.
	AND	
	Lower limb amputation	
	AND	
	CC condition	*See* appendix B.
618	Diabetes with certain manifestations	*See* DRG 616.
	AND	
	Lower limb amputation	
907	Traumatic amputation of upper or lower limb, crushing injuries	
	AND	
	Upper limb amputation except finger or thumb	
	OR	
	Lower limb amputation except toes	
	AND	
	MCC condition	*See* appendix B.
908	Traumatic amputation of upper or lower limb, crushing injuries	
	AND	
	Upper limb amputation except finger or thumb	
	OR	
	Lower limb amputation except toes	
	AND	
	CC condition	*See* appendix B.
909	Traumatic amputation of upper or lower limb, crushing injuries	
	AND	
	Upper limb amputation except finger or thumb	
	OR	
	Lower limb amputation except toes	

DRG 258 Cardiac Pacemaker Device Replacement with MCC — RW 2.7086

Potential DRGs

228	Other Cardiothoracic Procedures with MCC	5.0387
242	Permanent Cardiac Pacemaker Implant with MCC	3.4551
245	AICD Generator Procedures	4.5314
275	Cardiac Defibrillator Implant with Cardiac Catheterization and MCC	7.0358
276	Cardiac Defibrillator Implant with MCC	6.2102

DRG	PDx/SDx/Procedure	Tips
228	Leadless pacemaker insertion or replacement	Review the operative report carefully. Leadless or transcatheter pacemakers do not require a subcutaneous pocket or a tunneled lead. The device is placed within the heart chamber (intracardiac), typically the right ventricle, via a peripheral vessel.
	AND	
	MCC condition	*See* appendix B.
242	Permanent pacemaker implant (initial)	At least two codes must be reported—for both the pacemaker and lead(s).
	AND	
	MCC condition	*See* appendix B.
245	AICD generator implant	
275	Cardiac defibrillator implant	Two codes must be reported—insertion of generator and lead(s).
	AND	
	Cardiac catheterization	Measurement of cardiac sampling and pressure (right, left, bilateral).
	Coronary angiography	
	AND	
	MCC condition	*See* appendix B.
276	Cardiac defibrillator implant	*See* DRG 275.
	AND	
	MCC condition	*See* appendix B.

DRG 259 Cardiac Pacemaker Device Replacement without MCC — RW 1.8666

Potential DRGs

228	Other Cardiothoracic Procedures with MCC	5.0387
229	Other Cardiothoracic Procedures without MCC	3.1796
242	Permanent Cardiac Pacemaker Implant with MCC	3.4551
243	Permanent Cardiac Pacemaker Implant with CC	2.2776
245	AICD Generator Procedures	4.5314
258	Cardiac Pacemaker Device Replacement with MCC	2.7086
275	Cardiac Defibrillator Implant with Cardiac Catheterization and MCC	7.0358
276	Cardiac Defibrillator Implant with MCC	6.2102
277	Cardiac Defibrillator Implant without MCC	4.7824

DRG	PDx/SDx/Procedure	Tips
228	Leadless pacemaker insertion, replacement, or revision	Review the operative report carefully. Leadless or transcatheter pacemakers do not require a subcutaneous pocket or a tunneled lead. The device is placed within the heart chamber (intracardiac), typically the right ventricle, via a peripheral vessel.
	AND	
	MCC condition	*See* appendix B.
229	Leadless pacemaker insertion	*See* DRG 228.
242	Permanent pacemaker implant (initial)	At least two codes must be reported—for both the pacemaker and lead(s).
	AND	
	MCC condition	*See* appendix B.
243	Permanent pacemaker implant (initial)	*See* DRG 242.
	AND	
	CC condition	*See* appendix B.
245	AICD generator implant	
258	MCC condition	*See* appendix B.
275	Cardiac defibrillator implant	Two codes must be reported—insertion of generator and lead(s).
	AND	
	Cardiac catheterization	Measurement of cardiac sampling and pressure (right, left, bilateral).
	Coronary angiography	
	AND	
	MCC condition	*See* appendix B.
276	Cardiac defibrillator implant	*See* DRG 275.
	AND	
	MCC condition	*See* appendix B.
277	Cardiac defibrillator implant	*See* DRG 275.

DRG 260 Cardiac Pacemaker Revision Except Device Replacement with MCC — RW 3.3152

Potential DRGs

228	Other Cardiothoracic Procedures with MCC	5.0387
245	AICD Generator Procedures	4.5314
275	Cardiac Defibrillator Implant with Cardiac Catheterization and MCC	7.0358
276	Cardiac Defibrillator Implant with MCC	6.2102

DRG	PDx/SDx/Procedure	Tips
228	Leadless pacemaker insertion or replacement	Review the operative report carefully. Leadless or transcatheter pacemakers do not require a subcutaneous pocket or a tunneled lead. The device is placed within the heart chamber (intracardiac), typically the right ventricle, via a peripheral vessel.
	AND	
	MCC condition	*See* appendix B.
245	AICD generator implant	
275	Cardiac defibrillator implant	Two codes must be reported—insertion of generator and lead(s).
	AND	
	Cardiac catheterization	Measurement of cardiac sampling and pressure (right, left, bilateral).
	Coronary angiography	
	AND	
	MCC condition	*See* appendix B.
276	Cardiac defibrillator implant	*See* DRG 275.
	AND	
	MCC condition	*See* appendix B.

DRG 261 Cardiac Pacemaker Revision Except Device Replacement with CC — RW 1.8818

Potential DRGs

228	Other Cardiothoracic Procedures with MCC	5.0387
229	Other Cardiothoracic Procedures without MCC	3.1796
242	Permanent Cardiac Pacemaker Implant with MCC	3.4551
243	Permanent Cardiac Pacemaker Implant with CC	2.2776
245	AICD Generator Procedures	4.5314
258	Cardiac Pacemaker Device Replacement with MCC	2.7086
260	Cardiac Pacemaker Revision Except Device Replacement with MCC	3.3152
275	Cardiac Defibrillator Implant with Cardiac Catheterization and MCC	7.0358
276	Cardiac Defibrillator Implant with MCC	6.2102
277	Cardiac Defibrillator Implant without MCC	4.7824

DRG	PDx/SDx/Procedure	Tips
228	Leadless pacemaker insertion, replacement, or revision	Review the operative report carefully. Leadless or transcatheter pacemakers do not require a subcutaneous pocket or a tunneled lead. The device is placed within the heart chamber (intracardiac), typically the right ventricle, via a peripheral vessel.
	AND	
	MCC condition	*See* appendix B.
229	Leadless pacemaker insertion	*See* DRG 228.
242	Permanent pacemaker implant (initial)	At least two codes must be reported—for both the pacemaker and lead(s).
	AND	
	MCC condition	*See* appendix B.
243	Permanent pacemaker implant (initial)	*See* DRG 242.
	AND	
	CC condition	*See* appendix B.
245	AICD generator implant	
258	Pacemaker device replacement—insertion with removal of old device	Review record for pacemaker replacement procedure. Two codes must be reported—both removal and insertion.
	AND	
	MCC condition	*See* appendix B.
260	MCC condition	*See* appendix B.
275	Cardiac defibrillator implant	Two codes must be reported—insertion of generator and lead(s).
	AND	
	Cardiac catheterization	Measurement of cardiac sampling and pressure (right, left, bilateral).
	Coronary angiography	
	AND	
	MCC condition	*See* appendix B.
276	Cardiac defibrillator implant	*See* DRG 275.
	AND	
	MCC condition	*See* appendix B.
277	Cardiac defibrillator implant	*See* DRG 275.

DRG 262 Cardiac Pacemaker Revision Except Device Replacement without CC/MCC — RW 1.6453

Potential DRGs

228	Other Cardiothoracic Procedures with MCC	5.0387
229	Other Cardiothoracic Procedures without MCC	3.1796
242	Permanent Cardiac Pacemaker Implant with MCC	3.4551
243	Permanent Cardiac Pacemaker Implant with CC	2.2776
244	Permanent Cardiac Pacemaker Implant without CC/MCC	1.8295
245	AICD Generator Procedures	4.5314
258	Cardiac Pacemaker Device Replacement with MCC	2.7086
259	Cardiac Pacemaker Device Replacement without MCC	1.8666
260	Cardiac Pacemaker Revision Except Device Replacement with MCC	3.3152
261	Cardiac Pacemaker Revision Except Device Replacement with CC	1.8818
275	Cardiac Defibrillator Implant with Cardiac Catheterization and MCC	7.0358
276	Cardiac Defibrillator Implant with MCC	6.2102
277	Cardiac Defibrillator Implant without MCC	4.7824

DRG	PDx/SDx/Procedure	Tips
228	Leadless pacemaker insertion, replacement, or revision	Review the operative report carefully. Leadless or transcatheter pacemakers do not require a subcutaneous pocket or a tunneled lead. The device is placed within the heart chamber (intracardiac), typically the right ventricle, via a peripheral vessel.
	AND	
	MCC condition	*See* appendix B.
229	Leadless pacemaker insertion	*See* DRG 228.
242	Permanent pacemaker implant (initial)	At least two codes must be reported—for both the pacemaker and lead(s).
	AND	
	MCC condition	*See* appendix B.
243	Permanent pacemaker implant (initial)	At least two codes must be reported—for both the pacemaker and lead(s).
	AND	
	CC condition	*See* appendix B.
244	Permanent pacemaker implant (initial)	At least two codes must be reported—for both the pacemaker and lead(s).
245	AICD generator implant	
258	Pacemaker device replacement—insertion with removal of old device	Review record for pacemaker replacement procedure. Two codes must be reported—both removal and insertion.
	AND	
	MCC condition	*See* appendix B.
259	Pacemaker device replacement—insertion with removal of old device	Review record for pacemaker replacement procedure. Two codes must be reported—both removal and insertion.
260	MCC condition	*See* appendix B.
261	CC condition	*See* appendix B.
275	Cardiac defibrillator implant	Two codes must be reported—insertion of generator and lead(s).
	AND	
	Cardiac catheterization	Measurement of cardiac sampling and pressure (right, left, bilateral).
	Coronary angiography	
	AND	
	MCC condition	*See* appendix B.
276	Cardiac defibrillator implant	*See* DRG 275.
	AND	
	MCC condition	*See* appendix B.
277	Cardiac defibrillator implant	*See* DRG 275.

DRG 263 Vein Ligation and Stripping — RW 2.8252

Potential DRGs

252	Other Vascular Procedures with MCC	3.3538

DRG	PDx/SDx/Procedure	Tips
252	Extirpation, supplement, or occlusion of lower limb artery	Review operative report carefully to determine extent and anatomic site of all procedures.
	AND	
	MCC condition	*See* appendix B.

DRG 264 Other Circulatory System O.R. Procedures — RW 3.2660

Potential DRGs

252	Other Vascular Procedures with MCC	3.3538

DRG	PDx/SDx/Procedure	Tips
252	Extirpation, supplement, or occlusion of lower limb artery	Review operative report carefully to determine extent and anatomic site of all procedures.
	AND	
	MCC condition	*See* appendix B.

DRG 265 AICD Lead Procedures RW 3.5341

Potential DRGs

245	AICD Generator Procedures	4.5314
275	Cardiac Defibrillator Implant with Cardiac Catheterization and MCC	7.0358
276	Cardiac Defibrillator Implant with MCC	6.2102
277	Cardiac Defibrillator Implant without MCC	4.7824

DRG	PDx/SDx/Procedure	Tips
245	AIDC generator implant	
275	Cardiac defibrillator implant	Two codes must be reported—insertion of generator and lead(s).
	AND	
	Cardiac catheterization	Measurement of cardiac sampling and pressure (right, left, bilateral).
	Coronary angiography	
	AND	
	MCC condition	*See* appendix B.
276	Cardiac defibrillator implant	*See* DRG 275.
	AND	
	MCC condition	*See* appendix B.
277	Cardiac defibrillator implant	*See* DRG 275.

DRG 266 Endovascular Cardiac Valve Replacement and Supplement Procedures with MCC RW 6.2461

Potential DRGs

212	Concomitant Aortic and Mitral Valve Procedures	10.7707
216	Cardiac Valve and Other Major Cardiothoracic Procedures with Cardiac Catheterization with MCC	9.7053
219	Cardiac Valve and Other Major Cardiothoracic Procedures without Cardiac Catheterization with MCC	7.7112

DRG	PDx/SDx/Procedure	Tips
212	Repair or Replacement aortic valve	Open or percutaneous endoscopic approach.
	AND	
	Repair or Replacement mitral valve	Open or percutaneous endoscopic approach.
	AND	
	Insertion of short-term external heart assist system	Includes Impella® devices. Two codes must be reported. A code from root operation table 02H with a seventh character value of J Intraoperative, and a code from root operation table 5A0 with a seventh character of 6 Other Pump or D Impeller Pump.
	Cardiac catheterization	Measurement of cardiac sampling and pressure (right, left, bilateral).
216	Dilation (with or without device) of cardiac valve	Approach must be open. The objective of root operation Dilation is to enlarge the diameter of a tubular body part or orifice. If a device remains at the end of the procedure to maintain the new diameter, the device is captured using a sixth-character device value.
	Release of cardiac valve	Approach must be open. The objective of the root operation Release is to free a body part without cutting the body part. The body part value coded is the body part being freed, not the tissue being manipulated or cut to free the body part.
	OR	
	Replacement, Repair, or Supplement of cardiac valve	Approach must be open or percutaneous endoscopic only.
	AND	
	Cardiac catheterization	Measurement of cardiac sampling and pressure (right, left, bilateral).
	Coronary angiography	
	AND	
	MCC condition	*See* appendix B.
219	Dilation (with or without device) of cardiac valve	*See* DRG 216.
	Release of cardiac valve	*See* DRG 216.
	OR	
	Replacement, Repair, or Supplement of cardiac valve	*See* DRG 216.
	AND	
	MCC condition	*See* appendix B.

DRG 267 Endovascular Cardiac Valve Replacement and Supplement Procedures without MCC RW 4.8802

Potential DRGs

212	Concomitant Aortic and Mitral Valve Procedures	10.7707
216	Cardiac Valve and Other Major Cardiothoracic Procedures with Cardiac Catheterization with MCC	9.7053
217	Cardiac Valve and Other Major Cardiothoracic Procedures with Cardiac Catheterization with CC	6.3653
219	Cardiac Valve and Other Major Cardiothoracic Procedures without Cardiac Catheterization with MCC	7.7112
220	Cardiac Valve and Other Major Cardiothoracic Procedures without Cardiac Catheterization with CC	5.2446
266	Endovascular Cardiac Valve Replacement and Supplement Procedures with MCC	6.2461

DRG	PDx/SDx/Procedure	Tips
212	Repair or Replacement aortic valve	Open or percutaneous endoscopic approach.
	AND	
	Repair or Replacement mitral valve	Open or percutaneous endoscopic approach.
	AND	
	Insertion of short-term external heart assist system	Includes Impella® devices. Two codes must be reported. A code from root operation table 02H with a seventh character value of J Intraoperative, and a code from root operation table 5A0 with a seventh character of 6 Other Pump or D Impeller Pump.
	Cardiac catheterization	Measurement of cardiac sampling and pressure (right, left, bilateral).
216	Dilation (with or without device) of cardiac valve	Approach must be open. The objective of root operation Dilation is to enlarge the diameter of a tubular body part or orifice. If a device remains at the end of the procedure to maintain the new diameter, the device is captured using a sixth-character device value.
	Release of cardiac valve	Approach must be open. The objective of the root operation Release is to free a body part without cutting the body part. The body part value coded is the body part being freed, not the tissue being manipulated or cut to free the body part.
	OR	
	Replacement, Repair, or Supplement of cardiac valve	Approach must be open or percutaneous endoscopic only.
	AND	
	Cardiac catheterization	Measurement of cardiac sampling and pressure (right, left, bilateral).
	Coronary angiography	
	AND	
	MCC condition	*See* appendix B.
217	Dilation (with or without device) of cardiac valve	*See* DRG 216.
	Release of cardiac valve	*See* DRG 216.
	OR	
	Replacement, Repair, or Supplement of cardiac valve	*See* DRG 216.
	AND	
	Cardiac catheterization	Measurement of cardiac sampling and pressure (right, left, bilateral).
	Coronary angiography	
	AND	
	CC condition	*See* appendix B.
219	Dilation (with or without device) of cardiac valve	*See* DRG 216.
	Release of cardiac valve	*See* DRG 216.
	OR	
	Replacement, Repair, or Supplement of cardiac valve	*See* DRG 216.
	AND	
	MCC condition	*See* appendix B.
220	Dilation (with or without device) of cardiac valve	*See* DRG 216.
	Release of cardiac valve	*See* DRG 216.
	OR	
	Replacement, Repair, or Supplement of cardiac valve	*See* DRG 216.
	AND	
	CC condition	*See* appendix B.
266	MCC condition	*See* appendix B.

DRG 268 Aortic and Heart Assist Procedures Except Pulsation Balloon with MCC RW 6.8547

Potential DRGs

215	Other Heart Assist System Implant	10.2148
216	Cardiac Valve and Other Major Cardiothoracic Procedures with Cardiac Catheterization with MCC	9.7053
219	Cardiac Valve and Other Major Cardiothoracic Procedures without Cardiac Catheterization with MCC	7.7112

DRG	PDx/SDx/Procedure	Tips
215	Insertion of short-term external heart assist system, open or percutaneous approach	Review the surgical consent, operative reports, and nurse's notes carefully to determine the exact surgical procedure that was performed. It is important to clearly differentiate between insertion, revision, or removal to ensure the correct root operation is reported. It is equally important to differentiate between implantable or external heart assist systems to ensure the correct device character is reported.
	Revision of implantable or external heart assist system, open or percutaneous approach	
216	Supplement aortic valve, open, percutaneous endoscopic, autologous, zooplastic, synthetic, nonautologous tissue substitute	Review the surgical consent, operative reports, and nurse's notes carefully to determine the exact surgical procedure that was performed. It is important to clearly understand and select the correct body part character, e.g., aortic valve (F) versus heart (A) and the device character to accurately report the procedure performed and result in the appropriate MS-DRG assignment.
	Replacement thoracic aorta, open or percutaneous endoscopic, autologous, zooplastic, synthetic, nonautologous tissue substitute Supplement thoracic aorta, percutaneous or percutaneous endoscopic, synthetic tissue substitute	Review the surgical consent, operative reports, and nurse's notes carefully to determine the exact surgical procedure that was performed. It is important to clearly differentiate the root operation, e.g., Replacement (R), Supplement (U), or Restriction (V) versus Excision (B), Extirpation (C), or Repair (Q) to accurately report the procedure performed and result in the appropriate MS-DRG assignment.
	Restriction thoracic aorta, open, percutaneous, percutaneous endoscopic, intraluminal device	
	AND	
	Cardiac catheterization	Measurement of cardiac sampling and pressure (right, left, bilateral).
	Coronary angiography	
	AND	
	MCC condition	*See* appendix B.
219	Supplement aortic valve, open, percutaneous endoscopic, autologous, zooplastic, synthetic, nonautologous tissue substitute.	*See* DRG 216.
	Replacement thoracic aorta, open or percutaneous endoscopic, autologous, zooplastic, synthetic, nonautologous tissue substitute Supplement thoracic aorta, percutaneous or percutaneous endoscopic, synthetic tissue substitute	*See* DRG 216.
	Restriction thoracic aorta, open, percutaneous, percutaneous endoscopic, intraluminal device	
	AND	
	MCC condition	*See* appendix B.

DRG 269 Aortic and Heart Assist Procedures Except Pulsation Balloon without MCC — RW 4.1586

Potential DRGs

215	Other Heart Assist System Implant	10.2148
216	Cardiac Valve and Other Major Cardiothoracic Procedures with Cardiac Catheterization with MCC	9.7053
217	Cardiac Valve and Other Major Cardiothoracic Procedures with Cardiac Catheterization with CC	6.3653
219	Cardiac Valve and Other Major Cardiothoracic Procedures without Cardiac Catheterization with MCC	7.7112
220	Cardiac Valve and Other Major Cardiothoracic Procedures without Cardiac Catheterization with CC	5.2446
268	Aortic and Heart Assist Procedures Except Pulsation Balloon with MCC	6.8547

DRG	PDx/SDx/Procedure	Tips
215	Insertion of external short-term heart assist system, open or percutaneous approach	Review the surgical consent, operative reports, and nurse's notes carefully to determine the exact surgical procedure that was performed. It is important to clearly differentiate between insertion, revision, or removal to ensure the correct root operation is reported. It is equally important to differentiate between implantable or external heart assist systems to ensure the correct device character is reported.
	Revision of implantable or external heart assist system, open or percutaneous approach	
216	Supplement aortic valve, open, percutaneous endoscopic, autologous, zooplastic, synthetic, nonautologous tissue substitute	Review the surgical consent, operative reports, and nurse's notes carefully to determine the exact surgical procedure that was performed. It is important to clearly understand and select the correct body part character, e.g., aortic valve (F) versus heart (A) and the device character to accurately report the procedure performed and result in the appropriate MS-DRG assignment.
	Replacement thoracic aorta, open or percutaneous endoscopic, autologous, zooplastic, synthetic, nonautologous tissue substitute Supplement thoracic aorta, percutaneous or percutaneous endoscopic, synthetic tissue substitute	Review the surgical consent, operative reports, and nurse's notes carefully to determine the exact surgical procedure that was performed. It is important to clearly differentiate the root operation, e.g., Replacement (Ø2R), Supplement (U), or Restriction (V) versus Excision (B), Extirpation (C), or Repair (Q) to accurately report the procedure performed and result in the appropriate MS-DRG assignment.
	Restriction thoracic aorta, open, percutaneous, percutaneous endoscopic, intraluminal device	
	AND	
	Cardiac catheterization	Measurement of cardiac sampling and pressure (right, left, bilateral).
	Coronary angiography	
	AND	
	MCC condition	*See* appendix B.
217	Supplement aortic valve, open, percutaneous endoscopic, autologous, zooplastic, synthetic, nonautologous tissue substitute	*See* DRG 216.
	Replacement thoracic aorta, open or percutaneous endoscopic, autologous, zooplastic, synthetic, nonautologous tissue substitute Supplement thoracic aorta, percutaneous or percutaneous endoscopic, synthetic tissue substitute	*See* DRG 216.
	Restriction thoracic aorta, open, percutaneous, percutaneous endoscopic, intraluminal device	
	AND	
	Cardiac catheterization	*See* DRG 216.
	Coronary angiography	
	AND	
	CC condition	*See* appendix B.
219	Supplement aortic valve, open, percutaneous endoscopic, autologous, zooplastic, synthetic, nonautologous tissue substitute	*See* DRG 216.
	Replacement thoracic aorta, open or percutaneous endoscopic, autologous, zooplastic, synthetic, nonautologous tissue substitute Supplement thoracic aorta, percutaneous or percutaneous endoscopic, synthetic tissue substitute	*See* DRG 216.
	Restriction thoracic aorta, open, percutaneous, percutaneous endoscopic, intraluminal device	
	AND	
	MCC condition	*See* appendix B.
220	Supplement aortic valve, open, percutaneous endoscopic, autologous, zooplastic, synthetic, nonautologous tissue substitute	*See* DRG 216.
	Replacement thoracic aorta, open or percutaneous endoscopic, autologous, zooplastic, synthetic, nonautologous tissue substitute	*See* DRG 216.
	Supplement thoracic aorta, percutaneous or percutaneous endoscopic, synthetic tissue substitute	
	Restriction thoracic aorta, open, percutaneous, percutaneous endoscopic, intraluminal device	
	AND	
	MCC condition	*See* appendix B.
268	MCC condition	*See* appendix B.

DRG 270 Other Major Cardiovascular Procedures with MCC

RW 5.0569

Potential DRGs

216	Cardiac Valve and Other Major Cardiothoracic Procedures with Cardiac Catheterization with MCC	9.7053
219	Cardiac Valve and Other Major Cardiothoracic Procedures without Cardiac Catheterization with MCC	7.7112
268	Aortic and Heart Assist Procedures Except Pulsation Balloon with MCC	6.8547

DRG	PDx/SDx/Procedure	Tips
216	Release aortic, mitral, tricuspid valve, open approach	Review the operative report carefully to determine the exact surgical procedure that was performed. It is important to clearly differentiate the root operation, e.g., Release (N) versus Extirpation (C) and correctly identify the approach to accurately report the procedure performed and result in the appropriate MS-DRG assignment.
	Replacement pulmonary trunk, pulmonary artery [right, left], pulmonary vein [right, left], superior vena cava, thoracic aorta, open, percutaneous endoscopic approach, autologous tissue, zooplastic tissue, synthetic, nonautologous tissue substitute	Review the surgical consent, operative report, and nurse's notes carefully to determine the exact surgical procedure that was performed. It is important to clearly differentiate the root operation, e.g., Replacement (R) versus Destruction (5) and correctly identify the device character to accurately report the procedure performed and result in the appropriate MS-DRG assignment.
	Replacement internal mammary artery [right, left], innominate artery, subclavian artery [right, left], open, percutaneous endoscopic, autologous tissue, synthetic, nonautologous tissue substitute	Review the surgical consent, operative report, and nurse's notes carefully to determine the exact surgical procedure that was performed. It is important to clearly differentiate the root operation, e.g., Replacement (R) versus Destruction (5) or Excision (B) and correctly identify the device character to accurately report the procedure performed and result in the appropriate MS-DRG assignment.
	AND	
	Cardiac catheterization	Measurement of cardiac sampling and pressure (right, left, bilateral).
	Coronary angiography	
	AND	
	MCC condition	*See* appendix B.
219	Release aortic, mitral, tricuspid valve, open approach	*See* DRG 216.
	Replacement pulmonary trunk, pulmonary artery [right, left], pulmonary vein [right, left], superior vena cava, thoracic aorta, open, percutaneous endoscopic approach, autologous tissue, zooplastic tissue, synthetic, nonautologous tissue substitute	*See* DRG 216.
	Replacement internal mammary artery [right, left], innominate artery, subclavian artery [right, left], open, percutaneous endoscopic, autologous tissue, synthetic, nonautologous tissue substitute	*See* DRG 216.
	AND	
	MCC condition	*See* appendix B.
268	Bypass abdominal aorta, open, autologous venous tissue, autologous arterial tissue, synthetic substitute, nonautologous tissue substitute, renal artery right, left, bilateral	Review the operative report carefully to identify the exact vessel(s) the abdominal aorta was bypassed to. Verify the code assignment to ensure the correct qualifier character was assigned. Only the qualifiers of 3, 4, and 5 (renal artery, right, left, bilateral) are assigned to MS-DRG 268.
	Bypass abdominal aorta, percutaneous endoscopic, autologous venous tissue, autologous arterial tissue, synthetic substitute, nonautologous tissue substitute, renal artery [right, left, bilateral]	
	Excision thoracic aorta, open, percutaneous endoscopic	Review the surgical consent, operative report, and nurse's notes carefully to determine the exact surgical procedure that was performed. It is important to clearly differentiate the root operation, e.g., Excision (B) versus Bypass (1) to accurately report the procedure performed and result in the appropriate MS-DRG assignment.
	Repair thoracic aorta, open, percutaneous, percutaneous endoscopic	Review the surgical consent, operative report, and nurse's notes carefully to determine the exact surgical procedure that was performed. It is important to clearly differentiate the root operation, e.g., Repair (Q) versus Bypass (1) to accurately report the procedure performed and result in the appropriate MS-DRG assignment.
	AND	
	MCC condition	*See* appendix B.

Optimizing Tips

DRG 271 Other Major Cardiovascular Procedures with CC RW 3.4562

Potential DRGs

216	Cardiac Valve and Other Major Cardiothoracic Procedures with Cardiac Catheterization with MCC	9.7053
217	Cardiac Valve and Other Major Cardiothoracic Procedures with Cardiac Catheterization with CC	6.3653
219	Cardiac Valve and Other Major Cardiothoracic Procedures without Cardiac Catheterization with MCC	7.7112
220	Cardiac Valve and Other Major Cardiothoracic Procedures without Cardiac Catheterization with CC	5.2446
228	Other Cardiothoracic Procedures with MCC	5.0387
268	Aortic and Heart Assist Procedures Except Pulsation Balloon with MCC	6.8547
270	Other Major Cardiovascular Procedures with MCC	5.0569

DRG	PDx/SDx/Procedure	Tips
216	Release aortic, mitral, tricuspid valve, open approach	Review the operative report carefully to determine the exact surgical procedure that was performed. It is important to clearly differentiate the root operation, e.g., Release (N) versus Extirpation (C) and correctly identify the approach to accurately report the procedure performed and result in the appropriate MS-DRG assignment.
	Replacement pulmonary trunk, pulmonary artery [right, left], pulmonary vein [right, left], superior vena cava, thoracic aorta, open, percutaneous endoscopic approach, autologous tissue, zooplastic tissue, synthetic, nonautologous tissue substitute	Review the surgical consent, operative report, and nurse's notes carefully to determine the exact surgical procedure that was performed. It is important to clearly differentiate the root operation, e.g., Replacement (R) versus Destruction (5) and correctly identify the device character to accurately report the procedure performed and result in the appropriate MS-DRG assignment.
	Replacement internal mammary artery [right, left], innominate artery, subclavian artery [right, left], open, percutaneous endoscopic, autologous tissue, synthetic, nonautologous tissue substitute	Review the surgical consent, operative report, and nurse's notes carefully to determine the exact surgical procedure that was performed. It is important to clearly differentiate the root operation, e.g., Replacement (R) versus Destruction (5) or Excision (B) and correctly identify the device character to accurately report the procedure performed and result in the appropriate MS-DRG assignment.
	AND	
	Cardiac catheterization	Measurement of cardiac sampling and pressure (right, left, bilateral).
	Coronary angiography	
	AND	
	MCC condition	*See* appendix B.
217	Release aortic, mitral, tricuspid valve, open approach	*See* DRG 216.
	Replacement pulmonary trunk, pulmonary artery [right, left], pulmonary vein [right, left], superior vena cava, thoracic aorta, open, percutaneous endoscopic approach, autologous tissue, zooplastic tissue, synthetic, nonautologous tissue substitute	*See* DRG 216.
	Replacement internal mammary artery [right, left], innominate artery, subclavian artery [right, left], open, percutaneous endoscopic, autologous tissue, synthetic, nonautologous tissue substitute	*See* DRG 216.
	AND	
	Cardiac catheterization	*See* DRG 216.
	Coronary angiography	
	AND	
	CC condition	*See* appendix B.
219	Release aortic, mitral, tricuspid valve, open approach	*See* DRG 216.
	Replacement pulmonary trunk, pulmonary artery [right, left], pulmonary vein [right, left], superior vena cava, thoracic aorta, open, percutaneous endoscopic approach, autologous tissue, zooplastic tissue, synthetic, nonautologous tissue substitute	*See* DRG 216.
	Replacement internal mammary artery [right, left], innominate artery, subclavian artery [right, left], open, percutaneous endoscopic, autologous tissue, synthetic, nonautologous tissue substitute	*See* DRG 216.
	AND	
	MCC condition	*See* appendix B.
220	Release aortic, mitral, tricuspid valve, open approach	*See* DRG 216.
	Replacement pulmonary trunk, pulmonary artery [right, left], pulmonary vein [right, left], superior vena cava, thoracic aorta, open, percutaneous endoscopic approach, autologous tissue, zooplastic tissue, synthetic, nonautologous tissue substitute	*See* DRG 216.
	Replacement internal mammary artery [right, left], innominate artery, subclavian artery [right, left], open, percutaneous endoscopic, autologous tissue, synthetic, nonautologous tissue substitute	*See* DRG 216.
	AND	
	CC condition	*See* appendix B.

DRG 271 (Continued)

DRG	PDx/SDx/Procedure	Tips
228	Bypass right atrium, open, percutaneous endoscopic, autologous venous tissue, autologous arterial tissue, synthetic substitute, nonautologous tissue substitute, pulmonary trunk, pulmonary artery, right, left	Review the operative report carefully to identify the exact site(s) bypassed, specifically the qualifier character, e.g., pulmonary trunk, right, or left pulmonary artery versus left atrium. Verify the code assignment to ensure the correct qualifier character was assigned. Only the qualifiers of P, Q, and R (pulmonary trunk, pulmonary artery, right, left) are assigned to MS-DRG 228.
	Destruction of lesion or tissue of heart, open or percutaneous endoscopic	Numerous codes representing destruction of the heart and great vessels are divided amongst MS-DRGs 228 and 271. Review the surgical consent, operative reports, and nurse's notes carefully to determine the exact surgical procedure that was performed. It is important to clearly understand the body part key and select the correct body part character to accurately report the procedure performed and result in the appropriate MS-DRG assignment.
	AND	
	MCC condition	*See* appendix B.
268	Bypass abdominal aorta, open, autologous venous tissue, autologous arterial tissue, synthetic substitute, nonautologous tissue substitute, renal artery right, left, bilateral	Review the operative report carefully to identify the exact vessel(s) the abdominal aorta was bypassed to. Verify the code assignment to ensure the correct qualifier character was assigned. Only the qualifiers of 3, 4, and 5 (renal artery, right, left, bilateral) are assigned to MS-DRG 268.
	Bypass abdominal aorta, percutaneous endoscopic, autologous venous tissue, autologous arterial tissue, synthetic substitute, nonautologous tissue substitute, renal artery [right, left, bilateral]	
	Excision thoracic aorta, open, percutaneous endoscopic	Review the surgical consent, operative report, and nurse's notes carefully to determine the exact surgical procedure that was performed. It is important to clearly differentiate the root operation, e.g., Excision (B) versus Bypass (1) to accurately report the procedure performed and result in the appropriate MS-DRG assignment.
	Repair thoracic aorta, open, percutaneous, percutaneous endoscopic	Review the surgical consent, operative report, and nurse's notes carefully to determine the exact surgical procedure that was performed. It is important to clearly differentiate the root operation, e.g., Repair (Q) versus Bypass (1) to accurately report the procedure performed and result in the appropriate MS-DRG assignment.
	AND	
	MCC condition	*See* appendix B.
270	MCC condition	*See* appendix B.

DRG 272 Other Major Cardiovascular Procedures without CC/MCC — RW 2.4395

Potential DRGs

216	Cardiac Valve and Other Major Cardiothoracic Procedures with Cardiac Catheterization with MCC	9.7053
217	Cardiac Valve and Other Major Cardiothoracic Procedures with Cardiac Catheterization with CC	6.3653
218	Cardiac Valve and Other Major Cardiothoracic Procedures with Cardiac Catheterization without CC/MCC	5.6967
219	Cardiac Valve and Other Major Cardiothoracic Procedures without Cardiac Catheterization with MCC	7.7112
220	Cardiac Valve and Other Major Cardiothoracic Procedures without Cardiac Catheterization with CC	5.2446
228	Other Cardiothoracic Procedures with MCC	5.0387
268	Aortic and Heart Assist Procedures Except Pulsation Balloon with MCC	6.8547
270	Other Major Cardiovascular Procedures with MCC	5.0569
271	Other Major Cardiovascular Procedures with CC	3.4562

DRG	PDx/SDx/Procedure	Tips
216	Release aortic, mitral, tricuspid valve, open approach	Review the operative report carefully to determine the exact surgical procedure that was performed. It is important to clearly differentiate the root operation, e.g., Release (N) versus Extirpation (C) and correctly identify the approach to accurately report the procedure performed and result in the appropriate MS-DRG assignment.
	Replacement pulmonary trunk, pulmonary artery [right, left], pulmonary vein [right, left], superior vena cava, thoracic aorta, open, percutaneous endoscopic approach, autologous tissue, zooplastic tissue, synthetic, nonautologous tissue substitute	Review the surgical consent, operative report, and nurse's notes carefully to determine the exact surgical procedure that was performed. It is important to clearly differentiate the root operation, e.g., Replacement (R) versus Destruction (5) and correctly identify the device character to accurately report the procedure performed and result in the appropriate MS-DRG assignment.
	Replacement internal mammary artery [right, left], innominate artery, subclavian artery [right, left], open, percutaneous endoscopic, autologous tissue, synthetic, nonautologous tissue substitute	Review the surgical consent, operative report, and nurse's notes carefully to determine the exact surgical procedure that was performed. It is important to clearly differentiate the root operation, e.g., Replacement (R) versus Destruction (5) or Excision (B) and correctly identify the device character to accurately report the procedure performed and result in the appropriate MS-DRG assignment.
	AND	
	Cardiac catheterization	Measurement of cardiac sampling and pressure (right, left, bilateral).
	Coronary angiography	
	AND	
	MCC condition	*See* appendix B.

DRG 272 (Continued)

DRG	PDx/SDx/Procedure	Tips
217	Release aortic, mitral, tricuspid valve, open approach	*See* DRG 216.
	Replacement pulmonary trunk, pulmonary artery [right, left], pulmonary vein [right, left], superior vena cava, thoracic aorta, open, percutaneous endoscopic approach, autologous tissue, zooplastic tissue, synthetic, nonautologous tissue substitute	*See* DRG 216.
	Replacement internal mammary artery [right, left], innominate artery, subclavian artery [right, left], open, percutaneous endoscopic, autologous tissue, synthetic, nonautologous tissue substitute	*See* DRG 216.
	AND	
	Cardiac catheterization	*See* DRG 216.
	Coronary angiography	
	AND	
	CC condition	*See* appendix B.
218	Release aortic, mitral, tricuspid valve, open approach	*See* DRG 216.
	Replacement pulmonary trunk, pulmonary artery [right, left], pulmonary vein [right, left], superior vena cava, thoracic aorta, open, percutaneous endoscopic approach, autologous tissue, zooplastic tissue, synthetic, nonautologous tissue substitute	*See* DRG 216.
	Replacement internal mammary artery [right, left], innominate artery, subclavian artery [right, left], open, percutaneous endoscopic, autologous tissue, synthetic, nonautologous tissue substitute	*See* DRG 216.
	AND	
	Cardiac catheterization (right, left, bilateral) for measurement of cardiac sampling and pressure, or with angiocardiography (coronary angiography)	
219	Release aortic, mitral, tricuspid valve, open approach	*See* DRG 216.
	Replacement pulmonary trunk, pulmonary artery [right, left], pulmonary vein [right, left], superior vena cava, thoracic aorta, open, percutaneous endoscopic approach, autologous tissue, zooplastic tissue, synthetic, nonautologous tissue substitute	*See* DRG 216.
	Replacement internal mammary artery [right, left], innominate artery, subclavian artery [right, left], open, percutaneous endoscopic, autologous tissue, synthetic, nonautologous tissue substitute	*See* DRG 216.
	AND	
	MCC condition	*See* appendix B.
220	Release aortic, mitral, tricuspid valve, open approach	*See* DRG 216.
	Replacement pulmonary trunk, pulmonary artery [right, left], pulmonary vein [right, left], superior vena cava, thoracic aorta, open, percutaneous endoscopic approach, autologous tissue, zooplastic tissue, synthetic, nonautologous tissue substitute	*See* DRG 216.
	Replacement internal mammary artery [right, left], innominate artery, subclavian artery [right, left], open, percutaneous endoscopic, autologous tissue, synthetic, nonautologous tissue substitute	*See* DRG 216.
	AND	
	CC condition	*See* appendix B.
228	Bypass right atrium, open, percutaneous endoscopic, autologous venous tissue, autologous arterial tissue, synthetic substitute, nonautologous tissue substitute, pulmonary trunk, pulmonary artery, right, left	**Review the operative report carefully to identify the exact site(s) bypassed, specifically the qualifier character, e.g., pulmonary trunk, right, or left pulmonary artery versus left atrium. Verify the code assignment to ensure the correct qualifier character was assigned. Only the qualifiers of P, Q, and R (pulmonary trunk, pulmonary artery, right, left) are assigned to MS-DRG 228.**
	Destruction of lesion or tissue of heart, open or percutaneous endoscopic	**Numerous codes representing destruction of the heart and great vessels are divided amongst MS-DRGs 228 and 272. Review the surgical consent, operative reports, and nurse's notes carefully to determine the exact surgical procedure that was performed. It is important to clearly understand the body part key and select the correct body part character to accurately report the procedure performed and result in the appropriate MS-DRG assignment.**
	AND	
	MCC condition	*See* appendix B.

DRG 272 (Continued)

DRG	PDx/SDx/Procedure	Tips
268	Bypass abdominal aorta, open, autologous venous tissue, autologous arterial tissue, synthetic substitute, nonautologous tissue substitute, renal artery right, left, bilateral	Review the operative report carefully to identify the exact vessel(s) the abdominal aorta was bypassed to. Verify the code assignment to ensure the correct qualifier character was assigned. Only the qualifiers of 3, 4, and 5 (renal artery, right, left, bilateral) are assigned to MS-DRG 268.
	Bypass abdominal aorta, percutaneous endoscopic, autologous venous tissue, autologous arterial tissue, synthetic substitute, nonautologous tissue substitute, renal artery [right, left, bilateral]	
	Excision thoracic aorta, open, percutaneous endoscopic	Review the surgical consent, operative report, and nurse's notes carefully to determine the exact surgical procedure that was performed. It is important to clearly differentiate the root operation, e.g., Excision (B) versus Bypass (1) to accurately report the procedure performed and result in the appropriate MS-DRG assignment.
	Repair thoracic aorta, open, percutaneous, percutaneous endoscopic	Review the surgical consent, operative report, and nurse's notes carefully to determine the exact surgical procedure that was performed. It is important to clearly differentiate the root operation, e.g., Repair (Q) versus Bypass (1) to accurately report the procedure performed and result in the appropriate MS-DRG assignment.
	AND	
	MCC condition	*See* appendix B.
270	MCC condition	*See* appendix B.
271	CC condition	*See* appendix B.

DRG 273 Percutaneous Intracardiac Procedures with MCC — RW 3.8970

Potential DRGs

216	Cardiac Valve and Other Major Cardiothoracic Procedures with Cardiac Catheterization with MCC	9.7053
219	Cardiac Valve and Other Major Cardiothoracic Procedures without Cardiac Catheterization with MCC	7.7112
228	Other Cardiothoracic Procedures with MCC	5.0387
233	Coronary Bypass with Cardiac Catheterization or Open Ablation with MCC	7.7996
235	Coronary Bypass without Cardiac Catheterization with MCC	5.8806
245	AICD Generator Procedures	4.5314
266	Endovascular Cardiac Valve Replacement and Supplement Procedures with MCC	6.2461
270	Other Major Cardiovascular Procedures with MCC	5.0569

DRG	PDx/SDx/Procedure	Tips
216	Replacement of aortic, mitral, or pulmonary valve—open or percutaneous endoscopic	Review the surgical consent, operative reports, and nurse's notes carefully to determine the exact surgical procedure that was performed. Pay careful attention to the approach.
	Supplement of aortic, mitral, pulmonary or tricuspid valve—open or percutaneous endoscopic approach	
	AND	
	Cardiac catheterization	Measurement of cardiac sampling and pressure (right, left, bilateral).
	Coronary angiography	
	AND	
	MCC condition	*See* appendix B.
219	Replacement of aortic, mitral or pulmonary valve—open or percutaneous endoscopic	*See* DRG 216.
	Supplement of aortic, mitral, pulmonary or tricuspid valve—open or percutaneous endoscopic approach	
	AND	
	MCC condition	*See* appendix B.
228	Percutaneous endoscopic Destruction or Excision of: Atrial septum Conduction mechanism Chordae tendineae Ventricular septum Atrium, right/left Ventricle, right/left Heart valves—aortic/mitral/pulmonary/tricuspid	Review the surgical consent, operative reports, and nurse's notes carefully to determine the exact surgical procedure that was performed. It is important to correctly identify the body part character (including laterality) and differentiate between the approach 4 (Percutaneous Endoscopic) versus 3 (Percutaneous), to accurately report the procedure performed and result in the appropriate MS-DRG assignment.
	AND	
	MCC condition	*See* appendix B.
233	Bypass coronary artery, one, two, three, four or more arteries, percutaneous endoscopic	Review the surgical consent, operative reports, and nurse's notes carefully to determine the exact surgical procedure that was performed.
	AND	
	Cardiac catheterization	Measurement of cardiac sampling and pressure (right, left, bilateral).
	Coronary angiography	
	AND	
	MCC condition	*See* appendix B.
235	Bypass coronary artery, one, two, three, four or more arteries, percutaneous endoscopic	*See* DRG 233.
	AND	
	MCC condition	*See* appendix B.
245	AICD generator procedures	It is important to review the entire medical record carefully to capture and report an accurate principal diagnosis, secondary diagnoses, and all procedures performed during the inpatient stay. The MS-DRG surgical hierarchy ensures patients who undergo multiple procedures related to the principal diagnosis during the same inpatient stay are assigned to the MS-DRG associated with the most resource-intensive surgical class. MS-DRG 245 is higher in the surgical hierarchy than MS-DRG 273.
266	Replacement or supplement, aortic valve, mitral valve, pulmonary valve, percutaneous, autologous tissue substitute, zooplastic tissue, synthetic substitute, nonautologous tissue substitute	Review the surgical consent, operative reports, and nurse's notes carefully to determine the exact surgical procedure that was performed. It is important to clearly differentiate between the root operation Replace (R) or Supplement (U) versus Destruction (5) or Excision (B) to ensure the correct root operation is reported. Verify the final code selection carefully to ensure the correct selection was made.
	AND	
	MCC condition	*See* appendix B.

DRG 273 (Continued)

DRG	PDx/SDx/Procedure	Tips
270	Division conduction mechanism, percutaneous	Review the surgical consent, operative reports, and nurse's notes carefully to determine the exact surgical procedure that was performed. It is important to clearly differentiate between the root operations Division (8), Release (N) and Repair (Q) versus Excision (B) to ensure the correct root operation is reported and correctly identify the approach to accurately report the procedure performed and result in the appropriate MS-DRG assignment.
	Release conduction mechanism	
	Repair conduction mechanism, percutaneous	
	Extirpation, aortic valve, mitral valve, pulmonary valve, tricuspid valve, percutaneous	Review the surgical consent, operative reports, and nurse's notes carefully to determine the exact surgical procedure that was performed. It is important to clearly differentiate between the root operations Extirpation (C) and Release (N) versus Destruction (5) and Excision (B) to ensure the correct root operation is reported and correctly identify the approach to accurately report the procedure performed and result in the appropriate MS-DRG assignment.
	Release, aortic valve, mitral valve, pulmonary valve, tricuspid valve, percutaneous	
	Repair, right atrium, left atrium, percutaneous	Review the surgical consent, operative reports, and nurse's notes carefully to determine the exact surgical procedure that was performed. It is important to clearly differentiate between the root operations Repair (Q) and Supplement (U) versus Destruction (5) and Excision (B) to ensure the correct root operation is reported. Report the device character and correctly identify the approach to result in the appropriate MS-DRG assignment.
	Supplement right atrium, percutaneous, autologous tissue substitute, zooplastic tissue, synthetic substitute, nonautologous tissue substitute	
	Repair right ventricle, left ventricle, percutaneous	Review the surgical consent, operative reports, and nurse's notes carefully to determine the exact surgical procedure that was performed. It is important to clearly differentiate between the root operations Repair (Q) and Supplement (U) versus Destruction (5) to ensure the correct root operation is reported. Report the device character and correctly identify the approach to result in the appropriate MS-DRG assignment.
	Supplement right ventricle, left ventricle, percutaneous, autologous tissue substitute, zooplastic tissue, synthetic substitute	
	Replacement atrial septum, percutaneous endoscopic, autologous tissue substitute, zooplastic tissue, synthetic substitute, nonautologous tissue substitute	Review the surgical consent, operative reports, and nurse's notes carefully to determine the exact surgical procedure that was performed. It is important to clearly differentiate between the root operations Replacement (R) versus Destruction (5) and Excision (B) to ensure the correct root operation is reported. Report the device character and correctly identify the approach to result in the appropriate MS-DRG assignment.
	AND	
	MCC condition	*See* appendix B.

DRG 274 Percutaneous Intracardiac Procedures without MCC RW 3.2408

Potential DRGs

216	Cardiac Valve and Other Major Cardiothoracic Procedures with Cardiac Catheterization with MCC	9.7053
217	Cardiac Valve and Other Major Cardiothoracic Procedures with Cardiac Catheterization with CC	6.3653
218	Cardiac Valve and Other Major Cardiothoracic Procedures with Cardiac Catheterization without CC/MCC	5.6967
219	Cardiac Valve and Other Major Cardiothoracic Procedures without Cardiac Catheterization with MCC	7.7112
220	Cardiac Valve and Other Major Cardiothoracic Procedures without Cardiac Catheterization with CC	5.2446
221	Cardiac Valve and Other Major Cardiothoracic Procedures without Cardiac Catheterization without CC/MCC	4.6486
228	Other Cardiothoracic Procedures with MCC	5.0387
233	Coronary Bypass with Cardiac Catheterization or Open Ablation with MCC	7.7996
234	Coronary Bypass with Cardiac Catheterization or Open Ablation without MCC	5.1979
235	Coronary Bypass without Cardiac Catheterization with MCC	5.8806
236	Coronary Bypass without Cardiac Catheterization without MCC	4.0412
242	Permanent Cardiac Pacemaker Implant with MCC	3.4551
245	AICD Generator Procedures	4.5314
266	Endovascular Cardiac Valve Replacement and Supplement Procedures with MCC	6.2461
267	Endovascular Cardiac Valve Replacement and Supplement Procedures without MCC	4.8802
270	Other Major Cardiovascular Procedures with MCC	5.0569
273	Percutaneous Intracardiac Procedures with MCC	3.8970

DRG	PDx/SDx/Procedure	Tips
216	Replacement of aortic, mitral, or pulmonary valve—open or percutaneous endoscopic	Review the surgical consent, operative reports, and nurse's notes carefully to determine the exact surgical procedure that was performed. Pay careful attention to the approach.
	Supplement of aortic, mitral, pulmonary or tricuspid valve—open or percutaneous endoscopic approach	
	AND	
	Cardiac catheterization	Measurement of cardiac sampling and pressure (right, left, bilateral).
	Coronary angiography	
	AND	
	MCC condition	*See* appendix B.
217	Replacement of aortic, mitral or pulmonary valve—open or percutaneous endoscopic	*See* DRG 216.
	Supplement of aortic, mitral, pulmonary or tricuspid valve—open or percutaneous endoscopic approach	
	AND	
	Cardiac catheterization	*See* DRG 216.
	Coronary angiography	
	AND	
	CC condition	*See* appendix B.
218	Replacement of aortic, mitral or pulmonary valve—open or percutaneous endoscopic	*See* DRG 216.
	Supplement of aortic, mitral, pulmonary or tricuspid valve—open or percutaneous endoscopic approach	
	AND	
	Cardiac catheterization	*See* DRG 216.
	Coronary angiography	
219	Replacement of aortic, mitral or pulmonary valve—open or percutaneous endoscopic	*See* DRG 216.
	Supplement of aortic, mitral, pulmonary or tricuspid valve—open or percutaneous endoscopic approach	
	AND	
	MCC condition	*See* appendix B.
220	Replacement of aortic, mitral or pulmonary valve—open or percutaneous endoscopic	*See* DRG 216.
	Supplement of aortic, mitral, pulmonary or tricuspid valve—open or percutaneous endoscopic approach	
	AND	
	CC condition	*See* appendix B.
221	Replacement of aortic, mitral or pulmonary valve—open or percutaneous endoscopic	*See* DRG 216.
	Supplement of aortic, mitral, pulmonary or tricuspid valve—open or percutaneous endoscopic approach	
228	Percutaneous endoscopic Destruction or Excision of: Atrial septum Conduction mechanism Chordae tendineae Ventricular septum Atrium, right/left Ventricle, right/left Heart valves—aortic/mitral/pulmonary/tricuspid	Review the surgical consent, operative reports, and nurse's notes carefully to determine the exact surgical procedure that was performed. It is important to correctly identify the body part character (including laterality) and differentiate between the approach 4 (Percutaneous Endoscopic) versus 3 (Percutaneous), to accurately report the procedure performed and result in the appropriate MS-DRG assignment.
	AND	
	MCC condition	*See* appendix B.

DRG 274 (Continued)

DRG	PDx/SDx/Procedure	Tips
233	Bypass coronary artery, one, two, three, four or more arteries, percutaneous endoscopic	Review the surgical consent, operative reports, and nurse's notes carefully to determine the exact surgical procedure that was performed.
	AND	
	Cardiac catheterization	Measurement of cardiac sampling and pressure (right, left, bilateral).
	Coronary angiography	
	OR	
	Open ablation of: Coronary vein Atrial septum Atrium, right/left Conduction mechanism Chordae tendineae Pulmonary vein, right/left Left atrial appendage	Review operative report carefully to determine the extent of all procedures. Open ablation procedures are coded to the root operation Destruction. Accurate MS-DRG assignment depends on correctly identifying the body part character and approach value.
	AND	
	MCC condition	*See* appendix B.
234	Bypass coronary artery, one, two, three, four or more arteries, percutaneous endoscopic	*See* DRG 233.
	AND	
	Cardiac catheterization	*See* DRG 233.
	Coronary angiography	
	OR	
	Open ablation of: Coronary vein Atrial septum Atrium, right/left Conduction mechanism Chordae tendineae Pulmonary vein, right/left Left atrial appendage	*See* DRG 233
	AND	
	CC condition	*See* appendix B.
235	Bypass coronary artery, one, two, three, four or more arteries, percutaneous endoscopic	*See* DRG 233.
	AND	
	MCC condition	*See* appendix B.
236	Bypass coronary artery, one, two, three, four or more arteries, percutaneous endoscopic	*See* DRG 233.
242	Permanent pacemaker implant	It is important to review the entire medical record carefully to capture and report an accurate principal diagnosis, secondary diagnoses, and all procedures performed during the inpatient stay. The MS-DRG surgical hierarchy ensures patients who undergo multiple procedures related to the principal diagnosis during the same inpatient stay are assigned to the MS-DRG associated with the most resource-intensive surgical class. This DRG is higher in the surgical hierarchy than MS-DRG 274.
	AND	
	MCC condition	*See* appendix B.
245	AICD generator procedures	*See* DRG 242.
266	Replacement or supplement, aortic valve, mitral valve, pulmonary valve, percutaneous, autologous tissue substitute, zooplastic tissue, synthetic substitute, nonautologous tissue substitute	Review the surgical consent, operative reports, and nurse's notes carefully to determine the exact surgical procedure that was performed. It is important to clearly differentiate between the root operation Replace (R), Supplement (U) versus Destruction (5) or Excision (B) to ensure the correct root operation is reported. Verify the final code selection carefully to ensure the correct selection was made.
	AND	
	MCC condition	*See* appendix B.
267	Replacement or supplement, aortic valve, mitral valve, pulmonary valve, percutaneous, autologous tissue substitute, zooplastic tissue, synthetic substitute, nonautologous tissue substitute	*See* DRG 266.

Optimizing Tips

DRG 274 (Continued)

DRG	PDx/SDx/Procedure	Tips
270	Division conduction mechanism, percutaneous	Review the surgical consent, operative reports, and nurse's notes carefully to determine the exact surgical procedure that was performed. It is important to clearly differentiate between the root operations Division (8), Release (N) and Repair (Q) versus Excision (B) to ensure the correct root operation is reported and correctly identify the approach to accurately report the procedure performed and result in the appropriate MS-DRG assignment.
	Release conduction mechanism	
	Repair conduction mechanism, percutaneous	
	Extirpation, aortic valve, mitral valve, pulmonary valve, tricuspid valve, percutaneous	Review the surgical consent, operative reports, and nurse's notes carefully to determine the exact surgical procedure that was performed. It is important to clearly differentiate between the root operations Extirpation (C) and Release (N) versus Destruction (5) and Excision (B) to ensure the correct root operation is reported and correctly identify the approach to accurately report the procedure performed and result in the appropriate MS-DRG assignment.
	Release, aortic valve, mitral valve, pulmonary valve, tricuspid valve, percutaneous	
	Repair, right atrium, left atrium, percutaneous	Review the surgical consent, operative reports, and nurse's notes carefully to determine the exact surgical procedure that was performed. It is important to clearly differentiate between the root operations Repair (Q) and Supplement (U) versus Destruction (5) and Excision (B) to ensure the correct root operation is reported. Report the device character and correctly identify the approach to result in the appropriate MS-DRG assignment.
	Supplement right atrium, percutaneous, autologous tissue substitute, zooplastic tissue, synthetic substitute, nonautologous tissue substitute	
	Repair right ventricle, left ventricle, percutaneous	Review the surgical consent, operative reports, and nurse's notes carefully to determine the exact surgical procedure that was performed. It is important to clearly differentiate between the root operations Repair (Q) and Supplement (U) versus Destruction (5) to ensure the correct root operation is reported. Report the device character and correctly identify the approach to result in the appropriate MS-DRG assignment.
	Supplement right ventricle, left ventricle, percutaneous, autologous tissue substitute, zooplastic tissue, synthetic substitute	
	Replacement atrial septum, percutaneous endoscopic, autologous tissue substitute, zooplastic tissue, synthetic substitute, nonautologous tissue substitute	Review the surgical consent, operative reports, and nurse's notes carefully to determine the exact surgical procedure that was performed. It is important to clearly differentiate between the root operations Replacement (R) versus Destruction (5) and Excision (B) to ensure the correct root operation is reported. Report the device character and correctly identify the approach to result in the appropriate MS-DRG assignment.
	AND	
	MCC condition	*See* appendix B.
273	MCC condition	*See* appendix B.

DRG 275 Cardiac Defibrillator Implant with Cardiac Catheterization and MCC — RW 7.0358

No Potential DRGs

DRG 276 Cardiac Defibrillator Implant with MCC — RW 6.2102

Potential DRGs

275 Cardiac Defibrillator Implant with Cardiac Catheterization and MCC 7.0358

DRG	PDx/SDx/Procedure	Tips
275	Cardiac defibrillator implant	
	AND	
	Cardiac catheterization	Measurement of cardiac sampling and pressure (right, left, bilateral).
	Coronary angiography	
	AND	
	MCC condition	*See* appendix B.

DRG 277 Cardiac Defibrillator Implant without MCC — RW 4.7824

Potential DRGs

275	Cardiac Defibrillator Implant with Cardiac Catheterization and MCC	7.0358
276	Cardiac Defibrillator Implant with MCC	6.2102

DRG	PDx/SDx/Procedure	Tips
275	Cardiac defibrillator implant	
	AND	
	Cardiac catheterization	Measurement of cardiac sampling and pressure (right, left, bilateral).
	Coronary angiography	
	AND	
	MCC condition	*See* appendix B.
276	MCC condition	*See* appendix B.

DRG 278 Ultrasound Accelerated and Other Thrombolysis of Peripheral Vascular Structures with MCC — RW 4.4604

Potential DRGs

270	Other Major Cardiovascular Procedures with MCC	5.0569

DRG	PDx/SDx/Procedure	Tips
270	Peripheral: Atherectomy Endarterectomy Thrombectomy (arterial or venous)	The objective of the root operation Extirpation is to remove solid matter from a body part. This may require the solid matter to be broken up (Fragmentation) prior to removal. Only extirpation should be reported when the solid matter is fragmented and removed from the same body part.
	AND	
	MCC condition	*See* appendix B.

DRG 279 Ultrasound Accelerated and Other Thrombolysis of Peripheral Vascular Structures without MCC — RW 3.2006

Potential DRGs

270	Other Major Cardiovascular Procedures with MCC	5.0569
271	Other Major Cardiovascular Procedures with CC	3.4562
278	Ultrasound Accelerated and Other Thrombolysis of Peripheral Vascular Structures with MCC	4.4604

DRG	PDx/SDx/Procedure	Tips
270	Peripheral: Atherectomy Endarterectomy Thrombectomy (arterial or venous)	The objective of the root operation Extirpation is to remove solid matter from a body part. This may require the solid matter to be broken up (Fragmentation) prior to removal. Only extirpation should be reported when the solid matter is fragmented and removed from the same body part.
	AND	
	MCC condition	*See* appendix B.
271	Peripheral: Atherectomy Endarterectomy Thrombectomy (arterial or venous)	*See* DRG 270.
	AND	
	CC condition	*See* appendix B.
278	MCC condition	*See* appendix B.

DRG 280 Acute Myocardial Infarction, Discharged Alive with MCC RW 1.5865

Potential DRGs

250	Percutaneous Cardiovascular Procedures without Intraluminal Device with MCC	2.3508
270	Other Major Cardiovascular Procedures with MCC	5.0569
314	Other Circulatory System Diagnoses with MCC	2.0935
321	Percutaneous Cardiovascular Procedures with Intraluminal Device with MCC or 4+ Arteries/Intraluminal Devices	2.8747
323	Coronary Intravascular Lithotripsy with Intraluminal Device with MCC	4.1400

DRG	PDx/SDx/Procedure	Tips
250	Coronary atherectomy	The objective of the root operation Extirpation is to remove solid matter from a body part.
	Coronary angioplasty without insertion of intraluminal device	
	AND	
	MCC condition	*See* appendix B.
270	Major cardiovascular procedure	
	AND	
	MCC condition	*See* appendix B.
314	Principal diagnosis of postinfarction angina or other complications following AMI	Includes those conditions found in category I23.-.
	AND	
	MCC condition	*See* appendix B.
321	Insertion of intraluminal device(s)	Device may be drug-eluting or non-drug-eluting
	AND	
	MCC condition	*See* appendix B.
	OR	
	Procedure on four or more arteries or placement of four or more intraluminal devices	
323	Coronary intravascular lithotripsy	The objective of root operation Fragmentation is to break solid matter within a body part into pieces. The pieces are not removed.
	AND	
	Insertion of intraluminal device	Device may be drug-eluting or non-drug-eluting.
	AND	
	MCC condition	*See* appendix B.

DRG 281 Acute Myocardial Infarction, Discharged Alive with CC RW 0.9130

Potential DRGs

250	Percutaneous Cardiovascular Procedures without Intraluminal Device with MCC	2.3508
251	Percutaneous Cardiovascular Procedures without Intraluminal Device without MCC 1.5869	
270	Other Major Cardiovascular Procedures with MCC	5.0569
271	Other Major Cardiovascular Procedures with CC	3.4562
280	Acute Myocardial Infarction, Discharged Alive with MCC	1.5865
314	Other Circulatory System Diagnoses with MCC	2.0935
315	Other Circulatory System Diagnoses with CC	0.9673
321	Percutaneous Cardiovascular Procedures with Intraluminal Device with MCC or 4+ Arteries/Intraluminal Devices	2.8747
322	Percutaneous Cardiovascular Procedures with Intraluminal Device without MCC	1.8234
323	Coronary Intravascular Lithotripsy with Intraluminal Device with MCC	4.1400
324	Coronary Intravascular Lithotripsy with Intraluminal Device without MCC	2.9686

DRG	PDx/SDx/Procedure	Tips
250	Coronary atherectomy	The objective of the root operation Extirpation is to remove solid matter from a body part.
	Coronary angioplasty without insertion of intraluminal device	
	AND	
	MCC condition	*See* appendix B.
251	Coronary atherectomy	*See* DRG 250.
	Coronary angioplasty without insertion of intraluminal device	
270	Major cardiovascular procedure	
	AND	
	MCC condition	*See* appendix B.
271	Major cardiovascular procedure	
	AND	
	CC condition	*See* appendix B.
280	MCC condition	*See* appendix B.
314	Principal diagnosis of postinfarction angina or other complications following AMI	Includes those conditions found in category I23.-.
	AND	
	MCC condition	*See* appendix B.
315	Principal diagnosis of postinfarction angina or other complications following AMI	Includes those conditions found in category I23.-.
	AND	
	CC condition	*See* appendix B.

Optimizing Tips

DRG 281 (Continued)

DRG	PDx/SDx/Procedure	Tips
321	Insertion of intraluminal device(s)	Device may be drug-eluting or non-drug-eluting
	AND	
	MCC condition	*See* appendix B.
	OR	
	Procedure on four or more arteries or placement of four or more intraluminal devices	
322	Insertion of intraluminal device(s)	*See* DRG 321.
323	Coronary intravascular lithotripsy	The objective of root operation Fragmentation is to break solid matter, within a body part, into pieces. The pieces are not removed.
	AND	
	Insertion of intraluminal device	Device may be drug-eluting or non-drug-eluting.
	AND	
	MCC condition	*See* appendix B.
324	Coronary intravascular lithotripsy	*See* DRG 323.
	AND	
	Insertion of intraluminal device	*See* DRG 323.

DRG 282 Acute Myocardial Infarction, Discharged Alive without CC/MCC

RW 0.7181

Potential DRGs

250	Percutaneous Cardiovascular Procedures without Intraluminal Device with MCC	2.3508
251	Percutaneous Cardiovascular Procedures without Intraluminal Device without MCC	1.5869
270	Other Major Cardiovascular Procedures with MCC	5.0569
271	Other Major Cardiovascular Procedures with CC	3.4562
272	Other Major Cardiovascular Procedures without CC/MCC	2.4395
280	Acute Myocardial Infarction, Discharged Alive with MCC	1.5865
281	Acute Myocardial Infarction, Discharged Alive with CC	0.9130
314	Other Circulatory System Diagnoses with MCC	2.0935
315	Other Circulatory System Diagnoses with CC	0.9673
321	Percutaneous Cardiovascular Procedures with Intraluminal Device with MCC or 4+ Arteries/Intraluminal Devices	2.8747
322	Percutaneous Cardiovascular Procedures with Intraluminal Device without MCC	1.8234
323	Coronary Intravascular Lithotripsy with Intraluminal Device with MCC	4.1400
324	Coronary Intravascular Lithotripsy with Intraluminal Device without MCC	2.9686

DRG	PDx/SDx/Procedure	Tips
250	Coronary atherectomy	The objective of the root operation Extirpation is to remove solid matter from a body part.
	Coronary angioplasty without insertion of intraluminal device	
	AND	
	MCC condition	*See* appendix B.
251	Coronary atherectomy	*See* DRG 250.
	Coronary angioplasty without insertion of intraluminal device	
270	Major cardiovascular procedure	
	AND	
	MCC condition	*See* appendix B.
271	Major cardiovascular procedure	
	AND	
	CC condition	*See* appendix B.
272	Major cardiovascular procedure	
280	MCC condition	*See* appendix B.
281	CC condition	*See* appendix B.
314	Principal diagnosis of postinfarction angina or other complications following AMI	Includes those conditions found in category I23.-.
	AND	
	MCC condition	*See* appendix B.
315	Principal diagnosis of postinfarction angina or other complications following AMI	Includes those conditions found in category I23.-.
	AND	
	CC condition	*See* appendix B.
321	Insertion of intraluminal device(s)	Device may be drug-eluting or non-drug-eluting
	AND	
	MCC condition	*See* appendix B.
	OR	
	Procedure on four or more arteries or placement of four or more intraluminal devices	
322	Insertion of intraluminal device(s)	*See* DRG 321.

DRG 282 (Continued)

DRG	PDx/SDx/Procedure	Tips
323	Coronary intravascular lithotripsy	The objective of root operation Fragmentation is to break solid matter within a body part into pieces. The pieces are not removed.
	AND	
	Insertion of intraluminal device	Device may be drug-eluting or non-drug-eluting.
	AND	
	MCC condition	*See* appendix B.
324	Coronary intravascular lithotripsy	*See* DRG 323.
	AND	
	Insertion of intraluminal device	*See* DRG 323.

DRG 283 Acute Myocardial Infarction, Expired with MCC RW 1.9714

Potential DRGs

250	Percutaneous Cardiovascular Procedures without Intraluminal Device with MCC	2.3508
270	Other Major Cardiovascular Procedures with MCC	5.0569
314	Other Circulatory System Diagnoses with MCC	2.0935
321	Percutaneous Cardiovascular Procedures with Intraluminal Device with MCC or 4+ Arteries/Intraluminal Devices	2.8747
323	Coronary Intravascular Lithotripsy with Intraluminal Device with MCC	4.1400

DRG	PDx/SDx/Procedure	Tips
250	Coronary atherectomy	The objective of the root operation Extirpation is to remove solid matter from a body part.
	Coronary angioplasty without insertion of intraluminal device	
	AND	
	MCC condition	*See* appendix B.
270	Major cardiovascular procedure	
	AND	
	MCC condition	*See* appendix B.
314	Principal diagnosis of postinfarction angina or other complications following AMI	Includes those conditions found in category I23.-.
	AND	
	MCC condition	*See* appendix B.
321	Insertion of intraluminal device(s)	Device may be drug-eluting or non-drug-eluting
	AND	
	MCC condition	*See* appendix B.
	OR	
	Procedure on four or more arteries or placement of four or more intraluminal devices	
323	Coronary intravascular lithotripsy	The objective of root operation Fragmentation is to break solid matter within a body part into pieces. The pieces are not removed.
	AND	
	Insertion of intraluminal device	Device may be drug-eluting or non-drug-eluting.
	AND	
	MCC condition	*See* appendix B.

DRG 284 Acute Myocardial Infarction, Expired with CC

RW 0.7397

Potential DRGs

250	Percutaneous Cardiovascular Procedures without Intraluminal Device with MCC	2.3508
251	Percutaneous Cardiovascular Procedures without Intraluminal Device without MCC	1.5869
270	Other Major Cardiovascular Procedures with MCC	5.0569
271	Other Major Cardiovascular Procedures with CC	3.4562
280	Acute Myocardial Infarction, Discharged Alive with MCC	1.5865
281	Acute Myocardial Infarction, Discharged Alive with CC	0.9130
283	Acute Myocardial Infarction, Expired with MCC	1.9714
314	Other Circulatory System Diagnoses with MCC	2.0935
315	Other Circulatory System Diagnoses with CC	0.9673
321	Percutaneous Cardiovascular Procedures with Intraluminal Device with MCC or 4+ Arteries/Intraluminal Devices	2.8747
322	Percutaneous Cardiovascular Procedures with Intraluminal Device without MCC	1.8234
323	Coronary Intravascular Lithotripsy with Intraluminal Device with MCC	4.1400
324	Coronary Intravascular Lithotripsy with Intraluminal Device without MCC	2.9686

DRG	PDx/SDx/Procedure	Tips
250	Coronary atherectomy	The objective of the root operation Extirpation is to remove solid matter from a body part.
	Coronary angioplasty without insertion of intraluminal device	
	AND	
	MCC condition	*See* appendix B.
251	Coronary atherectomy	*See* DRG 250.
	Coronary angioplasty without insertion of intraluminal device	
270	Major cardiovascular procedure	
	AND	
	MCC condition	*See* appendix B.
271	Major cardiovascular procedure	
	AND	
	CC condition	*See* appendix B.
280	Discharge status alive	
	AND	
	MCC condition	*See* appendix B.
281	Discharge status alive	
	AND	
	CC condition	*See* appendix B.
283	MCC condition	*See* appendix B.
314	Principal diagnosis of postinfarction angina or other complications following AMI	Includes those conditions found in category I23.-.
	AND	
	MCC condition	*See* appendix B.
315	Principal diagnosis of postinfarction angina or other complications following AMI	Includes those conditions found in category I23.-.
	AND	
	CC condition	*See* appendix B.
321	Insertion of intraluminal device(s)	Device may be drug-eluting or non-drug-eluting
	AND	
	MCC condition	*See* appendix B.
	OR	
	Procedure on four or more arteries or placement of four or more intraluminal devices	
322	Insertion of intraluminal device(s)	*See* DRG 321.
323	Coronary intravascular lithotripsy	The objective of root operation Fragmentation is to break solid matter within a body part into pieces. The pieces are not removed.
	AND	
	Insertion of intraluminal device	Device may be drug-eluting or non-drug-eluting.
	AND	
	MCC condition	*See* appendix B.
324	Coronary intravascular lithotripsy	*See* DRG 323.
	AND	
	Insertion of intraluminal device	*See* DRG 323.

DRG 285 Acute Myocardial Infarction, Expired without CC/MCC — RW 0.4887

Potential DRGs

250	Percutaneous Cardiovascular Procedures without Intraluminal Device with MCC	2.3508
251	Percutaneous Cardiovascular Procedures without Intraluminal Device without MCC	1.5869
270	Other Major Cardiovascular Procedures with MCC	5.0569
271	Other Major Cardiovascular Procedures with CC	3.4562
272	Other Major Cardiovascular Procedures without CC/MCC	2.4395
280	Acute Myocardial Infarction, Discharged Alive with MCC	1.5865
281	Acute Myocardial Infarction, Discharged Alive with CC	0.9130
282	Acute Myocardial Infarction, Discharged Alive without CC/MCC	0.7181
283	Acute Myocardial Infarction, Expired with MCC	1.9714
284	Acute Myocardial Infarction, Expired with CC	0.7397
314	Other Circulatory System Diagnoses with MCC	2.0935
315	Other Circulatory System Diagnoses with CC	0.9673
321	Percutaneous Cardiovascular Procedures with Intraluminal Device with MCC or 4+ Arteries/Intraluminal Devices	2.8747
322	Percutaneous Cardiovascular Procedures with Intraluminal Device without MCC	1.8234
323	Coronary Intravascular Lithotripsy with Intraluminal Device with MCC	4.1400
324	Coronary Intravascular Lithotripsy with Intraluminal Device without MCC	2.9686

DRG	PDx/SDx/Procedure	Tips
250	Coronary atherectomy	The objective of the root operation Extirpation is to remove solid matter from a body part.
	Coronary angioplasty without insertion of intraluminal device	
	AND	
	MCC condition	*See* appendix B.
251	Coronary atherectomy	*See* DRG 250.
	Coronary angioplasty without insertion of intraluminal device	
270	Major cardiovascular procedure	
	AND	
	MCC condition	*See* appendix B.
271	Major cardiovascular procedure	
	AND	
	CC condition	*See* appendix B.
272	Major cardiovascular procedure	
280	Discharge status alive	
	AND	
	MCC condition	*See* appendix B.
281	Discharge status alive	
	AND	
	CC condition	*See* appendix B.
282	Discharge status alive	
283	MCC condition	*See* appendix B.
284	CC condition	*See* appendix B.
314	Principal diagnosis of postinfarction angina or other complications following AMI	Includes those conditions found in category I23.-.
	AND	
	MCC condition	*See* appendix B.
315	Principal diagnosis of postinfarction angina or other complications following AMI	Includes those conditions found in category I23.-.
	AND	
	CC condition	*See* appendix B.
321	Insertion of intraluminal device(s)	Device may be drug-eluting or non-drug-eluting
	AND	
	MCC condition	*See* appendix B.
	OR	
	Procedure on four or more arteries or placement of four or more intraluminal devices	
322	Insertion of intraluminal device(s)	*See* DRG 321.
323	Coronary intravascular lithotripsy	The objective of root operation Fragmentation is to break solid matter within a body part into pieces. The pieces are not removed.
	AND	
	Insertion of intraluminal device	Device may be drug-eluting or non-drug-eluting.
	AND	
	MCC condition	*See* appendix B.
324	Coronary intravascular lithotripsy	*See* DRG 323.
	AND	
	Insertion of intraluminal device	*See* DRG 323.

DRG 286 Circulatory Disorders Except Acute Myocardial Infarction, with Cardiac Catheterization with MCC — RW 2.1556

228	Other Cardiothoracic Procedures with MCC	5.0387
242	Permanent Cardiac Pacemaker Implant with MCC	3.4551
245	AICD Generator Procedures	4.5314
270	Other Major Cardiovascular Procedures with MCC	5.0569
275	Cardiac Defibrillator Implant with Cardiac Catheterization and MCC	7.0358
276	Cardiac Defibrillator Implant with MCC	6.2102
321	Percutaneous Cardiovascular Procedures with Intraluminal Device with MCC or 4+ Arteries/Intraluminal Devices	2.8747

DRG	PDx/SDx/Procedure	Tips
228	Insertion of intracardiac pacemaker	Single- or dual-chamber device. The dual-chamber device is coded from the New Technology section.
	AND	
	MCC condition	*See* appendix B.
242	Permanent pacemaker implant (initial)	At least two codes must be reported—for both the pacemaker and the lead(s).
	AND	
	MCC condition	*See* appendix B.
245	AICD generator implant	
270	Major cardiovascular procedure	
	AND	
	MCC condition	*See* appendix B.
275	Cardiac defibrillator implant	Two codes must be reported—insertion of generator and lead(s).
	AND	
	Cardiac catheterization	Measurement of cardiac sampling and pressure (right, left, bilateral).
	Coronary angiography	
	AND	
	MCC condition	*See* appendix B.
276	Cardiac defibrillator implant	*See* DRG 275.
	AND	
	MCC condition	*See* appendix B.
321	Insertion of intraluminal device(s)	Device may be drug-eluting or non-drug-eluting
	AND	
	MCC condition	*See* appendix B.
	OR	
	Procedure on four or more arteries or placement of four or more intraluminal devices	

DRG 287 Circulatory Disorders Except Acute Myocardial Infarction, with Cardiac Catheterization without MCC — RW 1.0816

Potential DRGs

228	Other Cardiothoracic Procedures with MCC	5.0387
229	Other Cardiothoracic Procedures without MCC	3.1796
242	Permanent Cardiac Pacemaker Implant with MCC	3.4551
243	Permanent Cardiac Pacemaker Implant with CC	2.2776
244	Permanent Cardiac Pacemaker Implant without CC/MCC	1.8295
245	AICD Generator Procedures	4.5314
270	Other Major Cardiovascular Procedures with MCC	5.0569
271	Other Major Cardiovascular Procedures with CC	3.4562
272	Other Major Cardiovascular Procedures without CC/MCC	2.4395
275	Cardiac Defibrillator Implant with Cardiac Catheterization and MCC	7.0358
276	Cardiac Defibrillator Implant with MCC	6.2102
277	Cardiac Defibrillator Implant without MCC	4.7824
280	Acute Myocardial Infarction, Discharged Alive with MCC	1.5865
286	Circulatory Disorders Except Acute Myocardial Infarction, with Cardiac Catheterization with MCC	2.1556
321	Percutaneous Cardiovascular Procedures with Intraluminal Device with MCC or 4+ Arteries/Intraluminal Devices	2.8747
322	Percutaneous Cardiovascular Procedures with Intraluminal Device without MCC	1.8234

DRG	PDx/SDx/Procedure	Tips
228	Insertion of intracardiac pacemaker	Single- or dual-chamber device. The dual chamber device is coded from the New Technology section.
	AND	
	MCC condition	*See* appendix B.
229	Insertion of intracardiac pacemaker	*See* DRG 228.
242	Permanent pacemaker implant (initial)	At least two codes must be reported—for both the pacemaker and lead(s).
	AND	
	MCC condition	*See* appendix B.
243	Permanent pacemaker implant (initial)	*See* DRG 242.
	AND	
	CC condition	*See* appendix B.
244	Permanent pacemaker implant (initial)	*See* DRG 242.
245	AICD generator implant	
270	Major cardiovascular procedure	
	AND	
	MCC condition	*See* appendix B.
271	Major cardiovascular procedure	
	AND	
	CC condition	*See* appendix B.
272	Major cardiovascular procedure	
275	Cardiac defibrillator implant	Two codes must be reported—insertion of generator and lead(s).
	AND	
	Cardiac catheterization	Measurement of cardiac sampling and pressure (right, left, bilateral).
	Coronary angiography	
	AND	
	MCC condition	*See* appendix B.
276	Cardiac defibrillator implant	*See* DRG 275.
	AND	
	MCC condition	*See* appendix B.
277	Cardiac defibrillator implant	*See* DRG 275.
280	Acute myocardial infarction	
	AND	
	MCC condition	*See* appendix B.
286	MCC condition	*See* appendix B.
321	Insertion of intraluminal device(s)	Device may be drug-eluting or non-drug-eluting
	AND	
	MCC condition	*See* appendix B.
	OR	
	Procedure on four or more arteries or placement of four or more intraluminal devices	
322	Insertion of intraluminal device(s)	Device may be drug-eluting or non-drug-eluting

DRG 288 Acute and Subacute Endocarditis with MCC — RW 2.5930

No Potential DRGs

DRG 289 Acute and Subacute Endocarditis with CC — RW 1.4777

Potential DRGs

288	Acute and Subacute Endocarditis with MCC	2.5930
306	Cardiac Congenital and Valvular Disorders with MCC	1.5368

DRG	PDx/SDx/Procedure	Tips
288	MCC condition	*See* appendix B.
306	Viral endocarditis	
	Acute rheumatic endocarditis	
	Rheumatic valve disease	
	Congenital valve malformations	
	Mechanical complication of heart valve prosthesis	
	AND	
	MCC condition	*See* appendix B.

DRG 290 Acute and Subacute Endocarditis without CC/MCC — RW 1.0252

Potential DRGs

288	Acute and Subacute Endocarditis with MCC	2.5930
289	Acute and Subacute Endocarditis with CC	1.4777
306	Cardiac Congenital and Valvular Disorders with MCC	1.5368

DRG	PDx/SDx/Procedure	Tips
288	MCC condition	*See* appendix B.
289	CC condition	*See* appendix B.
306	Viral endocarditis	
	Acute rheumatic endocarditis	
	Rheumatic valve disease	
	Congenital valve malformations	
	Mechanical complication of heart valve prosthesis	
	AND	
	MCC condition	*See* appendix B.

DRG 291 Heart Failure and Shock with MCC — RW 1.2839

Potential DRGs

175	Pulmonary Embolism with MCC or Acute Cor Pulmonale	1.4030
177	Respiratory Infections and Inflammations with MCC	1.6964
264	Other Circulatory System O.R. Procedures	3.2660
270	Other Major Cardiovascular Procedures with MCC	5.0569
280	Acute Myocardial Infarction, Discharged Alive with MCC	1.5865
283	Acute Myocardial Infarction, Expired with MCC	1.9714
286	Circulatory Disorders Except Acute Myocardial Infarction, with Cardiac Catheterization with MCC	2.1556
871	Septicemia or Severe Sepsis without Mechanical Ventilation > 96 Hours with MCC	1.9826
919	Complications of Treatment with MCC	1.8247

DRG	PDx/SDx/Procedure	Tips
175	Septic pulmonary embolism with or without acute cor pulmonale	
	Saddle embolus of pulmonary artery with or without acute cor pulmonale	
	Other pulmonary embolism with or without acute cor pulmonale	
	Chronic pulmonary embolism	
	Air or fat embolism, including that following infusion, transfusion, and therapeutic injection, initial encounter	
	AND	
	MCC condition	*See* appendix B.
177	Pneumonia with causative organism: Salmonella Klebsiella pneumoniae Pseudomonas Staphylococcus Proteus or other gram-negative organisms	Bacterial pneumonia should be assigned based on physician documentation.
	COVID-19	Sequence UØ7.1 before J12.82 According to the ICD-10-CM guidelines, documentation by the provider that the individual has COVID-19 is sufficient and does not require additional documentation of a positive test result.
	Aspiration pneumonia	If both aspiration pneumonia and bacterial pneumonia or pneumonia due to COVID-19 are documented, code both. Sequencing will depend on the circumstances of admission. Elderly patients with acute stroke, cerebrovascular and degenerative neurologic diseases associated with dysphagia and impaired cough reflex are at increased risk of oropharyngeal aspiration. Review records for documentation of swallow studies, swallow therapy, assessment of cough and gag reflexes, increased oral care, and dietary modification. Diagnosis of aspiration pneumonia may be based on clinical presentation and/or chest x-ray findings.
	AND	
	MCC condition	*See* appendix B.

DRG 291 (Continued)

DRG	PDx/SDx/Procedure	Tips
264	Insertion of implantable pressure sensor for intracardiac or great vessel hemodynamic monitoring	Two codes must be reported.
270	Major cardiovascular procedure	
	AND	
	MCC condition	*See* appendix B.
280	Acute myocardial infarction, discharged alive	
	AND	
	MCC condition	*See* appendix B.
283	Acute myocardial infarction, expired	
	AND	
	MCC condition	*See* appendix B.
286	Circulatory system principal diagnosis except acute myocardial infarction	
	AND	
	Cardiac catheterization	Measurement of cardiac sampling and pressure (right, left, bilateral).
	Coronary angiography	
	AND	
	MCC condition	*See* appendix B.
871	Septic, hypovolemic or other specified shock	For cases of septic shock, the code for the systemic infection should be sequenced first, followed by code R65.21, Severe sepsis with septic shock. The code for septic shock cannot be assigned as a principal diagnosis.
	AND	
	MCC condition	*See* appendix B.
919	Postoperative shock, initial encounter	
	AND	
	MCC condition	*See* appendix B.

DRG 292 Heart Failure and Shock with CC

RW 0.8565

Potential DRGs

175	Pulmonary Embolism with MCC or Acute Cor Pulmonale	1.4030
177	Respiratory Infections and Inflammations with MCC	1.6964
178	Respiratory Infections and Inflammations with CC	0.9867
264	Other Circulatory System O.R. Procedures	3.2660
270	Other Major Cardiovascular Procedures with MCC	5.0569
271	Other Major Cardiovascular Procedures with CC	3.4562
280	Acute Myocardial Infarction, Discharged Alive with MCC	1.5865
281	Acute Myocardial Infarction, Discharged Alive with CC	0.9130
283	Acute Myocardial Infarction, Expired with MCC	1.9714
286	Circulatory Disorders Except Acute Myocardial Infarction, with Cardiac Catheterization with MCC	2.1556
287	Circulatory Disorders Except Acute Myocardial Infarction, with Cardiac Catheterization without MCC	1.0816
291	Heart Failure and Shock with MCC	1.2839
871	Septicemia or Severe Sepsis without Mechanical Ventilation > 96 Hours with MCC	1.9826
872	Septicemia or Severe Sepsis without Mechanical Ventilation > 96 Hours without MCC	1.0299
915	Allergic Reactions with MCC	1.7740
919	Complications of Treatment with MCC	1.8247
922	Other Injury, Poisoning and Toxic Effect Diagnoses with MCC	1.7449

DRG	PDx/SDx/Procedure	Tips
175	Septic pulmonary embolism with or without acute cor pulmonale	
	Saddle embolus of pulmonary artery with or without acute cor pulmonale	
	Other pulmonary embolism with or without acute cor pulmonale	
	Chronic pulmonary embolism	
	Air or fat embolism, including that following infusion, transfusion, and therapeutic injection, initial encounter	
	AND	
	MCC condition	*See* appendix B.
177	Pneumonia with causative organism: *Salmonella* *Klebsiella pneumoniae* *Pseudomonas* *Staphylococcus* *Proteus* or other gram-negative organisms	Bacterial pneumonia should be assigned based on physician documentation.
	COVID-19	Sequence UØ7.1 before J12.82 According to the ICD-10-CM guidelines, documentation by the provider that the individual has COVID-19 is sufficient and does not require additional documentation of a positive test result.
	Aspiration pneumonia	If both aspiration pneumonia and bacterial pneumonia or pneumonia due to COVID-19 are documented, code both. Sequencing will depend on the circumstances of admission. Elderly patients with acute stroke, cerebrovascular and degenerative neurologic diseases associated with dysphagia and impaired cough reflex are at increased risk of oropharyngeal aspiration. Review records for documentation of swallow studies, swallow therapy, assessment of cough and gag reflexes, increased oral care, and dietary modification. Diagnosis of aspiration pneumonia may be based on clinical presentation and/or chest x-ray findings.
	AND	
	MCC condition	*See* appendix B.
178	Pneumonia due to: *Salmonella* *Klebsiella pneumoniae* *Pseudomonas* *Staphylococcus* *Proteus* or other gram-negative pneumonia	Bacterial pneumonia should be assigned based on physician documentation. If both aspiration and bacterial pneumonia are documented, code both.
	COVID-19	*See* DRG 177.
	Aspiration pneumonia	*See* DRG 177.
	AND	
	CC condition	*See* appendix B.
264	Insertion of implantable pressure sensor for intracardiac or great vessel hemodynamic monitoring	Two codes must be reported.
270	Major cardiovascular procedure	
	AND	
	MCC condition	*See* appendix B.
271	Major cardiovascular procedure	
	AND	
	CC condition	*See* appendix B.
280	Acute myocardial infarction, discharged alive	
	AND	
	MCC condition	*See* appendix B.

DRG 292 (Continued)

DRG	PDx/SDx/Procedure	Tips
281	Acute myocardial infarction, discharged alive	
	AND	
	CC condition	*See* appendix B.
283	Acute myocardial infarction, expired	
	AND	
	MCC condition	*See* appendix B.
286	Circulatory system principal diagnosis except acute myocardial infarction	
	AND	
	Cardiac catheterization	Measurement of cardiac sampling and pressure (right, left, bilateral).
	Coronary angiography	
	AND	
	MCC condition	*See* appendix B.
287	Circulatory system principal diagnosis except acute myocardial infarction	
	AND	
	Cardiac catheterization	*See* DRG 286.
	Coronary angiography	
291	MCC condition	*See* appendix B.
871	Septic, hypovolemic or other specified shock	For cases of septic shock, the code for the systemic infection should be sequenced first, followed by code R65.21, Severe sepsis with septic shock. The code for septic shock cannot be assigned as a principal diagnosis.
	AND	
	MCC condition	*See* appendix B.
872	Septic, hypovolemic or other specified shock	*See* DRG 871.
	AND	
	CC condition	*See* appendix B.
915	Anaphylactic reaction due to food, initial encounter	
	Anaphylactic shock unspecified, initial encounter	
	Anaphylactic reaction due to serum, initial encounter	
	Anaphylactic reaction due to adverse effect of correct drug or medicament properly administered, initial encounter	
919	Postoperative shock, initial encounter	
	AND	
	MCC condition	*See* appendix B.
922	Traumatic shock, initial encounter	
	AND	
	MCC condition	*See* appendix B.

DRG 293 Heart Failure and Shock without CC/MCC RW 0.5615

Potential DRGs

175	Pulmonary Embolism with MCC or Acute Cor Pulmonale	1.4030
176	Pulmonary Embolism without MCC	0.8156
177	Respiratory Infections and Inflammations with MCC	1.6964
178	Respiratory Infections and Inflammations with CC	0.9867
179	Respiratory Infections and Inflammations without CC/MCC	0.7633
190	Chronic Obstructive Pulmonary Disease with MCC	1.1020
191	Chronic Obstructive Pulmonary Disease with CC	0.8490
192	Chronic Obstructive Pulmonary Disease without CC/MCC	0.6418
264	Other Circulatory System O.R. Procedures	3.2660
270	Other Major Cardiovascular Procedures with MCC	5.0569
271	Other Major Cardiovascular Procedures with CC	3.4562
272	Other Major Cardiovascular Procedures without CC/MCC	2.4395
280	Acute Myocardial Infarction, Discharged Alive with MCC	1.5865
281	Acute Myocardial Infarction, Discharged Alive with CC	0.9130
282	Acute Myocardial Infarction, Discharged Alive without CC/MCC	0.7181
283	Acute Myocardial Infarction, Expired with MCC	1.9714
284	Acute Myocardial Infarction, Expired with CC	0.7397
286	Circulatory Disorders Except Acute Myocardial Infarction, with Cardiac Catheterization with MCC	2.1556
287	Circulatory Disorders Except Acute Myocardial Infarction, with Cardiac Catheterization without MCC	1.0816
291	Heart Failure and Shock with MCC	1.2839
292	Heart Failure and Shock with CC	0.8565
304	Hypertension with MCC	1.1490
309	Cardiac Arrhythmia and Conduction Disorders with CC	0.7447
871	Septicemia or Severe Sepsis without Mechanical Ventilation > 96 Hours with MCC	1.9826
872	Septicemia or Severe Sepsis without Mechanical Ventilation > 96 Hours without MCC	1.0299
915	Allergic Reactions with MCC	1.7740
919	Complications of Treatment with MCC	1.8247
920	Complications of Treatment with CC	1.0338
922	Other Injury, Poisoning and Toxic Effect Diagnoses with MCC	1.7449

DRG	PDx/SDx/Procedure	Tips
175	Septic pulmonary embolism with or without acute cor pulmonale	
	Saddle embolus of pulmonary artery with or without acute cor pulmonale	
	Other pulmonary embolism with or without acute cor pulmonale	
	Chronic pulmonary embolism	
	Air or fat embolism, including that following infusion, transfusion, and therapeutic injection, initial encounter	
	AND	
	MCC condition	*See* appendix B.
176	Septic pulmonary embolism with or without acute cor pulmonale	
	Saddle embolus of pulmonary artery with or without acute cor pulmonale	
	Other pulmonary embolism with or without acute cor pulmonale	
	Chronic pulmonary embolism	
	Air or fat embolism, including that following infusion, transfusion, and therapeutic injection, initial encounter	
177	Pneumonia with causative organism: *Salmonella* *Klebsiella pneumoniae* *Pseudomonas* *Staphylococcus* *Proteus* or other gram-negative organisms	Bacterial pneumonia should be assigned based on physician documentation.
	COVID-19	Sequence UØ7.1 before J12.82 According to the ICD-10-CM guidelines, documentation by the provider that the individual has COVID-19 is sufficient and does not require additional documentation of a positive test result.
	Aspiration pneumonia	If both aspiration pneumonia and bacterial pneumonia or pneumonia due to COVID-19 are documented, code both. Sequencing will depend on the circumstances of admission. Elderly patients with acute stroke, cerebrovascular and degenerative neurologic diseases associated with dysphagia and impaired cough reflex are at increased risk of oropharyngeal aspiration. Review records for documentation of swallow studies, swallow therapy, assessment of cough and gag reflexes, increased oral care, and dietary modification. Diagnosis of aspiration pneumonia may be based on clinical presentation and/or chest x-ray findings.
	AND	
	MCC condition	*See* appendix B.

DRG 293 (Continued)

DRG	PDx/SDx/Procedure	Tips
178	Pneumonia with causative organism: *Salmonella* *Klebsiella pneumoniae* *Pseudomonas* *Staphylococcus* *Proteus* or other gram-negative organisms	Bacterial pneumonia should be assigned based on physician documentation.
	COVID-19	*See* DRG 177.
	Aspiration pneumonia	*See* DRG 177.
	AND	
	CC condition	*See* appendix B.
179	Pneumonia with causative organism: *Salmonella* *Klebsiella pneumoniae* *Pseudomonas* *Staphylococcus* *Proteus* or other gram-negative organisms	Bacterial pneumonia should be assigned based on physician documentation.
	COVID-19	*See* DRG 177.
	Aspiration pneumonia	*See* DRG 177.
190	COPD, NEC	
	Chronic asthmatic (obstructive) bronchitis	
	Chronic bronchitis with airways obstruction	
	Chronic bronchitis with emphysema	
	Chronic emphysematous bronchitis	
	Chronic obstructive asthma	
	Chronic obstructive bronchitis	
	Chronic obstructive tracheobronchitis	
	Emphysema	
	Bronchiectasis	
	AND	
	MCC condition	*See* appendix B.
191	COPD, NEC	
	Chronic asthmatic (obstructive) bronchitis	
	Chronic bronchitis with airways obstruction	
	Chronic bronchitis with emphysema	
	Chronic emphysematous bronchitis	
	Chronic obstructive asthma	
	Chronic obstructive bronchitis	
	Chronic obstructive tracheobronchitis	
	Emphysema	
	Bronchiectasis	
	AND	
	CC condition	*See* appendix B.
192	COPD, NEC	
	Chronic asthmatic (obstructive) bronchitis	
	Chronic bronchitis with airways obstruction	
	Chronic bronchitis with emphysema	
	Chronic emphysematous bronchitis	
	Chronic obstructive asthma	
	Chronic obstructive bronchitis	
	Chronic obstructive tracheobronchitis	
	Emphysema	
	Bronchiectasis	
264	Insertion of implantable pressure sensor for intracardiac or great vessel hemodynamic monitoring	Two codes must be reported.
270	Major cardiovascular procedure	
	AND	
	MCC condition	*See* appendix B.
271	Major cardiovascular procedure	
	AND	
	CC condition	*See* appendix B.
272	Major cardiovascular procedure	
280	Acute myocardial infarction, discharged alive	
	AND	
	MCC condition	*See* appendix B.
281	Acute myocardial infarction, discharged alive	
	AND	
	CC condition	*See* appendix B.

DRG 293 (Continued)

DRG	PDx/SDx/Procedure	Tips
282	Acute myocardial infarction, discharged alive	
283	Acute myocardial infarction, expired	
	AND	
	MCC condition	*See* appendix B.
284	Acute myocardial infarction, expired	
	AND	
	CC condition	*See* appendix B.
286	Circulatory system principal diagnosis except acute myocardial infarction	
	AND	
	Cardiac catheterization	Measurement of cardiac sampling and pressure (right, left, bilateral).
	Coronary angiography	
	AND	
	MCC condition	*See* appendix B.
287	Circulatory system principal diagnosis except acute myocardial infarction	
	AND	
	Cardiac catheterization	*See* DRG 286.
	Coronary angiography	
291	MCC condition	*See* appendix B.
292	CC condition	*See* appendix B.
304	Essential (primary) hypertension	
	Hypertensive heart disease without heart failure	
	Hypertensive heart and kidney disease without heart failure, with CKD stage 1-4 or unspecified	
	Secondary hypertension	
	AND	
	MCC condition	*See* appendix B.
309	Cardiac arrhythmia (e.g., SVT, atrial fibrillation)	
	Conduction Disorders	
	AND	
	CC condition	*See* appendix B.
871	Septic, hypovolemic or other specified shock	For cases of septic shock, the code for the systemic infection should be sequenced first, followed by code R65.21, Severe sepsis with septic shock. The code for septic shock cannot be assigned as a principal diagnosis.
	AND	
	MCC condition	*See* appendix B.
872	Septic, hypovolemic or other specified shock	*See* DRG 871.
915	Anaphylactic reaction due to food, initial encounter	
	Anaphylactic shock unspecified, initial encounter	
	Anaphylactic reaction due to serum, initial encounter	
	Anaphylactic reaction due to adverse effect of correct drug or medicament properly administered, initial encounter	
	AND	
	MCC condition	*See* appendix B.
919	Postoperative shock, initial encounter	
	AND	
	MCC condition	*See* appendix B.
920	Postoperative shock, initial encounter	
	AND	
	CC condition	*See* appendix B.
922	Traumatic shock, initial encounter	
	AND	
	MCC condition	*See* appendix B.

DRG 294 Deep Vein Thrombophlebitis with CC/MCC — RW 1.0937

Potential DRGs

252	Other Vascular Procedures with MCC	3.3538
253	Other Vascular Procedures with CC	2.5511
299	Peripheral Vascular Disorders with MCC	1.5762

DRG	PDx/SDx/Procedure	Tips
252	Interruption of the vena cava by insertion of implant or sieve (IVC filter) Total interruption (Occlusion) of the vena cava Partial interruption (Restriction) of the vena cava	Root operation Insertion is defined as: "Putting in a non-biological device that monitors, assists, performs, or prevents a physiological function but does not physically take the place of a body part." Root operations Occlusion and Restriction both have the objective of altering the diameter of an orifice or tubular body part. In order to code these root operations correctly, it must be understood whether the objective is to merely narrow or to block the opening or lumen completely.
	AND	
	MCC condition	*See* appendix B.
253	Interruption of the vena cava by insertion of implant or sieve (IVC filter) Total interruption (Occlusion) of the vena cava Partial interruption (Restriction) of the vena cava	*See* DRG 252.
	AND	
	CC condition	*See* appendix B.
299	Phlebitis and thrombophlebitis superficial vessels of lower extremity and other and unspecified sites	The physician should be queried to qualify differences between deep vein thrombosis and phlebitis and thrombophlebitis.
	AND	
	MCC condition	*See* appendix B.

DRG 295 Deep Vein Thrombophlebitis without CC/MCC — RW 0.6315

Potential DRGs

252	Other Vascular Procedures with MCC	3.3538
253	Other Vascular Procedures with CC	2.5511
254	Other Vascular Procedures without CC/MCC	1.7351
294	Deep Vein Thrombophlebitis with CC/MCC	1.0937
299	Peripheral Vascular Disorders with MCC	1.5762
300	Peripheral Vascular Disorders with CC	1.0670

DRG	PDx/SDx/Procedure	Tips
252	Interruption of the vena cava by insertion of implant or sieve (IVC filter) Total interruption (Occlusion) of the vena cava Partial interruption (Restriction) of the vena cava	Root operation Insertion is defined as: "Putting in a non-biological device that monitors, assists, performs, or prevents a physiological function but does not physically take the place of a body part." Root operations Occlusion and Restriction both have the objective of altering the diameter of an orifice or tubular body part. In order to code these root operations correctly, it must be understood whether the objective is to merely narrow or to block the opening or lumen completely.
	AND	
	MCC condition	*See* appendix B.
253	Interruption of the vena cava by insertion of implant or sieve (IVC filter) Total interruption (Occlusion) of the vena cava Partial interruption (Restriction) of the vena cava	*See* DRG 252.
	AND	
	CC condition	*See* appendix B.
254	Interruption of the vena cava by insertion of implant or sieve (IVC filter) Total interruption (Occlusion) of the vena cava Partial interruption (Restriction) of the vena cava	*See* DRG 252.
294	CC/MCC condition	*See* appendix B.
299	Phlebitis and thrombophlebitis superficial vessels of lower extremity and other and unspecified sites	The physician should be queried to qualify differences between deep vein thrombosis and phlebitis and thrombophlebitis.
	AND	
	MCC condition	*See* appendix B.
300	Phlebitis and thrombophlebitis superficial vessels of lower extremity and other and unspecified sites	The physician should be queried to qualify differences between deep vein thrombosis and phlebitis and thrombophlebitis.
	AND	
	CC condition	*See* appendix B.

DRG 296 Cardiac Arrest, Unexplained with MCC

RW 1.6032

Potential DRGs

283	Acute Myocardial Infarction, Expired with MCC	1.9714

DRG	PDx/SDx/Procedure	Tips
283	Acute myocardial infarction	If AMI is determined to be the cause of the cardiac arrest, it should be sequenced as PDX.
	AND	
	Discharge status expired	
	AND	
	MCC condition	*See* appendix B.

DRG 297 Cardiac Arrest, Unexplained with CC

RW 0.7286

Potential DRGs

280	Acute Myocardial Infarction, Discharged Alive with MCC	1.5865
281	Acute Myocardial Infarction, Discharged Alive with CC	0.9130
283	Acute Myocardial Infarction, Expired with MCC	1.9714
284	Acute Myocardial Infarction, Expired with CC	0.7397
296	Cardiac Arrest, Unexplained with MCC	1.6032

DRG	PDx/SDx/Procedure	Tips
280	Acute myocardial infarction	If AMI is determined to be the cause of the cardiac arrest, it should be sequenced as PDX.
	AND	
	Discharged alive	
	AND	
	MCC condition	*See* appendix B.
281	Acute myocardial infarction	*See* DRG 280.
	AND	
	Discharged alive	
	AND	
	CC condition	*See* appendix B.
283	Acute myocardial infarction	If AMI is determined to be the cause of the cardiac arrest, it should be sequenced as PDX.
	AND	
	Discharge status expired	
	AND	
	MCC condition	*See* appendix B.
284	Acute myocardial infarction	If AMI is determined to be the cause of the cardiac arrest, it should be sequenced as PDX.
	AND	
	Discharge status expired	
	AND	
	CC condition	*See* appendix B.
296	MCC condition	*See* appendix B.

DRG 298 Cardiac Arrest, Unexplained without CC/MCC RW 0.4389

Potential DRGs

280	Acute Myocardial Infarction, Discharged Alive with MCC	1.5865
281	Acute Myocardial Infarction, Discharged Alive with CC	0.9130
282	Acute Myocardial Infarction, Discharged Alive without CC/MCC	0.7181
283	Acute Myocardial Infarction, Expired with MCC	1.9714
284	Acute Myocardial Infarction, Expired with CC	0.7397
285	Acute Myocardial Infarction, Expired without CC/MCC	0.4887
296	Cardiac Arrest, Unexplained with MCC	1.6032
297	Cardiac Arrest, Unexplained with CC	0.7286

DRG	PDx/SDx/Procedure	Tips
280	Acute myocardial infarction	If AMI is determined to be the cause of the cardiac arrest, it should be sequenced as PDX.
	AND	
	Discharged alive	
	AND	
	MCC condition	*See* appendix B.
281	Acute myocardial infarction	*See* DRG 280.
	AND	
	Discharged alive	
	AND	
	CC condition	*See* appendix B.
282	Acute myocardial infarction	*See* DRG 280.
	AND	
	Discharged alive	
283	Acute myocardial infarction	If AMI is determined to be the cause of the cardiac arrest, it should be sequenced as PDX.
	AND	
	Discharge status expired	
	AND	
	MCC condition	*See* appendix B.
284	Acute myocardial infarction	*See* DRG 283.
	AND	
	Discharge status expired	
	AND	
	CC condition	*See* appendix B.
285	Acute myocardial infarction	*See* DRG 283.
	AND	
	Discharge status expired	
296	MCC condition	*See* appendix B.
297	CC condition	*See* appendix B.

DRG 299 Peripheral Vascular Disorders with MCC RW 1.5762

Potential DRGs

252	Other Vascular Procedures with MCC	3.3538
270	Other Major Cardiovascular Procedures with MCC	5.0569
278	Ultrasound Accelerated and Other Thrombolysis of Peripheral Vascular Structures with MCC	4.4604

DRG	PDx/SDx/Procedure	Tips
252	Occlusion or Supplement of lower extremity artery	
	Extirpation of lower extremity artery	Open or percutaneous endoscopic approach only.
	AND	
	MCC condition	*See* appendix B.
270	Extirpation of lower extremity artery	Percutaneous approach only.
	AND	
	MCC condition	*See* appendix B.
278	Thrombolysis of lower extremity artery or vein	The objective of root operation Fragmentation is to break solid matter within a body part into pieces. The pieces are not removed. This root operation is also found in DRGs 252–254. Based on the surgical hierarchy, DRGs 278–279 always takes precedence over DRGs 252–254.
	AND	
	MCC condition	See appendix B.

DRG 300 Peripheral Vascular Disorders with CC

RW 1.0670

Potential DRGs

175	Pulmonary Embolism with MCC or Acute Cor Pulmonale	1.4030
252	Other Vascular Procedures with MCC	3.3538
253	Other Vascular Procedures with CC	2.5511
270	Other Major Cardiovascular Procedures with MCC	5.0569
271	Other Major Cardiovascular Procedures with CC	3.4562
278	Ultrasound Accelerated and Other Thrombolysis of Peripheral Vascular Structures with MCC	4.4604
279	Ultrasound Accelerated and Other Thrombolysis of Peripheral Vascular Structures without MCC	3.2006
299	Peripheral Vascular Disorders with MCC	1.5762

DRG	PDx/SDx/Procedure	Tips
175	Septic pulmonary embolism with or without acute cor pulmonale	
	Saddle embolus of pulmonary artery with or without acute cor pulmonale	
	Other pulmonary embolism with or without acute cor pulmonale	
	Chronic pulmonary embolism	
	Air or fat embolism, including that following infusion, transfusion, and therapeutic injection, initial encounter	
	AND	
	MCC condition	*See* appendix B.
252	Occlusion or Supplement of lower extremity artery	
	Extirpation of lower extremity artery	Open or percutaneous endoscopic approach only.
	AND	
	MCC condition	*See* appendix B.
253	Occlusion or Supplement of lower extremity artery	
	Extirpation of lower extremity artery	*See* DRG 252.
270	Extirpation of lower extremity artery	Percutaneous approach only.
	AND	
	MCC condition	*See* appendix B.
271	Extirpation of lower extremity artery	Percutaneous approach only.
	AND	
	CC condition	*See* appendix B.
278	Thrombolysis of lower extremity artery or vein	The objective of root operation Fragmentation is to break solid matter within a body part into pieces. The pieces are not removed. This root operation is also found in DRGs 252–254. Based on the surgical hierarchy, DRGs 278–279 always takes precedence over DRGs 252–254.
	AND	
	MCC condition	*See* appendix B.
279	Thrombolysis of lower extremity artery or vein	*See* DRG 278.
299	MCC condition	*See* appendix B.

DRG 301 Peripheral Vascular Disorders without CC/MCC — RW 0.7098

Potential DRGs

175	Pulmonary Embolism with MCC or Acute Cor Pulmonale	1.4030
176	Pulmonary Embolism without MCC	0.8156
252	Other Vascular Procedures with MCC	3.3538
253	Other Vascular Procedures with CC	2.5511
254	Other Vascular Procedures without CC/MCC	1.7351
270	Other Major Cardiovascular Procedures with MCC	5.0569
271	Other Major Cardiovascular Procedures with CC	3.4562
272	Other Major Cardiovascular Procedures without CC/MCC	2.4395
278	Ultrasound Accelerated and Other Thrombolysis of Peripheral Vascular Structures with MCC	4.4604
279	Ultrasound Accelerated and Other Thrombolysis of Peripheral Vascular Structures without MCC	3.2006
299	Peripheral Vascular Disorders with MCC	1.5762
300	Peripheral Vascular Disorders with CC	1.0670

DRG	PDx/SDx/Procedure	Tips
175	Septic pulmonary embolism with or without acute cor pulmonale	
	Saddle embolus of pulmonary artery with or without acute cor pulmonale	
	Other pulmonary embolism with or without acute cor pulmonale	
	Chronic pulmonary embolism	
	Air or fat embolism, including that following infusion, transfusion, and therapeutic injection, initial encounter	
	AND	
	MCC condition	*See* appendix B.
176	Septic pulmonary embolism with or without acute cor pulmonale	
	Saddle embolus of pulmonary artery with or without acute cor pulmonale	
	Other pulmonary embolism with or without acute cor pulmonale	
	Chronic pulmonary embolism	
	Air or fat embolism, including that following infusion, transfusion, and therapeutic injection, initial encounter	
252	Occlusion or Supplement of lower extremity artery	
	Extirpation of lower extremity artery	Open or percutaneous endoscopic approach only.
	AND	
	MCC condition	*See* appendix B.
253	Occlusion or Supplement of lower extremity artery	
	Extirpation of lower extremity artery	*See* DRG 252.
	AND	
	CC condition	*See* appendix B.
254	Occlusion or Supplement of lower extremity artery	
	Extirpation of lower extremity artery	*See* DRG 252.
270	Extirpation of lower extremity artery	Percutaneous approach only.
	AND	
	MCC condition	*See* appendix B.
271	Extirpation of lower extremity artery	Percutaneous approach only.
	AND	
	CC condition	*See* appendix B.
272	Extirpation of lower extremity artery	Percutaneous approach only.
278	Thrombolysis of lower extremity artery or vein	The objective of root operation Fragmentation is to break solid matter within a body part into pieces. The pieces are not removed. This root operation is also found in DRGs 252–254. Based on the surgical hierarchy, DRGs 278–279 always takes precedence over DRGs 252–254.
	AND	
	MCC condition	*See* appendix B.
279	Thrombolysis of lower extremity artery or vein	*See* DRG 278.
299	MCC condition	*See* appendix B.
300	CC condition	*See* appendix B.

DRG 302 Atherosclerosis with MCC — RW 1.1211

Potential DRGs

286	Circulatory Disorders Except Acute Myocardial Infarction, with Cardiac Catheterization with MCC	2.1556

DRG	PDx/SDx/Procedure	Tips
286	Cardiac catheterization (right, left, bilateral) for measurement of cardiac sampling and pressure, or with angiocardiography (coronary angiography)	
	AND	
	MCC condition	*See* appendix B.

DRG 303 Atherosclerosis without MCC — RW 0.6581

Potential DRGs

286	Circulatory Disorders Except Acute Myocardial Infarction, with Cardiac Catheterization with MCC	2.1556
287	Circulatory Disorders Except Acute Myocardial Infarction, with Cardiac Catheterization without MCC	1.0816
302	Atherosclerosis with MCC	1.1211
308	Cardiac Arrhythmia and Conduction Disorders with MCC	1.2022
309	Cardiac Arrhythmia and Conduction Disorders with CC	0.7447

DRG	PDx/SDx/Procedure	Tips
286	Cardiac catheterization (right, left, bilateral) for measurement of cardiac sampling and pressure, or with angiocardiography (coronary angiography)	
	AND	
	MCC condition	*See* appendix B.
287	Cardiac catheterization (right, left, bilateral) for measurement of cardiac sampling and pressure, or with angiocardiography (coronary angiography)	
302	MCC condition	*See* appendix B.
308	Cardiac arrhythmia (e.g., SVT, atrial fibrillation)	
	Conduction Disorders	
	AND	
	MCC condition	*See* appendix B.
309	Cardiac arrhythmia (e.g., SVT, atrial fibrillation)	
	Conduction Disorders	
	AND	
	CC condition	*See* appendix B.

DRG 304 Hypertension with MCC — RW 1.1490

Potential DRGs

280	Acute Myocardial Infarction, Discharged Alive with MCC	1.5865
291	Heart Failure and Shock with MCC	1.2839
682	Renal Failure with MCC	1.5008

DRG	PDx/SDx/Procedure	Tips
280	Acute myocardial infarction, discharged alive	
	AND	
	MCC condition	*See* appendix B.
291	Heart failure, all types	
	Hypertensive heart disease with heart failure Hypertensive heart and kidney disease with heart failure	According to the ICD-10-CM guidelines the classification presumes a causal relationship between hypertension and heart and kidney involvement, as these terms are linked by the term "with" in the alphabetic index (either under a main term or subterm). Heart and kidney disease should be coded as related to hypertension unless the documentation clearly states the conditions are unrelated, in which case they may be coded separately. These conditions do not require provider documentation linking them to hypertension.
	AND	
	MCC condition	*See* appendix B.
682	Hypertensive chronic kidney disease with stage 1-5 chronic kidney disease or end stage renal disease Hypertensive heart and chronic kidney disease without heart failure	According to the ICD-10-CM guidelines the classification presumes a causal relationship between hypertension and heart and kidney involvement, as these terms are linked by the term "with" in the alphabetic index (either under a main term or subterm). Heart and kidney disease should be coded as related to hypertension unless the documentation clearly states the conditions are unrelated, in which case they may be coded separately. These conditions do not require provider documentation linking them to hypertension.
	AND	
	MCC condition	*See* appendix B.

DRG 305 Hypertension without MCC — RW 0.7535

Potential DRGs

280	Acute Myocardial Infarction, Discharged Alive with MCC	1.5865
281	Acute Myocardial Infarction, Discharged Alive with CC	0.9130
291	Heart Failure and Shock with MCC	1.2839
292	Heart Failure and Shock with CC	0.8565
304	Hypertension with MCC	1.1490
682	Renal Failure with MCC	1.5008
683	Renal Failure with CC	0.9008

DRG	PDx/SDx/Procedure	Tips
280	Acute myocardial infarction, discharged alive	
	AND	
	MCC condition	*See* appendix B.
281	Acute myocardial infarction, discharged alive	
	AND	
	CC condition	*See* appendix B.
291	Heart failure, all types	
	Hypertensive heart disease with heart failure Hypertensive heart and kidney disease with heart failure	According to the ICD-10-CM guidelines the classification presumes a causal relationship between hypertension and heart and kidney involvement, as these terms are linked by the term "with" in the alphabetic index (either under a main term or subterm). Heart and kidney disease should be coded as related to hypertension unless the documentation clearly states the conditions are unrelated, in which case they may be coded separately. These conditions do not require provider documentation linking them to hypertension.
	AND	
	MCC condition	*See* appendix B.
292	Heart failure, all types	
	Hypertensive heart disease with heart failure Hypertensive heart and kidney disease with heart failure	*See* DRG 291.
	AND	
	CC condition	*See* appendix B.
304	MCC condition	*See* appendix B.
682	Hypertensive chronic kidney disease with stage 1-5 chronic kidney disease or end stage renal disease Hypertensive heart and chronic kidney disease without heart failure	According to the ICD-10-CM guidelines the classification presumes a causal relationship between hypertension and heart and kidney involvement, as these terms are linked by the term "with" in the alphabetic index (either under a main term or subterm). Heart and kidney disease should be coded as related to hypertension unless the documentation clearly states the conditions are unrelated, in which case they may be coded separately. These conditions do not require provider documentation linking them to hypertension.
	AND	
	MCC condition	*See* appendix B.
683	Hypertensive chronic kidney disease with stage 1-5 chronic kidney disease or end stage renal disease	*See* DRG 682.
	Hypertensive heart and chronic kidney disease without heart failure	
	AND	
	CC condition	*See* appendix B.

DRG 306 Cardiac Congenital and Valvular Disorders with MCC — RW 1.5368

Potential DRGs

288	Acute and Subacute Endocarditis with MCC	2.5930

DRG	PDx/SDx/Procedure	Tips
288	Acute or subacute endocarditis	
	Meningococcal or syphilitic endocarditis	
	AND	
	MCC condition	*See* appendix B.

DRG 307 Cardiac Congenital and Valvular Disorders without MCC — RW 0.9426

Potential DRGs

288	Acute and Subacute Endocarditis with MCC	2.5930
289	Acute and Subacute Endocarditis with CC	1.4777
306	Cardiac Congenital and Valvular Disorders with MCC	1.5368

DRG	PDx/SDx/Procedure	Tips
288	Acute or subacute endocarditis	
	Meningococcal or syphilitic endocarditis	
	AND	
	MCC condition	*See* appendix B.
289	Acute or subacute endocarditis	
	Meningococcal or syphilitic endocarditis	
	AND	
	CC condition	*See* appendix B.
306	MCC condition	*See* appendix B.

DRG 308 Cardiac Arrhythmia and Conduction Disorders with MCC — RW 1.2022

Potential DRGs

280	Acute Myocardial Infarction, Discharged Alive with MCC	1.5865
291	Heart Failure and Shock with MCC	1.2839

DRG	PDx/SDx/Procedure	Tips
280	Acute myocardial infarction, discharged alive	
	AND	
	MCC condition	*See* appendix B.
291	Heart failure, all types	
	Hypertensive heart disease with heart failure Hypertensive heart and kidney disease with heart failure	According to the ICD-10-CM guidelines the classification presumes a causal relationship between hypertension and heart and kidney involvement, as these terms are linked by the term "with" in the alphabetic index (either under a main term or subterm). Heart and kidney disease should be coded as related to hypertension unless the documentation clearly states the conditions are unrelated, in which case they may be coded separately. These conditions do not require provider documentation linking them to hypertension.
	AND	
	MCC condition	*See* appendix B.

DRG 309 Cardiac Arrhythmia and Conduction Disorders with CC — RW 0.7447

Potential DRGs

280	Acute Myocardial Infarction, Discharged Alive with MCC	1.5865
281	Acute Myocardial Infarction, Discharged Alive with CC	0.9130
291	Heart Failure and Shock with MCC	1.2839
292	Heart Failure and Shock with CC	0.8565
308	Cardiac Arrhythmia and Conduction Disorders with MCC	1.2022

DRG	PDx/SDx/Procedure	Tips
280	Acute myocardial infarction, discharged alive	
	AND	
	MCC condition	*See* appendix B.
281	Acute myocardial infarction, discharged alive	
	AND	
	CC condition	*See* appendix B.
291	Heart failure, all types	
	Hypertensive heart disease with heart failure Hypertensive heart and kidney disease with heart failure	According to the ICD-10-CM guidelines the classification presumes a causal relationship between hypertension and heart and kidney involvement, as these terms are linked by the term "with" in the alphabetic index (either under a main term or subterm). Heart and kidney disease should be coded as related to hypertension unless the documentation clearly states the conditions are unrelated, in which case they may be coded separately. These conditions do not require provider documentation linking them to hypertension.
	AND	
	MCC condition	*See* appendix B.
292	Heart failure, all types	
	Hypertensive heart disease with heart failure	*See* DRG 291.
	Hypertensive heart and kidney disease with heart failure	
	AND	
	CC condition	*See* appendix B.
308	MCC condition	*See* appendix B.

DRG 310 Cardiac Arrhythmia and Conduction Disorders without CC/MCC RW 0.5530

Potential DRGs

280	Acute Myocardial Infarction, Discharged Alive with MCC	1.5865
281	Acute Myocardial Infarction, Discharged Alive with CC	0.9130
282	Acute Myocardial Infarction, Discharged Alive without CC/MCC	0.7181
291	Heart Failure and Shock with MCC	1.2839
292	Heart Failure and Shock with CC	0.8565
293	Heart Failure and Shock without CC/MCC	0.5615
308	Cardiac Arrhythmia and Conduction Disorders with MCC	1.2022
309	Cardiac Arrhythmia and Conduction Disorders with CC	0.7447
311	Angina Pectoris	0.6981

DRG	PDx/SDx/Procedure	Tips
280	Acute myocardial infarction, discharged alive	
	AND	
	MCC condition	*See* appendix B.
281	Acute myocardial infarction, discharged alive	
	AND	
	CC condition	*See* appendix B.
282	Acute myocardial infarction, discharged alive	
291	Heart failure, all types	
	Hypertensive heart disease with heart failure Hypertensive heart and kidney disease with heart failure	According to the ICD-10-CM guidelines the classification presumes a causal relationship between hypertension and heart and kidney involvement, as these terms are linked by the term "with" in the alphabetic index (either under a main term or subterm). Heart and kidney disease should be coded as related to hypertension unless the documentation clearly states the conditions are unrelated, in which case they may be coded separately. These conditions do not require provider documentation linking them to hypertension.
	AND	
	MCC condition	*See* appendix B.
292	Heart failure, all types	
	Hypertensive heart disease with heart failure	*See* DRG 291.
	Hypertensive heart and kidney disease with heart failure	
	AND	
	CC condition	*See* appendix B.
293	Heart failure, all types	
	Hypertensive heart disease with heart failure	*See* DRG 291.
	Hypertensive heart and kidney disease with heart failure	
308	MCC condition	*See* appendix B.
309	CC condition	*See* appendix B.
311	Angina without indication of underlying cause	

DRG 311 Angina Pectoris RW 0.6981

Potential DRGs

280	Acute Myocardial Infarction, Discharged Alive with MCC	1.5865
281	Acute Myocardial Infarction, Discharged Alive with CC	0.9130
282	Acute Myocardial Infarction, Discharged Alive without CC/MCC	0.7181
291	Heart Failure and Shock with MCC	1.2839
292	Heart Failure and Shock with CC	0.8565
302	Atherosclerosis with MCC	1.1211
308	Cardiac Arrhythmia and Conduction Disorders with MCC	1.2022
309	Cardiac Arrhythmia and Conduction Disorders with CC	0.7447
313	Chest Pain	0.7236
314	Other Circulatory System Diagnoses with MCC	2.0935
315	Other Circulatory System Diagnoses with CC	0.9673

DRG	PDx/SDx/Procedure	Tips
280	Acute myocardial infarction, discharged alive	
	AND	
	MCC condition	*See* appendix B.
281	Acute myocardial infarction, discharged alive	
	AND	
	CC condition	*See* appendix B.
282	Acute myocardial infarction, discharged alive	
291	Heart failure, all types	
	Hypertensive heart disease with heart failure Hypertensive heart and kidney disease with heart failure	According to the ICD-10-CM guidelines the classification presumes a causal relationship between hypertension and heart and kidney involvement, as these terms are linked by the term "with" in the alphabetic index (either under a main term or subterm). Heart and kidney disease should be coded as related to hypertension unless the documentation clearly states the conditions are unrelated, in which case they may be coded separately. These conditions do not require provider documentation linking them to hypertension.
	AND	
	MCC condition	*See* appendix B.

Optimizing Tips

DRG 311 (Continued)

DRG	PDx/SDx/Procedure	Tips
292	Heart failure, all types	
	Hypertensive heart disease with heart failure	*See* DRG 291.
	Hypertensive heart and kidney disease with heart failure	
	AND	
	CC condition	*See* appendix B.
302	Angina due to or associated with chronic heart disease of native or transplanted heart (e.g. ASHD)	ICD-10-CM combination codes capture both coronary artery disease and angina pectoris.
	AND	
	MCC condition	*See* appendix B.
308	Cardiac arrhythmia (e.g., SVT, atrial fibrillation)	
	Conduction Disorders	
	AND	
	MCC condition	*See* appendix B.
309	Cardiac arrhythmia (e.g., SVT, atrial fibrillation)	
	Conduction Disorders	
	AND	
	CC condition	*See* appendix B.
313	Chest pain with no indication of underlying cause	
314	Cardiomyopathy	
	Takotsubo syndrome	
	Intra or post-procedural cardiac complication or cardiac function abnormality	Review the documentation carefully; code assignment is based on the provider's documentation of a relationship between the condition and the procedure. Unless the classification instructs otherwise, only when there is a clear cause-and-effect relationship between the care provided and the condition and the documentation indicates the condition is a complication, can the condition be coded as such. Query the provider for clarification if the relationship/complication is not clearly documented. See guideline I.B.16.
	Nonspecific abnormal cardiovascular function study	
	Various cardiac device, implant and graft complications	
	AND	
	MCC condition	*See* appendix B.
315	Cardiomyopathy	
	Takotsubo syndrome	
	Intra or post-procedural cardiac complication or cardiac function abnormality	*See* DRG 314.
	Nonspecific abnormal cardiovascular function study	
	Various cardiac device, implant and graft complications	
	AND	
	CC condition	*See* appendix B.

DRG 312 Syncope and Collapse RW 0.8635

Potential DRGs

067	Nonspecific Cerebrovascular Accident and Precerebral Occlusion without Infarction with MCC	1.4169
068	Nonspecific Cerebrovascular Accident and Precerebral Occlusion without Infarction without MCC	0.8710
308	Cardiac Arrhythmia and Conduction Disorders with MCC	1.2022
314	Other Circulatory System Diagnoses with MCC	2.0935
315	Other Circulatory System Diagnoses with CC	0.9673
637	Diabetes with MCC	1.4493
638	Diabetes with CC	0.8994
640	Miscellaneous Disorders of Nutrition, Metabolism, and Fluids and Electrolytes with MCC	1.3152

DRG	PDx/SDx/Procedure	Tips
067	Nonspecific cerebrovascular and precerebral occlusion without infarction	
	AND	
	MCC condition	*See* appendix B.
068	Nonspecific cerebrovascular and precerebral occlusion without infarction	
308	Cardiac arrhythmia (e.g., SVT, atrial fibrillation)	
	Conduction Disorders	
	AND	
	MCC condition	*See* appendix B.
314	Cardiomyopathy	
	Takotsubo syndrome	
	Intra or post-procedural cardiac complication or cardiac function abnormality	Review the documentation carefully; code assignment is based on the provider's documentation of a relationship between the condition and the procedure. Unless the classification instructs otherwise, only when there is a clear cause-and-effect relationship between the care provided and the condition and the documentation indicates the condition is a complication, can the condition be coded as such. Query the provider for clarification if the relationship/complication is not clearly documented. See guideline I.B.16.
	Nonspecific abnormal cardiovascular function study	
	Various cardiac device, implant and graft complications	
	AND	
	MCC condition	*See* appendix B.
315	Cardiomyopathy	
	Takotsubo syndrome	
	Intra or post-procedural cardiac complication or cardiac function abnormality	*See* DRG 314.
	Nonspecific abnormal cardiovascular function study	
	Various cardiac device, implant and graft complications	
	AND	
	CC condition	*See* appendix B.
637	Diabetes mellitus with ketoacidosis, hyperosmolarity, other specified, unspecified or no complications	According to ICD-10-CM guidelines, the classification presumes a causal relationship between diabetes and certain associated manifestations and/or conditions when these terms are linked by the term "with" in the alphabetic index (either under a main term or subterm). These conditions should be coded as related to the diabetes unless the documentation clearly states the conditions are unrelated, in which case they may be coded separately. These conditions do not require provider documentation linking them to diabetes. Review the record and/or query the physician if it is unclear whether a condition is related to diabetes mellitus or the ICD-10-CM classification does not provide instruction.
	AND	
	MCC condition	*See* appendix B.
638	Diabetes mellitus with ketoacidosis, hyperosmolarity, other specified, unspecified or no complications	*See* DRG 637.
	AND	
	CC condition	*See* appendix B.
640	Disorders of fluid, electrolyte, and acid-base balance	
	Nondiabetic hypoglycemic coma and hypoglycemia unspecified	
	Elevated blood glucose level	
	Nutritional deficiencies	
	AND	
	MCC condition	*See* appendix B.

DRG 313 Chest Pain

RW 0.7236

Potential DRGs

204	Respiratory Signs and Symptoms	0.8229
280	Acute Myocardial Infarction, Discharged Alive with MCC	1.5865
281	Acute Myocardial Infarction, Discharged Alive with CC	0.9130
291	Heart Failure and Shock with MCC	1.2839
292	Heart Failure and Shock with CC	0.8565
302	Atherosclerosis with MCC	1.1211
308	Cardiac Arrhythmia and Conduction Disorders with MCC	1.2022
309	Cardiac Arrhythmia and Conduction Disorders with CC	0.7447
314	Other Circulatory System Diagnoses with MCC	2.0935
315	Other Circulatory System Diagnoses with CC	0.9673
391	Esophagitis, Gastroenteritis and Miscellaneous Digestive Disorders with MCC	1.2757
392	Esophagitis, Gastroenteritis and Miscellaneous Digestive Disorders without MCC	0.7856

DRG	PDx/SDx/Procedure	Tips
204	Chest pain on breathing, pleurodynia Dyspnea and respiratory abnormalities	Codes that describe symptoms and signs are acceptable for reporting purposes when a related definitive diagnosis has not been established (confirmed) by the provider.
280	Acute myocardial infarction, discharged alive	
	AND	
	MCC condition	*See* appendix B.
281	Acute myocardial infarction, discharged alive	
	AND	
	CC condition	*See* appendix B.
291	Heart failure, all types	
	Hypertensive heart disease with heart failure Hypertensive heart and kidney disease with heart failure	According to the ICD-10-CM guidelines the classification presumes a causal relationship between hypertension and heart and kidney involvement, as these terms are linked by the term "with" in the alphabetic index (either under a main term or subterm). Heart and kidney disease should be coded as related to hypertension unless the documentation clearly states the conditions are unrelated, in which case they may be coded separately. These conditions do not require provider documentation linking them to hypertension.
	AND	
	MCC condition	*See* appendix B.
292	Heart failure, all types	
	Hypertensive heart disease with heart failure Hypertensive heart and kidney disease with heart failure	*See* DRG 291.
	AND	
	CC condition	*See* appendix B.
302	Angina due to or associated with chronic heart disease of native or transplanted heart (e.g. ASHD)	ICD-10-CM combination codes capture both coronary artery disease and angina pectoris.
	AND	
	MCC condition	*See* appendix B.
308	Cardiac arrhythmia (e.g., SVT, atrial fibrillation)	
	Conduction Disorders	
	AND	
	MCC condition	*See* appendix B.
309	Cardiac arrhythmia (e.g., SVT, atrial fibrillation)	
	Conduction Disorders	
	AND	
	CC condition	*See* appendix B.
314	Cardiomyopathy	
	Takotsubo syndrome	
	Intra or post-procedural cardiac complication or cardiac function abnormality	Review the documentation carefully; code assignment is based on the provider's documentation of a relationship between the condition and the procedure. Unless the classification instructs otherwise, only when there is a clear cause-and-effect relationship between the care provided and the condition and the documentation indicates the condition is a complication, can the condition be coded as such. Query the provider for clarification if the relationship/complication is not clearly documented. See guideline I.B.16.
	Nonspecific abnormal cardiovascular function study	
	Various cardiac device, implant and graft complications	
	AND	
	MCC condition	*See* appendix B.
315	Cardiomyopathy	
	Takotsubo syndrome	
	Intra or post-procedural cardiac complication or cardiac function abnormality	*See* DRG 314.
	Nonspecific abnormal cardiovascular function study	
	Various cardiac device, implant and graft complications	
	AND	
	CC condition	*See* appendix B.

DRG 313 (Continued)

DRG	PDx/SDx/Procedure	Tips
391	Esophagitis	Query physician for etiology of noncardiac chest pain.
	Gastroesophageal reflux disease	
	Dyspepsia	
	Hiatal hernia	
	Abdominal pain or tenderness	
	AND	
	MCC condition	*See* appendix B.
392	Esophagitis	Query physician for etiology of noncardiac chest pain.
	Gastroesophageal reflux disease	
	Dyspepsia	
	Hiatal hernia	
	Abdominal pain or tenderness	

DRG 314 Other Circulatory System Diagnoses with MCC RW 2.0935

Potential DRGs

286	Circulatory Disorders Except Acute Myocardial Infarction, with Cardiac Catheterization with MCC	2.1556

DRG	PDx/SDx/Procedure	Tips
286	Circulatory system principal diagnosis except acute myocardial infarction	
	AND	
	Cardiac catheterization (right, left, bilateral) for measurement of cardiac sampling and pressure, or with angiocardiography (coronary angiography)	
	AND	
	MCC condition	*See* appendix B.

DRG 315 Other Circulatory System Diagnoses with CC RW 0.9673

Potential DRGs

280	Acute Myocardial Infarction, Discharged Alive with MCC	1.5865
286	Circulatory Disorders Except Acute Myocardial Infarction, with Cardiac Catheterization with MCC	2.1556
287	Circulatory Disorders Except Acute Myocardial Infarction, with Cardiac Catheterization without MCC	1.0816
314	Other Circulatory System Diagnoses with MCC	2.0935

DRG	PDx/SDx/Procedure	Tips
280	Acute myocardial infarction, discharged alive	
	AND	
	MCC condition	*See* appendix B.
286	Circulatory system principal diagnosis except acute myocardial infarction	
	AND	
	Cardiac catheterization (right, left, bilateral) for measurement of cardiac sampling and pressure, or with angiocardiography (coronary angiography)	
	AND	
	MCC condition	*See* appendix B.
287	Circulatory system principal diagnosis except acute myocardial infarction	
	AND	
	Cardiac catheterization (right, left, bilateral) for measurement of cardiac sampling and pressure, or with angiocardiography (coronary angiography)	
314	MCC condition	*See* appendix B.

DRG 316 Other Circulatory System Diagnoses without CC/MCC RW 0.6927

Potential DRGs

280	Acute Myocardial Infarction, Discharged Alive with MCC	1.5865
281	Acute Myocardial Infarction, Discharged Alive with CC	0.9130
286	Circulatory Disorders Except Acute Myocardial Infarction, with Cardiac Catheterization with MCC	2.1556
287	Circulatory Disorders Except Acute Myocardial Infarction, with Cardiac Catheterization without MCC	1.0816
312	Syncope and Collapse	0.8635
314	Other Circulatory System Diagnoses with MCC	2.0935
315	Other Circulatory System Diagnoses with CC	0.9673

DRG	PDx/SDx/Procedure	Tips
280	Acute myocardial infarction, discharged alive	
	AND	
	MCC condition	*See* appendix B.
281	Acute myocardial infarction, discharged alive	
	AND	
	CC condition	*See* appendix B.
286	Circulatory system principal diagnosis except acute myocardial infarction	
	AND	
	Cardiac catheterization (right, left, bilateral) for measurement of cardiac sampling and pressure, or with angiocardiography (coronary angiography)	
	AND	
	MCC condition	*See* appendix B.
287	Circulatory system principal diagnosis except acute myocardial infarction	
	AND	
	Cardiac catheterization (right, left, bilateral) for measurement of cardiac sampling and pressure, or with angiocardiography (coronary angiography)	
312	Orthostatic or iatrogenic hypotension	
	Syncope and collapse	
314	MCC condition	*See* appendix B.
315	CC condition	*See* appendix B.

DRG 319 Other Endovascular Cardiac Valve Procedures with MCC RW 4.3619

Potential DRGs

212	Concomitant Aortic and Mitral Valve Procedures	10.7707
216	Cardiac Valve and Other Major Cardiothoracic Procedures with Cardiac Catheterization with MCC	9.7053
219	Cardiac Valve and Other Major Cardiothoracic Procedures without Cardiac Catheterization with MCC	7.7112
266	Endovascular Cardiac Valve Replacement and Supplement Procedures with MCC	6.2461

DRG	PDx/SDx/Procedure	Tips
212	Repair or Replacement aortic valve	Open or percutaneous endoscopic approach.
	AND	
	Repair or Replacement mitral valve	Open or percutaneous endoscopic approach.
	AND	
	Cardiac catheterization	Measurement of cardiac sampling and pressure (right, left, bilateral) or cardiac rhythm.
	Coronary angiography	
216	Open valvuloplasty without replacement	Dilation with or without a device, or release. Approach must be open. The objective of root operation Dilation is to enlarge the diameter of a tubular body part or orifice. If a device remains at the end of the procedure to maintain the new diameter, this is an integral part of the procedure and captured with a sixth-character device value.
		If the sole objective of the procedure is freeing a body part without cutting the body part, the root operation is Release. In the root operation Release, the body part value coded is the body part being freed, not the tissue being manipulated or cut to free the body part.
	OR	
	Cardiac valve replacement, repair, supplement	Open or percutaneous endoscopic approach only
	AND	
	Cardiac catheterization (right, left, bilateral) for measurement of cardiac sampling and pressure, or with angiocardiography (coronary angiography)	
	AND	
	MCC condition	*See* appendix B.
219	Open valvuloplasty without replacement	*See* DRG 216.
	OR	
	Cardiac valve replacement, repair, supplement	*See* DRG 216.
	AND	
	MCC condition	*See* appendix B.
266	Transapical percutaneous transcatheter aortic, mitral, or pulmonary valve replacement or percutaneous endovascular transcatheter aortic or pulmonary valve replacement (TAVR, TAVI)	In a transcatheter valve replacement, a bioprosthetic valve made of bovine (cow) pericardium and supported with a metal stent is inserted via catheter through the femoral artery (percutaneous endovascular approach) or through the apex of the heart by means of a minor thoracotomy incision between the ribs (percutaneous transapical approach). The bioprosthetic valve is placed on the balloon catheter, positioned directly inside the diseased valve, and the balloon is inflated to secure the valve in place.
		Approach for an aortic or pulmonary valve replacement may be percutaneous transapical OR percutaneous endovascular. Mitral valve replacement procedures in this DRG are by percutaneous transapical approach only. Angioplasty is not reported separately.
	OR	
	Transcatheter aortic, mitral, pulmonary, or tricuspid valve supplement	Percutaneous approach.
	AND	
	MCC condition	*See* appendix B.

DRG 320 Other Endovascular Cardiac Valve Procedures without MCC RW 2.2260

Potential DRGs

212	Concomitant Aortic and Mitral Valve Procedures	10.7707
216	Cardiac Valve and Other Major Cardiothoracic Procedures with Cardiac Catheterization with MCC	9.7053
217	Cardiac Valve and Other Major Cardiothoracic Procedures with Cardiac Catheterization with CC	6.3653
218	Cardiac Valve and Other Major Cardiothoracic Procedures with Cardiac Catheterization without CC/MCC	5.6967
219	Cardiac Valve and Other Major Cardiothoracic Procedures without Cardiac Catheterization with MCC	7.7112
220	Cardiac Valve and Other Major Cardiothoracic Procedures without Cardiac Catheterization with CC	5.2446
221	Cardiac Valve and Other Major Cardiothoracic Procedures without Cardiac Catheterization without CC/MCC	4.6486
266	Endovascular Cardiac Valve Replacement and Supplement Procedures with MCC	6.2461
267	Endovascular Cardiac Valve Replacement and Supplement Procedures without MCC	4.8802
319	Other Endovascular Cardiac Valve Procedures with MCC	4.3619

DRG	PDx/SDx/Procedure	Tips
212	Repair or Replacement aortic valve	Open or percutaneous endoscopic approach.
	AND	
	Repair or Replacement mitral valve	Open or percutaneous endoscopic approach.
	AND	
	Cardiac catheterization	Measurement of cardiac sampling and pressure (right, left, bilateral) or cardiac rhythm.
	Coronary angiography	
216	Open valvuloplasty without replacement	Dilation with or without a device, or release.
		Approach must be open. The objective of root operation Dilation is to enlarge the diameter of a tubular body part or orifice. A device's remaining at the end of the procedure to maintain the new diameter is an integral part of the procedure and captured with a sixth-character device value.
		If the sole objective of the procedure is freeing a body part without cutting the body part, the root operation is Release. In the root operation Release, the body part value coded is the body part being freed, not the tissue being manipulated or cut to free the body part.
	OR	
	Cardiac valve replacement, repair, supplement	Open or percutaneous endoscopic approach only
	AND	
	Cardiac catheterization (right, left, bilateral) for measurement of cardiac sampling and pressure, or with angiocardiography (coronary angiography)	
	AND	
	MCC condition	*See* appendix B.
217	Open valvuloplasty without replacement	*See* DRG 216.
	OR	
	Cardiac valve replacement, repair, supplement	*See* DRG 216.
	AND	
	CC condition	*See* appendix B.
218	Open valvuloplasty without replacement	*See* DRG 216.
	OR	
	Cardiac valve replacement, repair, supplement	*See* DRG 216.
219	Open valvuloplasty without replacement	*See* DRG 216.
	OR	
	Cardiac valve replacement, repair, supplement	*See* DRG 216.
	AND	
	MCC condition	*See* appendix B.
220	Open valvuloplasty without replacement	*See* DRG 216.
	OR	
	Cardiac valve replacement, repair, supplement	*See* DRG 216.
	AND	
	CC condition	*See* appendix B.
221	Open valvuloplasty without replacement	*See* DRG 216.
	OR	
	Cardiac valve replacement, repair, supplement	*See* DRG 216.

DRG 320 (Continued)

DRG	PDx/SDx/Procedure	Tips
266	Transapical percutaneous transcatheter aortic, mitral, or pulmonary valve replacement or percutaneous endovascular transcatheter aortic or pulmonary valve replacement (TAVR, TAVI)	In a transcatheter valve replacement, a bioprosthetic valve made of bovine (cow) pericardium and supported with a metal stent is inserted via catheter through the femoral artery (percutaneous endovascular approach) or through the apex of the heart by means of a minor thoracotomy incision between the ribs (percutaneous transapical approach). The bioprosthetic valve is placed on the balloon catheter, positioned directly inside the diseased valve, and the balloon is inflated to secure the valve in place.
		Approach for an aortic or pulmonary valve replacement may be percutaneous transapical OR percutaneous endovascular. Mitral valve replacement procedures in this DRG are by percutaneous transapical approach only. Angioplasty is not reported separately.
	OR	
	Transcatheter aortic, mitral, pulmonary, or tricuspid valve supplement	Percutaneous approach.
	AND	
	MCC condition	*See* appendix B.
267	Transapical percutaneous transcatheter aortic, mitral, or pulmonary valve replacement or percutaneous endovascular transcatheter aortic or pulmonary valve replacement (TAVR, TAVI)	*See* DRG 266.
	OR	
	Transcatheter aortic, mitral, pulmonary, or tricuspid valve supplement	*See* DRG 266.
319	MCC condition	*See* appendix B.

DRG 321 Percutaneous Cardiovascular Procedures with Intraluminal Device with MCC or 4+ Arteries/Intraluminal Devices RW 2.8747

Potential DRGs

228	Other Cardiothoracic Procedures with MCC	5.0387
231	Coronary Bypass with PTCA with MCC	8.1152
323	Coronary Intravascular Lithotripsy with Intraluminal Device with MCC	4.1400

DRG	PDx/SDx/Procedure	Tips
228	Percutaneous in situ coronary venous arterialization (PICVA)	PICVA is a catheter-based bypass procedure where an intraluminal device (drug-eluting or non-drug-eluting) is inserted through the wall of the diseased coronary artery into an adjacent coronary vein, diverting the blood flow past the blockage.
	AND	
	MCC condition	*See* appendix B.
231	Coronary artery bypass procedure with arterial or vein graft	Open or percutaneous endoscopic approach.
	AND	
	PTCA	Dilation with or without intraluminal device(s).
	AND	
	MCC condition	*See* appendix B.
323	Coronary intravascular lithotripsy	The objective of root operation Fragmentation is to break solid matter within a body part into pieces. The pieces are not removed.
	AND	
	Insertion of intraluminal device	
	AND	
	MCC condition	*See* appendix B.

DRG 322 Percutaneous Cardiovascular Procedures with Intraluminal Device without MCC — RW 1.8234

Potential DRGs

228	Other Cardiothoracic Procedures with MCC	5.0387
229	Other Cardiothoracic Procedures without MCC	3.1796
231	Coronary Bypass with PTCA with MCC	8.1152
232	Coronary Bypass with PTCA without MCC	5.9486
321	Percutaneous Cardiovascular Procedures with Intraluminal Device with MCC or 4+ Arteries/Intraluminal Devices	2.8747
323	Coronary Intravascular Lithotripsy with Intraluminal Device with MCC	4.1400
324	Coronary Intravascular Lithotripsy with Intraluminal Device without MCC	2.9686

DRG	PDx/SDx/Procedure	Tips
228	Percutaneous in situ coronary venous arterialization (PICVA)	PICVA is a catheter-based bypass procedure where an intraluminal device (drug-eluting or non-drug-eluting) is inserted through the wall of the diseased coronary artery into an adjacent coronary vein, diverting the blood flow past the blockage.
	AND	
	MCC condition	*See* appendix B.
229	Percutaneous in situ coronary venous arterialization (PICVA)	*See* DRG 228.
231	Coronary artery bypass procedure with arterial or vein graft	Open or percutaneous endoscopic approach.
	AND	
	PTCA	Dilation with or without intraluminal device(s).
	AND	
	MCC condition	*See* appendix B.
232	Coronary artery bypass procedure with arterial or vein graft	Open or percutaneous endoscopic approach.
	AND	
	PTCA	Dilation with or without intraluminal device(s).
321	Insertion of intraluminal device	
	AND	
	MCC condition	*See* appendix B.
	OR	
	Procedures on four or more arteries or placement of four or more intraluminal devices	
323	Coronary intravascular lithotripsy	The objective of root operation Fragmentation is to break solid matter within a body part into pieces. The pieces are not removed.
	AND	
	Insertion of intraluminal device	
	AND	
	MCC condition	*See* appendix B.
324	Coronary intravascular lithotripsy	*See* DRG 323.
	AND	
	Insertion of intraluminal device	

DRG 323 Coronary Intravascular Lithotripsy with Intraluminal Device with MCC — RW 4.1400

No Potential DRGs

DRG 324 Coronary Intravascular Lithotripsy with Intraluminal Device without MCC — RW 2.9686

Potential DRGs

323	Coronary Intravascular Lithotripsy with Intraluminal Device with MCC	4.1400

DRG	PDx/SDx/Procedure	Tips
323	MCC condition	*See* appendix B.

DRG 325 Coronary Intravascular Lithotripsy without Intraluminal Device — RW 2.6443

Potential DRGs

323	Coronary Intravascular Lithotripsy with Intraluminal Device with MCC	4.1400
324	Coronary Intravascular Lithotripsy with Intraluminal Device without MCC	2.9686

DRG	PDx/SDx/Procedure	Tips
323	Coronary intravascular lithotripsy	
	AND	
	Insertion of intraluminal device	Percutaneous or percutaneous endoscopic approach.
	AND	
	MCC condition	*See* appendix B.
324	Coronary intravascular lithotripsy	
	AND	
	Insertion of intraluminal device	Percutaneous or percutaneous endoscopic approach.

Diseases And Disorders Of The Digestive System

DRG 326 Stomach, Esophageal and Duodenal Procedures with MCC — RW 5.0790

No Potential DRGs

DRG 327 Stomach, Esophageal and Duodenal Procedures with CC — RW 2.4974

Potential DRGs

326 Stomach, Esophageal and Duodenal Procedures with MCC 5.0790

DRG	PDx/SDx/Procedure	Tips
326	MCC condition	*See* appendix B.

DRG 328 Stomach, Esophageal and Duodenal Procedures without CC/MCC — RW 1.5973

Potential DRGs

326 Stomach, Esophageal and Duodenal Procedures with MCC 5.0790
327 Stomach, Esophageal and Duodenal Procedures with CC 2.4974

DRG	PDx/SDx/Procedure	Tips
326	MCC condition	*See* appendix B.
327	CC condition	*See* appendix B.

DRG 329 Major Small and Large Bowel Procedures with MCC — RW 4.5168

Potential DRGs

326 Stomach, Esophageal and Duodenal Procedures with MCC 5.0790

DRG	PDx/SDx/Procedure	Tips
326	Suture of duodenal ulcer site or suture of laceration of duodenum	Code the entire scope of the procedure(s) documented in the operative record, including resections that involve multiple sites (small and large bowel) or additional procedures performed, such as an adjunct repair (suture or ligation) or biopsy.
	Local excision of lesion of duodenum	
	Destruction of lesion of duodenum	Laser interstitial thermal therapy (LITT) performed via open, percutaneous, or percutaneous endoscopic approach or destruction using other method with any approach except percutaneous endoscopic.
	Repair of diaphragmatic (hiatal) hernia, abdominal or thoracic approach (with or without mesh)	Diaphragmatic (hiatal) hernias are considered digestive system disorders even though the repair of these hernias is coded to the Respiratory body system in ICD-10-PCS. Hernia repair without mesh is coded to root operation Repair (0BQ). Hernia repair with mesh is coded to the root operation Supplement (0BU).
	AND	
	MCC condition	*See* appendix B.

DRG 330 Major Small and Large Bowel Procedures with CC — RW 2.3721

Potential DRGs

326 Stomach, Esophageal and Duodenal Procedures with MCC 5.0790
329 Major Small and Large Bowel Procedures with MCC 4.5168

DRG	PDx/SDx/Procedure	Tips
326	Suture of duodenal ulcer site or suture of laceration of duodenum	Code the entire scope of the procedure(s) documented in the operative record, including resections that involve multiple sites (small and large bowel) or additional procedures performed, such as an adjunct repair (suture or ligation) or biopsy.
	Local excision of lesion of duodenum	
	Destruction of lesion of duodenum	Laser interstitial thermal therapy (LITT) performed via open, percutaneous, or percutaneous endoscopic approach or destruction using other method with any approach except percutaneous endoscopic.
	Repair of diaphragmatic (hiatal) hernia, abdominal or thoracic approach (with or without mesh)	Diaphragmatic (hiatal) hernias are considered digestive system disorders even though the repair of these hernias is coded to the Respiratory body system in ICD-10-PCS. Hernia repair without mesh is coded to root operation Repair (0BQ). Hernia repair with mesh is coded to the root operation Supplement (0BU).
	AND	
	MCC condition	*See* appendix B.
329	MCC condition	*See* appendix B.

DRG 331 Major Small and Large Bowel Procedures without CC/MCC

RW 1.6720

Potential DRGs

326	Stomach, Esophageal and Duodenal Procedures with MCC	5.0790
327	Stomach, Esophageal and Duodenal Procedures with CC	2.4974
329	Major Small and Large Bowel Procedures with MCC	4.5168
330	Major Small and Large Bowel Procedures with CC	2.3721

DRG	PDx/SDx/Procedure	Tips
326	Suture of duodenal ulcer site or suture of laceration of duodenum	Code the entire scope of the procedure(s) documented in the operative record, including resections that involve multiple sites (small and large bowel) or additional procedures performed, such as an adjunct repair (suture or ligation) or biopsy.
	Local excision or destruction of lesion of duodenum	
	Repair of diaphragmatic (hiatal) hernia, abdominal or thoracic approach (with or without mesh)	Diaphragmatic (hiatal) hernias are considered digestive system disorders even though the repair of these hernias is coded to the Respiratory body system in ICD-10-PCS. Hernia repair without mesh is coded to root operation Repair (ØBQ). Hernia repair with mesh is coded to the root operation Supplement (ØBU).
	AND	
	MCC condition	*See* appendix B.
327	Suture of duodenal ulcer site or suture of laceration of duodenum	*See* DRG 326.
	Local excision or destruction of lesion of duodenum	
	Repair of diaphragmatic (hiatal) hernia, abdominal or thoracic approach (with or without mesh)	*See* DRG 326.
	AND	
	CC condition	*See* appendix B.
329	MCC condition	*See* appendix B.
330	CC condition	*See* appendix B.

DRG 332 Rectal Resection with MCC

RW 3.6276

Potential DRGs

329	Major Small and Large Bowel Procedures with MCC	4.5168

DRG	PDx/SDx/Procedure	Tips
329	Colostomy (temporary, permanent or NOS), root operation Bypass	Information about the anastomotic technique used to complete a colectomy procedure (e.g., side to end) is not specified in ICD-10-PCS. Only the specific Excision or Resection code is assigned. The anastomosis is inherent to the surgery and not coded separately. *ICD-10-PCS Official Guidelines for Coding and Reporting*, guideline B3.1b states: "Procedural steps necessary to reach the operative site and close the operative site, including anastomosis of a tubular body part, are also not coded separately." Code the entire scope of the procedure(s) documented in the operative record, including resections that involve multiple sites (colorectal) or resections performed as part of a greater repair (proctopexy) or take-down procedure.
	Ileostomy (temporary, continent, permanent or NOS)	
	Revision or repair of anastomosis of small or large intestine	
	Proctostomy	
	Closure of proctostomy	
	Abdominal or other proctopexy	
	Repair of colovaginal, rectovaginal or other vaginoenteric fistula	
	AND	
	MCC condition	*See* appendix B.

DRG 333 Rectal Resection with CC — RW 2.0795

Potential DRGs

329	Major Small and Large Bowel Procedures with MCC	4.5168
330	Major Small and Large Bowel Procedures with CC	2.3721
332	Rectal Resection with MCC	3.6276

DRG	PDx/SDx/Procedure	Tips
329	Colostomy (temporary, permanent or NOS), root operation Bypass	Information about the anastomotic technique used to complete a colectomy procedure (e.g., side to end) is not specified in ICD-10-PCS. Only the specific Excision or Resection code is assigned. The anastomosis is inherent to the surgery and not coded separately. *ICD-10-PCS Official Guidelines for Coding and Reporting*, guideline B3.1b states: "Procedural steps necessary to reach the operative site and close the operative site, including anastomosis of a tubular body part, are also not coded separately." Code the entire scope of the procedure(s) documented in the operative record, including resections that involve multiple sites (colorectal) or resections performed as part of a greater repair (proctopexy) or take-down procedure.
	Ileostomy (temporary, continent, permanent or NOS)	
	Revision or repair of anastomosis of small or large intestine	
	Proctostomy	
	Closure of proctostomy	
	Abdominal or other proctopexy	
	Repair of colovaginal, rectovaginal or other vaginoenteric fistula	
	AND	
	MCC condition	*See* appendix B.
330	Colostomy (temporary, permanent or NOS), root operation Bypass	*See* DRG 329.
	Ileostomy (temporary, continent, permanent or NOS)	
	Revision or repair of anastomosis of small or large intestine	
	Proctostomy	
	Closure of proctostomy	
	Abdominal or other proctopexy	
	Repair of colovaginal, rectovaginal or other vaginoenteric fistula	
	AND	
	CC condition	*See* appendix B.
332	MCC condition	*See* appendix B.

DRG 334 Rectal Resection without CC/MCC — RW 1.6051

Potential DRGs

329	Major Small and Large Bowel Procedures with MCC	4.5168
330	Major Small and Large Bowel Procedures with CC	2.3721
332	Rectal Resection with MCC	3.6276
333	Rectal Resection with CC	2.0795

DRG	PDx/SDx/Procedure	Tips
329	Colostomy (temporary, permanent or NOS), root operation Bypass	Information about the anastomotic technique used to complete a colectomy procedure (e.g., side to end) is not specified in ICD-10-PCS. Only the specific Excision or Resection code is assigned. The anastomosis is inherent to the surgery and not coded separately. *ICD-10-PCS Official Guidelines for Coding and Reporting*, guideline B3.1b states: "Procedural steps necessary to reach the operative site and close the operative site, including anastomosis of a tubular body part, are also not coded separately." Code the entire scope of the procedure(s) documented in the operative record, including resections that involve multiple sites (colorectal) or resections performed as part of a greater repair (proctopexy) or take-down procedure.
	Ileostomy (temporary, continent, permanent or NOS)	
	Revision or repair of anastomosis of small or large intestine	
	Proctostomy	
	Closure of proctostomy	
	Abdominal or other proctopexy	
	Repair of colovaginal, rectovaginal or other vaginoenteric fistula	
	AND	
	MCC condition	*See* appendix B.
330	Colostomy (temporary, permanent or NOS), root operation Bypass	*See* DRG 329.
	Ileostomy (temporary, continent, permanent or NOS)	
	Revision or repair of anastomosis of small or large intestine	
	Proctostomy	
	Closure of proctostomy	
	Abdominal or other proctopexy	
	Repair of colovaginal, rectovaginal or other vaginoenteric fistula	
	AND	
	CC condition	*See* appendix B.
332	MCC condition	*See* appendix B.
333	CC condition	*See* appendix B.

DRG 335 Peritoneal Adhesiolysis with MCC RW 3.5750

Potential DRGs

329	Major small or large bowel procedures with MCC	4.5168

DRG	PDx/SDx/Procedure	Tips
329	Repair of intraoperative laceration of intestine	Review operative report for enterotomies during surgery that are documented as clinically significant and a complication of the procedure.
	AND	
	MCC condition	*See* appendix B.

DRG 336 Peritoneal Adhesiolysis with CC RW 2.1053

Potential DRGs

329	Major Small and Large Bowel Procedures with MCC	4.5168
330	Major Small and Large Bowel Procedures with CC	2.3721
335	Peritoneal Adhesiolysis with MCC	3.5750

DRG	PDx/SDx/Procedure	Tips
329	Repair of intraoperative laceration of intestine	Review operative report for enterotomies during surgery that are documented as clinically significant and a complication of the procedure.
	AND	
	MCC condition	*See* appendix B.
330	Repair of intraoperative laceration of intestine	*See* DRG 329.
	AND	
	CC condition	*See* appendix B.
335	MCC condition	*See* appendix B.

DRG 337 Peritoneal Adhesiolysis without CC/MCC RW 1.4964

Potential DRGs

329	Major Small and Large Bowel Procedures with MCC	4.5168
330	Major Small and Large Bowel Procedures with CC	2.3721
331	Major Small and Large Bowel Procedures without CC/MCC	1.6720
335	Peritoneal Adhesiolysis with MCC	3.5750
336	Peritoneal Adhesiolysis with CC	2.1053

DRG	PDx/SDx/Procedure	Tips
329	Repair of intraoperative laceration of intestine	Review operative report for enterotomies during surgery that are documented as clinically significant and a complication of the procedure
	AND	
	MCC condition	*See* appendix B.
330	Repair of intraoperative laceration of intestine	*See* DRG 329.
	AND	
	CC condition	*See* appendix B.
331	Repair of intraoperative laceration of intestine	*See* DRG 329.
335	MCC condition	*See* appendix B.
336	CC condition	*See* appendix B.

DRG 344 Minor Small and Large Bowel Procedures with MCC RW 2.7404

Potential DRGs

329	Major Small and Large Bowel Procedures with MCC	4.5168

DRG	PDx/SDx/Procedure	Tips
329	Colostomy (temporary, permanent or NOS), root operation Bypass	Information about the anastomotic technique used to complete a colectomy procedure (e.g., side to end) is not specified in ICD-10-PCS. Only the specific Excision or Resection code is assigned. The anastomosis is inherent to the surgery and not coded separately. *ICD-10-PCS Official Guidelines for Coding and Reporting*, guideline B3.1b states: "Procedural steps necessary to reach the operative site and close the operative site, including anastomosis of a tubular body part, are also not coded separately." Code the entire scope of the procedure(s) documented in the operative record, including resections that involve multiple sites (colorectal) or resections performed as part of a greater repair (proctopexy) or take-down procedure.
	Ileostomy (temporary, continent, permanent or NOS)	
	Revision or repair of anastomosis of small or large intestine	
	Proctostomy	
	Closure of proctostomy	
	Abdominal or other proctopexy	
	Repair of colovaginal, rectovaginal or other vaginoenteric fistula	
	AND	
	MCC condition	*See* appendix B.

DRG 345 Minor Small and Large Bowel Procedures with CC RW 1.5406

Potential DRGs

329	Major Small and Large Bowel Procedures with MCC	4.5168
330	Major Small and Large Bowel Procedures with CC	2.3721
344	Minor Small and Large Bowel Procedures with MCC	2.7404

DRG	PDx/SDx/Procedure	Tips
329	Colostomy (temporary, permanent or NOS), root operation Bypass	Information about the anastomotic technique used to complete a colectomy procedure (e.g., side to end) is not specified in ICD-10-PCS. Only the specific Excision or Resection code is assigned. The anastomosis is inherent to the surgery and not coded separately. *ICD-10-PCS Official Guidelines for Coding and Reporting*, guideline B3.1b states: "Procedural steps necessary to reach the operative site and close the operative site, including anastomosis of a tubular body part, are also not coded separately." Code the entire scope of the procedure(s) documented in the operative record, including resections that involve multiple sites (colorectal) or resections performed as part of a greater repair (proctopexy) or take-down procedure.
	Ileostomy (temporary, continent, permanent or NOS)	
	Revision or repair of anastomosis of small or large intestine	
	Proctostomy	
	Closure of proctostomy	
	Abdominal or other proctopexy	
	Repair of colovaginal, rectovaginal or other vaginoenteric fistula	
	AND	
	MCC condition	*See* appendix B.
330	Colostomy (temporary, permanent or NOS), root operation Bypass	*See* DRG 329.
	Ileostomy (temporary, continent, permanent or NOS)	
	Revision or repair of anastomosis of small or large intestine	
	Proctostomy	
	Closure of proctostomy	
	Abdominal or other proctopexy	
	Repair of colovaginal, rectovaginal or other vaginoenteric fistula	
	AND	
	CC condition	*See* appendix B.
344	MCC condition	*See* appendix B.

DRG 346 Minor Small and Large Bowel Procedures without CC/MCC RW 1.2878

Potential DRGs

329	Major Small and Large Bowel Procedures with MCC	4.5168
330	Major Small and Large Bowel Procedures with CC	2.3721
331	Major Small and Large Bowel Procedures without CC/MCC	1.6720
344	Minor Small and Large Bowel Procedures with MCC	2.7404
345	Minor Small and Large Bowel Procedures with CC	1.5406

DRG	PDx/SDx/Procedure	Tips
329	Colostomy (temporary, permanent or NOS), root operation Bypass	Information about the anastomotic technique used to complete a colectomy procedure (e.g., side to end) is not specified in ICD-10-PCS. Only the specific Excision or Resection code is assigned. The anastomosis is inherent to the surgery and not coded separately. *ICD-10-PCS Official Guidelines for Coding and Reporting*, guideline B3.1b states: "Procedural steps necessary to reach the operative site and close the operative site, including anastomosis of a tubular body part, are also not coded separately." Code the entire scope of the procedure(s) documented in the operative record, including resections that involve multiple sites (colorectal) or resections performed as part of a greater repair (proctopexy) or take-down procedure.
	Ileostomy (temporary, continent, permanent or NOS)	
	Revision or repair of anastomosis of small or large intestine	
	Proctostomy	
	Closure of proctostomy	
	Abdominal or other proctopexy	
	Repair of colovaginal, rectovaginal or other vaginoenteric fistula	
	AND	
	MCC condition	*See* appendix B.
330	Colostomy (temporary, permanent or NOS), root operation Bypass	*See* DRG 329.
	Ileostomy (temporary, continent, permanent or NOS)	
	Revision or repair of anastomosis of small or large intestine	
	Proctostomy	
	Closure of proctostomy	
	Abdominal or other proctopexy	
	Repair of colovaginal, rectovaginal or other vaginoenteric fistula	
	AND	
	CC condition	*See* appendix B.
331	Colostomy (temporary, permanent or NOS), root operation Bypass	*See* DRG 329.
	Ileostomy (temporary, continent, permanent or NOS)	
	Revision or repair of anastomosis of small or large intestine	
	Proctostomy	
	Closure of proctostomy	
	Abdominal or other proctopexy	
	Repair of colovaginal, rectovaginal or other vaginoenteric fistula	
344	MCC condition	*See* appendix B.
345	CC condition	*See* appendix B.

DRG 347 Anal and Stomal Procedures with MCC RW 2.5491

Potential DRGs

329	Major Small and Large Bowel Procedures with MCC	4.5168
332	Rectal Resection with MCC	3.6276
335	Peritoneal Adhesiolysis with MCC	3.5750

DRG	PDx/SDx/Procedure	Tips
329	Colostomy (temporary, permanent or NOS), root operation Bypass	Information about the anastomotic technique used to complete a colectomy procedure (e.g., side to end) is not specified in ICD-10-PCS. Only the specific Excision or Resection code is assigned. The anastomosis is inherent to the surgery and not coded separately. *ICD-10-PCS Official Guidelines for Coding and Reporting*, guideline B3.1b states: "Procedural steps necessary to reach the operative site and close the operative site, including anastomosis of a tubular body part, are also not coded separately." Code the entire scope of the procedure(s) documented in the operative record, including resections that involve multiple sites (colorectal) or resections performed as part of a greater repair (proctopexy) or take-down procedure.
	Ileostomy (temporary, continent, permanent or NOS)	
	Revision or repair of anastomosis of small or large intestine	
	Proctostomy	
	Closure of proctostomy	
	Abdominal or other proctopexy	
	Repair of colovaginal, rectovaginal or other vaginoenteric fistula	
	AND	
	MCC condition	*See* appendix B.
332	Insertion, removal, or revision of artificial anal sphincter	
	AND	
	MCC condition	*See* appendix B.
335	Lysis of intra-abdominal adhesions	Adhesiolysis is reported with root operation Release which is defined as "Freeing a body part from an abnormal physical constraint by cutting or by use of force." Release procedures are coded to the body part being freed. In cases of extensive intra-abdominal adhesions, multiple sites may be reported if they are defined by distinct body part values, according to ICD-10-PCS Guideline B3.2: "During the same operative episode, multiple procedures are coded if: a. The same root operation is performed on different body parts as defined by distinct values of the body part character." Adhesions and lysis must be determined by the physician as significant enough to code and report.
	AND	
	MCC condition	*See* appendix B.

DRG 348 Anal and Stomal Procedures with CC — RW 1.3014

Potential DRGs

329	Major Small and Large Bowel Procedures with MCC	4.5168
330	Major Small and Large Bowel Procedures with CC	2.3721
332	Rectal Resection with MCC	3.6276
333	Rectal Resection with CC	2.0795
335	Peritoneal Adhesiolysis with MCC	3.5750
336	Peritoneal Adhesiolysis with CC	2.1053
347	Anal and Stomal Procedures with MCC	2.5491

DRG	PDx/SDx/Procedure	Tips
329	Colostomy (temporary, permanent or NOS), root operation Bypass	Information about the anastomotic technique used to complete a colectomy procedure (e.g., side to end) is not specified in ICD-10-PCS. Only the specific Excision or Resection code is assigned. The anastomosis is inherent to the surgery and not coded separately. *ICD-10-PCS Official Guidelines for Coding and Reporting*, guideline B3.1b states: "Procedural steps necessary to reach the operative site and close the operative site, including anastomosis of a tubular body part, are also not coded separately." Code the entire scope of the procedure(s) documented in the operative record, including resections that involve multiple sites (colorectal) or resections performed as part of a greater repair (proctopexy) or take-down procedure.
	Ileostomy (temporary, continent, permanent or NOS	
	Revision or repair of anastomosis of small or large intestine	
	Proctostomy	
	Closure of proctostomy	
	Abdominal or other proctopexy	
	Repair of colovaginal, rectovaginal or other vaginoenteric fistula	
	AND	
	MCC condition	*See* appendix B.
330	Colostomy (temporary, permanent or NOS), root operation Bypass	*See* DRG 329.
	Ileostomy (temporary, continent, permanent or NOS)	
	Revision or repair of anastomosis of small or large intestine	
	Proctostomy	
	Closure of proctostomy	
	Abdominal or other proctopexy	
	Repair of colovaginal, rectovaginal or other vaginoenteric fistula	
	AND	
	CC condition	*See* appendix B.
332	Insertion, removal, or revision of artificial anal sphincter	
	AND	
	MCC condition	*See* appendix B.
333	Insertion, removal, or revision of artificial anal sphincter	
	AND	
	CC condition	*See* appendix B.
335	Lysis of intra-abdominal adhesions	Adhesiolysis is reported with root operation Release which is defined as "Freeing a body part from an abnormal physical constraint by cutting or by use of force." Release procedures are coded to the body part being freed. In cases of extensive intra-abdominal adhesions, multiple sites may be reported if they are defined by distinct body part values, according to ICD-10-PCS Guideline B3.2: "During the same operative episode, multiple procedures are coded if: a. The same root operation is performed on different body parts as defined by distinct values of the body part character." Adhesions and lysis must be determined by the physician as significant enough to code and report.
	AND	
	MCC condition	*See* appendix B.
336	Lysis of intra-abdominal adhesions	*See* DRG 335.
	AND	
	CC condition	*See* appendix B.
347	MCC condition	*See* appendix B.

DRG 349 Anal and Stomal Procedures without CC/MCC — RW 0.9758

Potential DRGs

329	Major Small and Large Bowel Procedures with MCC	4.5168
330	Major Small and Large Bowel Procedures with CC	2.3721
331	Major Small and Large Bowel Procedures without CC/MCC	1.6720
332	Rectal Resection with MCC	3.6276
333	Rectal Resection with CC	2.0795
334	Rectal Resection without CC/MCC	1.6051
335	Peritoneal Adhesiolysis with MCC	3.5750
336	Peritoneal Adhesiolysis with CC	2.1053
337	Peritoneal Adhesiolysis without CC/MCC	1.4964
347	Anal and Stomal Procedures with MCC	2.5491
348	Anal and Stomal Procedures with CC	1.3014

DRG	PDx/SDx/Procedure	Tips
329	Colostomy (temporary, permanent or NOS), root operation Bypass	Information about the anastomotic technique used to complete a colectomy procedure (e.g., side to end) is not specified in ICD-10-PCS. Only the specific Excision or Resection code is assigned. The anastomosis is inherent to the surgery and not coded separately. *ICD-10-PCS Official Guidelines for Coding and Reporting*, guideline B3.1b states: "Procedural steps necessary to reach the operative site and close the operative site, including anastomosis of a tubular body part, are also not coded separately." Code the entire scope of the procedure(s) documented in the operative record, including resections that involve multiple sites (colorectal) or resections performed as part of a greater repair (proctopexy) or take-down procedure.
	Ileostomy (temporary, continent, permanent or NOS)	
	Revision or repair of anastomosis of small or large intestine	
	Proctostomy	
	Closure of proctostomy	
	Abdominal or other proctopexy	
	Repair of colovaginal, rectovaginal or other vaginoenteric fistula	
	AND	
	MCC condition	*See* appendix B.
330	Colostomy (temporary, permanent or NOS), root operation Bypass	*See* DRG 329.
	Ileostomy (temporary, continent, permanent or NOS)	
	Revision or repair of anastomosis of small or large intestine	
	Proctostomy	
	Closure of proctostomy	
	Abdominal or other proctopexy	
	Repair of colovaginal, rectovaginal or other vaginoenteric fistula	
	AND	
	CC condition	*See* appendix B.
331	Colostomy (temporary, permanent or NOS), root operation Bypass	*See* DRG 329.
	Ileostomy (temporary, continent, permanent or NOS)	
	Revision or repair of anastomosis of small or large intestine	
	Proctostomy	
	Closure of proctostomy	
	Abdominal or other proctopexy	
	Repair of colovaginal, rectovaginal or other vaginoenteric fistula	
332	Insertion, removal, or revision of artificial anal sphincter	
	AND	
	MCC condition	*See* appendix B.
333	Insertion, removal, or revision of artificial anal sphincter	
	AND	
	CC condition	*See* appendix B.
334	Insertion, removal, or revision of artificial anal sphincter	
335	Lysis of intra-abdominal adhesions	Adhesiolysis is reported with root operation Release which is defined as "Freeing a body part from an abnormal physical constraint by cutting or by use of force." Release procedures are coded to the body part being freed. In cases of extensive intra-abdominal adhesions, multiple sites may be reported if they are defined by distinct body part values, according to ICD-10-PCS Guideline B3.2: "During the same operative episode, multiple procedures are coded if: a. The same root operation is performed on different body parts as defined by distinct values of the body part character." Adhesions and lysis must be determined by the physician as significant enough to code and report.
	AND	
	MCC condition	*See* appendix B.
336	Lysis of intra-abdominal adhesions	*See* DRG 335.
	AND	
	CC condition	*See* appendix B.
337	Lysis of intra-abdominal adhesions	*See* DRG 335.
347	MCC condition	*See* appendix B.
348	CC condition	*See* appendix B.

DRG 350 Inguinal and Femoral Hernia Procedures with MCC — RW 2.4000

Potential DRGs

335	Peritoneal Adhesiolysis with MCC	3.5750

DRG	PDx/SDx/Procedure	Tips
335	Lysis of intra-abdominal adhesions	Adhesiolysis is reported with root operation Release which is defined as "Freeing a body part from an abnormal physical constraint by cutting or by use of force." Release procedures are coded to the body part being freed. In cases of extensive intra-abdominal adhesions, multiple sites may be reported if they are defined by distinct body part values, according to ICD-10-PCS Guideline B3.2: "During the same operative episode, multiple procedures are coded if: a. The same root operation is performed on different body parts as defined by distinct values of the body part character." Adhesions and lysis must be determined by the physician as significant enough to code and report.
	AND	
	MCC condition	*See* appendix B.

DRG 351 Inguinal and Femoral Hernia Procedures with CC — RW 1.4556

Potential DRGs

335	Peritoneal Adhesiolysis with MCC	3.5750
336	Peritoneal Adhesiolysis with CC	2.1053
350	Inguinal and Femoral Hernia Procedures with MCC	2.4000

DRG	PDx/SDx/Procedure	Tips
335	Lysis of intra-abdominal adhesions	Adhesiolysis is reported with root operation Release which is defined as "Freeing a body part from an abnormal physical constraint by cutting or by use of force." Release procedures are coded to the body part being freed. In cases of extensive intra-abdominal adhesions, multiple sites may be reported if they are defined by distinct body part values, according to ICD-10-PCS Guideline B3.2: "During the same operative episode, multiple procedures are coded if: a. The same root operation is performed on different body parts as defined by distinct values of the body part character." Adhesions and lysis must be determined by the physician as significant enough to code and report.
	AND	
	MCC condition	*See* appendix B.
336	Lysis of intra-abdominal adhesions	*See* DRG 335.
	AND	
	CC condition	*See* appendix B.
350	MCC condition	*See* appendix B.

DRG 352 Inguinal and Femoral Hernia Procedures without CC/MCC — RW 1.1090

Potential DRGs

335	Peritoneal Adhesiolysis with MCC	3.5750
336	Peritoneal Adhesiolysis with CC	2.1053
337	Peritoneal Adhesiolysis without CC/MCC	1.4964
350	Inguinal and Femoral Hernia Procedures with MCC	2.4000
351	Inguinal and Femoral Hernia Procedures with CC	1.4556

DRG	PDx/SDx/Procedure	Tips
335	Lysis of intra-abdominal adhesions	Adhesiolysis is reported with root operation Release which is defined as "Freeing a body part from an abnormal physical constraint by cutting or by use of force." Release procedures are coded to the body part being freed. In cases of extensive intra-abdominal adhesions, multiple sites may be reported if they are defined by distinct body part values, according to ICD-10-PCS Guideline B3.2: "During the same operative episode, multiple procedures are coded if: a. The same root operation is performed on different body parts as defined by distinct values of the body part character." Adhesions and lysis must be determined by the physician as significant enough to code and report.
	AND	
	MCC condition	*See* appendix B.
336	Lysis of intra-abdominal adhesions	*See* DRG 335.
	AND	
	CC condition	*See* appendix B.
337	Lysis of intra-abdominal adhesions	*See* DRG 335.
350	MCC condition	*See* appendix B.
351	CC condition	*See* appendix B.

DRG 353 Hernia Procedures Except Inguinal and Femoral with MCC — RW 2.9243

Potential DRGs

326	Stomach, Esophageal and Duodenal Procedures with MCC	5.0790
335	Peritoneal Adhesiolysis with MCC	3.5750

DRG	PDx/SDx/Procedure	Tips
326	Repair of diaphragmatic (hiatal) hernia, abdominal or thoracic (with or without mesh)	Diaphragmatic (hiatal) hernias are considered digestive system disorders even though the repair of these hernias is coded to the Respiratory body system in ICD-10-PCS. Hernia repair without mesh is coded to root operation Repair (ØBQ). Hernia repair with mesh is coded to the root operation Supplement (ØBU).
	AND	
	MCC condition	*See* appendix B.
335	Lysis of intra-abdominal adhesions	Adhesiolysis is reported with root operation Release which is defined as "Freeing a body part from an abnormal physical constraint by cutting or by use of force." Release procedures are coded to the body part being freed. In cases of extensive intra-abdominal adhesions, multiple sites may be reported if they are defined by distinct body part values, according to ICD-10-PCS Guideline B3.2: "During the same operative episode, multiple procedures are coded if: a. The same root operation is performed on different body parts as defined by distinct values of the body part character." Adhesions and lysis must be determined by the physician as significant enough to code and report.
	AND	
	MCC condition	*See* appendix B.

Optimizing Tips

DRG 354 Hernia Procedures Except Inguinal and Femoral with CC — RW 1.7178

Potential DRGs

326	Stomach, Esophageal and Duodenal Procedures with MCC	5.0790
327	Stomach, Esophageal and Duodenal Procedures with CC	2.4974
335	Peritoneal Adhesiolysis with MCC	3.5750
336	Peritoneal Adhesiolysis with CC	2.1053
353	Hernia Procedures Except Inguinal and Femoral with MCC	2.9243

DRG	PDx/SDx/Procedure	Tips
326	Repair of diaphragmatic (hiatal) hernia, abdominal or thoracic (with or without mesh)	Diaphragmatic (hiatal) hernias are considered digestive system disorders even though the repair of these hernias is coded to the Respiratory body system in ICD-10-PCS. Hernia repair without mesh is coded to root operation Repair (ØBQ). Hernia repair with mesh is coded to the root operation Supplement (ØBU).
	AND	
	MCC condition	*See* appendix B.
327	Repair of diaphragmatic (hiatal) hernia, abdominal or thoracic (with or without mesh)	*See* DRG 326.
	AND	
	CC condition	*See* appendix B.
335	Lysis of intra-abdominal adhesions	Adhesiolysis is reported with root operation Release which is defined as "Freeing a body part from an abnormal physical constraint by cutting or by use of force." Release procedures are coded to the body part being freed. In cases of extensive intra-abdominal adhesions, multiple sites may be reported if they are defined by distinct body part values, according to ICD-10-PCS Guideline B3.2: "During the same operative episode, multiple procedures are coded if: a. The same root operation is performed on different body parts as defined by distinct values of the body part character." Adhesions and lysis must be determined by the physician as significant enough to code and report.
	AND	
	MCC condition	*See* appendix B.
336	Lysis of intra-abdominal adhesions	*See* DRG 335.
	AND	
	CC condition	*See* appendix B.
353	MCC condition	*See* appendix B.

DRG 355 Hernia Procedures Except Inguinal and Femoral without CC/MCC RW 1.3626

Potential DRGs

326	Stomach, Esophageal and Duodenal Procedures with MCC	5.0790
327	Stomach, Esophageal and Duodenal Procedures with CC	2.4974
328	Stomach, Esophageal and Duodenal Procedures without CC/MCC	1.5973
335	Peritoneal Adhesiolysis with MCC	3.5750
336	Peritoneal Adhesiolysis with CC	2.1053
337	Peritoneal Adhesiolysis without CC/MCC	1.4964
353	Hernia Procedures Except Inguinal and Femoral with MCC	2.9243
354	Hernia Procedures Except Inguinal and Femoral with CC	1.7178

DRG	PDx/SDx/Procedure	Tips
326	Repair of diaphragmatic (hiatal) hernia, abdominal or thoracic (with or without mesh)	Diaphragmatic (hiatal) hernias are considered digestive system disorders even though the repair of these hernias is coded to the Respiratory body system in ICD-10-PCS. Hernia repair without mesh is coded to root operation Repair (ØBQ). Hernia repair with mesh is coded to the root operation Supplement (ØBU).
	AND	
	MCC condition	*See* appendix B.
327	Repair of diaphragmatic (hiatal) hernia, abdominal or thoracic (with or without mesh)	*See* DRG 326.
	AND	
	CC condition	*See* appendix B.
328	Repair of diaphragmatic (hiatal) hernia, abdominal or thoracic (with or without mesh)	*See* DRG 326.
335	Lysis of intra-abdominal adhesions	Adhesiolysis is reported with root operation Release which is defined as "Freeing a body part from an abnormal physical constraint by cutting or by use of force." Release procedures are coded to the body part being freed. In cases of extensive intra-abdominal adhesions, multiple sites may be reported if they are defined by distinct body part values, according to ICD-10-PCS Guideline B3.2: "During the same operative episode, multiple procedures are coded if: a. The same root operation is performed on different body parts as defined by distinct values of the body part character." Adhesions and lysis must be determined by the physician as significant enough to code and report.
	AND	
	MCC condition	*See* appendix B.
336	Lysis of intra-abdominal adhesions	*See* DRG 335.
	AND	
	CC condition	*See* appendix B.
337	Lysis of intra-abdominal adhesions	*See* DRG 335.
353	MCC condition	*See* appendix B.
354	CC condition	*See* appendix B.

DRG 356 Other Digestive System O.R. Procedures with MCC RW 4.2787

Potential DRGs

326	Stomach, Esophageal and Duodenal Procedures with MCC	5.0790

DRG	PDx/SDx/Procedure	Tips
326	Inspection of stomach or upper intestinal tract, percutaneous endoscopic approach	
	Removal of infusion or other device from the stomach	Review the documentation carefully for body part specificity.
	AND	
	MCC condition	*See* appendix B.

DRG 357 Other Digestive System O.R. Procedures with CC RW 2.1968

Potential DRGs

326	Stomach, Esophageal and Duodenal Procedures with MCC	5.0790
327	Stomach, Esophageal and Duodenal Procedures with CC	2.4974
335	Peritoneal Adhesiolysis with MCC	3.5750
356	Other Digestive System O.R. Procedures with MCC	4.2787

DRG	PDx/SDx/Procedure	Tips
326	Inspection of stomach or upper intestinal tract, percutaneous endoscopic approach	
	Removal of infusion or other device from the stomach	Review the documentation carefully for body part specificity.
	AND	
	MCC condition	*See* appendix B.
327	Inspection of stomach or upper intestinal tract, percutaneous endoscopic approach	
	Removal of infusion or other device from the stomach	Review the documentation carefully for body part specificity.
	AND	
	CC condition	*See* appendix B.
335	Lysis of intra-abdominal adhesions	Adhesiolysis is reported with root operation Release which is defined as "Freeing a body part from an abnormal physical constraint by cutting or by use of force." Release procedures are coded to the body part being freed. In cases of extensive intra-abdominal adhesions, multiple sites may be reported if they are defined by distinct body part values, according to ICD-10-PCS Guideline B3.2: "During the same operative episode, multiple procedures are coded if: a. The same root operation is performed on different body parts as defined by distinct values of the body part character." Adhesions and lysis must be determined by the physician as significant enough to code and report.
	AND	
	MCC condition	*See* appendix B.
356	MCC condition	*See* appendix B.

DRG 358 Other Digestive System O.R. Procedures without CC/MCC RW 1.2811

Potential DRGs

326	Stomach, Esophageal and Duodenal Procedures with MCC	5.0790
327	Stomach, Esophageal and Duodenal Procedures with CC	2.4974
328	Stomach, Esophageal and Duodenal Procedures without CC/MCC	1.5973
335	Peritoneal Adhesiolysis with MCC	3.5750
336	Peritoneal Adhesiolysis with CC	2.1053
337	Peritoneal Adhesiolysis without CC/MCC	1.4964
356	Other Digestive System O.R. Procedures with MCC	4.2787
357	Other Digestive System O.R. Procedures with CC	2.1968

DRG	PDx/SDx/Procedure	Tips
326	Inspection of stomach or upper intestinal tract, percutaneous endoscopic approach	
	Removal of infusion or other device from the stomach	Review the documentation carefully for body part specificity.
	AND	
	MCC condition	*See* appendix B.
327	Inspection of stomach or upper intestinal tract, percutaneous endoscopic approach	
	Removal of infusion or other device from the stomach	Review the documentation carefully for body part specificity.
	AND	
	CCC condition	*See* appendix B.
328	Inspection of stomach or upper intestinal tract, percutaneous endoscopic approach	
	Removal of infusion or other device from the stomach	Review the documentation carefully for body part specificity.
335	Lysis of intra-abdominal adhesions	Adhesiolysis is reported with root operation Release which is defined as "Freeing a body part from an abnormal physical constraint by cutting or by use of force." Release procedures are coded to the body part being freed. In cases of extensive intra-abdominal adhesions, multiple sites may be reported if they are defined by distinct body part values, according to ICD-10-PCS Guideline B3.2: "During the same operative episode, multiple procedures are coded if: a. The same root operation is performed on different body parts as defined by distinct values of the body part character." Adhesions and lysis must be determined by the physician as significant enough to code and report.
	AND	
	MCC condition	*See* appendix B.
336	Lysis of intra-abdominal adhesions	*See* DRG 335.
	AND	
	CC condition	*See* appendix B.
337	Lysis of intra-abdominal adhesions	*See* DRG 335.
356	MCC condition	*See* appendix B.
357	CC condition	*See* appendix B.

DRG 368 Major Esophageal Disorders with MCC

RW 1.6520

Potential DRGs

326	Stomach, Esophageal and Duodenal Procedures with MCC	5.0790
374	Digestive Malignancy with MCC	2.0990

DRG	PDx/SDx/Procedure	Tips
326	Intra-abdominal venous shunt	
	Local excision of lesion, tissue, or diverticulum of esophagus, open esophageal biopsy, or partial esophagectomy	
	Other repair of esophagus	
	Ligation of esophageal varices, open approach	
	AND	
	MCC condition	*See* appendix B.
374	Malignant neoplasm of esophagus	
	AND	
	MCC condition	*See* appendix B.

DRG 369 Major Esophageal Disorders with CC

RW 0.9883

Potential DRGs

326	Stomach, Esophageal and Duodenal Procedures with MCC	5.0790
327	Stomach, Esophageal and Duodenal Procedures with CC	2.4974
368	Major Esophageal Disorders with MCC	1.6520
374	Digestive Malignancy with MCC	2.0990
375	Digestive Malignancy with CC	1.1983
380	Complicated Peptic Ulcer with MCC	1.9485

DRG	PDx/SDx/Procedure	Tips
326	Intra-abdominal venous shunt	
	Local excision of lesion, tissue, or diverticulum of esophagus, open esophageal biopsy, or partial esophagectomy	
	Other repair of esophagus	
	Ligation of esophageal varices, open approach	
	AND	
	MCC condition	*See* appendix B.
327	Intra-abdominal venous shunt	
	Local excision of lesion, tissue, or diverticulum of esophagus, open esophageal biopsy, or partial esophagectomy	
	Other repair of esophagus	
	Ligation of esophageal varices, open approach	
	AND	
	CC condition	*See* appendix B.
368	MCC condition	*See* appendix B.
374	Malignant neoplasm of esophagus	
	AND	
	MCC condition	*See* appendix B.
375	Malignant neoplasm of esophagus	
	AND	
	CC condition	*See* appendix B.
380	Ulcer of esophagus	
	Barrett's esophagus	
	AND	
	MCC condition	*See* appendix B.

DRG 370 Major Esophageal Disorders without CC/MCC — RW 0.7437

Potential DRGs

326	Stomach, Esophageal and Duodenal Procedures with MCC	5.0790
327	Stomach, Esophageal and Duodenal Procedures with CC	2.4974
328	Stomach, Esophageal and Duodenal Procedures without CC/MCC	1.5973
368	Major Esophageal Disorders with MCC	1.6520
369	Major Esophageal Disorders with CC	0.9883
374	Digestive Malignancy with MCC	2.0990
375	Digestive Malignancy with CC	1.1983
376	Digestive Malignancy without CC/MCC	0.8914
380	Complicated Peptic Ulcer with MCC	1.9485
381	Complicated Peptic Ulcer with CC	1.0730
382	Complicated Peptic Ulcer without CC/MCC	0.7571

DRG	PDx/SDx/Procedure	Tips
326	Intra-abdominal venous shunt	
	Local excision of lesion, tissue, or diverticulum of esophagus, open esophageal biopsy, or partial esophagectomy	
	Other repair of esophagus	
	Ligation of esophageal varices, open approach	
	AND	
	MCC condition	*See* appendix B.
327	Intra-abdominal venous shunt	
	Local excision of lesion, tissue, or diverticulum of esophagus, open esophageal biopsy, or partial esophagectomy	
	Other repair of esophagus	
	Ligation of esophageal varices, open approach	
	AND	
	CC condition	*See* appendix B.
328	Intra-abdominal venous shunt	
	Local excision of lesion, tissue, or diverticulum of esophagus, open esophageal biopsy, or partial esophagectomy	
	Other repair of esophagus	
	Ligation of esophageal varices, open approach	
368	MCC condition	*See* appendix B.
369	CC condition	*See* appendix B.
374	Malignant neoplasm of esophagus	
	AND	
	MCC condition	*See* appendix B.
375	Malignant neoplasm of esophagus	
	AND	
	CC condition	*See* appendix B.
376	Malignant neoplasm of esophagus	
380	Ulcer of esophagus	
	Barrett's esophagus	
	AND	
	MCC condition	*See* appendix B.
381	Ulcer of esophagus	
	Barrett's esophagus	
	AND	
	CC condition	*See* appendix B.
382	Ulcer of esophagus	
	Barrett's esophagus	

DRG 371 Major Gastrointestinal Disorders and Peritoneal Infections with MCC — RW 1.7477

Potential DRGs

326	Stomach, Esophageal and Duodenal Procedures with MCC	5.0790
344	Minor Small and Large Bowel Procedures with MCC	2.7404
356	Other Digestive System O.R. Procedures with MCC	4.2787
374	Digestive Malignancy with MCC	2.0990
397	Appendix Procedures with MCC	2.2466

DRG	PDx/SDx/Procedure	Tips
326	Partial or total gastrectomy	
	Vagotomy	
	Pyloroplasty	
	AND	
	MCC condition	*See* appendix B.
344	Open biopsy of large or small intestine, or of rectum	
	Other destruction of lesion of large or small intestine, (except duodenum)	
	Closure or takedown of intestinal end stoma without excision of intestine	"Reposition" is the appropriate root operation for takedown of an end stoma because it captures the specific objective of the procedure. Root operation Reposition is defined as "Moving some or all of a body part to a normal or other suitable location."
	Repair of parastomal hernia of abdominal wall with intestinal repair	Requires two codes in combination: one code for repair of the parastomal hernia of the abdominal wall, and another code to report repair of intestine. Root operation Repair is defined as "Restoring, to the extent possible, a body part to its normal anatomic structure and function."
	AND	
	MCC condition	*See* appendix B.
356	Drainage of peritoneal abscess	Drainage of peritoneal cavity via an open approach, with or without drainage device, therapeutic or diagnostic, or by percutaneous endoscopic approach, diagnostic only.
	Diagnostic laparotomy or laparoscopy (inspection only)	Inspection of a body part(s) performed in order to achieve the objective of a procedure is not coded separately. However, when both an Inspection procedure and another procedure are performed on the same body part during the same episode, if the Inspection procedure is performed using a different approach than the other procedure, the Inspection procedure is coded separately. If a separate inspection is carried out, it is coded. Exploratory laparotomy with general inspection of abdominal contents is coded to the peritoneal cavity body part value.
	AND	
	MCC condition	*See* appendix B.
374	Digestive malignancy: Esophagus Stomach Small intestine Colon Rectum, rectosigmoid junction, anus	
	AND	
	MCC condition	*See* appendix B.
397	Appendectomy	
	Drainage of appendiceal abscess	Percutaneous drainage must have a seventh character qualifier of X Diagnostic.
	Other operations on the appendix	
	AND	
	MCC condition	*See* appendix B.

DRG 372 Major Gastrointestinal Disorders and Peritoneal Infections with CC RW 1.0423

Potential DRGs

326	Stomach, Esophageal and Duodenal Procedures with MCC	5.0790
327	Stomach, Esophageal and Duodenal Procedures with CC	2.4974
344	Minor Small and Large Bowel Procedures with MCC	2.7404
345	Minor Small and Large Bowel Procedures with CC	1.5406
356	Other Digestive System O.R. Procedures with MCC	4.2787
357	Other Digestive System O.R. Procedures with CC	2.1968
371	Major Gastrointestinal Disorders and Peritoneal Infections with MCC	1.7477
374	Digestive Malignancy with MCC	2.0990
375	Digestive Malignancy with CC	1.1983
393	Other Digestive System Diagnoses with MCC	1.6196
397	Appendix Procedures with MCC	2.2466
398	Appendix Procedures with CC	1.5133

DRG	PDx/SDx/Procedure	Tips
326	Partial or total gastrectomy	
	Vagotomy	
	Pyloroplasty	
	AND	
	MCC condition	*See* appendix B.
327	Partial or total gastrectomy	
	Vagotomy	
	Pyloroplasty	
	AND	
	CC condition	*See* appendix B.
344	Open biopsy of large or small intestine, or of rectum	
	Other destruction of lesion of large or small intestine, (except duodenum)	
	Closure or takedown of intestinal end stoma without excision of intestine	"Reposition" is the appropriate root operation for takedown of an end stoma because it captures the specific objective of the procedure. Root operation Reposition is defined as "Moving some or all of a body part to a normal or other suitable location."
	Repair of parastomal hernia of abdominal wall with intestinal repair	Requires two codes in combination: one code for repair of the parastomal hernia of the abdominal wall, and another code to report repair of intestine. Root operation Repair is defined as "Restoring, to the extent possible, a body part to its normal anatomic structure and function."
	AND	
	MCC condition	*See* appendix B.
345	Open biopsy of large or small intestine, or of rectum	
	Other destruction of lesion of large or small intestine, (except duodenum)	
	Closure or takedown of intestinal end stoma without excision of intestine	*See* DRG 344.
	Repair of parastomal hernia of abdominal wall with intestinal repair	*See* DRG 344.
	AND	
	CC condition	*See* appendix B.
356	Drainage of peritoneal abscess	Drainage of peritoneal cavity via an open approach, with or without drainage device, therapeutic or diagnostic, or by percutaneous endoscopic approach, diagnostic only.
	Diagnostic laparotomy or laparoscopy (inspection only)	Inspection of a body part(s) performed in order to achieve the objective of a procedure is not coded separately. However, when both an Inspection procedure and another procedure are performed on the same body part during the same episode, if the Inspection procedure is performed using a different approach than the other procedure, the Inspection procedure is coded separately. If a separate inspection is carried out, it is coded. Exploratory laparotomy with general inspection of abdominal contents is coded to the peritoneal cavity body part value.
	AND	
	MCC condition	*See* appendix B.
357	Drainage of peritoneal abscess	*See* DRG 356.
	Diagnostic laparotomy or laparoscopy (inspection only)	*See* DRG 356.
	AND	
	CC condition	*See* appendix B.
371	MCC condition	*See* appendix B.
374	Digestive malignancy: Esophagus Stomach Small intestine Colon Rectum, rectosigmoid junction, anus	
	AND	
	MCC condition	*See* appendix B.

DRG 372 (Continued)

DRG	PDx/SDx/Procedure	Tips
375	Digestive malignancy: Esophagus Stomach Small intestine Colon Rectum, rectosigmoid junction, anus	
	AND	
	CC condition	*See* appendix B.
393	Hernia, with or without obstruction	
	Gastric band and other bariatric procedure complications	Review the documentation carefully; code assignment is based on the provider's documentation of a relationship between the condition and the procedure. Unless the classification instructs otherwise, only when there is a clear cause-and-effect relationship between the care provided and the condition and the documentation indicates the condition is a complication, can the condition be coded as such. Query the provider for clarification if the relationship/complication is not clearly documented. See guideline I.B.16.
	AND	
	MCC condition	*See* appendix B.
397	Appendectomy	
	Drainage of appendiceal abscess	Percutaneous drainage must have a seventh character qualifier of X Diagnostic.
	Other operations on the appendix	
	AND	
	MCC condition	*See* appendix B.
398	Appendectomy	
	Drainage of appendiceal abscess	*See* DRG 397.
	Other operations on the appendix	
	AND	
	CC condition	*See* appendix B.

DRG 373 Major Gastrointestinal Disorders and Peritoneal Infections without CC/MCC RW 0.7165

Potential DRGs

326	Stomach, Esophageal and Duodenal Procedures with MCC	5.0790
327	Stomach, Esophageal and Duodenal Procedures with CC	2.4974
328	Stomach, Esophageal and Duodenal Procedures without CC/MCC	1.5973
344	Minor Small and Large Bowel Procedures with MCC	2.7404
345	Minor Small and Large Bowel Procedures with CC	1.5406
346	Minor Small and Large Bowel Procedures without CC/MCC	1.2878
356	Other Digestive System O.R. Procedures with MCC	4.2787
357	Other Digestive System O.R. Procedures with CC	2.1968
358	Other Digestive System O.R. Procedures without CC/MCC	1.2811
371	Major Gastrointestinal Disorders and Peritoneal Infections with MCC	1.7477
372	Major Gastrointestinal Disorders and Peritoneal Infections with CC	1.0423
374	Digestive Malignancy with MCC	2.0990
375	Digestive Malignancy with CC	1.1983
376	Digestive Malignancy without CC/MCC	0.8914
393	Other Digestive System Diagnoses with MCC	1.6196
394	Other Digestive System Diagnoses with CC	0.9369
397	Appendix Procedures with MCC	2.2466
398	Appendix Procedures with CC	1.5133
399	Appendix Procedures without CC/MCC	1.1131

DRG	PDx/SDx/Procedure	Tips
326	Partial or total gastrectomy	
	Vagotomy	
	Pyloroplasty	
	AND	
	MCC condition	*See* appendix B.
327	Partial or total gastrectomy	
	Vagotomy	
	Pyloroplasty	
	AND	
	CC condition	*See* appendix B.
328	Partial or total gastrectomy	
	Vagotomy	
	Pyloroplasty	
344	Open biopsy of large or small intestine, or of rectum	
	Other destruction of lesion of large or small intestine, (except duodenum)	
	Closure or takedown of intestinal end stoma without excision of intestine	"Reposition" is the appropriate root operation for takedown of an end stoma because it captures the specific objective of the procedure. Root operation Reposition is defined as "Moving some or all of a body part to a normal or other suitable location."
	Repair of parastomal hernia of abdominal wall with intestinal repair	Requires two codes in combination: one code for repair of the parastomal hernia of the abdominal wall, and another code to report repair of intestine. Root operation Repair is defined as "Restoring, to the extent possible, a body part to its normal anatomic structure and function."
	AND	
	MCC condition	*See* appendix B.
345	Open biopsy of large or small intestine, or of rectum	
	Other destruction of lesion of large or small intestine, (except duodenum)	
	Closure or takedown of intestinal end stoma without excision of intestine	*See* DRG 344.
	Repair of parastomal hernia of abdominal wall with intestinal repair	*See* DRG 344.
	AND	
	CC condition	*See* appendix B.
346	Open biopsy of large or small intestine, or of rectum	
	Other destruction of lesion of large or small intestine, (except duodenum)	
	Closure or takedown of intestinal end stoma without excision of intestine	*See* DRG 344.
	Repair of parastomal hernia of abdominal wall with intestinal repair	*See* DRG 344.

DRG 373 (Continued)

DRG	PDx/SDx/Procedure	Tips
356	Drainage of peritoneal abscess	Drainage of peritoneal cavity via an open approach, with or without drainage device, therapeutic or diagnostic, or by percutaneous endoscopic approach, diagnostic only.
	Diagnostic laparotomy or laparoscopy (inspection only)	Inspection of a body part(s) performed in order to achieve the objective of a procedure is not coded separately. However, when both an Inspection procedure and another procedure are performed on the same body part during the same episode, if the Inspection procedure is performed using a different approach than the other procedure, the Inspection procedure is coded separately. If a separate inspection is carried out, it is coded. Exploratory laparotomy with general inspection of abdominal contents is coded to the peritoneal cavity body part value.
	AND	
	MCC condition	*See* appendix B.
357	Drainage of peritoneal abscess	*See* DRG 356.
	Diagnostic laparotomy or laparoscopy (inspection only)	*See* DRG 356.
	AND	
	CC condition	*See* appendix B.
358	Drainage of peritoneal abscess	*See* DRG 356.
	Diagnostic laparotomy or laparoscopy (inspection only)	*See* DRG 356.
371	MCC condition	*See* appendix B.
372	CC condition	*See* appendix B.
374	Digestive malignancy: Esophagus Stomach Small intestine Colon Rectum, rectosigmoid junction, anus	
	AND	
	MCC condition	*See* appendix B.
375	Digestive malignancy: Esophagus Stomach Small intestine Colon Rectum, rectosigmoid junction, anus	
	AND	
	CC condition	*See* appendix B.
376	Digestive malignancy: Esophagus Stomach Small intestine Colon Rectum, rectosigmoid junction, anus	
393	Hernia, with or without obstruction	
	Gastric band and other bariatric procedure complications	Review the documentation carefully; code assignment is based on the provider's documentation of a relationship between the condition and the procedure. Unless the classification instructs otherwise, only when there is a clear cause-and-effect relationship between the care provided and the condition and the documentation indicates the condition is a complication, can the condition be coded as such. Query the provider for clarification if the relationship/complication is not clearly documented. See guideline I.B.16.
	AND	
	MCC condition	*See* appendix B.
394	Hernia, with or without obstruction	
	Gastric band and other bariatric procedure complications	*See* DRG 393.
	AND	
	CC condition	*See* appendix B.
397	Appendectomy	
	Drainage of appendiceal abscess	Percutaneous drainage must have a seventh character qualifier of X Diagnostic.
	Other operations on the appendix	
	AND	
	MCC condition	*See* appendix B.
398	Appendectomy	
	Drainage of appendiceal abscess	*See* DRG 397.
	Other operations on the appendix	
	AND	
	CC condition	*See* appendix B.
399	Appendectomy	
	Drainage of appendiceal abscess	*See* DRG 397.
	Other operations on the appendix	

Optimizing Tips

DRG 374 Digestive Malignancy with MCC — RW 2.0990

Potential DRGs

326	Stomach, Esophageal and Duodenal Procedures with MCC	5.0790
335	Peritoneal Adhesiolysis with MCC	3.5750
356	Other Digestive System O.R. Procedures with MCC	4.2787

DRG	PDx/SDx/Procedure	Tips
326	Local excision of lesion, tissue, or diverticulum of esophagus, open esophageal biopsy	
	Local excision of lesion or tissue of stomach, open stomach biopsy	
	Local excision of lesion or tissue of duodenum, open or percutaneous	
	AND	
	MCC condition	*See* appendix B.
335	Lysis of intra-abdominal adhesions	Adhesiolysis is reported with root operation Release which is defined as "Freeing a body part from an abnormal physical constraint by cutting or by use of force." Release procedures are coded to the body part being freed. In cases of extensive intra-abdominal adhesions, multiple sites may be reported if they are defined by distinct body part values, according to ICD-10-PCS Guideline B3.2: "During the same operative episode, multiple procedures are coded if: a. The same root operation is performed on different body parts as defined by distinct values of the body part character." Adhesions and lysis must be determined by the physician as significant enough to code and report.
	AND	
	MCC condition	*See* appendix B.
356	Mesenteric, pelvic, or aortic lymphatic biopsy	Lymph node excision implies that only a portion of the node or one node from a group or chain of nodes is removed. Lymph node resection implies that a particular group or chain of lymph nodes is completely removed. The root operation Excision is "cutting out or off, without replacement, a portion of a body part." Root operation Resection is "cutting out or off, without replacement, all of a body part." It includes all of a body part or any subdivision of body part having its own body part value in ICD-10-PCS. Review the description of the procedure for confirmation of removal of the entire group or chain, or if the intent was to remove the entire chain.
	Lymph node excision (neck, axillary, mesenteric, pelvic, aortic, inguinal)	
	Lymph node chain or group resection (head, upper extremity, axillary, thorax, internal mammary, mesenteric, pelvis, aortic, lower extremity, inguinal)	
	Peritoneal biopsy	
	AND	
	MCC condition	*See* appendix B.

DRG 375 Digestive Malignancy with CC

RW 1.1983

Potential DRGs

326	Stomach, Esophageal and Duodenal Procedures with MCC	5.0790
327	Stomach, Esophageal and Duodenal Procedures with CC	2.4974
335	Peritoneal Adhesiolysis with MCC	3.5750
336	Peritoneal Adhesiolysis with CC	2.1053
356	Other Digestive System O.R. Procedures with MCC	4.2787
357	Other Digestive System O.R. Procedures with CC	2.1968
371	Major Gastrointestinal Disorders and Peritoneal Infections with MCC	1.7477
374	Digestive Malignancy with MCC	2.0990
393	Other Digestive System Diagnoses with MCC	1.6196

DRG	PDx/SDx/Procedure	Tips
326	Local excision of lesion, tissue, or diverticulum of esophagus, open esophageal biopsy	
	Local excision of lesion or tissue of stomach, open stomach biopsy	
	Local excision of lesion or tissue of duodenum, open or percutaneous	
	AND	
	MCC condition	*See* appendix B.
327	Local excision of lesion, tissue, or diverticulum of esophagus, open esophageal biopsy	
	Local excision of lesion or tissue of stomach, open stomach biopsy	
	Local excision of lesion or tissue of duodenum, open or percutaneous	
	AND	
	CC condition	*See* appendix B.
335	Lysis of intra-abdominal adhesions	Adhesiolysis is reported with root operation Release which is defined as "Freeing a body part from an abnormal physical constraint by cutting or by use of force." Release procedures are coded to the body part being freed. In cases of extensive intra-abdominal adhesions, multiple sites may be reported if they are defined by distinct body part values, according to ICD-10-PCS Guideline B3.2: "During the same operative episode, multiple procedures are coded if: a. The same root operation is performed on different body parts as defined by distinct values of the body part character." Adhesions and lysis must be determined by the physician as significant enough to code and report.
	AND	
	MCC condition	*See* appendix B.
336	Lysis of intra-abdominal adhesions	*See* DRG 335.
	AND	
	CC condition	*See* appendix B.
356	Mesenteric, pelvic, or aortic lymphatic biopsy	Lymph node excision implies that only a portion of the node or one node from a group or chain of nodes is removed. Lymph node resection implies that a particular group or chain of lymph nodes is completely removed. The root operation Excision is "cutting out or off, without replacement, a portion of a body part." Root operation Resection is "cutting out or off, without replacement, all of a body part." It includes all of a body part or any subdivision of body part having its own body part value in ICD-10-PCS. Review the description of the procedure for confirmation of removal of the entire group or chain, or if the intent was to remove the entire chain.
	Lymph node excision (neck, axillary, mesenteric, pelvic, aortic, inguinal)	
	Lymph node chain or group resection (head, upper extremity, axillary, thorax, internal mammary, mesenteric, pelvis, aortic, lower extremity, inguinal)	
	Peritoneal biopsy	
	AND	
	MCC condition	*See* appendix B.
357	Mesenteric, pelvic, or aortic lymphatic biopsy	*See* DRG 356.
	Lymph node excision (neck, axillary, mesenteric, pelvic, aortic, inguinal)	
	Lymph node chain or group resection (head, upper extremity, axillary, thorax, internal mammary, mesenteric, pelvis, aortic, lower extremity, inguinal)	
	Peritoneal biopsy	
	AND	
	CC condition	*See* appendix B.
371	Intestinal infection due to identified organism	
	Bacterial food poisoning	
	Peritonitis or peritoneal, retroperitoneal abscess	
	AND	
	MCC condition	*See* appendix B.
374	MCC condition	*See* appendix B.
393	Hernia, with or without obstruction	
	Gastric band and other bariatric procedure complications	Review the documentation carefully; code assignment is based on the provider's documentation of a relationship between the condition and the procedure. Unless the classification instructs otherwise, only when there is a clear cause-and-effect relationship between the care provided and the condition and the documentation indicates the condition is a complication, can the condition be coded as such. Query the provider for clarification if the relationship/complication is not clearly documented. See guideline I.B.16.
	AND	
	MCC condition	*See* appendix B.

DRG 376 Digestive Malignancy without CC/MCC RW 0.8914

Potential DRGs

326	Stomach, Esophageal and Duodenal Procedures with MCC	5.0790
327	Stomach, Esophageal and Duodenal Procedures with CC	2.4974
328	Stomach, Esophageal and Duodenal Procedures without CC/MCC	1.5973
335	Peritoneal Adhesiolysis with MCC	3.5750
336	Peritoneal Adhesiolysis with CC	2.1053
337	Peritoneal Adhesiolysis without CC/MCC	1.4964
356	Other Digestive System O.R. Procedures with MCC	4.2787
357	Other Digestive System O.R. Procedures with CC	2.1968
358	Other Digestive System O.R. Procedures without CC/MCC	1.2811
371	Major Gastrointestinal Disorders and Peritoneal Infections with MCC	1.7477
372	Major Gastrointestinal Disorders and Peritoneal Infections with CC	1.0423
374	Digestive Malignancy with MCC	2.0990
375	Digestive Malignancy with CC	1.1983
377	GI Hemorrhage with MCC	1.7903
393	Other Digestive System Diagnoses with MCC	1.6196

DRG	PDx/SDx/Procedure	Tips
326	Local excision of lesion, tissue, or diverticulum of esophagus, open esophageal biopsy	
	Local excision of lesion or tissue of stomach, open stomach biopsy	
	Local excision of lesion or tissue of duodenum, open or percutaneous	
	AND	
	MCC condition	*See* appendix B.
327	Local excision of lesion, tissue, or diverticulum of esophagus, open esophageal biopsy	
	Local excision of lesion or tissue of stomach, open stomach biopsy	
	Local excision of lesion or tissue of duodenum, open or percutaneous	
	AND	
	CC condition	*See* appendix B.
328	Local excision of lesion, tissue, or diverticulum of esophagus, open esophageal biopsy	
	Local excision of lesion or tissue of stomach, open stomach biopsy	
	Local excision of lesion or tissue of duodenum, open or percutaneous	
335	Lysis of intra-abdominal adhesions	Adhesiolysis is reported with root operation Release which is defined as "Freeing a body part from an abnormal physical constraint by cutting or by use of force." Release procedures are coded to the body part being freed. In cases of extensive intra-abdominal adhesions, multiple sites may be reported if they are defined by distinct body part values, according to ICD-10-PCS Guideline B3.2: "During the same operative episode, multiple procedures are coded if: a. The same root operation is performed on different body parts as defined by distinct values of the body part character." Adhesions and lysis must be determined by the physician as significant enough to code and report.
	AND	
	MCC condition	*See* appendix B.
336	Lysis of intra-abdominal adhesions	*See* DRG 335.
	AND	
	CC condition	*See* appendix B.
337	Lysis of intra-abdominal adhesions	*See* DRG 335.
356	Mesenteric, pelvic, or aortic lymphatic biopsy	Lymph node excision implies that only a portion of the node or one node from a group or chain of nodes is removed. Lymph node resection implies that a particular group or chain of lymph nodes is completely removed. The root operation Excision is "cutting out or off, without replacement, a portion of a body part." Root operation Resection is "cutting out or off, without replacement, all of a body part." It includes all of a body part or any subdivision of body part having its own body part value in ICD-10-PCS. Review the description of the procedure for confirmation of removal of the entire group or chain, or if the intent was to remove the entire chain.
	Lymph node excision (neck, axillary, mesenteric, pelvic, aortic, inguinal)	
	Lymph node chain or group resection (head, upper extremity, axillary, thorax, internal mammary, mesenteric, pelvis, aortic, lower extremity, inguinal)	
	Peritoneal biopsy	
	AND	
	MCC condition	*See* appendix B.
357	Mesenteric, pelvic, or aortic lymphatic biopsy	*See* DRG 356.
	Lymph node excision (neck, axillary, mesenteric, pelvic, aortic, inguinal)	
	Lymph node chain or group resection (head, upper extremity, axillary, thorax, internal mammary, mesenteric, pelvis, aortic, lower extremity, inguinal)	
	Peritoneal biopsy	
	AND	
	CC condition	*See* appendix B.

DRG 376 (Continued)

DRG	PDx/SDx/Procedure	Tips
358	Mesenteric, pelvic, or aortic lymphatic biopsy	*See* DRG 356.
	Lymph node excision (neck, axillary, mesenteric, pelvic, aortic, inguinal)	
	Lymph node chain or group resection (head, upper extremity, axillary, thorax, internal mammary, mesenteric, pelvis, aortic, lower extremity, inguinal)	
	Peritoneal biopsy	
371	Intestinal infection due to identified organism	
	Bacterial food poisoning	
	Peritonitis or peritoneal, retroperitoneal abscess	
	AND	
	MCC condition	*See* appendix B.
372	Intestinal infection due to identified organism	
	Bacterial food poisoning	
	Peritonitis or peritoneal, retroperitoneal abscess	
	AND	
	CC condition	*See* appendix B.
374	MCC condition	*See* appendix B.
375	CC condition	*See* appendix B.
377	Any digestive ulcers with hemorrhage or hemorrhage and perforation	Review the alphabetic index and tabular list for gastrointestinal conditions linked by the terms "with hemorrhage" or "with bleeding" as the classification presumes a causal relationship between two conditions linked by these terms in the alphabetic index or tabular list. Unless the provider documents a different cause of the bleeding or states the conditions are unrelated, assign the combination code for these conditions.
	Gastritis and duodenitis with hemorrhage	
	Rectal or anal hemorrhage, hematemesis, melena	
	Gastrointestinal hemorrhage	
	AND	
	MCC condition	*See* appendix B.
393	Hernia, with or without obstruction	
	Gastric band and other bariatric procedure complications	Review the documentation carefully; code assignment is based on the provider's documentation of a relationship between the condition and the procedure. Unless the classification instructs otherwise, only when there is a clear cause-and-effect relationship between the care provided and the condition and the documentation indicates the condition is a complication, can the condition be coded as such. Query the provider for clarification if the relationship/complication is not clearly documented. See guideline I.B.16.
	AND	
	MCC condition	*See* appendix B.

DRG 377 GI Hemorrhage with MCC — RW 1.7903

Potential DRGs

326	Stomach, Esophageal and Duodenal Procedures with MCC	5.0790
374	Digestive Malignancy with MCC	2.0990
380	Complicated Peptic Ulcer with MCC	1.9485

DRG	PDx/SDx/Procedure	Tips
326	Suture of laceration of esophagus, stomach, or duodenum or peptic gastric, or duodenal ulcer	
	Ligation of esophageal or gastric varices (esophageal open approach only)	
	AND	
	MCC condition	*See* appendix B.
374	Digestive malignancy: Esophagus Stomach Small intestine Colon Rectum, rectosigmoid junction, anus	
	AND	
	MCC condition	*See* appendix B.
380	Ulcer of esophagus or Barrett's esophagus	
	Acute, chronic or unspecified gastric ulcer with perforation	
	Acute, chronic or unspecified duodenal ulcer with perforation	
	Acute, chronic or unspecified peptic ulcer with perforation	
	Acute, chronic or unspecified gastrojejunal ulcer without hemorrhage, with or without perforation	
	AND	
	MCC condition	*See* appendix B.

DRG 378 GI Hemorrhage with CC RW 0.9838

Potential DRGs

326	Stomach, Esophageal and Duodenal Procedures with MCC	5.0790
327	Stomach, Esophageal and Duodenal Procedures with CC	2.4974
374	Digestive Malignancy with MCC	2.0990
375	Digestive Malignancy with CC	1.1983
377	GI Hemorrhage with MCC	1.7903
380	Complicated Peptic Ulcer with MCC	1.9485
381	Complicated Peptic Ulcer with CC	1.0730

DRG	PDx/SDx/Procedure	Tips
326	Suture of laceration of esophagus, stomach, or duodenum or peptic gastric, or duodenal ulcer	
	Ligation of esophageal or gastric varices (esophageal open approach only)	
	AND	
	MCC condition	*See* appendix B.
327	Suture of laceration of esophagus, stomach, or duodenum or peptic gastric, or duodenal ulcer	
	Ligation of esophageal or gastric varices (esophageal open approach only)	
	AND	
	CC condition	*See* appendix B.
374	Digestive malignancy: Esophagus Stomach Small intestine Colon Rectum, rectosigmoid junction, anus	
	AND	
	MCC condition	*See* appendix B.
375	Digestive malignancy: Esophagus Stomach Small intestine Colon Rectum, rectosigmoid junction, anus	
	AND	
	CC condition	*See* appendix B.
377	MCC condition	*See* appendix B.
380	Ulcer of esophagus or Barrett's esophagus	
	Acute, chronic or unspecified gastric ulcer with perforation	
	Acute, chronic or unspecified duodenal ulcer with perforation	
	Acute, chronic or unspecified peptic ulcer with perforation	
	Acute, chronic or unspecified gastrojejunal ulcer without hemorrhage, with or without perforation	
	AND	
	MCC condition	*See* appendix B.
381	Ulcer of esophagus or Barrett's esophagus	
	Acute, chronic or unspecified gastric ulcer with perforation	
	Acute, chronic or unspecified duodenal ulcer with perforation	
	Acute, chronic or unspecified peptic ulcer with perforation	
	Acute, chronic or unspecified gastrojejunal ulcer without hemorrhage, with or without perforation	
	AND	
	CC condition	*See* appendix B.

DRG 379 GI Hemorrhage without CC/MCC

RW 0.6332

Potential DRGs

326	Stomach, Esophageal and Duodenal Procedures with MCC	5.0790
327	Stomach, Esophageal and Duodenal Procedures with CC	2.4974
328	Stomach, Esophageal and Duodenal Procedures without CC/MCC	1.5973
374	Digestive Malignancy with MCC	2.0990
375	Digestive Malignancy with CC	1.1983
376	Digestive Malignancy without CC/MCC	0.8914
377	GI Hemorrhage with MCC	1.7903
378	GI Hemorrhage with CC	0.9838
380	Complicated Peptic Ulcer with MCC	1.9485
381	Complicated Peptic Ulcer with CC	1.0730
382	Complicated Peptic Ulcer without CC/MCC	0.7571

DRG	PDx/SDx/Procedure	Tips
326	Suture of laceration of esophagus, stomach, or duodenum or peptic gastric, or duodenal ulcer	
	Ligation of esophageal or gastric varices (esophageal open approach only)	
	AND	
	MCC condition	*See* appendix B.
327	Suture of laceration of esophagus, stomach, or duodenum or peptic gastric, or duodenal ulcer	
	Ligation of esophageal or gastric varices (esophageal open approach only)	
	AND	
	CC condition	*See* appendix B.
328	Suture of laceration of esophagus, stomach, or duodenum or peptic gastric, or duodenal ulcer	
	Ligation of esophageal or gastric varices (esophageal open approach only)	
374	Digestive malignancy: Esophagus Stomach Small intestine Colon Rectum, rectosigmoid junction, anus	
	AND	
	MCC condition	*See* appendix B.
375	Digestive malignancy: Esophagus Stomach Small intestine Colon Rectum, rectosigmoid junction, anus	
	AND	
	CC condition	*See* appendix B.
376	Digestive malignancy: Esophagus Stomach Small intestine Colon Rectum, rectosigmoid junction, anus	
377	MCC condition	*See* appendix B.
378	CC condition	*See* appendix B.
380	Ulcer of esophagus or Barrett's esophagus	
	Acute, chronic or unspecified gastric ulcer with perforation	
	Acute, chronic or unspecified duodenal ulcer with perforation	
	Acute, chronic or unspecified peptic ulcer with perforation	
	Acute, chronic or unspecified gastrojejunal ulcer without hemorrhage, with or without perforation	
	AND	
	MCC condition	*See* appendix B.
381	Ulcer of esophagus or Barrett's esophagus	
	Acute, chronic or unspecified gastric ulcer with perforation	
	Acute, chronic or unspecified duodenal ulcer with perforation	
	Acute, chronic or unspecified peptic ulcer with perforation	
	Acute, chronic or unspecified gastrojejunal ulcer without hemorrhage, with or without perforation	
	AND	
	CC condition	*See* appendix B.
382	Ulcer of esophagus or Barrett's esophagus	
	Acute, chronic or unspecified gastric ulcer with perforation	
	Acute, chronic or unspecified duodenal ulcer with perforation	
	Acute, chronic or unspecified peptic ulcer with perforation	
	Acute, chronic or unspecified gastrojejunal ulcer without hemorrhage, with or without perforation	

DRG 380 Complicated Peptic Ulcer with MCC

RW 1.9485

Potential DRGs

326	Stomach, Esophageal and Duodenal Procedures with MCC	5.0790

DRG	PDx/SDx/Procedure	Tips
326	Suture of laceration of esophagus, stomach, or duodenum or peptic gastric, or duodenal ulcer	
	Ligation of esophageal or gastric varices (esophageal open approach only)	
	AND	
	MCC condition	*See* appendix B.

DRG 381 Complicated Peptic Ulcer with CC

RW 1.0730

Potential DRGs

326	Stomach, Esophageal and Duodenal Procedures with MCC	5.0790
327	Stomach, Esophageal and Duodenal Procedures with CC	2.4974
380	Complicated Peptic Ulcer with MCC	1.9485

DRG	PDx/SDx/Procedure	Tips
326	Suture of laceration of esophagus, stomach, or duodenum or peptic gastric, or duodenal ulcer	
	Ligation of esophageal or gastric varices (esophageal open approach only)	
	AND	
	MCC condition	*See* appendix B.
327	Suture of laceration of esophagus, stomach, or duodenum or peptic gastric, or duodenal ulcer	
	Ligation of esophageal or gastric varices (esophageal open approach only)	
	AND	
	CC condition	*See* appendix B.
380	MCC condition	*See* appendix B.

DRG 382 Complicated Peptic Ulcer without CC/MCC

RW 0.7571

Potential DRGs

326	Stomach, Esophageal and Duodenal Procedures with MCC	5.0790
327	Stomach, Esophageal and Duodenal Procedures with CC	2.4974
328	Stomach, Esophageal and Duodenal Procedures without CC/MCC	1.5973
380	Complicated Peptic Ulcer with MCC	1.9485
381	Complicated Peptic Ulcer with CC	1.0730

DRG	PDx/SDx/Procedure	Tips
326	Suture of laceration of esophagus, stomach, or duodenum or peptic gastric, or duodenal ulcer	
	Ligation of esophageal or gastric varices (esophageal open approach only)	
	AND	
	MCC condition	*See* appendix B.
327	Suture of laceration of esophagus, stomach, or duodenum or peptic gastric, or duodenal ulcer	
	Ligation of esophageal or gastric varices (esophageal open approach only)	
	AND	
	CC condition	*See* appendix B.
328	Suture of laceration of esophagus, stomach, or duodenum or peptic gastric, or duodenal ulcer	
	Ligation of esophageal or gastric varices (esophageal open approach only)	
380	MCC condition	*See* appendix B.
381	CC condition	*See* appendix B.

DRG 383 Uncomplicated Peptic Ulcer with MCC

RW 1.3982

Potential DRGs

326	Stomach, Esophageal and Duodenal Procedures with MCC	5.0790
377	GI Hemorrhage with MCC	1.7903
380	Complicated Peptic Ulcer with MCC	1.9485

DRG	PDx/SDx/Procedure	Tips
326	Suture of laceration of esophagus, stomach, or duodenum or peptic gastric, or duodenal ulcer	
	Ligation of esophageal or gastric varices (esophageal open approach only)	
	AND	
	MCC condition	*See* appendix B.
377	Any digestive ulcers with hemorrhage or hemorrhage and perforation	Review the alphabetic index and tabular list for gastrointestinal conditions linked by the terms "with hemorrhage" or "with bleeding" as the classification presumes a causal relationship between two conditions linked by these terms in the alphabetic index or tabular list. Unless the provider documents a different cause of the bleeding or states that the conditions are unrelated, assign the combination code for these conditions.
	Gastritis and duodenitis with hemorrhage	
	Rectal or anal hemorrhage, hematemesis, melena	
	Gastrointestinal hemorrhage	
	AND	
	MCC condition	*See* appendix B.
380	Ulcer of esophagus or Barrett's esophagus	
	Acute, chronic or unspecified gastric ulcer with perforation	
	Acute, chronic or unspecified duodenal ulcer with perforation	
	Acute, chronic or unspecified peptic ulcer with perforation	
	Acute, chronic or unspecified gastrojejunal ulcer without hemorrhage, with or without perforation	
	AND	
	MCC condition	*See* appendix B.

DRG 384 Uncomplicated Peptic Ulcer without MCC

RW 0.8757

Potential DRGs

326	Stomach, Esophageal and Duodenal Procedures with MCC	5.0790
327	Stomach, Esophageal and Duodenal Procedures with CC	2.4974
328	Stomach, Esophageal and Duodenal Procedures without CC/MCC	1.5973
377	GI Hemorrhage with MCC	1.7903
378	GI Hemorrhage with CC	0.9838
380	Complicated Peptic Ulcer with MCC	1.9485
381	Complicated Peptic Ulcer with CC	1.0730
383	Uncomplicated Peptic Ulcer with MCC	1.3982

DRG	PDx/SDx/Procedure	Tips
326	Suture of laceration of esophagus, stomach, or duodenum or peptic gastric, or duodenal ulcer	
	Ligation of esophageal or gastric varices (esophageal open approach only)	
	AND	
	MCC condition	*See* appendix B.
327	Suture of laceration of esophagus, stomach, or duodenum or peptic gastric, or duodenal ulcer	
	Ligation of esophageal or gastric varices (esophageal open approach only)	
	AND	
	CC condition	*See* appendix B.
328	Suture of laceration of esophagus, stomach, or duodenum or peptic gastric, or duodenal ulcer	
	Ligation of esophageal or gastric varices (esophageal open approach only)	
377	Any digestive ulcers with hemorrhage or hemorrhage and perforation	Review the alphabetic index and tabular list for gastrointestinal conditions linked by the terms "with hemorrhage" or "with bleeding" as the classification presumes a causal relationship between two conditions linked by these terms in the alphabetic index or tabular list. Unless the provider documents a different cause of the bleeding or states that the conditions are unrelated, assign the combination code for these conditions.
	Gastritis and duodenitis with hemorrhage	
	Rectal or anal hemorrhage, hematemesis, melena	
	Gastrointestinal hemorrhage	
	AND	
	MCC condition	*See* appendix B.
378	Any digestive ulcers with hemorrhage or hemorrhage and perforation	*See* DRG 377.
	Gastritis and duodenitis with hemorrhage	
	Rectal or anal hemorrhage, hematemesis, melena	
	Gastrointestinal hemorrhage	
	AND	
	CC condition	*See* appendix B.
380	Ulcer of esophagus or Barrett's esophagus	
	Acute, chronic or unspecified gastric ulcer with perforation	
	Acute, chronic or unspecified duodenal ulcer with perforation	
	Acute, chronic or unspecified peptic ulcer with perforation	
	Acute, chronic or unspecified gastrojejunal ulcer without hemorrhage, with or without perforation	
	AND	
	MCC condition	*See* appendix B.
381	Ulcer of esophagus or Barrett's esophagus	
	Acute, chronic or unspecified gastric ulcer with perforation	
	Acute, chronic or unspecified duodenal ulcer with perforation	
	Acute, chronic or unspecified peptic ulcer with perforation	
	Acute, chronic or unspecified gastrojejunal ulcer without hemorrhage, with or without perforation	
	AND	
	CC condition	*See* appendix B.
383	MCC condition	*See* appendix B.

DRG 385 Inflammatory Bowel Disease with MCC RW 1.5669

Potential DRGs

326	Stomach, Esophageal and Duodenal Procedures with MCC	5.0790
335	Peritoneal Adhesiolysis with MCC	3.5750
371	Major Gastrointestinal Disorders and Peritoneal Infections with MCC	1.7477

DRG	PDx/SDx/Procedure	Tips
326	Local excision of lesion, tissue, or diverticulum of esophagus, open esophageal biopsy	
	Local excision of lesion or tissue of stomach, open stomach biopsy	
	Local excision of lesion or tissue of duodenum, open or percutaneous	
	AND	
	MCC condition	*See* appendix B.
335	Lysis of intra-abdominal adhesions	Adhesiolysis is reported with root operation Release which is defined as "Freeing a body part from an abnormal physical constraint by cutting or by use of force." Release procedures are coded to the body part being freed. In cases of extensive intra-abdominal adhesions, multiple sites may be reported if they are defined by distinct body part values, according to ICD-10-PCS Guideline B3.2: "During the same operative episode, multiple procedures are coded if: a. The same root operation is performed on different body parts as defined by distinct values of the body part character." Adhesions and lysis must be determined by the physician as significant enough to code and report.
	AND	
	MCC condition	*See* appendix B.
371	Intestinal infection due to identified organism	
	Bacterial food poisoning	
	Peritonitis or peritoneal, retroperitoneal abscess	
	AND	
	CC condition	*See* appendix B.

DRG 386 Inflammatory Bowel Disease with CC RW 0.9716

Potential DRGs

326	Stomach, Esophageal and Duodenal Procedures with MCC	5.0790
327	Stomach, Esophageal and Duodenal Procedures with CC	2.4974
335	Peritoneal Adhesiolysis with MCC	3.5750
336	Peritoneal Adhesiolysis with CC	2.1053
371	Major Gastrointestinal Disorders and Peritoneal Infections with MCC	1.7477
372	Major Gastrointestinal Disorders and Peritoneal Infections with CC	1.0423
385	Inflammatory Bowel Disease with MCC	1.5669
391	Esophagitis, Gastroenteritis and Miscellaneous Digestive Disorders with MCC	1.2757

DRG	PDx/SDx/Procedure	Tips
326	Local excision of lesion, tissue, or diverticulum of esophagus, open esophageal biopsy	
	Local excision of lesion or tissue of stomach, open stomach biopsy	
	Local excision of lesion or tissue of duodenum, open or percutaneous	
	AND	
	MCC condition	*See* appendix B.
327	Local excision of lesion, tissue, or diverticulum of esophagus, open esophageal biopsy	
	Local excision of lesion or tissue of stomach, open stomach biopsy	
	Local excision of lesion or tissue of duodenum, open or percutaneous	
	AND	
	CC condition	*See* appendix B.
335	Lysis of intra-abdominal adhesions	Adhesiolysis is reported with root operation Release which is defined as "Freeing a body part from an abnormal physical constraint by cutting or by use of force." Release procedures are coded to the body part being freed. In cases of extensive intra-abdominal adhesions, multiple sites may be reported if they are defined by distinct body part values, according to ICD-10-PCS Guideline B3.2: "During the same operative episode, multiple procedures are coded if: a. The same root operation is performed on different body parts as defined by distinct values of the body part character." Adhesions and lysis must be determined by the physician as significant enough to code and report.
	AND	
	MCC condition	*See* appendix B.
336	Lysis of intra-abdominal adhesions	*See* DRG 335.
	AND	
	CC condition	*See* appendix B.
371	Intestinal infection due to identified organism	
	Bacterial food poisoning	
	Peritonitis or peritoneal, retroperitoneal abscess	
	AND	
	MCC condition	*See* appendix B.
372	Intestinal infection due to identified organism	
	Bacterial food poisoning	
	Peritonitis or peritoneal, retroperitoneal abscess	
	AND	
	CC condition	*See* appendix B.
385	MCC condition	*See* appendix B.
391	Esophagitis	
	Esophageal stricture/stenosis, dyskinesia, diverticulum, reflux, leukoplakia, other and unspecified disorders of esophagus	
	Gastritis/duodenitis without mention of hemorrhage	
	Chronic duodenal ileus	
	Diverticulosis/diverticulitis of intestine without hemorrhage	
	AND	
	MCC condition	*See* appendix B.

DRG 387 Inflammatory Bowel Disease without CC/MCC

RW 0.6841

Potential DRGs

326	Stomach, Esophageal and Duodenal Procedures with MCC	5.0790
327	Stomach, Esophageal and Duodenal Procedures with CC	2.4974
328	Stomach, Esophageal and Duodenal Procedures without CC/MCC	1.5973
335	Peritoneal Adhesiolysis with MCC	3.5750
336	Peritoneal Adhesiolysis with CC	2.1053
337	Peritoneal Adhesiolysis without CC/MCC	1.4964
371	Major Gastrointestinal Disorders and Peritoneal Infections with MCC	1.7477
372	Major Gastrointestinal Disorders and Peritoneal Infections with CC	1.0423
373	Major Gastrointestinal Disorders and Peritoneal Infections without CC/MCC	0.7165
385	Inflammatory Bowel Disease with MCC	1.5669
386	Inflammatory Bowel Disease with CC	0.9716
391	Esophagitis, Gastroenteritis and Miscellaneous Digestive Disorders with MCC	1.2757

DRG	PDx/SDx/Procedure	Tips
326	Local excision of lesion, tissue, or diverticulum of esophagus, open esophageal biopsy	
	Local excision of lesion or tissue of stomach, open stomach biopsy	
	Local excision of lesion or tissue of duodenum, open or percutaneous	
	AND	
	MCC condition	*See* appendix B.
327	Local excision of lesion, tissue, or diverticulum of esophagus, open esophageal biopsy	
	Local excision of lesion or tissue of stomach, open stomach biopsy	
	Local excision of lesion or tissue of duodenum, open or percutaneous	
	AND	
	CC condition	*See* appendix B.
328	Local excision of lesion, tissue, or diverticulum of esophagus, open esophageal biopsy	
	Local excision of lesion or tissue of stomach, open stomach biopsy	
	Local excision of lesion or tissue of duodenum, open or percutaneous	
335	Lysis of intra-abdominal adhesions	Adhesiolysis is reported with root operation Release which is defined as "Freeing a body part from an abnormal physical constraint by cutting or by use of force." Release procedures are coded to the body part being freed. In cases of extensive intra-abdominal adhesions, multiple sites may be reported if they are defined by distinct body part values, according to ICD-10-PCS Guideline B3.2: "During the same operative episode, multiple procedures are coded if: a. The same root operation is performed on different body parts as defined by distinct values of the body part character." Adhesions and lysis must be determined by the physician as significant enough to code and report.
	AND	
	MCC condition	*See* appendix B.
336	Lysis of intra-abdominal adhesions	*See* DRG 335.
	AND	
	CC condition	*See* appendix B.
337	Lysis of intra-abdominal adhesions	*See* DRG 335.
371	Intestinal infection due to identified organism	
	Bacterial food poisoning	
	Peritonitis or peritoneal, retroperitoneal abscess	
	AND	
	MCC condition	*See* appendix B.
372	Intestinal infection due to identified organism	
	Bacterial food poisoning	
	Peritonitis or peritoneal, retroperitoneal abscess	
	AND	
	CC condition	*See* appendix B.
373	Intestinal infection due to identified organism	
	Bacterial food poisoning	
	Peritonitis or peritoneal, retroperitoneal abscess	
385	MCC condition	*See* appendix B.
386	CC condition	*See* appendix B.
391	Esophagitis	
	Esophageal stricture/stenosis, dyskinesia, diverticulum, reflux, leukoplakia, other and unspecified disorders of esophagus	
	Gastritis/duodenitis without mention of hemorrhage	
	Chronic duodenal ileus	
	Diverticulosis/diverticulitis of intestine without hemorrhage	
	AND	
	MCC condition	*See* appendix B.

DRG 388 GI Obstruction with MCC RW 1.4535

Potential DRGs

326	Stomach, Esophageal and Duodenal Procedures with MCC	5.0790
380	Complicated Peptic Ulcer with MCC	1.9485
393	Other Digestive System Diagnoses with MCC	1.6196

DRG	PDx/SDx/Procedure	Tips
326	Pyloroplasty or pyloromyotomy	Dilation or division (incision) of pyloric stenosis for obstruction. Dilation is accomplished by stretching a tubular body part using intraluminal pressure or by cutting part of the orifice or wall of the tubular body part. Incision for the purpose of dilation is inherent to the dilation as the objective of the procedure is to open the tubular body part (pylorus). Incision performed in order to separate or transect a body part is reported as division.
	AND	
	MCC condition	*See* appendix B.
380	Pyloric and duodenal stenosis, except congenital	
	AND	
	MCC condition	*See* appendix B.
393	Hernia, with or without obstruction	
	Gastric band and other bariatric procedure complications	Review the documentation carefully; code assignment is based on the provider's documentation of a relationship between the condition and the procedure. Unless the classification instructs otherwise, only when there is a clear cause-and-effect relationship between the care provided and the condition and the documentation indicates the condition is a complication, can the condition be coded as such. Query the provider for clarification if the relationship/complication is not clearly documented. See guideline I.B.16.
	Congenital pyloric and duodenal stenosis	
	AND	
	MCC condition	*See* appendix B.

DRG 389 GI Obstruction with CC RW 0.7964

Potential DRGs

326	Stomach, Esophageal and Duodenal Procedures with MCC	5.0790
327	Stomach, Esophageal and Duodenal Procedures with CC	2.4974
380	Complicated Peptic Ulcer with MCC	1.9485
381	Complicated Peptic Ulcer with CC	1.0730
388	GI Obstruction with MCC	1.4535
391	Esophagitis, Gastroenteritis and Miscellaneous Digestive Disorders with MCC	1.2757
393	Other Digestive System Diagnoses with MCC	1.6196
394	Other Digestive System Diagnoses with CC	0.9369

DRG	PDx/SDx/Procedure	Tips
326	Pyloroplasty or pyloromyotomy	Dilation or division (incision) of pyloric stenosis for obstruction. Dilation is accomplished by stretching a tubular body part using intraluminal pressure or by cutting part of the orifice or wall of the tubular body part. Incision for the purpose of dilation is inherent to the dilation as the objective of the procedure is to open the tubular body part (pylorus). Incision performed in order to separate or transect a body part is reported as division.
	AND	
	MCC condition	*See* appendix B.
327	Pyloroplasty or pyloromyotomy	*See* DRG 326.
	AND	
	CC condition	*See* appendix B.
380	Pyloric and duodenal stenosis, except congenital	
	AND	
	MCC condition	*See* appendix B.
381	Pyloric and duodenal stenosis, except congenital	
	AND	
	CC condition	*See* appendix B.
388	MCC condition	*See* appendix B.
391	Esophagitis	
	Esophageal obstruction, dyskinesia, diverticulum, reflux, leukoplakia, other and unspecified disorders of esophagus	
	Gastritis, duodenitis without mention of hemorrhage	
	Diverticulosis, diverticulitis of intestine without hemorrhage	
	AND	
	MCC condition	*See* appendix B.
393	Hernia, with or without obstruction	
	Gastric band and other bariatric procedure complications	Review the documentation carefully; code assignment is based on the provider's documentation of a relationship between the condition and the procedure. Unless the classification instructs otherwise, only when there is a clear cause-and-effect relationship between the care provided and the condition and the documentation indicates the condition is a complication, can it be coded as such. Query the provider for clarification if the relationship/complication is not clearly documented. See guideline I.B.16.
	Congenital pyloric and duodenal stenosis	
	AND	
	MCC condition	*See* appendix B.
394	Hernia, with or without obstruction	
	Gastric band and other bariatric procedure complications	*See* DRG 393.
	Congenital pyloric and duodenal stenosis	
	AND	
	CC condition	*See* appendix B.

DRG 390 GI Obstruction without CC/MCC RW 0.5590

Potential DRGs

326	Stomach, Esophageal and Duodenal Procedures with MCC	5.0790
327	Stomach, Esophageal and Duodenal Procedures with CC	2.4974
328	Stomach, Esophageal and Duodenal Procedures without CC/MCC	1.5973
380	Complicated Peptic Ulcer with MCC	1.9485
381	Complicated Peptic Ulcer with CC	1.0730
382	Complicated Peptic Ulcer without CC/MCC	0.7571
388	GI Obstruction with MCC	1.4535
389	GI Obstruction with CC	0.7964
391	Esophagitis, Gastroenteritis and Miscellaneous Digestive Disorders with MCC	1.2757
392	Esophagitis, Gastroenteritis and Miscellaneous Digestive Disorders without MCC	0.7856
393	Other Digestive System Diagnoses with MCC	1.6196
394	Other Digestive System Diagnoses with CC	0.9369
395	Other Digestive System Diagnoses without CC/MCC	0.6475

DRG	PDx/SDx/Procedure	Tips
326	Pyloroplasty or pyloromyotomy	Dilation or division (incision) of pyloric stenosis for obstruction. Dilation is accomplished by stretching a tubular body part using intraluminal pressure or by cutting part of the orifice or wall of the tubular body part. Incision for the purpose of dilation is inherent to the dilation as the objective of the procedure is to open the tubular body part (pylorus). Incision performed in order to separate or transect a body part is reported as division.
	AND	
	MCC condition	*See* appendix B.
327	Pyloroplasty or pyloromyotomy	*See* DRG 326.
	AND	
	CC condition	*See* appendix B.
328	Pyloroplasty or pyloromyotomy	*See* DRG 326.
380	Pyloric and duodenal stenosis, except congenital	
	AND	
	MCC condition	*See* appendix B.
381	Pyloric and duodenal stenosis, except congenital	
	AND	
	CC condition	*See* appendix B.
382	Pyloric and duodenal stenosis, except congenital	
388	MCC condition	*See* appendix B.
389	CC condition	*See* appendix B.
391	Esophagitis	
	Esophageal obstruction, dyskinesia, diverticulum, reflux, leukoplakia, other and unspecified disorders of esophagus	
	Gastritis, duodenitis without mention of hemorrhage	
	Diverticulosis, diverticulitis of intestine without hemorrhage	
	AND	
	MCC condition	*See* appendix B.
392	Esophagitis	
	Esophageal obstruction, dyskinesia, diverticulum, reflux, leukoplakia, other and unspecified disorders of esophagus	
	Gastritis, duodenitis without mention of hemorrhage	
	Diverticulosis, diverticulitis of intestine without hemorrhage	
393	Hernia, with or without obstruction	
	Gastric band and other bariatric procedure complications	Review the documentation carefully; code assignment is based on the provider's documentation of a relationship between the condition and the procedure. Unless the classification instructs otherwise, only when there is a clear cause-and-effect relationship between the care provided and the condition and the documentation indicates the condition is a complication, can it be coded as such. Query the provider for clarification if the relationship/complication is not clearly documented. See guideline I.B.16.
	Congenital pyloric and duodenal stenosis	
	AND	
	MCC condition	*See* appendix B.
394	Hernia, with or without obstruction	
	Gastric band and other bariatric procedure complications	*See* DRG 393.
	Congenital pyloric and duodenal stenosis	
	AND	
	CC condition	*See* appendix B.
395	Hernia, with or without obstruction	
	Gastric band and other bariatric procedure complications	*See* DRG 393.
	Congenital pyloric and duodenal stenosis	

DRG 391 Esophagitis, Gastroenteritis and Miscellaneous Digestive Disorders with MCC — RW 1.2757

Potential DRGs

377	GI Hemorrhage with MCC	1.7903
380	Complicated Peptic Ulcer with MCC	1.9485
385	Inflammatory Bowel Disease with MCC	1.5669
388	GI Obstruction with MCC	1.4535

DRG	PDx/SDx/Procedure	Tips
377	Any digestive ulcers with hemorrhage or hemorrhage and perforation	Review the alphabetic index and tabular list for gastrointestinal conditions linked by the terms "with hemorrhage" or "with bleeding" as the classification presumes a causal relationship between two conditions linked by these terms in the alphabetic index (either under a main term or subterm) or tabular list. Unless the provider documents a different cause of the bleeding or states that the conditions are unrelated, assign the combination code for these conditions.
	Gastritis and duodenitis with hemorrhage	
	Rectal or anal hemorrhage, hematemesis, melena	
	Gastrointestinal hemorrhage	
	AND	
	MCC condition	*See* appendix B.
380	Ulcer of esophagus or Barrett's esophagus	
	Acute, chronic or unspecified gastric ulcer with perforation	
	Acute, chronic or unspecified duodenal ulcer with perforation	
	Acute, chronic or unspecified peptic ulcer with perforation	
	Acute, chronic or unspecified gastrojejunal ulcer without hemorrhage, with or without perforation	
	AND	
	MCC condition	*See* appendix B.
385	Regional enteritis (Crohn's disease)	
	AND	
	MCC condition	*See* appendix B.
388	Abdominal pain due to small bowel obstruction	
	AND	
	MCC condition	*See* appendix B.

DRG 392 Esophagitis, Gastroenteritis and Miscellaneous Digestive Disorders without MCC RW 0.7856

Potential DRGs

377	GI Hemorrhage with MCC	1.7903
378	GI Hemorrhage with CC	0.9838
380	Complicated Peptic Ulcer with MCC	1.9485
381	Complicated Peptic Ulcer with CC	1.0730
385	Inflammatory Bowel Disease with MCC	1.5669
386	Inflammatory Bowel Disease with CC	0.9716
388	GI Obstruction with MCC	1.4535
389	GI Obstruction with CC	0.7964
391	Esophagitis, Gastroenteritis and Miscellaneous Digestive Disorders with MCC	1.2757

DRG	PDx/SDx/Procedure	Tips
377	Any digestive ulcers with hemorrhage or hemorrhage and perforation	Review the alphabetic index and tabular list for gastrointestinal conditions linked by the terms "with hemorrhage" or "with bleeding" as the classification presumes a causal relationship between two conditions linked by these terms in the alphabetic index (either under a main term or subterm) or tabular list. Unless the provider documents a different cause of the bleeding or states that the conditions are unrelated, assign the combination code for these conditions.
	Gastritis and duodenitis with hemorrhage	
	Rectal or anal hemorrhage, hematemesis, melena	
	Gastrointestinal hemorrhage	
	AND	
	MCC condition	*See* appendix B.
378	Any digestive ulcers with hemorrhage or hemorrhage and perforation	*See* DRG 377.
	Gastritis and duodenitis with hemorrhage	
	Rectal or anal hemorrhage, hematemesis, melena	
	Gastrointestinal hemorrhage	
	AND	
	CC condition	*See* appendix B.
380	Ulcer of esophagus or Barrett's esophagus	
	Acute, chronic or unspecified gastric ulcer with perforation	
	Acute, chronic or unspecified duodenal ulcer with perforation	
	Acute, chronic or unspecified peptic ulcer with perforation	
	Acute, chronic or unspecified gastrojejunal ulcer without hemorrhage, with or without perforation	
	AND	
	MCC condition	*See* appendix B.
381	Ulcer of esophagus or Barrett's esophagus	
	Acute, chronic or unspecified gastric ulcer with perforation	
	Acute, chronic or unspecified duodenal ulcer with perforation	
	Acute, chronic or unspecified peptic ulcer with perforation	
	Acute, chronic or unspecified gastrojejunal ulcer without hemorrhage, with or without perforation	
	AND	
	CC condition	*See* appendix B.
385	Regional enteritis (Crohn's disease)	
	AND	
	MCC condition	*See* appendix B.
386	Regional enteritis (Crohn's disease)	
	AND	
	CC condition	*See* appendix B.
388	Abdominal pain due to small bowel obstruction	
	AND	
	MCC condition	*See* appendix B.
389	Abdominal pain due to small bowel obstruction	
	AND	
	CC condition	*See* appendix B.
391	MCC condition	*See* appendix B.

DRG 393 Other Digestive System Diagnoses with MCC

RW 1.6196

Potential DRGs

371	Major Gastrointestinal Disorders and Peritoneal Infections with MCC	1.7477
374	Digestive Malignancy with MCC	2.0990

DRG	PDx/SDx/Procedure	Tips
371	Intestinal infection due to identified organism	
	Bacterial food poisoning	
	Peritonitis or peritoneal, retroperitoneal abscess	
	AND	
	MCC condition	*See* appendix B.
374	Digestive malignancy: Esophagus Stomach Small intestine Colon Rectum, rectosigmoid junction, anus	
	AND	
	MCC condition	*See* appendix B.

DRG 394 Other Digestive System Diagnoses with CC

RW 0.9369

Potential DRGs

371	Major Gastrointestinal Disorders and Peritoneal Infections with MCC	1.7477
372	Major Gastrointestinal Disorders and Peritoneal Infections with CC	1.0423
374	Digestive Malignancy with MCC	2.0990
375	Digestive Malignancy with CC	1.1983
385	Inflammatory Bowel Disease with MCC	1.5669
386	Inflammatory Bowel Disease with CC	0.9716
393	Other Digestive System Diagnoses with MCC	1.6196

DRG	PDx/SDx/Procedure	Tips
371	Intestinal infection due to identified organism	
	Bacterial food poisoning	
	Peritonitis or peritoneal, retroperitoneal abscess	
	AND	
	MCC condition	*See* appendix B.
372	Intestinal infection due to identified organism	
	Bacterial food poisoning	
	Peritonitis or peritoneal, retroperitoneal abscess	
	AND	
	CC condition	*See* appendix B.
374	Digestive malignancy: Esophagus Stomach Small intestine Colon Rectum, rectosigmoid junction, anus	
	AND	
	MCC condition	*See* appendix B.
375	Digestive malignancy: Esophagus Stomach Small intestine Colon Rectum, rectosigmoid junction, anus	
	AND	
	CC condition	*See* appendix B.
385	Regional enteritis (Crohn's disease)	
	AND	
	MCC condition	*See* appendix B.
386	Regional enteritis (Crohn's disease)	
	AND	
	CC condition	*See* appendix B.
393	MCC condition	*See* appendix B.

DRG 395 Other Digestive System Diagnoses without CC/MCC RW 0.6475

Potential DRGs

371	Major Gastrointestinal Disorders and Peritoneal Infections with MCC	1.7477
372	Major Gastrointestinal Disorders and Peritoneal Infections with CC	1.0423
373	Major Gastrointestinal Disorders and Peritoneal Infections without CC/MCC	0.7165
374	Digestive Malignancy with MCC	2.0990
375	Digestive Malignancy with CC	1.1983
376	Digestive Malignancy without CC/MCC	0.8914
385	Inflammatory Bowel Disease with MCC	1.5669
386	Inflammatory Bowel Disease with CC	0.9716
387	Inflammatory Bowel Disease without CC/MCC	0.6841
393	Other Digestive System Diagnoses with MCC	1.6196
394	Other Digestive System Diagnoses with CC	0.9369

DRG	PDx/SDx/Procedure	Tips
371	Intestinal infection due to identified organism	
	Bacterial food poisoning	
	Peritonitis or peritoneal, retroperitoneal abscess	
	AND	
	MCC condition	*See* appendix B.
372	Intestinal infection due to identified organism	
	Bacterial food poisoning	
	Peritonitis or peritoneal, retroperitoneal abscess	
	AND	
	CC condition	*See* appendix B.
373	Intestinal infection due to identified organism	
	Bacterial food poisoning	
	Peritonitis or peritoneal, retroperitoneal abscess	
374	Digestive malignancy: Esophagus Stomach Small intestine Colon Rectum, rectosigmoid junction, anus	
	AND	
	MCC condition	*See* appendix B.
375	Digestive malignancy: Esophagus Stomach Small intestine Colon Rectum, rectosigmoid junction, anus	
	AND	
	CC condition	*See* appendix B.
376	Digestive malignancy: Esophagus Stomach Small intestine Colon Rectum, rectosigmoid junction, anus	
385	Regional enteritis (Crohn's disease)	
	AND	
	MCC condition	*See* appendix B.
386	Regional enteritis (Crohn's disease)	
	AND	
	CC condition	*See* appendix B.
387	Regional enteritis (Crohn's disease)	
393	MCC condition	*See* appendix B.
394	CC condition	*See* appendix B.

DRG 397 Appendix Procedures with MCC — RW 2.2466

Potential DRGs

329	Major Small and Large Bowel Procedures with MCC	4.5168
335	Peritoneal Adhesiolysis with MCC	3.5750

DRG	PDx/SDx/Procedure	Tips
329	Partial cecectomy	Any minor trimming or excision of the cecum to facilitate the removal of the appendix is incidental to the procedure, but if the extent of the disease process involves the cecum, as indicated by the documentation, a code for excision of cecum may be applied.
	AND	
	MCC condition	*See* appendix B.
335	Lysis of intra-abdominal adhesions	Adhesiolysis is reported with root operation Release, defined as "Freeing a body part from an abnormal physical constraint by cutting or by use of force." Release procedures are coded to the body part being freed. In cases of extensive intra-abdominal adhesions, multiple sites may be reported if they are defined by distinct body part values; according to ICD-10-PCS Guideline B3.2: "During the same operative episode, multiple procedures are coded if: a. The same root operation is performed on different body parts as defined by distinct values of the body part character." Adhesions and lysis must be determined by the physician as significant enough to code and report.
	AND	
	MCC condition	*See* appendix B.

DRG 398 Appendix Procedures with CC — RW 1.5133

Potential DRGs

329	Major Small and Large Bowel Procedures with MCC	4.5168
330	Major Small and Large Bowel Procedures with CC	2.3721
335	Peritoneal Adhesiolysis with MCC	3.5750
336	Peritoneal Adhesiolysis with CC	2.1053
397	Appendix Procedures with MCC	2.2466

DRG	PDx/SDx/Procedure	Tips
329	Partial cecectomy	Any minor trimming or excision of the cecum to facilitate the removal of the appendix is incidental to the procedure, but if the extent of the disease process involves the cecum, as indicated by the documentation, a code for excision of cecum may be applied.
	AND	
	MCC condition	*See* appendix B.
330	Partial cecectomy	*See* DRG 329.
	AND	
	CC condition	*See* appendix B.
335	Lysis of intra-abdominal adhesions	Adhesiolysis is reported with root operation Release, defined as "Freeing a body part from an abnormal physical constraint by cutting or by use of force." Release procedures are coded to the body part being freed. In cases of extensive intra-abdominal adhesions, multiple sites may be reported if they are defined by distinct body part values; according to ICD-10-PCS Guideline B3.2: "During the same operative episode, multiple procedures are coded if: a. The same root operation is performed on different body parts as defined by distinct values of the body part character." Adhesions and lysis must be determined by the physician as significant enough to code and report.
	AND	
	MCC condition	*See* appendix B.
336	Lysis of intra-abdominal adhesions	*See* DRG 335.
	AND	
	CC condition	*See* appendix B.
397	MCC condition	*See* appendix B.

DRG 399 Appendix Procedures without CC/MCC — RW 1.1311

Potential DRGs

329	Major Small and Large Bowel Procedures with MCC	4.5168
330	Major Small and Large Bowel Procedures with CC	2.3721
331	Major Small and Large Bowel Procedures without CC/MCC	1.6720
335	Peritoneal Adhesiolysis with MCC	3.5750
336	Peritoneal Adhesiolysis with CC	2.1053
337	Peritoneal Adhesiolysis without CC/MCC	1.4964
397	Appendix Procedures with MCC	2.2466
398	Appendix Procedures with CC	1.5133

DRG	PDx/SDx/Procedure	Tips
329	Partial cecectomy	Any minor trimming or excision of the cecum to facilitate the removal of the appendix is incidental to the procedure, but if the extent of the disease process involves the cecum, as indicated by the documentation, a code for excision of cecum may be applied.
	AND	
	MCC condition	*See* appendix B.
330	Partial cecectomy	*See* DRG 329.
	AND	
	CC condition	*See* appendix B.
331	Partial cecectomy	*See* DRG 329.
335	Lysis of intra-abdominal adhesions	Adhesiolysis is reported with root operation Release, defined as "Freeing a body part from an abnormal physical constraint by cutting or by use of force." Release procedures are coded to the body part being freed. In cases of extensive intra-abdominal adhesions, multiple sites may be reported if they are defined by distinct body part values; according to ICD-10-PCS Guideline B3.2: "During the same operative episode, multiple procedures are coded if: a. The same root operation is performed on different body parts as defined by distinct values of the body part character." Adhesions and lysis must be determined by the physician as significant enough to code and report.
	AND	
	MCC condition	*See* appendix B.
336	Lysis of intra-abdominal adhesions	*See* DRG 335.
	AND	
	CC condition	*See* appendix B.
337	Lysis of intra-abdominal adhesions	*See* DRG 335.
397	MCC condition	*See* appendix B.
398	CC condition	*See* appendix B.

Diseases And Disorders Of The Hepatobiliary System And Pancreas

DRG 405 Pancreas, Liver and Shunt Procedures with MCC — RW 5.5052

No Potential DRGs

DRG 406 Pancreas, Liver and Shunt Procedures with CC — RW 2.8874

Potential DRGs

405 Pancreas, Liver and Shunt Procedures with MCC 5.5052

DRG	PDx/SDx/Procedure	Tips
405	MCC condition	*See* appendix B.

DRG 407 Pancreas, Liver and Shunt Procedures without CC/MCC — RW 2.1510

Potential DRGs

405 Pancreas, Liver and Shunt Procedures with MCC 5.5052
406 Pancreas, Liver and Shunt Procedures with CC 2.8874

DRG	PDx/SDx/Procedure	Tips
405	MCC condition	*See* appendix B.
406	CC condition	*See* appendix B.

DRG 408 Biliary Tract Procedures Except Only Cholecystectomy with or without C.D.E. with MCC — RW 3.7222

No Potential DRGs

DRG 409 Biliary Tract Procedures Except Only Cholecystectomy with or without C.D.E. with CC — RW 1.9573

Potential DRGs

408 Biliary Tract Procedures Except Only Cholecystectomy with or without C.D.E. with MCC 3.7222

DRG	PDx/SDx/Procedure	Tips
408	MCC condition	*See* appendix B.

DRG 410 Biliary Tract Procedures Except Only Cholecystectomy with or without C.D.E. without CC/MCC — RW 1.5652

Potential DRGs

408 Biliary Tract Procedures Except Only Cholecystectomy with or without C.D.E. with MCC 3.7222
409 Biliary Tract Procedures Except Only Cholecystectomy with or without C.D.E. with CC 1.9573

DRG	PDx/SDx/Procedure	Tips
408	MCC condition	*See* appendix B.
409	CC condition	*See* appendix B.

DRG 411 Cholecystectomy with C.D.E. with MCC — RW 2.8805

No Potential DRGs

DRG 412 Cholecystectomy with C.D.E. with CC — RW 2.0455

Potential DRGs

408 Biliary Tract Procedures Except Only Cholecystectomy with or without C.D.E. with MCC 3.7222
411 Cholecystectomy with C.D.E. with MCC 2.8805

DRG	PDx/SDx/Procedure	Tips
408	Additional biliary tract procedure (excision or repair of bile ducts)	
	AND	
	MCC condition	*See* appendix B.
411	MCC condition	*See* appendix B.

DRG 413 Cholecystectomy with C.D.E. without CC/MCC — RW 1.5096

Potential DRGs

408 Biliary Tract Procedures Except Only Cholecystectomy with or without C.D.E. with MCC 3.7222
409 Biliary Tract Procedures Except Only Cholecystectomy with or without C.D.E. with CC 1.9573
411 Cholecystectomy with C.D.E. with MCC 2.8805
412 Cholecystectomy with C.D.E. with CC 2.0455

DRG	PDx/SDx/Procedure	Tips
408	Additional biliary tract procedure (excision or repair of bile ducts)	
	AND	
	MCC condition	*See* appendix B.
409	Additional biliary tract procedure (excision or repair of bile ducts)	
	AND	
	CC condition	*See* appendix B.
411	MCC condition	*See* appendix B.
412	CC condition	*See* appendix B.

DRG 414 Cholecystectomy Except by Laparoscope without C.D.E. with MCC RW 3.5252

Potential DRGs

408	Biliary Tract Procedures Except Only Cholecystectomy with or without C.D.E. with MCC	3.7222

DRG	PDx/SDx/Procedure	Tips
408	Additional biliary tract procedure (excision or repair of bile ducts)	
	AND	
	MCC condition	*See* appendix B.

DRG 415 Cholecystectomy Except by Laparoscope without C.D.E. with CC RW 1.9758

Potential DRGs

408	Biliary Tract Procedures Except Only Cholecystectomy with or without C.D.E. with MCC	3.7222
411	Cholecystectomy with C.D.E. with MCC	2.8805
412	Cholecystectomy with C.D.E. with CC	2.0455
414	Cholecystectomy Except by Laparoscope without C.D.E. with MCC	3.5252

DRG	PDx/SDx/Procedure	Tips
408	Additional biliary tract procedure (excision or repair of bile ducts)	
	AND	
	MCC condition	*See* appendix B.
411	Common bile duct exploration	
	AND	
	MCC condition	*See* appendix B.
412	Common bile duct exploration	
	AND	
	CC condition	*See* appendix B.
414	MCC condition	*See* appendix B.

DRG 416 Cholecystectomy Except by Laparoscope without C.D.E. without CC/MCC RW 1.3392

Potential DRGs

408	Biliary Tract Procedures Except Only Cholecystectomy with or without C.D.E. with MCC	3.7222
409	Biliary Tract Procedures Except Only Cholecystectomy with or without C.D.E. with CC	1.9573
410	Biliary Tract Procedures Except Only Cholecystectomy with or without C.D.E. without CC/MCC	1.5652
411	Cholecystectomy with C.D.E. with MCC	2.8805
412	Cholecystectomy with C.D.E. with CC	2.0455
413	Cholecystectomy with C.D.E. without CC/MCC	1.5096
414	Cholecystectomy Except by Laparoscope without C.D.E. with MCC	3.5252
415	Cholecystectomy Except by Laparoscope without C.D.E. with CC	1.9758

DRG	PDx/SDx/Procedure	Tips
408	Additional biliary tract procedure (excision or repair of bile ducts)	
	AND	
	MCC condition	*See* appendix B.
409	Additional biliary tract procedure (excision or repair of bile ducts)	
	AND	
	CC condition	*See* appendix B.
410	Additional biliary tract procedure (excision or repair of bile ducts)	
411	Common bile duct exploration	
	AND	
	MCC condition	*See* appendix B.
412	Common bile duct exploration	
	AND	
	CC condition	*See* appendix B.
413	Common bile duct exploration	
414	MCC condition	*See* appendix B.
415	CC condition	*See* appendix B.

DRG 417 Laparoscopic Cholecystectomy without C.D.E. with MCC RW 2.3178

Potential DRGs

411	Cholecystectomy with C.D.E. with MCC	2.8805
414	Cholecystectomy Except by Laparoscope without C.D.E. with MCC	3.5252

DRG	PDx/SDx/Procedure	Tips
411	Common bile duct exploration	
	AND	
	MCC condition	*See* appendix B.
414	Open cholecystectomy	
	AND	
	MCC condition	*See* appendix B.

DRG 418 Laparoscopic Cholecystectomy without C.D.E. with CC — RW 1.6347

Potential DRGs

411	Cholecystectomy with C.D.E. with MCC	2.8805
412	Cholecystectomy with C.D.E. with CC	2.0455
414	Cholecystectomy Except by Laparoscope without C.D.E. with MCC	3.5252
415	Cholecystectomy Except by Laparoscope without C.D.E. with CC	1.9758
417	Laparoscopic Cholecystectomy without C.D.E. with MCC	2.3178

DRG	PDx/SDx/Procedure	Tips
411	Common bile duct exploration	
	AND	
	MCC condition	*See* appendix B.
412	Common bile duct exploration	
	AND	
	CC condition	*See* appendix B.
414	Open cholecystectomy	
	AND	
	MCC condition	*See* appendix B.
415	Open cholecystectomy	
	AND	
	CC condition	*See* appendix B.
417	MCC condition	*See* appendix B.

DRG 419 Laparoscopic Cholecystectomy without C.D.E. without CC/MCC — RW 1.3132

Potential DRGs

411	Cholecystectomy with C.D.E. with MCC	2.8805
412	Cholecystectomy with C.D.E. with CC	2.0455
413	Cholecystectomy with C.D.E. without CC/MCC	1.5096
414	Cholecystectomy Except by Laparoscope without C.D.E. with MCC	3.5252
415	Cholecystectomy Except by Laparoscope without C.D.E. with CC	1.9758
416	Cholecystectomy Except by Laparoscope without C.D.E. without CC/MCC	1.3392
417	Laparoscopic Cholecystectomy without C.D.E. with MCC	2.3178
418	Laparoscopic Cholecystectomy without C.D.E. with CC	1.6347

DRG	PDx/SDx/Procedure	Tips
411	Common bile duct exploration	
	AND	
	MCC condition	*See* appendix B.
412	Common bile duct exploration	
	AND	
	CC condition	*See* appendix B.
413	Common bile duct exploration	
414	Open cholecystectomy	
	AND	
	MCC condition	*See* appendix B.
415	Open cholecystectomy	
	AND	
	CC condition	*See* appendix B.
416	Open cholecystectomy	
417	MCC condition	*See* appendix B.
418	CC condition	*See* appendix B.

DRG 420 Hepatobiliary Diagnostic Procedures with MCC — RW 3.2008

Potential DRGs

405	Pancreas, Liver and Shunt Procedures with MCC	5.5052

DRG	PDx/SDx/Procedure	Tips
405	Percutaneous, laparoscopic or other ablation/destruction of liver lesion or tissue	
	Dilation of pancreatic duct	
	AND	
	MCC condition	*See* appendix B.

Optimizing Tips

DRG 421 Hepatobiliary Diagnostic Procedures with CC RW 1.7096

Potential DRGs

405	Pancreas, Liver and Shunt Procedures with MCC	5.5052
406	Pancreas, Liver and Shunt Procedures with CC	2.8874
420	Hepatobiliary Diagnostic Procedures with MCC	3.2008

DRG	PDx/SDx/Procedure	Tips
405	Percutaneous, laparoscopic or other ablation/destruction of liver lesion or tissue	
	Dilation of pancreatic duct	
	AND	
	MCC condition	*See* appendix B.
406	Percutaneous, laparoscopic or other ablation/destruction of liver lesion or tissue	
	Dilation of pancreatic duct	
	AND	
	CC condition	*See* appendix B.
420	MCC condition	*See* appendix B.

DRG 422 Hepatobiliary Diagnostic Procedures without CC/MCC RW 1.4110

Potential DRGs

405	Pancreas, Liver and Shunt Procedures with MCC	5.5052
406	Pancreas, Liver and Shunt Procedures with CC	2.8874
407	Pancreas, Liver and Shunt Procedures without CC/MCC	2.1510
420	Hepatobiliary Diagnostic Procedures with MCC	3.2008
421	Hepatobiliary Diagnostic Procedures with CC	1.7096

DRG	PDx/SDx/Procedure	Tips
405	Percutaneous, laparoscopic or other ablation/destruction of liver lesion or tissue	
	Dilation of pancreatic duct	
	AND	
	MCC condition	*See* appendix B.
406	Percutaneous, laparoscopic or other ablation/destruction of liver lesion or tissue	
	Dilation of pancreatic duct	
	AND	
	CC condition	*See* appendix B.
407	Percutaneous, laparoscopic or other ablation/destruction of liver lesion or tissue	
	Dilation of pancreatic duct	
420	MCC condition	*See* appendix B.
421	CC condition	*See* appendix B.

DRG 423 Other Hepatobiliary or Pancreas O.R. Procedures with MCC RW 3.9109

Potential DRGs

405	Pancreas, Liver and Shunt Procedures with MCC	5.5052

DRG	PDx/SDx/Procedure	Tips
405	Percutaneous, laparoscopic or other ablation/destruction of liver lesion or tissue	
	Dilation of pancreatic duct	
	AND	
	MCC condition	*See* appendix B.

DRG 424 Other Hepatobiliary or Pancreas O.R. Procedures with CC RW 2.0873

Potential DRGs

405	Pancreas, Liver and Shunt Procedures with MCC	5.5052
406	Pancreas, Liver and Shunt Procedures with CC	2.8874
423	Other Hepatobiliary or Pancreas O.R. Procedures with MCC	3.9109

DRG	PDx/SDx/Procedure	Tips
405	Percutaneous, laparoscopic or other ablation/destruction of liver lesion or tissue	
	Dilation of pancreatic duct	
	AND	
	MCC condition	*See* appendix B.
406	Percutaneous, laparoscopic or other ablation/destruction of liver lesion or tissue	
	Dilation of pancreatic duct	
	AND	
	CC condition	*See* appendix B.
423	MCC condition	*See* appendix B.

DRG 425 Other Hepatobiliary or Pancreas O.R. Procedures without CC/MCC — RW 1.6019

Potential DRGs

405	Pancreas, Liver and Shunt Procedures with MCC	5.5052
406	Pancreas, Liver and Shunt Procedures with CC	2.8874
407	Pancreas, Liver and Shunt Procedures without CC/MCC	2.1510
423	Other Hepatobiliary or Pancreas O.R. Procedures with MCC	3.9109
424	Other Hepatobiliary or Pancreas O.R. Procedures with CC	2.0873

DRG	PDx/SDx/Procedure	Tips
405	Percutaneous, laparoscopic or other ablation/destruction of liver lesion or tissue	
	Dilation of pancreatic duct	
	AND	
	MCC condition	*See* appendix B.
406	Percutaneous, laparoscopic or other ablation/destruction of liver lesion or tissue	
	Dilation of pancreatic duct	
	AND	
	CC condition	*See* appendix B.
407	Percutaneous, laparoscopic or other ablation/destruction of liver lesion or tissue	
	Dilation of pancreatic duct	
423	MCC condition	*See* appendix B.
424	CC condition	*See* appendix B.

DRG 432 Cirrhosis and Alcoholic Hepatitis with MCC — RW 1.9160

Potential DRGs

405	Pancreas, Liver and Shunt Procedures with MCC	5.5052
420	Hepatobiliary Diagnostic Procedures with MCC	3.2008
423	Other Hepatobiliary or Pancreas O.R. Procedures with MCC	3.9109

DRG	PDx/SDx/Procedure	Tips
405	Intraabdominal shunt (open, percutaneous endoscopic approach)	
	Creation of peritoneovascular shunt (open, percutaneous endoscopic approach)	
	Insertion of choledochohepatic tube for decompression (Via Natural or Artificial Opening)	
	AND	
	MCC condition	*See* appendix B.
420	Open or laparoscopic liver biopsy	
	AND	
	MCC condition	*See* appendix B.
423	Ligation of esophageal varices, open	
	AND	
	MCC condition	*See* appendix B.

DRG 433 Cirrhosis and Alcoholic Hepatitis with CC RW 1.0310

Potential DRGs

405	Pancreas, Liver and Shunt Procedures with MCC	5.5052
406	Pancreas, Liver and Shunt Procedures with CC	2.8874
420	Hepatobiliary Diagnostic Procedures with MCC	3.2008
421	Hepatobiliary Diagnostic Procedures with CC	1.7096
423	Other Hepatobiliary or Pancreas O.R. Procedures with MCC	3.9109
424	Other Hepatobiliary or Pancreas O.R. Procedures with CC	2.0873
432	Cirrhosis and Alcoholic Hepatitis with MCC	1.9160
441	Disorders of Liver Except Malignancy, Cirrhosis, Alcoholic Hepatitis with MCC	1.8282
444	Disorders of the Biliary Tract with MCC	1.6332
445	Disorders of the Biliary Tract with CC	1.0868
895	Alcohol, Drug Abuse or Dependence with Rehabilitation Therapy	1.6088
896	Alcohol/Drug Abuse or Dependence without Rehabilitation Therapy with MCC	1.7781

DRG	PDx/SDx/Procedure	Tips
405	Intraabdominal shunt (open, percutaneous endoscopic approach)	
	Creation of peritoneovascular shunt (open, percutaneous endoscopic approach)	
	Insertion of choledochohepatic tube for decompression (Via Natural or Artificial Opening)	
	AND	
	MCC condition	*See* appendix B.
406	Intraabdominal shunt (open, percutaneous endoscopic approach)	
	Creation of peritoneovascular shunt (open, percutaneous endoscopic approach)	
	Insertion of choledochohepatic tube for decompression (Via Natural or Artificial Opening)	
	AND	
	CC condition	*See* appendix B.
420	Open or laparoscopic liver biopsy	
	AND	
	MCC condition	*See* appendix B.
421	Open or laparoscopic liver biopsy	
	AND	
	CC condition	*See* appendix B.
423	Ligation of esophageal varices, open	
	AND	
	MCC condition	*See* appendix B.
424	Ligation of esophageal varices, open	
	AND	
	CC condition	*See* appendix B.
432	MCC condition	*See* appendix B.
441	Benign neoplasm of liver and biliary passages	
	Chronic hepatitis	
	Unspecified and other chronic nonalcoholic liver disease	
	Liver abscess	
	AND	
	MCC condition	*See* appendix B.
444	Cholelithiasis, cholecystitis, other disorders of gallbladder or biliary tract	
	AND	
	MCC condition	*See* appendix B.
445	Cholelithiasis, cholecystitis, other disorders of gallbladder or biliary tract	
	AND	
	CC condition	*See* appendix B.
895	Alcohol-induced mental disorders	
	Acute alcoholic intoxication or other/unspecified alcohol dependence	
	Nondependent alcohol abuse	
	Excessive blood level of alcohol	
	AND	
	Rehabilitation therapy	Review therapy and other documentation carefully to differentiate therapy from detoxification.
896	Alcohol-induced mental disorders	
	Acute alcoholic intoxication or other/unspecified alcohol dependence	
	Nondependent alcohol abuse	
	Excessive blood level of alcohol	
	AND	
	MCC condition	*See* appendix B.

DRG 434 Cirrhosis and Alcoholic Hepatitis without CC/MCC RW 0.6695

Potential DRGs

405	Pancreas, Liver and Shunt Procedures with MCC	5.5052
406	Pancreas, Liver and Shunt Procedures with CC	2.8874
407	Pancreas, Liver and Shunt Procedures without CC/MCC	2.1510
420	Hepatobiliary Diagnostic Procedures with MCC	3.2008
421	Hepatobiliary Diagnostic Procedures with CC	1.7096
422	Hepatobiliary Diagnostic Procedures without CC/MCC	1.4110
423	Other Hepatobiliary or Pancreas O.R. Procedures with MCC	3.9109
424	Other Hepatobiliary or Pancreas O.R. Procedures with CC	2.0873
425	Other Hepatobiliary or Pancreas O.R. Procedures without CC/MCC	1.6019
432	Cirrhosis and Alcoholic Hepatitis with MCC	1.9160
433	Cirrhosis and Alcoholic Hepatitis with CC	1.0310
441	Disorders of Liver Except Malignancy, Cirrhosis, Alcoholic Hepatitis with MCC	1.8282
442	Disorders of Liver Except Malignancy, Cirrhosis, Alcoholic Hepatitis with CC	0.9515
443	Disorders of Liver Except Malignancy, Cirrhosis, Alcoholic Hepatitis without CC/MCC	0.7147
444	Disorders of the Biliary Tract with MCC	1.6332
445	Disorders of the Biliary Tract with CC	1.0868
446	Disorders of the Biliary Tract without CC/MCC	0.8015
895	Alcohol/Drug Abuse or Dependence with Rehabilitation Therapy	1.6088
896	Alcohol/Drug Abuse or Dependence without Rehabilitation Therapy with MCC	1.7781

DRG	PDx/SDx/Procedure	Tips
405	Intraabdominal shunt (open, percutaneous endoscopic approach)	
	Creation of peritoneovascular shunt (open, percutaneous endoscopic approach)	
	Insertion of choledochohepatic tube for decompression (Via Natural or Artificial Opening)	
	AND	
	MCC condition	*See* appendix B.
406	Intraabdominal shunt (open, percutaneous endoscopic approach)	
	Creation of peritoneovascular shunt (open, percutaneous endoscopic approach)	
	Insertion of choledochohepatic tube for decompression (Via Natural or Artificial Opening)	
	AND	
	CC condition	*See* appendix B.
407	Intraabdominal shunt (open, percutaneous endoscopic approach)	
	Creation of peritoneovascular shunt (open, percutaneous endoscopic approach)	
	Insertion of choledochohepatic tube for decompression (Via Natural or Artificial Opening)	
420	Open or laparoscopic liver biopsy	
	AND	
	MCC condition	*See* appendix B.
421	Open or laparoscopic liver biopsy	
	AND	
	CC condition	*See* appendix B.
422	Open or laparoscopic liver biopsy	
423	Ligation of esophageal varices, open	
	AND	
	MCC condition	*See* appendix B.
424	Ligation of esophageal varices, open	
	AND	
	CC condition	*See* appendix B.
425	Ligation of esophageal varices, open	
432	MCC condition	*See* appendix B.
433	CC condition	*See* appendix B.
441	Benign neoplasm of liver and biliary passages	
	Chronic hepatitis	
	Unspecified and other chronic nonalcoholic liver disease	
	Liver abscess	
	AND	
	MCC condition	*See* appendix B.
442	Benign neoplasm of liver and biliary passages	
	Chronic hepatitis	
	Unspecified and other chronic nonalcoholic liver disease	
	Liver abscess	
	AND	
	CC condition	*See* appendix B.
443	Benign neoplasm of liver and biliary passages	
	Chronic hepatitis	
	Unspecified and other chronic nonalcoholic liver disease	
	Liver abscess	

DRG 434 (Continued)

DRG	PDx/SDx/Procedure	Tips
444	Cholelithiasis, cholecystitis, other disorders of gallbladder or biliary tract	
	AND	
	MCC condition	*See* appendix B.
445	Cholelithiasis, cholecystitis, other disorders of gallbladder or biliary tract	
	AND	
	CC condition	*See* appendix B.
446	Cholelithiasis, cholecystitis, other disorders of gallbladder or biliary tract	
895	Alcohol-induced mental disorders	
	Acute alcoholic intoxication or other/unspecified alcohol dependence	
	Nondependent alcohol abuse	
	Excessive blood level of alcohol	
	AND	
	Rehabilitation therapy	Review therapy and other documentation carefully to differentiate therapy from detoxification.
896	Alcohol-induced mental disorders	
	Acute alcoholic intoxication or other/unspecified alcohol dependence	
	Nondependent alcohol abuse	
	Excessive blood level of alcohol	
	AND	
	MCC condition	*See* appendix B.

DRG 435 Malignancy of Hepatobiliary System or Pancreas with MCC RW 1.7599

Potential DRGs

420 Hepatobiliary Diagnostic Procedures with MCC 3.2008

DRG	PDx/SDx/Procedure	Tips
420	Open or laparoscopic liver biopsy	
	Open pancreas biopsy	
	Open biopsy of peritoneum	
	AND	
	MCC condition	*See* appendix B.

DRG 436 Malignancy of Hepatobiliary System or Pancreas with CC RW 1.1007

Potential DRGs

420 Hepatobiliary Diagnostic Procedures with MCC 3.2008
421 Hepatobiliary Diagnostic Procedures with CC 1.7096
435 Malignancy of Hepatobiliary System or Pancreas with MCC 1.7599

DRG	PDx/SDx/Procedure	Tips
420	Open or laparoscopic liver biopsy	
	Open pancreas biopsy	
	Open biopsy of peritoneum	
	AND	
	MCC condition	*See* appendix B.
421	Open or laparoscopic liver biopsy	
	Open pancreas biopsy	
	Open biopsy of peritoneum	
	AND	
	CC condition	*See* appendix B.
435	MCC condition	*See* appendix B.

DRG 437 Malignancy of Hepatobiliary System or Pancreas without CC/MCC — RW 0.8311

Potential DRGs

420	Hepatobiliary Diagnostic Procedures with MCC	3.2008
421	Hepatobiliary Diagnostic Procedures with CC	1.7096
422	Hepatobiliary Diagnostic Procedures without CC/MCC	1.4110
435	Malignancy of Hepatobiliary System or Pancreas with MCC	1.7599
436	Malignancy of Hepatobiliary System or Pancreas with CC	1.1007
444	Disorders of the Biliary Tract with MCC	1.6332
445	Disorders of the Biliary Tract with CC	1.0868

DRG	PDx/SDx/Procedure	Tips
420	Open or laparoscopic liver biopsy	
	Open pancreas biopsy	
	Open biopsy of peritoneum	
	AND	
	MCC condition	*See* appendix B.
421	Open or laparoscopic liver biopsy	
	Open pancreas biopsy	
	Open biopsy of peritoneum	
	AND	
	CC condition	*See* appendix B.
422	Open or laparoscopic liver biopsy	
	Open pancreas biopsy	
	Open biopsy of peritoneum	
435	MCC condition	*See* appendix B.
436	CC condition	*See* appendix B.
444	Cholelithiasis, cholecystitis, other disorders of gallbladder or biliary tract	
	AND	
	MCC condition	*See* appendix B.
445	Cholelithiasis, cholecystitis, other disorders of gallbladder or biliary tract	
	AND	
	CC condition	*See* appendix B.

DRG 438 Disorders of Pancreas Except Malignancy with MCC — RW 1.6688

Potential DRGs

420	Hepatobiliary Diagnostic Procedures with MCC	3.2008
435	Malignancy of Hepatobiliary System or Pancreas with MCC	1.7599

DRG	PDx/SDx/Procedure	Tips
420	Open pancreas biopsy	
	Inspection of pancreas, open or percutaneous endoscopic approach	
	AND	
	MCC condition	*See* appendix B.
435	Malignant neoplasm of pancreas	
	AND	
	MCC condition	*See* appendix B.

DRG 439 Disorders of Pancreas Except Malignancy with CC — RW 0.8552

Potential DRGs

420	Hepatobiliary Diagnostic Procedures with MCC	3.2008
421	Hepatobiliary Diagnostic Procedures with CC	1.7096
435	Malignancy of Hepatobiliary System or Pancreas with MCC	1.7599
436	Malignancy of Hepatobiliary System or Pancreas with CC	1.1007
438	Disorders of Pancreas Except Malignancy with MCC	1.6688

DRG	PDx/SDx/Procedure	Tips
420	Open pancreas biopsy	
	Inspection of pancreas	
	AND	
	MCC condition	*See* appendix B.
421	Open pancreas biopsy	
	Inspection of pancreas, open or percutaneous endoscopic approach	
	AND	
	CC condition	*See* appendix B.
435	Malignant neoplasm of pancreas	
	AND	
	MCC condition	*See* appendix B.
436	Malignant neoplasm of pancreas	
	AND	
	CC condition	*See* appendix B.
438	MCC condition	*See* appendix B.

DRG 440 Disorders of Pancreas Except Malignancy without CC/MCC — RW 0.6156

Potential DRGs

420	Hepatobiliary Diagnostic Procedures with MCC	3.2008
421	Hepatobiliary Diagnostic Procedures with CC	1.7096
422	Hepatobiliary Diagnostic Procedures without CC/MCC	1.4110
435	Malignancy of Hepatobiliary System or Pancreas with MCC	1.7599
436	Malignancy of Hepatobiliary System or Pancreas with CC	1.1007
437	Malignancy of Hepatobiliary System or Pancreas without CC/MCC	0.8311
438	Disorders of Pancreas Except Malignancy with MCC	1.6688
439	Disorders of Pancreas Except Malignancy with CC	0.8552

DRG	PDx/SDx/Procedure	Tips
420	Open pancreas biopsy	
	Inspection of pancreas, open or percutaneous endoscopic approach	
	AND	
	MCC condition	*See* appendix B.
421	Open pancreas biopsy	
	Inspection of pancreas, open or percutaneous endoscopic approach	
	AND	
	CC condition	*See* appendix B.
422	Open pancreas biopsy	
	Inspection of pancreas, open or percutaneous endoscopic approach	
435	Malignant neoplasm of pancreas	
	AND	
	MCC condition	*See* appendix B.
436	Malignant neoplasm of pancreas	
	AND	
	CC condition	*See* appendix B.
437	Malignant neoplasm of pancreas	
438	MCC condition	*See* appendix B.
439	CC condition	*See* appendix B.

DRG 441 Disorders of Liver Except Malignancy, Cirrhosis, Alcoholic Hepatitis with MCC — RW 1.8282

Potential DRGs

420	Hepatobiliary Diagnostic Procedures with MCC	3.2008

DRG	PDx/SDx/Procedure	Tips
420	Open or laparoscopic liver biopsy	
	Open diagnostic drainage of liver	The qualifier Diagnostic is used to identify drainage procedures that are biopsies.
	Inspection of liver, open or percutaneous endoscopic approach	
	AND	
	MCC condition	*See* appendix B.

DRG 442 Disorders of Liver Except Malignancy, Cirrhosis, Alcoholic Hepatitis with CC RW 0.9515

Potential DRGs

393	Other Digestive System Diagnoses with MCC	1.6196
420	Hepatobiliary Diagnostic Procedures with MCC	3.2008
421	Hepatobiliary Diagnostic Procedures with CC	1.7096
432	Cirrhosis and Alcoholic Hepatitis with MCC	1.9160
433	Cirrhosis and Alcoholic Hepatitis with CC	1.0310
435	Malignancy of Hepatobiliary System or Pancreas with MCC	1.7599
436	Malignancy of Hepatobiliary System or Pancreas with CC	1.1007
441	Disorders of Liver Except Malignancy, Cirrhosis, Alcoholic Hepatitis with MCC	1.8282

DRG	PDx/SDx/Procedure	Tips
393	Postprocedural hepatorenal syndrome or hepatic failure	
	AND	
	MCC condition	*See* appendix B.
420	Open or laparoscopic liver biopsy	
	Open diagnostic drainage of liver	The qualifier Diagnostic is used to identify drainage procedures that are biopsies.
	Inspection of liver, open or percutaneous endoscopic approach	
	AND	
	MCC condition	*See* appendix B.
421	Open or laparoscopic liver biopsy	
	Open diagnostic drainage of liver	*See* DRG 420.
	Inspection of liver, open or percutaneous endoscopic approach	
	AND	
	CC condition	*See* appendix B.
432	Acute alcoholic hepatitis	
	Cirrhosis with and w/o mention of alcohol	
	Unspecified alcoholic liver damage	
	Biliary cirrhosis	
	AND	
	MCC condition	*See* appendix B.
433	Acute alcoholic hepatitis	
	Cirrhosis with and w/o mention of alcohol	
	Unspecified alcoholic liver damage	
	Biliary cirrhosis	
	AND	
	CC condition	*See* appendix B.
435	Malignant neoplasm of the liver, intrahepatic bile ducts	
	Secondary malignant neoplasm, carcinoma in-situ, and neoplasm of uncertain behavior of liver and biliary passages	
	AND	
	MCC condition	*See* appendix B.
436	Malignant neoplasm of the liver, intrahepatic bile ducts	
	Secondary malignant neoplasm, carcinoma in-situ, and neoplasm of uncertain behavior of liver and biliary passages	
	AND	
	CC condition	*See* appendix B.
441	MCC condition	*See* appendix B.

Optimizing Tips

DRG 443 Disorders of Liver Except Malignancy, Cirrhosis, Alcoholic Hepatitis without CC/MCC — RW 0.7147

Potential DRGs

393	Other Digestive System Diagnoses with MCC	1.6196
394	Other Digestive System Diagnoses with CC	0.9369
420	Hepatobiliary Diagnostic Procedures with MCC	3.2008
421	Hepatobiliary Diagnostic Procedures with CC	1.7096
422	Hepatobiliary Diagnostic Procedures without CC/MCC	1.4110
432	Cirrhosis and Alcoholic Hepatitis with MCC	1.9160
433	Cirrhosis and Alcoholic Hepatitis with CC	1.0310
435	Malignancy of Hepatobiliary System or Pancreas with MCC	1.7599
436	Malignancy of Hepatobiliary System or Pancreas with CC	1.1007
437	Malignancy of Hepatobiliary System or Pancreas without CC/MCC	0.8311
441	Disorders of Liver Except Malignancy, Cirrhosis, Alcoholic Hepatitis with MCC	1.8282
442	Disorders of Liver Except Malignancy, Cirrhosis, Alcoholic Hepatitis with CC	0.9515
444	Disorders of the Biliary Tract with MCC	1.6332
445	Disorders of the Biliary Tract with CC	1.0868
446	Disorders of the Biliary Tract without CC/MCC	0.8015

DRG	PDx/SDx/Procedure	Tips
393	Postprocedural hepatorenal syndrome or hepatic failure	
	AND	
	MCC condition	*See* appendix B.
394	Postprocedural hepatorenal syndrome or hepatic failure	
	AND	
	CC condition	*See* appendix B.
420	Open or laparoscopic liver biopsy	
	Open diagnostic drainage of liver	The qualifier Diagnostic is used to identify drainage procedures that are biopsies.
	Inspection of liver, open or percutaneous endoscopic approach	
	AND	
	MCC condition	*See* appendix B.
421	Open or laparoscopic liver biopsy	*See* DRG 420.
	Open diagnostic drainage of liver	
	Inspection of liver, open or percutaneous endoscopic approach	
	AND	
	CC condition	*See* appendix B.
422	Open or laparoscopic liver biopsy	*See* DRG 420.
	Open diagnostic drainage of liver	
	Inspection of liver, open or percutaneous endoscopic approach	
432	Acute alcoholic hepatitis	
	Cirrhosis with and w/o mention of alcohol	
	Unspecified alcoholic liver damage	
	Biliary cirrhosis	
	AND	
	MCC condition	*See* appendix B.
433	Acute alcoholic hepatitis	
	Cirrhosis with and w/o mention of alcohol	
	Unspecified alcoholic liver damage	
	Biliary cirrhosis	
	AND	
	CC condition	*See* appendix B.
435	Malignant neoplasm of the liver, intrahepatic bile ducts	
	Secondary malignant neoplasm, carcinoma in-situ, and neoplasm of uncertain behavior of liver and biliary passages	
	AND	
	MCC condition	*See* appendix B.
436	Malignant neoplasm of the liver, intrahepatic bile ducts	
	Secondary malignant neoplasm, carcinoma in-situ, and neoplasm of uncertain behavior of liver and biliary passages	
	AND	
	CC condition	*See* appendix B.
437	Malignant neoplasm of the liver, intrahepatic bile ducts	
	Secondary malignant neoplasm, carcinoma in-situ, and neoplasm of uncertain behavior of liver and biliary passages	
441	MCC condition	*See* appendix B.
442	CC condition	*See* appendix B.
444	Cholelithiasis, cholecystitis, other disorders of gallbladder or biliary tract	
	AND	
	MCC condition	*See* appendix B.
445	Cholelithiasis, cholecystitis, other disorders of gallbladder or biliary tract	
	AND	
	CC condition	*See* appendix B.
446	Cholelithiasis, cholecystitis, other disorders of gallbladder or biliary tract	

DRG 444 Disorders of the Biliary Tract with MCC RW 1.6332

Potential DRGs

420	Hepatobiliary Diagnostic Procedures with MCC	3.2008
432	Cirrhosis and Alcoholic Hepatitis with MCC	1.9160
435	Malignancy of Hepatobiliary System or Pancreas with MCC	1.7599
441	Disorders of Liver Except Malignancy, Cirrhosis, Alcoholic Hepatitis with MCC	1.8282

DRG	PDx/SDx/Procedure	Tips
420	Open or laparoscopic liver biopsy	
	Open diagnostic drainage of liver	The qualifier Diagnostic is used to identify drainage procedures that are biopsies.
	Inspection of liver, open or percutaneous endoscopic approach	
	AND	
	MCC condition	*See* appendix B.
432	Acute alcoholic hepatitis	
	Cirrhosis with and w/o mention of alcohol	
	Unspecified alcoholic liver damage	
	Biliary cirrhosis	
	AND	
	MCC condition	*See* appendix B.
435	Malignant neoplasm of the liver, intrahepatic bile ducts	
	Secondary malignant neoplasm, carcinoma in-situ, and neoplasm of uncertain behavior of liver and biliary passages	
	AND	
	MCC condition	*See* appendix B.
441	Benign neoplasm of liver and biliary passages	
	Chronic hepatitis	
	Unspecified and other chronic nonalcoholic liver disease	
	Liver abscess	
	AND	
	MCC condition	*See* appendix B.

DRG 445 Disorders of the Biliary Tract with CC RW 1.0868

Potential DRGs

393	Other Digestive System Diagnoses with MCC	1.6196
420	Hepatobiliary Diagnostic Procedures with MCC	3.2008
421	Hepatobiliary Diagnostic Procedures with CC	1.7096
432	Cirrhosis and Alcoholic Hepatitis with MCC	1.9160
435	Malignancy of Hepatobiliary System or Pancreas with MCC	1.7599
436	Malignancy of Hepatobiliary System or Pancreas with CC	1.1007
441	Disorders of Liver Except Malignancy, Cirrhosis, Alcoholic Hepatitis with MCC	1.8282
444	Disorders of the Biliary Tract with MCC	1.6332

DRG	PDx/SDx/Procedure	Tips
393	Retained cholelithiasis following cholecystectomy	
	AND	
	MCC condition	*See* appendix B.
420	Open or laparoscopic liver biopsy	
	Open diagnostic drainage of liver	The qualifier Diagnostic is used to identify drainage procedures that are biopsies.
	Inspection of liver, open or percutaneous endoscopic approach	
	AND	
	MCC condition	*See* appendix B.
421	Open or laparoscopic liver biopsy	
	Open diagnostic drainage of liver	*See* DRG 420.
	Inspection of liver, open or percutaneous endoscopic approach	
	AND	
	CC condition	*See* appendix B.
432	Acute alcoholic hepatitis	
	Cirrhosis with and w/o mention of alcohol	
	Unspecified alcoholic liver damage	
	Biliary cirrhosis	
	AND	
	MCC condition	*See* appendix B.
435	Malignant neoplasm of the liver, intrahepatic bile ducts	
	Secondary malignant neoplasm, carcinoma in-situ, and neoplasm of uncertain behavior of liver and biliary passages	
	AND	
	MCC condition	*See* appendix B.
436	Malignant neoplasm of the liver, intrahepatic bile ducts	
	Secondary malignant neoplasm, carcinoma in-situ, and neoplasm of uncertain behavior of liver and biliary passages	
	AND	
	CC condition	*See* appendix B.
441	Benign neoplasm of liver and biliary passages	
	Chronic hepatitis	
	Unspecified and other chronic nonalcoholic liver disease	
	Liver abscess	
	AND	
	MCC condition	*See* appendix B.
444	MCC condition	*See* appendix B.

DRG 446 Disorders of the Biliary Tract without CC/MCC

RW 0.8015

Potential DRGs

393	Other Digestive System Diagnoses with MCC	1.6196
394	Other Digestive System Diagnoses with CC	0.9369
420	Hepatobiliary Diagnostic Procedures with MCC	3.2008
421	Hepatobiliary Diagnostic Procedures with CC	1.7096
422	Hepatobiliary Diagnostic Procedures without CC/MCC	1.4110
432	Cirrhosis and Alcoholic Hepatitis with MCC	1.9160
433	Cirrhosis and Alcoholic Hepatitis with CC	1.0310
435	Malignancy of Hepatobiliary System or Pancreas with MCC	1.7599
436	Malignancy of Hepatobiliary System or Pancreas with CC	1.1007
437	Malignancy of Hepatobiliary System or Pancreas without CC/MCC	0.8311
441	Disorders of Liver Except Malignancy, Cirrhosis, Alcoholic Hepatitis with MCC	1.8282
442	Disorders of Liver Except Malignancy, Cirrhosis, Alcoholic Hepatitis with CC	0.9515
444	Disorders of the Biliary Tract with MCC	1.6332
445	Disorders of the Biliary Tract with CC	1.0868

DRG	PDx/SDx/Procedure	Tips
393	Retained cholelithiasis following cholecystectomy	
	AND	
	MCC condition	*See* appendix B.
394	Retained cholelithiasis following cholecystectomy	
	AND	
	CC condition	*See* appendix B.
420	Open biopsy of gallbladder or bile ducts	
	Open diagnostic drainage of gallbladder or bile ducts	The qualifier Diagnostic is used to identify drainage procedures that are biopsies.
	Inspection of gallbladder, open or percutaneous endoscopic approach	
	AND	
	MCC condition	*See* appendix B.
421	Open biopsy of gallbladder or bile ducts	
	Open diagnostic drainage of gallbladder or bile ducts	*See* DRG 420.
	Inspection of gallbladder, open or percutaneous endoscopic approach	
	AND	
	CC condition	
422	Open biopsy of gallbladder or bile ducts	
	Open diagnostic drainage of gallbladder or bile ducts	*See* DRG 420.
	Inspection of gallbladder	
432	Acute alcoholic hepatitis	
	Cirrhosis with and w/o mention of alcohol	
	Unspecified alcoholic liver damage	
	Biliary cirrhosis	
	AND	
	MCC condition	*See* appendix B.
433	Acute alcoholic hepatitis	
	Cirrhosis with and w/o mention of alcohol	
	Unspecified alcoholic liver damage	
	Biliary cirrhosis	
	AND	
	CC condition	*See* appendix B.
435	Malignant neoplasm of the liver, intrahepatic bile ducts	
	Secondary malignant neoplasm, carcinoma in-situ, and neoplasm of uncertain behavior of liver and biliary passages	
	AND	
	MCC condition	*See* appendix B.
436	Malignant neoplasm of the liver, intrahepatic bile ducts	
	Secondary malignant neoplasm, carcinoma in-situ, and neoplasm of uncertain behavior of liver and biliary passages	
	AND	
	CC condition	*See* appendix B.
437	Malignant neoplasm of the liver, intrahepatic bile ducts	
	Secondary malignant neoplasm, carcinoma in-situ, and neoplasm of uncertain behavior of liver and biliary passages	
441	Benign neoplasm of liver and biliary passages	
	Chronic hepatitis	
	Unspecified and other chronic nonalcoholic liver disease	
	Liver abscess	
	AND	
	MCC condition	*See* appendix B.
442	Benign neoplasm of liver and biliary passages	
	Chronic hepatitis	
	Unspecified and other chronic nonalcoholic liver disease	
	Liver abscess	
	AND	
	CC condition	*See* appendix B.
444	MCC condition	*See* appendix B.
445	CC condition	*See* appendix B.

Diseases And Disorders Of The Musculoskeletal System And Connective Tissue

DRG 453 Combined Anterior/Posterior Spinal Fusion with MCC — RW 8.8614

No Potential DRGs

DRG 454 Combined Anterior/Posterior Spinal Fusion with CC — RW 6.1163

Potential DRGs

453 Combined Anterior/Posterior Spinal Fusion with MCC — 8.8614

DRG	PDx/SDx/Procedure	Tips
453	MCC condition	*See* appendix B.

DRG 455 Combined Anterior/Posterior Spinal Fusion without CC/MCC — RW 4.6056

Potential DRGs

453 Combined Anterior/Posterior Spinal Fusion with MCC — 8.8614
454 Combined Anterior/Posterior Spinal Fusion with CC — 6.1163

DRG	PDx/SDx/Procedure	Tips
453	MCC condition	*See* appendix B.
454	CC condition	*See* appendix B.

DRG 456 Spinal Fusion Except Cervical with Spinal Curvature/Malignancy/Infection or Extensive Fusions with MCC — RW 8.4294

Potential DRGs

453 Combined Anterior/Posterior Spinal Fusion with MCC — 8.8614

DRG	PDx/SDx/Procedure	Tips
453	Combination of anterior and posterior spinal fusion or refusion techniques	The anterior column may be fused using an anterior, lateral, or posterior technique. The posterior column may be fused using a posterior, posterolateral, or lateral transverse technique. Two operative notes may be dictated for different incisions/approaches. ICD-10-PCS Coding Guideline B3.10c states "if an interbody fusion device is used to render the joint immobile (containing bone graft or bone graft substitute), the procedure is coded with the device value Interbody Fusion Device." The fixation instrumentation (i.e., rods, plates, screws, etc.) is included in the Fusion root operation, and no additional code is assigned.
	AND	
	MCC condition	*See* appendix B.

DRG 457 Spinal Fusion Except Cervical with Spinal Curvature/Malignancy/Infection or Extensive Fusions with CC — RW 6.0753

Potential DRGs

453 Combined Anterior/Posterior Spinal Fusion with MCC — 8.8614
456 Spinal Fusion Except Cervical with Spinal Curvature/Malignancy/Infection or Extensive Fusions with MCC — 8.4294

DRG	PDx/SDx/Procedure	Tips
453	Combination of anterior and posterior spinal fusion or refusion techniques	The anterior column may be fused using an anterior, lateral, or posterior technique. The posterior column may be fused using a posterior, posterolateral, or lateral transverse technique. Two operative notes may be dictated for different incisions/approaches. ICD-10-PCS Coding Guideline B3.10c states "if an interbody fusion device is used to render the joint immobile (containing bone graft or bone graft substitute), the procedure is coded with the device value Interbody Fusion Device." The fixation instrumentation (i.e., rods, plates, screws, etc.) is included in the Fusion root operation, and no additional code is assigned.
	AND	
	MCC condition	*See* appendix B.
456	MCC condition	*See* appendix B.

DRG 458 Spinal Fusion Except Cervical with Spinal Curvature/Malignancy/Infection or Extensive Fusions without CC/MCC

RW 4.5310

Potential DRGs

028	Spinal Procedures with MCC	6.0261
453	Combined Anterior/Posterior Spinal Fusion with MCC	8.8614
454	Combined Anterior/Posterior Spinal Fusion with CC	6.1163
456	Spinal Fusion Except Cervical with Spinal Curvature/Malignancy/Infection or Extensive Fusions with MCC	8.4294
457	Spinal Fusion Except Cervical with Spinal Curvature/Malignancy/Infection or Extensive Fusions with CC	6.0753
459	Spinal Fusion Except Cervical with MCC	6.6323

DRG	PDx/SDx/Procedure	Tips
028	Diagnosis from MDC 1 Nervous System	Review the history and physical, surgical consent, physician progress notes, OP reports, and nurse's notes to determine the underlying reason for the procedure. The procedure codes assigned to MS-DRG 458 are also assigned to MS-DRG 028. The DRGs are differentiated based on principal diagnosis. It is important to clearly understand the official guidelines to accurately report the principal diagnosis.
	AND	
	MCC condition	*See* appendix B.
453	Combination of anterior and posterior spinal fusion or refusion techniques	The anterior column may be fused using an anterior, lateral, or posterior technique. The posterior column may be fused using a posterior, posterolateral, or lateral transverse technique. Two operative notes may be dictated for different incisions/approaches. ICD-10-PCS Coding Guideline B3.10c states "if an interbody fusion device is used to render the joint immobile (containing bone graft or bone graft substitute), the procedure is coded with the device value Interbody Fusion Device." The fixation instrumentation (i.e., rods, plates, screws, etc.) is included in the Fusion root operation, and no additional code is assigned.
	AND	
	MCC condition	*See* appendix B.
454	Combination of anterior and posterior spinal fusion or refusion techniques	*See* DRG 453.
	AND	
	CC condition	*See* appendix B.
456	MCC condition	*See* appendix B.
457	CC condition	*See* appendix B.
459	Any diagnosis in MDC 8 other than spinal curvature, malignancy, or infection	
	AND	
	Any spinal fusion or refusion except cervical, any technique	
	AND	
	MCC condition	*See* appendix B.

DRG 459 Spinal Fusion Except Cervical with MCC RW 6.6323

Potential DRGs

453	Combined Anterior/Posterior Spinal Fusion with MCC	8.8614
456	Spinal Fusion Except Cervical with Spinal Curvature/Malignancy/Infection or Extensive Fusions with MCC	8.4294

DRG	PDx/SDx/Procedure	Tips
453	Combination of anterior and posterior spinal fusion or refusion techniques	The anterior column may be fused using an anterior, lateral, or posterior technique. The posterior column may be fused using a posterior, posterolateral, or lateral transverse technique. Two operative notes may be dictated for different incisions/approaches. ICD-10-PCS Coding Guideline B3.10c states "if an interbody fusion device is used to render the joint immobile (containing bone graft or bone graft substitute), the procedure is coded with the device value Interbody Fusion Device." The fixation instrumentation (i.e., rods, plates, screws, etc.) is included in the Fusion root operation, and no additional code is assigned.
	AND	
	MCC condition	*See* appendix B.
456	Noncervical spinal fusions with principal diagnosis of noncervical curvature of spine, infection, or malignancy	Review operative report for indication of metastasis. Clarify with physician if pathological fracture is noted whether it is due to metastasis when patient has previous history of malignancy.
	OR	
	Principal or secondary diagnosis of secondary kyphosis, secondary or neuromuscular scoliosis	A code for the underlying disease or condition must be reported first before the code for secondary kyphosis or secondary scoliosis, per the "code first underlying disease" instructional note. Neuromuscular scoliosis can be assigned as principal diagnosis with the underlying condition coded as a secondary diagnosis.
	OR	
	Fusion of 8 or more thoracic vertebral segments	
	OR	
	Fusion of 2-7 thoracic vertebral segments	
	AND	
	Fusion of 2 or more lumbar vertebral segments	
	AND	
	MCC condition	*See* appendix B.

DRG 460 Spinal Fusion Except Cervical without MCC — RW 3.6579

Potential DRGs

453	Combined Anterior/Posterior Spinal Fusion with MCC	8.8614
454	Combined Anterior/Posterior Spinal Fusion with CC	6.1163
455	Combined Anterior/Posterior Spinal Fusion without CC/MCC	4.6056
456	Spinal Fusion Except Cervical with Spinal Curvature/Malignancy/Infection or Extensive Fusions with MCC	8.4294
457	Spinal Fusion Except Cervical with Spinal Curvature/Malignancy/Infection or Extensive Fusions with CC	6.0753
458	Spinal Fusion Except Cervical with Spinal Curvature/Malignancy/Infection or Extensive Fusions without CC/MCC	4.5310
459	Spinal Fusion Except Cervical with MCC	6.6323

DRG	PDx/SDx/Procedure	Tips
453	Combination of anterior and posterior spinal fusion or refusion techniques	The anterior column may be fused using an anterior, lateral, or posterior technique. The posterior column may be fused using a posterior, posterolateral, or lateral transverse technique. Two operative notes may be dictated for different incisions/approaches. ICD-10-PCS Coding Guideline B3.10c states "if an interbody fusion device is used to render the joint immobile (containing bone graft or bone graft substitute), the procedure is coded with the device value Interbody Fusion Device." The fixation instrumentation (i.e., rods, plates, screws, etc.) is included in the Fusion root operation, and no additional code is assigned.
	AND	
	MCC condition	*See* appendix B.
454	Combination of anterior and posterior spinal fusion or refusion techniques	*See* DRG 453.
	AND	
	CC condition	*See* appendix B.
455	Combination of anterior and posterior spinal fusion or refusion techniques	*See* DRG 453.
456	Noncervical spinal fusions with principal diagnosis of noncervical curvature of spine, infection, or malignancy	Review operative report for indication of metastasis. Clarify with physician if pathological fracture is noted whether it is due to metastasis when patient has previous history of malignancy.
	OR	
	Principal or secondary diagnosis of secondary kyphosis, secondary or neuromuscular scoliosis	A code for the underlying disease or condition must be reported first before the code for secondary kyphosis or secondary scoliosis, per the "code first underlying disease" instructional note. Neuromuscular scoliosis can be assigned as principal diagnosis with the underlying condition coded as a secondary diagnosis.
	OR	
	Fusion of 8 or more thoracic vertebral segments	
	OR	
	Fusion of 2-7 thoracic vertebral segments	
	AND	
	Fusion of 2 or more lumbar vertebral segments	
	AND	
	MCC condition	*See* appendix B.
457	Noncervical spinal fusions with principal diagnosis of noncervical curvature of spine, infection, or malignancy	*See* DRG 456.
	OR	
	Principal or secondary diagnosis of secondary kyphosis, secondary or neuromuscular scoliosis	*See* DRG 456.
	OR	
	Fusion of 8 or more thoracic vertebral segments	
	OR	
	Fusion of 2-7 thoracic vertebral segments	
	AND	
	Fusion of 2 or more lumbar vertebral segments	
	AND	
	CC condition	*See* appendix B.
458	Noncervical spinal fusions with principal diagnosis of noncervical curvature of spine, infection, or malignancy	*See* DRG 456.
	OR	
	Principal or secondary diagnosis of secondary kyphosis, secondary or neuromuscular scoliosis	*See* DRG 456.
	OR	
	Fusion of 8 or more thoracic vertebral segments	
	OR	
	Fusion of 2-7 thoracic vertebral segments	
	AND	
	Fusion of 2 or more lumbar vertebral segments	
459	MCC condition	*See* appendix B.

DRG 461 Bilateral or Multiple Major Joint Procedures of Lower Extremity with MCC — RW 6.8185

No Potential DRGs

DRG 462 Bilateral or Multiple Major Joint Procedures of Lower Extremity without MCC RW 2.8463

Potential DRGs

461	Bilateral or Multiple Major Joint Procedures of Lower Extremity with MCC	6.8185

DRG	PDx/SDx/Procedure	Tips
461	MCC condition	*See* appendix B.

DRG 463 Wound Debridement and Skin Graft Except Hand for Musculoskeletal and Connective Tissue Disorders with MCC RW 5.6637

573	Skin Graft for Skin Ulcer or Cellulitis with MCC	6.2181

DRG	PDx/SDx/Procedure	Tips
573	Skin ulcer or cellulitis principal diagnosis	
	AND	
	Skin grafting procedure	
	AND	
	MCC condition	*See* appendix B.

DRG 464 Wound Debridement and Skin Graft Except Hand for Musculoskeletal and Connective Tissue Disorders with CC RW 3.0014

Potential DRGs

463	Wound Debridement and Skin Graft Except Hand for Musculoskeletal and Connective Tissue Disorders with MCC	5.6637
573	Skin Graft for Skin Ulcer or Cellulitis with MCC	6.2181
574	Skin Graft for Skin Ulcer or Cellulitis with CC	3.4058
576	Skin Graft Except for Skin Ulcer or Cellulitis with MCC	5.6831
622	Skin Grafts and Wound Debridement for Endocrine, Nutritional and Metabolic Disorders with MCC	3.8256
901	Wound Debridements for Injuries with MCC	4.3278
904	Skin Grafts for Injuries with CC/MCC	3.2562

DRG	PDx/SDx/Procedure	Tips
463	MCC condition	
573	Skin ulcer or cellulitis principal diagnosis	
	AND	
	Skin grafting procedure	
	AND	
	MCC condition	*See* appendix B.
574	Skin ulcer or cellulitis principal diagnosis	
	AND	
	Skin grafting procedure	
	AND	
	CC condition	*See* appendix B.
576	Diagnosis from MDC 9 other than skin ulcer or cellulitis	
	AND	
	Skin grafting procedure	
	AND	
	MCC condition	*See* appendix B.
622	Diabetes (type 1, type 2, other specified) with ketoacidosis, hyperosmolarity, other coma, other and unspecified complications Diabetic foot or other skin ulcer principal diagnosis	
	AND	
	Excisional debridement of wound, infection, or burn	The ICD-10-PCS definition of the root operation Excision is "Cutting out or off, without replacement, a portion of a body part." Debridement by excision involves cutting with a sharp instrument such as a scalpel or other methods such as a hot knife or laser. Non-excisional debridement of skin is coded to root operation Extraction. Ensure that documentation includes instruments used, technique, and depth of debridement procedure.
	AND	
	MCC condition	*See* appendix B.
901	Injury diagnosis from MDC 21	
	AND	
	Excisional debridement of wound, infection, or burn	*See* DRG 622.
	AND	
	MCC condition	*See* appendix B.
904	Injury diagnosis from MDC 21	
	AND	
	Skin grafting procedure	
	AND	
	CC/MCC condition	*See* appendix B.

DRG 465 Wound Debridement and Skin Graft Except Hand for Musculoskeletal and Connective Tissue Disorders without CC/MCC RW 1.8708

Potential DRGs

463	Wound Debridement and Skin Graft Except Hand for Musculoskeletal and Connective Tissue Disorders with MCC	5.6637
464	Wound Debridement and Skin Graft Except Hand for Musculoskeletal and Connective Tissue Disorders with CC	3.0014
570	Skin Debridement with MCC	2.9222
573	Skin Graft for Skin Ulcer or Cellulitis with MCC	6.2181
574	Skin Graft for Skin Ulcer or Cellulitis with CC	3.4058
576	Skin Graft Except for Skin Ulcer or Cellulitis with MCC	5.6831
577	Skin Graft Except for Skin Ulcer or Cellulitis with CC	2.6491
622	Skin Grafts and Wound Debridement for Endocrine, Nutritional and Metabolic Disorders with MCC	3.8256
901	Wound Debridements for Injuries with MCC	4.3278
904	Skin Grafts for Injuries with CC/MCC	3.2562

DRG	PDx/SDx/Procedure	Tips
463	MCC condition	*See* appendix B.
464	CC condition	*See* appendix B.
570	Diagnosis from MDC 9 other than skin ulcer or cellulitis	
	AND	
	Excisional debridement of wound, infection, or burn	The ICD-10-PCS definition of the root operation Excision is "Cutting out or off, without replacement, a portion of a body part." Debridement by excision involves cutting with a sharp instrument such as a scalpel or other methods such as a hot knife or laser. Non-excisional debridement of skin is coded to root operation Extraction. Ensure that documentation includes instruments used, technique, and depth of debridement procedure.
	AND	
	MCC condition	*See* appendix B.
573	Skin ulcer or cellulitis principal diagnosis	
	AND	
	Skin grafting procedure	
	AND	
	MCC condition	*See* appendix B.
574	Skin ulcer or cellulitis principal diagnosis	
	AND	
	Skin grafting procedure	
	AND	
	CC condition	*See* appendix B.
576	Diagnosis from MDC 9 other than skin ulcer or cellulitis	
	AND	
	Skin grafting procedure	
	AND	
	MCC condition	*See* appendix B.
577	Diagnosis from MDC 9 other than skin ulcer or cellulitis	
	AND	
	Skin grafting procedure	
	AND	
	CC condition	*See* appendix B.
622	Diabetes (type 1, type 2, other specified) with ketoacidosis, hyperosmolarity, other coma, other and unspecified complications Diabetic foot or other skin ulcer principal diagnosis	
	AND	
	Excisional debridement of wound, infection, or burn	*See* DRG 570.
	AND	
	MCC condition	*See* appendix B.
901	Injury diagnosis from MDC 21	
	AND	
	Excisional debridement of wound, infection, or burn	*See* DRG 570.
	AND	
	MCC condition	*See* appendix B.
904	Injury diagnosis from MDC 21	
	AND	
	Skin grafting procedure	
	AND	
	CC/MCC condition	*See* appendix B.

DRG 466 Revision of Hip or Knee Replacement with MCC — RW 5.1866

Potential DRGs

461 Bilateral or Multiple Major Joint Procedures of Lower Extremity with MCC 6.8185

DRG	PDx/SDx/Procedure	Tips
461	Any combination of partial or total knee, hip or ankle joint replacement procedures	
	AND	
	MCC condition	*See* appendix B.

DRG 467 Revision of Hip or Knee Replacement with CC — RW 3.4863

Potential DRGs

461 Bilateral or Multiple Major Joint Procedures of Lower Extremity with MCC 6.8185
466 Revision of Hip or Knee Replacement with MCC 5.1866

DRG	PDx/SDx/Procedure	Tips
461	Any combination of partial or total knee, hip or ankle joint replacement procedures	
	AND	
	MCC condition	*See* appendix B.
466	MCC condition	*See* appendix B.

DRG 468 Revision of Hip or Knee Replacement without CC/MCC — RW 2.6696

Potential DRGs

461 Bilateral or Multiple Major Joint Procedures of Lower Extremity with MCC 6.8185
462 Bilateral or Multiple Major Joint Procedures of Lower Extremity without MCC 2.8463
466 Revision of Hip or Knee Replacement with MCC 5.1866
467 Revision of Hip or Knee Replacement with CC 3.4863

DRG	PDx/SDx/Procedure	Tips
461	Any combination of partial or total knee, hip or ankle joint replacement procedures	
	AND	
	MCC condition	*See* appendix B.
462	Any combination of partial or total knee, hip or ankle joint replacement procedures	
466	MCC condition	*See* appendix B.
467	CC condition	*See* appendix B.

DRG 469 Major Hip and Knee Joint Replacement or Reattachment of Lower Extremity with MCC or Total Ankle Replacement — RW 3.3298

Potential DRGs

461 Bilateral or Multiple Major Joint Procedures of Lower Extremity with MCC 6.8185
466 Revision of Hip or Knee Replacement with MCC 5.1866

DRG	PDx/SDx/Procedure	Tips
461	Any combination of partial or total knee, hip or ankle joint replacement procedures	
	AND	
	MCC condition	*See* appendix B.
466	Revision of hip or knee replacement procedure	ICD-10-PCS root operation Revision is defined as: "Correcting, to the extent possible, a portion of a malfunctioning device or the position of a displaced device." Explanation: Revision can include correcting a malfunctioning or displaced device by taking out or putting in components of the device such as a screw or pin. Example: recementing of hip prosthesis.
	OR	
	Removal and replacement of hip or knee prosthesis	Joint revisions involving the removal of a joint prosthesis, liner, resurfacing device, or spacer and subsequent insertion of a new joint prosthesis (Replacement) or liner (Supplement), either cemented or uncemented, open approach.
	AND	
	MCC condition	*See* appendix B.

DRG 470 Major Hip and Knee Joint Replacement or Reattachment of Lower Extremity without MCC — RW 1.8817

Potential DRGs

461	Bilateral or Multiple Major Joint Procedures of Lower Extremity with MCC	6.8185
462	Bilateral or Multiple Major Joint Procedures of Lower Extremity without MCC	2.8463
466	Revision of Hip or Knee Replacement with MCC	5.1866
467	Revision of Hip or Knee Replacement with CC	3.4863
468	Revision of Hip or Knee Replacement without CC/MCC	2.6696
469	Major Hip and Knee Joint Replacement or Reattachment of Lower Extremity with MCC or Total Ankle Replacement	3.3298

DRG	PDx/SDx/Procedure	Tips
461	Any combination of partial or total knee, hip or ankle joint replacement procedures	
	AND	
	MCC condition	*See* appendix B.
462	Any combination of partial or total knee, hip or ankle joint replacement procedures	
466	Revision of hip or knee replacement procedure	ICD-10-PCS root operation Revision is defined as: "Correcting, to the extent possible, a portion of a malfunctioning device or the position of a displaced device." Explanation: Revision can include correcting a malfunctioning or displaced device by taking out or putting in components of the device such as a screw or pin. Example: recementing of hip prosthesis.
	OR	
	Removal and replacement of hip or knee prosthesis	Joint revisions involving the removal of a joint prosthesis, liner, resurfacing device, or spacer and subsequent insertion of a new joint prosthesis (Replacement) or liner (Supplement), either cemented or uncemented, open approach.
	AND	
	MCC condition	*See* appendix B.
467	Revision of hip or knee replacement procedure	*See* DRG 466.
	OR	
	Removal and replacement of hip or knee prosthesis	
	AND	
	CC condition	*See* appendix B.
468	Revision of hip or knee replacement procedure	*See* DRG 466.
	OR	
	Removal and replacement of hip or knee prosthesis	
469	MCC condition	*See* appendix B.
	OR	
	Total ankle replacement	

DRG 471 Cervical Spinal Fusion with MCC — RW 4.9190

Potential DRGs

453	Combined Anterior/Posterior Spinal Fusion with MCC	8.8614

DRG	PDx/SDx/Procedure	Tips
453	Combination of anterior and posterior spinal fusion or refusion techniques	The anterior column may be fused using an anterior, lateral, or posterior technique. The posterior column may be fused using a posterior, posterolateral, or lateral transverse technique. Two operative notes may be dictated for different incisions/approaches. ICD-10-PCS Coding Guideline B3.10c states "if an interbody fusion device is used to render the joint immobile (containing bone graft or bone graft substitute), the procedure is coded with the device value Interbody Fusion Device." The fixation instrumentation (i.e., rods, plates, screws, etc.) is included in the Fusion root operation, and no additional code is assigned.
	AND	
	MCC condition	*See* appendix B.

DRG 472 Cervical Spinal Fusion with CC RW 2.9554

Potential DRGs

453	Combined Anterior/Posterior Spinal Fusion with MCC	8.8614
454	Combined Anterior/Posterior Spinal Fusion with CC	6.1163
471	Cervical Spinal Fusion with MCC	4.9190

DRG	PDx/SDx/Procedure	Tips
453	Combination of anterior and posterior spinal fusion or refusion techniques	The anterior column may be fused using an anterior, lateral, or posterior technique. The posterior column may be fused using a posterior, posterolateral, or lateral transverse technique. Two operative notes may be dictated for different incisions/approaches. ICD-10-PCS Coding Guideline B3.10c states "if an interbody fusion device is used to render the joint immobile (containing bone graft or bone graft substitute), the procedure is coded with the device value Interbody Fusion Device." The fixation instrumentation (i.e., rods, plates, screws, etc.) is included in the Fusion root operation, and no additional code is assigned.
	AND	
	MCC condition	*See* appendix B.
454	Combination of anterior and posterior spinal fusion or refusion techniques	*See* DRG 453.
	AND	
	CC condition	*See* appendix B.
471	MCC condition	*See* appendix B.

DRG 473 Cervical Spinal Fusion without CC/MCC RW 2.4606

Potential DRGs

453	Combined Anterior/Posterior Spinal Fusion with MCC	8.8614
454	Combined Anterior/Posterior Spinal Fusion with CC	6.1163
455	Combined Anterior/Posterior Spinal Fusion without CC/MCC	4.6056
471	Cervical Spinal Fusion with MCC	4.9190
472	Cervical Spinal Fusion with CC	2.9554

DRG	PDx/SDx/Procedure	Tips
453	Combination of anterior and posterior spinal fusion or refusion techniques	The anterior column may be fused using an anterior, lateral, or posterior technique. The posterior column may be fused using a posterior, posterolateral, or lateral transverse technique. Two operative notes may be dictated for different incisions/approaches. ICD-10-PCS Coding Guideline B3.10c states "if an interbody fusion device is used to render the joint immobile (containing bone graft or bone graft substitute), the procedure is coded with the device value Interbody Fusion Device." The fixation instrumentation (i.e., rods, plates, screws, etc.) is included in the Fusion root operation, and no additional code is assigned.
	AND	
	MCC condition	*See* appendix B.
454	Combination of anterior and posterior spinal fusion or refusion techniques	*See* DRG 453.
	AND	
	CC condition	*See* appendix B.
455	Combination of anterior and posterior spinal fusion or refusion techniques	*See* DRG 453.
471	MCC condition	*See* appendix B.
472	CC condition	*See* appendix B.

DRG 474 Amputation for Musculoskeletal System and Connective Tissue Disorders with MCC RW 4.3028

Potential DRGs

239	Amputation for Circulatory System Disorders Except Upper Limb and Toe with MCC	4.8068
957	Other O.R. Procedures for Multiple Significant Trauma with MCC	7.2325

DRG	PDx/SDx/Procedure	Tips
239	Diabetes with circulatory complications (e.g., peripheral angiopathy, with or without gangrene)	According to ICD-10-CM guidelines, the classification presumes a causal relationship between diabetes and certain associated manifestations and/or conditions when these terms are linked by the term "with" in the alphabetic index (either a main term or subterm). These conditions should be coded as related to the diabetes unless the documentation clearly states the conditions are unrelated, in which case they may be coded separately. These conditions do not require provider documentation linking them to diabetes. Review the record and/or query the physician if it is unclear whether a condition is related to diabetes mellitus or the ICD-10-CM classification does not provide instruction.
	AND	
	MCC condition	*See* appendix B.
957	Multiple significant trauma	Principal diagnosis of trauma and two or more different dx from two different body site categories in MS-DRG 963.
	AND	
	Amputation EXCEPT fingers or toes	
	AND	
	MCC condition	*See* appendix B.

DRG 475 Amputation for Musculoskeletal System and Connective Tissue Disorders with CC RW 2.1447

Potential DRGs

040	Peripheral/Cranial Nerve and Other Nervous System Procedures with MCC	3.8505
041	Peripheral/Cranial Nerve and Other Nervous System Procedures with CC or Peripheral Neurostimulator	2.2307
239	Amputation for Circulatory System Disorders Except Upper Limb and Toe with MCC	4.8068
240	Amputation for Circulatory System Disorders Except Upper Limb and Toe with CC	2.8092
474	Amputation for Musculoskeletal System and Connective Tissue Disorders with MCC	4.3028
616	Amputation of Lower Limb for Endocrine, Nutritional, and Metabolic Disorders with MCC	3.9577
957	Other O.R. Procedures for Multiple Significant Trauma with MCC	7.2325
958	Other O.R. Procedures for Multiple Significant Trauma with CC	4.0448

DRG	PDx/SDx/Procedure	Tips
040	Diabetes with neurological manifestations (e.g., neurogenic arthropathy, peripheral autonomic neuropathy, polyneuropathy)	According to ICD-10-CM guidelines, the classification presumes a causal relationship between diabetes and certain associated manifestations and/or conditions when these terms are linked by the term "with" in the alphabetic index (either a main term or subterm). These conditions should be coded as related to the diabetes unless the documentation clearly states the conditions are unrelated, in which case they may be coded separately. These conditions do not require provider documentation linking them to diabetes. Review the record and/or query the physician if it is unclear whether a condition is related to diabetes mellitus or the ICD-10-CM classification does not provide instruction.
	AND	
	MCC condition	*See* appendix B.
041	Diabetes with neurological manifestations (e.g., neurogenic arthropathy, peripheral autonomic neuropathy, polyneuropathy)	*See* DRG 040.
	AND	
	CC condition	*See* appendix B.
239	Diabetes with circulatory complications (e.g., peripheral angiopathy, with or without gangrene)	*See* DRG 040.
	AND	
	MCC condition	*See* appendix B.
240	Diabetes with circulatory complications (e.g., peripheral angiopathy, with or without gangrene)	*See* DRG 040.
	AND	
	CC condition	*See* appendix B.
474	MCC condition	*See* appendix B.
616	Diabetes with osteomyelitis	
	AND	
	MCC condition	*See* appendix B.
957	Multiple significant trauma	Principal diagnosis of trauma and two or more different dx from two different body site categories in MS-DRG 963.
	AND	
	Amputation EXCEPT fingers or toes	
	AND	
	MCC condition	*See* appendix B.
958	Multiple significant trauma	*See* DRG 957.
	AND	
	Amputation EXCEPT fingers or toes	
	AND	
	CC condition	*See* appendix B.

DRG 476 Amputation for Musculoskeletal System and Connective Tissue Disorders without CC/MCC — RW 1.1769

Potential DRGs

040	Peripheral/Cranial Nerve and Other Nervous System Procedures with MCC	3.8505
041	Peripheral/Cranial Nerve and Other Nervous System Procedures with CC or Peripheral Neurostimulator	2.2307
042	Peripheral/Cranial Nerve and Other Nervous System Procedures without CC/MCC	1.7398
239	Amputation for Circulatory System Disorders Except Upper Limb and Toe with MCC	4.8068
240	Amputation for Circulatory System Disorders Except Upper Limb and Toe with CC	2.8092
241	Amputation for Circulatory System Disorders Except Upper Limb and Toe without CC/MCC	1.3898
474	Amputation for Musculoskeletal System and Connective Tissue Disorders with MCC	4.3028
475	Amputation for Musculoskeletal System and Connective Tissue Disorders with CC	2.1447
616	Amputation of Lower Limb for Endocrine, Nutritional, and Metabolic Disorders with MCC	3.9577
617	Amputation of Lower Limb for Endocrine, Nutritional, and Metabolic Disorders with CC	1.9845
957	Other O.R. Procedures for Multiple Significant Trauma with MCC	7.2325
958	Other O.R. Procedures for Multiple Significant Trauma with CC	4.0448
959	Other O.R. Procedures for Multiple Significant Trauma without CC/MCC	2.5324

DRG	PDx/SDx/Procedure	Tips
040	Diabetes with neurological manifestations (e.g., neurogenic arthropathy, peripheral autonomic neuropathy, polyneuropathy)	According to ICD-10-CM guidelines, the classification presumes a causal relationship between diabetes and certain associated manifestations and/or conditions when these terms are linked by the term "with" in the alphabetic index (either a main term or subterm). These conditions should be coded as related to the diabetes unless the documentation clearly states the conditions are unrelated, in which case they may be coded separately. These conditions do not require provider documentation linking them to diabetes. Review the record and/or query the physician if it is unclear whether a condition is related to diabetes mellitus or the ICD-10-CM classification does not provide instruction.
	AND	
	MCC condition	*See* appendix B.
041	Diabetes with neurological manifestations (e.g., neurogenic arthropathy, peripheral autonomic neuropathy, polyneuropathy)	*See* DRG 040.
	AND	
	CC condition	*See* appendix B.
042	Diabetes with neurological manifestations (e.g., neurogenic arthropathy, peripheral autonomic neuropathy, polyneuropathy)	*See* DRG 040.
239	Diabetes with circulatory complications (e.g., peripheral angiopathy, with or without gangrene)	*See* DRG 040.
	AND	
	MCC condition	*See* appendix B.
240	Diabetes with circulatory complications (e.g., peripheral angiopathy, with or without gangrene)	*See* DRG 040.
	AND	
	CC condition	*See* appendix B.
241	Diabetes with circulatory complications (e.g., peripheral angiopathy, with or without gangrene)	*See* DRG 040.
474	MCC condition	*See* appendix B.
475	CC condition	*See* appendix B.
616	Diabetes with osteomyelitis	
	AND	
	MCC condition	*See* appendix B.
617	Diabetes with osteomyelitis	
	AND	
	CC condition	*See* appendix B.
957	Multiple significant trauma	Principal diagnosis of trauma and two or more different dx from two different body site categories in MS-DRG 963.
	AND	
	Amputation EXCEPT fingers or toes	
	AND	
	MCC condition	*See* appendix B.
958	Multiple significant trauma	*See* DRG 957.
	AND	
	Amputation EXCEPT fingers or toes	
	AND	
	CC condition	*See* appendix B.
959	Multiple significant trauma	*See* DRG 957.
	AND	
	Amputation EXCEPT fingers or toes	

DRG 477 Biopsies of Musculoskeletal System and Connective Tissue with MCC RW 3.3690

No Potential DRGs

DRG 478 Biopsies of Musculoskeletal System and Connective Tissue with CC RW 2.3837

Potential DRGs

477 Biopsies of Musculoskeletal System and Connective Tissue with MCC 3.3690

DRG	PDx/SDx/Procedure	Tips
477	MCC condition	*See* appendix B.

DRG 479 Biopsies of Musculoskeletal System and Connective Tissue without CC/MCC RW 1.8640

Potential DRGs

477 Biopsies of Musculoskeletal System and Connective Tissue with MCC 3.3690
478 Biopsies of Musculoskeletal System and Connective Tissue with CC 2.3837

DRG	PDx/SDx/Procedure	Tips
477	MCC condition	*See* appendix B.
478	CC condition	*See* appendix B.

DRG 480 Hip and Femur Procedures Except Major Joint with MCC RW 2.9489

Potential DRGs

463 Wound Debridement and Skin Graft Except Hand for Musculoskeletal and Connective Tissue Disorders with MCC 5.6637
466 Revision of Hip or Knee Replacement with MCC 5.1866
469 Major Hip and Knee Joint Replacement or Reattachment of Lower Extremity with MCC or Total Ankle Replacement 3.3298
956 Limb Reattachment, Hip and Femur Procedures for Multiple Significant Trauma 3.8782

DRG	PDx/SDx/Procedure	Tips
463	Arthrotomy for removal of hip prosthesis or liner without replacement	Review history and physical for previous joint replacement, and carefully review the operative report for removal of the prosthesis or liner without replacement. When a (cement) (joint) (methylmethacrylate) spacer is inserted, ØSH9[Ø,3,4]8Z, ØSHB[Ø,3,4]8Z must also be coded.
	AND	
	MCC condition	*See* appendix B.
466	Revision of hip replacement procedure	ICD-10-PCS root operation Revision is defined as: "Correcting, to the extent possible, a portion of a malfunctioning device or the position of a displaced device." Explanation: Revision can include correcting a malfunctioning or displaced device by taking out or putting in components of the device such as a screw or pin. Example: recementing of hip prosthesis.
	OR	
	Removal and replacement of hip prosthesis	Joint revisions must include both the removal of a joint prosthesis, liner, resurfacing device, or spacer and the subsequent insertion of a new joint prosthesis (Replacement) or liner (Supplement), either cemented or uncemented, performed via an open approach.
	AND	
	MCC condition	*See* appendix B.
469	Resurfacing procedure, total or partial hip replacement	
	AND	
	MCC condition	*See* appendix B.
956	Multiple significant trauma	Principal diagnosis of trauma and two or more different dx from two different body site categories in MS-DRG 963.
	AND	
	Reduction of femur fracture (reposition) with or without internal/external fixation, open approach	
	Reduction of femur fracture with internal/external fixation, percutaneous or percutaneous endoscopic approach	

DRG 481 Hip and Femur Procedures Except Major Joint with CC RW 2.0749

Potential DRGs

463	Wound Debridement and Skin Graft Except Hand for Musculoskeletal and Connective Tissue Disorders with MCC	5.6637
464	Wound Debridement and Skin Graft Except Hand for Musculoskeletal and Connective Tissue Disorders with CC	3.0014
466	Revision of Hip or Knee Replacement with MCC	5.1866
467	Revision of Hip or Knee Replacement with CC	3.4863
469	Major Hip and Knee Joint Replacement or Reattachment of Lower Extremity with MCC or Total Ankle Replacement	3.3298
480	Hip and Femur Procedures Except Major Joint with MCC	2.9489
956	Limb Reattachment, Hip and Femur Procedures for Multiple Significant Trauma	3.8782

DRG	PDx/SDx/Procedure	Tips
463	Arthrotomy for removal of hip prosthesis or liner without replacement	Review history and physical for previous joint replacement, and carefully review the operative report for removal of the prosthesis or liner without replacement. When a (cement) (joint) (methylmethacrylate) spacer is inserted, ØSH9[Ø,3,4]8Z, ØSHB[Ø,3,4]8Z must also be coded.
	AND	
	MCC condition	*See* appendix B.
464	Arthrotomy for removal of hip prosthesis or liner without replacement	*See* DRG 463.
	AND	
	CC condition	*See* appendix B.
466	Revision of hip replacement procedure	ICD-10-PCS root operation Revision is defined as: "Correcting, to the extent possible, a portion of a malfunctioning device or the position of a displaced device." Explanation: Revision can include correcting a malfunctioning or displaced device by taking out or putting in components of the device such as a screw or pin. Example: recementing of hip prosthesis.
	OR	
	Removal and replacement of hip prosthesis	Joint revisions must include both the removal of a joint prosthesis, liner, resurfacing device, or spacer and the subsequent insertion of a new joint prosthesis (Replacement) or liner (Supplement), either cemented or uncemented, performed via an open approach.
	AND	
	MCC condition	*See* appendix B.
467	Revision of hip replacement procedure	*See* DRG 466.
	OR	
	Removal and replacement of hip prosthesis	*See* DRG 466.
	AND	
	CC condition	*See* appendix B.
469	Resurfacing procedure, total or partial hip replacement	
	AND	
	MCC condition	*See* appendix B.
480	MCC condition	*See* appendix B.
956	Multiple significant trauma	Principal diagnosis of trauma and two or more different dx from two different body site categories in MS-DRG 963.
	AND	
	Reduction of femur fracture (reposition) with or without internal/external fixation, open approach	
	Reduction of femur fracture with internal/external fixation, percutaneous or percutaneous endoscopic approach	

DRG 482 Hip and Femur Procedures Except Major Joint without CC/MCC — RW 1.5884

Potential DRGs

463	Wound Debridement and Skin Graft Except Hand for Musculoskeletal and Connective Tissue Disorders with MCC	5.6637
464	Wound Debridement and Skin Graft Except Hand for Musculoskeletal and Connective Tissue Disorders with CC	3.0014
465	Wound Debridement and Skin Graft Except Hand for Musculoskeletal and Connective Tissue Disorders without CC/MCC	1.8708
466	Revision of Hip or Knee Replacement with MCC	5.1866
467	Revision of Hip or Knee Replacement with CC	3.4863
468	Revision of Hip or Knee Replacement without CC/MCC	2.6696
469	Major Hip and Knee Joint Replacement or Reattachment of Lower Extremity with MCC or Total Ankle Replacement	3.3298
470	Major Hip and Knee Joint Replacement or Reattachment of Lower Extremity without MCC	1.8817
480	Hip and Femur Procedures Except Major Joint with MCC	2.9489
481	Hip and Femur Procedures Except Major Joint with CC	2.0749
956	Limb Reattachment, Hip and Femur Procedures for Multiple Significant Trauma	3.8782

DRG	PDx/SDx/Procedure	Tips
463	Arthrotomy for removal of hip prosthesis or liner without replacement	Review history and physical for previous joint replacement, and carefully review the operative report for removal of the prosthesis or liner without replacement. When a (cement) (joint) (methylmethacrylate) spacer is inserted, ØSH9[Ø,3,4]8Z, ØSHB[Ø,3,4]8Z must also be coded.
	AND	
	MCC condition	*See* appendix B.
464	Arthrotomy for removal of hip prosthesis or liner without replacement	*See* DRG 463.
	AND	
	CC condition	*See* appendix B.
465	Arthrotomy for removal of hip prosthesis or liner without replacement	*See* DRG 463.
466	Revision of hip replacement procedure	ICD-10-PCS root operation Revision is defined as: "Correcting, to the extent possible, a portion of a malfunctioning device or the position of a displaced device." Explanation: Revision can include correcting a malfunctioning or displaced device by taking out or putting in components of the device such as a screw or pin. Example: recementing of hip prosthesis.
	OR	
	Removal and replacement of hip prosthesis	Joint revisions must include both the removal of a joint prosthesis, liner, resurfacing device, or spacer and the subsequent insertion of a new joint prosthesis (Replacement) or liner (Supplement), either cemented or uncemented, performed via an open approach.
	AND	
	MCC condition	*See* appendix B.
467	Revision of hip replacement procedure	*See* DRG 466.
	OR	
	Removal and replacement of hip prosthesis	*See* DRG 466.
	AND	
	CC condition	*See* appendix B.
468	Revision of hip replacement procedure	*See* DRG 466.
	OR	
	Removal and replacement of hip prosthesis	*See* DRG 466.
469	Resurfacing procedure, total or partial hip replacement	
	AND	
	MCC condition	*See* appendix B.
470	Resurfacing procedure, total or partial hip replacement	
480	MCC condition	*See* appendix B.
481	CC condition	*See* appendix B.
956	Multiple significant trauma	Principal diagnosis of trauma and two or more different dx from two different body site categories in MS-DRG 963.
	AND	
	Reduction of femur fracture (reposition) with or without internal/external fixation, open approach	
	Reduction of femur fracture with internal/external fixation, percutaneous or percutaneous endoscopic approach	

DRG 483 Major Joint/Limb Reattachment Procedure of Upper Extremities — RW 2.4842

Potential DRGs

957	Other O.R. Procedures for Multiple Significant Trauma with MCC	7.2325
958	Other O.R. Procedures for Multiple Significant Trauma with CC	4.0448

DRG	PDx/SDx/Procedure	Tips
957	Multiple significant trauma	Principal diagnosis of trauma and two or more different dx from two different body site categories in MS-DRG 963.
	AND	
	MCC condition	*See* appendix B.
958	Multiple significant trauma	*See* DRG 957.
	AND	
	CC condition	*See* appendix B.

Optimizing Tips

DRG 485 Knee Procedures with Principal Diagnosis of Infection with MCC — RW 3.2940

Potential DRGs

461	Bilateral or Multiple Major Joint Procedures of Lower Extremity with MCC	6.8185
466	Revision of Hip or Knee Replacement with MCC	5.1866

DRG	PDx/SDx/Procedure	Tips
461	Any combination of partial or total knee, hip or ankle joint replacement procedures	
	AND	
	MCC condition	*See* appendix B.
466	Revision of knee replacement procedure	
	OR	
	Removal and replacement of knee prosthesis	Joint revisions must include both the removal of a joint prosthesis, liner, resurfacing device, or spacer using an open or arthroscopic approach and the subsequent insertion of a new joint prosthesis (Replacement), either cemented or uncemented, performed via an open approach.
	AND	
	MCC condition	*See* appendix B.

DRG 486 Knee Procedures with Principal Diagnosis of Infection with CC — RW 2.0083

Potential DRGs

461	Bilateral or Multiple Major Joint Procedures of Lower Extremity with MCC	6.8185
462	Bilateral or Multiple Major Joint Procedures of Lower Extremity without MCC	2.8463
466	Revision of Hip or Knee Replacement with MCC	5.1866
467	Revision of Hip or Knee Replacement with CC	3.4863
469	Major Hip and Knee Joint Replacement or Reattachment of Lower Extremity with MCC or Total Ankle Replacement	3.3298
485	Knee Procedures with Principal Diagnosis of Infection with MCC	3.2940

DRG	PDx/SDx/Procedure	Tips
461	Any combination of partial or total knee, hip or ankle joint replacement procedures	
	AND	
	MCC condition	*See* appendix B.
462	Any combination of partial or total knee, hip or ankle joint replacement procedures	
466	Revision of knee replacement procedure	
	OR	
	Removal and replacement of knee prosthesis	Joint revisions must include both the removal of a joint prosthesis, liner, resurfacing device, or spacer using an open or arthroscopic approach and the subsequent insertion of a new joint prosthesis (Replacement), either cemented or uncemented, performed via an open approach.
	AND	
	MCC condition	*See* appendix B.
467	Revision of knee replacement procedure	
	OR	
	Removal and replacement of knee prosthesis	*See* DRG 466.
	AND	
	CC condition	*See* appendix B.
469	Knee replacement	
	AND	
	MCC condition	*See* appendix B.
485	MCC condition	*See* appendix B.

DRG 487 Knee Procedures with Principal Diagnosis of Infection without CC/MCC — RW 1.5449

Potential DRGs

461	Bilateral or Multiple Major Joint Procedures of Lower Extremity with MCC	6.8185
462	Bilateral or Multiple Major Joint Procedures of Lower Extremity without MCC	2.8463
466	Revision of Hip or Knee Replacement with MCC	5.1866
467	Revision of Hip or Knee Replacement with CC	3.4863
468	Revision of Hip or Knee Replacement without CC/MCC	2.6696
469	Major Hip and Knee Joint Replacement or Reattachment of Lower Extremity with MCC or Total Ankle Replacement	3.3298
470	Major Hip and Knee Joint Replacement or Reattachment of Lower Extremity without MCC	1.8817
485	Knee Procedures with Principal Diagnosis of Infection with MCC	3.2940
486	Knee Procedures with Principal Diagnosis of Infection with CC	2.0083

DRG	PDx/SDx/Procedure	Tips
461	Any combination of partial or total knee, hip or ankle joint replacement procedures	
	AND	
	MCC condition	*See* appendix B.
462	Any combination of partial or total knee, hip or ankle joint replacement procedures	
466	Revision of knee replacement procedure	
	OR	
	Removal and replacement of knee prosthesis	Joint revisions must include both the removal of a joint prosthesis, liner, resurfacing device, or spacer using an open or arthroscopic approach and the subsequent insertion of a new joint prosthesis (Replacement), either cemented or uncemented, performed via an open approach.
	AND	
	MCC condition	*See* appendix B.
467	Revision of knee replacement procedure	
	OR	
	Removal and replacement of knee prosthesis	*See* DRG 466.
	AND	
	CC condition	*See* appendix B.
468	Revision of knee replacement procedure	
	OR	
	Removal and replacement of knee prosthesis	*See* DRG 466.
469	Knee replacement	
	AND	
	MCC condition	*See* appendix B.
470	Knee replacement	
485	MCC condition	*See* appendix B.
486	CC condition	*See* appendix B.

DRG 488 Knee Procedures without Principal Diagnosis of Infection with CC/MCC — RW 2.1066

Potential DRGs

461	Bilateral or Multiple Major Joint Procedures of Lower Extremity with MCC	6.8185
462	Bilateral or Multiple Major Joint Procedures of Lower Extremity without MCC	2.8463
466	Revision of Hip or Knee Replacement with MCC	5.1866
467	Revision of Hip or Knee Replacement with CC	3.4863
469	Major Hip and Knee Joint Replacement or Reattachment of Lower Extremity with MCC or Total Ankle Replacement	3.3298
485	Knee Procedures with Principal Diagnosis of Infection with MCC	3.2940

DRG	PDx/SDx/Procedure	Tips
461	Any combination of partial or total knee, hip or ankle joint replacement procedures	
	AND	
	MCC condition	*See* appendix B.
462	Any combination of partial or total knee, hip or ankle joint replacement procedures	
466	Revision of knee replacement procedure	
	OR	
	Removal and replacement of knee prosthesis	Joint revisions must include both the removal of a joint prosthesis, liner, resurfacing device, or spacer using an open or arthroscopic approach and the subsequent insertion of a new joint prosthesis (Replacement), either cemented or uncemented, performed via an open approach.
	AND	
	MCC condition	*See* appendix B.
467	Revision of knee replacement procedure	
	OR	
	Removal and replacement of knee prosthesis	*See* DRG 466.
	AND	
	CC condition	*See* appendix B.
469	Knee replacement	
	AND	
	MCC condition	*See* appendix B.
485	Knee procedure with principal diagnosis of infection	
	AND	
	MCC condition	*See* appendix B.

DRG 489 Knee Procedures without Principal Diagnosis of Infection without CC/MCC RW 1.2377

Potential DRGs

461	Bilateral or Multiple Major Joint Procedures of Lower Extremity with MCC	6.8185
462	Bilateral or Multiple Major Joint Procedures of Lower Extremity without MCC	2.8463
466	Revision of Hip or Knee Replacement with MCC	5.1866
467	Revision of Hip or Knee Replacement with CC	3.4863
468	Revision of Hip or Knee Replacement without CC/MCC	2.6696
469	Major Hip and Knee Joint Replacement or Reattachment of Lower Extremity with MCC or Total Ankle Replacement	3.3298
470	Major Hip and Knee Joint Replacement or Reattachment of Lower Extremity without MCC	1.8817
485	Knee Procedures with Principal Diagnosis of Infection with MCC	3.2940
486	Knee Procedures with Principal Diagnosis of Infection with CC	2.0083
487	Knee Procedures with Principal Diagnosis of Infection without CC/MCC	1.5449
488	Knee Procedures without Principal Diagnosis of Infection with CC/MCC	2.1066

DRG	PDx/SDx/Procedure	Tips
461	Any combination of partial or total knee, hip or ankle joint replacement procedures	
	AND	
	MCC condition	*See* appendix B.
462	Any combination of partial or total knee, hip or ankle joint replacement procedures	
466	Revision of knee replacement procedure	
	OR	
	Removal and replacement of knee prosthesis	Joint revisions must include both the removal of a joint prosthesis, liner, resurfacing device, or spacer using an open or arthroscopic approach and the subsequent insertion of a new joint prosthesis (Replacement), either cemented or uncemented, performed via an open approach.
	AND	
	MCC condition	*See* appendix B.
467	Revision of knee replacement procedure	
	OR	
	Removal and replacement of knee prosthesis	*See* DRG 466.
	AND	
	CC condition	*See* appendix B.
468	Revision of knee replacement procedure	
	OR	*See* DRG 466.
	Removal and replacement of knee prosthesis	
469	Knee replacement	
	AND	
	MCC condition	*See* appendix B.
470	Knee replacement	
485	Knee procedure with principal diagnosis of infection	
	AND	
	MCC condition	*See* appendix B.
486	Knee procedure with principal diagnosis of infection	
	AND	
	CC condition	*See* appendix B.
487	Knee procedure with principal diagnosis of infection	
488	CC/MCC condition	*See* appendix B.

DRG 492 Lower Extremity and Humerus Procedures Except Hip, Foot, Femur with MCC RW 3.4621

Potential DRGs

461	Bilateral or Multiple Major Joint Procedures of Lower Extremity with MCC	6.8185

DRG	PDx/SDx/Procedure	Tips
461	Any combination of partial or total knee, hip or ankle joint replacement procedures	
	AND	
	MCC condition	*See* appendix B.

DRG 493 Lower Extremity and Humerus Procedures Except Hip, Foot, Femur with CC RW 2.4017

Potential DRGs

461	Bilateral or Multiple Major Joint Procedures of Lower Extremity with MCC	6.8185
462	Bilateral or Multiple Major Joint Procedures of Lower Extremity without MCC	2.8463
469	Major Hip and Knee Joint Replacement or Reattachment of Lower Extremity with MCC or Total Ankle Replacement	3.3298
477	Biopsies of Musculoskeletal System and Connective Tissue with MCC	3.3690
492	Lower Extremity and Humerus Procedures Except Hip, Foot, Femur with MCC	3.4621

DRG	PDx/SDx/Procedure	Tips
461	Any combination of partial or total knee, hip or ankle joint replacement procedures	
	AND	
	MCC condition	*See* appendix B.
462	Any combination of partial or total knee, hip or ankle joint replacement procedures	
469	Knee or ankle replacement	
	AND	
	MCC condition	*See* appendix B.
477	Biopsy of bone	Review the medical record carefully to determine the exact procedure that was performed. The ICD-10-PCS index instructs the coder to *see* Drainage with qualifier Diagnostic, *see* Excision with qualifier Diagnostic or *see* Extraction with qualifier Diagnostic to report a biopsy. It is important to always review the full definition of the root operation in the PCS table to accurately report the procedure performed.
	AND	
	MCC condition	*See* appendix B.
492	MCC condition	*See* appendix B.

DRG 494 Lower Extremity and Humerus Procedures Except Hip, Foot, Femur without CC/MCC RW 1.8692

Potential DRGs

461	Bilateral or Multiple Major Joint Procedures of Lower Extremity with MCC	6.8185
462	Bilateral or Multiple Major Joint Procedures of Lower Extremity without MCC	2.8463
469	Major Hip and Knee Joint Replacement or Reattachment of Lower Extremity with MCC or Total Ankle Replacement	3.3298
470	Major Hip and Knee Joint Replacement or Reattachment of Lower Extremity without MCC	1.8817
477	Biopsies of Musculoskeletal System and Connective Tissue with MCC	3.3690
478	Biopsies of Musculoskeletal System and Connective Tissue with CC	2.3837
492	Lower Extremity and Humerus Procedures Except Hip, Foot, Femur with MCC	3.4621
493	Lower Extremity and Humerus Procedures Except Hip, Foot, Femur with CC	2.4017

DRG	PDx/SDx/Procedure	Tips
461	Any combination of partial or total knee, hip or ankle joint replacement procedures	
	AND	
	MCC condition	*See* appendix B.
462	Any combination of partial or total knee, hip or ankle joint replacement procedures	
469	Knee or ankle replacement	
	AND	
	MCC condition	*See* appendix B.
470	Knee or ankle replacement	
477	Biopsy of bone	Review the medical record carefully to determine the exact procedure that was performed. The ICD-10-PCS index instructs the coder to *see* Drainage with qualifier Diagnostic, *see* Excision with qualifier Diagnostic or *see* Extraction with qualifier Diagnostic to report a biopsy. It is important to always review the full definition of the root operation in the PCS table to accurately report the procedure performed.
	AND	
	MCC condition	*See* appendix B.
478	Biopsy of bone	*See* DRG 477.
	AND	
	CC condition	*See* appendix B.
492	MCC condition	*See* appendix B.
493	CC condition	*See* appendix B.

DRG 495 Local Excision and Removal Internal Fixation Devices Except Hip and Femur with MCC — RW 3.5812

Potential DRGs

463	Wound Debridement and Skin Graft Except Hand for Musculoskeletal and Connective Tissue Disorders with MCC	5.6637

DRG	PDx/SDx/Procedure	Tips
463	Arthrotomy for removal of knee prosthesis or liner without replacement	Review history and physical for previous joint replacement, and carefully review the operative report for removal of the prosthesis or liner without replacement. When a (cement) (joint) (methylmethacrylate) spacer is inserted, 0SHC[0,3,4]8Z, 0SHD[0,3,4]8Z must also be coded.
	AND	
	MCC condition	*See* appendix B.

DRG 496 Local Excision and Removal Internal Fixation Devices Except Hip and Femur with CC — RW 1.9875

Potential DRGs

463	Wound Debridement and Skin Graft Except Hand for Musculoskeletal and Connective Tissue Disorders with MCC	5.6637
464	Wound Debridement and Skin Graft Except Hand for Musculoskeletal and Connective Tissue Disorders with CC	3.0014
477	Biopsies of Musculoskeletal System and Connective Tissue with MCC	3.3690
478	Biopsies of Musculoskeletal System and Connective Tissue with CC	2.3837
495	Local Excision and Removal Internal Fixation Devices Except Hip and Femur with MCC	3.5812

DRG	PDx/SDx/Procedure	Tips
463	Arthrotomy for removal of knee prosthesis or liner without replacement	Review history and physical for previous joint replacement, and carefully review the operative report for removal of the prosthesis or liner without replacement. When a (cement) (joint) (methylmethacrylate) spacer is inserted, ØSHC[Ø,3,4]8Z, ØSHD[Ø,3,4]8Z must also be coded.
	AND	
	MCC condition	*See* appendix B.
464	Arthrotomy for removal of knee prosthesis or liner without replacement	*See* DRG 463.
	AND	
	CC condition	*See* appendix B.
477	Biopsy of bone	Review the medical record carefully to determine the exact procedure that was performed. The ICD-10-PCS index instructs the coder to *see* Drainage with qualifier Diagnostic, *see* Excision with qualifier Diagnostic or *see* Extraction with qualifier Diagnostic to report a biopsy. It is important to always review the full definition of the root operation in the PCS table to accurately report the procedure performed.
	AND	
	MCC condition	*See* appendix B.
478	Biopsy of bone	*See* DRG 477.
	AND	
	CC condition	*See* appendix B.
495	MCC condition	*See* appendix B.

DRG 497 Local Excision and Removal Internal Fixation Devices Except Hip and Femur without CC/MCC

RW 1.4274

Potential DRGs

463	Wound Debridement and Skin Graft Except Hand for Musculoskeletal and Connective Tissue Disorders with MCC	5.6637
464	Wound Debridement and Skin Graft Except Hand for Musculoskeletal and Connective Tissue Disorders with CC	3.0014
465	Wound Debridement and Skin Graft Except Hand for Musculoskeletal and Connective Tissue Disorders without CC/MCC	1.8708
477	Biopsies of Musculoskeletal System and Connective Tissue with MCC	3.3690
478	Biopsies of Musculoskeletal System and Connective Tissue with CC	2.3837
479	Biopsies of Musculoskeletal System and Connective Tissue without CC/MCC	1.8640
495	Local Excision and Removal Internal Fixation Devices Except Hip and Femur with MCC	3.5812
496	Local Excision and Removal Internal Fixation Devices Except Hip and Femur with CC	1.9875

DRG	PDx/SDx/Procedure	Tips
463	Arthrotomy for removal of knee prosthesis or liner without replacement	Review history and physical for previous joint replacement, and carefully review the operative report for removal of the prosthesis or liner without replacement. When a (cement) (joint) (methylmethacrylate) spacer is inserted, ØSHC[Ø,3,4]8Z, ØSHD[Ø,3,4]8Z must also be coded.
	AND	
	MCC condition	*See* appendix B.
464	Arthrotomy for removal of knee prosthesis or liner without replacement	*See* DRG 463.
	AND	
	CC condition	*See* appendix B.
465	Arthrotomy for removal of knee prosthesis or liner without replacement	*See* DRG 463.
477	Biopsy of bone	Review the medical record carefully to determine the exact procedure that was performed. The ICD-10-PCS index instructs the coder to *see* Drainage with qualifier Diagnostic, *see* Excision with qualifier Diagnostic or *see* Extraction with qualifier Diagnostic to report a biopsy. It is important to always review the full definition of the root operation in the PCS table to accurately report the procedure performed.
	AND	
	MCC condition	*See* appendix B.
478	Biopsy of bone	*See* DRG 477.
	AND	
	CC condition	*See* appendix B.
479	Biopsy of bone	*See* DRG 477.
495	MCC condition	*See* appendix B.
496	CC condition	*See* appendix B.

DRG 498 Local Excision and Removal Internal Fixation Devices of Hip and Femur with CC/MCC

RW 2.6110

Potential DRGs

463	Wound Debridement and Skin Graft Except Hand for Musculoskeletal and Connective Tissue Disorders with MCC	5.6637
464	Wound Debridement and Skin Graft Except Hand for Musculoskeletal and Connective Tissue Disorders with CC	3.0014
466	Revision of Hip or Knee Replacement with MCC	5.1866
467	Revision of Hip or Knee Replacement with CC	3.4863

DRG	PDx/SDx/Procedure	Tips
463	Arthrotomy for removal of hip prosthesis or liner without replacement	Review history and physical for previous joint replacement, and carefully review the operative report for removal of the prosthesis or liner without replacement. When a (cement) (joint) (methylmethacrylate) spacer is inserted, ØSH9[Ø,3,4]8Z, ØSHB[Ø,3,4]8Z must also be coded.
	AND	
	MCC condition	*See* appendix B.
464	Arthrotomy for removal of hip prosthesis or liner without replacement	*See* DRG 463.
	AND	
	CC condition	*See* appendix B.
466	Revision of hip replacement procedure	
	OR	
	Removal and replacement of hip prosthesis	
	AND	
	MCC condition	*See* appendix B.
467	Revision of hip replacement procedure	
	OR	
	Removal and replacement of knee prosthesis	
	AND	
	CC condition	*See* appendix B.

DRG 499 Local Excision and Removal Internal Fixation Devices of Hip and Femur without CC/MCC RW 1.2898

Potential DRGs

463	Wound Debridement and Skin Graft Except Hand for Musculoskeletal and Connective Tissue Disorders with MCC	5.6637
464	Wound Debridement and Skin Graft Except Hand for Musculoskeletal and Connective Tissue Disorders with CC	3.0014
465	Wound Debridement and Skin Graft Except Hand for Musculoskeletal and Connective Tissue Disorders without CC/MCC	1.8708
466	Revision of Hip or Knee Replacement with MCC	5.1866
467	Revision of Hip or Knee Replacement with CC	3.4863
468	Revision of Hip or Knee Replacement without CC/MCC	2.6696
498	Local Excision and Removal Internal Fixation Devices of Hip and Femur with CC/MCC	2.6110

DRG	PDx/SDx/Procedure	Tips
463	Arthrotomy for removal of hip prosthesis or liner without replacement	Review history and physical for previous joint replacement, and carefully review the operative report for removal of the prosthesis or liner without replacement. When a (cement) (joint) (methylmethacrylate) spacer is inserted, ØSH9[Ø,3,4]8Z, ØSHB[Ø,3,4]8Z must also be coded.
	AND	
	MCC condition	*See* appendix B.
464	Arthrotomy for removal of hip prosthesis or liner without replacement	*See* DRG 463.
	AND	
	CC condition	*See* appendix B.
465	Arthrotomy for removal of hip prosthesis or liner without replacement	*See* DRG 463.
466	Revision of hip replacement procedure	
	OR	
	Removal and replacement of hip prosthesis	
	AND	
	MCC condition	*See* appendix B.
467	Revision of hip replacement procedure	
	OR	
	Removal and replacement of hip prosthesis	
	AND	
	CC condition	*See* appendix B.
468	Revision of hip replacement procedure	
	OR	
	Removal and replacement of hip prosthesis	
498	CC/MCC condition	*See* appendix B.

DRG 500 Soft Tissue Procedures with MCC RW 3.2428

Potential DRGs

463	Wound Debridement and Skin Graft Except Hand for Musculoskeletal and Connective Tissue Disorders with MCC	5.6637
622	Skin Grafts and Wound Debridement for Endocrine, Nutritional and Metabolic Disorders with MCC	3.8256

DRG	PDx/SDx/Procedure	Tips
463	Musculoskeletal and connective tissue principal diagnosis	
	Osteomyelitis, all types (except diabetic)	
	Open wounds (lacerations) with tendon involvement	Laceration tendon —*see* Injury, muscle, by site, laceration
	AND	
	Excisional debridement of wound, infection, or burn	The ICD-10-PCS definition of the root operation Excision is "Cutting out or off, without replacement, a portion of a body part." Debridement by excision involves cutting with a sharp instrument such as a scalpel or other methods such as a hot knife or laser. Non-excisional debridement of skin is coded to root operation Extraction. Ensure that documentation includes instruments used, technique, and depth of debridement procedure.
	OR	
	Skin grafting procedure	Skin grafting includes root operations Replacement of skin with a free graft of autologous (partial or full thickness), nonautologous or synthetic tissue; and Transfer of skin, and/or subcutaneous tissue and fascia which remains attached to its vascular and nervous supply. Other procedures include Excision and Supplement of tissues and Insertion of tissue expander.
	AND	
	MCC condition	*See* appendix B.
622	Diabetes with osteomyelitis	
	AND	
	Excisional debridement of wound, infection or burn	
	OR	
	Skin grafting procedure	*See* DRG 463.
	AND	
	MCC condition	*See* appendix B.

DRG 501 Soft Tissue Procedures with CC

RW 1.7357

Potential DRGs

463	Wound Debridement and Skin Graft Except Hand for Musculoskeletal and Connective Tissue Disorders with MCC	5.6637
464	Wound Debridement and Skin Graft Except Hand for Musculoskeletal and Connective Tissue Disorders with CC	3.0014
500	Soft Tissue Procedures with MCC	3.2428
622	Skin Grafts and Wound Debridement for Endocrine, Nutritional and Metabolic Disorders with MCC	3.8256
623	Skin Grafts and Wound Debridement for Endocrine, Nutritional and Metabolic Disorders with CC	1.8614

DRG	PDx/SDx/Procedure	Tips
463	Musculoskeletal and connective tissue principal diagnosis	
	Osteomyelitis, all types (except diabetic)	
	Open wounds (lacerations) with tendon involvement	Laceration tendon —*see* Injury, muscle, by site, laceration
	AND	
	Excisional debridement of wound, infection, or burn	The ICD-10-PCS definition of the root operation Excision is "Cutting out or off, without replacement, a portion of a body part." Debridement by excision involves cutting with a sharp instrument such as a scalpel or other methods such as a hot knife or laser. Non-excisional debridement of skin is coded to root operation Extraction. Ensure that documentation includes instruments used, technique, and depth of debridement procedure.
	OR	
	Skin grafting procedure	Skin grafting includes root operations Replacement of skin with a free graft of autologous (partial or full thickness), nonautologous or synthetic tissue; and Transfer of skin, and/or subcutaneous tissue and fascia which remains attached to its vascular and nervous supply. Other procedures include Excision and Supplement of tissues and Insertion of tissue expander.
	AND	
	MCC condition	*See* appendix B.
464	Musculoskeletal and connective tissue principal diagnosis	
	Osteomyelitis, all types (except diabetic)	
	Open wounds (lacerations) with tendon involvement	Laceration tendon —*see* Injury, muscle, by site, laceration
	AND	
	Excisional debridement of wound, infection, or burn	*See* DRG 463.
	OR	
	Skin grafting procedure	*See* DRG 463.
	AND	
	CC condition	*See* appendix B.
500	MCC condition	*See* appendix B.
622	Diabetes with osteomyelitis	
	AND	
	Excisional debridement of wound, infection or burn	The ICD-10-PCS definition of the root operation Excision is "Cutting out or off, without replacement, a portion of a body part." Debridement by excision involves cutting with a sharp instrument such as a scalpel or other methods such as a hot knife or laser. Nonexcisional debridement of skin is coded to root operation Extraction. Ensure that documentation includes instruments used, technique, and depth of debridement procedure.
	OR	
	Skin grafting procedure	Skin grafting includes root operations Replacement of skin with a free graft of autologous (partial or full thickness), nonautologous or synthetic tissue; and Transfer of skin, and/or subcutaneous tissue and fascia which remains attached to its vascular and nervous supply. Other procedures include Excision and Supplement of tissues and Insertion of tissue expander.
	AND	
	MCC condition	*See* appendix B.
623	Diabetes with osteomyelitis	
	AND	
	Excisional debridement of wound, infection or burn	*See* DRG 622.
	OR	
	Skin grafting procedure	*See* DRG 622.
	AND	
	CC condition	*See* appendix B.

DRG 502 Soft Tissue Procedures without CC/MCC — RW 1.3827

Potential DRGs

463	Wound Debridement and Skin Graft Except Hand for Musculoskeletal and Connective Tissue Disorders with MCC	5.6637
464	Wound Debridement and Skin Graft Except Hand for Musculoskeletal and Connective Tissue Disorders with CC	3.0014
465	Wound Debridement and Skin Graft Except Hand for Musculoskeletal and Connective Tissue Disorders without CC/MCC	1.8708
500	Soft Tissue Procedures with MCC	3.2428
501	Soft Tissue Procedures with CC	1.7357
622	Skin Grafts and Wound Debridement for Endocrine, Nutritional and Metabolic Disorders with MCC	3.8256
623	Skin Grafts and Wound Debridement for Endocrine, Nutritional and Metabolic Disorders with CC	1.8614

DRG	PDx/SDx/Procedure	Tips
463	Musculoskeletal and connective tissue principal diagnosis	
	Osteomyelitis, all types (except diabetic)	
	Open wounds (lacerations) with tendon involvement	Laceration tendon—*see* Injury, muscle, by site, laceration
	AND	
	Excisional debridement of wound, infection, or burn	The ICD-10-PCS definition of the root operation Excision is "Cutting out or off, without replacement, a portion of a body part." Debridement by excision involves cutting with a sharp instrument such as a scalpel or other methods such as a hot knife or laser. Non-excisional debridement of skin is coded to root operation Extraction. Ensure that documentation includes instruments used, technique, and depth of debridement procedure.
	OR	
	Skin grafting procedure	Skin grafting includes root operations Replacement of skin with a free graft of autologous (partial or full thickness), nonautologous or synthetic tissue; and Transfer of skin, and/or subcutaneous tissue and fascia which remains attached to its vascular and nervous supply. Other procedures include Excision and Supplement of tissues and Insertion of tissue expander.
	AND	
	MCC condition	*See* appendix B.
464	Musculoskeletal and connective tissue principal diagnosis	
	Osteomyelitis, all types (except diabetic)	
	Open wounds (lacerations) with tendon involvement	Laceration tendon—*see* Injury, muscle, by site, laceration
	AND	
	Excisional debridement of wound, infection, or burn	*See* DRG 463.
	OR	
	Skin grafting procedure	*See* DRG 463.
	AND	
	CC condition	*See* appendix B.
465	Musculoskeletal and connective tissue principal diagnosis	
	Osteomyelitis, all types (except diabetic)	
	Open wounds (lacerations) with tendon involvement	Laceration tendon—*see* Injury, muscle, by site, laceration
	AND	
	Excisional debridement of wound, infection, or burn	*See* DRG 463.
	OR	
	Skin grafting procedure	*See* DRG 463.
500	MCC condition	*See* appendix B.
501	CC condition	*See* appendix B.
622	Diabetes with osteomyelitis	
	AND	
	Excisional debridement of wound, infection or burn	The ICD-10-PCS definition of the root operation Excision is "Cutting out or off, without replacement, a portion of a body part." Debridement by excision involves cutting with a sharp instrument such as a scalpel or other methods such as a hot knife or laser. Nonexcisional debridement of skin is coded to root operation Extraction. Ensure that documentation includes instruments used, technique, and depth of debridement procedure.
	OR	
	Skin grafting procedure	Skin grafting includes root operations Replacement of skin with a free graft of autologous (partial or full thickness), nonautologous or synthetic tissue; and Transfer of skin, and/or subcutaneous tissue and fascia which remains attached to its vascular and nervous supply. Other procedures include Excision and Supplement of tissues and Insertion of tissue expander.
	AND	
	MCC condition	*See* appendix B.
623	Diabetes with osteomyelitis	
	AND	
	Excisional debridement of wound, infection or burn	*See* DRG 622.
	OR	
	Skin grafting procedure	*See* DRG 622.
	AND	
	CC condition	*See* appendix B.

DRG 503 Foot Procedures with MCC

RW 2.6819

Potential DRGs

040	Peripheral/Cranial Nerve and Other Nervous System Procedures with MCC	3.8505
239	Amputation for Circulatory System Disorders Except Upper Limb and Toe with MCC	4.8068
463	Wound Debridement and Skin Graft Except Hand for Musculoskeletal and Connective Tissue Disorders with MCC	5.6637
474	Amputation for Musculoskeletal System and Connective Tissue Disorders with MCC	4.3028
616	Amputation of Lower Limb for Endocrine, Nutritional, and Metabolic Disorders with MCC	3.9577

DRG	PDx/SDx/Procedure	Tips
040	Diabetes with neurological manifestations (e.g., neurogenic arthropathy, peripheral autonomic neuropathy, polyneuropathy)	According to ICD-10-CM guidelines, the classification presumes a causal relationship between diabetes and certain associated manifestations and/or conditions when these terms are linked by the term "with" in the alphabetic index (either under a main term or subterm). These conditions should be coded as related to the diabetes unless the documentation clearly states the conditions are unrelated, in which case they may be coded separately. These conditions do not require provider documentation linking them to diabetes. Review the record and/or query the physician if it is unclear whether a condition is related to diabetes mellitus or the ICD-10-CM classification does not provide instruction.
	AND	
	Amputation of toe	
	AND	
	MCC condition	*See* appendix B.
239	Diabetes with circulatory complications (e.g., peripheral angiopathy, with or without gangrene)	*See* DRG 040.
	AND	
	Amputation of foot complete or complete or partial ray	
	AND	
	MCC condition	*See* appendix B.
463	Musculoskeletal and connective tissue principal diagnosis	Ensure that documentation includes underlying cause of condition requiring debridement and depth of debridement procedure.
	Osteomyelitis, all types (except diabetic)	
	Open wounds (lacerations) with tendon involvement	Laceration tendon—*see* Injury, muscle, by site, laceration
	AND	
	Excisional debridement of wound, infection, or burn	The ICD-10-PCS definition of the root operation Excision is "Cutting out or off, without replacement, a portion of a body part." Debridement by excision involves cutting with a sharp instrument such as a scalpel or other methods such as a hot knife or laser. Non-excisional debridement of skin is coded to root operation Extraction. Ensure that documentation includes instruments used, technique, and depth of debridement procedure.
	OR	
	Skin grafting procedure	Skin grafting includes root operations Replacement of skin with a free graft of autologous (partial or full thickness), nonautologous or synthetic tissue; and Transfer of skin, and/or subcutaneous tissue and fascia which remains attached to its vascular and nervous supply. Other procedures include Excision and Supplement of tissues and Insertion of tissue expander.
	AND	
	MCC condition	*See* appendix B.
474	Upper and lower limb amputations	
	AND	
	MCC condition	*See* appendix B.
616	Diabetes (type 1, type 2, other specified) with ketoacidosis, hyperosmolarity, other coma, other and unspecified complications	
	Diabetic foot or other skin ulcer principal diagnosis	
	AND	
	Amputation of toe	
	AND	
	MCC condition	*See* appendix B.

DRG 504 Foot Procedures with CC RW 1.7271

Potential DRGs

040	Peripheral/Cranial Nerve and Other Nervous System Procedures with MCC	3.8505
041	Peripheral/Cranial Nerve and Other Nervous System Procedures with CC or Peripheral Neurostimulator	2.2307
239	Amputation for Circulatory System Disorders Except Upper Limb and Toe with MCC	4.8068
240	Amputation for Circulatory System Disorders Except Upper Limb and Toe with CC	2.8092
255	Upper Limb and Toe Amputation for Circulatory System Disorders with MCC	2.7474
463	Wound Debridement and Skin Graft Except Hand for Musculoskeletal and Connective Tissue Disorders with MCC	5.6637
464	Wound Debridement and Skin Graft Except Hand for Musculoskeletal and Connective Tissue Disorders with CC	3.0014
474	Amputation for Musculoskeletal System and Connective Tissue Disorders with MCC	4.3028
475	Amputation for Musculoskeletal System and Connective Tissue Disorders with CC	2.1447
503	Foot Procedures with MCC	2.6819
616	Amputation of Lower Limb for Endocrine, Nutritional, and Metabolic Disorders with MCC	3.9577
617	Amputation of Lower Limb for Endocrine, Nutritional, and Metabolic Disorders with CC	1.9845

DRG	PDx/SDx/Procedure	Tips
040	Diabetes with neurological manifestations (e.g., neurogenic arthropathy, peripheral autonomic neuropathy, polyneuropathy)	According to ICD-10-CM guidelines, the classification presumes a causal relationship between diabetes and certain associated manifestations and/or conditions when these terms are linked by the term "with" in the alphabetic index (either under a main term or subterm). These conditions should be coded as related to the diabetes unless the documentation clearly states the conditions are unrelated, in which case they may be coded separately. These conditions do not require provider documentation linking them to diabetes. Review the record and/or query the physician if it is unclear whether a condition is related to diabetes mellitus or the ICD-10-CM classification does not provide instruction.
	AND	
	Amputation of toe	
	AND	
	MCC condition	*See* appendix B.
041	Diabetes with neurological manifestations (e.g., neurogenic arthropathy, peripheral autonomic neuropathy, polyneuropathy)	*See* DRG 040.
	AND	
	Amputation of toe	
	AND	
	CC condition	*See* appendix B.
239	Diabetes with circulatory complications (e.g., peripheral angiopathy, with or without gangrene)	*See* DRG 040.
	AND	
	Amputation of foot complete or complete or partial ray	
	AND	
	MCC condition	*See* appendix B.
240	Diabetes with circulatory complications (e.g., peripheral angiopathy, with or without gangrene)	*See* DRG 040.
	AND	
	Amputation of foot complete or complete or partial ray	
	AND	
	CC condition	*See* appendix B.
255	Diabetes with circulatory complications (e.g., peripheral angiopathy, with or without gangrene)	*See* DRG 040.
	AND	
	Amputation of toe	
	AND	
	MCC condition	*See* appendix B.
463	Musculoskeletal and connective tissue principal diagnosis	
	Osteomyelitis, all types (except diabetic)	
	Open wounds (lacerations) with tendon involvement	Laceration tendon—*see* Injury, muscle, by site, laceration
	AND	
	Excisional debridement of skin wound, infection, or burn	The ICD-10-PCS definition of the root operation Excision is "Cutting out or off, without replacement, a portion of a body part." Debridement by excision involves cutting with a sharp instrument such as a scalpel or other methods such as a hot knife or laser. Non-excisional debridement of skin is coded to root operation Extraction. Ensure that documentation includes instruments used, technique, and depth of debridement procedure.
	OR	
	Skin grafting procedure	Skin grafting includes root operations Replacement of skin with a free graft of autologous (partial or full thickness), nonautologous or synthetic tissue; and Transfer of skin, and/or subcutaneous tissue and fascia which remains attached to its vascular and nervous supply. Other procedures include Excision and Supplement of tissues and Insertion of tissue expander.
	AND	
	MCC condition	*See* appendix B.

DRG 504 (Continued)

DRG	PDx/SDx/Procedure	Tips
464	Musculoskeletal and connective tissue principal diagnosis	
	Osteomyelitis, all types (except diabetic)	
	Open wounds (lacerations) with tendon involvement	Laceration tendon—*see* Injury, muscle, by site, laceration
	AND	
	Excisional debridement of skin wound, infection, or burn	*See* DRG 463.
	OR	
	Skin grafting procedure	*See* DRG 463.
	AND	
	CC condition	*See* appendix B.
474	Upper and lower limb amputations	
	AND	
	MCC condition	*See* appendix B.
475	Upper and lower limb amputations	
	AND	
	CC condition	*See* appendix B.
503	MCC condition	*See* appendix B.
616	Diabetes (type 1, type 2, other specified) with ketoacidosis, hyperosmolarity, other coma, other and unspecified complications	
	Diabetic foot or other skin ulcer principal diagnosis	
	AND	
	Amputation of toe	
	AND	
	MCC condition	*See* appendix B.
617	Diabetes (type 1, type 2, other specified) with ketoacidosis, hyperosmolarity, other coma, other and unspecified complications	
	Diabetic foot or other skin ulcer principal diagnosis	
	AND	
	Amputation of toe	
	AND	
	CC condition	*See* appendix B.

DRG 505 Foot Procedures without CC/MCC RW 1.7057

Potential DRGs

040	Peripheral/Cranial Nerve and Other Nervous System Procedures with MCC	3.8505
041	Peripheral/Cranial Nerve and Other Nervous System Procedures with CC or Peripheral Neurostimulator	2.2307
042	Peripheral/Cranial Nerve and Other Nervous System Procedures without CC/MCC	1.7398
239	Amputation for Circulatory System Disorders Except Upper Limb and Toe with MCC	4.8068
240	Amputation for Circulatory System Disorders Except Upper Limb and Toe with CC	2.8092
255	Upper Limb and Toe Amputation for Circulatory System Disorders with MCC	2.7474
463	Wound Debridement and Skin Graft Except Hand for Musculoskeletal and Connective Tissue Disorders with MCC	5.6637
464	Wound Debridement and Skin Graft Except Hand for Musculoskeletal and Connective Tissue Disorders with CC	3.0014
465	Wound Debridement and Skin Graft Except Hand for Musculoskeletal and Connective Tissue Disorders without CC/MCC	1.8708
474	Amputation for Musculoskeletal System and Connective Tissue Disorders with MCC	4.3028
475	Amputation for Musculoskeletal System and Connective Tissue Disorders with CC	2.1447
503	Foot Procedures with MCC	2.6819
504	Foot Procedures with CC	1.7271
616	Amputation of Lower Limb for Endocrine, Nutritional, and Metabolic Disorders with MCC	3.9577
617	Amputation of Lower Limb for Endocrine, Nutritional, and Metabolic Disorders with CC	1.9845

DRG	PDx/SDx/Procedure	Tips
040	Diabetes with neurological manifestations (e.g., neurogenic arthropathy, peripheral autonomic, neuropathy, polyneuropathy)	According to ICD-10-CM guidelines, the classification presumes a causal relationship between diabetes and certain associated manifestations and/or conditions when these terms are linked by the term "with" in the alphabetic index (either under a main term or subterm). These conditions should be coded as related to the diabetes unless the documentation clearly states the conditions are unrelated, in which case they may be coded separately. These conditions do not require provider documentation linking them to diabetes. Review the record and/or query the physician if it is unclear whether a condition is related to diabetes mellitus or the ICD-10-CM classification does not provide instruction.
	AND	
	Amputation of toe	
	AND	
	MCC condition	*See* appendix B.
041	Diabetes with neurological manifestations (e.g., neurogenic arthropathy, peripheral autonomic neuropathy, polyneuropathy)	*See* DRG 040.
	AND	
	Amputation of toe	
	AND	
	CC condition	*See* appendix B.
042	Diabetes with neurological manifestations (e.g., neurogenic arthropathy, peripheral autonomic neuropathy, polyneuropathy)	*See* DRG 040.
	AND	
	Amputation of toe	
239	Diabetes with circulatory complications (e.g., peripheral angiopathy, with or without gangrene)	*See* DRG 040.
	AND	
	Amputation of foot complete or complete or partial ray	
	AND	
	MCC condition	*See* appendix B.
240	Diabetes with circulatory complications (e.g., peripheral angiopathy, with or without gangrene)	*See* DRG 040.
	AND	
	Amputation of foot complete or complete or partial ray	
	AND	
	CC condition	*See* appendix B.
255	Diabetes with circulatory complications (e.g., peripheral angiopathy, with or without gangrene)	*See* DRG 040.
	AND	
	Amputation of toe	
	AND	
	MCC condition	*See* appendix B.

DRG 505 (Continued)

DRG	PDx/SDx/Procedure	Tips
463	Musculoskeletal and connective tissue principal diagnosis	
	Osteomyelitis, all types (except diabetic)	
	Open wounds (lacerations) with tendon involvement	Laceration tendon—*see* Injury, muscle, by site, laceration
	AND	
	Excisional debridement of skin wound, infection, or burn	The ICD-10-PCS definition of the root operation Excision is "Cutting out or off, without replacement, a portion of a body part." Debridement by excision involves cutting with a sharp instrument such as a scalpel or other methods such as a hot knife or laser. Non-excisional debridement of skin is coded to root operation Extraction. Ensure that documentation includes instruments used, technique, and depth of debridement procedure.
	OR	
	Skin grafting procedure	Skin grafting includes root operations Replacement of skin with a free graft of autologous (partial or full thickness), nonautologous or synthetic tissue; and Transfer of skin, and/or subcutaneous tissue and fascia which remains attached to its vascular and nervous supply. Other procedures include Excision and Supplement of tissues and Insertion of tissue expander.
	AND	
	MCC condition	*See* appendix B.
464	Musculoskeletal and connective tissue principal diagnosis	
	Osteomyelitis, all types (except diabetic)	
	Open wounds (lacerations) with tendon involvement	Laceration tendon—*see* Injury, muscle, by site, laceration
	AND	
	Excisional debridement of skin wound, infection, or burn	*See* DRG 463.
	OR	
	Skin grafting procedure	*See* DRG 463.
	AND	
	CC condition	*See* appendix B.
465	Musculoskeletal and connective tissue principal diagnosis	
	Osteomyelitis, all types (except diabetic)	
	Open wounds (lacerations) with tendon involvement	Laceration tendon—*see* Injury, muscle, by site, laceration
	AND	
	Excisional debridement of skin wound, infection, or burn	*See* DRG 463.
	OR	
	Skin grafting procedure	*See* DRG 463.
474	Upper and lower limb amputations	
	AND	
	MCC condition	*See* appendix B.
475	Upper and lower limb amputations	
	AND	
	CC condition	*See* appendix B.
503	MCC condition	*See* appendix B.
504	CC condition	*See* appendix B.
616	Diabetes (type 1, type 2, other specified) with ketoacidosis, hyperosmolarity, other coma, other and unspecified complications	
	Diabetic foot or other skin ulcer principal diagnosis	
	AND	
	Amputation of toe	
	AND	
	MCC condition	*See* appendix B.
617	Diabetes (type 1, type 2, other specified) with ketoacidosis, hyperosmolarity, other coma, other and unspecified complications	
	Diabetic foot or other skin ulcer principal diagnosis	
	AND	
	Amputation of toe	
	AND	
	CC condition	*See* appendix B.

DRG 506 Major Thumb or Joint Procedures — RW 1.4626

Potential DRGs

477	Biopsies of Musculoskeletal System and Connective Tissue with MCC	3.3690
478	Biopsies of Musculoskeletal System and Connective Tissue with CC	2.3837
479	Biopsies of Musculoskeletal System and Connective Tissue without CC/MCC	1.8640
500	Soft Tissue Procedures with MCC	3.2428
501	Soft Tissue Procedures with CC	1.7357

DRG	PDx/SDx/Procedure	Tips
477	Biopsy of bone	
	AND	
	MCC condition	*See* appendix B.
478	Biopsy of bone	
	AND	
	CC condition	*See* appendix B.
479	Biopsy of bone	
500	Diagnostic drainage of hand muscle or tendon	
	Excisional biopsy of hand muscle or tendon	
	Hand bursa or ligament suture (repair)	
	Hand subcutaneous tissue and fascia or bursa/ligament graft (transfer)	
	AND	
	MCC condition	*See* appendix B.
501	Diagnostic drainage of hand muscle or tendon	
	Excisional biopsy of hand muscle or tendon	
	Hand bursa or ligament suture (repair)	
	Hand subcutaneous tissue and fascia or bursa/ligament graft (transfer)	
	AND	
	CC condition	*See* appendix B.

DRG 507 Major Shoulder or Elbow Joint Procedures with CC/MCC — RW 2.1317

Potential DRGs

483	Major Joint/Limb Reattachment Procedure of Upper Extremities	2.4842

DRG	PDx/SDx/Procedure	Tips
483	Total, partial or reverse shoulder replacement	
	Total elbow replacement procedure	

DRG 508 Major Shoulder or Elbow Joint Procedures without CC/MCC — RW 1.4340

Potential DRGs

483	Major Joint/Limb Reattachment Procedure of Upper Extremities	2.4842
507	Major Shoulder or Elbow Joint Procedures with CC/MCC	2.1317

DRG	PDx/SDx/Procedure	Tips
483	Total, partial or reverse shoulder replacement	
	Total elbow replacement procedure	
507	CC/MCC condition	*See* appendix B.

DRG 509 Arthroscopy — RW 1.3262

Potential DRGs

485	Knee Procedures with Principal Diagnosis of Infection with MCC	3.2940
486	Knee Procedures with Principal Diagnosis of Infection with CC	2.0083
488	Knee Procedures without Principal Diagnosis of Infection with CC/MCC	2.1066
507	Major Shoulder or Elbow Joint Procedures with CC/MCC	2.1317
508	Major Shoulder or Elbow Joint Procedures without CC/MCC	1.4340

DRG	PDx/SDx/Procedure	Tips
485	Principal diagnosis of infection	Ensure that all procedures performed arthroscopically are coded.
	Arthroscopic knee procedures: meniscectomy, synovectomy, drainage (with device) of bursa or ligament, repair of knee joint structure or bursa or ligament	
	Arthroscopic lysis of knee joint adhesions or removal of foreign body from knee joint	
	AND	
	MCC condition	*See* appendix B.
486	Principal diagnosis of infection	Ensure that all procedures performed arthroscopically are coded.
	Arthroscopic knee procedures: meniscectomy, synovectomy, drainage (with device) of bursa or ligament, repair of knee joint structure or bursa or ligament	
	Arthroscopic lysis of knee joint adhesions or removal of foreign body from knee joint	
	AND	
	CC condition	*See* appendix B.
488	Arthroscopic knee procedures: meniscectomy, synovectomy, drainage (with device) of bursa or ligament, repair of knee joint structure or bursa or ligament	*See* DRG 486.
	Arthroscopic lysis of knee joint adhesions or removal of foreign body from knee joint	
507	Arthroscopic drainage of shoulder bursa or ligament	
	Arthroscopic removal of foreign body from sternoclavicular, acromioclavicular, or shoulder joint (Extirpation)	
	Arthroscopic repair of shoulder joint, sternoclavicular joint, or acromioclavicular joint	
	AND	
	CC/MCC condition	*See* appendix B.
508	Arthroscopic drainage of shoulder bursa or ligament	
	Arthroscopic removal of foreign body from sternoclavicular, acromioclavicular, or shoulder joint (Extirpation)	
	Arthroscopic repair of shoulder joint, sternoclavicular joint, or acromioclavicular joint	

DRG 510 Shoulder, Elbow or Forearm Procedure, Except Major Joint Procedure with MCC — RW 2.7206

No Potential DRGs

DRG 511 Shoulder, Elbow or Forearm Procedure, Except Major Joint Procedure with CC — RW 1.9938

Potential DRGs

483	Major Joint/Limb Reattachment Procedure of Upper Extremities	2.4842
510	Shoulder, Elbow or Forearm Procedure, Except Major Joint Procedure with MCC	2.7206

DRG	PDx/SDx/Procedure	Tips
483	Total, partial or reverse shoulder replacement	
	Total elbow replacement procedure	
510	MCC condition	*See* appendix B.

DRG 512 Shoulder, Elbow or Forearm Procedure, Except Major Joint Procedure without CC/MCC — RW 1.6138

Potential DRGs

483	Major Joint/Limb Reattachment Procedure of Upper Extremities	2.4842
507	Major Shoulder or Elbow Joint Procedures with CC/MCC	2.1317
510	Shoulder, Elbow or Forearm Procedure, Except Major Joint Procedure with MCC	2.7206
511	Shoulder, Elbow or Forearm Procedure, Except Major Joint Procedure with CC	1.9938

DRG	PDx/SDx/Procedure	Tips
483	Total, partial or reverse shoulder replacement	
	Total elbow replacement procedure	
507	Arthroscopic drainage of shoulder bursa or ligament	
	Arthroscopic removal of foreign body from sternoclavicular, acromioclavicular, or shoulder joint (Extirpation)	
	Arthroscopic repair of shoulder joint, sternoclavicular joint, or acromioclavicular joint	
	AND	
	CC/MCC condition	*See* appendix B.
510	MCC condition	*See* appendix B.
511	CC condition	*See* appendix B.

DRG 513 Hand or Wrist Procedures, Except Major Thumb or Joint Procedures with CC/MCC — RW 1.6210

Potential DRGs

255	Upper Limb and Toe Amputation for Circulatory System Disorders with MCC	2.7474
256	Upper Limb and Toe Amputation for Circulatory System Disorders with CC	1.6397

DRG	PDx/SDx/Procedure	Tips
255	Diabetes with circulatory complications (e.g., peripheral angiopathy, with or without gangrene)	According to ICD-10-CM guidelines, the classification presumes a causal relationship between diabetes and certain associated manifestations and/or conditions when these terms are linked by the term "with" in the alphabetic index (either under a main term or subterm). These conditions should be coded as related to the diabetes unless the documentation clearly states the conditions are unrelated, in which case they may be coded separately. These conditions do not require provider documentation linking them to diabetes. Review the record and/or query the physician if it is unclear whether a condition is related to diabetes mellitus or the ICD-10-CM classification does not provide instruction.
	AND	
	Finger or thumb amputation	
	AND	
	MCC condition	*See* appendix B.
256	Diabetes with circulatory complications (e.g., peripheral angiopathy, with or without gangrene)	*See* DRG 255.
	AND	
	Finger or thumb amputation	
	AND	
	CC condition	*See* appendix B.

DRG 514 Hand or Wrist Procedures, Except Major Thumb or Joint Procedures without CC/MCC — RW 1.0415

Potential DRGs

255	Upper Limb and Toe Amputation for Circulatory System Disorders with MCC	2.7474
256	Upper Limb and Toe Amputation for Circulatory System Disorders with CC	1.6397
506	Major Thumb or Joint Procedures	1.4626
513	Hand or Wrist Procedures, Except Major Thumb or Joint Procedures with CC/MCC	1.6210

DRG	PDx/SDx/Procedure	Tips
255	Diabetes with circulatory complications (e.g., peripheral angiopathy, with or without gangrene)	According to ICD-10-CM guidelines, the classification presumes a causal relationship between diabetes and certain associated manifestations and/or conditions when these terms are linked by the term "with" in the alphabetic index (either under a main term or subterm). These conditions should be coded as related to the diabetes unless the documentation clearly states the conditions are unrelated, in which case they may be coded separately. These conditions do not require provider documentation linking them to diabetes. Review the record and/or query the physician if it is unclear whether a condition is related to diabetes mellitus or the ICD-10-CM classification does not provide instruction.
	AND	
	Finger or thumb amputation	
	AND	
	MCC condition	*See* appendix B.
256	Diabetes with circulatory complications (e.g., peripheral angiopathy, with or without gangrene)	*See* DRG 255.
	AND	
	Finger or thumb amputation	
	AND	
	CC condition	*See* appendix B.
506	Arthroplasty and repair of hand, fingers and wrist	
	Reconstruction of thumb	
513	CC/MCC condition	*See* appendix B.

DRG 515 Other Musculoskeletal System and Connective Tissue O.R. Procedure with MCC — RW 3.1615

No Potential DRGs

DRG 516 Other Musculoskeletal System and Connective Tissue O.R. Procedure with CC — RW 2.0408

Potential DRGs

515	Other Musculoskeletal System and Connective Tissue O.R. Procedure with MCC	3.1615

DRG	PDx/SDx/Procedure	Tips
515	MCC condition	*See* appendix B.

DRG 517 Other Musculoskeletal System and Connective Tissue O.R. Procedure without CC/MCC

RW 1.4944

Potential DRGs

515	Other Musculoskeletal System and Connective Tissue O.R. Procedure with MCC	3.1615
516	Other Musculoskeletal System and Connective Tissue O.R. Procedure with CC	2.0408

DRG	PDx/SDx/Procedure	Tips
515	MCC condition	*See* appendix B.
516	CC condition	*See* appendix B.

DRG 518 Back and Neck Procedures Except Spinal Fusion with MCC or Disc Device/Neurostimulator

RW 3.6518

Potential DRGs

453	Combined Anterior/Posterior Spinal Fusion with MCC	8.8614
456	Spinal Fusion Except Cervical with Spinal Curvature/Malignancy/Infection or Extensive Fusions with MCC	8.4294
459	Spinal Fusion Except Cervical with MCC	6.6323
471	Cervical Spinal Fusion with MCC	4.9190

DRG	PDx/SDx/Procedure	Tips
453	Combination of anterior and posterior spinal fusion or refusion techniques	The anterior column may be fused using an anterior, lateral, or posterior technique. The posterior column may be fused using a posterior, posterolateral, or lateral transverse technique. Two operative notes may be dictated for different incisions/approaches. ICD-10-PCS Coding Guideline B3.10c states "if an interbody fusion device is used to render the joint immobile (containing bone graft or bone graft substitute), the procedure is coded with the device value Interbody Fusion Device." The fixation instrumentation (i.e., rods, plates, screws, etc.) is included in the fusion root operation, and no additional code is assigned.
	AND	
	MCC condition	*See* appendix B.
456	Noncervical spinal fusions with principal diagnosis of noncervical curvature of spine, infection, or malignancy	Review operative report for indication of metastasis. Clarify with physician if pathological fracture is noted and whether it was possibly due to metastasis when patient has previous history of malignancy.
	OR	
	Principal or secondary diagnosis of secondary kyphosis, lordosis, scoliosis, or other specific deforming dorsopathies	A code for the underlying disease or condition must be reported first before the code for secondary kyphosis or secondary scoliosis, per the "code first underlying disease" instructional note. Neuromuscular scoliosis can be assigned as principal diagnosis with the underlying condition coded as a secondary diagnosis.
	OR	
	Fusion of 8 or more thoracic vertebral segments	
	OR	
	Fusion of 2-7 thoracic vertebral segments	
	AND	
	Fusion of 2 or more lumbar vertebral segments	
	AND	
	MCC condition	*See* appendix B.
459	Any diagnosis in MDC 8 other than spinal curvature, malignancy, or infection	
	AND	
	Any spinal fusion or refusion except cervical, any technique	
	AND	
	MCC condition	*See* appendix B.
471	Fusion of cervical vertebral segments	
	AND	
	MCC condition	*See* appendix B.

DRG 519 Back and Neck Procedures Except Spinal Fusion with CC RW 1.9686

Potential DRGs

453	Combined Anterior/Posterior Spinal Fusion with MCC	8.8614
454	Combined Anterior/Posterior Spinal Fusion with CC	6.1163
456	Spinal Fusion Except Cervical with Spinal Curvature/Malignancy/Infection or Extensive Fusions with MCC	8.4294
457	Spinal Fusion Except Cervical with Spinal Curvature/Malignancy/Infection or Extensive Fusions with CC	6.0753
459	Spinal Fusion Except Cervical with MCC	6.6323
460	Spinal Fusion Except Cervical without MCC	3.6579
471	Cervical Spinal Fusion with MCC	4.9190
472	Cervical Spinal Fusion with CC	2.9554
518	Back and Neck Procedures Except Spinal Fusion with MCC or Disc Device/Neurostimulator	3.6518

DRG	PDx/SDx/Procedure	Tips
453	Combination of anterior and posterior spinal fusion or refusion techniques	The anterior column may be fused using an anterior, lateral, or posterior technique. The posterior column may be fused using a posterior, posterolateral, or lateral transverse technique. Two operative notes may be dictated for different incisions/approaches. ICD-10-PCS Coding Guideline B3.10c states "if an interbody fusion device is used to render the joint immobile (containing bone graft or bone graft substitute), the procedure is coded with the device value Interbody Fusion Device." The fixation instrumentation (i.e., rods, plates, screws, etc.) is included in the Fusion root operation, and no additional code is assigned.
	AND	
	MCC condition	*See* appendix B.
454	Combination of anterior and posterior spinal fusion or refusion techniques	*See* DRG 453.
	AND	
	CC condition	*See* appendix B.
456	Noncervical spinal fusions with principal diagnosis of noncervical curvature of spine, infection, or malignancy	Review operative report for indication of metastasis. Clarify with physician if pathological fracture is noted and whether it was possibly due to metastasis when patient has previous history of malignancy.
	OR	
	Principal or secondary diagnosis of secondary kyphosis, lordosis, scoliosis, or other specific deforming dorsopathies	A code for the underlying disease or condition must be reported first before the code for secondary kyphosis or secondary scoliosis, per the "code first underlying disease" instructional note. Neuromuscular scoliosis can be assigned as principal diagnosis with the underlying condition coded as a secondary diagnosis.
	OR	
	Fusion of 8 or more thoracic vertebral segments	
	OR	
	Fusion of 2-7 thoracic vertebral segments	
	AND	
	Fusion of 2 or more lumbar vertebral segments	
	AND	
	MCC condition	*See* appendix B.
457	Noncervical spinal fusions with principal diagnosis of noncervical curvature of spine, infection, or malignancy	*See* DRG 456.
	OR	
	Principal or secondary diagnosis of secondary kyphosis, lordosis, scoliosis, or other specific deforming dorsopathies	*See* DRG 456.
	OR	
	Fusion of 8 or more thoracic vertebral segments	
	OR	
	Fusion of 2-7 thoracic vertebral segments	
	AND	
	Fusion of 2 or more lumbar vertebral segments	
	AND	
	CC condition	*See* appendix B.
459	Any diagnosis in MDC 8 other than spinal curvature, malignancy, or infection	
	AND	
	Any spinal fusion or refusion except cervical, any technique	
	AND	
	MCC condition	*See* appendix B.
460	Any diagnosis in MDC 8 other than spinal curvature, malignancy, or infection	
	AND	
	Any spinal fusion or refusion except cervical, any technique	
471	Fusion of cervical vertebral segments	
	AND	
	MCC condition	*See* appendix B.
472	Fusion of cervical vertebral segments	
	AND	
	CC condition	*See* appendix B.
518	MCC condition	*See* appendix B.
	OR	
	Disc device or neurostimulator implant	

DRG 520 Back and Neck Procedures Except Spinal Fusion without CC/MCC RW 1.4315

Potential DRGs

453	Combined Anterior/Posterior Spinal Fusion with MCC	8.8614
454	Combined Anterior/Posterior Spinal Fusion with CC	6.1163
455	Combined Anterior/Posterior Spinal Fusion without CC/MCC	4.6056
456	Spinal Fusion Except Cervical with Spinal Curvature/Malignancy/Infection or Extensive Fusions with MCC	8.4294
457	Spinal Fusion Except Cervical with Spinal Curvature/Malignancy/Infection or Extensive Fusions with CC	6.0753
458	Spinal Fusion Except Cervical with Spinal Curvature/Malignancy/Infection or Extensive Fusions without CC/MCC	4.5310
459	Spinal Fusion Except Cervical with MCC	6.6323
460	Spinal Fusion Except Cervical without MCC	3.6579
471	Cervical Spinal Fusion with MCC	4.9190
472	Cervical Spinal Fusion with CC	2.9554
473	Cervical Spinal Fusion without CC/MCC	2.4606
518	Back and Neck Procedures Except Spinal Fusion with MCC or Disc Device/Neurostimulator	3.6518
519	Back and Neck Procedures Except Spinal Fusion with CC	1.9686

DRG	PDx/SDx/Procedure	Tips
453	Combination of anterior and posterior spinal fusion or refusion techniques	The anterior column may be fused using an anterior, lateral, or posterior technique. The posterior column may be fused using a posterior, posterolateral, or lateral transverse technique. Two operative notes may be dictated for different incisions/approaches. ICD-10-PCS Coding Guideline B3.10c states "if an interbody fusion device is used to render the joint immobile (containing bone graft or bone graft substitute), the procedure is coded with the device value Interbody Fusion Device." The fixation instrumentation (i.e., rods, plates, screws, etc.) is included in the Fusion root operation, and no additional code is assigned.
	AND	
	MCC condition	*See* appendix B.
454	Combination of anterior and posterior spinal fusion or refusion techniques	*See* DRG 453.
	AND	
	CC condition	*See* appendix B.
455	Combination of anterior and posterior spinal fusion or refusion techniques	*See* DRG 453.
456	Noncervical spinal fusions with principal diagnosis of noncervical curvature of spine, infection, or malignancy	Review operative report for indication of metastasis. Clarify with physician if pathological fracture is noted and whether it was possibly due to metastasis when patient has previous history of malignancy.
	OR	
	Principal or secondary diagnosis of secondary kyphosis, lordosis, scoliosis, or other specific deforming dorsopathies	A code for the underlying disease or condition must be reported first before the code for secondary kyphosis or secondary scoliosis, per the "code first underlying disease" instructional note. Neuromuscular scoliosis can be assigned as principal diagnosis with the underlying condition coded as a secondary diagnosis.
	OR	
	Fusion of 8 or more thoracic vertebral segments	
	OR	
	Fusion of 2-7 thoracic vertebral segments	
	AND	
	Fusion of 2 or more lumbar vertebral segments	
	AND	
	MCC condition	*See* appendix B.
457	Noncervical spinal fusions with principal diagnosis of noncervical curvature of spine, infection, or malignancy	*See* DRG 456.
	OR	
	Principal or secondary diagnosis of secondary kyphosis, lordosis, scoliosis, or other specific deforming dorsopathies	*See* DRG 456.
	OR	
	Fusion of 8 or more thoracic vertebral segments	
	OR	
	Fusion of 2-7 thoracic vertebral segments	
	AND	
	Fusion of 2 or more lumbar vertebral segments	
	AND	
	CC condition	*See* appendix B.
458	Noncervical spinal fusions with principal diagnosis of noncervical curvature of spine, infection, or malignancy	*See* DRG 456.
	OR	
	Principal or secondary diagnosis of secondary kyphosis, lordosis, scoliosis, or other specific deforming dorsopathies	*See* DRG 456.
	OR	
	Fusion of 8 or more thoracic vertebral segments	
	OR	
	Fusion of 2-7 thoracic vertebral segments	
	AND	
	Fusion of 2 or more lumbar vertebral segments	

DRG 520 (Continued)

DRG	PDx/SDx/Procedure	Tips
459	Any diagnosis in MDC 8 other than spinal curvature, malignancy, or infection	
	AND	
	Any spinal fusion or refusion except cervical, any technique	
	AND	
	MCC condition	*See* appendix B.
460	Any diagnosis in MDC 8 other than spinal curvature, malignancy, or infection	
	AND	
	Any spinal fusion or refusion except cervical, any technique	
471	Fusion of cervical vertebral segments	
	AND	
	MCC condition	*See* appendix B.
472	Fusion of cervical vertebral segments	
	AND	
	CC condition	*See* appendix B.
473	Fusion of cervical vertebral segments	
518	MCC condition	*See* appendix B.
	OR	
	Disc device or neurostimulator implant	
519	CC condition	*See* appendix B.

DRG 521 Hip Replacement with Principal Diagnosis of Hip Fracture with MCC — RW 2.9942

Potential DRGs

461 Bilateral or Multiple Major Joint Procedures of Lower Extremity with MCC 6.8185

DRG	PDx/SDx/Procedure	Tips
461	Any combination of partial or total knee, hip or ankle joint replacement procedures	
	AND	
	MCC condition	*See* appendix B.

DRG 522 Hip Replacement with Principal Diagnosis of Hip Fracture without MCC — RW 2.1122

Potential DRGs

461 Bilateral or Multiple Major Joint Procedures of Lower Extremity with MCC 6.8185
462 Bilateral or Multiple Major Joint Procedures of Lower Extremity without MCC 2.8463
521 Hip Replacement with Principal Diagnosis of Hip Fracture with MCC 2.9942

DRG	PDx/SDx/Procedure	Tips
461	Any combination of partial or total knee, hip or ankle joint replacement procedures	
	AND	
	MCC condition	*See* appendix B.
462	Any combination of partial or total knee, hip or ankle joint replacement procedures	
521	MCC condition	*See* appendix B.

DRG 533 Fractures of Femur with MCC — RW 1.6314

Potential DRGs

480 Hip and Femur Procedures Except Major Joint with MCC 2.9489
956 Limb Reattachment, Hip and Femur Procedures for Multiple Significant Trauma 3.8782
963 Other Multiple Significant Trauma with MCC 2.7343

DRG	PDx/SDx/Procedure	Tips
480	Reduction of femur fracture (reposition) with or without internal/external fixation, open approach	
	Reduction of femur fracture with internal/external fixation, percutaneous or percutaneous endoscopic approach	
	AND	
	MCC condition	*See* appendix B.
956	Multiple significant trauma	Principal diagnosis of trauma and two or more different dx from two different body site categories in MS-DRG 963.
	AND	
	Reduction of femur fracture (reposition) with or without internal/external fixation, open approach	
	Reduction of femur fracture with internal/external fixation, percutaneous or percutaneous endoscopic approach	
963	Multiple significant trauma	Principal diagnosis of trauma and two or more different dx from two different body site categories in MS-DRG 963.
	AND	
	MCC condition	*See* appendix B.

DRG 534 Fractures of Femur without MCC

RW 0.8100

Potential DRGs

480	Hip and Femur Procedures Except Major Joint with MCC	2.9489
481	Hip and Femur Procedures Except Major Joint with CC	2.0749
482	Hip and Femur Procedures Except Major Joint without CC/MCC	1.5884
533	Fractures of Femur with MCC	1.6314
956	Limb Reattachment, Hip and Femur Procedures for Multiple Significant Trauma	3.8782
963	Other Multiple Significant Trauma with MCC	2.7343
964	Other Multiple Significant Trauma with CC	1.5010
965	Other Multiple Significant Trauma without CC/MCC	0.9559

DRG	PDx/SDx/Procedure	Tips
480	Reduction of femur fracture (reposition) with or without internal/external fixation, open approach	
	Reduction of femur fracture with internal/external fixation, percutaneous or percutaneous endoscopic approach	
	AND	
	MCC condition	*See* appendix B.
481	Reduction of femur fracture (reposition) with or without internal/external fixation, open approach	
	Reduction of femur fracture with internal/external fixation, percutaneous or percutaneous endoscopic approach	
	AND	
	CC condition	*See* appendix B.
482	Reduction of femur fracture (reposition) with or without internal/external fixation, open approach	
	Reduction of femur fracture with internal/external fixation, percutaneous or percutaneous endoscopic approach	
533	MCC condition	*See* appendix B.
956	Multiple significant trauma	Principal diagnosis of trauma and two or more different dx from two different body site categories in MS-DRG 963.
	AND	
	Reduction of femur fracture (reposition) with or without internal/external fixation, open approach	
	Reduction of femur fracture with internal/external fixation, percutaneous or percutaneous endoscopic approach	
963	Multiple significant trauma	Principal diagnosis of trauma and two or more different dx from two different body site categories in MS-DRG 963.
	AND	
	MCC condition	*See* appendix B.
964	Multiple significant trauma	Principal diagnosis of trauma and two or more different dx from two different body site categories in MS-DRG 963.
	AND	
	CC condition	*See* appendix B.
965	Multiple significant trauma	Principal diagnosis of trauma and two or more different dx from two different body site categories in MS-DRG 963.

DRG 535 Fractures of Hip and Pelvis with MCC RW 1.2967

Potential DRGs

466	Revision of Hip or Knee Replacement with MCC	5.1866
469	Major Hip and Knee Joint Replacement or Reattachment of Lower Extremity with MCC or Total Ankle Replacement	3.3298
515	Other Musculoskeletal System and Connective Tissue O.R. Procedures with MCC	3.1615
542	Pathological Fractures and Musculoskeletal and Connective Tissue Malignancy with MCC	1.8237
956	Limb Reattachment, Hip and Femur Procedures for Multiple Significant Trauma	3.8782
963	Other Multiple Significant Trauma with MCC	2.7343

DRG	PDx/SDx/Procedure	Tips
466	Revision of hip replacement procedure	ICD-10-PCS root operation Revision is defined as: "Correcting, to the extent possible, a portion of a malfunctioning device or the position of a displaced device." Explanation: Revision can include correcting a malfunctioning or displaced device by taking out or putting in components of the device such as a screw or pin. Example: recementing of hip prosthesis.
	OR	
	Removal and replacement of hip prosthesis	Joint revisions must include both the removal of a joint prosthesis, liner, resurfacing device, or spacer and the subsequent insertion of a new joint prosthesis (Replacement) or liner (Supplement), either cemented or uncemented, performed via an open approach.
	AND	
	MCC condition	*See* appendix B.
469	Resurfacing procedure, total or partial hip replacement	
	AND	
	MCC condition	*See* appendix B.
515	Reposition of pelvic/acetabulum with or without internal/external fixation, open approach	
	Reposition of pelvic/acetabulum with internal/external fixation, percutaneous or percutaneous endoscopic approach	
	Insertion of internal/external fixation (without repositioning) in pelvic bone or acetabulum	
	AND	
	MCC condition	*See* appendix B.
542	Fatigue, stress or pathologic fracture	
	AND	
	MCC condition	*See* appendix B.
956	Multiple significant trauma	Principal diagnosis of trauma and two or more different dx from two different body site categories in MS-DRG 963.
	AND	
	Reduction of femur fracture (reposition) with or without internal/external fixation, open approach	
	Reduction of femur fracture with internal/external fixation, percutaneous or percutaneous endoscopic approach	
963	Multiple significant trauma	Principal diagnosis of trauma and two or more different dx from two different body site categories in MS-DRG 963.
	AND	
	MCC condition	*See* appendix B.

DRG 536 Fractures of Hip and Pelvis without MCC

RW 0.7871

Potential DRGs

466	Revision of Hip or Knee Replacement with MCC	5.1866
467	Revision of Hip or Knee Replacement with CC	3.4863
468	Revision of Hip or Knee Replacement without CC/MCC	2.6696
469	Major Hip and Knee Joint Replacement or Reattachment of Lower Extremity with MCC or Total Ankle Replacement	3.3298
470	Major Hip and Knee Joint Replacement or Reattachment of Lower Extremity without MCC	1.8817
515	Other Musculoskeletal System and Connective Tissue O.R. Procedures with MCC	3.1615
516	Other Musculoskeletal System and Connective Tissue O.R. Procedures with CC	2.0408
517	Other Musculoskeletal System and Connective Tissue O.R. Procedures without CC/MCC	1.4944
535	Fractures of Hip and Pelvis with MCC	1.2967
542	Pathological Fractures and Musculoskeletal and Connective Tissue Malignancy with MCC	1.8237
543	Pathological Fractures and Musculoskeletal and Connective Tissue Malignancy with CC	1.0907
956	Limb Reattachment, Hip and Femur Procedures for Multiple Significant Trauma	3.8782
963	Other Multiple Significant Trauma with MCC	2.7343
964	Other Multiple Significant Trauma with CC	1.5010
965	Other Multiple Significant Trauma without CC/MCC	0.9559

DRG	PDx/SDx/Procedure	Tips
466	Revision of hip replacement procedure	ICD-10-PCS root operation Revision is defined as: "Correcting, to the extent possible, a portion of a malfunctioning device or the position of a displaced device." Explanation: Revision can include correcting a malfunctioning or displaced device by taking out or putting in components of the device such as a screw or pin. Example: recementing of hip prosthesis.
	OR	
	Removal and replacement of hip prosthesis	Joint revisions must include both the removal of a joint prosthesis, liner, resurfacing device, or spacer and the subsequent insertion of a new joint prosthesis (Replacement) or liner (Supplement), either cemented or uncemented, performed via an open approach.
	AND	
	MCC condition	*See* appendix B.
467	Revision of hip replacement procedure	*See* DRG 466.
	OR	
	Removal and replacement of hip prosthesis	*See* DRG 466.
	AND	
	CC condition	*See* appendix B.
468	Revision of hip replacement procedure	*See* DRG 466.
	OR	
	Removal and replacement of hip prosthesis	*See* DRG 466.
469	Resurfacing procedure, total or partial hip replacement	
	AND	
	MCC condition	*See* appendix B.
470	Resurfacing procedure, total or partial hip replacement	
515	Reposition of pelvic/acetabulum with or without internal/external fixation, open approach	
	Reposition of pelvic/acetabulum with internal/external fixation, percutaneous or percutaneous endoscopic approach	
	Insertion of internal/external fixation (without repositioning) in pelvic bone or acetabulum	
	AND	
	MCC condition	*See* appendix B.
516	Reposition of pelvic/acetabulum with or without internal/external fixation, open approach	
	Reposition of pelvic/acetabulum with internal/external fixation, percutaneous or percutaneous endoscopic approach	
	Insertion of internal/external fixation (without repositioning) in pelvic bone or acetabulum	
	AND	
	CC condition	*See* appendix B.
517	Reposition of pelvic/acetabulum with or without internal/external fixation, open approach	
	Reposition of pelvic/acetabulum with internal/external fixation, percutaneous or percutaneous endoscopic approach	
	Insertion of internal/external fixation (without repositioning) in pelvic bone or acetabulum	
535	MCC condition	*See* appendix B.
542	Fatigue, stress or pathologic fracture	
	AND	
	MCC condition	*See* appendix B.
543	Fatigue, stress or pathologic fracture	
	AND	
	CC condition	*See* appendix B.
956	Multiple significant trauma	Principal diagnosis of trauma and two or more different dx from two different body site categories in MS-DRG 963.
	AND	
	Reduction of femur fracture (reposition) with or without internal/external fixation, open approach	
	Reduction of femur fracture with internal/external fixation, percutaneous or percutaneous endoscopic approach	

DRG 536 (Continued)

DRG	PDx/SDx/Procedure	Tips
963	Multiple significant trauma	*See* DRG 956.
	AND	
	MCC condition	*See* appendix B.
964	Multiple significant trauma	*See* DRG 956.
	AND	
	CC condition	*See* appendix B.
965	Multiple significant trauma	*See* DRG 956.

DRG 537 Sprains, Strains, and Dislocations of Hip, Pelvis and Thigh with CC/MCC RW 0.9670

Potential DRGs

466	Revision of Hip or Knee Replacement with MCC	5.1866
467	Revision of Hip or Knee Replacement with CC	3.4863
469	Major Hip and Knee Joint Replacement or Reattachment of Lower Extremity with MCC or Total Ankle Replacement	3.3298
470	Major Hip and Knee Joint Replacement or Reattachment of Lower Extremity without MCC	1.8817
480	Hip and Femur Procedures Except Major Joint with MCC	2.9489
481	Hip and Femur Procedures Except Major Joint with CC	2.0749
535	Fractures of Hip and Pelvis with MCC	1.2967
542	Pathological Fractures and Musculoskeletal and Connective Tissue Malignancy with MCC	1.8237
543	Pathological Fractures and Musculoskeletal and Connective Tissue Malignancy with CC	1.0907

DRG	PDx/SDx/Procedure	Tips
466	Revision of hip replacement procedure	ICD-10-PCS root operation Revision is defined as: "Correcting, to the extent possible, a portion of a malfunctioning device or the position of a displaced device." Explanation: Revision can include correcting a malfunctioning or displaced device by taking out or putting in components of the device such as a screw or pin. Example: recementing of hip prosthesis.
	OR	
	Removal and replacement of hip prosthesis	Joint revisions must include both the removal of a joint prosthesis, liner, resurfacing device, or spacer and the subsequent insertion of a new joint prosthesis (Replacement) or liner (Supplement), either cemented or uncemented, performed via an open approach.
	AND	
	MCC condition	*See* appendix B.
467	Revision of hip replacement procedure	*See* DRG 466.
	OR	
	Removal and replacement of hip prosthesis	*See* DRG 466.
	AND	
	CC condition	*See* appendix B.
469	Resurfacing procedure, total or partial hip replacement	
	AND	
	MCC condition	*See* appendix B.
470	Resurfacing procedure, total or partial hip replacement	
480	Reposition hip joint	
	Fusion of hip joint	
	Insertion of internal/external fixation into hip joint	
	AND	
	MCC condition	*See* appendix B.
481	Reposition hip joint	
	Fusion of hip joint	
	Insertion of internal/external fixation into hip joint	
	AND	
	CC condition	*See* appendix B.
535	Fracture of hip and pelvis	
	AND	
	MCC condition	*See* appendix B.
542	Fatigue, stress or pathologic fracture	A code from category M80 Osteoporosis with current pathological fracture, not a traumatic fracture code, should be used for any patient with known osteoporosis who suffers a fracture, even if the patient had a minor fall or trauma, if that fall or trauma would not usually break a normal, healthy bone.
	AND	
	MCC condition	*See* appendix B.
543	Fatigue, stress or pathologic fracture	*See* DRG 542.
	AND	
	CC condition	*See* appendix B.

DRG 538 Sprains, Strains, and Dislocations of Hip, Pelvis and Thigh without CC/MCC RW 0.7091

Potential DRGs

466	Revision of Hip or Knee Replacement with MCC	5.1866
467	Revision of Hip or Knee Replacement with CC	3.4863
468	Revision of Hip or Knee Replacement without CC/MCC	2.6696
469	Major Hip and Knee Joint Replacement or Reattachment of Lower Extremity with MCC or Total Ankle Replacement	3.3298
470	Major Hip and Knee Joint Replacement or Reattachment of Lower Extremity without MCC	1.8817
480	Hip and Femur Procedures Except Major Joint with MCC	2.9489
481	Hip and Femur Procedures Except Major Joint with CC	2.0749
482	Hip and Femur Procedures Except Major Joint without CC/MCC	1.5884
535	Fractures of Hip and Pelvis with MCC	1.2967
536	Fractures of Hip and Pelvis without MCC	0.7871
537	Sprains, Strains, and Dislocations of Hip, Pelvis and Thigh with CC/MCC	0.9670
542	Pathological Fractures and Musculoskeletal and Connective Tissue Malignancy with MCC	1.8237
543	Pathological Fractures and Musculoskeletal and Connective Tissue Malignancy with CC	1.0907
544	Pathological Fractures and Musculoskeletal and Connective Tissue Malignancy without CC/MCC	0.7675

DRG	PDx/SDx/Procedure	Tips
466	Revision of hip replacement procedure	ICD-10-PCS root operation Revision is defined as: "Correcting, to the extent possible, a portion of a malfunctioning device or the position of a displaced device." Explanation: Revision can include correcting a malfunctioning or displaced device by taking out or putting in components of the device such as a screw or pin. Example: recementing of hip prosthesis.
	OR	
	Removal and replacement of hip prosthesis	Joint revisions must include both the removal of a joint prosthesis, liner, resurfacing device, or spacer and the subsequent insertion of a new joint prosthesis (Replacement) or liner (Supplement), either cemented or uncemented, performed via an open approach.
	AND	
	MCC condition	*See* appendix B.
467	Revision of hip replacement procedure	*See* DRG 466.
	OR	
	Removal and replacement of hip prosthesis	*See* DRG 466.
	AND	
	CC condition	*See* appendix B.
468	Revision of hip replacement procedure	*See* DRG 466.
	OR	
	Removal and replacement of hip prosthesis	*See* DRG 466.
469	Resurfacing procedure, total or partial hip replacement	
	AND	
	MCC condition	*See* appendix B.
470	Resurfacing procedure, total or partial hip replacement	
480	Reposition hip joint	
	Fusion of hip joint	
	Insertion of internal/external fixation into hip joint	
	AND	
	MCC condition	*See* appendix B.
481	Reposition hip joint	
	Fusion of hip joint	
	Insertion of internal/external fixation into hip joint	
	AND	
	CC condition	*See* appendix B.
482	Reposition hip joint	
	Fusion of hip joint	
	Insertion of internal/external fixation into hip joint	
535	Fracture of hip and pelvis	
	AND	
	MCC condition	*See* appendix B.
536	Fracture of hip and pelvis	
537	CC/MCC condition	*See* appendix B.
542	Fatigue, stress or pathologic fracture	A code from category M8Ø, Osteoporosis with current pathological fracture, not a traumatic fracture code, should be used for any patient with known osteoporosis who suffers a fracture, even if the patient had a minor fall or trauma, if that fall or trauma would not usually break a normal, healthy bone.
	AND	
	MCC condition	*See* appendix B.
543	Fatigue, stress or pathologic fracture	*See* DRG 542.
	AND	
	CC condition	*See* appendix B.
544	Fatigue, stress or pathologic fracture	*See* DRG 542.

DRG 539 Osteomyelitis with MCC — RW 1.9844

Potential DRGs

463	Wound Debridement and Skin Graft Except Hand for Musculoskeletal and Connective Tissue Disorders with MCC	5.6637
477	Biopsies of Musculoskeletal System and Connective Tissue with MCC	3.3690
480	Hip and Femur Procedures Except Major Joint with MCC	2.9489
492	Lower Extremity and Humerus Procedures Except Hip, Foot, Femur with MCC	3.4621
498	Local Excision and Removal Internal Fixation Devices of Hip and Femur with CC/MCC	2.6110
503	Foot Procedures with MCC	2.6819
510	Shoulder, Elbow or Forearm Procedures, Except Major Joint Procedures with MCC	2.7206
515	Other Musculoskeletal System and Connective Tissue O.R. Procedures with MCC	3.1615

DRG	PDx/SDx/Procedure	Tips
463	Musculoskeletal and connective tissue principal diagnosis	
	Osteomyelitis, all types (except diabetic)	
	Open wounds (lacerations) with tendon involvement	
	AND	
	Excisional debridement of skin wound, infection, or burn	The ICD-10-PCS definition of the root operation Excision is "Cutting out or off, without replacement, a portion of a body part." Debridement by excision involves cutting with a sharp instrument such as a scalpel or other methods such as a hot knife or laser. Non-excisional debridement of skin is coded to root operation Extraction. Ensure that documentation includes instruments used, technique, and depth of debridement procedure.
	AND	
	MCC condition	*See* appendix B.
477	Biopsy of bone	
	AND	
	MCC condition	*See* appendix B.
480	Sequestrectomy of femur	A sequestrum is infected dead bone resulting from osteomyelitis; sequestrectomy is removal of necrotic bone. The ICD-10-PCS index entry for Sequestrectomy, bone directs the coder to *see* Extirpation.
	AND	
	MCC condition	*See* appendix B.
492	Excisional debridement of humerus, tibia, fibula	
	Sequestrectomy of humerus, tibia, fibula	*See* DRG 480.
	AND	
	MCC condition	*See* appendix B.
498	Excisional debridement femur	
	AND	
	CC/MCC condition	*See* appendix B.
503	Excisional debridement metatarsal, tarsal	
	Sequestrectomy of metatarsal, tarsal	*See* DRG 480.
	AND	
	MCC condition	*See* appendix B.
510	Excisional debridement radius, ulna	
	Sequestrectomy of radius, ulna	*See* DRG 480.
	AND	
	MCC condition	*See* appendix B.
515	Excisional debridement skull and facial bones, clavicle, scapula, sternum, ribs, vertebra, toe and finger phalanx	
	Sequestrectomy of clavicle, scapula, sternum, ribs, vertebra, toe and finger phalanx	A sequestrum is infected dead bone resulting from osteomyelitis; sequestrectomy is removal of necrotic bone. The ICD-10-PCS index entry for Sequestrectomy, bone directs the coder to *see* Extirpation. Sequestrectomy of skull or facial bones will not result in reassignment to MS-DRG 515.
	AND	
	MCC condition	*See* appendix B.

DRG 540 Osteomyelitis with CC — RW 1.2982

Potential DRGs

463	Wound Debridement and Skin Graft Except Hand for Musculoskeletal and Connective Tissue Disorders with MCC	5.6637
464	Wound Debridement and Skin Graft Except Hand for Musculoskeletal and Connective Tissue Disorders with CC	3.0014
477	Biopsies of Musculoskeletal System and Connective Tissue with MCC	3.3690
478	Biopsies of Musculoskeletal System and Connective Tissue with CC	2.3837
480	Hip and Femur Procedures Except Major Joint with MCC	2.9489
481	Hip and Femur Procedures Except Major Joint with CC	2.0749
492	Lower Extremity and Humerus Procedures Except Hip, Foot, Femur with MCC	3.4621
493	Lower Extremity and Humerus Procedures Except Hip, Foot, Femur with CC	2.4017
498	Local Excision and Removal Internal Fixation Devices of Hip and Femur with CC/MCC	2.6110
503	Foot Procedures with MCC	2.6819
504	Foot Procedures with CC	1.7271
510	Shoulder, Elbow or Forearm Procedures, Except Major Joint Procedures with MCC	2.7206
511	Shoulder, Elbow or Forearm Procedures, Except Major Joint Procedures with CC	1.9938
515	Other Musculoskeletal System and Connective Tissue O.R. Procedures with MCC	3.1615
516	Other Musculoskeletal System and Connective Tissue O.R. Procedures with CC	2.0408
539	Osteomyelitis with MCC	1.9844

DRG	PDx/SDx/Procedure	Tips
463	Musculoskeletal and connective tissue principal diagnosis	
	Osteomyelitis, all types (except diabetic)	
	Open wounds (lacerations) with tendon involvement	
	AND	
	Excisional debridement of skin wound, infection, or burn	The ICD-10-PCS definition of the root operation Excision is "Cutting out or off, without replacement, a portion of a body part." Debridement by excision involves cutting with a sharp instrument such as a scalpel or other methods such as a hot knife or laser. Non-excisional debridement of skin is coded to root operation Extraction. Ensure that documentation includes instruments used, technique, and depth of debridement procedure.
	AND	
	MCC condition	*See* appendix B.
464	Musculoskeletal and connective tissue principal diagnosis	
	Osteomyelitis, all types (except diabetic)	
	Open wounds (lacerations) with tendon involvement	
	AND	
	Excisional debridement of skin wound, infection, or burn	*See* DRG 463.
	AND	
	CC condition	*See* appendix B.
477	Biopsy of bone	
	AND	
	MCC condition	*See* appendix B.
478	Biopsy of bone	
	AND	
	CC condition	*See* appendix B.
480	Sequestrectomy of femur	A sequestrum is infected dead bone resulting from osteomyelitis; sequestrectomy is removal of necrotic bone. The ICD-10-PCS index entry for Sequestrectomy, bone directs the coder to *see* Extirpation.
	AND	
	MCC condition	*See* appendix B.
481	Sequestrectomy of femur	*See* DRG 480.
	AND	
	CC condition	*See* appendix B.
492	Excisional debridement of humerus, tibia, fibula	
	Sequestrectomy of humerus, tibia, fibula	*See* DRG 480.
	AND	
	MCC condition	*See* appendix B.
493	Excisional debridement of humerus, tibia, fibula	
	Sequestrectomy of humerus, tibia, fibula	*See* DRG 480.
	AND	
	CC condition	*See* appendix B.
498	Excisional debridement femur	
	AND	
	CC/MCC condition	*See* appendix B.
503	Excisional debridement metatarsal, tarsal	
	Sequestrectomy of metatarsal, tarsal	*See* DRG 480.
	AND	
	MCC condition	*See* appendix B.
504	Excisional debridement metatarsal, tarsal	
	Sequestrectomy of metatarsal, tarsal	*See* DRG 480.
	AND	
	CC condition	*See* appendix B.

DRG 540 (Continued)

DRG	PDx/SDx/Procedure	Tips
510	Excisional debridement radius, ulna	
	Sequestrectomy of radius, ulna	*See* DRG 480.
	AND	
	MCC condition	*See* appendix B.
511	Sequestrectomy of radius, ulna	*See* DRG 480.
	AND	
	CC condition	*See* appendix B.
515	Excisional debridement skull and facial bones, clavicle, scapula, sternum, ribs, vertebra, toe and finger phalanx	
	Sequestrectomy of clavicle, scapula, sternum, ribs, vertebra, toe and finger phalanx	A sequestrum is infected dead bone resulting from osteomyelitis; sequestrectomy is removal of necrotic bone. The ICD-10-PCS index entry for Sequestrectomy, bone directs the coder to *see* Extirpation. Sequestrectomy of skull or facial bones will not result in reassignment to MS-DRG 515.
	AND	
	MCC condition	*See* appendix B.
516	Excisional debridement skull and facial bones, clavicle, scapula, sternum, ribs, vertebra, toe and finger phalanx	
	Sequestrectomy of clavicle, scapula, sternum, ribs, vertebra, toe and finger phalanx	*See* DRG 515.
	AND	
	CC condition	*See* appendix B.
539	MCC condition	*See* appendix B.

DRG 541 Osteomyelitis without CC/MCC — RW 0.8579

Potential DRGs

463	Wound Debridement and Skin Graft Except Hand for Musculoskeletal and Connective Tissue Disorders with MCC	5.6637
464	Wound Debridement and Skin Graft Except Hand for Musculoskeletal and Connective Tissue Disorders with CC	3.0014
465	Wound Debridement and Skin Graft Except Hand for Musculoskeletal and Connective Tissue Disorders without CC/MCC	1.8708
477	Biopsies of Musculoskeletal System and Connective Tissue with MCC	3.3690
478	Biopsies of Musculoskeletal System and Connective Tissue with CC	2.3837
479	Biopsies of Musculoskeletal System and Connective Tissue without CC/MCC	1.8640
480	Hip and Femur Procedures Except Major Joint with MCC	2.9489
481	Hip and Femur Procedures Except Major Joint with CC	2.0749
482	Hip and Femur Procedures Except Major Joint without CC/MCC	1.5884
492	Lower Extremity and Humerus Procedures Except Hip, Foot, Femur with MCC	3.4621
493	Lower Extremity and Humerus Procedures Except Hip, Foot, Femur with CC	2.4017
494	Lower Extremity and Humerus Procedures Except Hip, Foot, Femur without CC/MCC	1.8692
498	Local Excision and Removal Internal Fixation Devices of Hip and Femur with CC/MCC	2.6110
499	Local Excision and Removal Internal Fixation Devices of Hip and Femur without CC/MCC	1.2898
503	Foot Procedures with MCC	2.6819
504	Foot Procedures with CC	1.7271
505	Foot Procedures without CC/MCC	1.7057
510	Shoulder, Elbow or Forearm Procedures, Except Major Joint Procedures with MCC	2.7206
511	Shoulder, Elbow or Forearm Procedures, Except Major Joint Procedures with CC	1.9938
512	Shoulder, Elbow or Forearm Procedures, Except Major Joint Procedures without CC/MCC	1.6138
515	Other Musculoskeletal System and Connective Tissue O.R. Procedures with MCC	3.1615
516	Other Musculoskeletal System and Connective Tissue O.R. Procedures with CC	2.0408
517	Other Musculoskeletal System and Connective Tissue O.R. Procedures without CC/MCC	1.4944
539	Osteomyelitis with MCC	1.9844
540	Osteomyelitis with CC	1.2982

DRG	PDx/SDx/Procedure	Tips
463	Musculoskeletal and connective tissue principal diagnosis	
	Osteomyelitis, all types (except diabetic)	
	Open wounds (lacerations) with tendon involvement	
	AND	
	Excisional debridement of skin wound, infection, or burn	The ICD-10-PCS definition of the root operation Excision is "Cutting out or off, without replacement, a portion of a body part." Debridement by excision involves cutting with a sharp instrument such as a scalpel or other methods such as a hot knife or laser. Non-excisional debridement of skin is coded to root operation Extraction. Ensure that documentation includes instruments used, technique, and depth of debridement procedure.
	AND	
	MCC condition	*See* appendix B.
464	Musculoskeletal and connective tissue principal diagnosis	
	Osteomyelitis, all types (except diabetic)	
	Open wounds (lacerations) with tendon involvement	
	AND	
	Excisional debridement of skin wound, infection, or burn	*See* DRG 463.
	AND	
	CC condition	*See* appendix B.

DRG 541 (Continued)

DRG	PDx/SDx/Procedure	Tips
465	Musculoskeletal and connective tissue principal diagnosis	
	Osteomyelitis, all types (except diabetic)	
	Open wounds (lacerations) with tendon involvement	
	AND	
	Excisional debridement of skin wound, infection, or burn	*See* DRG 463.
477	Biopsy of bone	
	AND	
	MCC condition	*See* appendix B.
478	Biopsy of bone	
	AND	
	CC condition	*See* appendix B.
479	Biopsy of bone	
480	Sequestrectomy of femur	A sequestrum is infected dead bone resulting from osteomyelitis; sequestrectomy is removal of necrotic bone. The ICD-10-PCS index entry for Sequestrectomy, bone directs the coder to *see* Extirpation.
	AND	
	MCC condition	*See* appendix B.
481	Sequestrectomy of femur	*See* DRG 480.
	AND	
	CC condition	*See* appendix B.
482	Sequestrectomy of femur	*See* DRG 480.
492	Excisional debridement of humerus, tibia, fibula	
	Sequestrectomy of humerus, tibia, fibula	*See* DRG 480.
	AND	
	MCC condition	*See* appendix B.
493	Excisional debridement of humerus, tibia, fibula	
	Sequestrectomy of humerus, tibia, fibula	*See* DRG 480.
	AND	
	CC condition	*See* appendix B.
494	Excisional debridement of humerus, tibia, fibula	
	Sequestrectomy of humerus, tibia, fibula	*See* DRG 480.
498	Excisional debridement femur	
	AND	
	CC/MCC condition	*See* appendix B.
499	Excisional debridement femur	
503	Excisional debridement metatarsal, tarsal	
	Sequestrectomy of metatarsal, tarsal	*See* DRG 480.
	AND	
	MCC condition	*See* appendix B.
504	Excisional debridement metatarsal, tarsal	
	Sequestrectomy of metatarsal, tarsal	*See* DRG 480.
	AND	
	CC condition	*See* appendix B.
505	Excisional debridement metatarsal, tarsal	
	Sequestrectomy of metatarsal, tarsal	*See* DRG 480.
510	Excisional debridement radius, ulna	
	Sequestrectomy of radius, ulna	*See* DRG 480.
	AND	
	MCC condition	*See* appendix B.
511	Excisional debridement radius, ulna	
	Sequestrectomy of radius, ulna	*See* DRG 480.
	AND	
	CC condition	*See* appendix B.
512	Excisional debridement radius, ulna	
	Sequestrectomy of radius, ulna	*See* DRG 480.
515	Excisional debridement skull and facial bones, clavicle, scapula, sternum, ribs, vertebra, toe and finger phalanx	
	Sequestrectomy of clavicle, scapula, sternum, ribs, vertebra, toe and finger phalanx	A sequestrum is infected dead bone resulting from osteomyelitis; sequestrectomy is removal of necrotic bone. The ICD-10-PCS index entry for Sequestrectomy, bone directs the coder to *see* Extirpation. Sequestrectomy of skull or facial bones will not result in reassignment to MS-DRG 515.
	AND	
	MCC condition	*See* appendix B.

DRG 541 (Continued)

DRG	PDx/SDx/Procedure	Tips
516	Excisional debridement skull and facial bones, clavicle, scapula, sternum, ribs, vertebra, toe and finger phalanx	
	Sequestrectomy of clavicle, scapula, sternum, ribs, vertebra, toe and finger phalanx	*See* DRG 515.
	AND	
	CC condition	*See* appendix B.
517	Excisional debridement skull and facial bones, clavicle, scapula, sternum, ribs, vertebra, toe and finger phalanx	
	Sequestrectomy of clavicle, scapula, sternum, ribs, vertebra, toe and finger phalanx	*See* DRG 515.
539	MCC condition	*See* appendix B.
540	CC condition	*See* appendix B.

DRG 542 Pathological Fractures and Musculoskeletal and Connective Tissue Malignancy with MCC RW 1.8237

Potential DRGs

477	Biopsies of Musculoskeletal System and Connective Tissue with MCC	3.3690
515	Other Musculoskeletal System and Connective Tissue O.R. Procedure with MCC	3.1615

DRG	PDx/SDx/Procedure	Tips
477	Vertebral or other bone biopsy (diagnostic e.g. to confirm malignancy)	Review the medical record carefully to determine the exact procedure that was performed. The ICD-10-PCS index instructs the coder to *see* Drainage with qualifier Diagnostic, *see* Excision with qualifier Diagnostic or *see* Extraction with qualifier Diagnostic to report a biopsy. It is important to always review the full definition of the root operation in the PCS table to accurately report the procedure performed.
	AND	
	MCC condition	*See* appendix B.
515	Kyphoplasty or vertebroplasty	
	Percutaneous vertebral augmentation	
	AND	
	MCC condition	*See* appendix B.

DRG 543 Pathological Fractures and Musculoskeletal and Connective Tissue Malignancy with CC RW 1.0907

Potential DRGs

477	Biopsies of Musculoskeletal System and Connective Tissue with MCC	3.3690
478	Biopsies of Musculoskeletal System and Connective Tissue with CC	2.3837
515	Other Musculoskeletal System and Connective Tissue O.R. Procedure with MCC	3.1615
516	Other Musculoskeletal System and Connective Tissue O.R. Procedure with CC	2.0408
535	Fractures of Hip and Pelvis with MCC	1.2967
542	Pathological Fractures and Musculoskeletal and Connective Tissue Malignancy with MCC	1.8237

DRG	PDx/SDx/Procedure	Tips
477	Vertebral or other bone biopsy (diagnostic e.g. to confirm malignancy)	Review the medical record carefully to determine the exact procedure that was performed. The ICD-10-PCS index instructs the coder to *see* Drainage with qualifier Diagnostic, *see* Excision with qualifier Diagnostic or *see* Extraction with qualifier Diagnostic to report a biopsy. It is important to always review the full definition of the root operation in the PCS table to accurately report the procedure performed.
	AND	
	MCC condition	*See* appendix B.
478	Vertebral or other bone biopsy (diagnostic e.g. to confirm malignancy)	*See* DRG 477.
	AND	
	CC condition	*See* appendix B.
515	Kyphoplasty or vertebroplasty	
	Percutaneous vertebral augmentation	
	AND	
	MCC condition	*See* appendix B.
516	Kyphoplasty or vertebroplasty	
	Percutaneous vertebral augmentation	
	AND	
	CC condition	*See* appendix B.
535	Fracture of hip and pelvis	The physician must document whether the fracture is due to trauma or an underlying disease process.
	AND	
	MCC condition	*See* appendix B.
542	MCC condition	*See* appendix B.

DRG 544 Pathological Fractures and Musculoskeletal and Connective Tissue Malignancy without CC/MCC — RW 0.7675

Potential DRGs

477	Biopsies of Musculoskeletal System and Connective Tissue with MCC	3.3690
478	Biopsies of Musculoskeletal System and Connective Tissue with CC	2.3837
479	Biopsies of Musculoskeletal System and Connective Tissue without CC/MCC	1.8640
515	Other Musculoskeletal System and Connective Tissue O.R. Procedure with MCC	3.1615
516	Other Musculoskeletal System and Connective Tissue O.R. Procedure with CC	2.0408
517	Other Musculoskeletal System and Connective Tissue O.R. Procedure without CC/MCC	1.4944
535	Fractures of Hip and Pelvis with MCC	1.2967
542	Pathological Fractures and Musculoskeletal and Connective Tissue Malignancy with MCC	1.8237
543	Pathological Fractures and Musculoskeletal and Connective Tissue Malignancy with CC	1.0907

DRG	PDx/SDx/Procedure	Tips
477	Vertebral or other bone biopsy (diagnostic e.g. to confirm malignancy)	Review the medical record carefully to determine the exact procedure that was performed. The ICD-10-PCS index instructs the coder to *see* Drainage with qualifier Diagnostic, *see* Excision with qualifier Diagnostic or *see* Extraction with qualifier Diagnostic to report a biopsy. It is important to always review the full definition of the root operation in the PCS table to accurately report the procedure performed.
	AND	
	MCC condition	*See* appendix B.
478	Vertebral or other bone biopsy (diagnostic e.g. to confirm malignancy)	*See* DRG 477.
	AND	
	CC condition	*See* appendix B.
479	Vertebral or other bone biopsy (diagnostic e.g. to confirm malignancy)	*See* DRG 477.
515	Kyphoplasty or vertebroplasty	
	Percutaneous vertebral augmentation	
	AND	
	MCC condition	*See* appendix B.
516	Kyphoplasty or vertebroplasty	
	Percutaneous vertebral augmentation	
	AND	
	CC condition	*See* appendix B.
517	Kyphoplasty or vertebroplasty	
	Percutaneous vertebral augmentation	
535	Fracture of hip and pelvis	The physician must document whether the fracture is due to trauma or an underlying disease process.
	AND	
	MCC condition	*See* appendix B.
542	MCC condition	*See* appendix B.
543	CC condition	*See* appendix B.

DRG 545 Connective Tissue Disorders with MCC — RW 2.4932

No Potential DRGs

DRG 546 Connective Tissue Disorders with CC — RW 1.1993

Potential DRGs

545	Connective Tissue Disorders with MCC	2.4932

DRG	PDx/SDx/Procedure	Tips
545	MCC condition	*See* appendix B.

DRG 547 Connective Tissue Disorders without CC/MCC — RW 0.8134

Potential DRGs

545	Connective Tissue Disorders with MCC	2.4932
546	Connective Tissue Disorders with CC	1.1993

DRG	PDx/SDx/Procedure	Tips
545	MCC condition	*See* appendix B.
546	CC condition	*See* appendix B.

DRG 548 Septic Arthritis with MCC — RW 1.9498

Potential DRGs

463	Wound Debridement and Skin Graft Except Hand for Musculoskeletal and Connective Tissue Disorders with MCC	5.6637
466	Revision of Hip or Knee Replacement with MCC	5.1866
477	Biopsies of Musculoskeletal System and Connective Tissue with MCC	3.3690
483	Major Joint/Limb Reattachment Procedure of Upper Extremities	2.4842
495	Local Excision and Removal Internal Fixation Devices Except Hip and Femur with MCC	3.5812

DRG	PDx/SDx/Procedure	Tips
463	Musculoskeletal and connective tissue principal diagnosis	
	Osteomyelitis, all types (except diabetic)	
	Open wounds (lacerations) with tendon involvement	
	AND	
	Removal of knee or hip prosthesis, any or all components	
	AND	
	MCC condition	*See* appendix B.
466	Removal and immediate replacement of hip or knee prosthesis, any or all components	
	AND	
	MCC condition	*See* appendix B.
477	Biopsy of bone	
	AND	
	MCC condition	*See* appendix B.
483	Removal and immediate replacement of shoulder prosthesis, any or all components	
495	Removal of shoulder prosthesis	
	AND	
	MCC condition	*See* appendix B.

DRG 549 Septic Arthritis with CC — RW 1.2062

Potential DRGs

463	Wound Debridement and Skin Graft Except Hand for Musculoskeletal and Connective Tissue Disorders with MCC	5.6637
464	Wound Debridement and Skin Graft Except Hand for Musculoskeletal and Connective Tissue Disorders with CC	3.0014
466	Revision of Hip or Knee Replacement with MCC	5.1866
467	Revision of Hip or Knee Replacement with CC	3.4863
477	Biopsies of Musculoskeletal System and Connective Tissue with MCC	3.3690
478	Biopsies of Musculoskeletal System and Connective Tissue with CC	2.3837
483	Major Joint/Limb Reattachment Procedure of Upper Extremities	2.4842
495	Local Excision and Removal Internal Fixation Devices Except Hip and Femur with MCC	3.5812
496	Local Excision and Removal Internal Fixation Devices Except Hip and Femur with CC	1.9875
548	Septic Arthritis with MCC	1.9498

DRG	PDx/SDx/Procedure	Tips
463	Musculoskeletal and connective tissue principal diagnosis	
	Osteomyelitis, all types (except diabetic)	
	Open wounds (lacerations) with tendon involvement	
	AND	
	Removal of hip or knee prosthesis, any or all components	
	AND	
	MCC condition	*See* appendix B.
464	Musculoskeletal and connective tissue principal diagnosis	
	Osteomyelitis, all types (except diabetic)	
	Open wounds (lacerations) with tendon involvement	
	AND	
	Removal of hip or knee prosthesis, any or all components	
	AND	
	CC condition	*See* appendix B.
466	Removal and immediate replacement of shoulder prosthesis, any or all components	
	AND	
	MCC condition	*See* appendix B.
467	Removal and immediate replacement of shoulder prosthesis, any or all components	
	AND	
	CC condition	*See* appendix B.
477	Biopsy of bone	
	AND	
	MCC condition	*See* appendix B.
478	Biopsy of bone	
	AND	
	CC condition	*See* appendix B.
483	Removal and immediate replacement of shoulder prosthesis, any or all components	
495	Removal of shoulder prosthesis	
	AND	
	MCC condition	*See* appendix B.
496	Removal of shoulder prosthesis	
	AND	
	CC condition	*See* appendix B.
548	MCC condition	*See* appendix B.

DRG 550 Septic Arthritis without CC/MCC

RW 0.9208

Potential DRGs

463	Wound Debridement and Skin Graft Except Hand for Musculoskeletal and Connective Tissue Disorders with MCC	5.6637
464	Wound Debridement and Skin Graft Except Hand for Musculoskeletal and Connective Tissue Disorders with CC	3.0014
465	Wound Debridement and Skin Graft Except Hand for Musculoskeletal and Connective Tissue Disorders without CC/MCC	1.8708
466	Revision of Hip or Knee Replacement with MCC	5.1866
467	Revision of Hip or Knee Replacement with CC	3.4863
468	Revision of Hip or Knee Replacement without CC/MCC	2.6696
477	Biopsies of Musculoskeletal System and Connective Tissue with MCC	3.3690
478	Biopsies of Musculoskeletal System and Connective Tissue with CC	2.3837
479	Biopsies of Musculoskeletal System and Connective Tissue without CC/MCC	1.8640
483	Major Joint/Limb Reattachment Procedure of Upper Extremities	2.4842
495	Local Excision and Removal Internal Fixation Devices Except Hip and Femur with MCC	3.5812
496	Local Excision and Removal Internal Fixation Devices Except Hip and Femur with CC	1.9875
497	Local Excision and Removal Internal Fixation Devices Except Hip and Femur without CC/MCC	1.4274
548	Septic Arthritis with MCC	1.9498
549	Septic Arthritis with CC	1.2062

DRG	PDx/SDx/Procedure	Tips
463	Musculoskeletal and connective tissue principal diagnosis	
	Osteomyelitis, all types (except diabetic)	
	Open wounds (lacerations) with tendon involvement	
	AND	
	Removal of hip or knee prosthesis, any or all components	
	AND	
	MCC condition	*See* appendix B.
464	Musculoskeletal and connective tissue principal diagnosis	
	Osteomyelitis, all types (except diabetic)	
	Open wounds (lacerations) with tendon involvement	
	AND	
	Removal of hip or knee prosthesis, any or all components	
	AND	
	CC condition	*See* appendix B.
465	Musculoskeletal and connective tissue principal diagnosis	
	Osteomyelitis, all types (except diabetic)	
	Open wounds (lacerations) with tendon involvement	
	AND	
	Removal of hip or knee prosthesis, any or all components	
466	Removal and immediate replacement of hip or knee prosthesis, any or all components	
	AND	
	MCC condition	*See* appendix B.
467	Removal and immediate replacement of hip or knee prosthesis, any or all components	
	AND	
	CC condition	*See* appendix B.
468	Removal and immediate replacement of hip or knee prosthesis, any or all components	
477	Biopsy of bone	
	AND	
	MCC condition	*See* appendix B.
478	Biopsy of bone	
	AND	
	CC condition	*See* appendix B.
479	Biopsy of bone	
483	Removal and immediate replacement of shoulder prosthesis, any or all components	
495	Removal of shoulder prosthesis	
	AND	
	MCC condition	*See* appendix B.
496	Removal of shoulder prosthesis	
	AND	
	CC condition	*See* appendix B.
497	Removal of shoulder prosthesis	
548	MCC condition	*See* appendix B.
549	CC condition	*See* appendix B.

DRG 551 Medical Back Problems with MCC RW 1.7019

Potential DRGs

515	Other Musculoskeletal System and Connective Tissue O.R. Procedure with MCC	3.1615
518	Back and Neck Procedures Except Spinal Fusion with MCC or Disc Device/Neurostimulator	3.6518
542	Pathological Fractures and Musculoskeletal and Connective Tissue Malignancy with MCC	1.8237

DRG	PDx/SDx/Procedure	Tips
515	Kyphoplasty or vertebroplasty	
	Percutaneous vertebral augmentation	
	AND	
	MCC condition	*See* appendix B.
518	Spinal cord decompression	The ICD-10-PCS index entry "Laminectomy" instructs the coder to see Excision, but a laminectomy done as the operative approach for spinal fusion is not coded separately. However, a decompressive laminectomy is reported with root operation Release because the objective of the procedure is to release/free up the spinal cord. Release procedures are coded to the body part being freed. Multiple decompression procedures in the same anatomical area, e.g., cervical spinal cord, thoracic spinal cord, or lumbar spinal cord, are coded only once regardless of the number of vertebral levels decompressed. Unlike the vertebral joints, the vertebral level designations at each spinal level of the spinal cord are not considered separate and distinct body parts with distinct body part values. Therefore, the multiple procedures guideline B3.2b would not apply.
	AND	
	MCC condition	*See* appendix B.
	OR	
	Spinal neurostimulator and lead (s) implant	
542	Fatigue, stress or pathologic fracture	A code from category M8Ø, Osteoporosis with current pathological fracture, not a traumatic fracture code, should be used for any patient with known osteoporosis who suffers a fracture, even if the patient had a minor fall or trauma, if that fall or trauma would not usually break a normal, healthy bone.
	AND	
	MCC condition	*See* appendix B.

DRG 552 Medical Back Problems without MCC

RW 0.9663

Potential DRGs

515	Other Musculoskeletal System and Connective Tissue O.R. Procedure with MCC	3.1615
516	Other Musculoskeletal System and Connective Tissue O.R. Procedure with CC	2.0408
517	Other Musculoskeletal System and Connective Tissue O.R. Procedure without CC/MCC	1.4944
518	Back and Neck Procedures Except Spinal Fusion with MCC or Disc Device/Neurostimulator	3.6518
519	Back and Neck Procedures Except Spinal Fusion with CC	1.9686
520	Back and Neck Procedures Except Spinal Fusion without CC/MCC	1.4315
542	Pathological Fractures and Musculoskeletal and Connective Tissue Malignancy with MCC	1.8237
543	Pathological Fractures and Musculoskeletal and Connective Tissue Malignancy with CC	1.0907
551	Medical Back Problems with MCC	1.7019

DRG	PDx/SDx/Procedure	Tips
515	Kyphoplasty or vertebroplasty	
	Percutaneous vertebral augmentation	
	AND	
	MCC condition	*See* appendix B.
516	Kyphoplasty or vertebroplasty	
	Percutaneous vertebral augmentation	
	AND	
	CC condition	*See* appendix B.
517	Kyphoplasty or vertebroplasty	
	Percutaneous vertebral augmentation	
518	Spinal cord decompression	The ICD-10-PCS index entry "Laminectomy" instructs the coder to see Excision, but a laminectomy done as the operative approach for spinal fusion is not coded separately. However, a decompressive laminectomy is reported with root operation Release because the objective of the procedure is to release/free up the spinal cord. Release procedures are coded to the body part being freed. Multiple decompression procedures in the same anatomical area, e.g., cervical spinal cord, thoracic spinal cord, or lumbar spinal cord, are coded only once regardless of the number of vertebral levels decompressed. Unlike the vertebral joints, the vertebral level designations at each spinal level of the spinal cord are not considered separate and distinct body parts with distinct body part values. Therefore, the multiple procedures guideline B3.2b would not apply.
	AND	
	MCC condition	*See* appendix B.
	OR	
	Spinal neurostimulator and lead (s) implant	
519	Spinal cord decompression	*See* DRG 518.
	AND	
	CC condition	*See* appendix B.
520	Spinal cord decompression	*See* DRG 518.
542	Fatigue, stress or pathologic fracture, initial encounter	A code from category M8Ø, Osteoporosis with current pathological fracture, not a traumatic fracture code, should be used for any patient with known osteoporosis who suffers a fracture, even if the patient had a minor fall or trauma, if that fall or trauma would not usually break a normal, healthy bone.
	AND	
	MCC condition	*See* appendix B.
543	Fatigue, stress or pathologic fracture, initial encounter	*See* DRG 542.
	AND	
	CC condition	*See* appendix B.
551	MCC condition	*See* appendix B.

DRG 553 Bone Diseases and Arthropathies with MCC — RW 1.3515

Potential DRGs

477	Biopsies of Musculoskeletal System and Connective Tissue with MCC	3.3690
545	Connective Tissue Disorders with MCC	2.4932

DRG	PDx/SDx/Procedure	Tips
477	Biopsy of bone	
	AND	
	MCC condition	*See* appendix B.
545	Felty's Syndrome	
	Rheumatoid vasculitis with rheumatoid arthritis	
	Rheumatoid heart disease with rheumatoid arthritis	
	Rheumatoid myopathy with rheumatoid arthritis	
	Rheumatoid polyneuropathy with rheumatoid arthritis	
	Rheumatoid arthritis with involvement of other organs and systems	
	Rheumatoid arthritis with rheumatoid factor without organ or systems involvement	
	Other and unspecified rheumatoid arthritis with rheumatoid factor	
	AND	
	MCC condition	*See* appendix B.

DRG 554 Bone Diseases and Arthropathies without MCC — RW 0.8218

Potential DRGs

477	Biopsies of Musculoskeletal System and Connective Tissue with MCC	3.3690
478	Biopsies of Musculoskeletal System and Connective Tissue with CC	2.3837
479	Biopsies of Musculoskeletal System and Connective Tissue without CC/MCC	1.8640
545	Connective Tissue Disorders with MCC	2.4932
546	Connective Tissue Disorders with CC	1.1993
553	Bone Diseases and Arthropathies with MCC	1.3515

DRG	PDx/SDx/Procedure	Tips
477	Biopsy of bone	
	AND	
	MCC condition	*See* appendix B.
478	Biopsy of bone	
	AND	
	CC condition	*See* appendix B.
479	Biopsy of bone	
545	Felty's Syndrome	
	Rheumatoid vasculitis with rheumatoid arthritis	
	Rheumatoid heart disease with rheumatoid arthritis	
	Rheumatoid myopathy with rheumatoid arthritis	
	Rheumatoid polyneuropathy with rheumatoid arthritis	
	Rheumatoid arthritis with involvement of other organs and systems	
	Rheumatoid arthritis with rheumatoid factor without organ or systems involvement	
	Other and unspecified rheumatoid arthritis with rheumatoid factor	
	AND	
	MCC condition	*See* appendix B.
546	Felty's Syndrome	
	Rheumatoid vasculitis with rheumatoid arthritis	
	Rheumatoid heart disease with rheumatoid arthritis	
	Rheumatoid myopathy with rheumatoid arthritis	
	Rheumatoid polyneuropathy with rheumatoid arthritis	
	Rheumatoid arthritis with involvement of other organs and systems	
	Rheumatoid arthritis with rheumatoid factor without organ or systems involvement	
	Other and unspecified rheumatoid arthritis with rheumatoid factor	
	AND	
	CC condition	*See* appendix B.
553	MCC condition	*See* appendix B.

DRG 555 Signs and Symptoms of Musculoskeletal System and Connective Tissue with MCC — RW 1.3990

Potential DRGs

542	Pathological Fractures and Musculoskeletal and Connective Tissue Malignancy with MCC	1.8237
545	Connective Tissue Disorders with MCC	2.4932
557	Tendonitis, Myositis and Bursitis with MCC	1.5568
564	Other Musculoskeletal System and Connective Tissue Diagnoses with MCC	1.5619

DRG	PDx/SDx/Procedure	Tips
542	Fatigue, stress or pathologic fracture, initial encounter	A code from category M80 Osteoporosis with current pathological fracture, not a traumatic fracture code, should be used for any patient with known osteoporosis who suffers a fracture, even if the patient had a minor fall or trauma, if that fall or trauma would not usually break a normal, healthy bone.
	AND	
	MCC condition	*See* appendix B.
545	Felty's Syndrome	
	Rheumatoid vasculitis with rheumatoid arthritis	
	Rheumatoid heart disease with rheumatoid arthritis	
	Rheumatoid myopathy with rheumatoid arthritis	
	Rheumatoid polyneuropathy with rheumatoid arthritis	
	Rheumatoid arthritis with involvement of other organs and systems	
	Rheumatoid arthritis with rheumatoid factor without organ or systems involvement	
	Other and unspecified rheumatoid arthritis with rheumatoid factor	
	AND	
	MCC condition	*See* appendix B.
557	Cause of musculoskeletal difficulty or pain such as: Adhesive capsulitis of shoulder or rotator cuff tear Synovitis and tenosynovitis Bursitis and bursal cyst Ganglion of joint or tendon sheath Disorders of muscle	
	AND	
	MCC condition	*See* appendix B.
564	Cause of musculoskeletal difficulty or pain such as: Benign neoplasm of any bone except lower jaw bone and ribs, sternum, and clavicle Loose body in joint Joint contracture Other and unspecified joint derangement Joint effusion	
	AND	
	MCC condition	*See* appendix B.

DRG 556 Signs and Symptoms of Musculoskeletal System and Connective Tissue without MCC RW 0.8244

Potential DRGs

542	Pathological Fractures and Musculoskeletal and Connective Tissue Malignancy with MCC	1.8237
543	Pathological Fractures and Musculoskeletal and Connective Tissue Malignancy with CC	1.0907
545	Connective Tissue Disorders with MCC	2.4932
546	Connective Tissue Disorders with CC	1.1993
555	Signs and Symptoms of Musculoskeletal System and Connective Tissue with MCC	1.3990
557	Tendonitis, Myositis and Bursitis with MCC	1.5568
558	Tendonitis, Myositis and Bursitis without MCC	0.8784
564	Other Musculoskeletal System and Connective Tissue Diagnoses with MCC	1.5619
565	Other Musculoskeletal System and Connective Tissue Diagnoses with CC	0.9994

DRG	PDx/SDx/Procedure	Tips
542	Fatigue, stress or pathologic fracture, initial encounter	A code from category M80 Osteoporosis with current pathological fracture, not a traumatic fracture code, should be used for any patient with known osteoporosis who suffers a fracture, even if the patient had a minor fall or trauma, if that fall or trauma would not usually break a normal, healthy bone.
	AND	
	MCC condition	*See* appendix B.
543	Fatigue, stress or pathologic fracture, initial encounter	*See* DRG 542.
	AND	
	CC condition	*See* appendix B.
545	Felty's Syndrome	
	Rheumatoid vasculitis with rheumatoid arthritis	
	Rheumatoid heart disease with rheumatoid arthritis	
	Rheumatoid myopathy with rheumatoid arthritis	
	Rheumatoid polyneuropathy with rheumatoid arthritis	
	Rheumatoid arthritis with involvement of other organs and systems	
	Rheumatoid arthritis with rheumatoid factor without organ or systems involvement	
	Other and unspecified rheumatoid arthritis with rheumatoid factor	
	AND	
	MCC condition	*See* appendix B.
546	Felty's Syndrome	
	Rheumatoid vasculitis with rheumatoid arthritis	
	Rheumatoid heart disease with rheumatoid arthritis	
	Rheumatoid myopathy with rheumatoid arthritis	
	Rheumatoid polyneuropathy with rheumatoid arthritis	
	Rheumatoid arthritis with involvement of other organs and systems	
	Rheumatoid arthritis with rheumatoid factor without organ or systems involvement	
	Other and unspecified rheumatoid arthritis with rheumatoid factor	
	AND	
	CC condition	*See* appendix B.
555	MCC condition	*See* appendix B.
557	Cause of musculoskeletal difficulty or pain such as: Adhesive capsulitis of shoulder or rotator cuff tear Synovitis and tenosynovitis Bursitis and bursal cyst Ganglion of joint or tendon sheath Disorders of muscle	
	AND	
	MCC condition	*See* appendix B.
558	Cause of musculoskeletal difficulty or pain such as: Adhesive capsulitis of shoulder or rotator cuff tear Synovitis and tenosynovitis Bursitis and bursal cyst Ganglion of joint or tendon sheath Disorders of muscle	

DRG 556 (Continued)

DRG	PDx/SDx/Procedure	Tips
564	Cause of musculoskeletal difficulty or pain such as: Benign neoplasm of any bone except lower jaw bone and ribs, sternum, and clavicle Loose body in joint Joint contracture Other and unspecified joint derangement Joint effusion	
	AND	
	MCC condition	*See* appendix B.
565	Cause of musculoskeletal difficulty or pain such as: Benign neoplasm of any bone except lower jaw bone and ribs, sternum, and clavicle Loose body in joint Joint contracture Other and unspecified joint derangement Joint effusion	
	AND	
	CC condition	*See* appendix B.

DRG 557 Tendonitis, Myositis and Bursitis with MCC

RW 1.5568

Potential DRGs

500	Soft Tissue Procedures with MCC	3.2428
510	Shoulder, Elbow or Forearm Procedure, Except Major Joint Procedure with MCC	2.7206

DRG	PDx/SDx/Procedure	Tips
500	Nontraumatic compartment syndrome, any site	
	AND	
	Fasciotomy	Fasciotomy done for release of compartment syndrome is reported with root operation Release (N) and the body part being freed is a muscle.
	AND	
	MCC condition	*See* appendix B.
510	Arthroscopic Repair of shoulder tendon Arthroscopic excision of sternoclavicular, acromioclavicular, or shoulder joint structure Arthroscopic lysis of adhesions (Release) of sternoclavicular, acromioclavicular, or shoulder joint	
	AND	
	MCC condition	*See* appendix B.

DRG 558 Tendonitis, Myositis and Bursitis without MCC — RW 0.8784

Potential DRGs

500	Soft Tissue Procedures with MCC	3.2428
501	Soft Tissue Procedures with CC	1.7357
502	Soft Tissue Procedures without CC/MCC	1.3827
510	Shoulder, Elbow or Forearm Procedure, Except Major Joint Procedure with MCC	2.7206
511	Shoulder, Elbow or Forearm Procedure, Except Major Joint Procedure with CC	1.9938
512	Shoulder, Elbow or Forearm Procedure, Except Major Joint Procedure without CC/MCC	1.6138
557	Tendonitis, Myositis and Bursitis with MCC	1.5568

DRG	PDx/SDx/Procedure	Tips
500	Nontraumatic compartment syndrome, any site	
	AND	
	Fasciotomy	Fasciotomy done for release of compartment syndrome is reported with root operation Release (N) and the body part being freed is a muscle.
	AND	
	MCC condition	*See* appendix B.
501	Nontraumatic compartment syndrome, any site	
	AND	
	Fasciotomy	*See* DRG 500.
	AND	
	CC condition	*See* appendix B.
502	Nontraumatic compartment syndrome, any site	
	AND	
	Fasciotomy	*See* DRG 500.
510	Arthroscopic Repair of shoulder tendon Arthroscopic excision of sternoclavicular, acromioclavicular, or shoulder joint structure Arthroscopic lysis of adhesions (Release) of sternoclavicular, acromioclavicular, or shoulder joint	
	AND	
	MCC condition	*See* appendix B.
511	Arthroscopic repair of shoulder tendon Arthroscopic excision of sternoclavicular, acromioclavicular, or shoulder joint structure Arthroscopic lysis of adhesions (Release) of sternoclavicular, acromioclavicular, or shoulder joint	
	AND	
	CC condition	*See* appendix B.
512	Arthroscopic repair of shoulder tendon Arthroscopic excision of sternoclavicular, acromioclavicular, or shoulder joint structure Arthroscopic lysis of adhesions (Release) of sternoclavicular, acromioclavicular, or shoulder joint	
557	MCC condition	*See* appendix B.

DRG 559 Aftercare, Musculoskeletal System and Connective Tissue with MCC — RW 1.8505

Potential DRGs

495	Local Excision and Removal Internal Fixation Devices Except Hip and Femur with MCC	3.5812
498	Local Excision and Removal Internal Fixation Devices of Hip and Femur with CC/MCC	2.6110

DRG	PDx/SDx/Procedure	Tips
495	Complications of internal orthopedic device (mechanical, infection, other)	
	OR	
	Encounter for removal of internal fixation device	
	AND	
	Removal of implanted device from any bone except femur	
	AND	
	MCC condition	*See* appendix B.
498	Complication of internal orthopedic device (mechanical, infection, other)	
	OR	
	Encounter for removal of internal fixation device	
	AND	
	Removal of implanted device from femur	
	AND	
	CC/MCC condition	*See* appendix B.

DRG 560 Aftercare, Musculoskeletal System and Connective Tissue with CC — RW 1.1321

Potential DRGs

495	Local Excision and Removal Internal Fixation Devices Except Hip and Femur with MCC	3.5812
496	Local Excision and Removal Internal Fixation Devices Except Hip and Femur with CC	1.9875
498	Local Excision and Removal Internal Fixation Devices of Hip and Femur with CC/MCC	2.6110
559	Aftercare, Musculoskeletal System and Connective Tissue with MCC	1.8505

DRG	PDx/SDx/Procedure	Tips
495	Complications of internal orthopedic device (mechanical, infection, other)	
	OR	
	Encounter for removal of internal fixation device	
	AND	
	Removal of implanted device from any bone except femur	
	AND	
	MCC condition	*See* appendix B.
496	Complications of internal orthopedic device (mechanical, infection, other)	
	OR	
	Encounter for removal of internal fixation device	
	AND	
	Removal of implanted device from any bone except femur	
	AND	
	CC condition	*See* appendix B.
498	Complication of internal orthopedic device (mechanical, infection, other)	
	OR	
	Encounter for removal of internal fixation device	
	AND	
	Removal of implanted device from femur	
	AND	
	CC/MCC condition	*See* appendix B.
559	MCC condition	*See* appendix B.

DRG 561 Aftercare, Musculoskeletal System and Connective Tissue without CC/MCC — RW 0.7802

Potential DRGs

495	Local Excision and Removal Internal Fixation Devices Except Hip and Femur with MCC	3.5812
496	Local Excision and Removal Internal Fixation Devices Except Hip and Femur with CC	1.9875
497	Local Excision and Removal Internal Fixation Devices Except Hip and Femur without CC/MCC	1.4274
498	Local Excision and Removal Internal Fixation Devices of Hip and Femur with CC/MCC	2.6110
499	Local Excision and Removal Internal Fixation Devices of Hip and Femur without CC/MCC	1.2898
559	Aftercare, Musculoskeletal System and Connective Tissue with MCC	1.8505
560	Aftercare, Musculoskeletal System and Connective Tissue with CC	1.1321

DRG	PDx/SDx/Procedure	Tips
495	Complications of internal orthopedic device (mechanical, infection, other)	
	OR	
	Encounter for removal of internal fixation device	
	AND	
	Removal of implanted device from any bone except femur	
	AND	
	MCC condition	*See* appendix B.
496	Complications of internal orthopedic device (mechanical, infection, other)	
	OR	
	Encounter for removal of internal fixation device	
	AND	
	Removal of implanted device from any bone except femur	
	AND	
	CC condition	*See* appendix B.
497	Complications of internal orthopedic device (mechanical, infection, other)	
	OR	
	Encounter for removal of internal fixation device	
	AND	
	Removal of implanted device from any bone except femur	
498	Complication of internal orthopedic device (mechanical, infection, other)	
	OR	
	Encounter for removal of internal fixation device	
	AND	
	Removal of implanted device from femur	
	AND	
	CC/MCC condition	*See* appendix B.
499	Complication of internal orthopedic device (mechanical, infection, other)	
	OR	
	Encounter for removal of internal fixation device	
	AND	
	Removal of implanted device from femur	
559	MCC condition	*See* appendix B.
560	CC condition	*See* appendix B.

DRG 562 Fractures, Sprains, Strains and Dislocations Except Femur, Hip, Pelvis and Thigh with MCC RW 1.5207

Potential DRGs

488	Knee Procedures without Principal Diagnosis of Infection with CC/MCC	2.1066
542	Pathological Fractures and Musculoskeletal and Connective Tissue Malignancy with MCC	1.8237
963	Other Multiple Significant Trauma with MCC	2.7343

DRG	PDx/SDx/Procedure	Tips
488	Meniscal and other internal derangement of knee	
	AND	
	Meniscectomy, synovectomy or other repair of knee	
	AND	
	CC/MCC condition	*See* appendix B.
542	Fatigue, stress or pathologic fracture	A code from category M80 Osteoporosis with current pathological fracture, not a traumatic fracture code, should be used for any patient with known osteoporosis who suffers a fracture, even if the patient had a minor fall or trauma, if that fall or trauma would not usually break a normal, healthy bone.
	AND	
	MCC condition	*See* appendix B.
963	Multiple significant trauma	Principal diagnosis of trauma and two or more different dx from two different body site categories in MS-DRG 963.
	AND	
	MCC condition	*See* appendix B.

DRG 563 Fractures, Sprains, Strains and Dislocations Except Femur, Hip, Pelvis and Thigh without MCC RW 0.8956

Potential DRGs

488	Knee Procedures without Principal Diagnosis of Infection with CC/MCC	2.1066
489	Knee Procedures without Principal Diagnosis of Infection without CC/MCC	1.2377
542	Pathological Fractures and Musculoskeletal and Connective Tissue Malignancy with MCC	1.8237
543	Pathological Fractures and Musculoskeletal and Connective Tissue Malignancy with CC	1.0907
562	Fractures, Sprains, Strains and Dislocations Except Femur, Hip, Pelvis and Thigh with MCC	1.5207
963	Other Multiple Significant Trauma with MCC	2.7343
964	Other Multiple Significant Trauma with CC	1.5010
965	Other Multiple Significant Trauma without CC/MCC	0.9559

DRG	PDx/SDx/Procedure	Tips
488	Meniscal and other internal derangement of knee	
	AND	
	Meniscectomy, synovectomy or other repair of knee	
	AND	
	CC/MCC condition	*See* appendix B.
489	Meniscal and other internal derangement of knee	
	AND	
	Meniscectomy, synovectomy or other repair of knee	
542	Fatigue, stress or pathologic fracture	A code from category M80 Osteoporosis with current pathological fracture, not a traumatic fracture code, should be used for any patient with known osteoporosis who suffers a fracture, even if the patient had a minor fall or trauma, if that fall or trauma would not usually break a normal, healthy bone.
	AND	
	MCC condition	*See* appendix B.
543	Fatigue, stress or pathologic fracture	*See* DRG 542.
	AND	
	CC condition	*See* appendix B.
562	MCC condition	*See* appendix B.
963	Multiple significant trauma	Principal diagnosis of trauma and two or more different dx from two different body site categories in MS-DRG 963.
	AND	
	MCC condition	*See* appendix B.
964	Multiple significant trauma	Principal diagnosis of trauma and two or more different dx from two different body site categories in MS-DRG 963.
	AND	
	CC condition	*See* appendix B.
965	Multiple significant trauma	Principal diagnosis of trauma and two or more different dx from two different body site categories in MS-DRG 963.

DRG 564 Other Musculoskeletal System and Connective Tissue Diagnoses with MCC — RW 1.5619

Potential DRGs

477	Biopsies of Musculoskeletal System and Connective Tissue with MCC	3.3690
503	Foot Procedures with MCC	2.6819

DRG	PDx/SDx/Procedure	Tips
477	Biopsy of bone	
	AND	
	MCC condition	*See* appendix B.
503	Acquired deformities of foot and toes	
	Congenital deformities of foot	
	AND	
	Osteotomy or other incision/division of tarsals and metatarsals	
	Reposition of tarsals and metatarsals	
	Excision or partial ostectomy of tarsals and metatarsals or local excision of lesion (nondiagnostic)	
	Excision of tarsal or metatarsal joint structure or local excision of joint lesion (nondiagnostic)	
	Fusion of foot	
	AND	
	MCC condition	*See* appendix B.

DRG 565 Other Musculoskeletal System and Connective Tissue Diagnoses with CC — RW 0.9994

Potential DRGs

477	Biopsies of Musculoskeletal System and Connective Tissue with MCC	3.3690
478	Biopsies of Musculoskeletal System and Connective Tissue with CC	2.3837
503	Foot Procedures with MCC	2.6819
504	Foot Procedures with CC	1.7271
564	Other Musculoskeletal System and Connective Tissue Diagnoses with MCC	1.5619

DRG	PDx/SDx/Procedure	Tips
477	Biopsy of bone	
	AND	
	MCC condition	*See* appendix B.
478	Biopsy of bone	
	AND	
	CC condition	*See* appendix B.
503	Acquired deformities of foot and toes	
	Congenital deformities of foot	
	AND	
	Osteotomy or other incision/division of tarsals and metatarsals	
	Reposition of tarsals and metatarsals	
	Excision or partial ostectomy of tarsals and metatarsals or local excision of lesion (nondiagnostic)	
	Excision of tarsal or metatarsal joint structure or local excision of joint lesion (nondiagnostic)	
	Fusion of foot	
	AND	
	MCC condition	*See* appendix B.
504	Acquired deformities of foot and toes	
	Congenital deformities of foot	
	AND	
	Osteotomy or other incision/division of tarsals and metatarsals	
	Reposition of tarsals and metatarsals	
	Excision or partial ostectomy of tarsals and metatarsals or local excision of lesion (nondiagnostic)	
	Excision of tarsal or metatarsal joint structure or local excision of joint lesion (nondiagnostic)	
	Fusion of foot	
	AND	
	CC condition	*See* appendix B.
564	MCC condition	*See* appendix B.

DRG 566 Other Musculoskeletal System and Connective Tissue Diagnoses without CC/MCC RW 0.7505

Potential DRGs

477	Biopsies of Musculoskeletal System and Connective Tissue with MCC	3.3690
478	Biopsies of Musculoskeletal System and Connective Tissue with CC RW	2.3837
479	Biopsies of Musculoskeletal System and Connective Tissue without CC/MCC	1.8640
503	Foot Procedures with MCC	2.6819
504	Foot Procedures with CC	1.7271
505	Foot Procedures without CC/MCC	1.7057
564	Other Musculoskeletal System and Connective Tissue Diagnoses with MCC	1.5619
565	Other Musculoskeletal System and Connective Tissue Diagnoses with CC	0.9994

DRG	PDx/SDx/Procedure	Tips
477	Biopsy of bone	
	AND	
	MCC condition	*See* appendix B.
478	Biopsy of bone	
	AND	
	CC condition	*See* appendix B.
479	Biopsy of bone	
503	Acquired deformities of foot and toes	
	Congenital deformities of foot	
	AND	
	Osteotomy or other incision/division of tarsals and metatarsals	
	Reposition of tarsals and metatarsals	
	Excision or partial ostectomy of tarsals and metatarsals or local excision of lesion (nondiagnostic)	
	Excision of tarsal or metatarsal joint structure or local excision of joint lesion (nondiagnostic)	
	Fusion of foot	
	AND	
	MCC condition	*See* appendix B.
504	Acquired deformities of foot and toes	
	Congenital deformities of foot	
	AND	
	Osteotomy or other incision/division of tarsals and metatarsals	
	Reposition of tarsals and metatarsals	
	Excision or partial ostectomy of tarsals and metatarsals or local excision of lesion (nondiagnostic)	
	Excision of tarsal or metatarsal joint structure or local excision of joint lesion (nondiagnostic)	
	Fusion of foot	
	AND	
	CC condition	*See* appendix B.
505	Acquired deformities of foot and toes	
	Congenital deformities of foot	
	AND	
	Osteotomy or other incision/division of tarsals and metatarsals	
	Reposition of tarsals and metatarsals	
	Excision or partial ostectomy of tarsals and metatarsals or local excision of lesion (nondiagnostic)	
	Excision of tarsal or metatarsal joint structure or local excision of joint lesion (nondiagnostic)	
	Fusion of foot	
564	MCC condition	*See* appendix B.
565	CC condition	*See* appendix B.

Diseases And Disorders Of The Skin, Subcutaneous Tissue And Breast

DRG 570 Skin Debridement with MCC — RW 2.9222

Potential DRGs

463	Wound Debridement and Skin Graft Except Hand for Musculoskeletal and Connective Tissue Disorders with MCC	5.6637
573	Skin Graft for Skin Ulcer or Cellulitis with MCC	6.2181
576	Skin Graft Except for Skin Ulcer or Cellulitis with MCC	5.6831
622	Skin Grafts and Wound Debridement for Endocrine, Nutritional and Metabolic Disorders with MCC	3.8256
901	Wound Debridements for Injuries with MCC	4.3278

DRG	PDx/SDx/Procedure	Tips
463	Musculoskeletal and connective tissue principal diagnosis	Ensure that documentation includes underlying cause of condition requiring debridement and depth of debridement procedure.
	Osteomyelitis, all types (except diabetic)	
	Open wounds (lacerations) with tendon involvement	Laceration tendon—*see* Injury, muscle, by site, laceration
	AND	
	MCC condition	*See* appendix B.
573	Skin ulcer or cellulitis principal diagnosis	
	AND	
	Skin grafting procedure	Skin grafting includes root operations Replacement of skin with a free graft of autologous (partial or full thickness), nonautologous or synthetic tissue; and Transfer of skin, and/or subcutaneous tissue and fascia which remains attached to its vascular and nervous supply. Other procedures include Excision and Supplement of tissues and Insertion of tissue expander.
	AND	
	MCC condition	*See* appendix B.
576	Diagnosis from MDC 9 other than skin ulcer or cellulitis	
	AND	
	Skin grafting procedure	*See* DRG 573.
	AND	
	MCC condition	*See* appendix B.
622	Diabetic foot or other skin ulcer principal diagnosis	
	AND	
	MCC condition	*See* appendix B.
901	Injury diagnosis from MDC 21	
	Excisional debridement of wound, infection, or burn	The ICD-10-PCS definition of the root operation Excision is "Cutting out or off, without replacement, a portion of a body part." Debridement by excision involves cutting with a sharp instrument such as a scalpel or other methods such as a hot knife or laser. Non-excisional debridement of skin is coded to root operation Extraction. Ensure that documentation includes instruments used, technique, and depth of debridement procedure.
	AND	
	MCC condition	*See* appendix B.

DRG 571 Skin Debridement with CC — RW 1.6919

Potential DRGs

463	Wound Debridement and Skin Graft Except Hand for Musculoskeletal and Connective Tissue Disorders with MCC	5.6637
464	Wound Debridement and Skin Graft Except Hand for Musculoskeletal and Connective Tissue Disorders with CC	3.0014
570	Skin Debridement with MCC	2.9222
573	Skin Graft for Skin Ulcer or Cellulitis with MCC	6.2181
574	Skin Graft for Skin Ulcer or Cellulitis with CC	3.4058
576	Skin Graft Except for Skin Ulcer or Cellulitis with MCC	5.6831
577	Skin Graft Except for Skin Ulcer or Cellulitis with CC	2.6491
622	Skin Grafts and Wound Debridement for Endocrine, Nutritional and Metabolic Disorders with MCC	3.8256
623	Skin Grafts and Wound Debridement for Endocrine, Nutritional and Metabolic Disorders with CC	1.8614
901	Wound Debridements for Injuries with MCC	4.3278
902	Wound Debridements for Injuries with CC	1.8847

DRG	PDx/SDx/Procedure	Tips
463	Musculoskeletal and connective tissue principal diagnosis	Ensure that documentation includes underlying cause of condition requiring debridement and depth of debridement procedure.
	Osteomyelitis, all types (except diabetic)	
	Open wounds (lacerations) with tendon involvement	Laceration tendon—*see* Injury, muscle, by site, laceration
	AND	
	MCC condition	*See* appendix B.
464	Musculoskeletal and connective tissue principal diagnosis	Ensure that documentation includes underlying cause of condition requiring debridement and depth of debridement procedure.
	Osteomyelitis, all types (except diabetic)	
	Open wounds (lacerations) with tendon involvement	Laceration tendon—*see* Injury, muscle, by site, laceration
	AND	
	CC condition	*See* appendix B.

DRG 571 (Continued)

DRG	PDx/SDx/Procedure	Tips
570	MCC condition	*See* appendix B.
573	Skin ulcer or cellulitis principal diagnosis	
	AND	
	Skin grafting procedure	Skin grafting includes root operations Replacement of skin with a free graft of autologous (partial or full thickness), nonautologous or synthetic tissue; and Transfer of skin, and/or subcutaneous tissue and fascia which remains attached to its vascular and nervous supply. Other procedures include Excision and Supplement of tissues and Insertion of tissue expander.
	AND	
	MCC condition	*See* appendix B.
574	Skin ulcer or cellulitis principal diagnosis	
	AND	
	Skin grafting procedure	*See* DRG 573.
	AND	
	CC condition	*See* appendix B.
576	Diagnosis from MDC 9 other than skin ulcer or cellulitis	
	AND	
	Skin grafting procedure	*See* DRG 573.
	AND	
	MCC condition	*See* appendix B.
577	Diagnosis from MDC 9 other than skin ulcer or cellulitis	
	AND	
	Skln grafting procedure	*See* DRG 573.
	AND	
	CC condition	*See* appendix B.
622	Diabetic foot or other skin ulcer principal diagnosis	
	AND	
	MCC condition	*See* appendix B.
623	Diabetic foot or other skin ulcer principal diagnosis	
	AND	
	CC condition	*See* appendix B.
901	Injury diagnosis from MDC 21	
	Excisional debridement of wound, infection, or burn	The ICD-10-PCS definition of the root operation Excision is "Cutting out or off, without replacement, a portion of a body part." Debridement by excision involves cutting with a sharp instrument such as a scalpel or other methods such as a hot knife or laser. Non-excisional debridement of skin is coded to root operation Extraction. Ensure that documentation includes instruments used, technique, and depth of debridement procedure.
	AND	
	MCC condition	*See* appendix B.
902	Injury diagnosis from MDC 21	
	Excisional debridement of wound, infection, or burn	*See* DRG 901.
	AND	
	CC condition	*See* appendix B.

DRG 572 Skin Debridement without CC/MCC

RW 1.1396

Potential DRGs

463	Wound Debridement and Skin Graft Except Hand for Musculoskeletal and Connective Tissue Disorders with MCC	5.6637
464	Wound Debridement and Skin Graft Except Hand for Musculoskeletal and Connective Tissue Disorders with CC	3.0014
465	Wound Debridement and Skin Graft Except Hand for Musculoskeletal and Connective Tissue Disorders without CC/MCC	1.8708
570	Skin Debridement with MCC	2.9222
571	Skin Debridement with CC	1.6919
573	Skin Graft for Skin Ulcer or Cellulitis with MCC	6.2181
574	Skin Graft for Skin Ulcer or Cellulitis with CC	3.4058
575	Skin Graft for Skin Ulcer or Cellulitis without CC/MCC	2.0460
576	Skin Graft Except for Skin Ulcer or Cellulitis with MCC	5.6831
577	Skin Graft Except for Skin Ulcer or Cellulitis with CC	2.6491
578	Skin Graft Except for Skin Ulcer or Cellulitis without CC/MCC	1.6105
622	Skin Grafts and Wound Debridement for Endocrine, Nutritional and Metabolic Disorders with MCC	3.8256
623	Skin Grafts and Wound Debridement for Endocrine, Nutritional and Metabolic Disorders with CC	1.8614
901	Wound Debridements for Injuries with MCC	4.3278
902	Wound Debridements for Injuries with CC	1.8847

DRG	PDx/SDx/Procedure	Tips
463	Musculoskeletal and connective tissue principal diagnosis	Ensure that documentation includes underlying cause of condition requiring debridement and depth of debridement procedure.
	Osteomyelitis, all types (except diabetic)	
	Open wounds (lacerations) with tendon involvement	Laceration tendon—*see* Injury, muscle, by site, laceration
	AND	
	MCC condition	*See* appendix B.
464	Musculoskeletal and connective tissue principal diagnosis	Ensure that documentation includes underlying cause of condition requiring debridement and depth of debridement procedure.
	Osteomyelitis, all types (except diabetic)	
	Open wounds (lacerations) with tendon involvement	Laceration tendon—*see* Injury, muscle, by site, laceration
	AND	
	CC condition	*See* appendix B.
465	Musculoskeletal and connective tissue principal diagnosis	Ensure that documentation includes underlying cause of condition requiring debridement and depth of debridement procedure.
	Osteomyelitis, all types (except diabetic)	
	Open wounds (lacerations) with tendon involvement	Laceration tendon—*see* Injury, muscle, by site, laceration
570	MCC condition	*See* appendix B.
571	CC condition	*See* appendix B.
573	Skin ulcer or cellulitis principal diagnosis	
	AND	
	Skin grafting procedure	Skin grafting includes root operations Replacement of skin with a free graft of autologous (partial or full thickness), nonautologous or synthetic tissue; and Transfer of skin, and/or subcutaneous tissue and fascia which remains attached to its vascular and nervous supply. Other procedures include Excision and Supplement of tissues and Insertion of tissue expander.
	AND	
	MCC condition	*See* appendix B.
574	Skin ulcer or cellulitis principal diagnosis	
	AND	
	Skin grafting procedure	*See* DRG 573.
	AND	
	CC condition	*See* appendix B.
575	Skin ulcer or cellulitis principal diagnosis	
	AND	
	Skin grafting procedure	*See* DRG 573.
576	Diagnosis from MDC 9 other than skin ulcer or cellulitis	
	AND	
	Skin grafting procedure	*See* DRG 573.
	AND	
	MCC condition	*See* appendix B.
577	Diagnosis from MDC 9 other than skin ulcer or cellulitis	
	AND	
	Skin grafting procedure	*See* DRG 573.
	AND	
	CC condition	*See* appendix B.
578	Diagnosis from MDC 9 other than skin ulcer or cellulitis	
	AND	
	Skin grafting procedure	*See* DRG 573.

DRG 572 (Continued)

DRG	PDx/SDx/Procedure	Tips
622	Diabetic foot or other skin ulcer principal diagnosis	
	AND	
	MCC condition	*See* appendix B.
623	Diabetic foot or other skin ulcer principal diagnosis	
	AND	
	CC condition	*See* appendix B.
901	Injury diagnosis from MDC 21	
	Excisional debridement of wound, infection, or burn	The ICD-10-PCS definition of the root operation Excision is "Cutting out or off, without replacement, a portion of a body part." Debridement by excision involves cutting with a sharp instrument such as a scalpel or other methods such as a hot knife or laser. Non-excisional debridement of skin is coded to root operation Extraction. Ensure that documentation includes instruments used, technique, and depth of debridement procedure.
	AND	
	MCC condition	*See* appendix B.
902	Injury diagnosis from MDC 21	
	Excisional debridement of wound, infection, or burn	*See* DRG 901.
	AND	
	CC condition	*See* appendix B.

DRG 573 Skin Graft for Skin Ulcer or Cellulitis with MCC — RW 6.2181

No Potential DRGs

DRG 574 Skin Graft for Skin Ulcer or Cellulitis with CC — RW 3.4058

Potential DRGs

463	Wound Debridement and Skin Graft Except Hand for Musculoskeletal and Connective Tissue Disorders with MCC	5.6637
573	Skin Graft for Skin Ulcer or Cellulitis with MCC	6.2181
622	Skin Grafts and Wound Debridement for Endocrine, Nutritional and Metabolic Disorders with MCC	3.8256

DRG	PDx/SDx/Procedure	Tips
463	Musculoskeletal and connective tissue principal diagnosis	Ensure that documentation includes underlying cause of condition requiring debridement and depth of debridement procedure.
	Osteomyelitis, all types (except diabetic)	
	Open wounds (lacerations) with tendon involvement	Laceration tendon—*see* Injury, muscle, by site, laceration.
	AND	
	MCC condition	*See* appendix B.
573	MCC condition	*See* appendix B.
622	Diabetic foot or other skin ulcer principal diagnosis	
	AND	
	MCC condition	*See* appendix B.

DRG 575 Skin Graft for Skin Ulcer or Cellulitis without CC/MCC RW 2.0460

Potential DRGs

463	Wound Debridement and Skin Graft Except Hand for Musculoskeletal and Connective Tissue Disorders with MCC	5.6637
464	Wound Debridement and Skin Graft Except Hand for Musculoskeletal and Connective Tissue Disorders with CC	3.0014
573	Skin Graft for Skin Ulcer or Cellulitis with MCC	6.2181
574	Skin Graft for Skin Ulcer or Cellulitis with CC	3.4058
622	Skin Grafts and Wound Debridement for Endocrine, Nutritional and Metabolic Disorders with MCC	3.8256

DRG	PDx/SDx/Procedure	Tips
463	Musculoskeletal and connective tissue principal diagnosis	Ensure that documentation includes underlying cause of condition requiring debridement and depth of debridement procedure.
	Osteomyelitis, all types (except diabetic)	
	Open wounds (lacerations) with tendon involvement	Laceration tendon—*see* Injury, muscle, by site, laceration.
	AND	
	MCC condition	*See* appendix B.
464	Musculoskeletal and connective tissue principal diagnosis	*See* DRG 463.
	Osteomyelitis, all types (except diabetic)	
	Open wounds (lacerations) with tendon involvement	Laceration tendon—*see* Injury, muscle, by site, laceration.
	AND	
	CC condition	*See* appendix B.
573	MCC condition	*See* appendix B.
574	CC condition	*See* appendix B.
622	Diabetic foot or other skin ulcer principal diagnosis	
	AND	
	MCC condition	*See* appendix B.

DRG 576 Skin Graft Except for Skin Ulcer or Cellulitis with MCC RW 5.6831

573	Skin Graft for Skin Ulcer or Cellulitis with MCC	6.2181

DRG	PDx/SDx/Procedure	Tips
573	Skin ulcer or cellulitis principal diagnosis	
	AND	
	MCC condition	*See* appendix B.

DRG 577 Skin Graft Except for Skin Ulcer or Cellulitis with CC RW 2.6491

Potential DRGs

463	Wound Debridement and Skin Graft Except Hand for Musculoskeletal and Connective Tissue Disorders with MCC	5.6637
464	Wound Debridement and Skin Graft Except Hand for Musculoskeletal and Connective Tissue Disorders with CC	3.0014
573	Skin Graft for Skin Ulcer or Cellulitis with MCC	6.2181
574	Skin Graft for Skin Ulcer or Cellulitis with CC	3.4058
576	Skin Graft Except for Skin Ulcer or Cellulitis with MCC	5.6831
622	Skin Grafts and Wound Debridement for Endocrine, Nutritional and Metabolic Disorders with MCC	3.8256

DRG	PDx/SDx/Procedure	Tips
463	Musculoskeletal and connective tissue principal diagnosis	Ensure that documentation includes underlying cause of condition requiring debridement and depth of debridement procedure.
	Osteomyelitis, all types (except diabetic)	
	Open wounds (lacerations) with tendon involvement	Laceration tendon—*see* Injury, muscle, by site, laceration.
	AND	
	MCC condition	*See* appendix B.
464	Musculoskeletal and connective tissue principal diagnosis	*See* DRG 463.
	Osteomyelitis, all types (except diabetic)	
	Open wounds (lacerations) with tendon involvement	Laceration tendon—*see* Injury, muscle, by site, laceration.
	AND	
	CC condition	*See* appendix B.
573	Skin ulcer or cellulitis principal diagnosis	
	AND	
	MCC condition	*See* appendix B.
574	Skin ulcer or cellulitis principal diagnosis	
	AND	
	CC condition	*See* appendix B.
576	MCC condition	*See* appendix B.
622	Diabetic foot or other skin ulcer principal diagnosis	
	AND	
	MCC condition	*See* appendix B.

DRG 578 Skin Graft Except for Skin Ulcer or Cellulitis without CC/MCC RW 1.6105

Potential DRGs

463	Wound Debridement and Skin Graft Except Hand for Musculoskeletal and Connective Tissue Disorders with MCC	5.6637
464	Wound Debridement and Skin Graft Except Hand for Musculoskeletal and Connective Tissue Disorders with CC	3.0014
465	Wound Debridement and Skin Graft Except Hand for Musculoskeletal and Connective Tissue Disorders without CC/MCC	1.8708
573	Skin Graft for Skin Ulcer or Cellulitis with MCC	6.2181
574	Skin Graft for Skin Ulcer or Cellulitis with CC	3.4058
575	Skin Graft for Skin Ulcer or Cellulitis without CC/MCC	2.0460
576	Skin Graft Except for Skin Ulcer or Cellulitis with MCC	5.6831
577	Skin Graft Except for Skin Ulcer or Cellulitis with CC	2.6491
622	Skin Grafts and Wound Debridement for Endocrine, Nutritional and Metabolic Disorders with MCC	3.8256
623	Skin Grafts and Wound Debridement for Endocrine, Nutritional and Metabolic Disorders with CC	1.8614

DRG	PDx/SDx/Procedure	Tips
463	Musculoskeletal and connective tissue principal diagnosis	Ensure that documentation includes underlying cause of condition requiring debridement and depth of debridement procedure.
	Osteomyelitis, all types (except diabetic)	
	Open wounds (lacerations) with tendon involvement	Laceration tendon—*see* Injury, muscle, by site, laceration.
	AND	
	MCC condition	*See* appendix B.
464	Musculoskeletal and connective tissue principal diagnosis	Ensure that documentation includes underlying cause of condition requiring debridement and depth of debridement procedure.
	Osteomyelitis, all types (except diabetic)	
	Open wounds (lacerations) with tendon involvement	Laceration tendon—*see* Injury, muscle, by site, laceration.
	AND	
	CC condition	*See* appendix B.
465	Musculoskeletal and connective tissue principal diagnosis	*See* DRG 464.
	Osteomyelitis, all types (except diabetic)	
	Open wounds (lacerations) with tendon involvement	Laceration tendon—*see* Injury, muscle, by site, laceration.
573	Skin ulcer or cellulitis principal diagnosis	
	AND	
	MCC condition	*See* appendix B.
574	Skin ulcer or cellulitis principal diagnosis	
	AND	
	CC condition	*See* appendix B.
575	Skin ulcer or cellulitis principal diagnosis	
576	MCC condition	*See* appendix B.
577	CC condition	*See* appendix B.
622	Diabetic foot or other skin ulcer principal diagnosis	
	AND	
	MCC condition	*See* appendix B.
623	Diabetic foot or other skin ulcer principal diagnosis	
	AND	
	CC condition	*See* appendix B.

DRG 579 Other Skin, Subcutaneous Tissue and Breast Procedures with MCC RW 3.3422

Potential DRGs

573	Skin Graft for Skin Ulcer or Cellulitis with MCC	6.2181

DRG	PDx/SDx/Procedure	Tips
573	Skin ulcer or cellulitis principal diagnosis	
	AND	
	Skin grafting procedure	Skin grafting includes root operations Replacement of skin with a free graft of autologous (partial or full thickness), nonautologous or synthetic tissue; and Transfer of skin, and/or subcutaneous tissue and fascia which remains attached to its vascular and nervous supply. Other procedures include Excision and Supplement of tissues and Insertion of tissue expander.
	AND	
	MCC condition	*See* appendix B.

DRG 580 Other Skin, Subcutaneous Tissue and Breast Procedures with CC

RW 1.7466

Potential DRGs

570	Skin Debridement with MCC	2.9222
573	Skin Graft for Skin Ulcer or Cellulitis with MCC	6.2181
574	Skin Graft for Skin Ulcer or Cellulitis with CC	3.4058
579	Other Skin, Subcutaneous Tissue and Breast Procedures with MCC	3.3422
904	Skin Grafts for Injuries with CC/MCC	3.2562

DRG	PDx/SDx/Procedure	Tips
570	Excisional debridement of skin	The ICD-10-PCS definition of the root operation Excision is "Cutting out or off, without replacement, a portion of a body part." Debridement by excision involves cutting with a sharp instrument such as a scalpel or other methods such as a hot knife or laser. Non-excisional debridement of skin is coded to root operation Extraction. Ensure that documentation includes instruments used, technique, and depth of debridement procedure.
	AND	
	MCC condition	*See* appendix B.
573	Skin ulcer or cellulitis principal diagnosis	
	AND	
	Skin grafting procedure	Skin grafting includes root operations Replacement of skin with a free graft of autologous (partial or full thickness), nonautologous or synthetic tissue; and Transfer of skin, and/or subcutaneous tissue and fascia which remains attached to its vascular and nervous supply. Other procedures include Excision and Supplement of tissues and Insertion of tissue expander.
	AND	
	MCC condition	*See* appendix B.
574	Skin ulcer or cellulitis principal diagnosis	
	AND	
	Skin grafting procedure	*See* DRG 573.
	AND	
	CC condition	*See* appendix B.
579	MCC condition	*See* appendix B.
904	Injury diagnosis from MDC 21	
	AND	
	Skin grafting procedure	*See* DRG 573.
	AND	
	CC/MCC condition	*See* appendix B.

DRG 581 Other Skin, Subcutaneous Tissue and Breast Procedures without CC/MCC — RW 1.3467

Potential DRGs

570	Skin Debridement with MCC	2.9222
571	Skin Debridement with CC	1.6919
573	Skin Graft for Skin Ulcer or Cellulitis with MCC	6.2181
574	Skin Graft for Skin Ulcer or Cellulitis with CC	3.4058
575	Skin Graft for Skin Ulcer or Cellulitis without CC/MCC	2.0460
579	Other Skin, Subcutaneous Tissue and Breast Procedures with MCC	3.3422
580	Other Skin, Subcutaneous Tissue and Breast Procedures with CC	1.7466
904	Skin Grafts for Injuries with CC/MCC	3.2562
905	Skin Grafts for Injuries without CC/MCC	1.5837

DRG	PDx/SDx/Procedure	Tips
570	Excisional debridement of skin	The ICD-10-PCS definition of the root operation Excision is "Cutting out or off, without replacement, a portion of a body part." Debridement by excision involves cutting with a sharp instrument such as a scalpel or other methods such as a hot knife or laser. Non-excisional debridement of skin is coded to root operation Extraction. Ensure that documentation includes instruments used, technique, and depth of debridement procedure.
	AND	
	MCC condition	*See* appendix B.
571	Excisional debridement of skin	*See* DRG 570.
	AND	
	CC condition	*See* appendix B.
573	Skin ulcer or cellulitis principal diagnosis	
	AND	
	Skin grafting procedure	Skin grafting includes root operations Replacement of skin with a free graft of autologous (partial or full thickness), nonautologous or synthetic tissue; and Transfer of skin, and/or subcutaneous tissue and fascia which remains attached to its vascular and nervous supply. Other procedures include Excision and Supplement of tissues and Insertion of tissue expander.
	AND	
	MCC condition	*See* appendix B.
574	Skin ulcer or cellulitis principal diagnosis	
	AND	
	Skin grafting procedure	*See* DRG 573.
	AND	
	CC condition	*See* appendix B.
575	Skin ulcer or cellulitis principal diagnosis	
	AND	
	Skin grafting procedure	*See* DRG 573.
579	MCC condition	*See* appendix B.
580	CC condition	*See* appendix B.
904	Injury diagnosis from MDC 21	
	AND	
	Skin grafting procedure	*See* DRG 573.
	AND	
	CC/MCC condition	*See* appendix B.
905	Injury diagnosis from MDC 21	
	AND	
	Skin grafting procedure	*See* DRG 573.

DRG 582 Mastectomy for Malignancy with CC/MCC — RW 1.6671

Potential DRGs

579	Other Skin, Subcutaneous Tissue and Breast Procedures with MCC	3.3422

DRG	PDx/SDx/Procedure	Tips
579	Lymph node excisions	
	OR	
	Insertion of infusion pump in subcutaneous tissue and fascia	
	AND	
	MCC condition	*See* appendix B.

DRG 583 Mastectomy for Malignancy without CC/MCC RW 1.5219

Potential DRGs

579	Other Skin, Subcutaneous Tissue and Breast Procedures with MCC	3.3422
580	Other Skin, Subcutaneous Tissue and Breast Procedures with CC	1.7466
582	Mastectomy for Malignancy with CC/MCC	1.6671

DRG	PDx/SDx/Procedure	Tips
579	Lymph node excisions	
	OR	
	Insertion of infusion pump in subcutaneous tissue and fascia	
	AND	
	MCC condition	*See* appendix B.
580	Lymph node excisions	
	OR	
	Insertion of infusion pump in subcutaneous tissue and fascia	
	AND	
	CC condition	*See* appendix B.
582	MCC condition	*See* appendix B.
	OR	
	CC condition	*See* appendix B.

DRG 584 Breast Biopsy, Local Excision and Other Breast Procedures with CC/MCC RW 1.9586

Potential DRGs

579	Other Skin, Subcutaneous Tissue and Breast Procedures with MCC	3.3422
619	O.R. Procedures for Obesity with MCC	2.5885

DRG	PDx/SDx/Procedure	Tips
579	Lymph node excisions	
	OR	
	Insertion of infusion pump in subcutaneous tissue and fascia	
	AND	
	MCC condition	*See* appendix B.
619	Obesity	
	AND	
	Reduction mammoplasty (unilateral or bilateral)	Excision only, not by liposuction (Alteration or Extraction)
	AND	
	MCC condition	*See* appendix B.

DRG 585 Breast Biopsy, Local Excision and Other Breast Procedures without CC/MCC RW 1.6840

Potential DRGs

579	Other Skin, Subcutaneous Tissue and Breast Procedures with MCC	3.3422
584	Breast Biopsy, Local Excision and Other Breast Procedures with CC/MCC	1.9586
619	O.R. Procedures for Obesity with MCC	2.5885

DRG	PDx/SDx/Procedure	Tips
579	Lymph node excisions	
	OR	
	Insertion of infusion pump in subcutaneous tissue and fascia	
	AND	
	MCC condition	*See* appendix B.
584	MCC condition	
	OR	
	CC condition	*See* appendix B.
619	Obesity	
	AND	
	Reduction mammoplasty (unilateral or bilateral)	Excision only, not by liposuction (Alteration or Extraction)
	AND	
	MCC condition	*See* appendix B.

DRG 592 Skin Ulcers with MCC — RW 2.0901

Potential DRGs

570	Skin Debridement with MCC	2.9222
573	Skin Graft for Skin Ulcer or Cellulitis with MCC	6.2181
622	Skin Grafts and Wound Debridement for Endocrine, Nutritional and Metabolic Disorders with MCC	3.8256

DRG	PDx/SDx/Procedure	Tips
570	Excisional debridement of skin	The ICD-10-PCS definition of the root operation Excision is "Cutting out or off, without replacement, a portion of a body part." Debridement by excision involves cutting with a sharp instrument such as a scalpel or other methods such as a hot knife or laser. Non-excisional debridement of skin is coded to root operation Extraction. Ensure that documentation includes instruments used, technique, and depth of debridement procedure.
	AND	
	MCC condition	*See* appendix B.
573	Skin grafting procedure	Skin grafting includes root operations Replacement of skin with a free graft of autologous (partial or full thickness), nonautologous or synthetic tissue; and Transfer of skin, and/or subcutaneous tissue and fascia which remains attached to its vascular and nervous supply. Other procedures include Excision and Supplement of tissues and Insertion of tissue expander.
	AND	
	MCC condition	*See* appendix B.
622	Diabetic foot or other skin ulcer principal diagnosis	
	AND	
	MCC condition	*See* appendix B.

DRG 593 Skin Ulcers with CC — RW 1.2099

Potential DRGs

570	Skin Debridement with MCC	2.9222
571	Skin Debridement with CC	1.6919
573	Skin Graft for Skin Ulcer or Cellulitis with MCC	6.2181
574	Skin Graft for Skin Ulcer or Cellulitis with CC	3.4058
592	Skin Ulcers with MCC	2.0901
602	Cellulitis with MCC	1.4875
622	Skin Grafts and Wound Debridement for Endocrine, Nutritional and Metabolic Disorders with MCC	3.8256
623	Skin Grafts and Wound Debridement for Endocrine, Nutritional and Metabolic Disorders with CC	1.8614

DRG	PDx/SDx/Procedure	Tips
570	Excisional debridement of skin	The ICD-10-PCS definition of the root operation Excision is "Cutting out or off, without replacement, a portion of a body part." Debridement by excision involves cutting with a sharp instrument such as a scalpel or other methods such as a hot knife or laser. Non-excisional debridement of skin is coded to root operation Extraction. Ensure that documentation includes instruments used, technique, and depth of debridement procedure.
	AND	
	MCC condition	*See* appendix B.
571	Excisional debridement of skin	*See* DRG 570.
	AND	
	CC condition	*See* appendix B.
573	Skin grafting procedure	Skin grafting includes root operations Replacement of skin with a free graft of autologous (partial or full thickness), nonautologous or synthetic tissue; and Transfer of skin, and/or subcutaneous tissue and fascia which remains attached to its vascular and nervous supply. Other procedures include Excision and Supplement of tissues and Insertion of tissue expander.
	AND	
	MCC condition	*See* appendix B.
574	Skin grafting procedure	*See* DRG 573.
	AND	
	CC condition	*See* appendix B.
592	MCC condition	*See* appendix B.
602	Cutaneous abscess and cellulitis Other local infection of skin and subcutaneous tissue	
	AND	
	MCC condition	*See* appendix B.
622	Diabetic foot or other skin ulcer principal diagnosis	
	AND	
	MCC condition	*See* appendix B.
623	Diabetic foot or other skin ulcer principal diagnosis	
	AND	
	CC condition	*See* appendix B.

DRG 594 Skin Ulcers without CC/MCC

RW 0.7874

Potential DRGs

570	Skin Debridement with MCC	2.9222
571	Skin Debridement with CC	1.6919
572	Skin Debridement without CC/MCC	1.1396
573	Skin Graft for Skin Ulcer or Cellulitis with MCC	6.2181
574	Skin Graft for Skin Ulcer or Cellulitis with CC	3.4058
575	Skin Graft for Skin Ulcer or Cellulitis without CC/MCC	2.0460
592	Skin Ulcers with MCC	2.0901
593	Skin Ulcers with CC	1.2099
602	Cellulitis with MCC	1.4875
603	Cellulitis without MCC	0.8847
622	Skin Grafts and Wound Debridement for Endocrine, Nutritional and Metabolic Disorders with MCC	3.8256
623	Skin Grafts and Wound Debridement for Endocrine, Nutritional and Metabolic Disorders with CC	1.8614
624	Skin Grafts and Wound Debridement for Endocrine, Nutritional and Metabolic Disorders without CC/MCC	1.1145

DRG	PDx/SDx/Procedure	Tips
570	Excisional debridement of skin	The ICD-10-PCS definition of the root operation Excision is "Cutting out or off, without replacement, a portion of a body part." Debridement by excision involves cutting with a sharp instrument such as a scalpel or other methods such as a hot knife or laser. Non-excisional debridement of skin is coded to root operation Extraction. Ensure that documentation includes instruments used, technique, and depth of debridement procedure.
	AND	
	MCC condition	*See* appendix B.
571	Excisional debridement of skin	*See* DRG 570.
	AND	
	CC condition	*See* appendix B.
572	Excisional debridement of skin	*See* DRG 570.
573	Skin grafting procedure	Skin grafting includes root operations Replacement of skin with a free graft of autologous (partial or full thickness), nonautologous or synthetic tissue; and Transfer of skin, and/or subcutaneous tissue and fascia which remains attached to its vascular and nervous supply. Other procedures include Excision and Supplement of tissues and Insertion of tissue expander.
	AND	
	MCC condition	*See* appendix B.
574	Skin grafting procedure	*See* DRG 573.
	AND	
	CC condition	*See* appendix B.
575	Skin grafting procedure	*See* DRG 573.
592	MCC condition	*See* appendix B.
593	CC condition	*See* appendix B.
602	Cutaneous abscess and cellulitis Other local infection of skin and subcutaneous tissue	
	AND	
	MCC condition	*See* appendix B.
603	Cutaneous abscess and cellulitis Other local infection of skin and subcutaneous tissue	
	AND	
	CC condition	*See* appendix B.
622	Diabetic foot or other skin ulcer principal diagnosis	
	AND	
	MCC condition	*See* appendix B.
623	Diabetic foot or other skin ulcer principal diagnosis	
	AND	
	CC condition	*See* appendix B.
624	Diabetic foot or other skin ulcer principal diagnosis	

DRG 595 Major Skin Disorders with MCC — RW 2.1750

Potential DRGs

576	Skin Graft Except for Skin Ulcer or Cellulitis with MCC	5.6831
579	Other Skin, Subcutaneous Tissue and Breast Procedures with MCC	3.3422

DRG	PDx/SDx/Procedure	Tips
576	Skin grafting procedure	Skin grafting includes root operations Replacement of skin with a free graft of autologous (partial or full thickness), nonautologous or synthetic tissue; and Transfer of skin, and/or subcutaneous tissue and fascia which remains attached to its vascular and nervous supply. Other procedures include Excision and Supplement of tissues and Insertion of tissue expander.
	AND	
	MCC condition	*See* appendix B.
579	Lymph node excisions	
	OR	
	Insertion of infusion pump in subcutaneous tissue and fascia	
	AND	
	MCC condition	*See* appendix B.

DRG 596 Major Skin Disorders without MCC — RW 1.0090

Potential DRGs

576	Skin Graft Except for Skin Ulcer or Cellulitis with MCC	5.6831
577	Skin Graft Except for Skin Ulcer or Cellulitis with CC	2.6491
578	Skin Graft Except for Skin Ulcer or Cellulitis without CC/MCC	1.6105
579	Other Skin, Subcutaneous Tissue and Breast Procedures with MCC	3.3422
580	Other Skin, Subcutaneous Tissue and Breast Procedures with CC	1.7466
581	Other Skin, Subcutaneous Tissue and Breast Procedures without CC/MCC	1.3467
595	Major Skin Disorders with MCC	2.1750

DRG	PDx/SDx/Procedure	Tips
576	Skin grafting procedure	Skin grafting includes root operations Replacement of skin with a free graft of autologous (partial or full thickness), nonautologous or synthetic tissue; and Transfer of skin, and/or subcutaneous tissue and fascia which remains attached to its vascular and nervous supply. Other procedures include Excision and Supplement of tissues and Insertion of tissue expander.
	AND	
	MCC condition	*See* appendix B.
577	Skin grafting procedure	*See* DRG 576.
	AND	
	CC condition	*See* appendix B.
578	Skin grafting procedure	*See* DRG 576.
579	Lymph node excisions	
	OR	
	Insertion of infusion pump in subcutaneous tissue and fascia	
	AND	
	MCC condition	*See* appendix B.
580	Lymph node excisions	
	OR	
	Insertion of infusion pump in subcutaneous tissue and fascia	
	AND	
	CC condition	*See* appendix B.
581	Lymph node excisions	
	OR	
	Insertion of infusion pump in subcutaneous tissue and fascia	
595	MCC condition	*See* appendix B.

DRG 597 Malignant Breast Disorders with MCC — RW 1.6005

Potential DRGs

579	Other Skin, Subcutaneous Tissue and Breast Procedures with MCC	3.3422
584	Breast Biopsy, Local Excision and Other Breast Procedures with CC/MCC	1.9586

DRG	PDx/SDx/Procedure	Tips
579	Lymph node excisions	
	OR	
	Insertion of infusion pump in subcutaneous tissue and fascia	
	AND	
	MCC condition	*See* appendix B.
584	Open excisional biopsy of breast	
	OR	
	Insertion of breast tissue expander(s)	
	AND	
	CC/MCC condition	*See* appendix B.

DRG 598 Malignant Breast Disorders with CC — RW 1.1988

Potential DRGs

579	Other Skin, Subcutaneous Tissue and Breast Procedures with MCC	3.3422
580	Other Skin, Subcutaneous Tissue and Breast Procedures with CC	1.7466
582	Mastectomy for Malignancy with CC/MCC	1.6671
584	Breast Biopsy, Local Excision and Other Breast Procedures with CC/MCC	1.9586
597	Malignant Breast Disorders with MCC	1.6005

DRG	PDx/SDx/Procedure	Tips
579	Lymph node excisions	
	OR	
	Insertion of infusion pump in subcutaneous tissue and fascia	
	AND	
	MCC condition	*See* appendix B.
580	Lymph node excisions	
	OR	
	Insertion of infusion pump in subcutaneous tissue and fascia	
	AND	
	CC condition	*See* appendix B.
582	Mastectomy, partial or total	
	AND	
	MCC condition	*See* appendix B.
	OR	
	CC condition	*See* appendix B.
584	Open excisional biopsy of breast	
	OR	
	Insertion of breast tissue expander(s)	
	AND	
	CC/MCC condition	*See* appendix B.
597	MCC condition	*See* appendix B.

DRG 599 Malignant Breast Disorders without CC/MCC — RW 0.6214

Potential DRGs

579	Other Skin, Subcutaneous Tissue and Breast Procedures with MCC	3.3422
580	Other Skin, Subcutaneous Tissue and Breast Procedures with CC	1.7466
581	Other Skin, Subcutaneous Tissue and Breast Procedures without CC/MCC	1.3467
582	Mastectomy for Malignancy with CC/MCC	1.6671
583	Mastectomy for Malignancy without CC/MCC	1.5219
584	Breast Biopsy, Local Excision and Other Breast Procedures with CC/MCC	1.9586
585	Breast Biopsy, Local Excision and Other Breast Procedures without CC/MCC	1.6840
597	Malignant Breast Disorders with MCC	1.6005
598	Malignant Breast Disorders with CC	1.1988

DRG	PDx/SDx/Procedure	Tips
579	Lymph node excisions	
	OR	
	Insertion of infusion pump in subcutaneous tissue and fascia	
	AND	
	MCC condition	*See* appendix B.
580	Lymph node excisions	
	OR	
	Insertion of infusion pump in subcutaneous tissue and fascia	
	AND	
	CC condition	*See* appendix B.
581	Lymph node excisions	
	OR	
	Insertion of infusion pump in subcutaneous tissue and fascia	
582	Mastectomy, partial or total	
	AND	
	CC/MCC condition	*See* appendix B.
583	Mastectomy, partial or total	
584	Open excisional biopsy of breast	
	OR	
	Insertion of breast tissue expander(s)	
	AND	
	CC/MCC condition	*See* appendix B.
585	Open excisional biopsy of breast	
	OR	
	Insertion of breast tissue expander(s)	
597	MCC condition	*See* appendix B.
598	CC condition	*See* appendix B.

DRG 600 Nonmalignant Breast Disorders with CC/MCC — RW 1.0255

Potential DRGs

579	Other Skin, Subcutaneous Tissue and Breast Procedures with MCC	3.3422
580	Other Skin, Subcutaneous Tissue and Breast Procedures with CC	1.7466
584	Breast Biopsy, Local Excision and Other Breast Procedures with CC/MCC	1.9586
597	Malignant Breast Disorders with MCC	1.6005
598	Malignant Breast Disorders with CC	1.1988

DRG	PDx/SDx/Procedure	Tips
579	Lymph node excisions	
	OR	
	Insertion of infusion pump in subcutaneous tissue and fascia	
	AND	
	MCC condition	*See* appendix B.
580	Lymph node excisions	
	OR	
	Insertion of infusion pump in subcutaneous tissue and fascia	
	AND	
	CC condition	*See* appendix B.
584	Open excisional biopsy of breast	
	OR	
	Insertion of breast tissue expander(s)	
	AND	
	CC/MCC condition	*See* appendix B.
597	Malignant primary or secondary neoplasm of female or male breast	
	OR	
	Carcinoma in situ or neoplasm of uncertain behavior of breast	
	AND	
	MCC condition	*See* appendix B.
598	Malignant primary or secondary neoplasm of female or male breast	
	OR	
	Carcinoma in situ or neoplasm of uncertain behavior of breast	
	AND	
	CC condition	*See* appendix B.

DRG 601 Nonmalignant Breast Disorders without CC/MCC

RW 0.6226

Potential DRGs

579	Other Skin, Subcutaneous Tissue and Breast Procedures with MCC	3.3422
580	Other Skin, Subcutaneous Tissue and Breast Procedures with CC	1.7466
581	Other Skin, Subcutaneous Tissue and Breast Procedures without CC/MCC	1.3467
584	Breast Biopsy, Local Excision and Other Breast Procedures with CC/MCC	1.9586
585	Breast Biopsy, Local Excision and Other Breast Procedures without CC/MCC	1.6840
597	Malignant Breast Disorders with MCC	1.6005
598	Malignant Breast Disorders with CC	1.1988
600	Nonmalignant Breast Disorders with CC/MCC	1.0255

DRG	PDx/SDx/Procedure	Tips
579	Lymph node excisions	
	OR	
	Insertion of infusion pump in subcutaneous tissue and fascia	
	AND	
	MCC condition	*See* appendix B.
580	Lymph node excisions	
	OR	
	Insertion of infusion pump in subcutaneous tissue and fascia	
	AND	
	CC condition	*See* appendix B.
581	Lymph node excisions	
	OR	
	Insertion of infusion pump in subcutaneous tissue and fascia	
584	Open excisional biopsy of breast	
	OR	
	Insertion of breast tissue expander(s)	
	AND	
	CC/MCC condition	*See* appendix B.
585	Open excisional biopsy of breast	
	OR	
	Insertion of breast tissue expander(s)	
597	Malignant primary or secondary neoplasm of female or male breast	
	OR	
	Carcinoma in situ or neoplasm of uncertain behavior of breast	
	AND	
	MCC condition	*See* appendix B.
598	Malignant primary or secondary neoplasm of female or male breast	
	OR	
	Carcinoma in situ or neoplasm of uncertain behavior of breast	
	AND	
	CC condition	*See* appendix B.
600	CC/MCC condition	*See* appendix B.

DRG 602 Cellulitis with MCC RW 1.4875

Potential DRGs

314	Other Circulatory System Diagnoses with MCC	2.0935
570	Skin Debridement with MCC	2.9222
573	Skin Graft for Skin Ulcer or Cellulitis with MCC	6.2181
579	Other Skin, Subcutaneous Tissue and Breast Procedures with MCC	3.3422
622	Skin Grafts and Wound Debridement for Endocrine, Nutritional and Metabolic Disorders with MCC	3.8256

DRG	PDx/SDx/Procedure	Tips
314	Cellulitis due to central venous catheter	When the provider documents a causal relationship between the catheter and cellulitis, the complication code should be reported first.
	AND	
	MCC condition	*See* appendix B.
570	Excisional debridement of skin	The ICD-10-PCS definition of the root operation Excision is "Cutting out or off, without replacement, a portion of a body part." Debridement by excision involves cutting with a sharp instrument such as a scalpel or other methods such as a hot knife or laser. Non-excisional debridement of skin is coded to root operation Extraction. Ensure that documentation includes instruments used, technique, and depth of debridement procedure.
	AND	
	MCC condition	*See* appendix B.
573	Skin grafting procedure	Skin grafting includes root operations Replacement of skin with a free graft of autologous (partial or full thickness), nonautologous or synthetic tissue; and Transfer of skin, and/or subcutaneous tissue and fascia which remains attached to its vascular and nervous supply. Other procedures include Excision and Supplement of tissues and Insertion of tissue expander.
	AND	
	MCC condition	*See* appendix B.
579	Insertion of infusion pump in subcutaneous tissue and fascia	
	AND	
	MCC condition	*See* appendix B.
622	Diabetes (type 1, type 2, other specified) with ketoacidosis, hyperosmolarity, other coma, other and unspecified complications Diabetic foot or other skin ulcer principal diagnosis	
	AND	
	Excisional debridement	
	AND	
	MCC condition	*See* appendix B.

DRG 603 Cellulitis without MCC RW 0.8847

Potential DRGs

314	Other Circulatory System Diagnoses with MCC	2.0935
315	Other Circulatory System Diagnoses with CC	0.9673
570	Skin Debridement with MCC	2.9222
571	Skin Debridement with CC	1.6919
572	Skin Debridement without CC/MCC	1.1396
573	Skin Graft for Skin Ulcer or Cellulitis with MCC	6.2181
574	Skin Graft for Skin Ulcer or Cellulitis with CC	3.4058
575	Skin Graft for Skin Ulcer or Cellulitis without CC/MCC	2.0460
579	Other Skin, Subcutaneous Tissue and Breast Procedures with MCC	3.3422
580	Other Skin, Subcutaneous Tissue and Breast Procedures with CC	1.7466
581	Other Skin, Subcutaneous Tissue and Breast Procedures without CC/MCC	1.3467
592	Skin Ulcers with MCC	2.0901
593	Skin Ulcers with CC	1.2099
602	Cellulitis with MCC	1.4875
622	Skin Grafts and Wound Debridement for Endocrine, Nutritional and Metabolic Disorders with MCC	3.8256
623	Skin Grafts and Wound Debridement for Endocrine, Nutritional and Metabolic Disorders with CC	1.8614
624	Skin Grafts and Wound Debridement for Endocrine, Nutritional and Metabolic Disorders without CC/MCC	1.1145

DRG	PDx/SDx/Procedure	Tips
314	Cellulitis due to central venous catheter	When the provider documents a causal relationship between the catheter and cellulitis, the complication code should be reported first.
	AND	
	MCC condition	*See* appendix B.
315	Cellulitis due to central venous catheter	*See* DRG 314.
	AND	
	CC condition	*See* appendix B.
570	Excisional debridement of skin	The ICD-10-PCS definition of the root operation Excision is "Cutting out or off, without replacement, a portion of a body part." Debridement by excision involves cutting with a sharp instrument such as a scalpel or other methods such as a hot knife or laser. Non-excisional debridement of skin is coded to root operation Extraction. Ensure that documentation includes instruments used, technique, and depth of debridement procedure.
	AND	
	MCC condition	*See* appendix B.

DRG 603 (Continued)

DRG	PDx/SDx/Procedure	Tips
571	Excisional debridement of skin	*See* DRG 570.
	AND	
	CC condition	*See* appendix B.
572	Excisional debridement of skin	*See* DRG 570.
573	Skin grafting procedure	Skin grafting includes root operations Replacement of skin with a free graft of autologous (partial or full thickness), nonautologous or synthetic tissue; and Transfer of skin, and/or subcutaneous tissue and fascia which remains attached to its vascular and nervous supply. Other procedures include Excision and Supplement of tissues and Insertion of tissue expander.
	AND	
	MCC condition	*See* appendix B.
574	Skin grafting procedure	*See* DRG 573.
	AND	
	CC condition	*See* appendix B.
575	Skin grafting procedure	*See* DRG 573.
579	Insertion of infusion pump in subcutaneous tissue and fascia	
	AND	
	MCC condition	*See* appendix B.
580	Insertion of infusion pump in subcutaneous tissue and fascia	
	AND	
	CC condition	*See* appendix B.
581	Insertion of infusion pump in subcutaneous tissue and fascia	
592	Skin ulcer	
	AND	
	MCC condition	*See* appendix B.
593	Skin ulcer	
	AND	
	CC condition	*See* appendix B.
602	MCC condition	*See* appendix B.
622	Diabetes (type 1, type 2, other specified) with ketoacidosis, hyperosmolarity, other coma, other and unspecified complications	
	Diabetic foot or other skin ulcer principal diagnosis	
	AND	
	MCC condition	*See* appendix B.
623	Diabetes (type 1, type 2, other specified) with ketoacidosis, hyperosmolarity, other coma, other and unspecified complications	
	Diabetic foot or other skin ulcer principal diagnosis	
	AND	
	CC condition	*See* appendix B.
624	Diabetes (type 1, type 2, other specified) with ketoacidosis, hyperosmolarity, other coma, other and unspecified complications	
	Diabetic foot or other skin ulcer principal diagnosis	

DRG 604 Trauma to the Skin, Subcutaneous Tissue and Breast with MCC — RW 1.5062

Potential DRGs

901	Wound Debridements for Injuries with MCC	4.3278
904	Skin Grafts for Injuries with CC/MCC	3.2562
922	Other Injury, Poisoning and Toxic Effect Diagnoses with MCC	1.7449

DRG	PDx/SDx/Procedure	Tips
901	Injury diagnosis from MDC 21	
	Excisional debridement of wound, infection, or burn	The ICD-10-PCS definition of the root operation Excision is "Cutting out or off, without replacement, a portion of a body part." Debridement by excision involves cutting with a sharp instrument such as a scalpel or other methods such as a hot knife or laser. Non-excisional debridement of skin is coded to root operation Extraction. Ensure that documentation includes instruments used, technique, and depth of debridement procedure.
	AND	
	MCC condition	*See* appendix B.
904	Injury diagnosis from MDC 21	
	AND	
	Skin grafting procedure	Skin grafting for injuries includes the root operations Replacement of skin with a free graft of autologous (partial or full thickness), nonautologous or synthetic tissue; and Transfer of skin, and/or subcutaneous tissue and fascia which remains attached to its vascular and nervous supply. Insertion of tissue expander is also included.
	AND	
	CC/MCC condition	*See* appendix B.
922	Observation following accident	Assign Z04.1, Z04.2, or Z04.3 only if there are no findings after diagnostic testing and a suspected diagnosis or injury is ruled out.
	AND	
	MCC condition	*See* appendix B.

DRG 605 Trauma to the Skin, Subcutaneous Tissue & Breast without MCC RW 0.9088

Potential DRGs

604	Trauma to the Skin, Subcutaneous Tissue and Breast with MCC	1.5062
901	Wound Debridements for Injuries with MCC	4.3278
902	Wound Debridements for Injuries with CC	1.8847
903	Wound Debridements for Injuries without CC/MCC	1.2415
904	Skin Grafts for Injuries with CC/MCC	3.2562
905	Skin Grafts for Injuries without CC/MCC	1.5837
913	Traumatic Injury with MCC	1.4945
922	Other Injury, Poisoning and Toxic Effect Diagnoses with MCC	1.7449

DRG	PDx/SDx/Procedure	Tips
604	MCC condition	*See* appendix B.
901	Injury diagnosis from MDC 21	
	Excisional debridement of wound, infection, or burn	The ICD-10-PCS definition of the root operation Excision is "Cutting out or off, without replacement, a portion of a body part." Debridement by excision involves cutting with a sharp instrument such as a scalpel or other methods such as a hot knife or laser. Non-excisional debridement of skin is coded to root operation Extraction. Ensure that documentation includes instruments used, technique, and depth of debridement procedure.
	AND	
	MCC condition	*See* appendix B.
902	Injury diagnosis from MDC 21	
	Excisional debridement of wound, infection, or burn	*See* DRG 901.
	AND	
	CC condition	*See* appendix B.
903	Injury diagnosis from MDC 21	
	Excisional debridement of wound, infection, or burn	*See* DRG 901.
904	Injury diagnosis from MDC 21	
	AND	
	Skin grafting procedure	Skin grafting for injuries includes the root operations Replacement of skin with a free graft of autologous (partial or full thickness), nonautologous or synthetic tissue; and Transfer of skin, and/or subcutaneous tissue and fascia which remains attached to its vascular and nervous supply. Insertion of tissue expander is also included.
	AND	
	CC/MCC condition	*See* appendix B.
905	Injury diagnosis from MDC 21	
	AND	
	Skin grafting procedure	*See* DRG 904.
913	Laceration or puncture wound of trunk with foreign body and/or penetration into thoracic cavity (initial encounter)	
	OR	
	Laceration or puncture wound of upper limb with foreign body (initial encounter)	
	OR	
	Laceration or puncture wound of lower limb with foreign body (initial encounter)	
	AND	
	MCC condition	*See* appendix B.
922	Observation following accident	Assign Z04.1, Z04.2, or Z04.3 only if there are no findings after diagnostic testing and a suspected diagnosis or injury is ruled out.
	AND	
	MCC condition	*See* appendix B.

DRG 606 Minor Skin Disorders with MCC RW 1.5858

Potential DRGs

595	Major Skin Disorders with MCC	2.1750

DRG	PDx/SDx/Procedure	Tips
595	Malignant melanoma	
	AND	
	MCC condition	*See* appendix B.

DRG 607 Minor Skin Disorders without MCC RW 0.8935

Potential DRGs

595	Major Skin Disorders with MCC	2.1750
596	Major Skin Disorders without MCC	1.0090
606	Minor Skin Disorders with MCC	1.5858

DRG	PDx/SDx/Procedure	Tips
595	Malignant melanoma	
	AND	
	MCC condition	*See* appendix B.
596	Malignant melanoma	
606	MCC condition	*See* appendix B.

Endocrine, Nutritional And Metabolic Diseases And Disorders

DRG 614 Adrenal and Pituitary Procedures with CC/MCC — RW 2.2524

No Potential DRGs

DRG 615 Adrenal and Pituitary Procedures without CC/MCC — RW 1.4711

Potential DRGs

614	Adrenal and Pituitary Procedures with CC/MCC	2.2524

DRG	PDx/SDx/Procedure	Tips
614	MCC condition	*See* appendix B.
	OR	
	CC condition	*See* appendix B.

DRG 616 Amputation of Lower Limb for Endocrine, Nutritional, and Metabolic Disorders with MCC — RW 3.9577

Potential DRGs

239	Amputation for Circulatory System Disorders Except Upper Limb and Toe with MCC	4.8068
474	Amputation for Musculoskeletal System and Connective Tissue Disorders with MCC	4.3028

DRG	PDx/SDx/Procedure	Tips
239	Diabetes with circulatory complications (e.g., peripheral angiopathy, with or without gangrene)	According to ICD-10-CM guidelines, the classification presumes a causal relationship between diabetes and certain associated manifestations and/or conditions when these terms are linked by the term "with" in the alphabetic index (either under a main term or subterm). These conditions should be coded as related to the diabetes unless the documentation clearly states the conditions are unrelated, in which case they may be coded separately. These conditions do not require provider documentation linking them to diabetes. Review the record and/or query the physician if it is unclear whether a condition is related to diabetes mellitus or the ICD-10-CM classification does not provide instruction.
	AND	
	MCC condition	*See* appendix B.
474	Musculoskeletal/connective tissue disorder: Osteomyelitis, acute, subacute, chronic, other, and unspecified Bone infections Pathologic fractures Osteonecrosis (aseptic necrosis) Malunion or nonunion of fracture	
	AND	
	MCC condition	*See* appendix B.

DRG 617 Amputation of Lower Limb for Endocrine, Nutritional, and Metabolic Disorders with CC

RW 1.9845

Potential DRGs

040	Peripheral/Cranial Nerve and Other Nervous System Procedures with MCC	3.8505
041	Peripheral/Cranial Nerve and Other Nervous System Procedures with CC or Peripheral Neurostimulator	2.2307
239	Amputation for Circulatory System Disorders Except Upper Limb and Toe with MCC	4.8068
240	Amputation for Circulatory System Disorders Except Upper Limb and Toe with CC	2.8092
255	Upper Limb and Toe Amputation for Circulatory System Disorders with MCC	2.7474
474	Amputation for Musculoskeletal System and Connective Tissue Disorders with MCC	4.3028
475	Amputation for Musculoskeletal System and Connective Tissue Disorders with CC	2.1447
503	Foot Procedures with MCC	2.6819
616	Amputation of Lower Limb for Endocrine, Nutritional, and Metabolic Disorders with MCC	3.9577

DRG	PDx/SDx/Procedure	Tips
040	Diabetes with neurological manifestations (e.g., neurogenic arthropathy, peripheral autonomic neuropathy, polyneuropathy)	According to ICD-10-CM guidelines, the classification presumes a causal relationship between diabetes and certain associated manifestations and/or conditions when these terms are linked by the term "with" in the alphabetic index (either under a main term or subterm). These conditions should be coded as related to the diabetes unless the documentation clearly states the conditions are unrelated, in which case they may be coded separately. These conditions do not require provider documentation linking them to diabetes. Review the record and/or query the physician if it is unclear whether a condition is related to diabetes mellitus or the ICD-10-CM classification does not provide instruction.
	AND	
	MCC condition	*See* appendix B.
041	Diabetes with neurological manifestations (e.g., neurogenic arthropathy, peripheral autonomic neuropathy, polyneuropathy)	*See* DRG 040.
	AND	
	CC condition	*See* appendix B.
239	Diabetes with circulatory complications (e.g., peripheral angiopathy, with or without gangrene)	*See* DRG 040.
	AND	
	MCC condition	*See* appendix B.
240	Diabetes with circulatory complications (e.g., peripheral angiopathy, with or without gangrene)	*See* DRG 239.
	AND	
	CC condition	*See* appendix B.
255	Diabetes with circulatory complications (e.g., peripheral angiopathy, with or without gangrene)	*See* DRG 239.
	AND	
	Amputation of toe	
	AND	
	MCC condition	*See* appendix B.
474	Musculoskeletal/connective tissue disorder: Osteomyelitis, acute, subacute, chronic, other, and unspecified Bone infections Pathologic fractures Osteonecrosis (aseptic necrosis) Malunion or nonunion of fracture	
	AND	
	MCC condition	*See* appendix B.
475	Musculoskeletal/connective tissue disorder: Osteomyelitis, acute, subacute, chronic, other, and unspecified Bone infections Pathologic fractures Osteonecrosis (aseptic necrosis) Malunion or nonunion of fracture	
	AND	
	CC condition	*See* appendix B.
503	Musculoskeletal/connective tissue disorder:	
	Osteomyelitis, acute, subacute, chronic, other, and unspecified	
	AND	
	Amputation of toe	
	AND	
	MCC condition	*See* appendix B.
616	MCC condition	*See* appendix B.

DRG 618 Amputation of Lower Limb for Endocrine, Nutritional, and Metabolic Disorders without CC/MCC

RW 1.1615

Potential DRGs

040	Peripheral/Cranial Nerve and Other Nervous System Procedures with MCC	3.8505
041	Peripheral/Cranial Nerve and Other Nervous System Procedures with CC or Peripheral Neurostimulator	2.2307
042	Peripheral/Cranial Nerve and Other Nervous System Procedures without CC/MCC	1.7398
239	Amputation for Circulatory System Disorders Except Upper Limb and Toe with MCC	4.8068
240	Amputation for Circulatory System Disorders Except Upper Limb and Toe with CC	2.8092
241	Amputation for Circulatory System Disorders Except Upper Limb and Toe without CC/MCC	1.3898
255	Upper Limb and Toe Amputation for Circulatory System Disorders with MCC	2.7474
256	Upper Limb and Toe Amputation for Circulatory System Disorders with CC	1.6397
474	Amputation for Musculoskeletal System and Connective Tissue Disorders with MCC	4.3028
475	Amputation for Musculoskeletal System and Connective Tissue Disorders with CC	2.1447
503	Foot Procedures with MCC	2.6819
504	Foot Procedures with CC	1.7271
505	Foot Procedures without CC/MCC	1.7057
616	Amputation of Lower Limb for Endocrine, Nutritional, and Metabolic Disorders with MCC	3.9577
617	Amputation of Lower Limb for Endocrine, Nutritional, and Metabolic Disorders with CC	1.9845

DRG	PDx/SDx/Procedure	Tips
040	Diabetes with neurological manifestations (e.g., neurogenic arthropathy, peripheral autonomic neuropathy, polyneuropathy)	According to ICD-10-CM guidelines, the classification presumes a causal relationship between diabetes and certain associated manifestations and/or conditions when these terms are linked by the term "with" in the alphabetic index (either under a main term or subterm). These conditions should be coded as related to the diabetes unless the documentation clearly states the conditions are unrelated, in which case they may be coded separately. These conditions do not require provider documentation linking them to diabetes. Review the record and/or query the physician if it is unclear whether a condition is related to diabetes mellitus or the ICD-10-CM classification does not provide instruction.
	AND	
	MCC condition	*See* appendix B.
041	Diabetes with neurological manifestations (e.g., neurogenic arthropathy, peripheral autonomic neuropathy, polyneuropathy)	*See* DRG 040.
	AND	
	CC condition	*See* appendix B.
042	Diabetes with neurological manifestations (e.g., neurogenic arthropathy, peripheral autonomic neuropathy, polyneuropathy)	*See* DRG 040.
239	Diabetes with circulatory complications (e.g., peripheral angiopathy, with or without gangrene)	*See* DRG 040.
	AND	
	MCC condition	*See* appendix B.
240	Diabetes with circulatory complications (e.g., peripheral angiopathy, with or without gangrene)	*See* DRG 239.
	AND	
	CC condition	*See* appendix B.
241	Diabetes with circulatory complications (e.g., peripheral angiopathy, with or without gangrene)	*See* DRG 239.
255	Diabetes with circulatory complications (e.g., peripheral angiopathy, with or without gangrene)	*See* DRG 040.
	AND	
	Amputation of toe	
	AND	
	MCC condition	*See* appendix B.
256	Diabetes with circulatory complications (e.g., peripheral angiopathy, with or without gangrene)	*See* DRG 255.
	AND	
	Amputation of toe	
	AND	
	CC condition	*See* appendix B.
474	Musculoskeletal/connective tissue disorder: Osteomyelitis, acute, subacute, chronic, other, and unspecified Bone infections Pathologic fractures Osteonecrosis (aseptic necrosis) Malunion or nonunion of fracture	
	AND	
	MCC condition	*See* appendix B.
475	Musculoskeletal/connective tissue disorder: Osteomyelitis, acute, subacute, chronic, other, and unspecified Bone infections Pathologic fractures Osteonecrosis (aseptic necrosis) Malunion or nonunion of fracture	
	AND	
	CC condition	*See* appendix B.

DRG 618 (Continued)

DRG	PDx/SDx/Procedure	Tips
503	Musculoskeletal/connective tissue disorder:	
	Osteomyelitis, acute, subacute, chronic, other, and unspecified	
	AND	
	Amputation of toe	
	AND	
	MCC condition	*See* appendix B.
504	Musculoskeletal/connective tissue disorder:	
	Osteomyelitis, acute, subacute, chronic, other, and unspecified	
	AND	
	Amputation of toe	
	AND	
	CC condition	*See* appendix B.
505	Musculoskeletal/connective tissue disorder:	
	Osteomyelitis, acute, subacute, chronic, other, and unspecified	
	AND	
	Amputation of toe	
616	MCC condition	*See* appendix B.
617	CC condition	*See* appendix B.

DRG 619 O.R. Procedures for Obesity with MCC RW 2.5885

No Potential DRGs

DRG 620 O.R. Procedures for Obesity with CC RW 1.6222

Potential DRGs

619 O.R. Procedures for Obesity with MCC 2.5885

DRG	PDx/SDx/Procedure	Tips
619	MCC condition	*See* appendix B.

DRG 621 O.R. Procedures for Obesity without CC/MCC RW 1.5173

Potential DRGs

619 O.R. Procedures for Obesity with MCC 2.5885
620 O.R. Procedures for Obesity with CC 1.6222

DRG	PDx/SDx/Procedure	Tips
619	MCC condition	*See* appendix B.
620	CC condition	*See* appendix B.

DRG 622 Skin Grafts and Wound Debridement for Endocrine, Nutritional and Metabolic Disorders with MCC

RW 3.8256

Potential DRGs

463	Wound Debridement and Skin Graft Except Hand for Musculoskeletal and Connective Tissue Disorders with MCC	5.6637
573	Skin Graft for Skin Ulcer or Cellulitis with MCC	6.2181
576	Skin Graft Except for Skin Ulcer or Cellulitis with MCC	5.6831
901	Wound Debridements for Injuries with MCC	4.3278

DRG	PDx/SDx/Procedure	Tips
463	Musculoskeletal and connective tissue principal diagnosis	Ensure that documentation includes underlying cause of condition requiring debridement and depth of debridement procedure.
	Osteomyelitis, all types (except diabetic)	
	Open wounds (lacerations) with tendon involvement	Laceration tendon—*see* Injury, muscle, by site, laceration.
	AND	
	MCC condition	*See* appendix B.
573	Skin ulcer or cellulitis principal diagnosis	
	AND	
	Skin grafting procedure	Skin grafting includes root operations Replacement of skin with a free graft of autologous (partial or full thickness), nonautologous or synthetic tissue; and Transfer of skin, and/or subcutaneous tissue and fascia which remains attached to its vascular and nervous supply. Other procedures include Excision and Supplement of tissues and Insertion of tissue expander.
	AND	
	MCC condition	*See* appendix B.
576	Malignant melanoma or neoplasm of skin (excluding eyelids)	
	Melanoma in-situ of skin (excluding eyelids)	
	Carcinoma in-situ of skin (excluding eyelids)	
	Benign neoplasm of skin (excluding eyelids)	
	Neoplasm of uncertain behavior of skin	
	AND	
	Skin grafting procedure	*See* DRG 573.
	AND	
	MCC condition	*See* appendix B.
901	Injury diagnosis from MDC 21	
	Excisional debridement of wound, infection, or burn	
	AND	
	MCC condition	*See* appendix B.

DRG 623 Skin Grafts and Wound Debridement for Endocrine, Nutritional and Metabolic Disorders with CC RW 1.8614

Potential DRGs

463	Wound Debridement and Skin Graft Except Hand for Musculoskeletal and Connective Tissue Disorders with MCC	5.6637
464	Wound Debridement and Skin Graft Except Hand for Musculoskeletal and Connective Tissue Disorders with CC	3.0014
570	Skin Debridement with MCC	2.9222
573	Skin Graft for Skin Ulcer or Cellulitis with MCC	6.2181
574	Skin Graft for Skin Ulcer or Cellulitis with CC	3.4058
576	Skin Graft Except for Skin Ulcer or Cellulitis with MCC	5.6831
577	Skin Graft Except for Skin Ulcer or Cellulitis with CC	2.6491
622	Skin Grafts and Wound Debridement for Endocrine, Nutritional and Metabolic Disorders with MCC	3.8256
901	Wound Debridements for Injuries with MCC	4.3278

DRG	PDx/SDx/Procedure	Tips
463	Musculoskeletal and connective tissue principal diagnosis	Ensure that documentation includes underlying cause of condition requiring debridement and depth of debridement procedure.
	Osteomyelitis, all types (except diabetic)	
	Open wounds (lacerations) with tendon involvement	Laceration tendon—*see* Injury, muscle, by site, laceration.
	AND	
	MCC condition	*See* appendix B.
464	Musculoskeletal and connective tissue principal diagnosis	*See* DRG 463.
	Osteomyelitis, all types (except diabetic)	
	Open wounds (lacerations) with tendon involvement	Laceration tendon—*see* Injury, muscle, by site, laceration.
	AND	
	CC condition	*See* appendix B.
570	Skin ulcer or cellulitis principal diagnosis	
	AND	
	Excisional debridement of skin	The ICD-10-PCS definition of the root operation Excision is "Cutting out or off, without replacement, a portion of a body part." Debridement by excision involves cutting with a sharp instrument such as a scalpel or other methods such as a hot knife or laser. Non-excisional debridement of skin is coded to root operation Extraction. Ensure that documentation includes instruments used, technique, and depth of debridement procedure.
	AND	
	MCC condition	*See* appendix B.
573	Skin ulcer or cellulitis principal diagnosis	
	AND	
	Skin grafting procedure	Skin grafting includes root operations Replacement of skin with a free graft of autologous (partial or full thickness), nonautologous or synthetic tissue; and Transfer of skin, and/or subcutaneous tissue and fascia which remains attached to its vascular and nervous supply. Other procedures include Excision and Supplement of tissues and Insertion of tissue expander.
	AND	
	MCC condition	*See* appendix B.
574	Skin ulcer or cellulitis principal diagnosis	
	AND	
	Skin grafting procedure	*See* DRG 573.
	AND	
	CC condition	*See* appendix B.
576	Malignant melanoma or neoplasm of skin (excluding eyelids)	
	Melanoma in-situ of skin (excluding eyelids)	
	Carcinoma in-situ of skin (excluding eyelids)	
	Benign neoplasm of skin (excluding eyelids)	
	Neoplasm of uncertain behavior of skin	
	AND	
	Skin grafting procedure	*See* DRG 573.
	AND	
	MCC condition	*See* appendix B.
577	Malignant melanoma or neoplasm of skin (excluding eyelids)	
	Melanoma in-situ of skin (excluding eyelids)	
	Carcinoma in-situ of skin (excluding eyelids)	
	Benign neoplasm of skin (excluding eyelids)	
	Neoplasm of uncertain behavior of skin	
	AND	
	Skin grafting procedure	*See* DRG 573.
	AND	
	CC condition	*See* appendix B.
622	MCC condition	*See* appendix B.
901	Injury diagnosis from MDC 21	
	Excisional debridement of wound, infection, or burn	*See* DRG 570.
	AND	
	MCC condition	*See* appendix B.

DRG 624 Skin Grafts and Wound Debridement for Endocrine, Nutritional and Metabolic Disorders without CC/MCC

RW 1.1145

Potential DRGs

463	Wound Debridement and Skin Graft Except Hand for Musculoskeletal and Connective Tissue Disorders with MCC	5.6637
464	Wound Debridement and Skin Graft Except Hand for Musculoskeletal and Connective Tissue Disorders with CC	3.0014
465	Wound Debridement and Skin Graft Except Hand for Musculoskeletal and Connective Tissue Disorders without CC/MCC	1.8708
570	Skin Debridement with MCC	2.9222
571	Skin Debridement with CC	1.6919
573	Skin Graft for Skin Ulcer or Cellulitis with MCC	6.2181
574	Skin Graft for Skin Ulcer or Cellulitis with CC	3.4058
575	Skin Graft for Skin Ulcer or Cellulitis without CC/MCC	2.0460
622	Skin Grafts and Wound Debridement for Endocrine, Nutritional and Metabolic Disorders with MCC	3.8256
623	Skin Grafts and Wound Debridement for Endocrine, Nutritional and Metabolic Disorders with CC	1.8614
901	Wound Debridements for Injuries with MCC	4.3278
902	Wound Debridements for Injuries with CC	1.8847
903	Wound Debridements for Injuries without CC/MCC	1.2415

DRG	PDx/SDx/Procedure	Tips
463	Musculoskeletal and connective tissue principal diagnosis	Ensure that documentation includes underlying cause of condition requiring debridement and depth of debridement procedure.
	Osteomyelitis, all types (except diabetic)	
	Open wounds (lacerations) with tendon involvement	Laceration tendon—*see* Injury, muscle, by site, laceration.
	AND	
	MCC condition	*See* appendix B.
464	Musculoskeletal and connective tissue principal diagnosis	*See* DRG 463.
	Osteomyelitis, all types (except diabetic)	
	Open wounds (lacerations) with tendon involvement	Laceration tendon—*see* Injury, muscle, by site, laceration.
	AND	
	CC condition	*See* appendix B.
465	Musculoskeletal and connective tissue principal diagnosis	*See* DRG 463.
	Osteomyelitis, all types (except diabetic)	
	Open wounds (lacerations) with tendon involvement	Laceration tendon—*see* Injury, muscle, by site, laceration.
570	Skin ulcer or cellulitis principal diagnosis	
	AND	
	Excisional debridement of skin	The ICD-10-PCS definition of the root operation Excision is "Cutting out or off, without replacement, a portion of a body part." Debridement by excision involves cutting with a sharp instrument such as a scalpel or other methods such as a hot knife or laser. Non-excisional debridement of skin is coded to root operation Extraction. Ensure that documentation includes instruments used, technique, and depth of debridement procedure.
	AND	
	MCC condition	*See* appendix B.
571	Skin ulcer or cellulitis principal diagnosis	
	AND	
	Excisional debridement of skin	*See* DRG 570.
	AND	
	CC condition	*See* appendix B.
573	Skin ulcer or cellulitis principal diagnosis	
	AND	
	Skin grafting procedure	Skin grafting includes root operations Replacement of skin with a free graft of autologous (partial or full thickness), nonautologous or synthetic tissue; and Transfer of skin, and/or subcutaneous tissue and fascia which remains attached to its vascular and nervous supply. Other procedures include Excision and Supplement of tissues and Insertion of tissue expander.
	AND	
	MCC condition	*See* appendix B.
574	Skin ulcer or cellulitis principal diagnosis	
	AND	
	Skin grafting procedure	*See* DRG 573.
	AND	
	CC condition	*See* appendix B.
575	Skin ulcer or cellulitis principal diagnosis	
	AND	
	Skin grafting procedure	*See* DRG 573.
622	MCC condition	*See* appendix B.
623	CC condition	*See* appendix B.
901	Injury diagnosis from MDC 21	
	Excisional debridement of wound, infection, or burn	*See* DRG 570.
	AND	
	MCC condition	*See* appendix B.

DRG 624 (Continued)

DRG	PDx/SDx/Procedure	Tips
902	Injury diagnosis from MDC 21	
	Excisional debridement of wound, infection, or burn	*See* DRG 570.
	AND	
	CC condition	*See* appendix B.
903	Injury diagnosis from MDC 21	
	Excisional debridement of wound, infection, or burn	*See* DRG 570.

DRG 625 Thyroid, Parathyroid and Thyroglossal Procedures with MCC RW 2.9212

No Potential DRGs

DRG 626 Thyroid, Parathyroid and Thyroglossal Procedures with CC RW 1.4919

Potential DRGs

625 Thyroid, Parathyroid and Thyroglossal Procedures with MCC 2.9212

DRG	PDx/SDx/Procedure	Tips
625	MCC condition	*See* appendix B.

DRG 627 Thyroid, Parathyroid and Thyroglossal Procedures without CC/MCC RW 1.2360

Potential DRGs

625 Thyroid, Parathyroid and Thyroglossal Procedures with MCC 2.9212
626 Thyroid, Parathyroid and Thyroglossal Procedures with CC 1.4919

DRG	PDx/SDx/Procedure	Tips
625	MCC condition	*See* appendix B.
626	CC condition	*See* appendix B.

DRG 628 Other Endocrine, Nutritional and Metabolic O.R. Procedures with MCC RW 4.0145

No Potential DRGs

DRG 629 Other Endocrine, Nutritional and Metabolic O.R. Procedures with CC RW 2.2628

Potential DRGs

264 Other Circulatory System O.R. Procedures 3.2660
622 Skin Grafts and Wound Debridement for Endocrine, Nutritional and Metabolic Disorders with MCC 3.8256
628 Other Endocrine, Nutritional and Metabolic O.R. Procedures with MCC 4.0145

DRG	PDx/SDx/Procedure	Tips
264	Diabetes with circulatory complications (e.g., peripheral angiopathy, with or without gangrene)	According to ICD-10-CM guidelines, the classification presumes a causal relationship between diabetes and certain associated manifestations and/or conditions when these terms are linked by the term "with" in the alphabetic index (either under a main term or subterm). These conditions should be coded as related to the diabetes unless the documentation clearly states the conditions are unrelated, in which case they may be coded separately. These conditions do not require provider documentation linking them to diabetes. Review the record and/or query the physician if it is unclear whether a condition is related to diabetes mellitus or the ICD-10-CM classification does not provide instruction.
	AND	
	Creation or revision of arteriovenostomy for renal dialysis	
	Removal of arteriovenostomy for renal dialysis	
622	Skin grafting procedures	Skin grafting includes root operations Replacement of skin with a free graft of autologous (partial or full thickness), nonautologous or synthetic tissue; and Transfer of skin, and/or subcutaneous tissue and fascia which remains attached to its vascular and nervous supply. Other procedures include Excision and Supplement of tissues and Insertion of tissue expander.
	OR	
	Excisional debridement	The ICD-10-PCS definition of the root operation Excision is "cutting out or off, without replacement, a portion of a body part." Debridement by excision involves cutting with a sharp instrument such as a scalp or other methods such as hot knife or laser. Nonexcisional debridement of skin is coded to root operation Extraction. Ensure that documentation includes instruments used, technique, and depth of debridement procedure.
	AND	
	MCC condition	*See* appendix B.
628	MCC condition	*See* appendix B.

DRG 630 Other Endocrine, Nutritional and Metabolic O.R. Procedures without CC/MCC — RW 1.3963

Potential DRGs

264	Other Circulatory System O.R. Procedures	3.2660
622	Skin Grafts and Wound Debridement for Endocrine, Nutritional and Metabolic Disorders with MCC	3.8256
623	Skin Grafts and Wound Debridement for Endocrine, Nutritional and Metabolic Disorders with CC	1.8614
628	Other Endocrine, Nutritional and Metabolic O.R. Procedures with MCC	4.0145
629	Other Endocrine, Nutritional and Metabolic O.R. Procedures with CC	2.2628
673	Other Kidney and Urinary Tract Procedures with MCC	3.6980
674	Other Kidney and Urinary Tract Procedures with CC	2.3822
675	Other Kidney and Urinary Tract Procedures without CC/MCC	1.5865

DRG	PDx/SDx/Procedure	Tips
264	Diabetes with circulatory complications (e.g., peripheral angiopathy, with or without gangrene)	According to ICD-10-CM guidelines, the classification presumes a causal relationship between diabetes and certain associated manifestations and/or conditions when these terms are linked by the term "with" in the alphabetic index (either under a main term or subterm). These conditions should be coded as related to the diabetes unless the documentation clearly states the conditions are unrelated, in which case they may be coded separately. These conditions do not require provider documentation linking them to diabetes. Review the record and/or query the physician if it is unclear whether a condition is related to diabetes mellitus or the ICD-10-CM classification does not provide instruction.
	AND	
	Creation or revision of arteriovenostomy for renal dialysis	
	Removal of arteriovenostomy for renal dialysis	
622	Skin grafting procedures	Skin grafting includes root operations Replacement of skin with a free graft of autologous (partial or full thickness), nonautologous or synthetic tissue; and Transfer of skin, and/or subcutaneous tissue and fascia which remains attached to its vascular and nervous supply. Other procedures include Excision and Supplement of tissues and Insertion of tissue expander.
	OR	
	Excisional debridement	The ICD-10-PCS definition of the root operation Excision is "cutting out or off, without replacement, a portion of a body part." Debridement by excision involves cutting with a sharp instrument such as a scalp or other methods such as hot knife or laser. Nonexcisional debridement of skin is coded to root operation Extraction. Ensure that documentation includes instruments used, technique, and depth of debridement procedure.
	AND	
	MCC condition	*See* appendix B.
623	Skin grafting procedures	*See* DRG 622.
	OR	
	Excisional debridement	*See* DRG 622.
	AND	
	CC condition	*See* appendix B.
628	MCC condition	*See* appendix B.
629	CC section	*See* appendix B.
673	Diabetes with renal manifestations	According to ICD-10-CM guidelines, the classification presumes a causal relationship between diabetes and certain associated manifestations and/or conditions when these terms are linked by the term "with" in the alphabetic index (either under a main term or subterm). These conditions should be coded as related to the diabetes unless the documentation clearly states the conditions are unrelated, in which case they may be coded separately. These conditions do not require provider documentation linking them to diabetes. Review the record and/or query the physician if it is unclear whether a condition is related to diabetes mellitus or the ICD-10-CM classification does not provide instruction.
	AND	
	Creation or revision of arteriovenostomy for renal dialysis	
	Removal of arteriovenostomy for renal dialysis	
	AND	
	MCC condition	*See* appendix B.
674	Diabetes with renal manifestations	*See* DRG 673.
	AND	
	Creation or revision of arteriovenostomy for renal dialysis	
	Removal of arteriovenostomy for renal dialysis	
	AND	
	CC condition	*See* appendix B.
675	Diabetes with renal manifestations	*See* DRG 673.
	AND	
	Creation or revision of arteriovenostomy for renal dialysis	
	Removal of arteriovenostomy for renal dialysis	

DRG 637 Diabetes with MCC — RW 1.4493

Potential DRGs

073	Cranial and Peripheral Nerve Disorders with MCC	1.5130
299	Peripheral Vascular Disorders with MCC	1.5762
622	Skin Grafts and Wound Debridement for Endocrine, Nutritional and Metabolic Disorders with MCC	3.8256
698	Other Kidney and Urinary Tract Diagnoses with MCC	1.6544

DRG	PDx/SDx/Procedure	Tips
073	Diabetes with neurological manifestations (e.g., neurogenic arthropathy, peripheral autonomic neuropathy, polyneuropathy)	According to ICD-10-CM guidelines, the classification presumes a causal relationship between diabetes and certain associated manifestations and/or conditions when these terms are linked by the term "with" in the alphabetic index (either under a main term or subterm). These conditions should be coded as related to the diabetes unless the documentation clearly states the conditions are unrelated, in which case they may be coded separately. These conditions do not require provider documentation linking them to diabetes. Review the record and/or query the physician if it is unclear whether a condition is related to diabetes mellitus or the ICD-10-CM classification does not provide instruction.
	AND	
	MCC condition	*See* appendix B.
299	Diabetes with circulatory complications (e.g., peripheral angiopathy, with or without gangrene)	*See* DRG 073.
	AND	
	MCC condition	*See* appendix B.
622	Diabetes with other specified manifestations (diabetic ulcer)	*See* DRG 073.
	AND	
	Excisional debridement of skin	The ICD-10-PCS definition of the root operation Excision is "Cutting out or off, without replacement, a portion of a body part." Debridement by excision involves cutting with a sharp instrument such as a scalpel or other methods such as a hot knife or laser. Nonexcisional debridement of skin is coded to root operation Extraction. Ensure that documentation includes instruments used, technique, and depth of debridement procedure.
	AND	
	MCC condition	*See* appendix B.
698	Diabetes with renal manifestations	*See* DRG 073.
	AND	
	MCC condition	*See* appendix B.

DRG 638 Diabetes with CC

RW 0.8994

Potential DRGs

073	Cranial and Peripheral Nerve Disorders with MCC	1.5130
074	Cranial and Peripheral Nerve Disorders without MCC	1.0262
299	Peripheral Vascular Disorders with MCC	1.5762
300	Peripheral Vascular Disorders with CC	1.0670
622	Skin Grafts and Wound Debridement for Endocrine, Nutritional and Metabolic Disorders with MCC	3.8256
623	Skin Grafts and Wound Debridement for Endocrine, Nutritional and Metabolic Disorders with CC	1.8614
637	Diabetes with MCC	1.4493
640	Miscellaneous Disorders of Nutrition, Metabolism, and Fluids and Electrolytes with MCC	1.3152
698	Other Kidney and Urinary Tract Diagnoses with MCC	1.6544
699	Other Kidney and Urinary Tract Diagnoses with CC	1.0208

DRG	PDx/SDx/Procedure	Tips
073	Diabetes with neurological manifestations (e.g., neurogenic arthropathy, peripheral autonomic neuropathy, polyneuropathy)	According to ICD-10-CM guidelines, the classification presumes a causal relationship between diabetes and certain associated manifestations and/or conditions when these terms are linked by the term "with" in the alphabetic index (either under a main term or subterm). These conditions should be coded as related to the diabetes unless the documentation clearly states the conditions are unrelated, in which case they may be coded separately. These conditions do not require provider documentation linking them to diabetes. Review the record and/or query the physician if it is unclear whether a condition is related to diabetes mellitus or the ICD-10-CM classification does not provide instruction.
	AND	
	MCC condition	*See* appendix B.
074	Diabetes with neurological manifestations (e.g., neurogenic arthropathy, peripheral autonomic neuropathy, polyneuropathy)	*See* DRG 073.
299	Diabetes with circulatory complications (e.g., peripheral angiopathy, with or without gangrene)	*See* DRG 073.
	AND	
	MCC condition	*See* appendix B.
300	Diabetes with circulatory complications (e.g., peripheral angiopathy, with or without gangrene)	*See* DRG 073.
	AND	
	CC condition	*See* appendix B.
622	Diabetes with other specified manifestations (diabetic ulcer)	*See* DRG 073.
	AND	
	Excisional debridement of skin	The ICD-10-PCS definition of the root operation Excision is "Cutting out or off, without replacement, a portion of a body part." Debridement by excision involves cutting with a sharp instrument such as a scalpel or other methods such as a hot knife or laser. Non-excisional debridement of skin is coded to root operation Extraction. Ensure that documentation includes instruments used, technique, and depth of debridement procedure.
	AND	
	MCC condition	*See* appendix B.
623	Diabetes with other specified manifestations (diabetic ulcer)	*See* DRG 073.
	AND	
	Excisional debridement of skin	*See* DRG 622.
	AND	
	CC condition	*See* appendix B.
637	MCC condition	*See* appendix B.
640	Dehydration, volume depletion, other disorders of fluid, electrolyte and acid-base balance	
	AND	
	MCC condition	*See* appendix B.
698	Diabetes with renal manifestations	*See* DRG 073.
	AND	
	MCC condition	*See* appendix B.
699	Diabetes with renal manifestations	*See* DRG 073.
	AND	
	CC condition	*See* appendix B.

Optimizing Tips

DRG 639 Diabetes without CC/MCC RW 0.6225

Potential DRGs

073	Cranial and Peripheral Nerve Disorders with MCC	1.5130
074	Cranial and Peripheral Nerve Disorders without MCC	1.0262
299	Peripheral Vascular Disorders with MCC	1.5762
300	Peripheral Vascular Disorders with CC	1.0670
301	Peripheral Vascular Disorders without CC/MCC	0.7098
622	Skin Grafts and Wound Debridement for Endocrine, Nutritional and Metabolic Disorders with MCC	3.8256
623	Skin Grafts and Wound Debridement for Endocrine, Nutritional and Metabolic Disorders with CC	1.8614
624	Skin Grafts and Wound Debridement for Endocrine, Nutritional and Metabolic Disorders without CC/MCC	1.1145
637	Diabetes with MCC	1.4493
638	Diabetes with CC	0.8994
640	Miscellaneous Disorders of Nutrition, Metabolism, and Fluids and Electrolytes with MCC	1.3152
641	Miscellaneous Disorders of Nutrition, Metabolism, and Fluids and Electrolytes without MCC	0.7814
698	Other Kidney and Urinary Tract Diagnoses with MCC	1.6544
699	Other Kidney and Urinary Tract Diagnoses with CC	1.0208
700	Other Kidney and Urinary Tract Diagnoses without CC/MCC	0.7083

DRG	PDx/SDx/Procedure	Tips
073	Diabetes with neurological manifestations (e.g., neurogenic arthropathy, peripheral autonomic neuropathy, polyneuropathy)	According to ICD-10-CM guidelines, the classification presumes a causal relationship between diabetes and certain associated manifestations and/or conditions when these terms are linked by the term "with" in the alphabetic index (either under a main term or subterm). These conditions should be coded as related to the diabetes unless the documentation clearly states the conditions are unrelated, in which case they may be coded separately. These conditions do not require provider documentation linking them to diabetes. Review the record and/or query the physician if it is unclear whether a condition is related to diabetes mellitus or the ICD-10-CM classification does not provide instruction.
	AND	
	MCC condition	*See* appendix B.
074	Diabetes with neurological manifestations (e.g., neurogenic arthropathy, peripheral autonomic neuropathy, polyneuropathy)	*See* DRG 073.
299	Diabetes with circulatory complications (e.g., peripheral angiopathy, with or without gangrene)	*See* DRG 073.
	AND	
	MCC condition	*See* appendix B.
300	Diabetes with circulatory complications (e.g., peripheral angiopathy, with or without gangrene)	*See* DRG 073.
	AND	
	CC condition	*See* appendix B.
301	Diabetes with circulatory complications (e.g., peripheral angiopathy, with or without gangrene)	*See* DRG 073.
622	Diabetes with other specified manifestations (diabetic ulcer)	*See* DRG 073.
	AND	
	Excisional debridement of skin	The ICD-10-PCS definition of the root operation Excision is "Cutting out or off, without replacement, a portion of a body part." Debridement by excision involves cutting with a sharp instrument such as a scalpel or other methods such as a hot knife or laser. Non-excisional debridement of skin is coded to root operation Extraction. Ensure that documentation includes instruments used, technique, and depth of debridement procedure.
	AND	
	MCC condition	*See* appendix B.
623	Diabetes with other specified manifestations (diabetic ulcer)	*See* DRG 073.
	AND	
	Excisional debridement of skin	*See* DRG 622.
	AND	
	CC condition	*See* appendix B.
624	Diabetes with other specified manifestations (diabetic ulcer)	*See* DRG 073.
	AND	
	Excisional debridement of skin	*See* DRG 622.
637	MCC condition	*See* appendix B.
638	CC condition	*See* appendix B.
640	Dehydration, volume depletion, other disorders of fluid, electrolyte and acid-base balance	
	AND	
	MCC condition	*See* appendix B.
641	Dehydration, volume depletion, other disorders of fluid, electrolyte and acid-base balance	
698	Diabetes with renal manifestations	*See* DRG 073.
	AND	
	MCC condition	*See* appendix B.
699	Diabetes with renal manifestations	*See* DRG 073.
	AND	
	CC condition	*See* appendix B.
700	Diabetes with renal manifestations	*See* DRG 073.

DRG 640 Miscellaneous Disorders of Nutrition, Metabolism, and Fluids and Electrolytes with MCC — RW 1.3152

Potential DRGs

619	O.R. Procedures for Obesity with MCC	2.5885

DRG	PDx/SDx/Procedure	Tips
619	Any laparoscopic procedure performed for obesity:	
	Laparoscopic banding (vertical banded gastroplasty—VBG)	
	Gastric restrictive procedure	
	Revision of gastric restrictive procedure	
	Removal of gastric restrictive device	
	Adjustment of size of adjustable gastric restrictive device	
	Vertical (sleeve) gastrectomy	
	AND	
	MCC condition	*See* appendix B.

DRG 641 Miscellaneous Disorders of Nutrition, Metabolism, and Fluids and Electrolytes without MCC — RW 0.7814

Potential DRGs

312	Syncope and Collapse	0.8635
619	O.R. Procedures for Obesity with MCC	2.5885
620	O.R. Procedures for Obesity with CC	1.6222
621	O.R. Procedures for Obesity without CC/MCC	1.5173
640	Miscellaneous Disorders of Nutrition, Metabolism, and Fluids and Electrolytes with MCC	1.3152
689	Kidney and Urinary Tract Infections with MCC	1.1744
690	Kidney and Urinary Tract Infections without MCC	0.8069

DRG	PDx/SDx/Procedure	Tips
312	Orthostatic and iatrogenic hypotension	
	Syncope and collapse	
619	Any laparoscopic procedure performed for obesity:	
	Laparoscopic banding (vertical banded gastroplasty—VBG)	
	Gastric restrictive procedure	
	Revision of gastric restrictive procedure	
	Removal of gastric restrictive device	
	Adjustment of size of adjustable gastric restrictive device	
	Vertical (sleeve) gastrectomy	
	AND	
	MCC condition	*See* appendix B.
620	Any laparoscopic procedure performed for obesity:	
	Laparoscopic banding (vertical banded gastroplasty—VBG)	
	Gastric restrictive procedure	
	Revision of gastric restrictive procedure	
	Removal of gastric restrictive device	
	Adjustment of size of adjustable gastric restrictive device	
	Vertical (sleeve) gastrectomy	
	AND	
	CC condition	*See* appendix B.
621	Any laparoscopic procedure performed for obesity:	
	Laparoscopic banding (vertical banded gastroplasty—VBG)	
	Gastric restrictive procedure	
	Revision of gastric restrictive procedure	
	Removal of gastric restrictive device	
	Adjustment of size of adjustable gastric restrictive device	
	Vertical (sleeve) gastrectomy	
640	MCC condition	*See* appendix B.
689	Urinary tract infection with co-existing dehydration or other volume depletion disorder	
	AND	
	MCC condition	*See* appendix B.
690	Urinary tract infection with co-existing dehydration or other volume depletion disorder	

DRG 642 Inborn and Other Disorders of Metabolism — RW 1.3033

No Potential DRGs

DRG 643 Endocrine Disorders with MCC — RW 1.6451

Potential DRGs

625	Thyroid, Parathyroid and Thyroglossal Procedures with MCC	2.9212

DRG	PDx/SDx/Procedure	Tips
625	Thyroidectomy, partial or total, any approach	
	OR	
	Parathyroidectomy, partial or total, any approach	
	AND	
	MCC condition	*See* appendix B.

DRG 644 Endocrine Disorders with CC — RW 1.0617

Potential DRGs

054	Nervous System Neoplasms with MCC	1.4735
625	Thyroid, Parathyroid and Thyroglossal Procedures with MCC	2.9212
626	Thyroid, Parathyroid and Thyroglossal Procedures with CC	1.4919
643	Endocrine Disorders with MCC	1.6451

DRG	PDx/SDx/Procedure	Tips
054	Malignant or benign neoplasm, pineal gland	
	AND	
	MCC condition	*See* appendix B.
625	Thyroidectomy, partial or total, any approach	
	OR	
	Parathyroidectomy, partial or total, any approach	
	AND	
	MCC condition	*See* appendix B.
626	Thyroidectomy, partial or total, any approach	
	OR	
	Parathyroidectomy, partial or total, any approach	
	AND	
	CC condition	*See* appendix B.
643	MCC condition	*See* appendix B.

DRG 645 Endocrine Disorders without CC/MCC — RW 0.7609

Potential DRGs

054	Nervous System Neoplasms with MCC	1.4735
055	Nervous System Neoplasms without MCC	1.0732
625	Thyroid, Parathyroid and Thyroglossal Procedures with MCC	2.9212
626	Thyroid, Parathyroid and Thyroglossal Procedures with CC	1.4919
627	Thyroid, Parathyroid and Thyroglossal Procedures without CC/MCC	1.2360
643	Endocrine Disorders with MCC	1.6451
644	Endocrine Disorders with CC	1.0617

DRG	PDx/SDx/Procedure	Tips
054	Malignant or benign neoplasm, pineal gland	
	AND	
	MCC condition	*See* appendix B.
055	Malignant or benign neoplasm, pineal gland	
625	Thyroidectomy, partial or total, any approach	
	OR	
	Parathyroidectomy, partial or total, any approach	
	AND	
	MCC condition	*See* appendix B.
626	Thyroidectomy, partial or total, any approach	
	OR	
	Parathyroidectomy, partial or total, any approach	
	AND	
	CC condition	*See* appendix B.
627	Thyroidectomy, partial or total, any approach	
	OR	
	Parathyroidectomy, partial or total, any approach	
643	MCC condition	*See* appendix B.
644	CC condition	*See* appendix B.

Diseases And Disorders Of The Kidney And Urinary Tract

DRG 650 Kidney Transplant with Hemodialysis with MCC RW 4.4975

Potential DRGs

019 Simultaneous Pancreas and Kidney Transplant with Hemodialysis 7.9935

DRG	PDx/SDx/Procedure	Tips
019	Principal and secondary diagnosis of diabetes, type 1, type 2, due to underlying condition, drug or chemical induced, or other specified diabetes, with any complications	According to ICD-10-CM guidelines, the classification presumes a causal relationship between diabetes and certain associated manifestations and/or conditions when these terms are linked by the term "with" in the alphabetic index (either under a main term or subterm). These conditions should be coded as related to the diabetes unless the documentation clearly states the conditions are unrelated, in which case they may be coded separately. These conditions do not require provider documentation linking them to diabetes. Review the record and/or query the physician if it is unclear whether a condition is related to diabetes mellitus or the ICD-10-CM classification does not provide instruction.
	AND	
	Principal or secondary diagnosis hypertensive chronic or end-stage kidney disease (with or without heart disease or heart failure), chronic or end-stage kidney disease, kidney transplant status or presence of endocrine or other unspecified functional implants	
	AND	
	Pancreas and kidney transplant procedure combinations	
	AND	
	Hemodialysis	Some patients require hemodialysis while waiting for a donor kidney, or after the kidney has been implanted but has not returned to optimal function.

DRG 651 Kidney Transplant with Hemodialysis without MCC RW 3.4584

Potential DRGs

019 Simultaneous Pancreas and Kidney Transplant with Hemodialysis 7.9935
650 Kidney Transplant with Hemodialysis with MCC 4.4975

DRG	PDx/SDx/Procedure	Tips
019	Principal and secondary diagnosis of diabetes, type 1, type 2, due to underlying condition, drug or chemical induced, or other specified diabetes, with any complications	According to ICD-10-CM guidelines, the classification presumes a causal relationship between diabetes and certain associated manifestations and/or conditions when these terms are linked by the term "with" in the alphabetic index (either under a main term or subterm). These conditions should be coded as related to the diabetes unless the documentation clearly states the conditions are unrelated, in which case they may be coded separately. These conditions do not require provider documentation linking them to diabetes. Review the record and/or query the physician if it is unclear whether a condition is related to diabetes mellitus or the ICD-10-CM classification does not provide instruction.
	AND	
	Principal or secondary diagnosis hypertensive chronic or end-stage kidney disease (with or without heart disease or heart failure), chronic or end-stage kidney disease, kidney transplant status or presence of endocrine or other unspecified functional implants	
	AND	
	Pancreas and kidney transplant procedure combinations	
	AND	
	Hemodialysis	Some patients require hemodialysis while waiting for a donor kidney, or after the kidney has been implanted but has not returned to optimal function.
650	MCC condition	*See* appendix B.

DRG 652 Kidney Transplant — RW 3.0044

Potential DRGs

008	Simultaneous Pancreas/Kidney Transplant	5.2617
019	Simultaneous Pancreas and Kidney Transplant with Hemodialysis	7.9935
650	Kidney Transplant with Hemodialysis with MCC	4.4975
651	Kidney Transplant with Hemodialysis without MCC	3.4584

DRG	PDx/SDx/Procedure	Tips
008	Principal or secondary diagnosis of diabetes, type 1, type 2, due to underlying condition, drug or chemical induced, or other specified diabetes, with any complications	According to ICD-10-CM guidelines, the classification presumes a causal relationship between diabetes and certain associated manifestations and/or conditions when these terms are linked by the term "with" in the alphabetic index (either under a main term or subterm). These conditions should be coded as related to the diabetes unless the documentation clearly states the conditions are unrelated, in which case they may be coded separately. These conditions do not require provider documentation linking them to diabetes. Review the record and/or query the physician if it is unclear whether a condition is related to diabetes mellitus or the ICD-10-CM classification does not provide instruction.
	AND	
	Principal or secondary diagnosis hypertensive chronic or end-stage kidney disease (with or without heart disease or heart failure), chronic or end-stage kidney disease, kidney transplant status or presence of endocrine or other unspecified functional implants	
	AND	
	Pancreas and kidney transplant procedure combinations	
019	Principal and secondary diagnosis of diabetes, type 1, type 2, due to underlying condition, drug or chemical induced, or other specified diabetes, with any complications	According to ICD-10-CM guidelines, the classification presumes a causal relationship between diabetes and certain associated manifestations and/or conditions when these terms are linked by the term "with" in the alphabetic index (either under a main term or subterm). These conditions should be coded as related to the diabetes unless the documentation clearly states the conditions are unrelated, in which case they may be coded separately. These conditions do not require provider documentation linking them to diabetes. Review the record and/or query the physician if it is unclear whether a condition is related to diabetes mellitus or the ICD-10-CM classification does not provide instruction.
	AND	
	Principal or secondary diagnosis hypertensive chronic or end-stage kidney disease (with or without heart disease or heart failure), chronic or end-stage kidney disease, kidney transplant status or presence of endocrine or other unspecified functional implants	
	AND	
	Pancreas and kidney transplant procedure combinations	
	AND	
	Hemodialysis	Some patients require hemodialysis while waiting for a donor kidney, or after the kidney has been implanted but has not returned to optimal function.
650	Kidney transplant	
	WITH	
	Hemodialysis	Some patients require hemodialysis while waiting for a donor kidney, or after the kidney has been implanted but has not returned to optimal function.
	AND	
	MCC condition	*See* appendix B.
651	Kidney transplant	
	WITH	
	Hemodialysis	See DRG 650.

DRG 653 Major Bladder Procedures with MCC — RW 5.4136

No Potential DRGs

DRG 654 Major Bladder Procedures with CC — RW 2.7375

Potential DRGs

653	Major Bladder Procedures with MCC	5.4136

DRG	PDx/SDx/Procedure	Tips
653	MCC condition	*See* appendix B.

DRG 655 Major Bladder Procedures without CC/MCC — RW 2.1078

Potential DRGs

653	Major Bladder Procedures with MCC	5.4136
654	Major Bladder Procedures with CC	2.7375

DRG	PDx/SDx/Procedure	Tips
653	MCC condition	*See* appendix B.
654	CC condition	*See* appendix B.

DRG 656 Kidney and Ureter Procedures for Neoplasm with MCC — RW 3.1376

Potential DRGs

653	Major Bladder Procedures with MCC	5.4136

DRG	PDx/SDx/Procedure	Tips
653	Bladder excision or resection	
	Bladder fistula repair	
	Reconstruction, anastomosis, or other repair of urinary bladder	
	AND	
	MCC condition	*See* appendix B.

DRG 657 Kidney and Ureter Procedures for Neoplasm with CC — RW 1.8442

Potential DRGs

653	Major Bladder Procedures with MCC	5.4136
654	Major Bladder Procedures with CC	2.7375
656	Kidney and Ureter Procedures for Neoplasm with MCC	3.1376

DRG	PDx/SDx/Procedure	Tips
653	Bladder excision or resection	
	Bladder fistula repair	
	Reconstruction, anastomosis, or other repair of urinary bladder	
	AND	
	MCC condition	*See* appendix B.
654	Bladder excision or resection	
	Bladder fistula repair	
	Reconstruction, anastomosis, or other repair of urinary bladder	
	AND	
	CC condition	*See* appendix B.
656	MCC condition	*See* appendix B.

DRG 658 Kidney and Ureter Procedures for Neoplasm without CC/MCC — RW 1.4804

Potential DRGs

653	Major Bladder Procedures with MCC	5.4136
654	Major Bladder Procedures with CC	2.7375
655	Major Bladder Procedures without CC/MCC	2.1078
656	Kidney and Ureter Procedures for Neoplasm with MCC	3.1376
657	Kidney and Ureter Procedures for Neoplasm with CC	1.8442

DRG	PDx/SDx/Procedure	Tips
653	Bladder excision or resection	
	Bladder fistula repair	
	Reconstruction, anastomosis, or other repair of urinary bladder	
	AND	
	MCC condition	*See* appendix B.
654	Bladder excision or resection	
	Bladder fistula repair	
	Reconstruction, anastomosis, or other repair of urinary bladder	
	AND	
	CC condition	*See* appendix B.
655	Bladder excision or resection	
	Bladder fistula repair	
	Reconstruction, anastomosis, or other repair of urinary bladder	
656	MCC condition	*See* appendix B.
657	CC condition	*See* appendix B.

DRG 659 Kidney and Ureter Procedures for Non-neoplasm with MCC — RW 2.5889

Potential DRGs

653	Major Bladder Procedures with MCC	5.4136
656	Kidney and Ureter Procedures for Neoplasm with MCC	3.1376

DRG	PDx/SDx/Procedure	Tips
653	Bladder excision or resection	
	Bladder fistula repair	
	Reconstruction, anastomosis, or other repair of urinary bladder	
	AND	
	MCC condition	*See* appendix B.
656	Neoplasm diagnosis	
	Kidney and ureter procedures: Nephrotomy and nephrostomy Pyelotomy and pyelostomy Local excision/destruction of lesion or tissue of kidney Partial or complete nephrectomy	Root operations Bypass, Dilation, Destruction, Drainage, Excision, Extirpation, Fragmentation, Repair, Reposition, Resection, Restriction, Revision
	AND	
	MCC condition	*See* appendix B.

DRG 660 Kidney and Ureter Procedures for Non-neoplasm with CC RW 1.3459

Potential DRGs

653	Major Bladder Procedures with MCC	5.4136
654	Major Bladder Procedures with CC	2.7375
656	Kidney and Ureter Procedures for Neoplasm with MCC	3.1376
657	Kidney and Ureter Procedures for Neoplasm with CC	1.8442
659	Kidney and Ureter Procedures for Non-neoplasm with MCC	2.5889

DRG	PDx/SDx/Procedure	Tips
653	Bladder excision or resection	
	Bladder fistula repair	
	Reconstruction, anastomosis, or other repair of urinary bladder	
	AND	
	MCC condition	*See* appendix B.
654	Bladder excision or resection	
	Bladder fistula repair	
	Reconstruction, anastomosis, or other repair of urinary bladder	
	AND	
	CC condition	*See* appendix B.
656	Neoplasm diagnosis	
	Kidney and ureter procedures: Nephrotomy and nephrostomy Pyelotomy and pyelostomy Local excision/destruction of lesion or tissue of kidney Partial or complete nephrectomy	Root operations Bypass, Dilation, Destruction, Drainage, Excision, Extirpation, Fragmentation, Repair, Reposition, Resection, Restriction, Revision
	AND	
	MCC condition	*See* appendix B.
657	Neoplasm diagnosis	
	Kidney and ureter procedures: Nephrotomy and nephrostomy Pyelotomy and pyelostomy Local excision/destruction of lesion or tissue of kidney Partial or complete nephrectomy	Root operations Bypass, Dilation, Destruction, Drainage, Excision, Extirpation, Fragmentation, Repair, Reposition, Resection, Restriction, Revision
	AND	
	CC condition	*See* appendix B.
659	MCC condition	*See* appendix B.

DRG 661 Kidney and Ureter Procedures for Non-neoplasm without CC/MCC — RW 1.0484

Potential DRGs

653	Major Bladder Procedures with MCC	5.4136
654	Major Bladder Procedures with CC	2.7375
655	Major Bladder Procedures without CC/MCC	2.1078
656	Kidney and Ureter Procedures for Neoplasm with MCC	3.1376
657	Kidney and Ureter Procedures for Neoplasm with CC	1.8442
658	Kidney and Ureter Procedures for Neoplasm without CC/MCC	1.4804
659	Kidney and Ureter Procedures for Non-neoplasm with MCC	2.5889
660	Kidney and Ureter Procedures for Non-neoplasm with CC	1.3459

DRG	PDx/SDx/Procedure	Tips
653	Bladder excision or resection	
	Bladder fistula repair	
	Reconstruction, anastomosis, or other repair of urinary bladder	
	AND	
	MCC condition	*See* appendix B.
654	Bladder excision or resection	
	Bladder fistula repair	
	Reconstruction, anastomosis, or other repair of urinary bladder	
	AND	
	CC condition	*See* appendix B.
655	Bladder excision or resection	
	Bladder fistula repair	
	Reconstruction, anastomosis, or other repair of urinary bladder	
656	Neoplasm diagnosis	
	Kidney and ureter procedures: Nephrotomy and nephrostomy Pyelotomy and pyelostomy Local excision/destruction of lesion or tissue of kidney Partial or complete nephrectomy	Root operations Bypass, Dilation, Destruction, Drainage, Excision, Extirpation, Fragmentation, Repair, Reposition, Resection, Restriction, Revision
	AND	
	MCC condition	*See* appendix B.
657	Neoplasm diagnosis	
	Kidney and ureter procedures: Nephrotomy and nephrostomy Pyelotomy and pyelostomy Local excision/destruction of lesion or tissue of kidney Partial or complete nephrectomy	Root operations Bypass, Dilation, Destruction, Drainage, Excision, Extirpation, Fragmentation, Repair, Reposition, Resection, Restriction, Revision
	AND	
	CC condition	*See* appendix B.
658	Neoplasm diagnosis	
	Kidney and ureter procedures: Nephrotomy and nephrostomy Pyelotomy and pyelostomy Local excision/destruction of lesion or tissue of kidney Partial or complete nephrectomy	Root operations Bypass, Dilation, Destruction, Drainage, Excision, Extirpation, Fragmentation, Repair, Reposition, Resection, Restriction, Revision
659	MCC condition	*See* appendix B.
660	CC condition	*See* appendix B.

DRG 662 Minor Bladder Procedures with MCC — RW 2.9967

Potential DRGs

653	Major Bladder Procedures with MCC	5.4136
656	Kidney and Ureter Procedures for Neoplasm with MCC	3.1376

DRG	PDx/SDx/Procedure	Tips
653	Repair of cystocele with graft or prosthesis	The root operation Repair of pelvic region subcutaneous tissue and fascia is reported for procedures performed to treat cystocele, rectocele, and enterocele. However, repair of cystocele with a tissue graft or device (autologous, synthetic, or nonautologous) to reinforce and increase support of the pelvic region subcutaneous tissue and fascia is reported with root operation Supplement (U).
	AND	
	MCC condition	*See* appendix B.
656	Urinary neoplasm principal diagnosis	
	AND	
	Kidney and ureter procedures: Nephrotomy and nephrostomy Pyelotomy and pyelostomy Local excision/destruction of lesion or tissue of kidney Partial or complete nephrectomy	Root operations Bypass, Dilation, Destruction, Drainage, Excision, Extirpation, Fragmentation, Repair, Reposition, Resection, Restriction, Revision.
	AND	
	MCC condition	*See* appendix B.

DRG 663 Minor Bladder Procedures with CC RW 1.4590

Potential DRGs

653	Major Bladder Procedures with MCC	5.4136
654	Major Bladder Procedures with CC	2.7375
656	Kidney and Ureter Procedures for Neoplasm with MCC	3.1376
657	Kidney and Ureter Procedures for Neoplasm with CC	1.8442
659	Kidney and Ureter Procedures for Non-neoplasm with MCC	2.5889
662	Minor Bladder Procedures with MCC	2.9967

DRG	PDx/SDx/Procedure	Tips
653	Repair of cystocele with graft or prosthesis	The root operation Repair of pelvic region subcutaneous tissue and fascia is reported for procedures performed to treat cystocele, rectocele, and enterocele. However, repair of cystocele with a tissue graft or device (autologous, synthetic, or nonautologous) to reinforce and increase support of the pelvic region subcutaneous tissue and fascia is reported with root operation Supplement (U).
	AND	
	MCC condition	*See* appendix B.
654	Repair of cystocele with graft or prosthesis	*See* DRG 653.
	AND	
	CC condition	*See* appendix B.
656	Urinary neoplasm principal diagnosis	
	AND	
	Kidney and ureter procedures: Nephrotomy and nephrostomy Pyelotomy and pyelostomy Local excision/destruction of lesion or tissue of kidney Partial or complete nephrectomy	Root operations Bypass, Dilation, Destruction, Drainage, Excision, Extirpation, Fragmentation, Repair, Reposition, Resection, Restriction, Revision.
	AND	
	MCC condition	*See* appendix B.
657	Urinary neoplasm principal diagnosis	
	AND	
	Kidney and ureter procedures: Nephrotomy and nephrostomy Pyelotomy and pyelostomy Local excision/destruction of lesion or tissue of kidney Partial or complete nephrectomy	Root operations Bypass, Dilation, Destruction, Drainage, Excision, Extirpation, Fragmentation, Repair, Reposition, Resection, Restriction, Revision.
	AND	
	CC condition	*See* appendix B.
659	Any urinary system diagnosis except malignant, benign, uncertain behavior and carcinoma-in-situ neoplasms	
	AND	
	Kidney and ureter procedures: Nephrotomy and nephrostomy Pyelotomy and pyelostomy Local excision/destruction of lesion or tissue of kidney Partial or complete nephrectomy	Root operations Bypass, Dilation, Destruction, Drainage, Excision, Extirpation, Fragmentation, Repair, Reposition, Resection, Restriction, Revision.
	AND	
	MCC condition	*See* appendix B.
662	MCC condition	*See* appendix B.

DRG 664 Minor Bladder Procedures without CC/MCC RW 1.0616

Potential DRGs

653	Major Bladder Procedures with MCC	5.4136
654	Major Bladder Procedures with CC	2.7375
655	Major Bladder Procedures without CC/MCC	2.1078
656	Kidney and Ureter Procedures for Neoplasm with MCC	3.1376
657	Kidney and Ureter Procedures for Neoplasm with CC	1.8442
658	Kidney and Ureter Procedures for Neoplasm without CC/MCC	1.4804
659	Kidney and Ureter Procedures for Non-neoplasm with MCC	2.5889
660	Kidney and Ureter Procedures for Non-neoplasm with CC	1.3459
662	Minor Bladder Procedures with MCC	2.9967
663	Minor Bladder Procedures with CC	1.4590

DRG	PDx/SDx/Procedure	Tips
653	Repair of cystocele with graft or prosthesis	The root operation Repair of pelvic region subcutaneous tissue and fascia is reported for procedures performed to treat cystocele, rectocele, and enterocele. However, repair of cystocele with a tissue graft or device (autologous, synthetic, or nonautologous) to reinforce and increase support of the pelvic region subcutaneous tissue and fascia is reported with root operation Supplement (U).
	AND	
	MCC condition	*See* appendix B.
654	Repair of cystocele with graft or prosthesis	*See* DRG 653.
	AND	
	CC condition	*See* appendix B.
655	Repair of cystocele with graft or prosthesis	*See* DRG 653.
656	Urinary neoplasm principal diagnosis	
	AND	
	Kidney and ureter procedures: Nephrotomy and nephrostomy Pyelotomy and pyelostomy Local excision/destruction of lesion or tissue of kidney Partial or complete nephrectomy	Root operations Bypass, Dilation, Destruction, Drainage, Excision, Extirpation, Fragmentation, Repair, Reposition, Resection, Restriction, Revision.
	AND	
	MCC condition	*See* appendix B.
657	Urinary neoplasm principal diagnosis	
	AND	
	Kidney and ureter procedures: Nephrotomy and nephrostomy Pyelotomy and pyelostomy Local excision/destruction of lesion or tissue of kidney Partial or complete nephrectomy	Root operations Bypass, Dilation, Destruction, Drainage, Excision, Extirpation, Fragmentation, Repair, Reposition, Resection, Restriction, Revision.
	AND	
	CC condition	*See* appendix B.
658	Urinary neoplasm principal diagnosis	
	AND	
	Kidney and ureter procedures: Nephrotomy and nephrostomy Pyelotomy and pyelostomy Local excision/destruction of lesion or tissue of kidney Partial or complete nephrectomy	Root operations Bypass, Dilation, Destruction, Drainage, Excision, Extirpation, Fragmentation, Repair, Reposition, Resection, Restriction, Revision.
659	Any urinary system diagnosis except malignant, benign, uncertain behavior and carcinoma-in-situ neoplasms	
	AND	
	Kidney and ureter procedures: Nephrotomy and nephrostomy Pyelotomy and pyelostomy Local excision/destruction of lesion or tissue of kidney Partial or complete nephrectomy	Root operations Bypass, Dilation, Destruction, Drainage, Excision, Extirpation, Fragmentation, Repair, Reposition, Resection, Restriction, Revision.
	AND	
	MCC condition	*See* appendix B.
660	Any urinary system diagnosis except malignant, benign, uncertain behavior and carcinoma-in-situ neoplasms	
	AND	
	Kidney and ureter procedures: Nephrotomy and nephrostomy Pyelotomy and pyelostomy Local excision/destruction of lesion or tissue of kidney Partial or complete nephrectomy	Root operations Bypass, Dilation, Destruction, Drainage, Excision, Extirpation, Fragmentation, Repair, Reposition, Resection, Restriction, Revision.
	AND	
	CC condition	*See* appendix B.
662	MCC condition	*See* appendix B.
663	CC condition	*See* appendix B.

DRG 665 Prostatectomy with MCC RW 3.0891

No Potential DRGs

DRG 666 Prostatectomy with CC — RW 1.7174

Potential DRGs

659	Kidney and Ureter Procedures for Non-neoplasm with MCC	2.5889
665	Prostatectomy with MCC	3.0891
715	Other Male Reproductive System O.R. Procedures for Malignancy with CC/MCC	2.2075

DRG	PDx/SDx/Procedure	Tips
659	Any urinary system diagnosis except malignant, benign, uncertain behavior and carcinoma-in-situ neoplasms	
	AND	
	Ureteral meatotomy	
	AND	
	MCC condition	*See* appendix B.
665	MCC condition	*See* appendix B.
715	Primary or secondary malignant neoplasm carcinoma-in-situ and neoplasm of uncertain behavior of male reproductive system	
	AND	
	Transurethral excision or destruction of bladder tissue/lesion	
	AND	
	CC/MCC condition	*See* appendix B.

DRG 667 Prostatectomy without CC/MCC — RW 1.0496

Potential DRGs

659	Kidney and Ureter Procedures for Non-neoplasm with MCC	2.5889
660	Kidney and Ureter Procedures for Non-neoplasm with CC	1.3459
665	Prostatectomy with MCC	3.0891
666	Prostatectomy with CC	1.7174
715	Other Male Reproductive System O.R. Procedures for Malignancy with CC/MCC	2.2075
716	Other Male Reproductive System O.R. Procedures for Malignancy without CC/MCC	1.4222

DRG	PDx/SDx/Procedure	Tips
659	Any urinary system diagnosis except malignant, benign, uncertain behavior and carcinoma-in-situ neoplasms	
	AND	
	Ureteral meatotomy	
	AND	
	MCC condition	*See* appendix B.
660	Any urinary system diagnosis except malignant, benign, uncertain behavior and carcinoma-in-situ neoplasms	
	AND	
	Ureteral meatotomy	
	AND	
	CC condition	*See* appendix B.
665	MCC condition	*See* appendix B.
666	CC condition	*See* appendix B.
715	Primary or secondary malignant neoplasm, carcinoma-in-situ and neoplasm of uncertain behavior of male reproductive system	
	AND	
	Transurethral excision or destruction of bladder tissue/lesion	
	AND	
	CC/MCC condition	*See* appendix B.
716	Primary or secondary malignant neoplasm, carcinoma-in-situ and neoplasm of uncertain behavior of male reproductive system	
	AND	
	Transurethral excision or destruction of bladder tissue/lesion	

DRG 668 Transurethral Procedures with MCC — RW 2.8180

Potential DRGs

665	Prostatectomy with MCC	3.0891

DRG	PDx/SDx/Procedure	Tips
665	Excision, destruction or resection of prostate, via natural or artificial opening, or via natural or artificial opening endoscopic	Review the surgical consent, OP reports, and nurse's notes carefully to determine the exact surgical procedure that was performed. It is important to clearly identify the approach used, for example via natural or artificial opening (7) or via natural or artificial opening endoscopic (8) versus open (Ø), and to determine whether the procedure was performed for diagnostic purposes to ensure the qualifier character is correctly assigned to accurately report the procedure performed and result in the appropriate MS-DRG assignment.
	AND	
	MCC condition	*See* appendix B.

DRG 669 Transurethral Procedures with CC — RW 1.5346

Potential DRGs

665	Prostatectomy with MCC	3.0891
666	Prostatectomy with CC	1.7174
668	Transurethral Procedures with MCC	2.8180

DRG	PDx/SDx/Procedure	Tips
665	Excision, destruction or resection of prostate, via natural or artificial opening, or via natural or artificial opening endoscopic	Review the surgical consent, OP reports, and nurse's notes carefully to determine the exact surgical procedure that was performed. It is important to clearly identify the approach used, for example via natural or artificial opening (7) or via natural or artificial opening endoscopic (8) versus open (Ø), and to determine whether the procedure was performed for diagnostic purposes to ensure the qualifier character is correctly assigned to accurately report the procedure performed and result in the appropriate MS-DRG assignment.
	AND	
	MCC condition	*See* appendix B.
666	Excision, destruction or resection of prostate, via natural or artificial opening, or via natural or artificial opening endoscopic	*See* DRG 665.
	AND	
	CC condition	*See* appendix B.
668	MCC condition	*See* appendix B.

DRG 670 Transurethral Procedures without CC/MCC — RW 0.9626

Potential DRGs

665	Prostatectomy with MCC	3.0891
666	Prostatectomy with CC	1.7174
668	Transurethral Procedures with MCC	2.8180
669	Transurethral Procedures with CC	1.5346

DRG	PDx/SDx/Procedure	Tips
665	Excision, destruction or resection of prostate, via natural or artificial opening, or via natural or artificial opening endoscopic	Review the surgical consent, OP reports, and nurse's notes carefully to determine the exact surgical procedure that was performed. It is important to clearly identify the approach used, for example via natural or artificial opening (7) or via natural or artificial opening endoscopic (8) versus open (Ø), and to determine whether the procedure was performed for diagnostic purposes to ensure the qualifier character is correctly assigned to accurately report the procedure performed and result in the appropriate MS-DRG assignment.
	AND	
	MCC condition	
666	Excision, destruction or resection of prostate, via natural or artificial opening, or via natural or artificial opening endoscopic	*See* DRG 665.
	AND	
	CC condition	*See* appendix B.
668	MCC condition	*See* appendix B.
669	CC condition	*See* appendix B.

DRG 671 Urethral Procedures with CC/MCC — RW 1.7119

Potential DRGs

662	Minor Bladder Procedures with MCC	2.9967
668	Transurethral Procedures with MCC	2.8180

DRG	PDx/SDx/Procedure	Tips
662	Planned urethral procedure extending into the bladder, with sphincterotomy of bladder	
	AND	
	MCC condition	*See* appendix B.
668	Transurethral biopsy of bladder	Root operation Excision, approach "Via Natural or Artificial Opening Endoscopic" with qualifier "diagnostic" is reported for transurethral biopsy of bladder.
	AND	
	MCC condition	*See* appendix B.

DRG 672 Urethral Procedures without CC/MCC — RW 0.9227

Potential DRGs

662	Minor Bladder Procedures with MCC	2.9967
663	Minor Bladder Procedures with CC	1.4590
664	Minor Bladder Procedures without CC/MCC	1.0616
668	Transurethral Procedures with MCC	2.8180
669	Transurethral Procedures with CC	1.5346
671	Urethral Procedures with CC/MCC	1.7119

DRG	PDx/SDx/Procedure	Tips
662	Planned urethral procedure extending into the bladder, with sphincterotomy of bladder	
	AND	
	MCC condition	*See* appendix B.
663	Planned urethral procedure extending into the bladder, with sphincterotomy of bladder	
	AND	
	CC condition	*See* appendix B.
664	Planned urethral procedure extending into the bladder, with sphincterotomy of bladder	
668	Transurethral biopsy of bladder	Root operation Excision, approach "Via Natural or Artificial Opening Endoscopic" with qualifier "diagnostic" are reported for transurethral biopsy of bladder.
	AND	
	MCC condition	*See* appendix B.
669	Transurethral biopsy of bladder	*See* DRG 668.
	AND	
	CC condition	*See* appendix B.
671	CC/MCC condition	*See* appendix B.

DRG 673 Other Kidney and Urinary Tract Procedures with MCC — RW 3.6980

No Potential DRGs

DRG 674 Other Kidney and Urinary Tract Procedures with CC — RW 2.3822

Potential DRGs

656	Kidney and Ureter Procedures for Neoplasm with MCC	3.1376
673	Other Kidney and Urinary Tract Procedures with MCC	3.6980

DRG	PDx/SDx/Procedure	Tips
656	Neoplasm diagnosis	
	Kidney and ureter procedures: Nephrotomy and nephrostomy Pyelotomy and pyelostomy Local excision/destruction of lesion or tissue of kidney Partial or complete nephrectomy	Root operations Bypass, Dilation, Destruction, Drainage, Excision, Extirpation, Fragmentation, Repair, Reposition, Resection, Restriction, Revision.
	AND	
	MCC condition	*See* appendix B.
673	MCC condition	*See* appendix B.

DRG 675 Other Kidney and Urinary Tract Procedures without CC/MCC — RW 1.5865

Potential DRGs

656	Kidney and Ureter Procedures for Neoplasm with MCC	3.1376
657	Kidney and Ureter Procedures for Neoplasm with CC	1.8442
673	Other Kidney and Urinary Tract Procedures with MCC	3.6980
674	Other Kidney and Urinary Tract Procedures with CC	2.3822

DRG	PDx/SDx/Procedure	Tips
656	Neoplasm diagnosis	
	Kidney and ureter procedures: Nephrotomy and nephrostomy Pyelotomy and pyelostomy Local excision/destruction of lesion or tissue of kidney Partial or complete nephrectomy	Root operations Bypass, Dilation, Destruction, Drainage, Excision, Extirpation, Fragmentation, Repair, Reposition, Resection, Restriction, Revision.
	AND	
	MCC condition	*See* appendix B.
657	Neoplasm diagnosis	
	Kidney and ureter procedures: Nephrotomy and nephrostomy Pyelotomy and pyelostomy Local excision/destruction of lesion or tissue of kidney Partial or complete nephrectomy	Root operations Bypass, Dilation, Destruction, Drainage, Excision, Extirpation, Fragmentation, Repair, Reposition, Resection, Restriction, Revision.
	AND	
	CC condition	*See* appendix B.
673	MCC condition	*See* appendix B.
674	CC condition	*See* appendix B.

DRG 682 Renal Failure with MCC

RW 1.5008

Potential DRGs

673	Other Kidney and Urinary Tract Procedures with MCC	3.6980
698	Other Kidney and Urinary Tract Diagnoses with MCC	1.6544

DRG	PDx/SDx/Procedure	Tips
673	Operative procedure in preparation for renal dialysis	Internal formation of arteriovenous shunt or external vessel-to-vessel cannula.
	AND	
	MCC condition	*See* appendix B.
698	Type 1, Type 2, or other specified diabetes with renal manifestations	According to ICD-10-CM guidelines, the classification presumes a causal relationship between diabetes and certain associated manifestations and/or conditions when these terms are linked by the term "with" in the alphabetic index (either under a main term or subterm). These conditions should be coded as related to the diabetes unless the documentation clearly states the conditions are unrelated, in which case they may be coded separately. These conditions do not require provider documentation linking them to diabetes. Review the record and/or query the physician if it is unclear whether a condition is related to diabetes mellitus or the ICD-10-CM classification does not provide instruction. Use an additional code to identify the stage of chronic kidney disease if known/present.
	Atrophy of kidney, renal sclerosis	
	Complications of urinary device	
	Cystostomy infection or other complication	
	Complications of transplanted kidney	Report only when a complication is documented, such as failure or rejection.
	AND	
	MCC condition	*See* appendix B.

DRG 683 Renal Failure with CC

RW 0.9008

Potential DRGs

673	Other Kidney and Urinary Tract Procedures with MCC	3.6980
674	Other Kidney and Urinary Tract Procedures with CC	2.3822
682	Renal Failure with MCC	1.5008
698	Other Kidney and Urinary Tract Diagnoses with MCC	1.6544
699	Other Kidney and Urinary Tract Diagnoses with CC	1.0208

DRG	PDx/SDx/Procedure	Tips
673	Operative procedure in preparation for renal dialysis	Internal formation of arteriovenous shunt or external vessel-to-vessel cannula.
	AND	
	MCC condition	*See* appendix B.
674	Operative procedure in preparation for renal dialysis	*See* DRG 673.
	AND	
	CC condition	*See* appendix B.
682	MCC condition	*See* appendix B.
698	Type 1, Type 2, or other specified diabetes with renal manifestations	According to ICD-10-CM guidelines, the classification presumes a causal relationship between diabetes and certain associated manifestations and/or conditions when these terms are linked by the term "with" in the alphabetic index (either under a main term or subterm). These conditions should be coded as related to the diabetes unless the documentation clearly states the conditions are unrelated, in which case they may be coded separately. These conditions do not require provider documentation linking them to diabetes. Review the record and/or query the physician if it is unclear whether a condition is related to diabetes mellitus or the ICD-10-CM classification does not provide instruction. Use an additional code to identify the stage of chronic kidney disease if known/present.
	Atrophy of kidney, renal sclerosis	
	Complications of urinary device	
	Cystostomy infection or other complication	
	Complications of transplanted kidney	Report only when a complication is documented, such as failure or rejection.
	AND	
	MCC condition	*See* appendix B.
699	Type 1, Type 2, or other specified diabetes with renal manifestations	*See* DRG 698.
	Atrophy of kidney, renal sclerosis	
	Complications of urinary device	
	Cystostomy infection or other complication	
	Complications of transplanted kidney	*See* DRG 698.
	AND	
	CC condition	*See* appendix B.

DRG 684 Renal Failure without CC/MCC

RW 0.6085

Potential DRGs

673	Other Kidney and Urinary Tract Procedures with MCC	3.6980
674	Other Kidney and Urinary Tract Procedures with CC	2.3822
675	Other Kidney and Urinary Tract Procedures without CC/MCC	1.5865
682	Renal Failure with MCC	1.5008
683	Renal Failure with CC	0.9008
698	Other Kidney and Urinary Tract Diagnoses with MCC	1.6544
699	Other Kidney and Urinary Tract Diagnoses with CC	1.0208
700	Other Kidney and Urinary Tract Diagnoses without CC/MCC	0.7083

DRG	PDx/SDx/Procedure	Tips
673	Operative procedure in preparation for renal dialysis	Internal formation of arteriovenous shunt or external vessel-to-vessel cannula.
	AND	
	MCC condition	*See* appendix B.
674	Operative procedure in preparation for renal dialysis	*See* DRG 673.
	AND	
	CC condition	*See* appendix B.
675	Operative procedure in preparation for renal dialysis	*See* DRG 673.
682	MCC condition	*See* appendix B.
683	CC condition	*See* appendix B.
698	Type 1, Type 2, or other specified diabetes with renal manifestations	According to ICD-10-CM guidelines, the classification presumes a causal relationship between diabetes and certain associated manifestations and/or conditions when these terms are linked by the term "with" in the alphabetic index (either under a main term or subterm). These conditions should be coded as related to the diabetes unless the documentation clearly states the conditions are unrelated, in which case they may be coded separately. These conditions do not require provider documentation linking them to diabetes. Review the record and/or query the physician if it is unclear whether a condition is related to diabetes mellitus or the ICD-10-CM classification does not provide instruction. Use an additional code to identify the stage of chronic kidney disease if known/present.
	Atrophy of kidney, renal sclerosis	
	Complications of urinary device	
	Cystostomy infection or other complication	
	Complications of transplanted kidney	Report only when a complication is documented, such as failure or rejection.
	AND	
	MCC condition	*See* appendix B.
699	Type 1, Type 2, or other specified diabetes with renal manifestations	*See* DRG 698.
	Atrophy of kidney, renal sclerosis	
	Complications of urinary device	
	Cystostomy infection or other complication	
	Complications of transplanted kidney	*See* DRG 698.
	AND	
	CC condition	*See* appendix B.
700	Type 1, Type 2, or other specified diabetes with renal manifestations	*See* DRG 698.
	Atrophy of kidney, renal sclerosis	
	Complications of urinary device	
	Cystostomy infection or other complication	
	Complications of transplanted kidney	*See* DRG 698.

DRG 686 Kidney and Urinary Tract Neoplasms with MCC

RW 1.8394

Potential DRGs

656	Kidney and Ureter Procedures for Neoplasm with MCC	3.1376
668	Transurethral Procedures with MCC	2.8180

DRG	PDx/SDx/Procedure	Tips
656	Urinary neoplasm principal diagnosis	
	AND	
	Kidney and ureter procedures: Nephrotomy and nephrostomy Pyelotomy and pyelostomy Local excision/destruction of lesion or tissue of kidney Partial or complete nephrectomy	Root operations Bypass, Dilation, Destruction, Drainage, Excision, Extirpation, Fragmentation, Repair, Reposition, Resection, Restriction, Revision.
	AND	
	MCC condition	*See* appendix B.
668	Transurethral bladder and bladder neck procedures	
	AND	
	MCC condition	*See* appendix B.

DRG 687 Kidney and Urinary Tract Neoplasms with CC

RW 1.0453

Potential DRGs

656	Kidney and Ureter Procedures for Neoplasm with MCC	3.1376
657	Kidney and Ureter Procedures for Neoplasm with CC	1.8442
668	Transurethral Procedures with MCC	2.8180
669	Transurethral Procedures with CC	1.5346
686	Kidney and Urinary Tract Neoplasms with MCC	1.8394

DRG	PDx/SDx/Procedure	Tips
656	Urinary neoplasm principal diagnosis	
	AND	
	Kidney and ureter procedures: Nephrotomy and nephrostomy Pyelotomy and pyelostomy Local excision/destruction of lesion or tissue of kidney Partial or complete nephrectomy	Root operations Bypass, Dilation, Destruction, Drainage, Excision, Extirpation, Fragmentation, Repair, Reposition, Resection, Restriction, Revision.
	AND	
	MCC condition	*See* appendix B.
657	Urinary neoplasm principal diagnosis	
	AND	
	Kidney and ureter procedures: Nephrotomy and nephrostomy Pyelotomy and pyelostomy Local excision/destruction of lesion or tissue of kidney Partial or complete nephrectomy	Root operations Bypass, Dilation, Destruction, Drainage, Excision, Extirpation, Fragmentation, Repair, Reposition, Resection, Restriction, Revision.
	AND	
	CC condition	*See* appendix B.
668	Transurethral bladder and bladder neck procedures	
	AND	
	MCC condition	*See* appendix B.
669	Transurethral bladder and bladder neck procedures	
	AND	
	CC condition	*See* appendix B.
686	MCC condition	*See* appendix B.

DRG 688 Kidney and Urinary Tract Neoplasms without CC/MCC — RW 0.7809

Potential DRGs

656	Kidney and Ureter Procedures for Neoplasm with MCC	3.1376
657	Kidney and Ureter Procedures for Neoplasm with CC	1.8442
658	Kidney and Ureter Procedures for Neoplasm without CC/MCC	1.4804
668	Transurethral Procedures with MCC	2.8180
669	Transurethral Procedures with CC	1.5346
670	Transurethral Procedures without CC/MCC	0.9626
686	Kidney and Urinary Tract Neoplasms with MCC	1.8394
687	Kidney and Urinary Tract Neoplasms with CC	1.0453

DRG	PDx/SDx/Procedure	Tips
656	Urinary neoplasm principal diagnosis	
	AND	
	Kidney and ureter procedures: Nephrotomy and nephrostomy Pyelotomy and pyelostomy Local excision/destruction of lesion or tissue of kidney Partial or complete nephrectomy	Root operations Bypass, Dilation, Destruction, Drainage, Excision, Extirpation, Fragmentation, Repair, Reposition, Resection, Restriction, Revision.
	AND	
	MCC condition	*See* appendix B.
657	Urinary neoplasm principal diagnosis	
	AND	
	Kidney and ureter procedures: Nephrotomy and nephrostomy Pyelotomy and pyelostomy Local excision/destruction of lesion or tissue of kidney Partial or complete nephrectomy	Root operations Bypass, Dilation, Destruction, Drainage, Excision, Extirpation, Fragmentation, Repair, Reposition, Resection, Restriction, Revision.
	AND	
	CC condition	*See* appendix B.
658	Urinary neoplasm principal diagnosis	
	AND	
	Kidney and ureter procedures: Nephrotomy and nephrostomy Pyelotomy and pyelostomy Local excision/destruction of lesion or tissue of kidney Partial or complete nephrectomy	Root operations Bypass, Dilation, Destruction, Drainage, Excision, Extirpation, Fragmentation, Repair, Reposition, Resection, Restriction, Revision.
668	Transurethral bladder and bladder neck procedures	
	AND	
	MCC condition	*See* appendix B.
669	Transurethral bladder and bladder neck procedures	
	AND	
	CC condition	*See* appendix B.
670	Transurethral bladder and bladder neck procedures	
686	MCC condition	*See* appendix B.
687	CC condition	*See* appendix B.

DRG 689 Kidney and Urinary Tract Infections with MCC — RW 1.1744

Potential DRGs

698	Other Kidney and Urinary Tract Diagnoses with MCC	1.6544

DRG	PDx/SDx/Procedure	Tips
698	Infection due to indwelling urinary catheter or other genitourinary device, implant and graft	When an infection is caused by a complication of care (e.g. due to an implanted device), the complication code must be sequenced as the principal diagnosis with additional codes for the infectious process.
	Cystostomy infection or other complication	
	AND	
	MCC condition	*See* appendix B.

DRG 690 Kidney and Urinary Tract Infections without MCC — RW 0.8069

Potential DRGs

689	Kidney and Urinary Tract Infections with MCC	1.1744
697	Urethral Stricture	1.1131
698	Other Kidney and Urinary Tract Diagnoses with MCC	1.6544
699	Other Kidney and Urinary Tract Diagnoses with CC	1.0208

DRG	PDx/SDx/Procedure	Tips
689	MCC condition	*See* appendix B.
697	Urethral stricture	
698	Infection due to indwelling urinary catheter or other genitourinary device, implant and graft	When an infection is caused by a complication of care (e.g. due to an implanted device), the complication code must be sequenced as the principal diagnosis with additional codes for the infectious process.
	Cystostomy infection or other complication	
	AND	
	MCC condition	*See* appendix B.
699	Infection due to indwelling urinary catheter or other genitourinary device, implant and graft	*See* DRG 698.
	Cystostomy infection or other complication	
	AND	
	CC condition	*See* appendix B.

DRG 693 Urinary Stones with MCC — RW 1.4163

Potential DRGs

659	Kidney and Ureter Procedures for Non-neoplasm with MCC	2.5889
668	Transurethral Procedures with MCC	2.8180

DRG	PDx/SDx/Procedure	Tips
659	Percutaneous nephrostomy with or without fragmentation	Key terms: nephroscopic nephrostolithotomy, percutaneous pyelostolithotomy. Percutaneous nephrostomy with kidney stone disruption, with placement of catheter, with fluoroscopic guidance. NOTE: Extracorporeal shock wave lithotripsy (ESWL) does not affect the DRG.
	AND	
	MCC condition	*See* appendix B.
668	Transurethral removal of urinary stones from ureter and renal pelvis	
	AND	
	MCC condition	*See* appendix B.

DRG 694 Urinary Stones without MCC — RW 0.7827

Potential DRGs

659	Kidney and Ureter Procedures for Non-neoplasm with MCC	2.5889
660	Kidney and Ureter Procedures for Non-neoplasm with CC	1.3459
661	Kidney and Ureter Procedures for Non-neoplasm without CC/MCC	1.0484
668	Transurethral Procedures with MCC	2.8180
669	Transurethral Procedures with CC	1.5346
670	Transurethral Procedures without CC/MCC	0.9626
693	Urinary Stones with MCC	1.4163

DRG	PDx/SDx/Procedure	Tips
659	Percutaneous nephrostomy with or without fragmentation	Key terms: nephroscopic nephrostolithotomy, percutaneous pyelostolithotomy. Percutaneous nephrostomy with kidney stone disruption, with placement of catheter, with fluoroscopic guidance. NOTE: Extracorporeal shock wave lithotripsy (ESWL) does not affect the DRG.
	AND	
	MCC condition	*See* appendix B.
660	Percutaneous nephrostomy with or without fragmentation	*See* DRG 659.
	AND	
	CC condition	*See* appendix B.
661	Percutaneous nephrostomy with or without fragmentation	*See* DRG 659.
668	Transurethral removal of urinary stones from ureter and renal pelvis	
	AND	
	MCC condition	*See* appendix B.
669	Transurethral removal of urinary stones from ureter and renal pelvis	
	AND	
	CC condition	*See* appendix B.
670	Transurethral removal of urinary stones from ureter and renal pelvis	
693	MCC condition	*See* appendix B.

DRG 695 Kidney and Urinary Tract Signs and Symptoms with MCC RW 1.1960

Potential DRGs

682	Renal Failure with MCC	1.5008
698	Other Kidney and Urinary Tract Diagnoses with MCC	1.6544

DRG	PDx/SDx/Procedure	Tips
682	Tumor lysis syndrome, hypertensive CKD, hypertensive heart and CKD without heart failure, with stage 5 CKD or ESRD, acute kidney failure, CKD, unspecified kidney failure, anuria and oliguria, traumatic anuria	
	AND	
	MCC condition	*See* appendix B.
698	Underlying disease causing the signs and symptoms (e.g. nephritic syndrome with an unspecified pathological lesion)	
	AND	
	MCC condition	*See* appendix B.

DRG 696 Kidney and Urinary Tract Signs and Symptoms without MCC RW 0.6921

Potential DRGs

682	Renal Failure with MCC	1.5008
683	Renal Failure with CC	0.9008
689	Kidney and Urinary Tract Infections with MCC	1.1744
690	Kidney and Urinary Tract Infections without MCC	0.8069
695	Kidney and Urinary Tract Signs and Symptoms with MCC	1.1960
698	Other Kidney and Urinary Tract Diagnoses with MCC	1.6544
699	Other Kidney and Urinary Tract Diagnoses with CC	1.0208
700	Other Kidney and Urinary Tract Diagnoses without CC/MCC	0.7083

DRG	PDx/SDx/Procedure	Tips
682	Tumor lysis syndrome, hypertensive CKD, hypertensive heart and CKD without heart failure, with stage 5 CKD or ESRD, acute kidney failure, CKD, unspecified kidney failure, anuria and oliguria, traumatic anuria	
	AND	
	MCC condition	*See* appendix B.
683	Tumor lysis syndrome, hypertensive CKD, hypertensive heart and CKD without heart failure, with stage 5 CKD or ESRD, acute kidney failure, CKD, unspecified kidney failure, anuria and oliguria, traumatic anuria	
	AND	
	CC condition	*See* appendix B.
689	Kidney infection, urinary tract infection	
	AND	
	MCC condition	*See* appendix B.
690	Kidney infection, urinary tract infection	
695	MCC condition	*See* appendix B.
698	Underlying disease causing the signs and symptoms (e.g. nephritic syndrome with an unspecified pathological lesion)	
	AND	
	MCC condition	*See* appendix B.
699	Underlying disease causing the signs and symptoms (e.g. nephritic syndrome with an unspecified pathological lesion)	
	AND	
	CC condition	*See* appendix B.
700	Underlying disease causing the signs and symptoms (e.g. nephritic syndrome with an unspecified pathological lesion)	

DRG 697 Urethral Stricture — RW 1.1131

Potential DRGs

662	Minor Bladder Procedures with MCC	2.9967
663	Minor Bladder Procedures with CC	1.4590
668	Transurethral Procedures with MCC	2.8180
669	Transurethral Procedures with CC	1.5346
689	Kidney and Urinary Tract Infections with MCC	1.1744
698	Other Kidney and Urinary Tract Diagnoses with MCC	1.6544

DRG	PDx/SDx/Procedure	Tips
662	Suprapubic cystostomy	
	AND	
	MCC condition	*See* appendix B.
663	Suprapubic cystostomy	
	AND	
	CC condition	*See* appendix B.
668	Transurethral procedures	
	AND	
	MCC condition	*See* appendix B.
669	Transurethral procedures	
	AND	
	CC condition	*See* appendix B.
689	Kidney infection, urinary tract infection	
	AND	
	MCC condition	*See* appendix B.
698	Infection due to indwelling urinary catheter or other genitourinary device, implant and graft	When an infection is caused by a complication of care (e.g. due to an implanted device), the complication code must be sequenced as the principal diagnosis with additional codes for the infectious process.
	Cystostomy infection or other complication	
	Congenital urethral stricture	
	AND	
	MCC condition	*See* appendix B.

DRG 698 Other Kidney and Urinary Tract Diagnoses with MCC — RW 1.6544

Potential DRGs

668	Transurethral Procedures with MCC	2.8180

DRG	PDx/SDx/Procedure	Tips
668	Urinary obstruction	Key terms: Hydronephrosis, pyonephrosis, obstructive uropathy.
	AND	
	Transurethral procedures	
	AND	
	MCC condition	*See* appendix B.

DRG 699 Other Kidney and Urinary Tract Diagnoses with CC — RW 1.0208

Potential DRGs

668	Transurethral Procedures with MCC	2.8180
669	Transurethral Procedures with CC	1.5346
682	Renal Failure with MCC	1.5008
689	Kidney and Urinary Tract Infections with MCC	1.1744
698	Other Kidney and Urinary Tract Diagnoses with MCC	1.6544

DRG	PDx/SDx/Procedure	Tips
668	Urinary obstruction	Key terms: Hydronephrosis, pyonephrosis, obstructive uropathy.
	AND	
	Transurethral removal of obstruction from ureter and renal pelvis	
	AND	
	MCC condition	*See* appendix B.
669	Urinary obstruction	Key terms: Hydronephrosis, pyonephrosis, obstructive uropathy.
	AND	
	Transurethral removal of obstruction from ureter and renal pelvis	
	AND	
	CC condition	*See* appendix B.
682	Tumor lysis syndrome, hypertensive CKD, hypertensive heart and CKD without heart failure, with stage 5 CKD or ESRD, acute kidney failure, CKD, unspecified kidney failure, anuria and oliguria, traumatic anuria	
	AND	
	MCC condition	*See* appendix B.
689	Cystitis, urinary tract infection, site not specified	
	AND	
	MCC condition	*See* appendix B.
698	MCC condition	*See* appendix B.

DRG 700 Other Kidney and Urinary Tract Diagnoses without CC/MCC RW 0.7083

Potential DRGs

668	Transurethral Procedures with MCC	2.8180
669	Transurethral Procedures with CC	1.5346
670	Transurethral Procedures without CC/MCC	0.9626
682	Renal Failure with MCC	1.5008
683	Renal Failure with CC	0.9008
689	Kidney and Urinary Tract Infections with MCC	1.1744
690	Kidney and Urinary Tract Infections without MCC	0.8069
695	Kidney and Urinary Tract Signs and Symptoms with MCC	1.1960
697	Urethral Stricture	1.1131
698	Other Kidney and Urinary Tract Diagnoses with MCC	1.6544
699	Other Kidney and Urinary Tract Diagnoses with CC	1.0208

DRG	PDx/SDx/Procedure	Tips
668	Urinary obstruction	Key terms: Hydronephrosis, pyonephrosis, obstructive uropathy.
	AND	
	Transurethral removal of obstruction from ureter and renal pelvis	
	AND	
	MCC condition	*See* appendix B.
669	Urinary obstruction	Key terms: Hydronephrosis, pyonephrosis, obstructive uropathy.
	AND	
	Transurethral removal of obstruction from ureter and renal pelvis	
	AND	
	CC condition	*See* appendix B.
670	Urinary obstruction	Key terms: Hydronephrosis, pyonephrosis, obstructive uropathy.
	AND	
	Transurethral removal of obstruction from ureter and renal pelvis	
682	Tumor lysis syndrome, hypertensive CKD, hypertensive heart and CKD without heart failure, with stage 5 CKD or ESRD, acute kidney failure, CKD, unspecified kidney failure, anuria and oliguria, traumatic anuria	
	AND	
	MCC condition	*See* appendix B.
683	Tumor lysis syndrome, hypertensive CKD, hypertensive heart and CKD without heart failure, with stage 5 CKD or ESRD, acute kidney failure, CKD, unspecified kidney failure, anuria and oliguria, traumatic anuria	
	AND	
	CC condition	*See* appendix B.
689	Cystitis, urinary tract infection, site not specified	
	AND	
	MCC condition	*See* appendix B.
690	Cystitis, urinary tract infection, site not specified	
695	Urinary incontinence, urinary symptoms such as hematuria, urinary retention, abnormal findings in urine	
	AND	
	MCC condition	*See* appendix B.
697	Urethral stricture	
698	MCC condition	*See* appendix B.
699	CC condition	*See* appendix B.

Diseases And Disorders Of The Male Reproductive System

DRG 707 Major Male Pelvic Procedures with CC/MCC RW 1.9619

Potential DRGs

659	Kidney and Ureter Procedures for Non-neoplasm with MCC	2.5889
665	Prostatectomy with MCC	3.0891

DRG	PDx/SDx/Procedure	Tips
659	Open renal biopsy	
	AND	
	MCC condition	*See* appendix B.
665	Urinary obstruction	
	AND	
	Destruction, Excision or Resection of Prostate	
	AND	
	MCC condition	*See* appendix B.
	OR	
	Resection of Prostate	
	AND	
	Resection of Seminal Vesicles	
	AND	
	MCC condition	*See* appendix B.

DRG 708 Major Male Pelvic Procedures without CC/MCC RW 1.4585

Potential DRGs

659	Kidney and Ureter Procedures for Non-neoplasm with MCC	2.5889
665	Prostatectomy with MCC	3.0891
666	Prostatectomy with CC	1.7174
707	Major Male Pelvic Procedures with CC/MCC	1.9619

DRG	PDx/SDx/Procedure	Tips
659	Open renal biopsy	
	AND	
	MCC condition	*See* appendix B.
665	Urinary obstruction	Principal diagnosis is that condition established after study to be chiefly responsible for occasioning the admission of the patient to the hospital for care.
	AND	
	Destruction, Excision or Resection of Prostate	
	AND	
	MCC condition	*See* appendix B.
	OR	
	Resection of Prostate	
	AND	
	Resection of Seminal Vesicles	
	AND	
	MCC condition	*See* appendix B.
666	Urinary obstruction	Principal diagnosis is that condition established after study to be chiefly responsible for occasioning the admission of the patient to the hospital for care.
	AND	
	Destruction, Excision or Resection of Prostate	
	AND	
	CC condition	*See* appendix B.
	OR	
	Resection of Prostate	
	AND	
	Resection of Seminal Vesicles	
	AND	
	CC condition	*See* appendix B.
707	CC/MCC condition	*See* appendix B.

DRG 709 Penis Procedures with CC/MCC — RW 2.1200

Potential DRGs

668 Transurethral Procedures with MCC — 2.8180

DRG	PDx/SDx/Procedure	Tips
668	Urethral stricture	
	AND	
	Transurethral procedures	
	AND	
	MCC condition	*See* appendix B.

DRG 710 Penis Procedures without CC/MCC — RW 1.2343

Potential DRGs

668 Transurethral Procedures with MCC — 2.8180
709 Penis Procedures with CC/MCC — 2.1200

DRG	PDx/SDx/Procedure	Tips
668	Urethral stricture	
	AND	
	Transurethral procedures	
	AND	
	MCC condition	*See* appendix B.
709	CC/MCC condition	*See* appendix B.

DRG 711 Testes Procedures with CC/MCC — RW 2.1229

No Potential DRGs

DRG 712 Testes Procedures without CC/MCC — RW 1.1884

Potential DRGs

711 Testes Procedures with CC/MCC — 2.1229

DRG	PDx/SDx/Procedure	Tips
711	CC/MCC condition	*See* appendix B.

DRG 713 Transurethral Prostatectomy with CC/MCC — RW 1.4507

Potential DRGs

665 Prostatectomy with MCC — 3.0891
666 Prostatectomy with CC — 1.7174

DRG	PDx/SDx/Procedure	Tips
665	Urinary obstruction	
	AND	
	Destruction, Excision or Resection of Prostate	
	OR	
	Resection of Prostate	
	AND	
	Resection of Seminal Vesicles	
	AND	
	MCC condition	*See* appendix B.
666	Urinary obstruction	
	AND	
	Destruction, Excision or Resection of Prostate	
	OR	
	Resection of Prostate	
	AND	
	Resection of Seminal Vesicles	
	AND	
	CC condition	*See* appendix B.

DRG 714 Transurethral Prostatectomy without CC/MCC — RW 0.9585

Potential DRGs

665	Prostatectomy with MCC	3.0891
666	Prostatectomy with CC	1.7174
667	Prostatectomy without CC/MCC	1.0496
713	Transurethral Prostatectomy with CC/MCC	1.4507

DRG	PDx/SDx/Procedure	Tips
665	Urinary obstruction	
	AND	
	Destruction, Excision or Resection of Prostate	
	OR	
	Resection of Prostate	
	AND	
	Resection of Seminal Vesicles	
	AND	
	MCC condition	*See* appendix B.
666	Urinary obstruction	
	AND	
	Destruction, Excision or Resection of Prostate	
	OR	
	Resection of Prostate	
	AND	
	Resection of Seminal Vesicles	
	AND	
	CC condition	*See* appendix B.
667	Urinary obstruction	
	AND	
	Destruction, Excision or Resection of Prostate	
	OR	
	Resection of Prostate	
	AND	
	Resection of Seminal Vesicles	
713	CC/MCC condition	*See* appendix B.

DRG 715 Other Male Reproductive System O.R. Procedures for Malignancy with CC/MCC — RW 2.2075

No Potential DRGs

DRG 716 Other Male Reproductive System O.R. Procedures for Malignancy without CC/MCC — RW 1.4222

Potential DRGs

707	Major Male Pelvic Procedures with CC/MCC	1.9619
711	Testes Procedures with CC/MCC	2.1229
715	Other Male Reproductive System O.R. Procedures for Malignancy with CC/MCC	2.2075

DRG	PDx/SDx/Procedure	Tips
707	Radical resection of lymph nodes	Lymph node excision implies that only a portion of the node or one node from a group or chain of nodes is removed. Lymph node resection implies that a particular group or chain of lymph nodes is completely removed. The root operation Excision is "cutting out or off, without replacement, a portion of a body part." Root operation Resection is "cutting out or off, without replacement, all of a body part." It includes all of a body part or any subdivision of body part having its own body part value in ICD-10-PCS. Review the description of the procedure for confirmation of removal of the entire group or chain, or if the intent was to remove the entire chain.
	OR	
	Resection of Prostate	
	AND	
	Resection of Seminal Vesicles	
	AND	
	CC/MCC condition	*See* appendix B.
711	Unilateral or bilateral orchiectomy	
	AND	
	CC/MCC condition	*See* appendix B.
715	CC/MCC condition	*See* appendix B.

DRG 717 Other Male Reproductive System O.R. Procedures Except Malignancy with CC/MCC RW 1.8137

Potential DRGs

711	Testes Procedures with CC/MCC	2.1229

DRG	PDx/SDx/Procedure	Tips
711	Excision of hydrocele (of tunica vaginalis)	
	Excision of cyst of epididymis	
	Reconstruction of surgically divided vas deferens	
	AND	
	CC/MCC condition	*See* appendix B.

DRG 718 Other Male Reproductive System O.R. Procedures Except Malignancy without CC/MCC RW 1.1758

Potential DRGs

711	Testes Procedures with CC/MCC	2.1229
717	Other Male Reproductive System O.R. Procedures Except Malignancy with CC/MCC	1.8137

DRG	PDx/SDx/Procedure	Tips
711	Excision of hydrocele (of tunica vaginalis)	
	Excision of cyst of epididymis	
	Reconstruction of surgically divided vas deferens	
	AND	
	CC/MCC condition	*See* appendix B.
717	CC/MCC condition	*See* appendix B.

DRG 722 Malignancy, Male Reproductive System with MCC RW 1.8748

Potential DRGs

707	Major Male Pelvic Procedures with CC/MCC	1.9619
709	Penis Procedures with CC/MCC	2.1200
711	Testes Procedures with CC/MCC	2.1229
715	Other Male Reproductive System O.R. Procedures for Malignancy with CC/MCC	2.2075

DRG	PDx/SDx/Procedure	Tips
707	Radical resection of lymph nodes	Lymph node excision implies that only a portion of the node or one node from a group or chain of nodes is removed. Lymph node resection implies that a particular group or chain of lymph nodes is completely removed. The root operation Excision is "cutting out or off, without replacement, a portion of a body part." Root operation Resection is "cutting out or off, without replacement, all of a body part." It includes all of a body part or any subdivision of body part having its own body part value in ICD-10-PCS. Review the description of the procedure for confirmation of removal of the entire group or chain, or if the intent was to remove the entire chain.
	OR	
	Resection of prostate	
	AND	
	Resection of seminal vesicles	
	AND	
	CC/MCC condition	*See* appendix B.
709	Release of urethral stricture	
	AND	
	CC/MCC condition	*See* appendix B.
711	Unilateral or bilateral orchiectomy	
	AND	
	CC/MCC condition	*See* appendix B.
715	Transurethral excision or destruction of lesion or tissue of bladder	
	AND	
	CC/MCC condition	*See* appendix B.

DRG 723 Malignancy, Male Reproductive System with CC

RW 1.1143

Potential DRGs

707	Major Male Pelvic Procedures with CC/MCC	1.9619
709	Penis Procedures with CC/MCC	2.1200
711	Testes Procedures with CC/MCC	2.1229
715	Other Male Reproductive System O.R. Procedures for Malignancy with CC/MCC	2.2075
722	Malignancy, Male Reproductive System with MCC	1.8748

DRG	PDx/SDx/Procedure	Tips
707	Radical resection of lymph nodes	Lymph node excision implies that only a portion of the node or one node from a group or chain of nodes is removed. Lymph node resection implies that a particular group or chain of lymph nodes is completely removed. The root operation Excision is "cutting out or off, without replacement, a portion of a body part." Root operation Resection is "cutting out or off, without replacement, all of a body part." It includes all of a body part or any subdivision of body part having its own body part value in ICD-10-PCS. Review the description of the procedure for confirmation of removal of the entire group or chain, or if the intent was to remove the entire chain.
	OR	
	Resection of Prostate	
	AND	
	Resection of Seminal Vesicles	
	AND	
	CC/MCC condition	*See* appendix B.
709	Release of urethral stricture	
	AND	
	CC/MCC condition	*See* appendix B.
711	Unilateral or bilateral orchiectomy	
	AND	
	CC/MCC condition	*See* appendix B.
715	Transurethral excision or destruction of lesion or tissue of bladder	
	AND	
	CC/MCC condition	*See* appendix B.
722	MCC condition	*See* appendix B.

DRG 724 Malignancy, Male Reproductive System without CC/MCC RW 0.8095

Potential DRGs

707	Major Male Pelvic Procedures with CC/MCC	1.9619
708	Major Male Pelvic Procedures without CC/MCC	1.4585
709	Penis Procedures with CC/MCC	2.1200
710	Penis Procedures without CC/MCC	1.2343
711	Testes Procedures with CC/MCC	2.1229
712	Testes Procedures without CC/MCC	1.1884
715	Other Male Reproductive System O.R. Procedures for Malignancy with CC/MCC	2.2075
716	Other Male Reproductive System O.R. Procedures for Malignancy without CC/MCC	1.4222
722	Malignancy, Male Reproductive System with MCC	1.8748
723	Malignancy, Male Reproductive System with CC	1.1143
729	Other Male Reproductive System Diagnoses with CC/MCC	1.0039

DRG	PDx/SDx/Procedure	Tips
707	Radical resection of lymph nodes	Lymph node excision implies that only a portion of the node or one node from a group or chain of nodes is removed. Lymph node resection implies that a particular group or chain of lymph nodes is completely removed. The root operation Excision is "cutting out or off, without replacement, a portion of a body part." Root operation Resection is "cutting out or off, without replacement, all of a body part." It includes all of a body part or any subdivision of body part having its own body part value in ICD-10-PCS. Review the description of the procedure for confirmation of removal of the entire group or chain, or if the intent was to remove the entire chain.
	OR	
	Resection of Prostate	
	AND	
	Resection of Seminal Vesicles	
	AND	
	CC/MCC condition	*See* appendix B.
708	Radical resection of lymph nodes	*See* DRG 707.
	OR	
	Resection of Prostate	
	AND	
	Resection of Seminal Vesicles	
709	Release of urethral stricture	
	AND	
	CC/MCC condition	*See* appendix B.
710	Release of urethral stricture	
711	Unilateral or bilateral orchiectomy	
	AND	
	CC/MCC condition	*See* appendix B.
712	Unilateral or bilateral orchiectomy	
715	Transurethral excision or destruction of lesion or tissue of bladder	
	AND	
	CC/MCC condition	*See* appendix B.
716	Transurethral excision or destruction of lesion or tissue of bladder	
722	MCC condition	*See* appendix B.
723	CC condition	*See* appendix B.
729	Benign neoplasm of genital organs	
	AND	
	CC/MCC condition	*See* appendix B.

DRG 725 Benign Prostatic Hypertrophy with MCC RW 1.2409

Potential DRGs

713	Transurethral Prostatectomy with CC/MCC	1.4507
727	Inflammation of the Male Reproductive System with MCC	1.6210

DRG	PDx/SDx/Procedure	Tips
713	Transurethral prostatectomy	
	AND	
	CC/MCC condition	*See* appendix B.
727	Inflammatory disease of prostate	
	AND	
	MCC condition	*See* appendix B.

DRG 726 Benign Prostatic Hypertrophy without MCC RW 0.7309

Potential DRGs

713	Transurethral Prostatectomy with CC/MCC	1.4507
714	Transurethral Prostatectomy without CC/MCC	0.9585
725	Benign Prostatic Hypertrophy with MCC	1.2409
727	Inflammation of the Male Reproductive System with MCC	1.6210
728	Inflammation of the Male Reproductive System without MCC	0.8001

DRG	PDx/SDx/Procedure	Tips
713	Transurethral Prostatectomy	
	AND	
	CC/MCC condition	
714	Transurethral prostatectomy	
725	MCC condition	*See* appendix B.
727	Inflammatory disease of prostate	
	AND	
	MCC condition	*See* appendix B.
728	Inflammatory disease of prostate	

DRG 727 Inflammation of the Male Reproductive System with MCC RW 1.6210

Potential DRGs

722	Malignancy, Male Reproductive System with MCC	1.8748

DRG	PDx/SDx/Procedure	Tips
722	Malignancy male reproductive system	
	AND	
	MCC condition	*See* appendix B.

DRG 728 Inflammation of the Male Reproductive System without MCC RW 0.8001

Potential DRGs

713	Transurethral Prostatectomy with CC/MCC	1.4507
722	Malignancy, Male Reproductive System with MCC	1.8748
723	Malignancy, Male Reproductive System with CC	1.1143
727	Inflammation of the Male Reproductive System with MCC	1.6210

DRG	PDx/SDx/Procedure	Tips
713	Transurethral Prostatectomy	
	AND	
	CC/MCC condition	*See* appendix B.
722	Malignancy male reproductive system	
	AND	
	MCC condition	*See* appendix B.
723	Malignancy male reproductive system	
	AND	
	CC condition	*See* appendix B.
727	MCC condition	*See* appendix B.

DRG 729 Other Male Reproductive System Diagnoses with CC/MCC RW 1.0039

Potential DRGs

722	Malignancy, Male Reproductive System with MCC	1.8748

DRG	PDx/SDx/Procedure	Tips
722	Malignancy male reproductive system	
	AND	
	MCC condition	*See* appendix B.

DRG 730 Other Male Reproductive System Diagnoses without CC/MCC RW 0.6216

Potential DRGs

722	Malignancy, Male Reproductive System with MCC	1.8748
723	Malignancy, Male Reproductive System with CC	1.1143
729	Other Male Reproductive System Diagnoses with CC/MCC	1.0039

DRG	PDx/SDx/Procedure	Tips
722	Malignancy male reproductive system	
	AND	
	MCC condition	*See* appendix B.
723	Malignancy male reproductive system	
	AND	
	CC condition	*See* appendix B.
729	CC/MCC condition	*See* appendix B.

Diseases And Disorders Of The Female Reproductive System

DRG 734 Pelvic Evisceration, Radical Hysterectomy and Radical Vulvectomy with CC/MCC RW 2.1736

Potential DRGs

736	Uterine and Adnexa Procedures for Ovarian or Adnexal Malignancy with MCC	3.8872
739	Uterine and Adnexa Procedures for Non-Ovarian and Non-Adnexal Malignancy with MCC	3.6163

DRG	PDx/SDx/Procedure	Tips
736	Principal diagnosis of primary or secondary neoplasm of ovary, neoplasm of uncertain behavior of ovary	Review pathology reports and query physician if necessary to ensure accurate code assignment of all malignancies.
	Primary neoplasm of fallopian tube, broad ligament, round ligament, parametrium, and other unspecified site of uterine adnexa	
	AND	
	Subtotal abdominal hysterectomy, laparoscopic or, other total abdominal hysterectomy, vaginal and, other and unspecified hysterectomy	A total hysterectomy includes the complete removal of the uterus and the cervix. Only one code for resection of the uterus (without a qualifier) is required when documentation supports a total hysterectomy; do not report an additional code for resection of the cervix. Resection of just the uterus with retention of the cervix is considered a supracervical (partial/subtotal) hysterectomy. When only the uterus is removed, report a code for resection of the uterus with a qualifier value of L Supracervical. If the ovaries and/or fallopian tubes are also resected, additional codes may be reported for the resection of these organs, according to the *ICD-10-PCS Official Guidelines for Coding and Reporting,* which state: "During the same operative episode, multiple procedures are coded if: The same root operation is performed on different body parts as defined by distinct values of the body part character."
	Partial removal (excision) or diagnostic biopsy of ovary, fallopian tube, uterus or uterine adnexa	Review operative report carefully to differentiate all types of procedures on ovaries, fallopian tubes, uterus or uterine adnexa.
	AND	
	MCC condition	*See* appendix B.
739	Any primary or secondary malignant neoplasm or neoplasm of uncertain behavior of female reproductive system OTHER THAN ovary and other uterine adnexa	Review pathology reports and query physician if necessary to ensure accurate code assignment of all malignancies.
	AND	
	Subtotal abdominal hysterectomy, laparoscopic or, other total abdominal hysterectomy, vaginal and, other and unspecified hysterectomy	*See* DRG 736.
	Partial removal (excision) or diagnostic biopsy of ovary, fallopian tube, uterus or uterine adnexa	Review operative report carefully to differentiate all types of procedures on ovaries, fallopian tubes, uterus or uterine adnexa.
	AND	
	MCC condition	*See* appendix B.

DRG 735 Pelvic Evisceration, Radical Hysterectomy and Radical Vulvectomy without CC/MCC RW 1.2602

Potential DRGs

734	Pelvic Evisceration, Radical Hysterectomy and Radical Vulvectomy with CC/MCC	2.1736
736	Uterine and Adnexa Procedures for Ovarian or Adnexal Malignancy with MCC	3.8872
737	Uterine and Adnexa Procedures for Ovarian or Adnexal Malignancy with CC	1.9738
738	Uterine and Adnexa Procedures for Ovarian or Adnexal Malignancy without CC/MCC	1.3646
739	Uterine and Adnexa Procedures for Non-Ovarian and Non-Adnexal Malignancy with MCC	3.6163
740	Uterine and Adnexa Procedures for Non-Ovarian and Non-Adnexal Malignancy with CC	1.7870

DRG	PDx/SDx/Procedure	Tips
734	CC/MCC condition	*See* appendix B.
736	Principal diagnosis of primary or secondary neoplasm of ovary, neoplasm of uncertain behavior of ovary	Review pathology reports and query physician if necessary to ensure accurate code assignment of all malignancies.
	Primary neoplasm of fallopian tube, broad ligament, round ligament, parametrium, and other unspecified site of uterine adnexa	
	AND	
	Subtotal abdominal hysterectomy, laparoscopic or, other total abdominal hysterectomy, vaginal and, other and unspecified hysterectomy	A total hysterectomy includes the complete removal of the uterus and the cervix. Only one code for resection of the uterus (without a qualifier) is required when documentation supports a total hysterectomy; do not report an additional code for resection of the cervix. Resection of just the uterus with retention of the cervix is considered a supracervical (partial/subtotal) hysterectomy. When only the uterus is removed, report a code for resection of the uterus with a qualifier value of L Supracervical. If the ovaries and/or fallopian tubes are also resected, additional codes may be reported for the resection of these organs, according to the *ICD-10-PCS Official Guidelines for Coding and Reporting,* which state: "During the same operative episode, multiple procedures are coded if: The same root operation is performed on different body parts as defined by distinct values of the body part character."
	Partial removal (excision) or diagnostic biopsy of ovary, fallopian tube, uterus or uterine adnexa	Review operative report carefully to differentiate all types of procedures on ovaries, fallopian tubes, uterus, or uterine adnexa.
	AND	
	MCC condition	*See* appendix B.

DRG 735 (Continued)

DRG	PDx/SDx/Procedure	Tips
737	Principal diagnosis of primary or secondary neoplasm of ovary, neoplasm of uncertain behavior of ovary	Review pathology reports and query physician if necessary to ensure accurate code assignment of all malignancies.
	Primary neoplasm of fallopian tube, broad ligament, round ligament, parametrium, and other unspecified site of uterine adnexa	
	AND	
	Subtotal abdominal hysterectomy, laparoscopic or, other total abdominal hysterectomy, vaginal and, other and unspecified hysterectomy	*See* DRG 736.
	Partial removal (excision) or diagnostic biopsy of ovary, fallopian tube, uterus or uterine adnexa	*See* DRG 736.
	AND	
	CC condition	*See* appendix B.
738	Principal diagnosis of primary or secondary neoplasm of ovary, neoplasm of uncertain behavior of ovary	*See* DRG 737.
	Primary neoplasm of fallopian tube, broad ligament, round ligament, parametrium, and other unspecified site of uterine adnexa	
	AND	
	Subtotal abdominal hysterectomy, laparoscopic or, other total abdominal hysterectomy, vaginal and, other and unspecified hysterectomy	*See* DRG 736.
	Partial removal (excision) or diagnostic biopsy of ovary, fallopian tube, uterus or uterine adnexa	*See* DRG 736.
739	Any primary or secondary malignant neoplasm or neoplasm of uncertain behavior of female reproductive system OTHER THAN ovary and other uterine adnexa	Review pathology reports and query physician if necessary to ensure accurate code assignment of all malignancies.
	AND	
	Subtotal abdominal hysterectomy, laparoscopic or, other total abdominal hysterectomy, vaginal and, other and unspecified hysterectomy	*See* DRG 736.
	Partial removal (excision) or diagnostic biopsy of ovary, fallopian tube, uterus or uterine adnexa	
	AND	
	MCC condition	*See* appendix B.
740	Any primary or secondary malignant neoplasm or neoplasm of uncertain behavior of female reproductive system OTHER THAN ovary and other uterine adnexa	Review pathology reports and query physician if necessary to ensure accurate code assignment of all malignancies.
	AND	
	Subtotal abdominal hysterectomy, laparoscopic or, other total abdominal hysterectomy, vaginal and, other and unspecified hysterectomy	*See* DRG 736.
	Partial removal (excision) or diagnostic biopsy of ovary, fallopian tube, uterus, or uterine adnexa	
	AND	
	CC condition	*See* appendix B.

DRG 736 Uterine and Adnexa Procedures for Ovarian or Adnexal Malignancy with MCC RW 3.8872

No Potential DRGs

DRG 737 Uterine and Adnexa Procedures for Ovarian or Adnexal Malignancy with CC RW 1.9738

Potential DRGs

734	Pelvic Evisceration, Radical Hysterectomy and Radical Vulvectomy with CC/MCC	2.1736
736	Uterine and Adnexa Procedures for Ovarian or Adnexal Malignancy with MCC	3.8872

DRG	PDx/SDx/Procedure	Tips
734	Resection of group or chain of lymph nodes	Lymph node excision implies that only a portion of the node or one node from a group or chain of nodes is removed. Lymph node resection implies that a particular group or chain of lymph nodes is completely removed. The root operation Excision is "cutting out or off, without replacement, a portion of a body part." Root operation Resection is "cutting out or off, without replacement, all of a body part." It includes all of a body part or any subdivision of body part having its own body part value in ICD-10-PCS. Review the description of the procedure for confirmation of removal of the entire group or chain, or if the intent was to remove the entire chain.
	OR	
	Excision of lymph node(s)	Excision of only a portion of a lymph node or one node from a group or chain of nodes.
	AND	
	Radical vulvectomy	Review the description of the operative report for removal of the entire vulva.
	AND	
	CC/MCC condition	*See* appendix B.
736	MCC condition	*See* appendix B.

DRG 738 Uterine and Adnexa Procedures for Ovarian or Adnexal Malignancy without CC/MCC RW 1.3646

Potential DRGs

734	Pelvic Evisceration, Radical Hysterectomy and Radical Vulvectomy with CC/MCC	2.1736
736	Uterine and Adnexa Procedures for Ovarian or Adnexal Malignancy with MCC	3.8872
737	Uterine and Adnexa Procedures for Ovarian or Adnexal Malignancy with CC	1.9738

DRG	PDx/SDx/Procedure	Tips
734	Resection of group or chain of lymph nodes	Lymph node excision implies that only a portion of the node or one node from a group or chain of nodes is removed. Lymph node resection implies that a particular group or chain of lymph nodes is completely removed. The root operation Excision is "cutting out or off, without replacement, a portion of a body part." Root operation Resection is "cutting out or off, without replacement, all of a body part." It includes all of a body part or any subdivision of body part having its own body part value in ICD-10-PCS. Review the description of the procedure for confirmation of removal of the entire group or chain, or if the intent was to remove the entire chain.
	OR	
	Excision of lymph node(s)	Excision of only a portion of a lymph node or one node from a group or chain of nodes.
	AND	
	Radical vulvectomy	Review the description of the operative report for removal of the entire vulva.
	AND	
	CC/MCC condition	*See* appendix B.
736	MCC condition	*See* appendix B.
737	CC condition	*See* appendix B.

DRG 739 Uterine and Adnexa Procedures for Non-Ovarian and Non-Adnexal Malignancy with MCC

RW 3.6163

Potential DRGs

736 Uterine and Adnexa Procedures for Ovarian or Adnexal Malignancy with MCC 3.8872

DRG	PDx/SDx/Procedure	Tips
736	Principal diagnosis of primary or secondary neoplasm of ovary, neoplasm of uncertain behavior of ovary, primary neoplasm of fallopian tube, broad ligament, round ligament, parametrium, and other unspecified site of uterine adnexa	Review pathology reports and query physician if necessary to ensure accurate code assignment of all malignancies.
	AND	
	Subtotal abdominal hysterectomy, laparoscopic or, other total abdominal hysterectomy, vaginal and, other and unspecified hysterectomy	A total hysterectomy includes the complete removal of the uterus and the cervix. Only one code for resection of the uterus (without a qualifier) is required when documentation supports a total hysterectomy; do not report an additional code for resection of the cervix. Resection of just the uterus with retention of the cervix is considered a supracervical (partial/subtotal) hysterectomy. When only the uterus is removed, report a code for resection of the uterus with a qualifier value of L Supracervical. If the ovaries and/or fallopian tubes are also resected, additional codes may be reported for the resection of these organs, according to the *ICD-10-PCS Official Guidelines for Coding and Reporting,* which state: "During the same operative episode, multiple procedures are coded if: The same root operation is performed on different body parts as defined by distinct values of the body part character."
	Partial removal (excision) or diagnostic biopsy of ovary, fallopian tube, uterus or uterine adnexa	Review operative report carefully to differentiate all types of procedures on ovaries, fallopian tubes, uterus or uterine adnexa.
	AND	
	MCC condition	*See* appendix B.

DRG 740 Uterine and Adnexa Procedures for Non-Ovarian and Non-Adnexal Malignancy with CC RW 1.7870

Potential DRGs

734	Pelvic Evisceration, Radical Hysterectomy and Radical Vulvectomy with CC/MCC	2.1736
736	Uterine and Adnexa Procedures for Ovarian or Adnexal Malignancy with MCC	3.8872
737	Uterine and Adnexa Procedures for Ovarian or Adnexal Malignancy with CC	1.9738
739	Uterine and Adnexa Procedures for Non-Ovarian and Non-Adnexal Malignancy with MCC	3.6163

DRG	PDx/SDx/Procedure	Tips
734	Resection of group or chain of lymph nodes	Lymph node excision implies that only a portion of the node or one node from a group or chain of nodes is removed. Lymph node resection implies that a particular group or chain of lymph nodes is completely removed. The root operation Excision is "cutting out or off, without replacement, a portion of a body part." Root operation Resection is "cutting out or off, without replacement, all of a body part." It includes all of a body part or any subdivision of body part having its own body part value in ICD-10-PCS. Review the description of the procedure for confirmation of removal of the entire group or chain, or if the intent was to remove the entire chain.
	OR	
	Excision of lymph node(s)	Excision of only a portion of a lymph node or one node from a group or chain of nodes.
	AND	
	Radical vulvectomy	Review the description of the operative report for removal of the entire vulva.
	AND	
	CC/MCC condition	*See* appendix B.
736	Principal diagnosis of primary or secondary neoplasm of ovary, neoplasm of uncertain behavior of ovary, primary neoplasm of fallopian tube, broad ligament, round ligament, parametrium, and other unspecified site of uterine adnexa	Review pathology reports and query physician if necessary to ensure accurate code assignment of all malignancies.
	AND	
	Subtotal abdominal hysterectomy, laparoscopic or, other total abdominal hysterectomy, vaginal and, other and unspecified hysterectomy	A total hysterectomy includes the complete removal of the uterus and the cervix. Only one code for resection of the uterus (without a qualifier) is required when documentation supports a total hysterectomy; do not report an additional code for resection of the cervix. Resection of just the uterus with retention of the cervix is considered a supracervical (partial/subtotal) hysterectomy. When only the uterus is removed, report a code for resection of the uterus with a qualifier value of L Supracervical. If the ovaries and/or fallopian tubes are also resected, additional codes may be reported for the resection of these organs, according to the *ICD-10-PCS Official Guidelines for Coding and Reporting,* which state: "During the same operative episode, multiple procedures are coded if: The same root operation is performed on different body parts as defined by distinct values of the body part character."
	Partial removal (excision) or diagnostic biopsy of ovary, fallopian tube, uterus or uterine adnexa	Review operative report carefully to differentiate all types of procedures on ovaries, fallopian tubes, uterus or uterine adnexa.
	AND	
	MCC condition	*See* appendix B.
737	Principal diagnosis of primary or secondary neoplasm of ovary, neoplasm of uncertain behavior of ovary, primary neoplasm of fallopian tube, broad ligament, round ligament, parametrium, and other unspecified site of uterine adnexa	Review pathology reports and query physician if necessary to ensure accurate code assignment of all malignancies.
	AND	
	Subtotal abdominal hysterectomy, laparoscopic or, other total abdominal hysterectomy, vaginal and, other and unspecified hysterectomy	*See* DRG 736.
	Partial removal (excision) or diagnostic biopsy of ovary, fallopian tube, uterus or uterine adnexa	Review operative report carefully to differentiate all types of procedures on ovaries, fallopian tubes, uterus or uterine adnexa.
	AND	
	CC condition	*See* appendix B.
739	MCC condition	*See* appendix B.

DRG 741 Uterine and Adnexa Procedures for Non-Ovarian and Non-Adnexal Malignancy without CC/MCC

RW 1.2993

Potential DRGs

734	Pelvic Evisceration, Radical Hysterectomy and Radical Vulvectomy with CC/MCC	2.1736
736	Uterine and Adnexa Procedures for Ovarian or Adnexal Malignancy with MCC	3.8872
737	Uterine and Adnexa Procedures for Ovarian or Adnexal Malignancy with CC	1.9738
738	Uterine and Adnexa Procedures for Ovarian or Adnexal Malignancy without CC/MCC	1.3646
739	Uterine and Adnexa Procedures for Non-Ovarian and Non-Adnexal Malignancy with MCC	3.6163
740	Uterine and Adnexa Procedures for Non-Ovarian and Non-Adnexal Malignancy with CC	1.7870

DRG	PDx/SDx/Procedure	Tips
734	Resection of group or chain of lymph nodes	Lymph node excision implies that only a portion of the node or one node from a group or chain of nodes is removed. Lymph node resection implies that a particular group or chain of lymph nodes is completely removed. The root operation Excision is "cutting out or off, without replacement, a portion of a body part." Root operation Resection is "cutting out or off, without replacement, all of a body part." It includes all of a body part or any subdivision of body part having its own body part value in ICD-10-PCS. Review the description of the procedure for confirmation of removal of the entire group or chain, or if the intent was to remove the entire chain.
	OR	
	Excision of lymph node(s)	Excision of only a portion of a lymph node or one node from a group or chain of nodes.
	AND	
	Radical vulvectomy	Review the description of the operative report for removal of the entire vulva.
	AND	
	CC/MCC condition	*See* appendix B.
736	Principal diagnosis of primary or secondary neoplasm of ovary, neoplasm of uncertain behavior of ovary, primary neoplasm of fallopian tube, broad ligament, round ligament, parametrium, and other unspecified site of uterine adnexa	Review pathology reports and query physician if necessary to ensure accurate code assignment of all malignancies.
	AND	
	Subtotal abdominal hysterectomy, laparoscopic or, other total abdominal hysterectomy, vaginal and, other and unspecified hysterectomy	A total hysterectomy includes the complete removal of the uterus and the cervix. Only one code for resection of the uterus (without a qualifier) is required when documentation supports a total hysterectomy; do not report an additional code for resection of the cervix. Resection of just the uterus with retention of the cervix is considered a supracervical (partial/subtotal) hysterectomy. When only the uterus is removed, report a code for resection of the uterus with a qualifier value of L Supracervical. If the ovaries and/or fallopian tubes are also resected, additional codes may be reported for the resection of these organs, according to the *ICD-10-PCS Official Guidelines for Coding and Reporting,* which state: "During the same operative episode, multiple procedures are coded if: The same root operation is performed on different body parts as defined by distinct values of the body part character."
	Partial removal (excision) or diagnostic biopsy of ovary, fallopian tube, uterus or uterine adnexa	Review operative report carefully to differentiate all types of procedures on ovaries, fallopian tubes, uterus or uterine adnexa.
	AND	
	MCC condition	*See* appendix B.
737	Principal diagnosis of primary or secondary neoplasm of ovary, neoplasm of uncertain behavior of ovary, primary neoplasm of fallopian tube, broad ligament, round ligament, parametrium, and other unspecified site of uterine adnexa	*See* DRG 736.
	AND	
	Subtotal abdominal hysterectomy, laparoscopic or, other total abdominal hysterectomy, vaginal and, other and unspecified hysterectomy	*See* DRG 736.
	Partial removal (excision) or diagnostic biopsy of ovary, fallopian tube, uterus or uterine adnexa	*See* DRG 736.
	AND	
	CC condition	*See* appendix B.
738	Principal diagnosis of primary or secondary neoplasm of ovary, neoplasm of uncertain behavior of ovary, primary neoplasm of fallopian tube, broad ligament, round ligament, parametrium, and other unspecified site of uterine adnexa	*See* DRG 736.
	AND	
	Subtotal abdominal hysterectomy, laparoscopic or, other total abdominal hysterectomy, vaginal and, other and unspecified hysterectomy	*See* DRG 736.
	Partial removal (excision) or diagnostic biopsy of ovary, fallopian tube, uterus or uterine adnexa	*See* DRG 736.
739	MCC condition	*See* appendix B.
740	CC condition	*See* appendix B.

Optimizing Tips

DRG 742 Uterine and Adnexa Procedures for Nonmalignancy with CC/MCC — RW 1.7819

Potential DRGs

736	Uterine and Adnexa Procedures for Ovarian or Adnexal Malignancy with MCC	3.8872
737	Uterine and Adnexa Procedures for Ovarian or Adnexal Malignancy with CC	1.9738
739	Uterine and Adnexa Procedures for Non-Ovarian and Non-Adnexal Malignancy with MCC	3.6163
740	Uterine and Adnexa Procedures for Non-Ovarian and Non-Adnexal Malignancy with CC	1.7870

DRG	PDx/SDx/Procedure	Tips
736	Principal diagnosis of primary or secondary neoplasm of ovary, neoplasm of uncertain behavior of ovary, primary neoplasm of fallopian tube, broad ligament, round ligament, parametrium, and other unspecified site of uterine adnexa	Review pathology reports and query physician if necessary to ensure accurate code assignment of all malignancies.
	AND	
	Subtotal abdominal hysterectomy, laparoscopic or, other total abdominal hysterectomy, vaginal and, other and unspecified hysterectomy	A total hysterectomy includes the complete removal of the uterus and the cervix. Only one code for resection of the uterus (without a qualifier) is required when documentation supports a total hysterectomy; do not report an additional code for resection of the cervix. Resection of just the uterus with retention of the cervix is considered a supracervical (partial/subtotal) hysterectomy. When only the uterus is removed, report a code for resection of the uterus with a qualifier value of L Supracervical. If the ovaries and/or fallopian tubes are also resected, additional codes may be reported for the resection of these organs, according to the *ICD-10-PCS Official Guidelines for Coding and Reporting,* which state: "During the same operative episode, multiple procedures are coded if: The same root operation is performed on different body parts as defined by distinct values of the body part character."
	Partial removal (excision) or diagnostic biopsy of ovary, fallopian tube, uterus or uterine adnexa	Review operative report carefully to differentiate all types of procedures on ovaries, fallopian tubes, uterus or uterine adnexa.
	AND	
	MCC condition	*See* appendix B.
737	Principal diagnosis of primary or secondary neoplasm of ovary, neoplasm of uncertain behavior of ovary, primary neoplasm of fallopian tube, broad ligament, round ligament, parametrium, and other unspecified site of uterine adnexa	*See* DRG 736.
	AND	
	Subtotal abdominal hysterectomy, laparoscopic or, other total abdominal hysterectomy, vaginal and, other and unspecified hysterectomy	*See* DRG 736.
	Partial removal (excision) or diagnostic biopsy of ovary, fallopian tube, uterus or uterine adnexa	*See* DRG 736.
	AND	
	CC condition	*See* appendix B.
739	Malignant neoplasm of uterus, cervix, placenta, other and unspecified female genital organs	Review pathology reports and query physician if necessary to ensure accurate code assignment of all malignancies.
	AND	
	Subtotal abdominal hysterectomy, laparoscopic or, other total abdominal hysterectomy, vaginal and, other and unspecified hysterectomy	*See* DRG 736.
	Partial removal (excision) or diagnostic biopsy of ovary, fallopian tube, uterus or uterine adnexa	Review operative report carefully to differentiate all types of procedures on ovaries, fallopian tubes, uterus or uterine adnexa.
	AND	
	MCC condition	*See* appendix B.
740	Malignant neoplasm of uterus, cervix, placenta, other and unspecified female genital organs	*See* DRG 739.
	AND	
	Subtotal abdominal hysterectomy, laparoscopic or, other total abdominal hysterectomy, vaginal and, other and unspecified hysterectomy	*See* DRG 739.
	Partial removal (excision) or diagnostic biopsy of ovary, fallopian tube, uterus or uterine adnexa	*See* DRG 739.
	AND	
	CC condition	*See* appendix B.

DRG 743 Uterine and Adnexa Procedures for Nonmalignancy without CC/MCC RW 1.1620

Potential DRGs

736	Uterine and Adnexa Procedures for Ovarian or Adnexal Malignancy with MCC	3.8872
737	Uterine and Adnexa Procedures for Ovarian or Adnexal Malignancy with CC	1.9738
738	Uterine and Adnexa Procedures for Ovarian or Adnexal Malignancy without CC/MCC	1.3646
739	Uterine and Adnexa Procedures for Non-Ovarian and Non-Adnexal Malignancy with MCC	3.6163
740	Uterine and Adnexa Procedures for Non-Ovarian and Non-Adnexal Malignancy with CC	1.7870
741	Uterine and Adnexa Procedures for Non-Ovarian and Non-Adnexal Malignancy without CC/MCC	1.2993
742	Uterine and Adnexa Procedures for Nonmalignancy with CC/MCC	1.7819

DRG	PDx/SDx/Procedure	Tips
736	Principal diagnosis of primary or secondary neoplasm of ovary, neoplasm of uncertain behavior of ovary, primary neoplasm of fallopian tube, broad ligament, round ligament, parametrium, and other unspecified site of uterine adnexa	Review pathology reports and query physician if necessary to ensure accurate code assignment of all malignancies.
	AND	
	Subtotal abdominal hysterectomy, laparoscopic or, other total abdominal hysterectomy, vaginal and, other and unspecified hysterectomy	A total hysterectomy includes the complete removal of the uterus and the cervix. Only one code for resection of the uterus (without a qualifier) is required when documentation supports a total hysterectomy; do not report an additional code for resection of the cervix. Resection of just the uterus with retention of the cervix is considered a supracervical (partial/subtotal) hysterectomy. When only the uterus is removed, report a code for resection of the uterus with a qualifier value of L Supracervical. If the ovaries and/or fallopian tubes are also resected, additional codes may be reported for the resection of these organs, according to the *ICD-10-PCS Official Guidelines for Coding and Reporting,* which state: "During the same operative episode, multiple procedures are coded if: The same root operation is performed on different body parts as defined by distinct values of the body part character."
	Partial removal (excision) or diagnostic biopsy of ovary, fallopian tube, uterus or uterine adnexa	Review operative report carefully to differentiate all types of procedures on ovaries, fallopian tubes, uterus or uterine adnexa.
	AND	
	MCC condition	*See* appendix B.
737	Principal diagnosis of primary or secondary neoplasm of ovary, neoplasm of uncertain behavior of ovary, primary neoplasm of fallopian tube, broad ligament, round ligament, parametrium, and other unspecified site of uterine adnexa	*See* DRG 736.
	AND	
	Subtotal abdominal hysterectomy, laparoscopic or, other total abdominal hysterectomy, vaginal and, other and unspecified hysterectomy	*See* DRG 736.
	Partial removal (excision) or diagnostic biopsy of ovary, fallopian tube, uterus or uterine adnexa	*See* DRG 736.
	AND	
	CC condition	*See* appendix B.
738	Principal diagnosis of primary or secondary neoplasm of ovary, neoplasm of uncertain behavior of ovary, primary neoplasm of fallopian tube, broad ligament, round ligament, parametrium, and other unspecified site of uterine adnexa	*See* DRG 736.
	AND	
	Subtotal abdominal hysterectomy, laparoscopic or, other total abdominal hysterectomy, vaginal and, other and unspecified hysterectomy	*See* DRG 736.
	Partial removal (excision) or diagnostic biopsy of ovary, fallopian tube, uterus or uterine adnexa	*See* DRG 736.
739	Malignant neoplasm of uterus, cervix, placenta, other and unspecified female genital organs	Review pathology reports and query physician if necessary to ensure accurate code assignment of all malignancies.
	AND	
	Subtotal abdominal hysterectomy, laparoscopic or, other total abdominal hysterectomy, vaginal and, other and unspecified hysterectomy	A total hysterectomy includes the complete removal of the uterus and the cervix. Only one code for resection of the uterus (without a qualifier) is required when documentation supports a total hysterectomy; do not report an additional code for resection of the cervix. Resection of just the uterus with retention of the cervix is considered a supracervical (partial/subtotal) hysterectomy. When only the uterus is removed, report a code for resection of the uterus with a qualifier value of L Supracervical. If the ovaries and/or fallopian tubes are also resected, additional codes may be reported for the resection of these organs, according to the *ICD-10-PCS Official Guidelines for Coding and Reporting,* which state: "During the same operative episode, multiple procedures are coded if: The same root operation is performed on different body parts as defined by distinct values of the body part character."
	Partial removal (excision) or diagnostic biopsy of ovary, fallopian tube, uterus or uterine adnexa	Review operative report carefully to differentiate all types of procedures on ovaries, fallopian tubes, uterus or uterine adnexa.
	AND	
	MCC condition	*See* appendix B.

DRG 743 (Continued)

DRG	PDx/SDx/Procedure	Tips
740	Malignant neoplasm of uterus, cervix, placenta, other and unspecified female genital organs	*See* DRG 739.
	AND	
	Subtotal abdominal hysterectomy, laparoscopic or, other total abdominal hysterectomy, vaginal and, other and unspecified hysterectomy	*See* DRG 739.
	Partial removal (excision) or diagnostic biopsy of ovary, fallopian tube, uterus or uterine adnexa	*See* DRG 739.
	AND	
	CC condition	*See* appendix B.
741	Malignant neoplasm of uterus, cervix, placenta, other and unspecified female genital organs	*See* DRG 739.
	AND	
	Subtotal abdominal hysterectomy, laparoscopic or, other total abdominal hysterectomy, vaginal and, other and unspecified hysterectomy	*See* DRG 739.
	Partial removal (excision) or diagnostic biopsy of ovary, fallopian tube, uterus or uterine adnexa	*See* DRG 739.
742	CC/MCC condition	*See* appendix B.

DRG 744 D&C, Conization, Laparoscopy and Tubal Interruption with CC/MCC — RW 1.8824

No Potential DRGs

DRG 745 D&C, Conization, Laparoscopy and Tubal Interruption without CC/MCC — RW 1.0359

Potential DRGs

742	Uterine and Adnexa Procedures for Nonmalignancy with CC/MCC	1.7819
744	D&C, Conization, Laparoscopy and Tubal Interruption with CC/MCC	1.8824

DRG	PDx/SDx/Procedure	Tips
742	Principal diagnosis of infection, sexually transmitted diseases, salpingitis, benign neoplasm, female infertility	
	AND	
	Total unilateral or bilateral salpingectomy (complete resection of fallopian tubes)	Review operative report carefully to differentiate all types of procedures on fallopian tubes.
	Excision or destruction of lesion of single fallopian tube, salpingectomy with removal of tubal pregnancy, other partial single salpingectomy, repair of one fallopian tube	
	Endometrial ablation	
	AND	
	CC/MCC condition	*See* appendix B.
744	CC/MCC condition	*See* appendix B.

DRG 746 Vagina, Cervix and Vulva Procedures with CC/MCC — RW 1.6761

Potential DRGs

744	D&C, Conization, Laparoscopy and Tubal Interruption with CC/MCC	1.8824

DRG	PDx/SDx/Procedure	Tips
744	Laparoscopy for inspection	Includes inspection of peritoneal and pelvic cavities and contents and GI and genitourinary tract.
	Laparoscopic or open bilateral salpingectomy	Includes excision, destruction or occlusion of both fallopian tubes.
	Insertion of radioactive element into cervix or vagina	
	Conization of cervix	Includes excision or extraction.
	AND	
	CC/MCC Condition	*See* appendix B.

DRG 747 Vagina, Cervix and Vulva Procedures without CC/MCC — RW 0.8872

Potential DRGs

744	D&C, Conization, Laparoscopy and Tubal Interruption with CC/MCC	1.8824
745	D&C, Conization, Laparoscopy and Tubal Interruption without CC/MCC	1.0359
746	Vagina, Cervix and Vulva Procedures with CC/MCC	1.6761

DRG	PDx/SDx/Procedure	Tips
744	Laparoscopy for inspection	Includes inspection of peritoneal and pelvic cavities and contents and GI and genitourinary tract.
	Laparoscopic or open bilateral salpingectomy	Includes excision, destruction or occlusion of both fallopian tubes.
	Insertion of radioactive element into cervix or vagina	
	Conization of cervix	Includes excision or extraction.
	AND	
	CC/MCC Condition	*See* appendix B.
745	Laparoscopy for inspection	*See* DRG 744.
	Laparoscopic or open bilateral salpingectomy	*See* DRG 744.
	Insertion of radioactive element into cervix or vagina	
	Conization of cervix	Includes excision or extraction.
746	CC/MCC condition	*See* appendix B.

DRG 748 Female Reproductive System Reconstructive Procedures — RW 1.4049

Potential DRGs

653	Major Bladder Procedures with MCC	5.4136
654	Major Bladder Procedures with CC	2.7375
655	Major Bladder Procedures without CC/MCC	2.1078

DRG	PDx/SDx/Procedure	Tips
653	Urinary incontinence, all types	Review documentation for underlying cause of incontinence, if possible.
	OR	
	Any diagnosis from MDC 11 (Kidney and Urinary Tract)	
	AND	
	Repair of cystocele and rectocele with graft or prosthesis	
	AND	
	MCC condition	*See* appendix B.
654	Urinary incontinence, all types	*See* DRG 653.
	OR	
	Any diagnosis from MDC 11 (Kidney and Urinary Tract)	
	AND	
	Repair of cystocele and rectocele with graft or prosthesis	
	AND	
	CC condition	*See* appendix B.
655	Urinary incontinence, all types	*See* DRG 653.
	OR	
	Any diagnosis from MDC 11 (Kidney and Urinary Tract)	
	AND	
	Repair of cystocele and rectocele with graft or prosthesis	

DRG 749 Other Female Reproductive System O.R. Procedures with CC/MCC — RW 2.5172

No Potential DRGs

DRG 750 Other Female Reproductive System O.R. Procedures without CC/MCC — RW 1.3600

Potential DRGs

749	Other Female Reproductive System O.R. Procedures with CC/MCC	2.5172

DRG	PDx/SDx/Procedure	Tips
749	CC/MCC condition	*See* appendix B.

DRG 754 Malignancy, Female Reproductive System with MCC RW 1.8525

Potential DRGs

736	Uterine and Adnexa Procedures for Ovarian or Adnexal Malignancy with MCC	3.8872
739	Uterine and Adnexa Procedures for Non-Ovarian and Non-Adnexal Malignancy with MCC	3.6163
749	Other Female Reproductive System O.R. Procedures with CC/MCC	2.5172

DRG	PDx/SDx/Procedure	Tips
736	Principal diagnosis of primary or secondary neoplasm of ovary, neoplasm of uncertain behavior of ovary, primary neoplasm of fallopian tube, broad ligament, round ligament, parametrium, and other unspecified site of uterine adnexa	Review pathology reports and query physician if necessary to ensure accurate code assignment of all malignancies.
	AND	
	Subtotal abdominal hysterectomy, laparoscopic or, other total abdominal hysterectomy, vaginal and, other and unspecified hysterectomy	A total hysterectomy includes the complete removal of the uterus and the cervix. Only one code for resection of the uterus (without a qualifier) is required when documentation supports a total hysterectomy; do not report an additional code for resection of the cervix. Resection of just the uterus with retention of the cervix is considered a supracervical (partial/subtotal) hysterectomy. When only the uterus is removed, report a code for resection of the uterus with a qualifier value of L Supracervical. If the ovaries and/or fallopian tubes are also resected, additional codes may be reported for the resection of these organs, according to the *ICD-10-PCS Official Guidelines for Coding and Reporting,* which state: "During the same operative episode, multiple procedures are coded if: The same root operation is performed on different body parts as defined by distinct values of the body part character."
	Partial removal (excision) or diagnostic biopsy of ovary, fallopian tube, uterus or uterine adnexa	Review operative report carefully to differentiate all types of procedures on ovaries, fallopian tubes, uterus or uterine adnexa.
	AND	
	MCC condition	*See* appendix B.
739	Malignant neoplasm of uterus, cervix, placenta, other and unspecified female genital organs	Review pathology reports and query physician if necessary to ensure accurate code assignment of all malignancies.
	AND	
	Subtotal abdominal hysterectomy, laparoscopic or, other total abdominal hysterectomy, vaginal and, other and unspecified hysterectomy	*See* DRG 736.
	Partial removal (excision) or diagnostic biopsy of ovary, fallopian tube, uterus or uterine adnexa	Review operative report carefully to differentiate all types of procedures on ovaries, fallopian tubes, uterus or uterine adnexa.
	AND	
	MCC condition	*See* appendix B.
749	Uterine artery embolization (UAE) with or without coils (e.g., for fibroids)	This procedure is most frequently done via percutaneous approach and may be performed in an interventional radiology area.
	AND	
	CC/MCC condition	*See* appendix B.

DRG 755 Malignancy, Female Reproductive System with CC

RW 1.0847

Potential DRGs

736	Uterine and Adnexa Procedures for Ovarian or Adnexal Malignancy with MCC	3.8872
737	Uterine and Adnexa Procedures for Ovarian or Adnexal Malignancy with CC	1.9738
739	Uterine and Adnexa Procedures for Non-Ovarian and Non-Adnexal Malignancy with MCC	3.6163
740	Uterine and Adnexa Procedures for Non-Ovarian and Non-Adnexal Malignancy with CC	1.7870
749	Other Female Reproductive System O.R. Procedures with CC/MCC	2.5172
754	Malignancy, Female Reproductive System with MCC	1.8525

DRG	PDx/SDx/Procedure	Tips
736	Principal diagnosis of primary or secondary neoplasm of ovary, neoplasm of uncertain behavior of ovary, primary neoplasm of fallopian tube, broad ligament, round ligament, parametrium, and other unspecified site of uterine adnexa	Review pathology reports and query physician if necessary to ensure accurate code assignment of all malignancies.
	AND	
	Subtotal abdominal hysterectomy, laparoscopic or, other total abdominal hysterectomy, vaginal and, other and unspecified hysterectomy	A total hysterectomy includes the complete removal of the uterus and the cervix. Only one code for resection of the uterus (without a qualifier) is required when documentation supports a total hysterectomy; do not report an additional code for resection of the cervix. Resection of just the uterus with retention of the cervix is considered a supracervical (partial/subtotal) hysterectomy. When only the uterus is removed, report a code for resection of the uterus with a qualifier value of L Supracervical. If the ovaries and/or fallopian tubes are also resected, additional codes may be reported for the resection of these organs, according to the *ICD-10-PCS Official Guidelines for Coding and Reporting,* which state: "During the same operative episode, multiple procedures are coded if: The same root operation is performed on different body parts as defined by distinct values of the body part character."
	Partial removal (excision) or diagnostic biopsy of ovary, fallopian tube, uterus or uterine adnexa	Review operative report carefully to differentiate all types of procedures on ovaries, fallopian tubes, uterus or uterine adnexa.
	AND	
	MCC condition	*See* appendix B.
737	Principal diagnosis of primary or secondary neoplasm of ovary, neoplasm of uncertain behavior of ovary, primary neoplasm of fallopian tube, broad ligament, round ligament, parametrium, and other unspecified site of uterine adnexa	Review pathology reports and query physician if necessary to ensure accurate code assignment of all malignancies.
	AND	
	Subtotal abdominal hysterectomy, laparoscopic or, other total abdominal hysterectomy, vaginal and, other and unspecified hysterectomy	*See* DRG 736.
	Partial removal (excision) or diagnostic biopsy of ovary, fallopian tube, uterus or uterine adnexa	Review operative report carefully to differentiate all types of procedures on ovaries, fallopian tubes, uterus or uterine adnexa.
	AND	
	CC condition	*See* appendix B.
739	Malignant neoplasm of uterus, cervix, placenta, other and unspecified female genital organs	Review pathology reports and query physician if necessary to ensure accurate code assignment of all malignancies.
	AND	
	Subtotal abdominal hysterectomy, laparoscopic or, other total abdominal hysterectomy, vaginal and, other and unspecified hysterectomy	*See* DRG 736.
	Partial removal (excision) or diagnostic biopsy of ovary, fallopian tube, uterus or uterine adnexa	Review operative report carefully to differentiate all types of procedures on ovaries, fallopian tubes, uterus or uterine adnexa.
	AND	
	MCC condition	*See* appendix B.
740	Malignant neoplasm of uterus, cervix, placenta, other and unspecified female genital organs	Review pathology reports and query physician if necessary to ensure accurate code assignment of all malignancies.
	AND	
	Subtotal abdominal hysterectomy, laparoscopic or, other total abdominal hysterectomy, vaginal and, other and unspecified hysterectomy	*See* DRG 736.
	Partial removal (excision) or diagnostic biopsy of ovary, fallopian tube, uterus or uterine adnexa	Review operative report carefully to differentiate all types of procedures on ovaries, fallopian tubes, uterus or uterine adnexa.
	AND	
	CC condition	*See* appendix B.
749	Uterine artery embolization (UAE) with or without coils (e.g., for fibroids)	This procedure is most frequently done via percutaneous approach and may be performed in an interventional radiology area.
	AND	
	CC/MCC condition	*See* appendix B.
754	MCC condition	*See* appendix B.

DRG 756 Malignancy, Female Reproductive System without CC/MCC RW 0.9897

Potential DRGs

736	Uterine and Adnexa Procedures for Ovarian or Adnexal Malignancy with MCC	3.8872
737	Uterine and Adnexa Procedures for Ovarian or Adnexal Malignancy with CC	1.9738
738	Uterine and Adnexa Procedures for Ovarian or Adnexal Malignancy without CC/MCC	1.3646
739	Uterine and Adnexa Procedures for Non-Ovarian and Non-Adnexal Malignancy with MCC	3.6163
740	Uterine and Adnexa Procedures for Non-Ovarian and Non-Adnexal Malignancy with CC	1.7870
741	Uterine and Adnexa Procedures for Non-Ovarian and Non-Adnexal Malignancy without CC/MCC	1.2993
749	Other Female Reproductive System O.R. Procedures with CC/MCC	2.5172
750	Other Female Reproductive System O.R. Procedures without CC/MCC	1.3600
754	Malignancy, Female Reproductive System with MCC	1.8525
755	Malignancy, Female Reproductive System with CC	1.0847

DRG	PDx/SDx/Procedure	Tips
736	Principal diagnosis of primary or secondary neoplasm of ovary, neoplasm of uncertain behavior of ovary, primary neoplasm of fallopian tube, broad ligament, round ligament, parametrium, and other unspecified site of uterine adnexa	Review pathology reports and query physician if necessary to ensure accurate code assignment of all malignancies.
	AND	
	Subtotal abdominal hysterectomy, laparoscopic or, other total abdominal hysterectomy, vaginal and, other and unspecified hysterectomy	A total hysterectomy includes the complete removal of the uterus and the cervix. Only one code for resection of the uterus (without a qualifier) is required when documentation supports a total hysterectomy; do not report an additional code for resection of the cervix. Resection of just the uterus with retention of the cervix is considered a supracervical (partial/subtotal) hysterectomy. When only the uterus is removed, report a code for resection of the uterus with a qualifier value of L Supracervical. If the ovaries and/or fallopian tubes are also resected, additional codes may be reported for the resection of these organs, according to the *ICD-10-PCS Official Guidelines for Coding and Reporting,* which state: "During the same operative episode, multiple procedures are coded if: The same root operation is performed on different body parts as defined by distinct values of the body part character."
	Partial removal (excision) or diagnostic biopsy of ovary, fallopian tube, uterus or uterine adnexa	Review operative report carefully to differentiate all types of procedures on ovaries, fallopian tubes, uterus or uterine adnexa.
	AND	
	MCC condition	*See* appendix B.
737	Principal diagnosis of primary or secondary neoplasm of ovary, neoplasm of uncertain behavior of ovary, primary neoplasm of fallopian tube, broad ligament, round ligament, parametrium, and other unspecified site of uterine adnexa	*See* DRG 736.
	AND	
	Subtotal abdominal hysterectomy, laparoscopic or, other total abdominal hysterectomy, vaginal and, other and unspecified hysterectomy	*See* DRG 736.
	Partial removal (excision) or diagnostic biopsy of ovary, fallopian tube, uterus or uterine adnexa	*See* DRG 736.
	AND	
	CC condition	*See* appendix B.
738	Principal diagnosis of primary or secondary neoplasm of ovary, neoplasm of uncertain behavior of ovary, primary neoplasm of fallopian tube, broad ligament, round ligament, parametrium, and other unspecified site of uterine adnexa	*See* DRG 736.
	AND	
	Subtotal abdominal hysterectomy, laparoscopic or, other total abdominal hysterectomy, vaginal and, other and unspecified hysterectomy	*See* DRG 736.
	Partial removal (excision) or diagnostic biopsy of ovary, fallopian tube, uterus or uterine adnexa	*See* DRG 736.
739	Malignant neoplasm of uterus, cervix, placenta, other and unspecified female genital organs	*See* DRG 736.
	AND	
	Subtotal abdominal hysterectomy, laparoscopic or, other total abdominal hysterectomy, vaginal and, other and unspecified hysterectomy	*See* DRG 736.
	Partial removal (excision) or diagnostic biopsy of ovary, fallopian tube, uterus or uterine adnexa	*See* DRG 736.
	AND	
	MCC condition	*See* appendix B.

DRG 756 (Continued)

DRG	PDx/SDx/Procedure	Tips
740	Malignant neoplasm of uterus, cervix, placenta, other and unspecified female genital organs	*See* DRG 736.
	AND	
	Subtotal abdominal hysterectomy, laparoscopic or, other total abdominal hysterectomy, vaginal and, other and unspecified hysterectomy	*See* DRG 736.
	Partial removal (excision) or diagnostic biopsy of ovary, fallopian tube, uterus or uterine adnexa	*See* DRG 736.
	AND	
	CC condition	*See* appendix B.
741	Malignant neoplasm of uterus, cervix, placenta, other and unspecified female genital organs	*See* DRG 736.
	AND	
	Subtotal abdominal hysterectomy, laparoscopic or, other total abdominal hysterectomy, vaginal and, other and unspecified hysterectomy	*See* DRG 736.
	Partial removal (excision) or diagnostic biopsy of ovary, fallopian tube, uterus or uterine adnexa	*See* DRG 736.
749	Uterine artery embolization (UAE) with or without coils (e.g., for fibroids)	This procedure is most frequently done via percutaneous approach and may be performed in an interventional radiology area.
	AND	
	CC/MCC condition	*See* appendix B.
750	Uterine artery embolization (UAE) with or without coils (e.g., for fibroids)	This procedure is most frequently done via percutaneous approach and may be performed in an interventional radiology area.
754	MCC condition	*See* appendix B.
755	CC condition	*See* appendix B.

Optimizing Tips

DRG 757 Infections, Female Reproductive System with MCC — RW 1.4916

Potential DRGs

749	Other Female Reproductive System O.R. Procedures with CC/MCC	2.5172

DRG	PDx/SDx/Procedure	Tips
749	Insertion of totally implantable infusion pump	Implantable infusion pumps are self-contained infusion devices that are surgically implanted into the patient. The pumps are intended to provide long-term, continuous or intermittent drug infusion using drug reservoirs with a slow-release mechanism that can be refilled as necessary through a needle injection port in the pump.
	AND	
	CC/MCC condition	*See* appendix B.

DRG 758 Infections, Female Reproductive System with CC — RW 0.9926

Potential DRGs

749	Other Female Reproductive System O.R. Procedures with CC/MCC	2.5172
757	Infections, Female Reproductive System with MCC	1.4916

DRG	PDx/SDx/Procedure	Tips
749	Insertion of totally implantable infusion pump	Implantable infusion pumps are self-contained infusion devices that are surgically implanted into the patient. The pumps are intended to provide long-term, continuous or intermittent drug infusion using drug reservoirs with a slow-release mechanism that can be refilled as necessary through a needle injection port in the pump.
	AND	
	CC/MCC condition	*See* appendix B.
757	MCC condition	*See* appendix B.

DRG 759 Infections, Female Reproductive System without CC/MCC — RW 0.6462

Potential DRGs

749	Other Female Reproductive System O.R. Procedures with CC/MCC	2.5172
750	Other Female Reproductive System O.R. Procedures without CC/MCC	1.3600
757	Infections, Female Reproductive System with MCC	1.4916
758	Infections, Female Reproductive System with CC	0.9926

DRG	PDx/SDx/Procedure	Tips
749	Insertion of totally implantable infusion pump	Implantable infusion pumps are self-contained infusion devices that are surgically implanted into the patient. The pumps are intended to provide long-term, continuous or intermittent drug infusion using drug reservoirs with a slow-release mechanism that can be refilled as necessary through a needle injection port in the pump.
	AND	
	CC/MCC condition	*See* appendix B.
750	Insertion of totally implantable infusion pump	*See* DRG 749.
757	MCC condition	*See* appendix B.
758	CC condition	*See* appendix B.

DRG 760 Menstrual and Other Female Reproductive System Disorders with CC/MCC RW 0.9954

Potential DRGs

744	D&C, Conization, Laparoscopy and Tubal Interruption with CC/MCC	1.8824
749	Other Female Reproductive System O.R. Procedures with CC/MCC	2.5172
754	Malignancy, Female Reproductive System with MCC	1.8525
755	Malignancy, Female Reproductive System with CC	1.0847

DRG	PDx/SDx/Procedure	Tips
744	Laparoscopy for inspection	Includes inspection of peritoneal and pelvic cavities and contents and GI and genitourinary tract.
	Laparoscopic or open bilateral salpingectomy	Includes excision, destruction or occlusion of both fallopian tubes.
	Insertion of radioactive element into cervix or vagina	
	Conization of cervix	Includes excision or extraction.
	AND	
	CC/MCC Condition	*See* appendix B.
749	Uterine artery embolization (UAE) with or without coils (e.g., for fibroids)	This procedure is most frequently done via percutaneous approach and may be performed in an interventional radiology area.
	AND	
	CC/MCC condition	*See* appendix B.
754	Any female reproductive system neoplasm	
	AND	
	MCC condition	*See* appendix B.
755	Any female reproductive system neoplasm	
	AND	
	CC condition	*See* appendix B.

DRG 761 Menstrual and Other Female Reproductive System Disorders without CC/MCC RW 0.6056

Potential DRGs

744	D&C, Conization, Laparoscopy and Tubal Interruption with CC/MCC	1.8824
745	D&C, Conization, Laparoscopy and Tubal Interruption without CC/MCC	1.0359
749	Other Female Reproductive System O.R. Procedures with CC/MCC	2.5172
750	Other Female Reproductive System O.R. Procedures without CC/MCC	1.3600
754	Malignancy, Female Reproductive System with MCC	1.8525
755	Malignancy, Female Reproductive System with CC	1.0847
756	Malignancy, Female Reproductive System without CC/MCC	0.9897
760	Menstrual and Other Female Reproductive System Disorders with CC/MCC	0.9954

DRG	PDx/SDx/Procedure	Tips
744	Laparoscopy for inspection	Includes inspection of peritoneal and pelvic cavities and contents and GI and genitourinary tract.
	Laparoscopic or open bilateral salpingectomy	Includes excision, destruction or occlusion of both fallopian tubes.
	Insertion of radioactive element into cervix or vagina	
	Conization of cervix	Includes excision or extraction.
	AND	
	CC/MCC condition	*See* appendix B.
745	Laparoscopy for inspection	*See* DRG 744.
	Laparoscopic or open bilateral salpingectomy	*See* DRG 744.
	Insertion of radioactive element into cervix or vagina	
	Conization of cervix	Includes excision or extraction.
749	Uterine artery embolization (UAE) with or without coils (e.g., for fibroids)	This procedure is most frequently done via percutaneous approach and may be performed in an interventional radiology area.
	AND	
	CC/MCC condition	*See* appendix B.
750	Uterine artery embolization (UAE) with or without coils (e.g., for fibroids)	This procedure is most frequently done via percutaneous approach and may be performed in an interventional radiology area.
754	Any female reproductive system neoplasm	Review pathology reports and query physician if necessary to ensure accurate code assignment of all malignancies.
	AND	
	MCC condition	*See* appendix B.
755	Any female reproductive system neoplasm	*See* DRG 754.
	AND	
	CC condition	*See* appendix B.
756	Any female reproductive system neoplasm	*See* DRG 754.
760	CC/MCC condition	*See* appendix B.

Pregnancy, Childbirth And The Puerperium

DRG 768 Vaginal Delivery with O.R. Procedure Except Sterilization and/or D&C — RW 1.2181

No Potential DRGs

DRG 769 Postpartum and Postabortion Diagnoses with O.R. Procedure — RW 1.5439

No Potential DRGs

DRG 770 Abortion with D&C, Aspiration Curettage or Hysterotomy — RW 0.7987

Potential DRGs

769 Postpartum and Postabortion Diagnoses with O.R. Procedure 1.5439

DRG	PDx/SDx/Procedure	Tips
769	Complications following abortion or ectopic and molar pregnancies	
	AND	
	Any operating room procedures, except repair of obstetric injury Examples:	
	Salpingectomy with removal of tubal pregnancy	
	Removal of extratubal ectopic pregnancy	

DRG 776 Postpartum and Postabortion Diagnoses without O.R. Procedure — RW 0.7167

Potential DRGs

769 Postpartum and Postabortion Diagnoses with O.R. Procedure 1.5439

DRG	PDx/SDx/Procedure	Tips
769	Complications following abortion or ectopic and molar pregnancies.	
	AND	
	Any operating room procedure, except repair of obstetric injury	

DRG 779 Abortion without D&C — RW 0.9892

No Potential DRGs

DRG 783 Cesarean Section with Sterilization with MCC — RW 1.7718

No Potential DRGs

DRG 784 Cesarean Section with Sterilization with CC — RW 1.0241

Potential DRGs

783 Cesarean Section with Sterilization with MCC 1.7718

DRG	PDx/SDx/Procedure	Tips
783	MCC condition	*See* appendix B.

DRG 785 Cesarean Section with Sterilization without CC/MCC — RW 0.8663

Potential DRGs

783 Cesarean Section with Sterilization with MCC 1.7718
784 Cesarean Section with Sterilization with CC 1.0241

DRG	PDx/SDx/Procedure	Tips
783	MCC condition	*See* appendix B.
784	CC condition	*See* appendix B.

DRG 786 Cesarean Section without Sterilization with MCC — RW 1.7495

Potential DRGs

783 Cesarean Section with Sterilization with MCC 1.7718

DRG	PDx/SDx/Procedure	Tips
783	Female sterilization procedure	
	AND	
	MCC condition	*See* appendix B.

DRG 787 Cesarean Section without Sterilization with CC — RW 1.0511

Potential DRGs

783 Cesarean Section with Sterilization with MCC 1.7718
786 Cesarean Section without Sterilization with MCC 1.7495

DRG	PDx/SDx/Procedure	Tips
783	Female sterilization procedure	
	AND	
	MCC condition	*See* appendix B.
786	MCC condition	*See* appendix B.

DRG 788 Cesarean Section without Sterilization without CC/MCC — RW 0.8550

Potential DRGs

783	Cesarean Section with Sterilization with MCC	1.7718
784	Cesarean Section with Sterilization with CC	1.0241
786	Cesarean Section without Sterilization with MCC	1.7495
787	Cesarean Section without Sterilization with CC	1.0511

DRG	PDx/SDx/Procedure	Tips
783	Female sterilization procedure	
	AND	
	MCC condition	*See* appendix B.
784	Female sterilization procedure	
	AND	
	CC condition	*See* appendix B.
786	MCC condition	*See* appendix B.
787	CC condition	*See* appendix B.

DRG 796 Vaginal Delivery with Sterilization/D&C with MCC — RW 1.4184

No Potential DRGs

DRG 797 Vaginal Delivery with Sterilization/D&C with CC — RW 0.9959

Potential DRGs

796	Vaginal Delivery with Sterilization/D&C with MCC	1.4184

DRG	PDx/SDx/Procedure	Tips
796	MCC condition	*See* appendix B.

DRG 798 Vaginal Delivery with Sterilization/D&C without CC/MCC — RW 0.8112

Potential DRGs

796	Vaginal Delivery with Sterilization/D&C with MCC	1.4184
797	Vaginal Delivery with Sterilization and/or D&C with CC	0.9959

DRG	PDx/SDx/Procedure	Tips
796	MCC condition	*See* appendix B.
797	CC condition	*See* appendix B.

DRG 805 Vaginal Delivery without Sterilization/D&C with MCC — RW 1.0082

Potential DRGs

796	Vaginal Delivery with Sterilization/D&C with MCC	1.4184

DRG	PDx/SDx/Procedure	Tips
796	D&C	D&C extraction for retained products of conception.
	Aspiration curettage	
	OR	
	Female sterilization procedure	
	AND	
	MCC condition	*See* appendix B.

DRG 806 Vaginal Delivery without Sterilization/D&C with CC — RW 0.7467

Potential DRGs

796	Vaginal Delivery with Sterilization/D&C with MCC	1.4184
797	Vaginal Delivery with Sterilization/D&C with CC	0.9959
805	Vaginal Delivery without Sterilization/D&C with MCC	1.0082

DRG	PDx/SDx/Procedure	Tips
796	D&C	D&C extraction for retained products of conception.
	Aspiration curettage	
	OR	
	Female sterilization procedure	
	AND	
	MCC condition	*See* appendix B.
797	D&C	*See* DRG 796.
	Aspiration curettage	
	OR	
	Female sterilization procedure	
	AND	
	CC condition	*See* appendix B.
805	MCC condition	*See* appendix B.

DRG 807 Vaginal Delivery without Sterilization/D&C without CC/MCC — RW 0.6543

Potential DRGs

796	Vaginal Delivery with Sterilization/D&C with MCC	1.4184
797	Vaginal Delivery with Sterilization/D&C with CC	0.9959
798	Vaginal Delivery with Sterilization/D&C without CC/MCC	0.8112
805	Vaginal Delivery without Sterilization/D&C with MCC	1.0082
806	Vaginal Delivery without Sterilization/D&C with CC	0.7467

DRG	PDx/SDx/Procedure	Tips
796	D&C	D&C extraction for retained products of conception.
	Aspiration curettage	
	OR	
	Female sterilization procedure	
	AND	
	MCC condition	*See* appendix B.
797	D&C	*See* DRG 796.
	Aspiration curettage	
	OR	
	Female sterilization procedure	
	AND	
	CC condition	*See* appendix B.
798	D&C	*See* DRG 796.
	Aspiration curettage	
	OR	
	Female sterilization procedure	
805	MCC condition	*See* appendix B.
806	CC condition	*See* appendix B.

DRG 817 Other Antepartum Diagnoses with O.R. Procedure with MCC — RW 2.2550

No Potential DRGs

DRG 818 Other Antepartum Diagnoses with O.R. Procedure with CC — RW 1.1731

Potential DRGs

817	Other Antepartum Diagnoses with O.R. Procedure with MCC	2.2550

DRG	PDx/SDx/Procedure	Tips
817	MCC condition	*See* appendix B.

DRG 819 Other Antepartum Diagnoses with O.R. Procedure without CC/MCC — RW 0.9072

Potential DRGs

817	Other Antepartum Diagnoses with O.R. Procedure with MCC	2.2550
818	Other Antepartum Diagnoses with O.R. Procedure with CC	1.1731

DRG	PDx/SDx/Procedure	Tips
817	MCC condition	*See* appendix B.
818	CC condition	*See* appendix B.

DRG 831 Other Antepartum Diagnoses without O.R. Procedure with MCC — RW 1.0098

Potential DRGs

817	Other Antepartum Diagnoses with O.R. Procedure with MCC	2.2550

DRG	PDx/SDx/Procedure	Tips
817	Any operating room procedure	
	AND	
	MCC condition	*See* appendix B.

DRG 832 Other Antepartum Diagnoses without O.R. Procedure with CC — RW 0.7377

Potential DRGs

817	Other Antepartum Diagnoses with O.R. Procedure with MCC	2.2550
818	Other Antepartum Diagnoses with O.R. Procedure with CC	1.1731
831	Other Antepartum Diagnoses without O.R. Procedure with MCC	1.0098

DRG	PDx/SDx/Procedure	Tips
817	Any operating room procedure	
	AND	
	MCC condition	*See* appendix B.
818	Any operating room procedure	
	AND	
	CC condition	*See* appendix B.
831	MCC condition	*See* appendix B.

DRG 833 Other Antepartum Diagnoses without O.R. Procedure without CC/MCC RW 0.5118

Potential DRGs

817	Other Antepartum Diagnoses with O.R. Procedure with MCC	2.2550
818	Other Antepartum Diagnoses with O.R. Procedure with CC	1.1731
819	Other Antepartum Diagnoses with O.R. Procedure without CC/MCC	0.9072
831	Other Antepartum Diagnoses without O.R. Procedure with MCC	1.0098
832	Other Antepartum Diagnoses without O.R. Procedure with CC	0.7377

DRG	PDx/SDx/Procedure	Tips
817	Any operating room procedure	
	AND	
	MCC condition	*See* appendix B.
818	Any operating room procedure	
	AND	
	CC condition	*See* appendix B.
819	Any operating room procedure	
831	MCC condition	*See* appendix B.
832	CC condition	*See* appendix B.

Newborns And Other Neonates With Conditions Originating In Perinatal Period

DRG 789 Neonates, Died or Transferred to Another Acute Care Facility — RW 1.8194

No Potential DRGs

DRG 790 Extreme Immaturity or Respiratory Distress Syndrome, Neonate — RW 6.0001

No Potential DRGs

DRG 791 Prematurity with Major Problems — RW 4.0977

Potential DRGs

790	Extreme Immaturity or Respiratory Distress Syndrome, Neonate	6.0001

DRG	PDx/SDx/Procedure	Tips
790	Principal or secondary diagnosis of: Extremely low birth weight [< 500 to 999 grams] Extreme immaturity [< 23 to 28 completed weeks of gestation]	Sequence birth weight code (PØ7.Ø-) before weeks of gestation code (PØ7.2-) when both are available.
	OR	
	Respiratory distress syndrome (RDS)	Also known as hyaline membrane disease and respiratory distress syndrome (RDS) Type 1, this condition occurs primarily in premature infants due to insufficient surfactant in the lungs, which are not fully developed, with symptoms of respiratory distress apparent immediately following the birth of the newborn. While symptoms of respiratory distress and tachypnea may be documented, this condition is not to be confused with respiratory distress or transient tachypnea of newborn (TTN)(RDS type 2). Review documentation carefully for haziness on chest x-ray consistent with surfactant deficiency, surfactant administration, mechanical ventilation, or support with continuous positive airway pressure (CPAP) or oxygen by high-flow nasal cannula (HFNC) for > 24 hours. The code for respiratory distress syndrome (P22.Ø) is not assigned unless the provider specifically documents this condition.

DRG 792 Prematurity without Major Problems — RW 2.4725

Potential DRGs

790	Extreme Immaturity or Respiratory Distress Syndrome, Neonate	6.0001
791	Prematurity with Major Problems	4.0977

DRG	PDx/SDx/Procedure	Tips
790	Principal or secondary diagnosis of: Extremely low birth weight [< 500 to 999 grams] Extreme immaturity [< 23 to 28 completed weeks of gestation]	Sequence birth weight code (PØ7.Ø-) before weeks of gestation code (PØ7.2-) when both are available.
	OR	
	Respiratory distress syndrome (RDS)	Also known as hyaline membrane disease and respiratory distress syndrome (RDS) Type 1, this condition occurs primarily in premature infants due to insufficient surfactant in the lungs, which are not fully developed, with symptoms of respiratory distress apparent immediately following the birth of the newborn. While symptoms of respiratory distress and tachypnea may be documented, this condition is not to be confused with respiratory distress or transient tachypnea of newborn (TTN)(RDS type 2). Review documentation carefully for haziness on chest x-ray consistent with surfactant deficiency, surfactant administration, mechanical ventilation, or support with continuous positive airway pressure (CPAP) or oxygen by high-flow nasal cannula (HFNC) for > 24 hours. The code for respiratory distress syndrome (P22.Ø) is not assigned unless the provider specifically documents this condition.
791	Principal or secondary diagnosis of: Low birth weight [1000 to 2499 grams] Preterm (prematurity NOS) [28 to 36 completed weeks of gestation]	Sequence birth weight code (PØ7.1-) before weeks of gestation code (PØ7.3-) when both are available.
	AND	
	Major problems	*See* appendix D. Key terms: neonatal abstinence syndrome, GBS sepsis, anemia of prematurity, congenital hydrocephalus, spina bifida, IVH, necrotizing enterocolitis (stages 1, 2, 3), PDA.

DRG 793 Full Term Neonate with Major Problems RW 4.2093

Potential DRGs

790	Extreme Immaturity or Respiratory Distress Syndrome, Neonate	6.0001

DRG	PDx/SDx/Procedure	Tips
790	Principal or secondary diagnosis of: Extremely low birth weight [< 500 to 999 grams] Extreme immaturity [< 23 to 28 completed weeks of gestation]	Sequence birth weight code (PØ7.Ø-) before weeks of gestation code (PØ7.2-) when both are available.
	OR	
	Respiratory distress syndrome (RDS)	Also known as hyaline membrane disease and respiratory distress syndrome (RDS) Type 1, this condition occurs primarily in premature infants due to insufficient surfactant in the lungs, which are not fully developed, with symptoms of respiratory distress apparent immediately following the birth of the newborn. While symptoms of respiratory distress and tachypnea may be documented, this condition is not to be confused with respiratory distress or transient tachypnea of newborn (TTN)(RDS type 2). Review documentation carefully for haziness on chest x-ray consistent with surfactant deficiency, surfactant administration, mechanical ventilation, or support with continuous positive airway pressure (CPAP) or oxygen by high-flow nasal cannula (HFNC) for > 24 hours. The code for respiratory distress syndrome (P22.Ø) is not assigned unless the provider specifically documents this condition.

DRG 794 Neonate with Other Significant Problems RW 1.4899

Potential DRGs

791	Prematurity with Major Problems	4.0977
793	Full Term Neonate with Major Problems	4.2093

DRG	PDx/SDx/Procedure	Tips
791	Principal or secondary diagnosis of: Low birth weight [1000 to 2499 grams] Preterm (prematurity NOS) [28 to 36 completed weeks of gestation]	Sequence birth weight code (PØ7.1-) before weeks of gestation code (PØ7.3-) when both are available.
	AND	
	Major problems	*See* appendix D. Key terms: neonatal abstinence syndrome, GBS sepsis, anemia of prematurity, congenital hydrocephalus, spina bifida, IVH, necrotizing enterocolitis (stages 1, 2, 3), PDA.
793	Full term neonate or newborn [> 36 completed weeks of gestation]	
	AND	
	Major problems	*See* DRG 791.

DRG 795 Normal Newborn

RW 0.2017

Potential DRGs

790	Extreme Immaturity or Respiratory Distress Syndrome, Neonate	6.0001
791	Prematurity with Major Problems	4.0977
792	Prematurity without Major Problems	2.4725
793	Full Term Neonate with Major Problems	4.2093
794	Neonate with Other Significant Problems	1.4899

DRG	PDx/SDx/Procedure	Tips
790	Principal or secondary diagnosis of: Extremely low birth weight [< 500 to 999 grams] Extreme immaturity [< 23 to 28 completed weeks of gestation]	Sequence birth weight code (PØ7.Ø-) before weeks of gestation code (PØ7.2-) when both are available.
	OR	
	Respiratory distress syndrome (RDS)	Also known as hyaline membrane disease and respiratory distress syndrome (RDS) Type 1, this condition occurs primarily in premature infants due to insufficient surfactant in the lungs, which are not fully developed, with symptoms of respiratory distress apparent immediately following the birth of the newborn. While symptoms of respiratory distress and tachypnea may be documented, this condition is not to be confused with respiratory distress or transient tachypnea of newborn (TTN)(RDS type 2). Review documentation carefully for haziness on chest x-ray consistent with surfactant deficiency, surfactant administration, mechanical ventilation, or support with continuous positive airway pressure (CPAP) or oxygen by high-flow nasal cannula (HFNC) for > 24 hours. The code for respiratory distress syndrome (P22.Ø) is not assigned unless the provider specifically documents this condition.
791	Principal or secondary diagnosis of: Low birth weight [1000 to 2499 grams] Preterm (prematurity NOS) [28 to 36 completed weeks of gestation]	Sequence birth weight code (PØ7.1-) before weeks of gestation code (PØ7.3-) when both are available.
	AND	
	Major problems	*See* appendix D. Key terms: neonatal abstinence syndrome, GBS sepsis, anemia of prematurity, congenital hydrocephalus, spina bifida, IVH, necrotizing enterocolitis (stages 1, 2, 3), PDA.
792	Principal or secondary diagnosis of: Low birth weight [1000 to 2499 grams] Preterm (prematurity NOS) [28 to 36 completed weeks of gestation]	Sequence birth weight code (PØ7.1-) before weeks of gestation code (PØ7.3-) when both are available.
793	Full term neonate or newborn [> 36 completed weeks of gestation]	
	AND	
	Major problems	*See* DRG 791.
794	Principal or secondary diagnosis of neonate or newborn with other significant problem	*See* appendix E. Review code assignment carefully; in addition to codes in appendix E, codes not assigned to DRGs 789-793 or 795 and codes from other ICD-10-CM chapters can group to DRG 794.

Diseases And Disorders Of Blood, Blood-Forming Organs And Immunologic Disorders

DRG 799 Splenic Procedures with MCC — RW 4.9546

Potential DRGs

820	Lymphoma and Leukemia with Major O.R. Procedure with MCC	6.0467
957	Other O.R. Procedures for Multiple Significant Trauma with MCC	7.2325

DRG	PDx/SDx/Procedure	Tips
820	PDx of lymphoma or leukemia	
	AND	
	Major O.R. procedure on spleen for lymphoma or leukemia	
	AND	
	MCC condition	*See* appendix B.
957	Other O.R. procedures for multiple significant trauma	PDx of trauma and at least two injuries (assigned as PDx or SDx) that are defined as significant trauma from different body site categories located under MS-DRG 963 and O.R. Procedure other than craniotomy or limb reattachment, hip and femur procedures.
	AND	
	MCC condition	*See* appendix B.

DRG 800 Splenic Procedures with CC — RW 2.8177

Potential DRGs

799	Splenic Procedures with MCC	4.9546
820	Lymphoma and Leukemia with Major O.R. Procedure with MCC	6.0467
826	Myeloproliferative Disorders or Poorly Differentiated Neoplasms with Major O.R. Procedure with MCC	4.3888
957	Other O.R. Procedures for Multiple Significant Trauma with MCC	7.2325
958	Other O.R. Procedures for Multiple Significant Trauma with CC	4.0448

DRG	PDx/SDx/Procedure	Tips
799	MCC condition	*See* appendix B.
820	PDx of lymphoma or leukemia	
	AND	
	Major O.R. procedure on spleen for lymphoma or leukemia	
	AND	
	MCC condition	*See* appendix B.
826	Principal diagnosis of myeloproliferative disorder or poorly differentiated neoplasm	
	AND	
	Major O.R. procedure on spleen for myeloproliferative disorders or poorly differentiated neoplasms	
	AND	
	MCC condition	*See* appendix B.
957	Other O.R. procedures for multiple significant trauma	PDx of trauma and at least two injuries (assigned as PDx or SDx) that are defined as significant trauma from different body site categories located under MS-DRG 963 and O.R. Procedure other than craniotomy or limb reattachment, hip and femur procedures.
	AND	
	MCC condition	*See* appendix B.
958	Other O.R. procedures for multiple significant trauma	*See* DRG 957.
	AND	
	CC condition	*See* appendix B.

DRG 801 Splenic Procedures without CC/MCC

RW 1.7897

Potential DRGs

799	Splenic Procedures with MCC	4.9546
800	Splenic Procedures with CC	2.8177
820	Lymphoma and Leukemia with Major O.R. Procedure with MCC	6.0467
821	Lymphoma and Leukemia with Major O.R. Procedure with CC	2.2321
826	Myeloproliferative Disorders or Poorly Differentiated Neoplasms with Major O.R. Procedure with MCC	4.3888
827	Myeloproliferative Disorders or Poorly Differentiated Neoplasms with Major O.R. Procedure with CC	2.3172
957	Other O.R. Procedures for Multiple Significant Trauma with MCC	7.2325
958	Other O.R. Procedures for Multiple Significant Trauma with CC	4.0448
959	Other O.R. Procedures for Multiple Significant Trauma without CC/MCC	2.5324

DRG	PDx/SDx/Procedure	Tips
799	MCC condition	*See* appendix B.
800	CC condition	*See* appendix B.
820	PDx of lymphoma or leukemia	
	AND	
	Major O.R. procedure on spleen for lymphoma or leukemia	
	AND	
	MCC condition	*See* appendix B.
821	PDx of lymphoma or leukemia	
	AND	
	Major O.R. procedure on spleen for lymphoma or leukemia	
	AND	
	CC condition	*See* appendix B.
826	Principal diagnosis of myeloproliferative disorder or poorly differentiated neoplasm	
	AND	
	Major O.R. procedure on spleen for myeloproliferative disorders or poorly differentiated neoplasms	
	AND	
	MCC condition	*See* appendix B.
827	Principal diagnosis of myeloproliferative disorder or poorly differentiated neoplasm	
	AND	
	Major O.R. procedure on spleen for myeloproliferative disorders or poorly differentiated neoplasms	
	AND	
	CC condition	*See* appendix B.
957	Other O.R. procedures for multiple significant trauma	PDx of trauma and at least two injuries (assigned as PDx or SDx) that are defined as significant trauma from different body site categories located under MS-DRG 963 and O.R. Procedure other than craniotomy or limb reattachment, hip and femur procedures.
	AND	
	MCC condition	*See* appendix B.
958	Other O.R. procedures for multiple significant trauma	*See* DRG 957.
	AND	
	CC condition	*See* appendix B.
959	Other O.R. procedures for multiple significant trauma	*See* DRG 957.

DRG 802 Other O.R. Procedures of the Blood and Blood-Forming Organs with MCC RW 3.3903

Potential DRGs

163	Major Chest Procedures with MCC	4.7136
356	Other Digestive System O.R. Procedures with MCC	4.2787
423	Other Hepatobiliary or Pancreas O.R. Procedures with MCC	3.9109
799	Splenic Procedures with MCC	4.9546
957	Other O.R. Procedures for Multiple Significant Trauma with MCC	7.2325

DRG	PDx/SDx/Procedure	Tips
163	PDx of disease/disorder of the respiratory system	
	Non-diagnostic drainage of thoracic duct or cisterna chyli with or without drainage device	Review operative report for indications of therapeutic, nondiagnostic indications for drainage rather than diagnostic.
	AND	
	MCC condition	*See* appendix B.
356	PDx of disease/disorder of the digestive system	
	AND	
	Insertion of a monitoring device or intraluminal device in the superior vena cava, open, percutaneous or percutaneous endoscopic approach	
	AND	
	MCC condition	*See* appendix B.
423	PDx of disease/disorder of the hepatobiliary system or pancreas	
	AND	
	Insertion of a monitoring device or intraluminal device in the superior vena cava, open, percutaneous or percutaneous endoscopic approach	
	Diagnostic drainage of cisterna chyli, any approach	
	AND	
	MCC condition	*See* appendix B.
799	Open biopsy of spleen	
	Excision/Destruction of lesion or tissue of spleen	
	Resection of spleen	
	Repair of spleen	
	Open drainage of spleen	
	Extirpation of spleen	
	Release of spleen	
	Open reposition of spleen	
	Removal or revision of a drainage, infusion or other device in spleen	
	AND	
	MCC condition	*See* appendix B.
957	Other O.R. procedures for multiple significant trauma	PDx of trauma and at least two injuries (assigned as PDx or SDx) that are defined as significant trauma from different body site categories located under MS-DRG 963 and O.R. Procedure other than craniotomy or limb reattachment, hip and femur procedures.
	Nondiagnostic drainage of thoracic duct or cisterna chyli with or without drainage device	Review operative report for indications of therapeutic, nondiagnostic indications for drainage rather than diagnostic.
	AND	
	MCC condition	*See* appendix B.

DRG 803 Other O.R. Procedures of the Blood and Blood-Forming Organs with CC — RW 1.8582

Potential DRGs

040	Peripheral/Cranial Nerve and Other Nervous System Procedures with MCC	3.8505
041	Peripheral/Cranial Nerve and Other Nervous System Procedures with CC or Peripheral Neurostimulator	2.2307
163	Major Chest Procedures with MCC	4.7136
164	Major Chest Procedures with CC	2.5504
166	Other Respiratory System O.R. Procedures with MCC	4.0578
356	Other Digestive System O.R. Procedures with MCC	4.2787
357	Other Digestive System O.R. Procedures with CC	2.1968
423	Other Hepatobiliary or Pancreas O.R. Procedures with MCC	3.9109
424	Other Hepatobiliary or Pancreas O.R. Procedures with CC	2.0873
799	Splenic Procedures with MCC	4.9546
800	Splenic Procedures with CC	2.8177
802	Other O.R. Procedures of the Blood and Blood-Forming Organs with MCC	3.3903
957	Other O.R. Procedures for Multiple Significant Trauma with MCC	7.2325
958	Other O.R. Procedures for Multiple Significant Trauma with CC	4.0448

DRG	PDx/SDx/Procedure	Tips
040	PDx of disease/disorder of the nervous system	
	AND	
	Insertion of a monitoring device or intraluminal device in the superior vena cava, open, percutaneous or percutaneous endoscopic approach	
	Diagnostic drainage of thoracic duct or cisterna chyli, any approach	
	AND	
	MCC condition	*See* appendix B.
041	PDx of disease/disorder of the nervous system	
	AND	
	Insertion of a monitoring device or intraluminal device in the superior vena cava, open, percutaneous or percutaneous endoscopic approach	
	Diagnostic drainage of thoracic duct or cisterna chyli, any approach	
	AND	
	CC condition	*See* appendix B.
163	PDx of disease/disorder of the respiratory system	
	Non-diagnostic drainage of thoracic duct or cisterna chyli with or without drainage device	Review operative report for indications of therapeutic, nondiagnostic indications for drainage rather than diagnostic.
	AND	
	MCC condition	*See* appendix B.
164	PDx of disease/disorder of the respiratory system	
	Non-diagnostic drainage of thoracic duct or cisterna chyli with or without drainage device	*See* DRG 163.
	AND	
	CC condition	*See* appendix B.
166	PDx of disease/disorder of the respiratory system	
	AND	
	Insertion of a monitoring device or intraluminal device in the superior vena cava, open, percutaneous or percutaneous endoscopic approach	
	Diagnostic drainage of thoracic duct, any approach	
	AND	
	MCC condition	*See* appendix B.
356	PDx of disease/disorder of the digestive system	
	AND	
	Insertion of a monitoring device or intraluminal device in the superior vena cava, open, percutaneous or percutaneous endoscopic approach	
	AND	
	MCC condition	*See* appendix B.
357	PDx of disease/disorder of the digestive system	
	AND	
	Insertion of a monitoring device or intraluminal device in the superior vena cava, open, percutaneous or percutaneous endoscopic approach	
	AND	
	CC condition	*See* appendix B.
423	PDx of disease/disorder of the hepatobiliary system or pancreas	
	AND	
	Insertion of a monitoring device or intraluminal device in the superior vena cava, open, percutaneous or percutaneous endoscopic approach	
	Diagnostic drainage of cisterna chyli, any approach	
	AND	
	MCC condition	*See* appendix B.

DRG 803 (Continued)

DRG	PDx/SDx/Procedure	Tips
424	PDx of disease/disorder of the hepatobiliary system or pancreas	
	AND	
	Insertion of a monitoring device or intraluminal device in the superior vena cava, open, percutaneous or percutaneous endoscopic approach	
	Diagnostic drainage of cisterna chyli, any approach	
	AND	
	CC condition	*See* appendix B.
799	Open biopsy of spleen	
	Excision/Destruction of lesion or tissue of spleen	
	Resection of spleen	
	Repair of spleen	
	Open drainage of spleen	
	Extirpation of spleen	
	Release of spleen	
	Open reposition of spleen	
	Removal or revision of a drainage, infusion or other device in spleen	
	AND	
	MCC condition	*See* appendix B.
800	Open biopsy of spleen	
	Excision/Destruction of lesion or tissue of spleen	
	Resection of spleen	
	Repair of spleen	
	Open drainage of spleen	
	Extirpation of spleen	
	Release of spleen	
	Open reposition of spleen	
	Removal or revision of a drainage, infusion or other device in spleen	
	AND	
	CC condition	*See* appendix B.
802	MCC condition	*See* appendix B.
957	Other O.R. procedures for multiple significant trauma	PDx of trauma and at least two injuries (assigned as PDx or SDx) that are defined as significant trauma from different body site categories located under MS-DRG 963 and O.R. Procedure other than craniotomy or limb reattachment, hip and femur procedures.
	Nondiagnostic drainage of thoracic duct or cisterna chyli with or without drainage device	Review operative report for indications of therapeutic, nondiagnostic indications for drainage rather than diagnostic.
	AND	
	MCC condition	*See* appendix B.
958	Other O.R. procedures for multiple significant trauma	*See* DRG 957.
	Nondiagnostic drainage of thoracic duct or cisterna chyli with or without drainage device	*See* DRG 957.
	AND	
	CC condition	*See* appendix B.

DRG 804 Other O.R. Procedures of the Blood and Blood-Forming Organs without CC/MCC RW 1.2104

Potential DRGs

040	Peripheral/Cranial Nerve and Other Nervous System Procedures with MCC	3.8505
041	Peripheral/Cranial Nerve and Other Nervous System Procedures with CC or Peripheral Neurostimulator	2.2307
042	Peripheral/Cranial Nerve and Other Nervous System Procedures without CC/MCC	1.7398
163	Major Chest Procedures with MCC	4.7136
164	Major Chest Procedures with CC	2.5504
165	Major Chest Procedures without CC/MCC	1.8764
166	Other Respiratory System O.R. Procedures with MCC	4.0578
167	Other Respiratory System O.R. Procedures with CC	1.8198
356	Other Digestive System O.R. Procedures with MCC	4.2787
357	Other Digestive System O.R. Procedures with CC	2.1968
423	Other Hepatobiliary or Pancreas O.R. Procedures with MCC	3.9109
424	Other Hepatobiliary or Pancreas O.R. Procedures with CC	2.0873
425	Other Hepatobiliary or Pancreas O.R. Procedures without CC/MCC	1.6019
799	Splenic Procedures with MCC	4.9546
800	Splenic Procedures with CC	2.8177
801	Splenic Procedures without CC/MCC	1.7897
802	Other O.R. Procedures of the Blood and Blood-Forming Organs with MCC	3.3903
803	Other O.R. Procedures of the Blood and Blood-Forming Organs with CC	1.8582
957	Other O.R. Procedures for Multiple Significant Trauma with MCC	7.2325
958	Other O.R. Procedures for Multiple Significant Trauma with CC	4.0448
959	Other O.R. Procedures for Multiple Significant Trauma without CC/MCC	2.5324

DRG	PDx/SDx/Procedure	Tips
040	PDx of disease/disorder of the nervous system	
	AND	
	Insertion of a monitoring device or intraluminal device in the superior vena cava, open, percutaneous or percutaneous endoscopic approach	
	Diagnostic drainage of thoracic duct or cisterna chyli, any approach	
	AND	
	MCC condition	*See* appendix B.
041	PDx of disease/disorder of the nervous system	
	AND	
	Insertion of a monitoring device or intraluminal device in the superior vena cava, open, percutaneous or percutaneous endoscopic approach	
	Diagnostic drainage of thoracic duct or cisterna chyli, any approach	
	AND	
	CC condition	*See* appendix B.
042	PDx of disease/disorder of the nervous system	
	AND	
	Insertion of a monitoring device or intraluminal device in the superior vena cava, open, percutaneous or percutaneous endoscopic approach	
	Diagnostic drainage of thoracic duct or cisterna chyli, any approach	
163	PDx of disease/disorder of the respiratory system	
	Non-diagnostic drainage of thoracic duct or cisterna chyli with or without drainage device	Review operative report for indications of therapeutic, nondiagnostic indications for drainage rather than diagnostic.
	AND	
	MCC condition	*See* appendix B.
164	PDx of disease/disorder of the respiratory system	
	Non-diagnostic drainage of thoracic duct or cisterna chyli with or without drainage device	*See* DRG 163.
	AND	
	CC condition	*See* appendix B.
165	PDx of disease/disorder of the respiratory system	
	Non-diagnostic drainage of thoracic duct or cisterna chyli with or without drainage device	*See* DRG 163.
166	PDx of disease/disorder of the respiratory system	
	AND	
	Insertion of a monitoring device or intraluminal device in the superior vena cava, open, percutaneous or percutaneous endoscopic approach	
	Diagnostic drainage of thoracic duct, any approach	
	AND	
	MCC condition	*See* appendix B.
167	PDx of disease/disorder of the respiratory system	
	AND	
	Insertion of a monitoring device or intraluminal device in the superior vena cava, open, percutaneous or percutaneous endoscopic approach	
	Diagnostic drainage of thoracic duct, any approach	
	AND	
	CC condition	*See* appendix B.

DRG 804 (Continued)

DRG	PDx/SDx/Procedure	Tips
356	PDx of disease/disorder of the digestive system	
	AND	
	Insertion of a monitoring device or intraluminal device in the superior vena cava, open, percutaneous or percutaneous endoscopic approach	
	AND	
	MCC condition	*See* appendix B.
357	PDx of disease/disorder of the digestive system	
	AND	
	Insertion of a monitoring device or intraluminal device in the superior vena cava, open, percutaneous or percutaneous endoscopic approach	
	AND	
	CC condition	*See* appendix B.
423	PDx of disease/disorder of the hepatobiliary system or pancreas	
	AND	
	Insertion of a monitoring device or intraluminal device in the superior vena cava, open, percutaneous or percutaneous endoscopic approach	
	Diagnostic drainage of cisterna chyli, any approach	
	AND	
	MCC condition	*See* appendix B.
424	PDx of disease/disorder of the hepatobiliary system or pancreas	
	AND	
	Insertion of a monitoring device or intraluminal device in the superior vena cava, open, percutaneous or percutaneous endoscopic approach	
	Diagnostic drainage of cisterna chyli, any approach	
	AND	
	CC condition	*See* appendix B.
425	PDx of disease/disorder of the hepatobiliary system or pancreas	
	AND	
	Insertion of a monitoring device or intraluminal device in the superior vena cava, open, percutaneous or percutaneous endoscopic approach	
	Diagnostic drainage of cisterna chyli, any approach	
799	Open biopsy of spleen	
	Excision/Destruction of lesion or tissue of spleen	
	Resection of spleen	
	Repair of spleen	
	Open drainage of spleen	
	Extirpation of spleen	
	Release of spleen	
	Open reposition of spleen	
	Removal or revision of a drainage, infusion or other device in spleen	
	AND	
	MCC condition	*See* appendix B.
800	Open biopsy of spleen	
	Excision/Destruction of lesion or tissue of spleen	
	Resection of spleen	
	Repair of spleen	
	Open drainage of spleen	
	Extirpation of spleen	
	Release of spleen	
	Open reposition of spleen	
	Removal or revision of a drainage, infusion or other device in spleen	
	AND	
	CC condition	*See* appendix B.
801	Open biopsy of spleen	
	Excision/Destruction of lesion or tissue of spleen	
	Resection of spleen	
	Repair of spleen	
	Open drainage of spleen	
	Extirpation of spleen	
	Release of spleen	
	Open reposition of spleen	
	Removal or revision of a drainage, infusion or other device in spleen	
802	MCC condition	*See* appendix B.
803	CC condition	*See* appendix B.

DRG 804 (Continued)

DRG	PDx/SDx/Procedure	Tips
957	Other O.R. procedures for multiple significant trauma	PDx of trauma and at least two injuries (assigned as PDx or SDx) that are defined as significant trauma from different body site categories located under MS-DRG 963 and O.R. Procedure other than craniotomy or limb reattachment, hip and femur procedures.
	Non-diagnostic drainage of thoracic duct or cisterna chyli with or without drainage device	Review operative report for indications of therapeutic, nondiagnostic indications for drainage rather than diagnostic.
	AND	
	MCC condition	*See* appendix B.
958	Other O.R. procedures for multiple significant trauma	*See* DRG 957.
	Non-diagnostic drainage of thoracic duct or cisterna chyli with or without drainage device	*See* DRG 957.
	AND	
	CC condition	*See* appendix B.
959	Other O.R. procedures for multiple significant trauma	*See* DRG 957.
	Non-diagnostic drainage of thoracic duct or cisterna chyli with or without drainage device	*See* DRG 957.

DRG 808 Major Hematologic/Immunologic Diagnoses Except Sickle Cell Crisis and Coagulation with MCC — RW 2.1901

No Potential DRGs

DRG 809 Major Hematologic/Immunologic Diagnoses Except Sickle Cell Crisis and Coagulation with CC — RW 1.2044

Potential DRGs

808 Major Hematologic/Immunologic Diagnoses Except Sickle Cell Crisis and Coagulation with MCC 2.1901

DRG	PDx/SDx/Procedure	Tips
808	MCC condition	*See* appendix B.

DRG 810 Major Hematologic/Immunologic Diagnoses Except Sickle Cell Crisis and Coagulation without CC/MCC — RW 1.0045

Potential DRGs

808 Major Hematologic/Immunologic Diagnoses Except Sickle Cell Crisis and Coagulation with MCC 2.1901
809 Major Hematologic/Immunologic Diagnoses Except Sickle Cell Crisis and Coagulation with CC 1.2044

DRG	PDx/SDx/Procedure	Tips
808	MCC condition	*See* appendix B.
809	CC condition	*See* appendix B.

DRG 811 Red Blood Cell Disorders with MCC RW 1.4036

Potential DRGs

377	GI Hemorrhage with MCC	1.7903
808	Major Hematologic/Immunologic Diagnoses Except Sickle Cell Crisis and Coagulation with MCC	2.1901
813	Coagulation Disorders	1.5600

DRG	PDx/SDx/Procedure	Tips
377	Any G.I. ulcer with hemorrhage	Review the alphabetic index and tabular list for gastrointestinal conditions linked by the terms "with hemorrhage" or "with bleeding" as the classification presumes a causal relationship between two conditions linked by these terms (either under a main term or subterm). Unless the provider documents a different cause of the bleeding or states that the conditions are unrelated, assign the combination code for these conditions.
	Gastritis, duodenitis, and diverticulitis with hemorrhage	
	Hemorrhage of anus and rectum, hematemesis, melena, gastrointestinal hemorrhage unspecified	
	AND	
	MCC condition	*See* appendix B.
808	Constitutional aplastic anemia, other specified and unspecified aplastic anemias	
	Neutropenia	Neutropenia is defined as an abnormally low level of neutrophils, a phagocytic type of white blood cell (WBC). Neutropenia is distinctly different from neutropenic fever, a potentially serious clinical condition. In the case of neutropenic fever, sequence the neutropenia code first, followed by a code for the associated fever.
	Pancytopenia	Pancytopenia is an abnormally low level of all blood cell types, red blood cells (RBCs) (anemia), white blood cells (WBCs) (leukopenia or neutropenia), and platelets (thrombocytopenia). Generally, a code is not reported for each individual blood cell type when pancytopenia is documented; only the code for the pancytopenia would be assigned. However, there are clinical scenarios in which a code for the low-level blood cell type may need to be reported in addition to the code for pancytopenia. Review the documentation carefully and query the physician, when appropriate.
	AND	
	MCC condition	*See* appendix B.
813	Coagulation defects, purpura and other hemorrhagic condition	
	Spontaneous ecchymoses	

DRG 812 Red Blood Cell Disorders without MCC

RW 0.9007

Potential DRGs

377	GI Hemorrhage with MCC	1.7903
378	GI Hemorrhage with CC	0.9838
808	Major Hematologic/Immunologic Diagnoses Except Sickle Cell Crisis and Coagulation with MCC	2.1901
809	Major Hematologic/Immunologic Diagnoses Except Sickle Cell Crisis and Coagulation with CC	1.2044
810	Major Hematologic/Immunologic Diagnoses Except Sickle Cell Crisis and Coagulation without CC/MCC	1.0045
811	Red Blood Cell Disorders with MCC	1.4036
813	Coagulation Disorders	1.5600

DRG	PDx/SDx/Procedure	Tips
377	Any G.I. ulcer with hemorrhage	Review the alphabetic index and tabular list for gastrointestinal conditions linked by the terms "with hemorrhage" or "with bleeding" as the classification presumes a causal relationship between two conditions linked by these terms (either under a main term or subterm). Unless the provider documents a different cause of the bleeding or states that the conditions are unrelated, assign the combination code for these conditions.
	Gastritis, duodenitis, and diverticulitis with hemorrhage	
	Hemorrhage of anus and rectum, hematemesis, melena, gastrointestinal hemorrhage unspecified	
	AND	
	MCC condition	*See* appendix B.
378	Any G.I. ulcer with hemorrhage	*See* DRG 377.
	Gastritis, duodenitis, and diverticulitis with hemorrhage	
	Hemorrhage of anus and rectum, hematemesis, melena, gastrointestinal hemorrhage unspecified	
	AND	
	CC condition	*See* appendix B.
808	Constitutional aplastic anemia, other specified and unspecified aplastic anemias	
	Neutropenia	Neutropenia is defined as an abnormally low level of neutrophils, a phagocytic type of white blood cell (WBC). Neutropenia is distinctly different from neutropenic fever, a potentially serious clinical condition. In the case of neutropenic fever, sequence the neutropenia code first, followed by a code for the associated fever.
	Pancytopenia	Pancytopenia is an abnormally low level of all blood cell types, red blood cells (RBCs) (anemia), white blood cells (WBCs) (leukopenia or neutropenia), and platelets (thrombocytopenia). Generally, a code is not reported for each individual blood cell type when pancytopenia is documented; only the code for the pancytopenia would be assigned. However, there are clinical scenarios in which a code for the low-level blood cell type may need to be reported in addition to the code for pancytopenia. Review the documentation carefully and query the physician, when appropriate.
	AND	
	MCC condition	*See* appendix B.
809	Constitutional aplastic anemia, other specified and unspecified aplastic anemias	
	Neutropenia	*See* DRG 808.
	Pancytopenia	*See* DRG 808.
	AND	
	CC condition	*See* appendix B.
810	Constitutional aplastic anemia, other specified and unspecified aplastic anemias	
	Neutropenia	*See* DRG 808.
	Pancytopenia	*See* DRG 808.
811	MCC condition	*See* appendix B.
813	Coagulation defects, purpura and other hemorrhagic conditions	
	Spontaneous ecchymoses	

DRG 813 Coagulation Disorders RW 1.5600

Potential DRGs

545	Connective Tissue Disorders with MCC	2.4932
799	Splenic Procedures with MCC	4.9546
800	Splenic Procedures with CC	2.8177

DRG	PDx/SDx/Procedure	Tips
545	Thrombotic microangiopathy (unspecified, secondary to hematopoietic stem cell transplantation, other)	Key terms: thrombotic thrombocytopenic purpura (M31.19), thrombotic microangiopathy secondary to bone marrow or stem cell transplant (M31.11)
	AND	
	MCC condition	*See* appendix B.
799	Open biopsy of spleen	
	Excision/Destruction of lesion or tissue of spleen	
	Resection of spleen	
	Repair of spleen	
	Open drainage of spleen	
	Extirpation of spleen	
	Release of spleen	
	Open reposition of spleen	
	Removal or revision of a drainage, infusion or other device in spleen	
	AND	
	MCC condition	*See* appendix B.
800	Open biopsy of spleen	
	Excision/Destruction of lesion or tissue of spleen	
	Resection of spleen	
	Repair of spleen	
	Open drainage of spleen	
	Extirpation of spleen	
	Release of spleen	
	Open reposition of spleen	
	Removal or revision of a drainage, infusion or other device in spleen	
	AND	
	CC condition	*See* appendix B.

DRG 814 Reticuloendothelial and Immunity Disorders with MCC RW 2.1281

Potential DRGs

799	Splenic Procedures with MCC	4.9546
957	Other O.R. Procedures for Multiple Significant Trauma with MCC	7.2325
969	HIV with Extensive O.R. Procedure with MCC	6.8726
974	HIV with Major Related Condition with MCC	2.9165

DRG	PDx/SDx/Procedure	Tips
799	Open biopsy of spleen	
	Excision/Destruction of lesion or tissue of spleen	
	Resection of spleen	
	Repair of spleen	
	Open drainage of spleen	
	Extirpation of spleen	
	Release of spleen	
	Open reposition of spleen	
	Removal or revision of a drainage, infusion or other device in spleen	
	AND	
	MCC condition	*See* appendix B.
957	Other O.R. procedures for multiple significant trauma	PDx of trauma and at least two injuries (assigned as PDx or SDx) that are defined as significant trauma from different body site categories located under MS-DRG 963 and O.R. Procedure other than craniotomy or limb reattachment, hip and femur procedures.
	Nondiagnostic drainage of thoracic duct or cisterna chyli with or without drainage	Review operative report for indications of therapeutic, nondiagnostic indications for drainage rather than diagnostic.
	AND	
	MCC condition	*See* appendix B.
969	HIV infection	Report B2Ø for confirmed cases only; provider's clinical diagnostic statement is sufficient. Admission for HIV-related condition: sequence B2Ø first followed by the HIV-related condition code except Chapter 15 codes which take sequencing priority. Admission due to complication of HIV-related condition: sequence B2Ø first followed by the HIV-related condition and the associated manifestation (i.e. acute respiratory failure due to AIDS related pneumonia).
	AND	
	Extensive O.R. procedure	Any O.R. procedure not listed in DRGs 987-989.
	AND	
	MCC condition	*See* appendix B.
974	Principal diagnosis of HIV infection	*See* DRG 969.
	AND	
	Major HIV-related diagnosis	*See* appendix C. A diagnosis from this list should not be assumed as HIV-related unless specifically documented as such by the provider. Admission for HIV-related condition: sequence B20 first followed by the HIV-related condition code except for chapter 15 codes, which take sequencing priority. Admission due to complication of HIV-related condition: sequence B20 first followed by the HIV-related condition and the associated manifestation (e.g., acute respiratory failure due to AIDS-related pneumonia).
	AND	
	MCC condition	*See* appendix B.

DRG 815 Reticuloendothelial and Immunity Disorders with CC — RW 0.9942

Potential DRGs

799	Splenic Procedures with MCC	4.9546
800	Splenic Procedures with CC	2.8177
814	Reticuloendothelial and Immunity Disorders with MCC	2.1281
957	Other O.R. Procedures for Multiple Significant Trauma with MCC	7.2325
958	Other O.R. Procedures for Multiple Significant Trauma with CC	4.0448
969	HIV with Extensive O.R. Procedure with MCC	6.8726
970	HIV with Extensive O.R. Procedure without MCC	2.4044
974	HIV with Major Related Condition with MCC	2.9165
975	HIV with Major Related Condition with CC	1.3633

DRG	PDx/SDx/Procedure	Tips
799	Open biopsy of spleen	
	Excision/Destruction of lesion or tissue of spleen	
	Resection of spleen	
	Repair of spleen	
	Open drainage of spleen	
	Extirpation of spleen	
	Release of spleen	
	Open reposition of spleen	
	Removal or revision of a drainage, infusion or other device in spleen	
	AND	
	MCC condition	*See* appendix B.
800	Open biopsy of spleen	
	Excision/Destruction of lesion or tissue of spleen	
	Resection of spleen	
	Repair of spleen	
	Open drainage of spleen	
	Extirpation of spleen	
	Release of spleen	
	Open reposition of spleen	
	Removal or revision of a drainage, infusion or other device in spleen	
	AND	
	CC condition	*See* appendix B.
814	MCC condition	*See* appendix B.
957	Other O.R. procedures for multiple significant trauma	PDx of trauma and at least two injuries (assigned as PDx or SDx) that are defined as significant trauma from different body site categories located under MS-DRG 963 and O.R. Procedure other than craniotomy or limb reattachment, hip and femur procedures.
	Nondiagnostic drainage of thoracic duct or cisterna chyli with or without drainage	Review operative report for indications of therapeutic, nondiagnostic indications for drainage rather than diagnostic.
	AND	
	MCC condition	*See* appendix B.
958	Other O.R. procedures for multiple significant trauma	*See* DRG 957.
	Nondiagnostic drainage of thoracic duct or cisterna chyli with or without drainage	*See* DRG 957.
	AND	
	CC condition	*See* appendix B.
969	HIV infection	Report B20 for confirmed cases only; provider's clinical diagnostic statement is sufficient. Admission for HIV-related condition: sequence B2Ø first followed by the HIV-related condition code except Chapter 15 codes which take sequencing priority. Admission due to complication of HIV-related condition: sequence B2Ø first followed by the HIV-related condition and the associated manifestation (i.e. acute respiratory failure due to AIDS related pneumonia).
	AND	
	Extensive O.R. procedure	Any O.R. procedure not listed in DRGs 987-989.
	AND	
	MCC condition	*See* appendix B.
970	HIV infection	*See* DRG 969.
	AND	
	Extensive O.R. procedure	Any O.R. procedure not listed in DRGs 987-989.

Optimizing Tips

DRG 815 (Continued)

DRG	PDx/SDx/Procedure	Tips
974	Principal diagnosis of HIV infection	*See* DRG 969.
	AND	
	Major HIV-related diagnosis	*See* appendix C. A diagnosis from this list should not be assumed as HIV-related unless specifically documented as such by the provider. Admission for HIV-related condition: sequence B20 first followed by the HIV-related condition code except for chapter 15 codes, which take sequencing priority. Admission due to complication of HIV-related condition: sequence B20 first followed by the HIV-related condition and the associated manifestation (e.g., acute respiratory failure due to AIDS-related pneumonia).
	AND	
	MCC condition	*See* appendix B.
975	Principal diagnosis of HIV infection	*See* DRG 969.
	AND	
	Major HIV-related diagnosis	*See* DRG 974.
	AND	
	CC condition	*See* appendix B.

DRG 816 Reticuloendothelial and Immunity Disorders without CC/MCC RW 0.7102

Potential DRGs

799	Splenic Procedures with MCC	4.9546
800	Splenic Procedures with CC	2.8177
801	Splenic Procedures without CC/MCC	1.7897
814	Reticuloendothelial and Immunity Disorders with MCC	2.1281
815	Reticuloendothelial and Immunity Disorders with CC	0.9942
957	Other O.R. Procedures for Multiple Significant Trauma with MCC	7.2325
958	Other O.R. Procedures for Multiple Significant Trauma with CC	4.0448
959	Other O.R. Procedures for Multiple Significant Trauma without CC/MCC	2.5324
969	HIV with Extensive O.R. Procedure with MCC	6.8726
970	HIV with Extensive O.R. Procedure without MCC	2.4044
974	HIV with Major Related Condition with MCC	2.9165
975	HIV with Major Related Condition with CC	1.3633
976	HIV with Major Related Condition without CC/MCC	0.8453

DRG	PDx/SDx/Procedure	Tips
799	Open biopsy of spleen	
	Excision/Destruction of lesion or tissue of spleen	
	Resection of spleen	
	Repair of spleen	
	Open drainage of spleen	
	Extirpation of spleen	
	Release of spleen	
	Open reposition of spleen	
	Removal or revision of a drainage, infusion or other device in spleen	
	AND	
	MCC condition	*See* appendix B.
800	Open biopsy of spleen	
	Excision/Destruction of lesion or tissue of spleen	
	Resection of spleen	
	Repair of spleen	
	Open drainage of spleen	
	Extirpation of spleen	
	Release of spleen	
	Open reposition of spleen	
	Removal or revision of a drainage, infusion or other device in spleen	
	AND	
	CC condition	*See* appendix B.
801	Open biopsy of spleen	
	Excision/Destruction of lesion or tissue of spleen	
	Resection of spleen	
	Repair of spleen	
	Open drainage of spleen	
	Extirpation of spleen	
	Release of spleen	
	Open reposition of spleen	
	Removal or revision of a drainage, infusion or other device in spleen	

DRG 816 (Continued)

DRG	PDx/SDx/Procedure	Tips
814	MCC condition	*See* appendix B.
815	CC condition	*See* appendix B.
957	Other O.R. procedures for multiple significant trauma	PDx of trauma and at least two injuries (assigned as PDx or SDx) that are defined as significant trauma from different body site categories located under MS-DRG 963 and O.R. Procedure other than craniotomy or limb reattachment, hip and femur procedures.
	Nondiagnostic drainage of thoracic duct or cisterna chyli with or without drainage	Review operative report for indications of therapeutic, nondiagnostic indications for drainage rather than diagnostic.
	AND	
	MCC condition	*See* appendix B.
958	Other O.R. procedures for multiple significant trauma	*See* DRG 957.
	Nondiagnostic drainage of thoracic duct or cisterna chyli with or without drainage	*See* DRG 957.
	AND	
	CC condition	*See* appendix B.
959	Other O.R. procedures for multiple significant trauma	*See* DRG 957.
	Nondiagnostic drainage of thoracic duct or cisterna chyli with or without drainage	*See* DRG 957.
969	HIV infection	Report B2Ø for confirmed cases only; provider's clinical diagnostic statement is sufficient. Admission for HIV-related condition: sequence B2Ø first followed by the HIV-related condition code except for chapter 15 codes, which take sequencing priority. Admission due to complication of HIV-related condition: sequence B2Ø first followed by the HIV-related condition and the associated manifestation (e.g., acute respiratory failure due to AIDS-related pneumonia).
	AND	
	Extensive O.R. procedure	Any O.R. procedure not listed in DRGs 987-989.
	AND	
	MCC condition	*See* appendix B.
970	HIV infection	*See* DRG 969.
	AND	
	Extensive O.R. procedure	*See* DRG 969.
974	Principal diagnosis of HIV infection	*See* DRG 969.
	AND	
	Major HIV-related diagnosis	*See* appendix C. A diagnosis from this list should not be assumed as HIV-related unless specifically documented as such by the provider. Admission for HIV-related condition: sequence B2Ø first followed by the HIV-related condition code except for chapter 15 codes, which take sequencing priority. Admission due to complication of HIV-related condition: sequence B2Ø first followed by the HIV-related condition and the associated manifestation (e.g., acute respiratory failure due to AIDS-related pneumonia).
	AND	
	MCC condition	*See* appendix B.
975	Principal diagnosis of HIV infection	*See* DRG 969.
	AND	
	Major HIV-related diagnosis	*See* DRG 974.
	AND	
	CC condition	*See* appendix B.
976	Principal diagnosis of HIV infection	*See* DRG 969.
	AND	
	Major HIV-related diagnosis	*See* DRG 974.

Myeloproliferative Diseases And Disorders, Poorly Differentiated Neoplasms

DRG 820 Lymphoma and Leukemia with Major O.R. Procedure with MCC — RW 6.0467

No Potential DRGs

DRG 821 Lymphoma and Leukemia with Major O.R. Procedure with CC — RW 2.2321

Potential DRGs

820	Lymphoma and Leukemia with Major O.R. Procedure with MCC	6.0467

DRG	PDx/SDx/Procedure	Tips
820	MCC condition	*See* appendix B.

DRG 822 Lymphoma and Leukemia with Major O.R. Procedure without CC/MCC — RW 1.2388

Potential DRGs

820	Lymphoma and Leukemia with Major O.R. Procedure with MCC	6.0467
821	Lymphoma and Leukemia with Major O.R. Procedure with CC	2.2321

DRG	PDx/SDx/Procedure	Tips
820	MCC condition	*See* appendix B.
821	CC condition	*See* appendix B.

DRG 823 Lymphoma and Nonacute Leukemia with Other Procedure with MCC — RW 4.5019

Potential DRGs

018	Chimeric Antigen Receptor (CAR) T-cell and Other Immunotherapies	36.8427
820	Lymphoma and Leukemia with Major O.R. Procedure with MCC	6.0467

DRG	PDx/SDx/Procedure	Tips
018	Immunotherapy: CAR T-cell (autologous or allogeneic) Afamitresgene Axicabtagene ciloleucel Brexucabtagene autoleucel Ciltacabtagene Idecabtagene vicleucel Lifileucel Lisocabtagene maraleucel Tabelecleucel Tisagenlecleucel	These substances are used to treat specific types of cancers that have relapsed or are refractory to treatment. All the codes are located in the New Technology section of ICD-10-PCS.
820	Insertion, revision or removal of neurostimulator lead(s)	
	Mediastinoscopy	
	Regional and radical lymph node procedures (Non-diagnostic excision and resection of lymph nodes)	Lymph node excision implies that only a portion of the node or one node from a group or chain of nodes is removed. Lymph node resection implies that a particular group or chain of lymph nodes is completely removed. Review the description of the procedure for confirmation of removal of single node(s) from a group or chain, or if the intent was to remove the entire chain.
	Other insertion of suprapubic catheter (open)	Review the documentation for specific information regarding the procedure. Procedure must be OPEN surgical creation of an opening (cystostomy) into the bladder via incision (cystotomy) through the skin, muscle, fat and fascia, with a cystostomy tube or catheter left at the end of the procedure.
	AND	
	MCC condition	*See* appendix B.

DRG 824 Lymphoma and Nonacute Leukemia with Other Procedure with CC RW 2.2329

Potential DRGs

018	Chimeric Antigen Receptor (CAR) T-cell and Other Immunotherapies	36.8427
820	Lymphoma and Leukemia with Major O.R. Procedure with MCC	6.0467
823	Lymphoma and Nonacute Leukemia with Other Procedure with MCC	4.5019

DRG	PDx/SDx/Procedure	Tips
018	Immunotherapy: CAR T-cell (autologous or allogeneic) Afamitresgene Axicabtagene ciloleucel Brexucabtagene autoleucel Ciltacabtagene Idecabtagene vicleucel Lifileucel Lisocabtagene maraleucel Tabelecleucel Tisagenlecleucel	These substances are used to treat specific types of cancers that have relapsed or are refractory to treatment. All the codes are located in the New Technology section of ICD-10-PCS.
820	Insertion, revision or removal of neurostimulator lead(s)	
	Mediastinoscopy	
	Regional and radical lymph node procedures (Non-diagnostic excision and resection of lymph nodes)	Lymph node excision implies that only a portion of the node or one node from a group or chain of nodes is removed. Lymph node resection implies that a particular group or chain of lymph nodes is completely removed. Review the description of the procedure for confirmation of removal of single node(s) from a group or chain, or if the intent was to remove the entire chain.
	Other insertion of suprapubic catheter (open)	Review the documentation for specific information regarding the procedure. Procedure must be OPEN surgical creation of an opening (cystostomy) into the bladder via incision (cystotomy) through the skin, muscle, fat and fascia, with a cystostomy tube or catheter left at the end of the procedure.
	AND	
	MCC condition	*See* appendix B.
823	MCC condition	*See* appendix B.

DRG 825 Lymphoma and Nonacute Leukemia with Other Procedure without CC/MCC RW 1.2914

Potential DRGs

018	Chimeric Antigen Receptor (CAR) T-cell and Other Immunotherapies	36.8427
820	Lymphoma and Leukemia with Major O.R. Procedure with MCC	6.0467
821	Lymphoma and Leukemia with Major O.R. Procedure with CC	2.2321
823	Lymphoma and Nonacute Leukemia with Other Procedure with MCC	4.5019
824	Lymphoma and Nonacute Leukemia with Other Procedure with CC	2.2329

DRG	PDx/SDx/Procedure	Tips
018	Immunotherapy: CAR T-cell (autologous or allogeneic) Afamitresgene Axicabtagene ciloleucel Brexucabtagene autoleucel Ciltacabtagene Idecabtagene vicleucel Lifileucel Lisocabtagene maraleucel Tabelecleucel Tisagenlecleucel	These substances are used to treat specific types of cancers that have relapsed or are refractory to treatment. All the codes are located in the New Technology section of ICD-10-PCS.
820	Insertion, revision or removal of neurostimulator lead(s)	
	Mediastinoscopy	
	Regional and radical lymph node procedures (Non-diagnostic excision and resection of lymph nodes)	Lymph node excision implies that only a portion of the node or one node from a group or chain of nodes is removed. Lymph node resection implies that a particular group or chain of lymph nodes is completely removed. Review the description of the procedure for confirmation of removal of single node(s) from a group or chain, or if the intent was to remove the entire chain.
	Other insertion of suprapubic catheter (open)	Review the documentation for specific information regarding the procedure. Procedure must be OPEN surgical creation of an opening (cystostomy) into the bladder via incision (cystotomy) through the skin, muscle, fat and fascia, with a cystostomy tube or catheter left at the end of the procedure.
	AND	
	MCC condition	*See* appendix B.
821	Insertion, revision or removal of neurostimulator lead(s)	
	Mediastinoscopy	
	Regional and radical lymph node procedures (Non-diagnostic excision and resection of lymph nodes)	*See* DRG 820.
	Other insertion of suprapubic catheter (open)	*See* DRG 820.
	AND	
	CC condition	*See* appendix B.
823	MCC condition	*See* appendix B.
824	CC condition	*See* appendix B.

DRG 826 Myeloproliferative Disorders or Poorly Differentiated Neoplasms with Major O.R. Procedure with MCC — RW 4.3888

No Potential DRGs

DRG 827 Myeloproliferative Disorders or Poorly Differentiated Neoplasms with Major O.R. Procedure with CC — RW 2.3172

Potential DRGs

356 Other Digestive System O.R. Procedures with MCC 4.2787
826 Myeloproliferative Disorders or Poorly Differentiated Neoplasms with Major O.R. Procedure with MCC 4.3888

DRG	PDx/SDx/Procedure	Tips
356	PDx of disease/disorder of the digestive system	
	AND	
	Control of hemorrhage	
	Total splenectomy (resection of spleen)	
	Diagnostic drainage or biopsy (diagnostic excision) procedure on liver or pancreas	
	Exploratory laparotomy or laparoscopy (inspection only)	Review the documentation for specific information regarding the procedure. Examination/Inspection only without definitive procedure.
	AND	
	MCC condition	*See* appendix B.
826	MCC condition	*See* appendix B.

DRG 828 Myeloproliferative Disorders or Poorly Differentiated Neoplasms with Major O.R. Procedure without CC/MCC — RW 1.6404

Potential DRGs

356 Other Digestive System O.R. Procedures with MCC 4.2787
357 Other Digestive System O.R. Procedures with CC 2.1968
826 Myeloproliferative Disorders or Poorly Differentiated Neoplasms with Major O.R. Procedure with MCC 4.3888
827 Myeloproliferative Disorders or Poorly Differentiated Neoplasms with Major O.R. Procedure with CC 2.3172

DRG	PDx/SDx/Procedure	Tips
356	PDx of disease/disorder of the digestive system	
	AND	
	Total splenectomy (resection of spleen)	
	Diagnostic drainage or biopsy (diagnostic excision) procedure on liver or pancreas	
	Exploratory laparotomy or laparoscopy (inspection only)	Review the documentation for specific information regarding the procedure. Examination/Inspection only without definitive procedure.
	AND	
	MCC condition	*See* appendix B.
357	PDx of disease/disorder of the digestive system	
	AND	
	Total splenectomy (resection of spleen)	
	Diagnostic drainage or biopsy (diagnostic excision) procedure on liver or pancreas	
	Exploratory laparotomy or laparoscopy (inspection only)	*See* DRG 356.
	AND	
	CC condition	*See* appendix B.
826	MCC condition	*See* appendix B.
827	CC condition	*See* appendix B.

DRG 829 Myeloproliferative Disorders or Poorly Differentiated Neoplasms with Other Procedure with CC/MCC — RW 3.1538

Potential DRGs

826 Myeloproliferative Disorders or Poorly Differentiated Neoplasms with Major O.R. Procedure with MCC 4.3888

DRG	PDx/SDx/Procedure	Tips
826	Implant, replacement or removal of neurostimulator lead(s)	
	Mediastinoscopy	
	Regional and radical lymph node procedures (Non-diagnostic excision and resection of lymph nodes)	Lymph node excision implies that only a portion of the node or one node from a group or chain of nodes is removed. Lymph node resection implies that a particular group or chain of lymph nodes is completely removed. Review the description of the procedure for confirmation of removal of single node(s) from a group or chain, or if the intent was to remove the entire chain.
	Other insertion of suprapubic catheter (open)	Review the documentation for specific information regarding the procedure. Procedure must be OPEN surgical creation of an opening (cystostomy) into the bladder via incision (cystotomy) through the skin, muscle, fat and fascia, with a cystostomy tube or catheter left at the end of the procedure.
	AND	
	MCC condition	*See* appendix B.

DRG 830 Myeloproliferative Disorders or Poorly Differentiated Neoplasms with Other Procedure without CC/MCC — RW 1.5812

Potential DRGs

826	Myeloproliferative Disorders or Poorly Differentiated Neoplasms with Major O.R. Procedure with MCC	4.3888
827	Myeloproliferative Disorders or Poorly Differentiated Neoplasms with Major O.R. Procedure with CC	2.3172
828	Myeloproliferative Disorders or Poorly Differentiated Neoplasms with Major O.R. Procedure without CC/MCC	1.6404
829	Myeloproliferative Disorders or Poorly Differentiated Neoplasms with Other Procedure with CC/MCC	3.1538

DRG	PDx/SDx/Procedure	Tips
826	Implant, replacement or removal of neurostimulator lead(s)	
	Mediastinoscopy	
	Regional and radical lymph node procedures (Non-diagnostic excision and resection of lymph nodes)	Lymph node excision implies that only a portion of the node or one node from a group or chain of nodes is removed. Lymph node resection implies that a particular group or chain of lymph nodes is completely removed. Review the description of the procedure for confirmation of removal of single node(s) from a group or chain, or if the intent was to remove the entire chain.
	Other insertion of suprapubic catheter (open)	Review the documentation for specific information regarding the procedure. Procedure must be OPEN surgical creation of an opening (cystostomy) into the bladder via incision (cystotomy) through the skin, muscle, fat and fascia, with a cystostomy tube or catheter left at the end of the procedure.
	AND	
	MCC condition	*See* appendix B.
827	Implant, replacement or removal of neurostimulator lead(s)	
	Mediastinoscopy	
	Regional and radical lymph node procedures (Non-diagnostic excision and resection of lymph nodes)	*See* DRG 826.
	Other insertion of suprapubic catheter (open)	*See* DRG 826.
	AND	
	CC condition	*See* appendix B.
828	Implant, replacement or removal of neurostimulator lead(s)	
	Mediastinoscopy	
	Regional and radical lymph node procedures (Non-diagnostic excision and resection of lymph nodes)	*See* DRG 826.
	Other insertion of suprapubic catheter (open)	*See* DRG 826.
829	CC/MCC condition	*See* appendix B.

DRG 834 Acute Leukemia without Major O.R. Procedure with MCC — RW 5.5990

No Potential DRGs

DRG 835 Acute Leukemia without Major O.R. Procedure with CC — RW 2.2355

Potential DRGs

820	Lymphoma and Leukemia with Major O.R. Procedure with MCC	6.0467
834	Acute Leukemia without Major O.R. Procedure with MCC	5.5990
837	Chemotherapy with Acute Leukemia as Secondary Diagnosis or with High Dose Chemotherapy Agent with MCC	4.7566

DRG	PDx/SDx/Procedure	Tips
820	Insertion, revision or removal of neurostimulator lead(s)	
	Mediastinoscopy	
	Regional and radical lymph node procedures (Non-diagnostic excision and resection of lymph nodes)	Lymph node excision implies that only a portion of the node or one node from a group or chain of nodes is removed. Lymph node resection implies that a particular group or chain of lymph nodes is completely removed. Review the description of the procedure for confirmation of removal of single node(s) from a group or chain, or if the intent was to remove the entire chain.
	Other insertion of suprapubic catheter (open)	Review the documentation for specific information regarding the procedure. Procedure must be OPEN surgical creation of an opening (cystostomy) into the bladder via incision (cystotomy) through the skin, muscle, fat and fascia, with a cystostomy tube or catheter left at the end of the procedure.
	AND	
	MCC condition	*See* appendix B.
834	MCC condition	*See* appendix B.
837	Chemotherapy encounter with acute leukemia as secondary diagnosis	Key terms: acute lymphoblastic leukemia, acute promyelocytic leukemia, myeloblastic, myelogenous, myelomonocytic.
	OR	
	High-dose chemotherapy agent (Interleukin-2)	High dose Interleukin-2 is administered via intravenous (IV) injection, usually 600,000–720,000 units/kg. High-dose interleukin-2 is highly toxic and must be given in a hospital setting where the patient can be closely monitored. Key terms: Interleukin-2, IL-2, aldesleukin, Proleukin, cytokine, T-cell growth factor, TCGF.
	AND	
	MCC condition	*See* appendix B.

DRG 836 Acute Leukemia without Major O.R. Procedure without CC/MCC — RW 1.1973

Potential DRGs

820	Lymphoma and Leukemia with Major O.R. Procedure with MCC	6.0467
821	Lymphoma and Leukemia with Major O.R. Procedure with CC	2.2321
834	Acute Leukemia without Major O.R. Procedure with MCC	5.5990
835	Acute Leukemia without Major O.R. Procedure with CC	2.2355
837	Chemotherapy with Acute Leukemia as Secondary Diagnosis or with High Dose Chemotherapy Agent with MCC	4.7566
838	Chemotherapy with Acute Leukemia as Secondary Diagnosis with CC or High Dose Chemotherapy Agent	1.9524

DRG	PDx/SDx/Procedure	Tips
820	Insertion, revision or removal of neurostimulator lead(s)	
	Mediastinoscopy	
	Regional and radical lymph node procedures (Non-diagnostic excision and resection of lymph nodes)	Lymph node excision implies that only a portion of the node or one node from a group or chain of nodes is removed. Lymph node resection implies that a particular group or chain of lymph nodes is completely removed. Review the description of the procedure for confirmation of removal of single node(s) from a group or chain, or if the intent was to remove the entire chain.
	Other insertion of suprapubic catheter (open)	Review the documentation for specific information regarding the procedure. Procedure must be OPEN surgical creation of an opening (cystostomy) into the bladder via incision (cystotomy) through the skin, muscle, fat and fascia, with a cystostomy tube or catheter left at the end of the procedure.
	AND	
	MCC condition	*See* appendix B.
821	Insertion, revision or removal of neurostimulator lead(s)	
	Mediastinoscopy	
	Regional and radical lymph node procedures (Non-diagnostic excision and resection of lymph nodes)	*See* DRG 820.
	Other insertion of suprapubic catheter (open)	*See* DRG 820.
	AND	
	CC condition	*See* appendix B.
834	MCC condition	*See* appendix B.
835	CC condition	*See* appendix B.
837	Chemotherapy encounter with acute leukemia as secondary diagnosis	Key terms: acute lymphoblastic leukemia, acute promyelocytic leukemia, myeloblastic, myelogenous, myelomonocytic.
	OR	
	High-dose chemotherapy agent (Interleukin-2)	High dose Interleukin-2 is administered via intravenous (IV) injection, usually 600,000–720,000 units/kg. High-dose interleukin-2 is highly toxic and must be given in a hospital setting where the patient can be closely monitored. Key terms: Interleukin-2, IL-2, aldesleukin, Proleukin, cytokine, T-cell growth factor, TCGF.
	AND	
	MCC condition	*See* appendix B.
838	Chemotherapy encounter with acute leukemia as secondary diagnosis	*See* DRG 837.
	AND	
	CC condition	*See* appendix B.
	OR	
	High-dose chemotherapy agent (Interleukin-2)	*See* DRG 837.

DRG 837 Chemotherapy with Acute Leukemia as Secondary Diagnosis or with High Dose Chemotherapy Agent with MCC — RW 4.7566

No Potential DRGs

DRG 838 Chemotherapy with Acute Leukemia as Secondary Diagnosis with CC or High Dose Chemotherapy Agent — RW 1.9524

Potential DRGs

820	Lymphoma and Leukemia with Major O.R. Procedure with MCC	6.0467
837	Chemotherapy with Acute Leukemia as Secondary Diagnosis or with High Dose Chemotherapy Agent with MCC	4.7566

DRG	PDx/SDx/Procedure	Tips
820	Insertion, revision or removal of neurostimulator lead(s)	
	Mediastinoscopy	
	Regional and radical lymph node procedures (Non-diagnostic excision and resection of lymph nodes)	Lymph node excision implies that only a portion of the node or one node from a group or chain of nodes is removed. Lymph node resection implies that a particular group or chain of lymph nodes is completely removed. Review the description of the procedure for confirmation of removal of single node(s) from a group or chain, or if the intent was to remove the entire chain.
	Other insertion of suprapubic catheter (open)	Review the documentation for specific information regarding the procedure. Procedure must be OPEN surgical creation of an opening (cystostomy) into the bladder via incision (cystotomy) through the skin, muscle, fat and fascia, with a cystostomy tube or catheter left at the end of the procedure.
	AND	
	MCC condition	*See* appendix B.
837	MCC condition	*See* appendix B.

DRG 839 Chemotherapy with Acute Leukemia as Secondary Diagnosis without CC/MCC — RW 1.3031

Potential DRGs

820	Lymphoma and Leukemia with Major O.R. Procedure with MCC	6.0467
821	Lymphoma and Leukemia with Major O.R. Procedure with CC	2.2321
837	Chemotherapy with Acute Leukemia as Secondary Diagnosis or with High Dose Chemotherapy Agent with MCC	4.7566
838	Chemotherapy with Acute Leukemia as Secondary Diagnosis with CC or High Dose Chemotherapy Agent	1.9524
849	Radiotherapy	2.6914

DRG	PDx/SDx/Procedure	Tips
820	Insertion, revision or removal of neurostimulator lead(s)	
	Mediastinoscopy	
	Regional and radical lymph node procedures (Non-diagnostic excision and resection of lymph nodes)	Lymph node excision implies that only a portion of the node or one node from a group or chain of nodes is removed. Lymph node resection implies that a particular group or chain of lymph nodes is completely removed. Review the description of the procedure for confirmation of removal of single node(s) from a group or chain, or if the intent was to remove the entire chain.
	Other insertion of suprapubic catheter (open)	Review the documentation for specific information regarding the procedure. Procedure must be OPEN surgical creation of an opening (cystostomy) into the bladder via incision (cystotomy) through the skin, muscle, fat and fascia, with a cystostomy tube or catheter left at the end of the procedure.
	AND	
	MCC condition	*See* appendix B.
821	Insertion, revision or removal of neurostimulator lead(s)	
	Mediastinoscopy	
	Regional and radical lymph node procedures (Non-diagnostic excision and resection of lymph nodes)	*See* DRG 820.
	Other insertion of suprapubic catheter (open)	*See* DRG 820.
	AND	
	CC condition	*See* appendix B.
837	MCC condition	*See* appendix B.
838	CC condition	*See* appendix B.
	OR	
	High-dose chemotherapy agent (Interleukin-2)	High dose Interleukin-2 is administered via intravenous (IV) injection, usually 600,000 – 720,000 units/kg. High-dose interleukin-2 is highly toxic and must be given in a hospital setting where the patient can be closely monitored. Key terms: Interleukin-2, IL-2, aldesleukin, Proleukin, cytokine, T-cell growth factor, TCGF
849	Principal diagnosis encounter for radiotherapy concomitant with chemotherapy	Official coding guideline (I.C.2.e.) states that if an admission/encounter is chiefly for the administration of chemotherapy, immunotherapy or radiation therapy and the patient receives more than one of these therapies during the same admission, more than one code may be assigned, in any sequence.

DRG 840 Lymphoma and Nonacute Leukemia with MCC

RW 3.1252

Potential DRGs

018	Chimeric Antigen Receptor (CAR) T-cell and Other Immunotherapies	36.8427
820	Lymphoma and Leukemia with Major Procedure with MCC	6.0467
823	Lymphoma and Nonacute Leukemia with Other Procedure with MCC	4.5019
834	Acute Leukemia without Major O.R. Procedure with MCC	5.5990

DRG	PDx/SDx/Procedure	Tips
018	Immunotherapy: CAR T-cell (autologous or allogeneic) Afamitresgene Axicabtagene ciloleucel Brexucabtagene autoleucel Ciltacabtagene Idecabtagene vicleucel Lifileucel Lisocabtagene maraleucel Tabelecleucel Tisagenlecleucel	These substances are used to treat specific types of cancers that have relapsed or are refractory to treatment. All the codes are located in the New Technology section of ICD-10-PCS.
820	Insertion, revision or removal of neurostimulator lead(s)	
	Mediastinoscopy	
	Regional and radical lymph node procedures (Non-diagnostic excision and resection of lymph nodes)	Lymph node excision implies that only a portion of the node or one node from a group or chain of nodes is removed. Lymph node resection implies that a particular group or chain of lymph nodes is completely removed. Review the description of the procedure for confirmation of removal of single node(s) from a group or chain, or if the intent was to remove the entire chain.
	Other insertion of suprapubic catheter (open)	Review the documentation for specific information regarding the procedure. Procedure must be OPEN surgical creation of an opening (cystostomy) into the bladder via incision (cystotomy) through the skin, muscle, fat and fascia, with a cystostomy tube or catheter left at the end of the procedure.
	AND	
	MCC condition	*See* appendix B.
823	Stereotactic radiosurgery	Review interventional radiology reports. Stereotactic radiosurgery delivers numerous precisely focused beams of high doses of radiation to a tumor located using CT, MRI or angiogram, usually in the brain. A stereotactic head or face frame may be used to immobilize the head. Stereotactic radiosurgery is actually a special form of radiation therapy, rather than surgery. It does not require an incision or opening into the body. Key terms: Gamma Knife, Linear Accelerators (LINAC) with brand names such as Peacock®, X-Knife®, CyberKnife®, Clinac®, etc.
	OR	
	Any other O.R. procedure not listed under MS-DRG 820	
	AND	
	MCC condition	*See* appendix B.
834	Principal diagnosis acute leukemia	
	AND	
	MCC condition	*See* appendix B.

DRG 841 Lymphoma and Nonacute Leukemia with CC — RW 1.5735

Potential DRGs

018	Chimeric Antigen Receptor (CAR) T-cell and Other Immunotherapies	36.8427
820	Lymphoma and Leukemia with Major Procedure with MCC	6.0467
821	Lymphoma and Leukemia with Major Procedure with CC	2.2321
823	Lymphoma and Nonacute Leukemia with Other Procedure with MCC	4.5019
824	Lymphoma and Nonacute Leukemia with Other Procedure with CC	2.2329
834	Acute Leukemia without Major O.R. Procedure with MCC	5.5990
835	Acute Leukemia without Major O.R. Procedure with CC	2.2355
840	Lymphoma and Nonacute Leukemia with MCC	3.1252

DRG	PDx/SDx/Procedure	Tips
018	Immunotherapy: CAR T-cell (autologous or allogeneic) Afamitresgene Axicabtagene ciloleucel Brexucabtagene autoleucel Ciltacabtagene Idecabtagene vicleucel Lifileucel Lisocabtagene maraleucel Tabelecleucel Tisagenlecleucel	These substances are used to treat specific types of cancers that have relapsed or are refractory to treatment. All the codes are located in the New Technology section of ICD-10-PCS.
820	Insertion, revision or removal of neurostimulator lead(s)	
	Mediastinoscopy	
	Regional and radical lymph node procedures (Non-diagnostic excision and resection of lymph nodes)	Lymph node excision implies that only a portion of the node or one node from a group or chain of nodes is removed. Lymph node resection implies that a particular group or chain of lymph nodes is completely removed. Review the description of the procedure for confirmation of removal of single node(s) from a group or chain, or if the intent was to remove the entire chain.
	Other insertion of suprapubic catheter (open)	Review the documentation for specific information regarding the procedure. Procedure must be OPEN surgical creation of an opening (cystostomy) into the bladder via incision (cystotomy) through the skin, muscle, fat and fascia, with a cystostomy tube or catheter left at the end of the procedure.
	AND	
	MCC condition	*See* appendix B.
821	Insertion, revision or removal of neurostimulator lead(s)	
	Mediastinoscopy	
	Regional and radical lymph node procedures (Non-diagnostic excision and resection of lymph nodes)	*See* DRG 820.
	Other insertion of suprapubic catheter (open)	*See* DRG 820.
	AND	
	CC condition	*See* appendix B.
823	Stereotactic radiosurgery	Review interventional radiology reports. Stereotactic radiosurgery delivers numerous precisely focused beams of high doses of radiation to a tumor located using CT, MRI or angiogram, usually in the brain. A stereotactic head or face frame may be used to immobilize the head. Stereotactic radiosurgery is actually a special form of radiation therapy, rather than surgery. It does not require an incision or opening into the body. Key terms: Gamma Knife, Linear Accelerators (LINAC) with brand names such as Peacock®, X-Knife®, CyberKnife®, Clinac®, etc.
	OR	
	Any other O.R. procedure not listed under MS-DRG 820	
	AND	
	MCC condition	*See* appendix B.
824	Stereotactic radiosurgery	*See* DRG 823.
	OR	
	Any other O.R. procedure not listed under MS-DRG 820	
	AND	
	CC condition	*See* appendix B.
834	Principal diagnosis acute leukemia	
	AND	
	MCC condition	*See* appendix B.
835	Principal diagnosis acute leukemia	
	AND	
	CC condition	*See* appendix B.
840	MCC condition	*See* appendix B.

DRG 842 Lymphoma and Nonacute Leukemia without CC/MCC

RW 1.0664

Potential DRGs

018	Chimeric Antigen Receptor (CAR) T-cell and Other Immunotherapies	36.8427
820	Lymphoma and Leukemia with Major O.R. Procedure with MCC	6.0467
821	Lymphoma and Leukemia with Major O.R. Procedure with CC	2.2321
822	Lymphoma and Leukemia with Major O.R. Procedure without CC/MCC	1.2388
823	Lymphoma and Nonacute Leukemia with Other Procedure with MCC	4.5019
824	Lymphoma and Nonacute Leukemia with Other Procedure with CC	2.2329
825	Lymphoma and Nonacute Leukemia with Other Procedure without CC/MCC	1.2914
834	Acute Leukemia without Major O.R. Procedure with MCC	5.5990
835	Acute Leukemia without Major O.R. Procedure with CC	2.2355
836	Acute Leukemia without Major O.R. Procedure without CC/MCC	1.1973
840	Lymphoma and Nonacute Leukemia with MCC	3.1252
841	Lymphoma and Nonacute Leukemia with CC	1.5735

DRG	PDx/SDx/Procedure	Tips
018	Immunotherapy: CAR T-cell (autologous or allogeneic) Afamitresgene Axicabtagene ciloleucel Brexucabtagene autoleucel Ciltacabtagene Idecabtagene vicleucel Lifileucel Lisocabtagene maraleucel Tabelecleucel Tisagenlecleucel	These substances are used to treat specific types of cancers that have relapsed or are refractory to treatment. All the codes are located in the New Technology section of ICD-10-PCS.
820	Insertion, revision or removal of neurostimulator lead(s)	
	Mediastinoscopy	
	Regional and radical lymph node procedures (Non-diagnostic excision and resection of lymph nodes)	Lymph node excision implies that only a portion of the node or one node from a group or chain of nodes is removed. Lymph node resection implies that a particular group or chain of lymph nodes is completely removed. Review the description of the procedure for confirmation of removal of single node(s) from a group or chain, or if the intent was to remove the entire chain.
	Other insertion of suprapubic catheter (open)	Review the documentation for specific information regarding the procedure. Procedure must be OPEN surgical creation of an opening (cystostomy) into the bladder via incision (cystotomy) through the skin, muscle, fat and fascia, with a cystostomy tube or catheter left at the end of the procedure.
	AND	
	MCC condition	*See* appendix B.
821	Insertion, revision or removal of neurostimulator lead(s)	
	Mediastinoscopy	
	Regional and radical lymph node procedures (Non-diagnostic excision and resection of lymph nodes)	*See* DRG 820.
	Other insertion of suprapubic catheter (open)	*See* DRG 820.
	AND	
	CC condition	*See* appendix B.
822	Insertion, revision or removal of neurostimulator lead(s)	
	Mediastinoscopy	
	Regional and radical lymph node procedures (Non-diagnostic excision and resection of lymph nodes)	*See* DRG 820.
	Other insertion of suprapubic catheter (open)	*See* DRG 820.
823	Stereotactic radiosurgery	Review interventional radiology reports. Stereotactic radiosurgery delivers numerous precisely focused beams of high doses of radiation to a tumor located using CT, MRI or angiogram, usually in the brain. A stereotactic head or face frame may be used to immobilize the head. Stereotactic radiosurgery is actually a special form of radiation therapy, rather than surgery. It does not require an incision or opening into the body. Key terms: Gamma Knife, Linear Accelerators (LINAC) with brand names such as Peacock®, X-Knife®, CyberKnife®, Clinac®, etc.
	OR	
	Any other O.R. procedure not listed under MS-DRG 820	
	AND	
	MCC condition	*See* appendix B.
824	Stereotactic radiosurgery	*See* DRG 823.
	OR	
	Any other O.R. procedure not listed under MS-DRG 820	
	AND	
	CC condition	*See* appendix B.
825	Stereotactic radiosurgery	*See* DRG 823.
	OR	
	Any other O.R. procedure not listed under MS-DRG 820	
834	Principal diagnosis acute leukemia	
	AND	
	MCC condition	*See* appendix B.

DRG 842 (Continued)

DRG	PDx/SDx/Procedure	Tips
835	Principal diagnosis acute leukemia	
	AND	
	CC condition	*See* appendix B.
836	Principal diagnosis acute leukemia	
840	MCC condition	*See* appendix B.
841	CC condition	*See* appendix B.

DRG 843 Other Myeloproliferative Disorders or Poorly Differentiated Neoplasm Diagnoses with MCC RW 1.8606

Potential DRGs

826	Myeloproliferative Disorders or Poorly Differentiated Neoplasms with Major O.R. Procedure with MCC	4.3888
829	Myeloproliferative Disorders or Poorly Differentiated Neoplasms with Other Procedure with CC/MCC	3.1538

DRG	PDx/SDx/Procedure	Tips
826	Implant, replacement or removal of neurostimulator lead(s)	
	Mediastinoscopy	
	Regional and radical lymph node procedures (Non-diagnostic excision and resection of lymph nodes)	Lymph node excision implies that only a portion of the node or one node from a group or chain of nodes is removed. Lymph node resection implies that a particular group or chain of lymph nodes is completely removed. Review the description of the procedure for confirmation of removal of single node(s) from a group or chain, or if the intent was to remove the entire chain.
	Other insertion of suprapubic catheter (open)	Review the documentation for specific information regarding the procedure. Procedure must be OPEN surgical creation of an opening (cystostomy) into the bladder via incision (cystotomy) through the skin, muscle, fat and fascia, with a cystostomy tube or catheter left at the end of the procedure.
	AND	
	MCC condition	*See* appendix B.
829	Stereotactic radiosurgery	Review interventional radiology reports. Stereotactic radiosurgery delivers numerous precisely focused beams of high doses of radiation to a tumor located using CT, MRI or angiogram, usually in the brain. A stereotactic head or face frame may be used to immobilize the head. Stereotactic radiosurgery is actually a special form of radiation therapy, rather than surgery. It does not require an incision or opening into the body. Key terms: Gamma Knife, Linear Accelerators (LINAC) with brand names such as Peacock®, X-Knife®, CyberKnife®, Clinac®, etc.
	OR	
	Any other O.R. procedure not listed under MS-DRG 820	
	AND	
	CC/MCC condition	*See* appendix B.

DRG 844 Other Myeloproliferative Disorders or Poorly Differentiated Neoplasm Diagnoses with CC

RW 1.1572

Potential DRGs

826	Myeloproliferative Disorders or Poorly Differentiated Neoplasms with Major O.R. Procedure with MCC	4.3888
827	Myeloproliferative Disorders or Poorly Differentiated Neoplasms with Major O.R. Procedure with CC	2.3172
829	Myeloproliferative Disorders or Poorly Differentiated Neoplasms with Other Procedure with CC/MCC	3.1538
843	Other Myeloproliferative Disorders or Poorly Differentiated Neoplasm Diagnoses with MCC	1.8606

DRG	PDx/SDx/Procedure	Tips
826	Implant, replacement or removal of neurostimulator lead(s)	
	Mediastinoscopy	
	Regional and radical lymph node procedures (Non-diagnostic excision and resection of lymph nodes)	Lymph node excision implies that only a portion of the node or one node from a group or chain of nodes is removed. Lymph node resection implies that a particular group or chain of lymph nodes is completely removed. Review the description of the procedure for confirmation of removal of single node(s) from a group or chain, or if the intent was to remove the entire chain.
	Other insertion of suprapubic catheter (open)	Review the documentation for specific information regarding the procedure. Procedure must be OPEN surgical creation of an opening (cystostomy) into the bladder via incision (cystotomy) through the skin, muscle, fat and fascia, with a cystostomy tube or catheter left at the end of the procedure.
	AND	
	MCC condition	*See* appendix B.
827	Implant, replacement or removal of neurostimulator lead(s)	
	Mediastinoscopy	
	Regional and radical lymph node procedures (Non-diagnostic excision and resection of lymph nodes)	*See* DRG 826.
	Other insertion of suprapubic catheter (open)	*See* DRG 826.
	AND	
	CC condition	*See* appendix B.
829	Stereotactic radiosurgery	Review interventional radiology reports. Stereotactic radiosurgery delivers numerous precisely focused beams of high doses of radiation to a tumor located using CT, MRI or angiogram, usually in the brain. A stereotactic head or face frame may be used to immobilize the head. Stereotactic radiosurgery is actually a special form of radiation therapy, rather than surgery. It does not require an incision or opening into the body. Key terms: Gamma Knife, Linear Accelerators (LINAC) with brand names such as Peacock®, X-Knife®, CyberKnife®, Clinac®, etc.
	OR	
	Any other O.R. procedure not listed under MS-DRG 820	
	AND	
	CC/MCC condition	*See* appendix B.
843	MCC condition	*See* appendix B.

DRG 845 Other Myeloproliferative Disorders or Poorly Differentiated Neoplasm Diagnoses without CC/MCC — RW 0.8649

Potential DRGs

826	Myeloproliferative Disorders or Poorly Differentiated Neoplasms with Major O.R. Procedure with MCC	4.3888
827	Myeloproliferative Disorders or Poorly Differentiated Neoplasms with Major O.R. Procedure with CC	2.3172
828	Myeloproliferative Disorders or Poorly Differentiated Neoplasms with Major O.R. Procedure without CC/MCC	1.6404
829	Myeloproliferative Disorders or Poorly Differentiated Neoplasms with Other Procedure with CC/MCC	3.1538
830	Myeloproliferative Disorders or Poorly Differentiated Neoplasms with Other Procedure without CC/MCC	1.5812
843	Other Myeloproliferative Disorders or Poorly Differentiated Neoplasm Diagnoses with MCC	1.8606
844	Other Myeloproliferative Disorders or Poorly Differentiated Neoplasm Diagnoses with CC	1.1572

DRG	PDx/SDx/Procedure	Tips
826	Implant, replacement or removal of neurostimulator lead(s)	
	Mediastinoscopy	
	Regional and radical lymph node procedures (Non-diagnostic excision and resection of lymph nodes)	Lymph node excision implies that only a portion of the node or one node from a group or chain of nodes is removed. Lymph node resection implies that a particular group or chain of lymph nodes is completely removed. Review the description of the procedure for confirmation of removal of single node(s) from a group or chain, or if the intent was to remove the entire chain.
	Other insertion of suprapubic catheter (open)	Review the documentation for specific information regarding the procedure. Procedure must be OPEN surgical creation of an opening (cystostomy) into the bladder via incision (cystotomy) through the skin, muscle, fat and fascia, with a cystostomy tube or catheter left at the end of the procedure.
	AND	
	MCC condition	*See* appendix B.
827	Implant, replacement or removal of neurostimulator lead(s)	
	Mediastinoscopy	
	Regional and radical lymph node procedures (Non-diagnostic excision and resection of lymph nodes)	*See* DRG 826.
	Other insertion of suprapubic catheter (open)	*See* DRG 826.
	AND	
	CC condition	*See* appendix B.
828	Implant, replacement or removal of neurostimulator lead(s)	
	Mediastinoscopy	
	Regional and radical lymph node procedures (Non-diagnostic excision and resection of lymph nodes)	*See* DRG 826.
	Other insertion of suprapubic catheter (open)	*See* DRG 826.
829	Stereotactic radiosurgery	Review interventional radiology reports. Stereotactic radiosurgery delivers numerous precisely focused beams of high doses of radiation to a tumor located using CT, MRI or angiogram, usually in the brain. A stereotactic head or face frame may be used to immobilize the head. Stereotactic radiosurgery is actually a special form of radiation therapy, rather than surgery. It does not require an incision or opening into the body. Key terms: Gamma Knife, Linear Accelerators (LINAC) with brand names such as Peacock®, X-Knife®, CyberKnife®, Clinac®, etc.
	OR	
	Any other O.R. procedure not listed under MS-DRG 820	
	AND	
	CC/MCC condition	*See* appendix B.
830	Stereotactic radiosurgery	*See* DRG 829.
	OR	
	Any other O.R. procedure not listed under MS-DRG 820	
843	MCC condition	*See* appendix B.
844	CC condition	*See* appendix B.

DRG 846 Chemotherapy without Acute Leukemia as Secondary Diagnosis with MCC — RW 2.4440

Potential DRGs

837	Chemotherapy with Acute Leukemia as Secondary Diagnosis or with High Dose Chemotherapy Agent with MCC	4.7566

DRG	PDx/SDx/Procedure	Tips
837	Acute leukemia as secondary diagnosis	Key terms: acute lymphoblastic leukemia, acute promyelocytic leukemia, myeloblastic, myelogenous, myelomonocytic
	OR	
	High-dose chemotherapy agent (Interleukin-2)	High dose Interleukin-2 is administered via intravenous (IV) injection, usually 600,000 – 720,000 units/kg. High-dose interleukin-2 is highly toxic and must be given in a hospital setting where the patient can be closely monitored. Key terms: Interleukin-2, IL-2, aldesleukin, Proleukin, cytokine, T-cell growth factor, TCGF
	AND	
	MCC condition	*See* appendix B.

DRG 847 Chemotherapy without Acute Leukemia as Secondary Diagnosis with CC — RW 1.2126

Potential DRGs

837	Chemotherapy with Acute Leukemia as Secondary Diagnosis or with High Dose Chemotherapy Agent with MCC	4.7566
838	Chemotherapy with Acute Leukemia as Secondary Diagnosis with CC or High Dose Chemotherapy Agent	1.9524
846	Chemotherapy without Acute Leukemia as Secondary Diagnosis with MCC	2.4440
849	Radiotherapy	2.6914

DRG	PDx/SDx/Procedure	Tips
837	Acute leukemia as secondary diagnosis	Key terms: acute lymphoblastic leukemia, acute promyelocytic leukemia, myeloblastic, myelogenous, myelomonocytic
	OR	
	High-dose chemotherapy agent (Interleukin-2)	High dose Interleukin-2 is administered via intravenous (IV) injection, usually 600,000 – 720,000 units/kg. High-dose interleukin-2 is highly toxic and must be given in a hospital setting where the patient can be closely monitored. Key terms: Interleukin-2, IL-2, aldesleukin, Proleukin, cytokine, T-cell growth factor, TCGF
	AND	
	MCC condition	*See* appendix B.
838	Acute leukemia as secondary diagnosis	*See* DRG 837.
	AND	
	CC condition	*See* appendix B.
	OR	
	High-dose chemotherapy agent (Interleukin-2)	*See* DRG 837.
846	MCC condition	*See* appendix B.
849	Principal diagnosis encounter for radiotherapy concomitant with chemotherapy	Official coding guidelines (I.C.2.e.) state that if an admission/encounter is chiefly for the administration of chemotherapy, immunotherapy or radiation therapy and the patient receives more than one of these therapies during the same admission, more than one code may be assigned, in any sequence.

DRG 848 Chemotherapy without Acute Leukemia as Secondary Diagnosis without CC/MCC — RW 0.7595

Potential DRGs

837	Chemotherapy with Acute Leukemia as Secondary Diagnosis or with High Dose Chemotherapy Agent with MCC	4.7566
838	Chemotherapy with Acute Leukemia as Secondary Diagnosis with CC or High Dose Chemotherapy Agent	1.9524
839	Chemotherapy with Acute Leukemia as Secondary Diagnosis without CC/MCC	1.3031
846	Chemotherapy without Acute Leukemia as Secondary Diagnosis with MCC	2.4440
847	Chemotherapy without Acute Leukemia as Secondary Diagnosis with CC	1.2126
849	Radiotherapy	2.6914

DRG	PDx/SDx/Procedure	Tips
837	Acute leukemia as secondary diagnosis	Key terms: acute lymphoblastic leukemia, acute promyelocytic leukemia, myeloblastic, myelogenous, myelomonocytic
	OR	
	High-dose chemotherapy agent (Interleukin-2)	High dose Interleukin-2 is administered via intravenous (IV) injection, usually 600,000 – 720,000 units/kg. High-dose interleukin-2 is highly toxic and must be given in a hospital setting where the patient can be closely monitored. Key terms: Interleukin-2, IL-2, aldesleukin, Proleukin, cytokine, T-cell growth factor, TCGF
	AND	
	MCC condition	*See* appendix B.
838	Acute leukemia as secondary diagnosis	*See* DRG 837.
	AND	
	CC condition	*See* appendix B.
	OR	
	High-dose chemotherapy agent (Interleukin-2)	*See* DRG 837.
839	Acute leukemia as secondary diagnosis	Key terms: acute lymphoblastic leukemia, acute promyelocytic leukemia, myeloblastic, myelogenous, myelomonocytic
846	MCC condition	*See* appendix B.
847	CC condition	*See* appendix B.
849	Principal diagnosis encounter for radiotherapy concomitant with chemotherapy	Official coding guidelines (I.C.2.e.) states that if an admission/encounter is chiefly for the administration of chemotherapy, immunotherapy or radiation therapy and the patient receives more than one of these therapies during the same admission, more than one code may be assigned, in any sequence.

DRG 849 Radiotherapy RW 2.6914

Potential DRGs

837 Chemotherapy with Acute Leukemia as Secondary Diagnosis or with High Dose Chemotherapy Agent with MCC 4.7566

DRG	PDx/SDx/Procedure	Tips
837	Acute leukemia as secondary diagnosis	Key terms: acute lymphoblastic leukemia, acute promyelocytic leukemia, myeloblastic, myelogenous, myelomonocytic
	OR	
	High-dose chemotherapy agent (Interleukin-2)	High dose Interleukin-2 is administered via intravenous (IV) injection, usually 600,000 – 720,000 units/kg. High-dose interleukin-2 is highly toxic and must be given in a hospital setting where the patient can be closely monitored. Key terms: Interleukin-2, IL-2, aldesleukin, Proleukin, cytokine, T-cell growth factor, TCGF
	AND	
	MCC condition	*See* appendix B.

Infectious And Parasitic Diseases, Systemic or Unspecified Sites

DRG 853 Infectious and Parasitic Diseases with O.R. Procedure with MCC — RW 4.9993

No Potential DRGs

DRG 854 Infectious and Parasitic Diseases with O.R. Procedure with CC — RW 2.0382

Potential DRGs

853	Infectious and Parasitic Diseases with O.R. Procedure with MCC	4.9993

DRG	PDx/SDx/Procedure	Tips
853	MCC condition	Excludes: AIDS (B2Ø).
		Sequencing: See the ICD-10-CM Tabular index for guidance related to categories B9Ø-B97.
		Chronic current infections: report as active infections.
		See appendix B.

DRG 855 Infectious and Parasitic Diseases with O.R. Procedure without CC/MCC — RW 1.7018

Potential DRGs

853	Infectious and Parasitic Diseases with O.R. Procedure with MCC	4.9993
854	Infectious and Parasitic Diseases with O.R. Procedure with CC	2.0382

DRG	PDx/SDx/Procedure	Tips
853	MCC condition	Excludes: AIDS (B2Ø).
		Sequencing: See the ICD-1Ø-CM Tabular index for guidance related to categories B9Ø-B97.
		Chronic current infections: report as active infections.
		See appendix B.
854	CC condition	*See* DRG 853.

DRG 856 Postoperative or Posttraumatic Infections with O.R. Procedure with MCC — RW 4.4284

Potential DRGs

853	Infectious and Parasitic Diseases with O.R. Procedure with MCC	4.9993

DRG	PDx/SDx/Procedure	Tips
853	PDx of infection not related to a procedure	If there is no provider documentation of a relationship between the infection and the procedure, the complication code should not be assigned (Official coding guideline I.C.1.d.5.a).
	AND	
	MCC condition	*See* appendix B.

DRG 857 Postoperative or Posttraumatic Infections with O.R. Procedure with CC — RW 2.1357

Potential DRGs

853	Infectious and Parasitic Diseases with O.R. Procedure with MCC	4.9993
856	Postoperative or Posttraumatic Infections with O.R. Procedure with MCC	4.4284

DRG	PDx/SDx/Procedure	Tips
853	PDx of infection not related to a procedure	If there is no provider documentation of a relationship between the infection and the procedure, the complication code should not be assigned (Official coding guideline I.C.1.d.5.a).
	AND	
	MCC condition	*See* appendix B.
856	MCC condition	*See* appendix B.

DRG 858 Postoperative or Posttraumatic Infections with O.R. Procedure without CC/MCC — RW 1.2834

Potential DRGs

853	Infectious and Parasitic Diseases with O.R. Procedure with MCC	4.9993
854	Infectious and Parasitic Diseases with O.R. Procedure with CC	2.0382
855	Infectious and Parasitic Diseases with O.R. Procedure without CC/MCC	1.7018
856	Postoperative or Posttraumatic Infections with O.R. Procedure with MCC	4.4284
857	Postoperative or Posttraumatic Infections with O.R. Procedure with CC	2.1357

DRG	PDx/SDx/Procedure	Tips
853	PDx of infection not related to a procedure	If there is no provider documentation of a relationship between the infection and the procedure, the complication code should not be assigned (Official coding guideline I.C.1.d.5.a).
	AND	
	MCC condition	*See* appendix B.
854	PDx of infection not related to a procedure	*See* DRG 853.
	AND	
	CC condition	*See* appendix B.
855	PDx of infection not related to a procedure	*See* DRG 853.
856	MCC condition	*See* appendix B.
857	CC condition	*See* appendix B.

DRG 862 Postoperative and Posttraumatic Infections with MCC — RW 1.8420

Potential DRGs

314	Other Circulatory System Diagnoses with MCC	2.0935
853	Infectious and Parasitic Diseases with O.R. Procedure with MCC	4.9993
856	Postoperative or Posttraumatic Infections with O.R. Procedure with MCC	4.4284

DRG	PDx/SDx/Procedure	Tips
314	Infection: due to CVC, PICC, cardiac valve prosthesis, other cardiac and vascular devices, implants and grafts, heart transplant infection, heart/lung transplant infections	Key Terms: line bacteremia, Hickman cath infection, portacath cellulitis, pacer pocket abscess, lead infection, pulse generator infection, CMV due to cardiac transplant. Severe sepsis: report an additional code from subcategory R65.2; report an additional code to specify the acute organ dysfunction. Identify specific infection: report an additional code for the specific infection, organism or manifestation if not identified within principal diagnosis code.
	AND	
	MCC condition	*See* appendix B.
853	PDx of infection not related to a procedure	If there is no provider documentation of a relationship between the infection and the procedure, the complication code should not be assigned (Official coding guideline I.C.1.d.5.a).
	AND	
	Any operating room procedure	
	AND	
	MCC condition	*See* appendix B.
856	Any operating room procedure	
	AND	
	MCC condition	*See* appendix B.

DRG 863 Postoperative and Posttraumatic Infections without MCC — RW 1.0055

Potential DRGs

314	Other Circulatory System Diagnoses with MCC	2.0935
853	Infectious and Parasitic Diseases with O.R. Procedure with MCC	4.9993
854	Infectious and Parasitic Diseases with O.R. Procedure with CC	2.0382
855	Infectious and Parasitic Diseases with O.R. Procedure without CC/MCC	1.7018
856	Postoperative or Posttraumatic Infections with O.R. Procedure with MCC	4.4284
857	Postoperative or Posttraumatic Infections with O.R. Procedure with CC	2.1357
858	Postoperative or Posttraumatic Infections with O.R. Procedure without CC/MCC	1.2834
862	Postoperative and Posttraumatic Infections with MCC	1.8420

DRG	PDx/SDx/Procedure	Tips
314	Infection: due to CVC, PICC, cardiac valve prosthesis, other cardiac and vascular devices, implants and grafts, heart transplant infection, heart/lung transplant infections	Key Terms: line bacteremia, Hickman cath infection, portacath cellulitis, pacer pocket abscess, lead infection, pulse generator infection, CMV due to cardiac transplant. Severe sepsis: report an additional code from subcategory R65.2; report an additional code to specify the acute organ dysfunction. Identify specific infection: report an additional code for the specific infection, organism or manifestation if not identified within principal diagnosis code.
	AND	
	MCC condition	*See* appendix B.
853	PDx of infection not related to a procedure	If there is no provider documentation of a relationship between the infection and the procedure, the complication code should not be assigned (Official coding guideline I.C.1.d.5.a).
	AND	
	Any operating room procedure	
	AND	
	MCC condition	*See* appendix B.
854	PDx of infection not related to a procedure	*See* DRG 853.
	AND	
	Any operating room procedure	
	AND	
	CC condition	*See* appendix B.
855	PDx of infection not related to a procedure	*See* DRG 853.
	AND	
	Any operating room procedure	
856	Any operating room procedure	
	AND	
	MCC condition	*See* appendix B.
857	Any operating room procedure	
	AND	
	CC condition	*See* appendix B.
858	Any operating room procedure	
862	MCC condition	*See* appendix B.

DRG 864 Fever and Inflammatory Conditions

RW 0.8828

Potential DRGs

808	Major Hematological and Immunological Diagnoses Except Sickle Cell Crisis and Coagulation Disorders with MCC	2.1901
809	Major Hematological and Immunological Diagnoses Except Sickle Cell Crisis and Coagulation Disorders with CC	1.2044
810	Major Hematological and Immunological Diagnoses Except Sickle Cell Crisis and Coagulation Disorders without CC/MCC	1.0045
865	Viral Illness with MCC	1.6399
867	Other Infectious and Parasitic Diseases Diagnoses with MCC	2.0923
868	Other Infectious and Parasitic Diseases Diagnoses with CC	1.0855

DRG	PDx/SDx/Procedure	Tips
808	Febrile neutropenia or pancytopenia	The neutropenia or pancytopenia code should be sequenced as the principal diagnosis, followed by the code for the fever.
	AND	
	MCC condition	*See* appendix B.
809	Febrile neutropenia or pancytopenia	*See* DRG 8Ø8.
	AND	
	CC condition	*See* appendix B.
810	Febrile neutropenia or pancytopenia	*See* DRG 8Ø8.
865	Viral illness with or without complications (varicella, zoster, measles, mumps, infectious mononucleosis, flu virus, other complications following immunization)	Excludes: AIDS (B2Ø). Sequencing: See the ICD-10-CM Tabular index for guidance related to category B97. Chronic current infections: report as active infections.
	AND	
	MCC condition	*See* appendix B.
867	Other infectious and parasitic diseases (botulism food poisoning, trichomoniasis, toxoplasmosis, Lyme disease, infection following insemination, infusion, transfusion, injection, immunization)	Selection of Principal Diagnosis: review coding conventions, tabular and alphabetic indexes and the official coding guidelines. Sequencing: See the ICD-10-CM Tabular index for guidance related to categories B9Ø-B97. Chronic current infections: report as active infections. Category Z16: Report as an additional code when documented.
	AND	
	MCC condition	*See* appendix B.
868	Other infectious and parasitic diseases (botulism food poisoning, trichomoniasis, toxoplasmosis, Lyme disease, infection following insemination, infusion, transfusion, injection, immunization)	*See* DRG 867.
	AND	
	CC condition	*See* appendix B.

DRG 865 Viral Illness with MCC

RW 1.6399

Potential DRGs

177	Respiratory Infections and Inflammations with MCC	1.6964
853	Infectious and Parasitic Diseases with O.R. Procedure with MCC	4.9993
974	HIV with Major Related Condition with MCC	2.9165

DRG	PDx/SDx/Procedure	Tips
177	COVID-19 as principal diagnosis	According to the ICD-10-CM guidelines, documentation by the provider that the individual has COVID-19 is sufficient and does not require additional documentation of a positive test result.
	AND	
	MCC condition	*See* appendix B.
853	Any operating room procedure	
	AND	
	MCC condition	*See* appendix B.
974	Diagnosis of HIV	
	AND	
	HIV-related viral illness	Patients with asymptomatic HIV presenting with a viral illness that is considered a major HIV-related condition, such as viral pneumonia, cytomegalovirus, or herpes. *See* appendix C for the full list of major HIV-related conditions. A diagnosis from this list should not be assumed as HIV-related unless specifically documented as such by the provider.
	AND	
	MCC condition	*See* appendix B.

DRG 866 Viral Illness without MCC RW 0.9177

Potential DRGs

177	Respiratory Infections and Inflammations with MCC	1.6964
178	Respiratory Infections and Inflammations with CC	0.9867
193	Simple Pneumonia and Pleurisy with MCC	1.3266
853	Infectious and Parasitic Diseases with O.R. Procedure with MCC	4.9993
854	Infectious and Parasitic Diseases with O.R. Procedure with CC	2.0382
855	Infectious and Parasitic Diseases with O.R. Procedure without CC/MCC	1.7018
865	Viral Illness with MCC	1.6399
974	HIV with Major Related Condition with MCC	2.9165
975	HIV with Major Related Condition with CC	1.3633

DRG	PDx/SDx/Procedure	Tips
177	COVID-19 as principal diagnosis	According to the ICD-10-CM guidelines, documentation by the provider that the individual has COVID-19 is sufficient and does not require additional documentation of a positive test result.
	AND	
	MCC condition	*See* appendix B.
178	COVID-19 as principal diagnosis	*See* DRG 177.
	AND	
	CC condition	*See* appendix B.
193	Simple pneumonia or pleurisy (Flu with pneumonia or other respiratory manifestation, viral pneumonia, bacterial pneumonia, pleurisy)	Key terms: Avian influenza, Influenza A/H5N1, Swine influenza, bronchopneumonia, lobar pneumonia. Categories J09/J10: report only confirmed cases which may be based on provider diagnostic statement. Possible/suspected/probable avian, other novel influenza A or other identified influenza virus is reported from category J11. Categories J13, J14, J15 which specify an organism must be confirmed by clinical validation.
	AND	
	MCC condition	*See* appendix B.
853	Any operating room procedure	
	AND	
	MCC condition	*See* appendix B.
854	Any operating room procedure	
	AND	
	CC condition	*See* appendix B.
855	Any operating room procedure	
865	MCC condition	*See* appendix B.
974	Diagnosis of HIV	
	AND	
	HIV-related viral illness	Patients with asymptomatic HIV presenting with a viral illness that is considered a major HIV-related condition, such as viral pneumonia, cytomegalovirus, or herpes. *See* appendix C for the full list of major HIV-related conditions. A diagnosis from this list should not be assumed as HIV-related unless specifically documented as such by the provider.
	AND	
	MCC condition	*See* appendix B.
975	Diagnosis of HIV	
	AND	
	HIV-related viral illness	*See* DRG 974.
	AND	
	CC condition	*See* appendix B.

DRG 867 Other Infectious and Parasitic Diseases Diagnoses with MCC RW 2.0923

Potential DRGs

853	Infectious and Parasitic Diseases with O.R. Procedure with MCC	4.9993

DRG	PDx/SDx/Procedure	Tips
853	Any operating room procedure	
	AND	
	MCC condition	*See* appendix B.

DRG 868 Other Infectious and Parasitic Diseases Diagnoses with CC — RW 1.0855

Potential DRGs

853	Infectious and Parasitic Diseases with O.R. Procedure with MCC	4.9993
854	Infectious and Parasitic Diseases with O.R. Procedure with CC	2.0382
867	Other Infectious and Parasitic Diseases Diagnoses with MCC	2.0923

DRG	PDx/SDx/Procedure	Tips
853	Any operating room procedure	
	AND	
	MCC condition	*See* appendix B.
854	Any operating room procedure	
	AND	
	CC condition	*See* appendix B.
867	MCC condition	*See* appendix B.

DRG 869 Other Infectious and Parasitic Diseases Diagnoses without CC/MCC — RW 0.6907

Potential DRGs

853	Infectious and Parasitic Diseases with O.R. Procedure with MCC	4.9993
854	Infectious and Parasitic Diseases with O.R. Procedure with CC	2.0382
855	Infectious and Parasitic Diseases with O.R. Procedure without CC/MCC	1.7018
867	Other Infectious and Parasitic Diseases Diagnoses with MCC	2.0923
868	Other Infectious and Parasitic Diseases Diagnoses with CC	1.0855

DRG	PDx/SDx/Procedure	Tips
853	Any operating room procedure	
	AND	
	MCC condition	*See* appendix B.
854	Any operating room procedure	
	AND	
	CC condition	*See* appendix B.
855	Any operating room procedure	
867	MCC condition	*See* appendix B.
868	CC condition	*See* appendix B.

DRG 870 Septicemia or Severe Sepsis with Mechanical Ventilation > 96 Hours — RW 6.9649

Potential DRGs

003	ECMO or Tracheostomy with Mechanical Ventilation >96 Hours or Principal Diagnosis Except Face, Mouth and Neck with Major O.R. procedures	21.3203
004	Tracheostomy with Mechanical Ventilation >96 Hours or Principal Diagnosis Except Face, Mouth and Neck without Major O.R. procedures	14.7000

DRG	PDx/SDx/Procedure	Tips
003	Extracorporeal membrane oxygenation (ECMO), central or peripheral	Central ECMO provides cardiorespiratory support and involves direct surgical cannulation of the right atrium and aorta via sternotomy. Peripheral (percutaneous) ECMO is a less invasive procedure than central ECMO. Veno-arterial (VA) peripheral ECMO cannulas are inserted percutaneously into both the femoral artery and the femoral vein. This type of ECMO provides both respiratory and circulatory support. Veno-venous (VV) peripheral ECMO requires two venous insertions, one in the upper veins and one in the lower veins, and provides respiratory support only.
	OR	
	Tracheostomy	Tracheostomy carried out elsewhere before admission or in an ambulance before arrival should not be reported as a current procedure. A tracheostomy procedure may be performed at the bedside and documented in the progress notes or in the operating room and documented in an operative report.
	WITH	
	Mechanical ventilation > 96 hours	Review record documentation for start and stop times. Calculation of mechanical ventilation hours begins when vent is initiated (or time of admission if patient already on a vent) and ends when it is turned off (or the time patient is discharged if still ventilated). The duration includes time spent to wean the patient from the vent. Do not assume that ventilation that spans four calendar days equals > 96 hours; count by the hour not day.
004	Tracheostomy	*See* DRG 003.
	WITH	
	Mechanical ventilation > 96 hours	*See* DRG 003.

DRG 871 Septicemia or Severe Sepsis without Mechanical Ventilation > 96 Hours with MCC RW 1.9826

Potential DRGs

003	ECMO or Tracheostomy with Mechanical Ventilation >96 Hours or Principal Diagnosis Except Face, Mouth and Neck with Major O.R. procedures	21.3203
004	Tracheostomy with Mechanical Ventilation >96 Hours or Principal Diagnosis Except Face, Mouth and Neck without Major O.R. procedure	14.7000
314	Other Circulatory System Diagnoses with MCC	2.0935
853	Infectious and Parasitic Diseases with O.R. Procedure with MCC	4.9993
856	Postoperative or Posttraumatic Infections with O.R. Procedure with MCC	4.4284
870	Septicemia or Severe Sepsis with Mechanical Ventilation > 96 Hours	6.9649

DRG	PDx/SDx/Procedure	Tips
003	Extracorporeal membrane oxygenation (ECMO), central or peripheral	Central ECMO provides cardiorespiratory support and involves direct surgical cannulation of the right atrium and aorta via sternotomy. Peripheral (percutaneous) ECMO is a less invasive procedure than central ECMO. Veno-arterial (VA) peripheral ECMO cannulas are inserted percutaneously into both the femoral artery and the femoral vein. This type of ECMO provides both respiratory and circulatory support. Veno-venous (VV) peripheral ECMO requires two venous insertions, one in the upper veins and one in the lower veins, and provides respiratory support only.
	OR	
	Tracheostomy	Tracheostomy carried out elsewhere before admission or in an ambulance before arrival should not be reported as a current procedure. A tracheostomy procedure may be performed at the bedside and documented in the progress notes or in the operating room and documented in an operative report.
	WITH	
	Mechanical ventilation > 96 hours	Review record documentation for start and stop times. Calculation of mechanical ventilation hours begins when vent is initiated (or time of admission if patient already on a vent) and ends when it is turned off (or the time patient is discharged if still ventilated). The duration includes time spent to wean the patient from the vent. Do not assume that ventilation that spans four calendar days equals > 96 hours; count by the hour not day.
004	Tracheostomy	*See* DRG 003.
	WITH	
	Mechanical ventilation > 96 hours	*See* DRG 003.
314	Infection: due to CVC, PICC, cardiac valve prosthesis, other cardiac and vascular devices, implants, and grafts, heart transplant infection, heart/lung transplant infections	Key Terms: line bacteremia, Hickman cath infection, portacath cellulitis, pacer pocket abscess, lead infection, pulse generator infection, CMV due to cardiac transplant. Severe sepsis: report an additional code from subcategory R65.2; report an additional code to specify the acute organ dysfunction. Identify specific infection: report an additional code for the specific infection, organism, or manifestation if not identified within principal diagnosis code.
	AND	
	MCC condition	*See* appendix B.
853	Any operating room procedure	
	AND	
	MCC condition	*See* appendix B.
856	PDx of postprocedural sepsis or infection	Excludes sepsis or infections due to devices listed in DRG 314 Documentation should provide a clear relationship between the procedure and the sepsis/infection (Official coding guideline I.C.1.d.5.a).
	AND	
	Any operating room procedure	
	AND	
	MCC condition	*See* appendix B.
870	Mechanical Ventilation > 96 hours	*See* DRG 003.

DRG 872 Septicemia or Severe Sepsis without Mechanical Ventilation > 96 Hours without MCC

RW 1.0299

Potential DRGs

003	ECMO or Tracheostomy with Mechanical Ventilation >96 Hours or Principal Diagnosis Except Face, Mouth and Neck with Major O.R. procedures	21.3203
004	Tracheostomy with Mechanical Ventilation >96 Hours or Principal Diagnosis Except Face, Mouth and Neck without Major O.R. procedures	14.7000
314	Other Circulatory System Diagnoses with MCC	2.0935
853	Infectious and Parasitic Diseases with O.R. Procedure with MCC	4.9993
854	Infectious and Parasitic Diseases with O.R. Procedure with CC	2.0382
855	Infectious and Parasitic Diseases with O.R. Procedure without CC/MCC	1.7018
856	Postoperative or Posttraumatic Infections with O.R. Procedure with MCC	4.4284
857	Postoperative or Posttraumatic Infections with O.R. Procedure with CC	2.1357
858	Postoperative or Posttraumatic Infections with O.R. Procedure without CC/MCC	1.2834
862	Postoperative and Posttraumatic Infections with MCC	1.8420
870	Septicemia or Severe Sepsis with Mechanical Ventilation > 96 Hours	6.9649
871	Septicemia or Severe Sepsis without Mechanical Ventilation > 96 Hours with MCC	1.9826

DRG	PDx/SDx/Procedure	Tips
003	Extracorporeal membrane oxygenation (ECMO), central or peripheral	Central ECMO provides cardiorespiratory support and involves direct surgical cannulation of the right atrium and aorta via sternotomy. Peripheral (percutaneous) ECMO is a less invasive procedure than central ECMO. Veno-arterial (VA) peripheral ECMO cannulas are inserted percutaneously into both the femoral artery and the femoral vein. This type of ECMO provides both respiratory and circulatory support. Veno-venous (VV) peripheral ECMO requires two venous insertions, one in the upper veins and one in the lower veins, and provides respiratory support only.
	OR	
	Tracheostomy	Tracheostomy carried out elsewhere before admission or in an ambulance before arrival should not be reported as a current procedure. A tracheostomy procedure may be performed at the bedside and documented in the progress notes or in the operating room and documented in an operative report.
	WITH	
	Mechanical ventilation > 96 hours	Review record documentation for start and stop times. Calculation of mechanical ventilation hours begins when vent is initiated (or time of admission if patient already on a vent) and ends when it is turned off (or the time patient is discharged if still ventilated). The duration includes time spent to wean the patient from the vent. Do not assume that ventilation that spans four calendar days equals > 96 hours; count by the hour not day.
004	Tracheostomy	*See* DRG 003.
	WITH	
	Mechanical ventilation > 96 hours	*See* DRG 003.
314	Infection: due to CVC, PICC, cardiac valve prosthesis, other cardiac and vascular devices, implants and grafts, heart transplant infection, heart/lung transplant infections	Key Terms: line bacteremia, Hickman cath infection, portacath cellulitis, pacer pocket abscess, lead infection, pulse generator infection, CMV due to cardiac transplant. Severe sepsis: report an additional code from subcategory R65.2; report an additional code to specify the acute organ dysfunction. Identify specific infection: report an additional code for the specific infection, organism or manifestation if not identified within principal diagnosis code.
	AND	
	MCC condition	*See* appendix B.
853	Any operating room procedure	
	AND	
	MCC condition	*See* appendix B.
854	Any operating room procedure	
	AND	
	CC condition	*See* appendix B.
855	Any operating room procedure	
856	PDx of postprocedural sepsis or infection	Excludes sepsis or infections due to devices listed in DRG 314 Documentation should provide a clear relationship between the procedure and the sepsis/infection (Official coding guideline I.C.1.d.5.a).
	AND	
	Any operating room procedure	
	AND	
	MCC condition	*See* appendix B.
857	PDx of postprocedural sepsis or infection	*See* DRG 856.
	AND	
	Any operating room procedure	
	AND	
	CC condition	*See* appendix B.
858	PDx of postprocedural sepsis or infection	*See* DRG 856.
	AND	
	Any operating room procedure	
862	PDx of postprocedural sepsis or infection	*See* DRG 856.
870	Mechanical Ventilation > 96 hours	*See* DRG 003.
871	MCC condition	*See* appendix B.

MDC 19

Mental Diseases And Disorders

DRG 876 O.R. Procedure with Principal Diagnoses of Mental Illness RW 3.7315

No Potential DRGs

DRG 880 Acute Adjustment Reaction and Psychosocial Dysfunction RW 0.9546

Potential DRGs

884 Organic Disturbances and Intellectual Disability 1.7569
885 Psychoses 1.3664

DRG	PDx/SDx/Procedure	Tips
884	Principal diagnosis - conditions such as: dementia (vascular, in other diseases, unspecified), mental, psychological, personality or behavioral disorders due to known physiological condition.	Review record documentation for underlying cause of dementia in other diseases, disorders due to known physiological condition, and review Includes and Excludes notes for sequencing guidelines.
	Puerperal psychosis (post-partum depression)	
	Mild, moderate, severe, profound, or other unspecified intellectual disabilities	
	Autistic disorder or other childhood disintegrative disorder	
	Trisomy 21, Down syndrome unspecified	
	Trisomy 18, 13, other specified chromosome deletion syndromes including fragile X chromosome	
	Transient alteration of awareness	
	Age-related cognitive decline	
885	Delusional disorders, psychotic disorders not due to substance or known physiological condition, schizoaffective disorders	
	Manic episode, bipolar disorder	
	Major depressive disorder, single episode, mild, moderate, severe with or without psychotic features, in partial or full remission, or other depressive episodes	
	Major depressive disorder, recurrent, mild, moderate, severe with or without psychotic features, in partial or full or unspecified remission, or other unspecified recurrent depressive disorders	
	Asperger's syndrome	

DRG 881 Depressive Neuroses

RW 0.9065

Potential DRGs

883	Disorders of Personality and Impulse Control	1.8754
884	Organic Disturbances and Intellectual Disability	1.7569
885	Psychoses	1.3664

DRG	PDx/SDx/Procedure	Tips
883	Schizotypal disorder	Key terms: dissociative identity disorder, fanatic personality
	Cyclothymic disorder	
	Dissociative identity disorder	
	Anorexia nervosa	
	Paranoid personality disorder, Schizoid personality disorder, Antisocial personality disorder, Borderline personality disorder, Histrionic personality disorder, Obsessive-compulsive personality disorder, Avoidant personality disorder, Dependent personality disorder, Narcissistic personality disorder	
	Pathological gambling	
	Kleptomania	
	Intermittent and other impulse disorders	
	Factitious disorder, unspecified/with predominantly physical signs/symptoms	
	Unspecified disorder of adult personality and behavior	
	Emotional lability	
	Nonsuicidal self-harm	
884	Principal diagnosis - conditions such as: dementia (vascular, in other diseases, unspecified), mental, psychological, personality or behavioral disorders due to known physiological condition.	Review record documentation for underlying cause of dementia in other diseases, disorders due to known physiological condition, and review Includes and Excludes notes for sequencing guidelines.
	Puerperal psychosis (post-partum depression)	
	Mild, moderate, severe, profound, or other unspecified intellectual disabilities	
	Autistic disorder or other childhood disintegrative disorder	
	Trisomy 21, Down syndrome unspecified	
	Trisomy 18, 13, other specified chromosome deletion syndromes including fragile X chromosome	
	Transient alteration of awareness	
	Age-related cognitive decline	
885	Delusional disorders, psychotic disorders not due to substance or known physiological condition, schizoaffective disorders	
	Manic episode, Bipolar disorder	
	Major depressive disorder, single episode, mild, moderate, severe with or without psychotic features, in partial or full remission, or other depressive episodes	
	Major depressive disorder, recurrent, mild, moderate, severe with or without psychotic features, in partial or full or unspecified remission, or other unspecified recurrent depressive disorders	
	Asperger's syndrome	

DRG 882 Neuroses Except Depressive RW 0.9393

Potential DRGs

883	Disorders of Personality and Impulse Control	1.8754
884	Organic Disturbances and Intellectual Disability	1.7569
885	Psychoses	1.3664
887	Other Mental Disorder Diagnoses	1.2956

DRG	PDx/SDx/Procedure	Tips
883	Schizotypal disorder	Key terms: dissociative identity disorder, fanatic personality
	Cyclothymic disorder	
	Dissociative identity disorder	
	Anorexia nervosa	
	Paranoid personality disorder, Schizoid personality disorder, Antisocial personality disorder, Borderline personality disorder, Histrionic personality disorder, Obsessive-compulsive personality disorder, Avoidant personality disorder, Dependent personality disorder, Narcissistic personality disorder	
	Pathological gambling	
	Kleptomania	
	Intermittent and other impulse disorders	
	Factitious disorder, unspecified/with predominantly physical signs/symptoms	
	Unspecified disorder of adult personality and behavior	
	Emotional lability	
	Nonsuicidal self-harm	
884	Principal diagnosis - conditions such as: dementia (vascular, in other diseases, unspecified), mental, psychological, personality or behavioral disorders due to known physiological condition.	Review record documentation for underlying cause of dementia in other diseases, disorders due to known physiological condition, and review Includes and Excludes notes for sequencing guidelines.
	Puerperal psychosis (post-partum depression)	
	Mild, moderate, severe, profound, or other unspecified intellectual disabilities	
	Autistic disorder or other childhood disintegrative disorder	
	Trisomy 21, Down syndrome unspecified	
	Trisomy 18, 13, other specified chromosome deletion syndromes including fragile X chromosome	
	Transient alteration of awareness	
	Age-related cognitive decline	
885	Delusional disorders, psychotic disorders not due to substance or known physiological condition, schizoaffective disorders	
	Manic episode, bipolar disorder	
	Major depressive disorder, single episode, mild, moderate, severe with or without psychotic features, in partial or full remission, or other depressive episodes	
	Major depressive disorder, recurrent, mild, moderate, severe with or without psychotic features, in partial or full or unspecified remission, or other unspecified recurrent depressive disorders	
	Asperger's syndrome	
887	Other mental disorders such as: Sleep disorders of nonorganic origin, Eating disorders, Sleep disorders not involving sleep apnea Sexual disorders/dysfunctions	

DRG 883 Disorders of Personality and Impulse Control RW 1.8754

No Potential DRGs

DRG 884 Organic Disturbances and Intellectual Disability — RW 1.7569

Potential DRGs

056	Degenerative Nervous System Disorders with MCC	2.3940
091	Other Disorders of Nervous System with MCC	1.7892
100	Seizures with MCC	1.9825
545	Connective Tissue Disorders with MCC	2.4932
867	Other Infectious and Parasitic Diseases Diagnoses with MCC	2.0923
974	HIV with Major Related Condition with MCC	2.9165

DRG	PDx/SDx/Procedure	Tips
056	Dementia due to underlying cause such as: Neurosyphilis (dementia paralytica) Creutzfeldt-Jakob disease (Jakob-Creutzfeldt disease) Cerebral lipidosis Parkinson's disease Alzheimer's disease Pick's disease Frontotemporal dementia Dementia with Lewy bodies	Review record documentation for underlying cause of dementia in other diseases, disorders due to known physiological condition, and review Includes and Excludes notes for sequencing guidelines.
	AND	
	MCC condition	*See* appendix B.
091	Late effect of contusion/laceration cerebrum, skull/face fracture, or intracranial injury	When coding late effects (sequela) of injuries, the complication or condition that arose as a direct result of the injury would be sequenced first followed by the injury (chapter 19) code as a secondary diagnosis. The injury code should have a 7th character "S" (Official coding guideline I.C.19.a).
	Nonruptured cerebral aneurysm	
	Mechanical complication of implanted electronic neurostimulator	
	AND	
	MCC condition	*See* appendix B.
100	Dementia due to epilepsy and recurrent seizures	Review record documentation for underlying cause of dementia in other diseases, disorders due to known physiological condition, and review Includes and Excludes notes for sequencing guidelines.
	AND	
	MCC condition	*See* appendix B.
545	Dementia due to polyarteritis nodosa or systemic lupus erythematosus (SLE)	*See* DRG 100.
	AND	
	MCC condition	*See* appendix B.
867	Dementia due to parasitic infections such as: Trypanosomiasis, malaria	*See* DRG 100.
	AND	
	MCC condition	*See* appendix B.
974	Dementia due to major HIV-related condition such as: Sepsis Tuberculosis/Mycobacterium avium complex (MAC) Herpes zoster Herpes simplex Human herpesvirus 6 or other human herpesvirus encephalitis Candidiasis of mouth, skin & nails, lung, other sites Kaposi's sarcoma Lymphomas Encephalopathy Pneumonia, various types	Admission for HIV-related condition: sequence B2Ø first followed by the HIV-related condition code except Chapter 15 codes which take sequencing priority. Admission due to complication of HIV-related condition: sequence B2Ø first followed by the HIV-related condition and the associated manifestation (i.e. acute respiratory failure due to AIDS related pneumonia). See appendix C for the full list of major HIV-related conditions. A diagnosis from this list should not be assumed as HIV-related unless specifically documented as such by the provider.
	AND	
	MCC condition	*See* appendix B.

DRG 885 Psychoses — RW 1.3664

No Potential DRGs

DRG 886 Behavioral and Developmental Disorders — RW 1.6817

No Potential DRGs

DRG 887 Other Mental Disorder Diagnoses — RW 1.2956

Potential DRGs

154	Other Ear, Nose, Mouth and Throat Diagnoses with MCC	1.5382

DRG	PDx/SD/Procedure	Tips
154	Sleep apnea and organic sleep disorders	Review sleep study documentation for sleep apnea diagnosis; clarify with physician.
	AND	
	MCC condition	*See* appendix B.

MDC 20

Alcohol Or Drug Use Or Induced Organic Mental Disorders

DRG 894 Alcohol/Drug Abuse or Dependence, Left Against Medical Advice RW 0.5745

Potential DRGs

432	Cirrhosis and Alcoholic Hepatitis with MCC	1.9160
433	Cirrhosis and Alcoholic Hepatitis with CC	1.0310
434	Cirrhosis and Alcoholic Hepatitis without CC/MCC	0.6695
441	Disorders of Liver Except Malignancy, Cirrhosis, Alcoholic Hepatitis with MCC	1.8282
442	Disorders of Liver Except Malignancy, Cirrhosis, Alcoholic Hepatitis with CC	0.9515
443	Disorders of Liver Except Malignancy, Cirrhosis, Alcoholic Hepatitis without CC/MCC	0.7147
895	Alcohol/Drug Abuse or Dependence with Rehabilitation Therapy	1.6088
896	Alcohol/Drug Abuse or Dependence without Rehabilitation Therapy with MCC	1.7781
897	Alcohol/Drug Abuse or Dependence without Rehabilitation Therapy without MCC	0.8556

DRG	PDx/SDx/Procedure	Tips
432	Alcoholic hepatitis with/without ascites	Key terms: acute alcoholic liver disease, florid cirrhosis, Laennec's cirrhosis.
	Alcoholic fibrosis and sclerosis of liver	
	Alcoholic cirrhosis of liver with/without ascites	
	Alcoholic hepatic failure with coma	
	Alcoholic liver disease, unspecified	
	AND	
	MCC condition	*See* appendix B.
433	Alcoholic hepatitis with/without ascites	Key terms: acute alcoholic liver disease, florid cirrhosis, Laennec's cirrhosis.
	Alcoholic fibrosis and sclerosis of liver	
	Alcoholic cirrhosis of liver with/without ascites	
	Alcoholic hepatic failure with coma	
	Alcoholic liver disease, unspecified	
	AND	
	CC condition	*See* appendix B.
434	Alcoholic hepatitis with/without ascites	Key terms: acute alcoholic liver disease, florid cirrhosis, Laennec's cirrhosis.
	Alcoholic fibrosis and sclerosis of liver	
	Alcoholic cirrhosis of liver with/without ascites	
	Alcoholic hepatic failure with coma	
	Alcoholic liver disease, unspecified	
441	Alcoholic fatty liver	Key terms: fatty cirrhosis, alcoholic fatty cirrhosis.
	Hepatic encephalopathy with SDx alcoholic hepatic failure without coma	Hepatic encephalopathy is not synonymous with hepatic coma. As the most severe stage of hepatic encephalopathy, hepatic coma requires explicit documentation. If hepatic coma is documented, only code K70.41 Alcoholic hepatic failure with coma, is reported and the case will be assigned to MS-DRGs 432–434.
	AND	
	MCC condition	*See* appendix B.
442	Alcoholic fatty liver	Key terms: fatty cirrhosis, alcoholic fatty cirrhosis.
	Hepatic encephalopathy with SDx alcoholic hepatic failure without coma	*See* DRG 441.
	AND	
	CC condition	*See* appendix B.
443	Alcoholic fatty liver	Key terms: fatty cirrhosis, alcoholic fatty cirrhosis.
	Hepatic encephalopathy with SDx alcoholic hepatic failure without coma	*See* DRG 441.
895	Patient disposition other than Left AMA	
	AND	
	Rehabilitation therapy	Review therapy and other documentation carefully to differentiate therapy from detoxification.
896	Patient disposition other than Left AMA	
	AND	
	MCC condition	*See* appendix B.
897	Patient disposition other than Left AMA	

DRG 895 Alcohol/Drug Abuse or Dependence with Rehabilitation Therapy — RW 1.6088

Potential DRGs

432	Cirrhosis and Alcoholic Hepatitis with MCC	1.9160
441	Disorders of Liver Except Malignancy, Cirrhosis, Alcoholic Hepatitis with MCC	1.8282
896	Alcohol/Drug Abuse or Dependence without Rehabilitation Therapy with MCC	1.7781

DRG	PDx/SDx/Procedure	Tips
432	Alcoholic hepatitis with/without ascites	Key terms: acute alcoholic liver disease, florid cirrhosis, Laennec's cirrhosis.
	Alcoholic fibrosis and sclerosis of liver	
	Alcoholic cirrhosis of liver with/without ascites	
	Alcoholic hepatic failure with coma	
	Alcoholic liver disease, unspecified	
	AND	
	MCC condition	*See* appendix B.
441	Alcoholic fatty liver	Key terms: fatty cirrhosis, alcoholic fatty cirrhosis.
	Hepatic encephalopathy with SDx alcoholic hepatic failure without coma	Hepatic encephalopathy is not synonymous with hepatic coma. As the most severe stage of hepatic encephalopathy, hepatic coma requires explicit documentation. If hepatic coma is documented, only code K70.41 Alcoholic hepatic failure with coma, is reported and the case will be assigned to MS-DRGs 432–434.
	AND	
	MCC condition	*See* appendix B.
896	No rehabilitation therapy	Review therapy and other documentation carefully to differentiate therapy from detoxification.
	AND	
	MCC condition	*See* appendix B.

DRG 896 Alcohol/Drug Abuse or Dependence without Rehabilitation Therapy with MCC — RW 1.7781

Potential DRGs

432	Cirrhosis and Alcoholic Hepatitis with MCC	1.9160
441	Disorders of Liver Except Malignancy, Cirrhosis, Alcoholic Hepatitis with MCC	1.8282

DRG	PDx/SDx/Procedure	Tips
432	Alcoholic hepatitis with/without ascites	Key terms: acute alcoholic liver disease, florid cirrhosis, Laennec's cirrhosis.
	Alcoholic fibrosis and sclerosis of liver	
	Alcoholic cirrhosis of liver with/without ascites	
	Alcoholic hepatic failure with coma	
	Alcoholic liver disease, unspecified	
	AND	
	MCC condition	*See* appendix B.
441	Alcoholic fatty liver	Key terms: fatty cirrhosis, alcoholic fatty cirrhosis.
	Hepatic encephalopathy with SDx alcoholic hepatic failure without coma	Hepatic encephalopathy is not synonymous with hepatic coma. As the most severe stage of hepatic encephalopathy, hepatic coma requires explicit documentation. If hepatic coma is documented, only code K70.41 Alcoholic hepatic failure with coma, is reported and the case will be assigned to MS-DRGs 432–434.
	AND	
	MCC condition	*See* appendix B.

DRG 897 Alcohol/Drug Abuse or Dependence without Rehabilitation Therapy without MCC RW 0.8556

Potential DRGs

432	Cirrhosis and Alcoholic Hepatitis with MCC	1.9160
433	Cirrhosis and Alcoholic Hepatitis with CC	1.0310
441	Disorders of Liver Except Malignancy, Cirrhosis, Alcoholic Hepatitis with MCC	1.8282
442	Disorders of Liver Except Malignancy, Cirrhosis, Alcoholic Hepatitis with CC	0.9515
895	Alcohol/Drug Abuse or Dependence with Rehabilitation Therapy	1.6088
896	Alcohol/Drug Abuse or Dependence without Rehabilitation Therapy with MCC	1.7781

DRG	PDx/SDx/Procedure	Tips
432	Alcoholic hepatitis with/without ascites	Key terms: acute alcoholic liver disease, florid cirrhosis, Laennec's cirrhosis.
	Alcoholic fibrosis and sclerosis of liver	
	Alcoholic cirrhosis of liver with/without ascites	
	Alcoholic hepatic failure with coma	
	Alcoholic liver disease, unspecified	
	AND	
	MCC condition	*See* appendix B.
433	Alcoholic hepatitis with/without ascites	Key terms: acute alcoholic liver disease, florid cirrhosis, Laennec's cirrhosis.
	Alcoholic fibrosis and sclerosis of liver	
	Alcoholic cirrhosis of liver with/without ascites	
	Alcoholic hepatic failure with coma	
	Alcoholic liver disease, unspecified	
	AND	
	CC condition	*See* appendix B.
441	Alcoholic fatty liver	Key terms: fatty cirrhosis, alcoholic fatty cirrhosis.
	Hepatic encephalopathy with SDx alcoholic hepatic failure without coma	Hepatic encephalopathy is not synonymous with hepatic coma. As the most severe stage of hepatic encephalopathy, hepatic coma requires explicit documentation. If hepatic coma is documented, only code K70.41 Alcoholic hepatic failure with coma, is reported and the case will be assigned to MS-DRGs 432–434.
	AND	
	MCC condition	*See* appendix B.
442	Alcoholic fatty liver	Key terms: fatty cirrhosis, alcoholic fatty cirrhosis.
	Hepatic encephalopathy with SDx alcoholic hepatic failure without coma	*See* DRG 441.
	AND	
	CC condition	*See* appendix B.
895	Rehabilitation therapy	
896	MCC condition	*See* appendix B.

Injuries, Poisonings And Toxic Effects Of Drugs

DRG 901 Wound Debridements for Injuries with MCC — RW 4.3278

Potential DRGs

463	Wound Debridement and Skin Graft Except Hand for Musculoskeletal and Connective Tissue Disorders with MCC	5.6637
957	Other O.R. Procedures for Multiple Significant Trauma with MCC	7.2325

DRG	PDx/SDx/Procedure	Tips
463	Fracture and dislocation injuries from MDC 8	Many fracture and dislocation injuries have overlying skin and soft tissue injuries that should be coded separately. These skin/soft tissue injuries do not necessarily constitute open fracture or dislocations. Note that the ICD-10-CM dislocation codes have a "Code Also" note to code also any associated open wounds. A "code also" note instructs that two codes may be required to fully describe a condition, but does not provide sequencing direction. Depending on the severity of the injury, circumstances of admission, diagnostic workup and therapy provided, either of these codes may be reported first.
	AND	
	Excisional wound debridement (e.g., of overlying skin, subcutaneous tissue or fascia)	
	AND	
	MCC condition	*See* appendix B.
957	Multiple significant trauma diagnosis	Principal diagnosis of trauma and two or more different dx from two different body site categories in MS-DRG 963.
	AND	
	Excisional debridement of wound, infection, or burn	The ICD-10-PCS definition of the root operation Excision is "Cutting out or off, without replacement, a portion of a body part." Debridement by excision involves cutting with a sharp instrument such as a scalpel or other methods such as a hot knife or laser. Non-excisional debridement of skin is coded to root operation Extraction. Ensure that documentation includes instruments used, technique, and depth of debridement procedure.
	AND	
	MCC condition	*See* appendix B.

DRG 902 Wound Debridements for Injuries with CC — RW 1.8847

Potential DRGs

040	Peripheral/Cranial Nerve and Other Nervous System Procedures with MCC	3.8505
041	Peripheral/Cranial Nerve and Other Nervous System Procedures with CC or Peripheral Neurostimulator	2.2307
463	Wound Debridement and Skin Graft Except Hand for Musculoskeletal and Connective Tissue Disorders with MCC	5.6637
464	Wound Debridement and Skin Graft Except Hand for Musculoskeletal and Connective Tissue Disorders with CC	3.0014
570	Skin Debridement with MCC	2.9222
901	Wound Debridements for Injuries with MCC	4.3278
957	Other O.R. Procedures for Multiple Significant Trauma with MCC	7.2325
958	Other O.R. Procedures for Multiple Significant Trauma with CC	4.0448

DRG	PDx/SDx/Procedure	Tips
040	Nerve injury	When the primary injury is to the blood vessels or nerves, that injury should be sequenced first.
	AND	
	Excisional debridement of wound, infection, or burn	The ICD-10-PCS definition of the root operation Excision is "Cutting out or off, without replacement, a portion of a body part." Debridement by excision involves cutting with a sharp instrument such as a scalpel or other methods such as a hot knife or laser. Non-excisional debridement of skin is coded to root operation Extraction. Ensure that documentation includes instruments used, technique, and depth of debridement procedure.
	AND	
	MCC condition	*See* appendix B.
041	Nerve injury	*See* DRG 040.
	AND	
	Excisional debridement of wound, infection, or burn	*See* DRG 040.
	AND	
	CC condition	*See* appendix B.

DRG 902 (Continued)

DRG	PDx/SDx/Procedure	Tips
463	Fracture and dislocation injuries from MDC 8	Many fracture and dislocation injuries have overlying skin and soft tissue injuries that should be coded separately. These skin/soft tissue injuries do not necessarily constitute open fracture or dislocations. Note that the ICD-10-CM dislocation codes have a "Code Also" note to code also any associated open wounds. A "code also" note instructs that two codes may be required to fully describe a condition, but does not provide sequencing direction. Depending on the severity of the injury, circumstances of admission, diagnostic workup and therapy provided, either of these codes may be reported first.
	AND	
	Excisional wound debridement (e.g., of overlying skin, subcutaneous tissue or fascia)	
	AND	
	MCC condition	*See* appendix B.
464	Fracture and dislocation injuries from MDC 8	*See* DRG 463.
	AND	
	Excisional wound debridement (e.g., of overlying skin, subcutaneous tissue or fascia)	
	AND	
	CC condition	*See* appendix B.
570	Cellulitis or skin ulcer	
	AND	
	Excisional debridement of skin	The ICD-10-PCS definition of the root operation Excision is "Cutting out or off, without replacement, a portion of a body part." Debridement by excision involves cutting with a sharp instrument such as a scalpel or other methods such as a hot knife or laser. Non-excisional debridement of skin is coded to root operation Extraction. Ensure that documentation includes instruments used, technique, and depth of debridement procedure.
	AND	
	MCC condition	*See* appendix B.
901	MCC condition	*See* appendix B.
957	Multiple significant trauma diagnosis	Principal diagnosis of trauma and two or more different dx from two different body site categories in MS-DRG 963.
	AND	
	Excisional debridement of wound, infection, or burn	The ICD-10-PCS definition of the root operation Excision is "Cutting out or off, without replacement, a portion of a body part." Debridement by excision involves cutting with a sharp instrument such as a scalpel or other methods such as a hot knife or laser. Non-excisional debridement of skin is coded to root operation Extraction. Ensure that documentation includes instruments used, technique, and depth of debridement procedure.
	AND	
	MCC condition	*See* appendix B.
958	Multiple significant trauma diagnosis	*See* DRG 957.
	AND	
	Excisional debridement of wound, infection, or burn	*See* DRG 957.
	AND	
	CC condition	*See* appendix B.

DRG 903 Wound Debridements for Injuries without CC/MCC

RW 1.2415

Potential DRGs

040	Peripheral/Cranial Nerve and Other Nervous System Procedures with MCC	3.8505
041	Peripheral/Cranial Nerve and Other Nervous System Procedures with CC or Peripheral Neurostimulator	2.2307
042	Peripheral/Cranial Nerve and Other Nervous System Procedures without CC/MCC	1.7398
463	Wound Debridement and Skin Graft Except Hand for Musculoskeletal and Connective Tissue Disorders with MCC	5.6637
464	Wound Debridement and Skin Graft Except Hand for Musculoskeletal and Connective Tissue Disorders with CC	3.0014
465	Wound Debridement and Skin Graft Except Hand for Musculoskeletal and Connective Tissue Disorders without CC/MCC	1.8708
570	Skin Debridement with MCC	2.9222
571	Skin Debridement with CC	1.6919
901	Wound Debridements for Injuries with MCC	4.3278
902	Wound Debridements for Injuries with CC	1.8847
957	Other O.R. Procedures for Multiple Significant Trauma with MCC	7.2325
958	Other O.R. Procedures for Multiple Significant Trauma with CC	4.0448
959	Other O.R. Procedures for Multiple Significant Trauma without CC/MCC	2.5324

DRG	PDx/SDx/Procedure	Tips
040	Nerve injury	When the primary injury is to the blood vessels or nerves, that injury should be sequenced first.
	AND	
	Excisional debridement of wound, infection, or burn	The ICD-10-PCS definition of the root operation Excision is "Cutting out or off, without replacement, a portion of a body part." Debridement by excision involves cutting with a sharp instrument such as a scalpel or other methods such as a hot knife or laser. Non-excisional debridement of skin is coded to root operation Extraction. Ensure that documentation includes instruments used, technique, and depth of debridement procedure.
	AND	
	MCC condition	*See* appendix B.
041	Nerve injury	*See* DRG 040.
	AND	
	Excisional debridement of wound, infection, or burn	*See* DRG 040.
	AND	
	CC condition	*See* appendix B.
042	Nerve injury	*See* DRG 040.
	AND	
	Excisional debridement of wound, infection, or burn	*See* DRG 040.
463	Fracture and dislocation injuries from MDC 8	Many fracture and dislocation injuries have overlying skin and soft tissue injuries that should be coded separately. These skin/soft tissue injuries do not necessarily constitute open fracture or dislocations. Note that the ICD-10-CM dislocation codes have a "Code Also" note to code also any associated open wounds. A "code also" note instructs that two codes may be required to fully describe a condition, but does not provide sequencing direction. Depending on the severity of the injury, circumstances of admission, diagnostic workup and therapy provided, either of these codes may be reported first.
	AND	
	Excisional wound debridement (e.g., of overlying skin, subcutaneous tissue or fascia)	
	AND	
	MCC condition	*See* appendix B.
464	Fracture and dislocation injuries from MDC 8	*See* DRG 463.
	AND	
	Excisional wound debridement (e.g., of overlying skin, subcutaneous tissue or fascia)	
	AND	
	CC condition	*See* appendix B.
465	Fracture and dislocation injuries from MDC 8	*See* DRG 463.
	AND	
	Excisional wound debridement (e.g., of overlying skin, subcutaneous tissue or fascia)	
570	Cellulitis or skin ulcer	
	AND	
	Excisional debridement of skin	The ICD-10-PCS definition of the root operation Excision is "Cutting out or off, without replacement, a portion of a body part." Debridement by excision involves cutting with a sharp instrument such as a scalpel or other methods such as a hot knife or laser. Non-excisional debridement of skin is coded to root operation Extraction. Ensure that documentation includes instruments used, technique, and depth of debridement procedure.
	AND	
	MCC condition	*See* appendix B.

DRG 903 (Continued)

DRG	PDx/SDx/Procedure	Tips
571	Cellulitis or skin ulcer	
	AND	
	Excisional debridement of skin	*See* DRG 570.
	AND	
	CC condition	*See* appendix B.
901	MCC condition	*See* appendix B.
902	CC condition	*See* appendix B.
957	Multiple significant trauma diagnosis	Principal diagnosis of trauma and two or more different dx from two different body site categories in MS-DRG 963.
	AND	
	Excisional debridement of wound, infection, or burn	The ICD-10-PCS definition of the root operation Excision is "Cutting out or off, without replacement, a portion of a body part." Debridement by excision involves cutting with a sharp instrument such as a scalpel or other methods such as a hot knife or laser. Non-excisional debridement of skin is coded to root operation Extraction. Ensure that documentation includes instruments used, technique, and depth of debridement procedure.
	AND	
	MCC condition	*See* appendix B.
958	Multiple significant trauma diagnosis	*See* DRG 957.
	AND	
	Excisional debridement of wound, infection, or burn	*See* DRG 957.
	AND	
	CC condition	*See* appendix B.
959	Multiple significant trauma diagnosis	*See* DRG 957.
	AND	
	Excisional debridement of wound, infection, or burn	*See* DRG 957.

DRG 904 Skin Grafts for Injuries with CC/MCC

RW 3.2562

Potential DRGs

040	Peripheral/Cranial Nerve and Other Nervous System Procedures with MCC	3.8505
463	Wound Debridement and Skin Graft Except Hand for Musculoskeletal and Connective Tissue Disorders with MCC	5.6637
901	Wound Debridements for Injuries with MCC	4.3278
957	Other O.R. Procedures for Multiple Significant Trauma with MCC	7.2325
958	Other O.R. Procedures for Multiple Significant Trauma with CC	4.0448

DRG	PDx/SDx/Procedure	Tips
040	Nerve injury	When the primary injury is to the blood vessels or nerves; that injury should be sequenced first.
	AND	
	Skin grafting procedure	
	AND	
	MCC condition	*See* appendix B.
463	Fracture and dislocation injuries from MDC 8	Many fracture and dislocation injuries have overlying skin and soft tissue injuries that should be coded separately. These skin/soft tissue injuries do not necessarily constitute open fracture or dislocations. Note that the ICD-10-CM dislocation codes have a "Code Also" note to code also any associated open wounds. A "code also" note instructs that two codes may be required to fully describe a condition, but does not provide sequencing direction. Depending on the severity of the injury, circumstances of admission, diagnostic workup and therapy provided, either of these codes may be reported first.
	AND	
	Skin grafting procedure	
	AND	
	MCC condition	*See* appendix B.
901	Excisional debridement of subcutaneous tissue or fascia in conjunction with skin grafting	If a graft is applied only at skin level and excisional debridement is of a deeper layer such as subcutaneous tissue and/or fascia excisional debridement is coded separately. ICD-10-PCS Official Guideline B3.5 states, "If root operations such as Excision, Extraction, Repair or Inspection are performed on overlapping layers of the musculoskeletal system, the body part specifying the deepest layer is coded." Excisional debridement that includes skin and subcutaneous tissue is coded to the subcutaneous tissue and fascia body part. The ICD-10-PCS definition of the root operation Excision is "Cutting out or off, without replacement, a portion of a body part." Debridement by excision involves cutting with a sharp instrument such as a scalpel or other methods such as a hot knife or laser. Ensure that documentation includes instruments used, technique, and depth of debridement procedure.
	AND	
	MCC condition	*See* appendix B.
957	Multiple significant trauma diagnosis	Principal diagnosis of trauma and two or more different dx from two different body site categories in MS-DRG 963.
	AND	
	Skin grafting procedure	
	AND	
	MCC condition	*See* appendix B.
958	Multiple significant trauma diagnosis	*See* DRG 957.
	AND	
	Skin grafting procedure	
	AND	
	CC condition	*See* appendix B.

Optimizing Tips

DRG 905 Skin Grafts for Injuries without CC/MCC RW 1.5837

Potential DRGs

040	Peripheral/Cranial Nerve and Other Nervous System Procedures with MCC	3.8505
041	Peripheral/Cranial Nerve and Other Nervous System Procedures with CC or Peripheral Neurostimulator	2.2307
042	Peripheral/Cranial Nerve and Other Nervous System Procedures without CC/MCC	1.7398
463	Wound Debridement and Skin Graft Except Hand for Musculoskeletal and Connective Tissue Disorders with MCC	5.6637
464	Wound Debridement and Skin Graft Except Hand for Musculoskeletal and Connective Tissue Disorders with CC	3.0014
465	Wound Debridement and Skin Graft Except Hand for Musculoskeletal and Connective Tissue Disorders without CC/MCC	1.8708
901	Wound Debridements for Injuries with MCC	4.3278
902	Wound Debridements for Injuries with CC	1.8847
904	Skin Grafts for Injuries with CC/MCC	3.2562
957	Other O.R. Procedures for Multiple Significant Trauma with MCC	7.2325
958	Other O.R. Procedures for Multiple Significant Trauma with CC	4.0448
959	Other O.R. Procedures for Multiple Significant Trauma without CC/MCC	2.5324

DRG	PDx/SDx/Procedure	Tips
040	Nerve injury	When the primary injury is to the blood vessels or nerves, that injury should be sequenced first.
	AND	
	Skin grafting procedure	
	AND	
	MCC condition	*See* appendix B.
041	Nerve injury	*See* DRG 040.
	AND	
	Skin grafting procedure	
	AND	
	CC condition	*See* appendix B.
042	Nerve injury	*See* DRG 040.
	AND	
	Skin grafting procedure	
463	Fracture and dislocation injuries from MDC 8	Many fracture and dislocation injuries have overlying skin and soft tissue injuries that should be coded separately. These skin/soft tissue injuries do not necessarily constitute open fracture or dislocations. Note that the ICD-10-CM dislocation codes have a "Code Also" note to code also any associated open wounds. A "code also" note instructs that two codes may be required to fully describe a condition, but does not provide sequencing direction. Depending on the severity of the injury, circumstances of admission, diagnostic workup and therapy provided, either of these codes may be reported first.
	AND	
	Skin grafting procedure	
	AND	
	MCC condition	*See* appendix B.
464	Fracture and dislocation injuries from MDC 8	*See* DRG 463.
	AND	
	Skin grafting procedure	
	AND	
	CC condition	*See* appendix B.
465	Fracture and dislocation injuries from MDC 8	*See* DRG 463.
	AND	
	Skin grafting procedure	
901	Excisional debridement of subcutaneous tissue or fascia in conjunction with skin grafting	If a graft is applied only at skin level and excisional debridement is of a deeper layer such as subcutaneous tissue and/or fascia excisional debridement is coded separately. ICD-10-PCS Official Guideline B3.5 states, "If root operations such as Excision, Extraction, Repair or Inspection are performed on overlapping layers of the musculoskeletal system, the body part specifying the deepest layer is coded." Excisional debridement that includes skin and subcutaneous tissue is coded to the subcutaneous tissue and fascia body part. The ICD-10-PCS definition of the root operation Excision is "Cutting out or off, without replacement, a portion of a body part." Debridement by excision involves cutting with a sharp instrument such as a scalpel or other methods such as a hot knife or laser. Ensure that documentation includes instruments used, technique, and depth of debridement procedure.
	AND	
	MCC condition	*See* appendix B.
902	Excisional debridement of subcutaneous tissue or fascia in conjunction with skin grafting	*See* DRG 901.
	AND	
	CC condition	*See* appendix B.
904	CC/MCC condition	*See* appendix B.

DRG 905 (Continued)

DRG	PDx/SDx/Procedure	Tips
957	Multiple significant trauma diagnosis	Principal diagnosis of trauma and two or more different dx from two different body site categories in MS-DRG 963.
	AND	
	Skin grafting procedure	
	AND	
	MCC condition	*See* appendix B.
958	Multiple significant trauma diagnosis	*See* DRG 957.
	AND	
	Skin grafting procedure	
	AND	
	CC condition	*See* appendix B.
959	Multiple significant trauma diagnosis	*See* DRG 957.
	AND	
	Skin grafting procedure	

DRG 906 Hand Procedures for Injuries RW 1.8816

Potential DRGs

957	Other O.R. Procedures for Multiple Significant Trauma with MCC	7.2325
958	Other O.R. Procedures for Multiple Significant Trauma with CC	4.0448
959	Other O.R. Procedures for Multiple Significant Trauma without CC/MCC	2.5324

DRG	PDx/SDx/Procedure	Tips
957	Multiple significant trauma diagnosis	Principal diagnosis of trauma and two or more different dx from two different body site categories in MS-DRG 963.
	AND	
	Operating room procedures related to hand, thumb or fingers	
	AND	
	MCC condition	*See* appendix B.
958	Multiple significant trauma diagnosis	*See* DRG 957.
	AND	
	Operating room procedures related to hand, thumb or fingers	
	AND	
	CC condition	*See* appendix B.
959	Multiple significant trauma diagnosis	*See* DRG 957.
	AND	
	Operating room procedures related to hand, thumb or fingers	

DRG 907 Other O.R. Procedures for Injuries with MCC RW 3.7195

Potential DRGs

901	Wound Debridements for Injuries with MCC	4.3278
955	Craniotomy for Multiple Significant Trauma	6.0902
957	Other O.R. Procedures for Multiple Significant Trauma with MCC	7.2325

DRG	PDx/SDx/Procedure	Tips
901	Excisional debridement of wound, infection, or burn	The ICD-10-PCS definition of the root operation Excision is "Cutting out or off, without replacement, a portion of a body part." Debridement by excision involves cutting with a sharp instrument such as a scalpel or other methods such as a hot knife or laser. Nonexcisional debridement of skin is coded to root operation Extraction. Ensure that documentation includes instruments used, technique, and depth of debridement procedure.
	AND	
	MCC condition	*See* appendix B.
955	Craniotomy for multiple significant trauma such as: Repair, reposition head and facial bones Repair traumatic injury to brain, cerebral meninges, dura mater, cerebral ventricle, basal ganglia, thalamus, hypothalamus, pons, cerebellum, medulla oblongata	Craniotomy and PDx of trauma and at least two injuries (assigned as PDx or SDx) that are defined as significant trauma from different body site categories listed under MS-DRG 963.
957	Multiple significant trauma diagnosis	Principal diagnosis of trauma and two or more different dx from two different body site categories in MS-DRG 963.
	AND	
	Operating room procedures from MDC 21 excluding pacemakers and devices	
	AND	
	MCC condition	*See* appendix B.

DRG 908 Other O.R. Procedures for Injuries with CC RW 2.0041

Potential DRGs

901	Wound Debridements for Injuries with MCC	4.3278
904	Skin Grafts for Injuries with CC/MCC	3.2562
907	Other O.R. Procedures for Injuries with MCC	3.7195
955	Craniotomy for Multiple Significant Trauma	6.0902
956	Limb Reattachment, Hip and Femur Procedures for Multiple Significant Trauma	3.8782
957	Other O.R. Procedures for Multiple Significant Trauma with MCC	7.2325
958	Other O.R. Procedures for Multiple Significant Trauma with CC	4.0448

DRG	PDx/SDx/Procedure	Tips
901	Excisional debridement of wound, infection, or burn	The ICD-10-PCS definition of the root operation Excision is "Cutting out or off, without replacement, a portion of a body part." Debridement by excision involves cutting with a sharp instrument such as a scalpel or other methods such as a hot knife or laser. Non-excisional debridement of skin is coded to root operation Extraction. Ensure that documentation includes instruments used, technique, and depth of debridement procedure.
	AND	
	MCC condition	*See* appendix B.
904	Skin grafting procedure	
	AND	
	CC/MCC condition	*See* appendix B.
907	MCC condition	*See* appendix B.
955	Craniotomy for multiple significant trauma such as: Repair, reposition head and facial bones Repair traumatic injury to brain, cerebral meninges, dura mater, cerebral ventricle, basal ganglia, thalamus, hypothalamus, pons, cerebellum, medulla oblongata	Craniotomy and PDx of trauma and at least two injuries (assigned as PDx or SDx) that are defined as significant trauma from different body site categories listed under MS-DRG 963.
956	Limb reattachment (excluding fingers and toes)	Principal diagnosis of trauma and two or more different dx from two different body site categories in MS-DRG 963.
	Hip and femur procedures for multiple significant trauma	
957	Multiple significant trauma diagnosis	Principal diagnosis of trauma and two or more different dx from two different body site categories in MS-DRG 963.
	AND	
	Operating room procedures from MDC 21 excluding pacemakers and devices	
	AND	
	MCC condition	*See* appendix B.
958	Multiple significant trauma diagnosis	*See* DRG 957.
	AND	
	Operating room procedures from MDC 21 excluding pacemaker leads and devices	
	AND	
	CC condition	*See* appendix B.

DRG 909 Other O.R. Procedures for Injuries without CC/MCC

RW 1.3563

Potential DRGs

901	Wound Debridements for Injuries with MCC	4.3278
902	Wound Debridements for Injuries with CC	1.8847
904	Skin Grafts for Injuries with CC/MCC	3.2562
905	Skin Grafts for Injuries without CC/MCC	1.5837
907	Other O.R. Procedures for Injuries with MCC	3.7195
908	Other O.R. Procedures for Injuries with CC	2.0041
955	Craniotomy for Multiple Significant Trauma	6.0902
956	Limb Reattachment, Hip and Femur Procedures for Multiple Significant Trauma	3.8782
957	Other O.R. Procedures for Multiple Significant Trauma with MCC	7.2325
958	Other O.R. Procedures for Multiple Significant Trauma with CC	4.0448
959	Other O.R. Procedures for Multiple Significant Trauma without CC/MCC	2.5324

DRG	PDx/SDx/Procedure	Tips
901	Excisional debridement of wound, infection, or burn	The ICD-10-PCS definition of the root operation Excision is "Cutting out or off, without replacement, a portion of a body part." Debridement by excision involves cutting with a sharp instrument such as a scalpel or other methods such as a hot knife or laser. Non-excisional debridement of skin is coded to root operation Extraction. Ensure that documentation includes instruments used, technique, and depth of debridement procedure.
	AND	
	MCC condition	*See* appendix B.
902	Excisional debridement of wound, infection, or burn	*See* DRG 901.
	AND	
	CC condition	*See* appendix B.
904	Skin grafting procedure	
	AND	
	CC/MCC condition	*See* appendix B.
905	Skin grafting procedure	
907	MCC condition	*See* appendix B.
908	CC condition	*See* appendix B.
955	Craniotomy for multiple significant trauma such as: Repair, reposition head and facial bones Repair traumatic injury to brain, cerebral meninges, dura mater, cerebral ventricle, basal ganglia, thalamus, hypothalamus, pons, cerebellum, medulla oblongata	Craniotomy and PDx of trauma and at least two injuries (assigned as PDx or SDx) that are defined as significant trauma from different body site categories listed under MS-DRG 963.
956	Limb reattachment (excluding fingers and toes)	Principal diagnosis of trauma and two or more different dx from two different body site categories in MS-DRG 963.
	Hip and femur procedures for multiple significant trauma	
957	Multiple significant trauma diagnosis	*See* DRG 956.
	AND	
	Operating room procedures from MDC 21 excluding pacemaker leads and devices	
	AND	
	MCC condition	*See* appendix B.
958	Multiple significant trauma diagnosis	*See* DRG 956.
	AND	
	Operating room procedures from MDC 21 excluding pacemaker leads and devices	
	AND	
	CC condition	*See* appendix B.
959	Multiple significant trauma diagnosis	*See* DRG 956.
	AND	
	Operating room procedures from MDC 21 excluding pacemaker leads and devices	

DRG 913 Traumatic Injury with MCC RW 1.4945

Potential DRGs

570	Skin Debridement with MCC	2.9222
901	Wound Debridements for Injuries with MCC	4.3278
907	Other O.R. Procedures for Injuries with MCC	3.7195
956	Limb Reattachment, Hip and Femur Procedures for Multiple Significant Trauma	3.8782
957	Other O.R. Procedures for Multiple Significant Trauma with MCC	7.2325
963	Other Multiple Significant Trauma with MCC	2.7343

DRG	PDx/SDx/Procedure	Tips
570	Skin ulcer or cellulitis principal diagnosis	
	AND	
	Excisional debridement of wound, infection, or burn	The ICD-10-PCS definition of the root operation Excision is "Cutting out or off, without replacement, a portion of a body part." Debridement by excision involves cutting with a sharp instrument such as a scalpel or other methods such as a hot knife or laser. Non-excisional debridement of skin is coded to root operation Extraction. Ensure that documentation includes instruments used, technique, and depth of debridement procedure.
	AND	
	MCC condition	*See* appendix B.
901	Excisional debridement of wound, infection, or burn	*See* DRG 570.
	AND	
	MCC condition	*See* appendix B.
907	Operative procedure for injury, such as: Exploratory laparotomy, laparoscopy Facial bone repair Open reduction facial fractures Open fracture bone debridement, all sites except carpals/metacarpals and phalanges Open reduction of joint dislocation, all sites except wrist & hand	
	AND	
	MCC condition	*See* appendix B.
956	Limb reattachment (excluding fingers and toes)	Principal diagnosis of trauma and two or more different dx from two different body site categories in MS-DRG 963.
	Hip and femur procedures for multiple significant trauma	
957	Multiple significant trauma diagnosis	Principal diagnosis of trauma and two or more different dx from two different body site categories in MS-DRG 963.
	AND	
	Operating room procedures from MDC 21 excluding pacemaker leads and devices	
	AND	
	MCC condition	*See* appendix B.
963	Other multiple significant trauma	
	AND	
	MCC condition	*See* appendix B.

DRG 914 Traumatic Injury without MCC

RW 0.9077

Potential DRGs

570	Skin Debridement with MCC	2.9222
571	Skin Debridement with CC	1.6919
572	Skin Debridement without CC/MCC	1.1396
901	Wound Debridements for Injuries with MCC	4.3278
902	Wound Debridements for Injuries with CC	1.8847
903	Wound Debridements for Injuries without CC/MCC	1.2415
907	Other O.R. Procedures for Injuries with MCC	3.7195
908	Other O.R. Procedures for Injuries with CC	2.0041
909	Other O.R. Procedures for Injuries without CC/MCC	1.3563
913	Traumatic Injury with MCC	1.4945
956	Limb Reattachment, Hip and Femur Procedures for Multiple Significant Trauma	3.8782
957	Other O.R. Procedures for Multiple Significant Trauma with MCC	7.2325
958	Other O.R. Procedures for Multiple Significant Trauma with CC	4.0448
959	Other O.R. Procedures for Multiple Significant Trauma without CC/MCC	2.5324
963	Other Multiple Significant Trauma with MCC	2.7343
964	Other Multiple Significant Trauma with CC	1.5010
965	Other Multiple Significant Trauma without CC/MCC	0.9559

DRG	PDx/SDx/Procedure	Tips
570	Skin ulcer or cellulitis principal diagnosis	
	AND	
	Excisional debridement of wound, infection, or burn	The ICD-10-PCS definition of the root operation Excision is "Cutting out or off, without replacement, a portion of a body part." Debridement by excision involves cutting with a sharp instrument such as a scalpel or other methods such as a hot knife or laser. Non-excisional debridement of skin is coded to root operation Extraction. Ensure that documentation includes instruments used, technique, and depth of debridement procedure.
	AND	
	MCC condition	*See* appendix B.
571	Skin ulcer or cellulitis principal diagnosis	
	AND	
	Excisional debridement of wound, infection, or burn	*See* DRG 570.
	AND	
	CC condition	*See* appendix B.
572	Skin ulcer or cellulitis principal diagnosis	
	AND	
	Excisional debridement of wound, infection, or burn	*See* DRG 570.
901	Excisional debridement of wound, infection, or burn	*See* DRG 570.
	AND	
	MCC condition	*See* appendix B.
902	Excisional debridement of wound, infection, or burn	*See* DRG 570.
	AND	
	CC condition	*See* appendix B.
903	Excisional debridement of wound, infection, or burn	*See* DRG 570.
907	Operative procedure for injury, such as: Exploratory laparotomy, laparoscopy Facial bone repair Open reduction facial fractures Open fracture bone debridement, all sites except carpals/metacarpals and phalanges Open reduction of joint dislocation, all sites except wrist & hand	
	AND	
	MCC condition	*See* appendix B.
908	Operative procedure for injury, such as: Exploratory laparotomy, laparoscopy Facial bone repair Open reduction facial fractures Open fracture bone debridement, all sites except carpals/metacarpals and phalanges Open reduction of joint dislocation, all sites except wrist & hand	
	AND	
	CC condition	*See* appendix B.
909	Operative procedure for injury, such as: Exploratory laparotomy, laparoscopy Facial bone repair Open reduction facial fractures Open fracture bone debridement, all sites except carpals/metacarpals and phalanges Open reduction of joint dislocation, all sites except wrist & hand	
913	MCC condition	*See* appendix B.

DRG 914 (Continued)

DRG	PDx/SDx/Procedure	Tips
956	Limb reattachment (excluding fingers and toes)	Principal diagnosis of trauma and two or more different dx from two different body site categories in MS-DRG 963.
	Hip and femur procedures for multiple significant trauma	
957	Multiple significant trauma diagnosis	Principal diagnosis of trauma and two or more different dx from two different body site categories in MS-DRG 963.
	AND	
	Operating room procedures from MDC 21 excluding pacemaker leads and devices	
	AND	
	MCC condition	*See* appendix B.
958	Multiple significant trauma diagnosis	*See* DRG 957.
	AND	
	Operating room procedures from MDC 21 excluding pacemaker leads and devices	
	AND	
	CC condition	*See* appendix B.
959	Multiple significant trauma diagnosis	*See* DRG 957.
	AND	
	Operating room procedures from MDC 21 excluding pacemaker leads and devices	
963	Other multiple significant trauma	Principal diagnosis of trauma and two or more different dx from two different body site categories in MS-DRG 963.
	AND	
	MCC condition	*See* appendix B.
964	Other multiple significant trauma	*See* DRG 963.
	AND	
	CC condition	*See* appendix B.
965	Other multiple significant trauma	*See* DRG 963.

DRG 915 Allergic Reactions with MCC RW 1.7740

No Potential DRGs

DRG 916 Allergic Reactions without MCC RW 0.6588

Potential DRGs

915	Allergic Reactions with MCC	1.7740
917	Poisoning and Toxic Effects of Drugs with MCC	1.5959
918	Poisoning and Toxic Effects of Drugs without MCC	0.8609
922	Other Injury, Poisoning and Toxic Effect Diagnoses with MCC	1.7449
923	Other Injury, Poisoning and Toxic Effect Diagnoses without MCC	1.0114

DRG	PDx/SDx/Procedure	Tips
915	MCC condition	*See* appendix B.
917	Poisoning by drugs, medicaments and biological substances, initial encounter	Codes in categories T36-T65 are combination codes that include the substance that was taken as well as the intent. No additional external cause code is required for poisonings, toxic effects, and adverse effects codes. When coding an adverse effect of a drug that has been correctly prescribed and properly administered, assign the appropriate code for the nature of the adverse effect followed by the appropriate code for the adverse effect of the drug (T36-T5Ø). The code for the drug should have a 6th character "5".
	Toxic effects of substances chiefly nonmedicinal as to source	
	AND	
	MCC condition	*See* appendix B.
918	Poisoning by drugs, medicaments and biological substances, initial encounter	*See* DRG 917.
	Toxic effects of substances chiefly nonmedicinal as to source	
	AND	
	CC condition	*See* appendix B.
922	Late effect of allergic reactions	When coding late effects (sequela) of allergic reactions, the complication or condition that arose as a direct result of the allergic reaction would be sequenced first followed by the injury (chapter 19) code as a secondary diagnosis. The injury code should have a 7th character "S" (Official coding guideline I.C.19.a).
	AND	
	MCC condition	*See* appendix B.
923	Sequela of allergic reactions	*See* DRG 922.

DRG 917 Poisoning and Toxic Effects of Drugs with MCC — RW 1.5959

Potential DRGs

377	GI Hemorrhage with MCC	1.7903
915	Allergic Reactions with MCC	1.7740

DRG	PDx/SDx/Procedure	Tips
377	Gastrointestinal bleeding due to adverse drug reaction	When coding an adverse effect of a drug that has been correctly prescribed and properly administered, assign the appropriate code for the nature of the adverse effect followed by the appropriate code for the adverse effect of the drug (T36-T5Ø). The code for the drug should have a 6th character "5".
	AND	
	MCC condition	*See* appendix B.
915	Anaphylactic reaction, angioneurotic edema, or other and unspecified allergy	
	AND	
	MCC condition	*See* appendix B.

DRG 918 Poisoning and Toxic Effects of Drugs without MCC — RW 0.8609

Potential DRGs

308	Cardiac Arrhythmia and Conduction Disorders with MCC	1.2022
377	GI Hemorrhage with MCC	1.7903
378	GI Hemorrhage with CC	0.9838
915	Allergic Reactions with MCC	1.7740
917	Poisoning and Toxic Effects of Drugs with MCC	1.5959

DRG	PDx/SDx/Procedure	Tips
308	Cardiac arrhythmia as an adverse effect of digitalis	Review medical record to determine if the toxicity is a poisoning or an adverse effect. When coding an adverse effect of a drug that has been correctly prescribed and properly administered, assign the appropriate code for the nature of the adverse effect followed by the appropriate code for the adverse effect of the drug (T36-T5Ø). The code for the drug should have a 6th character "5".
	AND	
	MCC condition	*See* appendix B.
377	Gastrointestinal bleeding due to adverse drug reaction	When coding an adverse effect of a drug that has been correctly prescribed and properly administered, assign the appropriate code for the nature of the adverse effect followed by the appropriate code for the adverse effect of the drug (T36-T5Ø). The code for the drug should have a 6th character "5".
	AND	
	MCC condition	*See* appendix B.
378	Gastrointestinal bleeding due to adverse drug reaction	*See* DRG 377.
	AND	
	CC condition	*See* appendix B.
915	Anaphylactic reaction, angioneurotic edema, or other and unspecified allergy	
	AND	
	MCC condition	*See* appendix B.
917	MCC condition	*See* appendix B.

DRG 919 Complications of Treatment with MCC — RW 1.8247

Potential DRGs

495	Local Excision and Removal Internal Fixation Devices Except Hip and Femur with MCC	3.5812
498	Local Excision and Removal Internal Fixation Devices of Hip and Femur with CC/MCC	2.6110
907	Other O.R. Procedures for Injuries with MCC	3.7195

DRG	PDx/SDx/Procedure	Tips
495	Infection, mechanical complication of other orthopedic internal fixation device, except hip and femur	
	AND	
	Removal of implanted device (all sites except hip and femur)	
	AND	
	MCC condition	*See* appendix B.
498	Infection, mechanical complication of hip and femur orthopedic internal fixation device	
	AND	
	Removal of implanted device (femur only)	
	AND	
	CC/MCC condition	*See* appendix B.
907	Disruption of external operative wound	
	AND	
	Reclosure of postoperative abdominal dehiscence	
	AND	
	MCC condition	*See* appendix B.

DRG 920 Complications of Treatment with CC RW 1.0338

Potential DRGs

393	Other Digestive System Diagnoses with MCC	1.6196
495	Local Excision and Removal Internal Fixation Devices Except Hip and Femur with MCC	3.5812
496	Local Excision and Removal Internal Fixation Devices Except Hip and Femur with CC	1.9875
498	Local Excision and Removal Internal Fixation Devices of Hip and Femur with CC/MCC	2.6110
907	Other O.R. Procedures for Injuries with MCC	3.7195
908	Other O.R. Procedures for Injuries with CC	2.0041
919	Complications of Treatment with MCC	1.8247

DRG	PDx/SDx/Procedure	Tips
393	Gastric band and other bariatric procedure complications and infections	
	AND	
	MCC condition	*See* appendix B.
495	Infection, mechanical complication of other orthopedic internal fixation device, except hip and femur	
	AND	
	Removal of implanted device (all sites except hip and femur)	
	AND	
	MCC condition	*See* appendix B.
496	Infection, mechanical complication of other orthopedic internal fixation device, except hip and femur	
	AND	
	Removal of implanted device (all sites except hip and femur)	
	AND	
	CC condition	*See* appendix B.
498	Infection, mechanical complication of hip and femur orthopedic internal fixation device	
	AND	
	Removal of implanted device (femur only)	
	AND	
	CC/MCC condition	*See* appendix B.
907	Disruption of external operative wound	
	AND	
	Reclosure of postoperative abdominal dehiscence	
	AND	
	MCC condition	*See* appendix B.
908	Disruption of external operative wound	
	AND	
	Reclosure of postoperative abdominal dehiscence	
	AND	
	CC condition	*See* appendix B.
919	MCC condition	*See* appendix B.

DRG 921 Complications of Treatment without CC/MCC

RW 0.6978

Potential DRGs

393	Other Digestive System Diagnoses with MCC	1.6196
394	Other Digestive System Diagnoses with CC	0.9369
495	Local Excision and Removal Internal Fixation Devices Except Hip and Femur with MCC	3.5812
496	Local Excision and Removal Internal Fixation Devices Except Hip and Femur with CC	1.9875
497	Local Excision and Removal Internal Fixation Devices Except Hip and Femur without CC/MCC	1.4274
498	Local Excision and Removal Internal Fixation Devices of Hip and Femur with CC/MCC	2.6110
499	Local Excision and Removal Internal Fixation Devices of Hip and Femur without CC/MCC	1.2898
907	Other O.R. Procedures for Injuries with MCC	3.7195
908	Other O.R. Procedures for Injuries with CC	2.0041
909	Other O.R. Procedures for Injuries without CC/MCC	1.3563
919	Complications of Treatment with MCC	1.8247
920	Complications of Treatment with CC	1.0338

DRG	PDx/SDx/Procedure	Tips
393	Gastric band and other bariatric procedure complications and infections	
	AND	
	MCC condition	*See* appendix B.
394	Gastric band and other bariatric procedure complications and infections	
	AND	
	CC condition	*See* appendix B.
495	Infection, mechanical complication of other orthopedic internal fixation device, except hip and femur	
	AND	
	Removal of implanted device (all sites except hip and femur)	
	AND	
	MCC condition	*See* appendix B.
496	Infection, mechanical complication of other orthopedic internal fixation device, except hip and femur	
	AND	
	Removal of implanted device (all sites except hip and femur)	
	AND	
	CC condition	*See* appendix B.
497	Infection, mechanical complication of other orthopedic internal fixation device, except hip and femur	
	AND	
	Removal of implanted device (all sites except hip and femur)	
498	Infection, mechanical complication of hip and femur orthopedic internal fixation device	
	AND	
	Removal of implanted device (femur only)	
	AND	
	CC/MCC condition	*See* appendix B.
499	Infection, mechanical complication of hip and femur orthopedic internal fixation device	
	AND	
	Removal of implanted device (femur only)	
907	Disruption of external operative wound	
	AND	
	Reclosure of postoperative abdominal dehiscence	
	AND	
	MCC condition	*See* appendix B.
908	Disruption of external operative wound	
	AND	
	Reclosure of postoperative abdominal dehiscence	
	AND	
	CC condition	*See* appendix B.
909	Disruption of external operative wound	
	AND	
	Reclosure of postoperative abdominal dehiscence	
919	MCC condition	*See* appendix B.
920	CC condition	*See* appendix B.

DRG 922 Other Injury, Poisoning and Toxic Effect Diagnoses with MCC — RW 1.7449

Potential DRGs

907	Other O.R. Procedures for Injuries with MCC	3.7195

DRG	PDx/SDx/Procedure	Tips
907	Traumatic compartment syndrome, all sites	
	AND	
	Fasciotomy	
	AND	
	MCC condition	*See* appendix B.

DRG 923 Other Injury, Poisoning and Toxic Effect Diagnoses without MCC — RW 1.0114

Potential DRGs

907	Other O.R. Procedures for Injuries with MCC	3.7195
908	Other O.R. Procedures for Injuries with CC	2.0041
909	Other O.R. Procedures for Injuries without CC/MCC	1.3563
922	Other Injury, Poisoning and Toxic Effect Diagnoses with MCC	1.7449

DRG	PDx/SDx/Procedure	Tips
907	Traumatic compartment syndrome, all sites	
	AND	
	Fasciotomy	
	AND	
	MCC condition	*See* appendix B.
908	Traumatic compartment syndrome, all sites	
	AND	
	Fasciotomy	
	AND	
	CC condition	*See* appendix B.
909	Traumatic compartment syndrome, all sites	
	AND	
	Fasciotomy	
922	MCC condition	*See* appendix B.

Burns

DRG 927 Extensive Burns or Full Thickness Burns with Mechanical Ventilation > 96 Hours with Skin Graft — RW 26.3587

No Potential DRGs

DRG 928 Full Thickness Burn with Skin Graft or Inhalation Injury with CC/MCC — RW 6.9197

Potential DRGs

003	ECMO or Tracheostomy with Mechanical Ventilation >96 Hours or Principal Diagnosis Except Face, Mouth and Neck with Major O.R. procedures	21.3203
004	Tracheostomy with Mechanical Ventilation >96 Hours or Principal Diagnosis Except Face, Mouth and Neck without Major O.R. procedures	14.7000
927	Extensive Burns or Full Thickness Burns with Mechanical Ventilation > 96 Hours with Skin Graft	26.3587

DRG	PDx/SDx/Procedure	Tips
003	Full thickness burns	Full thickness: third degree; deep necrosis of underlying tissue Burn: thermal from heat source, electricity and radiation, except sunburns Corrosions: due to chemicals. Report separate codes for each site; report only the highest degree of burn for varying degrees of the same local site. Include codes from categories T31 and T32 for burn mortality/burn unit reporting. Rule of nines: adjust for infants, children and large adults.
	AND	
	Tracheostomy	Tracheostomy carried out elsewhere prior to admission or in an ambulance prior to arrival should not be reported as a current procedure. A tracheostomy procedure may be performed at the bedside and documented in the progress notes or in the operating room and documented in an operative note.
	WITH	
	Mechanical ventilation > 96 consecutive hours	Review record documentation for start and stop times. Calculation of mechanical ventilation hours begins when vent is initiated (or time of admission if patient already on a vent) and ends when it is turned off (or the time patient is discharged if still ventilated). The duration includes time spent to wean the patient from the vent. Do not assume that ventilation that spans four calendar days equals > 96 hours; count by the hour not day.
	AND	
	Skin graft	Example: free skin graft—Replacement (putting in or on biological or synthetic material that physically takes the place and/or function of all or a portion of a body part.) Advancement flap graft—Transfer (moving, without taking out, all or a portion of a body part to another location to take over the function of all or a portion of a body part.)
004	Full thickness burns	*See* DRG 003.
	AND	
	Tracheostomy	*See* DRG 003.
	WITH	
	Mechanical ventilation > 96 consecutive hours	*See* DRG 003.
927	Extensive burn	Extensive: involves >= 20% body surface and >= 10% third degree burn. Burn: thermal from heat source, electricity and radiation, except sunburns. Corrosions: due to chemicals. Report separate codes for each site; report only the highest degree of burn for varying degrees of the same local site. Include codes from categories T31 and T32 for burn mortality/burn unit reporting. Rule of nines: adjust for infants, children and large adults.
	OR	
	Full thickness burns	Full thickness: third degree; deep necrosis of underlying tissue Burn: thermal from heat source, electricity and radiation, except sunburns Corrosions: due to chemicals. Report separate codes for each site; report only the highest degree of burn for varying degrees of the same local site. Include codes from categories T31 and T32 for burn mortality/burn unit reporting. Rule of nines: adjust for infants, children and large adults.
	AND	
	Mechanical ventilation > 96 consecutive hours	*See* DRG 003.
	AND	
	Skin graft	*See* DRG 003.

DRG 929 Full Thickness Burn with Skin Graft or Inhalation Injury without CC/MCC — RW 3.2155

Potential DRGs

003	ECMO or Tracheostomy with Mechanical Ventilation >96 Hours or Principal Diagnosis Except Face, Mouth and Neck with Major O.R. procedures	21.3203
004	Tracheostomy with Mechanical Ventilation >96 Hours or Principal Diagnosis Except Face, Mouth and Neck without Major O.R. procedures	14.7000
927	Extensive Burns or Full Thickness Burns with Mechanical Ventilation > 96 Hours with Skin Graft	26.3587
928	Full Thickness Burn with Skin Graft or Inhalation Injury with CC/MCC	6.9197

DRG	PDx/SDx/Procedure	Tips
003	Full thickness burns	Full thickness: third degree; deep necrosis of underlying tissue Burn: thermal from heat source, electricity and radiation, except sunburns Corrosions: due to chemicals. Report separate codes for each site; report only the highest degree of burn for varying degrees of the same local site. Include codes from categories T31 and T32 for burn mortality/burn unit reporting. Rule of nines: adjust for infants, children and large adults.
	AND	
	Tracheostomy	Tracheostomy carried out elsewhere prior to admission or in an ambulance prior to arrival should not be reported as a current procedure. A tracheostomy procedure may be performed at the bedside and documented in the progress notes or in the operating room and documented in an operative note.
	WITH	
	Mechanical ventilation > 96 consecutive hours	Review record documentation for start and stop times. Calculation of mechanical ventilation hours begins when vent is initiated (or time of admission if patient already on a vent) and ends when it is turned off (or the time patient is discharged if still ventilated). The duration includes time spent to wean the patient from the vent. Do not assume that ventilation that spans four calendar days equals > 96 hours; count by the hour not day.
	AND	
	Skin graft	Example: free skin graft—Replacement (putting in or on biological or synthetic material that physically takes the place and/or function of all or a portion of a body part.) Advancement flap graft—Transfer (moving, without taking out, all or a portion of a body part to another location to take over the function of all or a portion of a body part.)
004	Full thickness burns	*See* DRG 003.
	AND	
	Tracheostomy	*See* DRG 003.
	WITH	
	Mechanical ventilation > 96 consecutive hours	*See* DRG 003.
927	Extensive burn	Extensive: involves >= 20% body surface and >= 10% third degree burn. Burn: thermal from heat source, electricity and radiation, except sunburns. Corrosions: due to chemicals. Report separate codes for each site; report only the highest degree of burn for varying degrees of the same local site. Include codes from categories T31 and T32 for burn mortality/burn unit reporting. Rule of nines: adjust for infants, children and large adults.
	OR	
	Full thickness burns	*See* DRG 003.
	AND	
	Mechanical ventilation > 96 consecutive hours	*See* DRG 003.
	AND	
	Skin graft	*See* DRG 003.
928	CC/MCC condition	*See* appendix B.

DRG 933 Extensive Burns or Full Thickness Burns with Mechanical Ventilation > 96 Hours without Skin Graft

RW 3.0320

Potential DRGs

003	ECMO or Tracheostomy with Mechanical Ventilation >96 Hours or Principal Diagnosis Except Face, Mouth and Neck with Major O.R. procedures	21.3203
004	Tracheostomy with Mechanical Ventilation >96 Hours or Principal Diagnosis Except Face, Mouth and Neck without Major O.R. procedures	14.7000
927	Extensive Burns or Full Thickness Burns with Mechanical Ventilation > 96 Hours with Skin Graft	26.3587
928	Full Thickness Burn with Skin Graft or Inhalation Injury with CC/MCC	6.9197

DRG	PDx/SDx/Procedure	Tips
003	Full thickness burns	Full thickness: third degree; deep necrosis of underlying tissue Burn: thermal from heat source, electricity and radiation, except sunburns Corrosions: due to chemicals. Report separate codes for each site; report only the highest degree of burn for varying degrees of the same local site. Include codes from categories T31 and T32 for burn mortality/burn unit reporting. Rule of nines: adjust for infants, children and large adults.
	AND	
	Tracheostomy	Tracheostomy carried out elsewhere prior to admission or in an ambulance prior to arrival should not be reported as a current procedure. A tracheostomy procedure may be performed at the bedside and documented in the progress notes or in the operating room and documented in an operative note.
	WITH	
	Mechanical ventilation > 96 consecutive hours	Review record documentation for start and stop times. Calculation of mechanical ventilation hours begins when vent is initiated (or time of admission if patient already on a vent) and ends when it is turned off (or the time patient is discharged if still ventilated). The duration includes time spent to wean the patient from the vent. Do not assume that ventilation that spans four calendar days equals > 96 hours; count by the hour not day.
	AND	
	Skin graft	Example: free skin graft—Replacement (putting in or on biological or synthetic material that physically takes the place and/or function of all or a portion of a body part.) Advancement flap graft—Transfer (moving, without taking out, all or a portion of a body part to another location to take over the function of all or a portion of a body part.)
004	Full thickness burns	*See* DRG 003.
	AND	
	Tracheostomy	*See* DRG 003.
	WITH	
	Mechanical ventilation > 96 consecutive hours	*See* DRG 003.
927	Extensive burn	Extensive: involves >= 20% body surface and >= 10% third degree burn. Burn: thermal from heat source, electricity and radiation, except sunburns. Corrosions: due to chemicals. Report separate codes for each site; report only the highest degree of burn for varying degrees of the same local site. Include codes from categories T31 and T32 for burn mortality/burn unit reporting. Rule of nines: adjust for infants, children and large adults.
	OR	
	Full thickness burns	Full thickness: third degree; deep necrosis of underlying tissue. Burn: thermal from heat source, electricity and radiation, except sunburns. Corrosions: due to chemicals. Report separate codes for each site; report only the highest degree of burn for varying degrees of the same local site. Include codes from categories T31 and T32 for burn mortality/burn unit reporting. Rule of nines: adjust for infants, children and large adults.
	AND	
	Mechanical ventilation > 96 consecutive hours	*See* DRG 003.
	AND	
	Skin graft	*See* DRG 003.

DRG 933 (Continued)

DRG	PDx/SDx/Procedure	Tips
928	Full thickness burn	Burn/corrosion of eye and internal organs: report to site; degree is not a component of internal burns. Sequence internal and external burns and related conditions (i.e. respiratory failure) according to the circumstance of admission.
	AND	
	Skin graft	*See* DRG 003.
	OR	
	Full thickness burn	Burn/corrosion of eye and internal organs: report to site; degree is not a component of internal burns. Sequence internal and external burns and related conditions (i.e. respiratory failure) according to the circumstance of admission.
	AND	
	Secondary diagnosis of inhalation injury	Inhalation injury: corrosion/burn of internal organ such as: heat inhalation; toxic effect, such as: smoke intoxication, toxin inhalation (ex. carbon monoxide). Report acute pulmonary edema due to chemicals, gases, fumes and vapors as an additional code when documented due to smoke, gases, fumes, or vapors.
	AND	
	CC/MCC condition	*See* appendix B.

DRG 934 Full Thickness Burn without Skin Graft or Inhalation Injury — RW 2.0925

Potential DRGs

003	ECMO or Tracheostomy with Mechanical Ventilation >96 Hours or Principal Diagnosis Except Face, Mouth and Neck with Major O.R. procedures	21.3203
004	Tracheostomy with Mechanical Ventilation >96 Hours or Principal Diagnosis Except Face, Mouth and Neck without Major O.R. procedures	14.7000
927	Extensive Burns or Full Thickness Burns with Mechanical Ventilation > 96 Hours with Skin Graft	26.3587
928	Full Thickness Burn with Skin Graft or Inhalation Injury with CC/MCC	6.9197
929	Full Thickness Burn with Skin Graft or Inhalation Injury without CC/MCC	3.2155
933	Extensive Burns or Full Thickness Burns with Mechanical Ventilation > 96 Hours without Skin Graft	3.0320

DRG	PDx/SDx/Procedure	Tips
003	Full thickness burns	Full thickness: third degree; deep necrosis of underlying tissue Burn: thermal from heat source, electricity and radiation, except sunburns Corrosions: due to chemicals. Report separate codes for each site; report only the highest degree of burn for varying degrees of the same local site. Include codes from categories T31 and T32 for burn mortality/burn unit reporting. Rule of nines: adjust for infants, children and large adults.
	AND	
	Tracheostomy	Tracheostomy carried out elsewhere prior to admission or in an ambulance prior to arrival should not be reported as a current procedure. A tracheostomy procedure may be performed at the bedside and documented in the progress notes or in the operating room and documented in an operative note.
	WITH	
	Mechanical ventilation > 96 consecutive hours	Review record documentation for start and stop times. Calculation of mechanical ventilation hours begins when vent is initiated (or time of admission if patient already on a vent) and ends when it is turned off (or the time patient is discharged if still ventilated). The duration includes time spent to wean the patient from the vent. Do not assume that ventilation that spans four calendar days equals > 96 hours; count by the hour not day.
	AND	
	Skin graft	Example: free skin graft—Replacement (putting in or on biological or synthetic material that physically takes the place and/or function of all or a portion of a body part.) Advancement flap graft—Transfer (moving, without taking out, all or a portion of a body part to another location to take over the function of all or a portion of a body part.)
004	Full thickness burns	*See* DRG 003.
	AND	
	Tracheostomy	*See* DRG 003.
	WITH	
	Mechanical ventilation > 96 consecutive hours	*See* DRG 003.

DRG 934 (Continued)

DRG	PDx/SDx/Procedure	Tips
927	Extensive burn	Extensive: involves >= 20% body surface and >= 10% third degree burn. Burn: thermal from heat source, electricity and radiation, except sunburns. Corrosions: due to chemicals. Report separate codes for each site; report only the highest degree of burn for varying degrees of the same local site. Include codes from categories T31 and T32 for burn mortality/burn unit reporting. Rule of nines: adjust for infants, children and large adults.
	OR	
	Full thickness burns	*See* DRG 003.
	AND	
	Mechanical ventilation > 96 consecutive hours	*See* DRG 003.
	AND	
	Skin graft	*See* DRG 003.
928	Full thickness burn	Burn/corrosion of eye and internal organs: report to site; degree is not a component of internal burns. Sequence internal and external burns and related conditions (i.e. respiratory failure) according to the circumstance of admission.
	AND	
	Skin graft	*See* DRG 003.
	OR	
	Full thickness burn	Burn/corrosion of eye and internal organs: report to site; degree is not a component of internal burns. Sequence internal and external burns and related conditions (i.e. respiratory failure) according to the circumstance of admission.
	AND	
	Secondary diagnosis of inhalation injury	Inhalation injury: corrosion/burn of internal organ such as: heat inhalation; toxic effect, such as: smoke intoxication, toxin inhalation (ex. carbon monoxide). Report acute pulmonary edema due to chemicals, gases, fumes and vapors as an additional code when documented due to smoke, gases, fumes, or vapors.
	AND	
	CC/MCC condition	*See* appendix B.
929	Full thickness burn	*See* DRG 928.
	AND	
	Skin graft	*See* DRG 003.
	OR	
	Full thickness burn	*See* DRG 928.
	AND	
	Secondary diagnosis of inhalation injury	*See* DRG 928.
933	Extensive burn	*See* DRG 927.
	OR	
	Full thickness burn	*See* DRG 927.
	AND	
	Mechanical ventilation > 96 hours	*See* DRG 003.

DRG 935 Nonextensive Burns RW 2.0411

Potential DRGs

927	Extensive Burns or Full Thickness Burns with Mechanical Ventilation > 96 Hours with Skin Graft	26.3587
928	Full Thickness Burn with Skin Graft or Inhalation Injury with CC/MCC	6.9197
929	Full Thickness Burn with Skin Graft or Inhalation Injury without CC/MCC	3.2155
933	Extensive Burns or Full Thickness Burns with Mechanical Ventilation > 96 Hours without Skin Graft	3.0320

DRG	PDx/SDx/Procedure	Tips
927	Extensive burn	Extensive: involves >= 20% body surface and >= 10% third degree burn. Burn: thermal from heat source, electricity and radiation, except sunburns. Corrosions: due to chemicals. Report separate codes for each site; report only the highest degree of burn for varying degrees of the same local site. Include codes from categories T31 and T32 for burn mortality/burn unit reporting. Rule of nines: adjust for infants, children and large adults.
	OR	
	Full thickness burns	Full thickness: third degree; deep necrosis of underlying tissue. Burn: thermal from heat source, electricity and radiation, except sunburns. Corrosions: due to chemicals. Report separate codes for each site; report only the highest degree of burn for varying degrees of the same local site. Include codes from categories T31 and T32 for burn mortality/burn unit reporting. Rule of nines: adjust for infants, children and large adults.
	AND	
	Mechanical ventilation > 96 consecutive hours	Review record documentation for start and stop times. Calculation of mechanical ventilation hours begins when vent is initiated (or time of admission if patient already on a vent) and ends when it is turned off (or the time patient is discharged if still ventilated). The duration includes time spent to wean the patient from the vent. Do not assume that ventilation that spans four calendar days equals > 96 hours; count by the hour not day.
	AND	
	Skin graft	Example: Free skin graft - replacement (putting in or on biological or synthetic material that physically takes the place and/or function of all or a portion of a body part.) Advancement flap graft - transfer (moving, without taking out, all or a portion of a body part to another location to take over the function of all or a portion of a body part.)
928	Full thickness burn	Burn/corrosion of eye and internal organs: report to site; degree is not a component of internal burns.Sequence internal and external burns and related conditions (i.e. respiratory failure) according to the circumstance of admission.
	AND	
	Skin graft	*See* DRG 927.
	OR	
	Full thickness burn	Burn/corrosion of eye and internal organs: report to site; degree is not a component of internal burns. Sequence internal and external burns and related conditions (i.e. respiratory failure) according to the circumstance of admission.
	AND	
	Secondary diagnosis of inhalation injury	Inhalation injury: corrosion/burn of internal organ such as: heat inhalation; toxic effect, such as: smoke intoxication, toxin inhalation (ex. carbon monoxide). Report acute pulmonary edema due to chemicals, gases, fumes and vapors as an additional code when documented due to smoke, gases, fumes, or vapors.
	AND	
	CC/MCC condition	*See* appendix B.
929	Full thickness burn	*See* DRG 928.
	AND	
	Skin graft	*See* DRG 927.
	OR	
	Full thickness burn	*See* DRG 928.
	AND	
	Secondary diagnosis of inhalation injury	*See* DRG 928.
933	Extensive burn	*See* DRG 927.
	OR	
	Full thickness burn	*See* DRG 928.
	AND	
	Mechanical ventilation > 96 consecutive hours	*See* DRG 927.

Factors Influencing Health Status And Other Contacts With Health Services

DRG 939 O.R. Procedure with Diagnoses of Other Contact with Health Services with MCC — RW 3.2153

No Potential DRGs

DRG 940 O.R. Procedure with Diagnoses of Other Contact with Health Services with CC — RW 2.1666

Potential DRGs

939 O.R. Procedure with Diagnoses of Other Contact with Health Services with MCC — 3.2153

DRG	PDx/SDx/Procedure	Tips
939	MCC condition	*See* appendix B.

DRG 941 O.R. Procedure with Diagnoses of Other Contact with Health Services without CC/MCC — RW 1.8560

Potential DRGs

939 O.R. Procedure with Diagnoses of Other Contact with Health Services with MCC — 3.2153
940 O.R. Procedure with Diagnoses of Other Contact with Health Services with CC — 2.1666

DRG	PDx/SDx/Procedure	Tips
939	MCC condition	*See* appendix B.
940	CC condition	*See* appendix B.

DRG 945 Rehabilitation with CC/MCC — RW 1.5095

Potential DRGs

939 O.R. Procedure with Diagnoses of Other Contact with Health Services with MCC — 3.2153
940 O.R. Procedure with Diagnoses of Other Contact with Health Services with CC — 2.1666

DRG	PDx/SDx/Procedure	Tips
939	Encounter for planned postoperative wound closure	
	AND	
	Delayed closure abdominal wound	Example: Root operation Repair (suture).
	AND	
	MCC condition	*See* appendix B.
940	Encounter for planned postoperative wound closure	
	AND	
	Delayed closure abdominal wound	*See* DRG 939.
	AND	
	CC condition	*See* appendix B.

DRG 946 Rehabilitation without CC/MCC — RW 1.0127

Potential DRGs

939 O.R. Procedure with Diagnoses of Other Contact with Health Services with MCC — 3.2153
940 O.R. Procedure with Diagnoses of Other Contact with Health Services with CC — 2.1666
941 O.R. Procedure with Diagnoses of Other Contact with Health Services without CC/MCC — 1.8560
945 Rehabilitation with CC/MCC — 1.5095

DRG	PDx/SDx/Procedure	Tips
939	Encounter for planned postoperative wound closure	
	AND	
	Delayed closure abdominal wound	Example: Root operation Repair (suture).
	AND	
	MCC condition	*See* appendix B.
940	Encounter for planned postoperative wound closure	
	AND	
	Delayed closure abdominal wound	*See* DRG 939.
	AND	
	CC condition	*See* appendix B.
941	Encounter for planned postoperative wound closure	
	AND	
	Delayed closure abdominal wound	*See* DRG 939.
945	CC/MCC condition	*See* appendix B.

DRG 947 Signs and Symptoms with MCC — RW 1.2516

Potential DRGs

542	Pathological Fractures and Musculoskeletal and Connective Tissue Malignancy with MCC	1.8237
939	O.R. Procedure with Diagnoses of Other Contact with Health Services with MCC	3.2153

DRG	PDx/SDx/Procedure	Tips
542	Bone malignancy causing neoplasm related pain	Code G89.3 is assigned to pain documented as being related, associated or due to cancer, primary or secondary malignancy, or tumor, regardless of whether the pain is acute or chronic. Code G89.3 may be assigned as principal diagnosis when the reason for the encounter is pain control/pain management, with the underlying neoplasm reported as additional diagnosis. However, when the reason for the admission is management of both the neoplasm and associated pain, assign the neoplasm code as principal diagnosis with G89.3 as additional diagnosis. It is not necessary to assign an additional code for the site of the pain.
	AND	
	MCC condition	*See* appendix B.
939	Spinal neurostimulator implant (e.g. for treatment of acute or chronic pain)	When a patient is admitted for the insertion of a neurostimulator for pain control, assign the appropriate pain code as the principal or first-listed diagnosis. When an admission or encounter is for a procedure aimed at treating the underlying condition and a neurostimulator is inserted for pain control during the same admission/encounter, a code for the underlying condition should be assigned as the principal diagnosis and the appropriate pain code should be assigned as a secondary diagnosis.
	AND	
	MCC condition	*See* appendix B.

DRG 948 Signs and Symptoms without MCC — RW 0.8010

Potential DRGs

542	Pathological Fractures and Musculoskeletal and Connective Tissue Malignancy with MCC	1.8237
543	Pathological Fractures and Musculoskeletal and Connective Tissue Malignancy with CC	1.0907
640	Miscellaneous Disorders of Nutrition, Metabolism, and Fluids and Electrolytes with MCC	1.3152
939	O.R. Procedure with Diagnoses of Other Contact with Health Services with MCC	3.2153
940	O.R. Procedure with Diagnoses of Other Contact with Health Services with CC	2.1666
941	O.R. Procedure with Diagnoses of Other Contact with Health Services without CC/MCC	1.8560
947	Signs and Symptoms with MCC	1.2516

DRG	PDx/SDx/Procedure	Tips
542	Bone malignancy causing neoplasm related pain	Code G89.3 is assigned to pain documented as being related, associated or due to cancer, primary or secondary malignancy, or tumor, regardless of whether the pain is acute or chronic. Code G89.3 may be assigned as principal diagnosis when the reason for the encounter is pain control/pain management, with the underlying neoplasm reported as additional diagnosis. However, when the reason for the admission is management of both the neoplasm and associated pain, assign the neoplasm code as principal diagnosis with G89.3 as additional diagnosis. It is not necessary to assign an additional code for the site of the pain.
	AND	
	MCC condition	*See* appendix B.
543	Bone malignancy causing neoplasm related pain	*See* DRG 542.
	AND	
	CC condition	*See* appendix B.
640	Volume depletion, dehydration, hypovolemia	
	Fluid retention, abnormal glucose	
	Malnutrition	
	AND	
	MCC condition	*See* appendix B.
939	Spinal neurostimulator implant (e.g. for treatment of acute or chronic pain)	When a patient is admitted for the insertion of a neurostimulator for pain control, assign the appropriate pain code as the principal or first-listed diagnosis. When an admission or encounter is for a procedure aimed at treating the underlying condition and a neurostimulator is inserted for pain control during the same admission/encounter, a code for the underlying condition should be assigned as the principal diagnosis and the appropriate pain code should be assigned as a secondary diagnosis.
	AND	
	MCC condition	*See* appendix B.
940	Spinal neurostimulator implant (e.g. for treatment of acute or chronic pain)	See DRG 939.
	AND	
	CC condition	*See* appendix B.
941	Spinal neurostimulator implant (e.g. for treatment of acute or chronic pain)	See DRG 939.
947	MCC condition	*See* appendix B.

DRG 949 Aftercare with CC/MCC

RW 1.0361

Potential DRGs

056	Degenerative Nervous System Disorders with MCC	2.3940
280	Acute Myocardial Infarction, Discharged Alive with MCC	1.5865
283	Acute Myocardial Infarction, Expired with MCC	1.9714
939	O.R. Procedure with Diagnoses of Other Contact with Health Services with MCC	3.2153
940	O.R. Procedure with Diagnoses of Other Contact with Health Services with CC	2.1666

DRG	PDx/SDx/Procedure	Tips
056	Principal diagnosis sequela(e) of cerebrovascular disease	Admission for rehabilitation or continued care for persistent neurologic deficits such as hemiplegia following the initial onset of conditions such as a cerebrovascular infarction or disease classifiable to categories I60-I67. Codes from I60-I67 are reserved for the initial (first) episode of care for the acute cerebrovascular disease. Please refer to the Official Guidelines for Coding and Reporting for guidance as to the use of dominant/nondominant side for codes from category I69.
	AND	
	MCC condition	*See* appendix B.
280	Aftercare of myocardial infarction with a stated duration of 4 weeks (28 days) or less from onset.	If the patient requires continued care for an MI that is equal to or less than four weeks old, codes from category I21 may continue to be reported. For encounters after the four-week time frame, the appropriate aftercare code should be assigned, rather than a code from category I21. A code from category I22 Subsequent MI, is reported when a patient who has suffered a type 1 or unspecified AMI has a new type 1 or unspecified AMI within the four-week time frame of the initial AMI. For subsequent type 2, AMI assign only code I21.A1. For subsequent type 4 or type 5 AMI, assign only code I21.A9.
	AND	
	Discharged alive	
	AND	
	MCC condition	*See* appendix B.
283	Aftercare of myocardial infarction with a stated duration of 4 weeks (28 days) or less from onset.	*See* DRG 280.
	AND	
	Expired	Discharge status of 20.
	AND	
	MCC condition	*See* appendix B.
939	Encounter for planned postoperative wound closure	
	AND	
	Delayed closure abdominal wound	Example: Root operation Repair (suture).
	AND	
	MCC condition	*See* appendix B.
940	Encounter for planned postoperative wound closure	
	AND	
	Delayed closure abdominal wound	*See* DRG 939.
	AND	
	CC condition	*See* appendix B.

DRG 950 Aftercare without CC/MCC RW 0.6282

Potential DRGs

056	Degenerative Nervous System Disorders with MCC	2.3940
057	Degenerative Nervous System Disorders without MCC	1.3632
280	Acute Myocardial Infarction, Discharged Alive with MCC	1.5865
281	Acute Myocardial Infarction, Discharged Alive with CC	0.9130
283	Acute Myocardial Infarction, Expired with MCC	1.9714
939	O.R. Procedure with Diagnoses of Other Contact with Health Services with MCC	3.2153
940	O.R. Procedure with Diagnoses of Other Contact with Health Services with CC	2.1666
941	O.R. Procedure with Diagnoses of Other Contact with Health Services without CC/MCC	1.8560
949	Aftercare with CC/MCC	1.0361

DRG	PDx/SDx/Procedure	Tips
056	Principal diagnosis sequela(e) of cerebrovascular disease	Admission for rehabilitation or continued care for persistent neurologic deficits such as hemiplegia following the initial onset of conditions such as a cerebrovascular infarction or disease classifiable to categories I6Ø-I67. Codes from I6Ø-I67 are reserved for the initial (first) episode of care for the acute cerebrovascular disease. Please refer to the Official Guidelines for Coding and Reporting for guidance as to the use of dominant/nondominant side for codes from category I69.
	AND	
	MCC condition	*See* appendix B.
057	Principal diagnosis sequela(e) of cerebrovascular disease	*See* DRG 056.
280	Aftercare of myocardial infarction with a stated duration of 4 weeks (28 days) or less from onset.	If the patient requires continued care for an MI that is equal to or less than four weeks old, codes from category I21 may continue to be reported. For encounters after the four-week time frame the appropriate aftercare code should be assigned, rather than a code from category I21. A code from category I22 Subsequent MI, is reported when a patient who has suffered a type 1 or unspecified AMI has a new type 1 or unspecified AMI within the four-week time frame of the initial AMI. For subsequent type 2 AMI, assign only code I21.A1. For subsequent type 4 or type 5 AMI, assign only code I21.A9.
	AND	
	Discharged alive	
	AND	
	MCC condition	*See* appendix B.
281	Aftercare of myocardial infarction with a stated duration of 4 weeks (28 days) or less from onset.	*See* DRG 280.
	AND	
	Discharged alive	
	AND	
	CC condition	*See* appendix B.
283	Aftercare of myocardial infarction with a stated duration of 4 weeks (28 days) or less from onset.	*See* DRG 280.
	AND	
	Expired	Discharge status of 20.
	AND	
	MCC condition	*See* appendix B.
939	Encounter for planned postoperative wound closure	
	AND	
	Delayed closure abdominal wound	Example: Root operation Repair (suture).
	AND	
	MCC condition	*See* appendix B.
940	Encounter for planned postoperative wound closure	
	AND	
	Delayed closure abdominal wound	*See* DRG 939.
	AND	
	CC condition	*See* appendix B.
941	Encounter for planned postoperative wound closure	
	AND	
	Delayed closure abdominal wound	*See* DRG 939.
949	CC/MCC condition	*See* appendix B.

DRG 951 Other Factors Influencing Health Status

RW 0.5900

Potential DRGs

175	Pulmonary Embolism with MCC or Acute Cor Pulmonale	1.4030
176	Pulmonary Embolism without MCC	0.8156
177	Respiratory Infections and Inflammations with MCC	1.6964
178	Respiratory Infections and Inflammations with CC	0.9867
179	Respiratory Infections and Inflammations with CC	0.7633
196	Interstitial Lung Disease with MCC	1.8954
197	Interstitial Lung Disease with CC	0.9975
198	Interstitial Lung Disease without CC/MCC	0.7782
207	Respiratory System Diagnosis with Ventilator Support >96 Hours	6.9080
208	Respiratory System Diagnosis with Ventilator Support < = 96 Hours	2.7038
545	Connective Tissue Disorders with MCC	2.4932
546	Connective Tissue Disorders with CC	1.1993
547	Connective Tissue Disorders without CC/MCC	0.8134
922	Other Injury, Poisoning and Toxic Effect Diagnoses with MCC	1.7449
923	Other Injury, Poisoning and Toxic Effect Diagnoses without MCC	1.0114
939	O.R. Procedure with Diagnoses of Other Contact with Health Services with MCC	3.2153
940	O.R. Procedure with Diagnoses of Other Contact with Health Services with CC	2.1666
941	O.R. Procedure with Diagnoses of Other Contact with Health Services without CC/MCC	1.8560
945	Rehabilitation with CC/MCC	1.5095
946	Rehabilitation without CC/MCC	1.0127

DRG	PDx/SDx/Procedure	Tips
175	Pulmonary embolism as a post COVID-19 condition	If the pulmonary embolism is a residual effect of previous COVID-19, report the code for pulmonary embolism as principal diagnosis, followed by UØ9.9.
	AND	
	MCC condition	*See* appendix B.
176	Pulmonary embolism as a post COVID-19 condition	*See* DRG 175.
177	Acute COVID-19	Review documentation carefully to determine whether the patient has acute, current COVID-19 infection instead of post COVID-19 condition.
	AND	
	MCC condition	*See* appendix B.
178	Acute COVID-19	*See* DRG 177.
	AND	
	CC condition	*See* appendix B.
179	Acute COVID-19	*See* DRG 177.
196	Pulmonary fibrosis as a post COVID-19 condition	If the pulmonary fibrosis is a residual effect of previous COVID-19, report the code for pulmonary fibrosis as principal diagnosis, followed by UØ9.9.
	AND	
	MCC condition	*See* appendix B.
197	Pulmonary fibrosis as a post COVID-19 condition	*See* DRG 196.
	AND	
	CC condition	*See* appendix B.
198	Pulmonary fibrosis as a post COVID-19 condition	*See* DRG 196.
207	Encounter for weaning from mechanical ventilator	For encounters for weaning from a mechanical ventilator, assign a code from subcategory J96.1, Chronic respiratory failure, followed by code Z99.11, Dependence on respirator [ventilator] status.
	AND	
	Ventilator support > 96 hours	For a patient admitted still on a ventilator, the duration of mechanical ventilation is counted starting from the time of admission. The weaning period ends when the mechanical ventilation is turned off.
208	Encounter for weaning from mechanical ventilator	*See* DRG 207.
	AND	
	Ventilator support ≤ 96 hours	*See* DRG 207.
545	Multisystem inflammatory syndrome (MIS) as a post COVID-19 condition	If the MIS is a residual effect of previous COVID-19, report the code for MIS as principal diagnosis, followed by UØ9.9.
	AND	
	MCC condition	*See* appendix B.
546	Multisystem inflammatory syndrome (MIS) as a post COVID-19 condition	*See* DRG 545.
	AND	
	CC condition	*See* appendix B.
547	Multisystem inflammatory syndrome (MIS) as a post COVID-19 condition	*See* DRG 545.
922	Observation following motor vehicle, work, or other accident	Assign code(s) ZØ4.1, ZØ4.2, and ZØ4.3 when no evidence of the suspected condition is found and no treatment is required. The suspected condition is ruled out.
	AND	
	MCC condition	*See* appendix B.
923	Observation following motor vehicle, work, or other accident	*See* DRG 922.

DRG 951 (Continued)

DRG	PDx/SDx/Procedure	Tips
939	Fitting and adjustment of breast prosthesis and implant	
	AND	
	Breast prosthesis procedure	
	AND	
	MCC condition	*See* appendix B.
940	Fitting and adjustment of breast prosthesis and implant	
	AND	
	Breast prosthesis procedure	
	AND	
	CC condition	*See* appendix B.
941	Fitting and adjustment of breast prosthesis and implant	
	AND	
	Breast prosthesis procedure	
945	Principal diagnosis encounter for fitting and adjustment of other and unspecified external prosthetic device	
	OR	
	Any principal diagnosis from MDC 23 except the following:	
	Encounter for adjustment and management of infusion pump, vascular access device, fitting and adjustment of non-vascular catheter, change or removal of drains, planned postprocedural wound closure, aftercare following organ transplant, bone marrow transplant, aftercare following surgery, and therapeutic drug level-monitoring.	
	AND	
	Rehabilitation procedures	
	AND	
	CC/MCC condition	*See* appendix B.
946	Principal diagnosis encounter for fitting and adjustment of other and unspecified external prosthetic devices	
	OR	
	Any principal diagnosis from MDC 23 except the following: Encounter for adjustment and management of infusion pump, vascular access device, fitting and adjustment of non-vascular catheter, change or removal of drains, planned postprocedural wound closure, aftercare following organ transplant, bone marrow transplant, aftercare following surgery, and therapeutic drug level-monitoring.	
	AND	
	Rehabilitation procedures	

Multiple Significant Trauma

DRG 955 Craniotomy for Multiple Significant Trauma — RW 6.0902

No Potential DRGs

DRG 956 Limb Reattachment, Hip and Femur Procedures for Multiple Significant Trauma — RW 3.8782

Potential DRGs

955 Craniotomy for Multiple Significant Trauma 6.0902

DRG	PDx/SDx/Procedure	Tips
955	Craniotomy for multiple significant trauma such as: Repair, reposition head and facial bones Repair traumatic injury to brain, cerebral meninges, dura mater, cerebral ventricle, basal ganglia, thalamus, hypothalamus, pons, cerebellum, medulla oblongata	Craniotomy and PDx of trauma and at least two injuries (assigned as PDx or SDx) that are defined as significant trauma from different body site categories listed under MS-DRG 963.

DRG 957 Other O.R. Procedures for Multiple Significant Trauma with MCC — RW 7.2325

No Potential DRGs

DRG 958 Other O.R. Procedures for Multiple Significant Trauma with CC — RW 4.0448

Potential DRGs

955 Craniotomy for Multiple Significant Trauma 6.0902
957 Other O.R. Procedures for Multiple Significant Trauma with MCC 7.2325

DRG	PDx/SDx/Procedure	Tips
955	Craniotomy for multiple significant trauma such as: Repair, reposition head and facial bones Repair traumatic injury to brain, cerebral meninges, dura mater, cerebral ventricle, basal ganglia, thalamus, hypothalamus, pons, cerebellum, medulla oblongata	Craniotomy and PDx of trauma and at least two injuries (assigned as PDx or SDx) that are defined as significant trauma from different body site categories listed under MS-DRG 963.
957	MCC condition	*See* appendix B.

DRG 959 Other O.R. Procedures for Multiple Significant Trauma without CC/MCC — RW 2.5324

Potential DRGs

955 Craniotomy for Multiple Significant Trauma 6.0902
956 Limb Reattachment, Hip and Femur Procedures for Multiple Significant Trauma 3.8782
957 Other O.R. Procedures for Multiple Significant Trauma with MCC 7.2325
958 Other O.R. Procedures for Multiple Significant Trauma with CC 4.0448

DRG	PDx/SDx/Procedure	Tips
955	Craniotomy for multiple significant trauma such as: Repair, reposition head and facial bones Repair traumatic injury to brain, cerebral meninges, dura mater, cerebral ventricle, basal ganglia, thalamus, hypothalamus, pons, cerebellum, medulla oblongata	Craniotomy and PDx of trauma and at least two injuries (assigned as PDx or SDx) that are defined as significant trauma from different body site categories listed under MS-DRG 963.
956	Limb reattachment, hip/femur O.R. procedures	Joint replacement includes resection of the joint. Reduction of displaced fracture: reposition. Principal procedure: procedure most related to principal diagnosis, whether definitive treatment or diagnostic.
957	MCC condition	*See* appendix B.
958	CC condition	*See* appendix B.

DRG 963 Other Multiple Significant Trauma with MCC — RW 2.7343

Potential DRGs

955 Craniotomy for Multiple Significant Trauma 6.0902
956 Limb Reattachment, Hip and Femur Procedures for Multiple Significant Trauma 3.8782
957 Other O.R. Procedures for Multiple Significant Trauma with MCC 7.2325

DRG	PDx/SDx/Procedure	Tips
955	Craniotomy for multiple significant trauma such as: Repair, reposition head and facial bones Repair traumatic injury to brain, cerebral meninges, dura mater, cerebral ventricle, basal ganglia, thalamus, hypothalamus, pons, cerebellum, medulla oblongata	Craniotomy and PDx of trauma and at least two injuries (assigned as PDx or SDx) that are defined as significant trauma from different body site categories listed under MS-DRG 963.
956	Limb reattachment, hip/femur O.R. procedures	Joint replacement includes resection of the joint. Reduction of displaced fracture: reposition. Principal procedure: procedure most related to principal diagnosis, whether definitive treatment or diagnostic.
957	Other O.R. procedures for multiple significant trauma, excluding craniotomy, limb reattachment and hip/femur procedures	PDx of trauma and at least two injuries (assigned as PDx or SDx) that are defined as significant trauma from different body site categories located under MS-DRG 963 and O.R. procedure other than craniotomy or limb reattachment, hip and femur procedures.
	AND	
	MCC condition	*See* appendix B.

DRG 964 Other Multiple Significant Trauma with CC — RW 1.5010

Potential DRGs

955	Craniotomy for Multiple Significant Trauma	6.0902
956	Limb Reattachment, Hip and Femur Procedures for Multiple Significant Trauma	3.8782
957	Other O.R. Procedures for Multiple Significant Trauma with MCC	7.2325
958	Other O.R. Procedures for Multiple Significant Trauma with CC	4.0448
963	Other Multiple Significant Trauma with MCC	2.7343

DRG	PDx/SDx/Procedure	Tips
955	Craniotomy for multiple significant trauma such as: Repair, reposition head and facial bones Repair traumatic injury to brain, cerebral meninges, dura mater, cerebral ventricle, basal ganglia, thalamus, hypothalamus, pons, cerebellum, medulla oblongata	Craniotomy and PDx of trauma and at least two injuries (assigned as PDx or SDx) that are defined as significant trauma from different body site categories listed under MS-DRG 963.
956	Limb reattachment, hip/femur O.R. procedures	Joint replacement includes resection of the joint. Reduction of displaced fracture: reposition. Principal procedure: procedure most related to principal diagnosis, whether definitive treatment or diagnostic.
957	Other O.R. procedures for multiple significant trauma, excluding craniotomy, limb reattachment and hip/femur procedures	PDx of trauma and at least two injuries (assigned as PDx or SDx) that are defined as significant trauma from different body site categories located under MS-DRG 963 and O.R. procedure other than craniotomy or limb reattachment, hip and femur procedures.
	AND	
	MCC condition	*See* appendix B.
958	Other O.R. procedures for multiple significant trauma, excluding craniotomy, limb reattachment and hip/femur procedures	*See* DRG 957.
	AND	
	CC condition	*See* appendix B.
963	MCC condition	*See* appendix B.

DRG 965 Other Multiple Significant Trauma without CC/MCC — RW 0.9559

Potential DRGs

955	Craniotomy for Multiple Significant Trauma	6.0902
956	Limb Reattachment, Hip and Femur Procedures for Multiple Significant Trauma	3.8782
957	Other O.R. Procedures for Multiple Significant Trauma with MCC	7.2325
958	Other O.R. Procedures for Multiple Significant Trauma with CC	4.0448
959	Other O.R. Procedures for Multiple Significant Trauma without CC/MCC	2.5324
963	Other Multiple Significant Trauma with MCC	2.7343
964	Other Multiple Significant Trauma with CC	1.5010

DRG	PDx/SDx/Procedure	Tips
955	Craniotomy for multiple significant trauma such as: Repair, reposition head and facial bones Repair traumatic injury to brain, cerebral meninges, dura mater, cerebral ventricle, basal ganglia, thalamus, hypothalamus, pons, cerebellum, medulla oblongata	Craniotomy and PDx of trauma and at least two injuries (assigned as PDx or SDx) that are defined as significant trauma from different body site categories listed under MS-DRG 963.
956	Limb reattachment, hip/femur O.R. procedures	Joint replacement includes resection of the joint. Reduction of displaced fracture: reposition. Principal procedure: procedure most related to principal diagnosis, whether definitive treatment or diagnostic.
957	Other O.R. procedures for multiple significant trauma, excluding craniotomy, limb reattachment and hip/femur procedures	PDx of trauma and at least two injuries (assigned as PDx or SDx) that are defined as significant trauma from different body site categories located under MS-DRG 963 and O.R. procedure other than craniotomy or limb reattachment, hip and femur procedures.
	AND	
	MCC condition	*See* appendix B.
958	Other O.R. procedures for multiple significant trauma, excluding craniotomy, limb reattachment and hip/femur procedures	*See* DRG 957.
	AND	
	CC condition	*See* appendix B.
959	Other O.R. procedures for multiple significant trauma, excluding craniotomy, limb reattachment and hip/femur procedures	*See* DRG 957.
963	MCC condition	*See* appendix B.
964	CC condition	*See* appendix B.

Human Immunodeficiency Virus Infections

DRG 969 HIV with Extensive O.R. Procedure with MCC — RW 6.8726

No Potential DRGs

DRG 970 HIV with Extensive O.R. Procedure without MCC — RW 2.4044

Potential DRGs

969	HIV with Extensive O.R. Procedure with MCC	6.8726

DRG	PDx/SDx/Procedure	Tips
969	MCC condition	*See* appendix B.

DRG 974 HIV with Major Related Condition with MCC — RW 2.9165

Potential DRGs

969	HIV with Extensive O.R. Procedure with MCC	6.8726

DRG	PDx/SDx/Procedure	Tips
969	Extensive O.R procedure	Any procedure not listed in DRGs 987–989
	AND	
	MCC condition	*See* appendix B.

DRG 975 HIV with Major Related Condition with CC — RW 1.3633

Potential DRGs

969	HIV with Extensive O.R. Procedure with MCC	6.8726
970	HIV with Extensive O.R. Procedure without MCC	2.4044
974	HIV with Major Related Condition with MCC	2.9165

DRG	PDx/SDx/Procedure	Tips
969	Extensive O.R procedure	Any procedure not listed in DRGs 987–989
	OR	
	MCC condition	*See* appendix B.
970	Extensive O.R procedure	Any procedure not listed in DRGs 987–989
974	MCC condition	*See* appendix B.

DRG 976 HIV with Major Related Condition without CC/MCC — RW 0.8453

Potential DRGs

969	HIV with Extensive O.R. Procedure with MCC	6.8726
970	HIV with Extensive O.R. Procedure without MCC	2.4044
974	HIV with Major Related Condition with MCC	2.9165
975	HIV with Major Related Condition with CC	1.3633

DRG	PDx/SDx/Procedure	Tips
969	Extensive O.R procedure	Any procedure not listed in DRGs 987–989
	AND	
	MCC condition	*See* appendix B.
970	Extensive O.R procedure	Any procedure not listed in DRGs 987–989
974	MCC condition	*See* appendix B.
975	CC condition	*See* appendix B.

DRG 977 HIV with or without Other Related Condition — RW 1.4161

Potential DRGs

969	HIV with Extensive O.R. Procedure with MCC	6.8726
970	HIV with Extensive O.R. Procedure without MCC	2.4044
974	HIV with Major Related Condition with MCC	2.9165

DRG	PDx/SDx/Procedure	Tips
969	Extensive O.R procedure	Any procedure not listed in DRGs 987–989
	AND	
	MCC condition	*See* appendix B.
970	Extensive O.R procedure	Any procedure not listed in DRGs 987–989
974	Major HIV-related condition	See appendix C for the full list of major HIV-related conditions. A diagnosis from this list should not be assumed as HIV-related unless specifically documented as such by the provider. Admission for HIV-related condition: sequence B2Ø first followed by the HIV-related condition code; except Chapter 15 codes which take sequencing priority. Admission due to complication of HIV-related condition: sequence B2Ø first followed by the HIV-related condition and the associated manifestation (i.e. acute respiratory failure due to AIDS related pneumonia).
	AND	
	MCC condition	*See* appendix B.

ALL MDCs

DRG 981 Extensive O.R. Procedure Unrelated to Principal Diagnosis with MCC — RW 4.7404

No Potential DRGs

DRG 982 Extensive O.R. Procedure Unrelated to Principal Diagnosis with CC — RW 2.4860

Potential DRGs

981 Extensive O.R. Procedure Unrelated to Principal Diagnosis with MCC 4.7404

DRG	PDx/SDx/Procedure	Tips
981	MCC condition	*See* appendix B.

DRG 983 Extensive O.R. Procedure Unrelated to Principal Diagnosis without CC/MCC — RW 1.6352

Potential DRGs

981 Extensive O.R. Procedure Unrelated to Principal Diagnosis with MCC 4.7404
982 Extensive O.R. Procedure Unrelated to Principal Diagnosis with CC 2.4860

DRG	PDx/SDx/Procedure	Tips
981	MCC condition	*See* appendix B.
982	CC condition	*See* appendix B.

DRG 987 Nonextensive O.R. Procedure Unrelated to Principal Diagnosis with MCC — RW 3.3767

Potential DRGs

981 Extensive O.R. Procedure Unrelated to Principal Diagnosis with MCC 4.7404

DRG	PDx/SDx/Procedure	Tips
981	Extensive O.R. procedure unrelated to principal diagnosis	Principal diagnosis is that condition established after study to be chiefly responsible for occasioning the admission of the patient to the hospital for care.
	AND	
	MCC condition	*See* appendix B.

DRG 988 Nonextensive O.R. Procedure Unrelated to Principal Diagnosis with CC — RW 1.6970

Potential DRGs

981 Extensive O.R. Procedure Unrelated to Principal Diagnosis with MCC 4.7404
982 Extensive O.R. Procedure Unrelated to Principal Diagnosis with CC 2.4860
987 Nonextensive O.R. Procedure Unrelated to Principal Diagnosis with MCC 3.3767

DRG	PDx/SDx/Procedure	Tips
981	Extensive O.R. procedure unrelated to principal diagnosis	Principal diagnosis is that condition established after study to be chiefly responsible for occasioning the admission of the patient to the hospital for care.
	AND	
	MCC condition	*See* appendix B.
982	Extensive O.R. procedure unrelated to principal diagnosis	*See* DRG 981.
	AND	
	CC condition	*See* appendix B.
987	MCC condition	*See* appendix B.

DRG 989 Nonextensive O.R. Procedure Unrelated to Principal Diagnosis without CC/MCC — RW 1.0803

Potential DRGs

981 Extensive O.R. Procedure Unrelated to Principal Diagnosis with MCC 4.7404
982 Extensive O.R. Procedure Unrelated to Principal Diagnosis with CC 2.4860
983 Extensive O.R. Procedure Unrelated to Principal Diagnosis without CC/MCC 1.6352
987 Nonextensive O.R. Procedure Unrelated to Principal Diagnosis with MCC 3.3767
988 Nonextensive O.R. Procedure Unrelated to Principal Diagnosis with CC 1.6970

DRG	PDx/SDx/Procedure	Tips
981	Extensive O.R. procedure unrelated to principal diagnosis	Principal diagnosis is that condition established after study to be chiefly responsible for occasioning the admission of the patient to the hospital for care.
	AND	
	MCC condition	*See* appendix B.
982	Extensive O.R. procedure unrelated to principal diagnosis	*See* DRG 981.
	AND	
	CC condition	*See* appendix B.
983	Extensive O.R. procedure unrelated to principal diagnosis	*See* DRG 981.
987	MCC condition	*See* appendix B.
988	CC condition	*See* appendix B.

DRG 998 Principal Diagnosis Invalid as Discharge Diagnosis — RW 0.0000

No Potential DRGs

DRG 999 Ungroupable — RW 0.0000

No Potential DRGs

ICD-10-CM/PCS Codes by MS-DRG

This section lists each MS-DRG and includes a list of diagnosis and procedure codes specific to that MS-DRG. This list of codes is for data purposes only and does not include the full complex DRG logic. For full MS-DRG logic with associated codes and descriptions, see Optum's *2024 DRG Expert*.

Some numeric codes are followed by an asterisk, which indicates that the ICD-10 code is incomplete and represents a sequence or range of codes. Refer to the ICD-10-CM or ICD-10-PCS code book for the specific codes included in the range.

MDC PRE

DRG 001
Heart Transplant Operating Room Procedures
Ø2YAØZØ
Ø2YAØZ1
Ø2YAØZ2
OR
Ø2RKØJZ
AND
Ø2RLØJZ
OR
Implant of Heart Assist System Operating Room Procedures
Ø2HAØQZ
Ø2HAØRZ
Ø2HA3QZ
Ø2HA4QZ
Ø2RAØLZ
Ø2RAØMZ
OR
Ø2HAØRS
Ø2HAØRZ
Ø2HA3RS
Ø2HA4RS
Ø2HA4RZ
Ø2WAØQZ
Ø2WAØRZ
Ø2WA3QZ
Ø2WA3RZ
Ø2WA4QZ
Ø2WA4RZ
AND
Ø2PAØRZ
Ø2PA3RZ
Ø2PA4RZ
Ø2PW3RZ
OR
Ø2WW3RZ
AND
Ø2PAØRZ
Ø2PA3RZ
Ø2PA4RZ
OR
Ø2HAØRZ
AND
X2HXØF9
OR
Ø3HYØYZ
AND
X2HLØF9
X2HMØF9
X2HXØF9
OR
Ø2HA3RZ
AND
X2HLØF9
X2HMØF9

DRG 002
Select operating room procedures OR any procedure combinations listed under DRG 001

DRG 003
ECMO Operating Room Procedure
5A1522F
OR
Nonoperating Room Procedures
5A1522G
5A1522H
OR
Tracheostomy Operating Room Procedures
ØB11ØF4
ØB11ØZ4
ØB114F4
ØB114Z4
OR
Nonoperating Room Procedures
ØB113F4
ØB113Z4
AND EITHER
Principal Diagnosis
Any diagnosis EXCEPT mouth, larynx and pharynx disorders listed under DRG 011
OR
Nonoperating Room Procedure
5A1955Z
AND
Operating Room Procedures
Any O.R. procedure not listed in DRGs 987-989

DRG 004
Tracheostomy Operating Room Procedures
ØB11ØF4
ØB11ØZ4
ØB114F4
ØB114Z4
OR
Nonoperating Room Procedure
ØB113F4
ØB113Z4
AND EITHER
Principal Diagnosis
Any diagnosis EXCEPT mouth, larynx and pharynx disorders listed under DRG 011
OR
Nonoperating Room Procedure
5A1955Z

DRG 005
Intestinal Transplant Operating Room Procedures
ØDY8ØZØ
ØDY8ØZ1
ØDY8ØZ2
ØDYEØZØ
ØDYEØZ1
ØDYEØZ2
Liver Transplant Operating Room Procedures
ØFYØØZØ
ØFYØØZ1
ØFYØØZ2

DRG 006
Operating Room Procedures
ØFYØØZØ
ØFYØØZ1
ØFYØØZ2

DRG 007
Operating Room Procedures
ØBYCØZØ
ØBYCØZ1
ØBYCØZ2
ØBYDØZØ
ØBYDØZ1
ØBYDØZ2
ØBYFØZØ
ØBYFØZ1
ØBYFØZ2
ØBYGØZØ
ØBYGØZ1
ØBYGØZ2
ØBYHØZØ
ØBYHØZ1
ØBYHØZ2
ØBYJØZØ
ØBYJØZ1
ØBYJØZ2
ØBYKØZØ
ØBYKØZ1
ØBYKØZ2
ØBYLØZØ
ØBYLØZ1
ØBYLØZ2
ØBYMØZØ
ØBYMØZ1
ØBYMØZ2

DRG 008
Principal or Secondary Diagnosis
EØ8*
EØ9*
E1Ø*
E11*
E13*
E89.1
AND
Principal or Secondary Diagnosis
I12.Ø
I13.11
I13.2
N18*
Z94.Ø
Z96.49
Z96.89
Z96.9
AND
Operating Room Procedures
ØTYØØZØ
ØTYØØZ1
ØTYØØZ2
ØTY1ØZØ
ØTY1ØZ1
ØTY1ØZ2
AND
Operating Room Procedures
ØFYG*

DRG 010
Principal or Secondary Diagnosis
EØ8*
EØ9*
E1Ø*
E11*
E13*
E89.1
AND
Operating Room Procedures
ØFYG*

DRG 011
Laryngectomy Operating Room Procedures
ØCTSØZZ
ØCTS4ZZ
ØCTS7ZZ
ØCTS8ZZ
OR
Principal Diagnosis
A36.Ø
A36.1
A36.2
A54.5
A56.4
A66.5
A69.Ø
A69.1
BØØ.2
BØ8.5
B37.Ø
B37.83
CØØ*
CØ1
CØ2*
CØ3*
CØ4*
CØ5*
CØ6*
CØ7
CØ8*
CØ9*
C1Ø*
C11*
C12
C13*
C14*
C3Ø*
C31*
C32*
C39.Ø
C41.1
C44.Ø*
C46.2
C73
C76.Ø
C77.Ø
C81.Ø1
C81.11
C81.21
C81.31
C81.41
C81.71
C81.91
C82.Ø1
C82.11
C82.21
C82.31
C82.41
C82.51
C82.61
C82.81
C82.91
C83.Ø1
C83.31
C83.51
C83.71
C83.81
C83.91
C84.Ø1
C84.11
C84.91
C84.A1
C84.Z1
C85.11
C85.21
C85.81
C85.91
C86.Ø
C91.4Ø
C96.Ø
C96.2*
C96.9
C96.A
DØØ.Ø*
DØ2.Ø
D1Ø*
D11*
D14.Ø
D14.1
D16.4
D16.5
D18.ØØ
D18.Ø1
D18.Ø9
D34
D37.Ø*
D38.Ø
EØ3.4
EØ4.1
EØ5*
EØ6*
EØ7.89
EØ7.9
E35
G47.2*
G47.3*
G47.5*
G47.6*
G47.8
JØØ
JØ2*
JØ3*
JØ4.Ø
JØ4.2
JØ4.3*
JØ5*
JØ6*
J31.1
J31.2
J34.2
J35.Ø*
J35.1
J35.2
J35.3
J35.8
J35.9
J36
J37.Ø
J37.1
J38.Ø*
J38.1
J38.2
J38.3
J38.4
J38.5
J38.6
J38.7
J39.Ø
J39.1
J39.2
J39.3
J39.8
J39.9
J95.Ø*
J98.Ø*
KØØ*
KØ1*
KØ2.3
KØ2.5*
KØ2.6*
KØ2.7
KØ2.9
KØ3*
KØ4*
KØ5*
KØ6*
KØ8.Ø
KØ8.1*
KØ8.2*
KØ8.3
KØ8.4*
KØ8.5*
KØ8.8*
KØ8.9
KØ9*
K11*
K12.Ø
K12.1
K12.2
K12.3*
K13.Ø
K13.1
K13.2*
K13.3
K13.4
K13.5
K13.6
K13.7*
K14.Ø
K14.1
K14.2
K14.3
K14.4
K14.5
K14.6
K14.8
K14.9
LØ2.Ø1
LØ2.11
LØ3.2*
M26.Ø*
M26.1*
M26.2*
M26.3*
M26.4
M26.5*
M26.6*
M26.7*
M26.8*
M26.9
M27.Ø
M27.1
M27.2
M27.3
M27.4*
M27.5*
M27.6*
M27.8
M27.9
Q31.Ø
Q31.1
Q31.2
Q31.3
Q31.5
Q31.8
Q31.9
Q32.Ø
Q32.1
Q32.2
Q32.3
Q32.4
Q35.1
Q35.3
Q35.5
Q35.7
Q35.9
Q36.Ø
Q36.1
Q36.9
Q37.Ø
Q37.1
Q37.2
Q37.3
Q37.4
Q37.5
Q37.8
Q37.9
Q38.Ø
Q38.1
Q38.2
Q38.3
Q38.4
Q38.6
Q38.7
Q38.8
RØ4.1
R68.2
R68.84
SØ1.2ØXA
SØ1.21XA
SØ1.22XA
SØ1.23XA
SØ1.24XA
SØ1.25XA
SØ1.4Ø1A
SØ1.4Ø2A
SØ1.4Ø9A
SØ1.411A
SØ1.412A
SØ1.419A
SØ1.421A
SØ1.422A
SØ1.429A
SØ1.431A
SØ1.432A
SØ1.439A
SØ1.441A
SØ1.442A
SØ1.449A
SØ1.451A
SØ1.452A
SØ1.459A
SØ1.5Ø1A
SØ1.5Ø2A
SØ1.511A
SØ1.512A
SØ1.521A
SØ1.522A
SØ1.531A
SØ1.532A
SØ1.541A
SØ1.542A
SØ1.551A
SØ1.552A
SØ2.3ØXA
SØ2.3ØXB
SØ2.31XA
SØ2.31XB
SØ2.32XA
SØ2.32XB
SØ2.4ØØA
SØ2.4ØØB
SØ2.4Ø1A
SØ2.4Ø1B
SØ2.4Ø2A
SØ2.4Ø2B
SØ2.4ØAA
SØ2.4ØAB
SØ2.4ØBA
SØ2.4ØBB
SØ2.4ØCA
SØ2.4ØCB
SØ2.4ØDA
SØ2.4ØDB
SØ2.4ØEA
SØ2.4ØEB
SØ2.4ØFA
SØ2.4ØFB
SØ2.411A
SØ2.411B
SØ2.412A
SØ2.412B
SØ2.413A
SØ2.413B
SØ2.42XA
SØ2.42XB
SØ2.6ØØA
SØ2.6ØØB
SØ2.6Ø1A
SØ2.6Ø1B
SØ2.6Ø2A
SØ2.6Ø2B
SØ2.6Ø9A
SØ2.6Ø9B
SØ2.61ØA
SØ2.61ØB
SØ2.611A
SØ2.611B
SØ2.612A
SØ2.612B
SØ2.62ØA
SØ2.62ØB
SØ2.621A
SØ2.621B
SØ2.622A
SØ2.622B
SØ2.63ØA
SØ2.63ØB
SØ2.631A
SØ2.631B
SØ2.632A
SØ2.632B
SØ2.64ØA
SØ2.64ØB
SØ2.641A
SØ2.641B
SØ2.642A
SØ2.642B
SØ2.65ØA
SØ2.65ØB
SØ2.651A
SØ2.651B
SØ2.652A
SØ2.652B
SØ2.66XA
SØ2.66XB
SØ2.67ØA
SØ2.67ØB
SØ2.671A
SØ2.671B
SØ2.672A
SØ2.672B
SØ2.69XA
SØ2.69XB
SØ2.8ØXA
SØ2.8ØXB
SØ2.81XA
SØ2.81XB
SØ2.82XA
SØ2.82XB
SØ2.831A
SØ2.831B
SØ2.832A
SØ2.832B
SØ2.839A
SØ2.839B
SØ2.841A
SØ2.841B
SØ2.842A
SØ2.842B
SØ2.849A
SØ2.849B
SØ2.85XA
SØ2.85XB
SØ2.92XA
SØ2.92XB
SØ3.ØØXA
SØ3.Ø1XA
SØ3.Ø2XA
SØ3.Ø3XA
SØ6.AØXA
SØ6.A1XA
SØ7.ØXXA
SØ7.1XXA
SØ7.8XXA
SØ7.9XXA
SØ8.811A
SØ8.812A
SØ9.ØXXA
SØ9.1ØXA
SØ9.11XA
SØ9.19XA
SØ9.8XXA
SØ9.9ØXA
SØ9.92XA
SØ9.93XA
S11.Ø11A
S11.Ø12A
S11.Ø13A
S11.Ø14A
S11.Ø15A
S11.Ø19A
S11.Ø21A
S11.Ø22A
S11.Ø23A
S11.Ø24A
S11.Ø25A
S11.Ø29A
S11.Ø31A
S11.Ø32A
S11.Ø33A
S11.Ø34A
S11.Ø35A
S11.Ø39A
S11.1ØXA
S11.11XA
S11.12XA
S11.13XA
S11.14XA
S11.15XA
S11.2ØXA
S11.21XA
S11.22XA
S11.23XA
S11.24XA
S11.25XA
S11.8ØXA
S11.81XA
S11.82XA
S11.83XA
S11.84XA
S11.85XA
S11.89XA
S11.9ØXA
S11.91XA
S11.92XA
S11.93XA
S11.94XA
S11.95XA
S12.8XXA
S15.1Ø1A
S15.1Ø2A
S15.1Ø9A
S15.111A
S15.112A
S15.119A
S15.121A
S15.122A
S15.129A
S15.191A
S15.192A
S15.199A
S15.8XXA
S15.9XXA
S16.2XXA
S16.8XXA
S16.9XXA
S17.ØXXA
S17.8XXA
S17.9XXA
S19.8ØXA
S19.81XA
S19.82XA
S19.83XA
S19.84XA
S19.85XA
S19.89XA
S19.9XXA
T17.2ØØA
T17.2Ø8A
T17.21ØA
T17.218A
T17.22ØA
T17.228A
T17.29ØA
T17.298A
T17.3ØØA
T17.3Ø8A
T17.31ØA
T17.318A
T17.32ØA
T17.328A
T17.39ØA
T17.398A
T18.ØXXA
T28.ØXXA
T28.5XXA
Z85.21
Z85.81Ø
Z85.818
Z85.819
AND EITHER
Tracheostomy Operating Room Procedures
ØB11ØF4

ØB11ØZ4
ØB114F4
ØB114Z4

OR

Nonoperating Room Procedures

ØB113F4
ØB113Z4

DRG 012

Select laryngectomy operating room procedures OR principal diagnosis AND tracheostomy operating or nonoperating room procedures listed under DRG 011

DRG 013

Select laryngectomy operating room procedures OR principal diagnosis AND tracheostomy operating or nonoperating room procedures listed under DRG 011

DRG 019

Principal or Secondary Diagnosis

EØ8*
EØ9*
E1Ø*
E11*
E13*
E89.1

AND

Principal or Secondary Diagnosis

I12.Ø
I13.11
I13.2
N18*
Z94.Ø
Z96.49
Z96.89
Z96.9

AND

Operating Room Procedures

ØTYØØZØ
ØTYØØZ1
ØTYØØZ2
ØTY1ØZØ
ØTY1ØZ1
ØTY1ØZ2

AND

Operating Room Procedures

ØFYG*

AND

Nonoperating Room Procedures

5A1D7ØZ
5A1D8ØZ
5A1D9ØZ

DRG 014

Non-Operating Room Procedures

3Ø233G2
3Ø233G3
3Ø233G4
3Ø233U2
3Ø233U3
3Ø233U4
3Ø233X2
3Ø233X3
3Ø233X4
3Ø233Y2
3Ø233Y3
3Ø233Y4
3Ø243G2
3Ø243G3
3Ø243G4
3Ø243U2
3Ø243U3
3Ø243U4
3Ø243X2
3Ø243X3
3Ø243X4
3Ø243Y2
3Ø243Y3
3Ø243Y4
XW133C8
XW143C8

DRG 016

Bone Marrow Transplant Nonoperating Room Procedures

3Ø233AZ
3Ø233CØ
3Ø233GØ
3Ø233XØ
3Ø233YØ
3Ø243AZ
3Ø243CØ
3Ø243GØ
3Ø243XØ
3Ø243YØ
XW133B8
XW133F8
XW133G8
XW133H9
XW133J8
XW143B8
XW143F8
XW143G8
XW143H9
XW143J8

DRG 017

Select nonoperating room procedures listed under DRG 016

DRG 018

Immunotherapy Nonoperating Room Procedures

XWØ3368
XWØ3378
XWØ33A7
XWØ33C7
XWØ33G7
XWØ33H7
XWØ33J7
XWØ33K7
XWØ33L7
XWØ33M7
XWØ33N7
XWØ4368
XWØ4378
XWØ43A7
XWØ43C7
XWØ43G7
XWØ43H7
XWØ43J7
XWØ43K7
XWØ43L7
XWØ43M7
XWØ43N7

MDC 1

DRG 020

Principal Diagnosis

I6Ø.Ø*
I6Ø.1*
I6Ø.2
I6Ø.3*
I6Ø.4
I6Ø.5*
I6Ø.6
I6Ø.7
I6Ø.8
I6Ø.9
I61.Ø
I61.1
I61.2
I61.3
I61.4
I61.5
I61.6
I61.8
I61.9
I62.Ø*
I62.1
I62.9

AND

Operating Room Procedures

Ø31HØ9G
Ø31HØAG
Ø31HØJG
Ø31HØKG
Ø31HØZG
Ø31JØ9G
Ø31JØAG
Ø31JØJG
Ø31JØKG
Ø31JØZG
Ø31SØ9G
Ø31SØAG
Ø31SØJG
Ø31SØKG
Ø31SØZG
Ø31TØ9G
Ø31TØAG
Ø31TØJG
Ø31TØKG
Ø31TØZG
Ø35GØZZ
Ø35G3ZZ
Ø35G4ZZ
Ø3BGØZZ
Ø3BG3ZZ
Ø3BG4ZZ
Ø3CGØZZ
Ø3CG4ZZ
Ø3LGØBZ
Ø3LGØCZ
Ø3LGØDZ
Ø3LGØZZ
Ø3LG3BZ
Ø3LG3CZ
Ø3LG3DZ
Ø3LG3ZZ
Ø3LG4BZ
Ø3LG4CZ
Ø3LG4DZ
Ø3LG4ZZ
Ø3LHØBZ
Ø3LHØDZ
Ø3LH3BZ
Ø3LH3DZ
Ø3LH4BZ
Ø3LH4DZ
Ø3LJØBZ
Ø3LJØDZ
Ø3LJ3BZ
Ø3LJ3DZ
Ø3LJ4BZ
Ø3LJ4DZ
Ø3LKØBZ
Ø3LKØCZ
Ø3LKØDZ
Ø3LKØZZ
Ø3LK3BZ
Ø3LK3CZ
Ø3LK3DZ
Ø3LK3ZZ
Ø3LK4BZ
Ø3LK4CZ
Ø3LK4DZ
Ø3LK4ZZ
Ø3LLØBZ
Ø3LLØCZ
Ø3LLØDZ
Ø3LLØZZ
Ø3LL3BZ
Ø3LL3CZ
Ø3LL3DZ
Ø3LL3ZZ
Ø3LL4BZ
Ø3LL4CZ
Ø3LL4DZ
Ø3LL4ZZ
Ø3LMØBZ
Ø3LMØDZ
Ø3LM3BZ
Ø3LM3DZ
Ø3LM4BZ
Ø3LM4DZ
Ø3LNØBZ
Ø3LNØDZ
Ø3LN3BZ
Ø3LN3DZ
Ø3LN4BZ
Ø3LN4DZ
Ø3LPØBZ
Ø3LPØDZ
Ø3LP3BZ
Ø3LP3DZ
Ø3LP4BZ
Ø3LP4DZ
Ø3LQØBZ
Ø3LQØDZ
Ø3LQ3BZ
Ø3LQ3DZ
Ø3LQ4BZ
Ø3LQ4DZ
Ø3LRØDZ
Ø3LR3DZ
Ø3LR4DZ
Ø3LSØDZ
Ø3LS3DZ
Ø3LS4DZ
Ø3LTØDZ
Ø3LT3DZ
Ø3LT4DZ
Ø3RGØ7Z
Ø3RGØJZ
Ø3RGØKZ
Ø3RG47Z
Ø3RG4JZ
Ø3RG4KZ
Ø3VGØBZ
Ø3VGØCZ
Ø3VGØDZ
Ø3VGØHZ
Ø3VGØZZ
Ø3VG3BZ
Ø3VG3CZ
Ø3VG3DZ
Ø3VG3HZ
Ø3VG3ZZ
Ø3VG4BZ
Ø3VG4CZ
Ø3VG4DZ
Ø3VG4HZ
Ø3VG4ZZ
Ø3VHØBZ
Ø3VHØDZ
Ø3VH3BZ
Ø3VH3DZ
Ø3VH4BZ
Ø3VH4DZ
Ø3VJØBZ
Ø3VJØDZ
Ø3VJ3BZ
Ø3VJ3DZ
Ø3VJ4BZ
Ø3VJ4DZ
Ø3VKØBZ
Ø3VKØCZ
Ø3VKØDZ
Ø3VK3BZ
Ø3VK3CZ
Ø3VK3DZ
Ø3VK4BZ
Ø3VK4CZ
Ø3VK4DZ
Ø3VLØBZ
Ø3VLØCZ
Ø3VLØDZ
Ø3VL3BZ
Ø3VL3CZ
Ø3VL3DZ
Ø3VL4BZ
Ø3VL4CZ
Ø3VL4DZ
Ø3VMØBZ
Ø3VMØDZ
Ø3VM3BZ
Ø3VM3DZ
Ø3VM4BZ
Ø3VM4DZ
Ø3VNØBZ
Ø3VNØDZ
Ø3VN3BZ
Ø3VN3DZ
Ø3VN4BZ
Ø3VN4DZ
Ø3VPØBZ
Ø3VPØDZ
Ø3VP3BZ
Ø3VP3DZ
Ø3VP4BZ
Ø3VP4DZ
Ø3VQØBZ
Ø3VQØDZ
Ø3VQ3BZ
Ø3VQ3DZ
Ø3VQ4BZ
Ø3VQ4DZ
Ø3VRØDZ
Ø3VR3DZ
Ø3VR4DZ
Ø3VSØDZ
Ø3VS3DZ
Ø3VS4DZ
Ø3VTØDZ
Ø3VT3DZ
Ø3VT4DZ
Ø3VUØDZ
Ø3VU3DZ
Ø3VU4DZ
Ø3VVØDZ
Ø3VV3DZ
Ø3VV4DZ
Ø55LØZZ
Ø55L3ZZ
Ø55L4ZZ
Ø5BLØZZ
Ø5BL3ZZ
Ø5BL4ZZ
Ø5CLØZZ
Ø5CL4ZZ
Ø5LLØCZ
Ø5LLØDZ
Ø5LLØZZ
Ø5LL3CZ
Ø5LL3DZ
Ø5LL3ZZ
Ø5LL4CZ
Ø5LL4DZ
Ø5LL4ZZ
Ø5RLØ7Z
Ø5RLØJZ
Ø5RLØKZ
Ø5RL47Z
Ø5RL4JZ
Ø5RL4KZ
Ø5VLØCZ
Ø5VLØDZ
Ø5VLØZZ
Ø5VL3CZ
Ø5VL3DZ
Ø5VL3ZZ
Ø5VL4CZ
Ø5VL4DZ
Ø5VL4ZZ

DRG 021

Select principal diagnosis AND operating room procedures listed under DRG 020

DRG 022

Select principal diagnosis AND operating room procedures listed under DRG 020

DRG 023

Craniotomy Operating Room Procedures

ØØ16Ø7A
ØØ16Ø7B
ØØ16ØJA
ØØ16ØJB
ØØ16ØKA
ØØ16ØKB
ØØ16ØZB
ØØ1637A
ØØ1637B
ØØ163JA
ØØ163JB
ØØ163KA
ØØ163KB
ØØ163ZB
ØØ1647A
ØØ1647B
ØØ164JA
ØØ164JB
ØØ164KA
ØØ164KB
ØØ164ZB
ØØ5ØØZZ
ØØ5Ø3ZZ
ØØ5Ø4ZZ
ØØ51*
ØØ52*
ØØ56*
ØØ57*
ØØ58*
ØØ59*
ØØ5A*
ØØ5B*
ØØ5C*
ØØ5D*
ØØ76ØZZ
ØØ763ZZ
ØØ764ZZ
ØØ8Ø*
ØØ87*
ØØ88*
ØØ8P*
ØØ9ØØØZ
ØØ9ØØZX
ØØ9ØØZZ
ØØ9Ø3ØZ
ØØ9Ø3ZZ
ØØ9Ø4ØZ
ØØ9Ø4ZZ
ØØ91ØØZ
ØØ91ØZX
ØØ91ØZZ
ØØ913ØZ
ØØ913ZZ
ØØ914ØZ
ØØ914ZZ
ØØ92ØØZ
ØØ92ØZX
ØØ92ØZZ
ØØ923ØZ
ØØ923ZZ
ØØ924ØZ
ØØ924ZZ
ØØ93ØØZ
ØØ93ØZX
ØØ93ØZZ
ØØ933ØZ
ØØ933ZZ
ØØ934ØZ
ØØ934ZZ
ØØ94ØØZ
ØØ94ØZX
ØØ94ØZZ
ØØ943ØZ
ØØ943ZZ
ØØ944ØZ
ØØ944ZZ
ØØ95ØØZ
ØØ95ØZX
ØØ95ØZZ
ØØ953ØZ
ØØ953ZZ
ØØ954ØZ
ØØ954ZZ
ØØ96ØØZ
ØØ96ØZX
ØØ96ØZZ
ØØ963ØZ
ØØ963ZZ
ØØ964ØZ
ØØ964ZZ
ØØ97ØØZ
ØØ97ØZX
ØØ97ØZZ
ØØ973ØZ
ØØ973ZZ
ØØ974ØZ
ØØ974ZZ
ØØ98ØØZ
ØØ98ØZX
ØØ98ØZZ
ØØ983ØZ
ØØ983ZZ
ØØ984ØZ
ØØ984ZZ
ØØ99ØØZ
ØØ99ØZX
ØØ99ØZZ
ØØ993ØZ
ØØ993ZZ
ØØ994ØZ
ØØ994ZZ
ØØ9AØØZ
ØØ9AØZX
ØØ9AØZZ
ØØ9A3ØZ
ØØ9A3ZZ
ØØ9A4ØZ
ØØ9A4ZZ
ØØ9BØØZ
ØØ9BØZX
ØØ9BØZZ
ØØ9B3ØZ
ØØ9B3ZZ
ØØ9B4ØZ
ØØ9B4ZZ
ØØ9CØØZ
ØØ9CØZX
ØØ9CØZZ
ØØ9C3ØZ
ØØ9C3ZZ
ØØ9C4ØZ
ØØ9C4ZZ
ØØ9DØØZ
ØØ9DØZX
ØØ9DØZZ
ØØ9D3ØZ
ØØ9D3ZZ
ØØ9D4ØZ
ØØ9D4ZZ
ØØBØØZX
ØØBØØZZ
ØØBØ3ZX
ØØBØ3ZZ
ØØBØ4ZX
ØØBØ4ZZ
ØØB1ØZX
ØØB1ØZZ
ØØB13ZX
ØØB13ZZ
ØØB14ZX
ØØB14ZZ
ØØB2ØZX
ØØB2ØZZ
ØØB23ZX
ØØB23ZZ
ØØB24ZX
ØØB24ZZ
ØØB6ØZX
ØØB6ØZZ
ØØB63ZX
ØØB63ZZ
ØØB64ZX
ØØB64ZZ
ØØB7ØZX
ØØB7ØZZ
ØØB73ZX
ØØB73ZZ
ØØB74ZX
ØØB74ZZ
ØØB8ØZX
ØØB8ØZZ
ØØB83ZX
ØØB83ZZ
ØØB84ZX
ØØB84ZZ
ØØB9ØZX
ØØB9ØZZ
ØØB93ZX
ØØB93ZZ
ØØB94ZX
ØØB94ZZ
ØØBAØZX
ØØBAØZZ
ØØBA3ZX
ØØBA3ZZ
ØØBA4ZX
ØØBA4ZZ
ØØBBØZX
ØØBBØZZ
ØØBB3ZX
ØØBB3ZZ
ØØBB4ZX
ØØBB4ZZ
ØØBCØZX
ØØBCØZZ
ØØBC3ZX
ØØBC3ZZ
ØØBC4ZX
ØØBC4ZZ
ØØBDØZX
ØØBDØZZ
ØØBD3ZX
ØØBD3ZZ
ØØBD4ZX
ØØBD4ZZ
ØØBNØZZ
ØØCØØZZ
ØØCØ3ZZ
ØØCØ4ZZ
ØØC1ØZZ
ØØC13ZZ
ØØC14ZZ
ØØC2ØZZ
ØØC23ZZ
ØØC24ZZ
ØØC3ØZZ
ØØC33ZZ
ØØC34ZZ
ØØC4ØZZ
ØØC43ZZ
ØØC44ZZ
ØØC5ØZZ
ØØC53ZZ
ØØC54ZZ
ØØC6ØZZ
ØØC63ZZ
ØØC64ZZ
ØØC7ØZZ
ØØC73ZZ
ØØC74ZZ
ØØC8ØZZ
ØØC83ZZ
ØØC84ZZ
ØØC9ØZZ
ØØC93ZZ
ØØC94ZZ
ØØCAØZZ
ØØCA3ZZ
ØØCA4ZZ
ØØCBØZZ
ØØCB3ZZ
ØØCB4ZZ
ØØCCØZZ
ØØCC3ZZ
ØØCC4ZZ
ØØCDØZZ
ØØCD3ZZ
ØØCD4ZZ
ØØDØØZZ
ØØDØ3ZZ
ØØDØ4ZZ
ØØD1ØZZ
ØØD13ZZ
ØØD14ZZ
ØØD2ØZZ
ØØD23ZZ
ØØD24ZZ
ØØD7ØZZ
ØØD73ZZ
ØØD74ZZ
ØØDCØZZ
ØØDC3ZZ
ØØDC4ZZ
ØØF3ØZZ
ØØF33ZZ
ØØF34ZZ
ØØF4ØZZ
ØØF43ZZ
ØØF44ZZ
ØØF5ØZZ
ØØF53ZZ
ØØF54ZZ
ØØF6ØZZ
ØØF63ZZ
ØØF64ZZ
ØØHØØ1Z
ØØHØØ2Z
ØØHØØ3Z
ØØHØØMZ
ØØHØØYZ
ØØHØ31Z
ØØHØ32Z
ØØHØ33Z
ØØHØ3MZ
ØØHØ3YZ
ØØHØ41Z
ØØHØ42Z
ØØHØ43Z
ØØHØ4MZ
ØØHØ4YZ
ØØH6Ø1Z
ØØH6Ø2Z
ØØH6Ø3Z
ØØH6ØMZ
ØØH6ØYZ
ØØH631Z
ØØH632Z
ØØH633Z
ØØH63MZ
ØØH63YZ
ØØH641Z
ØØH642Z
ØØH643Z
ØØH64MZ
ØØH64YZ
ØØJØØZZ
ØØJØ4ZZ
ØØKØØZZ
ØØKØ3ZZ
ØØKØ4ZZ
ØØK7ØZZ
ØØK73ZZ
ØØK74ZZ
ØØK8ØZZ
ØØK83ZZ
ØØK84ZZ
ØØK9ØZZ
ØØK93ZZ
ØØK94ZZ
ØØKAØZZ
ØØKA3ZZ
ØØKA4ZZ
ØØKBØZZ
ØØKB3ZZ
ØØKB4ZZ
ØØKCØZZ
ØØKC3ZZ
ØØKC4ZZ
ØØKDØZZ
ØØKD3ZZ
ØØKD4ZZ
ØØNØØZZ
ØØNØ3ZZ
ØØNØ4ZZ
ØØN1ØZZ
ØØN13ZZ
ØØN14ZZ
ØØN2ØZZ
ØØN23ZZ
ØØN24ZZ
ØØN6ØZZ
ØØN63ZZ
ØØN64ZZ
ØØN7ØZZ
ØØN73ZZ
ØØN74ZZ
ØØN8ØZZ
ØØN83ZZ
ØØN84ZZ
ØØN9ØZZ
ØØN93ZZ
ØØN94ZZ
ØØNAØZZ
ØØNA3ZZ
ØØNA4ZZ
ØØNBØZZ
ØØNB3ZZ
ØØNB4ZZ
ØØNCØZZ
ØØNC3ZZ
ØØNC4ZZ

ØØNDØZZ
ØØND3ZZ
ØØND4ZZ
ØØNKØZZ
ØØNK3ZZ
ØØNK4ZZ
ØØPØØØZ
ØØPØØ2Z
ØØPØØ3Z
ØØPØØ7Z
ØØPØØJZ
ØØPØØKZ
ØØPØØMZ
ØØPØØYZ
ØØPØ37Z
ØØPØ3JZ
ØØPØ3KZ
ØØPØ3MZ
ØØPØ4ØZ
ØØPØ42Z
ØØPØ43Z
ØØPØ47Z
ØØPØ4JZ
ØØPØ4KZ
ØØPØ4MZ
ØØP6ØØZ
ØØP6Ø2Z
ØØP6Ø3Z
ØØP6ØMZ
ØØP6ØYZ
ØØP63MZ
ØØP64ØZ
ØØP642Z
ØØP643Z
ØØP64MZ
ØØQØØZZ
ØØQØ3ZZ
ØØQØ4ZZ
ØØQ1ØZZ
ØØQ13ZZ
ØØQ14ZZ
ØØQ2ØZZ
ØØQ23ZZ
ØØQ24ZZ
ØØQ6ØZZ
ØØQ63ZZ
ØØQ64ZZ
ØØQ7ØZZ
ØØQ73ZZ
ØØQ74ZZ
ØØQ8ØZZ
ØØQ83ZZ
ØØQ84ZZ
ØØQ9ØZZ
ØØQ93ZZ
ØØQ94ZZ
ØØQAØZZ
ØØQA3ZZ
ØØQA4ZZ
ØØQBØZZ
ØØQB3ZZ
ØØQB4ZZ
ØØQCØZZ
ØØQC3ZZ
ØØQC4ZZ
ØØQDØZZ
ØØQD3ZZ
ØØQD4ZZ
ØØR1Ø7Z
ØØR1ØJZ
ØØR1ØKZ
ØØR147Z
ØØR14JZ
ØØR14KZ
ØØR2Ø7Z
ØØR2ØJZ
ØØR2ØKZ
ØØR247Z
ØØR24JZ
ØØR24KZ
ØØR6Ø7Z
ØØR6ØJZ
ØØR6ØKZ
ØØR647Z
ØØR64JZ
ØØR64KZ
ØØT7ØZZ
ØØT73ZZ
ØØT74ZZ
ØØU1Ø7Z
ØØU1ØJZ
ØØU1ØKZ
ØØU137Z
ØØU13JZ
ØØU13KZ
ØØU147Z
ØØU14JZ
ØØU14KZ
ØØU2Ø7Z
ØØU2ØJZ
ØØU2ØKZ
ØØU237Z
ØØU23JZ
ØØU23KZ
ØØU247Z
ØØU24JZ
ØØU24KZ
ØØU6Ø7Z
ØØU6ØJZ
ØØU6ØKZ
ØØU637Z
ØØU63JZ
ØØU63KZ
ØØU647Z
ØØU64JZ
ØØU64KZ
ØØWØØØZ
ØØWØØ2Z
ØØWØØ3Z
ØØWØØ7Z
ØØWØØJZ
ØØWØØKZ
ØØWØØMZ
ØØWØØYZ
ØØWØ3ØZ
ØØWØ32Z
ØØWØ33Z
ØØWØ37Z
ØØWØ3JZ
ØØWØ3KZ
ØØWØ3MZ
ØØWØ4ØZ
ØØWØ42Z
ØØWØ43Z
ØØWØ47Z
ØØWØ4JZ
ØØWØ4KZ
ØØWØ4MZ
ØØW6ØØZ
ØØW6Ø2Z
ØØW6Ø3Z
ØØW6ØMZ
ØØW6ØYZ
ØØW63ØZ
ØØW632Z
ØØW633Z
ØØW63MZ
ØØW64ØZ
ØØW642Z
ØØW643Z
ØØW64MZ
Ø31HØ9G
Ø31HØAG
Ø31HØJG
Ø31HØKG
Ø31HØZG
Ø31JØ9G
Ø31JØAG
Ø31JØJG
Ø31JØKG
Ø31JØZG
Ø31SØ9G
Ø31SØAG
Ø31SØJG
Ø31SØKG
Ø31SØZG
Ø31TØ9G
Ø31TØAG
Ø31TØJG
Ø31TØKG
Ø31TØZG
Ø35GØZZ
Ø35G3ZZ
Ø35G4ZZ
Ø37G34Z
Ø37G35Z
Ø37G36Z
Ø37G37Z
Ø37G3DZ
Ø37G3EZ
Ø37G3FZ
Ø37G3GZ
Ø37G3ZZ
Ø37G44Z
Ø37G45Z
Ø37G46Z
Ø37G47Z
Ø37G4DZ
Ø37G4EZ
Ø37G4FZ
Ø37G4GZ
Ø37G4ZZ
Ø3BGØZZ
Ø3BG3ZZ
Ø3BG4ZZ
Ø3CGØZZ
Ø3CG3Z7
Ø3CG3ZZ
Ø3CG4ZZ
Ø3CH3Z7
Ø3CH3ZZ
Ø3CH4ZZ
Ø3CJ3Z7
Ø3CJ3ZZ
Ø3CJ4ZZ
Ø3CK3Z7
Ø3CK3ZZ
Ø3CK4ZZ
Ø3CL3Z7
Ø3CL3ZZ
Ø3CL4ZZ
Ø3CM3Z7
Ø3CM3ZZ
Ø3CM4ZZ
Ø3CN3Z7
Ø3CN3ZZ
Ø3CN4ZZ
Ø3CP3Z7
Ø3CP3ZZ
Ø3CP4ZZ
Ø3CQ3Z7
Ø3CQ3ZZ
Ø3CQ4ZZ
Ø3CR3ZZ
Ø3CR4ZZ
Ø3CS3ZZ
Ø3CS4ZZ
Ø3CT3ZZ
Ø3CT4ZZ
Ø3CU3ZZ
Ø3CU4ZZ
Ø3CV3ZZ
Ø3CV4ZZ
Ø3LGØBZ
Ø3LGØCZ
Ø3LGØDZ
Ø3LGØZZ
Ø3LG3BZ
Ø3LG3CZ
Ø3LG3DZ
Ø3LG3ZZ
Ø3LG4BZ
Ø3LG4CZ
Ø3LG4DZ
Ø3LG4ZZ
Ø3LHØBZ
Ø3LHØDZ
Ø3LH3BZ
Ø3LH3DZ
Ø3LH4BZ
Ø3LH4DZ
Ø3LJØBZ
Ø3LJØDZ
Ø3LJ3BZ
Ø3LJ3DZ
Ø3LJ4BZ
Ø3LJ4DZ
Ø3LKØBZ
Ø3LKØCZ
Ø3LKØDZ
Ø3LKØZZ
Ø3LK3BZ
Ø3LK3CZ
Ø3LK3DZ
Ø3LK3ZZ
Ø3LK4BZ
Ø3LK4CZ
Ø3LK4DZ
Ø3LK4ZZ
Ø3LLØBZ
Ø3LLØCZ
Ø3LLØDZ
Ø3LLØZZ
Ø3LL3BZ
Ø3LL3CZ
Ø3LL3DZ
Ø3LL3ZZ
Ø3LL4BZ
Ø3LL4CZ
Ø3LL4DZ
Ø3LL4ZZ
Ø3LMØBZ
Ø3LMØDZ
Ø3LM3BZ
Ø3LM3DZ
Ø3LM4BZ
Ø3LM4DZ
Ø3LNØBZ
Ø3LNØDZ
Ø3LN3BZ
Ø3LN3DZ
Ø3LN4BZ
Ø3LN4DZ
Ø3LPØBZ
Ø3LPØDZ
Ø3LP3BZ
Ø3LP3DZ
Ø3LP4BZ
Ø3LP4DZ
Ø3LQØBZ
Ø3LQØDZ
Ø3LQ3BZ
Ø3LQ3DZ
Ø3LQ4BZ
Ø3LQ4DZ
Ø3LRØDZ
Ø3LR3DZ
Ø3LR4DZ
Ø3LSØDZ
Ø3LS3DZ
Ø3LS4DZ
Ø3LTØDZ
Ø3LT3DZ
Ø3LT4DZ
Ø3RGØ7Z
Ø3RGØJZ
Ø3RGØKZ
Ø3RG47Z
Ø3RG4JZ
Ø3RG4KZ
Ø3VGØBZ
Ø3VGØCZ
Ø3VGØDZ
Ø3VGØHZ
Ø3VGØZZ
Ø3VG3BZ
Ø3VG3CZ
Ø3VG3DZ
Ø3VG3HZ
Ø3VG3ZZ
Ø3VG4BZ
Ø3VG4CZ
Ø3VG4DZ
Ø3VG4HZ
Ø3VG4ZZ
Ø3VHØBZ
Ø3VHØDZ
Ø3VH3BZ
Ø3VH3DZ
Ø3VH4BZ
Ø3VH4DZ
Ø3VJØBZ
Ø3VJØDZ
Ø3VJ3BZ
Ø3VJ3DZ
Ø3VJ4BZ
Ø3VJ4DZ
Ø3VKØBZ
Ø3VKØCZ
Ø3VKØDZ
Ø3VK3BZ
Ø3VK3CZ
Ø3VK3DZ
Ø3VK4BZ
Ø3VK4CZ
Ø3VK4DZ
Ø3VLØBZ
Ø3VLØCZ
Ø3VLØDZ
Ø3VL3BZ
Ø3VL3CZ
Ø3VL3DZ
Ø3VL4BZ
Ø3VL4CZ
Ø3VL4DZ
Ø3VMØBZ
Ø3VMØDZ
Ø3VM3BZ
Ø3VM3DZ
Ø3VM4BZ
Ø3VM4DZ
Ø3VNØBZ
Ø3VNØDZ
Ø3VN3BZ
Ø3VN3DZ
Ø3VN4BZ
Ø3VN4DZ
Ø3VPØBZ
Ø3VPØDZ
Ø3VP3BZ
Ø3VP3DZ
Ø3VP4BZ
Ø3VP4DZ
Ø3VQØBZ
Ø3VQØDZ
Ø3VQ3BZ
Ø3VQ3DZ
Ø3VQ4BZ
Ø3VQ4DZ
Ø3VRØDZ
Ø3VR3DZ
Ø3VR4DZ
Ø3VSØDZ
Ø3VS3DZ
Ø3VS4DZ
Ø3VTØDZ
Ø3VT3DZ
Ø3VT4DZ
Ø3VUØDZ
Ø3VU3DZ
Ø3VU4DZ
Ø3VVØDZ
Ø3VV3DZ
Ø3VV4DZ
Ø55LØZZ
Ø55L3ZZ
Ø55L4ZZ
Ø57L3DZ
Ø57L4DZ
Ø5BLØZZ
Ø5BL3ZZ
Ø5BL4ZZ
Ø5CLØZZ
Ø5CL3ZZ
Ø5CL4ZZ
Ø5LLØCZ
Ø5LLØDZ
Ø5LLØZZ
Ø5LL3CZ
Ø5LL3DZ
Ø5LL3ZZ
Ø5LL4CZ
Ø5LL4DZ
Ø5LL4ZZ
Ø5RLØ7Z
Ø5RLØJZ
Ø5RLØKZ
Ø5RL47Z
Ø5RL4JZ
Ø5RL4KZ
Ø5VLØCZ
Ø5VLØDZ
Ø5VLØZZ
Ø5VL3CZ
Ø5VL3DZ
Ø5VL3ZZ
Ø5VL4CZ
Ø5VL4DZ
Ø5VL4ZZ
ØG5ØØZ3
ØG5ØØZZ
ØG5Ø3Z3
ØG5Ø3ZZ
ØG5Ø4Z3
ØG5Ø4ZZ
ØG51ØZ3
ØG51ØZZ
ØG513Z3
ØG513ZZ
ØG514Z3
ØG514ZZ
ØG8ØØZZ
ØG8Ø3ZZ
ØG8Ø4ZZ
ØG9ØØØZ
ØG9ØØZX
ØG9ØØZZ
ØG9Ø3ZX
ØG9Ø4ØZ
ØG9Ø4ZX
ØG9Ø4ZZ
ØG91ØØZ
ØG91ØZX
ØG91ØZZ
ØG913ZX
ØG914ØZ
ØG914ZX
ØG914ZZ
ØGBØØZX
ØGBØØZZ
ØGBØ3ZX
ØGBØ3ZZ
ØGBØ4ZX
ØGBØ4ZZ
ØGB1ØZX
ØGB1ØZZ
ØGB13ZX
ØGB13ZZ
ØGB14ZX
ØGB14ZZ
ØGCØØZZ
ØGCØ3ZZ
ØGCØ4ZZ
ØGC1ØZZ
ØGC13ZZ
ØGC14ZZ
ØGJØØZZ
ØGJØ4ZZ
ØGJ1ØZZ
ØGJ14ZZ
ØGNØØZZ
ØGNØ3ZZ
ØGNØ4ZZ
ØGN1ØZZ
ØGN13ZZ
ØGN14ZZ
ØGPØØØZ
ØGPØ3ØZ
ØGPØ4ØZ
ØGP1ØØZ
ØGP13ØZ
ØGP14ØZ
ØGQØØZZ
ØGQØ3ZZ
ØGQØ4ZZ
ØGQ1ØZZ
ØGQ13ZZ
ØGQ14ZZ
ØGTØØZZ
ØGTØ4ZZ
ØGT1ØZZ
ØGT14ZZ
ØGWØØØZ
ØGWØ3ØZ
ØGWØ4ØZ
ØGW1ØØZ
ØGW13ØZ
ØGW14ØZ
ØN5ØØZZ
ØN5Ø3ZZ
ØN5Ø4ZZ
ØN51ØZZ
ØN513ZZ
ØN514ZZ
ØN53ØZZ
ØN533ZZ
ØN534ZZ
ØN54ØZZ
ØN543ZZ
ØN544ZZ
ØN55ØZZ
ØN553ZZ
ØN554ZZ
ØN56ØZZ
ØN563ZZ
ØN564ZZ
ØN57ØZZ
ØN573ZZ
ØN574ZZ
ØN8ØØZZ
ØN8Ø3ZZ
ØN8Ø4ZZ
ØN81ØZZ
ØN813ZZ
ØN814ZZ
ØN83ØZZ
ØN833ZZ
ØN834ZZ
ØN84ØZZ
ØN843ZZ
ØN844ZZ
ØN85ØZZ
ØN853ZZ
ØN854ZZ
ØN86ØZZ
ØN863ZZ
ØN864ZZ
ØN87ØZZ
ØN873ZZ
ØN874ZZ
ØN9ØØØZ
ØN9ØØZX
ØN9ØØZZ
ØN9Ø3ZX
ØN9Ø4ØZ
ØN9Ø4ZX
ØN9Ø4ZZ
ØN91ØØZ
ØN91ØZX
ØN91ØZZ
ØN913ZX
ØN914ØZ
ØN914ZX
ØN914ZZ
ØN93ØØZ
ØN93ØZX
ØN93ØZZ
ØN933ZX
ØN934ØZ
ØN934ZX
ØN934ZZ
ØN94ØØZ
ØN94ØZX
ØN94ØZZ
ØN943ZX
ØN944ØZ
ØN944ZX
ØN944ZZ
ØN95ØØZ
ØN95ØZX
ØN95ØZZ
ØN953ZX
ØN954ØZ
ØN954ZX
ØN954ZZ
ØN96ØØZ
ØN96ØZX
ØN96ØZZ
ØN963ZX
ØN964ØZ
ØN964ZX
ØN964ZZ
ØN97ØØZ
ØN97ØZX
ØN97ØZZ
ØN973ZX
ØN974ØZ
ØN974ZX
ØN974ZZ
ØNBØ*
ØNB1*
ØNB3*
ØNB4*
ØNB5*
ØNB6*
ØNB7*
ØNC1*
ØNC3*
ØNC4*
ØNC5*
ØNC6*
ØNC7*
ØNHØØ3Z
ØNHØØ4Z
ØNHØØMZ
ØNHØ33Z
ØNHØ34Z
ØNHØ3MZ
ØNHØ43Z
ØNHØ44Z
ØNHØ4MZ
ØNH1*
ØNH3*
ØNH4*
ØNH5Ø4Z
ØNH534Z
ØNH544Z
ØNH6Ø4Z
ØNH634Z
ØNH644Z
ØNH7*
ØNJØØZZ
ØNJØ4ZZ
ØNN1*
ØNN3*
ØNN4*
ØNN5*
ØNN6*
ØNN7*
ØNPØØØZ
ØNPØØ3Z
ØNPØØ4Z
ØNPØØ5Z
ØNPØØ7Z
ØNPØØJZ
ØNPØØKZ
ØNPØØMZ
ØNPØØSZ
ØNPØ3ØZ
ØNPØ33Z
ØNPØ34Z
ØNPØ37Z
ØNPØ3JZ
ØNPØ3KZ
ØNPØ3MZ
ØNPØ3SZ
ØNPØ4ØZ
ØNPØ43Z
ØNPØ44Z
ØNPØ47Z
ØNPØ4JZ
ØNPØ4KZ
ØNPØ4MZ
ØNPØ4SZ
ØNPØX4Z
ØNPØXMZ
ØNPØXSZ
ØNQØØZZ
ØNQØ3ZZ
ØNQØ4ZZ
ØNQ1ØZZ
ØNQ13ZZ
ØNQ14ZZ
ØNQ3ØZZ
ØNQ33ZZ
ØNQ34ZZ
ØNQ4ØZZ
ØNQ43ZZ
ØNQ44ZZ
ØNQ5ØZZ
ØNQ53ZZ
ØNQ54ZZ
ØNQ6ØZZ
ØNQ63ZZ
ØNQ64ZZ
ØNQ7ØZZ
ØNQ73ZZ
ØNQ74ZZ
ØNRØ*
ØNR1*
ØNR3*
ØNR4*
ØNR5*
ØNR6*
ØNR7*
ØNSØØ4Z
ØNSØØ5Z
ØNSØØZZ
ØNSØ34Z
ØNSØ35Z
ØNSØ3ZZ
ØNSØ44Z
ØNSØ45Z
ØNSØ4ZZ
ØNS1Ø4Z
ØNS1ØZZ
ØNS134Z
ØNS13ZZ
ØNS144Z
ØNS14ZZ
ØNS3Ø4Z
ØNS3ØZZ
ØNS334Z
ØNS33ZZ
ØNS344Z
ØNS34ZZ
ØNS4Ø4Z
ØNS4ØZZ
ØNS434Z
ØNS43ZZ
ØNS444Z
ØNS44ZZ
ØNS5Ø4Z
ØNS5ØZZ
ØNS534Z
ØNS53ZZ
ØNS544Z
ØNS54ZZ
ØNS6Ø4Z
ØNS6ØZZ
ØNS634Z
ØNS63ZZ
ØNS644Z
ØNS64ZZ
ØNS7Ø4Z
ØNS7ØZZ
ØNS734Z
ØNS73ZZ
ØNS744Z
ØNS74ZZ
ØNT1ØZZ
ØNT3ØZZ
ØNT4ØZZ
ØNT5ØZZ
ØNT6ØZZ
ØNT7ØZZ
ØNUØ*
ØNU1*
ØNU3Ø7Z
ØNU3ØJZ
ØNU3ØKZ
ØNU337Z
ØNU33JZ
ØNU33KZ
ØNU347Z
ØNU34JZ
ØNU34KZ
ØNU4*
ØNU5*
ØNU6*
ØNU7*
ØNWØØØZ
ØNWØØ3Z
ØNWØØ4Z
ØNWØØ5Z
ØNWØØ7Z
ØNWØØJZ
ØNWØØKZ
ØNWØØMZ
ØNWØØNZ
ØNWØØSZ
ØNWØ3ØZ
ØNWØ33Z
ØNWØ34Z
ØNWØ35Z
ØNWØ37Z
ØNWØ3JZ
ØNWØ3KZ
ØNWØ3MZ
ØNWØ3SZ
ØNWØ4ØZ
ØNWØ43Z
ØNWØ44Z
ØNWØ45Z
ØNWØ47Z
ØNWØ4JZ
ØNWØ4KZ
ØNWØ4MZ
ØNWØ4SZ
ØW31ØZZ
ØW313ZZ
ØW314ZZ
ØW91ØØZ
ØW91ØZX
ØW91ØZZ
ØWC1ØZZ
ØWC13ZZ
ØWC14ZZ
ØWF1ØZZ
ØWF13ZZ
ØWF14ZZ
ØWH1ØYZ
ØWH13YZ
ØWH14YZ
ØWJ1ØZZ
ØWJ14ZZ
ØWP1ØØZ
ØWP1Ø1Z
ØWP1ØJZ
ØWP1ØYZ
ØWP13ØZ
ØWP131Z
ØWP13JZ
ØWP13YZ
ØWP14ØZ
ØWP141Z
ØWP14JZ
ØWP14YZ
ØWW1ØØZ
ØWW1Ø1Z
ØWW1Ø3Z
ØWW1ØJZ
ØWW1ØYZ
ØWW13ØZ
ØWW131Z
ØWW133Z
ØWW13JZ
ØWW13YZ
ØWW14ØZ
ØWW141Z
ØWW143Z
ØWW14JZ
ØWW14YZ
XNR8ØD9

AND

Acute Complex CNS Principal Diagnosis

AØ2.21
AØ6.6
A17.Ø
A17.1
A17.8*
A27.8*
A39.Ø
A39.81

A51.41
A52.13
A52.14
A54.81
A8Ø.Ø
A8Ø.1
A8Ø.2
A8Ø.3*
A8Ø.9
A82.Ø
A82.1
A82.9
A83.Ø
A83.1
A83.2
A83.3
A83.4
A83.5
A83.6
A83.8
A83.9
A84.Ø
A84.1
A84.8*
A84.9
A85.2
A92.2
BØØ.3
BØØ.4
BØØ.82
BØ1.12
BØ2.24
BØ5.Ø
B1Ø.Ø*
B26.1
B26.2
B37.5
B38.4
B45.1
B58.2
GØØ.Ø
GØØ.1
GØØ.2
GØØ.3
GØØ.8
GØØ.9
GØ1
GØ2
GØ4.Ø*
GØ4.2
GØ4.3*
GØ4.8*
GØ4.9*
GØ5.3
GØ5.4
GØ6.Ø
GØ6.1
GØ6.2
GØ7
GØ8
G37.3
G37.4
G92*
I6Ø.Ø*
I6Ø.1*
I6Ø.2
I6Ø.3*
I6Ø.4
I6Ø.5*
I6Ø.6
I6Ø.7
I6Ø.8
I6Ø.9
I61.Ø
I61.1
I61.2
I61.3
I61.4
I61.5
I61.6
I61.8
I61.9
I62.9
I63.Ø*
I63.1*
I63.2*
I63.3*
I63.4*
I63.5*
I63.6
I63.81
I63.89
I63.9
SØ6.31ØA
SØ6.311A
SØ6.312A
SØ6.313A
SØ6.314A
SØ6.315A
SØ6.316A
SØ6.317A
SØ6.318A
SØ6.319A
SØ6.31AA
SØ6.32ØA
SØ6.321A
SØ6.322A
SØ6.323A
SØ6.324A
SØ6.325A
SØ6.326A
SØ6.327A
SØ6.328A
SØ6.329A
SØ6.32AA
SØ6.33ØA
SØ6.331A
SØ6.332A
SØ6.333A
SØ6.334A
SØ6.335A
SØ6.336A
SØ6.337A
SØ6.338A
SØ6.339A
SØ6.33AA
SØ6.34ØA
SØ6.341A
SØ6.342A
SØ6.343A
SØ6.344A
SØ6.345A
SØ6.346A
SØ6.347A
SØ6.348A
SØ6.349A
SØ6.34AA
SØ6.35ØA
SØ6.351A
SØ6.352A
SØ6.353A
SØ6.354A
SØ6.355A
SØ6.356A
SØ6.357A
SØ6.358A
SØ6.359A
SØ6.35AA
SØ6.36ØA
SØ6.361A
SØ6.362A
SØ6.363A
SØ6.364A
SØ6.365A
SØ6.366A
SØ6.367A
SØ6.368A
SØ6.369A
SØ6.36AA
SØ6.37ØA
SØ6.371A
SØ6.372A
SØ6.373A
SØ6.374A
SØ6.375A
SØ6.376A
SØ6.377A
SØ6.378A
SØ6.379A
SØ6.37AA
SØ6.38ØA
SØ6.381A
SØ6.382A
SØ6.383A
SØ6.384A
SØ6.385A
SØ6.386A
SØ6.387A
SØ6.388A
SØ6.389A
SØ6.38AA
SØ6.6XØA
SØ6.6X1A
SØ6.6X2A
SØ6.6X3A
SØ6.6X4A
SØ6.6X5A
SØ6.6X6A
SØ6.6X7A
SØ6.6X8A
SØ6.6X9A
SØ6.6XAA

OR

The following major device procedure combinations

ØØHØØMZ
ØØHØ3MZ
ØØHØ4MZ
ØØH6ØMZ
ØØH63MZ
ØØH64MZ

AND

ØJH6ØDZ
ØJH6ØEZ
ØJH63DZ
ØJH63EZ
ØJH7ØDZ
ØJH7ØEZ
ØJH73DZ
ØJH73EZ
ØJH8ØDZ
ØJH8ØEZ
ØJH83DZ
ØJH83EZ
ØNHØØNZ

OR

Chemotherapy Implant Nonoperating Room Procedures

ØØHØØ4Z
3EØQØØ5
3EØQ3Ø5
3EØQ7Ø5

OR

Epilepsy Principal Diagnosis

G4Ø.Ø*
G4Ø.1Ø1
G4Ø.1Ø9
G4Ø.111
G4Ø.119
G4Ø.2*
G4Ø.3*
G4Ø.4*
G4Ø.5*
G4Ø.8*
G4Ø.9*
G4Ø.A*
G4Ø.B*
G4Ø.C*

AND

The following neurostimulator procedure combinations

ØNHØØNZ

AND

ØØHØØMZ
ØØHØ3MZ
ØØHØ4MZ

DRG 024

Select craniotomy operating room procedures listed under DRG 023

AND

Select acute complex CNS principal diagnosis listed under DRG 023

OR

Select major device procedure combinations listed under DRG 023

DRG 025

Operating Room Procedures

ØØ16Ø7A
ØØ16Ø7B
ØØ16ØJA
ØØ16ØJB
ØØ16ØKA
ØØ16ØKB
ØØ16ØZB
ØØ1637A
ØØ1637B
ØØ163JA
ØØ163JB
ØØ163KA
ØØ163KB
ØØ163ZB
ØØ1647A
ØØ1647B
ØØ164JA
ØØ164JB
ØØ164KA
ØØ164KB
ØØ164ZB
ØØ5ØØZ3
ØØ5ØØZZ
ØØ5Ø3Z3
ØØ5Ø3ZZ
ØØ5Ø4Z3
ØØ5Ø4ZZ
ØØ51ØZZ
ØØ513ZZ
ØØ514ZZ
ØØ52ØZZ
ØØ523ZZ
ØØ524ZZ
ØØ56ØZZ
ØØ563ZZ
ØØ564ZZ
ØØ57ØZZ
ØØ573ZZ
ØØ574ZZ
ØØ58ØZZ
ØØ583ZZ
ØØ584ZZ
ØØ59ØZZ
ØØ593ZZ
ØØ594ZZ
ØØ5AØZZ
ØØ5A3ZZ
ØØ5A4ZZ
ØØ5BØZZ
ØØ5B3ZZ
ØØ5B4ZZ
ØØ5CØZZ
ØØ5C3ZZ
ØØ5C4ZZ
ØØ5DØZZ
ØØ5D3ZZ
ØØ5D4ZZ
ØØ76ØZZ
ØØ763ZZ
ØØ764ZZ
ØØ8ØØZZ
ØØ8Ø3ZZ
ØØ8Ø4ZZ
ØØ87ØZZ
ØØ873ZZ
ØØ874ZZ
ØØ88ØZZ
ØØ883ZZ
ØØ884ZZ
ØØ8PØZZ
ØØ8P3ZZ
ØØ8P4ZZ
ØØ9ØØØZ
ØØ9ØØZX
ØØ9ØØZZ
ØØ9Ø3ØZ
ØØ9Ø3ZZ
ØØ9Ø4ØZ
ØØ9Ø4ZZ
ØØ91ØØZ
ØØ91ØZX
ØØ91ØZZ
ØØ913ØZ
ØØ913ZZ
ØØ914ØZ
ØØ914ZZ
ØØ92ØØZ
ØØ92ØZX
ØØ92ØZZ
ØØ923ØZ
ØØ923ZZ
ØØ924ØZ
ØØ924ZZ
ØØ93ØØZ
ØØ93ØZX
ØØ93ØZZ
ØØ933ØZ
ØØ933ZZ
ØØ934ØZ
ØØ934ZZ
ØØ94ØØZ
ØØ94ØZX
ØØ94ØZZ
ØØ943ØZ
ØØ943ZZ
ØØ944ØZ
ØØ944ZZ
ØØ95ØØZ
ØØ95ØZX
ØØ95ØZZ
ØØ953ØZ
ØØ953ZZ
ØØ954ØZ
ØØ954ZZ
ØØ96ØØZ
ØØ96ØZX
ØØ96ØZZ
ØØ963ØZ
ØØ963ZZ
ØØ964ØZ
ØØ964ZZ
ØØ97ØØZ
ØØ97ØZX
ØØ97ØZZ
ØØ973ØZ
ØØ973ZZ
ØØ974ØZ
ØØ974ZZ
ØØ98ØØZ
ØØ98ØZX
ØØ98ØZZ
ØØ983ØZ
ØØ983ZZ
ØØ984ØZ
ØØ984ZZ
ØØ99ØØZ
ØØ99ØZX
ØØ99ØZZ
ØØ993ØZ
ØØ993ZZ
ØØ994ØZ
ØØ994ZZ
ØØ9AØØZ
ØØ9AØZX
ØØ9AØZZ
ØØ9A3ØZ
ØØ9A3ZZ
ØØ9A4ØZ
ØØ9A4ZZ
ØØ9BØØZ
ØØ9BØZX
ØØ9BØZZ
ØØ9B3ØZ
ØØ9B3ZZ
ØØ9B4ØZ
ØØ9B4ZZ
ØØ9CØØZ
ØØ9CØZX
ØØ9CØZZ
ØØ9C3ØZ
ØØ9C3ZZ
ØØ9C4ØZ
ØØ9C4ZZ
ØØ9DØØZ
ØØ9DØZX
ØØ9DØZZ
ØØ9D3ØZ
ØØ9D3ZZ
ØØ9D4ØZ
ØØ9D4ZZ
ØØBØØZX
ØØBØØZZ
ØØBØ3ZX
ØØBØ3ZZ
ØØBØ4ZX
ØØBØ4ZZ
ØØB1ØZX
ØØB1ØZZ
ØØB13ZX
ØØB13ZZ
ØØB14ZX
ØØB14ZZ
ØØB2ØZX
ØØB2ØZZ
ØØB23ZX
ØØB23ZZ
ØØB24ZX
ØØB24ZZ
ØØB6ØZX
ØØB6ØZZ
ØØB63ZX
ØØB63ZZ
ØØB64ZX
ØØB64ZZ
ØØB7ØZX
ØØB7ØZZ
ØØB73ZX
ØØB73ZZ
ØØB74ZX
ØØB74ZZ
ØØB8ØZX
ØØB8ØZZ
ØØB83ZX
ØØB83ZZ
ØØB84ZX
ØØB84ZZ
ØØB9ØZX
ØØB9ØZZ
ØØB93ZX
ØØB93ZZ
ØØB94ZX
ØØB94ZZ
ØØBAØZX
ØØBAØZZ
ØØBA3ZX
ØØBA3ZZ
ØØBA4ZX
ØØBA4ZZ
ØØBBØZX
ØØBBØZZ
ØØBB3ZX
ØØBB3ZZ
ØØBB4ZX
ØØBB4ZZ
ØØBCØZX
ØØBCØZZ
ØØBC3ZX
ØØBC3ZZ
ØØBC4ZX
ØØBC4ZZ
ØØBDØZX
ØØBDØZZ
ØØBD3ZX
ØØBD3ZZ
ØØBD4ZX
ØØBD4ZZ
ØØBNØZZ
ØØCØØZZ
ØØCØ3ZZ
ØØCØ4ZZ
ØØC1ØZZ
ØØC13ZZ
ØØC14ZZ
ØØC2ØZZ
ØØC23ZZ
ØØC24ZZ
ØØC3ØZZ
ØØC33ZZ
ØØC34ZZ
ØØC4ØZZ
ØØC43ZZ
ØØC44ZZ
ØØC5ØZZ
ØØC53ZZ
ØØC54ZZ
ØØC6ØZZ
ØØC63ZZ
ØØC64ZZ
ØØC7ØZZ
ØØC73ZZ
ØØC74ZZ
ØØC8ØZZ
ØØC83ZZ
ØØC84ZZ
ØØC9ØZZ
ØØC93ZZ
ØØC94ZZ
ØØCAØZZ
ØØCA3ZZ
ØØCA4ZZ
ØØCBØZZ
ØØCB3ZZ
ØØCB4ZZ
ØØCCØZZ
ØØCC3ZZ
ØØCC4ZZ
ØØCDØZZ
ØØCD3ZZ
ØØCD4ZZ
ØØDØØZZ
ØØDØ3ZZ
ØØDØ4ZZ
ØØD1ØZZ
ØØD13ZZ
ØØD14ZZ
ØØD2ØZZ
ØØD23ZZ
ØØD24ZZ
ØØD7ØZZ
ØØD73ZZ
ØØD74ZZ
ØØDCØZZ
ØØDC3ZZ
ØØDC4ZZ
ØØF3ØZZ
ØØF33ZZ
ØØF34ZZ
ØØF4ØZZ
ØØF43ZZ
ØØF44ZZ
ØØF5ØZZ
ØØF53ZZ
ØØF54ZZ
ØØF6ØZZ
ØØF63ZZ
ØØF64ZZ
ØØHØØ1Z
ØØHØØ2Z
ØØHØØ3Z
ØØHØØMZ
ØØHØØYZ
ØØHØ31Z
ØØHØ32Z
ØØHØ33Z
ØØHØ3MZ
ØØHØ3YZ
ØØHØ41Z
ØØHØ42Z
ØØHØ43Z
ØØHØ4MZ
ØØHØ4YZ
ØØH6Ø1Z
ØØH6Ø2Z
ØØH6Ø3Z
ØØH6ØMZ
ØØH6ØYZ
ØØH631Z
ØØH632Z
ØØH633Z
ØØH63MZ
ØØH63YZ
ØØH641Z
ØØH642Z
ØØH643Z
ØØH64MZ
ØØH64YZ
ØØJØØZZ
ØØJØ4ZZ
ØØKØØZZ
ØØKØ3ZZ
ØØKØ4ZZ
ØØK7ØZZ
ØØK73ZZ
ØØK74ZZ
ØØK8ØZZ
ØØK83ZZ
ØØK84ZZ
ØØK9ØZZ
ØØK93ZZ
ØØK94ZZ
ØØKAØZZ
ØØKA3ZZ
ØØKA4ZZ
ØØKBØZZ
ØØKB3ZZ
ØØKB4ZZ
ØØKCØZZ
ØØKC3ZZ
ØØKC4ZZ
ØØKDØZZ
ØØKD3ZZ
ØØKD4ZZ
ØØNØØZZ
ØØNØ3ZZ
ØØNØ4ZZ
ØØN1ØZZ
ØØN13ZZ
ØØN14ZZ
ØØN2ØZZ
ØØN23ZZ
ØØN24ZZ
ØØN6ØZZ
ØØN63ZZ
ØØN64ZZ
ØØN7ØZZ
ØØN73ZZ
ØØN74ZZ
ØØN8ØZZ
ØØN83ZZ
ØØN84ZZ
ØØN9ØZZ
ØØN93ZZ
ØØN94ZZ
ØØNAØZZ
ØØNA3ZZ
ØØNA4ZZ
ØØNBØZZ
ØØNB3ZZ
ØØNB4ZZ
ØØNCØZZ
ØØNC3ZZ
ØØNC4ZZ
ØØNDØZZ
ØØND3ZZ
ØØND4ZZ
ØØNKØZZ
ØØNK3ZZ
ØØNK4ZZ
ØØPØØØZ
ØØPØØ2Z
ØØPØØ3Z
ØØPØØ7Z
ØØPØØJZ
ØØPØØKZ
ØØPØØMZ
ØØPØØYZ
ØØPØ37Z
ØØPØ3JZ
ØØPØ3KZ
ØØPØ3MZ
ØØPØ4ØZ
ØØPØ42Z
ØØPØ43Z
ØØPØ47Z
ØØPØ4JZ
ØØPØ4KZ
ØØPØ4MZ
ØØP6ØØZ
ØØP6Ø2Z
ØØP6Ø3Z
ØØP6ØMZ
ØØP6ØYZ
ØØP63MZ
ØØP64ØZ
ØØP642Z
ØØP643Z
ØØP64MZ
ØØQØØZZ
ØØQØ3ZZ
ØØQØ4ZZ
ØØQ1ØZZ
ØØQ13ZZ
ØØQ14ZZ
ØØQ2ØZZ
ØØQ23ZZ
ØØQ24ZZ
ØØQ6ØZZ
ØØQ63ZZ
ØØQ64ZZ
ØØQ7ØZZ
ØØQ73ZZ
ØØQ74ZZ
ØØQ8ØZZ
ØØQ83ZZ
ØØQ84ZZ
ØØQ9ØZZ
ØØQ93ZZ
ØØQ94ZZ
ØØQAØZZ
ØØQA3ZZ
ØØQA4ZZ
ØØQBØZZ
ØØQB3ZZ
ØØQB4ZZ
ØØQCØZZ
ØØQC3ZZ
ØØQC4ZZ
ØØQDØZZ
ØØQD3ZZ
ØØQD4ZZ
ØØR1Ø7Z
ØØR1ØJZ
ØØR1ØKZ
ØØR147Z
ØØR14JZ
ØØR14KZ
ØØR2Ø7Z
ØØR2ØJZ
ØØR2ØKZ
ØØR247Z
ØØR24JZ
ØØR24KZ
ØØR6Ø7Z
ØØR6ØJZ
ØØR6ØKZ
ØØR647Z
ØØR64JZ
ØØR64KZ
ØØT7ØZZ
ØØT73ZZ
ØØT74ZZ
ØØU1Ø7Z
ØØU1ØJZ
ØØU1ØKZ
ØØU137Z
ØØU13JZ
ØØU13KZ
ØØU147Z
ØØU14JZ
ØØU14KZ
ØØU2Ø7Z
ØØU2ØJZ
ØØU2ØKZ
ØØU237Z
ØØU23JZ
ØØU23KZ
ØØU247Z
ØØU24JZ
ØØU24KZ
ØØU6Ø7Z
ØØU6ØJZ
ØØU6ØKZ
ØØU637Z
ØØU63JZ
ØØU63KZ
ØØU647Z
ØØU64JZ
ØØU64KZ
ØØWØØØZ
ØØWØØ2Z
ØØWØØ3Z
ØØWØØ7Z
ØØWØØJZ
ØØWØØKZ
ØØWØØMZ
ØØWØØYZ
ØØWØ3ØZ
ØØWØ32Z
ØØWØ33Z
ØØWØ37Z
ØØWØ3JZ
ØØWØ3KZ
ØØWØ3MZ
ØØWØ4ØZ
ØØWØ42Z
ØØWØ43Z
ØØWØ47Z
ØØWØ4JZ
ØØWØ4KZ
ØØWØ4MZ
ØØW6ØØZ
ØØW6Ø2Z
ØØW6Ø3Z
ØØW6ØMZ
ØØW6ØYZ
ØØW63ØZ
ØØW632Z
ØØW633Z
ØØW63MZ
ØØW64ØZ
ØØW642Z
ØØW643Z
ØØW64MZ
Ø31HØ9G
Ø31HØAG
Ø31HØJG
Ø31HØKG
Ø31HØZG
Ø31JØ9G
Ø31JØAG
Ø31JØJG
Ø31JØKG
Ø31JØZG
Ø31SØ9G
Ø31SØAG
Ø31SØJG
Ø31SØKG
Ø31SØZG
Ø31TØ9G
Ø31TØAG
Ø31TØJG
Ø31TØKG
Ø31TØZG
Ø35GØZZ
Ø35G3ZZ
Ø35G4ZZ
Ø37G34Z
Ø37G35Z
Ø37G36Z
Ø37G37Z
Ø37G3DZ
Ø37G3EZ
Ø37G3FZ
Ø37G3GZ
Ø37G3ZZ
Ø37G44Z
Ø37G45Z
Ø37G46Z
Ø37G47Z
Ø37G4DZ
Ø37G4EZ
Ø37G4FZ

Ø37G4GZ
Ø37G4ZZ
Ø3BGØZZ
Ø3BG3ZZ
Ø3BG4ZZ
Ø3CGØZZ
Ø3CG3Z7
Ø3CG3ZZ
Ø3CG4ZZ
Ø3CH3Z7
Ø3CH3ZZ
Ø3CH4ZZ
Ø3CJ3Z7
Ø3CJ3ZZ
Ø3CJ4ZZ
Ø3CK3Z7
Ø3CK3ZZ
Ø3CK4ZZ
Ø3CL3Z7
Ø3CL3ZZ
Ø3CL4ZZ
Ø3CM3Z7
Ø3CM3ZZ
Ø3CM4ZZ
Ø3CN3Z7
Ø3CN3ZZ
Ø3CN4ZZ
Ø3CP3Z7
Ø3CP3ZZ
Ø3CP4ZZ
Ø3CQ3Z7
Ø3CQ3ZZ
Ø3CQ4ZZ
Ø3CR3ZZ
Ø3CR4ZZ
Ø3CS3ZZ
Ø3CS4ZZ
Ø3CT3ZZ
Ø3CT4ZZ
Ø3CU3ZZ
Ø3CU4ZZ
Ø3CV3ZZ
Ø3CV4ZZ
Ø3LGØBZ
Ø3LGØCZ
Ø3LGØDZ
Ø3LGØZZ
Ø3LG3BZ
Ø3LG3CZ
Ø3LG3DZ
Ø3LG3ZZ
Ø3LG4BZ
Ø3LG4CZ
Ø3LG4DZ
Ø3LG4ZZ
Ø3LHØBZ
Ø3LHØDZ
Ø3LH3BZ
Ø3LH3DZ
Ø3LH4BZ
Ø3LH4DZ
Ø3LJØBZ
Ø3LJØDZ
Ø3LJ3BZ
Ø3LJ3DZ
Ø3LJ4BZ
Ø3LJ4DZ
Ø3LKØBZ
Ø3LKØCZ
Ø3LKØDZ
Ø3LKØZZ
Ø3LK3BZ
Ø3LK3CZ
Ø3LK3DZ
Ø3LK3ZZ
Ø3LK4BZ
Ø3LK4CZ
Ø3LK4DZ
Ø3LK4ZZ
Ø3LLØBZ
Ø3LLØCZ
Ø3LLØDZ
Ø3LLØZZ
Ø3LL3BZ
Ø3LL3CZ
Ø3LL3DZ
Ø3LL3ZZ
Ø3LL4BZ
Ø3LL4CZ
Ø3LL4DZ
Ø3LL4ZZ
Ø3LMØBZ
Ø3LMØDZ
Ø3LM3BZ
Ø3LM3DZ
Ø3LM4BZ
Ø3LM4DZ
Ø3LNØBZ
Ø3LNØDZ
Ø3LN3BZ
Ø3LN3DZ
Ø3LN4BZ
Ø3LN4DZ
Ø3LPØBZ
Ø3LPØDZ
Ø3LP3BZ
Ø3LP3DZ
Ø3LP4BZ
Ø3LP4DZ
Ø3LQØBZ
Ø3LQØDZ
Ø3LQ3BZ
Ø3LQ3DZ
Ø3LQ4BZ
Ø3LQ4DZ
Ø3LRØDZ
Ø3LR3DZ
Ø3LR4DZ
Ø3LSØDZ
Ø3LS3DZ
Ø3LS4DZ
Ø3LTØDZ
Ø3LT3DZ
Ø3LT4DZ
Ø3RGØ7Z
Ø3RGØJZ
Ø3RGØKZ
Ø3RG47Z
Ø3RG4JZ
Ø3RG4KZ
Ø3VGØBZ
Ø3VGØCZ
Ø3VGØDZ
Ø3VGØHZ
Ø3VGØZZ
Ø3VG3BZ
Ø3VG3CZ
Ø3VG3DZ
Ø3VG3HZ
Ø3VG3ZZ
Ø3VG4BZ
Ø3VG4CZ
Ø3VG4DZ
Ø3VG4HZ
Ø3VG4ZZ
Ø3VHØBZ
Ø3VHØDZ
Ø3VH3BZ
Ø3VH3DZ
Ø3VH4BZ
Ø3VH4DZ
Ø3VJØBZ
Ø3VJØDZ
Ø3VJ3BZ
Ø3VJ3DZ
Ø3VJ4BZ
Ø3VJ4DZ
Ø3VKØBZ
Ø3VKØCZ
Ø3VKØDZ
Ø3VK3BZ
Ø3VK3CZ
Ø3VK3DZ
Ø3VK4BZ
Ø3VK4CZ
Ø3VK4DZ
Ø3VLØBZ
Ø3VLØCZ
Ø3VLØDZ
Ø3VL3BZ
Ø3VL3CZ
Ø3VL3DZ
Ø3VL4BZ
Ø3VL4CZ
Ø3VL4DZ
Ø3VMØBZ
Ø3VMØDZ
Ø3VM3BZ
Ø3VM3DZ
Ø3VM4BZ
Ø3VM4DZ
Ø3VNØBZ
Ø3VNØDZ
Ø3VN3BZ
Ø3VN3DZ
Ø3VN4BZ
Ø3VN4DZ
Ø3VPØBZ
Ø3VPØDZ
Ø3VP3BZ
Ø3VP3DZ
Ø3VP4BZ
Ø3VP4DZ
Ø3VQØBZ
Ø3VQØDZ
Ø3VQ3BZ
Ø3VQ3DZ
Ø3VQ4BZ
Ø3VQ4DZ
Ø3VRØDZ
Ø3VR3DZ
Ø3VR4DZ
Ø3VSØDZ
Ø3VS3DZ
Ø3VS4DZ
Ø3VTØDZ
Ø3VT3DZ
Ø3VT4DZ
Ø3VUØDZ
Ø3VU3DZ
Ø3VU4DZ
Ø3VVØDZ
Ø3VV3DZ
Ø3VV4DZ
Ø55LØZZ
Ø55L3ZZ
Ø55L4ZZ
Ø57L3DZ
Ø57L4DZ
Ø5BLØZZ
Ø5BL3ZZ
Ø5BL4ZZ
Ø5CLØZZ
Ø5CL3ZZ
Ø5CL4ZZ
Ø5LLØCZ
Ø5LLØDZ
Ø5LLØZZ
Ø5LL3CZ
Ø5LL3DZ
Ø5LL3ZZ
Ø5LL4CZ
Ø5LL4DZ
Ø5LL4ZZ
Ø5RLØ7Z
Ø5RLØJZ
Ø5RLØKZ
Ø5RL47Z
Ø5RL4JZ
Ø5RL4KZ
Ø5VLØCZ
Ø5VLØDZ
Ø5VLØZZ
Ø5VL3CZ
Ø5VL3DZ
Ø5VL3ZZ
Ø5VL4CZ
Ø5VL4DZ
Ø5VL4ZZ
ØG5ØØZ3
ØG5ØØZZ
ØG5Ø3Z3
ØG5Ø3ZZ
ØG5Ø4Z3
ØG5Ø4ZZ
ØG51ØZ3
ØG51ØZZ
ØG513Z3
ØG513ZZ
ØG514Z3
ØG514ZZ
ØG8ØØZZ
ØG8Ø3ZZ
ØG8Ø4ZZ
ØG9ØØØZ
ØG9ØØZX
ØG9ØØZZ
ØG9Ø3ZX
ØG9Ø4ØZ
ØG9Ø4ZX
ØG9Ø4ZZ
ØG91ØØZ
ØG91ØZX
ØG91ØZZ
ØG913ZX
ØG914ØZ
ØG914ZX
ØG914ZZ
ØGBØØZX
ØGBØØZZ
ØGBØ3ZX
ØGBØ3ZZ
ØGBØ4ZX
ØGBØ4ZZ
ØGB1ØZX
ØGB1ØZZ
ØGB13ZX
ØGB13ZZ
ØGB14ZX
ØGB14ZZ
ØGCØØZZ
ØGCØ3ZZ
ØGCØ4ZZ
ØGC1ØZZ
ØGC13ZZ
ØGC14ZZ
ØGJØØZZ
ØGJØ4ZZ
ØGJ1ØZZ
ØGJ14ZZ
ØGNØØZZ
ØGNØ3ZZ
ØGNØ4ZZ
ØGN1ØZZ
ØGN13ZZ
ØGN14ZZ
ØGPØØØZ
ØGPØ3ØZ
ØGPØ4ØZ
ØGP1ØØZ
ØGP13ØZ
ØGP14ØZ
ØGQØØZZ
ØGQØ3ZZ
ØGQØ4ZZ
ØGQ1ØZZ
ØGQ13ZZ
ØGQ14ZZ
ØGTØØZZ
ØGTØ4ZZ
ØGT1ØZZ
ØGT14ZZ
ØGWØØØZ
ØGWØ3ØZ
ØGWØ4ØZ
ØGW1ØØZ
ØGW13ØZ
ØGW14ØZ
ØN5ØØZZ
ØN5Ø3ZZ
ØN5Ø4ZZ
ØN51ØZZ
ØN513ZZ
ØN514ZZ
ØN53ØZZ
ØN533ZZ
ØN534ZZ
ØN54ØZZ
ØN543ZZ
ØN544ZZ
ØN55ØZZ
ØN553ZZ
ØN554ZZ
ØN56ØZZ
ØN563ZZ
ØN564ZZ
ØN57ØZZ
ØN573ZZ
ØN574ZZ
ØN8ØØZZ
ØN8Ø3ZZ
ØN8Ø4ZZ
ØN81ØZZ
ØN813ZZ
ØN814ZZ
ØN83ØZZ
ØN833ZZ
ØN834ZZ
ØN84ØZZ
ØN843ZZ
ØN844ZZ
ØN85ØZZ
ØN853ZZ
ØN854ZZ
ØN86ØZZ
ØN863ZZ
ØN864ZZ
ØN87ØZZ
ØN873ZZ
ØN874ZZ
ØN9ØØØZ
ØN9ØØZX
ØN9ØØZZ
ØN9Ø3ZX
ØN9Ø4ØZ
ØN9Ø4ZX
ØN9Ø4ZZ
ØN91ØØZ
ØN91ØZX
ØN91ØZZ
ØN913ZX
ØN914ØZ
ØN914ZX
ØN914ZZ
ØN93ØØZ
ØN93ØZX
ØN93ØZZ
ØN933ZX
ØN934ØZ
ØN934ZX
ØN934ZZ
ØN94ØØZ
ØN94ØZX
ØN94ØZZ
ØN943ZX
ØN944ØZ
ØN944ZX
ØN944ZZ
ØN95ØØZ
ØN95ØZX
ØN95ØZZ
ØN953ZX
ØN954ØZ
ØN954ZX
ØN954ZZ
ØN96ØØZ
ØN96ØZX
ØN96ØZZ
ØN963ZX
ØN964ØZ
ØN964ZX
ØN964ZZ
ØN97ØØZ
ØN97ØZX
ØN97ØZZ
ØN973ZX
ØN974ØZ
ØN974ZX
ØN974ZZ
ØNBØØZX
ØNBØØZZ
ØNBØ3ZX
ØNBØ3ZZ
ØNBØ4ZX
ØNBØ4ZZ
ØNB1ØZX
ØNB1ØZZ
ØNB13ZX
ØNB13ZZ
ØNB14ZX
ØNB14ZZ
ØNB3ØZX
ØNB3ØZZ
ØNB33ZX
ØNB33ZZ
ØNB34ZX
ØNB34ZZ
ØNB4ØZX
ØNB4ØZZ
ØNB43ZX
ØNB43ZZ
ØNB44ZX
ØNB44ZZ
ØNB5ØZX
ØNB5ØZZ
ØNB53ZX
ØNB53ZZ
ØNB54ZX
ØNB54ZZ
ØNB6ØZX
ØNB6ØZZ
ØNB63ZX
ØNB63ZZ
ØNB64ZX
ØNB64ZZ
ØNB7ØZX
ØNB7ØZZ
ØNB73ZX
ØNB73ZZ
ØNB74ZX
ØNB74ZZ
ØNC1ØZZ
ØNC13ZZ
ØNC14ZZ
ØNC3ØZZ
ØNC33ZZ
ØNC34ZZ
ØNC4ØZZ
ØNC43ZZ
ØNC44ZZ
ØNC5ØZZ
ØNC53ZZ
ØNC54ZZ
ØNC6ØZZ
ØNC63ZZ
ØNC64ZZ
ØNC7ØZZ
ØNC73ZZ
ØNC74ZZ
ØNHØØ3Z
ØNHØØ4Z
ØNHØØMZ
ØNHØ33Z
ØNHØ34Z
ØNHØ3MZ
ØNHØ43Z
ØNHØ44Z
ØNHØ4MZ
ØNH1Ø4Z
ØNH134Z
ØNH144Z
ØNH3Ø4Z
ØNH334Z
ØNH344Z
ØNH4Ø4Z
ØNH434Z
ØNH444Z
ØNH5Ø4Z
ØNH534Z
ØNH544Z
ØNH6Ø4Z
ØNH634Z
ØNH644Z
ØNH7Ø4Z
ØNH734Z
ØNH744Z
ØNJØØZZ
ØNJØ4ZZ
ØNN1ØZZ
ØNN13ZZ
ØNN14ZZ
ØNN3ØZZ
ØNN33ZZ
ØNN34ZZ
ØNN4ØZZ
ØNN43ZZ
ØNN44ZZ
ØNN5ØZZ
ØNN53ZZ
ØNN54ZZ
ØNN6ØZZ
ØNN63ZZ
ØNN64ZZ
ØNN7ØZZ
ØNN73ZZ
ØNN74ZZ
ØNPØØØZ
ØNPØØ3Z
ØNPØØ4Z
ØNPØØ5Z
ØNPØØ7Z
ØNPØØJZ
ØNPØØKZ
ØNPØØMZ
ØNPØØSZ
ØNPØ3ØZ
ØNPØ33Z
ØNPØ34Z
ØNPØ37Z
ØNPØ3JZ
ØNPØ3KZ
ØNPØ3MZ
ØNPØ3SZ
ØNPØ4ØZ
ØNPØ43Z
ØNPØ44Z
ØNPØ47Z
ØNPØ4JZ
ØNPØ4KZ
ØNPØ4MZ
ØNPØ4SZ
ØNPØX4Z
ØNPØXMZ
ØNPØXSZ
ØNQØØZZ
ØNQØ3ZZ
ØNQØ4ZZ
ØNQ1ØZZ
ØNQ13ZZ
ØNQ14ZZ
ØNQ3ØZZ
ØNQ33ZZ
ØNQ34ZZ
ØNQ4ØZZ
ØNQ43ZZ
ØNQ44ZZ
ØNQ5ØZZ
ØNQ53ZZ
ØNQ54ZZ
ØNQ6ØZZ
ØNQ63ZZ
ØNQ64ZZ
ØNQ7ØZZ
ØNQ73ZZ
ØNQ74ZZ
ØNRØØ7Z
ØNRØØJZ
ØNRØØKZ
ØNRØ37Z
ØNRØ3JZ
ØNRØ3KZ
ØNRØ47Z
ØNRØ4JZ
ØNRØ4KZ
ØNR1Ø7Z
ØNR1ØJZ
ØNR1ØKZ
ØNR137Z
ØNR13JZ
ØNR13KZ
ØNR147Z
ØNR14JZ
ØNR14KZ
ØNR3Ø7Z
ØNR3ØJZ
ØNR3ØKZ
ØNR337Z
ØNR33JZ
ØNR33KZ
ØNR347Z
ØNR34JZ
ØNR34KZ
ØNR4Ø7Z
ØNR4ØJZ
ØNR4ØKZ
ØNR437Z
ØNR43JZ
ØNR43KZ
ØNR447Z
ØNR44JZ
ØNR44KZ
ØNR5Ø7Z
ØNR5ØJZ
ØNR5ØKZ
ØNR537Z
ØNR53JZ
ØNR53KZ
ØNR547Z
ØNR54JZ
ØNR54KZ
ØNR6Ø7Z
ØNR6ØJZ
ØNR6ØKZ
ØNR637Z
ØNR63JZ
ØNR63KZ
ØNR647Z
ØNR64JZ
ØNR64KZ
ØNR7Ø7Z
ØNR7ØJZ
ØNR7ØKZ
ØNR737Z
ØNR73JZ
ØNR73KZ
ØNR747Z
ØNR74JZ
ØNR74KZ
ØNSØØ4Z
ØNSØØ5Z
ØNSØØZZ
ØNSØ34Z
ØNSØ35Z
ØNSØ3ZZ
ØNSØ44Z
ØNSØ45Z
ØNSØ4ZZ
ØNS1Ø4Z
ØNS1ØZZ
ØNS134Z
ØNS13ZZ
ØNS144Z
ØNS14ZZ
ØNS3Ø4Z
ØNS3ØZZ
ØNS334Z
ØNS33ZZ
ØNS344Z
ØNS34ZZ
ØNS4Ø4Z
ØNS4ØZZ
ØNS434Z
ØNS43ZZ
ØNS444Z
ØNS44ZZ
ØNS5Ø4Z
ØNS5ØZZ
ØNS534Z
ØNS53ZZ
ØNS544Z
ØNS54ZZ
ØNS6Ø4Z
ØNS6ØZZ
ØNS634Z
ØNS63ZZ
ØNS644Z
ØNS64ZZ
ØNS7Ø4Z
ØNS7ØZZ
ØNS734Z
ØNS73ZZ
ØNS744Z
ØNS74ZZ
ØNT1ØZZ
ØNT3ØZZ
ØNT4ØZZ
ØNT5ØZZ
ØNT6ØZZ
ØNT7ØZZ
ØNUØØ7Z
ØNUØØJZ
ØNUØØKZ
ØNUØ37Z
ØNUØ3JZ
ØNUØ3KZ
ØNUØ47Z
ØNUØ4JZ
ØNUØ4KZ
ØNU1Ø7Z
ØNU1ØJZ
ØNU1ØKZ
ØNU137Z
ØNU13JZ
ØNU13KZ
ØNU147Z
ØNU14JZ
ØNU14KZ
ØNU3Ø7Z
ØNU3ØJZ
ØNU3ØKZ
ØNU337Z
ØNU33JZ
ØNU33KZ
ØNU347Z
ØNU34JZ
ØNU34KZ
ØNU4Ø7Z
ØNU4ØJZ
ØNU4ØKZ
ØNU437Z
ØNU43JZ
ØNU43KZ
ØNU447Z
ØNU44JZ
ØNU44KZ
ØNU5Ø7Z
ØNU5ØJZ
ØNU5ØKZ
ØNU537Z
ØNU53JZ
ØNU53KZ
ØNU547Z
ØNU54JZ
ØNU54KZ
ØNU6Ø7Z
ØNU6ØJZ
ØNU6ØKZ
ØNU637Z
ØNU63JZ
ØNU63KZ
ØNU647Z
ØNU64JZ
ØNU64KZ
ØNU7Ø7Z
ØNU7ØJZ
ØNU7ØKZ
ØNU737Z
ØNU73JZ
ØNU73KZ
ØNU747Z
ØNU74JZ
ØNU74KZ
ØNWØØØZ
ØNWØØ3Z
ØNWØØ4Z
ØNWØØ5Z
ØNWØØ7Z
ØNWØØJZ
ØNWØØKZ
ØNWØØMZ
ØNWØØNZ
ØNWØØSZ
ØNWØ3ØZ
ØNWØ33Z
ØNWØ34Z
ØNWØ35Z
ØNWØ37Z
ØNWØ3JZ
ØNWØ3KZ
ØNWØ3MZ
ØNWØ3SZ
ØNWØ4ØZ
ØNWØ43Z
ØNWØ44Z
ØNWØ45Z
ØNWØ47Z
ØNWØ4JZ
ØNWØ4KZ
ØNWØ4MZ
ØNWØ4SZ
ØW31ØZZ
ØW313ZZ
ØW314ZZ
ØW91ØØZ
ØW91ØZX
ØW91ØZZ
ØWC1ØZZ
ØWC13ZZ
ØWC14ZZ
ØWF1ØZZ
ØWF13ZZ
ØWF14ZZ
ØWH1ØYZ
ØWH13YZ
ØWH14YZ
ØWJ1ØZZ
ØWJ14ZZ
ØWP1ØØZ
ØWP1Ø1Z
ØWP1ØJZ
ØWP1ØYZ
ØWP13ØZ
ØWP131Z
ØWP13JZ
ØWP13YZ
ØWP14ØZ
ØWP141Z
ØWP14JZ
ØWP14YZ
ØWW1ØØZ
ØWW1Ø1Z
ØWW1Ø3Z
ØWW1ØJZ
ØWW1ØYZ
ØWW13ØZ
ØWW131Z
ØWW133Z
ØWW13JZ
ØWW13YZ
ØWW14ØZ
ØWW141Z
ØWW143Z
ØWW14JZ
ØWW14YZ
XNR8ØD9

DRG 026

Select operating room procedures listed under DRG 025

DRG 027

Select operating room procedures listed under DRG 025

DRG 028

Operating Room Procedures

ØØ1UØ72
ØØ1UØ74
ØØ1UØ76
ØØ1UØ77
ØØ1UØ79
ØØ1UØJ2
ØØ1UØJ4
ØØ1UØJ6
ØØ1UØJ7
ØØ1UØJ9
ØØ1UØK2
ØØ1UØK4
ØØ1UØK6
ØØ1UØK7
ØØ1UØK9
ØØ1U372

001U374
001U376
001U377
001U379
001U3J2
001U3J4
001U3J6
001U3J7
001U3J9
001U3K2
001U3K4
001U3K6
001U3K7
001U3K9
001U472
001U474
001U476
001U477
001U479
001U4J2
001U4J4
001U4J6
001U4J7
001U4J9
001U4K2
001U4K4
001U4K6
001U4K7
001U4K9
005T0ZZ
005T3ZZ
005T4ZZ
005W0Z3
005W0ZZ
005W3Z3
005W3ZZ
005W4Z3
005W4ZZ
005X0Z3
005X0ZZ
005X3Z3
005X3ZZ
005X4Z3
005X4ZZ
005Y0Z3
005Y0ZZ
005Y3Z3
005Y3ZZ
005Y4Z3
005Y4ZZ
008W0ZZ
008W3ZZ
008W4ZZ
008X0ZZ
008X3ZZ
008X4ZZ
008Y0ZZ
008Y3ZZ
008Y4ZZ
009T00Z
009T0ZX
009T0ZZ
009T40Z
009T4ZX
009T4ZZ
009U00Z
009U0ZX
009U0ZZ
009W00Z
009W0ZX
009W0ZZ
009W40Z
009W4ZX
009W4ZZ
009X00Z
009X0ZX
009X0ZZ
009X40Z
009X4ZX
009X4ZZ
009Y00Z
009Y0ZX
009Y0ZZ
009Y40Z
009Y4ZX
009Y4ZZ
00BT0ZX
00BT0ZZ
00BT3ZX
00BT3ZZ
00BT4ZX
00BT4ZZ
00BW0ZX
00BW0ZZ
00BW3ZX
00BW3ZZ
00BW4ZX
00BW4ZZ
00BX0ZX
00BX0ZZ
00BX3ZX
00BX3ZZ
00BX4ZX
00BX4ZZ
00BY0ZX
00BY0ZZ
00BY3ZX
00BY3ZZ
00BY4ZX
00BY4ZZ
00CT0ZZ
00CT3ZZ
00CT4ZZ
00CU0ZZ
00CU3ZZ
00CU4ZZ
00CW0ZZ
00CW3ZZ
00CW4ZZ
00CX0ZZ
00CX3ZZ
00CX4ZZ
00CY0ZZ
00CY3ZZ
00CY4ZZ
00DT0ZZ
00DT3ZZ
00DT4ZZ
00FU0ZZ
00FU3ZZ
00FU4ZZ
00FUXZZ
00HU01Z
00HU02Z
00HU0MZ
00HU0YZ
00HU31Z
00HU3MZ
00HU41Z
00HU42Z
00HU4MZ
00HV01Z
00HV02Z
00HV0MZ
00HV0YZ
00HV31Z
00HV3MZ
00HV3YZ
00HV41Z
00HV42Z
00HV4MZ
00HV4YZ
00JU0ZZ
00JU4ZZ
00JV0ZZ
00JV4ZZ
00NT0ZZ
00NT3ZZ
00NT4ZZ
00NW0ZZ
00NW3ZZ
00NW4ZZ
00NX0ZZ
00NX3ZZ
00NX4ZZ
00NY0ZZ
00NY3ZZ
00NY4ZZ
00PU00Z
00PU02Z
00PU03Z
00PU0JZ
00PU0MZ
00PU0YZ
00PU3JZ
00PU3MZ
00PU40Z
00PU42Z
00PU43Z
00PU4JZ
00PU4MZ
00PV00Z
00PV02Z
00PV03Z
00PV07Z
00PV0JZ
00PV0KZ
00PV0MZ
00PV0YZ
00PV37Z
00PV3JZ
00PV3KZ
00PV3MZ
00PV40Z
00PV42Z
00PV43Z
00PV47Z
00PV4JZ
00PV4KZ
00PV4MZ
00QT0ZZ
00QT3ZZ
00QT4ZZ
00QW0ZZ
00QW3ZZ
00QW4ZZ
00QX0ZZ
00QX3ZZ
00QX4ZZ
00QY0ZZ
00QY3ZZ
00QY4ZZ
00RT07Z
00RT0JZ
00RT0KZ
00RT47Z
00RT4JZ
00RT4KZ
00SW0ZZ
00SW3ZZ
00SW4ZZ
00SX0ZZ
00SX3ZZ
00SX4ZZ
00SY0ZZ
00SY3ZZ
00SY4ZZ
00UT07Z
00UT0JZ
00UT0KZ
00UT37Z
00UT3JZ
00UT3KZ
00UT47Z
00UT4JZ
00UT4KZ
00WU00Z
00WU02Z
00WU03Z
00WU0JZ
00WU0MZ
00WU0YZ
00WU30Z
00WU32Z
00WU33Z
00WU3JZ
00WU3MZ
00WU40Z
00WU42Z
00WU43Z
00WU4JZ
00WU4MZ
00WV00Z
00WV02Z
00WV03Z
00WV07Z
00WV0JZ
00WV0KZ
00WV0MZ
00WV0YZ
00WV30Z
00WV32Z
00WV33Z
00WV37Z
00WV3JZ
00WV3KZ
00WV3MZ
00WV40Z
00WV42Z
00WV43Z
00WV47Z
00WV4JZ
00WV4KZ
00WV4MZ
01510ZZ
01514ZZ
01580ZZ
01584ZZ
015B0ZZ
015B4ZZ
015R0ZZ
015R4ZZ
01810ZZ
01813ZZ
01814ZZ
01880ZZ
01883ZZ
01884ZZ
018B0ZZ
018B3ZZ
018B4ZZ
018R0ZZ
018R3ZZ
018R4ZZ
0PB00ZZ
0PB03ZZ
0PB04ZZ
0PB10ZZ
0PB13ZZ
0PB14ZZ
0PB20ZZ
0PB23ZZ
0PB24ZZ
0PB50ZZ
0PB53ZZ
0PB54ZZ
0PB60ZZ
0PB63ZZ
0PB64ZZ
0PB70ZZ
0PB73ZZ
0PB74ZZ
0PB80ZZ
0PB83ZZ
0PB84ZZ
0PB90ZZ
0PB93ZZ
0PB94ZZ
0PBB0ZZ
0PBB3ZZ
0PBB4ZZ
0PS304Z
0PS30ZZ
0PS334Z
0PS344Z
0PS34ZZ
0PS403Z
0PS404Z
0PS40ZZ
0PS434Z
0PS443Z
0PS444Z
0PS44ZZ
0PT00ZZ
0PT10ZZ
0PT20ZZ
0PT50ZZ
0PT60ZZ
0PT70ZZ
0PT80ZZ
0PT90ZZ
0PTB0ZZ
0QS003Z
0QS004Z
0QS00ZZ
0QS034Z
0QS043Z
0QS044Z
0QS04ZZ
0QS104Z
0QS10ZZ
0QS134Z
0QS144Z
0QS14ZZ
0QSS04Z
0QSS0ZZ
0QSS34Z
0QSS3ZZ
0QSS44Z
0QSS4ZZ
0R530ZZ
0R550ZZ
0R590ZZ
0R5B0ZZ
0RB00ZZ
0RB03ZZ
0RB04ZZ
0RB10ZZ
0RB13ZZ
0RB14ZZ
0RB30ZZ
0RB33ZZ
0RB34ZZ
0RB40ZZ
0RB43ZZ
0RB44ZZ
0RB50ZZ
0RB53ZZ
0RB54ZZ
0RB60ZZ
0RB63ZZ
0RB64ZZ
0RB90ZZ
0RB93ZZ
0RB94ZZ
0RBA0ZZ
0RBA3ZZ
0RBA4ZZ
0RBB0ZZ
0RBB3ZZ
0RBB4ZZ
0RG0070
0RG0071
0RG007J
0RG00A0
0RG00AJ
0RG00J0
0RG00J1
0RG00JJ
0RG00K0
0RG00K1
0RG00KJ
0RG0370
0RG0371
0RG037J
0RG03A0
0RG03AJ
0RG03J0
0RG03J1
0RG03JJ
0RG03K0
0RG03K1
0RG03KJ
0RG0470
0RG0471
0RG047J
0RG04A0
0RG04AJ
0RG04J0
0RG04J1
0RG04JJ
0RG04K0
0RG04K1
0RG04KJ
0RG1070
0RG1071
0RG107J
0RG10A0
0RG10AJ
0RG10J0
0RG10J1
0RG10JJ
0RG10K0
0RG10K1
0RG10KJ
0RG1370
0RG1371
0RG137J
0RG13A0
0RG13AJ
0RG13J0
0RG13J1
0RG13JJ
0RG13K0
0RG13K1
0RG13KJ
0RG1470
0RG1471
0RG147J
0RG14A0
0RG14AJ
0RG14J0
0RG14J1
0RG14JJ
0RG14K0
0RG14K1
0RG14KJ
0RG2070
0RG2071
0RG207J
0RG20A0
0RG20AJ
0RG20J0
0RG20J1
0RG20JJ
0RG20K0
0RG20K1
0RG20KJ
0RG2370
0RG2371
0RG237J
0RG23A0
0RG23AJ
0RG23J0
0RG23J1
0RG23JJ
0RG23K0
0RG23K1
0RG23KJ
0RG2470
0RG2471
0RG247J
0RG24A0
0RG24AJ
0RG24J0
0RG24J1
0RG24JJ
0RG24K0
0RG24K1
0RG24KJ
0RG4070
0RG4071
0RG407J
0RG40A0
0RG40AJ
0RG40J0
0RG40J1
0RG40JJ
0RG40K0
0RG40K1
0RG40KJ
0RG4370
0RG4371
0RG437J
0RG43A0
0RG43AJ
0RG43J0
0RG43J1
0RG43JJ
0RG43K0
0RG43K1
0RG43KJ
0RG4470
0RG4471
0RG447J
0RG44A0
0RG44AJ
0RG44J0
0RG44J1
0RG44JJ
0RG44K0
0RG44K1
0RG44KJ
0RG6070
0RG6071
0RG607J
0RG60A0
0RG60AJ
0RG60J0
0RG60J1
0RG60JJ
0RG60K0
0RG60K1
0RG60KJ
0RG6370
0RG6371
0RG637J
0RG63A0
0RG63AJ
0RG63J0
0RG63J1
0RG63JJ
0RG63K0
0RG63K1
0RG63KJ
0RG6470
0RG6471
0RG647J
0RG64A0
0RG64AJ
0RG64J0
0RG64J1
0RG64JJ
0RG64K0
0RG64K1
0RG64KJ
0RG7070
0RG7071
0RG707J
0RG70A0
0RG70AJ
0RG70J0
0RG70J1
0RG70JJ
0RG70K0
0RG70K1
0RG70KJ
0RG7370
0RG7371
0RG737J
0RG73A0
0RG73AJ
0RG73J0
0RG73J1
0RG73JJ
0RG73K0
0RG73K1
0RG73KJ
0RG7470
0RG7471
0RG747J
0RG74A0
0RG74AJ
0RG74J0
0RG74J1
0RG74JJ
0RG74K0
0RG74K1
0RG74KJ
0RG8070
0RG8071
0RG807J
0RG80A0
0RG80AJ
0RG80J0
0RG80J1
0RG80JJ
0RG80K0
0RG80K1
0RG80KJ
0RG8370
0RG8371
0RG837J
0RG83A0
0RG83AJ
0RG83J0
0RG83J1
0RG83JJ
0RG83K0
0RG83K1
0RG83KJ
0RG8470
0RG8471
0RG847J
0RG84A0
0RG84AJ
0RG84J0
0RG84J1
0RG84JJ
0RG84K0
0RG84K1
0RG84KJ
0RGA070
0RGA071
0RGA07J
0RGA0A0
0RGA0AJ
0RGA0J0
0RGA0J1
0RGA0JJ
0RGA0K0
0RGA0K1
0RGA0KJ
0RGA370
0RGA371
0RGA37J
0RGA3A0
0RGA3AJ
0RGA3J0
0RGA3J1
0RGA3JJ
0RGA3K0
0RGA3K1
0RGA3KJ
0RGA470
0RGA471
0RGA47J
0RGA4A0
0RGA4AJ
0RGA4J0
0RGA4J1
0RGA4JJ
0RGA4K0
0RGA4K1
0RGA4KJ
0RH00BZ
0RH00CZ
0RH00DZ
0RH03BZ
0RH03CZ
0RH03DZ
0RH04BZ
0RH04CZ
0RH04DZ
0RH10BZ
0RH10CZ
0RH10DZ
0RH13BZ
0RH13CZ
0RH13DZ
0RH14BZ
0RH14CZ
0RH14DZ
0RH40BZ
0RH40CZ
0RH40DZ
0RH43BZ
0RH43CZ
0RH43DZ
0RH44BZ
0RH44CZ
0RH44DZ
0RH60BZ
0RH60CZ
0RH60DZ
0RH63BZ
0RH63CZ
0RH63DZ
0RH64BZ
0RH64CZ
0RH64DZ
0RHA0BZ
0RHA0CZ
0RHA0DZ
0RHA3BZ
0RHA3CZ
0RHA3DZ
0RHA4BZ
0RHA4CZ
0RHA4DZ
0RQ30ZZ
0RQ90ZZ
0RQB0ZZ
0RR30JZ
0RR50JZ
0RR90JZ
0RRB0JZ
0RT30ZZ
0RT40ZZ
0RT50ZZ
0RT90ZZ
0RTB0ZZ
0RU00JZ
0RU03JZ
0RU04JZ
0RU10JZ
0RU13JZ
0RU14JZ
0RU307Z
0RU30JZ
0RU30KZ
0RU337Z
0RU33JZ
0RU33KZ
0RU347Z
0RU34JZ
0RU34KZ
0RU40JZ
0RU43JZ
0RU44JZ
0RU50JZ
0RU53JZ
0RU54JZ
0RU60JZ
0RU63JZ
0RU64JZ
0RU907Z
0RU90JZ
0RU90KZ
0RU937Z
0RU93JZ
0RU93KZ
0RU947Z
0RU94JZ
0RU94KZ
0RUA0JZ
0RUA3JZ
0RUA4JZ
0RUB07Z
0RUB0JZ
0RUB0KZ
0RUB37Z
0RUB3JZ
0RUB3KZ
0RUB47Z
0RUB4JZ
0RUB4KZ
0RW30JZ
0RW33JZ
0RW34JZ
0RW50JZ
0RW53JZ
0RW54JZ
0RW90JZ
0RW93JZ
0RW94JZ
0RWB0JZ
0RWB3JZ
0RWB4JZ
0S520ZZ
0S523ZZ
0S524ZZ
0S540ZZ
0S543ZZ
0S544ZZ
0SB00ZZ
0SB03ZZ
0SB04ZZ
0SB20ZZ
0SB23ZZ
0SB24ZZ
0SB30ZZ
0SB33ZZ
0SB34ZZ
0SB40ZZ
0SB43ZZ
0SB44ZZ
0SB50ZZ
0SB53ZZ
0SB54ZZ
0SB60ZZ
0SB63ZZ
0SB64ZZ
0SB70ZZ
0SB73ZZ
0SB74ZZ
0SB80ZZ
0SB83ZZ
0SB84ZZ
0SG0070
0SG0071
0SG007J
0SG00A0
0SG00AJ
0SG00J0
0SG00J1
0SG00JJ
0SG00K0
0SG00K1
0SG00KJ
0SG0370
0SG0371
0SG037J
0SG03A0
0SG03AJ
0SG03J0
0SG03J1
0SG03JJ
0SG03K0
0SG03K1
0SG03KJ
0SG0470
0SG0471
0SG047J
0SG04A0
0SG04AJ
0SG04J0
0SG04J1
0SG04JJ
0SG04K0
0SG04K1
0SG04KJ
0SG1070
0SG1071
0SG107J
0SG10A0
0SG10AJ
0SG10J0
0SG10J1
0SG10JJ
0SG10K0
0SG10K1
0SG10KJ
0SG1370
0SG1371
0SG137J
0SG13A0
0SG13AJ
0SG13J0
0SG13J1
0SG13JJ
0SG13K0
0SG13K1
0SG13KJ
0SG1470

0SG1471
0SG147J
0SG14A0
0SG14AJ
0SG14J0
0SG14J1
0SG14JJ
0SG14K0
0SG14K1
0SG14KJ
0SG3070
0SG3071
0SG307J
0SG30A0
0SG30AJ
0SG30J0
0SG30J1
0SG30JJ
0SG30K0
0SG30K1
0SG30KJ
0SG3370
0SG3371
0SG337J
0SG33A0
0SG33AJ
0SG33J0
0SG33J1
0SG33JJ
0SG33K0
0SG33K1
0SG33KJ
0SG3470
0SG3471
0SG347J
0SG34A0
0SG34AJ
0SG34J0
0SG34J1
0SG34JJ
0SG34K0
0SG34K1
0SG34KJ
0SG504Z
0SG507Z
0SG50JZ
0SG50KZ
0SG534Z
0SG537Z
0SG53JZ
0SG53KZ
0SG544Z
0SG547Z
0SG54JZ
0SG54KZ
0SG604Z
0SG607Z
0SG60JZ
0SG60KZ
0SG634Z
0SG637Z
0SG63JZ
0SG63KZ
0SG644Z
0SG647Z
0SG64JZ
0SG64KZ
0SG704Z
0SG707Z
0SG70JZ
0SG70KZ
0SG734Z
0SG737Z
0SG73JZ
0SG73KZ
0SG744Z
0SG747Z
0SG74JZ
0SG74KZ
0SG804Z
0SG807Z
0SG80JZ
0SG80KZ
0SG834Z
0SG837Z
0SG83JZ
0SG83KZ
0SG844Z
0SG847Z
0SG84JZ
0SG84KZ
0SH00BZ
0SH00CZ
0SH00DZ
0SH03BZ
0SH03CZ
0SH03DZ
0SH04BZ
0SH04CZ
0SH04DZ
0SH30BZ
0SH30CZ
0SH30DZ
0SH33BZ
0SH33CZ
0SH33DZ
0SH34BZ
0SH34CZ
0SH34DZ
0SQ20ZZ
0SQ40ZZ
0SR20JZ
0SR40JZ
0ST20ZZ
0ST40ZZ
0SU00JZ
0SU03JZ
0SU04JZ
0SU207Z
0SU20JZ
0SU20KZ
0SU237Z
0SU23JZ
0SU23KZ
0SU247Z
0SU24JZ
0SU24KZ
0SU30JZ
0SU33JZ
0SU34JZ
0SU407Z
0SU40JZ
0SU40KZ
0SU437Z
0SU43JZ
0SU43KZ
0SU447Z
0SU44JZ
0SU44KZ
0SU50JZ
0SU53JZ
0SU54JZ
0SU60JZ
0SU63JZ
0SU64JZ
0SW20JZ
0SW23JZ
0SW24JZ
0SW40JZ
0SW43JZ
0SW44JZ
XNS0032
XNS00C7
XNS0332
XNS03C7
XNS3032
XNS3332
XNS4032
XNS40C7
XNS4332
XNS43C7
XRGA0R7
XRGA3R7
XRGA4R7
XRGB0R7
XRGB3R7
XRGB4R7
XRGC0R7
XRGC3R7
XRGC4R7
XRGD0R7
XRGD3R7
XRGD4R7
XRGE058
XRGE358
XRGF058
XRGF358
XRHB018
XRHD018

DRG 029

Select operating room procedures listed under DRG 028

OR

Any of the following procedure combinations

0JH60BZ
0JH60CZ
0JH60DZ
0JH60EZ
0JH63BZ
0JH63CZ
0JH63DZ
0JH63EZ
0JH70BZ
0JH70CZ
0JH70DZ
0JH70EZ
0JH73BZ
0JH73CZ
0JH73DZ
0JH73EZ
0JH80BZ
0JH80CZ
0JH80DZ
0JH80EZ
0JH83BZ
0JH83CZ
0JH83DZ
0JH83EZ

AND

00HU0MZ
00HU3MZ
00HU4MZ
00HV0MZ
00HV3MZ
00HV4MZ

DRG 030

Select operating room procedures listed under DRG 028

DRG 031

Operating Room Procedures

16070
16071
16072
16073
16074
16075
16076
16077
16078
00160J0
00160J1
00160J2
00160J3
00160J4
00160J5
00160J6
00160J7
00160J8
00160K0
00160K1
00160K2
00160K3
00160K4
00160K5
00160K6
00160K7
00160K8
16370
16371
16372
16373
16374
16375
16376
16377
16378
00163J0
00163J1
00163J2
00163J3
00163J4
00163J5
00163J6
00163J7
00163J8
00163K0
00163K1
00163K2
00163K3
00163K4
00163K5
00163K6
00163K7
00163K8
16470
16471
16472
16473
16474
16475
16476
16477
16478
00164J0
00164J1
00164J2
00164J3
00164J4
00164J5
00164J6
00164J7
00164J8
00164K0
00164K1
00164K2
00164K3
00164K4
00164K5
00164K6
00164K7
00164K8
00P60JZ
00P63JZ
00P64JZ
00W60JZ
00W63JZ
00W64JZ
0W11*
0WPG0JZ
0WWG0JZ
0WWG4JZ

DRG 032

Select operating room procedures listed under DRG 031

DRG 033

Select operating room procedures listed under DRG 031

DRG 034

Operating Room Procedures Only

037H04Z
037H05Z
037H06Z
037H07Z
037H0DZ
037H0EZ
037H0FZ
037H0GZ
037H34Z
037H35Z
037H36Z
037H37Z
037H3DZ
037H3EZ
037H3FZ
037H3GZ
037H44Z
037H45Z
037H46Z
037H47Z
037H4DZ
037H4EZ
037H4FZ
037H4GZ
037J04Z
037J05Z
037J06Z
037J07Z
037J0DZ
037J0EZ
037J0FZ
037J0GZ
037J34Z
037J35Z
037J36Z
037J37Z
037J3DZ
037J3EZ
037J3FZ
037J3GZ
037J44Z
037J45Z
037J46Z
037J47Z
037J4DZ
037J4EZ
037J4FZ
037J4GZ
037K04Z
037K05Z
037K06Z
037K07Z
037K0DZ
037K0EZ
037K0FZ
037K0GZ
037K34Z
037K35Z
037K36Z
037K37Z
037K3DZ
037K3EZ
037K3FZ
037K3GZ
037K44Z
037K45Z
037K46Z
037K47Z
037K4DZ
037K4EZ
037K4FZ
037K4GZ
037L04Z
037L05Z
037L06Z
037L07Z
037L0DZ
037L0EZ
037L0FZ
037L0GZ
037L34Z
037L35Z
037L36Z
037L37Z
037L3DZ
037L3EZ
037L3FZ
037L3GZ
037L44Z
037L45Z
037L46Z
037L47Z
037L4DZ
037L4EZ
037L4FZ
037L4GZ
037M04Z
037M05Z
037M06Z
037M07Z
037M0DZ
037M0EZ
037M0FZ
037M0GZ
037M34Z
037M35Z
037M36Z
037M37Z
037M3DZ
037M3EZ
037M3FZ
037M3GZ
037M44Z
037M45Z
037M46Z
037M47Z
037M4DZ
037M4EZ
037M4FZ
037M4GZ
037N04Z
037N05Z
037N06Z
037N07Z
037N0DZ
037N0EZ
037N0FZ
037N0GZ
037N34Z
037N35Z
037N36Z
037N37Z
037N3DZ
037N3EZ
037N3FZ
037N3GZ
037N44Z
037N45Z
037N46Z
037N47Z
037N4DZ
037N4EZ
037N4FZ
037N4GZ

DRG 035

Select operating procedures or procedure combinations listed under DRG 034

DRG 036

Select operating procedure or procedure combinations listed under DRG 034

DRG 037

Operating Room Procedures

021W08A
021W08B
021W08D
021W08G
021W08H
021W09A
021W09B
021W09D
021W09G
021W09H
021W0AA
021W0AB
021W0AD
021W0AG
021W0AH
021W0JA
021W0JB
021W0JD
021W0JG
021W0JH
021W0KA
021W0KB
021W0KD
021W0KG
021W0KH
021W0ZA
021W0ZB
021W0ZD
021W48A
021W48B
021W48D
021W49A
021W49B
021W49D
021W4AA
021W4AB
021W4AD
021W4JA
021W4JB
021W4JD
021W4KA
021W4KB
021W4KD
021W4ZA
021W4ZB
021W4ZD
021X08A
021X08B
021X08D
021X09A
021X09B
021X09D
021X0AA
021X0AB
021X0AD
021X0JA
021X0JB
021X0JD
021X0KA
021X0KB
021X0KD
021X0ZA
021X0ZB
021X0ZD
021X48A
021X48B
021X48D
021X49A
021X49B
021X49D
021X4AA
021X4AB
021X4AD
021X4JA
021X4JB
021X4JD
021X4KA
021X4KB
021X4KD
021X4ZA
021X4ZB
021X4ZD
315090
03150A0
03150J0
03150K0
03150Z0
316091
03160A1
03160J1
03160K1
03160Z1
031H09J
031H09K
031H09Y
031H0AJ
031H0AK
031H0AY
031H0JJ
031H0JK
031H0JY
031H0KJ
031H0KK
031H0KY
031H0ZJ
031H0ZK
031H0ZY
031J09J
031J09K
031J09Y
031J0AJ
031J0AK
031J0AY
031J0JJ
031J0JK
031J0JY
031J0KJ
031J0KK
031J0KY
031J0ZJ
031J0ZK
031J0ZY
031K09J
031K09K
031K0AJ
031K0AK
031K0JJ
031K0JK
031K0KJ
031K0KK
031K0ZJ
031K0ZK
031L09J
031L09K
031L0AJ
031L0AK
031L0JJ
031L0JK
031L0KJ
031L0KK
031L0ZJ
031L0ZK
031M09J
031M09K
031M0AJ
031M0AK
031M0JJ
031M0JK
031M0KJ
031M0KK
031M0ZJ
031M0ZK
031N09J
031N09K
031N0AJ
031N0AK
031N0JJ
031N0JK
031N0KJ
031N0KK
031N0ZJ
031N0ZK
035H*
035J*
035K*
035L*
035M*
035N*
035P*
035Q*
035R*
035S*
035T*
035U*
035V*
037334Z
037335Z
037336Z
037337Z
03733D1
03733DZ
03733EZ
03733FZ
03733GZ
03733Z1
03733ZZ
037434Z
037435Z
037436Z
037437Z
03743D1
03743DZ
03743EZ
03743FZ
03743GZ
03743Z1
03743ZZ
037734Z
037735Z
037736Z
037737Z
03773D1
03773DZ
03773EZ
03773FZ
03773GZ
03773Z1
03773ZZ
037834Z
037835Z
037836Z
037837Z
03783D1
03783DZ
03783EZ
03783FZ
03783GZ
03783Z1
03783ZZ
037934Z
037935Z
037936Z
037937Z
03793D1
03793DZ
03793EZ
03793FZ
03793GZ
03793Z1
03793ZZ
037A34Z
037A35Z
037A36Z
037A37Z
037A3D1
037A3DZ
037A3EZ
037A3FZ
037A3GZ
037A3Z1
037A3ZZ
037H0ZZ
037H3ZZ
037H4ZZ
037J0ZZ
037J3ZZ
037J4ZZ
037K0ZZ
037K3ZZ
037K4ZZ
037L0ZZ
037L3ZZ
037L4ZZ
037M0ZZ
037M3ZZ
037M4ZZ
037N0ZZ
037N3ZZ
037N4ZZ
037P04Z
037P0DZ
037P0ZZ
037P34Z
037P35Z
037P36Z
037P37Z
037P3DZ
037P3EZ
037P3FZ
037P3GZ
037P3ZZ
037P44Z
037P45Z
037P46Z
037P47Z
037P4DZ
037P4EZ
037P4FZ
037P4GZ
037P4ZZ
037Q04Z
037Q0DZ
037Q0ZZ
037Q34Z
037Q35Z
037Q36Z
037Q37Z
037Q3DZ
037Q3EZ
037Q3FZ
037Q3GZ
037Q3ZZ
037Q44Z
037Q45Z
037Q46Z
037Q47Z
037Q4DZ
037Q4EZ
037Q4FZ
037Q4GZ
037Q4ZZ
037Y04Z
037Y0DZ
037Y0ZZ
037Y34Z
037Y35Z
037Y36Z
037Y37Z
037Y3DZ
037Y3EZ
037Y3FZ
037Y3GZ
037Y3ZZ
03BH0ZZ
03BH3ZZ
03BH4ZZ
03BJ0ZZ
03BJ3ZZ
03BJ4ZZ
03BK0ZZ
03BK3ZZ
03BK4ZZ
03BL0ZZ
03BL3ZZ
03BL4ZZ
03BM0ZZ
03BM3ZZ
03BM4ZZ
03BN0ZZ
03BN3ZZ
03BN4ZZ
03BP0ZZ
03BP3ZZ
03BP4ZZ
03BQ0ZZ
03BQ3ZZ
03BQ4ZZ
03BR0ZZ
03BR3ZZ
03BR4ZZ
03BS0ZZ
03BS3ZZ
03BS4ZZ
03BT0ZZ
03BT3ZZ
03BT4ZZ
03BU0ZZ
03BU3ZZ
03BU4ZZ
03BV0ZZ
03BV3ZZ
03BV4ZZ
03CH0ZZ
03CJ0ZZ
03CK0ZZ
03CL0ZZ
03CM0ZZ
03CN0ZZ
03CP0ZZ
03CQ0ZZ

Ø3CRØZZ
Ø3CSØZZ
Ø3CTØZZ
Ø3CUØZZ
Ø3CVØZZ
Ø3CY*
Ø3QH*
Ø3QJ*
Ø3QK*
Ø3QL*
Ø3QM*
Ø3QN*
Ø3QP*
Ø3QQ*
Ø3QR*
Ø3QS*
Ø3QT*
Ø3SH*
Ø3SJ*
Ø3SK*
Ø3SL*
Ø3SM*
Ø3SN*
Ø3SP*
Ø3SQ*
Ø3SR*
Ø3SS*
Ø3ST*
Ø3UHØ7Z
Ø3UHØJZ
Ø3UH37Z
Ø3UH3JZ
Ø3UH47Z
Ø3UH4JZ
Ø3UJØ7Z
Ø3UJØJZ
Ø3UJ37Z
Ø3UJ3JZ
Ø3UJ47Z
Ø3UJ4JZ
Ø3UKØ7Z
Ø3UKØJZ
Ø3UK37Z
Ø3UK3JZ
Ø3UK47Z
Ø3UK4JZ
Ø3ULØ7Z
Ø3ULØJZ
Ø3UL37Z
Ø3UL3JZ
Ø3UL47Z
Ø3UL4JZ
Ø3UMØ7Z
Ø3UMØJZ
Ø3UM37Z
Ø3UM3JZ
Ø3UM47Z
Ø3UM4JZ
Ø3UNØ7Z
Ø3UNØJZ
Ø3UN37Z
Ø3UN3JZ
Ø3UN47Z
Ø3UN4JZ
Ø3UPØ7Z
Ø3UPØJZ
Ø3UP37Z
Ø3UP3JZ
Ø3UP47Z
Ø3UP4JZ
Ø3UQØ7Z
Ø3UQØJZ
Ø3UQ37Z
Ø3UQ3JZ
Ø3UQ47Z
Ø3UQ4JZ
Ø3VHØHZ
Ø3VH3HZ
Ø3VH4HZ
Ø3VJØHZ
Ø3VJ3HZ
Ø3VJ4HZ
Ø3VKØHZ
Ø3VK3HZ
Ø3VK4HZ
Ø3VLØHZ
Ø3VL3HZ
Ø3VL4HZ
Ø3VMØHZ
Ø3VM3HZ
Ø3VM4HZ
Ø3VNØHZ
Ø3VN3HZ
Ø3VN4HZ
Ø3VPØHZ
Ø3VP3HZ
Ø3VP4HZ
Ø3VQØHZ
Ø3VQ3HZ
Ø3VQ4HZ
Ø41KØ9H
Ø41KØ9J
Ø41KØ9K
Ø41KØ9L
Ø41KØAH
Ø41KØAJ
Ø41KØAK
Ø41KØAL
Ø41KØJH
Ø41KØJJ
Ø41KØJK
Ø41KØJL
Ø41KØKH
Ø41KØKJ
Ø41KØKK
Ø41KØKL
Ø41KØZH
Ø41KØZJ
Ø41KØZK
Ø41KØZL
Ø41K49H
Ø41K49J
Ø41K49K
Ø41K49L
Ø41K4AH
Ø41K4AJ
Ø41K4AK
Ø41K4AL
Ø41K4JH
Ø41K4JJ
Ø41K4JK
Ø41K4JL
Ø41K4KH
Ø41K4KJ
Ø41K4KK
Ø41K4KL
Ø41K4ZH
Ø41K4ZJ
Ø41K4ZK
Ø41K4ZL
Ø41LØ9H
Ø41LØ9J
Ø41LØ9K
Ø41LØ9L
Ø41LØAH
Ø41LØAJ
Ø41LØAK
Ø41LØAL
Ø41LØJH
Ø41LØJJ
Ø41LØJK
Ø41LØJL
Ø41LØKH
Ø41LØKJ
Ø41LØKK
Ø41LØKL
Ø41LØZH
Ø41LØZJ
Ø41LØZK
Ø41LØZL
Ø41L49H
Ø41L49J
Ø41L49K
Ø41L49L
Ø41L4AH
Ø41L4AJ
Ø41L4AK
Ø41L4AL
Ø41L4JH
Ø41L4JJ
Ø41L4JK
Ø41L4JL
Ø41L4KH
Ø41L4KJ
Ø41L4KK
Ø41L4KL
Ø41L4ZH
Ø41L4ZJ
Ø41L4ZK
Ø41L4ZL
47Ø341
Ø47Ø34Z
Ø47Ø35Z
Ø47Ø36Z
Ø47Ø37Z
Ø47Ø3D1
Ø47Ø3DZ
Ø47Ø3EZ
Ø47Ø3FZ
Ø47Ø3GZ
Ø47Ø3Z1
Ø47Ø3ZZ
471341
Ø47134Z
Ø47135Z
Ø47136Z
Ø47137Z
Ø4713D1
Ø4713DZ
Ø4713EZ
Ø4713FZ
Ø4713GZ
Ø4713Z1
Ø4713ZZ
472341
Ø47234Z
Ø47235Z
Ø47236Z
Ø47237Z
Ø4723D1
Ø4723DZ
Ø4723EZ
Ø4723FZ
Ø4723GZ
Ø4723Z1
Ø4723ZZ
473341
Ø47334Z
Ø47335Z
Ø47336Z
Ø47337Z
Ø4733D1
Ø4733DZ
Ø4733EZ
Ø4733FZ
Ø4733GZ
Ø4733Z1
Ø4733ZZ
474341
Ø47434Z
Ø47435Z
Ø47436Z
Ø47437Z
Ø4743D1
Ø4743DZ
Ø4743EZ
Ø4743FZ
Ø4743GZ
Ø4743Z1
Ø4743ZZ
475341
Ø47534Z
Ø47535Z
Ø47536Z
Ø47537Z
Ø4753D1
Ø4753DZ
Ø4753EZ
Ø4753FZ
Ø4753GZ
Ø4753Z1
Ø4753ZZ
476341
Ø47634Z
Ø47635Z
Ø47636Z
Ø47637Z
Ø4763D1
Ø4763DZ
Ø4763EZ
Ø4763FZ
Ø4763GZ
Ø4763Z1
Ø4763ZZ
477341
Ø47734Z
Ø47735Z
Ø47736Z
Ø47737Z
Ø4773D1
Ø4773DZ
Ø4773EZ
Ø4773FZ
Ø4773GZ
Ø4773Z1
Ø4773ZZ
478341
Ø47834Z
Ø47835Z
Ø47836Z
Ø47837Z
Ø4783D1
Ø4783DZ
Ø4783EZ
Ø4783FZ
Ø4783GZ
Ø4783Z1
Ø4783ZZ
479341
Ø47934Z
Ø47935Z
Ø47936Z
Ø47937Z
Ø4793D1
Ø4793DZ
Ø4793EZ
Ø4793FZ
Ø4793GZ
Ø4793Z1
Ø4793ZZ
Ø47A341
Ø47A34Z
Ø47A35Z
Ø47A36Z
Ø47A37Z
Ø47A3D1
Ø47A3DZ
Ø47A3EZ
Ø47A3FZ
Ø47A3GZ
Ø47A3Z1
Ø47A3ZZ
Ø47B341
Ø47B34Z
Ø47B35Z
Ø47B36Z
Ø47B37Z
Ø47B3D1
Ø47B3DZ
Ø47B3EZ
Ø47B3FZ
Ø47B3GZ
Ø47B3Z1
Ø47B3ZZ
Ø47C341
Ø47C34Z
Ø47C35Z
Ø47C36Z
Ø47C37Z
Ø47C3D1
Ø47C3DZ
Ø47C3EZ
Ø47C3FZ
Ø47C3GZ
Ø47C3Z1
Ø47C3ZZ
Ø47D341
Ø47D34Z
Ø47D35Z
Ø47D36Z
Ø47D37Z
Ø47D3D1
Ø47D3DZ
Ø47D3EZ
Ø47D3FZ
Ø47D3GZ
Ø47D3Z1
Ø47D3ZZ
Ø47E341
Ø47E34Z
Ø47E35Z
Ø47E36Z
Ø47E37Z
Ø47E3D1
Ø47E3DZ
Ø47E3EZ
Ø47E3FZ
Ø47E3GZ
Ø47E3Z1
Ø47E3ZZ
Ø47F341
Ø47F34Z
Ø47F35Z
Ø47F36Z
Ø47F37Z
Ø47F3D1
Ø47F3DZ
Ø47F3EZ
Ø47F3FZ
Ø47F3GZ
Ø47F3Z1
Ø47F3ZZ
Ø47H341
Ø47H34Z
Ø47H35Z
Ø47H36Z
Ø47H37Z
Ø47H3D1
Ø47H3DZ
Ø47H3EZ
Ø47H3FZ
Ø47H3GZ
Ø47H3Z1
Ø47H3ZZ
Ø47J341
Ø47J34Z
Ø47J35Z
Ø47J36Z
Ø47J37Z
Ø47J3D1
Ø47J3DZ
Ø47J3EZ
Ø47J3FZ
Ø47J3GZ
Ø47J3Z1
Ø47J3ZZ
Ø47KØ41
Ø47KØD1
Ø47KØZ1
Ø47K341
Ø47K34Z
Ø47K35Z
Ø47K36Z
Ø47K37Z
Ø47K3D1
Ø47K3DZ
Ø47K3EZ
Ø47K3FZ
Ø47K3GZ
Ø47K3Z1
Ø47K3ZZ
Ø47K441
Ø47K4D1
Ø47K4Z1
Ø47LØ41
Ø47LØD1
Ø47LØZ1
Ø47L341
Ø47L34Z
Ø47L35Z
Ø47L36Z
Ø47L37Z
Ø47L3D1
Ø47L3DZ
Ø47L3EZ
Ø47L3FZ
Ø47L3GZ
Ø47L3Z1
Ø47L3ZZ
Ø47L441
Ø47L4D1
Ø47L4Z1
Ø47MØ41
Ø47MØD1
Ø47MØZ1
Ø47M341
Ø47M3D1
Ø47M3Z1
Ø47M441
Ø47M4D1
Ø47M4Z1
Ø47NØ41
Ø47NØD1
Ø47NØZ1
Ø47N341
Ø47N3D1
Ø47N3Z1
Ø47N441
Ø47N4D1
Ø47N4Z1
Ø47Y341
Ø47Y34Z
Ø47Y35Z
Ø47Y36Z
Ø47Y37Z
Ø47Y3D1
Ø47Y3DZ
Ø47Y3EZ
Ø47Y3FZ
Ø47Y3GZ
Ø47Y3Z1
Ø47Y3ZZ
Ø4CY*
Ø4VØØDJ
Ø4VØ3DJ
Ø4VØ4DJ
Ø55M*
Ø55N*
Ø55P*
Ø55Q*
Ø55R*
Ø55S*
Ø55T*
Ø55V*
Ø5793D1
Ø5793DZ
Ø5793Z1
Ø5793ZZ
Ø57A3D1
Ø57A3DZ
Ø57A3Z1
Ø57A3ZZ
Ø57B3D1
Ø57B3DZ
Ø57B3Z1
Ø57B3ZZ
Ø57C3D1
Ø57C3DZ
Ø57C3Z1
Ø57C3ZZ
Ø57D3D1
Ø57D3DZ
Ø57D3Z1
Ø57D3ZZ
Ø57F3D1
Ø57F3DZ
Ø57F3Z1
Ø57F3ZZ
Ø57MØDZ
Ø57MØZZ
Ø57M3DZ
Ø57M4DZ
Ø57NØDZ
Ø57NØZZ
Ø57N3DZ
Ø57N4DZ
Ø57PØDZ
Ø57PØZZ
Ø57P3DZ
Ø57P4DZ
Ø57QØDZ
Ø57QØZZ
Ø57Q3DZ
Ø57Q4DZ
Ø57RØDZ
Ø57RØZZ
Ø57R3DZ
Ø57R4DZ
Ø57SØDZ
Ø57SØZZ
Ø57S3DZ
Ø57S4DZ
Ø57TØDZ
Ø57TØZZ
Ø57T3DZ
Ø57T4DZ
Ø5BMØZZ
Ø5BM3ZZ
Ø5BM4ZZ
Ø5BNØZZ
Ø5BN3ZZ
Ø5BN4ZZ
Ø5BPØZZ
Ø5BP3ZZ
Ø5BP4ZZ
Ø5BQØZZ
Ø5BQ3ZZ
Ø5BQ4ZZ
Ø5BRØZZ
Ø5BR3ZZ
Ø5BR4ZZ
Ø5BSØZZ
Ø5BS3ZZ
Ø5BS4ZZ
Ø5BTØZZ
Ø5BT3ZZ
Ø5BT4ZZ
Ø5BVØZZ
Ø5BV3ZZ
Ø5BV4ZZ
Ø5QR*
Ø5QS*
Ø5URØ7Z
Ø5URØJZ
Ø5UR37Z
Ø5UR3JZ
Ø5UR47Z
Ø5UR4JZ
Ø5USØ7Z
Ø5USØJZ
Ø5US37Z
Ø5US3JZ
Ø5US47Z
Ø5US4JZ
Ø653*
Ø67Ø3DZ
Ø67Ø3ZZ
Ø6B3ØZZ
Ø6B33ZZ
Ø6B34ZZ
3EØ3ØTZ
3EØ4ØTZ

DRG 038

Select operating room procedures listed under DRG 037

DRG 039

Select operating room procedures listed under DRG 037

DRG 040

Operating Room Procedures

ØØ8F*
ØØ8G*
ØØ8H*
ØØ8J*
ØØ8K*
ØØ8L*
ØØ8M*
ØØ8N*
ØØ8Q*
ØØ8R*
ØØ8S*
ØØ9FØØZ
ØØ9FØZX
ØØ9FØZZ
ØØ9F3ØZ
ØØ9F3ZZ
ØØ9F4ØZ
ØØ9F4ZZ
ØØ9GØØZ
ØØ9GØZX
ØØ9GØZZ
ØØ9G3ØZ
ØØ9G3ZZ
ØØ9G4ØZ
ØØ9G4ZZ
ØØ9HØØZ
ØØ9HØZX
ØØ9HØZZ
ØØ9H3ØZ
ØØ9H3ZZ
ØØ9H4ØZ
ØØ9H4ZZ
ØØ9JØØZ
ØØ9JØZX
ØØ9JØZZ
ØØ9J3ØZ
ØØ9J3ZZ
ØØ9J4ØZ
ØØ9J4ZZ
ØØ9KØØZ
ØØ9KØZX
ØØ9KØZZ
ØØ9K3ØZ
ØØ9K3ZZ
ØØ9K4ØZ
ØØ9K4ZZ
ØØ9LØØZ
ØØ9LØZX
ØØ9LØZZ
ØØ9L3ØZ
ØØ9L3ZZ
ØØ9L4ØZ
ØØ9L4ZZ
ØØ9MØØZ
ØØ9MØZX
ØØ9MØZZ
ØØ9M3ØZ
ØØ9M3ZZ
ØØ9M4ØZ
ØØ9M4ZZ
ØØ9NØØZ
ØØ9NØZX
ØØ9NØZZ
ØØ9N3ØZ
ØØ9N3ZZ
ØØ9N4ØZ
ØØ9N4ZZ
ØØ9PØØZ
ØØ9PØZX
ØØ9PØZZ
ØØ9P3ØZ
ØØ9P3ZZ
ØØ9P4ØZ
ØØ9P4ZZ
ØØ9QØØZ
ØØ9QØZX
ØØ9QØZZ
ØØ9Q3ØZ
ØØ9Q3ZZ
ØØ9Q4ØZ
ØØ9Q4ZZ
ØØ9RØØZ
ØØ9RØZX
ØØ9RØZZ
ØØ9R3ØZ
ØØ9R3ZZ
ØØ9R4ØZ
ØØ9R4ZZ
ØØ9SØØZ
ØØ9SØZX
ØØ9SØZZ
ØØ9S3ØZ
ØØ9S3ZZ
ØØ9S4ØZ
ØØ9S4ZZ
ØØBFØZX
ØØBFØZZ
ØØBF3ZZ
ØØBF4ZZ
ØØBGØZX
ØØBGØZZ
ØØBG3ZZ
ØØBG4ZZ
ØØBHØZX
ØØBHØZZ
ØØBH3ZZ
ØØBH4ZZ
ØØBJØZX
ØØBJØZZ
ØØBJ3ZZ
ØØBJ4ZZ
ØØBKØZX
ØØBKØZZ
ØØBK3ZZ
ØØBK4ZZ
ØØBLØZX
ØØBLØZZ
ØØBL3ZZ
ØØBL4ZZ
ØØBMØZX
ØØBMØZZ
ØØBM3ZZ
ØØBM4ZZ
ØØBNØZX
ØØBN3ZZ
ØØBN4ZZ
ØØBPØZX
ØØBPØZZ
ØØBP3ZZ
ØØBP4ZZ
ØØBQØZX
ØØBQØZZ
ØØBQ3ZZ
ØØBQ4ZZ
ØØBRØZX
ØØBRØZZ
ØØBR3ZZ
ØØBR4ZZ
ØØBSØZX
ØØBSØZZ
ØØBS3ZZ
ØØBS4ZZ
ØØCF*
ØØCG*
ØØCH*
ØØCJ*
ØØCK*
ØØCL*
ØØCM*
ØØCN*
ØØCP*
ØØCQ*
ØØCR*
ØØCS*
ØØDF*
ØØDG*
ØØDH*
ØØDJ*
ØØDK*
ØØDL*
ØØDM*
ØØDN*
ØØDP*
ØØDQ*
ØØDR*
ØØDS*
ØØHEØ1Z
ØØHEØ2Z
ØØHEØ3Z
ØØHEØMZ
ØØHEØYZ
ØØHE31Z
ØØHE33Z
ØØHE3MZ
ØØHE41Z
ØØHE42Z
ØØHE43Z
ØØHE4MZ
ØØJEØZZ
ØØJE4ZZ
ØØNF*
ØØNG*
ØØNH*
ØØNJ*
ØØNL*
ØØNM*
ØØNN*
ØØNP*
ØØNQ*
ØØNR*
ØØNS*
ØØPEØØZ
ØØPEØ2Z
ØØPEØ3Z
ØØPEØ7Z
ØØPEØMZ
ØØPEØYZ
ØØPE37Z
ØØPE3MZ
ØØPE4ØZ
ØØPE42Z
ØØPE43Z
ØØPE47Z
ØØPE4MZ
ØØQF*
ØØQG*
ØØQH*
ØØQJ*
ØØQK*
ØØQL*
ØØQM*
ØØQN*
ØØQP*
ØØQQ*
ØØQR*
ØØQS*
ØØRFØ7Z
ØØRFØJZ
ØØRFØKZ
ØØRF47Z
ØØRF4JZ
ØØRF4KZ
ØØRGØ7Z
ØØRGØJZ
ØØRGØKZ
ØØRG47Z
ØØRG4JZ
ØØRG4KZ
ØØRHØ7Z
ØØRHØJZ
ØØRHØKZ
ØØRH47Z
ØØRH4JZ
ØØRH4KZ
ØØRJØ7Z
ØØRJØJZ
ØØRJØKZ
ØØRJ47Z
ØØRJ4JZ
ØØRJ4KZ
ØØRKØ7Z
ØØRKØJZ
ØØRKØKZ
ØØRK47Z
ØØRK4JZ
ØØRK4KZ
ØØRLØ7Z
ØØRLØJZ
ØØRLØKZ
ØØRL47Z
ØØRL4JZ
ØØRL4KZ
ØØRMØ7Z
ØØRMØJZ
ØØRMØKZ
ØØRM47Z
ØØRM4JZ
ØØRM4KZ
ØØRNØ7Z
ØØRNØJZ
ØØRNØKZ
ØØRN47Z
ØØRN4JZ
ØØRN4KZ
ØØRPØ7Z
ØØRPØJZ
ØØRPØKZ
ØØRP47Z
ØØRP4JZ

ØØRP4KZ
ØØRQØ7Z
ØØRQØJZ
ØØRQØKZ
ØØRQ47Z
ØØRQ4JZ
ØØRQ4KZ
ØØRRØ7Z
ØØRRØJZ
ØØRRØKZ
ØØRR47Z
ØØRR4JZ
ØØRR4KZ
ØØRSØ7Z
ØØRSØJZ
ØØRSØKZ
ØØRS47Z
ØØRS4JZ
ØØRS4KZ
ØØSF*
ØØSG*
ØØSH*
ØØSJ*
ØØSK*
ØØSL*
ØØSM*
ØØSN*
ØØSP*
ØØSQ*
ØØSR*
ØØSS*
ØØUF*
ØØUG*
ØØUH*
ØØUJ*
ØØUK*
ØØUL*
ØØUM*
ØØUN*
ØØUP*
ØØUQ*
ØØUR*
ØØUS*
ØØWEØØZ
ØØWEØ2Z
ØØWEØ3Z
ØØWEØ7Z
ØØWEØMZ
ØØWEØYZ
ØØWE3ØZ
ØØWE32Z
ØØWE33Z
ØØWE37Z
ØØWE3MZ
ØØWE4ØZ
ØØWE42Z
ØØWE43Z
ØØWE47Z
ØØWE4MZ
ØØX*
Ø15K*
Ø15L*
Ø15M*
Ø15N*
Ø15P*
Ø18Ø*
Ø182*
Ø183*
Ø184*
Ø185*
Ø186*
Ø189*
Ø18A*
Ø18C*
Ø18D*
Ø18F*
Ø18G*
Ø18H*
Ø18K*
Ø18L*
Ø18M*
Ø18N*
Ø18P*
Ø18Q*
Ø19ØØØZ
Ø19ØØZX
Ø19ØØZZ
Ø19Ø4ØZ
Ø19Ø4ZZ
Ø191ØØZ
Ø191ØZX
Ø191ØZZ
Ø1914ØZ
Ø1914ZZ
Ø192ØØZ
Ø192ØZX
Ø192ØZZ
Ø1924ØZ
Ø1924ZZ
Ø193ØØZ
Ø193ØZX
Ø193ØZZ
Ø1934ØZ
Ø1934ZZ
Ø194ØØZ
Ø194ØZX
Ø194ØZZ
Ø1944ØZ
Ø1944ZZ
Ø195ØØZ
Ø195ØZX
Ø195ØZZ
Ø1954ØZ
Ø1954ZZ
Ø196ØØZ
Ø196ØZX
Ø196ØZZ
Ø1964ØZ
Ø1964ZZ
Ø198ØØZ
Ø198ØZX
Ø198ØZZ
Ø1984ØZ
Ø1984ZZ
Ø199ØØZ
Ø199ØZX
Ø199ØZZ
Ø1994ØZ
Ø1994ZZ
Ø19AØØZ
Ø19AØZX
Ø19AØZZ
Ø19A4ØZ
Ø19A4ZZ
Ø19BØØZ
Ø19BØZX
Ø19BØZZ
Ø19B4ØZ
Ø19B4ZZ
Ø19CØØZ
Ø19CØZX
Ø19CØZZ
Ø19C4ØZ
Ø19C4ZZ
Ø19DØØZ
Ø19DØZX
Ø19DØZZ
Ø19D4ØZ
Ø19D4ZZ
Ø19FØØZ
Ø19FØZX
Ø19FØZZ
Ø19F4ØZ
Ø19F4ZZ
Ø19GØØZ
Ø19GØZX
Ø19GØZZ
Ø19G4ØZ
Ø19G4ZZ
Ø19HØØZ
Ø19HØZX
Ø19HØZZ
Ø19H4ØZ
Ø19H4ZZ
Ø19KØØZ
Ø19KØZX
Ø19KØZZ
Ø19K3ZX
Ø19K4ØZ
Ø19K4ZX
Ø19K4ZZ
Ø19LØØZ
Ø19LØZX
Ø19LØZZ
Ø19L3ZX
Ø19L4ØZ
Ø19L4ZX
Ø19L4ZZ
Ø19MØØZ
Ø19MØZX
Ø19MØZZ
Ø19M3ZX
Ø19M4ØZ
Ø19M4ZX
Ø19M4ZZ
Ø19NØØZ
Ø19NØZX
Ø19NØZZ
Ø19N3ZX
Ø19N4ØZ
Ø19N4ZX
Ø19N4ZZ
Ø19PØØZ
Ø19PØZX
Ø19PØZZ
Ø19P3ZX
Ø19P4ØZ
Ø19P4ZX
Ø19P4ZZ
Ø19QØØZ
Ø19QØZX
Ø19QØZZ
Ø19Q4ØZ
Ø19Q4ZZ
Ø19RØØZ
Ø19RØZX
Ø19RØZZ
Ø19R4ØZ
Ø19R4ZZ
Ø1BØØZX
Ø1BØØZZ
Ø1BØ3ZZ
Ø1BØ4ZZ
Ø1B1ØZX
Ø1B1ØZZ
Ø1B13ZZ
Ø1B14ZZ
Ø1B2ØZX
Ø1B2ØZZ
Ø1B23ZZ
Ø1B24ZZ
Ø1B3ØZX
Ø1B3ØZZ
Ø1B33ZZ
Ø1B34ZZ
Ø1B4ØZX
Ø1B4ØZZ
Ø1B43ZZ
Ø1B44ZZ
Ø1B5ØZX
Ø1B5ØZZ
Ø1B53ZZ
Ø1B54ZZ
Ø1B6ØZX
Ø1B6ØZZ
Ø1B63ZZ
Ø1B64ZZ
Ø1B8ØZX
Ø1B8ØZZ
Ø1B83ZZ
Ø1B84ZZ
Ø1B9ØZX
Ø1B9ØZZ
Ø1B93ZZ
Ø1B94ZZ
Ø1BAØZX
Ø1BAØZZ
Ø1BA3ZZ
Ø1BA4ZZ
Ø1BBØZX
Ø1BBØZZ
Ø1BB3ZZ
Ø1BB4ZZ
Ø1BCØZX
Ø1BCØZZ
Ø1BC3ZZ
Ø1BC4ZZ
Ø1BDØZX
Ø1BDØZZ
Ø1BD3ZZ
Ø1BD4ZZ
Ø1BFØZX
Ø1BFØZZ
Ø1BF3ZZ
Ø1BF4ZZ
Ø1BGØZX
Ø1BGØZZ
Ø1BG3ZZ
Ø1BG4ZZ
Ø1BHØZX
Ø1BHØZZ
Ø1BH3ZZ
Ø1BH4ZZ
Ø1BK*
Ø1BL*
Ø1BM*
Ø1BN*
Ø1BP*
Ø1BQØZX
Ø1BQØZZ
Ø1BQ3ZZ
Ø1BQ4ZZ
Ø1BRØZX
Ø1BRØZZ
Ø1BR3ZZ
Ø1BR4ZZ
Ø1C*
Ø1D*
Ø1HYØ1Z
Ø1HYØ2Z
Ø1HYØMZ
Ø1HYØYZ
Ø1HY32Z
Ø1HY3MZ
Ø1HY41Z
Ø1HY42Z
Ø1HY4MZ
Ø1JYØZZ
Ø1JY4ZZ
Ø1N*
Ø1PYØØZ
Ø1PYØ2Z
Ø1PYØ7Z
Ø1PYØMZ
Ø1PYØYZ
Ø1PY37Z
Ø1PY3MZ
Ø1PY4ØZ
Ø1PY42Z
Ø1PY47Z
Ø1PY4MZ
Ø1Q*
Ø1R1Ø7Z
Ø1R1ØJZ
Ø1R1ØKZ
Ø1R147Z
Ø1R14JZ
Ø1R14KZ
Ø1R2Ø7Z
Ø1R2ØJZ
Ø1R2ØKZ
Ø1R247Z
Ø1R24JZ
Ø1R24KZ
Ø1R4Ø7Z
Ø1R4ØJZ
Ø1R4ØKZ
Ø1R447Z
Ø1R44JZ
Ø1R44KZ
Ø1R5Ø7Z
Ø1R5ØJZ
Ø1R5ØKZ
Ø1R547Z
Ø1R54JZ
Ø1R54KZ
Ø1R6Ø7Z
Ø1R6ØJZ
Ø1R6ØKZ
Ø1R647Z
Ø1R64JZ
Ø1R64KZ
Ø1R8Ø7Z
Ø1R8ØJZ
Ø1R8ØKZ
Ø1R847Z
Ø1R84JZ
Ø1R84KZ
Ø1RBØ7Z
Ø1RBØJZ
Ø1RBØKZ
Ø1RB47Z
Ø1RB4JZ
Ø1RB4KZ
Ø1RCØ7Z
Ø1RCØJZ
Ø1RCØKZ
Ø1RC47Z
Ø1RC4JZ
Ø1RC4KZ
Ø1RDØ7Z
Ø1RDØJZ
Ø1RDØKZ
Ø1RD47Z
Ø1RD4JZ
Ø1RD4KZ
Ø1RFØ7Z
Ø1RFØJZ
Ø1RFØKZ
Ø1RF47Z
Ø1RF4JZ
Ø1RF4KZ
Ø1RGØ7Z
Ø1RGØJZ
Ø1RGØKZ
Ø1RG47Z
Ø1RG4JZ
Ø1RG4KZ
Ø1RHØ7Z
Ø1RHØJZ
Ø1RHØKZ
Ø1RH47Z
Ø1RH4JZ
Ø1RH4KZ
Ø1RRØ7Z
Ø1RRØJZ
Ø1RRØKZ
Ø1RR47Z
Ø1RR4JZ
Ø1RR4KZ
Ø1S*
Ø1U*
Ø1WYØØZ
Ø1WYØ2Z
Ø1WYØ7Z
Ø1WYØMZ
Ø1WYØYZ
Ø1WY3ØZ
Ø1WY32Z
Ø1WY37Z
Ø1WY3MZ
Ø1WY4ØZ
Ø1WY42Z
Ø1WY47Z
Ø1WY4MZ
Ø1X*
Ø2HVØ2Z
Ø2HVØDZ
Ø2HV3DZ
Ø2HV42Z
Ø2HV4DZ
Ø2LV*
Ø2PAØMZ
Ø2PA3MZ
Ø2PA4MZ
Ø2VV*
Ø2WAØMZ
Ø2WA3MZ
Ø2WA4MZ
Ø39SØZX
Ø39S4ZX
Ø39TØZX
Ø39T4ZX
Ø3BSØZX
Ø3BS3ZX
Ø3BS4ZX
Ø3BTØZX
Ø3BT3ZX
Ø3BT4ZX
Ø3LHØCZ
Ø3LHØZZ
Ø3LH3CZ
Ø3LH3ZZ
Ø3LH4CZ
Ø3LH4ZZ
Ø3LJØCZ
Ø3LJØZZ
Ø3LJ3CZ
Ø3LJ3ZZ
Ø3LJ4CZ
Ø3LJ4ZZ
Ø3LMØCZ
Ø3LMØZZ
Ø3LM3CZ
Ø3LM3ZZ
Ø3LM4CZ
Ø3LM4ZZ
Ø3LNØCZ
Ø3LNØZZ
Ø3LN3CZ
Ø3LN3ZZ
Ø3LN4CZ
Ø3LN4ZZ
Ø3LPØCZ
Ø3LPØZZ
Ø3LP3CZ
Ø3LP3ZZ
Ø3LP4CZ
Ø3LP4ZZ
Ø3LQØCZ
Ø3LQØZZ
Ø3LQ3CZ
Ø3LQ3ZZ
Ø3LQ4CZ
Ø3LQ4ZZ
Ø3LRØCZ
Ø3LRØZZ
Ø3LR3CZ
Ø3LR3ZZ
Ø3LR4CZ
Ø3LR4ZZ
Ø3LSØCZ
Ø3LSØZZ
Ø3LS3CZ
Ø3LS3ZZ
Ø3LS4CZ
Ø3LS4ZZ
Ø3LTØCZ
Ø3LTØZZ
Ø3LT3CZ
Ø3LT3ZZ
Ø3LT4CZ
Ø3LT4ZZ
Ø3RH*
Ø3RJ*
Ø3RK*
Ø3RL*
Ø3RM*
Ø3RN*
Ø3RP*
Ø3RQ*
Ø3RR*
Ø3RS*
Ø3RT*
Ø3RU*
Ø3RV*
Ø5CM*
Ø5CN*
Ø5CP*
Ø5CQ*
Ø5CR*
Ø5CS*
Ø5CT*
Ø5CV*
Ø5HØØ2Z
Ø5HØØMZ
Ø5HØ32Z
Ø5HØ3MZ
Ø5HØ42Z
Ø5HØ4MZ
Ø5H3ØMZ
Ø5H33MZ
Ø5H34MZ
Ø5H4ØMZ
Ø5H43MZ
Ø5H44MZ
Ø5HYØ2Z
Ø5HYØYZ
Ø5HY42Z
Ø5LM*
Ø5LN*
Ø5LP*
Ø5LQ*
Ø5LR*
Ø5LS*
Ø5LT*
Ø5LV*
Ø5PØØMZ
Ø5PØ3MZ
Ø5PØ4MZ
Ø5PØXMZ
Ø5P3ØMZ
Ø5P33MZ
Ø5P34MZ
Ø5P3XMZ
Ø5P4ØMZ
Ø5P43MZ
Ø5P44MZ
Ø5P4XMZ
Ø5RM*
Ø5RN*
Ø5RP*
Ø5RQ*
Ø5RR*
Ø5RS*
Ø5RT*
Ø5RV*
Ø5WØØMZ
Ø5WØ3MZ
Ø5WØ4MZ
Ø5W3ØMZ
Ø5W33MZ
Ø5W34MZ
Ø5W4ØMZ
Ø5W43MZ
Ø5W44MZ
Ø693ØØZ
Ø693ØZZ
Ø6934ØZ
Ø6934ZZ
Ø6C3*
Ø6HØØDZ
Ø6HØ4DZ
Ø6LØ*
Ø6R3*
Ø6VØ*
Ø75M*
Ø79ØØZX
Ø79Ø3ZX
Ø79Ø4ZX
Ø791ØZX
Ø7913ZX
Ø7914ZX
Ø792ØZX
Ø7923ZX
Ø7924ZX
Ø793ØZX
Ø7933ZX
Ø7934ZX
Ø794ØZX
Ø7943ZX
Ø7944ZX
Ø795ØZX
Ø7953ZX
Ø7954ZX
Ø796ØZX
Ø7963ZX
Ø7964ZX
Ø797ØZX
Ø7973ZX
Ø7974ZX
Ø798ØZX
Ø7983ZX
Ø7984ZX
Ø799ØZX
Ø7993ZX
Ø7994ZX
Ø79BØZX
Ø79B3ZX
Ø79B4ZX
Ø79CØZX
Ø79C3ZX
Ø79C4ZX
Ø79DØZX
Ø79D3ZX
Ø79D4ZX
Ø79FØZX
Ø79F3ZX
Ø79F4ZX
Ø79GØZX
Ø79G3ZX
Ø79G4ZX
Ø79HØZX
Ø79H3ZX
Ø79H4ZX
Ø79JØZX
Ø79J3ZX
Ø79J4ZX
Ø79KØZX
Ø79K3ZX
Ø79K4ZX
Ø79LØZX
Ø79L3ZX
Ø79L4ZX
Ø79M4ZZ
Ø7BØØZX
Ø7BØ3ZX
Ø7BØ4ZX
Ø7B1ØZX
Ø7B13ZX
Ø7B14ZX
Ø7B2ØZX
Ø7B23ZX
Ø7B24ZX
Ø7B3ØZX
Ø7B33ZX
Ø7B34ZX
Ø7B4ØZX
Ø7B43ZX
Ø7B44ZX
Ø7B5ØZX
Ø7B53ZX
Ø7B54ZX
Ø7B6ØZX
Ø7B63ZX
Ø7B64ZX
Ø7B7ØZX
Ø7B73ZX
Ø7B74ZX
Ø7B8ØZX
Ø7B83ZX
Ø7B84ZX
Ø7B9ØZX
Ø7B93ZX
Ø7B94ZX
Ø7BBØZX
Ø7BB3ZX
Ø7BB4ZX
Ø7BCØZX
Ø7BC3ZX
Ø7BC4ZX
Ø7BDØZX
Ø7BD3ZX
Ø7BD4ZX
Ø7BFØZX
Ø7BF3ZX
Ø7BF4ZX
Ø7BGØZX
Ø7BG3ZX
Ø7BG4ZX
Ø7BHØZX
Ø7BH3ZX
Ø7BH4ZX
Ø7BJØZX
Ø7BJ3ZX
Ø7BJ4ZX
Ø7BKØZX
Ø7BK3ZX
Ø7BK4ZX
Ø7BLØZX
Ø7BL3ZX
Ø7BL4ZX
Ø7BMØZZ
Ø7BM3ZZ
Ø7BM4ZZ
Ø7CM4ZZ
Ø7JM4ZZ
Ø7NM4ZZ
Ø7QM4ZZ
Ø7TM*
Ø8HØ31Z
Ø8HØX1Z
Ø8H131Z
Ø8H1X1Z
Ø8NN*
Ø8NP*
Ø8NQ*
Ø8NR*
Ø8SN*
Ø8SP*
Ø8SQ*
Ø8SR*
Ø9QN*
Ø9RN*
Ø9UN*
ØCQ2*
ØCQ3*
ØCQM*
ØCR2*
ØCR3*
ØCRM*
ØCS2*
ØCS3*
ØCU2Ø7Z
ØCU2ØKZ
ØCU237Z
ØCU23KZ
ØCU2X7Z
ØCU2XJZ
ØCU2XKZ
ØCU3*
ØCUM*
ØDH6ØMZ
ØDH63MZ
ØDH64MZ
ØDP6ØMZ
ØDP63MZ
ØDP64MZ
ØDPR*
ØDWWØJZ
ØDWW3JZ
ØDWW4JZ
ØHRØ*
ØHR1*
ØHR4*
ØHR5*
ØHR6*
ØHR7*
ØHR8*
ØHRA*
ØHRB*
ØHRC*
ØHRD*
ØHRE*
ØHRF*
ØHRG*
ØHRH*
ØHRJ*
ØHRK*
ØHRL*
ØHRM*
ØHRN*
ØHXØXZZ
ØHX1XZZ
ØHX4XZZ
ØHX5XZZ
ØHX6XZZ
ØHX7XZZ
ØHX8XZZ
ØHX9XZZ
ØHXAXZZ
ØHXBXZZ
ØHXCXZZ
ØHXDXZZ
ØHXEXZZ
ØHXFXZZ
ØHXGXZZ
ØHXHXZZ
ØHXJXZZ
ØHXKXZZ
ØHXLXZZ
ØHXMXZZ
ØHXNXZZ
ØJ8Ø*
ØJ84*
ØJ85*
ØJ86*
ØJ87*
ØJ88*
ØJ89*
ØJ8B*
ØJ8C*
ØJ8D*
ØJ8F*
ØJ8G*
ØJ8H*
ØJ8L*
ØJ8M*
ØJ8N*
ØJ8P*
ØJ8Q*
ØJ8R*
ØJ8S*
ØJ8T*
ØJ8V*
ØJ8W*
ØJBØØZZ
ØJB1ØZZ
ØJB4ØZZ
ØJB5ØZZ
ØJB6ØZZ
ØJB7ØZZ
ØJB8ØZZ
ØJB9ØZZ
ØJBBØZZ
ØJBCØZZ
ØJBDØZZ
ØJBFØZZ
ØJBGØZZ
ØJBHØZZ
ØJBLØZZ
ØJBMØZZ
ØJBNØZZ
ØJBPØZZ
ØJBQØZZ
ØJBRØZZ
ØJDØØZZ
ØJD1ØZZ
ØJD4ØZZ
ØJD5ØZZ
ØJD6ØZZ
ØJD7ØZZ
ØJD8ØZZ
ØJD9ØZZ
ØJDBØZZ
ØJDCØZZ
ØJDDØZZ
ØJDFØZZ
ØJDGØZZ
ØJDHØZZ
ØJDLØZZ
ØJDMØZZ
ØJDNØZZ
ØJDPØZZ
ØJDQØZZ
ØJDRØZZ
ØJHØ*
ØJH1*
ØJH4*
ØJH5*
ØJH6Ø2Z
ØJH6ØBZ
ØJH6ØCZ
ØJH6ØDZ
ØJH6ØEZ
ØJH6ØMZ
ØJH6ØNZ
ØJH6ØVZ
ØJH6ØYZ
ØJH632Z
ØJH63BZ
ØJH63CZ
ØJH63DZ
ØJH63EZ
ØJH63MZ

ØJH63NZ
ØJH63VZ
ØJH7ØBZ
ØJH7ØCZ
ØJH7ØDZ
ØJH7ØEZ
ØJH7ØMZ
ØJH7ØNZ
ØJH7ØVZ
ØJH7ØYZ
ØJH73BZ
ØJH73CZ
ØJH73DZ
ØJH73EZ
ØJH73MZ
ØJH73NZ
ØJH73VZ
ØJH8ØBZ
ØJH8ØCZ
ØJH8ØDZ
ØJH8ØEZ
ØJH8ØMZ
ØJH8ØNZ
ØJH8ØVZ
ØJH8ØYZ
ØJH83BZ
ØJH83CZ
ØJH83DZ
ØJH83EZ
ØJH83MZ
ØJH83NZ
ØJH83VZ
ØJH9*
ØJHB*
ØJHC*
ØJHDØNZ
ØJHDØVZ
ØJHD3NZ
ØJHD3VZ
ØJHFØNZ
ØJHFØVZ
ØJHF3NZ
ØJHF3VZ
ØJHGØNZ
ØJHGØVZ
ØJHG3NZ
ØJHG3VZ
ØJHHØNZ
ØJHHØVZ
ØJHH3NZ
ØJHH3VZ
ØJHJ*
ØJHK*
ØJHLØNZ
ØJHLØVZ
ØJHL3NZ
ØJHL3VZ
ØJHMØNZ
ØJHMØVZ
ØJHM3NZ
ØJHM3VZ
ØJHNØNZ
ØJHNØVZ
ØJHN3NZ
ØJHN3VZ
ØJHPØNZ
ØJHPØVZ
ØJHP3NZ
ØJHP3VZ
ØJHQ*
ØJHR*
ØJHTØVZ
ØJHTØYZ
ØJHT3VZ
ØJPTØFZ
ØJPTØPZ
ØJPT3FZ
ØJPT3PZ
ØJQØØZZ
ØJQJØZZ
ØJQKØZZ
ØJRJØ7Z
ØJRJØJZ
ØJRJØKZ
ØJRJ3JZ
ØJRJ3KZ
ØJRKØ7Z
ØJRKØJZ
ØJRKØKZ
ØJRK3JZ
ØJRK3KZ
ØJUJ*
ØJUK*
ØJWTØ2Z
ØJWTØFZ
ØJWTØPZ
ØJWTØYZ
ØJWT32Z
ØJWT3FZ
ØJWT3PZ
ØJXØØZB
ØJXØØZC
ØJXØ3ZB
ØJXØ3ZC
ØJX1ØZB
ØJX1ØZC
ØJX13ZB
ØJX13ZC
ØJX4ØZB
ØJX4ØZC
ØJX43ZB
ØJX43ZC
ØJX5ØZB
ØJX5ØZC
ØJX53ZB
ØJX53ZC
ØJX6ØZB
ØJX6ØZC
ØJX63ZB
ØJX63ZC
ØJX7ØZB
ØJX7ØZC
ØJX73ZB
ØJX73ZC
ØJX8ØZB
ØJX8ØZC
ØJX83ZB
ØJX83ZC
ØJX9ØZB
ØJX9ØZC
ØJX93ZB
ØJX93ZC
ØJXBØZB
ØJXBØZC
ØJXB3ZB
ØJXB3ZC
ØJXCØZB
ØJXCØZC
ØJXC3ZB
ØJXC3ZC
ØJXDØZB
ØJXDØZC
ØJXD3ZB
ØJXD3ZC
ØJXFØZB
ØJXFØZC
ØJXF3ZB
ØJXF3ZC
ØJXGØZB
ØJXGØZC
ØJXG3ZB
ØJXG3ZC
ØJXHØZB
ØJXHØZC
ØJXH3ZB
ØJXH3ZC
ØJXJØZZ
ØJXJ3ZZ
ØJXLØZB
ØJXLØZC
ØJXL3ZB
ØJXL3ZC
ØJXMØZB
ØJXMØZC
ØJXM3ZB
ØJXM3ZC
ØJXNØZB
ØJXNØZC
ØJXN3ZB
ØJXN3ZC
ØJXPØZB
ØJXPØZC
ØJXP3ZB
ØJXP3ZC
ØJXQØZB
ØJXQØZC
ØJXQ3ZB
ØJXQ3ZC
ØJXRØZB
ØJXRØZC
ØJXR3ZB
ØJXR3ZC
ØK8Ø*
ØK81*
ØK82*
ØK83*
ØK85*
ØK86*
ØK87*
ØK88*
ØK89*
ØK8B*
ØK8F*
ØK8G*
ØK8H*
ØK8J*
ØK8K*
ØK8L*
ØK8M*
ØK8N*
ØK8P*
ØK8Q*
ØK8R*
ØK8S*
ØK8T*
ØK8V*
ØK8W*
ØK9ØØZX
ØK91ØZX
ØK92ØZX
ØK93ØZX
ØK94ØZX
ØK95ØZX
ØK96ØZX
ØK97ØZX
ØK98ØZX
ØK99ØZX
ØK9BØZX
ØK9CØZX
ØK9DØZX
ØK9FØZX
ØK9GØZX
ØK9HØZX
ØK9JØZX
ØK9KØZX
ØK9LØZX
ØK9MØZX
ØK9NØZX
ØK9PØZX
ØK9QØZX
ØK9RØZX
ØK9SØZX
ØK9TØZX
ØK9VØZX
ØK9WØZX
ØKBØØZX
ØKBØØZZ
ØKBØ3ZZ
ØKBØ4ZZ
ØKB1ØZX
ØKB1ØZZ
ØKB13ZZ
ØKB14ZZ
ØKB2ØZX
ØKB2ØZZ
ØKB23ZZ
ØKB24ZZ
ØKB3ØZX
ØKB3ØZZ
ØKB33ZZ
ØKB34ZZ
ØKB4ØZX
ØKB4ØZZ
ØKB43ZZ
ØKB44ZZ
ØKB5ØZX
ØKB5ØZZ
ØKB53ZZ
ØKB54ZZ
ØKB6ØZX
ØKB6ØZZ
ØKB63ZZ
ØKB64ZZ
ØKB7ØZX
ØKB7ØZZ
ØKB73ZZ
ØKB74ZZ
ØKB8ØZX
ØKB8ØZZ
ØKB83ZZ
ØKB84ZZ
ØKB9ØZX
ØKB9ØZZ
ØKB93ZZ
ØKB94ZZ
ØKBBØZX
ØKBBØZZ
ØKBB3ZZ
ØKBB4ZZ
ØKBCØZX
ØKBDØZX
ØKBFØZX
ØKBFØZZ
ØKBF3ZZ
ØKBF4ZZ
ØKBGØZX
ØKBGØZZ
ØKBG3ZZ
ØKBG4ZZ
ØKBHØZX
ØKBHØZZ
ØKBH3ZZ
ØKBH4ZZ
ØKBJØZX
ØKBJØZZ
ØKBJ3ZZ
ØKBJ4ZZ
ØKBKØZX
ØKBKØZZ
ØKBK3ZZ
ØKBK4ZZ
ØKBLØZX
ØKBLØZZ
ØKBL3ZZ
ØKBL4ZZ
ØKBMØZX
ØKBMØZZ
ØKBM3ZZ
ØKBM4ZZ
ØKBNØZX
ØKBNØZZ
ØKBN4ZZ
ØKBPØZX
ØKBPØZZ
ØKBP4ZZ
ØKBQØZX
ØKBQØZZ
ØKBQ3ZZ
ØKBQ4ZZ
ØKBRØZX
ØKBRØZZ
ØKBR3ZZ
ØKBR4ZZ
ØKBSØZX
ØKBSØZZ
ØKBS3ZZ
ØKBS4ZZ
ØKBTØZX
ØKBTØZZ
ØKBT3ZZ
ØKBT4ZZ
ØKBVØZX
ØKBVØZZ
ØKBV3ZZ
ØKBV4ZZ
ØKBWØZX
ØKBWØZZ
ØKBW3ZZ
ØKBW4ZZ
ØKDØØZZ
ØKD1ØZZ
ØKD2ØZZ
ØKD3ØZZ
ØKD4ØZZ
ØKD5ØZZ
ØKD6ØZZ
ØKD7ØZZ
ØKD8ØZZ
ØKD9ØZZ
ØKDBØZZ
ØKDFØZZ
ØKDGØZZ
ØKDHØZZ
ØKDJØZZ
ØKDKØZZ
ØKDLØZZ
ØKDMØZZ
ØKDNØZZ
ØKDPØZZ
ØKDQØZZ
ØKDRØZZ
ØKDSØZZ
ØKDTØZZ
ØKDVØZZ
ØKDWØZZ
ØKHXØMZ
ØKHXØYZ
ØKHX3MZ
ØKHX4MZ
ØKHYØMZ
ØKHYØYZ
ØKHY3MZ
ØKHY4MZ
ØKM*
ØKPXØMZ
ØKPX3MZ
ØKPX4MZ
ØKPYØMZ
ØKPY3MZ
ØKPY4MZ
ØKQØ*
ØKQ1*
ØKQ2*
ØKQ3*
ØKQ4*
ØKQ5*
ØKQ6*
ØKQ7*
ØKQ8*
ØKQ9*
ØKQB*
ØKQF*
ØKQG*
ØKQH*
ØKQJ*
ØKQK*
ØKQL*
ØKQM*
ØKQN*
ØKQP*
ØKQS*
ØKQT*
ØKQV*
ØKQW*
ØKRØØ7Z
ØKRØØJZ
ØKRØØKZ
ØKRØ47Z
ØKRØ4JZ
ØKRØ4KZ
ØKR1Ø7Z
ØKR1ØJZ
ØKR1ØKZ
ØKR147Z
ØKR14JZ
ØKR14KZ
ØKR2Ø7Z
ØKR2ØJZ
ØKR2ØKZ
ØKR247Z
ØKR24JZ
ØKR24KZ
ØKR3Ø7Z
ØKR3ØJZ
ØKR3ØKZ
ØKR347Z
ØKR34JZ
ØKR34KZ
ØKR4Ø7Z
ØKR4ØJZ
ØKR4ØKZ
ØKR447Z
ØKR44JZ
ØKR44KZ
ØKR5Ø7Z
ØKR5ØJZ
ØKR5ØKZ
ØKR547Z
ØKR54JZ
ØKR54KZ
ØKR6Ø7Z
ØKR6ØJZ
ØKR6ØKZ
ØKR647Z
ØKR64JZ
ØKR64KZ
ØKR7Ø7Z
ØKR7ØJZ
ØKR7ØKZ
ØKR747Z
ØKR74JZ
ØKR74KZ
ØKR8Ø7Z
ØKR8ØJZ
ØKR8ØKZ
ØKR847Z
ØKR84JZ
ØKR84KZ
ØKR9Ø7Z
ØKR9ØJZ
ØKR9ØKZ
ØKR947Z
ØKR94JZ
ØKR94KZ
ØKRBØ7Z
ØKRBØJZ
ØKRBØKZ
ØKRB47Z
ØKRB4JZ
ØKRB4KZ
ØKRFØ7Z
ØKRFØJZ
ØKRFØKZ
ØKRF47Z
ØKRF4JZ
ØKRF4KZ
ØKRGØ7Z
ØKRGØJZ
ØKRGØKZ
ØKRG47Z
ØKRG4JZ
ØKRG4KZ
ØKRHØ7Z
ØKRHØJZ
ØKRHØKZ
ØKRH47Z
ØKRH4JZ
ØKRH4KZ
ØKRJØ7Z
ØKRJØJZ
ØKRJØKZ
ØKRJ47Z
ØKRJ4JZ
ØKRJ4KZ
ØKRKØ7Z
ØKRKØJZ
ØKRKØKZ
ØKRK47Z
ØKRK4JZ
ØKRK4KZ
ØKRLØ7Z
ØKRLØJZ
ØKRLØKZ
ØKRL47Z
ØKRL4JZ
ØKRL4KZ
ØKRMØ7Z
ØKRMØJZ
ØKRMØKZ
ØKRM47Z
ØKRM4JZ
ØKRM4KZ
ØKRNØ7Z
ØKRNØJZ
ØKRNØKZ
ØKRN47Z
ØKRN4JZ
ØKRN4KZ
ØKRPØ7Z
ØKRPØJZ
ØKRPØKZ
ØKRP47Z
ØKRP4JZ
ØKRP4KZ
ØKRSØ7Z
ØKRSØJZ
ØKRSØKZ
ØKRS47Z
ØKRS4JZ
ØKRS4KZ
ØKRTØ7Z
ØKRTØJZ
ØKRTØKZ
ØKRT47Z
ØKRT4JZ
ØKRT4KZ
ØKRVØ7Z
ØKRVØJZ
ØKRVØKZ
ØKRV47Z
ØKRV4JZ
ØKRV4KZ
ØKRWØ7Z
ØKRWØJZ
ØKRWØKZ
ØKRW47Z
ØKRW4JZ
ØKRW4KZ
ØKS*
ØKTØ*
ØKT1*
ØKT2*
ØKT3*
ØKT4*
ØKT5*
ØKT6*
ØKT7*
ØKT8*
ØKT9*
ØKTB*
ØKTF*
ØKTG*
ØKTH*
ØKTJ*
ØKTK*
ØKTL*
ØKTM*
ØKTN*
ØKTP*
ØKTQ*
ØKTR*
ØKTS*
ØKTT*
ØKTV*
ØKTW*
ØKU*
ØKXØ*
ØKX1*
ØKX2*
ØKX3*
ØKX4*
ØKX5*
ØKX6*
ØKX7*
ØKX8*
ØKX9*
ØKXB*
ØKXC*
ØKXD*
ØKXFØZØ
ØKXFØZ1
ØKXFØZ2
ØKXFØZZ
ØKXF4ZØ
ØKXF4Z1
ØKXF4Z2
ØKXF4ZZ
ØKXGØZØ
ØKXGØZ1
ØKXGØZ2
ØKXGØZZ
ØKXG4ZØ
ØKXG4Z1
ØKXG4Z2
ØKXG4ZZ
ØKXHØZØ
ØKXHØZ1
ØKXHØZ2
ØKXH4ZØ
ØKXH4Z1
ØKXH4Z2
ØKXJØZØ
ØKXJØZ1
ØKXJØZ2
ØKXJ4ZØ
ØKXJ4Z1
ØKXJ4Z2
ØKXKØZØ
ØKXKØZ1
ØKXKØZ2
ØKXKØZZ
ØKXK4ZØ
ØKXK4Z1
ØKXK4Z2
ØKXK4ZZ
ØKXLØZØ
ØKXLØZ1
ØKXLØZ2
ØKXLØZZ
ØKXL4ZØ
ØKXL4Z1
ØKXL4Z2
ØKXL4ZZ
ØKXM*
ØKXN*
ØKXP*
ØKXQ*
ØKXR*
ØKXS*
ØKXT*
ØKXV*
ØKXW*
ØL8Ø*
ØL81*
ØL82*
ØL83*
ØL84*
ØL85*
ØL86*
ØL89*
ØL8B*
ØL8C*
ØL8D*
ØL8F*
ØL8G*
ØL8H*
ØL8L*
ØL8M*
ØL8Q*
ØL8R*
ØL8S*
ØL8T*
ØL8V*
ØL8W*
ØLBØØZZ
ØLBØ3ZZ
ØLBØ4ZZ
ØLB1ØZZ
ØLB13ZZ
ØLB14ZZ
ØLB2ØZZ
ØLB23ZZ
ØLB24ZZ
ØLB3ØZZ
ØLB33ZZ
ØLB34ZZ
ØLB4ØZZ
ØLB43ZZ
ØLB44ZZ
ØLB5ØZZ
ØLB53ZZ
ØLB54ZZ
ØLB6ØZZ
ØLB63ZZ
ØLB64ZZ
ØLB9ØZZ
ØLB93ZZ
ØLB94ZZ
ØLBBØZZ
ØLBB3ZZ
ØLBB4ZZ
ØLBCØZZ
ØLBC3ZZ
ØLBC4ZZ
ØLBDØZZ
ØLBD3ZZ
ØLBD4ZZ
ØLBFØZZ
ØLBF3ZZ
ØLBF4ZZ
ØLBGØZZ
ØLBG3ZZ
ØLBG4ZZ
ØLBHØZZ
ØLBH3ZZ
ØLBH4ZZ
ØLBJØZZ
ØLBJ3ZZ
ØLBJ4ZZ
ØLBKØZZ
ØLBK3ZZ
ØLBK4ZZ
ØLBLØZZ
ØLBL3ZZ
ØLBL4ZZ
ØLBMØZZ
ØLBM3ZZ
ØLBM4ZZ
ØLBNØZZ
ØLBN3ZZ
ØLBN4ZZ
ØLBPØZZ
ØLBP3ZZ
ØLBP4ZZ
ØLBQØZZ
ØLBQ3ZZ
ØLBQ4ZZ
ØLBRØZZ
ØLBR3ZZ
ØLBR4ZZ
ØLBSØZZ
ØLBS3ZZ
ØLBS4ZZ
ØLBTØZZ
ØLBT3ZZ
ØLBT4ZZ
ØLBVØZZ
ØLBV3ZZ
ØLBV4ZZ
ØLBWØZZ
ØLBW3ZZ
ØLBW4ZZ
ØLDØØZZ
ØLD1ØZZ
ØLD2ØZZ
ØLD3ØZZ
ØLD4ØZZ
ØLD5ØZZ
ØLD6ØZZ
ØLD9ØZZ
ØLDBØZZ
ØLDCØZZ
ØLDDØZZ
ØLDFØZZ
ØLDGØZZ
ØLDHØZZ
ØLDJØZZ
ØLDKØZZ
ØLDLØZZ
ØLDMØZZ
ØLDNØZZ
ØLDPØZZ
ØLDQØZZ
ØLDRØZZ
ØLDSØZZ
ØLDTØZZ
ØLDVØZZ
ØLDWØZZ
ØLHXØYZ
ØLHYØYZ
ØLM*
ØLQØ*
ØLQ3*
ØLQ4*
ØLQ5*
ØLQ6*
ØLQ7*
ØLQ8*
ØLQ9*
ØLQB*
ØLQC*
ØLQD*
ØLQF*
ØLQG*
ØLQH*
ØLQJ*
ØLQK*
ØLQL*
ØLQM*
ØLQN*
ØLQP*
ØLQV*
ØLQW*
ØLR7*
ØLR8*
ØLS*
ØLU7*
ØLU8*
ØLX*
ØMHXØYZ
ØMHYØYZ
ØNDØØZZ
ØND1ØZZ
ØND3ØZZ
ØND4ØZZ
ØND5ØZZ
ØND6ØZZ
ØND7ØZZ
ØNDBØZZ
ØNDCØZZ
ØNDFØZZ
ØNDGØZZ
ØNDHØZZ
ØNDJØZZ
ØNDKØZZ
ØNDLØZZ
ØNDMØZZ
ØNDNØZZ
ØNDPØZZ
ØNDQØZZ
ØNDRØZZ
ØNDTØZZ
ØNDVØZZ
ØNDXØZZ
ØNHØØNZ
ØNPØØNZ
ØPDØØZZ
ØPD1ØZZ
ØPD2ØZZ
ØPD3ØZZ
ØPD4ØZZ
ØPD5ØZZ
ØPD6ØZZ
ØPD7ØZZ
ØPD8ØZZ
ØPD9ØZZ
ØPDBØZZ
ØPDCØZZ
ØPDDØZZ
ØPDFØZZ
ØPDGØZZ
ØPDHØZZ
ØPDJØZZ
ØPDKØZZ
ØPDLØZZ
ØQDØØZZ
ØQD1ØZZ
ØQD2ØZZ
ØQD3ØZZ
ØQD4ØZZ
ØQD5ØZZ
ØQD6ØZZ
ØQD7ØZZ
ØQD8ØZZ
ØQD9ØZZ

ØQDBØZZ
ØQDCØZZ
ØQDDØZZ
ØQDFØZZ
ØQDGØZZ
ØQDHØZZ
ØQDJØZZ
ØQDKØZZ
ØQDLØZZ
ØQDMØZZ
ØQDNØZZ
ØQDPØZZ
ØQDQØZZ
ØQDRØZZ
ØQDSØZZ
ØRQNØZZ
ØRQN3ZZ
ØRQN4ZZ
ØRQPØZZ
ØRQP3ZZ
ØRQP4ZZ
ØRQQØZZ
ØRQQ3ZZ
ØRQQ4ZZ
ØRQRØZZ
ØRQR3ZZ
ØRQR4ZZ
ØRQSØZZ
ØRQS3ZZ
ØRQS4ZZ
ØRQTØZZ
ØRQT3ZZ
ØRQT4ZZ
ØRQUØZZ
ØRQU3ZZ
ØRQU4ZZ
ØRQVØZZ
ØRQV3ZZ
ØRQV4ZZ
ØRQWØZZ
ØRQW3ZZ
ØRQW4ZZ
ØRQXØZZ
ØRQX3ZZ
ØRQX4ZZ
ØRRQ*
ØRRR*
ØRRS*
ØRRT*
ØRRU*
ØRRV*
ØRRW*
ØRRX*
ØRUN*
ØRUP*
ØRUQ*
ØRUR*
ØRUS*
ØRUT*
ØRUU*
ØRUV*
ØRUW*
ØRUX*
ØW9JØØZ
ØW9JØZZ
ØW9J4ØZ
ØW9J4ZZ
ØWBØØZZ
ØWBØ3ZZ
ØWBØ4ZZ
ØWBØXZZ
ØWB2ØZZ
ØWB23ZZ
ØWB24ZZ
ØWB2XZZ
ØWB4ØZZ
ØWB43ZZ
ØWB44ZZ
ØWB4XZZ
ØWB5ØZZ
ØWB53ZZ
ØWB54ZZ
ØWB5XZZ
ØWB6ØZZ
ØWB63ZZ
ØWB64ZZ
ØWB6XZZ
ØWBKØZZ
ØWBK3ZZ
ØWBK4ZZ
ØWBKXZZ
ØWBLØZZ
ØWBL3ZZ
ØWBL4ZZ
ØWBLXZZ
ØWBMØZZ
ØWBM3ZZ
ØWBM4ZZ
ØWBMXZZ
ØWHØØ1Z
ØWHØ31Z
ØWHØ41Z
ØWH1Ø1Z
ØWH131Z
ØWH141Z
ØWH2Ø1Z
ØWH231Z
ØWH241Z
ØWPCØGZ
ØWPC3GZ
ØWPC4GZ
ØWQ3ØZZ
ØWQ33ZZ
ØWQ34ZZ
ØWQ3XZZ
ØWU2Ø7Z
ØWU247Z
ØWU4Ø7Z
ØWU447Z
ØWU5Ø7Z
ØWU547Z
ØWWCØGZ
ØWWC3GZ
ØWWC4GZ
ØXB2ØZZ
ØXB23ZZ
ØXB24ZZ
ØXB3ØZZ
ØXB33ZZ
ØXB34ZZ
ØXB4ØZZ
ØXB43ZZ
ØXB44ZZ
ØXB5ØZZ
ØXB53ZZ
ØXB54ZZ
ØXB6ØZZ
ØXB63ZZ
ØXB64ZZ
ØXB7ØZZ
ØXB73ZZ
ØXB74ZZ
ØXB8ØZZ
ØXB83ZZ
ØXB84ZZ
ØXB9ØZZ
ØXB93ZZ
ØXB94ZZ
ØXBBØZZ
ØXBB3ZZ
ØXBB4ZZ
ØXBCØZZ
ØXBC3ZZ
ØXBC4ZZ
ØXBDØZZ
ØXBD3ZZ
ØXBD4ZZ
ØXBFØZZ
ØXBF3ZZ
ØXBF4ZZ
ØXBGØZZ
ØXBG3ZZ
ØXBG4ZZ
ØXBHØZZ
ØXBH3ZZ
ØXBH4ZZ
ØXBJØZZ
ØXBJ3ZZ
ØXBJ4ZZ
ØXBKØZZ
ØXBK3ZZ
ØXBK4ZZ
ØXQJ*
ØXQK*
ØXQL*
ØXQM*
ØXQN*
ØXQP*
ØXQQ*
ØXQR*
ØXQS*
ØXQT*
ØXQV*
ØXQW*
ØXR*
ØXUJØ7Z
ØXUJ47Z
ØXUKØ7Z
ØXUK47Z
ØXULØ7Z
ØXUL47Z
ØXUMØ7Z
ØXUM47Z
ØXUNØ7Z
ØXUN47Z
ØXUPØ7Z
ØXUP47Z
ØXUQØ7Z
ØXUQ47Z
ØXURØ7Z
ØXUR47Z
ØXUSØ7Z
ØXUS47Z
ØXUTØ7Z
ØXUT47Z
ØXUVØ7Z
ØXUV47Z
ØXUWØ7Z
ØXUW47Z
ØXX*
ØXYJØZØ
ØXYJØZ1
ØXYKØZØ
ØXYKØZ1
ØY6C*
ØY6D*
ØY6FØZZ
ØY6GØZZ
ØY6H*
ØY6J*
ØY6M*
ØY6N*
ØY6P*
ØY6Q*
ØY6R*
ØY6S*
ØY6T*
ØY6U*
ØY6V*
ØY6W*
ØY6X*
ØY6Y*
ØYBØØZZ
ØYBØ3ZZ
ØYBØ4ZZ
ØYB1ØZZ
ØYB13ZZ
ØYB14ZZ
ØYB9ØZZ
ØYB93ZZ
ØYB94ZZ
ØYBBØZZ
ØYBB3ZZ
ØYBB4ZZ
ØYBCØZZ
ØYBC3ZZ
ØYBC4ZZ
ØYBDØZZ
ØYBD3ZZ
ØYBD4ZZ
ØYBFØZZ
ØYBF3ZZ
ØYBF4ZZ
ØYBGØZZ
ØYBG3ZZ
ØYBG4ZZ
ØYBHØZZ
ØYBH3ZZ
ØYBH4ZZ
ØYBJØZZ
ØYBJ3ZZ
ØYBJ4ZZ
ØYBKØZZ
ØYBK3ZZ
ØYBK4ZZ
ØYBLØZZ
ØYBL3ZZ
ØYBL4ZZ
ØYBMØZZ
ØYBM3ZZ
ØYBM4ZZ
ØYBNØZZ
ØYBN3ZZ
ØYBN4ZZ
XØ51329
XØHK3Q8
XØHQ3R8
X2H13R9
XHRPXF7
OR
Nonoperating Room Procedures
Ø2H63JZ
Ø2H73JZ
Ø2HK3JZ
Ø2HL3JZ
OR
Nonoperating Room Procedures
DØ2*
D72*
D82*
D92*
DB2*
DD2*
DF2*
DG2*
DM2*
DT2*
DU2*
DV2*
DW2*

DRG 041

Select operating room or nonoperating room procedures listed under DRG 040
OR
ØJH6ØBZ
ØJH6ØCZ
ØJH6ØDZ
ØJH6ØEZ
ØJH6ØMZ
ØJH63BZ
ØJH63CZ
ØJH63DZ
ØJH63EZ
ØJH63MZ
ØJH7ØBZ
ØJH7ØCZ
ØJH7ØDZ
ØJH7ØEZ
ØJH7ØMZ
ØJH73BZ
ØJH73CZ
ØJH73DZ
ØJH73EZ
ØJH73MZ
ØJH8ØBZ
ØJH8ØCZ
ØJH8ØDZ
ØJH8ØEZ
ØJH8ØMZ
ØJH83BZ
ØJH83CZ
ØJH83DZ
ØJH83EZ
ØJH83MZ
AND
ØØHEØMZ
ØØHE3MZ
ØØHE4MZ
Ø1HYØMZ
Ø1HY3MZ
Ø1HY4MZ
Ø5HØØMZ
Ø5HØ3MZ
Ø5HØ4MZ
Ø5H3ØMZ
Ø5H33MZ
Ø5H34MZ
Ø5H4ØMZ
Ø5H43MZ
Ø5H44MZ
ØDH6ØMZ
ØDH63MZ
ØDH64MZ
XØHQ3R8

DRG 042

Select operating room or nonoperating room procedures listed under DRG 040

DRG 052

Principal Diagnosis
GØ4.1
G8Ø.Ø
G8Ø.1
G8Ø.2
G82*
G83.Ø
S14.ØXXA
S14.ØXXS
S14.1Ø1A
S14.1Ø1S
S14.1Ø2A
S14.1Ø2S
S14.1Ø3A
S14.1Ø3S
S14.1Ø4A
S14.1Ø4S
S14.1Ø5A
S14.1Ø5S
S14.1Ø6A
S14.1Ø6S
S14.1Ø7A
S14.1Ø7S
S14.1Ø8A
S14.1Ø8S
S14.1Ø9A
S14.1Ø9S
S14.111A
S14.111S
S14.112A
S14.112S
S14.113A
S14.113S
S14.114A
S14.114S
S14.115A
S14.115S
S14.116A
S14.116S
S14.117A
S14.117S
S14.118A
S14.118S
S14.119A
S14.119S
S14.121A
S14.121S
S14.122A
S14.122S
S14.123A
S14.123S
S14.124A
S14.124S
S14.125A
S14.125S
S14.126A
S14.126S
S14.127A
S14.127S
S14.128A
S14.128S
S14.129A
S14.129S
S14.131A
S14.131S
S14.132A
S14.132S
S14.133A
S14.133S
S14.134A
S14.134S
S14.135A
S14.135S
S14.136A
S14.136S
S14.137A
S14.137S
S14.138A
S14.138S
S14.139A
S14.139S
S14.141A
S14.141S
S14.142A
S14.142S
S14.143A
S14.143S
S14.144A
S14.144S
S14.145A
S14.145S
S14.146A
S14.146S
S14.147A
S14.147S
S14.148A
S14.148S
S14.149A
S14.149S
S14.151A
S14.151S
S14.152A
S14.152S
S14.153A
S14.153S
S14.154A
S14.154S
S14.155A
S14.155S
S14.156A
S14.156S
S14.157A
S14.157S
S14.158A
S14.158S
S14.159A
S14.159S
S24.ØXXA
S24.ØXXS
S24.1Ø1A
S24.1Ø1S
S24.1Ø2A
S24.1Ø2S
S24.1Ø3A
S24.1Ø3S
S24.1Ø4A
S24.1Ø4S
S24.1Ø9A
S24.1Ø9S
S24.111A
S24.111S
S24.112A
S24.112S
S24.113A
S24.113S
S24.114A
S24.114S
S24.119A
S24.119S
S24.131A
S24.131S
S24.132A
S24.132S
S24.133A
S24.133S
S24.134A
S24.134S
S24.139A
S24.139S
S24.141A
S24.141S
S24.142A
S24.142S
S24.143A
S24.143S
S24.144A
S24.144S
S24.149A
S24.149S
S24.151A
S24.151S
S24.152A
S24.152S
S24.153A
S24.153S
S24.154A
S24.154S
S24.159A
S24.159S
S34.Ø1XA
S34.Ø1XS
S34.Ø2XA
S34.Ø2XS
S34.1Ø1A
S34.1Ø1S
S34.1Ø2A
S34.1Ø2S
S34.1Ø3A
S34.1Ø3S
S34.1Ø4A
S34.1Ø4S
S34.1Ø5A
S34.1Ø5S
S34.1Ø9A
S34.1Ø9S
S34.111A
S34.111S
S34.112A
S34.112S
S34.113A
S34.113S
S34.114A
S34.114S
S34.115A
S34.115S
S34.119A
S34.119S
S34.121A
S34.121S
S34.122A
S34.122S
S34.123A
S34.123S
S34.124A
S34.124S
S34.125A
S34.125S
S34.129A
S34.129S
S34.131A
S34.131S
S34.132A
S34.132S
S34.139A
S34.139S
S34.3XXA

DRG 053

Select principal diagnosis listed under DRG 052

DRG 054

Principal Diagnosis
C7Ø*
C71*
C72*
C75.3
C75.4
C75.5
C79.3*
C79.4*
D32*
D33*
D35.4
D35.5
D35.6
D42*
D43*
D44.5
D44.6
D44.7
D49.6

DRG 055

Select principal diagnosis listed under DRG 054

DRG 056

Principal Diagnosis
A52.1Ø
A52.11
A52.12
A52.15
A52.16
A52.17
A52.19
A52.3
A81*
E75.Ø*
E75.1*
E75.23
E75.25
E75.26
E75.27
E75.28
E75.29
E75.4
FØ7.89
F48.2
F84.2
G1Ø
G12*
G13.2
G13.8
G2Ø*
G21.1*
G21.2
G21.3
G21.4
G21.8
G21.9
G23*
G24.1
G25.4
G25.5
G25.7*
G25.81
G25.89
G25.9
G26
G3Ø*
G31*
G7Ø.Ø*
G7Ø.8Ø
G7Ø.81
G73.1
G73.3
G8Ø.3
G81*
G9Ø.3
G91*
G94
G95.Ø
H57.Ø1
I67.3
I69*

DRG 057

Select principal diagnosis listed under DRG 056

DRG 058

Principal Diagnosis
G11*
G32.81
G35
G36*
G37.Ø
G37.1
G37.2
G37.5
G37.8*
G37.9

DRG 059

Select principal diagnosis listed under DRG 058

DRG 060

Select principal diagnosis listed under DRG 058

DRG 061

Principal Diagnosis
G45.Ø
G45.1
G45.2
G45.8
G45.9
G46.Ø
G46.1
G46.2
I63.ØØ
I63.Ø11
I63.Ø12
I63.Ø13
I63.Ø19
I63.Ø2
I63.Ø31
I63.Ø32
I63.Ø33
I63.Ø39
I63.Ø9
I63.1Ø
I63.111
I63.112
I63.113
I63.119
I63.12
I63.131
I63.132
I63.133
I63.139
I63.19
I63.2Ø
I63.211
I63.212
I63.213
I63.219
I63.22
I63.231
I63.232
I63.233
I63.239
I63.29
I63.3Ø
I63.311
I63.312
I63.313
I63.319
I63.321
I63.322
I63.323
I63.329
I63.331
I63.332
I63.333
I63.339
I63.341
I63.342
I63.343
I63.349
I63.39
I63.4Ø
I63.411
I63.412
I63.413
I63.419
I63.421
I63.422
I63.423
I63.429
I63.431
I63.432
I63.433
I63.439
I63.441
I63.442
I63.443
I63.449
I63.49
I63.5Ø
I63.511
I63.512
I63.513
I63.519
I63.521
I63.522
I63.523
I63.529
I63.531
I63.532
I63.533
I63.539
I63.541
I63.542
I63.543
I63.549
I63.59
I63.6
I63.81
I63.89
I63.9
I65.Ø1
I65.Ø2
I65.Ø3
I65.Ø9
I65.1
I65.21
I65.22
I65.23
I65.29
I65.8
I65.9
I66.Ø1
I66.Ø2
I66.Ø3
I66.Ø9
I66.11
I66.12
I66.13
I66.19
I66.21
I66.22
I66.23
I66.29
I66.3
I66.8
I66.9
I67.81
I67.82
I67.841
I67.848
I67.89
AND
Nonoperating Room Procedure
3EØ3Ø17
3EØ3317
3EØ4Ø17
3EØ4317
3EØ5Ø17
3EØ5317
3EØ6Ø17
3EØ6317
3EØ8Ø17
3EØ8317

ICD-10-CM/PCS Codes by MS-DRG

DRG 062

Select principal diagnosis AND nonoperating room procedure listed under DRG 061

DRG 063

Select principal diagnosis AND nonoperating room procedure listed under DRG 061

DRG 064

Principal Diagnosis

I6Ø*
I61*
I62*
I63.ØØ
I63.Ø11
I63.Ø12
I63.Ø13
I63.Ø19
I63.Ø2
I63.Ø31
I63.Ø32
I63.Ø33
I63.Ø39
I63.Ø9
I63.1Ø
I63.111
I63.112
I63.113
I63.119
I63.12
I63.131
I63.132
I63.133
I63.139
I63.19
I63.2Ø
I63.211
I63.212
I63.213
I63.219
I63.22
I63.231
I63.232
I63.233
I63.239
I63.29
I63.3Ø
I63.311
I63.312
I63.313
I63.319
I63.321
I63.322
I63.323
I63.329
I63.331
I63.332
I63.333
I63.339
I63.341
I63.342
I63.343
I63.349
I63.39
I63.4Ø
I63.411
I63.412
I63.413
I63.419
I63.421
I63.422
I63.423
I63.429
I63.431
I63.432
I63.433
I63.439
I63.441
I63.442
I63.443
I63.449
I63.49
I63.5Ø
I63.511
I63.512
I63.513
I63.519
I63.521
I63.522
I63.523
I63.529
I63.531
I63.532
I63.533
I63.539
I63.541
I63.542
I63.543
I63.549
I63.59
I63.6
I63.81
I63.89
I63.9

DRG 065

Select principal diagnosis listed under DRG 064

AND

Secondary Diagnosis

Z92.82

DRG 066

Select principal diagnosis listed under DRG 064

DRG 067

Principal Diagnosis

I65*
I66*

DRG 068

Select principal diagnosis listed under DRG 067

DRG 069

Principal Diagnosis

G45.Ø
G45.1
G45.2
G45.8
G45.9
G46.Ø
G46.1
G46.2
I67.81
I67.82
I67.841
I67.848
I67.89

DRG 070

Principal Diagnosis

G32.89
G45.4
G46.3
G46.4
G46.5
G46.6
G46.7
G46.8
G93.4*
G93.81
G93.89
G93.9
G96.8*
G96.9
G98*
G99.8
I67.2
I67.83
I67.85Ø
I67.858
I67.9
I68.Ø
I68.8

DRG 071

Select principal diagnosis listed under DRG 070

DRG 072

Select principal diagnosis listed under DRG 070

DRG 073

Principal Diagnosis

BØ2.Ø
BØ2.21
BØ2.22
BØ2.23
BØ2.29
BØ6.ØØ
B26.84
EØ8.4*
EØ8.61Ø
EØ9.4*
EØ9.61Ø
E1Ø.4*
E1Ø.61Ø
E11.4*
E11.61Ø
E13.4*
E13.61Ø
G13.Ø
G13.1
G5Ø*
G51.Ø
G51.1
G51.2
G51.31
G51.32
G51.33
G51.39
G51.4
G51.8
G51.9
G52*
G53
G54*
G55
G56*
G57*
G58*
G59
G6Ø.Ø
G6Ø.2
G6Ø.3
G6Ø.8
G6Ø.9
G61.1
G61.8*
G61.9
G62*
G63
G64
G65*
G7Ø.1
G7Ø.2
G7Ø.89
G7Ø.9
G83.4
G9Ø.Ø*
G9Ø.2
G9Ø.4
G9Ø.5*
G9Ø.8
G9Ø.9
G9Ø.B
G99.Ø
M21.331
M21.332
M21.339
M21.511
M21.512
M21.519
M21.521
M21.522
M21.529
M21.531
M21.532
M21.539
M34.83
M53.Ø
M53.1
M54.1Ø
M54.11
M54.12
M54.13
M54.18
M79.2
SØ4.1ØXA
SØ4.11XA
SØ4.12XA
SØ4.2ØXA
SØ4.21XA
SØ4.22XA
SØ4.3ØXA
SØ4.31XA
SØ4.32XA
SØ4.4ØXA
SØ4.41XA
SØ4.42XA
SØ4.5ØXA
SØ4.51XA
SØ4.52XA
SØ4.7ØXA
SØ4.71XA
SØ4.72XA
SØ4.811A
SØ4.812A
SØ4.819A
SØ4.891A
SØ4.892A
SØ4.899A
SØ4.9XXA
S14.2XXA
S14.3XXA
S14.4XXA
S14.5XXA
S14.8XXA
S14.9XXA
S24.2XXA
S24.3XXA
S24.4XXA
S24.8XXA
S24.9XXA
S34.21XA
S34.22XA
S34.4XXA
S34.5XXA
S34.6XXA
S34.8XXA
S34.9XXA
S44.ØØXA
S44.Ø1XA
S44.Ø2XA
S44.1ØXA
S44.11XA
S44.12XA
S44.2ØXA
S44.21XA
S44.22XA
S44.3ØXA
S44.31XA
S44.32XA
S44.4ØXA
S44.41XA
S44.42XA
S44.5ØXA
S44.51XA
S44.52XA
S44.8X1A
S44.8X2A
S44.8X9A
S44.9ØXA
S44.91XA
S44.92XA
S54.ØØXA
S54.Ø1XA
S54.Ø2XA
S54.1ØXA
S54.11XA
S54.12XA
S54.2ØXA
S54.21XA
S54.22XA
S54.3ØXA
S54.31XA
S54.32XA
S54.8X1A
S54.8X2A
S54.8X9A
S54.9ØXA
S54.91XA
S54.92XA
S64.ØØXA
S64.Ø1XA
S64.Ø2XA
S64.1ØXA
S64.11XA
S64.12XA
S64.2ØXA
S64.21XA
S64.22XA
S64.3ØXA
S64.31XA
S64.32XA
S64.4ØXA
S64.49ØA
S64.491A
S64.492A
S64.493A
S64.494A
S64.495A
S64.496A
S64.497A
S64.498A
S64.8X1A
S64.8X2A
S64.8X9A
S64.9ØXA
S64.91XA
S64.92XA
S74.ØØXA
S74.Ø1XA
S74.Ø2XA
S74.1ØXA
S74.11XA
S74.12XA
S74.2ØXA
S74.21XA
S74.22XA
S74.8X1A
S74.8X2A
S74.8X9A
S74.9ØXA
S74.91XA
S74.92XA
S84.ØØXA
S84.Ø1XA
S84.Ø2XA
S84.1ØXA
S84.11XA
S84.12XA
S84.2ØXA
S84.21XA
S84.22XA
S84.8Ø1A
S84.8Ø2A
S84.8Ø9A
S84.9ØXA
S84.91XA
S84.92XA
S94.ØØXA
S94.Ø1XA
S94.Ø2XA
S94.1ØXA
S94.11XA
S94.12XA
S94.2ØXA
S94.21XA
S94.22XA
S94.3ØXA
S94.31XA
S94.32XA
S94.8X1A
S94.8X2A
S94.8X9A
S94.9ØXA
S94.91XA
S94.92XA

DRG 074

Select principal diagnosis listed under DRG 073

DRG 075

Principal Diagnosis

A87*
A88.Ø
BØØ.3
BØ2.1
B26.1
GØ3.2

DRG 076

Select principal diagnosis listed under DRG 075

DRG 077

Principal Diagnosis

I67.4

DRG 078

Select principal diagnosis listed under DRG 077

DRG 079

Select principal diagnosis listed under DRG 077

DRG 080

Principal Diagnosis

EØ3.5
G93.5
G93.6
G93.82
R4Ø.Ø
R4Ø.1
R4Ø.2Ø
R4Ø.211Ø
R4Ø.2111
R4Ø.2112
R4Ø.2113
R4Ø.2114
R4Ø.212Ø
R4Ø.2121
R4Ø.2122
R4Ø.2123
R4Ø.2124
R4Ø.221Ø
R4Ø.2211
R4Ø.2212
R4Ø.2213
R4Ø.2214
R4Ø.222Ø
R4Ø.2221
R4Ø.2222
R4Ø.2223
R4Ø.2224
R4Ø.231Ø
R4Ø.2311
R4Ø.2312
R4Ø.2313
R4Ø.2314
R4Ø.232Ø
R4Ø.2321
R4Ø.2322
R4Ø.2323
R4Ø.2324
R4Ø.234Ø
R4Ø.2341
R4Ø.2342
R4Ø.2343
R4Ø.2344
R4Ø.2A
R4Ø.3

DRG 081

Select principal diagnosis listed under DRG 080

DRG 082

Principal Diagnosis of Traumatic Stupor and Coma > 1 Hour

SØ6.1X3A
SØ6.1X4A
SØ6.1X5A
SØ6.1X6A
SØ6.1X7A
SØ6.1X8A
SØ6.1X9A
SØ6.1XAA
SØ6.2X3A
SØ6.2X4A
SØ6.2X5A
SØ6.2X6A
SØ6.2X7A
SØ6.2X8A
SØ6.2X9A
SØ6.2XAA
SØ6.3Ø3A
SØ6.3Ø4A
SØ6.3Ø5A
SØ6.3Ø6A
SØ6.3Ø7A
SØ6.3Ø8A
SØ6.3Ø9A
SØ6.3ØAA
SØ6.313A
SØ6.314A
SØ6.315A
SØ6.316A
SØ6.317A
SØ6.318A
SØ6.319A
SØ6.31AA
SØ6.323A
SØ6.324A
SØ6.325A
SØ6.326A
SØ6.327A
SØ6.328A
SØ6.329A
SØ6.32AA
SØ6.333A
SØ6.334A
SØ6.335A
SØ6.336A
SØ6.337A
SØ6.338A
SØ6.339A
SØ6.33AA
SØ6.343A
SØ6.344A
SØ6.345A
SØ6.346A
SØ6.347A
SØ6.348A
SØ6.349A
SØ6.34AA
SØ6.353A
SØ6.354A
SØ6.355A
SØ6.356A
SØ6.357A
SØ6.358A
SØ6.359A
SØ6.35AA
SØ6.363A
SØ6.364A
SØ6.365A
SØ6.366A
SØ6.367A
SØ6.368A
SØ6.369A
SØ6.36AA
SØ6.373A
SØ6.374A
SØ6.375A
SØ6.376A
SØ6.377A
SØ6.378A
SØ6.379A
SØ6.37AA
SØ6.383A
SØ6.384A
SØ6.385A
SØ6.386A
SØ6.387A
SØ6.388A
SØ6.389A
SØ6.38AA
SØ6.4X3A
SØ6.4X4A
SØ6.4X5A
SØ6.4X6A
SØ6.4X7A
SØ6.4X8A
SØ6.4X9A
SØ6.4XAA
SØ6.5X3A
SØ6.5X4A
SØ6.5X5A
SØ6.5X6A
SØ6.5X7A
SØ6.5X8A
SØ6.5X9A
SØ6.5XAA
SØ6.6X3A
SØ6.6X4A
SØ6.6X5A
SØ6.6X6A
SØ6.6X7A
SØ6.6X8A
SØ6.6X9A
SØ6.6XAA
SØ6.813A
SØ6.814A
SØ6.815A
SØ6.816A
SØ6.817A
SØ6.818A
SØ6.819A
SØ6.81AA
SØ6.823A
SØ6.824A
SØ6.825A
SØ6.826A
SØ6.827A
SØ6.828A
SØ6.829A
SØ6.82AA
SØ6.893A
SØ6.894A
SØ6.895A
SØ6.896A
SØ6.897A
SØ6.898A
SØ6.899A
SØ6.89AA
SØ6.8A3A
SØ6.8A4A
SØ6.8A5A
SØ6.8A6A
SØ6.8A7A
SØ6.8A8A
SØ6.8A9A
SØ6.8AAA
SØ6.9X3A
SØ6.9X4A
SØ6.9X5A
SØ6.9X6A
SØ6.9X7A
SØ6.9X8A
SØ6.9X9A
SØ6.9XAA

OR

Principal Diagnosis

SØ2.ØXXA
SØ2.ØXXB
SØ2.1Ø1A
SØ2.1Ø1B
SØ2.1Ø2A
SØ2.1Ø2B
SØ2.1Ø9A
SØ2.1Ø9B
SØ2.11ØA
SØ2.11ØB
SØ2.111A
SØ2.111B
SØ2.112A
SØ2.112B
SØ2.113A
SØ2.113B
SØ2.118A
SØ2.118B
SØ2.119A
SØ2.119B
SØ2.11AA
SØ2.11AB
SØ2.11BA
SØ2.11BB
SØ2.11CA
SØ2.11CB
SØ2.11DA
SØ2.11DB
SØ2.11EA
SØ2.11EB
SØ2.11FA
SØ2.11FB
SØ2.11GA
SØ2.11GB
SØ2.11HA
SØ2.11HB
SØ2.121A
SØ2.121B
SØ2.122A
SØ2.122B
SØ2.129A
SØ2.129B
SØ2.19XA
SØ2.19XB
SØ2.831A
SØ2.831B
SØ2.832A
SØ2.832B
SØ2.839A
SØ2.839B
SØ2.841A
SØ2.841B
SØ2.842A
SØ2.842B
SØ2.849A
SØ2.849B
SØ2.85XA
SØ2.85XB
SØ2.91XA
SØ2.91XB
SØ6.1XØA
SØ6.1X1A
SØ6.1X2A
SØ6.1X3A
SØ6.1X4A
SØ6.1X5A
SØ6.1X6A
SØ6.1X7A
SØ6.1X8A
SØ6.1X9A
SØ6.1XAA
SØ6.2XØA
SØ6.2X1A
SØ6.2X2A
SØ6.2X3A
SØ6.2X4A
SØ6.2X5A
SØ6.2X6A
SØ6.2X7A
SØ6.2X8A
SØ6.2X9A
SØ6.2XAA
SØ6.3ØØA
SØ6.3Ø1A
SØ6.3Ø2A
SØ6.3Ø3A
SØ6.3Ø4A
SØ6.3Ø5A
SØ6.3Ø6A
SØ6.3Ø7A
SØ6.3Ø8A
SØ6.3Ø9A
SØ6.3ØAA
SØ6.31ØA
SØ6.311A
SØ6.312A
SØ6.313A
SØ6.314A
SØ6.315A
SØ6.316A
SØ6.317A
SØ6.318A
SØ6.319A
SØ6.31AA
SØ6.32ØA
SØ6.321A
SØ6.322A
SØ6.323A
SØ6.324A
SØ6.325A
SØ6.326A
SØ6.327A
SØ6.328A
SØ6.329A
SØ6.32AA
SØ6.33ØA
SØ6.331A
SØ6.332A
SØ6.333A
SØ6.334A
SØ6.335A
SØ6.336A
SØ6.337A
SØ6.338A
SØ6.339A
SØ6.33AA
SØ6.34ØA
SØ6.341A
SØ6.342A
SØ6.343A
SØ6.344A
SØ6.345A
SØ6.346A
SØ6.347A
SØ6.348A
SØ6.349A
SØ6.34AA
SØ6.35ØA
SØ6.351A
SØ6.352A
SØ6.353A
SØ6.354A
SØ6.355A
SØ6.356A
SØ6.357A
SØ6.358A
SØ6.359A
SØ6.35AA
SØ6.36ØA
SØ6.361A
SØ6.362A
SØ6.363A
SØ6.364A
SØ6.365A
SØ6.366A
SØ6.367A
SØ6.368A
SØ6.369A
SØ6.36AA
SØ6.37ØA
SØ6.371A
SØ6.372A
SØ6.373A
SØ6.374A
SØ6.375A
SØ6.376A
SØ6.377A
SØ6.378A
SØ6.379A
SØ6.37AA
SØ6.38ØA
SØ6.381A
SØ6.382A
SØ6.383A
SØ6.384A
SØ6.385A
SØ6.386A
SØ6.387A
SØ6.388A

SØ6.389A
SØ6.38AA
SØ6.4XØA
SØ6.4X1A
SØ6.4X2A
SØ6.4X3A
SØ6.4X4A
SØ6.4X5A
SØ6.4X6A
SØ6.4X7A
SØ6.4X8A
SØ6.4X9A
SØ6.4XAA
SØ6.5XØA
SØ6.5X1A
SØ6.5X2A
SØ6.5X3A
SØ6.5X4A
SØ6.5X5A
SØ6.5X6A
SØ6.5X7A
SØ6.5X8A
SØ6.5X9A
SØ6.5XAA
SØ6.6XØA
SØ6.6X1A
SØ6.6X2A
SØ6.6X3A
SØ6.6X4A
SØ6.6X5A
SØ6.6X6A
SØ6.6X7A
SØ6.6X8A
SØ6.6X9A
SØ6.6XAA
SØ6.81ØA
SØ6.811A
SØ6.812A
SØ6.813A
SØ6.814A
SØ6.815A
SØ6.816A
SØ6.817A
SØ6.818A
SØ6.819A
SØ6.81AA
SØ6.82ØA
SØ6.821A
SØ6.822A
SØ6.823A
SØ6.824A
SØ6.825A
SØ6.826A
SØ6.827A
SØ6.828A
SØ6.829A
SØ6.82AA
SØ6.89ØA
SØ6.891A
SØ6.892A
SØ6.893A
SØ6.894A
SØ6.895A
SØ6.896A
SØ6.897A
SØ6.898A
SØ6.899A
SØ6.89AA
SØ6.8A3A
SØ6.8A4A
SØ6.8A5A
SØ6.8A6A
SØ6.8A7A
SØ6.8A8A
SØ6.8A9A
SØ6.8AAA
SØ6.9XØA
SØ6.9X1A
SØ6.9X2A
SØ6.9X3A
SØ6.9X4A
SØ6.9X5A
SØ6.9X6A
SØ6.9X7A
SØ6.9X8A
SØ6.9X9A
SØ6.9XAA

AND

Secondary Diagnosis of Traumatic Stupor and Coma > 1 Hour

Select from above list of diagnoses with description of loss of consciousness greater than one hour or of unspecified duration

DRG 083

Select principal diagnosis of coma greater than one hour OR principal diagnosis of traumatic stupor AND a secondary diagnosis of coma greater than one hour listed under DRG 082

DRG 084

Select principal diagnosis of coma greater than one hour OR principal diagnosis of traumatic stupor AND a secondary diagnosis of coma greater than one hour listed under DRG 082

DRG 085

Principal Diagnosis of Traumatic Stupor and Coma < 1 Hour

SØ2.ØXXA
SØ2.ØXXB
SØ2.1Ø1A
SØ2.1Ø1B
SØ2.1Ø2A
SØ2.1Ø2B
SØ2.1Ø9A
SØ2.1Ø9B
SØ2.11ØA
SØ2.11ØB
SØ2.111A
SØ2.111B
SØ2.112A
SØ2.112B
SØ2.113A
SØ2.113B
SØ2.118A
SØ2.118B
SØ2.119A
SØ2.119B
SØ2.11AA
SØ2.11AB
SØ2.11BA
SØ2.11BB
SØ2.11CA
SØ2.11CB
SØ2.11DA
SØ2.11DB
SØ2.11EA
SØ2.11EB
SØ2.11FA
SØ2.11FB
SØ2.11GA
SØ2.11GB
SØ2.11HA
SØ2.11HB
SØ2.121A
SØ2.121B
SØ2.122A
SØ2.122B
SØ2.129A
SØ2.129B
SØ2.19XA
SØ2.19XB
SØ2.831A
SØ2.831B
SØ2.832A
SØ2.832B
SØ2.839A
SØ2.839B
SØ2.841A
SØ2.841B
SØ2.842A
SØ2.842B
SØ2.849A
SØ2.849B
SØ2.85XA
SØ2.85XB
SØ2.91XA
SØ2.91XB
SØ6.1XØA
SØ6.1X1A
SØ6.1X2A
SØ6.2XØA
SØ6.2X1A
SØ6.2X2A
SØ6.3ØØA
SØ6.3Ø1A
SØ6.3Ø2A
SØ6.31ØA
SØ6.311A
SØ6.312A
SØ6.32ØA
SØ6.321A
SØ6.322A
SØ6.33ØA
SØ6.331A
SØ6.332A
SØ6.34ØA
SØ6.341A
SØ6.342A
SØ6.35ØA
SØ6.351A
SØ6.352A
SØ6.36ØA
SØ6.361A
SØ6.362A
SØ6.37ØA
SØ6.371A
SØ6.372A
SØ6.38ØA
SØ6.381A
SØ6.382A
SØ6.4XØA
SØ6.4X1A
SØ6.4X2A
SØ6.5XØA
SØ6.5X1A
SØ6.5X2A
SØ6.6XØA
SØ6.6X1A
SØ6.6X2A
SØ6.81ØA
SØ6.811A
SØ6.812A
SØ6.82ØA
SØ6.821A
SØ6.822A
SØ6.89ØA
SØ6.891A
SØ6.892A
SØ6.8AØA
SØ6.8A1A
SØ6.8A2A
SØ6.9XØA
SØ6.9X1A
SØ6.9X2A
SØ6.AØXA
SØ6.A1XA

DRG 086

Select principal diagnosis listed under DRG 085

DRG 087

Select principal diagnosis listed under DRG 085

DRG 088

Principal Diagnosis

SØ6.ØXØA
SØ6.ØX1A
SØ6.ØX9A
SØ6.ØXAA

DRG 089

Select principal diagnosis listed under DRG 088

DRG 090

Select principal diagnosis listed under DRG 088

DRG 091

Principal Diagnosis

A88.1
B9Ø.Ø
B91
B94.1
D18.Ø2
F8Ø.81
F95*
GØ8
GØ9
G14
G21.Ø
G24.Ø*
G24.2
G24.3
G24.4
G24.8
G24.9
G25.Ø
G25.1
G25.2
G25.3
G25.6*
G25.82
G25.83
G32.Ø
G47.2*
G47.31
G47.35
G47.37
G47.4*
G47.51
G47.53
G47.61
G47.62
G6Ø.1
G71.ØØ
G71.Ø1
G71.Ø2
G71.Ø31
G71.Ø32
G71.Ø33
G71.Ø34Ø
G71.Ø341
G71.Ø342
G71.Ø349
G71.Ø35
G71.Ø38
G71.Ø39
G71.Ø9
G71.11
G71.12
G71.13
G71.14
G71.19
G71.2*
G71.3
G71.8
G71.9
G72.Ø
G72.1
G72.2
G72.3
G72.8*
G72.9
G73.7
G8Ø.4
G8Ø.8
G8Ø.9
G83.1*
G83.2*
G83.3*
G83.5
G83.8*
G83.9
G89.Ø
G89.2*
G89.4
G9Ø.1
G9Ø.A
G92*
G93.Ø
G93.1
G93.7
G95.1*
G95.2*
G95.8*
G95.9
G96.Ø*
G96.12
G96.19*
G97.Ø
G97.2
G97.3*
G97.8*
G99.2
H47.1Ø
H47.11
H47.141
H47.142
H47.143
H47.149
H47.4*
H47.5*
H47.6*
H47.9
H51.2*
I67.1
I67.5
I67.6
I97.81Ø
I97.811
I97.82Ø
I97.821
P91.2
QØØ*
QØ1*
QØ2
QØ3*
QØ4*
QØ5*
QØ6*
QØ7*
Q28.2
Q28.3
Q76.Ø
Q85.Ø*
Q85.1
R2Ø*
R25*
R26.Ø
R26.1
R26.8*
R26.9
R27*
R29.1
R29.2
R29.3
R29.5
R29.6
R29.81Ø
R29.818
R29.89Ø
R29.9*
R41.4
R41.842
R43*
R47*
R83*
R9Ø.81
R9Ø.82
R93.Ø
R94.Ø*
R94.118
R94.128
R94.13Ø
R94.138
SØ2.ØXXS
SØ2.1Ø1S
SØ2.1Ø2S
SØ2.1Ø9S
SØ2.11ØS
SØ2.111S
SØ2.112S
SØ2.113S
SØ2.118S
SØ2.119S
SØ2.11AS
SØ2.11BS
SØ2.11CS
SØ2.11DS
SØ2.11ES
SØ2.11FS
SØ2.11GS
SØ2.11HS
SØ2.19XS
SØ2.2XXS
SØ2.3ØXS
SØ2.31XS
SØ2.32XS
SØ2.4ØØS
SØ2.4Ø1S
SØ2.4Ø2S
SØ2.4ØAS
SØ2.4ØBS
SØ2.4ØCS
SØ2.4ØDS
SØ2.4ØES
SØ2.4ØFS
SØ2.411S
SØ2.412S
SØ2.413S
SØ2.42XS
SØ2.5XXS
SØ2.6ØØS
SØ2.6Ø1S
SØ2.6Ø2S
SØ2.6Ø9S
SØ2.61ØS
SØ2.611S
SØ2.612S
SØ2.62ØS
SØ2.621S
SØ2.622S
SØ2.63ØS
SØ2.631S
SØ2.632S
SØ2.64ØS
SØ2.641S
SØ2.642S
SØ2.65ØS
SØ2.651S
SØ2.652S
SØ2.66XS
SØ2.67ØS
SØ2.671S
SØ2.672S
SØ2.69XS
SØ2.8ØXS
SØ2.81XS
SØ2.82XS
SØ2.91XS
SØ2.92XS
SØ4.Ø11S
SØ4.Ø12S
SØ4.Ø19S
SØ4.Ø2XA
SØ4.Ø2XS
SØ4.Ø31A
SØ4.Ø31S
SØ4.Ø32A
SØ4.Ø32S
SØ4.Ø39A
SØ4.Ø39S
SØ4.Ø41A
SØ4.Ø41S
SØ4.Ø42A
SØ4.Ø42S
SØ4.Ø49A
SØ4.Ø49S
SØ4.1ØXS
SØ4.11XS
SØ4.12XS
SØ4.2ØXS
SØ4.21XS
SØ4.22XS
SØ4.3ØXS
SØ4.31XS
SØ4.32XS
SØ4.4ØXS
SØ4.41XS
SØ4.42XS
SØ4.5ØXS
SØ4.51XS
SØ4.52XS
SØ4.6ØXS
SØ4.61XS
SØ4.62XS
SØ4.7ØXS
SØ4.71XS
SØ4.72XS
SØ4.811S
SØ4.812S
SØ4.819S
SØ4.891S
SØ4.892S
SØ4.899S
SØ4.9XXS
SØ6.ØXØS
SØ6.ØX1S
SØ6.ØX9S
SØ6.ØXAS
SØ6.1XØS
SØ6.1X1S
SØ6.1X2S
SØ6.1X3S
SØ6.1X4S
SØ6.1X5S
SØ6.1X6S
SØ6.1X9S
SØ6.1XAS
SØ6.2XØS
SØ6.2X1S
SØ6.2X2S
SØ6.2X3S
SØ6.2X4S
SØ6.2X5S
SØ6.2X6S
SØ6.2X9S
SØ6.2XAS
SØ6.3ØØS
SØ6.3Ø1S
SØ6.3Ø2S
SØ6.3Ø3S
SØ6.3Ø4S
SØ6.3Ø5S
SØ6.3Ø6S
SØ6.3Ø9S
SØ6.3ØAS
SØ6.31ØS
SØ6.311S
SØ6.312S
SØ6.313S
SØ6.314S
SØ6.315S
SØ6.316S
SØ6.319S
SØ6.31AS
SØ6.32ØS
SØ6.321S
SØ6.322S
SØ6.323S
SØ6.324S
SØ6.325S
SØ6.326S
SØ6.329S
SØ6.32AS
SØ6.33ØS
SØ6.331S
SØ6.332S
SØ6.333S
SØ6.334S
SØ6.335S
SØ6.336S
SØ6.339S
SØ6.33AS
SØ6.34ØS
SØ6.341S
SØ6.342S
SØ6.343S
SØ6.344S
SØ6.345S
SØ6.346S
SØ6.349S
SØ6.34AS
SØ6.35ØS
SØ6.351S
SØ6.352S
SØ6.353S
SØ6.354S
SØ6.355S
SØ6.356S
SØ6.359S
SØ6.35AS
SØ6.36ØS
SØ6.361S
SØ6.362S
SØ6.363S
SØ6.364S
SØ6.365S
SØ6.366S
SØ6.369S
SØ6.36AS
SØ6.37ØS
SØ6.371S
SØ6.372S
SØ6.373S
SØ6.374S
SØ6.375S
SØ6.376S
SØ6.379S
SØ6.37AS
SØ6.38ØS
SØ6.381S
SØ6.382S
SØ6.383S
SØ6.384S
SØ6.385S
SØ6.386S
SØ6.389S
SØ6.38AS
SØ6.4XØS
SØ6.4X1S
SØ6.4X2S
SØ6.4X3S
SØ6.4X4S
SØ6.4X5S
SØ6.4X6S
SØ6.4X9S
SØ6.4XAS
SØ6.5XØS
SØ6.5X1S
SØ6.5X2S
SØ6.5X3S
SØ6.5X4S
SØ6.5X5S
SØ6.5X6S
SØ6.5X9S
SØ6.5XAS
SØ6.6XØS
SØ6.6X1S
SØ6.6X2S
SØ6.6X3S
SØ6.6X4S
SØ6.6X5S
SØ6.6X6S
SØ6.6X9S
SØ6.6XAS
SØ6.81ØS
SØ6.811S
SØ6.812S
SØ6.813S
SØ6.814S
SØ6.815S
SØ6.816S
SØ6.819S
SØ6.81AS
SØ6.82ØS
SØ6.821S
SØ6.822S
SØ6.823S
SØ6.824S
SØ6.825S
SØ6.826S
SØ6.829S
SØ6.82AS
SØ6.89ØS
SØ6.891S
SØ6.892S
SØ6.893S
SØ6.894S
SØ6.895S
SØ6.896S
SØ6.899S
SØ6.89AS
SØ6.8AØS
SØ6.8A1S
SØ6.8A2S
SØ6.8A3S
SØ6.8A4S
SØ6.8A5S
SØ6.8A6S
SØ6.8A9S
SØ6.8AAS
SØ6.9XØS
SØ6.9X1S
SØ6.9X2S
SØ6.9X3S
SØ6.9X4S
SØ6.9X5S
SØ6.9X6S
SØ6.9X9S
SØ6.9XAS
S14.2XXS
S14.3XXS
S14.4XXS
S14.5XXS
S14.8XXS
S14.9XXS
S24.2XXS
S24.3XXS
S24.4XXS
S24.8XXS
S24.9XXS
S34.21XS
S34.22XS
S34.3XXS
S34.4XXS
S34.5XXS
S34.6XXS
S34.8XXS
S34.9XXS
S44.ØØXS
S44.Ø1XS
S44.Ø2XS
S44.1ØXS
S44.11XS
S44.12XS
S44.2ØXS
S44.21XS
S44.22XS
S44.3ØXS
S44.31XS
S44.32XS
S44.4ØXS
S44.41XS
S44.42XS
S44.5ØXS
S44.51XS
S44.52XS
S44.8X1S
S44.8X2S
S44.8X9S
S44.9ØXS
S44.91XS
S44.92XS
S54.ØØXS
S54.Ø1XS
S54.Ø2XS
S54.1ØXS
S54.11XS
S54.12XS
S54.2ØXS
S54.21XS
S54.22XS
S54.3ØXS
S54.31XS
S54.32XS
S54.8X1S
S54.8X2S
S54.8X9S
S54.9ØXS
S54.91XS
S54.92XS
S64.ØØXS
S64.Ø1XS
S64.Ø2XS
S64.1ØXS
S64.11XS
S64.12XS
S64.2ØXS
S64.21XS
S64.22XS
S64.3ØXS
S64.31XS
S64.32XS
S64.4ØXS
S64.49ØS
S64.491S
S64.492S
S64.493S
S64.494S
S64.495S
S64.496S
S64.497S
S64.498S
S64.8X1S
S64.8X2S
S64.8X9S
S64.9ØXS
S64.91XS
S64.92XS
S74.ØØXS
S74.Ø1XS
S74.Ø2XS
S74.1ØXS
S74.11XS
S74.12XS
S74.2ØXS
S74.21XS
S74.22XS
S74.8X1S
S74.8X2S
S74.8X9S
S74.9ØXS
S74.91XS
S74.92XS
S84.ØØXS
S84.Ø1XS
S84.Ø2XS
S84.1ØXS
S84.11XS
S84.12XS
S84.2ØXS
S84.21XS
S84.22XS
S84.8Ø1S
S84.8Ø2S
S84.8Ø9S
S84.9ØXS
S84.91XS
S84.92XS
S94.ØØXS
S94.Ø1XS
S94.Ø2XS
S94.1ØXS
S94.11XS
S94.12XS
S94.2ØXS
S94.21XS
S94.22XS
S94.3ØXS
S94.31XS

S94.32XS
S94.8X1S
S94.8X2S
S94.8X9S
S94.9ØXS
S94.91XS
S94.92XS
T85.Ø1XA
T85.Ø2XA
T85.Ø3XA
T85.Ø9XA
T85.11ØA
T85.111A
T85.112A
T85.113A
T85.118A
T85.12ØA
T85.121A
T85.122A
T85.123A
T85.128A
T85.19ØA
T85.191A
T85.192A
T85.193A
T85.199A
T85.61ØA
T85.615A
T85.62ØA
T85.625A
T85.63ØA
T85.635A
T85.69ØA
T85.695A
T85.73ØA
T85.731A
T85.732A
T85.733A
T85.734A
T85.735A
T85.738A
T85.81ØA
T85.82ØA
T85.83ØA
T85.84ØA
T85.85ØA
T85.86ØA
T85.89ØA
Z45.3*
Z45.4*
Z46.2

DRG 092
Select principal diagnosis listed under DRG 091

DRG 093
Select principal diagnosis listed under DRG 091

DRG 094
Principal Diagnosis
AØ2.21
A17.Ø
A17.1
A17.8*
A39.Ø
A39.81
A54.81
GØØ*
GØ1
GØ4.2
GØ6*
GØ7
G61.Ø

DRG 095
Select principal diagnosis listed under DRG 094

DRG 096
Select principal diagnosis listed under DRG 094

DRG 097
Principal Diagnosis
AØ6.6
A27.8*
A5Ø.4Ø
A5Ø.41
A5Ø.42
A5Ø.43
A5Ø.45
A5Ø.49
A51.41
A52.13
A52.14
A52.2
A8Ø.Ø
A8Ø.1
A8Ø.2
A8Ø.3*
A8Ø.9
A82*
A83*
A84*
A85*
A86
A88.8
A89
A92.2
BØØ.4
BØØ.82
BØ1.1*
BØ2.24
BØ5.Ø
BØ6.Ø1
BØ6.Ø2
BØ6.Ø9
B1Ø.Ø*
B26.2
B37.5
B38.4
B45.1
B58.2
GØ2
GØ3.Ø
GØ3.1
GØ3.8
GØ3.9
GØ4.Ø*
GØ4.3*
GØ4.8*
GØ4.9*
GØ5*
G37.3
G37.4

DRG 098
Select principal diagnosis listed under DRG 097

DRG 099
Select principal diagnosis listed under DRG 097

DRG 100
Principal Diagnosis
G4Ø*
R56*

DRG 101
Select principal diagnosis listed under DRG 100

DRG 102
Principal Diagnosis
FØ7.81
G43*
G44*
G93.2
G97.1
I67.7
I68.2
R51*

DRG 103
Select principal diagnosis listed under DRG 102

MDC 2

DRG 113
Operating Room Procedures
Ø8BØØZX
Ø8BØ3ZX
Ø8BØXZX
Ø8B1ØZX
Ø8B13ZX
Ø8B1XZX
Ø8PØØ3Z
Ø8PØØJZ
Ø8P1Ø3Z
Ø8P1ØJZ
Ø8QØXZZ
Ø8Q1XZZ
Ø8RØØ7Z
Ø8RØØJZ
Ø8RØ37Z
Ø8RØ3KZ
Ø8R1Ø7Z
Ø8R1ØJZ
Ø8R137Z
Ø8R13KZ
Ø8TØXZZ
Ø8T1XZZ
Ø8WØØJZ
Ø8WØ3JZ
Ø8W1ØJZ
Ø8W13JZ
ØJ81*
ØJR1Ø7Z
ØJR1ØKZ
ØJR137Z
ØJR13KZ
ØN8P*
ØN8Q*
ØN9PØØZ
ØN9PØZX
ØN9PØZZ
ØN9P3ZX
ØN9P4ØZ
ØN9P4ZX
ØN9P4ZZ
ØN9QØØZ
ØN9QØZX
ØN9QØZZ
ØN9Q3ZX
ØN9Q4ØZ
ØN9Q4ZX
ØN9Q4ZZ
ØNBP*
ØNBQ*
ØNPWØJZ
ØNPW3JZ
ØNPW4JZ
ØNQPØZZ
ØNQP3ZZ
ØNQP4ZZ
ØNQQØZZ
ØNQQ3ZZ
ØNQQ4ZZ
ØNRCØJZ
ØNRC3JZ
ØNRC4JZ
ØNRFØJZ
ØNRF3JZ
ØNRF4JZ
ØNRGØJZ
ØNRG3JZ
ØNRG4JZ
ØNRHØJZ
ØNRH3JZ
ØNRH4JZ
ØNRJØJZ
ØNRJ3JZ
ØNRJ4JZ
ØNRKØJZ
ØNRK3JZ
ØNRK4JZ
ØNRLØJZ
ØNRL3JZ
ØNRL4JZ
ØNRMØJZ
ØNRM3JZ
ØNRM4JZ
ØNRNØJZ
ØNRN3JZ
ØNRN4JZ
ØNRPØ7Z
ØNRPØJZ
ØNRP37Z
ØNRP3JZ
ØNRP47Z
ØNRP4JZ
ØNRQØ7Z
ØNRQØJZ
ØNRQ37Z
ØNRQ3JZ
ØNRQ47Z
ØNRQ4JZ
ØNRXØJZ
ØNRX3JZ
ØNRX4JZ
ØNSCØ4Z
ØNSCØZZ
ØNSFØ4Z
ØNSFØZZ
ØNSGØ4Z
ØNSGØZZ
ØNSHØ4Z
ØNSHØZZ
ØNSJØ4Z
ØNSJØZZ
ØNSKØ4Z
ØNSKØZZ
ØNSLØ4Z
ØNSLØZZ
ØNSPØ4Z
ØNSPØZZ
ØNSQØ4Z
ØNSQØZZ
ØNSXØ4Z
ØNSXØZZ
ØNUCØJZ
ØNUC3JZ
ØNUC4JZ
ØNUFØJZ
ØNUF3JZ
ØNUF4JZ
ØNUGØJZ
ØNUG3JZ
ØNUG4JZ
ØNUHØJZ
ØNUH3JZ
ØNUH4JZ
ØNUJØJZ
ØNUJ3JZ
ØNUJ4JZ
ØNUKØJZ
ØNUK3JZ
ØNUK4JZ
ØNULØJZ
ØNUL3JZ
ØNUL4JZ
ØNUMØJZ
ØNUM3JZ
ØNUM4JZ
ØNUNØJZ
ØNUN3JZ
ØNUN4JZ
ØNUPØJZ
ØNUP3JZ
ØNUP4JZ
ØNUQØJZ
ØNUQ3JZ
ØNUQ4JZ
ØNUXØJZ
ØNUX3JZ
ØNUX4JZ
ØWQ2XZZ

DRG 114
Select operating room procedures listed under DRG 113

DRG 115
Operating Room Procedures
Ø39SØZX
Ø39S4ZX
Ø39TØZX
Ø39T4ZX
Ø3BSØZX
Ø3BS3ZX
Ø3BS4ZX
Ø3BTØZX
Ø3BT3ZX
Ø3BT4ZX
Ø81X*
Ø81Y*
Ø85ØXZZ
Ø851XZZ
Ø856XZZ
Ø857XZZ
Ø858XZZ
Ø859XZZ
Ø85L*
Ø85M*
Ø85N*
Ø85P*
Ø85Q*
Ø85R*
Ø85SXZZ
Ø85TXZZ
Ø85V*
Ø85W*
Ø85X*
Ø85Y*
Ø87*
Ø89ØXØZ
Ø891XØZ
Ø896XØZ
Ø897XØZ
Ø89L*
Ø89M*
Ø89NØZX
Ø89PØZX
Ø89QØZX
Ø89RØZX
Ø89SXØZ
Ø89TXØZ
Ø89V*
Ø89W*
Ø89X*
Ø89Y*
Ø8BØØZZ
Ø8BØ3ZZ
Ø8BØXZZ
Ø8B1ØZZ
Ø8B13ZZ
Ø8B1XZZ
Ø8B6XZZ
Ø8B7XZZ
Ø8B8*
Ø8B9*
Ø8BL*
Ø8BM*
Ø8BN*
Ø8BP*
Ø8BQ*
Ø8BR*
Ø8BS*
Ø8BT*
Ø8BV*
Ø8BW*
Ø8BX*
Ø8BY*
Ø8C8XZZ
Ø8C9XZZ
Ø8CLØZZ
Ø8CL3ZZ
Ø8CMØZZ
Ø8CM3ZZ
Ø8CVØZZ
Ø8CV3ZZ
Ø8CWØZZ
Ø8CW3ZZ
Ø8CX*
Ø8CY*
Ø8D8*
Ø8D9*
Ø8HØ33Z
Ø8HØX3Z
Ø8H133Z
Ø8H1X3Z
Ø8JLØZZ
Ø8JMØZZ
Ø8L*
Ø8M*
Ø8NØXZZ
Ø8N1XZZ
Ø8N6XZZ
Ø8N7XZZ
Ø8NL*
Ø8NM*
Ø8NN*
Ø8NP*
Ø8NQ*
Ø8NR*
Ø8NSXZZ
Ø8NTXZZ
Ø8NV*
Ø8NW*
Ø8NX*
Ø8NY*
Ø8PØØØZ
Ø8PØØ1Z
Ø8PØØ7Z
Ø8PØØCZ
Ø8PØØDZ
Ø8PØØKZ
Ø8PØØYZ
Ø8PØ3ØZ
Ø8PØ31Z
Ø8PØ33Z
Ø8PØ37Z
Ø8PØ3CZ
Ø8PØ3DZ
Ø8PØ3JZ
Ø8PØ3KZ
Ø8PØ71Z
Ø8PØ77Z
Ø8PØ7CZ
Ø8PØ7JZ
Ø8PØ7KZ
Ø8PØ81Z
Ø8PØ87Z
Ø8PØ8CZ
Ø8PØ8JZ
Ø8PØ8KZ
Ø8PØX7Z
Ø8PØXKZ
Ø8P1ØØZ
Ø8P1Ø1Z
Ø8P1Ø7Z
Ø8P1ØCZ
Ø8P1ØDZ
Ø8P1ØKZ
Ø8P1ØYZ
Ø8P13ØZ
Ø8P131Z
Ø8P133Z
Ø8P137Z
Ø8P13CZ
Ø8P13DZ
Ø8P13JZ
Ø8P13KZ
Ø8P171Z
Ø8P177Z
Ø8P17CZ
Ø8P17JZ
Ø8P17KZ
Ø8P181Z
Ø8P187Z
Ø8P18CZ
Ø8P18JZ
Ø8P18KZ
Ø8P1X7Z
Ø8P1XKZ
Ø8PLØØZ
Ø8PLØ7Z
Ø8PLØJZ
Ø8PLØKZ
Ø8PLØYZ
Ø8PL3ØZ
Ø8PL37Z
Ø8PL3JZ
Ø8PL3KZ
Ø8PMØØZ
Ø8PMØ7Z
Ø8PMØJZ
Ø8PMØKZ
Ø8PMØYZ
Ø8PM3ØZ
Ø8PM37Z
Ø8PM3JZ
Ø8PM3KZ
Ø8QL*
Ø8QM*
Ø8QSXZZ
Ø8QTXZZ
Ø8QVØZZ
Ø8QV3ZZ
Ø8QW*
Ø8QX*
Ø8QY*
Ø8RØØKZ
Ø8RØ3JZ
Ø8R1ØKZ
Ø8R13JZ
Ø8R6*
Ø8R7*
Ø8R8X7Z
Ø8R9X7Z
Ø8RN*
Ø8RP*
Ø8RQ*
Ø8RR*
Ø8RS*
Ø8RT*
Ø8RX*
Ø8RY*
Ø8SL*
Ø8SM*
Ø8SN*
Ø8SP*
Ø8SQ*
Ø8SR*
Ø8SV*
Ø8SW*
Ø8SX*
Ø8SY*
Ø8TL*
Ø8TM*
Ø8TN*
Ø8TP*
Ø8TQ*
Ø8TR*
Ø8TV*
Ø8TW*
Ø8TX*
Ø8TY*
Ø8UØ*
Ø8U1*
Ø8U8X7Z
Ø8U9X7Z
Ø8UL*
Ø8UM*
Ø8UN*
Ø8UP*
Ø8UQ*
Ø8UR*
Ø8UX*
Ø8UY*
Ø8V*
Ø8WØØØZ
Ø8WØØ3Z
Ø8WØØ7Z
Ø8WØØCZ
Ø8WØØDZ
Ø8WØØKZ
Ø8WØØYZ
Ø8WØ3ØZ
Ø8WØ33Z
Ø8WØ37Z
Ø8WØ3CZ
Ø8WØ3DZ
Ø8WØ3KZ
Ø8WØ7ØZ
Ø8WØ73Z
Ø8WØ77Z
Ø8WØ7CZ
Ø8WØ7DZ
Ø8WØ7JZ
Ø8WØ7KZ
Ø8WØ8ØZ
Ø8WØ83Z
Ø8WØ87Z
Ø8WØ8CZ
Ø8WØ8DZ
Ø8WØ8JZ
Ø8WØ8KZ
Ø8W1ØØZ
Ø8W1Ø3Z
Ø8W1Ø7Z
Ø8W1ØCZ
Ø8W1ØDZ
Ø8W1ØKZ
Ø8W1ØYZ
Ø8W13ØZ
Ø8W133Z
Ø8W137Z
Ø8W13CZ
Ø8W13DZ
Ø8W13KZ
Ø8W17ØZ
Ø8W173Z
Ø8W177Z
Ø8W17CZ
Ø8W17DZ
Ø8W17JZ
Ø8W17KZ
Ø8W18ØZ
Ø8W183Z
Ø8W187Z
Ø8W18CZ
Ø8W18DZ
Ø8W18JZ
Ø8W18KZ
Ø8WLØØZ
Ø8WLØ7Z
Ø8WLØJZ
Ø8WLØKZ
Ø8WLØYZ
Ø8WL3ØZ
Ø8WL37Z
Ø8WL3JZ
Ø8WL3KZ
Ø8WMØØZ
Ø8WMØ7Z
Ø8WMØJZ
Ø8WMØKZ
Ø8WMØYZ
Ø8WM3ØZ
Ø8WM37Z
Ø8WM3JZ
Ø8WM3KZ
Ø8X*
ØJBØØZZ
ØJB1ØZZ
ØJB4ØZZ
ØJB5ØZZ
ØJB6ØZZ
ØJB7ØZZ
ØJB8ØZZ
ØJB9ØZZ
ØJBBØZZ
ØJBCØZZ
ØJBDØZZ
ØJBFØZZ
ØJBGØZZ
ØJBHØZZ
ØJBLØZZ
ØJBMØZZ
ØJBNØZZ
ØJBPØZZ
ØJBQØZZ
ØJBRØZZ
ØKS1*
ØWBØØZZ
ØWBØ3ZZ
ØWBØ4ZZ
ØWBØXZZ
ØWB2ØZZ
ØWB23ZZ
ØWB24ZZ
ØWB2XZZ

DRG 116
Operating Room Procedures
Ø812*
Ø813*
Ø8523ZZ
Ø8533ZZ
Ø8543ZZ
Ø8553ZZ
Ø85A*
Ø85B*
Ø85C3ZZ
Ø85D3ZZ
Ø85G3ZZ
Ø85H3ZZ
Ø85J3ZZ
Ø85K3ZZ
Ø892*
Ø893*
Ø894*
Ø895*
Ø898XØZ
Ø899XØZ
Ø89A*
Ø89B*
Ø89C*
Ø89D*
Ø89E*
Ø89F*
Ø89G*
Ø89H*
Ø89J*
Ø89K*
Ø8B4*
Ø8B5*
Ø8B6XZX
Ø8B7XZX
Ø8BA*
Ø8BB*
Ø8BC*
Ø8BD*
Ø8BE*
Ø8BF*
Ø8BJ*
Ø8BK*
Ø8C23ZZ
Ø8C33ZZ
Ø8C4*
Ø8C5*
Ø8CA*
Ø8CB*
Ø8CC*
Ø8CD*
Ø8CE*
Ø8CF*
Ø8CG*
Ø8CH*
Ø8CJ*
Ø8CK*
Ø8CLXZZ
Ø8CMXZZ
Ø8CVXZZ
Ø8CWXZZ
Ø8DJ3ZZ
Ø8DK3ZZ
Ø8F43ZZ
Ø8F53ZZ
Ø8HØØ5Z
Ø8HØØYZ
Ø8HØ31Z
Ø8HØX1Z
Ø8H1Ø5Z
Ø8H1ØYZ
Ø8H131Z
Ø8H1X1Z
Ø8N23ZZ
Ø8N33ZZ
Ø8N43ZZ
Ø8N53ZZ
Ø8N8XZZ
Ø8N9XZZ
Ø8NA*
Ø8NB*
Ø8NC3ZZ
Ø8ND3ZZ
Ø8NE3ZZ
Ø8NF3ZZ
Ø8NG3ZZ
Ø8NH3ZZ
Ø8NJ3ZZ
Ø8NK3ZZ
Ø8PJ3JZ
Ø8PK3JZ
Ø8Q23ZZ
Ø8Q33ZZ
Ø8Q43ZZ
Ø8Q53ZZ
Ø8Q6XZZ
Ø8Q7XZZ
Ø8Q8XZZ
Ø8Q9XZZ
Ø8QA*
Ø8QB*
Ø8QC3ZZ
Ø8QD3ZZ
Ø8QE3ZZ
Ø8QF3ZZ
Ø8QG3ZZ
Ø8QH3ZZ
Ø8QJ3ZZ
Ø8QK3ZZ
Ø8R4*
Ø8R5*
Ø8R837Z
Ø8R83JZ
Ø8R83KZ
Ø8R8XJZ
Ø8R8XKZ
Ø8R937Z
Ø8R93JZ
Ø8R93KZ
Ø8R9XJZ
Ø8R9XKZ
Ø8RA*
Ø8RB*
Ø8RC*
Ø8RD*
Ø8RG*
Ø8RH*

Ø8RJ*
Ø8RK*
Ø8SC3ZZ
Ø8SD3ZZ
Ø8SG3ZZ
Ø8SH3ZZ
Ø8SJ3ZZ
Ø8SK3ZZ
Ø8T43ZZ
Ø8T53ZZ
Ø8T8XZZ
Ø8T9XZZ
Ø8TC3ZZ
Ø8TD3ZZ
Ø8TJ3ZZ
Ø8TK3ZZ
Ø8U8Ø7Z
Ø8U8ØJZ
Ø8U8ØKZ
Ø8U837Z
Ø8U83JZ
Ø8U83KZ
Ø8U8XJZ
Ø8U8XKZ
Ø8U9Ø7Z
Ø8U9ØJZ
Ø8U9ØKZ
Ø8U937Z
Ø8U93JZ
Ø8U93KZ
Ø8U9XJZ
Ø8U9XKZ
Ø8UC*
Ø8UD*
Ø8UE*
Ø8UF*
Ø8UG*
Ø8UH*
Ø8WJ3JZ
Ø8WK3JZ

DRG 117

Select operating room procedures listed under DRG 116

DRG 121

Principal Diagnosis

HØ4.Ø11
HØ4.Ø12
HØ4.Ø13
HØ4.Ø19
HØ4.321
HØ4.322
HØ4.323
HØ4.329
HØ4.331
HØ4.332
HØ4.333
HØ4.339
HØ5.Ø11
HØ5.Ø12
HØ5.Ø13
HØ5.Ø19
HØ5.Ø21
HØ5.Ø22
HØ5.Ø23
HØ5.Ø29
HØ5.Ø31
HØ5.Ø32
HØ5.Ø33
HØ5.Ø39
HØ5.Ø41
HØ5.Ø42
HØ5.Ø43
HØ5.Ø49
H16.ØØ1
H16.ØØ2
H16.ØØ3
H16.ØØ9
H16.Ø11
H16.Ø12
H16.Ø13
H16.Ø19
H16.Ø31
H16.Ø32
H16.Ø33
H16.Ø39
H16.Ø61
H16.Ø62
H16.Ø63
H16.Ø69
H16.Ø71
H16.Ø72
H16.Ø73
H16.Ø79
H16.311
H16.312
H16.313
H16.319
H21.331
H21.332
H21.333
H21.339
H33.121
H33.122
H33.123
H33.129
H44.Ø*
H44.121
H44.122
H44.123
H44.129
H44.19

DRG 122

Select principal diagnosis listed under DRG 121

DRG 123

Principal Diagnosis

A39.82
G45.3
HØ2.4Ø1
HØ2.4Ø2
HØ2.4Ø3
HØ2.4Ø9
HØ2.421
HØ2.422
HØ2.423
HØ2.429
HØ2.431
HØ2.432
HØ2.433
HØ2.439
HØ2.59
HØ5.211
HØ5.212
HØ5.213
HØ5.219
HØ5.251
HØ5.252
HØ5.253
HØ5.259
HØ5.261
HØ5.262
HØ5.263
HØ5.269
HØ5.821
HØ5.822
HØ5.823
HØ5.829
H34.ØØ
H34.Ø1
H34.Ø2
H34.Ø3
H34.211
H34.212
H34.213
H34.219
H34.811Ø
H34.8111
H34.8112
H34.812Ø
H34.8121
H34.8122
H34.813Ø
H34.8131
H34.8132
H34.819Ø
H34.8191
H34.8192
H34.821
H34.822
H34.823
H34.829
H34.831Ø
H34.8311
H34.8312
H34.832Ø
H34.8321
H34.8322
H34.833Ø
H34.8331
H34.8332
H34.839Ø
H34.8391
H34.8392
H34.9
H4Ø.12*
H46*
H47.Ø*
H47.2Ø
H47.211
H47.212
H47.213
H47.219
H47.22
H47.291
H47.292
H47.293
H47.299
H47.321
H47.322
H47.323
H47.329
H47.331
H47.332
H47.333
H47.339
H49.Ø*
H49.1*
H49.2*
H49.3*
H49.4*
H49.881
H49.882
H49.883
H49.889
H49.9
H5Ø.89
H51.8
H52.511
H52.512
H52.513
H52.519
H53.121
H53.122
H53.123
H53.129
H53.131
H53.132
H53.133
H53.139
H53.2
H53.4Ø
H53.411
H53.412
H53.413
H53.419
H53.431
H53.432
H53.433
H53.439
H53.451
H53.452
H53.453
H53.459
H53.461
H53.462
H53.469
H53.47
H53.481
H53.482
H53.483
H53.489
H53.52
H55.ØØ
H55.Ø2
H55.Ø4
H55.81
H57.ØØ
H57.Ø2
H57.Ø3
H57.Ø4
H57.Ø51
H57.Ø52
H57.Ø53
H57.Ø59
H57.Ø9

DRG 124

Principal Diagnosis

A18.5*
A36.86
A5Ø.31
A51.43
A52.71
A54.3*
A71*
A74.Ø
BØØ.5*
BØ2.3*
BØ5.81
B3Ø*
B58.Ø1
B58.Ø9
B6Ø.12
B6Ø.13
B94.Ø
C43.1Ø
C43.111
C43.112
C43.121
C43.122
C44.1Ø1
C44.1Ø21
C44.1Ø22
C44.1Ø91
C44.1Ø92
C44.111
C44.1121
C44.1122
C44.1191
C44.1192
C44.121
C44.1221
C44.1222
C44.1291
C44.1292
C44.131
C44.1321
C44.1322
C44.1391
C44.1392
C44.191
C44.1921
C44.1922
C44.1991
C44.1992
C69*
DØ3.1Ø
DØ3.111
DØ3.112
DØ3.121
DØ3.122
DØ4.1Ø
DØ4.111
DØ4.112
DØ4.121
DØ4.122
DØ9.2*
D22.1Ø
D22.111
D22.112
D22.121
D22.122
D23.1Ø
D23.111
D23.112
D23.121
D23.122
D31*
EØ8.3*
EØ9.3*
E1Ø.3*
E11.3*
E13.3*
E5Ø.Ø
E5Ø.1
E5Ø.2
E5Ø.3
E5Ø.4
E5Ø.5
E5Ø.6
E5Ø.7
G24.5
HØØ*
HØ1.ØØ1
HØ1.ØØ2
HØ1.ØØ3
HØ1.ØØ4
HØ1.ØØ5
HØ1.ØØ6
HØ1.ØØ9
HØ1.ØØA
HØ1.ØØB
HØ1.Ø11
HØ1.Ø12
HØ1.Ø13
HØ1.Ø14
HØ1.Ø15
HØ1.Ø16
HØ1.Ø19
HØ1.Ø1A
HØ1.Ø1B
HØ1.Ø21
HØ1.Ø22
HØ1.Ø23
HØ1.Ø24
HØ1.Ø25
HØ1.Ø26
HØ1.Ø29
HØ1.Ø2A
HØ1.Ø2B
HØ1.111
HØ1.112
HØ1.113
HØ1.114
HØ1.115
HØ1.116
HØ1.119
HØ1.121
HØ1.122
HØ1.123
HØ1.124
HØ1.125
HØ1.126
HØ1.129
HØ1.131
HØ1.132
HØ1.133
HØ1.134
HØ1.135
HØ1.136
HØ1.139
HØ1.141
HØ1.142
HØ1.143
HØ1.144
HØ1.145
HØ1.146
HØ1.149
HØ1.8
HØ1.9
HØ2.Ø*
HØ2.1Ø1
HØ2.1Ø2
HØ2.1Ø3
HØ2.1Ø4
HØ2.1Ø5
HØ2.1Ø6
HØ2.1Ø9
HØ2.111
HØ2.112
HØ2.113
HØ2.114
HØ2.115
HØ2.116
HØ2.119
HØ2.121
HØ2.122
HØ2.123
HØ2.124
HØ2.125
HØ2.126
HØ2.129
HØ2.131
HØ2.132
HØ2.133
HØ2.134
HØ2.135
HØ2.136
HØ2.139
HØ2.141
HØ2.142
HØ2.143
HØ2.144
HØ2.145
HØ2.146
HØ2.149
HØ2.151
HØ2.152
HØ2.153
HØ2.154
HØ2.155
HØ2.156
HØ2.159
HØ2.2Ø1
HØ2.2Ø2
HØ2.2Ø3
HØ2.2Ø4
HØ2.2Ø5
HØ2.2Ø6
HØ2.2Ø9
HØ2.2ØA
HØ2.2ØB
HØ2.2ØC
HØ2.211
HØ2.212
HØ2.213
HØ2.214
HØ2.215
HØ2.216
HØ2.219
HØ2.21A
HØ2.21B
HØ2.21C
HØ2.221
HØ2.222
HØ2.223
HØ2.224
HØ2.225
HØ2.226
HØ2.229
HØ2.22A
HØ2.22B
HØ2.22C
HØ2.231
HØ2.232
HØ2.233
HØ2.234
HØ2.235
HØ2.236
HØ2.239
HØ2.23A
HØ2.23B
HØ2.23C
HØ2.3Ø
HØ2.31
HØ2.32
HØ2.33
HØ2.34
HØ2.35
HØ2.36
HØ2.411
HØ2.412
HØ2.413
HØ2.419
HØ2.51*
HØ2.52*
HØ2.53*
HØ2.7*
HØ2.811
HØ2.812
HØ2.813
HØ2.814
HØ2.815
HØ2.816
HØ2.819
HØ2.821
HØ2.822
HØ2.823
HØ2.824
HØ2.825
HØ2.826
HØ2.829
HØ2.831
HØ2.832
HØ2.833
HØ2.834
HØ2.835
HØ2.836
HØ2.839
HØ2.841
HØ2.842
HØ2.843
HØ2.844
HØ2.845
HØ2.846
HØ2.849
HØ2.851
HØ2.852
HØ2.853
HØ2.854
HØ2.855
HØ2.856
HØ2.859
HØ2.861
HØ2.862
HØ2.863
HØ2.864
HØ2.865
HØ2.866
HØ2.869
HØ2.871
HØ2.872
HØ2.873
HØ2.874
HØ2.875
HØ2.876
HØ2.879
HØ2.881
HØ2.882
HØ2.883
HØ2.884
HØ2.885
HØ2.886
HØ2.889
HØ2.88A
HØ2.88B
HØ2.89
HØ2.9
HØ4.ØØ1
HØ4.ØØ2
HØ4.ØØ3
HØ4.ØØ9
HØ4.Ø21
HØ4.Ø22
HØ4.Ø23
HØ4.Ø29
HØ4.Ø31
HØ4.Ø32
HØ4.Ø33
HØ4.Ø39
HØ4.1*
HØ4.2*
HØ4.3Ø1
HØ4.3Ø2
HØ4.3Ø3
HØ4.3Ø9
HØ4.311
HØ4.312
HØ4.313
HØ4.319
HØ4.4*
HØ4.5*
HØ4.6*
HØ4.8*
HØ4.9
HØ5.ØØ
HØ5.1*
HØ5.2Ø
HØ5.221
HØ5.222
HØ5.223
HØ5.229
HØ5.231
HØ5.232
HØ5.233
HØ5.239
HØ5.241
HØ5.242
HØ5.243
HØ5.249
HØ5.3*
HØ5.4*
HØ5.5*
HØ5.811
HØ5.812
HØ5.813
HØ5.819
HØ5.89
HØ5.9
H1Ø.Ø11
H1Ø.Ø12
H1Ø.Ø13
H1Ø.Ø19
H1Ø.Ø21
H1Ø.Ø22
H1Ø.Ø23
H1Ø.Ø29
H1Ø.1Ø
H1Ø.11
H1Ø.12
H1Ø.13
H1Ø.211
H1Ø.212
H1Ø.213
H1Ø.219
H1Ø.221
H1Ø.222
H1Ø.223
H1Ø.229
H1Ø.231
H1Ø.232
H1Ø.233
H1Ø.239
H1Ø.3Ø
H1Ø.31
H1Ø.32
H1Ø.33
H1Ø.4Ø1
H1Ø.4Ø2
H1Ø.4Ø3
H1Ø.4Ø9
H1Ø.411
H1Ø.412
H1Ø.413
H1Ø.419
H1Ø.421
H1Ø.422
H1Ø.423
H1Ø.429
H1Ø.431
H1Ø.432
H1Ø.433
H1Ø.439
H1Ø.44
H1Ø.45
H1Ø.5Ø1
H1Ø.5Ø2
H1Ø.5Ø3
H1Ø.5Ø9
H1Ø.511
H1Ø.512
H1Ø.513
H1Ø.519
H1Ø.521
H1Ø.522
H1Ø.523
H1Ø.529
H1Ø.531
H1Ø.532
H1Ø.533
H1Ø.539
H1Ø.811
H1Ø.812
H1Ø.813
H1Ø.819
H1Ø.821
H1Ø.822
H1Ø.823
H1Ø.829
H1Ø.89
H1Ø.9
H11*
H15*
H16.Ø21
H16.Ø22
H16.Ø23
H16.Ø29
H16.Ø41
H16.Ø42
H16.Ø43
H16.Ø49
H16.Ø51
H16.Ø52
H16.Ø53
H16.Ø59
H16.1*
H16.2*
H16.3Ø1
H16.3Ø2
H16.3Ø3
H16.3Ø9
H16.321
H16.322
H16.323
H16.329
H16.331
H16.332
H16.333
H16.339
H16.391
H16.392
H16.393
H16.399
H16.4*
H16.8
H16.9
H17*
H18*
H2Ø*
H21.Ø*
H21.1*
H21.2*
H21.3Ø1
H21.3Ø2
H21.3Ø3
H21.3Ø9
H21.311
H21.312
H21.313
H21.319
H21.321
H21.322
H21.323
H21.329
H21.341
H21.342
H21.343
H21.349
H21.351
H21.352
H21.353
H21.359
H21.4*
H21.5*
H21.8*
H21.9
H22
H25*
H26*
H27*
H28
H3Ø*
H31*
H32
H33.Ø*
H33.1Ø1
H33.1Ø2
H33.1Ø3
H33.1Ø9
H33.111
H33.112
H33.113
H33.119
H33.191
H33.192
H33.193
H33.199
H33.2*
H33.3*
H33.4*
H33.8
H34.1Ø
H34.11
H34.12
H34.13
H34.231
H34.232
H34.233
H34.239
H35.ØØ
H35.Ø11
H35.Ø12
H35.Ø13
H35.Ø19
H35.Ø21
H35.Ø22
H35.Ø23
H35.Ø29
H35.Ø31
H35.Ø32
H35.Ø33
H35.Ø39
H35.Ø41
H35.Ø42
H35.Ø43
H35.Ø49
H35.Ø51
H35.Ø52
H35.Ø53
H35.Ø59
H35.Ø61
H35.Ø62
H35.Ø63
H35.Ø69
H35.Ø71
H35.Ø72
H35.Ø73
H35.Ø79
H35.Ø9
H35.1Ø1
H35.1Ø2
H35.1Ø3
H35.1Ø9
H35.111
H35.112
H35.113
H35.119
H35.121
H35.122
H35.123
H35.129
H35.131
H35.132
H35.133
H35.139
H35.141
H35.142
H35.143
H35.149
H35.151
H35.152
H35.153
H35.159
H35.161
H35.162
H35.163
H35.169
H35.171
H35.172

H35.173
H35.179
H35.20
H35.21
H35.22
H35.23
H35.30
H35.3110
H35.3111
H35.3112
H35.3113
H35.3114
H35.3120
H35.3121
H35.3122
H35.3123
H35.3124
H35.3130
H35.3131
H35.3132
H35.3133
H35.3134
H35.3190
H35.3191
H35.3192
H35.3193
H35.3194
H35.3210
H35.3211
H35.3212
H35.3213
H35.3220
H35.3221
H35.3222
H35.3223
H35.3230
H35.3231
H35.3232
H35.3233
H35.3290
H35.3291
H35.3292
H35.3293
H35.33
H35.341
H35.342
H35.343
H35.349
H35.351
H35.352
H35.353
H35.359
H35.361
H35.362
H35.363
H35.369
H35.371
H35.372
H35.373
H35.379
H35.381
H35.382
H35.383
H35.389
H35.40
H35.411
H35.412
H35.413
H35.419
H35.421
H35.422
H35.423
H35.429
H35.431
H35.432
H35.433
H35.439
H35.441
H35.442
H35.443
H35.449
H35.451
H35.452
H35.453
H35.459
H35.461
H35.462
H35.463
H35.469
H35.50
H35.51
H35.52
H35.53
H35.54
H35.60
H35.61
H35.62
H35.63
H35.70
H35.711
H35.712
H35.713
H35.719
H35.721
H35.722
H35.723
H35.729
H35.731
H35.732
H35.733
H35.739
H35.81
H35.82
H35.89
H35.9
H36*
H40.0*
H40.10*
H40.1110
H40.1111
H40.1112
H40.1113
H40.1114
H40.1120
H40.1121
H40.1122
H40.1123
H40.1124
H40.1130
H40.1131
H40.1132
H40.1133
H40.1134
H40.1190
H40.1191
H40.1192
H40.1193
H40.1194
H40.13*
H40.14*
H40.15*
H40.2*
H40.3*
H40.4*
H40.5*
H40.6*
H40.8*
H40.9
H42
H43*
H44.11*
H44.13*
H44.2*
H44.3*
H44.4*
H44.5*
H44.6*
H44.7*
H44.8*
H44.9
H47.12
H47.13
H47.23*
H47.31*
H47.39*
H50.0*
H50.1*
H50.2*
H50.3*
H50.4*
H50.5*
H50.6*
H50.811
H50.812
H50.9
H51.0
H51.1*
H51.9
H52.0*
H52.1*
H52.2*
H52.3*
H52.4
H52.52*
H52.53*
H52.6
H52.7
H53.001
H53.002
H53.003
H53.009
H53.011
H53.012
H53.013
H53.019
H53.021
H53.022
H53.023
H53.029
H53.031
H53.032
H53.033
H53.039
H53.041
H53.042
H53.043
H53.049
H53.10
H53.11
H53.141
H53.142
H53.143
H53.149
H53.15
H53.16
H53.19
H53.3*
H53.42*
H53.50
H53.51
H53.53
H53.54
H53.55
H53.59
H53.6*
H53.7*
H53.8
H53.9
H54*
H55.01
H55.03
H55.09
H55.82
H55.89
H57.1*
H57.811
H57.812
H57.813
H57.819
H57.89
H57.8A1
H57.8A2
H57.8A3
H57.8A9
H57.9
H59.02*
H59.4*
Q10*
Q11*
Q12*
Q13*
Q14*
Q15*
R44.1
R48.3
R94.110
R94.111
R94.112
R94.113
S00.10XA
S00.11XA
S00.12XA
S00.201A
S00.202A
S00.209A
S00.211A
S00.212A
S00.219A
S00.221A
S00.222A
S00.229A
S00.241A
S00.242A
S00.249A
S00.251A
S00.252A
S00.259A
S00.261A
S00.262A
S00.269A
S00.271A
S00.272A
S00.279A
S01.101A
S01.102A
S01.109A
S01.111A
S01.112A
S01.119A
S01.121A
S01.122A
S01.129A
S01.131A
S01.132A
S01.139A
S01.141A
S01.142A
S01.149A
S01.151A
S01.152A
S01.159A
S02.30XA
S02.30XB
S02.31XA
S02.31XB
S02.32XA
S02.32XB
S04.011A
S04.012A
S04.019A
S05.00XA
S05.01XA
S05.02XA
S05.10XA
S05.11XA
S05.12XA
S05.20XA
S05.21XA
S05.22XA
S05.30XA
S05.31XA
S05.32XA
S05.40XA
S05.41XA
S05.42XA
S05.50XA
S05.51XA
S05.52XA
S05.60XA
S05.61XA
S05.62XA
S05.70XA
S05.71XA
S05.72XA
S05.8X1A
S05.8X2A
S05.8X9A
S05.90XA
S05.91XA
S05.92XA
T15.00XA
T15.01XA
T15.02XA
T15.10XA
T15.11XA
T15.12XA
T15.80XA
T15.81XA
T15.82XA
T15.90XA
T15.91XA
T15.92XA
T26.00XA
T26.01XA
T26.02XA
T26.10XA
T26.11XA
T26.12XA
T26.20XA
T26.21XA
T26.22XA
T26.30XA
T26.31XA
T26.32XA
T26.40XA
T26.41XA
T26.42XA
T26.50XA
T26.51XA
T26.52XA
T26.60XA
T26.61XA
T26.62XA
T26.70XA
T26.71XA
T26.72XA
T26.80XA
T26.81XA
T26.82XA
T26.90XA
T26.91XA
T26.92XA
T85.21XA
T85.22XA
T85.29XA
T85.318A
T85.328A
T85.398A
T86.840*
T86.841*
Z90.01
Z94.7
Z96.1
Z97.0

AND

Thrombolytic Agent Nonoperating Room Procedures

3E03017
3E03317
3E04017
3E04317
3E05017
3E05317
3E06017
3E06317
3E08017
3E08317

DRG 125

Select principal diagnosis listed under DRG 124

MDC 3

DRG 135

Operating Room Procedures

095B*
095C*
095P*
095Q*
095R*
095S*
095T*
095U*
095V*
095W*
095X*
099B00Z
099B0ZZ
099B40Z
099B4ZZ
099C00Z
099C0ZZ
099C40Z
099C4ZZ
099P00Z
099P0ZX
099P0ZZ
099Q00Z
099Q0ZX
099Q0ZZ
099R00Z
099R0ZX
099R0ZZ
099S00Z
099S0ZX
099S0ZZ
099T00Z
099T0ZX
099T0ZZ
099U00Z
099U0ZX
099U0ZZ
099V00Z
099V0ZX
099V0ZZ
099W00Z
099W0ZX
099W0ZZ
099X00Z
099X0ZX
099X0ZZ
09BB0ZZ
09BB3ZZ
09BB4ZZ
09BB8ZZ
09BC0ZZ
09BC3ZZ
09BC4ZZ
09BC8ZZ
09BP0ZX
09BP0ZZ
09BP3ZZ
09BP4ZZ
09BP8ZZ
09BQ0ZX
09BQ0ZZ
09BQ3ZZ
09BQ4ZZ
09BQ8ZZ
09BR0ZX
09BR0ZZ
09BR3ZZ
09BR4ZZ
09BR8ZZ
09BS0ZX
09BS0ZZ
09BS3ZZ
09BS4ZZ
09BS8ZZ
09BT0ZX
09BT0ZZ
09BT3ZZ
09BT4ZZ
09BT8ZZ
09BU0ZX
09BU0ZZ
09BU3ZZ
09BU4ZZ
09BU8ZZ
09BV0ZX
09BV0ZZ
09BV3ZZ
09BV4ZZ
09BV8ZZ
09BW0ZX
09BW0ZZ
09BW3ZZ
09BW4ZZ
09BW8ZZ
09BX0ZX
09BX0ZZ
09BX3ZZ
09BX4ZZ
09BX8ZZ
09CB*
09CC*
09CP*
09CQ*
09CR*
09CS*
09CT*
09CU*
09CV*
09CW*
09CX*
09DB*
09DC*
09DP*
09DQ*
09DR*
09DS*
09DT*
09DU*
09DV*
09DW*
09DX*
09HY01Z
09HY0YZ
09NP*
09NQ*
09NR*
09NS*
09NT*
09NU*
09NV*
09NW*
09NX*
09PY00Z
09PY0YZ
09PY30Z
09PY40Z
09QB*
09QC*
09QP*
09QQ*
09QR*
09QS*
09QT*
09QU*
09QV*
09QW*
09QX*
09TB*
09TC*
09TP*
09TQ*
09TR*
09TS*
09TT*
09TU*
09TV*
09TW*
09TX*
09UB07Z
09UB0JZ
09UB0KZ
09UB37Z
09UB3JZ
09UB3KZ
09UB47Z
09UB4JZ
09UB4KZ
09UB77Z
09UB7JZ
09UB7KZ
09UB87Z
09UB8JZ
09UB8KZ
09UC07Z
09UC0JZ
09UC0KZ
09UC37Z
09UC3JZ
09UC3KZ
09UC47Z
09UC4JZ
09UC4KZ
09UC77Z
09UC7JZ
09UC7KZ
09UC87Z
09UC8JZ
09UC8KZ
09UP07Z
09UP0JZ
09UP0KZ
09UP37Z
09UP3JZ
09UP3KZ
09UP47Z
09UP4JZ
09UP4KZ
09UP77Z
09UP7JZ
09UP7KZ
09UP87Z
09UP8JZ
09UP8KZ
09UQ07Z
09UQ0JZ
09UQ0KZ
09UQ37Z
09UQ3JZ
09UQ3KZ
09UQ47Z
09UQ4JZ
09UQ4KZ
09UQ77Z
09UQ7JZ
09UQ7KZ
09UQ87Z
09UQ8JZ
09UQ8KZ
09UR07Z
09UR0JZ
09UR0KZ
09UR37Z
09UR3JZ
09UR3KZ
09UR47Z
09UR4JZ
09UR4KZ
09UR77Z
09UR7JZ
09UR7KZ
09UR87Z
09UR8JZ
09UR8KZ
09US07Z
09US0JZ
09US0KZ
09US37Z
09US3JZ
09US3KZ
09US47Z
09US4JZ
09US4KZ
09US77Z
09US7JZ
09US7KZ
09US87Z
09US8JZ
09US8KZ
09UT07Z
09UT0JZ
09UT0KZ
09UT37Z
09UT3JZ
09UT3KZ
09UT47Z
09UT4JZ
09UT4KZ
09UT77Z
09UT7JZ
09UT7KZ
09UT87Z
09UT8JZ
09UT8KZ
09UU07Z
09UU0JZ
09UU0KZ
09UU37Z
09UU3JZ
09UU3KZ
09UU47Z
09UU4JZ
09UU4KZ
09UU77Z
09UU7JZ
09UU7KZ
09UU87Z
09UU8JZ
09UU8KZ
09UV07Z
09UV0JZ
09UV0KZ
09UV37Z
09UV3JZ
09UV3KZ
09UV47Z
09UV4JZ
09UV4KZ
09UV77Z
09UV7JZ
09UV7KZ
09UV87Z
09UV8JZ
09UV8KZ
09UW07Z
09UW0JZ
09UW0KZ
09UW37Z
09UW3JZ
09UW3KZ
09UW47Z
09UW4JZ
09UW4KZ
09UW77Z
09UW7JZ
09UW7KZ
09UW87Z
09UW8JZ
09UW8KZ
09UX07Z
09UX0JZ
09UX0KZ
09UX37Z
09UX3JZ
09UX3KZ
09UX47Z
09UX4JZ
09UX4KZ
09UX77Z
09UX7JZ
09UX7KZ
09UX87Z
09UX8JZ
09UX8KZ
09WY00Z
09WY0YZ
09WY30Z
09WY40Z

DRG 136

Select operating room procedures listed under DRG 135

DRG 137

Operating Room Procedures

0C0*
0C50*
0C51*
0C52*
0C53*
0C54*
0C57*
0C5N*
0C9000Z
0C900ZZ
0C90X0Z
0C90XZZ
0C9100Z
0C910ZZ
0C91X0Z
0C91XZZ
0C9200Z
0C920ZX
0C920ZZ
0C923ZX
0C92X0Z
0C92XZX
0C92XZZ
0C9300Z
0C930ZX
0C930ZZ
0C933ZX
0C93X0Z
0C93XZX
0C93XZZ
0C9400Z
0C940ZZ
0C94X0Z
0C94XZZ
0C9700Z
0C970ZX
0C970ZZ
0C97X0Z
0C97XZZ
0C9N00Z
0C9N0ZX
0C9N0ZZ
0C9N3ZX
0C9NX0Z
0C9NXZX
0C9NXZZ
0CB00ZZ
0CB03ZZ
0CB0XZZ
0CB10ZZ
0CB13ZZ
0CB1XZZ
0CB2*
0CB3*
0CB40ZZ
0CB43ZZ
0CB4XZZ
0CB70ZX
0CB70ZZ
0CB73ZZ
0CB7XZZ
0CBN*
0CC00ZZ
0CC03ZZ
0CC10ZZ

ØCC13ZZ
ØCC2ØZZ
ØCC23ZZ
ØCC3ØZZ
ØCC33ZZ
ØCC4ØZZ
ØCC43ZZ
ØCC7ØZZ
ØCC73ZZ
ØCCNØZZ
ØCCN3ZZ
ØCMØØZZ
ØCM1ØZZ
ØCM3ØZZ
ØCM7ØZZ
ØCMNØZZ
ØCN2*
ØCN3*
ØCN4ØZZ
ØCN43ZZ
ØCNN*
ØCPYØØZ
ØCPYØ1Z
ØCPYØ7Z
ØCPYØDZ
ØCPYØJZ
ØCPYØKZ
ØCPYØYZ
ØCPY3ØZ
ØCPY31Z
ØCPY37Z
ØCPY3DZ
ØCPY3JZ
ØCPY3KZ
ØCQØØZZ
ØCQØ3ZZ
ØCQ1ØZZ
ØCQ13ZZ
ØCQ4ØZZ
ØCQ43ZZ
ØCQ7ØZZ
ØCQ73ZZ
ØCQN*
ØCRØ*
ØCR1*
ØCR4*
ØCR5*
ØCR6*
ØCR7*
ØCRN*
ØCSØ*
ØCS1*
ØCS7*
ØCSN*
ØCTØ*
ØCT1*
ØCT3*
ØCTN*
ØCUØ*
ØCU1*
ØCU4*
ØCU5*
ØCU6*
ØCU7*
ØCUN*
ØCWYØØZ
ØCWYØ1Z
ØCWYØDZ
ØCWYØJZ
ØCWYØKZ
ØCWYØYZ
ØCWY3ØZ
ØCWY31Z
ØCWY37Z
ØCWY3DZ
ØCWY3JZ
ØCWY3KZ
ØCX*
ØNNX*
ØW92ØØZ
ØW92ØZZ
ØW924ØZ
ØW924ZZ
ØW93ØØZ
ØW93ØZZ
ØW934ØZ
ØW934ZZ
ØW94ØØZ
ØW94ØZZ
ØW944ØZ
ØW944ZZ
ØW95ØØZ
ØW95ØZZ
ØW954ØZ
ØW954ZZ
ØWB3ØZX
ØWB3ØZZ
ØWB33ZX
ØWB33ZZ
ØWB34ZX
ØWB34ZZ
ØWB3XZX
ØWB3XZZ
ØWC3ØZZ
ØWC33ZZ
ØWC34ZZ
ØWF3ØZZ
ØWF33ZZ
ØWF34ZZ
ØWH3Ø3Z
ØWH3ØYZ
ØWH333Z
ØWH33YZ
ØWH343Z
ØWH34YZ

DRG 138

Select operating room procedures listed under DRG 137

DRG 139

Operating Room Procedures

ØC58*
ØC59*
ØC5B*
ØC5C*
ØC5D*
ØC5F*
ØC5G*
ØC5H*
ØC5J*
ØC98ØZX
ØC98ØZZ
ØC99ØZX
ØC99ØZZ
ØC9BØZX
ØC9CØZX
ØC9DØZX
ØC9FØZX
ØC9GØZX
ØC9GØZZ
ØC9HØZX
ØC9HØZZ
ØC9JØZX
ØCB8ØZX
ØCB8ØZZ
ØCB83ZZ
ØCB9ØZX
ØCB9ØZZ
ØCB93ZZ
ØCBBØZX
ØCBBØZZ
ØCBB3ZZ
ØCBCØZX
ØCBCØZZ
ØCBC3ZZ
ØCBDØZX
ØCBDØZZ
ØCBD3ZZ
ØCBFØZX
ØCBFØZZ
ØCBF3ZZ
ØCBGØZX
ØCBGØZZ
ØCBG3ZZ
ØCBHØZX
ØCBHØZZ
ØCBH3ZZ
ØCBJØZX
ØCBJØZZ
ØCBJ3ZZ
ØCC8ØZZ
ØCC9ØZZ
ØCCGØZZ
ØCCHØZZ
ØCL*
ØCN8*
ØCN9*
ØCNB*
ØCNC*
ØCND*
ØCNF*
ØCNG*
ØCNH*
ØCNJ*
ØCQ8*
ØCQ9*
ØCQB*
ØCQC*
ØCQD*
ØCQF*
ØCQG*
ØCQH*
ØCQJ*
ØCRB*
ØCRC*
ØCSB*
ØCSC*
ØCT8ØZZ
ØCT9ØZZ
ØCTBØZZ
ØCTCØZZ
ØCTDØZZ
ØCTFØZZ
ØCTGØZZ
ØCTHØZZ
ØCTJØZZ
ØCV*

DRG 140

Operating Room Procedures

Ø3LHØCZ
Ø3LHØZZ
Ø3LH3CZ
Ø3LH3ZZ
Ø3LH4CZ
Ø3LH4ZZ
Ø3LJØCZ
Ø3LJØZZ
Ø3LJ3CZ
Ø3LJ3ZZ
Ø3LJ4CZ
Ø3LJ4ZZ
Ø3LMØCZ
Ø3LMØZZ
Ø3LM3CZ
Ø3LM3ZZ
Ø3LM4CZ
Ø3LM4ZZ
Ø3LNØCZ
Ø3LNØZZ
Ø3LN3CZ
Ø3LN3ZZ
Ø3LN4CZ
Ø3LN4ZZ
Ø3LRØCZ
Ø3LRØZZ
Ø3LR3CZ
Ø3LR3ZZ
Ø3LR4CZ
Ø3LR4ZZ
Ø3LSØCZ
Ø3LSØZZ
Ø3LS3CZ
Ø3LS3ZZ
Ø3LS4CZ
Ø3LS4ZZ
Ø3LTØCZ
Ø3LTØZZ
Ø3LT3CZ
Ø3LT3ZZ
Ø3LT4CZ
Ø3LT4ZZ
Ø7TØØZZ
Ø7TØ4ZZ
Ø7T1ØZZ
Ø7T14ZZ
Ø7T2ØZZ
Ø7T24ZZ
Ø8QØXZZ
Ø8Q1XZZ
Ø8TØXZZ
Ø8T1XZZ
Ø9HDØ1Z
Ø9HDØ5Z
Ø9HDØ6Z
Ø9HDØSZ
Ø9HD35Z
Ø9HD36Z
Ø9HD41Z
Ø9HD45Z
Ø9HD46Z
Ø9HD4SZ
Ø9HEØ1Z
Ø9HEØ5Z
Ø9HEØ6Z
Ø9HEØSZ
Ø9HE35Z
Ø9HE36Z
Ø9HE41Z
Ø9HE45Z
Ø9HE46Z
Ø9HE4SZ
ØB51ØZZ
ØB513ZZ
ØB514ZZ
ØB517ZZ
ØB518ZZ
ØBW1ØFZ
ØBW14FZ
ØCBSØZZ
ØCBS4ZZ
ØCT2ØZZ
ØCT2XZZ
ØCT7ØZZ
ØCT7XZZ
ØHR1X73
ØHR1X74
ØHR4X73
ØHR4XJZ
ØJR1Ø7Z
ØJR1ØKZ
ØJX4ØZB
ØJX4ØZC
ØJX5ØZB
ØJX5ØZC
ØNBTØZZ
ØNBT4ZZ
ØNBVØZZ
ØNBV4ZZ
ØNNPØZZ
ØNNP3ZZ
ØNNP4ZZ
ØNNQØZZ
ØNNQ3ZZ
ØNNQ4ZZ
ØNRTØ7Z
ØNRTØJZ
ØNRTØKZ
ØNRT37Z
ØNRT3JZ
ØNRT3KZ
ØNRT47Z
ØNRT4JZ
ØNRT4KZ
ØNRVØ7Z
ØNRVØJZ
ØNRVØKZ
ØNRV37Z
ØNRV3JZ
ØNRV3KZ
ØNRV47Z
ØNRV4JZ
ØNRV4KZ
ØNS1Ø4Z
ØNS1ØZZ
ØNS134Z
ØNS13ZZ
ØNS144Z
ØNS14ZZ
ØNS7Ø4Z
ØNS7ØZZ
ØNS734Z
ØNS73ZZ
ØNS744Z
ØNS74ZZ
ØNSBØ4Z
ØNSBØZZ
ØNSCØ4Z
ØNSCØZZ
ØNSFØ4Z
ØNSFØZZ
ØNSGØ4Z
ØNSGØZZ
ØNSHØ4Z
ØNSHØZZ
ØNSJØ4Z
ØNSJØZZ
ØNSKØ4Z
ØNSKØZZ
ØNSLØ4Z
ØNSLØZZ
ØNSMØ4Z
ØNSNØ4Z
ØNSPØ4Z
ØNSPØZZ
ØNSQØ4Z
ØNSQØZZ
ØNSRØ4Z
ØNSRØZZ
ØNSTØ4Z
ØNSVØ4Z
ØNTTØZZ
ØNTVØZZ
ØRBDØZZ
ØRBD3ZZ
ØRBD4ZZ
ØRRCØ7Z
ØRRCØJZ
ØRRCØKZ
ØRRDØ7Z
ØRRDØJZ
ØRRDØKZ
ØRSCØ4Z
ØRSCØZZ
ØRSDØ4Z
ØRSDØZZ
ØRTCØZZ
ØRTDØZZ
ØW91ØØZ
ØW91ØZZ
ØWC1ØZZ
ØWC13ZZ
ØWC14ZZ

DRG 141

Select operating room procedures listed under DRG 140

DRG 142

Select operating room procedures listed under DRG 140

DRG 143

Operating Room Procedures

ØØ8FØZZ
ØØ8F3ZZ
ØØ8F4ZZ
ØØ8GØZZ
ØØ8G3ZZ
ØØ8G4ZZ
ØØ8HØZZ
ØØ8H3ZZ
ØØ8H4ZZ
ØØ8JØZZ
ØØ8J3ZZ
ØØ8J4ZZ
ØØ8KØZZ
ØØ8K3ZZ
ØØ8K4ZZ
ØØ8LØZZ
ØØ8L3ZZ
ØØ8L4ZZ
ØØ8MØZZ
ØØ8M3ZZ
ØØ8M4ZZ
ØØ8NØZZ
ØØ8N3ZZ
ØØ8N4ZZ
ØØ8PØZZ
ØØ8P3ZZ
ØØ8P4ZZ
ØØ8QØZZ
ØØ8Q3ZZ
ØØ8Q4ZZ
ØØ8RØZZ
ØØ8R3ZZ
ØØ8R4ZZ
ØØ8SØZZ
ØØ8S3ZZ
ØØ8S4ZZ
ØØ9FØZX
ØØ9GØZX
ØØ9HØZX
ØØ9JØZX
ØØ9KØZX
ØØ9LØZX
ØØ9MØZX
ØØ9NØZX
ØØ9PØZX
ØØ9QØZX
ØØ9RØZX
ØØ9SØZX
ØØBFØZX
ØØBFØZZ
ØØBF3ZZ
ØØBF4ZZ
ØØBGØZX
ØØBGØZZ
ØØBG3ZZ
ØØBG4ZZ
ØØBHØZX
ØØBHØZZ
ØØBH3ZZ
ØØBH4ZZ
ØØBJØZX
ØØBJØZZ
ØØBJ3ZZ
ØØBJ4ZZ
ØØBKØZX
ØØBKØZZ
ØØBK3ZZ
ØØBK4ZZ
ØØBLØZX
ØØBLØZZ
ØØBL3ZZ
ØØBL4ZZ
ØØBMØZX
ØØBMØZZ
ØØBM3ZZ
ØØBM4ZZ
ØØBNØZX
ØØBNØZZ
ØØBN3ZZ
ØØBN4ZZ
ØØBPØZX
ØØBPØZZ
ØØBP3ZZ
ØØBP4ZZ
ØØBQØZX
ØØBQØZZ
ØØBQ3ZZ
ØØBQ4ZZ
ØØBRØZX
ØØBRØZZ
ØØBR3ZZ
ØØBR4ZZ
ØØBSØZX
ØØBSØZZ
ØØBS3ZZ
ØØBS4ZZ
ØØDFØZZ
ØØDF3ZZ
ØØDF4ZZ
ØØDGØZZ
ØØDG3ZZ
ØØDG4ZZ
ØØDHØZZ
ØØDH3ZZ
ØØDH4ZZ
ØØDJØZZ
ØØDJ3ZZ
ØØDJ4ZZ
ØØDKØZZ
ØØDK3ZZ
ØØDK4ZZ
ØØDLØZZ
ØØDL3ZZ
ØØDL4ZZ
ØØDMØZZ
ØØDM3ZZ
ØØDM4ZZ
ØØDNØZZ
ØØDN3ZZ
ØØDN4ZZ
ØØDPØZZ
ØØDP3ZZ
ØØDP4ZZ
ØØDQØZZ
ØØDQ3ZZ
ØØDQ4ZZ
ØØDRØZZ
ØØDR3ZZ
ØØDR4ZZ
ØØDSØZZ
ØØDS3ZZ
ØØDS4ZZ
ØØHEØMZ
ØØHE3MZ
ØØHE4MZ
ØØNFØZZ
ØØNF3ZZ
ØØNF4ZZ
ØØNGØZZ
ØØNG3ZZ
ØØNG4ZZ
ØØNHØZZ
ØØNH3ZZ
ØØNH4ZZ
ØØNJØZZ
ØØNJ3ZZ
ØØNJ4ZZ
ØØNKØZZ
ØØNK3ZZ
ØØNK4ZZ
ØØNLØZZ
ØØNL3ZZ
ØØNL4ZZ
ØØNMØZZ
ØØNM3ZZ
ØØNM4ZZ
ØØNNØZZ
ØØNN3ZZ
ØØNN4ZZ
ØØNPØZZ
ØØNP3ZZ
ØØNP4ZZ
ØØNQØZZ
ØØNQ3ZZ
ØØNQ4ZZ
ØØNRØZZ
ØØNR3ZZ
ØØNR4ZZ
ØØNSØZZ
ØØNS3ZZ
ØØNS4ZZ
ØØPEØMZ
ØØPE3MZ
ØØPE4MZ
ØØQFØZZ
ØØQF3ZZ
ØØQF4ZZ
ØØQGØZZ
ØØQG3ZZ
ØØQG4ZZ
ØØQHØZZ
ØØQH3ZZ
ØØQH4ZZ
ØØQJØZZ
ØØQJ3ZZ
ØØQJ4ZZ
ØØQKØZZ
ØØQK3ZZ
ØØQK4ZZ
ØØQLØZZ
ØØQL3ZZ
ØØQL4ZZ
ØØQMØZZ
ØØQM3ZZ
ØØQM4ZZ
ØØQNØZZ
ØØQN3ZZ
ØØQN4ZZ
ØØQPØZZ
ØØQP3ZZ
ØØQP4ZZ
ØØQQØZZ
ØØQQ3ZZ
ØØQQ4ZZ
ØØQRØZZ
ØØQR3ZZ
ØØQR4ZZ
ØØQSØZZ
ØØQS3ZZ
ØØQS4ZZ
ØØRFØ7Z
ØØRFØJZ
ØØRFØKZ
ØØRF47Z
ØØRF4JZ
ØØRF4KZ
ØØRGØ7Z
ØØRGØJZ
ØØRGØKZ
ØØRG47Z
ØØRG4JZ
ØØRG4KZ
ØØRHØ7Z
ØØRHØJZ
ØØRHØKZ
ØØRH47Z
ØØRH4JZ
ØØRH4KZ
ØØRJØ7Z
ØØRJØJZ
ØØRJØKZ
ØØRJ47Z
ØØRJ4JZ
ØØRJ4KZ
ØØRKØ7Z
ØØRKØJZ
ØØRKØKZ
ØØRK47Z
ØØRK4JZ
ØØRK4KZ
ØØRLØ7Z
ØØRLØJZ
ØØRLØKZ
ØØRL47Z
ØØRL4JZ
ØØRL4KZ
ØØRMØ7Z
ØØRMØJZ
ØØRMØKZ
ØØRM47Z
ØØRM4JZ
ØØRM4KZ
ØØRNØ7Z
ØØRNØJZ
ØØRNØKZ
ØØRN47Z
ØØRN4JZ
ØØRN4KZ
ØØRPØ7Z
ØØRPØJZ
ØØRPØKZ
ØØRP47Z
ØØRP4JZ
ØØRP4KZ
ØØRQØ7Z
ØØRQØJZ
ØØRQØKZ
ØØRQ47Z
ØØRQ4JZ
ØØRQ4KZ
ØØRRØ7Z
ØØRRØJZ
ØØRRØKZ
ØØRR47Z
ØØRR4JZ
ØØRR4KZ
ØØRSØ7Z
ØØRSØJZ
ØØRSØKZ
ØØRS47Z
ØØRS4JZ
ØØRS4KZ
ØØUFØJZ
ØØUFØKZ
ØØUF3JZ
ØØUF3KZ
ØØUF4JZ
ØØUF4KZ
ØØUGØJZ
ØØUGØKZ
ØØUG3JZ
ØØUG3KZ
ØØUG4JZ
ØØUG4KZ
ØØUHØJZ
ØØUHØKZ
ØØUH3JZ
ØØUH3KZ
ØØUH4JZ
ØØUH4KZ
ØØUJØJZ
ØØUJØKZ
ØØUJ3JZ
ØØUJ3KZ
ØØUJ4JZ
ØØUJ4KZ
ØØUKØJZ
ØØUKØKZ
ØØUK3JZ
ØØUK3KZ
ØØUK4JZ
ØØUK4KZ
ØØULØJZ
ØØULØKZ
ØØUL3JZ
ØØUL3KZ
ØØUL4JZ
ØØUL4KZ
ØØUMØJZ
ØØUMØKZ
ØØUM3JZ
ØØUM3KZ
ØØUM4JZ
ØØUM4KZ
ØØUNØJZ
ØØUNØKZ
ØØUN3JZ
ØØUN3KZ
ØØUN4JZ
ØØUN4KZ
ØØUPØJZ
ØØUPØKZ
ØØUP3JZ
ØØUP3KZ
ØØUP4JZ
ØØUP4KZ
ØØUQØJZ
ØØUQØKZ
ØØUQ3JZ
ØØUQ3KZ
ØØUQ4JZ
ØØUQ4KZ
ØØURØJZ
ØØURØKZ
ØØUR3JZ
ØØUR3KZ
ØØUR4JZ
ØØUR4KZ
ØØUSØJZ
ØØUSØKZ
ØØUS3JZ
ØØUS3KZ
ØØUS4JZ
ØØUS4KZ
ØØXRØZM
ØØXRØZS
ØØXR4ZM
ØØXR4ZS
ØØXSØZM
ØØXS4ZM
Ø15KØZZ
Ø15K3ZZ
Ø15K4ZZ
Ø1BKØZZ
Ø1BK3ZZ
Ø1BK4ZZ
Ø1DKØZZ
Ø1DK3ZZ
Ø1DK4ZZ
Ø1HYØMZ
Ø1HY3MZ
Ø1HY4MZ
Ø1PYØMZ
Ø1PY3MZ
Ø1PY4MZ
Ø2JA4ZZ
Ø2JY4ZZ
Ø39SØZX
Ø39S4ZX
Ø39TØZX
Ø39T4ZX
Ø3BHØZZ
Ø3BH3ZZ
Ø3BH4ZZ
Ø3BJØZZ
Ø3BJ3ZZ
Ø3BJ4ZZ
Ø3BKØZZ
Ø3BK3ZZ
Ø3BK4ZZ
Ø3BLØZZ
Ø3BL3ZZ
Ø3BL4ZZ
Ø3BMØZZ
Ø3BM3ZZ
Ø3BM4ZZ
Ø3BNØZZ
Ø3BN3ZZ
Ø3BN4ZZ
Ø3BPØZZ
Ø3BP3ZZ
Ø3BP4ZZ
Ø3BQØZZ
Ø3BQ3ZZ
Ø3BQ4ZZ
Ø3BRØZZ
Ø3BR3ZZ
Ø3BR4ZZ
Ø3BSØZX
Ø3BSØZZ
Ø3BS3ZX
Ø3BS3ZZ
Ø3BS4ZX
Ø3BS4ZZ
Ø3BTØZX
Ø3BTØZZ
Ø3BT3ZX
Ø3BT3ZZ
Ø3BT4ZX
Ø3BT4ZZ
Ø3BUØZZ
Ø3BU3ZZ
Ø3BU4ZZ
Ø3BVØZZ
Ø3BV3ZZ
Ø3BV4ZZ
Ø3CHØZZ
Ø3CJØZZ
Ø3CKØZZ
Ø3CLØZZ
Ø3CMØZZ
Ø3CNØZZ
Ø3CPØZZ
Ø3CQØZZ
Ø3CRØZZ
Ø3CSØZZ
Ø3CTØZZ
Ø3CUØZZ
Ø3CVØZZ
Ø3H2ØDZ
Ø3H23DZ
Ø3H24DZ
Ø3HJØDZ
Ø3HJ3DZ

Ø3HJ4DZ
Ø3HKØDZ
Ø3HK3DZ
Ø3HK4DZ
Ø3HMØDZ
Ø3HM3DZ
Ø3HM4DZ
Ø3HNØDZ
Ø3HN3DZ
Ø3HN4DZ
Ø3HPØDZ
Ø3HP3DZ
Ø3HP4DZ
Ø3HQØDZ
Ø3HQ3DZ
Ø3HQ4DZ
Ø3HRØDZ
Ø3HR3DZ
Ø3HR4DZ
Ø3HSØDZ
Ø3HS3DZ
Ø3HS4DZ
Ø3HTØDZ
Ø3HT3DZ
Ø3HT4DZ
Ø3HUØDZ
Ø3HU3DZ
Ø3HU4DZ
Ø3HVØDZ
Ø3HV3DZ
Ø3HV4DZ
Ø3HYØDZ
Ø3HY3DZ
Ø3HY4DZ
Ø3LM3DZ
Ø3LN3DZ
Ø3LPØCZ
Ø3LPØZZ
Ø3LP3CZ
Ø3LP3ZZ
Ø3LP4CZ
Ø3LP4ZZ
Ø3LQØCZ
Ø3LQØZZ
Ø3LQ3CZ
Ø3LQ3ZZ
Ø3LQ4CZ
Ø3LQ4ZZ
Ø3LR3DZ
Ø5BMØZZ
Ø5BM4ZZ
Ø5BNØZZ
Ø5BN4ZZ
Ø5BPØZZ
Ø5BP4ZZ
Ø5BQØZZ
Ø5BQ4ZZ
Ø5BRØZZ
Ø5BR4ZZ
Ø5BSØZZ
Ø5BS4ZZ
Ø5BTØZZ
Ø5BT4ZZ
Ø5BVØZZ
Ø5BV4ZZ
Ø5CMØZZ
Ø5CM3ZZ
Ø5CM4ZZ
Ø5CNØZZ
Ø5CN3ZZ
Ø5CN4ZZ
Ø5CPØZZ
Ø5CP3ZZ
Ø5CP4ZZ
Ø5CQØZZ
Ø5CQ3ZZ
Ø5CQ4ZZ
Ø5CRØZZ
Ø5CR3ZZ
Ø5CR4ZZ
Ø5CSØZZ
Ø5CS3ZZ
Ø5CS4ZZ
Ø5CTØZZ
Ø5CT3ZZ
Ø5CT4ZZ
Ø5CVØZZ
Ø5CV3ZZ
Ø5CV4ZZ
Ø5HØØMZ
Ø5HØ3MZ
Ø5HØ4MZ
Ø5H3ØMZ
Ø5H33MZ
Ø5H34MZ
Ø5H4ØMZ
Ø5H43MZ
Ø5H44MZ
Ø5HMØDZ
Ø5HM3DZ
Ø5HM4DZ
Ø5HNØDZ
Ø5HN3DZ
Ø5HN4DZ
Ø5HPØDZ
Ø5HP3DZ
Ø5HP4DZ
Ø5HQØDZ
Ø5HQ3DZ
Ø5HQ4DZ
Ø5HRØDZ
Ø5HR3DZ
Ø5HR4DZ
Ø5HSØDZ
Ø5HS3DZ
Ø5HS4DZ
Ø5HTØDZ
Ø5HT3DZ
Ø5HT4DZ
Ø5HVØDZ
Ø5HV3DZ
Ø5HV4DZ
Ø5HYØ2Z
Ø5HYØDZ
Ø5HYØYZ
Ø5HY3DZ
Ø5HY42Z
Ø5HY4DZ
Ø5LMØCZ
Ø5LMØDZ
Ø5LMØZZ
Ø5LM3CZ
Ø5LM3DZ
Ø5LM3ZZ
Ø5LM4CZ
Ø5LM4DZ
Ø5LM4ZZ
Ø5LNØCZ
Ø5LNØDZ
Ø5LNØZZ
Ø5LN3CZ
Ø5LN3DZ
Ø5LN3ZZ
Ø5LN4CZ
Ø5LN4DZ
Ø5LN4ZZ
Ø5LPØCZ
Ø5LPØDZ
Ø5LPØZZ
Ø5LP3CZ
Ø5LP3DZ
Ø5LP3ZZ
Ø5LP4CZ
Ø5LP4DZ
Ø5LP4ZZ
Ø5LQØCZ
Ø5LQØDZ
Ø5LQØZZ
Ø5LQ3CZ
Ø5LQ3DZ
Ø5LQ3ZZ
Ø5LQ4CZ
Ø5LQ4DZ
Ø5LQ4ZZ
Ø5LRØCZ
Ø5LRØDZ
Ø5LRØZZ
Ø5LR3CZ
Ø5LR3DZ
Ø5LR3ZZ
Ø5LR4CZ
Ø5LR4DZ
Ø5LR4ZZ
Ø5LSØCZ
Ø5LSØDZ
Ø5LSØZZ
Ø5LS3CZ
Ø5LS3DZ
Ø5LS3ZZ
Ø5LS4CZ
Ø5LS4DZ
Ø5LS4ZZ
Ø5LTØCZ
Ø5LTØDZ
Ø5LTØZZ
Ø5LT3CZ
Ø5LT3DZ
Ø5LT3ZZ
Ø5LT4CZ
Ø5LT4DZ
Ø5LT4ZZ
Ø5LVØCZ
Ø5LVØDZ
Ø5LVØZZ
Ø5LV3CZ
Ø5LV3DZ
Ø5LV3ZZ
Ø5LV4CZ
Ø5LV4DZ
Ø5LV4ZZ
Ø5PØØMZ
Ø5PØ3MZ
Ø5PØ4MZ
Ø5PØXMZ
Ø5P3ØMZ
Ø5P33MZ
Ø5P34MZ
Ø5P3XMZ
Ø5P4ØMZ
Ø5P43MZ
Ø5P44MZ
Ø5P4XMZ
Ø693ØØZ
Ø693ØZZ
Ø6934ØZ
Ø6934ZZ
Ø6C3ØZZ
Ø6C33ZZ
Ø6C34ZZ
Ø6H3ØDZ
Ø6H33DZ
Ø6H34DZ
Ø6HYØDZ
Ø6HY3DZ
Ø6HY4DZ
Ø79ØØZX
Ø79Ø3ZX
Ø79Ø4ZX
Ø791ØZX
Ø7913ZX
Ø7914ZX
Ø792ØZX
Ø7923ZX
Ø7924ZX
Ø7BØØZX
Ø7BØØZZ
Ø7BØ3ZX
Ø7BØ4ZX
Ø7BØ4ZZ
Ø7B1ØZX
Ø7B1ØZZ
Ø7B13ZX
Ø7B13ZZ
Ø7B14ZX
Ø7B14ZZ
Ø7B2ØZX
Ø7B2ØZZ
Ø7B23ZX
Ø7B23ZZ
Ø7B24ZX
Ø7B24ZZ
Ø7B5ØZZ
Ø7B53ZZ
Ø7B54ZZ
Ø7B6ØZZ
Ø7B63ZZ
Ø7B64ZZ
Ø7T3ØZZ
Ø7T34ZZ
Ø7T4ØZZ
Ø7T44ZZ
Ø7T7ØZZ
Ø7T74ZZ
Ø7T8ØZZ
Ø7T84ZZ
Ø7T9ØZZ
Ø7T94ZZ
Ø7TBØZZ
Ø7TB4ZZ
Ø7TFØZZ
Ø7TF4ZZ
Ø7TGØZZ
Ø7TG4ZZ
Ø81XØJ3
Ø81XØK3
Ø81XØZ3
Ø81X3J3
Ø81X3K3
Ø81X3Z3
Ø81YØJ3
Ø81YØK3
Ø81YØZ3
Ø81Y3J3
Ø81Y3K3
Ø81Y3Z3
Ø87XØDZ
Ø87XØZZ
Ø87X3DZ
Ø87X3ZZ
Ø87X7DZ
Ø87X7ZZ
Ø87X8DZ
Ø87X8ZZ
Ø87YØDZ
Ø87YØZZ
Ø87Y3DZ
Ø87Y3ZZ
Ø87Y7DZ
Ø87Y7ZZ
Ø87Y8DZ
Ø87Y8ZZ
Ø89XØZX
Ø89X3ZX
Ø89X7ZX
Ø89X8ZX
Ø89YØZX
Ø89Y3ZX
Ø89Y7ZX
Ø89Y8ZX
Ø8BXØZX
Ø8BX3ZX
Ø8BX7ZX
Ø8BX8ZX
Ø8BYØZX
Ø8BY3ZX
Ø8BY7ZX
Ø8BY8ZX
Ø8NXØZZ
Ø8NX3ZZ
Ø8NX7ZZ
Ø8NX8ZZ
Ø8NYØZZ
Ø8NY3ZZ
Ø8NY7ZZ
Ø8NY8ZZ
Ø8SXØZZ
Ø8SX3ZZ
Ø8SX7ZZ
Ø8SX8ZZ
Ø8SYØZZ
Ø8SY3ZZ
Ø8SY7ZZ
Ø8SY8ZZ
Ø8TXØZZ
Ø8TX3ZZ
Ø8TX7ZZ
Ø8TX8ZZ
Ø8TYØZZ
Ø8TY3ZZ
Ø8TY7ZZ
Ø8TY8ZZ
Ø8VXØCZ
Ø8VXØDZ
Ø8VXØZZ
Ø8VX3CZ
Ø8VX3DZ
Ø8VX3ZZ
Ø8VX7DZ
Ø8VX7ZZ
Ø8VX8DZ
Ø8VX8ZZ
Ø8VYØCZ
Ø8VYØDZ
Ø8VYØZZ
Ø8VY3CZ
Ø8VY3DZ
Ø8VY3ZZ
Ø8VY7DZ
Ø8VY7ZZ
Ø8VY8DZ
Ø8VY8ZZ
Ø9ØØØ7Z
Ø9ØØØJZ
Ø9ØØØKZ
Ø9ØØØZZ
Ø9ØØ37Z
Ø9ØØ3JZ
Ø9ØØ3KZ
Ø9ØØ3ZZ
Ø9ØØ47Z
Ø9ØØ4JZ
Ø9ØØ4KZ
Ø9ØØ4ZZ
Ø9ØØX7Z
Ø9ØØXJZ
Ø9ØØXKZ
Ø9ØØXZZ
Ø9Ø1Ø7Z
Ø9Ø1ØJZ
Ø9Ø1ØKZ
Ø9Ø1ØZZ
Ø9Ø137Z
Ø9Ø13JZ
Ø9Ø13KZ
Ø9Ø13ZZ
Ø9Ø147Z
Ø9Ø14JZ
Ø9Ø14KZ
Ø9Ø14ZZ
Ø9Ø1X7Z
Ø9Ø1XJZ
Ø9Ø1XKZ
Ø9Ø1XZZ
Ø9Ø2Ø7Z
Ø9Ø2ØJZ
Ø9Ø2ØKZ
Ø9Ø2ØZZ
Ø9Ø237Z
Ø9Ø23JZ
Ø9Ø23KZ
Ø9Ø23ZZ
Ø9Ø247Z
Ø9Ø24JZ
Ø9Ø24KZ
Ø9Ø24ZZ
Ø9Ø2X7Z
Ø9Ø2XJZ
Ø9Ø2XKZ
Ø9Ø2XZZ
Ø9ØKØ7Z
Ø9ØKØJZ
Ø9ØKØKZ
Ø9ØKØZZ
Ø9ØK37Z
Ø9ØK3JZ
Ø9ØK3KZ
Ø9ØK3ZZ
Ø9ØK47Z
Ø9ØK4JZ
Ø9ØK4KZ
Ø9ØK4ZZ
Ø9ØKX7Z
Ø9ØKXJZ
Ø9ØKXKZ
Ø9ØKXZZ
Ø91DØ7Ø
Ø91DØJØ
Ø91DØKØ
Ø91DØZØ
Ø91EØ7Ø
Ø91EØJØ
Ø91EØKØ
Ø91EØZØ
Ø955ØZZ
Ø9558ZZ
Ø956ØZZ
Ø9568ZZ
Ø957ØZZ
Ø9573ZZ
Ø9574ZZ
Ø9577ZZ
Ø9578ZZ
Ø958ØZZ
Ø9583ZZ
Ø9584ZZ
Ø9587ZZ
Ø9588ZZ
Ø959ØZZ
Ø9598ZZ
Ø95AØZZ
Ø95A8ZZ
Ø95DØZZ
Ø95D8ZZ
Ø95EØZZ
Ø95E8ZZ
Ø95LØZZ
Ø95L3ZZ
Ø95L4ZZ
Ø95L7ZZ
Ø95L8ZZ
Ø95NØZZ
Ø95N3ZZ
Ø95N4ZZ
Ø95N7ZZ
Ø95N8ZZ
Ø98LØZZ
Ø98L3ZZ
Ø98L4ZZ
Ø98L7ZZ
Ø98L8ZZ
Ø995ØØZ
Ø995ØZX
Ø9957ØZ
Ø996ØØZ
Ø996ØZX
Ø9967ØZ
Ø997ØØZ
Ø997ØZX
Ø9973ØZ
Ø9973ZX
Ø9974ØZ
Ø9974ZX
Ø9977ØZ
Ø9978ØZ
Ø998ØØZ
Ø998ØZX
Ø9983ØZ
Ø9983ZX
Ø9984ØZ
Ø9984ZX
Ø9987ØZ
Ø9988ØZ
Ø999ØØZ
Ø999ØZX
Ø999ØZZ
Ø99AØØZ
Ø99AØZX
Ø99AØZZ
Ø99BØZX
Ø99B3ZX
Ø99B4ZX
Ø99CØZX
Ø99C3ZX
Ø99C4ZX
Ø99DØØZ
Ø99DØZX
Ø99DØZZ
Ø99EØØZ
Ø99EØZX
Ø99EØZZ
Ø99FØZX
Ø99F3ZX
Ø99F4ZX
Ø99GØZX
Ø99G3ZX
Ø99G4ZX
Ø99NØØZ
Ø99NØZZ
Ø99N4ØZ
Ø99N4ZZ
Ø99N7ØZ
Ø99N7ZZ
Ø99N8ØZ
Ø99N8ZZ
Ø9B5ØZX
Ø9B5ØZZ
Ø9B58ZX
Ø9B58ZZ
Ø9B6ØZX
Ø9B6ØZZ
Ø9B68ZX
Ø9B68ZZ
Ø9B7ØZX
Ø9B7ØZZ
Ø9B73ZX
Ø9B73ZZ
Ø9B74ZX
Ø9B74ZZ
Ø9B77ZX
Ø9B77ZZ
Ø9B78ZX
Ø9B78ZZ
Ø9B8ØZX
Ø9B8ØZZ
Ø9B83ZX
Ø9B83ZZ
Ø9B84ZX
Ø9B84ZZ
Ø9B87ZX
Ø9B87ZZ
Ø9B88ZX
Ø9B88ZZ
Ø9B9ØZX
Ø9B9ØZZ
Ø9B98ZX
Ø9B98ZZ
Ø9BAØZX
Ø9BAØZZ
Ø9BA8ZX
Ø9BA8ZZ
Ø9BBØZX
Ø9BB3ZX
Ø9BB4ZX
Ø9BB8ZX
Ø9BCØZX
Ø9BC3ZX
Ø9BC4ZX
Ø9BC8ZX
Ø9BDØZX
Ø9BDØZZ
Ø9BD8ZX
Ø9BD8ZZ
Ø9BEØZX
Ø9BEØZZ
Ø9BE8ZX
Ø9BE8ZZ
Ø9BLØZZ
Ø9BL3ZZ
Ø9BL4ZZ
Ø9BL7ZZ
Ø9BL8ZZ
Ø9BMØZZ
Ø9BM3ZZ
Ø9BM4ZZ
Ø9BM8ZZ
Ø9BNØZZ
Ø9BN3ZZ
Ø9BN4ZZ
Ø9BN7ZZ
Ø9BN8ZZ
Ø9C5ØZZ
Ø9C58ZZ
Ø9C6ØZZ
Ø9C68ZZ
Ø9C9ØZZ
Ø9C98ZZ
Ø9CAØZZ
Ø9CA8ZZ
Ø9CDØZZ
Ø9CD8ZZ
Ø9CEØZZ
Ø9CE8ZZ
Ø9CNØZZ
Ø9CN3ZZ
Ø9CN4ZZ
Ø9CN7ZZ
Ø9CN8ZZ
Ø9D7ØZZ
Ø9D73ZZ
Ø9D74ZZ
Ø9D77ZZ
Ø9D78ZZ
Ø9D8ØZZ
Ø9D83ZZ
Ø9D84ZZ
Ø9D87ZZ
Ø9D88ZZ
Ø9D9ØZZ
Ø9DAØZZ
Ø9DLØZZ
Ø9DL3ZZ
Ø9DL4ZZ
Ø9DL7ZZ
Ø9DL8ZZ
Ø9DMØZZ
Ø9DM3ZZ
Ø9DM4ZZ
Ø9HDØ4Z
Ø9HD31Z
Ø9HD34Z
Ø9HD3SZ
Ø9HD44Z
Ø9HEØ4Z
Ø9HE31Z
Ø9HE34Z
Ø9HE3SZ
Ø9HE44Z
Ø9HHØYZ
Ø9HJØYZ
Ø9J7ØZZ
Ø9J74ZZ
Ø9J8ØZZ
Ø9J84ZZ
Ø9JDØZZ
Ø9JD4ZZ
Ø9JEØZZ
Ø9JE4ZZ
Ø9MØXZZ
Ø9M1XZZ
Ø9MKXZZ
Ø9NØØZZ
Ø9NØ3ZZ
Ø9NØ4ZZ
Ø9N1ØZZ
Ø9N13ZZ
Ø9N14ZZ
Ø9N3ØZZ
Ø9N33ZZ
Ø9N34ZZ
Ø9N37ZZ
Ø9N38ZZ
Ø9N4ØZZ
Ø9N43ZZ
Ø9N44ZZ
Ø9N47ZZ
Ø9N48ZZ
Ø9N5ØZZ
Ø9N58ZZ
Ø9N6ØZZ
Ø9N68ZZ
Ø9N7ØZZ
Ø9N73ZZ
Ø9N74ZZ
Ø9N77ZZ
Ø9N78ZZ
Ø9N8ØZZ
Ø9N83ZZ
Ø9N84ZZ
Ø9N87ZZ
Ø9N88ZZ
Ø9N9ØZZ
Ø9N98ZZ
Ø9NAØZZ
Ø9NA8ZZ
Ø9NBØZZ
Ø9NB3ZZ
Ø9NB4ZZ
Ø9NB8ZZ
Ø9NCØZZ
Ø9NC3ZZ
Ø9NC4ZZ
Ø9NC8ZZ
Ø9NDØZZ
Ø9ND8ZZ
Ø9NEØZZ
Ø9NE8ZZ
Ø9NNØZZ
Ø9NN3ZZ
Ø9NN4ZZ
Ø9NN7ZZ
Ø9NN8ZZ
Ø9PDØSZ
Ø9PD7SZ
Ø9PD8SZ
Ø9PEØSZ
Ø9PE7SZ
Ø9PE8SZ
Ø9PHØØZ
Ø9PHØ7Z
Ø9PHØDZ
Ø9PHØJZ
Ø9PHØKZ
Ø9PHØYZ
Ø9PH37Z
Ø9PH3DZ
Ø9PH47Z
Ø9PH4DZ
Ø9PH77Z
Ø9PH7JZ
Ø9PH7KZ
Ø9PH87Z
Ø9PH8JZ
Ø9PH8KZ
Ø9PJØØZ
Ø9PJØ7Z
Ø9PJØDZ
Ø9PJØJZ
Ø9PJØKZ
Ø9PJØYZ
Ø9PJ37Z
Ø9PJ3DZ
Ø9PJ47Z
Ø9PJ4DZ
Ø9PJ77Z
Ø9PJ7JZ
Ø9PJ7KZ
Ø9PJ87Z
Ø9PJ8JZ
Ø9PJ8KZ
Ø9QØØZZ
Ø9QØ3ZZ
Ø9QØ4ZZ
Ø9Q1ØZZ
Ø9Q13ZZ
Ø9Q14ZZ
Ø9Q2ØZZ
Ø9Q23ZZ
Ø9Q24ZZ
Ø9Q3ØZZ
Ø9Q33ZZ
Ø9Q34ZZ
Ø9Q37ZZ
Ø9Q38ZZ
Ø9Q4ØZZ
Ø9Q43ZZ
Ø9Q44ZZ
Ø9Q47ZZ
Ø9Q48ZZ
Ø9Q5ØZZ
Ø9Q58ZZ
Ø9Q6ØZZ
Ø9Q68ZZ
Ø9Q7ØZZ
Ø9Q73ZZ
Ø9Q74ZZ
Ø9Q77ZZ
Ø9Q78ZZ
Ø9Q8ØZZ
Ø9Q83ZZ
Ø9Q84ZZ
Ø9Q87ZZ
Ø9Q88ZZ
Ø9Q9ØZZ
Ø9Q98ZZ
Ø9QAØZZ
Ø9QA8ZZ
Ø9QDØZZ
Ø9QD8ZZ
Ø9QEØZZ
Ø9QE8ZZ
Ø9QKØZZ
Ø9QK3ZZ
Ø9QK4ZZ
Ø9QK8ZZ
Ø9QLØZZ
Ø9QL3ZZ
Ø9QL4ZZ
Ø9QL7ZZ
Ø9QL8ZZ
Ø9QMØZZ
Ø9QM3ZZ
Ø9QM4ZZ
Ø9QM8ZZ
Ø9QNØZZ
Ø9QN3ZZ
Ø9QN4ZZ
Ø9QN7ZZ
Ø9QN8ZZ
Ø9RØØ7Z
Ø9RØØJZ
Ø9RØØKZ
Ø9RØX7Z
Ø9RØXJZ
Ø9RØXKZ
Ø9R1Ø7Z
Ø9R1ØJZ
Ø9R1ØKZ
Ø9R1X7Z
Ø9R1XJZ
Ø9R1XKZ
Ø9R2Ø7Z
Ø9R2ØJZ
Ø9R2ØKZ
Ø9R2X7Z
Ø9R2XJZ
Ø9R2XKZ
Ø9R5Ø7Z
Ø9R5ØJZ
Ø9R5ØKZ
Ø9R6Ø7Z
Ø9R6ØJZ
Ø9R6ØKZ
Ø9R7Ø7Z
Ø9R7ØJZ
Ø9R7ØKZ
Ø9R777Z
Ø9R77JZ
Ø9R77KZ
Ø9R787Z
Ø9R78JZ
Ø9R78KZ
Ø9R8Ø7Z
Ø9R8ØJZ
Ø9R8ØKZ
Ø9R877Z
Ø9R87JZ
Ø9R87KZ
Ø9R887Z
Ø9R88JZ
Ø9R88KZ
Ø9R9Ø7Z
Ø9R9ØJZ
Ø9R9ØKZ
Ø9RAØ7Z
Ø9RAØJZ
Ø9RAØKZ
Ø9RDØ7Z
Ø9RDØJZ
Ø9RDØKZ
Ø9REØ7Z
Ø9REØJZ
Ø9REØKZ
Ø9RKØ7Z
Ø9RKØJZ
Ø9RKØKZ

Ø9RKX7Z
Ø9RKXJZ
Ø9RKXKZ
Ø9RLØ7Z
Ø9RLØJZ
Ø9RLØKZ
Ø9RL37Z
Ø9RL3JZ
Ø9RL3KZ
Ø9RL47Z
Ø9RL4JZ
Ø9RL4KZ
Ø9RL77Z
Ø9RL7JZ
Ø9RL7KZ
Ø9RL87Z
Ø9RL8JZ
Ø9RL8KZ
Ø9RMØ7Z
Ø9RMØJZ
Ø9RMØKZ
Ø9RM37Z
Ø9RM3JZ
Ø9RM3KZ
Ø9RM47Z
Ø9RM4JZ
Ø9RM4KZ
Ø9RNØ7Z
Ø9RNØJZ
Ø9RNØKZ
Ø9RN77Z
Ø9RN7JZ
Ø9RN7KZ
Ø9RN87Z
Ø9RN8JZ
Ø9RN8KZ
Ø9SØØZZ
Ø9SØ4ZZ
Ø9SØXZZ
Ø9S1ØZZ
Ø9S14ZZ
Ø9S1XZZ
Ø9S2ØZZ
Ø9S24ZZ
Ø9S2XZZ
Ø9S7ØZZ
Ø9S74ZZ
Ø9S77ZZ
Ø9S78ZZ
Ø9S8ØZZ
Ø9S84ZZ
Ø9S87ZZ
Ø9S88ZZ
Ø9S9ØZZ
Ø9S94ZZ
Ø9SAØZZ
Ø9SA4ZZ
Ø9SKØZZ
Ø9SK4ZZ
Ø9SKXZZ
Ø9SLØZZ
Ø9SL4ZZ
Ø9SL7ZZ
Ø9SL8ZZ
Ø9SMØZZ
Ø9SM4ZZ
Ø9TØØZZ
Ø9TØ4ZZ
Ø9TØXZZ
Ø9T1ØZZ
Ø9T14ZZ
Ø9T1XZZ
Ø9T5ØZZ
Ø9T58ZZ
Ø9T6ØZZ
Ø9T68ZZ
Ø9T7ØZZ
Ø9T74ZZ
Ø9T77ZZ
Ø9T78ZZ
Ø9T8ØZZ
Ø9T84ZZ
Ø9T87ZZ
Ø9T88ZZ
Ø9T9ØZZ
Ø9T98ZZ
Ø9TAØZZ
Ø9TA8ZZ
Ø9TDØZZ
Ø9TD8ZZ
Ø9TEØZZ
Ø9TE8ZZ
Ø9TKØZZ
Ø9TK4ZZ
Ø9TK8ZZ
Ø9TKXZZ
Ø9TLØZZ
Ø9TL4ZZ
Ø9TL7ZZ
Ø9TL8ZZ
Ø9TMØZZ
Ø9TM4ZZ
Ø9TM8ZZ
Ø9TNØZZ
Ø9TN4ZZ
Ø9TN7ZZ
Ø9TN8ZZ
Ø9UØØ7Z
Ø9UØØJZ
Ø9UØØKZ
Ø9UØX7Z
Ø9UØXJZ
Ø9UØXKZ
Ø9U1Ø7Z
Ø9U1ØJZ
Ø9U1ØKZ
Ø9U1X7Z
Ø9U1XJZ
Ø9U1XKZ
Ø9U2Ø7Z
Ø9U2ØJZ
Ø9U2ØKZ
Ø9U2X7Z
Ø9U2XJZ
Ø9U2XKZ
Ø9U5Ø7Z
Ø9U5ØJZ
Ø9U5ØKZ
Ø9U587Z
Ø9U58JZ
Ø9U58KZ
Ø9U6Ø7Z
Ø9U6ØJZ
Ø9U6ØKZ
Ø9U687Z
Ø9U68JZ
Ø9U68KZ
Ø9U7Ø7Z
Ø9U7ØJZ
Ø9U7ØKZ
Ø9U777Z
Ø9U77JZ
Ø9U77KZ
Ø9U787Z
Ø9U78JZ
Ø9U78KZ
Ø9U8Ø7Z
Ø9U8ØJZ
Ø9U8ØKZ
Ø9U877Z
Ø9U87JZ
Ø9U87KZ
Ø9U887Z
Ø9U88JZ
Ø9U88KZ
Ø9U9Ø7Z
Ø9U9ØJZ
Ø9U9ØKZ
Ø9U987Z
Ø9U98JZ
Ø9U98KZ
Ø9UAØ7Z
Ø9UAØJZ
Ø9UAØKZ
Ø9UA87Z
Ø9UA8JZ
Ø9UA8KZ
Ø9UDØ7Z
Ø9UDØJZ
Ø9UDØKZ
Ø9UD87Z
Ø9UD8JZ
Ø9UD8KZ
Ø9UEØ7Z
Ø9UEØJZ
Ø9UEØKZ
Ø9UE87Z
Ø9UE8JZ
Ø9UE8KZ
Ø9UKØ7Z
Ø9UKØJZ
Ø9UKØKZ
Ø9UK87Z
Ø9UK8JZ
Ø9UK8KZ
Ø9UKX7Z
Ø9UKXJZ
Ø9UKXKZ
Ø9ULØ7Z
Ø9ULØJZ
Ø9ULØKZ
Ø9UL37Z
Ø9UL3JZ
Ø9UL3KZ
Ø9UL47Z
Ø9UL4JZ
Ø9UL4KZ
Ø9UL77Z
Ø9UL7JZ
Ø9UL7KZ
Ø9UL87Z
Ø9UL8JZ
Ø9UL8KZ
Ø9UMØ7Z
Ø9UMØJZ
Ø9UMØKZ
Ø9UM37Z
Ø9UM3JZ
Ø9UM3KZ
Ø9UM47Z
Ø9UM4JZ
Ø9UM4KZ
Ø9UM87Z
Ø9UM8JZ
Ø9UM8KZ
Ø9UNØ7Z
Ø9UNØJZ
Ø9UNØKZ
Ø9UN77Z
Ø9UN7JZ
Ø9UN7KZ
Ø9UN87Z
Ø9UN8JZ
Ø9UN8KZ
Ø9W7Ø7Z
Ø9W7ØJZ
Ø9W7ØKZ
Ø9W777Z
Ø9W77JZ
Ø9W77KZ
Ø9W787Z
Ø9W78JZ
Ø9W78KZ
Ø9W8Ø7Z
Ø9W8ØJZ
Ø9W8ØKZ
Ø9W877Z
Ø9W87JZ
Ø9W87KZ
Ø9W887Z
Ø9W88JZ
Ø9W88KZ
Ø9W9Ø7Z
Ø9W9ØJZ
Ø9W9ØKZ
Ø9W977Z
Ø9W97JZ
Ø9W97KZ
Ø9W987Z
Ø9W98JZ
Ø9W98KZ
Ø9WAØ7Z
Ø9WAØJZ
Ø9WAØKZ
Ø9WA77Z
Ø9WA7JZ
Ø9WA7KZ
Ø9WA87Z
Ø9WA8JZ
Ø9WA8KZ
Ø9WDØSZ
Ø9WD7SZ
Ø9WD8SZ
Ø9WEØSZ
Ø9WE7SZ
Ø9WE8SZ
Ø9WHØØZ
Ø9WHØ7Z
Ø9WHØDZ
Ø9WHØJZ
Ø9WHØKZ
Ø9WHØYZ
Ø9WH3ØZ
Ø9WH37Z
Ø9WH3DZ
Ø9WH4ØZ
Ø9WH47Z
Ø9WH4DZ
Ø9WH7ØZ
Ø9WH77Z
Ø9WH7JZ
Ø9WH7KZ
Ø9WH8ØZ
Ø9WH87Z
Ø9WH8JZ
Ø9WH8KZ
Ø9WJØØZ
Ø9WJØ7Z
Ø9WJØDZ
Ø9WJØJZ
Ø9WJØKZ
Ø9WJØYZ
Ø9WJ3ØZ
Ø9WJ37Z
Ø9WJ3DZ
Ø9WJ4ØZ
Ø9WJ47Z
Ø9WJ4DZ
Ø9WJ7ØZ
Ø9WJ77Z
Ø9WJ7JZ
Ø9WJ7KZ
Ø9WJ8ØZ
Ø9WJ87Z
Ø9WJ8JZ
Ø9WJ8KZ
ØB52ØZZ
ØB523ZZ
ØB524ZZ
ØB527ZZ
ØB528ZZ
ØB71ØDZ
ØB71ØZZ
ØB713DZ
ØB713ZZ
ØB714DZ
ØB714ZZ
ØB717DZ
ØB717ZZ
ØB718DZ
ØB718ZZ
ØB72ØDZ
ØB72ØZZ
ØB723DZ
ØB723ZZ
ØB724DZ
ØB724ZZ
ØB727DZ
ØB727ZZ
ØB728DZ
ØB728ZZ
ØB91ØZX
ØB92ØZX
ØBB1ØZX
ØBB1ØZZ
ØBB13ZZ
ØBB14ZZ
ØBB17ZZ
ØBB18ZZ
ØBB2ØZX
ØBB2ØZZ
ØBB23ZZ
ØBB24ZZ
ØBB27ZZ
ØBB28ZZ
ØBF1ØZZ
ØBF13ZZ
ØBF14ZZ
ØBF17ZZ
ØBF18ZZ
ØBF2ØZZ
ØBF23ZZ
ØBF24ZZ
ØBF27ZZ
ØBF28ZZ
ØBL1ØCZ
ØBL1ØDZ
ØBL1ØZZ
ØBL13CZ
ØBL13DZ
ØBL13ZZ
ØBL14CZ
ØBL14DZ
ØBL14ZZ
ØBL17DZ
ØBL17ZZ
ØBL18DZ
ØBL18ZZ
ØBL2ØCZ
ØBL2ØDZ
ØBL2ØZZ
ØBL23CZ
ØBL23DZ
ØBL23ZZ
ØBL24CZ
ØBL24DZ
ØBL24ZZ
ØBL27DZ
ØBL27ZZ
ØBL28DZ
ØBL28ZZ
ØBM1ØZZ
ØBM2ØZZ
ØBN1ØZZ
ØBN13ZZ
ØBN14ZZ
ØBN17ZZ
ØBN18ZZ
ØBN2ØZZ
ØBN23ZZ
ØBN24ZZ
ØBN27ZZ
ØBN28ZZ
ØBQ1ØZZ
ØBQ13ZZ
ØBQ14ZZ
ØBQ17ZZ
ØBQ18ZZ
ØBQ2ØZZ
ØBQ23ZZ
ØBQ24ZZ
ØBQ27ZZ
ØBQ28ZZ
ØBR1Ø7Z
ØBR1ØJZ
ØBR1ØKZ
ØBR147Z
ØBR14JZ
ØBR14KZ
ØBR2Ø7Z
ØBR2ØJZ
ØBR2ØKZ
ØBR247Z
ØBR24JZ
ØBR24KZ
ØBS1ØZZ
ØBS2ØZZ
ØBT1ØZZ
ØBT14ZZ
ØBT2ØZZ
ØBT24ZZ
ØBU1Ø7Z
ØBU1ØJZ
ØBU1ØKZ
ØBU147Z
ØBU14JZ
ØBU14KZ
ØBU187Z
ØBU18JZ
ØBU18KZ
ØBU2Ø7Z
ØBU2ØJZ
ØBU2ØKZ
ØBU247Z
ØBU24JZ
ØBU24KZ
ØBU287Z
ØBU28JZ
ØBU28KZ
ØBV1ØCZ
ØBV1ØDZ
ØBV1ØZZ
ØBV13CZ
ØBV13DZ
ØBV13ZZ
ØBV14CZ
ØBV14DZ
ØBV14ZZ
ØBV17DZ
ØBV17ZZ
ØBV18DZ
ØBV18ZZ
ØBV2ØCZ
ØBV2ØDZ
ØBV2ØZZ
ØBV23CZ
ØBV23DZ
ØBV23ZZ
ØBV24CZ
ØBV24DZ
ØBV24ZZ
ØBV27DZ
ØBV27ZZ
ØBV28DZ
ØBV28ZZ
ØBW13FZ
ØC5MØZZ
ØC5M3ZZ
ØC5M4ZZ
ØC5M7ZZ
ØC5M8ZZ
ØC5PØZZ
ØC5P3ZZ
ØC5PXZZ
ØC5QØZZ
ØC5Q3ZZ
ØC5QXZZ
ØC5RØZZ
ØC5R3ZZ
ØC5R4ZZ
ØC5R7ZZ
ØC5R8ZZ
ØC5SØZZ
ØC5S3ZZ
ØC5S4ZZ
ØC5S7ZZ
ØC5S8ZZ
ØC5TØZZ
ØC5T3ZZ
ØC5T4ZZ
ØC5T7ZZ
ØC5T8ZZ
ØC5VØZZ
ØC5V3ZZ
ØC5V4ZZ
ØC5V7ZZ
ØC5V8ZZ
ØC7SØDZ
ØC7SØZZ
ØC7S3DZ
ØC7S3ZZ
ØC7S4DZ
ØC7S4ZZ
ØC7S7DZ
ØC7S7ZZ
ØC7S8DZ
ØC7S8ZZ
ØC9MØØZ
ØC9MØZZ
ØC9M4ØZ
ØC9M4ZZ
ØC9M7ØZ
ØC9M7ZZ
ØC9M8ØZ
ØC9M8ZZ
ØC9PØØZ
ØC9PØZX
ØC9PØZZ
ØC9P3ZX
ØC9PXØZ
ØC9PXZX
ØC9PXZZ
ØC9QØØZ
ØC9QØZX
ØC9QØZZ
ØC9Q3ZX
ØC9QXØZ
ØC9QXZX
ØC9QXZZ
ØC9RØØZ
ØC9RØZX
ØC9RØZZ
ØC9R4ØZ
ØC9R4ZZ
ØC9R7ØZ
ØC9R7ZZ
ØC9R8ØZ
ØC9R8ZZ
ØC9SØØZ
ØC9SØZX
ØC9SØZZ
ØC9S4ØZ
ØC9S4ZZ
ØC9S7ØZ
ØC9S7ZZ
ØC9S8ØZ
ØC9S8ZZ
ØC9TØØZ
ØC9TØZX
ØC9TØZZ
ØC9T4ØZ
ØC9T4ZZ
ØC9T7ØZ
ØC9T7ZZ
ØC9T8ØZ
ØC9T8ZZ
ØC9VØØZ
ØC9VØZX
ØC9VØZZ
ØC9V4ØZ
ØC9V4ZZ
ØC9V7ØZ
ØC9V7ZZ
ØC9V8ØZ
ØC9V8ZZ
ØCBMØZZ
ØCBM3ZZ
ØCBM4ZZ
ØCBM7ZZ
ØCBM8ZZ
ØCBPØZX
ØCBPØZZ
ØCBP3ZX
ØCBP3ZZ
ØCBPXZX
ØCBPXZZ
ØCBQØZX
ØCBQØZZ
ØCBQ3ZX
ØCBQ3ZZ
ØCBQXZX
ØCBQXZZ
ØCBRØZX
ØCBRØZZ
ØCBR3ZZ
ØCBR4ZZ
ØCBR7ZZ
ØCBR8ZZ
ØCBSØZX
ØCBS3ZZ
ØCBS7ZZ
ØCBS8ZZ
ØCBTØZX
ØCBTØZZ
ØCBT3ZZ
ØCBT4ZZ
ØCBT7ZZ
ØCBT8ZZ
ØCBVØZX
ØCBVØZZ
ØCBV3ZZ
ØCBV4ZZ
ØCBV7ZZ
ØCBV8ZZ
ØCCMØZZ
ØCCM3ZZ
ØCCM4ZZ
ØCCPØZZ
ØCCP3ZZ
ØCCQØZZ
ØCCQ3ZZ
ØCCRØZZ
ØCCR3ZZ
ØCCR4ZZ
ØCCR7ZZ
ØCCR8ZZ
ØCCSØZZ
ØCCS3ZZ
ØCCS4ZZ
ØCCTØZZ
ØCCT3ZZ
ØCCT4ZZ
ØCCT7ZZ
ØCCT8ZZ
ØCCVØZZ
ØCCV3ZZ
ØCCV4ZZ
ØCCV7ZZ
ØCCV8ZZ
ØCDTØZZ
ØCDT3ZZ
ØCDT4ZZ
ØCDT7ZZ
ØCDT8ZZ
ØCDVØZZ
ØCDV3ZZ
ØCDV4ZZ
ØCDV7ZZ
ØCDV8ZZ
ØCH7Ø1Z
ØCH731Z
ØCH7X1Z
ØCHAØYZ
ØCNMØZZ
ØCNM3ZZ
ØCNM4ZZ
ØCNM7ZZ
ØCNM8ZZ
ØCNPØZZ
ØCNP3ZZ
ØCNPXZZ
ØCNQØZZ
ØCNQ3ZZ
ØCNQXZZ
ØCNRØZZ
ØCNR3ZZ
ØCNR4ZZ
ØCNR7ZZ
ØCNR8ZZ
ØCNSØZZ
ØCNS3ZZ
ØCNS4ZZ
ØCNS7ZZ
ØCNS8ZZ
ØCNTØZZ
ØCNT3ZZ
ØCNT4ZZ
ØCNT7ZZ
ØCNT8ZZ
ØCNVØZZ
ØCNV3ZZ
ØCNV4ZZ
ØCNV7ZZ
ØCNV8ZZ
ØCPSØØZ
ØCPSØ7Z
ØCPSØDZ
ØCPSØJZ
ØCPSØKZ
ØCPSØYZ
ØCPS3ØZ
ØCPS37Z
ØCPS3DZ
ØCPS3JZ
ØCPS3KZ
ØCPS77Z
ØCPS7JZ
ØCPS7KZ
ØCPS87Z
ØCPS8JZ
ØCPS8KZ
ØCPY71Z
ØCPY77Z
ØCPY7JZ
ØCPY7KZ
ØCPY81Z
ØCPY87Z
ØCPY8JZ
ØCPY8KZ
ØCQ2ØZZ
ØCQ23ZZ
ØCQ2XZZ
ØCQ3ØZZ
ØCQ33ZZ
ØCQ3XZZ
ØCQMØZZ
ØCQM3ZZ
ØCQM4ZZ
ØCQM7ZZ
ØCQM8ZZ
ØCQPØZZ
ØCQP3ZZ
ØCQPXZZ
ØCQQØZZ
ØCQQ3ZZ
ØCQQXZZ
ØCQRØZZ
ØCQR3ZZ
ØCQR4ZZ
ØCQR7ZZ
ØCQR8ZZ
ØCQSØZZ
ØCQS3ZZ
ØCQS4ZZ
ØCQS7ZZ
ØCQS8ZZ
ØCQTØZZ
ØCQT3ZZ
ØCQT4ZZ
ØCQT7ZZ
ØCQT8ZZ
ØCQVØZZ
ØCQV3ZZ
ØCQV4ZZ
ØCQV7ZZ
ØCQV8ZZ
ØCR2Ø7Z
ØCR2ØJZ
ØCR2ØKZ
ØCR237Z
ØCR23JZ
ØCR23KZ
ØCR2X7Z
ØCR2XJZ
ØCR2XKZ
ØCR3Ø7Z
ØCR3ØJZ
ØCR3ØKZ
ØCR337Z
ØCR33JZ
ØCR33KZ
ØCR3X7Z
ØCR3XJZ
ØCR3XKZ
ØCRMØ7Z
ØCRMØJZ
ØCRMØKZ
ØCRM77Z
ØCRM7JZ
ØCRM7KZ
ØCRM87Z
ØCRM8JZ
ØCRM8KZ
ØCRRØ7Z
ØCRRØJZ
ØCRRØKZ
ØCRR77Z
ØCRR7JZ
ØCRR7KZ
ØCRR87Z
ØCRR8JZ
ØCRR8KZ
ØCRSØ7Z
ØCRSØJZ
ØCRSØKZ
ØCRS77Z
ØCRS7JZ
ØCRS7KZ
ØCRS87Z
ØCRS8JZ
ØCRS8KZ
ØCRTØ7Z
ØCRTØJZ
ØCRTØKZ
ØCRT77Z
ØCRT7JZ
ØCRT7KZ
ØCRT87Z
ØCRT8JZ
ØCRT8KZ
ØCRVØ7Z
ØCRVØJZ
ØCRVØKZ
ØCRV77Z
ØCRV7JZ
ØCRV7KZ
ØCRV87Z
ØCRV8JZ
ØCRV8KZ
ØCS2ØZZ
ØCS2XZZ
ØCS3ØZZ
ØCS3XZZ
ØCSRØZZ
ØCSR7ZZ
ØCSR8ZZ
ØCSSØZZ
ØCSS7ZZ
ØCSS8ZZ
ØCSTØZZ
ØCST7ZZ
ØCST8ZZ
ØCSVØZZ
ØCSV7ZZ
ØCSV8ZZ
ØCTMØZZ
ØCTM4ZZ
ØCTM7ZZ
ØCTM8ZZ
ØCTPØZZ
ØCTPXZZ
ØCTQØZZ
ØCTQXZZ
ØCTRØZZ
ØCTR4ZZ
ØCTR7ZZ
ØCTR8ZZ
ØCTTØZZ
ØCTT4ZZ
ØCTT7ZZ
ØCTT8ZZ
ØCTVØZZ
ØCTV4ZZ
ØCTV7ZZ
ØCTV8ZZ
ØCU2Ø7Z
ØCU2ØKZ
ØCU237Z
ØCU23KZ
ØCU2X7Z
ØCU2XJZ
ØCU2XKZ
ØCU3Ø7Z
ØCU3ØJZ
ØCU3ØKZ
ØCU337Z
ØCU33JZ
ØCU33KZ
ØCU3X7Z
ØCU3XJZ
ØCU3XKZ
ØCUMØ7Z
ØCUMØJZ
ØCUMØKZ
ØCUM77Z

ØCUM7JZ
ØCUM7KZ
ØCUM87Z
ØCUM8JZ
ØCUM8KZ
ØCURØ7Z
ØCURØJZ
ØCURØKZ
ØCUR77Z
ØCUR7JZ
ØCUR7KZ
ØCUR87Z
ØCUR8JZ
ØCUR8KZ
ØCUSØ7Z
ØCUSØJZ
ØCUSØKZ
ØCUS77Z
ØCUS7JZ
ØCUS7KZ
ØCUS87Z
ØCUS8JZ
ØCUS8KZ
ØCUTØ7Z
ØCUTØJZ
ØCUTØKZ
ØCUT77Z
ØCUT7JZ
ØCUT7KZ
ØCUT87Z
ØCUT8JZ
ØCUT8KZ
ØCUVØ7Z
ØCUVØJZ
ØCUVØKZ
ØCUV77Z
ØCUV7JZ
ØCUV7KZ
ØCUV87Z
ØCUV8JZ
ØCUV8KZ
ØCWSØØZ
ØCWSØ7Z
ØCWSØDZ
ØCWSØJZ
ØCWSØKZ
ØCWSØYZ
ØCWS3ØZ
ØCWS37Z
ØCWS3DZ
ØCWS3JZ
ØCWS3KZ
ØCWS7ØZ
ØCWS77Z
ØCWS7DZ
ØCWS7JZ
ØCWS7KZ
ØCWS8ØZ
ØCWS87Z
ØCWS8DZ
ØCWS8JZ
ØCWS8KZ
ØCWY7ØZ
ØCWY71Z
ØCWY77Z
ØCWY7DZ
ØCWY7JZ
ØCWY7KZ
ØCWY8ØZ
ØCWY81Z
ØCWY87Z
ØCWY8DZ
ØCWY8JZ
ØCWY8KZ
ØD84ØZZ
ØD843ZZ
ØD844ZZ
ØD847ZZ
ØD848ZZ
ØDB1ØZX
ØDB1ØZZ
ØDB13ZZ
ØDB17ZZ
ØDJØ4ZZ
ØDQ5ØZZ
ØDQ53ZZ
ØDQ54ZZ
ØDQ57ZZ
ØDQ58ZZ
ØDU1Ø7Z
ØDU1ØJZ
ØDU1ØKZ
ØDU147Z
ØDU14JZ
ØDU14KZ
ØDU177Z
ØDU17JZ
ØDU17KZ
ØDU187Z
ØDU18JZ
ØDU18KZ
ØF9ØØZX
ØF91ØZX
ØF92ØZX
ØFBØØZX
ØFB1ØZX
ØFB2ØZX
ØG9GØØZ
ØG9GØZZ
ØG9HØØZ
ØG9HØZZ
ØG9KØØZ
ØG9KØZZ
ØG9LØØZ
ØG9LØZZ
ØG9MØØZ
ØG9MØZZ
ØG9NØØZ
ØG9NØZZ
ØG9PØØZ
ØG9PØZZ
ØG9QØØZ
ØG9QØZZ
ØG9RØØZ
ØG9RØZZ
ØGCGØZZ
ØGCG3ZZ
ØGCG4ZZ
ØGCHØZZ
ØGCH3ZZ
ØGCH4ZZ
ØGCKØZZ
ØGCK3ZZ
ØGCK4ZZ
ØGCLØZZ
ØGCL3ZZ
ØGCL4ZZ
ØGCMØZZ
ØGCM3ZZ
ØGCM4ZZ
ØGCNØZZ
ØGCN3ZZ
ØGCN4ZZ
ØGCPØZZ
ØGCP3ZZ
ØGCP4ZZ
ØGCQØZZ
ØGCQ3ZZ
ØGCQ4ZZ
ØGCRØZZ
ØGCR3ZZ
ØGCR4ZZ
ØGHSØ1Z
ØGHSØ2Z
ØGHSØ3Z
ØGHSØYZ
ØGHS32Z
ØGHS33Z
ØGHS41Z
ØGHS42Z
ØGHS43Z
ØGJKØZZ
ØGJRØZZ
ØGJSØZZ
ØGPKØØZ
ØGPK3ØZ
ØGPK4ØZ
ØGPRØØZ
ØGPR3ØZ
ØGPR4ØZ
ØGWKØØZ
ØGWK3ØZ
ØGWK4ØZ
ØGWRØØZ
ØGWR3ØZ
ØGWR4ØZ
ØHM1XZZ
ØHM2XZZ
ØHM3XZZ
ØHM4XZZ
ØHM9XZZ
ØHNØXZZ
ØHN1XZZ
ØHN2XZZ
ØHN3XZZ
ØHN4XZZ
ØHRØX72
ØHRØX73
ØHRØX74
ØHRØXJ3
ØHRØXJ4
ØHRØXJZ
ØHRØXK3
ØHRØXK4
ØHR1X72
ØHR1XJ3
ØHR1XJ4
ØHR1XJZ
ØHR1XK3
ØHR1XK4
ØHR2X72
ØHR2X73
ØHR2X74
ØHR2XJ3
ØHR2XJ4
ØHR2XJZ
ØHR2XK3
ØHR2XK4
ØHR3X72
ØHR3X73
ØHR3X74
ØHR3XJ3
ØHR3XJ4
ØHR3XJZ
ØHR3XK3
ØHR3XK4
ØHR4X72
ØHR4X74
ØHR4XJ3
ØHR4XJ4
ØHR4XK3
ØHR4XK4
ØHR5XK3
ØHR5XK4
ØHR6XK3
ØHR6XK4
ØHR7XK3
ØHR7XK4
ØHR8XK3
ØHR8XK4
ØHXØXZZ
ØHX1XZZ
ØHX2XZZ
ØHX3XZZ
ØHX4XZZ
ØHX5XZZ
ØHX6XZZ
ØHX7XZZ
ØHX8XZZ
ØHXHXZZ
ØHXJXZZ
ØHXKXZZ
ØHXLXZZ
ØJØ1ØZZ
ØJØ13ZZ
ØJ81ØZZ
ØJ813ZZ
ØJBØØZZ
ØJB1ØZZ
ØJB13ZZ
ØJB4ØZZ
ØJB5ØZZ
ØJB6ØZZ
ØJB7ØZZ
ØJB8ØZZ
ØJB9ØZZ
ØJBBØZZ
ØJBCØZZ
ØJBDØZZ
ØJBFØZZ
ØJBGØZZ
ØJBHØZZ
ØJBLØZZ
ØJBMØZZ
ØJBNØZZ
ØJBPØZZ
ØJBQØZZ
ØJBRØZZ
ØJHØØNZ
ØJHØ3NZ
ØJH1ØNZ
ØJH13NZ
ØJH4ØNZ
ØJH43NZ
ØJH5ØNZ
ØJH53NZ
ØJRØ37Z
ØJR137Z
ØJR13KZ
ØJR437Z
ØJR537Z
ØJR637Z
ØJR737Z
ØJR837Z
ØJR937Z
ØJRB37Z
ØJRC37Z
ØJRD37Z
ØJRF37Z
ØJRG37Z
ØJRH37Z
ØJRJ37Z
ØJRK37Z
ØJRL37Z
ØJRM37Z
ØJRN37Z
ØJRP37Z
ØJRQ37Z
ØJRR37Z
ØJXØØZB
ØJXØØZC
ØJXØ3ZB
ØJXØ3ZC
ØJX1ØZB
ØJX1ØZC
ØJX13ZB
ØJX13ZC
ØJX43ZB
ØJX43ZC
ØJX53ZB
ØJX53ZC
ØK84ØZZ
ØK843ZZ
ØK844ZZ
ØK847ZZ
ØK848ZZ
ØK9ØØØZ
ØK9ØØZZ
ØK9Ø4ØZ
ØK9Ø4ZZ
ØK91ØØZ
ØK91ØZZ
ØK914ØZ
ØK914ZZ
ØK92ØØZ
ØK92ØZZ
ØK924ØZ
ØK924ZZ
ØK93ØØZ
ØK93ØZZ
ØK934ØZ
ØK934ZZ
ØKCØØZZ
ØKCØ3ZZ
ØKCØ4ZZ
ØKC1ØZZ
ØKC13ZZ
ØKC14ZZ
ØKC2ØZZ
ØKC23ZZ
ØKC24ZZ
ØKC3ØZZ
ØKC33ZZ
ØKC34ZZ
ØN5ØØZZ
ØN5Ø3ZZ
ØN5Ø4ZZ
ØN51ØZZ
ØN513ZZ
ØN514ZZ
ØN53ØZZ
ØN533ZZ
ØN534ZZ
ØN54ØZZ
ØN543ZZ
ØN544ZZ
ØN55ØZZ
ØN553ZZ
ØN554ZZ
ØN56ØZZ
ØN563ZZ
ØN564ZZ
ØN57ØZZ
ØN573ZZ
ØN574ZZ
ØN5BØZZ
ØN5B3ZZ
ØN5B4ZZ
ØN5CØZZ
ØN5C3ZZ
ØN5C4ZZ
ØN5FØZZ
ØN5F3ZZ
ØN5F4ZZ
ØN5GØZZ
ØN5G3ZZ
ØN5G4ZZ
ØN5HØZZ
ØN5H3ZZ
ØN5H4ZZ
ØN5JØZZ
ØN5J3ZZ
ØN5J4ZZ
ØN5KØZZ
ØN5K3ZZ
ØN5K4ZZ
ØN5LØZZ
ØN5L3ZZ
ØN5L4ZZ
ØN5MØZZ
ØN5M3ZZ
ØN5M4ZZ
ØN5NØZZ
ØN5N3ZZ
ØN5N4ZZ
ØN5PØZZ
ØN5P3ZZ
ØN5P4ZZ
ØN5QØZZ
ØN5Q3ZZ
ØN5Q4ZZ
ØN5RØZZ
ØN5R3ZZ
ØN5R4ZZ
ØN5TØZZ
ØN5T3ZZ
ØN5T4ZZ
ØN5VØZZ
ØN5V3ZZ
ØN5V4ZZ
ØN5XØZZ
ØN5X3ZZ
ØN5X4ZZ
ØN8CØZZ
ØN8C3ZZ
ØN8C4ZZ
ØN8FØZZ
ØN8F3ZZ
ØN8F4ZZ
ØN8GØZZ
ØN8G3ZZ
ØN8G4ZZ
ØN8HØZZ
ØN8H3ZZ
ØN8H4ZZ
ØN8JØZZ
ØN8J3ZZ
ØN8J4ZZ
ØN8KØZZ
ØN8K3ZZ
ØN8K4ZZ
ØN8LØZZ
ØN8L3ZZ
ØN8L4ZZ
ØN8MØZZ
ØN8M3ZZ
ØN8M4ZZ
ØN8NØZZ
ØN8N3ZZ
ØN8N4ZZ
ØN8PØZZ
ØN8P3ZZ
ØN8P4ZZ
ØN8QØZZ
ØN8Q3ZZ
ØN8Q4ZZ
ØN8RØZZ
ØN8R3ZZ
ØN8R4ZZ
ØN8TØZZ
ØN8T3ZZ
ØN8T4ZZ
ØN8VØZZ
ØN8V3ZZ
ØN8V4ZZ
ØN8XØZZ
ØN8X3ZZ
ØN8X4ZZ
ØN9CØØZ
ØN9CØZX
ØN9CØZZ
ØN9C3ZX
ØN9C4ØZ
ØN9C4ZX
ØN9C4ZZ
ØN9FØØZ
ØN9FØZX
ØN9FØZZ
ØN9F3ZX
ØN9F4ØZ
ØN9F4ZX
ØN9F4ZZ
ØN9GØØZ
ØN9GØZX
ØN9GØZZ
ØN9G3ZX
ØN9G4ØZ
ØN9G4ZX
ØN9G4ZZ
ØN9HØØZ
ØN9HØZX
ØN9HØZZ
ØN9H3ZX
ØN9H4ØZ
ØN9H4ZX
ØN9H4ZZ
ØN9JØØZ
ØN9JØZX
ØN9JØZZ
ØN9J3ZX
ØN9J4ØZ
ØN9J4ZX
ØN9J4ZZ
ØN9KØØZ
ØN9KØZX
ØN9KØZZ
ØN9K3ZX
ØN9K4ØZ
ØN9K4ZX
ØN9K4ZZ
ØN9LØØZ
ØN9LØZX
ØN9LØZZ
ØN9L3ZX
ØN9L4ØZ
ØN9L4ZX
ØN9L4ZZ
ØN9MØØZ
ØN9MØZX
ØN9MØZZ
ØN9M3ZX
ØN9M4ØZ
ØN9M4ZX
ØN9M4ZZ
ØN9NØØZ
ØN9NØZX
ØN9NØZZ
ØN9N3ZX
ØN9N4ØZ
ØN9N4ZX
ØN9N4ZZ
ØN9PØØZ
ØN9PØZZ
ØN9P4ØZ
ØN9P4ZZ
ØN9QØØZ
ØN9QØZZ
ØN9Q4ØZ
ØN9Q4ZZ
ØN9RØZX
ØN9R3ZX
ØN9R4ZX
ØN9TØZX
ØN9T3ZX
ØN9T4ZX
ØN9VØZX
ØN9V3ZX
ØN9V4ZX
ØN9XØØZ
ØN9XØZX
ØN9XØZZ
ØN9X3ZX
ØN9X4ØZ
ØN9X4ZX
ØN9X4ZZ
ØNBØØZZ
ØNBØ3ZZ
ØNBØ4ZZ
ØNB1ØZZ
ØNB13ZZ
ØNB14ZZ
ØNB3ØZZ
ØNB33ZZ
ØNB34ZZ
ØNB4ØZZ
ØNB43ZZ
ØNB44ZZ
ØNB5ØZZ
ØNB53ZZ
ØNB54ZZ
ØNB6ØZZ
ØNB63ZZ
ØNB64ZZ
ØNB7ØZZ
ØNB73ZZ
ØNB74ZZ
ØNBBØZZ
ØNBB3ZZ
ØNBB4ZZ
ØNBCØZX
ØNBCØZZ
ØNBC3ZX
ØNBC3ZZ
ØNBC4ZX
ØNBC4ZZ
ØNBFØZX
ØNBFØZZ
ØNBF3ZX
ØNBF3ZZ
ØNBF4ZX
ØNBF4ZZ
ØNBGØZX
ØNBGØZZ
ØNBG3ZX
ØNBG3ZZ
ØNBG4ZX
ØNBG4ZZ
ØNBHØZX
ØNBHØZZ
ØNBH3ZX
ØNBH3ZZ
ØNBH4ZX
ØNBH4ZZ
ØNBJØZX
ØNBJØZZ
ØNBJ3ZX
ØNBJ3ZZ
ØNBJ4ZX
ØNBJ4ZZ
ØNBKØZX
ØNBKØZZ
ØNBK3ZX
ØNBK3ZZ
ØNBK4ZX
ØNBK4ZZ
ØNBLØZX
ØNBLØZZ
ØNBL3ZX
ØNBL3ZZ
ØNBL4ZX
ØNBL4ZZ
ØNBMØZX
ØNBMØZZ
ØNBM3ZX
ØNBM3ZZ
ØNBM4ZX
ØNBM4ZZ
ØNBNØZX
ØNBNØZZ
ØNBN3ZX
ØNBN3ZZ
ØNBN4ZX
ØNBN4ZZ
ØNBPØZZ
ØNBP3ZZ
ØNBP4ZZ
ØNBQØZZ
ØNBQ3ZZ
ØNBQ4ZZ
ØNBRØZZ
ØNBR3ZZ
ØNBR4ZZ
ØNBT3ZZ
ØNBV3ZZ
ØNBXØZX
ØNBXØZZ
ØNBX3ZX
ØNBX3ZZ
ØNBX4ZX
ØNBX4ZZ
ØNC1ØZZ
ØNC13ZZ
ØNC14ZZ
ØNC3ØZZ
ØNC33ZZ
ØNC34ZZ
ØNC4ØZZ
ØNC43ZZ
ØNC44ZZ
ØNC5ØZZ
ØNC53ZZ
ØNC54ZZ
ØNC6ØZZ
ØNC63ZZ
ØNC64ZZ
ØNC7ØZZ
ØNC73ZZ
ØNC74ZZ
ØNCCØZZ
ØNCC3ZZ
ØNCC4ZZ
ØNCFØZZ
ØNCF3ZZ
ØNCF4ZZ
ØNCGØZZ
ØNCG3ZZ
ØNCG4ZZ
ØNCHØZZ
ØNCH3ZZ
ØNCH4ZZ
ØNCJØZZ
ØNCJ3ZZ
ØNCJ4ZZ
ØNCKØZZ
ØNCK3ZZ
ØNCK4ZZ
ØNCLØZZ
ØNCL3ZZ
ØNCL4ZZ
ØNCMØZZ
ØNCM3ZZ
ØNCM4ZZ
ØNCNØZZ
ØNCN3ZZ
ØNCN4ZZ
ØNCPØZZ
ØNCP3ZZ
ØNCP4ZZ
ØNCQØZZ
ØNCQ3ZZ
ØNCQ4ZZ
ØNCXØZZ
ØNCX3ZZ
ØNCX4ZZ
ØNH1Ø4Z
ØNH134Z
ØNH144Z
ØNH3Ø4Z
ØNH334Z
ØNH344Z
ØNH4Ø4Z
ØNH434Z
ØNH444Z
ØNH5Ø4Z
ØNH5ØSZ
ØNH534Z
ØNH53SZ
ØNH544Z
ØNH54SZ
ØNH6Ø4Z
ØNH6ØSZ
ØNH634Z
ØNH63SZ
ØNH644Z
ØNH64SZ
ØNH7Ø4Z
ØNH734Z
ØNH744Z
ØNHCØ4Z
ØNHC34Z
ØNHC44Z
ØNHFØ4Z
ØNHF34Z
ØNHF44Z
ØNHGØ4Z
ØNHG34Z
ØNHG44Z
ØNHHØ4Z
ØNHH34Z
ØNHH44Z
ØNHJØ4Z
ØNHJ34Z
ØNHJ44Z
ØNHKØ4Z
ØNHK34Z
ØNHK44Z
ØNHLØ4Z
ØNHL34Z
ØNHL44Z
ØNHMØ4Z
ØNHM34Z
ØNHM44Z
ØNHNØ4Z
ØNHN34Z
ØNHN44Z
ØNHPØ4Z
ØNHP34Z
ØNHP44Z
ØNHQØ4Z
ØNHQ34Z
ØNHQ44Z
ØNHRØ4Z
ØNHRØ5Z
ØNHR34Z
ØNHR35Z
ØNHR44Z
ØNHR45Z
ØNHTØ4Z
ØNHTØ5Z
ØNHT34Z
ØNHT35Z
ØNHT44Z
ØNHT45Z
ØNHVØ4Z
ØNHVØ5Z
ØNHV34Z
ØNHV35Z
ØNHV44Z
ØNHV45Z
ØNHWØMZ
ØNHW3MZ
ØNHW4MZ
ØNHXØ4Z
ØNHX34Z
ØNHX44Z
ØNJBØZZ
ØNJB4ZZ
ØNJWØZZ
ØNJW4ZZ
ØNN1ØZZ
ØNN13ZZ
ØNN14ZZ
ØNN3ØZZ
ØNN33ZZ
ØNN34ZZ
ØNN4ØZZ
ØNN43ZZ
ØNN44ZZ
ØNN5ØZZ
ØNN53ZZ
ØNN54ZZ
ØNN6ØZZ
ØNN63ZZ
ØNN64ZZ
ØNN7ØZZ
ØNN73ZZ
ØNN74ZZ
ØNNCØZZ
ØNNC3ZZ
ØNNC4ZZ
ØNNFØZZ
ØNNF3ZZ
ØNNF4ZZ
ØNNGØZZ
ØNNG3ZZ
ØNNG4ZZ
ØNNHØZZ
ØNNH3ZZ
ØNNH4ZZ
ØNNJØZZ
ØNNJ3ZZ
ØNNJ4ZZ
ØNNKØZZ
ØNNK3ZZ
ØNNK4ZZ
ØNNLØZZ
ØNNL3ZZ
ØNNL4ZZ
ØNNMØZZ
ØNNM3ZZ
ØNNM4ZZ
ØNNNØZZ
ØNNN3ZZ
ØNNN4ZZ
ØNNRØZZ
ØNNR3ZZ
ØNNR4ZZ
ØNNTØZZ
ØNNT3ZZ
ØNNT4ZZ
ØNNVØZZ
ØNNV3ZZ
ØNNV4ZZ
ØNPØØJZ
ØNPØ3JZ
ØNPØ4JZ
ØNPWØØZ
ØNPWØ4Z
ØNPWØ7Z
ØNPWØKZ
ØNPWØMZ
ØNPW3ØZ
ØNPW34Z
ØNPW37Z
ØNPW3KZ
ØNPW3MZ
ØNPW4ØZ
ØNPW44Z
ØNPW47Z
ØNPW4KZ
ØNPW4MZ
ØNPWX4Z
ØNQØØZZ
ØNQØ3ZZ
ØNQØ4ZZ

ØNQ1ØZZ
ØNQ13ZZ
ØNQ14ZZ
ØNQ3ØZZ
ØNQ33ZZ
ØNQ34ZZ
ØNQ4ØZZ
ØNQ43ZZ
ØNQ44ZZ
ØNQ5ØZZ
ØNQ53ZZ
ØNQ54ZZ
ØNQ6ØZZ
ØNQ63ZZ
ØNQ64ZZ
ØNQ7ØZZ
ØNQ73ZZ
ØNQ74ZZ
ØNQBØZZ
ØNQB3ZZ
ØNQB4ZZ
ØNQCØZZ
ØNQC3ZZ
ØNQC4ZZ
ØNQFØZZ
ØNQF3ZZ
ØNQF4ZZ
ØNQGØZZ
ØNQG3ZZ
ØNQG4ZZ
ØNQHØZZ
ØNQH3ZZ
ØNQH4ZZ
ØNQJØZZ
ØNQJ3ZZ
ØNQJ4ZZ
ØNQKØZZ
ØNQK3ZZ
ØNQK4ZZ
ØNQLØZZ
ØNQL3ZZ
ØNQL4ZZ
ØNQMØZZ
ØNQM3ZZ
ØNQM4ZZ
ØNQNØZZ
ØNQN3ZZ
ØNQN4ZZ
ØNQPØZZ
ØNQP3ZZ
ØNQP4ZZ
ØNQQØZZ
ØNQQ3ZZ
ØNQQ4ZZ
ØNQRØZZ
ØNQR3ZZ
ØNQR4ZZ
ØNQTØZZ
ØNQT3ZZ
ØNQT4ZZ
ØNQVØZZ
ØNQV3ZZ
ØNQV4ZZ
ØNQXØZZ
ØNQX3ZZ
ØNQX4ZZ
ØNRØØ7Z
ØNRØØJZ
ØNRØØKZ
ØNRØ37Z
ØNRØ3JZ
ØNRØ3KZ
ØNRØ47Z
ØNRØ4JZ
ØNRØ4KZ
ØNR1Ø7Z
ØNR1ØJZ
ØNR1ØKZ
ØNR137Z
ØNR13JZ
ØNR13KZ
ØNR147Z
ØNR14JZ
ØNR14KZ
ØNR3Ø7Z
ØNR3ØJZ
ØNR3ØKZ
ØNR337Z
ØNR33JZ
ØNR33KZ
ØNR347Z
ØNR34JZ
ØNR34KZ
ØNR4Ø7Z
ØNR4ØJZ
ØNR4ØKZ
ØNR437Z
ØNR43JZ
ØNR43KZ
ØNR447Z
ØNR44JZ
ØNR44KZ
ØNR5Ø7Z
ØNR5ØJZ
ØNR5ØKZ
ØNR537Z
ØNR53JZ
ØNR53KZ
ØNR547Z
ØNR54JZ
ØNR54KZ
ØNR6Ø7Z
ØNR6ØJZ
ØNR6ØKZ
ØNR637Z
ØNR63JZ
ØNR63KZ
ØNR647Z
ØNR64JZ
ØNR64KZ
ØNR7Ø7Z
ØNR7ØJZ
ØNR7ØKZ
ØNR737Z
ØNR73JZ
ØNR73KZ
ØNR747Z
ØNR74JZ
ØNR74KZ
ØNRBØ7Z
ØNRBØJZ
ØNRBØKZ
ØNRB37Z
ØNRB3JZ
ØNRB3KZ
ØNRB47Z
ØNRB4JZ
ØNRB4KZ
ØNRCØ7Z
ØNRCØJZ
ØNRCØKZ
ØNRC37Z
ØNRC3JZ
ØNRC3KZ
ØNRC47Z
ØNRC4JZ
ØNRC4KZ
ØNRFØ7Z
ØNRFØJZ
ØNRFØKZ
ØNRF37Z
ØNRF3JZ
ØNRF3KZ
ØNRF47Z
ØNRF4JZ
ØNRF4KZ
ØNRGØ7Z
ØNRGØJZ
ØNRGØKZ
ØNRG37Z
ØNRG3JZ
ØNRG3KZ
ØNRG47Z
ØNRG4JZ
ØNRG4KZ
ØNRHØ7Z
ØNRHØJZ
ØNRHØKZ
ØNRH37Z
ØNRH3JZ
ØNRH3KZ
ØNRH47Z
ØNRH4JZ
ØNRH4KZ
ØNRJØ7Z
ØNRJØJZ
ØNRJØKZ
ØNRJ37Z
ØNRJ3JZ
ØNRJ3KZ
ØNRJ47Z
ØNRJ4JZ
ØNRJ4KZ
ØNRKØ7Z
ØNRKØJZ
ØNRKØKZ
ØNRK37Z
ØNRK3JZ
ØNRK3KZ
ØNRK47Z
ØNRK4JZ
ØNRK4KZ
ØNRLØ7Z
ØNRLØJZ
ØNRLØKZ
ØNRL37Z
ØNRL3JZ
ØNRL3KZ
ØNRL47Z
ØNRL4JZ
ØNRL4KZ
ØNRMØ7Z
ØNRMØJZ
ØNRMØKZ
ØNRM37Z
ØNRM3JZ
ØNRM3KZ
ØNRM47Z
ØNRM4JZ
ØNRM4KZ
ØNRNØ7Z
ØNRNØJZ
ØNRNØKZ
ØNRN37Z
ØNRN3JZ
ØNRN3KZ
ØNRN47Z
ØNRN4JZ
ØNRN4KZ
ØNRPØ7Z
ØNRPØJZ
ØNRPØKZ
ØNRP37Z
ØNRP3JZ
ØNRP3KZ
ØNRP47Z
ØNRP4JZ
ØNRP4KZ
ØNRQØ7Z
ØNRQØJZ
ØNRQØKZ
ØNRQ37Z
ØNRQ3JZ
ØNRQ3KZ
ØNRQ47Z
ØNRQ4JZ
ØNRQ4KZ
ØNRRØ7Z
ØNRRØJZ
ØNRRØKZ
ØNRR37Z
ØNRR3JZ
ØNRR3KZ
ØNRR47Z
ØNRR4JZ
ØNRR4KZ
ØNRXØ7Z
ØNRXØJZ
ØNRXØKZ
ØNRX37Z
ØNRX3JZ
ØNRX3KZ
ØNRX47Z
ØNRX4JZ
ØNRX4KZ
ØNSØØ4Z
ØNSØØ5Z
ØNSØØZZ
ØNSØ34Z
ØNSØ35Z
ØNSØ3ZZ
ØNSØ44Z
ØNSØ45Z
ØNSØ4ZZ
ØNS3Ø4Z
ØNS3ØZZ
ØNS334Z
ØNS33ZZ
ØNS344Z
ØNS34ZZ
ØNS4Ø4Z
ØNS4ØZZ
ØNS434Z
ØNS43ZZ
ØNS444Z
ØNS44ZZ
ØNS5Ø4Z
ØNS5ØZZ
ØNS534Z
ØNS53ZZ
ØNS544Z
ØNS54ZZ
ØNS6Ø4Z
ØNS6ØZZ
ØNS634Z
ØNS63ZZ
ØNS644Z
ØNS64ZZ
ØNSMØZZ
ØNSNØZZ
ØNSRØ5Z
ØNSTØ5Z
ØNSTØZZ
ØNSVØ5Z
ØNSVØZZ
ØNSXØ4Z
ØNSXØZZ
ØNT1ØZZ
ØNT3ØZZ
ØNT4ØZZ
ØNT5ØZZ
ØNT6ØZZ
ØNT7ØZZ
ØNTBØZZ
ØNTCØZZ
ØNTFØZZ
ØNTGØZZ
ØNTHØZZ
ØNTJØZZ
ØNTKØZZ
ØNTLØZZ
ØNTMØZZ
ØNTNØZZ
ØNTPØZZ
ØNTQØZZ
ØNTRØZZ
ØNTXØZZ
ØNUØØ7Z
ØNUØØJZ
ØNUØØKZ
ØNUØ37Z
ØNUØ3JZ
ØNUØ3KZ
ØNUØ47Z
ØNUØ4JZ
ØNUØ4KZ
ØNU1Ø7Z
ØNU1ØJZ
ØNU1ØKZ
ØNU137Z
ØNU13JZ
ØNU13KZ
ØNU147Z
ØNU14JZ
ØNU14KZ
ØNU3Ø7Z
ØNU3ØJZ
ØNU3ØKZ
ØNU337Z
ØNU33JZ
ØNU33KZ
ØNU347Z
ØNU34JZ
ØNU34KZ
ØNU4Ø7Z
ØNU4ØJZ
ØNU4ØKZ
ØNU437Z
ØNU43JZ
ØNU43KZ
ØNU447Z
ØNU44JZ
ØNU44KZ
ØNU5Ø7Z
ØNU5ØJZ
ØNU5ØKZ
ØNU537Z
ØNU53JZ
ØNU53KZ
ØNU547Z
ØNU54JZ
ØNU54KZ
ØNU6Ø7Z
ØNU6ØJZ
ØNU6ØKZ
ØNU637Z
ØNU63JZ
ØNU63KZ
ØNU647Z
ØNU64JZ
ØNU64KZ
ØNU7Ø7Z
ØNU7ØJZ
ØNU7ØKZ
ØNU737Z
ØNU73JZ
ØNU73KZ
ØNU747Z
ØNU74JZ
ØNU74KZ
ØNUBØ7Z
ØNUBØJZ
ØNUBØKZ
ØNUB37Z
ØNUB3JZ
ØNUB3KZ
ØNUB47Z
ØNUB4JZ
ØNUB4KZ
ØNUCØ7Z
ØNUCØJZ
ØNUCØKZ
ØNUC37Z
ØNUC3JZ
ØNUC3KZ
ØNUC47Z
ØNUC4JZ
ØNUC4KZ
ØNUFØ7Z
ØNUFØJZ
ØNUFØKZ
ØNUF37Z
ØNUF3JZ
ØNUF3KZ
ØNUF47Z
ØNUF4JZ
ØNUF4KZ
ØNUGØ7Z
ØNUGØJZ
ØNUGØKZ
ØNUG37Z
ØNUG3JZ
ØNUG3KZ
ØNUG47Z
ØNUG4JZ
ØNUG4KZ
ØNUHØ7Z
ØNUHØJZ
ØNUHØKZ
ØNUH37Z
ØNUH3JZ
ØNUH3KZ
ØNUH47Z
ØNUH4JZ
ØNUH4KZ
ØNUJØ7Z
ØNUJØJZ
ØNUJØKZ
ØNUJ37Z
ØNUJ3JZ
ØNUJ3KZ
ØNUJ47Z
ØNUJ4JZ
ØNUJ4KZ
ØNUKØ7Z
ØNUKØJZ
ØNUKØKZ
ØNUK37Z
ØNUK3JZ
ØNUK3KZ
ØNUK47Z
ØNUK4JZ
ØNUK4KZ
ØNULØ7Z
ØNULØJZ
ØNULØKZ
ØNUL37Z
ØNUL3JZ
ØNUL3KZ
ØNUL47Z
ØNUL4JZ
ØNUL4KZ
ØNUMØ7Z
ØNUMØJZ
ØNUMØKZ
ØNUM37Z
ØNUM3JZ
ØNUM3KZ
ØNUM47Z
ØNUM4JZ
ØNUM4KZ
ØNUNØ7Z
ØNUNØJZ
ØNUNØKZ
ØNUN37Z
ØNUN3JZ
ØNUN3KZ
ØNUN47Z
ØNUN4JZ
ØNUN4KZ
ØNUPØ7Z
ØNUPØJZ
ØNUPØKZ
ØNUP37Z
ØNUP3JZ
ØNUP3KZ
ØNUP47Z
ØNUP4JZ
ØNUP4KZ
ØNUQØ7Z
ØNUQØJZ
ØNUQØKZ
ØNUQ37Z
ØNUQ3JZ
ØNUQ3KZ
ØNUQ47Z
ØNUQ4JZ
ØNUQ4KZ
ØNURØ7Z
ØNURØJZ
ØNURØKZ
ØNUR37Z
ØNUR3JZ
ØNUR3KZ
ØNUR47Z
ØNUR4JZ
ØNUR4KZ
ØNUTØ7Z
ØNUTØJZ
ØNUTØKZ
ØNUT37Z
ØNUT3JZ
ØNUT3KZ
ØNUT47Z
ØNUT4JZ
ØNUT4KZ
ØNUVØ7Z
ØNUVØJZ
ØNUVØKZ
ØNUV37Z
ØNUV3JZ
ØNUV3KZ
ØNUV47Z
ØNUV4JZ
ØNUV4KZ
ØNUXØ7Z
ØNUXØJZ
ØNUXØKZ
ØNUX37Z
ØNUX3JZ
ØNUX3KZ
ØNUX47Z
ØNUX4JZ
ØNUX4KZ
ØNWWØØZ
ØNWWØ4Z
ØNWWØ7Z
ØNWWØJZ
ØNWWØKZ
ØNWWØMZ
ØNWW3ØZ
ØNWW34Z
ØNWW37Z
ØNWW3JZ
ØNWW3KZ
ØNWW3MZ
ØNWW4ØZ
ØNWW44Z
ØNWW47Z
ØNWW4JZ
ØNWW4KZ
ØNWW4MZ
ØP53ØZ3
ØP53ØZZ
ØP533Z3
ØP533ZZ
ØP534Z3
ØP534ZZ
ØP93ØZX
ØP933ZX
ØP934ZX
ØPB3ØZX
ØPB3ØZZ
ØPB33ZX
ØPB33ZZ
ØPB34ZX
ØPB34ZZ
ØPB4ØZZ
ØPB43ZZ
ØPB44ZZ
ØPSBØ4Z
ØPSBØZZ
ØQBØØZZ
ØQBØ3ZZ
ØQBØ4ZZ
ØR5CØZZ
ØR5C3ZZ
ØR5C4ZZ
ØR5DØZZ
ØR5D3ZZ
ØR5D4ZZ
ØR9CØØZ
ØR9CØZX
ØR9CØZZ
ØR9C3ZX
ØR9C4ØZ
ØR9C4ZX
ØR9C4ZZ
ØR9DØØZ
ØR9DØZX
ØR9DØZZ
ØR9D3ZX
ØR9D4ØZ
ØR9D4ZX
ØR9D4ZZ
ØRBCØZX
ØRBCØZZ
ØRBC3ZX
ØRBC3ZZ
ØRBC4ZX
ØRBC4ZZ
ØRBDØZX
ØRBD3ZX
ØRBD4ZX
ØRCCØZZ
ØRCC3ZZ
ØRCC4ZZ
ØRCDØZZ
ØRCD3ZZ
ØRCD4ZZ
ØRGCØ4Z
ØRGCØ7Z
ØRGCØJZ
ØRGCØKZ
ØRGC34Z
ØRGC37Z
ØRGC3JZ
ØRGC3KZ
ØRGC44Z
ØRGC47Z
ØRGC4JZ
ØRGC4KZ
ØRGDØ4Z
ØRGDØ7Z
ØRGDØJZ
ØRGDØKZ
ØRGD34Z
ØRGD37Z
ØRGD3JZ
ØRGD3KZ
ØRGD44Z
ØRGD47Z
ØRGD4JZ
ØRGD4KZ
ØRHCØ3Z
ØRHCØ4Z
ØRHC34Z
ØRHC43Z
ØRHC44Z
ØRHDØ3Z
ØRHDØ4Z
ØRHD34Z
ØRHD43Z
ØRHD44Z
ØRJCØZZ
ØRJC4ZZ
ØRJDØZZ
ØRJD4ZZ
ØRNCØZZ
ØRNC3ZZ
ØRNC4ZZ
ØRNDØZZ
ØRND3ZZ
ØRND4ZZ
ØRPCØØZ
ØRPCØ3Z
ØRPCØ4Z
ØRPCØ7Z
ØRPCØJZ
ØRPCØKZ
ØRPC34Z
ØRPC37Z
ØRPC3JZ
ØRPC3KZ
ØRPC4ØZ
ØRPC43Z
ØRPC44Z
ØRPC47Z
ØRPC4JZ
ØRPC4KZ
ØRPCX4Z
ØRPDØØZ
ØRPDØ3Z
ØRPDØ4Z
ØRPDØ7Z
ØRPDØJZ
ØRPDØKZ
ØRPD34Z
ØRPD37Z
ØRPD3JZ
ØRPD3KZ
ØRPD4ØZ
ØRPD43Z
ØRPD44Z
ØRPD47Z
ØRPD4JZ
ØRPD4KZ
ØRPDX4Z
ØRQCØZZ
ØRQC3ZZ
ØRQC4ZZ
ØRQDØZZ
ØRQD3ZZ
ØRQD4ZZ
ØRUCØ7Z
ØRUCØJZ
ØRUCØKZ
ØRUC37Z
ØRUC3JZ
ØRUC3KZ
ØRUC47Z
ØRUC4JZ
ØRUC4KZ
ØRUDØ7Z
ØRUDØJZ
ØRUDØKZ
ØRUD37Z
ØRUD3JZ
ØRUD3KZ
ØRUD47Z
ØRUD4JZ
ØRUD4KZ
ØRWCØØZ
ØRWCØ3Z
ØRWCØ4Z
ØRWCØ7Z
ØRWCØ8Z
ØRWCØJZ
ØRWCØKZ
ØRWC3ØZ
ØRWC33Z
ØRWC34Z
ØRWC37Z
ØRWC38Z
ØRWC3JZ
ØRWC3KZ
ØRWC4ØZ
ØRWC43Z
ØRWC44Z
ØRWC47Z
ØRWC48Z
ØRWC4JZ
ØRWC4KZ
ØRWDØØZ
ØRWDØ3Z
ØRWDØ4Z
ØRWDØ7Z
ØRWDØ8Z
ØRWDØJZ
ØRWDØKZ
ØRWD3ØZ
ØRWD33Z
ØRWD34Z
ØRWD37Z
ØRWD38Z
ØRWD3JZ
ØRWD3KZ
ØRWD4ØZ
ØRWD43Z
ØRWD44Z
ØRWD47Z
ØRWD48Z
ØRWD4JZ
ØRWD4KZ
ØWØ2Ø7Z
ØWØ2ØJZ
ØWØ2ØKZ
ØWØ2ØZZ
ØWØ237Z
ØWØ23JZ
ØWØ23KZ
ØWØ23ZZ
ØWØ247Z
ØWØ24JZ
ØWØ24KZ
ØWØ24ZZ
ØWØ4Ø7Z
ØWØ4ØJZ
ØWØ4ØKZ
ØWØ4ØZZ
ØWØ437Z
ØWØ43JZ
ØWØ43KZ
ØWØ43ZZ
ØWØ447Z
ØWØ44JZ
ØWØ44KZ
ØWØ44ZZ
ØWØ5Ø7Z
ØWØ5ØJZ
ØWØ5ØKZ
ØWØ5ØZZ
ØWØ537Z
ØWØ53JZ
ØWØ53KZ
ØWØ53ZZ
ØWØ547Z
ØWØ54JZ
ØWØ54KZ
ØWØ54ZZ
ØWØ6Ø7Z
ØWØ6ØJZ
ØWØ6ØKZ
ØWØ6ØZZ
ØWØ637Z
ØWØ63JZ
ØWØ63KZ
ØWØ63ZZ
ØWØ647Z
ØWØ64JZ
ØWØ64KZ
ØWØ64ZZ
ØW3ØØZZ
ØW3Ø3ZZ
ØW3Ø4ZZ
ØW31ØZZ
ØW313ZZ
ØW314ZZ
ØW32ØZZ
ØW323ZZ
ØW324ZZ
ØW33ØZZ
ØW333ZZ
ØW334ZZ
ØW34ØZZ
ØW343ZZ
ØW344ZZ
ØW35ØZZ
ØW353ZZ
ØW354ZZ
ØW36ØZZ
ØW363ZZ
ØW364ZZ
ØW96ØØZ
ØW96ØZZ
ØW964ØZ
ØW964ZZ
ØWBØØZZ
ØWBØ3ZZ
ØWBØ4ZZ
ØWBØXZZ
ØWB2ØZZ
ØWB23ZZ
ØWB24ZZ
ØWB2XZZ
ØWB4ØZZ
ØWB43ZZ
ØWB44ZZ
ØWB4XZZ
ØWB5ØZZ
ØWB53ZZ
ØWB54ZZ
ØWB5XZZ
ØWB6ØZZ
ØWB63ZZ
ØWB64ZZ
ØWB6XZ2
ØWB6XZZ
ØWC4ØZZ
ØWC44ZZ
ØWC5ØZZ
ØWC54ZZ
ØWH3Ø1Z
ØWH331Z
ØWH341Z
ØWH4Ø1Z
ØWH431Z
ØWH441Z
ØWH5Ø1Z
ØWH531Z
ØWH541Z
ØWH6Ø1Z
ØWH631Z
ØWH641Z
ØWJ6ØZZ

ØWJC4ZZ
ØWJD4ZZ
ØWM2ØZZ
ØWM4ØZZ
ØWM5ØZZ
ØWM6ØZZ
ØWQ2ØZZ
ØWQ23ZZ
ØWQ24ZZ
ØWQ2XZZ
ØWQ3ØZZ
ØWQ33ZZ
ØWQ34ZZ
ØWQ3XZZ
ØWQ4ØZZ
ØWQ43ZZ
ØWQ44ZZ
ØWQ4XZZ
ØWQ5ØZZ
ØWQ53ZZ
ØWQ54ZZ
ØWQ5XZZ
ØWQ6ØZZ
ØWQ63ZZ
ØWQ64ZZ
ØWQ6XZ2
ØWQ6XZZ
ØWU2ØJZ
ØWU2ØKZ
ØWU24JZ
ØWU24KZ
ØWU4Ø7Z
ØWU4ØJZ
ØWU4ØKZ
ØWU447Z
ØWU44JZ
ØWU44KZ
ØWU5Ø7Z
ØWU5ØJZ
ØWU5ØKZ
ØWU547Z
ØWU54JZ
ØWU54KZ
ØWU6ØJZ
ØWU6ØKZ
ØWU64JZ
ØWU64KZ
ØWY2ØZØ
ØWY2ØZ1
XØHK3Q8
XØHQ3R8
XHRPXF7
XNR8ØD9

DRG 144
Select operating room procedures listed under DRG 143

DRG 145
Select operating room procedures listed under DRG 143

DRG 146
Principal Diagnosis
CØØ*
CØ1
CØ2*
CØ3*
CØ4*
CØ5*
CØ6*
CØ7
CØ8*
CØ9*
C1Ø*
C11*
C12
C13*
C14*
C3Ø*
C31*
C32*
C39.Ø
C46.2
C76.Ø
DØØ.Ø*
DØ2.Ø
D37.Ø*
D38.Ø

DRG 147
Select principal diagnosis listed under DRG 146

DRG 148
Select principal diagnosis listed under DRG 146

DRG 149
Principal Diagnosis
H81*
H82*
H83.Ø*
H83.2*
H83.8*
H83.9*
R42
T75.3XXA

DRG 150
Principal Diagnosis
RØ4.Ø

DRG 151
Select principal diagnosis listed under DRG 150

DRG 152
Principal Diagnosis
A54.5
A56.4
A69.1
BØ5.3
BØ8.5
H61.ØØ1
H61.ØØ2
H61.ØØ3
H61.ØØ9
H65*
H66*
H67*
H68.Ø*
H7Ø.Ø*
H7Ø.1*
H7Ø.2*
H7Ø.9*
H73.Ø*
H73.1*
H73.2*
JØØ
JØ1*
JØ2*
JØ3*
JØ4.Ø
JØ4.2
JØ4.3*
JØ5*
JØ6*
J11.1
J3Ø*
J31*
J32*
J35.Ø*
J36
J37*
J39.Ø
J39.1
J39.3
J39.9
T7Ø.ØXXA
T7Ø.1XXA

DRG 153
Select principal diagnosis listed under DRG 152

DRG 154
Principal Diagnosis
A18.6
A36.Ø
A36.1
A36.2
A66.5
BØØ.1
B37.84
D1Ø.4
D1Ø.5
D1Ø.6
D1Ø.7
D1Ø.9
D11*
D14.Ø
D14.1
G47.3Ø
G47.33
G47.34
G47.36
G47.39
G47.5Ø
G47.52
G47.54
G47.59
G47.63
G47.69
G47.8
H6Ø*
H61.1*
H61.2*
H61.3*
H61.8*
H61.9*
H62*
H68.1*
H69*
H7Ø.8*
H71*
H72*
H73.8*
H73.9*
H74*
H75*
H8Ø*
H83.1*
H83.3*
H9Ø*
H91*
H92*
H93.Ø*
H93.1*
H93.211
H93.212
H93.213
H93.219
H93.221
H93.222
H93.223
H93.229
H93.231
H93.232
H93.233
H93.239
H93.241
H93.242
H93.243
H93.249
H93.291
H93.292
H93.293
H93.299
H93.3*
H93.8*
H93.9*
H93.A1
H93.A2
H93.A3
H93.A9
H94*
H95.Ø*
H95.1*
J33*
J34*
J35.1
J35.2
J35.3
J35.8
J35.9
J38*
J39.2
K11*
M95.Ø
M95.1*
Q16*
Q17*
Q18.Ø
Q18.1
Q18.2
Q18.8
Q3Ø*
Q31*
Q32*
Q38.4
Q38.7
Q38.8
RØ4.1
RØ6.5
RØ6.7
RØ7.Ø
RØ9.81
RØ9.82
R19.6
R49*
R68.2
R94.12Ø
R94.121
SØ1.2ØXA
SØ1.21XA
SØ1.22XA
SØ1.23XA
SØ1.24XA
SØ1.25XA
SØ1.3Ø1A
SØ1.3Ø2A
SØ1.3Ø9A
SØ1.311A
SØ1.312A
SØ1.319A
SØ1.321A
SØ1.322A
SØ1.329A
SØ1.331A
SØ1.332A
SØ1.339A
SØ1.341A
SØ1.342A
SØ1.349A
SØ1.351A
SØ1.352A
SØ1.359A
SØ2.2XXA
SØ2.2XXB
SØ4.6ØXA
SØ4.61XA
SØ4.62XA
SØ8.111A
SØ8.112A
SØ8.119A
SØ8.121A
SØ8.122A
SØ8.129A
SØ8.811A
SØ8.812A
SØ9.2ØXA
SØ9.21XA
SØ9.22XA
SØ9.3Ø1A
SØ9.3Ø2A
SØ9.3Ø9A
SØ9.311A
SØ9.312A
SØ9.313A
SØ9.319A
SØ9.391A
SØ9.392A
SØ9.399A
SØ9.91XA
S11.Ø11A
S11.Ø12A
S11.Ø13A
S11.Ø14A
S11.Ø15A
S11.Ø19A
S11.Ø31A
S11.Ø32A
S11.Ø33A
S11.Ø34A
S11.Ø35A
S11.Ø39A
S11.2ØXA
S11.21XA
S11.22XA
S11.23XA
S11.24XA
S11.25XA
S12.8XXA
T16.1XXA
T16.2XXA
T16.9XXA
T17.ØXXA
T17.1XXA
T17.2ØØA
T17.2Ø8A
T17.21ØA
T17.218A
T17.22ØA
T17.228A
T17.29ØA
T17.298A
T17.3ØØA
T17.3Ø8A
T17.31ØA
T17.318A
T17.32ØA
T17.328A
T17.39ØA
T17.398A
T28.ØXXA
T28.5XXA

DRG 155
Select principal diagnosis listed under DRG 154

DRG 156
Select principal diagnosis listed under DRG 154

DRG 157
Principal Diagnosis
A69.Ø
BØØ.2
B37.Ø
B37.83
D1Ø.Ø
D1Ø.1
D1Ø.2
D1Ø.3*
D16.5
KØØ*
KØ1*
KØ2*
KØ3*
KØ4*
KØ5*
KØ6*
KØ8*
KØ9*
K12*
K13*
K14*
M26*
M27*
Q18.4
Q18.5
Q18.6
Q18.7
Q35*
Q36*
Q37*
Q38.Ø
Q38.1
Q38.2
Q38.3
Q38.6
R68.84
SØ1.5Ø1A
SØ1.5Ø2A
SØ1.511A
SØ1.512A
SØ1.521A
SØ1.522A
SØ1.531A
SØ1.532A
SØ1.541A
SØ1.542A
SØ1.551A
SØ1.552A
SØ2.4ØØA
SØ2.4ØØB
SØ2.4Ø1A
SØ2.4Ø1B
SØ2.4Ø2A
SØ2.4Ø2B
SØ2.4ØAA
SØ2.4ØAB
SØ2.4ØBA
SØ2.4ØBB
SØ2.4ØCA
SØ2.4ØCB
SØ2.4ØDA
SØ2.4ØDB
SØ2.4ØEA
SØ2.4ØEB
SØ2.4ØFA
SØ2.4ØFB
SØ2.411A
SØ2.411B
SØ2.412A
SØ2.412B
SØ2.413A
SØ2.413B
SØ2.5XXA
SØ2.5XXB
SØ2.6ØØA
SØ2.6ØØB
SØ2.6Ø1A
SØ2.6Ø1B
SØ2.6Ø2A
SØ2.6Ø2B
SØ2.6Ø9A
SØ2.6Ø9B
SØ2.61ØA
SØ2.61ØB
SØ2.611A
SØ2.611B
SØ2.612A
SØ2.612B
SØ2.62ØA
SØ2.62ØB
SØ2.621A
SØ2.621B
SØ2.622A
SØ2.622B
SØ2.63ØA
SØ2.63ØB
SØ2.631A
SØ2.631B
SØ2.632A
SØ2.632B
SØ2.64ØA
SØ2.64ØB
SØ2.641A
SØ2.641B
SØ2.642A
SØ2.642B
SØ2.65ØA
SØ2.65ØB
SØ2.651A
SØ2.651B
SØ2.652A
SØ2.652B
SØ2.66XA
SØ2.66XB
SØ2.67ØA
SØ2.67ØB
SØ2.671A
SØ2.671B
SØ2.672A
SØ2.672B
SØ2.69XA
SØ2.69XB
SØ3.ØØXA
SØ3.Ø1XA
SØ3.Ø2XA
SØ3.Ø3XA
SØ3.2XXA
SØ3.4ØXA
SØ3.41XA
SØ3.42XA
SØ3.43XA
T18.ØXXA

DRG 158
Select principal diagnosis listed under DRG 157

DRG 159
Select principal diagnosis listed under DRG 157

MDC 4

DRG 163
Operating Room Procedures
Ø25N*
Ø25P*
Ø25Q*
Ø25R*
Ø25S*
Ø25T*
Ø25V*
Ø25W*
Ø25XØZZ
Ø25X3ZZ
Ø25X4ZZ
Ø2BN*
Ø2BPØZZ
Ø2BP3ZZ
Ø2BP4ZZ
Ø2BQØZZ
Ø2BQ3ZZ
Ø2BQ4ZZ
Ø2BRØZZ
Ø2BR3ZZ
Ø2BR4ZZ
Ø2BSØZZ
Ø2BS3ZZ
Ø2BS4ZZ
Ø2BTØZZ
Ø2BT3ZZ
Ø2BT4ZZ
Ø2BVØZZ
Ø2BV3ZZ
Ø2BV4ZZ
Ø2BW3ZZ
Ø2BX3ZZ
Ø2CN*
Ø2CP*
Ø2CQ*
Ø2CR*
Ø2CS*
Ø2CT*
Ø2CV*
Ø2HNØØZ
Ø2HNØ2Z
Ø2HNØYZ
Ø2HN3ØZ
Ø2HN3YZ
Ø2HN4ØZ
Ø2HN42Z
Ø2HN4YZ
Ø2JAØZZ
Ø2JYØZZ
Ø2NN*
Ø2QAØZZ
Ø2QP4ZZ
Ø2QQØZZ
Ø2QQ4ZZ
Ø2QRØZZ
Ø2QR4ZZ
Ø2QWØZZ
Ø2QW4ZZ
Ø2QXØZZ
Ø2QX4ZZ
Ø2RP*
Ø2RQ*
Ø2RR*
Ø2RS*
Ø2RT*
Ø2RV*
Ø2RW*
Ø2RXØ7Z
Ø2RXØ8Z
Ø2RXØJZ
Ø2RXØKZ
Ø2RX47Z
Ø2RX48Z
Ø2RX4JZ
Ø2RX4KZ
Ø2TN*
Ø35Ø*
Ø351*
Ø352*
Ø353*
Ø354*
Ø3BØØZZ
Ø3BØ3ZZ
Ø3BØ4ZZ
Ø3B1ØZZ
Ø3B13ZZ
Ø3B14ZZ
Ø3B2ØZZ
Ø3B23ZZ
Ø3B24ZZ
Ø3B3ØZZ
Ø3B33ZZ
Ø3B34ZZ
Ø3B4ØZZ
Ø3B43ZZ
Ø3B44ZZ
Ø3CØ*
Ø3C1*
Ø3C2*
Ø3C3*
Ø3C4*
Ø3L2*
Ø3L3*
Ø3L4*
Ø3RØ*
Ø3R1*
Ø3R2*
Ø3R3*
Ø3R4*
Ø55Ø*
Ø551*
Ø553*
Ø554*
Ø555*
Ø556*
Ø5BØØZZ
Ø5BØ3ZZ
Ø5BØ4ZZ
Ø5B1ØZZ
Ø5B13ZZ
Ø5B14ZZ
Ø5B3ØZZ
Ø5B33ZZ
Ø5B34ZZ
Ø5B4ØZZ
Ø5B43ZZ
Ø5B44ZZ
Ø5B5ØZZ
Ø5B53ZZ
Ø5B54ZZ
Ø5B6ØZZ
Ø5B63ZZ
Ø5B64ZZ
Ø5CØ*
Ø5C1*
Ø5C3*
Ø5C4*
Ø5C5*
Ø5C6*
Ø5L3*
Ø5L4*
Ø5L5*
Ø5L6*
Ø5RØ*
Ø5R1*
Ø5R3*
Ø5R4*
Ø5R5*
Ø5R6*
Ø75K*
Ø75L*
Ø75M*
Ø79KØØZ
Ø79KØZZ
Ø79K4ØZ
Ø79K4ZZ
Ø79LØØZ
Ø79LØZZ
Ø79L4ØZ
Ø79L4ZZ
Ø79MØØZ
Ø79MØZX
Ø79MØZZ
Ø79M3ZX
Ø79M4ØZ
Ø79M4ZX
Ø79M4ZZ
Ø7B8ØZZ
Ø7B83ZZ
Ø7B84ZZ
Ø7B9ØZZ
Ø7B93ZZ
Ø7B94ZZ
Ø7BKØZZ
Ø7BK3ZZ
Ø7BK4ZZ
Ø7BLØZZ
Ø7BL3ZZ
Ø7BL4ZZ
Ø7BM*
Ø7CM*
Ø7HKØ1Z
Ø7HKØYZ
Ø7HK41Z
Ø7HK4YZ
Ø7HLØ1Z
Ø7HLØYZ
Ø7HL41Z
Ø7HL4YZ
Ø7HMØ1Z
Ø7HMØYZ
Ø7HM41Z
Ø7HM4YZ
Ø7JMØZZ
Ø7JM4ZZ
Ø7LK*
Ø7LL*
Ø7NK*
Ø7NL*
Ø7NM*
Ø7PKØØZ
Ø7PKØ3Z
Ø7PKØCZ
Ø7PKØDZ
Ø7PKØYZ
Ø7PK3ØZ
Ø7PK33Z
Ø7PK3CZ
Ø7PK3DZ
Ø7PK4ØZ
Ø7PK43Z
Ø7PK4CZ
Ø7PK4DZ
Ø7PLØØZ
Ø7PLØ3Z
Ø7PLØCZ
Ø7PLØDZ
Ø7PLØYZ
Ø7PL3ØZ
Ø7PL33Z
Ø7PL3CZ
Ø7PL3DZ
Ø7PL4ØZ
Ø7PL43Z
Ø7PL4CZ
Ø7PL4DZ
Ø7PMØØZ
Ø7PMØ3Z
Ø7PMØYZ
Ø7PM3ØZ
Ø7PM33Z
Ø7PM4ØZ
Ø7PM43Z
Ø7QK*
Ø7QL*
Ø7QM*
Ø7SMØZZ
Ø7TD*
Ø7TK*
Ø7TL*
Ø7TM*
Ø7UK*
Ø7UL*
Ø7VK*
Ø7VL*
Ø7WKØØZ
Ø7WKØ3Z
Ø7WKØCZ
Ø7WKØDZ
Ø7WKØYZ
Ø7WK3ØZ
Ø7WK33Z
Ø7WK3CZ
Ø7WK3DZ
Ø7WK4ØZ
Ø7WK43Z
Ø7WK4CZ
Ø7WK4DZ
Ø7WLØØZ
Ø7WLØ3Z
Ø7WLØCZ
Ø7WLØDZ
Ø7WLØYZ
Ø7WL3ØZ
Ø7WL33Z
Ø7WL3CZ

Ø7WL3DZ
Ø7WL4ØZ
Ø7WL43Z
Ø7WL4CZ
Ø7WL4DZ
Ø7WMØØZ
Ø7WMØ3Z
Ø7WMØYZ
Ø7WM3ØZ
Ø7WM33Z
Ø7WM4ØZ
Ø7WM43Z
Ø7YM*
ØB53ØZZ
ØB533ZZ
ØB537ZZ
ØB538ZZ
ØB54ØZZ
ØB543ZZ
ØB547ZZ
ØB548ZZ
ØB55ØZZ
ØB553ZZ
ØB557ZZ
ØB558ZZ
ØB56ØZZ
ØB563ZZ
ØB567ZZ
ØB568ZZ
ØB57ØZZ
ØB573ZZ
ØB577ZZ
ØB578ZZ
ØB58ØZZ
ØB583ZZ
ØB587ZZ
ØB588ZZ
ØB59ØZZ
ØB593ZZ
ØB597ZZ
ØB598ZZ
ØB5BØZZ
ØB5B3ZZ
ØB5B7ZZ
ØB5B8ZZ
ØB5CØZ3
ØB5CØZZ
ØB5C4Z3
ØB5C4ZZ
ØB5C7ZZ
ØB5DØZ3
ØB5DØZZ
ØB5D4Z3
ØB5D4ZZ
ØB5D7ZZ
ØB5FØZ3
ØB5FØZZ
ØB5F4Z3
ØB5F4ZZ
ØB5F7ZZ
ØB5GØZ3
ØB5GØZZ
ØB5G4Z3
ØB5G4ZZ
ØB5G7ZZ
ØB5HØZ3
ØB5HØZZ
ØB5H4Z3
ØB5H4ZZ
ØB5H7ZZ
ØB5JØZ3
ØB5JØZZ
ØB5J4Z3
ØB5J4ZZ
ØB5J7ZZ
ØB5KØZ3
ØB5KØZZ
ØB5K4Z3
ØB5K4ZZ
ØB5K7ZZ
ØB5LØZ3
ØB5LØZZ
ØB5L4Z3
ØB5L4ZZ
ØB5L7ZZ
ØB5MØZ3
ØB5MØZZ
ØB5M4Z3
ØB5M4ZZ
ØB5M7ZZ
ØB5N*
ØB5P*
ØB5TØZZ
ØB5T3ZZ
ØB5T4ZZ
ØB93ØØZ
ØB93ØZX
ØB93ØZZ
ØB933ØZ
ØB933ZZ
ØB934ØZ
ØB934ZZ
ØB94ØØZ
ØB94ØZX
ØB94ØZZ
ØB943ØZ
ØB943ZZ
ØB944ØZ
ØB944ZZ
ØB95ØØZ
ØB95ØZX
ØB95ØZZ
ØB953ØZ
ØB953ZZ
ØB954ØZ
ØB954ZZ
ØB96ØØZ
ØB96ØZX
ØB96ØZZ
ØB963ØZ
ØB963ZZ
ØB964ØZ
ØB964ZZ
ØB97ØØZ
ØB97ØZX
ØB97ØZZ
ØB973ØZ
ØB973ZZ
ØB974ØZ
ØB974ZZ
ØB98ØØZ
ØB98ØZX
ØB98ØZZ
ØB983ØZ
ØB983ZZ
ØB984ØZ
ØB984ZZ
ØB99ØØZ
ØB99ØZX
ØB99ØZZ
ØB993ØZ
ØB993ZZ
ØB994ØZ
ØB994ZZ
ØB9BØØZ
ØB9BØZX
ØB9BØZZ
ØB9B3ØZ
ØB9B3ZZ
ØB9B4ØZ
ØB9B4ZZ
ØB9CØØZ
ØB9CØZX
ØB9CØZZ
ØB9DØØZ
ØB9DØZX
ØB9DØZZ
ØB9FØØZ
ØB9FØZX
ØB9FØZZ
ØB9GØØZ
ØB9GØZX
ØB9GØZZ
ØB9HØØZ
ØB9HØZX
ØB9HØZZ
ØB9JØØZ
ØB9JØZX
ØB9JØZZ
ØB9KØØZ
ØB9KØZX
ØB9KØZZ
ØB9LØØZ
ØB9LØZX
ØB9LØZZ
ØB9MØØZ
ØB9MØZX
ØB9MØZZ
ØB9TØØZ
ØB9TØZX
ØB9TØZZ
ØBB3ØZX
ØBB3ØZZ
ØBB33ZZ
ØBB37ZZ
ØBB4ØZX
ØBB4ØZZ
ØBB43ZZ
ØBB47ZZ
ØBB5ØZX
ØBB5ØZZ
ØBB53ZZ
ØBB57ZZ
ØBB6ØZX
ØBB6ØZZ
ØBB63ZZ
ØBB67ZZ
ØBB7ØZX
ØBB7ØZZ
ØBB73ZZ
ØBB77ZZ
ØBB8ØZX
ØBB8ØZZ
ØBB83ZZ
ØBB87ZZ
ØBB9ØZX
ØBB9ØZZ
ØBB93ZZ
ØBB97ZZ
ØBBBØZX
ØBBBØZZ
ØBBB3ZZ
ØBBB7ZZ
ØBBCØZX
ØBBCØZZ
ØBBC3ZZ
ØBBC4ZZ
ØBBC7ZZ
ØBBDØZX
ØBBDØZZ
ØBBD3ZZ
ØBBD4ZZ
ØBBD7ZZ
ØBBFØZX
ØBBFØZZ
ØBBF3ZZ
ØBBF4ZZ
ØBBF7ZZ
ØBBGØZX
ØBBGØZZ
ØBBG3ZZ
ØBBG4ZZ
ØBBG7ZZ
ØBBHØZX
ØBBHØZZ
ØBBH3ZZ
ØBBH4ZZ
ØBBH7ZZ
ØBBJØZX
ØBBJØZZ
ØBBJ3ZZ
ØBBJ4ZZ
ØBBJ7ZZ
ØBBKØZX
ØBBKØZZ
ØBBK3ZZ
ØBBK4ZZ
ØBBK7ZZ
ØBBLØZX
ØBBLØZZ
ØBBL3ZZ
ØBBL4ZZ
ØBBL7ZZ
ØBBMØZX
ØBBMØZZ
ØBBM3ZZ
ØBBM7ZZ
ØBBNØZZ
ØBBN3ZZ
ØBBN4ZZ
ØBBN8ZZ
ØBBPØZZ
ØBBP3ZZ
ØBBP4ZZ
ØBBP8ZZ
ØBBTØZX
ØBBTØZZ
ØBBT3ZX
ØBBT3ZZ
ØBBT4ZX
ØBBT4ZZ
ØBC3ØZZ
ØBC33ZZ
ØBC34ZZ
ØBC4ØZZ
ØBC43ZZ
ØBC44ZZ
ØBC5ØZZ
ØBC53ZZ
ØBC54ZZ
ØBC6ØZZ
ØBC63ZZ
ØBC64ZZ
ØBC7ØZZ
ØBC73ZZ
ØBC74ZZ
ØBC8ØZZ
ØBC83ZZ
ØBC84ZZ
ØBC9ØZZ
ØBC93ZZ
ØBC94ZZ
ØBCBØZZ
ØBCB3ZZ
ØBCB4ZZ
ØBCCØZZ
ØBCC3ZZ
ØBCC4ZZ
ØBCC7ZZ
ØBCC8ZZ
ØBCD*
ØBCF*
ØBCG*
ØBCH*
ØBCJ*
ØBCK*
ØBCL*
ØBCM*
ØBCNØZZ
ØBCN4ZZ
ØBCPØZZ
ØBCP4ZZ
ØBCTØZZ
ØBCT3ZZ
ØBCT4ZZ
ØBDNØZX
ØBDNØZZ
ØBDN3ZX
ØBDN3ZZ
ØBDN4ZX
ØBDN4ZZ
ØBDPØZX
ØBDPØZZ
ØBDP3ZX
ØBDP3ZZ
ØBDP4ZX
ØBDP4ZZ
ØBF1ØZZ
ØBF13ZZ
ØBF14ZZ
ØBF17ZZ
ØBF18ZZ
ØBF2ØZZ
ØBF23ZZ
ØBF24ZZ
ØBF27ZZ
ØBF28ZZ
ØBF3ØZZ
ØBF33ZZ
ØBF34ZZ
ØBF4ØZZ
ØBF43ZZ
ØBF44ZZ
ØBF5ØZZ
ØBF53ZZ
ØBF54ZZ
ØBF6ØZZ
ØBF63ZZ
ØBF64ZZ
ØBF7ØZZ
ØBF73ZZ
ØBF74ZZ
ØBF8ØZZ
ØBF83ZZ
ØBF84ZZ
ØBF9ØZZ
ØBF93ZZ
ØBF94ZZ
ØBFBØZZ
ØBFB3ZZ
ØBFB4ZZ
ØBHØØ2Z
ØBHØØ3Z
ØBHØØDZ
ØBHØØYZ
ØBHØ32Z
ØBHØ33Z
ØBHØ3DZ
ØBHØ42Z
ØBHØ43Z
ØBHØ4DZ
ØBHØ4YZ
ØBH3ØGZ
ØBH33GZ
ØBH34GZ
ØBH37GZ
ØBH4ØGZ
ØBH43GZ
ØBH44GZ
ØBH47GZ
ØBH5ØGZ
ØBH53GZ
ØBH54GZ
ØBH57GZ
ØBH6ØGZ
ØBH63GZ
ØBH64GZ
ØBH67GZ
ØBH7ØGZ
ØBH73GZ
ØBH74GZ
ØBH77GZ
ØBH8ØGZ
ØBH83GZ
ØBH84GZ
ØBH87GZ
ØBH9ØGZ
ØBH93GZ
ØBH94GZ
ØBH97GZ
ØBHBØGZ
ØBHB3GZ
ØBHB4GZ
ØBHB7GZ
ØBHKØ2Z
ØBHKØ3Z
ØBHKØYZ
ØBHK32Z
ØBHK33Z
ØBHK42Z
ØBHK43Z
ØBHK4YZ
ØBHK8YZ
ØBHLØ2Z
ØBHLØ3Z
ØBHLØYZ
ØBHL32Z
ØBHL33Z
ØBHL42Z
ØBHL43Z
ØBHL4YZ
ØBHL8YZ
ØBHQØYZ
ØBHQ4YZ
ØBHQ8YZ
ØBHTØ2Z
ØBHTØMZ
ØBHTØYZ
ØBHT32Z
ØBHT3MZ
ØBHT42Z
ØBHT4MZ
ØBHT4YZ
ØBL3*
ØBL4*
ØBL5*
ØBL6*
ØBL7*
ØBL8*
ØBL9*
ØBLB*
ØBM*
ØBN3*
ØBN4*
ØBN5*
ØBN6*
ØBN7*
ØBN8*
ØBN9*
ØBNB*
ØBNC*
ØBND*
ØBNF*
ØBNG*
ØBNH*
ØBNJ*
ØBNK*
ØBNL*
ØBNM*
ØBNTØZZ
ØBNT3ZZ
ØBNT4ZZ
ØBPØØØZ
ØBPØØ1Z
ØBPØØ2Z
ØBPØØCZ
ØBPØØDZ
ØBPØØJZ
ØBPØØKZ
ØBPØØYZ
ØBPØ3ØZ
ØBPØ31Z
ØBPØ32Z
ØBPØ3CZ
ØBPØ3DZ
ØBPØ3JZ
ØBPØ3KZ
ØBPØ4ØZ
ØBPØ41Z
ØBPØ42Z
ØBPØ4CZ
ØBPØ4DZ
ØBPØ4JZ
ØBPØ4KZ
ØBPØ71Z
ØBPØ81Z
ØBPKØØZ
ØBPKØ1Z
ØBPKØ2Z
ØBPKØ3Z
ØBPKØYZ
ØBPK3ØZ
ØBPK31Z
ØBPK32Z
ØBPK33Z
ØBPK4ØZ
ØBPK41Z
ØBPK42Z
ØBPK43Z
ØBPK4YZ
ØBPK8YZ
ØBPLØØZ
ØBPLØ1Z
ØBPLØ2Z
ØBPLØ3Z
ØBPLØYZ
ØBPL3ØZ
ØBPL31Z
ØBPL32Z
ØBPL33Z
ØBPL4ØZ
ØBPL41Z
ØBPL42Z
ØBPL43Z
ØBPL4YZ
ØBPL71Z
ØBPL81Z
ØBPL8YZ
ØBPQØYZ
ØBPQ4YZ
ØBPQ8YZ
ØBPTØØZ
ØBPTØ2Z
ØBPTØ7Z
ØBPTØJZ
ØBPTØKZ
ØBPTØMZ
ØBPTØYZ
ØBPT3ØZ
ØBPT32Z
ØBPT37Z
ØBPT3JZ
ØBPT3KZ
ØBPT3MZ
ØBPT4ØZ
ØBPT42Z
ØBPT47Z
ØBPT4JZ
ØBPT4KZ
ØBPT4MZ
ØBPT4YZ
ØBPT77Z
ØBPT7JZ
ØBPT7KZ
ØBPT7MZ
ØBPT87Z
ØBPT8JZ
ØBPT8KZ
ØBPT8MZ
ØBQ*
ØBR1Ø7Z
ØBR1ØJZ
ØBR1ØKZ
ØBR147Z
ØBR14JZ
ØBR14KZ
ØBR2Ø7Z
ØBR2ØJZ
ØBR2ØKZ
ØBR247Z
ØBR24JZ
ØBR24KZ
ØBR3Ø7Z
ØBR3ØJZ
ØBR3ØKZ
ØBR347Z
ØBR34JZ
ØBR34KZ
ØBR4Ø7Z
ØBR4ØJZ
ØBR4ØKZ
ØBR447Z
ØBR44JZ
ØBR44KZ
ØBR5Ø7Z
ØBR5ØJZ
ØBR5ØKZ
ØBR547Z
ØBR54JZ
ØBR54KZ
ØBR6Ø7Z
ØBR6ØJZ
ØBR6ØKZ
ØBR647Z
ØBR64JZ
ØBR64KZ
ØBR7Ø7Z
ØBR7ØJZ
ØBR7ØKZ
ØBR747Z
ØBR74JZ
ØBR74KZ
ØBR8Ø7Z
ØBR8ØJZ
ØBR8ØKZ
ØBR847Z
ØBR84JZ
ØBR84KZ
ØBR9Ø7Z
ØBR9ØJZ
ØBR9ØKZ
ØBR947Z
ØBR94JZ
ØBR94KZ
ØBRBØ7Z
ØBRBØJZ
ØBRBØKZ
ØBRB47Z
ØBRB4JZ
ØBRB4KZ
ØBRTØ7Z
ØBRTØJZ
ØBRTØKZ
ØBRT47Z
ØBRT4JZ
ØBRT4KZ
ØBS*
ØBT1*
ØBT2*
ØBT3*
ØBT4*
ØBT5*
ØBT6*
ØBT7*
ØBT8*
ØBT9*
ØBTB*
ØBTC*
ØBTD*
ØBTF*
ØBTG*
ØBTH*
ØBTJ*
ØBTK*
ØBTL*
ØBTM*
ØBU*
ØBV*
ØBWØØØZ
ØBWØØ2Z
ØBWØØCZ
ØBWØØDZ
ØBWØØJZ
ØBWØØKZ
ØBWØØYZ
ØBWØ3ØZ
ØBWØ32Z
ØBWØ3CZ
ØBWØ3DZ
ØBWØ3JZ
ØBWØ3KZ
ØBWØ4ØZ
ØBWØ42Z
ØBWØ4CZ
ØBWØ4DZ
ØBWØ4JZ
ØBWØ4KZ
ØBWØ7ØZ
ØBWØ8ØZ
ØBWKØØZ
ØBWKØ2Z
ØBWKØ3Z
ØBWKØYZ
ØBWK3ØZ
ØBWK32Z
ØBWK33Z
ØBWK4ØZ
ØBWK42Z
ØBWK43Z
ØBWK4YZ
ØBWK8YZ
ØBWLØØZ
ØBWLØ2Z
ØBWLØ3Z
ØBWLØYZ
ØBWL3ØZ
ØBWL32Z
ØBWL33Z
ØBWL4ØZ
ØBWL42Z
ØBWL43Z
ØBWL4YZ
ØBWL8YZ
ØBWQ4YZ
ØBWQ8YZ
ØBWTØØZ
ØBWTØ2Z
ØBWTØ7Z
ØBWTØJZ
ØBWTØKZ
ØBWTØMZ
ØBWTØYZ
ØBWT3ØZ
ØBWT32Z
ØBWT37Z
ØBWT3JZ
ØBWT3KZ
ØBWT3MZ
ØBWT4ØZ
ØBWT42Z
ØBWT47Z
ØBWT4JZ
ØBWT4KZ
ØBWT4MZ
ØBWT4YZ
ØBWT7ØZ
ØBWT72Z
ØBWT77Z
ØBWT7JZ
ØBWT7KZ
ØBWT7MZ
ØBWT8ØZ
ØBWT82Z
ØBWT87Z
ØBWT8JZ
ØBWT8KZ
ØBWT8MZ
ØPHØØØZ
ØPHØØ4Z
ØPHØ4ØZ
ØPHØ44Z
ØPH144Z
ØPH2Ø4Z
ØPH244Z
ØPQØØZZ
ØPQØ4ZZ
ØPS1ØZZ
ØPS144Z
ØPS2Ø4Z
ØPS2ØZZ
ØPS244Z
ØPTØØZZ
ØPT1ØZZ
ØPT2ØZZ
ØW337ZZ
ØW338ZZ
ØW33XZZ
ØW38*
ØW39*
ØW3B*
ØW3D*
ØW3Q*
ØW9DØØZ
ØW9DØZX
ØW9DØZZ
ØW9D4ØZ
ØW9D4ZX
ØW9D4ZZ
ØWCDØZZ
ØWCD3ZZ
ØWCD4ZZ
ØWHDØ3Z
ØWHDØYZ
ØWHD33Z
ØWHD3YZ
ØWHD43Z
ØWHD4YZ
ØWJ9ØZZ
ØWJBØZZ
ØWJCØZZ
ØWJQØZZ
ØWPDØØZ
ØWPDØ1Z
ØWPDØ3Z
ØWPDØYZ
ØWPD3ØZ
ØWPD31Z
ØWPD33Z
ØWPD3YZ
ØWPD4ØZ
ØWPD41Z
ØWPD43Z
ØWPD4YZ
ØWU8*
ØWWDØØZ
ØWWDØ1Z
ØWWDØ3Z
ØWWDØYZ
ØWWD3ØZ
ØWWD31Z
ØWWD33Z
ØWWD3YZ
ØWWD4ØZ
ØWWD41Z
ØWWD43Z
ØWWD4YZ
X2CQ3T7
X2CR3T7
X2CY3T7
X2RXØN7

OR

Nonoperating Room Procedures

ØBH38GZ
ØBH48GZ
ØBH58GZ
ØBH68GZ
ØBH78GZ
ØBH88GZ
ØBH98GZ
ØBHB8GZ

DRG 164

Select operating room procedures OR nonoperating room procedures listed under DRG 163

DRG 165

Select operating room procedures OR nonoperating room procedures listed under DRG 163

DRG 166

Operating Room Procedures

ØØ8Q*
Ø21PØ8A
Ø21PØ8B
Ø21PØ8D
Ø21PØ9A
Ø21PØ9B
Ø21PØ9D
Ø21PØAA
Ø21PØAB
Ø21PØAD
Ø21PØJA
Ø21PØJB
Ø21PØJD
Ø21PØKA
Ø21PØKB
Ø21PØKD
Ø21PØZA
Ø21PØZB
Ø21PØZD
Ø21P48A
Ø21P48B
Ø21P48D
Ø21P49A
Ø21P49B
Ø21P49D
Ø21P4AA
Ø21P4AB
Ø21P4AD
Ø21P4JA
Ø21P4JB
Ø21P4JD
Ø21P4KA
Ø21P4KB
Ø21P4KD
Ø21P4ZA
Ø21P4ZB

Ø21P4ZD
Ø21QØ8A
Ø21QØ8B
Ø21QØ8D
Ø21QØ9A
Ø21QØ9B
Ø21QØ9D
Ø21QØAA
Ø21QØAB
Ø21QØAD
Ø21QØJA
Ø21QØJB
Ø21QØJD
Ø21QØKA
Ø21QØKB
Ø21QØKD
Ø21QØZA
Ø21QØZB
Ø21QØZD
Ø21Q48A
Ø21Q48B
Ø21Q48D
Ø21Q49A
Ø21Q49B
Ø21Q49D
Ø21Q4AA
Ø21Q4AB
Ø21Q4AD
Ø21Q4JA
Ø21Q4JB
Ø21Q4JD
Ø21Q4KA
Ø21Q4KB
Ø21Q4KD
Ø21Q4ZA
Ø21Q4ZB
Ø21Q4ZD
Ø21RØ8A
Ø21RØ8B
Ø21RØ8D
Ø21RØ9A
Ø21RØ9B
Ø21RØ9D
Ø21RØAA
Ø21RØAB
Ø21RØAD
Ø21RØJA
Ø21RØJB
Ø21RØJD
Ø21RØKA
Ø21RØKB
Ø21RØKD
Ø21RØZA
Ø21RØZB
Ø21RØZD
Ø21R48A
Ø21R48B
Ø21R48D
Ø21R49A
Ø21R49B
Ø21R49D
Ø21R4AA
Ø21R4AB
Ø21R4AD
Ø21R4JA
Ø21R4JB
Ø21R4JD
Ø21R4KA
Ø21R4KB
Ø21R4KD
Ø21R4ZA
Ø21R4ZB
Ø21R4ZD
Ø2FP3ZØ
Ø2FP3ZZ
Ø2FQ3ZØ
Ø2FQ3ZZ
Ø2FR3ZØ
Ø2FR3ZZ
Ø2FS3ZØ
Ø2FS3ZZ
Ø2FT3ZØ
Ø2FT3ZZ
Ø2HVØ2Z
Ø2HVØDZ
Ø2HV3DZ
Ø2HV42Z
Ø2HV4DZ
Ø2JA4ZZ
Ø2JY4ZZ
Ø2LPØCZ
Ø2LPØDZ
Ø2LPØZZ
Ø2LP3CZ
Ø2LP3DZ
Ø2LP3ZZ
Ø2LP4CZ
Ø2LP4DZ
Ø2LP4ZZ
Ø2LQØCZ
Ø2LQØDZ
Ø2LQØZZ
Ø2LQ3CZ
Ø2LQ3DZ
Ø2LQ3ZZ
Ø2LQ4CZ
Ø2LQ4DZ
Ø2LQ4ZZ
Ø2LRØCZ
Ø2LRØDZ
Ø2LRØZZ
Ø2LR3CZ
Ø2LR3DZ
Ø2LR3ZZ
Ø2LR4CZ
Ø2LR4DZ
Ø2LR4ZZ
Ø2LV*
Ø2QPØZZ
Ø2QP3ZZ
Ø2QQ3ZZ
Ø2QR3ZZ
Ø2QW3ZZ
Ø2QX3ZZ
Ø2VV*
315Ø9Ø
Ø315ØAØ
Ø315ØJØ
Ø315ØKØ
Ø315ØZØ
316Ø91
Ø316ØA1
Ø316ØJ1
Ø316ØK1
Ø316ØZ1
Ø31HØ9J
Ø31HØ9Y
Ø31HØAJ
Ø31HØAY
Ø31HØJJ
Ø31HØJY
Ø31HØKJ
Ø31HØKY
Ø31HØZJ
Ø31HØZY
Ø31JØ9K
Ø31JØ9Y
Ø31JØAK
Ø31JØAY
Ø31JØJK
Ø31JØJY
Ø31JØKK
Ø31JØKY
Ø31JØZK
Ø31JØZY
Ø31KØ9J
Ø31KØAJ
Ø31KØJJ
Ø31KØKJ
Ø31KØZJ
Ø31LØ9K
Ø31LØAK
Ø31LØJK
Ø31LØKK
Ø31LØZK
Ø31MØ9J
Ø31MØAJ
Ø31MØJJ
Ø31MØKJ
Ø31MØZJ
Ø31NØ9K
Ø31NØAK
Ø31NØJK
Ø31NØKK
Ø31NØZK
Ø37334Z
Ø37335Z
Ø37336Z
Ø37337Z
Ø3733D1
Ø3733DZ
Ø3733EZ
Ø3733FZ
Ø3733GZ
Ø3733Z1
Ø3733ZZ
Ø37434Z
Ø37435Z
Ø37436Z
Ø37437Z
Ø3743D1
Ø3743DZ
Ø3743EZ
Ø3743FZ
Ø3743GZ
Ø3743Z1
Ø3743ZZ
Ø37734Z
Ø37735Z
Ø37736Z
Ø37737Z
Ø3773D1
Ø3773DZ
Ø3773EZ
Ø3773FZ
Ø3773GZ
Ø3773Z1
Ø3773ZZ
Ø37834Z
Ø37835Z
Ø37836Z
Ø37837Z
Ø3783D1
Ø3783DZ
Ø3783EZ
Ø3783FZ
Ø3783GZ
Ø3783Z1
Ø3783ZZ
Ø37934Z
Ø37935Z
Ø37936Z
Ø37937Z
Ø3793D1
Ø3793DZ
Ø3793EZ
Ø3793FZ
Ø3793GZ
Ø3793Z1
Ø3793ZZ
Ø37A34Z
Ø37A35Z
Ø37A36Z
Ø37A37Z
Ø37A3D1
Ø37A3DZ
Ø37A3EZ
Ø37A3FZ
Ø37A3GZ
Ø37A3Z1
Ø37A3ZZ
Ø37Y34Z
Ø37Y35Z
Ø37Y36Z
Ø37Y37Z
Ø37Y3DZ
Ø37Y3EZ
Ø37Y3FZ
Ø37Y3GZ
Ø37Y3ZZ
Ø39SØZX
Ø39S4ZX
Ø39TØZX
Ø39T4ZX
Ø3BSØZX
Ø3BS3ZX
Ø3BS4ZX
Ø3BTØZX
Ø3BT3ZX
Ø3BT4ZX
Ø3F23ZØ
Ø3F23ZZ
Ø3HØØDZ
Ø3HØ3DZ
Ø3HØ4DZ
Ø3H1ØDZ
Ø3H13DZ
Ø3H14DZ
Ø3H3ØDZ
Ø3H33DZ
Ø3H34DZ
Ø3H4ØDZ
Ø3H43DZ
Ø3H44DZ
Ø3H5ØDZ
Ø3H53DZ
Ø3H54DZ
Ø3H6ØDZ
Ø3H63DZ
Ø3H64DZ
Ø3LYØDZ
Ø3LY3DZ
Ø3LY4DZ
Ø3QØ*
Ø3Q1*
Ø3Q2*
Ø3Q3*
Ø3Q4*
Ø41KØ9H
Ø41KØ9J
Ø41KØ9K
Ø41KØ9L
Ø41KØAH
Ø41KØAJ
Ø41KØAK
Ø41KØAL
Ø41KØJH
Ø41KØJJ
Ø41KØJK
Ø41KØJL
Ø41KØKH
Ø41KØKJ
Ø41KØKK
Ø41KØKL
Ø41KØZH
Ø41KØZJ
Ø41KØZK
Ø41KØZL
Ø41K49H
Ø41K49J
Ø41K49K
Ø41K49L
Ø41K4AH
Ø41K4AJ
Ø41K4AK
Ø41K4AL
Ø41K4JH
Ø41K4JJ
Ø41K4JK
Ø41K4JL
Ø41K4KH
Ø41K4KJ
Ø41K4KK
Ø41K4KL
Ø41K4ZH
Ø41K4ZJ
Ø41K4ZK
Ø41K4ZL
Ø41LØ9H
Ø41LØ9J
Ø41LØ9K
Ø41LØ9L
Ø41LØAH
Ø41LØAJ
Ø41LØAK
Ø41LØAL
Ø41LØJH
Ø41LØJJ
Ø41LØJK
Ø41LØJL
Ø41LØKH
Ø41LØKJ
Ø41LØKK
Ø41LØKL
Ø41LØZH
Ø41LØZJ
Ø41LØZK
Ø41LØZL
Ø41L49H
Ø41L49J
Ø41L49K
Ø41L49L
Ø41L4AH
Ø41L4AJ
Ø41L4AK
Ø41L4AL
Ø41L4JH
Ø41L4JJ
Ø41L4JK
Ø41L4JL
Ø41L4KH
Ø41L4KJ
Ø41L4KK
Ø41L4KL
Ø41L4ZH
Ø41L4ZJ
Ø41L4ZK
Ø41L4ZL
47Ø341
Ø47Ø34Z
Ø47Ø35Z
Ø47Ø36Z
Ø47Ø37Z
Ø47Ø3D1
Ø47Ø3DZ
Ø47Ø3EZ
Ø47Ø3FZ
Ø47Ø3GZ
Ø47Ø3Z1
Ø47Ø3ZZ
471341
Ø47134Z
Ø47135Z
Ø47136Z
Ø47137Z
Ø4713D1
Ø4713DZ
Ø4713EZ
Ø4713FZ
Ø4713GZ
Ø4713Z1
Ø4713ZZ
472341
Ø47234Z
Ø47235Z
Ø47236Z
Ø47237Z
Ø4723D1
Ø4723DZ
Ø4723EZ
Ø4723FZ
Ø4723GZ
Ø4723Z1
Ø4723ZZ
473341
Ø47334Z
Ø47335Z
Ø47336Z
Ø47337Z
Ø4733D1
Ø4733DZ
Ø4733EZ
Ø4733FZ
Ø4733GZ
Ø4733Z1
Ø4733ZZ
474341
Ø47434Z
Ø47435Z
Ø47436Z
Ø47437Z
Ø4743D1
Ø4743DZ
Ø4743EZ
Ø4743FZ
Ø4743GZ
Ø4743Z1
Ø4743ZZ
475341
Ø47534Z
Ø47535Z
Ø47536Z
Ø47537Z
Ø4753D1
Ø4753DZ
Ø4753EZ
Ø4753FZ
Ø4753GZ
Ø4753Z1
Ø4753ZZ
476341
Ø47634Z
Ø47635Z
Ø47636Z
Ø47637Z
Ø4763D1
Ø4763DZ
Ø4763EZ
Ø4763FZ
Ø4763GZ
Ø4763Z1
Ø4763ZZ
477341
Ø47734Z
Ø47735Z
Ø47736Z
Ø47737Z
Ø4773D1
Ø4773DZ
Ø4773EZ
Ø4773FZ
Ø4773GZ
Ø4773Z1
Ø4773ZZ
478341
Ø47834Z
Ø47835Z
Ø47836Z
Ø47837Z
Ø4783D1
Ø4783DZ
Ø4783EZ
Ø4783FZ
Ø4783GZ
Ø4783Z1
Ø4783ZZ
479341
Ø47934Z
Ø47935Z
Ø47936Z
Ø47937Z
Ø4793D1
Ø4793DZ
Ø4793EZ
Ø4793FZ
Ø4793GZ
Ø4793Z1
Ø4793ZZ
Ø47A341
Ø47A34Z
Ø47A35Z
Ø47A36Z
Ø47A37Z
Ø47A3D1
Ø47A3DZ
Ø47A3EZ
Ø47A3FZ
Ø47A3GZ
Ø47A3Z1
Ø47A3ZZ
Ø47B341
Ø47B34Z
Ø47B35Z
Ø47B36Z
Ø47B37Z
Ø47B3D1
Ø47B3DZ
Ø47B3EZ
Ø47B3FZ
Ø47B3GZ
Ø47B3Z1
Ø47B3ZZ
Ø47C341
Ø47C34Z
Ø47C35Z
Ø47C36Z
Ø47C37Z
Ø47C3D1
Ø47C3DZ
Ø47C3EZ
Ø47C3FZ
Ø47C3GZ
Ø47C3Z1
Ø47C3ZZ
Ø47D341
Ø47D34Z
Ø47D35Z
Ø47D36Z
Ø47D37Z
Ø47D3D1
Ø47D3DZ
Ø47D3EZ
Ø47D3FZ
Ø47D3GZ
Ø47D3Z1
Ø47D3ZZ
Ø47E341
Ø47E34Z
Ø47E35Z
Ø47E36Z
Ø47E37Z
Ø47E3D1
Ø47E3DZ
Ø47E3EZ
Ø47E3FZ
Ø47E3GZ
Ø47E3Z1
Ø47E3ZZ
Ø47F341
Ø47F34Z
Ø47F35Z
Ø47F36Z
Ø47F37Z
Ø47F3D1
Ø47F3DZ
Ø47F3EZ
Ø47F3FZ
Ø47F3GZ
Ø47F3Z1
Ø47F3ZZ
Ø47H341
Ø47H34Z
Ø47H35Z
Ø47H36Z
Ø47H37Z
Ø47H3D1
Ø47H3DZ
Ø47H3EZ
Ø47H3FZ
Ø47H3GZ
Ø47H3Z1
Ø47H3ZZ
Ø47J341
Ø47J34Z
Ø47J35Z
Ø47J36Z
Ø47J37Z
Ø47J3D1
Ø47J3DZ
Ø47J3EZ
Ø47J3FZ
Ø47J3GZ
Ø47J3Z1
Ø47J3ZZ
Ø47KØ41
Ø47KØD1
Ø47KØZ1
Ø47K341
Ø47K34Z
Ø47K35Z
Ø47K36Z
Ø47K37Z
Ø47K3D1
Ø47K3DZ
Ø47K3EZ
Ø47K3FZ
Ø47K3GZ
Ø47K3Z1
Ø47K3ZZ
Ø47K441
Ø47K4D1
Ø47K4Z1
Ø47LØ41
Ø47LØD1
Ø47LØZ1
Ø47L341
Ø47L34Z
Ø47L35Z
Ø47L36Z
Ø47L37Z
Ø47L3D1
Ø47L3DZ
Ø47L3EZ
Ø47L3FZ
Ø47L3GZ
Ø47L3Z1
Ø47L3ZZ
Ø47L441
Ø47L4D1
Ø47L4Z1
Ø47MØ41
Ø47MØD1
Ø47MØZ1
Ø47M341
Ø47M3D1
Ø47M3Z1
Ø47M441
Ø47M4D1
Ø47M4Z1
Ø47NØ41
Ø47NØD1
Ø47NØZ1
Ø47N341
Ø47N3D1
Ø47N3Z1
Ø47N441
Ø47N4D1
Ø47N4Z1
Ø47Y341
Ø47Y34Z
Ø47Y35Z
Ø47Y36Z
Ø47Y37Z
Ø47Y3D1
Ø47Y3DZ
Ø47Y3EZ
Ø47Y3FZ
Ø47Y3GZ
Ø47Y3Z1
Ø47Y3ZZ
Ø5793D1
Ø5793DZ
Ø5793Z1
Ø5793ZZ
Ø57A3D1
Ø57A3DZ
Ø57A3Z1
Ø57A3ZZ
Ø57B3D1
Ø57B3DZ
Ø57B3Z1
Ø57B3ZZ
Ø57C3D1
Ø57C3DZ
Ø57C3Z1
Ø57C3ZZ
Ø57D3D1
Ø57D3DZ
Ø57D3Z1
Ø57D3ZZ
Ø57F3D1
Ø57F3DZ
Ø57F3Z1
Ø57F3ZZ
Ø5HØØDZ
Ø5HØ3DZ
Ø5HØ4DZ
Ø5H1ØDZ
Ø5H13DZ
Ø5H14DZ
Ø5H3ØDZ
Ø5H33DZ
Ø5H34DZ
Ø5H4ØDZ
Ø5H43DZ
Ø5H44DZ
Ø5H5ØDZ
Ø5H53DZ
Ø5H54DZ
Ø5H6ØDZ
Ø5H63DZ
Ø5H64DZ
Ø5HYØDZ
Ø5HY3DZ
Ø5HY4DZ
Ø67Ø3DZ
Ø67Ø3ZZ
Ø6HØØDZ
Ø6HØ4DZ
Ø6HYØDZ
Ø6HY3DZ
Ø6HY4DZ
Ø6LØ*
Ø6VØ*
Ø797ØZX
Ø7973ZX
Ø7974ZX
Ø79KØZX
Ø79K3ZX
Ø79K4ZX
Ø7B1ØZZ
Ø7B13ZZ
Ø7B14ZZ
Ø7B2ØZZ
Ø7B23ZZ
Ø7B24ZZ
Ø7B5ØZZ
Ø7B53ZZ
Ø7B54ZZ
Ø7B6ØZZ
Ø7B63ZZ
Ø7B64ZZ
Ø7B7ØZX
Ø7B7ØZZ
Ø7B73ZX
Ø7B74ZX
Ø7B74ZZ
Ø7BHØZZ
Ø7BH3ZZ
Ø7BH4ZZ
Ø7BJØZZ
Ø7BJ3ZZ
Ø7BJ4ZZ
Ø7BKØZX
Ø7BK3ZX
Ø7BK4ZX
Ø7JPØZZ
Ø7TØ*
Ø7T1*
Ø7T2*
Ø7T3*
Ø7T4*
Ø7T7*
Ø7T8*
Ø7T9*
Ø7TB*
Ø7TF*
Ø7TG*
ØB51*
ØB52*
ØB5C3Z3
ØB5C3ZZ
ØB5D3Z3
ØB5D3ZZ
ØB5F3Z3
ØB5F3ZZ
ØB5G3Z3
ØB5G3ZZ
ØB5H3Z3
ØB5H3ZZ
ØB5J3Z3
ØB5J3ZZ
ØB5K3Z3
ØB5K3ZZ
ØB5L3Z3
ØB5L3ZZ
ØB5M3Z3
ØB5M3ZZ
ØB71*
ØB72*
ØB91ØØZ
ØB91ØZX
ØB91ØZZ
ØB913ØZ
ØB913ZZ
ØB914ØZ
ØB914ZZ
ØB92ØØZ
ØB92ØZX
ØB92ØZZ
ØB923ØZ
ØB923ZZ
ØB924ØZ
ØB924ZZ
ØB9C3ØZ
ØB9C3ZZ
ØB9C4ØZ
ØB9C4ZZ
ØB9C7ØZ
ØB9C7ZZ
ØB9C8ØZ
ØB9D3ØZ
ØB9D3ZZ
ØB9D4ØZ
ØB9D4ZZ
ØB9D7ØZ
ØB9D7ZZ
ØB9D8ØZ
ØB9F3ØZ
ØB9F3ZZ
ØB9F4ØZ
ØB9F4ZZ
ØB9F7ØZ
ØB9F7ZZ
ØB9F8ØZ
ØB9G3ØZ
ØB9G3ZZ
ØB9G4ØZ
ØB9G4ZZ
ØB9G7ØZ
ØB9G7ZZ
ØB9G8ØZ
ØB9H3ØZ
ØB9H3ZZ
ØB9H4ØZ
ØB9H4ZZ
ØB9H7ØZ
ØB9H7ZZ
ØB9H8ØZ
ØB9J3ØZ
ØB9J3ZZ
ØB9J4ØZ
ØB9J4ZZ
ØB9J7ØZ
ØB9J7ZZ
ØB9J8ØZ
ØB9K3ØZ
ØB9K3ZZ
ØB9K4ØZ
ØB9K4ZZ
ØB9K7ØZ
ØB9K7ZZ
ØB9K8ØZ
ØB9L3ØZ
ØB9L3ZZ
ØB9L4ØZ
ØB9L4ZZ
ØB9L7ØZ
ØB9L7ZZ
ØB9L8ØZ
ØB9M3ØZ
ØB9M3ZZ
ØB9M4ØZ
ØB9M4ZZ
ØB9M7ØZ
ØB9M7ZZ
ØB9M8ØZ
ØB9N4ØZ
ØB9N4ZZ
ØB9P4ØZ
ØB9P4ZZ
ØBB1ØZX
ØBB1ØZZ
ØBB13ZZ
ØBB14ZZ

ØBB17ZZ
ØBB18ZZ
ØBB2ØZX
ØBB2ØZZ
ØBB23ZZ
ØBB24ZZ
ØBB27ZZ
ØBB28ZZ
ØBBC4ZX
ØBBC7ZX
ØBBC8ZX
ØBBD4ZX
ØBBD7ZX
ØBBD8ZX
ØBBF4ZX
ØBBF7ZX
ØBBF8ZX
ØBBG4ZX
ØBBG7ZX
ØBBG8ZX
ØBBH4ZX
ØBBH7ZX
ØBBH8ZX
ØBBJ4ZX
ØBBJ7ZX
ØBBJ8ZX
ØBBK4ZX
ØBBK7ZX
ØBBK8ZX
ØBBL4ZX
ØBBL7ZX
ØBBL8ZX
ØBBM4ZX
ØBBM7ZX
ØBBM8ZX
ØBBNØZX
ØBBN4ZX
ØBBN8ZX
ØBBPØZX
ØBBP4ZX
ØBBP8ZX
ØBC1ØZZ
ØBC13ZZ
ØBC14ZZ
ØBC2ØZZ
ØBC23ZZ
ØBC24ZZ
ØBHØØ1Z
ØBHØ31Z
ØBHØ41Z
ØBHØ71Z
ØBHØ81Z
ØBH1Ø2Z
ØBH1ØDZ
ØBH1ØYZ
ØBH13DZ
ØBH14DZ
ØBH14YZ
ØBHKØ1Z
ØBHK31Z
ØBHK41Z
ØBHK71Z
ØBHK81Z
ØBHLØ1Z
ØBHL31Z
ØBHL41Z
ØBHL71Z
ØBHL81Z
ØBJØØZZ
ØBJØ4ZZ
ØBJ1ØZZ
ØBJKØZZ
ØBJK4ZZ
ØBJLØZZ
ØBJL4ZZ
ØBJQØZZ
ØBJQ4ZZ
ØBJTØZZ
ØBJT4ZZ
ØBL1*
ØBL2*
ØBN1*
ØBN2*
ØBNN*
ØBNP*
ØBPØØ3Z
ØBPØØ7Z
ØBPØ33Z
ØBPØ37Z
ØBPØ43Z
ØBPØ47Z
ØBPØ77Z
ØBPØ7CZ
ØBPØ7JZ
ØBPØ7KZ
ØBPØ87Z
ØBPØ8CZ
ØBPØ8JZ
ØBPØ8KZ
ØBP1ØØZ
ØBP1Ø2Z
ØBP1Ø7Z
ØBP1ØCZ
ØBP1ØDZ
ØBP1ØJZ
ØBP1ØKZ
ØBP13ØZ
ØBP132Z
ØBP137Z
ØBP13CZ
ØBP13DZ
ØBP13JZ
ØBP13KZ
ØBP14ØZ
ØBP142Z
ØBP147Z
ØBP14CZ
ØBP14DZ
ØBP14JZ
ØBP14KZ
ØBP177Z
ØBP17CZ
ØBP17JZ
ØBP17KZ
ØBP187Z
ØBP18CZ
ØBP18JZ
ØBP18KZ
ØBTTØZZ
ØBTT4ZZ
ØBWØØ3Z
ØBWØØ7Z
ØBWØ33Z
ØBWØ37Z
ØBWØ43Z
ØBWØ47Z
ØBWØ77Z
ØBWØ7CZ
ØBWØ7JZ
ØBWØ7KZ
ØBWØ87Z
ØBWØ8CZ
ØBWØ8JZ
ØBWØ8KZ
ØBW1ØØZ
ØBW1Ø2Z
ØBW1Ø7Z
ØBW1ØCZ
ØBW1ØDZ
ØBW1ØFZ
ØBW1ØJZ
ØBW1ØKZ
ØBW13ØZ
ØBW132Z
ØBW137Z
ØBW13CZ
ØBW13DZ
ØBW13FZ
ØBW13JZ
ØBW13KZ
ØBW14ØZ
ØBW142Z
ØBW147Z
ØBW14CZ
ØBW14DZ
ØBW14FZ
ØBW14JZ
ØBW14KZ
ØBW17ØZ
ØBW172Z
ØBW177Z
ØBW17CZ
ØBW17DZ
ØBW17FZ
ØBW17JZ
ØBW17KZ
ØBW18ØZ
ØBW182Z
ØBW187Z
ØBW18CZ
ØBW18DZ
ØBW18FZ
ØBW18JZ
ØBW18KZ
ØC5R*
ØC5S*
ØC5T*
ØC5V*
ØC7S*
ØC9RØZX
ØC9SØZX
ØC9TØZX
ØC9VØZX
ØCBRØZX
ØCBRØZZ
ØCBR3ZZ
ØCBR4ZZ
ØCBR7ZZ
ØCBR8ZZ
ØCBSØZX
ØCBSØZZ
ØCBS3ZZ
ØCBS4ZZ
ØCBS7ZZ
ØCBS8ZZ
ØCBTØZX
ØCBTØZZ
ØCBT3ZZ
ØCBT4ZZ
ØCBT7ZZ
ØCBT8ZZ
ØCBVØZX
ØCBVØZZ
ØCBV3ZZ
ØCBV4ZZ
ØCBV7ZZ
ØCBV8ZZ
ØCDT*
ØCDV*
ØCNR*
ØCNS*
ØCNT*
ØCNV*
ØCPSØJZ
ØCPS3JZ
ØCPS7JZ
ØCPS8JZ
ØCQR*
ØCQS*
ØCQT*
ØCQV*
ØCRR*
ØCRS*
ØCRT*
ØCRV*
ØCSR*
ØCSSØZZ
ØCSS7ZZ
ØCSS8ZZ
ØCST*
ØCSV*
ØCTR*
ØCTT*
ØCTV*
ØCUR*
ØCUS*
ØCUT*
ØCUV*
ØDJØØZZ
ØDJ6ØZZ
ØDJDØZZ
ØDJUØZZ
ØDJVØZZ
ØDJWØZZ
ØF9ØØZX
ØF91ØZX
ØF92ØZX
ØFBØØZX
ØFB1ØZX
ØFB2ØZX
ØFJØØZZ
ØHR5X72
ØHR5X74
ØHR6X72
ØHR6X74
ØHR7X72
ØHR7X74
ØJBØØZZ
ØJB1ØZZ
ØJB4ØZZ
ØJB5ØZZ
ØJB6ØZZ
ØJB7ØZZ
ØJB8ØZZ
ØJB9ØZZ
ØJBBØZZ
ØJBCØZZ
ØJBDØZZ
ØJBFØZZ
ØJBGØZZ
ØJBHØZZ
ØJBLØZZ
ØJBMØZZ
ØJBNØZZ
ØJBPØZZ
ØJBQØZZ
ØJBRØZZ
ØJH6ØVZ
ØJH6ØWZ
ØJH6ØYZ
ØJH63VZ
ØJH7ØVZ
ØJH7ØYZ
ØJH73VZ
ØJH8ØVZ
ØJH8ØWZ
ØJH8ØYZ
ØJH83VZ
ØJHDØVZ
ØJHDØWZ
ØJHD3VZ
ØJHFØVZ
ØJHFØWZ
ØJHF3VZ
ØJHGØVZ
ØJHGØWZ
ØJHG3VZ
ØJHHØVZ
ØJHHØWZ
ØJHH3VZ
ØJHLØVZ
ØJHLØWZ
ØJHL3VZ
ØJHMØVZ
ØJHMØWZ
ØJHM3VZ
ØJHNØVZ
ØJHN3VZ
ØJHPØVZ
ØJHPØWZ
ØJHP3VZ
ØJHTØVZ
ØJHTØYZ
ØJHT3VZ
ØK9HØZX
ØK9JØZX
ØKBHØZX
ØKBJØZX
ØP5Ø*
ØP51*
ØP52*
ØP55*
ØP56*
ØP57*
ØP58*
ØP59*
ØP5B*
ØP8Ø*
ØP81*
ØP82*
ØP85*
ØP86*
ØP87*
ØP88*
ØP89*
ØP8B*
ØP9ØØZX
ØP9Ø3ZX
ØP9Ø4ZX
ØP91ØZX
ØP913ZX
ØP914ZX
ØP92ØZX
ØP923ZX
ØP924ZX
ØP94ØZX
ØP943ZX
ØP944ZX
ØP95ØZX
ØP953ZX
ØP954ZX
ØP96ØZX
ØP963ZX
ØP964ZX
ØP97ØZX
ØP973ZX
ØP974ZX
ØP98ØZX
ØP983ZX
ØP984ZX
ØP99ØZX
ØP993ZX
ØP994ZX
ØP9BØZX
ØP9B3ZX
ØP9B4ZX
ØPBØ*
ØPB1*
ØPB2*
ØPB4ØZX
ØPB43ZX
ØPB44ZX
ØPB5*
ØPB6*
ØPB7*
ØPB8*
ØPB9*
ØPBB*
ØPCØ*
ØPC1*
ØPC2*
ØPC5*
ØPC6*
ØPC7*
ØPC8*
ØPC9*
ØPCB*
ØPHØ3ØZ
ØPHØ34Z
ØPH1Ø4Z
ØPH134Z
ØPH234Z
ØPH5*
ØPH6*
ØPH7*
ØPH8*
ØPH9*
ØPHB*
ØPHY*
ØPJYØZZ
ØPJY4ZZ
ØPNØ*
ØPN1*
ØPN2*
ØPN5*
ØPN6*
ØPN7*
ØPN8*
ØPN9*
ØPNB*
ØPQØ3ZZ
ØPQ1ØZZ
ØPQ13ZZ
ØPQ14ZZ
ØPQ2ØZZ
ØPQ23ZZ
ØPQ24ZZ
ØPQ5ØZZ
ØPQ53ZZ
ØPQ54ZZ
ØPQ6ØZZ
ØPQ63ZZ
ØPQ64ZZ
ØPQ7ØZZ
ØPQ73ZZ
ØPQ74ZZ
ØPQ8ØZZ
ØPQ83ZZ
ØPQ84ZZ
ØPQ9ØZZ
ØPQ93ZZ
ØPQ94ZZ
ØPQBØZZ
ØPQB3ZZ
ØPQB4ZZ
ØPRØØJZ
ØPRØ3JZ
ØPRØ4JZ
ØPR1ØJZ
ØPR13JZ
ØPR14JZ
ØPR2ØJZ
ØPR23JZ
ØPR24JZ
ØPR5ØJZ
ØPR53JZ
ØPR54JZ
ØPR6ØJZ
ØPR63JZ
ØPR64JZ
ØPR7ØJZ
ØPR73JZ
ØPR74JZ
ØPR8ØJZ
ØPR83JZ
ØPR84JZ
ØPR9ØJZ
ØPR93JZ
ØPR94JZ
ØPRBØJZ
ØPRB3JZ
ØPRB4JZ
ØPSØØØZ
ØPSØ3ØZ
ØPSØ4ØZ
ØPS1Ø4Z
ØPS134Z
ØPS234Z
ØPT5ØZZ
ØPT6ØZZ
ØPT7ØZZ
ØPT8ØZZ
ØPT9ØZZ
ØPTBØZZ
ØPUØØJZ
ØPUØ3JZ
ØPUØ4JZ
ØPU1ØJZ
ØPU13JZ
ØPU14JZ
ØPU2ØJZ
ØPU23JZ
ØPU24JZ
ØPU5ØJZ
ØPU53JZ
ØPU54JZ
ØPU6ØJZ
ØPU63JZ
ØPU64JZ
ØPU7ØJZ
ØPU73JZ
ØPU74JZ
ØPU8ØJZ
ØPU83JZ
ØPU84JZ
ØPU9ØJZ
ØPU93JZ
ØPU94JZ
ØPUBØJZ
ØPUB3JZ
ØPUB4JZ
ØW19ØJ9
ØW19ØJB
ØW19ØJJ
ØW193J9
ØW193JB
ØW193JJ
ØW194J9
ØW194JB
ØW194JJ
ØW1BØJ9
ØW1BØJB
ØW1BØJJ
ØW1B3J9
ØW1B3JB
ØW1B3JJ
ØW1B4J9
ØW1B4JB
ØW1B4JJ
ØW994ØZ
ØW994ZX
ØW994ZZ
ØW9B4ØZ
ØW9B4ZX
ØW9B4ZZ
ØW9CØØZ
ØW9CØZX
ØW9CØZZ
ØW9C4ØZ
ØW9C4ZZ
ØWB6XZ2
ØWB8ØZZ
ØWB83ZZ
ØWB84ZZ
ØWB8XZZ
ØWBCØZX
ØWBCØZZ
ØWBC3ZX
ØWBC3ZZ
ØWBC4ZX
ØWBC4ZZ
ØWCCØZZ
ØWCC3ZZ
ØWCC4ZZ
ØWCQ7ZZ
ØWCQ8ZZ
ØWF9ØZZ
ØWF93ZZ
ØWF94ZZ
ØWFBØZZ
ØWFB3ZZ
ØWFB4ZZ
ØWFCØZZ
ØWFC3ZZ
ØWFC4ZZ
ØWFQØZZ
ØWFQ3ZZ
ØWFQ4ZZ
ØWFQ7ZZ
ØWFQ8ZZ
ØWH8Ø1Z
ØWH831Z
ØWH841Z
ØWH9Ø1Z
ØWH931Z
ØWH941Z
ØWHBØ1Z
ØWHB31Z
ØWHB41Z
ØWHCØ3Z
ØWHCØYZ
ØWHC33Z
ØWHC3YZ
ØWHC43Z
ØWHC4YZ
ØWHQØ1Z
ØWHQ31Z
ØWHQ33Z
ØWHQ3YZ
ØWHQ41Z
ØWHQ43Z
ØWHQ4YZ
ØWHQ71Z
ØWHQ81Z
ØWJ8ØZZ
ØWJ84ZZ
ØWJ94ZZ
ØWJB4ZZ
ØWJC4ZZ
ØWJD4ZZ
ØWJGØZZ
ØWJJØZZ
ØWJPØZZ
ØWJQ4ZZ
ØWJRØZZ
ØWM8ØZZ
ØWPCØØZ
ØWPCØ1Z
ØWPCØ3Z
ØWPCØ7Z
ØWPCØJZ
ØWPCØKZ
ØWPCØYZ
ØWPC3ØZ
ØWPC31Z
ØWPC33Z
ØWPC37Z
ØWPC3JZ
ØWPC3KZ
ØWPC3YZ
ØWPC4ØZ
ØWPC41Z
ØWPC43Z
ØWPC47Z
ØWPC4JZ
ØWPC4KZ
ØWPC4YZ
ØWPQ31Z
ØWPQ33Z
ØWPQ3YZ
ØWPQ41Z
ØWPQ43Z
ØWPQ4YZ
ØWPQ71Z
ØWPQ7YZ
ØWPQ81Z
ØWQ6XZ2
ØWQ8*
ØWQC*
ØWUC*
ØWWCØØZ
ØWWCØ1Z
ØWWCØ3Z
ØWWCØ7Z
ØWWCØJZ
ØWWCØKZ
ØWWCØYZ
ØWWC3ØZ
ØWWC31Z
ØWWC33Z
ØWWC37Z
ØWWC3JZ
ØWWC3KZ
ØWWC3YZ
ØWWC4ØZ
ØWWC41Z
ØWWC43Z
ØWWC47Z
ØWWC4JZ
ØWWC4KZ
ØWWC4YZ
ØWWQ31Z
ØWWQ33Z
ØWWQ3YZ
ØWWQ41Z
ØWWQ43Z
ØWWQ4YZ
ØWWQ71Z
ØWWQ73Z
ØWWQ7YZ
ØWWQ81Z
ØWWQ83Z
ØWWQ8YZ
3EØL4GC
X27H385
X27H395
X27H3B5
X27H3C5
X27J385
X27J395
X27J3B5
X27J3C5
X2H13R9

DRG 167

Select operating room procedures listed under DRG 166

DRG 168

Select operating room procedures listed under DRG 166

DRG 173

Pulmonary Embolism Principal Diagnosis

I26.Ø1
I26.Ø2
I26.Ø9
I26.9Ø
I26.92
I26.93
I26.94
I26.99
I27.82

AND

Operating Room Procedures

Ø2FP3ZØ
Ø2FP3ZZ
Ø2FQ3ZØ
Ø2FQ3ZZ
Ø2FR3ZØ
Ø2FR3ZZ
Ø2FS3ZØ
Ø2FS3ZZ
Ø2FT3ZØ
Ø2FT3ZZ

DRG 175

Principal Diagnosis

I26.9Ø
I26.92
I26.93
I26.94
I26.99
I27.82
T79.ØXXA
T79.1XXA
T8Ø.ØXXA

OR

Acute Cor Pulmonale

I26.Ø1
I26.Ø2
I26.Ø9

DRG 176

Select principal diagnosis listed under DRG 175

DRG 177

Principal Diagnosis

J1Ø.ØØ
J1Ø.Ø1
J1Ø.Ø8
J11.ØØ
J11.Ø8

AND

Secondary Diagnosis

A48.1
J15.Ø
J15.1
J15.2*
J15.5
J15.6*
J15.8

OR

Principal Diagnosis

AØ2.22
AØ6.5
A15*
A2Ø.2
A21.2
A22.1
A31.Ø
A42.Ø
A43.Ø
A48.1
A52.72
BØ1.2
BØ5.2
B25.Ø
B37.1
B38.Ø
B38.1
B38.2
B39.Ø
B39.1
B39.2
B44.Ø
B58.3
B59
B66.4
B67.1
E84.Ø
J15.Ø
J15.1
J15.2*
J15.5
J15.6*
J15.8
J17
J69*
J85*
J86*
J98.5*
R76.1*
UØ7.1

DRG 178

Select principal diagnosis or principal diagnosis and secondary diagnosis combinations listed under DRG 177

DRG 179

Select principal diagnosis or principal diagnosis and secondary diagnosis combinations listed under DRG 177

DRG 180

Principal Diagnosis

C33
C34*
C38.1
C38.2
C38.3
C38.4
C38.8
C39.9
C45.Ø
C46.5*
C76.1
C78.Ø*
C78.1
C78.2
C78.3*
C7A.Ø9Ø
DØ2.1
DØ2.2*
DØ2.3
DØ2.4
D14.2
D14.3*
D14.4
D15.2
D15.7
D15.9
D16.7
D17.4
D19.Ø
D38.1
D38.2
D38.3

D38.4
D38.5
D38.6
D3A.Ø9Ø
D49.1
J91.Ø

DRG 181
Select principal diagnosis listed under DRG 180

DRG 182
Select principal diagnosis listed under DRG 180

DRG 183
Principal Diagnosis
M96.A4
M99.18
S11.Ø21A
S11.Ø22A
S11.Ø23A
S11.Ø24A
S11.Ø25A
S11.Ø29A
S22.31XB
S22.32XB
S22.39XB
S22.41XA
S22.41XB
S22.42XA
S22.42XB
S22.43XA
S22.43XB
S22.49XA
S22.49XB
S22.5XXA
S22.5XXB
S27.331A
S27.332A
S27.339A
S27.4Ø1A
S27.4Ø2A
S27.4Ø9A
S27.411A
S27.412A
S27.419A
S27.421A
S27.422A
S27.429A
S27.431A
S27.432A
S27.439A
S27.491A
S27.492A
S27.499A
S27.8Ø2A
S27.8Ø3A
S27.8Ø8A
S27.8Ø9A
S43.2Ø1A
S43.2Ø2A
S43.2Ø3A
S43.2Ø4A
S43.2Ø5A
S43.2Ø6A
S43.211A
S43.212A
S43.213A
S43.214A
S43.215A
S43.216A
S43.221A
S43.222A
S43.223A
S43.224A
S43.225A
S43.226A

DRG 184
Select principal diagnosis listed under DRG 183

DRG 185
Select principal diagnosis listed under DRG 183

DRG 186
Principal Diagnosis
J9Ø
J91.8
J94.Ø
J94.2
J94.8

DRG 187
Select principal diagnosis listed under DRG 186

DRG 188
Select principal diagnosis listed under DRG 186

DRG 189
Principal Diagnosis
J18.2
J68.1
J8Ø
J81*
J95.1
J95.2
J95.3
J95.82*
J96*

DRG 190
Principal Diagnosis
J41.1
J41.8
J42
J43*
J44*
J47*
J4A.Ø
J4A.8
J4A.9
J68.4
J68.8
J68.9
Q33.4

DRG 191
Select principal diagnosis listed under DRG 190

DRG 192
Select principal diagnosis listed under DRG 190

DRG 193
Principal Diagnosis
B33.Ø
JØ9.X1
JØ9.X2
J1Ø.ØØ
J1Ø.Ø1
J1Ø.Ø8
J1Ø.1
J11.Ø*
J12*
J13
J14
J15.3
J15.4
J15.7
J15.9
J16*
J18.Ø
J18.1
J18.8
J18.9
J92*
J94.1
J94.9
RØ9.1

DRG 194
Select principal diagnosis listed under DRG 193

DRG 195
Select principal diagnosis listed under DRG 193

DRG 196
Principal Diagnosis
B44.81
B9Ø.9
D86*
J6Ø
J61
J62*
J63*
J64
J65
J66*
J67*
J7Ø.1
J82*
J84*
J99
MØ5.1*
M34.81
P27*

DRG 197
Select principal diagnosis listed under DRG 196

DRG 198
Select principal diagnosis listed under DRG 196

DRG 199
Principal Diagnosis
J93*
J95.81*
J98.2
S27.ØXXA
S27.1XXA
S27.2XXA
T79.7XXA

DRG 200
Select principal diagnosis listed under DRG 199

DRG 201
Select principal diagnosis listed under DRG 199

DRG 202
Principal Diagnosis
A37*
JØ4.1*
J2Ø*
J21*
J39.8
J4Ø
J41.Ø
J45*
J98.Ø*

DRG 203
Select principal diagnosis listed under DRG 202

DRG 204
Principal Diagnosis
G47.32
RØ4.2
RØ4.8*
RØ4.9
RØ5*
RØ6.Ø*
RØ6.1
RØ6.2
RØ6.3
RØ6.4
RØ6.6
RØ6.8*
RØ6.9
RØ7.1
RØ7.81
RØ9.3
R91.8

DRG 205
Principal Diagnosis
E66.2
J22
J68.Ø
J68.2
J68.3
J7Ø.Ø
J7Ø.2
J7Ø.3
J7Ø.4
J7Ø.5
J7Ø.8
J7Ø.9
J95.Ø*
J95.4
J95.5
J95.84
J95.851
J95.859
J95.87
J95.88
J95.89
J98.1*
J98.3
J98.4
J98.6
J98.8
J98.9
K76.81
M94.Ø
N8Ø.B1
N8Ø.B2
N8Ø.B31
N8Ø.B32
N8Ø.B39
Q33.Ø
Q33.1
Q33.2
Q33.3
Q33.5
Q33.6
Q33.8
Q33.9
Q34*
Q79.Ø
Q79.1
RØ9.Ø*
RØ9.2
R68.3
R91.1
R94.2
S22.31XA
S22.32XA
S22.39XA
S23.41XA
S23.42ØA
S23.421A
S23.428A
S23.429A
S26.ØØXS
S26.Ø1XS
S26.Ø2ØS
S26.Ø21S
S26.Ø22S
S26.Ø9XS
S26.1ØXS
S26.11XS
S26.12XS
S26.19XS
S26.9ØXS
S26.91XS
S26.92XS
S26.99XS
S27.ØXXS
S27.1XXS
S27.2XXS
S27.3Ø1A
S27.3Ø1S
S27.3Ø2A
S27.3Ø2S
S27.3Ø9A
S27.3Ø9S
S27.311A
S27.311S
S27.312A
S27.312S
S27.319A
S27.319S
S27.321A
S27.321S
S27.322A
S27.322S
S27.329A
S27.329S
S27.331S
S27.332S
S27.339S
S27.391A
S27.391S
S27.392A
S27.392S
S27.399A
S27.399S
S27.4Ø1S
S27.4Ø2S
S27.4Ø9S
S27.411S
S27.412S
S27.419S
S27.421S
S27.422S
S27.429S
S27.431S
S27.432S
S27.439S
S27.491S
S27.492S
S27.499S
S27.5ØXA
S27.5ØXS
S27.51XA
S27.51XS
S27.52XA
S27.52XS
S27.53XA
S27.53XS
S27.59XA
S27.59XS
S27.6ØXA
S27.6ØXS
S27.63XA
S27.63XS
S27.69XA
S27.69XS
S27.8Ø2S
S27.8Ø3S
S27.8Ø8S
S27.8Ø9S
S27.812S
S27.813S
S27.818S
S27.819S
S27.892A
S27.892S
S27.893A
S27.893S
S27.898A
S27.898S
S27.899A
S27.899S
S27.9XXS
T17.4ØØA
T17.4Ø8A
T17.41ØA
T17.418A
T17.42ØA
T17.428A
T17.49ØA
T17.498A
T17.5ØØA
T17.5Ø8A
T17.51ØA
T17.518A
T17.52ØA
T17.528A
T17.59ØA
T17.598A
T17.8ØØA
T17.8Ø8A
T17.81ØA
T17.818A
T17.82ØA
T17.828A
T17.89ØA
T17.898A
T17.9ØØA
T17.9Ø8A
T17.91ØA
T17.918A
T17.92ØA
T17.928A
T17.99ØA
T17.998A
T27.ØXXA
T27.1XXA
T27.2XXA
T27.3XXA
T27.4XXA
T27.5XXA
T27.6XXA
T27.7XXA
T86.81Ø
T86.811
T86.812
T86.818
T86.819
UØ7.Ø
Z43.Ø
Z9Ø.2
Z94.2

DRG 206
Select principal diagnosis listed under DRG 205

DRG 207
Select principal diagnosis from MDC 4
AND
Nonoperating Room Procedure
5A1955Z

DRG 208
Select principal diagnosis from MDC 4
AND
Nonoperating Room Procedures
5A1935Z
5A1945Z

MDC 5

DRG 212
Aortic Valve Operating Room Procedures
Ø2QFØZJ
Ø2QFØZZ
Ø2QF4ZJ
Ø2QF4ZZ
Ø2RFØ7Z
Ø2RFØ8N
Ø2RFØ8Z
Ø2RFØJZ
Ø2RFØKZ
Ø2RF47Z
Ø2RF48N
Ø2RF48Z
Ø2RF4JZ
Ø2RF4KZ
AND
Mitral Valve Operating Room Procedures
Ø2QGØZE
Ø2QGØZZ
Ø2QG4ZE
Ø2QG4ZZ
Ø2RGØ7Z
Ø2RGØ8Z
Ø2RGØJZ
Ø2RGØKZ
Ø2RG47Z
Ø2RG48Z
Ø2RG4JZ
Ø2RG4KZ
AND EITHER
Concomitant Operating Room Procedures
21ØØ83
21ØØ88
21ØØ89
Ø21ØØ8C
Ø21ØØ8F
Ø21ØØ8W
21ØØ93
21ØØ98
21ØØ99
Ø21ØØ9C
Ø21ØØ9F
Ø21ØØ9W
Ø21ØØA3
Ø21ØØA8
Ø21ØØA9
Ø21ØØAC
Ø21ØØAF
Ø21ØØAW
Ø21ØØJ3
Ø21ØØJ8
Ø21ØØJ9
Ø21ØØJC
Ø21ØØJF
Ø21ØØJW
Ø21ØØK3
Ø21ØØK8
Ø21ØØK9
Ø21ØØKC
Ø21ØØKF
Ø21ØØKW
Ø21ØØZ3
Ø21ØØZ8
Ø21ØØZ9
Ø21ØØZC
Ø21ØØZF
211Ø83
211Ø88
211Ø89
Ø211Ø8C
Ø211Ø8F
Ø211Ø8W
211Ø93
211Ø98
211Ø99
Ø211Ø9C
Ø211Ø9F
Ø211Ø9W
Ø211ØA3
Ø211ØA8
Ø211ØA9
Ø211ØAC
Ø211ØAF
Ø211ØAW
Ø211ØJ3
Ø211ØJ8
Ø211ØJ9
Ø211ØJC
Ø211ØJF
Ø211ØJW
Ø211ØK3
Ø211ØK8
Ø211ØK9
Ø211ØKC
Ø211ØKF
Ø211ØKW
Ø211ØZ3
Ø211ØZ8
Ø211ØZ9
Ø211ØZC
Ø211ØZF
212Ø83
212Ø88
212Ø89
Ø212Ø8C
Ø212Ø8F
Ø212Ø8W
212Ø93
212Ø98
212Ø99
Ø212Ø9C
Ø212Ø9F
Ø212Ø9W
Ø212ØA3
Ø212ØA8
Ø212ØA9
Ø212ØAC
Ø212ØAF
Ø212ØAW
Ø212ØJ3
Ø212ØJ8
Ø212ØJ9
Ø212ØJC
Ø212ØJF
Ø212ØJW
Ø212ØK3
Ø212ØK8
Ø212ØK9
Ø212ØKC
Ø212ØKF
Ø212ØKW
Ø212ØZ3
Ø212ØZ8
Ø212ØZ9
Ø212ØZC
Ø212ØZF
213Ø83
213Ø88
213Ø89
Ø213Ø8C
Ø213Ø8F
Ø213Ø8W
213Ø93
213Ø98
213Ø99
Ø213Ø9C
Ø213Ø9F
Ø213Ø9W
Ø213ØA3
Ø213ØA8
Ø213ØA9
Ø213ØAC
Ø213ØAF
Ø213ØAW
Ø213ØJ3
Ø213ØJ8
Ø213ØJ9
Ø213ØJC
Ø213ØJF
Ø213ØJW
Ø213ØK3
Ø213ØK8
Ø213ØK9
Ø213ØKC
Ø213ØKF
Ø213ØKW
Ø213ØZ3
Ø213ØZ8
Ø213ØZ9
Ø213ØZC
Ø213ØZF
Ø24FØ7J
Ø24FØ8J
Ø24FØJJ
Ø24FØKJ
Ø24GØ72
Ø24GØ82
Ø24GØJ2
Ø24GØK2
Ø24JØ72
Ø24JØ82
Ø24JØJ2
Ø24JØK2
Ø254ØZZ
Ø255ØZZ
Ø256ØZZ
Ø257ØZZ
Ø258ØZZ
Ø259ØZZ
Ø25SØZZ
Ø25TØZZ
Ø27FØ4Z
Ø27FØDZ
Ø27FØZZ
Ø27GØ4Z
Ø27GØDZ
Ø27GØZZ
Ø27HØ4Z
Ø27HØDZ
Ø27HØZZ
Ø27JØ4Z
Ø27JØDZ
Ø27JØZZ
Ø2HAØRJ
Ø2HA3RJ
Ø2HA4RJ
Ø2NFØZZ
Ø2NGØZZ
Ø2NHØZZ
Ø2NJØZZ
Ø2QHØZZ
Ø2QH4ZZ
Ø2QJØZG
Ø2QJØZZ
Ø2QJ4ZG
Ø2QJ4ZZ
Ø2RHØ7Z
Ø2RHØ8Z
Ø2RHØJZ
Ø2RHØKZ
Ø2RH47Z
Ø2RH48Z
Ø2RH4JZ
Ø2RH4KZ
Ø2RJØ7Z
Ø2RJØ8Z
Ø2RJØJZ
Ø2RJØKZ
Ø2RJ47Z
Ø2RJ48Z
Ø2RJ4JZ
Ø2RJ4KZ
Ø2RPØ7Z
Ø2RPØ8Z
Ø2RPØJZ
Ø2RPØKZ
Ø2RP47Z
Ø2RP48Z
Ø2RP4JZ
Ø2RP4KZ
Ø2RQØ7Z
Ø2RQØ8Z
Ø2RQØJZ
Ø2RQØKZ
Ø2RQ47Z
Ø2RQ48Z
Ø2RQ4JZ
Ø2RQ4KZ
Ø2RRØ7Z
Ø2RRØ8Z
Ø2RRØJZ
Ø2RRØKZ
Ø2RR47Z
Ø2RR48Z
Ø2RR4JZ
Ø2RR4KZ
Ø2RSØ7Z
Ø2RSØ8Z
Ø2RSØJZ
Ø2RSØKZ
Ø2RS47Z
Ø2RS48Z
Ø2RS4JZ
Ø2RS4KZ
Ø2RTØ7Z
Ø2RTØ8Z
Ø2RTØJZ
Ø2RTØKZ
Ø2RT47Z
Ø2RT48Z
Ø2RT4JZ
Ø2RT4KZ
Ø2RVØ7Z
Ø2RVØ8Z
Ø2RVØJZ
Ø2RVØKZ
Ø2RV47Z
Ø2RV48Z
Ø2RV4JZ
Ø2RV4KZ
Ø2RWØ7Z
Ø2RWØ8Z
Ø2RWØJZ
Ø2RWØKZ
Ø2RW47Z
Ø2RW48Z
Ø2RW4JZ
Ø2RW4KZ
Ø2RXØ7Z
Ø2RXØ8Z
Ø2RXØJZ
Ø2RXØKZ
Ø2RX47Z
Ø2RX48Z
Ø2RX4JZ
Ø2RX4KZ
Ø2UFØ7J
Ø2UFØ7Z
Ø2UFØ8J
Ø2UFØ8Z
Ø2UFØJJ
Ø2UFØJZ
Ø2UFØKJ
Ø2UFØKZ
Ø2UF47J
Ø2UF47Z
Ø2UF48J
Ø2UF48Z

Ø2UF4JJ
Ø2UF4JZ
Ø2UF4KJ
Ø2UF4KZ
Ø2UGØ7E
Ø2UGØ7Z
Ø2UGØ8E
Ø2UGØ8Z
Ø2UGØJE
Ø2UGØJZ
Ø2UGØKE
Ø2UGØKZ
Ø2UG47E
Ø2UG47Z
Ø2UG48E
Ø2UG48Z
Ø2UG4JE
Ø2UG4JZ
Ø2UG4KE
Ø2UG4KZ
Ø2UHØ7Z
Ø2UHØ8Z
Ø2UHØJZ
Ø2UHØKZ
Ø2UH47Z
Ø2UH48Z
Ø2UH4JZ
Ø2UH4KZ
Ø2UJØ7G
Ø2UJØ7Z
Ø2UJØ8G
Ø2UJØ8Z
Ø2UJØJG
Ø2UJØJZ
Ø2UJØKG
Ø2UJØKZ
Ø2UJ47G
Ø2UJ47Z
Ø2UJ48G
Ø2UJ48Z
Ø2UJ4JG
Ø2UJ4JZ
Ø2UJ4KG
Ø2UJ4KZ
Ø2UW3JZ
Ø2UW4JZ
Ø2UX3JZ
Ø2UX4JZ
Ø2VGØZZ
Ø2VG4ZZ
Ø2VWØDZ
Ø2VWØEZ
Ø2VWØFZ
Ø2VW3DZ
Ø2VW3EZ
Ø2VW3FZ
Ø2VW4DZ
Ø2VW4EZ
Ø2VW4FZ
Ø2VXØDZ
Ø2VXØEZ
Ø2VXØFZ
Ø2VX3DZ
Ø2VX3EZ
Ø2VX3FZ
Ø2VX4DZ
Ø2VX4EZ
Ø2VX4FZ
Ø2WF37Z
Ø3RØØ7Z
Ø3RØØJZ
Ø3RØØKZ
Ø3RØ47Z
Ø3RØ4JZ
Ø3RØ4KZ
Ø3R1Ø7Z
Ø3R1ØJZ
Ø3R1ØKZ
Ø3R147Z
Ø3R14JZ
Ø3R14KZ
Ø3R2Ø7Z
Ø3R2ØJZ
Ø3R2ØKZ
Ø3R247Z
Ø3R24JZ
Ø3R24KZ
Ø3R3Ø7Z
Ø3R3ØJZ
Ø3R3ØKZ
Ø3R347Z
Ø3R34JZ
Ø3R34KZ
Ø3R4Ø7Z
Ø3R4ØJZ
Ø3R4ØKZ
Ø3R447Z
Ø3R44JZ
Ø3R44KZ
Ø5RØØ7Z
Ø5RØØJZ
Ø5RØØKZ
Ø5RØ47Z
Ø5RØ4JZ
Ø5RØ4KZ
Ø5R1Ø7Z
Ø5R1ØJZ
Ø5R1ØKZ
Ø5R147Z
Ø5R14JZ
Ø5R14KZ
Ø5R3Ø7Z
Ø5R3ØJZ
Ø5R3ØKZ
Ø5R347Z
Ø5R34JZ
Ø5R34KZ
Ø5R4Ø7Z
Ø5R4ØJZ
Ø5R4ØKZ
Ø5R447Z
Ø5R44JZ
Ø5R44KZ
Ø5R5Ø7Z
Ø5R5ØJZ
Ø5R5ØKZ
Ø5R547Z
Ø5R54JZ
Ø5R54KZ
Ø5R6Ø7Z
Ø5R6ØJZ
Ø5R6ØKZ
Ø5R647Z
Ø5R64JZ
Ø5R64KZ
5AØ2116
5AØ211D
5AØ2216
5AØ221D
X2RXØN7
X2VWØN7

OR

Nonoperating Room Procedures

Ø257ØZK
4AØ2ØN6
4AØ2ØN7
4AØ2ØN8
4AØ23FZ
4AØ23N6
4AØ23N7
4AØ23N8
4AØ27FZ
4AØ27N6
4AØ27N7
4AØ27N8
4AØ28FZ
4AØ28N6
4AØ28N7
4AØ28N8
B2ØØØZZ
B2ØØ1ZZ
B2ØØYZZ
B2Ø1ØZZ
B2Ø11ZZ
B2Ø1YZZ
B2Ø2ØZZ
B2Ø21ZZ
B2Ø2YZZ
B2Ø3ØZZ
B2Ø31ZZ
B2Ø3YZZ
B2Ø4ØZZ
B2Ø41ZZ
B2Ø4YZZ
B2Ø5ØZZ
B2Ø51ZZ
B2Ø5YZZ
B2Ø6ØZZ
B2Ø61ZZ
B2Ø6YZZ
B2Ø7ØZZ
B2Ø71ZZ
B2Ø7YZZ
B2Ø8ØZZ
B2Ø81ZZ
B2Ø8YZZ
B2ØFØZZ
B2ØF1ZZ
B2ØFYZZ
B21ØØZZ
B21Ø1ZZ
B21ØYZZ
B211ØZZ
B2111ZZ
B211YZZ
B212ØZZ
B2121ZZ
B212YZZ
B213ØZZ
B2131ZZ
B213YZZ
B214ØZZ
B2141ZZ
B214YZZ
B215ØZZ
B2151ZZ
B215YZZ
B216ØZZ
B2161ZZ
B216YZZ
B217ØZZ
B2171ZZ
B217YZZ
B218ØZZ
B2181ZZ
B218YZZ
B21FØZZ
B21F1ZZ
B21FYZZ

DRG 215

Operating Room Procedures

Ø2HAØRS
Ø2HA3RS
Ø2HA3RZ
Ø2HA4RS
Ø2HA4RZ
Ø2HW3RZ
Ø2WAØJZ
Ø2WAØQZ
Ø2WAØRS
Ø2WAØRZ
Ø2WA3QZ
Ø2WA3RS
Ø2WA3RZ
Ø2WA4QZ
Ø2WA4RS
Ø2WA4RZ
Ø2WW3RZ

DRG 216

Operating Room Procedures

Ø24F*
Ø24G*
Ø24J*
Ø27FØ4Z
Ø27FØDZ
Ø27FØZZ
Ø27GØ4Z
Ø27GØDZ
Ø27GØZZ
Ø27HØ4Z
Ø27HØDZ
Ø27HØZZ
Ø27JØ4Z
Ø27JØDZ
Ø27JØZZ
Ø2HAØRJ
Ø2HA3RJ
Ø2HA4RJ
Ø2NFØZZ
Ø2NGØZZ
Ø2NHØZZ
Ø2NJØZZ
Ø2QFØZJ
Ø2QFØZZ
Ø2QF4ZJ
Ø2QF4ZZ
Ø2QGØZE
Ø2QGØZZ
Ø2QG4ZE
Ø2QG4ZZ
Ø2QHØZZ
Ø2QH4ZZ
Ø2QJØZG
Ø2QJØZZ
Ø2QJ4ZG
Ø2QJ4ZZ
Ø2RFØ7Z
Ø2RFØ8N
Ø2RFØ8Z
Ø2RFØJZ
Ø2RFØKZ
Ø2RF47Z
Ø2RF48N
Ø2RF48Z
Ø2RF4JZ
Ø2RF4KZ
Ø2RGØ7Z
Ø2RGØ8Z
Ø2RGØJZ
Ø2RGØKZ
Ø2RG47Z
Ø2RG48Z
Ø2RG4JZ
Ø2RG4KZ
Ø2RHØ7Z
Ø2RHØ8Z
Ø2RHØJZ
Ø2RHØKZ
Ø2RH47Z
Ø2RH48Z
Ø2RH4JZ
Ø2RH4KZ
Ø2RJØ7Z
Ø2RJØ8Z
Ø2RJØJZ
Ø2RJØKZ
Ø2RJ47Z
Ø2RJ48Z
Ø2RJ4JZ
Ø2RJ4KZ
Ø2RPØ7Z
Ø2RPØ8Z
Ø2RPØJZ
Ø2RPØKZ
Ø2RP47Z
Ø2RP48Z
Ø2RP4JZ
Ø2RP4KZ
Ø2RQØ7Z
Ø2RQØ8Z
Ø2RQØJZ
Ø2RQØKZ
Ø2RQ47Z
Ø2RQ48Z
Ø2RQ4JZ
Ø2RQ4KZ
Ø2RRØ7Z
Ø2RRØ8Z
Ø2RRØJZ
Ø2RRØKZ
Ø2RR47Z
Ø2RR48Z
Ø2RR4JZ
Ø2RR4KZ
Ø2RSØ7Z
Ø2RSØ8Z
Ø2RSØJZ
Ø2RSØKZ
Ø2RS47Z
Ø2RS48Z
Ø2RS4JZ
Ø2RS4KZ
Ø2RTØ7Z
Ø2RTØ8Z
Ø2RTØJZ
Ø2RTØKZ
Ø2RT47Z
Ø2RT48Z
Ø2RT4JZ
Ø2RT4KZ
Ø2RVØ7Z
Ø2RVØ8Z
Ø2RVØJZ
Ø2RVØKZ
Ø2RV47Z
Ø2RV48Z
Ø2RV4JZ
Ø2RV4KZ
Ø2RWØ7Z
Ø2RWØ8Z
Ø2RWØJZ
Ø2RWØKZ
Ø2RW47Z
Ø2RW48Z
Ø2RW4JZ
Ø2RW4KZ
Ø2RX*
Ø2UFØ7J
Ø2UFØ7Z
Ø2UFØ8J
Ø2UFØ8Z
Ø2UFØJJ
Ø2UFØJZ
Ø2UFØKJ
Ø2UFØKZ
Ø2UF47J
Ø2UF47Z
Ø2UF48J
Ø2UF48Z
Ø2UF4JJ
Ø2UF4JZ
Ø2UF4KJ
Ø2UF4KZ
Ø2UGØ7E
Ø2UGØ7Z
Ø2UGØ8E
Ø2UGØ8Z
Ø2UGØJE
Ø2UGØJZ
Ø2UGØKE
Ø2UGØKZ
Ø2UG47E
Ø2UG47Z
Ø2UG48E
Ø2UG48Z
Ø2UG4JE
Ø2UG4JZ
Ø2UG4KE
Ø2UG4KZ
Ø2UHØ7Z
Ø2UHØ8Z
Ø2UHØJZ
Ø2UHØKZ
Ø2UH47Z
Ø2UH48Z
Ø2UH4JZ
Ø2UH4KZ
Ø2UJØ7G
Ø2UJØ7Z
Ø2UJØ8G
Ø2UJØ8Z
Ø2UJØJG
Ø2UJØJZ
Ø2UJØKG
Ø2UJØKZ
Ø2UJ47G
Ø2UJ47Z
Ø2UJ48G
Ø2UJ48Z
Ø2UJ4JG
Ø2UJ4JZ
Ø2UJ4KG
Ø2UJ4KZ
Ø2UW3JZ
Ø2UW4JZ
Ø2UX3JZ
Ø2UX4JZ
Ø2VGØZZ
Ø2VG4ZZ
Ø2VWØDZ
Ø2VWØEZ
Ø2VWØFZ
Ø2VW3DZ
Ø2VW3EZ
Ø2VW3FZ
Ø2VW4DZ
Ø2VW4EZ
Ø2VW4FZ
Ø2VXØDZ
Ø2VXØEZ
Ø2VXØFZ
Ø2VX3DZ
Ø2VX3EZ
Ø2VX3FZ
Ø2VX4DZ
Ø2VX4EZ
Ø2VX4FZ
Ø2WF37Z
Ø3RØØ7Z
Ø3RØØJZ
Ø3RØØKZ
Ø3RØ47Z
Ø3RØ4JZ
Ø3RØ4KZ
Ø3R1Ø7Z
Ø3R1ØJZ
Ø3R1ØKZ
Ø3R147Z
Ø3R14JZ
Ø3R14KZ
Ø3R2Ø7Z
Ø3R2ØJZ
Ø3R2ØKZ
Ø3R247Z
Ø3R24JZ
Ø3R24KZ
Ø3R3Ø7Z
Ø3R3ØJZ
Ø3R3ØKZ
Ø3R347Z
Ø3R34JZ
Ø3R34KZ
Ø3R4Ø7Z
Ø3R4ØJZ
Ø3R4ØKZ
Ø3R447Z
Ø3R44JZ
Ø3R44KZ
Ø5RØØ7Z
Ø5RØØJZ
Ø5RØØKZ
Ø5RØ47Z
Ø5RØ4JZ
Ø5RØ4KZ
Ø5R1Ø7Z
Ø5R1ØJZ
Ø5R1ØKZ
Ø5R147Z
Ø5R14JZ
Ø5R14KZ
Ø5R3Ø7Z
Ø5R3ØJZ
Ø5R3ØKZ
Ø5R347Z
Ø5R34JZ
Ø5R34KZ
Ø5R4Ø7Z
Ø5R4ØJZ
Ø5R4ØKZ
Ø5R447Z
Ø5R44JZ
Ø5R44KZ
Ø5R5Ø7Z
Ø5R5ØJZ
Ø5R5ØKZ
Ø5R547Z
Ø5R54JZ
Ø5R54KZ
Ø5R6Ø7Z
Ø5R6ØJZ
Ø5R6ØKZ
Ø5R647Z
Ø5R64JZ
Ø5R64KZ
5AØ2116
5AØ211D
5AØ2216
5AØ221D
X2RXØN7
X2VWØN7

AND

Nonoperating Room Procedures

4AØ2ØN6
4AØ2ØN7
4AØ2ØN8
4AØ23FZ
4AØ23N6
4AØ23N7
4AØ23N8
4AØ27FZ
4AØ27N6
4AØ27N7
4AØ27N8
4AØ28FZ
4AØ28N6
4AØ28N7
4AØ28N8
B2Ø*
B21ØØZZ
B21Ø1ZZ
B21ØYZZ
B211ØZZ
B2111ZZ
B211YZZ
B212ØZZ
B2121ZZ
B212YZZ
B213ØZZ
B2131ZZ
B213YZZ
B214*
B215*
B216*
B217*
B218*
B21F*

DRG 217

Select operating room procedures AND nonoperating room procedures listed under DRG 216

DRG 218

Select operating room procedures AND nonoperating room procedures listed under DRG 216

DRG 219

Select operating room procedures listed under DRG 216

DRG 220

Select operating room procedures listed under DRG 216

DRG 221

Select operating room procedures listed under DRG 216

DRG 228

Operating Room Procedures

21Ø344
Ø21Ø3D4
21Ø444
Ø21Ø4D4
211344
Ø2113D4
211444
Ø2114D4
212344
Ø2123D4
212444
Ø2124D4
213344
Ø2133D4
213444
Ø2134D4
Ø216Ø8P
Ø216Ø8Q
Ø216Ø8R
Ø216Ø9P
Ø216Ø9Q
Ø216Ø9R
Ø216ØAP
Ø216ØAQ
Ø216ØAR
Ø216ØJP
Ø216ØJQ
Ø216ØJR
Ø216ØKP
Ø216ØKQ
Ø216ØKR
Ø216ØZP
Ø216ØZQ
Ø216ØZR
Ø21648P
Ø21648Q
Ø21648R
Ø21649P
Ø21649Q
Ø21649R
Ø2164AP
Ø2164AQ
Ø2164AR
Ø2164JP
Ø2164JQ
Ø2164JR
Ø2164KP
Ø2164KQ
Ø2164KR
Ø2164ZP
Ø2164ZQ
Ø2164ZR
Ø217Ø8P
Ø217Ø8Q
Ø217Ø8R
Ø217Ø8S
Ø217Ø8T
Ø217Ø8U
Ø217Ø9P
Ø217Ø9Q
Ø217Ø9R
Ø217Ø9S
Ø217Ø9T
Ø217Ø9U
Ø217ØAP
Ø217ØAQ
Ø217ØAR
Ø217ØAS
Ø217ØAT
Ø217ØAU
Ø217ØJP
Ø217ØJQ
Ø217ØJR
Ø217ØJS
Ø217ØJT
Ø217ØJU
Ø217ØKP
Ø217ØKQ
Ø217ØKR
Ø217ØKS
Ø217ØKT
Ø217ØKU
Ø217ØZP
Ø217ØZQ
Ø217ØZR
Ø217ØZS
Ø217ØZT
Ø217ØZU
Ø21748P
Ø21748Q
Ø21748R
Ø21748S
Ø21748T
Ø21748U
Ø21749P
Ø21749Q
Ø21749R
Ø21749S
Ø21749T
Ø21749U
Ø2174AP
Ø2174AQ
Ø2174AR
Ø2174AS
Ø2174AT
Ø2174AU
Ø2174JP
Ø2174JQ
Ø2174JR
Ø2174JS
Ø2174JT
Ø2174JU
Ø2174KP
Ø2174KQ
Ø2174KR
Ø2174KS
Ø2174KT
Ø2174KU
Ø2174ZP
Ø2174ZQ
Ø2174ZR
Ø2174ZS
Ø2174ZT
Ø2174ZU
Ø21KØ8P
Ø21KØ8Q
Ø21KØ8R
Ø21KØ9P
Ø21KØ9Q
Ø21KØ9R
Ø21KØAP
Ø21KØAQ
Ø21KØAR
Ø21KØJP
Ø21KØJQ
Ø21KØJR
Ø21KØKP
Ø21KØKQ
Ø21KØKR
Ø21KØZ5
Ø21KØZ8
Ø21KØZ9
Ø21KØZC
Ø21KØZF
Ø21KØZP
Ø21KØZQ
Ø21KØZR
Ø21KØZW
Ø21K48P
Ø21K48Q
Ø21K48R
Ø21K49P
Ø21K49Q
Ø21K49R
Ø21K4AP
Ø21K4AQ
Ø21K4AR
Ø21K4JP
Ø21K4JQ
Ø21K4JR
Ø21K4KP
Ø21K4KQ
Ø21K4KR
Ø21K4Z5
Ø21K4Z8
Ø21K4Z9
Ø21K4ZC
Ø21K4ZF
Ø21K4ZP
Ø21K4ZQ
Ø21K4ZR
Ø21K4ZW
Ø21LØ8P
Ø21LØ8Q
Ø21LØ8R
Ø21LØ9P
Ø21LØ9Q
Ø21LØ9R
Ø21LØAP
Ø21LØAQ
Ø21LØAR
Ø21LØJP
Ø21LØJQ
Ø21LØJR
Ø21LØKP
Ø21LØKQ
Ø21LØKR
Ø21LØZ5
Ø21LØZ8
Ø21LØZ9
Ø21LØZC
Ø21LØZF
Ø21LØZP
Ø21LØZQ
Ø21LØZR
Ø21LØZW
Ø21L48P
Ø21L48Q
Ø21L48R
Ø21L49P
Ø21L49Q
Ø21L49R
Ø21L4AP
Ø21L4AQ
Ø21L4AR
Ø21L4JP
Ø21L4JQ
Ø21L4JR
Ø21L4KP
Ø21L4KQ
Ø21L4KR
Ø21L4Z5
Ø21L4Z8
Ø21L4Z9
Ø21L4ZC
Ø21L4ZF
Ø21L4ZP
Ø21L4ZQ
Ø21L4ZR
Ø21L4ZW
Ø21VØ8S
Ø21VØ8T
Ø21VØ8U
Ø21VØ9S
Ø21VØ9T
Ø21VØ9U
Ø21VØAS
Ø21VØAT
Ø21VØAU
Ø21VØJS
Ø21VØJT
Ø21VØJU
Ø21VØKS
Ø21VØKT
Ø21VØKU
Ø21VØZS
Ø21VØZT
Ø21VØZU
Ø21V48S
Ø21V48T
Ø21V48U
Ø21V49S
Ø21V49T
Ø21V49U
Ø21V4AS
Ø21V4AT
Ø21V4AU
Ø21V4JS
Ø21V4JT
Ø21V4JU
Ø21V4KS
Ø21V4KT
Ø21V4KU
Ø21V4ZS
Ø21V4ZT
Ø21V4ZU
Ø254ØZZ
Ø2543ZZ
Ø2544ZZ
Ø255ØZZ

02554ZZ
02560ZZ
02564ZZ
02570ZZ
02574ZZ
02580ZZ
02584ZZ
02590ZZ
02594ZZ
025D0ZZ
025D3ZZ
025D4ZZ
025F0ZZ
025F4ZZ
025G0ZZ
025G4ZZ
025H0ZZ
025H4ZZ
025J0ZZ
025J4ZZ
025K0ZZ
025K4ZZ
025L0ZZ
025L4ZZ
025M0ZZ
025M4ZZ
270046
027004Z
270056
027005Z
270066
027006Z
270076
027007Z
02700D6
02700DZ
02700E6
02700EZ
02700F6
02700FZ
02700G6
02700GZ
02700T6
02700TZ
02700Z6
02700ZZ
271046
027104Z
271056
027105Z
271066
027106Z
271076
027107Z
02710D6
02710DZ
02710E6
02710EZ
02710F6
02710FZ
02710G6
02710GZ
02710T6
02710TZ
02710Z6
02710ZZ
272046
027204Z
272056
027205Z
272066
027206Z
272076
027207Z
02720D6
02720DZ
02720E6
02720EZ
02720F6
02720FZ
02720G6
02720GZ
02720T6
02720TZ
02720Z6
02720ZZ
273046
027304Z
273056
027305Z
273066
027306Z
273076
027307Z
02730D6
02730DZ
02730E6
02730EZ
02730F6
02730FZ
02730G6
02730GZ
02730T6
02730TZ
02730Z6
02730ZZ
02890ZZ
02893ZZ
02894ZZ
028D0ZZ
028D3ZZ
028D4ZZ
02B40ZZ
02B43ZZ
02B44ZZ
02B50ZZ
02B54ZZ
02B60ZZ
02B64ZZ
02B70ZZ
02B74ZZ
02B80ZZ
02B84ZZ
02B90ZZ
02B94ZZ
02BD0ZZ
02BD3ZZ
02BD4ZZ
02BF0ZZ
02BF4ZZ
02BG0ZZ
02BG4ZZ
02BH0ZZ
02BH4ZZ
02BJ0ZZ
02BJ4ZZ
02BK0ZZ
02BK3ZZ
02BK4ZZ
02BL0ZZ
02BL3ZZ
02BL4ZZ
02BM0ZZ
02BM4ZZ
02C00Z6
02C00ZZ
02C10Z6
02C10ZZ
02C20Z6
02C20ZZ
02C30Z6
02C30ZZ
02C40ZZ
02C43ZZ
02C44ZZ
02C50ZZ
02C53ZZ
02C54ZZ
02C60ZZ
02C63ZZ
02C64ZZ
02C70ZZ
02C73ZZ
02C74ZZ
02C80ZZ
02C83ZZ
02C84ZZ
02C90ZZ
02C93ZZ
02C94ZZ
02CD0ZZ
02CD3ZZ
02CD4ZZ
02CF0ZZ
02CG0ZZ
02CH0ZZ
02CJ0ZZ
02CK0ZZ
02CK3ZZ
02CK4ZZ
02CL0ZZ
02CL3ZZ
02CL4ZZ
02CM0ZZ
02CM3ZZ
02CM4ZZ
02H00DZ
02H00YZ
02H04DZ
02H04YZ
02H10DZ
02H10YZ
02H14DZ
02H14YZ
02H20DZ
02H20YZ
02H24DZ
02H24YZ
02H30DZ
02H30YZ
02H34DZ
02H34YZ
02H402Z
02H403Z
02H40DZ
02H40NZ
02H43DZ
02H43NZ
02H442Z
02H443Z
02H44DZ
02H44NZ
02H602Z
02H603Z
02H60DZ
02H60NZ
02H63DZ
02H63NZ
02H642Z
02H643Z
02H64DZ
02H64NZ
02H702Z
02H703Z
02H70DZ
02H70NZ
02H73DZ
02H73NZ
02H742Z
02H743Z
02H74DZ
02H74NZ
02HK03Z
02HK0DZ
02HK0NZ
02HK3DZ
02HK3NZ
02HK43Z
02HK4DZ
02HK4NZ
02HL02Z
02HL03Z
02HL0DZ
02HL0NZ
02HL3DZ
02HL3NZ
02HL42Z
02HL43Z
02HL4DZ
02HL4NZ
02N00ZZ
02N03ZZ
02N04ZZ
02N10ZZ
02N13ZZ
02N14ZZ
02N20ZZ
02N23ZZ
02N24ZZ
02N30ZZ
02N33ZZ
02N34ZZ
02N50ZZ
02N53ZZ
02N54ZZ
02N60ZZ
02N63ZZ
02N64ZZ
02N70ZZ
02N73ZZ
02N74ZZ
02N90ZZ
02N93ZZ
02N94ZZ
02ND0ZZ
02ND3ZZ
02ND4ZZ
02NK0ZZ
02NK3ZZ
02NK4ZZ
02NL0ZZ
02NL3ZZ
02NL4ZZ
02NM0ZZ
02NM3ZZ
02NM4ZZ
02PA02Z
02PA03Z
02PA07Z
02PA08Z
02PA0CZ
02PA0DZ
02PA0JZ
02PA0KZ
02PA0NZ
02PA0YZ
02PA37Z
02PA38Z
02PA3CZ
02PA3JZ
02PA3KZ
02PA3NZ
02PA42Z
02PA43Z
02PA47Z
02PA48Z
02PA4CZ
02PA4DZ
02PA4JZ
02PA4KZ
02PA4NZ
02Q00ZZ
02Q03ZZ
02Q04ZZ
02Q10ZZ
02Q13ZZ
02Q14ZZ
02Q20ZZ
02Q23ZZ
02Q24ZZ
02Q30ZZ
02Q33ZZ
02Q34ZZ
02Q40ZZ
02Q43ZZ
02Q44ZZ
02Q50ZZ
02Q53ZZ
02Q54ZZ
02Q90ZZ
02Q93ZZ
02Q94ZZ
02QB0ZZ
02QB3ZZ
02QB4ZZ
02QC0ZZ
02QC3ZZ
02QC4ZZ
02QD0ZZ
02QD3ZZ
02QD4ZZ
02QM0ZZ
02QM3ZZ
02QM4ZZ
02R907Z
02R908Z
02R90JZ
02R90KZ
02R947Z
02R948Z
02R94JZ
02R94KZ
02RD07Z
02RD08Z
02RD0JZ
02RD0KZ
02RD47Z
02RD48Z
02RD4JZ
02RD4KZ
02RK07Z
02RK0KZ
02RK47Z
02RK4KZ
02RL07Z
02RL0KZ
02RL47Z
02RL4KZ
02RM07Z
02RM0JZ
02RM0KZ
02RM47Z
02RM4JZ
02RM4KZ
02T50ZZ
02T53ZZ
02T54ZZ
02T80ZZ
02T84ZZ
02T90ZZ
02T93ZZ
02T94ZZ
02TD0ZZ
02TD3ZZ
02TD4ZZ
02TH0ZZ
02TH4ZZ
02TM0ZZ
02TM3ZZ
02TM4ZZ
02U507Z
02U508Z
02U50JZ
02U50KZ
02U537Z
02U538Z
02U53KZ
02U547Z
02U548Z
02U54KZ
02U607Z
02U608Z
02U60KZ
02U707Z
02U708Z
02U70KZ
02U737Z
02U738Z
02U73KZ
02U747Z
02U748Z
02U74KZ
02U907Z
02U908Z
02U90JZ
02U90KZ
02U937Z
02U938Z
02U93JZ
02U93KZ
02U947Z
02U948Z
02U94JZ
02U94KZ
02UD07Z
02UD08Z
02UD0JZ
02UD0KZ
02UD37Z
02UD38Z
02UD3JZ
02UD3KZ
02UD47Z
02UD48Z
02UD4JZ
02UD4KZ
02UK0KZ
02UK3KZ
02UK4KZ
02UL0KZ
02UL3KZ
02UL4KZ
02UM07Z
02UM0JZ
02UM0KZ
02UM37Z
02UM38Z
02UM3JZ
02UM3KZ
02UM47Z
02UM48Z
02UM4JZ
02UM4KZ
02W50JZ
02W54JZ
02WA02Z
02WA03Z
02WA07Z
02WA08Z
02WA0CZ
02WA0DZ
02WA0KZ
02WA0NZ
02WA0YZ
02WA37Z
02WA38Z
02WA3CZ
02WA3JZ
02WA3KZ
02WA3NZ
02WA42Z
02WA43Z
02WA47Z
02WA48Z
02WA4CZ
02WA4DZ
02WA4JZ
02WA4KZ
02WA4NZ
02WF07Z
02WF08Z
02WF0JZ
02WF0KZ
02WF47Z
02WF48Z
02WF4JZ
02WF4KZ
02WG07Z
02WG08Z
02WG0JZ
02WG0KZ
02WG47Z
02WG48Z
02WG4JZ
02WG4KZ
02WH07Z
02WH08Z
02WH0JZ
02WH0KZ
02WH47Z
02WH48Z
02WH4JZ
02WH4KZ
02WJ07Z
02WJ08Z
02WJ0JZ
02WJ0KZ
02WJ47Z
02WJ48Z
02WJ4JZ
02WJ4KZ
02WM0JZ
02WM4JZ
061007P
061007Q
061007R
061009P
061009Q
061009R
06100AP
06100AQ
06100AR
06100JP
06100JQ
06100JR
06100KP
06100KQ
06100KR
06100ZP
06100ZQ
06100ZR
061047P
061047Q
061047R
061049P
061049Q
061049R
06104AP
06104AQ
06104AR
06104JP
06104JQ
06104JR
06104KP
06104KQ
06104KR
06104ZP
06104ZQ
06104ZR
X2H63V9
X2HK3V9
X2V73Q7

DRG 229

Select operating room procedures listed under DRG 228

DRG 231

Coronary bypass operating room procedures

210083
210088
210089
021008C
021008F
021008W
210093
210098
210099
021009C
021009F
021009W
02100A3
02100A8
02100A9
02100AC
02100AF
02100AW
02100J3
02100J8
02100J9
02100JC
02100JF
02100JW
02100K3
02100K8
02100K9
02100KC
02100KF
02100KW
02100Z3
02100Z8
02100Z9
02100ZC
02100ZF
210483
210488
210489
021048C
021048F
021048W
210493
210498
210499
021049C
021049F
021049W
02104A3
02104A8
02104A9
02104AC
02104AF
02104AW
02104J3
02104J8
02104J9
02104JC
02104JF
02104JW
02104K3
02104K8
02104K9
02104KC
02104KF
02104KW
02104Z3
02104Z8
02104Z9
02104ZC
02104ZF
211083
211088
211089
021108C
021108F
021108W
211093
211098
211099
021109C
021109F
021109W
02110A3
02110A8
02110A9
02110AC
02110AF
02110AW
02110J3
02110J8
02110J9
02110JC
02110JF
02110JW
02110K3
02110K8
02110K9
02110KC
02110KF
02110KW
02110Z3
02110Z8
02110Z9
02110ZC
02110ZF
211483
211488
211489
021148C
021148F
021148W
211493
211498
211499
021149C
021149F
021149W
02114A3
02114A8
02114A9
02114AC
02114AF
02114AW
02114J3
02114J8
02114J9
02114JC
02114JF
02114JW
02114K3
02114K8
02114K9
02114KC
02114KF
02114KW
02114Z3
02114Z8
02114Z9
02114ZC
02114ZF
212083
212088
212089
021208C
021208F
021208W
212093
212098
212099
021209C
021209F
021209W
02120A3
02120A8
02120A9
02120AC
02120AF
02120AW
02120J3
02120J8
02120J9
02120JC
02120JF
02120JW
02120K3
02120K8
02120K9
02120KC
02120KF
02120KW
02120Z3
02120Z8
02120Z9
02120ZC
02120ZF
212483
212488
212489
021248C
021248F
021248W
212493
212498
212499
021249C
021249F
021249W
02124A3
02124A8
02124A9
02124AC
02124AF
02124AW
02124J3
02124J8
02124J9
02124JC
02124JF
02124JW
02124K3
02124K8
02124K9
02124KC
02124KF
02124KW
02124Z3
02124Z8
02124Z9
02124ZC
02124ZF
213083
213088
213089
021308C
021308F
021308W
213093
213098
213099
021309C
021309F
021309W
02130A3
02130A8
02130A9
02130AC
02130AF
02130AW
02130J3
02130J8
02130J9
02130JC
02130JF
02130JW
02130K3
02130K8
02130K9
02130KC
02130KF
02130KW
02130Z3
02130Z8
02130Z9
02130ZC
02130ZF
213483
213488
213489
021348C
021348F
021348W
213493
213498
213499
021349C
021349F
021349W
02134A3
02134A8
02134A9
02134AC
02134AF
02134AW
02134J3
02134J8
02134J9
02134JC
02134JF
02134JW
02134K3
02134K8
02134K9
02134KC
02134KF
02134KW
02134Z3
02134Z8
02134Z9
02134ZC
02134ZF

AND

PTCA operating room procedures

270346
027034Z
270356
027035Z
270366
027036Z
270376
027037Z
02703D6
02703DZ

Ø27Ø3E6
Ø27Ø3EZ
Ø27Ø3F6
Ø27Ø3FZ
Ø27Ø3G6
Ø27Ø3GZ
Ø27Ø3T6
Ø27Ø3TZ
Ø27Ø3Z6
Ø27Ø3ZZ
27Ø446
Ø27Ø44Z
27Ø456
Ø27Ø45Z
27Ø466
Ø27Ø46Z
27Ø476
Ø27Ø47Z
Ø27Ø4D6
Ø27Ø4DZ
Ø27Ø4E6
Ø27Ø4EZ
Ø27Ø4F6
Ø27Ø4FZ
Ø27Ø4G6
Ø27Ø4GZ
Ø27Ø4T6
Ø27Ø4TZ
Ø27Ø4Z6
Ø27Ø4ZZ
271346
Ø27134Z
271356
Ø27135Z
271366
Ø27136Z
271376
Ø27137Z
Ø2713D6
Ø2713DZ
Ø2713E6
Ø2713EZ
Ø2713F6
Ø2713FZ
Ø2713G6
Ø2713GZ
Ø2713T6
Ø2713TZ
Ø2713Z6
Ø2713ZZ
271446
Ø27144Z
271456
Ø27145Z
271466
Ø27146Z
271476
Ø27147Z
Ø2714D6
Ø2714DZ
Ø2714E6
Ø2714EZ
Ø2714F6
Ø2714FZ
Ø2714G6
Ø2714GZ
Ø2714T6
Ø2714TZ
Ø2714Z6
Ø2714ZZ
272346
Ø27234Z
272356
Ø27235Z
272366
Ø27236Z
272376
Ø27237Z
Ø2723D6
Ø2723DZ
Ø2723E6
Ø2723EZ
Ø2723F6
Ø2723FZ
Ø2723G6
Ø2723GZ
Ø2723T6
Ø2723TZ
Ø2723Z6
Ø2723ZZ
272446
Ø27244Z
272456
Ø27245Z
272466
Ø27246Z
272476
Ø27247Z
Ø2724D6
Ø2724DZ
Ø2724E6
Ø2724EZ
Ø2724F6
Ø2724FZ
Ø2724G6
Ø2724GZ
Ø2724T6
Ø2724TZ
Ø2724Z6
Ø2724ZZ
273346
Ø27334Z
273356
Ø27335Z
273366
Ø27336Z
273376
Ø27337Z
Ø2733D6
Ø2733DZ
Ø2733E6
Ø2733EZ
Ø2733F6
Ø2733FZ
Ø2733G6
Ø2733GZ
Ø2733T6
Ø2733TZ
Ø2733Z6
Ø2733ZZ
273446
Ø27344Z
273456
Ø27345Z
273466
Ø27346Z
273476
Ø27347Z
Ø2734D6
Ø2734DZ
Ø2734E6
Ø2734EZ
Ø2734F6
Ø2734FZ
Ø2734G6
Ø2734GZ
Ø2734T6
Ø2734TZ
Ø2734Z6
Ø2734ZZ
Ø27F34Z
Ø27F3DZ
Ø27F3ZZ
Ø27F44Z
Ø27F4DZ
Ø27F4ZZ
Ø27G34Z
Ø27G3DZ
Ø27G3ZZ
Ø27G44Z
Ø27G4DZ
Ø27G4ZZ
Ø27H34Z
Ø27H3DZ
Ø27H3ZZ
Ø27H44Z
Ø27H4DZ
Ø27H4ZZ
Ø27J34Z
Ø27J3DZ
Ø27J3ZZ
Ø27J44Z
Ø27J4DZ
Ø27J4ZZ
Ø2CØ3Z6
Ø2CØ3Z7
Ø2CØ3ZZ
Ø2C13Z6
Ø2C13Z7
Ø2C13ZZ
Ø2C23Z6
Ø2C23Z7
Ø2C23ZZ
Ø2C33Z6
Ø2C33Z7
Ø2C33ZZ
Ø2FØ3ZZ
Ø2F13ZZ
Ø2F23ZZ
Ø2F33ZZ
Ø2HØ3DZ
Ø2HØ3YZ
Ø2H13DZ
Ø2H13YZ
Ø2H23DZ
Ø2H23YZ
Ø2H33DZ
Ø2H33YZ

DRG 232

Select coronary bypass operating room procedures AND PTCA operating room procedures listed under DRG 231

DRG 233

Select coronary bypass operating room procedures listed under DRG 231
AND
Cardiac catheterization nonoperating room procedures

4AØ2ØN6
4AØ2ØN7
4AØ2ØN8
4AØ23N6
4AØ23N7
4AØ23N8
4AØ27N6
4AØ27N7
4AØ27N8
4AØ28N6
4AØ28N7
4AØ28N8
B2Ø*
B21ØØZZ
B21Ø1ZZ
B21ØYZZ
B211ØZZ
B2111ZZ
B211YZZ
B212ØZZ
B2121ZZ
B212YZZ
B213ØZZ
B2131ZZ
B213YZZ
B214*
B215*
B216*
B217*
B218*
B21F*
OR
Open ablation operating room procedures

Ø254ØZZ
Ø255ØZZ
Ø256ØZZ
Ø257ØZZ
Ø258ØZZ
Ø259ØZZ
Ø25SØZZ
Ø25TØZZ
OR
Open ablation nonoperating room procedures

Ø257ØZK

DRG 234

Select coronary bypass operating room procedures listed under DRG 231 AND nonoperating room procedures OR ablation procedures listed under DRG 233

DRG 235

Select coronary bypass operating room procedures listed under DRG 231

DRG 236

Select coronary bypass operating room procedures listed under DRG 231

DRG 239

Operating Room Procedures

ØY62ØZZ
ØY63ØZZ
ØY64ØZZ
ØY67ØZZ
ØY68ØZZ
ØY6C*
ØY6D*
ØY6FØZZ
ØY6GØZZ
ØY6H*
ØY6J*
ØY6M*
ØY6N*

DRG 240

Select operating room procedures listed under DRG 239

DRG 241

Select operating room procedures listed under DRG 239

DRG 242

Cardiac pacemaker device operating room procedures

ØJH6Ø4Z
ØJH6Ø5Z
ØJH6Ø6Z
ØJH6Ø7Z
ØJH6ØPZ
ØJH634Z
ØJH635Z
ØJH636Z
ØJH637Z
ØJH63PZ
ØJH8Ø4Z
ØJH8Ø5Z
ØJH8Ø6Z
ØJH8Ø7Z
ØJH8ØPZ
ØJH834Z
ØJH835Z
ØJH836Z
ØJH837Z
ØJH83PZ
In combination WITH
Cardiac pacemaker lead(s) operating room procedures

Ø2H4ØJZ
Ø2H4ØMZ
Ø2H43JZ
Ø2H43MZ
Ø2H44JZ
Ø2H44MZ
Ø2H6ØJZ
Ø2H6ØMZ
Ø2H63JZ
Ø2H63MZ
Ø2H64JZ
Ø2H64MZ
Ø2H7ØJZ
Ø2H7ØMZ
Ø2H73JZ
Ø2H73MZ
Ø2H74JZ
Ø2H74MZ
Ø2HKØJZ
Ø2HKØMZ
Ø2HK3JZ
Ø2HK3MZ
Ø2HK4JZ
Ø2HK4MZ
Ø2HLØJZ
Ø2HLØMZ
Ø2HL3JZ
Ø2HL3MZ
Ø2HL4JZ
Ø2HL4MZ
Ø2HNØJZ
Ø2HNØMZ
Ø2HN3JZ
Ø2HN3MZ
Ø2HN4JZ
Ø2HN4MZ

DRG 243

Select operating room procedure combinations listed under DRG 242

DRG 244

Select operating room procedure combinations listed under DRG 242

DRG 245

Operating Room Procedures

ØJH6Ø8Z
ØJH6Ø9Z
ØJH6ØAZ
ØJH638Z
ØJH639Z
ØJH63AZ
ØJH8Ø8Z
ØJH8Ø9Z
ØJH8ØAZ
ØJH838Z
ØJH839Z
ØJH83AZ

DRG 250

Operating Room Procedures

Ø27Ø3Z6
Ø27Ø3ZZ
Ø27Ø4Z6
Ø27Ø4ZZ
Ø2713Z6
Ø2713ZZ
Ø2714Z6
Ø2714ZZ
Ø2723Z6
Ø2723ZZ
Ø2724Z6
Ø2724ZZ
Ø2733Z6
Ø2733ZZ
Ø2734Z6
Ø2734ZZ
Ø2CØ3Z6
Ø2CØ3Z7
Ø2CØ3ZZ
Ø2CØ4Z6
Ø2CØ4ZZ
Ø2C13Z6
Ø2C13Z7
Ø2C13ZZ
Ø2C14Z6
Ø2C14ZZ
Ø2C23Z6
Ø2C23Z7
Ø2C23ZZ
Ø2C24Z6
Ø2C24ZZ
Ø2C33Z6
Ø2C33Z7
Ø2C33ZZ
Ø2C34Z6
Ø2C34ZZ
Ø2FP3ZØ
Ø2FP3ZZ
Ø2FQ3ZØ
Ø2FQ3ZZ
Ø2FR3ZØ
Ø2FR3ZZ
Ø2FS3ZØ
Ø2FS3ZZ
Ø2FT3ZØ
Ø2FT3ZZ
Ø2UØ37Z
Ø2UØ38Z
Ø2UØ3JZ
Ø2UØ3KZ
Ø2U137Z
Ø2U138Z
Ø2U13JZ
Ø2U13KZ
Ø2U237Z
Ø2U238Z
Ø2U23JZ
Ø2U23KZ
Ø2U337Z
Ø2U338Z
Ø2U33JZ
Ø2U33KZ
OR
Nonoperating Room Procedures

Ø257ØZK
Ø2B7ØZK
Ø2U73JZ
Ø2U74JZ
X2A7358

DRG 251

Select operating room procedures OR nonoperating room procedures listed under DRG 250

DRG 252

Operating Room Procedures

ØØHEØMZ
ØØHE3MZ
ØØHE4MZ
Ø1HYØMZ
Ø1HY3MZ
Ø1HY4MZ
Ø21PØ8A
Ø21PØ8B
Ø21PØ8D
Ø21PØ9A
Ø21PØ9B
Ø21PØ9D
Ø21PØAA
Ø21PØAB
Ø21PØAD
Ø21PØJA
Ø21PØJB
Ø21PØJD
Ø21PØKA
Ø21PØKB
Ø21PØKD
Ø21PØZA
Ø21PØZB
Ø21PØZD
Ø21P48A
Ø21P48B
Ø21P48D
Ø21P49A
Ø21P49B
Ø21P49D
Ø21P4AA
Ø21P4AB
Ø21P4AD
Ø21P4JA
Ø21P4JB
Ø21P4JD
Ø21P4KA
Ø21P4KB
Ø21P4KD
Ø21P4ZA
Ø21P4ZB
Ø21P4ZD
Ø21QØ8A
Ø21QØ8B
Ø21QØ8D
Ø21QØ9A
Ø21QØ9B
Ø21QØ9D
Ø21QØAA
Ø21QØAB
Ø21QØAD
Ø21QØJA
Ø21QØJB
Ø21QØJD
Ø21QØKA
Ø21QØKB
Ø21QØKD
Ø21QØZA
Ø21QØZB
Ø21QØZD
Ø21Q48A
Ø21Q48B
Ø21Q48D
Ø21Q49A
Ø21Q49B
Ø21Q49D
Ø21Q4AA
Ø21Q4AB
Ø21Q4AD
Ø21Q4JA
Ø21Q4JB
Ø21Q4JD
Ø21Q4KA
Ø21Q4KB
Ø21Q4KD
Ø21Q4ZA
Ø21Q4ZB
Ø21Q4ZD
Ø21RØ8A
Ø21RØ8B
Ø21RØ8D
Ø21RØ9A
Ø21RØ9B
Ø21RØ9D
Ø21RØAA
Ø21RØAB
Ø21RØAD
Ø21RØJA
Ø21RØJB
Ø21RØJD
Ø21RØKA
Ø21RØKB
Ø21RØKD
Ø21RØZA
Ø21RØZB
Ø21RØZD
Ø21R48A
Ø21R48B
Ø21R48D
Ø21R49A
Ø21R49B
Ø21R49D
Ø21R4AA
Ø21R4AB
Ø21R4AD
Ø21R4JA
Ø21R4JB
Ø21R4JD
Ø21R4KA
Ø21R4KB
Ø21R4KD
Ø21R4ZA
Ø21R4ZB
Ø21R4ZD
Ø27P*
Ø27Q*
Ø27RØ4Z
Ø27RØDZ
Ø27RØZZ
Ø27R34Z
Ø27R3DZ
Ø27R3ZZ
Ø27R44Z
Ø27R4DZ
Ø27R4ZZ
Ø27S*
Ø27T*
Ø27V*
Ø27W*
Ø27XØ4Z
Ø27XØDZ
Ø27XØZZ
Ø27X34Z
Ø27X3DZ
Ø27X3ZZ
Ø27X44Z
Ø27X4DZ
Ø27X4ZZ
Ø2BPØZX
Ø2BP3ZX
Ø2BP4ZX
Ø2BQØZX
Ø2BQ3ZX
Ø2BQ4ZX
Ø2BRØZX
Ø2BR3ZX
Ø2BR4ZX
Ø2BSØZX
Ø2BS3ZX
Ø2BS4ZX
Ø2BTØZX
Ø2BT3ZX
Ø2BT4ZX
Ø2BVØZX
Ø2BV3ZX
Ø2BV4ZX
Ø2BWØZX
Ø2BW3ZX
Ø2BW4ZX
Ø2BXØZX
Ø2BX3ZX
Ø2BX4ZX
Ø2HVØ2Z
Ø2HVØDZ
Ø2HV3DZ
Ø2HV42Z
Ø2HV4DZ
Ø2LPØCZ
Ø2LPØDZ
Ø2LPØZZ
Ø2LP3CZ
Ø2LP3DZ
Ø2LP3ZZ
Ø2LP4CZ
Ø2LP4DZ
Ø2LP4ZZ
Ø2LQØCZ
Ø2LQØDZ
Ø2LQØZZ
Ø2LQ3CZ
Ø2LQ3DZ
Ø2LQ3ZZ
Ø2LQ4CZ
Ø2LQ4DZ
Ø2LQ4ZZ
Ø2LRØCZ
Ø2LRØDZ
Ø2LRØZZ
Ø2LR3CZ
Ø2LR3DZ
Ø2LR3ZZ
Ø2LR4CZ
Ø2LR4DZ
Ø2LR4ZZ
Ø2LV*
Ø2NP*
Ø2NQ*
Ø2NR*
Ø2NS*
Ø2NT*
Ø2NV*
Ø2NW*
Ø2NXØZZ
Ø2NX3ZZ
Ø2NX4ZZ
Ø2QP*
Ø2QQ*
Ø2QR*
Ø2S*
Ø2UP*
Ø2UQ*
Ø2UR*
Ø2US*
Ø2UT*
Ø2UV*
Ø2UWØ7Z
Ø2UWØ8Z
Ø2UWØJZ
Ø2UWØKZ
Ø2UW37Z
Ø2UW38Z
Ø2UW3KZ
Ø2UW47Z
Ø2UW48Z
Ø2UW4KZ
Ø2UXØ7Z
Ø2UXØ8Z
Ø2UXØJZ
Ø2UXØKZ
Ø2UX37Z
Ø2UX38Z
Ø2UX3KZ
Ø2UX47Z
Ø2UX48Z
Ø2UX4KZ
Ø2VPØCZ
Ø2VP3CZ
Ø2VP4CZ
Ø2VRØCT
Ø2VR3CT
Ø2VR4CT
Ø2VSØCZ
Ø2VS3CZ
Ø2VS4CZ
Ø2VTØCZ
Ø2VT3CZ
Ø2VT4CZ
Ø2VV*
Ø2VWØCZ
Ø2VW3CZ
Ø2VW4CZ
Ø2VXØCZ
Ø2VX3CZ
Ø2VX4CZ
Ø312*
313Ø9Ø
313Ø91
313Ø92
313Ø93
313Ø94
313Ø95
313Ø96
313Ø97
313Ø98
313Ø99
Ø313Ø9B
Ø313Ø9C
Ø313Ø9D
Ø313Ø9F
Ø313Ø9J
Ø313Ø9K
Ø313Ø9W
Ø313ØAØ
Ø313ØA1
Ø313ØA2
Ø313ØA3
Ø313ØA4
Ø313ØA5
Ø313ØA6
Ø313ØA7
Ø313ØA8
Ø313ØA9
Ø313ØAB
Ø313ØAC
Ø313ØAD
Ø313ØAF
Ø313ØAJ
Ø313ØAK
Ø313ØAW
Ø313ØJØ
Ø313ØJ1
Ø313ØJ2
Ø313ØJ3
Ø313ØJ4
Ø313ØJ5
Ø313ØJ6
Ø313ØJ7
Ø313ØJ8
Ø313ØJ9
Ø313ØJB
Ø313ØJC
Ø313ØJD
Ø313ØJF
Ø313ØJJ
Ø313ØJK
Ø313ØJW
Ø313ØKØ
Ø313ØK1
Ø313ØK2
Ø313ØK3
Ø313ØK4
Ø313ØK5
Ø313ØK6
Ø313ØK7
Ø313ØK8
Ø313ØK9
Ø313ØKB
Ø313ØKC
Ø313ØKD
Ø313ØKF
Ø313ØKJ
Ø313ØKK
Ø313ØKW
Ø313ØZØ
Ø313ØZ1
Ø313ØZ2
Ø313ØZ3
Ø313ØZ4
Ø313ØZ5
Ø313ØZ6
Ø313ØZ7
Ø313ØZ8
Ø313ØZ9
Ø313ØZB
Ø313ØZC
Ø313ØZD
Ø313ØZF
Ø313ØZJ
Ø313ØZK
Ø313ØZW
314Ø9Ø
314Ø91
314Ø92
314Ø93
314Ø94
314Ø95
314Ø96
314Ø97
314Ø98
314Ø99
Ø314Ø9B
Ø314Ø9C
Ø314Ø9D
Ø314Ø9F
Ø314Ø9J
Ø314Ø9K
Ø314Ø9W
Ø314ØAØ

03140A1
03140A2
03140A3
03140A4
03140A5
03140A6
03140A7
03140A8
03140A9
03140AB
03140AC
03140AD
03140AF
03140AJ
03140AK
03140AW
03140J0
03140J1
03140J2
03140J3
03140J4
03140J5
03140J6
03140J7
03140J8
03140J9
03140JB
03140JC
03140JD
03140JF
03140JJ
03140JK
03140JW
03140K0
03140K1
03140K2
03140K3
03140K4
03140K5
03140K6
03140K7
03140K8
03140K9
03140KB
03140KC
03140KD
03140KF
03140KJ
03140KK
03140KW
03140Z0
03140Z1
03140Z2
03140Z3
03140Z4
03140Z5
03140Z6
03140Z7
03140Z8
03140Z9
03140ZB
03140ZC
03140ZD
03140ZF
03140ZJ
03140ZK
03140ZW
0315*
0316*
317090
317093
031709W
03170A0
03170A3
03170AW
03170J0
03170J3
03170JW
03170K0
03170K3
03170KW
03170Z0
03170Z3
03170ZW
318091
318094
031809W
03180A1
03180A4
03180AW
03180J1
03180J4
03180JW
03180K1
03180K4
03180KW
03180Z1
03180Z4
03180ZW
319093
03190A3
03190J3
03190K3
03190Z3
031A094
031A0A4
031A0J4
031A0K4
031A0Z4
031B093
031B0A3
031B0J3
031B0K3
031B0Z3
031C094
031C0A4
031C0J4
031C0K4
031C0Z4
031G*
031H09J
031H09K
031H09Y
031H0AJ
031H0AK
031H0AY
031H0JJ
031H0JK
031H0JY
031H0KJ
031H0KK
031H0KY
031H0ZJ
031H0ZK
031H0ZY
031J09J
031J09K
031J09Y
031J0AJ
031J0AK
031J0AY
031J0JJ
031J0JK
031J0JY
031J0KJ
031J0KK
031J0KY
031J0ZJ
031J0ZK
031J0ZY
031K09J
031K09K
031K0AJ
031K0AK
031K0JJ
031K0JK
031K0KJ
031K0KK
031K0ZJ
031K0ZK
031L09J
031L09K
031L0AJ
031L0AK
031L0JJ
031L0JK
031L0KJ
031L0KK
031L0ZJ
031L0ZK
031M09J
031M09K
031M0AJ
031M0AK
031M0JJ
031M0JK
031M0KJ
031M0KK
031M0ZJ
031M0ZK
031N09J
031N09K
031N0AJ
031N0AK
031N0JJ
031N0JK
031N0KJ
031N0KK
031N0ZJ
031N0ZK
0355*
0356*
0357*
0358*
0359*
035A*
035B*
035C*
035D*
035F*
035H*
035J*
035K*
035L*
035M*
035N*
035P*
035Q*
035R*
035S*
035T*
035U*
035V*
035Y*
037*
03900ZX
03904ZX
03910ZX
03914ZX
03920ZX
03924ZX
03930ZX
03934ZX
03940ZX
03944ZX
03950ZX
03954ZX
03960ZX
03964ZX
03970ZX
03974ZX
03980ZX
03984ZX
03990ZX
03994ZX
039A0ZX
039A4ZX
039B0ZX
039B4ZX
039C0ZX
039C4ZX
039D0ZX
039D4ZX
039F0ZX
039F4ZX
039G0ZX
039G4ZX
039H0ZX
039H4ZX
039J0ZX
039J4ZX
039K0ZX
039K4ZX
039L0ZX
039L4ZX
039M0ZX
039M4ZX
039N0ZX
039N4ZX
039P0ZX
039P4ZX
039Q0ZX
039Q4ZX
039R0ZX
039R4ZX
039S0ZX
039S4ZX
039T0ZX
039T4ZX
039U0ZX
039U4ZX
039V0ZX
039V4ZX
039Y0ZX
039Y4ZX
03B00ZX
03B03ZX
03B04ZX
03B10ZX
03B13ZX
03B14ZX
03B20ZX
03B23ZX
03B24ZX
03B30ZX
03B33ZX
03B34ZX
03B40ZX
03B43ZX
03B44ZX
03B5*
03B6*
03B7*
03B8*
03B9*
03BA*
03BB*
03BC*
03BD*
03BF*
03BG0ZX
03BG3ZX
03BG4ZX
03BH*
03BJ*
03BK*
03BL*
03BM*
03BN*
03BP*
03BQ*
03BR*
03BS*
03BT*
03BU*
03BV*
03BY*
03C5*
03C6*
03C7*
03C8*
03C9*
03CA*
03CB*
03CC*
03CD*
03CF*
03CG3Z7
03CG3ZZ
03CH0ZZ
03CJ0ZZ
03CK0ZZ
03CL0ZZ
03CM0ZZ
03CN0ZZ
03CP0ZZ
03CQ0ZZ
03CR0ZZ
03CS0ZZ
03CT0ZZ
03CU0ZZ
03CV0ZZ
03CY*
03F23Z0
03F23ZZ
03F33Z0
03F33ZZ
03F43Z0
03F43ZZ
03F53Z0
03F53ZZ
03F63Z0
03F63ZZ
03F73Z0
03F73ZZ
03F83Z0
03F83ZZ
03F93Z0
03F93ZZ
03FA3Z0
03FA3ZZ
03FB3Z0
03FB3ZZ
03FC3Z0
03FC3ZZ
03FG3Z0
03FG3ZZ
03FY3Z0
03FY3ZZ
03H00DZ
03H03DZ
03H04DZ
03H10DZ
03H13DZ
03H14DZ
03H20DZ
03H23DZ
03H24DZ
03H30DZ
03H33DZ
03H34DZ
03H40DZ
03H43DZ
03H44DZ
03H50DZ
03H53DZ
03H54DZ
03H60DZ
03H63DZ
03H64DZ
03H70DZ
03H73DZ
03H74DZ
03H80DZ
03H83DZ
03H84DZ
03H90DZ
03H93DZ
03H94DZ
03HA0DZ
03HA3DZ
03HA4DZ
03HB0DZ
03HB3DZ
03HB4DZ
03HC0DZ
03HC3DZ
03HC4DZ
03HD0DZ
03HD3DZ
03HD4DZ
03HF0DZ
03HF3DZ
03HF4DZ
03HG0DZ
03HG3DZ
03HG4DZ
03HH0DZ
03HH3DZ
03HH4DZ
03HJ0DZ
03HJ3DZ
03HJ4DZ
03HK0DZ
03HK0MZ
03HK3DZ
03HK3MZ
03HK4DZ
03HK4MZ
03HL0DZ
03HL0MZ
03HL3DZ
03HL3MZ
03HL4DZ
03HL4MZ
03HM0DZ
03HM3DZ
03HM4DZ
03HN0DZ
03HN3DZ
03HN4DZ
03HP0DZ
03HP3DZ
03HP4DZ
03HQ0DZ
03HQ3DZ
03HQ4DZ
03HR0DZ
03HR3DZ
03HR4DZ
03HS0DZ
03HS3DZ
03HS4DZ
03HT0DZ
03HT3DZ
03HT4DZ
03HU0DZ
03HU3DZ
03HU4DZ
03HV0DZ
03HV3DZ
03HV4DZ
03HY02Z
03HY0DZ
03HY0YZ
03HY3DZ
03HY42Z
03HY4DZ
03JY0ZZ
03L50CZ
03L50DZ
03L50ZZ
03L53CZ
03L53DZ
03L53ZZ
03L54CZ
03L54DZ
03L54ZZ
03L60CZ
03L60DZ
03L60ZZ
03L63CZ
03L63DZ
03L63ZZ
03L64CZ
03L64DZ
03L64ZZ
03L70CZ
03L70DZ
03L70ZZ
03L73CZ
03L73DZ
03L73ZZ
03L74CZ
03L74DZ
03L74ZZ
03L80CZ
03L80DZ
03L80ZZ
03L83CZ
03L83DZ
03L83ZZ
03L84CZ
03L84DZ
03L84ZZ
03L90CZ
03L90DZ
03L90ZZ
03L93CZ
03L93DZ
03L93ZZ
03L94CZ
03L94DZ
03L94ZZ
03LA0CZ
03LA0DZ
03LA0ZZ
03LA3CZ
03LA3DZ
03LA3ZZ
03LA4CZ
03LA4DZ
03LA4ZZ
03LB0CZ
03LB0DZ
03LB0ZZ
03LB3CZ
03LB3DZ
03LB3ZZ
03LB4CZ
03LB4DZ
03LB4ZZ
03LC0CZ
03LC0DZ
03LC0ZZ
03LC3CZ
03LC3DZ
03LC3ZZ
03LC4CZ
03LC4DZ
03LC4ZZ
03LD0CZ
03LD0DZ
03LD0ZZ
03LD3CZ
03LD3DZ
03LD3ZZ
03LD4CZ
03LD4DZ
03LD4ZZ
03LF0CZ
03LF0DZ
03LF0ZZ
03LF3CZ
03LF3DZ
03LF3ZZ
03LF4CZ
03LF4DZ
03LF4ZZ
03LH0CZ
03LH0ZZ
03LH3CZ
03LH3ZZ
03LH4CZ
03LH4ZZ
03LJ0CZ
03LJ0ZZ
03LJ3CZ
03LJ3ZZ
03LJ4CZ
03LJ4ZZ
03LK0CZ
03LK0ZZ
03LK3CZ
03LK3ZZ
03LK4CZ
03LK4ZZ
03LL0CZ
03LL0ZZ
03LL3CZ
03LL3ZZ
03LL4CZ
03LL4ZZ
03LM0CZ
03LM0ZZ
03LM3CZ
03LM3ZZ
03LM4CZ
03LM4ZZ
03LN0CZ
03LN0ZZ
03LN3CZ
03LN3ZZ
03LN4CZ
03LN4ZZ
03LP0CZ
03LP0ZZ
03LP3CZ
03LP3ZZ
03LP4CZ
03LP4ZZ
03LQ0CZ
03LQ0ZZ
03LQ3CZ
03LQ3ZZ
03LQ4CZ
03LQ4ZZ
03LR0CZ
03LR0ZZ
03LR3CZ
03LR3ZZ
03LR4CZ
03LR4ZZ
03LS0CZ
03LS0ZZ
03LS3CZ
03LS3ZZ
03LS4CZ
03LS4ZZ
03LT0CZ
03LT0ZZ
03LT3CZ
03LT3ZZ
03LT4CZ
03LT4ZZ
03LY0CZ
03LY0DZ
03LY0ZZ
03LY3CZ
03LY3DZ
03LY3ZZ
03LY4CZ
03LY4DZ
03LY4ZZ
03N*
03PY00Z
03PY02Z
03PY03Z
03PY0CZ
03PY0DZ
03PY0MZ
03PY0YZ
03PY3CZ
03PY3MZ
03PY40Z
03PY42Z
03PY43Z
03PY4CZ
03PY4DZ
03PY4MZ
03Q*
03R5*
03R6*
03R7*
03R8*
03R9*
03RA*
03RB*
03RC*
03RD*
03RF*
03RH*
03RJ*
03RK*
03RL*
03RM*
03RN*
03RP*
03RQ*
03RR*
03RS*
03RT*
03RU*
03RV*
03RY*
03S*
03U*
03V00CZ
03V03CZ
03V04CZ
03V10CZ
03V13CZ
03V14CZ
03V20CZ
03V23CZ
03V24CZ
03V30CZ
03V33CZ
03V34CZ
03V40CZ
03V43CZ
03V44CZ
03V50CZ
03V53CZ
03V54CZ
03V60CZ
03V63CZ
03V64CZ
03V70CZ
03V73CZ
03V74CZ
03V80CZ
03V83CZ
03V84CZ
03V90CZ
03V93CZ
03V94CZ
03VA0CZ
03VA3CZ
03VA4CZ
03VB0CZ
03VB3CZ
03VB4CZ
03VC0CZ
03VC3CZ
03VC4CZ
03VD0CZ
03VD3CZ
03VD4CZ
03VF0CZ
03VF3CZ
03VF4CZ
03VG0CZ
03VG3CZ
03VG4CZ
03VH0CZ
03VH0HZ
03VH3CZ
03VH3HZ
03VH4CZ
03VH4HZ
03VJ0CZ
03VJ0HZ
03VJ3CZ
03VJ3HZ
03VJ4CZ
03VJ4HZ
03VK0CZ
03VK0HZ
03VK3CZ
03VK3HZ
03VK4CZ
03VK4HZ
03VL0CZ
03VL0HZ
03VL3CZ
03VL3HZ
03VL4CZ
03VL4HZ
03VM0CZ
03VM0HZ
03VM3CZ
03VM3HZ
03VM4CZ
03VM4HZ
03VN0CZ
03VN0HZ
03VN3CZ
03VN3HZ
03VN4CZ
03VN4HZ
03VP0CZ
03VP0HZ
03VP3CZ
03VP3HZ
03VP4CZ
03VP4HZ
03VQ0CZ
03VQ0HZ
03VQ3CZ
03VQ3HZ
03VQ4CZ
03VQ4HZ
03VR0CZ
03VR3CZ
03VR4CZ
03VS0CZ
03VS3CZ
03VS4CZ
03VT0CZ
03VT3CZ
03VT4CZ
03VU0CZ
03VU3CZ
03VU4CZ
03VV0CZ
03VV3CZ
03VV4CZ
03VY0CZ
03VY3CZ
03VY4CZ
03WY00Z
03WY02Z
03WY03Z
03WY07Z
03WY0CZ
03WY0DZ
03WY0JZ
03WY0KZ
03WY0MZ
03WY0YZ
03WY37Z
03WY3CZ
03WY3DZ
03WY3JZ
03WY3KZ
03WY3MZ
03WY40Z
03WY42Z
03WY43Z
03WY47Z
03WY4CZ
03WY4DZ
03WY4JZ
03WY4KZ
03WY4MZ
041K*
041L*
041M*
041N*
041P0JQ
041P0JS
041P3JQ
041P3JS
041P4JQ
041P4JS
041Q0JQ
041Q0JS
041Q3JQ
041Q3JS
041Q4JQ
041Q4JS
041R0JQ
041R0JS
041R3JQ
041R3JS
041R4JQ
041R4JS
041S0JQ
041S0JS
041S3JQ
041S3JS
041S4JQ
041S4JS
041T09P
041T09Q
041T09S
041T0AP
041T0AQ
041T0AS
041T0JP
041T0JQ
041T0JS
041T0KP
041T0KQ

Ø41TØKS
Ø41TØZP
Ø41TØZQ
Ø41TØZS
Ø41T3JQ
Ø41T3JS
Ø41T49P
Ø41T49Q
Ø41T49S
Ø41T4AP
Ø41T4AQ
Ø41T4AS
Ø41T4JP
Ø41T4JQ
Ø41T4JS
Ø41T4KP
Ø41T4KQ
Ø41T4KS
Ø41T4ZP
Ø41T4ZQ
Ø41T4ZS
Ø41UØ9P
Ø41UØ9Q
Ø41UØ9S
Ø41UØAP
Ø41UØAQ
Ø41UØAS
Ø41UØJP
Ø41UØJQ
Ø41UØJS
Ø41UØKP
Ø41UØKQ
Ø41UØKS
Ø41UØZP
Ø41UØZQ
Ø41UØZS
Ø41U3JQ
Ø41U3JS
Ø41U49P
Ø41U49Q
Ø41U49S
Ø41U4AP
Ø41U4AQ
Ø41U4AS
Ø41U4JP
Ø41U4JQ
Ø41U4JS
Ø41U4KP
Ø41U4KQ
Ø41U4KS
Ø41U4ZP
Ø41U4ZQ
Ø41U4ZS
Ø41VØ9P
Ø41VØ9Q
Ø41VØ9S
Ø41VØAP
Ø41VØAQ
Ø41VØAS
Ø41VØJP
Ø41VØJQ
Ø41VØJS
Ø41VØKP
Ø41VØKQ
Ø41VØKS
Ø41VØZP
Ø41VØZQ
Ø41VØZS
Ø41V3JQ
Ø41V3JS
Ø41V49P
Ø41V49Q
Ø41V49S
Ø41V4AP
Ø41V4AQ
Ø41V4AS
Ø41V4JP
Ø41V4JQ
Ø41V4JS
Ø41V4KP
Ø41V4KQ
Ø41V4KS
Ø41V4ZP
Ø41V4ZQ
Ø41V4ZS
Ø41WØ9P
Ø41WØ9Q
Ø41WØ9S
Ø41WØAP
Ø41WØAQ
Ø41WØAS
Ø41WØJP
Ø41WØJQ
Ø41WØJS
Ø41WØKP
Ø41WØKQ
Ø41WØKS
Ø41WØZP
Ø41WØZQ
Ø41WØZS
Ø41W3JQ
Ø41W3JS
Ø41W49P
Ø41W49Q
Ø41W49S
Ø41W4AP
Ø41W4AQ
Ø41W4AS
Ø41W4JP
Ø41W4JQ
Ø41W4JS
Ø41W4KP
Ø41W4KQ
Ø41W4KS
Ø41W4ZP
Ø41W4ZQ
Ø41W4ZS
Ø45K*
Ø45L*
Ø45M*
Ø45N*
Ø45P*
Ø45Q*
Ø45R*
Ø45S*
Ø45T*
Ø45U*
Ø45V*
Ø45W*
Ø45Y*
Ø47*
Ø49ØØZX
Ø49Ø4ZX
Ø491ØZX
Ø4914ZX
Ø492ØZX
Ø4924ZX
Ø493ØZX
Ø4934ZX
Ø494ØZX
Ø4944ZX
Ø495ØZX
Ø4954ZX
Ø496ØZX
Ø4964ZX
Ø497ØZX
Ø4974ZX
Ø498ØZX
Ø4984ZX
Ø499ØZX
Ø4994ZX
Ø49AØZX
Ø49A4ZX
Ø49BØZX
Ø49B4ZX
Ø49CØZX
Ø49C4ZX
Ø49DØZX
Ø49D4ZX
Ø49EØZX
Ø49E4ZX
Ø49FØZX
Ø49F4ZX
Ø49HØZX
Ø49H4ZX
Ø49JØZX
Ø49J4ZX
Ø49KØZX
Ø49K4ZX
Ø49LØZX
Ø49L4ZX
Ø49MØZX
Ø49M4ZX
Ø49NØZX
Ø49N4ZX
Ø49PØZX
Ø49P4ZX
Ø49QØZX
Ø49Q4ZX
Ø49RØZX
Ø49R4ZX
Ø49SØZX
Ø49S4ZX
Ø49TØZX
Ø49T4ZX
Ø49UØZX
Ø49U4ZX
Ø49VØZX
Ø49V4ZX
Ø49WØZX
Ø49W4ZX
Ø49YØZX
Ø49Y4ZX
Ø4BØØZX
Ø4BØ3ZX
Ø4BØ4ZX
Ø4B1ØZX
Ø4B13ZX
Ø4B14ZX
Ø4B2ØZX
Ø4B23ZX
Ø4B24ZX
Ø4B3ØZX
Ø4B33ZX
Ø4B34ZX
Ø4B4ØZX
Ø4B43ZX
Ø4B44ZX
Ø4B5ØZX
Ø4B53ZX
Ø4B54ZX
Ø4B6ØZX
Ø4B63ZX
Ø4B64ZX
Ø4B7ØZX
Ø4B73ZX
Ø4B74ZX
Ø4B8ØZX
Ø4B83ZX
Ø4B84ZX
Ø4B9ØZX
Ø4B93ZX
Ø4B94ZX
Ø4BAØZX
Ø4BA3ZX
Ø4BA4ZX
Ø4BBØZX
Ø4BB3ZX
Ø4BB4ZX
Ø4BCØZX
Ø4BC3ZX
Ø4BC4ZX
Ø4BDØZX
Ø4BD3ZX
Ø4BD4ZX
Ø4BEØZX
Ø4BE3ZX
Ø4BE4ZX
Ø4BFØZX
Ø4BF3ZX
Ø4BF4ZX
Ø4BHØZX
Ø4BH3ZX
Ø4BH4ZX
Ø4BJØZX
Ø4BJ3ZX
Ø4BJ4ZX
Ø4BK*
Ø4BL*
Ø4BM*
Ø4BN*
Ø4BP*
Ø4BQ*
Ø4BR*
Ø4BS*
Ø4BT*
Ø4BU*
Ø4BV*
Ø4BW*
Ø4BY*
Ø4CKØZZ
Ø4CK4ZZ
Ø4CLØZZ
Ø4CL4ZZ
Ø4CMØZZ
Ø4CM4ZZ
Ø4CNØZZ
Ø4CN4ZZ
Ø4CPØZZ
Ø4CP4ZZ
Ø4CQØZZ
Ø4CQ4ZZ
Ø4CRØZZ
Ø4CR4ZZ
Ø4CSØZZ
Ø4CS4ZZ
Ø4CTØZZ
Ø4CT4ZZ
Ø4CUØZZ
Ø4CU4ZZ
Ø4CVØZZ
Ø4CV4ZZ
Ø4CWØZZ
Ø4CW4ZZ
Ø4CYØZZ
Ø4CY4ZZ
Ø4FC3ZØ
Ø4FC3ZZ
Ø4FD3ZØ
Ø4FD3ZZ
Ø4FE3ZØ
Ø4FE3ZZ
Ø4FF3ZØ
Ø4FF3ZZ
Ø4FH3ZØ
Ø4FH3ZZ
Ø4FJ3ZØ
Ø4FJ3ZZ
Ø4FK3ZØ
Ø4FK3ZZ
Ø4FL3ZØ
Ø4FL3ZZ
Ø4FM3ZØ
Ø4FM3ZZ
Ø4FN3ZØ
Ø4FN3ZZ
Ø4FP3ZØ
Ø4FP3ZZ
Ø4FQ3ZØ
Ø4FQ3ZZ
Ø4FR3ZØ
Ø4FR3ZZ
Ø4FS3ZØ
Ø4FS3ZZ
Ø4FT3ZØ
Ø4FT3ZZ
Ø4FU3ZØ
Ø4FU3ZZ
Ø4FY3ZØ
Ø4FY3ZZ
Ø4HØØDZ
Ø4HØ3DZ
Ø4HØ4DZ
Ø4H1ØDZ
Ø4H13DZ
Ø4H14DZ
Ø4H2ØDZ
Ø4H23DZ
Ø4H24DZ
Ø4H3ØDZ
Ø4H33DZ
Ø4H34DZ
Ø4H4ØDZ
Ø4H43DZ
Ø4H44DZ
Ø4H5ØDZ
Ø4H53DZ
Ø4H54DZ
Ø4H6ØDZ
Ø4H63DZ
Ø4H64DZ
Ø4H7ØDZ
Ø4H73DZ
Ø4H74DZ
Ø4H8ØDZ
Ø4H83DZ
Ø4H84DZ
Ø4H9ØDZ
Ø4H93DZ
Ø4H94DZ
Ø4HAØDZ
Ø4HA3DZ
Ø4HA4DZ
Ø4HBØDZ
Ø4HB3DZ
Ø4HB4DZ
Ø4HCØDZ
Ø4HC3DZ
Ø4HC4DZ
Ø4HDØDZ
Ø4HD3DZ
Ø4HD4DZ
Ø4HEØDZ
Ø4HE3DZ
Ø4HE4DZ
Ø4HFØDZ
Ø4HF3DZ
Ø4HF4DZ
Ø4HHØDZ
Ø4HH3DZ
Ø4HH4DZ
Ø4HJØDZ
Ø4HJ3DZ
Ø4HJ4DZ
Ø4HKØDZ
Ø4HK3DZ
Ø4HK4DZ
Ø4HLØDZ
Ø4HL3DZ
Ø4HL4DZ
Ø4HMØDZ
Ø4HM3DZ
Ø4HM4DZ
Ø4HNØDZ
Ø4HN3DZ
Ø4HN4DZ
Ø4HPØDZ
Ø4HP3DZ
Ø4HP4DZ
Ø4HQØDZ
Ø4HQ3DZ
Ø4HQ4DZ
Ø4HRØDZ
Ø4HR3DZ
Ø4HR4DZ
Ø4HSØDZ
Ø4HS3DZ
Ø4HS4DZ
Ø4HTØDZ
Ø4HT3DZ
Ø4HT4DZ
Ø4HUØDZ
Ø4HU3DZ
Ø4HU4DZ
Ø4HVØDZ
Ø4HV3DZ
Ø4HV4DZ
Ø4HWØDZ
Ø4HW3DZ
Ø4HW4DZ
Ø4HYØ2Z
Ø4HYØDZ
Ø4HYØYZ
Ø4HY3DZ
Ø4HY42Z
Ø4HY4DZ
Ø4JYØZZ
Ø4LEØCV
Ø4LEØDV
Ø4LEØZV
Ø4LE4CV
Ø4LE4DV
Ø4LE4ZV
Ø4LFØCW
Ø4LFØDW
Ø4LFØZW
Ø4LF4CW
Ø4LF4DW
Ø4LF4ZW
Ø4LKØCZ
Ø4LKØDZ
Ø4LKØZZ
Ø4LK3CZ
Ø4LK3DZ
Ø4LK3ZZ
Ø4LK4CZ
Ø4LK4DZ
Ø4LK4ZZ
Ø4LLØCZ
Ø4LLØDZ
Ø4LLØZZ
Ø4LL3CZ
Ø4LL3DZ
Ø4LL3ZZ
Ø4LL4CZ
Ø4LL4DZ
Ø4LL4ZZ
Ø4LMØCZ
Ø4LMØDZ
Ø4LMØZZ
Ø4LM3CZ
Ø4LM3DZ
Ø4LM3ZZ
Ø4LM4CZ
Ø4LM4DZ
Ø4LM4ZZ
Ø4LNØCZ
Ø4LNØDZ
Ø4LNØZZ
Ø4LN3CZ
Ø4LN3DZ
Ø4LN3ZZ
Ø4LN4CZ
Ø4LN4DZ
Ø4LN4ZZ
Ø4LPØCZ
Ø4LPØDZ
Ø4LPØZZ
Ø4LP3CZ
Ø4LP3DZ
Ø4LP3ZZ
Ø4LP4CZ
Ø4LP4DZ
Ø4LP4ZZ
Ø4LQØCZ
Ø4LQØDZ
Ø4LQØZZ
Ø4LQ3CZ
Ø4LQ3DZ
Ø4LQ3ZZ
Ø4LQ4CZ
Ø4LQ4DZ
Ø4LQ4ZZ
Ø4LRØCZ
Ø4LRØDZ
Ø4LRØZZ
Ø4LR3CZ
Ø4LR3DZ
Ø4LR3ZZ
Ø4LR4CZ
Ø4LR4DZ
Ø4LR4ZZ
Ø4LSØCZ
Ø4LSØDZ
Ø4LSØZZ
Ø4LS3CZ
Ø4LS3DZ
Ø4LS3ZZ
Ø4LS4CZ
Ø4LS4DZ
Ø4LS4ZZ
Ø4LTØCZ
Ø4LTØDZ
Ø4LTØZZ
Ø4LT3CZ
Ø4LT3DZ
Ø4LT3ZZ
Ø4LT4CZ
Ø4LT4DZ
Ø4LT4ZZ
Ø4LUØCZ
Ø4LUØDZ
Ø4LUØZZ
Ø4LU3CZ
Ø4LU3DZ
Ø4LU3ZZ
Ø4LU4CZ
Ø4LU4DZ
Ø4LU4ZZ
Ø4LVØCZ
Ø4LVØDZ
Ø4LVØZZ
Ø4LV3CZ
Ø4LV3DZ
Ø4LV3ZZ
Ø4LV4CZ
Ø4LV4DZ
Ø4LV4ZZ
Ø4LWØCZ
Ø4LWØDZ
Ø4LWØZZ
Ø4LW3CZ
Ø4LW3DZ
Ø4LW3ZZ
Ø4LW4CZ
Ø4LW4DZ
Ø4LW4ZZ
Ø4LYØCZ
Ø4LYØDZ
Ø4LYØZZ
Ø4LY3CZ
Ø4LY3DZ
Ø4LY3ZZ
Ø4LY4CZ
Ø4LY4DZ
Ø4LY4ZZ
Ø4N*
Ø4PYØØZ
Ø4PYØ2Z
Ø4PYØ3Z
Ø4PYØ7Z
Ø4PYØCZ
Ø4PYØDZ
Ø4PYØJZ
Ø4PYØKZ
Ø4PYØYZ
Ø4PY37Z
Ø4PY3CZ
Ø4PY3JZ
Ø4PY3KZ
Ø4PY4ØZ
Ø4PY42Z
Ø4PY43Z
Ø4PY47Z
Ø4PY4CZ
Ø4PY4DZ
Ø4PY4JZ
Ø4PY4KZ
Ø4Q*
Ø4RK*
Ø4RL*
Ø4RM*
Ø4RN*
Ø4RP*
Ø4RQ*
Ø4RR*
Ø4RS*
Ø4RT*
Ø4RU*
Ø4RV*
Ø4RW*
Ø4RY*
Ø4S*
Ø4UØØ7Z
Ø4UØØJZ
Ø4UØØKZ
Ø4UØ37Z
Ø4UØ3KZ
Ø4UØ47Z
Ø4UØ4KZ
Ø4U1*
Ø4U2*
Ø4U3*
Ø4U4*
Ø4U5*
Ø4U6*
Ø4U7*
Ø4U8*
Ø4U9*
Ø4UA*
Ø4UB*
Ø4UC*
Ø4UD*
Ø4UE*
Ø4UF*
Ø4UH*
Ø4UJ*
Ø4UK*
Ø4UL*
Ø4UM*
Ø4UN*
Ø4UP*
Ø4UQ*
Ø4UR*
Ø4US*
Ø4UT*
Ø4UU*
Ø4UV*
Ø4UW*
Ø4UY*
Ø4VØØCZ
Ø4VØØDJ
Ø4VØ3CZ
Ø4VØ3DJ
Ø4VØ4CZ
Ø4VØ4DJ
Ø4V1ØCZ
Ø4V13CZ
Ø4V14CZ
Ø4V2ØCZ
Ø4V23CZ
Ø4V24CZ
Ø4V3ØCZ
Ø4V33CZ
Ø4V34CZ
Ø4V4ØCZ
Ø4V43CZ
Ø4V44CZ
Ø4V5ØCZ
Ø4V53CZ
Ø4V54CZ
Ø4V6ØCZ
Ø4V63CZ
Ø4V64CZ
Ø4V7ØCZ
Ø4V73CZ
Ø4V74CZ
Ø4V8ØCZ
Ø4V83CZ
Ø4V84CZ
Ø4V9ØCZ
Ø4V93CZ
Ø4V94CZ
Ø4VAØCZ
Ø4VA3CZ
Ø4VA4CZ
Ø4VBØCZ
Ø4VB3CZ
Ø4VB4CZ
Ø4VCØCZ
Ø4VC3CZ
Ø4VC4CZ
Ø4VDØCZ
Ø4VD3CZ
Ø4VD4CZ
Ø4VEØCZ
Ø4VE3CZ
Ø4VE4CZ
Ø4VFØCZ
Ø4VF3CZ
Ø4VF4CZ
Ø4VHØCZ
Ø4VH3CZ
Ø4VH4CZ
Ø4VJØCZ
Ø4VJ3CZ
Ø4VJ4CZ
Ø4VKØCZ
Ø4VK3CZ
Ø4VK4CZ
Ø4VLØCZ
Ø4VL3CZ
Ø4VL4CZ
Ø4VMØCZ
Ø4VM3CZ
Ø4VM4CZ
Ø4VNØCZ
Ø4VN3CZ
Ø4VN4CZ
Ø4VPØCZ
Ø4VP3CZ
Ø4VP4CZ
Ø4VQØCZ
Ø4VQ3CZ
Ø4VQ4CZ
Ø4VRØCZ
Ø4VR3CZ
Ø4VR4CZ
Ø4VSØCZ
Ø4VS3CZ
Ø4VS4CZ
Ø4VTØCZ
Ø4VT3CZ
Ø4VT4CZ
Ø4VUØCZ
Ø4VU3CZ
Ø4VU4CZ
Ø4VVØCZ
Ø4VV3CZ
Ø4VV4CZ
Ø4VWØCZ
Ø4VW3CZ
Ø4VW4CZ
Ø4VYØCZ
Ø4VY3CZ
Ø4VY4CZ
Ø4WYØØZ
Ø4WYØ2Z
Ø4WYØ3Z
Ø4WYØ7Z
Ø4WYØCZ
Ø4WYØDZ
Ø4WYØJZ
Ø4WYØKZ
Ø4WYØYZ
Ø4WY37Z
Ø4WY3CZ
Ø4WY3DZ
Ø4WY3JZ
Ø4WY3KZ
Ø4WY4ØZ
Ø4WY42Z
Ø4WY43Z
Ø4WY47Z
Ø4WY4CZ
Ø4WY4DZ
Ø4WY4JZ
Ø4WY4KZ
Ø517*
Ø518*
Ø519*
Ø51A*
Ø51B*
Ø51C*
Ø51D*
Ø51F*
Ø51G*
Ø51H*
Ø51L*
Ø51M*
Ø51N*
Ø51P*
Ø51Q*
Ø51R*
Ø51S*
Ø51T*
Ø51V*
Ø557*
Ø558*
Ø559*
Ø55A*
Ø55B*
Ø55C*
Ø55D*
Ø55F*
Ø55G*
Ø55H*
Ø55M*
Ø55N*
Ø55P*
Ø55Q*
Ø55R*
Ø55S*
Ø55T*
Ø55V*
Ø55Y*
Ø57*
Ø59ØØZX
Ø59Ø4ZX
Ø591ØZX
Ø5914ZX
Ø593ØZX
Ø5934ZX
Ø594ØZX
Ø5944ZX
Ø595ØZX
Ø5954ZX
Ø596ØZX
Ø5964ZX
Ø597ØZX
Ø5974ZX
Ø598ØZX
Ø5984ZX
Ø599ØZX
Ø5994ZX
Ø59AØZX
Ø59A4ZX
Ø59BØZX
Ø59B4ZX
Ø59CØZX
Ø59C4ZX
Ø59DØZX
Ø59D4ZX
Ø59FØZX
Ø59F4ZX
Ø59GØZX
Ø59G4ZX
Ø59HØZX
Ø59H4ZX
Ø59LØZX
Ø59L4ZX
Ø59MØZX
Ø59M4ZX
Ø59NØZX
Ø59N4ZX
Ø59PØZX
Ø59P4ZX
Ø59QØZX
Ø59Q4ZX
Ø59RØZX
Ø59R4ZX
Ø59SØZX
Ø59S4ZX
Ø59TØZX
Ø59T4ZX
Ø59VØZX
Ø59V4ZX
Ø59YØZX
Ø59Y4ZX
Ø5BØØZX
Ø5BØ3ZX
Ø5BØ4ZX
Ø5B1ØZX
Ø5B13ZX
Ø5B14ZX
Ø5B3ØZX
Ø5B33ZX
Ø5B34ZX
Ø5B4ØZX
Ø5B43ZX
Ø5B44ZX
Ø5B5ØZX
Ø5B53ZX
Ø5B54ZX
Ø5B6ØZX
Ø5B63ZX
Ø5B64ZX
Ø5B7*
Ø5B8*
Ø5B9*
Ø5BA*
Ø5BB*
Ø5BC*
Ø5BD*
Ø5BF*

Ø5BG*
Ø5BH*
Ø5BLØZX
Ø5BL3ZX
Ø5BL4ZX
Ø5BM*
Ø5BN*
Ø5BP*
Ø5BQ*
Ø5BR*
Ø5BS*
Ø5BT*
Ø5BV*
Ø5BY*
Ø5C7*
Ø5C8*
Ø5C9*
Ø5CA*
Ø5CB*
Ø5CC*
Ø5CD*
Ø5CF*
Ø5CG*
Ø5CH*
Ø5CL3ZZ
Ø5CM*
Ø5CN*
Ø5CP*
Ø5CQ*
Ø5CR*
Ø5CS*
Ø5CT*
Ø5CV*
Ø5CY*
Ø5F33ZØ
Ø5F33ZZ
Ø5F43ZØ
Ø5F43ZZ
Ø5F53ZØ
Ø5F53ZZ
Ø5F63ZØ
Ø5F63ZZ
Ø5F73ZØ
Ø5F73ZZ
Ø5F83ZØ
Ø5F83ZZ
Ø5F93ZØ
Ø5F93ZZ
Ø5FA3ZØ
Ø5FA3ZZ
Ø5FB3ZØ
Ø5FB3ZZ
Ø5FC3ZØ
Ø5FC3ZZ
Ø5FD3ZØ
Ø5FD3ZZ
Ø5FF3ZØ
Ø5FF3ZZ
Ø5FY3ZØ
Ø5FY3ZZ
Ø5HØØ2Z
Ø5HØØDZ
Ø5HØØMZ
Ø5HØ32Z
Ø5HØ3DZ
Ø5HØ3MZ
Ø5HØ42Z
Ø5HØ4DZ
Ø5HØ4MZ
Ø5H1ØDZ
Ø5H13DZ
Ø5H14DZ
Ø5H3ØDZ
Ø5H3ØMZ
Ø5H33DZ
Ø5H33MZ
Ø5H34DZ
Ø5H34MZ
Ø5H4ØDZ
Ø5H4ØMZ
Ø5H43DZ
Ø5H43MZ
Ø5H44DZ
Ø5H44MZ
Ø5H5ØDZ
Ø5H53DZ
Ø5H54DZ
Ø5H6ØDZ
Ø5H63DZ
Ø5H64DZ
Ø5H7ØDZ
Ø5H73DZ
Ø5H74DZ
Ø5H8ØDZ
Ø5H83DZ
Ø5H84DZ
Ø5H9ØDZ
Ø5H93DZ
Ø5H94DZ
Ø5HAØDZ
Ø5HA3DZ
Ø5HA4DZ
Ø5HBØDZ
Ø5HB3DZ
Ø5HB4DZ
Ø5HCØDZ
Ø5HC3DZ
Ø5HC4DZ
Ø5HDØDZ
Ø5HD3DZ
Ø5HD4DZ
Ø5HFØDZ
Ø5HF3DZ
Ø5HF4DZ
Ø5HGØDZ
Ø5HG3DZ
Ø5HG4DZ
Ø5HHØDZ
Ø5HH3DZ
Ø5HH4DZ
Ø5HLØDZ
Ø5HL3DZ
Ø5HL4DZ
Ø5HMØDZ
Ø5HM3DZ
Ø5HM4DZ
Ø5HNØDZ
Ø5HN3DZ
Ø5HN4DZ
Ø5HPØDZ
Ø5HP3DZ
Ø5HP4DZ
Ø5HQØDZ
Ø5HQ3DZ
Ø5HQ4DZ
Ø5HRØDZ
Ø5HR3DZ
Ø5HR4DZ
Ø5HSØDZ
Ø5HS3DZ
Ø5HS4DZ
Ø5HTØDZ
Ø5HT3DZ
Ø5HT4DZ
Ø5HVØDZ
Ø5HV3DZ
Ø5HV4DZ
Ø5HYØ2Z
Ø5HYØDZ
Ø5HYØYZ
Ø5HY3DZ
Ø5HY42Z
Ø5HY4DZ
Ø5JYØZZ
Ø5JY4ZZ
Ø5L7ØCZ
Ø5L7ØDZ
Ø5L7ØZZ
Ø5L73CZ
Ø5L73DZ
Ø5L73ZZ
Ø5L74CZ
Ø5L74DZ
Ø5L74ZZ
Ø5L8ØCZ
Ø5L8ØDZ
Ø5L8ØZZ
Ø5L83CZ
Ø5L83DZ
Ø5L83ZZ
Ø5L84CZ
Ø5L84DZ
Ø5L84ZZ
Ø5L9ØCZ
Ø5L9ØDZ
Ø5L9ØZZ
Ø5L93CZ
Ø5L93DZ
Ø5L93ZZ
Ø5L94CZ
Ø5L94DZ
Ø5L94ZZ
Ø5LAØCZ
Ø5LAØDZ
Ø5LAØZZ
Ø5LA3CZ
Ø5LA3DZ
Ø5LA3ZZ
Ø5LA4CZ
Ø5LA4DZ
Ø5LA4ZZ
Ø5LBØCZ
Ø5LBØDZ
Ø5LBØZZ
Ø5LB3CZ
Ø5LB3DZ
Ø5LB3ZZ
Ø5LB4CZ
Ø5LB4DZ
Ø5LB4ZZ
Ø5LCØCZ
Ø5LCØDZ
Ø5LCØZZ
Ø5LC3CZ
Ø5LC3DZ
Ø5LC3ZZ
Ø5LC4CZ
Ø5LC4DZ
Ø5LC4ZZ
Ø5LDØCZ
Ø5LDØDZ
Ø5LDØZZ
Ø5LD3CZ
Ø5LD3DZ
Ø5LD3ZZ
Ø5LD4CZ
Ø5LD4DZ
Ø5LD4ZZ
Ø5LFØCZ
Ø5LFØDZ
Ø5LFØZZ
Ø5LF3CZ
Ø5LF3DZ
Ø5LF3ZZ
Ø5LF4CZ
Ø5LF4DZ
Ø5LF4ZZ
Ø5LGØCZ
Ø5LGØDZ
Ø5LGØZZ
Ø5LG3CZ
Ø5LG3DZ
Ø5LG3ZZ
Ø5LG4CZ
Ø5LG4DZ
Ø5LG4ZZ
Ø5LHØCZ
Ø5LHØDZ
Ø5LHØZZ
Ø5LH3CZ
Ø5LH3DZ
Ø5LH3ZZ
Ø5LH4CZ
Ø5LH4DZ
Ø5LH4ZZ
Ø5LM*
Ø5LN*
Ø5LP*
Ø5LQ*
Ø5LR*
Ø5LS*
Ø5LT*
Ø5LV*
Ø5LYØCZ
Ø5LYØDZ
Ø5LYØZZ
Ø5LY3CZ
Ø5LY3DZ
Ø5LY3ZZ
Ø5LY4CZ
Ø5LY4DZ
Ø5LY4ZZ
Ø5N*
Ø5PYØØZ
Ø5PYØ2Z
Ø5PYØ3Z
Ø5PYØ7Z
Ø5PYØCZ
Ø5PYØDZ
Ø5PYØJZ
Ø5PYØKZ
Ø5PYØYZ
Ø5PY37Z
Ø5PY3CZ
Ø5PY3JZ
Ø5PY3KZ
Ø5PY4ØZ
Ø5PY42Z
Ø5PY43Z
Ø5PY47Z
Ø5PY4CZ
Ø5PY4DZ
Ø5PY4JZ
Ø5PY4KZ
Ø5QY*
Ø5R7*
Ø5R8*
Ø5R9*
Ø5RA*
Ø5RB*
Ø5RC*
Ø5RD*
Ø5RF*
Ø5RG*
Ø5RH*
Ø5RM*
Ø5RN*
Ø5RP*
Ø5RQ*
Ø5RR*
Ø5RS*
Ø5RT*
Ø5RV*
Ø5RY*
Ø5S*
Ø5U*
Ø5VØØCZ
Ø5VØ3CZ
Ø5VØ4CZ
Ø5V1ØCZ
Ø5V13CZ
Ø5V14CZ
Ø5V3ØCZ
Ø5V33CZ
Ø5V34CZ
Ø5V4ØCZ
Ø5V43CZ
Ø5V44CZ
Ø5V5ØCZ
Ø5V53CZ
Ø5V54CZ
Ø5V6ØCZ
Ø5V63CZ
Ø5V64CZ
Ø5V7ØCZ
Ø5V73CZ
Ø5V74CZ
Ø5V8ØCZ
Ø5V83CZ
Ø5V84CZ
Ø5V9ØCZ
Ø5V93CZ
Ø5V94CZ
Ø5VAØCZ
Ø5VA3CZ
Ø5VA4CZ
Ø5VBØCZ
Ø5VB3CZ
Ø5VB4CZ
Ø5VCØCZ
Ø5VC3CZ
Ø5VC4CZ
Ø5VDØCZ
Ø5VD3CZ
Ø5VD4CZ
Ø5VFØCZ
Ø5VF3CZ
Ø5VF4CZ
Ø5VGØCZ
Ø5VG3CZ
Ø5VG4CZ
Ø5VHØCZ
Ø5VH3CZ
Ø5VH4CZ
Ø5VLØCZ
Ø5VL3CZ
Ø5VL4CZ
Ø5VMØCZ
Ø5VM3CZ
Ø5VM4CZ
Ø5VNØCZ
Ø5VN3CZ
Ø5VN4CZ
Ø5VPØCZ
Ø5VP3CZ
Ø5VP4CZ
Ø5VQØCZ
Ø5VQ3CZ
Ø5VQ4CZ
Ø5VRØCZ
Ø5VR3CZ
Ø5VR4CZ
Ø5VSØCZ
Ø5VS3CZ
Ø5VS4CZ
Ø5VTØCZ
Ø5VT3CZ
Ø5VT4CZ
Ø5VVØCZ
Ø5VV3CZ
Ø5VV4CZ
Ø5VYØCZ
Ø5VY3CZ
Ø5VY4CZ
Ø5WØØ2Z
Ø5WØ32Z
Ø5WØ42Z
Ø5WØX2Z
Ø5WYØØZ
Ø5WYØ2Z
Ø5WYØ3Z
Ø5WYØ7Z
Ø5WYØCZ
Ø5WYØDZ
Ø5WYØJZ
Ø5WYØKZ
Ø5WYØYZ
Ø5WY37Z
Ø5WY3CZ
Ø5WY3DZ
Ø5WY3JZ
Ø5WY3KZ
Ø5WY4ØZ
Ø5WY42Z
Ø5WY43Z
Ø5WY47Z
Ø5WY4CZ
Ø5WY4DZ
Ø5WY4JZ
Ø5WY4KZ
Ø613*
Ø61C*
Ø61D*
Ø61F*
Ø61G*
Ø61H*
Ø61M*
Ø61N*
Ø61P*
Ø61Q*
Ø61T*
Ø61V*
Ø653*
Ø67*
Ø69ØØZX
Ø69Ø4ZX
Ø691ØZX
Ø6914ZX
Ø692ØZX
Ø6924ZX
Ø693ØØZ
Ø693ØZX
Ø693ØZZ
Ø6934ØZ
Ø6934ZX
Ø6934ZZ
Ø694ØZX
Ø6944ZX
Ø695ØZX
Ø6954ZX
Ø696ØZX
Ø6964ZX
Ø697ØZX
Ø6974ZX
Ø698ØZX
Ø6984ZX
Ø699ØZX
Ø6994ZX
Ø69BØZX
Ø69B4ZX
Ø69CØZX
Ø69C4ZX
Ø69DØZX
Ø69D4ZX
Ø69FØZX
Ø69F4ZX
Ø69GØZX
Ø69G4ZX
Ø69HØZX
Ø69H4ZX
Ø69JØZX
Ø69J4ZX
Ø69MØZX
Ø69M4ZX
Ø69NØZX
Ø69N4ZX
Ø69PØZX
Ø69P4ZX
Ø69QØZX
Ø69Q4ZX
Ø69TØZX
Ø69T4ZX
Ø69VØZX
Ø69V4ZX
Ø69YØZX
Ø69Y4ZX
Ø6BØØZX
Ø6BØ3ZX
Ø6BØ4ZX
Ø6B1ØZX
Ø6B13ZX
Ø6B14ZX
Ø6B2ØZX
Ø6B23ZX
Ø6B24ZX
Ø6B3*
Ø6B4ØZX
Ø6B43ZX
Ø6B44ZX
Ø6B5ØZX
Ø6B53ZX
Ø6B54ZX
Ø6B6ØZX
Ø6B63ZX
Ø6B64ZX
Ø6B7ØZX
Ø6B73ZX
Ø6B74ZX
Ø6B8ØZX
Ø6B83ZX
Ø6B84ZX
Ø6B9ØZX
Ø6B93ZX
Ø6B94ZX
Ø6BBØZX
Ø6BB3ZX
Ø6BB4ZX
Ø6BCØZX
Ø6BC3ZX
Ø6BC4ZX
Ø6BDØZX
Ø6BD3ZX
Ø6BD4ZX
Ø6BFØZX
Ø6BF3ZX
Ø6BF4ZX
Ø6BGØZX
Ø6BG3ZX
Ø6BG4ZX
Ø6BHØZX
Ø6BH3ZX
Ø6BH4ZX
Ø6BJØZX
Ø6BJ3ZX
Ø6BJ4ZX
Ø6BMØZX
Ø6BM3ZX
Ø6BM4ZX
Ø6BNØZX
Ø6BN3ZX
Ø6BN4ZX
Ø6BPØZX
Ø6BP3ZX
Ø6BP4ZX
Ø6BQØZX
Ø6BQ3ZX
Ø6BQ4ZX
Ø6BTØZX
Ø6BT3ZX
Ø6BT4ZX
Ø6BVØZX
Ø6BV3ZX
Ø6BV4ZX
Ø6BYØZX
Ø6BYØZZ
Ø6BY3ZX
Ø6BY3ZZ
Ø6BY4ZX
Ø6BY4ZZ
Ø6C3*
Ø6CYØZZ
Ø6CY4ZZ
Ø6FC3ZØ
Ø6FC3ZZ
Ø6FD3ZØ
Ø6FD3ZZ
Ø6FF3ZØ
Ø6FF3ZZ
Ø6FG3ZØ
Ø6FG3ZZ
Ø6FH3ZØ
Ø6FH3ZZ
Ø6FJ3ZØ
Ø6FJ3ZZ
Ø6FM3ZØ
Ø6FM3ZZ
Ø6FN3ZØ
Ø6FN3ZZ
Ø6FP3ZØ
Ø6FP3ZZ
Ø6FQ3ZØ
Ø6FQ3ZZ
Ø6FY3ZØ
Ø6FY3ZZ
Ø6HØØDZ
Ø6HØ4DZ
Ø6H1ØDZ
Ø6H13DZ
Ø6H14DZ
Ø6H2ØDZ
Ø6H23DZ
Ø6H24DZ
Ø6H3ØDZ
Ø6H33DZ
Ø6H34DZ
Ø6H4ØDZ
Ø6H43DZ
Ø6H44DZ
Ø6H5ØDZ
Ø6H53DZ
Ø6H54DZ
Ø6H6ØDZ
Ø6H63DZ
Ø6H64DZ
Ø6H7ØDZ
Ø6H73DZ
Ø6H74DZ
Ø6H8ØDZ
Ø6H83DZ
Ø6H84DZ
Ø6H9ØDZ
Ø6H93DZ
Ø6H94DZ
Ø6HBØDZ
Ø6HB3DZ
Ø6HB4DZ
Ø6HCØDZ
Ø6HC3DZ
Ø6HC4DZ
Ø6HDØDZ
Ø6HD3DZ
Ø6HD4DZ
Ø6HFØDZ
Ø6HF3DZ
Ø6HF4DZ
Ø6HGØDZ
Ø6HG3DZ
Ø6HG4DZ
Ø6HHØDZ
Ø6HH3DZ
Ø6HH4DZ
Ø6HJØDZ
Ø6HJ3DZ
Ø6HJ4DZ
Ø6HMØDZ
Ø6HM3DZ
Ø6HM4DZ
Ø6HNØDZ
Ø6HN3DZ
Ø6HN4DZ
Ø6HPØDZ
Ø6HP3DZ
Ø6HP4DZ
Ø6HQØDZ
Ø6HQ3DZ
Ø6HQ4DZ
Ø6HTØDZ
Ø6HT3DZ
Ø6HT4DZ
Ø6HVØDZ
Ø6HV3DZ
Ø6HV4DZ
Ø6HYØDZ
Ø6HY3DZ
Ø6HY4DZ
Ø6JYØZZ
Ø6JY4ZZ
Ø6LØ*
Ø6LYØCZ
Ø6LYØZZ
Ø6LY3CZ
Ø6LY3ZZ
Ø6LY4CZ
Ø6LY4ZZ
Ø6N*
Ø6PYØ7Z
Ø6PYØJZ
Ø6PYØKZ
Ø6PY37Z
Ø6PY3JZ
Ø6PY3KZ
Ø6PY47Z
Ø6PY4JZ
Ø6PY4KZ
Ø6QY*
Ø6R3*
Ø6S*
Ø6U*
Ø6VØ*
Ø6V1ØCZ
Ø6V13CZ
Ø6V14CZ
Ø6V2ØCZ
Ø6V23CZ
Ø6V24CZ
Ø6V3ØCZ
Ø6V33CZ
Ø6V34CZ
Ø6V4ØCZ
Ø6V43CZ
Ø6V44CZ
Ø6V5ØCZ
Ø6V53CZ
Ø6V54CZ
Ø6V6ØCZ
Ø6V63CZ
Ø6V64CZ
Ø6V7ØCZ
Ø6V73CZ
Ø6V74CZ
Ø6V8ØCZ
Ø6V83CZ
Ø6V84CZ
Ø6V9ØCZ
Ø6V93CZ
Ø6V94CZ
Ø6VBØCZ
Ø6VB3CZ
Ø6VB4CZ
Ø6VCØCZ
Ø6VC3CZ
Ø6VC4CZ
Ø6VDØCZ
Ø6VD3CZ
Ø6VD4CZ
Ø6VFØCZ
Ø6VF3CZ
Ø6VF4CZ
Ø6VGØCZ
Ø6VG3CZ
Ø6VG4CZ
Ø6VHØCZ
Ø6VH3CZ
Ø6VH4CZ
Ø6VJØCZ
Ø6VJ3CZ
Ø6VJ4CZ
Ø6VMØCZ
Ø6VM3CZ
Ø6VM4CZ
Ø6VNØCZ
Ø6VN3CZ
Ø6VN4CZ
Ø6VPØCZ
Ø6VP3CZ
Ø6VP4CZ
Ø6VQØCZ
Ø6VQ3CZ
Ø6VQ4CZ
Ø6VTØCZ
Ø6VT3CZ
Ø6VT4CZ
Ø6VVØCZ
Ø6VV3CZ
Ø6VV4CZ
Ø6VYØCZ
Ø6VY3CZ
Ø6VY4CZ
Ø6WYØ7Z
Ø6WYØJZ
Ø6WYØKZ
Ø6WY37Z
Ø6WY3DZ
Ø6WY3JZ
Ø6WY3KZ
Ø6WY47Z
Ø6WY4JZ
Ø6WY4KZ
ØDH6ØMZ
ØDH63MZ
ØDH64MZ
ØG56ØZ3
ØG56ØZZ
ØG563Z3
ØG563ZZ
ØG564Z3
ØG564ZZ
ØG57ØZ3
ØG57ØZZ
ØG573Z3
ØG573ZZ
ØG574Z3
ØG574ZZ
ØG58ØZ3
ØG58ØZZ
ØG583Z3
ØG583ZZ
ØG584Z3
ØG584ZZ
ØG59ØZ3
ØG59ØZZ
ØG593Z3
ØG593ZZ
ØG594Z3
ØG594ZZ
ØG5BØZ3
ØG5BØZZ
ØG5B3Z3
ØG5B3ZZ
ØG5B4Z3
ØG5B4ZZ
ØG5CØZ3
ØG5CØZZ
ØG5C3Z3
ØG5C3ZZ
ØG5C4Z3
ØG5C4ZZ
ØG5DØZ3
ØG5DØZZ
ØG5D3Z3
ØG5D3ZZ
ØG5D4Z3
ØG5D4ZZ
ØG5FØZ3
ØG5FØZZ
ØG5F3Z3
ØG5F3ZZ
ØG5F4Z3
ØG5F4ZZ
ØG96ØØZ
ØG96ØZX
ØG96ØZZ
ØG963ZX
ØG964ØZ
ØG964ZX
ØG964ZZ
ØG97ØØZ
ØG97ØZX
ØG97ØZZ
ØG973ZX
ØG974ØZ
ØG974ZX
ØG974ZZ
ØG98ØØZ
ØG98ØZX
ØG98ØZZ
ØG983ZX
ØG984ØZ
ØG984ZX
ØG984ZZ
ØG99ØØZ
ØG99ØZX
ØG99ØZZ
ØG993ZX
ØG994ØZ
ØG994ZX
ØG994ZZ
ØG9BØØZ
ØG9BØZX
ØG9BØZZ
ØG9B3ZX
ØG9B4ØZ
ØG9B4ZX
ØG9B4ZZ
ØG9CØØZ
ØG9CØZX
ØG9CØZZ
ØG9C3ZX
ØG9C4ØZ
ØG9C4ZX
ØG9C4ZZ
ØG9DØØZ
ØG9DØZX
ØG9DØZZ
ØG9D3ZX
ØG9D4ØZ
ØG9D4ZX
ØG9D4ZZ
ØG9FØØZ
ØG9FØZX
ØG9FØZZ
ØG9F3ZX
ØG9F4ØZ
ØG9F4ZX
ØG9F4ZZ

ØGB6ØZX
ØGB6ØZZ
ØGB63ZX
ØGB63ZZ
ØGB64ZX
ØGB64ZZ
ØGB7ØZX
ØGB7ØZZ
ØGB73ZX
ØGB73ZZ
ØGB74ZX
ØGB74ZZ
ØGB8ØZX
ØGB8ØZZ
ØGB83ZX
ØGB83ZZ
ØGB84ZX
ØGB84ZZ
ØGB9ØZX
ØGB9ØZZ
ØGB93ZX
ØGB93ZZ
ØGB94ZX
ØGB94ZZ
ØGBBØZX
ØGBBØZZ
ØGBB3ZX
ØGBB3ZZ
ØGBB4ZX
ØGBB4ZZ
ØGBCØZX
ØGBCØZZ
ØGBC3ZX
ØGBC3ZZ
ØGBC4ZX
ØGBC4ZZ
ØGBDØZX
ØGBDØZZ
ØGBD3ZX
ØGBD3ZZ
ØGBD4ZX
ØGBD4ZZ
ØGBFØZX
ØGBFØZZ
ØGBF3ZX
ØGBF3ZZ
ØGBF4ZX
ØGBF4ZZ
ØGC6ØZZ
ØGC63ZZ
ØGC64ZZ
ØGC7ØZZ
ØGC73ZZ
ØGC74ZZ
ØGC8ØZZ
ØGC83ZZ
ØGC84ZZ
ØGC9ØZZ
ØGC93ZZ
ØGC94ZZ
ØGCBØZZ
ØGCB3ZZ
ØGCB4ZZ
ØGCCØZZ
ØGCC3ZZ
ØGCC4ZZ
ØGCDØZZ
ØGCD3ZZ
ØGCD4ZZ
ØGCFØZZ
ØGCF3ZZ
ØGCF4ZZ
ØGN6ØZZ
ØGN63ZZ
ØGN64ZZ
ØGN7ØZZ
ØGN73ZZ
ØGN74ZZ
ØGN8ØZZ
ØGN83ZZ
ØGN84ZZ
ØGN9ØZZ
ØGN93ZZ
ØGN94ZZ
ØGNBØZZ
ØGNB3ZZ
ØGNB4ZZ
ØGNCØZZ
ØGNC3ZZ
ØGNC4ZZ
ØGNDØZZ
ØGND3ZZ
ØGND4ZZ
ØGNFØZZ
ØGNF3ZZ
ØGNF4ZZ
ØGPSØØZ
ØGPSØ2Z
ØGPSØ3Z
ØGPSØYZ
ØGPS3ØZ
ØGPS32Z
ØGPS33Z
ØGPS4ØZ
ØGPS42Z
ØGPS43Z
ØGQ6ØZZ
ØGQ63ZZ
ØGQ64ZZ
ØGQ7ØZZ
ØGQ73ZZ
ØGQ74ZZ
ØGQ8ØZZ
ØGQ83ZZ
ØGQ84ZZ
ØGQ9ØZZ
ØGQ93ZZ
ØGQ94ZZ
ØGQBØZZ
ØGQB3ZZ
ØGQB4ZZ
ØGQCØZZ
ØGQC3ZZ
ØGQC4ZZ
ØGQDØZZ
ØGQD3ZZ
ØGQD4ZZ
ØGQFØZZ
ØGQF3ZZ
ØGQF4ZZ
ØGT6ØZZ
ØGT64ZZ
ØGT7ØZZ
ØGT74ZZ
ØGT8ØZZ
ØGT84ZZ
ØGT9ØZZ
ØGT94ZZ
ØGTBØZZ
ØGTB4ZZ
ØGTCØZZ
ØGTC4ZZ
ØGTDØZZ
ØGTD4ZZ
ØGTFØZZ
ØGTF4ZZ
ØGWSØØZ
ØGWSØ2Z
ØGWSØ3Z
ØGWSØYZ
ØGWS3ØZ
ØGWS32Z
ØGWS33Z
ØGWS4ØZ
ØGWS42Z
ØGWS43Z
ØJH6ØBZ
ØJH6ØCZ
ØJH6ØDZ
ØJH6ØEZ
ØJH6ØMZ
ØJH63BZ
ØJH63CZ
ØJH63DZ
ØJH63EZ
ØJH63MZ
ØJH7ØBZ
ØJH7ØCZ
ØJH7ØDZ
ØJH7ØEZ
ØJH7ØMZ
ØJH73BZ
ØJH73CZ
ØJH73DZ
ØJH73EZ
ØJH73MZ
ØJH8ØBZ
ØJH8ØCZ
ØJH8ØDZ
ØJH8ØEZ
ØJH8ØMZ
ØJH83BZ
ØJH83CZ
ØJH83DZ
ØJH83EZ
ØJH83MZ
ØW3C*
XØHK3Q8
XØHQ3R8
X27H385
X27H395
X27H3B5
X27H3C5
X27J385
X27J395
X27J3B5
X27J3C5
X27K385
X27K395
X27K3B5
X27K3C5
X27L385
X27L395
X27L3B5
X27L3C5
X27M385
X27M395
X27M3B5
X27M3C5
X27N385
X27N395
X27N3B5
X27N3C5
X27P385
X27P395
X27P3B5
X27P3C5
X27Q385
X27Q395
X27Q3B5
X27Q3C5
X27R385
X27R395
X27R3B5
X27R3C5
X27S385
X27S395
X27S3B5
X27S3C5
X27T385
X27T395
X27T3B5
X27T3C5
X27U385
X27U395
X27U3B5
X27U3C5
X2H13R9
X2H2ØR9
X2H3ØR9
X2HLØF9
X2HMØF9
X2HXØF9
X2KH3D9
X2KH3E9
X2KJ3D9
X2KJ3E9
X2UQØP9
X2URØP9

OR

Nonoperating Room Procedures

ØJWTØMZ
ØJWT3MZ
ØJWTXMZ

DRG 253

Select operating room OR nonoperating room procedures listed under DRG 252

DRG 254

Select operating room OR nonoperating room procedures listed under DRG 252

DRG 255

Operating Room Procedures

ØX6*
ØY6P*
ØY6Q*
ØY6R*
ØY6S*
ØY6T*
ØY6U*
ØY6V*
ØY6W*
ØY6X*
ØY6Y*

DRG 256

Select operating room procedures listed under DRG 255

DRG 257

Select operating room procedures listed under DRG 255

DRG 258

Nonoperating Room Procedures

ØJH6Ø4Z
ØJH6Ø5Z
ØJH6Ø6Z
ØJH6Ø7Z
ØJH6ØPZ
ØJH634Z
ØJH635Z
ØJH636Z
ØJH637Z
ØJH63PZ
ØJH8Ø4Z
ØJH8Ø5Z
ØJH8Ø6Z
ØJH8Ø7Z
ØJH8ØPZ
ØJH834Z
ØJH835Z
ØJH836Z
ØJH837Z
ØJH83PZ

DRG 259

Select nonoperating room procedures listed under DRG 258

DRG 260

Operating Room Procedures

Ø2HKØØZ
Ø2HKØ2Z
Ø2HKØYZ
Ø2HK3YZ
Ø2HK4ØZ
Ø2HK42Z
Ø2HK4YZ
Ø2PAØMZ
Ø2PA3MZ
Ø2PA4MZ
Ø2WAØMZ
Ø2WA3MZ
Ø2WA4MZ
ØJH6ØØZ
ØJH6Ø2Z
ØJH63ØZ
ØJH632Z
ØJH8ØØZ
ØJH83ØZ
ØJPTØPZ
ØJPT3PZ
ØJWTØ2Z
ØJWTØPZ
ØJWTØYZ
ØJWT32Z
ØJWT3PZ

OR

Nonoperating Room Procedures

Ø2H4ØJZ
Ø2H4ØMZ
Ø2H43JZ
Ø2H43MZ
Ø2H44JZ
Ø2H44MZ
Ø2H6ØJZ
Ø2H6ØMZ
Ø2H63JZ
Ø2H63MZ
Ø2H64JZ
Ø2H64MZ
Ø2H7ØJZ
Ø2H7ØMZ
Ø2H73JZ
Ø2H73MZ
Ø2H74JZ
Ø2H74MZ
Ø2HKØJZ
Ø2HKØMZ
Ø2HK32Z
Ø2HK3JZ
Ø2HK3MZ
Ø2HK4JZ
Ø2HK4MZ
Ø2HLØJZ
Ø2HLØMZ
Ø2HL3JZ
Ø2HL3MZ
Ø2HL4JZ
Ø2HL4MZ
Ø2HNØJZ
Ø2HNØMZ
Ø2HN3JZ
Ø2HN3MZ
Ø2HN4JZ
Ø2HN4MZ

DRG 261

Select operating room or nonoperating room procedures listed under DRG 260

DRG 262

Select operating room procedures listed under DRG 260

DRG 263

Operating Room Procedures

Ø2QS*
Ø2QT*
Ø2QV*
Ø5D*
Ø5QØ*
Ø5Q1*
Ø5Q3*
Ø5Q4*
Ø5Q5*
Ø5Q6*
Ø5Q7*
Ø5Q8*
Ø5Q9*
Ø5QA*
Ø5QB*
Ø5QC*
Ø5QD*
Ø5QF*
Ø5QG*
Ø5QH*
Ø5QL*
Ø5QM*
Ø5QN*
Ø5QP*
Ø5QQ*
Ø5QR*
Ø5QS*
Ø5QT*
Ø5QV*
Ø65M*
Ø65N*
Ø65P*
Ø65Q*
Ø65T*
Ø65V*
Ø65YØZZ
Ø65Y3ZZ
Ø65Y4ZZ
Ø6BMØZZ
Ø6BM3ZZ
Ø6BM4ZZ
Ø6BNØZZ
Ø6BN3ZZ
Ø6BN4ZZ
Ø6BPØZZ
Ø6BP3ZZ
Ø6BP4ZZ
Ø6BQØZZ
Ø6BQ3ZZ
Ø6BQ4ZZ
Ø6BTØZZ
Ø6BT3ZZ
Ø6BT4ZZ
Ø6BVØZZ
Ø6BV3ZZ
Ø6BV4ZZ
Ø6CMØZZ
Ø6CM4ZZ
Ø6CNØZZ
Ø6CN4ZZ
Ø6CPØZZ
Ø6CP4ZZ
Ø6CQØZZ
Ø6CQ4ZZ
Ø6CTØZZ
Ø6CT4ZZ
Ø6CVØZZ
Ø6CV4ZZ
Ø6D*
Ø6HYØ2Z
Ø6HYØYZ
Ø6HY42Z
Ø6LM*
Ø6LN*
Ø6LP*
Ø6LQ*
Ø6LT*
Ø6LV*
Ø6LYØDZ
Ø6LY3DZ
Ø6LY4DZ
Ø6LY7CZ
Ø6LY7DZ
Ø6LY7ZZ
Ø6LY8CZ
Ø6LY8DZ
Ø6LY8ZZ
Ø6PYØØZ
Ø6PYØ2Z
Ø6PYØ3Z
Ø6PYØCZ
Ø6PYØDZ
Ø6PYØYZ
Ø6PY3CZ
Ø6PY4ØZ
Ø6PY42Z
Ø6PY43Z
Ø6PY4CZ
Ø6PY4DZ
Ø6QØ*
Ø6Q1*
Ø6Q2*
Ø6Q3*
Ø6Q4*
Ø6Q5*
Ø6Q6*
Ø6Q7*
Ø6Q8*
Ø6Q9*
Ø6QB*
Ø6QC*
Ø6QD*
Ø6QF*
Ø6QG*
Ø6QH*
Ø6QJ*
Ø6QM*
Ø6QN*
Ø6QP*
Ø6QQ*
Ø6QT*
Ø6QV*
Ø6RM*
Ø6RN*
Ø6RP*
Ø6RQ*
Ø6RT*
Ø6RV*
Ø6RY*
Ø6WYØØZ
Ø6WYØ2Z
Ø6WYØ3Z
Ø6WYØCZ
Ø6WYØDZ
Ø6WYØYZ
Ø6WY3CZ
Ø6WY4ØZ
Ø6WY42Z
Ø6WY43Z
Ø6WY4CZ
Ø6WY4DZ
3EØ3ØTZ
3EØ4ØTZ

DRG 264

Operating Room Procedures

Ø15K*
Ø15L*
Ø15M*
Ø15N*
Ø15P*
Ø18K*
Ø18L*
Ø18M*
Ø18N*
Ø18P*
Ø19KØØZ
Ø19KØZZ
Ø19K4ØZ
Ø19K4ZZ
Ø19LØØZ
Ø19LØZZ
Ø19L4ØZ
Ø19L4ZZ
Ø19MØØZ
Ø19MØZZ
Ø19M4ØZ
Ø19M4ZZ
Ø19NØØZ
Ø19NØZZ
Ø19N4ØZ
Ø19N4ZZ
Ø19PØØZ
Ø19PØZZ
Ø19P4ØZ
Ø19P4ZZ
Ø1BKØZZ
Ø1BK3ZZ
Ø1BK4ZZ
Ø1BLØZZ
Ø1BL3ZZ
Ø1BL4ZZ
Ø1BMØZZ
Ø1BM3ZZ
Ø1BM4ZZ
Ø1BNØZZ
Ø1BN3ZZ
Ø1BN4ZZ
Ø1BPØZZ
Ø1BP3ZZ
Ø1BP4ZZ
Ø1CK*
Ø1CL*
Ø1CM*
Ø1CN*
Ø1CP*
Ø1DK*
Ø1DL*
Ø1DM*
Ø1DN*
Ø1DP*
Ø2H4ØØZ
Ø2H4ØYZ
Ø2H43ØZ
Ø2H43YZ
Ø2H44ØZ
Ø2H44YZ
Ø2H6ØØZ
Ø2H6ØYZ
Ø2H63ØZ
Ø2H63YZ
Ø2H64ØZ
Ø2H64YZ
Ø2H7ØØZ
Ø2H7ØYZ
Ø2H73ØZ
Ø2H73YZ
Ø2H74ØZ
Ø2H74YZ
Ø2HLØØZ
Ø2HLØYZ
Ø2HL3ØZ
Ø2HL3YZ
Ø2HL4ØZ
Ø2HL4YZ
Ø2HQØØZ
Ø2HQØYZ
Ø2HQ3ØZ
Ø2HQ3YZ
Ø2HQ4ØZ
Ø2HQ4YZ
Ø2HRØØZ
Ø2HRØYZ
Ø2HR3ØZ
Ø2HR3YZ
Ø2HR4ØZ
Ø2HR4YZ
Ø2HSØØZ
Ø2HSØYZ
Ø2HS3ØZ
Ø2HS3YZ
Ø2HS4ØZ
Ø2HS4YZ
Ø2HTØØZ
Ø2HTØYZ
Ø2HT3ØZ
Ø2HT3YZ
Ø2HT4ØZ
Ø2HT4YZ
Ø2HVØØZ
Ø2HVØYZ
Ø2HV3ØZ
Ø2HV3YZ
Ø2HV4ØZ
Ø2HV4YZ
Ø2JAØZZ
Ø2JA4ZZ
Ø2JYØZZ
Ø2JY4ZZ
Ø317Ø9D
Ø317Ø9F
Ø317Ø9V
Ø317ØAD
Ø317ØAF
Ø317ØAV
Ø317ØJD
Ø317ØJF
Ø317ØJV
Ø317ØKD
Ø317ØKF
Ø317ØKV
Ø317ØZD
Ø317ØZF
Ø317ØZV
Ø3173ZF
Ø318Ø9D
Ø318Ø9F
Ø318Ø9V
Ø318ØAD
Ø318ØAF
Ø318ØAV
Ø318ØJD
Ø318ØJF
Ø318ØJV
Ø318ØKD
Ø318ØKF
Ø318ØKV
Ø318ØZD
Ø318ØZF
Ø318ØZV
Ø3183ZF
Ø319Ø9F
Ø319ØAF
Ø319ØJF
Ø319ØKF
Ø319ØZF
Ø3193ZF
Ø31AØ9F
Ø31AØAF
Ø31AØJF
Ø31AØKF
Ø31AØZF
Ø31A3ZF
Ø31BØ9F
Ø31BØAF
Ø31BØJF
Ø31BØKF
Ø31BØZF
Ø31B3ZF
Ø31CØ9F
Ø31CØAF
Ø31CØJF
Ø31CØKF
Ø31CØZF
Ø31C3ZF
Ø3PYØ7Z
Ø3PYØJZ
Ø3PYØKZ
Ø3PY37Z
Ø3PY3JZ
Ø3PY3KZ
Ø3PY47Z
Ø3PY4JZ
Ø3PY4KZ
Ø4LE3CV
Ø4LE3DV
Ø4LE3ZV
Ø4LF3CW
Ø4LF3DW
Ø4LF3ZW
Ø79ØØZX
Ø79Ø3ZX
Ø79Ø4ZX
Ø791ØZX
Ø7913ZX
Ø7914ZX
Ø792ØZX
Ø7923ZX
Ø7924ZX
Ø793ØZX
Ø7933ZX
Ø7934ZX
Ø794ØZX
Ø7943ZX
Ø7944ZX
Ø795ØZX
Ø7953ZX
Ø7954ZX
Ø796ØZX
Ø7963ZX
Ø7964ZX
Ø797ØZX
Ø7973ZX
Ø7974ZX
Ø798ØZX
Ø7983ZX
Ø7984ZX
Ø799ØZX
Ø7993ZX
Ø7994ZX
Ø79BØZX
Ø79B3ZX
Ø79B4ZX
Ø79CØZX
Ø79C3ZX
Ø79C4ZX
Ø79DØZX
Ø79D3ZX
Ø79D4ZX
Ø79FØZX
Ø79F3ZX
Ø79F4ZX
Ø79GØZX
Ø79G3ZX
Ø79G4ZX
Ø79HØZX
Ø79H3ZX
Ø79H4ZX
Ø79JØZX
Ø79J3ZX
Ø79J4ZX
Ø79KØZX
Ø79K3ZX
Ø79K4ZX
Ø79LØZX
Ø79L3ZX
Ø79L4ZX
Ø7BØØZX
Ø7BØ3ZX
Ø7BØ4ZX
Ø7B1*
Ø7B2*
Ø7B3ØZX
Ø7B3ØZZ
Ø7B33ZX
Ø7B34ZX
Ø7B34ZZ
Ø7B4ØZX
Ø7B4ØZZ
Ø7B43ZX
Ø7B44ZX
Ø7B44ZZ
Ø7B5*
Ø7B6*
Ø7B7ØZX
Ø7B7ØZZ
Ø7B73ZX
Ø7B74ZX
Ø7B74ZZ
Ø7B8ØZX
Ø7B83ZX
Ø7B84ZX
Ø7B9ØZX
Ø7B93ZX
Ø7B94ZX
Ø7BBØZX
Ø7BB3ZX
Ø7BB4ZX
Ø7BCØZX
Ø7BC3ZX
Ø7BC4ZX
Ø7BDØZX
Ø7BD3ZX
Ø7BD4ZX
Ø7BFØZX
Ø7BFØZZ
Ø7BF3ZX
Ø7BF4ZX
Ø7BF4ZZ
Ø7BGØZX
Ø7BGØZZ
Ø7BG3ZX
Ø7BG4ZX
Ø7BG4ZZ
Ø7BH*
Ø7BJ*
Ø7BKØZX
Ø7BK3ZX
Ø7BK4ZX
Ø7BLØZX
Ø7BL3ZX
Ø7BL4ZX
Ø7JPØZZ
Ø7TP*
Ø9RKØ7Z

ICD-10-CM/PCS Codes by MS-DRG

ØB9CØZX
ØB9DØZX
ØB9FØZX
ØB9GØZX
ØB9HØZX
ØB9JØZX
ØB9KØZX
ØB9LØZX
ØB9MØZX
ØBBCØZX
ØBBC4ZX
ØBBC7ZX
ØBBC8ZX
ØBBDØZX
ØBBD4ZX
ØBBD7ZX
ØBBD8ZX
ØBBFØZX
ØBBF4ZX
ØBBF7ZX
ØBBF8ZX
ØBBGØZX
ØBBG4ZX
ØBBG7ZX
ØBBG8ZX
ØBBHØZX
ØBBH4ZX
ØBBH7ZX
ØBBH8ZX
ØBBJØZX
ØBBJ4ZX
ØBBJ7ZX
ØBBJ8ZX
ØBBKØZX
ØBBK4ZX
ØBBK7ZX
ØBBK8ZX
ØBBLØZX
ØBBL4ZX
ØBBL7ZX
ØBBL8ZX
ØBBMØZX
ØBBM4ZX
ØBBM7ZX
ØBBM8ZX
ØBJØ4ZZ
ØBJK4ZZ
ØBJL4ZZ
ØBQ1*
ØBR1Ø7Z
ØBR1ØJZ
ØBR1ØKZ
ØBR147Z
ØBR14JZ
ØBR14KZ
ØBW1ØFZ
ØBW13FZ
ØBW14FZ
ØC57*
ØD16Ø79
ØD16Ø7A
ØD16Ø7B
ØD16Ø7L
ØD16ØJ9
ØD16ØJA
ØD16ØJB
ØD16ØJL
ØD16ØK9
ØD16ØKA
ØD16ØKB
ØD16ØKL
ØD16ØZ9
ØD16ØZA
ØD16ØZB
ØD16ØZL
ØD16479
ØD1647A
ØD1647B
ØD1647L
ØD164J9
ØD164JA
ØD164JB
ØD164JL
ØD164K9
ØD164KA
ØD164KB
ØD164KL
ØD164Z9
ØD164ZA
ØD164ZB
ØD164ZL
ØD16879
ØD1687A
ØD1687B
ØD1687L
ØD168J9
ØD168JA
ØD168JB
ØD168JL
ØD168K9
ØD168KA
ØD168KB
ØD168KL
ØD168Z9
ØD168ZA
ØD168ZB
ØD168ZL
ØD1887H
ØD188JH
ØD188KH
ØD1A87H
ØD1A8JH
ØD1A8KH
ØD1B87H
ØD1B8JH
ØD1B8KH
ØD1EØZ4
ØD1E4Z4
ØD1E8Z4
ØD1KØZ4
ØD1K4Z4
ØD1K8Z4
ØD1LØZ4
ØD1L4Z4
ØD1L8Z4
ØD9PØZX
ØDB6ØZ3
ØDB6ØZZ
ØDB63Z3
ØDB63ZZ
ØDB67Z3
ØDB67ZZ
ØDB68Z3
ØDB8ØZZ
ØDB84ZZ
ØDBEØZZ
ØDBE3ZZ
ØDBE4ZZ
ØDBFØZZ
ØDBF3ZZ
ØDBF4ZZ
ØDBGØZZ
ØDBG3ZZ
ØDBG4ZZ
ØDBHØZZ
ØDBH3ZZ
ØDBH4ZZ
ØDBKØZZ
ØDBK3ZZ
ØDBK4ZZ
ØDBLØZZ
ØDBL3ZZ
ØDBL4ZZ
ØDBMØZZ
ØDBM3ZZ
ØDBM4ZZ
ØDBNØZZ
ØDBN3ZZ
ØDBN4ZZ
ØDBPØZX
ØDBPØZZ
ØDBP3ZZ
ØDBP4ZZ
ØDBP7ZZ
ØDJØØZZ
ØDJ6ØZZ
ØDJDØZZ
ØDJUØZZ
ØDJVØZZ
ØDJWØZZ
ØDT6*
ØDT7*
ØDT9*
ØDTA*
ØDTB*
ØDTC*
ØDTE*
ØDTF*
ØDTG*
ØDTH*
ØDTJØZZ
ØDTJ7ZZ
ØDTJ8ZZ
ØDTK*
ØDTL*
ØDTM*
ØDTPØZZ
ØDTP4ZZ
ØDWWØJZ
ØDWW3JZ
ØDWW4JZ
ØF9ØØZX
ØF91ØZX
ØF92ØZX
ØFBØØZX
ØFB1ØZX
ØFB2ØZX
ØFJØØZZ
ØHRØXK3
ØHRØXK4
ØHR1XK3
ØHR1XK4
ØHR4XK3
ØHR4XK4
ØHR5*
ØHR6*
ØHR7*
ØHR8*
ØHRA*
ØHRB*
ØHRC*
ØHRD*
ØHRE*
ØHRF*
ØHRG*
ØHRH*
ØHRJ*
ØHRK*
ØHRL*
ØHRM*
ØHRN*
ØHXØXZZ
ØHX1XZZ
ØHX4XZZ
ØHX5XZZ
ØHX6XZZ
ØHX7XZZ
ØHX8XZZ
ØHX9XZZ
ØHXAXZZ
ØHXBXZZ
ØHXCXZZ
ØHXDXZZ
ØHXEXZZ
ØHXFXZZ
ØHXGXZZ
ØHXHXZZ
ØHXJXZZ
ØHXKXZZ
ØHXLXZZ
ØHXMXZZ
ØHXNXZZ
ØJBØØZZ
ØJB1ØZZ
ØJB4ØZZ
ØJB5ØZZ
ØJB6ØZZ
ØJB7ØZZ
ØJB8ØZZ
ØJB9ØZZ
ØJBBØZZ
ØJBCØZZ
ØJBDØZZ
ØJBFØZZ
ØJBGØZZ
ØJBHØZZ
ØJBLØZZ
ØJBMØZZ
ØJBNØZZ
ØJBPØZZ
ØJBQØZZ
ØJBRØZZ
ØJHØ*
ØJH1*
ØJH4*
ØJH5*
ØJH6ØNZ
ØJH6ØVZ
ØJH6ØYZ
ØJH63NZ
ØJH63VZ
ØJH7ØNZ
ØJH7ØVZ
ØJH7ØYZ
ØJH73NZ
ØJH73VZ
ØJH8ØNZ
ØJH8ØVZ
ØJH8ØYZ
ØJH83NZ
ØJH83VZ
ØJH9*
ØJHB*
ØJHC*
ØJHDØNZ
ØJHDØVZ
ØJHD3NZ
ØJHD3VZ
ØJHFØNZ
ØJHFØVZ
ØJHF3NZ
ØJHF3VZ
ØJHGØNZ
ØJHGØVZ
ØJHG3NZ
ØJHG3VZ
ØJHHØNZ
ØJHHØVZ
ØJHH3NZ
ØJHH3VZ
ØJHLØNZ
ØJHLØVZ
ØJHL3NZ
ØJHL3VZ
ØJHMØNZ
ØJHMØVZ
ØJHM3NZ
ØJHM3VZ
ØJHNØNZ
ØJHNØVZ
ØJHN3NZ
ØJHN3VZ
ØJHPØNZ
ØJHPØVZ
ØJHP3NZ
ØJHP3VZ
ØJHQ*
ØJHR*
ØJHTØVZ
ØJHTØYZ
ØJHT3VZ
ØJXØØZB
ØJXØØZC
ØJXØ3ZB
ØJXØ3ZC
ØJX1ØZB
ØJX1ØZC
ØJX13ZB
ØJX13ZC
ØJX4ØZB
ØJX4ØZC
ØJX43ZB
ØJX43ZC
ØJX5ØZB
ØJX5ØZC
ØJX53ZB
ØJX53ZC
ØJX6ØZB
ØJX6ØZC
ØJX63ZB
ØJX63ZC
ØJX7ØZB
ØJX7ØZC
ØJX73ZB
ØJX73ZC
ØJX8ØZB
ØJX8ØZC
ØJX83ZB
ØJX83ZC
ØJX9ØZB
ØJX9ØZC
ØJX93ZB
ØJX93ZC
ØJXBØZB
ØJXBØZC
ØJXB3ZB
ØJXB3ZC
ØJXCØZB
ØJXCØZC
ØJXC3ZB
ØJXC3ZC
ØJXDØZB
ØJXDØZC
ØJXD3ZB
ØJXD3ZC
ØJXFØZB
ØJXFØZC
ØJXF3ZB
ØJXF3ZC
ØJXGØZB
ØJXGØZC
ØJXG3ZB
ØJXG3ZC
ØJXHØZB
ØJXHØZC
ØJXH3ZB
ØJXH3ZC
ØJXLØZB
ØJXLØZC
ØJXL3ZB
ØJXL3ZC
ØJXMØZB
ØJXMØZC
ØJXM3ZB
ØJXM3ZC
ØJXNØZB
ØJXNØZC
ØJXN3ZB
ØJXN3ZC
ØJXPØZB
ØJXPØZC
ØJXP3ZB
ØJXP3ZC
ØJXQØZB
ØJXQØZC
ØJXQ3ZB
ØJXQ3ZC
ØJXRØZB
ØJXRØZC
ØJXR3ZB
ØJXR3ZC
ØKBØØZZ
ØKB1ØZZ
ØKB2ØZZ
ØKB3ØZZ
ØKB4ØZZ
ØKB5ØZZ
ØKB6ØZZ
ØKB7ØZZ
ØKB8ØZZ
ØKB9ØZZ
ØKBBØZZ
ØKBCØZZ
ØKBDØZZ
ØKBFØZZ
ØKBGØZZ
ØKBHØZZ
ØKBJØZZ
ØKBKØZZ
ØKBLØZZ
ØKBMØZZ
ØKBNØZZ
ØKBPØZZ
ØKBQØZZ
ØKBRØZZ
ØKBSØZZ
ØKBTØZZ
ØKBVØZZ
ØKBWØZZ
ØPHØØØZ
ØPHØ3ØZ
ØPHØ4ØZ
ØPSØØØZ
ØPSØ3ØZ
ØPSØ4ØZ
ØT768DZ
ØT778DZ
ØT788DZ
ØW1GØJ4
ØW1G3J4
ØW1G4J4
ØW3Ø*
ØW31*
ØW32*
ØW33*
ØW34*
ØW35*
ØW36*
ØW38*
ØW39*
ØW3B*
ØW3D*
ØW3F*
ØW3GØZZ
ØW3G3ZZ
ØW3G4ZZ
ØW3H3ZZ
ØW3H4ZZ
ØW3J*
ØW3K*
ØW3L*
ØW3M*
ØW3N*
ØW3P3ZZ
ØW3P4ZZ
ØW3Q*
ØW3R*
ØW9CØØZ
ØW9CØZX
ØW9CØZZ
ØW9C4ØZ
ØW9C4ZZ
ØW9FØØZ
ØW9FØZZ
ØW9GØØZ
ØW9GØZZ
ØW9HØØZ
ØW9HØZZ
ØW9H4ØZ
ØW9H4ZZ
ØW9JØØZ
ØW9JØZZ
ØW9J4ØZ
ØW9J4ZZ
ØWBØØZZ
ØWBØ3ZZ
ØWBØ4ZZ
ØWBØXZZ
ØWB2ØZZ
ØWB23ZZ
ØWB24ZZ
ØWB2XZZ
ØWB4ØZZ
ØWB43ZZ
ØWB44ZZ
ØWB4XZZ
ØWB5ØZZ
ØWB53ZZ
ØWB54ZZ
ØWB5XZZ
ØWB6ØZZ
ØWB63ZZ
ØWB64ZZ
ØWB6XZ2
ØWB6XZZ
ØWBCØZX
ØWBKØZZ
ØWBK3ZZ
ØWBK4ZZ
ØWBKXZZ
ØWBLØZZ
ØWBL3ZZ
ØWBL4ZZ
ØWBLXZZ
ØWBMØZZ
ØWBM3ZZ
ØWBM4ZZ
ØWBMXZZ
ØWCCØZZ
ØWCC3ZZ
ØWCC4ZZ
ØWCJØZZ
ØWCJ3ZZ
ØWCJ4ZZ
ØWCPØZZ
ØWCP3ZZ
ØWCP4ZZ
ØWCRØZZ
ØWCR3ZZ
ØWCR4ZZ
ØWHCØ1Z
ØWHCØ3Z
ØWHCØYZ
ØWHC31Z
ØWHC33Z
ØWHC3YZ
ØWHC41Z
ØWHC43Z
ØWHC4YZ
ØWHDØ1Z
ØWHD31Z
ØWHD41Z
ØWJ9ØZZ
ØWJ94ZZ
ØWJBØZZ
ØWJB4ZZ
ØWJCØZZ
ØWJC4ZZ
ØWJD4ZZ
ØWJFØZZ
ØWJGØZZ
ØWJHØZZ
ØWJJØZZ
ØWJPØZZ
ØWJQØZZ
ØWJQ4ZZ
ØWJRØZZ
ØWPCØØZ
ØWPCØ1Z
ØWPCØ3Z
ØWPCØ7Z
ØWPCØJZ
ØWPCØKZ
ØWPCØYZ
ØWPC3ØZ
ØWPC31Z
ØWPC33Z
ØWPC37Z
ØWPC3JZ
ØWPC3KZ
ØWPC3YZ
ØWPC4ØZ
ØWPC41Z
ØWPC43Z
ØWPC47Z
ØWPC4JZ
ØWPC4KZ
ØWPC4YZ
ØWQ6XZ2
ØWWCØØZ
ØWWCØ1Z
ØWWCØ3Z
ØWWCØ7Z
ØWWCØJZ
ØWWCØKZ
ØWWCØYZ
ØWWC3ØZ
ØWWC31Z
ØWWC33Z
ØWWC37Z
ØWWC3JZ
ØWWC3KZ
ØWWC3YZ
ØWWC4ØZ
ØWWC41Z
ØWWC43Z
ØWWC47Z
ØWWC4JZ
ØWWC4KZ
ØWWC4YZ
ØX3*
ØXB2ØZZ
ØXB23ZZ
ØXB24ZZ
ØXB3ØZZ
ØXB33ZZ
ØXB34ZZ
ØXB4ØZZ
ØXB43ZZ
ØXB44ZZ
ØXB5ØZZ
ØXB53ZZ
ØXB54ZZ
ØXB6ØZZ
ØXB63ZZ
ØXB64ZZ
ØXB7ØZZ
ØXB73ZZ
ØXB74ZZ
ØXB8ØZZ
ØXB83ZZ
ØXB84ZZ
ØXB9ØZZ
ØXB93ZZ
ØXB94ZZ
ØXBBØZZ
ØXBB3ZZ
ØXBB4ZZ
ØXBCØZZ
ØXBC3ZZ
ØXBC4ZZ
ØXBDØZZ
ØXBD3ZZ
ØXBD4ZZ
ØXBFØZZ
ØXBF3ZZ
ØXBF4ZZ
ØXBGØZZ
ØXBG3ZZ
ØXBG4ZZ
ØXBHØZZ
ØXBH3ZZ
ØXBH4ZZ
ØXBJØZZ
ØXBJ3ZZ
ØXBJ4ZZ
ØXBKØZZ
ØXBK3ZZ
ØXBK4ZZ
ØXUJØ7Z
ØXUJ47Z
ØXUKØ7Z
ØXUK47Z
ØXULØ7Z
ØXUL47Z
ØXUMØ7Z
ØXUM47Z
ØXUNØ7Z
ØXUN47Z
ØXUPØ7Z
ØXUP47Z
ØXUQØ7Z
ØXUQ47Z
ØXURØ7Z
ØXUR47Z
ØXUSØ7Z
ØXUS47Z
ØXUTØ7Z
ØXUT47Z
ØXUVØ7Z
ØXUV47Z
ØXUWØ7Z
ØXUW47Z
ØY3*
ØY95ØØZ
ØY95ØZZ
ØY954ØZ
ØY954ZZ
ØY96ØØZ
ØY96ØZZ
ØY964ØZ
ØY964ZZ
ØYBØØZZ
ØYBØ3ZZ
ØYBØ4ZZ
ØYB1ØZZ
ØYB13ZZ
ØYB14ZZ
ØYB9ØZZ
ØYB93ZZ
ØYB94ZZ
ØYBBØZZ
ØYBB3ZZ
ØYBB4ZZ
ØYBCØZZ
ØYBC3ZZ
ØYBC4ZZ
ØYBDØZZ
ØYBD3ZZ
ØYBD4ZZ
ØYBFØZZ
ØYBF3ZZ
ØYBF4ZZ
ØYBGØZZ
ØYBG3ZZ
ØYBG4ZZ
ØYBHØZZ
ØYBH3ZZ
ØYBH4ZZ
ØYBJØZZ
ØYBJ3ZZ
ØYBJ4ZZ
ØYBKØZZ
ØYBK3ZZ
ØYBK4ZZ
ØYBLØZZ
ØYBL3ZZ
ØYBL4ZZ
ØYBMØZZ
ØYBM3ZZ
ØYBM4ZZ
ØYBNØZZ
ØYBN3ZZ
ØYBN4ZZ
ØYJ5ØZZ
ØYJ6ØZZ
ØYJ7ØZZ
ØYJAØZZ
3EØL4GC
XØ51329
X2KB317
X2KC317
XHRPXF7

DRG 265

Operating Room Procedures

Ø2H4ØKZ
Ø2H43KZ
Ø2H44KZ
Ø2H6ØKZ
Ø2H63KZ
Ø2H64KZ
Ø2H7ØKZ
Ø2H73KZ
Ø2H74KZ
Ø2HKØKZ
Ø2HK3KZ
Ø2HK4KZ
Ø2HLØKZ
Ø2HL3KZ
Ø2HL4KZ
Ø2HNØKZ
Ø2HN3KZ
Ø2HN4KZ
ØJH6ØFZ
ØJH63FZ
ØJPTØFZ
ØJPT3FZ
ØJWTØFZ
ØJWT3FZ
ØWHCØGZ
ØWHC3GZ
ØWHC4GZ
ØWPCØGZ
ØWPC3GZ
ØWPC4GZ
ØWWCØGZ
ØWWC3GZ
ØWWC4GZ

DRG 266

Operating Room Procedures

Ø2RF37H
Ø2RF37Z
Ø2RF38H
Ø2RF38N
Ø2RF38Z
Ø2RF3JH
Ø2RF3JZ
Ø2RF3KH
Ø2RF3KZ
Ø2RG37H
Ø2RG37Z
Ø2RG38H
Ø2RG38Z
Ø2RG3JH
Ø2RG3JZ
Ø2RG3KH
Ø2RG3KZ
Ø2RH37H
Ø2RH37Z
Ø2RH38H
Ø2RH38L
Ø2RH38M
Ø2RH38Z
Ø2RH3JH
Ø2RH3JZ
Ø2RH3KH
Ø2RH3KZ
Ø2RJ37H
Ø2RJ37Z
Ø2RJ38H
Ø2RJ38Z
Ø2RJ3JH
Ø2RJ3JZ
Ø2RJ3KH
Ø2RJ3KZ
Ø2UF37J
Ø2UF37Z
Ø2UF38J
Ø2UF38Z
Ø2UF3JJ
Ø2UF3JZ
Ø2UF3KJ
Ø2UF3KZ
Ø2UG37E
Ø2UG37Z
Ø2UG38E
Ø2UG38Z
Ø2UG3JE
Ø2UG3JH
Ø2UG3JZ
Ø2UG3KE
Ø2UG3KZ
Ø2UH37Z
Ø2UH38Z
Ø2UH3JZ
Ø2UH3KZ
Ø2UJ37G
Ø2UJ37Z
Ø2UJ38G
Ø2UJ38Z
Ø2UJ3JG
Ø2UJ3JZ
Ø2UJ3KG
Ø2UJ3KZ

DRG 267

Select operating room procedures listed under DRG 266

DRG 268

Operating Room Procedures

Ø2BWØZZ
Ø2BW4ZZ
Ø2BXØZZ
Ø2BX4ZZ
Ø2CWØZZ
Ø2CW3ZZ
Ø2CW4ZZ
Ø2CXØZZ

Ø2CX3ZZ
Ø2CX4ZZ
Ø2PAØQZ
Ø2PAØRS
Ø2PAØRZ
Ø2PA3QZ
Ø2PA3RS
Ø2PA3RZ
Ø2PA4QZ
Ø2PA4RS
Ø2PA4RZ
Ø2PW3RZ
Ø2QWØZZ
Ø2QW3ZZ
Ø2QW4ZZ
Ø2QXØZZ
Ø2QX3ZZ
Ø2QX4ZZ
Ø2UØØJZ
Ø2UØ4JZ
Ø2U1ØJZ
Ø2U14JZ
Ø2U2ØJZ
Ø2U24JZ
Ø2U3ØJZ
Ø2U34JZ
Ø2UAØJZ
Ø2UA3JZ
Ø2UA4JZ
41Ø093
41Ø094
41Ø095
Ø41ØØA3
Ø41ØØA4
Ø41ØØA5
Ø41ØØJ3
Ø41ØØJ4
Ø41ØØJ5
Ø41ØØK3
Ø41ØØK4
Ø41ØØK5
Ø41ØØZ3
Ø41ØØZ4
Ø41ØØZ5
41Ø493
41Ø494
41Ø495
Ø41Ø4A3
Ø41Ø4A4
Ø41Ø4A5
Ø41Ø4J3
Ø41Ø4J4
Ø41Ø4J5
Ø41Ø4K3
Ø41Ø4K4
Ø41Ø4K5
Ø41Ø4Z3
Ø41Ø4Z4
Ø41Ø4Z5
413Ø93
413Ø94
413Ø95
Ø413ØA3
Ø413ØA4
Ø413ØA5
Ø413ØJ3
Ø413ØJ4
Ø413ØJ5
Ø413ØK3
Ø413ØK4
Ø413ØK5
Ø413ØZ3
Ø413ØZ4
Ø413ØZ5
413493
413494
413495
Ø4134A3
Ø4134A4
Ø4134A5
Ø4134J3
Ø4134J4
Ø4134J5
Ø4134K3
Ø4134K4
Ø4134K5
Ø4134Z3
Ø4134Z4
Ø4134Z5
Ø45ØØZZ
Ø45Ø3ZZ
Ø45Ø4ZZ
Ø4BØØZZ
Ø4BØ3ZZ
Ø4BØ4ZZ
Ø4CØØZZ
Ø4CØ3ZZ
Ø4CØ4ZZ
Ø4LØØCZ
Ø4LØØDJ
Ø4LØØDZ
Ø4LØØZZ
Ø4LØ3CZ
Ø4LØ3DJ
Ø4LØ3DZ
Ø4LØ3ZZ
Ø4LØ4CZ
Ø4LØ4DZ
Ø4LØ4ZZ
Ø4RØØ7Z
Ø4RØØJZ
Ø4RØØKZ
Ø4RØ47Z
Ø4RØ4JZ
Ø4RØ4KZ
Ø4UØ3JZ
Ø4UØ4JZ
Ø4VØ3DZ
Ø4VØ3EZ
Ø4VØ3FZ
Ø4VØ4DZ
Ø4VØ4EZ
Ø4VØ4FZ
X2CP3T7

DRG 269

Select operating room procedures listed under DRG 268

DRG 270

Operating Room Procedures

Ø216ØZ7
Ø2163Z7
Ø2164Z7
Ø2173J6
Ø21VØ8P
Ø21VØ8Q
Ø21VØ8R
Ø21VØ9P
Ø21VØ9Q
Ø21VØ9R
Ø21VØAP
Ø21VØAQ
Ø21VØAR
Ø21VØJP
Ø21VØJQ
Ø21VØJR
Ø21VØKP
Ø21VØKQ
Ø21VØKR
Ø21VØZP
Ø21VØZQ
Ø21VØZR
Ø21V48P
Ø21V48Q
Ø21V48R
Ø21V49P
Ø21V49Q
Ø21V49R
Ø21V4AP
Ø21V4AQ
Ø21V4AR
Ø21V4JP
Ø21V4JQ
Ø21V4JR
Ø21V4KP
Ø21V4KQ
Ø21V4KR
Ø21V4ZP
Ø21V4ZQ
Ø21V4ZR
Ø21WØ8A
Ø21WØ8B
Ø21WØ8D
Ø21WØ8F
Ø21WØ8G
Ø21WØ8H
Ø21WØ8P
Ø21WØ8Q
Ø21WØ8R
Ø21WØ8V
Ø21WØ9A
Ø21WØ9B
Ø21WØ9D
Ø21WØ9F
Ø21WØ9G
Ø21WØ9H
Ø21WØ9P
Ø21WØ9Q
Ø21WØ9R
Ø21WØ9V
Ø21WØAA
Ø21WØAB
Ø21WØAD
Ø21WØAF
Ø21WØAG
Ø21WØAH
Ø21WØAP
Ø21WØAQ
Ø21WØAR
Ø21WØAV
Ø21WØJA
Ø21WØJB
Ø21WØJD
Ø21WØJF
Ø21WØJG
Ø21WØJH
Ø21WØJP
Ø21WØJQ
Ø21WØJR
Ø21WØJV
Ø21WØKA
Ø21WØKB
Ø21WØKD
Ø21WØKF
Ø21WØKG
Ø21WØKH
Ø21WØKP
Ø21WØKQ
Ø21WØKR
Ø21WØKV
Ø21WØZA
Ø21WØZB
Ø21WØZD
Ø21WØZP
Ø21WØZQ
Ø21WØZR
Ø21W48A
Ø21W48B
Ø21W48D
Ø21W48P
Ø21W48Q
Ø21W48R
Ø21W49A
Ø21W49B
Ø21W49D
Ø21W49P
Ø21W49Q
Ø21W49R
Ø21W4AA
Ø21W4AB
Ø21W4AD
Ø21W4AP
Ø21W4AQ
Ø21W4AR
Ø21W4JA
Ø21W4JB
Ø21W4JD
Ø21W4JP
Ø21W4JQ
Ø21W4JR
Ø21W4KA
Ø21W4KB
Ø21W4KD
Ø21W4KP
Ø21W4KQ
Ø21W4KR
Ø21W4ZA
Ø21W4ZB
Ø21W4ZD
Ø21W4ZP
Ø21W4ZQ
Ø21W4ZR
Ø21XØ8A
Ø21XØ8B
Ø21XØ8D
Ø21XØ8P
Ø21XØ8Q
Ø21XØ8R
Ø21XØ9A
Ø21XØ9B
Ø21XØ9D
Ø21XØ9P
Ø21XØ9Q
Ø21XØ9R
Ø21XØAA
Ø21XØAB
Ø21XØAD
Ø21XØAP
Ø21XØAQ
Ø21XØAR
Ø21XØJA
Ø21XØJB
Ø21XØJD
Ø21XØJP
Ø21XØJQ
Ø21XØJR
Ø21XØKA
Ø21XØKB
Ø21XØKD
Ø21XØKP
Ø21XØKQ
Ø21XØKR
Ø21XØZA
Ø21XØZB
Ø21XØZD
Ø21XØZP
Ø21XØZQ
Ø21XØZR
Ø21X48A
Ø21X48B
Ø21X48D
Ø21X48P
Ø21X48Q
Ø21X48R
Ø21X49A
Ø21X49B
Ø21X49D
Ø21X49P
Ø21X49Q
Ø21X49R
Ø21X4AA
Ø21X4AB
Ø21X4AD
Ø21X4AP
Ø21X4AQ
Ø21X4AR
Ø21X4JA
Ø21X4JB
Ø21X4JD
Ø21X4JP
Ø21X4JQ
Ø21X4JR
Ø21X4KA
Ø21X4KB
Ø21X4KD
Ø21X4KP
Ø21X4KQ
Ø21X4KR
Ø21X4ZA
Ø21X4ZB
Ø21X4ZD
Ø21X4ZP
Ø21X4ZQ
Ø21X4ZR
Ø25N*
Ø25P*
Ø25Q*
Ø25R*
Ø25S*
Ø25T*
Ø25V*
Ø25W*
Ø25X*
Ø27K*
Ø27L*
Ø27RØ4T
Ø27RØDT
Ø27RØZT
Ø27R34T
Ø27R3DT
Ø27R3ZT
Ø27R44T
Ø27R4DT
Ø27R4ZT
Ø288*
Ø2BN*
Ø2BPØZZ
Ø2BP3ZZ
Ø2BP4ZZ
Ø2BQØZZ
Ø2BQ3ZZ
Ø2BQ4ZZ
Ø2BRØZZ
Ø2BR3ZZ
Ø2BR4ZZ
Ø2BSØZZ
Ø2BS3ZZ
Ø2BS4ZZ
Ø2BTØZZ
Ø2BT3ZZ
Ø2BT4ZZ
Ø2BVØZZ
Ø2BV3ZZ
Ø2BV4ZZ
Ø2BW3ZZ
Ø2BX3ZZ
Ø2CF3ZZ
Ø2CF4ZZ
Ø2CG3ZZ
Ø2CG4ZZ
Ø2CH3ZZ
Ø2CH4ZZ
Ø2CJ3ZZ
Ø2CJ4ZZ
Ø2CN*
Ø2CP*
Ø2CQ*
Ø2CR*
Ø2CS*
Ø2CT*
Ø2CV*
Ø2FNØZZ
Ø2FN3ZZ
Ø2FN4ZZ
Ø2HAØYZ
Ø2HA3YZ
Ø2HA4YZ
Ø2HNØØZ
Ø2HNØ2Z
Ø2HNØYZ
Ø2HN3ØZ
Ø2HN3YZ
Ø2HN4ØZ
Ø2HN42Z
Ø2HN4YZ
Ø2HPØDZ
Ø2HPØYZ
Ø2HP3DZ
Ø2HP3YZ
Ø2HP4DZ
Ø2HP4YZ
Ø2HQØDZ
Ø2HQ3DZ
Ø2HQ4DZ
Ø2HRØDZ
Ø2HR3DZ
Ø2HR4DZ
Ø2HSØ2Z
Ø2HSØDZ
Ø2HS3DZ
Ø2HS42Z
Ø2HS4DZ
Ø2HTØ2Z
Ø2HTØDZ
Ø2HT3DZ
Ø2HT42Z
Ø2HT4DZ
Ø2HWØ2Z
Ø2HWØDZ
Ø2HWØYZ
Ø2HW3DZ
Ø2HW3YZ
Ø2HW42Z
Ø2HW4DZ
Ø2HW4YZ
Ø2HXØ2Z
Ø2HXØDZ
Ø2HX32Z
Ø2HX3DZ
Ø2HX42Z
Ø2HX4DZ
Ø2LHØCZ
Ø2LHØDZ
Ø2LHØZZ
Ø2LH3CZ
Ø2LH3DZ
Ø2LH3ZZ
Ø2LH4CZ
Ø2LH4DZ
Ø2LH4ZZ
Ø2LRØCT
Ø2LRØDT
Ø2LRØZT
Ø2LR3CT
Ø2LR3DT
Ø2LR3ZT
Ø2LR4CT
Ø2LR4DT
Ø2LR4ZT
Ø2LS*
Ø2LT*
Ø2LWØDJ
Ø2LW3DJ
Ø2N4*
Ø2N8*
Ø2NF3ZZ
Ø2NF4ZZ
Ø2NG3ZZ
Ø2NG4ZZ
Ø2NH3ZZ
Ø2NH4ZZ
Ø2NJ3ZZ
Ø2NJ4ZZ
Ø2NN*
Ø2PYØ2Z
Ø2PYØ3Z
Ø2PYØ7Z
Ø2PYØ8Z
Ø2PYØCZ
Ø2PYØDZ
Ø2PYØJZ
Ø2PYØKZ
Ø2PYØYZ
Ø2PY37Z
Ø2PY38Z
Ø2PY3CZ
Ø2PY3JZ
Ø2PY3KZ
Ø2PY42Z
Ø2PY43Z
Ø2PY47Z
Ø2PY48Z
Ø2PY4CZ
Ø2PY4DZ
Ø2PY4JZ
Ø2PY4KZ
Ø2Q6*
Ø2Q7*
Ø2Q8*
Ø2QA*
Ø2QK*
Ø2QL*
Ø2QN*
Ø2R5Ø7Z
Ø2R5Ø8Z
Ø2R5ØJZ
Ø2R5ØKZ
Ø2R547Z
Ø2R548Z
Ø2R54JZ
Ø2R54KZ
Ø2R6Ø7Z
Ø2R6Ø8Z
Ø2R6ØJZ
Ø2R6ØKZ
Ø2R647Z
Ø2R648Z
Ø2R64JZ
Ø2R64KZ
Ø2R7Ø7Z
Ø2R7Ø8Z
Ø2R7ØJZ
Ø2R7ØKZ
Ø2R747Z
Ø2R748Z
Ø2R74JZ
Ø2R74KZ
Ø2RKØ8Z
Ø2RKØJZ
Ø2RK48Z
Ø2RK4JZ
Ø2RLØ8Z
Ø2RLØJZ
Ø2RL48Z
Ø2RL4JZ
Ø2RMØ8Z
Ø2RM48Z
Ø2RNØ7Z
Ø2RNØ8Z
Ø2RNØJZ
Ø2RNØKZ
Ø2RN47Z
Ø2RN48Z
Ø2RN4JZ
Ø2RN4KZ
Ø2TNØZZ
Ø2TN3ZZ
Ø2TN4ZZ
Ø2UØØ7Z
Ø2UØØ8Z
Ø2UØØKZ
Ø2UØ47Z
Ø2UØ48Z
Ø2UØ4KZ
Ø2U1Ø7Z
Ø2U1Ø8Z
Ø2U1ØKZ
Ø2U147Z
Ø2U148Z
Ø2U14KZ
Ø2U2Ø7Z
Ø2U2Ø8Z
Ø2U2ØKZ
Ø2U247Z
Ø2U248Z
Ø2U24KZ
Ø2U3Ø7Z
Ø2U3Ø8Z
Ø2U3ØKZ
Ø2U347Z
Ø2U348Z
Ø2U34KZ
Ø2U6ØJZ
Ø2U637Z
Ø2U638Z
Ø2U63JZ
Ø2U63KZ
Ø2U647Z
Ø2U648Z
Ø2U64JZ
Ø2U64KZ
Ø2U7ØJZ
Ø2UAØ7Z
Ø2UAØ8Z
Ø2UAØKZ
Ø2UA37Z
Ø2UA38Z
Ø2UA3KZ
Ø2UA47Z
Ø2UA48Z
Ø2UA4KZ
Ø2UKØ7Z
Ø2UKØ8Z
Ø2UKØJZ
Ø2UK37Z
Ø2UK38Z
Ø2UK3JZ
Ø2UK47Z
Ø2UK48Z
Ø2UK4JZ
Ø2ULØ7Z
Ø2ULØ8Z
Ø2ULØJZ
Ø2UL37Z
Ø2UL38Z
Ø2UL3JZ
Ø2UL47Z
Ø2UL48Z
Ø2UL4JZ
Ø2UMØ8Z
Ø2UNØ7Z
Ø2UNØ8Z
Ø2UNØJZ
Ø2UNØKZ
Ø2UN37Z
Ø2UN38Z
Ø2UN3JZ
Ø2UN3KZ
Ø2UN47Z
Ø2UN48Z
Ø2UN4JZ
Ø2UN4KZ
Ø2VAØCZ
Ø2VAØZZ
Ø2VA3CZ
Ø2VA3ZZ
Ø2VA4CZ
Ø2VA4ZZ
Ø2VLØCZ
Ø2VLØDZ
Ø2VLØZZ
Ø2VL3DZ
Ø2VL4CZ
Ø2VL4DZ
Ø2VL4ZZ
Ø2VPØDZ
Ø2VPØZZ
Ø2VP3DZ
Ø2VP3ZZ
Ø2VP4DZ
Ø2VP4ZZ
Ø2VQØCZ
Ø2VQØDZ
Ø2VQØZZ
Ø2VQ3CZ
Ø2VQ3DZ
Ø2VQ3ZZ
Ø2VQ4CZ
Ø2VQ4DZ
Ø2VQ4ZZ
Ø2VRØCZ
Ø2VRØDT
Ø2VRØDZ
Ø2VRØZT
Ø2VRØZZ
Ø2VR3CZ
Ø2VR3DT
Ø2VR3DZ
Ø2VR3ZT
Ø2VR3ZZ
Ø2VR4CZ
Ø2VR4DT
Ø2VR4DZ
Ø2VR4ZT
Ø2VR4ZZ
Ø2VSØDZ
Ø2VSØZZ
Ø2VS3DZ
Ø2VS3ZZ
Ø2VS4DZ
Ø2VS4ZZ
Ø2VTØDZ
Ø2VTØZZ
Ø2VT3DZ
Ø2VT3ZZ
Ø2VT4DZ
Ø2VT4ZZ
Ø2VWØZZ
Ø2VW3ZZ
Ø2VW4ZZ
Ø2VXØZZ
Ø2VX3ZZ
Ø2VX4ZZ
Ø2WYØ2Z
Ø2WYØ3Z
Ø2WYØ7Z
Ø2WYØ8Z
Ø2WYØCZ
Ø2WYØDZ
Ø2WYØJZ
Ø2WYØKZ
Ø2WYØYZ
Ø2WY37Z
Ø2WY38Z
Ø2WY3CZ
Ø2WY3DZ
Ø2WY3JZ
Ø2WY3KZ
Ø2WY42Z
Ø2WY43Z
Ø2WY47Z
Ø2WY48Z
Ø2WY4CZ
Ø2WY4DZ
Ø2WY4JZ
Ø2WY4KZ
Ø313Ø9M
Ø313Ø9N
Ø313ØAM
Ø313ØAN
Ø313ØJM
Ø313ØJN
Ø313ØKM
Ø313ØKN
Ø313ØZM
Ø313ØZN
Ø314Ø9M
Ø314Ø9N
Ø314ØAM
Ø314ØAN
Ø314ØJM
Ø314ØJN
Ø314ØKM
Ø314ØKN
Ø314ØZM
Ø314ØZN
Ø35ØØZZ
Ø35Ø3ZZ
Ø35Ø4ZZ
Ø351ØZZ
Ø3513ZZ
Ø3514ZZ
Ø352ØZZ
Ø3523ZZ
Ø3524ZZ
Ø353ØZZ
Ø3533ZZ
Ø3534ZZ
Ø354ØZZ
Ø3543ZZ
Ø3544ZZ
Ø3BØØZZ
Ø3BØ3ZZ
Ø3BØ4ZZ
Ø3B1ØZZ
Ø3B13ZZ
Ø3B14ZZ
Ø3B2ØZZ
Ø3B23ZZ
Ø3B24ZZ
Ø3B3ØZZ
Ø3B33ZZ
Ø3B34ZZ
Ø3B4ØZZ
Ø3B43ZZ
Ø3B44ZZ
Ø3CØØZZ
Ø3CØ3ZZ
Ø3CØ4ZZ
Ø3C1ØZZ
Ø3C13ZZ
Ø3C14ZZ
Ø3C2ØZZ
Ø3C23ZZ
Ø3C24ZZ
Ø3C3ØZZ
Ø3C33ZZ
Ø3C34ZZ
Ø3C4ØZZ
Ø3C43ZZ
Ø3C44ZZ
Ø3LØØCZ
Ø3LØØDZ
Ø3LØØZZ
Ø3LØ3CZ
Ø3LØ3DZ
Ø3LØ3ZZ
Ø3LØ4CZ
Ø3LØ4DZ
Ø3LØ4ZZ
Ø3L1ØCZ
Ø3L1ØDZ
Ø3L1ØZZ
Ø3L13CZ
Ø3L13DZ
Ø3L13ZZ
Ø3L14CZ
Ø3L14DZ
Ø3L14ZZ
Ø3L2ØCZ
Ø3L2ØDZ
Ø3L2ØZZ
Ø3L23CZ
Ø3L23DZ
Ø3L23ZZ
Ø3L24CZ
Ø3L24DZ
Ø3L24ZZ
Ø3L3ØCZ
Ø3L3ØDZ
Ø3L3ØZZ
Ø3L33CZ
Ø3L33DZ
Ø3L33ZZ
Ø3L34CZ
Ø3L34DZ
Ø3L34ZZ
Ø3L4ØCZ
Ø3L4ØDZ
Ø3L4ØZZ
Ø3L43CZ
Ø3L43DZ
Ø3L43ZZ
Ø3L44CZ
Ø3L44DZ
Ø3L44ZZ
Ø3LGØBZ
Ø3LGØDZ
Ø3LG3BZ
Ø3LG3DZ
Ø3LG4BZ
Ø3LG4DZ
Ø3LHØBZ
Ø3LHØDZ
Ø3LH3BZ
Ø3LH3DZ
Ø3LH4BZ
Ø3LH4DZ
Ø3LJØBZ
Ø3LJØDZ
Ø3LJ3BZ
Ø3LJ3DZ
Ø3LJ4BZ
Ø3LJ4DZ
Ø3LKØBZ
Ø3LKØDZ
Ø3LK3BZ
Ø3LK3DZ
Ø3LK4BZ
Ø3LK4DZ
Ø3LLØBZ
Ø3LLØDZ
Ø3LL3BZ
Ø3LL3DZ
Ø3LL4BZ
Ø3LL4DZ
Ø3LMØBZ
Ø3LMØDZ
Ø3LM3BZ
Ø3LM3DZ
Ø3LM4BZ
Ø3LM4DZ

03LN0BZ
03LN0DZ
03LN3BZ
03LN3DZ
03LN4BZ
03LN4DZ
03LP0BZ
03LP0DZ
03LP3BZ
03LP3DZ
03LP4BZ
03LP4DZ
03LQ0BZ
03LQ0DZ
03LQ3BZ
03LQ3DZ
03LQ4BZ
03LQ4DZ
03LR0DZ
03LR3DZ
03LR4DZ
03LS0DZ
03LS3DZ
03LS4DZ
03LT0DZ
03LT3DZ
03LT4DZ
03V00DZ
03V00ZZ
03V03DZ
03V03ZZ
03V04DZ
03V04ZZ
03V10DZ
03V10ZZ
03V13DZ
03V13ZZ
03V14DZ
03V14ZZ
03V20DZ
03V20ZZ
03V23DZ
03V23ZZ
03V24DZ
03V24ZZ
03V30DZ
03V30ZZ
03V33DZ
03V33ZZ
03V34DZ
03V34ZZ
03V40DZ
03V40ZZ
03V43DZ
03V43ZZ
03V44DZ
03V44ZZ
03V50DZ
03V50ZZ
03V53DZ
03V53ZZ
03V54DZ
03V54ZZ
03V60DZ
03V60ZZ
03V63DZ
03V63ZZ
03V64DZ
03V64ZZ
03V70DZ
03V70ZZ
03V73DZ
03V73ZZ
03V74DZ
03V74ZZ
03V80DZ
03V80ZZ
03V83DZ
03V83ZZ
03V84DZ
03V84ZZ
03V90DZ
03V90ZZ
03V93DZ
03V93ZZ
03V94DZ
03V94ZZ
03VA0DZ
03VA0ZZ
03VA3DZ
03VA3ZZ
03VA4DZ
03VA4ZZ
03VB0DZ
03VB0ZZ
03VB3DZ
03VB3ZZ
03VB4DZ
03VB4ZZ
03VC0DZ
03VC0ZZ
03VC3DZ
03VC3ZZ
03VC4DZ
03VC4ZZ
03VD0DZ
03VD0ZZ
03VD3DZ
03VD3ZZ
03VD4DZ
03VD4ZZ
03VF0DZ
03VF0ZZ
03VF3DZ
03VF3ZZ
03VF4DZ
03VF4ZZ
03VG0BZ
03VG0DZ
03VG0HZ
03VG0ZZ
03VG3BZ
03VG3DZ
03VG3HZ
03VG3ZZ
03VG4BZ
03VG4DZ
03VG4HZ
03VG4ZZ
03VH0BZ
03VH0DZ
03VH0ZZ
03VH3BZ
03VH3DZ
03VH3ZZ
03VH4BZ
03VH4DZ
03VH4ZZ
03VJ0BZ
03VJ0DZ
03VJ0ZZ
03VJ3BZ
03VJ3DZ
03VJ3ZZ
03VJ4BZ
03VJ4DZ
03VJ4ZZ
03VK0BZ
03VK0DZ
03VK0ZZ
03VK3BZ
03VK3DZ
03VK3ZZ
03VK4BZ
03VK4DZ
03VK4ZZ
03VL0BZ
03VL0DZ
03VL0ZZ
03VL3BZ
03VL3DZ
03VL3ZZ
03VL4BZ
03VL4DZ
03VL4ZZ
03VM0BZ
03VM0DZ
03VM0ZZ
03VM3BZ
03VM3DZ
03VM3ZZ
03VM4BZ
03VM4DZ
03VM4ZZ
03VN0BZ
03VN0DZ
03VN0ZZ
03VN3BZ
03VN3DZ
03VN3ZZ
03VN4BZ
03VN4DZ
03VN4ZZ
03VP0BZ
03VP0DZ
03VP0ZZ
03VP3BZ
03VP3DZ
03VP3ZZ
03VP4BZ
03VP4DZ
03VP4ZZ
03VQ0BZ
03VQ0DZ
03VQ0ZZ
03VQ3BZ
03VQ3DZ
03VQ3ZZ
03VQ4BZ
03VQ4DZ
03VQ4ZZ
03VR0DZ
03VR0ZZ
03VR3DZ
03VR3ZZ
03VR4DZ
03VR4ZZ
03VS0DZ
03VS0ZZ
03VS3DZ
03VS3ZZ
03VS4DZ
03VS4ZZ
03VT0DZ
03VT0ZZ
03VT3DZ
03VT3ZZ
03VT4DZ
03VT4ZZ
03VU0DZ
03VU0ZZ
03VU3DZ
03VU3ZZ
03VU4DZ
03VU4ZZ
03VV0DZ
03VV0ZZ
03VV3DZ
03VV3ZZ
03VV4DZ
03VV4ZZ
03VY0DZ
03VY0ZZ
03VY3DZ
03VY3ZZ
03VY4DZ
03VY4ZZ
410090
410091
410092
410096
410097
410098
410099
041009B
041009C
041009D
041009F
041009G
041009H
041009J
041009K
041009Q
041009R
04100A0
04100A1
04100A2
04100A6
04100A7
04100A8
04100A9
04100AB
04100AC
04100AD
04100AF
04100AG
04100AH
04100AJ
04100AK
04100AQ
04100AR
04100J0
04100J1
04100J2
04100J6
04100J7
04100J8
04100J9
04100JB
04100JC
04100JD
04100JF
04100JG
04100JH
04100JJ
04100JK
04100JQ
04100JR
04100K0
04100K1
04100K2
04100K6
04100K7
04100K8
04100K9
04100KB
04100KC
04100KD
04100KF
04100KG
04100KH
04100KJ
04100KK
04100KQ
04100KR
04100Z0
04100Z1
04100Z2
04100Z6
04100Z7
04100Z8
04100Z9
04100ZB
04100ZC
04100ZD
04100ZF
04100ZG
04100ZH
04100ZJ
04100ZK
04100ZQ
04100ZR
410490
410491
410492
410496
410497
410498
410499
041049B
041049C
041049D
041049F
041049G
041049H
041049J
041049K
041049Q
041049R
04104A0
04104A1
04104A2
04104A6
04104A7
04104A8
04104A9
04104AB
04104AC
04104AD
04104AF
04104AG
04104AH
04104AJ
04104AK
04104AQ
04104AR
04104J0
04104J1
04104J2
04104J6
04104J7
04104J8
04104J9
04104JB
04104JC
04104JD
04104JF
04104JG
04104JH
04104JJ
04104JK
04104JQ
04104JR
04104K0
04104K1
04104K2
04104K6
04104K7
04104K8
04104K9
04104KB
04104KC
04104KD
04104KF
04104KG
04104KH
04104KJ
04104KK
04104KQ
04104KR
04104Z0
04104Z1
04104Z2
04104Z6
04104Z7
04104Z8
04104Z9
04104ZB
04104ZC
04104ZD
04104ZF
04104ZG
04104ZH
04104ZJ
04104ZK
04104ZQ
04104ZR
414093
414094
414095
04140A3
04140A4
04140A5
04140J3
04140J4
04140J5
04140K3
04140K4
04140K5
04140Z3
04140Z4
04140Z5
414493
414494
414495
04144A3
04144A4
04144A5
04144J3
04144J4
04144J5
04144K3
04144K4
04144K5
04144Z3
04144Z4
04144Z5
041C*
041D*
041E*
041F*
041H*
041J*
0451*
0452*
0453*
0454*
0455*
0456*
0457*
0458*
0459*
045A*
045B*
045C*
045D*
045E*
045F*
045H*
045J*
04B10ZZ
04B13ZZ
04B14ZZ
04B20ZZ
04B23ZZ
04B24ZZ
04B30ZZ
04B33ZZ
04B34ZZ
04B40ZZ
04B43ZZ
04B44ZZ
04B50ZZ
04B53ZZ
04B54ZZ
04B60ZZ
04B63ZZ
04B64ZZ
04B70ZZ
04B73ZZ
04B74ZZ
04B80ZZ
04B83ZZ
04B84ZZ
04B90ZZ
04B93ZZ
04B94ZZ
04BA0ZZ
04BA3ZZ
04BA4ZZ
04BB0ZZ
04BB3ZZ
04BB4ZZ
04BC0ZZ
04BC3ZZ
04BC4ZZ
04BD0ZZ
04BD3ZZ
04BD4ZZ
04BE0ZZ
04BE3ZZ
04BE4ZZ
04BF0ZZ
04BF3ZZ
04BF4ZZ
04BH0ZZ
04BH3ZZ
04BH4ZZ
04BJ0ZZ
04BJ3ZZ
04BJ4ZZ
04C10ZZ
04C13ZZ
04C14ZZ
04C20ZZ
04C23ZZ
04C24ZZ
04C30ZZ
04C33ZZ
04C34ZZ
04C40ZZ
04C43ZZ
04C44ZZ
04C50ZZ
04C53ZZ
04C54ZZ
04C60ZZ
04C63ZZ
04C64ZZ
04C70ZZ
04C73ZZ
04C74ZZ
04C80ZZ
04C83ZZ
04C84ZZ
04C90ZZ
04C93ZZ
04C94ZZ
04CA0ZZ
04CA3ZZ
04CA4ZZ
04CB0ZZ
04CB3ZZ
04CB4ZZ
04CC0ZZ
04CC3ZZ
04CC4ZZ
04CD0ZZ
04CD3ZZ
04CD4ZZ
04CE0ZZ
04CE3ZZ
04CE4ZZ
04CF0ZZ
04CF3ZZ
04CF4ZZ
04CH0ZZ
04CH3ZZ
04CH4ZZ
04CJ0ZZ
04CJ3ZZ
04CJ4ZZ
04CK3ZZ
04CL3ZZ
04CM3ZZ
04CN3ZZ
04CP3ZZ
04CQ3ZZ
04CR3ZZ
04CS3ZZ
04CT3ZZ
04CU3ZZ
04CV3ZZ
04CW3ZZ
04CY3ZZ
04L10CZ
04L10DZ
04L10ZZ
04L13CZ
04L13DZ
04L13ZZ
04L14CZ
04L14DZ
04L14ZZ
04L20CZ
04L20DZ
04L20ZZ
04L23CZ
04L23DZ
04L23ZZ
04L24CZ
04L24DZ
04L24ZZ
04L30CZ
04L30DZ
04L30ZZ
04L33CZ
04L33DZ
04L33ZZ
04L34CZ
04L34DZ
04L34ZZ
04L40CZ
04L40DZ
04L40ZZ
04L43CZ
04L43DZ
04L43ZZ
04L44CZ
04L44DZ
04L44ZZ
04L50CZ
04L50DZ
04L50ZZ
04L53CZ
04L53DZ
04L53ZZ
04L54CZ
04L54DZ
04L54ZZ
04L60CZ
04L60DZ
04L60ZZ
04L63CZ
04L63DZ
04L63ZZ
04L64CZ
04L64DZ
04L64ZZ
04L70CZ
04L70DZ
04L70ZZ
04L73CZ
04L73DZ
04L73ZZ
04L74CZ
04L74DZ
04L74ZZ
04L80CZ
04L80DZ
04L80ZZ
04L83CZ
04L83DZ
04L83ZZ
04L84CZ
04L84DZ
04L84ZZ
04L90CZ
04L90DZ
04L90ZZ
04L93CZ
04L93DZ
04L93ZZ
04L94CZ
04L94DZ
04L94ZZ
04LA0CZ
04LA0DZ
04LA0ZZ
04LA3CZ
04LA3DZ
04LA3ZZ
04LA4CZ
04LA4DZ
04LA4ZZ
04LB0CZ
04LB0DZ
04LB0ZZ
04LB3CZ
04LB3DZ
04LB3ZZ
04LB4CZ
04LB4DZ
04LB4ZZ
04LC0CZ
04LC0DZ
04LC0ZZ
04LC3CZ
04LC3DZ
04LC3ZZ
04LC4CZ
04LC4DZ
04LC4ZZ
04LD0CZ
04LD0DZ
04LD0ZZ
04LD3CZ
04LD3DZ
04LD3ZZ
04LD4CZ
04LD4DZ
04LD4ZZ
04LE0CZ
04LE0DZ
04LE0ZZ
04LE3CZ
04LE3DZ
04LE3ZZ
04LE4CZ
04LE4DZ
04LE4ZZ
04LF0CZ
04LF0DZ
04LF0ZZ
04LF3CZ
04LF3DZ
04LF3ZZ
04LF4CZ
04LF4DZ
04LF4ZZ
04LH0CZ
04LH0DZ
04LH0ZZ
04LH3CZ
04LH3DZ
04LH3ZZ
04LH4CZ
04LH4DZ
04LH4ZZ
04LJ0CZ
04LJ0DZ
04LJ0ZZ
04LJ3CZ
04LJ3DZ
04LJ3ZZ
04LJ4CZ
04LJ4DZ
04LJ4ZZ
04R107Z
04R10JZ
04R10KZ
04R147Z
04R14JZ
04R14KZ
04R207Z
04R20JZ
04R20KZ
04R247Z
04R24JZ
04R24KZ
04R307Z
04R30JZ
04R30KZ
04R347Z
04R34JZ
04R34KZ
04R407Z
04R40JZ
04R40KZ
04R447Z
04R44JZ
04R44KZ
04R507Z
04R50JZ
04R50KZ
04R547Z
04R54JZ
04R54KZ
04R607Z
04R60JZ
04R60KZ
04R647Z
04R64JZ
04R64KZ
04R707Z
04R70JZ
04R70KZ
04R747Z
04R74JZ
04R74KZ
04R807Z
04R80JZ
04R80KZ
04R847Z
04R84JZ
04R84KZ
04R907Z
04R90JZ
04R90KZ
04R947Z
04R94JZ
04R94KZ
04RA07Z
04RA0JZ
04RA0KZ
04RA47Z
04RA4JZ
04RA4KZ
04RB07Z
04RB0JZ
04RB0KZ
04RB47Z
04RB4JZ
04RB4KZ
04RC07Z
04RC0JZ
04RC0KZ
04RC47Z
04RC4JZ
04RC4KZ
04RD07Z
04RD0JZ
04RD0KZ
04RD47Z
04RD4JZ
04RD4KZ
04RE07Z
04RE0JZ
04RE0KZ
04RE47Z
04RE4JZ
04RE4KZ
04RF07Z
04RF0JZ
04RF0KZ
04RF47Z
04RF4JZ
04RF4KZ
04RH07Z
04RH0JZ
04RH0KZ
04RH47Z
04RH4JZ
04RH4KZ
04RJ07Z
04RJ0JZ
04RJ0KZ
04RJ47Z
04RJ4JZ
04RJ4KZ
04V00DZ
04V00EZ
04V00FZ
04V00ZZ
04V03ZZ
04V04ZZ
04V10DZ
04V10ZZ
04V13DZ
04V13ZZ
04V14DZ
04V14ZZ
04V20DZ
04V20ZZ
04V23DZ
04V23ZZ
04V24DZ
04V24ZZ
04V30DZ
04V30ZZ
04V33DZ
04V33ZZ
04V34DZ
04V34ZZ
04V40DZ

Ø4V4ØZZ
Ø4V43DZ
Ø4V43ZZ
Ø4V44DZ
Ø4V44ZZ
Ø4V5ØDZ
Ø4V5ØZZ
Ø4V53DZ
Ø4V53ZZ
Ø4V54DZ
Ø4V54ZZ
Ø4V6ØDZ
Ø4V6ØZZ
Ø4V63DZ
Ø4V63ZZ
Ø4V64DZ
Ø4V64ZZ
Ø4V7ØDZ
Ø4V7ØZZ
Ø4V73DZ
Ø4V73ZZ
Ø4V74DZ
Ø4V74ZZ
Ø4V8ØDZ
Ø4V8ØZZ
Ø4V83DZ
Ø4V83ZZ
Ø4V84DZ
Ø4V84ZZ
Ø4V9ØDZ
Ø4V9ØZZ
Ø4V93DZ
Ø4V93ZZ
Ø4V94DZ
Ø4V94ZZ
Ø4VAØDZ
Ø4VAØZZ
Ø4VA3DZ
Ø4VA3ZZ
Ø4VA4DZ
Ø4VA4ZZ
Ø4VBØDZ
Ø4VBØZZ
Ø4VB3DZ
Ø4VB3ZZ
Ø4VB4DZ
Ø4VB4ZZ
Ø4VCØDZ
Ø4VCØEZ
Ø4VCØZZ
Ø4VC3DZ
Ø4VC3EZ
Ø4VC3ZZ
Ø4VC4DZ
Ø4VC4EZ
Ø4VC4ZZ
Ø4VDØDZ
Ø4VDØEZ
Ø4VDØZZ
Ø4VD3DZ
Ø4VD3EZ
Ø4VD3ZZ
Ø4VD4DZ
Ø4VD4EZ
Ø4VD4ZZ
Ø4VEØDZ
Ø4VEØZZ
Ø4VE3DZ
Ø4VE3ZZ
Ø4VE4DZ
Ø4VE4ZZ
Ø4VFØDZ
Ø4VFØZZ
Ø4VF3DZ
Ø4VF3ZZ
Ø4VF4DZ
Ø4VF4ZZ
Ø4VHØDZ
Ø4VHØZZ
Ø4VH3DZ
Ø4VH3ZZ
Ø4VH4DZ
Ø4VH4ZZ
Ø4VJØDZ
Ø4VJØZZ
Ø4VJ3DZ
Ø4VJ3ZZ
Ø4VJ4DZ
Ø4VJ4ZZ
Ø4VKØDZ
Ø4VKØZZ
Ø4VK3DZ
Ø4VK3ZZ
Ø4VK4DZ
Ø4VK4ZZ
Ø4VLØDZ
Ø4VLØZZ
Ø4VL3DZ
Ø4VL3ZZ
Ø4VL4DZ
Ø4VL4ZZ
Ø4VMØDZ
Ø4VMØZZ
Ø4VM3DZ
Ø4VM3ZZ
Ø4VM4DZ
Ø4VM4ZZ
Ø4VNØDZ
Ø4VNØZZ
Ø4VN3DZ
Ø4VN3ZZ
Ø4VN4DZ
Ø4VN4ZZ
Ø4VPØDZ
Ø4VPØZZ
Ø4VP3DZ
Ø4VP3ZZ
Ø4VP4DZ
Ø4VP4ZZ
Ø4VQØDZ
Ø4VQØZZ
Ø4VQ3DZ
Ø4VQ3ZZ
Ø4VQ4DZ
Ø4VQ4ZZ
Ø4VRØDZ
Ø4VRØZZ
Ø4VR3DZ
Ø4VR3ZZ
Ø4VR4DZ
Ø4VR4ZZ
Ø4VSØDZ
Ø4VSØZZ
Ø4VS3DZ
Ø4VS3ZZ
Ø4VS4DZ
Ø4VS4ZZ
Ø4VTØDZ
Ø4VTØZZ
Ø4VT3DZ
Ø4VT3ZZ
Ø4VT4DZ
Ø4VT4ZZ
Ø4VUØDZ
Ø4VUØZZ
Ø4VU3DZ
Ø4VU3ZZ
Ø4VU4DZ
Ø4VU4ZZ
Ø4VVØDZ
Ø4VVØZZ
Ø4VV3DZ
Ø4VV3ZZ
Ø4VV4DZ
Ø4VV4ZZ
Ø4VWØDZ
Ø4VWØZZ
Ø4VW3DZ
Ø4VW3ZZ
Ø4VW4DZ
Ø4VW4ZZ
Ø4VYØDZ
Ø4VYØZZ
Ø4VY3DZ
Ø4VY3ZZ
Ø4VY4DZ
Ø4VY4ZZ
Ø51ØØ7Y
Ø51ØØ9Y
Ø51ØØAY
Ø51ØØJY
Ø51ØØKY
Ø51ØØZY
Ø51Ø47Y
Ø51Ø49Y
Ø51Ø4AY
Ø51Ø4JY
Ø51Ø4KY
Ø51Ø4ZY
Ø511Ø7Y
Ø511Ø9Y
Ø511ØAY
Ø511ØJY
Ø511ØKY
Ø511ØZY
Ø51147Y
Ø51149Y
Ø5114AY
Ø5114JY
Ø5114KY
Ø5114ZY
Ø513Ø7Y
Ø513Ø9Y
Ø513ØAY
Ø513ØJY
Ø513ØKY
Ø513ØZY
Ø51347Y
Ø51349Y
Ø5134AY
Ø5134JY
Ø5134KY
Ø5134ZY
Ø514Ø7Y
Ø514Ø9Y
Ø514ØAY
Ø514ØJY
Ø514ØKY
Ø514ØZY
Ø51447Y
Ø51449Y
Ø5144AY
Ø5144JY
Ø5144KY
Ø5144ZY
Ø515Ø7Y
Ø515Ø9Y
Ø515ØAY
Ø515ØJY
Ø515ØKY
Ø515ØZY
Ø51547Y
Ø51549Y
Ø5154AY
Ø5154JY
Ø5154KY
Ø5154ZY
Ø516Ø7Y
Ø516Ø9Y
Ø516ØAY
Ø516ØJY
Ø516ØKY
Ø516ØZY
Ø51647Y
Ø51649Y
Ø5164AY
Ø5164JY
Ø5164KY
Ø5164ZY
Ø55ØØZZ
Ø55Ø3ZZ
Ø55Ø4ZZ
Ø551ØZZ
Ø5513ZZ
Ø5514ZZ
Ø553ØZZ
Ø5533ZZ
Ø5534ZZ
Ø554ØZZ
Ø5543ZZ
Ø5544ZZ
Ø555ØZZ
Ø5553ZZ
Ø5554ZZ
Ø556ØZZ
Ø5563ZZ
Ø5564ZZ
Ø5BØØZZ
Ø5BØ3ZZ
Ø5BØ4ZZ
Ø5B1ØZZ
Ø5B13ZZ
Ø5B14ZZ
Ø5B3ØZZ
Ø5B33ZZ
Ø5B34ZZ
Ø5B4ØZZ
Ø5B43ZZ
Ø5B44ZZ
Ø5B5ØZZ
Ø5B53ZZ
Ø5B54ZZ
Ø5B6ØZZ
Ø5B63ZZ
Ø5B64ZZ
Ø5CØØZZ
Ø5CØ3ZZ
Ø5CØ4ZZ
Ø5C1ØZZ
Ø5C13ZZ
Ø5C14ZZ
Ø5C3ØZZ
Ø5C33ZZ
Ø5C34ZZ
Ø5C4ØZZ
Ø5C43ZZ
Ø5C44ZZ
Ø5C5ØZZ
Ø5C53ZZ
Ø5C54ZZ
Ø5C6ØZZ
Ø5C63ZZ
Ø5C64ZZ
Ø5LØØCZ
Ø5LØØDZ
Ø5LØØZZ
Ø5LØ3CZ
Ø5LØ3DZ
Ø5LØ3ZZ
Ø5LØ4CZ
Ø5LØ4DZ
Ø5LØ4ZZ
Ø5L1ØCZ
Ø5L1ØDZ
Ø5L1ØZZ
Ø5L13CZ
Ø5L13DZ
Ø5L13ZZ
Ø5L14CZ
Ø5L14DZ
Ø5L14ZZ
Ø5L3ØCZ
Ø5L3ØDZ
Ø5L3ØZZ
Ø5L33CZ
Ø5L33DZ
Ø5L33ZZ
Ø5L34CZ
Ø5L34DZ
Ø5L34ZZ
Ø5L4ØCZ
Ø5L4ØDZ
Ø5L4ØZZ
Ø5L43CZ
Ø5L43DZ
Ø5L43ZZ
Ø5L44CZ
Ø5L44DZ
Ø5L44ZZ
Ø5L5ØCZ
Ø5L5ØDZ
Ø5L5ØZZ
Ø5L53CZ
Ø5L53DZ
Ø5L53ZZ
Ø5L54CZ
Ø5L54DZ
Ø5L54ZZ
Ø5L6ØCZ
Ø5L6ØDZ
Ø5L6ØZZ
Ø5L63CZ
Ø5L63DZ
Ø5L63ZZ
Ø5L64CZ
Ø5L64DZ
Ø5L64ZZ
Ø5VØØDZ
Ø5VØØZZ
Ø5VØ3DZ
Ø5VØ3ZZ
Ø5VØ4DZ
Ø5VØ4ZZ
Ø5V1ØDZ
Ø5V1ØZZ
Ø5V13DZ
Ø5V13ZZ
Ø5V14DZ
Ø5V14ZZ
Ø5V3ØDZ
Ø5V3ØZZ
Ø5V33DZ
Ø5V33ZZ
Ø5V34DZ
Ø5V34ZZ
Ø5V4ØDZ
Ø5V4ØZZ
Ø5V43DZ
Ø5V43ZZ
Ø5V44DZ
Ø5V44ZZ
Ø5V5ØDZ
Ø5V5ØZZ
Ø5V53DZ
Ø5V53ZZ
Ø5V54DZ
Ø5V54ZZ
Ø5V6ØDZ
Ø5V6ØZZ
Ø5V63DZ
Ø5V63ZZ
Ø5V64DZ
Ø5V64ZZ
Ø5V7ØDZ
Ø5V7ØZZ
Ø5V73DZ
Ø5V73ZZ
Ø5V74DZ
Ø5V74ZZ
Ø5V8ØDZ
Ø5V8ØZZ
Ø5V83DZ
Ø5V83ZZ
Ø5V84DZ
Ø5V84ZZ
Ø5V9ØDZ
Ø5V9ØZZ
Ø5V93DZ
Ø5V93ZZ
Ø5V94DZ
Ø5V94ZZ
Ø5VAØDZ
Ø5VAØZZ
Ø5VA3DZ
Ø5VA3ZZ
Ø5VA4DZ
Ø5VA4ZZ
Ø5VBØDZ
Ø5VBØZZ
Ø5VB3DZ
Ø5VB3ZZ
Ø5VB4DZ
Ø5VB4ZZ
Ø5VCØDZ
Ø5VCØZZ
Ø5VC3DZ
Ø5VC3ZZ
Ø5VC4DZ
Ø5VC4ZZ
Ø5VDØDZ
Ø5VDØZZ
Ø5VD3DZ
Ø5VD3ZZ
Ø5VD4DZ
Ø5VD4ZZ
Ø5VFØDZ
Ø5VFØZZ
Ø5VF3DZ
Ø5VF3ZZ
Ø5VF4DZ
Ø5VF4ZZ
Ø5VGØDZ
Ø5VGØZZ
Ø5VG3DZ
Ø5VG3ZZ
Ø5VG4DZ
Ø5VG4ZZ
Ø5VHØDZ
Ø5VHØZZ
Ø5VH3DZ
Ø5VH3ZZ
Ø5VH4DZ
Ø5VH4ZZ
Ø5VLØDZ
Ø5VLØZZ
Ø5VL3DZ
Ø5VL3ZZ
Ø5VL4DZ
Ø5VL4ZZ
Ø5VMØDZ
Ø5VMØZZ
Ø5VM3DZ
Ø5VM3ZZ
Ø5VM4DZ
Ø5VM4ZZ
Ø5VNØDZ
Ø5VNØZZ
Ø5VN3DZ
Ø5VN3ZZ
Ø5VN4DZ
Ø5VN4ZZ
Ø5VPØDZ
Ø5VPØZZ
Ø5VP3DZ
Ø5VP3ZZ
Ø5VP4DZ
Ø5VP4ZZ
Ø5VQØDZ
Ø5VQØZZ
Ø5VQ3DZ
Ø5VQ3ZZ
Ø5VQ4DZ
Ø5VQ4ZZ
Ø5VRØDZ
Ø5VRØZZ
Ø5VR3DZ
Ø5VR3ZZ
Ø5VR4DZ
Ø5VR4ZZ
Ø5VSØDZ
Ø5VSØZZ
Ø5VS3DZ
Ø5VS3ZZ
Ø5VS4DZ
Ø5VS4ZZ
Ø5VTØDZ
Ø5VTØZZ
Ø5VT3DZ
Ø5VT3ZZ
Ø5VT4DZ
Ø5VT4ZZ
Ø5VVØDZ
Ø5VVØZZ
Ø5VV3DZ
Ø5VV3ZZ
Ø5VV4DZ
Ø5VV4ZZ
Ø5VYØDZ
Ø5VYØZZ
Ø5VY3DZ
Ø5VY3ZZ
Ø5VY4DZ
Ø5VY4ZZ
61Ø075
61Ø076
Ø61ØØ7Y
61Ø095
61Ø096
Ø61ØØ9Y
Ø61ØØA5
Ø61ØØA6
Ø61ØØAY
Ø61ØØJ5
Ø61ØØJ6
Ø61ØØJY
Ø61ØØK5
Ø61ØØK6
Ø61ØØKY
Ø61ØØZ5
Ø61ØØZ6
Ø61ØØZY
61Ø475
61Ø476
Ø61Ø47Y
61Ø495
61Ø496
Ø61Ø49Y
Ø61Ø4A5
Ø61Ø4A6
Ø61Ø4AY
Ø61Ø4J5
Ø61Ø4J6
Ø61Ø4JY
Ø61Ø4K5
Ø61Ø4K6
Ø61Ø4KY
Ø61Ø4Z5
Ø61Ø4Z6
Ø61Ø4ZY
Ø611*
Ø612*
Ø614*
Ø615*
Ø616*
Ø617*
Ø618*
Ø619*
Ø61B*
Ø61J*
Ø65ØØZZ
Ø65Ø3ZZ
Ø65Ø4ZZ
Ø651ØZZ
Ø6513ZZ
Ø6514ZZ
Ø652ØZZ
Ø6523ZZ
Ø6524ZZ
Ø654ØZZ
Ø6543ZZ
Ø6544ZZ
Ø655ØZZ
Ø6553ZZ
Ø6554ZZ
Ø656ØZZ
Ø6563ZZ
Ø6564ZZ
Ø657ØZZ
Ø6573ZZ
Ø6574ZZ
Ø658ØZZ
Ø6583ZZ
Ø6584ZZ
Ø659ØZZ
Ø6593ZZ
Ø6594ZZ
Ø65BØZZ
Ø65B3ZZ
Ø65B4ZZ
Ø65CØZZ
Ø65C3ZZ
Ø65C4ZZ
Ø65DØZZ
Ø65D3ZZ
Ø65D4ZZ
Ø65FØZZ
Ø65F3ZZ
Ø65F4ZZ
Ø65GØZZ
Ø65G3ZZ
Ø65G4ZZ
Ø65HØZZ
Ø65H3ZZ
Ø65H4ZZ
Ø65JØZZ
Ø65J3ZZ
Ø65J4ZZ
Ø6BØØZZ
Ø6BØ3ZZ
Ø6BØ4ZZ
Ø6B1ØZZ
Ø6B13ZZ
Ø6B14ZZ
Ø6B2ØZZ
Ø6B23ZZ
Ø6B24ZZ
Ø6B4ØZZ
Ø6B43ZZ
Ø6B44ZZ
Ø6B5ØZZ
Ø6B53ZZ
Ø6B54ZZ
Ø6B6ØZZ
Ø6B63ZZ
Ø6B64ZZ
Ø6B7ØZZ
Ø6B73ZZ
Ø6B74ZZ
Ø6B8ØZZ
Ø6B83ZZ
Ø6B84ZZ
Ø6B9ØZZ
Ø6B93ZZ
Ø6B94ZZ
Ø6BBØZZ
Ø6BB3ZZ
Ø6BB4ZZ
Ø6BCØZZ
Ø6BC3ZZ
Ø6BC4ZZ
Ø6BDØZZ
Ø6BD3ZZ
Ø6BD4ZZ
Ø6BFØZZ
Ø6BF3ZZ
Ø6BF4ZZ
Ø6BGØZZ
Ø6BG3ZZ
Ø6BG4ZZ
Ø6BHØZZ
Ø6BH3ZZ
Ø6BH4ZZ
Ø6BJØZZ
Ø6BJ3ZZ
Ø6BJ4ZZ
Ø6CØØZZ
Ø6CØ3ZZ
Ø6CØ4ZZ
Ø6C1ØZZ
Ø6C13ZZ
Ø6C14ZZ
Ø6C2ØZZ
Ø6C23ZZ
Ø6C24ZZ
Ø6C4ØZZ
Ø6C43ZZ
Ø6C44ZZ
Ø6C5ØZZ
Ø6C53ZZ
Ø6C54ZZ
Ø6C6ØZZ
Ø6C63ZZ
Ø6C64ZZ
Ø6C7ØZZ
Ø6C73ZZ
Ø6C74ZZ
Ø6C8ØZZ
Ø6C83ZZ
Ø6C84ZZ
Ø6C9ØZZ
Ø6C93ZZ
Ø6C94ZZ
Ø6CBØZZ
Ø6CB3ZZ
Ø6CB4ZZ
Ø6CCØZZ
Ø6CC3ZZ
Ø6CC4ZZ
Ø6CDØZZ
Ø6CD3ZZ
Ø6CD4ZZ
Ø6CFØZZ
Ø6CF3ZZ
Ø6CF4ZZ
Ø6CGØZZ
Ø6CG3ZZ
Ø6CG4ZZ
Ø6CHØZZ
Ø6CH3ZZ
Ø6CH4ZZ
Ø6CJØZZ
Ø6CJ3ZZ
Ø6CJ4ZZ
Ø6CM3ZZ
Ø6CN3ZZ
Ø6CP3ZZ
Ø6CQ3ZZ
Ø6CT3ZZ
Ø6CV3ZZ
Ø6CY3ZZ
Ø6L1ØCZ
Ø6L1ØDZ
Ø6L1ØZZ
Ø6L13CZ
Ø6L13DZ
Ø6L13ZZ
Ø6L14CZ
Ø6L14DZ
Ø6L14ZZ
Ø6L2ØCZ
Ø6L2ØDZ
Ø6L2ØZZ
Ø6L23CZ
Ø6L23DZ
Ø6L23ZZ
Ø6L24CZ
Ø6L24DZ
Ø6L24ZZ
Ø6L3ØCZ
Ø6L3ØDZ
Ø6L3ØZZ
Ø6L4ØCZ
Ø6L4ØDZ
Ø6L4ØZZ
Ø6L43CZ
Ø6L43DZ
Ø6L43ZZ
Ø6L44CZ
Ø6L44DZ
Ø6L44ZZ
Ø6L5ØCZ
Ø6L5ØDZ
Ø6L5ØZZ
Ø6L53CZ
Ø6L53DZ
Ø6L53ZZ
Ø6L54CZ
Ø6L54DZ
Ø6L54ZZ
Ø6L6ØCZ
Ø6L6ØDZ
Ø6L6ØZZ
Ø6L63CZ
Ø6L63DZ
Ø6L63ZZ
Ø6L64CZ
Ø6L64DZ
Ø6L64ZZ
Ø6L7ØCZ
Ø6L7ØDZ
Ø6L7ØZZ
Ø6L73CZ
Ø6L73DZ
Ø6L73ZZ
Ø6L74CZ
Ø6L74DZ
Ø6L74ZZ
Ø6L8ØCZ
Ø6L8ØDZ
Ø6L8ØZZ
Ø6L83CZ
Ø6L83DZ
Ø6L83ZZ
Ø6L84CZ
Ø6L84DZ
Ø6L84ZZ
Ø6L9ØCZ
Ø6L9ØDZ
Ø6L9ØZZ
Ø6L93CZ
Ø6L93DZ
Ø6L93ZZ
Ø6L94CZ
Ø6L94DZ
Ø6L94ZZ
Ø6LBØCZ
Ø6LBØDZ
Ø6LBØZZ
Ø6LB3CZ
Ø6LB3DZ
Ø6LB3ZZ
Ø6LB4CZ
Ø6LB4DZ
Ø6LB4ZZ
Ø6LCØCZ
Ø6LCØDZ
Ø6LCØZZ
Ø6LC3CZ
Ø6LC3DZ
Ø6LC3ZZ
Ø6LC4CZ
Ø6LC4DZ
Ø6LC4ZZ
Ø6LDØCZ
Ø6LDØDZ
Ø6LDØZZ
Ø6LD3CZ
Ø6LD3DZ
Ø6LD3ZZ
Ø6LD4CZ
Ø6LD4DZ
Ø6LD4ZZ
Ø6LFØCZ
Ø6LFØDZ
Ø6LFØZZ
Ø6LF3CZ
Ø6LF3DZ
Ø6LF3ZZ
Ø6LF4CZ
Ø6LF4DZ
Ø6LF4ZZ
Ø6LGØCZ
Ø6LGØDZ
Ø6LGØZZ
Ø6LG3CZ
Ø6LG3DZ
Ø6LG3ZZ
Ø6LG4CZ
Ø6LG4DZ
Ø6LG4ZZ
Ø6LHØCZ
Ø6LHØDZ
Ø6LHØZZ
Ø6LH3CZ
Ø6LH3DZ
Ø6LH3ZZ
Ø6LH4CZ
Ø6LH4DZ
Ø6LH4ZZ
Ø6LJØCZ
Ø6LJØDZ
Ø6LJØZZ
Ø6LJ3CZ
Ø6LJ3DZ
Ø6LJ3ZZ
Ø6LJ4CZ
Ø6LJ4DZ
Ø6LJ4ZZ
Ø6RØØ7Z
Ø6RØØJZ
Ø6RØØKZ
Ø6RØ47Z
Ø6RØ4JZ
Ø6RØ4KZ
Ø6R1Ø7Z
Ø6R1ØJZ
Ø6R1ØKZ
Ø6R147Z
Ø6R14JZ
Ø6R14KZ
Ø6R2Ø7Z
Ø6R2ØJZ
Ø6R2ØKZ
Ø6R247Z
Ø6R24JZ

06R24KZ
06R407Z
06R40JZ
06R40KZ
06R447Z
06R44JZ
06R44KZ
06R507Z
06R50JZ
06R50KZ
06R547Z
06R54JZ
06R54KZ
06R607Z
06R60JZ
06R60KZ
06R647Z
06R64JZ
06R64KZ
06R707Z
06R70JZ
06R70KZ
06R747Z
06R74JZ
06R74KZ
06R807Z
06R80JZ
06R80KZ
06R847Z
06R84JZ
06R84KZ
06R907Z
06R90JZ
06R90KZ
06R947Z
06R94JZ
06R94KZ
06RB07Z
06RB0JZ
06RB0KZ
06RB47Z
06RB4JZ
06RB4KZ
06RC07Z
06RC0JZ
06RC0KZ
06RC47Z
06RC4JZ
06RC4KZ
06RD07Z
06RD0JZ
06RD0KZ
06RD47Z
06RD4JZ
06RD4KZ
06RF07Z
06RF0JZ
06RF0KZ
06RF47Z
06RF4JZ
06RF4KZ
06RG07Z
06RG0JZ
06RG0KZ
06RG47Z
06RG4JZ
06RG4KZ
06RH07Z
06RH0JZ
06RH0KZ
06RH47Z
06RH4JZ
06RH4KZ
06RJ07Z
06RJ0JZ
06RJ0KZ
06RJ47Z
06RJ4JZ
06RJ4KZ
06V10DZ
06V10ZZ
06V13DZ
06V13ZZ
06V14DZ
06V14ZZ
06V20DZ
06V20ZZ
06V23DZ
06V23ZZ
06V24DZ
06V24ZZ
06V30DZ
06V30ZZ
06V33DZ
06V33ZZ
06V34DZ
06V34ZZ
06V40DZ
06V40ZZ
06V43DZ
06V43ZZ
06V44DZ
06V44ZZ
06V50DZ
06V50ZZ
06V53DZ
06V53ZZ
06V54DZ
06V54ZZ
06V60DZ
06V60ZZ
06V63DZ
06V63ZZ
06V64DZ
06V64ZZ
06V70DZ
06V70ZZ
06V73DZ
06V73ZZ
06V74DZ
06V74ZZ
06V80DZ
06V80ZZ
06V83DZ
06V83ZZ
06V84DZ
06V84ZZ
06V90DZ
06V90ZZ
06V93DZ
06V93ZZ
06V94DZ
06V94ZZ
06VB0DZ
06VB0ZZ
06VB3DZ
06VB3ZZ
06VB4DZ
06VB4ZZ
06VC0DZ
06VC0ZZ
06VC3DZ
06VC3ZZ
06VC4DZ
06VC4ZZ
06VD0DZ
06VD0ZZ
06VD3DZ
06VD3ZZ
06VD4DZ
06VD4ZZ
06VF0DZ
06VF0ZZ
06VF3DZ
06VF3ZZ
06VF4DZ
06VF4ZZ
06VG0DZ
06VG0ZZ
06VG3DZ
06VG3ZZ
06VG4DZ
06VG4ZZ
06VH0DZ
06VH0ZZ
06VH3DZ
06VH3ZZ
06VH4DZ
06VH4ZZ
06VJ0DZ
06VJ0ZZ
06VJ3DZ
06VJ3ZZ
06VJ4DZ
06VJ4ZZ
06VM0DZ
06VM0ZZ
06VM3DZ
06VM3ZZ
06VM4DZ
06VM4ZZ
06VN0DZ
06VN0ZZ
06VN3DZ
06VN3ZZ
06VN4DZ
06VN4ZZ
06VP0DZ
06VP0ZZ
06VP3DZ
06VP3ZZ
06VP4DZ
06VP4ZZ
06VQ0DZ
06VQ0ZZ
06VQ3DZ
06VQ3ZZ
06VQ4DZ
06VQ4ZZ
06VT0DZ
06VT0ZZ
06VT3DZ
06VT3ZZ
06VT4DZ
06VT4ZZ
06VV0DZ
06VV0ZZ
06VV3DZ
06VV3ZZ
06VV4DZ
06VV4ZZ
06VY0DZ
06VY0ZZ
06VY3DZ
06VY3ZZ
06VY4DZ
06VY4ZZ
0W9D00Z
0W9D0ZX
0W9D0ZZ
0W9D40Z
0W9D4ZX
0W9D4ZZ
0WCD0ZZ
0WCD3ZZ
0WCD4ZZ
0WFD0ZZ
0WFD3ZZ
0WFD4ZZ
0WFDXZZ
0WHD03Z
0WHD0YZ
0WHD33Z
0WHD3YZ
0WHD43Z
0WHD4YZ
0WPD00Z
0WPD01Z
0WPD03Z
0WPD0YZ
0WPD30Z
0WPD31Z
0WPD33Z
0WPD3YZ
0WPD40Z
0WPD41Z
0WPD43Z
0WPD4YZ
0WWD00Z
0WWD01Z
0WWD03Z
0WWD0YZ
0WWD30Z
0WWD31Z
0WWD33Z
0WWD3YZ
0WWD40Z
0WWD41Z
0WWD43Z
0WWD4YZ
5A02110
5A02210
X2CQ3T7
X2CR3T7
X2CS3T7
X2CT3T7
X2CU3T7
X2CV3T7
X2CY3T7
X2U4079

DRG 271

Select operating room procedures listed under DRG 270

DRG 272

Select operating room procedures listed under DRG 270

DRG 273

Operating Room Procedures

02553ZZ
02563ZZ
02573ZZ
02583ZZ
02593ZZ
025K3ZZ
025L3ZZ
025M3ZZ
027F44Z
027F4DZ
027F4ZZ
027G44Z
027G4DZ
027G4ZZ
027H44Z
027H4DZ
027H4ZZ
027J44Z
027J4DZ
027J4ZZ
02B53ZZ
02B63ZZ
02B73ZZ
02B83ZZ
02B93ZZ
02BM3ZZ
02T83ZZ
02U53JZ
02U54JZ
02VL3CZ
02VL3ZZ

OR

Nonoperating Room Procedures

02573ZK
02574ZK
02B73ZK
02B74ZK
02K80ZZ
02K83ZZ
02K84ZZ
02L70CK
02L70DK
02L70ZK
02L73CK
02L73DK
02L73ZK
02L74CK
02L74DK
02L74ZK
4A023FZ
4A027FZ
4A028FZ

DRG 274

Select operating room procedures OR nonoperating room procedures listed under DRG 273

DRG 275

Defibrillator Implant Operating Room Procedure Combinations

0JH60AZ
0JH63AZ
0JH80AZ
0JH83AZ

AND

02H60MZ
02H63MZ
02H64MZ
02HK0MZ
02HK3MZ
02HK4MZ

OR

0JH609Z
0JH639Z
0JH809Z
0JH839Z

AND

02H40KZ
02H43JZ
02H43KZ
02H43MZ
02H44KZ
02H60KZ
02H63KZ
02H64KZ
02H70KZ
02H73KZ
02H74KZ
02HK0KZ
02HK3KZ
02HK4KZ
02HL0KZ
02HL3KZ
02HL4KZ
02HN0JZ
02HN0KZ
02HN0MZ
02HN3JZ
02HN3KZ
02HN3MZ
02HN4JZ
02HN4KZ
02HN4MZ

OR

0JH608Z
0JH638Z
0JH808Z
0JH838Z

AND

02H40KZ
02H44KZ
02H60KZ
02H63KZ
02H64KZ
02H70KZ
02H73KZ
02H74KZ
02HK0KZ
02HK3KZ
02HK4KZ
02HL0KZ
02HL3KZ
02HL4KZ
02HN0JZ
02HN0KZ
02HN0MZ
02HN3JZ
02HN3KZ
02HN3MZ
02HN4JZ
02HN4KZ
02HN4MZ

OR

0JH60FZ
0JH63FZ
0WHC0GZ
0WHC3GZ
0WHC4GZ

AND

0JH608Z
0JH609Z
0JH638Z
0JH639Z
0JH808Z
0JH809Z
0JH838Z
0JH839Z

AND

Cardiac Catheterization Nonoperating Room Procedures

4A020N6
4A020N7
4A020N8
4A023N6
4A023N7
4A023N8
4A027N6
4A027N7
4A027N8
4A028N6
4A028N7
4A028N8
B20*
B2100ZZ
B2101ZZ
B210YZZ
B2110ZZ
B2111ZZ
B211YZZ
B2120ZZ
B2121ZZ
B212YZZ
B2130ZZ
B2131ZZ
B213YZZ
B214*
B215*
B216*
B217*
B218*
B21F*

DRG 276

Select defibrillator implant procedure combinations listed under DRG 275

DRG 277

Select defibrillator implant procedure combinations listed under DRG 275

DRG 278

Operating Room Procedures

03F23Z0
03F23ZZ
03F33Z0
03F33ZZ
03F43Z0
03F43ZZ
03F53Z0
03F53ZZ
03F63Z0
03F63ZZ
03F73Z0
03F73ZZ
03F83Z0
03F83ZZ
03F93Z0
03F93ZZ
03FA3Z0
03FA3ZZ
03FB3Z0
03FB3ZZ
03FC3Z0
03FC3ZZ
03FY3Z0
04FC3Z0
04FC3ZZ
04FD3Z0
04FD3ZZ
04FE3Z0
04FE3ZZ
04FF3Z0
04FF3ZZ
04FH3Z0
04FH3ZZ
04FJ3Z0
04FJ3ZZ
04FK3Z0
04FK3ZZ
04FL3Z0
04FL3ZZ
04FM3Z0
04FM3ZZ
04FN3Z0
04FN3ZZ
04FP3Z0
04FP3ZZ
04FQ3Z0
04FQ3ZZ
04FR3Z0
04FR3ZZ
04FS3Z0
04FS3ZZ
04FT3Z0
04FT3ZZ
04FU3Z0
04FU3ZZ
04FY3Z0
04FY3ZZ
05F33Z0
05F33ZZ
05F43Z0
05F43ZZ
05F53Z0
05F53ZZ
05F63Z0
05F63ZZ
05F73Z0
05F73ZZ
05F83Z0
05F83ZZ
05F93Z0
05F93ZZ
05FA3Z0
05FA3ZZ
05FB3Z0
05FB3ZZ
05FC3Z0
05FC3ZZ
05FD3Z0
05FD3ZZ
05FF3Z0
05FF3ZZ
05FY3Z0
05FY3ZZ
06FC3Z0
06FC3ZZ
06FD3Z0
06FD3ZZ
06FF3Z0
06FF3ZZ
06FG3Z0
06FG3ZZ
06FH3Z0
06FH3ZZ
06FJ3Z0
06FJ3ZZ
06FM3Z0
06FM3ZZ
06FN3Z0
06FN3ZZ
06FP3Z0
06FP3ZZ
06FQ3Z0
06FQ3ZZ
06FY3Z0
06FY3ZZ

DRG 279

Select operating room procedures under DRG 278

DRG 319

Operating Room Procedures

025F3ZZ
025G3ZZ
025H3ZZ
025J3ZZ
027F34Z
027F3DZ
027F3ZZ
027G34Z
027G3DZ
027G3ZZ
027H34Z
027H3DZ
027H3ZZ
027J34Z
027J3DZ
027J3ZZ
02BF3ZZ
02BG3ZZ
02BH3ZZ
02BJ3ZZ
02QF3ZJ
02QF3ZZ
02QG3ZE
02QG3ZZ
02QH3ZZ
02QJ3ZG
02QJ3ZZ
02TH3ZZ
02VG3ZZ
02WF38Z
02WF3JZ
02WF3KZ
02WG37Z
02WG38Z
02WG3JZ
02WG3KZ
02WH37Z
02WH38Z
02WH3JZ
02WH3KZ
02WJ37Z
02WJ38Z
02WJ3JZ
02WJ3KZ

DRG 320

Select operating room procedures listed under DRG 319

DRG 321

Percutaneous Cardiovascular Operating Room Procedures without Intraluminal Device

02703Z6
02703ZZ
02704Z6
02704ZZ
02713Z6
02713ZZ
02714Z6
02714ZZ
02723Z6
02723ZZ
02724Z6
02724ZZ
02733Z6
02733ZZ
02734Z6
02734ZZ
02C03Z6
02C03Z7
02C03ZZ
02C04Z6
02C04ZZ
02C13Z6
02C13Z7
02C13ZZ
02C14Z6
02C14ZZ
02C23Z6
02C23Z7
02C23ZZ
02C24Z6
02C24ZZ
02C33Z6
02C33Z7
02C33ZZ
02C34Z6
02C34ZZ

AND

Drug-eluting Intraluminal Device

270346
027034Z
270356
027035Z
270366
027036Z
270376
027037Z
270446
027044Z
270456
027045Z
270466
027046Z
270476
027047Z
271346
027134Z
271356
027135Z
271366
027136Z
271376
027137Z
271446
027144Z
271456
027145Z
271466
027146Z
271476
027147Z
272346
027234Z
272356
027235Z
272366
027236Z
272376
027237Z
272446
027244Z
272456
027245Z
272466
027246Z
272476
027247Z
273346
027334Z
273356
027335Z
273366
027336Z
273376
027337Z
273446
027344Z
273456
027345Z
273466
027346Z
273476
027347Z

OR

Non Drug-eluting Intraluminal Device

02703D6
02703DZ
02703E6
02703EZ
02703F6
02703FZ
02703G6
02703GZ
02703T6
02703TZ
02704D6
02704DZ
02704E6
02704EZ
02704F6
02704FZ
02704G6
02704GZ
02704T6
02704TZ
02713D6
02713DZ
02713E6
02713EZ
02713F6
02713FZ
02713G6
02713GZ
02713T6
02713TZ
02714D6
02714DZ
02714E6
02714EZ
02714F6
02714FZ
02714G6
02714GZ
02714T6
02714TZ
02723D6
02723DZ
02723E6
02723EZ
02723F6
02723FZ
02723G6
02723GZ
02723T6
02723TZ
02724D6
02724DZ
02724E6
02724EZ
02724F6
02724FZ
02724G6
02724GZ
02724T6
02724TZ
02733D6
02733DZ
02733E6
02733EZ
02733F6
02733FZ
02733G6
02733GZ
02733T6
02733TZ
02734D6
02734DZ
02734E6
02734EZ
02734F6
02734FZ
02734G6
02734GZ
02734T6
02734TZ
02H03DZ
02H03YZ
02H13DZ
02H13YZ
02H23DZ
02H23YZ
02H33DZ
02H33YZ

OR

Any combination of codes in the next eight lists adding up to four or more arteries/intraluminal devices

One Intraluminal Device

27Ø346
Ø27Ø34Z
Ø27Ø3D6
Ø27Ø3DZ
Ø27Ø3T6
Ø27Ø3TZ
27Ø446
Ø27Ø44Z
Ø27Ø4D6
Ø27Ø4DZ
Ø27Ø4T6
Ø27Ø4TZ
271346
Ø27134Z
Ø2713D6
Ø2713DZ
Ø2713T6
Ø2713TZ
271446
Ø27144Z
Ø2714D6
Ø2714DZ
Ø2714T6
Ø2714TZ
272346
Ø27234Z
Ø2723D6
Ø2723DZ
Ø2723T6
Ø2723TZ
272446
Ø27244Z
Ø2724D6
Ø2724DZ
Ø2724T6
Ø2724TZ
273346
Ø27334Z
Ø2733D6
Ø2733DZ
Ø2733T6
Ø2733TZ
273446
Ø27344Z
Ø2734D6
Ø2734DZ
Ø2734T6
Ø2734TZ
Ø2HØ3DZ
Ø2HØ3YZ
Ø2H13DZ
Ø2H13YZ
Ø2H23DZ
Ø2H23YZ
Ø2H33DZ
Ø2H33YZ

Two Intraluminal Devices

27Ø356
Ø27Ø35Z
Ø27Ø3E6
Ø27Ø3EZ
27Ø456
Ø27Ø45Z
Ø27Ø4E6
Ø27Ø4EZ
271356
Ø27135Z
Ø2713E6
Ø2713EZ
271456
Ø27145Z
Ø2714E6
Ø2714EZ
272356
Ø27235Z
Ø2723E6
Ø2723EZ
272456
Ø27245Z
Ø2724E6
Ø2724EZ
273356
Ø27335Z
Ø2733E6
Ø2733EZ
273456
Ø27345Z
Ø2734E6
Ø2734EZ

Three Intraluminal Devices

27Ø366
Ø27Ø36Z
Ø27Ø3F6
Ø27Ø3FZ
27Ø466
Ø27Ø46Z
Ø27Ø4F6
Ø27Ø4FZ
271366
Ø27136Z
Ø2713F6
Ø2713FZ
271466
Ø27146Z
Ø2714F6
Ø2714FZ
272366
Ø27236Z
Ø2723F6
Ø2723FZ
272466
Ø27246Z
Ø2724F6
Ø2724FZ
273366
Ø27336Z
Ø2733F6
Ø2733FZ
273466
Ø27346Z
Ø2734F6
Ø2734FZ

Four or More Intraluminal Devices

27Ø376
Ø27Ø37Z
Ø27Ø3G6
Ø27Ø3GZ
27Ø476
Ø27Ø47Z
Ø27Ø4G6
Ø27Ø4GZ
271376
Ø27137Z
Ø2713G6
Ø2713GZ
271476
Ø27147Z
Ø2714G6
Ø2714GZ
272376
Ø27237Z
Ø2723G6
Ø2723GZ
272476
Ø27247Z
Ø2724G6
Ø2724GZ
273376
Ø27337Z
Ø2733G6
Ø2733GZ
273476
Ø27347Z
Ø2734G6
Ø2734GZ

One Artery

27Ø346
Ø27Ø34Z
27Ø356
Ø27Ø35Z
27Ø366
Ø27Ø36Z
27Ø376
Ø27Ø37Z
Ø27Ø3D6
Ø27Ø3DZ
Ø27Ø3E6
Ø27Ø3EZ
Ø27Ø3F6
Ø27Ø3FZ
Ø27Ø3G6
Ø27Ø3GZ
Ø27Ø3T6
Ø27Ø3TZ
Ø27Ø3Z6
Ø27Ø3ZZ
27Ø446
Ø27Ø44Z
27Ø456
Ø27Ø45Z
27Ø466
Ø27Ø46Z
27Ø476
Ø27Ø47Z
Ø27Ø4D6
Ø27Ø4DZ
Ø27Ø4E6
Ø27Ø4EZ
Ø27Ø4F6
Ø27Ø4FZ
Ø27Ø4G6
Ø27Ø4GZ
Ø27Ø4T6
Ø27Ø4TZ
Ø27Ø4Z6
Ø27Ø4ZZ
Ø2CØ3Z6
Ø2CØ3Z7
Ø2CØ3ZZ
Ø2CØ4Z6
Ø2CØ4ZZ
Ø2FØ3ZZ
Ø2HØ3DZ
Ø2HØ3YZ

Two Arteries

271346
Ø27134Z
271356
Ø27135Z
271366
Ø27136Z
271376
Ø27137Z
Ø2713D6
Ø2713DZ
Ø2713E6
Ø2713EZ
Ø2713F6
Ø2713FZ
Ø2713G6
Ø2713GZ
Ø2713T6
Ø2713TZ
Ø2713Z6
Ø2713ZZ
271446
Ø27144Z
271456
Ø27145Z
271466
Ø27146Z
271476
Ø27147Z
Ø2714D6
Ø2714DZ
Ø2714E6
Ø2714EZ
Ø2714F6
Ø2714FZ
Ø2714G6
Ø2714GZ
Ø2714T6
Ø2714TZ
Ø2714Z6
Ø2714ZZ
Ø2C13Z6
Ø2C13Z7
Ø2C13ZZ
Ø2C14Z6
Ø2C14ZZ
Ø2F13ZZ
Ø2H13DZ
Ø2H13YZ

Three Arteries

272346
Ø27234Z
272356
Ø27235Z
272366
Ø27236Z
272376
Ø27237Z
Ø2723D6
Ø2723DZ
Ø2723E6
Ø2723EZ
Ø2723F6
Ø2723FZ
Ø2723G6
Ø2723GZ
Ø2723T6
Ø2723TZ
Ø2723Z6
Ø2723ZZ
272446
Ø27244Z
272456
Ø27245Z
272466
Ø27246Z
272476
Ø27247Z
Ø2724D6
Ø2724DZ
Ø2724E6
Ø2724EZ
Ø2724F6
Ø2724FZ
Ø2724G6
Ø2724GZ
Ø2724T6
Ø2724TZ
Ø2724Z6
Ø2724ZZ
Ø2C23Z6
Ø2C23Z7
Ø2C23ZZ
Ø2C24Z6
Ø2C24ZZ
Ø2F23ZZ
Ø2H23DZ
Ø2H23YZ

Four or More Arteries

273346
Ø27334Z
273356
Ø27335Z
273366
Ø27336Z
273376
Ø27337Z
Ø2733D6
Ø2733DZ
Ø2733E6
Ø2733EZ
Ø2733F6
Ø2733FZ
Ø2733G6
Ø2733GZ
Ø2733T6
Ø2733TZ
Ø2733Z6
Ø2733ZZ
273446
Ø27344Z
273456
Ø27345Z
273466
Ø27346Z
273476
Ø27347Z
Ø2734D6
Ø2734DZ
Ø2734E6
Ø2734EZ
Ø2734F6
Ø2734FZ
Ø2734G6
Ø2734GZ
Ø2734T6
Ø2734TZ
Ø2734Z6
Ø2734ZZ
Ø2C33Z6
Ø2C33Z7
Ø2C33ZZ
Ø2C34Z6
Ø2C34ZZ
Ø2F33ZZ
Ø2H33DZ
Ø2H33YZ

DRG 322

Select percutaneous cardiovascular operating room procedures without intraluminal device AND drug-eluting or non drug-eluting intraluminal device procedures listed under DRG 321

DRG 323

Lithotripsy Operating Room Procedures

Ø2FØ3ZZ
Ø2F13ZZ
Ø2F23ZZ
Ø2F33ZZ

AND

Intraluminal Device Operating Room Procedures

27Ø346
Ø27Ø34Z
27Ø356
Ø27Ø35Z
27Ø366
Ø27Ø36Z
27Ø376
Ø27Ø37Z
Ø27Ø3D6
Ø27Ø3DZ
Ø27Ø3E6
Ø27Ø3EZ
Ø27Ø3F6
Ø27Ø3FZ
Ø27Ø3G6
Ø27Ø3GZ
Ø27Ø3T6
Ø27Ø3TZ
27Ø446
Ø27Ø44Z
27Ø456
Ø27Ø45Z
27Ø466
Ø27Ø46Z
27Ø476
Ø27Ø47Z
Ø27Ø4D6
Ø27Ø4DZ
Ø27Ø4E6
Ø27Ø4EZ
Ø27Ø4F6
Ø27Ø4FZ
Ø27Ø4G6
Ø27Ø4GZ
Ø27Ø4T6
Ø27Ø4TZ
271346
Ø27134Z
271356
Ø27135Z
271366
Ø27136Z
271376
Ø27137Z
Ø2713D6
Ø2713DZ
Ø2713E6
Ø2713EZ
Ø2713F6
Ø2713FZ
Ø2713G6
Ø2713GZ
Ø2713T6
Ø2713TZ
271446
Ø27144Z
271456
Ø27145Z
271466
Ø27146Z
271476
Ø27147Z
Ø2714D6
Ø2714DZ
Ø2714E6
Ø2714EZ
Ø2714F6
Ø2714FZ
Ø2714G6
Ø2714GZ
Ø2714T6
Ø2714TZ
272346
Ø27234Z
272356
Ø27235Z
272366
Ø27236Z
272376
Ø27237Z
Ø2723D6
Ø2723DZ
Ø2723E6
Ø2723EZ
Ø2723F6
Ø2723FZ
Ø2723G6
Ø2723GZ
Ø2723T6
Ø2723TZ
272446
Ø27244Z
272456
Ø27245Z
272466
Ø27246Z
272476
Ø27247Z
Ø2724D6
Ø2724DZ
Ø2724E6
Ø2724EZ
Ø2724F6
Ø2724FZ
Ø2724G6
Ø2724GZ
Ø2724T6
Ø2724TZ
273346
Ø27334Z
273356
Ø27335Z
273366
Ø27336Z
273376
Ø27337Z
Ø2733D6
Ø2733DZ
Ø2733E6
Ø2733EZ
Ø2733F6
Ø2733FZ
Ø2733G6
Ø2733GZ
Ø2733T6
Ø2733TZ
273446
Ø27344Z
273456
Ø27345Z
273466
Ø27346Z
273476
Ø27347Z
Ø2734D6
Ø2734DZ
Ø2734E6
Ø2734EZ
Ø2734F6
Ø2734FZ
Ø2734G6
Ø2734GZ
Ø2734T6
Ø2734TZ
Ø2HØ3DZ
Ø2HØ3YZ
Ø2H13DZ
Ø2H13YZ
Ø2H23DZ
Ø2H23YZ
Ø2H33DZ
Ø2H33YZ

DRG 324

Select lithotripsy AND intraluminal device operating room procedures listed under DRG 323

DRG 325

Select lithotripsy operating room procedures listed under DRG 323

DRG 280

Principal or Secondary Diagnosis

I21*
I22*

DRG 281

Select principal or secondary diagnosis listed under DRG 280

DRG 282

Select principal or secondary diagnosis listed under DRG 280

DRG 283

Select principal or secondary diagnosis listed under DRG 280

DRG 284

Select principal or secondary diagnosis listed under DRG 280

DRG 285

Select principal or secondary diagnosis listed under DRG 280

DRG 286

Select any principal diagnosis listed under MDC 5 excluding AMI codes listed under DRG 280

AND

Nonoperating Room Procedures

4AØ2ØN6
4AØ2ØN7
4AØ2ØN8
4AØ23N6
4AØ23N7
4AØ23N8
4AØ27N6
4AØ27N7
4AØ27N8
4AØ28N6
4AØ28N7
4AØ28N8
B2Ø*
B21ØØZZ
B21Ø1ZZ
B21ØYZZ
B211ØZZ
B2111ZZ
B211YZZ
B212ØZZ
B2121ZZ
B212YZZ
B213ØZZ
B2131ZZ
B213YZZ
B214*
B215*
B216*
B217*
B218*
B21F*

DRG 287

Select any principal diagnosis listed under MDC 5 excluding AMI codes listed under DRG 280

AND

Select any nonoperating procedure listed under DRG 286

DRG 288

Principal Diagnosis

A39.51
A52.Ø3
B37.6
I33.Ø
I33.9

DRG 289

Select principal diagnosis listed under DRG 288

DRG 290

Select principal diagnosis listed under DRG 288

DRG 291

Principal Diagnosis

IØ9.81
I11.Ø
I13.Ø
I13.2
I5Ø*
R57.Ø
R57.9

DRG 292

Select principal diagnosis listed under DRG 291

DRG 293

Select principal diagnosis listed under DRG 291

DRG 294

Principal Diagnosis

I8Ø.1*
I8Ø.2*
I8Ø.3
I82.22Ø
I82.221

DRG 295

Select principal diagnosis listed under DRG 294

DRG 296

Principal Diagnosis

I46*

DRG 297

Select principal diagnosis listed under DRG 296

DRG 298

Select principal diagnosis listed under DRG 296

DRG 299

Principal Diagnosis

EØ8.5*
EØ9.5*
E1Ø.5*
E11.5*
E13.5*
I67.Ø
I7Ø.Ø
I7Ø.2*
I7Ø.3*
I7Ø.4*
I7Ø.5*
I7Ø.6*
I7Ø.7*
I7Ø.8
I7Ø.9*
I71*
I72.Ø
I72.1
I72.3
I72.4
I72.5
I72.6
I72.8
I72.9
I73.1
I73.8*
I73.9
I74*
I75.Ø*
I75.89
I76
I77.Ø
I77.1
I77.2
I77.3
I77.5
I77.7Ø
I77.71
I77.72
I77.74
I77.75
I77.76
I77.77
I77.79
I77.8*
I77.9
I78.Ø
I78.8
I78.9
I79*
I8Ø.Ø*
I8Ø.8
I8Ø.9
I82.1
I82.21Ø
I82.211
I82.29Ø
I82.291
I82.4*
I82.5*
I82.6*
I82.7*
I82.8*
I82.9*
I82.A*
I82.B*
I82.C*
I83.Ø*
I83.1*
I83.2*
I83.8*
I83.9*
I86.Ø
I86.4
I86.8
I87.Ø*
I87.1
I87.2
I87.3*
I96
M31.8
M31.9
Q26.5
Q26.6
Q27*
Q28.Ø
Q28.1
Q28.8
Q28.9
SØ9.ØXXS
S15.ØØ1S
S15.ØØ2S
S15.ØØ9S
S15.Ø11S
S15.Ø12S
S15.Ø19S
S15.Ø21S
S15.Ø22S
S15.Ø29S
S15.Ø91S
S15.Ø92S
S15.Ø99S
S15.1Ø1S
S15.1Ø2S
S15.1Ø9S
S15.111S
S15.112S
S15.119S
S15.121S
S15.122S
S15.129S
S15.191S
S15.192S
S15.199S
S15.2Ø1S
S15.2Ø2S
S15.2Ø9S
S15.211S
S15.212S
S15.219S
S15.221S
S15.222S
S15.229S
S15.291S
S15.292S
S15.299S
S15.3Ø1S
S15.3Ø2S
S15.3Ø9S
S15.311S
S15.312S
S15.319S
S15.321S
S15.322S
S15.329S
S15.391S
S15.392S
S15.399S
S15.8XXS
S15.9XXS
S25.ØØXS
S25.Ø1XS
S25.Ø2XS
S25.Ø9XS
S25.1Ø1S
S25.1Ø2S

S25.1Ø9S
S25.111S
S25.112S
S25.119S
S25.121S
S25.122S
S25.129S
S25.191S
S25.192S
S25.199S
S25.2ØXS
S25.21XS
S25.22XS
S25.29XS
S25.3Ø1S
S25.3Ø2S
S25.3Ø9S
S25.311S
S25.312S
S25.319S
S25.321S
S25.322S
S25.329S
S25.391S
S25.392S
S25.399S
S25.4Ø1S
S25.4Ø2S
S25.4Ø9S
S25.411S
S25.412S
S25.419S
S25.421S
S25.422S
S25.429S
S25.491S
S25.492S
S25.499S
S25.5Ø1S
S25.5Ø2S
S25.5Ø9S
S25.511S
S25.512S
S25.519S
S25.591S
S25.592S
S25.599S
S25.8Ø1S
S25.8Ø2S
S25.8Ø9S
S25.811S
S25.812S
S25.819S
S25.891S
S25.892S
S25.899S
S25.9ØXS
S25.91XS
S25.99XS
S35.ØØXS
S35.Ø1XS
S35.Ø2XS
S35.Ø9XS
S35.1ØXS
S35.11XS
S35.12XS
S35.19XS
S35.211S
S35.212S
S35.218S
S35.219S
S35.221S
S35.222S
S35.228S
S35.229S
S35.231S
S35.232S
S35.238S
S35.239S
S35.291S
S35.292S
S35.298S
S35.299S
S35.311S
S35.318S
S35.319S
S35.321S
S35.328S
S35.329S
S35.331S
S35.338S
S35.339S
S35.341S
S35.348S
S35.349S
S35.4Ø1S
S35.4Ø2S
S35.4Ø3S
S35.4Ø4S
S35.4Ø5S
S35.4Ø6S
S35.411S
S35.412S
S35.413S
S35.414S
S35.415S
S35.416S
S35.491S
S35.492S
S35.493S
S35.494S
S35.495S
S35.496S
S35.5ØXS
S35.511S
S35.512S
S35.513S
S35.514S
S35.515S
S35.516S
S35.531S
S35.532S
S35.533S
S35.534S
S35.535S
S35.536S
S35.59XS
S35.8X1S
S35.8X8S
S35.8X9S
S35.9ØXS
S35.91XS
S35.99XS
S45.ØØ1S
S45.ØØ2S
S45.ØØ9S
S45.Ø11S
S45.Ø12S
S45.Ø19S
S45.Ø91S
S45.Ø92S
S45.Ø99S
S45.1Ø1S
S45.1Ø2S
S45.1Ø9S
S45.111S
S45.112S
S45.119S
S45.191S
S45.192S
S45.199S
S45.2Ø1S
S45.2Ø2S
S45.2Ø9S
S45.211S
S45.212S
S45.219S
S45.291S
S45.292S
S45.299S
S45.3Ø1S
S45.3Ø2S
S45.3Ø9S
S45.311S
S45.312S
S45.319S
S45.391S
S45.392S
S45.399S
S45.8Ø1S
S45.8Ø2S
S45.8Ø9S
S45.811S
S45.812S
S45.819S
S45.891S
S45.892S
S45.899S
S45.9Ø1S
S45.9Ø2S
S45.9Ø9S
S45.911S
S45.912S
S45.919S
S45.991S
S45.992S
S45.999S
S55.ØØ1S
S55.ØØ2S
S55.ØØ9S
S55.Ø11S
S55.Ø12S
S55.Ø19S
S55.Ø91S
S55.Ø92S
S55.Ø99S
S55.1Ø1S
S55.1Ø2S
S55.1Ø9S
S55.111S
S55.112S
S55.119S
S55.191S
S55.192S
S55.199S
S55.2Ø1S
S55.2Ø2S
S55.2Ø9S
S55.211S
S55.212S
S55.219S
S55.291S
S55.292S
S55.299S
S55.8Ø1S
S55.8Ø2S
S55.8Ø9S
S55.811S
S55.812S
S55.819S
S55.891S
S55.892S
S55.899S
S55.9Ø1S
S55.9Ø2S
S55.9Ø9S
S55.911S
S55.912S
S55.919S
S55.991S
S55.992S
S55.999S
S65.ØØ1S
S65.ØØ2S
S65.ØØ9S
S65.Ø11S
S65.Ø12S
S65.Ø19S
S65.Ø91S
S65.Ø92S
S65.Ø99S
S65.1Ø1S
S65.1Ø2S
S65.1Ø9S
S65.111S
S65.112S
S65.119S
S65.191S
S65.192S
S65.199S
S65.2Ø1S
S65.2Ø2S
S65.2Ø9S
S65.211S
S65.212S
S65.219S
S65.291S
S65.292S
S65.299S
S65.3Ø1S
S65.3Ø2S
S65.3Ø9S
S65.311S
S65.312S
S65.319S
S65.391S
S65.392S
S65.399S
S65.4Ø1S
S65.4Ø2S
S65.4Ø9S
S65.411S
S65.412S
S65.419S
S65.491S
S65.492S
S65.499S
S65.5ØØS
S65.5Ø1S
S65.5Ø2S
S65.5Ø3S
S65.5Ø4S
S65.5Ø5S
S65.5Ø6S
S65.5Ø7S
S65.5Ø8S
S65.5Ø9S
S65.51ØS
S65.511S
S65.512S
S65.513S
S65.514S
S65.515S
S65.516S
S65.517S
S65.518S
S65.519S
S65.59ØS
S65.591S
S65.592S
S65.593S
S65.594S
S65.595S
S65.596S
S65.597S
S65.598S
S65.599S
S65.8Ø1S
S65.8Ø2S
S65.8Ø9S
S65.811S
S65.812S
S65.819S
S65.891S
S65.892S
S65.899S
S65.9Ø1S
S65.9Ø2S
S65.9Ø9S
S65.911S
S65.912S
S65.919S
S65.991S
S65.992S
S65.999S
S75.ØØ1S
S75.ØØ2S
S75.ØØ9S
S75.Ø11S
S75.Ø12S
S75.Ø19S
S75.Ø21S
S75.Ø22S
S75.Ø29S
S75.Ø91S
S75.Ø92S
S75.Ø99S
S75.1Ø1S
S75.1Ø2S
S75.1Ø9S
S75.111S
S75.112S
S75.119S
S75.121S
S75.122S
S75.129S
S75.191S
S75.192S
S75.199S
S75.2Ø1S
S75.2Ø2S
S75.2Ø9S
S75.211S
S75.212S
S75.219S
S75.221S
S75.222S
S75.229S
S75.291S
S75.292S
S75.299S
S75.8Ø1S
S75.8Ø2S
S75.8Ø9S
S75.811S
S75.812S
S75.819S
S75.891S
S75.892S
S75.899S
S75.9Ø1S
S75.9Ø2S
S75.9Ø9S
S75.911S
S75.912S
S75.919S
S75.991S
S75.992S
S75.999S
S85.ØØ1S
S85.ØØ2S
S85.ØØ9S
S85.Ø11S
S85.Ø12S
S85.Ø19S
S85.Ø91S
S85.Ø92S
S85.Ø99S
S85.1Ø1S
S85.1Ø2S
S85.1Ø9S
S85.111S
S85.112S
S85.119S
S85.121S
S85.122S
S85.129S
S85.131S
S85.132S
S85.139S
S85.141S
S85.142S
S85.149S
S85.151S
S85.152S
S85.159S
S85.161S
S85.162S
S85.169S
S85.171S
S85.172S
S85.179S
S85.181S
S85.182S
S85.189S
S85.2Ø1S
S85.2Ø2S
S85.2Ø9S
S85.211S
S85.212S
S85.219S
S85.291S
S85.292S
S85.299S
S85.3Ø1S
S85.3Ø2S
S85.3Ø9S
S85.311S
S85.312S
S85.319S
S85.391S
S85.392S
S85.399S
S85.4Ø1S
S85.4Ø2S
S85.4Ø9S
S85.411S
S85.412S
S85.419S
S85.491S
S85.492S
S85.499S
S85.5Ø1S
S85.5Ø2S
S85.5Ø9S
S85.511S
S85.512S
S85.519S
S85.591S
S85.592S
S85.599S
S85.8Ø1S
S85.8Ø2S
S85.8Ø9S
S85.811S
S85.812S
S85.819S
S85.891S
S85.892S
S85.899S
S85.9Ø1S
S85.9Ø2S
S85.9Ø9S
S85.911S
S85.912S
S85.919S
S85.991S
S85.992S
S85.999S
S95.ØØ1S
S95.ØØ2S
S95.ØØ9S
S95.Ø11S
S95.Ø12S
S95.Ø19S
S95.Ø91S
S95.Ø92S
S95.Ø99S
S95.1Ø1S
S95.1Ø2S
S95.1Ø9S
S95.111S
S95.112S
S95.119S
S95.191S
S95.192S
S95.199S
S95.2Ø1S
S95.2Ø2S
S95.2Ø9S
S95.211S
S95.212S
S95.219S
S95.291S
S95.292S
S95.299S
S95.8Ø1S
S95.8Ø2S
S95.8Ø9S
S95.811S
S95.812S
S95.819S
S95.891S
S95.892S
S95.899S
S95.9Ø1S
S95.9Ø2S
S95.9Ø9S
S95.911S
S95.912S
S95.919S
S95.991S
S95.992S
S95.999S
T81.718A
T81.719A
T81.72XA

DRG 300

Select principal diagnosis listed under DRG 299

DRG 301

Select principal diagnosis listed under DRG 299

DRG 302

Principal Diagnosis

I25.1*
I25.2
I25.5
I25.6
I25.7*
I25.8*
I25.9
I51.3
I51.7
I51.89
I51.9
I52
I87.8
I87.9
I99*
R93.1

DRG 303

Select principal diagnosis listed under DRG 302

DRG 304

Principal Diagnosis

I1Ø
I11.9
I15*
I16.Ø
I16.1
I16.9
I1A.Ø
N26.2

DRG 305

Select principal diagnosis listed under DRG 304

DRG 306

Principal Diagnosis

A52.Ø1
A52.Ø2
B33.21
IØ1.1
IØ5*
IØ6*
IØ7*
IØ8*
IØ9.1
IØ9.89
I23.4
I23.5
I34*
I35*
I36*
I37*
I38
I39
I51.1
I51.2
Q2Ø*
Q21*
Q22*
Q23*
Q24.Ø
Q24.1
Q24.2
Q24.3
Q24.4
Q24.5
Q24.8
Q24.9
Q25*
Q26.Ø
Q26.1
Q26.2
Q26.3
Q26.4
Q26.8
Q26.9
Q87.4*
RØ1.Ø
RØ1.1
T82.Ø1XA
T82.Ø2XA
T82.Ø3XA
T82.Ø9XA

DRG 307

Select principal diagnosis listed under DRG 306

DRG 308

Principal Diagnosis

I44*
I45*
I47*
I48*
I49*
Q24.6
RØØ.Ø
RØØ.1
RØØ.2
T82.11ØA
T82.111A
T82.12ØA
T82.121A
T82.19ØA
T82.191A

DRG 309

Select principal diagnosis listed under DRG 308

DRG 310

Select principal diagnosis listed under DRG 308

DRG 311

Principal Diagnosis

I2Ø*
I24.Ø
I24.8*
I24.9

DRG 312

Principal Diagnosis

I95.1
I95.2
I95.3
I95.81
R55

DRG 313

Principal Diagnosis

RØ7.2
RØ7.82
RØ7.89
RØ7.9

DRG 314

Principal Diagnosis

A36.81
A39.5Ø
A39.52
A39.53
A52.ØØ
A52.Ø4
A52.Ø5
A52.Ø6
A52.Ø9
A54.83
B33.2Ø
B33.22
B33.23
B33.24
B57.Ø
B57.2
B58.81
C38.Ø
C45.2
D15.1
D18.ØØ
D18.Ø9
IØ1.Ø
IØ1.2
IØ1.8
IØ1.9
IØ2*
IØ9.Ø
IØ9.2
IØ9.9
I23.Ø
I23.1
I23.2
I23.3
I23.6
I23.7
I23.8
I24.1
I25.3
I25.4*
I27.Ø
I27.1
I27.2*
I27.81
I27.83
I27.89
I27.9
I28*
I3Ø*
I31*
I32
I4Ø*
I41
I42*
I43
I51.Ø
I51.4
I51.5
I51.81
I5A
I95.Ø
I95.89
I95.9
I97.Ø
I97.1*
I97.7*
I97.88
I97.89
RØØ.8
RØØ.9
RØ1.2
RØ3*
RØ9.89
RØ9.AØ
RØ9.A1
RØ9.A2
RØ9.A9
R58
R94.3*
S26.ØØXA
S26.Ø1XA
S26.Ø2ØA
S26.Ø21A
S26.Ø22A
S26.Ø9XA
S26.1ØXA
S26.11XA
S26.12XA
S26.19XA
S26.9ØXA
S26.91XA
S26.92XA
S26.99XA
T8Ø.1XXA
T8Ø.211A
T8Ø.212A
T8Ø.218A
T8Ø.219A
T8Ø.81ØA
T8Ø.818A
T8Ø.9ØXA
T82.118A
T82.119A
T82.128A
T82.129A
T82.198A
T82.199A
T82.211A
T82.212A
T82.213A
T82.218A
T82.221A
T82.222A
T82.223A
T82.228A
T82.31ØA
T82.311A
T82.312A
T82.318A
T82.319A
T82.32ØA
T82.321A
T82.322A
T82.328A
T82.329A
T82.33ØA
T82.331A
T82.332A
T82.338A
T82.339A
T82.39ØA
T82.391A
T82.392A
T82.398A
T82.399A
T82.51ØA
T82.511A
T82.512A
T82.513A
T82.514A
T82.515A
T82.518A
T82.519A
T82.52ØA
T82.521A
T82.522A
T82.523A
T82.524A
T82.525A
T82.528A
T82.529A
T82.53ØA
T82.531A
T82.532A
T82.533A
T82.534A
T82.535A
T82.538A
T82.539A
T82.59ØA
T82.591A
T82.592A
T82.593A
T82.594A
T82.595A
T82.598A
T82.599A
T82.6XXA
T82.7XXA
T82.817A
T82.818A
T82.827A
T82.828A
T82.837A
T82.838A
T82.847A
T82.848A
T82.855A
T82.856A
T82.857A

T82.858A
T82.867A
T82.868A
T82.897A
T82.898A
T82.9XXA
T86.2*
T86.3*
Z45.Ø*
Z94.1
Z94.3
Z95.2
Z95.3
Z95.4
Z95.811
Z95.812
Z95.82Ø
Z95.828

DRG 315

Select principal diagnosis listed under DRG 314

DRG 316

Select principal diagnosis listed under DRG 314

MDC 6

DRG 326

Operating Room Procedures

ØØ8Q*
Ø2BP3ZZ
Ø2BQ3ZZ
Ø2BR3ZZ
Ø2BS3ZZ
Ø2BT3ZZ
Ø2BV3ZZ
Ø2BW3ZZ
Ø2BX3ZZ
Ø3BØ3ZZ
Ø3B13ZZ
Ø3B23ZZ
Ø3B33ZZ
Ø3B43ZZ
Ø3L2*
Ø3L3*
Ø3L4*
Ø5L3*
Ø5L4*
Ø5L5*
Ø5L6*
Ø61ØØJ5
Ø61ØØJ6
Ø61ØØJY
Ø61ØØZ5
Ø61ØØZ6
Ø61ØØZY
Ø61Ø4J5
Ø61Ø4J6
Ø61Ø4JY
Ø61Ø4Z5
Ø61Ø4Z6
Ø61Ø4ZY
Ø611ØJ9
Ø611ØJB
Ø611ØJY
Ø611ØZ9
Ø611ØZB
Ø611ØZY
Ø6114J9
Ø6114JB
Ø6114JY
Ø6114Z9
Ø6114ZB
Ø6114ZY
Ø618ØJ9
Ø618ØJB
Ø618ØJY
Ø618ØZ9
Ø618ØZB
Ø618ØZY
Ø6184J4
Ø6184J9
Ø6184JB
Ø6184JY
Ø6184Z9
Ø6184ZB
Ø6184ZY
Ø6L2ØZZ
Ø6L23ZZ
Ø6L24ZZ
Ø6L3ØZZ
Ø95N*
Ø9BNØZZ
Ø9BN3ZZ
Ø9BN4ZZ
Ø9BN7ZZ
Ø9BN8ZZ
Ø9TN*
ØBQTØZZ
ØBQT3ZZ
ØBQT4ZZ
ØBRTØ7Z
ØBRTØJZ
ØBRTØKZ
ØBRT47Z
ØBRT4JZ
ØBRT4KZ
ØBUTØ7Z
ØBUTØJZ
ØBUTØKZ
ØBUT47Z
ØBUT4JZ
ØBUT4KZ
ØC5M*
ØCBMØZZ
ØCBM3ZZ
ØCBM4ZZ
ØCBM7ZZ
ØCBM8ZZ
ØCTM*
ØD11*
ØD12*
ØD13*
ØD15*
ØD16Ø79
ØD16Ø7A
ØD16Ø7B
ØD16Ø7L
ØD16ØJ9
ØD16ØJA
ØD16ØJB
ØD16ØJL
ØD16ØK9
ØD16ØKA
ØD16ØKB
ØD16ØKL
ØD16ØZ9
ØD16ØZA
ØD16ØZB
ØD16ØZL
ØD16479
ØD1647A
ØD1647B
ØD1647L
ØD164J9
ØD164JA
ØD164JB
ØD164JL
ØD164K9
ØD164KA
ØD164KB
ØD164KL
ØD164Z9
ØD164ZA
ØD164ZB
ØD164ZL
ØD16879
ØD1687A
ØD1687B
ØD1687L
ØD168J9
ØD168JA
ØD168JB
ØD168JL
ØD168K9
ØD168KA
ØD168KB
ØD168KL
ØD168Z9
ØD168ZA
ØD168ZB
ØD168ZL
ØD51ØZ3
ØD51ØZZ
ØD513Z3
ØD513ZZ
ØD517ZZ
ØD52ØZ3
ØD52ØZZ
ØD523Z3
ØD523ZZ
ØD527ZZ
ØD53ØZ3
ØD53ØZZ
ØD533Z3
ØD533ZZ
ØD537ZZ
ØD54ØZ3
ØD54ØZZ
ØD543Z3
ØD543ZZ
ØD547ZZ
ØD55ØZ3
ØD55ØZZ
ØD553Z3
ØD553ZZ
ØD557ZZ
ØD56ØZ3
ØD56ØZZ
ØD563Z3
ØD563ZZ
ØD567ZZ
ØD57ØZ3
ØD57ØZZ
ØD573Z3
ØD573ZZ
ØD577ZZ
ØD59ØZ3
ØD59ØZZ
ØD593Z3
ØD593ZZ
ØD597ZZ
ØD71ØDZ
ØD71ØZZ
ØD713DZ
ØD713ZZ
ØD714DZ
ØD714ZZ
ØD72ØDZ
ØD72ØZZ
ØD723DZ
ØD723ZZ
ØD724DZ
ØD724ZZ
ØD73ØDZ
ØD73ØZZ
ØD733DZ
ØD733ZZ
ØD734DZ
ØD734ZZ
ØD74ØDZ
ØD74ØZZ
ØD743DZ
ØD743ZZ
ØD744DZ
ØD744ZZ
ØD75ØDZ
ØD75ØZZ
ØD753DZ
ØD753ZZ
ØD754DZ
ØD754ZZ
ØD76ØDZ
ØD76ØZZ
ØD763DZ
ØD763ZZ
ØD764DZ
ØD764ZZ
ØD77ØDZ
ØD77ØZZ
ØD773DZ
ØD773ZZ
ØD774ZZ
ØD84*
ØD87ØZZ
ØD873ZZ
ØD874ZZ
ØD877ZZ
ØD878ZZ
ØD91ØØZ
ØD91ØZX
ØD91ØZZ
ØD914ØZ
ØD914ZZ
ØD917ØZ
ØD917ZZ
ØD918ØZ
ØD918ZZ
ØD92ØØZ
ØD92ØZX
ØD92ØZZ
ØD924ØZ
ØD924ZZ
ØD927ØZ
ØD927ZZ
ØD928ØZ
ØD928ZZ
ØD93ØØZ
ØD93ØZX
ØD93ØZZ
ØD934ØZ
ØD934ZZ
ØD937ØZ
ØD937ZZ
ØD938ØZ
ØD938ZZ
ØD94ØØZ
ØD94ØZX
ØD94ØZZ
ØD944ØZ
ØD944ZZ
ØD947ØZ
ØD947ZZ
ØD948ØZ
ØD948ZZ
ØD95ØØZ
ØD95ØZX
ØD95ØZZ
ØD954ØZ
ØD954ZZ
ØD957ØZ
ØD957ZZ
ØD958ØZ
ØD958ZZ
ØD96ØØZ
ØD96ØZX
ØD96ØZZ
ØD964ØZ
ØD964ZZ
ØD967ZZ
ØD968ZZ
ØD97ØØZ
ØD97ØZX
ØD97ØZZ
ØD974ØZ
ØD974ZZ
ØD977ZZ
ØD978ZZ
ØD99ØØZ
ØD99ØZZ
ØD994ØZ
ØD994ZZ
ØD997ZZ
ØD998ZZ
ØDB1ØZX
ØDB1ØZZ
ØDB13ZZ
ØDB17ZZ
ØDB2ØZX
ØDB2ØZZ
ØDB23ZZ
ØDB27ZZ
ØDB3ØZX
ØDB3ØZZ
ØDB33ZZ
ØDB37ZZ
ØDB4ØZX
ØDB4ØZZ
ØDB43ZZ
ØDB44ZZ
ØDB47ZZ
ØDB5ØZX
ØDB5ØZZ
ØDB53ZZ
ØDB57ZZ
ØDB6ØZ3
ØDB6ØZX
ØDB6ØZZ
ØDB63Z3
ØDB63ZZ
ØDB64Z3
ØDB64ZX
ØDB64ZZ
ØDB67Z3
ØDB67ZZ
ØDB68Z3
ØDB7ØZX
ØDB7ØZZ
ØDB73ZZ
ØDB77ZZ
ØDB9ØZZ
ØDB93ZZ
ØDC1ØZZ
ØDC13ZZ
ØDC14ZZ
ØDC2ØZZ
ØDC23ZZ
ØDC24ZZ
ØDC3ØZZ
ØDC33ZZ
ØDC34ZZ
ØDC4ØZZ
ØDC43ZZ
ØDC44ZZ
ØDC5ØZZ
ØDC53ZZ
ØDC54ZZ
ØDC6ØZZ
ØDC63ZZ
ØDC64ZZ
ØDC7ØZZ
ØDC73ZZ
ØDC74ZZ
ØDC9ØZZ
ØDC93ZZ
ØDC94ZZ
ØDF5ØZZ
ØDF53ZZ
ØDF54ZZ
ØDF57ZZ
ØDF58ZZ
ØDF6ØZZ
ØDF63ZZ
ØDF64ZZ
ØDF67ZZ
ØDF68ZZ
ØDH5Ø2Z
ØDH5Ø3Z
ØDH5ØYZ
ØDH532Z
ØDH533Z
ØDH542Z
ØDH543Z
ØDH6Ø1Z
ØDH6Ø2Z
ØDH6Ø3Z
ØDH6ØDZ
ØDH6ØYZ
ØDH632Z
ØDH633Z
ØDH63DZ
ØDH641Z
ØDH642Z
ØDH643Z
ØDH64DZ
ØDH9Ø2Z
ØDH9Ø3Z
ØDH932Z
ØDH933Z
ØDH942Z
ØDH943Z
ØDJØ4ZZ
ØDJ64ZZ
ØDL6*
ØDL7*
ØDM5*
ØDM6*
ØDN1*
ØDN2*
ØDN3*
ØDN4*
ØDN5*
ØDN6*
ØDN7*
ØDP5Ø1Z
ØDP5Ø2Z
ØDP5Ø3Z
ØDP5ØUZ
ØDP5ØYZ
ØDP531Z
ØDP532Z
ØDP533Z
ØDP53UZ
ØDP541Z
ØDP542Z
ØDP543Z
ØDP54UZ
ØDP6ØØZ
ØDP6Ø2Z
ØDP6Ø3Z
ØDP6Ø7Z
ØDP6ØCZ
ØDP6ØDZ
ØDP6ØJZ
ØDP6ØKZ
ØDP6ØUZ
ØDP6ØYZ
ØDP63ØZ
ØDP632Z
ØDP633Z
ØDP637Z
ØDP63CZ
ØDP63DZ
ØDP63JZ
ØDP63KZ
ØDP63UZ
ØDP64ØZ
ØDP642Z
ØDP647Z
ØDP64CZ
ØDP64DZ
ØDP64JZ
ØDP64KZ
ØDP64UZ
ØDP677Z
ØDP67CZ
ØDP67JZ
ØDP67KZ
ØDP687Z
ØDP68CZ
ØDP68JZ
ØDP68KZ
ØDQ1*
ØDQ2*
ØDQ3*
ØDQ4*
ØDQ5*
ØDQ6*
ØDQ7*
ØDQ9*
ØDR5*
ØDS5ØZZ
ØDS54ZZ
ØDS57ZZ
ØDS58ZZ
ØDS6ØZZ
ØDS64ZZ
ØDS67ZZ
ØDS68ZZ
ØDT1*
ØDT2*
ØDT3*
ØDT4*
ØDT5*
ØDT6*
ØDT7*
ØDU1*
ØDU2*
ØDU3*
ØDU4*
ØDU5*
ØDU6*
ØDU7*
ØDV1*
ØDV2*
ØDV3*
ØDV4*
ØDV5*
ØDV6ØCZ
ØDV6ØDZ
ØDV6ØZZ
ØDV63CZ
ØDV63DZ
ØDV63ZZ
ØDV64CZ
ØDV64DZ
ØDV64ZZ
ØDV67ZZ
ØDV68ZZ
ØDV7*
ØDWØ4UZ
ØDW57DZ
ØDW58DZ
ØDW6ØØZ
ØDW6Ø2Z
ØDW6Ø3Z
ØDW6Ø7Z
ØDW6ØCZ
ØDW6ØDZ
ØDW6ØJZ
ØDW6ØKZ
ØDW6ØMZ
ØDW6ØUZ
ØDW6ØYZ
ØDW63ØZ
ØDW632Z
ØDW633Z
ØDW637Z
ØDW63CZ
ØDW63DZ
ØDW63JZ
ØDW63KZ
ØDW63MZ
ØDW63UZ
ØDW64ØZ
ØDW642Z
ØDW647Z
ØDW64CZ
ØDW64DZ
ØDW64JZ
ØDW64KZ
ØDW64MZ
ØDW64UZ
ØDW67ØZ
ØDW672Z
ØDW673Z
ØDW677Z
ØDW67CZ
ØDW67DZ
ØDW67JZ
ØDW67KZ
ØDW67UZ
ØDW68ØZ
ØDW682Z
ØDW683Z
ØDW687Z
ØDW68CZ
ØDW68DZ
ØDW68JZ
ØDW68KZ
ØDX6ØZ5
ØDX64Z5
ØDX8ØZ5
ØDX84Z5
ØDXEØZ5
ØDXE4Z5
ØDY6*
ØF8GØZZ
ØF8G3ZZ
ØFCCØZZ
ØFQC*
ØK84*
ØWQ6XZ2
OR
ØDT9ØZZ
AND
ØFTGØZZ
OR

Nonoperating Room Procedures

ØD514Z3
ØD524Z3
ØD534Z3
ØD544Z3
ØD554Z3
ØD564Z3
ØD574Z3
ØD594Z3

DRG 327

Select operating room procedures OR procedure combination OR nonoperationg procedures listed under DRG 326

DRG 328

Select operating room procedures OR procedure combination OR nonoperating room procedures listed under DRG 326

DRG 329

Operating Room Procedures

ØD18Ø74
ØD18Ø78
ØD18Ø7H
ØD18Ø7K
ØD18Ø7L
ØD18Ø7M
ØD18Ø7N
ØD18Ø7P
ØD18Ø7Q
ØD18ØJ4
ØD18ØJ8
ØD18ØJH
ØD18ØJK
ØD18ØJL
ØD18ØJM
ØD18ØJN
ØD18ØJP
ØD18ØJQ
ØD18ØK4
ØD18ØK8
ØD18ØKH
ØD18ØKK
ØD18ØKL
ØD18ØKM
ØD18ØKN
ØD18ØKP
ØD18ØKQ
ØD18ØZ4
ØD18ØZ8
ØD18ØZH
ØD18ØZK
ØD18ØZL
ØD18ØZM
ØD18ØZN
ØD18ØZP
ØD18ØZQ
ØD18474
ØD18478
ØD1847H
ØD1847K
ØD1847L
ØD1847M
ØD1847N
ØD1847P
ØD1847Q
ØD184J4
ØD184J8
ØD184JH
ØD184JK
ØD184JL
ØD184JM
ØD184JN
ØD184JP
ØD184JQ
ØD184K4
ØD184K8
ØD184KH
ØD184KK
ØD184KL
ØD184KM
ØD184KN
ØD184KP
ØD184KQ
ØD184Z4
ØD184Z8
ØD184ZH
ØD184ZK
ØD184ZL
ØD184ZM
ØD184ZN
ØD184ZP
ØD184ZQ
ØD18874
ØD18878
ØD1887H
ØD1887K
ØD1887L
ØD1887M
ØD1887N
ØD1887P
ØD1887Q
ØD188J4
ØD188J8
ØD188JH
ØD188JK
ØD188JL
ØD188JM
ØD188JN
ØD188JP
ØD188JQ
ØD188K4
ØD188K8
ØD188KH
ØD188KK
ØD188KL
ØD188KM
ØD188KN
ØD188KP
ØD188KQ
ØD188Z4
ØD188Z8
ØD188ZH
ØD188ZK
ØD188ZL
ØD188ZM
ØD188ZN
ØD188ZP
ØD188ZQ
ØD19*
ØD1A*
ØD1B*
ØD1EØ74
ØD1EØ7E
ØD1EØ7P
ØD1EØJ4
ØD1EØJE
ØD1EØJP
ØD1EØK4
ØD1EØKE
ØD1EØKP
ØD1EØZ4
ØD1EØZE
ØD1EØZP
ØD1E474
ØD1E47E
ØD1E47P
ØD1E4J4
ØD1E4JE
ØD1E4JP
ØD1E4K4
ØD1E4KE
ØD1E4KP
ØD1E4Z4
ØD1E4ZE
ØD1E4ZP
ØD1E874
ØD1E87E
ØD1E87P
ØD1E8J4
ØD1E8JE
ØD1E8JP
ØD1E8K4
ØD1E8KE
ØD1E8KP
ØD1E8Z4
ØD1E8ZE
ØD1E8ZP
ØD1H*
ØD1K*
ØD1L*
ØD1M*
ØD1N*
ØD78ØZZ
ØD783ZZ
ØD784ZZ
ØD79ØZZ
ØD793ZZ
ØD794ZZ
ØD7AØZZ
ØD7A3ZZ
ØD7A4ZZ
ØD7BØZZ
ØD7B3ZZ
ØD7B4ZZ
ØD7CØZZ
ØD7C3ZZ
ØD7C4ZZ
ØD7EØZZ

ØD7E3ZZ
ØD7E4ZZ
ØD7FØZZ
ØD7F3ZZ
ØD7F4ZZ
ØD7GØZZ
ØD7G3ZZ
ØD7G4ZZ
ØD7HØZZ
ØD7H3ZZ
ØD7H4ZZ
ØD7KØZZ
ØD7K3ZZ
ØD7K4ZZ
ØD7LØZZ
ØD7L3ZZ
ØD7L4ZZ
ØD7MØZZ
ØD7M3ZZ
ØD7M4ZZ
ØD7NØZZ
ØD7N3ZZ
ØD7N4ZZ
ØD7PØDZ
ØD7PØZZ
ØD7P3DZ
ØD7P3ZZ
ØD7P4DZ
ØD7P4ZZ
ØD9PØØZ
ØD9P4ØZ
ØDB8ØZZ
ØDB84ZZ
ØDBAØZZ
ØDBBØZZ
ØDBEØZZ
ØDBE3ZZ
ØDBE4ZZ
ØDBFØZZ
ØDBF3ZZ
ØDBF4ZZ
ØDBGØZZ
ØDBG3ZZ
ØDBG4ZZ
ØDBHØZZ
ØDBH3ZZ
ØDBH4ZZ
ØDBKØZZ
ØDBK3ZZ
ØDBK4ZZ
ØDBLØZZ
ØDBL3ZZ
ØDBL4ZZ
ØDBMØZZ
ØDBM3ZZ
ØDBM4ZZ
ØDBNØZZ
ØDBN3ZZ
ØDBN4ZZ
ØDF8ØZZ
ØDF83ZZ
ØDF84ZZ
ØDF87ZZ
ØDF88ZZ
ØDF9ØZZ
ØDF93ZZ
ØDF94ZZ
ØDF97ZZ
ØDF98ZZ
ØDFAØZZ
ØDFA3ZZ
ØDFA4ZZ
ØDFA7ZZ
ØDFA8ZZ
ØDFBØZZ
ØDFB3ZZ
ØDFB4ZZ
ØDFB7ZZ
ØDFB8ZZ
ØDFEØZZ
ØDFE3ZZ
ØDFE4ZZ
ØDFE7ZZ
ØDFE8ZZ
ØDFFØZZ
ØDFF3ZZ
ØDFF4ZZ
ØDFF7ZZ
ØDFF8ZZ
ØDFGØZZ
ØDFG3ZZ
ØDFG4ZZ
ØDFG7ZZ
ØDFG8ZZ
ØDFHØZZ
ØDFH3ZZ
ØDFH4ZZ
ØDFH7ZZ
ØDFH8ZZ
ØDFKØZZ
ØDFK3ZZ
ØDFK4ZZ
ØDFK7ZZ
ØDFK8ZZ
ØDFLØZZ
ØDFL3ZZ
ØDFL4ZZ
ØDFL7ZZ
ØDFL8ZZ
ØDFMØZZ
ØDFM3ZZ
ØDFM4ZZ
ØDFM7ZZ
ØDFM8ZZ
ØDFNØZZ
ØDFN3ZZ
ØDFN4ZZ
ØDFN7ZZ
ØDFN8ZZ
ØDL8*
ØDL9*
ØDLA*
ØDLB*
ØDLC*
ØDLE*
ØDLF*
ØDLG*
ØDLH*
ØDLK*
ØDLL*
ØDLM*
ØDLN*
ØDM8*
ØDM9*
ØDMA*
ØDMB*
ØDME*
ØDMF*
ØDMG*
ØDMH*
ØDMK*
ØDML*
ØDMM*
ØDMN*
ØDMP*
ØDNC7ZZ
ØDNC8ZZ
ØDQ8*
ØDQA*
ØDQB*
ØDQC*
ØDQE*
ØDQFØZZ
ØDQF3ZZ
ØDQF4ZZ
ØDQF7ZZ
ØDQF8ZZ
ØDQGØZZ
ØDQG3ZZ
ØDQG4ZZ
ØDQG7ZZ
ØDQG8ZZ
ØDQH*
ØDQK*
ØDQLØZZ
ØDQL3ZZ
ØDQL4ZZ
ØDQL7ZZ
ØDQL8ZZ
ØDQMØZZ
ØDQM3ZZ
ØDQM4ZZ
ØDQM7ZZ
ØDQM8ZZ
ØDQN*
ØDQP*
ØDS8ØZZ
ØDS84ZZ
ØDS87ZZ
ØDS88ZZ
ØDSBØZZ
ØDSB4ZZ
ØDSB7ZZ
ØDSB8ZZ
ØDSEØZZ
ØDSE4ZZ
ØDSE7ZZ
ØDSE8ZZ
ØDSHØZZ
ØDSH4ZZ
ØDSH7ZZ
ØDSH8ZZ
ØDSPØZZ
ØDSP4ZZ
ØDSP7ZZ
ØDSP8ZZ
ØDT8*
ØDT9*
ØDTA*
ØDTB*
ØDTC*
ØDTE*
ØDTF*
ØDTG*
ØDTH*
ØDTK*
ØDTL*
ØDTM*
ØDTN*
ØDU8*
ØDU9*
ØDUA*
ØDUB*
ØDUC*
ØDUE*
ØDUF*
ØDUG*
ØDUH*
ØDUK*
ØDUL*
ØDUM*
ØDUN*
ØDV8*
ØDV9*
ØDVA*
ØDVB*
ØDVC*
ØDVE*
ØDVF*
ØDVG*
ØDVH*
ØDVK*
ØDVL*
ØDVM*
ØDVN*
ØDW8*
ØDWE*
ØJQCØZZ
ØJUC*
ØUQGØZZ
ØUQG3ZZ
ØUQG4ZZ

DRG 330

Select operating room procedures listed under DRG 329

DRG 331

Select operating room procedures listed under DRG 329

DRG 332

Operating Room Procedures

ØDBPØZZ
ØDBP4ZZ
ØDHQØLZ
ØDHQ3LZ
ØDHQ4LZ
ØDPQ*
ØDTP*
ØDWQ*

DRG 333

Select operating room procedures listed under DRG 332

DRG 334

Select operating room procedures listed under DRG 332

DRG 335

Operating Room Procedures

ØDN8ØZZ
ØDN83ZZ
ØDN84ZZ
ØDN9ØZZ
ØDN93ZZ
ØDN94ZZ
ØDNAØZZ
ØDNA3ZZ
ØDNA4ZZ
ØDNBØZZ
ØDNB3ZZ
ØDNB4ZZ
ØDNCØZZ
ØDNC3ZZ
ØDNC4ZZ
ØDNEØZZ
ØDNE3ZZ
ØDNE4ZZ
ØDNFØZZ
ØDNF3ZZ
ØDNF4ZZ
ØDNGØZZ
ØDNG3ZZ
ØDNG4ZZ
ØDNHØZZ
ØDNH3ZZ
ØDNH4ZZ
ØDNJØZZ
ØDNJ3ZZ
ØDNJ4ZZ
ØDNKØZZ
ØDNK3ZZ
ØDNK4ZZ
ØDNLØZZ
ØDNL3ZZ
ØDNL4ZZ
ØDNMØZZ
ØDNM3ZZ
ØDNM4ZZ
ØDNNØZZ
ØDNN3ZZ
ØDNN4ZZ
ØDNUØZZ
ØDNU3ZZ
ØDNU4ZZ
ØDNV*
ØDNW*
ØFN*

DRG 336

Select operating room procedures listed under DRG 335

DRG 337

Select operating room procedures listed under DRG 335

DRG 344

Operating Room Procedures

ØD58ØZ3
ØD58ØZZ
ØD583Z3
ØD583ZZ
ØD584Z3
ØD584ZZ
ØD587ZZ
ØD5AØZ3
ØD5AØZZ
ØD5A3Z3
ØD5A3ZZ
ØD5A4Z3
ØD5A4ZZ
ØD5A7ZZ
ØD5BØZ3
ØD5BØZZ
ØD5B3Z3
ØD5B3ZZ
ØD5B4Z3
ØD5B4ZZ
ØD5B7ZZ
ØD5CØZ3
ØD5CØZZ
ØD5C3Z3
ØD5C3ZZ
ØD5C4Z3
ØD5C4ZZ
ØD5C7ZZ
ØD5EØZ3
ØD5EØZZ
ØD5E3Z3
ØD5E3ZZ
ØD5E7ZZ
ØD5FØZ3
ØD5FØZZ
ØD5F3Z3
ØD5F3ZZ
ØD5F7ZZ
ØD5GØZ3
ØD5GØZZ
ØD5G3Z3
ØD5G3ZZ
ØD5G7ZZ
ØD5HØZ3
ØD5HØZZ
ØD5H3Z3
ØD5H3ZZ
ØD5H7ZZ
ØD5KØZ3
ØD5KØZZ
ØD5K3Z3
ØD5K3ZZ
ØD5K7ZZ
ØD5LØZ3
ØD5LØZZ
ØD5L3Z3
ØD5L3ZZ
ØD5L7ZZ
ØD5MØZ3
ØD5MØZZ
ØD5M3Z3
ØD5M3ZZ
ØD5M7ZZ
ØD5NØZ3
ØD5NØZZ
ØD5N3Z3
ØD5N3ZZ
ØD5N7ZZ
ØD98ØØZ
ØD98ØZX
ØD98ØZZ
ØD984ØZ
ØD984ZZ
ØD987ZZ
ØD988ZZ
ØD99ØZX
ØD9AØØZ
ØD9AØZX
ØD9AØZZ
ØD9A4ØZ
ØD9A4ZZ
ØD9A7ZZ
ØD9A8ZZ
ØD9BØØZ
ØD9BØZX
ØD9BØZZ
ØD9B4ØZ
ØD9B4ZZ
ØD9B7ZZ
ØD9B8ZZ
ØD9CØØZ
ØD9CØZX
ØD9CØZZ
ØD9C4ØZ
ØD9C4ZZ
ØD9C7ØZ
ØD9C7ZZ
ØD9C8ØZ
ØD9C8ZZ
ØD9EØØZ
ØD9EØZX
ØD9EØZZ
ØD9E4ØZ
ØD9E4ZZ
ØD9E7ZZ
ØD9E8ZZ
ØD9FØØZ
ØD9FØZX
ØD9FØZZ
ØD9F4ØZ
ØD9F4ZZ
ØD9F7ZZ
ØD9F8ZZ
ØD9GØØZ
ØD9GØZX
ØD9GØZZ
ØD9G4ØZ
ØD9G4ZZ
ØD9G7ZZ
ØD9G8ZZ
ØD9HØØZ
ØD9HØZX
ØD9HØZZ
ØD9H4ØZ
ØD9H4ZZ
ØD9H7ZZ
ØD9H8ZZ
ØD9KØØZ
ØD9KØZX
ØD9KØZZ
ØD9K4ØZ
ØD9K4ZZ
ØD9K7ZZ
ØD9K8ZZ
ØD9LØØZ
ØD9LØZX
ØD9LØZZ
ØD9L4ØZ
ØD9L4ZZ
ØD9L7ZZ
ØD9L8ZZ
ØD9MØØZ
ØD9MØZX
ØD9MØZZ
ØD9M4ØZ
ØD9M4ZZ
ØD9M7ZZ
ØD9M8ZZ
ØD9NØØZ
ØD9NØZX
ØD9NØZZ
ØD9N4ØZ
ØD9N4ZZ
ØD9N7ZZ
ØD9N8ZZ
ØD9PØZX
ØD9PØZZ
ØD9P4ZZ
ØD9P7ZZ
ØD9P8ZZ
ØDB8ØZX
ØDB9ØZX
ØDBAØZX
ØDBBØZX
ØDBCØZX
ØDBEØZX
ØDBFØZX
ØDBGØZX
ØDBHØZX
ØDBKØZX
ØDBLØZX
ØDBMØZX
ØDBNØZX
ØDBPØZX
ØDC8ØZZ
ØDC83ZZ
ØDC84ZZ
ØDCAØZZ
ØDCA3ZZ
ØDCA4ZZ
ØDCBØZZ
ØDCB3ZZ
ØDCB4ZZ
ØDCCØZZ
ØDCC3ZZ
ØDCC4ZZ
ØDCEØZZ
ØDCE3ZZ
ØDCE4ZZ
ØDCFØZZ
ØDCF3ZZ
ØDCF4ZZ
ØDCGØZZ
ØDCG3ZZ
ØDCG4ZZ
ØDCHØZZ
ØDCH3ZZ
ØDCH4ZZ
ØDCKØZZ
ØDCK3ZZ
ØDCK4ZZ
ØDCLØZZ
ØDCL3ZZ
ØDCL4ZZ
ØDCMØZZ
ØDCM3ZZ
ØDCM4ZZ
ØDCNØZZ
ØDCN3ZZ
ØDCN4ZZ
ØDCPØZZ
ØDCP3ZZ
ØDCP4ZZ
ØDH8Ø2Z
ØDH8Ø3Z
ØDH832Z
ØDH833Z
ØDH842Z
ØDH843Z
ØDHAØ2Z
ØDHAØ3Z
ØDHA32Z
ØDHA33Z
ØDHA42Z
ØDHA43Z
ØDHBØ2Z
ØDHBØ3Z
ØDHB32Z
ØDHB33Z
ØDHB42Z
ØDHB43Z
ØDJD4ZZ
ØDPØØØZ
ØDPØØ2Z
ØDPØØ3Z
ØDPØØ7Z
ØDPØØCZ
ØDPØØDZ
ØDPØØJZ
ØDPØØKZ
ØDPØØUZ
ØDPØØYZ
ØDPØ3ØZ
ØDPØ32Z
ØDPØ33Z
ØDPØ37Z
ØDPØ3CZ
ØDPØ3DZ
ØDPØ3JZ
ØDPØ3KZ
ØDPØ3UZ
ØDPØ4ØZ
ØDPØ42Z
ØDPØ43Z
ØDPØ47Z
ØDPØ4CZ
ØDPØ4DZ
ØDPØ4JZ
ØDPØ4KZ
ØDPØ4UZ
ØDPØ77Z
ØDPØ7CZ
ØDPØ7JZ
ØDPØ7KZ
ØDPØ87Z
ØDPØ8CZ
ØDPØ8JZ
ØDPØ8KZ
ØDPDØØZ
ØDPDØ2Z
ØDPDØ3Z
ØDPDØ7Z
ØDPDØCZ
ØDPDØDZ
ØDPDØJZ
ØDPDØKZ
ØDPDØUZ
ØDPDØYZ
ØDPD3ØZ
ØDPD32Z
ØDPD33Z
ØDPD37Z
ØDPD3CZ
ØDPD3DZ
ØDPD3JZ
ØDPD3KZ
ØDPD3UZ
ØDPD4ØZ
ØDPD42Z
ØDPD43Z
ØDPD47Z
ØDPD4CZ
ØDPD4DZ
ØDPD4JZ
ØDPD4KZ
ØDPD4UZ
ØDPD77Z
ØDPD7CZ
ØDPD7JZ
ØDPD7KZ
ØDPD87Z
ØDPD8CZ
ØDPD8JZ
ØDPD8KZ
ØDPPØ1Z
ØDPP31Z
ØDPP41Z
ØDS9ØZZ
ØDS94ZZ
ØDS97ZZ
ØDS98ZZ
ØDSAØZZ
ØDSA4ZZ
ØDSA7ZZ
ØDSA8ZZ
ØDSKØZZ
ØDSK4ZZ
ØDSK7ZZ
ØDSK8ZZ
ØDSLØZZ
ØDSL4ZZ
ØDSL7ZZ
ØDSL8ZZ
ØDSMØZZ
ØDSM4ZZ
ØDSM7ZZ
ØDSM8ZZ
ØDSNØZZ
ØDSN4ZZ
ØDSN7ZZ
ØDSN8ZZ
ØDWØØØZ
ØDWØØ2Z
ØDWØØ3Z
ØDWØØ7Z
ØDWØØCZ
ØDWØØDZ
ØDWØØJZ
ØDWØØKZ
ØDWØØUZ
ØDWØØYZ
ØDWØ3ØZ
ØDWØ32Z
ØDWØ33Z
ØDWØ37Z
ØDWØ3CZ
ØDWØ3DZ
ØDWØ3JZ
ØDWØ3KZ
ØDWØ3UZ
ØDWØ4ØZ
ØDWØ42Z
ØDWØ43Z
ØDWØ47Z
ØDWØ4CZ
ØDWØ4DZ
ØDWØ4JZ
ØDWØ4KZ
ØDWØ7ØZ
ØDWØ72Z
ØDWØ73Z
ØDWØ77Z
ØDWØ7CZ
ØDWØ7DZ
ØDWØ7JZ
ØDWØ7KZ
ØDWØ7UZ
ØDWØ8ØZ
ØDWØ82Z
ØDWØ83Z
ØDWØ87Z
ØDWØ8CZ
ØDWØ8DZ
ØDWØ8JZ
ØDWØ8KZ
ØDWDØØZ
ØDWDØ2Z
ØDWDØ3Z
ØDWDØ7Z
ØDWDØCZ
ØDWDØDZ
ØDWDØJZ
ØDWDØKZ
ØDWDØUZ
ØDWDØYZ
ØDWD3ØZ
ØDWD32Z
ØDWD33Z
ØDWD37Z
ØDWD3CZ
ØDWD3DZ
ØDWD3JZ
ØDWD3KZ
ØDWD3UZ
ØDWD4ØZ
ØDWD42Z
ØDWD43Z
ØDWD47Z
ØDWD4CZ
ØDWD4DZ
ØDWD4JZ
ØDWD4KZ
ØDWD4UZ
ØDWD7ØZ
ØDWD72Z
ØDWD73Z
ØDWD77Z
ØDWD7CZ
ØDWD7DZ
ØDWD7JZ
ØDWD7KZ
ØDWD7UZ
ØDWD8ØZ
ØDWD82Z
ØDWD83Z
ØDWD87Z
ØDWD8CZ
ØDWD8DZ
ØDWD8JZ
ØDWD8KZ
ØTQ6*
ØTQ7*
ØTQB*
ØUQ9*
ØUQMØZZ

OR

ØWQFXZ2

AND

ØDQ8ØZZ
ØDQ9ØZZ
ØDQAØZZ
ØDQBØZZ
ØDQEØZZ
ØDQFØZZ
ØDQGØZZ
ØDQHØZZ
ØDQKØZZ
ØDQLØZZ
ØDQMØZZ
ØDQNØZZ

OR

Nonoperating Room Procedures

ØD5E4Z3
ØD5F4Z3
ØD5G4Z3
ØD5H4Z3
ØD5K4Z3
ØD5L4Z3
ØD5M4Z3
ØD5N4Z3
ØD5PØZ3
ØD5P3Z3
ØD5P4Z3

DRG 345

Select operating room procedures OR procedure combinations OR nonoperating room procedures listed under DRG 344

DRG 346

Select operating room procedures OR procedure combinations OR nonoperating room procedures listed under DRG 344

DRG 347

Operating Room Procedures

Ø65YØZC
Ø65Y3ZC
Ø65Y4ZC
Ø6BYØZC
Ø6BY3ZC
Ø6BY4ZC
Ø6LYØCC
Ø6LYØDC
Ø6LYØZC
Ø6LY3CC
Ø6LY3DC
Ø6LY3ZC
Ø6LY4CC
Ø6LY4DC
Ø6LY4ZC
Ø6LY7CC
Ø6LY7DC
Ø6LY7ZC
Ø6LY8CC
Ø6LY8DC
Ø6LY8ZC
ØD5QØZ3
ØD5QØZZ
ØD5Q3Z3
ØD5Q3ZZ
ØD5Q7ZZ
ØD5QXZZ
ØD5RØZZ
ØD5R3ZZ
ØD7QØDZ
ØD7QØZZ
ØD7Q3DZ
ØD7Q3ZZ
ØD7Q4DZ
ØD7Q4ZZ
ØD8R*
ØD9QØØZ
ØD9QØZZ
ØD9Q4ØZ

ØD9Q4ZZ
ØD9Q7ØZ
ØD9Q7ZZ
ØD9Q8ØZ
ØD9Q8ZZ
ØD9QXØZ
ØD9QXZZ
ØD9RØØZ
ØD9RØZZ
ØD9R4ØZ
ØD9R4ZZ
ØDB83ZZ
ØDB87ZZ
ØDB88ZZ
ØDBA3ZZ
ØDBA4ZZ
ØDBA7ZZ
ØDBA8ZZ
ØDBB3ZZ
ØDBB4ZZ
ØDBB7ZZ
ØDBB8ZZ
ØDBCØZZ
ØDBC3ZZ
ØDBC4ZZ
ØDBC7ZZ
ØDBC8ZZ
ØDBE7ZZ
ØDBF7ZZ
ØDBG7ZZ
ØDBGFZZ
ØDBH7ZZ
ØDBK7ZZ
ØDBL7ZZ
ØDBLFZZ
ØDBM7ZZ
ØDBMFZZ
ØDBN7ZZ
ØDBNFZZ
ØDBP3ZZ
ØDBP7ZZ
ØDBQØZZ
ØDBQ3ZZ
ØDBQ4ZZ
ØDBQ7ZZ
ØDBQXZZ
ØDBRØZZ
ØDBR3ZZ
ØDBR4ZZ
ØDCQØZZ
ØDCQ3ZZ
ØDCQ4ZZ
ØDCR*
ØDFPØZZ
ØDFP3ZZ
ØDFP4ZZ
ØDFP7ZZ
ØDFP8ZZ
ØDFQØZZ
ØDFQ3ZZ
ØDFQ4ZZ
ØDFQ7ZZ
ØDFQ8ZZ
ØDHQØDZ
ØDHQ3DZ
ØDHQ4DZ
ØDHQ7DZ
ØDHQ8DZ
ØDHR*
ØDLP*
ØDLQ*
ØDNP*
ØDNQ*
ØDNR*
ØDQQ*
ØDQR*
ØDRR*
ØDSQØZZ
ØDSQ4ZZ
ØDSQ7ZZ
ØDSQ8ZZ
ØDTQ*
ØDTR*
ØDUP*
ØDUQ*
ØDUR*
ØDVP*
ØDVQ*
ØDWR*
ØW3P7ZZ
ØWQFXZ2

OR

Nonoperating Room Procedure

ØD5Q4Z3

DRG 348

Select operating room procedures OR nonoperating room procedure listed under DRG 347

DRG 349

Select operating room procedures OR nonoperating room procedure listed under DRG 347

DRG 350

Operating Room Procedures

ØYQ5ØZZ
ØYQ53ZZ
ØYQ54ZZ
ØYQ6ØZZ
ØYQ63ZZ
ØYQ64ZZ
ØYQ7ØZZ
ØYQ73ZZ
ØYQ74ZZ
ØYQ8ØZZ
ØYQ83ZZ
ØYQ84ZZ
ØYQAØZZ
ØYQA3ZZ
ØYQA4ZZ
ØYQEØZZ
ØYQE3ZZ
ØYQE4ZZ
ØYU5*
ØYU6*
ØYU7*
ØYU8*
ØYUA*
ØYUE*

DRG 351

Select operating room procedures listed under DRG 350

DRG 352

Select operating room procedures listed under DRG 350

DRG 353

Operating Room Procedures

ØDQU*
ØWMFØZZ
ØWQFØZZ
ØWQF3ZZ
ØWQF4ZZ
ØWQFXZZ
ØWUF*

DRG 354

Select operating room procedures listed under DRG 353

DRG 355

Select operating room procedures listed under DRG 353

DRG 356

Operating Room Procedures

Ø2BWØZZ
Ø2BW4ZZ
Ø2BXØZZ
Ø2BX4ZZ
Ø2CW*
Ø2CXØZZ
Ø2CX3ZZ
Ø2CX4ZZ
Ø2HVØ2Z
Ø2HVØDZ
Ø2HV3DZ
Ø2HV42Z
Ø2HV4DZ
Ø2LV*
Ø2VV*
Ø313ØZD
Ø314ØZD
Ø315ØZD
Ø315ØZT
Ø315ØZV
Ø316ØZD
Ø316ØZT
Ø316ØZV
Ø317ØZD
Ø317ØZV
Ø318ØZD
Ø318ØZV
Ø319ØZF
Ø3193ZF
Ø31AØZF
Ø31A3ZF
Ø31BØZF
Ø31B3ZF
Ø31CØZF
Ø31C3ZF
Ø37334Z
Ø37335Z
Ø37336Z
Ø37337Z
Ø3733D1
Ø3733DZ
Ø3733EZ
Ø3733FZ
Ø3733GZ
Ø3733Z1
Ø3733ZZ
Ø37434Z
Ø37435Z
Ø37436Z
Ø37437Z
Ø3743D1
Ø3743DZ
Ø3743EZ
Ø3743FZ
Ø3743GZ
Ø3743Z1
Ø3743ZZ
Ø37734Z
Ø37735Z
Ø37736Z
Ø37737Z
Ø3773D1
Ø3773DZ
Ø3773EZ
Ø3773FZ
Ø3773GZ
Ø3773Z1
Ø3773ZZ
Ø37834Z
Ø37835Z
Ø37836Z
Ø37837Z
Ø3783D1
Ø3783DZ
Ø3783EZ
Ø3783FZ
Ø3783GZ
Ø3783Z1
Ø3783ZZ
Ø37934Z
Ø37935Z
Ø37936Z
Ø37937Z
Ø3793D1
Ø3793DZ
Ø3793EZ
Ø3793FZ
Ø3793GZ
Ø3793Z1
Ø3793ZZ
Ø37A34Z
Ø37A35Z
Ø37A36Z
Ø37A37Z
Ø37A3D1
Ø37A3DZ
Ø37A3EZ
Ø37A3FZ
Ø37A3GZ
Ø37A3Z1
Ø37A3ZZ
Ø37Y34Z
Ø37Y35Z
Ø37Y36Z
Ø37Y37Z
Ø37Y3DZ
Ø37Y3EZ
Ø37Y3FZ
Ø37Y3GZ
Ø37Y3ZZ
Ø3CY*
Ø3QY*
Ø41ØØJ1
Ø41ØØJ2
Ø41ØØZ1
Ø41ØØZ2
Ø41CØJ3
Ø41CØJ4
Ø41CØJ5
Ø41CØZ3
Ø41CØZ4
Ø41CØZ5
Ø41C4J3
Ø41C4J4
Ø41C4J5
Ø41C4Z3
Ø41C4Z4
Ø41C4Z5
Ø41DØJ3
Ø41DØJ4
Ø41DØJ5
Ø41DØZ3
Ø41DØZ4
Ø41DØZ5
Ø41D4J3
Ø41D4J4
Ø41D4J5
Ø41D4Z3
Ø41D4Z4
Ø41D4Z5
Ø45Ø*
47Ø341
Ø47Ø34Z
Ø47Ø35Z
Ø47Ø36Z
Ø47Ø37Z
Ø47Ø3D1
Ø47Ø3DZ
Ø47Ø3EZ
Ø47Ø3FZ
Ø47Ø3GZ
Ø47Ø3Z1
Ø47Ø3ZZ
471341
Ø47134Z
Ø47135Z
Ø47136Z
Ø47137Z
Ø4713D1
Ø4713DZ
Ø4713EZ
Ø4713FZ
Ø4713GZ
Ø4713Z1
Ø4713ZZ
472341
Ø47234Z
Ø47235Z
Ø47236Z
Ø47237Z
Ø4723D1
Ø4723DZ
Ø4723EZ
Ø4723FZ
Ø4723GZ
Ø4723Z1
Ø4723ZZ
473341
Ø47334Z
Ø47335Z
Ø47336Z
Ø47337Z
Ø4733D1
Ø4733DZ
Ø4733EZ
Ø4733FZ
Ø4733GZ
Ø4733Z1
Ø4733ZZ
474341
Ø47434Z
Ø47435Z
Ø47436Z
Ø47437Z
Ø4743D1
Ø4743DZ
Ø4743EZ
Ø4743FZ
Ø4743GZ
Ø4743Z1
Ø4743ZZ
475341
Ø47534Z
Ø47535Z
Ø47536Z
Ø47537Z
Ø4753D1
Ø4753DZ
Ø4753EZ
Ø4753FZ
Ø4753GZ
Ø4753Z1
Ø4753ZZ
476341
Ø47634Z
Ø47635Z
Ø47636Z
Ø47637Z
Ø4763D1
Ø4763DZ
Ø4763EZ
Ø4763FZ
Ø4763GZ
Ø4763Z1
Ø4763ZZ
477341
Ø47734Z
Ø47735Z
Ø47736Z
Ø47737Z
Ø4773D1
Ø4773DZ
Ø4773EZ
Ø4773FZ
Ø4773GZ
Ø4773Z1
Ø4773ZZ
478341
Ø47834Z
Ø47835Z
Ø47836Z
Ø47837Z
Ø4783D1
Ø4783DZ
Ø4783EZ
Ø4783FZ
Ø4783GZ
Ø4783Z1
Ø4783ZZ
479341
Ø47934Z
Ø47935Z
Ø47936Z
Ø47937Z
Ø4793D1
Ø4793DZ
Ø4793EZ
Ø4793FZ
Ø4793GZ
Ø4793Z1
Ø4793ZZ
Ø47A341
Ø47A34Z
Ø47A35Z
Ø47A36Z
Ø47A37Z
Ø47A3D1
Ø47A3DZ
Ø47A3EZ
Ø47A3FZ
Ø47A3GZ
Ø47A3Z1
Ø47A3ZZ
Ø47B341
Ø47B34Z
Ø47B35Z
Ø47B36Z
Ø47B37Z
Ø47B3D1
Ø47B3DZ
Ø47B3EZ
Ø47B3FZ
Ø47B3GZ
Ø47B3Z1
Ø47B3ZZ
Ø47C341
Ø47C34Z
Ø47C35Z
Ø47C36Z
Ø47C37Z
Ø47C3D1
Ø47C3DZ
Ø47C3EZ
Ø47C3FZ
Ø47C3GZ
Ø47C3Z1
Ø47C3ZZ
Ø47D341
Ø47D34Z
Ø47D35Z
Ø47D36Z
Ø47D37Z
Ø47D3D1
Ø47D3DZ
Ø47D3EZ
Ø47D3FZ
Ø47D3GZ
Ø47D3Z1
Ø47D3ZZ
Ø47E341
Ø47E34Z
Ø47E35Z
Ø47E36Z
Ø47E37Z
Ø47E3D1
Ø47E3DZ
Ø47E3EZ
Ø47E3FZ
Ø47E3GZ
Ø47E3Z1
Ø47E3ZZ
Ø47F341
Ø47F34Z
Ø47F35Z
Ø47F36Z
Ø47F37Z
Ø47F3D1
Ø47F3DZ
Ø47F3EZ
Ø47F3FZ
Ø47F3GZ
Ø47F3Z1
Ø47F3ZZ
Ø47H341
Ø47H34Z
Ø47H35Z
Ø47H36Z
Ø47H37Z
Ø47H3D1
Ø47H3DZ
Ø47H3EZ
Ø47H3FZ
Ø47H3GZ
Ø47H3Z1
Ø47H3ZZ
Ø47J341
Ø47J34Z
Ø47J35Z
Ø47J36Z
Ø47J37Z
Ø47J3D1
Ø47J3DZ
Ø47J3EZ
Ø47J3FZ
Ø47J3GZ
Ø47J3Z1
Ø47J3ZZ
Ø47KØ41
Ø47KØD1
Ø47KØZ1
Ø47K341
Ø47K34Z
Ø47K35Z
Ø47K36Z
Ø47K37Z
Ø47K3D1
Ø47K3DZ
Ø47K3EZ
Ø47K3FZ
Ø47K3GZ
Ø47K3Z1
Ø47K3ZZ
Ø47K441
Ø47K4D1
Ø47K4Z1
Ø47LØ41
Ø47LØD1
Ø47LØZ1
Ø47L341
Ø47L34Z
Ø47L35Z
Ø47L36Z
Ø47L37Z
Ø47L3D1
Ø47L3DZ
Ø47L3EZ
Ø47L3FZ
Ø47L3GZ
Ø47L3Z1
Ø47L3ZZ
Ø47L441
Ø47L4D1
Ø47L4Z1
Ø47MØ41
Ø47MØD1
Ø47MØZ1
Ø47M341
Ø47M3D1
Ø47M3Z1
Ø47M441
Ø47M4D1
Ø47M4Z1
Ø47NØ41
Ø47NØD1
Ø47NØZ1
Ø47N341
Ø47N3D1
Ø47N3Z1
Ø47N441
Ø47N4D1
Ø47N4Z1
Ø47Y341
Ø47Y34Z
Ø47Y35Z
Ø47Y36Z
Ø47Y37Z
Ø47Y3D1
Ø47Y3DZ
Ø47Y3EZ
Ø47Y3FZ
Ø47Y3GZ
Ø47Y3Z1
Ø47Y3ZZ
Ø4BØØZZ
Ø4BØ3ZZ
Ø4BØ4ZZ
Ø4B1ØZZ
Ø4B14ZZ
Ø4B2ØZZ
Ø4B24ZZ
Ø4B3ØZZ
Ø4B34ZZ
Ø4B4ØZZ
Ø4B44ZZ
Ø4B5ØZZ
Ø4B54ZZ
Ø4B6ØZZ
Ø4B64ZZ
Ø4B7ØZZ
Ø4B74ZZ
Ø4B8ØZZ
Ø4B84ZZ
Ø4B9ØZZ
Ø4B94ZZ
Ø4BAØZZ
Ø4BA4ZZ
Ø4BBØZZ
Ø4BB4ZZ
Ø4BCØZZ
Ø4BC4ZZ
Ø4BDØZZ
Ø4BD4ZZ
Ø4BEØZZ
Ø4BE4ZZ
Ø4BFØZZ
Ø4BF4ZZ
Ø4BHØZZ
Ø4BH4ZZ
Ø4BJØZZ
Ø4BJ4ZZ
Ø4CØ*
Ø4C1*
Ø4C2*
Ø4C3*
Ø4C4*
Ø4C5*
Ø4C6*
Ø4C7*
Ø4C8*
Ø4C9*
Ø4CA*
Ø4CB*
Ø4CC*
Ø4CD*
Ø4CE*
Ø4CF*
Ø4CH*
Ø4CJ*
Ø4CY*
Ø4HØØDZ
Ø4HØ3DZ
Ø4HØ4DZ
Ø4LØ*
Ø4L1*
Ø4L2ØCZ
Ø4L2ØDZ
Ø4L2ØZZ
Ø4L23CZ
Ø4L23DZ
Ø4L23ZZ
Ø4L24CZ
Ø4L24DZ
Ø4L24ZZ
Ø4L3*
Ø4L4*
Ø4L5*
Ø4L6*
Ø4L7*
Ø4L8*
Ø4L9*
Ø4LA*
Ø4LB*
Ø4LCØCZ
Ø4LCØZZ
Ø4LC3CZ
Ø4LC3ZZ
Ø4LC4CZ
Ø4LC4ZZ
Ø4LDØCZ
Ø4LDØZZ
Ø4LD3CZ
Ø4LD3ZZ
Ø4LD4CZ
Ø4LD4ZZ
Ø4LEØCZ
Ø4LEØZZ
Ø4LE3CZ
Ø4LE3ZZ
Ø4LE4CZ
Ø4LE4ZZ
Ø4LFØCZ
Ø4LFØZZ
Ø4LF3CZ
Ø4LF3ZZ
Ø4LF4CZ
Ø4LF4ZZ
Ø4LHØCZ
Ø4LHØZZ
Ø4LH3CZ
Ø4LH3ZZ
Ø4LH4CZ
Ø4LH4ZZ
Ø4LJØCZ
Ø4LJØZZ
Ø4LJ3CZ
Ø4LJ3ZZ
Ø4LJ4CZ
Ø4LJ4ZZ
Ø4NØØZZ
Ø4NØ4ZZ
Ø4N1ØZZ
Ø4N14ZZ
Ø4N2ØZZ
Ø4N24ZZ
Ø4N3ØZZ
Ø4N34ZZ
Ø4N4ØZZ
Ø4N44ZZ
Ø4N5ØZZ
Ø4N54ZZ
Ø4N6ØZZ
Ø4N64ZZ
Ø4N7ØZZ
Ø4N74ZZ
Ø4N8ØZZ
Ø4N84ZZ
Ø4N9ØZZ
Ø4N94ZZ
Ø4NAØZZ
Ø4NA4ZZ
Ø4NBØZZ
Ø4NB4ZZ
Ø4NCØZZ
Ø4NC4ZZ
Ø4NDØZZ
Ø4ND4ZZ
Ø4NEØZZ
Ø4NE4ZZ
Ø4NFØZZ
Ø4NF4ZZ
Ø4NHØZZ
Ø4NH4ZZ
Ø4NJØZZ
Ø4NJ4ZZ
Ø4QY*
Ø5793D1
Ø5793DZ
Ø5793Z1
Ø5793ZZ
Ø57A3D1
Ø57A3DZ
Ø57A3Z1
Ø57A3ZZ
Ø57B3D1
Ø57B3DZ
Ø57B3Z1
Ø57B3ZZ
Ø57C3D1
Ø57C3DZ
Ø57C3Z1
Ø57C3ZZ
Ø57D3D1
Ø57D3DZ
Ø57D3Z1
Ø57D3ZZ
Ø57F3D1
Ø57F3DZ
Ø57F3Z1
Ø57F3ZZ
Ø5CY*
Ø5HYØDZ
Ø5HY3DZ
Ø5HY4DZ
Ø5QY*
Ø67Ø3DZ
Ø67Ø3ZZ
Ø6CY*
Ø6HØØDZ
Ø6HØ4DZ
Ø6H1ØDZ
Ø6H13DZ
Ø6H14DZ
Ø6H2ØDZ
Ø6H23DZ
Ø6H24DZ
Ø6H3ØDZ
Ø6H33DZ
Ø6H34DZ
Ø6H4ØDZ
Ø6H43DZ
Ø6H44DZ
Ø6H5ØDZ
Ø6H53DZ
Ø6H54DZ
Ø6H6ØDZ
Ø6H63DZ
Ø6H64DZ
Ø6H7ØDZ
Ø6H73DZ
Ø6H74DZ
Ø6H8ØDZ
Ø6H83DZ
Ø6H84DZ
Ø6HYØDZ
Ø6HY3DZ
Ø6HY4DZ
Ø6LØ*
Ø6L1*
Ø6L2ØCZ
Ø6L2ØDZ
Ø6L23CZ
Ø6L23DZ
Ø6L24CZ
Ø6L24DZ
Ø6L3ØCZ
Ø6L3ØDZ
Ø6L4*
Ø6L5*
Ø6L6*
Ø6L7*
Ø6L8*
Ø6L9*
Ø6LB*
Ø6LCØCZ
Ø6LCØZZ
Ø6LC3CZ
Ø6LC3ZZ
Ø6LC4CZ
Ø6LC4ZZ
Ø6LDØCZ
Ø6LDØZZ
Ø6LD3CZ
Ø6LD3ZZ
Ø6LD4CZ
Ø6LD4ZZ
Ø6LFØCZ
Ø6LFØZZ
Ø6LF3CZ
Ø6LF3ZZ
Ø6LF4CZ
Ø6LF4ZZ
Ø6LGØCZ
Ø6LGØZZ
Ø6LG3CZ
Ø6LG3ZZ
Ø6LG4CZ
Ø6LG4ZZ
Ø6LH*
Ø6LJ*
Ø6NØØZZ
Ø6NØ4ZZ
Ø6N1ØZZ
Ø6N14ZZ
Ø6N2ØZZ

Ø6N24ZZ
Ø6N3ØZZ
Ø6N34ZZ
Ø6N4ØZZ
Ø6N44ZZ
Ø6N5ØZZ
Ø6N54ZZ
Ø6N6ØZZ
Ø6N64ZZ
Ø6N7ØZZ
Ø6N74ZZ
Ø6N8ØZZ
Ø6N84ZZ
Ø6N9ØZZ
Ø6N94ZZ
Ø6NBØZZ
Ø6NB4ZZ
Ø6NCØZZ
Ø6NC4ZZ
Ø6NDØZZ
Ø6ND4ZZ
Ø6NFØZZ
Ø6NF4ZZ
Ø6NGØZZ
Ø6NG4ZZ
Ø6NHØZZ
Ø6NH4ZZ
Ø6NJØZZ
Ø6NJ4ZZ
Ø6QY*
Ø6VØ*
Ø79BØZX
Ø79B3ZX
Ø79B4ZX
Ø79CØZX
Ø79C3ZX
Ø79C4ZX
Ø79DØZX
Ø79D3ZX
Ø79D4ZX
Ø79LØZX
Ø79L3ZX
Ø79L4ZX
Ø7B1ØZZ
Ø7B13ZZ
Ø7B14ZZ
Ø7B2ØZZ
Ø7B23ZZ
Ø7B24ZZ
Ø7B5ØZZ
Ø7B53ZZ
Ø7B54ZZ
Ø7B6ØZZ
Ø7B63ZZ
Ø7B64ZZ
Ø7BB*
Ø7BC*
Ø7BD*
Ø7BHØZZ
Ø7BH3ZZ
Ø7BH4ZZ
Ø7BJØZZ
Ø7BJ3ZZ
Ø7BJ4ZZ
Ø7BLØZX
Ø7BL3ZX
Ø7BL4ZX
Ø7JNØZZ
Ø7JN4ZZ
Ø7JPØZZ
Ø7TØ*
Ø7T3*
Ø7T4*
Ø7T5*
Ø7T6*
Ø7T7*
Ø7T8*
Ø7T9*
Ø7TB*
Ø7TC*
Ø7TD*
Ø7TF*
Ø7TG*
Ø7TH*
Ø7TJ*
Ø7TP*
ØD5UØZZ
ØD5U3ZZ
ØD5U4ZZ
ØD5V*
ØD5W*
ØD9UØØZ
ØD9UØZX
ØD9UØZZ
ØD9U4ZX
ØD9VØØZ
ØD9VØZX
ØD9VØZZ
ØD9V4ZX
ØD9WØØZ
ØD9WØZX
ØD9WØZZ
ØD9W4ØZ
ØD9W4ZX
ØD9W4ZZ
ØDBUØZX
ØDBUØZZ
ØDBU3ZZ
ØDBU4ZZ
ØDBVØZX
ØDBVØZZ
ØDBV3ZZ
ØDBV4ZZ
ØDBWØZX
ØDBWØZZ
ØDBW3ZZ
ØDBW4ZZ
ØDCUØZZ
ØDCU3ZZ
ØDCU4ZZ
ØDCV*
ØDCW*
ØDH5Ø1Z
ØDH531Z
ØDH541Z
ØDH571Z
ØDH581Z
ØDHPØ1Z
ØDHP31Z
ØDHP41Z
ØDHP71Z
ØDHP81Z
ØDJØØZZ
ØDJ6ØZZ
ØDJDØZZ
ØDJUØZZ
ØDJU4ZZ
ØDJVØZZ
ØDJV4ZZ
ØDJWØZZ
ØDJW4ZZ
ØDPU*
ØDPV*
ØDPW*
ØDQV*
ØDQW*
ØDRUØ7Z
ØDRUØJZ
ØDRUØKZ
ØDRU47Z
ØDRU4JZ
ØDRU4KZ
ØDRV*
ØDRW*
ØDTUØZZ
ØDTU4ZZ
ØDUUØ7Z
ØDUUØJZ
ØDUUØKZ
ØDUU47Z
ØDUU4JZ
ØDUU4KZ
ØDUV*
ØDUW*
ØDWUØ7Z
ØDWUØJZ
ØDWUØKZ
ØDWU37Z
ØDWU3JZ
ØDWU3KZ
ØDWU47Z
ØDWU4JZ
ØDWU4KZ
ØDWVØ7Z
ØDWVØJZ
ØDWVØKZ
ØDWV37Z
ØDWV3JZ
ØDWV3KZ
ØDWV47Z
ØDWV4JZ
ØDWV4KZ
ØDWWØ7Z
ØDWWØJZ
ØDWWØKZ
ØDWW37Z
ØDWW3JZ
ØDWW3KZ
ØDWW47Z
ØDWW4JZ
ØDWW4KZ
ØF14ØD3
ØF14ØDB
ØF14ØZ3
ØF14ØZB
ØF144D3
ØF144DB
ØF144Z3
ØF144ZB
ØF15ØD3
ØF15ØD4
ØF15ØDB
ØF15ØZ3
ØF15ØZ4
ØF15ØZB
ØF154D3
ØF154D4
ØF154DB
ØF154Z3
ØF154Z4
ØF154ZB
ØF16ØD3
ØF16ØD4
ØF16ØDB
ØF16ØZ3
ØF16ØZ4
ØF16ØZB
ØF164D3
ØF164D4
ØF164DB
ØF164Z3
ØF164Z4
ØF164ZB
ØF17ØD3
ØF17ØD4
ØF17ØDB
ØF17ØZ3
ØF17ØZ4
ØF17ØZB
ØF174D3
ØF174D4
ØF174DB
ØF174Z3
ØF174Z4
ØF174ZB
ØF18ØD3
ØF18ØDB
ØF18ØZ3
ØF18ØZB
ØF184D3
ØF184DB
ØF184Z3
ØF184ZB
ØF19ØD3
ØF19ØDB
ØF19ØZ3
ØF19ØZB
ØF194D3
ØF194DB
ØF194Z3
ØF194ZB
ØF5Ø*
ØF51*
ØF52*
ØF55ØZ3
ØF55ØZZ
ØF553Z3
ØF553ZZ
ØF557ZZ
ØF56ØZ3
ØF56ØZZ
ØF563Z3
ØF563ZZ
ØF567ZZ
ØF57ØZ3
ØF57ØZZ
ØF573Z3
ØF573ZZ
ØF577ZZ
ØF58ØZ3
ØF58ØZZ
ØF583Z3
ØF583ZZ
ØF587ZZ
ØF59ØZ3
ØF59ØZZ
ØF593Z3
ØF593ZZ
ØF597ZZ
ØF5CØZ3
ØF5CØZZ
ØF5C3Z3
ØF5C3ZZ
ØF5C7ZZ
ØF7CØDZ
ØF7CØZZ
ØF7C3DZ
ØF7C3ZZ
ØF7C4DZ
ØF7C4ZZ
ØF7C7DZ
ØF7C7ZZ
ØF7DØDZ
ØF7DØZZ
ØF7D3DZ
ØF7D3ZZ
ØF7FØDZ
ØF7FØZZ
ØF7F3DZ
ØF7F3ZZ
ØF7F7DZ
ØF9ØØZX
ØF91ØZX
ØF92ØZX
ØF95ØØZ
ØF95ØZX
ØF95ØZZ
ØF954ØZ
ØF954ZZ
ØF957ØZ
ØF957ZZ
ØF96ØØZ
ØF96ØZX
ØF96ØZZ
ØF964ØZ
ØF964ZZ
ØF967ØZ
ØF967ZZ
ØF97ØØZ
ØF97ØZX
ØF97ØZZ
ØF98ØØZ
ØF98ØZX
ØF98ØZZ
ØF984ØZ
ØF984ZZ
ØF987ØZ
ØF987ZZ
ØF99ØZX
ØF9CØZX
ØF9DØZX
ØF9FØZX
ØF9GØZX
ØFBØØZX
ØFBØ4ZX
ØFB1ØZX
ØFB14ZX
ØFB2ØZX
ØFB24ZX
ØFB4ØZX
ØFB5ØZX
ØFB5ØZZ
ØFB53ZZ
ØFB57ZZ
ØFB6ØZX
ØFB6ØZZ
ØFB63ZZ
ØFB67ZZ
ØFB7ØZX
ØFB7ØZZ
ØFB73ZZ
ØFB77ZZ
ØFB8ØZX
ØFB9ØZX
ØFB9ØZZ
ØFB93ZZ
ØFB97ZZ
ØFBCØZX
ØFBCØZZ
ØFBC3ZZ
ØFBC7ZZ
ØFBDØZX
ØFBFØZX
ØFBGØZX
ØFDØ4ZX
ØFD14ZX
ØFD24ZX
ØFHBØDZ
ØFHB3DZ
ØFHB7DZ
ØFHDØDZ
ØFHD3DZ
ØFHD7DZ
ØFJØØZZ
ØFJØ4ZZ
ØFJ4ØZZ
ØFJ44ZZ
ØFJDØZZ
ØFJD4ZZ
ØFJGØZZ
ØFJG4ZZ
ØFLD*
ØFLF*
ØFT4*
ØFT5*
ØFT6*
ØFT7ØZZ
ØFT74ZZ
ØFT77ZZ
ØFT78ZZ
ØFT8*
ØFT9*
ØFTC*
ØFUD37Z
ØFUD47Z
ØFUD87Z
ØHR5X72
ØHR5X73
ØHR5X74
ØHR5XJ3
ØHR5XJ4
ØHR5XJZ
ØHR6X72
ØHR6X73
ØHR6X74
ØHR6XJ3
ØHR6XJ4
ØHR6XJZ
ØHR7X72
ØHR7X73
ØHR7X74
ØHR7XJ3
ØHR7XJ4
ØHR7XJZ
ØHR8X73
ØHR8XJ3
ØHR8XJ4
ØHR8XJZ
ØHXØXZZ
ØHX1XZZ
ØHX4XZZ
ØHX5XZZ
ØHX6XZZ
ØHX7XZZ
ØHX8XZZ
ØHX9XZZ
ØHXAXZZ
ØHXBXZZ
ØHXCXZZ
ØHXDXZZ
ØHXEXZZ
ØHXFXZZ
ØHXGXZZ
ØHXHXZZ
ØHXJXZZ
ØHXKXZZ
ØHXLXZZ
ØHXMXZZ
ØHXNXZZ
ØJBØØZZ
ØJB1ØZZ
ØJB4ØZZ
ØJB5ØZZ
ØJB6ØZZ
ØJB7ØZZ
ØJB8ØZZ
ØJB9ØZZ
ØJBBØZZ
ØJBCØZZ
ØJBDØZZ
ØJBFØZZ
ØJBGØZZ
ØJBHØZZ
ØJBLØZZ
ØJBMØZZ
ØJBNØZZ
ØJBPØZZ
ØJBQØZZ
ØJBRØZZ
ØJHØ*
ØJH1*
ØJH4*
ØJH5*
ØJH6ØNZ
ØJH6ØVZ
ØJH6ØWZ
ØJH6ØYZ
ØJH63NZ
ØJH63VZ
ØJH7ØNZ
ØJH7ØVZ
ØJH7ØYZ
ØJH73NZ
ØJH73VZ
ØJH8ØNZ
ØJH8ØVZ
ØJH8ØWZ
ØJH8ØYZ
ØJH83NZ
ØJH83VZ
ØJHDØVZ
ØJHDØWZ
ØJHD3VZ
ØJHFØVZ
ØJHFØWZ
ØJHF3VZ
ØJHGØVZ
ØJHGØWZ
ØJHG3VZ
ØJHHØVZ
ØJHHØWZ
ØJHH3VZ
ØJHLØVZ
ØJHLØWZ
ØJHL3VZ
ØJHMØVZ
ØJHMØWZ
ØJHM3VZ
ØJHNØVZ
ØJHN3VZ
ØJHPØVZ
ØJHPØWZ
ØJHP3VZ
ØJHTØVZ
ØJHTØYZ
ØJHT3VZ
ØJXØØZB
ØJXØØZC
ØJXØ3ZB
ØJXØ3ZC
ØJX1ØZB
ØJX1ØZC
ØJX13ZB
ØJX13ZC
ØJX4ØZB
ØJX4ØZC
ØJX43ZB
ØJX43ZC
ØJX5ØZB
ØJX5ØZC
ØJX53ZB
ØJX53ZC
ØJX6ØZB
ØJX6ØZC
ØJX63ZB
ØJX63ZC
ØJX7ØZB
ØJX7ØZC
ØJX73ZB
ØJX73ZC
ØJX8ØZB
ØJX8ØZC
ØJX83ZB
ØJX83ZC
ØJX9ØZB
ØJX9ØZC
ØJX93ZB
ØJX93ZC
ØJXBØZB
ØJXBØZC
ØJXB3ZB
ØJXB3ZC
ØJXCØZB
ØJXCØZC
ØJXC3ZB
ØJXC3ZC
ØJXDØZB
ØJXDØZC
ØJXD3ZB
ØJXD3ZC
ØJXFØZB
ØJXFØZC
ØJXF3ZB
ØJXF3ZC
ØJXGØZB
ØJXGØZC
ØJXG3ZB
ØJXG3ZC
ØJXHØZB
ØJXHØZC
ØJXH3ZB
ØJXH3ZC
ØJXLØZB
ØJXLØZC
ØJXL3ZB
ØJXL3ZC
ØJXMØZB
ØJXMØZC
ØJXM3ZB
ØJXM3ZC
ØJXNØZB
ØJXNØZC
ØJXN3ZB
ØJXN3ZC
ØJXPØZB
ØJXPØZC
ØJXP3ZB
ØJXP3ZC
ØJXQØZB
ØJXQØZC
ØJXQ3ZB
ØJXQ3ZC
ØJXRØZB
ØJXRØZC
ØJXR3ZB
ØJXR3ZC
ØW1GØJ4
ØW1GØJ6
ØW1GØJW
ØW1GØJY
ØW1G3J4
ØW1G3J6
ØW1G3JW
ØW1G3JY
ØW1G4J4
ØW1G4J6
ØW1G4JW
ØW1G4JY
ØW3F*
ØW3GØZZ
ØW3G3ZZ
ØW3G4ZZ
ØW3H*
ØW3J*
ØW3PØZZ
ØW3P3ZZ
ØW3P4ZZ
ØW9FØØZ
ØW9FØZX
ØW9FØZZ
ØW9F3ZX
ØW9F4ZX
ØW9GØØZ
ØW9GØZX
ØW9GØZZ
ØW9G4ØZ
ØW9G4ZX
ØW9G4ZZ
ØW9HØØZ
ØW9HØZX
ØW9HØZZ
ØW9H3ZX
ØW9H4ØZ
ØW9H4ZX
ØW9H4ZZ
ØW9JØØZ
ØW9JØZX
ØW9JØZZ
ØW9J4ØZ
ØW9J4ZX
ØW9J4ZZ
ØWBF*
ØWBHØZX
ØWBHØZZ
ØWBH3ZZ
ØWBH4ZZ
ØWCGØZZ
ØWCG3ZZ
ØWCG4ZZ
ØWCHØZZ
ØWCH3ZZ
ØWCH4ZZ
ØWCJØZZ
ØWCJ3ZZ
ØWCJ4ZZ
ØWCPØZZ
ØWCP3ZZ
ØWCP4ZZ
ØWCRØZZ
ØWCR3ZZ
ØWCR4ZZ
ØWFGØZZ
ØWFG3ZZ
ØWFG4ZZ
ØWHF*
ØWHGØ1Z
ØWHGØ3Z
ØWHGØYZ
ØWHG31Z
ØWHG3YZ
ØWHG41Z
ØWHG43Z
ØWHG4YZ
ØWHHØ3Z
ØWHHØYZ
ØWHH33Z
ØWHH3YZ
ØWHH43Z
ØWHH4YZ
ØWHJØ3Z
ØWHJØYZ
ØWHJ33Z
ØWHJ3YZ
ØWHJ43Z
ØWHJ4YZ
ØWHPØ1Z
ØWHPØ3Z
ØWHP31Z
ØWHP41Z
ØWHP71Z
ØWHP81Z
ØWJFØZZ
ØWJF4ZZ
ØWJGØZZ
ØWJG4ZZ
ØWJHØZZ
ØWJH4ZZ
ØWJJØZZ
ØWJJ4ZZ
ØWJPØZZ
ØWJP4ZZ
ØWJRØZZ
ØWJR4ZZ
ØWPFØØZ
ØWPFØ1Z
ØWPFØ3Z
ØWPFØ7Z
ØWPFØJZ
ØWPFØKZ
ØWPFØYZ
ØWPF3ØZ
ØWPF31Z
ØWPF33Z
ØWPF37Z
ØWPF3JZ
ØWPF3KZ
ØWPF3YZ
ØWPF4ØZ
ØWPF41Z
ØWPF43Z
ØWPF47Z
ØWPF4JZ
ØWPF4KZ
ØWPF4YZ
ØWPGØØZ
ØWPGØ1Z
ØWPGØ3Z
ØWPGØJZ
ØWPGØYZ
ØWPG3ØZ
ØWPG31Z
ØWPG33Z
ØWPG3JZ
ØWPG3YZ
ØWPG4ØZ
ØWPG41Z
ØWPG43Z
ØWPG4JZ
ØWPG4YZ
ØWPHØØZ
ØWPHØ1Z
ØWPHØ3Z
ØWPHØYZ
ØWPH3ØZ
ØWPH31Z
ØWPH33Z
ØWPH3YZ
ØWPH4ØZ
ØWPH41Z
ØWPH43Z
ØWPH4YZ
ØWPPØ1Z
ØWPPØ3Z
ØWPPØYZ
ØWWFØØZ
ØWWFØ1Z
ØWWFØ3Z
ØWWFØ7Z
ØWWFØJZ
ØWWFØKZ
ØWWFØYZ
ØWWF3ØZ
ØWWF31Z
ØWWF33Z
ØWWF37Z
ØWWF3JZ
ØWWF3KZ
ØWWF3YZ
ØWWF4ØZ
ØWWF41Z
ØWWF43Z
ØWWF47Z
ØWWF4JZ
ØWWF4KZ
ØWWF4YZ
ØWWGØØZ
ØWWGØ1Z
ØWWGØ3Z
ØWWGØJZ
ØWWGØYZ
ØWWG3ØZ
ØWWG31Z
ØWWG33Z
ØWWG3JZ
ØWWG3YZ
ØWWG4ØZ
ØWWG41Z
ØWWG43Z
ØWWG4JZ
ØWWG4YZ
ØWWHØØZ
ØWWHØ1Z
ØWWHØ3Z
ØWWHØYZ
ØWWH3ØZ
ØWWH31Z
ØWWH33Z
ØWWH3YZ
ØWWH4ØZ
ØWWH41Z
ØWWH43Z
ØWWH4YZ
ØWWJØØZ
ØWWJØ1Z
ØWWJØ3Z
ØWWJØJZ
ØWWJØYZ
ØWWJ3ØZ
ØWWJ31Z
ØWWJ33Z
ØWWJ3JZ
ØWWJ3YZ
ØWWJ4ØZ
ØWWJ41Z
ØWWJ43Z
ØWWJ4JZ
ØWWJ4YZ
ØWWPØ1Z
ØWWPØ3Z
ØWWPØYZ
ØY35*
ØY36*
ØY95ØØZ
ØY95ØZX
ØY95ØZZ
ØY953ZX
ØY954ØZ
ØY954ZX
ØY954ZZ
ØY96ØØZ
ØY96ØZX
ØY96ØZZ
ØY963ZX
ØY964ØZ
ØY964ZX
ØY964ZZ
ØYB5*
ØYB6*
ØYB7*
ØYB8*
ØYJ5ØZZ
ØYJ54ZZ
ØYJ6ØZZ
ØYJ64ZZ
ØYJ7ØZZ
ØYJ74ZZ
ØYJ84ZZ
ØYJAØZZ
ØYJA4ZZ
ØYJE4ZZ
4AØC45Z
4AØC4BZ
X27H385
X27H395
X27H3B5
X27H3C5
X27J385
X27J395
X27J3B5
X27J3C5
X2CP3T7
X2CS3T7
X2CT3T7
X2H13R9
X2KB317

X2KC317
OR
Nonoperating Room Procedures
ØF554Z3
ØF564Z3
ØF574Z3
ØF584Z3
ØF594Z3
ØF5C4Z3

DRG 357
Select operating room procedures OR nonoperating room procedures listed under DRG 356

DRG 358
Select operating room procedures OR nonoperating room procedures listed under DRG 356

DRG 397
Operating Room Procedures
ØD5JØZ3
ØD5JØZZ
ØD5J3Z3
ØD5J3ZZ
ØD5J4Z3
ØD5J4ZZ
ØD5J7ZZ
ØD5J8ZZ
ØD9JØØZ
ØD9JØZX
ØD9JØZZ
ØD9J3ZX
ØD9J4ØZ
ØD9J4ZX
ØD9J4ZZ
ØD9J7ØZ
ØD9J7ZX
ØD9J7ZZ
ØD9J8ØZ
ØD9J8ZX
ØD9J8ZZ
ØDBJØZX
ØDBJØZZ
ØDBJ3ZX
ØDBJ3ZZ
ØDBJ4ZX
ØDBJ4ZZ
ØDBJ7ZX
ØDBJ7ZZ
ØDBJ8ZX
ØDBJ8ZZ
ØDCJØZZ
ØDCJ3ZZ
ØDCJ4ZZ
ØDCJ7ZZ
ØDCJ8ZZ
ØDDJ3ZX
ØDDJ4ZX
ØDDJ8ZX
ØDFJØZZ
ØDFJ3ZZ
ØDFJ4ZZ
ØDFJ7ZZ
ØDFJ8ZZ
ØDNJ7ZZ
ØDNJ8ZZ
ØDQJØZZ
ØDQJ3ZZ
ØDQJ4ZZ
ØDQJ7ZZ
ØDQJ8ZZ
ØDTJØZZ
ØDTJ4ZZ
ØDTJ7ZZ
ØDTJ8ZZ

DRG 398
Select operating room procedures listed under DRG 397

DRG 399
Select operating room procedures listed under DRG 397

DRG 368
Principal Diagnosis
B37.81
I85.Ø*
I85.11
K2Ø.81
K2Ø.91
K21.Ø1
K22.3
K22.6
Q39*
S27.812A
S27.813A
S27.818A
S27.819A
T28.1XXA
T28.6XXA

DRG 369
Select principal diagnosis listed under DRG 368

DRG 370
Select principal diagnosis listed under DRG 368

DRG 371
Principal Diagnosis
AØØ*
AØ2.Ø
AØ3*
AØ4*
AØ5.Ø
AØ5.2
AØ5.3
AØ5.4
AØ5.5
AØ5.8
AØ6.Ø
AØ6.1
AØ6.2
AØ7*
A18.3*
A18.83
A21.3
A22.2
A42.1
A54.85
B69*
B7Ø.1
B71*
B76*
K35.2*
K35.3*
K35.89Ø
K35.891
K63.Ø
K65.Ø
K65.1
K65.2
K65.8
K65.9
K67
K68.12
K68.19
K68.2
K68.3
K68.9

DRG 372
Select principal diagnosis listed under DRG 371

DRG 373
Select principal diagnosis listed under DRG 371

DRG 374
Principal Diagnosis
C15.3
C15.4
C15.5
C15.8
C15.9
C16*
C17*
C18*
C19
C2Ø
C21*
C26.Ø
C26.9
C45.1
C46.4
C48.1
C48.2
C48.8
C49.AØ
C49.A1
C49.A2
C49.A3
C49.A4
C49.A5
C49.A9
C76.2
C78.4
C78.5
C78.6
C78.8*
C7A.Ø1Ø
C7A.Ø11
C7A.Ø12
C7A.Ø19
C7A.Ø2Ø
C7A.Ø21
C7A.Ø22
C7A.Ø23
C7A.Ø24
C7A.Ø25
C7A.Ø26
C7A.Ø29
C7A.Ø92
C7A.Ø94
C7A.Ø95
C7A.Ø96
C7B.Ø4
DØØ.1
DØØ.2
DØ1.Ø
DØ1.1
DØ1.2
DØ1.3
DØ1.4*
DØ1.7
DØ1.9
D37.1
D37.2
D37.3
D37.4
D37.5
D37.8
D37.9
D48.3
D48.4
D49.Ø

DRG 375
Select principal diagnosis listed under DRG 374

DRG 376
Select principal diagnosis listed under DRG 374

DRG 377
Principal Diagnosis
K25.Ø
K25.2
K25.4
K25.6
K26.Ø
K26.2
K26.4
K26.6
K27.Ø
K27.2
K27.4
K27.6
K28.Ø
K28.2
K28.4
K28.6
K29.Ø1
K29.21
K29.31
K29.41
K29.51
K29.61
K29.71
K29.81
K29.91
K31.811
K31.82
K55.21
K57.Ø1
K57.11
K57.13
K57.21
K57.31
K57.33
K57.41
K57.51
K57.53
K57.81
K57.91
K57.93
K62.5
K92.Ø
K92.1
K92.2

DRG 378
Select principal diagnosis listed under DRG 377

DRG 379
Select principal diagnosis listed under DRG 377

DRG 380
Principal Diagnosis
E16.4
K22.1*
K22.7*
K25.1
K25.5
K26.1
K26.5
K27.1
K27.5
K28.1
K28.3
K28.5
K28.7
K28.9
K31.1
K31.5
Q43.Ø

DRG 381
Select principal diagnosis listed under DRG 380

DRG 382
Select principal diagnosis listed under DRG 380

DRG 383
Principal Diagnosis
K25.3
K25.7
K25.9
K26.3
K26.7
K26.9
K27.3
K27.7
K27.9

DRG 384
Select principal diagnosis listed under DRG 383

DRG 385
Principal Diagnosis
K5Ø*
K51*

DRG 386
Select principal diagnosis listed under DRG 385

DRG 387
Select principal diagnosis listed under DRG 385

DRG 388
Principal Diagnosis
K56*
K91.3Ø
K91.31
K91.32

DRG 389
Select principal diagnosis listed under DRG 388

DRG 390
Select principal diagnosis listed under DRG 388

DRG 391
Principal Diagnosis
AØ5.9
AØ8*
AØ9
B37.82
B68*
B7Ø.Ø
B77*
B78.Ø
B78.7
B78.9
B79
B8Ø
B81.Ø
B81.1
B81.2
B81.3
B81.8
B82*
D18.Ø3
E73*
E74.1*
E74.3*
I77.4
K2Ø.Ø
K2Ø.8Ø
K2Ø.9Ø
K21.ØØ
K21.9
K22.Ø
K22.2
K22.4
K22.5
K22.8*
K22.9
K23
K29.ØØ
K29.2Ø
K29.3Ø
K29.4Ø
K29.5Ø
K29.6Ø
K29.7Ø
K29.8Ø
K29.9Ø
K3Ø
K31.Ø
K31.2
K31.3
K31.4
K31.6
K31.819
K31.83
K31.84
K31.89
K31.9
K31.AØ
K31.A11
K31.A12
K31.A13
K31.A14
K31.A15
K31.A19
K31.A21
K31.A22
K31.A29
K44.Ø
K44.9
K52.2*
K52.3
K52.8*
K52.9
K57.ØØ
K57.1Ø
K57.12
K57.2Ø
K57.3Ø
K57.32
K57.4Ø
K57.5Ø
K57.52
K57.8Ø
K57.9Ø
K57.92
K58*
K59.Ø*
K59.1
K59.2
K59.4
K59.8*
K59.9
K9Ø.Ø
K9Ø.1
K9Ø.2
K9Ø.3
K9Ø.4*
K9Ø.821
K9Ø.822
K9Ø.829
K9Ø.83
K9Ø.89
K9Ø.9
K91.Ø
K91.1
K91.2
K92.81
N8Ø.5*
R1Ø*
R11.Ø
R11.1Ø
R11.11
R11.12
R11.14
R11.2
R12
R13*
R14*
R15*
R19.Ø*
R19.1*
R19.2
R19.4
R19.5
R19.7
R19.8
R93.3
R93.5

DRG 392
Select principal diagnosis listed under DRG 391

DRG 393
Principal Diagnosis
A51.1
A54.6
A56.3
BØØ.81
D12*
D13.Ø
D13.1
D13.2
D13.3*
D13.9*
D17.5
D19.1
D2Ø*
D3A.Ø1Ø
D3A.Ø11
D3A.Ø12
D3A.Ø19
D3A.Ø2Ø
D3A.Ø21
D3A.Ø22
D3A.Ø23
D3A.Ø24
D3A.Ø25
D3A.Ø26
D3A.Ø29
D3A.Ø92
D3A.Ø94
D3A.Ø95
D3A.Ø96
E84.19
I85.1Ø
I88.Ø
K31.7
K35.8Ø
K36
K37
K38*
K4Ø*
K41*
K42*
K43*
K44.1
K45*
K46*
K52.Ø
K52.1
K55.Ø*
K55.1
K55.2Ø
K55.3*
K55.8
K55.9
K59.3*
K6Ø*
K61.Ø
K61.1
K61.2
K61.31
K61.39
K61.4
K61.5
K62.Ø
K62.1
K62.2
K62.3
K62.4
K62.6
K62.7
K62.8*
K62.9
K63.1
K63.2
K63.3
K63.4
K63.5
K63.8*
K63.9
K64*
K65.3
K65.4
K66*
K9Ø.81
K91.81
K91.82
K91.83
K91.85Ø
K91.858
K91.86
K91.89
K92.89
K92.9
K94*
K95*
N82.2
N82.3
N82.4
N99.4
Q38.5
Q4Ø*
Q41*
Q42*
Q43.1
Q43.2
Q43.3
Q43.4
Q43.5
Q43.6
Q43.7
Q43.8
Q43.9
Q45.8
Q45.9
Q79.2
Q79.3
Q79.4
Q79.5*
Q89.3
Q89.4
R11.13
R11.15
R19.3*
R85.61*
R85.81
R85.82
S31.6ØØA
S31.6Ø1A
S31.6Ø2A
S31.6Ø3A
S31.6Ø4A
S31.6Ø5A
S31.6Ø9A
S31.61ØA
S31.611A
S31.612A
S31.613A
S31.614A
S31.615A
S31.619A
S31.62ØA
S31.621A
S31.622A
S31.623A
S31.624A
S31.625A
S31.629A
S31.63ØA
S31.631A
S31.632A
S31.633A
S31.634A
S31.635A
S31.639A
S31.64ØA
S31.641A
S31.642A
S31.643A
S31.644A
S31.645A
S31.649A
S31.65ØA
S31.651A
S31.652A
S31.653A
S31.654A
S31.655A
S31.659A
S36.ØØXS
S36.Ø2ØS
S36.Ø21S
S36.Ø29S
S36.Ø3ØS
S36.Ø31S
S36.Ø32S
S36.Ø39S
S36.Ø9XS
S36.112S
S36.113S
S36.114S
S36.115S
S36.116S
S36.118S
S36.119S
S36.122S
S36.123S
S36.128S
S36.129S
S36.13XS
S36.2ØØS
S36.2Ø1S
S36.2Ø2S
S36.2Ø9S
S36.22ØS
S36.221S
S36.222S
S36.229S
S36.23ØS
S36.231S
S36.232S
S36.239S
S36.24ØS
S36.241S
S36.242S
S36.249S
S36.25ØS
S36.251S
S36.252S
S36.259S
S36.26ØS
S36.261S
S36.262S
S36.269S
S36.29ØS
S36.291S
S36.292S
S36.299S
S36.3ØXA
S36.3ØXS
S36.32XA
S36.32XS
S36.33XA
S36.33XS
S36.39XA
S36.39XS
S36.4ØØA
S36.4ØØS
S36.4Ø8A
S36.4Ø8S
S36.4Ø9A
S36.4Ø9S
S36.41ØA
S36.41ØS
S36.418A
S36.418S
S36.419A
S36.419S
S36.42ØA
S36.42ØS
S36.428A
S36.428S
S36.429A
S36.429S
S36.43ØA
S36.43ØS
S36.438A
S36.438S
S36.439A
S36.439S
S36.49ØA
S36.49ØS
S36.498A
S36.498S
S36.499A
S36.499S
S36.5ØØA
S36.5ØØS
S36.5Ø1A
S36.5Ø1S
S36.5Ø2A
S36.5Ø2S
S36.5Ø3A
S36.5Ø3S
S36.5Ø8A
S36.5Ø8S
S36.5Ø9A
S36.5Ø9S
S36.51ØA
S36.51ØS
S36.511A
S36.511S
S36.512A
S36.512S
S36.513A
S36.513S
S36.518A
S36.518S
S36.519A
S36.519S
S36.52ØA
S36.52ØS
S36.521A
S36.521S
S36.522A
S36.522S
S36.523A
S36.523S
S36.528A
S36.528S
S36.529A
S36.529S
S36.53ØA
S36.53ØS
S36.531A
S36.531S
S36.532A
S36.532S
S36.533A
S36.533S
S36.538A
S36.538S
S36.539A
S36.539S
S36.59ØA
S36.59ØS
S36.591A
S36.591S
S36.592A
S36.592S
S36.593A
S36.593S
S36.598A
S36.598S
S36.599A
S36.599S
S36.6ØXA
S36.6ØXS
S36.61XA
S36.61XS
S36.62XA
S36.62XS
S36.63XA
S36.63XS
S36.69XA
S36.69XS
S36.81XA
S36.81XS
S36.892S
S36.893S
S36.898S

S36.899S
S36.9ØXA
S36.9ØXS
S36.92XA
S36.92XS
S36.93XA
S36.93XS
S36.99XA
S36.99XS
S37.ØØ1S
S37.ØØ2S
S37.ØØ9S
S37.Ø11S
S37.Ø12S
S37.Ø19S
S37.Ø21S
S37.Ø22S
S37.Ø29S
S37.Ø31S
S37.Ø32S
S37.Ø39S
S37.Ø41S
S37.Ø42S
S37.Ø49S
S37.Ø51S
S37.Ø52S
S37.Ø59S
S37.Ø61S
S37.Ø62S
S37.Ø69S
S37.Ø91S
S37.Ø92S
S37.Ø99S
T18.1ØØA
T18.1Ø8A
T18.11ØA
T18.118A
T18.12ØA
T18.128A
T18.19ØA
T18.198A
T18.2XXA
T18.3XXA
T18.4XXA
T18.5XXA
T18.8XXA
T18.9XXA
T28.2XXA
T28.7XXA
T81.71ØA
Z43.1
Z43.2
Z43.3
Z43.4
Z46.51
Z46.59

DRG 394

Select principal diagnosis listed under DRG 393

DRG 395

Select principal diagnosis listed under DRG 393

MDC 7

DRG 405

Operating Room Procedures

Ø61ØØJ5
Ø61ØØJ6
Ø61ØØJY
Ø61ØØZ5
Ø61ØØZ6
Ø61ØØZY
Ø61Ø4J5
Ø61Ø4J6
Ø61Ø4JY
Ø61Ø4Z5
Ø61Ø4Z6
Ø61Ø4ZY
Ø611ØJ9
Ø611ØJB
Ø611ØJY
Ø611ØZ9
Ø611ØZB
Ø611ØZY
Ø6114J9
Ø6114JB
Ø6114JY
Ø6114Z9
Ø6114ZB
Ø6114ZY
Ø618ØJ9
Ø618ØJB
Ø618ØJY
Ø618ØZ9
Ø618ØZB
Ø618ØZY
Ø6183J4
Ø6183JY
Ø6184J4
Ø6184J9
Ø6184JB
Ø6184JY
Ø6184Z9
Ø6184ZB
Ø6184ZY
ØF1D*
ØF1F*
ØF1G*
ØF5Ø*
ØF51*
ØF52*
ØF5DØZ3
ØF5DØZZ
ØF5D3Z3
ØF5D3ZZ
ØF5D7ZZ
ØF5FØZ3
ØF5FØZZ
ØF5F3Z3
ØF5F3ZZ
ØF5F7ZZ
ØF5GØZ3
ØF5GØZF
ØF5GØZZ
ØF5G3Z3
ØF5G3ZF
ØF5G3ZZ
ØF7DØDZ
ØF7DØZZ
ØF7D3DZ
ØF7D3ZZ
ØF7D7ZZ
ØF7FØDZ
ØF7FØZZ
ØF7F3DZ
ØF7F3ZZ
ØF7F7DZ
ØF7F7ZZ
ØF8ØØZZ
ØF8Ø4ZZ
ØF81ØZZ
ØF814ZZ
ØF82ØZZ
ØF824ZZ
ØF8GØZZ
ØF8G3ZZ
ØF8G4ZZ
ØF9ØØØZ
ØF9ØØZZ
ØF91ØØZ
ØF91ØZZ
ØF92ØØZ
ØF92ØZZ
ØF997ØZ
ØF9DØØZ
ØF9DØZZ
ØF9D4ØZ
ØF9D4ZZ
ØF9D7ØZ
ØF9D7ZZ
ØF9FØØZ
ØF9FØZZ
ØF9F4ØZ
ØF9F4ZZ
ØF9F7ØZ
ØF9F7ZZ
ØF9GØØZ
ØF9GØZZ
ØF9G4ØZ
ØF9G4ZZ
ØFBØØZZ
ØFBØ3ZZ
ØFBØ4ZZ
ØFB1ØZZ
ØFB13ZZ
ØFB14ZZ
ØFB2ØZZ
ØFB23ZZ
ØFB24ZZ
ØFBDØZZ
ØFBD3ZZ
ØFBD7ZZ
ØFBFØZZ
ØFBF3ZZ
ØFBF7ZZ
ØFBGØZZ
ØFBG3ZZ
ØFBG4ZZ
ØFBG8ZZ
ØFCØ*
ØFC1*
ØFC2*
ØFCCØZZ
ØFCDØZZ
ØFCD7ZZ
ØFCFØZZ
ØFCF7ZZ
ØFCG*
ØFFDØZZ
ØFFD3ZZ
ØFFD4ZZ
ØFFD7ZZ
ØFFFØZZ
ØFFF3ZZ
ØFFF4ZZ
ØFFF7ZZ
ØFHØØ1Z
ØFHØØ2Z
ØFHØØYZ
ØFHØ32Z
ØFHØ41Z
ØFHØ42Z
ØFH1Ø2Z
ØFH132Z
ØFH142Z
ØFH2Ø2Z
ØFH232Z
ØFH242Z
ØFHDØ2Z
ØFHDØDZ
ØFHDØYZ
ØFHD32Z
ØFHD3DZ
ØFHD42Z
ØFHD7DZ
ØFHGØ1Z
ØFHGØ2Z
ØFHGØYZ
ØFHG32Z
ØFHG41Z
ØFHG42Z
ØFLD*
ØFLF*
ØFMØ*
ØFM1*
ØFM2*
ØFMD*
ØFMF*
ØFMG*
ØFPØØØZ
ØFPØØ2Z
ØFPØØ3Z
ØFPØØYZ
ØFPØ3ØZ
ØFPØ32Z
ØFPØ33Z
ØFPØ4ØZ
ØFPØ42Z
ØFPØ43Z
ØFPDØØZ
ØFPDØ1Z
ØFPDØ2Z
ØFPDØ3Z
ØFPDØ7Z
ØFPDØCZ
ØFPDØDZ
ØFPDØJZ
ØFPDØKZ
ØFPDØYZ
ØFPD3ØZ
ØFPD31Z
ØFPD32Z
ØFPD33Z
ØFPD37Z
ØFPD3CZ
ØFPD3DZ
ØFPD3JZ
ØFPD3KZ
ØFPD4ØZ
ØFPD41Z
ØFPD42Z
ØFPD43Z
ØFPD47Z
ØFPD4CZ
ØFPD4DZ
ØFPD4JZ
ØFPD4KZ
ØFPD71Z
ØFPD77Z
ØFPD7CZ
ØFPD7JZ
ØFPD7KZ
ØFPD81Z
ØFPD87Z
ØFPD8CZ
ØFPD8JZ
ØFPD8KZ
ØFPGØØZ
ØFPGØ2Z
ØFPGØ3Z
ØFPGØDZ
ØFPGØYZ
ØFPG32Z
ØFPG33Z
ØFPG3DZ
ØFPG4ØZ
ØFPG42Z
ØFPG43Z
ØFPG4DZ
ØFPGXDZ
ØFQØ*
ØFQ1*
ØFQ2*
ØFQC*
ØFQD*
ØFQF*
ØFQG*
ØFRD*
ØFRF*
ØFSØ*
ØFSD*
ØFSF*
ØFSG*
ØFTØ*
ØFT1*
ØFT2*
ØFTDØZZ
ØFTD7ZZ
ØFTFØZZ
ØFTF7ZZ
ØFTG*
ØFUD*
ØFUF*
ØFVD*
ØFVF*
ØFWØØØZ
ØFWØØ2Z
ØFWØØ3Z
ØFWØØYZ
ØFWØ3ØZ
ØFWØ32Z
ØFWØ33Z
ØFWØ4ØZ
ØFWØ42Z
ØFWØ43Z
ØFWDØØZ
ØFWDØ2Z
ØFWDØ3Z
ØFWDØ7Z
ØFWDØCZ
ØFWDØDZ
ØFWDØJZ
ØFWDØKZ
ØFWDØYZ
ØFWD3ØZ
ØFWD32Z
ØFWD33Z
ØFWD37Z
ØFWD3CZ
ØFWD3DZ
ØFWD3JZ
ØFWD3KZ
ØFWD4ØZ
ØFWD42Z
ØFWD43Z
ØFWD47Z
ØFWD4CZ
ØFWD4DZ
ØFWD4JZ
ØFWD4KZ
ØFWD7ØZ
ØFWD72Z
ØFWD73Z
ØFWD77Z
ØFWD7CZ
ØFWD7DZ
ØFWD7JZ
ØFWD7KZ
ØFWD83Z
ØFWD87Z
ØFWD8CZ
ØFWD8JZ
ØFWD8KZ
ØFWGØØZ
ØFWGØ2Z
ØFWGØ3Z
ØFWGØDZ
ØFWGØYZ
ØFWG3ØZ
ØFWG32Z
ØFWG33Z
ØFWG3DZ
ØFWG4ØZ
ØFWG42Z
ØFWG43Z
ØFWG4DZ
ØFYG*
ØW1GØJW
ØW1GØJY
ØW1G3JW
ØW1G3JY
ØW1G4JW
ØW1G4JY

OR

Nonoperating Room Procedures

ØF5D4Z3
ØF5F4Z3
ØF5G4Z3
XF5ØXØ8
XF51XØ8
XF52XØ8

DRG 406

Select operating room procedures OR nonoperating room procedures listed under DRG 405

DRG 407

Select operating room procedures OR nonoperating room procedures listed under DRG 405

DRG 408

Operating Room Procedures

ØF14*
ØF15*
ØF16*
ØF17ØD3
ØF17ØD4
ØF17ØD5
ØF17ØD6
ØF17ØD7
ØF17ØD8
ØF17ØD9
ØF17ØDB
ØF17ØZ3
ØF17ØZ4
ØF17ØZ5
ØF17ØZ6
ØF17ØZ7
ØF17ØZ8
ØF17ØZ9
ØF17ØZB
ØF174D3
ØF174D4
ØF174D5
ØF174D6
ØF174D7
ØF174D8
ØF174D9
ØF174DB
ØF174Z3
ØF174Z4
ØF174Z5
ØF174Z6
ØF174Z7
ØF174Z8
ØF174Z9
ØF174ZB
ØF18*
ØF19*
ØF55ØZ3
ØF55ØZZ
ØF553Z3
ØF553ZZ
ØF557ZZ
ØF56ØZ3
ØF56ØZZ
ØF563Z3
ØF563ZZ
ØF567ZZ
ØF57ØZ3
ØF57ØZZ
ØF573Z3
ØF573ZZ
ØF577ZZ
ØF58ØZ3
ØF58ØZZ
ØF583Z3
ØF583ZZ
ØF587ZZ
ØF59ØZ3
ØF59ØZZ
ØF593Z3
ØF593ZZ
ØF597ZZ
ØF5CØZ3
ØF5CØZZ
ØF5C3Z3
ØF5C3ZZ
ØF5C7ZZ
ØF75ØDZ
ØF75ØZZ
ØF757ZZ
ØF76ØDZ
ØF76ØZZ
ØF767ZZ
ØF77ØDZ
ØF77ØZZ
ØF777ZZ
ØF78ØDZ
ØF78ØZZ
ØF787ZZ
ØF79ØDZ
ØF79ØZZ
ØF797ZZ
ØF7CØDZ
ØF7CØZZ
ØF7C3DZ
ØF7C3ZZ
ØF7C4DZ
ØF7C4ZZ
ØF7C7DZ
ØF7C7ZZ
ØF94ØØZ
ØF94ØZZ
ØF944ØZ
ØF944ZZ
ØF95ØØZ
ØF95ØZZ
ØF954ØZ
ØF954ZZ
ØF957ØZ
ØF957ZZ
ØF96ØØZ
ØF96ØZZ
ØF964ØZ
ØF964ZZ
ØF967ØZ
ØF967ZZ
ØF97ØØZ
ØF97ØZZ
ØF98ØØZ
ØF98ØZZ
ØF984ØZ
ØF984ZZ
ØF987ØZ
ØF987ZZ
ØF9CØØZ
ØF9CØZZ
ØF9C7ØZ
ØF9C7ZZ
ØFB5ØZZ
ØFB53ZZ
ØFB57ZZ
ØFB6ØZZ
ØFB63ZZ
ØFB67ZZ
ØFB7ØZZ
ØFB73ZZ
ØFB77ZZ
ØFB8ØZZ
ØFB83ZZ
ØFB87ZZ
ØFB9ØZZ
ØFB93ZZ
ØFB97ZZ
ØFBCØZZ
ØFBC3ZZ
ØFBC7ZZ
ØFC4*
ØFC5ØZZ
ØFC6ØZZ
ØFC7ØZZ
ØFC8ØZZ
ØFCC3ZZ
ØFCC7ZZ
ØFF4ØZZ
ØFF43ZZ
ØFF44ZZ
ØFF47ZZ
ØFF5ØZZ
ØFF53ZZ
ØFF54ZZ
ØFF57ZZ
ØFF6ØZZ
ØFF63ZZ
ØFF64ZZ
ØFF67ZZ
ØFF7ØZZ
ØFF73ZZ
ØFF74ZZ
ØFF77ZZ
ØFF8ØZZ
ØFF83ZZ
ØFF84ZZ
ØFF87ZZ
ØFF9ØZZ
ØFF93ZZ
ØFF94ZZ
ØFF97ZZ
ØFFCØZZ
ØFFC3ZZ
ØFFC4ZZ
ØFFC7ZZ
ØFH4Ø1Z
ØFH4Ø2Z
ØFH4ØYZ
ØFH432Z
ØFH441Z
ØFH442Z
ØFHBØ2Z
ØFHBØDZ
ØFHBØYZ
ØFHB32Z
ØFHB3DZ
ØFHB42Z
ØFHB7DZ
ØFL5ØCZ
ØFL5ØDZ
ØFL5ØZZ
ØFL6ØCZ
ØFL6ØDZ
ØFL6ØZZ
ØFL7ØCZ
ØFL7ØDZ
ØFL7ØZZ
ØFL8ØCZ
ØFL8ØDZ
ØFL8ØZZ
ØFL9ØCZ
ØFL9ØDZ
ØFL9ØZZ
ØFLC*
ØFM4ØZZ
ØFM5ØZZ
ØFM6ØZZ
ØFM7ØZZ
ØFM8ØZZ
ØFM9ØZZ
ØFMC*
ØFP4ØØZ
ØFP4Ø2Z
ØFP4Ø3Z
ØFP4ØDZ
ØFP4ØYZ
ØFP43ØZ
ØFP432Z
ØFP433Z
ØFP43DZ
ØFP44ØZ
ØFP442Z
ØFP443Z
ØFP44DZ
ØFPBØØZ
ØFPBØ1Z
ØFPBØ2Z
ØFPBØ3Z
ØFPBØ7Z
ØFPBØCZ
ØFPBØDZ
ØFPBØJZ
ØFPBØKZ
ØFPBØYZ
ØFPB3ØZ
ØFPB31Z
ØFPB32Z
ØFPB33Z
ØFPB37Z
ØFPB3CZ
ØFPB3DZ
ØFPB3JZ
ØFPB3KZ
ØFPB4ØZ
ØFPB41Z
ØFPB42Z
ØFPB43Z
ØFPB47Z
ØFPB4CZ
ØFPB4DZ
ØFPB4JZ
ØFPB4KZ
ØFPB71Z
ØFPB77Z
ØFPB7CZ
ØFPB7JZ
ØFPB7KZ
ØFPB81Z
ØFPB87Z
ØFPB8CZ
ØFPB8JZ
ØFPB8KZ
ØFQ4*
ØFQ5*
ØFQ6*
ØFQ7ØZZ
ØFQ73ZZ
ØFQ74ZZ
ØFQ77ZZ
ØFQ78ZZ
ØFQ8*
ØFQ9*
ØFR5*
ØFR6*
ØFR7Ø7Z
ØFR7ØJZ
ØFR7ØKZ
ØFR747Z
ØFR74JZ
ØFR74KZ
ØFR787Z
ØFR78JZ
ØFR78KZ
ØFR8*
ØFR9*
ØFRC*
ØFS4*
ØFS5*
ØFS6*
ØFS7ØZZ
ØFS74ZZ
ØFS8*
ØFS9*
ØFSC*
ØFT5*
ØFT6*
ØFT7ØZZ
ØFT74ZZ
ØFT77ZZ
ØFT78ZZ
ØFT8*
ØFT9*
ØFTC*
ØFU5*
ØFU6*
ØFU7Ø7Z
ØFU7ØJZ
ØFU7ØKZ
ØFU737Z
ØFU73JZ
ØFU73KZ
ØFU747Z
ØFU74JZ
ØFU74KZ
ØFU787Z
ØFU78JZ
ØFU78KZ
ØFU8*
ØFU9*
ØFUC*
ØFV5ØCZ
ØFV5ØDZ
ØFV5ØZZ
ØFV6ØCZ
ØFV6ØDZ
ØFV6ØZZ
ØFV7ØCZ
ØFV7ØDZ
ØFV7ØZZ
ØFV8ØCZ
ØFV8ØDZ
ØFV8ØZZ
ØFV9ØCZ
ØFV9ØDZ
ØFV9ØZZ
ØFVC*
ØFW4ØØZ
ØFW4Ø2Z
ØFW4Ø3Z
ØFW4ØDZ
ØFW4ØYZ
ØFW43ØZ
ØFW432Z
ØFW433Z
ØFW43DZ
ØFW44ØZ
ØFW442Z
ØFW443Z
ØFW44DZ
ØFWBØØZ
ØFWBØ2Z
ØFWBØ3Z
ØFWBØ7Z
ØFWBØCZ
ØFWBØDZ
ØFWBØJZ
ØFWBØKZ
ØFWBØYZ
ØFWB3ØZ
ØFWB32Z
ØFWB33Z
ØFWB37Z
ØFWB3CZ
ØFWB3DZ
ØFWB3JZ
ØFWB3KZ
ØFWB4ØZ
ØFWB42Z
ØFWB43Z
ØFWB47Z
ØFWB4CZ
ØFWB4DZ
ØFWB4JZ
ØFWB4KZ
ØFWB7ØZ
ØFWB72Z
ØFWB73Z
ØFWB77Z
ØFWB7CZ
ØFWB7DZ
ØFWB7JZ
ØFWB7KZ
ØFWB83Z
ØFWB87Z
ØFWB8CZ
ØFWB8JZ
ØFWB8KZ

OR

Nonoperating Room Procedures

ØF554Z3
ØF564Z3
ØF574Z3

OR
C.D.E. Operating Room Procedures
ØF99ØØZ
ØF99ØZZ
ØF994ØZ
ØFC9ØZZ
ØFC94ZZ
ØFJBØZZ
ØFJB4ZZ
Without Cholecystectomy ONLY Operating Room Procedures
ØF54*
ØFB4ØZZ
ØFB43ZZ
ØFB44ZZ
ØFB48ZZ
ØFT4*

DRG 409
Select operating room procedures EXCEPT choleystectomy only operating room procedures OR select nonoperating room procedures listed under DRG 408

DRG 410
Select operating room procedures EXCEPT choleystectomy only operating room procedures OR select nonoperating room procedures listed under DRG 408

DRG 411
Operating Room Procedures
ØF54*
ØFB4ØZZ
ØFB43ZZ
ØFB44ZZ
ØFB48ZZ
ØFT4*
AND
ØF99ØØZ
ØF99ØZZ
ØF994ØZ
ØFC9ØZZ
ØFC94ZZ
ØFJBØZZ
ØFJB4ZZ

DRG 412
Select operating room procedure combinations listed under DRG 411

DRG 413
Select operating room procedure combinations listed under DRG 411

DRG 414
Operating Room Procedures
ØF54ØZ3
ØF54ØZZ
ØF543Z3
ØF543ZZ
ØFB4ØZZ
ØFB43ZZ
ØFT4ØZZ

DRG 415
Select operating room procedures listed under DRG 414

DRG 416
Select operating room procedures listed under DRG 414

DRG 417
Operating Room Procedures
ØF544Z3
ØF544ZZ
ØF548ZZ
ØFB44ZZ
ØFB48ZZ
ØFT44ZZ

DRG 418
Select operating room procedures listed under DRG 417

DRG 419
Select operating room procedures listed under DRG 417

DRG 420
Operating Room Procedures
Ø7JPØZZ
ØD9UØZX
ØD9U4ZX
ØD9VØZX
ØD9V4ZX
ØD9WØZX
ØD9W4ZX
ØDBUØZX
ØDBVØZX
ØDBWØZX
ØDJØØZZ
ØDJ6ØZZ
ØDJ64ZZ
ØDJDØZZ
ØDJUØZZ
ØDJU4ZZ
ØDJVØZZ
ØDJV4ZZ
ØDJWØZZ
ØDJW4ZZ
ØF9ØØZX
ØF91ØZX
ØF92ØZX
ØF94ØZX
ØF944ZX
ØF95ØZX
ØF96ØZX
ØF97ØZX
ØF98ØZX
ØF99ØZX
ØF9CØZX
ØF9DØZX
ØF9FØZX
ØF9GØZX
ØFBØØZX
ØFBØ4ZX
ØFB1ØZX
ØFB14ZX
ØFB2ØZX
ØFB24ZX
ØFB4ØZX
ØFB5ØZX
ØFB6ØZX
ØFB7ØZX
ØFB8ØZX
ØFB9ØZX
ØFBCØZX
ØFBDØZX
ØFBFØZX
ØFBGØZX
ØFDØ4ZX
ØFD14ZX
ØFD24ZX
ØFJØØZZ
ØFJØ4ZZ
ØFJ4ØZZ
ØFJ44ZZ
ØFJDØZZ
ØFJD4ZZ
ØFJGØZZ
ØFJG4ZZ
ØW9GØØZ
ØW9GØZX
ØW9GØZZ
ØW9G4ØZ
ØW9G4ZX
ØW9G4ZZ
ØW9HØZX
ØW9H3ZX
ØW9H4ZX
ØW9JØZX
ØW9J4ZX
ØWBHØZX
ØWCJØZZ
ØWCPØZZ
ØWCRØZZ
ØWJF4ZZ
ØWJGØZZ
ØWJG4ZZ
ØWJH4ZZ
ØWJJØZZ
ØWJJ4ZZ
ØWJPØZZ
ØWJP4ZZ
ØWJRØZZ
ØWJR4ZZ
ØY95ØZX
ØY953ZX
ØY954ZX
ØY96ØZX
ØY963ZX
ØY964ZX
ØYB5ØZX
ØYB53ZX
ØYB54ZX
ØYB6ØZX
ØYB63ZX
ØYB64ZX
ØYB7ØZX
ØYB73ZX
ØYB74ZX
ØYB8ØZX
ØYB83ZX
ØYB84ZX
ØYJ54ZZ
ØYJ64ZZ
ØYJ74ZZ
ØYJ84ZZ
ØYJA4ZZ
ØYJE4ZZ
4AØC45Z
4AØC4BZ

DRG 421
Select operating room procedures listed under DRG 420

DRG 422
Select operating room procedures listed under DRG 420

DRG 423
Operating Room Procedures
ØØ8W*
ØØ8X*
ØØ8Y*
ØØPVØØZ
ØØPVØ2Z
ØØPVØ3Z
ØØPVØ7Z
ØØPVØJZ
ØØPVØKZ
ØØPVØYZ
ØØPV37Z
ØØPV3JZ
ØØPV3KZ
ØØPV4ØZ
ØØPV42Z
ØØPV43Z
ØØPV47Z
ØØPV4JZ
ØØPV4KZ
ØØWVØØZ
ØØWVØ2Z
ØØWVØ3Z
ØØWVØ7Z
ØØWVØJZ
ØØWVØKZ
ØØWVØMZ
ØØWVØYZ
ØØWV3ØZ
ØØWV32Z
ØØWV33Z
ØØWV37Z
ØØWV3JZ
ØØWV3KZ
ØØWV3MZ
ØØWV4ØZ
ØØWV42Z
ØØWV43Z
ØØWV47Z
ØØWV4JZ
ØØWV4KZ
ØØWV4MZ
Ø2HVØ2Z
Ø2HVØDZ
Ø2HV3DZ
Ø2HV42Z
Ø2HV4DZ
Ø2LV*
Ø2VV*
315Ø9Ø
Ø315ØAØ
Ø315ØJØ
Ø315ØKØ
Ø315ØZØ
316Ø91
Ø316ØA1
Ø316ØJ1
Ø316ØK1
Ø316ØZ1
Ø31HØ9J
Ø31HØ9Y
Ø31HØAJ
Ø31HØAY
Ø31HØJJ
Ø31HØJY
Ø31HØKJ
Ø31HØKY
Ø31HØZJ
Ø31HØZY
Ø31JØ9K
Ø31JØ9Y
Ø31JØAK
Ø31JØAY
Ø31JØJK
Ø31JØJY
Ø31JØKK
Ø31JØKY
Ø31JØZK
Ø31JØZY
Ø31KØ9J
Ø31KØAJ
Ø31KØJJ
Ø31KØKJ
Ø31KØZJ
Ø31LØ9K
Ø31LØAK
Ø31LØJK
Ø31LØKK
Ø31LØZK
Ø31MØ9J
Ø31MØAJ
Ø31MØJJ
Ø31MØKJ
Ø31MØZJ
Ø31NØ9K
Ø31NØAK
Ø31NØJK
Ø31NØKK
Ø31NØZK
Ø37334Z
Ø37335Z
Ø37336Z
Ø37337Z
Ø3733D1
Ø3733DZ
Ø3733EZ
Ø3733FZ
Ø3733GZ
Ø3733Z1
Ø3733ZZ
Ø37434Z
Ø37435Z
Ø37436Z
Ø37437Z
Ø3743D1
Ø3743DZ
Ø3743EZ
Ø3743FZ
Ø3743GZ
Ø3743Z1
Ø3743ZZ
Ø37734Z
Ø37735Z
Ø37736Z
Ø37737Z
Ø3773D1
Ø3773DZ
Ø3773EZ
Ø3773FZ
Ø3773GZ
Ø3773Z1
Ø3773ZZ
Ø37834Z
Ø37835Z
Ø37836Z
Ø37837Z
Ø3783D1
Ø3783DZ
Ø3783EZ
Ø3783FZ
Ø3783GZ
Ø3783Z1
Ø3783ZZ
Ø37934Z
Ø37935Z
Ø37936Z
Ø37937Z
Ø3793D1
Ø3793DZ
Ø3793EZ
Ø3793FZ
Ø3793GZ
Ø3793Z1
Ø3793ZZ
Ø37A34Z
Ø37A35Z
Ø37A36Z
Ø37A37Z
Ø37A3D1
Ø37A3DZ
Ø37A3EZ
Ø37A3FZ
Ø37A3GZ
Ø37A3Z1
Ø37A3ZZ
Ø37Y34Z
Ø37Y35Z
Ø37Y36Z
Ø37Y37Z
Ø37Y3DZ
Ø37Y3EZ
Ø37Y3FZ
Ø37Y3GZ
Ø37Y3ZZ
Ø3CY*
Ø3QY*
Ø41KØ9H
Ø41KØ9J
Ø41KØ9K
Ø41KØ9L
Ø41KØAH
Ø41KØAJ
Ø41KØAK
Ø41KØAL
Ø41KØJH
Ø41KØJJ
Ø41KØJK
Ø41KØJL
Ø41KØKH
Ø41KØKJ
Ø41KØKK
Ø41KØKL
Ø41KØZH
Ø41KØZJ
Ø41KØZK
Ø41KØZL
Ø41K49H
Ø41K49J
Ø41K49K
Ø41K49L
Ø41K4AH
Ø41K4AJ
Ø41K4AK
Ø41K4AL
Ø41K4JH
Ø41K4JJ
Ø41K4JK
Ø41K4JL
Ø41K4KH
Ø41K4KJ
Ø41K4KK
Ø41K4KL
Ø41K4ZH
Ø41K4ZJ
Ø41K4ZK
Ø41K4ZL
Ø41LØ9H
Ø41LØ9J
Ø41LØ9K
Ø41LØ9L
Ø41LØAH
Ø41LØAJ
Ø41LØAK
Ø41LØAL
Ø41LØJH
Ø41LØJJ
Ø41LØJK
Ø41LØJL
Ø41LØKH
Ø41LØKJ
Ø41LØKK
Ø41LØKL
Ø41LØZH
Ø41LØZJ
Ø41LØZK
Ø41LØZL
Ø41L49H
Ø41L49J
Ø41L49K
Ø41L49L
Ø41L4AH
Ø41L4AJ
Ø41L4AK
Ø41L4AL
Ø41L4JH
Ø41L4JJ
Ø41L4JK
Ø41L4JL
Ø41L4KH
Ø41L4KJ
Ø41L4KK
Ø41L4KL
Ø41L4ZH
Ø41L4ZJ
Ø41L4ZK
Ø41L4ZL
47Ø341
Ø47Ø34Z
Ø47Ø35Z
Ø47Ø36Z
Ø47Ø37Z
Ø47Ø3D1
Ø47Ø3DZ
Ø47Ø3EZ
Ø47Ø3FZ
Ø47Ø3GZ
Ø47Ø3Z1
Ø47Ø3ZZ
471341
Ø47134Z
Ø47135Z
Ø47136Z
Ø47137Z
Ø4713D1
Ø4713DZ
Ø4713EZ
Ø4713FZ
Ø4713GZ
Ø4713Z1
Ø4713ZZ
472341
Ø47234Z
Ø47235Z
Ø47236Z
Ø47237Z
Ø4723D1
Ø4723DZ
Ø4723EZ
Ø4723FZ
Ø4723GZ
Ø4723Z1
Ø4723ZZ
473341
Ø47334Z
Ø47335Z
Ø47336Z
Ø47337Z
Ø4733D1
Ø4733DZ
Ø4733EZ
Ø4733FZ
Ø4733GZ
Ø4733Z1
Ø4733ZZ
474341
Ø47434Z
Ø47435Z
Ø47436Z
Ø47437Z
Ø4743D1
Ø4743DZ
Ø4743EZ
Ø4743FZ
Ø4743GZ
Ø4743Z1
Ø4743ZZ
475341
Ø47534Z
Ø47535Z
Ø47536Z
Ø47537Z
Ø4753D1
Ø4753DZ
Ø4753EZ
Ø4753FZ
Ø4753GZ
Ø4753Z1
Ø4753ZZ
476341
Ø47634Z
Ø47635Z
Ø47636Z
Ø47637Z
Ø4763D1
Ø4763DZ
Ø4763EZ
Ø4763FZ
Ø4763GZ
Ø4763Z1
Ø4763ZZ
477341
Ø47734Z
Ø47735Z
Ø47736Z
Ø47737Z
Ø4773D1
Ø4773DZ
Ø4773EZ
Ø4773FZ
Ø4773GZ
Ø4773Z1
Ø4773ZZ
478341
Ø47834Z
Ø47835Z
Ø47836Z
Ø47837Z
Ø4783D1
Ø4783DZ
Ø4783EZ
Ø4783FZ
Ø4783GZ
Ø4783Z1
Ø4783ZZ
479341
Ø47934Z
Ø47935Z
Ø47936Z
Ø47937Z
Ø4793D1
Ø4793DZ
Ø4793EZ
Ø4793FZ
Ø4793GZ
Ø4793Z1
Ø4793ZZ
Ø47A341
Ø47A34Z
Ø47A35Z
Ø47A36Z
Ø47A37Z
Ø47A3D1
Ø47A3DZ
Ø47A3EZ
Ø47A3FZ
Ø47A3GZ
Ø47A3Z1
Ø47A3ZZ
Ø47B341
Ø47B34Z
Ø47B35Z
Ø47B36Z
Ø47B37Z
Ø47B3D1
Ø47B3DZ
Ø47B3EZ
Ø47B3FZ
Ø47B3GZ
Ø47B3Z1
Ø47B3ZZ
Ø47C341
Ø47C34Z
Ø47C35Z
Ø47C36Z
Ø47C37Z
Ø47C3D1
Ø47C3DZ
Ø47C3EZ
Ø47C3FZ
Ø47C3GZ
Ø47C3Z1
Ø47C3ZZ
Ø47D341
Ø47D34Z
Ø47D35Z
Ø47D36Z
Ø47D37Z
Ø47D3D1
Ø47D3DZ
Ø47D3EZ
Ø47D3FZ
Ø47D3GZ
Ø47D3Z1
Ø47D3ZZ
Ø47E341
Ø47E34Z
Ø47E35Z
Ø47E36Z
Ø47E37Z
Ø47E3D1
Ø47E3DZ
Ø47E3EZ
Ø47E3FZ
Ø47E3GZ
Ø47E3Z1
Ø47E3ZZ
Ø47F341
Ø47F34Z
Ø47F35Z
Ø47F36Z
Ø47F37Z
Ø47F3D1
Ø47F3DZ
Ø47F3EZ
Ø47F3FZ
Ø47F3GZ
Ø47F3Z1
Ø47F3ZZ
Ø47H341
Ø47H34Z
Ø47H35Z
Ø47H36Z
Ø47H37Z
Ø47H3D1
Ø47H3DZ
Ø47H3EZ
Ø47H3FZ
Ø47H3GZ
Ø47H3Z1
Ø47H3ZZ
Ø47J341
Ø47J34Z
Ø47J35Z
Ø47J36Z
Ø47J37Z
Ø47J3D1
Ø47J3DZ
Ø47J3EZ
Ø47J3FZ
Ø47J3GZ
Ø47J3Z1
Ø47J3ZZ
Ø47KØ41
Ø47KØD1
Ø47KØZ1
Ø47K341
Ø47K34Z
Ø47K35Z
Ø47K36Z
Ø47K37Z
Ø47K3D1
Ø47K3DZ
Ø47K3EZ
Ø47K3FZ
Ø47K3GZ
Ø47K3Z1
Ø47K3ZZ
Ø47K441
Ø47K4D1
Ø47K4Z1
Ø47LØ41
Ø47LØD1
Ø47LØZ1
Ø47L341
Ø47L34Z
Ø47L35Z
Ø47L36Z
Ø47L37Z
Ø47L3D1
Ø47L3DZ
Ø47L3EZ
Ø47L3FZ
Ø47L3GZ
Ø47L3Z1
Ø47L3ZZ
Ø47L441
Ø47L4D1
Ø47L4Z1
Ø47MØ41
Ø47MØD1
Ø47MØZ1
Ø47M341
Ø47M3D1
Ø47M3Z1
Ø47M441
Ø47M4D1
Ø47M4Z1
Ø47NØ41
Ø47NØD1
Ø47NØZ1
Ø47N341
Ø47N3D1
Ø47N3Z1
Ø47N441
Ø47N4D1
Ø47N4Z1
Ø47Y341
Ø47Y34Z
Ø47Y35Z
Ø47Y36Z
Ø47Y37Z
Ø47Y3D1
Ø47Y3DZ
Ø47Y3EZ
Ø47Y3FZ
Ø47Y3GZ
Ø47Y3Z1
Ø47Y3ZZ
Ø4CY*
Ø4L33DZ
Ø4QY*
Ø4V33DZ
Ø5793D1
Ø5793DZ
Ø5793Z1
Ø5793ZZ
Ø57A3D1
Ø57A3DZ
Ø57A3Z1
Ø57A3ZZ
Ø57B3D1
Ø57B3DZ
Ø57B3Z1
Ø57B3ZZ
Ø57C3D1
Ø57C3DZ
Ø57C3Z1
Ø57C3ZZ
Ø57D3D1
Ø57D3DZ
Ø57D3Z1
Ø57D3ZZ
Ø57F3D1
Ø57F3DZ
Ø57F3Z1
Ø57F3ZZ
Ø5CY*
Ø5QY*
Ø67Ø3DZ
Ø67Ø3ZZ
Ø6CY*
Ø6HØØDZ
Ø6HØ4DZ
Ø6LØ*
Ø6L2ØZZ
Ø6L23ZZ
Ø6L24ZZ
Ø6L3ØCZ
Ø6L3ØDZ
Ø6L3ØZZ
Ø6L43DZ
Ø6L83DZ
Ø6QY*
Ø6VØ*
Ø6V43DZ
Ø6V83DZ
Ø79BØZX
Ø79B3ZX
Ø79B4ZX
Ø79CØZX
Ø79C3ZX
Ø79C4ZX
Ø79DØZX
Ø79D3ZX
Ø79D4ZX
Ø79LØZX
Ø79L3ZX
Ø79L4ZX
Ø7BBØZX
Ø7BB3ZX
Ø7BB4ZX
Ø7BCØZX
Ø7BC3ZX
Ø7BC4ZX
Ø7BDØZX
Ø7BD3ZX
Ø7BD4ZX
Ø7BLØZX
Ø7BL3ZX
Ø7BL4ZX
ØD16Ø79
ØD16Ø7A

ØD16Ø7B
ØD16Ø7L
ØD16ØJ9
ØD16ØJA
ØD16ØJB
ØD16ØJL
ØD16ØK9
ØD16ØKA
ØD16ØKB
ØD16ØKL
ØD16ØZ9
ØD16ØZA
ØD16ØZB
ØD16ØZL
ØD16479
ØD1647A
ØD1647B
ØD1647L
ØD164J9
ØD164JA
ØD164JB
ØD164JL
ØD164K9
ØD164KA
ØD164KB
ØD164KL
ØD164Z9
ØD164ZA
ØD164ZB
ØD164ZL
ØD16879
ØD1687A
ØD1687B
ØD1687L
ØD168J9
ØD168JA
ØD168JB
ØD168JL
ØD168K9
ØD168KA
ØD168KB
ØD168KL
ØD168Z9
ØD168ZA
ØD168ZB
ØD168ZL
ØD59ØZ3
ØD59ØZZ
ØD593Z3
ØD593ZZ
ØD597ZZ
ØD5UØZZ
ØD5U3ZZ
ØD5U4ZZ
ØD5V*
ØD5W*
ØD96ØØZ
ØD96ØZZ
ØD964ØZ
ØD964ZZ
ØD967ZZ
ØD968ZZ
ØD99ØØZ
ØD99ØZZ
ØD994ØZ
ØD994ZZ
ØD997ZZ
ØD998ZZ
ØDB7ØZZ
ØDB73ZZ
ØDB77ZZ
ØDB9ØZZ
ØDB93ZZ
ØDBUØZZ
ØDBU3ZZ
ØDBU4ZZ
ØDBVØZZ
ØDBV3ZZ
ØDBV4ZZ
ØDBWØZZ
ØDBW3ZZ
ØDBW4ZZ
ØDC6ØZZ
ØDC63ZZ
ØDC64ZZ
ØDC9ØZZ
ØDC93ZZ
ØDC94ZZ
ØDH9Ø2Z
ØDH9Ø3Z
ØDH932Z
ØDH933Z
ØDH942Z
ØDH943Z
ØDL8*
ØDL9*
ØDN8ØZZ
ØDN83ZZ
ØDN84ZZ
ØDN9ØZZ
ØDN93ZZ
ØDN94ZZ
ØDNAØZZ
ØDNA3ZZ
ØDNA4ZZ
ØDNBØZZ
ØDNB3ZZ
ØDNB4ZZ
ØDNCØZZ
ØDNC3ZZ
ØDNC4ZZ
ØDNEØZZ
ØDNE3ZZ
ØDNE4ZZ
ØDNFØZZ
ØDNF3ZZ
ØDNF4ZZ
ØDNGØZZ
ØDNG3ZZ
ØDNG4ZZ
ØDNHØZZ
ØDNH3ZZ
ØDNH4ZZ
ØDNJØZZ
ØDNJ3ZZ
ØDNJ4ZZ
ØDNKØZZ
ØDNK3ZZ
ØDNK4ZZ
ØDNLØZZ
ØDNL3ZZ
ØDNL4ZZ
ØDNMØZZ
ØDNM3ZZ
ØDNM4ZZ
ØDNNØZZ
ØDNN3ZZ
ØDNN4ZZ
ØDNUØZZ
ØDNU3ZZ
ØDNU4ZZ
ØDNV*
ØDNW*
ØDQ6ØZZ
ØDQ63ZZ
ØDQ67ZZ
ØDQ68ZZ
ØDQV*
ØDQW*
ØDRUØ7Z
ØDRUØJZ
ØDRUØKZ
ØDRU47Z
ØDRU4JZ
ØDRU4KZ
ØDRV*
ØDRW*
ØDS67ZZ
ØDS68ZZ
ØDSBØZZ
ØDSB4ZZ
ØDSB7ZZ
ØDSB8ZZ
ØDSHØZZ
ØDSH4ZZ
ØDSH7ZZ
ØDSH8ZZ
ØDTUØZZ
ØDTU4ZZ
ØDUUØ7Z
ØDUUØJZ
ØDUUØKZ
ØDUU47Z
ØDUU4JZ
ØDUU4KZ
ØDUV*
ØDUW*
ØDWØ4UZ
ØDWWØJZ
ØDWW3JZ
ØDWW4JZ
ØFN*
ØJBØØZZ
ØJB1ØZZ
ØJB4ØZZ
ØJB5ØZZ
ØJB6ØZZ
ØJB7ØZZ
ØJB8ØZZ
ØJB9ØZZ
ØJBBØZZ
ØJBCØZZ
ØJBDØZZ
ØJBFØZZ
ØJBGØZZ
ØJBHØZZ
ØJBLØZZ
ØJBMØZZ
ØJBNØZZ
ØJBPØZZ
ØJBQØZZ
ØJBRØZZ
ØJH6ØVZ
ØJH6ØWZ
ØJH6ØYZ
ØJH63VZ
ØJH7ØVZ
ØJH7ØYZ
ØJH73VZ
ØJH8ØVZ
ØJH8ØWZ
ØJH8ØYZ
ØJH83VZ
ØJHDØVZ
ØJHDØWZ
ØJHD3VZ
ØJHFØVZ
ØJHFØWZ
ØJHF3VZ
ØJHGØVZ
ØJHGØWZ
ØJHG3VZ
ØJHHØVZ
ØJHHØWZ
ØJHH3VZ
ØJHLØVZ
ØJHLØWZ
ØJHL3VZ
ØJHMØVZ
ØJHMØWZ
ØJHM3VZ
ØJHNØVZ
ØJHN3VZ
ØJHPØVZ
ØJHPØWZ
ØJHP3VZ
ØJHTØVZ
ØJHTØYZ
ØJHT3VZ
ØW1GØJ4
ØW1GØJ6
ØW1G3J4
ØW1G3J6
ØW1G4J4
ØW1G4J6
ØW3F*
ØW3GØZZ
ØW3G3ZZ
ØW3G4ZZ
ØW3H*
ØW3J*
ØW3PØZZ
ØW3P3ZZ
ØW3P4ZZ
ØW9FØØZ
ØW9FØZZ
ØW9HØØZ
ØW9HØZZ
ØW9H4ØZ
ØW9H4ZZ
ØW9JØØZ
ØW9JØZZ
ØW9J4ØZ
ØW9J4ZZ
ØWCJ3ZZ
ØWCJ4ZZ
ØWCP3ZZ
ØWCP4ZZ
ØWCR3ZZ
ØWCR4ZZ
ØWFGØZZ
ØWFG3ZZ
ØWFG4ZZ
ØWJFØZZ
ØWJHØZZ
ØWMFØZZ
ØWQF3ZZ
ØWQF4ZZ
ØWQFXZZ
ØY35*
ØY36*
ØY95ØØZ
ØY95ØZZ
ØY954ØZ
ØY954ZZ
ØY96ØØZ
ØY96ØZZ
ØY964ØZ
ØY964ZZ
ØYJ5ØZZ
ØYJ6ØZZ
ØYJ7ØZZ
ØYJAØZZ
X27H385
X27H395
X27H3B5
X27H3C5
X27J385
X27J395
X27J3B5
X27J3C5
X2H13R9

OR

Nonoperating Room Procedure

ØD594Z3

DRG 424

Select operating room procedures OR nonoperating room procedure listed under DRG 423

DRG 425

Select operating room procedures OR nonoperating room procedure listed under DRG 423

DRG 432

Principal Diagnosis

K7Ø.1*
K7Ø.2
K7Ø.3*
K7Ø.4*
K7Ø.9
K74.Ø*
K74.3
K74.4
K74.5
K74.6*

DRG 433

Select principal diagnosis listed under DRG 432

DRG 434

Select principal diagnosis listed under DRG 432

DRG 435

Principal Diagnosis

C22*
C23
C24*
C25*
C78.7
C7B.Ø2
DØ1.5
D37.6

DRG 436

Select principal diagnosis listed under DRG 435

DRG 437

Select principal diagnosis listed under DRG 435

DRG 438

Principal Diagnosis

B25.2
B26.3
D13.6
K85*
K86*
Q45.Ø
Q45.1
Q45.2
Q45.3
S36.2ØØA
S36.2Ø1A
S36.2Ø2A
S36.2Ø9A
S36.22ØA
S36.221A
S36.222A
S36.229A
S36.23ØA
S36.231A
S36.232A
S36.239A
S36.24ØA
S36.241A
S36.242A
S36.249A
S36.25ØA
S36.251A
S36.252A
S36.259A
S36.26ØA
S36.261A
S36.262A
S36.269A
S36.29ØA
S36.291A
S36.292A
S36.299A
T86.89Ø
T86.891
T86.892
T86.898
T86.899
Z94.83

DRG 439

Select principal diagnosis listed under DRG 438

DRG 440

Select principal diagnosis listed under DRG 438

DRG 441

Principal Diagnosis

AØ6.4
A51.45
A52.74
B15*
B16*
B17*
B18*
B19*
B25.1
B26.81
B58.1
B65.1
B66.Ø
B66.1
B66.3
B66.5
B67.Ø
B67.5
B67.8
D13.4
D13.5
E8Ø.4
E8Ø.5
E8Ø.6
E8Ø.7
I81
I82.Ø
K7Ø.Ø
K71*
K72*
K73*
K74.1
K74.2
K75*
K76.Ø
K76.1
K76.2
K76.3
K76.4
K76.5
K76.6
K76.7
K76.82
K76.89
K76.9
K77
Q44.Ø
Q44.1
Q44.4
Q44.5
Q44.6
Q44.7*
R16.Ø
R16.2
R17
R82.2
R94.5
S36.112A
S36.113A
S36.114A
S36.115A
S36.116A
S36.118A
S36.119A
T86.4*
Z52.6
Z94.4

DRG 442

Select principal diagnosis listed under DRG 441

DRG 443

Select principal diagnosis listed under DRG 441

DRG 444

Principal Diagnosis

K8Ø*
K81*
K82*
K82.A1
K82.A2
K83*
K83.Ø1
K83.Ø9
K87
K91.5
Q44.2
Q44.3
R93.2
S36.122A
S36.123A
S36.128A
S36.129A
S36.13XA

DRG 445

Select principal diagnosis listed under DRG 444

DRG 446

Select principal diagnosis listed under DRG 444

MDC 8

DRG 453

Anterior Spinal Fusion Operating Room Procedures

ØRG1Ø7Ø
ØRG1Ø7J
ØRG1ØAØ
ØRG1ØAJ
ØRG1ØJØ
ØRG1ØJJ
ØRG1ØKØ
ØRG1ØKJ
ØRG137Ø
ØRG137J
ØRG13AØ
ØRG13AJ
ØRG13JØ
ØRG13JJ
ØRG13KØ
ØRG13KJ
ØRG147Ø
ØRG147J
ØRG14AØ
ØRG14AJ
ØRG14JØ
ØRG14JJ
ØRG14KØ
ØRG14KJ
ØRG2Ø7Ø
ØRG2Ø7J
ØRG2ØAØ
ØRG2ØAJ
ØRG2ØJØ
ØRG2ØJJ
ØRG2ØKØ
ØRG2ØKJ
ØRG237Ø
ØRG237J
ØRG23AØ
ØRG23AJ
ØRG23JØ
ØRG23JJ
ØRG23KØ
ØRG23KJ
ØRG247Ø
ØRG247J
ØRG24AØ
ØRG24AJ
ØRG24JØ
ØRG24JJ
ØRG24KØ
ØRG24KJ
ØRG4Ø7Ø
ØRG4Ø7J
ØRG4ØAØ
ØRG4ØAJ
ØRG4ØJØ
ØRG4ØJJ
ØRG4ØKØ
ØRG4ØKJ
ØRG437Ø
ØRG437J
ØRG43AØ
ØRG43AJ
ØRG43JØ
ØRG43JJ
ØRG43KØ
ØRG43KJ
ØRG447Ø
ØRG447J
ØRG44AØ
ØRG44AJ
ØRG44JØ
ØRG44JJ
ØRG44KØ
ØRG44KJ
ØRG6Ø7Ø
ØRG6Ø7J
ØRG6ØAØ
ØRG6ØAJ
ØRG6ØJØ
ØRG6ØJJ
ØRG6ØKØ
ØRG6ØKJ
ØRG637Ø
ØRG637J
ØRG63AØ
ØRG63AJ
ØRG63JØ
ØRG63JJ
ØRG63KØ
ØRG63KJ
ØRG647Ø
ØRG647J
ØRG64AØ
ØRG64AJ
ØRG64JØ
ØRG64JJ
ØRG64KØ
ØRG64KJ
ØRG7Ø7Ø
ØRG7Ø7J
ØRG7ØAØ
ØRG7ØAJ
ØRG7ØJØ
ØRG7ØJJ
ØRG7ØKØ
ØRG7ØKJ
ØRG737Ø
ØRG737J
ØRG73AØ
ØRG73AJ
ØRG73JØ
ØRG73JJ
ØRG73KØ
ØRG73KJ
ØRG747Ø
ØRG747J
ØRG74AØ
ØRG74AJ
ØRG74JØ
ØRG74JJ
ØRG74KØ
ØRG74KJ
ØRG8Ø7Ø
ØRG8Ø7J
ØRG8ØAØ
ØRG8ØAJ
ØRG8ØJØ
ØRG8ØJJ
ØRG8ØKØ
ØRG8ØKJ
ØRG837Ø
ØRG837J
ØRG83AØ
ØRG83AJ
ØRG83JØ
ØRG83JJ
ØRG83KØ
ØRG83KJ
ØRG847Ø
ØRG847J
ØRG84AØ
ØRG84AJ
ØRG84JØ
ØRG84JJ
ØRG84KØ
ØRG84KJ
ØRGAØ7Ø
ØRGAØ7J
ØRGAØAØ
ØRGAØAJ
ØRGAØJØ
ØRGAØJJ
ØRGAØKØ
ØRGAØKJ
ØRGA37Ø
ØRGA37J
ØRGA3AØ
ØRGA3AJ
ØRGA3JØ
ØRGA3JJ
ØRGA3KØ
ØRGA3KJ
ØRGA47Ø
ØRGA47J
ØRGA4AØ
ØRGA4AJ
ØRGA4JØ
ØRGA4JJ
ØRGA4KØ
ØRGA4KJ
ØSGØØ7Ø
ØSGØØ7J
ØSGØØAØ
ØSGØØAJ
ØSGØØJØ
ØSGØØJJ
ØSGØØKØ
ØSGØØKJ
ØSGØ37Ø
ØSGØ37J
ØSGØ3AØ
ØSGØ3AJ
ØSGØ3JØ
ØSGØ3JJ
ØSGØ3KØ
ØSGØ3KJ
ØSGØ47Ø
ØSGØ47J
ØSGØ4AØ
ØSGØ4AJ
ØSGØ4JØ
ØSGØ4JJ
ØSGØ4KØ
ØSGØ4KJ
ØSG1Ø7Ø
ØSG1Ø7J
ØSG1ØAØ
ØSG1ØAJ
ØSG1ØJØ
ØSG1ØJJ
ØSG1ØKØ
ØSG1ØKJ
ØSG137Ø
ØSG137J
ØSG13AØ
ØSG13AJ
ØSG13JØ
ØSG13JJ
ØSG13KØ
ØSG13KJ
ØSG147Ø
ØSG147J
ØSG14AØ
ØSG14AJ
ØSG14JØ
ØSG14JJ
ØSG14KØ
ØSG14KJ
ØSG3Ø7Ø
ØSG3Ø7J
ØSG3ØAØ
ØSG3ØAJ
ØSG3ØJØ
ØSG3ØJJ
ØSG3ØKØ
ØSG3ØKJ
ØSG337Ø
ØSG337J
ØSG33AØ
ØSG33AJ
ØSG33JØ
ØSG33JJ
ØSG33KØ
ØSG33KJ
ØSG347Ø
ØSG347J
ØSG34AØ
ØSG34AJ
ØSG34JØ
ØSG34JJ
ØSG34KØ
ØSG34KJ
XRGAØR7
XRGA3R7
XRGA4R7
XRGBØR7
XRGB3R7
XRGB4R7
XRGCØR7
XRGC3R7
XRGC4R7
XRGDØR7
XRGD3R7
XRGD4R7

AND

Posterior Spinal Fusion Operating Room Procedures

ØRG1Ø71
ØRG1ØJ1
ØRG1ØK1
ØRG1371
ØRG13J1
ØRG13K1
ØRG1471
ØRG14J1
ØRG14K1
ØRG2Ø71
ØRG2ØJ1
ØRG2ØK1
ØRG2371
ØRG23J1
ØRG23K1
ØRG2471
ØRG24J1
ØRG24K1

ØRG4Ø71
ØRG4ØJ1
ØRG4ØK1
ØRG4371
ØRG43J1
ØRG43K1
ØRG4471
ØRG44J1
ØRG44K1
ØRG6Ø71
ØRG6ØJ1
ØRG6ØK1
ØRG6371
ØRG63J1
ØRG63K1
ØRG6471
ØRG64J1
ØRG64K1
ØRG7Ø71
ØRG7ØJ1
ØRG7ØK1
ØRG7371
ØRG73J1
ØRG73K1
ØRG7471
ØRG74J1
ØRG74K1
ØRG8Ø71
ØRG8ØJ1
ØRG8ØK1
ØRG8371
ØRG83J1
ØRG83K1
ØRG8471
ØRG84J1
ØRG84K1
ØRGAØ71
ØRGAØJ1
ØRGAØK1
ØRGA371
ØRGA3J1
ØRGA3K1
ØRGA471
ØRGA4J1
ØRGA4K1
ØSGØØ71
ØSGØØJ1
ØSGØØK1
ØSGØ371
ØSGØ3J1
ØSGØ3K1
ØSGØ471
ØSGØ4J1
ØSGØ4K1
ØSG1Ø71
ØSG1ØJ1
ØSG1ØK1
ØSG1371
ØSG13J1
ØSG13K1
ØSG1471
ØSG14J1
ØSG14K1
ØSG3Ø71
ØSG3ØJ1
ØSG3ØK1
ØSG3371
ØSG33J1
ØSG33K1
ØSG3471
ØSG34J1
ØSG34K1
ØSG7Ø4Z
ØSG7Ø7Z
ØSG7ØJZ
ØSG7ØKZ
ØSG734Z
ØSG737Z
ØSG73JZ
ØSG73KZ
ØSG744Z
ØSG747Z
ØSG74JZ
ØSG74KZ
ØSG8Ø4Z
ØSG8Ø7Z
ØSG8ØJZ
ØSG8ØKZ
ØSG834Z
ØSG837Z
ØSG83JZ
ØSG83KZ
ØSG844Z
ØSG847Z
ØSG84JZ
ØSG84KZ
XRGEØ58
XRGE358
XRGFØ58
XRGF358

DRG 454

Select operating room procedure combinations listed under DRG 453

DRG 455

Select operating room procedure combinations listed under DRG 453

DRG 456

Principal Diagnosis
A18.Ø1
C41.2
C79.5*
C7B.Ø3
D16.6
D48.Ø
D49.2
M4Ø.ØØ
M4Ø.Ø4
M4Ø.Ø5
M4Ø.1Ø
M4Ø.14
M4Ø.15
M4Ø.2Ø4
M4Ø.2Ø5
M4Ø.2Ø9
M4Ø.294
M4Ø.295
M4Ø.299
M4Ø.3*
M4Ø.4*
M4Ø.5*
M41.ØØ
M41.Ø4
M41.Ø5
M41.Ø6
M41.Ø7
M41.Ø8
M41.114
M41.115
M41.116
M41.117
M41.119
M41.124
M41.125
M41.126
M41.127
M41.129
M41.2Ø
M41.24
M41.25
M41.26
M41.27
M41.3*
M41.4Ø
M41.44
M41.45
M41.46
M41.47
M41.5Ø
M41.54
M41.55
M41.56
M41.57
M41.8Ø
M41.84
M41.85
M41.86
M41.87
M41.9
M42.ØØ
M42.Ø4
M42.Ø5
M42.Ø6
M42.Ø7
M42.Ø8
M42.Ø9
M43.8X4
M43.8X5
M43.8X6
M43.8X7
M43.8X8
M43.8X9
M43.9
M46.2Ø
M46.24
M46.25
M46.26
M46.27
M46.28
M48.5ØXA
M48.54XA
M48.55XA
M48.56XA
M48.57XA
M48.58XA
M8Ø.Ø8XA
M8Ø.88XA
M84.58XA
M84.68XA
M86.Ø8
M86.18
M86.28
M86.38
M86.48
M86.58
M86.68
M86.8X8
M96.2
M96.3
M96.4
M96.5
Q67.5
Q76.3
Q76.42*
Q78.Ø
OR
Secondary Diagnosis
M4Ø.1Ø
M4Ø.14
M4Ø.15
M41.4Ø
M41.44
M41.45
M41.46
M41.47
M41.5Ø
M41.54
M41.55
M41.56
M41.57
M43.8X9
AND
Operating Room Procedures
ØRG6*
ØRG7*
ØRG8*
ØRGA*
ØSGØ*
ØSG1*
ØSG3*
ØSG5*
ØSG6*
ØSG7*
ØSG8*
XRGAØR7
XRGA3R7
XRGA4R7
XRGBØR7
XRGB3R7
XRGB4R7
XRGCØR7
XRGC3R7
XRGC4R7
XRGDØR7
XRGD3R7
XRGD4R7
XRGEØ58
XRGE358
XRGFØ58
XRGF358
OR
Operating Room Procedures
ØRG8*
OR
Operating Room Procedures
ØRG7Ø7Ø
ØRG7ØAØ
ØRG7ØJØ
ØRG7ØKØ
ØRG737Ø
ØRG73AØ
ØRG73JØ
ØRG73KØ
ØRG747Ø
ØRG74AØ
ØRG74JØ
ØRG74KØ
AND
Operating Room Procedures
ØSG1Ø7Ø
ØSG1ØAØ
ØSG1ØJØ
ØSG1ØKØ
ØSG137Ø
ØSG13AØ
ØSG13JØ
ØSG13KØ
ØSG147Ø
ØSG14AØ
ØSG14JØ
ØSG14KØ
XRGCØR7
XRGC3R7
XRGC4R7
OR
Operating Room Procedures
ØRG7Ø71
ØRG7Ø7J
ØRG7ØAJ
ØRG7ØJ1
ØRG7ØJJ
ØRG7ØK1
ØRG7ØKJ
ØRG7371
ØRG737J
ØRG73AJ
ØRG73J1
ØRG73JJ
ØRG73K1
ØRG73KJ
ØRG7471
ØRG747J
ØRG74AJ
ØRG74J1
ØRG74JJ
ØRG74K1
ØRG74KJ
AND
Operating Room Procedures
ØSG1Ø71
ØSG1Ø7J
ØSG1ØAJ
ØSG1ØJ1
ØSG1ØJJ
ØSG1ØK1
ØSG1ØKJ
ØSG1371
ØSG137J
ØSG13AJ
ØSG13J1
ØSG13JJ
ØSG13K1
ØSG13KJ
ØSG1471
ØSG147J
ØSG14AJ
ØSG14J1
ØSG14JJ
ØSG14K1
ØSG14KJ

DRG 457

Select principal OR secondary diagnosis AND operating room procedures listed under DRG 456

DRG 458

Select principal OR secondary diagnosis AND operating room procedures listed under DRG 456

DRG 459

Operating Room Procedures
ØRG6*
ØRG7*
ØRG8*
ØRGA*
ØSGØ*
ØSG1*
ØSG3*
ØSG5*
ØSG6*
ØSG7*
ØSG8*
XRGAØR7
XRGA3R7
XRGA4R7
XRGBØR7
XRGB3R7
XRGB4R7
XRGCØR7
XRGC3R7
XRGC4R7
XRGDØR7
XRGD3R7
XRGD4R7
XRGEØ58
XRGE358
XRGFØ58
XRGF358

DRG 460

Select operating room procedures listed under DRG 459

DRG 461

Any combination of two or more of the following operating room procedures or procedure combinations
ØSR9Ø19
ØSR9Ø1A
ØSR9Ø1Z
ØSR9Ø29
ØSR9Ø2A
ØSR9Ø2Z
ØSR9Ø39
ØSR9Ø3A
ØSR9Ø3Z
ØSR9Ø49
ØSR9Ø4A
ØSR9Ø4Z
ØSR9Ø69
ØSR9Ø6A
ØSR9Ø6Z
ØSR9Ø7Z
ØSR9ØJ9
ØSR9ØJA
ØSR9ØJZ
ØSR9ØKZ
ØSRA*
ØSRBØ19
ØSRBØ1A
ØSRBØ1Z
ØSRBØ29
ØSRBØ2A
ØSRBØ2Z
ØSRBØ39
ØSRBØ3A
ØSRBØ3Z
ØSRBØ49
ØSRBØ4A
ØSRBØ4Z
ØSRBØ69
ØSRBØ6A
ØSRBØ6Z
ØSRBØ7Z
ØSRBØJ9
ØSRBØJA
ØSRBØJZ
ØSRBØKZ
ØSRCØ69
ØSRCØ6A
ØSRCØ6Z
ØSRCØ7Z
ØSRCØJ9
ØSRCØJA
ØSRCØJZ
ØSRCØKZ
ØSRCØL9
ØSRCØLA
ØSRCØLZ
ØSRCØM9
ØSRCØMA
ØSRCØMZ
ØSRCØN9
ØSRCØNA
ØSRCØNZ
ØSRDØ69
ØSRDØ6A
ØSRDØ6Z
ØSRDØ7Z
ØSRDØJ9
ØSRDØJA
ØSRDØJZ
ØSRDØKZ
ØSRDØL9
ØSRDØLA
ØSRDØLZ
ØSRDØM9
ØSRDØMA
ØSRDØMZ
ØSRDØN9
ØSRDØNA
ØSRDØNZ
ØSRE*
ØSRF*
ØSRG*
ØSRR*
ØSRS*
ØSRT*
ØSRU*
ØSRV*
ØSRW*
ØSU9ØBZ
ØSUAØBZ
ØSUBØBZ
ØSUEØBZ
ØSURØBZ
ØSUSØBZ
XRRGØL8
XRRGØM8
XRRHØL8
XRRHØM8
OR
ØSP9Ø8Z
ØSP9Ø9Z
ØSP9ØBZ
ØSP9ØEZ
ØSP9ØJZ
ØSP948Z
ØSP94JZ
ØSPAØJZ
ØSPA4JZ
ØSPRØJZ
ØSPR4JZ
AND
ØSR9Ø19
ØSR9Ø1A
ØSR9Ø1Z
ØSR9Ø29
ØSR9Ø2A
ØSR9Ø2Z
ØSR9Ø39
ØSR9Ø3A
ØSR9Ø3Z
ØSR9Ø49
ØSR9Ø4A
ØSR9Ø4Z
ØSR9Ø69
ØSR9Ø6A
ØSR9Ø6Z
ØSR9ØJ9
ØSR9ØJA
ØSR9ØJZ
ØSRAØØ9
ØSRAØØA
ØSRAØØZ
ØSRAØ19
ØSRAØ1A
ØSRAØ1Z
ØSRAØ39
ØSRAØ3A
ØSRAØ3Z
ØSRAØJ9
ØSRAØJA
ØSRAØJZ
ØSRRØ19
ØSRRØ1A
ØSRRØ1Z
ØSRRØ39
ØSRRØ3A
ØSRRØ3Z
ØSRRØJ9
ØSRRØJA
ØSRRØJZ
OR
ØSPBØ8Z
ØSPBØ9Z
ØSPBØBZ
ØSPBØEZ
ØSPBØJZ
ØSPB48Z
ØSPB4JZ
ØSPEØJZ
ØSPE4JZ
ØSPSØJZ
ØSPS4JZ
AND
ØSRBØ19
ØSRBØ1A
ØSRBØ1Z
ØSRBØ29
ØSRBØ2A
ØSRBØ2Z
ØSRBØ39
ØSRBØ3A
ØSRBØ3Z
ØSRBØ49
ØSRBØ4A
ØSRBØ4Z
ØSRBØ69
ØSRBØ6A
ØSRBØ6Z
ØSRBØJ9
ØSRBØJA
ØSRBØJZ
ØSREØØ9
ØSREØØA
ØSREØØZ
ØSREØ19
ØSREØ1A
ØSREØ1Z
ØSREØ39
ØSREØ3A
ØSREØ3Z
ØSREØJ9
ØSREØJA
ØSREØJZ
ØSRSØ19
ØSRSØ1A
ØSRSØ1Z
ØSRSØ39
ØSRSØ3A
ØSRSØ3Z
ØSRSØJ9
ØSRSØJA
ØSRSØJZ
OR
ØSPC4JC
ØSPT4JZ
ØSPV4JZ
AND
ØSRCØ69
ØSRCØ6A
ØSRCØ6Z
ØSRCØJ9
ØSRCØJA
ØSRCØJZ
ØSRCØN9
ØSRCØNA
ØSRCØNZ
ØSRTØJ9
ØSRTØJA
ØSRVØJ9
ØSRVØJA
ØSRVØJZ
XRRGØL8
XRRGØM8
OR
ØSPCØ8Z
ØSPCØ9Z
ØSPCØJC
ØSPCØJZ
ØSPC38Z
ØSPC48Z
ØSPC4JZ
ØSPTØJZ
ØSPVØJZ
AND
ØSRCØN9
ØSRCØNA
ØSRCØNZ
OR
ØSPCØ9Z
ØSPCØJZ
ØSPCØLZ
ØSPCØMZ
ØSPCØNZ
ØSPC4JZ
ØSPC4LZ
ØSPC4MZ
ØSPC4NZ
AND
ØSRCØL9
ØSRCØLA
ØSRCØLZ
OR
ØSPCØ9Z
ØSPCØJZ
ØSPC4JZ
AND
ØSRCØM9
ØSRCØMA
ØSRCØMZ
OR
ØSPCØ8Z
ØSPCØ9Z
ØSPCØEZ
ØSPCØJC
ØSPCØJZ
ØSPCØLZ
ØSPCØMZ
ØSPCØNZ
ØSPC38Z
ØSPC48Z
ØSPC4JZ
ØSPC4LZ
ØSPC4MZ
ØSPC4NZ
ØSPTØJZ
ØSPVØJZ
AND
ØSRCØ69
ØSRCØ6A
ØSRCØ6Z
ØSRCØJ9
ØSRCØJA
ØSRCØJZ
ØSRTØJ9
ØSRTØJA
ØSRTØJZ
ØSRVØJ9
ØSRVØJA
ØSRVØJZ
XRRGØL8
XRRGØM8
OR
ØSPDØ8Z
ØSPDØ9Z
ØSPDØEZ
ØSPDØJC
ØSPDØJZ
ØSPDØLZ
ØSPDØMZ
ØSPDØNZ
ØSPD38Z
ØSPD48Z
ØSPD4JC
ØSPD4JZ
ØSPD4LZ
ØSPD4MZ
ØSPD4NZ
ØSPUØJZ
ØSPU4JZ
ØSPWØJZ
ØSPW4JZ
AND
ØSRDØ69
ØSRDØ6A
ØSRDØ6Z
ØSRDØJ9
ØSRDØJA
ØSRDØJZ
ØSRUØJ9
ØSRUØJA
ØSRWØJ9
ØSRWØJA
ØSRWØJZ
OR
ØSPDØ8Z
ØSPDØ9Z
ØSPDØJC
ØSPDØJZ
ØSPD38Z
ØSPD48Z
ØSPD4JC
ØSPD4JZ
ØSPUØJZ
ØSPU4JZ
ØSPWØJZ
ØSPW4JZ
AND
ØSRDØN9
ØSRDØNA
ØSRDØNZ
OR
ØSPDØ9Z
ØSPDØJZ
ØSPDØLZ
ØSPDØMZ
ØSPDØNZ
ØSPD4JZ
ØSPD4LZ
ØSPD4MZ
ØSPD4NZ
AND
ØSRDØL9
ØSRDØLA
ØSRDØLZ
OR
ØSPDØ9Z
ØSPDØJZ
ØSPD4JZ
AND
ØSRDØM9
ØSRDØMA
ØSRDØMZ
OR
ØSPDØ8Z
ØSPDØ9Z
ØSPDØEZ
ØSPDØJC
ØSPDØJZ
ØSPDØLZ
ØSPDØMZ
ØSPDØNZ
ØSPD38Z
ØSPD48Z
ØSPD4JZ
ØSPD4LZ
ØSPD4MZ
ØSPD4NZ
ØSPUØJZ
ØSPWØJZ
AND
ØSRUØJZ
XRRHØL8
XRRHØM8
OR
ØSPD4JC
ØSPU4JZ
ØSPW4JZ
AND
XRRHØL8
XRRHØM8

DRG 462

Select any combination of two or more operating room procedures listed under DRG 461

DRG 463

Operating Room Procedures
ØHRØ*
ØHR1*
ØHR4*
ØHR5*
ØHR6*
ØHR7*
ØHR8*
ØHRA*
ØHRB*
ØHRC*
ØHRD*
ØHRE*
ØHRH*
ØHRJ*
ØHRK*
ØHRL*
ØHRM*
ØHRN*
ØHXØXZZ
ØHX1XZZ
ØHX4XZZ
ØHX5XZZ
ØHX6XZZ
ØHX7XZZ
ØHX8XZZ
ØHX9XZZ
ØHXAXZZ
ØHXBXZZ
ØHXCXZZ
ØHXDXZZ
ØHXEXZZ
ØHXFXZZ
ØHXGXZZ
ØHXHXZZ
ØHXJXZZ
ØHXKXZZ
ØHXLXZZ
ØHXMXZZ
ØHXNXZZ
ØJBØØZZ
ØJB1ØZZ
ØJB4ØZZ
ØJB5ØZZ
ØJB6ØZZ
ØJB7ØZZ

ØJB8ØZZ
ØJB9ØZZ
ØJBBØZZ
ØJBCØZZ
ØJBDØZZ
ØJBFØZZ
ØJBGØZZ
ØJBHØZZ
ØJBLØZZ
ØJBMØZZ
ØJBNØZZ
ØJBPØZZ
ØJBQØZZ
ØJBRØZZ
ØJHØ*
ØJH1*
ØJH4*
ØJH5*
ØJH6ØNZ
ØJH63NZ
ØJH7ØNZ
ØJH73NZ
ØJH8ØNZ
ØJH83NZ
ØJH9*
ØJHB*
ØJHC*
ØJHDØNZ
ØJHD3NZ
ØJHFØNZ
ØJHF3NZ
ØJHGØNZ
ØJHG3NZ
ØJHHØNZ
ØJHH3NZ
ØJHLØNZ
ØJHL3NZ
ØJHMØNZ
ØJHM3NZ
ØJHNØNZ
ØJHN3NZ
ØJHPØNZ
ØJHP3NZ
ØJHQ*
ØJHR*
ØJXØØZB
ØJXØØZC
ØJXØ3ZB
ØJXØ3ZC
ØJX1ØZB
ØJX1ØZC
ØJX13ZB
ØJX13ZC
ØJX4ØZB
ØJX4ØZC
ØJX43ZB
ØJX43ZC
ØJX5ØZB
ØJX5ØZC
ØJX53ZB
ØJX53ZC
ØJX6ØZB
ØJX6ØZC
ØJX63ZB
ØJX63ZC
ØJX7ØZB
ØJX7ØZC
ØJX73ZB
ØJX73ZC
ØJX8ØZB
ØJX8ØZC
ØJX83ZB
ØJX83ZC
ØJX9ØZB
ØJX9ØZC
ØJX93ZB
ØJX93ZC
ØJXBØZB
ØJXBØZC
ØJXB3ZB
ØJXB3ZC
ØJXCØZB
ØJXCØZC
ØJXC3ZB
ØJXC3ZC
ØJXDØZB
ØJXDØZC
ØJXD3ZB
ØJXD3ZC
ØJXFØZB
ØJXFØZC
ØJXF3ZB
ØJXF3ZC
ØJXGØZB
ØJXGØZC
ØJXG3ZB
ØJXG3ZC
ØJXHØZB
ØJXHØZC
ØJXH3ZB
ØJXH3ZC
ØJXLØZB
ØJXLØZC
ØJXL3ZB
ØJXL3ZC
ØJXMØZB
ØJXMØZC
ØJXM3ZB
ØJXM3ZC
ØJXNØZB
ØJXNØZC
ØJXN3ZB
ØJXN3ZC
ØJXPØZB
ØJXPØZC
ØJXP3ZB
ØJXP3ZC
ØJXQØZB
ØJXQØZC
ØJXQ3ZB
ØJXQ3ZC
ØJXRØZB
ØJXRØZC
ØJXR3ZB
ØJXR3ZC
ØSP9Ø9Z
ØSP9ØJZ
ØSP93JZ
ØSP94JZ
ØSPAØJZ
ØSPA3JZ
ØSPA4JZ
ØSPBØ9Z
ØSPBØJZ
ØSPB3JZ
ØSPB4JZ
ØSPCØ9Z
ØSPCØJC
ØSPCØJZ
ØSPCØLZ
ØSPCØMZ
ØSPCØNZ
ØSPC3JC
ØSPC3JZ
ØSPC3LZ
ØSPC3MZ
ØSPC3NZ
ØSPC4JC
ØSPC4JZ
ØSPC4LZ
ØSPC4MZ
ØSPC4NZ
ØSPDØ9Z
ØSPDØJC
ØSPDØJZ
ØSPDØLZ
ØSPDØMZ
ØSPDØNZ
ØSPD3JC
ØSPD3JZ
ØSPD3LZ
ØSPD3MZ
ØSPD3NZ
ØSPD4JC
ØSPD4JZ
ØSPD4LZ
ØSPD4MZ
ØSPD4NZ
ØSPEØJZ
ØSPE3JZ
ØSPE4JZ
ØSPRØJZ
ØSPR3JZ
ØSPR4JZ
ØSPSØJZ
ØSPS3JZ
ØSPS4JZ
ØSPTØJZ
ØSPT3JZ
ØSPT4JZ
ØSPUØJZ
ØSPU3JZ
ØSPU4JZ
ØSPVØJZ
ØSPV3JZ
ØSPV4JZ
ØSPWØJZ
ØSPW3JZ
ØSPW4JZ
ØWUØØ7Z
ØWUØ47Z
ØWU2Ø7Z
ØWU247Z
ØWU6Ø7Z
ØWU647Z
ØWUKØ7Z
ØWUK47Z
ØWULØ7Z
ØWUL47Z
ØXU2Ø7Z
ØXU247Z
ØXU3Ø7Z
ØXU347Z
ØXU4Ø7Z
ØXU447Z
ØXU5Ø7Z
ØXU547Z
ØXU6Ø7Z
ØXU647Z
ØXU7Ø7Z
ØXU747Z
ØXU8Ø7Z
ØXU847Z
ØXU9Ø7Z
ØXU947Z
ØXUBØ7Z
ØXUB47Z
ØXUCØ7Z
ØXUC47Z
ØXUDØ7Z
ØXUD47Z
ØXUFØ7Z
ØXUF47Z
ØXUGØ7Z
ØXUG47Z
ØXUHØ7Z
ØXUH47Z
XHRPXF7

DRG 464

Select operating room procedures listed under DRG 463

DRG 465

Select operating room procedures listed under DRG 463

DRG 466

Operating Room Procedures

ØSPAØJZ
ØSPA4JZ
ØSPCØJC
ØSPC4JC
ØSPDØJC
ØSPD4JC
ØSPEØJZ
ØSPE4JZ
ØSPRØJZ
ØSPR4JZ
ØSPSØJZ
ØSPS4JZ
ØSPTØJZ
ØSPT4JZ
ØSPUØJZ
ØSPU4JZ
ØSPVØJZ
ØSPV4JZ
ØSPWØJZ
ØSPW4JZ
ØSW9ØJZ
ØSW93JZ
ØSW94JZ
ØSWAØJZ
ØSWA3JZ
ØSWA4JZ
ØSWBØJZ
ØSWB3JZ
ØSWB4JZ
ØSWCØJC
ØSWCØJZ
ØSWC3JC
ØSWC3JZ
ØSWC4JC
ØSWC4JZ
ØSWDØJC
ØSWDØJZ
ØSWD3JC
ØSWD3JZ
ØSWD4JC
ØSWD4JZ
ØSWEØJZ
ØSWE3JZ
ØSWE4JZ
ØSWRØJZ
ØSWR3JZ
ØSWR4JZ
ØSWSØJZ
ØSWS3JZ
ØSWS4JZ
ØSWTØJZ
ØSWT3JZ
ØSWT4JZ
ØSWUØJZ
ØSWU3JZ
ØSWU4JZ
ØSWVØJZ
ØSWV3JZ
ØSWV4JZ
ØSWWØJZ
ØSWW3JZ
ØSWW4JZ
OR
ØSPBØEZ
AND
ØSRBØ19
ØSRBØ1A
ØSRBØ1Z
ØSRBØ29
ØSRBØ2A
ØSRBØ2Z
ØSRBØ39
ØSRBØ3A
ØSRBØ3Z
ØSRBØ49
ØSRBØ4A
ØSRBØ4Z
ØSRBØ69
ØSRBØ6A
ØSRBØ6Z
ØSRBØJ9
ØSRBØJA
ØSRBØJZ
ØSREØØ9
ØSREØØA
ØSREØØZ
ØSREØ19
ØSREØ1A
ØSREØ1Z
ØSREØ39
ØSREØ3A
ØSREØ3Z
ØSREØJ9
ØSREØJA
ØSREØJZ
ØSRSØ19
ØSRSØ1A
ØSRSØ1Z
ØSRSØ39
ØSRSØ3A
ØSRSØ3Z
ØSRSØJ9
ØSRSØJA
ØSRSØJZ
ØSUBØ9Z
ØSUEØ9Z
ØSUSØ9Z
OR
ØSP9ØEZ
AND
ØSR9Ø19
ØSR9Ø1A
ØSR9Ø1Z
ØSR9Ø29
ØSR9Ø2A
ØSR9Ø2Z
ØSR9Ø39
ØSR9Ø3A
ØSR9Ø3Z
ØSR9Ø49
ØSR9Ø4A
ØSR9Ø4Z
ØSR9Ø69
ØSR9Ø6A
ØSR9Ø6Z
ØSR9ØJ9
ØSR9ØJA
ØSR9ØJZ
ØSRAØØ9
ØSRAØØA
ØSRAØØZ
ØSRAØ19
ØSRAØ1A
ØSRAØ1Z
ØSRAØ39
ØSRAØ3A
ØSRAØ3Z
ØSRAØJ9
ØSRAØJA
ØSRAØJZ
ØSRRØ19
ØSRRØ1A
ØSRRØ1Z
ØSRRØ39
ØSRRØ3A
ØSRRØ3Z
ØSRRØJ9
ØSRRØJA
ØSRRØJZ
ØSU9Ø9Z
ØSUAØ9Z
ØSURØ9Z
OR
ØSPBØ8Z
ØSPBØ9Z
ØSPBØBZ
ØSPB48Z
ØSPB4JZ
ØSPE4JZ
ØSPS4JZ
AND
ØSRBØ19
ØSRBØ1A
ØSRBØ1Z
ØSRBØ29
ØSRBØ2A
ØSRBØ2Z
ØSRBØ39
ØSRBØ3A
ØSRBØ3Z
ØSRBØ49
ØSRBØ4A
ØSRBØ4Z
ØSRBØ69
ØSRBØ6A
ØSRBØ6Z
ØSRBØEZ
ØSRBØJ9
ØSRBØJA
ØSRBØJZ
ØSREØØ9
ØSREØØA
ØSREØØZ
ØSREØ19
ØSREØ1A
ØSREØ1Z
ØSREØ39
ØSREØ3A
ØSREØ3Z
ØSREØJ9
ØSREØJA
ØSREØJZ
ØSRSØ19
ØSRSØ1A
ØSRSØ1Z
ØSRSØ39
ØSRSØ3A
ØSRSØ3Z
ØSRSØJ9
ØSRSØJA
ØSRSØJZ
ØSUBØ9Z
ØSUEØ9Z
ØSUSØ9Z
OR
ØSP9Ø8Z
ØSP9Ø9Z
ØSP9ØBZ
ØSP948Z
ØSP94JZ
ØSPA4JZ
ØSPR4JZ
AND
ØSR9Ø19
ØSR9Ø1A
ØSR9Ø1Z
ØSR9Ø29
ØSR9Ø2A
ØSR9Ø2Z
ØSR9Ø39
ØSR9Ø3A
ØSR9Ø3Z
ØSR9Ø49
ØSR9Ø4A
ØSR9Ø4Z
ØSR9Ø69
ØSR9Ø6A
ØSR9Ø6Z
ØSR9ØEZ
ØSR9ØJ9
ØSR9ØJA
ØSR9ØJZ
ØSRAØØ9
ØSRAØØA
ØSRAØØZ
ØSRAØ19
ØSRAØ1A
ØSRAØ1Z
ØSRAØ39
ØSRAØ3A
ØSRAØ3Z
ØSRAØJ9
ØSRAØJA
ØSRAØJZ
ØSRRØ19
ØSRRØ1A
ØSRRØ1Z
ØSRRØ39
ØSRRØ3A
ØSRRØ3Z
ØSRRØJ9
ØSRRØJA
ØSRRØJZ
ØSU9Ø9Z
ØSUAØ9Z
ØSURØ9Z
OR
ØSPBØJZ
ØSPEØJZ
ØSPSØJZ
AND
ØSRBØ19
ØSRBØ1A
ØSRBØ1Z
ØSRBØ29
ØSRBØ2A
ØSRBØ2Z
ØSRBØ39
ØSRBØ3A
ØSRBØ3Z
ØSRBØ49
ØSRBØ4A
ØSRBØ4Z
ØSRBØ69
ØSRBØ6A
ØSRBØ6Z
ØSRBØEZ
ØSRBØJ9
ØSRBØJA
ØSRBØJZ
ØSREØØ9
ØSREØØA
ØSREØØZ
ØSREØ19
ØSREØ1A
ØSREØ1Z
ØSREØ39
ØSREØ3A
ØSREØ3Z
ØSREØJ9
ØSREØJA
ØSREØJZ
ØSRSØ19
ØSRSØ1A
ØSRSØ1Z
ØSRSØ39
ØSRSØ3A
ØSRSØ3Z
ØSRSØJ9
ØSRSØJA
ØSRSØJZ
OR
ØSP9ØJZ
ØSPAØJZ
ØSPRØJZ
AND
ØSR9Ø19
ØSR9Ø1A
ØSR9Ø1Z
ØSR9Ø29
ØSR9Ø2A
ØSR9Ø2Z
ØSR9Ø39
ØSR9Ø3A
ØSR9Ø3Z
ØSR9Ø49
ØSR9Ø4A
ØSR9Ø4Z
ØSR9Ø69
ØSR9Ø6A
ØSR9Ø6Z
ØSR9ØEZ
ØSR9ØJ9
ØSR9ØJA
ØSR9ØJZ
ØSRAØØ9
ØSRAØØA
ØSRAØØZ
ØSRAØ19
ØSRAØ1A
ØSRAØ1Z
ØSRAØ39
ØSRAØ3A
ØSRAØ3Z
ØSRAØJ9
ØSRAØJA
ØSRAØJZ
ØSRRØ19
ØSRRØ1A
ØSRRØ1Z
ØSRRØ39
ØSRRØ3A
ØSRRØ3Z
ØSRRØJ9
ØSRRØJA
ØSRRØJZ
OR
ØSPDØEZ
AND
ØSRDØ69
ØSRDØ6A
ØSRDØ6Z
ØSRDØJ9
ØSRDØJA
ØSRDØJZ
ØSRUØJ9
ØSRUØJA
ØSRUØJZ
ØSRWØJ9
ØSRWØJA
ØSRWØJZ
XRRHØL8
XRRHØM8
OR
ØSPCØEZ
AND
ØSRCØ69
ØSRCØ6A
ØSRCØ6Z
ØSRCØJ9
ØSRCØJA
ØSRCØJZ
ØSRTØJ9
ØSRTØJA
ØSRTØJZ
ØSRVØJ9
ØSRVØJA
ØSRVØJZ
XRRGØL8
XRRGØM8
OR
ØSPDØ9Z
ØSPDØJZ
ØSPD4JZ
AND
ØSRDØ69
ØSRDØ6A
ØSRDØ6Z
ØSRDØEZ
ØSRDØJ9
ØSRDØJA
ØSRDØJZ
ØSRDØL9
ØSRDØLA
ØSRDØLZ
ØSRDØM9
ØSRDØMA
ØSRDØMZ
ØSRDØN9
ØSRDØNA
ØSRDØNZ
ØSRUØJ9
ØSRUØJA
ØSRUØJZ
ØSRWØJ9
ØSRWØJA
ØSRWØJZ
XRRHØL8
XRRHØM8
OR
ØSPCØ9Z
ØSPCØJZ
ØSPC4JZ
AND
ØSRCØ69
ØSRCØ6A
ØSRCØ6Z
ØSRCØEZ
ØSRCØJ9
ØSRCØJA
ØSRCØJZ
ØSRCØL9
ØSRCØLA
ØSRCØLZ
ØSRCØM9
ØSRCØMA
ØSRCØMZ
ØSRCØN9
ØSRCØNA
ØSRCØNZ
ØSRTØJ9
ØSRTØJA
ØSRTØJZ
ØSRVØJ9
ØSRVØJA
ØSRVØJZ
XRRGØL8
XRRGØM8
OR
ØSPDØLZ
ØSPDØMZ
ØSPDØNZ
ØSPD4LZ
ØSPD4MZ
ØSPD4NZ
AND
ØSRDØ69
ØSRDØ6A
ØSRDØ6Z
ØSRDØJ9
ØSRDØJA
ØSRDØJZ
ØSRDØL9
ØSRDØLA
ØSRDØLZ
ØSRUØJ9
ØSRUØJA
ØSRUØJZ
ØSRWØJ9
ØSRWØJA
ØSRWØJZ
XRRHØL8
XRRHØM8
OR
ØSPCØLZ
ØSPCØMZ
ØSPCØNZ
ØSPC4LZ
ØSPC4MZ
ØSPC4NZ
AND
ØSRCØ69
ØSRCØ6A
ØSRCØ6Z
ØSRCØJ9
ØSRCØJA
ØSRCØJZ
ØSRCØL9
ØSRCØLA
ØSRCØLZ
ØSRTØJ9
ØSRTØJA
ØSRTØJZ
ØSRVØJ9
ØSRVØJA
ØSRVØJZ
XRRGØL8
XRRGØM8
OR
ØSPDØ8Z
ØSPDØJC
ØSPD38Z
ØSPD48Z
ØSPUØJZ
ØSPWØJZ
AND
ØSRDØ69
ØSRDØ6A
ØSRDØ6Z
ØSRDØEZ
ØSRDØJ9
ØSRDØJA
ØSRDØJZ
ØSRDØN9
ØSRDØNA
ØSRDØNZ
ØSRUØJ9
ØSRUØJA
ØSRUØJZ
ØSRWØJ9
ØSRWØJA
ØSRWØJZ
XRRHØL8
XRRHØM8
OR
ØSPCØ8Z
ØSPCØJC
ØSPC38Z
ØSPC48Z
ØSPTØJZ
ØSPVØJZ
AND
ØSRCØ69
ØSRCØ6A
ØSRCØ6Z
ØSRCØEZ
ØSRCØJ9
ØSRCØJA
ØSRCØJZ
ØSRCØN9
ØSRCØNA
ØSRCØNZ
ØSRTØJ9
ØSRTØJA
ØSRTØJZ
ØSRVØJ9
ØSRVØJA
ØSRVØJZ
XRRGØL8
XRRGØM8
OR
ØSPD4JC
ØSPU4JZ
ØSPW4JZ
AND
ØSRDØ69
ØSRDØ6A
ØSRDØ6Z
ØSRDØEZ
ØSRDØJ9
ØSRDØJA
ØSRDØJZ
ØSRDØN9
ØSRDØNA
ØSRDØNZ
ØSRUØJ9
ØSRUØJA
ØSRWØJ9
ØSRWØJA
ØSRWØJZ
XRRHØL8
XRRHØM8
OR
ØSPC4JC
ØSPT4JZ
ØSPV4JZ
AND
ØSRCØ69
ØSRCØ6A
ØSRCØ6Z
ØSRCØEZ
ØSRCØJ9
ØSRCØJA
ØSRCØJZ
ØSRCØN9
ØSRCØNA
ØSRCØNZ
ØSRTØJ9
ØSRTØJA
ØSRVØJ9
ØSRVØJA
ØSRVØJZ
XRRGØL8
XRRGØM8

DRG 467

Select operating room procedures or procedure combinations listed under DRG 466

DRG 468

Select operating room procedures or procedure combinations listed under DRG 466

DRG 469

Major Hip/Knee Jt Replacement Operating Room Procedures

ØSR9Ø19
ØSR9Ø1A
ØSR9Ø1Z
ØSR9Ø29
ØSR9Ø2A
ØSR9Ø2Z
ØSR9Ø39

ØSR9Ø3A
ØSR9Ø3Z
ØSR9Ø49
ØSR9Ø4A
ØSR9Ø4Z
ØSR9Ø69
ØSR9Ø6A
ØSR9Ø6Z
ØSR9Ø7Z
ØSR9ØJ9
ØSR9ØJA
ØSR9ØJZ
ØSR9ØKZ
ØSRA*
ØSRBØ19
ØSRBØ1A
ØSRBØ1Z
ØSRBØ29
ØSRBØ2A
ØSRBØ2Z
ØSRBØ39
ØSRBØ3A
ØSRBØ3Z
ØSRBØ49
ØSRBØ4A
ØSRBØ4Z
ØSRBØ69
ØSRBØ6A
ØSRBØ6Z
ØSRBØ7Z
ØSRBØJ9
ØSRBØJA
ØSRBØJZ
ØSRBØKZ
ØSRCØ69
ØSRCØ6A
ØSRCØ6Z
ØSRCØ7Z
ØSRCØJ9
ØSRCØJA
ØSRCØJZ
ØSRCØKZ
ØSRCØL9
ØSRCØLA
ØSRCØLZ
ØSRCØM9
ØSRCØMA
ØSRCØMZ
ØSRCØN9
ØSRCØNA
ØSRCØNZ
ØSRDØ69
ØSRDØ6A
ØSRDØ6Z
ØSRDØ7Z
ØSRDØJ9
ØSRDØJA
ØSRDØJZ
ØSRDØKZ
ØSRDØL9
ØSRDØLA
ØSRDØLZ
ØSRDØM9
ØSRDØMA
ØSRDØMZ
ØSRDØN9
ØSRDØNA
ØSRDØNZ
ØSRE*
ØSRFØ7Z
ØSRFØKZ
ØSRGØ7Z
ØSRGØKZ
ØSRR*
ØSRS*
ØSRT*
ØSRU*
ØSRV*
ØSRW*
ØSU9ØBZ
ØSUAØBZ
ØSUBØBZ
ØSUEØBZ
ØSURØBZ
ØSUSØBZ
XRRGØL8
XRRGØM8
XRRHØL8
XRRHØM8

OR

Reattachment of Lower Extremity Operating Room Procedures

ØYM7ØZZ
ØYM8ØZZ
ØYMCØZZ
ØYMDØZZ
ØYMFØZZ
ØYMGØZZ
ØYMHØZZ
ØYMJØZZ
ØYMKØZZ
ØYMLØZZ
ØYMMØZZ
ØYMNØZZ

OR

Total Ankle Replacement Operating Room Procedures

ØSRFØJ9
ØSRFØJA
ØSRFØJZ
ØSRGØJ9
ØSRGØJA
ØSRGØJZ

DRG 470

Select major hip/knee joint replacement or reattachment of lower extremity operating room procedures listed under DRG 469

DRG 471

Operating Room Procedures

ØRGØ*
ØRG1*
ØRG2*
ØRG4*

DRG 472

Select operating room procedures listed under DRG 471

DRG 473

Select operating room procedures listed under DRG 471

DRG 474

Operating Room Procedures

ØX6ØØZZ
ØX61ØZZ
ØX62ØZZ
ØX63ØZZ
ØX68*
ØX69*
ØX6BØZZ
ØX6CØZZ
ØX6D*
ØX6F*
ØX6J*
ØX6K*
ØY62ØZZ
ØY63ØZZ
ØY64ØZZ
ØY67ØZZ
ØY68ØZZ
ØY6C*
ØY6D*
ØY6FØZZ
ØY6GØZZ
ØY6H*
ØY6J*
ØY6M*
ØY6N*

DRG 475

Select operating room procedures listed under DRG 474

DRG 476

Select operating room procedures listed under DRG 474

DRG 477

Operating Room Procedures

ØMJXØZZ
ØMJX4ZZ
ØMJYØZZ
ØMJY4ZZ
ØN9ØØZX
ØN9Ø3ZX
ØN9Ø4ZX
ØN91ØZX
ØN913ZX
ØN914ZX
ØN93ØZX
ØN933ZX
ØN934ZX
ØN94ØZX
ØN943ZX
ØN944ZX
ØN95ØZX
ØN953ZX
ØN954ZX
ØN96ØZX
ØN963ZX
ØN964ZX
ØN97ØZX
ØN973ZX
ØN974ZX
ØN9CØZX
ØN9C3ZX
ØN9C4ZX
ØN9FØZX
ØN9F3ZX
ØN9F4ZX
ØN9GØZX
ØN9G3ZX
ØN9G4ZX
ØN9HØZX
ØN9H3ZX
ØN9H4ZX
ØN9JØZX
ØN9J3ZX
ØN9J4ZX
ØN9KØZX
ØN9K3ZX
ØN9K4ZX
ØN9LØZX
ØN9L3ZX
ØN9L4ZX
ØN9MØZX
ØN9M3ZX
ØN9M4ZX
ØN9NØZX
ØN9N3ZX
ØN9N4ZX
ØN9RØZX
ØN9R3ZX
ØN9R4ZX
ØN9TØZX
ØN9T3ZX
ØN9T4ZX
ØN9VØZX
ØN9V3ZX
ØN9V4ZX
ØN9XØZX
ØN9X3ZX
ØN9X4ZX
ØNBØØZX
ØNBØ3ZX
ØNBØ4ZX
ØNB1ØZX
ØNB13ZX
ØNB14ZX
ØNB3ØZX
ØNB33ZX
ØNB34ZX
ØNB4ØZX
ØNB43ZX
ØNB44ZX
ØNB5ØZX
ØNB53ZX
ØNB54ZX
ØNB6ØZX
ØNB63ZX
ØNB64ZX
ØNB7ØZX
ØNB73ZX
ØNB74ZX
ØNBCØZX
ØNBC3ZX
ØNBC4ZX
ØNBFØZX
ØNBF3ZX
ØNBF4ZX
ØNBGØZX
ØNBG3ZX
ØNBG4ZX
ØNBHØZX
ØNBH3ZX
ØNBH4ZX
ØNBJØZX
ØNBJ3ZX
ØNBJ4ZX
ØNBKØZX
ØNBK3ZX
ØNBK4ZX
ØNBLØZX
ØNBL3ZX
ØNBL4ZX
ØNBMØZX
ØNBM3ZX
ØNBM4ZX
ØNBNØZX
ØNBN3ZX
ØNBN4ZX
ØNBXØZX
ØNBX3ZX
ØNBX4ZX
ØNJØØZZ
ØNJØ4ZZ
ØNJBØZZ
ØNJB4ZZ
ØNJWØZZ
ØNJW4ZZ
ØP9ØØZX
ØP9Ø3ZX
ØP9Ø4ZX
ØP91ØZX
ØP913ZX
ØP914ZX
ØP92ØZX
ØP923ZX
ØP924ZX
ØP93ØZX
ØP933ZX
ØP934ZX
ØP94ØZX
ØP943ZX
ØP944ZX
ØP95ØZX
ØP953ZX
ØP954ZX
ØP96ØZX
ØP963ZX
ØP964ZX
ØP97ØZX
ØP973ZX
ØP974ZX
ØP98ØZX
ØP983ZX
ØP984ZX
ØP99ØZX
ØP993ZX
ØP994ZX
ØP9BØZX
ØP9B3ZX
ØP9B4ZX
ØP9CØZX
ØP9C3ZX
ØP9C4ZX
ØP9DØZX
ØP9D3ZX
ØP9D4ZX
ØP9FØZX
ØP9F3ZX
ØP9F4ZX
ØP9GØZX
ØP9G3ZX
ØP9G4ZX
ØP9HØZX
ØP9H3ZX
ØP9H4ZX
ØP9JØZX
ØP9J3ZX
ØP9J4ZX
ØP9KØZX
ØP9K3ZX
ØP9K4ZX
ØP9LØZX
ØP9L3ZX
ØP9L4ZX
ØP9RØZX
ØP9R3ZX
ØP9R4ZX
ØP9SØZX
ØP9S3ZX
ØP9S4ZX
ØP9TØZX
ØP9T3ZX
ØP9T4ZX
ØP9VØZX
ØP9V3ZX
ØP9V4ZX
ØPBØØZX
ØPBØ3ZX
ØPBØ4ZX
ØPB1ØZX
ØPB13ZX
ØPB14ZX
ØPB2ØZX
ØPB23ZX
ØPB24ZX
ØPB3ØZX
ØPB33ZX
ØPB34ZX
ØPB4ØZX
ØPB43ZX
ØPB44ZX
ØPB5ØZX
ØPB53ZX
ØPB54ZX
ØPB6ØZX
ØPB63ZX
ØPB64ZX
ØPB7ØZX
ØPB73ZX
ØPB74ZX
ØPB8ØZX
ØPB83ZX
ØPB84ZX
ØPB9ØZX
ØPB93ZX
ØPB94ZX
ØPBBØZX
ØPBB3ZX
ØPBB4ZX
ØPBCØZX
ØPBC3ZX
ØPBC4ZX
ØPBDØZX
ØPBD3ZX
ØPBD4ZX
ØPBFØZX
ØPBF3ZX
ØPBF4ZX
ØPBGØZX
ØPBG3ZX
ØPBG4ZX
ØPBHØZX
ØPBH3ZX
ØPBH4ZX
ØPBJØZX
ØPBJ3ZX
ØPBJ4ZX
ØPBKØZX
ØPBK3ZX
ØPBK4ZX
ØPBLØZX
ØPBL3ZX
ØPBL4ZX
ØPBRØZX
ØPBR3ZX
ØPBR4ZX
ØPBSØZX
ØPBS3ZX
ØPBS4ZX
ØPBTØZX
ØPBT3ZX
ØPBT4ZX
ØPBVØZX
ØPBV3ZX
ØPBV4ZX
ØPJYØZZ
ØPJY4ZZ
ØQ9ØØZX
ØQ9Ø3ZX
ØQ9Ø4ZX
ØQ91ØZX
ØQ913ZX
ØQ914ZX
ØQ92ØZX
ØQ923ZX
ØQ924ZX
ØQ93ØZX
ØQ933ZX
ØQ934ZX
ØQ94ØZX
ØQ943ZX
ØQ944ZX
ØQ95ØZX
ØQ953ZX
ØQ954ZX
ØQ96ØZX
ØQ963ZX
ØQ964ZX
ØQ97ØZX
ØQ973ZX
ØQ974ZX
ØQ98ØZX
ØQ983ZX
ØQ984ZX
ØQ99ØZX
ØQ993ZX
ØQ994ZX
ØQ9BØZX
ØQ9B3ZX
ØQ9B4ZX
ØQ9CØZX
ØQ9C3ZX
ØQ9C4ZX
ØQ9DØZX
ØQ9D3ZX
ØQ9D4ZX
ØQ9FØZX
ØQ9F3ZX
ØQ9F4ZX
ØQ9GØZX
ØQ9G3ZX
ØQ9G4ZX
ØQ9HØZX
ØQ9H3ZX
ØQ9H4ZX
ØQ9JØZX
ØQ9J3ZX
ØQ9J4ZX
ØQ9KØZX
ØQ9K3ZX
ØQ9K4ZX
ØQ9LØZX
ØQ9L3ZX
ØQ9L4ZX
ØQ9MØZX
ØQ9M3ZX
ØQ9M4ZX
ØQ9NØZX
ØQ9N3ZX
ØQ9N4ZX
ØQ9PØZX
ØQ9P3ZX
ØQ9P4ZX
ØQ9QØZX
ØQ9Q3ZX
ØQ9Q4ZX
ØQ9RØZX
ØQ9R3ZX
ØQ9R4ZX
ØQ9SØZX
ØQ9S3ZX
ØQ9S4ZX
ØQBØØZX
ØQBØ3ZX
ØQBØ4ZX
ØQB1ØZX
ØQB13ZX
ØQB14ZX
ØQB2ØZX
ØQB23ZX
ØQB24ZX
ØQB3ØZX
ØQB33ZX
ØQB34ZX
ØQB4ØZX
ØQB43ZX
ØQB44ZX
ØQB5ØZX
ØQB53ZX
ØQB54ZX
ØQB6ØZX
ØQB63ZX
ØQB64ZX
ØQB7ØZX
ØQB73ZX
ØQB74ZX
ØQB8ØZX
ØQB83ZX
ØQB84ZX
ØQB9ØZX
ØQB93ZX
ØQB94ZX
ØQBBØZX
ØQBB3ZX
ØQBB4ZX
ØQBCØZX
ØQBC3ZX
ØQBC4ZX
ØQBDØZX
ØQBD3ZX
ØQBD4ZX
ØQBFØZX
ØQBF3ZX
ØQBF4ZX
ØQBGØZX
ØQBG3ZX
ØQBG4ZX
ØQBHØZX
ØQBH3ZX
ØQBH4ZX
ØQBJØZX
ØQBJ3ZX
ØQBJ4ZX
ØQBKØZX
ØQBK3ZX
ØQBK4ZX
ØQBLØZX
ØQBL3ZX
ØQBL4ZX
ØQBMØZX
ØQBM3ZX
ØQBM4ZX
ØQBNØZX
ØQBN3ZX
ØQBN4ZX
ØQBPØZX
ØQBP3ZX
ØQBP4ZX
ØQBQØZX
ØQBQ3ZX
ØQBQ4ZX
ØQBRØZX
ØQBR3ZX
ØQBR4ZX
ØQBSØZX
ØQBS3ZX
ØQBS4ZX
ØQJYØZZ
ØQJY4ZZ
ØR9CØZX
ØR9C3ZX
ØR9C4ZX
ØR9DØZX
ØR9D3ZX
ØR9D4ZX
ØRBCØZX
ØRBC3ZX
ØRBC4ZX
ØRBDØZX
ØRBD3ZX
ØRBD4ZX
ØRJCØZZ
ØRJC4ZZ
ØRJDØZZ
ØRJD4ZZ
ØSJ24ZZ
ØSJ44ZZ

DRG 478

Select operating room procedures listed under DRG 477

DRG 479

Select operating room procedures listed under DRG 477

DRG 480

Operating Room Procedures

ØL8J*
ØL8K*
ØM9L4ZZ
ØM9M4ZZ
ØQ86*
ØQ87*
ØQ88*
ØQ89*
ØQ8B*
ØQ8C*
ØQC6*
ØQC7*
ØQC8*
ØQC9*
ØQCB*
ØQCC*
ØQH6Ø4Z
ØQH6Ø5Z
ØQH6Ø6Z
ØQH6ØBZ
ØQH6ØCZ
ØQH6ØDZ
ØQH634Z
ØQH635Z
ØQH636Z
ØQH63BZ
ØQH63CZ
ØQH63DZ
ØQH644Z
ØQH645Z
ØQH646Z
ØQH64BZ
ØQH64CZ
ØQH64DZ
ØQH7Ø4Z
ØQH7Ø5Z
ØQH7Ø6Z
ØQH7ØBZ
ØQH7ØCZ
ØQH7ØDZ
ØQH734Z
ØQH735Z
ØQH736Z
ØQH73BZ
ØQH73CZ
ØQH73DZ
ØQH744Z
ØQH745Z
ØQH746Z
ØQH74BZ
ØQH74CZ
ØQH74DZ
ØQH8Ø4Z
ØQH8Ø5Z
ØQH8Ø6Z
ØQH8Ø7Z
ØQH8ØBZ
ØQH8ØCZ
ØQH8ØDZ
ØQH834Z
ØQH835Z
ØQH836Z
ØQH837Z
ØQH83BZ
ØQH83CZ
ØQH83DZ
ØQH844Z
ØQH845Z
ØQH846Z
ØQH847Z
ØQH84BZ
ØQH84CZ
ØQH84DZ
ØQH9Ø4Z
ØQH9Ø5Z
ØQH9Ø6Z
ØQH9Ø7Z
ØQH9ØBZ
ØQH9ØCZ
ØQH9ØDZ
ØQH934Z
ØQH935Z
ØQH936Z
ØQH937Z
ØQH93BZ
ØQH93CZ
ØQH93DZ
ØQH944Z
ØQH945Z
ØQH946Z
ØQH947Z
ØQH94BZ
ØQH94CZ
ØQH94DZ
ØQHBØ4Z
ØQHBØ5Z
ØQHBØ6Z
ØQHBØBZ
ØQHBØCZ
ØQHBØDZ
ØQHB34Z
ØQHB35Z
ØQHB36Z
ØQHB3BZ
ØQHB3CZ
ØQHB3DZ
ØQHB44Z
ØQHB45Z
ØQHB46Z
ØQHB4BZ
ØQHB4CZ
ØQHB4DZ
ØQHCØ4Z
ØQHCØ5Z
ØQHCØ6Z
ØQHCØBZ
ØQHCØCZ
ØQHCØDZ
ØQHC34Z
ØQHC35Z
ØQHC36Z
ØQHC3BZ
ØQHC3CZ
ØQHC3DZ
ØQHC44Z
ØQHC45Z
ØQHC46Z
ØQHC4BZ
ØQHC4CZ
ØQHC4DZ
ØQN6*
ØQN7*
ØQN8*
ØQN9*
ØQNB*
ØQNC*
ØQQ6ØZZ
ØQQ63ZZ
ØQQ64ZZ
ØQQ7ØZZ
ØQQ73ZZ
ØQQ74ZZ
ØQQ8ØZZ
ØQQ83ZZ
ØQQ84ZZ
ØQQ9ØZZ
ØQQ93ZZ
ØQQ94ZZ
ØQQBØZZ
ØQQB3ZZ
ØQQB4ZZ
ØQQCØZZ
ØQQC3ZZ
ØQQC4ZZ
ØQR6*
ØQR7*
ØQR8*
ØQR9*
ØQRB*
ØQRC*
ØQS6Ø4Z
ØQS6Ø5Z
ØQS6Ø6Z
ØQS6ØBZ
ØQS6ØCZ
ØQS6ØDZ
ØQS6ØZZ
ØQS634Z
ØQS635Z
ØQS636Z
ØQS63BZ
ØQS63CZ
ØQS63DZ
ØQS644Z
ØQS645Z
ØQS646Z
ØQS64BZ
ØQS64CZ
ØQS64DZ
ØQS7Ø4Z
ØQS7Ø5Z
ØQS7Ø6Z
ØQS7ØBZ
ØQS7ØCZ
ØQS7ØDZ
ØQS7ØZZ
ØQS734Z
ØQS735Z
ØQS736Z
ØQS73BZ
ØQS73CZ
ØQS73DZ
ØQS744Z
ØQS745Z
ØQS746Z
ØQS74BZ
ØQS74CZ
ØQS74DZ
ØQS8Ø4Z
ØQS8Ø5Z
ØQS8Ø6Z
ØQS8ØBZ
ØQS8ØCZ
ØQS8ØDZ
ØQS8ØZZ
ØQS834Z
ØQS835Z
ØQS836Z
ØQS83BZ
ØQS83CZ
ØQS83DZ
ØQS844Z
ØQS845Z
ØQS846Z
ØQS84BZ
ØQS84CZ
ØQS84DZ
ØQS9Ø4Z
ØQS9Ø5Z
ØQS9Ø6Z
ØQS9ØBZ
ØQS9ØCZ

ØQS9ØDZ
ØQS9ØZZ
ØQS934Z
ØQS935Z
ØQS936Z
ØQS93BZ
ØQS93CZ
ØQS93DZ
ØQS944Z
ØQS945Z
ØQS946Z
ØQS94BZ
ØQS94CZ
ØQS94DZ
ØQSBØ4Z
ØQSBØ5Z
ØQSBØ6Z
ØQSBØBZ
ØQSBØCZ
ØQSBØDZ
ØQSBØZZ
ØQSB34Z
ØQSB35Z
ØQSB36Z
ØQSB3BZ
ØQSB3CZ
ØQSB3DZ
ØQSB44Z
ØQSB45Z
ØQSB46Z
ØQSB4BZ
ØQSB4CZ
ØQSB4DZ
ØQSCØ4Z
ØQSCØ5Z
ØQSCØ6Z
ØQSCØBZ
ØQSCØCZ
ØQSCØDZ
ØQSCØZZ
ØQSC34Z
ØQSC35Z
ØQSC36Z
ØQSC3BZ
ØQSC3CZ
ØQSC3DZ
ØQSC44Z
ØQSC45Z
ØQSC46Z
ØQSC4BZ
ØQSC4CZ
ØQSC4DZ
ØQT6ØZZ
ØQT7ØZZ
ØQT8ØZZ
ØQT9ØZZ
ØQTBØZZ
ØQTCØZZ
ØQU6*
ØQU7*
ØQU8*
ØQU9*
ØQUB*
ØQUC*
ØS99ØØZ
ØS99ØZZ
ØS9BØØZ
ØS9BØZZ
ØSB9ØZZ
ØSB93ZZ
ØSB94ZZ
ØSBBØZZ
ØSBB3ZZ
ØSBB4ZZ
ØSC9*
ØSCB*
ØSG9*
ØSGB*
ØSH9Ø4Z
ØSH9Ø5Z
ØSH9Ø8Z
ØSH934Z
ØSH935Z
ØSH944Z
ØSH945Z
ØSHBØ4Z
ØSHBØ5Z
ØSHBØ8Z
ØSHB34Z
ØSHB35Z
ØSHB44Z
ØSHB45Z
ØSJ9ØZZ
ØSJBØZZ
ØSN9ØZZ
ØSN93ZZ
ØSN94ZZ
ØSNBØZZ
ØSNB3ZZ
ØSNB4ZZ
ØSP9ØØZ
ØSP9Ø3Z
ØSP9Ø4Z
ØSP9Ø5Z
ØSP9Ø7Z
ØSP9Ø8Z
ØSP9ØBZ
ØSP9ØEZ
ØSP9ØKZ
ØSP934Z
ØSP935Z
ØSP937Z
ØSP93KZ
ØSP94ØZ
ØSP943Z
ØSP944Z
ØSP945Z
ØSP947Z
ØSP94KZ
ØSPBØØZ
ØSPBØ3Z
ØSPBØ4Z
ØSPBØ5Z
ØSPBØ7Z
ØSPBØ8Z
ØSPBØBZ
ØSPBØEZ
ØSPBØKZ
ØSPB34Z
ØSPB35Z
ØSPB37Z
ØSPB3KZ
ØSPB4ØZ
ØSPB43Z
ØSPB44Z
ØSPB45Z
ØSPB47Z
ØSPB4KZ
ØSQ9ØZZ
ØSQ93ZZ
ØSQ94ZZ
ØSQBØZZ
ØSQB3ZZ
ØSQB4ZZ
ØSR9ØEZ
ØSRBØEZ
ØSS9Ø4Z
ØSS9Ø5Z
ØSS9ØZZ
ØSS934Z
ØSSBØ4Z
ØSSBØ5Z
ØSSBØZZ
ØSSB34Z
ØST9ØZZ
ØSTBØZZ
ØSW9ØØZ
ØSW9Ø3Z
ØSW9Ø4Z
ØSW9Ø5Z
ØSW9Ø7Z
ØSW9Ø8Z
ØSW9Ø9Z
ØSW9ØBZ
ØSW9ØKZ
ØSW93ØZ
ØSW933Z
ØSW934Z
ØSW935Z
ØSW937Z
ØSW938Z
ØSW93KZ
ØSW94ØZ
ØSW943Z
ØSW944Z
ØSW945Z
ØSW947Z
ØSW948Z
ØSW94KZ
ØSWBØØZ
ØSWBØ3Z
ØSWBØ4Z
ØSWBØ5Z
ØSWBØ7Z
ØSWBØ8Z
ØSWBØ9Z
ØSWBØBZ
ØSWBØKZ
ØSWB3ØZ
ØSWB33Z
ØSWB34Z
ØSWB35Z
ØSWB37Z
ØSWB38Z
ØSWB3KZ
ØSWB4ØZ
ØSWB43Z
ØSWB44Z
ØSWB45Z
ØSWB47Z
ØSWB48Z
ØSWB4KZ

DRG 481

Select operating room procedures listed under DRG 480

DRG 482

Select operating room procedures listed under DRG 480

DRG 483

Operating Room Procedures

ØRRE*
ØRRF*
ØRRG*
ØRRH*
ØRRJ*
ØRRK*
ØRRL*
ØRRM*
ØRRN*
ØRRP*
ØXMØØZZ
ØXM1ØZZ
ØXM2ØZZ
ØXM3ØZZ
ØXM4ØZZ
ØXM5ØZZ
ØXM6ØZZ
ØXM7ØZZ
ØXM8ØZZ
ØXM9ØZZ
ØXMBØZZ
ØXMCØZZ
ØXMDØZZ
ØXMFØZZ
ØXMGØZZ
ØXMHØZZ
ØXMJØZZ
ØXMKØZZ

DRG 485

Principal Diagnosis

A18.Ø2
A54.42
MØØ.Ø6*
MØØ.161
MØØ.162
MØØ.169
MØØ.261
MØØ.262
MØØ.269
MØØ.861
MØØ.862
MØØ.869
MØØ.9
MØ1.X61
MØ1.X62
MØ1.X69
M71.Ø61
M71.Ø62
M71.Ø69
M71.161
M71.162
M71.169
M86.Ø61
M86.Ø62
M86.Ø69
M86.161
M86.162
M86.169
M86.261
M86.262
M86.269
M86.361
M86.362
M86.369
M86.461
M86.462
M86.469
M86.561
M86.562
M86.569
M86.661
M86.662
M86.669
M86.8X6
T84.53XA
T84.54XA
T84.62ØA
T84.621A
T84.622A
T84.623A
T84.624A
T84.625A
T84.629A
T84.7XXA

AND

Operating Room Procedures

ØM9N4ØZ
ØM9P4ØZ
ØMQN*
ØMQP*
ØMRNØ7Z
ØMRNØJZ
ØMRNØKZ
ØMRN47Z
ØMRN4JZ
ØMRN4KZ
ØMRPØ7Z
ØMRPØJZ
ØMRPØKZ
ØMRP47Z
ØMRP4JZ
ØMRP4KZ
ØQ8D*
ØQ8F*
ØQBDØZZ
ØQBD3ZZ
ØQBD4ZZ
ØQBFØZZ
ØQBF3ZZ
ØQBF4ZZ
ØQCD*
ØQCF*
ØQHD*
ØQHF*
ØQND*
ØQNF*
ØQQDØZZ
ØQQD4ZZ
ØQQFØZZ
ØQQF4ZZ
ØQRD*
ØQRF*
ØQSDØ5Z
ØQSD35Z
ØQSD45Z
ØQSFØ5Z
ØQSF35Z
ØQSF45Z
ØQTDØZZ
ØQTFØZZ
ØQUD*
ØQUF*
ØS9CØØZ
ØS9CØZZ
ØS9DØØZ
ØS9DØZZ
ØSBCØZZ
ØSBC3ZZ
ØSBC4ZZ
ØSBDØZZ
ØSBD3ZZ
ØSBD4ZZ
ØSCC*
ØSCD*
ØSGC*
ØSGD*
ØSHCØ4Z
ØSHCØ5Z
ØSHCØ8Z
ØSHC34Z
ØSHC35Z
ØSHC44Z
ØSHC45Z
ØSHDØ4Z
ØSHDØ5Z
ØSHDØ8Z
ØSHD34Z
ØSHD35Z
ØSHD44Z
ØSHD45Z
ØSJCØZZ
ØSJDØZZ
ØSNCØZZ
ØSNC3ZZ
ØSNC4ZZ
ØSNDØZZ
ØSND3ZZ
ØSND4ZZ
ØSPCØØZ
ØSPCØ3Z
ØSPCØ4Z
ØSPCØ5Z
ØSPCØ7Z
ØSPCØ8Z
ØSPCØEZ
ØSPCØKZ
ØSPC34Z
ØSPC35Z
ØSPC37Z
ØSPC3KZ
ØSPC4ØZ
ØSPC43Z
ØSPC44Z
ØSPC45Z
ØSPC47Z
ØSPC4KZ
ØSPDØØZ
ØSPDØ3Z
ØSPDØ4Z
ØSPDØ5Z
ØSPDØ7Z
ØSPDØ8Z
ØSPDØEZ
ØSPDØKZ
ØSPD34Z
ØSPD35Z
ØSPD37Z
ØSPD3KZ
ØSPD4ØZ
ØSPD43Z
ØSPD44Z
ØSPD45Z
ØSPD47Z
ØSPD4KZ
ØSQCØZZ
ØSQC3ZZ
ØSQC4ZZ
ØSQDØZZ
ØSQD3ZZ
ØSQD4ZZ
ØSRCØEZ
ØSRDØEZ
ØSSCØ4Z
ØSSCØ5Z
ØSSCØZZ
ØSSDØ4Z
ØSSDØ5Z
ØSSDØZZ
ØSTCØZZ
ØSTDØZZ
ØSWCØØZ
ØSWCØ3Z
ØSWCØ4Z
ØSWCØ5Z
ØSWCØ7Z
ØSWCØ8Z
ØSWCØ9Z
ØSWCØKZ
ØSWC3ØZ
ØSWC33Z
ØSWC34Z
ØSWC35Z
ØSWC37Z
ØSWC38Z
ØSWC3KZ
ØSWC4ØZ
ØSWC43Z
ØSWC44Z
ØSWC45Z
ØSWC47Z
ØSWC48Z
ØSWC4KZ
ØSWDØØZ
ØSWDØ3Z
ØSWDØ4Z
ØSWDØ5Z
ØSWDØ7Z
ØSWDØ8Z
ØSWDØ9Z
ØSWDØKZ
ØSWD3ØZ
ØSWD33Z
ØSWD34Z
ØSWD35Z
ØSWD37Z
ØSWD38Z
ØSWD3KZ
ØSWD4ØZ
ØSWD43Z
ØSWD44Z
ØSWD45Z
ØSWD47Z
ØSWD48Z
ØSWD4KZ

OR

ØSUVØ9Z

AND

ØSPCØ9Z

OR

ØSUWØ9Z

AND

ØSPDØ9Z

DRG 486

Select principal diagnosis AND operating room procedures or procedure combinations listed under DRG 485

DRG 487

Select principal diagnosis AND operating room procedures or procedure combinations listed under DRG 485

DRG 488

Select only operating room procedures or procedure combinations under DRG 485

DRG 489

Select only operating room procedures or procedure combinations under DRG 485

DRG 492

Operating Room Procedures

ØM5Q*
ØM5R*
ØM9Q4ØZ
ØM9R4ØZ
ØP8C*
ØP8D*
ØP8F*
ØP8G*
ØPBCØZZ
ØPBC3ZZ
ØPBC4ZZ
ØPBDØZZ
ØPBD3ZZ
ØPBD4ZZ
ØPBFØZZ
ØPBF3ZZ
ØPBF4ZZ
ØPBGØZZ
ØPBG3ZZ
ØPBG4ZZ
ØPCC*
ØPCD*
ØPCF*
ØPCG*
ØPHCØ4Z
ØPHCØ5Z
ØPHCØ6Z
ØPHCØBZ
ØPHCØCZ
ØPHCØDZ
ØPHC34Z
ØPHC35Z
ØPHC36Z
ØPHC3BZ
ØPHC3CZ
ØPHC3DZ
ØPHC44Z
ØPHC45Z
ØPHC46Z
ØPHC4BZ
ØPHC4CZ
ØPHC4DZ
ØPHDØ4Z
ØPHDØ5Z
ØPHDØ6Z
ØPHDØBZ
ØPHDØCZ
ØPHDØDZ
ØPHD34Z
ØPHD35Z
ØPHD36Z
ØPHD3BZ
ØPHD3CZ
ØPHD3DZ
ØPHD44Z
ØPHD45Z
ØPHD46Z
ØPHD4BZ
ØPHD4CZ
ØPHD4DZ
ØPHFØ4Z
ØPHFØ5Z
ØPHFØ6Z
ØPHFØ7Z
ØPHFØBZ
ØPHFØCZ
ØPHFØDZ
ØPHF34Z
ØPHF35Z
ØPHF36Z
ØPHF37Z
ØPHF3BZ
ØPHF3CZ
ØPHF3DZ
ØPHF44Z
ØPHF45Z
ØPHF46Z
ØPHF47Z
ØPHF4BZ
ØPHF4CZ
ØPHF4DZ
ØPHGØ4Z
ØPHGØ5Z
ØPHGØ6Z
ØPHGØ7Z
ØPHGØBZ
ØPHGØCZ
ØPHGØDZ
ØPHG34Z
ØPHG35Z
ØPHG36Z
ØPHG37Z
ØPHG3BZ
ØPHG3CZ
ØPHG3DZ
ØPHG44Z
ØPHG45Z
ØPHG46Z
ØPHG47Z
ØPHG4BZ
ØPHG4CZ
ØPHG4DZ
ØPNC*
ØPND*
ØPNF*
ØPNG*
ØPQCØZZ
ØPQC3ZZ
ØPQC4ZZ
ØPQDØZZ
ØPQD3ZZ
ØPQD4ZZ
ØPQFØZZ
ØPQF3ZZ
ØPQF4ZZ
ØPQGØZZ
ØPQG3ZZ
ØPQG4ZZ
ØPRCØ7Z
ØPRCØJZ
ØPRCØKZ
ØPRC37Z
ØPRC3JZ
ØPRC3KZ
ØPRC47Z
ØPRC4JZ
ØPRC4KZ
ØPRDØ7Z
ØPRDØJZ
ØPRDØKZ
ØPRD37Z
ØPRD3JZ
ØPRD3KZ
ØPRD47Z
ØPRD4JZ
ØPRD4KZ
ØPRF*
ØPRG*
ØPSCØ4Z
ØPSCØ5Z
ØPSCØ6Z
ØPSCØBZ
ØPSCØCZ
ØPSCØDZ
ØPSCØZZ
ØPSC34Z
ØPSC35Z
ØPSC36Z
ØPSC3BZ
ØPSC3CZ
ØPSC3DZ
ØPSC44Z
ØPSC45Z
ØPSC46Z
ØPSC4BZ
ØPSC4CZ
ØPSC4DZ
ØPSDØ4Z
ØPSDØ5Z
ØPSDØ6Z
ØPSDØBZ
ØPSDØCZ
ØPSDØDZ
ØPSDØZZ
ØPSD34Z
ØPSD35Z
ØPSD36Z
ØPSD3BZ
ØPSD3CZ
ØPSD3DZ
ØPSD44Z
ØPSD45Z
ØPSD46Z
ØPSD4BZ
ØPSD4CZ
ØPSD4DZ
ØPSFØ4Z
ØPSFØ5Z
ØPSFØ6Z
ØPSFØBZ
ØPSFØCZ
ØPSFØDZ
ØPSFØZZ
ØPSF34Z
ØPSF35Z
ØPSF36Z
ØPSF3BZ
ØPSF3CZ
ØPSF3DZ
ØPSF44Z
ØPSF45Z
ØPSF46Z
ØPSF4BZ
ØPSF4CZ
ØPSF4DZ
ØPSGØ4Z
ØPSGØ5Z
ØPSGØ6Z
ØPSGØBZ
ØPSGØCZ
ØPSGØDZ
ØPSGØZZ
ØPSG34Z
ØPSG35Z
ØPSG36Z
ØPSG3BZ
ØPSG3CZ
ØPSG3DZ
ØPSG44Z
ØPSG45Z
ØPSG46Z
ØPSG4BZ
ØPSG4CZ
ØPSG4DZ
ØPTCØZZ
ØPTDØZZ
ØPTFØZZ
ØPTGØZZ
ØPUC*
ØPUD*
ØPUF*
ØPUG*
ØQ8G*
ØQ8H*
ØQ8J*
ØQ8K*
ØQBGØZZ
ØQBG3ZZ
ØQBG4ZZ
ØQBHØZZ
ØQBH3ZZ
ØQBH4ZZ
ØQBJØZZ
ØQBJ3ZZ
ØQBJ4ZZ
ØQBKØZZ
ØQBK3ZZ
ØQBK4ZZ
ØQCG*
ØQCH*
ØQCJ*
ØQCK*
ØQHGØ4Z
ØQHGØ5Z
ØQHGØ6Z
ØQHGØ7Z
ØQHGØBZ
ØQHGØCZ
ØQHGØDZ
ØQHG34Z
ØQHG35Z
ØQHG36Z
ØQHG37Z
ØQHG3BZ
ØQHG3CZ
ØQHG3DZ
ØQHG44Z
ØQHG45Z
ØQHG46Z
ØQHG47Z
ØQHG4BZ
ØQHG4CZ
ØQHG4DZ
ØQHHØ4Z
ØQHHØ5Z
ØQHHØ6Z
ØQHHØ7Z
ØQHHØBZ
ØQHHØCZ
ØQHHØDZ
ØQHH34Z
ØQHH35Z
ØQHH36Z
ØQHH37Z
ØQHH3BZ
ØQHH3CZ
ØQHH3DZ
ØQHH44Z
ØQHH45Z
ØQHH46Z
ØQHH47Z
ØQHH4BZ
ØQHH4CZ
ØQHH4DZ
ØQHJØ4Z
ØQHJØ5Z
ØQHJØ6Z
ØQHJØBZ
ØQHJØCZ
ØQHJØDZ
ØQHJ34Z
ØQHJ35Z
ØQHJ36Z
ØQHJ3BZ
ØQHJ3CZ
ØQHJ3DZ
ØQHJ44Z
ØQHJ45Z
ØQHJ46Z
ØQHJ4BZ
ØQHJ4CZ
ØQHJ4DZ
ØQHKØ4Z
ØQHKØ5Z
ØQHKØ6Z
ØQHKØBZ
ØQHKØCZ
ØQHKØDZ
ØQHK34Z
ØQHK35Z
ØQHK36Z
ØQHK3BZ
ØQHK3CZ
ØQHK3DZ
ØQHK44Z
ØQHK45Z
ØQHK46Z
ØQHK4BZ
ØQHK4CZ
ØQHK4DZ
ØQNG*
ØQNH*
ØQNJ*
ØQNK*
ØQQGØZZ
ØQQG3ZZ
ØQQG4ZZ

ØQQHØZZ
ØQQH3ZZ
ØQQH4ZZ
ØQQJØZZ
ØQQJ3ZZ
ØQQJ4ZZ
ØQQKØZZ
ØQQK3ZZ
ØQQK4ZZ
ØQRG*
ØQRH*
ØQRJ*
ØQRK*
ØQSGØ4Z
ØQSGØ5Z
ØQSGØ6Z
ØQSGØBZ
ØQSGØCZ
ØQSGØDZ
ØQSGØZZ
ØQSG34Z
ØQSG35Z
ØQSG36Z
ØQSG3BZ
ØQSG3CZ
ØQSG3DZ
ØQSG44Z
ØQSG45Z
ØQSG46Z
ØQSG4BZ
ØQSG4CZ
ØQSG4DZ
ØQSHØ4Z
ØQSHØ5Z
ØQSHØ6Z
ØQSHØBZ
ØQSHØCZ
ØQSHØDZ
ØQSHØZZ
ØQSH34Z
ØQSH35Z
ØQSH36Z
ØQSH3BZ
ØQSH3CZ
ØQSH3DZ
ØQSH44Z
ØQSH45Z
ØQSH46Z
ØQSH4BZ
ØQSH4CZ
ØQSH4DZ
ØQSJØ4Z
ØQSJØ5Z
ØQSJØ6Z
ØQSJØBZ
ØQSJØCZ
ØQSJØDZ
ØQSJØZZ
ØQSJ34Z
ØQSJ35Z
ØQSJ36Z
ØQSJ3BZ
ØQSJ3CZ
ØQSJ3DZ
ØQSJ44Z
ØQSJ45Z
ØQSJ46Z
ØQSJ4BZ
ØQSJ4CZ
ØQSJ4DZ
ØQSKØ4Z
ØQSKØ5Z
ØQSKØ6Z
ØQSKØBZ
ØQSKØCZ
ØQSKØDZ
ØQSKØZZ
ØQSK34Z
ØQSK35Z
ØQSK36Z
ØQSK3BZ
ØQSK3CZ
ØQSK3DZ
ØQSK44Z
ØQSK45Z
ØQSK46Z
ØQSK4BZ
ØQSK4CZ
ØQSK4DZ
ØQTGØZZ
ØQTHØZZ
ØQTJØZZ
ØQTKØZZ
ØQUG*
ØQUH*
ØQUJ*
ØQUK*
ØS5F*
ØS5G*
ØS9FØØZ
ØS9FØZZ
ØS9GØØZ
ØS9GØZZ
ØSBFØZZ
ØSBF3ZZ
ØSBF4ZZ
ØSBGØZZ
ØSBG3ZZ
ØSBG4ZZ
ØSCF*
ØSCG*
ØSGF*
ØSGG*
ØSHFØ4Z
ØSHFØ5Z
ØSHF34Z
ØSHF35Z
ØSHF44Z
ØSHF45Z
ØSHGØ4Z
ØSHGØ5Z
ØSHG34Z
ØSHG35Z
ØSHG44Z
ØSHG45Z
ØSJFØZZ
ØSJGØZZ
ØSNFØZZ
ØSNF3ZZ
ØSNF4ZZ
ØSNGØZZ
ØSNG3ZZ
ØSNG4ZZ
ØSPFØØZ
ØSPFØ3Z
ØSPFØ4Z
ØSPFØ5Z
ØSPFØ7Z
ØSPFØKZ
ØSPF34Z
ØSPF35Z
ØSPF37Z
ØSPF3KZ
ØSPF4ØZ
ØSPF43Z
ØSPF44Z
ØSPF45Z
ØSPF47Z
ØSPF4KZ
ØSPGØØZ
ØSPGØ3Z
ØSPGØ4Z
ØSPGØ5Z
ØSPGØ7Z
ØSPGØKZ
ØSPG34Z
ØSPG35Z
ØSPG37Z
ØSPG3KZ
ØSPG4ØZ
ØSPG43Z
ØSPG44Z
ØSPG45Z
ØSPG47Z
ØSPG4KZ
ØSQFØZZ
ØSQF3ZZ
ØSQF4ZZ
ØSQGØZZ
ØSQG3ZZ
ØSQG4ZZ
ØSSFØ4Z
ØSSFØ5Z
ØSSFØZZ
ØSSGØ4Z
ØSSGØ5Z
ØSSGØZZ
ØSTFØZZ
ØSTGØZZ
ØSWFØØZ
ØSWFØ3Z
ØSWFØ4Z
ØSWFØ5Z
ØSWFØ7Z
ØSWFØ8Z
ØSWFØKZ
ØSWF3ØZ
ØSWF33Z
ØSWF34Z
ØSWF35Z
ØSWF37Z
ØSWF38Z
ØSWF3KZ
ØSWF4ØZ
ØSWF43Z
ØSWF44Z
ØSWF45Z
ØSWF47Z
ØSWF48Z
ØSWF4KZ
ØSWGØØZ
ØSWGØ3Z
ØSWGØ4Z
ØSWGØ5Z
ØSWGØ7Z
ØSWGØ8Z
ØSWGØKZ
ØSWG3ØZ
ØSWG33Z
ØSWG34Z
ØSWG35Z
ØSWG37Z
ØSWG38Z
ØSWG3KZ
ØSWG4ØZ
ØSWG43Z
ØSWG44Z
ØSWG45Z
ØSWG47Z
ØSWG48Z
ØSWG4KZ
XRGJØB9
XRGKØB9

DRG 493

Select operating room procedures listed under DRG 492

DRG 494

Select operating room procedures listed under DRG 492

DRG 495

Operating Room Procedures

ØM5Ø*
ØM51*
ØM52*
ØM53*
ØM54*
ØM59*
ØM5B*
ØM5C*
ØM5D*
ØM5F*
ØM5G*
ØM5H*
ØM5J*
ØM5K*
ØM5N*
ØM5P*
ØM5V*
ØM5W*
ØN5B*
ØN5C*
ØN5F*
ØN5G*
ØN5H*
ØN5J*
ØN5K*
ØN5L*
ØN5M*
ØN5N*
ØN5P*
ØN5Q*
ØN5R*
ØN5T*
ØN5V*
ØN5X*
ØNPWØØZ
ØNPWØ4Z
ØNPWØ7Z
ØNPWØKZ
ØNPWØMZ
ØNPW3ØZ
ØNPW34Z
ØNPW37Z
ØNPW3KZ
ØNPW3MZ
ØNPW4ØZ
ØNPW44Z
ØNPW47Z
ØNPW4KZ
ØNPW4MZ
ØNPWX4Z
ØP5Ø*
ØP51*
ØP52*
ØP54*
ØP55*
ØP56*
ØP57*
ØP58*
ØP59*
ØP5B*
ØP5C*
ØP5D*
ØP5F*
ØP5G*
ØP5H*
ØP5J*
ØP5K*
ØP5L*
ØP5R*
ØP5S*
ØP5T*
ØP5V*
ØP9ØØØZ
ØP9ØØZZ
ØP9Ø4ØZ
ØP9Ø4ZZ
ØP91ØØZ
ØP91ØZZ
ØP914ØZ
ØP914ZZ
ØP92ØØZ
ØP92ØZZ
ØP924ØZ
ØP924ZZ
ØP93ØØZ
ØP93ØZZ
ØP934ØZ
ØP934ZZ
ØP94ØØZ
ØP94ØZZ
ØP944ØZ
ØP944ZZ
ØP95ØØZ
ØP95ØZZ
ØP954ØZ
ØP954ZZ
ØP96ØØZ
ØP96ØZZ
ØP964ØZ
ØP964ZZ
ØP97ØØZ
ØP97ØZZ
ØP974ØZ
ØP974ZZ
ØP98ØØZ
ØP98ØZZ
ØP984ØZ
ØP984ZZ
ØP99ØØZ
ØP99ØZZ
ØP994ØZ
ØP994ZZ
ØP9BØØZ
ØP9BØZZ
ØP9B4ØZ
ØP9B4ZZ
ØP9CØØZ
ØP9CØZZ
ØP9C4ØZ
ØP9C4ZZ
ØP9DØØZ
ØP9DØZZ
ØP9D4ØZ
ØP9D4ZZ
ØP9FØØZ
ØP9FØZZ
ØP9F4ØZ
ØP9F4ZZ
ØP9GØØZ
ØP9GØZZ
ØP9G4ØZ
ØP9G4ZZ
ØP9HØØZ
ØP9HØZZ
ØP9H4ØZ
ØP9H4ZZ
ØP9JØØZ
ØP9JØZZ
ØP9J4ØZ
ØP9J4ZZ
ØP9KØØZ
ØP9KØZZ
ØP9K4ØZ
ØP9K4ZZ
ØP9LØØZ
ØP9LØZZ
ØP9L4ØZ
ØP9L4ZZ
ØP9RØØZ
ØP9RØZZ
ØP9R4ØZ
ØP9R4ZZ
ØP9SØØZ
ØP9SØZZ
ØP9S4ØZ
ØP9S4ZZ
ØP9TØØZ
ØP9TØZZ
ØP9T4ØZ
ØP9T4ZZ
ØP9VØØZ
ØP9VØZZ
ØP9V4ØZ
ØP9V4ZZ
ØPPØØ4Z
ØPPØØ7Z
ØPPØØJZ
ØPPØØKZ
ØPPØ34Z
ØPPØ37Z
ØPPØ3JZ
ØPPØ3KZ
ØPPØ44Z
ØPPØ47Z
ØPPØ4JZ
ØPPØ4KZ
ØPP1Ø4Z
ØPP1Ø7Z
ØPP1ØJZ
ØPP1ØKZ
ØPP134Z
ØPP137Z
ØPP13JZ
ØPP13KZ
ØPP144Z
ØPP147Z
ØPP14JZ
ØPP14KZ
ØPP2Ø4Z
ØPP2Ø7Z
ØPP2ØJZ
ØPP2ØKZ
ØPP234Z
ØPP237Z
ØPP23JZ
ØPP23KZ
ØPP244Z
ØPP247Z
ØPP24JZ
ØPP24KZ
ØPP3Ø4Z
ØPP3Ø7Z
ØPP3ØJZ
ØPP3ØKZ
ØPP334Z
ØPP337Z
ØPP33JZ
ØPP33KZ
ØPP344Z
ØPP347Z
ØPP34JZ
ØPP34KZ
ØPP4Ø4Z
ØPP4Ø7Z
ØPP4ØJZ
ØPP4ØKZ
ØPP434Z
ØPP437Z
ØPP43JZ
ØPP43KZ
ØPP444Z
ØPP447Z
ØPP44JZ
ØPP44KZ
ØPP5Ø4Z
ØPP5Ø7Z
ØPP5ØJZ
ØPP5ØKZ
ØPP534Z
ØPP537Z
ØPP53JZ
ØPP53KZ
ØPP544Z
ØPP547Z
ØPP54JZ
ØPP54KZ
ØPP6Ø4Z
ØPP6Ø7Z
ØPP6ØJZ
ØPP6ØKZ
ØPP634Z
ØPP637Z
ØPP63JZ
ØPP63KZ
ØPP644Z
ØPP647Z
ØPP64JZ
ØPP64KZ
ØPP7Ø4Z
ØPP7Ø7Z
ØPP7ØJZ
ØPP7ØKZ
ØPP734Z
ØPP737Z
ØPP73JZ
ØPP73KZ
ØPP744Z
ØPP747Z
ØPP74JZ
ØPP74KZ
ØPP8Ø4Z
ØPP8Ø7Z
ØPP8ØJZ
ØPP8ØKZ
ØPP834Z
ØPP837Z
ØPP83JZ
ØPP83KZ
ØPP844Z
ØPP847Z
ØPP84JZ
ØPP84KZ
ØPP9Ø4Z
ØPP9Ø7Z
ØPP9ØJZ
ØPP9ØKZ
ØPP934Z
ØPP937Z
ØPP93JZ
ØPP93KZ
ØPP944Z
ØPP947Z
ØPP94JZ
ØPP94KZ
ØPPBØ4Z
ØPPBØ7Z
ØPPBØJZ
ØPPBØKZ
ØPPB34Z
ØPPB37Z
ØPPB3JZ
ØPPB3KZ
ØPPB44Z
ØPPB47Z
ØPPB4JZ
ØPPB4KZ
ØPPCØ4Z
ØPPCØ5Z
ØPPCØ7Z
ØPPCØJZ
ØPPCØKZ
ØPPC34Z
ØPPC35Z
ØPPC37Z
ØPPC3JZ
ØPPC3KZ
ØPPC44Z
ØPPC45Z
ØPPC47Z
ØPPC4JZ
ØPPC4KZ
ØPPDØ4Z
ØPPDØ5Z
ØPPDØ7Z
ØPPDØJZ
ØPPDØKZ
ØPPD34Z
ØPPD35Z
ØPPD37Z
ØPPD3JZ
ØPPD3KZ
ØPPD44Z
ØPPD45Z
ØPPD47Z
ØPPD4JZ
ØPPD4KZ
ØPPFØ4Z
ØPPFØ5Z
ØPPFØ7Z
ØPPFØJZ
ØPPFØKZ
ØPPF34Z
ØPPF35Z
ØPPF37Z
ØPPF3JZ
ØPPF3KZ
ØPPF44Z
ØPPF45Z
ØPPF47Z
ØPPF4JZ
ØPPF4KZ
ØPPGØ4Z
ØPPGØ5Z
ØPPGØ7Z
ØPPGØJZ
ØPPGØKZ
ØPPG34Z
ØPPG35Z
ØPPG37Z
ØPPG3JZ
ØPPG3KZ
ØPPG44Z
ØPPG45Z
ØPPG47Z
ØPPG4JZ
ØPPG4KZ
ØPPHØ4Z
ØPPHØ5Z
ØPPHØ7Z
ØPPHØJZ
ØPPHØKZ
ØPPH34Z
ØPPH35Z
ØPPH37Z
ØPPH3JZ
ØPPH3KZ
ØPPH44Z
ØPPH45Z
ØPPH47Z
ØPPH4JZ
ØPPH4KZ
ØPPJØ4Z
ØPPJØ5Z
ØPPJØ7Z
ØPPJØJZ
ØPPJØKZ
ØPPJ34Z
ØPPJ35Z
ØPPJ37Z
ØPPJ3JZ
ØPPJ3KZ
ØPPJ44Z
ØPPJ45Z
ØPPJ47Z
ØPPJ4JZ
ØPPJ4KZ
ØPPKØ4Z
ØPPKØ5Z
ØPPKØ7Z
ØPPKØJZ
ØPPKØKZ
ØPPK34Z
ØPPK35Z
ØPPK37Z
ØPPK3JZ
ØPPK3KZ
ØPPK44Z
ØPPK45Z
ØPPK47Z
ØPPK4JZ
ØPPK4KZ
ØPPLØ4Z
ØPPLØ5Z
ØPPLØ7Z
ØPPLØJZ
ØPPLØKZ
ØPPL34Z
ØPPL35Z
ØPPL37Z
ØPPL3JZ
ØPPL3KZ
ØPPL44Z
ØPPL45Z
ØPPL47Z
ØPPL4JZ
ØPPL4KZ
ØPPMØ4Z
ØPPMØ5Z
ØPPMØ7Z
ØPPMØJZ
ØPPMØKZ
ØPPM34Z
ØPPM35Z
ØPPM37Z
ØPPM3JZ
ØPPM3KZ
ØPPM44Z
ØPPM45Z
ØPPM47Z
ØPPM4JZ
ØPPM4KZ
ØPPNØ4Z
ØPPNØ5Z
ØPPNØ7Z
ØPPNØJZ
ØPPNØKZ
ØPPN34Z
ØPPN35Z
ØPPN37Z
ØPPN3JZ
ØPPN3KZ
ØPPN44Z
ØPPN45Z
ØPPN47Z
ØPPN4JZ
ØPPN4KZ
ØPPPØ4Z
ØPPPØ5Z
ØPPPØ7Z
ØPPPØJZ
ØPPPØKZ
ØPPP34Z
ØPPP35Z
ØPPP37Z
ØPPP3JZ
ØPPP3KZ
ØPPP44Z
ØPPP45Z
ØPPP47Z
ØPPP4JZ
ØPPP4KZ
ØPPQØ4Z
ØPPQØ5Z
ØPPQØ7Z
ØPPQØJZ
ØPPQØKZ
ØPPQ34Z
ØPPQ35Z
ØPPQ37Z
ØPPQ3JZ
ØPPQ3KZ
ØPPQ44Z
ØPPQ45Z
ØPPQ47Z
ØPPQ4JZ
ØPPQ4KZ
ØPPRØ4Z
ØPPRØ5Z
ØPPRØ7Z
ØPPRØJZ
ØPPRØKZ
ØPPR34Z
ØPPR35Z
ØPPR37Z
ØPPR3JZ
ØPPR3KZ
ØPPR44Z
ØPPR45Z
ØPPR47Z
ØPPR4JZ
ØPPR4KZ
ØPPSØ4Z
ØPPSØ5Z
ØPPSØ7Z
ØPPSØJZ
ØPPSØKZ
ØPPS34Z
ØPPS35Z
ØPPS37Z
ØPPS3JZ
ØPPS3KZ
ØPPS44Z
ØPPS45Z
ØPPS47Z
ØPPS4JZ
ØPPS4KZ
ØPPTØ4Z
ØPPTØ5Z
ØPPTØ7Z
ØPPTØJZ
ØPPTØKZ
ØPPT34Z
ØPPT35Z
ØPPT37Z
ØPPT3JZ
ØPPT3KZ
ØPPT44Z
ØPPT45Z
ØPPT47Z
ØPPT4JZ
ØPPT4KZ
ØPPVØ4Z
ØPPVØ5Z
ØPPVØ7Z
ØPPVØJZ
ØPPVØKZ
ØPPV34Z
ØPPV35Z
ØPPV37Z
ØPPV3JZ
ØPPV3KZ
ØPPV44Z
ØPPV45Z
ØPPV47Z
ØPPV4JZ
ØPPV4KZ
ØPPYØØZ
ØPPYØMZ
ØPPY3MZ
ØPPY4ØZ
ØPPY4MZ
ØPWØØ4Z
ØPWØØ7Z
ØPWØØJZ
ØPWØØKZ
ØPWØ34Z
ØPWØ37Z
ØPWØ3JZ
ØPWØ3KZ
ØPWØ44Z
ØPWØ47Z
ØPWØ4JZ
ØPWØ4KZ
ØPW1Ø4Z
ØPW1Ø7Z
ØPW1ØJZ
ØPW1ØKZ
ØPW134Z
ØPW137Z
ØPW13JZ
ØPW13KZ
ØPW144Z
ØPW147Z
ØPW14JZ
ØPW14KZ
ØPW2Ø4Z
ØPW2Ø7Z
ØPW2ØJZ
ØPW2ØKZ
ØPW234Z
ØPW237Z
ØPW23JZ
ØPW23KZ
ØPW244Z
ØPW247Z
ØPW24JZ
ØPW24KZ
ØPW3Ø4Z
ØPW3Ø7Z
ØPW3ØJZ
ØPW3ØKZ
ØPW334Z
ØPW337Z
ØPW33JZ
ØPW33KZ
ØPW344Z
ØPW347Z
ØPW34JZ
ØPW34KZ
ØPW4Ø4Z
ØPW4Ø7Z
ØPW4ØJZ
ØPW4ØKZ
ØPW434Z
ØPW437Z
ØPW43JZ
ØPW43KZ
ØPW444Z
ØPW447Z
ØPW44JZ
ØPW44KZ
ØPW5Ø4Z
ØPW5Ø7Z
ØPW5ØJZ
ØPW5ØKZ
ØPW534Z
ØPW537Z
ØPW53JZ
ØPW53KZ
ØPW544Z
ØPW547Z
ØPW54JZ
ØPW54KZ
ØPW6Ø4Z
ØPW6Ø7Z
ØPW6ØJZ
ØPW6ØKZ
ØPW634Z

ØPW637Z
ØPW63JZ
ØPW63KZ
ØPW644Z
ØPW647Z
ØPW64JZ
ØPW64KZ
ØPW7Ø4Z
ØPW7Ø7Z
ØPW7ØJZ
ØPW7ØKZ
ØPW734Z
ØPW737Z
ØPW73JZ
ØPW73KZ
ØPW744Z
ØPW747Z
ØPW74JZ
ØPW74KZ
ØPW8Ø4Z
ØPW8Ø7Z
ØPW8ØJZ
ØPW8ØKZ
ØPW834Z
ØPW837Z
ØPW83JZ
ØPW83KZ
ØPW844Z
ØPW847Z
ØPW84JZ
ØPW84KZ
ØPW9Ø4Z
ØPW9Ø7Z
ØPW9ØJZ
ØPW9ØKZ
ØPW934Z
ØPW937Z
ØPW93JZ
ØPW93KZ
ØPW944Z
ØPW947Z
ØPW94JZ
ØPW94KZ
ØPWBØ4Z
ØPWBØ7Z
ØPWBØJZ
ØPWBØKZ
ØPWB34Z
ØPWB37Z
ØPWB3JZ
ØPWB3KZ
ØPWB44Z
ØPWB47Z
ØPWB4JZ
ØPWB4KZ
ØPWCØ4Z
ØPWCØ5Z
ØPWCØ7Z
ØPWCØJZ
ØPWCØKZ
ØPWC34Z
ØPWC35Z
ØPWC37Z
ØPWC3JZ
ØPWC3KZ
ØPWC44Z
ØPWC45Z
ØPWC47Z
ØPWC4JZ
ØPWC4KZ
ØPWDØ4Z
ØPWDØ5Z
ØPWDØ7Z
ØPWDØJZ
ØPWDØKZ
ØPWD34Z
ØPWD35Z
ØPWD37Z
ØPWD3JZ
ØPWD3KZ
ØPWD44Z
ØPWD45Z
ØPWD47Z
ØPWD4JZ
ØPWD4KZ
ØPWFØ4Z
ØPWFØ5Z
ØPWFØ7Z
ØPWFØJZ
ØPWFØKZ
ØPWF34Z
ØPWF35Z
ØPWF37Z
ØPWF3JZ
ØPWF3KZ
ØPWF44Z
ØPWF45Z
ØPWF47Z
ØPWF4JZ
ØPWF4KZ
ØPWGØ4Z
ØPWGØ5Z
ØPWGØ7Z
ØPWGØJZ
ØPWGØKZ
ØPWG34Z
ØPWG35Z
ØPWG37Z
ØPWG3JZ
ØPWG3KZ
ØPWG44Z
ØPWG45Z
ØPWG47Z
ØPWG4JZ
ØPWG4KZ
ØPWHØ4Z
ØPWHØ5Z
ØPWHØ7Z
ØPWHØJZ
ØPWHØKZ
ØPWH34Z
ØPWH35Z
ØPWH37Z
ØPWH3JZ
ØPWH3KZ
ØPWH44Z
ØPWH45Z
ØPWH47Z
ØPWH4JZ
ØPWH4KZ
ØPWJØ4Z
ØPWJØ5Z
ØPWJØ7Z
ØPWJØJZ
ØPWJØKZ
ØPWJ34Z
ØPWJ35Z
ØPWJ37Z
ØPWJ3JZ
ØPWJ3KZ
ØPWJ44Z
ØPWJ45Z
ØPWJ47Z
ØPWJ4JZ
ØPWJ4KZ
ØPWKØ4Z
ØPWKØ5Z
ØPWKØ7Z
ØPWKØJZ
ØPWKØKZ
ØPWK34Z
ØPWK35Z
ØPWK37Z
ØPWK3JZ
ØPWK3KZ
ØPWK44Z
ØPWK45Z
ØPWK47Z
ØPWK4JZ
ØPWK4KZ
ØPWLØ4Z
ØPWLØ5Z
ØPWLØ7Z
ØPWLØJZ
ØPWLØKZ
ØPWL34Z
ØPWL35Z
ØPWL37Z
ØPWL3JZ
ØPWL3KZ
ØPWL44Z
ØPWL45Z
ØPWL47Z
ØPWL4JZ
ØPWL4KZ
ØPWRØ4Z
ØPWRØ5Z
ØPWRØ7Z
ØPWRØJZ
ØPWRØKZ
ØPWR34Z
ØPWR35Z
ØPWR37Z
ØPWR3JZ
ØPWR3KZ
ØPWR44Z
ØPWR45Z
ØPWR47Z
ØPWR4JZ
ØPWR4KZ
ØPWSØ4Z
ØPWSØ5Z
ØPWSØ7Z
ØPWSØJZ
ØPWSØKZ
ØPWS34Z
ØPWS35Z
ØPWS37Z
ØPWS3JZ
ØPWS3KZ
ØPWS44Z
ØPWS45Z
ØPWS47Z
ØPWS4JZ
ØPWS4KZ
ØPWTØ4Z
ØPWTØ5Z
ØPWTØ7Z
ØPWTØJZ
ØPWTØKZ
ØPWT34Z
ØPWT35Z
ØPWT37Z
ØPWT3JZ
ØPWT3KZ
ØPWT44Z
ØPWT45Z
ØPWT47Z
ØPWT4JZ
ØPWT4KZ
ØPWVØ4Z
ØPWVØ5Z
ØPWVØ7Z
ØPWVØJZ
ØPWVØKZ
ØPWV34Z
ØPWV35Z
ØPWV37Z
ØPWV3JZ
ØPWV3KZ
ØPWV44Z
ØPWV45Z
ØPWV47Z
ØPWV4JZ
ØPWV4KZ
ØPWYØØZ
ØPWYØMZ
ØPWY3ØZ
ØPWY3MZ
ØPWY4ØZ
ØPWY4MZ
ØQ5Ø*
ØQ51*
ØQ52*
ØQ53*
ØQ54*
ØQ55*
ØQ5D*
ØQ5F*
ØQ5G*
ØQ5H*
ØQ5J*
ØQ5K*
ØQ5Q*
ØQ5R*
ØQ5S*
ØQ9ØØØZ
ØQ9ØØZZ
ØQ9Ø4ØZ
ØQ9Ø4ZZ
ØQ91ØØZ
ØQ91ØZZ
ØQ914ØZ
ØQ914ZZ
ØQ92ØØZ
ØQ92ØZZ
ØQ924ØZ
ØQ924ZZ
ØQ93ØØZ
ØQ93ØZZ
ØQ934ØZ
ØQ934ZZ
ØQ94ØØZ
ØQ94ØZZ
ØQ944ØZ
ØQ944ZZ
ØQ95ØØZ
ØQ95ØZZ
ØQ954ØZ
ØQ954ZZ
ØQ9DØØZ
ØQ9DØZZ
ØQ9D4ØZ
ØQ9D4ZZ
ØQ9FØØZ
ØQ9FØZZ
ØQ9F4ØZ
ØQ9F4ZZ
ØQ9GØØZ
ØQ9GØZZ
ØQ9G4ØZ
ØQ9G4ZZ
ØQ9HØØZ
ØQ9HØZZ
ØQ9H4ØZ
ØQ9H4ZZ
ØQ9JØØZ
ØQ9JØZZ
ØQ9J4ØZ
ØQ9J4ZZ
ØQ9KØØZ
ØQ9KØZZ
ØQ9K4ØZ
ØQ9K4ZZ
ØQ9QØØZ
ØQ9QØZZ
ØQ9Q4ØZ
ØQ9Q4ZZ
ØQ9RØØZ
ØQ9RØZZ
ØQ9R4ØZ
ØQ9R4ZZ
ØQ9SØØZ
ØQ9SØZZ
ØQ9S4ØZ
ØQ9S4ZZ
ØQPØØ4Z
ØQPØØ5Z
ØQPØØ7Z
ØQPØØJZ
ØQPØØKZ
ØQPØ34Z
ØQPØ35Z
ØQPØ37Z
ØQPØ3JZ
ØQPØ3KZ
ØQPØ44Z
ØQPØ45Z
ØQPØ47Z
ØQPØ4JZ
ØQPØ4KZ
ØQP1Ø4Z
ØQP1Ø5Z
ØQP1Ø7Z
ØQP1ØJZ
ØQP1ØKZ
ØQP134Z
ØQP135Z
ØQP137Z
ØQP13JZ
ØQP13KZ
ØQP144Z
ØQP145Z
ØQP147Z
ØQP14JZ
ØQP14KZ
ØQP2Ø4Z
ØQP2Ø5Z
ØQP2Ø7Z
ØQP2ØJZ
ØQP2ØKZ
ØQP234Z
ØQP235Z
ØQP237Z
ØQP23JZ
ØQP23KZ
ØQP244Z
ØQP245Z
ØQP247Z
ØQP24JZ
ØQP24KZ
ØQP3Ø4Z
ØQP3Ø5Z
ØQP3Ø7Z
ØQP3ØJZ
ØQP3ØKZ
ØQP334Z
ØQP335Z
ØQP337Z
ØQP33JZ
ØQP33KZ
ØQP344Z
ØQP345Z
ØQP347Z
ØQP34JZ
ØQP34KZ
ØQP4Ø4Z
ØQP4Ø5Z
ØQP4Ø7Z
ØQP4ØJZ
ØQP4ØKZ
ØQP434Z
ØQP435Z
ØQP437Z
ØQP43JZ
ØQP43KZ
ØQP444Z
ØQP445Z
ØQP447Z
ØQP44JZ
ØQP44KZ
ØQP5Ø4Z
ØQP5Ø5Z
ØQP5Ø7Z
ØQP5ØJZ
ØQP5ØKZ
ØQP534Z
ØQP535Z
ØQP537Z
ØQP53JZ
ØQP53KZ
ØQP544Z
ØQP545Z
ØQP547Z
ØQP54JZ
ØQP54KZ
ØQPDØ4Z
ØQPDØ5Z
ØQPDØ7Z
ØQPDØJZ
ØQPDØKZ
ØQPD34Z
ØQPD35Z
ØQPD37Z
ØQPD3JZ
ØQPD3KZ
ØQPD44Z
ØQPD45Z
ØQPD47Z
ØQPD4JZ
ØQPD4KZ
ØQPFØ4Z
ØQPFØ5Z
ØQPFØ7Z
ØQPFØJZ
ØQPFØKZ
ØQPF34Z
ØQPF35Z
ØQPF37Z
ØQPF3JZ
ØQPF3KZ
ØQPF44Z
ØQPF45Z
ØQPF47Z
ØQPF4JZ
ØQPF4KZ
ØQPGØ4Z
ØQPGØ5Z
ØQPGØ7Z
ØQPGØJZ
ØQPGØKZ
ØQPG34Z
ØQPG35Z
ØQPG37Z
ØQPG3JZ
ØQPG3KZ
ØQPG44Z
ØQPG45Z
ØQPG47Z
ØQPG4JZ
ØQPG4KZ
ØQPHØ4Z
ØQPHØ5Z
ØQPHØ7Z
ØQPHØJZ
ØQPHØKZ
ØQPH34Z
ØQPH35Z
ØQPH37Z
ØQPH3JZ
ØQPH3KZ
ØQPH44Z
ØQPH45Z
ØQPH47Z
ØQPH4JZ
ØQPH4KZ
ØQPJØ4Z
ØQPJØ5Z
ØQPJØ7Z
ØQPJØJZ
ØQPJØKZ
ØQPJ34Z
ØQPJ35Z
ØQPJ37Z
ØQPJ3JZ
ØQPJ3KZ
ØQPJ44Z
ØQPJ45Z
ØQPJ47Z
ØQPJ4JZ
ØQPJ4KZ
ØQPKØ4Z
ØQPKØ5Z
ØQPKØ7Z
ØQPKØJZ
ØQPKØKZ
ØQPK34Z
ØQPK35Z
ØQPK37Z
ØQPK3JZ
ØQPK3KZ
ØQPK44Z
ØQPK45Z
ØQPK47Z
ØQPK4JZ
ØQPK4KZ
ØQPLØ4Z
ØQPLØ5Z
ØQPLØ7Z
ØQPLØJZ
ØQPLØKZ
ØQPL34Z
ØQPL35Z
ØQPL37Z
ØQPL3JZ
ØQPL3KZ
ØQPL44Z
ØQPL45Z
ØQPL47Z
ØQPL4JZ
ØQPL4KZ
ØQPMØ4Z
ØQPMØ5Z
ØQPMØ7Z
ØQPMØJZ
ØQPMØKZ
ØQPM34Z
ØQPM35Z
ØQPM37Z
ØQPM3JZ
ØQPM3KZ
ØQPM44Z
ØQPM45Z
ØQPM47Z
ØQPM4JZ
ØQPM4KZ
ØQPNØ4Z
ØQPNØ5Z
ØQPNØ7Z
ØQPNØJZ
ØQPNØKZ
ØQPN34Z
ØQPN35Z
ØQPN37Z
ØQPN3JZ
ØQPN3KZ
ØQPN44Z
ØQPN45Z
ØQPN47Z
ØQPN4JZ
ØQPN4KZ
ØQPPØ4Z
ØQPPØ5Z
ØQPPØ7Z
ØQPPØJZ
ØQPPØKZ
ØQPP34Z
ØQPP35Z
ØQPP37Z
ØQPP3JZ
ØQPP3KZ
ØQPP44Z
ØQPP45Z
ØQPP47Z
ØQPP4JZ
ØQPP4KZ
ØQPQØ4Z
ØQPQØ5Z
ØQPQØ7Z
ØQPQØJZ
ØQPQØKZ
ØQPQ34Z
ØQPQ35Z
ØQPQ37Z
ØQPQ3JZ
ØQPQ3KZ
ØQPQ44Z
ØQPQ45Z
ØQPQ47Z
ØQPQ4JZ
ØQPQ4KZ
ØQPRØ4Z
ØQPRØ5Z
ØQPRØ7Z
ØQPRØJZ
ØQPRØKZ
ØQPR34Z
ØQPR35Z
ØQPR37Z
ØQPR3JZ
ØQPR3KZ
ØQPR44Z
ØQPR45Z
ØQPR47Z
ØQPR4JZ
ØQPR4KZ
ØQPSØ4Z
ØQPSØ5Z
ØQPSØ7Z
ØQPSØJZ
ØQPSØKZ
ØQPS34Z
ØQPS35Z
ØQPS37Z
ØQPS3JZ
ØQPS3KZ
ØQPS44Z
ØQPS45Z
ØQPS47Z
ØQPS4JZ
ØQPS4KZ
ØQPYØØZ
ØQPYØMZ
ØQPY3MZ
ØQPY4ØZ
ØQPY4MZ
ØQWØØ4Z
ØQWØØ7Z
ØQWØØJZ
ØQWØØKZ
ØQWØ34Z
ØQWØ37Z
ØQWØ3JZ
ØQWØ3KZ
ØQWØ44Z
ØQWØ47Z
ØQWØ4JZ
ØQWØ4KZ
ØQW1Ø4Z
ØQW1Ø7Z
ØQW1ØJZ
ØQW1ØKZ
ØQW134Z
ØQW137Z
ØQW13JZ
ØQW13KZ
ØQW144Z
ØQW147Z
ØQW14JZ
ØQW14KZ
ØQW2Ø4Z
ØQW2Ø5Z
ØQW2Ø7Z
ØQW2ØJZ
ØQW2ØKZ
ØQW234Z
ØQW235Z
ØQW237Z
ØQW23JZ
ØQW23KZ
ØQW244Z
ØQW245Z
ØQW247Z
ØQW24JZ
ØQW24KZ
ØQW3Ø4Z
ØQW3Ø5Z
ØQW3Ø7Z
ØQW3ØJZ
ØQW3ØKZ
ØQW334Z
ØQW335Z
ØQW337Z
ØQW33JZ
ØQW33KZ
ØQW344Z
ØQW345Z
ØQW347Z
ØQW34JZ
ØQW34KZ
ØQW4Ø4Z
ØQW4Ø7Z
ØQW4ØJZ
ØQW4ØKZ
ØQW434Z
ØQW437Z
ØQW43JZ
ØQW43KZ
ØQW444Z
ØQW447Z
ØQW44JZ
ØQW44KZ
ØQW5Ø4Z
ØQW5Ø7Z
ØQW5ØJZ
ØQW5ØKZ
ØQW534Z
ØQW537Z
ØQW53JZ
ØQW53KZ
ØQW544Z
ØQW547Z
ØQW54JZ
ØQW54KZ
ØQWDØ4Z
ØQWDØ5Z
ØQWDØ7Z
ØQWDØJZ
ØQWDØKZ
ØQWD34Z
ØQWD35Z
ØQWD37Z
ØQWD3JZ
ØQWD3KZ
ØQWD44Z
ØQWD45Z
ØQWD47Z
ØQWD4JZ
ØQWD4KZ
ØQWFØ4Z
ØQWFØ5Z
ØQWFØ7Z
ØQWFØJZ
ØQWFØKZ
ØQWF34Z
ØQWF35Z
ØQWF37Z
ØQWF3JZ
ØQWF3KZ
ØQWF44Z
ØQWF45Z
ØQWF47Z
ØQWF4JZ
ØQWF4KZ
ØQWGØ4Z
ØQWGØ5Z
ØQWGØ7Z
ØQWGØJZ
ØQWGØKZ
ØQWG34Z
ØQWG35Z
ØQWG37Z
ØQWG3JZ
ØQWG3KZ
ØQWG44Z
ØQWG45Z
ØQWG47Z
ØQWG4JZ
ØQWG4KZ
ØQWHØ4Z
ØQWHØ5Z
ØQWHØ7Z
ØQWHØJZ
ØQWHØKZ
ØQWH34Z
ØQWH35Z
ØQWH37Z
ØQWH3JZ
ØQWH3KZ
ØQWH44Z
ØQWH45Z
ØQWH47Z
ØQWH4JZ
ØQWH4KZ
ØQWJØ4Z
ØQWJØ5Z
ØQWJØ7Z
ØQWJØJZ
ØQWJØKZ
ØQWJ34Z
ØQWJ35Z
ØQWJ37Z
ØQWJ3JZ
ØQWJ3KZ
ØQWJ44Z
ØQWJ45Z
ØQWJ47Z
ØQWJ4JZ
ØQWJ4KZ
ØQWKØ4Z
ØQWKØ5Z
ØQWKØ7Z
ØQWKØJZ
ØQWKØKZ
ØQWK34Z
ØQWK35Z
ØQWK37Z
ØQWK3JZ
ØQWK3KZ
ØQWK44Z
ØQWK45Z
ØQWK47Z
ØQWK4JZ
ØQWK4KZ
ØQWQØ4Z
ØQWQØ5Z
ØQWQØ7Z
ØQWQØJZ
ØQWQØKZ
ØQWQ34Z
ØQWQ35Z
ØQWQ37Z
ØQWQ3JZ
ØQWQ3KZ
ØQWQ44Z
ØQWQ45Z
ØQWQ47Z
ØQWQ4JZ
ØQWQ4KZ
ØQWRØ4Z
ØQWRØ5Z
ØQWRØ7Z
ØQWRØJZ
ØQWRØKZ
ØQWR34Z
ØQWR35Z
ØQWR37Z
ØQWR3JZ
ØQWR3KZ
ØQWR44Z
ØQWR45Z
ØQWR47Z
ØQWR4JZ
ØQWR4KZ
ØQWSØ4Z
ØQWSØ7Z
ØQWSØJZ
ØQWSØKZ
ØQWS34Z
ØQWS37Z
ØQWS3JZ
ØQWS3KZ
ØQWS44Z
ØQWS47Z
ØQWS4JZ
ØQWS4KZ
ØQWYØØZ
ØQWYØMZ
ØQWY3ØZ
ØQWY3MZ
ØQWY4ØZ
ØQWY4MZ
ØR5Ø*
ØR51*
ØR54*
ØR56*
ØR5A*
ØR5C*
ØR5D*
ØR5E*
ØR5F*
ØR5G*
ØR5H*
ØR5J*
ØR5K*
ØR5L*
ØR5M*
ØRBCØZZ
ØRBC3ZZ
ØRBC4ZZ
ØRBDØZZ
ØRBD3ZZ
ØRBD4ZZ
ØRPØØJZ
ØRPØ3JZ
ØRPØ4JZ
ØRP1ØJZ
ØRP13JZ
ØRP14JZ
ØRP3ØJZ
ØRP33JZ
ØRP34JZ
ØRP4ØJZ
ØRP43JZ
ØRP44JZ

ØRP5ØJZ
ØRP53JZ
ØRP54JZ
ØRP6ØJZ
ØRP63JZ
ØRP64JZ
ØRP9ØJZ
ØRP93JZ
ØRP94JZ
ØRPAØJZ
ØRPA3JZ
ØRPA4JZ
ØRPBØJZ
ØRPB3JZ
ØRPB4JZ
ØRPCØØZ
ØRPCØ3Z
ØRPCØ4Z
ØRPCØ7Z
ØRPCØJZ
ØRPCØKZ
ØRPC34Z
ØRPC37Z
ØRPC3JZ
ØRPC3KZ
ØRPC4ØZ
ØRPC43Z
ØRPC44Z
ØRPC47Z
ØRPC4JZ
ØRPC4KZ
ØRPCX4Z
ØRPDØØZ
ØRPDØ3Z
ØRPDØ4Z
ØRPDØ7Z
ØRPDØJZ
ØRPDØKZ
ØRPD34Z
ØRPD37Z
ØRPD3JZ
ØRPD3KZ
ØRPD4ØZ
ØRPD43Z
ØRPD44Z
ØRPD47Z
ØRPD4JZ
ØRPD4KZ
ØRPDX4Z
ØRPEØJZ
ØRPE3JZ
ØRPE4JZ
ØRPFØJZ
ØRPF3JZ
ØRPF4JZ
ØRPGØJZ
ØRPG3JZ
ØRPG4JZ
ØRPHØJZ
ØRPH3JZ
ØRPH4JZ
ØRPJØJ6
ØRPJØJ7
ØRPJØJZ
ØRPJ3J6
ØRPJ3J7
ØRPJ3JZ
ØRPJ4J6
ØRPJ4J7
ØRPJ4JZ
ØRPKØJ6
ØRPKØJ7
ØRPKØJZ
ØRPK3J6
ØRPK3J7
ØRPK3JZ
ØRPK4J6
ØRPK4J7
ØRPK4JZ
ØRPLØJZ
ØRPL3JZ
ØRPL4JZ
ØRPMØJZ
ØRPM3JZ
ØRPM4JZ
ØRPNØJZ
ØRPN3JZ
ØRPN4JZ
ØRPPØJZ
ØRPP3JZ
ØRPP4JZ
ØRPQØJZ
ØRPQ3JZ
ØRPQ4JZ
ØRPRØJZ
ØRPR3JZ
ØRPR4JZ
ØRPSØJZ
ØRPS3JZ
ØRPS4JZ
ØRPTØJZ
ØRPT3JZ
ØRPT4JZ
ØRPUØJZ
ØRPU3JZ
ØRPU4JZ
ØRPVØJZ
ØRPV3JZ
ØRPV4JZ
ØRPWØJZ
ØRPW3JZ
ØRPW4JZ
ØRPXØJZ
ØRPX3JZ
ØRPX4JZ
ØS5Ø*
ØS53*
ØS55*
ØS56*
ØS57*
ØS58*
ØS5C*
ØS5D*
ØSPØØJZ
ØSPØ3JZ
ØSPØ4JZ
ØSP2ØJZ
ØSP23JZ
ØSP24JZ
ØSP3ØJZ
ØSP33JZ
ØSP34JZ
ØSP4ØJZ
ØSP43JZ
ØSP44JZ
ØSP5ØJZ
ØSP53JZ
ØSP54JZ
ØSP6ØJZ
ØSP63JZ
ØSP64JZ
ØSP7ØJZ
ØSP73JZ
ØSP74JZ
ØSP8ØJZ
ØSP83JZ
ØSP84JZ
ØSPFØJZ
ØSPF3JZ
ØSPF4JZ
ØSPGØJZ
ØSPG3JZ
ØSPG4JZ
ØSPHØJZ
ØSPH3JZ
ØSPH4JZ
ØSPJØJZ
ØSPJ3JZ
ØSPJ4JZ
ØSPKØJZ
ØSPK3JZ
ØSPK4JZ
ØSPLØJZ
ØSPL3JZ
ØSPL4JZ
ØSPMØJZ
ØSPM3JZ
ØSPM4JZ
ØSPNØJZ
ØSPN3JZ
ØSPN4JZ
ØSPPØJZ
ØSPP3JZ
ØSPP4JZ
ØSPQØJZ
ØSPQ3JZ
ØSPQ4JZ
ØWB8ØZZ
ØWB83ZZ
ØWB84ZZ
ØWB8XZZ

DRG 496

Select operating room procedures listed under DRG 495

DRG 497

Select operating room procedures listed under DRG 495

DRG 498

Operating Room Procedures

ØM5L*
ØM5M*
ØQ56*
ØQ57*
ØQ58*
ØQ59*
ØQ5B*
ØQ5C*
ØQ96ØØZ
ØQ96ØZZ
ØQ964ØZ
ØQ964ZZ
ØQ97ØØZ
ØQ97ØZZ
ØQ974ØZ
ØQ974ZZ
ØQ98ØØZ
ØQ98ØZZ
ØQ984ØZ
ØQ984ZZ
ØQ99ØØZ
ØQ99ØZZ
ØQ994ØZ
ØQ994ZZ
ØQ9BØØZ
ØQ9BØZZ
ØQ9B4ØZ
ØQ9B4ZZ
ØQ9CØØZ
ØQ9CØZZ
ØQ9C4ØZ
ØQ9C4ZZ
ØQB6ØZZ
ØQB63ZZ
ØQB64ZZ
ØQB7ØZZ
ØQB73ZZ
ØQB74ZZ
ØQB8ØZZ
ØQB83ZZ
ØQB84ZZ
ØQB9ØZZ
ØQB93ZZ
ØQB94ZZ
ØQBBØZZ
ØQBB3ZZ
ØQBB4ZZ
ØQBCØZZ
ØQBC3ZZ
ØQBC4ZZ
ØQP6Ø4Z
ØQP6Ø5Z
ØQP6Ø7Z
ØQP6ØJZ
ØQP6ØKZ
ØQP634Z
ØQP635Z
ØQP637Z
ØQP63JZ
ØQP63KZ
ØQP644Z
ØQP645Z
ØQP647Z
ØQP64JZ
ØQP64KZ
ØQP7Ø4Z
ØQP7Ø5Z
ØQP7Ø7Z
ØQP7ØJZ
ØQP7ØKZ
ØQP734Z
ØQP735Z
ØQP737Z
ØQP73JZ
ØQP73KZ
ØQP744Z
ØQP745Z
ØQP747Z
ØQP74JZ
ØQP74KZ
ØQP8Ø4Z
ØQP8Ø5Z
ØQP8Ø7Z
ØQP8ØJZ
ØQP8ØKZ
ØQP834Z
ØQP835Z
ØQP837Z
ØQP83JZ
ØQP83KZ
ØQP844Z
ØQP845Z
ØQP847Z
ØQP84JZ
ØQP84KZ
ØQP9Ø4Z
ØQP9Ø5Z
ØQP9Ø7Z
ØQP9ØJZ
ØQP9ØKZ
ØQP934Z
ØQP935Z
ØQP937Z
ØQP93JZ
ØQP93KZ
ØQP944Z
ØQP945Z
ØQP947Z
ØQP94JZ
ØQP94KZ
ØQPBØ4Z
ØQPBØ5Z
ØQPBØ7Z
ØQPBØJZ
ØQPBØKZ
ØQPB34Z
ØQPB35Z
ØQPB37Z
ØQPB3JZ
ØQPB3KZ
ØQPB44Z
ØQPB45Z
ØQPB47Z
ØQPB4JZ
ØQPB4KZ
ØQPCØ4Z
ØQPCØ5Z
ØQPCØ7Z
ØQPCØJZ
ØQPCØKZ
ØQPC34Z
ØQPC35Z
ØQPC37Z
ØQPC3JZ
ØQPC3KZ
ØQPC44Z
ØQPC45Z
ØQPC47Z
ØQPC4JZ
ØQPC4KZ
ØQW6Ø4Z
ØQW6Ø5Z
ØQW6Ø7Z
ØQW6ØJZ
ØQW6ØKZ
ØQW634Z
ØQW635Z
ØQW637Z
ØQW63JZ
ØQW63KZ
ØQW644Z
ØQW645Z
ØQW647Z
ØQW64JZ
ØQW64KZ
ØQW7Ø4Z
ØQW7Ø5Z
ØQW7Ø7Z
ØQW7ØJZ
ØQW7ØKZ
ØQW734Z
ØQW735Z
ØQW737Z
ØQW73JZ
ØQW73KZ
ØQW744Z
ØQW745Z
ØQW747Z
ØQW74JZ
ØQW74KZ
ØQW8Ø4Z
ØQW8Ø5Z
ØQW8Ø7Z
ØQW8ØJZ
ØQW8ØKZ
ØQW834Z
ØQW835Z
ØQW837Z
ØQW83JZ
ØQW83KZ
ØQW844Z
ØQW845Z
ØQW847Z
ØQW84JZ
ØQW84KZ
ØQW9Ø4Z
ØQW9Ø5Z
ØQW9Ø7Z
ØQW9ØJZ
ØQW9ØKZ
ØQW934Z
ØQW935Z
ØQW937Z
ØQW93JZ
ØQW93KZ
ØQW944Z
ØQW945Z
ØQW947Z
ØQW94JZ
ØQW94KZ
ØQWBØ4Z
ØQWBØ5Z
ØQWBØ7Z
ØQWBØJZ
ØQWBØKZ
ØQWB34Z
ØQWB35Z
ØQWB37Z
ØQWB3JZ
ØQWB3KZ
ØQWB44Z
ØQWB45Z
ØQWB47Z
ØQWB4JZ
ØQWB4KZ
ØQWCØ4Z
ØQWCØ5Z
ØQWCØ7Z
ØQWCØJZ
ØQWCØKZ
ØQWC34Z
ØQWC35Z
ØQWC37Z
ØQWC3JZ
ØQWC3KZ
ØQWC44Z
ØQWC45Z
ØQWC47Z
ØQWC4JZ
ØQWC4KZ
ØS59*
ØS5B*

DRG 499

Select operating room procedures listed under DRG 498

DRG 500

Operating Room Procedures

ØHDTØZZ
ØHDUØZZ
ØHDVØZZ
ØHDYØZZ
ØJ8Ø*
ØJ84*
ØJ85*
ØJ86*
ØJ87*
ØJ88*
ØJ89*
ØJ8B*
ØJ8C*
ØJ8D*
ØJ8F*
ØJ8G*
ØJ8H*
ØJ8L*
ØJ8M*
ØJ8N*
ØJ8P*
ØJ8Q*
ØJ8R*
ØJ8S*
ØJ8T*
ØJ8V*
ØJ8W*
ØJDØØZZ
ØJD1ØZZ
ØJD4ØZZ
ØJD5ØZZ
ØJD6ØZZ
ØJD7ØZZ
ØJD8ØZZ
ØJD9ØZZ
ØJDBØZZ
ØJDCØZZ
ØJDDØZZ
ØJDFØZZ
ØJDGØZZ
ØJDHØZZ
ØJDLØZZ
ØJDMØZZ
ØJDNØZZ
ØJDPØZZ
ØJDQØZZ
ØJDRØZZ
ØJNØØZZ
ØJNØ3ZZ
ØJN1ØZZ
ØJN13ZZ
ØJN4ØZZ
ØJN43ZZ
ØJN5ØZZ
ØJN53ZZ
ØJN6ØZZ
ØJN63ZZ
ØJN7ØZZ
ØJN73ZZ
ØJN8ØZZ
ØJN83ZZ
ØJN9ØZZ
ØJN93ZZ
ØJNBØZZ
ØJNB3ZZ
ØJNCØZZ
ØJNC3ZZ
ØJNDØZZ
ØJND3ZZ
ØJNFØZZ
ØJNF3ZZ
ØJNGØZZ
ØJNG3ZZ
ØJNHØZZ
ØJNH3ZZ
ØJNLØZZ
ØJNL3ZZ
ØJNMØZZ
ØJNM3ZZ
ØJNNØZZ
ØJNN3ZZ
ØJNPØZZ
ØJNP3ZZ
ØJNQØZZ
ØJNQ3ZZ
ØJNRØZZ
ØJNR3ZZ
ØJQØØZZ
ØJQ1ØZZ
ØJQ4ØZZ
ØJQ5ØZZ
ØJQ6ØZZ
ØJQ7ØZZ
ØJQ8ØZZ
ØJQ9ØZZ
ØJQBØZZ
ØJQCØZZ
ØJQDØZZ
ØJQFØZZ
ØJQGØZZ
ØJQHØZZ
ØJQLØZZ
ØJQMØZZ
ØJQNØZZ
ØJQPØZZ
ØJQQØZZ
ØJQRØZZ
ØJRØ*
ØJR1*
ØJR4*
ØJR5*
ØJR6*
ØJR7*
ØJR8*
ØJR9*
ØJRB*
ØJRC*
ØJRD*
ØJRF*
ØJRG*
ØJRH*
ØJRL*
ØJRM*
ØJRN*
ØJRP*
ØJRQ*
ØJRR*
ØJUØ*
ØJU1*
ØJU4*
ØJU5*
ØJU6*
ØJU7*
ØJU8*
ØJU9*
ØJUB*
ØJUC*
ØJUD*
ØJUF*
ØJUG*
ØJUH*
ØJUL*
ØJUM*
ØJUN*
ØJUP*
ØJUQ*
ØJUR*
ØJXØØZZ
ØJXØ3ZZ
ØJX1ØZZ
ØJX13ZZ
ØJX4ØZZ
ØJX43ZZ
ØJX5ØZZ
ØJX53ZZ
ØJX6ØZZ
ØJX63ZZ
ØJX7ØZZ
ØJX73ZZ
ØJX8ØZZ
ØJX83ZZ
ØJX9ØZZ
ØJX93ZZ
ØJXBØZZ
ØJXB3ZZ
ØJXCØZZ
ØJXC3ZZ
ØJXDØZZ
ØJXD3ZZ
ØJXFØZZ
ØJXF3ZZ
ØJXGØZZ
ØJXG3ZZ
ØJXHØZZ
ØJXH3ZZ
ØJXJØZZ
ØJXJ3ZZ
ØJXKØZZ
ØJXK3ZZ
ØJXLØZZ
ØJXL3ZZ
ØJXMØZZ
ØJXM3ZZ
ØJXNØZZ
ØJXN3ZZ
ØJXPØZZ
ØJXP3ZZ
ØJXQØZZ
ØJXQ3ZZ
ØJXRØZZ
ØJXR3ZZ
ØK5Ø*
ØK51*
ØK52*
ØK53*
ØK54*
ØK55*
ØK56*
ØK57*
ØK58*
ØK59*
ØK5B*
ØK5F*
ØK5G*
ØK5H*
ØK5J*
ØK5K*
ØK5L*
ØK5M*
ØK5N*
ØK5P*
ØK5Q*
ØK5R*
ØK5S*
ØK5T*
ØK5V*
ØK5W*
ØK8Ø*
ØK81*
ØK82*
ØK83*
ØK85*
ØK86*
ØK87*
ØK88*
ØK89*
ØK8B*
ØK8F*
ØK8G*
ØK8H*
ØK8J*
ØK8K*
ØK8L*
ØK8M*
ØK8N*
ØK8P*
ØK8Q*
ØK8R*
ØK8S*
ØK8T*
ØK8V*
ØK8W*
ØK9ØØØZ
ØK9ØØZX
ØK9ØØZZ
ØK9Ø3ZX
ØK9Ø4ØZ
ØK9Ø4ZX
ØK9Ø4ZZ
ØK91ØØZ
ØK91ØZX
ØK91ØZZ
ØK913ZX
ØK914ØZ
ØK914ZX
ØK914ZZ
ØK92ØØZ
ØK92ØZX
ØK92ØZZ
ØK923ZX
ØK924ØZ
ØK924ZX
ØK924ZZ
ØK93ØØZ
ØK93ØZX
ØK93ØZZ
ØK933ZX
ØK934ØZ
ØK934ZX
ØK934ZZ
ØK94ØØZ
ØK94ØZX
ØK94ØZZ
ØK943ZX
ØK944ØZ
ØK944ZX
ØK944ZZ
ØK95ØØZ
ØK95ØZX
ØK95ØZZ
ØK953ZX
ØK954ØZ
ØK954ZX
ØK954ZZ
ØK96ØØZ
ØK96ØZX
ØK96ØZZ
ØK963ZX
ØK964ØZ
ØK964ZX
ØK964ZZ
ØK97ØØZ
ØK97ØZX
ØK97ØZZ
ØK973ZX
ØK974ØZ
ØK974ZX
ØK974ZZ
ØK98ØØZ
ØK98ØZX
ØK98ØZZ
ØK983ZX
ØK984ØZ
ØK984ZX
ØK984ZZ
ØK99ØØZ
ØK99ØZX
ØK99ØZZ
ØK993ZX
ØK994ØZ
ØK994ZX
ØK994ZZ
ØK9BØØZ
ØK9BØZX
ØK9BØZZ
ØK9B3ZX
ØK9B4ØZ
ØK9B4ZX
ØK9B4ZZ
ØK9CØZX
ØK9C3ZX
ØK9C4ZX
ØK9DØZX
ØK9D3ZX
ØK9D4ZX
ØK9FØØZ
ØK9FØZX
ØK9FØZZ
ØK9F3ZX
ØK9F4ØZ
ØK9F4ZX
ØK9F4ZZ
ØK9GØØZ
ØK9GØZX
ØK9GØZZ
ØK9G3ZX
ØK9G4ØZ
ØK9G4ZX
ØK9G4ZZ
ØK9HØØZ
ØK9HØZX
ØK9HØZZ
ØK9H3ZX
ØK9H4ØZ
ØK9H4ZX
ØK9H4ZZ
ØK9JØØZ
ØK9JØZX
ØK9JØZZ
ØK9J3ZX
ØK9J4ØZ
ØK9J4ZX
ØK9J4ZZ
ØK9KØØZ
ØK9KØZX
ØK9KØZZ
ØK9K3ZX
ØK9K4ØZ
ØK9K4ZX
ØK9K4ZZ
ØK9LØØZ
ØK9LØZX
ØK9LØZZ
ØK9L3ZX
ØK9L4ØZ
ØK9L4ZX
ØK9L4ZZ
ØK9MØØZ
ØK9MØZX
ØK9MØZZ
ØK9M3ZX
ØK9M4ØZ
ØK9M4ZX
ØK9M4ZZ
ØK9NØØZ
ØK9NØZX
ØK9NØZZ
ØK9N3ZX
ØK9N4ØZ
ØK9N4ZX
ØK9N4ZZ
ØK9PØØZ
ØK9PØZX
ØK9PØZZ
ØK9P3ZX
ØK9P4ØZ
ØK9P4ZX
ØK9P4ZZ
ØK9QØØZ
ØK9QØZX
ØK9QØZZ
ØK9Q3ZX
ØK9Q4ØZ
ØK9Q4ZX
ØK9Q4ZZ
ØK9RØØZ
ØK9RØZX
ØK9RØZZ
ØK9R3ZX
ØK9R4ØZ
ØK9R4ZX
ØK9R4ZZ
ØK9SØØZ
ØK9SØZX
ØK9SØZZ
ØK9S3ZX
ØK9S4ØZ
ØK9S4ZX
ØK9S4ZZ
ØK9TØØZ
ØK9TØZX
ØK9TØZZ
ØK9T3ZX
ØK9T4ØZ
ØK9T4ZX

ØK9T4ZZ
ØK9VØØZ
ØK9VØZX
ØK9VØZZ
ØK9V3ZX
ØK9V4ØZ
ØK9V4ZX
ØK9V4ZZ
ØK9WØØZ
ØK9WØZX
ØK9WØZZ
ØK9W3ZX
ØK9W4ØZ
ØK9W4ZX
ØK9W4ZZ
ØKBØ*
ØKB1*
ØKB2*
ØKB3*
ØKB4*
ØKB5*
ØKB6*
ØKB7*
ØKB8*
ØKB9*
ØKBB*
ØKBCØZX
ØKBC3ZX
ØKBC4ZX
ØKBDØZX
ØKBD3ZX
ØKBD4ZX
ØKBF*
ØKBG*
ØKBH*
ØKBJ*
ØKBK*
ØKBL*
ØKBM*
ØKBNØZX
ØKBNØZZ
ØKBN4ZX
ØKBN4ZZ
ØKBPØZX
ØKBPØZZ
ØKBP4ZX
ØKBP4ZZ
ØKBQ*
ØKBR*
ØKBS*
ØKBT*
ØKBV*
ØKBW*
ØKCØ*
ØKC1*
ØKC2*
ØKC3*
ØKC4*
ØKC5*
ØKC6*
ØKC7*
ØKC8*
ØKC9*
ØKCB*
ØKCF*
ØKCG*
ØKCH*
ØKCJ*
ØKCK*
ØKCL*
ØKCM*
ØKCN*
ØKCP*
ØKCQ*
ØKCR*
ØKCS*
ØKCT*
ØKCV*
ØKCW*
ØKDØØZZ
ØKD1ØZZ
ØKD2ØZZ
ØKD3ØZZ
ØKD4ØZZ
ØKD5ØZZ
ØKD6ØZZ
ØKD7ØZZ
ØKD8ØZZ
ØKD9ØZZ
ØKDBØZZ
ØKDFØZZ
ØKDGØZZ
ØKDHØZZ
ØKDJØZZ
ØKDKØZZ
ØKDLØZZ
ØKDMØZZ
ØKDNØZZ
ØKDPØZZ
ØKDQØZZ
ØKDRØZZ
ØKDSØZZ
ØKDTØZZ
ØKDVØZZ
ØKDWØZZ
ØKHXØMZ
ØKHXØYZ
ØKHX3MZ
ØKHX4MZ
ØKHYØMZ
ØKHYØYZ
ØKHY3MZ
ØKHY4MZ
ØKJXØZZ
ØKJX4ZZ
ØKJYØZZ
ØKJY4ZZ
ØKMØ*
ØKM1*
ØKM2*
ØKM3*
ØKM4*
ØKM5*
ØKM6*
ØKM7*
ØKM8*
ØKM9*
ØKMB*
ØKMF*
ØKMG*
ØKMH*
ØKMJ*
ØKMK*
ØKML*
ØKMM*
ØKMN*
ØKMP*
ØKMQ*
ØKMR*
ØKMS*
ØKMT*
ØKMV*
ØKMW*
ØKNØØZZ
ØKNØ3ZZ
ØKNØ4ZZ
ØKN1ØZZ
ØKN13ZZ
ØKN14ZZ
ØKN2ØZZ
ØKN23ZZ
ØKN24ZZ
ØKN3ØZZ
ØKN33ZZ
ØKN34ZZ
ØKN4ØZZ
ØKN43ZZ
ØKN44ZZ
ØKN5ØZZ
ØKN53ZZ
ØKN54ZZ
ØKN6ØZZ
ØKN63ZZ
ØKN64ZZ
ØKN7ØZZ
ØKN73ZZ
ØKN74ZZ
ØKN8ØZZ
ØKN83ZZ
ØKN84ZZ
ØKN9ØZZ
ØKN93ZZ
ØKN94ZZ
ØKNBØZZ
ØKNB3ZZ
ØKNB4ZZ
ØKNFØZZ
ØKNF3ZZ
ØKNF4ZZ
ØKNGØZZ
ØKNG3ZZ
ØKNG4ZZ
ØKNHØZZ
ØKNH3ZZ
ØKNH4ZZ
ØKNJØZZ
ØKNJ3ZZ
ØKNJ4ZZ
ØKNKØZZ
ØKNK3ZZ
ØKNK4ZZ
ØKNLØZZ
ØKNL3ZZ
ØKNL4ZZ
ØKNMØZZ
ØKNM3ZZ
ØKNM4ZZ
ØKNNØZZ
ØKNN3ZZ
ØKNN4ZZ
ØKNPØZZ
ØKNP3ZZ
ØKNP4ZZ
ØKNQØZZ
ØKNQ3ZZ
ØKNQ4ZZ
ØKNRØZZ
ØKNR3ZZ
ØKNR4ZZ
ØKNSØZZ
ØKNS3ZZ
ØKNS4ZZ
ØKNTØZZ
ØKNT3ZZ
ØKNT4ZZ
ØKNVØZZ
ØKNV3ZZ
ØKNV4ZZ
ØKNWØZZ
ØKNW3ZZ
ØKNW4ZZ
ØKPXØØZ
ØKPXØ7Z
ØKPXØJZ
ØKPXØKZ
ØKPXØMZ
ØKPXØYZ
ØKPX3ØZ
ØKPX37Z
ØKPX3JZ
ØKPX3KZ
ØKPX3MZ
ØKPX4ØZ
ØKPX47Z
ØKPX4JZ
ØKPX4KZ
ØKPX4MZ
ØKPYØØZ
ØKPYØ7Z
ØKPYØJZ
ØKPYØKZ
ØKPYØMZ
ØKPYØYZ
ØKPY3ØZ
ØKPY37Z
ØKPY3JZ
ØKPY3KZ
ØKPY3MZ
ØKPY4ØZ
ØKPY47Z
ØKPY4JZ
ØKPY4KZ
ØKPY4MZ
ØKQØ*
ØKQ1*
ØKQ2*
ØKQ3*
ØKQ4*
ØKQ5*
ØKQ6*
ØKQ7*
ØKQ8*
ØKQ9*
ØKQB*
ØKQF*
ØKQG*
ØKQH*
ØKQJ*
ØKQK*
ØKQL*
ØKQM*
ØKQN*
ØKQP*
ØKQQ*
ØKQR*
ØKQS*
ØKQT*
ØKQV*
ØKQW*
ØKRØØ7Z
ØKRØØJZ
ØKRØØKZ
ØKRØ47Z
ØKRØ4JZ
ØKRØ4KZ
ØKR1Ø7Z
ØKR1ØJZ
ØKR1ØKZ
ØKR147Z
ØKR14JZ
ØKR14KZ
ØKR2Ø7Z
ØKR2ØJZ
ØKR2ØKZ
ØKR247Z
ØKR24JZ
ØKR24KZ
ØKR3Ø7Z
ØKR3ØJZ
ØKR3ØKZ
ØKR347Z
ØKR34JZ
ØKR34KZ
ØKR4Ø7Z
ØKR4ØJZ
ØKR4ØKZ
ØKR447Z
ØKR44JZ
ØKR44KZ
ØKR5Ø7Z
ØKR5ØJZ
ØKR5ØKZ
ØKR547Z
ØKR54JZ
ØKR54KZ
ØKR6Ø7Z
ØKR6ØJZ
ØKR6ØKZ
ØKR647Z
ØKR64JZ
ØKR64KZ
ØKR7Ø7Z
ØKR7ØJZ
ØKR7ØKZ
ØKR747Z
ØKR74JZ
ØKR74KZ
ØKR8Ø7Z
ØKR8ØJZ
ØKR8ØKZ
ØKR847Z
ØKR84JZ
ØKR84KZ
ØKR9Ø7Z
ØKR9ØJZ
ØKR9ØKZ
ØKR947Z
ØKR94JZ
ØKR94KZ
ØKRBØ7Z
ØKRBØJZ
ØKRBØKZ
ØKRB47Z
ØKRB4JZ
ØKRB4KZ
ØKRFØ7Z
ØKRFØJZ
ØKRFØKZ
ØKRF47Z
ØKRF4JZ
ØKRF4KZ
ØKRGØ7Z
ØKRGØJZ
ØKRGØKZ
ØKRG47Z
ØKRG4JZ
ØKRG4KZ
ØKRHØ7Z
ØKRHØJZ
ØKRHØKZ
ØKRH47Z
ØKRH4JZ
ØKRH4KZ
ØKRJØ7Z
ØKRJØJZ
ØKRJØKZ
ØKRJ47Z
ØKRJ4JZ
ØKRJ4KZ
ØKRKØ7Z
ØKRKØJZ
ØKRKØKZ
ØKRK47Z
ØKRK4JZ
ØKRK4KZ
ØKRLØ7Z
ØKRLØJZ
ØKRLØKZ
ØKRL47Z
ØKRL4JZ
ØKRL4KZ
ØKRMØ7Z
ØKRMØJZ
ØKRMØKZ
ØKRM47Z
ØKRM4JZ
ØKRM4KZ
ØKRNØ7Z
ØKRNØJZ
ØKRNØKZ
ØKRN47Z
ØKRN4JZ
ØKRN4KZ
ØKRPØ7Z
ØKRPØJZ
ØKRPØKZ
ØKRP47Z
ØKRP4JZ
ØKRP4KZ
ØKRQØ7Z
ØKRQØJZ
ØKRQØKZ
ØKRQ47Z
ØKRQ4JZ
ØKRQ4KZ
ØKRRØ7Z
ØKRRØJZ
ØKRRØKZ
ØKRR47Z
ØKRR4JZ
ØKRR4KZ
ØKRSØ7Z
ØKRSØJZ
ØKRSØKZ
ØKRS47Z
ØKRS4JZ
ØKRS4KZ
ØKRTØ7Z
ØKRTØJZ
ØKRTØKZ
ØKRT47Z
ØKRT4JZ
ØKRT4KZ
ØKRVØ7Z
ØKRVØJZ
ØKRVØKZ
ØKRV47Z
ØKRV4JZ
ØKRV4KZ
ØKRWØ7Z
ØKRWØJZ
ØKRWØKZ
ØKRW47Z
ØKRW4JZ
ØKRW4KZ
ØKSØ*
ØKS1*
ØKS2*
ØKS3*
ØKS4*
ØKS5*
ØKS6*
ØKS7*
ØKS8*
ØKS9*
ØKSB*
ØKSF*
ØKSG*
ØKSH*
ØKSJ*
ØKSK*
ØKSL*
ØKSM*
ØKSN*
ØKSP*
ØKSQ*
ØKSR*
ØKSS*
ØKST*
ØKSV*
ØKSW*
ØKTØ*
ØKT1*
ØKT2*
ØKT3*
ØKT4*
ØKT5*
ØKT6*
ØKT7*
ØKT8*
ØKT9*
ØKTB*
ØKTF*
ØKTG*
ØKTH*
ØKTJ*
ØKTK*
ØKTL*
ØKTM*
ØKTN*
ØKTP*
ØKTQ*
ØKTR*
ØKTS*
ØKTT*
ØKTV*
ØKTW*
ØKUØ*
ØKU1*
ØKU2*
ØKU3*
ØKU4*
ØKU5*
ØKU6*
ØKU7*
ØKU8*
ØKU9*
ØKUB*
ØKUF*
ØKUG*
ØKUH*
ØKUJ*
ØKUK*
ØKUL*
ØKUM*
ØKUN*
ØKUP*
ØKUQ*
ØKUR*
ØKUS*
ØKUT*
ØKUV*
ØKUW*
ØKWXØØZ
ØKWXØ7Z
ØKWXØJZ
ØKWXØKZ
ØKWXØMZ
ØKWXØYZ
ØKWX3ØZ
ØKWX37Z
ØKWX3JZ
ØKWX3KZ
ØKWX3MZ
ØKWX4ØZ
ØKWX47Z
ØKWX4JZ
ØKWX4KZ
ØKWX4MZ
ØKWYØØZ
ØKWYØ7Z
ØKWYØJZ
ØKWYØKZ
ØKWYØMZ
ØKWYØYZ
ØKWY3ØZ
ØKWY37Z
ØKWY3JZ
ØKWY3KZ
ØKWY3MZ
ØKWY4ØZ
ØKWY47Z
ØKWY4JZ
ØKWY4KZ
ØKWY4MZ
ØKXØ*
ØKX1*
ØKX2*
ØKX3*
ØKX4*
ØKX5*
ØKX6*
ØKX7*
ØKX8*
ØKX9*
ØKXB*
ØKXFØZØ
ØKXFØZ1
ØKXFØZ2
ØKXFØZZ
ØKXF4ZØ
ØKXF4Z1
ØKXF4Z2
ØKXF4ZZ
ØKXGØZØ
ØKXGØZ1
ØKXGØZ2
ØKXGØZZ
ØKXG4ZØ
ØKXG4Z1
ØKXG4Z2
ØKXG4ZZ
ØKXHØZØ
ØKXHØZ1
ØKXHØZ2
ØKXH4ZØ
ØKXH4Z1
ØKXH4Z2
ØKXJØZØ
ØKXJØZ1
ØKXJØZ2
ØKXJ4ZØ
ØKXJ4Z1
ØKXJ4Z2
ØKXKØZØ
ØKXKØZ1
ØKXKØZ2
ØKXKØZZ
ØKXK4ZØ
ØKXK4Z1
ØKXK4Z2
ØKXK4ZZ
ØKXLØZØ
ØKXLØZ1
ØKXLØZ2
ØKXLØZZ
ØKXL4ZØ
ØKXL4Z1
ØKXL4Z2
ØKXL4ZZ
ØKXM*
ØKXN*
ØKXP*
ØKXQ*
ØKXR*
ØKXS*
ØKXT*
ØKXV*
ØKXW*
ØL5Ø*
ØL51*
ØL52*
ØL53*
ØL54*
ØL55*
ØL56*
ØL59*
ØL5B*
ØL5C*
ØL5D*
ØL5F*
ØL5G*
ØL5H*
ØL5J*
ØL5K*
ØL5L*
ØL5M*
ØL5N*
ØL5P*
ØL5Q*
ØL5R*
ØL5S*
ØL5T*
ØL5V*
ØL5W*
ØL8Ø*
ØL81*
ØL82*
ØL83*
ØL84*
ØL85*
ØL86*
ØL89*
ØL8B*
ØL8C*
ØL8D*
ØL8F*
ØL8G*
ØL8H*
ØL8L*
ØL8M*
ØL8Q*
ØL8R*
ØL8S*
ØL8T*
ØL8V*
ØL8W*
ØL9ØØØZ
ØL9ØØZX
ØL9ØØZZ
ØL9Ø3ZX
ØL9Ø4ØZ
ØL9Ø4ZX
ØL9Ø4ZZ
ØL91ØØZ
ØL91ØZX
ØL91ØZZ
ØL913ZX
ØL914ØZ
ØL914ZX
ØL914ZZ
ØL92ØØZ
ØL92ØZX
ØL92ØZZ
ØL923ZX
ØL924ØZ
ØL924ZX
ØL924ZZ
ØL93ØØZ
ØL93ØZX
ØL93ØZZ
ØL933ZX
ØL934ØZ
ØL934ZX
ØL934ZZ
ØL94ØØZ
ØL94ØZX
ØL94ØZZ
ØL943ZX
ØL944ØZ
ØL944ZX
ØL944ZZ
ØL95ØØZ
ØL95ØZX
ØL95ØZZ
ØL953ZX
ØL954ØZ
ØL954ZX
ØL954ZZ
ØL96ØØZ
ØL96ØZX
ØL96ØZZ
ØL963ZX
ØL964ØZ
ØL964ZX
ØL964ZZ
ØL97ØZX
ØL973ZX
ØL974ZX
ØL98ØZX
ØL983ZX
ØL984ZX
ØL99ØØZ
ØL99ØZX
ØL99ØZZ
ØL993ZX
ØL994ØZ
ØL994ZX
ØL994ZZ
ØL9BØØZ
ØL9BØZX
ØL9BØZZ
ØL9B3ZX
ØL9B4ØZ
ØL9B4ZX
ØL9B4ZZ
ØL9CØØZ
ØL9CØZX
ØL9CØZZ
ØL9C3ZX
ØL9C4ØZ
ØL9C4ZX
ØL9C4ZZ
ØL9DØØZ
ØL9DØZX
ØL9DØZZ
ØL9D3ZX
ØL9D4ØZ
ØL9D4ZX
ØL9D4ZZ
ØL9FØØZ
ØL9FØZX
ØL9FØZZ
ØL9F3ZX
ØL9F4ØZ
ØL9F4ZX
ØL9F4ZZ
ØL9GØØZ
ØL9GØZX
ØL9GØZZ
ØL9G3ZX
ØL9G4ØZ
ØL9G4ZX
ØL9G4ZZ
ØL9HØØZ
ØL9HØZX
ØL9HØZZ
ØL9H3ZX
ØL9H4ØZ
ØL9H4ZX
ØL9H4ZZ
ØL9JØØZ
ØL9JØZX
ØL9JØZZ
ØL9J3ZX
ØL9J4ØZ
ØL9J4ZX
ØL9J4ZZ
ØL9KØØZ
ØL9KØZX
ØL9KØZZ
ØL9K3ZX
ØL9K4ØZ
ØL9K4ZX
ØL9K4ZZ
ØL9LØØZ
ØL9LØZX
ØL9LØZZ
ØL9L3ZX
ØL9L4ØZ
ØL9L4ZX
ØL9L4ZZ
ØL9MØØZ
ØL9MØZX
ØL9MØZZ
ØL9M3ZX
ØL9M4ØZ
ØL9M4ZX
ØL9M4ZZ
ØL9NØØZ
ØL9NØZX
ØL9NØZZ
ØL9N3ZX
ØL9N4ØZ
ØL9N4ZX
ØL9N4ZZ
ØL9PØØZ
ØL9PØZX
ØL9PØZZ
ØL9P3ZX
ØL9P4ØZ
ØL9P4ZX
ØL9P4ZZ
ØL9QØØZ
ØL9QØZX
ØL9QØZZ
ØL9Q3ZX
ØL9Q4ØZ
ØL9Q4ZX
ØL9Q4ZZ
ØL9RØØZ
ØL9RØZX
ØL9RØZZ
ØL9R3ZX
ØL9R4ØZ
ØL9R4ZX
ØL9R4ZZ
ØL9SØØZ
ØL9SØZX
ØL9SØZZ
ØL9S3ZX
ØL9S4ØZ
ØL9S4ZX
ØL9S4ZZ
ØL9TØØZ
ØL9TØZX
ØL9TØZZ
ØL9T3ZX
ØL9T4ØZ
ØL9T4ZX
ØL9T4ZZ
ØL9VØØZ
ØL9VØZX
ØL9VØZZ
ØL9V3ZX
ØL9V4ØZ
ØL9V4ZX
ØL9V4ZZ
ØL9WØØZ
ØL9WØZX
ØL9WØZZ
ØL9W3ZX
ØL9W4ØZ
ØL9W4ZX
ØL9W4ZZ
ØLBØ*
ØLB1*
ØLB2*
ØLB3*
ØLB4*
ØLB5*
ØLB6*
ØLB7ØZX
ØLB73ZX
ØLB74ZX

ØLB8ØZX
ØLB83ZX
ØLB84ZX
ØLB9*
ØLBB*
ØLBC*
ØLBD*
ØLBF*
ØLBG*
ØLBH*
ØLBJ*
ØLBK*
ØLBL*
ØLBM*
ØLBN*
ØLBP*
ØLBQ*
ØLBR*
ØLBS*
ØLBT*
ØLBV*
ØLBW*
ØLCØ*
ØLC1*
ØLC2*
ØLC3*
ØLC4*
ØLC5*
ØLC6*
ØLC9*
ØLCB*
ØLCC*
ØLCD*
ØLCF*
ØLCG*
ØLCH*
ØLCJ*
ØLCK*
ØLCL*
ØLCM*
ØLCN*
ØLCP*
ØLCQ*
ØLCR*
ØLCS*
ØLCT*
ØLCV*
ØLCW*
ØLDØØZZ
ØLD1ØZZ
ØLD2ØZZ
ØLD3ØZZ
ØLD4ØZZ
ØLD5ØZZ
ØLD6ØZZ
ØLD9ØZZ
ØLDBØZZ
ØLDCØZZ
ØLDDØZZ
ØLDFØZZ
ØLDGØZZ
ØLDHØZZ
ØLDJØZZ
ØLDKØZZ
ØLDLØZZ
ØLDMØZZ
ØLDNØZZ
ØLDPØZZ
ØLDQØZZ
ØLDRØZZ
ØLDSØZZ
ØLDTØZZ
ØLDVØZZ
ØLDWØZZ
ØLHXØYZ
ØLHYØYZ
ØLJYØZZ
ØLJY4ZZ
ØLMØ*
ØLM1*
ØLM2*
ØLM3*
ØLM4*
ØLM5*
ØLM6*
ØLM9*
ØLMB*
ØLMC*
ØLMD*
ØLMF*
ØLMG*
ØLMH*
ØLMJ*
ØLMK*
ØLML*
ØLMM*
ØLMN*
ØLMP*
ØLMQ*
ØLMR*
ØLMS*
ØLMT*
ØLMV*
ØLMW*
ØLNØØZZ
ØLNØ3ZZ
ØLNØ4ZZ
ØLN1ØZZ
ØLN13ZZ
ØLN14ZZ
ØLN2ØZZ
ØLN23ZZ
ØLN24ZZ
ØLN3ØZZ
ØLN33ZZ
ØLN34ZZ
ØLN4ØZZ
ØLN43ZZ
ØLN44ZZ
ØLN5ØZZ
ØLN53ZZ
ØLN54ZZ
ØLN6ØZZ
ØLN63ZZ
ØLN64ZZ
ØLN9ØZZ
ØLN93ZZ
ØLN94ZZ
ØLNBØZZ
ØLNB3ZZ
ØLNB4ZZ
ØLNCØZZ
ØLNC3ZZ
ØLNC4ZZ
ØLNDØZZ
ØLND3ZZ
ØLND4ZZ
ØLNFØZZ
ØLNF3ZZ
ØLNF4ZZ
ØLNGØZZ
ØLNG3ZZ
ØLNG4ZZ
ØLNHØZZ
ØLNH3ZZ
ØLNH4ZZ
ØLNJØZZ
ØLNJ3ZZ
ØLNJ4ZZ
ØLNKØZZ
ØLNK3ZZ
ØLNK4ZZ
ØLNLØZZ
ØLNL3ZZ
ØLNL4ZZ
ØLNMØZZ
ØLNM3ZZ
ØLNM4ZZ
ØLNNØZZ
ØLNN3ZZ
ØLNN4ZZ
ØLNPØZZ
ØLNP3ZZ
ØLNP4ZZ
ØLNQØZZ
ØLNQ3ZZ
ØLNQ4ZZ
ØLNRØZZ
ØLNR3ZZ
ØLNR4ZZ
ØLNSØZZ
ØLNS3ZZ
ØLNS4ZZ
ØLNTØZZ
ØLNT3ZZ
ØLNT4ZZ
ØLNVØZZ
ØLNV3ZZ
ØLNV4ZZ
ØLNWØZZ
ØLNW3ZZ
ØLNW4ZZ
ØLPXØØZ
ØLPXØ7Z
ØLPXØJZ
ØLPXØKZ
ØLPXØYZ
ØLPX37Z
ØLPX3JZ
ØLPX3KZ
ØLPX4ØZ
ØLPX47Z
ØLPX4JZ
ØLPX4KZ
ØLPYØØZ
ØLPYØ7Z
ØLPYØJZ
ØLPYØKZ
ØLPYØYZ
ØLPY37Z
ØLPY3JZ
ØLPY3KZ
ØLPY4ØZ
ØLPY47Z
ØLPY4JZ
ØLPY4KZ
ØLQØ*
ØLQ3*
ØLQ4*
ØLQ5*
ØLQ6*
ØLQ9*
ØLQB*
ØLQC*
ØLQD*
ØLQF*
ØLQG*
ØLQH*
ØLQJ*
ØLQK*
ØLQL*
ØLQM*
ØLQN*
ØLQP*
ØLQQ*
ØLQR*
ØLQS*
ØLQT*
ØLQV*
ØLQW*
ØLRØ*
ØLR1*
ØLR2*
ØLR3*
ØLR4*
ØLR5*
ØLR6*
ØLR9*
ØLRB*
ØLRC*
ØLRD*
ØLRF*
ØLRG*
ØLRH*
ØLRJ*
ØLRK*
ØLRL*
ØLRM*
ØLRN*
ØLRP*
ØLRQ*
ØLRR*
ØLRS*
ØLRT*
ØLRV*
ØLRW*
ØLSØ*
ØLS1*
ØLS2*
ØLS3*
ØLS4*
ØLS5*
ØLS6*
ØLS9*
ØLSB*
ØLSC*
ØLSD*
ØLSF*
ØLSG*
ØLSH*
ØLSJ*
ØLSK*
ØLSL*
ØLSM*
ØLSN*
ØLSP*
ØLSQ*
ØLSR*
ØLSS*
ØLST*
ØLSV*
ØLSW*
ØLTØ*
ØLT1*
ØLT2*
ØLT3*
ØLT4*
ØLT5*
ØLT6*
ØLT9*
ØLTB*
ØLTC*
ØLTD*
ØLTF*
ØLTG*
ØLTH*
ØLTJ*
ØLTK*
ØLTL*
ØLTM*
ØLTN*
ØLTP*
ØLTQ*
ØLTR*
ØLTS*
ØLTT*
ØLTV*
ØLTW*
ØLUØ*
ØLU1*
ØLU2*
ØLU3*
ØLU4*
ØLU5*
ØLU6*
ØLU9*
ØLUB*
ØLUC*
ØLUD*
ØLUF*
ØLUG*
ØLUH*
ØLUJ*
ØLUK*
ØLUL*
ØLUM*
ØLUN*
ØLUP*
ØLUQ*
ØLUR*
ØLUS*
ØLUT*
ØLUV*
ØLUW*
ØLWXØØZ
ØLWXØ7Z
ØLWXØJZ
ØLWXØKZ
ØLWXØYZ
ØLWX3ØZ
ØLWX37Z
ØLWX3JZ
ØLWX3KZ
ØLWX4ØZ
ØLWX47Z
ØLWX4JZ
ØLWX4KZ
ØLWYØØZ
ØLWYØ7Z
ØLWYØJZ
ØLWYØKZ
ØLWYØYZ
ØLWY3ØZ
ØLWY37Z
ØLWY3JZ
ØLWY3KZ
ØLWY4ØZ
ØLWY47Z
ØLWY4JZ
ØLWY4KZ
ØLXØ*
ØLX1*
ØLX2*
ØLX3*
ØLX4*
ØLX5*
ØLX6*
ØLX9*
ØLXB*
ØLXC*
ØLXD*
ØLXF*
ØLXG*
ØLXH*
ØLXJ*
ØLXK*
ØLXL*
ØLXM*
ØLXN*
ØLXP*
ØLXQ*
ØLXR*
ØLXS*
ØLXT*
ØLXV*
ØLXW*
ØM8Ø*
ØM81*
ØM82*
ØM83*
ØM84*
ØM85ØZZ
ØM853ZZ
ØM854ZZ
ØM86ØZZ
ØM863ZZ
ØM864ZZ
ØM89*
ØM8B*
ØM8C*
ØM8D*
ØM8F*
ØM8G*
ØM8H*
ØM8J*
ØM8K*
ØM8L*
ØM8M*
ØM8N*
ØM8P*
ØM8Q*
ØM8R*
ØM8S*
ØM8T*
ØM8V*
ØM8W*
ØM9ØØØZ
ØM9ØØZZ
ØM91ØØZ
ØM91ØZZ
ØM92ØØZ
ØM92ØZZ
ØM93ØØZ
ØM93ØZZ
ØM94ØØZ
ØM94ØZZ
ØM99ØØZ
ØM99ØZX
ØM99ØZZ
ØM993ZX
ØM994ZX
ØM9BØØZ
ØM9BØZX
ØM9BØZZ
ØM9B3ZX
ØM9B4ZX
ØM9CØØZ
ØM9CØZZ
ØM9DØØZ
ØM9DØZZ
ØM9FØØZ
ØM9FØZZ
ØM9GØØZ
ØM9GØZZ
ØM9HØØZ
ØM9HØZX
ØM9HØZZ
ØM9H3ZX
ØM9H4ZX
ØM9JØØZ
ØM9JØZX
ØM9JØZZ
ØM9J3ZX
ØM9J4ZX
ØM9KØØZ
ØM9KØZX
ØM9KØZZ
ØM9K3ZX
ØM9K4ZX
ØM9LØØZ
ØM9LØZZ
ØM9MØØZ
ØM9MØZZ
ØM9NØØZ
ØM9NØZZ
ØM9PØØZ
ØM9PØZZ
ØM9QØØZ
ØM9QØZZ
ØM9RØØZ
ØM9RØZZ
ØM9SØØZ
ØM9SØZZ
ØM9TØØZ
ØM9TØZZ
ØM9VØØZ
ØM9VØZX
ØM9VØZZ
ØM9V3ZX
ØM9V4ZX
ØM9WØØZ
ØM9WØZX
ØM9WØZZ
ØM9W3ZX
ØM9W4ZX
ØMBØØZZ
ØMBØ3ZZ
ØMBØ4ZZ
ØMB1ØZZ
ØMB13ZZ
ØMB14ZZ
ØMB2ØZZ
ØMB23ZZ
ØMB24ZZ
ØMB3ØZZ
ØMB33ZZ
ØMB34ZZ
ØMB4ØZZ
ØMB43ZZ
ØMB44ZZ
ØMB5ØZZ
ØMB53ZZ
ØMB54ZZ
ØMB6ØZZ
ØMB63ZZ
ØMB64ZZ
ØMB9ØZX
ØMB9ØZZ
ØMB93ZX
ØMB93ZZ
ØMB94ZZ
ØMBBØZZ
ØMBB3ZZ
ØMBB4ZZ
ØMBCØZZ
ØMBC3ZZ
ØMBC4ZZ
ØMBDØZZ
ØMBD3ZZ
ØMBD4ZZ
ØMBFØZZ
ØMBF3ZZ
ØMBF4ZZ
ØMBGØZZ
ØMBG3ZZ
ØMBG4ZZ
ØMBH*
ØMBJ*
ØMBK*
ØMBLØZZ
ØMBL3ZZ
ØMBL4ZZ
ØMBMØZZ
ØMBM3ZZ
ØMBM4ZZ
ØMBNØZZ
ØMBN3ZZ
ØMBN4ZZ
ØMBPØZZ
ØMBP3ZZ
ØMBP4ZZ
ØMBQØZZ
ØMBQ3ZZ
ØMBQ4ZZ
ØMBRØZZ
ØMBR3ZZ
ØMBR4ZZ
ØMBSØZZ
ØMBS3ZZ
ØMBS4ZZ
ØMBTØZZ
ØMBT3ZZ
ØMBT4ZZ
ØMBV*
ØMBW*
ØMCØ*
ØMC1*
ØMC2*
ØMC3*
ØMC4*
ØMC9*
ØMCB*
ØMCC*
ØMCD*
ØMCF*
ØMCG*
ØMCH*
ØMCJ*
ØMCK*
ØMCL*
ØMCM*
ØMCN*
ØMCP*
ØMCQ*
ØMCR*
ØMCS*
ØMCT*
ØMCV*
ØMCW*
ØMDØ*
ØMD1*
ØMD2*
ØMD3*
ØMD4*
ØMD5*
ØMD6*
ØMD9*
ØMDB*
ØMDC*
ØMDD*
ØMDF*
ØMDG*
ØMDH*
ØMDJ*
ØMDK*
ØMDL*
ØMDM*
ØMDN*
ØMDP*
ØMDQ*
ØMDR*
ØMDS*
ØMDT*
ØMDV*
ØMDW*
ØMHXØYZ
ØMHYØYZ
ØMNØØZZ
ØMNØ3ZZ
ØMNØ4ZZ
ØMN1ØZZ
ØMN13ZZ
ØMN14ZZ
ØMN2ØZZ
ØMN23ZZ
ØMN24ZZ
ØMN3ØZZ
ØMN33ZZ
ØMN34ZZ
ØMN4ØZZ
ØMN43ZZ
ØMN44ZZ
ØMN5ØZZ
ØMN53ZZ
ØMN54ZZ
ØMN6ØZZ
ØMN63ZZ
ØMN64ZZ
ØMN9ØZZ
ØMN93ZZ
ØMN94ZZ
ØMNBØZZ
ØMNB3ZZ
ØMNB4ZZ
ØMNCØZZ
ØMNC3ZZ
ØMNC4ZZ
ØMNDØZZ
ØMND3ZZ
ØMND4ZZ
ØMNFØZZ
ØMNF3ZZ
ØMNF4ZZ
ØMNGØZZ
ØMNG3ZZ
ØMNG4ZZ
ØMNHØZZ
ØMNH3ZZ
ØMNH4ZZ
ØMNJØZZ
ØMNJ3ZZ
ØMNJ4ZZ
ØMNKØZZ
ØMNK3ZZ
ØMNK4ZZ
ØMNLØZZ
ØMNL3ZZ
ØMNL4ZZ
ØMNMØZZ
ØMNM3ZZ
ØMNM4ZZ
ØMNNØZZ
ØMNN3ZZ
ØMNN4ZZ
ØMNPØZZ
ØMNP3ZZ
ØMNP4ZZ
ØMNQØZZ
ØMNQ3ZZ
ØMNQ4ZZ
ØMNRØZZ
ØMNR3ZZ
ØMNR4ZZ
ØMNSØZZ
ØMNS3ZZ
ØMNS4ZZ
ØMNTØZZ
ØMNT3ZZ
ØMNT4ZZ
ØMNVØZZ
ØMNV3ZZ
ØMNV4ZZ
ØMNWØZZ
ØMNW3ZZ
ØMNW4ZZ
ØMPXØ7Z
ØMPXØKZ
ØMPX37Z
ØMPX3KZ
ØMPX47Z
ØMPX4KZ
ØMPYØ7Z
ØMPYØKZ
ØMPY37Z
ØMPY3KZ
ØMPY47Z
ØMPY4KZ
ØMQØ*
ØMQ1*
ØMQ2*
ØMQ3*
ØMQ4*
ØMQ5*
ØMQ6*
ØMQ7*
ØMQ8*
ØMQ9*
ØMQB*
ØMQC*
ØMQD*
ØMQF*
ØMQG*
ØMQH*
ØMQJ*
ØMQK*
ØMQL*
ØMQM*
ØMQQ*
ØMQR*
ØMQV*
ØMQW*
ØMRØØ7Z
ØMRØØJZ
ØMRØØKZ
ØMRØ47Z
ØMRØ4JZ
ØMRØ4KZ
ØMR1Ø7Z
ØMR1ØJZ
ØMR1ØKZ
ØMR147Z
ØMR14JZ
ØMR14KZ
ØMR2Ø7Z
ØMR2ØJZ
ØMR2ØKZ
ØMR247Z
ØMR24JZ
ØMR24KZ
ØMR3Ø7Z
ØMR3ØJZ
ØMR3ØKZ
ØMR347Z
ØMR34JZ
ØMR34KZ
ØMR4Ø7Z
ØMR4ØJZ
ØMR4ØKZ
ØMR447Z
ØMR44JZ
ØMR44KZ
ØMR5Ø7Z
ØMR5ØJZ
ØMR5ØKZ
ØMR547Z
ØMR54JZ
ØMR54KZ
ØMR6Ø7Z
ØMR6ØJZ
ØMR6ØKZ
ØMR647Z
ØMR64JZ
ØMR64KZ
ØMR7Ø7Z
ØMR7ØJZ
ØMR7ØKZ
ØMR747Z
ØMR74JZ
ØMR74KZ
ØMR8Ø7Z
ØMR8ØJZ
ØMR8ØKZ
ØMR847Z
ØMR84JZ
ØMR84KZ
ØMR9Ø7Z
ØMR9ØJZ
ØMR9ØKZ
ØMR947Z
ØMR94JZ
ØMR94KZ
ØMRBØ7Z
ØMRBØJZ
ØMRBØKZ
ØMRB47Z
ØMRB4JZ
ØMRB4KZ
ØMRCØ7Z
ØMRCØJZ
ØMRCØKZ
ØMRC47Z
ØMRC4JZ
ØMRC4KZ
ØMRDØ7Z
ØMRDØJZ
ØMRDØKZ
ØMRD47Z
ØMRD4JZ
ØMRD4KZ
ØMRFØ7Z
ØMRFØJZ
ØMRFØKZ
ØMRF47Z
ØMRF4JZ
ØMRF4KZ
ØMRGØ7Z
ØMRGØJZ
ØMRGØKZ
ØMRG47Z
ØMRG4JZ
ØMRG4KZ
ØMRHØ7Z
ØMRHØJZ
ØMRHØKZ
ØMRH47Z
ØMRH4JZ
ØMRH4KZ
ØMRJØ7Z
ØMRJØJZ
ØMRJØKZ
ØMRJ47Z
ØMRJ4JZ
ØMRJ4KZ
ØMRKØ7Z
ØMRKØJZ
ØMRKØKZ
ØMRK47Z
ØMRK4JZ
ØMRK4KZ
ØMRLØ7Z
ØMRLØJZ
ØMRLØKZ
ØMRL47Z
ØMRL4JZ
ØMRL4KZ
ØMRMØ7Z
ØMRMØJZ
ØMRMØKZ
ØMRM47Z
ØMRM4JZ
ØMRM4KZ
ØMRQØ7Z
ØMRQØJZ
ØMRQØKZ
ØMRQ47Z
ØMRQ4JZ
ØMRQ4KZ
ØMRRØ7Z
ØMRRØJZ
ØMRRØKZ
ØMRR47Z
ØMRR4JZ
ØMRR4KZ
ØMRVØ7Z
ØMRVØJZ

ØMRVØKZ
ØMRV47Z
ØMRV4JZ
ØMRV4KZ
ØMRWØ7Z
ØMRWØJZ
ØMRWØKZ
ØMRW47Z
ØMRW4JZ
ØMRW4KZ
ØMS9*
ØMSB*
ØMSV*
ØMSW*
ØMTØ*
ØMT1*
ØMT2*
ØMT3*
ØMT4*
ØMT5*
ØMT6*
ØMT9*
ØMTB*
ØMTC*
ØMTD*
ØMTF*
ØMTG*
ØMTH*
ØMTJ*
ØMTK*
ØMTL*
ØMTM*
ØMTN*
ØMTP*
ØMTQ*
ØMTR*
ØMTS*
ØMTT*
ØMTV*
ØMTW*
ØMU9*
ØMUB*
ØMUV*
ØMUW*
ØMWXØØZ
ØMWXØ7Z
ØMWXØJZ
ØMWXØKZ
ØMWXØYZ
ØMWX3ØZ
ØMWX37Z
ØMWX3JZ
ØMWX3KZ
ØMWX4ØZ
ØMWX47Z
ØMWX4JZ
ØMWX4KZ
ØMWYØØZ
ØMWYØ7Z
ØMWYØJZ
ØMWYØKZ
ØMWYØYZ
ØMWY3ØZ
ØMWY37Z
ØMWY3JZ
ØMWY3KZ
ØMWY4ØZ
ØMWY47Z
ØMWY4JZ
ØMWY4KZ
ØMX*
ØNDØØZZ
ØND1ØZZ
ØND3ØZZ
ØND4ØZZ
ØND5ØZZ
ØND6ØZZ
ØND7ØZZ
ØNDBØZZ
ØNDCØZZ
ØNDFØZZ
ØNDGØZZ
ØNDHØZZ
ØNDJØZZ
ØNDKØZZ
ØNDLØZZ
ØNDMØZZ
ØNDNØZZ
ØNDPØZZ
ØNDQØZZ
ØNDRØZZ
ØNDTØZZ
ØNDVØZZ
ØNDXØZZ
ØPDØØZZ
ØPD1ØZZ
ØPD2ØZZ
ØPD3ØZZ
ØPD4ØZZ
ØPD5ØZZ
ØPD6ØZZ
ØPD7ØZZ
ØPD8ØZZ
ØPD9ØZZ
ØPDBØZZ
ØPDCØZZ
ØPDDØZZ
ØPDFØZZ
ØPDGØZZ
ØPDHØZZ
ØPDJØZZ
ØPDKØZZ
ØPDLØZZ
ØQDØØZZ
ØQD1ØZZ
ØQD2ØZZ
ØQD3ØZZ
ØQD4ØZZ
ØQD5ØZZ
ØQD6ØZZ
ØQD7ØZZ
ØQD8ØZZ
ØQD9ØZZ
ØQDBØZZ
ØQDCØZZ
ØQDDØZZ
ØQDFØZZ
ØQDGØZZ
ØQDHØZZ
ØQDJØZZ
ØQDKØZZ
ØQDLØZZ
ØQDMØZZ
ØQDNØZZ
ØQDPØZZ
ØQDQØZZ
ØQDRØZZ
ØQDSØZZ
ØWBØØZZ
ØWBØ3ZZ
ØWBØ4ZZ
ØWBØXZZ
ØWB2ØZZ
ØWB23ZZ
ØWB24ZZ
ØWB2XZZ
ØWB4ØZZ
ØWB43ZZ
ØWB44ZZ
ØWB4XZZ
ØWB5ØZZ
ØWB53ZZ
ØWB54ZZ
ØWB5XZZ
ØWB6ØZZ
ØWB63ZZ
ØWB64ZZ
ØWB6XZZ
ØWBFØZZ
ØWBF3ZZ
ØWBF4ZZ
ØWBFXZ2
ØWBFXZZ
ØWBKØZZ
ØWBK3ZZ
ØWBK4ZZ
ØWBKXZZ
ØWBLØZZ
ØWBL3ZZ
ØWBL4ZZ
ØWBLXZZ
ØWBMØZZ
ØWBM3ZZ
ØWBM4ZZ
ØWBMXZZ
ØXB2ØZZ
ØXB23ZZ
ØXB24ZZ
ØXB3ØZZ
ØXB33ZZ
ØXB34ZZ
ØXB4ØZZ
ØXB43ZZ
ØXB44ZZ
ØXB5ØZZ
ØXB53ZZ
ØXB54ZZ
ØXB6ØZZ
ØXB63ZZ
ØXB64ZZ
ØXB7ØZZ
ØXB73ZZ
ØXB74ZZ
ØXB8ØZZ
ØXB83ZZ
ØXB84ZZ
ØXB9ØZZ
ØXB93ZZ
ØXB94ZZ
ØXBBØZZ
ØXBB3ZZ
ØXBB4ZZ
ØXBCØZZ
ØXBC3ZZ
ØXBC4ZZ
ØXBDØZZ
ØXBD3ZZ
ØXBD4ZZ
ØXBFØZZ
ØXBF3ZZ
ØXBF4ZZ
ØXBGØZZ
ØXBG3ZZ
ØXBG4ZZ
ØXBHØZZ
ØXBH3ZZ
ØXBH4ZZ
ØXBJØZZ
ØXBJ3ZZ
ØXBJ4ZZ
ØXBKØZZ
ØXBK3ZZ
ØXBK4ZZ
ØXJJ4ZZ
ØXJK4ZZ
ØYBØØZZ
ØYBØ3ZZ
ØYBØ4ZZ
ØYB1ØZZ
ØYB13ZZ
ØYB14ZZ
ØYB5ØZZ
ØYB53ZZ
ØYB54ZZ
ØYB6ØZZ
ØYB63ZZ
ØYB64ZZ
ØYB7ØZZ
ØYB73ZZ
ØYB74ZZ
ØYB8ØZZ
ØYB83ZZ
ØYB84ZZ
ØYB9ØZZ
ØYB93ZZ
ØYB94ZZ
ØYBBØZZ
ØYBB3ZZ
ØYBB4ZZ
ØYBCØZZ
ØYBC3ZZ
ØYBC4ZZ
ØYBDØZZ
ØYBD3ZZ
ØYBD4ZZ
ØYBFØZZ
ØYBF3ZZ
ØYBF4ZZ
ØYBGØZZ
ØYBG3ZZ
ØYBG4ZZ
ØYBHØZZ
ØYBH3ZZ
ØYBH4ZZ
ØYBJØZZ
ØYBJ3ZZ
ØYBJ4ZZ
ØYBKØZZ
ØYBK3ZZ
ØYBK4ZZ
ØYBLØZZ
ØYBL3ZZ
ØYBL4ZZ
ØYBMØZZ
ØYBM3ZZ
ØYBM4ZZ
ØYBNØZZ
ØYBN3ZZ
ØYBN4ZZ

DRG 501

Select operating room procedures listed under DRG 500

DRG 502

Select operating room procedures listed under DRG 500

DRG 503

Operating Room Procedures

Ø1NG*
ØL8N*
ØL8P*
ØM5S*
ØM5T*
ØM9S4ØZ
ØM9T4ØZ
ØMQS*
ØMQT*
ØMRSØ7Z
ØMRSØJZ
ØMRSØKZ
ØMRS47Z
ØMRS4JZ
ØMRS4KZ
ØMRTØ7Z
ØMRTØJZ
ØMRTØKZ
ØMRT47Z
ØMRT4JZ
ØMRT4KZ
ØQ5L*
ØQ5M*
ØQ5N*
ØQ5P*
ØQ8L*
ØQ8M*
ØQ8N*
ØQ8P*
ØQ9LØØZ
ØQ9LØZZ
ØQ9L4ØZ
ØQ9L4ZZ
ØQ9MØØZ
ØQ9MØZZ
ØQ9M4ØZ
ØQ9M4ZZ
ØQ9NØØZ
ØQ9NØZZ
ØQ9N4ØZ
ØQ9N4ZZ
ØQ9PØØZ
ØQ9PØZZ
ØQ9P4ØZ
ØQ9P4ZZ
ØQBLØZZ
ØQBL3ZZ
ØQBL4ZZ
ØQBMØZZ
ØQBM3ZZ
ØQBM4ZZ
ØQBNØZ2
ØQBNØZZ
ØQBN3Z2
ØQBN3ZZ
ØQBN4Z2
ØQBN4ZZ
ØQBPØZ2
ØQBPØZZ
ØQBP3Z2
ØQBP3ZZ
ØQBP4Z2
ØQBP4ZZ
ØQCL*
ØQCM*
ØQCN*
ØQCP*
ØQHL*
ØQHM*
ØQHN*
ØQHP*
ØQNL*
ØQNM*
ØQNN*
ØQNP*
ØQQLØZZ
ØQQL3ZZ
ØQQL4ZZ
ØQQMØZZ
ØQQM3ZZ
ØQQM4ZZ
ØQQNØZZ
ØQQN3ZZ
ØQQN4ZZ
ØQQPØZZ
ØQQP3ZZ
ØQQP4ZZ
ØQRL*
ØQRM*
ØQRN*
ØQRP*
ØQSLØ4Z
ØQSLØ5Z
ØQSLØZZ
ØQSL34Z
ØQSL35Z
ØQSL44Z
ØQSL45Z
ØQSMØ4Z
ØQSMØ5Z
ØQSMØZZ
ØQSM34Z
ØQSM35Z
ØQSM44Z
ØQSM45Z
ØQSNØ42
ØQSNØ4Z
ØQSNØ52
ØQSNØ5Z
ØQSNØZ2
ØQSNØZZ
ØQSN342
ØQSN34Z
ØQSN352
ØQSN35Z
ØQSN442
ØQSN44Z
ØQSN452
ØQSN45Z
ØQSPØ42
ØQSPØ4Z
ØQSPØ52
ØQSPØ5Z
ØQSPØZ2
ØQSPØZZ
ØQSP342
ØQSP34Z
ØQSP352
ØQSP35Z
ØQSP442
ØQSP44Z
ØQSP452
ØQSP45Z
ØQSQØ4Z
ØQSQØZZ
ØQSQ34Z
ØQSQ44Z
ØQSRØ4Z
ØQSRØZZ
ØQSR34Z
ØQSR44Z
ØQTLØZZ
ØQTMØZZ
ØQTNØZZ
ØQTPØZZ
ØQUL*
ØQUM*
ØQUN*
ØQUP*
ØQWLØ4Z
ØQWLØ5Z
ØQWLØ7Z
ØQWLØJZ
ØQWLØKZ
ØQWL34Z
ØQWL35Z
ØQWL37Z
ØQWL3JZ
ØQWL3KZ
ØQWL44Z
ØQWL45Z
ØQWL47Z
ØQWL4JZ
ØQWL4KZ
ØQWMØ4Z
ØQWMØ5Z
ØQWMØ7Z
ØQWMØJZ
ØQWMØKZ
ØQWM34Z
ØQWM35Z
ØQWM37Z
ØQWM3JZ
ØQWM3KZ
ØQWM44Z
ØQWM45Z
ØQWM47Z
ØQWM4JZ
ØQWM4KZ
ØQWNØ4Z
ØQWNØ5Z
ØQWNØ7Z
ØQWNØJZ
ØQWNØKZ
ØQWN34Z
ØQWN35Z
ØQWN37Z
ØQWN3JZ
ØQWN3KZ
ØQWN44Z
ØQWN45Z
ØQWN47Z
ØQWN4JZ
ØQWN4KZ
ØQWPØ4Z
ØQWPØ5Z
ØQWPØ7Z
ØQWPØJZ
ØQWPØKZ
ØQWP34Z
ØQWP35Z
ØQWP37Z
ØQWP3JZ
ØQWP3KZ
ØQWP44Z
ØQWP45Z
ØQWP47Z
ØQWP4JZ
ØQWP4KZ
ØS5H*
ØS5J*
ØS5K*
ØS5L*
ØS5M*
ØS5N*
ØS5P*
ØS5Q*
ØS9HØØZ
ØS9HØZZ
ØS9JØØZ
ØS9JØZZ
ØS9KØØZ
ØS9KØZZ
ØS9LØØZ
ØS9LØZZ
ØS9MØØZ
ØS9MØZZ
ØS9NØØZ
ØS9NØZZ
ØS9PØØZ
ØS9PØZZ
ØS9QØØZ
ØS9QØZZ
ØSBHØZZ
ØSBH3ZZ
ØSBH4ZZ
ØSBJØZZ
ØSBJ3ZZ
ØSBJ4ZZ
ØSBKØZZ
ØSBK3ZZ
ØSBK4ZZ
ØSBLØZZ
ØSBL3ZZ
ØSBL4ZZ
ØSBMØZZ
ØSBM3ZZ
ØSBM4ZZ
ØSBNØZZ
ØSBN3ZZ
ØSBN4ZZ
ØSBPØZZ
ØSBP3ZZ
ØSBP4ZZ
ØSBQØZZ
ØSBQ3ZZ
ØSBQ4ZZ
ØSCH*
ØSCJ*
ØSCK*
ØSCL*
ØSCM*
ØSCN*
ØSCP*
ØSCQ*
ØSGH*
ØSGJ*
ØSGK*
ØSGL*
ØSGM*
ØSGN*
ØSGP*
ØSGQ*
ØSHHØ4Z
ØSHHØ5Z
ØSHH34Z
ØSHH35Z
ØSHH44Z
ØSHH45Z
ØSHJØ4Z
ØSHJØ5Z
ØSHJ34Z
ØSHJ35Z
ØSHJ44Z
ØSHJ45Z
ØSHKØ4Z
ØSHKØ5Z
ØSHK34Z
ØSHK35Z
ØSHK44Z
ØSHK45Z
ØSHLØ4Z
ØSHLØ5Z
ØSHL34Z
ØSHL35Z
ØSHL44Z
ØSHL45Z
ØSHMØ4Z
ØSHMØ5Z
ØSHM34Z
ØSHM35Z
ØSHM44Z
ØSHM45Z
ØSHNØ4Z
ØSHNØ5Z
ØSHN34Z
ØSHN35Z
ØSHN44Z
ØSHN45Z
ØSHPØ4Z
ØSHPØ5Z
ØSHP34Z
ØSHP35Z
ØSHP44Z
ØSHP45Z
ØSHQØ4Z
ØSHQØ5Z
ØSHQ34Z
ØSHQ35Z
ØSHQ44Z
ØSHQ45Z
ØSJHØZZ
ØSJJØZZ
ØSJKØZZ
ØSJLØZZ
ØSJMØZZ
ØSJNØZZ
ØSJPØZZ
ØSJQØZZ
ØSNHØZZ
ØSNH3ZZ
ØSNH4ZZ
ØSNJØZZ
ØSNJ3ZZ
ØSNJ4ZZ
ØSNKØZZ
ØSNK3ZZ
ØSNK4ZZ
ØSNLØZZ
ØSNL3ZZ
ØSNL4ZZ
ØSNMØZZ
ØSNM3ZZ
ØSNM4ZZ
ØSNNØZZ
ØSNN3ZZ
ØSNN4ZZ
ØSNPØZZ
ØSNP3ZZ
ØSNP4ZZ
ØSNQØZZ
ØSNQ3ZZ
ØSNQ4ZZ
ØSPHØØZ
ØSPHØ3Z
ØSPHØ4Z
ØSPHØ5Z
ØSPHØ7Z
ØSPHØKZ
ØSPH34Z
ØSPH35Z
ØSPH37Z
ØSPH3KZ
ØSPH4ØZ
ØSPH43Z
ØSPH44Z
ØSPH45Z
ØSPH47Z
ØSPH4KZ
ØSPJØØZ
ØSPJØ3Z
ØSPJØ4Z
ØSPJØ5Z
ØSPJØ7Z
ØSPJØKZ
ØSPJ34Z
ØSPJ35Z
ØSPJ37Z
ØSPJ3KZ
ØSPJ4ØZ
ØSPJ43Z
ØSPJ44Z
ØSPJ45Z
ØSPJ47Z
ØSPJ4KZ
ØSPKØØZ
ØSPKØ3Z
ØSPKØ4Z
ØSPKØ5Z
ØSPKØ7Z
ØSPKØKZ
ØSPK34Z
ØSPK35Z
ØSPK37Z
ØSPK3KZ
ØSPK4ØZ
ØSPK43Z
ØSPK44Z
ØSPK45Z
ØSPK47Z
ØSPK4KZ
ØSPLØØZ
ØSPLØ3Z
ØSPLØ4Z
ØSPLØ5Z
ØSPLØ7Z
ØSPLØKZ
ØSPL34Z
ØSPL35Z
ØSPL37Z
ØSPL3KZ
ØSPL4ØZ
ØSPL43Z
ØSPL44Z
ØSPL45Z
ØSPL47Z
ØSPL4KZ
ØSPMØØZ
ØSPMØ3Z
ØSPMØ4Z
ØSPMØ5Z
ØSPMØ7Z
ØSPMØKZ
ØSPM34Z
ØSPM35Z
ØSPM37Z
ØSPM3KZ
ØSPM4ØZ
ØSPM43Z
ØSPM44Z
ØSPM45Z
ØSPM47Z
ØSPM4KZ
ØSPNØØZ
ØSPNØ3Z
ØSPNØ4Z
ØSPNØ5Z
ØSPNØ7Z
ØSPNØKZ
ØSPN34Z
ØSPN35Z
ØSPN37Z
ØSPN3KZ
ØSPN4ØZ
ØSPN43Z
ØSPN44Z
ØSPN45Z
ØSPN47Z
ØSPN4KZ
ØSPPØØZ
ØSPPØ3Z
ØSPPØ4Z
ØSPPØ5Z
ØSPPØ7Z
ØSPPØKZ
ØSPP34Z
ØSPP35Z
ØSPP37Z
ØSPP3KZ
ØSPP4ØZ
ØSPP43Z
ØSPP44Z
ØSPP45Z
ØSPP47Z
ØSPP4KZ
ØSPQØØZ
ØSPQØ3Z
ØSPQØ4Z
ØSPQØ5Z
ØSPQØ7Z
ØSPQØKZ
ØSPQ34Z
ØSPQ35Z
ØSPQ37Z
ØSPQ3KZ
ØSPQ4ØZ
ØSPQ43Z
ØSPQ44Z
ØSPQ45Z
ØSPQ47Z
ØSPQ4KZ
ØSRH*
ØSRJ*
ØSRK*
ØSRL*
ØSRM*
ØSRN*
ØSRP*
ØSRQ*
ØSSHØ4Z
ØSSHØ5Z
ØSSHØZZ
ØSSJØ4Z
ØSSJØ5Z
ØSSJØZZ
ØSSKØ4Z
ØSSKØ5Z
ØSSKØZZ
ØSSLØ4Z
ØSSLØ5Z
ØSSLØZZ
ØSSMØ4Z
ØSSMØ5Z
ØSSMØZZ
ØSSNØ4Z
ØSSNØ5Z
ØSSNØZZ
ØSSPØ4Z
ØSSPØ5Z
ØSSPØZZ
ØSSQØ4Z
ØSSQØ5Z
ØSSQØZZ
ØSTHØZZ
ØSTJØZZ
ØSTKØZZ
ØSTLØZZ
ØSTMØZZ
ØSTNØZZ
ØSTPØZZ
ØSTQØZZ
ØSWHØØZ
ØSWHØ3Z
ØSWHØ4Z
ØSWHØ5Z
ØSWHØ7Z
ØSWHØ8Z
ØSWHØKZ
ØSWH3ØZ
ØSWH33Z
ØSWH34Z
ØSWH35Z
ØSWH37Z
ØSWH38Z
ØSWH3KZ
ØSWH4ØZ
ØSWH43Z
ØSWH44Z
ØSWH45Z
ØSWH47Z
ØSWH48Z
ØSWH4KZ
ØSWJØØZ
ØSWJØ3Z
ØSWJØ4Z
ØSWJØ5Z
ØSWJØ7Z
ØSWJØ8Z
ØSWJØKZ
ØSWJ3ØZ
ØSWJ33Z
ØSWJ34Z
ØSWJ35Z
ØSWJ37Z
ØSWJ38Z
ØSWJ3KZ
ØSWJ4ØZ
ØSWJ43Z
ØSWJ44Z
ØSWJ45Z
ØSWJ47Z

ØSWJ48Z
ØSWJ4KZ
ØSWKØØZ
ØSWKØ3Z
ØSWKØ4Z
ØSWKØ5Z
ØSWKØ7Z
ØSWKØ8Z
ØSWKØKZ
ØSWK3ØZ
ØSWK33Z
ØSWK34Z
ØSWK35Z
ØSWK37Z
ØSWK38Z
ØSWK3KZ
ØSWK4ØZ
ØSWK43Z
ØSWK44Z
ØSWK45Z
ØSWK47Z
ØSWK48Z
ØSWK4KZ
ØSWLØØZ
ØSWLØ3Z
ØSWLØ4Z
ØSWLØ5Z
ØSWLØ7Z
ØSWLØ8Z
ØSWLØKZ
ØSWL3ØZ
ØSWL33Z
ØSWL34Z
ØSWL35Z
ØSWL37Z
ØSWL38Z
ØSWL3KZ
ØSWL4ØZ
ØSWL43Z
ØSWL44Z
ØSWL45Z
ØSWL47Z
ØSWL48Z
ØSWL4KZ
ØSWMØØZ
ØSWMØ3Z
ØSWMØ4Z
ØSWMØ5Z
ØSWMØ7Z
ØSWMØ8Z
ØSWMØKZ
ØSWM3ØZ
ØSWM33Z
ØSWM34Z
ØSWM35Z
ØSWM37Z
ØSWM38Z
ØSWM3KZ
ØSWM4ØZ
ØSWM43Z
ØSWM44Z
ØSWM45Z
ØSWM47Z
ØSWM48Z
ØSWM4KZ
ØSWNØØZ
ØSWNØ3Z
ØSWNØ4Z
ØSWNØ5Z
ØSWNØ7Z
ØSWNØ8Z
ØSWNØKZ
ØSWN3ØZ
ØSWN33Z
ØSWN34Z
ØSWN35Z
ØSWN37Z
ØSWN38Z
ØSWN3KZ
ØSWN4ØZ
ØSWN43Z
ØSWN44Z
ØSWN45Z
ØSWN47Z
ØSWN48Z
ØSWN4KZ
ØSWPØØZ
ØSWPØ3Z
ØSWPØ4Z
ØSWPØ5Z
ØSWPØ7Z
ØSWPØ8Z
ØSWPØKZ
ØSWP3ØZ
ØSWP33Z
ØSWP34Z
ØSWP35Z
ØSWP37Z
ØSWP38Z
ØSWP3KZ
ØSWP4ØZ
ØSWP43Z
ØSWP44Z
ØSWP45Z
ØSWP47Z
ØSWP48Z
ØSWP4KZ
ØSWQØØZ
ØSWQØ3Z
ØSWQØ4Z
ØSWQØ5Z
ØSWQØ7Z
ØSWQØ8Z
ØSWQØKZ
ØSWQ3ØZ
ØSWQ33Z
ØSWQ34Z
ØSWQ35Z
ØSWQ37Z
ØSWQ38Z
ØSWQ3KZ
ØSWQ4ØZ
ØSWQ43Z
ØSWQ44Z
ØSWQ45Z
ØSWQ47Z
ØSWQ48Z
ØSWQ4KZ
ØY6P*
ØY6Q*
ØY6R*
ØY6S*
ØY6T*
ØY6U*
ØY6V*
ØY6W*
ØY6X*
ØY6Y*
ØYMPØZZ
ØYMQØZZ
ØYMRØZZ
ØYMSØZZ
ØYMTØZZ
ØYMUØZZ
ØYMVØZZ
ØYMWØZZ
ØYMXØZZ
ØYMYØZZ
XNRLØ99
XNRMØ99
XRGLØB9
XRGMØB9

DRG 504

Select operating room procedures listed under DRG 503

DRG 505

Select operating room procedures listed under DRG 503

DRG 506

Operating Room Procedures

ØM95ØØZ
ØM95ØZZ
ØM954ØZ
ØM96ØØZ
ØM96ØZZ
ØM964ØZ
ØMC5*
ØMC6*
ØR9NØØZ
ØR9NØZZ
ØR9PØØZ
ØR9PØZZ
ØR9QØØZ
ØR9QØZZ
ØR9RØØZ
ØR9RØZZ
ØR9SØØZ
ØR9SØZZ
ØR9TØØZ
ØR9TØZZ
ØR9UØØZ
ØR9UØZZ
ØR9VØØZ
ØR9VØZZ
ØR9WØØZ
ØR9WØZZ
ØR9XØØZ
ØR9XØZZ
ØRCN*
ØRCP*
ØRCQ*
ØRCR*
ØRCS*
ØRCT*
ØRCU*
ØRCV*
ØRCW*
ØRCX*
ØRHNØ4Z
ØRHNØ5Z
ØRHN34Z
ØRHN35Z
ØRHN44Z
ØRHN45Z
ØRHPØ4Z
ØRHPØ5Z
ØRHP34Z
ØRHP35Z
ØRHP44Z
ØRHP45Z
ØRHQØ4Z
ØRHQØ5Z
ØRHQ34Z
ØRHQ35Z
ØRHQ44Z
ØRHQ45Z
ØRHRØ4Z
ØRHRØ5Z
ØRHR34Z
ØRHR35Z
ØRHR44Z
ØRHR45Z
ØRHSØ4Z
ØRHSØ5Z
ØRHS34Z
ØRHS35Z
ØRHS44Z
ØRHS45Z
ØRHTØ4Z
ØRHTØ5Z
ØRHT34Z
ØRHT35Z
ØRHT44Z
ØRHT45Z
ØRHUØ4Z
ØRHUØ5Z
ØRHU34Z
ØRHU35Z
ØRHU44Z
ØRHU45Z
ØRHVØ4Z
ØRHVØ5Z
ØRHV34Z
ØRHV35Z
ØRHV44Z
ØRHV45Z
ØRHWØ4Z
ØRHWØ5Z
ØRHW34Z
ØRHW35Z
ØRHW44Z
ØRHW45Z
ØRHXØ4Z
ØRHXØ5Z
ØRHX34Z
ØRHX35Z
ØRHX44Z
ØRHX45Z
ØRJNØZZ
ØRJPØZZ
ØRJQØZZ
ØRJRØZZ
ØRJSØZZ
ØRJTØZZ
ØRJUØZZ
ØRJVØZZ
ØRJWØZZ
ØRJXØZZ
ØRPNØØZ
ØRPNØ3Z
ØRPNØ4Z
ØRPNØ5Z
ØRPNØ7Z
ØRPNØKZ
ØRPN34Z
ØRPN35Z
ØRPN37Z
ØRPN3KZ
ØRPN4ØZ
ØRPN43Z
ØRPN44Z
ØRPN45Z
ØRPN47Z
ØRPN4KZ
ØRPPØØZ
ØRPPØ3Z
ØRPPØ4Z
ØRPPØ5Z
ØRPPØ7Z
ØRPPØKZ
ØRPP34Z
ØRPP35Z
ØRPP37Z
ØRPP3KZ
ØRPP4ØZ
ØRPP43Z
ØRPP44Z
ØRPP45Z
ØRPP47Z
ØRPP4KZ
ØRPQØØZ
ØRPQØ3Z
ØRPQØ4Z
ØRPQØ5Z
ØRPQØ7Z
ØRPQØKZ
ØRPQ34Z
ØRPQ35Z
ØRPQ37Z
ØRPQ3KZ
ØRPQ4ØZ
ØRPQ43Z
ØRPQ44Z
ØRPQ45Z
ØRPQ47Z
ØRPQ4KZ
ØRPRØØZ
ØRPRØ3Z
ØRPRØ4Z
ØRPRØ5Z
ØRPRØ7Z
ØRPRØKZ
ØRPR34Z
ØRPR35Z
ØRPR37Z
ØRPR3KZ
ØRPR4ØZ
ØRPR43Z
ØRPR44Z
ØRPR45Z
ØRPR47Z
ØRPR4KZ
ØRPSØØZ
ØRPSØ3Z
ØRPSØ4Z
ØRPSØ5Z
ØRPSØ7Z
ØRPSØKZ
ØRPS34Z
ØRPS35Z
ØRPS37Z
ØRPS3KZ
ØRPS4ØZ
ØRPS43Z
ØRPS44Z
ØRPS45Z
ØRPS47Z
ØRPS4KZ
ØRPTØØZ
ØRPTØ3Z
ØRPTØ4Z
ØRPTØ5Z
ØRPTØ7Z
ØRPTØKZ
ØRPT34Z
ØRPT35Z
ØRPT37Z
ØRPT3KZ
ØRPT4ØZ
ØRPT43Z
ØRPT44Z
ØRPT45Z
ØRPT47Z
ØRPT4KZ
ØRPUØØZ
ØRPUØ3Z
ØRPUØ4Z
ØRPUØ5Z
ØRPUØ7Z
ØRPUØKZ
ØRPU34Z
ØRPU35Z
ØRPU37Z
ØRPU3KZ
ØRPU4ØZ
ØRPU43Z
ØRPU44Z
ØRPU45Z
ØRPU47Z
ØRPU4KZ
ØRPVØØZ
ØRPVØ3Z
ØRPVØ4Z
ØRPVØ5Z
ØRPVØ7Z
ØRPVØKZ
ØRPV34Z
ØRPV35Z
ØRPV37Z
ØRPV3KZ
ØRPV4ØZ
ØRPV43Z
ØRPV44Z
ØRPV45Z
ØRPV47Z
ØRPV4KZ
ØRPWØØZ
ØRPWØ3Z
ØRPWØ4Z
ØRPWØ5Z
ØRPWØ7Z
ØRPWØKZ
ØRPW34Z
ØRPW35Z
ØRPW37Z
ØRPW3KZ
ØRPW4ØZ
ØRPW43Z
ØRPW44Z
ØRPW45Z
ØRPW47Z
ØRPW4KZ
ØRPXØØZ
ØRPXØ3Z
ØRPXØ4Z
ØRPXØ5Z
ØRPXØ7Z
ØRPXØKZ
ØRPX34Z
ØRPX35Z
ØRPX37Z
ØRPX3KZ
ØRPX4ØZ
ØRPX43Z
ØRPX44Z
ØRPX45Z
ØRPX47Z
ØRPX4KZ
ØRQNØZZ
ØRQN3ZZ
ØRQN4ZZ
ØRQPØZZ
ØRQP3ZZ
ØRQP4ZZ
ØRQQØZZ
ØRQQ3ZZ
ØRQQ4ZZ
ØRQRØZZ
ØRQR3ZZ
ØRQR4ZZ
ØRQSØZZ
ØRQS3ZZ
ØRQS4ZZ
ØRQTØZZ
ØRQT3ZZ
ØRQT4ZZ
ØRQUØZZ
ØRQU3ZZ
ØRQU4ZZ
ØRQVØZZ
ØRQV3ZZ
ØRQV4ZZ
ØRQWØZZ
ØRQW3ZZ
ØRQW4ZZ
ØRQXØZZ
ØRQX3ZZ
ØRQX4ZZ
ØRRQ*
ØRRR*
ØRRS*
ØRRT*
ØRRU*
ØRRV*
ØRRW*
ØRRX*
ØRUN*
ØRUP*
ØRUQ*
ØRUR*
ØRUS*
ØRUT*
ØRUU*
ØRUV*
ØRUW*
ØRUX*
ØRWNØØZ
ØRWNØ3Z
ØRWNØ4Z
ØRWNØ5Z
ØRWNØ7Z
ØRWNØ8Z
ØRWNØKZ
ØRWN3ØZ
ØRWN33Z
ØRWN34Z
ØRWN35Z
ØRWN37Z
ØRWN38Z
ØRWN3KZ
ØRWN4ØZ
ØRWN43Z
ØRWN44Z
ØRWN45Z
ØRWN47Z
ØRWN48Z
ØRWN4KZ
ØRWPØØZ
ØRWPØ3Z
ØRWPØ4Z
ØRWPØ5Z
ØRWPØ7Z
ØRWPØ8Z
ØRWPØKZ
ØRWP3ØZ
ØRWP33Z
ØRWP34Z
ØRWP35Z
ØRWP37Z
ØRWP38Z
ØRWP3KZ
ØRWP4ØZ
ØRWP43Z
ØRWP44Z
ØRWP45Z
ØRWP47Z
ØRWP48Z
ØRWP4KZ
ØRWQØØZ
ØRWQØ3Z
ØRWQØ4Z
ØRWQØ5Z
ØRWQØ7Z
ØRWQØ8Z
ØRWQØKZ
ØRWQ3ØZ
ØRWQ33Z
ØRWQ34Z
ØRWQ35Z
ØRWQ37Z
ØRWQ38Z
ØRWQ3KZ
ØRWQ4ØZ
ØRWQ43Z
ØRWQ44Z
ØRWQ45Z
ØRWQ47Z
ØRWQ48Z
ØRWQ4KZ
ØRWRØØZ
ØRWRØ3Z
ØRWRØ4Z
ØRWRØ5Z
ØRWRØ7Z
ØRWRØ8Z
ØRWRØKZ
ØRWR3ØZ
ØRWR33Z
ØRWR34Z
ØRWR35Z
ØRWR37Z
ØRWR38Z
ØRWR3KZ
ØRWR4ØZ
ØRWR43Z
ØRWR44Z
ØRWR45Z
ØRWR47Z
ØRWR48Z
ØRWR4KZ
ØRWSØØZ
ØRWSØ3Z
ØRWSØ4Z
ØRWSØ5Z
ØRWSØ7Z
ØRWSØ8Z
ØRWSØKZ
ØRWS3ØZ
ØRWS33Z
ØRWS34Z
ØRWS35Z
ØRWS37Z
ØRWS38Z
ØRWS3KZ
ØRWS4ØZ
ØRWS43Z
ØRWS44Z
ØRWS45Z
ØRWS47Z
ØRWS48Z
ØRWS4KZ
ØRWTØØZ
ØRWTØ3Z
ØRWTØ4Z
ØRWTØ5Z
ØRWTØ7Z
ØRWTØ8Z
ØRWTØKZ
ØRWT3ØZ
ØRWT33Z
ØRWT34Z
ØRWT35Z
ØRWT37Z
ØRWT38Z
ØRWT3KZ
ØRWT4ØZ
ØRWT43Z
ØRWT44Z
ØRWT45Z
ØRWT47Z
ØRWT48Z
ØRWT4KZ
ØRWUØØZ
ØRWUØ3Z
ØRWUØ4Z
ØRWUØ5Z
ØRWUØ7Z
ØRWUØ8Z
ØRWUØKZ
ØRWU3ØZ
ØRWU33Z
ØRWU34Z
ØRWU35Z
ØRWU37Z
ØRWU38Z
ØRWU3KZ
ØRWU4ØZ
ØRWU43Z
ØRWU44Z
ØRWU45Z
ØRWU47Z
ØRWU48Z
ØRWU4KZ
ØRWVØØZ
ØRWVØ3Z
ØRWVØ4Z
ØRWVØ5Z
ØRWVØ7Z
ØRWVØ8Z
ØRWVØKZ
ØRWV3ØZ
ØRWV33Z
ØRWV34Z
ØRWV35Z
ØRWV37Z
ØRWV38Z
ØRWV3KZ
ØRWV4ØZ
ØRWV43Z
ØRWV44Z
ØRWV45Z
ØRWV47Z
ØRWV48Z
ØRWV4KZ
ØRWWØØZ
ØRWWØ3Z
ØRWWØ4Z
ØRWWØ5Z
ØRWWØ7Z
ØRWWØ8Z
ØRWWØKZ
ØRWW3ØZ
ØRWW33Z
ØRWW34Z
ØRWW35Z
ØRWW37Z
ØRWW38Z
ØRWW3KZ
ØRWW4ØZ
ØRWW43Z
ØRWW44Z
ØRWW45Z
ØRWW47Z
ØRWW48Z
ØRWW4KZ
ØRWXØØZ
ØRWXØ3Z
ØRWXØ4Z
ØRWXØ5Z
ØRWXØ7Z
ØRWXØ8Z
ØRWXØKZ
ØRWX3ØZ
ØRWX33Z
ØRWX34Z
ØRWX35Z
ØRWX37Z
ØRWX38Z
ØRWX3KZ
ØRWX4ØZ
ØRWX43Z
ØRWX44Z
ØRWX45Z
ØRWX47Z
ØRWX48Z
ØRWX4KZ
ØXRLØ7N
ØXRLØ7P
ØXRL47N
ØXRL47P
ØXRMØ7N
ØXRMØ7P
ØXRM47N
ØXRM47P
ØXXNØZL
ØXXPØZM

DRG 507

Operating Room Procedures

ØM914ZZ
ØM924ZZ
ØM934ZZ
ØM944ZZ
ØR9EØØZ
ØR9EØZZ
ØR9FØØZ
ØR9FØZZ
ØR9GØØZ
ØR9GØZZ
ØR9HØØZ
ØR9HØZZ
ØR9JØØZ
ØR9JØZZ
ØR9KØØZ
ØR9KØZZ
ØR9LØØZ
ØR9LØZZ
ØR9MØØZ
ØR9MØZZ
ØRCE*
ØRCF*
ØRCG*
ØRCH*
ØRCJ*
ØRCK*
ØRCL*
ØRCM*
ØRGE*
ØRGF*
ØRGG*
ØRGH*
ØRGJ*
ØRGK*
ØRGL*
ØRGM*
ØRHEØ4Z
ØRHE34Z
ØRHE44Z
ØRHFØ4Z
ØRHF34Z
ØRHF44Z
ØRHGØ4Z
ØRHG34Z
ØRHG44Z
ØRHHØ4Z
ØRHH34Z
ØRHH44Z
ØRHJØ4Z
ØRHJ34Z
ØRHJ44Z
ØRHKØ4Z
ØRHK34Z
ØRHK44Z
ØRHLØ4Z
ØRHLØ5Z
ØRHL34Z
ØRHL35Z
ØRHL44Z
ØRHL45Z
ØRHMØ4Z
ØRHMØ5Z
ØRHM34Z
ØRHM35Z
ØRHM44Z
ØRHM45Z
ØRJEØZZ
ØRJFØZZ
ØRJGØZZ
ØRJHØZZ
ØRJJØZZ
ØRJKØZZ
ØRJLØZZ
ØRJMØZZ
ØRPEØØZ
ØRPEØ3Z
ØRPEØ4Z
ØRPEØ7Z
ØRPEØKZ
ØRPE34Z
ØRPE37Z
ØRPE3KZ
ØRPE4ØZ
ØRPE43Z
ØRPE44Z
ØRPE47Z
ØRPE4KZ
ØRPFØØZ
ØRPFØ3Z
ØRPFØ4Z
ØRPFØ7Z
ØRPFØKZ
ØRPF34Z
ØRPF37Z
ØRPF3KZ
ØRPF4ØZ
ØRPF43Z
ØRPF44Z
ØRPF47Z
ØRPF4KZ
ØRPGØØZ
ØRPGØ3Z
ØRPGØ4Z
ØRPGØ7Z
ØRPGØKZ
ØRPG34Z
ØRPG37Z
ØRPG3KZ
ØRPG4ØZ
ØRPG43Z
ØRPG44Z
ØRPG47Z
ØRPG4KZ
ØRPHØØZ
ØRPHØ3Z
ØRPHØ4Z
ØRPHØ7Z
ØRPHØKZ
ØRPH34Z
ØRPH37Z
ØRPH3KZ
ØRPH4ØZ
ØRPH43Z
ØRPH44Z
ØRPH47Z
ØRPH4KZ
ØRPJØØZ
ØRPJØ3Z
ØRPJØ4Z
ØRPJØ7Z
ØRPJØKZ
ØRPJ34Z
ØRPJ37Z
ØRPJ3KZ
ØRPJ4ØZ
ØRPJ43Z
ØRPJ44Z
ØRPJ47Z
ØRPJ4KZ
ØRPKØØZ
ØRPKØ3Z
ØRPKØ4Z
ØRPKØ7Z
ØRPKØKZ
ØRPK34Z
ØRPK37Z
ØRPK3KZ
ØRPK4ØZ
ØRPK43Z

ØRPK44Z
ØRPK47Z
ØRPK4KZ
ØRPLØØZ
ØRPLØ3Z
ØRPLØ4Z
ØRPLØ5Z
ØRPLØ7Z
ØRPLØKZ
ØRPL34Z
ØRPL35Z
ØRPL37Z
ØRPL3KZ
ØRPL4ØZ
ØRPL43Z
ØRPL44Z
ØRPL45Z
ØRPL47Z
ØRPL4KZ
ØRPMØØZ
ØRPMØ3Z
ØRPMØ4Z
ØRPMØ5Z
ØRPMØ7Z
ØRPMØKZ
ØRPM34Z
ØRPM35Z
ØRPM37Z
ØRPM3KZ
ØRPM4ØZ
ØRPM43Z
ØRPM44Z
ØRPM45Z
ØRPM47Z
ØRPM4KZ
ØRQEØZZ
ØRQE3ZZ
ØRQE4ZZ
ØRQFØZZ
ØRQF3ZZ
ØRQF4ZZ
ØRQGØZZ
ØRQG3ZZ
ØRQG4ZZ
ØRQHØZZ
ØRQH3ZZ
ØRQH4ZZ
ØRQJØZZ
ØRQJ3ZZ
ØRQJ4ZZ
ØRQKØZZ
ØRQK3ZZ
ØRQK4ZZ
ØRQLØZZ
ØRQL3ZZ
ØRQL4ZZ
ØRQMØZZ
ØRQM3ZZ
ØRQM4ZZ
ØRUE*
ØRUF*
ØRUG*
ØRUH*
ØRUJ*
ØRUK*
ØRUL*
ØRUM*
ØRWEØØZ
ØRWEØ3Z
ØRWEØ4Z
ØRWEØ7Z
ØRWEØ8Z
ØRWEØJZ
ØRWEØKZ
ØRWE3ØZ
ØRWE33Z
ØRWE34Z
ØRWE37Z
ØRWE38Z
ØRWE3JZ
ØRWE3KZ
ØRWE4ØZ
ØRWE43Z
ØRWE44Z
ØRWE47Z
ØRWE48Z
ØRWE4JZ
ØRWE4KZ
ØRWFØØZ
ØRWFØ3Z
ØRWFØ4Z
ØRWFØ7Z
ØRWFØ8Z
ØRWFØJZ
ØRWFØKZ
ØRWF3ØZ
ØRWF33Z
ØRWF34Z
ØRWF37Z
ØRWF38Z
ØRWF3JZ
ØRWF3KZ
ØRWF4ØZ
ØRWF43Z
ØRWF44Z
ØRWF47Z
ØRWF48Z
ØRWF4JZ
ØRWF4KZ
ØRWGØØZ
ØRWGØ3Z
ØRWGØ4Z
ØRWGØ7Z
ØRWGØ8Z
ØRWGØKZ
ØRWG3ØZ
ØRWG33Z
ØRWG34Z
ØRWG37Z
ØRWG38Z
ØRWG3KZ
ØRWG4ØZ
ØRWG43Z
ØRWG44Z
ØRWG47Z
ØRWG48Z
ØRWG4KZ
ØRWHØØZ
ØRWHØ3Z
ØRWHØ4Z
ØRWHØ7Z
ØRWHØ8Z
ØRWHØKZ
ØRWH3ØZ
ØRWH33Z
ØRWH34Z
ØRWH37Z
ØRWH38Z
ØRWH3KZ
ØRWH4ØZ
ØRWH43Z
ØRWH44Z
ØRWH47Z
ØRWH48Z
ØRWH4KZ
ØRWJØØZ
ØRWJØ3Z
ØRWJØ4Z
ØRWJØ7Z
ØRWJØ8Z
ØRWJØKZ
ØRWJ3ØZ
ØRWJ33Z
ØRWJ34Z
ØRWJ37Z
ØRWJ38Z
ØRWJ3KZ
ØRWJ4ØZ
ØRWJ43Z
ØRWJ44Z
ØRWJ47Z
ØRWJ48Z
ØRWJ4KZ
ØRWKØØZ
ØRWKØ3Z
ØRWKØ4Z
ØRWKØ7Z
ØRWKØ8Z
ØRWKØKZ
ØRWK3ØZ
ØRWK33Z
ØRWK34Z
ØRWK37Z
ØRWK38Z
ØRWK3KZ
ØRWK4ØZ
ØRWK43Z
ØRWK44Z
ØRWK47Z
ØRWK48Z
ØRWK4KZ
ØRWLØØZ
ØRWLØ3Z
ØRWLØ4Z
ØRWLØ5Z
ØRWLØ7Z
ØRWLØ8Z
ØRWLØKZ
ØRWL3ØZ
ØRWL33Z
ØRWL34Z
ØRWL35Z
ØRWL37Z
ØRWL38Z
ØRWL3KZ
ØRWL4ØZ
ØRWL43Z
ØRWL44Z
ØRWL45Z
ØRWL47Z
ØRWL48Z
ØRWL4KZ
ØRWMØØZ
ØRWMØ3Z
ØRWMØ4Z
ØRWMØ5Z
ØRWMØ7Z
ØRWMØ8Z
ØRWMØKZ
ØRWM3ØZ
ØRWM33Z
ØRWM34Z
ØRWM35Z
ØRWM37Z
ØRWM38Z
ØRWM3KZ
ØRWM4ØZ
ØRWM43Z
ØRWM44Z
ØRWM45Z
ØRWM47Z
ØRWM48Z
ØRWM4KZ

DRG 508

Select operating room procedures listed under DRG 507

DRG 509

Operating Room Procedures

ØRJØ4ZZ
ØRJ14ZZ
ØRJ34ZZ
ØRJ44ZZ
ØRJ54ZZ
ØRJ64ZZ
ØRJ94ZZ
ØRJA4ZZ
ØRJB4ZZ
ØRJE4ZZ
ØRJF4ZZ
ØRJG4ZZ
ØRJH4ZZ
ØRJJ4ZZ
ØRJK4ZZ
ØRJL4ZZ
ØRJM4ZZ
ØRJN4ZZ
ØRJP4ZZ
ØRJQ4ZZ
ØRJR4ZZ
ØRJS4ZZ
ØRJT4ZZ
ØRJU4ZZ
ØRJV4ZZ
ØRJW4ZZ
ØRJX4ZZ
ØSJØ4ZZ
ØSJ34ZZ
ØSJ54ZZ
ØSJ64ZZ
ØSJ74ZZ
ØSJ84ZZ
ØSJ94ZZ
ØSJB4ZZ
ØSJC4ZZ
ØSJD4ZZ
ØSJF4ZZ
ØSJG4ZZ
ØSJH4ZZ
ØSJJ4ZZ
ØSJK4ZZ
ØSJL4ZZ
ØSJM4ZZ
ØSJN4ZZ
ØSJP4ZZ
ØSJQ4ZZ

DRG 510

Operating Room Procedures

ØLQ1*
ØLQ2*
ØP8H*
ØP8J*
ØP8K*
ØP8L*
ØPBHØZZ
ØPBH3ZZ
ØPBH4ZZ
ØPBJØZZ
ØPBJ3ZZ
ØPBJ4ZZ
ØPBKØZZ
ØPBK3ZZ
ØPBK4ZZ
ØPBLØZZ
ØPBL3ZZ
ØPBL4ZZ
ØPCH*
ØPCJ*
ØPCK*
ØPCL*
ØPHHØ4Z
ØPHHØ5Z
ØPHHØ6Z
ØPHHØBZ
ØPHHØCZ
ØPHHØDZ
ØPHH34Z
ØPHH35Z
ØPHH36Z
ØPHH3BZ
ØPHH3CZ
ØPHH3DZ
ØPHH44Z
ØPHH45Z
ØPHH46Z
ØPHH4BZ
ØPHH4CZ
ØPHH4DZ
ØPHJØ4Z
ØPHJØ5Z
ØPHJØ6Z
ØPHJØBZ
ØPHJØCZ
ØPHJØDZ
ØPHJ34Z
ØPHJ35Z
ØPHJ36Z
ØPHJ3BZ
ØPHJ3CZ
ØPHJ3DZ
ØPHJ44Z
ØPHJ45Z
ØPHJ46Z
ØPHJ4BZ
ØPHJ4CZ
ØPHJ4DZ
ØPHKØ4Z
ØPHKØ5Z
ØPHKØ6Z
ØPHKØBZ
ØPHKØCZ
ØPHKØDZ
ØPHK34Z
ØPHK35Z
ØPHK36Z
ØPHK3BZ
ØPHK3CZ
ØPHK3DZ
ØPHK44Z
ØPHK45Z
ØPHK46Z
ØPHK4BZ
ØPHK4CZ
ØPHK4DZ
ØPHLØ4Z
ØPHLØ5Z
ØPHLØ6Z
ØPHLØBZ
ØPHLØCZ
ØPHLØDZ
ØPHL34Z
ØPHL35Z
ØPHL36Z
ØPHL3BZ
ØPHL3CZ
ØPHL3DZ
ØPHL44Z
ØPHL45Z
ØPHL46Z
ØPHL4BZ
ØPHL4CZ
ØPHL4DZ
ØPNH*
ØPNJ*
ØPNK*
ØPNL*
ØPQHØZZ
ØPQH3ZZ
ØPQH4ZZ
ØPQJØZZ
ØPQJ3ZZ
ØPQJ4ZZ
ØPQKØZZ
ØPQK3ZZ
ØPQK4ZZ
ØPQLØZZ
ØPQL3ZZ
ØPQL4ZZ
ØPRH*
ØPRJ*
ØPRK*
ØPRL*
ØPSHØ4Z
ØPSHØ5Z
ØPSHØ6Z
ØPSHØBZ
ØPSHØCZ
ØPSHØDZ
ØPSHØZZ
ØPSH34Z
ØPSH35Z
ØPSH36Z
ØPSH3BZ
ØPSH3CZ
ØPSH3DZ
ØPSH44Z
ØPSH45Z
ØPSH46Z
ØPSH4BZ
ØPSH4CZ
ØPSH4DZ
ØPSJØ4Z
ØPSJØ5Z
ØPSJØ6Z
ØPSJØBZ
ØPSJØCZ
ØPSJØDZ
ØPSJØZZ
ØPSJ34Z
ØPSJ35Z
ØPSJ36Z
ØPSJ3BZ
ØPSJ3CZ
ØPSJ3DZ
ØPSJ44Z
ØPSJ45Z
ØPSJ46Z
ØPSJ4BZ
ØPSJ4CZ
ØPSJ4DZ
ØPSKØ4Z
ØPSKØ5Z
ØPSKØ6Z
ØPSKØBZ
ØPSKØCZ
ØPSKØDZ
ØPSKØZZ
ØPSK34Z
ØPSK35Z
ØPSK36Z
ØPSK3BZ
ØPSK3CZ
ØPSK3DZ
ØPSK44Z
ØPSK45Z
ØPSK46Z
ØPSK4BZ
ØPSK4CZ
ØPSK4DZ
ØPSLØ4Z
ØPSLØ5Z
ØPSLØ6Z
ØPSLØBZ
ØPSLØCZ
ØPSLØDZ
ØPSLØZZ
ØPSL34Z
ØPSL35Z
ØPSL36Z
ØPSL3BZ
ØPSL3CZ
ØPSL3DZ
ØPSL44Z
ØPSL45Z
ØPSL46Z
ØPSL4BZ
ØPSL4CZ
ØPSL4DZ
ØPTHØZZ
ØPTJØZZ
ØPTKØZZ
ØPTLØZZ
ØPUH*
ØPUJ*
ØPUK*
ØPUL*
ØRBEØZZ
ØRBE3ZZ
ØRBE4ZZ
ØRBFØZZ
ØRBF3ZZ
ØRBF4ZZ
ØRBGØZZ
ØRBG3ZZ
ØRBG4ZZ
ØRBHØZZ
ØRBH3ZZ
ØRBH4ZZ
ØRBJØZZ
ØRBJ3ZZ
ØRBJ4ZZ
ØRBKØZZ
ØRBK3ZZ
ØRBK4ZZ
ØRBLØZZ
ØRBL3ZZ
ØRBL4ZZ
ØRBMØZZ
ØRBM3ZZ
ØRBM4ZZ
ØRHJØ8Z
ØRHJ48Z
ØRHKØ8Z
ØRHK48Z
ØRNEØZZ
ØRNE3ZZ
ØRNE4ZZ
ØRNFØZZ
ØRNF3ZZ
ØRNF4ZZ
ØRNGØZZ
ØRNG3ZZ
ØRNG4ZZ
ØRNHØZZ
ØRNH3ZZ
ØRNH4ZZ
ØRNJØZZ
ØRNJ3ZZ
ØRNJ4ZZ
ØRNKØZZ
ØRNK3ZZ
ØRNK4ZZ
ØRNLØZZ
ØRNL3ZZ
ØRNL4ZZ
ØRNMØZZ
ØRNM3ZZ
ØRNM4ZZ
ØRPJØ8Z
ØRPJ48Z
ØRPKØ8Z
ØRPK48Z
ØRSEØ4Z
ØRSEØZZ
ØRSFØ4Z
ØRSFØZZ
ØRSGØ4Z
ØRSGØZZ
ØRSHØ4Z
ØRSHØZZ
ØRSJØ4Z
ØRSJØZZ
ØRSKØ4Z
ØRSKØZZ
ØRSLØ4Z
ØRSLØ5Z
ØRSLØZZ
ØRSMØ4Z
ØRSMØ5Z
ØRSMØZZ
ØRTEØZZ
ØRTFØZZ
ØRTGØZZ
ØRTHØZZ
ØRTJØZZ
ØRTKØZZ
ØRTLØZZ
ØRTMØZZ

DRG 511

Select operating room procedures listed under DRG 510

DRG 512

Select operating room procedures listed under DRG 510

DRG 513

Operating Room Procedures

Ø1N5*
ØHRF*
ØHRG*
ØJ8J*
ØJ8K*
ØJBJØZZ
ØJBJ3ZZ
ØJBKØZZ
ØJBK3ZZ
ØJDJØZZ
ØJDKØZZ
ØJHJ*
ØJHK*
ØJNJØZZ
ØJNJ3ZZ
ØJNKØZZ
ØJNK3ZZ
ØJQJØZZ
ØJQKØZZ
ØJRJØ7Z
ØJRJØJZ
ØJRJØKZ
ØJRJ3JZ
ØJRJ3KZ
ØJRKØ7Z
ØJRKØJZ
ØJRKØKZ
ØJRK3JZ
ØJRK3KZ
ØJUJ*
ØJUK*
ØJXJØZB
ØJXJØZC
ØJXJ3ZB
ØJXJ3ZC
ØJXKØZB
ØJXKØZC
ØJXK3ZB
ØJXK3ZC
ØK5C*
ØK5D*
ØK8C*
ØK8D*
ØK9CØØZ
ØK9CØZZ
ØK9C4ØZ
ØK9DØØZ
ØK9DØZZ
ØK9D4ØZ
ØKBCØZZ
ØKBC3ZZ
ØKBC4ZZ
ØKBDØZZ
ØKBD3ZZ
ØKBD4ZZ
ØKCC*
ØKCD*
ØKDCØZZ
ØKDDØZZ
ØKMC*
ØKMD*
ØKNCØZZ
ØKNC3ZZ
ØKNC4ZZ
ØKNDØZZ
ØKND3ZZ
ØKND4ZZ
ØKQC*
ØKQD*
ØKRCØ7Z
ØKRCØJZ
ØKRCØKZ
ØKRC47Z
ØKRC4JZ
ØKRC4KZ
ØKRDØ7Z
ØKRDØJZ
ØKRDØKZ
ØKRD47Z
ØKRD4JZ
ØKRD4KZ
ØKSC*
ØKSD*
ØKTC*
ØKTD*
ØKUC*
ØKUD*
ØKXC*
ØKXD*
ØL57*
ØL58*
ØL87*
ØL88*
ØL97ØØZ
ØL97ØZZ
ØL974ØZ
ØL98ØØZ
ØL98ØZZ
ØL984ØZ
ØLB7ØZZ
ØLB73ZZ
ØLB74ZZ
ØLB8ØZZ
ØLB83ZZ
ØLB84ZZ
ØLC7*
ØLC8*
ØLD7ØZZ
ØLD8ØZZ
ØLJXØZZ
ØLJX4ZZ
ØLM7*
ØLM8*
ØLN7ØZZ
ØLN73ZZ
ØLN74ZZ
ØLN8ØZZ
ØLN83ZZ
ØLN84ZZ
ØLQ7*
ØLQ8*
ØLR7*
ØLR8*
ØLS7*
ØLS8*
ØLT7*
ØLT8*
ØLU7*
ØLU8*
ØLX7*
ØLX8*
ØM55*
ØM56*
ØM57*
ØM58*
ØM87*
ØM88*
ØM97ØØZ
ØM97ØZZ
ØM98ØØZ
ØM98ØZZ
ØMB7ØZZ
ØMB73ZZ
ØMB74ZZ
ØMB8ØZZ
ØMB83ZZ
ØMB84ZZ
ØMC7*
ØMC8*
ØMD7*
ØMD8*
ØMN7ØZZ
ØMN73ZZ
ØMN74ZZ
ØMN8ØZZ
ØMN83ZZ
ØMN84ZZ
ØMT7*
ØMT8*
ØP5M*
ØP5N*
ØP5P*
ØP5Q*
ØP8M*
ØP8N*
ØP8P*
ØP8Q*
ØP9MØØZ
ØP9MØZX
ØP9MØZZ
ØP9M3ZX
ØP9M4ØZ
ØP9M4ZX
ØP9M4ZZ
ØP9NØØZ
ØP9NØZX
ØP9NØZZ
ØP9N3ZX
ØP9N4ØZ
ØP9N4ZX
ØP9N4ZZ
ØP9PØØZ
ØP9PØZX
ØP9PØZZ
ØP9P3ZX
ØP9P4ØZ
ØP9P4ZX
ØP9P4ZZ
ØP9QØØZ
ØP9QØZX
ØP9QØZZ
ØP9Q3ZX
ØP9Q4ØZ
ØP9Q4ZX
ØP9Q4ZZ
ØPBM*
ØPBN*
ØPBP*
ØPBQ*
ØPCM*
ØPCN*
ØPCP*
ØPCQ*
ØPDMØZZ
ØPDNØZZ
ØPDPØZZ
ØPDQØZZ
ØPDRØZZ
ØPDSØZZ
ØPDTØZZ
ØPDVØZZ
ØPHM*
ØPHN*
ØPHP*
ØPHQ*
ØPNM*
ØPNN*
ØPNP*
ØPNQ*
ØPQMØZZ
ØPQM3ZZ
ØPQM4ZZ
ØPQNØZZ
ØPQN3ZZ
ØPQN4ZZ
ØPQPØZZ
ØPQP3ZZ
ØPQP4ZZ
ØPQQØZZ
ØPQQ3ZZ
ØPQQ4ZZ
ØPRM*
ØPRN*
ØPRP*
ØPRQ*
ØPSMØ4Z
ØPSMØ5Z
ØPSMØZZ
ØPSM34Z
ØPSM35Z
ØPSM44Z
ØPSM45Z
ØPSNØ4Z
ØPSNØ5Z
ØPSNØZZ
ØPSN34Z
ØPSN35Z
ØPSN44Z
ØPSN45Z
ØPSPØ4Z
ØPSPØ5Z
ØPSPØZZ
ØPSP34Z
ØPSP35Z
ØPSP44Z
ØPSP45Z
ØPSQØ4Z
ØPSQØ5Z
ØPSQØZZ
ØPSQ34Z
ØPSQ35Z
ØPSQ44Z
ØPSQ45Z
ØPSRØ4Z
ØPSRØZZ
ØPSR34Z
ØPSR44Z
ØPSSØ4Z
ØPSSØZZ
ØPSS34Z
ØPSS44Z
ØPSTØ4Z
ØPSTØZZ
ØPST34Z
ØPST44Z
ØPSVØ4Z

ØPSVØZZ
ØPSV34Z
ØPSV44Z
ØPTMØZZ
ØPTNØZZ
ØPTPØZZ
ØPTQØZZ
ØPUM*
ØPUN*
ØPUP*
ØPUQ*
ØPWMØ4Z
ØPWMØ5Z
ØPWMØ7Z
ØPWMØJZ
ØPWMØKZ
ØPWM34Z
ØPWM35Z
ØPWM37Z
ØPWM3JZ
ØPWM3KZ
ØPWM44Z
ØPWM45Z
ØPWM47Z
ØPWM4JZ
ØPWM4KZ
ØPWNØ4Z
ØPWNØ5Z
ØPWNØ7Z
ØPWNØJZ
ØPWNØKZ
ØPWN34Z
ØPWN35Z
ØPWN37Z
ØPWN3JZ
ØPWN3KZ
ØPWN44Z
ØPWN45Z
ØPWN47Z
ØPWN4JZ
ØPWN4KZ
ØPWPØ4Z
ØPWPØ5Z
ØPWPØ7Z
ØPWPØJZ
ØPWPØKZ
ØPWP34Z
ØPWP35Z
ØPWP37Z
ØPWP3JZ
ØPWP3KZ
ØPWP44Z
ØPWP45Z
ØPWP47Z
ØPWP4JZ
ØPWP4KZ
ØPWQØ4Z
ØPWQØ5Z
ØPWQØ7Z
ØPWQØJZ
ØPWQØKZ
ØPWQ34Z
ØPWQ35Z
ØPWQ37Z
ØPWQ3JZ
ØPWQ3KZ
ØPWQ44Z
ØPWQ45Z
ØPWQ47Z
ØPWQ4JZ
ØPWQ4KZ
ØR5N*
ØR5P*
ØR5Q*
ØR5R*
ØR5S*
ØR5T*
ØR5U*
ØR5V*
ØR5W*
ØR5X*
ØRBNØZZ
ØRBN3ZZ
ØRBN4ZZ
ØRBPØZZ
ØRBP3ZZ
ØRBP4ZZ
ØRBQØZZ
ØRBQ3ZZ
ØRBQ4ZZ
ØRBRØZZ
ØRBR3ZZ
ØRBR4ZZ
ØRBSØZZ
ØRBS3ZZ
ØRBS4ZZ
ØRBTØZZ
ØRBT3ZZ
ØRBT4ZZ
ØRBUØZZ
ØRBU3ZZ
ØRBU4ZZ
ØRBVØZZ
ØRBV3ZZ
ØRBV4ZZ
ØRBWØZZ
ØRBW3ZZ
ØRBW4ZZ
ØRBXØZZ
ØRBX3ZZ
ØRBX4ZZ
ØRGN*
ØRGP*
ØRGQ*
ØRGR*
ØRGS*
ØRGT*
ØRGU*
ØRGV*
ØRGW*
ØRGX*
ØRNNØZZ
ØRNN3ZZ
ØRNN4ZZ
ØRNPØZZ
ØRNP3ZZ
ØRNP4ZZ
ØRNQØZZ
ØRNQ3ZZ
ØRNQ4ZZ
ØRNRØZZ
ØRNR3ZZ
ØRNR4ZZ
ØRNSØZZ
ØRNS3ZZ
ØRNS4ZZ
ØRNTØZZ
ØRNT3ZZ
ØRNT4ZZ
ØRNUØZZ
ØRNU3ZZ
ØRNU4ZZ
ØRNVØZZ
ØRNV3ZZ
ØRNV4ZZ
ØRNWØZZ
ØRNW3ZZ
ØRNW4ZZ
ØRNXØZZ
ØRNX3ZZ
ØRNX4ZZ
ØRSNØ4Z
ØRSNØ5Z
ØRSNØZZ
ØRSPØ4Z
ØRSPØ5Z
ØRSPØZZ
ØRSQØ4Z
ØRSQØ5Z
ØRSQØZZ
ØRSRØ4Z
ØRSRØ5Z
ØRSRØZZ
ØRSSØ4Z
ØRSSØ5Z
ØRSSØZZ
ØRSTØ4Z
ØRSTØ5Z
ØRSTØZZ
ØRSUØ4Z
ØRSUØ5Z
ØRSUØZZ
ØRSVØ4Z
ØRSVØ5Z
ØRSVØZZ
ØRSWØ4Z
ØRSWØ5Z
ØRSWØZZ
ØRSXØ4Z
ØRSXØ5Z
ØRSXØZZ
ØRTNØZZ
ØRTPØZZ
ØRTQØZZ
ØRTRØZZ
ØRTSØZZ
ØRTTØZZ
ØRTUØZZ
ØRTVØZZ
ØRTWØZZ
ØRTXØZZ
ØX6L*
ØX6M*
ØX6N*
ØX6P*
ØX6Q*
ØX6R*
ØX6S*
ØX6T*
ØX6V*
ØX6W*
ØXMLØZZ
ØXMMØZZ
ØXMNØZZ
ØXMPØZZ
ØXMQØZZ
ØXMRØZZ
ØXMSØZZ
ØXMTØZZ
ØXMVØZZ
ØXMWØZZ
ØXUJØ7Z
ØXUJ47Z
ØXUKØ7Z
ØXUK47Z
ØXULØ7Z
ØXUL47Z
ØXUMØ7Z
ØXUM47Z
ØXUNØ7Z
ØXUN47Z
ØXUPØ7Z
ØXUP47Z
ØXUQØ7Z
ØXUQ47Z
ØXURØ7Z
ØXUR47Z
ØXUSØ7Z
ØXUS47Z
ØXUTØ7Z
ØXUT47Z
ØXUVØ7Z
ØXUV47Z
ØXUWØ7Z
ØXUW47Z

DRG 514

Select operating room procedures listed under DRG 513

DRG 515

Operating Room Procedures

ØØ8F*
ØØ8G*
ØØ8H*
ØØ8J*
ØØ8L*
ØØ8M*
ØØ8N*
ØØ8R*
ØØ8S*
ØØ9FØZX
ØØ9GØZX
ØØ9HØZX
ØØ9JØZX
ØØ9KØZX
ØØ9LØZX
ØØ9MØZX
ØØ9NØZX
ØØ9PØZX
ØØ9QØZX
ØØ9RØZX
ØØ9SØZX
ØØBFØZX
ØØBFØZZ
ØØBF3ZZ
ØØBF4ZZ
ØØBGØZX
ØØBGØZZ
ØØBG3ZZ
ØØBG4ZZ
ØØBHØZX
ØØBHØZZ
ØØBH3ZZ
ØØBH4ZZ
ØØBJØZX
ØØBJØZZ
ØØBJ3ZZ
ØØBJ4ZZ
ØØBKØZX
ØØBKØZZ
ØØBK3ZZ
ØØBK4ZZ
ØØBLØZX
ØØBLØZZ
ØØBL3ZZ
ØØBL4ZZ
ØØBMØZX
ØØBMØZZ
ØØBM3ZZ
ØØBM4ZZ
ØØBNØZX
ØØBN3ZZ
ØØBN4ZZ
ØØBPØZX
ØØBPØZZ
ØØBP3ZZ
ØØBP4ZZ
ØØBQØZX
ØØBQØZZ
ØØBQ3ZZ
ØØBQ4ZZ
ØØBRØZX
ØØBRØZZ
ØØBR3ZZ
ØØBR4ZZ
ØØBSØZX
ØØBSØZZ
ØØBS3ZZ
ØØBS4ZZ
ØØDF*
ØØDG*
ØØDH*
ØØDJ*
ØØDK*
ØØDL*
ØØDM*
ØØDN*
ØØDP*
ØØDQ*
ØØDR*
ØØDS*
ØØHEØMZ
ØØHE3MZ
ØØHE4MZ
ØØPEØMZ
ØØPE3MZ
ØØPE4MZ
Ø18Ø*
Ø182*
Ø183*
Ø184*
Ø185*
Ø186*
Ø189*
Ø18A*
Ø18C*
Ø18D*
Ø18F*
Ø18G*
Ø18H*
Ø18Q*
Ø19ØØZX
Ø191ØZX
Ø192ØZX
Ø193ØZX
Ø194ØZX
Ø195ØZX
Ø196ØZX
Ø198ØZX
Ø199ØZX
Ø19AØZX
Ø19BØZX
Ø19CØZX
Ø19DØZX
Ø19FØZX
Ø19GØZX
Ø19HØZX
Ø19QØZX
Ø19RØZX
Ø1BØØZX
Ø1BØØZZ
Ø1BØ3ZZ
Ø1BØ4ZZ
Ø1B1ØZX
Ø1B1ØZZ
Ø1B13ZZ
Ø1B14ZZ
Ø1B2ØZX
Ø1B2ØZZ
Ø1B23ZZ
Ø1B24ZZ
Ø1B3ØZX
Ø1B3ØZZ
Ø1B33ZZ
Ø1B34ZZ
Ø1B4ØZX
Ø1B4ØZZ
Ø1B43ZZ
Ø1B44ZZ
Ø1B5ØZX
Ø1B5ØZZ
Ø1B53ZZ
Ø1B54ZZ
Ø1B6ØZX
Ø1B6ØZZ
Ø1B63ZZ
Ø1B64ZZ
Ø1B8ØZX
Ø1B8ØZZ
Ø1B83ZZ
Ø1B84ZZ
Ø1B9ØZX
Ø1B9ØZZ
Ø1B93ZZ
Ø1B94ZZ
Ø1BAØZX
Ø1BAØZZ
Ø1BA3ZZ
Ø1BA4ZZ
Ø1BBØZX
Ø1BBØZZ
Ø1BB3ZZ
Ø1BB4ZZ
Ø1BCØZX
Ø1BCØZZ
Ø1BC3ZZ
Ø1BC4ZZ
Ø1BDØZX
Ø1BDØZZ
Ø1BD3ZZ
Ø1BD4ZZ
Ø1BFØZX
Ø1BFØZZ
Ø1BF3ZZ
Ø1BF4ZZ
Ø1BGØZX
Ø1BGØZZ
Ø1BG3ZZ
Ø1BG4ZZ
Ø1BHØZX
Ø1BHØZZ
Ø1BH3ZZ
Ø1BH4ZZ
Ø1BQØZX
Ø1BQØZZ
Ø1BQ3ZZ
Ø1BQ4ZZ
Ø1BRØZX
Ø1BRØZZ
Ø1BR3ZZ
Ø1BR4ZZ
Ø1DØ*
Ø1D1*
Ø1D2*
Ø1D3*
Ø1D4*
Ø1D5*
Ø1D6*
Ø1D8*
Ø1D9*
Ø1DA*
Ø1DB*
Ø1DC*
Ø1DD*
Ø1DF*
Ø1DG*
Ø1DH*
Ø1DQ*
Ø1DR*
Ø1HYØMZ
Ø1HY3MZ
Ø1HY4MZ
Ø1NØ*
Ø1N1*
Ø1N2*
Ø1N3*
Ø1N4*
Ø1N6*
Ø1N8*
Ø1N9*
Ø1NA*
Ø1NB*
Ø1NC*
Ø1ND*
Ø1NF*
Ø1NH*
Ø1NQ*
Ø1NR*
Ø1PYØMZ
Ø1PY3MZ
Ø1PY4MZ
Ø1QØ*
Ø1Q1*
Ø1Q2*
Ø1Q3*
Ø1Q4*
Ø1Q5*
Ø1Q6*
Ø1Q8*
Ø1Q9*
Ø1QA*
Ø1QB*
Ø1QC*
Ø1QD*
Ø1QF*
Ø1QG*
Ø1QH*
Ø1QQ*
Ø1R1Ø7Z
Ø1R1ØJZ
Ø1R1ØKZ
Ø1R147Z
Ø1R14JZ
Ø1R14KZ
Ø1R2Ø7Z
Ø1R2ØJZ
Ø1R2ØKZ
Ø1R247Z
Ø1R24JZ
Ø1R24KZ
Ø1R4Ø7Z
Ø1R4ØJZ
Ø1R4ØKZ
Ø1R447Z
Ø1R44JZ
Ø1R44KZ
Ø1R5Ø7Z
Ø1R5ØJZ
Ø1R5ØKZ
Ø1R547Z
Ø1R54JZ
Ø1R54KZ
Ø1R6Ø7Z
Ø1R6ØJZ
Ø1R6ØKZ
Ø1R647Z
Ø1R64JZ
Ø1R64KZ
Ø1R8Ø7Z
Ø1R8ØJZ
Ø1R8ØKZ
Ø1R847Z
Ø1R84JZ
Ø1R84KZ
Ø1RBØ7Z
Ø1RBØJZ
Ø1RBØKZ
Ø1RB47Z
Ø1RB4JZ
Ø1RB4KZ
Ø1RCØ7Z
Ø1RCØJZ
Ø1RCØKZ
Ø1RC47Z
Ø1RC4JZ
Ø1RC4KZ
Ø1RDØ7Z
Ø1RDØJZ
Ø1RDØKZ
Ø1RD47Z
Ø1RD4JZ
Ø1RD4KZ
Ø1RFØ7Z
Ø1RFØJZ
Ø1RFØKZ
Ø1RF47Z
Ø1RF4JZ
Ø1RF4KZ
Ø1RGØ7Z
Ø1RGØJZ
Ø1RGØKZ
Ø1RG47Z
Ø1RG4JZ
Ø1RG4KZ
Ø1RHØ7Z
Ø1RHØJZ
Ø1RHØKZ
Ø1RH47Z
Ø1RH4JZ
Ø1RH4KZ
Ø1U1ØJZ
Ø1U1ØKZ
Ø1U13JZ
Ø1U13KZ
Ø1U14JZ
Ø1U14KZ
Ø1U2ØJZ
Ø1U2ØKZ
Ø1U23JZ
Ø1U23KZ
Ø1U24JZ
Ø1U24KZ
Ø1U4ØJZ
Ø1U4ØKZ
Ø1U43JZ
Ø1U43KZ
Ø1U44JZ
Ø1U44KZ
Ø1U5ØJZ
Ø1U5ØKZ
Ø1U53JZ
Ø1U53KZ
Ø1U54JZ
Ø1U54KZ
Ø1U6ØJZ
Ø1U6ØKZ
Ø1U63JZ
Ø1U63KZ
Ø1U64JZ
Ø1U64KZ
Ø1U8ØJZ
Ø1U8ØKZ
Ø1U83JZ
Ø1U83KZ
Ø1U84JZ
Ø1U84KZ
Ø1UBØJZ
Ø1UBØKZ
Ø1UB3JZ
Ø1UB3KZ
Ø1UB4JZ
Ø1UB4KZ
Ø1UCØJZ
Ø1UCØKZ
Ø1UC3JZ
Ø1UC3KZ
Ø1UC4JZ
Ø1UC4KZ
Ø1UDØJZ
Ø1UDØKZ
Ø1UD3JZ
Ø1UD3KZ
Ø1UD4JZ
Ø1UD4KZ
Ø1UFØJZ
Ø1UFØKZ
Ø1UF3JZ
Ø1UF3KZ
Ø1UF4JZ
Ø1UF4KZ
Ø1UGØJZ
Ø1UGØKZ
Ø1UG3JZ
Ø1UG3KZ
Ø1UG4JZ
Ø1UG4KZ
Ø1UHØJZ
Ø1UHØKZ
Ø1UH3JZ
Ø1UH3KZ
Ø1UH4JZ
Ø1UH4KZ
Ø2HVØ2Z
Ø2HVØDZ
Ø2HV3DZ
Ø2HV42Z
Ø2HV4DZ
Ø2LV*
Ø2VV*
Ø37334Z
Ø37335Z
Ø37336Z
Ø37337Z
Ø3733D1
Ø3733DZ
Ø3733EZ
Ø3733FZ
Ø3733GZ
Ø3733Z1
Ø3733ZZ
Ø37434Z
Ø37435Z
Ø37436Z
Ø37437Z
Ø3743D1
Ø3743DZ
Ø3743EZ
Ø3743FZ
Ø3743GZ
Ø3743Z1
Ø3743ZZ
Ø37734Z
Ø37735Z
Ø37736Z
Ø37737Z
Ø3773D1
Ø3773DZ
Ø3773EZ
Ø3773FZ
Ø3773GZ
Ø3773Z1
Ø3773ZZ
Ø37834Z
Ø37835Z
Ø37836Z
Ø37837Z
Ø3783D1
Ø3783DZ
Ø3783EZ
Ø3783FZ
Ø3783GZ
Ø3783Z1
Ø3783ZZ
Ø37934Z
Ø37935Z
Ø37936Z
Ø37937Z
Ø3793D1
Ø3793DZ
Ø3793EZ
Ø3793FZ
Ø3793GZ
Ø3793Z1
Ø3793ZZ
Ø37A34Z
Ø37A35Z
Ø37A36Z
Ø37A37Z
Ø37A3D1
Ø37A3DZ
Ø37A3EZ
Ø37A3FZ
Ø37A3GZ
Ø37A3Z1
Ø37A3ZZ
Ø37Y34Z
Ø37Y35Z
Ø37Y36Z
Ø37Y37Z
Ø37Y3DZ
Ø37Y3EZ
Ø37Y3FZ
Ø37Y3GZ
Ø37Y3ZZ
Ø39SØZX
Ø39S4ZX
Ø39TØZX
Ø39T4ZX
Ø3BSØZX
Ø3BS3ZX
Ø3BS4ZX
Ø3BTØZX
Ø3BT3ZX
Ø3BT4ZX
47Ø341
Ø47Ø34Z
Ø47Ø35Z
Ø47Ø36Z
Ø47Ø37Z
Ø47Ø3D1
Ø47Ø3DZ
Ø47Ø3EZ
Ø47Ø3FZ
Ø47Ø3GZ
Ø47Ø3Z1
Ø47Ø3ZZ
471341
Ø47134Z
Ø47135Z
Ø47136Z
Ø47137Z
Ø4713D1
Ø4713DZ
Ø4713EZ
Ø4713FZ
Ø4713GZ
Ø4713Z1
Ø4713ZZ
472341
Ø47234Z
Ø47235Z
Ø47236Z
Ø47237Z
Ø4723D1
Ø4723DZ
Ø4723EZ
Ø4723FZ
Ø4723GZ
Ø4723Z1
Ø4723ZZ
473341
Ø47334Z
Ø47335Z
Ø47336Z
Ø47337Z
Ø4733D1
Ø4733DZ
Ø4733EZ
Ø4733FZ
Ø4733GZ
Ø4733Z1
Ø4733ZZ
474341
Ø47434Z
Ø47435Z
Ø47436Z
Ø47437Z
Ø4743D1
Ø4743DZ
Ø4743EZ
Ø4743FZ
Ø4743GZ
Ø4743Z1
Ø4743ZZ
475341
Ø47534Z
Ø47535Z
Ø47536Z
Ø47537Z
Ø4753D1
Ø4753DZ
Ø4753EZ
Ø4753FZ
Ø4753GZ
Ø4753Z1
Ø4753ZZ
476341
Ø47634Z
Ø47635Z
Ø47636Z
Ø47637Z
Ø4763D1
Ø4763DZ
Ø4763EZ
Ø4763FZ
Ø4763GZ
Ø4763Z1
Ø4763ZZ
477341
Ø47734Z
Ø47735Z
Ø47736Z
Ø47737Z
Ø4773D1
Ø4773DZ
Ø4773EZ
Ø4773FZ
Ø4773GZ
Ø4773Z1
Ø4773ZZ
478341
Ø47834Z
Ø47835Z
Ø47836Z
Ø47837Z
Ø4783D1
Ø4783DZ
Ø4783EZ
Ø4783FZ
Ø4783GZ
Ø4783Z1
Ø4783ZZ
479341
Ø47934Z
Ø47935Z
Ø47936Z
Ø47937Z
Ø4793D1
Ø4793DZ
Ø4793EZ
Ø4793FZ
Ø4793GZ
Ø4793Z1
Ø4793ZZ
Ø47A341
Ø47A34Z
Ø47A35Z
Ø47A36Z
Ø47A37Z
Ø47A3D1
Ø47A3DZ
Ø47A3EZ

ICD-10-CM/PCS Codes by MS-DRG

Ø47A3FZ
Ø47A3GZ
Ø47A3Z1
Ø47A3ZZ
Ø47B341
Ø47B34Z
Ø47B35Z
Ø47B36Z
Ø47B37Z
Ø47B3D1
Ø47B3DZ
Ø47B3EZ
Ø47B3FZ
Ø47B3GZ
Ø47B3Z1
Ø47B3ZZ
Ø47C341
Ø47C34Z
Ø47C35Z
Ø47C36Z
Ø47C37Z
Ø47C3D1
Ø47C3DZ
Ø47C3EZ
Ø47C3FZ
Ø47C3GZ
Ø47C3Z1
Ø47C3ZZ
Ø47D341
Ø47D34Z
Ø47D35Z
Ø47D36Z
Ø47D37Z
Ø47D3D1
Ø47D3DZ
Ø47D3EZ
Ø47D3FZ
Ø47D3GZ
Ø47D3Z1
Ø47D3ZZ
Ø47E341
Ø47E34Z
Ø47E35Z
Ø47E36Z
Ø47E37Z
Ø47E3D1
Ø47E3DZ
Ø47E3EZ
Ø47E3FZ
Ø47E3GZ
Ø47E3Z1
Ø47E3ZZ
Ø47F341
Ø47F34Z
Ø47F35Z
Ø47F36Z
Ø47F37Z
Ø47F3D1
Ø47F3DZ
Ø47F3EZ
Ø47F3FZ
Ø47F3GZ
Ø47F3Z1
Ø47F3ZZ
Ø47H341
Ø47H34Z
Ø47H35Z
Ø47H36Z
Ø47H37Z
Ø47H3D1
Ø47H3DZ
Ø47H3EZ
Ø47H3FZ
Ø47H3GZ
Ø47H3Z1
Ø47H3ZZ
Ø47J341
Ø47J34Z
Ø47J35Z
Ø47J36Z
Ø47J37Z
Ø47J3D1
Ø47J3DZ
Ø47J3EZ
Ø47J3FZ
Ø47J3GZ
Ø47J3Z1
Ø47J3ZZ
Ø47KØ41
Ø47KØD1
Ø47KØZ1
Ø47K341
Ø47K34Z
Ø47K35Z
Ø47K36Z
Ø47K37Z
Ø47K3D1
Ø47K3DZ
Ø47K3EZ
Ø47K3FZ
Ø47K3GZ
Ø47K3Z1
Ø47K3ZZ
Ø47K441
Ø47K4D1
Ø47K4Z1
Ø47LØ41
Ø47LØD1
Ø47LØZ1
Ø47L341
Ø47L34Z
Ø47L35Z
Ø47L36Z
Ø47L37Z
Ø47L3D1
Ø47L3DZ
Ø47L3EZ
Ø47L3FZ
Ø47L3GZ
Ø47L3Z1
Ø47L3ZZ
Ø47L441
Ø47L4D1
Ø47L4Z1
Ø47MØ41
Ø47MØD1
Ø47MØZ1
Ø47M341
Ø47M3D1
Ø47M3Z1
Ø47M441
Ø47M4D1
Ø47M4Z1
Ø47NØ41
Ø47NØD1
Ø47NØZ1
Ø47N341
Ø47N3D1
Ø47N3Z1
Ø47N441
Ø47N4D1
Ø47N4Z1
Ø47Y341
Ø47Y34Z
Ø47Y35Z
Ø47Y36Z
Ø47Y37Z
Ø47Y3D1
Ø47Y3DZ
Ø47Y3EZ
Ø47Y3FZ
Ø47Y3GZ
Ø47Y3Z1
Ø47Y3ZZ
Ø5793D1
Ø5793Z1
Ø5793ZZ
Ø57A3D1
Ø57A3DZ
Ø57A3Z1
Ø57A3ZZ
Ø57B3D1
Ø57B3DZ
Ø57B3Z1
Ø57B3ZZ
Ø57C3D1
Ø57C3DZ
Ø57C3Z1
Ø57C3ZZ
Ø57D3D1
Ø57D3DZ
Ø57D3Z1
Ø57D3ZZ
Ø57F3D1
Ø57F3DZ
Ø57F3Z1
Ø57F3ZZ
Ø5HØØMZ
Ø5HØ3MZ
Ø5HØ4MZ
Ø5H3ØMZ
Ø5H33MZ
Ø5H34MZ
Ø5H4ØMZ
Ø5H43MZ
Ø5H44MZ
Ø5PØØMZ
Ø5PØ3MZ
Ø5PØ4MZ
Ø5PØXMZ
Ø5P3ØMZ
Ø5P33MZ
Ø5P34MZ
Ø5P3XMZ
Ø5P4ØMZ
Ø5P43MZ
Ø5P44MZ
Ø5P4XMZ
Ø67Ø3DZ
Ø67Ø3ZZ
Ø6HØØDZ
Ø6HØ4DZ
Ø6LØ*
Ø6VØ*
Ø79ØØZX
Ø79Ø3ZX
Ø79Ø4ZX
Ø791ØZX
Ø7913ZX
Ø7914ZX
Ø792ØZX
Ø7923ZX
Ø7924ZX
Ø793ØZX
Ø7933ZX
Ø7934ZX
Ø794ØZX
Ø7943ZX
Ø7944ZX
Ø795ØZX
Ø7953ZX
Ø7954ZX
Ø796ØZX
Ø7963ZX
Ø7964ZX
Ø797ØZX
Ø7973ZX
Ø7974ZX
Ø798ØZX
Ø7983ZX
Ø7984ZX
Ø799ØZX
Ø7993ZX
Ø7994ZX
Ø79BØZX
Ø79B3ZX
Ø79B4ZX
Ø79CØZX
Ø79C3ZX
Ø79C4ZX
Ø79DØZX
Ø79D3ZX
Ø79D4ZX
Ø79FØZX
Ø79F3ZX
Ø79F4ZX
Ø79GØZX
Ø79G3ZX
Ø79G4ZX
Ø79HØZX
Ø79H3ZX
Ø79H4ZX
Ø79JØZX
Ø79J3ZX
Ø79J4ZX
Ø79KØZX
Ø79K3ZX
Ø79K4ZX
Ø79LØZX
Ø79L3ZX
Ø79L4ZX
Ø7BØØZX
Ø7BØ3ZX
Ø7BØ4ZX
Ø7B1*
Ø7B2*
Ø7B3ØZX
Ø7B3ØZZ
Ø7B33ZX
Ø7B34ZX
Ø7B34ZZ
Ø7B4ØZX
Ø7B4ØZZ
Ø7B43ZX
Ø7B44ZX
Ø7B44ZZ
Ø7B5*
Ø7B6*
Ø7B7ØZX
Ø7B7ØZZ
Ø7B73ZX
Ø7B74ZX
Ø7B74ZZ
Ø7B8ØZX
Ø7B83ZX
Ø7B84ZX
Ø7B9ØZX
Ø7B93ZX
Ø7B94ZX
Ø7BBØZX
Ø7BB3ZX
Ø7BB4ZX
Ø7BCØZX
Ø7BC3ZX
Ø7BC4ZX
Ø7BDØZX
Ø7BD3ZX
Ø7BD4ZX
Ø7BFØZX
Ø7BFØZZ
Ø7BF3ZX
Ø7BF4ZX
Ø7BF4ZZ
Ø7BGØZX
Ø7BGØZZ
Ø7BG3ZX
Ø7BG4ZX
Ø7BG4ZZ
Ø7BH*
Ø7BJ*
Ø7BKØZX
Ø7BK3ZX
Ø7BK4ZX
Ø7BLØZX
Ø7BL3ZX
Ø7BL4ZX
Ø7BPØZZ
Ø7BP3ZZ
Ø7BP4ZZ
Ø7T5*
Ø7T6*
Ø7T8*
Ø7T9*
Ø7TC*
Ø7TD*
Ø7TH*
Ø7TJ*
Ø7TP*
Ø8TØXZZ
Ø8T1XZZ
Ø9ØK*
Ø9BQØZZ
Ø9BQ3ZZ
Ø9BQ4ZZ
Ø9BQ8ZZ
Ø9BRØZZ
Ø9BR3ZZ
Ø9BR4ZZ
Ø9BR8ZZ
Ø9MKXZZ
Ø9QKØZZ
Ø9QK3ZZ
Ø9QK4ZZ
Ø9QK8ZZ
Ø9QM*
Ø9RK*
Ø9RM*
Ø9SK*
Ø9SM*
Ø9TQ*
Ø9TR*
Ø9UK*
Ø9UM*
ØB5TØZZ
ØB5T3ZZ
ØB5T4ZZ
ØB9CØZX
ØB9DØZX
ØB9FØZX
ØB9GØZX
ØB9HØZX
ØB9JØZX
ØB9KØZX
ØB9LØZX
ØB9MØZX
ØBBCØZX
ØBBC4ZX
ØBBDØZX
ØBBD4ZX
ØBBFØZX
ØBBF4ZX
ØBBGØZX
ØBBG4ZX
ØBBHØZX
ØBBH4ZX
ØBBJØZX
ØBBJ4ZX
ØBBKØZX
ØBBK4ZX
ØBBLØZX
ØBBL4ZX
ØBBMØZX
ØBBTØZZ
ØBBT3ZZ
ØBBT4ZZ
ØDH6ØMZ
ØDH63MZ
ØDH64MZ
ØDP6ØMZ
ØDP63MZ
ØDP64MZ
ØDPR*
ØF9ØØZX
ØF91ØZX
ØF92ØZX
ØFBØØZX
ØFB1ØZX
ØFB2ØZX
ØG9LØZX
ØG9L3ZX
ØG9L4ZX
ØG9MØZX
ØG9M3ZX
ØG9M4ZX
ØG9NØZX
ØG9N3ZX
ØG9N4ZX
ØG9PØZX
ØG9P3ZX
ØG9P4ZX
ØG9QØZX
ØG9Q3ZX
ØG9Q4ZX
ØG9RØZX
ØG9R3ZX
ØG9R4ZX
ØGBLØZX
ØGBL3ZX
ØGBL4ZX
ØGBMØZX
ØGBM3ZX
ØGBM4ZX
ØGBNØZX
ØGBN3ZX
ØGBN4ZX
ØGBPØZX
ØGBP3ZX
ØGBP4ZX
ØGBQØZX
ØGBQ3ZX
ØGBQ4ZX
ØGBRØZX
ØGBR3ZX
ØGBR4ZX
ØGJK4ZZ
ØGJR4ZZ
ØGJS4ZZ
ØJH6ØVZ
ØJH6ØWZ
ØJH6ØYZ
ØJH63VZ
ØJH7ØVZ
ØJH7ØYZ
ØJH73VZ
ØJH8ØVZ
ØJH8ØWZ
ØJH8ØYZ
ØJH83VZ
ØJHDØVZ
ØJHDØWZ
ØJHD3VZ
ØJHFØVZ
ØJHFØWZ
ØJHF3VZ
ØJHGØVZ
ØJHGØWZ
ØJHG3VZ
ØJHHØVZ
ØJHHØWZ
ØJHH3VZ
ØJHLØVZ
ØJHLØWZ
ØJHL3VZ
ØJHMØVZ
ØJHMØWZ
ØJHM3VZ
ØJHNØVZ
ØJHN3VZ
ØJHPØVZ
ØJHPØWZ
ØJHP3VZ
ØJHTØVZ
ØJHTØYZ
ØJHT3VZ
ØM9Ø4ØZ
ØMM*
ØMPXØØZ
ØMPXØJZ
ØMPXØYZ
ØMPX3JZ
ØMPX4ØZ
ØMPX4JZ
ØMPYØØZ
ØMPYØJZ
ØMPYØYZ
ØMPY3JZ
ØMPY4ØZ
ØMPY4JZ
ØMSØ*
ØMS1*
ØMS2*
ØMS3*
ØMS4*
ØMS5*
ØMS6*
ØMS7*
ØMS8*
ØMSC*
ØMSD*
ØMSF*
ØMSG*
ØMSH*
ØMSJ*
ØMSK*
ØMSL*
ØMSM*
ØMSN*
ØMSP*
ØMSQ*
ØMSR*
ØMSS*
ØMST*
ØMUØ*
ØMU1*
ØMU2*
ØMU3*
ØMU4*
ØMU5*
ØMU6*
ØMU7*
ØMU8*
ØMUC*
ØMUD*
ØMUF*
ØMUG*
ØMUH*
ØMUJ*
ØMUK*
ØMUL*
ØMUM*
ØMUN*
ØMUP*
ØMUQ*
ØMUR*
ØMUS*
ØMUT*
ØN5Ø*
ØN51*
ØN53*
ØN54*
ØN55*
ØN56*
ØN57*
ØNBØØZZ
ØNBØ3ZZ
ØNBØ4ZZ
ØNB1ØZZ
ØNB13ZZ
ØNB14ZZ
ØNB3ØZZ
ØNB33ZZ
ØNB34ZZ
ØNB4ØZZ
ØNB43ZZ
ØNB44ZZ
ØNB5ØZZ
ØNB53ZZ
ØNB54ZZ
ØNB6ØZZ
ØNB63ZZ
ØNB64ZZ
ØNB7ØZZ
ØNB73ZZ
ØNB74ZZ
ØNBBØZZ
ØNBB3ZZ
ØNBB4ZZ
ØNBCØZZ
ØNBC3ZZ
ØNBC4ZZ
ØNBFØZZ
ØNBF3ZZ
ØNBF4ZZ
ØNBGØZZ
ØNBG3ZZ
ØNBG4ZZ
ØNBHØZZ
ØNBH3ZZ
ØNBH4ZZ
ØNBJØZZ
ØNBJ3ZZ
ØNBJ4ZZ
ØNBKØZZ
ØNBK3ZZ
ØNBK4ZZ
ØNBLØZZ
ØNBL3ZZ
ØNBL4ZZ
ØNBMØZZ
ØNBM3ZZ
ØNBM4ZZ
ØNBNØZZ
ØNBN3ZZ
ØNBN4ZZ
ØNBRØZZ
ØNBR3ZZ
ØNBR4ZZ
ØNBTØZZ
ØNBT3ZZ
ØNBT4ZZ
ØNBVØZZ
ØNBV3ZZ
ØNBV4ZZ
ØNBXØZZ
ØNBX3ZZ
ØNBX4ZZ
ØNHØØ4Z
ØNHØ34Z
ØNHØ44Z
ØNH1*
ØNH3*
ØNH4*
ØNH5Ø4Z
ØNH534Z
ØNH544Z
ØNH6Ø4Z
ØNH634Z
ØNH644Z
ØNH7*
ØNN1*
ØNN3*
ØNN4*
ØNN5*
ØNN6*
ØNN7*
ØNPØØJZ
ØNPØ3JZ
ØNPØ4JZ
ØNQØØZZ
ØNQØ3ZZ
ØNQØ4ZZ
ØNQ1ØZZ
ØNQ13ZZ
ØNQ14ZZ
ØNQ3ØZZ
ØNQ33ZZ
ØNQ34ZZ
ØNQ4ØZZ
ØNQ43ZZ
ØNQ44ZZ
ØNQ5ØZZ
ØNQ53ZZ
ØNQ54ZZ
ØNQ6ØZZ
ØNQ63ZZ
ØNQ64ZZ
ØNQ7ØZZ
ØNQ73ZZ
ØNQ74ZZ
ØNQBØZZ
ØNQB3ZZ
ØNQB4ZZ
ØNQRØZZ
ØNQR3ZZ
ØNQR4ZZ
ØNQTØZZ
ØNQT3ZZ
ØNQT4ZZ
ØNQVØZZ
ØNQV3ZZ
ØNQV4ZZ
ØNRØ*
ØNR1*
ØNR3*
ØNR4*
ØNR5*
ØNR6*
ØNR7*
ØNRB*
ØNRCØJZ
ØNRC3JZ
ØNRC4JZ
ØNRFØJZ
ØNRF3JZ
ØNRF4JZ
ØNRGØJZ
ØNRG3JZ
ØNRG4JZ
ØNRHØJZ
ØNRH3JZ
ØNRH4JZ
ØNRJØJZ
ØNRJ3JZ
ØNRJ4JZ
ØNRKØJZ
ØNRK3JZ
ØNRK4JZ
ØNRLØJZ
ØNRL3JZ
ØNRL4JZ
ØNRMØJZ
ØNRM3JZ
ØNRM4JZ
ØNRNØJZ
ØNRN3JZ
ØNRN4JZ
ØNRT*
ØNRV*
ØNRXØJZ
ØNRX3JZ
ØNRX4JZ
ØNSØØ4Z
ØNSØØ5Z
ØNSØØZZ
ØNSØ34Z
ØNSØ35Z
ØNSØ3ZZ
ØNSØ44Z
ØNSØ45Z
ØNSØ4ZZ
ØNS1Ø4Z
ØNS1ØZZ
ØNS134Z
ØNS13ZZ
ØNS144Z
ØNS14ZZ
ØNS3Ø4Z
ØNS3ØZZ
ØNS334Z
ØNS33ZZ
ØNS344Z
ØNS34ZZ
ØNS4Ø4Z
ØNS4ØZZ
ØNS434Z
ØNS43ZZ
ØNS444Z
ØNS44ZZ
ØNS5Ø4Z
ØNS5ØZZ
ØNS534Z
ØNS53ZZ
ØNS544Z
ØNS54ZZ
ØNS6Ø4Z
ØNS6ØZZ
ØNS634Z
ØNS63ZZ
ØNS644Z
ØNS64ZZ
ØNS7Ø4Z
ØNS7ØZZ
ØNS734Z
ØNS73ZZ
ØNS744Z
ØNS74ZZ
ØNSBØ4Z
ØNSBØZZ
ØNSCØ4Z
ØNSCØZZ
ØNSFØ4Z
ØNSFØZZ
ØNSGØ4Z
ØNSGØZZ
ØNSHØ4Z
ØNSHØZZ
ØNSJØ4Z
ØNSJØZZ
ØNSKØ4Z
ØNSKØZZ
ØNSLØ4Z
ØNSLØZZ
ØNSMØ4Z
ØNSMØZZ
ØNSNØ4Z
ØNSNØZZ
ØNSPØ4Z
ØNSPØZZ
ØNSQØ4Z
ØNSQØZZ
ØNSRØ4Z
ØNSRØ5Z
ØNSRØZZ
ØNSTØ4Z
ØNSTØ5Z
ØNSTØZZ
ØNSVØ4Z
ØNSVØ5Z
ØNSVØZZ
ØNSXØ4Z
ØNSXØZZ
ØNT*
ØNUØ*
ØNU1*
ØNU3*
ØNU4*
ØNU5*
ØNU6*
ØNU7*
ØNUB*
ØNUCØJZ
ØNUC3JZ
ØNUC4JZ
ØNUFØJZ
ØNUF3JZ
ØNUF4JZ
ØNUGØJZ
ØNUG3JZ
ØNUG4JZ
ØNUHØJZ
ØNUH3JZ
ØNUH4JZ
ØNUJØJZ
ØNUJ3JZ
ØNUJ4JZ
ØNUKØJZ
ØNUK3JZ
ØNUK4JZ
ØNULØJZ
ØNUL3JZ
ØNUL4JZ
ØNUMØJZ
ØNUM3JZ
ØNUM4JZ
ØNUNØJZ
ØNUN3JZ
ØNUN4JZ
ØNUT*
ØNUV*
ØNUXØJZ
ØNUX3JZ
ØNUX4JZ
ØP8Ø*
ØP81*
ØP82*
ØP83*
ØP84*
ØP85*
ØP86*
ØP87*
ØP88*
ØP89*
ØP8B*
ØP8R*
ØP8S*
ØP8T*
ØP8V*
ØPBØØZZ
ØPBØ3ZZ
ØPBØ4ZZ
ØPB1ØZZ
ØPB13ZZ
ØPB14ZZ
ØPB2ØZZ
ØPB23ZZ
ØPB24ZZ
ØPB3ØZZ
ØPB33ZZ
ØPB34ZZ
ØPB4ØZZ
ØPB43ZZ
ØPB44ZZ
ØPB5ØZZ
ØPB53ZZ

ØPB54ZZ
ØPB6ØZZ
ØPB63ZZ
ØPB64ZZ
ØPB7ØZZ
ØPB73ZZ
ØPB74ZZ
ØPB8ØZZ
ØPB83ZZ
ØPB84ZZ
ØPB9ØZZ
ØPB93ZZ
ØPB94ZZ
ØPBBØZZ
ØPBB3ZZ
ØPBB4ZZ
ØPBRØZZ
ØPBR3ZZ
ØPBR4ZZ
ØPBSØZZ
ØPBS3ZZ
ØPBS4ZZ
ØPBTØZZ
ØPBT3ZZ
ØPBT4ZZ
ØPBVØZZ
ØPBV3ZZ
ØPBV4ZZ
ØPCØ*
ØPC1*
ØPC2*
ØPC3*
ØPC4*
ØPC5*
ØPC6*
ØPC7*
ØPC8*
ØPC9*
ØPCB*
ØPCR*
ØPCS*
ØPCT*
ØPCV*
ØPHØ*
ØPH1*
ØPH2*
ØPH3*
ØPH4*
ØPH5*
ØPH6*
ØPH7*
ØPH8*
ØPH9*
ØPHB*
ØPHR*
ØPHS*
ØPHT*
ØPHV*
ØPHY*
ØPNØ*
ØPN1*
ØPN2*
ØPN3*
ØPN4*
ØPN5*
ØPN6*
ØPN7*
ØPN8*
ØPN9*
ØPNB*
ØPNR*
ØPNS*
ØPNT*
ØPNV*
ØPQØØZZ
ØPQØ3ZZ
ØPQØ4ZZ
ØPQ1ØZZ
ØPQ13ZZ
ØPQ14ZZ
ØPQ2ØZZ
ØPQ23ZZ
ØPQ24ZZ
ØPQ3ØZZ
ØPQ33ZZ
ØPQ34ZZ
ØPQ4ØZZ
ØPQ43ZZ
ØPQ44ZZ
ØPQ5ØZZ
ØPQ53ZZ
ØPQ54ZZ
ØPQ6ØZZ
ØPQ63ZZ
ØPQ64ZZ
ØPQ7ØZZ
ØPQ73ZZ
ØPQ74ZZ
ØPQ8ØZZ
ØPQ83ZZ
ØPQ84ZZ
ØPQ9ØZZ
ØPQ93ZZ
ØPQ94ZZ
ØPQBØZZ
ØPQB3ZZ
ØPQB4ZZ
ØPQRØZZ
ØPQR3ZZ
ØPQR4ZZ
ØPQSØZZ
ØPQS3ZZ
ØPQS4ZZ
ØPQTØZZ
ØPQT3ZZ
ØPQT4ZZ
ØPQVØZZ
ØPQV3ZZ
ØPQV4ZZ
ØPRØ*
ØPR1*
ØPR2*
ØPR3*
ØPR4*
ØPR5*
ØPR6*
ØPR7*
ØPR8*
ØPR9*
ØPRB*
ØPRR*
ØPRS*
ØPRT*
ØPRV*
ØPSØØØZ
ØPSØØ4Z
ØPSØØZZ
ØPSØ3ØZ
ØPSØ34Z
ØPSØ4ØZ
ØPSØ44Z
ØPS1Ø4Z
ØPS1ØZZ
ØPS134Z
ØPS144Z
ØPS2Ø4Z
ØPS2ØZZ
ØPS234Z
ØPS244Z
ØPS33ZZ
ØPS43ZZ
ØPS5Ø4Z
ØPS5ØZZ
ØPS534Z
ØPS544Z
ØPS6Ø4Z
ØPS6ØZZ
ØPS634Z
ØPS644Z
ØPS7Ø4Z
ØPS7ØZZ
ØPS734Z
ØPS744Z
ØPS8Ø4Z
ØPS8ØZZ
ØPS834Z
ØPS844Z
ØPS9Ø4Z
ØPS9ØZZ
ØPS934Z
ØPS944Z
ØPSBØ4Z
ØPSBØZZ
ØPSB34Z
ØPSB44Z
ØPSRØ5Z
ØPSR35Z
ØPSR45Z
ØPSSØ5Z
ØPSS35Z
ØPSS45Z
ØPSTØ5Z
ØPST35Z
ØPST45Z
ØPSVØ5Z
ØPSV35Z
ØPSV45Z
ØPTØØZZ
ØPT1ØZZ
ØPT2ØZZ
ØPT5ØZZ
ØPT6ØZZ
ØPT7ØZZ
ØPT8ØZZ
ØPT9ØZZ
ØPTBØZZ
ØPTRØZZ
ØPTSØZZ
ØPTTØZZ
ØPTVØZZ
ØPUØ*
ØPU1*
ØPU2*
ØPU3Ø7Z
ØPU3ØJZ
ØPU3ØKZ
ØPU337Z
ØPU33JZ
ØPU33KZ
ØPU347Z
ØPU34JZ
ØPU34KZ
ØPU4*
ØPU5*
ØPU6*
ØPU7*
ØPU8*
ØPU9*
ØPUB*
ØPUR*
ØPUS*
ØPUT*
ØPUV*
ØQ8Ø*
ØQ81*
ØQ82*
ØQ83*
ØQ84*
ØQ85*
ØQ8Q*
ØQ8R*
ØQ8S*
ØQBØØZZ
ØQBØ3ZZ
ØQBØ4ZZ
ØQB1ØZZ
ØQB13ZZ
ØQB14ZZ
ØQB2ØZZ
ØQB23ZZ
ØQB24ZZ
ØQB3ØZZ
ØQB33ZZ
ØQB34ZZ
ØQB4ØZZ
ØQB43ZZ
ØQB44ZZ
ØQB5ØZZ
ØQB53ZZ
ØQB54ZZ
ØQBQØZZ
ØQBQ3ZZ
ØQBQ4ZZ
ØQBRØZZ
ØQBR3ZZ
ØQBR4ZZ
ØQBSØZZ
ØQBS3ZZ
ØQBS4ZZ
ØQCØ*
ØQC1*
ØQC2*
ØQC3*
ØQC4*
ØQC5*
ØQCQ*
ØQCR*
ØQCS*
ØQHØ*
ØQH1*
ØQH2*
ØQH3*
ØQH4*
ØQH5*
ØQHQ*
ØQHR*
ØQHS*
ØQHY*
ØQNØ*
ØQN1*
ØQN2*
ØQN3*
ØQN4*
ØQN5*
ØQNQ*
ØQNR*
ØQNS*
ØQQØØZZ
ØQQØ3ZZ
ØQQØ4ZZ
ØQQ1ØZZ
ØQQ13ZZ
ØQQ14ZZ
ØQQ2ØZZ
ØQQ23ZZ
ØQQ24ZZ
ØQQ3ØZZ
ØQQ33ZZ
ØQQ34ZZ
ØQQ4ØZZ
ØQQ43ZZ
ØQQ44ZZ
ØQQ5ØZZ
ØQQ53ZZ
ØQQ54ZZ
ØQQD3ZZ
ØQQF3ZZ
ØQQQØZZ
ØQQQ3ZZ
ØQQQ4ZZ
ØQQRØZZ
ØQQR3ZZ
ØQQR4ZZ
ØQQSØZZ
ØQQS3ZZ
ØQQS4ZZ
ØQRØ*
ØQR1*
ØQR2*
ØQR3*
ØQR4*
ØQR5*
ØQRQ*
ØQRR*
ØQRS*
ØQSØ3ZZ
ØQS13ZZ
ØQS2Ø4Z
ØQS2Ø5Z
ØQS2ØZZ
ØQS234Z
ØQS235Z
ØQS244Z
ØQS245Z
ØQS3Ø4Z
ØQS3Ø5Z
ØQS3ØZZ
ØQS334Z
ØQS335Z
ØQS344Z
ØQS345Z
ØQS4Ø4Z
ØQS4ØZZ
ØQS434Z
ØQS444Z
ØQS5Ø4Z
ØQS5ØZZ
ØQS534Z
ØQS544Z
ØQSDØ4Z
ØQSDØZZ
ØQSD34Z
ØQSD44Z
ØQSFØ4Z
ØQSFØZZ
ØQSF34Z
ØQSF44Z
ØQSQØ5Z
ØQSQ35Z
ØQSQ45Z
ØQSRØ5Z
ØQSR35Z
ØQSR45Z
ØQT2ØZZ
ØQT3ØZZ
ØQT4ØZZ
ØQT5ØZZ
ØQTQØZZ
ØQTRØZZ
ØQTSØZZ
ØQUØ*
ØQU1*
ØQU2*
ØQU3*
ØQU4*
ØQU5*
ØQUQ*
ØQUR*
ØQUS*
ØR9ØØØZ
ØR9ØØZZ
ØR91ØØZ
ØR91ØZZ
ØR93ØØZ
ØR93ØZZ
ØR94ØØZ
ØR94ØZZ
ØR95ØØZ
ØR95ØZZ
ØR96ØØZ
ØR96ØZZ
ØR99ØØZ
ØR99ØZZ
ØR9AØØZ
ØR9AØZZ
ØR9BØØZ
ØR9BØZZ
ØRCØ*
ØRC1*
ØRC3*
ØRC4*
ØRC5*
ØRC6*
ØRC9*
ØRCA*
ØRCB*
ØRCC*
ØRCD*
ØRGC*
ØRGD*
ØRHØØ4Z
ØRHØ34Z
ØRHØ44Z
ØRH1Ø4Z
ØRH134Z
ØRH144Z
ØRH4Ø4Z
ØRH434Z
ØRH444Z
ØRH6Ø4Z
ØRH634Z
ØRH644Z
ØRHAØ4Z
ØRHA34Z
ØRHA44Z
ØRJØØZZ
ØRJ1ØZZ
ØRJ3ØZZ
ØRJ4ØZZ
ØRJ5ØZZ
ØRJ6ØZZ
ØRJ9ØZZ
ØRJAØZZ
ØRJBØZZ
ØRPØØØZ
ØRPØØ3Z
ØRPØØ4Z
ØRPØØ7Z
ØRPØØAZ
ØRPØØKZ
ØRPØ34Z
ØRPØ37Z
ØRPØ3AZ
ØRPØ3KZ
ØRPØ4ØZ
ØRPØ43Z
ØRPØ44Z
ØRPØ47Z
ØRPØ4AZ
ØRPØ4KZ
ØRP1ØØZ
ØRP1Ø3Z
ØRP1Ø4Z
ØRP1Ø7Z
ØRP1ØAZ
ØRP1ØKZ
ØRP134Z
ØRP137Z
ØRP13AZ
ØRP13KZ
ØRP14ØZ
ØRP143Z
ØRP144Z
ØRP147Z
ØRP14AZ
ØRP14KZ
ØRP3ØØZ
ØRP3Ø3Z
ØRP3Ø7Z
ØRP3ØKZ
ØRP337Z
ØRP33KZ
ØRP34ØZ
ØRP343Z
ØRP347Z
ØRP34KZ
ØRP4ØØZ
ØRP4Ø3Z
ØRP4Ø4Z
ØRP4Ø7Z
ØRP4ØAZ
ØRP4ØKZ
ØRP434Z
ØRP437Z
ØRP43AZ
ØRP43KZ
ØRP44ØZ
ØRP443Z
ØRP444Z
ØRP447Z
ØRP44AZ
ØRP44KZ
ØRP5ØØZ
ØRP5Ø3Z
ØRP5Ø7Z
ØRP5ØKZ
ØRP537Z
ØRP53KZ
ØRP54ØZ
ØRP543Z
ØRP547Z
ØRP54KZ
ØRP6ØØZ
ØRP6Ø3Z
ØRP6Ø4Z
ØRP6Ø7Z
ØRP6ØAZ
ØRP6ØKZ
ØRP634Z
ØRP637Z
ØRP63AZ
ØRP63KZ
ØRP64ØZ
ØRP643Z
ØRP644Z
ØRP647Z
ØRP64AZ
ØRP64KZ
ØRP9ØØZ
ØRP9Ø3Z
ØRP9Ø7Z
ØRP9ØKZ
ØRP937Z
ØRP93KZ
ØRP94ØZ
ØRP943Z
ØRP947Z
ØRP94KZ
ØRPAØØZ
ØRPAØ3Z
ØRPAØ4Z
ØRPAØ7Z
ØRPAØAZ
ØRPAØKZ
ØRPA34Z
ØRPA37Z
ØRPA3AZ
ØRPA3KZ
ØRPA4ØZ
ØRPA43Z
ØRPA44Z
ØRPA47Z
ØRPA4AZ
ØRPA4KZ
ØRPBØØZ
ØRPBØ3Z
ØRPBØ7Z
ØRPBØKZ
ØRPB37Z
ØRPB3KZ
ØRPB4ØZ
ØRPB43Z
ØRPB47Z
ØRPB4KZ
ØRQØØZZ
ØRQØ3ZZ
ØRQØ4ZZ
ØRQ1ØZZ
ØRQ13ZZ
ØRQ14ZZ
ØRQ33ZZ
ØRQ34ZZ
ØRQ4ØZZ
ØRQ43ZZ
ØRQ44ZZ
ØRQ5ØZZ
ØRQ53ZZ
ØRQ54ZZ
ØRQ6ØZZ
ØRQ63ZZ
ØRQ64ZZ
ØRQ93ZZ
ØRQ94ZZ
ØRQAØZZ
ØRQA3ZZ
ØRQA4ZZ
ØRQB3ZZ
ØRQB4ZZ
ØRQCØZZ
ØRQC3ZZ
ØRQC4ZZ
ØRQDØZZ
ØRQD3ZZ
ØRQD4ZZ
ØRRØØ7Z
ØRRØØJZ
ØRRØØKZ
ØRR1Ø7Z
ØRR1ØJZ
ØRR1ØKZ
ØRR3Ø7Z
ØRR3ØKZ
ØRR4Ø7Z
ØRR4ØJZ
ØRR4ØKZ
ØRR5Ø7Z
ØRR5ØKZ
ØRR6Ø7Z
ØRR6ØJZ
ØRR6ØKZ
ØRR9Ø7Z
ØRR9ØKZ
ØRRAØ7Z
ØRRAØJZ
ØRRAØKZ
ØRRBØ7Z
ØRRBØKZ
ØRRC*
ØRRD*
ØRSØØ4Z
ØRSØØZZ
ØRS1Ø4Z
ØRS1ØZZ
ØRS4Ø4Z
ØRS4ØZZ
ØRS6Ø4Z
ØRS6ØZZ
ØRSAØ4Z
ØRSAØZZ
ØRSCØ4Z
ØRSCØZZ
ØRSDØ4Z
ØRSDØZZ
ØRTCØZZ
ØRTDØZZ
ØRUØØ7Z
ØRUØØKZ
ØRUØ37Z
ØRUØ3KZ
ØRUØ47Z
ØRUØ4KZ
ØRU1Ø7Z
ØRU1ØKZ
ØRU137Z
ØRU13KZ
ØRU147Z
ØRU14KZ
ØRU4Ø7Z
ØRU4ØKZ
ØRU437Z
ØRU43KZ
ØRU447Z
ØRU44KZ
ØRU5Ø7Z
ØRU5ØKZ
ØRU537Z
ØRU53KZ
ØRU547Z
ØRU54KZ
ØRU6Ø7Z
ØRU6ØKZ
ØRU637Z
ØRU63KZ
ØRU647Z
ØRU64KZ
ØRUAØ7Z
ØRUAØKZ
ØRUA37Z
ØRUA3KZ
ØRUA47Z
ØRUA4KZ
ØRUC*
ØRUD*
ØRWØØØZ
ØRWØØ3Z
ØRWØØ4Z
ØRWØØ7Z
ØRWØØ8Z
ØRWØØAZ
ØRWØØJZ
ØRWØØKZ
ØRWØ3ØZ
ØRWØ33Z
ØRWØ34Z
ØRWØ37Z
ØRWØ38Z
ØRWØ3AZ
ØRWØ3JZ
ØRWØ3KZ
ØRWØ4ØZ
ØRWØ43Z
ØRWØ44Z
ØRWØ47Z
ØRWØ48Z
ØRWØ4AZ
ØRWØ4JZ
ØRWØ4KZ
ØRW1ØØZ
ØRW1Ø3Z
ØRW1Ø4Z
ØRW1Ø7Z
ØRW1Ø8Z
ØRW1ØAZ
ØRW1ØJZ
ØRW1ØKZ
ØRW13ØZ
ØRW133Z
ØRW134Z
ØRW137Z
ØRW138Z
ØRW13AZ
ØRW13JZ
ØRW13KZ
ØRW14ØZ
ØRW143Z
ØRW144Z
ØRW147Z
ØRW148Z
ØRW14AZ
ØRW14JZ
ØRW14KZ
ØRW3ØØZ
ØRW3Ø3Z
ØRW3Ø7Z
ØRW3ØKZ
ØRW33ØZ
ØRW333Z
ØRW337Z
ØRW33KZ
ØRW34ØZ
ØRW343Z
ØRW347Z
ØRW34KZ
ØRW4ØØZ
ØRW4Ø3Z
ØRW4Ø4Z
ØRW4Ø7Z
ØRW4Ø8Z
ØRW4ØAZ
ØRW4ØJZ
ØRW4ØKZ
ØRW43ØZ
ØRW433Z
ØRW434Z
ØRW437Z
ØRW438Z
ØRW43AZ
ØRW43JZ
ØRW43KZ
ØRW44ØZ
ØRW443Z
ØRW444Z
ØRW447Z
ØRW448Z
ØRW44AZ
ØRW44JZ
ØRW44KZ
ØRW5ØØZ
ØRW5Ø3Z
ØRW5Ø7Z
ØRW5ØKZ
ØRW53ØZ
ØRW533Z
ØRW537Z
ØRW53KZ
ØRW54ØZ
ØRW543Z
ØRW547Z
ØRW54KZ
ØRW6ØØZ
ØRW6Ø3Z
ØRW6Ø4Z
ØRW6Ø7Z
ØRW6Ø8Z
ØRW6ØAZ
ØRW6ØJZ
ØRW6ØKZ
ØRW63ØZ
ØRW633Z
ØRW634Z
ØRW637Z
ØRW638Z
ØRW63AZ
ØRW63JZ
ØRW63KZ
ØRW64ØZ
ØRW643Z
ØRW644Z
ØRW647Z
ØRW648Z
ØRW64AZ
ØRW64JZ
ØRW64KZ
ØRW9ØØZ
ØRW9Ø3Z
ØRW9Ø7Z
ØRW9ØKZ
ØRW93ØZ
ØRW933Z
ØRW937Z
ØRW93KZ
ØRW94ØZ
ØRW943Z
ØRW947Z
ØRW94KZ
ØRWAØØZ
ØRWAØ3Z
ØRWAØ4Z
ØRWAØ7Z
ØRWAØ8Z
ØRWAØAZ
ØRWAØJZ
ØRWAØKZ
ØRWA3ØZ
ØRWA33Z
ØRWA34Z
ØRWA37Z
ØRWA38Z
ØRWA3AZ
ØRWA3JZ
ØRWA3KZ
ØRWA4ØZ
ØRWA43Z
ØRWA44Z
ØRWA47Z
ØRWA48Z
ØRWA4AZ
ØRWA4JZ
ØRWA4KZ
ØRWBØØZ
ØRWBØ3Z
ØRWBØ7Z
ØRWBØKZ
ØRWB3ØZ
ØRWB33Z
ØRWB37Z
ØRWB3KZ
ØRWB4ØZ
ØRWB43Z
ØRWB47Z
ØRWB4KZ
ØRWGØJZ
ØRWG3JZ
ØRWG4JZ
ØRWHØJZ
ØRWH3JZ
ØRWH4JZ
ØRWJØJ6
ØRWJØJ7
ØRWJØJZ
ØRWJ3J6
ØRWJ3J7
ØRWJ3JZ
ØRWJ4J6
ØRWJ4J7
ØRWJ4JZ
ØRWKØJ6
ØRWKØJ7
ØRWKØJZ
ØRWK3J6
ØRWK3J7
ØRWK3JZ
ØRWK4J6
ØRWK4J7
ØRWK4JZ

ØRWLØJZ
ØRWL3JZ
ØRWL4JZ
ØRWMØJZ
ØRWM3JZ
ØRWM4JZ
ØRWNØJZ
ØRWN3JZ
ØRWN4JZ
ØRWPØJZ
ØRWP3JZ
ØRWP4JZ
ØRWQØJZ
ØRWQ3JZ
ØRWQ4JZ
ØRWRØJZ
ØRWR3JZ
ØRWR4JZ
ØRWSØJZ
ØRWS3JZ
ØRWS4JZ
ØRWTØJZ
ØRWT3JZ
ØRWT4JZ
ØRWUØJZ
ØRWU3JZ
ØRWU4JZ
ØRWVØJZ
ØRWV3JZ
ØRWV4JZ
ØRWWØJZ
ØRWW3JZ
ØRWW4JZ
ØRWXØJZ
ØRWX3JZ
ØRWX4JZ
ØS9ØØØZ
ØS9ØØZZ
ØS92ØØZ
ØS92ØZZ
ØS93ØØZ
ØS93ØZZ
ØS94ØØZ
ØS94ØZZ
ØS95ØØZ
ØS95ØZZ
ØS96ØØZ
ØS96ØZZ
ØS97ØØZ
ØS97ØZZ
ØS98ØØZ
ØS98ØZZ
ØSCØ*
ØSC2*
ØSC3*
ØSC4*
ØSC5*
ØSC6*
ØSC7*
ØSC8*
ØSHØØ4Z
ØSHØ34Z
ØSHØ44Z
ØSH3Ø4Z
ØSH334Z
ØSH344Z
ØSH5Ø4Z
ØSH534Z
ØSH544Z
ØSH6Ø4Z
ØSH634Z
ØSH644Z
ØSH7Ø4Z
ØSH734Z
ØSH744Z
ØSH8Ø4Z
ØSH834Z
ØSH844Z
ØSJØØZZ
ØSJ2ØZZ
ØSJ3ØZZ
ØSJ4ØZZ
ØSJ5ØZZ
ØSJ6ØZZ
ØSJ7ØZZ
ØSJ8ØZZ
ØSPØØØZ
ØSPØØ3Z
ØSPØØ4Z
ØSPØØ7Z
ØSPØØAZ
ØSPØØKZ
ØSPØ34Z
ØSPØ37Z
ØSPØ3AZ
ØSPØ3KZ
ØSPØ4ØZ
ØSPØ43Z
ØSPØ44Z
ØSPØ47Z
ØSPØ4AZ
ØSPØ4KZ
ØSP2ØØZ
ØSP2Ø3Z
ØSP2Ø7Z
ØSP2ØKZ
ØSP237Z
ØSP23KZ
ØSP24ØZ
ØSP243Z
ØSP247Z
ØSP24KZ
ØSP3ØØZ
ØSP3Ø3Z
ØSP3Ø4Z
ØSP3Ø7Z
ØSP3ØAZ
ØSP3ØKZ
ØSP334Z
ØSP337Z
ØSP33AZ
ØSP33KZ
ØSP34ØZ
ØSP343Z
ØSP344Z
ØSP347Z
ØSP34AZ
ØSP34KZ
ØSP4ØØZ
ØSP4Ø3Z
ØSP4Ø7Z
ØSP4ØKZ
ØSP437Z
ØSP43KZ
ØSP44ØZ
ØSP443Z
ØSP447Z
ØSP44KZ
ØSP5ØØZ
ØSP5Ø3Z
ØSP5Ø4Z
ØSP5Ø7Z
ØSP5ØKZ
ØSP534Z
ØSP537Z
ØSP53KZ
ØSP54ØZ
ØSP543Z
ØSP544Z
ØSP547Z
ØSP54KZ
ØSP6ØØZ
ØSP6Ø3Z
ØSP6Ø4Z
ØSP6Ø7Z
ØSP6ØKZ
ØSP634Z
ØSP637Z
ØSP63KZ
ØSP64ØZ
ØSP643Z
ØSP644Z
ØSP647Z
ØSP64KZ
ØSP7ØØZ
ØSP7Ø3Z
ØSP7Ø4Z
ØSP7Ø7Z
ØSP7ØKZ
ØSP734Z
ØSP737Z
ØSP73KZ
ØSP74ØZ
ØSP743Z
ØSP744Z
ØSP747Z
ØSP74KZ
ØSP8ØØZ
ØSP8Ø3Z
ØSP8Ø4Z
ØSP8Ø7Z
ØSP8ØKZ
ØSP834Z
ØSP837Z
ØSP83KZ
ØSP84ØZ
ØSP843Z
ØSP844Z
ØSP847Z
ØSP84KZ
ØSQØØZZ
ØSQØ3ZZ
ØSQØ4ZZ
ØSQ23ZZ
ØSQ24ZZ
ØSQ3ØZZ
ØSQ33ZZ
ØSQ34ZZ
ØSQ43ZZ
ØSQ44ZZ
ØSQ5ØZZ
ØSQ53ZZ
ØSQ54ZZ
ØSQ6ØZZ
ØSQ63ZZ
ØSQ64ZZ
ØSQ7ØZZ
ØSQ73ZZ
ØSQ74ZZ
ØSQ8ØZZ
ØSQ83ZZ
ØSQ84ZZ
ØSQHØZZ
ØSQH3ZZ
ØSQH4ZZ
ØSQJØZZ
ØSQJ3ZZ
ØSQJ4ZZ
ØSQKØZZ
ØSQK3ZZ
ØSQK4ZZ
ØSQLØZZ
ØSQL3ZZ
ØSQL4ZZ
ØSQMØZZ
ØSQM3ZZ
ØSQM4ZZ
ØSQNØZZ
ØSQN3ZZ
ØSQN4ZZ
ØSQPØZZ
ØSQP3ZZ
ØSQP4ZZ
ØSQQØZZ
ØSQQ3ZZ
ØSQQ4ZZ
ØSRØØ7Z
ØSRØØJZ
ØSRØØKZ
ØSR2Ø7Z
ØSR2ØKZ
ØSR3Ø7Z
ØSR3ØJZ
ØSR3ØKZ
ØSR4Ø7Z
ØSR4ØKZ
ØSR5*
ØSR6*
ØSR7*
ØSR8*
ØSSØØ4Z
ØSSØØZZ
ØSS3Ø4Z
ØSS3ØZZ
ØSS5Ø4Z
ØSS5ØZZ
ØSS6Ø4Z
ØSS6ØZZ
ØSS7Ø4Z
ØSS7ØZZ
ØSS734Z
ØSS8Ø4Z
ØSS8ØZZ
ØSS834Z
ØST5ØZZ
ØST6ØZZ
ØST7ØZZ
ØST8ØZZ
ØSUØØ7Z
ØSUØØKZ
ØSUØ37Z
ØSUØ3KZ
ØSUØ47Z
ØSUØ4KZ
ØSU3Ø7Z
ØSU3ØKZ
ØSU337Z
ØSU33KZ
ØSU347Z
ØSU34KZ
ØSU5Ø7Z
ØSU5ØKZ
ØSU537Z
ØSU53KZ
ØSU547Z
ØSU54KZ
ØSU6Ø7Z
ØSU6ØKZ
ØSU637Z
ØSU63KZ
ØSU647Z
ØSU64KZ
ØSU7*
ØSU8*
ØSU9Ø7Z
ØSU9Ø9Z
ØSU9ØJZ
ØSU9ØKZ
ØSU937Z
ØSU93JZ
ØSU93KZ
ØSU947Z
ØSU94JZ
ØSU94KZ
ØSUAØ9Z
ØSUBØ7Z
ØSUBØ9Z
ØSUBØJZ
ØSUBØKZ
ØSUB37Z
ØSUB3JZ
ØSUB3KZ
ØSUB47Z
ØSUB4JZ
ØSUB4KZ
ØSUC*
ØSUD*
ØSUEØ9Z
ØSUF*
ØSUG*
ØSUH*
ØSUJ*
ØSUK*
ØSUL*
ØSUM*
ØSUN*
ØSUP*
ØSUQ*
ØSURØ9Z
ØSUSØ9Z
ØSUTØ9Z
ØSUUØ9Z
ØSUVØ9Z
ØSUWØ9Z
ØSWØØØZ
ØSWØØ3Z
ØSWØØ4Z
ØSWØØ7Z
ØSWØØ8Z
ØSWØØAZ
ØSWØØJZ
ØSWØØKZ
ØSWØ3ØZ
ØSWØ33Z
ØSWØ34Z
ØSWØ37Z
ØSWØ38Z
ØSWØ3AZ
ØSWØ3JZ
ØSWØ3KZ
ØSWØ4ØZ
ØSWØ43Z
ØSWØ44Z
ØSWØ47Z
ØSWØ48Z
ØSWØ4AZ
ØSWØ4JZ
ØSWØ4KZ
ØSW2ØØZ
ØSW2Ø3Z
ØSW2Ø7Z
ØSW2ØKZ
ØSW23ØZ
ØSW233Z
ØSW237Z
ØSW23KZ
ØSW24ØZ
ØSW243Z
ØSW247Z
ØSW24KZ
ØSW3ØØZ
ØSW3Ø3Z
ØSW3Ø4Z
ØSW3Ø7Z
ØSW3Ø8Z
ØSW3ØAZ
ØSW3ØJZ
ØSW3ØKZ
ØSW33ØZ
ØSW333Z
ØSW334Z
ØSW337Z
ØSW338Z
ØSW33AZ
ØSW33JZ
ØSW33KZ
ØSW34ØZ
ØSW343Z
ØSW344Z
ØSW347Z
ØSW348Z
ØSW34AZ
ØSW34JZ
ØSW34KZ
ØSW4ØØZ
ØSW4Ø3Z
ØSW4Ø7Z
ØSW4ØKZ
ØSW43ØZ
ØSW433Z
ØSW437Z
ØSW43KZ
ØSW44ØZ
ØSW443Z
ØSW447Z
ØSW44KZ
ØSW5ØØZ
ØSW5Ø3Z
ØSW5Ø4Z
ØSW5Ø7Z
ØSW5Ø8Z
ØSW5ØJZ
ØSW5ØKZ
ØSW53ØZ
ØSW533Z
ØSW534Z
ØSW537Z
ØSW538Z
ØSW53JZ
ØSW53KZ
ØSW54ØZ
ØSW543Z
ØSW544Z
ØSW547Z
ØSW548Z
ØSW54JZ
ØSW54KZ
ØSW6ØØZ
ØSW6Ø3Z
ØSW6Ø4Z
ØSW6Ø7Z
ØSW6Ø8Z
ØSW6ØJZ
ØSW6ØKZ
ØSW63ØZ
ØSW633Z
ØSW634Z
ØSW637Z
ØSW638Z
ØSW63JZ
ØSW63KZ
ØSW64ØZ
ØSW643Z
ØSW644Z
ØSW647Z
ØSW648Z
ØSW64JZ
ØSW64KZ
ØSW7ØØZ
ØSW7Ø3Z
ØSW7Ø4Z
ØSW7Ø7Z
ØSW7Ø8Z
ØSW7ØJZ
ØSW7ØKZ
ØSW73ØZ
ØSW733Z
ØSW734Z
ØSW737Z
ØSW738Z
ØSW73JZ
ØSW73KZ
ØSW74ØZ
ØSW743Z
ØSW744Z
ØSW747Z
ØSW748Z
ØSW74JZ
ØSW74KZ
ØSW8ØØZ
ØSW8Ø3Z
ØSW8Ø4Z
ØSW8Ø7Z
ØSW8Ø8Z
ØSW8ØJZ
ØSW8ØKZ
ØSW83ØZ
ØSW833Z
ØSW834Z
ØSW837Z
ØSW838Z
ØSW83JZ
ØSW83KZ
ØSW84ØZ
ØSW843Z
ØSW844Z
ØSW847Z
ØSW848Z
ØSW84JZ
ØSW84KZ
ØSWFØJZ
ØSWF3JZ
ØSWF4JZ
ØSWGØJZ
ØSWG3JZ
ØSWG4JZ
ØSWHØJZ
ØSWH3JZ
ØSWH4JZ
ØSWJØJZ
ØSWJ3JZ
ØSWJ4JZ
ØSWKØJZ
ØSWK3JZ
ØSWK4JZ
ØSWLØJZ
ØSWL3JZ
ØSWL4JZ
ØSWMØJZ
ØSWM3JZ
ØSWM4JZ
ØSWNØJZ
ØSWN3JZ
ØSWN4JZ
ØSWPØJZ
ØSWP3JZ
ØSWP4JZ
ØSWQØJZ
ØSWQ3JZ
ØSWQ4JZ
ØT9ØØZX
ØT91ØZX
ØT93ØZX
ØT94ØZX
ØTBØØZX
ØTB1ØZX
ØTB3ØZX
ØTB4ØZX
ØVTC*
ØWØ4*
ØWØ5*
ØW38*
ØW3F*
ØW3K*
ØW3L*
ØWBHØZZ
ØWBH3ZZ
ØWBH4ZZ
ØWJ64ZZ
ØWM8ØZZ
ØWQ8*
ØWU4*
ØWU5*
ØWU8Ø7Z
ØWU8ØJZ
ØWU8ØKZ
ØWU84JZ
ØX3*
ØY3*
ØYM2ØZZ
ØYM3ØZZ
ØYM4ØZZ
ØYM5ØZZ
ØYM6ØZZ
ØYM9ØZZ
ØYMBØZZ
XØHK3Q8
XØHQ3R8
X27H385
X27H395
X27H3B5
X27H3C5
X27J385
X27J395
X27J3B5
X27J3C5
X2H13R9
XKUCØ68
XKUDØ68
XNH6Ø58
XNH6358
XNH7Ø58
XNH7358
XNR8ØD9
XNUØ356
XNU4356
OR
ØQSS3ZZ
AND
ØQUS3JZ
OR
ØPS33ZZ
AND
ØPU33JZ
OR
ØPS43ZZ
AND
ØPU43JZ
OR
ØQSØ3ZZ
AND
ØQUØ3JZ
OR
ØQS13ZZ
AND
ØQU13JZ

DRG 516

Select operating room procedures or procedure combinations listed under DRG 515

DRG 517

Select operating room procedures or procedure combinations listed under DRG 515

DRG 518

Back and neck except disc devices operating room procedures

ØØ5TØZZ
ØØ5T3ZZ
ØØ5T4ZZ
ØØ5WØZ3
ØØ5WØZZ
ØØ5W3Z3
ØØ5W3ZZ
ØØ5W4Z3
ØØ5W4ZZ
ØØ5XØZ3
ØØ5XØZZ
ØØ5X3Z3
ØØ5X3ZZ
ØØ5X4Z3
ØØ5X4ZZ
ØØ5YØZ3
ØØ5YØZZ
ØØ5Y3Z3
ØØ5Y3ZZ
ØØ5Y4Z3
ØØ5Y4ZZ
ØØ9TØØZ
ØØ9TØZX
ØØ9TØZZ
ØØ9T4ØZ
ØØ9T4ZX
ØØ9T4ZZ
ØØ9UØØZ
ØØ9UØZX
ØØ9UØZZ
ØØ9WØØZ
ØØ9WØZX
ØØ9WØZZ
ØØ9W4ØZ
ØØ9W4ZX
ØØ9W4ZZ
ØØ9XØØZ
ØØ9XØZX
ØØ9XØZZ
ØØ9X4ØZ
ØØ9X4ZX
ØØ9X4ZZ
ØØ9YØØZ
ØØ9YØZX
ØØ9YØZZ
ØØ9Y4ØZ
ØØ9Y4ZX
ØØ9Y4ZZ
ØØBTØZX
ØØBTØZZ
ØØBT3ZX
ØØBT3ZZ
ØØBT4ZX
ØØBT4ZZ
ØØBWØZX
ØØBWØZZ
ØØBW3ZX
ØØBW3ZZ
ØØBW4ZX
ØØBW4ZZ
ØØBXØZX
ØØBXØZZ
ØØBX3ZX
ØØBX3ZZ
ØØBX4ZX
ØØBX4ZZ
ØØBYØZX
ØØBYØZZ
ØØBY3ZX
ØØBY3ZZ
ØØBY4ZX
ØØBY4ZZ
ØØDTØZZ
ØØDT3ZZ
ØØDT4ZZ
ØØFUØZZ
ØØFU3ZZ
ØØFU4ZZ
ØØFUXZZ
ØØHUØ1Z
ØØHUØ2Z
ØØHUØMZ
ØØHUØYZ
ØØHU31Z
ØØHU3MZ
ØØHU41Z
ØØHU42Z
ØØHU4MZ
ØØHVØ1Z
ØØHVØ2Z
ØØHVØMZ
ØØHVØYZ
ØØHV31Z
ØØHV3MZ
ØØHV3YZ
ØØHV41Z
ØØHV42Z
ØØHV4MZ
ØØHV4YZ
ØØJUØZZ
ØØJU4ZZ
ØØJVØZZ
ØØJV4ZZ
ØØNTØZZ
ØØNT3ZZ
ØØNT4ZZ
ØØNWØZZ
ØØNW3ZZ
ØØNW4ZZ
ØØNXØZZ
ØØNX3ZZ
ØØNX4ZZ
ØØNYØZZ
ØØNY3ZZ
ØØNY4ZZ
ØØPUØØZ
ØØPUØ2Z
ØØPUØ3Z
ØØPUØJZ
ØØPUØMZ
ØØPUØYZ
ØØPU3JZ
ØØPU3MZ
ØØPU4ØZ
ØØPU42Z
ØØPU43Z
ØØPU4JZ
ØØPU4MZ
ØØPVØMZ
ØØPV3MZ
ØØPV4MZ
ØØQTØZZ
ØØQT3ZZ
ØØQT4ZZ
ØØQWØZZ
ØØQW3ZZ
ØØQW4ZZ
ØØQXØZZ
ØØQX3ZZ
ØØQX4ZZ
ØØQYØZZ
ØØQY3ZZ
ØØQY4ZZ
ØØRTØ7Z
ØØRTØJZ
ØØRTØKZ
ØØRT47Z
ØØRT4JZ
ØØRT4KZ
ØØSWØZZ
ØØSW3ZZ
ØØSW4ZZ
ØØSXØZZ
ØØSX3ZZ
ØØSX4ZZ
ØØSYØZZ
ØØSY3ZZ
ØØSY4ZZ
ØØUTØ7Z
ØØUTØJZ
ØØUTØKZ
ØØUT37Z
ØØUT3JZ
ØØUT3KZ
ØØUT47Z
ØØUT4JZ
ØØUT4KZ
ØØWUØØZ
ØØWUØ2Z
ØØWUØ3Z
ØØWUØJZ
ØØWUØMZ
ØØWUØYZ
ØØWU3ØZ
ØØWU32Z
ØØWU33Z
ØØWU3JZ
ØØWU3MZ
ØØWU4ØZ
ØØWU42Z
ØØWU43Z
ØØWU4JZ
ØØWU4MZ
Ø151ØZZ
Ø1514ZZ
Ø158ØZZ
Ø1584ZZ
Ø15BØZZ
Ø15B4ZZ
Ø15RØZZ
Ø15R4ZZ
Ø181ØZZ
Ø1813ZZ
Ø1814ZZ
Ø188ØZZ
Ø1883ZZ
Ø1884ZZ
Ø18BØZZ
Ø18B3ZZ
Ø18B4ZZ
Ø18RØZZ
Ø18R3ZZ
Ø18R4ZZ
ØPS3Ø4Z
ØPS3ØZZ
ØPS334Z
ØPS344Z
ØPS34ZZ
ØPS4Ø3Z
ØPS4Ø4Z
ØPS4ØZZ
ØPS434Z
ØPS443Z
ØPS444Z
ØPS44ZZ
ØQSØØ3Z
ØQSØØ4Z
ØQSØØZZ
ØQSØ34Z
ØQSØ43Z
ØQSØ44Z
ØQSØ4ZZ
ØQS1Ø4Z
ØQS1ØZZ
ØQS134Z
ØQS144Z
ØQS14ZZ
ØQSSØ4Z
ØQSSØZZ
ØQSS34Z
ØQSS3ZZ
ØQSS44Z
ØQSS4ZZ
ØR53ØZZ
ØR55ØZZ
ØR59ØZZ
ØR5BØZZ
ØRBØØZZ

ØRBØ3ZZ
ØRBØ4ZZ
ØRB1ØZZ
ØRB13ZZ
ØRB14ZZ
ØRB3ØZZ
ØRB33ZZ
ØRB34ZZ
ØRB4ØZZ
ØRB43ZZ
ØRB44ZZ
ØRB5ØZZ
ØRB53ZZ
ØRB54ZZ
ØRB6ØZZ
ØRB63ZZ
ØRB64ZZ
ØRB9ØZZ
ØRB93ZZ
ØRB94ZZ
ØRBAØZZ
ØRBA3ZZ
ØRBA4ZZ
ØRBBØZZ
ØRBB3ZZ
ØRBB4ZZ
ØRQ3ØZZ
ØRQ9ØZZ
ØRQBØZZ
ØRR9ØJZ
ØRRBØJZ
ØRT3ØZZ
ØRT4ØZZ
ØRT5ØZZ
ØRT9ØZZ
ØRTBØZZ
ØRU3Ø7Z
ØRU3ØJZ
ØRU3ØKZ
ØRU337Z
ØRU33JZ
ØRU33KZ
ØRU347Z
ØRU34JZ
ØRU34KZ
ØRU9Ø7Z
ØRU9ØJZ
ØRU9ØKZ
ØRU937Z
ØRU93JZ
ØRU93KZ
ØRU947Z
ØRU94JZ
ØRU94KZ
ØRUBØ7Z
ØRUBØJZ
ØRUBØKZ
ØRUB37Z
ØRUB3JZ
ØRUB3KZ
ØRUB47Z
ØRUB4JZ
ØRUB4KZ
ØRW3ØJZ
ØRW33JZ
ØRW34JZ
ØRW5ØJZ
ØRW53JZ
ØRW54JZ
ØRW9ØJZ
ØRW93JZ
ØRW94JZ
ØRWBØJZ
ØRWB3JZ
ØRWB4JZ
ØS52ØZZ
ØS523ZZ
ØS524ZZ
ØS54ØZZ
ØS543ZZ
ØS544ZZ
ØSBØØZZ
ØSBØ3ZZ
ØSBØ4ZZ
ØSB2ØZZ
ØSB23ZZ
ØSB24ZZ
ØSB3ØZZ
ØSB33ZZ
ØSB34ZZ
ØSB4ØZZ
ØSB43ZZ
ØSB44ZZ
ØSB5ØZZ
ØSB53ZZ
ØSB54ZZ
ØSB6ØZZ
ØSB63ZZ
ØSB64ZZ
ØSB7ØZZ
ØSB73ZZ
ØSB74ZZ
ØSB8ØZZ
ØSB83ZZ
ØSB84ZZ
ØSQ2ØZZ
ØSQ4ØZZ
ØST2ØZZ
ØST4ØZZ
ØSU2Ø7Z
ØSU2ØJZ
ØSU2ØKZ
ØSU237Z
ØSU23JZ
ØSU23KZ
ØSU247Z
ØSU24JZ
ØSU24KZ
ØSU4Ø7Z
ØSU4ØJZ
ØSU4ØKZ
ØSU437Z
ØSU43JZ
ØSU43KZ
ØSU447Z
ØSU44JZ
ØSU44KZ
ØSW2ØJZ
ØSW23JZ
ØSW24JZ
ØSW4ØJZ
ØSW43JZ
ØSW44JZ
XNSØØ32
XNSØØC7
XNSØ332
XNSØ3C7
XNS3Ø32
XNS3332
XNS4Ø32
XNS4ØC7
XNS4332
XNS43C7

OR

Disc devices operating room procedures

ØRHØØBZ
ØRHØØCZ
ØRHØØDZ
ØRHØ3BZ
ØRHØ3CZ
ØRHØ3DZ
ØRHØ4BZ
ØRHØ4CZ
ØRHØ4DZ
ØRH1ØBZ
ØRH1ØCZ
ØRH1ØDZ
ØRH13BZ
ØRH13CZ
ØRH13DZ
ØRH14BZ
ØRH14CZ
ØRH14DZ
ØRH4ØBZ
ØRH4ØCZ
ØRH4ØDZ
ØRH43BZ
ØRH43CZ
ØRH43DZ
ØRH44BZ
ØRH44CZ
ØRH44DZ
ØRH6ØBZ
ØRH6ØCZ
ØRH6ØDZ
ØRH63BZ
ØRH63CZ
ØRH63DZ
ØRH64BZ
ØRH64CZ
ØRH64DZ
ØRHAØBZ
ØRHAØCZ
ØRHAØDZ
ØRHA3BZ
ØRHA3CZ
ØRHA3DZ
ØRHA4BZ
ØRHA4CZ
ØRHA4DZ
ØRR3ØJZ
ØRR5ØJZ
ØRUØØJZ
ØRUØ3JZ
ØRUØ4JZ
ØRU1ØJZ
ØRU13JZ
ØRU14JZ
ØRU4ØJZ
ØRU43JZ
ØRU44JZ
ØRU5ØJZ
ØRU53JZ
ØRU54JZ
ØRU6ØJZ
ØRU63JZ
ØRU64JZ
ØRUAØJZ
ØRUA3JZ
ØRUA4JZ
ØSHØØBZ
ØSHØØCZ
ØSHØØDZ
ØSHØ3BZ
ØSHØ3CZ
ØSHØ3DZ
ØSHØ4BZ
ØSHØ4CZ
ØSHØ4DZ
ØSH3ØBZ
ØSH3ØCZ
ØSH3ØDZ
ØSH33BZ
ØSH33CZ
ØSH33DZ
ØSH34BZ
ØSH34CZ
ØSH34DZ
ØSR2ØJZ
ØSR4ØJZ
ØSUØØJZ
ØSUØ3JZ
ØSUØ4JZ
ØSU3ØJZ
ØSU33JZ
ØSU34JZ
ØSU5ØJZ
ØSU53JZ
ØSU54JZ
ØSU6ØJZ
ØSU63JZ
ØSU64JZ
XRHBØ18
XRHDØ18

OR

The following neurostimulator device procedure combinations

ØØHUØMZ
ØØHU3MZ
ØØHU4MZ
ØØHVØMZ
ØØHV3MZ
ØØHV4MZ

AND

ØJH6ØBZ
ØJH6ØCZ
ØJH6ØDZ
ØJH6ØEZ
ØJH63BZ
ØJH63CZ
ØJH63DZ
ØJH63EZ
ØJH7ØBZ
ØJH7ØCZ
ØJH7ØDZ
ØJH7ØEZ
ØJH73BZ
ØJH73CZ
ØJH73DZ
ØJH73EZ
ØJH8ØBZ
ØJH8ØCZ
ØJH8ØDZ
ØJH8ØEZ
ØJH83BZ
ØJH83CZ
ØJH83DZ
ØJH83EZ

DRG 519

Select back and neck except disc devices operating room procedures listed under DRG 518

DRG 520

Select back and neck except disc devices operating room procedures listed under DRG 518

DRG 521

Principal Diagnosis

M8Ø.Ø51A
M8Ø.Ø51G
M8Ø.Ø51K
M8Ø.Ø51P
M8Ø.Ø52A
M8Ø.Ø52G
M8Ø.Ø52K
M8Ø.Ø52P
M8Ø.Ø59A
M8Ø.Ø59G
M8Ø.Ø59K
M8Ø.Ø59P
M8Ø.ØAXA
M8Ø.ØAXD
M8Ø.ØAXG
M8Ø.ØAXK
M8Ø.ØAXP
M8Ø.ØB1A
M8Ø.ØB1D
M8Ø.ØB1G
M8Ø.ØB1K
M8Ø.ØB1P
M8Ø.ØB2A
M8Ø.ØB2D
M8Ø.ØB2G
M8Ø.ØB2K
M8Ø.ØB2P
M8Ø.ØB9A
M8Ø.ØB9D
M8Ø.ØB9G
M8Ø.ØB9K
M8Ø.ØB9P
M8Ø.851A
M8Ø.851G
M8Ø.851K
M8Ø.851P
M8Ø.852A
M8Ø.852G
M8Ø.852K
M8Ø.852P
M8Ø.859A
M8Ø.859G
M8Ø.859K
M8Ø.859P
M8Ø.8AXA
M8Ø.8AXD
M8Ø.8AXG
M8Ø.8AXK
M8Ø.8AXP
M8Ø.8B1A
M8Ø.8B1D
M8Ø.8B1G
M8Ø.8B1K
M8Ø.8B1P
M8Ø.8B2A
M8Ø.8B2D
M8Ø.8B2G
M8Ø.8B2K
M8Ø.8B2P
M8Ø.8B9A
M8Ø.8B9D
M8Ø.8B9G
M8Ø.8B9K
M8Ø.8B9P
M84.351A
M84.351K
M84.351P
M84.352A
M84.352K
M84.352P
M84.353A
M84.353K
M84.353P
M84.359A
M84.359K
M84.359P
M84.451A
M84.451K
M84.451P
M84.452A
M84.452K
M84.452P
M84.453A
M84.453K
M84.453P
M84.459A
M84.459K
M84.459P
M84.551A
M84.551K
M84.551P
M84.552A
M84.552K
M84.552P
M84.553A
M84.553K
M84.553P
M84.559A
M84.559K
M84.559P
M84.651A
M84.651K
M84.651P
M84.652A
M84.652K
M84.652P
M84.653A
M84.653K
M84.653P
M84.659A
M84.659K
M84.659P
M84.75ØA
M84.75ØG
M84.75ØK
M84.75ØP
M84.751A
M84.751G
M84.751K
M84.751P
M84.752A
M84.752G
M84.752K
M84.752P
M84.753A
M84.753G
M84.753K
M84.753P
M84.754A
M84.754G
M84.754K
M84.754P
M84.755A
M84.755G
M84.755K
M84.755P
M84.756A
M84.756G
M84.756K
M84.756P
M84.757A
M84.757G
M84.757K
M84.757P
M84.758A
M84.758G
M84.758K
M84.758P
M84.759A
M84.759G
M84.759K
M84.759P
S32.4Ø1A
S32.4Ø1B
S32.4Ø1G
S32.4Ø1K
S32.4Ø2A
S32.4Ø2B
S32.4Ø2G
S32.4Ø2K
S32.4Ø9A
S32.4Ø9B
S32.4Ø9G
S32.4Ø9K
S32.411A
S32.411B
S32.411G
S32.411K
S32.412A
S32.412B
S32.412G
S32.412K
S32.413A
S32.413B
S32.413G
S32.413K
S32.414A
S32.414B
S32.414G
S32.414K
S32.415A
S32.415B
S32.415G
S32.415K
S32.416A
S32.416B
S32.416G
S32.416K
S32.421A
S32.421B
S32.421G
S32.421K
S32.422A
S32.422B
S32.422G
S32.422K
S32.423A
S32.423B
S32.423G
S32.423K
S32.424A
S32.424B
S32.424G
S32.424K
S32.425A
S32.425B
S32.425G
S32.425K
S32.426A
S32.426B
S32.426G
S32.426K
S32.431A
S32.431B
S32.431G
S32.431K
S32.432A
S32.432B
S32.432G
S32.432K
S32.433A
S32.433B
S32.433G
S32.433K
S32.434A
S32.434B
S32.434G
S32.434K
S32.435A
S32.435B
S32.435G
S32.435K
S32.436A
S32.436B
S32.436G
S32.436K
S32.441A
S32.441B
S32.441G
S32.441K
S32.442A
S32.442B
S32.442G
S32.442K
S32.443A
S32.443B
S32.443G
S32.443K
S32.444A
S32.444B
S32.444G
S32.444K
S32.445A
S32.445B
S32.445G
S32.445K
S32.446A
S32.446B
S32.446G
S32.446K
S32.451A
S32.451B
S32.451G
S32.451K
S32.452A
S32.452B
S32.452G
S32.452K
S32.453A
S32.453B
S32.453G
S32.453K
S32.454A
S32.454B
S32.454G
S32.454K
S32.455A
S32.455B
S32.455G
S32.455K
S32.456A
S32.456B
S32.456G
S32.456K
S32.461A
S32.461B
S32.461G
S32.461K
S32.462A
S32.462B
S32.462G
S32.462K
S32.463A
S32.463B
S32.463G
S32.463K
S32.464A
S32.464B
S32.464G
S32.464K
S32.465A
S32.465B
S32.465G
S32.465K
S32.466A
S32.466B
S32.466G
S32.466K
S32.471A
S32.471B
S32.471G
S32.471K
S32.472A
S32.472B
S32.472G
S32.472K
S32.473A
S32.473B
S32.473G
S32.473K
S32.474A
S32.474B
S32.474G
S32.474K
S32.475A
S32.475B
S32.475G
S32.475K
S32.476A
S32.476B
S32.476G
S32.476K
S32.481A
S32.481B
S32.481G
S32.481K
S32.482A
S32.482B
S32.482G
S32.482K
S32.483A
S32.483B
S32.483G
S32.483K
S32.484A
S32.484B
S32.484G
S32.484K
S32.485A
S32.485B
S32.485G
S32.485K
S32.486A
S32.486B
S32.486G
S32.486K
S32.491A
S32.491B
S32.491G
S32.491K
S32.492A
S32.492B
S32.492G
S32.492K
S32.499A
S32.499B
S32.499G
S32.499K
S72.ØØ1A
S72.ØØ1B
S72.ØØ1C
S72.ØØ1G
S72.ØØ1H
S72.ØØ1J
S72.ØØ1K
S72.ØØ1M
S72.ØØ1N
S72.ØØ1P
S72.ØØ1Q
S72.ØØ1R
S72.ØØ2A
S72.ØØ2B
S72.ØØ2C
S72.ØØ2G
S72.ØØ2H
S72.ØØ2J
S72.ØØ2K
S72.ØØ2M
S72.ØØ2N
S72.ØØ2P
S72.ØØ2Q
S72.ØØ2R
S72.ØØ9A
S72.ØØ9B
S72.ØØ9C
S72.ØØ9G
S72.ØØ9H
S72.ØØ9J
S72.ØØ9K
S72.ØØ9M
S72.ØØ9N
S72.ØØ9P
S72.ØØ9Q
S72.ØØ9R
S72.Ø11A
S72.Ø11B
S72.Ø11C
S72.Ø11G
S72.Ø11H
S72.Ø11J
S72.Ø11K
S72.Ø11M
S72.Ø11N
S72.Ø11P
S72.Ø11Q
S72.Ø11R
S72.Ø12A
S72.Ø12B
S72.Ø12C
S72.Ø12G
S72.Ø12H
S72.Ø12J
S72.Ø12K
S72.Ø12M
S72.Ø12N
S72.Ø12P
S72.Ø12Q
S72.Ø12R
S72.Ø19A
S72.Ø19B
S72.Ø19C
S72.Ø19G
S72.Ø19H
S72.Ø19J
S72.Ø19K
S72.Ø19M
S72.Ø19N
S72.Ø19P
S72.Ø19Q
S72.Ø19R
S72.Ø21A
S72.Ø21B
S72.Ø21C
S72.Ø21G
S72.Ø21H
S72.Ø21J
S72.Ø21K
S72.Ø21M
S72.Ø21N
S72.Ø21P
S72.Ø21Q
S72.Ø21R
S72.Ø22A
S72.Ø22B
S72.Ø22C
S72.Ø22G
S72.Ø22H
S72.Ø22J
S72.Ø22K
S72.Ø22M
S72.Ø22N
S72.Ø22P
S72.Ø22Q
S72.Ø22R
S72.Ø23A
S72.Ø23B
S72.Ø23C
S72.Ø23G
S72.Ø23H
S72.Ø23J
S72.Ø23K
S72.Ø23M
S72.Ø23N
S72.Ø23P
S72.Ø23Q
S72.Ø23R
S72.Ø24A
S72.Ø24B
S72.Ø24C
S72.Ø24G
S72.Ø24H
S72.Ø24J
S72.Ø24K
S72.Ø24M
S72.Ø24N
S72.Ø24P
S72.Ø24Q
S72.Ø24R
S72.Ø25A
S72.Ø25B
S72.Ø25C
S72.Ø25G
S72.Ø25H
S72.Ø25J
S72.Ø25K
S72.Ø25M
S72.Ø25N
S72.Ø25P
S72.Ø25Q
S72.Ø25R
S72.Ø26A
S72.Ø26B
S72.Ø26C
S72.Ø26G
S72.Ø26H
S72.Ø26J
S72.Ø26K
S72.Ø26M
S72.Ø26N
S72.Ø26P
S72.Ø26Q
S72.Ø26R
S72.Ø31A
S72.Ø31B
S72.Ø31C
S72.Ø31G
S72.Ø31H
S72.Ø31J
S72.Ø31K
S72.Ø31M
S72.Ø31N
S72.Ø31P
S72.Ø31Q
S72.Ø31R
S72.Ø32A
S72.Ø32B
S72.Ø32C
S72.Ø32G
S72.Ø32H
S72.Ø32J
S72.Ø32K
S72.Ø32M
S72.Ø32N
S72.Ø32P
S72.Ø32Q
S72.Ø32R
S72.Ø33A
S72.Ø33B
S72.Ø33C
S72.Ø33G
S72.Ø33H
S72.Ø33J
S72.Ø33K
S72.Ø33M
S72.Ø33N
S72.Ø33P
S72.Ø33Q
S72.Ø33R
S72.Ø34A
S72.Ø34B
S72.Ø34C
S72.Ø34G
S72.Ø34H

S72.Ø34J
S72.Ø34K
S72.Ø34M
S72.Ø34N
S72.Ø34P
S72.Ø34Q
S72.Ø34R
S72.Ø35A
S72.Ø35B
S72.Ø35C
S72.Ø35G
S72.Ø35H
S72.Ø35J
S72.Ø35K
S72.Ø35M
S72.Ø35N
S72.Ø35P
S72.Ø35Q
S72.Ø35R
S72.Ø36A
S72.Ø36B
S72.Ø36C
S72.Ø36G
S72.Ø36H
S72.Ø36J
S72.Ø36K
S72.Ø36M
S72.Ø36N
S72.Ø36P
S72.Ø36Q
S72.Ø36R
S72.Ø41A
S72.Ø41B
S72.Ø41C
S72.Ø41G
S72.Ø41H
S72.Ø41J
S72.Ø41K
S72.Ø41M
S72.Ø41N
S72.Ø41P
S72.Ø41Q
S72.Ø41R
S72.Ø42A
S72.Ø42B
S72.Ø42C
S72.Ø42G
S72.Ø42H
S72.Ø42J
S72.Ø42K
S72.Ø42M
S72.Ø42N
S72.Ø42P
S72.Ø42Q
S72.Ø42R
S72.Ø43A
S72.Ø43B
S72.Ø43C
S72.Ø43G
S72.Ø43H
S72.Ø43J
S72.Ø43K
S72.Ø43M
S72.Ø43N
S72.Ø43P
S72.Ø43Q
S72.Ø43R
S72.Ø44A
S72.Ø44B
S72.Ø44C
S72.Ø44G
S72.Ø44H
S72.Ø44J
S72.Ø44K
S72.Ø44M
S72.Ø44N
S72.Ø44P
S72.Ø44Q
S72.Ø44R
S72.Ø45A
S72.Ø45B
S72.Ø45C
S72.Ø45G
S72.Ø45H
S72.Ø45J
S72.Ø45K
S72.Ø45M
S72.Ø45N
S72.Ø45P
S72.Ø45Q
S72.Ø45R
S72.Ø46A
S72.Ø46B
S72.Ø46C
S72.Ø46G
S72.Ø46H
S72.Ø46J
S72.Ø46K
S72.Ø46M
S72.Ø46N
S72.Ø46P
S72.Ø46Q
S72.Ø46R
S72.Ø51A
S72.Ø51B
S72.Ø51C
S72.Ø51G
S72.Ø51H
S72.Ø51J
S72.Ø51K
S72.Ø51M
S72.Ø51N
S72.Ø51P
S72.Ø51Q
S72.Ø51R
S72.Ø52A
S72.Ø52B
S72.Ø52C
S72.Ø52G
S72.Ø52H
S72.Ø52J
S72.Ø52K
S72.Ø52M
S72.Ø52N
S72.Ø52P
S72.Ø52Q
S72.Ø52R
S72.Ø59A
S72.Ø59B
S72.Ø59C
S72.Ø59G
S72.Ø59H
S72.Ø59J
S72.Ø59K
S72.Ø59M
S72.Ø59N
S72.Ø59P
S72.Ø59Q
S72.Ø59R
S72.Ø61A
S72.Ø61B
S72.Ø61C
S72.Ø61G
S72.Ø61H
S72.Ø61J
S72.Ø61K
S72.Ø61M
S72.Ø61N
S72.Ø61P
S72.Ø61Q
S72.Ø61R
S72.Ø62A
S72.Ø62B
S72.Ø62C
S72.Ø62G
S72.Ø62H
S72.Ø62J
S72.Ø62K
S72.Ø62M
S72.Ø62N
S72.Ø62P
S72.Ø62Q
S72.Ø62R
S72.Ø63A
S72.Ø63B
S72.Ø63C
S72.Ø63G
S72.Ø63H
S72.Ø63J
S72.Ø63K
S72.Ø63M
S72.Ø63N
S72.Ø63P
S72.Ø63Q
S72.Ø63R
S72.Ø64A
S72.Ø64B
S72.Ø64C
S72.Ø64G
S72.Ø64H
S72.Ø64J
S72.Ø64K
S72.Ø64M
S72.Ø64N
S72.Ø64P
S72.Ø64Q
S72.Ø64R
S72.Ø65A
S72.Ø65B
S72.Ø65C
S72.Ø65G
S72.Ø65H
S72.Ø65J
S72.Ø65K
S72.Ø65M
S72.Ø65N
S72.Ø65P
S72.Ø65Q
S72.Ø65R
S72.Ø66A
S72.Ø66B
S72.Ø66C
S72.Ø66G
S72.Ø66H
S72.Ø66J
S72.Ø66K
S72.Ø66M
S72.Ø66N
S72.Ø66P
S72.Ø66Q
S72.Ø66R
S72.Ø91A
S72.Ø91B
S72.Ø91C
S72.Ø91G
S72.Ø91H
S72.Ø91J
S72.Ø91K
S72.Ø91M
S72.Ø91N
S72.Ø91P
S72.Ø91Q
S72.Ø91R
S72.Ø92A
S72.Ø92B
S72.Ø92C
S72.Ø92G
S72.Ø92H
S72.Ø92J
S72.Ø92K
S72.Ø92M
S72.Ø92N
S72.Ø92P
S72.Ø92Q
S72.Ø92R
S72.Ø99A
S72.Ø99B
S72.Ø99C
S72.Ø99G
S72.Ø99H
S72.Ø99J
S72.Ø99K
S72.Ø99M
S72.Ø99N
S72.Ø99P
S72.Ø99Q
S72.Ø99R
S72.1Ø1A
S72.1Ø1B
S72.1Ø1C
S72.1Ø1G
S72.1Ø1H
S72.1Ø1J
S72.1Ø1K
S72.1Ø1M
S72.1Ø1N
S72.1Ø1P
S72.1Ø1Q
S72.1Ø1R
S72.1Ø2A
S72.1Ø2B
S72.1Ø2C
S72.1Ø2G
S72.1Ø2H
S72.1Ø2J
S72.1Ø2K
S72.1Ø2M
S72.1Ø2N
S72.1Ø2P
S72.1Ø2Q
S72.1Ø2R
S72.1Ø9A
S72.1Ø9B
S72.1Ø9C
S72.1Ø9G
S72.1Ø9H
S72.1Ø9J
S72.1Ø9K
S72.1Ø9M
S72.1Ø9N
S72.1Ø9P
S72.1Ø9Q
S72.1Ø9R
S72.111A
S72.111B
S72.111C
S72.111G
S72.111H
S72.111J
S72.111K
S72.111M
S72.111N
S72.111P
S72.111Q
S72.111R
S72.112A
S72.112B
S72.112C
S72.112G
S72.112H
S72.112J
S72.112K
S72.112M
S72.112N
S72.112P
S72.112Q
S72.112R
S72.113A
S72.113B
S72.113C
S72.113G
S72.113H
S72.113J
S72.113K
S72.113M
S72.113N
S72.113P
S72.113Q
S72.113R
S72.114A
S72.114B
S72.114C
S72.114G
S72.114H
S72.114J
S72.114K
S72.114M
S72.114N
S72.114P
S72.114Q
S72.114R
S72.115A
S72.115B
S72.115C
S72.115G
S72.115H
S72.115J
S72.115K
S72.115M
S72.115N
S72.115P
S72.115Q
S72.115R
S72.116A
S72.116B
S72.116C
S72.116G
S72.116H
S72.116J
S72.116K
S72.116M
S72.116N
S72.116P
S72.116Q
S72.116R
S72.121A
S72.121B
S72.121C
S72.121G
S72.121H
S72.121J
S72.121K
S72.121M
S72.121N
S72.121P
S72.121Q
S72.121R
S72.122A
S72.122B
S72.122C
S72.122G
S72.122H
S72.122J
S72.122K
S72.122M
S72.122N
S72.122P
S72.122Q
S72.122R
S72.123A
S72.123B
S72.123C
S72.123G
S72.123H
S72.123J
S72.123K
S72.123M
S72.123N
S72.123P
S72.123Q
S72.123R
S72.124A
S72.124B
S72.124C
S72.124G
S72.124H
S72.124J
S72.124K
S72.124M
S72.124N
S72.124P
S72.124Q
S72.124R
S72.125A
S72.125B
S72.125C
S72.125G
S72.125H
S72.125J
S72.125K
S72.125M
S72.125N
S72.125P
S72.125Q
S72.125R
S72.126A
S72.126B
S72.126C
S72.126G
S72.126H
S72.126J
S72.126K
S72.126M
S72.126N
S72.126P
S72.126Q
S72.126R
S72.131A
S72.131B
S72.131C
S72.131G
S72.131H
S72.131J
S72.131K
S72.131M
S72.131N
S72.131P
S72.131Q
S72.131R
S72.132A
S72.132B
S72.132C
S72.132G
S72.132H
S72.132J
S72.132K
S72.132M
S72.132N
S72.132P
S72.132Q
S72.132R
S72.133A
S72.133B
S72.133C
S72.133G
S72.133H
S72.133J
S72.133K
S72.133M
S72.133N
S72.133P
S72.133Q
S72.133R
S72.134A
S72.134B
S72.134C
S72.134G
S72.134H
S72.134J
S72.134K
S72.134M
S72.134N
S72.134P
S72.134Q
S72.134R
S72.135A
S72.135B
S72.135C
S72.135G
S72.135H
S72.135J
S72.135K
S72.135M
S72.135N
S72.135P
S72.135Q
S72.135R
S72.136A
S72.136B
S72.136C
S72.136G
S72.136H
S72.136J
S72.136K
S72.136M
S72.136N
S72.136P
S72.136Q
S72.136R
S72.141A
S72.141B
S72.141C
S72.141G
S72.141H
S72.141J
S72.141K
S72.141M
S72.141N
S72.141P
S72.141Q
S72.141R
S72.142A
S72.142B
S72.142C
S72.142G
S72.142H
S72.142J
S72.142K
S72.142M
S72.142N
S72.142P
S72.142Q
S72.142R
S72.143A
S72.143B
S72.143C
S72.143G
S72.143H
S72.143J
S72.143K
S72.143M
S72.143N
S72.143P
S72.143Q
S72.143R
S72.144A
S72.144B
S72.144C
S72.144G
S72.144H
S72.144J
S72.144K
S72.144M
S72.144N
S72.144P
S72.144Q
S72.144R
S72.145A
S72.145B
S72.145C
S72.145G
S72.145H
S72.145J
S72.145K
S72.145M
S72.145N
S72.145P
S72.145Q
S72.145R
S72.146A
S72.146B
S72.146C
S72.146G
S72.146H
S72.146J
S72.146K
S72.146M
S72.146N
S72.146P
S72.146Q
S72.146R
S72.21XA
S72.21XB
S72.21XC
S72.21XG
S72.21XH
S72.21XJ
S72.21XK
S72.21XM
S72.21XN
S72.21XP
S72.21XQ
S72.21XR
S72.22XA
S72.22XB
S72.22XC
S72.22XG
S72.22XH
S72.22XJ
S72.22XK
S72.22XM
S72.22XN
S72.22XP
S72.22XQ
S72.22XR
S72.23XA
S72.23XB
S72.23XC
S72.23XG
S72.23XH
S72.23XJ
S72.23XK
S72.23XM
S72.23XN
S72.23XP
S72.23XQ
S72.23XR
S72.24XA
S72.24XB
S72.24XC
S72.24XG
S72.24XH
S72.24XJ
S72.24XK
S72.24XM
S72.24XN
S72.24XP
S72.24XQ
S72.24XR
S72.25XA
S72.25XB
S72.25XC
S72.25XG
S72.25XH
S72.25XJ
S72.25XK
S72.25XM
S72.25XN
S72.25XP
S72.25XQ
S72.25XR
S72.26XA
S72.26XB
S72.26XC
S72.26XG
S72.26XH
S72.26XJ
S72.26XK
S72.26XM
S72.26XN
S72.26XP
S72.26XQ
S72.26XR
S79.ØØ1A
S79.ØØ1G
S79.ØØ1K
S79.ØØ1P
S79.ØØ2A
S79.ØØ2G
S79.ØØ2K
S79.ØØ2P
S79.ØØ9A
S79.ØØ9G
S79.ØØ9K
S79.ØØ9P
S79.Ø11A
S79.Ø11G
S79.Ø11K
S79.Ø11P
S79.Ø12A
S79.Ø12G
S79.Ø12K
S79.Ø12P
S79.Ø19A
S79.Ø19G
S79.Ø19K
S79.Ø19P
S79.Ø91A
S79.Ø91G
S79.Ø91K
S79.Ø91P
S79.Ø92A
S79.Ø92G
S79.Ø92K
S79.Ø92P
S79.Ø99A
S79.Ø99G
S79.Ø99K
S79.Ø99P

AND

Operating Room Procedures

ØSR9Ø19
ØSR9Ø1A
ØSR9Ø1Z
ØSR9Ø29
ØSR9Ø2A
ØSR9Ø2Z
ØSR9Ø39
ØSR9Ø3A
ØSR9Ø3Z
ØSR9Ø49
ØSR9Ø4A
ØSR9Ø4Z
ØSR9Ø69
ØSR9Ø6A
ØSR9Ø6Z
ØSR9Ø7Z
ØSR9ØJ9
ØSR9ØJA
ØSR9ØJZ
ØSR9ØKZ
ØSRAØØ9
ØSRAØØA
ØSRAØØZ
ØSRAØ19
ØSRAØ1A
ØSRAØ1Z
ØSRAØ39
ØSRAØ3A
ØSRAØ3Z
ØSRAØ7Z
ØSRAØJ9
ØSRAØJA
ØSRAØJZ
ØSRAØKZ
ØSRBØ19
ØSRBØ1A
ØSRBØ1Z
ØSRBØ29
ØSRBØ2A
ØSRBØ2Z
ØSRBØ39
ØSRBØ3A
ØSRBØ3Z
ØSRBØ49
ØSRBØ4A
ØSRBØ4Z
ØSRBØ69
ØSRBØ6A
ØSRBØ6Z
ØSRBØ7Z
ØSRBØJ9
ØSRBØJA
ØSRBØJZ
ØSRBØKZ
ØSREØØ9
ØSREØØA
ØSREØØZ
ØSREØ19
ØSREØ1A
ØSREØ1Z
ØSREØ39
ØSREØ3A
ØSREØ3Z
ØSREØ7Z
ØSREØJ9
ØSREØJA
ØSREØJZ
ØSREØKZ
ØSRRØ19
ØSRRØ1A
ØSRRØ1Z
ØSRRØ39
ØSRRØ3A
ØSRRØ3Z
ØSRRØ7Z
ØSRRØJ9
ØSRRØJA
ØSRRØJZ
ØSRRØKZ
ØSRSØ19
ØSRSØ1A
ØSRSØ1Z
ØSRSØ39
ØSRSØ3A
ØSRSØ3Z
ØSRSØ7Z
ØSRSØJ9
ØSRSØJA
ØSRSØJZ
ØSRSØKZ
ØSU9ØBZ
ØSUAØBZ
ØSUBØBZ
ØSUEØBZ
ØSURØBZ
ØSUSØBZ

DRG 522

Select principal diagnosis AND operating room procedures listed under DRG 521

DRG 533

Principal Diagnosis

S72.3Ø1A
S72.3Ø1B
S72.3Ø1C
S72.3Ø2A
S72.3Ø2B
S72.3Ø2C
S72.3Ø9A
S72.3Ø9B
S72.3Ø9C
S72.321A
S72.321B
S72.321C
S72.322A
S72.322B
S72.322C
S72.323A
S72.323B
S72.323C
S72.324A
S72.324B
S72.324C
S72.325A
S72.325B
S72.325C
S72.326A
S72.326B
S72.326C
S72.331A
S72.331B
S72.331C
S72.332A
S72.332B
S72.332C
S72.333A
S72.333B
S72.333C
S72.334A
S72.334B
S72.334C
S72.335A
S72.335B
S72.335C
S72.336A
S72.336B
S72.336C
S72.341A
S72.341B
S72.341C
S72.342A
S72.342B
S72.342C
S72.343A
S72.343B
S72.343C
S72.344A
S72.344B
S72.344C
S72.345A
S72.345B
S72.345C
S72.346A
S72.346B
S72.346C
S72.351A
S72.351B
S72.351C
S72.352A

ICD-10-CM/PCS Codes by MS-DRG

S72.352B
S72.352C
S72.353A
S72.353B
S72.353C
S72.354A
S72.354B
S72.354C
S72.355A
S72.355B
S72.355C
S72.356A
S72.356B
S72.356C
S72.361A
S72.361B
S72.361C
S72.362A
S72.362B
S72.362C
S72.363A
S72.363B
S72.363C
S72.364A
S72.364B
S72.364C
S72.365A
S72.365B
S72.365C
S72.366A
S72.366B
S72.366C
S72.391A
S72.391B
S72.391C
S72.392A
S72.392B
S72.392C
S72.399A
S72.399B
S72.399C
S72.401A
S72.401B
S72.401C
S72.402A
S72.402B
S72.402C
S72.409A
S72.409B
S72.409C
S72.411A
S72.411B
S72.411C
S72.412A
S72.412B
S72.412C
S72.413A
S72.413B
S72.413C
S72.414A
S72.414B
S72.414C
S72.415A
S72.415B
S72.415C
S72.416A
S72.416B
S72.416C
S72.421A
S72.421B
S72.421C
S72.422A
S72.422B
S72.422C
S72.423A
S72.423B
S72.423C
S72.424A
S72.424B
S72.424C
S72.425A
S72.425B
S72.425C
S72.426A
S72.426B
S72.426C
S72.431A
S72.431B
S72.431C
S72.432A
S72.432B
S72.432C
S72.433A
S72.433B
S72.433C
S72.434A
S72.434B
S72.434C
S72.435A
S72.435B
S72.435C
S72.436A
S72.436B
S72.436C
S72.441A
S72.441B
S72.441C
S72.442A
S72.442B
S72.442C
S72.443A
S72.443B
S72.443C
S72.444A
S72.444B
S72.444C
S72.445A
S72.445B
S72.445C
S72.446A
S72.446B
S72.446C
S72.451A
S72.451B
S72.451C
S72.452A
S72.452B
S72.452C
S72.453A
S72.453B
S72.453C
S72.454A
S72.454B
S72.454C
S72.455A
S72.455B
S72.455C
S72.456A
S72.456B
S72.456C
S72.461A
S72.461B
S72.461C
S72.462A
S72.462B
S72.462C
S72.463A
S72.463B
S72.463C
S72.464A
S72.464B
S72.464C
S72.465A
S72.465B
S72.465C
S72.466A
S72.466B
S72.466C
S72.471A
S72.472A
S72.479A
S72.491A
S72.491B
S72.491C
S72.492A
S72.492B
S72.492C
S72.499A
S72.499B
S72.499C
S72.8X1A
S72.8X1B
S72.8X1C
S72.8X2A
S72.8X2B
S72.8X2C
S72.8X9A
S72.8X9B
S72.8X9C
S72.90XA
S72.90XB
S72.90XC
S72.91XA
S72.91XB
S72.91XC
S72.92XA
S72.92XB
S72.92XC
S79.101A
S79.102A
S79.109A
S79.111A
S79.112A
S79.119A
S79.121A
S79.122A
S79.129A
S79.131A
S79.132A
S79.139A
S79.141A
S79.142A
S79.149A
S79.191A
S79.192A
S79.199A

DRG 534

Select principal diagnosis listed under DRG 533

DRG 535

Principal Diagnosis

S32.301A
S32.301B
S32.302A
S32.302B
S32.309A
S32.309B
S32.311A
S32.311B
S32.312A
S32.312B
S32.313A
S32.313B
S32.314A
S32.314B
S32.315A
S32.315B
S32.316A
S32.316B
S32.391A
S32.391B
S32.392A
S32.392B
S32.399A
S32.399B
S32.401A
S32.401B
S32.402A
S32.402B
S32.409A
S32.409B
S32.411A
S32.411B
S32.412A
S32.412B
S32.413A
S32.413B
S32.414A
S32.414B
S32.415A
S32.415B
S32.416A
S32.416B
S32.421A
S32.421B
S32.422A
S32.422B
S32.423A
S32.423B
S32.424A
S32.424B
S32.425A
S32.425B
S32.426A
S32.426B
S32.431A
S32.431B
S32.432A
S32.432B
S32.433A
S32.433B
S32.434A
S32.434B
S32.435A
S32.435B
S32.436A
S32.436B
S32.441A
S32.441B
S32.442A
S32.442B
S32.443A
S32.443B
S32.444A
S32.444B
S32.445A
S32.445B
S32.446A
S32.446B
S32.451A
S32.451B
S32.452A
S32.452B
S32.453A
S32.453B
S32.454A
S32.454B
S32.455A
S32.455B
S32.456A
S32.456B
S32.461A
S32.461B
S32.462A
S32.462B
S32.463A
S32.463B
S32.464A
S32.464B
S32.465A
S32.465B
S32.466A
S32.466B
S32.471A
S32.471B
S32.472A
S32.472B
S32.473A
S32.473B
S32.474A
S32.474B
S32.475A
S32.475B
S32.476A
S32.476B
S32.481A
S32.481B
S32.482A
S32.482B
S32.483A
S32.483B
S32.484A
S32.484B
S32.485A
S32.485B
S32.486A
S32.486B
S32.491A
S32.491B
S32.492A
S32.492B
S32.499A
S32.499B
S32.501A
S32.501B
S32.502A
S32.502B
S32.509A
S32.509B
S32.511A
S32.511B
S32.512A
S32.512B
S32.519A
S32.519B
S32.591A
S32.591B
S32.592A
S32.592B
S32.599A
S32.599B
S32.601A
S32.601B
S32.602A
S32.602B
S32.609A
S32.609B
S32.611A
S32.611B
S32.612A
S32.612B
S32.613A
S32.613B
S32.614A
S32.614B
S32.615A
S32.615B
S32.616A
S32.616B
S32.691A
S32.691B
S32.692A
S32.692B
S32.699A
S32.699B
S32.810A
S32.810B
S32.811A
S32.811B
S32.82XA
S32.82XB
S32.89XA
S32.89XB
S32.9XXA
S32.9XXB
S72.001A
S72.001B
S72.001C
S72.002A
S72.002B
S72.002C
S72.009A
S72.009B
S72.009C
S72.011A
S72.011B
S72.011C
S72.012A
S72.012B
S72.012C
S72.019A
S72.019B
S72.019C
S72.021A
S72.021B
S72.021C
S72.022A
S72.022B
S72.022C
S72.023A
S72.023B
S72.023C
S72.024A
S72.024B
S72.024C
S72.025A
S72.025B
S72.025C
S72.026A
S72.026B
S72.026C
S72.031A
S72.031B
S72.031C
S72.032A
S72.032B
S72.032C
S72.033A
S72.033B
S72.033C
S72.034A
S72.034B
S72.034C
S72.035A
S72.035B
S72.035C
S72.036A
S72.036B
S72.036C
S72.041A
S72.041B
S72.041C
S72.042A
S72.042B
S72.042C
S72.043A
S72.043B
S72.043C
S72.044A
S72.044B
S72.044C
S72.045A
S72.045B
S72.045C
S72.046A
S72.046B
S72.046C
S72.051A
S72.051B
S72.051C
S72.052A
S72.052B
S72.052C
S72.059A
S72.059B
S72.059C
S72.061A
S72.061B
S72.061C
S72.062A
S72.062B
S72.062C
S72.063A
S72.063B
S72.063C
S72.064A
S72.064B
S72.064C
S72.065A
S72.065B
S72.065C
S72.066A
S72.066B
S72.066C
S72.091A
S72.091B
S72.091C
S72.092A
S72.092B
S72.092C
S72.099A
S72.099B
S72.099C
S72.101A
S72.101B
S72.101C
S72.102A
S72.102B
S72.102C
S72.109A
S72.109B
S72.109C
S72.111A
S72.111B
S72.111C
S72.112A
S72.112B
S72.112C
S72.113A
S72.113B
S72.113C
S72.114A
S72.114B
S72.114C
S72.115A
S72.115B
S72.115C
S72.116A
S72.116B
S72.116C
S72.121A
S72.121B
S72.121C
S72.122A
S72.122B
S72.122C
S72.123A
S72.123B
S72.123C
S72.124A
S72.124B
S72.124C
S72.125A
S72.125B
S72.125C
S72.126A
S72.126B
S72.126C
S72.131A
S72.131B
S72.131C
S72.132A
S72.132B
S72.132C
S72.133A
S72.133B
S72.133C
S72.134A
S72.134B
S72.134C
S72.135A
S72.135B
S72.135C
S72.136A
S72.136B
S72.136C
S72.141A
S72.141B
S72.141C
S72.142A
S72.142B
S72.142C
S72.143A
S72.143B
S72.143C
S72.144A
S72.144B
S72.144C
S72.145A
S72.145B
S72.145C
S72.146A
S72.146B
S72.146C
S72.21XA
S72.21XB
S72.21XC
S72.22XA
S72.22XB
S72.22XC
S72.23XA
S72.23XB
S72.23XC
S72.24XA
S72.24XB
S72.24XC
S72.25XA
S72.25XB
S72.25XC
S72.26XA
S72.26XB
S72.26XC
S79.001A
S79.002A
S79.009A
S79.011A
S79.012A
S79.019A
S79.091A
S79.092A
S79.099A

DRG 536

Select principal diagnosis listed under DRG 535

DRG 537

Principal Diagnosis

S33.4XXA
S73.001A
S73.002A
S73.003A
S73.004A
S73.005A
S73.006A
S73.011A
S73.012A
S73.013A
S73.014A
S73.015A
S73.016A
S73.021A
S73.022A
S73.023A
S73.024A
S73.025A
S73.026A
S73.031A
S73.032A
S73.033A
S73.034A
S73.035A
S73.036A
S73.041A
S73.042A
S73.043A
S73.044A
S73.045A
S73.046A
S73.101A
S73.102A
S73.109A
S73.111A
S73.112A
S73.119A
S73.121A
S73.122A
S73.129A
S73.191A
S73.192A
S73.199A
S76.011A
S76.012A
S76.019A
S76.111A
S76.112A
S76.119A
S76.211A
S76.212A
S76.219A
S76.311A
S76.312A
S76.319A
S76.811A
S76.812A
S76.819A
S76.911A
S76.912A
S76.919A

DRG 538

Select principal diagnosis listed under DRG 537

DRG 539

Principal Diagnosis

A02.24
A18.01
A18.03
A51.46
A52.77
A54.41
M46.2*
M46.3*
M86*

DRG 540

Select principal diagnosis listed under DRG 539

DRG 541

Select principal diagnosis listed under DRG 539

DRG 542

Principal Diagnosis

C40*
C41*
C47*
C49.0
C49.10
C49.11
C49.12
C49.20
C49.21
C49.22
C49.3
C49.4
C49.5
C49.6
C49.8
C49.9
C79.5*
C7B.03
D48.0
M30.1
M31.2
M31.3*
M48.40XA
M48.41XA
M48.42XA
M48.43XA
M48.44XA
M48.45XA
M48.46XA
M48.47XA
M48.48XA
M48.50XA
M48.51XA
M48.52XA
M48.53XA
M48.54XA
M48.55XA
M48.56XA
M48.57XA
M48.58XA
M80.00XA
M80.011A
M80.012A
M80.019A
M80.021A
M80.022A
M80.029A
M80.031A
M80.032A
M80.039A
M80.041A
M80.042A
M80.049A
M80.051A
M80.052A
M80.059A
M80.061A
M80.062A
M80.069A
M80.071A
M80.072A
M80.079A
M80.08XA
M80.0AXA
M80.0B1A
M80.0B2A
M80.0B9A
M80.80XA
M80.811A
M80.812A
M80.819A
M80.821A
M80.822A
M80.829A
M80.831A
M80.832A
M80.839A
M80.841A
M80.842A
M80.849A
M80.851A
M80.852A
M80.859A
M80.861A
M80.862A
M80.869A
M80.871A
M80.872A
M80.879A
M80.88XA
M80.8AXA
M80.8B1A
M80.8B2A
M80.8B9A
M84.30XA
M84.311A
M84.312A
M84.319A
M84.321A
M84.322A
M84.329A
M84.331A
M84.332A
M84.333A
M84.334A
M84.339A
M84.341A
M84.342A
M84.343A
M84.344A
M84.345A
M84.346A
M84.350A
M84.351A
M84.352A
M84.353A
M84.359A
M84.361A
M84.362A
M84.363A
M84.364A
M84.369A
M84.371A
M84.372A
M84.373A
M84.374A
M84.375A
M84.376A
M84.377A
M84.378A
M84.379A
M84.38XA
M84.40XA
M84.411A
M84.412A
M84.419A
M84.421A
M84.422A
M84.429A
M84.431A
M84.432A
M84.433A

M84.434A
M84.439A
M84.441A
M84.442A
M84.443A
M84.444A
M84.445A
M84.446A
M84.451A
M84.452A
M84.453A
M84.454A
M84.459A
M84.461A
M84.462A
M84.463A
M84.464A
M84.469A
M84.471A
M84.472A
M84.473A
M84.474A
M84.475A
M84.476A
M84.477A
M84.478A
M84.479A
M84.48XA
M84.5ØXA
M84.511A
M84.512A
M84.519A
M84.521A
M84.522A
M84.529A
M84.531A
M84.532A
M84.533A
M84.534A
M84.539A
M84.541A
M84.542A
M84.549A
M84.55ØA
M84.551A
M84.552A
M84.553A
M84.559A
M84.561A
M84.562A
M84.563A
M84.564A
M84.569A
M84.571A
M84.572A
M84.573A
M84.574A
M84.575A
M84.576A
M84.58XA
M84.6ØXA
M84.611A
M84.612A
M84.619A
M84.621A
M84.622A
M84.629A
M84.631A
M84.632A
M84.633A
M84.634A
M84.639A
M84.641A
M84.642A
M84.649A
M84.65ØA
M84.651A
M84.652A
M84.653A
M84.659A
M84.661A
M84.662A
M84.663A
M84.664A
M84.669A
M84.671A
M84.672A
M84.673A
M84.674A
M84.675A
M84.676A
M84.68XA
M84.75ØA
M84.751A
M84.752A
M84.753A
M84.754A
M84.755A
M84.756A
M84.757A
M84.758A
M84.759A

DRG 543

Select principal diagnosis listed under DRG 542

DRG 544

Select principal diagnosis listed under DRG 542

DRG 545

Principal Diagnosis

D89.82
E85*
G72.4*
IØØ
I73.Ø*
I77.6
L4Ø.5*
MØ2.3*
MØ4*
MØ5.Ø*
MØ5.2*
MØ5.3*
MØ5.4*
MØ5.5*
MØ5.6*
MØ5.7*
MØ5.8*
MØ5.9
MØ6.Ø*
MØ6.1
MØ6.2*
MØ6.3*
MØ6.8*
MØ6.9
MØ8*
M3Ø.Ø
M3Ø.2
M3Ø.3
M3Ø.8
M31.Ø
M31.1*
M31.4
M31.5
M31.6
M31.7
M32*
M33*
M34.Ø
M34.1
M34.2
M34.82
M34.89
M34.9
M35.Ø*
M35.1
M35.2
M35.3
M35.5
M35.8*
M35.9
M36.Ø
M36.8
M45*
M48.8*

DRG 546

Select principal diagnosis listed under DRG 545

DRG 547

Select principal diagnosis listed under DRG 545

DRG 548

Principal Diagnosis

AØ2.23
A18.Ø2
A18.Ø9
A39.83
A39.84
A54.4Ø
A54.42
A54.43
A54.49
A66.6
MØØ.ØØ
MØØ.Ø11
MØØ.Ø12
MØØ.Ø19
MØØ.Ø21
MØØ.Ø22
MØØ.Ø29
MØØ.Ø31
MØØ.Ø32
MØØ.Ø39
MØØ.Ø41
MØØ.Ø42
MØØ.Ø49
MØØ.Ø51
MØØ.Ø52
MØØ.Ø59
MØØ.Ø61
MØØ.Ø62
MØØ.Ø69
MØØ.Ø71
MØØ.Ø72
MØØ.Ø79
MØØ.Ø8
MØØ.Ø9
MØØ.1*
MØØ.2*
MØØ.8*
MØØ.9
MØ1*
MØ2.8*

DRG 549

Select principal diagnosis listed under DRG 548

DRG 550

Select principal diagnosis listed under DRG 548

DRG 551

Principal Diagnosis

M25.78
M4Ø*
M41*
M43.Ø*
M43.1*
M43.2*
M43.6
M43.8*
M43.9
M46.Ø*
M46.1
M46.4*
M46.5*
M46.8*
M46.9*
M47*
M48.Ø*
M48.1*
M48.2*
M48.3*
M48.4ØXS
M48.41XS
M48.42XS
M48.43XS
M48.44XS
M48.45XS
M48.46XS
M48.47XS
M48.48XS
M48.5ØXS
M48.51XS
M48.52XS
M48.53XS
M48.54XS
M48.55XS
M48.56XS
M48.57XS
M48.58XS
M48.9
M49*
M5Ø.Ø*
M5Ø.1Ø
M5Ø.11
M5Ø.12*
M5Ø.13
M5Ø.2*
M5Ø.3*
M5Ø.8*
M5Ø.9*
M51*
M53.2X7
M53.2X8
M53.3
M53.8*
M53.9
M54.Ø3
M54.Ø4
M54.Ø5
M54.Ø6
M54.Ø7
M54.Ø8
M54.Ø9
M54.14
M54.15
M54.16
M54.17
M54.2
M54.3*
M54.4*
M54.5*
M54.6
M54.8*
M54.9
M62.83Ø
M8Ø.Ø8XS
M8Ø.88XS
M84.35ØS
M84.454S
M84.55ØS
M84.58XS
M84.65ØS
M96.1
M96.2
M96.3
M96.4
M96.5
M99.Ø1
M99.Ø2
M99.Ø3
M99.Ø4
M99.1Ø
M99.11
M99.12
M99.13
M99.14
M99.15
M99.2*
M99.3*
M99.4*
M99.5*
M99.6*
M99.7*
M99.83
M99.84
Q76.2
Q76.411
Q76.412
Q76.413
Q76.414
Q76.415
Q76.419
Q76.49
R29.891
S12.ØØØA
S12.ØØØB
S12.ØØØS
S12.ØØ1A
S12.ØØ1B
S12.ØØ1S
S12.Ø1XA
S12.Ø1XB
S12.Ø1XS
S12.Ø2XA
S12.Ø2XB
S12.Ø2XS
S12.Ø3ØA
S12.Ø3ØB
S12.Ø3ØS
S12.Ø31A
S12.Ø31B
S12.Ø31S
S12.Ø4ØA
S12.Ø4ØB
S12.Ø4ØS
S12.Ø41A
S12.Ø41B
S12.Ø41S
S12.Ø9ØA
S12.Ø9ØB
S12.Ø9ØS
S12.Ø91A
S12.Ø91B
S12.Ø91S
S12.1ØØA
S12.1ØØB
S12.1ØØS
S12.1Ø1A
S12.1Ø1B
S12.1Ø1S
S12.11ØA
S12.11ØB
S12.11ØS
S12.111A
S12.111B
S12.111S
S12.112A
S12.112B
S12.112S
S12.12ØA
S12.12ØB
S12.12ØS
S12.121A
S12.121B
S12.121S
S12.13ØA
S12.13ØB
S12.13ØS
S12.131A
S12.131B
S12.131S
S12.14XA
S12.14XB
S12.14XS
S12.15ØA
S12.15ØB
S12.15ØS
S12.151A
S12.151B
S12.151S
S12.19ØA
S12.19ØB
S12.19ØS
S12.191A
S12.191B
S12.191S
S12.2ØØA
S12.2ØØB
S12.2ØØS
S12.2Ø1A
S12.2Ø1B
S12.2Ø1S
S12.23ØA
S12.23ØB
S12.23ØS
S12.231A
S12.231B
S12.231S
S12.24XA
S12.24XB
S12.24XS
S12.25ØA
S12.25ØB
S12.25ØS
S12.251A
S12.251B
S12.251S
S12.29ØA
S12.29ØB
S12.29ØS
S12.291A
S12.291B
S12.291S
S12.3ØØA
S12.3ØØB
S12.3ØØS
S12.3Ø1A
S12.3Ø1B
S12.3Ø1S
S12.33ØA
S12.33ØB
S12.33ØS
S12.331A
S12.331B
S12.331S
S12.34XA
S12.34XB
S12.34XS
S12.35ØA
S12.35ØB
S12.35ØS
S12.351A
S12.351B
S12.351S
S12.39ØA
S12.39ØB
S12.39ØS
S12.391A
S12.391B
S12.391S
S12.4ØØA
S12.4ØØB
S12.4ØØS
S12.4Ø1A
S12.4Ø1B
S12.4Ø1S
S12.43ØA
S12.43ØB
S12.43ØS
S12.431A
S12.431B
S12.431S
S12.44XA
S12.44XB
S12.44XS
S12.45ØA
S12.45ØB
S12.45ØS
S12.451A
S12.451B
S12.451S
S12.49ØA
S12.49ØB
S12.49ØS
S12.491A
S12.491B
S12.491S
S12.5ØØA
S12.5ØØB
S12.5ØØS
S12.5Ø1A
S12.5Ø1B
S12.5Ø1S
S12.53ØA
S12.53ØB
S12.53ØS
S12.531A
S12.531B
S12.531S
S12.54XA
S12.54XB
S12.54XS
S12.55ØA
S12.55ØB
S12.55ØS
S12.551A
S12.551B
S12.551S
S12.59ØA
S12.59ØB
S12.59ØS
S12.591A
S12.591B
S12.591S
S12.6ØØA
S12.6ØØB
S12.6ØØS
S12.6Ø1A
S12.6Ø1B
S12.6Ø1S
S12.63ØA
S12.63ØB
S12.63ØS
S12.631A
S12.631B
S12.631S
S12.64XA
S12.64XB
S12.64XS
S12.65ØA
S12.65ØB
S12.65ØS
S12.651A
S12.651B
S12.651S
S12.69ØA
S12.69ØB
S12.69ØS
S12.691A
S12.691B
S12.691S
S12.8XXS
S12.9XXA
S12.9XXS
S13.ØXXA
S13.1ØØA
S13.1Ø1A
S13.11ØA
S13.111A
S13.12ØA
S13.121A
S13.13ØA
S13.131A
S13.14ØA
S13.141A
S13.15ØA
S13.151A
S13.16ØA
S13.161A
S13.17ØA
S13.171A
S13.18ØA
S13.181A
S13.2ØXA
S13.29XA
S13.4XXA
S13.8XXA
S13.9XXA
S16.1XXA
S22.ØØØA
S22.ØØØB
S22.ØØØS
S22.ØØ1A
S22.ØØ1B
S22.ØØ1S
S22.ØØ2A
S22.ØØ2B
S22.ØØ2S
S22.ØØ8A
S22.ØØ8B
S22.ØØ8S
S22.ØØ9A
S22.ØØ9B
S22.ØØ9S
S22.Ø1ØA
S22.Ø1ØB
S22.Ø1ØS
S22.Ø11A
S22.Ø11B
S22.Ø11S
S22.Ø12A
S22.Ø12B
S22.Ø12S
S22.Ø18A
S22.Ø18B
S22.Ø18S
S22.Ø19A
S22.Ø19B
S22.Ø19S
S22.Ø2ØA
S22.Ø2ØB
S22.Ø2ØS
S22.Ø21A
S22.Ø21B
S22.Ø21S
S22.Ø22A
S22.Ø22B
S22.Ø22S
S22.Ø28A
S22.Ø28B
S22.Ø28S
S22.Ø29A
S22.Ø29B
S22.Ø29S
S22.Ø3ØA
S22.Ø3ØB
S22.Ø3ØS
S22.Ø31A
S22.Ø31B
S22.Ø31S
S22.Ø32A
S22.Ø32B
S22.Ø32S
S22.Ø38A
S22.Ø38B
S22.Ø38S
S22.Ø39A
S22.Ø39B
S22.Ø39S
S22.Ø4ØA
S22.Ø4ØB
S22.Ø4ØS
S22.Ø41A
S22.Ø41B
S22.Ø41S
S22.Ø42A
S22.Ø42B
S22.Ø42S
S22.Ø48A
S22.Ø48B
S22.Ø48S
S22.Ø49A
S22.Ø49B
S22.Ø49S
S22.Ø5ØA
S22.Ø5ØB
S22.Ø5ØS
S22.Ø51A
S22.Ø51B
S22.Ø51S
S22.Ø52A
S22.Ø52B
S22.Ø52S
S22.Ø58A
S22.Ø58B
S22.Ø58S
S22.Ø59A
S22.Ø59B
S22.Ø59S
S22.Ø6ØA
S22.Ø6ØB
S22.Ø6ØS
S22.Ø61A
S22.Ø61B
S22.Ø61S
S22.Ø62A
S22.Ø62B
S22.Ø62S
S22.Ø68A
S22.Ø68B
S22.Ø68S
S22.Ø69A
S22.Ø69B
S22.Ø69S
S22.Ø7ØA
S22.Ø7ØB
S22.Ø7ØS
S22.Ø71A
S22.Ø71B
S22.Ø71S
S22.Ø72A
S22.Ø72B
S22.Ø72S
S22.Ø78A
S22.Ø78B
S22.Ø78S
S22.Ø79A
S22.Ø79B
S22.Ø79S
S22.Ø8ØA
S22.Ø8ØB
S22.Ø8ØS
S22.Ø81A
S22.Ø81B
S22.Ø81S
S22.Ø82A
S22.Ø82B
S22.Ø82S
S22.Ø88A
S22.Ø88B
S22.Ø88S
S22.Ø89A
S22.Ø89B
S22.Ø89S
S22.2ØXS
S22.21XS
S22.22XS
S22.23XS
S22.24XS
S22.31XS
S22.32XS
S22.39XS
S22.41XS
S22.42XS
S22.43XS
S22.49XS
S22.5XXS
S22.9XXS
S23.ØXXA
S23.1ØØA
S23.1Ø1A
S23.11ØA
S23.111A
S23.12ØA
S23.121A
S23.122A
S23.123A
S23.13ØA
S23.131A
S23.132A
S23.133A
S23.14ØA
S23.141A
S23.142A
S23.143A
S23.15ØA
S23.151A
S23.152A
S23.153A
S23.16ØA
S23.161A
S23.162A
S23.163A
S23.17ØA
S23.171A
S23.2ØXA
S23.29XA
S23.3XXA
S23.8XXA
S23.9XXA
S32.ØØØA
S32.ØØØB
S32.ØØØS
S32.ØØ1A
S32.ØØ1B
S32.ØØ1S
S32.ØØ2A
S32.ØØ2B
S32.ØØ2S
S32.ØØ8A
S32.ØØ8B
S32.ØØ8S
S32.ØØ9A
S32.ØØ9B
S32.ØØ9S
S32.Ø1ØA
S32.Ø1ØB
S32.Ø1ØS
S32.Ø11A
S32.Ø11B
S32.Ø11S
S32.Ø12A
S32.Ø12B
S32.Ø12S
S32.Ø18A
S32.Ø18B
S32.Ø18S
S32.Ø19A
S32.Ø19B
S32.Ø19S
S32.Ø2ØA
S32.Ø2ØB
S32.Ø2ØS
S32.Ø21A
S32.Ø21B
S32.Ø21S
S32.Ø22A
S32.Ø22B
S32.Ø22S
S32.Ø28A
S32.Ø28B
S32.Ø28S
S32.Ø29A
S32.Ø29B
S32.Ø29S
S32.Ø3ØA
S32.Ø3ØB
S32.Ø3ØS
S32.Ø31A
S32.Ø31B
S32.Ø31S
S32.Ø32A
S32.Ø32B
S32.Ø32S
S32.Ø38A
S32.Ø38B
S32.Ø38S
S32.Ø39A
S32.Ø39B
S32.Ø39S
S32.Ø4ØA
S32.Ø4ØB
S32.Ø4ØS
S32.Ø41A
S32.Ø41B
S32.Ø41S
S32.Ø42A
S32.Ø42B
S32.Ø42S
S32.Ø48A
S32.Ø48B
S32.Ø48S
S32.Ø49A
S32.Ø49B
S32.Ø49S
S32.Ø5ØA
S32.Ø5ØB
S32.Ø5ØS
S32.Ø51A
S32.Ø51B
S32.Ø51S
S32.Ø52A
S32.Ø52B
S32.Ø52S
S32.Ø58A
S32.Ø58B
S32.Ø58S
S32.Ø59A
S32.Ø59B
S32.Ø59S
S32.1ØXA

S32.1ØXB
S32.1ØXS
S32.11ØA
S32.11ØB
S32.11ØS
S32.111A
S32.111B
S32.111S
S32.112A
S32.112B
S32.112S
S32.119A
S32.119B
S32.119S
S32.12ØA
S32.12ØB
S32.12ØS
S32.121A
S32.121B
S32.121S
S32.122A
S32.122B
S32.122S
S32.129A
S32.129B
S32.129S
S32.13ØA
S32.13ØB
S32.13ØS
S32.131A
S32.131B
S32.131S
S32.132A
S32.132B
S32.132S
S32.139A
S32.139B
S32.139S
S32.14XA
S32.14XB
S32.14XS
S32.15XA
S32.15XB
S32.15XS
S32.16XA
S32.16XB
S32.16XS
S32.17XA
S32.17XB
S32.17XS
S32.19XA
S32.19XB
S32.19XS
S32.2XXA
S32.2XXB
S32.2XXS
S32.3Ø1S
S32.3Ø2S
S32.3Ø9S
S32.311S
S32.312S
S32.313S
S32.314S
S32.315S
S32.316S
S32.391S
S32.392S
S32.399S
S32.4Ø1S
S32.4Ø2S
S32.4Ø9S
S32.411S
S32.412S
S32.413S
S32.414S
S32.415S
S32.416S
S32.421S
S32.422S
S32.423S
S32.424S
S32.425S
S32.426S
S32.431S
S32.432S
S32.433S
S32.434S
S32.435S
S32.436S
S32.441S
S32.442S
S32.443S
S32.444S
S32.445S
S32.446S
S32.451S
S32.452S
S32.453S
S32.454S
S32.455S
S32.456S
S32.461S
S32.462S
S32.463S
S32.464S
S32.465S
S32.466S
S32.471S
S32.472S
S32.473S
S32.474S
S32.475S
S32.476S
S32.481S
S32.482S
S32.483S
S32.484S
S32.485S
S32.486S
S32.491S
S32.492S
S32.499S
S32.5Ø1S
S32.5Ø2S
S32.5Ø9S
S32.511S
S32.512S
S32.519S
S32.591S
S32.592S
S32.599S
S32.6Ø1S
S32.6Ø2S
S32.6Ø9S
S32.611S
S32.612S
S32.613S
S32.614S
S32.615S
S32.616S
S32.691S
S32.692S
S32.699S
S32.81ØS
S32.811S
S32.82XS
S32.89XS
S32.9XXS
S33.ØXXA
S33.1ØØA
S33.1Ø1A
S33.11ØA
S33.111A
S33.12ØA
S33.121A
S33.13ØA
S33.131A
S33.14ØA
S33.141A
S33.2XXA
S33.5XXA
S33.6XXA
S33.8XXA
S33.9XXA

DRG 552

Select principal diagnosis listed under DRG 551

DRG 553

Principal Diagnosis

BØ6.82
E55.Ø
E64.3
MØ2.Ø*
MØ2.1*
MØ2.2*
MØ2.9
MØ6.4
MØ7*
M1Ø.Ø*
M1Ø.1*
M1Ø.2*
M1Ø.4*
M1Ø.9
M11*
M12*
M13*
M14*
M15*
M16*
M17*
M18*
M19*
M1A.Ø*
M1A.2*
M1A.3*
M1A.4*
M1A.9*
M24.6*
M25.Ø*
M36.1
M36.2
M36.3
M36.4
M42*
M81*
M83*
M85.Ø*
M85.3*
M85.4*
M85.5*
M85.6*
M87*
M88*
M89.4*
M89.7*
M9Ø*
M91*
M92*
M93*
M94.2*

DRG 554

Select principal diagnosis listed under DRG 553

DRG 555

Principal Diagnosis

M25.1*
M25.5*
M25.6*
M25.8*
M25.9
M6Ø.8*
M6Ø.9
M62.4*
M62.81
M62.831
M62.838
M7Ø.8*
M7Ø.9*
M79.Ø
M79.1Ø
M79.11
M79.12
M79.18
M79.6*
M79.7
M79.8*
M79.9
M99.ØØ
M99.Ø5
M99.Ø6
M99.Ø7
M99.Ø8
M99.Ø9
R26.2
R29.4
R29.898

DRG 556

Select principal diagnosis listed under DRG 555

DRG 557

Principal Diagnosis

A52.78
M24.2*
M25.7Ø
M25.711
M25.712
M25.719
M25.721
M25.722
M25.729
M25.731
M25.732
M25.739
M25.741
M25.742
M25.749
M25.751
M25.752
M25.759
M25.761
M25.762
M25.769
M25.771
M25.772
M25.773
M25.774
M25.775
M25.776
M35.4
M35.7
M6Ø.Ø*
M6Ø.1*
M6Ø.2*
M61*
M62.Ø*
M62.1*
M62.2*
M62.3
M62.5*
M62.82
M62.84
M62.89
M62.9
M63*
M65*
M66*
M67*
M7Ø.Ø*
M7Ø.1*
M7Ø.2*
M7Ø.3*
M7Ø.4*
M7Ø.5*
M7Ø.6*
M7Ø.7*
M71*
M72*
M75*
M76*
M77.Ø*
M77.1*
M77.2*
M77.4*
M77.5*
M77.8
M77.9
M79.A*

DRG 558

Select principal diagnosis listed under DRG 557

DRG 559

Principal Diagnosis

M48.4ØXD
M48.4ØXG
M48.41XD
M48.41XG
M48.42XD
M48.42XG
M48.43XD
M48.43XG
M48.44XD
M48.44XG
M48.45XD
M48.45XG
M48.46XD
M48.46XG
M48.47XD
M48.47XG
M48.48XD
M48.48XG
M48.5ØXD
M48.5ØXG
M48.51XD
M48.51XG
M48.52XD
M48.52XG
M48.53XD
M48.53XG
M48.54XD
M48.54XG
M48.55XD
M48.55XG
M48.56XD
M48.56XG
M48.57XD
M48.57XG
M48.58XD
M48.58XG
M8Ø.ØØXD
M8Ø.ØØXG
M8Ø.ØØXS
M8Ø.Ø11D
M8Ø.Ø11G
M8Ø.Ø11S
M8Ø.Ø12D
M8Ø.Ø12G
M8Ø.Ø12S
M8Ø.Ø19D
M8Ø.Ø19G
M8Ø.Ø19S
M8Ø.Ø21D
M8Ø.Ø21G
M8Ø.Ø21S
M8Ø.Ø22D
M8Ø.Ø22G
M8Ø.Ø22S
M8Ø.Ø29D
M8Ø.Ø29G
M8Ø.Ø29S
M8Ø.Ø31D
M8Ø.Ø31G
M8Ø.Ø31S
M8Ø.Ø32D
M8Ø.Ø32G
M8Ø.Ø32S
M8Ø.Ø39D
M8Ø.Ø39G
M8Ø.Ø39S
M8Ø.Ø41D
M8Ø.Ø41G
M8Ø.Ø41S
M8Ø.Ø42D
M8Ø.Ø42G
M8Ø.Ø42S
M8Ø.Ø49D
M8Ø.Ø49G
M8Ø.Ø49S
M8Ø.Ø51D
M8Ø.Ø51G
M8Ø.Ø51S
M8Ø.Ø52D
M8Ø.Ø52G
M8Ø.Ø52S
M8Ø.Ø59D
M8Ø.Ø59G
M8Ø.Ø59S
M8Ø.Ø61D
M8Ø.Ø61G
M8Ø.Ø61S
M8Ø.Ø62D
M8Ø.Ø62G
M8Ø.Ø62S
M8Ø.Ø69D
M8Ø.Ø69G
M8Ø.Ø69S
M8Ø.Ø71D
M8Ø.Ø71G
M8Ø.Ø71S
M8Ø.Ø72D
M8Ø.Ø72G
M8Ø.Ø72S
M8Ø.Ø79D
M8Ø.Ø79G
M8Ø.Ø79S
M8Ø.Ø8XD
M8Ø.Ø8XG
M8Ø.ØAXD
M8Ø.ØAXG
M8Ø.ØAXS
M8Ø.ØB1D
M8Ø.ØB1G
M8Ø.ØB1S
M8Ø.ØB2D
M8Ø.ØB2G
M8Ø.ØB2S
M8Ø.ØB9D
M8Ø.ØB9G
M8Ø.ØB9S
M8Ø.8ØXD
M8Ø.8ØXG
M8Ø.8ØXS
M8Ø.811D
M8Ø.811G
M8Ø.811S
M8Ø.812D
M8Ø.812G
M8Ø.812S
M8Ø.819D
M8Ø.819G
M8Ø.819S
M8Ø.821D
M8Ø.821G
M8Ø.821S
M8Ø.822D
M8Ø.822G
M8Ø.822S
M8Ø.829D
M8Ø.829G
M8Ø.829S
M8Ø.831D
M8Ø.831G
M8Ø.831S
M8Ø.832D
M8Ø.832G
M8Ø.832S
M8Ø.839D
M8Ø.839G
M8Ø.839S
M8Ø.841D
M8Ø.841G
M8Ø.841S
M8Ø.842D
M8Ø.842G
M8Ø.842S
M8Ø.849D
M8Ø.849G
M8Ø.849S
M8Ø.851D
M8Ø.851G
M8Ø.851S
M8Ø.852D
M8Ø.852G
M8Ø.852S
M8Ø.859D
M8Ø.859G
M8Ø.859S
M8Ø.861D
M8Ø.861G
M8Ø.861S
M8Ø.862D
M8Ø.862G
M8Ø.862S
M8Ø.869D
M8Ø.869G
M8Ø.869S
M8Ø.871D
M8Ø.871G
M8Ø.871S
M8Ø.872D
M8Ø.872G
M8Ø.872S
M8Ø.879D
M8Ø.879G
M8Ø.879S
M8Ø.88XD
M8Ø.88XG
M8Ø.8AXD
M8Ø.8AXG
M8Ø.8AXS
M8Ø.8B1D
M8Ø.8B1G
M8Ø.8B1S
M8Ø.8B2D
M8Ø.8B2G
M8Ø.8B2S
M8Ø.8B9D
M8Ø.8B9G
M8Ø.8B9S
M84.3ØXD
M84.3ØXG
M84.3ØXS
M84.311D
M84.311G
M84.311S
M84.312D
M84.312G
M84.312S
M84.319D
M84.319G
M84.319S
M84.321D
M84.321G
M84.321S
M84.322D
M84.322G
M84.322S
M84.329D
M84.329G
M84.329S
M84.331D
M84.331G
M84.331S
M84.332D
M84.332G
M84.332S
M84.333D
M84.333G
M84.333S
M84.334D
M84.334G
M84.334S
M84.339D
M84.339G
M84.339S
M84.341D
M84.341G
M84.341S
M84.342D
M84.342G
M84.342S
M84.343D
M84.343G
M84.343S
M84.344D
M84.344G
M84.344S
M84.345D
M84.345G
M84.345S
M84.346D
M84.346G
M84.346S
M84.35ØD
M84.35ØG
M84.351D
M84.351G
M84.351S
M84.352D
M84.352G
M84.352S
M84.353D
M84.353G
M84.353S
M84.359D
M84.359G
M84.359S
M84.361D
M84.361G
M84.361S
M84.362D
M84.362G
M84.362S
M84.363D
M84.363G
M84.363S
M84.364D
M84.364G
M84.364S
M84.369D
M84.369G
M84.369S
M84.371D
M84.371G
M84.371S
M84.372D
M84.372G
M84.372S
M84.373D
M84.373G
M84.373S
M84.374D
M84.374G
M84.374S
M84.375D
M84.375G
M84.375S
M84.376D
M84.376G
M84.376S
M84.377D
M84.377G
M84.377S
M84.378D
M84.378G
M84.378S
M84.379D
M84.379G
M84.379S
M84.38XD
M84.38XG
M84.38XS
M84.4ØXD
M84.4ØXG
M84.4ØXS
M84.411D
M84.411G
M84.411S
M84.412D
M84.412G
M84.412S
M84.419D
M84.419G
M84.419S
M84.421D
M84.421G
M84.421S
M84.422D
M84.422G
M84.422S
M84.429D
M84.429G
M84.429S
M84.431D
M84.431G
M84.431S
M84.432D
M84.432G
M84.432S
M84.433D
M84.433G
M84.433S
M84.434D
M84.434G
M84.434S
M84.439D
M84.439G
M84.439S
M84.441D
M84.441G
M84.441S
M84.442D
M84.442G
M84.442S
M84.443D
M84.443G
M84.443S
M84.444D
M84.444G
M84.444S
M84.445D
M84.445G
M84.445S
M84.446D
M84.446G
M84.446S
M84.451D
M84.451G
M84.451S
M84.452D
M84.452G
M84.452S
M84.453D
M84.453G
M84.453S
M84.454D
M84.454G
M84.454S
M84.459D
M84.459G
M84.459S
M84.461D
M84.461G
M84.461S
M84.462D
M84.462G
M84.462S
M84.463D
M84.463G
M84.463S
M84.464D
M84.464G
M84.464S
M84.469D
M84.469G
M84.469S
M84.471D
M84.471G
M84.471S
M84.472D
M84.472G
M84.472S
M84.473D
M84.473G
M84.473S
M84.474D
M84.474G
M84.474S
M84.475D
M84.475G
M84.475S
M84.476D
M84.476G
M84.476S
M84.477D
M84.477G
M84.477S
M84.478D
M84.478G
M84.478S
M84.479D
M84.479G
M84.479S
M84.48XD
M84.48XG
M84.48XS
M84.5ØXD
M84.5ØXG
M84.5ØXS
M84.511D
M84.511G
M84.511S
M84.512D
M84.512G
M84.512S
M84.519D
M84.519G
M84.519S
M84.521D
M84.521G
M84.521S
M84.522D
M84.522G
M84.522S
M84.529D
M84.529G
M84.529S
M84.531D
M84.531G
M84.531S
M84.532D
M84.532G
M84.532S
M84.533D
M84.533G
M84.533S
M84.534D
M84.534G
M84.534S
M84.539D
M84.539G
M84.539S
M84.541D
M84.541G
M84.541S
M84.542D
M84.542G
M84.542S
M84.549D
M84.549G
M84.549S
M84.55ØD
M84.55ØG
M84.551D
M84.551G
M84.551S
M84.552D
M84.552G
M84.552S
M84.553D
M84.553G
M84.553S
M84.559D
M84.559G
M84.559S
M84.561D
M84.561G
M84.561S
M84.562D
M84.562G
M84.562S
M84.563D
M84.563G
M84.563S
M84.564D
M84.564G
M84.564S
M84.569D
M84.569G
M84.569S
M84.571D
M84.571G
M84.571S
M84.572D
M84.572G
M84.572S
M84.573D
M84.573G
M84.573S
M84.574D
M84.574G
M84.574S
M84.575D
M84.575G
M84.575S

M84.576D
M84.576G
M84.576S
M84.58XD
M84.58XG
M84.6ØXD
M84.6ØXG
M84.6ØXS
M84.611D
M84.611G
M84.611S
M84.612D
M84.612G
M84.612S
M84.619D
M84.619G
M84.619S
M84.621D
M84.621G
M84.621S
M84.622D
M84.622G
M84.622S
M84.629D
M84.629G
M84.629S
M84.631D
M84.631G
M84.631S
M84.632D
M84.632G
M84.632S
M84.633D
M84.633G
M84.633S
M84.634D
M84.634G
M84.634S
M84.639D
M84.639G
M84.639S
M84.641D
M84.641G
M84.641S
M84.642D
M84.642G
M84.642S
M84.649D
M84.649G
M84.649S
M84.65ØD
M84.65ØG
M84.651D
M84.651G
M84.651S
M84.652D
M84.652G
M84.652S
M84.653D
M84.653G
M84.653S
M84.659D
M84.659G
M84.659S
M84.661D
M84.661G
M84.661S
M84.662D
M84.662G
M84.662S
M84.663D
M84.663G
M84.663S
M84.664D
M84.664G
M84.664S
M84.669D
M84.669G
M84.669S
M84.671D
M84.671G
M84.671S
M84.672D
M84.672G
M84.672S
M84.673D
M84.673G
M84.673S
M84.674D
M84.674G
M84.674S
M84.675D
M84.675G
M84.675S
M84.676D
M84.676G
M84.676S
M84.68XD
M84.68XG
M84.68XS
M84.75ØD
M84.75ØG
M84.75ØS
M84.751D
M84.751G
M84.751S
M84.752D
M84.752G
M84.752S
M84.753D
M84.753G
M84.753S
M84.754D
M84.754G
M84.754S
M84.755D
M84.755G
M84.755S
M84.756D
M84.756G
M84.756S
M84.757D
M84.757G
M84.757S
M84.758D
M84.758G
M84.758S
M84.759D
M84.759G
M84.759S
M96.Ø
M96.621
M96.622
M96.629
M96.631
M96.632
M96.639
M96.65
M96.661
M96.662
M96.669
M96.671
M96.672
M96.679
M96.69
M97.Ø1XA
M97.Ø1XD
M97.Ø2XA
M97.Ø2XD
M97.11XA
M97.11XD
M97.12XA
M97.12XD
M97.21XA
M97.21XD
M97.22XA
M97.22XD
M97.31XA
M97.31XD
M97.32XA
M97.32XD
M97.41XA
M97.41XD
M97.42XA
M97.42XD
M97.8XXA
M97.8XXD
M97.9XXA
M97.9XXD
SØ2.ØXXD
SØ2.ØXXG
SØ2.1Ø1D
SØ2.1Ø1G
SØ2.1Ø2D
SØ2.1Ø2G
SØ2.1Ø9D
SØ2.1Ø9G
SØ2.11ØD
SØ2.11ØG
SØ2.111D
SØ2.111G
SØ2.112D
SØ2.112G
SØ2.113D
SØ2.113G
SØ2.118D
SØ2.118G
SØ2.119D
SØ2.119G
SØ2.11AD
SØ2.11AG
SØ2.11BD
SØ2.11BG
SØ2.11CD
SØ2.11CG
SØ2.11DD
SØ2.11DG
SØ2.11ED
SØ2.11EG
SØ2.11FD
SØ2.11FG
SØ2.11GD
SØ2.11GG
SØ2.11HD
SØ2.11HG
SØ2.19XD
SØ2.19XG
SØ2.2XXD
SØ2.2XXG
SØ2.3ØXD
SØ2.3ØXG
SØ2.31XD
SØ2.31XG
SØ2.32XD
SØ2.32XG
SØ2.4ØØD
SØ2.4ØØG
SØ2.4Ø1D
SØ2.4Ø1G
SØ2.4Ø2D
SØ2.4Ø2G
SØ2.4ØAD
SØ2.4ØAG
SØ2.4ØBD
SØ2.4ØBG
SØ2.4ØCD
SØ2.4ØCG
SØ2.4ØDD
SØ2.4ØDG
SØ2.4ØED
SØ2.4ØEG
SØ2.4ØFD
SØ2.4ØFG
SØ2.411D
SØ2.411G
SØ2.412D
SØ2.412G
SØ2.413D
SØ2.413G
SØ2.42XD
SØ2.42XG
SØ2.5XXD
SØ2.5XXG
SØ2.6ØØD
SØ2.6ØØG
SØ2.6Ø1D
SØ2.6Ø1G
SØ2.6Ø2D
SØ2.6Ø2G
SØ2.6Ø9D
SØ2.6Ø9G
SØ2.61ØD
SØ2.61ØG
SØ2.611D
SØ2.611G
SØ2.612D
SØ2.612G
SØ2.62ØD
SØ2.62ØG
SØ2.621D
SØ2.621G
SØ2.622D
SØ2.622G
SØ2.63ØD
SØ2.63ØG
SØ2.631D
SØ2.631G
SØ2.632D
SØ2.632G
SØ2.64ØD
SØ2.64ØG
SØ2.641D
SØ2.641G
SØ2.642D
SØ2.642G
SØ2.65ØD
SØ2.65ØG
SØ2.651D
SØ2.651G
SØ2.652D
SØ2.652G
SØ2.66XD
SØ2.66XG
SØ2.67ØD
SØ2.67ØG
SØ2.671D
SØ2.671G
SØ2.672D
SØ2.672G
SØ2.69XD
SØ2.69XG
SØ2.8ØXD
SØ2.8ØXG
SØ2.81XD
SØ2.81XG
SØ2.82XD
SØ2.82XG
SØ2.91XD
SØ2.91XG
SØ2.92XD
SØ2.92XG
S12.ØØØD
S12.ØØØG
S12.ØØ1D
S12.ØØ1G
S12.Ø1XD
S12.Ø1XG
S12.Ø2XD
S12.Ø2XG
S12.Ø3ØD
S12.Ø3ØG
S12.Ø31D
S12.Ø31G
S12.Ø4ØD
S12.Ø4ØG
S12.Ø41D
S12.Ø41G
S12.Ø9ØD
S12.Ø9ØG
S12.Ø91D
S12.Ø91G
S12.1ØØD
S12.1ØØG
S12.1Ø1D
S12.1Ø1G
S12.11ØD
S12.11ØG
S12.111D
S12.111G
S12.112D
S12.112G
S12.12ØD
S12.12ØG
S12.121D
S12.121G
S12.13ØD
S12.13ØG
S12.131D
S12.131G
S12.14XD
S12.14XG
S12.15ØD
S12.15ØG
S12.151D
S12.151G
S12.19ØD
S12.19ØG
S12.191D
S12.191G
S12.2ØØD
S12.2ØØG
S12.2Ø1D
S12.2Ø1G
S12.23ØD
S12.23ØG
S12.231D
S12.231G
S12.24XD
S12.24XG
S12.25ØD
S12.25ØG
S12.251D
S12.251G
S12.29ØD
S12.29ØG
S12.291D
S12.291G
S12.3ØØD
S12.3ØØG
S12.3Ø1D
S12.3Ø1G
S12.33ØD
S12.33ØG
S12.331D
S12.331G
S12.34XD
S12.34XG
S12.35ØD
S12.35ØG
S12.351D
S12.351G
S12.39ØD
S12.39ØG
S12.391D
S12.391G
S12.4ØØD
S12.4ØØG
S12.4Ø1D
S12.4Ø1G
S12.43ØD
S12.43ØG
S12.431D
S12.431G
S12.44XD
S12.44XG
S12.45ØD
S12.45ØG
S12.451D
S12.451G
S12.49ØD
S12.49ØG
S12.491D
S12.491G
S12.5ØØD
S12.5ØØG
S12.5Ø1D
S12.5Ø1G
S12.53ØD
S12.53ØG
S12.531D
S12.531G
S12.54XD
S12.54XG
S12.55ØD
S12.55ØG
S12.551D
S12.551G
S12.59ØD
S12.59ØG
S12.591D
S12.591G
S12.6ØØD
S12.6ØØG
S12.6Ø1D
S12.6Ø1G
S12.63ØD
S12.63ØG
S12.631D
S12.631G
S12.64XD
S12.64XG
S12.65ØD
S12.65ØG
S12.651D
S12.651G
S12.69ØD
S12.69ØG
S12.691D
S12.691G
S12.8XXD
S12.9XXD
S22.ØØØD
S22.ØØØG
S22.ØØ1D
S22.ØØ1G
S22.ØØ2D
S22.ØØ2G
S22.ØØ8D
S22.ØØ8G
S22.ØØ9D
S22.ØØ9G
S22.Ø1ØD
S22.Ø1ØG
S22.Ø11D
S22.Ø11G
S22.Ø12D
S22.Ø12G
S22.Ø18D
S22.Ø18G
S22.Ø19D
S22.Ø19G
S22.Ø2ØD
S22.Ø2ØG
S22.Ø21D
S22.Ø21G
S22.Ø22D
S22.Ø22G
S22.Ø28D
S22.Ø28G
S22.Ø29D
S22.Ø29G
S22.Ø3ØD
S22.Ø3ØG
S22.Ø31D
S22.Ø31G
S22.Ø32D
S22.Ø32G
S22.Ø38D
S22.Ø38G
S22.Ø39D
S22.Ø39G
S22.Ø4ØD
S22.Ø4ØG
S22.Ø41D
S22.Ø41G
S22.Ø42D
S22.Ø42G
S22.Ø48D
S22.Ø48G
S22.Ø49D
S22.Ø49G
S22.Ø5ØD
S22.Ø5ØG
S22.Ø51D
S22.Ø51G
S22.Ø52D
S22.Ø52G
S22.Ø58D
S22.Ø58G
S22.Ø59D
S22.Ø59G
S22.Ø6ØD
S22.Ø6ØG
S22.Ø61D
S22.Ø61G
S22.Ø62D
S22.Ø62G
S22.Ø68D
S22.Ø68G
S22.Ø69D
S22.Ø69G
S22.Ø7ØD
S22.Ø7ØG
S22.Ø71D
S22.Ø71G
S22.Ø72D
S22.Ø72G
S22.Ø78D
S22.Ø78G
S22.Ø79D
S22.Ø79G
S22.Ø8ØD
S22.Ø8ØG
S22.Ø81D
S22.Ø81G
S22.Ø82D
S22.Ø82G
S22.Ø88D
S22.Ø88G
S22.Ø89D
S22.Ø89G
S22.2ØXD
S22.2ØXG
S22.21XD
S22.21XG
S22.22XD
S22.22XG
S22.23XD
S22.23XG
S22.24XD
S22.24XG
S22.31XD
S22.31XG
S22.32XD
S22.32XG
S22.39XD
S22.39XG
S22.41XD
S22.41XG
S22.42XD
S22.42XG
S22.43XD
S22.43XG
S22.49XD
S22.49XG
S22.5XXD
S22.5XXG
S22.9XXD
S22.9XXG
S32.ØØØD
S32.ØØØG
S32.ØØ1D
S32.ØØ1G
S32.ØØ2D
S32.ØØ2G
S32.ØØ8D
S32.ØØ8G
S32.ØØ9D
S32.ØØ9G
S32.Ø1ØD
S32.Ø1ØG
S32.Ø11D
S32.Ø11G
S32.Ø12D
S32.Ø12G
S32.Ø18D
S32.Ø18G
S32.Ø19D
S32.Ø19G
S32.Ø2ØD
S32.Ø2ØG
S32.Ø21D
S32.Ø21G
S32.Ø22D
S32.Ø22G
S32.Ø28D
S32.Ø28G
S32.Ø29D
S32.Ø29G
S32.Ø3ØD
S32.Ø3ØG
S32.Ø31D
S32.Ø31G
S32.Ø32D
S32.Ø32G
S32.Ø38D
S32.Ø38G
S32.Ø39D
S32.Ø39G
S32.Ø4ØD
S32.Ø4ØG
S32.Ø41D
S32.Ø41G
S32.Ø42D
S32.Ø42G
S32.Ø48D
S32.Ø48G
S32.Ø49D
S32.Ø49G
S32.Ø5ØD
S32.Ø5ØG
S32.Ø51D
S32.Ø51G
S32.Ø52D
S32.Ø52G
S32.Ø58D
S32.Ø58G
S32.Ø59D
S32.Ø59G
S32.1ØXD
S32.1ØXG
S32.11ØD
S32.11ØG
S32.111D
S32.111G
S32.112D
S32.112G
S32.119D
S32.119G
S32.12ØD
S32.12ØG
S32.121D
S32.121G
S32.122D
S32.122G
S32.129D
S32.129G
S32.13ØD
S32.13ØG
S32.131D
S32.131G
S32.132D
S32.132G
S32.139D
S32.139G
S32.14XD
S32.14XG
S32.15XD
S32.15XG
S32.16XD
S32.16XG
S32.17XD
S32.17XG
S32.19XD
S32.19XG
S32.2XXD
S32.2XXG
S32.3Ø1D
S32.3Ø1G
S32.3Ø2D
S32.3Ø2G
S32.3Ø9D
S32.3Ø9G
S32.311D
S32.311G
S32.312D
S32.312G
S32.313D
S32.313G
S32.314D
S32.314G
S32.315D
S32.315G
S32.316D
S32.316G
S32.391D
S32.391G
S32.392D
S32.392G
S32.399D
S32.399G
S32.4Ø1D
S32.4Ø1G
S32.4Ø2D
S32.4Ø2G
S32.4Ø9D
S32.4Ø9G
S32.411D
S32.411G
S32.412D
S32.412G
S32.413D
S32.413G
S32.414D
S32.414G
S32.415D
S32.415G
S32.416D
S32.416G
S32.421D
S32.421G
S32.422D
S32.422G
S32.423D
S32.423G
S32.424D
S32.424G
S32.425D
S32.425G
S32.426D
S32.426G
S32.431D
S32.431G
S32.432D
S32.432G
S32.433D
S32.433G
S32.434D
S32.434G
S32.435D
S32.435G
S32.436D
S32.436G
S32.441D
S32.441G
S32.442D
S32.442G
S32.443D
S32.443G
S32.444D
S32.444G
S32.445D
S32.445G
S32.446D
S32.446G
S32.451D
S32.451G
S32.452D
S32.452G
S32.453D
S32.453G
S32.454D
S32.454G
S32.455D
S32.455G
S32.456D
S32.456G
S32.461D
S32.461G
S32.462D
S32.462G
S32.463D
S32.463G
S32.464D
S32.464G
S32.465D
S32.465G
S32.466D
S32.466G
S32.471D
S32.471G
S32.472D
S32.472G
S32.473D
S32.473G
S32.474D
S32.474G
S32.475D
S32.475G
S32.476D
S32.476G
S32.481D
S32.481G
S32.482D
S32.482G
S32.483D
S32.483G
S32.484D
S32.484G
S32.485D
S32.485G
S32.486D
S32.486G
S32.491D
S32.491G
S32.492D
S32.492G
S32.499D
S32.499G
S32.5Ø1D
S32.5Ø1G
S32.5Ø2D
S32.5Ø2G
S32.5Ø9D
S32.5Ø9G
S32.511D
S32.511G
S32.512D
S32.512G
S32.519D
S32.519G
S32.591D
S32.591G
S32.592D
S32.592G
S32.599D
S32.599G
S32.6Ø1D
S32.6Ø1G
S32.6Ø2D
S32.6Ø2G
S32.6Ø9D
S32.6Ø9G
S32.611D
S32.611G
S32.612D
S32.612G
S32.613D
S32.613G
S32.614D
S32.614G
S32.615D
S32.615G
S32.616D
S32.616G
S32.691D
S32.691G
S32.692D
S32.692G
S32.699D
S32.699G
S32.81ØD
S32.81ØG
S32.811D
S32.811G
S32.82XD
S32.82XG
S32.89XD
S32.89XG
S32.9XXD
S32.9XXG
S42.ØØ1D
S42.ØØ1G
S42.ØØ1S
S42.ØØ2D
S42.ØØ2G
S42.ØØ2S
S42.ØØ9D
S42.ØØ9G
S42.ØØ9S
S42.Ø11D
S42.Ø11G
S42.Ø11S
S42.Ø12D
S42.Ø12G

S42.012S
S42.013D
S42.013G
S42.013S
S42.014D
S42.014G
S42.014S
S42.015D
S42.015G
S42.015S
S42.016D
S42.016G
S42.016S
S42.017D
S42.017G
S42.017S
S42.018D
S42.018G
S42.018S
S42.019D
S42.019G
S42.019S
S42.021D
S42.021G
S42.021S
S42.022D
S42.022G
S42.022S
S42.023D
S42.023G
S42.023S
S42.024D
S42.024G
S42.024S
S42.025D
S42.025G
S42.025S
S42.026D
S42.026G
S42.026S
S42.031D
S42.031G
S42.031S
S42.032D
S42.032G
S42.032S
S42.033D
S42.033G
S42.033S
S42.034D
S42.034G
S42.034S
S42.035D
S42.035G
S42.035S
S42.036D
S42.036G
S42.036S
S42.101D
S42.101G
S42.101S
S42.102D
S42.102G
S42.102S
S42.109D
S42.109G
S42.109S
S42.111D
S42.111G
S42.111S
S42.112D
S42.112G
S42.112S
S42.113D
S42.113G
S42.113S
S42.114D
S42.114G
S42.114S
S42.115D
S42.115G
S42.115S
S42.116D
S42.116G
S42.116S
S42.121D
S42.121G
S42.121S
S42.122D
S42.122G
S42.122S
S42.123D
S42.123G
S42.123S
S42.124D
S42.124G
S42.124S
S42.125D
S42.125G
S42.125S
S42.126D
S42.126G
S42.126S
S42.131D
S42.131G
S42.131S
S42.132D
S42.132G
S42.132S
S42.133D
S42.133G
S42.133S
S42.134D
S42.134G
S42.134S
S42.135D
S42.135G
S42.135S
S42.136D
S42.136G
S42.136S
S42.141D
S42.141G
S42.141S
S42.142D
S42.142G
S42.142S
S42.143D
S42.143G
S42.143S
S42.144D
S42.144G
S42.144S
S42.145D
S42.145G
S42.145S
S42.146D
S42.146G
S42.146S
S42.151D
S42.151G
S42.151S
S42.152D
S42.152G
S42.152S
S42.153D
S42.153G
S42.153S
S42.154D
S42.154G
S42.154S
S42.155D
S42.155G
S42.155S
S42.156D
S42.156G
S42.156S
S42.191D
S42.191G
S42.191S
S42.192D
S42.192G
S42.192S
S42.199D
S42.199G
S42.199S
S42.201D
S42.201G
S42.201S
S42.202D
S42.202G
S42.202S
S42.209D
S42.209G
S42.209S
S42.211D
S42.211G
S42.211S
S42.212D
S42.212G
S42.212S
S42.213D
S42.213G
S42.213S
S42.214D
S42.214G
S42.214S
S42.215D
S42.215G
S42.215S
S42.216D
S42.216G
S42.216S
S42.221D
S42.221G
S42.221S
S42.222D
S42.222G
S42.222S
S42.223D
S42.223G
S42.223S
S42.224D
S42.224G
S42.224S
S42.225D
S42.225G
S42.225S
S42.226D
S42.226G
S42.226S
S42.231D
S42.231G
S42.231S
S42.232D
S42.232G
S42.232S
S42.239D
S42.239G
S42.239S
S42.241D
S42.241G
S42.241S
S42.242D
S42.242G
S42.242S
S42.249D
S42.249G
S42.249S
S42.251D
S42.251G
S42.251S
S42.252D
S42.252G
S42.252S
S42.253D
S42.253G
S42.253S
S42.254D
S42.254G
S42.254S
S42.255D
S42.255G
S42.255S
S42.256D
S42.256G
S42.256S
S42.261D
S42.261G
S42.261S
S42.262D
S42.262G
S42.262S
S42.263D
S42.263G
S42.263S
S42.264D
S42.264G
S42.264S
S42.265D
S42.265G
S42.265S
S42.266D
S42.266G
S42.266S
S42.271D
S42.271G
S42.271S
S42.272D
S42.272G
S42.272S
S42.279D
S42.279G
S42.279S
S42.291D
S42.291G
S42.291S
S42.292D
S42.292G
S42.292S
S42.293D
S42.293G
S42.293S
S42.294D
S42.294G
S42.294S
S42.295D
S42.295G
S42.295S
S42.296D
S42.296G
S42.296S
S42.301D
S42.301G
S42.301S
S42.302D
S42.302G
S42.302S
S42.309D
S42.309G
S42.309S
S42.311D
S42.311G
S42.311S
S42.312D
S42.312G
S42.312S
S42.319D
S42.319G
S42.319S
S42.321D
S42.321G
S42.321S
S42.322D
S42.322G
S42.322S
S42.323D
S42.323G
S42.323S
S42.324D
S42.324G
S42.324S
S42.325D
S42.325G
S42.325S
S42.326D
S42.326G
S42.326S
S42.331D
S42.331G
S42.331S
S42.332D
S42.332G
S42.332S
S42.333D
S42.333G
S42.333S
S42.334D
S42.334G
S42.334S
S42.335D
S42.335G
S42.335S
S42.336D
S42.336G
S42.336S
S42.341D
S42.341G
S42.341S
S42.342D
S42.342G
S42.342S
S42.343D
S42.343G
S42.343S
S42.344D
S42.344G
S42.344S
S42.345D
S42.345G
S42.345S
S42.346D
S42.346G
S42.346S
S42.351D
S42.351G
S42.351S
S42.352D
S42.352G
S42.352S
S42.353D
S42.353G
S42.353S
S42.354D
S42.354G
S42.354S
S42.355D
S42.355G
S42.355S
S42.356D
S42.356G
S42.356S
S42.361D
S42.361G
S42.361S
S42.362D
S42.362G
S42.362S
S42.363D
S42.363G
S42.363S
S42.364D
S42.364G
S42.364S
S42.365D
S42.365G
S42.365S
S42.366D
S42.366G
S42.366S
S42.391D
S42.391G
S42.391S
S42.392D
S42.392G
S42.392S
S42.399D
S42.399G
S42.399S
S42.401D
S42.401G
S42.401S
S42.402D
S42.402G
S42.402S
S42.409D
S42.409G
S42.409S
S42.411D
S42.411G
S42.411S
S42.412D
S42.412G
S42.412S
S42.413D
S42.413G
S42.413S
S42.414D
S42.414G
S42.414S
S42.415D
S42.415G
S42.415S
S42.416D
S42.416G
S42.416S
S42.421D
S42.421G
S42.421S
S42.422D
S42.422G
S42.422S
S42.423D
S42.423G
S42.423S
S42.424D
S42.424G
S42.424S
S42.425D
S42.425G
S42.425S
S42.426D
S42.426G
S42.426S
S42.431D
S42.431G
S42.431S
S42.432D
S42.432G
S42.432S
S42.433D
S42.433G
S42.433S
S42.434D
S42.434G
S42.434S
S42.435D
S42.435G
S42.435S
S42.436D
S42.436G
S42.436S
S42.441D
S42.441G
S42.441S
S42.442D
S42.442G
S42.442S
S42.443D
S42.443G
S42.443S
S42.444D
S42.444G
S42.444S
S42.445D
S42.445G
S42.445S
S42.446D
S42.446G
S42.446S
S42.447D
S42.447G
S42.447S
S42.448D
S42.448G
S42.448S
S42.449D
S42.449G
S42.449S
S42.451D
S42.451G
S42.451S
S42.452D
S42.452G
S42.452S
S42.453D
S42.453G
S42.453S
S42.454D
S42.454G
S42.454S
S42.455D
S42.455G
S42.455S
S42.456D
S42.456G
S42.456S
S42.461D
S42.461G
S42.461S
S42.462D
S42.462G
S42.462S
S42.463D
S42.463G
S42.463S
S42.464D
S42.464G
S42.464S
S42.465D
S42.465G
S42.465S
S42.466D
S42.466G
S42.466S
S42.471D
S42.471G
S42.471S
S42.472D
S42.472G
S42.472S
S42.473D
S42.473G
S42.473S
S42.474D
S42.474G
S42.474S
S42.475D
S42.475G
S42.475S
S42.476D
S42.476G
S42.476S
S42.481D
S42.481G
S42.481S
S42.482D
S42.482G
S42.482S
S42.489D
S42.489G
S42.489S
S42.491D
S42.491G
S42.491S
S42.492D
S42.492G
S42.492S
S42.493D
S42.493G
S42.493S
S42.494D
S42.494G
S42.494S
S42.495D
S42.495G
S42.495S
S42.496D
S42.496G
S42.496S
S42.90XD
S42.90XG
S42.90XS
S42.91XD
S42.91XG
S42.91XS
S42.92XD
S42.92XG
S42.92XS
S48.011S
S48.012S
S48.019S
S48.021S
S48.022S
S48.029S
S48.111S
S48.112S
S48.119S
S48.121S
S48.122S
S48.129S
S48.911S
S48.912S
S48.919S
S48.921S
S48.922S
S48.929S
S49.001D
S49.001G
S49.001S
S49.002D
S49.002G
S49.002S
S49.009D
S49.009G
S49.009S
S49.011D
S49.011G
S49.011S
S49.012D
S49.012G
S49.012S
S49.019D
S49.019G
S49.019S
S49.021D
S49.021G
S49.021S
S49.022D
S49.022G
S49.022S
S49.029D
S49.029G
S49.029S
S49.031D
S49.031G
S49.031S
S49.032D
S49.032G
S49.032S
S49.039D
S49.039G
S49.039S
S49.041D
S49.041G
S49.041S
S49.042D
S49.042G
S49.042S
S49.049D
S49.049G
S49.049S
S49.091D
S49.091G
S49.091S
S49.092D
S49.092G
S49.092S
S49.099D
S49.099G
S49.099S
S49.101D
S49.101G
S49.101S
S49.102D
S49.102G
S49.102S
S49.109D
S49.109G
S49.109S
S49.111D
S49.111G
S49.111S
S49.112D
S49.112G
S49.112S
S49.119D
S49.119G
S49.119S
S49.121D
S49.121G
S49.121S
S49.122D
S49.122G
S49.122S
S49.129D
S49.129G
S49.129S
S49.131D
S49.131G
S49.131S
S49.132D
S49.132G
S49.132S
S49.139D
S49.139G
S49.139S
S49.141D
S49.141G
S49.141S
S49.142D
S49.142G
S49.142S
S49.149D
S49.149G
S49.149S
S49.191D
S49.191G
S49.191S
S49.192D
S49.192G
S49.192S
S49.199D
S49.199G
S49.199S
S52.001D
S52.001E
S52.001F
S52.001G
S52.001H
S52.001J
S52.001S
S52.002D
S52.002E
S52.002F
S52.002G
S52.002H
S52.002J
S52.002S
S52.009D
S52.009E
S52.009F
S52.009G
S52.009H
S52.009J
S52.009S
S52.011D
S52.011G
S52.011S
S52.012D
S52.012G
S52.012S
S52.019D
S52.019G
S52.019S
S52.021D
S52.021E
S52.021F
S52.021G
S52.021H
S52.021J
S52.021S
S52.022D
S52.022E
S52.022F
S52.022G
S52.022H
S52.022J
S52.022S
S52.023D
S52.023E
S52.023F
S52.023G
S52.023H
S52.023J
S52.023S
S52.024D
S52.024E
S52.024F
S52.024G
S52.024H
S52.024J
S52.024S
S52.025D
S52.025E
S52.025F
S52.025G
S52.025H
S52.025J
S52.025S
S52.026D
S52.026E
S52.026F
S52.026G
S52.026H
S52.026J
S52.026S
S52.031D
S52.031E
S52.031F
S52.031G
S52.031H
S52.031J
S52.031S
S52.032D
S52.032E
S52.032F
S52.032G
S52.032H
S52.032J
S52.032S
S52.033D
S52.033E
S52.033F
S52.033G
S52.033H
S52.033J
S52.033S
S52.034D
S52.034E
S52.034F
S52.034G
S52.034H
S52.034J
S52.034S
S52.035D
S52.035E
S52.035F
S52.035G
S52.035H
S52.035J
S52.035S
S52.036D
S52.036E
S52.036F
S52.036G
S52.036H
S52.036J
S52.036S
S52.041D
S52.041E
S52.041F
S52.041G
S52.041H
S52.041J
S52.041S
S52.042D
S52.042E
S52.042F
S52.042G
S52.042H
S52.042J
S52.042S
S52.043D
S52.043E
S52.043F
S52.043G
S52.043H
S52.043J
S52.043S
S52.044D
S52.044E
S52.044F
S52.044G
S52.044H

S52.044J
S52.044S
S52.045D
S52.045E
S52.045F
S52.045G
S52.045H
S52.045J
S52.045S
S52.046D
S52.046E
S52.046F
S52.046G
S52.046H
S52.046J
S52.046S
S52.091D
S52.091E
S52.091F
S52.091G
S52.091H
S52.091J
S52.091S
S52.092D
S52.092E
S52.092F
S52.092G
S52.092H
S52.092J
S52.092S
S52.099D
S52.099E
S52.099F
S52.099G
S52.099H
S52.099J
S52.099S
S52.101D
S52.101E
S52.101F
S52.101G
S52.101H
S52.101J
S52.101S
S52.102D
S52.102E
S52.102F
S52.102G
S52.102H
S52.102J
S52.102S
S52.109D
S52.109E
S52.109F
S52.109G
S52.109H
S52.109J
S52.109S
S52.111D
S52.111G
S52.111S
S52.112D
S52.112G
S52.112S
S52.119D
S52.119G
S52.119S
S52.121D
S52.121E
S52.121F
S52.121G
S52.121H
S52.121J
S52.121S
S52.122D
S52.122E
S52.122F
S52.122G
S52.122H
S52.122J
S52.122S
S52.123D
S52.123E
S52.123F
S52.123G
S52.123H
S52.123J
S52.123S
S52.124D
S52.124E
S52.124F
S52.124G
S52.124H
S52.124J
S52.124S
S52.125D
S52.125E
S52.125F
S52.125G
S52.125H
S52.125J
S52.125S
S52.126D
S52.126E
S52.126F
S52.126G
S52.126H
S52.126J
S52.126S
S52.131D
S52.131E
S52.131F
S52.131G
S52.131H
S52.131J
S52.131S
S52.132D
S52.132E
S52.132F
S52.132G
S52.132H
S52.132J
S52.132S
S52.133D
S52.133E
S52.133F
S52.133G
S52.133H
S52.133J
S52.133S
S52.134D
S52.134E
S52.134F
S52.134G
S52.134H
S52.134J
S52.134S
S52.135D
S52.135E
S52.135F
S52.135G
S52.135H
S52.135J
S52.135S
S52.136D
S52.136E
S52.136F
S52.136G
S52.136H
S52.136J
S52.136S
S52.181D
S52.181E
S52.181F
S52.181G
S52.181H
S52.181J
S52.181S
S52.182D
S52.182E
S52.182F
S52.182G
S52.182H
S52.182J
S52.182S
S52.189D
S52.189E
S52.189F
S52.189G
S52.189H
S52.189J
S52.189S
S52.201D
S52.201E
S52.201F
S52.201G
S52.201H
S52.201J
S52.201S
S52.202D
S52.202E
S52.202F
S52.202G
S52.202H
S52.202J
S52.202S
S52.209D
S52.209E
S52.209F
S52.209G
S52.209H
S52.209J
S52.209S
S52.211D
S52.211G
S52.211S
S52.212D
S52.212G
S52.212S
S52.219D
S52.219G
S52.219S
S52.221D
S52.221E
S52.221F
S52.221G
S52.221H
S52.221J
S52.221S
S52.222D
S52.222E
S52.222F
S52.222G
S52.222H
S52.222J
S52.222S
S52.223D
S52.223E
S52.223F
S52.223G
S52.223H
S52.223J
S52.223S
S52.224D
S52.224E
S52.224F
S52.224G
S52.224H
S52.224J
S52.224S
S52.225D
S52.225E
S52.225F
S52.225G
S52.225H
S52.225J
S52.225S
S52.226D
S52.226E
S52.226F
S52.226G
S52.226H
S52.226J
S52.226S
S52.231D
S52.231E
S52.231F
S52.231G
S52.231H
S52.231J
S52.231S
S52.232D
S52.232E
S52.232F
S52.232G
S52.232H
S52.232J
S52.232S
S52.233D
S52.233E
S52.233F
S52.233G
S52.233H
S52.233J
S52.233S
S52.234D
S52.234E
S52.234F
S52.234G
S52.234H
S52.234J
S52.234S
S52.235D
S52.235E
S52.235F
S52.235G
S52.235H
S52.235J
S52.235S
S52.236D
S52.236E
S52.236F
S52.236G
S52.236H
S52.236J
S52.236S
S52.241D
S52.241E
S52.241F
S52.241G
S52.241H
S52.241J
S52.241S
S52.242D
S52.242E
S52.242F
S52.242G
S52.242H
S52.242J
S52.242S
S52.243D
S52.243E
S52.243F
S52.243G
S52.243H
S52.243J
S52.243S
S52.244D
S52.244E
S52.244F
S52.244G
S52.244H
S52.244J
S52.244S
S52.245D
S52.245E
S52.245F
S52.245G
S52.245H
S52.245J
S52.245S
S52.246D
S52.246E
S52.246F
S52.246G
S52.246H
S52.246J
S52.246S
S52.251D
S52.251E
S52.251F
S52.251G
S52.251H
S52.251J
S52.251S
S52.252D
S52.252E
S52.252F
S52.252G
S52.252H
S52.252J
S52.252S
S52.253D
S52.253E
S52.253F
S52.253G
S52.253H
S52.253J
S52.253S
S52.254D
S52.254E
S52.254F
S52.254G
S52.254H
S52.254J
S52.254S
S52.255D
S52.255E
S52.255F
S52.255G
S52.255H
S52.255J
S52.255S
S52.256D
S52.256E
S52.256F
S52.256G
S52.256H
S52.256J
S52.256S
S52.261D
S52.261E
S52.261F
S52.261G
S52.261H
S52.261J
S52.261S
S52.262D
S52.262E
S52.262F
S52.262G
S52.262H
S52.262J
S52.262S
S52.263D
S52.263E
S52.263F
S52.263G
S52.263H
S52.263J
S52.263S
S52.264D
S52.264E
S52.264F
S52.264G
S52.264H
S52.264J
S52.264S
S52.265D
S52.265E
S52.265F
S52.265G
S52.265H
S52.265J
S52.265S
S52.266D
S52.266E
S52.266F
S52.266G
S52.266H
S52.266J
S52.266S
S52.271D
S52.271E
S52.271F
S52.271G
S52.271H
S52.271J
S52.271S
S52.272D
S52.272E
S52.272F
S52.272G
S52.272H
S52.272J
S52.272S
S52.279D
S52.279E
S52.279F
S52.279G
S52.279H
S52.279J
S52.279S
S52.281D
S52.281E
S52.281F
S52.281G
S52.281H
S52.281J
S52.281S
S52.282D
S52.282E
S52.282F
S52.282G
S52.282H
S52.282J
S52.282S
S52.283D
S52.283E
S52.283F
S52.283G
S52.283H
S52.283J
S52.283S
S52.291D
S52.291E
S52.291F
S52.291G
S52.291H
S52.291J
S52.291S
S52.292D
S52.292E
S52.292F
S52.292G
S52.292H
S52.292J
S52.292S
S52.299D
S52.299E
S52.299F
S52.299G
S52.299H
S52.299J
S52.299S
S52.301D
S52.301E
S52.301F
S52.301G
S52.301H
S52.301J
S52.301S
S52.302D
S52.302E
S52.302F
S52.302G
S52.302H
S52.302J
S52.302S
S52.309D
S52.309E
S52.309F
S52.309G
S52.309H
S52.309J
S52.309S
S52.311D
S52.311G
S52.311S
S52.312D
S52.312G
S52.312S
S52.319D
S52.319G
S52.319S
S52.321D
S52.321E
S52.321F
S52.321G
S52.321H
S52.321J
S52.321S
S52.322D
S52.322E
S52.322F
S52.322G
S52.322H
S52.322J
S52.322S
S52.323D
S52.323E
S52.323F
S52.323G
S52.323H
S52.323J
S52.323S
S52.324D
S52.324E
S52.324F
S52.324G
S52.324H
S52.324J
S52.324S
S52.325D
S52.325E
S52.325F
S52.325G
S52.325H
S52.325J
S52.325S
S52.326D
S52.326E
S52.326F
S52.326G
S52.326H
S52.326J
S52.326S
S52.331D
S52.331E
S52.331F
S52.331G
S52.331H
S52.331J
S52.331S
S52.332D
S52.332E
S52.332F
S52.332G
S52.332H
S52.332J
S52.332S
S52.333D
S52.333E
S52.333F
S52.333G
S52.333H
S52.333J
S52.333S
S52.334D
S52.334E
S52.334F
S52.334G
S52.334H
S52.334J
S52.334S
S52.335D
S52.335E
S52.335F
S52.335G
S52.335H
S52.335J
S52.335S
S52.336D
S52.336E
S52.336F
S52.336G
S52.336H
S52.336J
S52.336S
S52.341D
S52.341E
S52.341F
S52.341G
S52.341H
S52.341J
S52.341S
S52.342D
S52.342E
S52.342F
S52.342G
S52.342H
S52.342J
S52.342S
S52.343D
S52.343E
S52.343F
S52.343G
S52.343H
S52.343J
S52.343S
S52.344D
S52.344E
S52.344F
S52.344G
S52.344H
S52.344J
S52.344S
S52.345D
S52.345E
S52.345F
S52.345G
S52.345H
S52.345J
S52.345S
S52.346D
S52.346E
S52.346F
S52.346G
S52.346H
S52.346J
S52.346S
S52.351D
S52.351E
S52.351F
S52.351G
S52.351H
S52.351J
S52.351S
S52.352D
S52.352E
S52.352F
S52.352G
S52.352H
S52.352J
S52.352S
S52.353D
S52.353E
S52.353F
S52.353G
S52.353H
S52.353J
S52.353S
S52.354D
S52.354E
S52.354F
S52.354G
S52.354H
S52.354J
S52.354S
S52.355D
S52.355E
S52.355F
S52.355G
S52.355H
S52.355J
S52.355S
S52.356D
S52.356E
S52.356F
S52.356G
S52.356H
S52.356J
S52.356S
S52.361D
S52.361E
S52.361F
S52.361G
S52.361H
S52.361J
S52.361S
S52.362D
S52.362E
S52.362F
S52.362G
S52.362H
S52.362J
S52.362S
S52.363D
S52.363E
S52.363F
S52.363G
S52.363H
S52.363J
S52.363S
S52.364D
S52.364E
S52.364F
S52.364G
S52.364H
S52.364J
S52.364S
S52.365D
S52.365E
S52.365F
S52.365G
S52.365H
S52.365J
S52.365S
S52.366D
S52.366E
S52.366F
S52.366G
S52.366H
S52.366J
S52.366S
S52.371D
S52.371E
S52.371F
S52.371G
S52.371H
S52.371J
S52.371S
S52.372D
S52.372E
S52.372F
S52.372G
S52.372H
S52.372J
S52.372S
S52.379D
S52.379E
S52.379F
S52.379G
S52.379H
S52.379J
S52.379S
S52.381D
S52.381E
S52.381F
S52.381G
S52.381H
S52.381J
S52.381S
S52.382D
S52.382E
S52.382F
S52.382G
S52.382H
S52.382J
S52.382S
S52.389D
S52.389E
S52.389F
S52.389G
S52.389H
S52.389J
S52.389S
S52.391D
S52.391E
S52.391F
S52.391G
S52.391H
S52.391J
S52.391S
S52.392D
S52.392E
S52.392F
S52.392G
S52.392H
S52.392J
S52.392S
S52.399D
S52.399E
S52.399F
S52.399G
S52.399H
S52.399J
S52.399S
S52.501D
S52.501E
S52.501F
S52.501G
S52.501H
S52.501J
S52.501S
S52.502D
S52.502E
S52.502F
S52.502G
S52.502H
S52.502J
S52.502S
S52.509D
S52.509E
S52.509F
S52.509G
S52.509H
S52.509J
S52.509S
S52.511D
S52.511E
S52.511F
S52.511G
S52.511H
S52.511J
S52.511S
S52.512D
S52.512E
S52.512F
S52.512G
S52.512H
S52.512J
S52.512S
S52.513D
S52.513E
S52.513F
S52.513G
S52.513H
S52.513J
S52.513S
S52.514D
S52.514E
S52.514F
S52.514G
S52.514H
S52.514J
S52.514S
S52.515D
S52.515E
S52.515F
S52.515G
S52.515H
S52.515J
S52.515S
S52.516D
S52.516E
S52.516F
S52.516G
S52.516H
S52.516J
S52.516S
S52.521D
S52.521G
S52.521S
S52.522D
S52.522G
S52.522S
S52.529D
S52.529G
S52.529S
S52.531D
S52.531E
S52.531F
S52.531G
S52.531H

S52.531J
S52.531S
S52.532D
S52.532E
S52.532F
S52.532G
S52.532H
S52.532J
S52.532S
S52.539D
S52.539E
S52.539F
S52.539G
S52.539H
S52.539J
S52.539S
S52.541D
S52.541E
S52.541F
S52.541G
S52.541H
S52.541J
S52.541S
S52.542D
S52.542E
S52.542F
S52.542G
S52.542H
S52.542J
S52.542S
S52.549D
S52.549E
S52.549F
S52.549G
S52.549H
S52.549J
S52.549S
S52.551D
S52.551E
S52.551F
S52.551G
S52.551H
S52.551J
S52.551S
S52.552D
S52.552E
S52.552F
S52.552G
S52.552H
S52.552J
S52.552S
S52.559D
S52.559E
S52.559F
S52.559G
S52.559H
S52.559J
S52.559S
S52.561D
S52.561E
S52.561F
S52.561G
S52.561H
S52.561J
S52.561S
S52.562D
S52.562E
S52.562F
S52.562G
S52.562H
S52.562J
S52.562S
S52.569D
S52.569E
S52.569F
S52.569G
S52.569H
S52.569J
S52.569S
S52.571D
S52.571E
S52.571F
S52.571G
S52.571H
S52.571J
S52.571S
S52.572D
S52.572E
S52.572F
S52.572G
S52.572H
S52.572J
S52.572S
S52.579D
S52.579E
S52.579F
S52.579G
S52.579H
S52.579J
S52.579S
S52.591D
S52.591E
S52.591F
S52.591G
S52.591H
S52.591J
S52.591S
S52.592D
S52.592E
S52.592F
S52.592G
S52.592H
S52.592J
S52.592S
S52.599D
S52.599E
S52.599F
S52.599G
S52.599H
S52.599J
S52.599S
S52.601D
S52.601E
S52.601F
S52.601G
S52.601H
S52.601J
S52.601S
S52.602D
S52.602E
S52.602F
S52.602G
S52.602H
S52.602J
S52.602S
S52.609D
S52.609E
S52.609F
S52.609G
S52.609H
S52.609J
S52.609S
S52.611D
S52.611E
S52.611F
S52.611G
S52.611H
S52.611J
S52.611S
S52.612D
S52.612E
S52.612F
S52.612G
S52.612H
S52.612J
S52.612S
S52.613D
S52.613E
S52.613F
S52.613G
S52.613H
S52.613J
S52.613S
S52.614D
S52.614E
S52.614F
S52.614G
S52.614H
S52.614J
S52.614S
S52.615D
S52.615E
S52.615F
S52.615G
S52.615H
S52.615J
S52.615S
S52.616D
S52.616E
S52.616F
S52.616G
S52.616H
S52.616J
S52.616S
S52.621D
S52.621G
S52.621S
S52.622D
S52.622G
S52.622S
S52.629D
S52.629G
S52.629S
S52.691D
S52.691E
S52.691F
S52.691G
S52.691H
S52.691J
S52.691S
S52.692D
S52.692E
S52.692F
S52.692G
S52.692H
S52.692J
S52.692S
S52.699D
S52.699E
S52.699F
S52.699G
S52.699H
S52.699J
S52.699S
S52.90XD
S52.90XE
S52.90XF
S52.90XG
S52.90XH
S52.90XJ
S52.90XS
S52.91XD
S52.91XE
S52.91XF
S52.91XG
S52.91XH
S52.91XJ
S52.91XS
S52.92XD
S52.92XE
S52.92XF
S52.92XG
S52.92XH
S52.92XJ
S52.92XS
S58.011S
S58.012S
S58.019S
S58.021S
S58.022S
S58.029S
S58.111S
S58.112S
S58.119S
S58.121S
S58.122S
S58.129S
S58.911S
S58.912S
S58.919S
S58.921S
S58.922S
S58.929S
S59.001D
S59.001G
S59.001S
S59.002D
S59.002G
S59.002S
S59.009D
S59.009G
S59.009S
S59.011D
S59.011G
S59.011S
S59.012D
S59.012G
S59.012S
S59.019D
S59.019G
S59.019S
S59.021D
S59.021G
S59.021S
S59.022D
S59.022G
S59.022S
S59.029D
S59.029G
S59.029S
S59.031D
S59.031G
S59.031S
S59.032D
S59.032G
S59.032S
S59.039D
S59.039G
S59.039S
S59.041D
S59.041G
S59.041S
S59.042D
S59.042G
S59.042S
S59.049D
S59.049G
S59.049S
S59.091D
S59.091G
S59.091S
S59.092D
S59.092G
S59.092S
S59.099D
S59.099G
S59.099S
S59.101D
S59.101G
S59.101S
S59.102D
S59.102G
S59.102S
S59.109D
S59.109G
S59.109S
S59.111D
S59.111G
S59.111S
S59.112D
S59.112G
S59.112S
S59.119D
S59.119G
S59.119S
S59.121D
S59.121G
S59.121S
S59.122D
S59.122G
S59.122S
S59.129D
S59.129G
S59.129S
S59.131D
S59.131G
S59.131S
S59.132D
S59.132G
S59.132S
S59.139D
S59.139G
S59.139S
S59.141D
S59.141G
S59.141S
S59.142D
S59.142G
S59.142S
S59.149D
S59.149G
S59.149S
S59.191D
S59.191G
S59.191S
S59.192D
S59.192G
S59.192S
S59.199D
S59.199G
S59.199S
S59.201D
S59.201G
S59.201S
S59.202D
S59.202G
S59.202S
S59.209D
S59.209G
S59.209S
S59.211D
S59.211G
S59.211S
S59.212D
S59.212G
S59.212S
S59.219D
S59.219G
S59.219S
S59.221D
S59.221G
S59.221S
S59.222D
S59.222G
S59.222S
S59.229D
S59.229G
S59.229S
S59.231D
S59.231G
S59.231S
S59.232D
S59.232G
S59.232S
S59.239D
S59.239G
S59.239S
S59.241D
S59.241G
S59.241S
S59.242D
S59.242G
S59.242S
S59.249D
S59.249G
S59.249S
S59.291D
S59.291G
S59.291S
S59.292D
S59.292G
S59.292S
S59.299D
S59.299G
S59.299S
S62.001D
S62.001G
S62.001S
S62.002D
S62.002G
S62.002S
S62.009D
S62.009G
S62.009S
S62.011D
S62.011G
S62.011S
S62.012D
S62.012G
S62.012S
S62.013D
S62.013G
S62.013S
S62.014D
S62.014G
S62.014S
S62.015D
S62.015G
S62.015S
S62.016D
S62.016G
S62.016S
S62.021D
S62.021G
S62.021S
S62.022D
S62.022G
S62.022S
S62.023D
S62.023G
S62.023S
S62.024D
S62.024G
S62.024S
S62.025D
S62.025G
S62.025S
S62.026D
S62.026G
S62.026S
S62.031D
S62.031G
S62.031S
S62.032D
S62.032G
S62.032S
S62.033D
S62.033G
S62.033S
S62.034D
S62.034G
S62.034S
S62.035D
S62.035G
S62.035S
S62.036D
S62.036G
S62.036S
S62.101D
S62.101G
S62.101S
S62.102D
S62.102G
S62.102S
S62.109D
S62.109G
S62.109S
S62.111D
S62.111G
S62.111S
S62.112D
S62.112G
S62.112S
S62.113D
S62.113G
S62.113S
S62.114D
S62.114G
S62.114S
S62.115D
S62.115G
S62.115S
S62.116D
S62.116G
S62.116S
S62.121D
S62.121G
S62.121S
S62.122D
S62.122G
S62.122S
S62.123D
S62.123G
S62.123S
S62.124D
S62.124G
S62.124S
S62.125D
S62.125G
S62.125S
S62.126D
S62.126G
S62.126S
S62.131D
S62.131G
S62.131S
S62.132D
S62.132G
S62.132S
S62.133D
S62.133G
S62.133S
S62.134D
S62.134G
S62.134S
S62.135D
S62.135G
S62.135S
S62.136D
S62.136G
S62.136S
S62.141D
S62.141G
S62.141S
S62.142D
S62.142G
S62.142S
S62.143D
S62.143G
S62.143S
S62.144D
S62.144G
S62.144S
S62.145D
S62.145G
S62.145S
S62.146D
S62.146G
S62.146S
S62.151D
S62.151G
S62.151S
S62.152D
S62.152G
S62.152S
S62.153D
S62.153G
S62.153S
S62.154D
S62.154G
S62.154S
S62.155D
S62.155G
S62.155S
S62.156D
S62.156G
S62.156S
S62.161D
S62.161G
S62.161S
S62.162D
S62.162G
S62.162S
S62.163D
S62.163G
S62.163S
S62.164D
S62.164G
S62.164S
S62.165D
S62.165G
S62.165S
S62.166D
S62.166G
S62.166S
S62.171D
S62.171G
S62.171S
S62.172D
S62.172G
S62.172S
S62.173D
S62.173G
S62.173S
S62.174D
S62.174G
S62.174S
S62.175D
S62.175G
S62.175S
S62.176D
S62.176G
S62.176S
S62.181D
S62.181G
S62.181S
S62.182D
S62.182G
S62.182S
S62.183D
S62.183G
S62.183S
S62.184D
S62.184G
S62.184S
S62.185D
S62.185G
S62.185S
S62.186D
S62.186G
S62.186S
S62.201D
S62.201G
S62.201S
S62.202D
S62.202G
S62.202S
S62.209D
S62.209G
S62.209S
S62.211D
S62.211G
S62.211S
S62.212D
S62.212G
S62.212S
S62.213D
S62.213G
S62.213S
S62.221D
S62.221G
S62.221S
S62.222D
S62.222G
S62.222S
S62.223D
S62.223G
S62.223S
S62.224D
S62.224G
S62.224S
S62.225D
S62.225G
S62.225S
S62.226D
S62.226G
S62.226S
S62.231D
S62.231G
S62.231S
S62.232D
S62.232G
S62.232S
S62.233D
S62.233G
S62.233S
S62.234D
S62.234G
S62.234S
S62.235D
S62.235G
S62.235S
S62.236D
S62.236G
S62.236S
S62.241D
S62.241G
S62.241S
S62.242D
S62.242G
S62.242S
S62.243D
S62.243G
S62.243S
S62.244D
S62.244G
S62.244S
S62.245D
S62.245G
S62.245S
S62.246D
S62.246G
S62.246S
S62.251D
S62.251G
S62.251S
S62.252D
S62.252G
S62.252S
S62.253D
S62.253G
S62.253S
S62.254D
S62.254G
S62.254S
S62.255D
S62.255G
S62.255S
S62.256D
S62.256G
S62.256S
S62.291D
S62.291G
S62.291S
S62.292D
S62.292G
S62.292S
S62.299D
S62.299G
S62.299S
S62.300D
S62.300G
S62.300S
S62.301D
S62.301G
S62.301S
S62.302D
S62.302G
S62.302S
S62.303D
S62.303G
S62.303S
S62.304D
S62.304G
S62.304S
S62.305D
S62.305G
S62.305S
S62.306D
S62.306G
S62.306S
S62.307D
S62.307G
S62.307S
S62.308D
S62.308G
S62.308S
S62.309D
S62.309G
S62.309S
S62.310D
S62.310G
S62.310S
S62.311D
S62.311G
S62.311S
S62.312D
S62.312G
S62.312S
S62.313D
S62.313G
S62.313S
S62.314D
S62.314G
S62.314S
S62.315D
S62.315G
S62.315S
S62.316D
S62.316G
S62.316S
S62.317D
S62.317G
S62.317S
S62.318D
S62.318G
S62.318S
S62.319D
S62.319G
S62.319S
S62.320D
S62.320G
S62.320S
S62.321D
S62.321G
S62.321S
S62.322D
S62.322G
S62.322S
S62.323D
S62.323G
S62.323S
S62.324D
S62.324G
S62.324S
S62.325D
S62.325G
S62.325S
S62.326D
S62.326G
S62.326S
S62.327D
S62.327G
S62.327S
S62.328D
S62.328G
S62.328S
S62.329D
S62.329G
S62.329S
S62.330D
S62.330G
S62.330S
S62.331D
S62.331G
S62.331S
S62.332D
S62.332G
S62.332S
S62.333D
S62.333G
S62.333S
S62.334D
S62.334G
S62.334S
S62.335D
S62.335G
S62.335S
S62.336D
S62.336G
S62.336S
S62.337D
S62.337G
S62.337S
S62.338D
S62.338G
S62.338S
S62.339D
S62.339G
S62.339S
S62.340D
S62.340G
S62.340S
S62.341D
S62.341G

S62.341S
S62.342D
S62.342G
S62.342S
S62.343D
S62.343G
S62.343S
S62.344D
S62.344G
S62.344S
S62.345D
S62.345G
S62.345S
S62.346D
S62.346G
S62.346S
S62.347D
S62.347G
S62.347S
S62.348D
S62.348G
S62.348S
S62.349D
S62.349G
S62.349S
S62.350D
S62.350G
S62.350S
S62.351D
S62.351G
S62.351S
S62.352D
S62.352G
S62.352S
S62.353D
S62.353G
S62.353S
S62.354D
S62.354G
S62.354S
S62.355D
S62.355G
S62.355S
S62.356D
S62.356G
S62.356S
S62.357D
S62.357G
S62.357S
S62.358D
S62.358G
S62.358S
S62.359D
S62.359G
S62.359S
S62.360D
S62.360G
S62.360S
S62.361D
S62.361G
S62.361S
S62.362D
S62.362G
S62.362S
S62.363D
S62.363G
S62.363S
S62.364D
S62.364G
S62.364S
S62.365D
S62.365G
S62.365S
S62.366D
S62.366G
S62.366S
S62.367D
S62.367G
S62.367S
S62.368D
S62.368G
S62.368S
S62.369D
S62.369G
S62.369S
S62.390D
S62.390G
S62.390S
S62.391D
S62.391G
S62.391S
S62.392D
S62.392G
S62.392S
S62.393D
S62.393G
S62.393S
S62.394D
S62.394G
S62.394S
S62.395D
S62.395G
S62.395S
S62.396D
S62.396G
S62.396S
S62.397D
S62.397G
S62.397S
S62.398D
S62.398G
S62.398S
S62.399D
S62.399G
S62.399S
S62.501D
S62.501G
S62.501S
S62.502D
S62.502G
S62.502S
S62.509D
S62.509G
S62.509S
S62.511D
S62.511G
S62.511S
S62.512D
S62.512G
S62.512S
S62.513D
S62.513G
S62.513S
S62.514D
S62.514G
S62.514S
S62.515D
S62.515G
S62.515S
S62.516D
S62.516G
S62.516S
S62.521D
S62.521G
S62.521S
S62.522D
S62.522G
S62.522S
S62.523D
S62.523G
S62.523S
S62.524D
S62.524G
S62.524S
S62.525D
S62.525G
S62.525S
S62.526D
S62.526G
S62.526S
S62.600D
S62.600G
S62.600S
S62.601D
S62.601G
S62.601S
S62.602D
S62.602G
S62.602S
S62.603D
S62.603G
S62.603S
S62.604D
S62.604G
S62.604S
S62.605D
S62.605G
S62.605S
S62.606D
S62.606G
S62.606S
S62.607D
S62.607G
S62.607S
S62.608D
S62.608G
S62.608S
S62.609D
S62.609G
S62.609S
S62.610D
S62.610G
S62.610S
S62.611D
S62.611G
S62.611S
S62.612D
S62.612G
S62.612S
S62.613D
S62.613G
S62.613S
S62.614D
S62.614G
S62.614S
S62.615D
S62.615G
S62.615S
S62.616D
S62.616G
S62.616S
S62.617D
S62.617G
S62.617S
S62.618D
S62.618G
S62.618S
S62.619D
S62.619G
S62.619S
S62.620D
S62.620G
S62.620S
S62.621D
S62.621G
S62.621S
S62.622D
S62.622G
S62.622S
S62.623D
S62.623G
S62.623S
S62.624D
S62.624G
S62.624S
S62.625D
S62.625G
S62.625S
S62.626D
S62.626G
S62.626S
S62.627D
S62.627G
S62.627S
S62.628D
S62.628G
S62.628S
S62.629D
S62.629G
S62.629S
S62.630D
S62.630G
S62.630S
S62.631D
S62.631G
S62.631S
S62.632D
S62.632G
S62.632S
S62.633D
S62.633G
S62.633S
S62.634D
S62.634G
S62.634S
S62.635D
S62.635G
S62.635S
S62.636D
S62.636G
S62.636S
S62.637D
S62.637G
S62.637S
S62.638D
S62.638G
S62.638S
S62.639D
S62.639G
S62.639S
S62.640D
S62.640G
S62.640S
S62.641D
S62.641G
S62.641S
S62.642D
S62.642G
S62.642S
S62.643D
S62.643G
S62.643S
S62.644D
S62.644G
S62.644S
S62.645D
S62.645G
S62.645S
S62.646D
S62.646G
S62.646S
S62.647D
S62.647G
S62.647S
S62.648D
S62.648G
S62.648S
S62.649D
S62.649G
S62.649S
S62.650D
S62.650G
S62.650S
S62.651D
S62.651G
S62.651S
S62.652D
S62.652G
S62.652S
S62.653D
S62.653G
S62.653S
S62.654D
S62.654G
S62.654S
S62.655D
S62.655G
S62.655S
S62.656D
S62.656G
S62.656S
S62.657D
S62.657G
S62.657S
S62.658D
S62.658G
S62.658S
S62.659D
S62.659G
S62.659S
S62.660D
S62.660G
S62.660S
S62.661D
S62.661G
S62.661S
S62.662D
S62.662G
S62.662S
S62.663D
S62.663G
S62.663S
S62.664D
S62.664G
S62.664S
S62.665D
S62.665G
S62.665S
S62.666D
S62.666G
S62.666S
S62.667D
S62.667G
S62.667S
S62.668D
S62.668G
S62.668S
S62.669D
S62.669G
S62.669S
S62.90XD
S62.90XG
S62.90XS
S62.91XD
S62.91XG
S62.91XS
S62.92XD
S62.92XG
S62.92XS
S68.011S
S68.012S
S68.019S
S68.021S
S68.022S
S68.029S
S68.110S
S68.111S
S68.112S
S68.113S
S68.114S
S68.115S
S68.116S
S68.117S
S68.118S
S68.119S
S68.120S
S68.121S
S68.122S
S68.123S
S68.124S
S68.125S
S68.126S
S68.127S
S68.128S
S68.129S
S68.411S
S68.412S
S68.419S
S68.421S
S68.422S
S68.429S
S68.511S
S68.512S
S68.519S
S68.521S
S68.522S
S68.529S
S68.610S
S68.611S
S68.612S
S68.613S
S68.614S
S68.615S
S68.616S
S68.617S
S68.618S
S68.619S
S68.620S
S68.621S
S68.622S
S68.623S
S68.624S
S68.625S
S68.626S
S68.627S
S68.628S
S68.629S
S68.711S
S68.712S
S68.719S
S68.721S
S68.722S
S68.729S
S72.001D
S72.001E
S72.001F
S72.001G
S72.001H
S72.001J
S72.001S
S72.002D
S72.002E
S72.002F
S72.002G
S72.002H
S72.002J
S72.002S
S72.009D
S72.009E
S72.009F
S72.009G
S72.009H
S72.009J
S72.009S
S72.011D
S72.011E
S72.011F
S72.011G
S72.011H
S72.011J
S72.011S
S72.012D
S72.012E
S72.012F
S72.012G
S72.012H
S72.012J
S72.012S
S72.019D
S72.019E
S72.019F
S72.019G
S72.019H
S72.019J
S72.019S
S72.021D
S72.021E
S72.021F
S72.021G
S72.021H
S72.021J
S72.021S
S72.022D
S72.022E
S72.022F
S72.022G
S72.022H
S72.022J
S72.022S
S72.023D
S72.023E
S72.023F
S72.023G
S72.023H
S72.023J
S72.023S
S72.024D
S72.024E
S72.024F
S72.024G
S72.024H
S72.024J
S72.024S
S72.025D
S72.025E
S72.025F
S72.025G
S72.025H
S72.025J
S72.025S
S72.026D
S72.026E
S72.026F
S72.026G
S72.026H
S72.026J
S72.026S
S72.031D
S72.031E
S72.031F
S72.031G
S72.031H
S72.031J
S72.031S
S72.032D
S72.032E
S72.032F
S72.032G
S72.032H
S72.032J
S72.032S
S72.033D
S72.033E
S72.033F
S72.033G
S72.033H
S72.033J
S72.033S
S72.034D
S72.034E
S72.034F
S72.034G
S72.034H
S72.034J
S72.034S
S72.035D
S72.035E
S72.035F
S72.035G
S72.035H
S72.035J
S72.035S
S72.036D
S72.036E
S72.036F
S72.036G
S72.036H
S72.036J
S72.036S
S72.041D
S72.041E
S72.041F
S72.041G
S72.041H
S72.041J
S72.041S
S72.042D
S72.042E
S72.042F
S72.042G
S72.042H
S72.042J
S72.042S
S72.043D
S72.043E
S72.043F
S72.043G
S72.043H
S72.043J
S72.043S
S72.044D
S72.044E
S72.044F
S72.044G
S72.044H
S72.044J
S72.044S
S72.045D
S72.045E
S72.045F
S72.045G
S72.045H
S72.045J
S72.045S
S72.046D
S72.046E
S72.046F
S72.046G
S72.046H
S72.046J
S72.046S
S72.051D
S72.051E
S72.051F
S72.051G
S72.051H
S72.051J
S72.051S
S72.052D
S72.052E
S72.052F
S72.052G
S72.052H
S72.052J
S72.052S
S72.059D
S72.059E
S72.059F
S72.059G
S72.059H
S72.059J
S72.059S
S72.061D
S72.061E
S72.061F
S72.061G
S72.061H
S72.061J
S72.061S
S72.062D
S72.062E
S72.062F
S72.062G
S72.062H
S72.062J
S72.062S
S72.063D
S72.063E
S72.063F
S72.063G
S72.063H
S72.063J
S72.063S
S72.064D
S72.064E
S72.064F
S72.064G
S72.064H
S72.064J
S72.064S
S72.065D
S72.065E
S72.065F
S72.065G
S72.065H
S72.065J
S72.065S
S72.066D
S72.066E
S72.066F
S72.066G
S72.066H
S72.066J
S72.066S
S72.091D
S72.091E
S72.091F
S72.091G
S72.091H
S72.091J
S72.091S
S72.092D
S72.092E
S72.092F
S72.092G
S72.092H
S72.092J
S72.092S
S72.099D
S72.099E
S72.099F
S72.099G
S72.099H
S72.099J
S72.099S
S72.101D
S72.101E
S72.101F
S72.101G
S72.101H
S72.101J
S72.101S
S72.102D
S72.102E
S72.102F
S72.102G
S72.102H
S72.102J
S72.102S
S72.109D
S72.109E
S72.109F
S72.109G
S72.109H
S72.109J
S72.109S
S72.111D
S72.111E
S72.111F
S72.111G
S72.111H
S72.111J
S72.111S
S72.112D
S72.112E
S72.112F
S72.112G
S72.112H
S72.112J
S72.112S
S72.113D
S72.113E
S72.113F
S72.113G
S72.113H
S72.113J
S72.113S
S72.114D
S72.114E
S72.114F
S72.114G
S72.114H
S72.114J
S72.114S
S72.115D
S72.115E
S72.115F
S72.115G
S72.115H
S72.115J
S72.115S
S72.116D
S72.116E
S72.116F
S72.116G
S72.116H
S72.116J
S72.116S
S72.121D
S72.121E
S72.121F
S72.121G
S72.121H
S72.121J
S72.121S
S72.122D
S72.122E
S72.122F
S72.122G
S72.122H
S72.122J
S72.122S
S72.123D
S72.123E
S72.123F
S72.123G
S72.123H
S72.123J
S72.123S
S72.124D
S72.124E
S72.124F
S72.124G
S72.124H
S72.124J
S72.124S
S72.125D
S72.125E
S72.125F
S72.125G
S72.125H
S72.125J
S72.125S
S72.126D
S72.126E
S72.126F
S72.126G
S72.126H
S72.126J
S72.126S
S72.131D
S72.131E
S72.131F
S72.131G
S72.131H
S72.131J
S72.131S
S72.132D
S72.132E
S72.132F
S72.132G
S72.132H
S72.132J
S72.132S
S72.133D
S72.133E
S72.133F
S72.133G
S72.133H
S72.133J
S72.133S
S72.134D
S72.134E
S72.134F
S72.134G
S72.134H
S72.134J
S72.134S
S72.135D
S72.135E
S72.135F
S72.135G
S72.135H
S72.135J
S72.135S
S72.136D
S72.136E
S72.136F
S72.136G
S72.136H
S72.136J
S72.136S
S72.141D
S72.141E
S72.141F
S72.141G
S72.141H
S72.141J
S72.141S
S72.142D
S72.142E
S72.142F
S72.142G
S72.142H
S72.142J

S72.142S
S72.143D
S72.143E
S72.143F
S72.143G
S72.143H
S72.143J
S72.143S
S72.144D
S72.144E
S72.144F
S72.144G
S72.144H
S72.144J
S72.144S
S72.145D
S72.145E
S72.145F
S72.145G
S72.145H
S72.145J
S72.145S
S72.146D
S72.146E
S72.146F
S72.146G
S72.146H
S72.146J
S72.146S
S72.21XD
S72.21XE
S72.21XF
S72.21XG
S72.21XH
S72.21XJ
S72.21XS
S72.22XD
S72.22XE
S72.22XF
S72.22XG
S72.22XH
S72.22XJ
S72.22XS
S72.23XD
S72.23XE
S72.23XF
S72.23XG
S72.23XH
S72.23XJ
S72.23XS
S72.24XD
S72.24XE
S72.24XF
S72.24XG
S72.24XH
S72.24XJ
S72.24XS
S72.25XD
S72.25XE
S72.25XF
S72.25XG
S72.25XH
S72.25XJ
S72.25XS
S72.26XD
S72.26XE
S72.26XF
S72.26XG
S72.26XH
S72.26XJ
S72.26XS
S72.3Ø1D
S72.3Ø1E
S72.3Ø1F
S72.3Ø1G
S72.3Ø1H
S72.3Ø1J
S72.3Ø1S
S72.3Ø2D
S72.3Ø2E
S72.3Ø2F
S72.3Ø2G
S72.3Ø2H
S72.3Ø2J
S72.3Ø2S
S72.3Ø9D
S72.3Ø9E
S72.3Ø9F
S72.3Ø9G
S72.3Ø9H
S72.3Ø9J
S72.3Ø9S
S72.321D
S72.321E
S72.321F
S72.321G
S72.321H
S72.321J
S72.321S
S72.322D
S72.322E
S72.322F
S72.322G
S72.322H
S72.322J
S72.322S
S72.323D
S72.323E
S72.323F
S72.323G
S72.323H
S72.323J
S72.323S
S72.324D
S72.324E
S72.324F
S72.324G
S72.324H
S72.324J
S72.324S
S72.325D
S72.325E
S72.325F
S72.325G
S72.325H
S72.325J
S72.325S
S72.326D
S72.326E
S72.326F
S72.326G
S72.326H
S72.326J
S72.326S
S72.331D
S72.331E
S72.331F
S72.331G
S72.331H
S72.331J
S72.331S
S72.332D
S72.332E
S72.332F
S72.332G
S72.332H
S72.332J
S72.332S
S72.333D
S72.333E
S72.333F
S72.333G
S72.333H
S72.333J
S72.333S
S72.334D
S72.334E
S72.334F
S72.334G
S72.334H
S72.334J
S72.334S
S72.335D
S72.335E
S72.335F
S72.335G
S72.335H
S72.335J
S72.335S
S72.336D
S72.336E
S72.336F
S72.336G
S72.336H
S72.336J
S72.336S
S72.341D
S72.341E
S72.341F
S72.341G
S72.341H
S72.341J
S72.341S
S72.342D
S72.342E
S72.342F
S72.342G
S72.342H
S72.342J
S72.342S
S72.343D
S72.343E
S72.343F
S72.343G
S72.343H
S72.343J
S72.343S
S72.344D
S72.344E
S72.344F
S72.344G
S72.344H
S72.344J
S72.344S
S72.345D
S72.345E
S72.345F
S72.345G
S72.345H
S72.345J
S72.345S
S72.346D
S72.346E
S72.346F
S72.346G
S72.346H
S72.346J
S72.346S
S72.351D
S72.351E
S72.351F
S72.351G
S72.351H
S72.351J
S72.351S
S72.352D
S72.352E
S72.352F
S72.352G
S72.352H
S72.352J
S72.352S
S72.353D
S72.353E
S72.353F
S72.353G
S72.353H
S72.353J
S72.353S
S72.354D
S72.354E
S72.354F
S72.354G
S72.354H
S72.354J
S72.354S
S72.355D
S72.355E
S72.355F
S72.355G
S72.355H
S72.355J
S72.355S
S72.356D
S72.356E
S72.356F
S72.356G
S72.356H
S72.356J
S72.356S
S72.361D
S72.361E
S72.361F
S72.361G
S72.361H
S72.361J
S72.361S
S72.362D
S72.362E
S72.362F
S72.362G
S72.362H
S72.362J
S72.362S
S72.363D
S72.363E
S72.363F
S72.363G
S72.363H
S72.363J
S72.363S
S72.364D
S72.364E
S72.364F
S72.364G
S72.364H
S72.364J
S72.364S
S72.365D
S72.365E
S72.365F
S72.365G
S72.365H
S72.365J
S72.365S
S72.366D
S72.366E
S72.366F
S72.366G
S72.366H
S72.366J
S72.366S
S72.391D
S72.391E
S72.391F
S72.391G
S72.391H
S72.391J
S72.391S
S72.392D
S72.392E
S72.392F
S72.392G
S72.392H
S72.392J
S72.392S
S72.399D
S72.399E
S72.399F
S72.399G
S72.399H
S72.399J
S72.399S
S72.4Ø1D
S72.4Ø1E
S72.4Ø1F
S72.4Ø1G
S72.4Ø1H
S72.4Ø1J
S72.4Ø1S
S72.4Ø2D
S72.4Ø2E
S72.4Ø2F
S72.4Ø2G
S72.4Ø2H
S72.4Ø2J
S72.4Ø2S
S72.4Ø9D
S72.4Ø9E
S72.4Ø9F
S72.4Ø9G
S72.4Ø9H
S72.4Ø9J
S72.4Ø9S
S72.411D
S72.411E
S72.411F
S72.411G
S72.411H
S72.411J
S72.411S
S72.412D
S72.412E
S72.412F
S72.412G
S72.412H
S72.412J
S72.412S
S72.413D
S72.413E
S72.413F
S72.413G
S72.413H
S72.413J
S72.413S
S72.414D
S72.414E
S72.414F
S72.414G
S72.414H
S72.414J
S72.414S
S72.415D
S72.415E
S72.415F
S72.415G
S72.415H
S72.415J
S72.415S
S72.416D
S72.416E
S72.416F
S72.416G
S72.416H
S72.416J
S72.416S
S72.421D
S72.421E
S72.421F
S72.421G
S72.421H
S72.421J
S72.421S
S72.422D
S72.422E
S72.422F
S72.422G
S72.422H
S72.422J
S72.422S
S72.423D
S72.423E
S72.423F
S72.423G
S72.423H
S72.423J
S72.423S
S72.424D
S72.424E
S72.424F
S72.424G
S72.424H
S72.424J
S72.424S
S72.425D
S72.425E
S72.425F
S72.425G
S72.425H
S72.425J
S72.425S
S72.426D
S72.426E
S72.426F
S72.426G
S72.426H
S72.426J
S72.426S
S72.431D
S72.431E
S72.431F
S72.431G
S72.431H
S72.431J
S72.431S
S72.432D
S72.432E
S72.432F
S72.432G
S72.432H
S72.432J
S72.432S
S72.433D
S72.433E
S72.433F
S72.433G
S72.433H
S72.433J
S72.433S
S72.434D
S72.434E
S72.434F
S72.434G
S72.434H
S72.434J
S72.434S
S72.435D
S72.435E
S72.435F
S72.435G
S72.435H
S72.435J
S72.435S
S72.436D
S72.436E
S72.436F
S72.436G
S72.436H
S72.436J
S72.436S
S72.441D
S72.441E
S72.441F
S72.441G
S72.441H
S72.441J
S72.441S
S72.442D
S72.442E
S72.442F
S72.442G
S72.442H
S72.442J
S72.442S
S72.443D
S72.443E
S72.443F
S72.443G
S72.443H
S72.443J
S72.443S
S72.444D
S72.444E
S72.444F
S72.444G
S72.444H
S72.444J
S72.444S
S72.445D
S72.445E
S72.445F
S72.445G
S72.445H
S72.445J
S72.445S
S72.446D
S72.446E
S72.446F
S72.446G
S72.446H
S72.446J
S72.446S
S72.451D
S72.451E
S72.451F
S72.451G
S72.451H
S72.451J
S72.451S
S72.452D
S72.452E
S72.452F
S72.452G
S72.452H
S72.452J
S72.452S
S72.453D
S72.453E
S72.453F
S72.453G
S72.453H
S72.453J
S72.453S
S72.454D
S72.454E
S72.454F
S72.454G
S72.454H
S72.454J
S72.454S
S72.455D
S72.455E
S72.455F
S72.455G
S72.455H
S72.455J
S72.455S
S72.456D
S72.456E
S72.456F
S72.456G
S72.456H
S72.456J
S72.456S
S72.461D
S72.461E
S72.461F
S72.461G
S72.461H
S72.461J
S72.461S
S72.462D
S72.462E
S72.462F
S72.462G
S72.462H
S72.462J
S72.462S
S72.463D
S72.463E
S72.463F
S72.463G
S72.463H
S72.463J
S72.463S
S72.464D
S72.464E
S72.464F
S72.464G
S72.464H
S72.464J
S72.464S
S72.465D
S72.465E
S72.465F
S72.465G
S72.465H
S72.465J
S72.465S
S72.466D
S72.466E
S72.466F
S72.466G
S72.466H
S72.466J
S72.466S
S72.471D
S72.471G
S72.471S
S72.472D
S72.472G
S72.472S
S72.479D
S72.479G
S72.479S
S72.491D
S72.491E
S72.491F
S72.491G
S72.491H
S72.491J
S72.491S
S72.492D
S72.492E
S72.492F
S72.492G
S72.492H
S72.492J
S72.492S
S72.499D
S72.499E
S72.499F
S72.499G
S72.499H
S72.499J
S72.499S
S72.8X1D
S72.8X1E
S72.8X1F
S72.8X1G
S72.8X1H
S72.8X1J
S72.8X1S
S72.8X2D
S72.8X2E
S72.8X2F
S72.8X2G
S72.8X2H
S72.8X2J
S72.8X2S
S72.8X9D
S72.8X9E
S72.8X9F
S72.8X9G
S72.8X9H
S72.8X9J
S72.8X9S
S72.9ØXD
S72.9ØXE
S72.9ØXF
S72.9ØXG
S72.9ØXH
S72.9ØXJ
S72.9ØXS
S72.91XD
S72.91XE
S72.91XF
S72.91XG
S72.91XH
S72.91XJ
S72.91XS
S72.92XD
S72.92XE
S72.92XF
S72.92XG
S72.92XH
S72.92XJ
S72.92XS
S78.Ø11S
S78.Ø12S
S78.Ø19S
S78.Ø21S
S78.Ø22S
S78.Ø29S
S78.111S
S78.112S
S78.119S
S78.121S
S78.122S
S78.129S
S78.911S
S78.912S
S78.919S
S78.921S
S78.922S
S78.929S
S79.ØØ1D
S79.ØØ1G
S79.ØØ1S
S79.ØØ2D
S79.ØØ2G
S79.ØØ2S
S79.ØØ9D
S79.ØØ9G
S79.ØØ9S
S79.Ø11D
S79.Ø11G
S79.Ø11S
S79.Ø12D
S79.Ø12G
S79.Ø12S
S79.Ø19D
S79.Ø19G
S79.Ø19S
S79.Ø91D
S79.Ø91G
S79.Ø91S
S79.Ø92D
S79.Ø92G
S79.Ø92S
S79.Ø99D
S79.Ø99G
S79.Ø99S
S79.1Ø1D
S79.1Ø1G
S79.1Ø1S
S79.1Ø2D
S79.1Ø2G
S79.1Ø2S
S79.1Ø9D
S79.1Ø9G
S79.1Ø9S
S79.111D
S79.111G
S79.111S
S79.112D
S79.112G
S79.112S
S79.119D
S79.119G
S79.119S
S79.121D
S79.121G
S79.121S
S79.122D
S79.122G
S79.122S
S79.129D
S79.129G
S79.129S
S79.131D
S79.131G
S79.131S
S79.132D
S79.132G
S79.132S
S79.139D
S79.139G
S79.139S
S79.141D
S79.141G
S79.141S
S79.142D
S79.142G
S79.142S
S79.149D
S79.149G
S79.149S
S79.191D
S79.191G
S79.191S
S79.192D
S79.192G
S79.192S
S79.199D
S79.199G
S79.199S
S82.ØØ1D
S82.ØØ1E
S82.ØØ1F
S82.ØØ1G
S82.ØØ1H
S82.ØØ1J
S82.ØØ1S
S82.ØØ2D
S82.ØØ2E
S82.ØØ2F
S82.ØØ2G
S82.ØØ2H
S82.ØØ2J
S82.ØØ2S
S82.ØØ9D
S82.ØØ9E
S82.ØØ9F
S82.ØØ9G
S82.ØØ9H
S82.ØØ9J
S82.ØØ9S
S82.Ø11D
S82.Ø11E
S82.Ø11F
S82.Ø11G
S82.Ø11H
S82.Ø11J
S82.Ø11S
S82.Ø12D
S82.Ø12E
S82.Ø12F
S82.Ø12G
S82.Ø12H
S82.Ø12J
S82.Ø12S
S82.Ø13D
S82.Ø13E
S82.Ø13F
S82.Ø13G
S82.Ø13H
S82.Ø13J
S82.Ø13S
S82.Ø14D
S82.Ø14E
S82.Ø14F
S82.Ø14G
S82.Ø14H
S82.Ø14J
S82.Ø14S
S82.Ø15D
S82.Ø15E
S82.Ø15F
S82.Ø15G
S82.Ø15H
S82.Ø15J
S82.Ø15S
S82.Ø16D
S82.Ø16E
S82.Ø16F
S82.Ø16G
S82.Ø16H
S82.Ø16J
S82.Ø16S
S82.Ø21D
S82.Ø21E
S82.Ø21F
S82.Ø21G
S82.Ø21H
S82.Ø21J
S82.Ø21S
S82.Ø22D
S82.Ø22E
S82.Ø22F
S82.Ø22G
S82.Ø22H
S82.Ø22J
S82.Ø22S
S82.Ø23D
S82.Ø23E
S82.Ø23F
S82.Ø23G
S82.Ø23H
S82.Ø23J
S82.Ø23S
S82.Ø24D
S82.Ø24E
S82.Ø24F
S82.Ø24G

S82.024H
S82.024J
S82.024S
S82.025D
S82.025E
S82.025F
S82.025G
S82.025H
S82.025J
S82.025S
S82.026D
S82.026E
S82.026F
S82.026G
S82.026H
S82.026J
S82.026S
S82.031D
S82.031E
S82.031F
S82.031G
S82.031H
S82.031J
S82.031S
S82.032D
S82.032E
S82.032F
S82.032G
S82.032H
S82.032J
S82.032S
S82.033D
S82.033E
S82.033F
S82.033G
S82.033H
S82.033J
S82.033S
S82.034D
S82.034E
S82.034F
S82.034G
S82.034H
S82.034J
S82.034S
S82.035D
S82.035E
S82.035F
S82.035G
S82.035H
S82.035J
S82.035S
S82.036D
S82.036E
S82.036F
S82.036G
S82.036H
S82.036J
S82.036S
S82.041D
S82.041E
S82.041F
S82.041G
S82.041H
S82.041J
S82.041S
S82.042D
S82.042E
S82.042F
S82.042G
S82.042H
S82.042J
S82.042S
S82.043D
S82.043E
S82.043F
S82.043G
S82.043H
S82.043J
S82.043S
S82.044D
S82.044E
S82.044F
S82.044G
S82.044H
S82.044J
S82.044S
S82.045D
S82.045E
S82.045F
S82.045G
S82.045H
S82.045J
S82.045S
S82.046D
S82.046E
S82.046F
S82.046G
S82.046H
S82.046J
S82.046S
S82.091D
S82.091E
S82.091F
S82.091G
S82.091H
S82.091J
S82.091S
S82.092D
S82.092E
S82.092F
S82.092G
S82.092H
S82.092J
S82.092S
S82.099D
S82.099E
S82.099F
S82.099G
S82.099H
S82.099J
S82.099S
S82.101D
S82.101E
S82.101F
S82.101G
S82.101H
S82.101J
S82.101S
S82.102D
S82.102E
S82.102F
S82.102G
S82.102H
S82.102J
S82.102S
S82.109D
S82.109E
S82.109F
S82.109G
S82.109H
S82.109J
S82.109S
S82.111D
S82.111E
S82.111F
S82.111G
S82.111H
S82.111J
S82.111S
S82.112D
S82.112E
S82.112F
S82.112G
S82.112H
S82.112J
S82.112S
S82.113D
S82.113E
S82.113F
S82.113G
S82.113H
S82.113J
S82.113S
S82.114D
S82.114E
S82.114F
S82.114G
S82.114H
S82.114J
S82.114S
S82.115D
S82.115E
S82.115F
S82.115G
S82.115H
S82.115J
S82.115S
S82.116D
S82.116E
S82.116F
S82.116G
S82.116H
S82.116J
S82.116S
S82.121D
S82.121E
S82.121F
S82.121G
S82.121H
S82.121J
S82.121S
S82.122D
S82.122E
S82.122F
S82.122G
S82.122H
S82.122J
S82.122S
S82.123D
S82.123E
S82.123F
S82.123G
S82.123H
S82.123J
S82.123S
S82.124D
S82.124E
S82.124F
S82.124G
S82.124H
S82.124J
S82.124S
S82.125D
S82.125E
S82.125F
S82.125G
S82.125H
S82.125J
S82.125S
S82.126D
S82.126E
S82.126F
S82.126G
S82.126H
S82.126J
S82.126S
S82.131D
S82.131E
S82.131F
S82.131G
S82.131H
S82.131J
S82.131S
S82.132D
S82.132E
S82.132F
S82.132G
S82.132H
S82.132J
S82.132S
S82.133D
S82.133E
S82.133F
S82.133G
S82.133H
S82.133J
S82.133S
S82.134D
S82.134E
S82.134F
S82.134G
S82.134H
S82.134J
S82.134S
S82.135D
S82.135E
S82.135F
S82.135G
S82.135H
S82.135J
S82.135S
S82.136D
S82.136E
S82.136F
S82.136G
S82.136H
S82.136J
S82.136S
S82.141D
S82.141E
S82.141F
S82.141G
S82.141H
S82.141J
S82.141S
S82.142D
S82.142E
S82.142F
S82.142G
S82.142H
S82.142J
S82.142S
S82.143D
S82.143E
S82.143F
S82.143G
S82.143H
S82.143J
S82.143S
S82.144D
S82.144E
S82.144F
S82.144G
S82.144H
S82.144J
S82.144S
S82.145D
S82.145E
S82.145F
S82.145G
S82.145H
S82.145J
S82.145S
S82.146D
S82.146E
S82.146F
S82.146G
S82.146H
S82.146J
S82.146S
S82.151D
S82.151E
S82.151F
S82.151G
S82.151H
S82.151J
S82.151S
S82.152D
S82.152E
S82.152F
S82.152G
S82.152H
S82.152J
S82.152S
S82.153D
S82.153E
S82.153F
S82.153G
S82.153H
S82.153J
S82.153S
S82.154D
S82.154E
S82.154F
S82.154G
S82.154H
S82.154J
S82.154S
S82.155D
S82.155E
S82.155F
S82.155G
S82.155H
S82.155J
S82.155S
S82.156D
S82.156E
S82.156F
S82.156G
S82.156H
S82.156J
S82.156S
S82.161D
S82.161G
S82.161S
S82.162D
S82.162G
S82.162S
S82.169D
S82.169G
S82.169S
S82.191D
S82.191E
S82.191F
S82.191G
S82.191H
S82.191J
S82.191S
S82.192D
S82.192E
S82.192F
S82.192G
S82.192H
S82.192J
S82.192S
S82.199D
S82.199E
S82.199F
S82.199G
S82.199H
S82.199J
S82.199S
S82.201D
S82.201E
S82.201F
S82.201G
S82.201H
S82.201J
S82.201S
S82.202D
S82.202E
S82.202F
S82.202G
S82.202H
S82.202J
S82.202S
S82.209D
S82.209E
S82.209F
S82.209G
S82.209H
S82.209J
S82.209S
S82.221D
S82.221E
S82.221F
S82.221G
S82.221H
S82.221J
S82.221S
S82.222D
S82.222E
S82.222F
S82.222G
S82.222H
S82.222J
S82.222S
S82.223D
S82.223E
S82.223F
S82.223G
S82.223H
S82.223J
S82.223S
S82.224D
S82.224E
S82.224F
S82.224G
S82.224H
S82.224J
S82.224S
S82.225D
S82.225E
S82.225F
S82.225G
S82.225H
S82.225J
S82.225S
S82.226D
S82.226E
S82.226F
S82.226G
S82.226H
S82.226J
S82.226S
S82.231D
S82.231E
S82.231F
S82.231G
S82.231H
S82.231J
S82.231S
S82.232D
S82.232E
S82.232F
S82.232G
S82.232H
S82.232J
S82.232S
S82.233D
S82.233E
S82.233F
S82.233G
S82.233H
S82.233J
S82.233S
S82.234D
S82.234E
S82.234F
S82.234G
S82.234H
S82.234J
S82.234S
S82.235D
S82.235E
S82.235F
S82.235G
S82.235H
S82.235J
S82.235S
S82.236D
S82.236E
S82.236F
S82.236G
S82.236H
S82.236J
S82.236S
S82.241D
S82.241E
S82.241F
S82.241G
S82.241H
S82.241J
S82.241S
S82.242D
S82.242E
S82.242F
S82.242G
S82.242H
S82.242J
S82.242S
S82.243D
S82.243E
S82.243F
S82.243G
S82.243H
S82.243J
S82.243S
S82.244D
S82.244E
S82.244F
S82.244G
S82.244H
S82.244J
S82.244S
S82.245D
S82.245E
S82.245F
S82.245G
S82.245H
S82.245J
S82.245S
S82.246D
S82.246E
S82.246F
S82.246G
S82.246H
S82.246J
S82.246S
S82.251D
S82.251E
S82.251F
S82.251G
S82.251H
S82.251J
S82.251S
S82.252D
S82.252E
S82.252F
S82.252G
S82.252H
S82.252J
S82.252S
S82.253D
S82.253E
S82.253F
S82.253G
S82.253H
S82.253J
S82.253S
S82.254D
S82.254E
S82.254F
S82.254G
S82.254H
S82.254J
S82.254S
S82.255D
S82.255E
S82.255F
S82.255G
S82.255H
S82.255J
S82.255S
S82.256D
S82.256E
S82.256F
S82.256G
S82.256H
S82.256J
S82.256S
S82.261D
S82.261E
S82.261F
S82.261G
S82.261H
S82.261J
S82.261S
S82.262D
S82.262E
S82.262F
S82.262G
S82.262H
S82.262J
S82.262S
S82.263D
S82.263E
S82.263F
S82.263G
S82.263H
S82.263J
S82.263S
S82.264D
S82.264E
S82.264F
S82.264G
S82.264H
S82.264J
S82.264S
S82.265D
S82.265E
S82.265F
S82.265G
S82.265H
S82.265J
S82.265S
S82.266D
S82.266E
S82.266F
S82.266G
S82.266H
S82.266J
S82.266S
S82.291D
S82.291E
S82.291F
S82.291G
S82.291H
S82.291J
S82.291S
S82.292D
S82.292E
S82.292F
S82.292G
S82.292H
S82.292J
S82.292S
S82.299D
S82.299E
S82.299F
S82.299G
S82.299H
S82.299J
S82.299S
S82.301D
S82.301E
S82.301F
S82.301G
S82.301H
S82.301J
S82.301S
S82.302D
S82.302E
S82.302F
S82.302G
S82.302H
S82.302J
S82.302S
S82.309D
S82.309E
S82.309F
S82.309G
S82.309H
S82.309J
S82.309S
S82.311D
S82.311G
S82.311S
S82.312D
S82.312G
S82.312S
S82.319D
S82.319G
S82.319S
S82.391D
S82.391E
S82.391F
S82.391G
S82.391H
S82.391J
S82.391S
S82.392D
S82.392E
S82.392F
S82.392G
S82.392H
S82.392J
S82.392S
S82.399D
S82.399E
S82.399F
S82.399G
S82.399H
S82.399J
S82.399S
S82.401D
S82.401E
S82.401F
S82.401G
S82.401H
S82.401J
S82.401S
S82.402D
S82.402E
S82.402F
S82.402G
S82.402H
S82.402J
S82.402S
S82.409D
S82.409E
S82.409F
S82.409G
S82.409H
S82.409J
S82.409S
S82.421D
S82.421E
S82.421F
S82.421G
S82.421H
S82.421J
S82.421S
S82.422D
S82.422E
S82.422F
S82.422G
S82.422H
S82.422J
S82.422S
S82.423D
S82.423E
S82.423F
S82.423G
S82.423H
S82.423J
S82.423S
S82.424D
S82.424E
S82.424F
S82.424G
S82.424H
S82.424J
S82.424S
S82.425D
S82.425E
S82.425F
S82.425G
S82.425H
S82.425J
S82.425S
S82.426D
S82.426E
S82.426F
S82.426G
S82.426H
S82.426J
S82.426S
S82.431D
S82.431E
S82.431F
S82.431G
S82.431H
S82.431J
S82.431S
S82.432D
S82.432E
S82.432F
S82.432G
S82.432H
S82.432J
S82.432S
S82.433D
S82.433E
S82.433F
S82.433G
S82.433H
S82.433J
S82.433S
S82.434D
S82.434E
S82.434F
S82.434G
S82.434H
S82.434J
S82.434S
S82.435D
S82.435E
S82.435F
S82.435G
S82.435H
S82.435J
S82.435S
S82.436D
S82.436E
S82.436F
S82.436G
S82.436H
S82.436J
S82.436S
S82.441D
S82.441E
S82.441F
S82.441G
S82.441H
S82.441J
S82.441S
S82.442D
S82.442E
S82.442F
S82.442G
S82.442H
S82.442J
S82.442S
S82.443D
S82.443E
S82.443F
S82.443G
S82.443H
S82.443J
S82.443S
S82.444D
S82.444E
S82.444F
S82.444G
S82.444H
S82.444J
S82.444S
S82.445D
S82.445E
S82.445F
S82.445G
S82.445H
S82.445J
S82.445S
S82.446D
S82.446E
S82.446F
S82.446G
S82.446H
S82.446J
S82.446S
S82.451D
S82.451E
S82.451F
S82.451G
S82.451H
S82.451J
S82.451S
S82.452D
S82.452E
S82.452F
S82.452G
S82.452H
S82.452J
S82.452S
S82.453D
S82.453E
S82.453F
S82.453G
S82.453H
S82.453J
S82.453S
S82.454D

S82.454E
S82.454F
S82.454G
S82.454H
S82.454J
S82.454S
S82.455D
S82.455E
S82.455F
S82.455G
S82.455H
S82.455J
S82.455S
S82.456D
S82.456E
S82.456F
S82.456G
S82.456H
S82.456J
S82.456S
S82.461D
S82.461E
S82.461F
S82.461G
S82.461H
S82.461J
S82.461S
S82.462D
S82.462E
S82.462F
S82.462G
S82.462H
S82.462J
S82.462S
S82.463D
S82.463E
S82.463F
S82.463G
S82.463H
S82.463J
S82.463S
S82.464D
S82.464E
S82.464F
S82.464G
S82.464H
S82.464J
S82.464S
S82.465D
S82.465E
S82.465F
S82.465G
S82.465H
S82.465J
S82.465S
S82.466D
S82.466E
S82.466F
S82.466G
S82.466H
S82.466J
S82.466S
S82.491D
S82.491E
S82.491F
S82.491G
S82.491H
S82.491J
S82.491S
S82.492D
S82.492E
S82.492F
S82.492G
S82.492H
S82.492J
S82.492S
S82.499D
S82.499E
S82.499F
S82.499G
S82.499H
S82.499J
S82.499S
S82.51XD
S82.51XE
S82.51XF
S82.51XG
S82.51XH
S82.51XJ
S82.51XS
S82.52XD
S82.52XE
S82.52XF
S82.52XG
S82.52XH
S82.52XJ
S82.52XS
S82.53XD
S82.53XE
S82.53XF
S82.53XG
S82.53XH
S82.53XJ
S82.53XS
S82.54XD
S82.54XE
S82.54XF
S82.54XG
S82.54XH
S82.54XJ
S82.54XS
S82.55XD
S82.55XE
S82.55XF
S82.55XG
S82.55XH
S82.55XJ
S82.55XS
S82.56XD
S82.56XE
S82.56XF
S82.56XG
S82.56XH
S82.56XJ
S82.56XS
S82.61XD
S82.61XE
S82.61XF
S82.61XG
S82.61XH
S82.61XJ
S82.61XS
S82.62XD
S82.62XE
S82.62XF
S82.62XG
S82.62XH
S82.62XJ
S82.62XS
S82.63XD
S82.63XE
S82.63XF
S82.63XG
S82.63XH
S82.63XJ
S82.63XS
S82.64XD
S82.64XE
S82.64XF
S82.64XG
S82.64XH
S82.64XJ
S82.64XS
S82.65XD
S82.65XE
S82.65XF
S82.65XG
S82.65XH
S82.65XJ
S82.65XS
S82.66XD
S82.66XE
S82.66XF
S82.66XG
S82.66XH
S82.66XJ
S82.66XS
S82.811D
S82.811G
S82.811S
S82.812D
S82.812G
S82.812S
S82.819D
S82.819G
S82.819S
S82.821D
S82.821G
S82.821S
S82.822D
S82.822G
S82.822S
S82.829D
S82.829G
S82.829S
S82.831D
S82.831E
S82.831F
S82.831G
S82.831H
S82.831J
S82.831S
S82.832D
S82.832E
S82.832F
S82.832G
S82.832H
S82.832J
S82.832S
S82.839D
S82.839E
S82.839F
S82.839G
S82.839H
S82.839J
S82.839S
S82.841D
S82.841E
S82.841F
S82.841G
S82.841H
S82.841J
S82.841S
S82.842D
S82.842E
S82.842F
S82.842G
S82.842H
S82.842J
S82.842S
S82.843D
S82.843E
S82.843F
S82.843G
S82.843H
S82.843J
S82.843S
S82.844D
S82.844E
S82.844F
S82.844G
S82.844H
S82.844J
S82.844S
S82.845D
S82.845E
S82.845F
S82.845G
S82.845H
S82.845J
S82.845S
S82.846D
S82.846E
S82.846F
S82.846G
S82.846H
S82.846J
S82.846S
S82.851D
S82.851E
S82.851F
S82.851G
S82.851H
S82.851J
S82.851S
S82.852D
S82.852E
S82.852F
S82.852G
S82.852H
S82.852J
S82.852S
S82.853D
S82.853E
S82.853F
S82.853G
S82.853H
S82.853J
S82.853S
S82.854D
S82.854E
S82.854F
S82.854G
S82.854H
S82.854J
S82.854S
S82.855D
S82.855E
S82.855F
S82.855G
S82.855H
S82.855J
S82.855S
S82.856D
S82.856E
S82.856F
S82.856G
S82.856H
S82.856J
S82.856S
S82.861D
S82.861E
S82.861F
S82.861G
S82.861H
S82.861J
S82.861S
S82.862D
S82.862E
S82.862F
S82.862G
S82.862H
S82.862J
S82.862S
S82.863D
S82.863E
S82.863F
S82.863G
S82.863H
S82.863J
S82.863S
S82.864D
S82.864E
S82.864F
S82.864G
S82.864H
S82.864J
S82.864S
S82.865D
S82.865E
S82.865F
S82.865G
S82.865H
S82.865J
S82.865S
S82.866D
S82.866E
S82.866F
S82.866G
S82.866H
S82.866J
S82.866S
S82.871D
S82.871E
S82.871F
S82.871G
S82.871H
S82.871J
S82.871S
S82.872D
S82.872E
S82.872F
S82.872G
S82.872H
S82.872J
S82.872S
S82.873D
S82.873E
S82.873F
S82.873G
S82.873H
S82.873J
S82.873S
S82.874D
S82.874E
S82.874F
S82.874G
S82.874H
S82.874J
S82.874S
S82.875D
S82.875E
S82.875F
S82.875G
S82.875H
S82.875J
S82.875S
S82.876D
S82.876E
S82.876F
S82.876G
S82.876H
S82.876J
S82.876S
S82.891D
S82.891E
S82.891F
S82.891G
S82.891H
S82.891J
S82.891S
S82.892D
S82.892E
S82.892F
S82.892G
S82.892H
S82.892J
S82.892S
S82.899D
S82.899E
S82.899F
S82.899G
S82.899H
S82.899J
S82.899S
S82.9ØXD
S82.9ØXE
S82.9ØXF
S82.9ØXG
S82.9ØXH
S82.9ØXJ
S82.9ØXS
S82.91XD
S82.91XE
S82.91XF
S82.91XG
S82.91XH
S82.91XJ
S82.91XS
S82.92XD
S82.92XE
S82.92XF
S82.92XG
S82.92XH
S82.92XJ
S82.92XS
S88.Ø11S
S88.Ø12S
S88.Ø19S
S88.Ø21S
S88.Ø22S
S88.Ø29S
S88.111S
S88.112S
S88.119S
S88.121S
S88.122S
S88.129S
S88.911S
S88.912S
S88.919S
S88.921S
S88.922S
S88.929S
S89.ØØ1D
S89.ØØ1G
S89.ØØ1S
S89.ØØ2D
S89.ØØ2G
S89.ØØ2S
S89.ØØ9D
S89.ØØ9G
S89.ØØ9S
S89.Ø11D
S89.Ø11G
S89.Ø11S
S89.Ø12D
S89.Ø12G
S89.Ø12S
S89.Ø19D
S89.Ø19G
S89.Ø19S
S89.Ø21D
S89.Ø21G
S89.Ø21S
S89.Ø22D
S89.Ø22G
S89.Ø22S
S89.Ø29D
S89.Ø29G
S89.Ø29S
S89.Ø31D
S89.Ø31G
S89.Ø31S
S89.Ø32D
S89.Ø32G
S89.Ø32S
S89.Ø39D
S89.Ø39G
S89.Ø39S
S89.Ø41D
S89.Ø41G
S89.Ø41S
S89.Ø42D
S89.Ø42G
S89.Ø42S
S89.Ø49D
S89.Ø49G
S89.Ø49S
S89.Ø91D
S89.Ø91G
S89.Ø91S
S89.Ø92D
S89.Ø92G
S89.Ø92S
S89.Ø99D
S89.Ø99G
S89.Ø99S
S89.1Ø1D
S89.1Ø1G
S89.1Ø1S
S89.1Ø2D
S89.1Ø2G
S89.1Ø2S
S89.1Ø9D
S89.1Ø9G
S89.1Ø9S
S89.111D
S89.111G
S89.111S
S89.112D
S89.112G
S89.112S
S89.119D
S89.119G
S89.119S
S89.121D
S89.121G
S89.121S
S89.122D
S89.122G
S89.122S
S89.129D
S89.129G
S89.129S
S89.131D
S89.131G
S89.131S
S89.132D
S89.132G
S89.132S
S89.139D
S89.139G
S89.139S
S89.141D
S89.141G
S89.141S
S89.142D
S89.142G
S89.142S
S89.149D
S89.149G
S89.149S
S89.191D
S89.191G
S89.191S
S89.192D
S89.192G
S89.192S
S89.199D
S89.199G
S89.199S
S89.2Ø1D
S89.2Ø1G
S89.2Ø1S
S89.2Ø2D
S89.2Ø2G
S89.2Ø2S
S89.2Ø9D
S89.2Ø9G
S89.2Ø9S
S89.211D
S89.211G
S89.211S
S89.212D
S89.212G
S89.212S
S89.219D
S89.219G
S89.219S
S89.221D
S89.221G
S89.221S
S89.222D
S89.222G
S89.222S
S89.229D
S89.229G
S89.229S
S89.291D
S89.291G
S89.291S
S89.292D
S89.292G
S89.292S
S89.299D
S89.299G
S89.299S
S89.3Ø1D
S89.3Ø1G
S89.3Ø1S
S89.3Ø2D
S89.3Ø2G
S89.3Ø2S
S89.3Ø9D
S89.3Ø9G
S89.3Ø9S
S89.311D
S89.311G
S89.311S
S89.312D
S89.312G
S89.312S
S89.319D
S89.319G
S89.319S
S89.321D
S89.321G
S89.321S
S89.322D
S89.322G
S89.322S
S89.329D
S89.329G
S89.329S
S89.391D
S89.391G
S89.391S
S89.392D
S89.392G
S89.392S
S89.399D
S89.399G
S89.399S
S92.ØØ1D
S92.ØØ1G
S92.ØØ1S
S92.ØØ2D
S92.ØØ2G
S92.ØØ2S
S92.ØØ9D
S92.ØØ9G
S92.ØØ9S
S92.Ø11D
S92.Ø11G
S92.Ø11S
S92.Ø12D
S92.Ø12G
S92.Ø12S
S92.Ø13D
S92.Ø13G
S92.Ø13S
S92.Ø14D
S92.Ø14G
S92.Ø14S
S92.Ø15D
S92.Ø15G
S92.Ø15S
S92.Ø16D
S92.Ø16G
S92.Ø16S
S92.Ø21D
S92.Ø21G
S92.Ø21S
S92.Ø22D
S92.Ø22G
S92.Ø22S
S92.Ø23D
S92.Ø23G
S92.Ø23S
S92.Ø24D
S92.Ø24G
S92.Ø24S
S92.Ø25D
S92.Ø25G
S92.Ø25S
S92.Ø26D
S92.Ø26G
S92.Ø26S
S92.Ø31D
S92.Ø31G
S92.Ø31S
S92.Ø32D
S92.Ø32G
S92.Ø32S
S92.Ø33D
S92.Ø33G
S92.Ø33S
S92.Ø34D
S92.Ø34G
S92.Ø34S
S92.Ø35D
S92.Ø35G
S92.Ø35S
S92.Ø36D
S92.Ø36G
S92.Ø36S
S92.Ø41D
S92.Ø41G
S92.Ø41S
S92.Ø42D
S92.Ø42G
S92.Ø42S
S92.Ø43D
S92.Ø43G
S92.Ø43S
S92.Ø44D
S92.Ø44G
S92.Ø44S
S92.Ø45D
S92.Ø45G
S92.Ø45S
S92.Ø46D
S92.Ø46G
S92.Ø46S
S92.Ø51D
S92.Ø51G
S92.Ø51S
S92.Ø52D
S92.Ø52G
S92.Ø52S
S92.Ø53D
S92.Ø53G
S92.Ø53S
S92.Ø54D
S92.Ø54G
S92.Ø54S
S92.Ø55D
S92.Ø55G
S92.Ø55S
S92.Ø56D
S92.Ø56G
S92.Ø56S
S92.Ø61D
S92.Ø61G
S92.Ø61S
S92.Ø62D
S92.Ø62G
S92.Ø62S
S92.Ø63D
S92.Ø63G
S92.Ø63S
S92.Ø64D
S92.Ø64G
S92.Ø64S
S92.Ø65D
S92.Ø65G
S92.Ø65S
S92.Ø66D
S92.Ø66G
S92.Ø66S
S92.1Ø1D
S92.1Ø1G
S92.1Ø1S
S92.1Ø2D
S92.1Ø2G
S92.1Ø2S
S92.1Ø9D
S92.1Ø9G
S92.1Ø9S
S92.111D
S92.111G
S92.111S
S92.112D
S92.112G
S92.112S
S92.113D
S92.113G
S92.113S
S92.114D
S92.114G
S92.114S
S92.115D
S92.115G
S92.115S
S92.116D
S92.116G
S92.116S
S92.121D
S92.121G
S92.121S
S92.122D
S92.122G
S92.122S
S92.123D
S92.123G
S92.123S
S92.124D
S92.124G
S92.124S
S92.125D
S92.125G
S92.125S
S92.126D
S92.126G
S92.126S
S92.131D
S92.131G
S92.131S
S92.132D
S92.132G
S92.132S
S92.133D
S92.133G
S92.133S
S92.134D
S92.134G
S92.134S
S92.135D
S92.135G
S92.135S
S92.136D
S92.136G
S92.136S
S92.141D
S92.141G
S92.141S
S92.142D
S92.142G
S92.142S
S92.143D
S92.143G
S92.143S
S92.144D
S92.144G
S92.144S
S92.145D
S92.145G
S92.145S
S92.146D
S92.146G
S92.146S
S92.151D
S92.151G
S92.151S
S92.152D
S92.152G
S92.152S
S92.153D
S92.153G
S92.153S
S92.154D
S92.154G
S92.154S
S92.155D
S92.155G
S92.155S
S92.156D
S92.156G
S92.156S
S92.191D
S92.191G
S92.191S
S92.192D
S92.192G
S92.192S
S92.199D
S92.199G
S92.199S
S92.2Ø1D
S92.2Ø1G
S92.2Ø1S
S92.2Ø2D
S92.2Ø2G
S92.2Ø2S
S92.2Ø9D
S92.2Ø9G
S92.2Ø9S
S92.211D
S92.211G
S92.211S
S92.212D
S92.212G
S92.212S
S92.213D

S92.213G
S92.213S
S92.214D
S92.214G
S92.214S
S92.215D
S92.215G
S92.215S
S92.216D
S92.216G
S92.216S
S92.221D
S92.221G
S92.221S
S92.222D
S92.222G
S92.222S
S92.223D
S92.223G
S92.223S
S92.224D
S92.224G
S92.224S
S92.225D
S92.225G
S92.225S
S92.226D
S92.226G
S92.226S
S92.231D
S92.231G
S92.231S
S92.232D
S92.232G
S92.232S
S92.233D
S92.233G
S92.233S
S92.234D
S92.234G
S92.234S
S92.235D
S92.235G
S92.235S
S92.236D
S92.236G
S92.236S
S92.241D
S92.241G
S92.241S
S92.242D
S92.242G
S92.242S
S92.243D
S92.243G
S92.243S
S92.244D
S92.244G
S92.244S
S92.245D
S92.245G
S92.245S
S92.246D
S92.246G
S92.246S
S92.251D
S92.251G
S92.251S
S92.252D
S92.252G
S92.252S
S92.253D
S92.253G
S92.253S
S92.254D
S92.254G
S92.254S
S92.255D
S92.255G
S92.255S
S92.256D
S92.256G
S92.256S
S92.301D
S92.301G
S92.301S
S92.302D
S92.302G
S92.302S
S92.309D
S92.309G
S92.309S
S92.311D
S92.311G
S92.311S
S92.312D
S92.312G
S92.312S
S92.313D
S92.313G
S92.313S
S92.314D
S92.314G
S92.314S
S92.315D
S92.315G
S92.315S
S92.316D
S92.316G
S92.316S
S92.321D
S92.321G
S92.321S
S92.322D
S92.322G
S92.322S
S92.323D
S92.323G
S92.323S
S92.324D
S92.324G
S92.324S
S92.325D
S92.325G
S92.325S
S92.326D
S92.326G
S92.326S
S92.331D
S92.331G
S92.331S
S92.332D
S92.332G
S92.332S
S92.333D
S92.333G
S92.333S
S92.334D
S92.334G
S92.334S
S92.335D
S92.335G
S92.335S
S92.336D
S92.336G
S92.336S
S92.341D
S92.341G
S92.341S
S92.342D
S92.342G
S92.342S
S92.343D
S92.343G
S92.343S
S92.344D
S92.344G
S92.344S
S92.345D
S92.345G
S92.345S
S92.346D
S92.346G
S92.346S
S92.351D
S92.351G
S92.351S
S92.352D
S92.352G
S92.352S
S92.353D
S92.353G
S92.353S
S92.354D
S92.354G
S92.354S
S92.355D
S92.355G
S92.355S
S92.356D
S92.356G
S92.356S
S92.401D
S92.401G
S92.401S
S92.402D
S92.402G
S92.402S
S92.403D
S92.403G
S92.403S
S92.404D
S92.404G
S92.404S
S92.405D
S92.405G
S92.405S
S92.406D
S92.406G
S92.406S
S92.411D
S92.411G
S92.411S
S92.412D
S92.412G
S92.412S
S92.413D
S92.413G
S92.413S
S92.414D
S92.414G
S92.414S
S92.415D
S92.415G
S92.415S
S92.416D
S92.416G
S92.416S
S92.421D
S92.421G
S92.421S
S92.422D
S92.422G
S92.422S
S92.423D
S92.423G
S92.423S
S92.424D
S92.424G
S92.424S
S92.425D
S92.425G
S92.425S
S92.426D
S92.426G
S92.426S
S92.491D
S92.491G
S92.491S
S92.492D
S92.492G
S92.492S
S92.499D
S92.499G
S92.499S
S92.501D
S92.501G
S92.501S
S92.502D
S92.502G
S92.502S
S92.503D
S92.503G
S92.503S
S92.504D
S92.504G
S92.504S
S92.505D
S92.505G
S92.505S
S92.506D
S92.506G
S92.506S
S92.511D
S92.511G
S92.511S
S92.512D
S92.512G
S92.512S
S92.513D
S92.513G
S92.513S
S92.514D
S92.514G
S92.514S
S92.515D
S92.515G
S92.515S
S92.516D
S92.516G
S92.516S
S92.521D
S92.521G
S92.521S
S92.522D
S92.522G
S92.522S
S92.523D
S92.523G
S92.523S
S92.524D
S92.524G
S92.524S
S92.525D
S92.525G
S92.525S
S92.526D
S92.526G
S92.526S
S92.531D
S92.531G
S92.531S
S92.532D
S92.532G
S92.532S
S92.533D
S92.533G
S92.533S
S92.534D
S92.534G
S92.534S
S92.535D
S92.535G
S92.535S
S92.536D
S92.536G
S92.536S
S92.591D
S92.591G
S92.591S
S92.592D
S92.592G
S92.592S
S92.599D
S92.599G
S92.599S
S92.811D
S92.811G
S92.811S
S92.812D
S92.812G
S92.812S
S92.819D
S92.819G
S92.819S
S92.901D
S92.901G
S92.901S
S92.902D
S92.902G
S92.902S
S92.909D
S92.909G
S92.909S
S92.911D
S92.911G
S92.911S
S92.912D
S92.912G
S92.912S
S92.919D
S92.919G
S92.919S
S98.011S
S98.012S
S98.019S
S98.021S
S98.022S
S98.029S
S98.111S
S98.112S
S98.119S
S98.121S
S98.122S
S98.129S
S98.131S
S98.132S
S98.139S
S98.141S
S98.142S
S98.149S
S98.211S
S98.212S
S98.219S
S98.221S
S98.222S
S98.229S
S98.311S
S98.312S
S98.319S
S98.321S
S98.322S
S98.329S
S98.911S
S98.912S
S98.919S
S98.921S
S98.922S
S98.929S
T84.010A
T84.011A
T84.012A
T84.013A
T84.018A
T84.019A
T84.020A
T84.021A
T84.022A
T84.023A
T84.028A
T84.029A
T84.030A
T84.031A
T84.032A
T84.033A
T84.038A
T84.039A
T84.050A
T84.051A
T84.052A
T84.053A
T84.058A
T84.059A
T84.060A
T84.061A
T84.062A
T84.063A
T84.068A
T84.069A
T84.090A
T84.091A
T84.092A
T84.093A
T84.098A
T84.099A
T84.110A
T84.111A
T84.112A
T84.113A
T84.114A
T84.115A
T84.116A
T84.117A
T84.119A
T84.120A
T84.121A
T84.122A
T84.123A
T84.124A
T84.125A
T84.126A
T84.127A
T84.129A
T84.190A
T84.191A
T84.192A
T84.193A
T84.194A
T84.195A
T84.196A
T84.197A
T84.199A
T84.210A
T84.213A
T84.216A
T84.218A
T84.220A
T84.223A
T84.226A
T84.228A
T84.290A
T84.293A
T84.296A
T84.298A
T84.310A
T84.318A
T84.320A
T84.328A
T84.390A
T84.398A
T84.410A
T84.418A
T84.420A
T84.428A
T84.490A
T84.498A
T84.50XA
T84.51XA
T84.52XA
T84.53XA
T84.54XA
T84.59XA
T84.60XA
T84.610A
T84.611A
T84.612A
T84.613A
T84.614A
T84.615A
T84.619A
T84.620A
T84.621A
T84.622A
T84.623A
T84.624A
T84.625A
T84.629A
T84.63XA
T84.69XA
T84.7XXA
T84.81XA
T84.82XA
T84.83XA
T84.84XA
T84.85XA
T84.86XA
T84.89XA
T84.9XXA
T87.0X1
T87.0X2
T87.0X9
T87.1X1
T87.1X2
T87.1X9
T87.2
Z44.001
Z44.002
Z44.009
Z44.011
Z44.012
Z44.019
Z44.021
Z44.022
Z44.029
Z44.101
Z44.102
Z44.109
Z44.111
Z44.112
Z44.119
Z44.121
Z44.122
Z44.129
Z47.1
Z47.2
Z47.3*
Z47.81
Z47.82
Z47.89

DRG 560

Select principal diagnosis listed under DRG 559

DRG 561

Select principal diagnosis listed under DRG 559

DRG 562

Principal Diagnosis

M22*
M23.0*
M23.2*
M23.3*
M23.6*
M23.8*
M23.9*
M24.111
M24.112
M24.119
M24.121
M24.122
M24.129
M24.131
M24.132
M24.139
M24.141
M24.142
M24.149
M24.171
M24.172
M24.173
M24.174
M24.175
M24.176
M24.30
M24.311
M24.312
M24.319
M24.321
M24.322
M24.329
M24.331
M24.332
M24.339
M24.341
M24.342
M24.349
M24.361
M24.362
M24.369
M24.371
M24.372
M24.373
M24.374
M24.375
M24.376
M24.39
M24.411
M24.412
M24.419
M24.421
M24.422
M24.429
M24.431
M24.432
M24.439
M24.441
M24.442
M24.443
M24.444
M24.445
M24.446
M24.461
M24.462
M24.469
M24.471
M24.472
M24.473
M24.474
M24.475
M24.476
M24.477
M24.478
M24.479
M99.16
M99.17
M99.19
Q68.6
S03.00XS
S03.01XS
S03.02XS
S03.03XS
S03.1XXA
S03.1XXS
S03.40XS
S03.41XS
S03.42XS
S03.43XS
S03.8XXS
S03.9XXA
S03.9XXS
S09.11XS
S13.0XXS
S13.100S
S13.101S
S13.110S
S13.111S
S13.120S
S13.121S
S13.130S
S13.131S
S13.140S
S13.141S
S13.150S
S13.151S
S13.160S
S13.161S
S13.170S
S13.171S
S13.180S
S13.181S
S13.20XS
S13.29XS
S13.4XXS
S13.5XXS
S13.8XXS
S13.9XXS
S16.1XXS
S23.0XXS
S23.100S
S23.101S
S23.110S
S23.111S
S23.120S
S23.121S
S23.122S
S23.123S
S23.130S
S23.131S
S23.132S
S23.133S
S23.140S
S23.141S
S23.142S
S23.143S
S23.150S
S23.151S
S23.152S
S23.153S
S23.160S
S23.161S
S23.162S
S23.163S
S23.170S
S23.171S
S23.20XS
S23.29XS
S23.3XXS
S23.41XS
S23.420S
S23.421S
S23.428S
S23.429S
S23.8XXS
S23.9XXS
S29.011A
S29.011S
S29.012A
S29.012S
S29.019A
S29.019S
S33.0XXS
S33.100S
S33.101S
S33.110S
S33.111S
S33.120S
S33.121S
S33.130S
S33.131S
S33.140S
S33.141S
S33.2XXS
S33.30XA
S33.30XS
S33.39XA
S33.39XS
S33.4XXS
S33.5XXS
S33.6XXS
S33.8XXS
S33.9XXS
S39.011A
S39.011S
S39.012A
S39.012S
S39.013A
S39.013S
S42.001A
S42.001B
S42.002A
S42.002B
S42.009A
S42.009B
S42.011A
S42.011B
S42.012A
S42.012B
S42.013A
S42.013B
S42.014A
S42.014B
S42.015A
S42.015B
S42.016A
S42.016B
S42.017A
S42.017B
S42.018A
S42.018B
S42.019A
S42.019B
S42.021A
S42.021B
S42.022A
S42.022B
S42.023A
S42.023B
S42.024A
S42.024B
S42.025A
S42.025B
S42.026A
S42.026B
S42.031A
S42.031B
S42.032A
S42.032B
S42.033A
S42.033B
S42.034A
S42.034B
S42.035A
S42.035B
S42.036A
S42.036B
S42.101A
S42.101B
S42.102A
S42.102B
S42.109A
S42.109B
S42.121A
S42.121B
S42.122A
S42.122B
S42.123A
S42.123B
S42.124A
S42.124B
S42.125A
S42.125B
S42.126A
S42.126B
S42.131A
S42.131B
S42.132A
S42.132B
S42.133A
S42.133B
S42.134A
S42.134B
S42.135A
S42.135B
S42.136A
S42.136B
S42.141A
S42.141B
S42.142A
S42.142B
S42.143A
S42.143B
S42.144A
S42.144B
S42.145A
S42.145B
S42.146A
S42.146B
S42.151A
S42.151B
S42.152A
S42.152B
S42.153A
S42.153B
S42.154A
S42.154B
S42.155A
S42.155B
S42.156A
S42.156B
S42.201A
S42.201B
S42.202A
S42.202B
S42.209A
S42.209B
S42.211A
S42.211B
S42.212A
S42.212B
S42.213A
S42.213B

S42.214A
S42.214B
S42.215A
S42.215B
S42.216A
S42.216B
S42.221A
S42.221B
S42.222A
S42.222B
S42.223A
S42.223B
S42.224A
S42.224B
S42.225A
S42.225B
S42.226A
S42.226B
S42.231A
S42.231B
S42.232A
S42.232B
S42.239A
S42.239B
S42.241A
S42.241B
S42.242A
S42.242B
S42.249A
S42.249B
S42.251A
S42.251B
S42.252A
S42.252B
S42.253A
S42.253B
S42.254A
S42.254B
S42.255A
S42.255B
S42.256A
S42.256B
S42.261A
S42.261B
S42.262A
S42.262B
S42.263A
S42.263B
S42.264A
S42.264B
S42.265A
S42.265B
S42.266A
S42.266B
S42.271A
S42.272A
S42.279A
S42.291A
S42.291B
S42.292A
S42.292B
S42.293A
S42.293B
S42.294A
S42.294B
S42.295A
S42.295B
S42.296A
S42.296B
S42.301A
S42.301B
S42.302A
S42.302B
S42.309A
S42.309B
S42.311A
S42.312A
S42.319A
S42.321A
S42.321B
S42.322A
S42.322B
S42.323A
S42.323B
S42.324A
S42.324B
S42.325A
S42.325B
S42.326A
S42.326B
S42.331A
S42.331B
S42.332A
S42.332B
S42.333A
S42.333B
S42.334A
S42.334B
S42.335A
S42.335B
S42.336A
S42.336B
S42.341A
S42.341B
S42.342A
S42.342B
S42.343A
S42.343B
S42.344A
S42.344B
S42.345A
S42.345B
S42.346A
S42.346B
S42.351A
S42.351B
S42.352A
S42.352B
S42.353A
S42.353B
S42.354A
S42.354B
S42.355A
S42.355B
S42.356A
S42.356B
S42.361A
S42.361B
S42.362A
S42.362B
S42.363A
S42.363B
S42.364A
S42.364B
S42.365A
S42.365B
S42.366A
S42.366B
S42.391A
S42.391B
S42.392A
S42.392B
S42.399A
S42.399B
S42.401A
S42.401B
S42.402A
S42.402B
S42.409A
S42.409B
S42.411A
S42.411B
S42.412A
S42.412B
S42.413A
S42.413B
S42.414A
S42.414B
S42.415A
S42.415B
S42.416A
S42.416B
S42.421A
S42.421B
S42.422A
S42.422B
S42.423A
S42.423B
S42.424A
S42.424B
S42.425A
S42.425B
S42.426A
S42.426B
S42.431A
S42.431B
S42.432A
S42.432B
S42.433A
S42.433B
S42.434A
S42.434B
S42.435A
S42.435B
S42.436A
S42.436B
S42.441A
S42.441B
S42.442A
S42.442B
S42.443A
S42.443B
S42.444A
S42.444B
S42.445A
S42.445B
S42.446A
S42.446B
S42.447A
S42.447B
S42.448A
S42.448B
S42.449A
S42.449B
S42.451A
S42.451B
S42.452A
S42.452B
S42.453A
S42.453B
S42.454A
S42.454B
S42.455A
S42.455B
S42.456A
S42.456B
S42.461A
S42.461B
S42.462A
S42.462B
S42.463A
S42.463B
S42.464A
S42.464B
S42.465A
S42.465B
S42.466A
S42.466B
S42.471A
S42.471B
S42.472A
S42.472B
S42.473A
S42.473B
S42.474A
S42.474B
S42.475A
S42.475B
S42.476A
S42.476B
S42.481A
S42.482A
S42.489A
S42.491A
S42.491B
S42.492A
S42.492B
S42.493A
S42.493B
S42.494A
S42.494B
S42.495A
S42.495B
S42.496A
S42.496B
S42.90XA
S42.90XB
S42.91XA
S42.91XB
S42.92XA
S42.92XB
S43.001A
S43.001S
S43.002A
S43.002S
S43.003A
S43.003S
S43.004A
S43.004S
S43.005A
S43.005S
S43.006A
S43.006S
S43.011A
S43.011S
S43.012A
S43.012S
S43.013A
S43.013S
S43.014A
S43.014S
S43.015A
S43.015S
S43.016A
S43.016S
S43.021A
S43.021S
S43.022A
S43.022S
S43.023A
S43.023S
S43.024A
S43.024S
S43.025A
S43.025S
S43.026A
S43.026S
S43.031A
S43.031S
S43.032A
S43.032S
S43.033A
S43.033S
S43.034A
S43.034S
S43.035A
S43.035S
S43.036A
S43.036S
S43.081A
S43.081S
S43.082A
S43.082S
S43.083A
S43.083S
S43.084A
S43.084S
S43.085A
S43.085S
S43.086A
S43.086S
S43.101A
S43.101S
S43.102A
S43.102S
S43.109A
S43.109S
S43.111A
S43.111S
S43.112A
S43.112S
S43.119A
S43.119S
S43.121A
S43.121S
S43.122A
S43.122S
S43.129A
S43.129S
S43.131A
S43.131S
S43.132A
S43.132S
S43.139A
S43.139S
S43.141A
S43.141S
S43.142A
S43.142S
S43.149A
S43.149S
S43.151A
S43.151S
S43.152A
S43.152S
S43.159A
S43.159S
S43.201S
S43.202S
S43.203S
S43.204S
S43.205S
S43.206S
S43.211S
S43.212S
S43.213S
S43.214S
S43.215S
S43.216S
S43.221S
S43.222S
S43.223S
S43.224S
S43.225S
S43.226S
S43.301A
S43.301S
S43.302A
S43.302S
S43.303A
S43.303S
S43.304A
S43.304S
S43.305A
S43.305S
S43.306A
S43.306S
S43.311A
S43.311S
S43.312A
S43.312S
S43.313A
S43.313S
S43.314A
S43.314S
S43.315A
S43.315S
S43.316A
S43.316S
S43.391A
S43.391S
S43.392A
S43.392S
S43.393A
S43.393S
S43.394A
S43.394S
S43.395A
S43.395S
S43.396A
S43.396S
S43.401A
S43.401S
S43.402A
S43.402S
S43.409A
S43.409S
S43.411A
S43.411S
S43.412A
S43.412S
S43.419A
S43.419S
S43.421A
S43.421S
S43.422A
S43.422S
S43.429A
S43.429S
S43.431A
S43.431S
S43.432A
S43.432S
S43.439A
S43.439S
S43.491A
S43.491S
S43.492A
S43.492S
S43.499A
S43.499S
S43.50XA
S43.50XS
S43.51XA
S43.51XS
S43.52XA
S43.52XS
S43.60XA
S43.60XS
S43.61XA
S43.61XS
S43.62XA
S43.62XS
S43.80XA
S43.80XS
S43.81XA
S43.81XS
S43.82XA
S43.82XS
S43.90XA
S43.90XS
S43.91XA
S43.91XS
S43.92XA
S43.92XS
S46.011A
S46.011S
S46.012A
S46.012S
S46.019A
S46.019S
S46.111A
S46.111S
S46.112A
S46.112S
S46.119A
S46.119S
S46.211A
S46.211S
S46.212A
S46.212S
S46.219A
S46.219S
S46.311A
S46.311S
S46.312A
S46.312S
S46.319A
S46.319S
S46.811A
S46.811S
S46.812A
S46.812S
S46.819A
S46.819S
S46.911A
S46.911S
S46.912A
S46.912S
S46.919A
S46.919S
S49.001A
S49.002A
S49.009A
S49.011A
S49.012A
S49.019A
S49.021A
S49.022A
S49.029A
S49.031A
S49.032A
S49.039A
S49.041A
S49.042A
S49.049A
S49.091A
S49.092A
S49.099A
S49.101A
S49.102A
S49.109A
S49.111A
S49.112A
S49.119A
S49.121A
S49.122A
S49.129A
S49.131A
S49.132A
S49.139A
S49.141A
S49.142A
S49.149A
S49.191A
S49.192A
S49.199A
S52.001A
S52.001B
S52.001C
S52.002A
S52.002B
S52.002C
S52.009A
S52.009B
S52.009C
S52.011A
S52.012A
S52.019A
S52.021A
S52.021B
S52.021C
S52.022A
S52.022B
S52.022C
S52.023A
S52.023B
S52.023C
S52.024A
S52.024B
S52.024C
S52.025A
S52.025B
S52.025C
S52.026A
S52.026B
S52.026C
S52.031A
S52.031B
S52.031C
S52.032A
S52.032B
S52.032C
S52.033A
S52.033B
S52.033C
S52.034A
S52.034B
S52.034C
S52.035A
S52.035B
S52.035C
S52.036A
S52.036B
S52.036C
S52.041A
S52.041B
S52.041C
S52.042A
S52.042B
S52.042C
S52.043A
S52.043B
S52.043C
S52.044A
S52.044B
S52.044C
S52.045A
S52.045B
S52.045C
S52.046A
S52.046B
S52.046C
S52.091A
S52.091B
S52.091C
S52.092A
S52.092B
S52.092C
S52.099A
S52.099B
S52.099C
S52.101A
S52.101B
S52.101C
S52.102A
S52.102B
S52.102C
S52.109A
S52.109B
S52.109C
S52.111A
S52.112A
S52.119A
S52.121A
S52.121B
S52.121C
S52.122A
S52.122B
S52.122C
S52.123A
S52.123B
S52.123C
S52.124A
S52.124B
S52.124C
S52.125A
S52.125B
S52.125C
S52.126A
S52.126B
S52.126C
S52.131A
S52.131B
S52.131C
S52.132A
S52.132B
S52.132C
S52.133A
S52.133B
S52.133C
S52.134A
S52.134B
S52.134C
S52.135A
S52.135B
S52.135C
S52.136A
S52.136B
S52.136C
S52.181A
S52.181B
S52.181C
S52.182A
S52.182B
S52.182C
S52.189A
S52.189B
S52.189C
S52.201A
S52.201B
S52.201C
S52.202A
S52.202B
S52.202C
S52.209A
S52.209B
S52.209C
S52.211A
S52.212A
S52.219A
S52.221A
S52.221B
S52.221C
S52.222A
S52.222B
S52.222C
S52.223A
S52.223B
S52.223C
S52.224A
S52.224B
S52.224C
S52.225A
S52.225B
S52.225C
S52.226A
S52.226B
S52.226C
S52.231A
S52.231B
S52.231C
S52.232A
S52.232B
S52.232C
S52.233A
S52.233B
S52.233C
S52.234A
S52.234B
S52.234C
S52.235A
S52.235B
S52.235C
S52.236A
S52.236B
S52.236C
S52.241A
S52.241B
S52.241C
S52.242A
S52.242B
S52.242C
S52.243A
S52.243B
S52.243C
S52.244A
S52.244B
S52.244C
S52.245A
S52.245B
S52.245C
S52.246A
S52.246B
S52.246C
S52.251A
S52.251B
S52.251C
S52.252A
S52.252B
S52.252C
S52.253A
S52.253B
S52.253C
S52.254A
S52.254B
S52.254C
S52.255A
S52.255B
S52.255C
S52.256A
S52.256B
S52.256C
S52.261A
S52.261B
S52.261C
S52.262A
S52.262B
S52.262C
S52.263A
S52.263B
S52.263C
S52.264A
S52.264B
S52.264C
S52.265A
S52.265B
S52.265C
S52.266A
S52.266B
S52.266C
S52.271A
S52.271B
S52.271C
S52.272A
S52.272B
S52.272C
S52.279A
S52.279B
S52.279C
S52.281A
S52.281B
S52.281C
S52.282A
S52.282B
S52.282C
S52.283A
S52.283B
S52.283C
S52.291A
S52.291B
S52.291C
S52.292A
S52.292B
S52.292C
S52.299A
S52.299B
S52.299C
S52.301A
S52.301B
S52.301C
S52.302A
S52.302B
S52.302C
S52.309A
S52.309B
S52.309C
S52.311A
S52.312A
S52.319A
S52.321A
S52.321B
S52.321C
S52.322A
S52.322B
S52.322C
S52.323A
S52.323B
S52.323C
S52.324A
S52.324B
S52.324C
S52.325A
S52.325B
S52.325C
S52.326A
S52.326B
S52.326C
S52.331A
S52.331B
S52.331C
S52.332A
S52.332B
S52.332C
S52.333A
S52.333B
S52.333C
S52.334A
S52.334B
S52.334C
S52.335A
S52.335B
S52.335C
S52.336A
S52.336B
S52.336C
S52.341A
S52.341B
S52.341C
S52.342A
S52.342B
S52.342C
S52.343A
S52.343B
S52.343C

S52.344A
S52.344B
S52.344C
S52.345A
S52.345B
S52.345C
S52.346A
S52.346B
S52.346C
S52.351A
S52.351B
S52.351C
S52.352A
S52.352B
S52.352C
S52.353A
S52.353B
S52.353C
S52.354A
S52.354B
S52.354C
S52.355A
S52.355B
S52.355C
S52.356A
S52.356B
S52.356C
S52.361A
S52.361B
S52.361C
S52.362A
S52.362B
S52.362C
S52.363A
S52.363B
S52.363C
S52.364A
S52.364B
S52.364C
S52.365A
S52.365B
S52.365C
S52.366A
S52.366B
S52.366C
S52.371A
S52.371B
S52.371C
S52.372A
S52.372B
S52.372C
S52.379A
S52.379B
S52.379C
S52.381A
S52.381B
S52.381C
S52.382A
S52.382B
S52.382C
S52.389A
S52.389B
S52.389C
S52.391A
S52.391B
S52.391C
S52.392A
S52.392B
S52.392C
S52.399A
S52.399B
S52.399C
S52.5Ø1A
S52.5Ø1B
S52.5Ø1C
S52.5Ø2A
S52.5Ø2B
S52.5Ø2C
S52.5Ø9A
S52.5Ø9B
S52.5Ø9C
S52.511A
S52.511B
S52.511C
S52.512A
S52.512B
S52.512C
S52.513A
S52.513B
S52.513C
S52.514A
S52.514B
S52.514C
S52.515A
S52.515B
S52.515C
S52.516A
S52.516B
S52.516C
S52.521A
S52.522A
S52.529A
S52.531A
S52.531B
S52.531C
S52.532A
S52.532B
S52.532C
S52.539A
S52.539B
S52.539C
S52.541A
S52.541B
S52.541C
S52.542A
S52.542B
S52.542C
S52.549A
S52.549B
S52.549C
S52.551A
S52.551B
S52.551C
S52.552A
S52.552B
S52.552C
S52.559A
S52.559B
S52.559C
S52.561A
S52.561B
S52.561C
S52.562A
S52.562B
S52.562C
S52.569A
S52.569B
S52.569C
S52.571A
S52.571B
S52.571C
S52.572A
S52.572B
S52.572C
S52.579A
S52.579B
S52.579C
S52.591A
S52.591B
S52.591C
S52.592A
S52.592B
S52.592C
S52.599A
S52.599B
S52.599C
S52.6Ø1A
S52.6Ø1B
S52.6Ø1C
S52.6Ø2A
S52.6Ø2B
S52.6Ø2C
S52.6Ø9A
S52.6Ø9B
S52.6Ø9C
S52.611A
S52.611B
S52.611C
S52.612A
S52.612B
S52.612C
S52.613A
S52.613B
S52.613C
S52.614A
S52.614B
S52.614C
S52.615A
S52.615B
S52.615C
S52.616A
S52.616B
S52.616C
S52.621A
S52.622A
S52.629A
S52.691A
S52.691B
S52.691C
S52.692A
S52.692B
S52.692C
S52.699A
S52.699B
S52.699C
S52.9ØXA
S52.9ØXB
S52.9ØXC
S52.91XA
S52.91XB
S52.91XC
S52.92XA
S52.92XB
S52.92XC
S53.ØØ1A
S53.ØØ1S
S53.ØØ2A
S53.ØØ2S
S53.ØØ3A
S53.ØØ3S
S53.ØØ4A
S53.ØØ4S
S53.ØØ5A
S53.ØØ5S
S53.ØØ6A
S53.ØØ6S
S53.Ø11A
S53.Ø11S
S53.Ø12A
S53.Ø12S
S53.Ø13A
S53.Ø13S
S53.Ø14A
S53.Ø14S
S53.Ø15A
S53.Ø15S
S53.Ø16A
S53.Ø16S
S53.Ø21A
S53.Ø21S
S53.Ø22A
S53.Ø22S
S53.Ø23A
S53.Ø23S
S53.Ø24A
S53.Ø24S
S53.Ø25A
S53.Ø25S
S53.Ø26A
S53.Ø26S
S53.Ø31A
S53.Ø31S
S53.Ø32A
S53.Ø32S
S53.Ø33A
S53.Ø33S
S53.Ø91A
S53.Ø91S
S53.Ø92A
S53.Ø92S
S53.Ø93A
S53.Ø93S
S53.Ø94A
S53.Ø94S
S53.Ø95A
S53.Ø95S
S53.Ø96A
S53.Ø96S
S53.1Ø1A
S53.1Ø1S
S53.1Ø2A
S53.1Ø2S
S53.1Ø3A
S53.1Ø3S
S53.1Ø4A
S53.1Ø4S
S53.1Ø5A
S53.1Ø5S
S53.1Ø6A
S53.1Ø6S
S53.111A
S53.111S
S53.112A
S53.112S
S53.113A
S53.113S
S53.114A
S53.114S
S53.115A
S53.115S
S53.116A
S53.116S
S53.121A
S53.121S
S53.122A
S53.122S
S53.123A
S53.123S
S53.124A
S53.124S
S53.125A
S53.125S
S53.126A
S53.126S
S53.131A
S53.131S
S53.132A
S53.132S
S53.133A
S53.133S
S53.134A
S53.134S
S53.135A
S53.135S
S53.136A
S53.136S
S53.141A
S53.141S
S53.142A
S53.142S
S53.143A
S53.143S
S53.144A
S53.144S
S53.145A
S53.145S
S53.146A
S53.146S
S53.191A
S53.191S
S53.192A
S53.192S
S53.193A
S53.193S
S53.194A
S53.194S
S53.195A
S53.195S
S53.196A
S53.196S
S53.2ØXA
S53.2ØXS
S53.21XA
S53.21XS
S53.22XA
S53.22XS
S53.3ØXA
S53.3ØXS
S53.31XA
S53.31XS
S53.32XA
S53.32XS
S53.4Ø1A
S53.4Ø1S
S53.4Ø2A
S53.4Ø2S
S53.4Ø9A
S53.4Ø9S
S53.411A
S53.411S
S53.412A
S53.412S
S53.419A
S53.419S
S53.421A
S53.421S
S53.422A
S53.422S
S53.429A
S53.429S
S53.431A
S53.431S
S53.432A
S53.432S
S53.439A
S53.439S
S53.441A
S53.441S
S53.442A
S53.442S
S53.449A
S53.449S
S53.491A
S53.491S
S53.492A
S53.492S
S53.499A
S53.499S
S56.Ø11A
S56.Ø11S
S56.Ø12A
S56.Ø12S
S56.Ø19A
S56.Ø19S
S56.111A
S56.111S
S56.112A
S56.112S
S56.113A
S56.113S
S56.114A
S56.114S
S56.115A
S56.115S
S56.116A
S56.116S
S56.117A
S56.117S
S56.118A
S56.118S
S56.119A
S56.119S
S56.211A
S56.211S
S56.212A
S56.212S
S56.219A
S56.219S
S56.311A
S56.311S
S56.312A
S56.312S
S56.319A
S56.319S
S56.411A
S56.411S
S56.412A
S56.412S
S56.413A
S56.413S
S56.414A
S56.414S
S56.415A
S56.415S
S56.416A
S56.416S
S56.417A
S56.417S
S56.418A
S56.418S
S56.419A
S56.419S
S56.511A
S56.511S
S56.512A
S56.512S
S56.519A
S56.519S
S56.811A
S56.811S
S56.812A
S56.812S
S56.819A
S56.819S
S56.911A
S56.911S
S56.912A
S56.912S
S56.919A
S56.919S
S59.ØØ1A
S59.ØØ2A
S59.ØØ9A
S59.Ø11A
S59.Ø12A
S59.Ø19A
S59.Ø21A
S59.Ø22A
S59.Ø29A
S59.Ø31A
S59.Ø32A
S59.Ø39A
S59.Ø41A
S59.Ø42A
S59.Ø49A
S59.Ø91A
S59.Ø92A
S59.Ø99A
S59.1Ø1A
S59.1Ø2A
S59.1Ø9A
S59.111A
S59.112A
S59.119A
S59.121A
S59.122A
S59.129A
S59.131A
S59.132A
S59.139A
S59.141A
S59.142A
S59.149A
S59.191A
S59.192A
S59.199A
S59.2Ø1A
S59.2Ø2A
S59.2Ø9A
S59.211A
S59.212A
S59.219A
S59.221A
S59.222A
S59.229A
S59.231A
S59.232A
S59.239A
S59.241A
S59.242A
S59.249A
S59.291A
S59.292A
S59.299A
S62.ØØ1A
S62.ØØ1B
S62.ØØ2A
S62.ØØ2B
S62.ØØ9A
S62.ØØ9B
S62.Ø11A
S62.Ø11B
S62.Ø12A
S62.Ø12B
S62.Ø13A
S62.Ø13B
S62.Ø14A
S62.Ø14B
S62.Ø15A
S62.Ø15B
S62.Ø16A
S62.Ø16B
S62.Ø21A
S62.Ø21B
S62.Ø22A
S62.Ø22B
S62.Ø23A
S62.Ø23B
S62.Ø24A
S62.Ø24B
S62.Ø25A
S62.Ø25B
S62.Ø26A
S62.Ø26B
S62.Ø31A
S62.Ø31B
S62.Ø32A
S62.Ø32B
S62.Ø33A
S62.Ø33B
S62.Ø34A
S62.Ø34B
S62.Ø35A
S62.Ø35B
S62.Ø36A
S62.Ø36B
S62.1Ø1A
S62.1Ø1B
S62.1Ø2A
S62.1Ø2B
S62.1Ø9A
S62.1Ø9B
S62.111A
S62.111B
S62.112A
S62.112B
S62.113A
S62.113B
S62.114A
S62.114B
S62.115A
S62.115B
S62.116A
S62.116B
S62.121A
S62.121B
S62.122A
S62.122B
S62.123A
S62.123B
S62.124A
S62.124B
S62.125A
S62.125B
S62.126A
S62.126B
S62.131A
S62.131B
S62.132A
S62.132B
S62.133A
S62.133B
S62.134A
S62.134B
S62.135A
S62.135B
S62.136A
S62.136B
S62.141A
S62.141B
S62.142A
S62.142B
S62.143A
S62.143B
S62.144A
S62.144B
S62.145A
S62.145B
S62.146A
S62.146B
S62.151A
S62.151B
S62.152A
S62.152B
S62.153A
S62.153B
S62.154A
S62.154B
S62.155A
S62.155B
S62.156A
S62.156B
S62.161A
S62.161B
S62.162A
S62.162B
S62.163A
S62.163B
S62.164A
S62.164B
S62.165A
S62.165B
S62.166A
S62.166B
S62.171A
S62.171B
S62.172A
S62.172B
S62.173A
S62.173B
S62.174A
S62.174B
S62.175A
S62.175B
S62.176A
S62.176B
S62.181A
S62.181B
S62.182A
S62.182B
S62.183A
S62.183B
S62.184A
S62.184B
S62.185A
S62.185B
S62.186A
S62.186B
S62.2Ø1A
S62.2Ø1B
S62.2Ø2A
S62.2Ø2B
S62.2Ø9A
S62.2Ø9B
S62.211A
S62.211B
S62.212A
S62.212B
S62.213A
S62.213B
S62.221A
S62.221B
S62.222A
S62.222B
S62.223A
S62.223B
S62.224A
S62.224B
S62.225A
S62.225B
S62.226A
S62.226B
S62.231A
S62.231B
S62.232A
S62.232B
S62.233A
S62.233B
S62.234A
S62.234B
S62.235A
S62.235B
S62.236A
S62.236B
S62.241A
S62.241B
S62.242A
S62.242B
S62.243A
S62.243B
S62.244A
S62.244B
S62.245A
S62.245B
S62.246A
S62.246B
S62.251A
S62.251B
S62.252A
S62.252B
S62.253A
S62.253B
S62.254A
S62.254B
S62.255A
S62.255B
S62.256A
S62.256B
S62.291A
S62.291B
S62.292A
S62.292B
S62.299A
S62.299B
S62.3ØØA
S62.3ØØB
S62.3Ø1A
S62.3Ø1B
S62.3Ø2A
S62.3Ø2B
S62.3Ø3A
S62.3Ø3B
S62.3Ø4A
S62.3Ø4B
S62.3Ø5A
S62.3Ø5B
S62.3Ø6A
S62.3Ø6B
S62.3Ø7A
S62.3Ø7B
S62.3Ø8A
S62.3Ø8B
S62.3Ø9A
S62.3Ø9B
S62.31ØA
S62.31ØB
S62.311A
S62.311B
S62.312A
S62.312B
S62.313A
S62.313B
S62.314A
S62.314B
S62.315A
S62.315B
S62.316A
S62.316B
S62.317A
S62.317B
S62.318A
S62.318B
S62.319A
S62.319B
S62.32ØA
S62.32ØB
S62.321A
S62.321B
S62.322A
S62.322B
S62.323A
S62.323B
S62.324A
S62.324B
S62.325A
S62.325B
S62.326A
S62.326B
S62.327A
S62.327B
S62.328A
S62.328B
S62.329A
S62.329B
S62.33ØA
S62.33ØB
S62.331A
S62.331B
S62.332A
S62.332B
S62.333A
S62.333B
S62.334A
S62.334B
S62.335A
S62.335B
S62.336A
S62.336B
S62.337A
S62.337B
S62.338A
S62.338B
S62.339A
S62.339B
S62.34ØA
S62.34ØB
S62.341A
S62.341B
S62.342A
S62.342B
S62.343A
S62.343B
S62.344A
S62.344B
S62.345A
S62.345B
S62.346A
S62.346B
S62.347A
S62.347B
S62.348A
S62.348B
S62.349A
S62.349B
S62.35ØA
S62.35ØB
S62.351A
S62.351B
S62.352A
S62.352B
S62.353A
S62.353B
S62.354A
S62.354B
S62.355A
S62.355B
S62.356A
S62.356B
S62.357A
S62.357B
S62.358A
S62.358B
S62.359A
S62.359B
S62.36ØA
S62.36ØB
S62.361A
S62.361B
S62.362A
S62.362B
S62.363A
S62.363B
S62.364A
S62.364B
S62.365A
S62.365B
S62.366A
S62.366B
S62.367A
S62.367B
S62.368A
S62.368B
S62.369A
S62.369B
S62.39ØA

S62.390B
S62.391A
S62.391B
S62.392A
S62.392B
S62.393A
S62.393B
S62.394A
S62.394B
S62.395A
S62.395B
S62.396A
S62.396B
S62.397A
S62.397B
S62.398A
S62.398B
S62.399A
S62.399B
S62.501A
S62.501B
S62.502A
S62.502B
S62.509A
S62.509B
S62.511A
S62.511B
S62.512A
S62.512B
S62.513A
S62.513B
S62.514A
S62.514B
S62.515A
S62.515B
S62.516A
S62.516B
S62.521A
S62.521B
S62.522A
S62.522B
S62.523A
S62.523B
S62.524A
S62.524B
S62.525A
S62.525B
S62.526A
S62.526B
S62.600A
S62.600B
S62.601A
S62.601B
S62.602A
S62.602B
S62.603A
S62.603B
S62.604A
S62.604B
S62.605A
S62.605B
S62.606A
S62.606B
S62.607A
S62.607B
S62.608A
S62.608B
S62.609A
S62.609B
S62.610A
S62.610B
S62.611A
S62.611B
S62.612A
S62.612B
S62.613A
S62.613B
S62.614A
S62.614B
S62.615A
S62.615B
S62.616A
S62.616B
S62.617A
S62.617B
S62.618A
S62.618B
S62.619A
S62.619B
S62.620A
S62.620B
S62.621A
S62.621B
S62.622A
S62.622B
S62.623A
S62.623B
S62.624A
S62.624B
S62.625A
S62.625B
S62.626A
S62.626B
S62.627A
S62.627B
S62.628A
S62.628B
S62.629A
S62.629B
S62.630A
S62.630B
S62.631A
S62.631B
S62.632A
S62.632B
S62.633A
S62.633B
S62.634A
S62.634B
S62.635A
S62.635B
S62.636A
S62.636B
S62.637A
S62.637B
S62.638A
S62.638B
S62.639A
S62.639B
S62.640A
S62.640B
S62.641A
S62.641B
S62.642A
S62.642B
S62.643A
S62.643B
S62.644A
S62.644B
S62.645A
S62.645B
S62.646A
S62.646B
S62.647A
S62.647B
S62.648A
S62.648B
S62.649A
S62.649B
S62.650A
S62.650B
S62.651A
S62.651B
S62.652A
S62.652B
S62.653A
S62.653B
S62.654A
S62.654B
S62.655A
S62.655B
S62.656A
S62.656B
S62.657A
S62.657B
S62.658A
S62.658B
S62.659A
S62.659B
S62.660A
S62.660B
S62.661A
S62.661B
S62.662A
S62.662B
S62.663A
S62.663B
S62.664A
S62.664B
S62.665A
S62.665B
S62.666A
S62.666B
S62.667A
S62.667B
S62.668A
S62.668B
S62.669A
S62.669B
S62.90XA
S62.90XB
S62.91XA
S62.91XB
S62.92XA
S62.92XB
S63.001A
S63.001S
S63.002A
S63.002S
S63.003A
S63.003S
S63.004A
S63.004S
S63.005A
S63.005S
S63.006A
S63.006S
S63.011A
S63.011S
S63.012A
S63.012S
S63.013A
S63.013S
S63.014A
S63.014S
S63.015A
S63.015S
S63.016A
S63.016S
S63.021A
S63.021S
S63.022A
S63.022S
S63.023A
S63.023S
S63.024A
S63.024S
S63.025A
S63.025S
S63.026A
S63.026S
S63.031A
S63.031S
S63.032A
S63.032S
S63.033A
S63.033S
S63.034A
S63.034S
S63.035A
S63.035S
S63.036A
S63.036S
S63.041A
S63.041S
S63.042A
S63.042S
S63.043A
S63.043S
S63.044A
S63.044S
S63.045A
S63.045S
S63.046A
S63.046S
S63.051A
S63.051S
S63.052A
S63.052S
S63.053A
S63.053S
S63.054A
S63.054S
S63.055A
S63.055S
S63.056A
S63.056S
S63.061A
S63.061S
S63.062A
S63.062S
S63.063A
S63.063S
S63.064A
S63.064S
S63.065A
S63.065S
S63.066A
S63.066S
S63.071A
S63.071S
S63.072A
S63.072S
S63.073A
S63.073S
S63.074A
S63.074S
S63.075A
S63.075S
S63.076A
S63.076S
S63.091A
S63.091S
S63.092A
S63.092S
S63.093A
S63.093S
S63.094A
S63.094S
S63.095A
S63.095S
S63.096A
S63.096S
S63.101A
S63.101S
S63.102A
S63.102S
S63.103A
S63.103S
S63.104A
S63.104S
S63.105A
S63.105S
S63.106A
S63.106S
S63.111A
S63.111S
S63.112A
S63.112S
S63.113A
S63.113S
S63.114A
S63.114S
S63.115A
S63.115S
S63.116A
S63.116S
S63.121A
S63.121S
S63.122A
S63.122S
S63.123A
S63.123S
S63.124A
S63.124S
S63.125A
S63.125S
S63.126A
S63.126S
S63.200A
S63.200S
S63.201A
S63.201S
S63.202A
S63.202S
S63.203A
S63.203S
S63.204A
S63.204S
S63.205A
S63.205S
S63.206A
S63.206S
S63.207A
S63.207S
S63.208A
S63.208S
S63.209A
S63.209S
S63.210A
S63.210S
S63.211A
S63.211S
S63.212A
S63.212S
S63.213A
S63.213S
S63.214A
S63.214S
S63.215A
S63.215S
S63.216A
S63.216S
S63.217A
S63.217S
S63.218A
S63.218S
S63.219A
S63.219S
S63.220A
S63.220S
S63.221A
S63.221S
S63.222A
S63.222S
S63.223A
S63.223S
S63.224A
S63.224S
S63.225A
S63.225S
S63.226A
S63.226S
S63.227A
S63.227S
S63.228A
S63.228S
S63.229A
S63.229S
S63.230A
S63.230S
S63.231A
S63.231S
S63.232A
S63.232S
S63.233A
S63.233S
S63.234A
S63.234S
S63.235A
S63.235S
S63.236A
S63.236S
S63.237A
S63.237S
S63.238A
S63.238S
S63.239A
S63.239S
S63.240A
S63.240S
S63.241A
S63.241S
S63.242A
S63.242S
S63.243A
S63.243S
S63.244A
S63.244S
S63.245A
S63.245S
S63.246A
S63.246S
S63.247A
S63.247S
S63.248A
S63.248S
S63.249A
S63.249S
S63.250A
S63.250S
S63.251A
S63.251S
S63.252A
S63.252S
S63.253A
S63.253S
S63.254A
S63.254S
S63.255A
S63.255S
S63.256A
S63.256S
S63.257A
S63.257S
S63.258A
S63.258S
S63.259A
S63.259S
S63.260A
S63.260S
S63.261A
S63.261S
S63.262A
S63.262S
S63.263A
S63.263S
S63.264A
S63.264S
S63.265A
S63.265S
S63.266A
S63.266S
S63.267A
S63.267S
S63.268A
S63.268S
S63.269A
S63.269S
S63.270A
S63.270S
S63.271A
S63.271S
S63.272A
S63.272S
S63.273A
S63.273S
S63.274A
S63.274S
S63.275A
S63.275S
S63.276A
S63.276S
S63.277A
S63.277S
S63.278A
S63.278S
S63.279A
S63.279S
S63.280A
S63.280S
S63.281A
S63.281S
S63.282A
S63.282S
S63.283A
S63.283S
S63.284A
S63.284S
S63.285A
S63.285S
S63.286A
S63.286S
S63.287A
S63.287S
S63.288A
S63.288S
S63.289A
S63.289S
S63.290A
S63.290S
S63.291A
S63.291S
S63.292A
S63.292S
S63.293A
S63.293S
S63.294A
S63.294S
S63.295A
S63.295S
S63.296A
S63.296S
S63.297A
S63.297S
S63.298A
S63.298S
S63.299A
S63.299S
S63.301A
S63.301S
S63.302A
S63.302S
S63.309A
S63.309S
S63.311A
S63.311S
S63.312A
S63.312S
S63.319A
S63.319S
S63.321A
S63.321S
S63.322A
S63.322S
S63.329A
S63.329S
S63.331A
S63.331S
S63.332A
S63.332S
S63.339A
S63.339S
S63.391A
S63.391S
S63.392A
S63.392S
S63.399A
S63.399S
S63.400A
S63.400S
S63.401A
S63.401S
S63.402A
S63.402S
S63.403A
S63.403S
S63.404A
S63.404S
S63.405A
S63.405S
S63.406A
S63.406S
S63.407A
S63.407S
S63.408A
S63.408S
S63.409A
S63.409S
S63.410A
S63.410S
S63.411A
S63.411S
S63.412A
S63.412S
S63.413A
S63.413S
S63.414A
S63.414S
S63.415A
S63.415S
S63.416A
S63.416S
S63.417A
S63.417S
S63.418A
S63.418S
S63.419A
S63.419S
S63.420A
S63.420S
S63.421A
S63.421S
S63.422A
S63.422S
S63.423A
S63.423S
S63.424A
S63.424S
S63.425A
S63.425S
S63.426A
S63.426S
S63.427A
S63.427S
S63.428A
S63.428S
S63.429A
S63.429S
S63.430A
S63.430S
S63.431A
S63.431S
S63.432A
S63.432S
S63.433A
S63.433S
S63.434A
S63.434S
S63.435A
S63.435S
S63.436A
S63.436S
S63.437A
S63.437S
S63.438A
S63.438S
S63.439A
S63.439S
S63.490A
S63.490S
S63.491A
S63.491S
S63.492A
S63.492S
S63.493A
S63.493S
S63.494A
S63.494S
S63.495A
S63.495S
S63.496A
S63.496S
S63.497A
S63.497S
S63.498A
S63.498S
S63.499A
S63.499S
S63.501A
S63.501S
S63.502A
S63.502S
S63.509A
S63.509S
S63.511A
S63.511S
S63.512A
S63.512S
S63.519A
S63.519S
S63.521A
S63.521S
S63.522A
S63.522S
S63.529A
S63.529S
S63.591A
S63.591S
S63.592A
S63.592S
S63.599A
S63.599S
S63.601A
S63.601S
S63.602A
S63.602S
S63.609A
S63.609S
S63.610A
S63.610S
S63.611A
S63.611S
S63.612A
S63.612S
S63.613A
S63.613S
S63.614A
S63.614S
S63.615A
S63.615S
S63.616A
S63.616S
S63.617A
S63.617S
S63.618A
S63.618S
S63.619A
S63.619S
S63.621A
S63.621S
S63.622A
S63.622S
S63.629A
S63.629S
S63.630A
S63.630S
S63.631A
S63.631S
S63.632A
S63.632S
S63.633A
S63.633S
S63.634A
S63.634S
S63.635A
S63.635S
S63.636A
S63.636S
S63.637A
S63.637S
S63.638A
S63.638S
S63.639A
S63.639S
S63.641A
S63.641S
S63.642A
S63.642S
S63.649A
S63.649S
S63.650A
S63.650S
S63.651A
S63.651S
S63.652A
S63.652S
S63.653A
S63.653S
S63.654A
S63.654S
S63.655A
S63.655S
S63.656A
S63.656S
S63.657A
S63.657S
S63.658A
S63.658S
S63.659A
S63.659S
S63.681A
S63.681S
S63.682A
S63.682S
S63.689A
S63.689S
S63.690A
S63.690S
S63.691A
S63.691S
S63.692A
S63.692S
S63.693A
S63.693S
S63.694A
S63.694S
S63.695A
S63.695S
S63.696A
S63.696S
S63.697A
S63.697S
S63.698A
S63.698S
S63.699A
S63.699S
S63.8X1A
S63.8X1S
S63.8X2A
S63.8X2S
S63.8X9A
S63.8X9S
S63.90XA
S63.90XS
S63.91XA
S63.91XS
S63.92XA
S63.92XS
S66.011A
S66.011S
S66.012A
S66.012S
S66.019A
S66.019S
S66.110A
S66.110S
S66.111A
S66.111S
S66.112A
S66.112S
S66.113A
S66.113S
S66.114A
S66.114S
S66.115A
S66.115S
S66.116A
S66.116S
S66.117A
S66.117S
S66.118A
S66.118S
S66.119A
S66.119S
S66.211A
S66.211S
S66.212A
S66.212S
S66.219A
S66.219S
S66.310A
S66.310S
S66.311A
S66.311S
S66.312A
S66.312S
S66.313A
S66.313S
S66.314A
S66.314S
S66.315A
S66.315S
S66.316A
S66.316S

S66.317A
S66.317S
S66.318A
S66.318S
S66.319A
S66.319S
S66.411A
S66.411S
S66.412A
S66.412S
S66.419A
S66.419S
S66.51ØA
S66.51ØS
S66.511A
S66.511S
S66.512A
S66.512S
S66.513A
S66.513S
S66.514A
S66.514S
S66.515A
S66.515S
S66.516A
S66.516S
S66.517A
S66.517S
S66.518A
S66.518S
S66.519A
S66.519S
S66.811A
S66.811S
S66.812A
S66.812S
S66.819A
S66.819S
S66.911A
S66.911S
S66.912A
S66.912S
S66.919A
S66.919S
S73.ØØ1S
S73.ØØ2S
S73.ØØ3S
S73.ØØ4S
S73.ØØ5S
S73.ØØ6S
S73.Ø11S
S73.Ø12S
S73.Ø13S
S73.Ø14S
S73.Ø15S
S73.Ø16S
S73.Ø21S
S73.Ø22S
S73.Ø23S
S73.Ø24S
S73.Ø25S
S73.Ø26S
S73.Ø31S
S73.Ø32S
S73.Ø33S
S73.Ø34S
S73.Ø35S
S73.Ø36S
S73.Ø41S
S73.Ø42S
S73.Ø43S
S73.Ø44S
S73.Ø45S
S73.Ø46S
S73.1Ø1S
S73.1Ø2S
S73.1Ø9S
S73.111S
S73.112S
S73.119S
S73.121S
S73.122S
S73.129S
S73.191S
S73.192S
S73.199S
S76.Ø11S
S76.Ø12S
S76.Ø19S
S76.111S
S76.112S
S76.119S
S76.211S
S76.212S
S76.219S
S76.311S
S76.312S
S76.319S
S76.811S
S76.812S
S76.819S
S76.911S
S76.912S
S76.919S
S82.ØØ1A
S82.ØØ1B
S82.ØØ1C
S82.ØØ2A
S82.ØØ2B
S82.ØØ2C
S82.ØØ9A
S82.ØØ9B
S82.ØØ9C
S82.Ø11A
S82.Ø11B
S82.Ø11C
S82.Ø12A
S82.Ø12B
S82.Ø12C
S82.Ø13A
S82.Ø13B
S82.Ø13C
S82.Ø14A
S82.Ø14B
S82.Ø14C
S82.Ø15A
S82.Ø15B
S82.Ø15C
S82.Ø16A
S82.Ø16B
S82.Ø16C
S82.Ø21A
S82.Ø21B
S82.Ø21C
S82.Ø22A
S82.Ø22B
S82.Ø22C
S82.Ø23A
S82.Ø23B
S82.Ø23C
S82.Ø24A
S82.Ø24B
S82.Ø24C
S82.Ø25A
S82.Ø25B
S82.Ø25C
S82.Ø26A
S82.Ø26B
S82.Ø26C
S82.Ø31A
S82.Ø31B
S82.Ø31C
S82.Ø32A
S82.Ø32B
S82.Ø32C
S82.Ø33A
S82.Ø33B
S82.Ø33C
S82.Ø34A
S82.Ø34B
S82.Ø34C
S82.Ø35A
S82.Ø35B
S82.Ø35C
S82.Ø36A
S82.Ø36B
S82.Ø36C
S82.Ø41A
S82.Ø41B
S82.Ø41C
S82.Ø42A
S82.Ø42B
S82.Ø42C
S82.Ø43A
S82.Ø43B
S82.Ø43C
S82.Ø44A
S82.Ø44B
S82.Ø44C
S82.Ø45A
S82.Ø45B
S82.Ø45C
S82.Ø46A
S82.Ø46B
S82.Ø46C
S82.Ø91A
S82.Ø91B
S82.Ø91C
S82.Ø92A
S82.Ø92B
S82.Ø92C
S82.Ø99A
S82.Ø99B
S82.Ø99C
S82.1Ø1A
S82.1Ø1B
S82.1Ø1C
S82.1Ø2A
S82.1Ø2B
S82.1Ø2C
S82.1Ø9A
S82.1Ø9B
S82.1Ø9C
S82.111A
S82.111B
S82.111C
S82.112A
S82.112B
S82.112C
S82.113A
S82.113B
S82.113C
S82.114A
S82.114B
S82.114C
S82.115A
S82.115B
S82.115C
S82.116A
S82.116B
S82.116C
S82.121A
S82.121B
S82.121C
S82.122A
S82.122B
S82.122C
S82.123A
S82.123B
S82.123C
S82.124A
S82.124B
S82.124C
S82.125A
S82.125B
S82.125C
S82.126A
S82.126B
S82.126C
S82.131A
S82.131B
S82.131C
S82.132A
S82.132B
S82.132C
S82.133A
S82.133B
S82.133C
S82.134A
S82.134B
S82.134C
S82.135A
S82.135B
S82.135C
S82.136A
S82.136B
S82.136C
S82.141A
S82.141B
S82.141C
S82.142A
S82.142B
S82.142C
S82.143A
S82.143B
S82.143C
S82.144A
S82.144B
S82.144C
S82.145A
S82.145B
S82.145C
S82.146A
S82.146B
S82.146C
S82.151A
S82.151B
S82.151C
S82.152A
S82.152B
S82.152C
S82.153A
S82.153B
S82.153C
S82.154A
S82.154B
S82.154C
S82.155A
S82.155B
S82.155C
S82.156A
S82.156B
S82.156C
S82.161A
S82.162A
S82.169A
S82.191A
S82.191B
S82.191C
S82.192A
S82.192B
S82.192C
S82.199A
S82.199B
S82.199C
S82.2Ø1A
S82.2Ø1B
S82.2Ø1C
S82.2Ø2A
S82.2Ø2B
S82.2Ø2C
S82.2Ø9A
S82.2Ø9B
S82.2Ø9C
S82.221A
S82.221B
S82.221C
S82.222A
S82.222B
S82.222C
S82.223A
S82.223B
S82.223C
S82.224A
S82.224B
S82.224C
S82.225A
S82.225B
S82.225C
S82.226A
S82.226B
S82.226C
S82.231A
S82.231B
S82.231C
S82.232A
S82.232B
S82.232C
S82.233A
S82.233B
S82.233C
S82.234A
S82.234B
S82.234C
S82.235A
S82.235B
S82.235C
S82.236A
S82.236B
S82.236C
S82.241A
S82.241B
S82.241C
S82.242A
S82.242B
S82.242C
S82.243A
S82.243B
S82.243C
S82.244A
S82.244B
S82.244C
S82.245A
S82.245B
S82.245C
S82.246A
S82.246B
S82.246C
S82.251A
S82.251B
S82.251C
S82.252A
S82.252B
S82.252C
S82.253A
S82.253B
S82.253C
S82.254A
S82.254B
S82.254C
S82.255A
S82.255B
S82.255C
S82.256A
S82.256B
S82.256C
S82.261A
S82.261B
S82.261C
S82.262A
S82.262B
S82.262C
S82.263A
S82.263B
S82.263C
S82.264A
S82.264B
S82.264C
S82.265A
S82.265B
S82.265C
S82.266A
S82.266B
S82.266C
S82.291A
S82.291B
S82.291C
S82.292A
S82.292B
S82.292C
S82.299A
S82.299B
S82.299C
S82.3Ø1A
S82.3Ø1B
S82.3Ø1C
S82.3Ø2A
S82.3Ø2B
S82.3Ø2C
S82.3Ø9A
S82.3Ø9B
S82.3Ø9C
S82.311A
S82.312A
S82.319A
S82.391A
S82.391B
S82.391C
S82.392A
S82.392B
S82.392C
S82.399A
S82.399B
S82.399C
S82.4Ø1A
S82.4Ø1B
S82.4Ø1C
S82.4Ø2A
S82.4Ø2B
S82.4Ø2C
S82.4Ø9A
S82.4Ø9B
S82.4Ø9C
S82.421A
S82.421B
S82.421C
S82.422A
S82.422B
S82.422C
S82.423A
S82.423B
S82.423C
S82.424A
S82.424B
S82.424C
S82.425A
S82.425B
S82.425C
S82.426A
S82.426B
S82.426C
S82.431A
S82.431B
S82.431C
S82.432A
S82.432B
S82.432C
S82.433A
S82.433B
S82.433C
S82.434A
S82.434B
S82.434C
S82.435A
S82.435B
S82.435C
S82.436A
S82.436B
S82.436C
S82.441A
S82.441B
S82.441C
S82.442A
S82.442B
S82.442C
S82.443A
S82.443B
S82.443C
S82.444A
S82.444B
S82.444C
S82.445A
S82.445B
S82.445C
S82.446A
S82.446B
S82.446C
S82.451A
S82.451B
S82.451C
S82.452A
S82.452B
S82.452C
S82.453A
S82.453B
S82.453C
S82.454A
S82.454B
S82.454C
S82.455A
S82.455B
S82.455C
S82.456A
S82.456B
S82.456C
S82.461A
S82.461B
S82.461C
S82.462A
S82.462B
S82.462C
S82.463A
S82.463B
S82.463C
S82.464A
S82.464B
S82.464C
S82.465A
S82.465B
S82.465C
S82.466A
S82.466B
S82.466C
S82.491A
S82.491B
S82.491C
S82.492A
S82.492B
S82.492C
S82.499A
S82.499B
S82.499C
S82.51XA
S82.51XB
S82.51XC
S82.52XA
S82.52XB
S82.52XC
S82.53XA
S82.53XB
S82.53XC
S82.54XA
S82.54XB
S82.54XC
S82.55XA
S82.55XB
S82.55XC
S82.56XA
S82.56XB
S82.56XC
S82.61XA
S82.61XB
S82.61XC
S82.62XA
S82.62XB
S82.62XC
S82.63XA
S82.63XB
S82.63XC
S82.64XA
S82.64XB
S82.64XC
S82.65XA
S82.65XB
S82.65XC
S82.66XA
S82.66XB
S82.66XC
S82.811A
S82.812A
S82.819A
S82.821A
S82.822A
S82.829A
S82.831A
S82.831B
S82.831C
S82.832A
S82.832B
S82.832C
S82.839A
S82.839B
S82.839C
S82.841A
S82.841B
S82.841C
S82.842A
S82.842B
S82.842C
S82.843A
S82.843B
S82.843C
S82.844A
S82.844B
S82.844C
S82.845A
S82.845B
S82.845C
S82.846A
S82.846B
S82.846C
S82.851A
S82.851B
S82.851C
S82.852A
S82.852B
S82.852C
S82.853A
S82.853B
S82.853C
S82.854A
S82.854B
S82.854C
S82.855A
S82.855B
S82.855C
S82.856A
S82.856B
S82.856C
S82.861A
S82.861B
S82.861C
S82.862A
S82.862B
S82.862C
S82.863A
S82.863B
S82.863C
S82.864A
S82.864B
S82.864C
S82.865A
S82.865B
S82.865C
S82.866A
S82.866B
S82.866C
S82.871A
S82.871B
S82.871C
S82.872A
S82.872B
S82.872C
S82.873A
S82.873B
S82.873C
S82.874A
S82.874B
S82.874C
S82.875A
S82.875B
S82.875C
S82.876A
S82.876B
S82.876C
S82.891A
S82.891B
S82.891C
S82.892A
S82.892B
S82.892C
S82.899A
S82.899B
S82.899C
S82.9ØXA
S82.9ØXB
S82.9ØXC
S82.91XA
S82.91XB
S82.91XC
S82.92XA
S82.92XB
S82.92XC
S83.ØØ1A
S83.ØØ1S
S83.ØØ2A
S83.ØØ2S
S83.ØØ3A
S83.ØØ3S
S83.ØØ4A
S83.ØØ4S
S83.ØØ5A
S83.ØØ5S
S83.ØØ6A
S83.ØØ6S
S83.Ø11A
S83.Ø11S
S83.Ø12A
S83.Ø12S
S83.Ø13A
S83.Ø13S
S83.Ø14A
S83.Ø14S
S83.Ø15A
S83.Ø15S
S83.Ø16A
S83.Ø16S
S83.Ø91A
S83.Ø91S
S83.Ø92A
S83.Ø92S
S83.Ø93A
S83.Ø93S
S83.Ø94A
S83.Ø94S
S83.Ø95A
S83.Ø95S
S83.Ø96A
S83.Ø96S
S83.1Ø1A
S83.1Ø1S
S83.1Ø2A
S83.1Ø2S
S83.1Ø3A
S83.1Ø3S
S83.1Ø4A
S83.1Ø4S
S83.1Ø5A
S83.1Ø5S
S83.1Ø6A
S83.1Ø6S
S83.111A
S83.111S
S83.112A
S83.112S
S83.113A
S83.113S
S83.114A
S83.114S
S83.115A
S83.115S
S83.116A
S83.116S
S83.121A
S83.121S
S83.122A
S83.122S
S83.123A
S83.123S
S83.124A
S83.124S
S83.125A
S83.125S
S83.126A
S83.126S
S83.131A
S83.131S
S83.132A
S83.132S
S83.133A
S83.133S
S83.134A
S83.134S
S83.135A
S83.135S
S83.136A
S83.136S
S83.141A
S83.141S
S83.142A
S83.142S
S83.143A
S83.143S
S83.144A
S83.144S
S83.145A
S83.145S
S83.146A
S83.146S
S83.191A
S83.191S
S83.192A
S83.192S
S83.193A
S83.193S
S83.194A
S83.194S
S83.195A
S83.195S
S83.196A
S83.196S
S83.2ØØA
S83.2ØØS
S83.2Ø1A
S83.2Ø1S
S83.2Ø2A
S83.2Ø2S
S83.2Ø3A
S83.2Ø3S
S83.2Ø4A
S83.2Ø4S
S83.2Ø5A
S83.2Ø5S
S83.2Ø6A
S83.2Ø6S
S83.2Ø7A
S83.2Ø7S
S83.2Ø9A
S83.2Ø9S
S83.211A
S83.211S
S83.212A
S83.212S
S83.219A
S83.219S
S83.221A
S83.221S
S83.222A
S83.222S
S83.229A
S83.229S
S83.231A
S83.231S
S83.232A
S83.232S
S83.239A
S83.239S
S83.241A
S83.241S
S83.242A
S83.242S
S83.249A
S83.249S
S83.251A
S83.251S
S83.252A
S83.252S
S83.259A
S83.259S
S83.261A
S83.261S
S83.262A
S83.262S
S83.269A
S83.269S
S83.271A
S83.271S
S83.272A
S83.272S
S83.279A
S83.279S
S83.281A
S83.281S
S83.282A
S83.282S

S83.289A
S83.289S
S83.3ØXA
S83.3ØXS
S83.31XA
S83.31XS
S83.32XA
S83.32XS
S83.4Ø1A
S83.4Ø1S
S83.4Ø2A
S83.4Ø2S
S83.4Ø9A
S83.4Ø9S
S83.411A
S83.411S
S83.412A
S83.412S
S83.419A
S83.419S
S83.421A
S83.421S
S83.422A
S83.422S
S83.429A
S83.429S
S83.5Ø1A
S83.5Ø1S
S83.5Ø2A
S83.5Ø2S
S83.5Ø9A
S83.5Ø9S
S83.511A
S83.511S
S83.512A
S83.512S
S83.519A
S83.519S
S83.521A
S83.521S
S83.522A
S83.522S
S83.529A
S83.529S
S83.6ØXA
S83.6ØXS
S83.61XA
S83.61XS
S83.62XA
S83.62XS
S83.8X1A
S83.8X1S
S83.8X2A
S83.8X2S
S83.8X9A
S83.8X9S
S83.9ØXA
S83.9ØXS
S83.91XA
S83.91XS
S83.92XA
S83.92XS
S86.Ø11A
S86.Ø11S
S86.Ø12A
S86.Ø12S
S86.Ø19A
S86.Ø19S
S86.111A
S86.111S
S86.112A
S86.112S
S86.119A
S86.119S
S86.211A
S86.211S
S86.212A
S86.212S
S86.219A
S86.219S
S86.311A
S86.311S
S86.312A
S86.312S
S86.319A
S86.319S
S86.811A
S86.811S
S86.812A
S86.812S
S86.819A
S86.819S
S86.911A
S86.911S
S86.912A
S86.912S
S86.919A
S86.919S
S89.ØØ1A
S89.ØØ2A
S89.ØØ9A
S89.Ø11A
S89.Ø12A
S89.Ø19A
S89.Ø21A
S89.Ø22A
S89.Ø29A
S89.Ø31A
S89.Ø32A
S89.Ø39A
S89.Ø41A
S89.Ø42A
S89.Ø49A
S89.Ø91A
S89.Ø92A
S89.Ø99A
S89.1Ø1A
S89.1Ø2A
S89.1Ø9A
S89.111A
S89.112A
S89.119A
S89.121A
S89.122A
S89.129A
S89.131A
S89.132A
S89.139A
S89.141A
S89.142A
S89.149A
S89.191A
S89.192A
S89.199A
S89.2Ø1A
S89.2Ø2A
S89.2Ø9A
S89.211A
S89.212A
S89.219A
S89.221A
S89.222A
S89.229A
S89.291A
S89.292A
S89.299A
S89.3Ø1A
S89.3Ø2A
S89.3Ø9A
S89.311A
S89.312A
S89.319A
S89.321A
S89.322A
S89.329A
S89.391A
S89.392A
S89.399A
S92.ØØ1A
S92.ØØ1B
S92.ØØ2A
S92.ØØ2B
S92.ØØ9A
S92.ØØ9B
S92.Ø11A
S92.Ø11B
S92.Ø12A
S92.Ø12B
S92.Ø13A
S92.Ø13B
S92.Ø14A
S92.Ø14B
S92.Ø15A
S92.Ø15B
S92.Ø16A
S92.Ø16B
S92.Ø21A
S92.Ø21B
S92.Ø22A
S92.Ø22B
S92.Ø23A
S92.Ø23B
S92.Ø24A
S92.Ø24B
S92.Ø25A
S92.Ø25B
S92.Ø26A
S92.Ø26B
S92.Ø31A
S92.Ø31B
S92.Ø32A
S92.Ø32B
S92.Ø33A
S92.Ø33B
S92.Ø34A
S92.Ø34B
S92.Ø35A
S92.Ø35B
S92.Ø36A
S92.Ø36B
S92.Ø41A
S92.Ø41B
S92.Ø42A
S92.Ø42B
S92.Ø43A
S92.Ø43B
S92.Ø44A
S92.Ø44B
S92.Ø45A
S92.Ø45B
S92.Ø46A
S92.Ø46B
S92.Ø51A
S92.Ø51B
S92.Ø52A
S92.Ø52B
S92.Ø53A
S92.Ø53B
S92.Ø54A
S92.Ø54B
S92.Ø55A
S92.Ø55B
S92.Ø56A
S92.Ø56B
S92.Ø61A
S92.Ø61B
S92.Ø62A
S92.Ø62B
S92.Ø63A
S92.Ø63B
S92.Ø64A
S92.Ø64B
S92.Ø65A
S92.Ø65B
S92.Ø66A
S92.Ø66B
S92.1Ø1A
S92.1Ø1B
S92.1Ø2A
S92.1Ø2B
S92.1Ø9A
S92.1Ø9B
S92.111A
S92.111B
S92.112A
S92.112B
S92.113A
S92.113B
S92.114A
S92.114B
S92.115A
S92.115B
S92.116A
S92.116B
S92.121A
S92.121B
S92.122A
S92.122B
S92.123A
S92.123B
S92.124A
S92.124B
S92.125A
S92.125B
S92.126A
S92.126B
S92.131A
S92.131B
S92.132A
S92.132B
S92.133A
S92.133B
S92.134A
S92.134B
S92.135A
S92.135B
S92.136A
S92.136B
S92.141A
S92.141B
S92.142A
S92.142B
S92.143A
S92.143B
S92.144A
S92.144B
S92.145A
S92.145B
S92.146A
S92.146B
S92.151A
S92.151B
S92.152A
S92.152B
S92.153A
S92.153B
S92.154A
S92.154B
S92.155A
S92.155B
S92.156A
S92.156B
S92.191A
S92.191B
S92.192A
S92.192B
S92.199A
S92.199B
S92.2Ø1A
S92.2Ø1B
S92.2Ø2A
S92.2Ø2B
S92.2Ø9A
S92.2Ø9B
S92.211A
S92.211B
S92.212A
S92.212B
S92.213A
S92.213B
S92.214A
S92.214B
S92.215A
S92.215B
S92.216A
S92.216B
S92.221A
S92.221B
S92.222A
S92.222B
S92.223A
S92.223B
S92.224A
S92.224B
S92.225A
S92.225B
S92.226A
S92.226B
S92.231A
S92.231B
S92.232A
S92.232B
S92.233A
S92.233B
S92.234A
S92.234B
S92.235A
S92.235B
S92.236A
S92.236B
S92.241A
S92.241B
S92.242A
S92.242B
S92.243A
S92.243B
S92.244A
S92.244B
S92.245A
S92.245B
S92.246A
S92.246B
S92.251A
S92.251B
S92.252A
S92.252B
S92.253A
S92.253B
S92.254A
S92.254B
S92.255A
S92.255B
S92.256A
S92.256B
S92.3Ø1A
S92.3Ø1B
S92.3Ø2A
S92.3Ø2B
S92.3Ø9A
S92.3Ø9B
S92.311A
S92.311B
S92.312A
S92.312B
S92.313A
S92.313B
S92.314A
S92.314B
S92.315A
S92.315B
S92.316A
S92.316B
S92.321A
S92.321B
S92.322A
S92.322B
S92.323A
S92.323B
S92.324A
S92.324B
S92.325A
S92.325B
S92.326A
S92.326B
S92.331A
S92.331B
S92.332A
S92.332B
S92.333A
S92.333B
S92.334A
S92.334B
S92.335A
S92.335B
S92.336A
S92.336B
S92.341A
S92.341B
S92.342A
S92.342B
S92.343A
S92.343B
S92.344A
S92.344B
S92.345A
S92.345B
S92.346A
S92.346B
S92.351A
S92.351B
S92.352A
S92.352B
S92.353A
S92.353B
S92.354A
S92.354B
S92.355A
S92.355B
S92.356A
S92.356B
S92.4Ø1A
S92.4Ø1B
S92.4Ø2A
S92.4Ø2B
S92.4Ø3A
S92.4Ø3B
S92.4Ø4A
S92.4Ø4B
S92.4Ø5A
S92.4Ø5B
S92.4Ø6A
S92.4Ø6B
S92.411A
S92.411B
S92.412A
S92.412B
S92.413A
S92.413B
S92.414A
S92.414B
S92.415A
S92.415B
S92.416A
S92.416B
S92.421A
S92.421B
S92.422A
S92.422B
S92.423A
S92.423B
S92.424A
S92.424B
S92.425A
S92.425B
S92.426A
S92.426B
S92.491A
S92.491B
S92.492A
S92.492B
S92.499A
S92.499B
S92.5Ø1A
S92.5Ø1B
S92.5Ø2A
S92.5Ø2B
S92.5Ø3A
S92.5Ø3B
S92.5Ø4A
S92.5Ø4B
S92.5Ø5A
S92.5Ø5B
S92.5Ø6A
S92.5Ø6B
S92.511A
S92.511B
S92.512A
S92.512B
S92.513A
S92.513B
S92.514A
S92.514B
S92.515A
S92.515B
S92.516A
S92.516B
S92.521A
S92.521B
S92.522A
S92.522B
S92.523A
S92.523B
S92.524A
S92.524B
S92.525A
S92.525B
S92.526A
S92.526B
S92.531A
S92.531B
S92.532A
S92.532B
S92.533A
S92.533B
S92.534A
S92.534B
S92.535A
S92.535B
S92.536A
S92.536B
S92.591A
S92.591B
S92.592A
S92.592B
S92.599A
S92.599B
S92.811A
S92.811B
S92.812A
S92.812B
S92.819A
S92.819B
S92.9Ø1A
S92.9Ø1B
S92.9Ø2A
S92.9Ø2B
S92.9Ø9A
S92.9Ø9B
S92.911A
S92.911B
S92.912A
S92.912B
S92.919A
S92.919B
S93.Ø1XA
S93.Ø1XS
S93.Ø2XA
S93.Ø2XS
S93.Ø3XA
S93.Ø3XS
S93.Ø4XA
S93.Ø4XS
S93.Ø5XA
S93.Ø5XS
S93.Ø6XA
S93.Ø6XS
S93.1Ø1A
S93.1Ø1S
S93.1Ø2A
S93.1Ø2S
S93.1Ø3A
S93.1Ø3S
S93.1Ø4A
S93.1Ø4S
S93.1Ø5A
S93.1Ø5S
S93.1Ø6A
S93.1Ø6S
S93.111A
S93.111S
S93.112A
S93.112S
S93.113A
S93.113S
S93.114A
S93.114S
S93.115A
S93.115S
S93.116A
S93.116S
S93.119A
S93.119S
S93.121A
S93.121S
S93.122A
S93.122S
S93.123A
S93.123S
S93.124A
S93.124S
S93.125A
S93.125S
S93.126A
S93.126S
S93.129A
S93.129S
S93.131A
S93.131S
S93.132A
S93.132S
S93.133A
S93.133S
S93.134A
S93.134S
S93.135A
S93.135S
S93.136A
S93.136S
S93.139A
S93.139S
S93.141A
S93.141S
S93.142A
S93.142S
S93.143A
S93.143S
S93.144A
S93.144S
S93.145A
S93.145S
S93.146A
S93.146S
S93.149A
S93.149S
S93.3Ø1A
S93.3Ø1S
S93.3Ø2A
S93.3Ø2S
S93.3Ø3A
S93.3Ø3S
S93.3Ø4A
S93.3Ø4S
S93.3Ø5A
S93.3Ø5S
S93.3Ø6A
S93.3Ø6S
S93.311A
S93.311S
S93.312A
S93.312S
S93.313A
S93.313S
S93.314A
S93.314S
S93.315A
S93.315S
S93.316A
S93.316S
S93.321A
S93.321S
S93.322A
S93.322S
S93.323A
S93.323S
S93.324A
S93.324S
S93.325A
S93.325S
S93.326A
S93.326S
S93.331A
S93.331S
S93.332A
S93.332S
S93.333A
S93.333S
S93.334A
S93.334S
S93.335A
S93.335S
S93.336A
S93.336S
S93.4Ø1A
S93.4Ø1S
S93.4Ø2A
S93.4Ø2S
S93.4Ø9A
S93.4Ø9S
S93.411A
S93.411S
S93.412A
S93.412S
S93.419A
S93.419S
S93.421A
S93.421S
S93.422A
S93.422S
S93.429A
S93.429S
S93.431A
S93.431S
S93.432A
S93.432S
S93.439A
S93.439S
S93.491A
S93.491S
S93.492A
S93.492S
S93.499A
S93.499S
S93.5Ø1A
S93.5Ø1S
S93.5Ø2A
S93.5Ø2S
S93.5Ø3A
S93.5Ø3S
S93.5Ø4A
S93.5Ø4S
S93.5Ø5A
S93.5Ø5S
S93.5Ø6A
S93.5Ø6S
S93.5Ø9A
S93.5Ø9S
S93.511A
S93.511S
S93.512A
S93.512S
S93.513A
S93.513S
S93.514A
S93.514S
S93.515A
S93.515S
S93.516A
S93.516S
S93.519A
S93.519S
S93.521A
S93.521S
S93.522A
S93.522S
S93.523A
S93.523S
S93.524A
S93.524S
S93.525A
S93.525S
S93.526A
S93.526S
S93.529A
S93.529S
S93.6Ø1A
S93.6Ø1S
S93.6Ø2A
S93.6Ø2S
S93.6Ø9A
S93.6Ø9S
S93.611A
S93.611S
S93.612A
S93.612S
S93.619A
S93.619S
S93.621A
S93.621S
S93.622A
S93.622S
S93.629A
S93.629S
S93.691A
S93.691S
S93.692A
S93.692S
S93.699A
S93.699S
S96.Ø11A
S96.Ø11S
S96.Ø12A
S96.Ø12S
S96.Ø19A
S96.Ø19S
S96.111A
S96.111S
S96.112A
S96.112S
S96.119A
S96.119S
S96.211A
S96.211S
S96.212A
S96.212S
S96.219A
S96.219S
S96.811A
S96.811S
S96.812A
S96.812S
S96.819A
S96.819S
S96.911A
S96.911S
S96.912A
S96.912S
S96.919A
S96.919S

DRG 563

Select principal diagnosis listed under DRG 562

DRG 564

Principal Diagnosis

B9Ø.2
D16.ØØ
D16.Ø1
D16.Ø2
D16.1Ø
D16.11
D16.12
D16.2Ø
D16.21
D16.22
D16.3Ø
D16.31
D16.32
D16.4
D16.6
D16.8
D16.9
D21.Ø
D21.1Ø
D21.11
D21.12
D21.2Ø
D21.21
D21.22
D21.3
D21.4
D21.5
D21.6
D21.9
D36.1Ø
D36.11
D36.12
D36.13
D36.14
D36.15
D36.16
D36.17
D48.1*
D48.2

D49.2
E78.71
E78.72
H61.Ø11
H61.Ø12
H61.Ø13
H61.Ø19
H61.Ø21
H61.Ø22
H61.Ø23
H61.Ø29
H61.Ø31
H61.Ø32
H61.Ø33
H61.Ø39
M2Ø.ØØ1
M2Ø.ØØ2
M2Ø.ØØ9
M2Ø.Ø11
M2Ø.Ø12
M2Ø.Ø19
M2Ø.Ø21
M2Ø.Ø22
M2Ø.Ø29
M2Ø.Ø31
M2Ø.Ø32
M2Ø.Ø39
M2Ø.Ø91
M2Ø.Ø92
M2Ø.Ø99
M2Ø.1Ø
M2Ø.11
M2Ø.12
M2Ø.2Ø
M2Ø.21
M2Ø.22
M2Ø.3Ø
M2Ø.31
M2Ø.32
M2Ø.4Ø
M2Ø.41
M2Ø.42
M2Ø.5X1
M2Ø.5X2
M2Ø.5X9
M2Ø.6Ø
M2Ø.61
M2Ø.62
M21.ØØ
M21.Ø21
M21.Ø22
M21.Ø29
M21.Ø51
M21.Ø52
M21.Ø59
M21.Ø61
M21.Ø62
M21.Ø69
M21.Ø71
M21.Ø72
M21.Ø79
M21.1Ø
M21.121
M21.122
M21.129
M21.151
M21.152
M21.159
M21.161
M21.162
M21.169
M21.171
M21.172
M21.179
M21.2Ø
M21.211
M21.212
M21.219
M21.221
M21.222
M21.229
M21.231
M21.232
M21.239
M21.241
M21.242
M21.249
M21.251
M21.252
M21.259
M21.261
M21.262
M21.269
M21.271
M21.272
M21.279
M21.371
M21.372
M21.379
M21.4Ø
M21.41
M21.42
M21.541
M21.542
M21.549
M21.611
M21.612
M21.619
M21.621
M21.622
M21.629
M21.6X1
M21.6X2
M21.6X9
M21.7Ø
M21.721
M21.722
M21.729
M21.731
M21.732
M21.733
M21.734
M21.739
M21.751
M21.752
M21.759
M21.761
M21.762
M21.763
M21.764
M21.769
M21.8Ø
M21.821
M21.822
M21.829
M21.831
M21.832
M21.839
M21.851
M21.852
M21.859
M21.861
M21.862
M21.869
M21.9Ø
M21.921
M21.922
M21.929
M21.931
M21.932
M21.939
M21.941
M21.942
M21.949
M21.951
M21.952
M21.959
M21.961
M21.962
M21.969
M23.4*
M23.5*
M24.Ø*
M24.1Ø
M24.151
M24.152
M24.159
M24.19
M24.351
M24.352
M24.359
M24.4Ø
M24.451
M24.452
M24.459
M24.49
M24.5*
M24.7
M24.8*
M24.9
M25.2*
M25.3*
M25.4*
M43.3
M43.4
M43.5*
M53.2X1
M53.2X2
M53.2X3
M53.2X4
M53.2X5
M53.2X6
M53.2X9
M77.3*
M79.5
M8Ø.ØØXK
M8Ø.ØØXP
M8Ø.Ø11K
M8Ø.Ø11P
M8Ø.Ø12K
M8Ø.Ø12P
M8Ø.Ø19K
M8Ø.Ø19P
M8Ø.Ø21K
M8Ø.Ø21P
M8Ø.Ø22K
M8Ø.Ø22P
M8Ø.Ø29K
M8Ø.Ø29P
M8Ø.Ø31K
M8Ø.Ø31P
M8Ø.Ø32K
M8Ø.Ø32P
M8Ø.Ø39K
M8Ø.Ø39P
M8Ø.Ø41K
M8Ø.Ø41P
M8Ø.Ø42K
M8Ø.Ø42P
M8Ø.Ø49K
M8Ø.Ø49P
M8Ø.Ø51K
M8Ø.Ø51P
M8Ø.Ø52K
M8Ø.Ø52P
M8Ø.Ø59K
M8Ø.Ø59P
M8Ø.Ø61K
M8Ø.Ø61P
M8Ø.Ø62K
M8Ø.Ø62P
M8Ø.Ø69K
M8Ø.Ø69P
M8Ø.Ø71K
M8Ø.Ø71P
M8Ø.Ø72K
M8Ø.Ø72P
M8Ø.Ø79K
M8Ø.Ø79P
M8Ø.Ø8XK
M8Ø.Ø8XP
M8Ø.ØAXK
M8Ø.ØAXP
M8Ø.ØB1K
M8Ø.ØB1P
M8Ø.ØB2K
M8Ø.ØB2P
M8Ø.ØB9K
M8Ø.ØB9P
M8Ø.8ØXK
M8Ø.8ØXP
M8Ø.811K
M8Ø.811P
M8Ø.812K
M8Ø.812P
M8Ø.819K
M8Ø.819P
M8Ø.821K
M8Ø.821P
M8Ø.822K
M8Ø.822P
M8Ø.829K
M8Ø.829P
M8Ø.831K
M8Ø.831P
M8Ø.832K
M8Ø.832P
M8Ø.839K
M8Ø.839P
M8Ø.841K
M8Ø.841P
M8Ø.842K
M8Ø.842P
M8Ø.849K
M8Ø.849P
M8Ø.851K
M8Ø.851P
M8Ø.852K
M8Ø.852P
M8Ø.859K
M8Ø.859P
M8Ø.861K
M8Ø.861P
M8Ø.862K
M8Ø.862P
M8Ø.869K
M8Ø.869P
M8Ø.871K
M8Ø.871P
M8Ø.872K
M8Ø.872P
M8Ø.879K
M8Ø.879P
M8Ø.88XK
M8Ø.88XP
M8Ø.8AXK
M8Ø.8AXP
M8Ø.8B1K
M8Ø.8B1P
M8Ø.8B2K
M8Ø.8B2P
M8Ø.8B9K
M8Ø.8B9P
M84.3ØXK
M84.3ØXP
M84.311K
M84.311P
M84.312K
M84.312P
M84.319K
M84.319P
M84.321K
M84.321P
M84.322K
M84.322P
M84.329K
M84.329P
M84.331K
M84.331P
M84.332K
M84.332P
M84.333K
M84.333P
M84.334K
M84.334P
M84.339K
M84.339P
M84.341K
M84.341P
M84.342K
M84.342P
M84.343K
M84.343P
M84.344K
M84.344P
M84.345K
M84.345P
M84.346K
M84.346P
M84.35ØK
M84.35ØP
M84.351K
M84.351P
M84.352K
M84.352P
M84.353K
M84.353P
M84.359K
M84.359P
M84.361K
M84.361P
M84.362K
M84.362P
M84.363K
M84.363P
M84.364K
M84.364P
M84.369K
M84.369P
M84.371K
M84.371P
M84.372K
M84.372P
M84.373K
M84.373P
M84.374K
M84.374P
M84.375K
M84.375P
M84.376K
M84.376P
M84.377K
M84.377P
M84.378K
M84.378P
M84.379K
M84.379P
M84.38XK
M84.38XP
M84.4ØXK
M84.4ØXP
M84.411K
M84.411P
M84.412K
M84.412P
M84.419K
M84.419P
M84.421K
M84.421P
M84.422K
M84.422P
M84.429K
M84.429P
M84.431K
M84.431P
M84.432K
M84.432P
M84.433K
M84.433P
M84.434K
M84.434P
M84.439K
M84.439P
M84.441K
M84.441P
M84.442K
M84.442P
M84.443K
M84.443P
M84.444K
M84.444P
M84.445K
M84.445P
M84.446K
M84.446P
M84.451K
M84.451P
M84.452K
M84.452P
M84.453K
M84.453P
M84.454K
M84.454P
M84.459K
M84.459P
M84.461K
M84.461P
M84.462K
M84.462P
M84.463K
M84.463P
M84.464K
M84.464P
M84.469K
M84.469P
M84.471K
M84.471P
M84.472K
M84.472P
M84.473K
M84.473P
M84.474K
M84.474P
M84.475K
M84.475P
M84.476K
M84.476P
M84.477K
M84.477P
M84.478K
M84.478P
M84.479K
M84.479P
M84.48XK
M84.48XP
M84.5ØXK
M84.5ØXP
M84.511K
M84.511P
M84.512K
M84.512P
M84.519K
M84.519P
M84.521K
M84.521P
M84.522K
M84.522P
M84.529K
M84.529P
M84.531K
M84.531P
M84.532K
M84.532P
M84.533K
M84.533P
M84.534K
M84.534P
M84.539K
M84.539P
M84.541K
M84.541P
M84.542K
M84.542P
M84.549K
M84.549P
M84.55ØK
M84.55ØP
M84.551K
M84.551P
M84.552K
M84.552P
M84.553K
M84.553P
M84.559K
M84.559P
M84.561K
M84.561P
M84.562K
M84.562P
M84.563K
M84.563P
M84.564K
M84.564P
M84.569K
M84.569P
M84.571K
M84.571P
M84.572K
M84.572P
M84.573K
M84.573P
M84.574K
M84.574P
M84.575K
M84.575P
M84.576K
M84.576P
M84.58XK
M84.58XP
M84.6ØXK
M84.6ØXP
M84.611K
M84.611P
M84.612K
M84.612P
M84.619K
M84.619P
M84.621K
M84.621P
M84.622K
M84.622P
M84.629K
M84.629P
M84.631K
M84.631P
M84.632K
M84.632P
M84.633K
M84.633P
M84.634K
M84.634P
M84.639K
M84.639P
M84.641K
M84.641P
M84.642K
M84.642P
M84.649K
M84.649P
M84.65ØK
M84.65ØP
M84.651K
M84.651P
M84.652K
M84.652P
M84.653K
M84.653P
M84.659K
M84.659P
M84.661K
M84.661P
M84.662K
M84.662P
M84.663K
M84.663P
M84.664K
M84.664P
M84.669K
M84.669P
M84.671K
M84.671P
M84.672K
M84.672P
M84.673K
M84.673P
M84.674K
M84.674P
M84.675K
M84.675P
M84.676K
M84.676P
M84.68XK
M84.68XP
M84.75ØK
M84.75ØP
M84.751K
M84.751P
M84.752K
M84.752P
M84.753K
M84.753P
M84.754K
M84.754P
M84.755K
M84.755P
M84.756K
M84.756P
M84.757K
M84.757P
M84.758K
M84.758P
M84.759K
M84.759P
M84.8*
M84.9
M85.1*
M85.2
M85.8*
M85.9
M89.Ø*
M89.1*
M89.2*
M89.3*
M89.5*
M89.6*
M89.8*
M89.9
M94.1
M94.3*
M94.8*
M94.9
M95.2
M95.3
M95.4
M95.5
M95.8
M95.9
M96.A1
M96.A2
M96.A3
M96.A9
M99.8Ø
M99.81
M99.82
M99.85
M99.86
M99.87
M99.88
M99.89
M99.9
Q65*
Q66*
Q67.Ø
Q67.1
Q67.2
Q67.3
Q67.4
Q67.5
Q67.6
Q67.7
Q67.8
Q68.Ø
Q68.1
Q68.2
Q68.3
Q68.4
Q68.5
Q68.8
Q69*
Q7Ø*
Q71*
Q72*
Q73*
Q74*
Q75*
Q76.1
Q76.3
Q76.425
Q76.426
Q76.427
Q76.428
Q76.429
Q76.5
Q76.6
Q76.7
Q76.8
Q76.9
Q77.Ø
Q77.1
Q77.2
Q77.3
Q77.4
Q77.5
Q77.6
Q77.7
Q77.8
Q77.9
Q78.Ø
Q78.1
Q78.2
Q78.3
Q78.4
Q78.5
Q78.6
Q78.8
Q78.9
Q79.6*
Q79.8
Q79.9
Q87.Ø
Q87.1*
Q87.2
Q87.3
Q87.5
Q87.8*
Q89.7
Q89.8
R93.6
R93.7
R94.131
SØ2.ØXXK
SØ2.1Ø1K
SØ2.1Ø2K
SØ2.1Ø9K
SØ2.11ØK
SØ2.111K
SØ2.112K
SØ2.113K
SØ2.118K
SØ2.119K
SØ2.11AK
SØ2.11BK
SØ2.11CK
SØ2.11DK
SØ2.11EK
SØ2.11FK
SØ2.11GK
SØ2.11HK
SØ2.19XK
SØ2.2XXK
SØ2.3ØXK
SØ2.31XK
SØ2.32XK
SØ2.4ØØK
SØ2.4Ø1K
SØ2.4Ø2K
SØ2.4ØAK
SØ2.4ØBK
SØ2.4ØCK
SØ2.4ØDK
SØ2.4ØEK
SØ2.4ØFK
SØ2.411K
SØ2.412K
SØ2.413K
SØ2.42XA
SØ2.42XB
SØ2.42XK
SØ2.5XXK
SØ2.6ØØK
SØ2.6Ø1K
SØ2.6Ø2K
SØ2.6Ø9K
SØ2.61ØK
SØ2.611K
SØ2.612K
SØ2.62ØK
SØ2.621K
SØ2.622K
SØ2.63ØK
SØ2.631K
SØ2.632K
SØ2.64ØK
SØ2.641K
SØ2.642K
SØ2.65ØK
SØ2.651K
SØ2.652K
SØ2.66XK
SØ2.67ØK
SØ2.671K
SØ2.672K
SØ2.69XK
SØ2.8ØXA
SØ2.8ØXB
SØ2.8ØXK
SØ2.81XA
SØ2.81XB
SØ2.81XK
SØ2.82XA
SØ2.82XB
SØ2.82XK
SØ2.91XK
SØ2.92XA
SØ2.92XB
SØ2.92XK
SØ3.8XXA
S12.ØØØK
S12.ØØ1K
S12.Ø1XK
S12.Ø2XK
S12.Ø3ØK
S12.Ø31K
S12.Ø4ØK
S12.Ø41K
S12.Ø9ØK
S12.Ø91K
S12.1ØØK
S12.1Ø1K
S12.11ØK
S12.111K
S12.112K
S12.12ØK
S12.121K
S12.13ØK
S12.131K
S12.14XK
S12.15ØK
S12.151K
S12.19ØK
S12.191K
S12.2ØØK
S12.2Ø1K
S12.23ØK
S12.231K
S12.24XK
S12.25ØK
S12.251K
S12.29ØK
S12.291K
S12.3ØØK
S12.3Ø1K
S12.33ØK
S12.331K
S12.34XK
S12.35ØK
S12.351K
S12.39ØK
S12.391K
S12.4ØØK
S12.4Ø1K
S12.43ØK
S12.431K
S12.44XK
S12.45ØK
S12.451K
S12.49ØK
S12.491K
S12.5ØØK
S12.5Ø1K
S12.53ØK
S12.531K
S12.54XK
S12.55ØK
S12.551K
S12.59ØK
S12.591K
S12.6ØØK
S12.6Ø1K
S12.63ØK
S12.631K
S12.64XK
S12.65ØK
S12.651K
S12.69ØK

S12.691K
S13.5XXA
S22.ØØØK
S22.ØØ1K
S22.ØØ2K
S22.ØØ8K
S22.ØØ9K
S22.Ø1ØK
S22.Ø11K
S22.Ø12K
S22.Ø18K
S22.Ø19K
S22.Ø2ØK
S22.Ø21K
S22.Ø22K
S22.Ø28K
S22.Ø29K
S22.Ø3ØK
S22.Ø31K
S22.Ø32K
S22.Ø38K
S22.Ø39K
S22.Ø4ØK
S22.Ø41K
S22.Ø42K
S22.Ø48K
S22.Ø49K
S22.Ø5ØK
S22.Ø51K
S22.Ø52K
S22.Ø58K
S22.Ø59K
S22.Ø6ØK
S22.Ø61K
S22.Ø62K
S22.Ø68K
S22.Ø69K
S22.Ø7ØK
S22.Ø71K
S22.Ø72K
S22.Ø78K
S22.Ø79K
S22.Ø8ØK
S22.Ø81K
S22.Ø82K
S22.Ø88K
S22.Ø89K
S22.2ØXA
S22.2ØXB
S22.2ØXK
S22.21XA
S22.21XB
S22.21XK
S22.22XA
S22.22XB
S22.22XK
S22.23XA
S22.23XB
S22.23XK
S22.24XA
S22.24XB
S22.24XK
S22.31XK
S22.32XK
S22.39XK
S22.41XK
S22.42XK
S22.43XK
S22.49XK
S22.5XXK
S22.9XXA
S22.9XXB
S22.9XXK
S32.ØØØK
S32.ØØ1K
S32.ØØ2K
S32.ØØ8K
S32.ØØ9K
S32.Ø1ØK
S32.Ø11K
S32.Ø12K
S32.Ø18K
S32.Ø19K
S32.Ø2ØK
S32.Ø21K
S32.Ø22K
S32.Ø28K
S32.Ø29K
S32.Ø3ØK
S32.Ø31K
S32.Ø32K
S32.Ø38K
S32.Ø39K
S32.Ø4ØK
S32.Ø41K
S32.Ø42K
S32.Ø48K
S32.Ø49K
S32.Ø5ØK
S32.Ø51K
S32.Ø52K
S32.Ø58K
S32.Ø59K
S32.1ØXK
S32.11ØK
S32.111K
S32.112K
S32.119K
S32.12ØK
S32.121K
S32.122K
S32.129K
S32.13ØK
S32.131K
S32.132K
S32.139K
S32.14XK
S32.15XK
S32.16XK
S32.17XK
S32.19XK
S32.2XXK
S32.3Ø1K
S32.3Ø2K
S32.3Ø9K
S32.311K
S32.312K
S32.313K
S32.314K
S32.315K
S32.316K
S32.391K
S32.392K
S32.399K
S32.4Ø1K
S32.4Ø2K
S32.4Ø9K
S32.411K
S32.412K
S32.413K
S32.414K
S32.415K
S32.416K
S32.421K
S32.422K
S32.423K
S32.424K
S32.425K
S32.426K
S32.431K
S32.432K
S32.433K
S32.434K
S32.435K
S32.436K
S32.441K
S32.442K
S32.443K
S32.444K
S32.445K
S32.446K
S32.451K
S32.452K
S32.453K
S32.454K
S32.455K
S32.456K
S32.461K
S32.462K
S32.463K
S32.464K
S32.465K
S32.466K
S32.471K
S32.472K
S32.473K
S32.474K
S32.475K
S32.476K
S32.481K
S32.482K
S32.483K
S32.484K
S32.485K
S32.486K
S32.491K
S32.492K
S32.499K
S32.5Ø1K
S32.5Ø2K
S32.5Ø9K
S32.511K
S32.512K
S32.519K
S32.591K
S32.592K
S32.599K
S32.6Ø1K
S32.6Ø2K
S32.6Ø9K
S32.611K
S32.612K
S32.613K
S32.614K
S32.615K
S32.616K
S32.691K
S32.692K
S32.699K
S32.81ØK
S32.811K
S32.82XK
S32.89XK
S32.9XXK
S42.ØØ1K
S42.ØØ1P
S42.ØØ2K
S42.ØØ2P
S42.ØØ9K
S42.ØØ9P
S42.Ø11K
S42.Ø11P
S42.Ø12K
S42.Ø12P
S42.Ø13K
S42.Ø13P
S42.Ø14K
S42.Ø14P
S42.Ø15K
S42.Ø15P
S42.Ø16K
S42.Ø16P
S42.Ø17K
S42.Ø17P
S42.Ø18K
S42.Ø18P
S42.Ø19K
S42.Ø19P
S42.Ø21K
S42.Ø21P
S42.Ø22K
S42.Ø22P
S42.Ø23K
S42.Ø23P
S42.Ø24K
S42.Ø24P
S42.Ø25K
S42.Ø25P
S42.Ø26K
S42.Ø26P
S42.Ø31K
S42.Ø31P
S42.Ø32K
S42.Ø32P
S42.Ø33K
S42.Ø33P
S42.Ø34K
S42.Ø34P
S42.Ø35K
S42.Ø35P
S42.Ø36K
S42.Ø36P
S42.1Ø1K
S42.1Ø1P
S42.1Ø2K
S42.1Ø2P
S42.1Ø9K
S42.1Ø9P
S42.111A
S42.111B
S42.111K
S42.111P
S42.112A
S42.112B
S42.112K
S42.112P
S42.113A
S42.113B
S42.113K
S42.113P
S42.114A
S42.114B
S42.114K
S42.114P
S42.115A
S42.115B
S42.115K
S42.115P
S42.116A
S42.116B
S42.116K
S42.116P
S42.121K
S42.121P
S42.122K
S42.122P
S42.123K
S42.123P
S42.124K
S42.124P
S42.125K
S42.125P
S42.126K
S42.126P
S42.131K
S42.131P
S42.132K
S42.132P
S42.133K
S42.133P
S42.134K
S42.134P
S42.135K
S42.135P
S42.136K
S42.136P
S42.141K
S42.141P
S42.142K
S42.142P
S42.143K
S42.143P
S42.144K
S42.144P
S42.145K
S42.145P
S42.146K
S42.146P
S42.151K
S42.151P
S42.152K
S42.152P
S42.153K
S42.153P
S42.154K
S42.154P
S42.155K
S42.155P
S42.156K
S42.156P
S42.191A
S42.191B
S42.191K
S42.191P
S42.192A
S42.192B
S42.192K
S42.192P
S42.199A
S42.199B
S42.199K
S42.199P
S42.2Ø1K
S42.2Ø1P
S42.2Ø2K
S42.2Ø2P
S42.2Ø9K
S42.2Ø9P
S42.211K
S42.211P
S42.212K
S42.212P
S42.213K
S42.213P
S42.214K
S42.214P
S42.215K
S42.215P
S42.216K
S42.216P
S42.221K
S42.221P
S42.222K
S42.222P
S42.223K
S42.223P
S42.224K
S42.224P
S42.225K
S42.225P
S42.226K
S42.226P
S42.231K
S42.231P
S42.232K
S42.232P
S42.239K
S42.239P
S42.241K
S42.241P
S42.242K
S42.242P
S42.249K
S42.249P
S42.251K
S42.251P
S42.252K
S42.252P
S42.253K
S42.253P
S42.254K
S42.254P
S42.255K
S42.255P
S42.256K
S42.256P
S42.261K
S42.261P
S42.262K
S42.262P
S42.263K
S42.263P
S42.264K
S42.264P
S42.265K
S42.265P
S42.266K
S42.266P
S42.271K
S42.271P
S42.272K
S42.272P
S42.279K
S42.279P
S42.291K
S42.291P
S42.292K
S42.292P
S42.293K
S42.293P
S42.294K
S42.294P
S42.295K
S42.295P
S42.296K
S42.296P
S42.3Ø1K
S42.3Ø1P
S42.3Ø2K
S42.3Ø2P
S42.3Ø9K
S42.3Ø9P
S42.311K
S42.311P
S42.312K
S42.312P
S42.319K
S42.319P
S42.321K
S42.321P
S42.322K
S42.322P
S42.323K
S42.323P
S42.324K
S42.324P
S42.325K
S42.325P
S42.326K
S42.326P
S42.331K
S42.331P
S42.332K
S42.332P
S42.333K
S42.333P
S42.334K
S42.334P
S42.335K
S42.335P
S42.336K
S42.336P
S42.341K
S42.341P
S42.342K
S42.342P
S42.343K
S42.343P
S42.344K
S42.344P
S42.345K
S42.345P
S42.346K
S42.346P
S42.351K
S42.351P
S42.352K
S42.352P
S42.353K
S42.353P
S42.354K
S42.354P
S42.355K
S42.355P
S42.356K
S42.356P
S42.361K
S42.361P
S42.362K
S42.362P
S42.363K
S42.363P
S42.364K
S42.364P
S42.365K
S42.365P
S42.366K
S42.366P
S42.391K
S42.391P
S42.392K
S42.392P
S42.399K
S42.399P
S42.4Ø1K
S42.4Ø1P
S42.4Ø2K
S42.4Ø2P
S42.4Ø9K
S42.4Ø9P
S42.411K
S42.411P
S42.412K
S42.412P
S42.413K
S42.413P
S42.414K
S42.414P
S42.415K
S42.415P
S42.416K
S42.416P
S42.421K
S42.421P
S42.422K
S42.422P
S42.423K
S42.423P
S42.424K
S42.424P
S42.425K
S42.425P
S42.426K
S42.426P
S42.431K
S42.431P
S42.432K
S42.432P
S42.433K
S42.433P
S42.434K
S42.434P
S42.435K
S42.435P
S42.436K
S42.436P
S42.441K
S42.441P
S42.442K
S42.442P
S42.443K
S42.443P
S42.444K
S42.444P
S42.445K
S42.445P
S42.446K
S42.446P
S42.447K
S42.447P
S42.448K
S42.448P
S42.449K
S42.449P
S42.451K
S42.451P
S42.452K
S42.452P
S42.453K
S42.453P
S42.454K
S42.454P
S42.455K
S42.455P
S42.456K
S42.456P
S42.461K
S42.461P
S42.462K
S42.462P
S42.463K
S42.463P
S42.464K
S42.464P
S42.465K
S42.465P
S42.466K
S42.466P
S42.471K
S42.471P
S42.472K
S42.472P
S42.473K
S42.473P
S42.474K
S42.474P
S42.475K
S42.475P
S42.476K
S42.476P
S42.481K
S42.481P
S42.482K
S42.482P
S42.489K
S42.489P
S42.491K
S42.491P
S42.492K
S42.492P
S42.493K
S42.493P
S42.494K
S42.494P
S42.495K
S42.495P
S42.496K
S42.496P
S42.9ØXK
S42.9ØXP
S42.91XK
S42.91XP
S42.92XK
S42.92XP
S46.Ø21A
S46.Ø22A
S46.Ø29A
S46.121A
S46.122A
S46.129A
S46.221A
S46.222A
S46.229A
S46.321A
S46.322A
S46.329A
S46.821A
S46.822A
S46.829A
S46.921A
S46.922A
S46.929A
S49.ØØ1K
S49.ØØ1P
S49.ØØ2K
S49.ØØ2P
S49.ØØ9K
S49.ØØ9P
S49.Ø11K
S49.Ø11P
S49.Ø12K
S49.Ø12P
S49.Ø19K
S49.Ø19P
S49.Ø21K
S49.Ø21P
S49.Ø22K
S49.Ø22P
S49.Ø29K
S49.Ø29P
S49.Ø31K
S49.Ø31P
S49.Ø32K
S49.Ø32P
S49.Ø39K
S49.Ø39P
S49.Ø41K
S49.Ø41P
S49.Ø42K
S49.Ø42P
S49.Ø49K
S49.Ø49P
S49.Ø91K
S49.Ø91P
S49.Ø92K
S49.Ø92P
S49.Ø99K
S49.Ø99P
S49.1Ø1K
S49.1Ø1P
S49.1Ø2K
S49.1Ø2P
S49.1Ø9K
S49.1Ø9P
S49.111K
S49.111P
S49.112K
S49.112P
S49.119K
S49.119P
S49.121K
S49.121P
S49.122K
S49.122P
S49.129K
S49.129P
S49.131K
S49.131P
S49.132K
S49.132P
S49.139K
S49.139P
S49.141K
S49.141P
S49.142K
S49.142P
S49.149K
S49.149P
S49.191K
S49.191P
S49.192K
S49.192P
S49.199K
S49.199P
S52.ØØ1K
S52.ØØ1M
S52.ØØ1N
S52.ØØ1P
S52.ØØ1Q
S52.ØØ1R
S52.ØØ2K
S52.ØØ2M
S52.ØØ2N
S52.ØØ2P
S52.ØØ2Q
S52.ØØ2R
S52.ØØ9K
S52.ØØ9M
S52.ØØ9N
S52.ØØ9P
S52.ØØ9Q
S52.ØØ9R
S52.Ø11K
S52.Ø11P
S52.Ø12K
S52.Ø12P
S52.Ø19K
S52.Ø19P
S52.Ø21K
S52.Ø21M
S52.Ø21N
S52.Ø21P
S52.Ø21Q
S52.Ø21R
S52.Ø22K
S52.Ø22M
S52.Ø22N
S52.Ø22P
S52.Ø22Q
S52.Ø22R
S52.Ø23K
S52.Ø23M
S52.Ø23N
S52.Ø23P
S52.Ø23Q
S52.Ø23R
S52.Ø24K
S52.Ø24M
S52.Ø24N
S52.Ø24P
S52.Ø24Q
S52.Ø24R
S52.Ø25K
S52.Ø25M
S52.Ø25N
S52.Ø25P
S52.Ø25Q
S52.Ø25R
S52.Ø26K
S52.Ø26M
S52.Ø26N
S52.Ø26P
S52.Ø26Q
S52.Ø26R
S52.Ø31K
S52.Ø31M
S52.Ø31N
S52.Ø31P
S52.Ø31Q
S52.Ø31R
S52.Ø32K
S52.Ø32M
S52.Ø32N
S52.Ø32P
S52.Ø32Q
S52.Ø32R
S52.Ø33K
S52.Ø33M
S52.Ø33N
S52.Ø33P
S52.Ø33Q
S52.Ø33R
S52.Ø34K
S52.Ø34M
S52.Ø34N
S52.Ø34P
S52.Ø34Q
S52.Ø34R
S52.Ø35K
S52.Ø35M
S52.Ø35N
S52.Ø35P
S52.Ø35Q
S52.Ø35R
S52.Ø36K
S52.Ø36M
S52.Ø36N
S52.Ø36P
S52.Ø36Q
S52.Ø36R
S52.Ø41K
S52.Ø41M
S52.Ø41N
S52.Ø41P
S52.Ø41Q
S52.Ø41R
S52.Ø42K
S52.Ø42M
S52.Ø42N
S52.Ø42P
S52.Ø42Q
S52.Ø42R
S52.Ø43K
S52.Ø43M
S52.Ø43N
S52.Ø43P
S52.Ø43Q
S52.Ø43R
S52.Ø44K
S52.Ø44M
S52.Ø44N
S52.Ø44P
S52.Ø44Q
S52.Ø44R
S52.Ø45K
S52.Ø45M
S52.Ø45N
S52.Ø45P
S52.Ø45Q
S52.Ø45R
S52.Ø46K
S52.Ø46M
S52.Ø46N
S52.Ø46P
S52.Ø46Q

ICD-10-CM/PCS Codes by MS-DRG

S52.046R
S52.091K
S52.091M
S52.091N
S52.091P
S52.091Q
S52.091R
S52.092K
S52.092M
S52.092N
S52.092P
S52.092Q
S52.092R
S52.099K
S52.099M
S52.099N
S52.099P
S52.099Q
S52.099R
S52.101K
S52.101M
S52.101N
S52.101P
S52.101Q
S52.101R
S52.102K
S52.102M
S52.102N
S52.102P
S52.102Q
S52.102R
S52.109K
S52.109M
S52.109N
S52.109P
S52.109Q
S52.109R
S52.111K
S52.111P
S52.112K
S52.112P
S52.119K
S52.119P
S52.121K
S52.121M
S52.121N
S52.121P
S52.121Q
S52.121R
S52.122K
S52.122M
S52.122N
S52.122P
S52.122Q
S52.122R
S52.123K
S52.123M
S52.123N
S52.123P
S52.123Q
S52.123R
S52.124K
S52.124M
S52.124N
S52.124P
S52.124Q
S52.124R
S52.125K
S52.125M
S52.125N
S52.125P
S52.125Q
S52.125R
S52.126K
S52.126M
S52.126N
S52.126P
S52.126Q
S52.126R
S52.131K
S52.131M
S52.131N
S52.131P
S52.131Q
S52.131R
S52.132K
S52.132M
S52.132N
S52.132P
S52.132Q
S52.132R
S52.133K
S52.133M
S52.133N
S52.133P
S52.133Q
S52.133R
S52.134K
S52.134M
S52.134N
S52.134P
S52.134Q
S52.134R
S52.135K
S52.135M
S52.135N
S52.135P
S52.135Q
S52.135R
S52.136K
S52.136M
S52.136N
S52.136P
S52.136Q
S52.136R
S52.181K
S52.181M
S52.181N
S52.181P
S52.181Q
S52.181R
S52.182K
S52.182M
S52.182N
S52.182P
S52.182Q
S52.182R
S52.189K
S52.189M
S52.189N
S52.189P
S52.189Q
S52.189R
S52.201K
S52.201M
S52.201N
S52.201P
S52.201Q
S52.201R
S52.202K
S52.202M
S52.202N
S52.202P
S52.202Q
S52.202R
S52.209K
S52.209M
S52.209N
S52.209P
S52.209Q
S52.209R
S52.211K
S52.211P
S52.212K
S52.212P
S52.219K
S52.219P
S52.221K
S52.221M
S52.221N
S52.221P
S52.221Q
S52.221R
S52.222K
S52.222M
S52.222N
S52.222P
S52.222Q
S52.222R
S52.223K
S52.223M
S52.223N
S52.223P
S52.223Q
S52.223R
S52.224K
S52.224M
S52.224N
S52.224P
S52.224Q
S52.224R
S52.225K
S52.225M
S52.225N
S52.225P
S52.225Q
S52.225R
S52.226K
S52.226M
S52.226N
S52.226P
S52.226Q
S52.226R
S52.231K
S52.231M
S52.231N
S52.231P
S52.231Q
S52.231R
S52.232K
S52.232M
S52.232N
S52.232P
S52.232Q
S52.232R
S52.233K
S52.233M
S52.233N
S52.233P
S52.233Q
S52.233R
S52.234K
S52.234M
S52.234N
S52.234P
S52.234Q
S52.234R
S52.235K
S52.235M
S52.235N
S52.235P
S52.235Q
S52.235R
S52.236K
S52.236M
S52.236N
S52.236P
S52.236Q
S52.236R
S52.241K
S52.241M
S52.241N
S52.241P
S52.241Q
S52.241R
S52.242K
S52.242M
S52.242N
S52.242P
S52.242Q
S52.242R
S52.243K
S52.243M
S52.243N
S52.243P
S52.243Q
S52.243R
S52.244K
S52.244M
S52.244N
S52.244P
S52.244Q
S52.244R
S52.245K
S52.245M
S52.245N
S52.245P
S52.245Q
S52.245R
S52.246K
S52.246M
S52.246N
S52.246P
S52.246Q
S52.246R
S52.251K
S52.251M
S52.251N
S52.251P
S52.251Q
S52.251R
S52.252K
S52.252M
S52.252N
S52.252P
S52.252Q
S52.252R
S52.253K
S52.253M
S52.253N
S52.253P
S52.253Q
S52.253R
S52.254K
S52.254M
S52.254N
S52.254P
S52.254Q
S52.254R
S52.255K
S52.255M
S52.255N
S52.255P
S52.255Q
S52.255R
S52.256K
S52.256M
S52.256N
S52.256P
S52.256Q
S52.256R
S52.261K
S52.261M
S52.261N
S52.261P
S52.261Q
S52.261R
S52.262K
S52.262M
S52.262N
S52.262P
S52.262Q
S52.262R
S52.263K
S52.263M
S52.263N
S52.263P
S52.263Q
S52.263R
S52.264K
S52.264M
S52.264N
S52.264P
S52.264Q
S52.264R
S52.265K
S52.265M
S52.265N
S52.265P
S52.265Q
S52.265R
S52.266K
S52.266M
S52.266N
S52.266P
S52.266Q
S52.266R
S52.271K
S52.271M
S52.271N
S52.271P
S52.271Q
S52.271R
S52.272K
S52.272M
S52.272N
S52.272P
S52.272Q
S52.272R
S52.279K
S52.279M
S52.279N
S52.279P
S52.279Q
S52.279R
S52.281K
S52.281M
S52.281N
S52.281P
S52.281Q
S52.281R
S52.282K
S52.282M
S52.282N
S52.282P
S52.282Q
S52.282R
S52.283K
S52.283M
S52.283N
S52.283P
S52.283Q
S52.283R
S52.291K
S52.291M
S52.291N
S52.291P
S52.291Q
S52.291R
S52.292K
S52.292M
S52.292N
S52.292P
S52.292Q
S52.292R
S52.299K
S52.299M
S52.299N
S52.299P
S52.299Q
S52.299R
S52.301K
S52.301M
S52.301N
S52.301P
S52.301Q
S52.301R
S52.302K
S52.302M
S52.302N
S52.302P
S52.302Q
S52.302R
S52.309K
S52.309M
S52.309N
S52.309P
S52.309Q
S52.309R
S52.311K
S52.311P
S52.312K
S52.312P
S52.319K
S52.319P
S52.321K
S52.321M
S52.321N
S52.321P
S52.321Q
S52.321R
S52.322K
S52.322M
S52.322N
S52.322P
S52.322Q
S52.322R
S52.323K
S52.323M
S52.323N
S52.323P
S52.323Q
S52.323R
S52.324K
S52.324M
S52.324N
S52.324P
S52.324Q
S52.324R
S52.325K
S52.325M
S52.325N
S52.325P
S52.325Q
S52.325R
S52.326K
S52.326M
S52.326N
S52.326P
S52.326Q
S52.326R
S52.331K
S52.331M
S52.331N
S52.331P
S52.331Q
S52.331R
S52.332K
S52.332M
S52.332N
S52.332P
S52.332Q
S52.332R
S52.333K
S52.333M
S52.333N
S52.333P
S52.333Q
S52.333R
S52.334K
S52.334M
S52.334N
S52.334P
S52.334Q
S52.334R
S52.335K
S52.335M
S52.335N
S52.335P
S52.335Q
S52.335R
S52.336K
S52.336M
S52.336N
S52.336P
S52.336Q
S52.336R
S52.341K
S52.341M
S52.341N
S52.341P
S52.341Q
S52.341R
S52.342K
S52.342M
S52.342N
S52.342P
S52.342Q
S52.342R
S52.343K
S52.343M
S52.343N
S52.343P
S52.343Q
S52.343R
S52.344K
S52.344M
S52.344N
S52.344P
S52.344Q
S52.344R
S52.345K
S52.345M
S52.345N
S52.345P
S52.345Q
S52.345R
S52.346K
S52.346M
S52.346N
S52.346P
S52.346Q
S52.346R
S52.351K
S52.351M
S52.351N
S52.351P
S52.351Q
S52.351R
S52.352K
S52.352M
S52.352N
S52.352P
S52.352Q
S52.352R
S52.353K
S52.353M
S52.353N
S52.353P
S52.353Q
S52.353R
S52.354K
S52.354M
S52.354N
S52.354P
S52.354Q
S52.354R
S52.355K
S52.355M
S52.355N
S52.355P
S52.355Q
S52.355R
S52.356K
S52.356M
S52.356N
S52.356P
S52.356Q
S52.356R
S52.361K
S52.361M
S52.361N
S52.361P
S52.361Q
S52.361R
S52.362K
S52.362M
S52.362N
S52.362P
S52.362Q
S52.362R
S52.363K
S52.363M
S52.363N
S52.363P
S52.363Q
S52.363R
S52.364K
S52.364M
S52.364N
S52.364P
S52.364Q
S52.364R
S52.365K
S52.365M
S52.365N
S52.365P
S52.365Q
S52.365R
S52.366K
S52.366M
S52.366N
S52.366P
S52.366Q
S52.366R
S52.371K
S52.371M
S52.371N
S52.371P
S52.371Q
S52.371R
S52.372K
S52.372M
S52.372N
S52.372P
S52.372Q
S52.372R
S52.379K
S52.379M
S52.379N
S52.379P
S52.379Q
S52.379R
S52.381K
S52.381M
S52.381N
S52.381P
S52.381Q
S52.381R
S52.382K
S52.382M
S52.382N
S52.382P
S52.382Q
S52.382R
S52.389K
S52.389M
S52.389N
S52.389P
S52.389Q
S52.389R
S52.391K
S52.391M
S52.391N
S52.391P
S52.391Q
S52.391R
S52.392K
S52.392M
S52.392N
S52.392P
S52.392Q
S52.392R
S52.399K
S52.399M
S52.399N
S52.399P
S52.399Q
S52.399R
S52.501K
S52.501M
S52.501N
S52.501P
S52.501Q
S52.501R
S52.502K
S52.502M
S52.502N
S52.502P
S52.502Q
S52.502R
S52.509K
S52.509M
S52.509N
S52.509P
S52.509Q
S52.509R
S52.511K
S52.511M
S52.511N
S52.511P
S52.511Q
S52.511R
S52.512K
S52.512M
S52.512N
S52.512P
S52.512Q
S52.512R
S52.513K
S52.513M
S52.513N
S52.513P
S52.513Q
S52.513R
S52.514K
S52.514M
S52.514N
S52.514P
S52.514Q
S52.514R
S52.515K
S52.515M
S52.515N
S52.515P
S52.515Q
S52.515R
S52.516K
S52.516M
S52.516N
S52.516P
S52.516Q
S52.516R
S52.521K
S52.521P
S52.522K
S52.522P
S52.529K
S52.529P
S52.531K
S52.531M
S52.531N
S52.531P
S52.531Q
S52.531R
S52.532K
S52.532M
S52.532N
S52.532P
S52.532Q
S52.532R
S52.539K
S52.539M
S52.539N
S52.539P
S52.539Q
S52.539R
S52.541K
S52.541M
S52.541N
S52.541P
S52.541Q
S52.541R
S52.542K
S52.542M
S52.542N
S52.542P
S52.542Q
S52.542R
S52.549K
S52.549M
S52.549N
S52.549P
S52.549Q
S52.549R
S52.551K
S52.551M
S52.551N
S52.551P
S52.551Q
S52.551R
S52.552K
S52.552M
S52.552N
S52.552P
S52.552Q
S52.552R
S52.559K
S52.559M
S52.559N
S52.559P
S52.559Q
S52.559R
S52.561K
S52.561M
S52.561N
S52.561P
S52.561Q
S52.561R
S52.562K
S52.562M
S52.562N
S52.562P
S52.562Q
S52.562R
S52.569K
S52.569M
S52.569N
S52.569P
S52.569Q
S52.569R
S52.571K
S52.571M
S52.571N
S52.571P
S52.571Q
S52.571R
S52.572K
S52.572M
S52.572N
S52.572P
S52.572Q
S52.572R
S52.579K
S52.579M
S52.579N
S52.579P
S52.579Q
S52.579R
S52.591K
S52.591M
S52.591N
S52.591P
S52.591Q
S52.591R
S52.592K
S52.592M
S52.592N
S52.592P
S52.592Q
S52.592R
S52.599K
S52.599M
S52.599N
S52.599P
S52.599Q
S52.599R
S52.601K
S52.601M
S52.601N
S52.601P
S52.601Q
S52.601R
S52.602K
S52.602M
S52.602N
S52.602P
S52.602Q
S52.602R
S52.609K
S52.609M
S52.609N
S52.609P
S52.609Q
S52.609R
S52.611K
S52.611M
S52.611N
S52.611P
S52.611Q
S52.611R
S52.612K
S52.612M
S52.612N
S52.612P
S52.612Q
S52.612R
S52.613K
S52.613M
S52.613N
S52.613P
S52.613Q
S52.613R
S52.614K
S52.614M

S52.614N
S52.614P
S52.614Q
S52.614R
S52.615K
S52.615M
S52.615N
S52.615P
S52.615Q
S52.615R
S52.616K
S52.616M
S52.616N
S52.616P
S52.616Q
S52.616R
S52.621K
S52.621P
S52.622K
S52.622P
S52.629K
S52.629P
S52.691K
S52.691M
S52.691N
S52.691P
S52.691Q
S52.691R
S52.692K
S52.692M
S52.692N
S52.692P
S52.692Q
S52.692R
S52.699K
S52.699M
S52.699N
S52.699P
S52.699Q
S52.699R
S52.90XK
S52.90XM
S52.90XN
S52.90XP
S52.90XQ
S52.90XR
S52.91XK
S52.91XM
S52.91XN
S52.91XP
S52.91XQ
S52.91XR
S52.92XK
S52.92XM
S52.92XN
S52.92XP
S52.92XQ
S52.92XR
S56.021A
S56.022A
S56.029A
S56.121A
S56.122A
S56.123A
S56.124A
S56.125A
S56.126A
S56.127A
S56.128A
S56.129A
S56.221A
S56.222A
S56.229A
S56.321A
S56.322A
S56.329A
S56.421A
S56.422A
S56.423A
S56.424A
S56.425A
S56.426A
S56.427A
S56.428A
S56.429A
S56.521A
S56.522A
S56.529A
S56.821A
S56.822A
S56.829A
S56.921A
S56.922A
S56.929A
S59.001K
S59.001P
S59.002K
S59.002P
S59.009K
S59.009P
S59.011K
S59.011P
S59.012K
S59.012P
S59.019K
S59.019P
S59.021K
S59.021P
S59.022K
S59.022P
S59.029K
S59.029P
S59.031K
S59.031P
S59.032K
S59.032P
S59.039K
S59.039P
S59.041K
S59.041P
S59.042K
S59.042P
S59.049K
S59.049P
S59.091K
S59.091P
S59.092K
S59.092P
S59.099K
S59.099P
S59.101K
S59.101P
S59.102K
S59.102P
S59.109K
S59.109P
S59.111K
S59.111P
S59.112K
S59.112P
S59.119K
S59.119P
S59.121K
S59.121P
S59.122K
S59.122P
S59.129K
S59.129P
S59.131K
S59.131P
S59.132K
S59.132P
S59.139K
S59.139P
S59.141K
S59.141P
S59.142K
S59.142P
S59.149K
S59.149P
S59.191K
S59.191P
S59.192K
S59.192P
S59.199K
S59.199P
S59.201K
S59.201P
S59.202K
S59.202P
S59.209K
S59.209P
S59.211K
S59.211P
S59.212K
S59.212P
S59.219K
S59.219P
S59.221K
S59.221P
S59.222K
S59.222P
S59.229K
S59.229P
S59.231K
S59.231P
S59.232K
S59.232P
S59.239K
S59.239P
S59.241K
S59.241P
S59.242K
S59.242P
S59.249K
S59.249P
S59.291K
S59.291P
S59.292K
S59.292P
S59.299K
S59.299P
S62.001K
S62.001P
S62.002K
S62.002P
S62.009K
S62.009P
S62.011K
S62.011P
S62.012K
S62.012P
S62.013K
S62.013P
S62.014K
S62.014P
S62.015K
S62.015P
S62.016K
S62.016P
S62.021K
S62.021P
S62.022K
S62.022P
S62.023K
S62.023P
S62.024K
S62.024P
S62.025K
S62.025P
S62.026K
S62.026P
S62.031K
S62.031P
S62.032K
S62.032P
S62.033K
S62.033P
S62.034K
S62.034P
S62.035K
S62.035P
S62.036K
S62.036P
S62.101K
S62.101P
S62.102K
S62.102P
S62.109K
S62.109P
S62.111K
S62.111P
S62.112K
S62.112P
S62.113K
S62.113P
S62.114K
S62.114P
S62.115K
S62.115P
S62.116K
S62.116P
S62.121K
S62.121P
S62.122K
S62.122P
S62.123K
S62.123P
S62.124K
S62.124P
S62.125K
S62.125P
S62.126K
S62.126P
S62.131K
S62.131P
S62.132K
S62.132P
S62.133K
S62.133P
S62.134K
S62.134P
S62.135K
S62.135P
S62.136K
S62.136P
S62.141K
S62.141P
S62.142K
S62.142P
S62.143K
S62.143P
S62.144K
S62.144P
S62.145K
S62.145P
S62.146K
S62.146P
S62.151K
S62.151P
S62.152K
S62.152P
S62.153K
S62.153P
S62.154K
S62.154P
S62.155K
S62.155P
S62.156K
S62.156P
S62.161K
S62.161P
S62.162K
S62.162P
S62.163K
S62.163P
S62.164K
S62.164P
S62.165K
S62.165P
S62.166K
S62.166P
S62.171K
S62.171P
S62.172K
S62.172P
S62.173K
S62.173P
S62.174K
S62.174P
S62.175K
S62.175P
S62.176K
S62.176P
S62.181K
S62.181P
S62.182K
S62.182P
S62.183K
S62.183P
S62.184K
S62.184P
S62.185K
S62.185P
S62.186K
S62.186P
S62.201K
S62.201P
S62.202K
S62.202P
S62.209K
S62.209P
S62.211K
S62.211P
S62.212K
S62.212P
S62.213K
S62.213P
S62.221K
S62.221P
S62.222K
S62.222P
S62.223K
S62.223P
S62.224K
S62.224P
S62.225K
S62.225P
S62.226K
S62.226P
S62.231K
S62.231P
S62.232K
S62.232P
S62.233K
S62.233P
S62.234K
S62.234P
S62.235K
S62.235P
S62.236K
S62.236P
S62.241K
S62.241P
S62.242K
S62.242P
S62.243K
S62.243P
S62.244K
S62.244P
S62.245K
S62.245P
S62.246K
S62.246P
S62.251K
S62.251P
S62.252K
S62.252P
S62.253K
S62.253P
S62.254K
S62.254P
S62.255K
S62.255P
S62.256K
S62.256P
S62.291K
S62.291P
S62.292K
S62.292P
S62.299K
S62.299P
S62.300K
S62.300P
S62.301K
S62.301P
S62.302K
S62.302P
S62.303K
S62.303P
S62.304K
S62.304P
S62.305K
S62.305P
S62.306K
S62.306P
S62.307K
S62.307P
S62.308K
S62.308P
S62.309K
S62.309P
S62.310K
S62.310P
S62.311K
S62.311P
S62.312K
S62.312P
S62.313K
S62.313P
S62.314K
S62.314P
S62.315K
S62.315P
S62.316K
S62.316P
S62.317K
S62.317P
S62.318K
S62.318P
S62.319K
S62.319P
S62.320K
S62.320P
S62.321K
S62.321P
S62.322K
S62.322P
S62.323K
S62.323P
S62.324K
S62.324P
S62.325K
S62.325P
S62.326K
S62.326P
S62.327K
S62.327P
S62.328K
S62.328P
S62.329K
S62.329P
S62.330K
S62.330P
S62.331K
S62.331P
S62.332K
S62.332P
S62.333K
S62.333P
S62.334K
S62.334P
S62.335K
S62.335P
S62.336K
S62.336P
S62.337K
S62.337P
S62.338K
S62.338P
S62.339K
S62.339P
S62.340K
S62.340P
S62.341K
S62.341P
S62.342K
S62.342P
S62.343K
S62.343P
S62.344K
S62.344P
S62.345K
S62.345P
S62.346K
S62.346P
S62.347K
S62.347P
S62.348K
S62.348P
S62.349K
S62.349P
S62.350K
S62.350P
S62.351K
S62.351P
S62.352K
S62.352P
S62.353K
S62.353P
S62.354K
S62.354P
S62.355K
S62.355P
S62.356K
S62.356P
S62.357K
S62.357P
S62.358K
S62.358P
S62.359K
S62.359P
S62.360K
S62.360P
S62.361K
S62.361P
S62.362K
S62.362P
S62.363K
S62.363P
S62.364K
S62.364P
S62.365K
S62.365P
S62.366K
S62.366P
S62.367K
S62.367P
S62.368K
S62.368P
S62.369K
S62.369P
S62.390K
S62.390P
S62.391K
S62.391P
S62.392K
S62.392P
S62.393K
S62.393P
S62.394K
S62.394P
S62.395K
S62.395P
S62.396K
S62.396P
S62.397K
S62.397P
S62.398K
S62.398P
S62.399K
S62.399P
S62.501K
S62.501P
S62.502K
S62.502P
S62.509K
S62.509P
S62.511K
S62.511P
S62.512K
S62.512P
S62.513K
S62.513P
S62.514K
S62.514P
S62.515K
S62.515P
S62.516K
S62.516P
S62.521K
S62.521P
S62.522K
S62.522P
S62.523K
S62.523P
S62.524K
S62.524P
S62.525K
S62.525P
S62.526K
S62.526P
S62.600K
S62.600P
S62.601K
S62.601P
S62.602K
S62.602P
S62.603K
S62.603P
S62.604K
S62.604P
S62.605K
S62.605P
S62.606K
S62.606P
S62.607K
S62.607P
S62.608K
S62.608P
S62.609K
S62.609P
S62.610K
S62.610P
S62.611K
S62.611P
S62.612K
S62.612P
S62.613K
S62.613P
S62.614K
S62.614P
S62.615K
S62.615P
S62.616K
S62.616P
S62.617K
S62.617P
S62.618K
S62.618P
S62.619K
S62.619P
S62.620K
S62.620P
S62.621K
S62.621P
S62.622K
S62.622P
S62.623K
S62.623P
S62.624K
S62.624P
S62.625K
S62.625P
S62.626K
S62.626P
S62.627K
S62.627P
S62.628K
S62.628P
S62.629K
S62.629P
S62.630K
S62.630P
S62.631K
S62.631P
S62.632K
S62.632P
S62.633K
S62.633P
S62.634K
S62.634P
S62.635K
S62.635P
S62.636K
S62.636P
S62.637K
S62.637P
S62.638K
S62.638P
S62.639K
S62.639P
S62.640K
S62.640P
S62.641K
S62.641P
S62.642K
S62.642P
S62.643K
S62.643P
S62.644K
S62.644P
S62.645K
S62.645P
S62.646K
S62.646P
S62.647K
S62.647P
S62.648K
S62.648P
S62.649K
S62.649P
S62.650K
S62.650P
S62.651K
S62.651P
S62.652K
S62.652P
S62.653K
S62.653P
S62.654K
S62.654P
S62.655K
S62.655P
S62.656K
S62.656P
S62.657K
S62.657P
S62.658K
S62.658P
S62.659K
S62.659P
S62.660K
S62.660P
S62.661K
S62.661P
S62.662K
S62.662P
S62.663K
S62.663P
S62.664K
S62.664P
S62.665K
S62.665P
S62.666K
S62.666P
S62.667K
S62.667P
S62.668K
S62.668P
S62.669K
S62.669P
S62.90XK
S62.90XP
S62.91XK
S62.91XP
S62.92XK
S62.92XP
S66.021A
S66.022A
S66.029A
S66.120A
S66.121A
S66.122A
S66.123A
S66.124A
S66.125A
S66.126A
S66.127A
S66.128A
S66.129A
S66.221A
S66.222A
S66.229A
S66.320A
S66.321A
S66.322A
S66.323A
S66.324A
S66.325A
S66.326A
S66.327A
S66.328A
S66.329A
S66.421A
S66.422A
S66.429A
S66.520A
S66.521A
S66.522A
S66.523A
S66.524A
S66.525A
S66.526A
S66.527A
S66.528A
S66.529A
S66.821A
S66.822A
S66.829A
S66.921A
S66.922A
S66.929A
S72.001K
S72.001M
S72.001N
S72.001P
S72.001Q
S72.001R
S72.002K
S72.002M
S72.002N
S72.002P
S72.002Q
S72.002R
S72.009K
S72.009M
S72.009N
S72.009P
S72.009Q
S72.009R
S72.011K
S72.011M
S72.011N
S72.011P
S72.011Q
S72.011R
S72.012K
S72.012M
S72.012N
S72.012P
S72.012Q
S72.012R
S72.019K
S72.019M
S72.019N
S72.019P
S72.019Q
S72.019R
S72.021K
S72.021M
S72.021N
S72.021P
S72.021Q
S72.021R
S72.022K
S72.022M
S72.022N
S72.022P
S72.022Q
S72.022R
S72.023K
S72.023M
S72.023N
S72.023P
S72.023Q
S72.023R
S72.024K
S72.024M
S72.024N
S72.024P
S72.024Q
S72.024R
S72.025K
S72.025M

ICD-10-CM/PCS Codes by MS-DRG

S72.025N
S72.025P
S72.025Q
S72.025R
S72.026K
S72.026M
S72.026N
S72.026P
S72.026Q
S72.026R
S72.031K
S72.031M
S72.031N
S72.031P
S72.031Q
S72.031R
S72.032K
S72.032M
S72.032N
S72.032P
S72.032Q
S72.032R
S72.033K
S72.033M
S72.033N
S72.033P
S72.033Q
S72.033R
S72.034K
S72.034M
S72.034N
S72.034P
S72.034Q
S72.034R
S72.035K
S72.035M
S72.035N
S72.035P
S72.035Q
S72.035R
S72.036K
S72.036M
S72.036N
S72.036P
S72.036Q
S72.036R
S72.041K
S72.041M
S72.041N
S72.041P
S72.041Q
S72.041R
S72.042K
S72.042M
S72.042N
S72.042P
S72.042Q
S72.042R
S72.043K
S72.043M
S72.043N
S72.043P
S72.043Q
S72.043R
S72.044K
S72.044M
S72.044N
S72.044P
S72.044Q
S72.044R
S72.045K
S72.045M
S72.045N
S72.045P
S72.045Q
S72.045R
S72.046K
S72.046M
S72.046N
S72.046P
S72.046Q
S72.046R
S72.051K
S72.051M
S72.051N
S72.051P
S72.051Q
S72.051R
S72.052K
S72.052M
S72.052N
S72.052P
S72.052Q
S72.052R
S72.059K
S72.059M
S72.059N
S72.059P
S72.059Q
S72.059R
S72.061K
S72.061M
S72.061N
S72.061P
S72.061Q
S72.061R
S72.062K
S72.062M
S72.062N
S72.062P
S72.062Q
S72.062R
S72.063K
S72.063M
S72.063N
S72.063P
S72.063Q
S72.063R
S72.064K
S72.064M
S72.064N
S72.064P
S72.064Q
S72.064R
S72.065K
S72.065M
S72.065N
S72.065P
S72.065Q
S72.065R
S72.066K
S72.066M
S72.066N
S72.066P
S72.066Q
S72.066R
S72.091K
S72.091M
S72.091N
S72.091P
S72.091Q
S72.091R
S72.092K
S72.092M
S72.092N
S72.092P
S72.092Q
S72.092R
S72.099K
S72.099M
S72.099N
S72.099P
S72.099Q
S72.099R
S72.101K
S72.101M
S72.101N
S72.101P
S72.101Q
S72.101R
S72.102K
S72.102M
S72.102N
S72.102P
S72.102Q
S72.102R
S72.109K
S72.109M
S72.109N
S72.109P
S72.109Q
S72.109R
S72.111K
S72.111M
S72.111N
S72.111P
S72.111Q
S72.111R
S72.112K
S72.112M
S72.112N
S72.112P
S72.112Q
S72.112R
S72.113K
S72.113M
S72.113N
S72.113P
S72.113Q
S72.113R
S72.114K
S72.114M
S72.114N
S72.114P
S72.114Q
S72.114R
S72.115K
S72.115M
S72.115N
S72.115P
S72.115Q
S72.115R
S72.116K
S72.116M
S72.116N
S72.116P
S72.116Q
S72.116R
S72.121K
S72.121M
S72.121N
S72.121P
S72.121Q
S72.121R
S72.122K
S72.122M
S72.122N
S72.122P
S72.122Q
S72.122R
S72.123K
S72.123M
S72.123N
S72.123P
S72.123Q
S72.123R
S72.124K
S72.124M
S72.124N
S72.124P
S72.124Q
S72.124R
S72.125K
S72.125M
S72.125N
S72.125P
S72.125Q
S72.125R
S72.126K
S72.126M
S72.126N
S72.126P
S72.126Q
S72.126R
S72.131K
S72.131M
S72.131N
S72.131P
S72.131Q
S72.131R
S72.132K
S72.132M
S72.132N
S72.132P
S72.132Q
S72.132R
S72.133K
S72.133M
S72.133N
S72.133P
S72.133Q
S72.133R
S72.134K
S72.134M
S72.134N
S72.134P
S72.134Q
S72.134R
S72.135K
S72.135M
S72.135N
S72.135P
S72.135Q
S72.135R
S72.136K
S72.136M
S72.136N
S72.136P
S72.136Q
S72.136R
S72.141K
S72.141M
S72.141N
S72.141P
S72.141Q
S72.141R
S72.142K
S72.142M
S72.142N
S72.142P
S72.142Q
S72.142R
S72.143K
S72.143M
S72.143N
S72.143P
S72.143Q
S72.143R
S72.144K
S72.144M
S72.144N
S72.144P
S72.144Q
S72.144R
S72.145K
S72.145M
S72.145N
S72.145P
S72.145Q
S72.145R
S72.146K
S72.146M
S72.146N
S72.146P
S72.146Q
S72.146R
S72.21XK
S72.21XM
S72.21XN
S72.21XP
S72.21XQ
S72.21XR
S72.22XK
S72.22XM
S72.22XN
S72.22XP
S72.22XQ
S72.22XR
S72.23XK
S72.23XM
S72.23XN
S72.23XP
S72.23XQ
S72.23XR
S72.24XK
S72.24XM
S72.24XN
S72.24XP
S72.24XQ
S72.24XR
S72.25XK
S72.25XM
S72.25XN
S72.25XP
S72.25XQ
S72.25XR
S72.26XK
S72.26XM
S72.26XN
S72.26XP
S72.26XQ
S72.26XR
S72.301K
S72.301M
S72.301N
S72.301P
S72.301Q
S72.301R
S72.302K
S72.302M
S72.302N
S72.302P
S72.302Q
S72.302R
S72.309K
S72.309M
S72.309N
S72.309P
S72.309Q
S72.309R
S72.321K
S72.321M
S72.321N
S72.321P
S72.321Q
S72.321R
S72.322K
S72.322M
S72.322N
S72.322P
S72.322Q
S72.322R
S72.323K
S72.323M
S72.323N
S72.323P
S72.323Q
S72.323R
S72.324K
S72.324M
S72.324N
S72.324P
S72.324Q
S72.324R
S72.325K
S72.325M
S72.325N
S72.325P
S72.325Q
S72.325R
S72.326K
S72.326M
S72.326N
S72.326P
S72.326Q
S72.326R
S72.331K
S72.331M
S72.331N
S72.331P
S72.331Q
S72.331R
S72.332K
S72.332M
S72.332N
S72.332P
S72.332Q
S72.332R
S72.333K
S72.333M
S72.333N
S72.333P
S72.333Q
S72.333R
S72.334K
S72.334M
S72.334N
S72.334P
S72.334Q
S72.334R
S72.335K
S72.335M
S72.335N
S72.335P
S72.335Q
S72.335R
S72.336K
S72.336M
S72.336N
S72.336P
S72.336Q
S72.336R
S72.341K
S72.341M
S72.341N
S72.341P
S72.341Q
S72.341R
S72.342K
S72.342M
S72.342N
S72.342P
S72.342Q
S72.342R
S72.343K
S72.343M
S72.343N
S72.343P
S72.343Q
S72.343R
S72.344K
S72.344M
S72.344N
S72.344P
S72.344Q
S72.344R
S72.345K
S72.345M
S72.345N
S72.345P
S72.345Q
S72.345R
S72.346K
S72.346M
S72.346N
S72.346P
S72.346Q
S72.346R
S72.351K
S72.351M
S72.351N
S72.351P
S72.351Q
S72.351R
S72.352K
S72.352M
S72.352N
S72.352P
S72.352Q
S72.352R
S72.353K
S72.353M
S72.353N
S72.353P
S72.353Q
S72.353R
S72.354K
S72.354M
S72.354N
S72.354P
S72.354Q
S72.354R
S72.355K
S72.355M
S72.355N
S72.355P
S72.355Q
S72.355R
S72.356K
S72.356M
S72.356N
S72.356P
S72.356Q
S72.356R
S72.361K
S72.361M
S72.361N
S72.361P
S72.361Q
S72.361R
S72.362K
S72.362M
S72.362N
S72.362P
S72.362Q
S72.362R
S72.363K
S72.363M
S72.363N
S72.363P
S72.363Q
S72.363R
S72.364K
S72.364M
S72.364N
S72.364P
S72.364Q
S72.364R
S72.365K
S72.365M
S72.365N
S72.365P
S72.365Q
S72.365R
S72.366K
S72.366M
S72.366N
S72.366P
S72.366Q
S72.366R
S72.391K
S72.391M
S72.391N
S72.391P
S72.391Q
S72.391R
S72.392K
S72.392M
S72.392N
S72.392P
S72.392Q
S72.392R
S72.399K
S72.399M
S72.399N
S72.399P
S72.399Q
S72.399R
S72.401K
S72.401M
S72.401N
S72.401P
S72.401Q
S72.401R
S72.402K
S72.402M
S72.402N
S72.402P
S72.402Q
S72.402R
S72.409K
S72.409M
S72.409N
S72.409P
S72.409Q
S72.409R
S72.411K
S72.411M
S72.411N
S72.411P
S72.411Q
S72.411R
S72.412K
S72.412M
S72.412N
S72.412P
S72.412Q
S72.412R
S72.413K
S72.413M
S72.413N
S72.413P
S72.413Q
S72.413R
S72.414K
S72.414M
S72.414N
S72.414P
S72.414Q
S72.414R
S72.415K
S72.415M
S72.415N
S72.415P
S72.415Q
S72.415R
S72.416K
S72.416M
S72.416N
S72.416P
S72.416Q
S72.416R
S72.421K
S72.421M
S72.421N
S72.421P
S72.421Q
S72.421R
S72.422K
S72.422M
S72.422N
S72.422P
S72.422Q
S72.422R
S72.423K
S72.423M
S72.423N
S72.423P
S72.423Q
S72.423R
S72.424K
S72.424M
S72.424N
S72.424P
S72.424Q
S72.424R
S72.425K
S72.425M
S72.425N
S72.425P
S72.425Q
S72.425R
S72.426K
S72.426M
S72.426N
S72.426P
S72.426Q
S72.426R
S72.431K
S72.431M
S72.431N
S72.431P
S72.431Q
S72.431R
S72.432K
S72.432M
S72.432N
S72.432P
S72.432Q
S72.432R
S72.433K
S72.433M
S72.433N
S72.433P
S72.433Q
S72.433R
S72.434K
S72.434M
S72.434N
S72.434P
S72.434Q
S72.434R
S72.435K
S72.435M
S72.435N
S72.435P
S72.435Q
S72.435R
S72.436K
S72.436M
S72.436N
S72.436P
S72.436Q
S72.436R
S72.441K
S72.441M
S72.441N
S72.441P
S72.441Q
S72.441R
S72.442K
S72.442M
S72.442N
S72.442P
S72.442Q
S72.442R
S72.443K
S72.443M
S72.443N
S72.443P
S72.443Q
S72.443R
S72.444K
S72.444M
S72.444N
S72.444P
S72.444Q
S72.444R
S72.445K
S72.445M
S72.445N
S72.445P
S72.445Q
S72.445R
S72.446K
S72.446M
S72.446N
S72.446P
S72.446Q
S72.446R
S72.451K
S72.451M
S72.451N
S72.451P
S72.451Q
S72.451R
S72.452K
S72.452M
S72.452N
S72.452P
S72.452Q
S72.452R
S72.453K
S72.453M
S72.453N
S72.453P
S72.453Q
S72.453R
S72.454K
S72.454M
S72.454N
S72.454P
S72.454Q
S72.454R
S72.455K
S72.455M
S72.455N
S72.455P
S72.455Q
S72.455R
S72.456K
S72.456M
S72.456N
S72.456P
S72.456Q
S72.456R
S72.461K
S72.461M
S72.461N
S72.461P
S72.461Q
S72.461R
S72.462K
S72.462M
S72.462N
S72.462P
S72.462Q
S72.462R
S72.463K
S72.463M
S72.463N
S72.463P
S72.463Q
S72.463R
S72.464K
S72.464M
S72.464N
S72.464P
S72.464Q
S72.464R
S72.465K
S72.465M
S72.465N
S72.465P
S72.465Q
S72.465R
S72.466K
S72.466M
S72.466N
S72.466P
S72.466Q
S72.466R
S72.471K
S72.471P
S72.472K
S72.472P
S72.479K
S72.479P
S72.491K
S72.491M
S72.491N
S72.491P
S72.491Q
S72.491R
S72.492K
S72.492M
S72.492N
S72.492P
S72.492Q
S72.492R
S72.499K
S72.499M
S72.499N
S72.499P
S72.499Q
S72.499R
S72.8X1K
S72.8X1M
S72.8X1N
S72.8X1P
S72.8X1Q
S72.8X1R
S72.8X2K
S72.8X2M
S72.8X2N
S72.8X2P
S72.8X2Q
S72.8X2R
S72.8X9K
S72.8X9M
S72.8X9N
S72.8X9P
S72.8X9Q
S72.8X9R
S72.90XK
S72.90XM
S72.90XN
S72.90XP
S72.90XQ
S72.90XR
S72.91XK
S72.91XM
S72.91XN
S72.91XP
S72.91XQ

S72.91XR
S72.92XK
S72.92XM
S72.92XN
S72.92XP
S72.92XQ
S72.92XR
S76.021A
S76.022A
S76.029A
S76.121A
S76.122A
S76.129A
S76.221A
S76.222A
S76.229A
S76.321A
S76.322A
S76.329A
S76.821A
S76.822A
S76.829A
S76.921A
S76.922A
S76.929A
S79.001K
S79.001P
S79.002K
S79.002P
S79.009K
S79.009P
S79.011K
S79.011P
S79.012K
S79.012P
S79.019K
S79.019P
S79.091K
S79.091P
S79.092K
S79.092P
S79.099K
S79.099P
S79.101K
S79.101P
S79.102K
S79.102P
S79.109K
S79.109P
S79.111K
S79.111P
S79.112K
S79.112P
S79.119K
S79.119P
S79.121K
S79.121P
S79.122K
S79.122P
S79.129K
S79.129P
S79.131K
S79.131P
S79.132K
S79.132P
S79.139K
S79.139P
S79.141K
S79.141P
S79.142K
S79.142P
S79.149K
S79.149P
S79.191K
S79.191P
S79.192K
S79.192P
S79.199K
S79.199P
S82.001K
S82.001M
S82.001N
S82.001P
S82.001Q
S82.001R
S82.002K
S82.002M
S82.002N
S82.002P
S82.002Q
S82.002R
S82.009K
S82.009M
S82.009N
S82.009P
S82.009Q
S82.009R
S82.011K
S82.011M
S82.011N
S82.011P
S82.011Q
S82.011R
S82.012K
S82.012M
S82.012N
S82.012P
S82.012Q
S82.012R
S82.013K
S82.013M
S82.013N
S82.013P
S82.013Q
S82.013R
S82.014K
S82.014M
S82.014N
S82.014P
S82.014Q
S82.014R
S82.015K
S82.015M
S82.015N
S82.015P
S82.015Q
S82.015R
S82.016K
S82.016M
S82.016N
S82.016P
S82.016Q
S82.016R
S82.021K
S82.021M
S82.021N
S82.021P
S82.021Q
S82.021R
S82.022K
S82.022M
S82.022N
S82.022P
S82.022Q
S82.022R
S82.023K
S82.023M
S82.023N
S82.023P
S82.023Q
S82.023R
S82.024K
S82.024M
S82.024N
S82.024P
S82.024Q
S82.024R
S82.025K
S82.025M
S82.025N
S82.025P
S82.025Q
S82.025R
S82.026K
S82.026M
S82.026N
S82.026P
S82.026Q
S82.026R
S82.031K
S82.031M
S82.031N
S82.031P
S82.031Q
S82.031R
S82.032K
S82.032M
S82.032N
S82.032P
S82.032Q
S82.032R
S82.033K
S82.033M
S82.033N
S82.033P
S82.033Q
S82.033R
S82.034K
S82.034M
S82.034N
S82.034P
S82.034Q
S82.034R
S82.035K
S82.035M
S82.035N
S82.035P
S82.035Q
S82.035R
S82.036K
S82.036M
S82.036N
S82.036P
S82.036Q
S82.036R
S82.041K
S82.041M
S82.041N
S82.041P
S82.041Q
S82.041R
S82.042K
S82.042M
S82.042N
S82.042P
S82.042Q
S82.042R
S82.043K
S82.043M
S82.043N
S82.043P
S82.043Q
S82.043R
S82.044K
S82.044M
S82.044N
S82.044P
S82.044Q
S82.044R
S82.045K
S82.045M
S82.045N
S82.045P
S82.045Q
S82.045R
S82.046K
S82.046M
S82.046N
S82.046P
S82.046Q
S82.046R
S82.091K
S82.091M
S82.091N
S82.091P
S82.091Q
S82.091R
S82.092K
S82.092M
S82.092N
S82.092P
S82.092Q
S82.092R
S82.099K
S82.099M
S82.099N
S82.099P
S82.099Q
S82.099R
S82.101K
S82.101M
S82.101N
S82.101P
S82.101Q
S82.101R
S82.102K
S82.102M
S82.102N
S82.102P
S82.102Q
S82.102R
S82.109K
S82.109M
S82.109N
S82.109P
S82.109Q
S82.109R
S82.111K
S82.111M
S82.111N
S82.111P
S82.111Q
S82.111R
S82.112K
S82.112M
S82.112N
S82.112P
S82.112Q
S82.112R
S82.113K
S82.113M
S82.113N
S82.113P
S82.113Q
S82.113R
S82.114K
S82.114M
S82.114N
S82.114P
S82.114Q
S82.114R
S82.115K
S82.115M
S82.115N
S82.115P
S82.115Q
S82.115R
S82.116K
S82.116M
S82.116N
S82.116P
S82.116Q
S82.116R
S82.121K
S82.121M
S82.121N
S82.121P
S82.121Q
S82.121R
S82.122K
S82.122M
S82.122N
S82.122P
S82.122Q
S82.122R
S82.123K
S82.123M
S82.123N
S82.123P
S82.123Q
S82.123R
S82.124K
S82.124M
S82.124N
S82.124P
S82.124Q
S82.124R
S82.125K
S82.125M
S82.125N
S82.125P
S82.125Q
S82.125R
S82.126K
S82.126M
S82.126N
S82.126P
S82.126Q
S82.126R
S82.131K
S82.131M
S82.131N
S82.131P
S82.131Q
S82.131R
S82.132K
S82.132M
S82.132N
S82.132P
S82.132Q
S82.132R
S82.133K
S82.133M
S82.133N
S82.133P
S82.133Q
S82.133R
S82.134K
S82.134M
S82.134N
S82.134P
S82.134Q
S82.134R
S82.135K
S82.135M
S82.135N
S82.135P
S82.135Q
S82.135R
S82.136K
S82.136M
S82.136N
S82.136P
S82.136Q
S82.136R
S82.141K
S82.141M
S82.141N
S82.141P
S82.141Q
S82.141R
S82.142K
S82.142M
S82.142N
S82.142P
S82.142Q
S82.142R
S82.143K
S82.143M
S82.143N
S82.143P
S82.143Q
S82.143R
S82.144K
S82.144M
S82.144N
S82.144P
S82.144Q
S82.144R
S82.145K
S82.145M
S82.145N
S82.145P
S82.145Q
S82.145R
S82.146K
S82.146M
S82.146N
S82.146P
S82.146Q
S82.146R
S82.151K
S82.151M
S82.151N
S82.151P
S82.151Q
S82.151R
S82.152K
S82.152M
S82.152N
S82.152P
S82.152Q
S82.152R
S82.153K
S82.153M
S82.153N
S82.153P
S82.153Q
S82.153R
S82.154K
S82.154M
S82.154N
S82.154P
S82.154Q
S82.154R
S82.155K
S82.155M
S82.155N
S82.155P
S82.155Q
S82.155R
S82.156K
S82.156M
S82.156N
S82.156P
S82.156Q
S82.156R
S82.161K
S82.161P
S82.162K
S82.162P
S82.169K
S82.169P
S82.191K
S82.191M
S82.191N
S82.191P
S82.191Q
S82.191R
S82.192K
S82.192M
S82.192N
S82.192P
S82.192Q
S82.192R
S82.199K
S82.199M
S82.199N
S82.199P
S82.199Q
S82.199R
S82.201K
S82.201M
S82.201N
S82.201P
S82.201Q
S82.201R
S82.202K
S82.202M
S82.202N
S82.202P
S82.202Q
S82.202R
S82.209K
S82.209M
S82.209N
S82.209P
S82.209Q
S82.209R
S82.221K
S82.221M
S82.221N
S82.221P
S82.221Q
S82.221R
S82.222K
S82.222M
S82.222N
S82.222P
S82.222Q
S82.222R
S82.223K
S82.223M
S82.223N
S82.223P
S82.223Q
S82.223R
S82.224K
S82.224M
S82.224N
S82.224P
S82.224Q
S82.224R
S82.225K
S82.225M
S82.225N
S82.225P
S82.225Q
S82.225R
S82.226K
S82.226M
S82.226N
S82.226P
S82.226Q
S82.226R
S82.231K
S82.231M
S82.231N
S82.231P
S82.231Q
S82.231R
S82.232K
S82.232M
S82.232N
S82.232P
S82.232Q
S82.232R
S82.233K
S82.233M
S82.233N
S82.233P
S82.233Q
S82.233R
S82.234K
S82.234M
S82.234N
S82.234P
S82.234Q
S82.234R
S82.235K
S82.235M
S82.235N
S82.235P
S82.235Q
S82.235R
S82.236K
S82.236M
S82.236N
S82.236P
S82.236Q
S82.236R
S82.241K
S82.241M
S82.241N
S82.241P
S82.241Q
S82.241R
S82.242K
S82.242M
S82.242N
S82.242P
S82.242Q
S82.242R
S82.243K
S82.243M
S82.243N
S82.243P
S82.243Q
S82.243R
S82.244K
S82.244M
S82.244N
S82.244P
S82.244Q
S82.244R
S82.245K
S82.245M
S82.245N
S82.245P
S82.245Q
S82.245R
S82.246K
S82.246M
S82.246N
S82.246P
S82.246Q
S82.246R
S82.251K
S82.251M
S82.251N
S82.251P
S82.251Q
S82.251R
S82.252K
S82.252M
S82.252N
S82.252P
S82.252Q
S82.252R
S82.253K
S82.253M
S82.253N
S82.253P
S82.253Q
S82.253R
S82.254K
S82.254M
S82.254N
S82.254P
S82.254Q
S82.254R
S82.255K
S82.255M
S82.255N
S82.255P
S82.255Q
S82.255R
S82.256K
S82.256M
S82.256N
S82.256P
S82.256Q
S82.256R
S82.261K
S82.261M
S82.261N
S82.261P
S82.261Q
S82.261R
S82.262K
S82.262M
S82.262N
S82.262P
S82.262Q
S82.262R
S82.263K
S82.263M
S82.263N
S82.263P
S82.263Q
S82.263R
S82.264K
S82.264M
S82.264N
S82.264P
S82.264Q
S82.264R
S82.265K
S82.265M
S82.265N
S82.265P
S82.265Q
S82.265R
S82.266K
S82.266M
S82.266N
S82.266P
S82.266Q
S82.266R
S82.291K
S82.291M
S82.291N
S82.291P
S82.291Q
S82.291R
S82.292K
S82.292M
S82.292N
S82.292P
S82.292Q
S82.292R
S82.299K
S82.299M
S82.299N
S82.299P
S82.299Q
S82.299R
S82.301K
S82.301M
S82.301N
S82.301P
S82.301Q
S82.301R
S82.302K
S82.302M
S82.302N
S82.302P
S82.302Q
S82.302R
S82.309K
S82.309M
S82.309N
S82.309P
S82.309Q
S82.309R
S82.311K
S82.311P
S82.312K
S82.312P
S82.319K
S82.319P
S82.391K
S82.391M
S82.391N
S82.391P
S82.391Q
S82.391R
S82.392K
S82.392M
S82.392N
S82.392P
S82.392Q
S82.392R
S82.399K
S82.399M
S82.399N
S82.399P
S82.399Q
S82.399R
S82.401K
S82.401M
S82.401N
S82.401P
S82.401Q
S82.401R
S82.402K
S82.402M
S82.402N
S82.402P
S82.402Q
S82.402R
S82.409K
S82.409M
S82.409N
S82.409P
S82.409Q
S82.409R
S82.421K
S82.421M
S82.421N
S82.421P
S82.421Q
S82.421R
S82.422K
S82.422M
S82.422N
S82.422P
S82.422Q
S82.422R
S82.423K
S82.423M
S82.423N
S82.423P
S82.423Q
S82.423R
S82.424K
S82.424M
S82.424N
S82.424P
S82.424Q
S82.424R
S82.425K
S82.425M
S82.425N
S82.425P
S82.425Q
S82.425R
S82.426K
S82.426M
S82.426N
S82.426P
S82.426Q
S82.426R
S82.431K
S82.431M
S82.431N
S82.431P
S82.431Q
S82.431R
S82.432K
S82.432M
S82.432N
S82.432P
S82.432Q
S82.432R
S82.433K
S82.433M
S82.433N
S82.433P
S82.433Q
S82.433R
S82.434K
S82.434M
S82.434N
S82.434P
S82.434Q
S82.434R
S82.435K
S82.435M
S82.435N
S82.435P
S82.435Q
S82.435R
S82.436K
S82.436M
S82.436N
S82.436P
S82.436Q
S82.436R
S82.441K
S82.441M
S82.441N
S82.441P
S82.441Q
S82.441R
S82.442K
S82.442M
S82.442N
S82.442P
S82.442Q
S82.442R
S82.443K
S82.443M
S82.443N
S82.443P
S82.443Q
S82.443R
S82.444K
S82.444M
S82.444N
S82.444P
S82.444Q
S82.444R
S82.445K
S82.445M

S82.445N
S82.445P
S82.445Q
S82.445R
S82.446K
S82.446M
S82.446N
S82.446P
S82.446Q
S82.446R
S82.451K
S82.451M
S82.451N
S82.451P
S82.451Q
S82.451R
S82.452K
S82.452M
S82.452N
S82.452P
S82.452Q
S82.452R
S82.453K
S82.453M
S82.453N
S82.453P
S82.453Q
S82.453R
S82.454K
S82.454M
S82.454N
S82.454P
S82.454Q
S82.454R
S82.455K
S82.455M
S82.455N
S82.455P
S82.455Q
S82.455R
S82.456K
S82.456M
S82.456N
S82.456P
S82.456Q
S82.456R
S82.461K
S82.461M
S82.461N
S82.461P
S82.461Q
S82.461R
S82.462K
S82.462M
S82.462N
S82.462P
S82.462Q
S82.462R
S82.463K
S82.463M
S82.463N
S82.463P
S82.463Q
S82.463R
S82.464K
S82.464M
S82.464N
S82.464P
S82.464Q
S82.464R
S82.465K
S82.465M
S82.465N
S82.465P
S82.465Q
S82.465R
S82.466K
S82.466M
S82.466N
S82.466P
S82.466Q
S82.466R
S82.491K
S82.491M
S82.491N
S82.491P
S82.491Q
S82.491R
S82.492K
S82.492M
S82.492N
S82.492P
S82.492Q
S82.492R
S82.499K
S82.499M
S82.499N
S82.499P
S82.499Q
S82.499R
S82.51XK
S82.51XM
S82.51XN
S82.51XP
S82.51XQ
S82.51XR
S82.52XK
S82.52XM
S82.52XN
S82.52XP
S82.52XQ
S82.52XR
S82.53XK
S82.53XM
S82.53XN
S82.53XP
S82.53XQ
S82.53XR
S82.54XK
S82.54XM
S82.54XN
S82.54XP
S82.54XQ
S82.54XR
S82.55XK
S82.55XM
S82.55XN
S82.55XP
S82.55XQ
S82.55XR
S82.56XK
S82.56XM
S82.56XN
S82.56XP
S82.56XQ
S82.56XR
S82.61XK
S82.61XM
S82.61XN
S82.61XP
S82.61XQ
S82.61XR
S82.62XK
S82.62XM
S82.62XN
S82.62XP
S82.62XQ
S82.62XR
S82.63XK
S82.63XM
S82.63XN
S82.63XP
S82.63XQ
S82.63XR
S82.64XK
S82.64XM
S82.64XN
S82.64XP
S82.64XQ
S82.64XR
S82.65XK
S82.65XM
S82.65XN
S82.65XP
S82.65XQ
S82.65XR
S82.66XK
S82.66XM
S82.66XN
S82.66XP
S82.66XQ
S82.66XR
S82.811K
S82.811P
S82.812K
S82.812P
S82.819K
S82.819P
S82.821K
S82.821P
S82.822K
S82.822P
S82.829K
S82.829P
S82.831K
S82.831M
S82.831N
S82.831P
S82.831Q
S82.831R
S82.832K
S82.832M
S82.832N
S82.832P
S82.832Q
S82.832R
S82.839K
S82.839M
S82.839N
S82.839P
S82.839Q
S82.839R
S82.841K
S82.841M
S82.841N
S82.841P
S82.841Q
S82.841R
S82.842K
S82.842M
S82.842N
S82.842P
S82.842Q
S82.842R
S82.843K
S82.843M
S82.843N
S82.843P
S82.843Q
S82.843R
S82.844K
S82.844M
S82.844N
S82.844P
S82.844Q
S82.844R
S82.845K
S82.845M
S82.845N
S82.845P
S82.845Q
S82.845R
S82.846K
S82.846M
S82.846N
S82.846P
S82.846Q
S82.846R
S82.851K
S82.851M
S82.851N
S82.851P
S82.851Q
S82.851R
S82.852K
S82.852M
S82.852N
S82.852P
S82.852Q
S82.852R
S82.853K
S82.853M
S82.853N
S82.853P
S82.853Q
S82.853R
S82.854K
S82.854M
S82.854N
S82.854P
S82.854Q
S82.854R
S82.855K
S82.855M
S82.855N
S82.855P
S82.855Q
S82.855R
S82.856K
S82.856M
S82.856N
S82.856P
S82.856Q
S82.856R
S82.861K
S82.861M
S82.861N
S82.861P
S82.861Q
S82.861R
S82.862K
S82.862M
S82.862N
S82.862P
S82.862Q
S82.862R
S82.863K
S82.863M
S82.863N
S82.863P
S82.863Q
S82.863R
S82.864K
S82.864M
S82.864N
S82.864P
S82.864Q
S82.864R
S82.865K
S82.865M
S82.865N
S82.865P
S82.865Q
S82.865R
S82.866K
S82.866M
S82.866N
S82.866P
S82.866Q
S82.866R
S82.871K
S82.871M
S82.871N
S82.871P
S82.871Q
S82.871R
S82.872K
S82.872M
S82.872N
S82.872P
S82.872Q
S82.872R
S82.873K
S82.873M
S82.873N
S82.873P
S82.873Q
S82.873R
S82.874K
S82.874M
S82.874N
S82.874P
S82.874Q
S82.874R
S82.875K
S82.875M
S82.875N
S82.875P
S82.875Q
S82.875R
S82.876K
S82.876M
S82.876N
S82.876P
S82.876Q
S82.876R
S82.891K
S82.891M
S82.891N
S82.891P
S82.891Q
S82.891R
S82.892K
S82.892M
S82.892N
S82.892P
S82.892Q
S82.892R
S82.899K
S82.899M
S82.899N
S82.899P
S82.899Q
S82.899R
S82.90XK
S82.90XM
S82.90XN
S82.90XP
S82.90XQ
S82.90XR
S82.91XK
S82.91XM
S82.91XN
S82.91XP
S82.91XQ
S82.91XR
S82.92XK
S82.92XM
S82.92XN
S82.92XP
S82.92XQ
S82.92XR
S86.021A
S86.022A
S86.029A
S86.121A
S86.122A
S86.129A
S86.221A
S86.222A
S86.229A
S86.321A
S86.322A
S86.329A
S86.821A
S86.822A
S86.829A
S86.921A
S86.922A
S86.929A
S89.001K
S89.001P
S89.002K
S89.002P
S89.009K
S89.009P
S89.011K
S89.011P
S89.012K
S89.012P
S89.019K
S89.019P
S89.021K
S89.021P
S89.022K
S89.022P
S89.029K
S89.029P
S89.031K
S89.031P
S89.032K
S89.032P
S89.039K
S89.039P
S89.041K
S89.041P
S89.042K
S89.042P
S89.049K
S89.049P
S89.091K
S89.091P
S89.092K
S89.092P
S89.099K
S89.099P
S89.101K
S89.101P
S89.102K
S89.102P
S89.109K
S89.109P
S89.111K
S89.111P
S89.112K
S89.112P
S89.119K
S89.119P
S89.121K
S89.121P
S89.122K
S89.122P
S89.129K
S89.129P
S89.131K
S89.131P
S89.132K
S89.132P
S89.139K
S89.139P
S89.141K
S89.141P
S89.142K
S89.142P
S89.149K
S89.149P
S89.191K
S89.191P
S89.192K
S89.192P
S89.199K
S89.199P
S89.201K
S89.201P
S89.202K
S89.202P
S89.209K
S89.209P
S89.211K
S89.211P
S89.212K
S89.212P
S89.219K
S89.219P
S89.221K
S89.221P
S89.222K
S89.222P
S89.229K
S89.229P
S89.291K
S89.291P
S89.292K
S89.292P
S89.299K
S89.299P
S89.301K
S89.301P
S89.302K
S89.302P
S89.309K
S89.309P
S89.311K
S89.311P
S89.312K
S89.312P
S89.319K
S89.319P
S89.321K
S89.321P
S89.322K
S89.322P
S89.329K
S89.329P
S89.391K
S89.391P
S89.392K
S89.392P
S89.399K
S89.399P
S92.001K
S92.001P
S92.002K
S92.002P
S92.009K
S92.009P
S92.011K
S92.011P
S92.012K
S92.012P
S92.013K
S92.013P
S92.014K
S92.014P
S92.015K
S92.015P
S92.016K
S92.016P
S92.021K
S92.021P
S92.022K
S92.022P
S92.023K
S92.023P
S92.024K
S92.024P
S92.025K
S92.025P
S92.026K
S92.026P
S92.031K
S92.031P
S92.032K
S92.032P
S92.033K
S92.033P
S92.034K
S92.034P
S92.035K
S92.035P
S92.036K
S92.036P
S92.041K
S92.041P
S92.042K
S92.042P
S92.043K
S92.043P
S92.044K
S92.044P
S92.045K
S92.045P
S92.046K
S92.046P
S92.051K
S92.051P
S92.052K
S92.052P
S92.053K
S92.053P
S92.054K
S92.054P
S92.055K
S92.055P
S92.056K
S92.056P
S92.061K
S92.061P
S92.062K
S92.062P
S92.063K
S92.063P
S92.064K
S92.064P
S92.065K
S92.065P
S92.066K
S92.066P
S92.101K
S92.101P
S92.102K
S92.102P
S92.109K
S92.109P
S92.111K
S92.111P
S92.112K
S92.112P
S92.113K
S92.113P
S92.114K
S92.114P
S92.115K
S92.115P
S92.116K
S92.116P
S92.121K
S92.121P
S92.122K
S92.122P
S92.123K
S92.123P
S92.124K
S92.124P
S92.125K
S92.125P
S92.126K
S92.126P
S92.131K
S92.131P
S92.132K
S92.132P
S92.133K
S92.133P
S92.134K
S92.134P
S92.135K
S92.135P
S92.136K
S92.136P
S92.141K
S92.141P
S92.142K
S92.142P
S92.143K
S92.143P
S92.144K
S92.144P
S92.145K
S92.145P
S92.146K
S92.146P
S92.151K
S92.151P
S92.152K
S92.152P
S92.153K
S92.153P
S92.154K
S92.154P
S92.155K
S92.155P
S92.156K
S92.156P
S92.191K
S92.191P
S92.192K
S92.192P
S92.199K
S92.199P
S92.201K
S92.201P
S92.202K
S92.202P
S92.209K
S92.209P
S92.211K
S92.211P
S92.212K
S92.212P
S92.213K
S92.213P
S92.214K
S92.214P
S92.215K
S92.215P
S92.216K
S92.216P
S92.221K
S92.221P
S92.222K
S92.222P
S92.223K
S92.223P
S92.224K
S92.224P
S92.225K
S92.225P
S92.226K
S92.226P
S92.231K
S92.231P
S92.232K
S92.232P
S92.233K
S92.233P
S92.234K
S92.234P
S92.235K
S92.235P
S92.236K
S92.236P
S92.241K
S92.241P
S92.242K
S92.242P
S92.243K
S92.243P
S92.244K
S92.244P
S92.245K
S92.245P
S92.246K
S92.246P
S92.251K
S92.251P
S92.252K
S92.252P
S92.253K
S92.253P
S92.254K
S92.254P
S92.255K
S92.255P
S92.256K
S92.256P
S92.301K
S92.301P
S92.302K
S92.302P
S92.309K
S92.309P
S92.311K
S92.311P
S92.312K
S92.312P
S92.313K
S92.313P
S92.314K
S92.314P
S92.315K
S92.315P
S92.316K
S92.316P
S92.321K
S92.321P
S92.322K
S92.322P
S92.323K
S92.323P
S92.324K
S92.324P
S92.325K
S92.325P
S92.326K
S92.326P
S92.331K
S92.331P
S92.332K
S92.332P
S92.333K
S92.333P
S92.334K
S92.334P
S92.335K
S92.335P
S92.336K
S92.336P
S92.341K
S92.341P
S92.342K
S92.342P
S92.343K
S92.343P
S92.344K
S92.344P
S92.345K
S92.345P
S92.346K
S92.346P
S92.351K
S92.351P
S92.352K
S92.352P
S92.353K
S92.353P
S92.354K
S92.354P
S92.355K
S92.355P
S92.356K
S92.356P
S92.401K
S92.401P
S92.402K
S92.402P
S92.403K
S92.403P
S92.404K
S92.404P
S92.405K
S92.405P
S92.406K
S92.406P
S92.411K
S92.411P
S92.412K
S92.412P
S92.413K
S92.413P
S92.414K
S92.414P
S92.415K
S92.415P
S92.416K
S92.416P
S92.421K
S92.421P
S92.422K
S92.422P
S92.423K
S92.423P
S92.424K
S92.424P
S92.425K
S92.425P
S92.426K
S92.426P
S92.491K
S92.491P
S92.492K
S92.492P
S92.499K
S92.499P
S92.501K
S92.501P
S92.502K
S92.502P
S92.503K
S92.503P
S92.504K
S92.504P
S92.505K
S92.505P
S92.506K

S92.5Ø6P
S92.511K
S92.511P
S92.512K
S92.512P
S92.513K
S92.513P
S92.514K
S92.514P
S92.515K
S92.515P
S92.516K
S92.516P
S92.521K
S92.521P
S92.522K
S92.522P
S92.523K
S92.523P
S92.524K
S92.524P
S92.525K
S92.525P
S92.526K
S92.526P
S92.531K
S92.531P
S92.532K
S92.532P
S92.533K
S92.533P
S92.534K
S92.534P
S92.535K
S92.535P
S92.536K
S92.536P
S92.591K
S92.591P
S92.592K
S92.592P
S92.599K
S92.599P
S92.811K
S92.811P
S92.812K
S92.812P
S92.819K
S92.819P
S92.9Ø1K
S92.9Ø1P
S92.9Ø2K
S92.9Ø2P
S92.9Ø9K
S92.9Ø9P
S92.911K
S92.911P
S92.912K
S92.912P
S92.919K
S92.919P
S96.Ø21A
S96.Ø22A
S96.Ø29A
S96.121A
S96.122A
S96.129A
S96.221A
S96.222A
S96.229A
S96.821A
S96.822A
S96.829A
S96.921A
S96.922A
S96.929A
T79.6XXA
T87.3*
T87.4*
T87.5*
T87.8*
T87.9
Z52.2*
Z94.6
Z96.6*
Z96.7
Z97.1*

DRG 565

Select principal diagnosis listed under DRG 564

DRG 566

Select principal diagnosis listed under DRG 564

MDC 9

DRG 570

Operating Room Procedures

ØJBØØZZ
ØJB1ØZZ
ØJB4ØZZ
ØJB5ØZZ
ØJB6ØZZ
ØJB7ØZZ
ØJB8ØZZ
ØJB9ØZZ
ØJBBØZZ
ØJBCØZZ
ØJBDØZZ
ØJBFØZZ
ØJBGØZZ
ØJBHØZZ
ØJBLØZZ
ØJBMØZZ
ØJBNØZZ
ØJBPØZZ
ØJBQØZZ
ØJBRØZZ

DRG 571

Select operating room procedures listed under DRG 570

DRG 572

Select operating room procedures listed under DRG 570

DRG 573

Principal Diagnosis

LØ2.Ø1
LØ2.11
LØ2.21*
LØ2.31
LØ2.41*
LØ2.51*
LØ2.61*
LØ2.81*
LØ2.91
LØ3*
L89*
L97*
L98.3
L98.4*

AND

Operating Room Procedures

ØHRØ*
ØHR1*
ØHR4*
ØHR5*
ØHR6*
ØHR7*
ØHR8*
ØHRA*
ØHRB*
ØHRC*
ØHRD*
ØHRE*
ØHRF*
ØHRG*
ØHRH*
ØHRJ*
ØHRK*
ØHRL*
ØHRM*
ØHRN*
ØHXØXZZ
ØHX1XZZ
ØHX4XZZ
ØHX5XZZ
ØHX6XZZ
ØHX7XZZ
ØHX8XZZ
ØHX9XZZ
ØHXAXZZ
ØHXBXZZ
ØHXCXZZ
ØHXDXZZ
ØHXEXZZ
ØHXFXZZ
ØHXGXZZ
ØHXHXZZ
ØHXJXZZ
ØHXKXZZ
ØHXLXZZ
ØHXMXZZ
ØHXNXZZ
ØJHØ*
ØJH1*
ØJH4*
ØJH5*
ØJH6ØNZ
ØJH63NZ
ØJH7ØNZ
ØJH73NZ
ØJH8ØNZ
ØJH83NZ
ØJH9*
ØJHB*
ØJHC*
ØJHDØNZ
ØJHD3NZ
ØJHFØNZ
ØJHF3NZ
ØJHGØNZ
ØJHG3NZ
ØJHHØNZ
ØJHH3NZ
ØJHJ*
ØJHK*
ØJHLØNZ
ØJHL3NZ
ØJHMØNZ
ØJHM3NZ
ØJHNØNZ
ØJHN3NZ
ØJHPØNZ
ØJHP3NZ
ØJHQ*
ØJHR*
ØJXØØZB
ØJXØØZC
ØJXØ3ZB
ØJXØ3ZC
ØJX1ØZB
ØJX1ØZC
ØJX13ZB
ØJX13ZC
ØJX4ØZB
ØJX4ØZC
ØJX43ZB
ØJX43ZC
ØJX5ØZB
ØJX5ØZC
ØJX53ZB
ØJX53ZC
ØJX6ØZB
ØJX6ØZC
ØJX63ZB
ØJX63ZC
ØJX7ØZB
ØJX7ØZC
ØJX73ZB
ØJX73ZC
ØJX8ØZB
ØJX8ØZC
ØJX83ZB
ØJX83ZC
ØJX9ØZB
ØJX9ØZC
ØJX93ZB
ØJX93ZC
ØJXBØZB
ØJXBØZC
ØJXB3ZB
ØJXB3ZC
ØJXCØZB
ØJXCØZC
ØJXC3ZB
ØJXC3ZC
ØJXDØZB
ØJXDØZC
ØJXD3ZB
ØJXD3ZC
ØJXFØZB
ØJXFØZC
ØJXF3ZB
ØJXF3ZC
ØJXGØZB
ØJXGØZC
ØJXG3ZB
ØJXG3ZC
ØJXHØZB
ØJXHØZC
ØJXH3ZB
ØJXH3ZC
ØJXJØZB
ØJXJØZC
ØJXJ3ZB
ØJXJ3ZC
ØJXKØZB
ØJXKØZC
ØJXK3ZB
ØJXK3ZC
ØJXLØZB
ØJXLØZC
ØJXL3ZB
ØJXL3ZC
ØJXMØZB
ØJXMØZC
ØJXM3ZB
ØJXM3ZC
ØJXNØZB
ØJXNØZC
ØJXN3ZB
ØJXN3ZC
ØJXPØZB
ØJXPØZC
ØJXP3ZB
ØJXP3ZC
ØJXQØZB
ØJXQØZC
ØJXQ3ZB
ØJXQ3ZC
ØJXRØZB
ØJXRØZC
ØJXR3ZB
ØJXR3ZC
ØKXHØZZ
ØKXH4ZZ
ØKXJØZZ
ØKXJ4ZZ
ØKXNØZZ
ØKXPØZZ
ØWBØØZZ
ØWBØ3ZZ
ØWBØ4ZZ
ØWBØXZZ
ØWB2ØZZ
ØWB23ZZ
ØWB24ZZ
ØWB2XZZ
ØWB4ØZZ
ØWB43ZZ
ØWB44ZZ
ØWB4XZZ
ØWB5ØZZ
ØWB53ZZ
ØWB54ZZ
ØWB5XZZ
ØWB6ØZZ
ØWB63ZZ
ØWB64ZZ
ØWB6XZZ
ØWBKØZZ
ØWBK3ZZ
ØWBK4ZZ
ØWBKXZZ
ØWBLØZZ
ØWBL3ZZ
ØWBL4ZZ
ØWBLXZZ
ØWBMØZZ
ØWBM3ZZ
ØWBM4ZZ
ØWBMXZZ
ØXB2ØZZ
ØXB23ZZ
ØXB24ZZ
ØXB3ØZZ
ØXB33ZZ
ØXB34ZZ
ØXB4ØZZ
ØXB43ZZ
ØXB44ZZ
ØXB5ØZZ
ØXB53ZZ
ØXB54ZZ
ØXB6ØZZ
ØXB63ZZ
ØXB64ZZ
ØXB7ØZZ
ØXB73ZZ
ØXB74ZZ
ØXB8ØZZ
ØXB83ZZ
ØXB84ZZ
ØXB9ØZZ
ØXB93ZZ
ØXB94ZZ
ØXBBØZZ
ØXBB3ZZ
ØXBB4ZZ
ØXBCØZZ
ØXBC3ZZ
ØXBC4ZZ
ØXBDØZZ
ØXBD3ZZ
ØXBD4ZZ
ØXBFØZZ
ØXBF3ZZ
ØXBF4ZZ
ØXBGØZZ
ØXBG3ZZ
ØXBG4ZZ
ØXBHØZZ
ØXBH3ZZ
ØXBH4ZZ
ØXBJØZZ
ØXBJ3ZZ
ØXBJ4ZZ
ØXBKØZZ
ØXBK3ZZ
ØXBK4ZZ
ØXUJØ7Z
ØXUJ47Z
ØXUKØ7Z
ØXUK47Z
ØXULØ7Z
ØXUL47Z
ØXUMØ7Z
ØXUM47Z
ØXUNØ7Z
ØXUN47Z
ØXUPØ7Z
ØXUP47Z
ØXUQØ7Z
ØXUQ47Z
ØXURØ7Z
ØXUR47Z
ØXUSØ7Z
ØXUS47Z
ØXUTØ7Z
ØXUT47Z
ØXUVØ7Z
ØXUV47Z
ØXUWØ7Z
ØXUW47Z
ØYBØØZZ
ØYBØ3ZZ
ØYBØ4ZZ
ØYB1ØZZ
ØYB13ZZ
ØYB14ZZ
ØYB9ØZZ
ØYB93ZZ
ØYB94ZZ
ØYBBØZZ
ØYBB3ZZ
ØYBB4ZZ
ØYBCØZZ
ØYBC3ZZ
ØYBC4ZZ
ØYBDØZZ
ØYBD3ZZ
ØYBD4ZZ
ØYBFØZZ
ØYBF3ZZ
ØYBF4ZZ
ØYBGØZZ
ØYBG3ZZ
ØYBG4ZZ
ØYBHØZZ
ØYBH3ZZ
ØYBH4ZZ
ØYBJØZZ
ØYBJ3ZZ
ØYBJ4ZZ
ØYBKØZZ
ØYBK3ZZ
ØYBK4ZZ
ØYBLØZZ
ØYBL3ZZ
ØYBL4ZZ
ØYBMØZZ
ØYBM3ZZ
ØYBM4ZZ
ØYBNØZZ
ØYBN3ZZ
ØYBN4ZZ
XHRPXF7

DRG 574

Select principal diagnosis AND operating room procedures listed under DRG 573

DRG 575

Select principal diagnosis AND operating room procedures listed under DRG 573

DRG 576

Select principal diagnosis in MDC 9 EXCEPT skin ulcer or cellulitis AND operating room procedures listed under DRG 573

DRG 577

Select principal diagnosis in MDC 9 EXCEPT skin ulcer or cellulitis AND operating room procedures listed under DRG 573

DRG 578

Select principal diagnosis in MDC 9 EXCEPT skin ulcer or cellulitis AND operating room procedures listed under DRG 573

DRG 579

Operating Room Procedures

315Ø9Ø
Ø315Ø9W
Ø315ØAØ
Ø315ØAW
Ø315ØJØ
Ø315ØJW
Ø315ØKØ
Ø315ØKW
Ø315ØZØ
Ø315ØZW
316Ø91
Ø316Ø9W
Ø316ØA1
Ø316ØAW
Ø316ØJ1
Ø316ØJW
Ø316ØK1
Ø316ØKW
Ø316ØZ1
Ø316ØZW
Ø317Ø9W
Ø317ØAW
Ø317ØJW
Ø317ØKW
Ø317ØZW
Ø318Ø9W
Ø318ØAW
Ø318ØJW
Ø318ØKW
Ø318ØZW
Ø31HØ9J
Ø31HØ9Y
Ø31HØAJ
Ø31HØAY
Ø31HØJJ
Ø31HØJY
Ø31HØKJ
Ø31HØKY
Ø31HØZJ
Ø31HØZY
Ø31JØ9K
Ø31JØ9Y
Ø31JØAK
Ø31JØAY
Ø31JØJK
Ø31JØJY
Ø31JØKK
Ø31JØKY
Ø31JØZK
Ø31JØZY
Ø31KØ9J
Ø31KØAJ
Ø31KØJJ
Ø31KØKJ
Ø31KØZJ
Ø31LØ9K
Ø31LØAK
Ø31LØJK
Ø31LØKK
Ø31LØZK
Ø31MØ9J
Ø31MØAJ
Ø31MØJJ
Ø31MØKJ
Ø31MØZJ
Ø31NØ9K
Ø31NØAK
Ø31NØJK
Ø31NØKK
Ø31NØZK
Ø37334Z
Ø37335Z
Ø37336Z
Ø37337Z
Ø3733D1
Ø3733DZ
Ø3733EZ
Ø3733FZ
Ø3733GZ
Ø3733Z1
Ø3733ZZ
Ø37434Z
Ø37435Z
Ø37436Z
Ø37437Z
Ø3743D1
Ø3743DZ
Ø3743EZ
Ø3743FZ
Ø3743GZ
Ø3743Z1
Ø3743ZZ
Ø37734Z
Ø37735Z
Ø37736Z
Ø37737Z
Ø3773D1
Ø3773DZ
Ø3773EZ
Ø3773FZ
Ø3773GZ
Ø3773Z1
Ø3773ZZ
Ø37834Z
Ø37835Z
Ø37836Z
Ø37837Z
Ø3783D1
Ø3783DZ
Ø3783EZ
Ø3783FZ
Ø3783GZ
Ø3783Z1
Ø3783ZZ
Ø37934Z
Ø37935Z
Ø37936Z
Ø37937Z
Ø3793D1
Ø3793DZ
Ø3793EZ
Ø3793FZ
Ø3793GZ
Ø3793Z1
Ø3793ZZ
Ø37A34Z
Ø37A35Z
Ø37A36Z
Ø37A37Z
Ø37A3D1
Ø37A3DZ
Ø37A3EZ
Ø37A3FZ
Ø37A3GZ
Ø37A3Z1
Ø37A3ZZ
Ø37Y34Z
Ø37Y35Z
Ø37Y36Z
Ø37Y37Z
Ø37Y3DZ
Ø37Y3EZ
Ø37Y3FZ
Ø37Y3GZ
Ø37Y3ZZ
Ø3Q5ØZZ
Ø3Q53ZZ
Ø3Q54ZZ
Ø3Q6ØZZ
Ø3Q63ZZ
Ø3Q64ZZ
Ø3Q7ØZZ
Ø3Q73ZZ
Ø3Q74ZZ
Ø3Q8ØZZ
Ø3Q83ZZ
Ø3Q84ZZ
Ø3Q9ØZZ
Ø3Q93ZZ
Ø3Q94ZZ
Ø3QAØZZ
Ø3QA3ZZ
Ø3QA4ZZ
Ø3QBØZZ
Ø3QB3ZZ
Ø3QB4ZZ
Ø3QCØZZ
Ø3QC3ZZ
Ø3QC4ZZ
Ø3QDØZZ
Ø3QD3ZZ
Ø3QD4ZZ
Ø3QFØZZ
Ø3QF3ZZ
Ø3QF4ZZ
Ø3S5ØZZ
Ø3S53ZZ
Ø3S54ZZ
Ø3S6ØZZ
Ø3S63ZZ
Ø3S64ZZ
Ø3S7ØZZ
Ø3S73ZZ
Ø3S74ZZ
Ø3S8ØZZ
Ø3S83ZZ
Ø3S84ZZ
Ø3S9ØZZ
Ø3S93ZZ
Ø3S94ZZ
Ø3SAØZZ
Ø3SA3ZZ
Ø3SA4ZZ
Ø3SBØZZ
Ø3SB3ZZ
Ø3SB4ZZ
Ø3SCØZZ
Ø3SC3ZZ
Ø3SC4ZZ
Ø3SDØZZ
Ø3SD3ZZ
Ø3SD4ZZ
Ø3SFØZZ
Ø3SF3ZZ
Ø3SF4ZZ
41ØØ96
41ØØ97
41ØØ98
41ØØ99
Ø41ØØ9B
Ø41ØØ9C
Ø41ØØ9D
Ø41ØØ9F
Ø41ØØ9G
Ø41ØØ9H
Ø41ØØ9J
Ø41ØØ9K
Ø41ØØ9Q
Ø41ØØ9R
Ø41ØØA6
Ø41ØØA7
Ø41ØØA8
Ø41ØØA9
Ø41ØØAB
Ø41ØØAC
Ø41ØØAD
Ø41ØØAF
Ø41ØØAG
Ø41ØØAH
Ø41ØØAJ
Ø41ØØAK
Ø41ØØAQ
Ø41ØØAR
Ø41ØØJ6
Ø41ØØJ7
Ø41ØØJ8
Ø41ØØJ9
Ø41ØØJB
Ø41ØØJC
Ø41ØØJD
Ø41ØØJF
Ø41ØØJG
Ø41ØØJH
Ø41ØØJJ
Ø41ØØJK
Ø41ØØJQ
Ø41ØØJR
Ø41ØØK6
Ø41ØØK7
Ø41ØØK8
Ø41ØØK9
Ø41ØØKB
Ø41ØØKC
Ø41ØØKD
Ø41ØØKF
Ø41ØØKG
Ø41ØØKH
Ø41ØØKJ
Ø41ØØKK
Ø41ØØKQ
Ø41ØØKR
Ø41ØØZ6
Ø41ØØZ7
Ø41ØØZ8
Ø41ØØZ9
Ø41ØØZB
Ø41ØØZC
Ø41ØØZD
Ø41ØØZF
Ø41ØØZG
Ø41ØØZH
Ø41ØØZJ
Ø41ØØZK
Ø41ØØZQ
Ø41ØØZR
41Ø496
41Ø497
41Ø498
41Ø499
Ø41Ø49B
Ø41Ø49C
Ø41Ø49D
Ø41Ø49F
Ø41Ø49G
Ø41Ø49H
Ø41Ø49J
Ø41Ø49K
Ø41Ø49Q
Ø41Ø49R
Ø41Ø4A6
Ø41Ø4A7
Ø41Ø4A8
Ø41Ø4A9
Ø41Ø4AB
Ø41Ø4AC
Ø41Ø4AD
Ø41Ø4AF
Ø41Ø4AG
Ø41Ø4AH
Ø41Ø4AJ
Ø41Ø4AK
Ø41Ø4AQ
Ø41Ø4AR
Ø41Ø4J6
Ø41Ø4J7
Ø41Ø4J8
Ø41Ø4J9

Ø41Ø4JB
Ø41Ø4JC
Ø41Ø4JD
Ø41Ø4JF
Ø41Ø4JG
Ø41Ø4JH
Ø41Ø4JJ
Ø41Ø4JK
Ø41Ø4JQ
Ø41Ø4JR
Ø41Ø4K6
Ø41Ø4K7
Ø41Ø4K8
Ø41Ø4K9
Ø41Ø4KB
Ø41Ø4KC
Ø41Ø4KD
Ø41Ø4KF
Ø41Ø4KG
Ø41Ø4KH
Ø41Ø4KJ
Ø41Ø4KK
Ø41Ø4KQ
Ø41Ø4KR
Ø41Ø4Z6
Ø41Ø4Z7
Ø41Ø4Z8
Ø41Ø4Z9
Ø41Ø4ZB
Ø41Ø4ZC
Ø41Ø4ZD
Ø41Ø4ZF
Ø41Ø4ZG
Ø41Ø4ZH
Ø41Ø4ZJ
Ø41Ø4ZK
Ø41Ø4ZQ
Ø41Ø4ZR
Ø41CØ9H
Ø41CØ9J
Ø41CØ9K
Ø41CØAH
Ø41CØAJ
Ø41CØAK
Ø41CØJH
Ø41CØJJ
Ø41CØJK
Ø41CØKH
Ø41CØKJ
Ø41CØKK
Ø41CØZH
Ø41CØZJ
Ø41CØZK
Ø41C49H
Ø41C49J
Ø41C49K
Ø41C4AH
Ø41C4AJ
Ø41C4AK
Ø41C4JH
Ø41C4JJ
Ø41C4JK
Ø41C4KH
Ø41C4KJ
Ø41C4KK
Ø41C4ZH
Ø41C4ZJ
Ø41C4ZK
Ø41DØ9H
Ø41DØ9J
Ø41DØ9K
Ø41DØAH
Ø41DØAJ
Ø41DØAK
Ø41DØJH
Ø41DØJJ
Ø41DØJK
Ø41DØKH
Ø41DØKJ
Ø41DØKK
Ø41DØZH
Ø41DØZJ
Ø41DØZK
Ø41D49H
Ø41D49J
Ø41D49K
Ø41D4AH
Ø41D4AJ
Ø41D4AK
Ø41D4JH
Ø41D4JJ
Ø41D4JK
Ø41D4KH
Ø41D4KJ
Ø41D4KK
Ø41D4ZH
Ø41D4ZJ
Ø41D4ZK
Ø41EØ9H
Ø41EØ9J
Ø41EØ9K
Ø41EØAH
Ø41EØAJ
Ø41EØAK
Ø41EØJH
Ø41EØJJ
Ø41EØJK
Ø41EØKH
Ø41EØKJ
Ø41EØKK
Ø41EØZH
Ø41EØZJ
Ø41EØZK
Ø41E49H
Ø41E49J
Ø41E49K
Ø41E4AH
Ø41E4AJ
Ø41E4AK
Ø41E4JH
Ø41E4JJ
Ø41E4JK
Ø41E4KH
Ø41E4KJ
Ø41E4KK
Ø41E4ZH
Ø41E4ZJ
Ø41E4ZK
Ø41FØ9H
Ø41FØ9J
Ø41FØ9K
Ø41FØAH
Ø41FØAJ
Ø41FØAK
Ø41FØJH
Ø41FØJJ
Ø41FØJK
Ø41FØKH
Ø41FØKJ
Ø41FØKK
Ø41FØZH
Ø41FØZJ
Ø41FØZK
Ø41F49H
Ø41F49J
Ø41F49K
Ø41F4AH
Ø41F4AJ
Ø41F4AK
Ø41F4JH
Ø41F4JJ
Ø41F4JK
Ø41F4KH
Ø41F4KJ
Ø41F4KK
Ø41F4ZH
Ø41F4ZJ
Ø41F4ZK
Ø41HØ9H
Ø41HØ9J
Ø41HØ9K
Ø41HØAH
Ø41HØAJ
Ø41HØAK
Ø41HØJH
Ø41HØJJ
Ø41HØJK
Ø41HØKH
Ø41HØKJ
Ø41HØKK
Ø41HØZH
Ø41HØZJ
Ø41HØZK
Ø41H49H
Ø41H49J
Ø41H49K
Ø41H4AH
Ø41H4AJ
Ø41H4AK
Ø41H4JH
Ø41H4JJ
Ø41H4JK
Ø41H4KH
Ø41H4KJ
Ø41H4KK
Ø41H4ZH
Ø41H4ZJ
Ø41H4ZK
Ø41JØ9H
Ø41JØ9J
Ø41JØ9K
Ø41JØAH
Ø41JØAJ
Ø41JØAK
Ø41JØJH
Ø41JØJJ
Ø41JØJK
Ø41JØKH
Ø41JØKJ
Ø41JØKK
Ø41JØZH
Ø41JØZJ
Ø41JØZK
Ø41J49H
Ø41J49J
Ø41J49K
Ø41J4AH
Ø41J4AJ
Ø41J4AK
Ø41J4JH
Ø41J4JJ
Ø41J4JK
Ø41J4KH
Ø41J4KJ
Ø41J4KK
Ø41J4ZH
Ø41J4ZJ
Ø41J4ZK
Ø41KØ9H
Ø41KØ9J
Ø41KØ9K
Ø41KØ9L
Ø41KØAH
Ø41KØAJ
Ø41KØAK
Ø41KØAL
Ø41KØJH
Ø41KØJJ
Ø41KØJK
Ø41KØJL
Ø41KØKH
Ø41KØKJ
Ø41KØKK
Ø41KØKL
Ø41KØZH
Ø41KØZJ
Ø41KØZK
Ø41KØZL
Ø41K49H
Ø41K49J
Ø41K49K
Ø41K49L
Ø41K4AH
Ø41K4AJ
Ø41K4AK
Ø41K4AL
Ø41K4JH
Ø41K4JJ
Ø41K4JK
Ø41K4JL
Ø41K4KH
Ø41K4KJ
Ø41K4KK
Ø41K4KL
Ø41K4ZH
Ø41K4ZJ
Ø41K4ZK
Ø41K4ZL
Ø41LØ9H
Ø41LØ9J
Ø41LØ9K
Ø41LØ9L
Ø41LØAH
Ø41LØAJ
Ø41LØAK
Ø41LØAL
Ø41LØJH
Ø41LØJJ
Ø41LØJK
Ø41LØJL
Ø41LØKH
Ø41LØKJ
Ø41LØKK
Ø41LØKL
Ø41LØZH
Ø41LØZJ
Ø41LØZK
Ø41LØZL
Ø41L49H
Ø41L49J
Ø41L49K
Ø41L49L
Ø41L4AH
Ø41L4AJ
Ø41L4AK
Ø41L4AL
Ø41L4JH
Ø41L4JJ
Ø41L4JK
Ø41L4JL
Ø41L4KH
Ø41L4KJ
Ø41L4KK
Ø41L4KL
Ø41L4ZH
Ø41L4ZJ
Ø41L4ZK
Ø41L4ZL
47Ø341
Ø47Ø34Z
Ø47Ø35Z
Ø47Ø36Z
Ø47Ø37Z
Ø47Ø3D1
Ø47Ø3DZ
Ø47Ø3EZ
Ø47Ø3FZ
Ø47Ø3GZ
Ø47Ø3Z1
Ø47Ø3ZZ
471341
Ø47134Z
Ø47135Z
Ø47136Z
Ø47137Z
Ø4713D1
Ø4713DZ
Ø4713EZ
Ø4713FZ
Ø4713GZ
Ø4713Z1
Ø4713ZZ
472341
Ø47234Z
Ø47235Z
Ø47236Z
Ø47237Z
Ø4723D1
Ø4723DZ
Ø4723EZ
Ø4723FZ
Ø4723GZ
Ø4723Z1
Ø4723ZZ
473341
Ø47334Z
Ø47335Z
Ø47336Z
Ø47337Z
Ø4733D1
Ø4733DZ
Ø4733EZ
Ø4733FZ
Ø4733GZ
Ø4733Z1
Ø4733ZZ
474341
Ø47434Z
Ø47435Z
Ø47436Z
Ø47437Z
Ø4743D1
Ø4743DZ
Ø4743EZ
Ø4743FZ
Ø4743GZ
Ø4743Z1
Ø4743ZZ
475341
Ø47534Z
Ø47535Z
Ø47536Z
Ø47537Z
Ø4753D1
Ø4753DZ
Ø4753EZ
Ø4753FZ
Ø4753GZ
Ø4753Z1
Ø4753ZZ
476341
Ø47634Z
Ø47635Z
Ø47636Z
Ø47637Z
Ø4763D1
Ø4763DZ
Ø4763EZ
Ø4763FZ
Ø4763GZ
Ø4763Z1
Ø4763ZZ
477341
Ø47734Z
Ø47735Z
Ø47736Z
Ø47737Z
Ø4773D1
Ø4773DZ
Ø4773EZ
Ø4773FZ
Ø4773GZ
Ø4773Z1
Ø4773ZZ
478341
Ø47834Z
Ø47835Z
Ø47836Z
Ø47837Z
Ø4783D1
Ø4783DZ
Ø4783EZ
Ø4783FZ
Ø4783GZ
Ø4783Z1
Ø4783ZZ
479341
Ø47934Z
Ø47935Z
Ø47936Z
Ø47937Z
Ø4793D1
Ø4793DZ
Ø4793EZ
Ø4793FZ
Ø4793GZ
Ø4793Z1
Ø4793ZZ
Ø47A341
Ø47A34Z
Ø47A35Z
Ø47A36Z
Ø47A37Z
Ø47A3D1
Ø47A3DZ
Ø47A3EZ
Ø47A3FZ
Ø47A3GZ
Ø47A3Z1
Ø47A3ZZ
Ø47B341
Ø47B34Z
Ø47B35Z
Ø47B36Z
Ø47B37Z
Ø47B3D1
Ø47B3DZ
Ø47B3EZ
Ø47B3FZ
Ø47B3GZ
Ø47B3Z1
Ø47B3ZZ
Ø47C341
Ø47C34Z
Ø47C35Z
Ø47C36Z
Ø47C37Z
Ø47C3D1
Ø47C3DZ
Ø47C3EZ
Ø47C3FZ
Ø47C3GZ
Ø47C3Z1
Ø47C3ZZ
Ø47D341
Ø47D34Z
Ø47D35Z
Ø47D36Z
Ø47D37Z
Ø47D3D1
Ø47D3DZ
Ø47D3EZ
Ø47D3FZ
Ø47D3GZ
Ø47D3Z1
Ø47D3ZZ
Ø47E341
Ø47E34Z
Ø47E35Z
Ø47E36Z
Ø47E37Z
Ø47E3D1
Ø47E3DZ
Ø47E3EZ
Ø47E3FZ
Ø47E3GZ
Ø47E3Z1
Ø47E3ZZ
Ø47F341
Ø47F34Z
Ø47F35Z
Ø47F36Z
Ø47F37Z
Ø47F3D1
Ø47F3DZ
Ø47F3EZ
Ø47F3FZ
Ø47F3GZ
Ø47F3Z1
Ø47F3ZZ
Ø47H341
Ø47H34Z
Ø47H35Z
Ø47H36Z
Ø47H37Z
Ø47H3D1
Ø47H3DZ
Ø47H3EZ
Ø47H3FZ
Ø47H3GZ
Ø47H3Z1
Ø47H3ZZ
Ø47J341
Ø47J34Z
Ø47J35Z
Ø47J36Z
Ø47J37Z
Ø47J3D1
Ø47J3DZ
Ø47J3EZ
Ø47J3FZ
Ø47J3GZ
Ø47J3Z1
Ø47J3ZZ
Ø47KØ41
Ø47KØD1
Ø47KØZ1
Ø47K341
Ø47K34Z
Ø47K35Z
Ø47K36Z
Ø47K37Z
Ø47K3D1
Ø47K3DZ
Ø47K3EZ
Ø47K3FZ
Ø47K3GZ
Ø47K3Z1
Ø47K3ZZ
Ø47K441
Ø47K4D1
Ø47K4Z1
Ø47LØ41
Ø47LØD1
Ø47LØZ1
Ø47L341
Ø47L34Z
Ø47L35Z
Ø47L36Z
Ø47L37Z
Ø47L3D1
Ø47L3DZ
Ø47L3EZ
Ø47L3FZ
Ø47L3GZ
Ø47L3Z1
Ø47L3ZZ
Ø47L441
Ø47L4D1
Ø47L4Z1
Ø47MØ41
Ø47MØD1
Ø47MØZ1
Ø47M341
Ø47M3D1
Ø47M3Z1
Ø47M441
Ø47M4D1
Ø47M4Z1
Ø47NØ41
Ø47NØD1
Ø47NØZ1
Ø47N341
Ø47N3D1
Ø47N3Z1
Ø47N441
Ø47N4D1
Ø47N4Z1
Ø47Y341
Ø47Y34Z
Ø47Y35Z
Ø47Y36Z
Ø47Y37Z
Ø47Y3D1
Ø47Y3DZ
Ø47Y3EZ
Ø47Y3FZ
Ø47Y3GZ
Ø47Y3Z1
Ø47Y3ZZ
Ø4QCØZZ
Ø4QC3ZZ
Ø4QC4ZZ
Ø4QDØZZ
Ø4QD3ZZ
Ø4QD4ZZ
Ø4QEØZZ
Ø4QE3ZZ
Ø4QE4ZZ
Ø4QFØZZ
Ø4QF3ZZ
Ø4QF4ZZ
Ø4QHØZZ
Ø4QH3ZZ
Ø4QH4ZZ
Ø4QJØZZ
Ø4QJ3ZZ
Ø4QJ4ZZ
Ø4QKØZZ
Ø4QK3ZZ
Ø4QK4ZZ
Ø4QLØZZ
Ø4QL3ZZ
Ø4QL4ZZ
Ø4QMØZZ
Ø4QM3ZZ
Ø4QM4ZZ
Ø4QNØZZ
Ø4QN3ZZ
Ø4QN4ZZ
Ø4QPØZZ
Ø4QP3ZZ
Ø4QP4ZZ
Ø4QQØZZ
Ø4QQ3ZZ
Ø4QQ4ZZ
Ø4QRØZZ
Ø4QR3ZZ
Ø4QR4ZZ
Ø4QSØZZ
Ø4QS3ZZ
Ø4QS4ZZ
Ø4QTØZZ
Ø4QT3ZZ
Ø4QT4ZZ
Ø4QUØZZ
Ø4QU3ZZ
Ø4QU4ZZ
Ø4QVØZZ
Ø4QV3ZZ
Ø4QV4ZZ
Ø4QWØZZ
Ø4QW3ZZ
Ø4QW4ZZ
Ø4SKØZZ
Ø4SK3ZZ
Ø4SK4ZZ
Ø4SLØZZ
Ø4SL3ZZ
Ø4SL4ZZ
Ø4SMØZZ
Ø4SM3ZZ
Ø4SM4ZZ
Ø4SNØZZ
Ø4SN3ZZ
Ø4SN4ZZ
Ø4SPØZZ
Ø4SP3ZZ
Ø4SP4ZZ
Ø4SQØZZ
Ø4SQ3ZZ
Ø4SQ4ZZ
Ø4SRØZZ
Ø4SR3ZZ
Ø4SR4ZZ
Ø4SSØZZ
Ø4SS3ZZ
Ø4SS4ZZ
Ø4STØZZ
Ø4ST3ZZ
Ø4ST4ZZ
Ø4SUØZZ
Ø4SU3ZZ
Ø4SU4ZZ
Ø4SVØZZ
Ø4SV3ZZ
Ø4SV4ZZ
Ø4SWØZZ
Ø4SW3ZZ
Ø4SW4ZZ
Ø4SYØZZ
Ø4SY3ZZ
Ø4SY4ZZ
Ø5793D1
Ø5793DZ
Ø5793Z1
Ø5793ZZ
Ø57A3D1
Ø57A3DZ
Ø57A3Z1
Ø57A3ZZ
Ø57B3D1
Ø57B3DZ
Ø57B3Z1
Ø57B3ZZ
Ø57C3D1
Ø57C3DZ
Ø57C3Z1
Ø57C3ZZ
Ø57D3D1
Ø57D3DZ
Ø57D3Z1
Ø57D3ZZ
Ø57F3D1
Ø57F3DZ
Ø57F3Z1
Ø57F3ZZ
Ø5S7ØZZ
Ø5S73ZZ
Ø5S74ZZ
Ø5S8ØZZ
Ø5S83ZZ
Ø5S84ZZ
Ø5S9ØZZ
Ø5S93ZZ
Ø5S94ZZ
Ø5SAØZZ
Ø5SA3ZZ
Ø5SA4ZZ
Ø5SBØZZ
Ø5SB3ZZ
Ø5SB4ZZ
Ø5SCØZZ
Ø5SC3ZZ
Ø5SC4ZZ
Ø5SDØZZ
Ø5SD3ZZ
Ø5SD4ZZ
Ø5SFØZZ
Ø5SF3ZZ
Ø5SF4ZZ
Ø5SGØZZ
Ø5SG3ZZ
Ø5SG4ZZ
Ø5SHØZZ
Ø5SH3ZZ
Ø5SH4ZZ
Ø67Ø3DZ
Ø67Ø3ZZ
Ø6SMØZZ
Ø6SM3ZZ
Ø6SM4ZZ
Ø6SNØZZ
Ø6SN3ZZ
Ø6SN4ZZ
Ø6SPØZZ
Ø6SP3ZZ
Ø6SP4ZZ
Ø6SQØZZ
Ø6SQ3ZZ
Ø6SQ4ZZ
Ø6STØZZ
Ø6ST3ZZ
Ø6ST4ZZ
Ø6SVØZZ
Ø6SV3ZZ
Ø6SV4ZZ
Ø6SYØZZ
Ø6SY3ZZ
Ø6SY4ZZ
Ø79ØØØZ
Ø79ØØZX
Ø79ØØZZ
Ø79Ø3ZX
Ø79Ø4ØZ
Ø79Ø4ZX
Ø79Ø4ZZ
Ø791ØØZ
Ø791ØZX
Ø791ØZZ
Ø7913ZX
Ø7914ØZ
Ø7914ZX
Ø7914ZZ
Ø792ØØZ
Ø792ØZX
Ø792ØZZ
Ø7923ZX
Ø7924ØZ
Ø7924ZX
Ø7924ZZ
Ø793ØØZ
Ø793ØZX
Ø793ØZZ
Ø7933ZX
Ø7934ØZ
Ø7934ZX
Ø7934ZZ
Ø794ØØZ
Ø794ØZX
Ø794ØZZ
Ø7943ZX
Ø7944ØZ
Ø7944ZX
Ø7944ZZ
Ø795ØØZ
Ø795ØZX
Ø795ØZZ
Ø7953ZX
Ø7954ØZ
Ø7954ZX
Ø7954ZZ
Ø796ØØZ
Ø796ØZX
Ø796ØZZ
Ø7963ZX
Ø7964ØZ
Ø7964ZX
Ø7964ZZ
Ø797ØØZ
Ø797ØZX
Ø797ØZZ
Ø7973ZX
Ø7974ØZ
Ø7974ZX
Ø7974ZZ
Ø798ØØZ
Ø798ØZX
Ø798ØZZ
Ø7983ZX
Ø7984ØZ
Ø7984ZX
Ø7984ZZ
Ø799ØØZ
Ø799ØZX
Ø799ØZZ
Ø7993ZX
Ø7994ØZ
Ø7994ZX
Ø7994ZZ
Ø79BØØZ
Ø79BØZX
Ø79BØZZ
Ø79B3ZX
Ø79B4ØZ
Ø79B4ZX
Ø79B4ZZ
Ø79CØØZ
Ø79CØZX
Ø79CØZZ
Ø79C3ZX
Ø79C4ØZ
Ø79C4ZX
Ø79C4ZZ
Ø79DØØZ
Ø79DØZX
Ø79DØZZ
Ø79D3ZX
Ø79D4ØZ
Ø79D4ZX
Ø79D4ZZ
Ø79FØØZ
Ø79FØZX
Ø79FØZZ
Ø79F3ZX
Ø79F4ØZ
Ø79F4ZX
Ø79F4ZZ
Ø79GØØZ
Ø79GØZX
Ø79GØZZ
Ø79G3ZX
Ø79G4ØZ
Ø79G4ZX
Ø79G4ZZ

ICD-10-CM/PCS Codes by MS-DRG

Ø79HØØZ
Ø79HØZX
Ø79HØZZ
Ø79H3ZX
Ø79H4ØZ
Ø79H4ZX
Ø79H4ZZ
Ø79JØØZ
Ø79JØZX
Ø79JØZZ
Ø79J3ZX
Ø79J4ØZ
Ø79J4ZX
Ø79J4ZZ
Ø79KØZX
Ø79K3ZX
Ø79K4ZX
Ø79LØZX
Ø79L3ZX
Ø79L4ZX
Ø7BØØZX
Ø7BØØZZ
Ø7BØ3ZX
Ø7BØ3ZZ
Ø7BØ4ZX
Ø7BØ4ZZ
Ø7B1ØZX
Ø7B1ØZZ
Ø7B13ZX
Ø7B13ZZ
Ø7B14ZX
Ø7B14ZZ
Ø7B2ØZX
Ø7B2ØZZ
Ø7B23ZX
Ø7B23ZZ
Ø7B24ZX
Ø7B24ZZ
Ø7B3ØZX
Ø7B3ØZZ
Ø7B33ZX
Ø7B33ZZ
Ø7B34ZX
Ø7B34ZZ
Ø7B4ØZX
Ø7B4ØZZ
Ø7B43ZX
Ø7B43ZZ
Ø7B44ZX
Ø7B44ZZ
Ø7B5ØZX
Ø7B5ØZZ
Ø7B53ZX
Ø7B53ZZ
Ø7B54ZX
Ø7B54ZZ
Ø7B6ØZX
Ø7B6ØZZ
Ø7B63ZX
Ø7B63ZZ
Ø7B64ZX
Ø7B64ZZ
Ø7B7ØZX
Ø7B7ØZZ
Ø7B73ZX
Ø7B73ZZ
Ø7B74ZX
Ø7B74ZZ
Ø7B8ØZX
Ø7B8ØZZ
Ø7B83ZX
Ø7B83ZZ
Ø7B84ZX
Ø7B84ZZ
Ø7B9ØZX
Ø7B9ØZZ
Ø7B93ZX
Ø7B93ZZ
Ø7B94ZX
Ø7B94ZZ
Ø7BBØZX
Ø7BBØZZ
Ø7BB3ZX
Ø7BB3ZZ
Ø7BB4ZX
Ø7BB4ZZ
Ø7BCØZX
Ø7BCØZZ
Ø7BC3ZX
Ø7BC3ZZ
Ø7BC4ZX
Ø7BC4ZZ
Ø7BDØZX
Ø7BDØZZ
Ø7BD3ZX
Ø7BD3ZZ
Ø7BD4ZX
Ø7BD4ZZ
Ø7BFØZX
Ø7BFØZZ
Ø7BF3ZX
Ø7BF3ZZ
Ø7BF4ZX
Ø7BF4ZZ
Ø7BGØZX
Ø7BGØZZ
Ø7BG3ZX
Ø7BG3ZZ
Ø7BG4ZX
Ø7BG4ZZ
Ø7BHØZX
Ø7BHØZZ
Ø7BH3ZX
Ø7BH3ZZ
Ø7BH4ZX
Ø7BH4ZZ
Ø7BJØZX
Ø7BJØZZ
Ø7BJ3ZX
Ø7BJ3ZZ
Ø7BJ4ZX
Ø7BJ4ZZ
Ø7BKØZX
Ø7BK3ZX
Ø7BK4ZX
Ø7BLØZX
Ø7BL3ZX
Ø7BL4ZX
Ø7CØØZZ
Ø7CØ3ZZ
Ø7CØ4ZZ
Ø7C1ØZZ
Ø7C13ZZ
Ø7C14ZZ
Ø7C2ØZZ
Ø7C23ZZ
Ø7C24ZZ
Ø7C3ØZZ
Ø7C33ZZ
Ø7C34ZZ
Ø7C4ØZZ
Ø7C43ZZ
Ø7C44ZZ
Ø7C5ØZZ
Ø7C53ZZ
Ø7C54ZZ
Ø7C6ØZZ
Ø7C63ZZ
Ø7C64ZZ
Ø7C7ØZZ
Ø7C73ZZ
Ø7C74ZZ
Ø7C8ØZZ
Ø7C83ZZ
Ø7C84ZZ
Ø7C9ØZZ
Ø7C93ZZ
Ø7C94ZZ
Ø7CBØZZ
Ø7CB3ZZ
Ø7CB4ZZ
Ø7CCØZZ
Ø7CC3ZZ
Ø7CC4ZZ
Ø7CDØZZ
Ø7CD3ZZ
Ø7CD4ZZ
Ø7CFØZZ
Ø7CF3ZZ
Ø7CF4ZZ
Ø7CGØZZ
Ø7CG3ZZ
Ø7CG4ZZ
Ø7CHØZZ
Ø7CH3ZZ
Ø7CH4ZZ
Ø7CJØZZ
Ø7CJ3ZZ
Ø7CJ4ZZ
Ø7CKØZZ
Ø7CK3ZZ
Ø7CK4ZZ
Ø7CLØZZ
Ø7CL3ZZ
Ø7CL4ZZ
Ø7HNØ1Z
Ø7HNØYZ
Ø7HN41Z
Ø7JKØZZ
Ø7JK4ZZ
Ø7JLØZZ
Ø7JL4ZZ
Ø7JNØZZ
Ø7JN4ZZ
Ø7JPØZZ
Ø7PNØØZ
Ø7PNØ3Z
Ø7PNØCZ
Ø7PNØDZ
Ø7PNØYZ
Ø7PN3ØZ
Ø7PN33Z
Ø7PN3CZ
Ø7PN3DZ
Ø7PN4ØZ
Ø7PN43Z
Ø7PN4CZ
Ø7PN4DZ
Ø7TØØZZ
Ø7TØ4ZZ
Ø7T1ØZZ
Ø7T14ZZ
Ø7T2ØZZ
Ø7T24ZZ
Ø7T3ØZZ
Ø7T34ZZ
Ø7T4ØZZ
Ø7T44ZZ
Ø7T5ØZZ
Ø7T54ZZ
Ø7T6ØZZ
Ø7T64ZZ
Ø7T7ØZZ
Ø7T74ZZ
Ø7T8ØZZ
Ø7T84ZZ
Ø7T9ØZZ
Ø7T94ZZ
Ø7TBØZZ
Ø7TB4ZZ
Ø7TCØZZ
Ø7TC4ZZ
Ø7TDØZZ
Ø7TD4ZZ
Ø7TFØZZ
Ø7TF4ZZ
Ø7TGØZZ
Ø7TG4ZZ
Ø7THØZZ
Ø7TH4ZZ
Ø7TJØZZ
Ø7TJ4ZZ
Ø7WNØØZ
Ø7WNØ3Z
Ø7WNØCZ
Ø7WNØDZ
Ø7WNØYZ
Ø7WN3ØZ
Ø7WN33Z
Ø7WN3CZ
Ø7WN3DZ
Ø7WN4ØZ
Ø7WN43Z
Ø7WN4CZ
Ø7WN4DZ
Ø85NØZZ
Ø85N3ZZ
Ø85NXZZ
Ø85PØZZ
Ø85P3ZZ
Ø85PXZZ
Ø85QØZZ
Ø85Q3ZZ
Ø85QXZZ
Ø85RØZZ
Ø85R3ZZ
Ø85RXZZ
Ø8BØØZZ
Ø8BØ3ZZ
Ø8BØXZZ
Ø8B1ØZZ
Ø8B13ZZ
Ø8B1XZZ
Ø8BNØZZ
Ø8BN3ZZ
Ø8BNXZZ
Ø8BPØZZ
Ø8BP3ZZ
Ø8BPXZZ
Ø8BQØZZ
Ø8BQ3ZZ
Ø8BQXZZ
Ø8BRØZZ
Ø8BR3ZZ
Ø8BRXZZ
Ø8MNXZZ
Ø8MPXZZ
Ø8MQXZZ
Ø8MRXZZ
Ø8NNØZZ
Ø8NN3ZZ
Ø8NNXZZ
Ø8NPØZZ
Ø8NP3ZZ
Ø8NPXZZ
Ø8NQØZZ
Ø8NQ3ZZ
Ø8NQXZZ
Ø8NRØZZ
Ø8NR3ZZ
Ø8NRXZZ
Ø8QX7ZZ
Ø8QX8ZZ
Ø8QY7ZZ
Ø8QY8ZZ
Ø8RNØ7Z
Ø8RNØJZ
Ø8RNØKZ
Ø8RN37Z
Ø8RN3JZ
Ø8RN3KZ
Ø8RNX7Z
Ø8RNXJZ
Ø8RNXKZ
Ø8RPØ7Z
Ø8RPØJZ
Ø8RPØKZ
Ø8RP37Z
Ø8RP3JZ
Ø8RP3KZ
Ø8RPX7Z
Ø8RPXJZ
Ø8RPXKZ
Ø8RQØ7Z
Ø8RQØJZ
Ø8RQØKZ
Ø8RQ37Z
Ø8RQ3JZ
Ø8RQ3KZ
Ø8RQX7Z
Ø8RQXJZ
Ø8RQXKZ
Ø8RRØ7Z
Ø8RRØJZ
Ø8RRØKZ
Ø8RR37Z
Ø8RR3JZ
Ø8RR3KZ
Ø8RRX7Z
Ø8RRXJZ
Ø8RRXKZ
Ø8RXØ7Z
Ø8RXØJZ
Ø8RXØKZ
Ø8RX37Z
Ø8RX3JZ
Ø8RX3KZ
Ø8RX77Z
Ø8RX7JZ
Ø8RX7KZ
Ø8RX87Z
Ø8RX8JZ
Ø8RX8KZ
Ø8RYØ7Z
Ø8RYØJZ
Ø8RYØKZ
Ø8RY37Z
Ø8RY3JZ
Ø8RY3KZ
Ø8RY77Z
Ø8RY7JZ
Ø8RY7KZ
Ø8RY87Z
Ø8RY8JZ
Ø8RY8KZ
Ø8SNØZZ
Ø8SN3ZZ
Ø8SNXZZ
Ø8SPØZZ
Ø8SP3ZZ
Ø8SPXZZ
Ø8SQØZZ
Ø8SQ3ZZ
Ø8SQXZZ
Ø8SRØZZ
Ø8SR3ZZ
Ø8SRXZZ
Ø8TNØZZ
Ø8TNXZZ
Ø8TPØZZ
Ø8TPXZZ
Ø8TQØZZ
Ø8TQXZZ
Ø8TRØZZ
Ø8TRXZZ
Ø8UNØ7Z
Ø8UNØJZ
Ø8UNØKZ
Ø8UN37Z
Ø8UN3JZ
Ø8UN3KZ
Ø8UNX7Z
Ø8UNXJZ
Ø8UNXKZ
Ø8UPØ7Z
Ø8UPØJZ
Ø8UPØKZ
Ø8UP37Z
Ø8UP3JZ
Ø8UP3KZ
Ø8UPX7Z
Ø8UPXJZ
Ø8UPXKZ
Ø8UQØ7Z
Ø8UQØJZ
Ø8UQØKZ
Ø8UQ37Z
Ø8UQ3JZ
Ø8UQ3KZ
Ø8UQX7Z
Ø8UQXJZ
Ø8UQXKZ
Ø8URØ7Z
Ø8URØJZ
Ø8URØKZ
Ø8UR37Z
Ø8UR3JZ
Ø8UR3KZ
Ø8URX7Z
Ø8URXJZ
Ø8URXKZ
Ø8UXØ7Z
Ø8UXØJZ
Ø8UXØKZ
Ø8UX37Z
Ø8UX3JZ
Ø8UX3KZ
Ø8UX77Z
Ø8UX7JZ
Ø8UX7KZ
Ø8UX87Z
Ø8UX8JZ
Ø8UX8KZ
Ø8UYØ7Z
Ø8UYØJZ
Ø8UYØKZ
Ø8UY37Z
Ø8UY3JZ
Ø8UY3KZ
Ø8UY77Z
Ø8UY7JZ
Ø8UY7KZ
Ø8UY87Z
Ø8UY8JZ
Ø8UY8KZ
Ø9ØØØ7Z
Ø9ØØØJZ
Ø9ØØØKZ
Ø9ØØØZZ
Ø9ØØ37Z
Ø9ØØ3JZ
Ø9ØØ3KZ
Ø9ØØ3ZZ
Ø9ØØ47Z
Ø9ØØ4JZ
Ø9ØØ4KZ
Ø9ØØ4ZZ
Ø9ØØX7Z
Ø9ØØXJZ
Ø9ØØXKZ
Ø9ØØXZZ
Ø9Ø1Ø7Z
Ø9Ø1ØJZ
Ø9Ø1ØKZ
Ø9Ø1ØZZ
Ø9Ø137Z
Ø9Ø13JZ
Ø9Ø13KZ
Ø9Ø13ZZ
Ø9Ø147Z
Ø9Ø14JZ
Ø9Ø14KZ
Ø9Ø14ZZ
Ø9Ø1X7Z
Ø9Ø1XJZ
Ø9Ø1XKZ
Ø9Ø1XZZ
Ø9Ø2Ø7Z
Ø9Ø2ØJZ
Ø9Ø2ØKZ
Ø9Ø2ØZZ
Ø9Ø237Z
Ø9Ø23JZ
Ø9Ø23KZ
Ø9Ø23ZZ
Ø9Ø247Z
Ø9Ø24JZ
Ø9Ø24KZ
Ø9Ø24ZZ
Ø9Ø2X7Z
Ø9Ø2XJZ
Ø9Ø2XKZ
Ø9Ø2XZZ
Ø9ØKØ7Z
Ø9ØKØJZ
Ø9ØKØKZ
Ø9ØKØZZ
Ø9ØK37Z
Ø9ØK3JZ
Ø9ØK3KZ
Ø9ØK3ZZ
Ø9ØK47Z
Ø9ØK4JZ
Ø9ØK4KZ
Ø9ØK4ZZ
Ø9ØKX7Z
Ø9ØKXJZ
Ø9ØKXKZ
Ø9ØKXZZ
Ø9DMØZZ
Ø9DM3ZZ
Ø9DM4ZZ
Ø9MKXZZ
Ø9NØØZZ
Ø9NØ3ZZ
Ø9NØ4ZZ
Ø9N1ØZZ
Ø9N13ZZ
Ø9N14ZZ
Ø9N3ØZZ
Ø9N33ZZ
Ø9N34ZZ
Ø9N37ZZ
Ø9N38ZZ
Ø9N4ØZZ
Ø9N43ZZ
Ø9N44ZZ
Ø9N47ZZ
Ø9N48ZZ
Ø9QØØZZ
Ø9QØ3ZZ
Ø9QØ4ZZ
Ø9Q1ØZZ
Ø9Q13ZZ
Ø9Q14ZZ
Ø9Q2ØZZ
Ø9Q23ZZ
Ø9Q24ZZ
Ø9Q3ØZZ
Ø9Q33ZZ
Ø9Q34ZZ
Ø9Q37ZZ
Ø9Q38ZZ
Ø9Q4ØZZ
Ø9Q43ZZ
Ø9Q44ZZ
Ø9Q47ZZ
Ø9Q48ZZ
Ø9QKØZZ
Ø9QK3ZZ
Ø9QK4ZZ
Ø9QK8ZZ
Ø9QLØZZ
Ø9QL3ZZ
Ø9QL4ZZ
Ø9QL7ZZ
Ø9QL8ZZ
Ø9QMØZZ
Ø9QM3ZZ
Ø9QM4ZZ
Ø9QM8ZZ
Ø9RØØ7Z
Ø9RØØJZ
Ø9RØØKZ
Ø9RØX7Z
Ø9RØXJZ
Ø9RØXKZ
Ø9R1Ø7Z
Ø9R1ØJZ
Ø9R1ØKZ
Ø9R1X7Z
Ø9R1XJZ
Ø9R1XKZ
Ø9R2Ø7Z
Ø9R2ØJZ
Ø9R2ØKZ
Ø9R2X7Z
Ø9R2XJZ
Ø9R2XKZ
Ø9RKØ7Z
Ø9RKØJZ
Ø9RKØKZ
Ø9RKX7Z
Ø9RKXJZ
Ø9RKXKZ
Ø9RLØ7Z
Ø9RLØJZ
Ø9RLØKZ
Ø9RL37Z
Ø9RL3JZ
Ø9RL3KZ
Ø9RL47Z
Ø9RL4JZ
Ø9RL4KZ
Ø9RL77Z
Ø9RL7JZ
Ø9RL7KZ
Ø9RL87Z
Ø9RL8JZ
Ø9RL8KZ
Ø9RMØ7Z
Ø9RMØJZ
Ø9RMØKZ
Ø9RM37Z
Ø9RM3JZ
Ø9RM3KZ
Ø9RM47Z
Ø9RM4JZ
Ø9RM4KZ
Ø9SØØZZ
Ø9SØ4ZZ
Ø9SØXZZ
Ø9S1ØZZ
Ø9S14ZZ
Ø9S1XZZ
Ø9S2ØZZ
Ø9S24ZZ
Ø9S2XZZ
Ø9SKØZZ
Ø9SK4ZZ
Ø9SKXZZ
Ø9SMØZZ
Ø9SM4ZZ
Ø9TØØZZ
Ø9TØ4ZZ
Ø9TØXZZ
Ø9T1ØZZ
Ø9T14ZZ
Ø9T1XZZ
Ø9TKØZZ
Ø9TK4ZZ
Ø9TK8ZZ
Ø9TKXZZ
Ø9UØØ7Z
Ø9UØØJZ
Ø9UØØKZ
Ø9UØX7Z
Ø9UØXJZ
Ø9UØXKZ
Ø9U1Ø7Z
Ø9U1ØJZ
Ø9U1ØKZ
Ø9U1X7Z
Ø9U1XJZ
Ø9U1XKZ
Ø9U2Ø7Z
Ø9U2ØJZ
Ø9U2ØKZ
Ø9U2X7Z
Ø9U2XJZ
Ø9U2XKZ
Ø9UKØ7Z
Ø9UKØJZ
Ø9UKØKZ
Ø9UK87Z
Ø9UK8JZ
Ø9UK8KZ
Ø9UKX7Z
Ø9UKXJZ
Ø9UKXKZ
Ø9ULØ7Z
Ø9ULØJZ
Ø9ULØKZ
Ø9UL37Z
Ø9UL3JZ
Ø9UL3KZ
Ø9UL47Z
Ø9UL4JZ
Ø9UL4KZ
Ø9UL77Z
Ø9UL7JZ
Ø9UL7KZ
Ø9UL87Z
Ø9UL8JZ
Ø9UL8KZ
Ø9UMØ7Z
Ø9UMØJZ
Ø9UMØKZ
Ø9UM37Z
Ø9UM3JZ
Ø9UM3KZ
Ø9UM47Z
Ø9UM4JZ
Ø9UM4KZ
Ø9UM87Z
Ø9UM8JZ
Ø9UM8KZ
ØBQ1ØZZ
ØBQ13ZZ
ØBQ14ZZ
ØBQ17ZZ
ØBQ18ZZ
ØBR1Ø7Z
ØBR1ØJZ
ØBR1ØKZ
ØBR147Z
ØBR14JZ
ØBR14KZ
ØBW1ØFZ
ØBW13FZ
ØBW14FZ
ØCØØX7Z
ØCØØXJZ
ØCØØXKZ
ØCØØXZZ
ØCØ1X7Z
ØCØ1XJZ
ØCØ1XKZ
ØCØ1XZZ
ØC5ØØZZ
ØC5Ø3ZZ
ØC5ØXZZ
ØC51ØZZ
ØC513ZZ
ØC51XZZ
ØC9ØØØZ
ØC9ØØZZ
ØC9ØXØZ
ØC9ØXZZ
ØC91ØØZ
ØC91ØZZ
ØC91XØZ
ØC91XZZ
ØC94ØØZ
ØC94ØZZ
ØC94XØZ
ØC94XZZ
ØCBØØZZ
ØCBØ3ZZ
ØCBØXZZ
ØCB1ØZZ
ØCB13ZZ
ØCB1XZZ
ØCCØØZZ
ØCCØ3ZZ
ØCC1ØZZ
ØCC13ZZ
ØCC4ØZZ
ØCC43ZZ
ØCMØØZZ
ØCM1ØZZ
ØCM3ØZZ
ØCN2ØZZ
ØCN23ZZ
ØCN2XZZ
ØCN3ØZZ
ØCN33ZZ
ØCN3XZZ
ØCN4ØZZ
ØCN43ZZ
ØCPYØØZ
ØCPYØ1Z
ØCPYØ7Z
ØCPYØDZ
ØCPYØJZ
ØCPYØKZ
ØCPYØYZ
ØCPY3ØZ
ØCPY31Z
ØCPY37Z
ØCPY3DZ
ØCPY3JZ
ØCPY3KZ
ØCQØØZZ
ØCQØ3ZZ
ØCQ1ØZZ
ØCQ13ZZ
ØCQ2ØZZ
ØCQ23ZZ
ØCQ2XZZ
ØCQ3ØZZ
ØCQ33ZZ
ØCQ3XZZ
ØCQ4ØZZ
ØCQ43ZZ
ØCQMØZZ
ØCQM3ZZ
ØCQM4ZZ
ØCQM7ZZ
ØCQM8ZZ
ØCRØØ7Z
ØCRØØJZ
ØCRØØKZ
ØCRØ37Z
ØCRØ3JZ
ØCRØ3KZ
ØCRØX7Z
ØCRØXJZ
ØCRØXKZ
ØCR1Ø7Z
ØCR1ØJZ
ØCR1ØKZ
ØCR137Z
ØCR13JZ
ØCR13KZ
ØCR1X7Z
ØCR1XJZ
ØCR1XKZ
ØCR2Ø7Z
ØCR2ØJZ
ØCR2ØKZ
ØCR237Z
ØCR23JZ
ØCR23KZ
ØCR2X7Z
ØCR2XJZ
ØCR2XKZ
ØCR3Ø7Z
ØCR3ØJZ
ØCR3ØKZ
ØCR337Z
ØCR33JZ
ØCR33KZ
ØCR3X7Z
ØCR3XJZ
ØCR3XKZ
ØCR4Ø7Z
ØCR4ØJZ
ØCR4ØKZ
ØCR437Z
ØCR43JZ
ØCR43KZ
ØCR4X7Z
ØCR4XJZ
ØCR4XKZ
ØCSØØZZ
ØCSØXZZ
ØCS1ØZZ
ØCS1XZZ
ØCS2ØZZ
ØCS2XZZ
ØCS3ØZZ
ØCS3XZZ
ØCUØØ7Z
ØCUØØJZ
ØCUØØKZ
ØCUØ37Z
ØCUØ3JZ
ØCUØ3KZ
ØCUØX7Z
ØCUØXJZ
ØCUØXKZ
ØCU1Ø7Z
ØCU1ØJZ
ØCU1ØKZ
ØCU137Z
ØCU13JZ
ØCU13KZ
ØCU1X7Z
ØCU1XJZ
ØCU1XKZ
ØCU2Ø7Z
ØCU2ØKZ
ØCU237Z
ØCU23KZ

ØCU2X7Z
ØCU2XKZ
ØCU307Z
ØCU30JZ
ØCU30KZ
ØCU337Z
ØCU33JZ
ØCU33KZ
ØCU3X7Z
ØCU3XJZ
ØCU3XKZ
ØCU407Z
ØCU40JZ
ØCU40KZ
ØCU437Z
ØCU43JZ
ØCU43KZ
ØCU4X7Z
ØCU4XJZ
ØCU4XKZ
ØCWYØØZ
ØCWYØ1Z
ØCWYØDZ
ØCWYØJZ
ØCWYØKZ
ØCWYØYZ
ØCWY3ØZ
ØCWY31Z
ØCWY37Z
ØCWY3DZ
ØCWY3JZ
ØCWY3KZ
ØCXØØZZ
ØCXØXZZ
ØCX1ØZZ
ØCX1XZZ
ØCX3ØZZ
ØCX3XZZ
ØCX4ØZZ
ØCX4XZZ
ØCX5ØZZ
ØCX5XZZ
ØCX6ØZZ
ØCX6XZZ
ØD5QØZ3
ØD5QØZZ
ØD5Q3Z3
ØD5Q3ZZ
ØD5Q7ZZ
ØD5QXZZ
ØD5RØZZ
ØD5R3ZZ
ØD9QØØZ
ØD9QØZZ
ØD9Q4ØZ
ØD9Q4ZZ
ØD9Q7ØZ
ØD9Q7ZZ
ØD9Q8ØZ
ØD9Q8ZZ
ØD9QXØZ
ØD9QXZZ
ØDBP3ZZ
ØDBP7ZZ
ØDBQØZZ
ØDBQ3ZZ
ØDBQ4ZZ
ØDHQØLZ
ØDHQ3LZ
ØDHQ4LZ
ØDJØØZZ
ØDJ6ØZZ
ØDJDØZZ
ØDJUØZZ
ØDJU4ZZ
ØDJVØZZ
ØDJV4ZZ
ØDJWØZZ
ØDJW4ZZ
ØDNPØZZ
ØDNP3ZZ
ØDNP4ZZ
ØDNP7ZZ
ØDNP8ZZ
ØDNRØZZ
ØDNR3ZZ
ØDNR4ZZ
ØDPQØLZ
ØDPQ3LZ
ØDPQ4LZ
ØDPQ7LZ
ØDPQ8LZ
ØDQPØZZ
ØDQP3ZZ
ØDQP4ZZ
ØDQP7ZZ
ØDQP8ZZ
ØDQQØZZ
ØDQQ3ZZ
ØDQQ4ZZ
ØDQQ7ZZ
ØDQQ8ZZ
ØDQQXZZ
ØDQRØZZ
ØDQR3ZZ
ØDQR4ZZ
ØDRRØ7Z
ØDRRØJZ
ØDRRØKZ
ØDRR47Z
ØDRR4JZ
ØDRR4KZ
ØDURØ7Z
ØDURØJZ
ØDURØKZ
ØDUR47Z
ØDUR4JZ
ØDUR4KZ
ØDVQØCZ
ØDVQØDZ
ØDVQØZZ
ØDVQ3CZ
ØDVQ3DZ
ØDVQ3ZZ
ØDVQ4CZ
ØDVQ4DZ
ØDVQ4ZZ
ØDVQ7DZ
ØDVQ7ZZ
ØDVQ8DZ
ØDVQ8ZZ
ØDVQXCZ
ØDVQXDZ
ØDVQXZZ
ØDWQØLZ
ØDWQ3LZ
ØDWQ4LZ
ØDWQ7LZ
ØDWQ8LZ
ØF9ØØZX
ØF91ØZX
ØF92ØZX
ØFBØØZX
ØFBØ4ZX
ØFB1ØZX
ØFB14ZX
ØFB2ØZX
ØFB24ZX
ØFDØ4ZX
ØFD14ZX
ØFD24ZX
ØFJØØZZ
ØFJØ4ZZ
ØFJ44ZZ
ØFJD4ZZ
ØFJG4ZZ
ØG5ØØZ3
ØG5ØØZZ
ØG5Ø3Z3
ØG5Ø3ZZ
ØG5Ø4Z3
ØG5Ø4ZZ
ØG9ØØØZ
ØG9ØØZZ
ØG9Ø4ØZ
ØG9Ø4ZZ
ØG9GØØZ
ØG9GØZZ
ØG9HØØZ
ØG9HØZZ
ØG9KØØZ
ØG9KØZZ
ØG9LØØZ
ØG9LØZZ
ØG9MØØZ
ØG9MØZZ
ØG9NØØZ
ØG9NØZZ
ØG9PØØZ
ØG9PØZZ
ØG9QØØZ
ØG9QØZZ
ØG9RØØZ
ØG9RØZZ
ØGBØØZZ
ØGBØ3ZZ
ØGBØ4ZZ
ØGCØØZZ
ØGCØ3ZZ
ØGCØ4ZZ
ØGCGØZZ
ØGCG3ZZ
ØGCG4ZZ
ØGCHØZZ
ØGCH3ZZ
ØGCH4ZZ
ØGCKØZZ
ØGCK3ZZ
ØGCK4ZZ
ØGCLØZZ
ØGCL3ZZ
ØGCL4ZZ
ØGCMØZZ
ØGCM3ZZ
ØGCM4ZZ
ØGCNØZZ
ØGCN3ZZ
ØGCN4ZZ
ØGCPØZZ
ØGCP3ZZ
ØGCP4ZZ
ØGCQØZZ
ØGCQ3ZZ
ØGCQ4ZZ
ØGCRØZZ
ØGCR3ZZ
ØGCR4ZZ
ØGHSØ1Z
ØGHSØ2Z
ØGHSØ3Z
ØGHSØYZ
ØGHS32Z
ØGHS33Z
ØGHS41Z
ØGHS42Z
ØGHS43Z
ØGJKØZZ
ØGJRØZZ
ØGJSØZZ
ØGNØØZZ
ØGNØ3ZZ
ØGNØ4ZZ
ØGPØØØZ
ØGPØ3ØZ
ØGPØ4ØZ
ØGPKØØZ
ØGPK3ØZ
ØGPK4ØZ
ØGPRØØZ
ØGPR3ØZ
ØGPR4ØZ
ØGQØØZZ
ØGQØ3ZZ
ØGQØ4ZZ
ØGTØØZZ
ØGTØ4ZZ
ØGT2ØZZ
ØGT24ZZ
ØGT3ØZZ
ØGT34ZZ
ØGT4ØZZ
ØGT44ZZ
ØGWØØØZ
ØGWØ3ØZ
ØGWØ4ØZ
ØGWKØØZ
ØGWK3ØZ
ØGWK4ØZ
ØGWRØØZ
ØGWR3ØZ
ØGWR4ØZ
ØH99XØZ
ØH99XZZ
ØHDTØZZ
ØHDUØZZ
ØHDVØZZ
ØHDYØZZ
ØHHTØ1Z
ØHHT31Z
ØHHT71Z
ØHHT81Z
ØHHUØ1Z
ØHHU31Z
ØHHU71Z
ØHHU81Z
ØHHVØ1Z
ØHHV31Z
ØHHV71Z
ØHHV81Z
ØHHWØ1Z
ØHHW31Z
ØHHW71Z
ØHHW81Z
ØHHWX1Z
ØHHXØ1Z
ØHHX31Z
ØHHX71Z
ØHHX81Z
ØHHXX1Z
ØHM1XZZ
ØHM2XZZ
ØHM3XZZ
ØHM4XZZ
ØHM5XZZ
ØHM6XZZ
ØHM7XZZ
ØHM8XZZ
ØHM9XZZ
ØHMAXZZ
ØHMBXZZ
ØHMCXZZ
ØHMDXZZ
ØHMEXZZ
ØHMFXZZ
ØHMGXZZ
ØHMHXZZ
ØHMJXZZ
ØHMKXZZ
ØHMLXZZ
ØHMMXZZ
ØHMNXZZ
ØHNØXZZ
ØHN1XZZ
ØHN2XZZ
ØHN3XZZ
ØHN4XZZ
ØHN5XZZ
ØHN6XZZ
ØHN7XZZ
ØHN8XZZ
ØHN9XZZ
ØHNAXZZ
ØHNBXZZ
ØHNCXZZ
ØHNDXZZ
ØHNEXZZ
ØHNFXZZ
ØHNGXZZ
ØHNHXZZ
ØHNJXZZ
ØHNKXZZ
ØHNLXZZ
ØHNMXZZ
ØHNNXZZ
ØHNQXZZ
ØHNRXZZ
ØHQQXZZ
ØHQRXZZ
ØHR2X72
ØHR2X73
ØHR2X74
ØHR2XJ3
ØHR2XJ4
ØHR2XJZ
ØHR2XK3
ØHR2XK4
ØHR3X72
ØHR3X73
ØHR3X74
ØHR3XJ3
ØHR3XJ4
ØHR3XJZ
ØHR3XK3
ØHR3XK4
ØHRQX7Z
ØHRQXJZ
ØHRQXKZ
ØHRRX7Z
ØHRRXJZ
ØHRRXKZ
ØHRSXJZ
ØHRSXKZ
ØHX2XZZ
ØHX3XZZ
ØJØ1ØZZ
ØJØ13ZZ
ØJØ4ØZZ
ØJØ43ZZ
ØJØ5ØZZ
ØJØ53ZZ
ØJØ6ØZZ
ØJØ63ZZ
ØJØ7ØZZ
ØJØ73ZZ
ØJØ8ØZZ
ØJØ83ZZ
ØJØ9ØZZ
ØJØ93ZZ
ØJØDØZZ
ØJØD3ZZ
ØJØFØZZ
ØJØF3ZZ
ØJØGØZZ
ØJØG3ZZ
ØJØHØZZ
ØJØH3ZZ
ØJØLØZZ
ØJØL3ZZ
ØJØMØZZ
ØJØM3ZZ
ØJØNØZZ
ØJØN3ZZ
ØJØPØZZ
ØJØP3ZZ
ØJ8ØØZZ
ØJ8Ø3ZZ
ØJ84ØZZ
ØJ843ZZ
ØJ85ØZZ
ØJ853ZZ
ØJ86ØZZ
ØJ863ZZ
ØJ87ØZZ
ØJ873ZZ
ØJ88ØZZ
ØJ883ZZ
ØJ89ØZZ
ØJ893ZZ
ØJ8BØZZ
ØJ8B3ZZ
ØJ8CØZZ
ØJ8C3ZZ
ØJ8DØZZ
ØJ8D3ZZ
ØJ8FØZZ
ØJ8F3ZZ
ØJ8GØZZ
ØJ8G3ZZ
ØJ8HØZZ
ØJ8H3ZZ
ØJ8JØZZ
ØJ8J3ZZ
ØJ8KØZZ
ØJ8K3ZZ
ØJ8LØZZ
ØJ8L3ZZ
ØJ8MØZZ
ØJ8M3ZZ
ØJ8NØZZ
ØJ8N3ZZ
ØJ8PØZZ
ØJ8P3ZZ
ØJ8QØZZ
ØJ8Q3ZZ
ØJ8RØZZ
ØJ8R3ZZ
ØJ8SØZZ
ØJ8S3ZZ
ØJ8TØZZ
ØJ8T3ZZ
ØJ8VØZZ
ØJ8V3ZZ
ØJ8WØZZ
ØJ8W3ZZ
ØJBJØZZ
ØJBJ3ZZ
ØJBKØZZ
ØJBK3ZZ
ØJCØØZZ
ØJC1ØZZ
ØJC4ØZZ
ØJC5ØZZ
ØJC6ØZZ
ØJC7ØZZ
ØJC8ØZZ
ØJC9ØZZ
ØJCBØZZ
ØJCCØZZ
ØJCDØZZ
ØJCFØZZ
ØJCGØZZ
ØJCHØZZ
ØJCJØZZ
ØJCKØZZ
ØJCLØZZ
ØJCMØZZ
ØJCNØZZ
ØJCPØZZ
ØJCQØZZ
ØJCRØZZ
ØJDØØZZ
ØJD1ØZZ
ØJD4ØZZ
ØJD5ØZZ
ØJD6ØZZ
ØJD7ØZZ
ØJD8ØZZ
ØJD9ØZZ
ØJDBØZZ
ØJDCØZZ
ØJDDØZZ
ØJDFØZZ
ØJDGØZZ
ØJDHØZZ
ØJDLØZZ
ØJDMØZZ
ØJDNØZZ
ØJDPØZZ
ØJDQØZZ
ØJDRØZZ
ØJH6Ø2Z
ØJH6ØVZ
ØJH6ØWZ
ØJH6ØYZ
ØJH632Z
ØJH63VZ
ØJH7ØVZ
ØJH7ØYZ
ØJH73VZ
ØJH8ØVZ
ØJH8ØWZ
ØJH8ØYZ
ØJH83VZ
ØJHDØVZ
ØJHDØWZ
ØJHD3VZ
ØJHFØVZ
ØJHFØWZ
ØJHF3VZ
ØJHGØVZ
ØJHGØWZ
ØJHG3VZ
ØJHHØVZ
ØJHHØWZ
ØJHH3VZ
ØJHLØVZ
ØJHLØWZ
ØJHL3VZ
ØJHMØVZ
ØJHMØWZ
ØJHM3VZ
ØJHNØVZ
ØJHNØWZ
ØJHN3VZ
ØJHPØVZ
ØJHPØWZ
ØJHP3VZ
ØJHSØ1Z
ØJHSØYZ
ØJHS31Z
ØJHTØ1Z
ØJHTØVZ
ØJHTØYZ
ØJHT31Z
ØJHT3VZ
ØJHVØ1Z
ØJHVØYZ
ØJHV31Z
ØJHWØ1Z
ØJHWØYZ
ØJHW31Z
ØJQØØZZ
ØJQ1ØZZ
ØJQ4ØZZ
ØJQ5ØZZ
ØJQ6ØZZ
ØJQ7ØZZ
ØJQ8ØZZ
ØJQ9ØZZ
ØJQBØZZ
ØJQCØZZ
ØJQDØZZ
ØJQFØZZ
ØJQGØZZ
ØJQHØZZ
ØJQJØZZ
ØJQKØZZ
ØJQLØZZ
ØJQMØZZ
ØJQNØZZ
ØJQPØZZ
ØJQQØZZ
ØJQRØZZ
ØJRØØ7Z
ØJRØØJZ
ØJRØØKZ
ØJRØ37Z
ØJRØ3JZ
ØJRØ3KZ
ØJR1Ø7Z
ØJR1ØJZ
ØJR1ØKZ
ØJR137Z
ØJR13JZ
ØJR13KZ
ØJR4Ø7Z
ØJR4ØJZ
ØJR4ØKZ
ØJR437Z
ØJR43JZ
ØJR43KZ
ØJR5Ø7Z
ØJR5ØJZ
ØJR5ØKZ
ØJR537Z
ØJR53JZ
ØJR53KZ
ØJR6Ø7Z
ØJR6ØJZ
ØJR6ØKZ
ØJR637Z
ØJR63JZ
ØJR63KZ
ØJR7Ø7Z
ØJR7ØJZ
ØJR7ØKZ
ØJR737Z
ØJR73JZ
ØJR73KZ
ØJR8Ø7Z
ØJR8ØJZ
ØJR8ØKZ
ØJR837Z
ØJR83JZ
ØJR83KZ
ØJR9Ø7Z
ØJR9ØJZ
ØJR9ØKZ
ØJR937Z
ØJR93JZ
ØJR93KZ
ØJRBØ7Z
ØJRBØJZ
ØJRBØKZ
ØJRB37Z
ØJRB3JZ
ØJRB3KZ
ØJRCØ7Z
ØJRCØJZ
ØJRCØKZ
ØJRC37Z
ØJRC3JZ
ØJRC3KZ
ØJRDØ7Z
ØJRDØJZ
ØJRDØKZ
ØJRD37Z
ØJRD3JZ
ØJRD3KZ
ØJRFØ7Z
ØJRFØJZ
ØJRFØKZ
ØJRF37Z
ØJRF3JZ
ØJRF3KZ
ØJRGØ7Z
ØJRGØJZ
ØJRGØKZ
ØJRG37Z
ØJRG3JZ
ØJRG3KZ
ØJRHØ7Z
ØJRHØJZ
ØJRHØKZ
ØJRH37Z
ØJRH3JZ
ØJRH3KZ
ØJRJØ7Z
ØJRJØJZ
ØJRJØKZ
ØJRJ37Z
ØJRJ3JZ
ØJRJ3KZ
ØJRKØ7Z
ØJRKØJZ
ØJRKØKZ
ØJRK37Z
ØJRK3JZ
ØJRK3KZ
ØJRLØ7Z
ØJRLØJZ
ØJRLØKZ
ØJRL37Z
ØJRL3JZ
ØJRL3KZ
ØJRMØ7Z
ØJRMØJZ
ØJRMØKZ
ØJRM37Z
ØJRM3JZ
ØJRM3KZ
ØJRNØ7Z
ØJRNØJZ
ØJRNØKZ
ØJRN37Z
ØJRN3JZ
ØJRN3KZ
ØJRPØ7Z
ØJRPØJZ
ØJRPØKZ
ØJRP37Z
ØJRP3JZ
ØJRP3KZ
ØJRQØ7Z
ØJRQØJZ
ØJRQØKZ
ØJRQ37Z
ØJRQ3JZ
ØJRQ3KZ
ØJRRØ7Z
ØJRRØJZ
ØJRRØKZ
ØJRR37Z
ØJRR3JZ
ØJRR3KZ
ØJUØØ7Z
ØJUØØJZ
ØJUØØKZ
ØJUØ37Z
ØJUØ3JZ
ØJUØ3KZ
ØJU1Ø7Z
ØJU1ØJZ
ØJU1ØKZ
ØJU137Z
ØJU13JZ
ØJU13KZ
ØJU4Ø7Z
ØJU4ØJZ
ØJU4ØKZ
ØJU437Z
ØJU43JZ
ØJU43KZ
ØJU5Ø7Z
ØJU5ØJZ
ØJU5ØKZ
ØJU537Z
ØJU53JZ
ØJU53KZ
ØJU6Ø7Z
ØJU6ØJZ
ØJU6ØKZ
ØJU637Z
ØJU63JZ
ØJU63KZ
ØJU7Ø7Z
ØJU7ØJZ
ØJU7ØKZ
ØJU737Z
ØJU73JZ
ØJU73KZ
ØJU8Ø7Z
ØJU8ØJZ
ØJU8ØKZ
ØJU837Z
ØJU83JZ
ØJU83KZ
ØJU9Ø7Z
ØJU9ØJZ
ØJU9ØKZ
ØJU937Z
ØJU93JZ
ØJU93KZ
ØJUBØ7Z
ØJUBØJZ
ØJUBØKZ
ØJUB37Z
ØJUB3JZ
ØJUB3KZ
ØJUCØ7Z
ØJUCØJZ
ØJUCØKZ
ØJUC37Z
ØJUC3JZ
ØJUC3KZ
ØJUDØ7Z
ØJUDØJZ
ØJUDØKZ
ØJUD37Z
ØJUD3JZ
ØJUD3KZ
ØJUFØ7Z
ØJUFØJZ
ØJUFØKZ
ØJUF37Z
ØJUF3JZ
ØJUF3KZ
ØJUGØ7Z
ØJUGØJZ
ØJUGØKZ
ØJUG37Z
ØJUG3JZ
ØJUG3KZ
ØJUHØ7Z
ØJUHØJZ
ØJUHØKZ
ØJUH37Z
ØJUH3JZ
ØJUH3KZ
ØJUJØ7Z
ØJUJØJZ
ØJUJØKZ
ØJUJ37Z
ØJUJ3JZ
ØJUJ3KZ
ØJUKØ7Z
ØJUKØJZ
ØJUKØKZ
ØJUK37Z
ØJUK3JZ
ØJUK3KZ
ØJULØ7Z
ØJULØJZ
ØJULØKZ
ØJUL37Z
ØJUL3JZ
ØJUL3KZ
ØJUMØ7Z
ØJUMØJZ
ØJUMØKZ
ØJUM37Z
ØJUM3JZ
ØJUM3KZ
ØJUNØ7Z
ØJUNØJZ
ØJUNØKZ
ØJUN37Z
ØJUN3JZ
ØJUN3KZ
ØJUPØ7Z
ØJUPØJZ
ØJUPØKZ
ØJUP37Z
ØJUP3JZ
ØJUP3KZ
ØJUQØ7Z
ØJUQØJZ
ØJUQØKZ
ØJUQ37Z
ØJUQ3JZ
ØJUQ3KZ
ØJURØ7Z
ØJURØJZ
ØJURØKZ
ØJUR37Z
ØJUR3JZ
ØJUR3KZ
ØJWTØ2Z
ØJWTØFZ
ØJWTØPZ
ØJWTØYZ
ØJWT32Z
ØJWT3FZ
ØJWT3PZ
ØJXØØZZ
ØJXØ3ZZ
ØJX1ØZZ
ØJX13ZZ
ØJX4ØZZ
ØJX43ZZ
ØJX5ØZZ
ØJX53ZZ
ØJX6ØZZ
ØJX63ZZ
ØJX7ØZZ
ØJX73ZZ
ØJX8ØZZ
ØJX83ZZ
ØJX9ØZZ
ØJX93ZZ
ØJXBØZZ
ØJXB3ZZ
ØJXCØZZ
ØJXC3ZZ
ØJXDØZZ

ØJXD3ZZ
ØJXFØZZ
ØJXF3ZZ
ØJXGØZZ
ØJXG3ZZ
ØJXHØZZ
ØJXH3ZZ
ØJXJØZZ
ØJXJ3ZZ
ØJXLØZZ
ØJXL3ZZ
ØJXMØZZ
ØJXM3ZZ
ØJXNØZZ
ØJXN3ZZ
ØJXPØZZ
ØJXP3ZZ
ØJXQØZZ
ØJXQ3ZZ
ØJXRØZZ
ØJXR3ZZ
ØK5ØØZZ
ØK5Ø3ZZ
ØK5Ø4ZZ
ØK51ØZZ
ØK513ZZ
ØK514ZZ
ØK52ØZZ
ØK523ZZ
ØK524ZZ
ØK53ØZZ
ØK533ZZ
ØK534ZZ
ØK54ØZZ
ØK543ZZ
ØK544ZZ
ØK55ØZZ
ØK553ZZ
ØK554ZZ
ØK56ØZZ
ØK563ZZ
ØK564ZZ
ØK57ØZZ
ØK573ZZ
ØK574ZZ
ØK58ØZZ
ØK583ZZ
ØK584ZZ
ØK59ØZZ
ØK593ZZ
ØK594ZZ
ØK5BØZZ
ØK5B3ZZ
ØK5B4ZZ
ØK5FØZZ
ØK5F3ZZ
ØK5F4ZZ
ØK5GØZZ
ØK5G3ZZ
ØK5G4ZZ
ØK5HØZZ
ØK5H3ZZ
ØK5H4ZZ
ØK5JØZZ
ØK5J3ZZ
ØK5J4ZZ
ØK5KØZZ
ØK5K3ZZ
ØK5K4ZZ
ØK5LØZZ
ØK5L3ZZ
ØK5L4ZZ
ØK5MØZZ
ØK5M3ZZ
ØK5M4ZZ
ØK5NØZZ
ØK5N3ZZ
ØK5N4ZZ
ØK5PØZZ
ØK5P3ZZ
ØK5P4ZZ
ØK5QØZZ
ØK5Q3ZZ
ØK5Q4ZZ
ØK5RØZZ
ØK5R3ZZ
ØK5R4ZZ
ØK5SØZZ
ØK5S3ZZ
ØK5S4ZZ
ØK5TØZZ
ØK5T3ZZ
ØK5T4ZZ
ØK5VØZZ
ØK5V3ZZ
ØK5V4ZZ
ØK5WØZZ
ØK5W3ZZ
ØK5W4ZZ
ØK9ØØØZ
ØK9ØØZX
ØK9ØØZZ
ØK9Ø4ØZ
ØK9Ø4ZZ
ØK91ØØZ
ØK91ØZX
ØK91ØZZ
ØK914ØZ
ØK914ZZ
ØK92ØØZ
ØK92ØZX
ØK92ØZZ
ØK924ØZ
ØK924ZZ
ØK93ØØZ
ØK93ØZX
ØK93ØZZ
ØK934ØZ
ØK934ZZ
ØK94ØØZ
ØK94ØZX
ØK94ØZZ
ØK944ØZ
ØK944ZZ
ØK95ØØZ
ØK95ØZX
ØK95ØZZ
ØK954ØZ
ØK954ZZ
ØK96ØØZ
ØK96ØZX
ØK96ØZZ
ØK964ØZ
ØK964ZZ
ØK97ØØZ
ØK97ØZX
ØK97ØZZ
ØK974ØZ
ØK974ZZ
ØK98ØØZ
ØK98ØZX
ØK98ØZZ
ØK984ØZ
ØK984ZZ
ØK99ØØZ
ØK99ØZX
ØK99ØZZ
ØK994ØZ
ØK994ZZ
ØK9BØØZ
ØK9BØZX
ØK9BØZZ
ØK9B4ØZ
ØK9B4ZZ
ØK9CØZX
ØK9DØZX
ØK9FØØZ
ØK9FØZX
ØK9FØZZ
ØK9F4ØZ
ØK9F4ZZ
ØK9GØØZ
ØK9GØZX
ØK9GØZZ
ØK9G4ØZ
ØK9G4ZZ
ØK9HØØZ
ØK9HØZX
ØK9HØZZ
ØK9H4ØZ
ØK9H4ZZ
ØK9JØØZ
ØK9JØZX
ØK9JØZZ
ØK9J4ØZ
ØK9J4ZZ
ØK9KØØZ
ØK9KØZX
ØK9KØZZ
ØK9K4ØZ
ØK9K4ZZ
ØK9LØØZ
ØK9LØZX
ØK9LØZZ
ØK9L4ØZ
ØK9L4ZZ
ØK9MØØZ
ØK9MØZX
ØK9MØZZ
ØK9M4ØZ
ØK9M4ZZ
ØK9NØØZ
ØK9NØZX
ØK9NØZZ
ØK9N4ØZ
ØK9N4ZZ
ØK9PØØZ
ØK9PØZX
ØK9PØZZ
ØK9P4ØZ
ØK9P4ZZ
ØK9QØØZ
ØK9QØZX
ØK9QØZZ
ØK9Q4ØZ
ØK9Q4ZZ
ØK9RØØZ
ØK9RØZX
ØK9RØZZ
ØK9R4ØZ
ØK9R4ZZ
ØK9SØØZ
ØK9SØZX
ØK9SØZZ
ØK9S4ØZ
ØK9S4ZZ
ØK9TØØZ
ØK9TØZX
ØK9TØZZ
ØK9T4ØZ
ØK9T4ZZ
ØK9VØØZ
ØK9VØZX
ØK9VØZZ
ØK9V4ØZ
ØK9V4ZZ
ØK9WØØZ
ØK9WØZX
ØK9WØZZ
ØK9W4ØZ
ØK9W4ZZ
ØKBØØZX
ØKBØØZZ
ØKBØ3ZZ
ØKBØ4ZZ
ØKB1ØZX
ØKB1ØZZ
ØKB13ZZ
ØKB14ZZ
ØKB2ØZX
ØKB2ØZZ
ØKB23ZZ
ØKB24ZZ
ØKB3ØZX
ØKB3ØZZ
ØKB33ZZ
ØKB34ZZ
ØKB4ØZX
ØKB4ØZZ
ØKB43ZZ
ØKB44ZZ
ØKB5ØZX
ØKB5ØZZ
ØKB53ZZ
ØKB54ZZ
ØKB6ØZX
ØKB6ØZZ
ØKB63ZZ
ØKB64ZZ
ØKB7ØZX
ØKB7ØZZ
ØKB73ZZ
ØKB74ZZ
ØKB8ØZX
ØKB8ØZZ
ØKB83ZZ
ØKB84ZZ
ØKB9ØZX
ØKB9ØZZ
ØKB93ZZ
ØKB94ZZ
ØKBBØZX
ØKBBØZZ
ØKBB3ZZ
ØKBB4ZZ
ØKBCØZX
ØKBDØZX
ØKBFØZX
ØKBFØZZ
ØKBF3ZZ
ØKBF4ZZ
ØKBGØZX
ØKBGØZZ
ØKBG3ZZ
ØKBG4ZZ
ØKBHØZX
ØKBHØZZ
ØKBH3ZZ
ØKBH4ZZ
ØKBJØZX
ØKBJØZZ
ØKBJ3ZZ
ØKBJ4ZZ
ØKBKØZX
ØKBKØZZ
ØKBK3ZZ
ØKBK4ZZ
ØKBLØZX
ØKBLØZZ
ØKBL3ZZ
ØKBL4ZZ
ØKBMØZX
ØKBMØZZ
ØKBM3ZZ
ØKBM4ZZ
ØKBNØZX
ØKBNØZZ
ØKBN4ZZ
ØKBPØZX
ØKBPØZZ
ØKBP4ZZ
ØKBQØZX
ØKBQØZZ
ØKBQ3ZZ
ØKBQ4ZZ
ØKBRØZX
ØKBRØZZ
ØKBR3ZZ
ØKBR4ZZ
ØKBSØZX
ØKBSØZZ
ØKBS3ZZ
ØKBS4ZZ
ØKBTØZX
ØKBTØZZ
ØKBT3ZZ
ØKBT4ZZ
ØKBVØZX
ØKBVØZZ
ØKBV3ZZ
ØKBV4ZZ
ØKBWØZX
ØKBWØZZ
ØKBW3ZZ
ØKBW4ZZ
ØKCØØZZ
ØKCØ3ZZ
ØKCØ4ZZ
ØKC1ØZZ
ØKC13ZZ
ØKC14ZZ
ØKC2ØZZ
ØKC23ZZ
ØKC24ZZ
ØKC3ØZZ
ØKC33ZZ
ØKC34ZZ
ØKC4ØZZ
ØKC43ZZ
ØKC44ZZ
ØKC5ØZZ
ØKC53ZZ
ØKC54ZZ
ØKC6ØZZ
ØKC63ZZ
ØKC64ZZ
ØKC7ØZZ
ØKC73ZZ
ØKC74ZZ
ØKC8ØZZ
ØKC83ZZ
ØKC84ZZ
ØKC9ØZZ
ØKC93ZZ
ØKC94ZZ
ØKCBØZZ
ØKCB3ZZ
ØKCB4ZZ
ØKCFØZZ
ØKCF3ZZ
ØKCF4ZZ
ØKCGØZZ
ØKCG3ZZ
ØKCG4ZZ
ØKCHØZZ
ØKCH3ZZ
ØKCH4ZZ
ØKCJØZZ
ØKCJ3ZZ
ØKCJ4ZZ
ØKCKØZZ
ØKCK3ZZ
ØKCK4ZZ
ØKCLØZZ
ØKCL3ZZ
ØKCL4ZZ
ØKCMØZZ
ØKCM3ZZ
ØKCM4ZZ
ØKCNØZZ
ØKCN3ZZ
ØKCN4ZZ
ØKCPØZZ
ØKCP3ZZ
ØKCP4ZZ
ØKCQØZZ
ØKCQ3ZZ
ØKCQ4ZZ
ØKCRØZZ
ØKCR3ZZ
ØKCR4ZZ
ØKCSØZZ
ØKCS3ZZ
ØKCS4ZZ
ØKCTØZZ
ØKCT3ZZ
ØKCT4ZZ
ØKCVØZZ
ØKCV3ZZ
ØKCV4ZZ
ØKCWØZZ
ØKCW3ZZ
ØKCW4ZZ
ØKDØØZZ
ØKD1ØZZ
ØKD2ØZZ
ØKD3ØZZ
ØKD4ØZZ
ØKD5ØZZ
ØKD6ØZZ
ØKD7ØZZ
ØKD8ØZZ
ØKD9ØZZ
ØKDBØZZ
ØKDFØZZ
ØKDGØZZ
ØKDHØZZ
ØKDJØZZ
ØKDKØZZ
ØKDLØZZ
ØKDMØZZ
ØKDNØZZ
ØKDPØZZ
ØKDQØZZ
ØKDRØZZ
ØKDSØZZ
ØKDTØZZ
ØKDVØZZ
ØKDWØZZ
ØKNCØZZ
ØKNC3ZZ
ØKNC4ZZ
ØKNDØZZ
ØKND3ZZ
ØKND4ZZ
ØKPXØØZ
ØKPXØ7Z
ØKPXØJZ
ØKPXØKZ
ØKPXØYZ
ØKPX3ØZ
ØKPX37Z
ØKPX3JZ
ØKPX3KZ
ØKPX4ØZ
ØKPX47Z
ØKPX4JZ
ØKPX4KZ
ØKPYØØZ
ØKPYØ7Z
ØKPYØJZ
ØKPYØKZ
ØKPYØYZ
ØKPY3ØZ
ØKPY37Z
ØKPY3JZ
ØKPY3KZ
ØKPY4ØZ
ØKPY47Z
ØKPY4JZ
ØKPY4KZ
ØKQØØZZ
ØKQØ3ZZ
ØKQØ4ZZ
ØKQ1ØZZ
ØKQ13ZZ
ØKQ14ZZ
ØKQ2ØZZ
ØKQ23ZZ
ØKQ24ZZ
ØKQ3ØZZ
ØKQ33ZZ
ØKQ34ZZ
ØKQ4ØZZ
ØKQ43ZZ
ØKQ44ZZ
ØKQ5ØZZ
ØKQ53ZZ
ØKQ54ZZ
ØKQ6ØZZ
ØKQ63ZZ
ØKQ64ZZ
ØKQ7ØZZ
ØKQ73ZZ
ØKQ74ZZ
ØKQ8ØZZ
ØKQ83ZZ
ØKQ84ZZ
ØKQ9ØZZ
ØKQ93ZZ
ØKQ94ZZ
ØKQBØZZ
ØKQB3ZZ
ØKQB4ZZ
ØKQFØZZ
ØKQF3ZZ
ØKQF4ZZ
ØKQGØZZ
ØKQG3ZZ
ØKQG4ZZ
ØKQHØZZ
ØKQH3ZZ
ØKQH4ZZ
ØKQJØZZ
ØKQJ3ZZ
ØKQJ4ZZ
ØKQKØZZ
ØKQK3ZZ
ØKQK4ZZ
ØKQLØZZ
ØKQL3ZZ
ØKQL4ZZ
ØKQMØZZ
ØKQM3ZZ
ØKQM4ZZ
ØKQNØZZ
ØKQN3ZZ
ØKQN4ZZ
ØKQPØZZ
ØKQP3ZZ
ØKQP4ZZ
ØKQSØZZ
ØKQS3ZZ
ØKQS4ZZ
ØKQTØZZ
ØKQT3ZZ
ØKQT4ZZ
ØKQVØZZ
ØKQV3ZZ
ØKQV4ZZ
ØKQWØZZ
ØKQW3ZZ
ØKQW4ZZ
ØKRØØ7Z
ØKRØØJZ
ØKRØØKZ
ØKRØ47Z
ØKRØ4JZ
ØKRØ4KZ
ØKR1Ø7Z
ØKR1ØJZ
ØKR1ØKZ
ØKR147Z
ØKR14JZ
ØKR14KZ
ØKR2Ø7Z
ØKR2ØJZ
ØKR2ØKZ
ØKR247Z
ØKR24JZ
ØKR24KZ
ØKR3Ø7Z
ØKR3ØJZ
ØKR3ØKZ
ØKR347Z
ØKR34JZ
ØKR34KZ
ØKR4Ø7Z
ØKR4ØJZ
ØKR4ØKZ
ØKR447Z
ØKR44JZ
ØKR44KZ
ØKR5Ø7Z
ØKR5ØJZ
ØKR5ØKZ
ØKR547Z
ØKR54JZ
ØKR54KZ
ØKR6Ø7Z
ØKR6ØJZ
ØKR6ØKZ
ØKR647Z
ØKR64JZ
ØKR64KZ
ØKR7Ø7Z
ØKR7ØJZ
ØKR7ØKZ
ØKR747Z
ØKR74JZ
ØKR74KZ
ØKR8Ø7Z
ØKR8ØJZ
ØKR8ØKZ
ØKR847Z
ØKR84JZ
ØKR84KZ
ØKR9Ø7Z
ØKR9ØJZ
ØKR9ØKZ
ØKR947Z
ØKR94JZ
ØKR94KZ
ØKRBØ7Z
ØKRBØJZ
ØKRBØKZ
ØKRB47Z
ØKRB4JZ
ØKRB4KZ
ØKRFØ7Z
ØKRFØJZ
ØKRFØKZ
ØKRF47Z
ØKRF4JZ
ØKRF4KZ
ØKRGØ7Z
ØKRGØJZ
ØKRGØKZ
ØKRG47Z
ØKRG4JZ
ØKRG4KZ
ØKRHØ7Z
ØKRHØJZ
ØKRHØKZ
ØKRH47Z
ØKRH4JZ
ØKRH4KZ
ØKRJØ7Z
ØKRJØJZ
ØKRJØKZ
ØKRJ47Z
ØKRJ4JZ
ØKRJ4KZ
ØKRKØ7Z
ØKRKØJZ
ØKRKØKZ
ØKRK47Z
ØKRK4JZ
ØKRK4KZ
ØKRLØ7Z
ØKRLØJZ
ØKRLØKZ
ØKRL47Z
ØKRL4JZ
ØKRL4KZ
ØKRMØ7Z
ØKRMØJZ
ØKRMØKZ
ØKRM47Z
ØKRM4JZ
ØKRM4KZ
ØKRNØ7Z
ØKRNØJZ
ØKRNØKZ
ØKRN47Z
ØKRN4JZ
ØKRN4KZ
ØKRPØ7Z
ØKRPØJZ
ØKRPØKZ
ØKRP47Z
ØKRP4JZ
ØKRP4KZ
ØKRSØ7Z
ØKRSØJZ
ØKRSØKZ
ØKRS47Z
ØKRS4JZ
ØKRS4KZ
ØKRTØ7Z
ØKRTØJZ
ØKRTØKZ
ØKRT47Z
ØKRT4JZ
ØKRT4KZ
ØKRVØ7Z
ØKRVØJZ
ØKRVØKZ
ØKRV47Z
ØKRV4JZ
ØKRV4KZ
ØKRWØ7Z
ØKRWØJZ
ØKRWØKZ
ØKRW47Z
ØKRW4JZ
ØKRW4KZ
ØKTØØZZ
ØKTØ4ZZ
ØKT1ØZZ
ØKT14ZZ
ØKT2ØZZ
ØKT24ZZ
ØKT3ØZZ
ØKT34ZZ
ØKT4ØZZ
ØKT44ZZ
ØKT5ØZZ
ØKT54ZZ
ØKT6ØZZ
ØKT64ZZ
ØKT7ØZZ
ØKT74ZZ
ØKT8ØZZ
ØKT84ZZ
ØKT9ØZZ
ØKT94ZZ
ØKTBØZZ
ØKTB4ZZ
ØKTFØZZ
ØKTF4ZZ
ØKTGØZZ
ØKTG4ZZ
ØKTHØZZ
ØKTH4ZZ
ØKTJØZZ
ØKTJ4ZZ
ØKTKØZZ
ØKTK4ZZ
ØKTLØZZ
ØKTL4ZZ
ØKTMØZZ
ØKTM4ZZ
ØKTNØZZ
ØKTN4ZZ
ØKTPØZZ
ØKTP4ZZ
ØKTQØZZ
ØKTQ4ZZ
ØKTRØZZ
ØKTR4ZZ
ØKTSØZZ
ØKTS4ZZ
ØKTTØZZ
ØKTT4ZZ
ØKTVØZZ
ØKTV4ZZ
ØKTWØZZ
ØKTW4ZZ
ØKUØØ7Z
ØKUØØJZ
ØKUØØKZ
ØKUØ47Z
ØKUØ4JZ
ØKUØ4KZ
ØKU1Ø7Z
ØKU1ØJZ
ØKU1ØKZ
ØKU147Z
ØKU14JZ
ØKU14KZ
ØKU2Ø7Z
ØKU2ØJZ
ØKU2ØKZ
ØKU247Z
ØKU24JZ
ØKU24KZ
ØKU3Ø7Z
ØKU3ØJZ
ØKU3ØKZ
ØKU347Z
ØKU34JZ
ØKU34KZ
ØKU4Ø7Z
ØKU4ØJZ
ØKU4ØKZ
ØKU447Z
ØKU44JZ
ØKU44KZ
ØKU5Ø7Z
ØKU5ØJZ
ØKU5ØKZ
ØKU547Z
ØKU54JZ
ØKU54KZ
ØKU6Ø7Z
ØKU6ØJZ
ØKU6ØKZ
ØKU647Z
ØKU64JZ
ØKU64KZ
ØKU7Ø7Z
ØKU7ØJZ
ØKU7ØKZ
ØKU747Z
ØKU74JZ
ØKU74KZ
ØKU8Ø7Z
ØKU8ØJZ
ØKU8ØKZ
ØKU847Z
ØKU84JZ
ØKU84KZ
ØKU9Ø7Z
ØKU9ØJZ
ØKU9ØKZ
ØKU947Z
ØKU94JZ
ØKU94KZ
ØKUBØ7Z
ØKUBØJZ
ØKUBØKZ
ØKUB47Z
ØKUB4JZ
ØKUB4KZ
ØKUCØ7Z
ØKUCØJZ
ØKUCØKZ
ØKUC47Z
ØKUC4JZ
ØKUC4KZ
ØKUDØ7Z
ØKUDØJZ
ØKUDØKZ
ØKUD47Z
ØKUD4JZ
ØKUD4KZ
ØKUFØ7Z
ØKUFØJZ
ØKUFØKZ
ØKUF47Z
ØKUF4JZ
ØKUF4KZ
ØKUGØ7Z
ØKUGØJZ
ØKUGØKZ
ØKUG47Z
ØKUG4JZ
ØKUG4KZ
ØKUHØ7Z
ØKUHØJZ
ØKUHØKZ
ØKUH47Z
ØKUH4JZ
ØKUH4KZ
ØKUJØ7Z
ØKUJØJZ
ØKUJØKZ
ØKUJ47Z
ØKUJ4JZ
ØKUJ4KZ
ØKUKØ7Z
ØKUKØJZ
ØKUKØKZ
ØKUK47Z
ØKUK4JZ
ØKUK4KZ
ØKULØ7Z
ØKULØJZ
ØKULØKZ
ØKUL47Z
ØKUL4JZ
ØKUL4KZ
ØKUMØ7Z
ØKUMØJZ

ØKUMØKZ
ØKUM47Z
ØKUM4JZ
ØKUM4KZ
ØKUNØ7Z
ØKUNØJZ
ØKUNØKZ
ØKUN47Z
ØKUN4JZ
ØKUN4KZ
ØKUPØ7Z
ØKUPØJZ
ØKUPØKZ
ØKUP47Z
ØKUP4JZ
ØKUP4KZ
ØKUQØ7Z
ØKUQØJZ
ØKUQØKZ
ØKUQ47Z
ØKUQ4JZ
ØKUQ4KZ
ØKURØ7Z
ØKURØJZ
ØKURØKZ
ØKUR47Z
ØKUR4JZ
ØKUR4KZ
ØKUSØ7Z
ØKUSØJZ
ØKUSØKZ
ØKUS47Z
ØKUS4JZ
ØKUS4KZ
ØKUTØ7Z
ØKUTØJZ
ØKUTØKZ
ØKUT47Z
ØKUT4JZ
ØKUT4KZ
ØKUVØ7Z
ØKUVØJZ
ØKUVØKZ
ØKUV47Z
ØKUV4JZ
ØKUV4KZ
ØKUWØ7Z
ØKUWØJZ
ØKUWØKZ
ØKUW47Z
ØKUW4JZ
ØKUW4KZ
ØKWXØØZ
ØKWXØ7Z
ØKWXØJZ
ØKWXØKZ
ØKWXØMZ
ØKWXØYZ
ØKWX3ØZ
ØKWX37Z
ØKWX3JZ
ØKWX3KZ
ØKWX3MZ
ØKWX4ØZ
ØKWX47Z
ØKWX4JZ
ØKWX4KZ
ØKWX4MZ
ØKWYØØZ
ØKWYØ7Z
ØKWYØJZ
ØKWYØKZ
ØKWYØMZ
ØKWYØYZ
ØKWY3ØZ
ØKWY37Z
ØKWY3JZ
ØKWY3KZ
ØKWY3MZ
ØKWY4ØZ
ØKWY47Z
ØKWY4JZ
ØKWY4KZ
ØKWY4MZ
ØL57ØZZ
ØL573ZZ
ØL574ZZ
ØL58ØZZ
ØL583ZZ
ØL584ZZ
ØL9ØØZX
ØL91ØZX
ØL92ØZX
ØL93ØZX
ØL94ØZX
ØL95ØZX
ØL96ØZX
ØL97ØZX
ØL98ØZX
ØL99ØZX
ØL9BØZX
ØL9CØZX
ØL9DØZX
ØL9FØZX
ØL9GØZX
ØL9HØZX
ØL9JØZX
ØL9KØZX
ØL9LØZX
ØL9MØZX
ØL9NØZX
ØL9PØZX
ØL9QØZX
ØL9RØZX
ØL9SØZX
ØL9TØZX
ØL9VØZX
ØL9WØZX
ØLBØØZX
ØLB1ØZX
ØLB2ØZX
ØLB3ØZX
ØLB4ØZX
ØLB5ØZX
ØLB6ØZX
ØLB7ØZX
ØLB8ØZX
ØLB9ØZX
ØLBBØZX
ØLBCØZX
ØLBDØZX
ØLBFØZX
ØLBGØZX
ØLBHØZX
ØLBJØZX
ØLBKØZX
ØLBLØZX
ØLBMØZX
ØLBNØZX
ØLBPØZX
ØLBQØZX
ØLBRØZX
ØLBSØZX
ØLBSØZZ
ØLBTØZX
ØLBTØZZ
ØLBVØZX
ØLBWØZX
ØLDØØZZ
ØLD1ØZZ
ØLD2ØZZ
ØLD3ØZZ
ØLD4ØZZ
ØLD5ØZZ
ØLD6ØZZ
ØLD9ØZZ
ØLDBØZZ
ØLDCØZZ
ØLDDØZZ
ØLDFØZZ
ØLDGØZZ
ØLDHØZZ
ØLDJØZZ
ØLDKØZZ
ØLDLØZZ
ØLDMØZZ
ØLDNØZZ
ØLDPØZZ
ØLDQØZZ
ØLDRØZZ
ØLDSØZZ
ØLDTØZZ
ØLDVØZZ
ØLDWØZZ
ØLN7ØZZ
ØLN73ZZ
ØLN74ZZ
ØLN8ØZZ
ØLN83ZZ
ØLN84ZZ
ØLQØØZZ
ØLQØ3ZZ
ØLQØ4ZZ
ØLQ3ØZZ
ØLQ33ZZ
ØLQ34ZZ
ØLQ4ØZZ
ØLQ43ZZ
ØLQ44ZZ
ØLQ5ØZZ
ØLQ53ZZ
ØLQ54ZZ
ØLQ6ØZZ
ØLQ63ZZ
ØLQ64ZZ
ØLQ7ØZZ
ØLQ73ZZ
ØLQ74ZZ
ØLQ8ØZZ
ØLQ83ZZ
ØLQ84ZZ
ØLQ9ØZZ
ØLQ93ZZ
ØLQ94ZZ
ØLQBØZZ
ØLQB3ZZ
ØLQB4ZZ
ØLQCØZZ
ØLQC3ZZ
ØLQC4ZZ
ØLQDØZZ
ØLQD3ZZ
ØLQD4ZZ
ØLQFØZZ
ØLQF3ZZ
ØLQF4ZZ
ØLQGØZZ
ØLQG3ZZ
ØLQG4ZZ
ØLQHØZZ
ØLQH3ZZ
ØLQH4ZZ
ØLQJØZZ
ØLQJ3ZZ
ØLQJ4ZZ
ØLQKØZZ
ØLQK3ZZ
ØLQK4ZZ
ØLQLØZZ
ØLQL3ZZ
ØLQL4ZZ
ØLQMØZZ
ØLQM3ZZ
ØLQM4ZZ
ØLQNØZZ
ØLQN3ZZ
ØLQN4ZZ
ØLQPØZZ
ØLQP3ZZ
ØLQP4ZZ
ØLQVØZZ
ØLQV3ZZ
ØLQV4ZZ
ØLQWØZZ
ØLQW3ZZ
ØLQW4ZZ
ØLR7Ø7Z
ØLR7ØJZ
ØLR7ØKZ
ØLR747Z
ØLR74JZ
ØLR74KZ
ØLR8Ø7Z
ØLR8ØJZ
ØLR8ØKZ
ØLR847Z
ØLR84JZ
ØLR84KZ
ØLSØØZZ
ØLSØ4ZZ
ØLS1ØZZ
ØLS14ZZ
ØLS2ØZZ
ØLS24ZZ
ØLS3ØZZ
ØLS34ZZ
ØLS4ØZZ
ØLS44ZZ
ØLS5ØZZ
ØLS54ZZ
ØLS6ØZZ
ØLS64ZZ
ØLS9ØZZ
ØLS94ZZ
ØLSBØZZ
ØLSB4ZZ
ØLSCØZZ
ØLSC4ZZ
ØLSDØZZ
ØLSD4ZZ
ØLSFØZZ
ØLSF4ZZ
ØLSGØZZ
ØLSG4ZZ
ØLSHØZZ
ØLSH4ZZ
ØLSJØZZ
ØLSJ4ZZ
ØLSKØZZ
ØLSK4ZZ
ØLSLØZZ
ØLSL4ZZ
ØLSMØZZ
ØLSM4ZZ
ØLSNØZZ
ØLSN4ZZ
ØLSPØZZ
ØLSP4ZZ
ØLSQØZZ
ØLSQ4ZZ
ØLSRØZZ
ØLSR4ZZ
ØLSSØZZ
ØLSS4ZZ
ØLSTØZZ
ØLST4ZZ
ØLSVØZZ
ØLSV4ZZ
ØLSWØZZ
ØLSW4ZZ
ØLU7Ø7Z
ØLU7ØJZ
ØLU7ØKZ
ØLU747Z
ØLU74JZ
ØLU74KZ
ØLU8Ø7Z
ØLU8ØJZ
ØLU8ØKZ
ØLU847Z
ØLU84JZ
ØLU84KZ
ØM55ØZZ
ØM553ZZ
ØM554ZZ
ØM56ØZZ
ØM563ZZ
ØM564ZZ
ØM99ØZX
ØM9BØZX
ØM9HØZX
ØM9JØZX
ØM9KØZX
ØM9VØZX
ØM9WØZX
ØMB9ØZX
ØMBHØZX
ØMBJØZX
ØMBKØZX
ØMBVØZX
ØMBWØZX
ØMN7ØZZ
ØMN73ZZ
ØMN74ZZ
ØMN8ØZZ
ØMN83ZZ
ØMN84ZZ
ØNDØØZZ
ØND1ØZZ
ØND3ØZZ
ØND4ØZZ
ØND5ØZZ
ØND6ØZZ
ØND7ØZZ
ØNDBØZZ
ØNDCØZZ
ØNDFØZZ
ØNDGØZZ
ØNDHØZZ
ØNDJØZZ
ØNDKØZZ
ØNDLØZZ
ØNDMØZZ
ØNDNØZZ
ØNDPØZZ
ØNDQØZZ
ØNDRØZZ
ØNDTØZZ
ØNDVØZZ
ØNDXØZZ
ØNNXØZZ
ØNNX3ZZ
ØNNX4ZZ
ØNQBØZZ
ØNQB3ZZ
ØNQB4ZZ
ØNRØØJZ
ØNRBØ7Z
ØNRBØJZ
ØNRBØKZ
ØNRB37Z
ØNRB3JZ
ØNRB3KZ
ØNRB47Z
ØNRB4JZ
ØNRB4KZ
ØNSBØ4Z
ØNSBØZZ
ØNUBØ7Z
ØNUBØJZ
ØNUBØKZ
ØNUB37Z
ØNUB3JZ
ØNUB3KZ
ØNUB47Z
ØNUB4JZ
ØNUB4KZ
ØNUTØ7Z
ØNUTØJZ
ØNUTØKZ
ØNUT37Z
ØNUT3JZ
ØNUT3KZ
ØNUT47Z
ØNUT4JZ
ØNUT4KZ
ØNUVØ7Z
ØNUVØJZ
ØNUVØKZ
ØNUV37Z
ØNUV3JZ
ØNUV3KZ
ØNUV47Z
ØNUV4JZ
ØNUV4KZ
ØP9ØØZX
ØP9Ø3ZX
ØP9Ø4ZX
ØP91ØZX
ØP913ZX
ØP914ZX
ØP92ØZX
ØP923ZX
ØP924ZX
ØP95ØZX
ØP953ZX
ØP954ZX
ØP96ØZX
ØP963ZX
ØP964ZX
ØP97ØZX
ØP973ZX
ØP974ZX
ØP98ØZX
ØP983ZX
ØP984ZX
ØP99ØZX
ØP993ZX
ØP994ZX
ØP9BØZX
ØP9B3ZX
ØP9B4ZX
ØP9CØZX
ØP9C3ZX
ØP9C4ZX
ØP9DØZX
ØP9D3ZX
ØP9D4ZX
ØP9FØZX
ØP9F3ZX
ØP9F4ZX
ØP9GØZX
ØP9G3ZX
ØP9G4ZX
ØP9HØZX
ØP9H3ZX
ØP9H4ZX
ØP9JØZX
ØP9J3ZX
ØP9J4ZX
ØP9KØZX
ØP9K3ZX
ØP9K4ZX
ØP9LØZX
ØP9L3ZX
ØP9L4ZX
ØP9MØZX
ØP9M3ZX
ØP9M4ZX
ØP9NØZX
ØP9N3ZX
ØP9N4ZX
ØP9PØZX
ØP9P3ZX
ØP9P4ZX
ØP9QØZX
ØP9Q3ZX
ØP9Q4ZX
ØP9RØZX
ØP9R3ZX
ØP9R4ZX
ØP9SØZX
ØP9S3ZX
ØP9S4ZX
ØP9TØZX
ØP9T3ZX
ØP9T4ZX
ØP9VØZX
ØP9V3ZX
ØP9V4ZX
ØPBØØZX
ØPBØ3ZX
ØPBØ4ZX
ØPB1ØZX
ØPB13ZX
ØPB14ZX
ØPB2ØZX
ØPB23ZX
ØPB24ZX
ØPB5ØZX
ØPB53ZX
ØPB54ZX
ØPB6ØZX
ØPB63ZX
ØPB64ZX
ØPB7ØZX
ØPB73ZX
ØPB74ZX
ØPB8ØZX
ØPB83ZX
ØPB84ZX
ØPB9ØZX
ØPB93ZX
ØPB94ZX
ØPBBØZX
ØPBB3ZX
ØPBB4ZX
ØPBCØZX
ØPBC3ZX
ØPBC4ZX
ØPBDØZX
ØPBD3ZX
ØPBD4ZX
ØPBFØZX
ØPBF3ZX
ØPBF4ZX
ØPBGØZX
ØPBG3ZX
ØPBG4ZX
ØPBHØZX
ØPBH3ZX
ØPBH4ZX
ØPBJØZX
ØPBJ3ZX
ØPBJ4ZX
ØPBKØZX
ØPBK3ZX
ØPBK4ZX
ØPBLØZX
ØPBL3ZX
ØPBL4ZX
ØPBMØZX
ØPBM3ZX
ØPBM4ZX
ØPBNØZX
ØPBN3ZX
ØPBN4ZX
ØPBPØZX
ØPBP3ZX
ØPBP4ZX
ØPBQØZX
ØPBQ3ZX
ØPBQ4ZX
ØPBRØZX
ØPBRØZZ
ØPBR3ZX
ØPBR3ZZ
ØPBR4ZX
ØPBR4ZZ
ØPBSØZX
ØPBSØZZ
ØPBS3ZX
ØPBS3ZZ
ØPBS4ZX
ØPBS4ZZ
ØPBTØZX
ØPBTØZZ
ØPBT3ZX
ØPBT3ZZ
ØPBT4ZX
ØPBT4ZZ
ØPBVØZX
ØPBVØZZ
ØPBV3ZX
ØPBV3ZZ
ØPBV4ZX
ØPBV4ZZ
ØPDØØZZ
ØPD1ØZZ
ØPD2ØZZ
ØPD3ØZZ
ØPD4ØZZ
ØPD5ØZZ
ØPD6ØZZ
ØPD7ØZZ
ØPD8ØZZ
ØPD9ØZZ
ØPDBØZZ
ØPDCØZZ
ØPDDØZZ
ØPDFØZZ
ØPDGØZZ
ØPDHØZZ
ØPDJØZZ
ØPDKØZZ
ØPDLØZZ
ØPTRØZZ
ØPTSØZZ
ØPTTØZZ
ØPTVØZZ
ØQ96ØZX
ØQ963ZX
ØQ964ZX
ØQ97ØZX
ØQ973ZX
ØQ974ZX
ØQ98ØZX
ØQ983ZX
ØQ984ZX
ØQ99ØZX
ØQ993ZX
ØQ994ZX
ØQ9BØZX
ØQ9B3ZX
ØQ9B4ZX
ØQ9CØZX
ØQ9C3ZX
ØQ9C4ZX
ØQ9DØZX
ØQ9D3ZX
ØQ9D4ZX
ØQ9FØZX
ØQ9F3ZX
ØQ9F4ZX
ØQ9GØZX
ØQ9G3ZX
ØQ9G4ZX
ØQ9HØZX
ØQ9H3ZX
ØQ9H4ZX
ØQ9JØZX
ØQ9J3ZX
ØQ9J4ZX
ØQ9KØZX
ØQ9K3ZX
ØQ9K4ZX
ØQ9LØZX
ØQ9L3ZX
ØQ9L4ZX
ØQ9MØZX
ØQ9M3ZX
ØQ9M4ZX
ØQ9NØZX
ØQ9N3ZX
ØQ9N4ZX
ØQ9PØZX
ØQ9P3ZX
ØQ9P4ZX
ØQ9QØZX
ØQ9Q3ZX
ØQ9Q4ZX
ØQ9RØZX
ØQ9R3ZX
ØQ9R4ZX
ØQB1ØZZ
ØQB2ØZZ
ØQB3ØZZ
ØQB6ØZX
ØQB63ZX
ØQB64ZX
ØQB7ØZX
ØQB73ZX
ØQB74ZX
ØQB8ØZX
ØQB83ZX
ØQB84ZX
ØQB9ØZX
ØQB93ZX
ØQB94ZX
ØQBBØZX
ØQBB3ZX
ØQBB4ZX
ØQBCØZX
ØQBC3ZX
ØQBC4ZX
ØQBDØZX
ØQBD3ZX
ØQBD4ZX
ØQBFØZX
ØQBF3ZX
ØQBF4ZX
ØQBGØZX
ØQBG3ZX
ØQBG4ZX
ØQBHØZX
ØQBH3ZX
ØQBH4ZX
ØQBJØZX
ØQBJ3ZX
ØQBJ4ZX
ØQBKØZX
ØQBK3ZX
ØQBK4ZX
ØQBLØZX
ØQBL3ZX
ØQBL4ZX
ØQBMØZX
ØQBM3ZX
ØQBM4ZX
ØQBNØZX
ØQBN3ZX
ØQBN4ZX
ØQBPØZX
ØQBP3ZX
ØQBP4ZX
ØQBQØZX
ØQBQ3ZX
ØQBQ4ZX
ØQBRØZX
ØQBR3ZX
ØQBR4ZX
ØQBSØZZ
ØQDØØZZ
ØQD1ØZZ
ØQD2ØZZ
ØQD3ØZZ
ØQD4ØZZ
ØQD5ØZZ
ØQD6ØZZ
ØQD7ØZZ
ØQD8ØZZ
ØQD9ØZZ
ØQDBØZZ
ØQDCØZZ
ØQDDØZZ
ØQDFØZZ
ØQDGØZZ
ØQDHØZZ
ØQDJØZZ
ØQDKØZZ
ØQDLØZZ
ØQDMØZZ
ØQDNØZZ
ØQDPØZZ
ØQDQØZZ
ØQDRØZZ
ØQDSØZZ
ØR5NØZZ
ØR5N3ZZ
ØR5N4ZZ
ØR5PØZZ
ØR5P3ZZ
ØR5P4ZZ
ØRTWØZZ
ØRTXØZZ
ØU5GØZZ
ØU5G3ZZ
ØU5G4ZZ
ØU5G7ZZ
ØU5G8ZZ
ØU5GXZZ
ØU5LØZZ
ØU5LXZZ
ØU5MØZZ
ØU5MXZZ
ØU9CØZX
ØU9C3ZX
ØU9C4ZX
ØU9C7ZX
ØU9C8ZX
ØU9GØZX
ØU9G3ZX
ØU9G4ZX
ØU9G7ZX
ØU9G8ZX
ØU9GXZX
ØU9JØZX
ØU9JXZX
ØU9MØØZ
ØU9MØZX
ØU9MØZZ
ØU9MXØZ
ØU9MXZX
ØU9MXZZ
ØUBCØZX
ØUBCØZZ
ØUBC3ZX
ØUBC3ZZ
ØUBC4ZX
ØUBC4ZZ
ØUBC7ZX
ØUBC7ZZ
ØUBC8ZX
ØUBC8ZZ
ØUBGØZX
ØUBGØZZ
ØUBG3ZX
ØUBG3ZZ
ØUBG4ZX
ØUBG4ZZ
ØUBG7ZX
ØUBG7ZZ
ØUBG8ZX
ØUBG8ZZ
ØUBGXZX
ØUBGXZZ
ØUBLØZZ
ØUBLXZZ
ØUBMØZX
ØUBMXZX
ØUCMØZZ
ØUJMØZZ
ØUPMØØZ
ØUPMØ7Z
ØUPMØJZ
ØUPMØKZ
ØUQG8ZZ
ØUQMØZZ
ØUTØØZZ
ØUTØ4ZZ
ØUTØ7ZZ
ØUTØ8ZZ
ØUTØFZZ
ØUT1ØZZ
ØUT14ZZ
ØUT17ZZ
ØUT18ZZ
ØUT1FZZ
ØUT2ØZZ
ØUT24ZZ
ØUT27ZZ
ØUT28ZZ
ØUT2FZZ
ØUTLØZZ
ØUTLXZZ
ØUTMØZZ
ØUTMXZZ
ØUWMØØZ
ØUWMØ7Z
ØUWMØJZ
ØUWMØKZ
ØV5SØZZ
ØV5S3ZZ
ØV5S4ZZ
ØV5SXZZ
ØV5TØZZ
ØV5T3ZZ
ØV5T4ZZ
ØV5TXZZ
ØV9SØZX
ØV9S3ZX
ØV9S4ZX
ØV9SXZX
ØV9TØZX
ØV9T3ZX
ØV9T4ZX
ØV9TXZX
ØVBSØZX
ØVBSØZZ
ØVBS3ZX
ØVBS3ZZ
ØVBS4ZX
ØVBS4ZZ
ØVBSXZX
ØVBSXZZ

ØVBTØZX
ØVBTØZZ
ØVBT3ZX
ØVBT3ZZ
ØVBT4ZX
ØVBT4ZZ
ØVBTXZX
ØVBTXZZ
ØVQSØZZ
ØVQS3ZZ
ØVQS4ZZ
ØVQTØZZ
ØVQT3ZZ
ØVQT4ZZ
ØVQTXZZ
ØVUTØ7Z
ØVUTØJZ
ØVUTØKZ
ØVUT47Z
ØVUT4JZ
ØVUT4KZ
ØVUTX7Z
ØVUTXJZ
ØVUTXKZ
ØVXTØZS
ØWØØØ7Z
ØWØØØJZ
ØWØØØKZ
ØWØØØZZ
ØWØØ37Z
ØWØØ3JZ
ØWØØ3KZ
ØWØØ3ZZ
ØWØØ47Z
ØWØØ4JZ
ØWØØ4KZ
ØWØØ4ZZ
ØWØ2Ø7Z
ØWØ2ØJZ
ØWØ2ØKZ
ØWØ2ØZZ
ØWØ237Z
ØWØ23JZ
ØWØ23KZ
ØWØ23ZZ
ØWØ247Z
ØWØ24JZ
ØWØ24KZ
ØWØ24ZZ
ØWØ6Ø7Z
ØWØ6ØJZ
ØWØ6ØKZ
ØWØ6ØZZ
ØWØ637Z
ØWØ63JZ
ØWØ63KZ
ØWØ63ZZ
ØWØ647Z
ØWØ64JZ
ØWØ64KZ
ØWØ64ZZ
ØWØ8Ø7Z
ØWØ8ØJZ
ØWØ8ØKZ
ØWØ8ØZZ
ØWØ837Z
ØWØ83JZ
ØWØ83KZ
ØWØ83ZZ
ØWØ847Z
ØWØ84JZ
ØWØ84KZ
ØWØ84ZZ
ØWØFØ7Z
ØWØFØJZ
ØWØFØKZ
ØWØFØZZ
ØWØF37Z
ØWØF3JZ
ØWØF3KZ
ØWØF3ZZ
ØWØF47Z
ØWØF4JZ
ØWØF4KZ
ØWØF4ZZ
ØWØKØ7Z
ØWØKØJZ
ØWØKØKZ
ØWØKØZZ
ØWØK37Z
ØWØK3JZ
ØWØK3KZ
ØWØK3ZZ
ØWØK47Z
ØWØK4JZ
ØWØK4KZ
ØWØK4ZZ
ØWØLØ7Z
ØWØLØJZ
ØWØLØKZ
ØWØLØZZ
ØWØL37Z
ØWØL3JZ
ØWØL3KZ
ØWØL3ZZ
ØWØL47Z
ØWØL4JZ
ØWØL4KZ
ØWØL4ZZ
ØWØMØ7Z
ØWØMØJZ
ØWØMØKZ
ØWØMØZZ
ØWØM37Z
ØWØM3JZ
ØWØM3KZ
ØWØM3ZZ
ØWØM47Z
ØWØM4JZ
ØWØM4KZ
ØWØM4ZZ
ØW38ØZZ
ØW383ZZ
ØW384ZZ
ØW3FØZZ
ØW3F3ZZ
ØW3F4ZZ
ØW3KØZZ
ØW3K3ZZ
ØW3K4ZZ
ØW3LØZZ
ØW3L3ZZ
ØW3L4ZZ
ØW92ØØZ
ØW92ØZZ
ØW924ØZ
ØW924ZZ
ØW93ØØZ
ØW93ØZZ
ØW934ØZ
ØW934ZZ
ØW94ØØZ
ØW94ØZZ
ØW944ØZ
ØW944ZZ
ØW95ØØZ
ØW95ØZZ
ØW954ØZ
ØW954ZZ
ØW96ØØZ
ØW96ØZZ
ØW964ØZ
ØW964ZZ
ØW9FØØZ
ØW9FØZX
ØW9FØZZ
ØW9F3ZX
ØW9F4ZX
ØW9HØØZ
ØW9HØZZ
ØW9H4ØZ
ØW9H4ZZ
ØW9NØØZ
ØW9NØZZ
ØW9N4ØZ
ØW9N4ZZ
ØWB6XZ2
ØWB8ØZZ
ØWB83ZZ
ØWB84ZZ
ØWB8XZZ
ØWBFØZX
ØWBFØZZ
ØWBF3ZX
ØWBF3ZZ
ØWBF4ZX
ØWBF4ZZ
ØWBFXZ2
ØWBFXZX
ØWBFXZZ
ØWBHØZZ
ØWBH3ZZ
ØWBH4ZZ
ØWBNØZX
ØWBNØZZ
ØWBN3ZX
ØWBN3ZZ
ØWBN4ZX
ØWBN4ZZ
ØWBNXZX
ØWBNXZZ
ØWC3ØZZ
ØWC33ZZ
ØWC34ZZ
ØWCJ3ZZ
ØWCJ4ZZ
ØWCP3ZZ
ØWCP4ZZ
ØWCR3ZZ
ØWCR4ZZ
ØWF3ØZZ
ØWF33ZZ
ØWF34ZZ
ØWH3Ø3Z
ØWH3ØYZ
ØWH333Z
ØWH33YZ
ØWH343Z
ØWH34YZ
ØWHNØ3Z
ØWHNØYZ
ØWHN33Z
ØWHN3YZ
ØWHN43Z
ØWHN4YZ
ØWJ6ØZZ
ØWJFØZZ
ØWJF4ZZ
ØWJGØZZ
ØWJG4ZZ
ØWJHØZZ
ØWJJØZZ
ØWJJ4ZZ
ØWJPØZZ
ØWJP4ZZ
ØWJRØZZ
ØWJR4ZZ
ØWM2ØZZ
ØWM4ØZZ
ØWM5ØZZ
ØWM6ØZZ
ØWM8ØZZ
ØWMFØZZ
ØWMKØZZ
ØWMLØZZ
ØWMMØZZ
ØWPNØØZ
ØWPNØ1Z
ØWPNØ3Z
ØWPNØ7Z
ØWPNØJZ
ØWPNØKZ
ØWPNØYZ
ØWPN3ØZ
ØWPN31Z
ØWPN33Z
ØWPN37Z
ØWPN3JZ
ØWPN3KZ
ØWPN3YZ
ØWPN4ØZ
ØWPN41Z
ØWPN43Z
ØWPN47Z
ØWPN4JZ
ØWPN4KZ
ØWPN4YZ
ØWQØØZZ
ØWQØ3ZZ
ØWQØ4ZZ
ØWQØXZZ
ØWQ2ØZZ
ØWQ23ZZ
ØWQ24ZZ
ØWQ2XZZ
ØWQ3ØZZ
ØWQ33ZZ
ØWQ34ZZ
ØWQ3XZZ
ØWQ4ØZZ
ØWQ43ZZ
ØWQ44ZZ
ØWQ4XZZ
ØWQ5ØZZ
ØWQ53ZZ
ØWQ54ZZ
ØWQ5XZZ
ØWQ6ØZZ
ØWQ63ZZ
ØWQ64ZZ
ØWQ6XZ2
ØWQ6XZZ
ØWQ8ØZZ
ØWQ83ZZ
ØWQ84ZZ
ØWQ8XZZ
ØWQF3ZZ
ØWQF4ZZ
ØWQFXZZ
ØWQKØZZ
ØWQK3ZZ
ØWQK4ZZ
ØWQKXZZ
ØWQLØZZ
ØWQL3ZZ
ØWQL4ZZ
ØWQLXZZ
ØWQMØZZ
ØWQM3ZZ
ØWQM4ZZ
ØWQMXZZ
ØWUØØJZ
ØWUØØKZ
ØWUØ4JZ
ØWUØ4KZ
ØWU2Ø7Z
ØWU2ØJZ
ØWU2ØKZ
ØWU247Z
ØWU24JZ
ØWU24KZ
ØWU4Ø7Z
ØWU447Z
ØWU5Ø7Z
ØWU547Z
ØWU6ØJZ
ØWU6ØKZ
ØWU64JZ
ØWU64KZ
ØWUKØJZ
ØWUKØKZ
ØWUK4JZ
ØWUK4KZ
ØWULØJZ
ØWULØKZ
ØWUL4JZ
ØWUL4KZ
ØWUMØJZ
ØWUMØKZ
ØWUM4JZ
ØWUM4KZ
ØWWCØGZ
ØWWC3GZ
ØWWC4GZ
ØWWNØØZ
ØWWNØ1Z
ØWWNØ3Z
ØWWNØ7Z
ØWWNØJZ
ØWWNØKZ
ØWWNØYZ
ØWWN3ØZ
ØWWN31Z
ØWWN33Z
ØWWN37Z
ØWWN3JZ
ØWWN3KZ
ØWWN3YZ
ØWWN4ØZ
ØWWN41Z
ØWWN43Z
ØWWN47Z
ØWWN4JZ
ØWWN4KZ
ØWWN4YZ
ØWY2ØZØ
ØWY2ØZ1
ØXØ2Ø7Z
ØXØ2ØJZ
ØXØ2ØKZ
ØXØ2ØZZ
ØXØ237Z
ØXØ23JZ
ØXØ23KZ
ØXØ23ZZ
ØXØ247Z
ØXØ24JZ
ØXØ24KZ
ØXØ24ZZ
ØXØ3Ø7Z
ØXØ3ØJZ
ØXØ3ØKZ
ØXØ3ØZZ
ØXØ337Z
ØXØ33JZ
ØXØ33KZ
ØXØ33ZZ
ØXØ347Z
ØXØ34JZ
ØXØ34KZ
ØXØ34ZZ
ØXØ4Ø7Z
ØXØ4ØJZ
ØXØ4ØKZ
ØXØ4ØZZ
ØXØ437Z
ØXØ43JZ
ØXØ43KZ
ØXØ43ZZ
ØXØ447Z
ØXØ44JZ
ØXØ44KZ
ØXØ44ZZ
ØXØ5Ø7Z
ØXØ5ØJZ
ØXØ5ØKZ
ØXØ5ØZZ
ØXØ537Z
ØXØ53JZ
ØXØ53KZ
ØXØ53ZZ
ØXØ547Z
ØXØ54JZ
ØXØ54KZ
ØXØ54ZZ
ØXØ6Ø7Z
ØXØ6ØJZ
ØXØ6ØKZ
ØXØ6ØZZ
ØXØ637Z
ØXØ63JZ
ØXØ63KZ
ØXØ63ZZ
ØXØ647Z
ØXØ64JZ
ØXØ64KZ
ØXØ64ZZ
ØXØ7Ø7Z
ØXØ7ØJZ
ØXØ7ØKZ
ØXØ7ØZZ
ØXØ737Z
ØXØ73JZ
ØXØ73KZ
ØXØ73ZZ
ØXØ747Z
ØXØ74JZ
ØXØ74KZ
ØXØ74ZZ
ØXØ8Ø7Z
ØXØ8ØJZ
ØXØ8ØKZ
ØXØ8ØZZ
ØXØ837Z
ØXØ83JZ
ØXØ83KZ
ØXØ83ZZ
ØXØ847Z
ØXØ84JZ
ØXØ84KZ
ØXØ84ZZ
ØXØ9Ø7Z
ØXØ9ØJZ
ØXØ9ØKZ
ØXØ9ØZZ
ØXØ937Z
ØXØ93JZ
ØXØ93KZ
ØXØ93ZZ
ØXØ947Z
ØXØ94JZ
ØXØ94KZ
ØXØ94ZZ
ØXØBØ7Z
ØXØBØJZ
ØXØBØKZ
ØXØBØZZ
ØXØB37Z
ØXØB3JZ
ØXØB3KZ
ØXØB3ZZ
ØXØB47Z
ØXØB4JZ
ØXØB4KZ
ØXØB4ZZ
ØXØCØ7Z
ØXØCØJZ
ØXØCØKZ
ØXØCØZZ
ØXØC37Z
ØXØC3JZ
ØXØC3KZ
ØXØC3ZZ
ØXØC47Z
ØXØC4JZ
ØXØC4KZ
ØXØC4ZZ
ØXØDØ7Z
ØXØDØJZ
ØXØDØKZ
ØXØDØZZ
ØXØD37Z
ØXØD3JZ
ØXØD3KZ
ØXØD3ZZ
ØXØD47Z
ØXØD4JZ
ØXØD4KZ
ØXØD4ZZ
ØXØFØ7Z
ØXØFØJZ
ØXØFØKZ
ØXØFØZZ
ØXØF37Z
ØXØF3JZ
ØXØF3KZ
ØXØF3ZZ
ØXØF47Z
ØXØF4JZ
ØXØF4KZ
ØXØF4ZZ
ØXØGØ7Z
ØXØGØJZ
ØXØGØKZ
ØXØGØZZ
ØXØG37Z
ØXØG3JZ
ØXØG3KZ
ØXØG3ZZ
ØXØG47Z
ØXØG4JZ
ØXØG4KZ
ØXØG4ZZ
ØXØHØ7Z
ØXØHØJZ
ØXØHØKZ
ØXØHØZZ
ØXØH37Z
ØXØH3JZ
ØXØH3KZ
ØXØH3ZZ
ØXØH47Z
ØXØH4JZ
ØXØH4KZ
ØXØH4ZZ
ØX32ØZZ
ØX323ZZ
ØX324ZZ
ØX33ØZZ
ØX333ZZ
ØX334ZZ
ØX34ØZZ
ØX343ZZ
ØX344ZZ
ØX35ØZZ
ØX353ZZ
ØX354ZZ
ØX36ØZZ
ØX363ZZ
ØX364ZZ
ØX37ØZZ
ØX373ZZ
ØX374ZZ
ØX38ØZZ
ØX383ZZ
ØX384ZZ
ØX39ØZZ
ØX393ZZ
ØX394ZZ
ØX3BØZZ
ØX3B3ZZ
ØX3B4ZZ
ØX3CØZZ
ØX3C3ZZ
ØX3C4ZZ
ØX3DØZZ
ØX3D3ZZ
ØX3D4ZZ
ØX3FØZZ
ØX3F3ZZ
ØX3F4ZZ
ØX3GØZZ
ØX3G3ZZ
ØX3G4ZZ
ØX3HØZZ
ØX3H3ZZ
ØX3H4ZZ
ØX3JØZZ
ØX3J3ZZ
ØX3J4ZZ
ØX3KØZZ
ØX3K3ZZ
ØX3K4ZZ
ØX6ØØZZ
ØX61ØZZ
ØX62ØZZ
ØX63ØZZ
ØX68ØZ1
ØX68ØZ2
ØX68ØZ3
ØX69ØZ1
ØX69ØZ2
ØX69ØZ3
ØX6BØZZ
ØX6CØZZ
ØX6DØZ1
ØX6DØZ2
ØX6DØZ3
ØX6FØZ1
ØX6FØZ2
ØX6FØZ3
ØX6JØZØ
ØX6JØZ4
ØX6JØZ5
ØX6JØZ6
ØX6JØZ7
ØX6JØZ8
ØX6JØZ9
ØX6JØZB
ØX6JØZC
ØX6JØZD
ØX6JØZF
ØX6KØZØ
ØX6KØZ4
ØX6KØZ5
ØX6KØZ6
ØX6KØZ7
ØX6KØZ8
ØX6KØZ9
ØX6KØZB
ØX6KØZC
ØX6KØZD
ØX6KØZF
ØX6LØZØ
ØX6LØZ1
ØX6LØZ2
ØX6LØZ3
ØX6MØZØ
ØX6MØZ1
ØX6MØZ2
ØX6MØZ3
ØX6NØZØ
ØX6NØZ1
ØX6NØZ2
ØX6NØZ3
ØX6PØZØ
ØX6PØZ1
ØX6PØZ2
ØX6PØZ3
ØX6QØZØ
ØX6QØZ1
ØX6QØZ2
ØX6QØZ3
ØX6RØZØ
ØX6RØZ1
ØX6RØZ2
ØX6RØZ3
ØX6SØZØ
ØX6SØZ1
ØX6SØZ2
ØX6SØZ3
ØX6TØZØ
ØX6TØZ1
ØX6TØZ2
ØX6TØZ3
ØX6VØZØ
ØX6VØZ1
ØX6VØZ2
ØX6VØZ3
ØX6WØZØ
ØX6WØZ1
ØX6WØZ2
ØX6WØZ3
ØXU2ØJZ
ØXU2ØKZ
ØXU24JZ
ØXU24KZ
ØXU3ØJZ
ØXU3ØKZ
ØXU34JZ
ØXU34KZ
ØXU4ØJZ
ØXU4ØKZ
ØXU44JZ
ØXU44KZ
ØXU5ØJZ
ØXU5ØKZ
ØXU54JZ
ØXU54KZ
ØXU6ØJZ
ØXU6ØKZ
ØXU64JZ
ØXU64KZ
ØXU7ØJZ
ØXU7ØKZ
ØXU74JZ
ØXU74KZ
ØXU8ØJZ
ØXU8ØKZ
ØXU84JZ
ØXU84KZ
ØXU9ØJZ
ØXU9ØKZ
ØXU94JZ
ØXU94KZ
ØXUBØJZ
ØXUBØKZ
ØXUB4JZ
ØXUB4KZ
ØXUCØJZ
ØXUCØKZ
ØXUC4JZ
ØXUC4KZ
ØXUDØJZ
ØXUDØKZ
ØXUD4JZ
ØXUD4KZ
ØXUFØJZ
ØXUFØKZ
ØXUF4JZ
ØXUF4KZ
ØXUGØJZ
ØXUGØKZ
ØXUG4JZ
ØXUG4KZ
ØXUHØJZ
ØXUHØKZ
ØXUH4JZ
ØXUH4KZ
ØXUJØJZ
ØXUJØKZ
ØXUJ4JZ
ØXUJ4KZ
ØXUKØJZ
ØXUKØKZ
ØXUK4JZ
ØXUK4KZ
ØXULØJZ
ØXULØKZ
ØXUL4JZ
ØXUL4KZ
ØXUMØJZ
ØXUMØKZ
ØXUM4JZ
ØXUM4KZ
ØXUNØJZ
ØXUNØKZ
ØXUN4JZ
ØXUN4KZ
ØXUPØJZ
ØXUPØKZ
ØXUP4JZ
ØXUP4KZ
ØXUQØJZ
ØXUQØKZ
ØXUQ4JZ
ØXUQ4KZ
ØXURØJZ
ØXURØKZ
ØXUR4JZ
ØXUR4KZ
ØXUSØJZ
ØXUSØKZ
ØXUS4JZ
ØXUS4KZ
ØXUTØJZ
ØXUTØKZ
ØXUT4JZ
ØXUT4KZ
ØXUVØJZ
ØXUVØKZ
ØXUV4JZ
ØXUV4KZ
ØXUWØJZ
ØXUWØKZ
ØXUW4JZ
ØXUW4KZ
ØYØØØ7Z
ØYØØØJZ
ØYØØØKZ
ØYØØØZZ
ØYØØ37Z
ØYØØ3JZ
ØYØØ3KZ
ØYØØ3ZZ
ØYØØ47Z
ØYØØ4JZ
ØYØØ4KZ
ØYØØ4ZZ
ØYØ1Ø7Z
ØYØ1ØJZ
ØYØ1ØKZ
ØYØ1ØZZ
ØYØ137Z
ØYØ13JZ
ØYØ13KZ
ØYØ13ZZ
ØYØ147Z
ØYØ14JZ
ØYØ14KZ
ØYØ14ZZ
ØYØ9Ø7Z
ØYØ9ØJZ
ØYØ9ØKZ
ØYØ9ØZZ
ØYØ937Z
ØYØ93JZ
ØYØ93KZ
ØYØ93ZZ
ØYØ947Z
ØYØ94JZ
ØYØ94KZ
ØYØ94ZZ
ØYØBØ7Z
ØYØBØJZ
ØYØBØKZ
ØYØBØZZ
ØYØB37Z
ØYØB3JZ
ØYØB3KZ
ØYØB3ZZ
ØYØB47Z
ØYØB4JZ
ØYØB4KZ
ØYØB4ZZ
ØYØCØ7Z
ØYØCØJZ
ØYØCØKZ
ØYØCØZZ
ØYØC37Z
ØYØC3JZ
ØYØC3KZ
ØYØC3ZZ
ØYØC47Z
ØYØC4JZ
ØYØC4KZ
ØYØC4ZZ
ØYØDØ7Z
ØYØDØJZ
ØYØDØKZ
ØYØDØZZ
ØYØD37Z
ØYØD3JZ
ØYØD3KZ
ØYØD3ZZ
ØYØD47Z
ØYØD4JZ
ØYØD4KZ
ØYØD4ZZ
ØYØFØ7Z
ØYØFØJZ
ØYØFØKZ
ØYØFØZZ
ØYØF37Z
ØYØF3JZ
ØYØF3KZ
ØYØF3ZZ
ØYØF47Z
ØYØF4JZ
ØYØF4KZ
ØYØF4ZZ
ØYØGØ7Z
ØYØGØJZ
ØYØGØKZ
ØYØGØZZ
ØYØG37Z
ØYØG3JZ
ØYØG3KZ
ØYØG3ZZ
ØYØG47Z
ØYØG4JZ
ØYØG4KZ
ØYØG4ZZ
ØYØHØ7Z
ØYØHØJZ

ØYØHØKZ
ØYØHØZZ
ØYØH37Z
ØYØH3JZ
ØYØH3KZ
ØYØH3ZZ
ØYØH47Z
ØYØH4JZ
ØYØH4KZ
ØYØH4ZZ
ØYØJØ7Z
ØYØJØJZ
ØYØJØKZ
ØYØJØZZ
ØYØJ37Z
ØYØJ3JZ
ØYØJ3KZ
ØYØJ3ZZ
ØYØJ47Z
ØYØJ4JZ
ØYØJ4KZ
ØYØJ4ZZ
ØYØKØ7Z
ØYØKØJZ
ØYØKØKZ
ØYØKØZZ
ØYØK37Z
ØYØK3JZ
ØYØK3KZ
ØYØK3ZZ
ØYØK47Z
ØYØK4JZ
ØYØK4KZ
ØYØK4ZZ
ØYØLØ7Z
ØYØLØJZ
ØYØLØKZ
ØYØLØZZ
ØYØL37Z
ØYØL3JZ
ØYØL3KZ
ØYØL3ZZ
ØYØL47Z
ØYØL4JZ
ØYØL4KZ
ØYØL4ZZ
ØY3ØØZZ
ØY3Ø3ZZ
ØY3Ø4ZZ
ØY31ØZZ
ØY313ZZ
ØY314ZZ
ØY35ØZZ
ØY353ZZ
ØY354ZZ
ØY36ØZZ
ØY363ZZ
ØY364ZZ
ØY37ØZZ
ØY373ZZ
ØY374ZZ
ØY38ØZZ
ØY383ZZ
ØY384ZZ
ØY39ØZZ
ØY393ZZ
ØY394ZZ
ØY3BØZZ
ØY3B3ZZ
ØY3B4ZZ
ØY3CØZZ
ØY3C3ZZ
ØY3C4ZZ
ØY3DØZZ
ØY3D3ZZ
ØY3D4ZZ
ØY3FØZZ
ØY3F3ZZ
ØY3F4ZZ
ØY3GØZZ
ØY3G3ZZ
ØY3G4ZZ
ØY3HØZZ
ØY3H3ZZ
ØY3H4ZZ
ØY3JØZZ
ØY3J3ZZ
ØY3J4ZZ
ØY3KØZZ
ØY3K3ZZ
ØY3K4ZZ
ØY3LØZZ
ØY3L3ZZ
ØY3L4ZZ
ØY3MØZZ
ØY3M3ZZ
ØY3M4ZZ
ØY3NØZZ
ØY3N3ZZ
ØY3N4ZZ
ØY62ØZZ
ØY63ØZZ
ØY64ØZZ
ØY67ØZZ
ØY68ØZZ
ØY6CØZ1
ØY6CØZ2
ØY6CØZ3
ØY6DØZ1
ØY6DØZ2
ØY6DØZ3
ØY6FØZZ
ØY6GØZZ
ØY6HØZ1
ØY6HØZ2
ØY6HØZ3
ØY6JØZ1
ØY6JØZ2
ØY6JØZ3
ØY6MØZØ
ØY6MØZ4
ØY6MØZ5
ØY6MØZ6
ØY6MØZ7
ØY6MØZ8
ØY6MØZ9
ØY6MØZB
ØY6MØZC
ØY6MØZD
ØY6MØZF
ØY6NØZØ
ØY6NØZ4
ØY6NØZ5
ØY6NØZ6
ØY6NØZ7
ØY6NØZ8
ØY6NØZ9
ØY6NØZB
ØY6NØZC
ØY6NØZD
ØY6NØZF
ØY6PØZØ
ØY6PØZ1
ØY6PØZ2
ØY6PØZ3
ØY6QØZØ
ØY6QØZ1
ØY6QØZ2
ØY6QØZ3
ØY6RØZØ
ØY6RØZ1
ØY6RØZ2
ØY6RØZ3
ØY6SØZØ
ØY6SØZ1
ØY6SØZ2
ØY6SØZ3
ØY6TØZØ
ØY6TØZ1
ØY6TØZ2
ØY6TØZ3
ØY6UØZØ
ØY6UØZ1
ØY6UØZ2
ØY6UØZ3
ØY6VØZØ
ØY6VØZ1
ØY6VØZ2
ØY6VØZ3
ØY6WØZØ
ØY6WØZ1
ØY6WØZ2
ØY6WØZ3
ØY6XØZØ
ØY6XØZ1
ØY6XØZ2
ØY6XØZ3
ØY6YØZØ
ØY6YØZ1
ØY6YØZ2
ØY6YØZ3
ØY95ØØZ
ØY95ØZZ
ØY954ØZ
ØY954ZZ
ØY96ØØZ
ØY96ØZZ
ØY964ØZ
ØY964ZZ
ØYB5ØZZ
ØYB53ZZ
ØYB54ZZ
ØYB6ØZZ
ØYB63ZZ
ØYB64ZZ
ØYB7ØZZ
ØYB73ZZ
ØYB74ZZ
ØYB8ØZZ
ØYB83ZZ
ØYB84ZZ
ØYJ5ØZZ
ØYJ6ØZZ
ØYJ7ØZZ
ØYJAØZZ
ØYMØØZZ
ØYM1ØZZ
ØYUØØ7Z
ØYUØØJZ
ØYUØØKZ
ØYUØ47Z
ØYUØ4JZ
ØYUØ4KZ
ØYU1Ø7Z
ØYU1ØJZ
ØYU1ØKZ
ØYU147Z
ØYU14JZ
ØYU14KZ
ØYU9Ø7Z
ØYU9ØJZ
ØYU9ØKZ
ØYU947Z
ØYU94JZ
ØYU94KZ
ØYUBØ7Z
ØYUBØJZ
ØYUBØKZ
ØYUB47Z
ØYUB4JZ
ØYUB4KZ
ØYUCØ7Z
ØYUCØJZ
ØYUCØKZ
ØYUC47Z
ØYUC4JZ
ØYUC4KZ
ØYUDØ7Z
ØYUDØJZ
ØYUDØKZ
ØYUD47Z
ØYUD4JZ
ØYUD4KZ
ØYUFØ7Z
ØYUFØJZ
ØYUFØKZ
ØYUF47Z
ØYUF4JZ
ØYUF4KZ
ØYUGØ7Z
ØYUGØJZ
ØYUGØKZ
ØYUG47Z
ØYUG4JZ
ØYUG4KZ
ØYUHØ7Z
ØYUHØJZ
ØYUHØKZ
ØYUH47Z
ØYUH4JZ
ØYUH4KZ
ØYUJØ7Z
ØYUJØJZ
ØYUJØKZ
ØYUJ47Z
ØYUJ4JZ
ØYUJ4KZ
ØYUKØ7Z
ØYUKØJZ
ØYUKØKZ
ØYUK47Z
ØYUK4JZ
ØYUK4KZ
ØYULØ7Z
ØYULØJZ
ØYULØKZ
ØYUL47Z
ØYUL4JZ
ØYUL4KZ
ØYUMØ7Z
ØYUMØJZ
ØYUMØKZ
ØYUM47Z
ØYUM4JZ
ØYUM4KZ
ØYUNØ7Z
ØYUNØJZ
ØYUNØKZ
ØYUN47Z
ØYUN4JZ
ØYUN4KZ
ØYUPØ7Z
ØYUPØJZ
ØYUPØKZ
ØYUP47Z
ØYUP4JZ
ØYUP4KZ
ØYUQØ7Z
ØYUQØJZ
ØYUQØKZ
ØYUQ47Z
ØYUQ4JZ
ØYUQ4KZ
ØYURØ7Z
ØYURØJZ
ØYURØKZ
ØYUR47Z
ØYUR4JZ
ØYUR4KZ
ØYUSØ7Z
ØYUSØJZ
ØYUSØKZ
ØYUS47Z
ØYUS4JZ
ØYUS4KZ
ØYUTØ7Z
ØYUTØJZ
ØYUTØKZ
ØYUT47Z
ØYUT4JZ
ØYUT4KZ
ØYUUØ7Z
ØYUUØJZ
ØYUUØKZ
ØYUU47Z
ØYUU4JZ
ØYUU4KZ
ØYUVØ7Z
ØYUVØJZ
ØYUVØKZ
ØYUV47Z
ØYUV4JZ
ØYUV4KZ
ØYUWØ7Z
ØYUWØJZ
ØYUWØKZ
ØYUW47Z
ØYUW4JZ
ØYUW4KZ
ØYUXØ7Z
ØYUXØJZ
ØYUXØKZ
ØYUX47Z
ØYUX4JZ
ØYUX4KZ
ØYUYØ7Z
ØYUYØJZ
ØYUYØKZ
ØYUY47Z
ØYUY4JZ
ØYUY4KZ
4AØ6Ø5Z
4AØ6ØBZ
4A16Ø5Z
4A16ØBZ
X27H385
X27H395
X27H3B5
X27H3C5
X27J385
X27J395
X27J3B5
X27J3C5
XNR8ØD9

OR

Nonoperating Room Procedures

ØH5ØXZD
ØH5ØXZZ
ØH51XZD
ØH51XZZ
ØH54XZD
ØH54XZZ
ØH55XZD
ØH55XZZ
ØH56XZD
ØH56XZZ
ØH57XZD
ØH57XZZ
ØH58XZD
ØH58XZZ
ØH59XZD
ØH59XZZ
ØH5AXZD
ØH5AXZZ
ØH5BXZD
ØH5BXZZ
ØH5CXZD
ØH5CXZZ
ØH5DXZD
ØH5DXZZ
ØH5EXZD
ØH5EXZZ
ØH5FXZD
ØH5FXZZ
ØH5GXZD
ØH5GXZZ
ØH5HXZD
ØH5HXZZ
ØH5JXZD
ØH5JXZZ
ØH5KXZD
ØH5KXZZ
ØH5LXZD
ØH5LXZZ
ØH5MXZD
ØH5MXZZ
ØH5NXZD
ØH5NXZZ
ØH5QXZZ
ØH5RXZZ
ØHB9XZZ
ØJ5ØØZZ
ØJ5Ø3ZZ
ØJ51ØZZ
ØJ513ZZ
ØJ54ØZZ
ØJ543ZZ
ØJ55ØZZ
ØJ553ZZ
ØJ56ØZZ
ØJ563ZZ
ØJ57ØZZ
ØJ573ZZ
ØJ58ØZZ
ØJ583ZZ
ØJ59ØZZ
ØJ593ZZ
ØJ5BØZZ
ØJ5B3ZZ
ØJ5CØZZ
ØJ5C3ZZ
ØJ5DØZZ
ØJ5D3ZZ
ØJ5FØZZ
ØJ5F3ZZ
ØJ5GØZZ
ØJ5G3ZZ
ØJ5HØZZ
ØJ5H3ZZ
ØJ5JØZZ
ØJ5J3ZZ
ØJ5KØZZ
ØJ5K3ZZ
ØJ5LØZZ
ØJ5L3ZZ
ØJ5MØZZ
ØJ5M3ZZ
ØJ5NØZZ
ØJ5N3ZZ
ØJ5PØZZ
ØJ5P3ZZ
ØJ5QØZZ
ØJ5Q3ZZ
ØJ5RØZZ
ØJ5R3ZZ
ØJBØ3ZZ
ØJB43ZZ
ØJB53ZZ
ØJB63ZZ
ØJB73ZZ
ØJB83ZZ
ØJB93ZZ
ØJBB3ZZ
ØJBC3ZZ
ØJBD3ZZ
ØJBF3ZZ
ØJBG3ZZ
ØJBH3ZZ
ØJBL3ZZ
ØJBM3ZZ
ØJBN3ZZ
ØJBP3ZZ
ØJBQ3ZZ
ØJBR3ZZ
ØJH6ØHZ
ØJH6ØXZ
ØJH63HZ
ØJH63WZ
ØJH63XZ
ØJH8Ø2Z
ØJH8ØHZ
ØJH8ØXZ
ØJH832Z
ØJH83HZ
ØJH83WZ
ØJH83XZ
ØJHDØXZ
ØJHD3WZ
ØJHD3XZ
ØJHFØXZ
ØJHF3WZ
ØJHF3XZ
ØJHGØXZ
ØJHG3WZ
ØJHG3XZ
ØJHHØXZ
ØJHH3WZ
ØJHH3XZ
ØJHLØXZ
ØJHL3WZ
ØJHL3XZ
ØJHMØXZ
ØJHM3WZ
ØJHM3XZ
ØJHNØXZ
ØJHN3HZ
ØJHN3WZ
ØJHN3XZ
ØJHPØHZ
ØJHPØXZ
ØJHP3HZ
ØJHP3WZ
ØJHP3XZ
ØJWSØØZ
ØJWSØ3Z
ØJWSØ7Z
ØJWSØJZ
ØJWSØKZ
ØJWSØNZ
ØJWSØYZ
ØJWS3ØZ
ØJWS33Z
ØJWS37Z
ØJWS3JZ
ØJWS3KZ
ØJWS3NZ
ØJWS3YZ
ØJWTØØZ
ØJWTØ3Z
ØJWTØ7Z
ØJWTØHZ
ØJWTØJZ
ØJWTØKZ
ØJWTØNZ
ØJWTØVZ
ØJWTØWZ
ØJWTØXZ
ØJWT3ØZ
ØJWT33Z
ØJWT37Z
ØJWT3HZ
ØJWT3JZ
ØJWT3KZ
ØJWT3NZ
ØJWT3VZ
ØJWT3WZ
ØJWT3XZ
ØJWVØØZ
ØJWVØ3Z
ØJWVØ7Z
ØJWVØHZ
ØJWVØJZ
ØJWVØKZ
ØJWVØNZ
ØJWVØVZ
ØJWVØWZ
ØJWVØXZ
ØJWVØYZ
ØJWV3ØZ
ØJWV33Z
ØJWV37Z
ØJWV3HZ
ØJWV3JZ
ØJWV3KZ
ØJWV3NZ
ØJWV3VZ
ØJWV3WZ
ØJWV3XZ
ØJWV3YZ
ØJWWØØZ
ØJWWØ3Z
ØJWWØ7Z
ØJWWØHZ
ØJWWØJZ
ØJWWØKZ
ØJWWØNZ
ØJWWØVZ
ØJWWØWZ
ØJWWØXZ
ØJWWØYZ
ØJWW3ØZ
ØJWW33Z
ØJWW37Z
ØJWW3HZ
ØJWW3JZ
ØJWW3KZ
ØJWW3NZ
ØJWW3VZ
ØJWW3WZ
ØJWW3XZ
ØJWW3YZ
ØWHØØ3Z
ØWHØØYZ
ØWHØ33Z
ØWHØ3YZ
ØWHØ43Z
ØWHØ4YZ
ØWH2Ø3Z
ØWH2ØYZ
ØWH233Z
ØWH23YZ
ØWH243Z
ØWH24YZ
ØWH4Ø3Z
ØWH4ØYZ
ØWH433Z
ØWH43YZ
ØWH443Z
ØWH44YZ
ØWH5Ø3Z
ØWH5ØYZ
ØWH533Z
ØWH53YZ
ØWH543Z
ØWH54YZ
ØWH6Ø3Z
ØWH6ØYZ
ØWH633Z
ØWH63YZ
ØWH643Z
ØWH64YZ
ØWHKØ3Z
ØWHKØYZ
ØWHK33Z
ØWHK3YZ
ØWHK43Z
ØWHK4YZ
ØWHLØ3Z
ØWHLØYZ
ØWHL33Z
ØWHL3YZ
ØWHL43Z
ØWHL4YZ
ØWHMØ3Z
ØWHMØYZ
ØWHM33Z
ØWHM3YZ
ØWHM43Z
ØWHM4YZ
ØWJØØZZ
ØWJ2ØZZ
ØWJ4ØZZ
ØWJ5ØZZ
ØWJKØZZ
ØWJLØZZ
ØWJMØZZ
ØWJM4ZZ
ØWWØØØZ
ØWWØØ1Z
ØWWØØ3Z
ØWWØØ7Z
ØWWØØJZ
ØWWØØKZ
ØWWØØYZ
ØWWØ3ØZ
ØWWØ31Z
ØWWØ33Z
ØWWØ37Z
ØWWØ3JZ
ØWWØ3KZ
ØWWØ3YZ
ØWWØ4ØZ
ØWWØ41Z
ØWWØ43Z
ØWWØ47Z
ØWWØ4JZ
ØWWØ4KZ
ØWWØ4YZ
ØWW2ØØZ
ØWW2Ø1Z
ØWW2Ø3Z
ØWW2Ø7Z
ØWW2ØJZ
ØWW2ØKZ
ØWW2ØYZ
ØWW23ØZ
ØWW231Z
ØWW233Z
ØWW237Z
ØWW23JZ
ØWW23KZ
ØWW23YZ
ØWW24ØZ
ØWW241Z
ØWW243Z
ØWW247Z
ØWW24JZ
ØWW24KZ
ØWW24YZ
ØWW4ØØZ
ØWW4Ø1Z
ØWW4Ø3Z
ØWW4Ø7Z
ØWW4ØJZ
ØWW4ØKZ
ØWW4ØYZ
ØWW43ØZ
ØWW431Z
ØWW433Z
ØWW437Z
ØWW43JZ
ØWW43KZ
ØWW43YZ
ØWW44ØZ
ØWW441Z
ØWW443Z
ØWW447Z
ØWW44JZ
ØWW44KZ
ØWW44YZ
ØWW5ØØZ
ØWW5Ø1Z
ØWW5Ø3Z
ØWW5Ø7Z
ØWW5ØJZ
ØWW5ØKZ
ØWW5ØYZ
ØWW53ØZ
ØWW531Z
ØWW533Z
ØWW537Z
ØWW53JZ
ØWW53KZ
ØWW53YZ
ØWW54ØZ
ØWW541Z
ØWW543Z
ØWW547Z
ØWW54JZ
ØWW54KZ
ØWW54YZ
ØWW6ØØZ
ØWW6Ø1Z
ØWW6Ø3Z
ØWW6Ø7Z
ØWW6ØJZ
ØWW6ØKZ
ØWW6ØYZ
ØWW63ØZ
ØWW631Z
ØWW633Z
ØWW637Z
ØWW63JZ
ØWW63KZ
ØWW63YZ
ØWW64ØZ
ØWW641Z
ØWW643Z
ØWW647Z
ØWW64JZ
ØWW64KZ
ØWW64YZ
ØWWKØØZ
ØWWKØ1Z
ØWWKØ3Z
ØWWKØ7Z
ØWWKØJZ
ØWWKØKZ
ØWWKØYZ
ØWWK3ØZ
ØWWK31Z
ØWWK33Z
ØWWK37Z
ØWWK3JZ
ØWWK3KZ
ØWWK3YZ
ØWWK4ØZ
ØWWK41Z
ØWWK43Z
ØWWK47Z
ØWWK4JZ
ØWWK4KZ
ØWWK4YZ
ØWWLØØZ
ØWWLØ1Z
ØWWLØ3Z
ØWWLØ7Z
ØWWLØJZ
ØWWLØKZ
ØWWLØYZ
ØWWL3ØZ
ØWWL31Z
ØWWL33Z
ØWWL37Z
ØWWL3JZ
ØWWL3KZ
ØWWL3YZ
ØWWL4ØZ
ØWWL41Z
ØWWL43Z
ØWWL47Z
ØWWL4JZ
ØWWL4KZ
ØWWL4YZ
ØWWMØØZ
ØWWMØ1Z
ØWWMØ3Z
ØWWMØJZ
ØWWMØYZ
ØWWM3ØZ
ØWWM31Z
ØWWM33Z
ØWWM3JZ
ØWWM3YZ
ØWWM4ØZ
ØWWM41Z
ØWWM43Z
ØWWM4JZ
ØWWM4YZ
ØXH2Ø3Z
ØXH2ØYZ
ØXH233Z
ØXH23YZ
ØXH243Z
ØXH24YZ
ØXH3Ø3Z
ØXH3ØYZ
ØXH333Z
ØXH33YZ
ØXH343Z
ØXH34YZ
ØXH4Ø3Z
ØXH4ØYZ
ØXH433Z
ØXH43YZ
ØXH443Z
ØXH44YZ
ØXH5Ø3Z
ØXH5ØYZ
ØXH533Z
ØXH53YZ
ØXH543Z
ØXH54YZ
ØXH6Ø3Z
ØXH6ØYZ
ØXH633Z
ØXH63YZ
ØXH643Z
ØXH64YZ
ØXH7Ø3Z
ØXH7ØYZ
ØXH733Z
ØXH73YZ
ØXH743Z
ØXH74YZ
ØXH8Ø3Z
ØXH8ØYZ
ØXH833Z
ØXH83YZ
ØXH843Z
ØXH84YZ
ØXH9Ø3Z
ØXH9ØYZ
ØXH933Z

ØXH93YZ
ØXH943Z
ØXH94YZ
ØXHBØ3Z
ØXHBØYZ
ØXHB33Z
ØXHB3YZ
ØXHB43Z
ØXHB4YZ
ØXHCØ3Z
ØXHCØYZ
ØXHC33Z
ØXHC3YZ
ØXHC43Z
ØXHC4YZ
ØXHDØ3Z
ØXHDØYZ
ØXHD33Z
ØXHD3YZ
ØXHD43Z
ØXHD4YZ
ØXHFØ3Z
ØXHFØYZ
ØXHF33Z
ØXHF3YZ
ØXHF43Z
ØXHF4YZ
ØXHGØ3Z
ØXHGØYZ
ØXHG33Z
ØXHG3YZ
ØXHG43Z
ØXHG4YZ
ØXHHØ3Z
ØXHHØYZ
ØXHH33Z
ØXHH3YZ
ØXHH43Z
ØXHH4YZ
ØXHJØ3Z
ØXHJØYZ
ØXHJ33Z
ØXHJ3YZ
ØXHJ43Z
ØXHJ4YZ
ØXHKØ3Z
ØXHKØYZ
ØXHK33Z
ØXHK3YZ
ØXHK43Z
ØXHK4YZ
ØXJ2ØZZ
ØXJ3ØZZ
ØXJ4ØZZ
ØXJ5ØZZ
ØXJ6ØZZ
ØXJ7ØZZ
ØXJ8ØZZ
ØXJ9ØZZ
ØXJBØZZ
ØXJCØZZ
ØXJDØZZ
ØXJFØZZ
ØXJGØZZ
ØXJHØZZ
ØXJJØZZ
ØXJKØZZ
ØXW6ØØZ
ØXW6Ø3Z
ØXW6Ø7Z
ØXW6ØJZ
ØXW6ØKZ
ØXW6ØYZ
ØXW63ØZ
ØXW633Z
ØXW637Z
ØXW63JZ
ØXW63KZ
ØXW63YZ
ØXW64ØZ
ØXW643Z
ØXW647Z
ØXW64JZ
ØXW64KZ
ØXW64YZ
ØXW7ØØZ
ØXW7Ø3Z
ØXW7Ø7Z
ØXW7ØJZ
ØXW7ØKZ
ØXW7ØYZ
ØXW73ØZ
ØXW733Z
ØXW737Z
ØXW73JZ
ØXW73KZ
ØXW73YZ
ØXW74ØZ
ØXW743Z
ØXW747Z
ØXW74JZ
ØXW74KZ
ØXW74YZ
ØYHØØ3Z
ØYHØØYZ
ØYHØ33Z
ØYHØ3YZ
ØYHØ43Z
ØYHØ4YZ
ØYH1Ø3Z
ØYH1ØYZ
ØYH133Z
ØYH13YZ
ØYH143Z
ØYH14YZ
ØYH5Ø3Z
ØYH5ØYZ
ØYH533Z
ØYH53YZ
ØYH543Z
ØYH54YZ
ØYH6Ø3Z
ØYH6ØYZ
ØYH633Z
ØYH63YZ
ØYH643Z
ØYH64YZ
ØYH7Ø3Z
ØYH7ØYZ
ØYH733Z
ØYH73YZ
ØYH743Z
ØYH74YZ
ØYH8Ø3Z
ØYH8ØYZ
ØYH833Z
ØYH83YZ
ØYH843Z
ØYH84YZ
ØYH9Ø3Z
ØYH9ØYZ
ØYH933Z
ØYH93YZ
ØYH943Z
ØYH94YZ
ØYHBØ3Z
ØYHBØYZ
ØYHB33Z
ØYHB3YZ
ØYHB43Z
ØYHB4YZ
ØYHCØ3Z
ØYHCØYZ
ØYHC33Z
ØYHC3YZ
ØYHC43Z
ØYHC4YZ
ØYHDØ3Z
ØYHDØYZ
ØYHD33Z
ØYHD3YZ
ØYHD43Z
ØYHD4YZ
ØYHFØ3Z
ØYHFØYZ
ØYHF33Z
ØYHF3YZ
ØYHF43Z
ØYHF4YZ
ØYHGØ3Z
ØYHGØYZ
ØYHG33Z
ØYHG3YZ
ØYHG43Z
ØYHG4YZ
ØYHHØ3Z
ØYHHØYZ
ØYHH33Z
ØYHH3YZ
ØYHH43Z
ØYHH4YZ
ØYHJØ3Z
ØYHJØYZ
ØYHJ33Z
ØYHJ3YZ
ØYHJ43Z
ØYHJ4YZ
ØYHKØ3Z
ØYHKØYZ
ØYHK33Z
ØYHK3YZ
ØYHK43Z
ØYHK4YZ
ØYHLØ3Z
ØYHLØYZ
ØYHL33Z
ØYHL3YZ
ØYHL43Z
ØYHL4YZ
ØYHMØ3Z
ØYHMØYZ
ØYHM33Z
ØYHM3YZ
ØYHM43Z
ØYHM4YZ
ØYHNØ3Z
ØYHNØYZ
ØYHN33Z
ØYHN3YZ
ØYHN43Z
ØYHN4YZ
ØYJØØZZ
ØYJ1ØZZ
ØYJ8ØZZ
ØYJ9ØZZ
ØYJBØZZ
ØYJCØZZ
ØYJDØZZ
ØYJEØZZ
ØYJFØZZ
ØYJGØZZ
ØYJHØZZ
ØYJJØZZ
ØYJKØZZ
ØYJLØZZ
ØYJMØZZ
ØYJNØZZ
ØYW9ØØZ
ØYW9Ø3Z
ØYW9Ø7Z
ØYW9ØJZ
ØYW9ØKZ
ØYW9ØYZ
ØYW93ØZ
ØYW933Z
ØYW937Z
ØYW93JZ
ØYW93KZ
ØYW93YZ
ØYW94ØZ
ØYW943Z
ØYW947Z
ØYW94JZ
ØYW94KZ
ØYW94YZ
ØYWBØØZ
ØYWBØ3Z
ØYWBØ7Z
ØYWBØJZ
ØYWBØKZ
ØYWBØYZ
ØYWB3ØZ
ØYWB33Z
ØYWB37Z
ØYWB3JZ
ØYWB3KZ
ØYWB3YZ
ØYWB4ØZ
ØYWB43Z
ØYWB47Z
ØYWB4JZ
ØYWB4KZ
ØYWB4YZ
XNHGØF9
XNHHØF9

DRG 580

Select operating room procedures OR nonoperating room procedures listed under DRG 579

DRG 581

Select operating room procedures OR nonoperating room procedures listed under DRG 579

DRG 582

Principal or Secondary Diagnosis

C5Ø.Ø11
C5Ø.Ø12
C5Ø.Ø19
C5Ø.Ø21
C5Ø.Ø22
C5Ø.Ø29
C5Ø.111
C5Ø.112
C5Ø.119
C5Ø.121
C5Ø.122
C5Ø.129
C5Ø.211
C5Ø.212
C5Ø.219
C5Ø.221
C5Ø.222
C5Ø.229
C5Ø.311
C5Ø.312
C5Ø.319
C5Ø.321
C5Ø.322
C5Ø.329
C5Ø.411
C5Ø.412
C5Ø.419
C5Ø.421
C5Ø.422
C5Ø.429
C5Ø.511
C5Ø.512
C5Ø.519
C5Ø.521
C5Ø.522
C5Ø.529
C5Ø.611
C5Ø.612
C5Ø.619
C5Ø.621
C5Ø.622
C5Ø.629
C5Ø.811
C5Ø.812
C5Ø.819
C5Ø.821
C5Ø.822
C5Ø.829
C5Ø.911
C5Ø.912
C5Ø.919
C5Ø.921
C5Ø.922
C5Ø.929
C79.2
C79.81
DØ5.ØØ
DØ5.Ø1
DØ5.Ø2
DØ5.1Ø
DØ5.11
DØ5.12
DØ5.8Ø
DØ5.81
DØ5.82
DØ5.9Ø
DØ5.91
DØ5.92
D48.6Ø
D48.61
D48.62
AND
Operating Room Procedures
ØHØVØJZ
ØHBTØZZ
ØHBT3ZZ
ØHBUØZZ
ØHBU3ZZ
ØHBVØZZ
ØHBV3ZZ
ØHRTØ75
ØHRTØ76
ØHRTØ77
ØHRTØ78
ØHRTØ79
ØHRTØ7Z
ØHRTØJZ
ØHRTØKZ
ØHRT3JZ
ØHRUØ75
ØHRUØ76
ØHRUØ77
ØHRUØ78
ØHRUØ79
ØHRUØ7Z
ØHRUØJZ
ØHRUØKZ
ØHRU3JZ
ØHRVØ75
ØHRVØ76
ØHRVØ77
ØHRVØ78
ØHRVØ79
ØHRVØJZ
ØHRV3JZ
ØHTTØZZ
ØHTUØZZ
ØHTVØZZ
ØKXFØZ5
ØKXFØZ7
ØKXFØZ8
ØKXFØZ9
ØKXF4Z5
ØKXF4Z7
ØKXF4Z8
ØKXF4Z9
ØKXGØZ5
ØKXGØZ7
ØKXGØZ8
ØKXGØZ9
ØKXG4Z5
ØKXG4Z7
ØKXG4Z8
ØKXG4Z9
ØKXKØZ6
ØKXK4Z6
ØKXLØZ6
ØKXL4Z6
OR
ØHTTØZZ
AND
Ø7T5ØZZ
OR
ØHTUØZZ
AND
Ø7T6ØZZ
OR
ØHTVØZZ
AND both
Ø7T5ØZZ
Ø7T6ØZZ
OR
ØHTTØZZ
AND both
Ø7T5ØZZ
ØKTHØZZ
OR
ØHTUØZZ
AND both
Ø7T6ØZZ
ØKTJØZZ
OR
ØHTVØZZ
AND all of the following
Ø7T5ØZZ
Ø7T6ØZZ
ØKTHØZZ
ØKTJØZZ
OR
ØHTTØZZ
AND all of the following
Ø7T5ØZZ
Ø7T7ØZZ
Ø7T8ØZZ
ØKTHØZZ
OR
ØHTUØZZ
AND all of the following
Ø7T6ØZZ
Ø7T7ØZZ
Ø7T9ØZZ
ØKTJØZZ
OR
ØHTVØZZ
AND all of the following
Ø7T5ØZZ
Ø7T6ØZZ
Ø7T7ØZZ
Ø7T8ØZZ
Ø7T9ØZZ
ØKTHØZZ
ØKTJØZZ

DRG 583

Select principal or secondary diagnosis AND operating room procedures or procedure combinations listed under DRG 582

DRG 584

Operating Room Procedures

ØHØTØ7Z
ØHØTØJZ
ØHØTØKZ
ØHØTØZZ
ØHØT37Z
ØHØT3KZ
ØHØT3ZZ
ØHØUØ7Z
ØHØUØJZ
ØHØUØKZ
ØHØUØZZ
ØHØU37Z
ØHØU3KZ
ØHØU3ZZ
ØHØVØ7Z
ØHØVØJZ
ØHØVØKZ
ØHØVØZZ
ØHØV37Z
ØHØV3KZ
ØHØV3ZZ
ØH5T*
ØH5U*
ØH5V*
ØH5W*
ØH5X*
ØH9TØZX
ØH9TØZZ
ØH9UØZX
ØH9UØZZ
ØH9VØZX
ØH9VØZZ
ØH9WØZX
ØH9WØZZ
ØH9XØZX
ØH9XØZZ
ØHBTØZX
ØHBTØZZ
ØHBT3ZZ
ØHBT7ZZ
ØHBT8ZZ
ØHBUØZX
ØHBUØZZ
ØHBU3ZZ
ØHBU7ZZ
ØHBU8ZZ
ØHBVØZX
ØHBVØZZ
ØHBV3ZZ
ØHBV7ZZ
ØHBV8ZZ
ØHBWØZX
ØHBWØZZ
ØHBW3ZZ
ØHBW7ZZ
ØHBW8ZZ
ØHBWXZZ
ØHBXØZX
ØHBXØZZ
ØHBX3ZZ
ØHBX7ZZ
ØHBX8ZZ
ØHBXXZZ
ØHBYØZX
ØHBYØZZ
ØHBY3ZZ
ØHBY7ZZ
ØHBY8ZZ
ØHCTØZZ
ØHCUØZZ
ØHCVØZZ
ØHCWØZZ
ØHCXØZZ
ØHHTØNZ
ØHHTØYZ
ØHHT3NZ
ØHHT7NZ
ØHHT8NZ
ØHHUØNZ
ØHHUØYZ
ØHHU3NZ
ØHHU7NZ
ØHHU8NZ
ØHHVØNZ
ØHHV3NZ
ØHHV7NZ
ØHHV8NZ
ØHHWØNZ
ØHHW3NZ
ØHHW7NZ
ØHHW8NZ
ØHHXØNZ
ØHHX3NZ
ØHHX7NZ
ØHHX8NZ
ØHMTXZZ
ØHMUXZZ
ØHMVXZZ
ØHMWXZZ
ØHMXXZZ
ØHNT*
ØHNU*
ØHNV*
ØHNW*
ØHNX*
ØHPTØJZ
ØHPTØNZ
ØHPTØYZ
ØHPT3JZ
ØHPT3NZ
ØHPUØJZ
ØHPUØNZ
ØHPUØYZ
ØHPU3JZ
ØHPU3NZ
ØHQTØZZ
ØHQT3ZZ
ØHQT7ZZ
ØHQT8ZZ
ØHQUØZZ
ØHQU3ZZ
ØHQU7ZZ
ØHQU8ZZ
ØHQVØZZ
ØHQV3ZZ
ØHQV7ZZ
ØHQV8ZZ
ØHQW*
ØHQX*
ØHQYØZZ
ØHQY3ZZ
ØHQY7ZZ
ØHQY8ZZ
ØHRTØ75
ØHRTØ76
ØHRTØ77
ØHRTØ78
ØHRTØ79
ØHRTØ7Z
ØHRTØJZ
ØHRTØKZ
ØHRT37Z
ØHRT3JZ
ØHRT3KZ
ØHRUØ75
ØHRUØ76
ØHRUØ77
ØHRUØ78
ØHRUØ79
ØHRUØ7Z
ØHRUØJZ
ØHRUØKZ
ØHRU37Z
ØHRU3JZ
ØHRU3KZ
ØHRVØ75
ØHRVØ76
ØHRVØ77
ØHRVØ78
ØHRVØ79
ØHRVØ7Z
ØHRVØJZ
ØHRVØKZ
ØHRV37Z
ØHRV3JZ
ØHRV3KZ
ØHRW*
ØHRX*
ØHSTØZZ
ØHSUØZZ
ØHSVØZZ
ØHSWXZZ
ØHSXXZZ
ØHTTØZZ
ØHTUØZZ
ØHTVØZZ
ØHTWXZZ
ØHTXXZZ
ØHTYØZZ
ØHUTØ7Z
ØHUTØJZ
ØHUTØKZ
ØHUT37Z
ØHUT3KZ
ØHUT77Z
ØHUT7JZ
ØHUT7KZ
ØHUT87Z
ØHUT8JZ
ØHUT8KZ
ØHUUØ7Z
ØHUUØJZ
ØHUUØKZ
ØHUU37Z
ØHUU3KZ
ØHUU77Z
ØHUU7JZ
ØHUU7KZ
ØHUU87Z
ØHUU8JZ
ØHUU8KZ
ØHUVØ7Z
ØHUVØJZ
ØHUVØKZ
ØHUV37Z
ØHUV3KZ
ØHUV77Z
ØHUV7JZ
ØHUV7KZ
ØHUV87Z
ØHUV8JZ
ØHUV8KZ
ØHUWØ7Z
ØHUWØJZ
ØHUWØKZ
ØHUW37Z
ØHUW3JZ
ØHUW3KZ
ØHUW77Z
ØHUW7JZ
ØHUW7KZ
ØHUW87Z
ØHUW8JZ
ØHUW8KZ
ØHUWX7Z
ØHUWXJZ
ØHUWXKZ
ØHUXØ7Z
ØHUXØJZ
ØHUXØKZ
ØHUX37Z
ØHUX3JZ
ØHUX3KZ
ØHUX77Z
ØHUX7JZ
ØHUX7KZ
ØHUX87Z
ØHUX8JZ
ØHUX8KZ
ØHUXX7Z
ØHUXXJZ
ØHUXXKZ
ØHWTØJZ
ØHWTØYZ
ØHWT3JZ
ØHWUØJZ
ØHWUØYZ
ØHWU3JZ
ØKXFØZ5
ØKXFØZ7
ØKXFØZ8
ØKXFØZ9
ØKXF4Z5
ØKXF4Z7
ØKXF4Z8
ØKXF4Z9
ØKXGØZ5
ØKXGØZ7
ØKXGØZ8
ØKXGØZ9
ØKXG4Z5
ØKXG4Z7
ØKXG4Z8
ØKXG4Z9
ØKXKØZ6
ØKXK4Z6
ØKXLØZ6
ØKXL4Z6
OR
ØHTTØZZ
AND
Ø7T5ØZZ
OR
ØHTUØZZ
AND
Ø7T6ØZZ
OR
ØHTVØZZ
AND both
Ø7T5ØZZ
Ø7T6ØZZ
OR
ØHTTØZZ
AND both
Ø7T5ØZZ
ØKTHØZZ
OR
ØHTUØZZ
AND both
Ø7T6ØZZ
ØKTJØZZ
OR
ØHTVØZZ
AND all of the following
Ø7T5ØZZ
Ø7T6ØZZ
ØKTHØZZ
ØKTJØZZ
OR
ØHTTØZZ
AND all of the following
Ø7T5ØZZ
Ø7T7ØZZ
Ø7T8ØZZ
ØKTHØZZ
OR
ØHTUØZZ
AND all of the following
Ø7T6ØZZ
Ø7T7ØZZ
Ø7T9ØZZ
ØKTJØZZ
OR
ØHTVØZZ
AND all of the following
Ø7T5ØZZ
Ø7T6ØZZ
Ø7T7ØZZ
Ø7T8ØZZ
Ø7T9ØZZ
ØKTHØZZ
ØKTJØZZ
OR
ØHRT37Z
ØHRU37Z
ØHRV37Z
AND
ØJD63ZZ
ØJD73ZZ
ØJD83ZZ
ØJD93ZZ
ØJDL3ZZ
ØJDM3ZZ

DRG 585

Select operating room procedures or procedure combinations listed under DRG 584

DRG 592

Principal Diagnosis

L89*
L97*
L98.4*

DRG 593

Select principal diagnosis listed under DRG 592

DRG 594

Select principal diagnosis listed under DRG 592

DRG 595

Principal Diagnosis

BØ2.9
C43.Ø
C43.2*
C43.3*

C43.4
C43.5*
C43.6*
C43.7*
C43.8
C43.9
C4A*
C4A.111
C4A.112
C4A.121
C4A.122
DØ3.Ø
DØ3.2*
DØ3.3*
DØ3.4
DØ3.5*
DØ3.6*
DØ3.7*
DØ3.8
DØ3.9
LØØ
L1Ø*
L12.Ø
L12.1
L12.3*
L12.8
L12.9
L13.8
L13.9
L14
L4Ø.Ø
L4Ø.2
L4Ø.3
L4Ø.4
L4Ø.8
L4Ø.9
L41*
L51*
L52
L53.Ø
L53.1
L53.2
L53.3
L93*
L94.5

DRG 596

Select principal diagnosis listed under DRG 595

DRG 597

Principal Diagnosis

C5Ø*
C79.2
C79.81
DØ5*
D48.6*

DRG 598

Select principal diagnosis listed under DRG 597

DRG 599

Select principal diagnosis listed under DRG 597

DRG 600

Principal Diagnosis

D49.3
I97.2
N6Ø*
N61*
N62
N63*
N64*
N65*
Q83*
R92*
T85.41XA
T85.42XA
T85.43XA
T85.44XA
T85.49XA
Z4Ø.Ø1

DRG 601

Select principal diagnosis listed under DRG 600

DRG 602

Principal Diagnosis

A46
B78.1
E83.2
I89.1
LØ1*
LØ2*
LØ3.Ø11
LØ3.Ø12
LØ3.Ø19
LØ3.Ø21
LØ3.Ø22
LØ3.Ø29
LØ3.Ø31
LØ3.Ø32
LØ3.Ø39
LØ3.Ø41
LØ3.Ø42
LØ3.Ø49
LØ3.111
LØ3.112
LØ3.113
LØ3.114
LØ3.115
LØ3.116
LØ3.119
LØ3.121
LØ3.122
LØ3.123
LØ3.124
LØ3.125
LØ3.126
LØ3.129
LØ3.211
LØ3.212
LØ3.213
LØ3.221
LØ3.222
LØ3.311
LØ3.312
LØ3.313
LØ3.314
LØ3.315
LØ3.316
LØ3.317
LØ3.319
LØ3.321
LØ3.322
LØ3.323
LØ3.324
LØ3.325
LØ3.326
LØ3.327
LØ3.329
LØ3.811
LØ3.818
LØ3.891
LØ3.898
LØ3.9Ø
LØ3.91
LØ5*
LØ8.Ø
LØ8.8*
LØ8.9
L88
L92.8
L98.Ø
L98.3

DRG 603

Select principal diagnosis listed under DRG 602

DRG 604

Principal Diagnosis

SØØ.ØØXA
SØØ.ØØXS
SØØ.Ø1XA
SØØ.Ø1XS
SØØ.Ø2XS
SØØ.Ø3XA
SØØ.Ø3XS
SØØ.Ø4XA
SØØ.Ø4XS
SØØ.Ø5XA
SØØ.Ø5XS
SØØ.Ø6XS
SØØ.Ø7XA
SØØ.Ø7XS
SØØ.1ØXS
SØØ.11XS
SØØ.12XS
SØØ.2Ø1S
SØØ.2Ø2S
SØØ.2Ø9S
SØØ.211S
SØØ.212S
SØØ.219S
SØØ.221S
SØØ.222S
SØØ.229S
SØØ.241S
SØØ.242S
SØØ.249S
SØØ.251S
SØØ.252S
SØØ.259S
SØØ.261S
SØØ.262S
SØØ.269S
SØØ.271S
SØØ.272S
SØØ.279S
SØØ.3ØXA
SØØ.3ØXS
SØØ.31XA
SØØ.31XS
SØØ.32XS
SØØ.33XA
SØØ.33XS
SØØ.34XA
SØØ.34XS
SØØ.35XA
SØØ.35XS
SØØ.36XS
SØØ.37XA
SØØ.37XS
SØØ.4Ø1A
SØØ.4Ø1S
SØØ.4Ø2A
SØØ.4Ø2S
SØØ.4Ø9A
SØØ.4Ø9S
SØØ.411A
SØØ.411S
SØØ.412A
SØØ.412S
SØØ.419A
SØØ.419S
SØØ.421S
SØØ.422S
SØØ.429S
SØØ.431A
SØØ.431S
SØØ.432A
SØØ.432S
SØØ.439A
SØØ.439S
SØØ.441A
SØØ.441S
SØØ.442A
SØØ.442S
SØØ.449A
SØØ.449S
SØØ.451A
SØØ.451S
SØØ.452A
SØØ.452S
SØØ.459A
SØØ.459S
SØØ.461S
SØØ.462S
SØØ.469S
SØØ.471A
SØØ.471S
SØØ.472A
SØØ.472S
SØØ.479A
SØØ.479S
SØØ.5Ø1A
SØØ.5Ø1S
SØØ.5Ø2A
SØØ.5Ø2S
SØØ.511A
SØØ.511S
SØØ.512A
SØØ.512S
SØØ.521S
SØØ.522S
SØØ.531A
SØØ.531S
SØØ.532A
SØØ.532S
SØØ.541A
SØØ.541S
SØØ.542A
SØØ.542S
SØØ.551A
SØØ.551S
SØØ.552A
SØØ.552S
SØØ.561S
SØØ.562S
SØØ.571A
SØØ.571S
SØØ.572A
SØØ.572S
SØØ.8ØXA
SØØ.8ØXS
SØØ.81XA
SØØ.81XS
SØØ.82XS
SØØ.83XA
SØØ.83XS
SØØ.84XA
SØØ.84XS
SØØ.85XA
SØØ.85XS
SØØ.86XS
SØØ.87XA
SØØ.87XS
SØØ.9ØXA
SØØ.9ØXS
SØØ.91XA
SØØ.91XS
SØØ.92XS
SØØ.93XA
SØØ.93XS
SØØ.94XA
SØØ.94XS
SØØ.95XA
SØØ.95XS
SØØ.96XS
SØØ.97XA
SØØ.97XS
SØ1.ØØXA
SØ1.ØØXS
SØ1.Ø1XA
SØ1.Ø1XS
SØ1.Ø2XA
SØ1.Ø2XS
SØ1.Ø3XA
SØ1.Ø3XS
SØ1.Ø4XA
SØ1.Ø4XS
SØ1.Ø5XA
SØ1.Ø5XS
SØ1.1Ø1S
SØ1.1Ø2S
SØ1.1Ø9S
SØ1.111S
SØ1.112S
SØ1.119S
SØ1.121S
SØ1.122S
SØ1.129S
SØ1.131S
SØ1.132S
SØ1.139S
SØ1.141S
SØ1.142S
SØ1.149S
SØ1.151S
SØ1.152S
SØ1.159S
SØ1.2ØXS
SØ1.21XS
SØ1.22XS
SØ1.23XS
SØ1.24XS
SØ1.25XS
SØ1.3Ø1S
SØ1.3Ø2S
SØ1.3Ø9S
SØ1.311S
SØ1.312S
SØ1.319S
SØ1.321S
SØ1.322S
SØ1.329S
SØ1.331S
SØ1.332S
SØ1.339S
SØ1.341S
SØ1.342S
SØ1.349S
SØ1.351S
SØ1.352S
SØ1.359S
SØ1.4Ø1A
SØ1.4Ø1S
SØ1.4Ø2A
SØ1.4Ø2S
SØ1.4Ø9A
SØ1.4Ø9S
SØ1.411A
SØ1.411S
SØ1.412A
SØ1.412S
SØ1.419A
SØ1.419S
SØ1.421A
SØ1.421S
SØ1.422A
SØ1.422S
SØ1.429A
SØ1.429S
SØ1.431A
SØ1.431S
SØ1.432A
SØ1.432S
SØ1.439A
SØ1.439S
SØ1.441A
SØ1.441S
SØ1.442A
SØ1.442S
SØ1.449A
SØ1.449S
SØ1.451A
SØ1.451S
SØ1.452A
SØ1.452S
SØ1.459A
SØ1.459S
SØ1.5Ø1S
SØ1.5Ø2S
SØ1.511S
SØ1.512S
SØ1.521S
SØ1.522S
SØ1.531S
SØ1.532S
SØ1.541S
SØ1.542S
SØ1.551S
SØ1.552S
SØ1.8ØXA
SØ1.8ØXS
SØ1.81XA
SØ1.81XS
SØ1.82XA
SØ1.82XS
SØ1.83XA
SØ1.83XS
SØ1.84XA
SØ1.84XS
SØ1.85XA
SØ1.85XS
SØ1.9ØXA
SØ1.9ØXS
SØ1.91XA
SØ1.91XS
SØ1.92XA
SØ1.92XS
SØ1.93XA
SØ1.93XS
SØ1.94XA
SØ1.94XS
SØ1.95XA
SØ1.95XS
SØ3.2XXS
SØ5.ØØXS
SØ5.Ø1XS
SØ5.Ø2XS
SØ5.1ØXS
SØ5.11XS
SØ5.12XS
SØ5.2ØXS
SØ5.21XS
SØ5.22XS
SØ5.3ØXS
SØ5.31XS
SØ5.32XS
SØ5.4ØXS
SØ5.41XS
SØ5.42XS
SØ5.5ØXS
SØ5.51XS
SØ5.52XS
SØ5.6ØXS
SØ5.61XS
SØ5.62XS
SØ7.ØXXS
SØ7.1XXS
SØ7.8XXS
SØ7.9XXS
SØ8.ØXXA
SØ8.ØXXS
SØ8.111S
SØ8.112S
SØ8.119S
SØ8.121S
SØ8.122S
SØ8.129S
SØ8.811S
SØ8.812S
SØ8.89XA
SØ8.89XS
SØ9.12XA
SØ9.12XS
SØ9.21XS
SØ9.22XS
SØ9.311S
SØ9.312S
SØ9.313S
SØ9.319S
S1Ø.ØXXA
S1Ø.ØXXS
S1Ø.1ØXA
S1Ø.1ØXS
S1Ø.11XA
S1Ø.11XS
S1Ø.12XS
S1Ø.14XA
S1Ø.14XS
S1Ø.15XA
S1Ø.15XS
S1Ø.16XS
S1Ø.17XA
S1Ø.17XS
S1Ø.8ØXA
S1Ø.8ØXS
S1Ø.81XA
S1Ø.81XS
S1Ø.82XS
S1Ø.83XA
S1Ø.83XS
S1Ø.84XA
S1Ø.84XS
S1Ø.85XA
S1Ø.85XS
S1Ø.86XS
S1Ø.87XA
S1Ø.87XS
S1Ø.9ØXA
S1Ø.9ØXS
S1Ø.91XA
S1Ø.91XS
S1Ø.92XS
S1Ø.93XA
S1Ø.93XS
S1Ø.94XA
S1Ø.94XS
S1Ø.95XA
S1Ø.95XS
S1Ø.96XS
S1Ø.97XA
S1Ø.97XS
S11.Ø11S
S11.Ø12S
S11.Ø13S
S11.Ø14S
S11.Ø15S
S11.Ø19S
S11.Ø21S
S11.Ø22S
S11.Ø23S
S11.Ø24S
S11.Ø25S
S11.Ø29S
S11.Ø31S
S11.Ø32S
S11.Ø33S
S11.Ø34S
S11.Ø35S
S11.Ø39S
S11.1ØXS
S11.11XS
S11.12XS
S11.13XS
S11.14XS
S11.15XS
S11.2ØXS
S11.21XS
S11.22XS
S11.23XS
S11.24XS
S11.25XS
S11.8ØXA
S11.8ØXS
S11.81XA
S11.81XS
S11.82XA
S11.82XS
S11.83XA
S11.83XS
S11.84XA
S11.84XS
S11.85XA
S11.85XS
S11.89XA
S11.89XS
S11.9ØXA
S11.9ØXS
S11.91XA
S11.91XS
S11.92XA
S11.92XS
S11.93XA
S11.93XS
S11.94XA
S11.94XS
S11.95XA
S11.95XS
S16.2XXA
S16.2XXS
S17.ØXXS
S17.8XXS
S17.9XXS
S2Ø.ØØXA
S2Ø.ØØXS
S2Ø.Ø1XA
S2Ø.Ø1XS
S2Ø.Ø2XA
S2Ø.Ø2XS
S2Ø.1Ø1A
S2Ø.1Ø1S
S2Ø.1Ø2A
S2Ø.1Ø2S
S2Ø.1Ø9A
S2Ø.1Ø9S
S2Ø.111A
S2Ø.111S
S2Ø.112A
S2Ø.112S
S2Ø.119A
S2Ø.119S
S2Ø.121S
S2Ø.122S
S2Ø.129S
S2Ø.141A
S2Ø.141S
S2Ø.142A
S2Ø.142S
S2Ø.149A
S2Ø.149S
S2Ø.151A
S2Ø.151S
S2Ø.152A
S2Ø.152S
S2Ø.159A
S2Ø.159S
S2Ø.161S
S2Ø.162S
S2Ø.169S
S2Ø.171A
S2Ø.171S
S2Ø.172A
S2Ø.172S
S2Ø.179A
S2Ø.179S
S2Ø.2ØXA
S2Ø.2ØXS
S2Ø.211A
S2Ø.211S
S2Ø.212A
S2Ø.212S
S2Ø.213A
S2Ø.213S
S2Ø.214A
S2Ø.214S
S2Ø.219A
S2Ø.219S
S2Ø.221A
S2Ø.221S
S2Ø.222A
S2Ø.222S
S2Ø.223A
S2Ø.223S
S2Ø.224A
S2Ø.224S
S2Ø.229A
S2Ø.229S
S2Ø.3Ø1A
S2Ø.3Ø1S
S2Ø.3Ø2A
S2Ø.3Ø2S
S2Ø.3Ø3A
S2Ø.3Ø3S
S2Ø.3Ø4A
S2Ø.3Ø4S
S2Ø.3Ø9A
S2Ø.3Ø9S
S2Ø.311A
S2Ø.311S
S2Ø.312A
S2Ø.312S
S2Ø.313A
S2Ø.313S
S2Ø.314A
S2Ø.314S
S2Ø.319A
S2Ø.319S
S2Ø.321S
S2Ø.322S
S2Ø.323S
S2Ø.324S
S2Ø.329S
S2Ø.341A
S2Ø.341S
S2Ø.342A
S2Ø.342S
S2Ø.343A
S2Ø.343S
S2Ø.344A
S2Ø.344S
S2Ø.349A
S2Ø.349S
S2Ø.351A
S2Ø.351S
S2Ø.352A
S2Ø.352S
S2Ø.353A
S2Ø.353S
S2Ø.354A
S2Ø.354S
S2Ø.359A
S2Ø.359S
S2Ø.361S
S2Ø.362S
S2Ø.363S
S2Ø.364S
S2Ø.369S
S2Ø.371A
S2Ø.371S
S2Ø.372A
S2Ø.372S
S2Ø.373A
S2Ø.373S
S2Ø.374A
S2Ø.374S
S2Ø.379A
S2Ø.379S
S2Ø.4Ø1A
S2Ø.4Ø1S
S2Ø.4Ø2A
S2Ø.4Ø2S
S2Ø.4Ø9A
S2Ø.4Ø9S
S2Ø.411A
S2Ø.411S
S2Ø.412A
S2Ø.412S
S2Ø.419A
S2Ø.419S
S2Ø.421S
S2Ø.422S
S2Ø.429S
S2Ø.441A
S2Ø.441S
S2Ø.442A
S2Ø.442S
S2Ø.449A
S2Ø.449S
S2Ø.451A
S2Ø.451S
S2Ø.452A
S2Ø.452S
S2Ø.459A
S2Ø.459S
S2Ø.461S
S2Ø.462S
S2Ø.469S
S2Ø.471A
S2Ø.471S
S2Ø.472A
S2Ø.472S
S2Ø.479A
S2Ø.479S
S2Ø.9ØXA
S2Ø.9ØXS
S2Ø.91XA
S2Ø.91XS
S2Ø.92XS
S2Ø.94XA
S2Ø.94XS
S2Ø.95XA
S2Ø.95XS
S2Ø.96XS
S2Ø.97XA
S2Ø.97XS
S21.ØØ1A
S21.ØØ1S
S21.ØØ2A
S21.ØØ2S
S21.ØØ9A
S21.ØØ9S
S21.Ø11A
S21.Ø11S
S21.Ø12A
S21.Ø12S
S21.Ø19A
S21.Ø19S
S21.Ø21A
S21.Ø21S
S21.Ø22A
S21.Ø22S
S21.Ø29A
S21.Ø29S
S21.Ø31A
S21.Ø31S
S21.Ø32A
S21.Ø32S
S21.Ø39A
S21.Ø39S
S21.Ø41A
S21.Ø41S
S21.Ø42A
S21.Ø42S
S21.Ø49A
S21.Ø49S
S21.Ø51A
S21.Ø51S
S21.Ø52A
S21.Ø52S
S21.Ø59A
S21.Ø59S
S21.1Ø1A
S21.1Ø1S
S21.1Ø2A
S21.1Ø2S
S21.1Ø9A
S21.1Ø9S
S21.111A
S21.111S
S21.112A
S21.112S
S21.119A
S21.119S
S21.121S
S21.122S
S21.129S
S21.131A
S21.131S
S21.132A
S21.132S
S21.139A
S21.139S
S21.141S
S21.142S
S21.149S
S21.151A
S21.151S
S21.152A
S21.152S
S21.159A
S21.159S
S21.2Ø1A
S21.2Ø1S
S21.2Ø2A
S21.2Ø2S
S21.2Ø9A
S21.2Ø9S
S21.211A
S21.211S
S21.212A
S21.212S
S21.219A
S21.219S
S21.221A
S21.221S
S21.222A
S21.222S
S21.229A
S21.229S
S21.231A
S21.231S
S21.232A
S21.232S
S21.239A

S21.239S
S21.241A
S21.241S
S21.242A
S21.242S
S21.249A
S21.249S
S21.251A
S21.251S
S21.252A
S21.252S
S21.259A
S21.259S
S21.301S
S21.302S
S21.309S
S21.311S
S21.312S
S21.319S
S21.321S
S21.322S
S21.329S
S21.331S
S21.332S
S21.339S
S21.341S
S21.342S
S21.349S
S21.351S
S21.352S
S21.359S
S21.401S
S21.402S
S21.409S
S21.411S
S21.412S
S21.419S
S21.421S
S21.422S
S21.429S
S21.431S
S21.432S
S21.439S
S21.441S
S21.442S
S21.449S
S21.451S
S21.452S
S21.459S
S21.90XA
S21.90XS
S21.91XA
S21.91XS
S21.92XS
S21.93XA
S21.93XS
S21.94XS
S21.95XA
S21.95XS
S28.0XXS
S28.1XXA
S28.1XXS
S28.211A
S28.211S
S28.212A
S28.212S
S28.219A
S28.219S
S28.221A
S28.221S
S28.222A
S28.222S
S28.229A
S28.229S
S29.021A
S29.021S
S29.022A
S29.022S
S29.029A
S29.029S
S30.0XXA
S30.0XXS
S30.1XXA
S30.1XXS
S30.201S
S30.202S
S30.21XS
S30.22XS
S30.23XS
S30.3XXA
S30.3XXS
S30.810A
S30.810S
S30.811A
S30.811S
S30.812A
S30.812S
S30.813A
S30.813S
S30.814A
S30.814S
S30.815A
S30.815S
S30.816A
S30.816S
S30.817A
S30.817S
S30.820S
S30.821S
S30.822S
S30.823S
S30.824S
S30.825S
S30.826S
S30.827S
S30.840A
S30.840S
S30.841A
S30.841S
S30.842A
S30.842S
S30.843A
S30.843S
S30.844A
S30.844S
S30.845A
S30.845S
S30.846A
S30.846S
S30.850A
S30.850S
S30.851A
S30.851S
S30.852A
S30.852S
S30.853A
S30.853S
S30.854A
S30.854S
S30.855A
S30.855S
S30.856A
S30.856S
S30.857A
S30.857S
S30.860S
S30.861S
S30.862S
S30.863S
S30.864S
S30.865S
S30.866S
S30.867S
S30.870A
S30.870S
S30.871A
S30.871S
S30.872A
S30.872S
S30.873A
S30.873S
S30.874A
S30.874S
S30.875A
S30.875S
S30.876A
S30.876S
S30.877A
S30.877S
S30.91XA
S30.91XS
S30.92XA
S30.92XS
S30.93XA
S30.93XS
S30.94XA
S30.94XS
S30.95XA
S30.95XS
S30.96XA
S30.96XS
S30.97XA
S30.97XS
S30.98XA
S30.98XS
S31.000A
S31.000S
S31.001S
S31.010A
S31.010S
S31.011S
S31.020A
S31.020S
S31.021S
S31.030A
S31.030S
S31.031S
S31.040A
S31.040S
S31.041S
S31.050A
S31.050S
S31.051S
S31.100A
S31.100S
S31.101A
S31.101S
S31.102A
S31.102S
S31.103A
S31.103S
S31.104A
S31.104S
S31.105A
S31.105S
S31.109A
S31.109S
S31.110A
S31.110S
S31.111A
S31.111S
S31.112A
S31.112S
S31.113A
S31.113S
S31.114A
S31.114S
S31.115A
S31.115S
S31.119A
S31.119S
S31.120S
S31.121S
S31.122S
S31.123S
S31.124S
S31.125S
S31.129S
S31.130A
S31.130S
S31.131A
S31.131S
S31.132A
S31.132S
S31.133A
S31.133S
S31.134A
S31.134S
S31.135A
S31.135S
S31.139A
S31.139S
S31.140S
S31.141S
S31.142S
S31.143S
S31.144S
S31.145S
S31.149S
S31.150A
S31.150S
S31.151A
S31.151S
S31.152A
S31.152S
S31.153A
S31.153S
S31.154A
S31.154S
S31.155A
S31.155S
S31.159A
S31.159S
S31.20XS
S31.21XS
S31.22XS
S31.23XS
S31.24XS
S31.25XS
S31.30XS
S31.31XS
S31.32XS
S31.33XS
S31.34XS
S31.35XS
S31.40XS
S31.41XS
S31.42XS
S31.43XS
S31.44XS
S31.45XS
S31.600S
S31.601S
S31.602S
S31.603S
S31.604S
S31.605S
S31.609S
S31.610S
S31.611S
S31.612S
S31.613S
S31.614S
S31.615S
S31.619S
S31.620S
S31.621S
S31.622S
S31.623S
S31.624S
S31.625S
S31.629S
S31.630S
S31.631S
S31.632S
S31.633S
S31.634S
S31.635S
S31.639S
S31.640S
S31.641S
S31.642S
S31.643S
S31.644S
S31.645S
S31.649S
S31.650S
S31.651S
S31.652S
S31.653S
S31.654S
S31.655S
S31.659S
S31.801A
S31.801S
S31.802A
S31.802S
S31.803A
S31.803S
S31.804A
S31.804S
S31.805A
S31.805S
S31.809A
S31.809S
S31.811A
S31.811S
S31.812A
S31.812S
S31.813A
S31.813S
S31.814A
S31.814S
S31.815A
S31.815S
S31.819A
S31.819S
S31.821A
S31.821S
S31.822A
S31.822S
S31.823A
S31.823S
S31.824A
S31.824S
S31.825A
S31.825S
S31.829A
S31.829S
S31.831A
S31.831S
S31.832S
S31.833A
S31.833S
S31.834S
S31.835A
S31.835S
S31.839A
S31.839S
S38.001S
S38.002S
S38.01XS
S38.02XS
S38.03XS
S38.1XXS
S38.211S
S38.212S
S38.221S
S38.222S
S38.231S
S38.232S
S38.3XXA
S38.3XXS
S39.021A
S39.021S
S39.022A
S39.022S
S39.023A
S39.023S
S40.011A
S40.011S
S40.012A
S40.012S
S40.019A
S40.019S
S40.021A
S40.021S
S40.022A
S40.022S
S40.029A
S40.029S
S40.211A
S40.211S
S40.212A
S40.212S
S40.219A
S40.219S
S40.221A
S40.221S
S40.222A
S40.222S
S40.229A
S40.229S
S40.241A
S40.241S
S40.242A
S40.242S
S40.249A
S40.249S
S40.251A
S40.251S
S40.252A
S40.252S
S40.259A
S40.259S
S40.261S
S40.262S
S40.269S
S40.271A
S40.271S
S40.272A
S40.272S
S40.279A
S40.279S
S40.811A
S40.811S
S40.812A
S40.812S
S40.819A
S40.819S
S40.821A
S40.821S
S40.822A
S40.822S
S40.829A
S40.829S
S40.841A
S40.841S
S40.842A
S40.842S
S40.849A
S40.849S
S40.851A
S40.851S
S40.852A
S40.852S
S40.859A
S40.859S
S40.861S
S40.862S
S40.869S
S40.871A
S40.871S
S40.872A
S40.872S
S40.879A
S40.879S
S40.911A
S40.911S
S40.912A
S40.912S
S40.919A
S40.919S
S40.921A
S40.921S
S40.922A
S40.922S
S40.929A
S40.929S
S41.001A
S41.001S
S41.002A
S41.002S
S41.009A
S41.009S
S41.011A
S41.011S
S41.012A
S41.012S
S41.019A
S41.019S
S41.021S
S41.022S
S41.029S
S41.031A
S41.031S
S41.032A
S41.032S
S41.039A
S41.039S
S41.041S
S41.042S
S41.049S
S41.051A
S41.051S
S41.052A
S41.052S
S41.059A
S41.059S
S41.101A
S41.101S
S41.102A
S41.102S
S41.109A
S41.109S
S41.111A
S41.111S
S41.112A
S41.112S
S41.119A
S41.119S
S41.121S
S41.122S
S41.129S
S41.131A
S41.131S
S41.132A
S41.132S
S41.139A
S41.139S
S41.141S
S41.142S
S41.149S
S41.151A
S41.151S
S41.152A
S41.152S
S41.159A
S41.159S
S46.021S
S46.022S
S46.029S
S46.121S
S46.122S
S46.129S
S46.221S
S46.222S
S46.229S
S46.321S
S46.322S
S46.329S
S46.821S
S46.822S
S46.829S
S46.921S
S46.922S
S46.929S
S47.1XXS
S47.2XXS
S47.9XXS
S50.00XA
S50.00XS
S50.01XA
S50.01XS
S50.02XA
S50.02XS
S50.10XA
S50.10XS
S50.11XA
S50.11XS
S50.12XA
S50.12XS
S50.311A
S50.311S
S50.312A
S50.312S
S50.319A
S50.319S
S50.321S
S50.322S
S50.329S
S50.341A
S50.341S
S50.342A
S50.342S
S50.349A
S50.349S
S50.351A
S50.351S
S50.352A
S50.352S
S50.359A
S50.359S
S50.361S
S50.362S
S50.369S
S50.371A
S50.371S
S50.372A
S50.372S
S50.379A
S50.379S
S50.811A
S50.811S
S50.812A
S50.812S
S50.819A
S50.819S
S50.821S
S50.822S
S50.829S
S50.841A
S50.841S
S50.842A
S50.842S
S50.849A
S50.849S
S50.851A
S50.851S
S50.852A
S50.852S
S50.859A
S50.859S
S50.861S
S50.862S
S50.869S
S50.871A
S50.871S
S50.872A
S50.872S
S50.879A
S50.879S
S50.901A
S50.901S
S50.902A
S50.902S
S50.909A
S50.909S
S50.911A
S50.911S
S50.912A
S50.912S
S50.919A
S50.919S
S51.001A
S51.001S
S51.002A
S51.002S
S51.009A
S51.009S
S51.011A
S51.011S
S51.012A
S51.012S
S51.019A
S51.019S
S51.021S
S51.022S
S51.029S
S51.031A
S51.031S
S51.032A
S51.032S
S51.039A
S51.039S
S51.041S
S51.042S
S51.049S
S51.051A
S51.051S
S51.052A
S51.052S
S51.059A
S51.059S
S51.801A
S51.801S
S51.802A
S51.802S
S51.809A
S51.809S
S51.811A
S51.811S
S51.812A
S51.812S
S51.819A
S51.819S
S51.821S
S51.822S
S51.829S
S51.831A
S51.831S
S51.832A
S51.832S
S51.839A
S51.839S
S51.841S
S51.842S
S51.849S
S51.851A
S51.851S
S51.852A
S51.852S
S51.859A
S51.859S
S56.021S
S56.022S
S56.029S
S56.121S
S56.122S
S56.123S
S56.124S
S56.125S
S56.126S
S56.127S
S56.128S
S56.129S
S56.221S
S56.222S
S56.229S
S56.321S
S56.322S
S56.329S
S56.421S
S56.422S
S56.423S
S56.424S
S56.425S
S56.426S
S56.427S
S56.428S
S56.429S
S56.521S
S56.522S
S56.529S
S56.821S
S56.822S
S56.829S
S56.921S
S56.922S
S56.929S
S57.00XS
S57.01XS
S57.02XS
S57.80XS
S57.81XS
S57.82XS
S60.00XA
S60.00XS
S60.011A
S60.011S
S60.012A
S60.012S
S60.019A
S60.019S
S60.021A
S60.021S
S60.022A
S60.022S
S60.029A
S60.029S
S60.031A
S60.031S
S60.032A
S60.032S
S60.039A
S60.039S
S60.041A
S60.041S
S60.042A
S60.042S
S60.049A
S60.049S
S60.051A
S60.051S
S60.052A
S60.052S
S60.059A
S60.059S
S60.10XA
S60.10XS
S60.111A
S60.111S
S60.112A
S60.112S
S60.119A
S60.119S
S60.121A
S60.121S
S60.122A
S60.122S
S60.129A
S60.129S
S60.131A
S60.131S
S60.132A
S60.132S
S60.139A
S60.139S
S60.141A
S60.141S
S60.142A
S60.142S
S60.149A
S60.149S
S60.151A
S60.151S
S60.152A
S60.152S
S60.159A
S60.159S
S60.211A
S60.211S
S60.212A
S60.212S
S60.219A
S60.219S
S60.221A
S60.221S
S60.222A
S60.222S
S60.229A
S60.229S
S60.311A
S60.311S
S60.312A
S60.312S
S60.319A
S60.319S
S60.321S
S60.322S
S60.329S
S60.341A
S60.341S
S60.342A
S60.342S
S60.349A
S60.349S
S60.351A
S60.351S
S60.352A
S60.352S
S60.359A
S60.359S
S60.361S
S60.362S

S60.369S
S60.371A
S60.371S
S60.372A
S60.372S
S60.379A
S60.379S
S60.391A
S60.391S
S60.392A
S60.392S
S60.399A
S60.399S
S60.410A
S60.410S
S60.411A
S60.411S
S60.412A
S60.412S
S60.413A
S60.413S
S60.414A
S60.414S
S60.415A
S60.415S
S60.416A
S60.416S
S60.417A
S60.417S
S60.418A
S60.418S
S60.419A
S60.419S
S60.420S
S60.421S
S60.422S
S60.423S
S60.424S
S60.425S
S60.426S
S60.427S
S60.428S
S60.429S
S60.440A
S60.440S
S60.441A
S60.441S
S60.442A
S60.442S
S60.443A
S60.443S
S60.444A
S60.444S
S60.445A
S60.445S
S60.446A
S60.446S
S60.447A
S60.447S
S60.448A
S60.448S
S60.449A
S60.449S
S60.450A
S60.450S
S60.451A
S60.451S
S60.452A
S60.452S
S60.453A
S60.453S
S60.454A
S60.454S
S60.455A
S60.455S
S60.456A
S60.456S
S60.457A
S60.457S
S60.458A
S60.458S
S60.459A
S60.459S
S60.460S
S60.461S
S60.462S
S60.463S
S60.464S
S60.465S
S60.466S
S60.467S
S60.468S
S60.469S
S60.470A
S60.470S
S60.471A
S60.471S
S60.472A
S60.472S
S60.473A
S60.473S
S60.474A
S60.474S
S60.475A
S60.475S
S60.476A
S60.476S
S60.477A
S60.477S
S60.478A
S60.478S
S60.479A
S60.479S
S60.511A
S60.511S
S60.512A
S60.512S
S60.519A
S60.519S
S60.521S
S60.522S
S60.529S
S60.541A
S60.541S
S60.542A
S60.542S
S60.549A
S60.549S
S60.551A
S60.551S
S60.552A
S60.552S
S60.559A
S60.559S
S60.561S
S60.562S
S60.569S
S60.571A
S60.571S
S60.572A
S60.572S
S60.579A
S60.579S
S60.811A
S60.811S
S60.812A
S60.812S
S60.819A
S60.819S
S60.821S
S60.822S
S60.829S
S60.841A
S60.841S
S60.842A
S60.842S
S60.849A
S60.849S
S60.851A
S60.851S
S60.852A
S60.852S
S60.859A
S60.859S
S60.861S
S60.862S
S60.869S
S60.871A
S60.871S
S60.872A
S60.872S
S60.879A
S60.879S
S60.911A
S60.911S
S60.912A
S60.912S
S60.919A
S60.919S
S60.921A
S60.921S
S60.922A
S60.922S
S60.929A
S60.929S
S60.931A
S60.931S
S60.932A
S60.932S
S60.939A
S60.939S
S60.940A
S60.940S
S60.941A
S60.941S
S60.942A
S60.942S
S60.943A
S60.943S
S60.944A
S60.944S
S60.945A
S60.945S
S60.946A
S60.946S
S60.947A
S60.947S
S60.948A
S60.948S
S60.949A
S60.949S
S61.001A
S61.001S
S61.002A
S61.002S
S61.009A
S61.009S
S61.011A
S61.011S
S61.012A
S61.012S
S61.019A
S61.019S
S61.021S
S61.022S
S61.029S
S61.031A
S61.031S
S61.032A
S61.032S
S61.039A
S61.039S
S61.041S
S61.042S
S61.049S
S61.051A
S61.051S
S61.052A
S61.052S
S61.059A
S61.059S
S61.101A
S61.101S
S61.102A
S61.102S
S61.109A
S61.109S
S61.111A
S61.111S
S61.112A
S61.112S
S61.119A
S61.119S
S61.121S
S61.122S
S61.129S
S61.131A
S61.131S
S61.132A
S61.132S
S61.139A
S61.139S
S61.141S
S61.142S
S61.149S
S61.151A
S61.151S
S61.152A
S61.152S
S61.159A
S61.159S
S61.200A
S61.200S
S61.201A
S61.201S
S61.202A
S61.202S
S61.203A
S61.203S
S61.204A
S61.204S
S61.205A
S61.205S
S61.206A
S61.206S
S61.207A
S61.207S
S61.208A
S61.208S
S61.209A
S61.209S
S61.210A
S61.210S
S61.211A
S61.211S
S61.212A
S61.212S
S61.213A
S61.213S
S61.214A
S61.214S
S61.215A
S61.215S
S61.216A
S61.216S
S61.217A
S61.217S
S61.218A
S61.218S
S61.219A
S61.219S
S61.220S
S61.221S
S61.222S
S61.223S
S61.224S
S61.225S
S61.226S
S61.227S
S61.228S
S61.229S
S61.230A
S61.230S
S61.231A
S61.231S
S61.232A
S61.232S
S61.233A
S61.233S
S61.234A
S61.234S
S61.235A
S61.235S
S61.236A
S61.236S
S61.237A
S61.237S
S61.238A
S61.238S
S61.239A
S61.239S
S61.240S
S61.241S
S61.242S
S61.243S
S61.244S
S61.245S
S61.246S
S61.247S
S61.248S
S61.249S
S61.250A
S61.250S
S61.251A
S61.251S
S61.252A
S61.252S
S61.253A
S61.253S
S61.254A
S61.254S
S61.255A
S61.255S
S61.256A
S61.256S
S61.257A
S61.257S
S61.258A
S61.258S
S61.259A
S61.259S
S61.300A
S61.300S
S61.301A
S61.301S
S61.302A
S61.302S
S61.303A
S61.303S
S61.304A
S61.304S
S61.305A
S61.305S
S61.306A
S61.306S
S61.307A
S61.307S
S61.308A
S61.308S
S61.309A
S61.309S
S61.310A
S61.310S
S61.311A
S61.311S
S61.312A
S61.312S
S61.313A
S61.313S
S61.314A
S61.314S
S61.315A
S61.315S
S61.316A
S61.316S
S61.317A
S61.317S
S61.318A
S61.318S
S61.319A
S61.319S
S61.320S
S61.321S
S61.322S
S61.323S
S61.324S
S61.325S
S61.326S
S61.327S
S61.328S
S61.329S
S61.330A
S61.330S
S61.331A
S61.331S
S61.332A
S61.332S
S61.333A
S61.333S
S61.334A
S61.334S
S61.335A
S61.335S
S61.336A
S61.336S
S61.337A
S61.337S
S61.338A
S61.338S
S61.339A
S61.339S
S61.340S
S61.341S
S61.342S
S61.343S
S61.344S
S61.345S
S61.346S
S61.347S
S61.348S
S61.349S
S61.350A
S61.350S
S61.351A
S61.351S
S61.352A
S61.352S
S61.353A
S61.353S
S61.354A
S61.354S
S61.355A
S61.355S
S61.356A
S61.356S
S61.357A
S61.357S
S61.358A
S61.358S
S61.359A
S61.359S
S61.401A
S61.401S
S61.402A
S61.402S
S61.409A
S61.409S
S61.411A
S61.411S
S61.412A
S61.412S
S61.419A
S61.419S
S61.421S
S61.422S
S61.429S
S61.431A
S61.431S
S61.432A
S61.432S
S61.439A
S61.439S
S61.441S
S61.442S
S61.449S
S61.451A
S61.451S
S61.452A
S61.452S
S61.459A
S61.459S
S61.501A
S61.501S
S61.502A
S61.502S
S61.509A
S61.509S
S61.511A
S61.511S
S61.512A
S61.512S
S61.519A
S61.519S
S61.521S
S61.522S
S61.529S
S61.531A
S61.531S
S61.532A
S61.532S
S61.539A
S61.539S
S61.541S
S61.542S
S61.549S
S61.551A
S61.551S
S61.552A
S61.552S
S61.559A
S61.559S
S66.021S
S66.022S
S66.029S
S66.120S
S66.121S
S66.122S
S66.123S
S66.124S
S66.125S
S66.126S
S66.127S
S66.128S
S66.129S
S66.221S
S66.222S
S66.229S
S66.320S
S66.321S
S66.322S
S66.323S
S66.324S
S66.325S
S66.326S
S66.327S
S66.328S
S66.329S
S66.421S
S66.422S
S66.429S
S66.520S
S66.521S
S66.522S
S66.523S
S66.524S
S66.525S
S66.526S
S66.527S
S66.528S
S66.529S
S66.821S
S66.822S
S66.829S
S66.921S
S66.922S
S66.929S
S67.00XS
S67.01XS
S67.02XS
S67.10XS
S67.190S
S67.191S
S67.192S
S67.193S
S67.194S
S67.195S
S67.196S
S67.197S
S67.198S
S67.20XS
S67.21XS
S67.22XS
S67.30XS
S67.31XS
S67.32XS
S67.40XS
S67.41XS
S67.42XS
S67.90XS
S67.91XS
S67.92XS
S70.00XA
S70.00XS
S70.01XA
S70.01XS
S70.02XA
S70.02XS
S70.10XA
S70.10XS
S70.11XA
S70.11XS
S70.12XA
S70.12XS
S70.211A
S70.211S
S70.212A
S70.212S
S70.219A
S70.219S
S70.221S
S70.222S
S70.229S
S70.241A
S70.241S
S70.242A
S70.242S
S70.249A
S70.249S
S70.251A
S70.251S
S70.252A
S70.252S
S70.259A
S70.259S
S70.261S
S70.262S
S70.269S
S70.271A
S70.271S
S70.272A
S70.272S
S70.279A
S70.279S
S70.311A
S70.311S
S70.312A
S70.312S
S70.319A
S70.319S
S70.321S
S70.322S
S70.329S
S70.341A
S70.341S
S70.342A
S70.342S
S70.349A
S70.349S
S70.351A
S70.351S
S70.352A
S70.352S
S70.359A
S70.359S
S70.361S
S70.362S
S70.369S
S70.371A
S70.371S
S70.372A
S70.372S
S70.379A
S70.379S
S70.911A
S70.911S
S70.912A
S70.912S
S70.919A
S70.919S
S70.921A
S70.921S
S70.922A
S70.922S
S70.929A
S70.929S
S71.001A
S71.001S
S71.002A
S71.002S
S71.009A
S71.009S
S71.011A
S71.011S
S71.012A
S71.012S
S71.019A
S71.019S
S71.021S
S71.022S
S71.029S
S71.031A
S71.031S
S71.032A
S71.032S
S71.039A
S71.039S
S71.041S
S71.042S
S71.049S
S71.051A
S71.051S
S71.052A
S71.052S
S71.059A
S71.059S
S71.101A
S71.101S
S71.102A
S71.102S
S71.109A
S71.109S
S71.111A
S71.111S
S71.112A
S71.112S
S71.119A
S71.119S
S71.121S
S71.122S
S71.129S
S71.131A
S71.131S
S71.132A
S71.132S
S71.139A
S71.139S
S71.141S
S71.142S
S71.149S
S71.151A
S71.151S
S71.152A
S71.152S
S71.159A
S71.159S
S76.021S
S76.022S
S76.029S
S76.121S
S76.122S
S76.129S
S76.221S
S76.222S
S76.229S
S76.321S
S76.322S
S76.329S
S76.821S
S76.822S
S76.829S
S76.921S
S76.922S
S76.929S
S77.00XS
S77.01XS
S77.02XS
S77.10XS
S77.11XS
S77.12XS
S77.20XS
S77.21XS
S77.22XS
S80.00XA
S80.00XS
S80.01XA
S80.01XS
S80.02XA
S80.02XS
S80.10XA
S80.10XS
S80.11XA
S80.11XS
S80.12XA
S80.12XS
S80.211A
S80.211S
S80.212A
S80.212S
S80.219A
S80.219S
S80.221S
S80.222S
S80.229S
S80.241A
S80.241S
S80.242A
S80.242S
S80.249A
S80.249S
S80.251A
S80.251S
S80.252A
S80.252S
S80.259A
S80.259S
S80.261S
S80.262S
S80.269S
S80.271A
S80.271S
S80.272A
S80.272S
S80.279A
S80.279S
S80.811A
S80.811S
S80.812A
S80.812S
S80.819A
S80.819S
S80.821S
S80.822S
S80.829S
S80.841A
S80.841S
S80.842A
S80.842S
S80.849A
S80.849S
S80.851A
S80.851S
S80.852A
S80.852S
S80.859A
S80.859S
S80.861S
S80.862S
S80.869S
S80.871A
S80.871S
S80.872A
S80.872S
S80.879A
S80.879S
S80.911A
S80.911S
S80.912A
S80.912S
S80.919A
S80.919S
S80.921A
S80.921S
S80.922A
S80.922S
S80.929A

S80.929S
S81.001A
S81.001S
S81.002A
S81.002S
S81.009A
S81.009S
S81.011A
S81.011S
S81.012A
S81.012S
S81.019A
S81.019S
S81.021S
S81.022S
S81.029S
S81.031A
S81.031S
S81.032A
S81.032S
S81.039A
S81.039S
S81.041S
S81.042S
S81.049S
S81.051A
S81.051S
S81.052A
S81.052S
S81.059A
S81.059S
S81.801A
S81.801S
S81.802A
S81.802S
S81.809A
S81.809S
S81.811A
S81.811S
S81.812A
S81.812S
S81.819A
S81.819S
S81.821S
S81.822S
S81.829S
S81.831A
S81.831S
S81.832A
S81.832S
S81.839A
S81.839S
S81.841S
S81.842S
S81.849S
S81.851A
S81.851S
S81.852A
S81.852S
S81.859A
S81.859S
S86.021S
S86.022S
S86.029S
S86.121S
S86.122S
S86.129S
S86.221S
S86.222S
S86.229S
S86.321S
S86.322S
S86.329S
S86.821S
S86.822S
S86.829S
S86.921S
S86.922S
S86.929S
S87.00XS
S87.01XS
S87.02XS
S87.80XS
S87.81XS
S87.82XS
S90.00XA
S90.00XS
S90.01XA
S90.01XS
S90.02XA
S90.02XS
S90.111A
S90.111S
S90.112A
S90.112S
S90.119A
S90.119S
S90.121A
S90.121S
S90.122A
S90.122S
S90.129A
S90.129S
S90.211A
S90.211S
S90.212A
S90.212S
S90.219A
S90.219S
S90.221A
S90.221S
S90.222A
S90.222S
S90.229A
S90.229S
S90.30XA
S90.30XS
S90.31XA
S90.31XS
S90.32XA
S90.32XS
S90.411A
S90.411S
S90.412A
S90.412S
S90.413A
S90.413S
S90.414A
S90.414S
S90.415A
S90.415S
S90.416A
S90.416S
S90.421S
S90.422S
S90.423S
S90.424S
S90.425S
S90.426S
S90.441A
S90.441S
S90.442A
S90.442S
S90.443A
S90.443S
S90.444A
S90.444S
S90.445A
S90.445S
S90.446A
S90.446S
S90.451A
S90.451S
S90.452A
S90.452S
S90.453A
S90.453S
S90.454A
S90.454S
S90.455A
S90.455S
S90.456A
S90.456S
S90.461S
S90.462S
S90.463S
S90.464S
S90.465S
S90.466S
S90.471A
S90.471S
S90.472A
S90.472S
S90.473A
S90.473S
S90.474A
S90.474S
S90.475A
S90.475S
S90.476A
S90.476S
S90.511A
S90.511S
S90.512A
S90.512S
S90.519A
S90.519S
S90.521S
S90.522S
S90.529S
S90.541A
S90.541S
S90.542A
S90.542S
S90.549A
S90.549S
S90.551A
S90.551S
S90.552A
S90.552S
S90.559A
S90.559S
S90.561S
S90.562S
S90.569S
S90.571A
S90.571S
S90.572A
S90.572S
S90.579A
S90.579S
S90.811A
S90.811S
S90.812A
S90.812S
S90.819A
S90.819S
S90.821S
S90.822S
S90.829S
S90.841A
S90.841S
S90.842A
S90.842S
S90.849A
S90.849S
S90.851A
S90.851S
S90.852A
S90.852S
S90.859A
S90.859S
S90.861S
S90.862S
S90.869S
S90.871A
S90.871S
S90.872A
S90.872S
S90.879A
S90.879S
S90.911A
S90.911S
S90.912A
S90.912S
S90.919A
S90.919S
S90.921A
S90.921S
S90.922A
S90.922S
S90.929A
S90.929S
S90.931A
S90.931S
S90.932A
S90.932S
S90.933A
S90.933S
S90.934A
S90.934S
S90.935A
S90.935S
S90.936A
S90.936S
S91.001A
S91.001S
S91.002A
S91.002S
S91.009A
S91.009S
S91.011A
S91.011S
S91.012A
S91.012S
S91.019A
S91.019S
S91.021S
S91.022S
S91.029S
S91.031A
S91.031S
S91.032A
S91.032S
S91.039A
S91.039S
S91.041S
S91.042S
S91.049S
S91.051A
S91.051S
S91.052A
S91.052S
S91.059A
S91.059S
S91.101A
S91.101S
S91.102A
S91.102S
S91.103A
S91.103S
S91.104A
S91.104S
S91.105A
S91.105S
S91.106A
S91.106S
S91.109A
S91.109S
S91.111A
S91.111S
S91.112A
S91.112S
S91.113A
S91.113S
S91.114A
S91.114S
S91.115A
S91.115S
S91.116A
S91.116S
S91.119A
S91.119S
S91.121S
S91.122S
S91.123S
S91.124S
S91.125S
S91.126S
S91.129S
S91.131A
S91.131S
S91.132A
S91.132S
S91.133A
S91.133S
S91.134A
S91.134S
S91.135A
S91.135S
S91.136A
S91.136S
S91.139A
S91.139S
S91.141S
S91.142S
S91.143S
S91.144S
S91.145S
S91.146S
S91.149S
S91.151A
S91.151S
S91.152A
S91.152S
S91.153A
S91.153S
S91.154A
S91.154S
S91.155A
S91.155S
S91.156A
S91.156S
S91.159A
S91.159S
S91.201A
S91.201S
S91.202A
S91.202S
S91.203A
S91.203S
S91.204A
S91.204S
S91.205A
S91.205S
S91.206A
S91.206S
S91.209A
S91.209S
S91.211A
S91.211S
S91.212A
S91.212S
S91.213A
S91.213S
S91.214A
S91.214S
S91.215A
S91.215S
S91.216A
S91.216S
S91.219A
S91.219S
S91.221S
S91.222S
S91.223S
S91.224S
S91.225S
S91.226S
S91.229S
S91.231A
S91.231S
S91.232A
S91.232S
S91.233A
S91.233S
S91.234A
S91.234S
S91.235A
S91.235S
S91.236A
S91.236S
S91.239A
S91.239S
S91.241S
S91.242S
S91.243S
S91.244S
S91.245S
S91.246S
S91.249S
S91.251A
S91.251S
S91.252A
S91.252S
S91.253A
S91.253S
S91.254A
S91.254S
S91.255A
S91.255S
S91.256A
S91.256S
S91.259A
S91.259S
S91.301A
S91.301S
S91.302A
S91.302S
S91.309A
S91.309S
S91.311A
S91.311S
S91.312A
S91.312S
S91.319A
S91.319S
S91.321S
S91.322S
S91.329S
S91.331A
S91.331S
S91.332A
S91.332S
S91.339A
S91.339S
S91.341S
S91.342S
S91.349S
S91.351A
S91.351S
S91.352A
S91.352S
S91.359A
S91.359S
S96.021S
S96.022S
S96.029S
S96.121S
S96.122S
S96.129S
S96.221S
S96.222S
S96.229S
S96.821S
S96.822S
S96.829S
S96.921S
S96.922S
S96.929S
S97.00XS
S97.01XS
S97.02XS
S97.101S
S97.102S
S97.109S
S97.111S
S97.112S
S97.119S
S97.121S
S97.122S
S97.129S
S97.80XS
S97.81XS
S97.82XS
T20.00XS
T20.011S
T20.012S
T20.019S
T20.02XS
T20.03XS
T20.04XS
T20.05XS
T20.06XS
T20.07XS
T20.09XS
T20.10XS
T20.111S
T20.112S
T20.119S
T20.12XS
T20.13XS
T20.14XS
T20.15XS
T20.16XS
T20.17XS
T20.19XS
T20.20XS
T20.211S
T20.212S
T20.219S
T20.22XS
T20.23XS
T20.24XS
T20.25XS
T20.26XS
T20.27XS
T20.29XS
T20.30XS
T20.311S
T20.312S
T20.319S
T20.32XS
T20.33XS
T20.34XS
T20.35XS
T20.36XS
T20.37XS
T20.39XS
T20.40XS
T20.411S
T20.412S
T20.419S
T20.42XS
T20.43XS
T20.44XS
T20.45XS
T20.46XS
T20.47XS
T20.49XS
T20.50XS
T20.511S
T20.512S
T20.519S
T20.52XS
T20.53XS
T20.54XS
T20.55XS
T20.56XS
T20.57XS
T20.59XS
T20.60XS
T20.611S
T20.612S
T20.619S
T20.62XS
T20.63XS
T20.64XS
T20.65XS
T20.66XS
T20.67XS
T20.69XS
T20.70XS
T20.711S
T20.712S
T20.719S
T20.72XS
T20.73XS
T20.74XS
T20.75XS
T20.76XS
T20.77XS
T20.79XS
T21.00XS
T21.01XS
T21.02XS
T21.03XS
T21.04XS
T21.05XS
T21.06XS
T21.07XS
T21.09XS
T21.10XS
T21.11XS
T21.12XS
T21.13XS
T21.14XS
T21.15XS
T21.16XS
T21.17XS
T21.19XS
T21.20XS
T21.21XS
T21.22XS
T21.23XS
T21.24XS
T21.25XS
T21.26XS
T21.27XS
T21.29XS
T21.30XS
T21.31XS
T21.32XS
T21.33XS
T21.34XS
T21.35XS
T21.36XS
T21.37XS
T21.39XS
T21.40XS
T21.41XS
T21.42XS
T21.43XS
T21.44XS
T21.45XS
T21.46XS
T21.47XS
T21.49XS
T21.50XS
T21.51XS
T21.52XS
T21.53XS
T21.54XS
T21.55XS
T21.56XS
T21.57XS
T21.59XS
T21.60XS
T21.61XS
T21.62XS
T21.63XS
T21.64XS
T21.65XS
T21.66XS
T21.67XS
T21.69XS
T21.70XS
T21.71XS
T21.72XS
T21.73XS
T21.74XS
T21.75XS
T21.76XS
T21.77XS
T21.79XS
T22.00XS
T22.011S
T22.012S
T22.019S
T22.021S
T22.022S
T22.029S
T22.031S
T22.032S
T22.039S
T22.041S
T22.042S
T22.049S
T22.051S
T22.052S
T22.059S
T22.061S
T22.062S
T22.069S
T22.091S
T22.092S
T22.099S
T22.10XS
T22.111S
T22.112S
T22.119S
T22.121S
T22.122S
T22.129S
T22.131S
T22.132S
T22.139S
T22.141S
T22.142S
T22.149S
T22.151S
T22.152S
T22.159S
T22.161S
T22.162S
T22.169S
T22.191S
T22.192S
T22.199S
T22.20XS
T22.211S
T22.212S
T22.219S
T22.221S
T22.222S
T22.229S
T22.231S
T22.232S
T22.239S
T22.241S
T22.242S
T22.249S
T22.251S
T22.252S
T22.259S
T22.261S
T22.262S
T22.269S
T22.291S
T22.292S
T22.299S
T22.30XS
T22.311S
T22.312S
T22.319S
T22.321S
T22.322S
T22.329S
T22.331S
T22.332S
T22.339S
T22.341S
T22.342S
T22.349S
T22.351S
T22.352S
T22.359S
T22.361S
T22.362S
T22.369S
T22.391S
T22.392S
T22.399S
T22.40XS
T22.411S
T22.412S
T22.419S
T22.421S
T22.422S
T22.429S
T22.431S
T22.432S
T22.439S
T22.441S
T22.442S
T22.449S
T22.451S
T22.452S
T22.459S
T22.461S
T22.462S
T22.469S
T22.491S
T22.492S
T22.499S
T22.50XS
T22.511S
T22.512S
T22.519S
T22.521S
T22.522S
T22.529S
T22.531S
T22.532S
T22.539S
T22.541S
T22.542S
T22.549S
T22.551S
T22.552S
T22.559S
T22.561S
T22.562S
T22.569S
T22.591S
T22.592S
T22.599S
T22.60XS
T22.611S
T22.612S
T22.619S
T22.621S
T22.622S
T22.629S
T22.631S
T22.632S
T22.639S
T22.641S
T22.642S
T22.649S
T22.651S
T22.652S
T22.659S
T22.661S
T22.662S
T22.669S
T22.691S
T22.692S
T22.699S
T22.70XS
T22.711S
T22.712S
T22.719S
T22.721S
T22.722S
T22.729S
T22.731S
T22.732S
T22.739S
T22.741S
T22.742S
T22.749S
T22.751S
T22.752S
T22.759S
T22.761S
T22.762S
T22.769S
T22.791S
T22.792S
T22.799S
T23.001S
T23.002S
T23.009S
T23.011S
T23.012S
T23.019S
T23.021S
T23.022S
T23.029S
T23.031S
T23.032S
T23.039S
T23.041S
T23.042S
T23.049S
T23.051S
T23.052S
T23.059S
T23.061S
T23.062S
T23.069S
T23.071S
T23.072S
T23.079S

ICD-10-CM/PCS Codes by MS-DRG

T23.Ø91S
T23.Ø92S
T23.Ø99S
T23.1Ø1S
T23.1Ø2S
T23.1Ø9S
T23.111S
T23.112S
T23.119S
T23.121S
T23.122S
T23.129S
T23.131S
T23.132S
T23.139S
T23.141S
T23.142S
T23.149S
T23.151S
T23.152S
T23.159S
T23.161S
T23.162S
T23.169S
T23.171S
T23.172S
T23.179S
T23.191S
T23.192S
T23.199S
T23.2Ø1S
T23.2Ø2S
T23.2Ø9S
T23.211S
T23.212S
T23.219S
T23.221S
T23.222S
T23.229S
T23.231S
T23.232S
T23.239S
T23.241S
T23.242S
T23.249S
T23.251S
T23.252S
T23.259S
T23.261S
T23.262S
T23.269S
T23.271S
T23.272S
T23.279S
T23.291S
T23.292S
T23.299S
T23.3Ø1S
T23.3Ø2S
T23.3Ø9S
T23.311S
T23.312S
T23.319S
T23.321S
T23.322S
T23.329S
T23.331S
T23.332S
T23.339S
T23.341S
T23.342S
T23.349S
T23.351S
T23.352S
T23.359S
T23.361S
T23.362S
T23.369S
T23.371S
T23.372S
T23.379S
T23.391S
T23.392S
T23.399S
T23.4Ø1S
T23.4Ø2S
T23.4Ø9S
T23.411S
T23.412S
T23.419S
T23.421S
T23.422S
T23.429S
T23.431S
T23.432S
T23.439S
T23.441S
T23.442S
T23.449S
T23.451S
T23.452S
T23.459S
T23.461S
T23.462S
T23.469S
T23.471S
T23.472S
T23.479S
T23.491S
T23.492S
T23.499S
T23.5Ø1S
T23.5Ø2S
T23.5Ø9S
T23.511S
T23.512S
T23.519S
T23.521S
T23.522S
T23.529S
T23.531S
T23.532S
T23.539S
T23.541S
T23.542S
T23.549S
T23.551S
T23.552S
T23.559S
T23.561S
T23.562S
T23.569S
T23.571S
T23.572S
T23.579S
T23.591S
T23.592S
T23.599S
T23.6Ø1S
T23.6Ø2S
T23.6Ø9S
T23.611S
T23.612S
T23.619S
T23.621S
T23.622S
T23.629S
T23.631S
T23.632S
T23.639S
T23.641S
T23.642S
T23.649S
T23.651S
T23.652S
T23.659S
T23.661S
T23.662S
T23.669S
T23.671S
T23.672S
T23.679S
T23.691S
T23.692S
T23.699S
T23.7Ø1S
T23.7Ø2S
T23.7Ø9S
T23.711S
T23.712S
T23.719S
T23.721S
T23.722S
T23.729S
T23.731S
T23.732S
T23.739S
T23.741S
T23.742S
T23.749S
T23.751S
T23.752S
T23.759S
T23.761S
T23.762S
T23.769S
T23.771S
T23.772S
T23.779S
T23.791S
T23.792S
T23.799S
T24.ØØ1S
T24.ØØ2S
T24.ØØ9S
T24.Ø11S
T24.Ø12S
T24.Ø19S
T24.Ø21S
T24.Ø22S
T24.Ø29S
T24.Ø31S
T24.Ø32S
T24.Ø39S
T24.Ø91S
T24.Ø92S
T24.Ø99S
T24.1Ø1S
T24.1Ø2S
T24.1Ø9S
T24.111S
T24.112S
T24.119S
T24.121S
T24.122S
T24.129S
T24.131S
T24.132S
T24.139S
T24.191S
T24.192S
T24.199S
T24.2Ø1S
T24.2Ø2S
T24.2Ø9S
T24.211S
T24.212S
T24.219S
T24.221S
T24.222S
T24.229S
T24.231S
T24.232S
T24.239S
T24.291S
T24.292S
T24.299S
T24.3Ø1S
T24.3Ø2S
T24.3Ø9S
T24.311S
T24.312S
T24.319S
T24.321S
T24.322S
T24.329S
T24.331S
T24.332S
T24.339S
T24.391S
T24.392S
T24.399S
T24.4Ø1S
T24.4Ø2S
T24.4Ø9S
T24.411S
T24.412S
T24.419S
T24.421S
T24.422S
T24.429S
T24.431S
T24.432S
T24.439S
T24.491S
T24.492S
T24.499S
T24.5Ø1S
T24.5Ø2S
T24.5Ø9S
T24.511S
T24.512S
T24.519S
T24.521S
T24.522S
T24.529S
T24.531S
T24.532S
T24.539S
T24.591S
T24.592S
T24.599S
T24.6Ø1S
T24.6Ø2S
T24.6Ø9S
T24.611S
T24.612S
T24.619S
T24.621S
T24.622S
T24.629S
T24.631S
T24.632S
T24.639S
T24.691S
T24.692S
T24.699S
T24.7Ø1S
T24.7Ø2S
T24.7Ø9S
T24.711S
T24.712S
T24.719S
T24.721S
T24.722S
T24.729S
T24.731S
T24.732S
T24.739S
T24.791S
T24.792S
T24.799S
T25.Ø11S
T25.Ø12S
T25.Ø19S
T25.Ø21S
T25.Ø22S
T25.Ø29S
T25.Ø31S
T25.Ø32S
T25.Ø39S
T25.Ø91S
T25.Ø92S
T25.Ø99S
T25.111S
T25.112S
T25.119S
T25.121S
T25.122S
T25.129S
T25.131S
T25.132S
T25.139S
T25.191S
T25.192S
T25.199S
T25.211S
T25.212S
T25.219S
T25.221S
T25.222S
T25.229S
T25.231S
T25.232S
T25.239S
T25.291S
T25.292S
T25.299S
T25.311S
T25.312S
T25.319S
T25.321S
T25.322S
T25.329S
T25.331S
T25.332S
T25.339S
T25.391S
T25.392S
T25.399S
T25.411S
T25.412S
T25.419S
T25.421S
T25.422S
T25.429S
T25.431S
T25.432S
T25.439S
T25.491S
T25.492S
T25.499S
T25.511S
T25.512S
T25.519S
T25.521S
T25.522S
T25.529S
T25.531S
T25.532S
T25.539S
T25.591S
T25.592S
T25.599S
T25.611S
T25.612S
T25.619S
T25.621S
T25.622S
T25.629S
T25.631S
T25.632S
T25.639S
T25.691S
T25.692S
T25.699S
T25.711S
T25.712S
T25.719S
T25.721S
T25.722S
T25.729S
T25.731S
T25.732S
T25.739S
T25.791S
T25.792S
T25.799S
T26.ØØXS
T26.Ø1XS
T26.Ø2XS
T26.1ØXS
T26.11XS
T26.12XS
T26.2ØXS
T26.21XS
T26.22XS
T26.3ØXS
T26.31XS
T26.32XS
T26.4ØXS
T26.41XS
T26.42XS
T26.5ØXS
T26.51XS
T26.52XS
T26.6ØXS
T26.61XS
T26.62XS
T26.7ØXS
T26.71XS
T26.72XS
T26.8ØXS
T26.81XS
T26.82XS
T26.9ØXS
T26.91XS
T26.92XS
T27.ØXXS
T27.1XXS
T27.2XXS
T27.3XXS
T27.4XXS
T27.5XXS
T27.6XXS
T27.7XXS
T28.ØXXS
T28.1XXS
T28.2XXS
T28.3XXS
T28.4ØXS
T28.411S
T28.412S
T28.419S
T28.49XS
T28.5XXS
T28.6XXS
T28.7XXS
T28.8XXS
T28.9ØXS
T28.911S
T28.912S
T28.919S
T28.99XS

DRG 605

Select principal diagnosis listed under DRG 604

DRG 606

Principal diagnosis

AØ6.7
A18.4
A22.Ø
A31.1
A36.3
A42.2
A43.1
A51.3*
A63.Ø
A66.Ø
A66.1
A66.2
A66.3
A66.4
A67.Ø
A67.1
A67.3
BØØ.Ø
BØØ.9
BØ7*
BØ8.Ø2
BØ8.Ø3
BØ8.1
B1Ø.8*
B35*
B36*
B37.2
B38.3
B38.81
B47.9
B55.1
B55.2
B65.3
B83.4
B85*
B86
B87*
B88*
C44.ØØ
C44.Ø1
C44.Ø2
C44.Ø9
C44.2Ø1
C44.2Ø2
C44.2Ø9
C44.211
C44.212
C44.219
C44.221
C44.222
C44.229
C44.291
C44.292
C44.299
C44.3*
C44.4Ø
C44.41
C44.42
C44.49
C44.5ØØ
C44.5Ø1
C44.5Ø9
C44.51Ø
C44.511
C44.519
C44.52Ø
C44.521
C44.529
C44.59Ø
C44.591
C44.599
C44.6Ø1
C44.6Ø2
C44.6Ø9
C44.611
C44.612
C44.619
C44.621
C44.622
C44.629
C44.691
C44.692
C44.699
C44.7Ø1
C44.7Ø2
C44.7Ø9
C44.711
C44.712
C44.719
C44.721
C44.722
C44.729
C44.791
C44.792
C44.799
C44.8Ø
C44.81
C44.82
C44.89
C44.9Ø
C44.91
C44.92
C44.99
C46.Ø
C46.1
C46.7
C46.9
DØ4.Ø
DØ4.2*
DØ4.3*
DØ4.4
DØ4.5
DØ4.6*
DØ4.7*
DØ4.8
DØ4.9
D17.Ø
D17.1
D17.2*
D17.3*
D17.79
D17.9
D18.Ø1
D22.Ø
D22.2*
D22.3*
D22.4
D22.5
D22.6*
D22.7*
D22.9
D23.Ø
D23.2*
D23.3*
D23.4
D23.5
D23.6*
D23.7*
D23.9
D24*
D48.5
HØ2.6*
I78.1
I89.Ø
LØ8.1
L11*
L12.2
L13.Ø
L13.1
L2Ø*
L21*
L22
L23*
L24*
L25*
L26
L27*
L28*
L29.Ø
L29.8
L29.9
L3Ø*
L4Ø.1
L42
L43*
L44.Ø
L44.1
L44.2
L44.3
L44.8
L44.9
L45
L49*
L5Ø*
L53.8
L53.9
L54
L55*
L56*
L57*
L58*
L59*
L6Ø*
L62
L63*
L64*
L65*
L66*
L67*
L68*
L7Ø*
L71*
L72*
L73*
L74*
L75*
L8Ø
L81*
L82*
L83
L84
L85*
L86
L87*
L9Ø*
L91*
L92.Ø
L92.1
L92.2
L92.3
L92.9
L94.Ø
L94.1
L94.2
L94.3
L94.4
L94.8
L94.9
L95*
L98.1
L98.2
L98.5
L98.6
L98.7
L98.8
L98.9
L99
M35.6
M54.ØØ
M54.Ø1
M54.Ø2
M79.3
M79.4
N8Ø.6
Q18.3
Q18.9
Q8Ø*
Q81*
Q82*
Q84*
R21
R22.Ø
R22.1
R22.2
R22.3*
R22.4*
R22.9
R23.4
R23.8
R23.9
R61
R9Ø.Ø
SØØ.Ø2XA
SØØ.Ø6XA
SØØ.32XA
SØØ.36XA
SØØ.421A
SØØ.422A
SØØ.429A
SØØ.461A
SØØ.462A
SØØ.469A
SØØ.521A
SØØ.522A
SØØ.561A
SØØ.562A
SØØ.82XA
SØØ.86XA
SØØ.92XA
SØØ.96XA
S1Ø.12XA
S1Ø.16XA
S1Ø.82XA
S1Ø.86XA
S1Ø.92XA
S1Ø.96XA
S2Ø.121A
S2Ø.122A
S2Ø.129A
S2Ø.161A
S2Ø.162A
S2Ø.169A
S2Ø.321A
S2Ø.322A
S2Ø.323A
S2Ø.324A
S2Ø.329A
S2Ø.361A
S2Ø.362A
S2Ø.363A
S2Ø.364A
S2Ø.369A
S2Ø.421A
S2Ø.422A
S2Ø.429A
S2Ø.461A
S2Ø.462A
S2Ø.469A
S2Ø.92XA
S2Ø.96XA
S3Ø.82ØA
S3Ø.821A
S3Ø.822A
S3Ø.823A
S3Ø.824A
S3Ø.825A
S3Ø.826A
S3Ø.827A
S3Ø.86ØA
S3Ø.861A
S3Ø.862A
S3Ø.863A
S3Ø.864A
S3Ø.865A
S3Ø.866A
S3Ø.867A
S4Ø.261A
S4Ø.262A
S4Ø.269A
S4Ø.861A
S4Ø.862A
S4Ø.869A
S5Ø.321A
S5Ø.322A
S5Ø.329A
S5Ø.361A
S5Ø.362A
S5Ø.369A
S5Ø.821A
S5Ø.822A
S5Ø.829A
S5Ø.861A
S5Ø.862A
S5Ø.869A
S6Ø.321A
S6Ø.322A
S6Ø.329A
S6Ø.361A
S6Ø.362A
S6Ø.369A
S6Ø.42ØA
S6Ø.421A
S6Ø.422A
S6Ø.423A
S6Ø.424A
S6Ø.425A
S6Ø.426A
S6Ø.427A
S6Ø.428A
S6Ø.429A
S6Ø.46ØA
S6Ø.461A
S6Ø.462A
S6Ø.463A
S6Ø.464A
S6Ø.465A
S6Ø.466A
S6Ø.467A
S6Ø.468A
S6Ø.469A
S6Ø.521A
S6Ø.522A
S6Ø.529A
S6Ø.561A
S6Ø.562A
S6Ø.569A
S6Ø.821A
S6Ø.822A
S6Ø.829A
S6Ø.861A
S6Ø.862A
S6Ø.869A
S7Ø.221A
S7Ø.222A
S7Ø.229A
S7Ø.261A
S7Ø.262A
S7Ø.269A
S7Ø.321A
S7Ø.322A
S7Ø.329A
S7Ø.361A
S7Ø.362A

S7Ø.369A
S8Ø.221A
S8Ø.222A
S8Ø.229A
S8Ø.261A
S8Ø.262A
S8Ø.269A
S8Ø.821A
S8Ø.822A
S8Ø.829A
S8Ø.861A
S8Ø.862A
S8Ø.869A
S9Ø.421A
S9Ø.422A
S9Ø.423A
S9Ø.424A
S9Ø.425A
S9Ø.426A
S9Ø.461A
S9Ø.462A
S9Ø.463A
S9Ø.464A
S9Ø.465A
S9Ø.466A
S9Ø.521A
S9Ø.522A
S9Ø.529A
S9Ø.561A
S9Ø.562A
S9Ø.569A
S9Ø.821A
S9Ø.822A
S9Ø.829A
S9Ø.861A
S9Ø.862A
S9Ø.869A
Z41.1
Z42*
Z52.1*
Z94.5

DRG 607
Select principal diagnosis listed under DRG 606

MDC 10

DRG 614
Operating Room Procedures
Ø18M*
Ø6L9ØZZ
Ø6L93ZZ
Ø6L94ZZ
Ø6LBØZZ
Ø6LB3ZZ
Ø6LB4ZZ
ØG5Ø*
ØG51*
ØG52*
ØG53*
ØG54*
ØG8Ø*
ØG9ØØØZ
ØG9ØØZX
ØG9ØØZZ
ØG9Ø3ZX
ØG9Ø4ØZ
ØG9Ø4ZX
ØG9Ø4ZZ
ØG91ØØZ
ØG91ØZX
ØG91ØZZ
ØG913ZX
ØG914ØZ
ØG914ZX
ØG914ZZ
ØG92ØØZ
ØG92ØZX
ØG92ØZZ
ØG924ØZ
ØG924ZZ
ØG93ØØZ
ØG93ØZX
ØG93ØZZ
ØG934ØZ
ØG934ZZ
ØG94ØØZ
ØG94ØZX
ØG94ØZZ
ØG944ØZ
ØG944ZZ
ØGBØ*
ØGB1*
ØGB2ØZX
ØGB2ØZZ
ØGB23ZZ
ØGB24ZZ
ØGB3ØZX
ØGB3ØZZ
ØGB33ZZ
ØGB34ZZ
ØGB4ØZX
ØGB4ØZZ
ØGB43ZZ
ØGB44ZZ
ØGCØ*
ØGC1*
ØGC2*
ØGC3*
ØGC4*
ØGJØØZZ
ØGJØ4ZZ
ØGJ1ØZZ
ØGJ14ZZ
ØGJ5ØZZ
ØGJ54ZZ
ØGM2*
ØGM3*
ØGNØ*
ØGN1*
ØGN2*
ØGN3*
ØGN4*
ØGPØØØZ
ØGPØ3ØZ
ØGPØ4ØZ
ØGP1ØØZ
ØGP13ØZ
ØGP14ØZ
ØGP5ØØZ
ØGP53ØZ
ØGP54ØZ
ØGQØ*
ØGQ1*
ØGQ2*
ØGQ3*
ØGQ4*
ØGS2*
ØGS3*
ØGTØ*
ØGT1*
ØGT2*
ØGT3*
ØGT4*
ØGWØØØZ
ØGWØ3ØZ
ØGWØ4ØZ
ØGW1ØØZ
ØGW13ØZ
ØGW14ØZ
ØGW5ØØZ
ØGW53ØZ
ØGW54ØZ

DRG 615
Select operating room procedures listed under DRG 614

DRG 616
Operating Room Procedures
ØY6C*
ØY6D*
ØY6FØZZ
ØY6GØZZ
ØY6H*
ØY6J*
ØY6M*
ØY6N*
ØY6P*
ØY6Q*
ØY6R*
ØY6S*
ØY6T*
ØY6U*
ØY6V*
ØY6W*
ØY6X*
ØY6Y*

DRG 617
Select operating room procedures listed under DRG 616

DRG 618
Select operating room procedures listed under DRG 616

DRG 619
Operating Room Procedures
ØD16Ø79
ØD16Ø7A
ØD16Ø7B
ØD16Ø7L
ØD16ØJ9
ØD16ØJA
ØD16ØJB
ØD16ØJL
ØD16ØK9
ØD16ØKA
ØD16ØKB
ØD16ØKL
ØD16ØZ9
ØD16ØZA
ØD16ØZB
ØD16ØZL
ØD16479
ØD1647A
ØD1647B
ØD1647L
ØD164J9
ØD164JA
ØD164JB
ØD164JL
ØD164K9
ØD164KA
ØD164KB
ØD164KL
ØD164Z9
ØD164ZA
ØD164ZB
ØD164ZL
ØD16879
ØD1687A
ØD1687B
ØD1687L
ØD168J9
ØD168JA
ØD168JB
ØD168JL
ØD168K9
ØD168KA
ØD168KB
ØD168KL
ØD168Z9
ØD168ZA
ØD168ZB
ØD168ZL
ØD18Ø78
ØD18ØJ8
ØD18ØK8
ØD18ØZ8
ØD18478
ØD184J8
ØD184K8
ØD184Z8
ØD18878
ØD188J8
ØD188K8
ØD188Z8
ØD188ZH
ØD19Ø79
ØD19Ø7A
ØD19Ø7B
ØD19ØJ9
ØD19ØJA
ØD19ØJB
ØD19ØK9
ØD19ØKA
ØD19ØKB
ØD19ØZ9
ØD19ØZA
ØD19ØZB
ØD19479
ØD1947A
ØD1947B
ØD194J9
ØD194JA
ØD194JB
ØD194K9
ØD194KA
ØD194KB
ØD194Z9
ØD194ZA
ØD194ZB
ØD19879
ØD1987A
ØD1987B
ØD198J9
ØD198JA
ØD198JB
ØD198K9
ØD198KA
ØD198KB
ØD198Z9
ØD198ZA
ØD198ZB
ØD1AØ7A
ØD1AØ7B
ØD1AØJA
ØD1AØJB
ØD1AØKA
ØD1AØKB
ØD1AØZA
ØD1AØZB
ØD1A47A
ØD1A47B
ØD1A4JA
ØD1A4JB
ØD1A4KA
ØD1A4KB
ØD1A4ZA
ØD1A4ZB
ØD1A87A
ØD1A87B
ØD1A8JA
ØD1A8JB
ØD1A8KA
ØD1A8KB
ØD1A8ZA
ØD1A8ZB
ØD1A8ZH
ØD1BØ7B
ØD1BØJB
ØD1BØKB
ØD1BØZB
ØD1B47B
ØD1B4JB
ØD1B4KB
ØD1B4ZB
ØD1B87B
ØD1B8JB
ØD1B8KB
ØD1B8ZB
ØD1B8ZH
ØD76ØDZ
ØD76ØZZ
ØD763DZ
ØD763ZZ
ØD764DZ
ØD764ZZ
ØDB6ØZ3
ØDB6ØZZ
ØDB63Z3
ØDB63ZZ
ØDB64Z3
ØDB64ZX
ØDB64ZZ
ØDB67Z3
ØDB67ZZ
ØDB68Z3
ØDF6ØZZ
ØDF63ZZ
ØDF64ZZ
ØDF67ZZ
ØDF68ZZ
ØDH6ØDZ
ØDH63DZ
ØDH64DZ
ØDL6*
ØDL7*
ØDM6*
ØDN6*
ØDP643Z
ØDP64CZ
ØDQ6*
ØDU6*
ØDV6ØCZ
ØDV6ØDZ
ØDV6ØZZ
ØDV63CZ
ØDV63DZ
ØDV63ZZ
ØDV64CZ
ØDV64DZ
ØDV64ZZ
ØDV67ZZ
ØDV68ZZ
ØDWØ4UZ
ØDW643Z
ØDW64CZ
ØDY6*
ØHBTØZZ
ØHBT3ZZ
ØHBUØZZ
ØHBU3ZZ
ØHBVØZZ
ØHBV3ZZ
ØHM7XZZ
ØHM9XZZ
ØJØ4*
ØJØ5*
ØJØ6*
ØJØ7*
ØJØ8*
ØJØ9*
ØJØD*
ØJØF*
ØJØG*
ØJØH*
ØJØL*
ØJØM*
ØJØN*
ØJØP*
ØJRØ37Z
ØJR137Z
ØJR437Z
ØJR537Z
ØJR637Z
ØJR737Z
ØJR837Z
ØJR937Z
ØJRB37Z
ØJRC37Z
ØJRD37Z
ØJRF37Z
ØJRG37Z
ØJRH37Z
ØJRJ37Z
ØJRK37Z
ØJRL37Z
ØJRM37Z
ØJRN37Z
ØJRP37Z
ØJRQ37Z
ØJRR37Z
ØWØF*

DRG 620
Select operating room procedures listed under DRG 619

DRG 621
Select operating room procedures listed under DRG 619

DRG 622
Operating Room Procedures
ØHRØX72
ØHRØX73
ØHRØX74
ØHRØXJ3
ØHRØXJ4
ØHRØXJZ
ØHRØXK3
ØHRØXK4
ØHR1X72
ØHR1X73
ØHR1X74
ØHR1XJ3
ØHR1XJ4
ØHR1XJZ
ØHR1XK3
ØHR1XK4
ØHR4X72
ØHR4X73
ØHR4X74
ØHR4XJ3
ØHR4XJ4
ØHR4XJZ
ØHR4XK3
ØHR4XK4
ØHR5X72
ØHR5X73
ØHR5X74
ØHR5XJ3
ØHR5XJ4
ØHR5XJZ
ØHR5XK3
ØHR5XK4
ØHR6X72
ØHR6X73
ØHR6X74
ØHR6XJ3
ØHR6XJ4
ØHR6XJZ
ØHR6XK3
ØHR6XK4
ØHR7X72
ØHR7X73
ØHR7X74
ØHR7XJ3
ØHR7XJ4
ØHR7XJZ
ØHR7XK3
ØHR7XK4
ØHR8X72
ØHR8X73
ØHR8X74
ØHR8XJ3
ØHR8XJ4
ØHR8XJZ
ØHR8XK3
ØHR8XK4
ØHRAX72
ØHRAX73
ØHRAX74
ØHRAXJ3
ØHRAXJ4
ØHRAXJZ
ØHRBX72
ØHRBX73
ØHRBX74
ØHRBXJ3
ØHRBXJ4
ØHRBXJZ
ØHRCX72
ØHRCX73
ØHRCX74
ØHRCXJ3
ØHRCXJ4
ØHRCXJZ
ØHRDX72
ØHRDX73
ØHRDX74
ØHRDXJ3
ØHRDXJ4
ØHRDXJZ
ØHREX72
ØHREX73
ØHREX74
ØHREXJ3
ØHREXJ4
ØHREXJZ
ØHRFXJ3
ØHRFXJ4
ØHRFXJZ
ØHRGXJ3
ØHRGXJ4
ØHRGXJZ
ØHRHX72
ØHRHX73
ØHRHX74
ØHRHXJ3
ØHRHXJ4
ØHRHXJZ
ØHRJX72
ØHRJX73
ØHRJX74
ØHRJXJ3
ØHRJXJ4
ØHRJXJZ
ØHRKX72
ØHRKX73
ØHRKX74
ØHRKXJ3
ØHRKXJ4
ØHRKXJZ
ØHRLX72
ØHRLX73
ØHRLX74
ØHRLXJ3
ØHRLXJ4
ØHRLXJZ
ØHRMX72
ØHRMX73
ØHRMX74
ØHRMXJ3
ØHRMXJ4
ØHRMXJZ
ØHRNX72
ØHRNX73
ØHRNX74
ØHRNXJ3
ØHRNXJ4
ØHRNXJZ
ØHXØXZZ
ØHX1XZZ
ØHX4XZZ
ØHX5XZZ
ØHX6XZZ
ØHX7XZZ
ØHX8XZZ
ØHX9XZZ
ØHXAXZZ
ØHXBXZZ
ØHXCXZZ
ØHXDXZZ
ØHXEXZZ
ØHXFXZZ
ØHXGXZZ
ØHXHXZZ
ØHXJXZZ
ØHXKXZZ
ØHXLXZZ
ØHXMXZZ
ØHXNXZZ
ØJBØØZZ
ØJB1ØZZ
ØJB4ØZZ
ØJB5ØZZ
ØJB6ØZZ
ØJB7ØZZ
ØJB8ØZZ
ØJB9ØZZ
ØJBBØZZ
ØJBCØZZ
ØJBDØZZ
ØJBFØZZ
ØJBGØZZ
ØJBHØZZ
ØJBLØZZ
ØJBMØZZ
ØJBNØZZ
ØJBPØZZ
ØJBQØZZ
ØJBRØZZ
ØJHØ*
ØJH1*
ØJH4*
ØJH5*
ØJH6ØNZ
ØJH63NZ
ØJH7ØNZ
ØJH73NZ
ØJH8ØNZ
ØJH83NZ
ØJH9*
ØJHB*
ØJHC*
ØJHDØNZ
ØJHD3NZ
ØJHFØNZ
ØJHF3NZ
ØJHGØNZ
ØJHG3NZ
ØJHHØNZ
ØJHH3NZ
ØJHJ*
ØJHK*
ØJHLØNZ
ØJHL3NZ
ØJHMØNZ
ØJHM3NZ
ØJHNØNZ
ØJHN3NZ
ØJHPØNZ
ØJHP3NZ
ØJHQ*
ØJHR*
ØJXØØZB
ØJXØØZC
ØJXØ3ZB
ØJXØ3ZC
ØJX1ØZB
ØJX1ØZC
ØJX13ZB
ØJX13ZC
ØJX4ØZB
ØJX4ØZC
ØJX43ZB
ØJX43ZC
ØJX5ØZB
ØJX5ØZC
ØJX53ZB
ØJX53ZC
ØJX6ØZB
ØJX6ØZC
ØJX63ZB
ØJX63ZC
ØJX7ØZB
ØJX7ØZC
ØJX73ZB
ØJX73ZC
ØJX8ØZB
ØJX8ØZC
ØJX83ZB
ØJX83ZC
ØJX9ØZB
ØJX9ØZC
ØJX93ZB
ØJX93ZC
ØJXBØZB
ØJXBØZC
ØJXB3ZB
ØJXB3ZC
ØJXCØZB
ØJXCØZC
ØJXC3ZB
ØJXC3ZC
ØJXDØZB
ØJXDØZC
ØJXD3ZB
ØJXD3ZC
ØJXFØZB
ØJXFØZC
ØJXF3ZB
ØJXF3ZC
ØJXGØZB
ØJXGØZC
ØJXG3ZB
ØJXG3ZC
ØJXHØZB
ØJXHØZC
ØJXH3ZB
ØJXH3ZC
ØJXLØZB
ØJXLØZC
ØJXL3ZB
ØJXL3ZC
ØJXMØZB
ØJXMØZC
ØJXM3ZB
ØJXM3ZC
ØJXNØZB
ØJXNØZC
ØJXN3ZB
ØJXN3ZC
ØJXPØZB
ØJXPØZC
ØJXP3ZB
ØJXP3ZC
ØJXQØZB
ØJXQØZC
ØJXQ3ZB
ØJXQ3ZC
ØJXRØZB
ØJXRØZC
ØJXR3ZB
ØJXR3ZC
ØKBNØZZ
ØKBPØZZ
ØKBSØZZ
ØKBTØZZ
ØKBVØZZ
ØKBWØZZ
ØLBVØZZ
ØLBWØZZ
XHRPXF7

DRG 623
Select operating room procedures listed under DRG 622

DRG 624
Select operating room procedures listed under DRG 622

DRG 625
Operating Room Procedures
Ø3LU*
Ø3LV*
ØCB7ØZZ
ØCB73ZZ
ØCB7XZZ
ØG5G*
ØG5H*
ØG5K*
ØG5L*
ØG5M*
ØG5N*
ØG5P*
ØG5Q*
ØG5R*
ØG8J*
ØG9GØØZ
ØG9GØZX
ØG9GØZZ
ØG9HØØZ
ØG9HØZX
ØG9HØZZ
ØG9KØØZ
ØG9KØZX
ØG9KØZZ
ØG9LØØZ
ØG9LØZX
ØG9LØZZ
ØG9L3ZX
ØG9L4ZX
ØG9MØØZ
ØG9MØZX
ØG9MØZZ
ØG9M3ZX
ØG9M4ZX
ØG9NØØZ
ØG9NØZX
ØG9NØZZ
ØG9N3ZX
ØG9N4ZX
ØG9PØØZ
ØG9PØZX
ØG9PØZZ
ØG9P3ZX
ØG9P4ZX
ØG9QØØZ
ØG9QØZX
ØG9QØZZ
ØG9Q3ZX
ØG9Q4ZX
ØG9RØØZ
ØG9RØZX
ØG9RØZZ
ØG9R3ZX
ØG9R4ZX
ØGBGØZX
ØGBGØZZ
ØGBG3ZZ
ØGBG4ZZ
ØGBHØZX
ØGBHØZZ
ØGBH3ZZ
ØGBH4ZZ
ØGBJØZX
ØGBJØZZ
ØGBJ3ZZ
ØGBJ4ZZ
ØGBL*
ØGBM*
ØGBN*
ØGBP*
ØGBQ*
ØGBR*

ØGCG*
ØGCH*
ØGCK*
ØGCL*
ØGCM*
ØGCN*
ØGCP*
ØGCQ*
ØGCR*
ØGHSØ1Z
ØGHSØ2Z
ØGHSØ3Z
ØGHSØYZ
ØGHS32Z
ØGHS33Z
ØGHS41Z
ØGHS42Z
ØGHS43Z
ØGJKØZZ
ØGJK4ZZ
ØGJRØZZ
ØGJR4ZZ
ØGJSØZZ
ØGJS4ZZ
ØGMG*
ØGMH*
ØGML*
ØGMM*
ØGMN*
ØGMP*
ØGMQ*
ØGMR*
ØGNG*
ØGNH*
ØGNK*
ØGNL*
ØGNM*
ØGNN*
ØGNP*
ØGNQ*
ØGNR*
ØGPKØØZ
ØGPK3ØZ
ØGPK4ØZ
ØGPRØØZ
ØGPR3ØZ
ØGPR4ØZ
ØGQG*
ØGQH*
ØGQJ*
ØGQK*
ØGQL*
ØGQM*
ØGQN*
ØGQP*
ØGQQ*
ØGQR*
ØGSG*
ØGSH*
ØGSL*
ØGSM*
ØGSN*
ØGSP*
ØGSQ*
ØGSR*
ØGTG*
ØGTH*
ØGTJØZZ
ØGTJ4ZZ
ØGTK*
ØGTL*
ØGTM*
ØGTN*
ØGTP*
ØGTQ*
ØGTR*
ØGWKØØZ
ØGWK3ØZ
ØGWK4ØZ
ØGWRØØZ
ØGWR3ØZ
ØGWR4ØZ
ØW96ØØZ
ØW96ØZZ
ØW964ØZ
ØW964ZZ
ØWJ6ØZZ
ØWJ64ZZ

DRG 626

Select operating room procedures listed under DRG 625

DRG 627

Select operating room procedures listed under DRG 625

DRG 628

Operating Room Procedures

Ø2HVØ2Z
Ø2HVØDZ
Ø2HV3DZ
Ø2HV42Z
Ø2HV4DZ
Ø2LV*
Ø2VV*
Ø313ØZD
Ø314ØZD
315Ø9Ø
Ø315Ø9W
Ø315ØAØ
Ø315ØAW
Ø315ØJØ
Ø315ØJW
Ø315ØKØ
Ø315ØKW
Ø315ØZØ
Ø315ØZD
Ø315ØZT
Ø315ØZV
Ø315ØZW
316Ø91
Ø316Ø9W
Ø316ØA1
Ø316ØAW
Ø316ØJ1
Ø316ØJW
Ø316ØK1
Ø316ØKW
Ø316ØZ1
Ø316ØZD
Ø316ØZT
Ø316ØZV
Ø316ØZW
Ø317Ø9D
Ø317Ø9F
Ø317Ø9V
Ø317Ø9W
Ø317ØAD
Ø317ØAF
Ø317ØAV
Ø317ØAW
Ø317ØJD
Ø317ØJF
Ø317ØJV
Ø317ØJW
Ø317ØKD
Ø317ØKF
Ø317ØKV
Ø317ØKW
Ø317ØZD
Ø317ØZF
Ø317ØZV
Ø317ØZW
Ø3173ZF
Ø318Ø9D
Ø318Ø9F
Ø318Ø9V
Ø318Ø9W
Ø318ØAD
Ø318ØAF
Ø318ØAV
Ø318ØAW
Ø318ØJD
Ø318ØJF
Ø318ØJV
Ø318ØJW
Ø318ØKD
Ø318ØKF
Ø318ØKV
Ø318ØKW
Ø318ØZD
Ø318ØZF
Ø318ØZV
Ø318ØZW
Ø3183ZF
Ø319Ø9F
Ø319ØAF
Ø319ØJF
Ø319ØKF
Ø319ØZF
Ø3193ZF
Ø31AØ9F
Ø31AØAF
Ø31AØJF
Ø31AØKF
Ø31AØZF
Ø31A3ZF
Ø31BØ9F
Ø31BØAF
Ø31BØJF
Ø31BØKF
Ø31BØZF
Ø31B3ZF
Ø31CØ9F
Ø31CØAF
Ø31CØJF
Ø31CØKF
Ø31CØZF
Ø31C3ZF
Ø31HØ9J
Ø31HØ9Y
Ø31HØAJ
Ø31HØAY
Ø31HØJJ
Ø31HØJY
Ø31HØKJ
Ø31HØKY
Ø31HØZJ
Ø31HØZY
Ø31JØ9K
Ø31JØ9Y
Ø31JØAK
Ø31JØAY
Ø31JØJK
Ø31JØJY
Ø31JØKK
Ø31JØKY
Ø31JØZK
Ø31JØZY
Ø31KØ9J
Ø31KØAJ
Ø31KØJJ
Ø31KØKJ
Ø31KØZJ
Ø31LØ9K
Ø31LØAK
Ø31LØJK
Ø31LØKK
Ø31LØZK
Ø31MØ9J
Ø31MØAJ
Ø31MØJJ
Ø31MØKJ
Ø31MØZJ
Ø31NØ9K
Ø31NØAK
Ø31NØJK
Ø31NØKK
Ø31NØZK
Ø355*
Ø356*
Ø357*
Ø358*
Ø359*
Ø35A*
Ø35B*
Ø35C*
Ø35D*
Ø35F*
Ø35Y*
Ø37334Z
Ø37335Z
Ø37336Z
Ø37337Z
Ø3733D1
Ø3733DZ
Ø3733EZ
Ø3733FZ
Ø3733GZ
Ø3733Z1
Ø3733ZZ
Ø37434Z
Ø37435Z
Ø37436Z
Ø37437Z
Ø3743D1
Ø3743DZ
Ø3743EZ
Ø3743FZ
Ø3743GZ
Ø3743Z1
Ø3743ZZ
Ø37734Z
Ø37735Z
Ø37736Z
Ø37737Z
Ø3773D1
Ø3773DZ
Ø3773EZ
Ø3773FZ
Ø3773GZ
Ø3773Z1
Ø3773ZZ
Ø37834Z
Ø37835Z
Ø37836Z
Ø37837Z
Ø3783D1
Ø3783DZ
Ø3783EZ
Ø3783FZ
Ø3783GZ
Ø3783Z1
Ø3783ZZ
Ø37934Z
Ø37935Z
Ø37936Z
Ø37937Z
Ø3793D1
Ø3793DZ
Ø3793EZ
Ø3793FZ
Ø3793GZ
Ø3793Z1
Ø3793ZZ
Ø37A34Z
Ø37A35Z
Ø37A36Z
Ø37A37Z
Ø37A3D1
Ø37A3DZ
Ø37A3EZ
Ø37A3FZ
Ø37A3GZ
Ø37A3Z1
Ø37A3ZZ
Ø37Y34Z
Ø37Y35Z
Ø37Y36Z
Ø37Y37Z
Ø37Y3DZ
Ø37Y3EZ
Ø37Y3FZ
Ø37Y3GZ
Ø37Y3ZZ
Ø39SØZX
Ø39S4ZX
Ø39TØZX
Ø39T4ZX
Ø3B5ØZZ
Ø3B53ZZ
Ø3B54ZZ
Ø3B6ØZZ
Ø3B63ZZ
Ø3B64ZZ
Ø3B7ØZZ
Ø3B73ZZ
Ø3B74ZZ
Ø3B8ØZZ
Ø3B83ZZ
Ø3B84ZZ
Ø3B9ØZZ
Ø3B93ZZ
Ø3B94ZZ
Ø3BAØZZ
Ø3BA3ZZ
Ø3BA4ZZ
Ø3BBØZZ
Ø3BB3ZZ
Ø3BB4ZZ
Ø3BCØZZ
Ø3BC3ZZ
Ø3BC4ZZ
Ø3BDØZZ
Ø3BD3ZZ
Ø3BD4ZZ
Ø3BFØZZ
Ø3BF3ZZ
Ø3BF4ZZ
Ø3BSØZX
Ø3BS3ZX
Ø3BS4ZX
Ø3BTØZX
Ø3BT3ZX
Ø3BT4ZX
Ø3BYØZZ
Ø3BY3ZZ
Ø3BY4ZZ
Ø3C5*
Ø3C6*
Ø3C7*
Ø3C8*
Ø3C9*
Ø3CA*
Ø3CB*
Ø3CC*
Ø3CD*
Ø3CF*
Ø3CHØZZ
Ø3CJØZZ
Ø3CKØZZ
Ø3CLØZZ
Ø3CMØZZ
Ø3CNØZZ
Ø3CPØZZ
Ø3CQØZZ
Ø3CRØZZ
Ø3CSØZZ
Ø3CTØZZ
Ø3CUØZZ
Ø3CVØZZ
Ø3CY*
Ø3L5ØCZ
Ø3L5ØZZ
Ø3L53CZ
Ø3L53ZZ
Ø3L54CZ
Ø3L54ZZ
Ø3L6ØCZ
Ø3L6ØZZ
Ø3L63CZ
Ø3L63ZZ
Ø3L64CZ
Ø3L64ZZ
Ø3L7ØCZ
Ø3L7ØZZ
Ø3L73CZ
Ø3L73ZZ
Ø3L74CZ
Ø3L74ZZ
Ø3L8ØCZ
Ø3L8ØZZ
Ø3L83CZ
Ø3L83ZZ
Ø3L84CZ
Ø3L84ZZ
Ø3L9ØCZ
Ø3L9ØZZ
Ø3L93CZ
Ø3L93ZZ
Ø3L94CZ
Ø3L94ZZ
Ø3LAØCZ
Ø3LAØZZ
Ø3LA3CZ
Ø3LA3ZZ
Ø3LA4CZ
Ø3LA4ZZ
Ø3LBØCZ
Ø3LBØZZ
Ø3LB3CZ
Ø3LB3ZZ
Ø3LB4CZ
Ø3LB4ZZ
Ø3LCØCZ
Ø3LCØZZ
Ø3LC3CZ
Ø3LC3ZZ
Ø3LC4CZ
Ø3LC4ZZ
Ø3LDØCZ
Ø3LDØZZ
Ø3LD3CZ
Ø3LD3ZZ
Ø3LD4CZ
Ø3LD4ZZ
Ø3LFØCZ
Ø3LFØZZ
Ø3LF3CZ
Ø3LF3ZZ
Ø3LF4CZ
Ø3LF4ZZ
Ø3Q5*
Ø3Q6*
Ø3Q7*
Ø3Q8*
Ø3Q9*
Ø3QA*
Ø3QB*
Ø3QC*
Ø3QD*
Ø3QF*
Ø3QY*
Ø41KØ9H
Ø41KØ9J
Ø41KØ9K
Ø41KØ9L
Ø41KØAH
Ø41KØAJ
Ø41KØAK
Ø41KØAL
Ø41KØJH
Ø41KØJJ
Ø41KØJK
Ø41KØJL
Ø41KØKH
Ø41KØKJ
Ø41KØKK
Ø41KØKL
Ø41KØZH
Ø41KØZJ
Ø41KØZK
Ø41KØZL
Ø41K49H
Ø41K49J
Ø41K49K
Ø41K49L
Ø41K4AH
Ø41K4AJ
Ø41K4AK
Ø41K4AL
Ø41K4JH
Ø41K4JJ
Ø41K4JK
Ø41K4JL
Ø41K4KH
Ø41K4KJ
Ø41K4KK
Ø41K4KL
Ø41K4ZH
Ø41K4ZJ
Ø41K4ZK
Ø41K4ZL
Ø41LØ9H
Ø41LØ9J
Ø41LØ9K
Ø41LØ9L
Ø41LØAH
Ø41LØAJ
Ø41LØAK
Ø41LØAL
Ø41LØJH
Ø41LØJJ
Ø41LØJK
Ø41LØJL
Ø41LØKH
Ø41LØKJ
Ø41LØKK
Ø41LØKL
Ø41LØZH
Ø41LØZJ
Ø41LØZK
Ø41LØZL
Ø41L49H
Ø41L49J
Ø41L49K
Ø41L49L
Ø41L4AH
Ø41L4AJ
Ø41L4AK
Ø41L4AL
Ø41L4JH
Ø41L4JJ
Ø41L4JK
Ø41L4JL
Ø41L4KH
Ø41L4KJ
Ø41L4KK
Ø41L4KL
Ø41L4ZH
Ø41L4ZJ
Ø41L4ZK
Ø41L4ZL
Ø45K*
Ø45L*
Ø45M*
Ø45N*
Ø45P*
Ø45Q*
Ø45R*
Ø45S*
Ø45T*
Ø45U*
Ø45V*
Ø45W*
Ø45Y*
47Ø341
Ø47Ø34Z
Ø47Ø35Z
Ø47Ø36Z
Ø47Ø37Z
Ø47Ø3D1
Ø47Ø3DZ
Ø47Ø3EZ
Ø47Ø3FZ
Ø47Ø3GZ
Ø47Ø3Z1
Ø47Ø3ZZ
471341
Ø47134Z
Ø47135Z
Ø47136Z
Ø47137Z
Ø4713D1
Ø4713DZ
Ø4713EZ
Ø4713FZ
Ø4713GZ
Ø4713Z1
Ø4713ZZ
472341
Ø47234Z
Ø47235Z
Ø47236Z
Ø47237Z
Ø4723D1
Ø4723DZ
Ø4723EZ
Ø4723FZ
Ø4723GZ
Ø4723Z1
Ø4723ZZ
473341
Ø47334Z
Ø47335Z
Ø47336Z
Ø47337Z
Ø4733D1
Ø4733DZ
Ø4733EZ
Ø4733FZ
Ø4733GZ
Ø4733Z1
Ø4733ZZ
474341
Ø47434Z
Ø47435Z
Ø47436Z
Ø47437Z
Ø4743D1
Ø4743DZ
Ø4743EZ
Ø4743FZ
Ø4743GZ
Ø4743Z1
Ø4743ZZ
475341
Ø47534Z
Ø47535Z
Ø47536Z
Ø47537Z
Ø4753D1
Ø4753DZ
Ø4753EZ
Ø4753FZ
Ø4753GZ
Ø4753Z1
Ø4753ZZ
476341
Ø47634Z
Ø47635Z
Ø47636Z
Ø47637Z
Ø4763D1
Ø4763DZ
Ø4763EZ
Ø4763FZ
Ø4763GZ
Ø4763Z1
Ø4763ZZ
477341
Ø47734Z
Ø47735Z
Ø47736Z
Ø47737Z
Ø4773D1
Ø4773DZ
Ø4773EZ
Ø4773FZ
Ø4773GZ
Ø4773Z1
Ø4773ZZ
478341
Ø47834Z
Ø47835Z
Ø47836Z
Ø47837Z
Ø4783D1
Ø4783DZ
Ø4783EZ
Ø4783FZ
Ø4783GZ
Ø4783Z1
Ø4783ZZ
479341
Ø47934Z
Ø47935Z
Ø47936Z
Ø47937Z
Ø4793D1
Ø4793DZ
Ø4793EZ
Ø4793FZ
Ø4793GZ
Ø4793Z1
Ø4793ZZ
Ø47A341
Ø47A34Z
Ø47A35Z
Ø47A36Z
Ø47A37Z
Ø47A3D1
Ø47A3DZ
Ø47A3EZ
Ø47A3FZ
Ø47A3GZ
Ø47A3Z1
Ø47A3ZZ
Ø47B341
Ø47B34Z
Ø47B35Z
Ø47B36Z
Ø47B37Z
Ø47B3D1
Ø47B3DZ
Ø47B3EZ
Ø47B3FZ
Ø47B3GZ
Ø47B3Z1
Ø47B3ZZ
Ø47C341
Ø47C34Z
Ø47C35Z
Ø47C36Z
Ø47C37Z
Ø47C3D1
Ø47C3DZ
Ø47C3EZ
Ø47C3FZ
Ø47C3GZ
Ø47C3Z1
Ø47C3ZZ
Ø47D341
Ø47D34Z
Ø47D35Z
Ø47D36Z
Ø47D37Z
Ø47D3D1
Ø47D3DZ
Ø47D3EZ
Ø47D3FZ
Ø47D3GZ
Ø47D3Z1
Ø47D3ZZ
Ø47E341
Ø47E34Z
Ø47E35Z
Ø47E36Z
Ø47E37Z
Ø47E3D1
Ø47E3DZ
Ø47E3EZ
Ø47E3FZ
Ø47E3GZ
Ø47E3Z1
Ø47E3ZZ
Ø47F341
Ø47F34Z
Ø47F35Z
Ø47F36Z
Ø47F37Z
Ø47F3D1
Ø47F3DZ
Ø47F3EZ
Ø47F3FZ
Ø47F3GZ
Ø47F3Z1
Ø47F3ZZ
Ø47H341
Ø47H34Z
Ø47H35Z
Ø47H36Z
Ø47H37Z
Ø47H3D1
Ø47H3DZ
Ø47H3EZ
Ø47H3FZ
Ø47H3GZ
Ø47H3Z1
Ø47H3ZZ
Ø47J341
Ø47J34Z
Ø47J35Z
Ø47J36Z
Ø47J37Z
Ø47J3D1
Ø47J3DZ
Ø47J3EZ
Ø47J3FZ
Ø47J3GZ
Ø47J3Z1
Ø47J3ZZ
Ø47KØ41
Ø47KØD1
Ø47KØZ1
Ø47K341
Ø47K34Z
Ø47K35Z
Ø47K36Z
Ø47K37Z
Ø47K3D1
Ø47K3DZ
Ø47K3EZ
Ø47K3FZ
Ø47K3GZ
Ø47K3Z1
Ø47K3ZZ
Ø47K441
Ø47K4D1
Ø47K4Z1
Ø47LØ41
Ø47LØD1
Ø47LØZ1
Ø47L341
Ø47L34Z
Ø47L35Z
Ø47L36Z
Ø47L37Z
Ø47L3D1
Ø47L3DZ
Ø47L3EZ
Ø47L3FZ
Ø47L3GZ
Ø47L3Z1
Ø47L3ZZ
Ø47L441
Ø47L4D1
Ø47L4Z1
Ø47MØ41
Ø47MØD1
Ø47MØZ1
Ø47M341
Ø47M3D1
Ø47M3Z1
Ø47M441
Ø47M4D1
Ø47M4Z1
Ø47NØ41
Ø47NØD1
Ø47NØZ1
Ø47N341
Ø47N3D1
Ø47N3Z1
Ø47N441
Ø47N4D1
Ø47N4Z1
Ø47Y341
Ø47Y34Z
Ø47Y35Z
Ø47Y36Z
Ø47Y37Z
Ø47Y3D1
Ø47Y3DZ
Ø47Y3EZ
Ø47Y3FZ
Ø47Y3GZ
Ø47Y3Z1
Ø47Y3ZZ
Ø4BKØZZ
Ø4BK3ZZ
Ø4BK4ZZ
Ø4BLØZZ
Ø4BL3ZZ
Ø4BL4ZZ
Ø4BMØZZ
Ø4BM3ZZ
Ø4BM4ZZ
Ø4BNØZZ
Ø4BN3ZZ

Ø4BN4ZZ
Ø4BPØZZ
Ø4BP3ZZ
Ø4BP4ZZ
Ø4BQØZZ
Ø4BQ3ZZ
Ø4BQ4ZZ
Ø4BRØZZ
Ø4BR3ZZ
Ø4BR4ZZ
Ø4BSØZZ
Ø4BS3ZZ
Ø4BS4ZZ
Ø4BTØZZ
Ø4BT3ZZ
Ø4BT4ZZ
Ø4BUØZZ
Ø4BU3ZZ
Ø4BU4ZZ
Ø4BVØZZ
Ø4BV3ZZ
Ø4BV4ZZ
Ø4BWØZZ
Ø4BW3ZZ
Ø4BW4ZZ
Ø4BYØZZ
Ø4BY3ZZ
Ø4BY4ZZ
Ø4CK*
Ø4CL*
Ø4CM*
Ø4CN*
Ø4CP*
Ø4CQ*
Ø4CR*
Ø4CS*
Ø4CT*
Ø4CU*
Ø4CV*
Ø4CW*
Ø4CY*
Ø4HYØ2Z
Ø4HYØYZ
Ø4HY42Z
Ø4PYØØZ
Ø4PYØ2Z
Ø4PYØ3Z
Ø4PYØCZ
Ø4PYØDZ
Ø4PYØYZ
Ø4PY3CZ
Ø4PY4ØZ
Ø4PY42Z
Ø4PY43Z
Ø4PY4CZ
Ø4PY4DZ
Ø4QC*
Ø4QD*
Ø4QE*
Ø4QF*
Ø4QH*
Ø4QJ*
Ø4QK*
Ø4QL*
Ø4QM*
Ø4QN*
Ø4QP*
Ø4QQ*
Ø4QR*
Ø4QS*
Ø4QT*
Ø4QU*
Ø4QV*
Ø4QW*
Ø4QY*
Ø4RK*
Ø4RL*
Ø4RM*
Ø4RN*
Ø4RP*
Ø4RQ*
Ø4RR*
Ø4RS*
Ø4RT*
Ø4RU*
Ø4RV*
Ø4RW*
Ø4RY*
Ø4SØ*
Ø4S1*
Ø4S2*
Ø4S3*
Ø4S4*
Ø4S5*
Ø4S6*
Ø4S7*
Ø4S8*
Ø4SB*
Ø4WYØØZ
Ø4WYØ2Z
Ø4WYØ3Z
Ø4WYØCZ
Ø4WYØDZ
Ø4WYØYZ
Ø4WY3CZ
Ø4WY4ØZ
Ø4WY42Z
Ø4WY43Z
Ø4WY4CZ
Ø4WY4DZ
Ø557*
Ø558*
Ø559*
Ø55A*
Ø55B*
Ø55C*
Ø55D*
Ø55F*
Ø55G*
Ø55H*
Ø55Y*
Ø5793D1
Ø5793DZ
Ø5793Z1
Ø5793ZZ
Ø57A3D1
Ø57A3DZ
Ø57A3Z1
Ø57A3ZZ
Ø57B3D1
Ø57B3DZ
Ø57B3Z1
Ø57B3ZZ
Ø57C3D1
Ø57C3DZ
Ø57C3Z1
Ø57C3ZZ
Ø57D3D1
Ø57D3DZ
Ø57D3Z1
Ø57D3ZZ
Ø57F3D1
Ø57F3DZ
Ø57F3Z1
Ø57F3ZZ
Ø5B7ØZZ
Ø5B73ZZ
Ø5B74ZZ
Ø5B8ØZZ
Ø5B83ZZ
Ø5B84ZZ
Ø5B9ØZZ
Ø5B93ZZ
Ø5B94ZZ
Ø5BAØZZ
Ø5BA3ZZ
Ø5BA4ZZ
Ø5BBØZZ
Ø5BB3ZZ
Ø5BB4ZZ
Ø5BCØZZ
Ø5BC3ZZ
Ø5BC4ZZ
Ø5BDØZZ
Ø5BD3ZZ
Ø5BD4ZZ
Ø5BFØZZ
Ø5BF3ZZ
Ø5BF4ZZ
Ø5BGØZZ
Ø5BG3ZZ
Ø5BG4ZZ
Ø5BHØZZ
Ø5BH3ZZ
Ø5BH4ZZ
Ø5BYØZZ
Ø5BY3ZZ
Ø5BY4ZZ
Ø5C7*
Ø5C8*
Ø5C9*
Ø5CA*
Ø5CB*
Ø5CC*
Ø5CD*
Ø5CF*
Ø5CG*
Ø5CH*
Ø5CM*
Ø5CN*
Ø5CP*
Ø5CQ*
Ø5CR*
Ø5CS*
Ø5CT*
Ø5CV*
Ø5CY*
Ø5HYØ2Z
Ø5HYØYZ
Ø5HY42Z
Ø5L7ØCZ
Ø5L7ØZZ
Ø5L73CZ
Ø5L73ZZ
Ø5L74CZ
Ø5L74ZZ
Ø5L8ØCZ
Ø5L8ØZZ
Ø5L83CZ
Ø5L83ZZ
Ø5L84CZ
Ø5L84ZZ
Ø5L9ØCZ
Ø5L9ØZZ
Ø5L93CZ
Ø5L93ZZ
Ø5L94CZ
Ø5L94ZZ
Ø5LAØCZ
Ø5LAØZZ
Ø5LA3CZ
Ø5LA3ZZ
Ø5LA4CZ
Ø5LA4ZZ
Ø5LBØCZ
Ø5LBØZZ
Ø5LB3CZ
Ø5LB3ZZ
Ø5LB4CZ
Ø5LB4ZZ
Ø5LCØCZ
Ø5LCØZZ
Ø5LC3CZ
Ø5LC3ZZ
Ø5LC4CZ
Ø5LC4ZZ
Ø5LDØCZ
Ø5LDØZZ
Ø5LD3CZ
Ø5LD3ZZ
Ø5LD4CZ
Ø5LD4ZZ
Ø5LFØCZ
Ø5LFØZZ
Ø5LF3CZ
Ø5LF3ZZ
Ø5LF4CZ
Ø5LF4ZZ
Ø5LGØCZ
Ø5LGØZZ
Ø5LG3CZ
Ø5LG3ZZ
Ø5LG4CZ
Ø5LG4ZZ
Ø5LHØCZ
Ø5LHØZZ
Ø5LH3CZ
Ø5LH3ZZ
Ø5LH4CZ
Ø5LH4ZZ
Ø5QY*
Ø67Ø3DZ
Ø67Ø3ZZ
Ø693ØØZ
Ø693ØZZ
Ø6934ØZ
Ø6934ZZ
Ø6BYØZZ
Ø6BY3ZZ
Ø6BY4ZZ
Ø6C3*
Ø6CY*
Ø6HØØDZ
Ø6HØ4DZ
Ø6LØ*
Ø6QY*
Ø6SØ*
Ø6S1*
Ø6S2*
Ø6S3*
Ø6S4*
Ø6S5*
Ø6S6*
Ø6S7*
Ø6S8*
Ø6VØ*
Ø75M*
Ø79ØØZX
Ø79Ø3ZX
Ø79Ø4ZX
Ø791ØZX
Ø7913ZX
Ø7914ZX
Ø792ØZX
Ø7923ZX
Ø7924ZX
Ø793ØZX
Ø7933ZX
Ø7934ZX
Ø794ØZX
Ø7943ZX
Ø7944ZX
Ø795ØZX
Ø7953ZX
Ø7954ZX
Ø796ØZX
Ø7963ZX
Ø7964ZX
Ø797ØZX
Ø7973ZX
Ø7974ZX
Ø798ØZX
Ø7983ZX
Ø7984ZX
Ø799ØZX
Ø7993ZX
Ø7994ZX
Ø79BØZX
Ø79B3ZX
Ø79B4ZX
Ø79CØZX
Ø79C3ZX
Ø79C4ZX
Ø79DØZX
Ø79D3ZX
Ø79D4ZX
Ø79FØZX
Ø79F3ZX
Ø79F4ZX
Ø79GØZX
Ø79G3ZX
Ø79G4ZX
Ø79HØZX
Ø79H3ZX
Ø79H4ZX
Ø79JØZX
Ø79J3ZX
Ø79J4ZX
Ø79KØZX
Ø79K3ZX
Ø79K4ZX
Ø79LØZX
Ø79L3ZX
Ø79L4ZX
Ø79MØØZ
Ø79MØZX
Ø79MØZZ
Ø79M3ZX
Ø79M4ØZ
Ø79M4ZX
Ø79M4ZZ
Ø7BØØZX
Ø7BØ3ZX
Ø7BØ4ZX
Ø7B1*
Ø7B2*
Ø7B3ØZX
Ø7B3ØZZ
Ø7B33ZX
Ø7B34ZX
Ø7B34ZZ
Ø7B4ØZX
Ø7B4ØZZ
Ø7B43ZX
Ø7B44ZX
Ø7B44ZZ
Ø7B5ØZX
Ø7B53ZX
Ø7B54ZX
Ø7B6ØZX
Ø7B63ZX
Ø7B64ZX
Ø7B7ØZX
Ø7B7ØZZ
Ø7B73ZX
Ø7B74ZX
Ø7B74ZZ
Ø7B8ØZX
Ø7B83ZX
Ø7B84ZX
Ø7B9ØZX
Ø7B93ZX
Ø7B94ZX
Ø7BBØZX
Ø7BBØZZ
Ø7BB3ZX
Ø7BB4ZX
Ø7BB4ZZ
Ø7BCØZX
Ø7BC3ZX
Ø7BC4ZX
Ø7BDØZX
Ø7BD3ZX
Ø7BD4ZX
Ø7BFØZX
Ø7BFØZZ
Ø7BF3ZX
Ø7BF4ZX
Ø7BF4ZZ
Ø7BGØZX
Ø7BGØZZ
Ø7BG3ZX
Ø7BG4ZX
Ø7BG4ZZ
Ø7BHØZX
Ø7BH3ZX
Ø7BH4ZX
Ø7BJØZX
Ø7BJ3ZX
Ø7BJ4ZX
Ø7BKØZX
Ø7BK3ZX
Ø7BK4ZX
Ø7BLØZX
Ø7BL3ZX
Ø7BL4ZX
Ø7BM*
Ø7CM*
Ø7HMØ1Z
Ø7HMØYZ
Ø7HM41Z
Ø7HM4YZ
Ø7JMØZZ
Ø7JM4ZZ
Ø7JPØZZ
Ø7NM*
Ø7PMØØZ
Ø7PMØ3Z
Ø7PMØYZ
Ø7PM3ØZ
Ø7PM33Z
Ø7PM4ØZ
Ø7PM43Z
Ø7QM*
Ø7SMØZZ
Ø7T1*
Ø7T2*
Ø7TC*
Ø7TD*
Ø7TM*
Ø7WMØØZ
Ø7WMØ3Z
Ø7WMØYZ
Ø7WM3ØZ
Ø7WM33Z
Ø7WM4ØZ
Ø7WM43Z
Ø7YM*
Ø8123Z4
Ø8133Z4
Ø85C3ZZ
Ø85D3ZZ
Ø8943ØZ
Ø8943ZZ
Ø8953ØZ
Ø8953ZZ
Ø8BNØZZ
Ø8BN3ZZ
Ø8BNXZZ
Ø8BPØZZ
Ø8BP3ZZ
Ø8BPXZZ
Ø8BQØZZ
Ø8BQ3ZZ
Ø8BQXZZ
Ø8BRØZZ
Ø8BR3ZZ
Ø8BRXZZ
Ø8DJ3ZZ
Ø8DK3ZZ
Ø8PØ3JZ
Ø8P13JZ
Ø8QC3ZZ
Ø8QD3ZZ
Ø8QE3ZZ
Ø8QF3ZZ
Ø8RØØKZ
Ø8RØ3JZ
Ø8R1ØKZ
Ø8R13JZ
Ø8R4*
Ø8R5*
Ø8RNØJZ
Ø8RN3JZ
Ø8RNXJZ
Ø8RPØJZ
Ø8RP3JZ
Ø8RPXJZ
Ø8RQØJZ
Ø8RQ3JZ
Ø8RQXJZ
Ø8RRØJZ
Ø8RR3JZ
Ø8RRXJZ
Ø8SN*
Ø8SP*
Ø8SQ*
Ø8SR*
Ø8UØ*
Ø8U1*
Ø8UNØJZ
Ø8UN3JZ
Ø8UNXJZ
Ø8UPØJZ
Ø8UP3JZ
Ø8UPXJZ
Ø8UQØJZ
Ø8UQ3JZ
Ø8UQXJZ
Ø8URØJZ
Ø8UR3JZ
Ø8URXJZ
ØD18Ø7H
ØD18Ø7K
ØD18Ø7L
ØD18Ø7M
ØD18Ø7N
ØD18ØJH
ØD18ØJK
ØD18ØJL
ØD18ØJM
ØD18ØJN
ØD18ØKH
ØD18ØKK
ØD18ØKL
ØD18ØKM
ØD18ØKN
ØD18ØZH
ØD18ØZK
ØD18ØZL
ØD18ØZM
ØD18ØZN
ØD1847H
ØD1847K
ØD1847L
ØD1847M
ØD1847N
ØD184JH
ØD184JK
ØD184JL
ØD184JM
ØD184JN
ØD184KH
ØD184KK
ØD184KL
ØD184KM
ØD184KN
ØD184ZH
ØD184ZK
ØD184ZL
ØD184ZM
ØD184ZN
ØD1887H
ØD1887K
ØD1887L
ØD1887M
ØD1887N
ØD188JH
ØD188JK
ØD188JL
ØD188JM
ØD188JN
ØD188KH
ØD188KK
ØD188KL
ØD188KM
ØD188KN
ØD188ZK
ØD188ZL
ØD188ZM
ØD188ZN
ØD19Ø7L
ØD19ØJL
ØD19ØKL
ØD19ØZL
ØD1947L
ØD194JL
ØD194KL
ØD194ZL
ØD1987L
ØD198JL
ØD198KL
ØD198ZL
ØD1AØ7H
ØD1AØ7K
ØD1AØ7L
ØD1AØ7M
ØD1AØ7N
ØD1AØJH
ØD1AØJK
ØD1AØJL
ØD1AØJM
ØD1AØJN
ØD1AØKH
ØD1AØKK
ØD1AØKL
ØD1AØKM
ØD1AØKN
ØD1AØZH
ØD1AØZK
ØD1AØZL
ØD1AØZM
ØD1AØZN
ØD1A47H
ØD1A47K
ØD1A47L
ØD1A47M
ØD1A47N
ØD1A4JH
ØD1A4JK
ØD1A4JL
ØD1A4JM
ØD1A4JN
ØD1A4KH
ØD1A4KK
ØD1A4KL
ØD1A4KM
ØD1A4KN
ØD1A4ZH
ØD1A4ZK
ØD1A4ZL
ØD1A4ZM
ØD1A4ZN
ØD1A87H
ØD1A87K
ØD1A87L
ØD1A87M
ØD1A87N
ØD1A8JH
ØD1A8JK
ØD1A8JL
ØD1A8JM
ØD1A8JN
ØD1A8KH
ØD1A8KK
ØD1A8KL
ØD1A8KM
ØD1A8KN
ØD1A8ZK
ØD1A8ZL
ØD1A8ZM
ØD1A8ZN
ØD1BØ7H
ØD1BØ7K
ØD1BØ7L
ØD1BØ7M
ØD1BØ7N
ØD1BØJH
ØD1BØJK
ØD1BØJL
ØD1BØJM
ØD1BØJN
ØD1BØKH
ØD1BØKK
ØD1BØKL
ØD1BØKM
ØD1BØKN
ØD1BØZH
ØD1BØZK
ØD1BØZL
ØD1BØZM
ØD1BØZN
ØD1B47H
ØD1B47K
ØD1B47L
ØD1B47M
ØD1B47N
ØD1B4JH
ØD1B4JK
ØD1B4JL
ØD1B4JM
ØD1B4JN
ØD1B4KH
ØD1B4KK
ØD1B4KL
ØD1B4KM
ØD1B4KN
ØD1B4ZH
ØD1B4ZK
ØD1B4ZL
ØD1B4ZM
ØD1B4ZN
ØD1B87H
ØD1B87K
ØD1B87L
ØD1B87M
ØD1B87N
ØD1B8JH
ØD1B8JK
ØD1B8JL
ØD1B8JM
ØD1B8JN
ØD1B8KH
ØD1B8KK
ØD1B8KL
ØD1B8KM
ØD1B8KN
ØD1B8ZK
ØD1B8ZL
ØD1B8ZM
ØD1B8ZN
ØD1EØ7E
ØD1EØ7P
ØD1EØJE
ØD1EØJP
ØD1EØKE
ØD1EØKP
ØD1EØZE
ØD1EØZP
ØD1E47E
ØD1E47P
ØD1E4JE
ØD1E4JP
ØD1E4KE
ØD1E4KP
ØD1E4ZE
ØD1E4ZP
ØD1E87E
ØD1E87P
ØD1E8JE
ØD1E8JP
ØD1E8KE
ØD1E8KP
ØD1E8ZE
ØD1E8ZP
ØD1HØ7H
ØD1HØ7K
ØD1HØ7L
ØD1HØ7M
ØD1HØ7N
ØD1HØ7P
ØD1HØJH
ØD1HØJK
ØD1HØJL
ØD1HØJM
ØD1HØJN
ØD1HØJP
ØD1HØKH
ØD1HØKK
ØD1HØKL
ØD1HØKM
ØD1HØKN
ØD1HØKP
ØD1HØZH
ØD1HØZK
ØD1HØZL
ØD1HØZM
ØD1HØZN
ØD1HØZP
ØD1H47H
ØD1H47K
ØD1H47L
ØD1H47M
ØD1H47N
ØD1H47P
ØD1H4JH
ØD1H4JK
ØD1H4JL
ØD1H4JM
ØD1H4JN
ØD1H4JP
ØD1H4KH
ØD1H4KK
ØD1H4KL
ØD1H4KM
ØD1H4KN
ØD1H4KP
ØD1H4ZH
ØD1H4ZK
ØD1H4ZL
ØD1H4ZM
ØD1H4ZN
ØD1H4ZP
ØD1H87H
ØD1H87K
ØD1H87L
ØD1H87M
ØD1H87N
ØD1H8JH
ØD1H8JK
ØD1H8JL
ØD1H8JM
ØD1H8JN
ØD1H8KH
ØD1H8KK
ØD1H8KL
ØD1H8KM
ØD1H8KN
ØD1H8ZH
ØD1H8ZK
ØD1H8ZL
ØD1H8ZM
ØD1H8ZN
ØD1KØ7K
ØD1KØ7L
ØD1KØ7M
ØD1KØ7N
ØD1KØ7P
ØD1KØJK
ØD1KØJL
ØD1KØJM
ØD1KØJN
ØD1KØJP
ØD1KØKK
ØD1KØKL
ØD1KØKM
ØD1KØKN
ØD1KØKP
ØD1KØZK
ØD1KØZL
ØD1KØZM
ØD1KØZN
ØD1KØZP
ØD1K47K
ØD1K47L
ØD1K47M
ØD1K47N
ØD1K47P
ØD1K4JK
ØD1K4JL
ØD1K4JM
ØD1K4JN
ØD1K4JP
ØD1K4KK
ØD1K4KL
ØD1K4KM
ØD1K4KN
ØD1K4KP
ØD1K4ZK
ØD1K4ZL
ØD1K4ZM
ØD1K4ZN
ØD1K4ZP
ØD1K87K
ØD1K87L
ØD1K87M
ØD1K87N
ØD1K87P
ØD1K8JK
ØD1K8JL
ØD1K8JM
ØD1K8JN
ØD1K8JP
ØD1K8KK
ØD1K8KL
ØD1K8KM
ØD1K8KN
ØD1K8KP
ØD1K8ZK
ØD1K8ZL
ØD1K8ZM
ØD1K8ZN
ØD1K8ZP
ØD1LØ7L
ØD1LØ7M

ØD1LØ7N
ØD1LØ7P
ØD1LØJL
ØD1LØJM
ØD1LØJN
ØD1LØJP
ØD1LØKL
ØD1LØKM
ØD1LØKN
ØD1LØKP
ØD1LØZL
ØD1LØZM
ØD1LØZN
ØD1LØZP
ØD1L47L
ØD1L47M
ØD1L47N
ØD1L47P
ØD1L4JL
ØD1L4JM
ØD1L4JN
ØD1L4JP
ØD1L4KL
ØD1L4KM
ØD1L4KN
ØD1L4KP
ØD1L4ZL
ØD1L4ZM
ØD1L4ZN
ØD1L4ZP
ØD1L87L
ØD1L87M
ØD1L87N
ØD1L87P
ØD1L8JL
ØD1L8JM
ØD1L8JN
ØD1L8JP
ØD1L8KL
ØD1L8KM
ØD1L8KN
ØD1L8KP
ØD1L8ZL
ØD1L8ZM
ØD1L8ZN
ØD1L8ZP
ØD1MØ7M
ØD1MØ7N
ØD1MØ7P
ØD1MØJM
ØD1MØJN
ØD1MØJP
ØD1MØKM
ØD1MØKN
ØD1MØKP
ØD1MØZM
ØD1MØZN
ØD1MØZP
ØD1M47M
ØD1M47N
ØD1M47P
ØD1M4JM
ØD1M4JN
ØD1M4JP
ØD1M4KM
ØD1M4KN
ØD1M4KP
ØD1M4ZM
ØD1M4ZN
ØD1M4ZP
ØD1M87M
ØD1M87N
ØD1M87P
ØD1M8JM
ØD1M8JN
ØD1M8JP
ØD1M8KM
ØD1M8KN
ØD1M8KP
ØD1M8ZM
ØD1M8ZN
ØD1M8ZP
ØD1NØ7N
ØD1NØ7P
ØD1NØJN
ØD1NØJP
ØD1NØKN
ØD1NØKP
ØD1NØZN
ØD1NØZP
ØD1N47N
ØD1N47P
ØD1N4JN
ØD1N4JP
ØD1N4KN
ØD1N4KP
ØD1N4ZN
ØD1N4ZP
ØD1N87N
ØD1N87P
ØD1N8JN
ØD1N8JP
ØD1N8KN
ØD1N8KP
ØD1N8ZN
ØD1N8ZP
ØD5UØZZ
ØD5U3ZZ
ØD5U4ZZ
ØD5V*
ØD5W*
ØDB7ØZZ
ØDB73ZZ
ØDB77ZZ
ØDB8ØZZ
ØDB84ZZ
ØDBEØZZ
ØDBE3ZZ
ØDBE7ZZ
ØDBFØZZ
ØDBF3ZZ
ØDBF7ZZ
ØDBGØZZ
ØDBG3ZZ
ØDBG7ZZ
ØDBGFZZ
ØDBHØZZ
ØDBH3ZZ
ØDBH7ZZ
ØDBKØZZ
ØDBK3ZZ
ØDBK7ZZ
ØDBLØZZ
ØDBL3ZZ
ØDBL7ZZ
ØDBLFZZ
ØDBMØZZ
ØDBM3ZZ
ØDBM7ZZ
ØDBMFZZ
ØDBNØZZ
ØDBN3ZZ
ØDBN7ZZ
ØDBNFZZ
ØDBUØZZ
ØDBU3ZZ
ØDBU4ZZ
ØDBVØZZ
ØDBV3ZZ
ØDBV4ZZ
ØDBWØZZ
ØDBW3ZZ
ØDBW4ZZ
ØDJØØZZ
ØDJ6ØZZ
ØDJDØZZ
ØDJUØZZ
ØDJVØZZ
ØDJWØZZ
ØDN8ØZZ
ØDN83ZZ
ØDN9ØZZ
ØDN93ZZ
ØDNAØZZ
ØDNA3ZZ
ØDNBØZZ
ØDNB3ZZ
ØDNCØZZ
ØDNC3ZZ
ØDNEØZZ
ØDNE3ZZ
ØDNFØZZ
ØDNF3ZZ
ØDNGØZZ
ØDNG3ZZ
ØDNHØZZ
ØDNH3ZZ
ØDNJØZZ
ØDNJ3ZZ
ØDNKØZZ
ØDNK3ZZ
ØDNLØZZ
ØDNL3ZZ
ØDNMØZZ
ØDNM3ZZ
ØDNNØZZ
ØDNN3ZZ
ØDNUØZZ
ØDNU3ZZ
ØDNVØZZ
ØDNV3ZZ
ØDNWØZZ
ØDNW3ZZ
ØDS67ZZ
ØDS68ZZ
ØDT9*
ØDTA*
ØDTB*
ØDTC*
ØDTG*
ØDTUØZZ
ØDTU4ZZ
ØF5DØZ3
ØF5DØZZ
ØF5D3Z3
ØF5D3ZZ
ØF5D7ZZ
ØF5FØZ3
ØF5FØZZ
ØF5F3Z3
ØF5F3ZZ
ØF5F7ZZ
ØF5GØZ3
ØF5GØZF
ØF5GØZZ
ØF5G3Z3
ØF5G3ZF
ØF5G3ZZ
ØF9ØØZX
ØF91ØZX
ØF92ØZX
ØF9FØZX
ØF9GØZX
ØFBØØZX
ØFB1ØZX
ØFB2ØZX
ØFBDØZX
ØFBDØZZ
ØFBD3ZZ
ØFBD7ZZ
ØFBFØZX
ØFBFØZZ
ØFBF3ZZ
ØFBF7ZZ
ØFBGØZX
ØFBGØZZ
ØFBG3ZZ
ØFBG4ZZ
ØFBG8ZZ
ØFJØØZZ
ØFJDØZZ
ØFJGØZZ
ØFNØØZZ
ØFNØ3ZZ
ØFN1ØZZ
ØFN13ZZ
ØFN2ØZZ
ØFN23ZZ
ØFN4ØZZ
ØFN43ZZ
ØFN5ØZZ
ØFN53ZZ
ØFN57ZZ
ØFN58ZZ
ØFN6ØZZ
ØFN63ZZ
ØFN67ZZ
ØFN68ZZ
ØFN7ØZZ
ØFN73ZZ
ØFN77ZZ
ØFN78ZZ
ØFN8ØZZ
ØFN83ZZ
ØFN87ZZ
ØFN88ZZ
ØFN9ØZZ
ØFN93ZZ
ØFN97ZZ
ØFN98ZZ
ØFNCØZZ
ØFNC3ZZ
ØFNC7ZZ
ØFNC8ZZ
ØFNDØZZ
ØFND3ZZ
ØFND7ZZ
ØFND8ZZ
ØFNFØZZ
ØFNF3ZZ
ØFNF7ZZ
ØFNF8ZZ
ØFNGØZZ
ØFNG3ZZ
ØFTDØZZ
ØFTD7ZZ
ØFTFØZZ
ØFTF7ZZ
ØFYG*
ØH9TØZX
ØH9TØZZ
ØH9UØZX
ØH9UØZZ
ØH9VØZX
ØH9VØZZ
ØH9WØZX
ØH9WØZZ
ØH9XØZX
ØH9XØZZ
ØHBTØZX
ØHBT7ZZ
ØHBT8ZZ
ØHBUØZX
ØHBU7ZZ
ØHBU8ZZ
ØHBVØZX
ØHBV7ZZ
ØHBV8ZZ
ØHBWØZX
ØHBXØZX
ØHBYØZX
ØHCTØZZ
ØHCUØZZ
ØHCVØZZ
ØHCWØZZ
ØHCXØZZ
ØJH6ØVZ
ØJH6ØYZ
ØJH63VZ
ØJH7ØVZ
ØJH7ØYZ
ØJH73VZ
ØJH8ØVZ
ØJH8ØYZ
ØJH83VZ
ØJHDØVZ
ØJHD3VZ
ØJHFØVZ
ØJHF3VZ
ØJHGØVZ
ØJHG3VZ
ØJHHØVZ
ØJHH3VZ
ØJHLØVZ
ØJHL3VZ
ØJHMØVZ
ØJHM3VZ
ØJHNØVZ
ØJHN3VZ
ØJHPØVZ
ØJHP3VZ
ØJHTØVZ
ØJHTØYZ
ØJHT3VZ
ØJQBØZZ
ØJQDØZZ
ØJQFØZZ
ØJQGØZZ
ØJQHØZZ
ØJQLØZZ
ØJQMØZZ
ØJQNØZZ
ØJQPØZZ
ØJQQØZZ
ØJQRØZZ
ØKQ5*
ØKQ6*
ØKQ7*
ØKQ8*
ØKQ9*
ØKQB*
ØKQN*
ØKQP*
ØKQS*
ØKQT*
ØKQV*
ØKQW*
ØKR5Ø7Z
ØKR5ØJZ
ØKR5ØKZ
ØKR547Z
ØKR54JZ
ØKR54KZ
ØKR6Ø7Z
ØKR6ØJZ
ØKR6ØKZ
ØKR647Z
ØKR64JZ
ØKR64KZ
ØKR7Ø7Z
ØKR7ØJZ
ØKR7ØKZ
ØKR747Z
ØKR74JZ
ØKR74KZ
ØKR8Ø7Z
ØKR8ØJZ
ØKR8ØKZ
ØKR847Z
ØKR84JZ
ØKR84KZ
ØKR9Ø7Z
ØKR9ØJZ
ØKR9ØKZ
ØKR947Z
ØKR94JZ
ØKR94KZ
ØKRBØ7Z
ØKRBØJZ
ØKRBØKZ
ØKRB47Z
ØKRB4JZ
ØKRB4KZ
ØKRNØ7Z
ØKRNØJZ
ØKRNØKZ
ØKRN47Z
ØKRN4JZ
ØKRN4KZ
ØKRPØ7Z
ØKRPØJZ
ØKRPØKZ
ØKRP47Z
ØKRP4JZ
ØKRP4KZ
ØKRSØ7Z
ØKRSØJZ
ØKRSØKZ
ØKRS47Z
ØKRS4JZ
ØKRS4KZ
ØKRTØ7Z
ØKRTØJZ
ØKRTØKZ
ØKRT47Z
ØKRT4JZ
ØKRT4KZ
ØKRVØ7Z
ØKRVØJZ
ØKRVØKZ
ØKRV47Z
ØKRV4JZ
ØKRV4KZ
ØKRWØ7Z
ØKRWØJZ
ØKRWØKZ
ØKRW47Z
ØKRW4JZ
ØKRW4KZ
ØKSØ*
ØKS1*
ØKS2*
ØKS3*
ØKS4*
ØKS5*
ØKS6*
ØKS7*
ØKS8*
ØKS9*
ØKSB*
ØKSF*
ØKSG*
ØKSH*
ØKSJ*
ØKSK*
ØKSL*
ØKSM*
ØKSN*
ØKSP*
ØKSQ*
ØKSR*
ØKSS*
ØKST*
ØKSV*
ØKSW*
ØL5*
ØL8Ø*
ØL81*
ØL82*
ØL83*
ØL84*
ØL85*
ØL86*
ØL89*
ØL8B*
ØL8C*
ØL8D*
ØL8F*
ØL8G*
ØL8H*
ØL8L*
ØL8M*
ØL8Q*
ØL8R*
ØL8S*
ØL8T*
ØL8V*
ØL8W*
ØLB7ØZZ
ØLB73ZZ
ØLB74ZZ
ØLB8ØZZ
ØLB83ZZ
ØLB84ZZ
ØLT7*
ØLT8*
ØLXØ*
ØLX1*
ØLX2*
ØLX3*
ØLX4*
ØLX5*
ØLX6*
ØLX9*
ØLXB*
ØLXC*
ØLXD*
ØLXF*
ØLXG*
ØLXH*
ØLXJ*
ØLXK*
ØLXL*
ØLXM*
ØLXN*
ØLXP*
ØLXQ*
ØLXR*
ØLXS*
ØLXT*
ØLXV*
ØLXW*
ØM53*
ØM54*
ØM5S*
ØM5T*
ØM934ZZ
ØM944ZZ
ØM9N4ØZ
ØM9P4ØZ
ØN9ØØZX
ØN9Ø3ZX
ØN9Ø4ZX
ØN91ØZX
ØN913ZX
ØN914ZX
ØN93ØZX
ØN933ZX
ØN934ZX
ØN94ØZX
ØN943ZX
ØN944ZX
ØN95ØZX
ØN953ZX
ØN954ZX
ØN96ØZX
ØN963ZX
ØN964ZX
ØN97ØZX
ØN973ZX
ØN974ZX
ØNBØØZX
ØNBØ3ZX
ØNBØ4ZX
ØNB1ØZX
ØNB13ZX
ØNB14ZX
ØNB3ØZX
ØNB33ZX
ØNB34ZX
ØNB4ØZX
ØNB43ZX
ØNB44ZX
ØNB5ØZX
ØNB53ZX
ØNB54ZX
ØNB6ØZX
ØNB63ZX
ØNB64ZX
ØNB7ØZX
ØNB73ZX
ØNB74ZX
ØP5Ø*
ØP51*
ØP52*
ØP55*
ØP56*
ØP57*
ØP58*
ØP59*
ØP5B*
ØP9ØØZX
ØP9Ø3ZX
ØP9Ø4ZX
ØP91ØZX
ØP913ZX
ØP914ZX
ØP92ØZX
ØP923ZX
ØP924ZX
ØP95ØZX
ØP953ZX
ØP954ZX
ØP96ØZX
ØP963ZX
ØP964ZX
ØP97ØZX
ØP973ZX
ØP974ZX
ØP98ØZX
ØP983ZX
ØP984ZX
ØP99ØZX
ØP993ZX
ØP994ZX
ØP9BØZX
ØP9B3ZX
ØP9B4ZX
ØP9CØZX
ØP9C3ZX
ØP9C4ZX
ØP9DØZX
ØP9D3ZX
ØP9D4ZX
ØP9FØZX
ØP9F3ZX
ØP9F4ZX
ØP9GØZX
ØP9G3ZX
ØP9G4ZX
ØP9HØZX
ØP9H3ZX
ØP9H4ZX
ØP9JØZX
ØP9J3ZX
ØP9J4ZX
ØP9KØZX
ØP9K3ZX
ØP9K4ZX
ØP9LØZX
ØP9L3ZX
ØP9L4ZX
ØP9MØZX
ØP9M3ZX
ØP9M4ZX
ØP9NØZX
ØP9N3ZX
ØP9N4ZX
ØP9PØZX
ØP9P3ZX
ØP9P4ZX
ØP9QØZX
ØP9Q3ZX
ØP9Q4ZX
ØPBØØZX
ØPBØ3ZX
ØPBØ4ZX
ØPB1ØZX
ØPB13ZX
ØPB14ZX
ØPB2ØZX
ØPB23ZX
ØPB24ZX
ØPB3ØZZ
ØPB33ZZ
ØPB34ZZ
ØPB4ØZZ
ØPB43ZZ
ØPB44ZZ
ØPB5ØZX
ØPB53ZX
ØPB54ZX
ØPB6ØZX
ØPB63ZX
ØPB64ZX
ØPB7ØZX
ØPB73ZX
ØPB74ZX
ØPB8ØZX
ØPB83ZX
ØPB84ZX
ØPB9ØZX
ØPB93ZX
ØPB94ZX
ØPBBØZX
ØPBB3ZX
ØPBB4ZX
ØPBCØZX
ØPBC3ZX
ØPBC4ZX
ØPBDØZX
ØPBD3ZX
ØPBD4ZX
ØPBFØZX
ØPBF3ZX
ØPBF4ZX
ØPBGØZX
ØPBG3ZX
ØPBG4ZX
ØPBHØZX
ØPBH3ZX
ØPBH4ZX
ØPBJØZX
ØPBJ3ZX
ØPBJ4ZX
ØPBKØZX
ØPBK3ZX
ØPBK4ZX
ØPBLØZX
ØPBL3ZX
ØPBL4ZX
ØPBMØZX
ØPBM3ZX
ØPBM4ZX
ØPBNØZX
ØPBN3ZX
ØPBN4ZX
ØPBPØZX
ØPBP3ZX
ØPBP4ZX
ØPBQØZX
ØPBQ3ZX
ØPBQ4ZX
ØPBRØZZ
ØPBR3ZZ
ØPBR4ZZ
ØPBSØZZ
ØPBS3ZZ
ØPBS4ZZ
ØPBTØZZ
ØPBT3ZZ
ØPBT4ZZ
ØPBVØZZ
ØPBV3ZZ
ØPBV4ZZ
ØQ5L*
ØQ5M*
ØQ5N*
ØQ5P*
ØQ8G*
ØQ8H*
ØQ8J*
ØQ8K*
ØQ8L*
ØQ8M*
ØQ8N*
ØQ8P*
ØQ9ØØZX
ØQ9Ø3ZX
ØQ9Ø4ZX
ØQ91ØZX
ØQ913ZX
ØQ914ZX
ØQ92ØZX
ØQ923ZX
ØQ924ZX
ØQ93ØZX
ØQ933ZX
ØQ934ZX
ØQ94ØZX
ØQ943ZX
ØQ944ZX
ØQ95ØZX
ØQ953ZX
ØQ954ZX
ØQ96ØZX
ØQ963ZX
ØQ964ZX
ØQ97ØZX
ØQ973ZX
ØQ974ZX
ØQ98ØZX
ØQ983ZX
ØQ984ZX
ØQ99ØZX
ØQ993ZX
ØQ994ZX
ØQ9BØZX
ØQ9B3ZX
ØQ9B4ZX
ØQ9CØZX
ØQ9C3ZX
ØQ9C4ZX
ØQ9DØZX
ØQ9D3ZX
ØQ9D4ZX
ØQ9FØZX
ØQ9F3ZX
ØQ9F4ZX
ØQ9GØZX
ØQ9G3ZX
ØQ9G4ZX
ØQ9HØZX
ØQ9H3ZX
ØQ9H4ZX
ØQ9JØZX
ØQ9J3ZX
ØQ9J4ZX
ØQ9KØZX
ØQ9K3ZX
ØQ9K4ZX
ØQ9LØZX
ØQ9L3ZX
ØQ9L4ZX
ØQ9MØZX
ØQ9M3ZX
ØQ9M4ZX
ØQ9NØZX
ØQ9N3ZX
ØQ9N4ZX
ØQ9PØZX
ØQ9P3ZX
ØQ9P4ZX
ØQ9SØZX
ØQ9S3ZX
ØQ9S4ZX
ØQBØ*
ØQB1*
ØQB2*
ØQB3*
ØQB4*
ØQB5*
ØQB6ØZX
ØQB63ZX
ØQB64ZX
ØQB7ØZX
ØQB73ZX
ØQB74ZX
ØQB8ØZX
ØQB83ZX
ØQB84ZX
ØQB9ØZX
ØQB93ZX
ØQB94ZX
ØQBBØZX
ØQBB3ZX
ØQBB4ZX
ØQBCØZX
ØQBC3ZX
ØQBC4ZX
ØQBDØZX
ØQBD3ZX
ØQBD4ZX
ØQBFØZX
ØQBF3ZX
ØQBF4ZX
ØQBGØZX
ØQBG3ZX
ØQBG4ZX
ØQBHØZX
ØQBH3ZX
ØQBH4ZX
ØQBJØZX
ØQBJ3ZX
ØQBJ4ZX
ØQBKØZX
ØQBK3ZX
ØQBK4ZX
ØQBL*
ØQBM*
ØQBN*
ØQBP*
ØQBQØZZ
ØQBQ3ZZ
ØQBQ4ZZ

ICD-10-CM/PCS Codes by MS-DRG

ØQBRØZZ
ØQBR3ZZ
ØQBR4ZZ
ØQBS*
ØQP6Ø4Z
ØQP6Ø5Z
ØQP6Ø7Z
ØQP6ØJZ
ØQP6ØKZ
ØQP634Z
ØQP635Z
ØQP637Z
ØQP63JZ
ØQP63KZ
ØQP644Z
ØQP645Z
ØQP647Z
ØQP64JZ
ØQP64KZ
ØQP7Ø4Z
ØQP7Ø5Z
ØQP7Ø7Z
ØQP7ØJZ
ØQP7ØKZ
ØQP734Z
ØQP735Z
ØQP737Z
ØQP73JZ
ØQP73KZ
ØQP744Z
ØQP745Z
ØQP747Z
ØQP74JZ
ØQP74KZ
ØQP8Ø4Z
ØQP8Ø5Z
ØQP8Ø7Z
ØQP8ØJZ
ØQP8ØKZ
ØQP834Z
ØQP835Z
ØQP837Z
ØQP83JZ
ØQP83KZ
ØQP844Z
ØQP845Z
ØQP847Z
ØQP84JZ
ØQP84KZ
ØQP9Ø4Z
ØQP9Ø5Z
ØQP9Ø7Z
ØQP9ØJZ
ØQP9ØKZ
ØQP934Z
ØQP935Z
ØQP937Z
ØQP93JZ
ØQP93KZ
ØQP944Z
ØQP945Z
ØQP947Z
ØQP94JZ
ØQP94KZ
ØQPBØ4Z
ØQPBØ5Z
ØQPBØ7Z
ØQPBØJZ
ØQPBØKZ
ØQPB34Z
ØQPB35Z
ØQPB37Z
ØQPB3JZ
ØQPB3KZ
ØQPB44Z
ØQPB45Z
ØQPB47Z
ØQPB4JZ
ØQPB4KZ
ØQPCØ4Z
ØQPCØ5Z
ØQPCØ7Z
ØQPCØJZ
ØQPCØKZ
ØQPC34Z
ØQPC35Z
ØQPC37Z
ØQPC3JZ
ØQPC3KZ
ØQPC44Z
ØQPC45Z
ØQPC47Z
ØQPC4JZ
ØQPC4KZ
ØQS6Ø4Z
ØQS6Ø6Z
ØQS7Ø4Z
ØQS7Ø6Z
ØQS8Ø4Z
ØQS8Ø6Z
ØQS9Ø4Z
ØQS9Ø6Z
ØQSBØ4Z
ØQSBØ6Z
ØQSCØ4Z
ØQSCØ6Z
ØQT4ØZZ
ØQT5ØZZ
ØR5L*
ØR5M*
ØR9LØØZ
ØR9LØZZ
ØR9MØØZ
ØR9MØZZ
ØRCL*
ØRCM*
ØS5H*
ØS5J*
ØS5K*
ØS5L*
ØS5M*
ØS5N*
ØS5P*
ØS5Q*
ØS9CØØZ
ØS9CØZZ
ØS9DØØZ
ØS9DØZZ
ØSBCØZZ
ØSBC3ZZ
ØSBC4ZZ
ØSBDØZZ
ØSBD3ZZ
ØSBD4ZZ
ØSCC*
ØSCD*
ØSGF*
ØSGG*
ØSJC4ZZ
ØSJD4ZZ
ØSRA*
ØSRE*
ØSRR*
ØSRS*
ØSTHØZZ
ØSTJØZZ
ØSTKØZZ
ØSTLØZZ
ØSTMØZZ
ØSTNØZZ
ØSTPØZZ
ØSTQØZZ
ØSUAØBZ
ØSUEØBZ
ØSURØBZ
ØSUSØBZ
ØSW9ØJZ
ØSW93JZ
ØSW94JZ
ØSWAØJZ
ØSWA3JZ
ØSWA4JZ
ØSWBØJZ
ØSWB3JZ
ØSWB4JZ
ØSWEØJZ
ØSWE3JZ
ØSWE4JZ
ØSWRØJZ
ØSWR3JZ
ØSWR4JZ
ØSWSØJZ
ØSWS3JZ
ØSWS4JZ
ØUBØØZZ
ØUBØ3ZZ
ØUBØ4ZZ
ØUBØ7ZZ
ØUBØ8ZZ
ØUB1ØZZ
ØUB13ZZ
ØUB14ZZ
ØUB17ZZ
ØUB18ZZ
ØUB2ØZZ
ØUB23ZZ
ØUB24ZZ
ØUB27ZZ
ØUB28ZZ
ØVR*
ØW3Ø*
ØW31*
ØW32*
ØW33*
ØW34*
ØW35*
ØW36*
ØW39*
ØW3B*
ØW3C*
ØW3K*
ØW3L*
ØW3Q3ZZ
ØW3Q4ZZ
ØW3Q7ZZ
ØW9CØZX
ØWB8ØZZ
ØWB83ZZ
ØWB84ZZ
ØWB8XZZ
ØWBCØZX
ØWBCØZZ
ØWBC3ZX
ØWBC3ZZ
ØWBC4ZX
ØWBC4ZZ
ØWBFØZZ
ØWBF3ZZ
ØWBF4ZZ
ØWBFXZ2
ØWBFXZZ
ØWH6Ø1Z
ØWH631Z
ØWH641Z
ØWHGØ1Z
ØWHG31Z
ØWHG41Z
ØWHHØ1Z
ØWHH31Z
ØWHH41Z
ØWJGØZZ
ØWJJØZZ
ØWJPØZZ
ØWJRØZZ
ØYB5ØZZ
ØYB53ZZ
ØYB54ZZ
ØYB6ØZZ
ØYB63ZZ
ØYB64ZZ
ØYB7ØZZ
ØYB73ZZ
ØYB74ZZ
ØYB8ØZZ
ØYB83ZZ
ØYB84ZZ
X27H385
X27H395
X27H3B5
X27H3C5
X27J385
X27J395
X27J3B5
X27J3C5
X2H13R9
X2KB317
X2KC317
XRGJØB9
XRGKØB9
XWØ2ØD8
XWØQ316
OR
ØSP9Ø8Z
ØSP9Ø9Z
ØSP9ØBZ
ØSP9ØJZ
ØSP948Z
ØSP94JZ
ØSPAØJZ
ØSPA4JZ
ØSPRØJZ
ØSPR4JZ
AND
ØSR9Ø19
ØSR9Ø1A
ØSR9Ø1Z
ØSR9Ø29
ØSR9Ø2A
ØSR9Ø2Z
ØSR9Ø39
ØSR9Ø3A
ØSR9Ø3Z
ØSR9Ø49
ØSR9Ø4A
ØSR9Ø4Z
ØSR9Ø69
ØSR9Ø6A
ØSR9Ø6Z
ØSR9ØJ9
ØSR9ØJA
ØSR9ØJZ
ØSRAØØ9
ØSRAØØA
ØSRAØØZ
ØSRAØ19
ØSRAØ1A
ØSRAØ1Z
ØSRAØ39
ØSRAØ3A
ØSRAØ3Z
ØSRAØJ9
ØSRAØJA
ØSRAØJZ
ØSRRØ19
ØSRRØ1A
ØSRRØ1Z
ØSRRØ39
ØSRRØ3A
ØSRRØ3Z
ØSRRØJ9
ØSRRØJA
ØSRRØJZ
OR
ØSP9Ø8Z
ØSP9Ø9Z
ØSP9ØBZ
ØSP948Z
ØSP94JZ
ØSPA4JZ
ØSPR4JZ
AND
ØSU9Ø9Z
ØSUAØ9Z
ØSURØ9Z
OR
ØSPBØ8Z
ØSPBØ9Z
ØSPBØBZ
ØSPBØJZ
ØSPB48Z
ØSPB4JZ
ØSPEØJZ
ØSPE4JZ
ØSPSØJZ
ØSPS4JZ
AND
ØSRBØ19
ØSRBØ1A
ØSRBØ1Z
ØSRBØ29
ØSRBØ2A
ØSRBØ2Z
ØSRBØ39
ØSRBØ3A
ØSRBØ3Z
ØSRBØ49
ØSRBØ4A
ØSRBØ4Z
ØSRBØ69
ØSRBØ6A
ØSRBØ6Z
ØSRBØJ9
ØSRBØJA
ØSRBØJZ
ØSREØØ9
ØSREØØA
ØSREØØZ
ØSREØ19
ØSREØ1A
ØSREØ1Z
ØSREØ39
ØSREØ3A
ØSREØ3Z
ØSREØJ9
ØSREØJA
ØSREØJZ
ØSRSØ19
ØSRSØ1A
ØSRSØ1Z
ØSRSØ39
ØSRSØ3A
ØSRSØ3Z
ØSRSØJ9
ØSRSØJA
ØSRSØJZ
OR
ØSPBØ8Z
ØSPBØ9Z
ØSPBØBZ
ØSPB48Z
ØSPB4JZ
ØSPE4JZ
ØSPS4JZ
AND
ØSUBØ9Z
ØSUEØ9Z
ØSUSØ9Z
OR
ØSPCØJC
ØSPCØJZ
ØSPCØLZ
ØSPCØMZ
ØSPCØNZ
ØSPC4JC
ØSPC4JZ
ØSPC4LZ
ØSPC4MZ
ØSPC4NZ
ØSPTØJZ
ØSPT4JZ
ØSPVØJZ
ØSPV4JZ
AND
ØSRTØJ9
ØSRTØJA
ØSRVØJ9
ØSRVØJA
ØSRVØJZ
OR
ØSPCØ9Z
AND
ØSRCØ69
ØSRCØ6A
ØSRCØ6Z
ØSRCØJ9
ØSRCØJA
ØSRCØJZ
ØSRCØL9
ØSRCØLA
ØSRCØLZ
ØSRCØM9
ØSRCØMA
ØSRCØMZ
ØSRCØN9
ØSRCØNA
ØSRCØNZ
ØSRTØJ9
ØSRTØJA
ØSRTØJZ
ØSRVØJ9
ØSRVØJA
ØSRVØJZ
XRRGØL8
XRRGØM8
OR
ØSPDØ9Z
AND
ØSRDØ69
ØSRDØ6A
ØSRDØ6Z
ØSRDØJ9
ØSRDØJA
ØSRDØJZ
ØSRDØL9
ØSRDØLA
ØSRDØLZ
ØSRDØM9
ØSRDØMA
ØSRDØMZ
ØSRDØN9
ØSRDØNA
ØSRDØNZ
ØSRUØJ9
ØSRUØJA
ØSRUØJZ
ØSRWØJ9
ØSRWØJA
ØSRWØJZ
XRRHØL8
XRRHØM8
OR
ØSPDØJC
ØSPDØJZ
ØSPDØLZ
ØSPDØMZ
ØSPDØNZ
ØSPD4JC
ØSPD4JZ
ØSPD4LZ
ØSPD4MZ
ØSPD4NZ
ØSPUØJZ
ØSPU4JZ
ØSPWØJZ
ØSPW4JZ
AND
ØSRUØJ9
ØSRUØJA
ØSRWØJ9
ØSRWØJA
ØSRWØJZ
OR

Nonoperating Room Procedures

DØ2*
D72*
D82*
D92*
DB2*
DD2*
DF2*
DG2*
DM2*
DT2*
DU2*
DV2*
DW2*

DRG 629

Select operating room procedures OR procedure combinations OR nonoperating room procedures listed under DRG 628

DRG 630

Select operating room procedures OR procedure combinations OR nonoperating room procedures listed under DRG 628

DRG 637

Principal Diagnosis

EØ8.Ø*
EØ8.1*
EØ8.618
EØ8.62*
EØ8.63*
EØ8.64*
EØ8.65
EØ8.69
EØ8.8
EØ8.9
EØ9.Ø*
EØ9.1*
EØ9.618
EØ9.62*
EØ9.63*
EØ9.64*
EØ9.65
EØ9.69
EØ9.8
EØ9.9
E1Ø.1*
E1Ø.618
E1Ø.62*
E1Ø.63*
E1Ø.64*
E1Ø.65
E1Ø.69
E1Ø.8
E1Ø.9
E11.Ø*
E11.1Ø
E11.11
E11.618
E11.62*
E11.63*
E11.64*
E11.65
E11.69
E11.8
E11.9
E13.Ø*
E13.1*
E13.618
E13.62*
E13.63*
E13.64*
E13.65
E13.69
E13.8
E13.9
R81

DRG 638

Select principal diagnosis listed under DRG 637

DRG 639

Select principal diagnosis listed under DRG 637

DRG 640

Principal Diagnosis

D81.818
D81.819
E15
E16.2
E2Ø.1
E4Ø
E41
E42
E43
E44*
E45
E46
E5Ø.8
E5Ø.9
E51*
E52
E53*
E54
E55.9
E56*
E58
E59
E6Ø
E61*
E63*
E64.Ø
E64.1
E64.2
E64.8
E64.9
E65
E66.Ø*
E66.1
E66.3
E66.8
E66.9
E67*
E68
E83.4*
E83.5*
E83.81
E84.8
E84.9
E86*
E87*
E89.1
P92.6
R29.Ø
R62*
R63*
R73*
R82.4
Z68.4*

DRG 641

Select principal diagnosis listed under DRG 640

DRG 642

Principal Diagnosis

C96.5
C96.6
D81.3*
D81.5
D81.81Ø
D84.1
E7Ø*
E71*
E72*
E74.Ø*
E74.2*
E74.4
E74.8*
E74.9
E75.21
E75.22
E75.24*
E75.3
E75.5
E75.6
E76*
E77*
E78.Ø*
E78.1
E78.2
E78.3
E78.4*
E78.5
E78.6
E78.7Ø
E78.79
E78.8*
E78.9
E79.1
E79.2
E79.8*
E79.9
E8Ø.Ø
E8Ø.1
E8Ø.2*
E8Ø.3
E83.Ø*
E83.1*
E83.3*
E83.89
E83.9
E88.Ø1
E88.1
E88.2
E88.4*
E88.8*
E88.9
E88.A
H49.81*

DRG 643

Principal Diagnosis

A18.7
A18.81
B67.31
C73
C74*
C75.Ø
C75.1
C75.2
C75.8
C75.9
C79.7*
D13.7
D34
D35.Ø*
D35.1
D35.2
D35.3
D35.7
D35.9
D44.Ø
D44.1*
D44.2
D44.3
D44.4
D44.9
D49.7
EØØ*
EØ1*
EØ2
EØ3.Ø
EØ3.1
EØ3.2
EØ3.3
EØ3.4
EØ3.8
EØ3.9
EØ4*
EØ5*
EØ6*
EØ7.Ø
EØ7.1
EØ7.89
EØ7.9
E16.Ø
E16.1
E16.3
E16.8
E16.9
E2Ø.Ø
E2Ø.8*
E2Ø.9
E21*
E22*
E23*
E24*
E25*
E26*
E27*
E29*
E3Ø*
E31*
E34*
E35
E89.Ø
E89.2
E89.3
E89.5
E89.6
Q89.1
Q89.2
R94.6
R94.7
S11.1ØXA
S11.11XA
S11.12XA
S11.13XA
S11.14XA
S11.15XA
S37.812A
S37.813A
S37.818A
S37.819A

DRG 644

Select principal diagnosis listed under DRG 643

DRG 645

Select principal diagnosis listed under DRG 643

MDC 11

DRG 650
Operating Room Procedures
ØTYØØZØ
ØTYØØZ1
ØTYØØZ2
ØTY1ØZØ
ØTY1ØZ1
ØTY1ØZ2
AND
Nonoperating Room Procedures
5A1D7ØZ
5A1D8ØZ
5A1D9ØZ

DRG 651
Select operating room procedure AND nonoperating room procedure under DRG 650

DRG 652
Operating Room Procedures
ØTY*

DRG 653
Operating Room Procedures
ØDX8ØZB
ØDX84ZB
ØDXEØZB
ØDXE4ZB
ØJUC*
ØT1BØ79
ØT1BØ7C
ØT1BØ7D
ØT1BØJ9
ØT1BØJC
ØT1BØJD
ØT1BØK9
ØT1BØKC
ØT1BØKD
ØT1BØZ9
ØT1BØZC
ØT1B3JD
ØT1B479
ØT1B47C
ØT1B47D
ØT1B4J9
ØT1B4JC
ØT1B4JD
ØT1B4K9
ØT1B4KC
ØT1B4KD
ØT1B4Z9
ØT1B4ZC
ØT7BØDZ
ØT7BØZZ
ØT7B3DZ
ØT7B3ZZ
ØT7B4DZ
ØT7B4ZZ
ØT7B8DZ
ØT7B8ZZ
ØTBBØZZ
ØTBB3ZZ
ØTBB4ZZ
ØTBCØZZ
ØTBC3ZZ
ØTBC4ZZ
ØTMB*
ØTMC*
ØTQB*
ØTQCØZZ
ØTQC3ZZ
ØTQC4ZZ
ØTQC7ZZ
ØTQC8ZZ
ØTRB*
ØTRC*
ØTSB*
ØTTB*
ØTTC*
ØTUB*
ØTVB*
ØTVC*

DRG 654
Select operating room procedures listed under DRG 653

DRG 655
Select operating room procedures listed under DRG 653

DRG 656
Principal Diagnosis
C64*
C65*
C66*
C67*
C68*
C79.Ø*
C79.1*
C7A.Ø93
DØ9.Ø
DØ9.1*
D17.71
D17.72
D3Ø*
D3A.Ø93
D41*
D49.4
D49.5*
AND
Operating Room Procedures
41ØØ93
41ØØ94
41ØØ95
Ø41ØØA3
Ø41ØØA4
Ø41ØØA5
Ø41ØØJ1
Ø41ØØJ2
Ø41ØØJ3
Ø41ØØJ4
Ø41ØØJ5
Ø41ØØK3
Ø41ØØK4
Ø41ØØK5
Ø41ØØZ1
Ø41ØØZ2
Ø41ØØZ3
Ø41ØØZ4
Ø41ØØZ5
41Ø493
41Ø494
41Ø495
Ø41Ø4A3
Ø41Ø4A4
Ø41Ø4A5
Ø41Ø4J3
Ø41Ø4J4
Ø41Ø4J5
Ø41Ø4K3
Ø41Ø4K4
Ø41Ø4K5
Ø41Ø4Z3
Ø41Ø4Z4
Ø41Ø4Z5
413Ø93
413Ø94
413Ø95
Ø413ØA3
Ø413ØA4
Ø413ØA5
Ø413ØJ3
Ø413ØJ4
Ø413ØJ5
Ø413ØK3
Ø413ØK4
Ø413ØK5
Ø413ØZ3
Ø413ØZ4
Ø413ØZ5
413493
413494
413495
Ø4134A3
Ø4134A4
Ø4134A5
Ø4134J3
Ø4134J4
Ø4134J5
Ø4134K3
Ø4134K4
Ø4134K5
Ø4134Z3
Ø4134Z4
Ø4134Z5
Ø41CØJ3
Ø41CØJ4
Ø41CØJ5
Ø41CØZ3
Ø41CØZ4
Ø41CØZ5
Ø41C4J3
Ø41C4J4
Ø41C4J5
Ø41C4Z3
Ø41C4Z4
Ø41C4Z5
Ø41DØJ3
Ø41DØJ4
Ø41DØJ5
Ø41DØZ3
Ø41DØZ4
Ø41DØZ5
Ø41D4J3
Ø41D4J4
Ø41D4J5
Ø41D4Z3
Ø41D4Z4
Ø41D4Z5
Ø4S9*
Ø4SA*
Ø6S9*
Ø6SB*
Ø7T8*
Ø7T9*
Ø7TC*
Ø7TD*
Ø7TH*
Ø7TJ*
ØDX8ØZC
ØDX8ØZD
ØDX8ØZF
ØDX84ZC
ØDX84ZD
ØDX84ZF
ØT13*
ØT14*
ØT16*
ØT17*
ØT18*
ØT5Ø*
ØT51*
ØT53*
ØT54*
ØT56*
ØT57*
ØT73*
ØT74*
ØT76ØZZ
ØT763ZZ
ØT764ZZ
ØT768DZ
ØT768ZZ
ØT77ØZZ
ØT773ZZ
ØT774ZZ
ØT778DZ
ØT778ZZ
ØT78ØZZ
ØT783ZZ
ØT784ZZ
ØT788DZ
ØT82*
ØT9ØØØZ
ØT9ØØZX
ØT9ØØZZ
ØT9Ø4ØZ
ØT9Ø7ØZ
ØT9Ø7ZZ
ØT9Ø8ØZ
ØT9Ø8ZZ
ØT91ØØZ
ØT91ØZX
ØT91ØZZ
ØT914ØZ
ØT917ØZ
ØT917ZZ
ØT918ØZ
ØT918ZZ
ØT93ØØZ
ØT93ØZX
ØT93ØZZ
ØT934ØZ
ØT937ØZ
ØT937ZZ
ØT938ØZ
ØT938ZZ
ØT94ØØZ
ØT94ØZX
ØT94ØZZ
ØT944ØZ
ØT947ØZ
ØT947ZZ
ØT948ØZ
ØT948ZZ
ØT96ØZX
ØT96ØZZ
ØT964ZZ
ØT967ZZ
ØT968ZZ
ØT97ØZX
ØT97ØZZ
ØT974ZZ
ØT977ZZ
ØT978ZZ
ØT98ØZX
ØT98ØZZ
ØT984ZZ
ØT987ZZ
ØT988ZZ
ØTBØØZX
ØTBØØZZ
ØTBØ3ZZ
ØTBØ4ZZ
ØTBØ7ZZ
ØTBØ8ZZ
ØTB1ØZX
ØTB1ØZZ
ØTB13ZZ
ØTB14ZZ
ØTB17ZZ
ØTB18ZZ
ØTB3ØZX
ØTB3ØZZ
ØTB33ZZ
ØTB34ZZ
ØTB37ZZ
ØTB38ZZ
ØTB4ØZX
ØTB4ØZZ
ØTB43ZZ
ØTB44ZZ
ØTB47ZZ
ØTB48ZZ
ØTB6ØZX
ØTB6ØZZ
ØTB63ZZ
ØTB64ZZ
ØTB67ZZ
ØTB68ZZ
ØTB7ØZX
ØTB7ØZZ
ØTB73ZZ
ØTB74ZZ
ØTB77ZZ
ØTB78ZZ
ØTCØØZZ
ØTCØ3ZZ
ØTCØ4ZZ
ØTCØ7ZZ
ØTC1ØZZ
ØTC13ZZ
ØTC14ZZ
ØTC17ZZ
ØTC3ØZZ
ØTC33ZZ
ØTC34ZZ
ØTC4ØZZ
ØTC43ZZ
ØTC44ZZ
ØTC6ØZZ
ØTC63ZZ
ØTC64ZZ
ØTC7ØZZ
ØTC73ZZ
ØTC74ZZ
ØTDØ*
ØTD1*
ØTF33ZZ
ØTF34ZZ
ØTF43ZZ
ØTF44ZZ
ØTH5Ø1Z
ØTH5Ø2Z
ØTH5ØYZ
ØTH532Z
ØTH541Z
ØTH542Z
ØTH581Z
ØTH58YZ
ØTH9Ø1Z
ØTH9Ø2Z
ØTH9ØMZ
ØTH9ØYZ
ØTH932Z
ØTH93MZ
ØTH941Z
ØTH942Z
ØTH94MZ
ØTH97MZ
ØTH981Z
ØTH98MZ
ØTH98YZ
ØTJ5ØZZ
ØTJ9ØZZ
ØTL3*
ØTL4*
ØTL6*
ØTL7*
ØTMØ*
ØTM1*
ØTM2*
ØTM3*
ØTM4*
ØTM6*
ØTM7*
ØTM8*
ØTNØ*
ØTN1*
ØTN3*
ØTN4*
ØTN6*
ØTN7*
ØTP5ØØZ
ØTP5Ø2Z
ØTP5Ø3Z
ØTP5Ø7Z
ØTP5ØCZ
ØTP5ØDZ
ØTP5ØJZ
ØTP5ØKZ
ØTP5ØYZ
ØTP53ØZ
ØTP532Z
ØTP533Z
ØTP537Z
ØTP53CZ
ØTP53DZ
ØTP53JZ
ØTP53KZ
ØTP54ØZ
ØTP542Z
ØTP543Z
ØTP547Z
ØTP54CZ
ØTP54DZ
ØTP54JZ
ØTP54KZ
ØTP577Z
ØTP57CZ
ØTP57JZ
ØTP57KZ
ØTP587Z
ØTP58CZ
ØTP58JZ
ØTP58KZ
ØTP58YZ
ØTP9ØØZ
ØTP9Ø2Z
ØTP9Ø3Z
ØTP9Ø7Z
ØTP9ØCZ
ØTP9ØDZ
ØTP9ØJZ
ØTP9ØKZ
ØTP9ØMZ
ØTP9ØYZ
ØTP93ØZ
ØTP932Z
ØTP933Z
ØTP937Z
ØTP93CZ
ØTP93DZ
ØTP93JZ
ØTP93KZ
ØTP93MZ
ØTP94ØZ
ØTP942Z
ØTP943Z
ØTP947Z
ØTP94CZ
ØTP94DZ
ØTP94JZ
ØTP94KZ
ØTP94MZ
ØTP977Z
ØTP97CZ
ØTP97JZ
ØTP97KZ
ØTP97MZ
ØTP987Z
ØTP98CZ
ØTP98JZ
ØTP98KZ
ØTP98MZ
ØTP98YZ
ØTP9XMZ
ØTQØ*
ØTQ1*
ØTQ3*
ØTQ4*
ØTQ6*
ØTQ7*
ØTR3*
ØTR4*
ØTR6*
ØTR7*
ØTSØ*
ØTS1*
ØTS2*
ØTS3*
ØTS4*
ØTS6*
ØTS7*
ØTS8*
ØTTØ*
ØTT1*
ØTT2*
ØTT3*
ØTT4*
ØTT6*
ØTT7*
ØTU3*
ØTU4*
ØTU6*
ØTU7*
ØTV3*
ØTV4*
ØTV6*
ØTV7*
ØTW5ØØZ
ØTW5Ø2Z
ØTW5Ø3Z
ØTW5Ø7Z
ØTW5ØCZ
ØTW5ØDZ
ØTW5ØJZ
ØTW5ØKZ
ØTW5ØYZ
ØTW53ØZ
ØTW532Z
ØTW533Z
ØTW537Z
ØTW53CZ
ØTW53DZ
ØTW53JZ
ØTW53KZ
ØTW54ØZ
ØTW542Z
ØTW543Z
ØTW547Z
ØTW54CZ
ØTW54DZ
ØTW54JZ
ØTW54KZ
ØTW57ØZ
ØTW572Z
ØTW573Z
ØTW577Z
ØTW57CZ
ØTW57DZ
ØTW57JZ
ØTW57KZ
ØTW58ØZ
ØTW582Z
ØTW583Z
ØTW587Z
ØTW58CZ
ØTW58DZ
ØTW58JZ
ØTW58KZ
ØTW58YZ
ØTW9ØØZ
ØTW9Ø2Z
ØTW9Ø3Z
ØTW9Ø7Z
ØTW9ØCZ
ØTW9ØDZ
ØTW9ØJZ
ØTW9ØKZ
ØTW9ØMZ
ØTW9ØYZ
ØTW93ØZ
ØTW932Z
ØTW933Z
ØTW937Z
ØTW93CZ
ØTW93DZ
ØTW93JZ
ØTW93KZ
ØTW93MZ
ØTW94ØZ
ØTW942Z
ØTW943Z
ØTW947Z
ØTW94CZ
ØTW94DZ
ØTW94JZ
ØTW94KZ
ØTW94MZ
ØTW97ØZ
ØTW972Z
ØTW973Z
ØTW977Z
ØTW97CZ
ØTW97DZ
ØTW97JZ
ØTW97KZ
ØTW97MZ
ØTW98ØZ
ØTW982Z
ØTW983Z
ØTW987Z
ØTW98CZ
ØTW98DZ
ØTW98JZ
ØTW98KZ
ØTW98MZ
ØTW98YZ
ØWBHØZZ
ØWBH3ZZ
ØWBH4ZZ
ØWQFØZZ
ØWQF3ZZ
ØWQF4ZZ

DRG 657
Select principal diagnosis AND operating room procedures listed under DRG 656

DRG 658
Select principal diagnosis AND operating room procedures listed under DRG 656

DRG 659
Select only operating room procedures listed under DRG 656

DRG 660
Select only operating room procedures listed under DRG 656

DRG 661
Select only operating room procedures listed under DRG 656

DRG 662
Operating Room Procedures
ØJQCØZZ
ØT1BØZD
ØT1B4ZD
ØT5BØZZ
ØT5B3ZZ
ØT5B4ZZ
ØT5CØZZ
ØT5C3ZZ
ØT5C4ZZ
ØT8C*
ØT9BØØZ
ØT9BØZX
ØT9BØZZ
ØT9CØØZ
ØT9CØZX
ØT9CØZZ
ØTBBØZX
ØTBCØZX
ØTCBØZZ
ØTCB3ZZ
ØTCB4ZZ
ØTCCØZZ
ØTCC3ZZ
ØTCC4ZZ
ØTHBØ1Z
ØTHBØ2Z
ØTHBØLZ
ØTHBØMZ
ØTHBØYZ
ØTHB32Z
ØTHB3LZ
ØTHB3MZ
ØTHB41Z
ØTHB42Z
ØTHB4LZ
ØTHB4MZ
ØTHB7LZ
ØTHB7MZ
ØTHB81Z
ØTHB8LZ
ØTHB8MZ
ØTHB8YZ
ØTHC*
ØTHDØLZ
ØTHD3LZ
ØTHD4LZ
ØTHD7LZ
ØTHD8LZ
ØTHDXLZ
ØTJBØZZ
ØTJB4ZZ
ØTLB*
ØTLC*
ØTNBØZZ
ØTNB3ZZ
ØTNB4ZZ
ØTNCØZZ
ØTNC3ZZ
ØTNC4ZZ
ØTPBØØZ
ØTPBØ2Z
ØTPBØ3Z
ØTPBØ7Z
ØTPBØCZ
ØTPBØDZ
ØTPBØJZ
ØTPBØKZ
ØTPBØLZ
ØTPBØMZ
ØTPBØYZ
ØTPB3ØZ
ØTPB32Z
ØTPB33Z
ØTPB37Z
ØTPB3CZ
ØTPB3DZ
ØTPB3JZ
ØTPB3KZ
ØTPB3LZ
ØTPB3MZ
ØTPB4ØZ
ØTPB42Z
ØTPB43Z
ØTPB47Z
ØTPB4CZ
ØTPB4DZ
ØTPB4JZ
ØTPB4KZ
ØTPB4LZ
ØTPB4MZ
ØTPB77Z
ØTPB7CZ
ØTPB7JZ
ØTPB7KZ
ØTPB7LZ
ØTPB7MZ
ØTPB87Z
ØTPB8CZ
ØTPB8JZ
ØTPB8KZ
ØTPB8LZ
ØTPB8MZ
ØTPB8YZ
ØTPBXMZ
ØTQDØZZ
ØTQD3ZZ
ØTQD4ZZ
ØTSC*
ØTSD*
ØTUC*
ØTWBØØZ
ØTWBØ2Z
ØTWBØ3Z
ØTWBØ7Z
ØTWBØCZ
ØTWBØDZ
ØTWBØJZ
ØTWBØKZ
ØTWBØLZ
ØTWBØMZ
ØTWBØYZ
ØTWB3ØZ
ØTWB32Z
ØTWB33Z
ØTWB37Z
ØTWB3CZ
ØTWB3DZ
ØTWB3JZ
ØTWB3KZ
ØTWB3LZ
ØTWB3MZ
ØTWB4ØZ
ØTWB42Z
ØTWB43Z
ØTWB47Z
ØTWB4CZ
ØTWB4DZ
ØTWB4JZ
ØTWB4KZ
ØTWB4LZ
ØTWB4MZ
ØTWB7ØZ
ØTWB72Z
ØTWB73Z
ØTWB77Z
ØTWB7CZ
ØTWB7DZ
ØTWB7JZ
ØTWB7KZ
ØTWB7LZ
ØTWB7MZ
ØTWB8ØZ
ØTWB82Z
ØTWB83Z
ØTWB87Z
ØTWB8CZ
ØTWB8DZ
ØTWB8JZ
ØTWB8KZ
ØTWB8LZ
ØTWB8MZ
ØTWB8YZ
ØUSG*
ØVXTØZD
ØW3R*
ØWQFXZ2
ØWQFXZZ
OR
ØTQBØZZ
ØTQB3ZZ
ØTQB4ZZ
AND
ØWQFXZ2
ØWQFXZZ

DRG 663
Select operating room procedures or procedure combination listed under DRG 662

DRG 664
Select operating room procedures or procedure combination listed under DRG 662

DRG 665
Operating Room Procedures

ØV5Ø*
ØVBØ7ZZ
ØVBØ8ZZ
ØVTØ*
OR
ØVTØ*
AND
ØVT3*

DRG 666
Select operating room procedures or procedure combination listed under DRG 665

DRG 667
Select operating room procedures or procedure combination listed under DRG 665

DRG 668
Operating Room Procedures

ØT5B7ZZ
ØT5B8ZZ
ØT5C7ZZ
ØT5C8ZZ
ØT9B3ZX
ØT9B4ZX
ØT9B7ZX
ØT9B8ZX
ØT9C3ZX
ØT9C4ZX
ØT9C7ZX
ØT9C8ZX
ØTBB3ZX
ØTBB4ZX
ØTBB7ZX
ØTBB7ZZ
ØTBB8ZX
ØTBB8ZZ
ØTBC3ZX
ØTBC4ZX
ØTBC7ZX
ØTBC7ZZ
ØTBC8ZX
ØTBC8ZZ
ØTC37ZZ
ØTC47ZZ
ØTC67ZZ
ØTC77ZZ
ØTNB7ZZ
ØTNB8ZZ
ØTNC7ZZ
ØTNC8ZZ
ØV9ØØZX
ØVBØØZX

DRG 669
Select operating room procedures listed under DRG 668

DRG 670
Select operating room procedures listed under DRG 668

DRG 671
Operating Room Procedures

ØT7DØZZ
ØT7D3ZZ
ØT7D4ZZ
ØT9DØØZ
ØT9DØZZ
ØT9D4ØZ
ØT9D4ZZ
ØT9D7ØZ
ØT9D7ZZ
ØT9D8ØZ
ØT9D8ZZ
ØT9DXØZ
ØT9DXZZ
ØTBDØZZ
ØTBD3ZZ
ØTBD4ZZ
ØTBD7ZZ
ØTBD8ZZ
ØTBDXZZ
ØTCDØZZ
ØTCD3ZZ
ØTCD4ZZ
ØTHDØ1Z
ØTHDØ2Z
ØTHDØYZ
ØTHD32Z
ØTHD41Z
ØTHD42Z
ØTHD81Z
ØTHDX2Z
ØTJDØZZ
ØTLD*
ØTMD*
ØTND*
ØTPDØØZ
ØTPDØ2Z
ØTPDØ3Z
ØTPDØ7Z
ØTPDØCZ
ØTPDØDZ
ØTPDØJZ
ØTPDØKZ
ØTPDØLZ
ØTPDØYZ
ØTPD3ØZ
ØTPD32Z
ØTPD33Z
ØTPD37Z
ØTPD3CZ
ØTPD3DZ
ØTPD3JZ
ØTPD3KZ
ØTPD3LZ
ØTPD4ØZ
ØTPD42Z
ØTPD43Z
ØTPD47Z
ØTPD4CZ
ØTPD4DZ
ØTPD4JZ
ØTPD4KZ
ØTPD4LZ
ØTPD77Z
ØTPD7CZ
ØTPD7JZ
ØTPD7KZ
ØTPD7LZ
ØTPD87Z
ØTPD8CZ
ØTPD8JZ
ØTPD8KZ
ØTPD8LZ
ØTPDXLZ
ØTQD7ZZ
ØTQD8ZZ
ØTQDXZZ
ØTRD*
ØTUD*
ØTVD*
ØTWDØØZ
ØTWDØ2Z
ØTWDØ3Z
ØTWDØ7Z
ØTWDØCZ
ØTWDØDZ
ØTWDØJZ
ØTWDØKZ
ØTWDØLZ
ØTWDØYZ
ØTWD3ØZ
ØTWD32Z
ØTWD33Z
ØTWD37Z
ØTWD3CZ
ØTWD3DZ
ØTWD3JZ
ØTWD3KZ
ØTWD3LZ
ØTWD4ØZ
ØTWD42Z
ØTWD43Z
ØTWD47Z
ØTWD4CZ
ØTWD4DZ
ØTWD4JZ
ØTWD4KZ
ØTWD4LZ
ØTWD7ØZ
ØTWD72Z
ØTWD73Z
ØTWD77Z
ØTWD7CZ
ØTWD7DZ
ØTWD7JZ
ØTWD7KZ
ØTWD7LZ
ØTWD8ØZ
ØTWD82Z
ØTWD83Z
ØTWD87Z
ØTWD8CZ
ØTWD8DZ
ØTWD8JZ
ØTWD8KZ
ØTWD8LZ
ØVXTXZD

DRG 672
Select operating room procedures listed under DRG 671

DRG 673
Operating Room Procedures

ØØHEØMZ
ØØHE3MZ
ØØHE4MZ
ØØHUØMZ
ØØHU3MZ
ØØHU4MZ
ØØHVØMZ
ØØHV3MZ
ØØHV4MZ
ØØPUØMZ
ØØPU3MZ
ØØPU4MZ
ØØPVØMZ
ØØPV3MZ
ØØPV4MZ
Ø1HYØMZ
Ø1HY3MZ
Ø1HY4MZ
Ø2HVØ2Z
Ø2HVØDZ
Ø2HV3DZ
Ø2HV42Z
Ø2HV4DZ
Ø2JAØZZ
Ø2JYØZZ
Ø2LV*
Ø2UW3JZ
Ø2UW4JZ
Ø2UX3JZ
Ø2UX4JZ
Ø2VV*
Ø2VWØDZ
Ø2VWØEZ
Ø2VWØFZ
Ø2VW3DZ
Ø2VW3EZ
Ø2VW3FZ
Ø2VW4DZ
Ø2VW4EZ
Ø2VW4FZ
Ø2VXØDZ
Ø2VXØEZ
Ø2VXØFZ
Ø2VX3DZ
Ø2VX3EZ
Ø2VX3FZ
Ø2VX4DZ
Ø2VX4EZ
Ø2VX4FZ
Ø313ØZD
Ø314ØZD
Ø315ØZD
Ø315ØZT
Ø315ØZV
Ø316ØZD
Ø316ØZT
Ø316ØZV
Ø317Ø9D
Ø317Ø9F
Ø317Ø9V
Ø317ØAD
Ø317ØAF
Ø317ØAV
Ø317ØJD
Ø317ØJF
Ø317ØJV
Ø317ØKD
Ø317ØKF
Ø317ØKV
Ø317ØZD
Ø317ØZF
Ø317ØZV
Ø3173ZF
Ø318Ø9D
Ø318Ø9F
Ø318Ø9V
Ø318ØAD
Ø318ØAF
Ø318ØAV
Ø318ØJD
Ø318ØJF
Ø318ØJV
Ø318ØKD
Ø318ØKF
Ø318ØKV
Ø318ØZD
Ø318ØZF
Ø318ØZV
Ø3183ZF
Ø319Ø9F
Ø319ØAF
Ø319ØJF
Ø319ØKF
Ø319ØZF
Ø3193ZF
Ø31AØ9F
Ø31AØAF
Ø31AØJF
Ø31AØKF
Ø31AØZF
Ø31A3ZF
Ø31BØ9F
Ø31BØAF
Ø31BØJF
Ø31BØKF
Ø31BØZF
Ø31B3ZF
Ø31CØ9F
Ø31CØAF
Ø31CØJF
Ø31CØKF
Ø31CØZF
Ø31C3ZF
Ø37334Z
Ø37335Z
Ø37336Z
Ø37337Z
Ø3733D1
Ø3733DZ
Ø3733EZ
Ø3733FZ
Ø3733GZ
Ø3733Z1
Ø3733ZZ
Ø37434Z
Ø37435Z
Ø37436Z
Ø37437Z
Ø3743D1
Ø3743DZ
Ø3743EZ
Ø3743FZ
Ø3743GZ
Ø3743Z1
Ø3743ZZ
Ø37734Z
Ø37735Z
Ø37736Z
Ø37737Z
Ø3773D1
Ø3773DZ
Ø3773EZ
Ø3773FZ
Ø3773GZ
Ø3773Z1
Ø3773ZZ
Ø37834Z
Ø37835Z
Ø37836Z
Ø37837Z
Ø3783D1
Ø3783DZ
Ø3783EZ
Ø3783FZ
Ø3783GZ
Ø3783Z1
Ø3783ZZ
Ø37934Z
Ø37935Z
Ø37936Z
Ø37937Z
Ø3793D1
Ø3793DZ
Ø3793EZ
Ø3793FZ
Ø3793GZ
Ø3793Z1
Ø3793ZZ
Ø37A34Z
Ø37A35Z
Ø37A36Z
Ø37A37Z
Ø37A3D1
Ø37A3DZ
Ø37A3EZ
Ø37A3FZ
Ø37A3GZ
Ø37A3Z1
Ø37A3ZZ
Ø37Y34Z
Ø37Y35Z
Ø37Y36Z
Ø37Y37Z
Ø37Y3DZ
Ø37Y3EZ
Ø37Y3FZ
Ø37Y3GZ
Ø37Y3ZZ
Ø39SØZX
Ø39S4ZX
Ø39TØZX
Ø39T4ZX
Ø3BSØZX
Ø3BS3ZX
Ø3BS4ZX
Ø3BTØZX
Ø3BT3ZX
Ø3BT4ZX
Ø3CY*
Ø3LGØBZ
Ø3LGØDZ
Ø3LG3BZ
Ø3LG3DZ
Ø3LG4BZ
Ø3LG4DZ
Ø3LHØBZ
Ø3LHØDZ
Ø3LH3BZ
Ø3LH3DZ
Ø3LH4BZ
Ø3LH4DZ
Ø3LJØBZ
Ø3LJØDZ
Ø3LJ3BZ
Ø3LJ3DZ
Ø3LJ4BZ
Ø3LJ4DZ
Ø3LKØBZ
Ø3LKØDZ
Ø3LK3BZ
Ø3LK3DZ
Ø3LK4BZ
Ø3LK4DZ
Ø3LLØBZ
Ø3LLØDZ
Ø3LL3BZ
Ø3LL3DZ
Ø3LL4BZ
Ø3LL4DZ
Ø3LMØBZ
Ø3LMØDZ
Ø3LM3BZ
Ø3LM3DZ
Ø3LM4BZ
Ø3LM4DZ
Ø3LNØBZ
Ø3LNØDZ
Ø3LN3BZ
Ø3LN3DZ
Ø3LN4BZ
Ø3LN4DZ
Ø3LPØBZ
Ø3LPØDZ
Ø3LP3BZ
Ø3LP3DZ
Ø3LP4BZ
Ø3LP4DZ
Ø3LQØBZ
Ø3LQØDZ
Ø3LQ3BZ
Ø3LQ3DZ
Ø3LQ4BZ
Ø3LQ4DZ
Ø3LRØDZ
Ø3LR3DZ
Ø3LR4DZ
Ø3LSØDZ
Ø3LS3DZ
Ø3LS4DZ
Ø3LTØDZ
Ø3LT3DZ
Ø3LT4DZ
Ø3PYØ7Z
Ø3PYØJZ
Ø3PYØKZ
Ø3PY37Z
Ø3PY3JZ
Ø3PY3KZ
Ø3PY47Z
Ø3PY4JZ
Ø3PY4KZ
Ø3QY*
Ø3VGØBZ
Ø3VGØDZ
Ø3VGØHZ
Ø3VG3BZ
Ø3VG3DZ
Ø3VG3HZ
Ø3VG4BZ
Ø3VG4DZ
Ø3VG4HZ
Ø3VHØBZ
Ø3VHØDZ
Ø3VH3BZ
Ø3VH3DZ
Ø3VH4BZ
Ø3VH4DZ
Ø3VJØBZ
Ø3VJØDZ
Ø3VJ3BZ
Ø3VJ3DZ
Ø3VJ4BZ
Ø3VJ4DZ
Ø3VKØBZ
Ø3VKØDZ
Ø3VK3BZ
Ø3VK3DZ
Ø3VK4BZ
Ø3VK4DZ
Ø3VLØBZ
Ø3VLØDZ
Ø3VL3BZ
Ø3VL3DZ
Ø3VL4BZ
Ø3VL4DZ
Ø3VMØBZ
Ø3VMØDZ
Ø3VM3BZ
Ø3VM3DZ
Ø3VM4BZ
Ø3VM4DZ
Ø3VNØBZ
Ø3VNØDZ
Ø3VN3BZ
Ø3VN3DZ
Ø3VN4BZ
Ø3VN4DZ
Ø3VPØBZ
Ø3VPØDZ
Ø3VP3BZ
Ø3VP3DZ
Ø3VP4BZ
Ø3VP4DZ
Ø3VQØBZ
Ø3VQØDZ
Ø3VQ3BZ
Ø3VQ3DZ
Ø3VQ4BZ
Ø3VQ4DZ
Ø3VRØDZ
Ø3VR3DZ
Ø3VR4DZ
Ø3VSØDZ
Ø3VS3DZ
Ø3VS4DZ
Ø3VTØDZ
Ø3VT3DZ
Ø3VT4DZ
Ø3VUØDZ
Ø3VU3DZ
Ø3VU4DZ
Ø3VVØDZ
Ø3VV3DZ
Ø3VV4DZ
Ø3WYØJZ
Ø3WY3JZ
Ø3WY4JZ
Ø459*
Ø45A*
47Ø341
Ø47Ø34Z
Ø47Ø35Z
Ø47Ø36Z
Ø47Ø37Z
Ø47Ø3D1
Ø47Ø3DZ
Ø47Ø3EZ
Ø47Ø3FZ
Ø47Ø3GZ
Ø47Ø3Z1
Ø47Ø3ZZ
471341
Ø47134Z
Ø47135Z
Ø47136Z
Ø47137Z
Ø4713D1
Ø4713DZ
Ø4713EZ
Ø4713FZ
Ø4713GZ
Ø4713Z1
Ø4713ZZ
472341
Ø47234Z
Ø47235Z
Ø47236Z
Ø47237Z
Ø4723D1
Ø4723DZ
Ø4723EZ
Ø4723FZ
Ø4723GZ
Ø4723Z1
Ø4723ZZ
473341
Ø47334Z
Ø47335Z
Ø47336Z
Ø47337Z
Ø4733D1
Ø4733DZ
Ø4733EZ
Ø4733FZ
Ø4733GZ
Ø4733Z1
Ø4733ZZ
474341
Ø47434Z
Ø47435Z
Ø47436Z
Ø47437Z
Ø4743D1
Ø4743DZ
Ø4743EZ
Ø4743FZ
Ø4743GZ
Ø4743Z1
Ø4743ZZ
475341
Ø47534Z
Ø47535Z
Ø47536Z
Ø47537Z
Ø4753D1
Ø4753DZ
Ø4753EZ
Ø4753FZ
Ø4753GZ
Ø4753Z1
Ø4753ZZ
476341
Ø47634Z
Ø47635Z
Ø47636Z
Ø47637Z
Ø4763D1
Ø4763DZ
Ø4763EZ
Ø4763FZ
Ø4763GZ
Ø4763Z1
Ø4763ZZ
477341
Ø47734Z
Ø47735Z
Ø47736Z
Ø47737Z
Ø4773D1
Ø4773DZ
Ø4773EZ
Ø4773FZ
Ø4773GZ
Ø4773Z1
Ø4773ZZ
478341
Ø47834Z
Ø47835Z
Ø47836Z
Ø47837Z
Ø4783D1
Ø4783DZ
Ø4783EZ
Ø4783FZ
Ø4783GZ
Ø4783Z1
Ø4783ZZ
479341
Ø47934Z
Ø47935Z
Ø47936Z
Ø47937Z
Ø4793D1
Ø4793DZ
Ø4793EZ
Ø4793FZ
Ø4793GZ
Ø4793Z1
Ø4793ZZ
Ø47A341
Ø47A34Z
Ø47A35Z
Ø47A36Z
Ø47A37Z
Ø47A3D1
Ø47A3DZ
Ø47A3EZ
Ø47A3FZ
Ø47A3GZ
Ø47A3Z1
Ø47A3ZZ
Ø47B341
Ø47B34Z
Ø47B35Z
Ø47B36Z
Ø47B37Z
Ø47B3D1
Ø47B3DZ
Ø47B3EZ
Ø47B3FZ
Ø47B3GZ
Ø47B3Z1
Ø47B3ZZ
Ø47C341
Ø47C34Z
Ø47C35Z
Ø47C36Z
Ø47C37Z
Ø47C3D1
Ø47C3DZ
Ø47C3EZ
Ø47C3FZ
Ø47C3GZ
Ø47C3Z1
Ø47C3ZZ
Ø47D341
Ø47D34Z
Ø47D35Z
Ø47D36Z
Ø47D37Z
Ø47D3D1
Ø47D3DZ
Ø47D3EZ
Ø47D3FZ
Ø47D3GZ
Ø47D3Z1
Ø47D3ZZ
Ø47E341
Ø47E34Z
Ø47E35Z
Ø47E36Z
Ø47E37Z
Ø47E3D1
Ø47E3DZ
Ø47E3EZ
Ø47E3FZ
Ø47E3GZ
Ø47E3Z1
Ø47E3ZZ
Ø47F341
Ø47F34Z
Ø47F35Z
Ø47F36Z
Ø47F37Z
Ø47F3D1
Ø47F3DZ
Ø47F3EZ
Ø47F3FZ
Ø47F3GZ
Ø47F3Z1
Ø47F3ZZ
Ø47H341
Ø47H34Z
Ø47H35Z
Ø47H36Z
Ø47H37Z
Ø47H3D1
Ø47H3DZ
Ø47H3EZ
Ø47H3FZ
Ø47H3GZ
Ø47H3Z1
Ø47H3ZZ
Ø47J341
Ø47J34Z
Ø47J35Z
Ø47J36Z
Ø47J37Z
Ø47J3D1
Ø47J3DZ
Ø47J3EZ
Ø47J3FZ
Ø47J3GZ
Ø47J3Z1
Ø47J3ZZ
Ø47KØ41
Ø47KØD1
Ø47KØZ1
Ø47K341
Ø47K34Z
Ø47K35Z
Ø47K36Z
Ø47K37Z
Ø47K3D1
Ø47K3DZ
Ø47K3EZ
Ø47K3FZ
Ø47K3GZ
Ø47K3Z1
Ø47K3ZZ
Ø47K441
Ø47K4D1
Ø47K4Z1
Ø47LØ41
Ø47LØD1
Ø47LØZ1
Ø47L341
Ø47L34Z
Ø47L35Z
Ø47L36Z
Ø47L37Z
Ø47L3D1
Ø47L3DZ
Ø47L3EZ
Ø47L3FZ
Ø47L3GZ
Ø47L3Z1
Ø47L3ZZ
Ø47L441
Ø47L4D1
Ø47L4Z1
Ø47MØ41
Ø47MØD1
Ø47MØZ1
Ø47M341
Ø47M3D1
Ø47M3Z1
Ø47M441
Ø47M4D1
Ø47M4Z1
Ø47NØ41
Ø47NØD1
Ø47NØZ1
Ø47N341
Ø47N3D1
Ø47N3Z1
Ø47N441
Ø47N4D1
Ø47N4Z1
Ø47Y341
Ø47Y34Z
Ø47Y35Z
Ø47Y36Z
Ø47Y37Z
Ø47Y3D1
Ø47Y3DZ
Ø47Y3EZ
Ø47Y3FZ
Ø47Y3GZ
Ø47Y3Z1
Ø47Y3ZZ
Ø4B1ØZZ
Ø4B14ZZ
Ø4B2ØZZ
Ø4B24ZZ
Ø4B3ØZZ

Ø4B34ZZ
Ø4B4ØZZ
Ø4B44ZZ
Ø4B5ØZZ
Ø4B54ZZ
Ø4B6ØZZ
Ø4B64ZZ
Ø4B7ØZZ
Ø4B74ZZ
Ø4B8ØZZ
Ø4B84ZZ
Ø4B9ØZZ
Ø4B94ZZ
Ø4BAØZZ
Ø4BA4ZZ
Ø4BBØZZ
Ø4BB4ZZ
Ø4BCØZZ
Ø4BC4ZZ
Ø4BDØZZ
Ø4BD4ZZ
Ø4BEØZZ
Ø4BE4ZZ
Ø4BFØZZ
Ø4BF4ZZ
Ø4BHØZZ
Ø4BH4ZZ
Ø4BJØZZ
Ø4BJ4ZZ
Ø4C1*
Ø4C2*
Ø4C3*
Ø4C4*
Ø4C5*
Ø4C6*
Ø4C7*
Ø4C8*
Ø4C9*
Ø4CA*
Ø4CB*
Ø4CC*
Ø4CD*
Ø4CE*
Ø4CF*
Ø4CH*
Ø4CJ*
Ø4CY*
Ø4L9*
Ø4LA*
Ø4QY*
Ø4R9*
Ø4RA*
Ø4SØ*
Ø4S1*
Ø4S2*
Ø4S3*
Ø4S4*
Ø4S5*
Ø4S6*
Ø4S7*
Ø4S8*
Ø4SB*
Ø4UØ3JZ
Ø4UØ4JZ
Ø4U9Ø7Z
Ø4U9ØJZ
Ø4U937Z
Ø4U93JZ
Ø4U947Z
Ø4U94JZ
Ø4UAØ7Z
Ø4UAØJZ
Ø4UA37Z
Ø4UA3JZ
Ø4UA47Z
Ø4UA4JZ
Ø4VØØDZ
Ø4VØØEZ
Ø4VØØFZ
Ø4VØØZZ
Ø4VØ3DZ
Ø4VØ3EZ
Ø4VØ3FZ
Ø4VØ3ZZ
Ø4VØ4DZ
Ø4VØ4EZ
Ø4VØ4FZ
Ø4VØ4ZZ
Ø4V1ØZZ
Ø4V13ZZ
Ø4V14ZZ
Ø4V2ØZZ
Ø4V23ZZ
Ø4V24ZZ
Ø4V3ØZZ
Ø4V33ZZ
Ø4V34ZZ
Ø4V4ØZZ
Ø4V43ZZ
Ø4V44ZZ
Ø4V5ØZZ
Ø4V53ZZ
Ø4V54ZZ
Ø4V6ØZZ
Ø4V63ZZ
Ø4V64ZZ
Ø4V7ØZZ
Ø4V73ZZ
Ø4V74ZZ
Ø4V8ØZZ
Ø4V83ZZ
Ø4V84ZZ
Ø4V9ØDZ
Ø4V9ØZZ
Ø4V93DZ
Ø4V93ZZ
Ø4V94DZ
Ø4V94ZZ
Ø4VAØDZ
Ø4VAØZZ
Ø4VA3DZ
Ø4VA3ZZ
Ø4VA4DZ
Ø4VA4ZZ
Ø4VBØZZ
Ø4VB3ZZ
Ø4VB4ZZ
Ø5793D1
Ø5793DZ
Ø5793Z1
Ø5793ZZ
Ø57A3D1
Ø57A3DZ
Ø57A3Z1
Ø57A3ZZ
Ø57B3D1
Ø57B3DZ
Ø57B3Z1
Ø57B3ZZ
Ø57C3D1
Ø57C3DZ
Ø57C3Z1
Ø57C3ZZ
Ø57D3D1
Ø57D3DZ
Ø57D3Z1
Ø57D3ZZ
Ø57F3D1
Ø57F3DZ
Ø57F3Z1
Ø57F3ZZ
Ø5CY*
Ø5HØØMZ
Ø5HØ3MZ
Ø5HØ4MZ
Ø5H3ØMZ
Ø5H33MZ
Ø5H34MZ
Ø5H4ØMZ
Ø5H43MZ
Ø5H44MZ
Ø5QY*
Ø5SBØZZ
Ø5SB3ZZ
Ø5SCØZZ
Ø5SC3ZZ
Ø67Ø3DZ
Ø67Ø3ZZ
Ø6C9*
Ø6CB*
Ø6CY*
Ø6HØØDZ
Ø6HØ4DZ
Ø6LØ*
Ø6L9ØCZ
Ø6L9ØZZ
Ø6L93CZ
Ø6L93ZZ
Ø6L94CZ
Ø6L94ZZ
Ø6LBØCZ
Ø6LBØZZ
Ø6LB3CZ
Ø6LB3ZZ
Ø6LB4CZ
Ø6LB4ZZ
Ø6QY*
Ø6SØ*
Ø6S1*
Ø6S2*
Ø6S3*
Ø6S4*
Ø6S5*
Ø6S6*
Ø6S7*
Ø6S8*
Ø6U9Ø7Z
Ø6U9ØJZ
Ø6U937Z
Ø6U93JZ
Ø6U947Z
Ø6U94JZ
Ø6UBØ7Z
Ø6UBØJZ
Ø6UB37Z
Ø6UB3JZ
Ø6UB47Z
Ø6UB4JZ
Ø6VØ*
Ø6V1ØZZ
Ø6V13ZZ
Ø6V14ZZ
Ø6V2ØZZ
Ø6V23ZZ
Ø6V24ZZ
Ø6V3ØZZ
Ø6V33ZZ
Ø6V34ZZ
Ø6V4ØZZ
Ø6V43ZZ
Ø6V44ZZ
Ø6V5ØZZ
Ø6V53ZZ
Ø6V54ZZ
Ø6V6ØZZ
Ø6V63ZZ
Ø6V64ZZ
Ø6V7ØZZ
Ø6V73ZZ
Ø6V74ZZ
Ø6V8ØZZ
Ø6V83ZZ
Ø6V84ZZ
Ø6V9ØDZ
Ø6V9ØZZ
Ø6V93DZ
Ø6V93ZZ
Ø6V94DZ
Ø6V94ZZ
Ø6VBØDZ
Ø6VBØZZ
Ø6VB3DZ
Ø6VB3ZZ
Ø6VB4DZ
Ø6VB4ZZ
Ø79CØZX
Ø79C3ZX
Ø79C4ZX
Ø79DØZX
Ø79D3ZX
Ø79D4ZX
Ø79LØZX
Ø79L3ZX
Ø79L4ZX
Ø7BCØZX
Ø7BC3ZX
Ø7BC4ZX
Ø7BDØZX
Ø7BD3ZX
Ø7BD4ZX
Ø7BHØZZ
Ø7BH3ZZ
Ø7BH4ZZ
Ø7BJØZZ
Ø7BJ3ZZ
Ø7BJ4ZZ
Ø7BLØZX
Ø7BL3ZX
Ø7BL4ZX
Ø7JPØZZ
Ø7TØ*
Ø7T3*
Ø7T4*
Ø7T7*
Ø7TB*
Ø7TF*
Ø7TG*
ØB9CØZX
ØB9DØZX
ØB9FØZX
ØB9GØZX
ØB9HØZX
ØB9JØZX
ØB9KØZX
ØB9LØZX
ØB9MØZX
ØBBCØZX
ØBBC4ZX
ØBBDØZX
ØBBD4ZX
ØBBFØZX
ØBBF4ZX
ØBBGØZX
ØBBG4ZX
ØBBHØZX
ØBBH4ZX
ØBBJØZX
ØBBJ4ZX
ØBBKØZX
ØBBK4ZX
ØBBLØZX
ØBBL4ZX
ØBBMØZX
ØDCUØZZ
ØDCU3ZZ
ØDCU4ZZ
ØDCV*
ØDCW*
ØDH6ØMZ
ØDH63MZ
ØDH64MZ
ØDJØØZZ
ØDJ6ØZZ
ØDJDØZZ
ØDJUØZZ
ØDJU4ZZ
ØDJVØZZ
ØDJV4ZZ
ØDJWØZZ
ØDJW4ZZ
ØDN8ØZZ
ØDN83ZZ
ØDN84ZZ
ØDN9ØZZ
ØDN93ZZ
ØDN94ZZ
ØDNAØZZ
ØDNA3ZZ
ØDNA4ZZ
ØDNBØZZ
ØDNB3ZZ
ØDNB4ZZ
ØDNCØZZ
ØDNC3ZZ
ØDNC4ZZ
ØDNEØZZ
ØDNE3ZZ
ØDNE4ZZ
ØDNFØZZ
ØDNF3ZZ
ØDNF4ZZ
ØDNGØZZ
ØDNG3ZZ
ØDNG4ZZ
ØDNHØZZ
ØDNH3ZZ
ØDNH4ZZ
ØDNJØZZ
ØDNJ3ZZ
ØDNJ4ZZ
ØDNKØZZ
ØDNK3ZZ
ØDNK4ZZ
ØDNLØZZ
ØDNL3ZZ
ØDNL4ZZ
ØDNMØZZ
ØDNM3ZZ
ØDNM4ZZ
ØDNNØZZ
ØDNN3ZZ
ØDNN4ZZ
ØDNUØZZ
ØDNU3ZZ
ØDNU4ZZ
ØDNV*
ØDNW*
ØDTNØZZ
ØDTN4ZZ
ØDWWØJZ
ØDWW3JZ
ØDWW4JZ
ØF9ØØZX
ØF91ØZX
ØF92ØZX
ØFBØØZX
ØFBØ4ZX
ØFB1ØZX
ØFB14ZX
ØFB2ØZX
ØFB24ZX
ØFDØ4ZX
ØFD14ZX
ØFD24ZX
ØFJØØZZ
ØFJØ4ZZ
ØFJ44ZZ
ØFJD4ZZ
ØFJG4ZZ
ØFN*
ØG5L*
ØG5M*
ØG5N*
ØG5P*
ØG5Q*
ØG5R*
ØGBLØZZ
ØGBL3ZZ
ØGBL4ZZ
ØGBMØZZ
ØGBM3ZZ
ØGBM4ZZ
ØGBNØZZ
ØGBN3ZZ
ØGBN4ZZ
ØGBPØZZ
ØGBP3ZZ
ØGBP4ZZ
ØGBQØZZ
ØGBQ3ZZ
ØGBQ4ZZ
ØGBRØZZ
ØGBR3ZZ
ØGBR4ZZ
ØGTL*
ØGTM*
ØGTN*
ØGTP*
ØGTQ*
ØGTR*
ØJBØØZZ
ØJB1ØZZ
ØJB4ØZZ
ØJB5ØZZ
ØJB6ØZZ
ØJB7ØZZ
ØJB8ØZZ
ØJB9ØZZ
ØJBBØZZ
ØJBCØZZ
ØJBDØZZ
ØJBFØZZ
ØJBGØZZ
ØJBHØZZ
ØJBLØZZ
ØJBMØZZ
ØJBNØZZ
ØJBPØZZ
ØJBQØZZ
ØJBRØZZ
ØJH6ØVZ
ØJH6ØWZ
ØJH6ØYZ
ØJH63VZ
ØJH7ØVZ
ØJH7ØYZ
ØJH73VZ
ØJH8ØVZ
ØJH8ØWZ
ØJH8ØYZ
ØJH83VZ
ØJHDØVZ
ØJHDØWZ
ØJHD3VZ
ØJHFØVZ
ØJHFØWZ
ØJHF3VZ
ØJHGØVZ
ØJHGØWZ
ØJHG3VZ
ØJHHØVZ
ØJHHØWZ
ØJHH3VZ
ØJHLØVZ
ØJHLØWZ
ØJHL3VZ
ØJHMØVZ
ØJHMØWZ
ØJHM3VZ
ØJHNØVZ
ØJHNØWZ
ØJHN3VZ
ØJHPØVZ
ØJHPØWZ
ØJHP3VZ
ØJHTØVZ
ØJHTØYZ
ØJHT3VZ
ØP9ØØZX
ØP9Ø3ZX
ØP9Ø4ZX
ØP91ØZX
ØP913ZX
ØP914ZX
ØP92ØZX
ØP923ZX
ØP924ZX
ØP95ØZX
ØP953ZX
ØP954ZX
ØP96ØZX
ØP963ZX
ØP964ZX
ØP97ØZX
ØP973ZX
ØP974ZX
ØP98ØZX
ØP983ZX
ØP984ZX
ØP99ØZX
ØP993ZX
ØP994ZX
ØP9BØZX
ØP9B3ZX
ØP9B4ZX
ØP9CØZX
ØP9C3ZX
ØP9C4ZX
ØP9DØZX
ØP9D3ZX
ØP9D4ZX
ØP9FØZX
ØP9F3ZX
ØP9F4ZX
ØP9GØZX
ØP9G3ZX
ØP9G4ZX
ØP9HØZX
ØP9H3ZX
ØP9H4ZX
ØP9JØZX
ØP9J3ZX
ØP9J4ZX
ØP9KØZX
ØP9K3ZX
ØP9K4ZX
ØP9LØZX
ØP9L3ZX
ØP9L4ZX
ØP9MØZX
ØP9M3ZX
ØP9M4ZX
ØP9NØZX
ØP9N3ZX
ØP9N4ZX
ØP9PØZX
ØP9P3ZX
ØP9P4ZX
ØP9QØZX
ØP9Q3ZX
ØP9Q4ZX
ØPBØØZX
ØPBØ3ZX
ØPBØ4ZX
ØPB1ØZX
ØPB13ZX
ØPB14ZX
ØPB2ØZX
ØPB23ZX
ØPB24ZX
ØPB5ØZX
ØPB53ZX
ØPB54ZX
ØPB6ØZX
ØPB63ZX
ØPB64ZX
ØPB7ØZX
ØPB73ZX
ØPB74ZX
ØPB8ØZX
ØPB83ZX
ØPB84ZX
ØPB9ØZX
ØPB93ZX
ØPB94ZX
ØPBBØZX
ØPBB3ZX
ØPBB4ZX
ØPBCØZX
ØPBC3ZX
ØPBC4ZX
ØPBDØZX
ØPBD3ZX
ØPBD4ZX
ØPBFØZX
ØPBF3ZX
ØPBF4ZX
ØPBGØZX
ØPBG3ZX
ØPBG4ZX
ØPBHØZX
ØPBH3ZX
ØPBH4ZX
ØPBJØZX
ØPBJ3ZX
ØPBJ4ZX
ØPBKØZX
ØPBK3ZX
ØPBK4ZX
ØPBLØZX
ØPBL3ZX
ØPBL4ZX
ØPBMØZX
ØPBM3ZX
ØPBM4ZX
ØPBNØZX
ØPBN3ZX
ØPBN4ZX
ØPBPØZX
ØPBP3ZX
ØPBP4ZX
ØPBQØZX
ØPBQ3ZX
ØPBQ4ZX
ØQ9ØØZX
ØQ9Ø3ZX
ØQ9Ø4ZX
ØQ91ØZX
ØQ913ZX
ØQ914ZX
ØQ92ØZX
ØQ923ZX
ØQ924ZX
ØQ93ØZX
ØQ933ZX
ØQ934ZX
ØQ94ØZX
ØQ943ZX
ØQ944ZX
ØQ95ØZX
ØQ953ZX
ØQ954ZX
ØQ96ØZX
ØQ963ZX
ØQ964ZX
ØQ97ØZX
ØQ973ZX
ØQ974ZX
ØQ98ØZX
ØQ983ZX
ØQ984ZX
ØQ99ØZX
ØQ993ZX
ØQ994ZX
ØQ9BØZX
ØQ9B3ZX
ØQ9B4ZX
ØQ9CØZX
ØQ9C3ZX
ØQ9C4ZX
ØQ9DØZX
ØQ9D3ZX
ØQ9D4ZX
ØQ9FØZX
ØQ9F3ZX
ØQ9F4ZX
ØQ9GØZX
ØQ9G3ZX
ØQ9G4ZX
ØQ9HØZX
ØQ9H3ZX
ØQ9H4ZX
ØQ9JØZX
ØQ9J3ZX
ØQ9J4ZX
ØQ9KØZX
ØQ9K3ZX
ØQ9K4ZX
ØQ9LØZX
ØQ9L3ZX
ØQ9L4ZX
ØQ9MØZX
ØQ9M3ZX
ØQ9M4ZX
ØQ9NØZX
ØQ9N3ZX
ØQ9N4ZX
ØQ9PØZX
ØQ9P3ZX
ØQ9P4ZX
ØQ9SØZX
ØQ9S3ZX
ØQ9S4ZX
ØQBØØZX
ØQBØ3ZX
ØQBØ4ZX
ØQB1ØZX
ØQB13ZX
ØQB14ZX
ØQB2ØZX
ØQB23ZX
ØQB24ZX
ØQB3ØZX
ØQB33ZX
ØQB34ZX
ØQB4ØZX
ØQB43ZX
ØQB44ZX
ØQB5ØZX
ØQB53ZX
ØQB54ZX
ØQB6ØZX
ØQB63ZX
ØQB64ZX
ØQB7ØZX
ØQB73ZX
ØQB74ZX
ØQB8ØZX
ØQB83ZX
ØQB84ZX
ØQB9ØZX
ØQB93ZX
ØQB94ZX
ØQBBØZX
ØQBB3ZX
ØQBB4ZX
ØQBCØZX
ØQBC3ZX
ØQBC4ZX
ØQBDØZX
ØQBD3ZX
ØQBD4ZX
ØQBFØZX
ØQBF3ZX
ØQBF4ZX
ØQBGØZX
ØQBG3ZX
ØQBG4ZX
ØQBHØZX
ØQBH3ZX
ØQBH4ZX
ØQBJØZX
ØQBJ3ZX
ØQBJ4ZX
ØQBKØZX
ØQBK3ZX
ØQBK4ZX
ØQBLØZX
ØQBL3ZX
ØQBL4ZX
ØQBMØZX
ØQBM3ZX
ØQBM4ZX
ØQBNØZX
ØQBN3ZX
ØQBN4ZX
ØQBPØZX
ØQBP3ZX
ØQBP4ZX
ØQBSØZX
ØQBS3ZX
ØQBS4ZX
ØVPSØJZ
ØVPS3JZ
ØVPS4JZ
ØVPS7JZ
ØVPS8JZ
ØVUSØJZ
ØVUS4JZ
ØW1GØJ4
ØW1GØJ6
ØW1G3J4
ØW1G3J6
ØW1G4J4
ØW1G4J6
ØW3F*
ØW3GØZZ
ØW3G3ZZ
ØW3G4ZZ
ØW3H*
ØW3J*
ØW3PØZZ
ØW3P3ZZ
ØW3P4ZZ
ØW9FØØZ
ØW9FØZZ
ØW9GØØZ
ØW9GØZZ
ØW9G4ØZ
ØW9G4ZZ
ØW9HØØZ
ØW9HØZZ
ØW9H4ØZ
ØW9H4ZZ
ØW9JØØZ
ØW9JØZZ
ØW9J4ØZ
ØW9J4ZZ
ØWCGØZZ
ØWCG3ZZ
ØWCG4ZZ
ØWCHØZZ
ØWCH3ZZ
ØWCH4ZZ
ØWCJØZZ
ØWCJ3ZZ
ØWCJ4ZZ
ØWCPØZZ
ØWCP3ZZ
ØWCP4ZZ
ØWCRØZZ
ØWCR3ZZ
ØWCR4ZZ
ØWHGØ3Z
ØWHG43Z
ØWHHØ1Z
ØWHH31Z
ØWHH41Z
ØWHRØ1Z
ØWHR31Z
ØWHR41Z
ØWHR71Z
ØWHR81Z
ØWJ9ØZZ
ØWJBØZZ
ØWJCØZZ
ØWJFØZZ
ØWJF4ZZ
ØWJGØZZ
ØWJG4ZZ
ØWJHØZZ
ØWJJØZZ
ØWJJ4ZZ
ØWJPØZZ
ØWJP4ZZ
ØWJQØZZ
ØWJRØZZ
ØWJR4ZZ
ØY35*
ØY36*
ØY95ØØZ
ØY95ØZZ
ØY954ØZ
ØY954ZZ
ØY96ØØZ
ØY96ØZZ
ØY964ØZ
ØY964ZZ
ØYJ5ØZZ
ØYJ6ØZZ
ØYJ7ØZZ
ØYJAØZZ
X27H385
X27H395
X27H3B5
X27H3C5
X27J385
X27J395
X27J3B5
X27J3C5
X2CS3T7
X2CT3T7
X2H13R9
X2KB317
X2KC317
X2VWØN7

OR

Principal Diagnosis

E88.3
I12.0
I13.11
N17*
N18.5
N18.6
N19

R34
T79.5XXA
T82.41XA
T82.42XA
T82.43XA
T82.49XA
T86.11
T86.12
T86.13
T86.19
AND
Nonoperating Room Procedures
ØJH6ØXZ
ØJH63WZ
ØJH63XZ
ØJH8ØXZ
ØJH83WZ
ØJH83XZ
ØJHDØXZ
ØJHD3WZ
ØJHD3XZ
ØJHFØXZ
ØJHF3WZ
ØJHF3XZ
ØJHGØXZ
ØJHG3WZ
ØJHG3XZ
ØJHHØXZ
ØJHH3WZ
ØJHH3XZ
ØJHLØXZ
ØJHL3WZ
ØJHL3XZ
ØJHMØXZ
ØJHM3WZ
ØJHM3XZ
ØJHNØXZ
ØJHN3WZ
ØJHN3XZ
ØJHPØXZ
ØJHP3WZ
ØJHP3XZ
OR
Principal Diagnosis
EØ9.22
E1Ø.22
E11.22
E13.22
WITH
Secondary Diagnosis
N18.5
N18.6
AND
Nonoperating Room Procedures
ØJH6ØXZ
ØJH63WZ
ØJH63XZ
ØJH8ØXZ
ØJH83WZ
ØJH83XZ
ØJHDØXZ
ØJHD3WZ
ØJHD3XZ
ØJHFØXZ
ØJHF3WZ
ØJHF3XZ
ØJHGØXZ
ØJHG3WZ
ØJHG3XZ
ØJHHØXZ
ØJHH3WZ
ØJHH3XZ
ØJHLØXZ
ØJHL3WZ
ØJHL3XZ
ØJHMØXZ
ØJHM3WZ
ØJHM3XZ
ØJHNØXZ
ØJHN3WZ
ØJHN3XZ
ØJHPØXZ
ØJHP3WZ
ØJHP3XZ
OR
Principal Diagnosis
E1Ø.2*
AND
Nonoperating Room Procedures
3EØ3ØUØ
3EØ3ØU1
3EØ33UØ
3EØ33U1
3EØJ3UØ
3EØJ3U1
3EØJ7UØ
3EØJ7U1
3EØJ8UØ
3EØJ8U1

DRG 674
Select operating room procedures OR principal diagnosis with/without secondary diagnosis and nonoperating room procedures listed under DRG 673

DRG 675
Select operating room procedures OR principal diagnosis with/without secondary diagnosis and nonoperating room procedures listed under DRG 673

DRG 682
Principal Diagnosis
E88.3
I12*
I13.1Ø
I13.11
N17*
N18*
N19
R34
T79.5XXA

DRG 683
Select principal diagnosis listed under DRG 682

DRG 684
Select principal diagnosis listed under DRG 682

DRG 686
Principal Diagnosis
C64*
C65*
C66*
C67*
C68*
C79.Ø*
C79.1*
C7A.Ø93
DØ9.Ø
DØ9.1*
D17.71
D17.72
D3Ø*
D3A.Ø93
D41*
D49.4
D49.5*

DRG 687
Select principal diagnosis listed under DRG 686

DRG 688
Select principal diagnosis listed under DRG 686

DRG 689
Principal Diagnosis
A18.1Ø
A18.11
A18.12
A18.13
A36.85
A52.75
A54.Ø1
A56.1*
A98.5
B65.Ø
B9Ø.1
N1Ø
N11.Ø
N11.8
N11.9
N12
N13.5
N13.6
N15.1
N28.84
N28.85
N28.86
N3Ø.Ø*
N3Ø.1*
N3Ø.2*
N3Ø.3*
N3Ø.8*
N3Ø.9*
N34.Ø
N34.2
N34.3
N39.Ø

DRG 690
Select principal diagnosis listed under DRG 689

DRG 693
Principal Diagnosis
N11.1
N13.Ø
N13.1
N13.2
N13.3Ø
N13.39
N13.4
N13.8
N2Ø.Ø
N2Ø.1
N2Ø.2
N2Ø.9
N21.Ø
N21.1
N21.8
N21.9
N22
N23

DRG 694
Select principal diagnosis listed under DRG 693

DRG 695
Principal Diagnosis
N39.3
N39.4*
R3Ø*
R31*
R32
R33*
R35*
R36.Ø
R36.9
R39*
R8Ø.Ø
R8Ø.1
R8Ø.3
R8Ø.8
R8Ø.9
R82.Ø
R82.3
R82.5
R82.6
R82.7*
R82.8*
R82.9Ø
R82.91
R82.991
R82.992
R82.993
R82.994
R82.998
R93.4*
R94.4
R94.8

DRG 696
Select principal diagnosis listed under DRG 695

DRG 697
Principal Diagnosis
N35.Ø1Ø
N35.Ø11
N35.Ø12
N35.Ø13
N35.Ø14
N35.Ø16
N35.Ø21
N35.Ø28
N35.111
N35.112
N35.113
N35.114
N35.116
N35.119
N35.12
N35.811
N35.812
N35.813
N35.814
N35.816
N35.819
N35.82
N35.911
N35.912
N35.913
N35.914
N35.916
N35.919
N35.92
N37
N99.11Ø
N99.111
N99.112
N99.113
N99.114
N99.115
N99.116
N99.12

DRG 698
Principal Diagnosis
EØ8.2*
EØ9.2*
E1Ø.2*
E11.2*
E13.2*
I7Ø.1
I72.2
I75.81
I77.73
I82.3
M1Ø.3*
NØØ*
NØ1*
NØ2*
NØ3*
NØ4*
NØ5*
NØ6*
NØ7*
NØ8
N13.7*
N13.9
N14*
N15.Ø
N15.8
N15.9
N16
N25*
N26.1
N26.9
N27*
N28.Ø
N28.1
N28.81
N28.82
N28.83
N28.89
N28.9
N29
N3Ø.4*
N31*
N32*
N33
N36*
N39.8
N39.9
N8Ø.AØ
N8Ø.A1
N8Ø.A2
N8Ø.A41
N8Ø.A42
N8Ø.A43
N8Ø.A49
N8Ø.A51
N8Ø.A52
N8Ø.A53
N8Ø.A59
N8Ø.A61
N8Ø.A62
N8Ø.A63
N8Ø.A69
N99.Ø
N99.5*
N99.81
N99.89
Q6Ø*
Q61*
Q62*
Q63*
Q64.1*
Q64.2
Q64.3*
Q64.4
Q64.5
Q64.6
Q64.7*
Q64.8
Q64.9
R8Ø.2
S31.ØØ1A
S31.Ø11A
S31.Ø21A
S31.Ø31A
S31.Ø41A
S31.Ø51A
S37.ØØ1A
S37.ØØ2A
S37.ØØ9A
S37.Ø11A
S37.Ø12A
S37.Ø19A
S37.Ø21A
S37.Ø22A
S37.Ø29A
S37.Ø31A
S37.Ø32A
S37.Ø39A
S37.Ø41A
S37.Ø42A
S37.Ø49A
S37.Ø51A
S37.Ø52A
S37.Ø59A
S37.Ø61A
S37.Ø62A
S37.Ø69A
S37.Ø91A
S37.Ø92A
S37.Ø99A
S37.1ØXA
S37.12XA
S37.13XA
S37.19XA
S37.2ØXA
S37.22XA
S37.23XA
S37.29XA
S37.3ØXA
S37.32XA
S37.33XA
S37.39XA
T19.ØXXA
T19.1XXA
T19.8XXA
T19.9XXA
T81.711A
T82.41XA
T82.42XA
T82.43XA
T82.49XA
T83.Ø1ØA
T83.Ø11A
T83.Ø12A
T83.Ø18A
T83.Ø2ØA
T83.Ø21A
T83.Ø22A
T83.Ø28A
T83.Ø3ØA
T83.Ø31A
T83.Ø32A
T83.Ø38A
T83.Ø9ØA
T83.Ø91A
T83.Ø92A
T83.Ø98A
T83.11ØA
T83.111A
T83.112A
T83.113A
T83.118A
T83.12ØA
T83.121A
T83.122A
T83.123A
T83.128A
T83.19ØA
T83.191A
T83.192A
T83.193A
T83.198A
T83.21XA
T83.22XA
T83.23XA
T83.24XA
T83.25XA
T83.29XA
T83.41ØA
T83.411A
T83.418A
T83.42ØA
T83.421A
T83.428A
T83.49ØA
T83.491A
T83.498A
T83.51ØA
T83.511A
T83.512A
T83.518A
T83.59ØA
T83.591A
T83.592A
T83.593A
T83.598A
T83.61XA
T83.62XA
T83.69XA
T83.712A
T83.713A
T83.714A
T83.718A
T83.719A
T83.722A
T83.723A
T83.724A
T83.728A
T83.729A
T83.79XA
T83.81XA
T83.82XA
T83.83XA
T83.84XA
T83.85XA
T83.86XA
T83.89XA
T83.9XXA
T86.1*
Z43.5
Z43.6
Z46.6
Z49.Ø1
Z49.Ø2
Z49.31
Z49.32
Z52.4
Z9Ø.6
Z94.Ø
Z96.Ø

DRG 699
Select principal diagnosis listed under DRG 698

DRG 700
Select principal diagnosis listed under DRG 698

MDC 12

DRG 707
Operating Room Procedures
Ø7JPØZZ
Ø7T8*
Ø7T9*
Ø7TC*
Ø7TD*
Ø7TH*
Ø7TJ*
ØDBPØZZ
ØDBP4ZZ
ØDJØØZZ
ØDJ6ØZZ
ØDJDØZZ
ØDJUØZZ
ØDJVØZZ
ØDJWØZZ
ØFJØØZZ
ØTBBØZZ
ØTBB3ZZ
ØTBB4ZZ
ØTBCØZZ
ØTBC3ZZ
ØTBC4ZZ
ØTTB*
ØTTC*
ØV5ØØZ3
ØV5ØØZZ
ØV5Ø3Z3
ØV5Ø3ZZ
ØV5Ø4Z3
ØV5Ø4ZZ
ØVTØØZZ
ØVTØ4ZZ
ØWBHØZZ
ØWBH3ZZ
ØWBH4ZZ
ØWJGØZZ
ØWJJØZZ
ØWJPØZZ
ØWJRØZZ
OR
ØVTØ*
AND
ØVT3*

DRG 708
Select operating room procedures or procedure combination listed under DRG 707

DRG 709
Operating Room Procedures
ØTMD*
ØTND*
ØTQD*
ØTRD*
ØTSD*
ØTUD*
ØTVD*
ØV5S*
ØV5T*
ØV9SØØZ
ØV9SØZX
ØV9SØZZ
ØV9S3ZX
ØV9S4ØZ
ØV9S4ZX
ØV9S4ZZ
ØV9SXØZ
ØV9SXZX
ØV9SXZZ
ØV9TØØZ
ØV9TØZX
ØV9TØZZ
ØV9T3ZX
ØV9T4ØZ
ØV9T4ZX
ØV9T4ZZ
ØV9TXØZ
ØV9TXZX
ØV9TXZZ
ØVBS*
ØVBT*
ØVCSØZZ
ØVCS3ZZ
ØVCS4ZZ
ØVCT*
ØVJSØZZ
ØVMSXZZ
ØVNS*
ØVPSØØZ
ØVPSØ3Z
ØVPSØ7Z
ØVPSØJZ
ØVPSØKZ
ØVPSØYZ
ØVPS3ØZ
ØVPS33Z
ØVPS37Z
ØVPS3JZ
ØVPS3KZ
ØVPS4ØZ
ØVPS43Z
ØVPS47Z
ØVPS4JZ
ØVPS4KZ
ØVPS77Z
ØVPS7JZ
ØVPS7KZ
ØVPS87Z
ØVPS8JZ
ØVPS8KZ
ØVQS*
ØVQT*
ØVTS*
ØVUSØ7Z
ØVUSØJZ
ØVUSØKZ
ØVUS47Z
ØVUS4JZ
ØVUS4KZ
ØVUTØ7Z
ØVUTØJZ
ØVUTØKZ
ØVUT47Z
ØVUT4JZ
ØVUT4KZ
ØVUTX7Z
ØVUTXJZ
ØVUTXKZ
ØVWSØØZ
ØVWSØ3Z
ØVWSØ7Z
ØVWSØJZ
ØVWSØKZ
ØVWSØYZ
ØVWS3ØZ
ØVWS33Z
ØVWS37Z
ØVWS3JZ
ØVWS3KZ
ØVWS4ØZ
ØVWS43Z
ØVWS47Z
ØVWS4JZ
ØVWS4KZ
ØVWS7ØZ
ØVWS73Z
ØVWS77Z
ØVWS7JZ
ØVWS7KZ
ØVWS8ØZ
ØVWS83Z
ØVWS87Z
ØVWS8JZ
ØVWS8KZ
ØVXTØZD
ØVXTØZS
ØVXTXZD
ØVXTXZS
ØVYSØZØ
ØVYSØZ1
ØVYSØZ2
ØW4M*
ØWPMØ7Z
ØWPMØKZ
ØWPM37Z
ØWPM3KZ
ØWPM47Z
ØWPM4KZ
ØWPMX7Z
ØWPMXJZ
ØWPMXKZ
ØWUMØ7Z
ØWUM47Z
ØWWMØ7Z
ØWWMØKZ
ØWWM37Z
ØWWM3KZ
ØWWM47Z
ØWWM4KZ

DRG 710
Select operating room procedures listed under DRG 709

DRG 711
Operating Room Procedures
ØV1*
ØV56*
ØV57*
ØV59*
ØV5B*
ØV5C*
ØV5F*
ØV5G*
ØV5H*
ØV5J*
ØV5K*
ØV5L*
ØV7*
ØV99ØØZ
ØV99ØZX
ØV99ØZZ
ØV9BØØZ
ØV9BØZX
ØV9BØZZ
ØV9CØØZ
ØV9CØZX
ØV9CØZZ
ØV9JØØZ
ØV9JØZZ
ØV9J4ØZ
ØV9J4ZZ
ØV9KØØZ
ØV9KØZZ
ØV9K4ØZ
ØV9K4ZZ
ØV9LØØZ
ØV9LØZZ
ØV9L4ØZ
ØV9L4ZZ
ØVB6ØZZ
ØVB63ZZ
ØVB64ZZ
ØVB7ØZZ
ØVB73ZZ
ØVB74ZZ
ØVB9ØZX
ØVB9ØZZ
ØVB93ZZ
ØVB94ZZ
ØVBBØZX
ØVBBØZZ
ØVBB3ZZ
ØVBB4ZZ
ØVBCØZX
ØVBCØZZ
ØVBC3ZZ
ØVBC4ZZ
ØVBFØZZ
ØVBF3ZZ
ØVBF4ZZ
ØVBF8ZZ
ØVBGØZZ
ØVBG3ZZ
ØVBG4ZZ
ØVBG8ZZ
ØVBHØZZ

ØVBH3ZZ
ØVBH4ZZ
ØVBH8ZZ
ØVBJØZZ
ØVBJ3ZZ
ØVBJ4ZZ
ØVBJ8ZZ
ØVBKØZZ
ØVBK3ZZ
ØVBK4ZZ
ØVBK8ZZ
ØVBLØZZ
ØVBL3ZZ
ØVBL4ZZ
ØVBL8ZZ
ØVC9*
ØVCB*
ØVCC*
ØVCF*
ØVCG*
ØVCH*
ØVCJ*
ØVCK*
ØVCL*
ØVJDØZZ
ØVJD4ZZ
ØVJMØZZ
ØVJM4ZZ
ØVJRØZZ
ØVJR4ZZ
ØVLNØDZ
ØVLN3DZ
ØVLN4DZ
ØVLN8DZ
ØVLPØDZ
ØVLP3DZ
ØVLP4DZ
ØVLP8DZ
ØVLQØDZ
ØVLQ3DZ
ØVLQ4DZ
ØVLQ8DZ
ØVM5XZZ
ØVM6*
ØVM7*
ØVM9*
ØVMB*
ØVMC*
ØVMF*
ØVMG*
ØVMH*
ØVN5*
ØVN6*
ØVN7*
ØVNF*
ØVNG*
ØVNH*
ØVNJ*
ØVNK*
ØVNL*
ØVNN*
ØVNP*
ØVNQ*
ØVPDØØZ
ØVPDØ3Z
ØVPDØ7Z
ØVPDØJZ
ØVPDØKZ
ØVPDØYZ
ØVPD3ØZ
ØVPD33Z
ØVPD37Z
ØVPD3JZ
ØVPD3KZ
ØVPD4ØZ
ØVPD43Z
ØVPD47Z
ØVPD4JZ
ØVPD4KZ
ØVPD77Z
ØVPD7JZ
ØVPD7KZ
ØVPD87Z
ØVPD8JZ
ØVPD8KZ
ØVPMØØZ
ØVPMØ3Z
ØVPMØ7Z
ØVPMØCZ
ØVPMØJZ
ØVPMØKZ
ØVPMØYZ
ØVPM3ØZ
ØVPM33Z
ØVPM37Z
ØVPM3CZ
ØVPM3JZ
ØVPM3KZ
ØVPM4ØZ
ØVPM43Z
ØVPM47Z
ØVPM4CZ
ØVPM4JZ
ØVPM4KZ
ØVPM77Z
ØVPM7CZ
ØVPM7JZ
ØVPM7KZ
ØVPM87Z
ØVPM8CZ
ØVPM8JZ
ØVPM8KZ
ØVPRØDZ
ØVPR3DZ
ØVPR4DZ
ØVQ9*
ØVQB*
ØVQC*
ØVQF*
ØVQG*
ØVQH*
ØVQJ*
ØVQK*
ØVQL*
ØVQN*
ØVQP*
ØVQQ*
ØVR*
ØVS*
ØVT6*
ØVT7*
ØVT9*
ØVTB*
ØVTC*
ØVTF*
ØVTG*
ØVTH*
ØVTJ*
ØVTK*
ØVTL*
ØVU5*
ØVU6*
ØVU7*
ØVU9*
ØVUB*
ØVUC*
ØVUF*
ØVUG*
ØVUH*
ØVUJ*
ØVUK*
ØVUL*
ØVUN*
ØVUP*
ØVUQ*
ØVWDØØZ
ØVWDØ3Z
ØVWDØ7Z
ØVWDØJZ
ØVWDØKZ
ØVWDØYZ
ØVWD3ØZ
ØVWD33Z
ØVWD37Z
ØVWD3JZ
ØVWD3KZ
ØVWD4ØZ
ØVWD43Z
ØVWD47Z
ØVWD4JZ
ØVWD4KZ
ØVWD7ØZ
ØVWD73Z
ØVWD77Z
ØVWD7JZ
ØVWD7KZ
ØVWD8ØZ
ØVWD83Z
ØVWD87Z
ØVWD8JZ
ØVWD8KZ
ØVWMØØZ
ØVWMØ3Z
ØVWMØ7Z
ØVWMØCZ
ØVWMØJZ
ØVWMØKZ
ØVWMØYZ
ØVWM3ØZ
ØVWM33Z
ØVWM37Z
ØVWM3CZ
ØVWM3JZ
ØVWM3KZ
ØVWM4ØZ
ØVWM43Z
ØVWM47Z
ØVWM4CZ
ØVWM4JZ
ØVWM4KZ
ØVWM7ØZ
ØVWM73Z
ØVWM77Z
ØVWM7CZ
ØVWM7JZ
ØVWM7KZ
ØVWM8ØZ
ØVWM83Z
ØVWM87Z
ØVWM8CZ
ØVWM8JZ
ØVWM8KZ
ØVY5ØZØ
ØVY5ØZ1
ØVY5ØZ2

DRG 712

Select operating room procedures listed under DRG 711

DRG 713

Operating Room Procedures

ØV5Ø7ZZ
ØV5Ø8ZZ
ØVBØ7ZZ
ØVBØ8ZZ
ØVTØ7ZZ
ØVTØ8ZZ

DRG 714

Select operating room procedures listed under DRG 713

DRG 715

Principal Diagnosis

C6Ø*
C61
C62*
C63*
C76.3
C79.82
DØ7.4
DØ7.5
DØ7.6*
D4Ø*

AND

Operating Room Procedures

ØØHEØMZ
ØØHE3MZ
ØØHE4MZ
ØØHUØMZ
ØØHU3MZ
ØØHU4MZ
ØØHVØMZ
ØØHV3MZ
ØØHV4MZ
ØØPEØMZ
ØØPE3MZ
ØØPE4MZ
ØØPUØMZ
ØØPU3MZ
ØØPU4MZ
ØØPVØMZ
ØØPV3MZ
ØØPV4MZ
Ø1HYØMZ
Ø1HY3MZ
Ø1HY4MZ
Ø1PYØMZ
Ø1PY3MZ
Ø1PY4MZ
Ø2HVØ2Z
Ø2HVØDZ
Ø2HV3DZ
Ø2HV42Z
Ø2HV4DZ
Ø2LV*
Ø2VV*
Ø4LEØCV
Ø4LEØDV
Ø4LEØZV
Ø4LE3CV
Ø4LE3DV
Ø4LE3ZV
Ø4LE4CV
Ø4LE4DV
Ø4LE4ZV
Ø4LFØCW
Ø4LFØDW
Ø4LFØZW
Ø4LF3CW
Ø4LF3DW
Ø4LF3ZW
Ø4LF4CW
Ø4LF4DW
Ø4LF4ZW
Ø5HØØMZ
Ø5HØ3MZ
Ø5HØ4MZ
Ø5H3ØMZ
Ø5H33MZ
Ø5H34MZ
Ø5H4ØMZ
Ø5H43MZ
Ø5H44MZ
Ø5PØØMZ
Ø5PØ3MZ
Ø5PØ4MZ
Ø5PØXMZ
Ø5P3ØMZ
Ø5P33MZ
Ø5P34MZ
Ø5P3XMZ
Ø5P4ØMZ
Ø5P43MZ
Ø5P44MZ
Ø5P4XMZ
Ø6HØØDZ
Ø6HØ4DZ
Ø6LØ*
Ø6LB3DZ
Ø6VØ*
Ø79CØZX
Ø79C3ZX
Ø79C4ZX
Ø79HØZX
Ø79H3ZX
Ø79H4ZX
Ø79JØZX
Ø79J3ZX
Ø79J4ZX
Ø7BCØZX
Ø7BC3ZX
Ø7BC4ZX
Ø7BH*
Ø7BJ*
Ø7TØ*
Ø7T3*
Ø7T4*
Ø7T7*
Ø7TB*
Ø7TF*
Ø7TG*
ØDH6ØMZ
ØDH63MZ
ØDH64MZ
ØDP6ØMZ
ØDP63MZ
ØDP64MZ
ØDPR*
ØF9ØØZX
ØF91ØZX
ØF92ØZX
ØFBØØZX
ØFB1ØZX
ØFB2ØZX
ØJBØØZZ
ØJB1ØZZ
ØJB4ØZZ
ØJB5ØZZ
ØJB6ØZZ
ØJB7ØZZ
ØJB8ØZZ
ØJB9ØZZ
ØJBBØZZ
ØJBCØZZ
ØJBDØZZ
ØJBFØZZ
ØJBGØZZ
ØJBHØZZ
ØJBLØZZ
ØJBMØZZ
ØJBNØZZ
ØJBPØZZ
ØJBQØZZ
ØJBRØZZ
ØJH6ØVZ
ØJH6ØYZ
ØJH63VZ
ØJH7ØVZ
ØJH7ØYZ
ØJH73VZ
ØJH8ØVZ
ØJH8ØYZ
ØJH83VZ
ØJHDØVZ
ØJHD3VZ
ØJHFØVZ
ØJHF3VZ
ØJHGØVZ
ØJHG3VZ
ØJHHØVZ
ØJHH3VZ
ØJHLØVZ
ØJHL3VZ
ØJHMØVZ
ØJHM3VZ
ØJHNØVZ
ØJHN3VZ
ØJHPØVZ
ØJHP3VZ
ØJHTØVZ
ØJHTØYZ
ØJHT3VZ
ØP9ØØZX
ØP9Ø3ZX
ØP9Ø4ZX
ØP91ØZX
ØP913ZX
ØP914ZX
ØP92ØZX
ØP923ZX
ØP924ZX
ØP95ØZX
ØP953ZX
ØP954ZX
ØP96ØZX
ØP963ZX
ØP964ZX
ØP97ØZX
ØP973ZX
ØP974ZX
ØP98ØZX
ØP983ZX
ØP984ZX
ØP99ØZX
ØP993ZX
ØP994ZX
ØP9BØZX
ØP9B3ZX
ØP9B4ZX
ØP9CØZX
ØP9C3ZX
ØP9C4ZX
ØP9DØZX
ØP9D3ZX
ØP9D4ZX
ØP9FØZX
ØP9F3ZX
ØP9F4ZX
ØP9GØZX
ØP9G3ZX
ØP9G4ZX
ØP9HØZX
ØP9H3ZX
ØP9H4ZX
ØP9JØZX
ØP9J3ZX
ØP9J4ZX
ØP9KØZX
ØP9K3ZX
ØP9K4ZX
ØP9LØZX
ØP9L3ZX
ØP9L4ZX
ØP9MØZX
ØP9M3ZX
ØP9M4ZX
ØP9NØZX
ØP9N3ZX
ØP9N4ZX
ØP9PØZX
ØP9P3ZX
ØP9P4ZX
ØP9QØZX
ØP9Q3ZX
ØP9Q4ZX
ØPBØØZX
ØPBØ3ZX
ØPBØ4ZX
ØPB1ØZX
ØPB13ZX
ØPB14ZX
ØPB2ØZX
ØPB23ZX
ØPB24ZX
ØPB5ØZX
ØPB53ZX
ØPB54ZX
ØPB6ØZX
ØPB63ZX
ØPB64ZX
ØPB7ØZX
ØPB73ZX
ØPB74ZX
ØPB8ØZX
ØPB83ZX
ØPB84ZX
ØPB9ØZX
ØPB93ZX
ØPB94ZX
ØPBBØZX
ØPBB3ZX
ØPBB4ZX
ØPBCØZX
ØPBC3ZX
ØPBC4ZX
ØPBDØZX
ØPBD3ZX
ØPBD4ZX
ØPBFØZX
ØPBF3ZX
ØPBF4ZX
ØPBGØZX
ØPBG3ZX
ØPBG4ZX
ØPBHØZX
ØPBH3ZX
ØPBH4ZX
ØPBJØZX
ØPBJ3ZX
ØPBJ4ZX
ØPBKØZX
ØPBK3ZX
ØPBK4ZX
ØPBLØZX
ØPBL3ZX
ØPBL4ZX
ØPBMØZX
ØPBM3ZX
ØPBM4ZX
ØPBNØZX
ØPBN3ZX
ØPBN4ZX
ØPBPØZX
ØPBP3ZX
ØPBP4ZX
ØPBQØZX
ØPBQ3ZX
ØPBQ4ZX
ØQ9ØØZX
ØQ9Ø3ZX
ØQ9Ø4ZX
ØQ91ØZX
ØQ913ZX
ØQ914ZX
ØQ92ØZX
ØQ923ZX
ØQ924ZX
ØQ93ØZX
ØQ933ZX
ØQ934ZX
ØQ94ØZX
ØQ943ZX
ØQ944ZX
ØQ95ØZX
ØQ953ZX
ØQ954ZX
ØQ96ØZX
ØQ963ZX
ØQ964ZX
ØQ97ØZX
ØQ973ZX
ØQ974ZX
ØQ98ØZX
ØQ983ZX
ØQ984ZX
ØQ99ØZX
ØQ993ZX
ØQ994ZX
ØQ9BØZX
ØQ9B3ZX
ØQ9B4ZX
ØQ9CØZX
ØQ9C3ZX
ØQ9C4ZX
ØQ9DØZX
ØQ9D3ZX
ØQ9D4ZX
ØQ9FØZX
ØQ9F3ZX
ØQ9F4ZX
ØQ9GØZX
ØQ9G3ZX
ØQ9G4ZX
ØQ9HØZX
ØQ9H3ZX
ØQ9H4ZX
ØQ9JØZX
ØQ9J3ZX
ØQ9J4ZX
ØQ9KØZX
ØQ9K3ZX
ØQ9K4ZX
ØQ9LØZX
ØQ9L3ZX
ØQ9L4ZX
ØQ9MØZX
ØQ9M3ZX
ØQ9M4ZX
ØQ9NØZX
ØQ9N3ZX
ØQ9N4ZX
ØQ9PØZX
ØQ9P3ZX
ØQ9P4ZX
ØQ9SØZX
ØQ9S3ZX
ØQ9S4ZX
ØQBØØZX
ØQBØ3ZX
ØQBØ4ZX
ØQB1ØZX
ØQB13ZX
ØQB14ZX
ØQB2ØZX
ØQB23ZX
ØQB24ZX
ØQB3ØZX
ØQB33ZX
ØQB34ZX
ØQB4ØZX
ØQB43ZX
ØQB44ZX
ØQB5ØZX
ØQB53ZX
ØQB54ZX
ØQB6ØZX
ØQB63ZX
ØQB64ZX
ØQB7ØZX
ØQB73ZX
ØQB74ZX
ØQB8ØZX
ØQB83ZX
ØQB84ZX
ØQB9ØZX
ØQB93ZX
ØQB94ZX
ØQBBØZX
ØQBB3ZX
ØQBB4ZX
ØQBCØZX
ØQBC3ZX
ØQBC4ZX
ØQBDØZX
ØQBD3ZX
ØQBD4ZX
ØQBFØZX
ØQBF3ZX
ØQBF4ZX
ØQBGØZX
ØQBG3ZX
ØQBG4ZX
ØQBHØZX
ØQBH3ZX
ØQBH4ZX
ØQBJØZX
ØQBJ3ZX
ØQBJ4ZX
ØQBKØZX
ØQBK3ZX
ØQBK4ZX
ØQBLØZX
ØQBL3ZX
ØQBL4ZX
ØQBMØZX
ØQBM3ZX
ØQBM4ZX
ØQBNØZX
ØQBN3ZX
ØQBN4ZX
ØQBPØZX
ØQBP3ZX
ØQBP4ZX
ØQBSØZX
ØQBS3ZX
ØQBS4ZX
ØT13Ø7B
ØT13ØJB
ØT13ØKB
ØT13ØZB
ØT1347B
ØT134JB
ØT134KB
ØT134ZB
ØT14Ø7B
ØT14ØJB
ØT14ØKB
ØT14ØZB
ØT1447B
ØT144JB
ØT144KB
ØT144ZB
ØT16Ø76
ØT16Ø77
ØT16Ø78
ØT16Ø79
ØT16Ø7A
ØT16Ø7C
ØT16Ø7D
ØT16ØJ6
ØT16ØJ7
ØT16ØJ8
ØT16ØJ9
ØT16ØJA
ØT16ØJC
ØT16ØJD
ØT16ØK6
ØT16ØK7
ØT16ØK8
ØT16ØK9
ØT16ØKA
ØT16ØKC
ØT16ØKD
ØT16ØZ6
ØT16ØZ7
ØT16ØZ8
ØT16ØZ9
ØT16ØZA
ØT16ØZC
ØT16ØZD
ØT163JD
ØT16476
ØT16477
ØT16478
ØT16479
ØT1647A
ØT1647C
ØT1647D
ØT164J6
ØT164J7
ØT164J8
ØT164J9
ØT164JA
ØT164JC
ØT164JD
ØT164K6
ØT164K7
ØT164K8
ØT164K9
ØT164KA
ØT164KC
ØT164KD
ØT164Z6
ØT164Z7
ØT164Z8
ØT164Z9
ØT164ZA
ØT164ZC
ØT164ZD
ØT17Ø76
ØT17Ø77
ØT17Ø78
ØT17Ø79
ØT17Ø7A
ØT17Ø7C
ØT17Ø7D
ØT17ØJ6
ØT17ØJ7
ØT17ØJ8
ØT17ØJ9
ØT17ØJA
ØT17ØJC
ØT17ØJD
ØT17ØK6
ØT17ØK7
ØT17ØK8
ØT17ØK9
ØT17ØKA
ØT17ØKC
ØT17ØKD
ØT17ØZ6
ØT17ØZ7
ØT17ØZ8
ØT17ØZ9
ØT17ØZA
ØT17ØZC
ØT17ØZD
ØT173JD
ØT17476
ØT17477
ØT17478
ØT17479
ØT1747A
ØT1747C
ØT1747D
ØT174J6
ØT174J7
ØT174J8
ØT174J9
ØT174JA
ØT174JC
ØT174JD
ØT174K6
ØT174K7
ØT174K8
ØT174K9
ØT174KA
ØT174KC
ØT174KD
ØT174Z6
ØT174Z7
ØT174Z8
ØT174Z9
ØT174ZA
ØT174ZC
ØT174ZD
ØT18Ø76
ØT18Ø77
ØT18Ø78
ØT18Ø79
ØT18Ø7A
ØT18Ø7C
ØT18Ø7D
ØT18ØJ6
ØT18ØJ7
ØT18ØJ8
ØT18ØJ9
ØT18ØJA
ØT18ØJC
ØT18ØJD
ØT18ØK6
ØT18ØK7
ØT18ØK8
ØT18ØK9
ØT18ØKA
ØT18ØKC
ØT18ØKD
ØT18ØZ6
ØT18ØZ7
ØT18ØZ8
ØT18ØZ9
ØT18ØZA
ØT18ØZC
ØT18ØZD
ØT183JD
ØT18476
ØT18477
ØT18478
ØT18479
ØT1847A
ØT1847C
ØT1847D
ØT184J6
ØT184J7
ØT184J8
ØT184J9
ØT184JA
ØT184JC
ØT184JD
ØT184K6
ØT184K7
ØT184K8
ØT184K9
ØT184KA
ØT184KC
ØT184KD
ØT184Z6
ØT184Z7
ØT184Z8

ØT184Z9
ØT184ZA
ØT184ZC
ØT184ZD
ØT1B*
ØT56*
ØT57*
ØT5B*
ØT5C*
ØT7DØZZ
ØT7D3ZZ
ØT7D4ZZ
ØT93ØØZ
ØT93ØZZ
ØT934ØZ
ØT94ØØZ
ØT94ØZZ
ØT944ØZ
ØT9BØØZ
ØT9BØZX
ØT9B3ZX
ØT9B4ZX
ØT9B7ZX
ØT9B8ZX
ØT9CØZX
ØT9C3ZX
ØT9C4ZX
ØT9C7ZX
ØT9C8ZX
ØTBØØZZ
ØTBØ3ZZ
ØTBØ4ZZ
ØTB1ØZZ
ØTB13ZZ
ØTB14ZZ
ØTB3ØZZ
ØTB33ZZ
ØTB34ZZ
ØTB4ØZZ
ØTB43ZZ
ØTB44ZZ
ØTB6ØZZ
ØTB63ZZ
ØTB64ZZ
ØTB67ZZ
ØTB68ZZ
ØTB7ØZZ
ØTB73ZZ
ØTB74ZZ
ØTB77ZZ
ØTB78ZZ
ØTBBØZX
ØTBB3ZX
ØTBB4ZX
ØTBB7ZX
ØTBB7ZZ
ØTBB8ZX
ØTBB8ZZ
ØTBCØZX
ØTBC3ZX
ØTBC4ZX
ØTBC7ZX
ØTBC7ZZ
ØTBC8ZX
ØTBC8ZZ
ØTJB4ZZ
ØTLD*
ØTNØ*
ØTN1*
ØTN3*
ØTN4*
ØTN6ØZZ
ØTN63ZZ
ØTN64ZZ
ØTN7ØZZ
ØTN73ZZ
ØTN74ZZ
ØTNB3ZZ
ØTNB4ZZ
ØTNC3ZZ
ØTNC4ZZ
ØTPDØLZ
ØTPD3LZ
ØTPD4LZ
ØTPD7LZ
ØTPD8LZ
ØTPDXLZ
ØTQØ*
ØTQ1*
ØTQ7*
ØTQB*
ØTWDØLZ
ØTWD3LZ
ØTWD4LZ
ØTWD7LZ
ØTWD8LZ
ØV51*
ØV52*
ØV53*
ØV9ØØØZ
ØV9ØØZX
ØV9ØØZZ
ØV9Ø7ØZ
ØV9Ø7ZZ
ØV9Ø8ØZ
ØV9Ø8ZZ
ØV91ØØZ
ØV91ØZX
ØV91ØZZ
ØV92ØØZ
ØV92ØZX
ØV92ØZZ
ØV93ØØZ
ØV93ØZX
ØV93ØZZ
ØV95ØZZ
ØVBØØZX
ØVBØØZZ
ØVBØ3ZZ
ØVBØ4ZZ
ØVB1ØZX
ØVB1ØZZ
ØVB13ZZ
ØVB14ZZ
ØVB2ØZX
ØVB2ØZZ
ØVB23ZZ
ØVB24ZZ
ØVB3ØZX
ØVB3ØZZ
ØVB33ZZ
ØVB34ZZ
ØVB5ØZZ
ØVCØ*
ØVC1*
ØVC2*
ØVC3*
ØVC5ØZZ
ØVHØ*
ØVJ4ØZZ
ØVJ44ZZ
ØVNØ*
ØVN1*
ØVN2*
ØVN3*
ØVP4ØØZ
ØVP4Ø1Z
ØVP4Ø3Z
ØVP4Ø7Z
ØVP4ØJZ
ØVP4ØKZ
ØVP4ØYZ
ØVP43ØZ
ØVP431Z
ØVP433Z
ØVP437Z
ØVP43JZ
ØVP43KZ
ØVP44ØZ
ØVP441Z
ØVP443Z
ØVP447Z
ØVP44JZ
ØVP44KZ
ØVP471Z
ØVP477Z
ØVP47JZ
ØVP47KZ
ØVP481Z
ØVP487Z
ØVP48JZ
ØVP48KZ
ØVQØ*
ØVQ1*
ØVQ2*
ØVQ3*
ØVT1*
ØVT2*
ØVT3*
ØVU1*
ØVU2*
ØVU3*
ØVW4ØØZ
ØVW4Ø3Z
ØVW4Ø7Z
ØVW4ØJZ
ØVW4ØKZ
ØVW4ØYZ
ØVW43ØZ
ØVW433Z
ØVW437Z
ØVW43JZ
ØVW43KZ
ØVW44ØZ
ØVW443Z
ØVW447Z
ØVW44JZ
ØVW44KZ
ØVW47ØZ
ØVW473Z
ØVW477Z
ØVW47JZ
ØVW47KZ
ØVW48ØZ
ØVW483Z
ØVW487Z
ØVW48JZ
ØVW48KZ
ØW3M*
ØW3R*
ØWHJØ1Z
ØWHJ31Z
ØWHJ41Z
ØWHMØ1Z
ØWHM31Z
ØWHM41Z
ØWHRØ1Z
ØWHR31Z
ØWHR41Z
ØWHR71Z
ØWHR81Z
ØWQFØZZ
ØWQF3ZZ
ØWQF4ZZ
ØWQFXZ2
ØWQFXZZ
X2H13R9

DRG 716

Select principal diagnosis AND operating room procedures listed under DRG 715

DRG 717

Select only operating room procedures listed under DRG 715

DRG 718

Select only operating room procedures listed under DRG 715

DRG 722

Principal Diagnosis

C6Ø*
C61
C62*
C63*
C76.3
C79.82
DØ7.4
DØ7.5
DØ7.6*
D4Ø*

DRG 723

Select principal diagnosis listed under DRG 722

DRG 724

Select principal diagnosis listed under DRG 722

DRG 725

Principal Diagnosis

N4Ø*
N42.83

DRG 726

Select principal diagnosis listed under DRG 725

DRG 727

Principal Diagnosis

A18.14
A18.15
A51.Ø
A54.ØØ
A54.Ø9
A54.1
A54.21
A54.22
A54.23
A54.29
A55
A56.ØØ
A56.Ø1
A56.Ø9
A56.2
A56.8
A57
A58
A59.ØØ
A59.Ø2
A59.Ø3
A59.Ø9
A6Ø.ØØ
A6Ø.Ø1
A6Ø.Ø2
A6Ø.Ø9
A6Ø.1
A6Ø.9
A63.8
A64
B26.Ø
B37.4*
N34.1
N41*
N43.1
N45*
N47*
N48.1
N48.2*
N49*
Z41.2

DRG 728

Select principal diagnosis listed under DRG 727

DRG 729

Principal Diagnosis

D17.6
D29*
I86.1
I86.2
L29.1
L29.3
N42.Ø
N42.1
N42.3*
N42.81
N42.82
N42.89
N42.9
N43.Ø
N43.2
N43.3
N43.4*
N44*
N46*
N48.Ø
N48.3*
N48.5
N48.6
N48.8*
N48.9
N5Ø*
N51
N52*
N53*
Q53*
Q54*
Q55*
Q56.Ø
Q56.1
Q56.3
Q56.4
Q64.Ø
Q98*
Q99.Ø
Q99.1
Q99.8
R36.1
R86*
R93.811
R93.812
R93.813
R93.819
S3Ø.2Ø1A
S3Ø.21XA
S3Ø.22XA
S31.2ØXA
S31.21XA
S31.22XA
S31.23XA
S31.24XA
S31.25XA
S31.3ØXA
S31.31XA
S31.32XA
S31.33XA
S31.34XA
S31.35XA
S31.5Ø1A
S31.5Ø1S
S31.511A
S31.511S
S31.521A
S31.521S
S31.531A
S31.531S
S31.541A
S31.541S
S31.551A
S31.551S
S37.1ØXS
S37.12XS
S37.13XS
S37.19XS
S37.2ØXS
S37.22XS
S37.23XS
S37.29XS
S37.3ØXS
S37.32XS
S37.33XS
S37.39XS
S37.812S
S37.813S
S37.818S
S37.819S
S37.822A
S37.822S
S37.823A
S37.823S
S37.828A
S37.828S
S37.829A
S37.829S
S37.892A
S37.892S
S37.893A
S37.893S
S37.898A
S37.898S
S37.899A
S37.899S
S37.9ØXA
S37.9ØXS
S37.92XA
S37.92XS
S37.93XA
S37.93XS
S37.99XA
S37.99XS
S38.ØØ1A
S38.Ø1XA
S38.Ø2XA
S38.221A
S38.222A
S38.231A
S38.232A
T19.4XXA
Z3Ø.2
Z31.Ø
Z9Ø.79

DRG 730

Select principal diagnosis listed under DRG 729

MDC 13

DRG 734

Operating Room Procedures

Ø7TØ*
Ø7T3*
Ø7T4*
Ø7T7*
Ø7T8*
Ø7T9*
Ø7TB*
Ø7TC*
Ø7TD*
Ø7TF*
Ø7TG*
Ø7TH*
Ø7TJ*
OR
ØUT94ZZ
ØUT9FZZ
AND both
ØUT44ZZ
ØUTC4ZZ
OR
ØUT9ØZZ
AND both
ØUT4ØZZ
ØUTCØZZ
OR
ØUTM*
AND
Ø7BHØZZ
Ø7BH4ZZ
Ø7BJØZZ
Ø7BJ4ZZ
OR
ØUT97ZZ
ØUT98ZZ
AND
ØUT47ZZ
ØUT48ZZ
AND
ØUTC7ZZ
ØUTC8ZZ
OR
ØTTBØZZ
AND ALL
ØTTDØZZ
ØUT2ØZZ
ØUT7ØZZ
ØUT9ØZZ
ØUTCØZZ
ØUTGØZZ

DRG 735

Select operating room procedures OR procedure combinations listed under DRG 734

DRG 736

Principal Diagnosis

C56*
C57.Ø*
C57.1*
C57.2*
C57.3
C57.4
C79.6*
D39.1*
AND
Operating Room Procedures
Ø15P*
ØU1*
ØU5Ø*
ØU51*
ØU52*
ØU54*
ØU55*
ØU56*
ØU59*
ØU5B*
ØU75*
ØU76*
ØU77*
ØU79*
ØU8Ø*
ØU81*
ØU82*
ØU9ØØØZ
ØU9ØØZX
ØU9ØØZZ
ØU9Ø3ZX
ØU9Ø4ØZ
ØU9Ø4ZX
ØU9Ø4ZZ
ØU9ØXZZ
ØU91ØØZ
ØU91ØZX
ØU91ØZZ
ØU913ZX
ØU914ØZ
ØU914ZX
ØU914ZZ
ØU91XZZ
ØU92ØØZ
ØU92ØZX
ØU92ØZZ
ØU923ZX
ØU924ØZ
ØU924ZX
ØU924ZZ
ØU92XZZ
ØU94ØZX
ØU95ØØZ
ØU95ØZX
ØU95ØZZ
ØU953ZX
ØU954ØZ
ØU954ZX
ØU957ØZ
ØU957ZX
ØU958ØZ
ØU958ZX
ØU96ØØZ
ØU96ØZX
ØU96ØZZ
ØU963ZX
ØU964ØZ
ØU964ZX
ØU967ØZ
ØU967ZX
ØU968ØZ
ØU968ZX
ØU97ØØZ
ØU97ØZX
ØU97ØZZ
ØU973ZX
ØU974ØZ
ØU974ZX
ØU977ØZ
ØU977ZX
ØU978ØZ
ØU978ZX
ØU99ØØZ
ØU99ØZX
ØU99ØZZ
ØU994ØZ
ØU994ZZ
ØU997ØZ
ØU997ZZ
ØU998ØZ
ØU998ZZ
ØUBØ*
ØUB1*
ØUB2*
ØUB4ØZX
ØUB4ØZZ
ØUB43ZZ
ØUB44ZZ
ØUB47ZZ
ØUB48ZZ
ØUB5*
ØUB6*
ØUB7ØZX
ØUB73ZX
ØUB74ZX
ØUB77ZX
ØUB78ZX
ØUB9ØZX
ØUB9ØZZ
ØUB93ZZ
ØUB94ZZ
ØUB97ZZ
ØUB98ZZ
ØUCØ*
ØUC1*
ØUC2*
ØUC5*
ØUC6*
ØUC7*
ØUC9ØZZ
ØUC93ZZ
ØUC94ZZ
ØUDN*
ØUF5ØZZ
ØUF53ZZ
ØUF54ZZ
ØUF57ZZ
ØUF58ZZ
ØUF6ØZZ
ØUF63ZZ
ØUF64ZZ
ØUF67ZZ
ØUF68ZZ
ØUF7ØZZ
ØUF73ZZ
ØUF74ZZ
ØUF77ZZ
ØUF78ZZ
ØUH3Ø1Z
ØUH341Z
ØUJ3ØZZ
ØUJ34ZZ
ØUJ8ØZZ
ØUJ84ZZ
ØUJDØZZ
ØUJD4ZZ
ØUL5*
ØUL6*
ØUMØ*
ØUM1*
ØUM2*
ØUM5*
ØUM6*
ØUM7*
ØUNØ*
ØUN1*
ØUN2*
ØUN5*
ØUN6*
ØUN7*
ØUP3ØØZ
ØUP3Ø3Z
ØUP3ØYZ
ØUP33ØZ
ØUP333Z
ØUP34ØZ
ØUP343Z
ØUP8ØØZ
ØUP8Ø3Z
ØUP8Ø7Z
ØUP8ØCZ
ØUP8ØDZ
ØUP8ØJZ
ØUP8ØKZ
ØUP8ØYZ
ØUP83ØZ
ØUP833Z
ØUP837Z
ØUP83CZ
ØUP83DZ
ØUP83JZ
ØUP83KZ
ØUP84ØZ
ØUP843Z
ØUP847Z
ØUP84CZ
ØUP84DZ
ØUP84JZ
ØUP84KZ
ØUP877Z
ØUP87CZ
ØUP87JZ
ØUP87KZ
ØUP887Z
ØUP88CZ
ØUP88JZ
ØUP88KZ
ØUPDØØZ
ØUPDØ1Z
ØUPDØ3Z
ØUPDØ7Z
ØUPDØDZ
ØUPDØHZ
ØUPDØJZ
ØUPDØKZ
ØUPDØYZ
ØUPD3ØZ
ØUPD31Z
ØUPD33Z
ØUPD37Z
ØUPD3DZ
ØUPD3HZ
ØUPD3JZ
ØUPD3KZ
ØUPD4ØZ
ØUPD41Z
ØUPD43Z
ØUPD47Z
ØUPD4DZ
ØUPD4HZ
ØUPD4JZ
ØUPD4KZ
ØUPD71Z
ØUPD77Z
ØUPD7JZ
ØUPD7KZ
ØUPD81Z
ØUPD87Z
ØUPD8JZ
ØUPD8KZ
ØUQØ*
ØUQ1*
ØUQ2*
ØUQ5*
ØUQ6*
ØUQ7*
ØUQ9*
ØUSØ*
ØUS1*
ØUS2*
ØUS5*
ØUS6*
ØUS7*
ØUSC*
ØUTØ*
ØUT1*
ØUT2*
ØUT5*
ØUT6*
ØUT7*
ØUT9*
ØUU5*
ØUU6*
ØUU7*
ØUW3ØØZ
ØUW3Ø3Z
ØUW3ØYZ
ØUW33ØZ
ØUW333Z
ØUW34ØZ
ØUW343Z
ØUW8ØØZ
ØUW8Ø3Z
ØUW8Ø7Z
ØUW8ØCZ
ØUW8ØDZ
ØUW8ØJZ
ØUW8ØKZ
ØUW8ØYZ
ØUW83ØZ
ØUW833Z
ØUW837Z
ØUW83CZ
ØUW83DZ
ØUW83JZ
ØUW83KZ
ØUW84ØZ
ØUW843Z
ØUW847Z
ØUW84CZ
ØUW84DZ
ØUW84JZ
ØUW84KZ
ØUW87ØZ
ØUW873Z
ØUW877Z
ØUW87CZ

ØUW87DZ
ØUW87JZ
ØUW87KZ
ØUW88ØZ
ØUW883Z
ØUW887Z
ØUW88CZ
ØUW88DZ
ØUW88JZ
ØUW88KZ
ØUWDØØZ
ØUWDØ1Z
ØUWDØ3Z
ØUWDØ7Z
ØUWDØDZ
ØUWDØHZ
ØUWDØJZ
ØUWDØKZ
ØUWDØYZ
ØUWD3ØZ
ØUWD31Z
ØUWD33Z
ØUWD37Z
ØUWD3DZ
ØUWD3HZ
ØUWD3JZ
ØUWD3KZ
ØUWD4ØZ
ØUWD41Z
ØUWD43Z
ØUWD47Z
ØUWD4DZ
ØUWD4HZ
ØUWD4JZ
ØUWD4KZ
ØUWD7ØZ
ØUWD71Z
ØUWD73Z
ØUWD77Z
ØUWD7DZ
ØUWD7HZ
ØUWD7JZ
ØUWD7KZ
ØUWD8ØZ
ØUWD81Z
ØUWD83Z
ØUWD87Z
ØUWD8DZ
ØUWD8HZ
ØUWD8JZ
ØUWD8KZ
ØUYØØZØ
ØUYØØZ1
ØUYØØZ2
ØUY1ØZØ
ØUY1ØZ1
ØUY1ØZ2
ØUY9ØZØ
ØUY9ØZ1
ØUY9ØZ2
1ØD2*
1ØT*

DRG 737

Select principal diagnosis AND operating room procedures listed under DRG 736

DRG 738

Select principal diagnosis AND operating room procedures listed under DRG 736

DRG 739

Principal Diagnosis

C51*
C52
C53*
C54*
C55
C57.7
C57.8
C57.9
C58
C76.3
C79.82
DØ6*
DØ7.Ø
DØ7.1
DØ7.2
DØ7.3*
D39.Ø
D39.2
D39.8
D39.9

AND

Operating room procedures listed under DRG 736

DRG 740

Select principal diagnosis listed under DRG 739 AND operating room procedures listed under DRG 736

DRG 741

Select principal diagnosis listed under DRG 739 AND operating room procedures listed under DRG 736

DRG 742

Principal Diagnosis

A18.16
A18.17
A18.18
A51.Ø
A54.ØØ
A54.Ø2
A54.Ø3
A54.Ø9
A54.1
A54.21
A54.24
A54.29
A55
A56.Ø*
A56.2
A56.8
A57
A58
A59.ØØ
A59.Ø1
A59.Ø3
A59.Ø9
A6Ø.ØØ
A6Ø.Ø3
A6Ø.Ø4
A6Ø.Ø9
A6Ø.1
A6Ø.9
A63.8
A64
B37.41
B37.49
D25*
D26*
D27*
D28*
E28*
E89.4*
F52.5
I86.2
I86.3
L29.2
L29.3
N34.1
N39.3
N7Ø*
N71*
N72
N73*
N74
N75*
N76*
N77*
N8Ø.Ø*
N8Ø.1*
N8Ø.2*
N8Ø.3*
N8Ø.4*
N8Ø.8
N8Ø.9
N8Ø.B4
N8Ø.B5
N8Ø.B6
N8Ø.C*
N8Ø.D*
N81*
N82.Ø
N82.1
N82.5
N82.8
N82.9
N83*
N84*
N85*
N86
N87*
N88*
N89*
N9Ø*
N91*
N92*
N93*
N94*
N95*
N96
N97*
N99.2
N99.3
N99.83
Q5Ø*
Q51.Ø
Q51.1Ø
Q51.11
Q51.21
Q51.22
Q51.28
Q51.3
Q51.4
Q51.5
Q51.6
Q51.7
Q51.81Ø
Q51.811
Q51.818
Q51.82Ø
Q51.821
Q51.828
Q51.9
Q52*
Q56.Ø
Q56.2
Q56.3
Q56.4
Q96*
Q97*
Q98.5
Q99.Ø
Q99.1
Q99.8
R87.61Ø
R87.611
R87.612
R87.613
R87.614
R87.615
R87.616
R87.62Ø
R87.621
R87.622
R87.623
R87.624
R87.625
R87.628
R87.81Ø
R87.811
R87.82Ø
R87.821
S3Ø.2Ø2A
S3Ø.23XA
S31.4ØXA
S31.41XA
S31.42XA
S31.43XA
S31.44XA
S31.45XA
S31.5Ø2A
S31.5Ø2S
S31.512A
S31.512S
S31.522A
S31.522S
S31.532A
S31.532S
S31.542A
S31.542S
S31.552A
S31.552S
S37.1ØXS
S37.12XS
S37.13XS
S37.19XS
S37.2ØXS
S37.22XS
S37.23XS
S37.29XS
S37.3ØXS
S37.32XS
S37.33XS
S37.39XS
S37.4Ø1A
S37.4Ø1S
S37.4Ø2A
S37.4Ø2S
S37.4Ø9A
S37.4Ø9S
S37.421A
S37.421S
S37.422A
S37.422S
S37.429A
S37.429S
S37.431A
S37.431S
S37.432A
S37.432S
S37.439A
S37.439S
S37.491A
S37.491S
S37.492A
S37.492S
S37.499A
S37.499S
S37.5Ø1A
S37.5Ø1S
S37.5Ø2A
S37.5Ø2S
S37.5Ø9A
S37.5Ø9S
S37.511A
S37.511S
S37.512A
S37.512S
S37.519A
S37.519S
S37.521A
S37.521S
S37.522A
S37.522S
S37.529A
S37.529S
S37.531A
S37.531S
S37.532A
S37.532S
S37.539A
S37.539S
S37.591A
S37.591S
S37.592A
S37.592S
S37.599A
S37.599S
S37.6ØXA
S37.6ØXS
S37.62XA
S37.62XS
S37.63XA
S37.63XS
S37.69XA
S37.69XS
S37.812S
S37.813S
S37.818S
S37.819S
S37.892A
S37.892S
S37.893A
S37.893S
S37.898A
S37.898S
S37.899A
S37.899S
S37.9ØXA
S37.9ØXS
S37.92XA
S37.92XS
S37.93XA
S37.93XS
S37.99XA
S37.99XS
S38.ØØ2A
S38.Ø3XA
S38.211A
S38.212A
T19.2XXA
T19.3XXA
T83.31XA
T83.32XA
T83.39XA
T83.711A
T83.721A
Z3Ø.2
Z31.Ø
Z4Ø.Ø2
Z4Ø.Ø3
Z43.7
Z64.1
Z9Ø.7*

AND

Operating room procedures listed under DRG 736

DRG 743

Select principal diagnosis listed under DRG 742 AND operating room procedures listed under DRG 736

DRG 744

Operating Room Procedures

ØDJU4ZZ
ØDJV4ZZ
ØDJW4ZZ
ØFJØ4ZZ
ØFJ44ZZ
ØFJD4ZZ
ØFJG4ZZ
ØU57*
ØU943ZX
ØU944ZX
ØU993ZX
ØU994ZX
ØU997ZX
ØU998ZX
ØU9CØZX
ØU9C3ZX
ØU9C4ZX
ØU9C7ZX
ØU9C8ZX
ØUB43ZX
ØUB44ZX
ØUB47ZX
ØUB48ZX
ØUB7ØZZ
ØUB73ZZ
ØUB74ZZ
ØUB77ZZ
ØUB78ZZ
ØUB93ZX
ØUB94ZX
ØUB97ZX
ØUB98ZX
ØUBCØZX
ØUBC3ZX
ØUBC4ZX
ØUBC7ZX
ØUBC8ZX
ØUDB*
ØUHCØ1Z
ØUHC31Z
ØUHC41Z
ØUHC71Z
ØUHC81Z
ØUHGØ1Z
ØUHG31Z
ØUHG41Z
ØUHG71Z
ØUHG81Z
ØUHGX1Z
ØUL7*
ØUN9*
ØWHJØ1Z
ØWHJ31Z
ØWHJ41Z
ØWHNØ1Z
ØWHN31Z
ØWHN41Z
ØWHRØ1Z
ØWHR31Z
ØWHR41Z
ØWHR71Z
ØWHR81Z
ØWJF4ZZ
ØWJG4ZZ
ØWJJ4ZZ
ØWJP4ZZ
ØWJR4ZZ

DRG 745

Select operating room procedures listed under DRG 744

DRG 746

Operating Room Procedures

ØH99XØZ
ØH99XZZ
ØHR9*
ØT1BØZD
ØT1B4ZD
ØT9BØØZ
ØU5C*
ØU5F*
ØU5G*
ØU5J*
ØU5K*
ØU5L*
ØU5M*
ØU7GØDZ
ØU7GØZZ
ØU7G3DZ
ØU7G3ZZ
ØU7G4DZ
ØU7G4ZZ
ØU9CØØZ
ØU9CØZZ
ØU9C4ØZ
ØU9C4ZZ
ØU9C7ØZ
ØU9C7ZZ
ØU9C8ØZ
ØU9C8ZZ
ØU9FØZX
ØU9F3ZX
ØU9F4ZX
ØU9F7ZX
ØU9F8ZX
ØU9GØØZ
ØU9GØZX
ØU9GØZZ
ØU9G3ZX
ØU9G4ØZ
ØU9G4ZX
ØU9G4ZZ
ØU9G7ØZ
ØU9G7ZX
ØU9G7ZZ
ØU9G8ØZ
ØU9G8ZX
ØU9G8ZZ
ØU9GXØZ
ØU9GXZX
ØU9GXZZ
ØU9J*
ØU9KØZX
ØU9K3ZX
ØU9K4ZX
ØU9K7ZX
ØU9K8ZX
ØU9KXZX
ØU9M*
ØUBCØZZ
ØUBC3ZZ
ØUBC4ZZ
ØUBC7ZZ
ØUBC8ZZ
ØUBF*
ØUBG*
ØUBJ*
ØUBK*
ØUBL*
ØUBMØZX
ØUBMØZZ
ØUBMXZX
ØUBMXZZ
ØUCC*
ØUCGØZZ
ØUCG3ZZ
ØUCG4ZZ
ØUCJ*
ØUCL*
ØUCMØZZ
ØUHHØ3Z
ØUHHØYZ
ØUHH33Z
ØUHH43Z
ØUJHØZZ
ØUJH4ZZ
ØUJMØZZ
ØULF*
ØUMF*
ØUMG*
ØUMJXZZ
ØUMK*
ØUMMXZZ
ØUNF*
ØUNG*
ØUNJ*
ØUNK*
ØUNL*
ØUNM*
ØUPDØCZ
ØUPHØØZ
ØUPHØ1Z
ØUPHØ3Z
ØUPHØ7Z
ØUPHØDZ
ØUPHØJZ
ØUPHØKZ
ØUPHØYZ
ØUPH3ØZ
ØUPH31Z
ØUPH33Z
ØUPH37Z
ØUPH3DZ
ØUPH3JZ
ØUPH3KZ
ØUPH4ØZ
ØUPH41Z
ØUPH43Z
ØUPH47Z
ØUPH4DZ
ØUPH4JZ
ØUPH4KZ
ØUPH71Z
ØUPH77Z
ØUPH7JZ
ØUPH7KZ
ØUPH81Z
ØUPH87Z
ØUPH8JZ
ØUPH8KZ
ØUPMØØZ
ØUPMØ7Z
ØUPMØJZ
ØUPMØKZ
ØUQC*
ØUQF*
ØUQGØZZ
ØUQG3ZZ
ØUQG4ZZ
ØUQJ*
ØUQKØZZ
ØUQK3ZZ
ØUQK4ZZ
ØUQK7ZZ
ØUQK8ZZ
ØUQL*
ØUQMØZZ
ØUSF*
ØUTC*
ØUTF*
ØUTJ*
ØUTK*
ØUTL*
ØUTM*
ØUUF*
ØUUJ*
ØUUM*
ØUV*
ØUWDØCZ
ØUWD3CZ
ØUWD4CZ
ØUWD7CZ
ØUWD8CZ
ØUWHØØZ
ØUWHØ1Z
ØUWHØ3Z
ØUWHØ7Z
ØUWHØDZ
ØUWHØJZ
ØUWHØKZ
ØUWHØYZ
ØUWH3ØZ
ØUWH31Z
ØUWH33Z
ØUWH37Z
ØUWH3DZ
ØUWH3JZ
ØUWH3KZ
ØUWH4ØZ
ØUWH41Z
ØUWH43Z
ØUWH47Z
ØUWH4DZ
ØUWH4JZ
ØUWH4KZ
ØUWH7ØZ
ØUWH71Z
ØUWH73Z
ØUWH77Z
ØUWH7DZ
ØUWH7JZ
ØUWH7KZ
ØUWH8ØZ
ØUWH81Z
ØUWH83Z
ØUWH87Z
ØUWH8DZ
ØUWH8JZ
ØUWH8KZ
ØUWMØØZ
ØUWMØ7Z
ØUWMØJZ
ØUWMØKZ
ØWØN*
ØW9NØØZ
ØW9NØZZ
ØW9N4ØZ
ØW9N4ZZ
ØWBN*
ØWHNØ3Z
ØWHNØYZ
ØWHN33Z
ØWHN3YZ
ØWHN43Z
ØWHN4YZ
ØWMNØZZ
ØWPNØØZ
ØWPNØ1Z
ØWPNØ3Z
ØWPNØ7Z
ØWPNØJZ
ØWPNØKZ
ØWPNØYZ
ØWPN3ØZ
ØWPN31Z
ØWPN33Z
ØWPN37Z
ØWPN3JZ
ØWPN3KZ
ØWPN3YZ
ØWPN4ØZ
ØWPN41Z
ØWPN43Z
ØWPN47Z
ØWPN4JZ
ØWPN4KZ
ØWPN4YZ
ØWQNØZZ
ØWQN3ZZ
ØWQN4ZZ
ØWUN*
ØWWNØØZ
ØWWNØ1Z
ØWWNØ3Z
ØWWNØ7Z
ØWWNØJZ
ØWWNØKZ
ØWWNØYZ
ØWWN3ØZ
ØWWN31Z
ØWWN33Z
ØWWN37Z
ØWWN3JZ
ØWWN3KZ
ØWWN3YZ
ØWWN4ØZ
ØWWN41Z
ØWWN43Z
ØWWN47Z
ØWWN4JZ
ØWWN4KZ
ØWWN4YZ

OR

Nonoperating Room Procedure

ØHQ9XZZ

DRG 747

Select procedures listed under DRG 746

DRG 748

Operating Room Procedures

ØDXEØZ7
ØDXE4Z7
ØJQCØZZ
ØJUC*
ØTSC*
ØTSD*
ØTUC*
ØTVC*
ØU7K*
ØU84*
ØU94ØØZ
ØU94ØZZ
ØU944ØZ
ØU944ZZ
ØUC4*
ØULG*
ØUM4*
ØUN4*
ØUQ4*
ØUS4*
ØUS9ØZZ
ØUS94ZZ
ØUS97ZZ
ØUS98ZZ
ØUSG*
ØUT4*
ØUTG*
ØUU4*
ØUUG*
ØW4N*

DRG 749

Operating Room Procedures

ØØHEØMZ
ØØHE3MZ
ØØHE4MZ
ØØHUØMZ
ØØHU3MZ
ØØHU4MZ
ØØHVØMZ
ØØHV3MZ
ØØHV4MZ
ØØPEØMZ
ØØPE3MZ
ØØPE4MZ
ØØPUØMZ
ØØPU3MZ
ØØPU4MZ
ØØPVØMZ
ØØPV3MZ
ØØPV4MZ
Ø1BPØZZ
Ø1BP3ZZ
Ø1BP4ZZ
Ø1DP*
Ø1HYØMZ
Ø1HY3MZ
Ø1HY4MZ
Ø1PYØMZ
Ø1PY3MZ
Ø1PY4MZ
Ø2HVØ2Z
Ø2HVØDZ
Ø2HV3DZ
Ø2HV42Z
Ø2HV4DZ
Ø2LV*
Ø2VV*
Ø4LEØCT
Ø4LEØDT
Ø4LEØZT
Ø4LE3CT
Ø4LE3DT
Ø4LE3ZT
Ø4LE4CT
Ø4LE4DT
Ø4LE4ZT
Ø4LFØCU
Ø4LFØDU
Ø4LFØZU
Ø4LF3CU
Ø4LF3DU
Ø4LF3ZU
Ø4LF4CU
Ø4LF4DU
Ø4LF4ZU
Ø5HØØMZ
Ø5HØ3MZ
Ø5HØ4MZ
Ø5H3ØMZ
Ø5H33MZ
Ø5H34MZ
Ø5H4ØMZ
Ø5H43MZ
Ø5H44MZ
Ø5PØØMZ
Ø5PØ3MZ
Ø5PØ4MZ
Ø5PØXMZ

Ø5P3ØMZ
Ø5P33MZ
Ø5P34MZ
Ø5P3XMZ
Ø5P4ØMZ
Ø5P43MZ
Ø5P44MZ
Ø5P4XMZ
Ø6HØØDZ
Ø6HØ4DZ
Ø6LØ*
Ø6LB3DZ
Ø6VØ*
Ø79CØZX
Ø79C3ZX
Ø79C4ZX
Ø79HØZX
Ø79H3ZX
Ø79H4ZX
Ø79JØZX
Ø79J3ZX
Ø79J4ZX
Ø7BCØZX
Ø7BC3ZX
Ø7BC4ZX
Ø7BH*
Ø7BJ*
Ø7JPØZZ
ØD5UØZZ
ØD5U3ZZ
ØD5U4ZZ
ØD5V*
ØD5W*
ØD9UØZX
ØD9U4ZX
ØD9VØZX
ØD9V4ZX
ØD9WØZX
ØD9W4ZX
ØDBUØZX
ØDBUØZZ
ØDBU3ZZ
ØDBU4ZZ
ØDBVØZX
ØDBVØZZ
ØDBV3ZZ
ØDBV4ZZ
ØDBWØZX
ØDBWØZZ
ØDBW3ZZ
ØDBW4ZZ
ØDH6ØMZ
ØDH63MZ
ØDH64MZ
ØDJØØZZ
ØDJ6ØZZ
ØDJDØZZ
ØDJUØZZ
ØDJVØZZ
ØDJWØZZ
ØDN8ØZZ
ØDN83ZZ
ØDN84ZZ
ØDN9ØZZ
ØDN93ZZ
ØDN94ZZ
ØDNAØZZ
ØDNA3ZZ
ØDNA4ZZ
ØDNBØZZ
ØDNB3ZZ
ØDNB4ZZ
ØDNCØZZ
ØDNC3ZZ
ØDNC4ZZ
ØDNEØZZ
ØDNE3ZZ
ØDNE4ZZ
ØDNFØZZ
ØDNF3ZZ
ØDNF4ZZ
ØDNGØZZ
ØDNG3ZZ
ØDNG4ZZ
ØDNHØZZ
ØDNH3ZZ
ØDNH4ZZ
ØDNJØZZ
ØDNJ3ZZ
ØDNJ4ZZ
ØDNKØZZ
ØDNK3ZZ
ØDNK4ZZ
ØDNLØZZ
ØDNL3ZZ
ØDNL4ZZ
ØDNMØZZ
ØDNM3ZZ
ØDNM4ZZ
ØDNNØZZ
ØDNN3ZZ
ØDNN4ZZ
ØDNUØZZ
ØDNU3ZZ
ØDNU4ZZ
ØDNV*
ØDNW*
ØDP6ØMZ
ØDP63MZ
ØDP64MZ
ØDPR*
ØDTJ*
ØDTUØZZ
ØDTU4ZZ
ØF9ØØZX
ØF91ØZX
ØF92ØZX
ØFBØØZX
ØFB1ØZX
ØFB2ØZX
ØFJØØZZ
ØFNØ*
ØFN1*
ØFN2*
ØFN4*
ØFN5*
ØFN6*
ØFN7ØZZ
ØFN73ZZ
ØFN74ZZ
ØFN77ZZ
ØFN78ZZ
ØFN8*
ØFN9*
ØFNC*
ØFND*
ØFNF*
ØFNG*
ØJBØØZZ
ØJB1ØZZ
ØJB4ØZZ
ØJB5ØZZ
ØJB6ØZZ
ØJB7ØZZ
ØJB8ØZZ
ØJB9ØZZ
ØJBBØZZ
ØJBCØZZ
ØJBDØZZ
ØJBFØZZ
ØJBGØZZ
ØJBHØZZ
ØJBLØZZ
ØJBMØZZ
ØJBNØZZ
ØJBPØZZ
ØJBQØZZ
ØJBRØZZ
ØJH6ØVZ
ØJH6ØWZ
ØJH6ØYZ
ØJH63VZ
ØJH7ØVZ
ØJH7ØYZ
ØJH73VZ
ØJH8ØVZ
ØJH8ØWZ
ØJH8ØYZ
ØJH83VZ
ØJHDØVZ
ØJHDØWZ
ØJHD3VZ
ØJHFØVZ
ØJHFØWZ
ØJHF3VZ
ØJHGØVZ
ØJHGØWZ
ØJHG3VZ
ØJHHØVZ
ØJHHØWZ
ØJHH3VZ
ØJHLØVZ
ØJHLØWZ
ØJHL3VZ
ØJHMØVZ
ØJHMØWZ
ØJHM3VZ
ØJHNØVZ
ØJHN3VZ
ØJHPØVZ
ØJHPØWZ
ØJHP3VZ
ØJHTØVZ
ØJHTØYZ
ØJHT3VZ
ØT13Ø7B
ØT13ØJB
ØT13ØKB
ØT13ØZB
ØT1347B
ØT134JB
ØT134KB
ØT134ZB
ØT14Ø7B
ØT14ØJB
ØT14ØKB
ØT14ØZB
ØT1447B
ØT144JB
ØT144KB
ØT144ZB
ØT16Ø76
ØT16Ø77
ØT16Ø78
ØT16Ø79
ØT16Ø7A
ØT16Ø7C
ØT16Ø7D
ØT16ØJ6
ØT16ØJ7
ØT16ØJ8
ØT16ØJ9
ØT16ØJA
ØT16ØJC
ØT16ØJD
ØT16ØK6
ØT16ØK7
ØT16ØK8
ØT16ØK9
ØT16ØKA
ØT16ØKC
ØT16ØKD
ØT16ØZ6
ØT16ØZ7
ØT16ØZ8
ØT16ØZ9
ØT16ØZA
ØT16ØZC
ØT16ØZD
ØT163JD
ØT16476
ØT16477
ØT16478
ØT16479
ØT1647A
ØT1647C
ØT1647D
ØT164J6
ØT164J7
ØT164J8
ØT164J9
ØT164JA
ØT164JC
ØT164JD
ØT164K6
ØT164K7
ØT164K8
ØT164K9
ØT164KA
ØT164KC
ØT164KD
ØT164Z6
ØT164Z7
ØT164Z8
ØT164Z9
ØT164ZA
ØT164ZC
ØT164ZD
ØT17Ø76
ØT17Ø77
ØT17Ø78
ØT17Ø79
ØT17Ø7A
ØT17Ø7C
ØT17Ø7D
ØT17ØJ6
ØT17ØJ7
ØT17ØJ8
ØT17ØJ9
ØT17ØJA
ØT17ØJC
ØT17ØJD
ØT17ØK6
ØT17ØK7
ØT17ØK8
ØT17ØK9
ØT17ØKA
ØT17ØKC
ØT17ØKD
ØT17ØZ6
ØT17ØZ7
ØT17ØZ8
ØT17ØZ9
ØT17ØZA
ØT17ØZC
ØT17ØZD
ØT173JD
ØT17476
ØT17477
ØT17478
ØT17479
ØT1747A
ØT1747C
ØT1747D
ØT174J6
ØT174J7
ØT174J8
ØT174J9
ØT174JA
ØT174JC
ØT174JD
ØT174K6
ØT174K7
ØT174K8
ØT174K9
ØT174KA
ØT174KC
ØT174KD
ØT174Z6
ØT174Z7
ØT174Z8
ØT174Z9
ØT174ZA
ØT174ZC
ØT174ZD
ØT18Ø76
ØT18Ø77
ØT18Ø78
ØT18Ø79
ØT18Ø7A
ØT18Ø7C
ØT18Ø7D
ØT18ØJ6
ØT18ØJ7
ØT18ØJ8
ØT18ØJ9
ØT18ØJA
ØT18ØJC
ØT18ØJD
ØT18ØK6
ØT18ØK7
ØT18ØK8
ØT18ØK9
ØT18ØKA
ØT18ØKC
ØT18ØKD
ØT18ØZ6
ØT18ØZ7
ØT18ØZ8
ØT18ØZ9
ØT18ØZA
ØT18ØZC
ØT18ØZD
ØT183JD
ØT18476
ØT18477
ØT18478
ØT18479
ØT1847A
ØT1847C
ØT1847D
ØT184J6
ØT184J7
ØT184J8
ØT184J9
ØT184JA
ØT184JC
ØT184JD
ØT184K6
ØT184K7
ØT184K8
ØT184K9
ØT184KA
ØT184KC
ØT184KD
ØT184Z6
ØT184Z7
ØT184Z8
ØT184Z9
ØT184ZA
ØT184ZC
ØT184ZD
ØT56*
ØT57*
ØT5BØZZ
ØT5B3ZZ
ØT5B4ZZ
ØT5CØZZ
ØT5C3ZZ
ØT5C4ZZ
ØT7BØDZ
ØT7BØZZ
ØT7B3DZ
ØT7B3ZZ
ØT7B4DZ
ØT7B4ZZ
ØT7B8DZ
ØT7B8ZZ
ØT93ØØZ
ØT93ØZZ
ØT934ØZ
ØT94ØØZ
ØT94ØZZ
ØT944ØZ
ØT9BØZX
ØT9B3ZX
ØT9B4ZX
ØT9B7ZX
ØT9B8ZX
ØT9CØZX
ØT9C3ZX
ØT9C4ZX
ØT9C7ZX
ØT9C8ZX
ØTB6ØZZ
ØTB63ZZ
ØTB64ZZ
ØTB67ZZ
ØTB68ZZ
ØTB7ØZZ
ØTB73ZZ
ØTB74ZZ
ØTB77ZZ
ØTB78ZZ
ØTBBØZX
ØTBBØZZ
ØTBB3ZX
ØTBB3ZZ
ØTBB4ZX
ØTBB4ZZ
ØTBB7ZX
ØTBB8ZX
ØTBCØZX
ØTBCØZZ
ØTBC3ZX
ØTBC3ZZ
ØTBC4ZX
ØTBC4ZZ
ØTBC7ZX
ØTBC8ZX
ØTJDØZZ
ØTLD*
ØTMB*
ØTMC*
ØTMD*
ØTNØ*
ØTN1*
ØTN3*
ØTN4*
ØTN6ØZZ
ØTN63ZZ
ØTN64ZZ
ØTN7ØZZ
ØTN73ZZ
ØTN74ZZ
ØTNB3ZZ
ØTNB4ZZ
ØTNC3ZZ
ØTNC4ZZ
ØTND*
ØTPDØLZ
ØTPD3LZ
ØTPD4LZ
ØTPD7LZ
ØTPD8LZ
ØTPDXLZ
ØTQ7*
ØTQB*
ØTQCØZZ
ØTQC3ZZ
ØTQC4ZZ
ØTQC7ZZ
ØTQC8ZZ
ØTTB*
ØTTC*
ØTVB*
ØTVD*
ØTWDØLZ
ØTWD3LZ
ØTWD4LZ
ØTWD7LZ
ØTWD8LZ
ØU9FØØZ
ØU9FØZZ
ØU9F7ØZ
ØU9F7ZZ
ØU9F8ØZ
ØU9F8ZZ
ØUCB*
ØUCF*
ØUF9ØZZ
ØUF93ZZ
ØUF94ZZ
ØUF97ZZ
ØUF98ZZ
ØUM9*
ØUMC*
ØUNC*
ØUUK*
ØW1JØJ9
ØW1JØJB
ØW1JØJG
ØW1JØJJ
ØW1J3J9
ØW1J3JB
ØW1J3JG
ØW1J3JJ
ØW1J4J9
ØW1J4JB
ØW1J4JG
ØW1J4JJ
ØW3HØZZ
ØW3N*
ØW3PØZZ
ØW3R*
ØW9GØØZ
ØW9GØZX
ØW9GØZZ
ØW9G4ØZ
ØW9G4ZX
ØW9G4ZZ
ØW9HØZX
ØW9H3ZX
ØW9H4ZX
ØW9JØZX
ØW9J4ZX
ØWBHØZX
ØWBHØZZ
ØWBH3ZZ
ØWBH4ZZ
ØWJGØZZ
ØWJH4ZZ
ØWJJØZZ
ØWJNØZZ
ØWJN4ZZ
ØWJPØZZ
ØWJRØZZ
ØWQF*
ØY95ØZX
ØY953ZX
ØY954ZX
ØY96ØZX
ØY963ZX
ØY964ZX
ØYB5ØZX
ØYB53ZX
ØYB54ZX
ØYB6ØZX
ØYB63ZX
ØYB64ZX
ØYB7ØZX
ØYB73ZX
ØYB74ZX
ØYB8ØZX
ØYB83ZX
ØYB84ZX
ØYJ54ZZ
ØYJ64ZZ
ØYJ74ZZ
ØYJ84ZZ
ØYJA4ZZ
ØYJE4ZZ
1ØS2*
3EØP3QØ
3EØP3Q1
3EØP7QØ
3EØP7Q1
X2H13R9

DRG 750

Select operating room procedures listed under DRG 749

DRG 754

Principal Diagnosis

C51*
C52
C53*
C54*
C55
C56*
C57*
C58
C76.3
C79.6*
C79.82
DØ6*
DØ7.Ø
DØ7.1
DØ7.2
DØ7.3*
D39*

DRG 755

Select principal diagnosis listed under DRG 754

DRG 756

Select principal diagnosis listed under DRG 754

DRG 757

Principal Diagnosis

A18.16
A18.17
A18.18
A51.Ø
A54.ØØ
A54.Ø2
A54.Ø3
A54.Ø9
A54.1
A54.21
A54.24
A54.29
A55
A56.Ø*
A56.2
A56.8
A57
A58
A59.ØØ
A59.Ø1
A59.Ø3
A59.Ø9
A6Ø.ØØ
A6Ø.Ø3
A6Ø.Ø4
A6Ø.Ø9
A6Ø.1
A6Ø.9
A63.8
A64
B37.3*
B37.41
B37.49
L29.2
L29.3
N34.1
N7Ø*
N71*
N72
N73.Ø
N73.1
N73.2
N73.3
N73.4
N73.5
N73.8
N73.9
N74
N75.1
N75.9
N76.Ø
N76.1
N76.2
N76.3
N76.4
N76.5
N76.8*
N77.1
N94.81Ø

DRG 758

Select principal diagnosis listed under DRG 757

DRG 759

Select principal diagnosis listed under DRG 757

DRG 760

Principal Diagnosis

D25*
D26*
D27*
D28*
E28*
E89.4*
F52.5
I86.2
I86.3
N39.3
N73.6
N75.Ø
N75.8
N76.6
N77.Ø
N8Ø.Ø*
N8Ø.1*
N8Ø.2*
N8Ø.3*
N8Ø.4*
N8Ø.8
N8Ø.9
N8Ø.B4
N8Ø.B5
N8Ø.B6
N8Ø.C*
N8Ø.D*
N81*
N82.Ø
N82.1
N82.5
N82.8
N82.9
N83*
N84*
N85*
N86
N87*
N88*
N89*
N9Ø*
N91*
N92*
N93*
N94.Ø
N94.1*
N94.2
N94.3
N94.4
N94.5
N94.6
N94.818
N94.819
N94.89
N94.9
N95*
N96
N97*
N99.2
N99.3
N99.83
N99.85
Q5Ø*
Q51.Ø
Q51.1Ø
Q51.11
Q51.21
Q51.22
Q51.28
Q51.3
Q51.4
Q51.5
Q51.6
Q51.7
Q51.81Ø
Q51.811
Q51.818
Q51.82Ø
Q51.821
Q51.828
Q51.9
Q52*
Q56.Ø
Q56.2
Q56.3
Q56.4
Q96*
Q97*
Q98.5
Q99.Ø
Q99.1
Q99.8
R87.61Ø
R87.611
R87.612
R87.613
R87.614
R87.615
R87.616
R87.62Ø
R87.621
R87.622
R87.623
R87.624
R87.625
R87.628
R87.81Ø
R87.811
R87.82Ø
R87.821
S3Ø.2Ø2A
S3Ø.23XA
S31.4ØXA
S31.41XA
S31.42XA
S31.43XA
S31.44XA
S31.45XA
S31.5Ø2A
S31.5Ø2S
S31.512A
S31.512S
S31.522A
S31.522S
S31.532A
S31.532S
S31.542A
S31.542S
S31.552A
S31.552S
S37.1ØXS
S37.12XS
S37.13XS
S37.19XS
S37.2ØXS
S37.22XS
S37.23XS
S37.29XS
S37.3ØXS
S37.32XS
S37.33XS
S37.39XS
S37.4Ø1A
S37.4Ø1S
S37.4Ø2A
S37.4Ø2S
S37.4Ø9A
S37.4Ø9S
S37.421A
S37.421S
S37.422A
S37.422S
S37.429A
S37.429S
S37.431A
S37.431S
S37.432A
S37.432S
S37.439A
S37.439S
S37.491A
S37.491S
S37.492A
S37.492S
S37.499A
S37.499S
S37.5Ø1A
S37.5Ø1S
S37.5Ø2A
S37.5Ø2S
S37.5Ø9A
S37.5Ø9S
S37.511A
S37.511S
S37.512A
S37.512S

S37.519A
S37.519S
S37.521A
S37.521S
S37.522A
S37.522S
S37.529A
S37.529S
S37.531A
S37.531S
S37.532A
S37.532S
S37.539A
S37.539S
S37.591A
S37.591S
S37.592A
S37.592S
S37.599A
S37.599S
S37.6ØXA
S37.6ØXS
S37.62XA
S37.62XS
S37.63XA
S37.63XS
S37.69XA
S37.69XS
S37.812S
S37.813S
S37.818S
S37.819S
S37.892A
S37.892S
S37.893A
S37.893S
S37.898A
S37.898S
S37.899A
S37.899S
S37.9ØXA
S37.9ØXS
S37.92XA
S37.92XS
S37.93XA
S37.93XS
S37.99XA
S37.99XS
S38.ØØ2A
S38.Ø3XA
S38.211A
S38.212A
T19.2XXA
T19.3XXA
T83.31XA
T83.32XA
T83.39XA
T83.711A
T83.721A
Z3Ø.2
Z31.Ø
Z4Ø.Ø2
Z4Ø.Ø3
Z43.7
Z64.1
Z9Ø.7*

DRG 761

Select principal diagnosis listed under DRG 760

MDC 14

DRG 768

Secondary Diagnosis
Z37*
AND
Delivery Operating Room Procedures
1ØD17Z9
1ØD18Z9
OR
Delivery Nonoperating Room Procedures
1ØDØ7Z3
1ØDØ7Z4
1ØDØ7Z5
1ØDØ7Z6
1ØDØ7Z7
1ØDØ7Z8
1ØEØXZZ
AND
Any Operating Room Procedures Except
ØKQMØZZ
ØU57ØZZ
ØU573ZZ
ØU574ZZ
ØU577ZZ
ØU578ZZ
ØUB5ØZZ
ØUB53ZZ
ØUB54ZZ
ØUB57ZZ
ØUB58ZZ
ØUB6ØZZ
ØUB63ZZ
ØUB64ZZ
ØUB67ZZ
ØUB68ZZ
ØUB7ØZZ
ØUB73ZZ
ØUB74ZZ
ØUB77ZZ
ØUB78ZZ
ØUJMØZZ
ØUL5ØCZ
ØUL5ØDZ
ØUL5ØZZ
ØUL53CZ
ØUL53DZ
ØUL53ZZ
ØUL54CZ
ØUL54DZ
ØUL54ZZ
ØUL57DZ
ØUL57ZZ
ØUL58DZ
ØUL58ZZ
ØUL6ØCZ
ØUL6ØDZ
ØUL6ØZZ
ØUL63CZ
ØUL63DZ
ØUL63ZZ
ØUL64CZ
ØUL64DZ
ØUL64ZZ
ØUL67DZ
ØUL67ZZ
ØUL68DZ
ØUL68ZZ
ØUL7ØCZ
ØUL7ØDZ
ØUL7ØZZ
ØUL73CZ
ØUL73DZ
ØUL73ZZ
ØUL74CZ
ØUL74DZ
ØUL74ZZ
ØUL77DZ
ØUL77ZZ
ØUL78DZ
ØUL78ZZ
ØUT5ØZZ
ØUT54ZZ
ØUT57ZZ
ØUT58ZZ
ØUT5FZZ
ØUT6ØZZ
ØUT64ZZ
ØUT67ZZ
ØUT68ZZ
ØUT6FZZ
ØUT7ØZZ
ØUT74ZZ
ØUT77ZZ
ØUT78ZZ
ØUT7FZZ
1ØD17Z9
1ØD17ZZ
1ØD18Z9
1ØD18ZZ

DRG 769

Principal Diagnosis
A34
OØ8*
O1Ø.Ø3
O1Ø.13
O1Ø.23
O1Ø.33
O1Ø.43
O1Ø.93
O11.5
O12.Ø5
O12.15
O12.25
O13.5
O14.Ø5
O14.15
O14.25
O14.95
O15.2
O16.5
O24.Ø3
O24.13
O24.33
O24.43Ø
O24.434
O24.435
O24.439
O24.83
O24.93
O25.3
O26.63
O26.73
O43.211
O43.212
O43.213
O43.219
O43.221
O43.222
O43.223
O43.229
O43.231
O43.232
O43.233
O43.239
O7Ø*
O71.2
O71.3
O71.4
O71.5
O71.6
O71.7
O71.82
O71.89
O71.9
O72.Ø
O72.1
O72.2
O72.3
O73*
O75.4
O85
O86.ØØ
O86.Ø1
O86.Ø2
O86.Ø3
O86.Ø4
O86.Ø9
O86.1*
O86.2*
O86.4
O86.8*
O87*
O88.Ø3
O88.13
O88.23
O88.33
O88.83
O89*
O9Ø.Ø
O9Ø.1
O9Ø.2
O9Ø.3
O9Ø.4*
O9Ø.5
O9Ø.6
O9Ø.8*
O9Ø.9
O91.Ø2
O91.Ø3
O91.12
O91.13
O91.22
O91.23
O92.Ø2
O92.Ø3
O92.12
O92.13
O92.2*
O92.3
O92.4
O92.5
O92.6
O92.7*
O94
O98.Ø3
O98.13
O98.23
O98.33
O98.43
O98.53
O98.63
O98.73
O98.83
O98.93
O99.Ø3
O99.13
O99.215
O99.285
O99.315
O99.325
O99.335
O99.345
O99.355
O99.43
O99.53
O99.63
O99.73
O99.815
O99.825
O99.835
O99.845
O99.893
O9A.13
O9A.23
O9A.33
O9A.43
O9A.53
Z39.Ø
AND
Select any operating room procedure

DRG 770

Principal Diagnosis
OØ2.1
OØ3*
OØ4*
OØ7*
Z33.2
Z64.Ø
AND
Operating Room Procedures
1ØAØØZZ
1ØAØ3ZZ
1ØAØ4ZZ
1ØAØ7ZZ
1ØAØ8ZZ
1ØD17ZZ
1ØD18ZZ

DRG 783

C-Section Delivery Operating Room Procedures
1ØDØØZØ
1ØDØØZ1
1ØDØØZ2
AND
Sterilization Operating Room Procedures
ØU57ØZZ
ØU573ZZ
ØU574ZZ
ØU577ZZ
ØU578ZZ
ØUB5ØZZ
ØUB53ZZ
ØUB54ZZ
ØUB57ZZ
ØUB58ZZ
ØUB6ØZZ
ØUB63ZZ
ØUB64ZZ
ØUB67ZZ
ØUB68ZZ
ØUB7ØZZ
ØUB73ZZ
ØUB74ZZ
ØUB77ZZ
ØUB78ZZ
ØUL5ØCZ
ØUL5ØDZ
ØUL5ØZZ
ØUL53CZ
ØUL53DZ
ØUL53ZZ
ØUL54CZ
ØUL54DZ
ØUL54ZZ
ØUL57DZ
ØUL57ZZ
ØUL58DZ
ØUL58ZZ
ØUL6ØCZ
ØUL6ØDZ
ØUL6ØZZ
ØUL63CZ
ØUL63DZ
ØUL63ZZ
ØUL64CZ
ØUL64DZ
ØUL64ZZ
ØUL67DZ
ØUL67ZZ
ØUL68DZ
ØUL68ZZ
ØUL7ØCZ
ØUL7ØDZ
ØUL7ØZZ
ØUL73CZ
ØUL73DZ
ØUL73ZZ
ØUL74CZ
ØUL74DZ
ØUL74ZZ
ØUL77DZ
ØUL77ZZ
ØUL78DZ
ØUL78ZZ
ØUT5ØZZ
ØUT54ZZ
ØUT57ZZ
ØUT58ZZ
ØUT5FZZ
ØUT6ØZZ
ØUT64ZZ
ØUT67ZZ
ØUT68ZZ
ØUT6FZZ
ØUT7ØZZ
ØUT74ZZ
ØUT77ZZ
ØUT78ZZ
ØUT7FZZ

DRG 784

Select C-section AND sterilization operating room procedures under DRG 783

DRG 785

Select C-section AND sterilization operating room procedures under DRG 783

DRG 786

C-Section delivery operating room procedures listed under DRG 783
Without sterilization operating room procedures listed under DRG 783

DRG 787

C-Section delivery operating room procedures listed under DRG 783
Without sterilization operating room procedures listed under DRG 783

DRG 788

C-Section delivery operating room procedures listed under DRG 783
Without sterilization operating room procedures listed under DRG 783

DRG 796

Secondary Diagnosis
Z37*
AND
Delivery Operating Room Procedures
1ØD17Z9
1ØD18Z9
OR
Delivery Nonoperating Room Procedures
1ØDØ7Z3
1ØDØ7Z4
1ØDØ7Z5
1ØDØ7Z6
1ØDØ7Z7
1ØDØ7Z8
1ØEØXZZ
AND
Sterilization Operating Room Procedures
ØU57ØZZ
ØU573ZZ
ØU574ZZ
ØU577ZZ
ØU578ZZ
ØUB5ØZZ
ØUB53ZZ
ØUB54ZZ
ØUB57ZZ
ØUB58ZZ
ØUB6ØZZ
ØUB63ZZ
ØUB64ZZ
ØUB67ZZ
ØUB68ZZ
ØUB7ØZZ
ØUB73ZZ
ØUB74ZZ
ØUB77ZZ
ØUB78ZZ
ØUL5ØCZ
ØUL5ØDZ
ØUL5ØZZ
ØUL53CZ
ØUL53DZ
ØUL53ZZ
ØUL54CZ
ØUL54DZ
ØUL54ZZ
ØUL57DZ
ØUL57ZZ
ØUL58DZ
ØUL58ZZ
ØUL6ØCZ
ØUL6ØDZ
ØUL6ØZZ
ØUL63CZ
ØUL63DZ
ØUL63ZZ
ØUL64CZ
ØUL64DZ
ØUL64ZZ
ØUL67DZ
ØUL67ZZ
ØUL68DZ
ØUL68ZZ
ØUL7ØCZ
ØUL7ØDZ
ØUL7ØZZ
ØUL73CZ
ØUL73DZ
ØUL73ZZ
ØUL74CZ
ØUL74DZ
ØUL74ZZ
ØUL77DZ
ØUL77ZZ
ØUL78DZ
ØUL78ZZ
ØUT5ØZZ
ØUT54ZZ
ØUT57ZZ
ØUT58ZZ
ØUT5FZZ
ØUT6ØZZ
ØUT64ZZ
ØUT67ZZ
ØUT68ZZ
ØUT6FZZ
ØUT7ØZZ
ØUT74ZZ
ØUT77ZZ
ØUT78ZZ
ØUT7FZZ
OR
D&C Operating Room Procedures
1ØD17ZZ
1ØD18ZZ

DRG 797

Select secondary diagnoses AND delivery procedures AND sterilization/D&C procedures listed under DRG 796

DRG 798

Select secondary diagnoses AND delivery procedures AND sterilization/D&C procedures listed under DRG 796

DRG 817

Principal Diagnosis
OØØ.ØØ
OØØ.Ø1
OØØ.1Ø1
OØØ.1Ø2
OØØ.1Ø9
OØØ.111
OØØ.112
OØØ.119
OØØ.2Ø1
OØØ.2Ø2
OØØ.2Ø9
OØØ.211
OØØ.212
OØØ.219
OØØ.8Ø
OØØ.81
OØØ.9Ø
OØØ.91
OØ1.Ø
OØ1.1
OØ1.9
OØ2.Ø
OØ2.81
OØ2.89
OØ2.9
O1Ø.Ø11
O1Ø.Ø12
O1Ø.Ø13
O1Ø.Ø19
O1Ø.111
O1Ø.112
O1Ø.113
O1Ø.119
O1Ø.211
O1Ø.212
O1Ø.213
O1Ø.219
O1Ø.311
O1Ø.312
O1Ø.313
O1Ø.319
O1Ø.411
O1Ø.412
O1Ø.413
O1Ø.419
O1Ø.911
O1Ø.912
O1Ø.913
O1Ø.919
O11.1
O11.2
O11.3
O11.9
O12.ØØ
O12.Ø1
O12.Ø2
O12.Ø3
O12.1Ø
O12.11
O12.12
O12.13
O12.2Ø
O12.21
O12.22
O12.23
O13.1
O13.2
O13.3
O13.9
O14.ØØ
O14.Ø2
O14.Ø3
O14.1Ø
O14.12
O14.13
O14.2Ø
O14.22
O14.23
O14.9Ø
O14.92
O14.93
O15.ØØ
O15.Ø2
O15.Ø3
O15.1
O15.9
O16.1
O16.2
O16.3
O16.9
O2Ø.Ø
O2Ø.8
O2Ø.9
O21.Ø
O21.1
O21.2
O21.8
O21.9
O22.ØØ
O22.Ø1
O22.Ø2
O22.Ø3
O22.1Ø
O22.11
O22.12
O22.13
O22.2Ø
O22.21
O22.22
O22.23
O22.3Ø
O22.31
O22.32
O22.33
O22.4Ø
O22.41
O22.42
O22.43
O22.5Ø
O22.51
O22.52
O22.53
O22.8X1
O22.8X2
O22.8X3
O22.8X9
O22.9Ø
O22.91
O22.92
O22.93
O23.ØØ
O23.Ø1
O23.Ø2
O23.Ø3
O23.1Ø
O23.11
O23.12
O23.13
O23.2Ø
O23.21
O23.22
O23.23
O23.3Ø
O23.31
O23.32
O23.33
O23.4Ø
O23.41
O23.42
O23.43
O23.511
O23.512
O23.513
O23.519
O23.521
O23.522
O23.523
O23.529
O23.591
O23.592
O23.593
O23.599
O23.9Ø
O23.91
O23.92
O23.93
O24.Ø11
O24.Ø12
O24.Ø13
O24.Ø19
O24.111
O24.112
O24.113
O24.119
O24.311
O24.312
O24.313
O24.319
O24.41Ø
O24.414
O24.415
O24.419
O24.811
O24.812
O24.813
O24.819
O24.911
O24.912
O24.913
O24.919
O25.1Ø
O25.11
O25.12
O25.13
O26.ØØ
O26.Ø1
O26.Ø2
O26.Ø3
O26.1Ø
O26.11
O26.12
O26.13
O26.2Ø
O26.21
O26.22
O26.23
O26.3Ø
O26.31
O26.32
O26.33
O26.4Ø
O26.41
O26.42
O26.43
O26.5Ø
O26.51
O26.52
O26.53
O26.611
O26.612
O26.613
O26.619
O26.641
O26.642
O26.643
O26.649

O26.711
O26.712
O26.713
O26.719
O26.811
O26.812
O26.813
O26.819
O26.821
O26.822
O26.823
O26.829
O26.831
O26.832
O26.833
O26.839
O26.841
O26.842
O26.843
O26.849
O26.851
O26.852
O26.853
O26.859
O26.86
O26.872
O26.873
O26.879
O26.891
O26.892
O26.893
O26.899
O26.90
O26.91
O26.92
O26.93
O28.0
O28.1
O28.2
O28.3
O28.4
O28.5
O28.8
O28.9
O29.011
O29.012
O29.013
O29.019
O29.021
O29.022
O29.023
O29.029
O29.091
O29.092
O29.093
O29.099
O29.111
O29.112
O29.113
O29.119
O29.121
O29.122
O29.123
O29.129
O29.191
O29.192
O29.193
O29.199
O29.211
O29.212
O29.213
O29.219
O29.291
O29.292
O29.293
O29.299
O29.3X1
O29.3X2
O29.3X3
O29.3X9
O29.40
O29.41
O29.42
O29.43
O29.5X1
O29.5X2
O29.5X3
O29.5X9
O29.60
O29.61
O29.62
O29.63
O29.8X1
O29.8X2
O29.8X3
O29.8X9
O29.90
O29.91
O29.92
O29.93
O30.001
O30.002
O30.003
O30.009
O30.011
O30.012
O30.013
O30.019
O30.021
O30.022
O30.023
O30.029
O30.031
O30.032
O30.033
O30.039
O30.041
O30.042
O30.043
O30.049
O30.091
O30.092
O30.093
O30.099
O30.101
O30.102
O30.103
O30.109
O30.111
O30.112
O30.113
O30.119
O30.121
O30.122
O30.123
O30.129
O30.131
O30.132
O30.133
O30.139
O30.191
O30.192
O30.193
O30.199
O30.201
O30.202
O30.203
O30.209
O30.211
O30.212
O30.213
O30.219
O30.221
O30.222
O30.223
O30.229
O30.231
O30.232
O30.233
O30.239
O30.291
O30.292
O30.293
O30.299
O30.801
O30.802
O30.803
O30.809
O30.811
O30.812
O30.813
O30.819
O30.821
O30.822
O30.823
O30.829
O30.831
O30.832
O30.833
O30.839
O30.891
O30.892
O30.893
O30.899
O30.90
O30.91
O30.92
O30.93
O31.00X0
O31.00X1
O31.00X2
O31.00X3
O31.00X4
O31.00X5
O31.00X9
O31.01X0
O31.01X1
O31.01X2
O31.01X3
O31.01X4
O31.01X5
O31.01X9
O31.02X0
O31.02X1
O31.02X2
O31.02X3
O31.02X4
O31.02X5
O31.02X9
O31.03X0
O31.03X1
O31.03X2
O31.03X3
O31.03X4
O31.03X5
O31.03X9
O31.10X0
O31.10X1
O31.10X2
O31.10X3
O31.10X4
O31.10X5
O31.10X9
O31.11X0
O31.11X1
O31.11X2
O31.11X3
O31.11X4
O31.11X5
O31.11X9
O31.12X0
O31.12X1
O31.12X2
O31.12X3
O31.12X4
O31.12X5
O31.12X9
O31.13X0
O31.13X1
O31.13X2
O31.13X3
O31.13X4
O31.13X5
O31.13X9
O31.20X0
O31.20X1
O31.20X2
O31.20X3
O31.20X4
O31.20X5
O31.20X9
O31.21X0
O31.21X1
O31.21X2
O31.21X3
O31.21X4
O31.21X5
O31.21X9
O31.22X0
O31.22X1
O31.22X2
O31.22X3
O31.22X4
O31.22X5
O31.22X9
O31.23X0
O31.23X1
O31.23X2
O31.23X3
O31.23X4
O31.23X5
O31.23X9
O31.30X0
O31.30X1
O31.30X2
O31.30X3
O31.30X4
O31.30X5
O31.30X9
O31.31X0
O31.31X1
O31.31X2
O31.31X3
O31.31X4
O31.31X5
O31.31X9
O31.32X0
O31.32X1
O31.32X2
O31.32X3
O31.32X4
O31.32X5
O31.32X9
O31.33X0
O31.33X1
O31.33X2
O31.33X3
O31.33X4
O31.33X5
O31.33X9
O31.8X10
O31.8X11
O31.8X12
O31.8X13
O31.8X14
O31.8X15
O31.8X19
O31.8X20
O31.8X21
O31.8X22
O31.8X23
O31.8X24
O31.8X25
O31.8X29
O31.8X30
O31.8X31
O31.8X32
O31.8X33
O31.8X34
O31.8X35
O31.8X39
O31.8X90
O31.8X91
O31.8X92
O31.8X93
O31.8X94
O31.8X95
O31.8X99
O32.0XX0
O32.0XX1
O32.0XX2
O32.0XX3
O32.0XX4
O32.0XX5
O32.0XX9
O32.1XX0
O32.1XX1
O32.1XX2
O32.1XX3
O32.1XX4
O32.1XX5
O32.1XX9
O32.2XX0
O32.2XX1
O32.2XX2
O32.2XX3
O32.2XX4
O32.2XX5
O32.2XX9
O32.3XX0
O32.3XX1
O32.3XX2
O32.3XX3
O32.3XX4
O32.3XX5
O32.3XX9
O32.4XX0
O32.4XX1
O32.4XX2
O32.4XX3
O32.4XX4
O32.4XX5
O32.4XX9
O32.6XX0
O32.6XX1
O32.6XX2
O32.6XX3
O32.6XX4
O32.6XX5
O32.6XX9
O32.8XX0
O32.8XX1
O32.8XX2
O32.8XX3
O32.8XX4
O32.8XX5
O32.8XX9
O32.9XX0
O32.9XX1
O32.9XX2
O32.9XX3
O32.9XX4
O32.9XX5
O32.9XX9
O33.0
O33.1
O33.2
O33.3XX0
O33.3XX1
O33.3XX2
O33.3XX3
O33.3XX4
O33.3XX5
O33.3XX9
O33.4XX0
O33.4XX1
O33.4XX2
O33.4XX3
O33.4XX4
O33.4XX5
O33.4XX9
O33.5XX0
O33.5XX1
O33.5XX2
O33.5XX3
O33.5XX4
O33.5XX5
O33.5XX9
O33.6XX0
O33.6XX1
O33.6XX2
O33.6XX3
O33.6XX4
O33.6XX5
O33.6XX9
O33.7XX0
O33.7XX1
O33.7XX2
O33.7XX3
O33.7XX4
O33.7XX5
O33.7XX9
O33.8
O33.9
O34.00
O34.01
O34.02
O34.03
O34.10
O34.11
O34.12
O34.13
O34.211
O34.212
O34.218
O34.219
O34.22
O34.29
O34.30
O34.31
O34.32
O34.33
O34.40
O34.41
O34.42
O34.43
O34.511
O34.512
O34.513
O34.519
O34.521
O34.522
O34.523
O34.529
O34.531
O34.532
O34.533
O34.539
O34.591
O34.592
O34.593
O34.599
O34.60
O34.61
O34.62
O34.63
O34.70
O34.71
O34.72
O34.73
O34.80
O34.81
O34.82
O34.83
O34.90
O34.91
O34.92
O34.93
O35.00X0
O35.00X1
O35.00X2
O35.00X3
O35.00X4
O35.00X5
O35.00X9
O35.01X0
O35.01X1
O35.01X2
O35.01X3
O35.01X4
O35.01X5
O35.01X9
O35.02X0
O35.02X1
O35.02X2
O35.02X3
O35.02X4
O35.02X5
O35.02X9
O35.03X0
O35.03X1
O35.03X2
O35.03X3
O35.03X4
O35.03X5
O35.03X9
O35.04X0
O35.04X1
O35.04X2
O35.04X3
O35.04X4
O35.04X5
O35.04X9
O35.05X0
O35.05X1
O35.05X2
O35.05X3
O35.05X4
O35.05X5
O35.05X9
O35.06X0
O35.06X1
O35.06X2
O35.06X3
O35.06X4
O35.06X5
O35.06X9
O35.07X0
O35.07X1
O35.07X2
O35.07X3
O35.07X4
O35.07X5
O35.07X9
O35.08X0
O35.08X1
O35.08X2
O35.08X3
O35.08X4
O35.08X5
O35.08X9
O35.09X0
O35.09X1
O35.09X2
O35.09X3
O35.09X4
O35.09X5
O35.09X9
O35.10X0
O35.10X1
O35.10X2
O35.10X3
O35.10X4
O35.10X5
O35.10X9
O35.11X0
O35.11X1
O35.11X2
O35.11X3
O35.11X4
O35.11X5
O35.11X9
O35.12X0
O35.12X1
O35.12X2
O35.12X3
O35.12X4
O35.12X5
O35.12X9
O35.13X0
O35.13X1
O35.13X2
O35.13X3
O35.13X4
O35.13X5
O35.13X9
O35.14X0
O35.14X1
O35.14X2
O35.14X3
O35.14X4
O35.14X5
O35.14X9
O35.15X0
O35.15X1
O35.15X2
O35.15X3
O35.15X4
O35.15X5
O35.15X9
O35.19X0
O35.19X1
O35.19X2
O35.19X3
O35.19X4
O35.19X5
O35.19X9
O35.2XX0
O35.2XX1
O35.2XX2
O35.2XX3
O35.2XX4
O35.2XX5
O35.2XX9
O35.3XX0
O35.3XX1
O35.3XX2
O35.3XX3
O35.3XX4
O35.3XX5
O35.3XX9
O35.4XX0
O35.4XX1
O35.4XX2
O35.4XX3
O35.4XX4
O35.4XX5
O35.4XX9
O35.5XX0
O35.5XX1
O35.5XX2
O35.5XX3
O35.5XX4
O35.5XX5
O35.5XX9
O35.6XX0
O35.6XX1
O35.6XX2
O35.6XX3
O35.6XX4
O35.6XX5
O35.6XX9
O35.7XX0
O35.7XX1
O35.7XX2
O35.7XX3
O35.7XX4
O35.7XX5
O35.7XX9
O35.8XX0
O35.8XX1
O35.8XX2
O35.8XX3
O35.8XX4
O35.8XX5
O35.8XX9
O35.9XX0
O35.9XX1
O35.9XX2
O35.9XX3
O35.9XX4
O35.9XX5
O35.9XX9
O35.AXX0
O35.AXX1
O35.AXX2
O35.AXX3
O35.AXX4
O35.AXX5
O35.AXX9
O35.BXX0
O35.BXX1
O35.BXX2
O35.BXX3
O35.BXX4
O35.BXX5
O35.BXX9
O35.CXX0
O35.CXX1
O35.CXX2
O35.CXX3
O35.CXX4
O35.CXX5
O35.CXX9
O35.DXX0
O35.DXX1
O35.DXX2
O35.DXX3
O35.DXX4
O35.DXX5
O35.DXX9
O35.EXX0
O35.EXX1
O35.EXX2
O35.EXX3
O35.EXX4
O35.EXX5
O35.EXX9
O35.FXX0
O35.FXX1
O35.FXX2
O35.FXX3
O35.FXX4
O35.FXX5
O35.FXX9
O35.GXX0
O35.GXX1
O35.GXX2
O35.GXX3
O35.GXX4
O35.GXX5
O35.GXX9
O35.HXX0
O35.HXX1
O35.HXX2
O35.HXX3
O35.HXX4
O35.HXX5
O35.HXX9
O36.0110
O36.0111
O36.0112
O36.0113
O36.0114
O36.0115
O36.0119
O36.0120
O36.0121
O36.0122
O36.0123
O36.0124
O36.0125
O36.0129
O36.0130
O36.0131
O36.0132
O36.0133
O36.0134
O36.0135
O36.0139
O36.0190
O36.0191
O36.0192
O36.0193
O36.0194
O36.0195
O36.0199
O36.0910
O36.0911
O36.0912
O36.0913
O36.0914
O36.0915
O36.0919
O36.0920
O36.0921
O36.0922
O36.0923
O36.0924
O36.0925
O36.0929
O36.0930
O36.0931
O36.0932
O36.0933
O36.0934
O36.0935
O36.0939
O36.0990
O36.0991
O36.0992
O36.0993
O36.0994
O36.0995
O36.0999
O36.1110
O36.1111
O36.1112
O36.1113
O36.1114
O36.1115
O36.1119
O36.1120
O36.1121
O36.1122
O36.1123
O36.1124
O36.1125
O36.1129
O36.1130
O36.1131
O36.1132
O36.1133
O36.1134
O36.1135
O36.1139
O36.1190
O36.1191
O36.1192
O36.1193
O36.1194
O36.1195
O36.1199
O36.1910
O36.1911
O36.1912
O36.1913
O36.1914
O36.1915
O36.1919
O36.1920
O36.1921
O36.1922
O36.1923
O36.1924
O36.1925
O36.1929
O36.1930
O36.1931
O36.1932
O36.1933
O36.1934
O36.1935
O36.1939
O36.1990
O36.1991
O36.1992
O36.1993
O36.1994
O36.1995
O36.1999
O36.20X0
O36.20X1
O36.20X2
O36.20X3
O36.20X4
O36.20X5
O36.20X9
O36.21X0
O36.21X1
O36.21X2
O36.21X3
O36.21X4
O36.21X5
O36.21X9
O36.22X0
O36.22X1
O36.22X2
O36.22X3
O36.22X4
O36.22X5
O36.22X9
O36.23X0
O36.23X1
O36.23X2
O36.23X3
O36.23X4
O36.23X5
O36.23X9
O36.4XX0
O36.4XX1
O36.4XX2
O36.4XX3
O36.4XX4
O36.4XX5

O36.4XX9
O36.5110
O36.5111
O36.5112
O36.5113
O36.5114
O36.5115
O36.5119
O36.5120
O36.5121
O36.5122
O36.5123
O36.5124
O36.5125
O36.5129
O36.5130
O36.5131
O36.5132
O36.5133
O36.5134
O36.5135
O36.5139
O36.5190
O36.5191
O36.5192
O36.5193
O36.5194
O36.5195
O36.5199
O36.5910
O36.5911
O36.5912
O36.5913
O36.5914
O36.5915
O36.5919
O36.5920
O36.5921
O36.5922
O36.5923
O36.5924
O36.5925
O36.5929
O36.5930
O36.5931
O36.5932
O36.5933
O36.5934
O36.5935
O36.5939
O36.5990
O36.5991
O36.5992
O36.5993
O36.5994
O36.5995
O36.5999
O36.60X0
O36.60X1
O36.60X2
O36.60X3
O36.60X4
O36.60X5
O36.60X9
O36.61X0
O36.61X1
O36.61X2
O36.61X3
O36.61X4
O36.61X5
O36.61X9
O36.62X0
O36.62X1
O36.62X2
O36.62X3
O36.62X4
O36.62X5
O36.62X9
O36.63X0
O36.63X1
O36.63X2
O36.63X3
O36.63X4
O36.63X5
O36.63X9
O36.70X0
O36.70X1
O36.70X2
O36.70X3
O36.70X4
O36.70X5
O36.70X9
O36.71X0
O36.71X1
O36.71X2
O36.71X3
O36.71X4
O36.71X5
O36.71X9
O36.72X0
O36.72X1
O36.72X2
O36.72X3
O36.72X4
O36.72X5
O36.72X9
O36.73X0
O36.73X1
O36.73X2
O36.73X3
O36.73X4
O36.73X5
O36.73X9
O36.80X0
O36.80X1
O36.80X2
O36.80X3
O36.80X4
O36.80X5
O36.80X9
O36.8120
O36.8121
O36.8122
O36.8123
O36.8124
O36.8125
O36.8129
O36.8130
O36.8131
O36.8132
O36.8133
O36.8134
O36.8135
O36.8139
O36.8190
O36.8191
O36.8192
O36.8193
O36.8194
O36.8195
O36.8199
O36.8210
O36.8211
O36.8212
O36.8213
O36.8214
O36.8215
O36.8219
O36.8220
O36.8221
O36.8222
O36.8223
O36.8224
O36.8225
O36.8229
O36.8230
O36.8231
O36.8232
O36.8233
O36.8234
O36.8235
O36.8239
O36.8290
O36.8291
O36.8292
O36.8293
O36.8294
O36.8295
O36.8299
O36.8310
O36.8311
O36.8312
O36.8313
O36.8314
O36.8315
O36.8319
O36.8320
O36.8321
O36.8322
O36.8323
O36.8324
O36.8325
O36.8329
O36.8330
O36.8331
O36.8332
O36.8333
O36.8334
O36.8335
O36.8339
O36.8390
O36.8391
O36.8392
O36.8393
O36.8394
O36.8395
O36.8399
O36.8910
O36.8911
O36.8912
O36.8913
O36.8914
O36.8915
O36.8919
O36.8920
O36.8921
O36.8922
O36.8923
O36.8924
O36.8925
O36.8929
O36.8930
O36.8931
O36.8932
O36.8933
O36.8934
O36.8935
O36.8939
O36.8990
O36.8991
O36.8992
O36.8993
O36.8994
O36.8995
O36.8999
O36.90X0
O36.90X1
O36.90X2
O36.90X3
O36.90X4
O36.90X5
O36.90X9
O36.91X0
O36.91X1
O36.91X2
O36.91X3
O36.91X4
O36.91X5
O36.91X9
O36.92X0
O36.92X1
O36.92X2
O36.92X3
O36.92X4
O36.92X5
O36.92X9
O36.93X0
O36.93X1
O36.93X2
O36.93X3
O36.93X4
O36.93X5
O36.93X9
O40.1XX0
O40.1XX1
O40.1XX2
O40.1XX3
O40.1XX4
O40.1XX5
O40.1XX9
O40.2XX0
O40.2XX1
O40.2XX2
O40.2XX3
O40.2XX4
O40.2XX5
O40.2XX9
O40.3XX0
O40.3XX1
O40.3XX2
O40.3XX3
O40.3XX4
O40.3XX5
O40.3XX9
O40.9XX0
O40.9XX1
O40.9XX2
O40.9XX3
O40.9XX4
O40.9XX5
O40.9XX9
O41.00X0
O41.00X1
O41.00X2
O41.00X3
O41.00X4
O41.00X5
O41.00X9
O41.01X0
O41.01X1
O41.01X2
O41.01X3
O41.01X4
O41.01X5
O41.01X9
O41.02X0
O41.02X1
O41.02X2
O41.02X3
O41.02X4
O41.02X5
O41.02X9
O41.03X0
O41.03X1
O41.03X2
O41.03X3
O41.03X4
O41.03X5
O41.03X9
O41.1010
O41.1011
O41.1012
O41.1013
O41.1014
O41.1015
O41.1019
O41.1020
O41.1021
O41.1022
O41.1023
O41.1024
O41.1025
O41.1029
O41.1030
O41.1031
O41.1032
O41.1033
O41.1034
O41.1035
O41.1039
O41.1090
O41.1091
O41.1092
O41.1093
O41.1094
O41.1095
O41.1099
O41.1210
O41.1211
O41.1212
O41.1213
O41.1214
O41.1215
O41.1219
O41.1220
O41.1221
O41.1222
O41.1223
O41.1224
O41.1225
O41.1229
O41.1230
O41.1231
O41.1232
O41.1233
O41.1234
O41.1235
O41.1239
O41.1290
O41.1291
O41.1292
O41.1293
O41.1294
O41.1295
O41.1299
O41.1410
O41.1411
O41.1412
O41.1413
O41.1414
O41.1415
O41.1419
O41.1420
O41.1421
O41.1422
O41.1423
O41.1424
O41.1425
O41.1429
O41.1430
O41.1431
O41.1432
O41.1433
O41.1434
O41.1435
O41.1439
O41.1490
O41.1491
O41.1492
O41.1493
O41.1494
O41.1495
O41.1499
O41.8X10
O41.8X11
O41.8X12
O41.8X13
O41.8X14
O41.8X15
O41.8X19
O41.8X20
O41.8X21
O41.8X22
O41.8X23
O41.8X24
O41.8X25
O41.8X29
O41.8X30
O41.8X31
O41.8X32
O41.8X33
O41.8X34
O41.8X35
O41.8X39
O41.8X90
O41.8X91
O41.8X92
O41.8X93
O41.8X94
O41.8X95
O41.8X99
O41.90X0
O41.90X1
O41.90X2
O41.90X3
O41.90X4
O41.90X5
O41.90X9
O41.91X0
O41.91X1
O41.91X2
O41.91X3
O41.91X4
O41.91X5
O41.91X9
O41.92X0
O41.92X1
O41.92X2
O41.92X3
O41.92X4
O41.92X5
O41.92X9
O41.93X0
O41.93X1
O41.93X2
O41.93X3
O41.93X4
O41.93X5
O41.93X9
O42.00
O42.011
O42.012
O42.013
O42.019
O42.02
O42.10
O42.111
O42.112
O42.113
O42.119
O42.12
O42.90
O42.911
O42.912
O42.913
O42.919
O42.92
O43.011
O43.012
O43.013
O43.019
O43.021
O43.022
O43.023
O43.029
O43.101
O43.102
O43.103
O43.109
O43.111
O43.112
O43.113
O43.119
O43.121
O43.122
O43.123
O43.129
O43.191
O43.192
O43.193
O43.199
O43.811
O43.812
O43.813
O43.819
O43.891
O43.892
O43.893
O43.899
O43.90
O43.91
O43.92
O43.93
O44.00
O44.01
O44.02
O44.03
O44.10
O44.11
O44.12
O44.13
O44.20
O44.21
O44.22
O44.23
O44.30
O44.31
O44.32
O44.33
O44.40
O44.41
O44.42
O44.43
O44.50
O44.51
O44.52
O44.53
O45.001
O45.002
O45.003
O45.009
O45.011
O45.012
O45.013
O45.019
O45.021
O45.022
O45.023
O45.029
O45.091
O45.092
O45.093
O45.099
O45.8X1
O45.8X2
O45.8X3
O45.8X9
O45.90
O45.91
O45.92
O45.93
O46.001
O46.002
O46.003
O46.009
O46.011
O46.012
O46.013
O46.019
O46.021
O46.022
O46.023
O46.029
O46.091
O46.092
O46.093
O46.099
O46.8X1
O46.8X2
O46.8X3
O46.8X9
O46.90
O46.91
O46.92
O46.93
O47.00
O47.02
O47.03
O47.1
O47.9
O48.0
O48.1
O60.00
O60.02
O60.03
O61.0
O61.1
O61.8
O61.9
O62.0
O62.1
O62.2
O62.3
O62.4
O62.8
O62.9
O63.0
O63.1
O63.9
O64.0XX0
O64.0XX1
O64.0XX2
O64.0XX3
O64.0XX4
O64.0XX5
O64.0XX9
O64.1XX0
O64.1XX1
O64.1XX2
O64.1XX3
O64.1XX4
O64.1XX5
O64.1XX9
O64.2XX0
O64.2XX1
O64.2XX2
O64.2XX3
O64.2XX4
O64.2XX5
O64.2XX9
O64.3XX0
O64.3XX1
O64.3XX2
O64.3XX3
O64.3XX4
O64.3XX5
O64.3XX9
O64.4XX0
O64.4XX1
O64.4XX2
O64.4XX3
O64.4XX4
O64.4XX5
O64.4XX9
O64.5XX0
O64.5XX1
O64.5XX2
O64.5XX3
O64.5XX4
O64.5XX5
O64.5XX9
O64.8XX0
O64.8XX1
O64.8XX2
O64.8XX3
O64.8XX4
O64.8XX5
O64.8XX9
O64.9XX0
O64.9XX1
O64.9XX2
O64.9XX3
O64.9XX4
O64.9XX5
O64.9XX9
O65.0
O65.1
O65.2
O65.3
O65.4
O65.5
O65.8
O65.9
O66.0
O66.1
O66.2
O66.3
O66.40
O66.5
O66.6
O66.8
O66.9
O71.00
O71.02
O71.03
O71.1
O71.81
O75.2
O75.3
O88.011
O88.012
O88.013
O88.019
O88.111
O88.112
O88.113
O88.119
O88.211
O88.212
O88.213
O88.219
O88.311
O88.312
O88.313
O88.319
O88.811
O88.812
O88.813
O88.819
O91.011
O91.012
O91.013
O91.019
O91.111
O91.112
O91.113
O91.119
O91.211
O91.212
O91.213
O91.219
O92.011
O92.012
O92.013
O92.019
O92.111
O92.112
O92.113
O92.119
O98.011
O98.012
O98.013
O98.019
O98.111
O98.112
O98.113
O98.119
O98.211
O98.212
O98.213
O98.219
O98.311
O98.312
O98.313
O98.319
O98.411
O98.412
O98.413
O98.419
O98.511
O98.512
O98.513
O98.519
O98.611
O98.612
O98.613
O98.619
O98.711
O98.712
O98.713
O98.719
O98.811
O98.812
O98.813
O98.819
O98.911
O98.912
O98.913
O98.919
O99.011
O99.012
O99.013
O99.019
O99.111
O99.112
O99.113
O99.119
O99.210
O99.211
O99.212
O99.213
O99.280
O99.281
O99.282
O99.283
O99.310
O99.311
O99.312
O99.313
O99.320
O99.321
O99.322
O99.323
O99.330
O99.331
O99.332
O99.333
O99.340
O99.341
O99.342
O99.343
O99.350
O99.351
O99.352
O99.353
O99.411
O99.412
O99.413
O99.419
O99.511
O99.512
O99.513
O99.519
O99.611
O99.612
O99.613
O99.619
O99.711
O99.712
O99.713
O99.719
O99.810
O99.820
O99.830
O99.840
O99.841
O99.842
O99.843
O99.891
O9A.111
O9A.112
O9A.113
O9A.119
O9A.211
O9A.212
O9A.213
O9A.219
O9A.311
O9A.312
O9A.313
O9A.319
O9A.411
O9A.412
O9A.413
O9A.419
O9A.511
O9A.512
O9A.513
O9A.519

AND

Any operating room procedure

DRG 818

Select principal diagnoses listed under DRG 817

AND

Any operating room procedure

DRG 819

Select principal diagnoses listed under DRG 817

AND
Any operating room procedure

DRG 776
Select principal diagnosis listed under DRG 769

DRG 779
Select principal diagnoses listed under DRG 770

DRG 805
Select secondary diagnoses and delivery procedures listed under DRG 796

DRG 806
Select secondary diagnoses and delivery procedures listed under DRG 796

DRG 807
Select secondary diagnoses and delivery procedures listed under DRG 796

DRG 831
Select principal diagnoses listed under DRG 817

DRG 832
Select principal diagnoses listed under DRG 817

DRG 833
Select principal diagnoses listed under DRG 817

DRG 998
Principal Diagnosis
OØ9.Ø*
OØ9.1*
OØ9.2*
OØ9.3*
OØ9.4Ø
OØ9.41
OØ9.42
OØ9.43
OØ9.5*
OØ9.6*
OØ9.7*
OØ9.8*
OØ9.9*
OØ9.AØ
OØ9.A1
OØ9.A2
OØ9.A3
O1Ø.Ø2
O1Ø.12
O1Ø.22
O1Ø.32
O1Ø.42
O1Ø.92
O11.4
O12.Ø4
O12.14
O12.24
O13.4
O14.Ø4
O14.14
O14.24
O14.94
O16.4
O24.Ø2
O24.12
O24.32
O24.42Ø
O24.424
O24.425
O24.429
O24.82
O24.92
O25.2
O26.62
O26.72
O6Ø.1ØXØ
O6Ø.1ØX1
O6Ø.1ØX2
O6Ø.1ØX3
O6Ø.1ØX4
O6Ø.1ØX5
O6Ø.1ØX9
O6Ø.12XØ
O6Ø.12X1
O6Ø.12X2
O6Ø.12X3
O6Ø.12X4
O6Ø.12X5
O6Ø.12X9
O6Ø.13XØ
O6Ø.13X1
O6Ø.13X2
O6Ø.13X3
O6Ø.13X4
O6Ø.13X5
O6Ø.13X9
O6Ø.14XØ
O6Ø.14X1
O6Ø.14X2
O6Ø.14X3
O6Ø.14X4
O6Ø.14X5
O6Ø.14X9
O6Ø.2ØXØ
O6Ø.2ØX1
O6Ø.2ØX2
O6Ø.2ØX3
O6Ø.2ØX4
O6Ø.2ØX5
O6Ø.2ØX9
O6Ø.22XØ
O6Ø.22X1
O6Ø.22X2
O6Ø.22X3
O6Ø.22X4
O6Ø.22X5
O6Ø.22X9
O6Ø.23XØ
O6Ø.23X1
O6Ø.23X2
O6Ø.23X3
O6Ø.23X4
O6Ø.23X5
O6Ø.23X9
O63.2
O66.41
O67.Ø
O67.8
O67.9
O68
O69.ØXXØ
O69.ØXX1
O69.ØXX2
O69.ØXX3
O69.ØXX4
O69.ØXX5
O69.ØXX9
O69.1XXØ
O69.1XX1
O69.1XX2
O69.1XX3
O69.1XX4
O69.1XX5
O69.1XX9
O69.2XXØ
O69.2XX1
O69.2XX2
O69.2XX3
O69.2XX4
O69.2XX5
O69.2XX9
O69.3XXØ
O69.3XX1
O69.3XX2
O69.3XX3
O69.3XX4
O69.3XX5
O69.3XX9
O69.4XXØ
O69.4XX1
O69.4XX2
O69.4XX3
O69.4XX4
O69.4XX5
O69.4XX9
O69.5XXØ
O69.5XX1
O69.5XX2
O69.5XX3
O69.5XX4
O69.5XX5
O69.5XX9
O69.81XØ
O69.81X1
O69.81X2
O69.81X3
O69.81X4
O69.81X5
O69.81X9
O69.82XØ
O69.82X1
O69.82X2
O69.82X3
O69.82X4
O69.82X5
O69.82X9
O69.89XØ
O69.89X1
O69.89X2
O69.89X3
O69.89X4
O69.89X5
O69.89X9
O69.9XXØ
O69.9XX1
O69.9XX2
O69.9XX3
O69.9XX4
O69.9XX5
O69.9XX9
O74.Ø
O74.1
O74.2
O74.3
O74.4
O74.5
O74.6
O74.7
O74.8
O74.9
O75.Ø
O75.1
O75.5
O75.81
O75.82
O75.89
O75.9
O76
O77.Ø
O77.1
O77.8
O77.9
O8Ø
O82
O88.Ø2
O88.12
O88.22
O88.32
O88.82
O98.Ø2
O98.12
O98.22
O98.32
O98.42
O98.52
O98.62
O98.72
O98.82
O98.92
O99.Ø2
O99.12
O99.214
O99.284
O99.314
O99.324
O99.334
O99.344
O99.354
O99.42
O99.52
O99.62
O99.72
O99.814
O99.824
O99.834
O99.844
O99.892
O9A.12
O9A.22
O9A.32
O9A.42
O9A.52

MDC 15

DRG 789
Discharge status disposition of transfer to an acute care facility or expired Discharge status
02 - Short term hospital
05 - Cancer center or children's hospital
20 - Expired (Died)
66 - Critical access hospital
82 - Short term hospital with planned readmission
85 - Cancer center or children's hospital with planned readmission
94 - Critical access hospital with planned readmission

DRG 790
Principal or Secondary Diagnosis
PØ7.ØØ
PØ7.Ø1
PØ7.Ø2
PØ7.Ø3
PØ7.2Ø
PØ7.21
PØ7.22
PØ7.23
PØ7.24
PØ7.25
PØ7.26
P22.Ø

DRG 791
Principal or Secondary Diagnosis
PØ7.1*
PØ7.3*
AND
Principal or secondary diagnosis listed under DRG 793

DRG 792
Principal or Secondary Diagnosis
PØ7.1*
PØ7.3*

DRG 793
Principal or Secondary Diagnosis
E84.11
PØ3.4
PØ5.11
PØ5.12
PØ5.13
PØ5.14
PØ5.15
PØ5.16
PØ5.17
PØ5.2
P1Ø*
P11.Ø
P11.2
P11.4
P11.5
P11.9
P12.2
P14.2
P14.8
P14.9
P23*
P24*
P25*
P26*
P28.Ø
P28.5
P29.3*
P29.81
P35.Ø
P35.1
P35.2
P35.3
P35.4
P35.8
P35.9
P36*
P37.Ø
P37.1
P37.2
P37.3
P37.4
P37.8
P37.9
P38*
P39.Ø
P39.2
P39.3
P39.4
P39.8
P39.9
P5Ø*
P52*
P53
P54.1
P54.2
P54.3
P54.4
P55.8
P55.9
P56*
P57*
P59.1
P59.2*
P6Ø
P61.Ø
P61.2
P61.6
P7Ø.2
P7Ø.3
P7Ø.4
P71*
P72.1
P74.Ø
P74.1
P74.21
P74.22
P74.31
P74.32
P74.421
P74.422
P74.49
P76.Ø
P76.2
P77*
P78.Ø
P83.2
P9Ø
P91.Ø
P91.1
P91.3
P91.4
P91.5
P91.62
P91.63
P91.8*
P91.9
P92.Ø1
P93*
P94.Ø
P96.1
P96.2
OR
Secondary Diagnosis
A35
A39.1
A39.5*
A39.82
A39.83
A39.84
A4Ø.9
A41*
A42.7
A48.Ø
A48.1
A48.51
A81.1
BØØ.Ø
BØØ.1
BØØ.2
BØØ.3
BØØ.4
BØØ.5*
BØØ.7
BØØ.81
BØØ.89
BØ1.Ø
BØ1.11
BØ1.2
BØ1.81
BØ1.89
BØ1.9
BØ2.Ø
BØ2.1
BØ2.21
BØ2.22
BØ2.23
BØ2.29
BØ2.3*
BØ2.7
BØ2.8
BØ2.9
BØ5.Ø
BØ5.1
BØ5.2
BØ5.3
BØ5.4
BØ5.8*
BØ6.Ø*
BØ6.8*
BØ8.2*
B1Ø.Ø*
B16*
B17*
B18*
B19.Ø
B19.1*
B19.9
B25.2
B26.Ø
B26.1
B26.2
B26.3
B26.8*
B37.1
B37.5
B37.6
B37.81
B37.82
B37.84
B38.4
B38.7
B38.89
B39.Ø
B39.1
B39.2
B4Ø*
B41*
B44.1
B44.2
B44.7
B44.89
B44.9
B45*
B46*
B47.Ø
B48.2
B48.4
B48.8
B58.Ø*
B58.1
B58.2
B58.3
B58.8*
B59
B97.4
D56.Ø
D56.1
D56.2
D56.5
D56.8
D56.9
D57.4*
D59.2
D59.3*
D59.4
D59.5
D59.6
D59.8
D59.9
D62
D65
D69.5*
D75.82*
D75.84
D78.1*
EØ3.5
E15
E2Ø.Ø
E2Ø.8*
E2Ø.9
E23.2
E32.1
E36.1*
E41
E43
E44*
E46
E64.Ø
E86*
E87*
E88.3
E89.2
F11.13
F11.23
F11.93
F13.13Ø
F13.131
F13.132
F13.139
F13.23Ø
F13.231
F13.232
F13.239
F13.93Ø
F13.931
F13.932
F13.939
F14.13
F14.23
F14.93
F15.13
F15.23
F15.93
F17.2Ø3
F17.213
F17.223
F17.293
F19.13Ø
F19.131
F19.132
F19.139
F19.23Ø
F19.231
F19.232
F19.239
F19.93Ø
F19.931
F19.932
F19.939
GØØ*
GØ1
GØ2
GØ3.Ø
GØ3.8
GØ3.9
GØ4.2
GØ6*
GØ7
G9Ø.1
G9Ø.A
G92*
G93.1
G96.Ø*
G96.11
G97.Ø
G97.1
G97.2
G97.4*
G97.8*
H47.1Ø
H47.11
H47.12
H59.2*
H7Ø.Ø11
H7Ø.Ø12
H7Ø.Ø13
H7Ø.Ø19
H7Ø.811
H7Ø.812
H7Ø.813
H7Ø.819
H95.3*
IØ9.81
I11.Ø
I13.Ø
I13.2
I25.3
I26*
I27.82
I31.2
I32
I33*
I38
I39
I4Ø.Ø
I41
I43
I44.2
I45.2
I45.3
I45.6
I45.89
I46*
I47.Ø
I47.2*
I48.Ø
I48.19
I48.21
I48.3
I48.4
I48.91
I48.92
I49.Ø1
I49.Ø2
I5Ø*
I6Ø*
I61*
I62*
I63.ØØ
I63.Ø11
I63.Ø12
I63.Ø13
I63.Ø19
I63.Ø2
I63.Ø31
I63.Ø32
I63.Ø33
I63.Ø39
I63.Ø9
I63.1Ø
I63.111
I63.112
I63.113
I63.119
I63.12
I63.131
I63.132
I63.133
I63.139
I63.19
I63.2Ø
I63.211
I63.212
I63.213
I63.219
I63.22
I63.231
I63.232
I63.233
I63.239
I63.29
I63.3Ø
I63.311
I63.312
I63.313
I63.319
I63.321
I63.322
I63.323
I63.329
I63.331
I63.332
I63.333
I63.339
I63.341
I63.342
I63.343
I63.349
I63.39
I63.4Ø
I63.411
I63.412
I63.413
I63.419
I63.421
I63.422
I63.423
I63.429
I63.431
I63.432
I63.433
I63.439
I63.441
I63.442
I63.443
I63.449
I63.49
I63.5Ø
I63.511
I63.512
I63.513
I63.519
I63.521
I63.522
I63.523
I63.529
I63.531
I63.532
I63.533
I63.539
I63.541
I63.542
I63.543
I63.549
I63.59
I63.6
I63.81
I63.89
I63.9
I66*
I7Ø.261
I7Ø.262
I7Ø.263
I7Ø.268
I7Ø.269
I74*
I76
I8Ø.1*
I8Ø.2*
I8Ø.3
I82.22Ø
I82.221
I89.1
I96
I97.Ø
I97.1*
I97.5*
I97.7*
I97.88
I97.89
JØ9.X1
JØ9.X2
J1Ø.Ø8
J1Ø.1
J13
J14
J15*
J16*
J18.Ø
J18.1
J18.8
J18.9
J38.Ø*
J38.5
J39.Ø
J45.22
J45.32
J45.42

J45.52
J45.902
J69.0
J69.8
J70.0
J81.0
J84.83
J84.84*
J85*
J86*
J90
J91.8
J94.0
J94.2
J94.8
J95.1
J95.2
J95.3
J95.4
J95.5
J95.7*
J95.851
J95.859
J95.87
J95.88
J95.89
J98.11
J98.19
J98.2
J98.5*
K22.3
K31.0
K40.00
K40.10
K40.30
K40.40
K41.00
K41.10
K41.30
K41.40
K42.0
K42.1
K43.0
K43.1
K43.3
K43.4
K43.6
K43.7
K44.0
K44.1
K45.0
K45.1
K46.0
K46.1
K52.1
K55.0*
K55.30
K55.31
K55.32
K55.33
K56.0
K56.1
K56.2
K56.41
K56.49
K56.600
K56.601
K56.609
K56.690
K56.691
K56.699
K56.7
K61.0
K61.1
K61.2
K61.31
K61.39
K61.4
K61.5
K62.5
K63.1
K65*
K66.1
K67
K68*
K71*
K72.0*
K72.9*
K75.0
K75.1
K75.2
K75.3
K75.8*
K75.9
K76.2
K76.3
K76.4
K76.7
K76.82
K83.01
K83.09
K85*
K86.2
K86.3
K91.2
K91.30
K91.31
K91.32
K91.7*
K91.81
K91.82
K91.83
K91.850
K91.858
K91.86
K91.89
K92.0
K92.1
K92.2
L02.01
L02.11
L02.21*
L02.31
L02.41*
L02.51*
L02.61*
L02.81*
L02.91
L03.1*
L03.2*
L03.3*
L03.8*
L03.9*
L04*
L27.0
L27.1
L50.0
L53.0
L53.1
L53.2
L53.3
L76.1*
L98.3
M48.50XA
M48.51XA
M48.52XA
M48.53XA
M48.54XA
M48.55XA
M48.56XA
M48.57XA
M48.58XA
M80.00XA
M80.011A
M80.012A
M80.019A
M80.021A
M80.022A
M80.029A
M80.031A
M80.032A
M80.039A
M80.041A
M80.042A
M80.049A
M80.051A
M80.052A
M80.059A
M80.061A
M80.062A
M80.069A
M80.071A
M80.072A
M80.079A
M80.08XA
M80.0AXA
M80.80XA
M80.811A
M80.812A
M80.819A
M80.821A
M80.822A
M80.829A
M80.831A
M80.832A
M80.839A
M80.841A
M80.842A
M80.849A
M80.851A
M80.852A
M80.859A
M80.861A
M80.862A
M80.869A
M80.871A
M80.872A
M80.879A
M80.88XA
M80.8AXA
M84.40XA
M84.411A
M84.412A
M84.419A
M84.421A
M84.422A
M84.429A
M84.431A
M84.432A
M84.433A
M84.434A
M84.439A
M84.441A
M84.442A
M84.443A
M84.444A
M84.445A
M84.446A
M84.451A
M84.452A
M84.453A
M84.454A
M84.459A
M84.461A
M84.462A
M84.463A
M84.464A
M84.469A
M84.471A
M84.472A
M84.473A
M84.474A
M84.475A
M84.476A
M84.477A
M84.478A
M84.479A
M84.48XA
M84.50XA
M84.511A
M84.512A
M84.519A
M84.521A
M84.522A
M84.529A
M84.531A
M84.532A
M84.533A
M84.534A
M84.539A
M84.541A
M84.542A
M84.549A
M84.550A
M84.551A
M84.552A
M84.553A
M84.559A
M84.561A
M84.562A
M84.563A
M84.564A
M84.569A
M84.571A
M84.572A
M84.573A
M84.574A
M84.575A
M84.576A
M84.58XA
M84.60XA
M84.611A
M84.612A
M84.619A
M84.621A
M84.622A
M84.629A
M84.631A
M84.632A
M84.633A
M84.634A
M84.639A
M84.641A
M84.642A
M84.649A
M84.650A
M84.651A
M84.652A
M84.653A
M84.659A
M84.661A
M84.662A
M84.663A
M84.664A
M84.669A
M84.671A
M84.672A
M84.673A
M84.674A
M84.675A
M84.676A
M84.68XA
M84.750A
M84.751A
M84.752A
M84.753A
M84.754A
M84.755A
M84.756A
M84.757A
M84.758A
M84.759A
M96.820
M96.821
N00*
N01*
N10
N11.9
N12
N13.0
N13.1
N13.2
N13.3*
N13.4
N13.6
N13.9
N15.1
N17*
N28.84
N28.85
N28.86
N30.0*
N30.8*
N30.9*
N31.2
N32.0
N32.1
N32.2
N34.0
N39.0
N82.2
N82.3
N82.4
N82.8
N83.7
N98.0
N99.0
N99.520
N99.521
N99.522
N99.523
N99.524
N99.528
N99.530
N99.531
N99.532
N99.533
N99.534
N99.538
N99.7*
N99.81
N99.89
P91.2
Q00*
Q01*
Q02
Q03*
Q04*
Q05*
Q06*
Q07*
Q21.0
Q79.2
Q79.3
Q89.4
R00.0
R09.2
R29.0
R31*
R33*
R39.14
R40.20
R40.2110
R40.2111
R40.2112
R40.2113
R40.2114
R40.2120
R40.2121
R40.2122
R40.2123
R40.2124
R40.2210
R40.2211
R40.2212
R40.2213
R40.2214
R40.2220
R40.2221
R40.2222
R40.2223
R40.2224
R40.2310
R40.2311
R40.2312
R40.2313
R40.2314
R40.2320
R40.2321
R40.2322
R40.2323
R40.2324
R40.2340
R40.2341
R40.2342
R40.2343
R40.2344
R40.2A
R40.3
R56.00
R56.9
R57.9
R58
R78.81
R82.0
S14.3XXA
S15.001A
S15.002A
S15.009A
S15.011A
S15.012A
S15.019A
S15.021A
S15.022A
S15.029A
S15.091A
S15.092A
S15.099A
S15.201A
S15.202A
S15.209A
S15.211A
S15.212A
S15.219A
S15.221A
S15.222A
S15.229A
S15.291A
S15.292A
S15.299A
S15.301A
S15.302A
S15.309A
S15.311A
S15.312A
S15.319A
S15.321A
S15.322A
S15.329A
S15.391A
S15.392A
S15.399A
S25.00XA
S25.01XA
S25.02XA
S25.09XA
S25.101A
S25.102A
S25.109A
S25.111A
S25.112A
S25.119A
S25.121A
S25.122A
S25.129A
S25.191A
S25.192A
S25.199A
S25.20XA
S25.21XA
S25.22XA
S25.29XA
S25.301A
S25.302A
S25.309A
S25.311A
S25.312A
S25.319A
S25.321A
S25.322A
S25.329A
S25.391A
S25.392A
S25.399A
S25.401A
S25.402A
S25.409A
S25.411A
S25.412A
S25.419A
S25.421A
S25.422A
S25.429A
S25.491A
S25.492A
S25.499A
S27.0XXA
S27.1XXA
S27.2XXA
S35.00XA
S35.01XA
S35.02XA
S35.09XA
S35.10XA
S35.11XA
S35.12XA
S35.19XA
S36.00XA
S36.020A
S36.021A
S36.029A
S36.030A
S36.031A
S36.032A
S36.039A
S36.09XA
S72.001A
S72.001B
S72.001C
S72.002A
S72.002B
S72.002C
S72.009A
S72.009B
S72.009C
S72.011A
S72.011B
S72.011C
S72.012A
S72.012B
S72.012C
S72.019A
S72.019B
S72.019C
S72.021A
S72.021B
S72.021C
S72.022A
S72.022B
S72.022C
S72.023A
S72.023B
S72.023C
S72.024A
S72.024B
S72.024C
S72.025A
S72.025B
S72.025C
S72.026A
S72.026B
S72.026C
S72.031A
S72.031B
S72.031C
S72.032A
S72.032B
S72.032C
S72.033A
S72.033B
S72.033C
S72.034A
S72.034B
S72.034C
S72.035A
S72.035B
S72.035C
S72.036A
S72.036B
S72.036C
S72.041A
S72.041B
S72.041C
S72.042A
S72.042B
S72.042C
S72.043A
S72.043B
S72.043C
S72.044A
S72.044B
S72.044C
S72.045A
S72.045B
S72.045C
S72.046A
S72.046B
S72.046C
S72.051A
S72.051B
S72.051C
S72.052A
S72.052B
S72.052C
S72.059A
S72.059B
S72.059C
S72.061A
S72.061B
S72.061C
S72.062A
S72.062B
S72.062C
S72.063A
S72.063B
S72.063C
S72.064A
S72.064B
S72.064C
S72.065A
S72.065B
S72.065C
S72.066A
S72.066B
S72.066C
S72.091A
S72.091B
S72.091C
S72.092A
S72.092B
S72.092C
S72.099A
S72.099B
S72.099C
S72.101A
S72.101B
S72.101C
S72.102A
S72.102B
S72.102C
S72.109A
S72.109B
S72.109C
S72.111A
S72.111B
S72.111C
S72.112A
S72.112B
S72.112C
S72.113A
S72.113B
S72.113C
S72.114A
S72.114B
S72.114C
S72.115A
S72.115B
S72.115C
S72.116A
S72.116B
S72.116C
S72.121A
S72.121B
S72.121C
S72.122A
S72.122B
S72.122C
S72.123A
S72.123B
S72.123C
S72.124A
S72.124B
S72.124C
S72.125A
S72.125B
S72.125C
S72.126A
S72.126B
S72.126C
S72.131A
S72.131B
S72.131C
S72.132A
S72.132B
S72.132C
S72.133A
S72.133B
S72.133C
S72.134A
S72.134B
S72.134C
S72.135A
S72.135B
S72.135C
S72.136A
S72.136B
S72.136C
S72.141A
S72.141B
S72.141C
S72.142A
S72.142B
S72.142C
S72.143A
S72.143B
S72.143C
S72.144A
S72.144B
S72.144C
S72.145A
S72.145B
S72.145C
S72.146A
S72.146B
S72.146C
S72.21XA
S72.21XB
S72.21XC
S72.22XA
S72.22XB
S72.22XC
S72.23XA
S72.23XB
S72.23XC
S72.24XA
S72.24XB
S72.24XC
S72.25XA
S72.25XB
S72.25XC
S72.26XA
S72.26XB
S72.26XC
S72.301A
S72.301B
S72.301C
S72.302A
S72.302B
S72.302C
S72.309A
S72.309B
S72.309C
S72.321A
S72.321B
S72.321C
S72.322A
S72.322B
S72.322C
S72.323A
S72.323B
S72.323C
S72.324A
S72.324B
S72.324C
S72.325A
S72.325B
S72.325C
S72.326A
S72.326B
S72.326C
S72.331A
S72.331B
S72.331C
S72.332A
S72.332B
S72.332C
S72.333A
S72.333B
S72.333C
S72.334A
S72.334B
S72.334C
S72.335A
S72.335B
S72.335C
S72.336A
S72.336B
S72.336C
S72.341A
S72.341B
S72.341C
S72.342A
S72.342B
S72.342C
S72.343A
S72.343B
S72.343C
S72.344A
S72.344B
S72.344C
S72.345A
S72.345B
S72.345C
S72.346A
S72.346B
S72.346C
S72.351A
S72.351B
S72.351C
S72.352A
S72.352B
S72.352C
S72.353A
S72.353B
S72.353C
S72.354A
S72.354B
S72.354C
S72.355A
S72.355B
S72.355C
S72.356A
S72.356B
S72.356C
S72.361A
S72.361B
S72.361C
S72.362A
S72.362B
S72.362C
S72.363A
S72.363B
S72.363C
S72.364A
S72.364B
S72.364C
S72.365A
S72.365B
S72.365C
S72.366A
S72.366B
S72.366C
S72.391A
S72.391B
S72.391C
S72.392A
S72.392B
S72.392C
S72.399A
S72.399B
S72.399C
S72.8X1A
S72.8X1B
S72.8X1C
S72.8X2A
S72.8X2B
S72.8X2C
S72.8X9A
S72.8X9B
S72.8X9C
S72.90XA
S72.90XB
S72.90XC
S72.91XA
S72.91XB

S72.91XC
S72.92XA
S72.92XB
S72.92XC
S79.ØØ1A
S79.ØØ2A
S79.ØØ9A
S79.Ø11A
S79.Ø12A
S79.Ø19A
S79.Ø91A
S79.Ø92A
S79.Ø99A
T36.ØX5A
T36.1X5A
T36.2X5A
T36.3X5A
T36.4X5A
T36.5X5A
T36.6X5A
T36.7X5A
T36.8X5A
T36.95XA
T37.ØX5A
T37.1X5A
T37.2X5A
T37.3X5A
T37.4X5A
T37.5X5A
T37.8X5A
T37.95XA
T38.ØX5A
T38.1X5A
T38.2X5A
T38.3X5A
T38.4X5A
T38.5X5A
T38.6X5A
T38.7X5A
T38.8Ø5A
T38.815A
T38.895A
T38.9Ø5A
T38.995A
T39.Ø15A
T39.Ø95A
T39.1X5A
T39.2X5A
T39.315A
T39.395A
T39.4X5A
T39.8X5A
T39.95XA
T4Ø.ØX5A
T4Ø.2X5A
T4Ø.3X5A
T4Ø.415A
T4Ø.425A
T4Ø.495A
T4Ø.5X5A
T4Ø.6Ø5A
T4Ø.695A
T4Ø.715A
T4Ø.725A
T4Ø.9Ø5A
T4Ø.995A
T41.ØX5A
T41.1X5A
T41.2Ø5A
T41.295A
T41.3X5A
T41.45XA
T41.5X5A
T42.ØX5A
T42.1X5A
T42.2X5A
T42.3X5A
T42.4X5A
T42.5X5A
T42.6X5A
T42.75XA
T42.8X5A
T43.Ø15A
T43.Ø25A
T43.1X5A
T43.2Ø5A
T43.215A
T43.225A
T43.295A
T43.3X5A
T43.4X5A
T43.5Ø5A
T43.595A
T43.6Ø5A
T43.615A
T43.625A
T43.635A
T43.655A
T43.695A
T43.8X5A
T43.95XA
T44.ØX5A
T44.1X5A
T44.2X5A
T44.3X5A
T44.4X5A
T44.5X5A
T44.6X5A
T44.7X5A
T44.8X5A
T44.9Ø5A
T44.995A
T45.ØX5A
T45.1X5A
T45.2X5A
T45.3X5A
T45.4X5A
T45.515A
T45.525A
T45.6Ø5A
T45.615A
T45.625A
T45.695A
T45.7X5A
T45.8X5A
T45.95XA
T46.ØX5A
T46.1X5A
T46.2X5A
T46.3X5A
T46.4X5A
T46.5X5A
T46.6X5A
T46.7X5A
T46.8X5A
T46.9Ø5A
T46.995A
T47.ØX5A
T47.1X5A
T47.2X5A
T47.3X5A
T47.4X5A
T47.5X5A
T47.6X5A
T47.7X5A
T47.8X5A
T47.95XA
T48.ØX5A
T48.1X5A
T48.2Ø5A
T48.295A
T48.3X5A
T48.4X5A
T48.5X5A
T48.6X5A
T48.9Ø5A
T48.995A
T49.ØX5A
T49.1X5A
T49.2X5A
T49.3X5A
T49.4X5A
T49.5X5A
T49.6X5A
T49.7X5A
T49.8X5A
T49.95XA
T5Ø.ØX5A
T5Ø.1X5A
T5Ø.2X5A
T5Ø.3X5A
T5Ø.4X5A
T5Ø.5X5A
T5Ø.6X5A
T5Ø.7X5A
T5Ø.8X5A
T5Ø.9Ø5A
T5Ø.915A
T5Ø.995A
T5Ø.A15A
T5Ø.A25A
T5Ø.A95A
T5Ø.B15A
T5Ø.B95A
T5Ø.Z15A
T5Ø.Z95A
T78.41XA
T79.ØXXA
T79.1XXA
T79.2XXA
T79.4XXA
T79.5XXA
T79.7XXA
T8Ø.ØXXA
T8Ø.1XXA
T8Ø.22XA
T8Ø.29XA
T8Ø.3ØXA
T8Ø.31ØA
T8Ø.311A
T8Ø.319A
T8Ø.39XA
T8Ø.4ØXA
T8Ø.41ØA
T8Ø.411A
T8Ø.419A
T8Ø.49XA
T8Ø.51XA
T8Ø.52XA
T8Ø.59XA
T8Ø.61XA
T8Ø.62XA
T8Ø.69XA
T8Ø.81ØA
T8Ø.818A
T8Ø.82XA
T8Ø.89XA
T8Ø.9ØXA
T8Ø.91ØA
T8Ø.911A
T8Ø.919A
T8Ø.92XA
T8Ø.AØXA
T8Ø.A1ØA
T8Ø.A11A
T8Ø.A19A
T8Ø.A9XA
T81.1ØXA
T81.11XA
T81.12XA
T81.19XA
T81.4ØXA
T81.41XA
T81.42XA
T81.43XA
T81.44XA
T81.49XA
T81.5ØØA
T81.5Ø1A
T81.5Ø2A
T81.5Ø3A
T81.5Ø4A
T81.5Ø5A
T81.5Ø6A
T81.5Ø7A
T81.5Ø8A
T81.5Ø9A
T81.51ØA
T81.511A
T81.512A
T81.513A
T81.514A
T81.515A
T81.516A
T81.517A
T81.518A
T81.519A
T81.52ØA
T81.521A
T81.522A
T81.523A
T81.524A
T81.525A
T81.526A
T81.527A
T81.528A
T81.529A
T81.53ØA
T81.531A
T81.532A
T81.533A
T81.534A
T81.535A
T81.536A
T81.537A
T81.538A
T81.539A
T81.59ØA
T81.591A
T81.592A
T81.593A
T81.594A
T81.595A
T81.596A
T81.597A
T81.598A
T81.599A
T81.6ØXA
T81.61XA
T81.69XA
T81.71ØA
T81.711A
T81.718A
T81.719A
T81.72XA
T81.83XA
T81.9XXA
T88.ØXXA
T88.2XXA
T88.53XA
T88.59XA
UØ7.1

DRG 794

Principal or secondary diagnosis of newborn or neonate, with other significant problems, not assigned to DRG 789 through 793 or 795

Principal or secondary diagnosis

A33
PØØ.Ø
PØØ.1
PØØ.4
PØØ.5
PØØ.6
PØØ.7
PØØ.81
PØ1*
PØ2.Ø
PØ2.1
PØ2.2*
PØ2.3
PØ2.7Ø
PØ2.78
PØ2.8
PØ2.9
PØ3.6
PØ3.8*
PØ4.Ø
PØ4.11
PØ4.12
PØ4.13
PØ4.14
PØ4.15
PØ4.16
PØ4.17
PØ4.18
PØ4.19
PØ4.1A
PØ4.2
PØ4.3
PØ4.4Ø
PØ4.41
PØ4.42
PØ4.49
PØ4.5
PØ4.6
PØ4.81
PØ4.89
PØ4.9
PØ5.ØØ
PØ5.Ø1
PØ5.Ø2
PØ5.Ø3
PØ5.Ø4
PØ5.Ø5
PØ5.Ø6
PØ5.Ø7
PØ5.Ø9
PØ5.1Ø
PØ5.19
PØ5.9
P11.1
P11.3
P13*
P14.Ø
P14.1
P14.3
P15*
P19*
P22.1
P22.8
P22.9
P28.1*
P28.2
P28.3*
P28.4*
P28.8*
P28.9
P29.Ø
P29.1*
P29.2
P29.4
P29.89
P29.9
P37.5
P39.1
P51*
P54.Ø
P54.6
P54.8
P54.9
P55.Ø
P55.1
P58*
P59.Ø
P61.1
P61.3
P61.4
P61.5
P61.8
P61.9
P7Ø.Ø
P7Ø.1
P7Ø.8
P7Ø.9
P72.Ø
P72.2
P72.8
P72.9
P74.41
P74.5
P74.6
P74.8
P74.9
P76.1
P76.8
P76.9
P78.1
P78.2
P78.3
P78.8*
P78.9
P8Ø.Ø
P8Ø.8
P8Ø.9
P81*
P83.Ø
P83.3*
P83.4
P83.5
P83.9
P84
P91.6Ø
P91.61
P94.1
P94.2
P94.8
P94.9
P95
P96.Ø
P96.3
P96.5
P96.81
P96.83
P96.89
P96.9
Q86*

DRG 795

Principal Diagnosis

PØØ.3
PØØ.9
PØ2.4
PØ2.5
PØ2.6Ø
PØ2.69
PØ3.Ø
PØ3.1
PØ3.2
PØ3.3
PØ3.5
PØ3.9
PØ5.Ø8
PØ5.18
PØ8.Ø
PØ8.1
PØ8.21
PØ8.22
P12.Ø
P12.1
P12.3
P12.4
P12.81
P12.89
P12.9
P54.5
P59.3
P59.8
P59.9
P83.1
P83.6
P83.8*
P92.Ø9
P92.1
P92.2
P92.3
P92.4
P92.5
P92.8
P92.9
P96.82
Z38.ØØ
Z38.Ø1
Z38.1
Z38.2
Z38.3Ø
Z38.31
Z38.4
Z38.5
Z38.61
Z38.62
Z38.63
Z38.64
Z38.65
Z38.66
Z38.68
Z38.69
Z38.7
Z38.8

AND

No secondary diagnoses

OR

Only secondary diagnoses

J34.Ø
J34.1
J34.81
J34.89
J34.9
KØØ.6
KØ1.Ø
KØ1.1
LØ8.9
L22
L57.3
L8Ø
L81.Ø
L81.1
L81.2
L81.3
L81.4
L81.5
L81.6
L81.7
L81.8
L81.9
N47.Ø
N47.1
N47.2
N47.3
N47.4
N47.5
N47.7
N47.8
N89.8
PØØ.2
PØØ.82
PØØ.89
Q17.Ø
Q53.ØØ
Q53.Ø1
Q53.Ø2
Q53.1Ø
Q53.11*
Q53.12
Q53.13
Q53.2Ø
Q53.21*
Q53.22
Q53.23
Q53.9
Q55.22
Q66.5Ø
Q66.51
Q66.52
Q66.8Ø
Q66.81
Q66.82
Q81.Ø
Q81.1
Q81.2
Q81.8
Q81.9
Q82.1
Q82.2
Q82.3
Q82.6
Q82.8
Q82.9
RØ9.81
R87.618
R87.619
R87.629
R89.7
R94.12Ø
ZØØ.11Ø
ZØØ.111
ZØØ.121
ZØØ.129
ZØ1.1Ø
ZØ1.11Ø
ZØ1.118
ZØ1.12
ZØ2.6
ZØ2.82
ZØ2.84
ZØ2.89
ZØ5*
Z13.228
Z2Ø.Ø1
Z2Ø.Ø9
Z2Ø.1
Z2Ø.2
Z2Ø.3
Z2Ø.4
Z2Ø.5
Z2Ø.6
Z2Ø.7
Z2Ø.81Ø
Z2Ø.811
Z2Ø.818
Z2Ø.82Ø
Z2Ø.821
Z2Ø.822
Z2Ø.828
Z2Ø.89
Z2Ø.9
Z23
Z28.Ø1
Z28.Ø2
Z28.Ø3
Z28.Ø4
Z28.Ø9
Z28.1
Z28.2Ø
Z28.21
Z28.29
Z28.81
Z28.82
Z28.83
Z28.89
Z28.9
Z41.2
Z41.3
Z53.Ø1
Z53.Ø9
Z53.1
Z53.2Ø
Z53.21
Z53.29
Z53.8
Z53.9
Z76.2
Z81.8
Z82.Ø
Z82.49
Z83.1
Z83.3
Z83.42
Z83.43Ø
Z83.438
Z83.49

MDC 16

DRG 799

Operating Room Procedures

Ø4L4ØCZ
Ø4L4ØDZ
Ø4L4ØZZ
Ø4L43CZ
Ø4L43DZ
Ø4L43ZZ
Ø4L44CZ
Ø4L44DZ
Ø4L44ZZ
Ø75P*
Ø79PØØZ
Ø79PØZX
Ø79PØZZ
Ø7BPØZX
Ø7BPØZZ
Ø7BP3ZZ
Ø7BP4ZZ
Ø7CPØZZ
Ø7HPØ1Z
Ø7HPØYZ
Ø7HP41Z
Ø7NP*
Ø7PPØØZ
Ø7PPØ3Z
Ø7PPØYZ
Ø7PP3ØZ
Ø7PP33Z
Ø7PP4ØZ
Ø7PP43Z
Ø7QP*
Ø7SPØZZ
Ø7TP*
Ø7WPØØZ
Ø7WPØ3Z
Ø7WPØYZ
Ø7WP3ØZ
Ø7WP33Z
Ø7WP4ØZ
Ø7WP43Z
Ø7YP*

DRG 800

Select operating room procedures listed under DRG 799

DRG 801

Select operating room procedures listed under DRG 799

DRG 802

Operating Room Procedures

Ø2HVØ2Z
Ø2HVØDZ
Ø2HV3DZ
Ø2HV42Z
Ø2HV4DZ
Ø2JA4ZZ
Ø2JY4ZZ
Ø2LV*
Ø2VV*
Ø6HØØDZ
Ø6HØ4DZ
Ø6LØ*
Ø6VØ*
Ø75Ø*
Ø751*
Ø752*
Ø753*
Ø754*
Ø755*
Ø756*
Ø757*
Ø758*
Ø759*
Ø75B*
Ø75C*
Ø75D*
Ø75F*
Ø75G*
Ø75H*
Ø75J*
Ø75M*
Ø79ØØØZ
Ø79ØØZX
Ø79ØØZZ
Ø79Ø3ZX
Ø79Ø4ØZ
Ø79Ø4ZX
Ø79Ø4ZZ
Ø791ØØZ
Ø791ØZX
Ø791ØZZ
Ø7913ZX
Ø7914ØZ
Ø7914ZX
Ø7914ZZ
Ø792ØØZ
Ø792ØZX
Ø792ØZZ
Ø7923ZX
Ø7924ØZ
Ø7924ZX
Ø7924ZZ
Ø793ØØZ
Ø793ØZX
Ø793ØZZ
Ø7933ZX
Ø7934ØZ
Ø7934ZX
Ø7934ZZ
Ø794ØØZ
Ø794ØZX
Ø794ØZZ
Ø7943ZX
Ø7944ØZ
Ø7944ZX
Ø7944ZZ
Ø795ØØZ
Ø795ØZX
Ø795ØZZ
Ø7953ZX
Ø7954ØZ
Ø7954ZX
Ø7954ZZ
Ø796ØØZ
Ø796ØZX
Ø796ØZZ
Ø7963ZX
Ø7964ØZ
Ø7964ZX
Ø7964ZZ
Ø797ØØZ
Ø797ØZX
Ø797ØZZ
Ø7973ZX
Ø7974ØZ
Ø7974ZX
Ø7974ZZ
Ø798ØØZ
Ø798ØZX
Ø798ØZZ
Ø7983ZX
Ø7984ØZ
Ø7984ZX

Ø7984ZZ
Ø799ØØZ
Ø799ØZX
Ø799ØZZ
Ø7993ZX
Ø7994ØZ
Ø7994ZX
Ø7994ZZ
Ø79BØØZ
Ø79BØZX
Ø79BØZZ
Ø79B3ZX
Ø79B4ØZ
Ø79B4ZX
Ø79B4ZZ
Ø79CØØZ
Ø79CØZX
Ø79CØZZ
Ø79C3ZX
Ø79C4ØZ
Ø79C4ZX
Ø79C4ZZ
Ø79DØØZ
Ø79DØZX
Ø79DØZZ
Ø79D3ZX
Ø79D4ØZ
Ø79D4ZX
Ø79D4ZZ
Ø79FØØZ
Ø79FØZX
Ø79FØZZ
Ø79F3ZX
Ø79F4ØZ
Ø79F4ZX
Ø79F4ZZ
Ø79GØØZ
Ø79GØZX
Ø79GØZZ
Ø79G3ZX
Ø79G4ØZ
Ø79G4ZX
Ø79G4ZZ
Ø79HØØZ
Ø79HØZX
Ø79HØZZ
Ø79H3ZX
Ø79H4ØZ
Ø79H4ZX
Ø79H4ZZ
Ø79JØØZ
Ø79JØZX
Ø79JØZZ
Ø79J3ZX
Ø79J4ØZ
Ø79J4ZX
Ø79J4ZZ
Ø79KØZX
Ø79K3ZX
Ø79K4ZX
Ø79LØZX
Ø79L3ZX
Ø79L4ZX
Ø79MØØZ
Ø79MØZX
Ø79MØZZ
Ø79M3ZX
Ø79M4ØZ
Ø79M4ZX
Ø79M4ZZ
Ø7BØ*
Ø7B1*
Ø7B2*
Ø7B3*
Ø7B4*
Ø7B5*
Ø7B6*
Ø7B7*
Ø7B8*
Ø7B9*
Ø7BB*
Ø7BC*
Ø7BD*
Ø7BF*
Ø7BG*
Ø7BH*
Ø7BJ*
Ø7BKØZX
Ø7BK3ZX
Ø7BK4ZX
Ø7BLØZX
Ø7BL3ZX
Ø7BL4ZX
Ø7BMØZX
Ø7BMØZZ
Ø7BM3ZX
Ø7BM3ZZ
Ø7BM4ZX
Ø7BM4ZZ
Ø7CØØZZ
Ø7CØ3ZZ
Ø7CØ4ZZ
Ø7C1ØZZ
Ø7C13ZZ
Ø7C14ZZ
Ø7C2ØZZ
Ø7C23ZZ
Ø7C24ZZ
Ø7C3ØZZ
Ø7C33ZZ
Ø7C34ZZ
Ø7C4ØZZ
Ø7C43ZZ
Ø7C44ZZ
Ø7C5ØZZ
Ø7C53ZZ
Ø7C54ZZ
Ø7C6ØZZ
Ø7C63ZZ
Ø7C64ZZ
Ø7C7ØZZ
Ø7C73ZZ
Ø7C74ZZ
Ø7C8ØZZ
Ø7C83ZZ
Ø7C84ZZ
Ø7C9ØZZ
Ø7C93ZZ
Ø7C94ZZ
Ø7CBØZZ
Ø7CB3ZZ
Ø7CB4ZZ
Ø7CCØZZ
Ø7CC3ZZ
Ø7CC4ZZ
Ø7CDØZZ
Ø7CD3ZZ
Ø7CD4ZZ
Ø7CFØZZ
Ø7CF3ZZ
Ø7CF4ZZ
Ø7CGØZZ
Ø7CG3ZZ
Ø7CG4ZZ
Ø7CHØZZ
Ø7CH3ZZ
Ø7CH4ZZ
Ø7CJØZZ
Ø7CJ3ZZ
Ø7CJ4ZZ
Ø7CKØZZ
Ø7CK3ZZ
Ø7CK4ZZ
Ø7CLØZZ
Ø7CL3ZZ
Ø7CL4ZZ
Ø7CMØZZ
Ø7CM3ZZ
Ø7CM4ZZ
Ø7HMØ1Z
Ø7HMØYZ
Ø7HM41Z
Ø7HM4YZ
Ø7HNØ1Z
Ø7HNØYZ
Ø7HN41Z
Ø7JKØZZ
Ø7JK4ZZ
Ø7JLØZZ
Ø7JL4ZZ
Ø7JMØZZ
Ø7JM4ZZ
Ø7JNØZZ
Ø7JN4ZZ
Ø7JPØZZ
Ø7LØØCZ
Ø7LØØDZ
Ø7LØØZZ
Ø7LØ3CZ
Ø7LØ3DZ
Ø7LØ3ZZ
Ø7LØ4CZ
Ø7LØ4DZ
Ø7LØ4ZZ
Ø7L1ØCZ
Ø7L1ØDZ
Ø7L1ØZZ
Ø7L13CZ
Ø7L13DZ
Ø7L13ZZ
Ø7L14CZ
Ø7L14DZ
Ø7L14ZZ
Ø7L2ØCZ
Ø7L2ØDZ
Ø7L2ØZZ
Ø7L23CZ
Ø7L23DZ
Ø7L23ZZ
Ø7L24CZ
Ø7L24DZ
Ø7L24ZZ
Ø7L3ØCZ
Ø7L3ØDZ
Ø7L3ØZZ
Ø7L33CZ
Ø7L33DZ
Ø7L33ZZ
Ø7L34CZ
Ø7L34DZ
Ø7L34ZZ
Ø7L4ØCZ
Ø7L4ØDZ
Ø7L4ØZZ
Ø7L43CZ
Ø7L43DZ
Ø7L43ZZ
Ø7L44CZ
Ø7L44DZ
Ø7L44ZZ
Ø7L5ØCZ
Ø7L5ØDZ
Ø7L5ØZZ
Ø7L53CZ
Ø7L53DZ
Ø7L53ZZ
Ø7L54CZ
Ø7L54DZ
Ø7L54ZZ
Ø7L6ØCZ
Ø7L6ØDZ
Ø7L6ØZZ
Ø7L63CZ
Ø7L63DZ
Ø7L63ZZ
Ø7L64CZ
Ø7L64DZ
Ø7L64ZZ
Ø7L7ØCZ
Ø7L7ØDZ
Ø7L7ØZZ
Ø7L73CZ
Ø7L73DZ
Ø7L73ZZ
Ø7L74CZ
Ø7L74DZ
Ø7L74ZZ
Ø7L8ØCZ
Ø7L8ØDZ
Ø7L8ØZZ
Ø7L83CZ
Ø7L83DZ
Ø7L83ZZ
Ø7L84CZ
Ø7L84DZ
Ø7L84ZZ
Ø7L9ØCZ
Ø7L9ØDZ
Ø7L9ØZZ
Ø7L93CZ
Ø7L93DZ
Ø7L93ZZ
Ø7L94CZ
Ø7L94DZ
Ø7L94ZZ
Ø7LBØCZ
Ø7LBØDZ
Ø7LBØZZ
Ø7LB3CZ
Ø7LB3DZ
Ø7LB3ZZ
Ø7LB4CZ
Ø7LB4DZ
Ø7LB4ZZ
Ø7LCØCZ
Ø7LCØDZ
Ø7LCØZZ
Ø7LC3CZ
Ø7LC3DZ
Ø7LC3ZZ
Ø7LC4CZ
Ø7LC4DZ
Ø7LC4ZZ
Ø7LDØCZ
Ø7LDØDZ
Ø7LDØZZ
Ø7LD3CZ
Ø7LD3DZ
Ø7LD3ZZ
Ø7LD4CZ
Ø7LD4DZ
Ø7LD4ZZ
Ø7LFØCZ
Ø7LFØDZ
Ø7LFØZZ
Ø7LF3CZ
Ø7LF3DZ
Ø7LF3ZZ
Ø7LF4CZ
Ø7LF4DZ
Ø7LF4ZZ
Ø7LGØCZ
Ø7LGØDZ
Ø7LGØZZ
Ø7LG3CZ
Ø7LG3DZ
Ø7LG3ZZ
Ø7LG4CZ
Ø7LG4DZ
Ø7LG4ZZ
Ø7LHØCZ
Ø7LHØDZ
Ø7LHØZZ
Ø7LH3CZ
Ø7LH3DZ
Ø7LH3ZZ
Ø7LH4CZ
Ø7LH4DZ
Ø7LH4ZZ
Ø7LJØCZ
Ø7LJØDZ
Ø7LJØZZ
Ø7LJ3CZ
Ø7LJ3DZ
Ø7LJ3ZZ
Ø7LJ4CZ
Ø7LJ4DZ
Ø7LJ4ZZ
Ø7NØØZZ
Ø7NØ3ZZ
Ø7NØ4ZZ
Ø7N1ØZZ
Ø7N13ZZ
Ø7N14ZZ
Ø7N2ØZZ
Ø7N23ZZ
Ø7N24ZZ
Ø7N3ØZZ
Ø7N33ZZ
Ø7N34ZZ
Ø7N4ØZZ
Ø7N43ZZ
Ø7N44ZZ
Ø7N5ØZZ
Ø7N53ZZ
Ø7N54ZZ
Ø7N6ØZZ
Ø7N63ZZ
Ø7N64ZZ
Ø7N7ØZZ
Ø7N73ZZ
Ø7N74ZZ
Ø7N8ØZZ
Ø7N83ZZ
Ø7N84ZZ
Ø7N9ØZZ
Ø7N93ZZ
Ø7N94ZZ
Ø7NBØZZ
Ø7NB3ZZ
Ø7NB4ZZ
Ø7NCØZZ
Ø7NC3ZZ
Ø7NC4ZZ
Ø7NDØZZ
Ø7ND3ZZ
Ø7ND4ZZ
Ø7NFØZZ
Ø7NF3ZZ
Ø7NF4ZZ
Ø7NGØZZ
Ø7NG3ZZ
Ø7NG4ZZ
Ø7NHØZZ
Ø7NH3ZZ
Ø7NH4ZZ
Ø7NJØZZ
Ø7NJ3ZZ
Ø7NJ4ZZ
Ø7NMØZZ
Ø7NM3ZZ
Ø7NM4ZZ
Ø7PKØ7Z
Ø7PKØJZ
Ø7PKØKZ
Ø7PK37Z
Ø7PK3JZ
Ø7PK3KZ
Ø7PK47Z
Ø7PK4JZ
Ø7PK4KZ
Ø7PLØ7Z
Ø7PLØJZ
Ø7PLØKZ
Ø7PL37Z
Ø7PL3JZ
Ø7PL3KZ
Ø7PL47Z
Ø7PL4JZ
Ø7PL4KZ
Ø7PMØØZ
Ø7PMØ3Z
Ø7PMØYZ
Ø7PM3ØZ
Ø7PM33Z
Ø7PM4ØZ
Ø7PM43Z
Ø7PNØØZ
Ø7PNØ3Z
Ø7PNØ7Z
Ø7PNØCZ
Ø7PNØDZ
Ø7PNØJZ
Ø7PNØKZ
Ø7PNØYZ
Ø7PN3ØZ
Ø7PN33Z
Ø7PN37Z
Ø7PN3CZ
Ø7PN3DZ
Ø7PN3JZ
Ø7PN3KZ
Ø7PN4ØZ
Ø7PN43Z
Ø7PN47Z
Ø7PN4CZ
Ø7PN4DZ
Ø7PN4JZ
Ø7PN4KZ
Ø7QØØZZ
Ø7QØ3ZZ
Ø7QØ4ZZ
Ø7QØ8ZZ
Ø7Q1ØZZ
Ø7Q13ZZ
Ø7Q14ZZ
Ø7Q18ZZ
Ø7Q2ØZZ
Ø7Q23ZZ
Ø7Q24ZZ
Ø7Q28ZZ
Ø7Q3ØZZ
Ø7Q33ZZ
Ø7Q34ZZ
Ø7Q38ZZ
Ø7Q4ØZZ
Ø7Q43ZZ
Ø7Q44ZZ
Ø7Q48ZZ
Ø7Q5ØZZ
Ø7Q53ZZ
Ø7Q54ZZ
Ø7Q58ZZ
Ø7Q6ØZZ
Ø7Q63ZZ
Ø7Q64ZZ
Ø7Q68ZZ
Ø7Q7ØZZ
Ø7Q73ZZ
Ø7Q74ZZ
Ø7Q78ZZ
Ø7Q8ØZZ
Ø7Q83ZZ
Ø7Q84ZZ
Ø7Q88ZZ
Ø7Q9ØZZ
Ø7Q93ZZ
Ø7Q94ZZ
Ø7Q98ZZ
Ø7QBØZZ
Ø7QB3ZZ
Ø7QB4ZZ
Ø7QB8ZZ
Ø7QCØZZ
Ø7QC3ZZ
Ø7QC4ZZ
Ø7QC8ZZ
Ø7QDØZZ
Ø7QD3ZZ
Ø7QD4ZZ
Ø7QD8ZZ
Ø7QFØZZ
Ø7QF3ZZ
Ø7QF4ZZ
Ø7QF8ZZ
Ø7QGØZZ
Ø7QG3ZZ
Ø7QG4ZZ
Ø7QG8ZZ
Ø7QHØZZ
Ø7QH3ZZ
Ø7QH4ZZ
Ø7QH8ZZ
Ø7QJØZZ
Ø7QJ3ZZ
Ø7QJ4ZZ
Ø7QJ8ZZ
Ø7QMØZZ
Ø7QM3ZZ
Ø7QM4ZZ
Ø7SMØZZ
Ø7TØØZZ
Ø7TØ4ZZ
Ø7T1ØZZ
Ø7T14ZZ
Ø7T2ØZZ
Ø7T24ZZ
Ø7T3ØZZ
Ø7T34ZZ
Ø7T4ØZZ
Ø7T44ZZ
Ø7T5ØZZ
Ø7T54ZZ
Ø7T6ØZZ
Ø7T64ZZ
Ø7T7ØZZ
Ø7T74ZZ
Ø7T8ØZZ
Ø7T84ZZ
Ø7T9ØZZ
Ø7T94ZZ
Ø7TBØZZ
Ø7TB4ZZ
Ø7TCØZZ
Ø7TC4ZZ
Ø7TDØZZ
Ø7TD4ZZ
Ø7TFØZZ
Ø7TF4ZZ
Ø7TGØZZ
Ø7TG4ZZ
Ø7THØZZ
Ø7TH4ZZ
Ø7TJØZZ
Ø7TJ4ZZ
Ø7TMØZZ
Ø7TM4ZZ
Ø7UØØ7Z
Ø7UØØJZ
Ø7UØØKZ
Ø7UØ47Z
Ø7UØ4JZ
Ø7UØ4KZ
Ø7U1Ø7Z
Ø7U1ØJZ
Ø7U1ØKZ
Ø7U147Z
Ø7U14JZ
Ø7U14KZ
Ø7U2Ø7Z
Ø7U2ØJZ
Ø7U2ØKZ
Ø7U247Z
Ø7U24JZ
Ø7U24KZ
Ø7U3Ø7Z
Ø7U3ØJZ
Ø7U3ØKZ
Ø7U347Z
Ø7U34JZ
Ø7U34KZ
Ø7U4Ø7Z
Ø7U4ØJZ
Ø7U4ØKZ
Ø7U447Z
Ø7U44JZ
Ø7U44KZ
Ø7U5Ø7Z
Ø7U5ØJZ
Ø7U5ØKZ
Ø7U547Z
Ø7U54JZ
Ø7U54KZ
Ø7U6Ø7Z
Ø7U6ØJZ
Ø7U6ØKZ
Ø7U647Z
Ø7U64JZ
Ø7U64KZ
Ø7U7Ø7Z
Ø7U7ØJZ
Ø7U7ØKZ
Ø7U747Z
Ø7U74JZ
Ø7U74KZ
Ø7U8Ø7Z
Ø7U8ØJZ
Ø7U8ØKZ
Ø7U847Z
Ø7U84JZ
Ø7U84KZ
Ø7U9Ø7Z
Ø7U9ØJZ
Ø7U9ØKZ
Ø7U947Z
Ø7U94JZ
Ø7U94KZ
Ø7UBØ7Z
Ø7UBØJZ
Ø7UBØKZ
Ø7UB47Z
Ø7UB4JZ
Ø7UB4KZ
Ø7UCØ7Z
Ø7UCØJZ
Ø7UCØKZ
Ø7UC47Z
Ø7UC4JZ
Ø7UC4KZ
Ø7UDØ7Z
Ø7UDØJZ
Ø7UDØKZ
Ø7UD47Z
Ø7UD4JZ
Ø7UD4KZ
Ø7UFØ7Z
Ø7UFØJZ
Ø7UFØKZ
Ø7UF47Z
Ø7UF4JZ
Ø7UF4KZ
Ø7UGØ7Z
Ø7UGØJZ
Ø7UGØKZ
Ø7UG47Z
Ø7UG4JZ
Ø7UG4KZ
Ø7UHØ7Z
Ø7UHØJZ
Ø7UHØKZ
Ø7UH47Z
Ø7UH4JZ
Ø7UH4KZ
Ø7UJØ7Z
Ø7UJØJZ
Ø7UJØKZ
Ø7UJ47Z
Ø7UJ4JZ
Ø7UJ4KZ
Ø7VØØCZ
Ø7VØØDZ
Ø7VØØZZ
Ø7VØ3CZ
Ø7VØ3DZ
Ø7VØ3ZZ
Ø7VØ4CZ
Ø7VØ4DZ
Ø7VØ4ZZ
Ø7V1ØCZ
Ø7V1ØDZ
Ø7V1ØZZ
Ø7V13CZ
Ø7V13DZ
Ø7V13ZZ
Ø7V14CZ
Ø7V14DZ
Ø7V14ZZ
Ø7V2ØCZ
Ø7V2ØDZ
Ø7V2ØZZ
Ø7V23CZ
Ø7V23DZ
Ø7V23ZZ
Ø7V24CZ
Ø7V24DZ
Ø7V24ZZ
Ø7V3ØCZ
Ø7V3ØDZ
Ø7V3ØZZ
Ø7V33CZ
Ø7V33DZ
Ø7V33ZZ
Ø7V34CZ
Ø7V34DZ
Ø7V34ZZ
Ø7V4ØCZ
Ø7V4ØDZ
Ø7V4ØZZ
Ø7V43CZ
Ø7V43DZ
Ø7V43ZZ
Ø7V44CZ
Ø7V44DZ
Ø7V44ZZ
Ø7V5ØCZ
Ø7V5ØDZ
Ø7V5ØZZ
Ø7V53CZ
Ø7V53DZ
Ø7V53ZZ
Ø7V54CZ
Ø7V54DZ
Ø7V54ZZ
Ø7V6ØCZ
Ø7V6ØDZ
Ø7V6ØZZ
Ø7V63CZ
Ø7V63DZ
Ø7V63ZZ
Ø7V64CZ
Ø7V64DZ
Ø7V64ZZ
Ø7V7ØCZ
Ø7V7ØDZ
Ø7V7ØZZ
Ø7V73CZ
Ø7V73DZ
Ø7V73ZZ
Ø7V74CZ
Ø7V74DZ
Ø7V74ZZ
Ø7V8ØCZ
Ø7V8ØDZ
Ø7V8ØZZ
Ø7V83CZ
Ø7V83DZ
Ø7V83ZZ
Ø7V84CZ
Ø7V84DZ
Ø7V84ZZ
Ø7V9ØCZ
Ø7V9ØDZ
Ø7V9ØZZ
Ø7V93CZ
Ø7V93DZ
Ø7V93ZZ
Ø7V94CZ
Ø7V94DZ
Ø7V94ZZ
Ø7VBØCZ
Ø7VBØDZ
Ø7VBØZZ
Ø7VB3CZ
Ø7VB3DZ
Ø7VB3ZZ
Ø7VB4CZ
Ø7VB4DZ
Ø7VB4ZZ
Ø7VCØCZ
Ø7VCØDZ
Ø7VCØZZ
Ø7VC3CZ
Ø7VC3DZ
Ø7VC3ZZ
Ø7VC4CZ
Ø7VC4DZ
Ø7VC4ZZ
Ø7VDØCZ
Ø7VDØDZ
Ø7VDØZZ
Ø7VD3CZ
Ø7VD3DZ
Ø7VD3ZZ
Ø7VD4CZ
Ø7VD4DZ
Ø7VD4ZZ
Ø7VFØCZ
Ø7VFØDZ
Ø7VFØZZ
Ø7VF3CZ
Ø7VF3DZ
Ø7VF3ZZ
Ø7VF4CZ
Ø7VF4DZ
Ø7VF4ZZ
Ø7VGØCZ
Ø7VGØDZ
Ø7VGØZZ
Ø7VG3CZ
Ø7VG3DZ
Ø7VG3ZZ
Ø7VG4CZ
Ø7VG4DZ
Ø7VG4ZZ
Ø7VHØCZ
Ø7VHØDZ
Ø7VHØZZ
Ø7VH3CZ
Ø7VH3DZ
Ø7VH3ZZ
Ø7VH4CZ
Ø7VH4DZ
Ø7VH4ZZ
Ø7VJØCZ
Ø7VJØDZ
Ø7VJØZZ
Ø7VJ3CZ
Ø7VJ3DZ
Ø7VJ3ZZ
Ø7VJ4CZ
Ø7VJ4DZ
Ø7VJ4ZZ
Ø7WKØ7Z
Ø7WKØJZ
Ø7WKØKZ
Ø7WK37Z
Ø7WK3JZ
Ø7WK3KZ
Ø7WK47Z
Ø7WK4JZ
Ø7WK4KZ
Ø7WLØ7Z
Ø7WLØJZ
Ø7WLØKZ
Ø7WL37Z
Ø7WL3JZ
Ø7WL3KZ
Ø7WL47Z
Ø7WL4JZ
Ø7WL4KZ
Ø7WMØØZ
Ø7WMØ3Z
Ø7WMØYZ
Ø7WM3ØZ
Ø7WM33Z
Ø7WM4ØZ
Ø7WM43Z
Ø7WNØØZ
Ø7WNØ3Z
Ø7WNØ7Z
Ø7WNØCZ
Ø7WNØDZ
Ø7WNØJZ
Ø7WNØKZ
Ø7WNØYZ
Ø7WN3ØZ
Ø7WN33Z
Ø7WN37Z
Ø7WN3CZ
Ø7WN3DZ
Ø7WN3JZ
Ø7WN3KZ
Ø7WN4ØZ
Ø7WN43Z
Ø7WN47Z
Ø7WN4CZ
Ø7WN4DZ
Ø7WN4JZ
Ø7WN4KZ
Ø7YMØZØ
Ø7YMØZ1
Ø7YMØZ2
ØD9UØZX
ØD9U4ZX
ØD9VØZX
ØD9V4ZX
ØD9WØZX
ØD9W4ZX
ØDBUØZX
ØDBVØZX
ØDBWØZX
ØDJØØZZ
ØDJ6ØZZ
ØDJDØZZ
ØDJUØZZ

ØDJU4ZZ
ØDJVØZZ
ØDJV4ZZ
ØDJWØZZ
ØDJW4ZZ
ØF9ØØZX
ØF91ØZX
ØF92ØZX
ØFBØØZX
ØFBØ4ZX
ØFB1ØZX
ØFB14ZX
ØFB2ØZX
ØFB24ZX
ØFDØ4ZX
ØFD14ZX
ØFD24ZX
ØFJØØZZ
ØFJØ4ZZ
ØFJ44ZZ
ØFJD4ZZ
ØFJG4ZZ
ØJBØØZZ
ØJB1ØZZ
ØJB4ØZZ
ØJB5ØZZ
ØJB6ØZZ
ØJB7ØZZ
ØJB8ØZZ
ØJB9ØZZ
ØJBBØZZ
ØJBCØZZ
ØJBDØZZ
ØJBFØZZ
ØJBGØZZ
ØJBHØZZ
ØJBLØZZ
ØJBMØZZ
ØJBNØZZ
ØJBPØZZ
ØJBQØZZ
ØJBRØZZ
ØJH6ØVZ
ØJH6ØWZ
ØJH6ØYZ
ØJH63VZ
ØJH7ØVZ
ØJH7ØYZ
ØJH73VZ
ØJH8ØVZ
ØJH8ØWZ
ØJH8ØYZ
ØJH83VZ
ØJHDØVZ
ØJHDØWZ
ØJHD3VZ
ØJHFØVZ
ØJHFØWZ
ØJHF3VZ
ØJHGØVZ
ØJHGØWZ
ØJHG3VZ
ØJHHØVZ
ØJHHØWZ
ØJHH3VZ
ØJHLØVZ
ØJHLØWZ
ØJHL3VZ
ØJHMØVZ
ØJHMØWZ
ØJHM3VZ
ØJHNØVZ
ØJHN3VZ
ØJHPØVZ
ØJHPØWZ
ØJHP3VZ
ØJHTØVZ
ØJHTØYZ
ØJHT3VZ
ØK9ØØZX
ØK91ØZX
ØK92ØZX
ØK93ØZX
ØK94ØZX
ØK95ØZX
ØK96ØZX
ØK97ØZX
ØK98ØZX
ØK99ØZX
ØK9BØZX
ØK9CØZX
ØK9DØZX
ØK9FØZX
ØK9GØZX
ØK9HØZX
ØK9JØZX
ØK9KØZX
ØK9LØZX
ØK9MØZX
ØK9NØZX
ØK9PØZX
ØK9QØZX
ØK9RØZX
ØK9SØZX
ØK9TØZX
ØK9VØZX
ØK9WØZX
ØKBØØZX
ØKB1ØZX
ØKB2ØZX
ØKB3ØZX
ØKB4ØZX
ØKB5ØZX
ØKB6ØZX
ØKB7ØZX
ØKB8ØZX
ØKB9ØZX
ØKBBØZX
ØKBCØZX
ØKBDØZX
ØKBFØZX
ØKBGØZX
ØKBHØZX
ØKBJØZX
ØKBKØZX
ØKBLØZX
ØKBMØZX
ØKBNØZX
ØKBPØZX
ØKBQØZX
ØKBRØZX
ØKBSØZX
ØKBTØZX
ØKBVØZX
ØKBWØZX
ØP93ØZX
ØP933ZX
ØP934ZX
ØP94ØZX
ØP943ZX
ØP944ZX
ØP9RØZX
ØP9R3ZX
ØP9R4ZX
ØP9SØZX
ØP9S3ZX
ØP9S4ZX
ØP9TØZX
ØP9T3ZX
ØP9T4ZX
ØP9VØZX
ØP9V3ZX
ØP9V4ZX
ØPB3ØZX
ØPB33ZX
ØPB34ZX
ØPB4ØZX
ØPB43ZX
ØPB44ZX
ØPBRØZX
ØPBR3ZX
ØPBR4ZX
ØPBSØZX
ØPBS3ZX
ØPBS4ZX
ØPBTØZX
ØPBT3ZX
ØPBT4ZX
ØPBVØZX
ØPBV3ZX
ØPBV4ZX
ØQ9ØØZX
ØQ9Ø3ZX
ØQ9Ø4ZX
ØQ91ØZX
ØQ913ZX
ØQ914ZX
ØQ92ØZX
ØQ923ZX
ØQ924ZX
ØQ93ØZX
ØQ933ZX
ØQ934ZX
ØQ94ØZX
ØQ943ZX
ØQ944ZX
ØQ95ØZX
ØQ953ZX
ØQ954ZX
ØQ9QØZX
ØQ9Q3ZX
ØQ9Q4ZX
ØQ9RØZX
ØQ9R3ZX
ØQ9R4ZX
ØQ9SØZX
ØQ9S3ZX
ØQ9S4ZX
ØQBØØZX
ØQBØ3ZX
ØQBØ4ZX
ØQB1ØZX
ØQB13ZX
ØQB14ZX
ØQB2ØZX
ØQB23ZX
ØQB24ZX
ØQB3ØZX
ØQB33ZX
ØQB34ZX
ØQB4ØZX
ØQB43ZX
ØQB44ZX
ØQB5ØZX
ØQB53ZX
ØQB54ZX
ØQBQØZX
ØQBQ3ZX
ØQBQ4ZX
ØQBRØZX
ØQBR3ZX
ØQBR4ZX
ØQBSØZX
ØQBS3ZX
ØQBS4ZX
ØT9ØØZX
ØT91ØZX
ØT93ØZX
ØT94ØZX
ØTBØØZX
ØTB1ØZX
ØTB3ØZX
ØTB4ØZX
ØW9CØZX
ØW9GØØZ
ØW9GØZX
ØW9GØZZ
ØW9G4ØZ
ØW9G4ZX
ØW9G4ZZ
ØW9HØZX
ØW9H3ZX
ØW9H4ZX
ØW9JØZX
ØW9J4ZX
ØWBCØZX
ØWBHØZX
ØWJC4ZZ
ØWJD4ZZ
ØWJF4ZZ
ØWJGØZZ
ØWJG4ZZ
ØWJH4ZZ
ØWJJØZZ
ØWJJ4ZZ
ØWJPØZZ
ØWJP4ZZ
ØWJRØZZ
ØWJR4ZZ
ØY95ØZX
ØY953ZX
ØY954ZX
ØY96ØZX
ØY963ZX
ØY964ZX
ØYB5ØZX
ØYB53ZX
ØYB54ZX
ØYB6ØZX
ØYB63ZX
ØYB64ZX
ØYB7ØZX
ØYB73ZX
ØYB74ZX
ØYB8ØZX
ØYB83ZX
ØYB84ZX
ØYJ54ZZ
ØYJ64ZZ
ØYJ74ZZ
ØYJ84ZZ
ØYJA4ZZ
ØYJE4ZZ
4AØ6Ø5Z
4AØ6ØBZ
4A16Ø5Z
4A16ØBZ
X2H13R9

DRG 803

Select operating room procedures listed under DRG 802

DRG 804

Select operating room procedures listed under DRG 802

DRG 808

Principal Diagnosis

D59.Ø
D59.1*
D59.2
D59.4
D59.5
D59.6
D59.8
D59.9
D6Ø*
D61.Ø*
D61.1
D61.2
D61.3
D61.81*
D61.89
D61.9
D7Ø.Ø
D7Ø.1
D7Ø.2
D7Ø.3
D7Ø.4
D7Ø.8
D7Ø.9
D71
D72.Ø
D8Ø.6
D8Ø.8
D8Ø.9
D81.Ø
D81.1
D81.2
D81.4
D81.6
D81.7
D81.82
D81.89
D81.9
D82.Ø
D82.1
D89.81Ø
D89.811
D89.812
D89.813
T86.Ø*

DRG 809

Select principal diagnosis listed under DRG 808

DRG 810

Select principal diagnosis listed under DRG 808

DRG 811

Principal Diagnosis

D46*
D5Ø*
D51*
D52*
D53*
D55*
D56*
D57*
D58*
D59.3*
D62
D63*
D64*
D74*
R71*
T8Ø.3ØXA
T8Ø.31ØA
T8Ø.311A
T8Ø.319A
T8Ø.39XA
T8Ø.4ØXA
T8Ø.41ØA
T8Ø.411A
T8Ø.419A
T8Ø.49XA
T8Ø.89XA
T8Ø.91ØA
T8Ø.911A
T8Ø.919A
T8Ø.92XA
T8Ø.AØXA
T8Ø.A1ØA
T8Ø.A11A
T8Ø.A19A
T8Ø.A9XA

DRG 812

Select principal diagnosis listed under DRG 811

DRG 813

Principal Diagnosis

D65
D66
D67
D68.Ø*
D68.1
D68.2
D68.311
D68.318
D68.32
D68.4
D68.8
D68.9
D69*
D75.82*
D75.84
R23.3

DRG 814

Principal Diagnosis

A18.2
A18.85
A28.1
D15.Ø
D18.1
D36.Ø
D3A.Ø91
D47.2
D47.3
D47.4
D68.312
D68.5*
D68.6*
D72.1*
D72.8*
D72.9
D73.Ø
D73.1
D73.2
D73.3
D73.4
D73.5
D73.8*
D73.9
D75.Ø
D75.1
D75.838
D75.839
D75.89
D75.9
D75.A
D76.1
D76.2
D76.3
D77
D8Ø.Ø
D8Ø.1
D8Ø.2
D8Ø.3
D8Ø.4
D8Ø.5
D8Ø.7
D82.2
D82.3
D82.4
D82.8
D82.9
D83.Ø
D83.1
D83.2
D83.8
D83.9
D84.Ø
D84.8*
D84.9
D89.Ø
D89.2
D89.3
D89.4Ø
D89.41
D89.42
D89.43
D89.44
D89.49
D89.831
D89.832
D89.833
D89.834
D89.835
D89.839
D89.84
D89.89
D89.9
E32.Ø
E32.1
E32.8
E32.9
I88.1
I88.8
I88.9
I89.8
I89.9
LØ4.Ø
LØ4.1
LØ4.2
LØ4.3
LØ4.8
LØ4.9
Q89.Ø*
R16.1
R59.Ø
R59.1
R59.9
R75
R76.Ø
R76.8
R76.9
S36.ØØXA
S36.Ø2ØA
S36.Ø21A
S36.Ø29A
S36.Ø3ØA
S36.Ø31A
S36.Ø32A
S36.Ø39A
S36.Ø9XA
T8Ø.82XA
Z94.81
Z94.84

DRG 815

Select principal diagnoses listed under DRG 814

DRG 816

Select principal diagnoses listed under DRG 814

MDC 17

DRG 820

Principal Diagnosis

C26.1
C46.3
C77*
C7B.Ø1
C81*
C82*
C83*
C84*
C85*
C86*
C88*
C9Ø*
C91*
C92*
C93*
C94*
C95*
C96.2*
C96.4
C96.9
C96.A
C96.Z
D45
D47.Ø*
D47.1
D47.9
D47.Z2
D47.Z9
D61.82
D75.81
D89.1

AND

Operating Room Procedures

ØØ16Ø7Ø
ØØ16Ø71
ØØ16Ø72
ØØ16Ø73
ØØ16Ø74
ØØ16Ø75
ØØ16Ø76
ØØ16Ø77
ØØ16Ø78
ØØ16Ø7B
ØØ16ØJØ
ØØ16ØJ1
ØØ16ØJ2
ØØ16ØJ3
ØØ16ØJ4
ØØ16ØJ5
ØØ16ØJ6
ØØ16ØJ7
ØØ16ØJ8
ØØ16ØJB
ØØ16ØKØ
ØØ16ØK1
ØØ16ØK2
ØØ16ØK3
ØØ16ØK4
ØØ16ØK5
ØØ16ØK6
ØØ16ØK7
ØØ16ØK8
ØØ16ØKB
ØØ1637Ø
ØØ16371
ØØ16372
ØØ16373
ØØ16374
ØØ16375
ØØ16376
ØØ16377
ØØ16378
ØØ1637B
ØØ163JØ
ØØ163J1
ØØ163J2
ØØ163J3
ØØ163J4
ØØ163J5
ØØ163J6
ØØ163J7
ØØ163J8
ØØ163JB
ØØ163KØ
ØØ163K1
ØØ163K2
ØØ163K3
ØØ163K4
ØØ163K5
ØØ163K6
ØØ163K7
ØØ163K8
ØØ163KB
ØØ1647Ø
ØØ16471
ØØ16472
ØØ16473
ØØ16474
ØØ16475
ØØ16476
ØØ16477
ØØ16478
ØØ1647B
ØØ164JØ
ØØ164J1
ØØ164J2
ØØ164J3
ØØ164J4
ØØ164J5
ØØ164J6
ØØ164J7
ØØ164J8
ØØ164JB
ØØ164KØ
ØØ164K1
ØØ164K2
ØØ164K3
ØØ164K4
ØØ164K5
ØØ164K6
ØØ164K7
ØØ164K8
ØØ164KB
ØØ1UØ72
ØØ1UØ74
ØØ1UØ76
ØØ1UØ77
ØØ1UØ79
ØØ1UØJ2
ØØ1UØJ4
ØØ1UØJ6
ØØ1UØJ7
ØØ1UØJ9
ØØ1UØK2
ØØ1UØK4
ØØ1UØK6
ØØ1UØK7
ØØ1UØK9
ØØ1U372
ØØ1U374
ØØ1U376
ØØ1U377
ØØ1U379
ØØ1U3J2
ØØ1U3J4
ØØ1U3J6
ØØ1U3J7
ØØ1U3J9
ØØ1U3K2
ØØ1U3K4
ØØ1U3K6
ØØ1U3K7
ØØ1U3K9
ØØ1U472
ØØ1U474
ØØ1U476
ØØ1U477
ØØ1U479
ØØ1U4J2
ØØ1U4J4
ØØ1U4J6
ØØ1U4J7
ØØ1U4J9
ØØ1U4K2
ØØ1U4K4
ØØ1U4K6
ØØ1U4K7
ØØ1U4K9
ØØ5ØØZ3
ØØ5ØØZZ
ØØ5Ø3Z3
ØØ5Ø3ZZ
ØØ5Ø4Z3
ØØ5Ø4ZZ
ØØ51ØZZ
ØØ513ZZ
ØØ514ZZ
ØØ52ØZZ
ØØ523ZZ
ØØ524ZZ
ØØ57ØZZ
ØØ573ZZ
ØØ574ZZ
ØØ58ØZZ
ØØ583ZZ
ØØ584ZZ
ØØ59ØZZ
ØØ593ZZ
ØØ594ZZ
ØØ5AØZZ
ØØ5A3ZZ
ØØ5A4ZZ
ØØ5BØZZ
ØØ5B3ZZ
ØØ5B4ZZ
ØØ5CØZZ
ØØ5C3ZZ
ØØ5C4ZZ
ØØ5DØZZ
ØØ5D3ZZ
ØØ5D4ZZ
ØØ5TØZZ
ØØ5T3ZZ
ØØ5T4ZZ
ØØ5WØZ3
ØØ5WØZZ
ØØ5W3Z3
ØØ5W3ZZ
ØØ5W4Z3
ØØ5W4ZZ
ØØ5XØZ3
ØØ5XØZZ
ØØ5X3Z3
ØØ5X3ZZ
ØØ5X4Z3
ØØ5X4ZZ
ØØ5YØZ3
ØØ5YØZZ
ØØ5Y3Z3
ØØ5Y3ZZ
ØØ5Y4Z3
ØØ5Y4ZZ
ØØ8ØØZZ
ØØ8Ø3ZZ
ØØ8Ø4ZZ
ØØ87ØZZ
ØØ873ZZ
ØØ874ZZ
ØØ88ØZZ
ØØ883ZZ
ØØ884ZZ
ØØ8WØZZ
ØØ8W3ZZ
ØØ8W4ZZ
ØØ8XØZZ
ØØ8X3ZZ
ØØ8X4ZZ
ØØ8YØZZ
ØØ8Y3ZZ
ØØ8Y4ZZ
ØØ9ØØZX
ØØ91ØØZ
ØØ91ØZX
ØØ91ØZZ
ØØ92ØØZ
ØØ92ØZX
ØØ92ØZZ
ØØ93ØZX
ØØ94ØØZ
ØØ94ØZX
ØØ94ØZZ
ØØ95ØØZ
ØØ95ØZX
ØØ95ØZZ
ØØ96ØØZ
ØØ96ØZX
ØØ963ØZ
ØØ964ØZ
ØØ97ØZX
ØØ98ØØZ
ØØ98ØZX
ØØ98ØZZ
ØØ983ØZ
ØØ983ZZ
ØØ984ØZ
ØØ984ZZ
ØØ99ØØZ

00990ZX
00990ZZ
009930Z
00993ZZ
009940Z
00994ZZ
009A00Z
009A0ZX
009A0ZZ
009A30Z
009A3ZZ
009A40Z
009A4ZZ
009B0ZX
009C0ZX
009D0ZX
009T00Z
009T0ZX
009T0ZZ
009T40Z
009T4ZX
009T4ZZ
009U00Z
009U0ZX
009U0ZZ
009W00Z
009W0ZX
009W0ZZ
009W40Z
009W4ZX
009W4ZZ
009X00Z
009X0ZX
009X0ZZ
009X40Z
009X4ZX
009X4ZZ
009Y00Z
009Y0ZX
009Y0ZZ
009Y40Z
009Y4ZX
009Y4ZZ
00B00ZX
00B00ZZ
00B03ZX
00B03ZZ
00B04ZX
00B04ZZ
00B10ZX
00B10ZZ
00B13ZX
00B13ZZ
00B14ZX
00B14ZZ
00B20ZX
00B20ZZ
00B23ZX
00B23ZZ
00B24ZX
00B24ZZ
00B60ZX
00B60ZZ
00B63ZX
00B63ZZ
00B64ZX
00B64ZZ
00B70ZX
00B70ZZ
00B73ZX
00B73ZZ
00B74ZX
00B74ZZ
00B80ZX
00B80ZZ
00B83ZX
00B83ZZ
00B84ZX
00B84ZZ
00B90ZX
00B90ZZ
00B93ZX
00B93ZZ
00B94ZX
00B94ZZ
00BA0ZX
00BA0ZZ
00BA3ZX
00BA3ZZ
00BA4ZX
00BA4ZZ
00BB0ZX
00BB0ZZ
00BB3ZX
00BB3ZZ
00BB4ZX
00BB4ZZ
00BC0ZX
00BC0ZZ
00BC3ZX
00BC3ZZ
00BC4ZX
00BC4ZZ
00BD0ZX
00BD0ZZ
00BD3ZX
00BD3ZZ
00BD4ZX
00BD4ZZ
00BT0ZX
00BT0ZZ
00BT3ZX
00BT3ZZ
00BT4ZX
00BT4ZZ
00BW0ZX
00BW0ZZ
00BW3ZX
00BW3ZZ
00BW4ZX
00BW4ZZ
00BX0ZX
00BX0ZZ
00BX3ZX
00BX3ZZ
00BX4ZX
00BX4ZZ
00BY0ZX
00BY0ZZ
00BY3ZX
00BY3ZZ
00BY4ZX
00BY4ZZ
00C10ZZ
00C13ZZ
00C14ZZ
00C20ZZ
00C23ZZ
00C24ZZ
00C40ZZ
00C43ZZ
00C44ZZ
00C50ZZ
00C53ZZ
00C54ZZ
00C80ZZ
00C83ZZ
00C84ZZ
00C90ZZ
00C93ZZ
00C94ZZ
00CA0ZZ
00CA3ZZ
00CA4ZZ
00D00ZZ
00D03ZZ
00D04ZZ
00D10ZZ
00D13ZZ
00D14ZZ
00D20ZZ
00D23ZZ
00D24ZZ
00D70ZZ
00D73ZZ
00D74ZZ
00DC0ZZ
00DC3ZZ
00DC4ZZ
00DT0ZZ
00DT3ZZ
00DT4ZZ
00FU0ZZ
00FU3ZZ
00FU4ZZ
00FUXZZ
00H00MZ
00H033Z
00H03MZ
00H04MZ
00H60MZ
00H63MZ
00H64MZ
00HU01Z
00HU02Z
00HU0MZ
00HU0YZ
00HU31Z
00HU3MZ
00HU41Z
00HU42Z
00HU4MZ
00HV01Z
00HV02Z
00HV0MZ
00HV0YZ
00HV31Z
00HV3MZ
00HV3YZ
00HV41Z
00HV42Z
00HV4MZ
00HV4YZ
00J00ZZ
00J04ZZ
00JU0ZZ
00JU4ZZ
00JV0ZZ
00JV4ZZ
00K00ZZ
00K03ZZ
00K04ZZ
00K70ZZ
00K73ZZ
00K74ZZ
00K80ZZ
00K83ZZ
00K84ZZ
00K90ZZ
00K93ZZ
00K94ZZ
00KA0ZZ
00KA3ZZ
00KA4ZZ
00KB0ZZ
00KB3ZZ
00KB4ZZ
00KC0ZZ
00KC3ZZ
00KC4ZZ
00KD0ZZ
00KD3ZZ
00KD4ZZ
00N00ZZ
00N03ZZ
00N04ZZ
00N10ZZ
00N13ZZ
00N14ZZ
00N20ZZ
00N23ZZ
00N24ZZ
00N70ZZ
00N73ZZ
00N74ZZ
00N90ZZ
00N93ZZ
00N94ZZ
00NA0ZZ
00NA3ZZ
00NA4ZZ
00NT0ZZ
00NT3ZZ
00NT4ZZ
00NW0ZZ
00NW3ZZ
00NW4ZZ
00NX0ZZ
00NX3ZZ
00NX4ZZ
00NY0ZZ
00NY3ZZ
00NY4ZZ
00P00MZ
00P03MZ
00P04MZ
00P60MZ
00P63MZ
00P64MZ
00PU00Z
00PU02Z
00PU03Z
00PU0YZ
00PU40Z
00PU42Z
00PU43Z
00PV00Z
00PV02Z
00PV03Z
00PV07Z
00PV0JZ
00PV0KZ
00PV0YZ
00PV37Z
00PV3JZ
00PV3KZ
00PV40Z
00PV42Z
00PV43Z
00PV47Z
00PV4JZ
00PV4KZ
00Q90ZZ
00Q93ZZ
00Q94ZZ
00QA0ZZ
00QA3ZZ
00QA4ZZ
00QT0ZZ
00QT3ZZ
00QT4ZZ
00QW0ZZ
00QW3ZZ
00QW4ZZ
00QX0ZZ
00QX3ZZ
00QX4ZZ
00QY0ZZ
00QY3ZZ
00QY4ZZ
00RT07Z
00RT0JZ
00RT0KZ
00RT47Z
00RT4JZ
00RT4KZ
00SW0ZZ
00SW3ZZ
00SW4ZZ
00SX0ZZ
00SX3ZZ
00SX4ZZ
00SY0ZZ
00SY3ZZ
00SY4ZZ
00T70ZZ
00T73ZZ
00T74ZZ
00UT07Z
00UT0JZ
00UT0KZ
00UT37Z
00UT3JZ
00UT3KZ
00UT47Z
00UT4JZ
00UT4KZ
00W60JZ
00W63JZ
00W64JZ
00WU00Z
00WU02Z
00WU03Z
00WU0JZ
00WU0MZ
00WU0YZ
00WU30Z
00WU32Z
00WU33Z
00WU3JZ
00WU3MZ
00WU40Z
00WU42Z
00WU43Z
00WU4JZ
00WU4MZ
00WV00Z
00WV02Z
00WV03Z
00WV07Z
00WV0JZ
00WV0KZ
00WV0MZ
00WV0YZ
00WV30Z
00WV32Z
00WV33Z
00WV37Z
00WV3JZ
00WV3KZ
00WV3MZ
00WV40Z
00WV42Z
00WV43Z
00WV47Z
00WV4JZ
00WV4KZ
00WV4MZ
01510ZZ
01514ZZ
01580ZZ
01584ZZ
015B0ZZ
015B4ZZ
015R0ZZ
015R4ZZ
01810ZZ
01813ZZ
01814ZZ
01880ZZ
01883ZZ
01884ZZ
018B0ZZ
018B3ZZ
018B4ZZ
018R0ZZ
018R3ZZ
018R4ZZ
025N0ZZ
025N3ZZ
025N4ZZ
02BN0ZX
02BN0ZZ
02BN3ZX
02BN3ZZ
02BN4ZX
02BN4ZZ
02CN0ZZ
02CN3ZZ
02CN4ZZ
02HN00Z
02HN02Z
02HN0YZ
02HN30Z
02HN3YZ
02HN40Z
02HN42Z
02HN4YZ
02JA0ZZ
02JA4ZZ
02JY0ZZ
02JY4ZZ
02NN0ZZ
02NN3ZZ
02NN4ZZ
02QA0ZZ
02TN0ZZ
02TN3ZZ
02TN4ZZ
03H00DZ
03H03DZ
03H04DZ
03H10DZ
03H13DZ
03H14DZ
03H20DZ
03H23DZ
03H24DZ
03H30DZ
03H33DZ
03H34DZ
03H40DZ
03H43DZ
03H44DZ
03H50DZ
03H53DZ
03H54DZ
03H60DZ
03H63DZ
03H64DZ
03H70DZ
03H73DZ
03H74DZ
03H80DZ
03H83DZ
03H84DZ
03H90DZ
03H93DZ
03H94DZ
03HA0DZ
03HA3DZ
03HA4DZ
03HB0DZ
03HB3DZ
03HB4DZ
03HC0DZ
03HC3DZ
03HC4DZ
03HD0DZ
03HD3DZ
03HD4DZ
03HF0DZ
03HF3DZ
03HF4DZ
03HG0DZ
03HG3DZ
03HG4DZ
03HH0DZ
03HH3DZ
03HH4DZ
03HJ0DZ
03HJ3DZ
03HJ4DZ
03HK0DZ
03HK3DZ
03HK4DZ
03HL0DZ
03HL3DZ
03HL4DZ
03HM0DZ
03HM3DZ
03HM4DZ
03HN0DZ
03HN3DZ
03HN4DZ
03HP0DZ
03HP3DZ
03HP4DZ
03HQ0DZ
03HQ3DZ
03HQ4DZ
03HR0DZ
03HR3DZ
03HR4DZ
03HS0DZ
03HS3DZ
03HS4DZ
03HT0DZ
03HT3DZ
03HT4DZ
03HU0DZ
03HU3DZ
03HU4DZ
03HV0DZ
03HV3DZ
03HV4DZ
03HY0DZ
03HY3DZ
03HY4DZ
04CK0ZZ
04CK3ZZ
04CK4ZZ
04CL0ZZ
04CL3ZZ
04CL4ZZ
04CM0ZZ
04CM3ZZ
04CM4ZZ
04CN0ZZ
04CN3ZZ
04CN4ZZ
04CP0ZZ
04CP3ZZ
04CP4ZZ
04CQ0ZZ
04CQ3ZZ
04CQ4ZZ
04CR0ZZ
04CR3ZZ
04CR4ZZ
04CS0ZZ
04CS3ZZ
04CS4ZZ
04CT0ZZ
04CT3ZZ
04CT4ZZ
04CU0ZZ
04CU3ZZ
04CU4ZZ
04CV0ZZ
04CV3ZZ
04CV4ZZ
04CW0ZZ
04CW3ZZ
04CW4ZZ
04CY0ZZ
04CY3ZZ
04CY4ZZ
04H00DZ
04H03DZ
04H04DZ
04H10DZ
04H13DZ
04H14DZ
04H20DZ
04H23DZ
04H24DZ
04H30DZ
04H33DZ
04H34DZ
04H40DZ
04H43DZ
04H44DZ
04H50DZ
04H53DZ
04H54DZ
04H60DZ
04H63DZ
04H64DZ
04H70DZ
04H73DZ
04H74DZ
04H80DZ
04H83DZ
04H84DZ
04H90DZ
04H93DZ
04H94DZ
04HA0DZ
04HA3DZ
04HA4DZ
04HB0DZ
04HB3DZ
04HB4DZ
04HC0DZ
04HC3DZ
04HC4DZ
04HD0DZ
04HD3DZ
04HD4DZ
04HE0DZ
04HE3DZ
04HE4DZ
04HF0DZ
04HF3DZ
04HF4DZ
04HH0DZ
04HH3DZ
04HH4DZ
04HJ0DZ
04HJ3DZ
04HJ4DZ
04HK0DZ
04HK3DZ
04HK4DZ
04HL0DZ
04HL3DZ
04HL4DZ
04HM0DZ
04HM3DZ
04HM4DZ
04HN0DZ
04HN3DZ
04HN4DZ
04HP0DZ
04HP3DZ
04HP4DZ
04HQ0DZ
04HQ3DZ
04HQ4DZ
04HR0DZ
04HR3DZ
04HR4DZ
04HS0DZ
04HS3DZ
04HS4DZ
04HT0DZ
04HT3DZ
04HT4DZ
04HU0DZ
04HU3DZ
04HU4DZ
04HV0DZ
04HV3DZ
04HV4DZ
04HW0DZ
04HW3DZ
04HW4DZ
04HY02Z
04HY0DZ
04HY0YZ
04HY3DZ
04HY42Z
04HY4DZ
04PY00Z
04PY02Z
04PY03Z
04PY0CZ
04PY0DZ
04PY0YZ
04PY3CZ
04PY40Z
04PY42Z
04PY43Z
04PY4CZ
04PY4DZ
04WY00Z
04WY02Z
04WY03Z
04WY0CZ
04WY0DZ
04WY0YZ
04WY3CZ
04WY40Z
04WY42Z
04WY43Z
04WY4CZ
04WY4DZ
05H00DZ
05H03DZ
05H04DZ
05H10DZ
05H13DZ
05H14DZ
05H30DZ
05H33DZ
05H34DZ
05H40DZ
05H43DZ
05H44DZ
05H50DZ
05H53DZ
05H54DZ
05H60DZ
05H63DZ
05H64DZ
05H70DZ
05H73DZ
05H74DZ
05H80DZ
05H83DZ
05H84DZ
05H90DZ
05H93DZ
05H94DZ
05HA0DZ
05HA3DZ
05HA4DZ
05HB0DZ
05HB3DZ
05HB4DZ
05HC0DZ
05HC3DZ
05HC4DZ
05HD0DZ
05HD3DZ
05HD4DZ
05HF0DZ
05HF3DZ
05HF4DZ
05HG0DZ
05HG3DZ
05HG4DZ
05HH0DZ
05HH3DZ
05HH4DZ
05HL0DZ
05HL3DZ
05HL4DZ
05HM0DZ
05HM3DZ
05HM4DZ
05HN0DZ
05HN3DZ
05HN4DZ
05HP0DZ
05HP3DZ
05HP4DZ
05HQ0DZ
05HQ3DZ
05HQ4DZ
05HR0DZ
05HR3DZ
05HR4DZ
05HS0DZ
05HS3DZ
05HS4DZ
05HT0DZ
05HT3DZ
05HT4DZ
05HV0DZ
05HV3DZ
05HV4DZ
05HY0DZ
05HY3DZ
05HY4DZ
06H10DZ
06H13DZ
06H14DZ
06H20DZ
06H23DZ
06H24DZ
06H30DZ
06H33DZ
06H34DZ
06H40DZ
06H43DZ
06H44DZ
06H50DZ
06H53DZ
06H54DZ
06H60DZ
06H63DZ
06H64DZ
06H70DZ
06H73DZ
06H74DZ
06H80DZ
06H83DZ
06H84DZ
06H90DZ
06H93DZ
06H94DZ
06HB0DZ
06HB3DZ
06HB4DZ
06HC0DZ
06HC3DZ
06HC4DZ
06HD0DZ
06HD3DZ
06HD4DZ
06HF0DZ
06HF3DZ
06HF4DZ
06HG0DZ
06HG3DZ
06HG4DZ
06HH0DZ
06HH3DZ
06HH4DZ
06HJ0DZ
06HJ3DZ
06HJ4DZ
06HM0DZ
06HM3DZ
06HM4DZ
06HN0DZ
06HN3DZ
06HN4DZ
06HP0DZ
06HP3DZ
06HP4DZ
06HQ0DZ
06HQ3DZ
06HQ4DZ
06HT0DZ
06HT3DZ
06HT4DZ
06HV0DZ
06HV3DZ
06HV4DZ
06HY0DZ
06HY3DZ
06HY4DZ
07500ZZ
07503ZZ
07504ZZ
07510ZZ
07513ZZ
07514ZZ
07520ZZ
07523ZZ
07524ZZ
07530ZZ
07533ZZ
07534ZZ
07540ZZ
07543ZZ
07544ZZ
07550ZZ
07553ZZ
07554ZZ
07560ZZ
07563ZZ
07564ZZ
07570ZZ
07573ZZ
07574ZZ
07580ZZ
07583ZZ
07584ZZ
07590ZZ
07593ZZ
07594ZZ

Ø75BØZZ
Ø75B3ZZ
Ø75B4ZZ
Ø75CØZZ
Ø75C3ZZ
Ø75C4ZZ
Ø75DØZZ
Ø75D3ZZ
Ø75D4ZZ
Ø75FØZZ
Ø75F3ZZ
Ø75F4ZZ
Ø75GØZZ
Ø75G3ZZ
Ø75G4ZZ
Ø75HØZZ
Ø75H3ZZ
Ø75H4ZZ
Ø75JØZZ
Ø75J3ZZ
Ø75J4ZZ
Ø75MØZZ
Ø75M3ZZ
Ø75M4ZZ
Ø75PØZZ
Ø75P3ZZ
Ø75P4ZZ
Ø79MØØZ
Ø79MØZX
Ø79MØZZ
Ø79M3ZX
Ø79M4ØZ
Ø79M4ZX
Ø79M4ZZ
Ø79PØØZ
Ø79PØZX
Ø79PØZZ
Ø7BØØZZ
Ø7BØ4ZZ
Ø7B3ØZZ
Ø7B34ZZ
Ø7B4ØZZ
Ø7B44ZZ
Ø7B7ØZZ
Ø7B74ZZ
Ø7BBØZZ
Ø7BB4ZZ
Ø7BFØZZ
Ø7BF4ZZ
Ø7BGØZZ
Ø7BG4ZZ
Ø7BMØZX
Ø7BMØZZ
Ø7BM3ZX
Ø7BM3ZZ
Ø7BM4ZX
Ø7BM4ZZ
Ø7BPØZX
Ø7BPØZZ
Ø7BP3ZZ
Ø7BP4ZZ
Ø7CMØZZ
Ø7CM3ZZ
Ø7CM4ZZ
Ø7CPØZZ
Ø7HMØ1Z
Ø7HMØYZ
Ø7HM41Z
Ø7HM4YZ
Ø7HPØ1Z
Ø7HPØYZ
Ø7HP41Z
Ø7JMØZZ
Ø7JM4ZZ
Ø7JPØZZ
Ø7LØØCZ
Ø7LØØDZ
Ø7LØØZZ
Ø7LØ3CZ
Ø7LØ3DZ
Ø7LØ3ZZ
Ø7LØ4CZ
Ø7LØ4DZ
Ø7LØ4ZZ
Ø7L1ØCZ
Ø7L1ØDZ
Ø7L1ØZZ
Ø7L13CZ
Ø7L13DZ
Ø7L13ZZ
Ø7L14CZ
Ø7L14DZ
Ø7L14ZZ
Ø7L2ØCZ
Ø7L2ØDZ
Ø7L2ØZZ
Ø7L23CZ
Ø7L23DZ
Ø7L23ZZ
Ø7L24CZ
Ø7L24DZ
Ø7L24ZZ
Ø7L3ØCZ
Ø7L3ØDZ
Ø7L3ØZZ
Ø7L33CZ
Ø7L33DZ
Ø7L33ZZ
Ø7L34CZ
Ø7L34DZ
Ø7L34ZZ
Ø7L4ØCZ
Ø7L4ØDZ
Ø7L4ØZZ
Ø7L43CZ
Ø7L43DZ
Ø7L43ZZ
Ø7L44CZ
Ø7L44DZ
Ø7L44ZZ
Ø7L5ØCZ
Ø7L5ØDZ
Ø7L5ØZZ
Ø7L53CZ
Ø7L53DZ
Ø7L53ZZ
Ø7L54CZ
Ø7L54DZ
Ø7L54ZZ
Ø7L6ØCZ
Ø7L6ØDZ
Ø7L6ØZZ
Ø7L63CZ
Ø7L63DZ
Ø7L63ZZ
Ø7L64CZ
Ø7L64DZ
Ø7L64ZZ
Ø7L7ØCZ
Ø7L7ØDZ
Ø7L7ØZZ
Ø7L73CZ
Ø7L73DZ
Ø7L73ZZ
Ø7L74CZ
Ø7L74DZ
Ø7L74ZZ
Ø7L8ØCZ
Ø7L8ØDZ
Ø7L8ØZZ
Ø7L83CZ
Ø7L83DZ
Ø7L83ZZ
Ø7L84CZ
Ø7L84DZ
Ø7L84ZZ
Ø7L9ØCZ
Ø7L9ØDZ
Ø7L9ØZZ
Ø7L93CZ
Ø7L93DZ
Ø7L93ZZ
Ø7L94CZ
Ø7L94DZ
Ø7L94ZZ
Ø7LBØCZ
Ø7LBØDZ
Ø7LBØZZ
Ø7LB3CZ
Ø7LB3DZ
Ø7LB3ZZ
Ø7LB4CZ
Ø7LB4DZ
Ø7LB4ZZ
Ø7LCØCZ
Ø7LCØDZ
Ø7LCØZZ
Ø7LC3CZ
Ø7LC3DZ
Ø7LC3ZZ
Ø7LC4CZ
Ø7LC4DZ
Ø7LC4ZZ
Ø7LDØCZ
Ø7LDØDZ
Ø7LDØZZ
Ø7LD3CZ
Ø7LD3DZ
Ø7LD3ZZ
Ø7LD4CZ
Ø7LD4DZ
Ø7LD4ZZ
Ø7LFØCZ
Ø7LFØDZ
Ø7LFØZZ
Ø7LF3CZ
Ø7LF3DZ
Ø7LF3ZZ
Ø7LF4CZ
Ø7LF4DZ
Ø7LF4ZZ
Ø7LGØCZ
Ø7LGØDZ
Ø7LGØZZ
Ø7LG3CZ
Ø7LG3DZ
Ø7LG3ZZ
Ø7LG4CZ
Ø7LG4DZ
Ø7LG4ZZ
Ø7LHØCZ
Ø7LHØDZ
Ø7LHØZZ
Ø7LH3CZ
Ø7LH3DZ
Ø7LH3ZZ
Ø7LH4CZ
Ø7LH4DZ
Ø7LH4ZZ
Ø7LJØCZ
Ø7LJØDZ
Ø7LJØZZ
Ø7LJ3CZ
Ø7LJ3DZ
Ø7LJ3ZZ
Ø7LJ4CZ
Ø7LJ4DZ
Ø7LJ4ZZ
Ø7NØØZZ
Ø7NØ3ZZ
Ø7NØ4ZZ
Ø7N1ØZZ
Ø7N13ZZ
Ø7N14ZZ
Ø7N2ØZZ
Ø7N23ZZ
Ø7N24ZZ
Ø7N3ØZZ
Ø7N33ZZ
Ø7N34ZZ
Ø7N4ØZZ
Ø7N43ZZ
Ø7N44ZZ
Ø7N5ØZZ
Ø7N53ZZ
Ø7N54ZZ
Ø7N6ØZZ
Ø7N63ZZ
Ø7N64ZZ
Ø7N7ØZZ
Ø7N73ZZ
Ø7N74ZZ
Ø7N8ØZZ
Ø7N83ZZ
Ø7N84ZZ
Ø7N9ØZZ
Ø7N93ZZ
Ø7N94ZZ
Ø7NBØZZ
Ø7NB3ZZ
Ø7NB4ZZ
Ø7NCØZZ
Ø7NC3ZZ
Ø7NC4ZZ
Ø7NDØZZ
Ø7ND3ZZ
Ø7ND4ZZ
Ø7NFØZZ
Ø7NF3ZZ
Ø7NF4ZZ
Ø7NGØZZ
Ø7NG3ZZ
Ø7NG4ZZ
Ø7NHØZZ
Ø7NH3ZZ
Ø7NH4ZZ
Ø7NJØZZ
Ø7NJ3ZZ
Ø7NJ4ZZ
Ø7NMØZZ
Ø7NM3ZZ
Ø7NM4ZZ
Ø7NPØZZ
Ø7NP3ZZ
Ø7NP4ZZ
Ø7PKØ7Z
Ø7PKØJZ
Ø7PKØKZ
Ø7PK37Z
Ø7PK3JZ
Ø7PK3KZ
Ø7PK47Z
Ø7PK4JZ
Ø7PK4KZ
Ø7PLØ7Z
Ø7PLØJZ
Ø7PLØKZ
Ø7PL37Z
Ø7PL3JZ
Ø7PL3KZ
Ø7PL47Z
Ø7PL4JZ
Ø7PL4KZ
Ø7PMØØZ
Ø7PMØ3Z
Ø7PMØYZ
Ø7PM3ØZ
Ø7PM33Z
Ø7PM4ØZ
Ø7PM43Z
Ø7PNØ7Z
Ø7PNØJZ
Ø7PNØKZ
Ø7PN37Z
Ø7PN3JZ
Ø7PN3KZ
Ø7PN47Z
Ø7PN4JZ
Ø7PN4KZ
Ø7PPØØZ
Ø7PPØ3Z
Ø7PPØYZ
Ø7PP3ØZ
Ø7PP33Z
Ø7PP4ØZ
Ø7PP43Z
Ø7QØØZZ
Ø7QØ3ZZ
Ø7QØ4ZZ
Ø7QØ8ZZ
Ø7Q1ØZZ
Ø7Q13ZZ
Ø7Q14ZZ
Ø7Q18ZZ
Ø7Q2ØZZ
Ø7Q23ZZ
Ø7Q24ZZ
Ø7Q28ZZ
Ø7Q3ØZZ
Ø7Q33ZZ
Ø7Q34ZZ
Ø7Q38ZZ
Ø7Q4ØZZ
Ø7Q43ZZ
Ø7Q44ZZ
Ø7Q48ZZ
Ø7Q5ØZZ
Ø7Q53ZZ
Ø7Q54ZZ
Ø7Q58ZZ
Ø7Q6ØZZ
Ø7Q63ZZ
Ø7Q64ZZ
Ø7Q68ZZ
Ø7Q7ØZZ
Ø7Q73ZZ
Ø7Q74ZZ
Ø7Q78ZZ
Ø7Q8ØZZ
Ø7Q83ZZ
Ø7Q84ZZ
Ø7Q88ZZ
Ø7Q9ØZZ
Ø7Q93ZZ
Ø7Q94ZZ
Ø7Q98ZZ
Ø7QBØZZ
Ø7QB3ZZ
Ø7QB4ZZ
Ø7QB8ZZ
Ø7QCØZZ
Ø7QC3ZZ
Ø7QC4ZZ
Ø7QC8ZZ
Ø7QDØZZ
Ø7QD3ZZ
Ø7QD4ZZ
Ø7QD8ZZ
Ø7QFØZZ
Ø7QF3ZZ
Ø7QF4ZZ
Ø7QF8ZZ
Ø7QGØZZ
Ø7QG3ZZ
Ø7QG4ZZ
Ø7QG8ZZ
Ø7QHØZZ
Ø7QH3ZZ
Ø7QH4ZZ
Ø7QH8ZZ
Ø7QJØZZ
Ø7QJ3ZZ
Ø7QJ4ZZ
Ø7QJ8ZZ
Ø7QMØZZ
Ø7QM3ZZ
Ø7QM4ZZ
Ø7QPØZZ
Ø7QP3ZZ
Ø7QP4ZZ
Ø7SMØZZ
Ø7SPØZZ
Ø7TØØZZ
Ø7TØ4ZZ
Ø7T1ØZZ
Ø7T14ZZ
Ø7T2ØZZ
Ø7T24ZZ
Ø7T3ØZZ
Ø7T34ZZ
Ø7T4ØZZ
Ø7T44ZZ
Ø7T5ØZZ
Ø7T54ZZ
Ø7T6ØZZ
Ø7T64ZZ
Ø7T7ØZZ
Ø7T74ZZ
Ø7T8ØZZ
Ø7T84ZZ
Ø7T9ØZZ
Ø7T94ZZ
Ø7TBØZZ
Ø7TB4ZZ
Ø7TCØZZ
Ø7TC4ZZ
Ø7TDØZZ
Ø7TD4ZZ
Ø7TFØZZ
Ø7TF4ZZ
Ø7TGØZZ
Ø7TG4ZZ
Ø7THØZZ
Ø7TH4ZZ
Ø7TJØZZ
Ø7TJ4ZZ
Ø7TMØZZ
Ø7TM4ZZ
Ø7TPØZZ
Ø7TP4ZZ
Ø7UØØ7Z
Ø7UØØJZ
Ø7UØØKZ
Ø7UØ47Z
Ø7UØ4JZ
Ø7UØ4KZ
Ø7U1Ø7Z
Ø7U1ØJZ
Ø7U1ØKZ
Ø7U147Z
Ø7U14JZ
Ø7U14KZ
Ø7U2Ø7Z
Ø7U2ØJZ
Ø7U2ØKZ
Ø7U247Z
Ø7U24JZ
Ø7U24KZ
Ø7U3Ø7Z
Ø7U3ØJZ
Ø7U3ØKZ
Ø7U347Z
Ø7U34JZ
Ø7U34KZ
Ø7U4Ø7Z
Ø7U4ØJZ
Ø7U4ØKZ
Ø7U447Z
Ø7U44JZ
Ø7U44KZ
Ø7U5Ø7Z
Ø7U5ØJZ
Ø7U5ØKZ
Ø7U547Z
Ø7U54JZ
Ø7U54KZ
Ø7U6Ø7Z
Ø7U6ØJZ
Ø7U6ØKZ
Ø7U647Z
Ø7U64JZ
Ø7U64KZ
Ø7U7Ø7Z
Ø7U7ØJZ
Ø7U7ØKZ
Ø7U747Z
Ø7U74JZ
Ø7U74KZ
Ø7U8Ø7Z
Ø7U8ØJZ
Ø7U8ØKZ
Ø7U847Z
Ø7U84JZ
Ø7U84KZ
Ø7U9Ø7Z
Ø7U9ØJZ
Ø7U9ØKZ
Ø7U947Z
Ø7U94JZ
Ø7U94KZ
Ø7UBØ7Z
Ø7UBØJZ
Ø7UBØKZ
Ø7UB47Z
Ø7UB4JZ
Ø7UB4KZ
Ø7UCØ7Z
Ø7UCØJZ
Ø7UCØKZ
Ø7UC47Z
Ø7UC4JZ
Ø7UC4KZ
Ø7UDØ7Z
Ø7UDØJZ
Ø7UDØKZ
Ø7UD47Z
Ø7UD4JZ
Ø7UD4KZ
Ø7UFØ7Z
Ø7UFØJZ
Ø7UFØKZ
Ø7UF47Z
Ø7UF4JZ
Ø7UF4KZ
Ø7UGØ7Z
Ø7UGØJZ
Ø7UGØKZ
Ø7UG47Z
Ø7UG4JZ
Ø7UG4KZ
Ø7UHØ7Z
Ø7UHØJZ
Ø7UHØKZ
Ø7UH47Z
Ø7UH4JZ
Ø7UH4KZ
Ø7UJØ7Z
Ø7UJØJZ
Ø7UJØKZ
Ø7UJ47Z
Ø7UJ4JZ
Ø7UJ4KZ
Ø7VØØCZ
Ø7VØØDZ
Ø7VØØZZ
Ø7VØ3CZ
Ø7VØ3DZ
Ø7VØ3ZZ
Ø7VØ4CZ
Ø7VØ4DZ
Ø7VØ4ZZ
Ø7V1ØCZ
Ø7V1ØDZ
Ø7V1ØZZ
Ø7V13CZ
Ø7V13DZ
Ø7V13ZZ
Ø7V14CZ
Ø7V14DZ
Ø7V14ZZ
Ø7V2ØCZ
Ø7V2ØDZ
Ø7V2ØZZ
Ø7V23CZ
Ø7V23DZ
Ø7V23ZZ
Ø7V24CZ
Ø7V24DZ
Ø7V24ZZ
Ø7V3ØCZ
Ø7V3ØDZ
Ø7V3ØZZ
Ø7V33CZ
Ø7V33DZ
Ø7V33ZZ
Ø7V34CZ
Ø7V34DZ
Ø7V34ZZ
Ø7V4ØCZ
Ø7V4ØDZ
Ø7V4ØZZ
Ø7V43CZ
Ø7V43DZ
Ø7V43ZZ
Ø7V44CZ
Ø7V44DZ
Ø7V44ZZ
Ø7V5ØCZ
Ø7V5ØDZ
Ø7V5ØZZ
Ø7V53CZ
Ø7V53DZ
Ø7V53ZZ
Ø7V54CZ
Ø7V54DZ
Ø7V54ZZ
Ø7V6ØCZ
Ø7V6ØDZ
Ø7V6ØZZ
Ø7V63CZ
Ø7V63DZ
Ø7V63ZZ
Ø7V64CZ
Ø7V64DZ
Ø7V64ZZ
Ø7V7ØCZ
Ø7V7ØDZ
Ø7V7ØZZ
Ø7V73CZ
Ø7V73DZ
Ø7V73ZZ
Ø7V74CZ
Ø7V74DZ
Ø7V74ZZ
Ø7V8ØCZ
Ø7V8ØDZ
Ø7V8ØZZ
Ø7V83CZ
Ø7V83DZ
Ø7V83ZZ
Ø7V84CZ
Ø7V84DZ
Ø7V84ZZ
Ø7V9ØCZ
Ø7V9ØDZ
Ø7V9ØZZ
Ø7V93CZ
Ø7V93DZ
Ø7V93ZZ
Ø7V94CZ
Ø7V94DZ
Ø7V94ZZ
Ø7VBØCZ
Ø7VBØDZ
Ø7VBØZZ
Ø7VB3CZ
Ø7VB3DZ
Ø7VB3ZZ
Ø7VB4CZ
Ø7VB4DZ
Ø7VB4ZZ
Ø7VCØCZ
Ø7VCØDZ
Ø7VCØZZ
Ø7VC3CZ
Ø7VC3DZ
Ø7VC3ZZ
Ø7VC4CZ
Ø7VC4DZ
Ø7VC4ZZ
Ø7VDØCZ
Ø7VDØDZ
Ø7VDØZZ
Ø7VD3CZ
Ø7VD3DZ
Ø7VD3ZZ
Ø7VD4CZ
Ø7VD4DZ
Ø7VD4ZZ
Ø7VFØCZ
Ø7VFØDZ
Ø7VFØZZ
Ø7VF3CZ
Ø7VF3DZ
Ø7VF3ZZ
Ø7VF4CZ
Ø7VF4DZ
Ø7VF4ZZ
Ø7VGØCZ
Ø7VGØDZ
Ø7VGØZZ
Ø7VG3CZ
Ø7VG3DZ
Ø7VG3ZZ
Ø7VG4CZ
Ø7VG4DZ
Ø7VG4ZZ
Ø7VHØCZ
Ø7VHØDZ
Ø7VHØZZ
Ø7VH3CZ
Ø7VH3DZ
Ø7VH3ZZ
Ø7VH4CZ
Ø7VH4DZ
Ø7VH4ZZ
Ø7VJØCZ
Ø7VJØDZ
Ø7VJØZZ
Ø7VJ3CZ
Ø7VJ3DZ
Ø7VJ3ZZ
Ø7VJ4CZ
Ø7VJ4DZ
Ø7VJ4ZZ
Ø7WKØ7Z
Ø7WKØJZ
Ø7WKØKZ
Ø7WK37Z
Ø7WK3JZ
Ø7WK3KZ
Ø7WK47Z
Ø7WK4JZ
Ø7WK4KZ
Ø7WLØ7Z
Ø7WLØJZ
Ø7WLØKZ
Ø7WL37Z
Ø7WL3JZ
Ø7WL3KZ
Ø7WL47Z
Ø7WL4JZ
Ø7WL4KZ
Ø7WMØØZ
Ø7WMØ3Z
Ø7WMØYZ
Ø7WM3ØZ
Ø7WM33Z
Ø7WM4ØZ
Ø7WM43Z
Ø7WNØ7Z
Ø7WNØJZ
Ø7WNØKZ
Ø7WN37Z
Ø7WN3JZ
Ø7WN3KZ
Ø7WN47Z
Ø7WN4JZ
Ø7WN4KZ
Ø7WPØØZ
Ø7WPØ3Z
Ø7WPØYZ
Ø7WP3ØZ
Ø7WP33Z
Ø7WP4ØZ
Ø7WP43Z
Ø7YMØZØ
Ø7YMØZ1
Ø7YMØZ2
Ø7YPØZØ
Ø7YPØZ1
Ø7YPØZ2
ØB5CØZ3
ØB5CØZZ
ØB5C4Z3
ØB5C4ZZ
ØB5DØZ3
ØB5DØZZ
ØB5D4Z3
ØB5D4ZZ
ØB5FØZ3
ØB5FØZZ
ØB5F4Z3
ØB5F4ZZ
ØB5GØZ3
ØB5GØZZ
ØB5G4Z3
ØB5G4ZZ
ØB5HØZ3
ØB5HØZZ
ØB5H4Z3
ØB5H4ZZ
ØB5JØZ3
ØB5JØZZ
ØB5J4Z3
ØB5J4ZZ
ØB5KØZ3
ØB5KØZZ
ØB5K4Z3
ØB5K4ZZ
ØB5LØZ3
ØB5LØZZ
ØB5L4Z3
ØB5L4ZZ
ØB5MØZ3
ØB5MØZZ
ØB5M4Z3
ØB5M4ZZ
ØB5NØZZ
ØB5N3ZZ
ØB5N4ZZ
ØB5PØZZ
ØB5P3ZZ
ØB5P4ZZ
ØB9CØZX
ØB9DØZX
ØB9FØZX
ØB9GØZX
ØB9HØZX
ØB9JØZX
ØB9KØZX
ØB9LØZX
ØB9MØZX
ØBBCØZX
ØBBCØZZ
ØBBC3ZZ
ØBBC4ZZ
ØBBC7ZZ
ØBBDØZX
ØBBDØZZ
ØBBD3ZZ
ØBBD4ZZ
ØBBD7ZZ
ØBBFØZX
ØBBFØZZ
ØBBF3ZZ
ØBBF4ZZ
ØBBF7ZZ
ØBBGØZX
ØBBGØZZ
ØBBG3ZZ
ØBBG4ZZ
ØBBG7ZZ
ØBBHØZX
ØBBHØZZ
ØBBH3ZZ
ØBBH4ZZ
ØBBH7ZZ
ØBBJØZX
ØBBJØZZ
ØBBJ3ZZ
ØBBJ4ZZ
ØBBJ7ZZ
ØBBKØZX
ØBBKØZZ
ØBBK3ZZ
ØBBK4ZZ
ØBBK7ZZ
ØBBLØZX
ØBBLØZZ
ØBBL3ZZ
ØBBL4ZZ
ØBBL7ZZ
ØBBMØZX
ØBBMØZZ
ØBBM3ZZ
ØBBM7ZZ
ØBDNØZX
ØBDNØZZ
ØBDN3ZX
ØBDN3ZZ
ØBDN4ZX
ØBDN4ZZ
ØBDPØZX
ØBDPØZZ
ØBDP3ZX
ØBDP3ZZ
ØBDP4ZX
ØBDP4ZZ
ØBTHØZZ
ØBTH4ZZ
ØD11Ø74
ØD11Ø76
ØD11ØJ4
ØD11ØJ6

ØD11ØK4
ØD11ØK6
ØD11ØZ4
ØD11ØZ6
ØD113J4
ØD11474
ØD11476
ØD114J4
ØD114J6
ØD114K4
ØD114K6
ØD114Z4
ØD114Z6
ØD11874
ØD11876
ØD118J4
ØD118J6
ØD118K4
ØD118K6
ØD118Z4
ØD118Z6
ØD12Ø74
ØD12Ø76
ØD12ØJ4
ØD12ØJ6
ØD12ØK4
ØD12ØK6
ØD12ØZ4
ØD12ØZ6
ØD123J4
ØD12474
ØD12476
ØD124J4
ØD124J6
ØD124K4
ØD124K6
ØD124Z4
ØD124Z6
ØD12874
ØD12876
ØD128J4
ØD128J6
ØD128K4
ØD128K6
ØD128Z4
ØD128Z6
ØD13Ø74
ØD13Ø76
ØD13ØJ4
ØD13ØJ6
ØD13ØK4
ØD13ØK6
ØD13ØZ4
ØD13ØZ6
ØD133J4
ØD13474
ØD13476
ØD134J4
ØD134J6
ØD134K4
ØD134K6
ØD134Z4
ØD134Z6
ØD13874
ØD13876
ØD138J4
ØD138J6
ØD138K4
ØD138K6
ØD138Z4
ØD138Z6
ØD15Ø74
ØD15Ø76
ØD15Ø79
ØD15Ø7A
ØD15Ø7B
ØD15ØJ4
ØD15ØJ6
ØD15ØJ9
ØD15ØJA
ØD15ØJB
ØD15ØK4
ØD15ØK6
ØD15ØK9
ØD15ØKA
ØD15ØKB
ØD15ØZ4
ØD15ØZ6
ØD15ØZ9
ØD15ØZA
ØD15ØZB
ØD153J4
ØD15474
ØD15476
ØD15479
ØD1547A
ØD1547B
ØD154J4
ØD154J6
ØD154J9
ØD154JA
ØD154JB
ØD154K4
ØD154K6
ØD154K9
ØD154KA
ØD154KB
ØD154Z4
ØD154Z6
ØD154Z9
ØD154ZA
ØD154ZB
ØD15874
ØD15876
ØD15879
ØD1587A
ØD1587B
ØD158J4
ØD158J6
ØD158J9
ØD158JA
ØD158JB
ØD158K4
ØD158K6
ØD158K9
ØD158KA
ØD158KB
ØD158Z4
ØD158Z6
ØD158Z9
ØD158ZA
ØD158ZB
ØD16Ø79
ØD16Ø7A
ØD16Ø7B
ØD16Ø7L
ØD16ØJ9
ØD16ØJA
ØD16ØJB
ØD16ØJL
ØD16ØK9
ØD16ØKA
ØD16ØKB
ØD16ØKL
ØD16ØZ9
ØD16ØZA
ØD16ØZB
ØD16ØZL
ØD16479
ØD1647A
ØD1647B
ØD1647L
ØD164J9
ØD164JA
ØD164JB
ØD164JL
ØD164K9
ØD164KA
ØD164KB
ØD164KL
ØD164Z9
ØD164ZA
ØD164ZB
ØD164ZL
ØD16879
ØD1687A
ØD1687B
ØD1687L
ØD168J9
ØD168JA
ØD168JB
ØD168JL
ØD168K9
ØD168KA
ØD168KB
ØD168KL
ØD168Z9
ØD168ZA
ØD168ZB
ØD168ZL
ØD18Ø74
ØD18Ø78
ØD18Ø7H
ØD18Ø7K
ØD18Ø7L
ØD18Ø7M
ØD18Ø7N
ØD18Ø7P
ØD18Ø7Q
ØD18ØJ4
ØD18ØJ8
ØD18ØJH
ØD18ØJK
ØD18ØJL
ØD18ØJM
ØD18ØJN
ØD18ØJP
ØD18ØJQ
ØD18ØK4
ØD18ØK8
ØD18ØKH
ØD18ØKK
ØD18ØKL
ØD18ØKM
ØD18ØKN
ØD18ØKP
ØD18ØKQ
ØD18ØZ4
ØD18ØZ8
ØD18ØZH
ØD18ØZK
ØD18ØZL
ØD18ØZM
ØD18ØZN
ØD18ØZP
ØD18ØZQ
ØD18474
ØD18478
ØD1847H
ØD1847K
ØD1847L
ØD1847M
ØD1847N
ØD1847P
ØD1847Q
ØD184J4
ØD184J8
ØD184JH
ØD184JK
ØD184JL
ØD184JM
ØD184JN
ØD184JP
ØD184JQ
ØD184K4
ØD184K8
ØD184KH
ØD184KK
ØD184KL
ØD184KM
ØD184KN
ØD184KP
ØD184KQ
ØD184Z4
ØD184Z8
ØD184ZH
ØD184ZK
ØD184ZL
ØD184ZM
ØD184ZN
ØD184ZP
ØD184ZQ
ØD18874
ØD18878
ØD1887H
ØD1887K
ØD1887L
ØD1887M
ØD1887N
ØD1887P
ØD1887Q
ØD188J4
ØD188J8
ØD188JH
ØD188JK
ØD188JL
ØD188JM
ØD188JN
ØD188JP
ØD188JQ
ØD188K4
ØD188K8
ØD188KH
ØD188KK
ØD188KL
ØD188KM
ØD188KN
ØD188KP
ØD188KQ
ØD188Z4
ØD188Z8
ØD188ZH
ØD188ZK
ØD188ZL
ØD188ZM
ØD188ZN
ØD188ZP
ØD188ZQ
ØD19Ø74
ØD19Ø79
ØD19Ø7A
ØD19Ø7B
ØD19Ø7L
ØD19ØJ4
ØD19ØJ9
ØD19ØJA
ØD19ØJB
ØD19ØJL
ØD19ØK4
ØD19ØK9
ØD19ØKA
ØD19ØKB
ØD19ØKL
ØD19ØZ4
ØD19ØZ9
ØD19ØZA
ØD19ØZB
ØD19ØZL
ØD193J4
ØD19474
ØD19479
ØD1947A
ØD1947B
ØD1947L
ØD194J4
ØD194J9
ØD194JA
ØD194JB
ØD194JL
ØD194K4
ØD194K9
ØD194KA
ØD194KB
ØD194KL
ØD194Z4
ØD194Z9
ØD194ZA
ØD194ZB
ØD194ZL
ØD19874
ØD19879
ØD1987A
ØD1987B
ØD1987L
ØD198J4
ØD198J9
ØD198JA
ØD198JB
ØD198JL
ØD198K4
ØD198K9
ØD198KA
ØD198KB
ØD198KL
ØD198Z4
ØD198Z9
ØD198ZA
ØD198ZB
ØD198ZL
ØD1AØ74
ØD1AØ7A
ØD1AØ7B
ØD1AØ7H
ØD1AØ7K
ØD1AØ7L
ØD1AØ7M
ØD1AØ7N
ØD1AØ7P
ØD1AØ7Q
ØD1AØJ4
ØD1AØJA
ØD1AØJB
ØD1AØJH
ØD1AØJK
ØD1AØJL
ØD1AØJM
ØD1AØJN
ØD1AØJP
ØD1AØJQ
ØD1AØK4
ØD1AØKA
ØD1AØKB
ØD1AØKH
ØD1AØKK
ØD1AØKL
ØD1AØKM
ØD1AØKN
ØD1AØKP
ØD1AØKQ
ØD1AØZ4
ØD1AØZA
ØD1AØZB
ØD1AØZH
ØD1AØZK
ØD1AØZL
ØD1AØZM
ØD1AØZN
ØD1AØZP
ØD1AØZQ
ØD1A3J4
ØD1A474
ØD1A47A
ØD1A47B
ØD1A47H
ØD1A47K
ØD1A47L
ØD1A47M
ØD1A47N
ØD1A47P
ØD1A47Q
ØD1A4J4
ØD1A4JA
ØD1A4JB
ØD1A4JH
ØD1A4JK
ØD1A4JL
ØD1A4JM
ØD1A4JN
ØD1A4JP
ØD1A4JQ
ØD1A4K4
ØD1A4KA
ØD1A4KB
ØD1A4KH
ØD1A4KK
ØD1A4KL
ØD1A4KM
ØD1A4KN
ØD1A4KP
ØD1A4KQ
ØD1A4Z4
ØD1A4ZA
ØD1A4ZB
ØD1A4ZH
ØD1A4ZK
ØD1A4ZL
ØD1A4ZM
ØD1A4ZN
ØD1A4ZP
ØD1A4ZQ
ØD1A874
ØD1A87A
ØD1A87B
ØD1A87H
ØD1A87K
ØD1A87L
ØD1A87M
ØD1A87N
ØD1A87P
ØD1A87Q
ØD1A8J4
ØD1A8JA
ØD1A8JB
ØD1A8JH
ØD1A8JK
ØD1A8JL
ØD1A8JM
ØD1A8JN
ØD1A8JP
ØD1A8JQ
ØD1A8K4
ØD1A8KA
ØD1A8KB
ØD1A8KH
ØD1A8KK
ØD1A8KL
ØD1A8KM
ØD1A8KN
ØD1A8KP
ØD1A8KQ
ØD1A8Z4
ØD1A8ZA
ØD1A8ZB
ØD1A8ZH
ØD1A8ZK
ØD1A8ZL
ØD1A8ZM
ØD1A8ZN
ØD1A8ZP
ØD1A8ZQ
ØD1BØ74
ØD1BØ7B
ØD1BØ7H
ØD1BØ7K
ØD1BØ7L
ØD1BØ7M
ØD1BØ7N
ØD1BØ7P
ØD1BØ7Q
ØD1BØJ4
ØD1BØJB
ØD1BØJH
ØD1BØJK
ØD1BØJL
ØD1BØJM
ØD1BØJN
ØD1BØJP
ØD1BØJQ
ØD1BØK4
ØD1BØKB
ØD1BØKH
ØD1BØKK
ØD1BØKL
ØD1BØKM
ØD1BØKN
ØD1BØKP
ØD1BØKQ
ØD1BØZ4
ØD1BØZB
ØD1BØZH
ØD1BØZK
ØD1BØZL
ØD1BØZM
ØD1BØZN
ØD1BØZP
ØD1BØZQ
ØD1B3J4
ØD1B474
ØD1B47B
ØD1B47H
ØD1B47K
ØD1B47L
ØD1B47M
ØD1B47N
ØD1B47P
ØD1B47Q
ØD1B4J4
ØD1B4JB
ØD1B4JH
ØD1B4JK
ØD1B4JL
ØD1B4JM
ØD1B4JN
ØD1B4JP
ØD1B4JQ
ØD1B4K4
ØD1B4KB
ØD1B4KH
ØD1B4KK
ØD1B4KL
ØD1B4KM
ØD1B4KN
ØD1B4KP
ØD1B4KQ
ØD1B4Z4
ØD1B4ZB
ØD1B4ZH
ØD1B4ZK
ØD1B4ZL
ØD1B4ZM
ØD1B4ZN
ØD1B4ZP
ØD1B4ZQ
ØD1B874
ØD1B87B
ØD1B87H
ØD1B87K
ØD1B87L
ØD1B87M
ØD1B87N
ØD1B87P
ØD1B87Q
ØD1B8J4
ØD1B8JB
ØD1B8JH
ØD1B8JK
ØD1B8JL
ØD1B8JM
ØD1B8JN
ØD1B8JP
ØD1B8JQ
ØD1B8K4
ØD1B8KB
ØD1B8KH
ØD1B8KK
ØD1B8KL
ØD1B8KM
ØD1B8KN
ØD1B8KP
ØD1B8KQ
ØD1B8Z4
ØD1B8ZB
ØD1B8ZH
ØD1B8ZK
ØD1B8ZL
ØD1B8ZM
ØD1B8ZN
ØD1B8ZP
ØD1B8ZQ
ØD1EØ74
ØD1EØJ4
ØD1EØK4
ØD1EØZ4
ØD1E474
ØD1E4J4
ØD1E4K4
ØD1E4Z4
ØD1E874
ØD1E87E
ØD1E87P
ØD1E8J4
ØD1E8JE
ØD1E8JP
ØD1E8K4
ØD1E8KE
ØD1E8KP
ØD1E8Z4
ØD1E8ZE
ØD1E8ZP
ØD1HØ74
ØD1HØJ4
ØD1HØK4
ØD1HØZ4
ØD1H3J4
ØD1H474
ØD1H4J4
ØD1H4K4
ØD1H4Z4
ØD1H874
ØD1H87P
ØD1H8J4
ØD1H8JP
ØD1H8K4
ØD1H8KP
ØD1H8Z4
ØD1H8ZP
ØD1KØ74
ØD1KØJ4
ØD1KØK4
ØD1KØZ4
ØD1K3J4
ØD1K474
ØD1K4J4
ØD1K4K4
ØD1K4Z4
ØD1K874
ØD1K8J4
ØD1K8K4
ØD1K8Z4
ØD1LØ74
ØD1LØJ4
ØD1LØK4
ØD1LØZ4
ØD1L3J4
ØD1L474
ØD1L4J4
ØD1L4K4
ØD1L4Z4
ØD1L874
ØD1L8J4
ØD1L8K4
ØD1L8Z4
ØD1MØ74
ØD1MØJ4
ØD1MØK4
ØD1MØZ4
ØD1M3J4
ØD1M474
ØD1M4J4
ØD1M4K4
ØD1M4Z4
ØD1M874
ØD1M8J4
ØD1M8K4
ØD1M8Z4
ØD1NØ74
ØD1NØJ4
ØD1NØK4
ØD1N3J4
ØD1N474
ØD1N4J4
ØD1N4K4
ØD1N4Z4
ØD1N874
ØD1N8J4
ØD1N8K4
ØD1N8Z4
ØD51ØZ3
ØD51ØZZ
ØD513Z3
ØD513ZZ
ØD517ZZ
ØD52ØZ3
ØD52ØZZ
ØD523Z3
ØD523ZZ
ØD527ZZ
ØD53ØZ3
ØD53ØZZ
ØD533Z3
ØD533ZZ
ØD537ZZ
ØD54ØZ3
ØD54ØZZ
ØD543Z3
ØD543ZZ
ØD547ZZ
ØD55ØZ3
ØD55ØZZ
ØD553Z3
ØD553ZZ
ØD557ZZ
ØD58ØZ3
ØD58ØZZ
ØD583Z3
ØD583ZZ
ØD584Z3
ØD584ZZ
ØD587ZZ
ØD59ØZ3
ØD59ØZZ
ØD593Z3
ØD593ZZ
ØD597ZZ
ØD5AØZ3
ØD5AØZZ
ØD5A3Z3
ØD5A3ZZ
ØD5A4Z3
ØD5A4ZZ
ØD5A7ZZ
ØD5BØZ3
ØD5BØZZ
ØD5B3Z3
ØD5B3ZZ
ØD5B4Z3
ØD5B4ZZ
ØD5B7ZZ
ØD5CØZ3
ØD5CØZZ
ØD5C3Z3
ØD5C3ZZ
ØD5C4Z3
ØD5C4ZZ
ØD5C7ZZ
ØD5EØZ3
ØD5EØZZ
ØD5E3Z3
ØD5E3ZZ
ØD5E7ZZ
ØD5FØZ3
ØD5FØZZ
ØD5F3Z3
ØD5F3ZZ
ØD5F7ZZ
ØD5GØZ3
ØD5GØZZ
ØD5G3Z3
ØD5G3ZZ
ØD5G7ZZ
ØD5HØZ3
ØD5HØZZ
ØD5H3Z3
ØD5H3ZZ
ØD5H7ZZ
ØD5KØZ3
ØD5KØZZ
ØD5K3Z3
ØD5K3ZZ
ØD5K7ZZ
ØD5LØZ3
ØD5LØZZ
ØD5L3Z3
ØD5L3ZZ
ØD5L7ZZ
ØD5MØZ3
ØD5MØZZ
ØD5M3Z3
ØD5M3ZZ
ØD5M7ZZ
ØD5NØZ3
ØD5NØZZ
ØD5N3Z3
ØD5N3ZZ
ØD5N7ZZ
ØD5UØZZ
ØD5U3ZZ
ØD5U4ZZ
ØD5VØZZ
ØD5V3ZZ
ØD5V4ZZ
ØD5WØZZ
ØD5W3ZZ
ØD5W4ZZ
ØD71ØDZ
ØD71ØZZ
ØD713DZ
ØD713ZZ
ØD714DZ
ØD714ZZ
ØD72ØDZ
ØD72ØZZ
ØD723DZ
ØD723ZZ
ØD724DZ
ØD724ZZ
ØD73ØDZ
ØD73ØZZ
ØD733DZ
ØD733ZZ
ØD734DZ
ØD734ZZ
ØD74ØDZ
ØD74ØZZ
ØD743DZ
ØD743ZZ
ØD744DZ
ØD744ZZ
ØD75ØDZ
ØD75ØZZ
ØD753DZ
ØD753ZZ
ØD754DZ
ØD754ZZ
ØD84ØZZ
ØD843ZZ
ØD844ZZ
ØD847ZZ
ØD848ZZ
ØD91ØZX
ØD92ØZX
ØD93ØZX
ØD94ØZX
ØD95ØZX
ØD98ØØZ
ØD98ØZZ
ØD984ØZ
ØD984ZZ
ØD987ZZ
ØD988ZZ
ØD9AØØZ
ØD9AØZZ
ØD9A4ØZ
ØD9A4ZZ
ØD9A7ZZ
ØD9A8ZZ
ØD9BØØZ
ØD9BØZZ
ØD9B4ØZ
ØD9B4ZZ
ØD9B7ZZ
ØD9B8ZZ
ØD9CØØZ
ØD9CØZZ
ØD9C4ØZ
ØD9C4ZZ
ØD9C7ØZ
ØD9C7ZZ
ØD9C8ØZ
ØD9C8ZZ
ØDB1ØZX
ØDB1ØZZ
ØDB13ZZ
ØDB17ZZ
ØDB2ØZX
ØDB2ØZZ
ØDB23ZZ
ØDB27ZZ
ØDB3ØZX
ØDB3ØZZ
ØDB33ZZ
ØDB37ZZ
ØDB4ØZX
ØDB4ØZZ
ØDB43ZZ

ØDB44ZZ
ØDB47ZZ
ØDB5ØZX
ØDB5ØZZ
ØDB53ZZ
ØDB57ZZ
ØDB6ØZ3
ØDB6ØZZ
ØDB63Z3
ØDB63ZZ
ØDB64Z3
ØDB64ZX
ØDB64ZZ
ØDB67Z3
ØDB67ZZ
ØDB68Z3
ØDB8ØZZ
ØDB83ZZ
ØDB84ZZ
ØDB87ZZ
ØDB88ZZ
ØDB9ØZZ
ØDB93ZZ
ØDBA7ZZ
ØDBB7ZZ
ØDBC7ZZ
ØDBEØZZ
ØDBE3ZZ
ØDBE4ZZ
ØDBFØZZ
ØDBF3ZZ
ØDBF4ZZ
ØDBGØZZ
ØDBG3ZZ
ØDBG4ZZ
ØDBHØZZ
ØDBH3ZZ
ØDBH4ZZ
ØDBKØZZ
ØDBK3ZZ
ØDBK4ZZ
ØDBLØZZ
ØDBL3ZZ
ØDBL4ZZ
ØDBMØZZ
ØDBM3ZZ
ØDBM4ZZ
ØDBNØZZ
ØDBN3ZZ
ØDBN4ZZ
ØDBPØZZ
ØDBP4ZZ
ØDBUØZZ
ØDBU3ZZ
ØDBU4ZZ
ØDBVØZZ
ØDBV3ZZ
ØDBV4ZZ
ØDBWØZZ
ØDBW3ZZ
ØDBW4ZZ
ØDC8ØZZ
ØDC83ZZ
ØDC84ZZ
ØDCAØZZ
ØDCA3ZZ
ØDCA4ZZ
ØDCBØZZ
ØDCB3ZZ
ØDCB4ZZ
ØDCCØZZ
ØDCC3ZZ
ØDCC4ZZ
ØDJØØZZ
ØDJØ4ZZ
ØDJ6ØZZ
ØDJ64ZZ
ØDJDØZZ
ØDJD4ZZ
ØDJUØZZ
ØDJVØZZ
ØDJWØZZ
ØDQ5ØZZ
ØDQ53ZZ
ØDQ54ZZ
ØDQ57ZZ
ØDQ58ZZ
ØDQ6ØZZ
ØDQ63ZZ
ØDQ67ZZ
ØDQ68ZZ
ØDQVØZZ
ØDQV3ZZ
ØDQV4ZZ
ØDQWØZZ
ØDQW3ZZ
ØDQW4ZZ
ØDR5Ø7Z
ØDR5ØJZ
ØDR5ØKZ
ØDR547Z
ØDR54JZ
ØDR54KZ
ØDR577Z
ØDR57JZ
ØDR57KZ
ØDR587Z
ØDR58JZ
ØDR58KZ
ØDRUØ7Z
ØDRUØJZ
ØDRUØKZ
ØDRU47Z
ØDRU4JZ
ØDRU4KZ
ØDRVØ7Z
ØDRVØJZ
ØDRVØKZ
ØDRV47Z
ØDRV4JZ
ØDRV4KZ
ØDRWØ7Z
ØDRWØJZ
ØDRWØKZ
ØDRW47Z
ØDRW4JZ
ØDRW4KZ
ØDSBØZZ
ØDSB4ZZ
ØDSB7ZZ
ØDSB8ZZ
ØDSHØZZ
ØDSH4ZZ
ØDSH7ZZ
ØDSH8ZZ
ØDT1ØZZ
ØDT14ZZ
ØDT17ZZ
ØDT18ZZ
ØDT2ØZZ
ØDT24ZZ
ØDT27ZZ
ØDT28ZZ
ØDT3ØZZ
ØDT34ZZ
ØDT37ZZ
ØDT38ZZ
ØDT4ØZZ
ØDT44ZZ
ØDT47ZZ
ØDT48ZZ
ØDT5ØZZ
ØDT54ZZ
ØDT57ZZ
ØDT58ZZ
ØDT6ØZZ
ØDT64ZZ
ØDT67ZZ
ØDT68ZZ
ØDT7ØZZ
ØDT74ZZ
ØDT77ZZ
ØDT78ZZ
ØDT8ØZZ
ØDT84ZZ
ØDT87ZZ
ØDT88ZZ
ØDT9ØZZ
ØDT94ZZ
ØDT97ZZ
ØDT98ZZ
ØDTAØZZ
ØDTA4ZZ
ØDTA7ZZ
ØDTA8ZZ
ØDTBØZZ
ØDTB4ZZ
ØDTB7ZZ
ØDTB8ZZ
ØDTCØZZ
ØDTC4ZZ
ØDTC7ZZ
ØDTC8ZZ
ØDTEØZZ
ØDTE4ZZ
ØDTE7ZZ
ØDTE8ZZ
ØDTFØZZ
ØDTF4ZZ
ØDTF7ZZ
ØDTF8ZZ
ØDTGØZZ
ØDTG4ZZ
ØDTG7ZZ
ØDTG8ZZ
ØDTGFZZ
ØDTKØZZ
ØDTK4ZZ
ØDTK7ZZ
ØDTK8ZZ
ØDTLØZZ
ØDTL4ZZ
ØDTL7ZZ
ØDTL8ZZ
ØDTLFZZ
ØDTMØZZ
ØDTM4ZZ
ØDTM7ZZ
ØDTM8ZZ
ØDTMFZZ
ØDTNØZZ
ØDTN4ZZ
ØDTN7ZZ
ØDTN8ZZ
ØDTNFZZ
ØDTPØZZ
ØDTP4ZZ
ØDTP7ZZ
ØDTP8ZZ
ØDTUØZZ
ØDTU4ZZ
ØDU1Ø7Z
ØDU1ØJZ
ØDU1ØKZ
ØDU147Z
ØDU14JZ
ØDU14KZ
ØDU177Z
ØDU17JZ
ØDU17KZ
ØDU187Z
ØDU18JZ
ØDU18KZ
ØDU2Ø7Z
ØDU2ØJZ
ØDU2ØKZ
ØDU247Z
ØDU24JZ
ØDU24KZ
ØDU277Z
ØDU27JZ
ØDU27KZ
ØDU287Z
ØDU28JZ
ØDU28KZ
ØDU3Ø7Z
ØDU3ØJZ
ØDU3ØKZ
ØDU347Z
ØDU34JZ
ØDU34KZ
ØDU377Z
ØDU37JZ
ØDU37KZ
ØDU387Z
ØDU38JZ
ØDU38KZ
ØDU5Ø7Z
ØDU5ØJZ
ØDU5ØKZ
ØDU547Z
ØDU54JZ
ØDU54KZ
ØDU577Z
ØDU57JZ
ØDU57KZ
ØDU587Z
ØDU58JZ
ØDU58KZ
ØDUUØ7Z
ØDUUØJZ
ØDUUØKZ
ØDUU47Z
ØDUU4JZ
ØDUU4KZ
ØDUVØ7Z
ØDUVØJZ
ØDUVØKZ
ØDUV47Z
ØDUV4JZ
ØDUV4KZ
ØDUWØ7Z
ØDUWØJZ
ØDUWØKZ
ØDUW47Z
ØDUW4JZ
ØDUW4KZ
ØDWØ4UZ
ØDX6ØZ5
ØDX64Z5
ØDX8ØZ5
ØDX84Z5
ØDXEØZ5
ØDXE4Z5
ØF14ØD3
ØF14ØD4
ØF14ØD5
ØF14ØD6
ØF14ØD7
ØF14ØD8
ØF14ØD9
ØF14ØDB
ØF14ØZ3
ØF14ØZ4
ØF14ØZ5
ØF14ØZ6
ØF14ØZ7
ØF14ØZ8
ØF14ØZ9
ØF14ØZB
ØF144D3
ØF144D4
ØF144D5
ØF144D6
ØF144D7
ØF144D8
ØF144D9
ØF144DB
ØF144Z3
ØF144Z4
ØF144Z5
ØF144Z6
ØF144Z7
ØF144Z8
ØF144Z9
ØF144ZB
ØF15ØD3
ØF15ØD4
ØF15ØD5
ØF15ØD6
ØF15ØD7
ØF15ØD8
ØF15ØD9
ØF15ØDB
ØF15ØZ3
ØF15ØZ4
ØF15ØZ5
ØF15ØZ6
ØF15ØZ7
ØF15ØZ8
ØF15ØZ9
ØF15ØZB
ØF154D3
ØF154D4
ØF154D5
ØF154D6
ØF154D7
ØF154D8
ØF154D9
ØF154DB
ØF154Z3
ØF154Z4
ØF154Z5
ØF154Z6
ØF154Z7
ØF154Z8
ØF154Z9
ØF154ZB
ØF16ØD3
ØF16ØD4
ØF16ØD5
ØF16ØD6
ØF16ØD7
ØF16ØD8
ØF16ØD9
ØF16ØDB
ØF16ØZ3
ØF16ØZ4
ØF16ØZ5
ØF16ØZ6
ØF16ØZ7
ØF16ØZ8
ØF16ØZ9
ØF16ØZB
ØF164D3
ØF164D4
ØF164D5
ØF164D6
ØF164D7
ØF164D8
ØF164D9
ØF164DB
ØF164Z3
ØF164Z4
ØF164Z5
ØF164Z6
ØF164Z7
ØF164Z8
ØF164Z9
ØF164ZB
ØF17ØD3
ØF17ØD4
ØF17ØD5
ØF17ØD6
ØF17ØD7
ØF17ØD8
ØF17ØD9
ØF17ØDB
ØF17ØZ3
ØF17ØZ4
ØF17ØZ5
ØF17ØZ6
ØF17ØZ7
ØF17ØZ8
ØF17ØZ9
ØF17ØZB
ØF174D3
ØF174D4
ØF174D5
ØF174D6
ØF174D7
ØF174D8
ØF174D9
ØF174DB
ØF174Z3
ØF174Z4
ØF174Z5
ØF174Z6
ØF174Z7
ØF174Z8
ØF174Z9
ØF174ZB
ØF18ØD3
ØF18ØD4
ØF18ØD5
ØF18ØD6
ØF18ØD7
ØF18ØD8
ØF18ØD9
ØF18ØDB
ØF18ØZ3
ØF18ØZ4
ØF18ØZ5
ØF18ØZ6
ØF18ØZ7
ØF18ØZ8
ØF18ØZ9
ØF18ØZB
ØF184D3
ØF184D4
ØF184D5
ØF184D6
ØF184D7
ØF184D8
ØF184D9
ØF184DB
ØF184Z3
ØF184Z4
ØF184Z5
ØF184Z6
ØF184Z7
ØF184Z8
ØF184Z9
ØF184ZB
ØF19ØD3
ØF19ØD4
ØF19ØD5
ØF19ØD6
ØF19ØD7
ØF19ØD8
ØF19ØD9
ØF19ØDB
ØF19ØZ3
ØF19ØZ4
ØF19ØZ5
ØF19ØZ6
ØF19ØZ7
ØF19ØZ8
ØF19ØZ9
ØF19ØZB
ØF194D3
ØF194D4
ØF194D5
ØF194D6
ØF194D7
ØF194D8
ØF194D9
ØF194DB
ØF194Z3
ØF194Z4
ØF194Z5
ØF194Z6
ØF194Z7
ØF194Z8
ØF194Z9
ØF194ZB
ØF54ØZ3
ØF54ØZZ
ØF543Z3
ØF543ZZ
ØF544Z3
ØF544ZZ
ØF548ZZ
ØF7DØDZ
ØF7D3DZ
ØF7FØDZ
ØF7F3DZ
ØF7F7DZ
ØF9ØØZX
ØF91ØZX
ØF92ØZX
ØF997ØZ
ØF9FØZX
ØF9GØZX
ØFBØØZX
ØFBØ4ZX
ØFB1ØZX
ØFB14ZX
ØFB2ØZX
ØFB24ZX
ØFB4ØZZ
ØFB43ZZ
ØFB44ZZ
ØFB48ZZ
ØFBDØZX
ØFBFØZX
ØFBGØZX
ØFC5ØZZ
ØFC6ØZZ
ØFC7ØZZ
ØFC8ØZZ
ØFC9ØZZ
ØFDØ4ZX
ØFD14ZX
ØFD24ZX
ØFF5ØZZ
ØFF53ZZ
ØFF54ZZ
ØFF57ZZ
ØFF6ØZZ
ØFF63ZZ
ØFF64ZZ
ØFF67ZZ
ØFF7ØZZ
ØFF73ZZ
ØFF74ZZ
ØFF77ZZ
ØFF8ØZZ
ØFF83ZZ
ØFF84ZZ
ØFF87ZZ
ØFF9ØZZ
ØFF93ZZ
ØFF94ZZ
ØFF97ZZ
ØFFCØZZ
ØFFC3ZZ
ØFFC4ZZ
ØFFC7ZZ
ØFHBØDZ
ØFHB3DZ
ØFHB7DZ
ØFHDØDZ
ØFHD3DZ
ØFHD7DZ
ØFJØØZZ
ØFJDØZZ
ØFJGØZZ
ØFL5ØCZ
ØFL5ØDZ
ØFL5ØZZ
ØFL6ØCZ
ØFL6ØDZ
ØFL6ØZZ
ØFL7ØCZ
ØFL7ØDZ
ØFL7ØZZ
ØFL8ØCZ
ØFL8ØDZ
ØFL8ØZZ
ØFL9ØCZ
ØFL9ØDZ
ØFL9ØZZ
ØFM4ØZZ
ØFP4ØDZ
ØFP43DZ
ØFP44DZ
ØFQ4ØZZ
ØFQ43ZZ
ØFQ44ZZ
ØFQ48ZZ
ØFQ5ØZZ
ØFQ53ZZ
ØFQ54ZZ
ØFQ57ZZ
ØFQ58ZZ
ØFQ6ØZZ
ØFQ63ZZ
ØFQ64ZZ
ØFQ67ZZ
ØFQ68ZZ
ØFQ7ØZZ
ØFQ73ZZ
ØFQ74ZZ
ØFQ77ZZ
ØFQ78ZZ
ØFQ8ØZZ
ØFQ83ZZ
ØFQ84ZZ
ØFQ87ZZ
ØFQ88ZZ
ØFQ9ØZZ
ØFQ93ZZ
ØFQ94ZZ
ØFQ97ZZ
ØFQ98ZZ
ØFR5ØJZ
ØFR54JZ
ØFR58JZ
ØFR6ØJZ
ØFR64JZ
ØFR68JZ
ØFR7ØJZ
ØFR74JZ
ØFR78JZ
ØFR8ØJZ
ØFR84JZ
ØFR88JZ
ØFR9ØJZ
ØFR94JZ
ØFR98JZ
ØFS4ØZZ
ØFS44ZZ
ØFT4ØZZ
ØFT44ZZ
ØFUD37Z
ØFUD47Z
ØFUD87Z
ØFV5ØCZ
ØFV5ØDZ
ØFV5ØZZ
ØFV6ØCZ
ØFV6ØDZ
ØFV6ØZZ
ØFV7ØCZ
ØFV7ØDZ
ØFV7ØZZ
ØFV8ØCZ
ØFV8ØDZ
ØFV8ØZZ
ØFV9ØCZ
ØFV9ØDZ
ØFV9ØZZ
ØN5ØØZZ
ØN5Ø3ZZ
ØN5Ø4ZZ
ØN51ØZZ
ØN513ZZ
ØN514ZZ
ØN53ØZZ
ØN533ZZ
ØN534ZZ
ØN54ØZZ
ØN543ZZ
ØN544ZZ
ØN55ØZZ
ØN553ZZ
ØN554ZZ
ØN56ØZZ
ØN563ZZ
ØN564ZZ
ØN57ØZZ
ØN573ZZ
ØN574ZZ
ØNBØØZZ
ØNBØ3ZZ
ØNBØ4ZZ
ØNB1ØZZ
ØNB13ZZ
ØNB14ZZ
ØNB3ØZZ
ØNB33ZZ
ØNB34ZZ
ØNB4ØZZ
ØNB43ZZ
ØNB44ZZ
ØNB5ØZZ
ØNB53ZZ
ØNB54ZZ
ØNB6ØZZ
ØNB63ZZ
ØNB64ZZ
ØNB7ØZZ
ØNB73ZZ
ØNB74ZZ
ØNC1ØZZ
ØNC13ZZ
ØNC14ZZ
ØNC3ØZZ
ØNC33ZZ
ØNC34ZZ
ØNC4ØZZ
ØNC43ZZ
ØNC44ZZ
ØNC5ØZZ
ØNC53ZZ
ØNC54ZZ
ØNC6ØZZ
ØNC63ZZ
ØNC64ZZ
ØNC7ØZZ
ØNC73ZZ
ØNC74ZZ
ØNPØØMZ
ØNPØ3MZ
ØNPØ4MZ
ØNPØXMZ
ØNT1ØZZ
ØNT3ØZZ
ØNT4ØZZ
ØNT5ØZZ
ØNT6ØZZ
ØNT7ØZZ
ØPS3Ø4Z
ØPS3ØZZ
ØPS334Z
ØPS344Z
ØPS34ZZ
ØPS4Ø3Z
ØPS4Ø4Z
ØPS4ØZZ
ØPS434Z
ØPS443Z
ØPS444Z
ØPS44ZZ
ØQSØØ3Z
ØQSØØ4Z
ØQSØØZZ
ØQSØ34Z
ØQSØ43Z
ØQSØ44Z
ØQSØ4ZZ
ØQS1Ø4Z
ØQS1ØZZ
ØQS134Z
ØQS144Z
ØQS14ZZ
ØQSSØ4Z
ØQSSØZZ
ØQSS34Z
ØQSS3ZZ
ØQSS44Z
ØQSS4ZZ
ØRBØØZZ
ØRBØ3ZZ
ØRBØ4ZZ
ØRB1ØZZ
ØRB13ZZ
ØRB14ZZ
ØRB4ØZZ
ØRB43ZZ
ØRB44ZZ
ØRB6ØZZ
ØRB63ZZ
ØRB64ZZ
ØRBAØZZ
ØRBA3ZZ
ØRBA4ZZ
ØRQ3ØZZ
ØRQ9ØZZ
ØRQBØZZ
ØRU3Ø7Z
ØRU3ØJZ
ØRU3ØKZ
ØRU337Z
ØRU33JZ
ØRU33KZ
ØRU347Z
ØRU34JZ
ØRU34KZ
ØRU9Ø7Z
ØRU9ØJZ
ØRU9ØKZ
ØRU937Z
ØRU93JZ
ØRU93KZ
ØRU947Z
ØRU94JZ
ØRU94KZ
ØRUBØ7Z
ØRUBØJZ
ØRUBØKZ
ØRUB37Z
ØRUB3JZ
ØRUB3KZ
ØRUB47Z
ØRUB4JZ
ØRUB4KZ
ØSBØØZZ
ØSBØ3ZZ
ØSBØ4ZZ
ØSB3ØZZ
ØSB33ZZ
ØSB34ZZ
ØSB5ØZZ
ØSB53ZZ
ØSB54ZZ
ØSB6ØZZ
ØSB63ZZ
ØSB64ZZ
ØSB7ØZZ
ØSB73ZZ
ØSB74ZZ
ØSB8ØZZ
ØSB83ZZ
ØSB84ZZ
ØSQ2ØZZ
ØSQ4ØZZ
ØSU2Ø7Z
ØSU2ØJZ
ØSU2ØKZ
ØSU237Z
ØSU23JZ
ØSU23KZ
ØSU247Z
ØSU24JZ
ØSU24KZ
ØSU4Ø7Z
ØSU4ØJZ
ØSU4ØKZ
ØSU437Z
ØSU43JZ
ØSU43KZ
ØSU447Z
ØSU44JZ
ØSU44KZ
ØT13Ø7B
ØT13ØJB
ØT13ØKB
ØT13ØZB
ØT1347B
ØT134JB
ØT134KB
ØT134ZB
ØT14Ø7B
ØT14ØJB
ØT14ØKB
ØT14ØZB
ØT1447B
ØT144JB
ØT144KB
ØT144ZB
ØT16Ø76
ØT16Ø77
ØT16Ø78
ØT16Ø79
ØT16Ø7A
ØT16Ø7C
ØT16Ø7D
ØT16ØJ6
ØT16ØJ7
ØT16ØJ8
ØT16ØJ9
ØT16ØJA
ØT16ØJC

ØT160JD
ØT160K6
ØT160K7
ØT160K8
ØT160K9
ØT160KA
ØT160KC
ØT160KD
ØT160Z6
ØT160Z7
ØT160Z8
ØT160Z9
ØT160ZA
ØT160ZC
ØT160ZD
ØT163JD
ØT16476
ØT16477
ØT16478
ØT16479
ØT1647A
ØT1647C
ØT1647D
ØT164J6
ØT164J7
ØT164J8
ØT164J9
ØT164JA
ØT164JC
ØT164JD
ØT164K6
ØT164K7
ØT164K8
ØT164K9
ØT164KA
ØT164KC
ØT164KD
ØT164Z6
ØT164Z7
ØT164Z8
ØT164Z9
ØT164ZA
ØT164ZC
ØT164ZD
ØT17076
ØT17077
ØT17078
ØT17079
ØT1707A
ØT1707C
ØT1707D
ØT170J6
ØT170J7
ØT170J8
ØT170J9
ØT170JA
ØT170JC
ØT170JD
ØT170K6
ØT170K7
ØT170K8
ØT170K9
ØT170KA
ØT170KC
ØT170KD
ØT170Z6
ØT170Z7
ØT170Z8
ØT170Z9
ØT170ZA
ØT170ZC
ØT170ZD
ØT173JD
ØT17476
ØT17477
ØT17478
ØT17479
ØT1747A
ØT1747C
ØT1747D
ØT174J6
ØT174J7
ØT174J8
ØT174J9
ØT174JA
ØT174JC
ØT174JD
ØT174K6
ØT174K7
ØT174K8
ØT174K9
ØT174KA
ØT174KC
ØT174KD
ØT174Z6
ØT174Z7
ØT174Z8
ØT174Z9
ØT174ZA
ØT174ZC
ØT174ZD
ØT18076
ØT18077
ØT18078
ØT18079
ØT1807A
ØT1807C
ØT1807D
ØT180J6
ØT180J7
ØT180J8
ØT180J9
ØT180JA
ØT180JC
ØT180JD
ØT180K6
ØT180K7
ØT180K8
ØT180K9
ØT180KA
ØT180KC
ØT180KD
ØT180Z6
ØT180Z7
ØT180Z8
ØT180Z9
ØT180ZA
ØT180ZC
ØT180ZD
ØT183JD
ØT18476
ØT18477
ØT18478
ØT18479
ØT1847A
ØT1847C
ØT1847D
ØT184J6
ØT184J7
ØT184J8
ØT184J9
ØT184JA
ØT184JC
ØT184JD
ØT184K6
ØT184K7
ØT184K8
ØT184K9
ØT184KA
ØT184KC
ØT184KD
ØT184Z6
ØT184Z7
ØT184Z8
ØT184Z9
ØT184ZA
ØT184ZC
ØT184ZD
ØT1BØ79
ØT1BØ7C
ØT1BØ7D
ØT1BØJ9
ØT1BØJC
ØT1BØJD
ØT1BØK9
ØT1BØKC
ØT1BØKD
ØT1BØZ9
ØT1BØZC
ØT1BØZD
ØT1B3JD
ØT1B479
ØT1B47C
ØT1B47D
ØT1B4J9
ØT1B4JC
ØT1B4JD
ØT1B4K9
ØT1B4KC
ØT1B4KD
ØT1B4Z9
ØT1B4ZC
ØT1B4ZD
ØT5BØZZ
ØT5B3ZZ
ØT5B4ZZ
ØT5CØZZ
ØT5C3ZZ
ØT5C4ZZ
ØT9ØØZX
ØT91ØZX
ØT93ØØZ
ØT93ØZX
ØT93ØZZ
ØT934ØZ
ØT94ØØZ
ØT94ØZX
ØT94ØZZ
ØT944ØZ
ØT9BØØZ
ØT9BØZX
ØT9CØZX
ØTBØØZX
ØTBØØZZ
ØTBØ3ZZ
ØTBØ4ZZ
ØTB1ØZX
ØTB1ØZZ
ØTB13ZZ
ØTB14ZZ
ØTB3ØZX
ØTB3ØZZ
ØTB33ZZ
ØTB34ZZ
ØTB4ØZX
ØTB4ØZZ
ØTB43ZZ
ØTB44ZZ
ØTBBØZX
ØTBBØZZ
ØTBB3ZZ
ØTBB4ZZ
ØTBCØZX
ØTBCØZZ
ØTBC3ZZ
ØTBC4ZZ
ØTJB4ZZ
ØTNØØZZ
ØTNØ3ZZ
ØTNØ4ZZ
ØTNØ7ZZ
ØTNØ8ZZ
ØTN1ØZZ
ØTN13ZZ
ØTN14ZZ
ØTN17ZZ
ØTN18ZZ
ØTN3ØZZ
ØTN33ZZ
ØTN34ZZ
ØTN37ZZ
ØTN38ZZ
ØTN4ØZZ
ØTN43ZZ
ØTN44ZZ
ØTN47ZZ
ØTN48ZZ
ØTN6ØZZ
ØTN63ZZ
ØTN64ZZ
ØTN7ØZZ
ØTN73ZZ
ØTN74ZZ
ØTNB3ZZ
ØTNB4ZZ
ØTNC3ZZ
ØTNC4ZZ
ØTQØØZZ
ØTQØ3ZZ
ØTQØ4ZZ
ØTQØ7ZZ
ØTQØ8ZZ
ØTQ1ØZZ
ØTQ13ZZ
ØTQ14ZZ
ØTQ17ZZ
ØTQ18ZZ
ØTQ7ØZZ
ØTQ73ZZ
ØTQ74ZZ
ØTQ77ZZ
ØTQ78ZZ
ØTQBØZZ
ØTQB3ZZ
ØTQB4ZZ
ØTQB7ZZ
ØTQB8ZZ
ØTQDØZZ
ØTQD3ZZ
ØTQD4ZZ
ØTQD7ZZ
ØTQD8ZZ
ØTQDXZZ
ØTTBØZZ
ØTTB4ZZ
ØTTB7ZZ
ØTTB8ZZ
ØTTCØZZ
ØTTC4ZZ
ØTTC7ZZ
ØTTC8ZZ
ØUQGØZZ
ØUQG3ZZ
ØUQG4ZZ
ØUQG8ZZ
ØVXTØZD
ØVXTXZD
ØW11ØJ9
ØW11ØJB
ØW11ØJG
ØW11ØJJ
ØW1GØJ4
ØW1GØJW
ØW1GØJY
ØW1G3J4
ØW1G3JW
ØW1G3JY
ØW1G4J4
ØW1G4JW
ØW1G4JY
ØW3ØØZZ
ØW3Ø3ZZ
ØW3Ø4ZZ
ØW31ØZZ
ØW313ZZ
ØW314ZZ
ØW32ØZZ
ØW323ZZ
ØW324ZZ
ØW33*
ØW34ØZZ
ØW343ZZ
ØW344ZZ
ØW35ØZZ
ØW353ZZ
ØW354ZZ
ØW36ØZZ
ØW363ZZ
ØW364ZZ
ØW38ØZZ
ØW383ZZ
ØW384ZZ
ØW39ØZZ
ØW393ZZ
ØW394ZZ
ØW3BØZZ
ØW3B3ZZ
ØW3B4ZZ
ØW3DØZZ
ØW3D3ZZ
ØW3D4ZZ
ØW3FØZZ
ØW3F3ZZ
ØW3F4ZZ
ØW3GØZZ
ØW3G3ZZ
ØW3G4ZZ
ØW3HØZZ
ØW3H3ZZ
ØW3H4ZZ
ØW3JØZZ
ØW3J3ZZ
ØW3J4ZZ
ØW3KØZZ
ØW3K3ZZ
ØW3K4ZZ
ØW3LØZZ
ØW3L3ZZ
ØW3L4ZZ
ØW3MØZZ
ØW3M3ZZ
ØW3M4ZZ
ØW3NØZZ
ØW3N3ZZ
ØW3N4ZZ
ØW3PØZZ
ØW3P3ZZ
ØW3P4ZZ
ØW3Q3ZZ
ØW3Q4ZZ
ØW3Q7ZZ
ØW3Q8ZZ
ØW3RØZZ
ØW3R3ZZ
ØW3R4ZZ
ØW3R7ZZ
ØW3R8ZZ
ØW91ØØZ
ØW91ØZX
ØW91ØZZ
ØW9CØZX
ØW9DØØZ
ØW9DØZX
ØW9DØZZ
ØW9D4ØZ
ØW9D4ZX
ØW9D4ZZ
ØW9FØØZ
ØW9FØZX
ØW9FØZZ
ØW9F3ZX
ØW9F4ZX
ØW9GØØZ
ØW9GØZX
ØW9GØZZ
ØW9G4ØZ
ØW9G4ZX
ØW9G4ZZ
ØW9HØØZ
ØW9HØZX
ØW9HØZZ
ØW9H3ZX
ØW9H4ØZ
ØW9H4ZX
ØW9H4ZZ
ØW9JØZX
ØW9J4ZX
ØWB8ØZZ
ØWB83ZZ
ØWB84ZZ
ØWB8XZZ
ØWBCØZX
ØWBCØZZ
ØWBC3ZX
ØWBC3ZZ
ØWBC4ZX
ØWBC4ZZ
ØWBFØZX
ØWBFØZZ
ØWBF3ZX
ØWBF3ZZ
ØWBF4ZX
ØWBF4ZZ
ØWBFXZ2
ØWBFXZX
ØWBFXZZ
ØWBHØZZ
ØWBH3ZZ
ØWBH4ZZ
ØWC1ØZZ
ØWC13ZZ
ØWC14ZZ
ØWCDØZZ
ØWCD3ZZ
ØWCD4ZZ
ØWCJØZZ
ØWCJ3ZZ
ØWCJ4ZZ
ØWCPØZZ
ØWCP3ZZ
ØWCP4ZZ
ØWCRØZZ
ØWCR3ZZ
ØWCR4ZZ
ØWFGØZZ
ØWFG3ZZ
ØWFG4ZZ
ØWHDØ3Z
ØWHDØYZ
ØWHD33Z
ØWHD3YZ
ØWHD43Z
ØWHD4YZ
ØWJ1ØZZ
ØWJ14ZZ
ØWJ9ØZZ
ØWJBØZZ
ØWJCØZZ
ØWJC4ZZ
ØWJD4ZZ
ØWJFØZZ
ØWJGØZZ
ØWJHØZZ
ØWJH4ZZ
ØWJJØZZ
ØWJPØZZ
ØWJQØZZ
ØWJRØZZ
ØWMFØZZ
ØWPDØØZ
ØWPDØ1Z
ØWPDØ3Z
ØWPDØYZ
ØWPD3ØZ
ØWPD31Z
ØWPD33Z
ØWPD3YZ
ØWPD4ØZ
ØWPD41Z
ØWPD43Z
ØWPD4YZ
ØWQ6XZ2
ØWQFØZZ
ØWQF3ZZ
ØWQF4ZZ
ØWQFXZ2
ØWQFXZZ
ØWWDØØZ
ØWWDØ1Z
ØWWDØ3Z
ØWWDØYZ
ØWWD3ØZ
ØWWD31Z
ØWWD33Z
ØWWD3YZ
ØWWD4ØZ
ØWWD41Z
ØWWD43Z
ØWWD4YZ
ØX32ØZZ
ØX323ZZ
ØX324ZZ
ØX33ØZZ
ØX333ZZ
ØX334ZZ
ØX34ØZZ
ØX343ZZ
ØX344ZZ
ØX35ØZZ
ØX353ZZ
ØX354ZZ
ØX36ØZZ
ØX363ZZ
ØX364ZZ
ØX37ØZZ
ØX373ZZ
ØX374ZZ
ØX38ØZZ
ØX383ZZ
ØX384ZZ
ØX39ØZZ
ØX393ZZ
ØX394ZZ
ØX3BØZZ
ØX3B3ZZ
ØX3B4ZZ
ØX3CØZZ
ØX3C3ZZ
ØX3C4ZZ
ØX3DØZZ
ØX3D3ZZ
ØX3D4ZZ
ØX3FØZZ
ØX3F3ZZ
ØX3F4ZZ
ØX3GØZZ
ØX3G3ZZ
ØX3G4ZZ
ØX3HØZZ
ØX3H3ZZ
ØX3H4ZZ
ØX3JØZZ
ØX3J3ZZ
ØX3J4ZZ
ØX3KØZZ
ØX3K3ZZ
ØX3K4ZZ
ØY3ØØZZ
ØY3Ø3ZZ
ØY3Ø4ZZ
ØY31ØZZ
ØY313ZZ
ØY314ZZ
ØY35ØZZ
ØY353ZZ
ØY354ZZ
ØY36ØZZ
ØY363ZZ
ØY364ZZ
ØY37ØZZ
ØY373ZZ
ØY374ZZ
ØY38ØZZ
ØY383ZZ
ØY384ZZ
ØY39ØZZ
ØY393ZZ
ØY394ZZ
ØY3BØZZ
ØY3B3ZZ
ØY3B4ZZ
ØY3CØZZ
ØY3C3ZZ
ØY3C4ZZ
ØY3DØZZ
ØY3D3ZZ
ØY3D4ZZ
ØY3FØZZ
ØY3F3ZZ
ØY3F4ZZ
ØY3GØZZ
ØY3G3ZZ
ØY3G4ZZ
ØY3HØZZ
ØY3H3ZZ
ØY3H4ZZ
ØY3JØZZ
ØY3J3ZZ
ØY3J4ZZ
ØY3KØZZ
ØY3K3ZZ
ØY3K4ZZ
ØY3LØZZ
ØY3L3ZZ
ØY3L4ZZ
ØY3MØZZ
ØY3M3ZZ
ØY3M4ZZ
ØY3NØZZ
ØY3N3ZZ
ØY3N4ZZ
ØY95ØØZ
ØY95ØZX
ØY95ØZZ
ØY953ZX
ØY954ØZ
ØY954ZX
ØY954ZZ
ØY96ØØZ
ØY96ØZX
ØY96ØZZ
ØY963ZX
ØY964ØZ
ØY964ZX
ØY964ZZ
ØYB5ØZX
ØYB5ØZZ
ØYB53ZX
ØYB53ZZ
ØYB54ZX
ØYB54ZZ
ØYB6ØZX
ØYB6ØZZ
ØYB63ZX
ØYB63ZZ
ØYB64ZX
ØYB64ZZ
ØYB7ØZX
ØYB7ØZZ
ØYB73ZX
ØYB73ZZ
ØYB74ZX
ØYB74ZZ
ØYB8ØZX
ØYB8ØZZ
ØYB83ZX
ØYB83ZZ
ØYB84ZX
ØYB84ZZ
ØYJ5ØZZ
ØYJ54ZZ
ØYJ6ØZZ
ØYJ64ZZ
ØYJ7ØZZ
ØYJ74ZZ
ØYJ84ZZ
ØYJAØZZ
ØYJA4ZZ
ØYJE4ZZ
X2H2ØR9
X2H3ØR9
XNSØØ32
XNSØØC7
XNSØ332
XNSØ3C7
XNS3Ø32
XNS3332
XNS4Ø32
XNS4ØC7
XNS4332
XNS43C7

DRG 821

Select principal diagnosis AND operating room procedures listed under DRG 820

DRG 822

Select principal diagnosis AND operating room procedures listed under DRG 820

DRG 823

Principal Diagnosis

C26.1
C46.3
C77*
C7B.Ø1
C81*
C82*
C83*
C84*
C85*
C86*
C88*
C9Ø*
C91.1*
C91.3*
C91.4*
C91.5*
C91.6*
C91.9*
C91.A*
C91.Z*
C92.1*
C92.2*
C92.3*
C92.9*
C92.Z*
C93.1*
C93.3*
C93.9*
C93.Z*
C94.2*
C94.3*
C94.4*
C94.6
C94.8*
C95.1*
C95.9*
C96.2*
C96.4
C96.9
C96.A
C96.Z
D45
D47.Ø*
D47.1
D47.9
D47.Z2
D47.Z9
D61.82
D75.81
D89.1

AND

Select any other operating room procedures not listed under DRG 820

OR

Nonoperating Room Procedures

DØ2*
D72*
D82*
D92*
DB2*
DD2*
DF2*
DG2*
DM2*
DT2*
DU2*
DV2*
DW2*

DRG 824

Select principal diagnosis listed under DRG 823

AND

Select any other operating room procedures not listed under DRG 820

OR

Select nonoperating room procedures listed under DRG 823

DRG 825

Select principal diagnosis listed under DRG 823

AND

Select any other operating room procedures not listed under DRG 820

OR

Select nonoperating room procedures listed under DRG 823

DRG 826

Principal Diagnosis

C37
C45.7
C45.9
C48.Ø
C76.4*
C76.5*
C76.8
C79.89
C79.9
C7A.ØØ
C7A.Ø91
C7A.Ø98
C7A.1
C7A.8
C7B.ØØ
C7B.Ø9
C7B.1
C7B.8
C8Ø.Ø
C8Ø.1
C8Ø.2
C96.Ø
DØ9.3
DØ9.8
DØ9.9
D19.7
D19.9
D36.7
D36.9
D3A.ØØ
D3A.Ø98
D3A.8
D48.7
D48.9
D49.8*
D49.9
E88.Ø2
E88.Ø9
Q85.8*
Q85.9
ZØ8
Z51.Ø
Z51.1*
Z85*
Z87.41Ø

AND

Select operating room procedures listed under DRG 820

DRG 827

Select principal diagnosis listed under DRG 826 AND operating room procedures listed under DRG 820

DRG 828

Select principal diagnosis listed under DRG 826 AND operating room procedures listed under DRG 820

DRG 829
Select principal diagnosis listed under DRG 826
AND
Select any other operating room procedures not listed under DRG 820
OR
Select nonoperating room procedures listed under DRG 823

DRG 830
Select principal diagnosis listed under DRG 826
AND
Select any other operating room procedures not listed under DRG 820
OR
Select nonoperating room procedures listed under DRG 823

DRG 834
Principal Diagnosis
C91.Ø*
C92.Ø*
C92.4*
C92.5*
C92.6*
C92.A*
C93.Ø*
C94.Ø*
C95.Ø*

DRG 835
Select principal diagnosis listed under DRG 834

DRG 836
Select principal diagnosis listed under DRG 834

DRG 837
Principal Diagnosis
ZØ8
Z51.1*
AND
Secondary Diagnosis
C91.Ø*
C92.Ø*
C92.4*
C92.5*
C92.6*
C92.A*
C93.Ø*
C94.Ø*
C95.Ø*
OR
Nonoperating Room Procedure
3EØ3ØØ2
3EØ33Ø2
3EØ4ØØ2
3EØ43Ø2
3EØ5ØØ2
3EØ53Ø2
3EØ6ØØ2
3EØ63Ø2
3EØR3Ø2
3EØS3Ø2

DRG 838
Select principal and secondary diagnosis OR nonoperating room procedure listed under DRG 837

DRG 839
Select principal diagnosis AND secondary diagnosis listed under DRG 837

DRG 840
Principal Diagnosis
C26.1
C46.3
C77*
C7B.Ø1
C81*
C82*
C83*
C84*
C85*
C86*
C88*
C9Ø*
C91.1*
C91.3*
C91.4*
C91.5*
C91.6*
C91.9*
C91.A*
C91.Z*
C92.1*
C92.2*
C92.3*
C92.9*
C92.Z*
C93.1*
C93.3*
C93.9*
C93.Z*
C94.2*
C94.3*
C94.4*
C94.6
C94.8*
C95.1*
C95.9*
C96.2*
C96.4
C96.9
C96.A
C96.Z
D45
D47.Ø*
D47.1
D47.9
D47.Z2
D47.Z9
D61.82
D75.81
D89.1

DRG 841
Select principal diagnosis listed under DRG 840

DRG 842
Select principal diagnosis listed under DRG 840

DRG 843
Principal Diagnosis
C37
C45.7
C45.9
C48.Ø
C76.4*
C76.5*
C76.8
C79.89
C79.9
C7A.ØØ
C7A.Ø91
C7A.Ø98
C7A.1
C7A.8
C7B.ØØ
C7B.Ø9
C7B.1
C7B.8
C8Ø.Ø
C8Ø.1
C8Ø.2
C96.Ø
DØ9.3
DØ9.8
DØ9.9
D19.7
D19.9
D36.7
D36.9
D3A.ØØ
D3A.Ø98
D3A.8
D48.7
D48.9
D49.8*
D49.9
E88.Ø2
E88.Ø9
Q85.8*
Q85.9
Z85.Ø*
Z85.1*
Z85.2*
Z85.3
Z85.4*
Z85.5*
Z85.6
Z85.7*
Z85.8*
Z85.9
Z87.41Ø

DRG 844
Select principal diagnosis listed under DRG 843

DRG 845
Select principal diagnosis listed under DRG 843

DRG 846
Principal Diagnosis
ZØ8
Z51.1*

DRG 847
Select principal diagnosis listed under DRG 846

DRG 848
Select principal diagnosis listed under DRG 846

DRG 849
Principal Diagnosis
Z51.Ø

MDC 18

DRG 853
Select any principal diagnosis from MDC 18 excluding
K68.11
N98.Ø
T8Ø.22XA
T8Ø.29XA
T81.4ØXA
T81.41XA
T81.42XA
T81.43XA
T81.44XA
T81.49XA
T88.ØXXA
AND
Select any operating room procedures

DRG 854
Select principal diagnosis AND operating room procedure under DRG 853

DRG 855
Select principal diagnosis AND operating room procedure under DRG 853

DRG 856
Principal Diagnosis
K68.11
N98.Ø
T8Ø.22XA
T8Ø.29XA
T81.4ØXA
T81.41XA
T81.42XA
T81.43XA
T81.44XA
T81.49XA
T88.ØXXA
AND
Select any operating room procedure

DRG 857
Select principal diagnosis AND operating room procedure under DRG 856

DRG 858
Select principal diagnosis AND operating room procedure under DRG 856

DRG 862
Principal Diagnosis
K68.11
T81.4ØXA
T81.41XA
T81.42XA
T81.43XA
T81.44XA
T81.49XA

DRG 863
Select principal diagnosis listed under DRG 862

DRG 864
Principal Diagnosis
R5Ø*
R65.1Ø
R65.11

DRG 865
Principal Diagnosis
A7Ø
A74.8*
A74.9
A8Ø.4
A9Ø
A91
A92.Ø
A92.1
A92.3*
A92.4
A92.5
A92.8
A92.9
A93*
A94
A95*
A96*
A98.Ø
A98.1
A98.2
A98.3
A98.4
A98.8
A99
BØØ.89
BØ1.Ø
BØ1.8*
BØ1.9
BØ2.7
BØ2.8
BØ3
BØ4
BØ5.1
BØ5.4
BØ5.89
BØ5.9
BØ6.81
BØ6.89
BØ6.9
BØ8.Ø1Ø
BØ8.Ø11
BØ8.Ø4
BØ8.Ø9
BØ8.2*
BØ8.3
BØ8.4
BØ8.6*
BØ8.7*
BØ8.8
BØ9
B25.8
B25.9
B26.82
B26.83
B26.85
B26.89
B26.9
B27*
B33.1
B33.3
B33.4
B33.8
B34*
B97*
JØ9.X3
JØ9.X9
J1Ø.2
J1Ø.8*
J11.2
J11.8*
L44.4
T88.1XXA
Z21

DRG 866
Select principal diagnosis listed under DRG 865

DRG 867
Principal Diagnosis
AØ1*
AØ2.2Ø
AØ2.25
AØ2.29
AØ2.8
AØ2.9
AØ5.1
AØ6.3
AØ6.8*
AØ6.9
A17.9
A18.82
A18.84
A18.89
A19*
A2Ø.Ø
A2Ø.1
A2Ø.3
A2Ø.8
A2Ø.9
A21.Ø
A21.1
A21.7
A21.8
A21.9
A22.8
A22.9
A23*
A24*
A25*
A26.Ø
A26.8
A26.9
A27.Ø
A27.9
A28.Ø
A28.2
A28.8
A28.9
A3Ø*
A31.2
A31.8
A31.9
A32.Ø
A32.1*
A32.8*
A32.9
A35
A36.82
A36.83
A36.84
A36.89
A36.9
A38*
A42.8*
A42.9
A43.8
A43.9
A44*
A48.Ø
A48.2
A48.3
A48.4
A48.5*
A48.8
A49*
A5Ø.Ø*
A5Ø.1
A5Ø.2
A5Ø.3Ø
A5Ø.32
A5Ø.39
A5Ø.44
A5Ø.5*
A5Ø.6
A5Ø.7
A5Ø.9
A51.2
A51.42
A51.44
A51.49
A51.5
A51.9
A52.73
A52.76
A52.79
A52.8
A52.9
A53*
A54.82
A54.84
A54.89
A54.9
A59.8
A59.9
A65
A66.7
A66.8
A66.9
A67.2
A67.9
A68*
A69.2*
A69.8
A69.9
A75*
A77*
A78
A79*
B37.89
B37.9
B38.7
B38.89
B38.9
B39.3
B39.4
B39.5
B39.9
B4Ø*
B41*
B42*
B43*
B44.1
B44.2
B44.7
B44.89
B44.9
B45.Ø
B45.2
B45.3
B45.7
B45.8
B45.9
B46*
B47.Ø
B47.1
B48*
B49
B5Ø*
B51*
B52*
B53*
B54
B55.Ø
B55.9
B56*
B57.1
B57.3*
B57.4*
B57.5
B58.ØØ
B58.82
B58.83
B58.89
B58.9
B6Ø.Ø*
B6Ø.1Ø
B6Ø.11
B6Ø.19
B6Ø.2
B6Ø.8
B64
B65.2
B65.8
B65.9
B66.2
B66.8
B66.9
B67.2
B67.32
B67.39
B67.4
B67.6*
B67.7
B67.9Ø
B67.99
B72
B73*
B74*
B75
B81.4
B83.Ø
B83.1
B83.2
B83.3
B83.8
B83.9
B89
B9Ø.8
B92
B94.2
B94.8
B94.9
B95*
B96*
B99*
L94.6
N98.Ø
R89.9
T8Ø.22XA
T8Ø.29XA
T88.ØXXA
Z16*

DRG 868
Select principal diagnosis listed under DRG 867

DRG 869
Select principal diagnosis listed under DRG 867

DRG 870
Principal Diagnosis
AØ2.1
A2Ø.7
A22.7
A26.7
A32.7
A39.1
A39.2
A39.3
A39.4
A39.89
A39.9
A4Ø*
A41*
A42.7
A54.86
BØØ.7
B37.7
R57.1
R57.8
R65.2Ø
R65.21
R78.81
AND
Nonoperating Room Procedure
5A1955Z

DRG 871
Select principal diagnosis listed under DRG 870

DRG 872
Select principal diagnosis listed under DRG 870

MDC 19

DRG 876
Select any operating room procedure

DRG 880
Principal Diagnosis
FØ5
F41*
F43.Ø
F44.Ø
F44.1
F44.2
F44.4
F44.5
F44.6
F44.7
F44.9
F48.9
F68.11
F68.13
F68.8
F99
R44.Ø
R44.2
R44.3
R45.Ø
R45.2
R45.3
R45.4
R45.5
R45.6
R45.7
R45.851
R45.89
Z72.81Ø
Z72.811

DRG 881
Principal Diagnosis
F32.9
F32.A
F34.1
F43.21
F53.Ø

DRG 882
Principal Diagnosis
F4Ø*
F42.2
F42.3
F42.4
F42.8
F42.9
F43.1*
F43.2Ø
F43.22
F43.23
F43.24
F43.25
F43.29
F43.8*
F43.9
F45*
F48.1
F48.8
F93.Ø
F98.21
R45.87

DRG 883
Principal Diagnosis
F21
F34.Ø
F44.81
F5Ø.Ø*
F6Ø*
F63.Ø
F63.2
F63.8*
F68.1Ø
F68.12
F68.A
F69
R45.86
R45.88

DRG 884
Principal Diagnosis
FØ1*
FØ2*
FØ3*
FØ4
FØ6*
FØ7.Ø
FØ7.9
FØ9
F54
F63.3
F7Ø
F71
F72
F73
F78*
F79

F84.Ø
F84.3
Q9Ø*
Q91*
Q93.3
Q93.4
Q93.51
Q93.52
Q93.59
Q93.7
Q93.8*
Q93.9
Q99.2
R4Ø.4
R41.81
R41.841
R41.843
R41.844
R41.89
R45.1
R45.81
R45.82
R54

DRG 885

Principal Diagnosis

F2Ø*
F22
F23
F24
F25*
F28
F29
F3Ø*
F31*
F32.Ø
F32.1
F32.2
F32.3
F32.4
F32.5
F32.81
F32.89
F33*
F34.81
F34.89
F34.9
F39
F53.1
F84.5
F84.8
F84.9

DRG 886

Principal Diagnosis

F63.1
F63.9
F8Ø.Ø
F8Ø.1
F8Ø.2
F8Ø.4
F8Ø.82
F8Ø.89
F8Ø.9
F81*
F82
F88
F89
F9Ø*
F91*
F93.8
F93.9
F94*
F98.Ø
F98.1
F98.3
F98.8
F98.9
H93.25
R41.84Ø
R48.Ø
R48.1
R48.2
R48.8

DRG 887

Principal Diagnosis

F44.89
F5Ø.2
F5Ø.8*
F5Ø.9
F51*
F52.Ø
F52.1
F52.2*
F52.3*
F52.4
F52.6
F52.8
F52.9
F59
F64*
F65*
F66
F98.29
F98.4
F98.5
G47.Ø*
G47.1*
G47.9
R37
R48.9
Z87.89Ø

MDC 20

DRG 894

Select principal diagnosis in MDC 20
AND
Discharge status of left against medical advice (AMA)

DRG 895

Select principal diagnosis in MDC 20
AND
Nonoperating Room Procedure

HZ3ØZZZ
HZ31ZZZ
HZ32ZZZ
HZ33ZZZ
HZ34ZZZ
HZ35ZZZ
HZ36ZZZ
HZ37ZZZ
HZ38ZZZ
HZ39ZZZ
HZ3BZZZ
HZ4ØZZZ
HZ41ZZZ
HZ42ZZZ
HZ43ZZZ
HZ44ZZZ
HZ45ZZZ
HZ46ZZZ
HZ47ZZZ
HZ48ZZZ
HZ49ZZZ
HZ4BZZZ
HZ5ØZZZ
HZ51ZZZ
HZ52ZZZ
HZ53ZZZ
HZ54ZZZ
HZ55ZZZ
HZ56ZZZ
HZ57ZZZ
HZ58ZZZ
HZ59ZZZ
HZ5BZZZ
HZ5CZZZ
HZ5DZZZ

DRG 896

Select principal diagnosis in MDC 20

DRG 897

Select principal diagnosis in MDC 20

MDC 21

DRG 901

Operating Room Procedures

ØJBØØZZ
ØJB1ØZZ
ØJB4ØZZ
ØJB5ØZZ
ØJB6ØZZ
ØJB7ØZZ
ØJB8ØZZ
ØJB9ØZZ
ØJBBØZZ
ØJBCØZZ
ØJBDØZZ
ØJBFØZZ
ØJBGØZZ
ØJBHØZZ
ØJBLØZZ
ØJBMØZZ
ØJBNØZZ
ØJBPØZZ
ØJBQØZZ
ØJBRØZZ

DRG 902

Select operating room procedures listed under DRG 901

DRG 903

Select operating room procedures listed under DRG 901

DRG 904

Operating Room Procedures

ØHRØX72
ØHRØX73
ØHRØX74
ØHRØXJ3
ØHRØXJ4
ØHRØXJZ
ØHRØXK3
ØHRØXK4
ØHR1X72
ØHR1X73
ØHR1X74
ØHR1XJ3
ØHR1XJ4
ØHR1XJZ
ØHR1XK3
ØHR1XK4
ØHR4X72
ØHR4X73
ØHR4X74
ØHR4XJ3
ØHR4XJ4
ØHR4XJZ
ØHR4XK3
ØHR4XK4
ØHR5X72
ØHR5X73
ØHR5X74
ØHR5XJ3
ØHR5XJ4
ØHR5XJZ
ØHR5XK3
ØHR5XK4
ØHR6X72
ØHR6X73
ØHR6X74
ØHR6XJ3
ØHR6XJ4
ØHR6XJZ
ØHR6XK3
ØHR6XK4
ØHR7X72
ØHR7X73
ØHR7X74
ØHR7XJ3
ØHR7XJ4
ØHR7XJZ
ØHR7XK3
ØHR7XK4
ØHR8X72
ØHR8X73
ØHR8X74
ØHR8XJ3
ØHR8XJ4
ØHR8XJZ
ØHR8XK3
ØHR8XK4
ØHRAX72
ØHRAX73
ØHRAX74
ØHRAXJ3
ØHRAXJ4
ØHRAXJZ
ØHRAXK3
ØHRAXK4
ØHRBX72
ØHRBX73
ØHRBX74
ØHRBXJ3
ØHRBXJ4
ØHRBXJZ
ØHRBXK3
ØHRBXK4
ØHRCX72
ØHRCX73
ØHRCX74
ØHRCXJ3
ØHRCXJ4
ØHRCXJZ
ØHRCXK3
ØHRCXK4
ØHRDX72
ØHRDX73
ØHRDX74
ØHRDXJ3
ØHRDXJ4
ØHRDXJZ
ØHRDXK3
ØHRDXK4
ØHREX72
ØHREX73
ØHREX74
ØHREXJ3
ØHREXJ4
ØHREXJZ
ØHREXK3
ØHREXK4
ØHRFXJ3
ØHRFXJ4
ØHRFXJZ
ØHRFXK3
ØHRFXK4
ØHRGXJ3
ØHRGXJ4
ØHRGXJZ
ØHRGXK3
ØHRGXK4
ØHRHX72
ØHRHX73
ØHRHX74
ØHRHXJ3
ØHRHXJ4
ØHRHXJZ
ØHRHXK3
ØHRHXK4
ØHRJX72
ØHRJX73
ØHRJX74
ØHRJXJ3
ØHRJXJ4
ØHRJXJZ
ØHRJXK3
ØHRJXK4
ØHRKX72
ØHRKX73
ØHRKX74
ØHRKXJ3
ØHRKXJ4
ØHRKXJZ
ØHRKXK3
ØHRKXK4
ØHRLX72
ØHRLX73
ØHRLX74
ØHRLXJ3
ØHRLXJ4
ØHRLXJZ
ØHRLXK3
ØHRLXK4
ØHRMX72
ØHRMX73
ØHRMX74
ØHRMXJ3
ØHRMXJ4
ØHRMXJZ
ØHRMXK3
ØHRMXK4
ØHRNX72
ØHRNX73
ØHRNX74
ØHRNXJ3
ØHRNXJ4
ØHRNXJZ
ØHRNXK3
ØHRNXK4
ØHXØXZZ
ØHX1XZZ
ØHX4XZZ
ØHX5XZZ
ØHX6XZZ
ØHX7XZZ
ØHX8XZZ
ØHX9XZZ
ØHXAXZZ
ØHXBXZZ
ØHXCXZZ
ØHXDXZZ
ØHXEXZZ
ØHXFXZZ
ØHXGXZZ
ØHXHXZZ
ØHXJXZZ
ØHXKXZZ
ØHXLXZZ
ØHXMXZZ
ØHXNXZZ
ØJHØØNZ
ØJHØ3NZ
ØJH1ØNZ
ØJH13NZ
ØJH4ØNZ
ØJH43NZ
ØJH5ØNZ
ØJH53NZ
ØJH6ØNZ
ØJH63NZ
ØJH7ØNZ
ØJH73NZ
ØJH8ØNZ
ØJH83NZ
ØJH9ØNZ
ØJH93NZ
ØJHBØNZ
ØJHB3NZ
ØJHCØNZ
ØJHC3NZ
ØJHDØNZ
ØJHD3NZ
ØJHFØNZ
ØJHF3NZ
ØJHGØNZ
ØJHG3NZ
ØJHHØNZ
ØJHH3NZ
ØJHJØNZ
ØJHJ3NZ
ØJHKØNZ
ØJHK3NZ
ØJHLØNZ
ØJHL3NZ
ØJHMØNZ
ØJHM3NZ
ØJHNØNZ
ØJHN3NZ
ØJHPØNZ
ØJHP3NZ
ØJHQØNZ
ØJHQ3NZ
ØJHRØNZ
ØJHR3NZ
ØJXØØZB
ØJXØØZC
ØJXØ3ZB
ØJXØ3ZC
ØJX1ØZB
ØJX1ØZC
ØJX13ZB
ØJX13ZC
ØJX4ØZB
ØJX4ØZC
ØJX43ZB
ØJX43ZC
ØJX5ØZB
ØJX5ØZC
ØJX53ZB
ØJX53ZC
ØJX6ØZB
ØJX6ØZC
ØJX63ZB
ØJX63ZC
ØJX7ØZB
ØJX7ØZC
ØJX73ZB
ØJX73ZC
ØJX8ØZB
ØJX8ØZC
ØJX83ZB
ØJX83ZC
ØJX9ØZB
ØJX9ØZC
ØJX93ZB
ØJX93ZC
ØJXBØZB
ØJXBØZC
ØJXB3ZB
ØJXB3ZC
ØJXCØZB
ØJXCØZC
ØJXC3ZB
ØJXC3ZC
ØJXDØZB
ØJXDØZC
ØJXD3ZB
ØJXD3ZC
ØJXFØZB
ØJXFØZC
ØJXF3ZB
ØJXF3ZC
ØJXGØZB
ØJXGØZC
ØJXG3ZB
ØJXG3ZC
ØJXHØZB
ØJXHØZC
ØJXH3ZB
ØJXH3ZC
ØJXLØZB
ØJXLØZC
ØJXL3ZB
ØJXL3ZC
ØJXMØZB
ØJXMØZC
ØJXM3ZB
ØJXM3ZC
ØJXNØZB
ØJXNØZC
ØJXN3ZB
ØJXN3ZC
ØJXPØZB
ØJXPØZC
ØJXP3ZB
ØJXP3ZC
ØJXQØZB
ØJXQØZC
ØJXQ3ZB
ØJXQ3ZC
ØJXRØZB
ØJXRØZC
ØJXR3ZB
ØJXR3ZC
XHRPXF7

DRG 905

Select operating room procedures listed under DRG 904

DRG 906

Operating Room Procedures

Ø1N5ØZZ
Ø1N53ZZ
Ø1N54ZZ
ØHRFX72
ØHRFX73
ØHRFX74
ØHRGX72
ØHRGX73
ØHRGX74
ØJ8JØZZ
ØJ8J3ZZ
ØJ8KØZZ
ØJ8K3ZZ
ØJBJØZZ
ØJBJ3ZZ
ØJBKØZZ
ØJBK3ZZ
ØJDJØZZ
ØJDKØZZ
ØJNJØZZ
ØJNJ3ZZ
ØJNKØZZ
ØJNK3ZZ
ØJQJØZZ
ØJQKØZZ
ØJRJØ7Z
ØJRJØJZ
ØJRJØKZ
ØJRJ3JZ
ØJRJ3KZ
ØJRKØ7Z
ØJRKØJZ
ØJRKØKZ
ØJRK3JZ
ØJRK3KZ
ØJUJØ7Z
ØJUJØJZ
ØJUJØKZ
ØJUJ37Z
ØJUJ3JZ
ØJUJ3KZ
ØJUKØ7Z
ØJUKØJZ
ØJUKØKZ
ØJUK37Z
ØJUK3JZ
ØJUK3KZ
ØJXJØZB
ØJXJØZC
ØJXJ3ZB
ØJXJ3ZC
ØJXKØZB
ØJXKØZC
ØJXK3ZB
ØJXK3ZC
ØK5CØZZ
ØK5C3ZZ
ØK5C4ZZ
ØK5DØZZ
ØK5D3ZZ
ØK5D4ZZ
ØK8CØZZ
ØK8C3ZZ
ØK8C4ZZ
ØK8DØZZ
ØK8D3ZZ
ØK8D4ZZ
ØK9CØØZ
ØK9CØZZ
ØK9C4ØZ
ØK9DØØZ
ØK9DØZZ
ØK9D4ØZ
ØKBCØZZ
ØKBC3ZZ
ØKBC4ZZ
ØKBDØZZ
ØKBD3ZZ
ØKBD4ZZ
ØKCCØZZ
ØKCC3ZZ
ØKCC4ZZ
ØKCDØZZ
ØKCD3ZZ
ØKCD4ZZ
ØKDCØZZ
ØKDDØZZ
ØKMCØZZ
ØKMC4ZZ
ØKMDØZZ
ØKMD4ZZ
ØKNCØZZ
ØKNC3ZZ
ØKNC4ZZ
ØKNDØZZ
ØKND3ZZ
ØKND4ZZ
ØKQCØZZ
ØKQC3ZZ
ØKQC4ZZ
ØKQDØZZ
ØKQD3ZZ
ØKQD4ZZ
ØKRCØ7Z
ØKRCØJZ
ØKRCØKZ
ØKRC47Z
ØKRC4JZ
ØKRC4KZ
ØKRDØ7Z
ØKRDØJZ
ØKRDØKZ
ØKRD47Z
ØKRD4JZ
ØKRD4KZ
ØKSCØZZ
ØKSC4ZZ
ØKSDØZZ
ØKSD4ZZ
ØKTCØZZ
ØKTC4ZZ
ØKTDØZZ
ØKTD4ZZ
ØKUCØ7Z
ØKUCØJZ
ØKUCØKZ
ØKUC47Z
ØKUC4JZ
ØKUC4KZ
ØKUDØ7Z
ØKUDØJZ
ØKUDØKZ
ØKUD47Z
ØKUD4JZ
ØKUD4KZ
ØKXCØZØ
ØKXCØZ1
ØKXCØZ2
ØKXCØZZ
ØKXC4ZØ
ØKXC4Z1
ØKXC4Z2
ØKXC4ZZ
ØKXDØZØ
ØKXDØZ1
ØKXDØZ2
ØKXDØZZ
ØKXD4ZØ
ØKXD4Z1
ØKXD4Z2
ØKXD4ZZ
ØL57ØZZ
ØL573ZZ
ØL574ZZ
ØL58ØZZ
ØL583ZZ
ØL584ZZ
ØL87ØZZ
ØL873ZZ
ØL874ZZ
ØL88ØZZ
ØL883ZZ
ØL884ZZ
ØL97ØØZ
ØL97ØZZ
ØL974ØZ
ØL98ØØZ
ØL98ØZZ
ØL984ØZ
ØLB7ØZZ
ØLB73ZZ
ØLB74ZZ
ØLB8ØZZ
ØLB83ZZ
ØLB84ZZ
ØLC7ØZZ
ØLC73ZZ
ØLC74ZZ
ØLC8ØZZ
ØLC83ZZ
ØLC84ZZ
ØLD7ØZZ
ØLD8ØZZ
ØLJXØZZ
ØLJX4ZZ
ØLM7ØZZ
ØLM74ZZ
ØLM8ØZZ
ØLM84ZZ
ØLN7ØZZ
ØLN73ZZ
ØLN74ZZ
ØLN8ØZZ
ØLN83ZZ
ØLN84ZZ
ØLQ7ØZZ
ØLQ73ZZ
ØLQ74ZZ
ØLQ8ØZZ
ØLQ83ZZ
ØLQ84ZZ
ØLR7Ø7Z
ØLR7ØJZ
ØLR7ØKZ
ØLR747Z
ØLR74JZ
ØLR74KZ
ØLR8Ø7Z
ØLR8ØJZ
ØLR8ØKZ
ØLR847Z
ØLR84JZ
ØLR84KZ
ØLS7ØZZ
ØLS74ZZ
ØLS8ØZZ
ØLS84ZZ
ØLT7ØZZ
ØLT74ZZ
ØLT8ØZZ
ØLT84ZZ
ØLU7Ø7Z
ØLU7ØJZ
ØLU7ØKZ
ØLU747Z
ØLU74JZ
ØLU74KZ
ØLU8Ø7Z
ØLU8ØJZ
ØLU8ØKZ
ØLU847Z
ØLU84JZ
ØLU84KZ
ØLX7ØZZ
ØLX74ZZ
ØLX8ØZZ
ØLX84ZZ
ØM55ØZZ
ØM553ZZ
ØM554ZZ
ØM56ØZZ
ØM563ZZ
ØM564ZZ
ØM57ØZZ
ØM573ZZ
ØM574ZZ
ØM58ØZZ
ØM583ZZ
ØM584ZZ
ØM87ØZZ
ØM873ZZ
ØM874ZZ
ØM88ØZZ
ØM883ZZ
ØM884ZZ
ØM95ØØZ
ØM95ØZZ

ØM954ØZ
ØM96ØØZ
ØM96ØZZ
ØM964ØZ
ØM97ØØZ
ØM97ØZZ
ØM98ØØZ
ØM98ØZZ
ØMB7ØZZ
ØMB73ZZ
ØMB74ZZ
ØMB8ØZZ
ØMB83ZZ
ØMB84ZZ
ØMC5ØZZ
ØMC53ZZ
ØMC54ZZ
ØMC6ØZZ
ØMC63ZZ
ØMC64ZZ
ØMC7ØZZ
ØMC73ZZ
ØMC74ZZ
ØMC8ØZZ
ØMC83ZZ
ØMC84ZZ
ØMD7ØZZ
ØMD73ZZ
ØMD74ZZ
ØMD8ØZZ
ØMD83ZZ
ØMD84ZZ
ØMN7ØZZ
ØMN73ZZ
ØMN74ZZ
ØMN8ØZZ
ØMN83ZZ
ØMN84ZZ
ØMT7ØZZ
ØMT74ZZ
ØMT8ØZZ
ØMT84ZZ
ØP5MØZZ
ØP5M3ZZ
ØP5M4ZZ
ØP5NØZZ
ØP5N3ZZ
ØP5N4ZZ
ØP5PØZZ
ØP5P3ZZ
ØP5P4ZZ
ØP5QØZZ
ØP5Q3ZZ
ØP5Q4ZZ
ØP8MØZZ
ØP8M3ZZ
ØP8M4ZZ
ØP8NØZZ
ØP8N3ZZ
ØP8N4ZZ
ØP8PØZZ
ØP8P3ZZ
ØP8P4ZZ
ØP8QØZZ
ØP8Q3ZZ
ØP8Q4ZZ
ØP9MØZX
ØP9M3ZX
ØP9M4ZX
ØP9NØZX
ØP9N3ZX
ØP9N4ZX
ØP9PØZX
ØP9P3ZX
ØP9P4ZX
ØP9QØZX
ØP9Q3ZX
ØP9Q4ZX
ØPBMØZX
ØPBMØZZ
ØPBM3ZX
ØPBM3ZZ
ØPBM4ZX
ØPBM4ZZ
ØPBNØZX
ØPBNØZZ
ØPBN3ZX
ØPBN3ZZ
ØPBN4ZX
ØPBN4ZZ
ØPBPØZX
ØPBPØZZ
ØPBP3ZX
ØPBP3ZZ
ØPBP4ZX
ØPBP4ZZ
ØPBQØZX
ØPBQØZZ
ØPBQ3ZX
ØPBQ3ZZ
ØPBQ4ZX
ØPBQ4ZZ
ØPCMØZZ
ØPCM3ZZ
ØPCM4ZZ
ØPCNØZZ
ØPCN3ZZ
ØPCN4ZZ
ØPCPØZZ
ØPCP3ZZ
ØPCP4ZZ
ØPCQØZZ
ØPCQ3ZZ
ØPCQ4ZZ
ØPDMØZZ
ØPDNØZZ
ØPDPØZZ
ØPDQØZZ
ØPDRØZZ
ØPDSØZZ
ØPDTØZZ
ØPDVØZZ
ØPHMØ4Z
ØPHMØ5Z
ØPHM34Z
ØPHM35Z
ØPHM44Z
ØPHM45Z
ØPHNØ4Z
ØPHNØ5Z
ØPHN34Z
ØPHN35Z
ØPHN44Z
ØPHN45Z
ØPHPØ4Z
ØPHPØ5Z
ØPHP34Z
ØPHP35Z
ØPHP44Z
ØPHP45Z
ØPHQØ4Z
ØPHQØ5Z
ØPHQ34Z
ØPHQ35Z
ØPHQ44Z
ØPHQ45Z
ØPNMØZZ
ØPNM3ZZ
ØPNM4ZZ
ØPNNØZZ
ØPNN3ZZ
ØPNN4ZZ
ØPNPØZZ
ØPNP3ZZ
ØPNP4ZZ
ØPNQØZZ
ØPNQ3ZZ
ØPNQ4ZZ
ØPPMØ4Z
ØPPMØ5Z
ØPPMØ7Z
ØPPMØJZ
ØPPMØKZ
ØPPM34Z
ØPPM35Z
ØPPM37Z
ØPPM3JZ
ØPPM3KZ
ØPPM44Z
ØPPM45Z
ØPPM47Z
ØPPM4JZ
ØPPM4KZ
ØPPNØ4Z
ØPPNØ5Z
ØPPNØ7Z
ØPPNØJZ
ØPPNØKZ
ØPPN34Z
ØPPN35Z
ØPPN37Z
ØPPN3JZ
ØPPN3KZ
ØPPN44Z
ØPPN45Z
ØPPN47Z
ØPPN4JZ
ØPPN4KZ
ØPPPØ4Z
ØPPPØ5Z
ØPPPØ7Z
ØPPPØJZ
ØPPPØKZ
ØPPP34Z
ØPPP35Z
ØPPP37Z
ØPPP3JZ
ØPPP3KZ
ØPPP44Z
ØPPP45Z
ØPPP47Z
ØPPP4JZ
ØPPP4KZ
ØPPQØ4Z
ØPPQØ5Z
ØPPQØ7Z
ØPPQØJZ
ØPPQØKZ
ØPPQ34Z
ØPPQ35Z
ØPPQ37Z
ØPPQ3JZ
ØPPQ3KZ
ØPPQ44Z
ØPPQ45Z
ØPPQ47Z
ØPPQ4JZ
ØPPQ4KZ
ØPQMØZZ
ØPQM3ZZ
ØPQM4ZZ
ØPQNØZZ
ØPQN3ZZ
ØPQN4ZZ
ØPQPØZZ
ØPQP3ZZ
ØPQP4ZZ
ØPQQØZZ
ØPQQ3ZZ
ØPQQ4ZZ
ØPRMØ7Z
ØPRMØJZ
ØPRMØKZ
ØPRM37Z
ØPRM3JZ
ØPRM3KZ
ØPRM47Z
ØPRM4JZ
ØPRM4KZ
ØPRNØ7Z
ØPRNØJZ
ØPRNØKZ
ØPRN37Z
ØPRN3JZ
ØPRN3KZ
ØPRN47Z
ØPRN4JZ
ØPRN4KZ
ØPRPØ7Z
ØPRPØJZ
ØPRPØKZ
ØPRP37Z
ØPRP3JZ
ØPRP3KZ
ØPRP47Z
ØPRP4JZ
ØPRP4KZ
ØPRQØ7Z
ØPRQØJZ
ØPRQØKZ
ØPRQ37Z
ØPRQ3JZ
ØPRQ3KZ
ØPRQ47Z
ØPRQ4JZ
ØPRQ4KZ
ØPSMØ4Z
ØPSMØ5Z
ØPSMØZZ
ØPSM34Z
ØPSM35Z
ØPSM44Z
ØPSM45Z
ØPSNØ4Z
ØPSNØ5Z
ØPSNØZZ
ØPSN34Z
ØPSN35Z
ØPSN44Z
ØPSN45Z
ØPSPØ4Z
ØPSPØ5Z
ØPSPØZZ
ØPSP34Z
ØPSP35Z
ØPSP44Z
ØPSP45Z
ØPSQØ4Z
ØPSQØ5Z
ØPSQØZZ
ØPSQ34Z
ØPSQ35Z
ØPSQ44Z
ØPSQ45Z
ØPSRØ4Z
ØPSRØZZ
ØPSR34Z
ØPSR44Z
ØPSSØ4Z
ØPSSØZZ
ØPSS34Z
ØPSS44Z
ØPSTØ4Z
ØPSTØZZ
ØPST34Z
ØPST44Z
ØPSVØ4Z
ØPSVØZZ
ØPSV34Z
ØPSV44Z
ØPTMØZZ
ØPTNØZZ
ØPTPØZZ
ØPTQØZZ
ØPUMØ7Z
ØPUMØJZ
ØPUMØKZ
ØPUM37Z
ØPUM3JZ
ØPUM3KZ
ØPUM47Z
ØPUM4JZ
ØPUM4KZ
ØPUNØ7Z
ØPUNØJZ
ØPUNØKZ
ØPUN37Z
ØPUN3JZ
ØPUN3KZ
ØPUN47Z
ØPUN4JZ
ØPUN4KZ
ØPUPØ7Z
ØPUPØJZ
ØPUPØKZ
ØPUP37Z
ØPUP3JZ
ØPUP3KZ
ØPUP47Z
ØPUP4JZ
ØPUP4KZ
ØPUQØ7Z
ØPUQØJZ
ØPUQØKZ
ØPUQ37Z
ØPUQ3JZ
ØPUQ3KZ
ØPUQ47Z
ØPUQ4JZ
ØPUQ4KZ
ØR5NØZZ
ØR5N3ZZ
ØR5N4ZZ
ØR5PØZZ
ØR5P3ZZ
ØR5P4ZZ
ØR5QØZZ
ØR5Q3ZZ
ØR5Q4ZZ
ØR5RØZZ
ØR5R3ZZ
ØR5R4ZZ
ØR5SØZZ
ØR5S3ZZ
ØR5S4ZZ
ØR5TØZZ
ØR5T3ZZ
ØR5T4ZZ
ØR5UØZZ
ØR5U3ZZ
ØR5U4ZZ
ØR5VØZZ
ØR5V3ZZ
ØR5V4ZZ
ØR5WØZZ
ØR5W3ZZ
ØR5W4ZZ
ØR5XØZZ
ØR5X3ZZ
ØR5X4ZZ
ØR9NØØZ
ØR9NØZZ
ØR9PØØZ
ØR9PØZZ
ØR9QØØZ
ØR9QØZZ
ØR9RØØZ
ØR9RØZZ
ØR9SØØZ
ØR9SØZZ
ØR9TØØZ
ØR9TØZZ
ØR9UØØZ
ØR9UØZZ
ØR9VØØZ
ØR9VØZZ
ØR9WØØZ
ØR9WØZZ
ØR9XØØZ
ØR9XØZZ
ØRBNØZZ
ØRBN3ZZ
ØRBN4ZZ
ØRBPØZZ
ØRBP3ZZ
ØRBP4ZZ
ØRBQØZZ
ØRBQ3ZZ
ØRBQ4ZZ
ØRBRØZZ
ØRBR3ZZ
ØRBR4ZZ
ØRBSØZZ
ØRBS3ZZ
ØRBS4ZZ
ØRBTØZZ
ØRBT3ZZ
ØRBT4ZZ
ØRBUØZZ
ØRBU3ZZ
ØRBU4ZZ
ØRBVØZZ
ØRBV3ZZ
ØRBV4ZZ
ØRBWØZZ
ØRBW3ZZ
ØRBW4ZZ
ØRBXØZZ
ØRBX3ZZ
ØRBX4ZZ
ØRCNØZZ
ØRCN3ZZ
ØRCN4ZZ
ØRCPØZZ
ØRCP3ZZ
ØRCP4ZZ
ØRCQØZZ
ØRCQ3ZZ
ØRCQ4ZZ
ØRCRØZZ
ØRCR3ZZ
ØRCR4ZZ
ØRCSØZZ
ØRCS3ZZ
ØRCS4ZZ
ØRCTØZZ
ØRCT3ZZ
ØRCT4ZZ
ØRCUØZZ
ØRCU3ZZ
ØRCU4ZZ
ØRCVØZZ
ØRCV3ZZ
ØRCV4ZZ
ØRCWØZZ
ØRCW3ZZ
ØRCW4ZZ
ØRCXØZZ
ØRCX3ZZ
ØRCX4ZZ
ØRGNØ3Z
ØRGNØ4Z
ØRGNØ5Z
ØRGNØ7Z
ØRGNØJZ
ØRGNØKZ
ØRGN33Z
ØRGN34Z
ØRGN35Z
ØRGN37Z
ØRGN3JZ
ØRGN3KZ
ØRGN43Z
ØRGN44Z
ØRGN45Z
ØRGN47Z
ØRGN4JZ
ØRGN4KZ
ØRGPØ3Z
ØRGPØ4Z
ØRGPØ5Z
ØRGPØ7Z
ØRGPØJZ
ØRGPØKZ
ØRGP33Z
ØRGP34Z
ØRGP35Z
ØRGP37Z
ØRGP3JZ
ØRGP3KZ
ØRGP43Z
ØRGP44Z
ØRGP45Z
ØRGP47Z
ØRGP4JZ
ØRGP4KZ
ØRGQØ3Z
ØRGQØ4Z
ØRGQØ5Z
ØRGQØ7Z
ØRGQØJZ
ØRGQØKZ
ØRGQ33Z
ØRGQ34Z
ØRGQ35Z
ØRGQ37Z
ØRGQ3JZ
ØRGQ3KZ
ØRGQ43Z
ØRGQ44Z
ØRGQ45Z
ØRGQ47Z
ØRGQ4JZ
ØRGQ4KZ
ØRGRØ3Z
ØRGRØ4Z
ØRGRØ5Z
ØRGRØ7Z
ØRGRØJZ
ØRGRØKZ
ØRGR33Z
ØRGR34Z
ØRGR35Z
ØRGR37Z
ØRGR3JZ
ØRGR3KZ
ØRGR43Z
ØRGR44Z
ØRGR45Z
ØRGR47Z
ØRGR4JZ
ØRGR4KZ
ØRGSØ3Z
ØRGSØ4Z
ØRGSØ5Z
ØRGSØ7Z
ØRGSØJZ
ØRGSØKZ
ØRGS33Z
ØRGS34Z
ØRGS35Z
ØRGS37Z
ØRGS3JZ
ØRGS3KZ
ØRGS43Z
ØRGS44Z
ØRGS45Z
ØRGS47Z
ØRGS4JZ
ØRGS4KZ
ØRGTØ3Z
ØRGTØ4Z
ØRGTØ5Z
ØRGTØ7Z
ØRGTØJZ
ØRGTØKZ
ØRGT33Z
ØRGT34Z
ØRGT35Z
ØRGT37Z
ØRGT3JZ
ØRGT3KZ
ØRGT43Z
ØRGT44Z
ØRGT45Z
ØRGT47Z
ØRGT4JZ
ØRGT4KZ
ØRGUØ3Z
ØRGUØ4Z
ØRGUØ5Z
ØRGUØ7Z
ØRGUØJZ
ØRGUØKZ
ØRGU33Z
ØRGU34Z
ØRGU35Z
ØRGU37Z
ØRGU3JZ
ØRGU3KZ
ØRGU43Z
ØRGU44Z
ØRGU45Z
ØRGU47Z
ØRGU4JZ
ØRGU4KZ
ØRGVØ3Z
ØRGVØ4Z
ØRGVØ5Z
ØRGVØ7Z
ØRGVØJZ
ØRGVØKZ
ØRGV33Z
ØRGV34Z
ØRGV35Z
ØRGV37Z
ØRGV3JZ
ØRGV3KZ
ØRGV43Z
ØRGV44Z
ØRGV45Z
ØRGV47Z
ØRGV4JZ
ØRGV4KZ
ØRGWØ3Z
ØRGWØ4Z
ØRGWØ5Z
ØRGWØ7Z
ØRGWØJZ
ØRGWØKZ
ØRGW33Z
ØRGW34Z
ØRGW35Z
ØRGW37Z
ØRGW3JZ
ØRGW3KZ
ØRGW43Z
ØRGW44Z
ØRGW45Z
ØRGW47Z
ØRGW4JZ
ØRGW4KZ
ØRGXØ3Z
ØRGXØ4Z
ØRGXØ5Z
ØRGXØ7Z
ØRGXØJZ
ØRGXØKZ
ØRGX33Z
ØRGX34Z
ØRGX35Z
ØRGX37Z
ØRGX3JZ
ØRGX3KZ
ØRGX43Z
ØRGX44Z
ØRGX45Z
ØRGX47Z
ØRGX4JZ
ØRGX4KZ
ØRHNØ4Z
ØRHNØ5Z
ØRHN34Z
ØRHN35Z
ØRHN44Z
ØRHN45Z
ØRHPØ4Z
ØRHPØ5Z
ØRHP34Z
ØRHP35Z
ØRHP44Z
ØRHP45Z
ØRHQØ4Z
ØRHQØ5Z
ØRHQ34Z
ØRHQ35Z
ØRHQ44Z
ØRHQ45Z
ØRHRØ4Z
ØRHRØ5Z
ØRHR34Z
ØRHR35Z
ØRHR44Z
ØRHR45Z
ØRHSØ4Z
ØRHSØ5Z
ØRHS34Z
ØRHS35Z
ØRHS44Z
ØRHS45Z
ØRHTØ4Z
ØRHTØ5Z
ØRHT34Z
ØRHT35Z
ØRHT44Z
ØRHT45Z
ØRHUØ4Z
ØRHUØ5Z
ØRHU34Z
ØRHU35Z
ØRHU44Z
ØRHU45Z
ØRHVØ4Z
ØRHVØ5Z
ØRHV34Z
ØRHV35Z
ØRHV44Z
ØRHV45Z
ØRHWØ4Z
ØRHWØ5Z
ØRHW34Z
ØRHW35Z
ØRHW44Z
ØRHW45Z
ØRHXØ4Z
ØRHXØ5Z
ØRHX34Z
ØRHX35Z
ØRHX44Z
ØRHX45Z
ØRJNØZZ
ØRJPØZZ
ØRJQØZZ
ØRJRØZZ
ØRJSØZZ
ØRJTØZZ
ØRJUØZZ
ØRJVØZZ
ØRJWØZZ
ØRJXØZZ
ØRNNØZZ
ØRNN3ZZ
ØRNN4ZZ
ØRNPØZZ
ØRNP3ZZ
ØRNP4ZZ
ØRNQØZZ
ØRNQ3ZZ
ØRNQ4ZZ
ØRNRØZZ
ØRNR3ZZ
ØRNR4ZZ
ØRNSØZZ
ØRNS3ZZ
ØRNS4ZZ
ØRNTØZZ
ØRNT3ZZ
ØRNT4ZZ
ØRNUØZZ
ØRNU3ZZ
ØRNU4ZZ
ØRNVØZZ
ØRNV3ZZ
ØRNV4ZZ
ØRNWØZZ
ØRNW3ZZ
ØRNW4ZZ
ØRNXØZZ
ØRNX3ZZ
ØRNX4ZZ
ØRPNØØZ
ØRPNØ3Z
ØRPNØ4Z
ØRPNØ5Z
ØRPNØ7Z
ØRPNØJZ
ØRPNØKZ
ØRPN34Z
ØRPN35Z
ØRPN37Z
ØRPN3JZ
ØRPN3KZ
ØRPN4ØZ
ØRPN43Z
ØRPN44Z
ØRPN45Z
ØRPN47Z
ØRPN4JZ
ØRPN4KZ
ØRPPØØZ
ØRPPØ3Z
ØRPPØ4Z
ØRPPØ5Z
ØRPPØ7Z
ØRPPØJZ
ØRPPØKZ
ØRPP34Z
ØRPP35Z
ØRPP37Z
ØRPP3JZ
ØRPP3KZ
ØRPP4ØZ
ØRPP43Z
ØRPP44Z
ØRPP45Z
ØRPP47Z
ØRPP4JZ
ØRPP4KZ
ØRPQØØZ
ØRPQØ3Z
ØRPQØ4Z
ØRPQØ5Z
ØRPQØ7Z
ØRPQØJZ
ØRPQØKZ
ØRPQ34Z
ØRPQ35Z
ØRPQ37Z
ØRPQ3JZ
ØRPQ3KZ
ØRPQ4ØZ
ØRPQ43Z
ØRPQ44Z
ØRPQ45Z
ØRPQ47Z
ØRPQ4JZ
ØRPQ4KZ
ØRPRØØZ
ØRPRØ3Z
ØRPRØ4Z
ØRPRØ5Z
ØRPRØ7Z
ØRPRØJZ
ØRPRØKZ
ØRPR34Z
ØRPR35Z
ØRPR37Z
ØRPR3JZ
ØRPR3KZ
ØRPR4ØZ
ØRPR43Z
ØRPR44Z
ØRPR45Z
ØRPR47Z
ØRPR4JZ
ØRPR4KZ
ØRPSØØZ
ØRPSØ3Z
ØRPSØ4Z
ØRPSØ5Z
ØRPSØ7Z
ØRPSØJZ
ØRPSØKZ
ØRPS34Z
ØRPS35Z
ØRPS37Z
ØRPS3JZ
ØRPS3KZ
ØRPS4ØZ
ØRPS43Z
ØRPS44Z
ØRPS45Z
ØRPS47Z
ØRPS4JZ
ØRPS4KZ
ØRPTØØZ
ØRPTØ3Z
ØRPTØ4Z
ØRPTØ5Z
ØRPTØ7Z
ØRPTØJZ
ØRPTØKZ
ØRPT34Z
ØRPT35Z
ØRPT37Z
ØRPT3JZ
ØRPT3KZ
ØRPT4ØZ
ØRPT43Z
ØRPT44Z
ØRPT45Z
ØRPT47Z
ØRPT4JZ
ØRPT4KZ
ØRPUØØZ

ØRPUØ3Z
ØRPUØ4Z
ØRPUØ5Z
ØRPUØ7Z
ØRPUØJZ
ØRPUØKZ
ØRPU34Z
ØRPU35Z
ØRPU37Z
ØRPU3JZ
ØRPU3KZ
ØRPU4ØZ
ØRPU43Z
ØRPU44Z
ØRPU45Z
ØRPU47Z
ØRPU4JZ
ØRPU4KZ
ØRPVØØZ
ØRPVØ3Z
ØRPVØ4Z
ØRPVØ5Z
ØRPVØ7Z
ØRPVØJZ
ØRPVØKZ
ØRPV34Z
ØRPV35Z
ØRPV37Z
ØRPV3JZ
ØRPV3KZ
ØRPV4ØZ
ØRPV43Z
ØRPV44Z
ØRPV45Z
ØRPV47Z
ØRPV4JZ
ØRPV4KZ
ØRPWØØZ
ØRPWØ3Z
ØRPWØ4Z
ØRPWØ5Z
ØRPWØ7Z
ØRPWØJZ
ØRPWØKZ
ØRPW34Z
ØRPW35Z
ØRPW37Z
ØRPW3JZ
ØRPW3KZ
ØRPW4ØZ
ØRPW43Z
ØRPW44Z
ØRPW45Z
ØRPW47Z
ØRPW4JZ
ØRPW4KZ
ØRPXØØZ
ØRPXØ3Z
ØRPXØ4Z
ØRPXØ5Z
ØRPXØ7Z
ØRPXØJZ
ØRPXØKZ
ØRPX34Z
ØRPX35Z
ØRPX37Z
ØRPX3JZ
ØRPX3KZ
ØRPX4ØZ
ØRPX43Z
ØRPX44Z
ØRPX45Z
ØRPX47Z
ØRPX4JZ
ØRPX4KZ
ØRQNØZZ
ØRQN3ZZ
ØRQN4ZZ
ØRQPØZZ
ØRQP3ZZ
ØRQP4ZZ
ØRQQØZZ
ØRQQ3ZZ
ØRQQ4ZZ
ØRQRØZZ
ØRQR3ZZ
ØRQR4ZZ
ØRQSØZZ
ØRQS3ZZ
ØRQS4ZZ
ØRQTØZZ
ØRQT3ZZ
ØRQT4ZZ
ØRQUØZZ
ØRQU3ZZ
ØRQU4ZZ
ØRQVØZZ
ØRQV3ZZ
ØRQV4ZZ
ØRQWØZZ
ØRQW3ZZ
ØRQW4ZZ
ØRQXØZZ
ØRQX3ZZ
ØRQX4ZZ
ØRRQØ7Z
ØRRQØJZ
ØRRQØKZ
ØRRRØ7Z
ØRRRØJZ
ØRRRØKZ
ØRRSØ7Z
ØRRSØJZ
ØRRSØKZ
ØRRTØ7Z
ØRRTØJZ
ØRRTØKZ
ØRRUØ7Z
ØRRUØJZ
ØRRUØKZ
ØRRVØ7Z
ØRRVØJZ
ØRRVØKZ
ØRRWØ7Z
ØRRWØJZ
ØRRWØKZ
ØRRXØ7Z
ØRRXØJZ
ØRRXØKZ
ØRSNØ4Z
ØRSNØ5Z
ØRSNØZZ
ØRSPØ4Z
ØRSPØ5Z
ØRSPØZZ
ØRSQØ4Z
ØRSQØ5Z
ØRSQØZZ
ØRSRØ4Z
ØRSRØ5Z
ØRSRØZZ
ØRSSØ4Z
ØRSSØ5Z
ØRSSØZZ
ØRSTØ4Z
ØRSTØ5Z
ØRSTØZZ
ØRSUØ4Z
ØRSUØ5Z
ØRSUØZZ
ØRSVØ4Z
ØRSVØ5Z
ØRSVØZZ
ØRSWØ4Z
ØRSWØ5Z
ØRSWØZZ
ØRSXØ4Z
ØRSXØ5Z
ØRSXØZZ
ØRTNØZZ
ØRTPØZZ
ØRTQØZZ
ØRTRØZZ
ØRTSØZZ
ØRTTØZZ
ØRTUØZZ
ØRTVØZZ
ØRTWØZZ
ØRTXØZZ
ØRUNØ7Z
ØRUNØJZ
ØRUNØKZ
ØRUN37Z
ØRUN3JZ
ØRUN3KZ
ØRUN47Z
ØRUN4JZ
ØRUN4KZ
ØRUPØ7Z
ØRUPØJZ
ØRUPØKZ
ØRUP37Z
ØRUP3JZ
ØRUP3KZ
ØRUP47Z
ØRUP4JZ
ØRUP4KZ
ØRUQØ7Z
ØRUQØJZ
ØRUQØKZ
ØRUQ37Z
ØRUQ3JZ
ØRUQ3KZ
ØRUQ47Z
ØRUQ4JZ
ØRUQ4KZ
ØRURØ7Z
ØRURØJZ
ØRURØKZ
ØRUR37Z
ØRUR3JZ
ØRUR3KZ
ØRUR47Z
ØRUR4JZ
ØRUR4KZ
ØRUSØ7Z
ØRUSØJZ
ØRUSØKZ
ØRUS37Z
ØRUS3JZ
ØRUS3KZ
ØRUS47Z
ØRUS4JZ
ØRUS4KZ
ØRUTØ7Z
ØRUTØJZ
ØRUTØKZ
ØRUT37Z
ØRUT3JZ
ØRUT3KZ
ØRUT47Z
ØRUT4JZ
ØRUT4KZ
ØRUUØ7Z
ØRUUØJZ
ØRUUØKZ
ØRUU37Z
ØRUU3JZ
ØRUU3KZ
ØRUU47Z
ØRUU4JZ
ØRUU4KZ
ØRUVØ7Z
ØRUVØJZ
ØRUVØKZ
ØRUV37Z
ØRUV3JZ
ØRUV3KZ
ØRUV47Z
ØRUV4JZ
ØRUV4KZ
ØRUWØ7Z
ØRUWØJZ
ØRUWØKZ
ØRUW37Z
ØRUW3JZ
ØRUW3KZ
ØRUW47Z
ØRUW4JZ
ØRUW4KZ
ØRUXØ7Z
ØRUXØJZ
ØRUXØKZ
ØRUX37Z
ØRUX3JZ
ØRUX3KZ
ØRUX47Z
ØRUX4JZ
ØRUX4KZ
ØRWNØØZ
ØRWNØ3Z
ØRWNØ4Z
ØRWNØ5Z
ØRWNØ7Z
ØRWNØ8Z
ØRWNØKZ
ØRWN3ØZ
ØRWN33Z
ØRWN34Z
ØRWN35Z
ØRWN37Z
ØRWN38Z
ØRWN3KZ
ØRWN4ØZ
ØRWN43Z
ØRWN44Z
ØRWN45Z
ØRWN47Z
ØRWN48Z
ØRWN4KZ
ØRWPØØZ
ØRWPØ3Z
ØRWPØ4Z
ØRWPØ5Z
ØRWPØ7Z
ØRWPØ8Z
ØRWPØKZ
ØRWP3ØZ
ØRWP33Z
ØRWP34Z
ØRWP35Z
ØRWP37Z
ØRWP38Z
ØRWP3KZ
ØRWP4ØZ
ØRWP43Z
ØRWP44Z
ØRWP45Z
ØRWP47Z
ØRWP48Z
ØRWP4KZ
ØRWQØØZ
ØRWQØ3Z
ØRWQØ4Z
ØRWQØ5Z
ØRWQØ7Z
ØRWQØ8Z
ØRWQØKZ
ØRWQ3ØZ
ØRWQ33Z
ØRWQ34Z
ØRWQ35Z
ØRWQ37Z
ØRWQ38Z
ØRWQ3KZ
ØRWQ4ØZ
ØRWQ43Z
ØRWQ44Z
ØRWQ45Z
ØRWQ47Z
ØRWQ48Z
ØRWQ4KZ
ØRWRØØZ
ØRWRØ3Z
ØRWRØ4Z
ØRWRØ5Z
ØRWRØ7Z
ØRWRØ8Z
ØRWRØKZ
ØRWR3ØZ
ØRWR33Z
ØRWR34Z
ØRWR35Z
ØRWR37Z
ØRWR38Z
ØRWR3KZ
ØRWR4ØZ
ØRWR43Z
ØRWR44Z
ØRWR45Z
ØRWR47Z
ØRWR48Z
ØRWR4KZ
ØRWSØØZ
ØRWSØ3Z
ØRWSØ4Z
ØRWSØ5Z
ØRWSØ7Z
ØRWSØ8Z
ØRWSØKZ
ØRWS3ØZ
ØRWS33Z
ØRWS34Z
ØRWS35Z
ØRWS37Z
ØRWS38Z
ØRWS3KZ
ØRWS4ØZ
ØRWS43Z
ØRWS44Z
ØRWS45Z
ØRWS47Z
ØRWS48Z
ØRWS4KZ
ØRWTØØZ
ØRWTØ3Z
ØRWTØ4Z
ØRWTØ5Z
ØRWTØ7Z
ØRWTØ8Z
ØRWTØKZ
ØRWT3ØZ
ØRWT33Z
ØRWT34Z
ØRWT35Z
ØRWT37Z
ØRWT38Z
ØRWT3KZ
ØRWT4ØZ
ØRWT43Z
ØRWT44Z
ØRWT45Z
ØRWT47Z
ØRWT48Z
ØRWT4KZ
ØRWUØØZ
ØRWUØ3Z
ØRWUØ4Z
ØRWUØ5Z
ØRWUØ7Z
ØRWUØ8Z
ØRWUØKZ
ØRWU3ØZ
ØRWU33Z
ØRWU34Z
ØRWU35Z
ØRWU37Z
ØRWU38Z
ØRWU3KZ
ØRWU4ØZ
ØRWU43Z
ØRWU44Z
ØRWU45Z
ØRWU47Z
ØRWU48Z
ØRWU4KZ
ØRWVØØZ
ØRWVØ3Z
ØRWVØ4Z
ØRWVØ5Z
ØRWVØ7Z
ØRWVØ8Z
ØRWVØKZ
ØRWV3ØZ
ØRWV33Z
ØRWV34Z
ØRWV35Z
ØRWV37Z
ØRWV38Z
ØRWV3KZ
ØRWV4ØZ
ØRWV43Z
ØRWV44Z
ØRWV45Z
ØRWV47Z
ØRWV48Z
ØRWV4KZ
ØRWWØØZ
ØRWWØ3Z
ØRWWØ4Z
ØRWWØ5Z
ØRWWØ7Z
ØRWWØ8Z
ØRWWØKZ
ØRWW3ØZ
ØRWW33Z
ØRWW34Z
ØRWW35Z
ØRWW37Z
ØRWW38Z
ØRWW3KZ
ØRWW4ØZ
ØRWW43Z
ØRWW44Z
ØRWW45Z
ØRWW47Z
ØRWW48Z
ØRWW4KZ
ØRWXØØZ
ØRWXØ3Z
ØRWXØ4Z
ØRWXØ5Z
ØRWXØ7Z
ØRWXØ8Z
ØRWXØKZ
ØRWX3ØZ
ØRWX33Z
ØRWX34Z
ØRWX35Z
ØRWX37Z
ØRWX38Z
ØRWX3KZ
ØRWX4ØZ
ØRWX43Z
ØRWX44Z
ØRWX45Z
ØRWX47Z
ØRWX48Z
ØRWX4KZ
ØX6LØZØ
ØX6LØZ1
ØX6LØZ2
ØX6LØZ3
ØX6MØZØ
ØX6MØZ1
ØX6MØZ2
ØX6MØZ3
ØX6NØZØ
ØX6NØZ1
ØX6NØZ2
ØX6NØZ3
ØX6PØZØ
ØX6PØZ1
ØX6PØZ2
ØX6PØZ3
ØX6QØZØ
ØX6QØZ1
ØX6QØZ2
ØX6QØZ3
ØX6RØZØ
ØX6RØZ1
ØX6RØZ2
ØX6RØZ3
ØX6SØZØ
ØX6SØZ1
ØX6SØZ2
ØX6SØZ3
ØX6TØZØ
ØX6TØZ1
ØX6TØZ2
ØX6TØZ3
ØX6VØZØ
ØX6VØZ1
ØX6VØZ2
ØX6VØZ3
ØX6WØZØ
ØX6WØZ1
ØX6WØZ2
ØX6WØZ3
ØXMLØZZ
ØXMMØZZ
ØXMNØZZ
ØXMPØZZ
ØXMQØZZ
ØXMRØZZ
ØXMSØZZ
ØXMTØZZ
ØXMVØZZ
ØXMWØZZ
ØXRLØ7N
ØXRLØ7P
ØXRL47N
ØXRL47P
ØXRMØ7N
ØXRMØ7P
ØXRM47N
ØXRM47P
ØXUJØ7Z
ØXUJ47Z
ØXUKØ7Z
ØXUK47Z
ØXULØ7Z
ØXUL47Z
ØXUMØ7Z
ØXUM47Z
ØXUNØ7Z
ØXUN47Z
ØXUPØ7Z
ØXUP47Z
ØXUQØ7Z
ØXUQ47Z
ØXURØ7Z
ØXUR47Z
ØXUSØ7Z
ØXUS47Z
ØXUTØ7Z
ØXUT47Z
ØXUVØ7Z
ØXUV47Z
ØXUWØ7Z
ØXUW47Z
ØXXNØZL
ØXXPØZM

DRG 907

Operating Room Procedures

ØØ16*
ØØ5Ø*
ØØ57*
ØØ59*
ØØ5A*
ØØ5B*
ØØ5C*
ØØ5D*
ØØ76ØZZ
ØØ763ZZ
ØØ764ZZ
ØØ8Ø*
ØØ87*
ØØ8F*
ØØ8G*
ØØ8H*
ØØ8J*
ØØ8K*
ØØ8L*
ØØ8M*
ØØ8N*
ØØ8R*
ØØ8S*
ØØ8W*
ØØ8X*
ØØ8Y*
ØØ9ØØØZ
ØØ9ØØZZ
ØØ9Ø3ØZ
ØØ9Ø3ZZ
ØØ9Ø4ØZ
ØØ9Ø4ZZ
ØØ91ØØZ
ØØ91ØZZ
ØØ92ØØZ
ØØ92ØZZ
ØØ93ØØZ
ØØ93ØZZ
ØØ933ØZ
ØØ933ZZ
ØØ934ØZ
ØØ934ZZ
ØØ94ØØZ
ØØ94ØZZ
ØØ95ØØZ
ØØ95ØZZ
ØØ96ØØZ
ØØ96ØZZ
ØØ963ØZ
ØØ964ØZ
ØØ97ØØZ
ØØ97ØZZ
ØØ973ØZ
ØØ973ZZ
ØØ974ØZ
ØØ974ZZ
ØØ99ØØZ
ØØ99ØZZ
ØØ993ØZ
ØØ993ZZ
ØØ994ØZ
ØØ994ZZ
ØØ9AØØZ
ØØ9AØZZ
ØØ9A3ØZ
ØØ9A3ZZ
ØØ9A4ØZ
ØØ9A4ZZ
ØØ9BØØZ
ØØ9BØZZ
ØØ9B3ØZ
ØØ9B3ZZ
ØØ9B4ØZ
ØØ9B4ZZ
ØØ9CØØZ
ØØ9CØZZ
ØØ9C3ØZ
ØØ9C3ZZ
ØØ9C4ØZ
ØØ9C4ZZ
ØØ9DØØZ
ØØ9DØZZ
ØØ9D3ØZ
ØØ9D3ZZ
ØØ9D4ØZ
ØØ9D4ZZ
ØØ9FØZX
ØØ9GØZX
ØØ9HØZX
ØØ9JØZX
ØØ9KØZX
ØØ9LØZX
ØØ9MØZX
ØØ9NØZX
ØØ9PØZX
ØØ9QØZX
ØØ9RØZX
ØØ9SØZX
ØØ9TØØZ
ØØ9TØZZ
ØØ9T4ØZ
ØØ9T4ZZ
ØØ9UØØZ
ØØ9UØZZ
ØØ9WØØZ
ØØ9WØZZ
ØØ9W4ØZ
ØØ9W4ZZ
ØØ9XØØZ
ØØ9XØZZ
ØØ9X4ØZ
ØØ9X4ZZ
ØØ9YØØZ
ØØ9YØZZ
ØØ9Y4ØZ
ØØ9Y4ZZ
ØØBØØZZ
ØØBØ3ZZ
ØØBØ4ZZ
ØØB6ØZZ
ØØB63ZZ
ØØB64ZZ
ØØB7ØZZ
ØØB73ZZ
ØØB74ZZ
ØØB9ØZZ
ØØB93ZZ
ØØB94ZZ
ØØBAØZZ
ØØBA3ZZ
ØØBA4ZZ
ØØBBØZZ
ØØBB3ZZ
ØØBB4ZZ
ØØBCØZZ
ØØBC3ZZ
ØØBC4ZZ
ØØBDØZZ
ØØBD3ZZ
ØØBD4ZZ
ØØBFØZX
ØØBFØZZ
ØØBF3ZZ
ØØBF4ZZ
ØØBGØZX
ØØBGØZZ
ØØBG3ZZ
ØØBG4ZZ
ØØBHØZX
ØØBHØZZ
ØØBH3ZZ
ØØBH4ZZ
ØØBJØZX
ØØBJØZZ
ØØBJ3ZZ
ØØBJ4ZZ
ØØBKØZX
ØØBKØZZ
ØØBK3ZZ
ØØBK4ZZ
ØØBLØZX
ØØBLØZZ
ØØBL3ZZ
ØØBL4ZZ
ØØBMØZX
ØØBMØZZ
ØØBM3ZZ
ØØBM4ZZ
ØØBNØZX
ØØBN3ZZ
ØØBN4ZZ
ØØBPØZX
ØØBPØZZ
ØØBP3ZZ
ØØBP4ZZ
ØØBQØZX
ØØBQØZZ
ØØBQ3ZZ
ØØBQ4ZZ
ØØBRØZX
ØØBRØZZ
ØØBR3ZZ
ØØBR4ZZ
ØØBSØZX
ØØBSØZZ
ØØBS3ZZ
ØØBS4ZZ
ØØCØ*
ØØC1*
ØØC2*
ØØC3*
ØØC4*
ØØC5*
ØØC6*
ØØC7*
ØØC9*
ØØCA*
ØØCB*
ØØCC*
ØØCD*
ØØCT*
ØØCUØZZ
ØØCU3ZZ
ØØCU4ZZ
ØØCW*
ØØCX*
ØØCY*
ØØDØØZZ
ØØDØ3ZZ
ØØDØ4ZZ
ØØD7ØZZ
ØØD73ZZ
ØØD74ZZ
ØØDCØZZ
ØØDC3ZZ
ØØDC4ZZ
ØØDF*
ØØDG*
ØØDH*
ØØDJ*
ØØDK*
ØØDL*
ØØDM*
ØØDN*
ØØDP*
ØØDQ*
ØØDR*
ØØDS*
ØØDT*
ØØF3ØZZ
ØØF33ZZ
ØØF34ZZ
ØØF4ØZZ
ØØF43ZZ
ØØF44ZZ
ØØF5ØZZ
ØØF53ZZ
ØØF54ZZ
ØØF6ØZZ
ØØF63ZZ
ØØF64ZZ
ØØFU*
ØØHØØ1Z
ØØHØØ2Z
ØØHØØ3Z
ØØHØØMZ
ØØHØØYZ
ØØHØ31Z
ØØHØ32Z
ØØHØ33Z
ØØHØ3MZ
ØØHØ3YZ
ØØHØ41Z
ØØHØ42Z
ØØHØ43Z
ØØHØ4MZ
ØØHØ4YZ
ØØH6Ø1Z
ØØH6Ø2Z
ØØH6Ø3Z
ØØH6ØMZ
ØØH6ØYZ
ØØH631Z
ØØH632Z
ØØH633Z
ØØH63MZ
ØØH63YZ
ØØH641Z
ØØH642Z
ØØH643Z
ØØH64MZ
ØØH64YZ
ØØHEØMZ
ØØHE3MZ
ØØHE4MZ
ØØHUØ1Z
ØØHUØ2Z
ØØHUØMZ
ØØHUØYZ
ØØHU31Z
ØØHU3MZ
ØØHU41Z
ØØHU42Z
ØØHU4MZ
ØØHVØ1Z
ØØHVØ2Z
ØØHVØMZ
ØØHVØYZ
ØØHV31Z
ØØHV3MZ
ØØHV3YZ
ØØHV41Z
ØØHV42Z
ØØHV4MZ
ØØHV4YZ
ØØJØØZZ
ØØJØ4ZZ
ØØJUØZZ

ØØJVØZZ
ØØK*
ØØN*
ØØPØØØZ
ØØPØØ2Z
ØØPØØ3Z
ØØPØØ7Z
ØØPØØJZ
ØØPØØKZ
ØØPØØYZ
ØØPØ37Z
ØØPØ3JZ
ØØPØ3KZ
ØØPØ4ØZ
ØØPØ42Z
ØØPØ43Z
ØØPØ47Z
ØØPØ4JZ
ØØPØ4KZ
ØØP6ØØZ
ØØP6Ø2Z
ØØP6Ø3Z
ØØP6ØJZ
ØØP6ØYZ
ØØP63JZ
ØØP64ØZ
ØØP642Z
ØØP643Z
ØØP64JZ
ØØPEØMZ
ØØPE3MZ
ØØPE4MZ
ØØPUØØZ
ØØPUØ2Z
ØØPUØ3Z
ØØPUØJZ
ØØPUØMZ
ØØPUØYZ
ØØPU3JZ
ØØPU3MZ
ØØPU4ØZ
ØØPU42Z
ØØPU43Z
ØØPU4JZ
ØØPU4MZ
ØØPVØØZ
ØØPVØ2Z
ØØPVØ3Z
ØØPVØ7Z
ØØPVØJZ
ØØPVØKZ
ØØPVØMZ
ØØPVØYZ
ØØPV37Z
ØØPV3JZ
ØØPV3KZ
ØØPV3MZ
ØØPV4ØZ
ØØPV42Z
ØØPV43Z
ØØPV47Z
ØØPV4JZ
ØØPV4KZ
ØØPV4MZ
ØØQ*
ØØR1Ø7Z
ØØR1ØJZ
ØØR1ØKZ
ØØR147Z
ØØR14JZ
ØØR14KZ
ØØR2Ø7Z
ØØR2ØJZ
ØØR2ØKZ
ØØR247Z
ØØR24JZ
ØØR24KZ
ØØR6Ø7Z
ØØR6ØJZ
ØØR6ØKZ
ØØR647Z
ØØR64JZ
ØØR64KZ
ØØRFØ7Z
ØØRFØJZ
ØØRFØKZ
ØØRF47Z
ØØRF4JZ
ØØRF4KZ
ØØRGØ7Z
ØØRGØJZ
ØØRGØKZ
ØØRG47Z
ØØRG4JZ
ØØRG4KZ
ØØRHØ7Z
ØØRHØJZ
ØØRHØKZ
ØØRH47Z
ØØRH4JZ
ØØRH4KZ
ØØRJØ7Z
ØØRJØJZ
ØØRJØKZ
ØØRJ47Z
ØØRJ4JZ
ØØRJ4KZ
ØØRKØ7Z
ØØRKØJZ
ØØRKØKZ
ØØRK47Z
ØØRK4JZ
ØØRK4KZ
ØØRLØ7Z
ØØRLØJZ
ØØRLØKZ
ØØRL47Z
ØØRL4JZ
ØØRL4KZ
ØØRMØ7Z
ØØRMØJZ
ØØRMØKZ
ØØRM47Z
ØØRM4JZ
ØØRM4KZ
ØØRNØ7Z
ØØRNØJZ
ØØRNØKZ
ØØRN47Z
ØØRN4JZ
ØØRN4KZ
ØØRPØ7Z
ØØRPØJZ
ØØRPØKZ
ØØRP47Z
ØØRP4JZ
ØØRP4KZ
ØØRQØ7Z
ØØRQØJZ
ØØRQØKZ
ØØRQ47Z
ØØRQ4JZ
ØØRQ4KZ
ØØRRØ7Z
ØØRRØJZ
ØØRRØKZ
ØØRR47Z
ØØRR4JZ
ØØRR4KZ
ØØRSØ7Z
ØØRSØJZ
ØØRSØKZ
ØØRS47Z
ØØRS4JZ
ØØRS4KZ
ØØRTØ7Z
ØØRTØJZ
ØØRTØKZ
ØØRT47Z
ØØRT4JZ
ØØRT4KZ
ØØSW*
ØØSX*
ØØSY*
ØØT*
ØØU*
ØØWØØØZ
ØØWØØ2Z
ØØWØØ3Z
ØØWØØ7Z
ØØWØØMZ
ØØWØØYZ
ØØWØ3ØZ
ØØWØ32Z
ØØWØ33Z
ØØWØ37Z
ØØWØ3JZ
ØØWØ3KZ
ØØWØ3MZ
ØØWØ4ØZ
ØØWØ42Z
ØØWØ43Z
ØØWØ47Z
ØØWØ4JZ
ØØWØ4KZ
ØØWØ4MZ
ØØW6ØØZ
ØØW6Ø2Z
ØØW6Ø3Z
ØØW6ØJZ
ØØW6ØMZ
ØØW6ØYZ
ØØW63ØZ
ØØW632Z
ØØW633Z
ØØW63JZ
ØØW63MZ
ØØW64ØZ
ØØW642Z
ØØW643Z
ØØW64JZ
ØØW64MZ
ØØWUØØZ
ØØWUØ2Z
ØØWUØ3Z
ØØWUØJZ
ØØWUØMZ
ØØWUØYZ
ØØWU3ØZ
ØØWU32Z
ØØWU33Z
ØØWU3JZ
ØØWU3MZ
ØØWU4ØZ
ØØWU42Z
ØØWU43Z
ØØWU4JZ
ØØWU4MZ
ØØWVØØZ
ØØWVØ2Z
ØØWVØ3Z
ØØWVØ7Z
ØØWVØJZ
ØØWVØKZ
ØØWVØMZ
ØØWVØYZ
ØØWV3ØZ
ØØWV32Z
ØØWV33Z
ØØWV37Z
ØØWV3JZ
ØØWV3KZ
ØØWV3MZ
ØØWV4ØZ
ØØWV42Z
ØØWV43Z
ØØWV47Z
ØØWV4JZ
ØØWV4KZ
ØØWV4MZ
ØØX*
Ø151ØZZ
Ø1514ZZ
Ø158ØZZ
Ø1584ZZ
Ø15BØZZ
Ø15B4ZZ
Ø15RØZZ
Ø15R4ZZ
Ø18Ø*
Ø181*
Ø182*
Ø183*
Ø184*
Ø185*
Ø186*
Ø188*
Ø189*
Ø18A*
Ø18B*
Ø18C*
Ø18D*
Ø18F*
Ø18G*
Ø18H*
Ø18Q*
Ø18R*
Ø19ØØZX
Ø191ØZX
Ø192ØZX
Ø193ØZX
Ø194ØZX
Ø195ØZX
Ø196ØZX
Ø198ØZX
Ø199ØZX
Ø19AØZX
Ø19BØZX
Ø19CØZX
Ø19DØZX
Ø19FØZX
Ø19GØZX
Ø19HØZX
Ø19QØZX
Ø19RØZX
Ø1BØØZX
Ø1BØØZZ
Ø1BØ3ZZ
Ø1BØ4ZZ
Ø1B1ØZX
Ø1B1ØZZ
Ø1B13ZZ
Ø1B14ZZ
Ø1B2ØZX
Ø1B2ØZZ
Ø1B23ZZ
Ø1B24ZZ
Ø1B3ØZX
Ø1B3ØZZ
Ø1B33ZZ
Ø1B34ZZ
Ø1B4ØZX
Ø1B4ØZZ
Ø1B43ZZ
Ø1B44ZZ
Ø1B5ØZX
Ø1B5ØZZ
Ø1B53ZZ
Ø1B54ZZ
Ø1B6ØZX
Ø1B6ØZZ
Ø1B63ZZ
Ø1B64ZZ
Ø1B8ØZX
Ø1B8ØZZ
Ø1B83ZZ
Ø1B84ZZ
Ø1B9ØZX
Ø1B9ØZZ
Ø1B93ZZ
Ø1B94ZZ
Ø1BAØZX
Ø1BAØZZ
Ø1BA3ZZ
Ø1BA4ZZ
Ø1BBØZX
Ø1BBØZZ
Ø1BB3ZZ
Ø1BB4ZZ
Ø1BCØZX
Ø1BCØZZ
Ø1BC3ZZ
Ø1BC4ZZ
Ø1BDØZX
Ø1BDØZZ
Ø1BD3ZZ
Ø1BD4ZZ
Ø1BFØZX
Ø1BFØZZ
Ø1BF3ZZ
Ø1BF4ZZ
Ø1BGØZX
Ø1BGØZZ
Ø1BG3ZZ
Ø1BG4ZZ
Ø1BHØZX
Ø1BHØZZ
Ø1BH3ZZ
Ø1BH4ZZ
Ø1BQØZX
Ø1BQØZZ
Ø1BQ3ZZ
Ø1BQ4ZZ
Ø1BRØZX
Ø1BRØZZ
Ø1BR3ZZ
Ø1BR4ZZ
Ø1DØ*
Ø1D1*
Ø1D2*
Ø1D3*
Ø1D4*
Ø1D5*
Ø1D6*
Ø1D8*
Ø1D9*
Ø1DA*
Ø1DB*
Ø1DC*
Ø1DD*
Ø1DF*
Ø1DG*
Ø1DH*
Ø1DQ*
Ø1DR*
Ø1HYØMZ
Ø1HY3MZ
Ø1HY4MZ
Ø1NØ*
Ø1N1*
Ø1N2*
Ø1N3*
Ø1N4*
Ø1N6*
Ø1N8*
Ø1N9*
Ø1NA*
Ø1NB*
Ø1NC*
Ø1ND*
Ø1NF*
Ø1NG*
Ø1NH*
Ø1NQ*
Ø1NR*
Ø1PYØMZ
Ø1PY3MZ
Ø1PY4MZ
Ø1QØ*
Ø1Q1*
Ø1Q2*
Ø1Q3*
Ø1Q4*
Ø1Q5*
Ø1Q6*
Ø1Q8*
Ø1Q9*
Ø1QA*
Ø1QB*
Ø1QC*
Ø1QD*
Ø1QF*
Ø1QG*
Ø1QH*
Ø1QQ*
Ø1QR*
Ø1R1Ø7Z
Ø1R1ØJZ
Ø1R1ØKZ
Ø1R147Z
Ø1R14JZ
Ø1R14KZ
Ø1R2Ø7Z
Ø1R2ØJZ
Ø1R2ØKZ
Ø1R247Z
Ø1R24JZ
Ø1R24KZ
Ø1R4Ø7Z
Ø1R4ØJZ
Ø1R4ØKZ
Ø1R447Z
Ø1R44JZ
Ø1R44KZ
Ø1R5Ø7Z
Ø1R5ØJZ
Ø1R5ØKZ
Ø1R547Z
Ø1R54JZ
Ø1R54KZ
Ø1R6Ø7Z
Ø1R6ØJZ
Ø1R6ØKZ
Ø1R647Z
Ø1R64JZ
Ø1R64KZ
Ø1R8Ø7Z
Ø1R8ØJZ
Ø1R8ØKZ
Ø1R847Z
Ø1R84JZ
Ø1R84KZ
Ø1RBØ7Z
Ø1RBØJZ
Ø1RBØKZ
Ø1RB47Z
Ø1RB4JZ
Ø1RB4KZ
Ø1RCØ7Z
Ø1RCØJZ
Ø1RCØKZ
Ø1RC47Z
Ø1RC4JZ
Ø1RC4KZ
Ø1RDØ7Z
Ø1RDØJZ
Ø1RDØKZ
Ø1RD47Z
Ø1RD4JZ
Ø1RD4KZ
Ø1RFØ7Z
Ø1RFØJZ
Ø1RFØKZ
Ø1RF47Z
Ø1RF4JZ
Ø1RF4KZ
Ø1RGØ7Z
Ø1RGØJZ
Ø1RGØKZ
Ø1RG47Z
Ø1RG4JZ
Ø1RG4KZ
Ø1RHØ7Z
Ø1RHØJZ
Ø1RHØKZ
Ø1RH47Z
Ø1RH4JZ
Ø1RH4KZ
Ø1RRØ7Z
Ø1RRØJZ
Ø1RRØKZ
Ø1RR47Z
Ø1RR4JZ
Ø1RR4KZ
Ø1U*
Ø216ØZ7
Ø2163Z7
Ø2164Z7
Ø217Ø8S
Ø217Ø8T
Ø217Ø8U
Ø217Ø9S
Ø217Ø9T
Ø217Ø9U
Ø217ØAS
Ø217ØAT
Ø217ØAU
Ø217ØJS
Ø217ØJT
Ø217ØJU
Ø217ØKS
Ø217ØKT
Ø217ØKU
Ø217ØZS
Ø217ØZT
Ø217ØZU
Ø2173J6
Ø21748S
Ø21748T
Ø21748U
Ø21749S
Ø21749T
Ø21749U
Ø2174AS
Ø2174AT
Ø2174AU
Ø2174JS
Ø2174JT
Ø2174JU
Ø2174KS
Ø2174KT
Ø2174KU
Ø2174ZS
Ø2174ZT
Ø2174ZU
Ø21PØ8A
Ø21PØ8B
Ø21PØ8D
Ø21PØ9A
Ø21PØ9B
Ø21PØ9D
Ø21PØAA
Ø21PØAB
Ø21PØAD
Ø21PØJA
Ø21PØJB
Ø21PØJD
Ø21PØKA
Ø21PØKB
Ø21PØKD
Ø21PØZA
Ø21PØZB
Ø21PØZD
Ø21P48A
Ø21P48B
Ø21P48D
Ø21P49A
Ø21P49B
Ø21P49D
Ø21P4AA
Ø21P4AB
Ø21P4AD
Ø21P4JA
Ø21P4JB
Ø21P4JD
Ø21P4KA
Ø21P4KB
Ø21P4KD
Ø21P4ZA
Ø21P4ZB
Ø21P4ZD
Ø21QØ8A
Ø21QØ8B
Ø21QØ8D
Ø21QØ9A
Ø21QØ9B
Ø21QØ9D
Ø21QØAA
Ø21QØAB
Ø21QØAD
Ø21QØJA
Ø21QØJB
Ø21QØJD
Ø21QØKA
Ø21QØKB
Ø21QØKD
Ø21QØZA
Ø21QØZB
Ø21QØZD
Ø21Q48A
Ø21Q48B
Ø21Q48D
Ø21Q49A
Ø21Q49B
Ø21Q49D
Ø21Q4AA
Ø21Q4AB
Ø21Q4AD
Ø21Q4JA
Ø21Q4JB
Ø21Q4JD
Ø21Q4KA
Ø21Q4KB
Ø21Q4KD
Ø21Q4ZA
Ø21Q4ZB
Ø21Q4ZD
Ø21RØ8A
Ø21RØ8B
Ø21RØ8D
Ø21RØ9A
Ø21RØ9B
Ø21RØ9D
Ø21RØAA
Ø21RØAB
Ø21RØAD
Ø21RØJA
Ø21RØJB
Ø21RØJD
Ø21RØKA
Ø21RØKB
Ø21RØKD
Ø21RØZA
Ø21RØZB
Ø21RØZD
Ø21R48A
Ø21R48B
Ø21R48D
Ø21R49A
Ø21R49B
Ø21R49D
Ø21R4AA
Ø21R4AB
Ø21R4AD
Ø21R4JA
Ø21R4JB
Ø21R4JD
Ø21R4KA
Ø21R4KB
Ø21R4KD
Ø21R4ZA
Ø21R4ZB
Ø21R4ZD
Ø21VØ8S
Ø21VØ8T
Ø21VØ8U
Ø21VØ9S
Ø21VØ9T
Ø21VØ9U
Ø21VØAS
Ø21VØAT
Ø21VØAU
Ø21VØJS
Ø21VØJT
Ø21VØJU
Ø21VØKS
Ø21VØKT
Ø21VØKU
Ø21VØZS
Ø21VØZT
Ø21VØZU
Ø21V48S
Ø21V48T
Ø21V48U
Ø21V49S
Ø21V49T
Ø21V49U
Ø21V4AS
Ø21V4AT
Ø21V4AU
Ø21V4JS
Ø21V4JT
Ø21V4JU
Ø21V4KS
Ø21V4KT
Ø21V4KU
Ø21V4ZS
Ø21V4ZT
Ø21V4ZU
Ø21WØ8A
Ø21WØ8B
Ø21WØ8D
Ø21WØ8G
Ø21WØ8H
Ø21WØ9A
Ø21WØ9B
Ø21WØ9D
Ø21WØ9G
Ø21WØ9H
Ø21WØAA
Ø21WØAB
Ø21WØAD
Ø21WØAG
Ø21WØAH
Ø21WØJA
Ø21WØJB
Ø21WØJD
Ø21WØJG
Ø21WØJH
Ø21WØKA
Ø21WØKB
Ø21WØKD
Ø21WØKG
Ø21WØKH
Ø21WØZA
Ø21WØZB
Ø21WØZD
Ø21W48A
Ø21W48B
Ø21W48D
Ø21W49A
Ø21W49B
Ø21W49D
Ø21W4AA
Ø21W4AB
Ø21W4AD
Ø21W4JA
Ø21W4JB
Ø21W4JD
Ø21W4KA
Ø21W4KB
Ø21W4KD
Ø21W4ZA
Ø21W4ZB
Ø21W4ZD
Ø21XØ8A
Ø21XØ8B
Ø21XØ8D
Ø21XØ9A
Ø21XØ9B
Ø21XØ9D
Ø21XØAA
Ø21XØAB
Ø21XØAD
Ø21XØJA
Ø21XØJB
Ø21XØJD
Ø21XØKA
Ø21XØKB
Ø21XØKD
Ø21XØZA
Ø21XØZB
Ø21XØZD
Ø21X48A
Ø21X48B
Ø21X48D
Ø21X49A
Ø21X49B
Ø21X49D
Ø21X4AA
Ø21X4AB
Ø21X4AD
Ø21X4JA
Ø21X4JB
Ø21X4JD
Ø21X4KA
Ø21X4KB
Ø21X4KD
Ø21X4ZA
Ø21X4ZB
Ø21X4ZD
Ø25N*
Ø27K*
Ø27LØ4Z
Ø27LØDZ
Ø27LØZZ
Ø27L34Z
Ø27L3DZ
Ø27L3ZZ
Ø27L44Z
Ø27L4DZ
Ø27L4ZZ
Ø27RØ4T
Ø27RØDT
Ø27RØZT
Ø27R34T
Ø27R3DT
Ø27R3ZT
Ø27R44T
Ø27R4DT
Ø27R4ZT
Ø2BNØZZ
Ø2BN3ZZ
Ø2BN4ZZ
Ø2BP3ZZ
Ø2BQ3ZZ
Ø2BR3ZZ
Ø2BS3ZZ
Ø2BT3ZZ
Ø2BV3ZZ
Ø2BWØZZ
Ø2BW3ZZ
Ø2BW4ZZ
Ø2BXØZZ
Ø2BX3ZZ
Ø2BX4ZZ
Ø2CN*
Ø2CP*
Ø2CQ*
Ø2CR*
Ø2CS*
Ø2CT*
Ø2CV*
Ø2CW*
Ø2CXØZZ
Ø2CX3ZZ
Ø2CX4ZZ
Ø2FNØZZ
Ø2FN3ZZ
Ø2FN4ZZ
Ø2H6Ø2Z
Ø2H642Z
Ø2H7Ø2Z
Ø2H742Z
Ø2HLØ2Z
Ø2HL42Z
Ø2HNØØZ
Ø2HNØ2Z
Ø2HNØYZ
Ø2HN3ØZ
Ø2HN3YZ
Ø2HN4ØZ
Ø2HN42Z
Ø2HN4YZ
Ø2HVØ2Z
Ø2HVØDZ
Ø2HV3DZ
Ø2HV42Z
Ø2HV4DZ
Ø2JAØZZ
Ø2JYØZZ
Ø2LHØCZ
Ø2LHØDZ
Ø2LHØZZ
Ø2LH3CZ
Ø2LH3DZ
Ø2LH3ZZ
Ø2LH4CZ
Ø2LH4DZ
Ø2LH4ZZ
Ø2LPØCZ
Ø2LPØDZ
Ø2LPØZZ
Ø2LP3CZ
Ø2LP3DZ
Ø2LP3ZZ
Ø2LP4CZ
Ø2LP4DZ
Ø2LP4ZZ
Ø2LQØCZ
Ø2LQØDZ
Ø2LQØZZ
Ø2LQ3CZ
Ø2LQ3DZ
Ø2LQ3ZZ

ICD-10-CM/PCS Codes by MS-DRG

Ø2LQ4CZ
Ø2LQ4DZ
Ø2LQ4ZZ
Ø2LRØCT
Ø2LRØCZ
Ø2LRØDT
Ø2LRØDZ
Ø2LRØZT
Ø2LRØZZ
Ø2LR3CT
Ø2LR3CZ
Ø2LR3DT
Ø2LR3DZ
Ø2LR3ZT
Ø2LR3ZZ
Ø2LR4CT
Ø2LR4CZ
Ø2LR4DT
Ø2LR4DZ
Ø2LR4ZT
Ø2LR4ZZ
Ø2LSØCZ
Ø2LSØDZ
Ø2LSØZZ
Ø2LS3CZ
Ø2LS3DZ
Ø2LS3ZZ
Ø2LS4CZ
Ø2LS4DZ
Ø2LS4ZZ
Ø2LTØCZ
Ø2LTØDZ
Ø2LTØZZ
Ø2LT3CZ
Ø2LT3DZ
Ø2LT3ZZ
Ø2LT4CZ
Ø2LT4DZ
Ø2LT4ZZ
Ø2LVØCZ
Ø2LVØDZ
Ø2LVØZZ
Ø2LV3CZ
Ø2LV3DZ
Ø2LV3ZZ
Ø2LV4CZ
Ø2LV4DZ
Ø2LV4ZZ
Ø2LWØDJ
Ø2LW3DJ
Ø2N4*
Ø2N8*
Ø2NN*
Ø2PAØMZ
Ø2PA3MZ
Ø2PA4MZ
Ø2Q6*
Ø2Q7*
Ø2Q8*
Ø2QA*
Ø2QK*
Ø2QL*
Ø2QN*
Ø2QP*
Ø2QQ*
Ø2QR*
Ø2QS*
Ø2QT*
Ø2QV*
Ø2QW*
Ø2QXØZZ
Ø2QX3ZZ
Ø2QX4ZZ
Ø2R5*
Ø2R6*
Ø2R7*
Ø2RKØ8Z
Ø2RKØJZ
Ø2RK48Z
Ø2RK4JZ
Ø2RLØ8Z
Ø2RLØJZ
Ø2RL48Z
Ø2RL4JZ
Ø2RMØ8Z
Ø2RM48Z
Ø2RN*
Ø2RP*
Ø2RQ*
Ø2RR*
Ø2RS*
Ø2RT*
Ø2RV*
Ø2RW*
Ø2RXØ7Z
Ø2RXØ8Z
Ø2RXØJZ
Ø2RXØKZ
Ø2RX47Z
Ø2RX48Z
Ø2RX4JZ
Ø2RX4KZ
Ø2S*
Ø2TN*
Ø2UØØ7Z
Ø2UØØ8Z
Ø2UØØKZ
Ø2UØ47Z
Ø2UØ48Z
Ø2UØ4KZ
Ø2U1Ø7Z
Ø2U1Ø8Z
Ø2U1ØKZ
Ø2U147Z
Ø2U148Z
Ø2U14KZ
Ø2U2Ø7Z
Ø2U2Ø8Z
Ø2U2ØKZ
Ø2U247Z
Ø2U248Z
Ø2U24KZ
Ø2U3Ø7Z
Ø2U3Ø8Z
Ø2U3ØKZ
Ø2U347Z
Ø2U348Z
Ø2U34KZ
Ø2U6ØJZ
Ø2U637Z
Ø2U638Z
Ø2U63JZ
Ø2U63KZ
Ø2U647Z
Ø2U648Z
Ø2U64JZ
Ø2U64KZ
Ø2U7ØJZ
Ø2UAØ7Z
Ø2UAØ8Z
Ø2UAØKZ
Ø2UA37Z
Ø2UA38Z
Ø2UA3KZ
Ø2UA47Z
Ø2UA48Z
Ø2UA4KZ
Ø2UKØ7Z
Ø2UKØ8Z
Ø2UKØJZ
Ø2UK37Z
Ø2UK38Z
Ø2UK3JZ
Ø2UK47Z
Ø2UK48Z
Ø2UK4JZ
Ø2ULØ7Z
Ø2ULØ8Z
Ø2ULØJZ
Ø2UL37Z
Ø2UL38Z
Ø2UL3JZ
Ø2UL47Z
Ø2UL48Z
Ø2UL4JZ
Ø2UMØ8Z
Ø2UN*
Ø2UP*
Ø2UQ*
Ø2UR*
Ø2US*
Ø2UT*
Ø2UV*
Ø2UW*
Ø2UXØ7Z
Ø2UXØ8Z
Ø2UXØJZ
Ø2UXØKZ
Ø2UX37Z
Ø2UX38Z
Ø2UX3JZ
Ø2UX3KZ
Ø2UX47Z
Ø2UX48Z
Ø2UX4JZ
Ø2UX4KZ
Ø2VA*
Ø2VLØCZ
Ø2VLØDZ
Ø2VLØZZ
Ø2VL3CZ
Ø2VL3DZ
Ø2VL3ZZ
Ø2VL4CZ
Ø2VL4DZ
Ø2VL4ZZ
Ø2VPØDZ
Ø2VPØZZ
Ø2VP3DZ
Ø2VP3ZZ
Ø2VP4DZ
Ø2VP4ZZ
Ø2VQØDZ
Ø2VQØZZ
Ø2VQ3DZ
Ø2VQ3ZZ
Ø2VQ4DZ
Ø2VQ4ZZ
Ø2VRØDT
Ø2VRØDZ
Ø2VRØZT
Ø2VRØZZ
Ø2VR3DT
Ø2VR3DZ
Ø2VR3ZT
Ø2VR3ZZ
Ø2VR4DT
Ø2VR4DZ
Ø2VR4ZT
Ø2VR4ZZ
Ø2VSØDZ
Ø2VSØZZ
Ø2VS3DZ
Ø2VS3ZZ
Ø2VS4DZ
Ø2VS4ZZ
Ø2VTØDZ
Ø2VTØZZ
Ø2VT3DZ
Ø2VT3ZZ
Ø2VT4DZ
Ø2VT4ZZ
Ø2VV*
Ø2VWØDZ
Ø2VWØEZ
Ø2VWØFZ
Ø2VWØZZ
Ø2VW3DZ
Ø2VW3EZ
Ø2VW3FZ
Ø2VW3ZZ
Ø2VW4DZ
Ø2VW4EZ
Ø2VW4FZ
Ø2VW4ZZ
Ø2VXØDZ
Ø2VXØEZ
Ø2VXØFZ
Ø2VXØZZ
Ø2VX3DZ
Ø2VX3EZ
Ø2VX3FZ
Ø2VX3ZZ
Ø2VX4DZ
Ø2VX4EZ
Ø2VX4FZ
Ø2VX4ZZ
Ø2WAØKZ
Ø2WAØMZ
Ø2WA3JZ
Ø2WA3KZ
Ø2WA3MZ
Ø2WA4JZ
Ø2WA4KZ
Ø2WA4MZ
Ø312Ø9W
Ø312ØAW
Ø312ØJW
Ø312ØKW
Ø312ØZW
Ø313Ø9W
Ø313ØAW
Ø313ØJW
Ø313ØKW
Ø313ØZD
Ø313ØZW
Ø314Ø9W
Ø314ØAW
Ø314ØJW
Ø314ØKW
Ø314ØZD
Ø314ØZW
31509Ø
Ø315Ø9W
Ø315ØAØ
Ø315ØAW
Ø315ØJØ
Ø315ØJW
Ø315ØKØ
Ø315ØKW
Ø315ØZØ
Ø315ØZD
Ø315ØZT
Ø315ØZV
Ø315ØZW
316091
Ø316Ø9W
Ø316ØA1
Ø316ØAW
Ø316ØJ1
Ø316ØJW
Ø316ØK1
Ø316ØKW
Ø316ØZ1
Ø316ØZD
Ø316ØZT
Ø316ØZV
Ø316ØZW
Ø317Ø9D
Ø317Ø9F
Ø317Ø9V
Ø317Ø9W
Ø317ØAD
Ø317ØAF
Ø317ØAV
Ø317ØAW
Ø317ØJD
Ø317ØJF
Ø317ØJV
Ø317ØJW
Ø317ØKD
Ø317ØKF
Ø317ØKV
Ø317ØKW
Ø317ØZD
Ø317ØZF
Ø317ØZV
Ø317ØZW
Ø3173ZF
Ø318Ø9D
Ø318Ø9F
Ø318Ø9V
Ø318Ø9W
Ø318ØAD
Ø318ØAF
Ø318ØAV
Ø318ØAW
Ø318ØJD
Ø318ØJF
Ø318ØJV
Ø318ØJW
Ø318ØKD
Ø318ØKF
Ø318ØKV
Ø318ØKW
Ø318ØZD
Ø318ØZF
Ø318ØZV
Ø318ØZW
Ø3183ZF
Ø319Ø9F
Ø319ØAF
Ø319ØJF
Ø319ØKF
Ø319ØZF
Ø3193ZF
Ø31AØ9F
Ø31AØAF
Ø31AØJF
Ø31AØKF
Ø31AØZF
Ø31A3ZF
Ø31BØ9F
Ø31BØAF
Ø31BØJF
Ø31BØKF
Ø31BØZF
Ø31B3ZF
Ø31CØ9F
Ø31CØAF
Ø31CØJF
Ø31CØKF
Ø31CØZF
Ø31C3ZF
Ø31HØ9G
Ø31HØ9J
Ø31HØ9K
Ø31HØ9Y
Ø31HØAG
Ø31HØAJ
Ø31HØAK
Ø31HØAY
Ø31HØJG
Ø31HØJJ
Ø31HØJK
Ø31HØJY
Ø31HØKG
Ø31HØKJ
Ø31HØKK
Ø31HØKY
Ø31HØZG
Ø31HØZJ
Ø31HØZK
Ø31HØZY
Ø31JØ9G
Ø31JØ9J
Ø31JØ9K
Ø31JØ9Y
Ø31JØAG
Ø31JØAJ
Ø31JØAK
Ø31JØAY
Ø31JØJG
Ø31JØJJ
Ø31JØJK
Ø31JØJY
Ø31JØKG
Ø31JØKJ
Ø31JØKK
Ø31JØKY
Ø31JØZG
Ø31JØZJ
Ø31JØZK
Ø31JØZY
Ø31K*
Ø31L*
Ø31M*
Ø31N*
Ø31S*
Ø31T*
Ø355*
Ø356*
Ø357*
Ø358*
Ø359*
Ø35A*
Ø35B*
Ø35C*
Ø35D*
Ø35F*
Ø35G*
Ø35H*
Ø35J*
Ø35K*
Ø35L*
Ø35M*
Ø35N*
Ø35P*
Ø35Q*
Ø35R*
Ø35S*
Ø35T*
Ø35U*
Ø35V*
Ø35Y*
Ø37334Z
Ø37335Z
Ø37336Z
Ø37337Z
Ø3733D1
Ø3733DZ
Ø3733EZ
Ø3733FZ
Ø3733GZ
Ø3733Z1
Ø3733ZZ
Ø37434Z
Ø37435Z
Ø37436Z
Ø37437Z
Ø3743D1
Ø3743DZ
Ø3743EZ
Ø3743FZ
Ø3743GZ
Ø3743Z1
Ø3743ZZ
Ø37734Z
Ø37735Z
Ø37736Z
Ø37737Z
Ø3773D1
Ø3773DZ
Ø3773EZ
Ø3773FZ
Ø3773GZ
Ø3773Z1
Ø3773ZZ
Ø37834Z
Ø37835Z
Ø37836Z
Ø37837Z
Ø3783D1
Ø3783DZ
Ø3783EZ
Ø3783FZ
Ø3783GZ
Ø3783Z1
Ø3783ZZ
Ø37934Z
Ø37935Z
Ø37936Z
Ø37937Z
Ø3793D1
Ø3793DZ
Ø3793EZ
Ø3793FZ
Ø3793GZ
Ø3793Z1
Ø3793ZZ
Ø37A34Z
Ø37A35Z
Ø37A36Z
Ø37A37Z
Ø37A3D1
Ø37A3DZ
Ø37A3EZ
Ø37A3FZ
Ø37A3GZ
Ø37A3Z1
Ø37A3ZZ
Ø37G34Z
Ø37G35Z
Ø37G36Z
Ø37G37Z
Ø37G3DZ
Ø37G3EZ
Ø37G3FZ
Ø37G3GZ
Ø37G3ZZ
Ø37G44Z
Ø37G45Z
Ø37G46Z
Ø37G47Z
Ø37G4DZ
Ø37G4EZ
Ø37G4FZ
Ø37G4GZ
Ø37G4ZZ
Ø37H34Z
Ø37H35Z
Ø37H36Z
Ø37H37Z
Ø37H3DZ
Ø37H3EZ
Ø37H3FZ
Ø37H3GZ
Ø37H3ZZ
Ø37H44Z
Ø37H45Z
Ø37H46Z
Ø37H47Z
Ø37H4DZ
Ø37H4EZ
Ø37H4FZ
Ø37H4GZ
Ø37H4ZZ
Ø37J34Z
Ø37J35Z
Ø37J36Z
Ø37J37Z
Ø37J3DZ
Ø37J3EZ
Ø37J3FZ
Ø37J3GZ
Ø37J3ZZ
Ø37J44Z
Ø37J45Z
Ø37J46Z
Ø37J47Z
Ø37J4DZ
Ø37J4EZ
Ø37J4FZ
Ø37J4GZ
Ø37J4ZZ
Ø37K34Z
Ø37K35Z
Ø37K36Z
Ø37K37Z
Ø37K3DZ
Ø37K3EZ
Ø37K3FZ
Ø37K3GZ
Ø37K3ZZ
Ø37K44Z
Ø37K45Z
Ø37K46Z
Ø37K47Z
Ø37K4DZ
Ø37K4EZ
Ø37K4FZ
Ø37K4GZ
Ø37K4ZZ
Ø37L34Z
Ø37L35Z
Ø37L36Z
Ø37L37Z
Ø37L3DZ
Ø37L3EZ
Ø37L3FZ
Ø37L3GZ
Ø37L3ZZ
Ø37L44Z
Ø37L45Z
Ø37L46Z
Ø37L47Z
Ø37L4DZ
Ø37L4EZ
Ø37L4FZ
Ø37L4GZ
Ø37L4ZZ
Ø37M34Z
Ø37M35Z
Ø37M36Z
Ø37M37Z
Ø37M3DZ
Ø37M3EZ
Ø37M3FZ
Ø37M3GZ
Ø37M3ZZ
Ø37M44Z
Ø37M45Z
Ø37M46Z
Ø37M47Z
Ø37M4DZ
Ø37M4EZ
Ø37M4FZ
Ø37M4GZ
Ø37M4ZZ
Ø37N34Z
Ø37N35Z
Ø37N36Z
Ø37N37Z
Ø37N3DZ
Ø37N3EZ
Ø37N3FZ
Ø37N3GZ
Ø37N3ZZ
Ø37N44Z
Ø37N45Z
Ø37N46Z
Ø37N47Z
Ø37N4DZ
Ø37N4EZ
Ø37N4FZ
Ø37N4GZ
Ø37N4ZZ
Ø37P34Z
Ø37P35Z
Ø37P36Z
Ø37P37Z
Ø37P3DZ
Ø37P3EZ
Ø37P3FZ
Ø37P3GZ
Ø37P3ZZ
Ø37P44Z
Ø37P45Z
Ø37P46Z
Ø37P47Z
Ø37P4DZ
Ø37P4EZ
Ø37P4FZ
Ø37P4GZ
Ø37P4ZZ
Ø37Q34Z
Ø37Q35Z
Ø37Q36Z
Ø37Q37Z
Ø37Q3DZ
Ø37Q3EZ
Ø37Q3FZ
Ø37Q3GZ
Ø37Q3ZZ
Ø37Q44Z
Ø37Q45Z
Ø37Q46Z
Ø37Q47Z
Ø37Q4DZ
Ø37Q4EZ
Ø37Q4FZ
Ø37Q4GZ
Ø37Q4ZZ
Ø37Y34Z
Ø37Y35Z
Ø37Y36Z
Ø37Y37Z
Ø37Y3DZ
Ø37Y3EZ
Ø37Y3FZ
Ø37Y3GZ
Ø37Y3ZZ
Ø3BØ3ZZ
Ø3B13ZZ
Ø3B23ZZ
Ø3B33ZZ
Ø3B43ZZ
Ø3B5ØZZ
Ø3B53ZZ
Ø3B54ZZ
Ø3B6ØZZ
Ø3B63ZZ
Ø3B64ZZ
Ø3B7ØZZ
Ø3B73ZZ
Ø3B74ZZ
Ø3B8ØZZ
Ø3B83ZZ
Ø3B84ZZ
Ø3B9ØZZ
Ø3B93ZZ
Ø3B94ZZ
Ø3BAØZZ
Ø3BA3ZZ
Ø3BA4ZZ
Ø3BBØZZ
Ø3BB3ZZ
Ø3BB4ZZ
Ø3BCØZZ
Ø3BC3ZZ
Ø3BC4ZZ
Ø3BDØZZ
Ø3BD3ZZ
Ø3BD4ZZ
Ø3BFØZZ
Ø3BF3ZZ
Ø3BF4ZZ
Ø3BGØZZ
Ø3BG3ZZ
Ø3BG4ZZ
Ø3BHØZZ
Ø3BH3ZZ
Ø3BH4ZZ
Ø3BJØZZ
Ø3BJ3ZZ
Ø3BJ4ZZ
Ø3BKØZZ
Ø3BK3ZZ
Ø3BK4ZZ
Ø3BLØZZ
Ø3BL3ZZ
Ø3BL4ZZ
Ø3BMØZZ
Ø3BM3ZZ
Ø3BM4ZZ
Ø3BNØZZ
Ø3BN3ZZ
Ø3BN4ZZ
Ø3BPØZZ
Ø3BP3ZZ
Ø3BP4ZZ
Ø3BQØZZ
Ø3BQ3ZZ
Ø3BQ4ZZ
Ø3BRØZZ
Ø3BR3ZZ
Ø3BR4ZZ
Ø3BSØZZ
Ø3BS3ZZ
Ø3BS4ZZ
Ø3BTØZZ
Ø3BT3ZZ
Ø3BT4ZZ
Ø3BUØZZ
Ø3BU3ZZ
Ø3BU4ZZ
Ø3BVØZZ
Ø3BV3ZZ
Ø3BV4ZZ
Ø3BYØZZ
Ø3BY3ZZ
Ø3BY4ZZ
Ø3CØØZZ
Ø3CØ3ZZ
Ø3CØ4ZZ
Ø3C1ØZZ
Ø3C13ZZ
Ø3C14ZZ
Ø3C2ØZZ
Ø3C23ZZ
Ø3C24ZZ
Ø3C3ØZZ
Ø3C33ZZ
Ø3C34ZZ
Ø3C4ØZZ
Ø3C43ZZ
Ø3C44ZZ
Ø3C5ØZZ
Ø3C53ZZ
Ø3C54ZZ
Ø3C6ØZZ
Ø3C63ZZ
Ø3C64ZZ
Ø3C7ØZZ
Ø3C73ZZ
Ø3C74ZZ
Ø3C8ØZZ
Ø3C83ZZ
Ø3C84ZZ
Ø3C9ØZZ
Ø3C93ZZ
Ø3C94ZZ
Ø3CAØZZ
Ø3CA3ZZ
Ø3CA4ZZ
Ø3CBØZZ
Ø3CB3ZZ
Ø3CB4ZZ
Ø3CCØZZ
Ø3CC3ZZ
Ø3CC4ZZ
Ø3CDØZZ
Ø3CD3ZZ
Ø3CD4ZZ
Ø3CFØZZ
Ø3CF3ZZ
Ø3CF4ZZ
Ø3CGØZZ
Ø3CG3Z7
Ø3CG3ZZ
Ø3CG4ZZ
Ø3CHØZZ
Ø3CH3Z7
Ø3CH3ZZ
Ø3CH4ZZ
Ø3CJØZZ
Ø3CJ3Z7
Ø3CJ3ZZ
Ø3CJ4ZZ
Ø3CKØZZ
Ø3CK3Z7
Ø3CK3ZZ
Ø3CK4ZZ
Ø3CLØZZ
Ø3CL3Z7
Ø3CL3ZZ
Ø3CL4ZZ
Ø3CMØZZ
Ø3CM3Z7
Ø3CM3ZZ
Ø3CM4ZZ
Ø3CNØZZ
Ø3CN3Z7
Ø3CN3ZZ
Ø3CN4ZZ
Ø3CPØZZ
Ø3CP3Z7
Ø3CP3ZZ
Ø3CP4ZZ
Ø3CQØZZ
Ø3CQ3Z7
Ø3CQ3ZZ
Ø3CQ4ZZ
Ø3CRØZZ
Ø3CR3ZZ
Ø3CR4ZZ
Ø3CSØZZ
Ø3CS3ZZ
Ø3CS4ZZ
Ø3CTØZZ
Ø3CT3ZZ
Ø3CT4ZZ
Ø3CUØZZ
Ø3CU3ZZ
Ø3CU4ZZ

Ø3CVØZZ
Ø3CV3ZZ
Ø3CV4ZZ
Ø3CYØZZ
Ø3CY3ZZ
Ø3CY4ZZ
Ø3HØØDZ
Ø3HØ3DZ
Ø3HØ4DZ
Ø3H1ØDZ
Ø3H13DZ
Ø3H14DZ
Ø3H2ØDZ
Ø3H23DZ
Ø3H24DZ
Ø3H3ØDZ
Ø3H33DZ
Ø3H34DZ
Ø3H4ØDZ
Ø3H43DZ
Ø3H44DZ
Ø3H5ØDZ
Ø3H53DZ
Ø3H54DZ
Ø3H6ØDZ
Ø3H63DZ
Ø3H64DZ
Ø3H7ØDZ
Ø3H73DZ
Ø3H74DZ
Ø3H8ØDZ
Ø3H83DZ
Ø3H84DZ
Ø3H9ØDZ
Ø3H93DZ
Ø3H94DZ
Ø3HAØDZ
Ø3HA3DZ
Ø3HA4DZ
Ø3HBØDZ
Ø3HB3DZ
Ø3HB4DZ
Ø3HCØDZ
Ø3HC3DZ
Ø3HC4DZ
Ø3HDØDZ
Ø3HD3DZ
Ø3HD4DZ
Ø3HFØDZ
Ø3HF3DZ
Ø3HF4DZ
Ø3HGØDZ
Ø3HG3DZ
Ø3HG4DZ
Ø3HHØDZ
Ø3HH3DZ
Ø3HH4DZ
Ø3HJØDZ
Ø3HJ3DZ
Ø3HJ4DZ
Ø3HKØDZ
Ø3HK3DZ
Ø3HK4DZ
Ø3HLØDZ
Ø3HL3DZ
Ø3HL4DZ
Ø3HMØDZ
Ø3HM3DZ
Ø3HM4DZ
Ø3HNØDZ
Ø3HN3DZ
Ø3HN4DZ
Ø3HPØDZ
Ø3HP3DZ
Ø3HP4DZ
Ø3HQØDZ
Ø3HQ3DZ
Ø3HQ4DZ
Ø3HRØDZ
Ø3HR3DZ
Ø3HR4DZ
Ø3HSØDZ
Ø3HS3DZ
Ø3HS4DZ
Ø3HTØDZ
Ø3HT3DZ
Ø3HT4DZ
Ø3HUØDZ
Ø3HU3DZ
Ø3HU4DZ
Ø3HVØDZ
Ø3HV3DZ
Ø3HV4DZ
Ø3HYØDZ
Ø3HY3DZ
Ø3HY4DZ
Ø3LØ*
Ø3L1*
Ø3L2*
Ø3L3*
Ø3L4*
Ø3L5*
Ø3L6*
Ø3L7*
Ø3L8*
Ø3L9*
Ø3LA*
Ø3LB*
Ø3LC*
Ø3LD*
Ø3LF*
Ø3LG*
Ø3LH*
Ø3LJ*
Ø3LKØBZ
Ø3LKØDZ
Ø3LK3BZ
Ø3LK3DZ
Ø3LK4BZ
Ø3LK4DZ
Ø3LLØBZ
Ø3LLØDZ
Ø3LL3BZ
Ø3LL3DZ
Ø3LL4BZ
Ø3LL4DZ
Ø3LM*
Ø3LN*
Ø3LP*
Ø3LQ*
Ø3LR*
Ø3LS*
Ø3LT*
Ø3LU*
Ø3LV*
Ø3LY*
Ø3PYØ7Z
Ø3PYØJZ
Ø3PYØKZ
Ø3PY37Z
Ø3PY3JZ
Ø3PY3KZ
Ø3PY47Z
Ø3PY4JZ
Ø3PY4KZ
Ø3Q*
Ø3RØ*
Ø3R1*
Ø3R2*
Ø3R3*
Ø3R4*
Ø3R5*
Ø3R6*
Ø3R7*
Ø3R8*
Ø3R9*
Ø3RA*
Ø3RB*
Ø3RC*
Ø3RD*
Ø3RF*
Ø3RG*
Ø3RY*
Ø3S*
Ø3UØØ7Z
Ø3UØØJZ
Ø3UØ37Z
Ø3UØ3JZ
Ø3UØ47Z
Ø3UØ4JZ
Ø3U1Ø7Z
Ø3U1ØJZ
Ø3U137Z
Ø3U13JZ
Ø3U147Z
Ø3U14JZ
Ø3U2Ø7Z
Ø3U2ØJZ
Ø3U237Z
Ø3U23JZ
Ø3U247Z
Ø3U24JZ
Ø3U3Ø7Z
Ø3U3ØJZ
Ø3U337Z
Ø3U33JZ
Ø3U347Z
Ø3U34JZ
Ø3U4Ø7Z
Ø3U4ØJZ
Ø3U437Z
Ø3U43JZ
Ø3U447Z
Ø3U44JZ
Ø3U5Ø7Z
Ø3U5ØJZ
Ø3U537Z
Ø3U53JZ
Ø3U547Z
Ø3U54JZ
Ø3U6Ø7Z
Ø3U6ØJZ
Ø3U637Z
Ø3U63JZ
Ø3U647Z
Ø3U64JZ
Ø3U7Ø7Z
Ø3U7ØJZ
Ø3U737Z
Ø3U73JZ
Ø3U747Z
Ø3U74JZ
Ø3U8Ø7Z
Ø3U8ØJZ
Ø3U837Z
Ø3U83JZ
Ø3U847Z
Ø3U84JZ
Ø3U9Ø7Z
Ø3U9ØJZ
Ø3U937Z
Ø3U93JZ
Ø3U947Z
Ø3U94JZ
Ø3UAØ7Z
Ø3UAØJZ
Ø3UA37Z
Ø3UA3JZ
Ø3UA47Z
Ø3UA4JZ
Ø3UBØ7Z
Ø3UBØJZ
Ø3UB37Z
Ø3UB3JZ
Ø3UB47Z
Ø3UB4JZ
Ø3UCØ7Z
Ø3UCØJZ
Ø3UC37Z
Ø3UC3JZ
Ø3UC47Z
Ø3UC4JZ
Ø3UDØ7Z
Ø3UDØJZ
Ø3UD37Z
Ø3UD3JZ
Ø3UD47Z
Ø3UD4JZ
Ø3UFØ7Z
Ø3UFØJZ
Ø3UF37Z
Ø3UF3JZ
Ø3UF47Z
Ø3UF4JZ
Ø3UGØ7Z
Ø3UGØJZ
Ø3UG37Z
Ø3UG3JZ
Ø3UG47Z
Ø3UG4JZ
Ø3UHØ7Z
Ø3UHØJZ
Ø3UH37Z
Ø3UH3JZ
Ø3UH47Z
Ø3UH4JZ
Ø3UJØ7Z
Ø3UJØJZ
Ø3UJ37Z
Ø3UJ3JZ
Ø3UJ47Z
Ø3UJ4JZ
Ø3UKØ7Z
Ø3UKØJZ
Ø3UK37Z
Ø3UK3JZ
Ø3UK47Z
Ø3UK4JZ
Ø3ULØ7Z
Ø3ULØJZ
Ø3UL37Z
Ø3UL3JZ
Ø3UL47Z
Ø3UL4JZ
Ø3UMØ7Z
Ø3UMØJZ
Ø3UM37Z
Ø3UM3JZ
Ø3UM47Z
Ø3UM4JZ
Ø3UNØ7Z
Ø3UNØJZ
Ø3UN37Z
Ø3UN3JZ
Ø3UN47Z
Ø3UN4JZ
Ø3UPØ7Z
Ø3UPØJZ
Ø3UP37Z
Ø3UP3JZ
Ø3UP47Z
Ø3UP4JZ
Ø3UQØ7Z
Ø3UQØJZ
Ø3UQ37Z
Ø3UQ3JZ
Ø3UQ47Z
Ø3UQ4JZ
Ø3URØ7Z
Ø3URØJZ
Ø3UR37Z
Ø3UR3JZ
Ø3UR47Z
Ø3UR4JZ
Ø3USØ7Z
Ø3USØJZ
Ø3US37Z
Ø3US3JZ
Ø3US47Z
Ø3US4JZ
Ø3UTØ7Z
Ø3UTØJZ
Ø3UT37Z
Ø3UT3JZ
Ø3UT47Z
Ø3UT4JZ
Ø3UUØ7Z
Ø3UUØJZ
Ø3UU37Z
Ø3UU3JZ
Ø3UU47Z
Ø3UU4JZ
Ø3UVØ7Z
Ø3UVØJZ
Ø3UV37Z
Ø3UV3JZ
Ø3UV47Z
Ø3UV4JZ
Ø3UYØ7Z
Ø3UYØJZ
Ø3UY37Z
Ø3UY3JZ
Ø3UY47Z
Ø3UY4JZ
Ø3VØØDZ
Ø3VØØZZ
Ø3VØ3DZ
Ø3VØ3ZZ
Ø3VØ4DZ
Ø3VØ4ZZ
Ø3V1ØDZ
Ø3V1ØZZ
Ø3V13DZ
Ø3V13ZZ
Ø3V14DZ
Ø3V14ZZ
Ø3V2ØDZ
Ø3V2ØZZ
Ø3V23DZ
Ø3V23ZZ
Ø3V24DZ
Ø3V24ZZ
Ø3V3ØDZ
Ø3V3ØZZ
Ø3V33DZ
Ø3V33ZZ
Ø3V34DZ
Ø3V34ZZ
Ø3V4ØDZ
Ø3V4ØZZ
Ø3V43DZ
Ø3V43ZZ
Ø3V44DZ
Ø3V44ZZ
Ø3V5ØDZ
Ø3V5ØZZ
Ø3V53DZ
Ø3V53ZZ
Ø3V54DZ
Ø3V54ZZ
Ø3V6ØDZ
Ø3V6ØZZ
Ø3V63DZ
Ø3V63ZZ
Ø3V64DZ
Ø3V64ZZ
Ø3V7ØDZ
Ø3V7ØZZ
Ø3V73DZ
Ø3V73ZZ
Ø3V74DZ
Ø3V74ZZ
Ø3V8ØDZ
Ø3V8ØZZ
Ø3V83DZ
Ø3V83ZZ
Ø3V84DZ
Ø3V84ZZ
Ø3V9ØDZ
Ø3V9ØZZ
Ø3V93DZ
Ø3V93ZZ
Ø3V94DZ
Ø3V94ZZ
Ø3VAØDZ
Ø3VAØZZ
Ø3VA3DZ
Ø3VA3ZZ
Ø3VA4DZ
Ø3VA4ZZ
Ø3VBØDZ
Ø3VBØZZ
Ø3VB3DZ
Ø3VB3ZZ
Ø3VB4DZ
Ø3VB4ZZ
Ø3VCØDZ
Ø3VCØZZ
Ø3VC3DZ
Ø3VC3ZZ
Ø3VC4DZ
Ø3VC4ZZ
Ø3VDØDZ
Ø3VDØZZ
Ø3VD3DZ
Ø3VD3ZZ
Ø3VD4DZ
Ø3VD4ZZ
Ø3VFØDZ
Ø3VFØZZ
Ø3VF3DZ
Ø3VF3ZZ
Ø3VF4DZ
Ø3VF4ZZ
Ø3VGØBZ
Ø3VGØDZ
Ø3VGØHZ
Ø3VGØZZ
Ø3VG3BZ
Ø3VG3DZ
Ø3VG3HZ
Ø3VG3ZZ
Ø3VG4BZ
Ø3VG4DZ
Ø3VG4HZ
Ø3VG4ZZ
Ø3VHØBZ
Ø3VHØDZ
Ø3VHØHZ
Ø3VHØZZ
Ø3VH3BZ
Ø3VH3DZ
Ø3VH3HZ
Ø3VH3ZZ
Ø3VH4BZ
Ø3VH4DZ
Ø3VH4HZ
Ø3VH4ZZ
Ø3VJØBZ
Ø3VJØDZ
Ø3VJØHZ
Ø3VJØZZ
Ø3VJ3BZ
Ø3VJ3DZ
Ø3VJ3HZ
Ø3VJ3ZZ
Ø3VJ4BZ
Ø3VJ4DZ
Ø3VJ4HZ
Ø3VJ4ZZ
Ø3VKØBZ
Ø3VKØDZ
Ø3VKØHZ
Ø3VKØZZ
Ø3VK3BZ
Ø3VK3DZ
Ø3VK3HZ
Ø3VK3ZZ
Ø3VK4BZ
Ø3VK4DZ
Ø3VK4HZ
Ø3VK4ZZ
Ø3VLØBZ
Ø3VLØDZ
Ø3VLØHZ
Ø3VLØZZ
Ø3VL3BZ
Ø3VL3DZ
Ø3VL3HZ
Ø3VL3ZZ
Ø3VL4BZ
Ø3VL4DZ
Ø3VL4HZ
Ø3VL4ZZ
Ø3VMØBZ
Ø3VMØDZ
Ø3VMØHZ
Ø3VMØZZ
Ø3VM3BZ
Ø3VM3DZ
Ø3VM3HZ
Ø3VM3ZZ
Ø3VM4BZ
Ø3VM4DZ
Ø3VM4HZ
Ø3VM4ZZ
Ø3VNØBZ
Ø3VNØDZ
Ø3VNØHZ
Ø3VNØZZ
Ø3VN3BZ
Ø3VN3DZ
Ø3VN3HZ
Ø3VN3ZZ
Ø3VN4BZ
Ø3VN4DZ
Ø3VN4HZ
Ø3VN4ZZ
Ø3VPØBZ
Ø3VPØDZ
Ø3VPØHZ
Ø3VPØZZ
Ø3VP3BZ
Ø3VP3DZ
Ø3VP3HZ
Ø3VP3ZZ
Ø3VP4BZ
Ø3VP4DZ
Ø3VP4HZ
Ø3VP4ZZ
Ø3VQØBZ
Ø3VQØDZ
Ø3VQØHZ
Ø3VQØZZ
Ø3VQ3BZ
Ø3VQ3DZ
Ø3VQ3HZ
Ø3VQ3ZZ
Ø3VQ4BZ
Ø3VQ4DZ
Ø3VQ4HZ
Ø3VQ4ZZ
Ø3VRØDZ
Ø3VRØZZ
Ø3VR3DZ
Ø3VR3ZZ
Ø3VR4DZ
Ø3VR4ZZ
Ø3VSØDZ
Ø3VSØZZ
Ø3VS3DZ
Ø3VS3ZZ
Ø3VS4DZ
Ø3VS4ZZ
Ø3VTØDZ
Ø3VTØZZ
Ø3VT3DZ
Ø3VT3ZZ
Ø3VT4DZ
Ø3VT4ZZ
Ø3VUØDZ
Ø3VUØZZ
Ø3VU3DZ
Ø3VU3ZZ
Ø3VU4DZ
Ø3VU4ZZ
Ø3VVØDZ
Ø3VVØZZ
Ø3VV3DZ
Ø3VV3ZZ
Ø3VV4DZ
Ø3VV4ZZ
Ø3VYØDZ
Ø3VYØZZ
Ø3VY3DZ
Ø3VY3ZZ
Ø3VY4DZ
Ø3VY4ZZ
41ØØ93
41ØØ94
41ØØ95
41ØØ96
41ØØ97
41ØØ98
41ØØ99
Ø41ØØ9B
Ø41ØØ9C
Ø41ØØ9D
Ø41ØØ9F
Ø41ØØ9G
Ø41ØØ9H
Ø41ØØ9J
Ø41ØØ9K
Ø41ØØ9Q
Ø41ØØ9R
Ø41ØØA3
Ø41ØØA4
Ø41ØØA5
Ø41ØØA6
Ø41ØØA7
Ø41ØØA8
Ø41ØØA9
Ø41ØØAB
Ø41ØØAC
Ø41ØØAD
Ø41ØØAF
Ø41ØØAG
Ø41ØØAH
Ø41ØØAJ
Ø41ØØAK
Ø41ØØAQ
Ø41ØØAR
Ø41ØØJ3
Ø41ØØJ4
Ø41ØØJ5
Ø41ØØJ6
Ø41ØØJ7
Ø41ØØJ8
Ø41ØØJ9
Ø41ØØJB
Ø41ØØJC
Ø41ØØJD
Ø41ØØJF
Ø41ØØJG
Ø41ØØJH
Ø41ØØJJ
Ø41ØØJK
Ø41ØØJQ
Ø41ØØJR
Ø41ØØK3
Ø41ØØK4
Ø41ØØK5
Ø41ØØK6
Ø41ØØK7
Ø41ØØK8
Ø41ØØK9
Ø41ØØKB
Ø41ØØKC
Ø41ØØKD
Ø41ØØKF
Ø41ØØKG
Ø41ØØKH
Ø41ØØKJ
Ø41ØØKK
Ø41ØØKQ
Ø41ØØKR
Ø41ØØZ3
Ø41ØØZ4
Ø41ØØZ5
Ø41ØØZ6
Ø41ØØZ7
Ø41ØØZ8
Ø41ØØZ9
Ø41ØØZB
Ø41ØØZC
Ø41ØØZD
Ø41ØØZF
Ø41ØØZG
Ø41ØØZH
Ø41ØØZJ
Ø41ØØZK
Ø41ØØZQ
Ø41ØØZR
41Ø493
41Ø494
41Ø495
41Ø496
41Ø497
41Ø498
41Ø499
Ø41Ø49B
Ø41Ø49C
Ø41Ø49D
Ø41Ø49F
Ø41Ø49G
Ø41Ø49H
Ø41Ø49J
Ø41Ø49K
Ø41Ø49Q
Ø41Ø49R
Ø41Ø4A3
Ø41Ø4A4
Ø41Ø4A5
Ø41Ø4A6
Ø41Ø4A7
Ø41Ø4A8
Ø41Ø4A9
Ø41Ø4AB
Ø41Ø4AC
Ø41Ø4AD
Ø41Ø4AF
Ø41Ø4AG
Ø41Ø4AH
Ø41Ø4AJ
Ø41Ø4AK
Ø41Ø4AQ
Ø41Ø4AR
Ø41Ø4J3
Ø41Ø4J4
Ø41Ø4J5
Ø41Ø4J6
Ø41Ø4J7
Ø41Ø4J8
Ø41Ø4J9
Ø41Ø4JB
Ø41Ø4JC
Ø41Ø4JD
Ø41Ø4JF
Ø41Ø4JG
Ø41Ø4JH
Ø41Ø4JJ
Ø41Ø4JK
Ø41Ø4JQ
Ø41Ø4JR
Ø41Ø4K3
Ø41Ø4K4
Ø41Ø4K5
Ø41Ø4K6
Ø41Ø4K7
Ø41Ø4K8
Ø41Ø4K9
Ø41Ø4KB
Ø41Ø4KC
Ø41Ø4KD
Ø41Ø4KF
Ø41Ø4KG
Ø41Ø4KH
Ø41Ø4KJ
Ø41Ø4KK
Ø41Ø4KQ
Ø41Ø4KR
Ø41Ø4Z3
Ø41Ø4Z4
Ø41Ø4Z5
Ø41Ø4Z6
Ø41Ø4Z7
Ø41Ø4Z8
Ø41Ø4Z9
Ø41Ø4ZB
Ø41Ø4ZC
Ø41Ø4ZD
Ø41Ø4ZF
Ø41Ø4ZG
Ø41Ø4ZH
Ø41Ø4ZJ
Ø41Ø4ZK
Ø41Ø4ZQ
Ø41Ø4ZR
413Ø93
413Ø94
413Ø95
Ø413ØA3
Ø413ØA4
Ø413ØA5
Ø413ØJ3
Ø413ØJ4
Ø413ØJ5
Ø413ØK3
Ø413ØK4
Ø413ØK5
Ø413ØZ3
Ø413ØZ4
Ø413ØZ5
413493
413494
413495
Ø4134A3
Ø4134A4
Ø4134A5
Ø4134J3
Ø4134J4
Ø4134J5
Ø4134K3
Ø4134K4
Ø4134K5
Ø4134Z3
Ø4134Z4
Ø4134Z5
Ø41CØ9H
Ø41CØ9J
Ø41CØ9K
Ø41CØAH
Ø41CØAJ
Ø41CØAK
Ø41CØJH
Ø41CØJJ
Ø41CØJK
Ø41CØKH
Ø41CØKJ
Ø41CØKK
Ø41CØZH
Ø41CØZJ
Ø41CØZK
Ø41C49H
Ø41C49J
Ø41C49K
Ø41C4AH
Ø41C4AJ
Ø41C4AK
Ø41C4JH
Ø41C4JJ
Ø41C4JK
Ø41C4KH
Ø41C4KJ
Ø41C4KK
Ø41C4ZH
Ø41C4ZJ
Ø41C4ZK
Ø41DØ9H
Ø41DØ9J
Ø41DØ9K
Ø41DØAH
Ø41DØAJ
Ø41DØAK
Ø41DØJH
Ø41DØJJ
Ø41DØJK
Ø41DØKH
Ø41DØKJ
Ø41DØKK
Ø41DØZH
Ø41DØZJ
Ø41DØZK
Ø41D49H
Ø41D49J
Ø41D49K
Ø41D4AH
Ø41D4AJ
Ø41D4AK
Ø41D4JH
Ø41D4JJ
Ø41D4JK
Ø41D4KH
Ø41D4KJ
Ø41D4KK
Ø41D4ZH
Ø41D4ZJ
Ø41D4ZK
Ø41EØ9H
Ø41EØ9J
Ø41EØ9K
Ø41EØAH
Ø41EØAJ
Ø41EØAK
Ø41EØJH
Ø41EØJJ
Ø41EØJK
Ø41EØKH
Ø41EØKJ
Ø41EØKK
Ø41EØZH
Ø41EØZJ
Ø41EØZK
Ø41E49H
Ø41E49J

041E49K
041E4AH
041E4AJ
041E4AK
041E4JH
041E4JJ
041E4JK
041E4KH
041E4KJ
041E4KK
041E4ZH
041E4ZJ
041E4ZK
041F09H
041F09J
041F09K
041F0AH
041F0AJ
041F0AK
041F0JH
041F0JJ
041F0JK
041F0KH
041F0KJ
041F0KK
041F0ZH
041F0ZJ
041F0ZK
041F49H
041F49J
041F49K
041F4AH
041F4AJ
041F4AK
041F4JH
041F4JJ
041F4JK
041F4KH
041F4KJ
041F4KK
041F4ZH
041F4ZJ
041F4ZK
041H09H
041H09J
041H09K
041H0AH
041H0AJ
041H0AK
041H0JH
041H0JJ
041H0JK
041H0KH
041H0KJ
041H0KK
041H0ZH
041H0ZJ
041H0ZK
041H49H
041H49J
041H49K
041H4AH
041H4AJ
041H4AK
041H4JH
041H4JJ
041H4JK
041H4KH
041H4KJ
041H4KK
041H4ZH
041H4ZJ
041H4ZK
041J09H
041J09J
041J09K
041J0AH
041J0AJ
041J0AK
041J0JH
041J0JJ
041J0JK
041J0KH
041J0KJ
041J0KK
041J0ZH
041J0ZJ
041J0ZK
041J49H
041J49J
041J49K
041J4AH
041J4AJ
041J4AK
041J4JH
041J4JJ
041J4JK
041J4KH
041J4KJ
041J4KK
041J4ZH
041J4ZJ
041J4ZK
041K09H
041K09J
041K09K
041K09L
041K0AH
041K0AJ
041K0AK
041K0AL
041K0JH
041K0JJ
041K0JK
041K0JL
041K0KH
041K0KJ
041K0KK
041K0KL
041K0ZH
041K0ZJ
041K0ZK
041K0ZL
041K49H
041K49J
041K49K
041K49L
041K4AH
041K4AJ
041K4AK
041K4AL
041K4JH
041K4JJ
041K4JK
041K4JL
041K4KH
041K4KJ
041K4KK
041K4KL
041K4ZH
041K4ZJ
041K4ZK
041K4ZL
041L09H
041L09J
041L09K
041L09L
041L0AH
041L0AJ
041L0AK
041L0AL
041L0JH
041L0JJ
041L0JK
041L0JL
041L0KH
041L0KJ
041L0KK
041L0KL
041L0ZH
041L0ZJ
041L0ZK
041L0ZL
041L49H
041L49J
041L49K
041L49L
041L4AH
041L4AJ
041L4AK
041L4AL
041L4JH
041L4JJ
041L4JK
041L4JL
041L4KH
041L4KJ
041L4KK
041L4KL
041L4ZH
041L4ZJ
041L4ZK
041L4ZL
0450*
045K*
045L*
045M*
045N*
045P*
045Q*
045R*
045S*
045T*
045U*
045V*
045W*
045Y*
470341
047034Z
047035Z
047036Z
047037Z
04703D1
04703DZ
04703EZ
04703FZ
04703GZ
04703Z1
04703ZZ
471341
047134Z
047135Z
047136Z
047137Z
04713D1
04713DZ
04713EZ
04713FZ
04713GZ
04713Z1
04713ZZ
472341
047234Z
047235Z
047236Z
047237Z
04723D1
04723DZ
04723EZ
04723FZ
04723GZ
04723Z1
04723ZZ
473341
047334Z
047335Z
047336Z
047337Z
04733D1
04733DZ
04733EZ
04733FZ
04733GZ
04733Z1
04733ZZ
474341
047434Z
047435Z
047436Z
047437Z
04743D1
04743DZ
04743EZ
04743FZ
04743GZ
04743Z1
04743ZZ
475341
047534Z
047535Z
047536Z
047537Z
04753D1
04753DZ
04753EZ
04753FZ
04753GZ
04753Z1
04753ZZ
476341
047634Z
047635Z
047636Z
047637Z
04763D1
04763DZ
04763EZ
04763FZ
04763GZ
04763Z1
04763ZZ
477341
047734Z
047735Z
047736Z
047737Z
04773D1
04773DZ
04773EZ
04773FZ
04773GZ
04773Z1
04773ZZ
478341
047834Z
047835Z
047836Z
047837Z
04783D1
04783DZ
04783EZ
04783FZ
04783GZ
04783Z1
04783ZZ
479341
047934Z
047935Z
047936Z
047937Z
04793D1
04793DZ
04793EZ
04793FZ
04793GZ
04793Z1
04793ZZ
047A341
047A34Z
047A35Z
047A36Z
047A37Z
047A3D1
047A3DZ
047A3EZ
047A3FZ
047A3GZ
047A3Z1
047A3ZZ
047B341
047B34Z
047B35Z
047B36Z
047B37Z
047B3D1
047B3DZ
047B3EZ
047B3FZ
047B3GZ
047B3Z1
047B3ZZ
047C341
047C34Z
047C35Z
047C36Z
047C37Z
047C3D1
047C3DZ
047C3EZ
047C3FZ
047C3GZ
047C3Z1
047C3ZZ
047D341
047D34Z
047D35Z
047D36Z
047D37Z
047D3D1
047D3DZ
047D3EZ
047D3FZ
047D3GZ
047D3Z1
047D3ZZ
047E341
047E34Z
047E35Z
047E36Z
047E37Z
047E3D1
047E3DZ
047E3EZ
047E3FZ
047E3GZ
047E3Z1
047E3ZZ
047F341
047F34Z
047F35Z
047F36Z
047F37Z
047F3D1
047F3DZ
047F3EZ
047F3FZ
047F3GZ
047F3Z1
047F3ZZ
047H341
047H34Z
047H35Z
047H36Z
047H37Z
047H3D1
047H3DZ
047H3EZ
047H3FZ
047H3GZ
047H3Z1
047H3ZZ
047J341
047J34Z
047J35Z
047J36Z
047J37Z
047J3D1
047J3DZ
047J3EZ
047J3FZ
047J3GZ
047J3Z1
047J3ZZ
047K041
047K0D1
047K0Z1
047K341
047K34Z
047K35Z
047K36Z
047K37Z
047K3D1
047K3DZ
047K3EZ
047K3FZ
047K3GZ
047K3Z1
047K3ZZ
047K441
047K4D1
047K4Z1
047L041
047L0D1
047L0Z1
047L341
047L34Z
047L35Z
047L36Z
047L37Z
047L3D1
047L3DZ
047L3EZ
047L3FZ
047L3GZ
047L3Z1
047L3ZZ
047L441
047L4D1
047L4Z1
047M041
047M0D1
047M0Z1
047M341
047M3D1
047M3Z1
047M441
047M4D1
047M4Z1
047N041
047N0D1
047N0Z1
047N341
047N3D1
047N3Z1
047N441
047N4D1
047N4Z1
047Y341
047Y34Z
047Y35Z
047Y36Z
047Y37Z
047Y3D1
047Y3DZ
047Y3EZ
047Y3FZ
047Y3GZ
047Y3Z1
047Y3ZZ
04B00ZZ
04B03ZZ
04B04ZZ
04B10ZZ
04B14ZZ
04B20ZZ
04B24ZZ
04B30ZZ
04B34ZZ
04B40ZZ
04B44ZZ
04B50ZZ
04B54ZZ
04B60ZZ
04B64ZZ
04B70ZZ
04B74ZZ
04B80ZZ
04B84ZZ
04B90ZZ
04B94ZZ
04BA0ZZ
04BA4ZZ
04BB0ZZ
04BB4ZZ
04BC0ZZ
04BC4ZZ
04BD0ZZ
04BD4ZZ
04BE0ZZ
04BE4ZZ
04BF0ZZ
04BF4ZZ
04BH0ZZ
04BH4ZZ
04BJ0ZZ
04BJ4ZZ
04BK0ZZ
04BK3ZZ
04BK4ZZ
04BL0ZZ
04BL3ZZ
04BL4ZZ
04BM0ZZ
04BM3ZZ
04BM4ZZ
04BN0ZZ
04BN3ZZ
04BN4ZZ
04BP0ZZ
04BP3ZZ
04BP4ZZ
04BQ0ZZ
04BQ3ZZ
04BQ4ZZ
04BR0ZZ
04BR3ZZ
04BR4ZZ
04BS0ZZ
04BS3ZZ
04BS4ZZ
04BT0ZZ
04BT3ZZ
04BT4ZZ
04BU0ZZ
04BU3ZZ
04BU4ZZ
04BV0ZZ
04BV3ZZ
04BV4ZZ
04BW0ZZ
04BW3ZZ
04BW4ZZ
04BY0ZZ
04BY3ZZ
04BY4ZZ
04C*
04H00DZ
04H03DZ
04H04DZ
04H10DZ
04H13DZ
04H14DZ
04H20DZ
04H23DZ
04H24DZ
04H30DZ
04H33DZ
04H34DZ
04H40DZ
04H43DZ
04H44DZ
04H50DZ
04H53DZ
04H54DZ
04H60DZ
04H63DZ
04H64DZ
04H70DZ
04H73DZ
04H74DZ
04H80DZ
04H83DZ
04H84DZ
04H90DZ
04H93DZ
04H94DZ
04HA0DZ
04HA3DZ
04HA4DZ
04HB0DZ
04HB3DZ
04HB4DZ
04HC0DZ
04HC3DZ
04HC4DZ
04HD0DZ
04HD3DZ
04HD4DZ
04HE0DZ
04HE3DZ
04HE4DZ
04HF0DZ
04HF3DZ
04HF4DZ
04HH0DZ
04HH3DZ
04HH4DZ
04HJ0DZ
04HJ3DZ
04HJ4DZ
04HK0DZ
04HK3DZ
04HK4DZ
04HL0DZ
04HL3DZ
04HL4DZ
04HM0DZ
04HM3DZ
04HM4DZ
04HN0DZ
04HN3DZ
04HN4DZ
04HP0DZ
04HP3DZ
04HP4DZ
04HQ0DZ
04HQ3DZ
04HQ4DZ
04HR0DZ
04HR3DZ
04HR4DZ
04HS0DZ
04HS3DZ
04HS4DZ
04HT0DZ
04HT3DZ
04HT4DZ
04HU0DZ
04HU3DZ
04HU4DZ
04HV0DZ
04HV3DZ
04HV4DZ
04HW0DZ
04HW3DZ
04HW4DZ
04HY02Z
04HY0DZ
04HY0YZ
04HY3DZ
04HY42Z
04HY4DZ
04L0*
04L1*
04L20CZ
04L20DZ
04L20ZZ
04L23CZ
04L23DZ
04L23ZZ
04L24CZ
04L24DZ
04L24ZZ
04L3*
04L4*
04L5*
04L6*
04L7*
04L8*
04L9*
04LA*
04LB*
04LC*
04LD*
04LE0CV
04LE0CZ
04LE0DV
04LE0DZ
04LE0ZV
04LE0ZZ
04LE3CV
04LE3CZ
04LE3DV
04LE3DZ
04LE3ZV
04LE3ZZ
04LE4CV
04LE4CZ
04LE4DV
04LE4DZ
04LE4ZV
04LE4ZZ
04LF0CW
04LF0CZ
04LF0DW
04LF0DZ
04LF0ZW
04LF0ZZ
04LF3CW
04LF3CZ
04LF3DW
04LF3DZ
04LF3ZW
04LF3ZZ
04LF4CW
04LF4CZ
04LF4DW
04LF4DZ
04LF4ZW
04LF4ZZ
04LH*
04LJ*
04LK*
04LL*
04LM*
04LN*
04LP*
04LQ*
04LR*
04LS*
04LT*
04LU*
04LV*
04LW*
04LY*
04PY00Z
04PY02Z
04PY03Z
04PY0CZ
04PY0DZ
04PY0YZ
04PY3CZ
04PY40Z
04PY42Z
04PY43Z
04PY4CZ
04PY4DZ
04Q*
04R0*
04R1*
04R2*
04R3*
04R4*
04R5*
04R6*
04R7*
04R8*
04RB*
04RC*
04RD*
04RE*
04RF*
04RH*
04RJ*
04RK*
04RL*
04RM*
04RN*
04RP*
04RQ*
04RR*
04RS*
04RT*
04RU*
04RV*
04RW*
04RY*
04S0*
04S1*
04S2*
04S3*
04S4*
04S5*
04S6*
04S7*
04S8*
04SB*
04SC*
04SD*
04SE*
04SF*
04SH*
04SJ*
04SK*
04SL*
04SM*
04SN*
04SP*
04SQ*
04SR*
04SS*
04ST*
04SU*
04SV*
04SW*
04SY*
04U007Z
04U00JZ
04U037Z
04U03JZ
04U047Z
04U04JZ
04U107Z
04U10JZ
04U137Z
04U13JZ
04U147Z
04U14JZ
04U207Z
04U20JZ
04U237Z
04U23JZ
04U247Z
04U24JZ
04U307Z
04U30JZ
04U337Z
04U33JZ
04U347Z
04U34JZ
04U407Z
04U40JZ
04U437Z
04U43JZ
04U447Z
04U44JZ
04U507Z
04U50JZ
04U537Z
04U53JZ
04U547Z
04U54JZ
04U607Z
04U60JZ
04U637Z
04U63JZ
04U647Z
04U64JZ
04U707Z
04U70JZ
04U737Z
04U73JZ
04U747Z
04U74JZ
04U807Z
04U80JZ
04U837Z
04U83JZ
04U847Z
04U84JZ
04U907Z
04U90JZ
04U937Z
04U93JZ
04U947Z

Ø4U94JZ
Ø4UAØ7Z
Ø4UAØJZ
Ø4UA37Z
Ø4UA3JZ
Ø4UA47Z
Ø4UA4JZ
Ø4UBØ7Z
Ø4UBØJZ
Ø4UB37Z
Ø4UB3JZ
Ø4UB47Z
Ø4UB4JZ
Ø4UCØ7Z
Ø4UCØJZ
Ø4UC37Z
Ø4UC3JZ
Ø4UC47Z
Ø4UC4JZ
Ø4UDØ7Z
Ø4UDØJZ
Ø4UD37Z
Ø4UD3JZ
Ø4UD47Z
Ø4UD4JZ
Ø4UEØ7Z
Ø4UEØJZ
Ø4UE37Z
Ø4UE3JZ
Ø4UE47Z
Ø4UE4JZ
Ø4UFØ7Z
Ø4UFØJZ
Ø4UF37Z
Ø4UF3JZ
Ø4UF47Z
Ø4UF4JZ
Ø4UHØ7Z
Ø4UHØJZ
Ø4UH37Z
Ø4UH3JZ
Ø4UH47Z
Ø4UH4JZ
Ø4UJØ7Z
Ø4UJØJZ
Ø4UJ37Z
Ø4UJ3JZ
Ø4UJ47Z
Ø4UJ4JZ
Ø4UKØ7Z
Ø4UKØJZ
Ø4UK37Z
Ø4UK3JZ
Ø4UK47Z
Ø4UK4JZ
Ø4ULØ7Z
Ø4ULØJZ
Ø4UL37Z
Ø4UL3JZ
Ø4UL47Z
Ø4UL4JZ
Ø4UMØ7Z
Ø4UMØJZ
Ø4UM37Z
Ø4UM3JZ
Ø4UM47Z
Ø4UM4JZ
Ø4UNØ7Z
Ø4UNØJZ
Ø4UN37Z
Ø4UN3JZ
Ø4UN47Z
Ø4UN4JZ
Ø4UPØ7Z
Ø4UPØJZ
Ø4UP37Z
Ø4UP3JZ
Ø4UP47Z
Ø4UP4JZ
Ø4UQØ7Z
Ø4UQØJZ
Ø4UQ37Z
Ø4UQ3JZ
Ø4UQ47Z
Ø4UQ4JZ
Ø4URØ7Z
Ø4URØJZ
Ø4UR37Z
Ø4UR3JZ
Ø4UR47Z
Ø4UR4JZ
Ø4USØ7Z
Ø4USØJZ
Ø4US37Z
Ø4US3JZ
Ø4US47Z
Ø4US4JZ
Ø4UTØ7Z
Ø4UTØJZ
Ø4UT37Z
Ø4UT3JZ
Ø4UT47Z
Ø4UT4JZ
Ø4UUØ7Z
Ø4UUØJZ
Ø4UU37Z
Ø4UU3JZ
Ø4UU47Z
Ø4UU4JZ
Ø4UVØ7Z
Ø4UVØJZ
Ø4UV37Z
Ø4UV3JZ
Ø4UV47Z
Ø4UV4JZ
Ø4UWØ7Z
Ø4UWØJZ
Ø4UW37Z
Ø4UW3JZ
Ø4UW47Z
Ø4UW4JZ
Ø4UYØ7Z
Ø4UYØJZ
Ø4UY37Z
Ø4UY3JZ
Ø4UY47Z
Ø4UY4JZ
Ø4VØØDJ
Ø4VØØDZ
Ø4VØØEZ
Ø4VØØFZ
Ø4VØØZZ
Ø4VØ3DJ
Ø4VØ3DZ
Ø4VØ3EZ
Ø4VØ3FZ
Ø4VØ3ZZ
Ø4VØ4DJ
Ø4VØ4DZ
Ø4VØ4EZ
Ø4VØ4FZ
Ø4VØ4ZZ
Ø4V1ØDZ
Ø4V1ØZZ
Ø4V13DZ
Ø4V13ZZ
Ø4V14DZ
Ø4V14ZZ
Ø4V2ØDZ
Ø4V2ØZZ
Ø4V23DZ
Ø4V23ZZ
Ø4V24DZ
Ø4V24ZZ
Ø4V3ØDZ
Ø4V3ØZZ
Ø4V33DZ
Ø4V33ZZ
Ø4V34DZ
Ø4V34ZZ
Ø4V4ØDZ
Ø4V4ØZZ
Ø4V43DZ
Ø4V43ZZ
Ø4V44DZ
Ø4V44ZZ
Ø4V5ØDZ
Ø4V5ØZZ
Ø4V53DZ
Ø4V53ZZ
Ø4V54DZ
Ø4V54ZZ
Ø4V6ØDZ
Ø4V6ØZZ
Ø4V63DZ
Ø4V63ZZ
Ø4V64DZ
Ø4V64ZZ
Ø4V7ØDZ
Ø4V7ØZZ
Ø4V73DZ
Ø4V73ZZ
Ø4V74DZ
Ø4V74ZZ
Ø4V8ØDZ
Ø4V8ØZZ
Ø4V83DZ
Ø4V83ZZ
Ø4V84DZ
Ø4V84ZZ
Ø4V9ØDZ
Ø4V9ØZZ
Ø4V93DZ
Ø4V93ZZ
Ø4V94DZ
Ø4V94ZZ
Ø4VAØDZ
Ø4VAØZZ
Ø4VA3DZ
Ø4VA3ZZ
Ø4VA4DZ
Ø4VA4ZZ
Ø4VBØDZ
Ø4VBØZZ
Ø4VB3DZ
Ø4VB3ZZ
Ø4VB4DZ
Ø4VB4ZZ
Ø4VCØDZ
Ø4VCØEZ
Ø4VCØZZ
Ø4VC3DZ
Ø4VC3EZ
Ø4VC3ZZ
Ø4VC4DZ
Ø4VC4EZ
Ø4VC4ZZ
Ø4VDØDZ
Ø4VDØEZ
Ø4VDØZZ
Ø4VD3DZ
Ø4VD3EZ
Ø4VD3ZZ
Ø4VD4DZ
Ø4VD4EZ
Ø4VD4ZZ
Ø4VEØDZ
Ø4VEØZZ
Ø4VE3DZ
Ø4VE3ZZ
Ø4VE4DZ
Ø4VE4ZZ
Ø4VFØDZ
Ø4VFØZZ
Ø4VF3DZ
Ø4VF3ZZ
Ø4VF4DZ
Ø4VF4ZZ
Ø4VHØDZ
Ø4VHØZZ
Ø4VH3DZ
Ø4VH3ZZ
Ø4VH4DZ
Ø4VH4ZZ
Ø4VJØDZ
Ø4VJØZZ
Ø4VJ3DZ
Ø4VJ3ZZ
Ø4VJ4DZ
Ø4VJ4ZZ
Ø4VKØDZ
Ø4VKØZZ
Ø4VK3DZ
Ø4VK3ZZ
Ø4VK4DZ
Ø4VK4ZZ
Ø4VLØDZ
Ø4VLØZZ
Ø4VL3DZ
Ø4VL3ZZ
Ø4VL4DZ
Ø4VL4ZZ
Ø4VMØDZ
Ø4VMØZZ
Ø4VM3DZ
Ø4VM3ZZ
Ø4VM4DZ
Ø4VM4ZZ
Ø4VNØDZ
Ø4VNØZZ
Ø4VN3DZ
Ø4VN3ZZ
Ø4VN4DZ
Ø4VN4ZZ
Ø4VPØDZ
Ø4VPØZZ
Ø4VP3DZ
Ø4VP3ZZ
Ø4VP4DZ
Ø4VP4ZZ
Ø4VQØDZ
Ø4VQØZZ
Ø4VQ3DZ
Ø4VQ3ZZ
Ø4VQ4DZ
Ø4VQ4ZZ
Ø4VRØDZ
Ø4VRØZZ
Ø4VR3DZ
Ø4VR3ZZ
Ø4VR4DZ
Ø4VR4ZZ
Ø4VSØDZ
Ø4VSØZZ
Ø4VS3DZ
Ø4VS3ZZ
Ø4VS4DZ
Ø4VS4ZZ
Ø4VTØDZ
Ø4VTØZZ
Ø4VT3DZ
Ø4VT3ZZ
Ø4VT4DZ
Ø4VT4ZZ
Ø4VUØDZ
Ø4VUØZZ
Ø4VU3DZ
Ø4VU3ZZ
Ø4VU4DZ
Ø4VU4ZZ
Ø4VVØDZ
Ø4VVØZZ
Ø4VV3DZ
Ø4VV3ZZ
Ø4VV4DZ
Ø4VV4ZZ
Ø4VWØDZ
Ø4VWØZZ
Ø4VW3DZ
Ø4VW3ZZ
Ø4VW4DZ
Ø4VW4ZZ
Ø4VYØDZ
Ø4VYØZZ
Ø4VY3DZ
Ø4VY3ZZ
Ø4VY4DZ
Ø4VY4ZZ
Ø4WYØØZ
Ø4WYØ2Z
Ø4WYØ3Z
Ø4WYØCZ
Ø4WYØDZ
Ø4WYØYZ
Ø4WY3CZ
Ø4WY4ØZ
Ø4WY42Z
Ø4WY43Z
Ø4WY4CZ
Ø4WY4DZ
Ø51Ø*
Ø511*
Ø513*
Ø514*
Ø515*
Ø516*
Ø557*
Ø558*
Ø559*
Ø55A*
Ø55B*
Ø55C*
Ø55D*
Ø55F*
Ø55G*
Ø55H*
Ø55L*
Ø55M*
Ø55N*
Ø55P*
Ø55Q*
Ø55R*
Ø55S*
Ø55T*
Ø55V*
Ø55Y*
Ø5793D1
Ø5793DZ
Ø5793Z1
Ø5793ZZ
Ø57A3D1
Ø57A3DZ
Ø57A3Z1
Ø57A3ZZ
Ø57B3D1
Ø57B3DZ
Ø57B3Z1
Ø57B3ZZ
Ø57C3D1
Ø57C3DZ
Ø57C3Z1
Ø57C3ZZ
Ø57D3D1
Ø57D3DZ
Ø57D3Z1
Ø57D3ZZ
Ø57F3D1
Ø57F3DZ
Ø57F3Z1
Ø57F3ZZ
Ø57L3DZ
Ø57L4DZ
Ø57M3DZ
Ø57M4DZ
Ø57N3DZ
Ø57N4DZ
Ø57P3DZ
Ø57P4DZ
Ø57Q3DZ
Ø57Q4DZ
Ø57R3DZ
Ø57R4DZ
Ø57S3DZ
Ø57S4DZ
Ø57T3DZ
Ø57T4DZ
Ø5B7ØZZ
Ø5B73ZZ
Ø5B74ZZ
Ø5B8ØZZ
Ø5B83ZZ
Ø5B84ZZ
Ø5B9ØZZ
Ø5B93ZZ
Ø5B94ZZ
Ø5BAØZZ
Ø5BA3ZZ
Ø5BA4ZZ
Ø5BBØZZ
Ø5BB3ZZ
Ø5BB4ZZ
Ø5BCØZZ
Ø5BC3ZZ
Ø5BC4ZZ
Ø5BDØZZ
Ø5BD3ZZ
Ø5BD4ZZ
Ø5BFØZZ
Ø5BF3ZZ
Ø5BF4ZZ
Ø5BGØZZ
Ø5BG3ZZ
Ø5BG4ZZ
Ø5BHØZZ
Ø5BH3ZZ
Ø5BH4ZZ
Ø5BLØZZ
Ø5BL3ZZ
Ø5BL4ZZ
Ø5BMØZZ
Ø5BM3ZZ
Ø5BM4ZZ
Ø5BNØZZ
Ø5BN3ZZ
Ø5BN4ZZ
Ø5BPØZZ
Ø5BP3ZZ
Ø5BP4ZZ
Ø5BQØZZ
Ø5BQ3ZZ
Ø5BQ4ZZ
Ø5BRØZZ
Ø5BR3ZZ
Ø5BR4ZZ
Ø5BSØZZ
Ø5BS3ZZ
Ø5BS4ZZ
Ø5BTØZZ
Ø5BT3ZZ
Ø5BT4ZZ
Ø5BVØZZ
Ø5BV3ZZ
Ø5BV4ZZ
Ø5BYØZZ
Ø5BY3ZZ
Ø5BY4ZZ
Ø5C7*
Ø5C8*
Ø5C9*
Ø5CA*
Ø5CB*
Ø5CC*
Ø5CD*
Ø5CF*
Ø5CG*
Ø5CH*
Ø5CL*
Ø5CM*
Ø5CN*
Ø5CP*
Ø5CQ*
Ø5CR*
Ø5CS*
Ø5CT*
Ø5CV*
Ø5CY*
Ø5HØØDZ
Ø5HØØMZ
Ø5HØ3DZ
Ø5HØ3MZ
Ø5HØ4DZ
Ø5HØ4MZ
Ø5H1ØDZ
Ø5H13DZ
Ø5H14DZ
Ø5H3ØDZ
Ø5H3ØMZ
Ø5H33DZ
Ø5H33MZ
Ø5H34DZ
Ø5H34MZ
Ø5H4ØDZ
Ø5H4ØMZ
Ø5H43DZ
Ø5H43MZ
Ø5H44DZ
Ø5H44MZ
Ø5H5ØDZ
Ø5H53DZ
Ø5H54DZ
Ø5H6ØDZ
Ø5H63DZ
Ø5H64DZ
Ø5H7ØDZ
Ø5H73DZ
Ø5H74DZ
Ø5H8ØDZ
Ø5H83DZ
Ø5H84DZ
Ø5H9ØDZ
Ø5H93DZ
Ø5H94DZ
Ø5HAØDZ
Ø5HA3DZ
Ø5HA4DZ
Ø5HBØDZ
Ø5HB3DZ
Ø5HB4DZ
Ø5HCØDZ
Ø5HC3DZ
Ø5HC4DZ
Ø5HDØDZ
Ø5HD3DZ
Ø5HD4DZ
Ø5HFØDZ
Ø5HF3DZ
Ø5HF4DZ
Ø5HGØDZ
Ø5HG3DZ
Ø5HG4DZ
Ø5HHØDZ
Ø5HH3DZ
Ø5HH4DZ
Ø5HLØDZ
Ø5HL3DZ
Ø5HL4DZ
Ø5HMØDZ
Ø5HM3DZ
Ø5HM4DZ
Ø5HNØDZ
Ø5HN3DZ
Ø5HN4DZ
Ø5HPØDZ
Ø5HP3DZ
Ø5HP4DZ
Ø5HQØDZ
Ø5HQ3DZ
Ø5HQ4DZ
Ø5HRØDZ
Ø5HR3DZ
Ø5HR4DZ
Ø5HSØDZ
Ø5HS3DZ
Ø5HS4DZ
Ø5HTØDZ
Ø5HT3DZ
Ø5HT4DZ
Ø5HVØDZ
Ø5HV3DZ
Ø5HV4DZ
Ø5HYØ2Z
Ø5HYØDZ
Ø5HYØYZ
Ø5HY3DZ
Ø5HY42Z
Ø5HY4DZ
Ø5L*
Ø5PØØMZ
Ø5PØ3MZ
Ø5PØ4MZ
Ø5PØXMZ
Ø5P3ØMZ
Ø5P33MZ
Ø5P34MZ
Ø5P3XMZ
Ø5P4ØMZ
Ø5P43MZ
Ø5P44MZ
Ø5P4XMZ
Ø5Q*
Ø5RØ*
Ø5R1*
Ø5R3*
Ø5R4*
Ø5R5*
Ø5R6*
Ø5R7*
Ø5R8*
Ø5R9*
Ø5RA*
Ø5RB*
Ø5RC*
Ø5RD*
Ø5RF*
Ø5RG*
Ø5RH*
Ø5RL*
Ø5RY*
Ø5S*
Ø5UØØ7Z
Ø5UØØJZ
Ø5UØ37Z
Ø5UØ3JZ
Ø5UØ47Z
Ø5UØ4JZ
Ø5U1Ø7Z
Ø5U1ØJZ
Ø5U137Z
Ø5U13JZ
Ø5U147Z
Ø5U14JZ
Ø5U3Ø7Z
Ø5U3ØJZ
Ø5U337Z
Ø5U33JZ
Ø5U347Z
Ø5U34JZ
Ø5U4Ø7Z
Ø5U4ØJZ
Ø5U437Z
Ø5U43JZ
Ø5U447Z
Ø5U44JZ
Ø5U5Ø7Z
Ø5U5ØJZ
Ø5U537Z
Ø5U53JZ
Ø5U547Z
Ø5U54JZ
Ø5U6Ø7Z
Ø5U6ØJZ
Ø5U637Z
Ø5U63JZ
Ø5U647Z
Ø5U64JZ
Ø5U7Ø7Z
Ø5U7ØJZ
Ø5U737Z
Ø5U73JZ
Ø5U747Z
Ø5U74JZ
Ø5U8Ø7Z
Ø5U8ØJZ
Ø5U837Z
Ø5U83JZ
Ø5U847Z
Ø5U84JZ
Ø5U9Ø7Z
Ø5U9ØJZ
Ø5U937Z
Ø5U93JZ
Ø5U947Z
Ø5U94JZ
Ø5UAØ7Z
Ø5UAØJZ
Ø5UA37Z
Ø5UA3JZ
Ø5UA47Z
Ø5UA4JZ
Ø5UBØ7Z
Ø5UBØJZ
Ø5UB37Z
Ø5UB3JZ
Ø5UB47Z
Ø5UB4JZ
Ø5UCØ7Z
Ø5UCØJZ
Ø5UC37Z
Ø5UC3JZ
Ø5UC47Z
Ø5UC4JZ
Ø5UDØ7Z
Ø5UDØJZ
Ø5UD37Z
Ø5UD3JZ
Ø5UD47Z
Ø5UD4JZ
Ø5UFØ7Z
Ø5UFØJZ
Ø5UF37Z
Ø5UF3JZ
Ø5UF47Z
Ø5UF4JZ
Ø5UGØ7Z
Ø5UGØJZ
Ø5UG37Z
Ø5UG3JZ
Ø5UG47Z
Ø5UG4JZ
Ø5UHØ7Z
Ø5UHØJZ
Ø5UH37Z
Ø5UH3JZ
Ø5UH47Z
Ø5UH4JZ
Ø5ULØ7Z
Ø5ULØJZ
Ø5UL37Z
Ø5UL3JZ
Ø5UL47Z
Ø5UL4JZ
Ø5UMØ7Z
Ø5UMØJZ
Ø5UM37Z
Ø5UM3JZ
Ø5UM47Z
Ø5UM4JZ
Ø5UNØ7Z
Ø5UNØJZ
Ø5UN37Z
Ø5UN3JZ
Ø5UN47Z
Ø5UN4JZ
Ø5UPØ7Z
Ø5UPØJZ
Ø5UP37Z
Ø5UP3JZ
Ø5UP47Z
Ø5UP4JZ
Ø5UQØ7Z
Ø5UQØJZ
Ø5UQ37Z
Ø5UQ3JZ
Ø5UQ47Z
Ø5UQ4JZ
Ø5URØ7Z
Ø5URØJZ
Ø5UR37Z
Ø5UR3JZ
Ø5UR47Z
Ø5UR4JZ
Ø5USØ7Z
Ø5USØJZ
Ø5US37Z
Ø5US3JZ
Ø5US47Z
Ø5US4JZ
Ø5UTØ7Z
Ø5UTØJZ
Ø5UT37Z
Ø5UT3JZ
Ø5UT47Z
Ø5UT4JZ
Ø5UVØ7Z
Ø5UVØJZ
Ø5UV37Z
Ø5UV3JZ
Ø5UV47Z
Ø5UV4JZ
Ø5UYØ7Z
Ø5UYØJZ
Ø5UY37Z
Ø5UY3JZ
Ø5UY47Z
Ø5UY4JZ
Ø5VØØDZ
Ø5VØØZZ
Ø5VØ3DZ
Ø5VØ3ZZ
Ø5VØ4DZ
Ø5VØ4ZZ
Ø5V1ØDZ
Ø5V1ØZZ
Ø5V13DZ
Ø5V13ZZ
Ø5V14DZ
Ø5V14ZZ
Ø5V3ØDZ
Ø5V3ØZZ
Ø5V33DZ
Ø5V33ZZ
Ø5V34DZ
Ø5V34ZZ
Ø5V4ØDZ
Ø5V4ØZZ
Ø5V43DZ
Ø5V43ZZ
Ø5V44DZ
Ø5V44ZZ
Ø5V5ØDZ
Ø5V5ØZZ
Ø5V53DZ
Ø5V53ZZ
Ø5V54DZ
Ø5V54ZZ
Ø5V6ØDZ
Ø5V6ØZZ
Ø5V63DZ
Ø5V63ZZ
Ø5V64DZ
Ø5V64ZZ
Ø5V7ØDZ
Ø5V7ØZZ
Ø5V73DZ
Ø5V73ZZ
Ø5V74DZ
Ø5V74ZZ
Ø5V8ØDZ
Ø5V8ØZZ
Ø5V83DZ
Ø5V83ZZ
Ø5V84DZ
Ø5V84ZZ
Ø5V9ØDZ
Ø5V9ØZZ
Ø5V93DZ
Ø5V93ZZ
Ø5V94DZ
Ø5V94ZZ
Ø5VAØDZ
Ø5VAØZZ
Ø5VA3DZ
Ø5VA3ZZ
Ø5VA4DZ
Ø5VA4ZZ
Ø5VBØDZ
Ø5VBØZZ
Ø5VB3DZ
Ø5VB3ZZ
Ø5VB4DZ
Ø5VB4ZZ
Ø5VCØDZ
Ø5VCØZZ
Ø5VC3DZ
Ø5VC3ZZ
Ø5VC4DZ
Ø5VC4ZZ
Ø5VDØDZ
Ø5VDØZZ
Ø5VD3DZ
Ø5VD3ZZ
Ø5VD4DZ
Ø5VD4ZZ
Ø5VFØDZ
Ø5VFØZZ
Ø5VF3DZ
Ø5VF3ZZ
Ø5VF4DZ
Ø5VF4ZZ
Ø5VGØDZ
Ø5VGØZZ
Ø5VG3DZ
Ø5VG3ZZ
Ø5VG4DZ
Ø5VG4ZZ

Ø5VHØDZ
Ø5VHØZZ
Ø5VH3DZ
Ø5VH3ZZ
Ø5VH4DZ
Ø5VH4ZZ
Ø5VLØDZ
Ø5VLØZZ
Ø5VL3DZ
Ø5VL3ZZ
Ø5VL4DZ
Ø5VL4ZZ
Ø5VMØDZ
Ø5VMØZZ
Ø5VM3DZ
Ø5VM3ZZ
Ø5VM4DZ
Ø5VM4ZZ
Ø5VNØDZ
Ø5VNØZZ
Ø5VN3DZ
Ø5VN3ZZ
Ø5VN4DZ
Ø5VN4ZZ
Ø5VPØDZ
Ø5VPØZZ
Ø5VP3DZ
Ø5VP3ZZ
Ø5VP4DZ
Ø5VP4ZZ
Ø5VQØDZ
Ø5VQØZZ
Ø5VQ3DZ
Ø5VQ3ZZ
Ø5VQ4DZ
Ø5VQ4ZZ
Ø5VRØDZ
Ø5VRØZZ
Ø5VR3DZ
Ø5VR3ZZ
Ø5VR4DZ
Ø5VR4ZZ
Ø5VSØDZ
Ø5VSØZZ
Ø5VS3DZ
Ø5VS3ZZ
Ø5VS4DZ
Ø5VS4ZZ
Ø5VTØDZ
Ø5VTØZZ
Ø5VT3DZ
Ø5VT3ZZ
Ø5VT4DZ
Ø5VT4ZZ
Ø5VVØDZ
Ø5VVØZZ
Ø5VV3DZ
Ø5VV3ZZ
Ø5VV4DZ
Ø5VV4ZZ
Ø5VYØDZ
Ø5VYØZZ
Ø5VY3DZ
Ø5VY3ZZ
Ø5VY4DZ
Ø5VY4ZZ
Ø653*
Ø65M*
Ø65N*
Ø65P*
Ø65Q*
Ø65T*
Ø65V*
Ø65YØZZ
Ø65Y3ZZ
Ø65Y4ZZ
Ø67Ø3DZ
Ø67Ø3ZZ
Ø693ØØZ
Ø693ØZZ
Ø6934ØZ
Ø6934ZZ
Ø6B3ØZZ
Ø6B33ZZ
Ø6B34ZZ
Ø6BMØZZ
Ø6BM3ZZ
Ø6BM4ZZ
Ø6BNØZZ
Ø6BN3ZZ
Ø6BN4ZZ
Ø6BPØZZ
Ø6BP3ZZ
Ø6BP4ZZ
Ø6BQØZZ
Ø6BQ3ZZ
Ø6BQ4ZZ
Ø6BTØZZ
Ø6BT3ZZ
Ø6BT4ZZ
Ø6BVØZZ
Ø6BV3ZZ
Ø6BV4ZZ
Ø6BYØZZ
Ø6BY3ZZ
Ø6BY4ZZ
Ø6C3*
Ø6CM*
Ø6CN*
Ø6CP*
Ø6CQ*
Ø6CT*
Ø6CV*
Ø6CY*
Ø6HØØDZ
Ø6HØ4DZ
Ø6H1ØDZ
Ø6H13DZ
Ø6H14DZ
Ø6H2ØDZ
Ø6H23DZ
Ø6H24DZ
Ø6H3ØDZ
Ø6H33DZ
Ø6H34DZ
Ø6H4ØDZ
Ø6H43DZ
Ø6H44DZ
Ø6H5ØDZ
Ø6H53DZ
Ø6H54DZ
Ø6H6ØDZ
Ø6H63DZ
Ø6H64DZ
Ø6H7ØDZ
Ø6H73DZ
Ø6H74DZ
Ø6H8ØDZ
Ø6H83DZ
Ø6H84DZ
Ø6H9ØDZ
Ø6H93DZ
Ø6H94DZ
Ø6HBØDZ
Ø6HB3DZ
Ø6HB4DZ
Ø6HCØDZ
Ø6HC3DZ
Ø6HC4DZ
Ø6HDØDZ
Ø6HD3DZ
Ø6HD4DZ
Ø6HFØDZ
Ø6HF3DZ
Ø6HF4DZ
Ø6HGØDZ
Ø6HG3DZ
Ø6HG4DZ
Ø6HHØDZ
Ø6HH3DZ
Ø6HH4DZ
Ø6HJØDZ
Ø6HJ3DZ
Ø6HJ4DZ
Ø6HMØDZ
Ø6HM3DZ
Ø6HM4DZ
Ø6HNØDZ
Ø6HN3DZ
Ø6HN4DZ
Ø6HPØDZ
Ø6HP3DZ
Ø6HP4DZ
Ø6HQØDZ
Ø6HQ3DZ
Ø6HQ4DZ
Ø6HTØDZ
Ø6HT3DZ
Ø6HT4DZ
Ø6HVØDZ
Ø6HV3DZ
Ø6HV4DZ
Ø6HYØ2Z
Ø6HYØDZ
Ø6HYØYZ
Ø6HY3DZ
Ø6HY42Z
Ø6HY4DZ
Ø6LØ*
Ø6L1*
Ø6L2ØCZ
Ø6L2ØDZ
Ø6L2ØZZ
Ø6L23CZ
Ø6L23DZ
Ø6L23ZZ
Ø6L24CZ
Ø6L24DZ
Ø6L24ZZ
Ø6L3ØCZ
Ø6L3ØDZ
Ø6L3ØZZ
Ø6L4*
Ø6L5*
Ø6L6*
Ø6L7*
Ø6L8*
Ø6L9*
Ø6LB*
Ø6LC*
Ø6LD*
Ø6LF*
Ø6LG*
Ø6LH*
Ø6LJ*
Ø6LM*
Ø6LN*
Ø6LP*
Ø6LQ*
Ø6LT*
Ø6LV*
Ø6LYØCZ
Ø6LYØDZ
Ø6LYØZZ
Ø6LY3CZ
Ø6LY3DZ
Ø6LY3ZZ
Ø6LY4CZ
Ø6LY4DZ
Ø6LY4ZZ
Ø6LY7CZ
Ø6LY7DZ
Ø6LY7ZZ
Ø6LY8CZ
Ø6LY8DZ
Ø6LY8ZZ
Ø6PYØØZ
Ø6PYØ2Z
Ø6PYØ3Z
Ø6PYØCZ
Ø6PYØDZ
Ø6PYØYZ
Ø6PY3CZ
Ø6PY4ØZ
Ø6PY42Z
Ø6PY43Z
Ø6PY4CZ
Ø6PY4DZ
Ø6Q*
Ø6RM*
Ø6RN*
Ø6RP*
Ø6RQ*
Ø6RT*
Ø6RV*
Ø6RY*
Ø6SØ*
Ø6S1*
Ø6S2*
Ø6S3*
Ø6S4*
Ø6S5*
Ø6S6*
Ø6S7*
Ø6S8*
Ø6SC*
Ø6SD*
Ø6SF*
Ø6SG*
Ø6SH*
Ø6SJ*
Ø6SM*
Ø6SN*
Ø6SP*
Ø6SQ*
Ø6ST*
Ø6SV*
Ø6SY*
Ø6UØØ7Z
Ø6UØØJZ
Ø6UØ37Z
Ø6UØ3JZ
Ø6UØ47Z
Ø6UØ4JZ
Ø6U1Ø7Z
Ø6U1ØJZ
Ø6U137Z
Ø6U13JZ
Ø6U147Z
Ø6U14JZ
Ø6U2Ø7Z
Ø6U2ØJZ
Ø6U237Z
Ø6U23JZ
Ø6U247Z
Ø6U24JZ
Ø6U3Ø7Z
Ø6U3ØJZ
Ø6U337Z
Ø6U33JZ
Ø6U347Z
Ø6U34JZ
Ø6U4Ø7Z
Ø6U4ØJZ
Ø6U437Z
Ø6U43JZ
Ø6U447Z
Ø6U44JZ
Ø6U5Ø7Z
Ø6U5ØJZ
Ø6U537Z
Ø6U53JZ
Ø6U547Z
Ø6U54JZ
Ø6U6Ø7Z
Ø6U6ØJZ
Ø6U637Z
Ø6U63JZ
Ø6U647Z
Ø6U64JZ
Ø6U7Ø7Z
Ø6U7ØJZ
Ø6U737Z
Ø6U73JZ
Ø6U747Z
Ø6U74JZ
Ø6U8Ø7Z
Ø6U8ØJZ
Ø6U837Z
Ø6U83JZ
Ø6U847Z
Ø6U84JZ
Ø6U9Ø7Z
Ø6U9ØJZ
Ø6U937Z
Ø6U93JZ
Ø6U947Z
Ø6U94JZ
Ø6UBØ7Z
Ø6UBØJZ
Ø6UB37Z
Ø6UB3JZ
Ø6UB47Z
Ø6UB4JZ
Ø6UCØ7Z
Ø6UCØJZ
Ø6UC37Z
Ø6UC3JZ
Ø6UC47Z
Ø6UC4JZ
Ø6UDØ7Z
Ø6UDØJZ
Ø6UD37Z
Ø6UD3JZ
Ø6UD47Z
Ø6UD4JZ
Ø6UFØ7Z
Ø6UFØJZ
Ø6UF37Z
Ø6UF3JZ
Ø6UF47Z
Ø6UF4JZ
Ø6UGØ7Z
Ø6UGØJZ
Ø6UG37Z
Ø6UG3JZ
Ø6UG47Z
Ø6UG4JZ
Ø6UHØ7Z
Ø6UHØJZ
Ø6UH37Z
Ø6UH3JZ
Ø6UH47Z
Ø6UH4JZ
Ø6UJØ7Z
Ø6UJØJZ
Ø6UJ37Z
Ø6UJ3JZ
Ø6UJ47Z
Ø6UJ4JZ
Ø6UMØ7Z
Ø6UMØJZ
Ø6UM37Z
Ø6UM3JZ
Ø6UM47Z
Ø6UM4JZ
Ø6UNØ7Z
Ø6UNØJZ
Ø6UN37Z
Ø6UN3JZ
Ø6UN47Z
Ø6UN4JZ
Ø6UPØ7Z
Ø6UPØJZ
Ø6UP37Z
Ø6UP3JZ
Ø6UP47Z
Ø6UP4JZ
Ø6UQØ7Z
Ø6UQØJZ
Ø6UQ37Z
Ø6UQ3JZ
Ø6UQ47Z
Ø6UQ4JZ
Ø6UTØ7Z
Ø6UTØJZ
Ø6UT37Z
Ø6UT3JZ
Ø6UT47Z
Ø6UT4JZ
Ø6UVØ7Z
Ø6UVØJZ
Ø6UV37Z
Ø6UV3JZ
Ø6UV47Z
Ø6UV4JZ
Ø6UYØ7Z
Ø6UYØJZ
Ø6UY37Z
Ø6UY3JZ
Ø6UY47Z
Ø6UY4JZ
Ø6VØ*
Ø6V1ØDZ
Ø6V1ØZZ
Ø6V13DZ
Ø6V13ZZ
Ø6V14DZ
Ø6V14ZZ
Ø6V2ØDZ
Ø6V2ØZZ
Ø6V23DZ
Ø6V23ZZ
Ø6V24DZ
Ø6V24ZZ
Ø6V3ØDZ
Ø6V3ØZZ
Ø6V33DZ
Ø6V33ZZ
Ø6V34DZ
Ø6V34ZZ
Ø6V4ØDZ
Ø6V4ØZZ
Ø6V43DZ
Ø6V43ZZ
Ø6V44DZ
Ø6V44ZZ
Ø6V5ØDZ
Ø6V5ØZZ
Ø6V53DZ
Ø6V53ZZ
Ø6V54DZ
Ø6V54ZZ
Ø6V6ØDZ
Ø6V6ØZZ
Ø6V63DZ
Ø6V63ZZ
Ø6V64DZ
Ø6V64ZZ
Ø6V7ØDZ
Ø6V7ØZZ
Ø6V73DZ
Ø6V73ZZ
Ø6V74DZ
Ø6V74ZZ
Ø6V8ØDZ
Ø6V8ØZZ
Ø6V83DZ
Ø6V83ZZ
Ø6V84DZ
Ø6V84ZZ
Ø6V9ØDZ
Ø6V9ØZZ
Ø6V93DZ
Ø6V93ZZ
Ø6V94DZ
Ø6V94ZZ
Ø6VBØDZ
Ø6VBØZZ
Ø6VB3DZ
Ø6VB3ZZ
Ø6VB4DZ
Ø6VB4ZZ
Ø6VCØDZ
Ø6VCØZZ
Ø6VC3DZ
Ø6VC3ZZ
Ø6VC4DZ
Ø6VC4ZZ
Ø6VDØDZ
Ø6VDØZZ
Ø6VD3DZ
Ø6VD3ZZ
Ø6VD4DZ
Ø6VD4ZZ
Ø6VFØDZ
Ø6VFØZZ
Ø6VF3DZ
Ø6VF3ZZ
Ø6VF4DZ
Ø6VF4ZZ
Ø6VGØDZ
Ø6VGØZZ
Ø6VG3DZ
Ø6VG3ZZ
Ø6VG4DZ
Ø6VG4ZZ
Ø6VHØDZ
Ø6VHØZZ
Ø6VH3DZ
Ø6VH3ZZ
Ø6VH4DZ
Ø6VH4ZZ
Ø6VJØDZ
Ø6VJØZZ
Ø6VJ3DZ
Ø6VJ3ZZ
Ø6VJ4DZ
Ø6VJ4ZZ
Ø6VMØDZ
Ø6VMØZZ
Ø6VM3DZ
Ø6VM3ZZ
Ø6VM4DZ
Ø6VM4ZZ
Ø6VNØDZ
Ø6VNØZZ
Ø6VN3DZ
Ø6VN3ZZ
Ø6VN4DZ
Ø6VN4ZZ
Ø6VPØDZ
Ø6VPØZZ
Ø6VP3DZ
Ø6VP3ZZ
Ø6VP4DZ
Ø6VP4ZZ
Ø6VQØDZ
Ø6VQØZZ
Ø6VQ3DZ
Ø6VQ3ZZ
Ø6VQ4DZ
Ø6VQ4ZZ
Ø6VTØDZ
Ø6VTØZZ
Ø6VT3DZ
Ø6VT3ZZ
Ø6VT4DZ
Ø6VT4ZZ
Ø6VVØDZ
Ø6VVØZZ
Ø6VV3DZ
Ø6VV3ZZ
Ø6VV4DZ
Ø6VV4ZZ
Ø6VYØDZ
Ø6VYØZZ
Ø6VY3DZ
Ø6VY3ZZ
Ø6VY4DZ
Ø6VY4ZZ
Ø6WYØØZ
Ø6WYØ2Z
Ø6WYØ3Z
Ø6WYØCZ
Ø6WYØDZ
Ø6WYØYZ
Ø6WY3CZ
Ø6WY4ØZ
Ø6WY42Z
Ø6WY43Z
Ø6WY4CZ
Ø6WY4DZ
Ø75Ø*
Ø751*
Ø752*
Ø753*
Ø754*
Ø755*
Ø756*
Ø757*
Ø758*
Ø759*
Ø75B*
Ø75C*
Ø75D*
Ø75F*
Ø75G*
Ø75H*
Ø75J*
Ø75M*
Ø75P*
Ø79KØØZ
Ø79KØZZ
Ø79K4ØZ
Ø79K4ZZ
Ø79LØØZ
Ø79LØZZ
Ø79L4ØZ
Ø79L4ZZ
Ø79MØØZ
Ø79MØZZ
Ø79M4ØZ
Ø79M4ZZ
Ø79PØØZ
Ø79PØZZ
Ø7BMØZZ
Ø7BM3ZZ
Ø7BM4ZZ
Ø7BPØZZ
Ø7BP3ZZ
Ø7BP4ZZ
Ø7CM*
Ø7CPØZZ
Ø7HKØ1Z
Ø7HKØYZ
Ø7HK41Z
Ø7HK4YZ
Ø7HLØ1Z
Ø7HLØYZ
Ø7HL41Z
Ø7HL4YZ
Ø7HMØ1Z
Ø7HMØYZ
Ø7HM41Z
Ø7HM4YZ
Ø7HPØ1Z
Ø7HPØYZ
Ø7HP41Z
Ø7JMØZZ
Ø7JM4ZZ
Ø7JPØZZ
Ø7L*
Ø7NØ*
Ø7N1*
Ø7N2*
Ø7N3*
Ø7N4*
Ø7N5*
Ø7N6*
Ø7N7*
Ø7N8*
Ø7N9*
Ø7NB*
Ø7NC*
Ø7ND*
Ø7NF*
Ø7NG*
Ø7NH*
Ø7NJ*
Ø7NM*
Ø7NP*
Ø7PKØ7Z
Ø7PKØJZ
Ø7PKØKZ
Ø7PK37Z
Ø7PK3JZ
Ø7PK3KZ
Ø7PK47Z
Ø7PK4JZ
Ø7PK4KZ
Ø7PLØ7Z
Ø7PLØJZ
Ø7PLØKZ
Ø7PL37Z
Ø7PL3JZ
Ø7PL3KZ
Ø7PL47Z
Ø7PL4JZ
Ø7PL4KZ
Ø7PMØØZ
Ø7PMØ3Z
Ø7PMØYZ
Ø7PM3ØZ
Ø7PM33Z
Ø7PM4ØZ
Ø7PM43Z
Ø7PNØ7Z
Ø7PNØJZ
Ø7PNØKZ
Ø7PN37Z
Ø7PN3JZ
Ø7PN3KZ
Ø7PN47Z
Ø7PN4JZ
Ø7PN4KZ
Ø7PPØØZ
Ø7PPØ3Z
Ø7PPØYZ
Ø7PP3ØZ
Ø7PP33Z
Ø7PP4ØZ
Ø7PP43Z
Ø7QØ*
Ø7Q1*
Ø7Q2*
Ø7Q3*
Ø7Q4*
Ø7Q5*
Ø7Q6*
Ø7Q7*
Ø7Q8*
Ø7Q9*
Ø7QB*
Ø7QC*
Ø7QD*
Ø7QF*
Ø7QG*
Ø7QH*
Ø7QJ*
Ø7QK*
Ø7QM*
Ø7QP*
Ø7S*
Ø7TM*
Ø7TP*
Ø7UØ*
Ø7U1*
Ø7U2*
Ø7U3*
Ø7U4*
Ø7U5*
Ø7U6*
Ø7U7*
Ø7U8*
Ø7U9*
Ø7UB*
Ø7UC*
Ø7UD*
Ø7UF*
Ø7UG*
Ø7UH*
Ø7UJ*
Ø7VØ*
Ø7V1*
Ø7V2*
Ø7V3*
Ø7V4*
Ø7V5*
Ø7V6*
Ø7V7*
Ø7V8*
Ø7V9*
Ø7VB*
Ø7VC*
Ø7VD*
Ø7VF*
Ø7VG*
Ø7VH*
Ø7VJ*
Ø7WKØ7Z
Ø7WKØJZ
Ø7WKØKZ
Ø7WK37Z
Ø7WK3JZ
Ø7WK3KZ
Ø7WK47Z
Ø7WK4JZ
Ø7WK4KZ
Ø7WLØ7Z
Ø7WLØJZ
Ø7WLØKZ
Ø7WL37Z
Ø7WL3JZ
Ø7WL3KZ
Ø7WL47Z
Ø7WL4JZ
Ø7WL4KZ
Ø7WMØØZ
Ø7WMØ3Z
Ø7WMØYZ
Ø7WM3ØZ
Ø7WM33Z
Ø7WM4ØZ
Ø7WM43Z
Ø7WNØ7Z
Ø7WNØJZ
Ø7WNØKZ
Ø7WN37Z
Ø7WN3JZ
Ø7WN3KZ
Ø7WN47Z
Ø7WN4JZ
Ø7WN4KZ
Ø7WPØØZ
Ø7WPØ3Z
Ø7WPØYZ
Ø7WP3ØZ
Ø7WP33Z
Ø7WP4ØZ
Ø7WP43Z
Ø81*
Ø8523ZZ
Ø8533ZZ
Ø8543ZZ
Ø8553ZZ
Ø856XZZ
Ø857XZZ
Ø858XZZ
Ø859XZZ
Ø85A*
Ø85B*
Ø85C3ZZ
Ø85D3ZZ
Ø85G3ZZ
Ø85H3ZZ
Ø85L*
Ø85M*
Ø85N*
Ø85P*
Ø85Q*
Ø85R*
Ø85SXZZ
Ø85TXZZ
Ø85V*
Ø85W*
Ø85X*
Ø85Y*
Ø87XØDZ
Ø87X3DZ
Ø87X7DZ
Ø87X8DZ
Ø87YØDZ
Ø87Y3DZ
Ø87Y7DZ
Ø87Y8DZ
Ø892*
Ø893*
Ø8943ØZ
Ø8943ZZ
Ø8953ØZ
Ø8953ZZ
Ø896XØZ
Ø897XØZ
Ø898XØZ
Ø899XØZ
Ø89AØØZ
Ø89AØZZ
Ø89A3ØZ
Ø89A3ZZ
Ø89BØØZ
Ø89BØZZ
Ø89B3ØZ
Ø89B3ZZ
Ø89C*
Ø89D*
Ø89E3ØZ
Ø89E3ZZ
Ø89F3ØZ
Ø89F3ZZ
Ø89G3ØZ
Ø89G3ZZ
Ø89H3ØZ
Ø89H3ZZ
Ø89J*

Ø89K*
Ø89LØØZ
Ø89LØZZ
Ø89L3ØZ
Ø89L3ZZ
Ø89MØØZ
Ø89MØZZ
Ø89M3ØZ
Ø89M3ZZ
Ø89NØZX
Ø89PØZX
Ø89QØZX
Ø89RØZX
Ø89VØZX
Ø89V3ZX
Ø89WØZX
Ø89W3ZX
Ø89X7ØZ
Ø89X7ZZ
Ø89X8ØZ
Ø89X8ZZ
Ø89Y7ØZ
Ø89Y7ZZ
Ø89Y8ØZ
Ø89Y8ZZ
Ø8BØØZZ
Ø8BØ3ZZ
Ø8BØXZZ
Ø8B1ØZZ
Ø8B13ZZ
Ø8B1XZZ
Ø8B43ZZ
Ø8B53ZZ
Ø8B6*
Ø8B7*
Ø8B8*
Ø8B9*
Ø8BAØZZ
Ø8BA3ZZ
Ø8BBØZZ
Ø8BB3ZZ
Ø8BC*
Ø8BD*
Ø8BJ3ZX
Ø8BK3ZX
Ø8BN*
Ø8BP*
Ø8BQ*
Ø8BR*
Ø8BSXZZ
Ø8BTXZZ
Ø8BV*
Ø8BW*
Ø8BXØZZ
Ø8BX3ZZ
Ø8BX7ZZ
Ø8BX8ZZ
Ø8BYØZZ
Ø8BY3ZZ
Ø8BY7ZZ
Ø8BY8ZZ
Ø8C23ZZ
Ø8C33ZZ
Ø8C4*
Ø8C5*
Ø8C8XZZ
Ø8C9XZZ
Ø8CA*
Ø8CB*
Ø8CC*
Ø8CD*
Ø8CE*
Ø8CF*
Ø8CG*
Ø8CH*
Ø8CJ*
Ø8CK*
Ø8CL*
Ø8CM*
Ø8CV3ZZ
Ø8CVXZZ
Ø8CW3ZZ
Ø8CWXZZ
Ø8F43ZZ
Ø8F53ZZ
Ø8HØØ5Z
Ø8HØØYZ
Ø8HØ31Z
Ø8HØX1Z
Ø8H1Ø5Z
Ø8H1ØYZ
Ø8H131Z
Ø8H1X1Z
Ø8L*
Ø8M*
Ø8N23ZZ
Ø8N33ZZ
Ø8N43ZZ
Ø8N53ZZ
Ø8N6XZZ
Ø8N7XZZ
Ø8N8XZZ
Ø8N9XZZ
Ø8NA*
Ø8NB*
Ø8NC3ZZ
Ø8ND3ZZ
Ø8NE3ZZ
Ø8NF3ZZ
Ø8NG3ZZ
Ø8NH3ZZ
Ø8NJ3ZZ
Ø8NK3ZZ
Ø8NL*
Ø8NM*
Ø8NN*
Ø8NP*
Ø8NQ*
Ø8NR*
Ø8NV*
Ø8NW*
Ø8NX*
Ø8NY*
Ø8PØØ3Z
Ø8PØØJZ
Ø8PØ3JZ
Ø8P1Ø3Z
Ø8P1ØJZ
Ø8P13JZ
Ø8PJ3JZ
Ø8PK3JZ
Ø8PLØØZ
Ø8PLØYZ
Ø8PL3ØZ
Ø8PMØØZ
Ø8PMØYZ
Ø8PM3ØZ
Ø8QØXZZ
Ø8Q1XZZ
Ø8Q23ZZ
Ø8Q33ZZ
Ø8Q43ZZ
Ø8Q53ZZ
Ø8Q6XZZ
Ø8Q7XZZ
Ø8Q8XZZ
Ø8Q9XZZ
Ø8QA*
Ø8QB*
Ø8QC3ZZ
Ø8QD3ZZ
Ø8QE3ZZ
Ø8QF3ZZ
Ø8QG3ZZ
Ø8QH3ZZ
Ø8QJ3ZZ
Ø8QK3ZZ
Ø8QL*
Ø8QM*
Ø8QSXZZ
Ø8QTXZZ
Ø8QV*
Ø8QW*
Ø8QX*
Ø8QY*
Ø8R*
Ø8SC3ZZ
Ø8SD3ZZ
Ø8SG3ZZ
Ø8SH3ZZ
Ø8SJ3ZZ
Ø8SK3ZZ
Ø8SN*
Ø8SP*
Ø8SQ*
Ø8SR*
Ø8SV*
Ø8SW*
Ø8SX*
Ø8SY*
Ø8TØXZZ
Ø8T1XZZ
Ø8T43ZZ
Ø8T53ZZ
Ø8T8XZZ
Ø8T9XZZ
Ø8TC3ZZ
Ø8TD3ZZ
Ø8TJ3ZZ
Ø8TK3ZZ
Ø8TN*
Ø8TP*
Ø8TQ*
Ø8TR*
Ø8TV*
Ø8TW*
Ø8TX*
Ø8TY*
Ø8UØ*
Ø8U1*
Ø8U8*
Ø8U9*
Ø8UC*
Ø8UD*
Ø8UEØJZ
Ø8UE3JZ
Ø8UFØJZ
Ø8UF3JZ
Ø8UG*
Ø8UH*
Ø8UL*
Ø8UM*
Ø8UN*
Ø8UP*
Ø8UQ*
Ø8UR*
Ø8UX*
Ø8UY*
Ø8V*
Ø8WØØJZ
Ø8WØ3JZ
Ø8W1ØJZ
Ø8W13JZ
Ø8WJ3JZ
Ø8WK3JZ
Ø8WLØØZ
Ø8WLØYZ
Ø8WL3ØZ
Ø8WMØØZ
Ø8WMØYZ
Ø8WM3ØZ
Ø9Ø*
Ø98L*
Ø99NØØZ
Ø99NØZZ
Ø99N4ØZ
Ø99N4ZZ
Ø99N7ØZ
Ø99N7ZZ
Ø99N8ØZ
Ø99N8ZZ
Ø9BLØZZ
Ø9BL3ZZ
Ø9BL4ZZ
Ø9BL7ZZ
Ø9BL8ZZ
Ø9BMØZZ
Ø9BM3ZZ
Ø9BM4ZZ
Ø9BM8ZZ
Ø9CN*
Ø9DL*
Ø9DM*
Ø9M*
Ø9NØØZZ
Ø9NØ3ZZ
Ø9NØ4ZZ
Ø9N1ØZZ
Ø9N13ZZ
Ø9N14ZZ
Ø9N3ØZZ
Ø9N33ZZ
Ø9N34ZZ
Ø9N37ZZ
Ø9N38ZZ
Ø9N4ØZZ
Ø9N43ZZ
Ø9N44ZZ
Ø9N47ZZ
Ø9N48ZZ
Ø9QØØZZ
Ø9QØ3ZZ
Ø9QØ4ZZ
Ø9Q1ØZZ
Ø9Q13ZZ
Ø9Q14ZZ
Ø9Q2ØZZ
Ø9Q23ZZ
Ø9Q24ZZ
Ø9Q3ØZZ
Ø9Q33ZZ
Ø9Q34ZZ
Ø9Q37ZZ
Ø9Q38ZZ
Ø9Q4ØZZ
Ø9Q43ZZ
Ø9Q44ZZ
Ø9Q47ZZ
Ø9Q48ZZ
Ø9QKØZZ
Ø9QK3ZZ
Ø9QK4ZZ
Ø9QK8ZZ
Ø9QL*
Ø9QM*
Ø9QN*
Ø9RØ*
Ø9R1*
Ø9R2*
Ø9RK*
Ø9RL*
Ø9RM*
Ø9RN*
Ø9SØ*
Ø9S1*
Ø9S2*
Ø9SK*
Ø9SL*
Ø9SM*
Ø9TØ*
Ø9T1*
Ø9TK*
Ø9TL*
Ø9TM*
Ø9UØ*
Ø9U1*
Ø9U2*
Ø9UK*
Ø9UL*
Ø9UM*
Ø9UN*
ØB5KØZ3
ØB5KØZZ
ØB5K4Z3
ØB5K7ZZ
ØB5LØZ3
ØB5LØZZ
ØB5L4Z3
ØB5L7ZZ
ØB5MØZ3
ØB5MØZZ
ØB5M4Z3
ØB5M7ZZ
ØB5N*
ØB5P*
ØB71*
ØB72*
ØB9CØØZ
ØB9CØZZ
ØB9DØØZ
ØB9DØZZ
ØB9FØØZ
ØB9FØZZ
ØB9GØØZ
ØB9GØZZ
ØB9HØØZ
ØB9HØZZ
ØB9JØØZ
ØB9JØZZ
ØB9KØØZ
ØB9KØZZ
ØB9LØØZ
ØB9LØZZ
ØB9MØØZ
ØB9MØZZ
ØBBC4ZZ
ØBBD4ZZ
ØBBF4ZZ
ØBBG4ZZ
ØBBH4ZZ
ØBBJ4ZZ
ØBBK4ZZ
ØBBL4ZZ
ØBBMØZZ
ØBBM3ZZ
ØBBM7ZZ
ØBBNØZZ
ØBBN3ZZ
ØBBN4ZZ
ØBBN8ZZ
ØBBPØZZ
ØBBP3ZZ
ØBBP4ZZ
ØBBP8ZZ
ØBCCØZZ
ØBCC3ZZ
ØBCC4ZZ
ØBCC7ZZ
ØBCC8ZZ
ØBCD*
ØBCF*
ØBCG*
ØBCH*
ØBCJ*
ØBCK*
ØBCL*
ØBCM*
ØBDNØZX
ØBDNØZZ
ØBDN3ZX
ØBDN3ZZ
ØBDN4ZX
ØBDN4ZZ
ØBDPØZX
ØBDPØZZ
ØBDP3ZX
ØBDP3ZZ
ØBDP4ZX
ØBDP4ZZ
ØBF1ØZZ
ØBF13ZZ
ØBF14ZZ
ØBF17ZZ
ØBF18ZZ
ØBF2ØZZ
ØBF23ZZ
ØBF24ZZ
ØBF27ZZ
ØBF28ZZ
ØBHØØ1Z
ØBHØ31Z
ØBHØ41Z
ØBHØ71Z
ØBHØ81Z
ØBHKØ1Z
ØBHKØ2Z
ØBHKØ3Z
ØBHKØYZ
ØBHK31Z
ØBHK32Z
ØBHK33Z
ØBHK41Z
ØBHK42Z
ØBHK43Z
ØBHK4YZ
ØBHK71Z
ØBHK81Z
ØBHK8YZ
ØBHLØ1Z
ØBHLØ2Z
ØBHLØ3Z
ØBHLØYZ
ØBHL31Z
ØBHL32Z
ØBHL33Z
ØBHL41Z
ØBHL42Z
ØBHL43Z
ØBHL4YZ
ØBHL71Z
ØBHL81Z
ØBHL8YZ
ØBHQØYZ
ØBHQ4YZ
ØBHQ8YZ
ØBHTØMZ
ØBHT3MZ
ØBHT4MZ
ØBHT4YZ
ØBJØ4ZZ
ØBJK4ZZ
ØBJL4ZZ
ØBL1*
ØBL2*
ØBM1ØZZ
ØBM2ØZZ
ØBN1*
ØBN2*
ØBNN*
ØBNP*
ØBPKØØZ
ØBPKØ1Z
ØBPKØ2Z
ØBPKØ3Z
ØBPKØYZ
ØBPK3ØZ
ØBPK31Z
ØBPK32Z
ØBPK33Z
ØBPK4ØZ
ØBPK41Z
ØBPK42Z
ØBPK43Z
ØBPK4YZ
ØBPK8YZ
ØBPLØØZ
ØBPLØ1Z
ØBPLØ2Z
ØBPLØ3Z
ØBPLØYZ
ØBPL3ØZ
ØBPL31Z
ØBPL32Z
ØBPL33Z
ØBPL4ØZ
ØBPL41Z
ØBPL42Z
ØBPL43Z
ØBPL4YZ
ØBPL71Z
ØBPL81Z
ØBPL8YZ
ØBPQØYZ
ØBPQ4YZ
ØBPQ8YZ
ØBQ1*
ØBQ2*
ØBQ3*
ØBQ4*
ØBQ5*
ØBQ6*
ØBQ7*
ØBQ8*
ØBQ9*
ØBQB*
ØBQK*
ØBQL*
ØBQM*
ØBQN*
ØBQP*
ØBQTØZZ
ØBQT3ZZ
ØBQT4ZZ
ØBR1Ø7Z
ØBR1ØJZ
ØBR1ØKZ
ØBR147Z
ØBR14JZ
ØBR14KZ
ØBR2Ø7Z
ØBR2ØJZ
ØBR2ØKZ
ØBR247Z
ØBR24JZ
ØBR24KZ
ØBR3Ø7Z
ØBR3ØJZ
ØBR3ØKZ
ØBR347Z
ØBR34JZ
ØBR34KZ
ØBR4Ø7Z
ØBR4ØJZ
ØBR4ØKZ
ØBR447Z
ØBR44JZ
ØBR44KZ
ØBR5Ø7Z
ØBR5ØJZ
ØBR5ØKZ
ØBR547Z
ØBR54JZ
ØBR54KZ
ØBR6Ø7Z
ØBR6ØJZ
ØBR6ØKZ
ØBR647Z
ØBR64JZ
ØBR64KZ
ØBR7Ø7Z
ØBR7ØJZ
ØBR7ØKZ
ØBR747Z
ØBR74JZ
ØBR74KZ
ØBR8Ø7Z
ØBR8ØJZ
ØBR8ØKZ
ØBR847Z
ØBR84JZ
ØBR84KZ
ØBR9Ø7Z
ØBR9ØJZ
ØBR9ØKZ
ØBR947Z
ØBR94JZ
ØBR94KZ
ØBRBØ7Z
ØBRBØJZ
ØBRBØKZ
ØBRB47Z
ØBRB4JZ
ØBRB4KZ
ØBRTØ7Z
ØBRTØJZ
ØBRTØKZ
ØBRT47Z
ØBRT4JZ
ØBRT4KZ
ØBS1ØZZ
ØBS2ØZZ
ØBT*
ØBU1*
ØBU2*
ØBUTØ7Z
ØBUTØJZ
ØBUTØKZ
ØBUT47Z
ØBUT4JZ
ØBUT4KZ
ØBV1*
ØBV2*
ØBW1ØFZ
ØBW13FZ
ØBW14FZ
ØBWKØØZ
ØBWKØ2Z
ØBWKØ3Z
ØBWKØYZ
ØBWK3ØZ
ØBWK32Z
ØBWK33Z
ØBWK4ØZ
ØBWK42Z
ØBWK43Z
ØBWK4YZ
ØBWK8YZ
ØBWLØØZ
ØBWLØ2Z
ØBWLØ3Z
ØBWLØYZ
ØBWL3ØZ
ØBWL32Z
ØBWL33Z
ØBWL4ØZ
ØBWL42Z
ØBWL43Z
ØBWL4YZ
ØBWL8YZ
ØBWQ4YZ
ØBWQ8YZ
ØCØ*
ØC53*
ØC54*
ØC5R*
ØC9ØØØZ
ØC9ØØZZ
ØC9ØXØZ
ØC9ØXZZ
ØC91ØØZ
ØC91ØZZ
ØC91XØZ
ØC91XZZ
ØC94ØØZ
ØC94ØZZ
ØC94XØZ
ØC94XZZ
ØC9MØØZ
ØC9MØZZ
ØC9M4ØZ
ØC9M4ZZ
ØC9M7ØZ
ØC9M7ZZ
ØC9M8ØZ
ØC9M8ZZ
ØCB3ØZZ
ØCB33ZZ
ØCB3XZZ
ØCB4ØZZ
ØCB43ZZ
ØCB4XZZ
ØCBRØZZ
ØCBR3ZZ
ØCBR4ZZ
ØCBR7ZZ
ØCBR8ZZ
ØCBSØZZ
ØCBS3ZZ
ØCBS4ZZ
ØCBS7ZZ
ØCBS8ZZ
ØCBTØZZ
ØCBT3ZZ
ØCBT4ZZ
ØCBT7ZZ
ØCBT8ZZ
ØCBVØZZ
ØCBV3ZZ
ØCBV4ZZ
ØCBV7ZZ
ØCBV8ZZ
ØCCØØZZ
ØCCØ3ZZ
ØCC1ØZZ
ØCC13ZZ
ØCC4ØZZ
ØCC43ZZ
ØCCMØZZ
ØCCM3ZZ
ØCCM4ZZ
ØCCPØZZ
ØCCP3ZZ
ØCCQØZZ
ØCCQ3ZZ
ØCH7*
ØCHAØYZ
ØCMØØZZ
ØCM1ØZZ
ØCM3ØZZ
ØCM7ØZZ
ØCN2*
ØCN3*
ØCN4ØZZ
ØCN43ZZ
ØCN8*
ØCN9*
ØCNB*
ØCNC*
ØCND*
ØCNF*
ØCNG*
ØCNH*
ØCNJ*
ØCNR*
ØCNS*
ØCNT*
ØCNV*
ØCPYØØZ
ØCPYØ1Z
ØCPYØ7Z
ØCPYØDZ
ØCPYØJZ
ØCPYØKZ
ØCPYØYZ
ØCPY3ØZ
ØCPY31Z
ØCPY37Z
ØCPY3DZ
ØCPY3JZ
ØCPY3KZ
ØCPY71Z
ØCPY77Z
ØCPY7JZ
ØCPY7KZ
ØCPY81Z
ØCPY87Z
ØCPY8JZ
ØCPY8KZ
ØCQØØZZ
ØCQØ3ZZ
ØCQ1ØZZ
ØCQ13ZZ
ØCQ2*
ØCQ3*
ØCQ4ØZZ
ØCQ43ZZ
ØCQ8*
ØCQ9*
ØCQB*
ØCQC*
ØCQD*
ØCQF*
ØCQG*
ØCQH*
ØCQJ*
ØCQM*
ØCQR*
ØCQS*
ØCQT*
ØCQV*
ØCRØ*
ØCR1*
ØCR4*
ØCR5*
ØCR6*
ØCR7*
ØCRB*
ØCRC*
ØCRM*
ØCRR*
ØCRS*
ØCRTØ7Z
ØCRTØKZ
ØCRT77Z
ØCRT7KZ
ØCRT87Z
ØCRT8KZ
ØCRVØ7Z
ØCRVØKZ
ØCRV77Z
ØCRV7KZ
ØCRV8JZ
ØCRV8KZ
ØCSØ*
ØCS1*
ØCS7*
ØCSB*
ØCSC*
ØCSR*
ØCSSØZZ
ØCSS7ZZ
ØCSS8ZZ
ØCST*
ØCSV*
ØCTØ*
ØCT1*
ØCT3*
ØCTR*
ØCTT*
ØCTV*
ØCUØ*
ØCU1*
ØCU4*
ØCU5*
ØCU6*
ØCU7*
ØCUM*
ØCUR*
ØCUS*
ØCUT*
ØCUV*
ØCVB7DZ
ØCVB7ZZ
ØCVB8DZ
ØCVB8ZZ
ØCVC7DZ
ØCVC7ZZ
ØCVC8DZ
ØCVC8ZZ
ØCWYØØZ
ØCWYØ1Z
ØCWYØDZ
ØCWYØJZ
ØCWYØKZ
ØCWYØYZ
ØCWY3ØZ
ØCWY31Z
ØCWY37Z
ØCWY3DZ
ØCWY3JZ
ØCWY3KZ
ØCWY7ØZ
ØCWY71Z
ØCWY77Z
ØCWY7DZ
ØCWY7JZ
ØCWY7KZ
ØCWY8ØZ
ØCWY81Z
ØCWY87Z
ØCWY8DZ
ØCWY8JZ
ØCWY8KZ
ØCX*
ØD11Ø74
ØD11Ø76
ØD11ØJ4
ØD11ØJ6
ØD11ØK4
ØD11ØK6
ØD11ØZ4
ØD11ØZ6
ØD113J4
ØD11474
ØD11476
ØD114J4
ØD114J6
ØD114K4
ØD114K6
ØD114Z4
ØD114Z6
ØD11874
ØD11876
ØD118J4
ØD118J6

ØD118K4
ØD118K6
ØD118Z4
ØD118Z6
ØD12Ø74
ØD12Ø76
ØD12ØJ4
ØD12ØJ6
ØD12ØK4
ØD12ØK6
ØD12ØZ4
ØD12ØZ6
ØD123J4
ØD12474
ØD12476
ØD124J4
ØD124J6
ØD124K4
ØD124K6
ØD124Z4
ØD124Z6
ØD12874
ØD12876
ØD128J4
ØD128J6
ØD128K4
ØD128K6
ØD128Z4
ØD128Z6
ØD13Ø74
ØD13Ø76
ØD13ØJ4
ØD13ØJ6
ØD13ØK4
ØD13ØK6
ØD13ØZ4
ØD13ØZ6
ØD133J4
ØD13474
ØD13476
ØD134J4
ØD134J6
ØD134K4
ØD134K6
ØD134Z4
ØD134Z6
ØD13874
ØD13876
ØD138J4
ØD138J6
ØD138K4
ØD138K6
ØD138Z4
ØD138Z6
ØD15*
ØD18Ø74
ØD18Ø78
ØD18Ø7H
ØD18Ø7K
ØD18Ø7L
ØD18Ø7M
ØD18Ø7N
ØD18Ø7P
ØD18Ø7Q
ØD18ØJ4
ØD18ØJ8
ØD18ØJH
ØD18ØJK
ØD18ØJL
ØD18ØJM
ØD18ØJN
ØD18ØJP
ØD18ØJQ
ØD18ØK4
ØD18ØK8
ØD18ØKH
ØD18ØKK
ØD18ØKL
ØD18ØKM
ØD18ØKN
ØD18ØKP
ØD18ØKQ
ØD18ØZ4
ØD18ØZ8
ØD18ØZH
ØD18ØZK
ØD18ØZL
ØD18ØZM
ØD18ØZN
ØD18ØZP
ØD18ØZQ
ØD18474
ØD18478
ØD1847H
ØD1847K
ØD1847L
ØD1847M
ØD1847N
ØD1847P
ØD1847Q
ØD184J4
ØD184J8
ØD184JH
ØD184JK
ØD184JL
ØD184JM
ØD184JN
ØD184JP
ØD184JQ
ØD184K4
ØD184K8
ØD184KH
ØD184KK
ØD184KL
ØD184KM
ØD184KN
ØD184KP
ØD184KQ
ØD184Z4
ØD184Z8
ØD184ZH
ØD184ZK
ØD184ZL
ØD184ZM
ØD184ZN
ØD184ZP
ØD184ZQ
ØD18874
ØD18878
ØD1887H
ØD1887K
ØD1887L
ØD1887M
ØD1887N
ØD1887P
ØD1887Q
ØD188J4
ØD188J8
ØD188JH
ØD188JK
ØD188JL
ØD188JM
ØD188JN
ØD188JP
ØD188JQ
ØD188K4
ØD188K8
ØD188KH
ØD188KK
ØD188KL
ØD188KM
ØD188KN
ØD188KP
ØD188KQ
ØD188Z4
ØD188Z8
ØD188ZH
ØD188ZK
ØD188ZL
ØD188ZM
ØD188ZN
ØD188ZP
ØD188ZQ
ØD19*
ØD1A*
ØD1B*
ØD1EØ74
ØD1EØ7E
ØD1EØ7P
ØD1EØJ4
ØD1EØJE
ØD1EØJP
ØD1EØK4
ØD1EØKE
ØD1EØKP
ØD1EØZ4
ØD1EØZE
ØD1EØZP
ØD1E474
ØD1E47E
ØD1E47P
ØD1E4J4
ØD1E4JE
ØD1E4JP
ØD1E4K4
ØD1E4KE
ØD1E4KP
ØD1E4Z4
ØD1E4ZE
ØD1E4ZP
ØD1E874
ØD1E87E
ØD1E87P
ØD1E8J4
ØD1E8JE
ØD1E8JP
ØD1E8K4
ØD1E8KE
ØD1E8KP
ØD1E8Z4
ØD1E8ZE
ØD1E8ZP
ØD1H*
ØD1K*
ØD1L*
ØD1M*
ØD1NØ74
ØD1NØ7N
ØD1NØ7P
ØD1NØJ4
ØD1NØJN
ØD1NØJP
ØD1NØK4
ØD1NØKN
ØD1NØKP
ØD1NØZN
ØD1NØZP
ØD1N3J4
ØD1N474
ØD1N47N
ØD1N47P
ØD1N4J4
ØD1N4JN
ØD1N4JP
ØD1N4K4
ØD1N4KN
ØD1N4KP
ØD1N4Z4
ØD1N4ZN
ØD1N4ZP
ØD1N874
ØD1N87N
ØD1N87P
ØD1N8J4
ØD1N8JN
ØD1N8JP
ØD1N8K4
ØD1N8KN
ØD1N8KP
ØD1N8Z4
ØD1N8ZN
ØD1N8ZP
ØD71ØDZ
ØD71ØZZ
ØD713DZ
ØD713ZZ
ØD714DZ
ØD714ZZ
ØD72ØDZ
ØD72ØZZ
ØD723DZ
ØD723ZZ
ØD724DZ
ØD724ZZ
ØD73ØDZ
ØD73ØZZ
ØD733DZ
ØD733ZZ
ØD734DZ
ØD734ZZ
ØD74ØDZ
ØD74ØZZ
ØD743DZ
ØD743ZZ
ØD744DZ
ØD744ZZ
ØD75ØDZ
ØD75ØZZ
ØD753DZ
ØD753ZZ
ØD754DZ
ØD754ZZ
ØD76ØDZ
ØD76ØZZ
ØD763DZ
ØD763ZZ
ØD764DZ
ØD764ZZ
ØD7QØDZ
ØD7QØZZ
ØD7Q3DZ
ØD7Q3ZZ
ØD7Q4DZ
ØD7Q4ZZ
ØD84*
ØD91ØØZ
ØD91ØZZ
ØD914ØZ
ØD914ZZ
ØD917ØZ
ØD917ZZ
ØD918ØZ
ØD918ZZ
ØD92ØØZ
ØD92ØZZ
ØD924ØZ
ØD924ZZ
ØD927ØZ
ØD927ZZ
ØD928ØZ
ØD928ZZ
ØD93ØØZ
ØD93ØZZ
ØD934ØZ
ØD934ZZ
ØD937ØZ
ØD937ZZ
ØD938ØZ
ØD938ZZ
ØD94ØØZ
ØD94ØZZ
ØD944ØZ
ØD944ZZ
ØD947ØZ
ØD947ZZ
ØD948ØZ
ØD948ZZ
ØD95ØØZ
ØD95ØZZ
ØD954ØZ
ØD954ZZ
ØD957ØZ
ØD957ZZ
ØD958ØZ
ØD958ZZ
ØD96ØØZ
ØD96ØZZ
ØD964ØZ
ØD964ZZ
ØD967ZZ
ØD968ZZ
ØD98ØØZ
ØD98ØZZ
ØD984ØZ
ØD984ZZ
ØD987ZZ
ØD988ZZ
ØD99ØØZ
ØD99ØZZ
ØD994ØZ
ØD994ZZ
ØD997ZZ
ØD998ZZ
ØD9AØØZ
ØD9AØZZ
ØD9A4ØZ
ØD9A4ZZ
ØD9A7ZZ
ØD9A8ZZ
ØD9BØØZ
ØD9BØZZ
ØD9B4ØZ
ØD9B4ZZ
ØD9B7ZZ
ØD9B8ZZ
ØD9CØØZ
ØD9CØZZ
ØD9C4ØZ
ØD9C4ZZ
ØD9C7ØZ
ØD9C7ZZ
ØD9C8ØZ
ØD9C8ZZ
ØD9EØØZ
ØD9EØZZ
ØD9E4ØZ
ØD9E4ZZ
ØD9E7ZZ
ØD9E8ZZ
ØD9FØØZ
ØD9FØZZ
ØD9F4ØZ
ØD9F4ZZ
ØD9F7ZZ
ØD9F8ZZ
ØD9GØØZ
ØD9GØZZ
ØD9G4ØZ
ØD9G4ZZ
ØD9G7ZZ
ØD9G8ZZ
ØD9HØØZ
ØD9HØZZ
ØD9H4ØZ
ØD9H4ZZ
ØD9H7ZZ
ØD9H8ZZ
ØD9KØØZ
ØD9KØZZ
ØD9K4ØZ
ØD9K4ZZ
ØD9K7ZZ
ØD9K8ZZ
ØD9LØØZ
ØD9LØZZ
ØD9L4ØZ
ØD9L4ZZ
ØD9L7ZZ
ØD9L8ZZ
ØD9MØØZ
ØD9MØZZ
ØD9M4ØZ
ØD9M4ZZ
ØD9M7ZZ
ØD9M8ZZ
ØD9NØØZ
ØD9NØZZ
ØD9N4ØZ
ØD9N4ZZ
ØD9N7ZZ
ØD9N8ZZ
ØD9PØØZ
ØD9PØZZ
ØD9P4ØZ
ØD9P4ZZ
ØD9P7ZZ
ØD9P8ZZ
ØD9UØØZ
ØD9UØZZ
ØD9VØØZ
ØD9VØZZ
ØD9WØØZ
ØD9WØZZ
ØD9W4ØZ
ØD9W4ZZ
ØDB1ØZZ
ØDB13ZZ
ØDB17ZZ
ØDB2ØZZ
ØDB23ZZ
ØDB27ZZ
ØDB3ØZZ
ØDB33ZZ
ØDB37ZZ
ØDB4ØZZ
ØDB43ZZ
ØDB44ZZ
ØDB47ZZ
ØDB5ØZZ
ØDB53ZZ
ØDB57ZZ
ØDB6ØZ3
ØDB6ØZZ
ØDB63Z3
ØDB63ZZ
ØDB67Z3
ØDB67ZZ
ØDB68Z3
ØDB8ØZZ
ØDB84ZZ
ØDB87ZZ
ØDB97ZZ
ØDBA7ZZ
ØDBB7ZZ
ØDBEØZZ
ØDBE3ZZ
ØDBE4ZZ
ØDBFØZZ
ØDBF3ZZ
ØDBF4ZZ
ØDBGØZZ
ØDBG3ZZ
ØDBG4ZZ
ØDBHØZZ
ØDBH3ZZ
ØDBH4ZZ
ØDBKØZZ
ØDBK3ZZ
ØDBK4ZZ
ØDBLØZZ
ØDBL3ZZ
ØDBL4ZZ
ØDBMØZZ
ØDBM3ZZ
ØDBM4ZZ
ØDBNØZZ
ØDBN3ZZ
ØDBN4ZZ
ØDBPØZZ
ØDBP3ZZ
ØDBP4ZZ
ØDBP7ZZ
ØDBQØZZ
ØDBQ3ZZ
ØDBQ4ZZ
ØDC1ØZZ
ØDC13ZZ
ØDC14ZZ
ØDC2ØZZ
ØDC23ZZ
ØDC24ZZ
ØDC3ØZZ
ØDC33ZZ
ØDC34ZZ
ØDC4ØZZ
ØDC43ZZ
ØDC44ZZ
ØDC5ØZZ
ØDC53ZZ
ØDC54ZZ
ØDC6ØZZ
ØDC63ZZ
ØDC64ZZ
ØDC8ØZZ
ØDC83ZZ
ØDC84ZZ
ØDC9ØZZ
ØDC93ZZ
ØDC94ZZ
ØDCAØZZ
ØDCA3ZZ
ØDCA4ZZ
ØDCBØZZ
ØDCB3ZZ
ØDCB4ZZ
ØDCCØZZ
ØDCC3ZZ
ØDCC4ZZ
ØDCEØZZ
ØDCE3ZZ
ØDCE4ZZ
ØDCFØZZ
ØDCF3ZZ
ØDCF4ZZ
ØDCGØZZ
ØDCG3ZZ
ØDCG4ZZ
ØDCHØZZ
ØDCH3ZZ
ØDCH4ZZ
ØDCKØZZ
ØDCK3ZZ
ØDCK4ZZ
ØDCLØZZ
ØDCL3ZZ
ØDCL4ZZ
ØDCMØZZ
ØDCM3ZZ
ØDCM4ZZ
ØDCNØZZ
ØDCN3ZZ
ØDCN4ZZ
ØDCPØZZ
ØDCP3ZZ
ØDCP4ZZ
ØDCUØZZ
ØDCU3ZZ
ØDCU4ZZ
ØDCV*
ØDCW*
ØDF5ØZZ
ØDF53ZZ
ØDF54ZZ
ØDF57ZZ
ØDF58ZZ
ØDF6ØZZ
ØDF63ZZ
ØDF64ZZ
ØDF67ZZ
ØDF68ZZ
ØDF8ØZZ
ØDF83ZZ
ØDF84ZZ
ØDF87ZZ
ØDF88ZZ
ØDF9ØZZ
ØDF93ZZ
ØDF94ZZ
ØDF97ZZ
ØDF98ZZ
ØDFAØZZ
ØDFA3ZZ
ØDFA4ZZ
ØDFA7ZZ
ØDFA8ZZ
ØDFBØZZ
ØDFB3ZZ
ØDFB4ZZ
ØDFB7ZZ
ØDFB8ZZ
ØDFEØZZ
ØDFE3ZZ
ØDFE4ZZ
ØDFE7ZZ
ØDFE8ZZ
ØDFFØZZ
ØDFF3ZZ
ØDFF4ZZ
ØDFF7ZZ
ØDFF8ZZ
ØDFGØZZ
ØDFG3ZZ
ØDFG4ZZ
ØDFG7ZZ
ØDFG8ZZ
ØDFHØZZ
ØDFH3ZZ
ØDFH4ZZ
ØDFH7ZZ
ØDFH8ZZ
ØDFKØZZ
ØDFK3ZZ
ØDFK4ZZ
ØDFK7ZZ
ØDFK8ZZ
ØDFLØZZ
ØDFL3ZZ
ØDFL4ZZ
ØDFL7ZZ
ØDFL8ZZ
ØDFMØZZ
ØDFM3ZZ
ØDFM4ZZ
ØDFM7ZZ
ØDFM8ZZ
ØDFNØZZ
ØDFN3ZZ
ØDFN4ZZ
ØDFN7ZZ
ØDFN8ZZ
ØDFPØZZ
ØDFP3ZZ
ØDFP4ZZ
ØDFP7ZZ
ØDFP8ZZ
ØDFQØZZ
ØDFQ3ZZ
ØDFQ4ZZ
ØDFQ7ZZ
ØDFQ8ZZ
ØDH5Ø1Z
ØDH5Ø2Z
ØDH5Ø3Z
ØDH5ØYZ
ØDH531Z
ØDH532Z
ØDH533Z
ØDH541Z
ØDH542Z
ØDH543Z
ØDH571Z
ØDH581Z
ØDH6Ø1Z
ØDH6Ø2Z
ØDH6Ø3Z
ØDH6ØDZ
ØDH6ØMZ
ØDH6ØYZ
ØDH632Z
ØDH633Z
ØDH63DZ
ØDH63MZ
ØDH641Z
ØDH642Z
ØDH643Z
ØDH64DZ
ØDH64MZ
ØDH8Ø2Z
ØDH8Ø3Z
ØDH832Z
ØDH833Z
ØDH842Z
ØDH843Z
ØDH9Ø2Z
ØDH9Ø3Z
ØDH932Z
ØDH933Z
ØDH942Z
ØDH943Z
ØDHAØ2Z
ØDHAØ3Z
ØDHA32Z
ØDHA33Z
ØDHA42Z
ØDHA43Z
ØDHBØ2Z
ØDHBØ3Z
ØDHB32Z
ØDHB33Z
ØDHB42Z
ØDHB43Z
ØDHPØ1Z
ØDHP31Z
ØDHP41Z
ØDHP71Z
ØDHP81Z
ØDHQ*
ØDJØØZZ
ØDJØ4ZZ
ØDJ6ØZZ
ØDJ64ZZ
ØDJDØZZ
ØDJD4ZZ
ØDJUØZZ
ØDJU4ZZ
ØDJVØZZ
ØDJV4ZZ
ØDJWØZZ
ØDJW4ZZ
ØDL6*
ØDL7*
ØDLQ*
ØDM*
ØDN1*
ØDN2*
ØDN3*
ØDN4*
ØDN5*
ØDN6*
ØDN8ØZZ
ØDN83ZZ
ØDN84ZZ
ØDN9ØZZ
ØDN93ZZ
ØDN94ZZ
ØDNAØZZ
ØDNA3ZZ
ØDNA4ZZ
ØDNBØZZ
ØDNB3ZZ
ØDNB4ZZ
ØDNC*
ØDNEØZZ
ØDNE3ZZ
ØDNE4ZZ
ØDNFØZZ
ØDNF3ZZ
ØDNF4ZZ
ØDNGØZZ
ØDNG3ZZ
ØDNG4ZZ
ØDNHØZZ
ØDNH3ZZ
ØDNH4ZZ
ØDNJØZZ
ØDNJ3ZZ
ØDNJ4ZZ
ØDNKØZZ
ØDNK3ZZ
ØDNK4ZZ
ØDNLØZZ
ØDNL3ZZ
ØDNL4ZZ
ØDNMØZZ
ØDNM3ZZ
ØDNM4ZZ
ØDNNØZZ
ØDNN3ZZ
ØDNN4ZZ
ØDNP*
ØDNR*
ØDNUØZZ
ØDNU3ZZ
ØDNU4ZZ
ØDNV*
ØDNW*
ØDPØØØZ
ØDPØØ2Z
ØDPØØ3Z
ØDPØØ7Z
ØDPØØCZ
ØDPØØDZ
ØDPØØJZ
ØDPØØKZ
ØDPØØUZ
ØDPØØYZ
ØDPØ3ØZ
ØDPØ32Z
ØDPØ33Z
ØDPØ37Z
ØDPØ3CZ
ØDPØ3DZ
ØDPØ3JZ
ØDPØ3KZ
ØDPØ3UZ
ØDPØ4ØZ
ØDPØ42Z
ØDPØ43Z
ØDPØ47Z
ØDPØ4CZ
ØDPØ4DZ
ØDPØ4JZ
ØDPØ4KZ
ØDPØ4UZ
ØDPØ77Z
ØDPØ7CZ
ØDPØ7JZ
ØDPØ7KZ
ØDPØ87Z
ØDPØ8CZ
ØDPØ8JZ
ØDPØ8KZ
ØDP5Ø1Z
ØDP5Ø2Z
ØDP5Ø3Z
ØDP5ØUZ
ØDP5ØYZ
ØDP531Z
ØDP532Z
ØDP533Z
ØDP53UZ
ØDP541Z
ØDP542Z
ØDP543Z
ØDP54UZ
ØDP6ØØZ
ØDP6Ø2Z
ØDP6Ø3Z
ØDP6Ø7Z
ØDP6ØCZ
ØDP6ØDZ
ØDP6ØJZ
ØDP6ØKZ
ØDP6ØMZ
ØDP6ØUZ
ØDP6ØYZ
ØDP63ØZ
ØDP632Z
ØDP633Z
ØDP637Z
ØDP63CZ
ØDP63DZ
ØDP63JZ
ØDP63KZ
ØDP63MZ
ØDP63UZ
ØDP64ØZ
ØDP642Z
ØDP647Z
ØDP64DZ
ØDP64JZ
ØDP64KZ
ØDP64MZ
ØDP64UZ
ØDP677Z
ØDP67CZ
ØDP67JZ
ØDP67KZ
ØDP687Z
ØDP68CZ
ØDP68JZ
ØDP68KZ
ØDPDØØZ
ØDPDØ2Z
ØDPDØ3Z
ØDPDØ7Z
ØDPDØCZ
ØDPDØDZ
ØDPDØJZ
ØDPDØKZ
ØDPDØUZ
ØDPDØYZ
ØDPD3ØZ
ØDPD32Z
ØDPD33Z

ØDPD37Z
ØDPD3CZ
ØDPD3DZ
ØDPD3JZ
ØDPD3KZ
ØDPD3UZ
ØDPD4ØZ
ØDPD42Z
ØDPD43Z
ØDPD47Z
ØDPD4CZ
ØDPD4DZ
ØDPD4JZ
ØDPD4KZ
ØDPD4UZ
ØDPD77Z
ØDPD7CZ
ØDPD7JZ
ØDPD7KZ
ØDPD87Z
ØDPD8CZ
ØDPD8JZ
ØDPD8KZ
ØDPPØ1Z
ØDPP31Z
ØDPP41Z
ØDPQ*
ØDPR*
ØDQ1*
ØDQ2*
ØDQ3*
ØDQ4*
ØDQ5*
ØDQ6*
ØDQ8*
ØDQ9*
ØDQA*
ØDQB*
ØDQC*
ØDQE*
ØDQF3ZZ
ØDQF4ZZ
ØDQF7ZZ
ØDQF8ZZ
ØDQG3ZZ
ØDQG4ZZ
ØDQG7ZZ
ØDQG8ZZ
ØDQH*
ØDQJ*
ØDQK*
ØDQL3ZZ
ØDQL4ZZ
ØDQL7ZZ
ØDQL8ZZ
ØDQM3ZZ
ØDQM4ZZ
ØDQM7ZZ
ØDQM8ZZ
ØDQN*
ØDQP*
ØDQQ*
ØDQR*
ØDQV*
ØDQW*
ØDR*
ØDS5ØZZ
ØDS54ZZ
ØDS57ZZ
ØDS58ZZ
ØDS6ØZZ
ØDS64ZZ
ØDS67ZZ
ØDS68ZZ
ØDS8ØZZ
ØDS84ZZ
ØDS87ZZ
ØDS88ZZ
ØDSBØZZ
ØDSB4ZZ
ØDSB7ZZ
ØDSB8ZZ
ØDSEØZZ
ØDSE4ZZ
ØDSE7ZZ
ØDSE8ZZ
ØDSHØZZ
ØDSH4ZZ
ØDSH7ZZ
ØDSH8ZZ
ØDSPØZZ
ØDSP4ZZ
ØDSP7ZZ
ØDSP8ZZ
ØDT1*
ØDT2*
ØDT3*
ØDT4*
ØDT5*
ØDT6*
ØDT7*
ØDT8*
ØDT9*
ØDTA*
ØDTB*
ØDTC*
ØDTE*
ØDTF*
ØDTG*
ØDTH*
ØDTJ*
ØDTK*
ØDTL*
ØDTM*
ØDTN*
ØDTPØZZ
ØDTP4ZZ
ØDU1*
ØDU2*
ØDU3*
ØDU4*
ØDU5*
ØDU6*
ØDU8*
ØDU9*
ØDUA*
ØDUB*
ØDUC*
ØDUE*
ØDUF*
ØDUG*
ØDUH*
ØDUK*
ØDUL*
ØDUM*
ØDUN*
ØDUP*
ØDUQ*
ØDUR*
ØDUUØ7Z
ØDUUØJZ
ØDUUØKZ
ØDUU47Z
ØDUU4JZ
ØDUU4KZ
ØDUV*
ØDUW*
ØDV1*
ØDV2*
ØDV3*
ØDV4*
ØDV5*
ØDV6ØCZ
ØDV6ØDZ
ØDV6ØZZ
ØDV63CZ
ØDV63DZ
ØDV63ZZ
ØDV64CZ
ØDV64DZ
ØDV64ZZ
ØDV67ZZ
ØDV68ZZ
ØDV8*
ØDV9*
ØDVA*
ØDVB*
ØDVC*
ØDVE*
ØDVF*
ØDVG*
ØDVH*
ØDVK*
ØDVL*
ØDVM*
ØDVN*
ØDVP*
ØDWØØØZ
ØDWØØ2Z
ØDWØØ3Z
ØDWØØ7Z
ØDWØØCZ
ØDWØØDZ
ØDWØØJZ
ØDWØØKZ
ØDWØØUZ
ØDWØØYZ
ØDWØ3ØZ
ØDWØ32Z
ØDWØ33Z
ØDWØ37Z
ØDWØ3CZ
ØDWØ3DZ
ØDWØ3JZ
ØDWØ3KZ
ØDWØ3UZ
ØDWØ4ØZ
ØDWØ42Z
ØDWØ43Z
ØDWØ47Z
ØDWØ4CZ
ØDWØ4DZ
ØDWØ4JZ
ØDWØ4KZ
ØDWØ7ØZ
ØDWØ72Z
ØDWØ73Z
ØDWØ77Z
ØDWØ7CZ
ØDWØ7DZ
ØDWØ7JZ
ØDWØ7KZ
ØDWØ7UZ
ØDWØ8ØZ
ØDWØ82Z
ØDWØ83Z
ØDWØ87Z
ØDWØ8CZ
ØDWØ8DZ
ØDWØ8JZ
ØDWØ8KZ
ØDW57DZ
ØDW58DZ
ØDW6ØØZ
ØDW6Ø2Z
ØDW6Ø3Z
ØDW6Ø7Z
ØDW6ØCZ
ØDW6ØDZ
ØDW6ØJZ
ØDW6ØKZ
ØDW6ØMZ
ØDW6ØUZ
ØDW6ØYZ
ØDW63ØZ
ØDW632Z
ØDW633Z
ØDW637Z
ØDW63CZ
ØDW63DZ
ØDW63JZ
ØDW63KZ
ØDW63MZ
ØDW63UZ
ØDW64ØZ
ØDW642Z
ØDW647Z
ØDW64DZ
ØDW64JZ
ØDW64KZ
ØDW64MZ
ØDW64UZ
ØDW67ØZ
ØDW672Z
ØDW673Z
ØDW677Z
ØDW67CZ
ØDW67DZ
ØDW67JZ
ØDW67KZ
ØDW67UZ
ØDW68ØZ
ØDW682Z
ØDW683Z
ØDW687Z
ØDW68CZ
ØDW68DZ
ØDW68JZ
ØDW68KZ
ØDW8*
ØDWDØØZ
ØDWDØ2Z
ØDWDØ3Z
ØDWDØ7Z
ØDWDØCZ
ØDWDØDZ
ØDWDØJZ
ØDWDØKZ
ØDWDØUZ
ØDWDØYZ
ØDWD3ØZ
ØDWD32Z
ØDWD33Z
ØDWD37Z
ØDWD3CZ
ØDWD3DZ
ØDWD3JZ
ØDWD3KZ
ØDWD3UZ
ØDWD4ØZ
ØDWD42Z
ØDWD43Z
ØDWD47Z
ØDWD4CZ
ØDWD4DZ
ØDWD4JZ
ØDWD4KZ
ØDWD4UZ
ØDWD7ØZ
ØDWD72Z
ØDWD73Z
ØDWD77Z
ØDWD7CZ
ØDWD7DZ
ØDWD7JZ
ØDWD7KZ
ØDWD7UZ
ØDWD8ØZ
ØDWD82Z
ØDWD83Z
ØDWD87Z
ØDWD8CZ
ØDWD8DZ
ØDWD8JZ
ØDWD8KZ
ØDWE*
ØDWQ*
ØDWWØJZ
ØDWW3JZ
ØDWW4JZ
ØDX*
ØDY6*
ØF1*
ØF54*
ØF75ØDZ
ØF75ØZZ
ØF757ZZ
ØF76ØDZ
ØF76ØZZ
ØF767ZZ
ØF77ØDZ
ØF77ØZZ
ØF777ZZ
ØF78ØDZ
ØF78ØZZ
ØF787ZZ
ØF79ØDZ
ØF79ØZZ
ØF797ZZ
ØF7CØDZ
ØF7CØZZ
ØF7C3DZ
ØF7C3ZZ
ØF7C4DZ
ØF7C4ZZ
ØF7C7DZ
ØF7C7ZZ
ØF7DØDZ
ØF7DØZZ
ØF7D3DZ
ØF7D3ZZ
ØF7D7ZZ
ØF7FØDZ
ØF7FØZZ
ØF7F3DZ
ØF7F3ZZ
ØF7F7DZ
ØF7F7ZZ
ØF8ØØZZ
ØF8Ø4ZZ
ØF81ØZZ
ØF814ZZ
ØF82ØZZ
ØF824ZZ
ØF8GØZZ
ØF8G3ZZ
ØF9ØØØZ
ØF9ØØZX
ØF9ØØZZ
ØF91ØØZ
ØF91ØZX
ØF91ØZZ
ØF92ØØZ
ØF92ØZX
ØF92ØZZ
ØF95ØØZ
ØF95ØZZ
ØF954ØZ
ØF954ZZ
ØF957ØZ
ØF957ZZ
ØF96ØØZ
ØF96ØZZ
ØF964ØZ
ØF964ZZ
ØF967ØZ
ØF967ZZ
ØF97ØØZ
ØF97ØZZ
ØF98ØØZ
ØF98ØZZ
ØF984ØZ
ØF984ZZ
ØF987ØZ
ØF987ZZ
ØF997ØZ
ØF9CØØZ
ØF9CØZZ
ØF9C7ØZ
ØF9C7ZZ
ØF9FØZX
ØF9GØZX
ØFBØØZX
ØFBØØZZ
ØFBØ3ZZ
ØFBØ4ZX
ØFBØ4ZZ
ØFB1ØZX
ØFB1ØZZ
ØFB13ZZ
ØFB14ZX
ØFB14ZZ
ØFB2ØZX
ØFB2ØZZ
ØFB23ZZ
ØFB24ZX
ØFB24ZZ
ØFB4ØZZ
ØFB43ZZ
ØFB44ZZ
ØFB48ZZ
ØFB8ØZZ
ØFB83ZZ
ØFB87ZZ
ØFBDØZX
ØFBFØZX
ØFBGØZX
ØFBGØZZ
ØFBG3ZZ
ØFBG4ZZ
ØFBG8ZZ
ØFCØ*
ØFC1*
ØFC2*
ØFC9ØZZ
ØFCCØZZ
ØFCC3ZZ
ØFCC7ZZ
ØFDØ4ZX
ØFD14ZX
ØFD24ZX
ØFHØØ1Z
ØFHØØ2Z
ØFHØØYZ
ØFHØ32Z
ØFHØ41Z
ØFHØ42Z
ØFH1Ø2Z
ØFH132Z
ØFH142Z
ØFH2Ø2Z
ØFH232Z
ØFH242Z
ØFHBØ1Z
ØFHBØ2Z
ØFHBØDZ
ØFHBØYZ
ØFHB31Z
ØFHB32Z
ØFHB3DZ
ØFHB41Z
ØFHB42Z
ØFHB71Z
ØFHB7DZ
ØFHB81Z
ØFHDØ1Z
ØFHDØDZ
ØFHD31Z
ØFHD3DZ
ØFHD41Z
ØFHD71Z
ØFHD7DZ
ØFHD81Z
ØFJØØZZ
ØFJØ4ZZ
ØFJ44ZZ
ØFJDØZZ
ØFJD4ZZ
ØFJGØZZ
ØFJG4ZZ
ØFL5ØCZ
ØFL5ØDZ
ØFL5ØZZ
ØFL6ØCZ
ØFL6ØDZ
ØFL6ØZZ
ØFL7ØCZ
ØFL7ØDZ
ØFL7ØZZ
ØFL8ØCZ
ØFL8ØDZ
ØFL8ØZZ
ØFL9ØCZ
ØFL9ØDZ
ØFL9ØZZ
ØFLC*
ØFLD*
ØFLF*
ØFMØ*
ØFM1*
ØFM2*
ØFM4ØZZ
ØFM5ØZZ
ØFM6ØZZ
ØFM7ØZZ
ØFM8ØZZ
ØFM9ØZZ
ØFMC*
ØFMD*
ØFMF*
ØFMG*
ØFN*
ØFPØØØZ
ØFPØØ2Z
ØFPØØ3Z
ØFPØØYZ
ØFPØ3ØZ
ØFPØ32Z
ØFPØ33Z
ØFPØ4ØZ
ØFPØ42Z
ØFPØ43Z
ØFP4ØDZ
ØFP43DZ
ØFP44DZ
ØFPBØØZ
ØFPBØ1Z
ØFPBØ2Z
ØFPBØ3Z
ØFPBØ7Z
ØFPBØCZ
ØFPBØDZ
ØFPBØJZ
ØFPBØKZ
ØFPBØYZ
ØFPB3ØZ
ØFPB31Z
ØFPB32Z
ØFPB33Z
ØFPB37Z
ØFPB3CZ
ØFPB3DZ
ØFPB3JZ
ØFPB3KZ
ØFPB4ØZ
ØFPB41Z
ØFPB42Z
ØFPB43Z
ØFPB47Z
ØFPB4CZ
ØFPB4DZ
ØFPB4JZ
ØFPB4KZ
ØFPB71Z
ØFPB77Z
ØFPB7CZ
ØFPB7JZ
ØFPB7KZ
ØFPB81Z
ØFPB87Z
ØFPB8CZ
ØFPB8JZ
ØFPB8KZ
ØFQ*
ØFR*
ØFSØ*
ØFS4*
ØFS5*
ØFS6*
ØFS7ØZZ
ØFS74ZZ
ØFS8*
ØFS9*
ØFSC*
ØFSD*
ØFSF*
ØFTØ*
ØFT1*
ØFT2*
ØFT4*
ØFTG*
ØFU*
ØFV5ØCZ
ØFV5ØDZ
ØFV5ØZZ
ØFV6ØCZ
ØFV6ØDZ
ØFV6ØZZ
ØFV7ØCZ
ØFV7ØDZ
ØFV7ØZZ
ØFV8ØCZ
ØFV8ØDZ
ØFV8ØZZ
ØFV9ØCZ
ØFV9ØDZ
ØFV9ØZZ
ØFVC*
ØFVD*
ØFVF*
ØFWØØØZ
ØFWØØ2Z
ØFWØØ3Z
ØFWØØYZ
ØFWØ3ØZ
ØFWØ32Z
ØFWØ33Z
ØFWØ4ØZ
ØFWØ42Z
ØFWØ43Z
ØFWBØØZ
ØFWBØ2Z
ØFWBØ3Z
ØFWBØ7Z
ØFWBØCZ
ØFWBØDZ
ØFWBØJZ
ØFWBØKZ
ØFWBØYZ
ØFWB3ØZ
ØFWB32Z
ØFWB33Z
ØFWB37Z
ØFWB3CZ
ØFWB3DZ
ØFWB3JZ
ØFWB3KZ
ØFWB4ØZ
ØFWB42Z
ØFWB43Z
ØFWB47Z
ØFWB4CZ
ØFWB4DZ
ØFWB4JZ
ØFWB4KZ
ØFWB7ØZ
ØFWB72Z
ØFWB73Z
ØFWB77Z
ØFWB7CZ
ØFWB7DZ
ØFWB7JZ
ØFWB7KZ
ØFWB83Z
ØFWB87Z
ØFWB8CZ
ØFWB8JZ
ØFWB8KZ
ØG9GØØZ
ØG9GØZZ
ØG9HØØZ
ØG9HØZZ
ØG9KØØZ
ØG9KØZZ
ØG9LØØZ
ØG9LØZZ
ØG9MØØZ
ØG9MØZZ
ØG9NØØZ
ØG9NØZZ
ØG9PØØZ
ØG9PØZZ
ØG9QØØZ
ØG9QØZZ
ØG9RØØZ
ØG9RØZZ
ØGCG*
ØGCH*
ØGCK*
ØGCL*
ØGCM*
ØGCN*
ØGCP*
ØGCQ*
ØGCR*
ØGHSØ1Z
ØGHSØ2Z
ØGHSØ3Z
ØGHSØYZ
ØGHS32Z
ØGHS33Z
ØGHS41Z
ØGHS42Z
ØGHS43Z
ØGJKØZZ
ØGJRØZZ
ØGJSØZZ
ØGM2*
ØGM3*
ØGN2*
ØGN3*
ØGN4*
ØGPKØØZ
ØGPK3ØZ
ØGPK4ØZ
ØGPRØØZ
ØGPR3ØZ
ØGPR4ØZ
ØGQ2*
ØGQ3*
ØGQ4*
ØGQG*
ØGQH*
ØGQJ*
ØGQK*
ØGS2*
ØGS3*
ØGWKØØZ
ØGWK3ØZ
ØGWK4ØZ
ØGWRØØZ
ØGWR3ØZ
ØGWR4ØZ
ØHØTØ7Z
ØHØT37Z
ØHØUØ7Z
ØHØU37Z
ØHØVØ7Z
ØHØVØJZ
ØHØVØKZ
ØHØV37Z
ØHØV3KZ
ØH5T*
ØH5U*
ØH5V*
ØH5W*
ØH5X*
ØH9TØZX
ØH9TØZZ
ØH9UØZX
ØH9UØZZ
ØH9VØZX
ØH9VØZZ
ØH9WØZX
ØH9WØZZ
ØH9XØZX
ØH9XØZZ
ØHBTØZX
ØHBTØZZ
ØHBT3ZZ
ØHBT7ZZ
ØHBT8ZZ
ØHBUØZX
ØHBUØZZ
ØHBU3ZZ
ØHBU7ZZ
ØHBU8ZZ
ØHBVØZX
ØHBVØZZ
ØHBV3ZZ
ØHBV7ZZ
ØHBV8ZZ
ØHBWØZX
ØHBWØZZ
ØHBW3ZZ
ØHBW7ZZ
ØHBW8ZZ
ØHBWXZZ
ØHBXØZX
ØHBXØZZ
ØHBX3ZZ
ØHBX7ZZ
ØHBX8ZZ
ØHBXXZZ
ØHBYØZX
ØHBYØZZ
ØHBY3ZZ
ØHBY7ZZ
ØHBY8ZZ
ØHCTØZZ
ØHCUØZZ
ØHCVØZZ
ØHCWØZZ
ØHCXØZZ
ØHDTØZZ
ØHDUØZZ
ØHDVØZZ
ØHDYØZZ
ØHHTØ1Z
ØHHTØNZ
ØHHTØYZ
ØHHT31Z
ØHHT3NZ
ØHHT71Z
ØHHT7NZ
ØHHT81Z
ØHHT8NZ
ØHHUØ1Z
ØHHUØNZ
ØHHUØYZ
ØHHU31Z
ØHHU3NZ
ØHHU71Z
ØHHU7NZ
ØHHU81Z
ØHHU8NZ
ØHHVØ1Z
ØHHVØNZ
ØHHV31Z
ØHHV3NZ
ØHHV71Z
ØHHV7NZ
ØHHV81Z
ØHHV8NZ
ØHHWØ1Z
ØHHWØNZ
ØHHW31Z
ØHHW3NZ
ØHHW71Z
ØHHW7NZ
ØHHW81Z
ØHHW8NZ
ØHHWX1Z
ØHHXØ1Z
ØHHXØNZ
ØHHX31Z
ØHHX3NZ
ØHHX71Z
ØHHX7NZ
ØHHX81Z
ØHHX8NZ
ØHHXX1Z
ØHM1XZZ
ØHM2XZZ
ØHM3XZZ
ØHM4XZZ
ØHM5XZZ
ØHM6XZZ
ØHM7XZZ
ØHM8XZZ
ØHM9XZZ
ØHMAXZZ
ØHMBXZZ
ØHMCXZZ
ØHMDXZZ
ØHMEXZZ
ØHMFXZZ
ØHMGXZZ
ØHMHXZZ
ØHMJXZZ
ØHMKXZZ
ØHMLXZZ
ØHMMXZZ
ØHMNXZZ
ØHMWXZZ
ØHMXXZZ
ØHNØXZZ
ØHN1XZZ
ØHN2XZZ
ØHN3XZZ
ØHN4XZZ
ØHN5XZZ
ØHN6XZZ
ØHN7XZZ
ØHN8XZZ

ØHN9XZZ
ØHNAXZZ
ØHNBXZZ
ØHNCXZZ
ØHNDXZZ
ØHNEXZZ
ØHNFXZZ
ØHNGXZZ
ØHNHXZZ
ØHNJXZZ
ØHNKXZZ
ØHNLXZZ
ØHNMXZZ
ØHNNXZZ
ØHNQXZZ
ØHNRXZZ
ØHPTØJZ
ØHPTØNZ
ØHPTØYZ
ØHPT3JZ
ØHPT3NZ
ØHPUØJZ
ØHPUØNZ
ØHPUØYZ
ØHPU3JZ
ØHPU3NZ
ØHQQXZZ
ØHQRXZZ
ØHQTØZZ
ØHQT3ZZ
ØHQT7ZZ
ØHQT8ZZ
ØHQUØZZ
ØHQU3ZZ
ØHQU7ZZ
ØHQU8ZZ
ØHQW*
ØHQX*
ØHR2*
ØHR3*
ØHR9*
ØHRQ*
ØHRR*
ØHRSXJZ
ØHRSXKZ
ØHRTØ75
ØHRTØ76
ØHRTØ77
ØHRTØ78
ØHRTØ79
ØHRTØ7Z
ØHRTØJZ
ØHRTØKZ
ØHRT3JZ
ØHRUØ75
ØHRUØ76
ØHRUØ77
ØHRUØ78
ØHRUØ79
ØHRUØ7Z
ØHRUØJZ
ØHRUØKZ
ØHRU3JZ
ØHRVØ75
ØHRVØ76
ØHRVØ77
ØHRVØ78
ØHRVØ79
ØHRVØJZ
ØHRV3JZ
ØHRW*
ØHRX*
ØHSTØZZ
ØHSUØZZ
ØHSVØZZ
ØHSWXZZ
ØHSXXZZ
ØHTTØZZ
ØHTUØZZ
ØHTVØZZ
ØHTWXZZ
ØHTXXZZ
ØHTYØZZ
ØHUW*
ØHUX*
ØHWTØJZ
ØHWTØYZ
ØHWT3JZ
ØHWUØJZ
ØHWUØYZ
ØHWU3JZ
ØHX2XZZ
ØHX3XZZ
ØJØ*
ØJ8Ø*
ØJ81*
ØJ84*
ØJ85*
ØJ86*
ØJ87*
ØJ88*
ØJ89*
ØJ8B*
ØJ8C*
ØJ8D*
ØJ8F*
ØJ8G*
ØJ8H*
ØJ8L*
ØJ8M*
ØJ8N*
ØJ8P*
ØJ8Q*
ØJ8R*
ØJ8S*
ØJ8T*
ØJ8V*
ØJ8W*
ØJCØØZZ
ØJC1ØZZ
ØJC4ØZZ
ØJC5ØZZ
ØJC6ØZZ
ØJC7ØZZ
ØJC8ØZZ
ØJC9ØZZ
ØJCBØZZ
ØJCCØZZ
ØJCDØZZ
ØJCFØZZ
ØJCGØZZ
ØJCHØZZ
ØJCJØZZ
ØJCKØZZ
ØJCLØZZ
ØJCMØZZ
ØJCNØZZ
ØJCPØZZ
ØJCQØZZ
ØJCRØZZ
ØJDØØZZ
ØJD1ØZZ
ØJD4ØZZ
ØJD5ØZZ
ØJD6ØZZ
ØJD7ØZZ
ØJD8ØZZ
ØJD9ØZZ
ØJDBØZZ
ØJDCØZZ
ØJDDØZZ
ØJDFØZZ
ØJDGØZZ
ØJDHØZZ
ØJDLØZZ
ØJDMØZZ
ØJDNØZZ
ØJDPØZZ
ØJDQØZZ
ØJDRØZZ
ØJH6Ø2Z
ØJH6ØVZ
ØJH6ØYZ
ØJH632Z
ØJH63VZ
ØJH7ØVZ
ØJH7ØYZ
ØJH73VZ
ØJH8ØVZ
ØJH8ØYZ
ØJH83VZ
ØJHDØVZ
ØJHD3VZ
ØJHFØVZ
ØJHF3VZ
ØJHGØVZ
ØJHG3VZ
ØJHHØVZ
ØJHH3VZ
ØJHLØVZ
ØJHL3VZ
ØJHMØVZ
ØJHM3VZ
ØJHNØVZ
ØJHN3VZ
ØJHPØVZ
ØJHP3VZ
ØJHSØ1Z
ØJHSØYZ
ØJHS31Z
ØJHTØ1Z
ØJHTØVZ
ØJHTØYZ
ØJHT31Z
ØJHT3VZ
ØJHVØ1Z
ØJHVØYZ
ØJHV31Z
ØJHWØ1Z
ØJHWØYZ
ØJHW31Z
ØJPTØFZ
ØJPTØPZ
ØJPT3FZ
ØJPT3PZ
ØJQØØZZ
ØJQ1ØZZ
ØJQ4ØZZ
ØJQ5ØZZ
ØJQ6ØZZ
ØJQ7ØZZ
ØJQ8ØZZ
ØJQ9ØZZ
ØJQBØZZ
ØJQCØZZ
ØJQDØZZ
ØJQFØZZ
ØJQGØZZ
ØJQHØZZ
ØJQLØZZ
ØJQMØZZ
ØJQNØZZ
ØJQPØZZ
ØJQQØZZ
ØJQRØZZ
ØJRØ*
ØJR1*
ØJR4*
ØJR5*
ØJR6*
ØJR7*
ØJR8*
ØJR9*
ØJRB*
ØJRC*
ØJRD*
ØJRF*
ØJRG*
ØJRH*
ØJRJ37Z
ØJRK37Z
ØJRL*
ØJRM*
ØJRN*
ØJRP*
ØJRQ*
ØJRR*
ØJUØ*
ØJU1*
ØJU4*
ØJU5*
ØJU6*
ØJU7*
ØJU8*
ØJU9*
ØJUB*
ØJUC*
ØJUD*
ØJUF*
ØJUG*
ØJUH*
ØJUL*
ØJUM*
ØJUN*
ØJUP*
ØJUQ*
ØJUR*
ØJWTØ2Z
ØJWTØFZ
ØJWTØPZ
ØJWTØYZ
ØJWT32Z
ØJWT3FZ
ØJWT3PZ
ØJXØØZZ
ØJXØ3ZZ
ØJX1ØZZ
ØJX13ZZ
ØJX4ØZZ
ØJX43ZZ
ØJX5ØZZ
ØJX53ZZ
ØJX6ØZZ
ØJX63ZZ
ØJX7ØZZ
ØJX73ZZ
ØJX8ØZZ
ØJX83ZZ
ØJX9ØZZ
ØJX93ZZ
ØJXBØZZ
ØJXB3ZZ
ØJXCØZZ
ØJXC3ZZ
ØJXDØZZ
ØJXD3ZZ
ØJXFØZZ
ØJXF3ZZ
ØJXGØZZ
ØJXG3ZZ
ØJXHØZZ
ØJXH3ZZ
ØJXJØZZ
ØJXJ3ZZ
ØJXKØZZ
ØJXK3ZZ
ØJXLØZZ
ØJXL3ZZ
ØJXMØZZ
ØJXM3ZZ
ØJXNØZZ
ØJXN3ZZ
ØJXPØZZ
ØJXP3ZZ
ØJXQØZZ
ØJXQ3ZZ
ØJXRØZZ
ØJXR3ZZ
ØK5Ø*
ØK51*
ØK52*
ØK53*
ØK54*
ØK55*
ØK56*
ØK57*
ØK58*
ØK59*
ØK5B*
ØK5F*
ØK5G*
ØK5H*
ØK5J*
ØK5K*
ØK5L*
ØK5M*
ØK5N*
ØK5P*
ØK5Q*
ØK5R*
ØK5S*
ØK5T*
ØK5V*
ØK5W*
ØK8Ø*
ØK81*
ØK82*
ØK83*
ØK85*
ØK86*
ØK87*
ØK88*
ØK89*
ØK8B*
ØK8F*
ØK8G*
ØK8H*
ØK8J*
ØK8K*
ØK8L*
ØK8M*
ØK8N*
ØK8P*
ØK8Q*
ØK8R*
ØK8S*
ØK8T*
ØK8V*
ØK8W*
ØK9ØØØZ
ØK9ØØZZ
ØK9Ø4ØZ
ØK9Ø4ZZ
ØK91ØØZ
ØK91ØZZ
ØK914ØZ
ØK914ZZ
ØK92ØØZ
ØK92ØZZ
ØK924ØZ
ØK924ZZ
ØK93ØØZ
ØK93ØZZ
ØK934ØZ
ØK934ZZ
ØK94ØØZ
ØK94ØZZ
ØK944ØZ
ØK944ZZ
ØK95ØØZ
ØK95ØZZ
ØK954ØZ
ØK954ZZ
ØK96ØØZ
ØK96ØZZ
ØK964ØZ
ØK964ZZ
ØK97ØØZ
ØK97ØZZ
ØK974ØZ
ØK974ZZ
ØK98ØØZ
ØK98ØZZ
ØK984ØZ
ØK984ZZ
ØK99ØØZ
ØK99ØZZ
ØK994ØZ
ØK994ZZ
ØK9BØØZ
ØK9BØZZ
ØK9B4ØZ
ØK9B4ZZ
ØK9FØØZ
ØK9FØZZ
ØK9F4ØZ
ØK9F4ZZ
ØK9GØØZ
ØK9GØZZ
ØK9G4ØZ
ØK9G4ZZ
ØK9HØØZ
ØK9HØZZ
ØK9H4ØZ
ØK9H4ZZ
ØK9JØØZ
ØK9JØZZ
ØK9J4ØZ
ØK9J4ZZ
ØK9KØØZ
ØK9KØZZ
ØK9K4ØZ
ØK9K4ZZ
ØK9LØØZ
ØK9LØZZ
ØK9L4ØZ
ØK9L4ZZ
ØK9MØØZ
ØK9MØZZ
ØK9M4ØZ
ØK9M4ZZ
ØK9NØØZ
ØK9NØZZ
ØK9N4ØZ
ØK9N4ZZ
ØK9PØØZ
ØK9PØZZ
ØK9P4ØZ
ØK9P4ZZ
ØK9QØØZ
ØK9QØZZ
ØK9Q4ØZ
ØK9Q4ZZ
ØK9RØØZ
ØK9RØZZ
ØK9R4ØZ
ØK9R4ZZ
ØK9SØØZ
ØK9SØZZ
ØK9S4ØZ
ØK9S4ZZ
ØK9TØØZ
ØK9TØZZ
ØK9T4ØZ
ØK9T4ZZ
ØK9VØØZ
ØK9VØZZ
ØK9V4ØZ
ØK9V4ZZ
ØK9WØØZ
ØK9WØZZ
ØK9W4ØZ
ØK9W4ZZ
ØKBØØZZ
ØKBØ3ZZ
ØKBØ4ZZ
ØKB1ØZZ
ØKB13ZZ
ØKB14ZZ
ØKB2ØZZ
ØKB23ZZ
ØKB24ZZ
ØKB3ØZZ
ØKB33ZZ
ØKB34ZZ
ØKB4ØZZ
ØKB43ZZ
ØKB44ZZ
ØKB5ØZZ
ØKB53ZZ
ØKB54ZZ
ØKB6ØZZ
ØKB63ZZ
ØKB64ZZ
ØKB7ØZZ
ØKB73ZZ
ØKB74ZZ
ØKB8ØZZ
ØKB83ZZ
ØKB84ZZ
ØKB9ØZZ
ØKB93ZZ
ØKB94ZZ
ØKBBØZZ
ØKBB3ZZ
ØKBB4ZZ
ØKBFØZZ
ØKBF3ZZ
ØKBF4ZZ
ØKBGØZZ
ØKBG3ZZ
ØKBG4ZZ
ØKBHØZZ
ØKBH3ZZ
ØKBH4ZZ
ØKBJØZZ
ØKBJ3ZZ
ØKBJ4ZZ
ØKBKØZZ
ØKBK3ZZ
ØKBK4ZZ
ØKBLØZZ
ØKBL3ZZ
ØKBL4ZZ
ØKBMØZZ
ØKBM3ZZ
ØKBM4ZZ
ØKBNØZZ
ØKBN4ZZ
ØKBPØZZ
ØKBP4ZZ
ØKBQØZZ
ØKBQ3ZZ
ØKBQ4ZZ
ØKBRØZZ
ØKBR3ZZ
ØKBR4ZZ
ØKBSØZZ
ØKBS3ZZ
ØKBS4ZZ
ØKBTØZZ
ØKBT3ZZ
ØKBT4ZZ
ØKBVØZZ
ØKBV3ZZ
ØKBV4ZZ
ØKBWØZZ
ØKBW3ZZ
ØKBW4ZZ
ØKCØ*
ØKC1*
ØKC2*
ØKC3*
ØKC4*
ØKC5*
ØKC6*
ØKC7*
ØKC8*
ØKC9*
ØKCB*
ØKCF*
ØKCG*
ØKCH*
ØKCJ*
ØKCK*
ØKCL*
ØKCM*
ØKCN*
ØKCP*
ØKCQ*
ØKCR*
ØKCS*
ØKCT*
ØKCV*
ØKCW*
ØKDØØZZ
ØKD1ØZZ
ØKD2ØZZ
ØKD3ØZZ
ØKD4ØZZ
ØKD5ØZZ
ØKD6ØZZ
ØKD7ØZZ
ØKD8ØZZ
ØKD9ØZZ
ØKDBØZZ
ØKDFØZZ
ØKDGØZZ
ØKDHØZZ
ØKDJØZZ
ØKDKØZZ
ØKDLØZZ
ØKDMØZZ
ØKDNØZZ
ØKDPØZZ
ØKDQØZZ
ØKDRØZZ
ØKDSØZZ
ØKDTØZZ
ØKDVØZZ
ØKDWØZZ
ØKHXØMZ
ØKHXØYZ
ØKHX3MZ
ØKHX4MZ
ØKHYØMZ
ØKHYØYZ
ØKHY3MZ
ØKHY4MZ
ØKMØ*
ØKM1*
ØKM2*
ØKM3*
ØKM4*
ØKM5*
ØKM6*
ØKM7*
ØKM8*
ØKM9*
ØKMB*
ØKMF*
ØKMG*
ØKMH*
ØKMJ*
ØKMK*
ØKML*
ØKMM*
ØKMN*
ØKMP*
ØKMQ*
ØKMR*
ØKMS*
ØKMT*
ØKMV*
ØKMW*
ØKPXØØZ
ØKPXØ7Z
ØKPXØJZ
ØKPXØKZ
ØKPXØMZ
ØKPXØYZ
ØKPX3ØZ
ØKPX37Z
ØKPX3JZ
ØKPX3KZ
ØKPX3MZ
ØKPX4ØZ
ØKPX47Z
ØKPX4JZ
ØKPX4KZ
ØKPX4MZ
ØKPYØØZ
ØKPYØ7Z
ØKPYØJZ
ØKPYØKZ
ØKPYØMZ
ØKPYØYZ
ØKPY3ØZ
ØKPY37Z
ØKPY3JZ
ØKPY3KZ
ØKPY3MZ
ØKPY4ØZ
ØKPY47Z
ØKPY4JZ
ØKPY4KZ
ØKPY4MZ
ØKQØ*
ØKQ1*
ØKQ2*
ØKQ3*
ØKQ4*
ØKQ5*
ØKQ6*
ØKQ7*
ØKQ8*
ØKQ9*
ØKQB*
ØKQF*
ØKQG*
ØKQH*
ØKQJ*
ØKQK*
ØKQL*
ØKQM*
ØKQN*
ØKQP*
ØKQQ*
ØKQR*
ØKQS*
ØKQT*
ØKQV*
ØKQW*
ØKRØØ7Z
ØKRØØJZ
ØKRØØKZ
ØKRØ47Z
ØKRØ4JZ
ØKRØ4KZ
ØKR1Ø7Z
ØKR1ØJZ
ØKR1ØKZ
ØKR147Z
ØKR14JZ
ØKR14KZ
ØKR2Ø7Z
ØKR2ØJZ
ØKR2ØKZ
ØKR247Z
ØKR24JZ
ØKR24KZ
ØKR3Ø7Z
ØKR3ØJZ
ØKR3ØKZ
ØKR347Z
ØKR34JZ
ØKR34KZ
ØKR4Ø7Z
ØKR4ØJZ
ØKR4ØKZ
ØKR447Z
ØKR44JZ
ØKR44KZ
ØKR5Ø7Z
ØKR5ØJZ
ØKR5ØKZ
ØKR547Z
ØKR54JZ
ØKR54KZ
ØKR6Ø7Z
ØKR6ØJZ
ØKR6ØKZ
ØKR647Z
ØKR64JZ
ØKR64KZ
ØKR7Ø7Z
ØKR7ØJZ
ØKR7ØKZ
ØKR747Z
ØKR74JZ
ØKR74KZ
ØKR8Ø7Z
ØKR8ØJZ
ØKR8ØKZ
ØKR847Z
ØKR84JZ
ØKR84KZ
ØKR9Ø7Z
ØKR9ØJZ
ØKR9ØKZ
ØKR947Z
ØKR94JZ
ØKR94KZ
ØKRBØ7Z
ØKRBØJZ
ØKRBØKZ
ØKRB47Z
ØKRB4JZ
ØKRB4KZ
ØKRFØ7Z
ØKRFØJZ
ØKRFØKZ
ØKRF47Z
ØKRF4JZ
ØKRF4KZ
ØKRGØ7Z
ØKRGØJZ
ØKRGØKZ
ØKRG47Z
ØKRG4JZ
ØKRG4KZ
ØKRHØ7Z
ØKRHØJZ
ØKRHØKZ
ØKRH47Z
ØKRH4JZ
ØKRH4KZ
ØKRJØ7Z
ØKRJØJZ
ØKRJØKZ
ØKRJ47Z
ØKRJ4JZ
ØKRJ4KZ
ØKRKØ7Z
ØKRKØJZ
ØKRKØKZ
ØKRK47Z
ØKRK4JZ
ØKRK4KZ
ØKRLØ7Z
ØKRLØJZ
ØKRLØKZ
ØKRL47Z
ØKRL4JZ
ØKRL4KZ
ØKRMØ7Z
ØKRMØJZ
ØKRMØKZ
ØKRM47Z
ØKRM4JZ
ØKRM4KZ
ØKRNØ7Z
ØKRNØJZ
ØKRNØKZ
ØKRN47Z
ØKRN4JZ
ØKRN4KZ
ØKRPØ7Z
ØKRPØJZ
ØKRPØKZ
ØKRP47Z
ØKRP4JZ
ØKRP4KZ
ØKRQØ7Z
ØKRQØJZ
ØKRQØKZ
ØKRQ47Z
ØKRQ4JZ
ØKRQ4KZ
ØKRRØ7Z
ØKRRØJZ
ØKRRØKZ
ØKRR47Z
ØKRR4JZ
ØKRR4KZ
ØKRSØ7Z
ØKRSØJZ
ØKRSØKZ
ØKRS47Z
ØKRS4JZ
ØKRS4KZ
ØKRTØ7Z
ØKRTØJZ
ØKRTØKZ
ØKRT47Z
ØKRT4JZ
ØKRT4KZ
ØKRVØ7Z
ØKRVØJZ
ØKRVØKZ
ØKRV47Z
ØKRV4JZ
ØKRV4KZ
ØKRWØ7Z
ØKRWØJZ
ØKRWØKZ
ØKRW47Z
ØKRW4JZ
ØKRW4KZ
ØKSØ*
ØKS1*
ØKS2*
ØKS3*
ØKS4*
ØKS5*

ØKS6*
ØKS7*
ØKS8*
ØKS9*
ØKSB*
ØKSF*
ØKSG*
ØKSH*
ØKSJ*
ØKSK*
ØKSL*
ØKSM*
ØKSN*
ØKSP*
ØKSQ*
ØKSR*
ØKSS*
ØKST*
ØKSV*
ØKSW*
ØKTØ*
ØKT1*
ØKT2*
ØKT3*
ØKT4*
ØKT5*
ØKT6*
ØKT7*
ØKT8*
ØKT9*
ØKTB*
ØKTF*
ØKTG*
ØKTH*
ØKTJ*
ØKTK*
ØKTL*
ØKTM*
ØKTN*
ØKTP*
ØKTQ*
ØKTR*
ØKTS*
ØKTT*
ØKTV*
ØKTW*
ØKUØ*
ØKU1*
ØKU2*
ØKU3*
ØKU4*
ØKU5*
ØKU6*
ØKU7*
ØKU8*
ØKU9*
ØKUB*
ØKUF*
ØKUG*
ØKUH*
ØKUJ*
ØKUK*
ØKUL*
ØKUM*
ØKUN*
ØKUP*
ØKUQ*
ØKUR*
ØKUS*
ØKUT*
ØKUV*
ØKUW*
ØKWXØØZ
ØKWXØ7Z
ØKWXØJZ
ØKWXØKZ
ØKWXØMZ
ØKWXØYZ
ØKWX3ØZ
ØKWX37Z
ØKWX3JZ
ØKWX3KZ
ØKWX3MZ
ØKWX4ØZ
ØKWX47Z
ØKWX4JZ
ØKWX4KZ
ØKWX4MZ
ØKWYØØZ
ØKWYØ7Z
ØKWYØJZ
ØKWYØKZ
ØKWYØMZ
ØKWYØYZ
ØKWY3ØZ
ØKWY37Z
ØKWY3JZ
ØKWY3KZ
ØKWY3MZ
ØKWY4ØZ
ØKWY47Z
ØKWY4JZ
ØKWY4KZ
ØKWY4MZ
ØKXFØZ5
ØKXFØZ7
ØKXFØZ8
ØKXFØZ9
ØKXF4Z5
ØKXF4Z7
ØKXF4Z8
ØKXF4Z9
ØKXGØZ5
ØKXGØZ7
ØKXGØZ8
ØKXGØZ9
ØKXG4Z5
ØKXG4Z7
ØKXG4Z8
ØKXG4Z9
ØKXHØZZ
ØKXH4ZZ
ØKXJØZZ
ØKXJ4ZZ
ØKXKØZ6
ØKXK4Z6
ØKXLØZ6
ØKXL4Z6
ØL5Ø*
ØL51*
ØL52*
ØL53*
ØL54*
ØL55*
ØL56*
ØL59*
ØL5B*
ØL5C*
ØL5D*
ØL5F*
ØL5G*
ØL5H*
ØL5J*
ØL5K*
ØL5L*
ØL5M*
ØL5N*
ØL5P*
ØL5Q*
ØL5R*
ØL5S*
ØL5T*
ØL5V*
ØL5W*
ØL8Ø*
ØL81*
ØL82*
ØL83*
ØL84*
ØL85*
ØL86*
ØL89*
ØL8B*
ØL8C*
ØL8D*
ØL8F*
ØL8G*
ØL8H*
ØL8J*
ØL8K*
ØL8L*
ØL8M*
ØL8N*
ØL8P*
ØL8Q*
ØL8R*
ØL8S*
ØL8T*
ØL8V*
ØL8W*
ØL9ØØØZ
ØL9ØØZZ
ØL9Ø4ØZ
ØL9Ø4ZZ
ØL91ØØZ
ØL91ØZZ
ØL914ØZ
ØL914ZZ
ØL92ØØZ
ØL92ØZZ
ØL924ØZ
ØL924ZZ
ØL93ØØZ
ØL93ØZZ
ØL934ØZ
ØL934ZZ
ØL94ØØZ
ØL94ØZZ
ØL944ØZ
ØL944ZZ
ØL95ØØZ
ØL95ØZZ
ØL954ØZ
ØL954ZZ
ØL96ØØZ
ØL96ØZZ
ØL964ØZ
ØL964ZZ
ØL99ØØZ
ØL99ØZZ
ØL994ØZ
ØL994ZZ
ØL9BØØZ
ØL9BØZZ
ØL9B4ØZ
ØL9B4ZZ
ØL9CØØZ
ØL9CØZZ
ØL9C4ØZ
ØL9C4ZZ
ØL9DØØZ
ØL9DØZZ
ØL9D4ØZ
ØL9D4ZZ
ØL9FØØZ
ØL9FØZZ
ØL9F4ØZ
ØL9F4ZZ
ØL9GØØZ
ØL9GØZZ
ØL9G4ØZ
ØL9G4ZZ
ØL9HØØZ
ØL9HØZZ
ØL9H4ØZ
ØL9H4ZZ
ØL9JØØZ
ØL9JØZZ
ØL9J4ØZ
ØL9J4ZZ
ØL9KØØZ
ØL9KØZZ
ØL9K4ØZ
ØL9K4ZZ
ØL9LØØZ
ØL9LØZZ
ØL9L4ØZ
ØL9L4ZZ
ØL9MØØZ
ØL9MØZZ
ØL9M4ØZ
ØL9M4ZZ
ØL9NØØZ
ØL9NØZZ
ØL9N4ØZ
ØL9N4ZZ
ØL9PØØZ
ØL9PØZZ
ØL9P4ØZ
ØL9P4ZZ
ØL9QØØZ
ØL9QØZZ
ØL9Q4ØZ
ØL9Q4ZZ
ØL9RØØZ
ØL9RØZZ
ØL9R4ØZ
ØL9R4ZZ
ØL9SØØZ
ØL9SØZZ
ØL9S4ØZ
ØL9S4ZZ
ØL9TØØZ
ØL9TØZZ
ØL9T4ØZ
ØL9T4ZZ
ØL9VØØZ
ØL9VØZZ
ØL9V4ØZ
ØL9V4ZZ
ØL9WØØZ
ØL9WØZZ
ØL9W4ØZ
ØL9W4ZZ
ØLBØØZZ
ØLBØ3ZZ
ØLBØ4ZZ
ØLB1ØZZ
ØLB13ZZ
ØLB14ZZ
ØLB2ØZZ
ØLB23ZZ
ØLB24ZZ
ØLB3ØZZ
ØLB33ZZ
ØLB34ZZ
ØLB4ØZZ
ØLB43ZZ
ØLB44ZZ
ØLB5ØZZ
ØLB53ZZ
ØLB54ZZ
ØLB6ØZZ
ØLB63ZZ
ØLB64ZZ
ØLB9ØZZ
ØLB93ZZ
ØLB94ZZ
ØLBBØZZ
ØLBB3ZZ
ØLBB4ZZ
ØLBCØZZ
ØLBC3ZZ
ØLBC4ZZ
ØLBDØZZ
ØLBD3ZZ
ØLBD4ZZ
ØLBFØZZ
ØLBF3ZZ
ØLBF4ZZ
ØLBGØZZ
ØLBG3ZZ
ØLBG4ZZ
ØLBHØZZ
ØLBH3ZZ
ØLBH4ZZ
ØLBJØZZ
ØLBJ3ZZ
ØLBJ4ZZ
ØLBKØZZ
ØLBK3ZZ
ØLBK4ZZ
ØLBLØZZ
ØLBL3ZZ
ØLBL4ZZ
ØLBMØZZ
ØLBM3ZZ
ØLBM4ZZ
ØLBNØZZ
ØLBN3ZZ
ØLBN4ZZ
ØLBPØZZ
ØLBP3ZZ
ØLBP4ZZ
ØLBQØZZ
ØLBQ3ZZ
ØLBQ4ZZ
ØLBRØZZ
ØLBR3ZZ
ØLBR4ZZ
ØLBSØZZ
ØLBS3ZZ
ØLBS4ZZ
ØLBTØZZ
ØLBT3ZZ
ØLBT4ZZ
ØLBVØZZ
ØLBV3ZZ
ØLBV4ZZ
ØLBWØZZ
ØLBW3ZZ
ØLBW4ZZ
ØLCØ*
ØLC1*
ØLC2*
ØLC3*
ØLC4*
ØLC5*
ØLC6*
ØLC9*
ØLCB*
ØLCC*
ØLCD*
ØLCF*
ØLCG*
ØLCH*
ØLCJ*
ØLCK*
ØLCL*
ØLCM*
ØLCN*
ØLCP*
ØLCQ*
ØLCR*
ØLCS*
ØLCT*
ØLCV*
ØLCW*
ØLDØØZZ
ØLD1ØZZ
ØLD2ØZZ
ØLD3ØZZ
ØLD4ØZZ
ØLD5ØZZ
ØLD6ØZZ
ØLD9ØZZ
ØLDBØZZ
ØLDCØZZ
ØLDDØZZ
ØLDFØZZ
ØLDGØZZ
ØLDHØZZ
ØLDJØZZ
ØLDKØZZ
ØLDLØZZ
ØLDMØZZ
ØLDNØZZ
ØLDPØZZ
ØLDQØZZ
ØLDRØZZ
ØLDSØZZ
ØLDTØZZ
ØLDVØZZ
ØLDWØZZ
ØLHXØYZ
ØLHYØYZ
ØLMØ*
ØLM1*
ØLM2*
ØLM3*
ØLM4*
ØLM5*
ØLM6*
ØLM9*
ØLMB*
ØLMC*
ØLMD*
ØLMF*
ØLMG*
ØLMH*
ØLMJ*
ØLMK*
ØLML*
ØLMM*
ØLMN*
ØLMP*
ØLMQ*
ØLMR*
ØLMS*
ØLMT*
ØLMV*
ØLMW*
ØLPXØØZ
ØLPXØ7Z
ØLPXØJZ
ØLPXØKZ
ØLPXØYZ
ØLPX37Z
ØLPX3JZ
ØLPX3KZ
ØLPX4ØZ
ØLPX47Z
ØLPX4JZ
ØLPX4KZ
ØLPYØØZ
ØLPYØ7Z
ØLPYØJZ
ØLPYØKZ
ØLPYØYZ
ØLPY37Z
ØLPY3JZ
ØLPY3KZ
ØLPY4ØZ
ØLPY47Z
ØLPY4JZ
ØLPY4KZ
ØLQØ*
ØLQ1*
ØLQ2*
ØLQ3*
ØLQ4*
ØLQ5*
ØLQ6*
ØLQ9*
ØLQB*
ØLQC*
ØLQD*
ØLQF*
ØLQG*
ØLQH*
ØLQJ*
ØLQK*
ØLQL*
ØLQM*
ØLQN*
ØLQP*
ØLQQ*
ØLQR*
ØLQS*
ØLQT*
ØLQV*
ØLQW*
ØLRØ*
ØLR1*
ØLR2*
ØLR3*
ØLR4*
ØLR5*
ØLR6*
ØLR9*
ØLRB*
ØLRC*
ØLRD*
ØLRF*
ØLRG*
ØLRH*
ØLRJ*
ØLRK*
ØLRL*
ØLRM*
ØLRN*
ØLRP*
ØLRQ*
ØLRR*
ØLRS*
ØLRT*
ØLRV*
ØLRW*
ØLSØ*
ØLS1*
ØLS2*
ØLS3*
ØLS4*
ØLS5*
ØLS6*
ØLS9*
ØLSB*
ØLSC*
ØLSD*
ØLSF*
ØLSG*
ØLSH*
ØLSJ*
ØLSK*
ØLSL*
ØLSM*
ØLSN*
ØLSP*
ØLSQ*
ØLSR*
ØLSS*
ØLST*
ØLSV*
ØLSW*
ØLTØ*
ØLT1*
ØLT2*
ØLT3*
ØLT4*
ØLT5*
ØLT6*
ØLT9*
ØLTB*
ØLTC*
ØLTD*
ØLTF*
ØLTG*
ØLTH*
ØLTJ*
ØLTK*
ØLTL*
ØLTM*
ØLTN*
ØLTP*
ØLTQ*
ØLTR*
ØLTS*
ØLTT*
ØLTV*
ØLTW*
ØLUØ*
ØLU1*
ØLU2*
ØLU3*
ØLU4*
ØLU5*
ØLU6*
ØLU9*
ØLUB*
ØLUC*
ØLUD*
ØLUF*
ØLUG*
ØLUH*
ØLUJ*
ØLUK*
ØLUL*
ØLUM*
ØLUN*
ØLUP*
ØLUQ*
ØLUR*
ØLUS*
ØLUT*
ØLUV*
ØLUW*
ØLWXØØZ
ØLWXØ7Z
ØLWXØJZ
ØLWXØKZ
ØLWXØYZ
ØLWX3ØZ
ØLWX37Z
ØLWX3JZ
ØLWX3KZ
ØLWX4ØZ
ØLWX47Z
ØLWX4JZ
ØLWX4KZ
ØLWYØØZ
ØLWYØ7Z
ØLWYØJZ
ØLWYØKZ
ØLWYØYZ
ØLWY3ØZ
ØLWY37Z
ØLWY3JZ
ØLWY3KZ
ØLWY4ØZ
ØLWY47Z
ØLWY4JZ
ØLWY4KZ
ØLXØ*
ØLX1*
ØLX2*
ØLX3*
ØLX4*
ØLX5*
ØLX6*
ØLX9*
ØLXB*
ØLXC*
ØLXD*
ØLXF*
ØLXG*
ØLXH*
ØLXJ*
ØLXK*
ØLXL*
ØLXM*
ØLXN*
ØLXP*
ØLXQ*
ØLXR*
ØLXS*
ØLXT*
ØLXV*
ØLXW*
ØM5Ø*
ØM51*
ØM52*
ØM53*
ØM54*
ØM59*
ØM5B*
ØM5C*
ØM5D*
ØM5F*
ØM5G*
ØM5H*
ØM5J*
ØM5K*
ØM5L*
ØM5M*
ØM5N*
ØM5P*
ØM5Q*
ØM5R*
ØM5S*
ØM5T*
ØM8Ø*
ØM81*
ØM82*
ØM83*
ØM84*
ØM89*
ØM8B*
ØM8C*
ØM8D*
ØM8F*
ØM8G*
ØM8H*
ØM8J*
ØM8K*
ØM8L*
ØM8M*
ØM8N*
ØM8P*
ØM8Q*
ØM8R*
ØM8S*
ØM8T*
ØM8V*
ØM8W*
ØM9ØØØZ
ØM9ØØZZ
ØM91ØØZ
ØM91ØZZ
ØM914ZZ
ØM92ØØZ
ØM92ØZZ
ØM924ZZ
ØM93ØØZ
ØM93ØZZ
ØM934ZZ
ØM94ØØZ
ØM94ØZZ
ØM944ZZ
ØM99ØØZ
ØM99ØZZ
ØM9BØØZ
ØM9BØZZ
ØM9CØØZ
ØM9CØZZ
ØM9DØØZ
ØM9DØZZ
ØM9FØØZ
ØM9FØZZ
ØM9GØØZ
ØM9GØZZ
ØM9HØØZ
ØM9HØZZ
ØM9JØØZ
ØM9JØZZ
ØM9KØØZ
ØM9KØZZ
ØM9LØØZ
ØM9LØZZ
ØM9L4ZZ
ØM9MØØZ
ØM9MØZZ
ØM9M4ZZ
ØM9NØØZ
ØM9NØZZ
ØM9N4ØZ
ØM9PØØZ
ØM9PØZZ
ØM9P4ØZ
ØM9QØØZ
ØM9QØZZ
ØM9Q4ØZ
ØM9RØØZ
ØM9RØZZ
ØM9R4ØZ
ØM9SØØZ
ØM9SØZZ
ØM9S4ØZ
ØM9TØØZ
ØM9TØZZ
ØM9T4ØZ
ØM9VØØZ
ØM9VØZZ
ØM9WØØZ
ØM9WØZZ
ØMBØØZZ
ØMBØ3ZZ
ØMBØ4ZZ
ØMB1ØZZ
ØMB13ZZ
ØMB14ZZ
ØMB2ØZZ
ØMB23ZZ
ØMB24ZZ
ØMB3ØZZ
ØMB33ZZ
ØMB34ZZ
ØMB4ØZZ
ØMB43ZZ
ØMB44ZZ
ØMB5ØZZ
ØMB53ZZ
ØMB54ZZ
ØMB6ØZZ
ØMB63ZZ
ØMB64ZZ
ØMB9ØZZ
ØMB93ZZ
ØMB94ZZ
ØMBBØZZ
ØMBB3ZZ
ØMBB4ZZ
ØMBCØZZ
ØMBC3ZZ
ØMBC4ZZ
ØMBDØZZ
ØMBD3ZZ
ØMBD4ZZ
ØMBFØZZ
ØMBF3ZZ
ØMBF4ZZ
ØMBGØZZ
ØMBG3ZZ
ØMBG4ZZ
ØMBHØZZ
ØMBH3ZZ
ØMBH4ZZ
ØMBJØZZ
ØMBJ3ZZ
ØMBJ4ZZ
ØMBKØZZ
ØMBK3ZZ
ØMBK4ZZ
ØMBLØZZ
ØMBL3ZZ
ØMBL4ZZ
ØMBMØZZ
ØMBM3ZZ
ØMBM4ZZ
ØMBNØZZ
ØMBN3ZZ
ØMBN4ZZ
ØMBPØZZ
ØMBP3ZZ
ØMBP4ZZ
ØMBQØZZ
ØMBQ3ZZ
ØMBQ4ZZ
ØMBRØZZ
ØMBR3ZZ
ØMBR4ZZ
ØMBSØZZ
ØMBS3ZZ
ØMBS4ZZ
ØMBTØZZ
ØMBT3ZZ
ØMBT4ZZ
ØMBVØZZ
ØMBV3ZZ
ØMBV4ZZ
ØMBWØZZ
ØMBW3ZZ
ØMBW4ZZ
ØMCØ*
ØMC1*
ØMC2*
ØMC3*
ØMC4*
ØMC9*
ØMCB*
ØMCC*
ØMCD*
ØMCF*
ØMCG*
ØMCH*
ØMCJ*
ØMCK*
ØMCL*
ØMCM*
ØMCN*
ØMCP*
ØMCQ*
ØMCR*
ØMCS*
ØMCT*
ØMCV*

ØMCW*
ØMDØ*
ØMD1*
ØMD2*
ØMD3*
ØMD4*
ØMD5*
ØMD6*
ØMD9*
ØMDB*
ØMDC*
ØMDD*
ØMDF*
ØMDG*
ØMDH*
ØMDJ*
ØMDK*
ØMDL*
ØMDM*
ØMDN*
ØMDP*
ØMDQ*
ØMDR*
ØMDS*
ØMDT*
ØMDV*
ØMDW*
ØMHXØYZ
ØMHYØYZ
ØMPXØ7Z
ØMPXØKZ
ØMPX37Z
ØMPX3KZ
ØMPX47Z
ØMPX4KZ
ØMPYØ7Z
ØMPYØKZ
ØMPY37Z
ØMPY3KZ
ØMPY47Z
ØMPY4KZ
ØMQ1*
ØMQ2*
ØMQ3*
ØMQ4*
ØMQ5*
ØMQ6*
ØMQ7*
ØMQ8*
ØMQN*
ØMQP*
ØMQQ*
ØMQR*
ØMQS*
ØMQT*
ØMR1Ø7Z
ØMR1ØJZ
ØMR1ØKZ
ØMR147Z
ØMR14JZ
ØMR14KZ
ØMR2Ø7Z
ØMR2ØJZ
ØMR2ØKZ
ØMR247Z
ØMR24JZ
ØMR24KZ
ØMR3Ø7Z
ØMR3ØJZ
ØMR3ØKZ
ØMR347Z
ØMR34JZ
ØMR34KZ
ØMR4Ø7Z
ØMR4ØJZ
ØMR4ØKZ
ØMR447Z
ØMR44JZ
ØMR44KZ
ØMR5Ø7Z
ØMR5ØJZ
ØMR5ØKZ
ØMR547Z
ØMR54JZ
ØMR54KZ
ØMR6Ø7Z
ØMR6ØJZ
ØMR6ØKZ
ØMR647Z
ØMR64JZ
ØMR64KZ
ØMR7Ø7Z
ØMR7ØJZ
ØMR7ØKZ
ØMR747Z
ØMR74JZ
ØMR74KZ
ØMR8Ø7Z
ØMR8ØJZ
ØMR8ØKZ
ØMR847Z
ØMR84JZ
ØMR84KZ
ØMRNØ7Z
ØMRNØJZ
ØMRNØKZ
ØMRN47Z
ØMRN4JZ
ØMRN4KZ
ØMRPØ7Z
ØMRPØJZ
ØMRPØKZ
ØMRP47Z
ØMRP4JZ
ØMRP4KZ
ØMRQØ7Z
ØMRQØJZ
ØMRQØKZ
ØMRQ47Z
ØMRQ4JZ
ØMRQ4KZ
ØMRRØ7Z
ØMRRØJZ
ØMRRØKZ
ØMRR47Z
ØMRR4JZ
ØMRR4KZ
ØMRSØ7Z
ØMRSØJZ
ØMRSØKZ
ØMRS47Z
ØMRS4JZ
ØMRS4KZ
ØMRTØ7Z
ØMRTØJZ
ØMRTØKZ
ØMRT47Z
ØMRT4JZ
ØMRT4KZ
ØMTØ*
ØMT1*
ØMT2*
ØMT3*
ØMT4*
ØMT5*
ØMT6*
ØMT9*
ØMTB*
ØMTC*
ØMTD*
ØMTF*
ØMTG*
ØMTH*
ØMTJ*
ØMTK*
ØMTL*
ØMTM*
ØMTN*
ØMTP*
ØMTQ*
ØMTR*
ØMTS*
ØMTT*
ØMTV*
ØMTW*
ØMWXØØZ
ØMWXØ7Z
ØMWXØJZ
ØMWXØKZ
ØMWXØYZ
ØMWX3ØZ
ØMWX37Z
ØMWX3JZ
ØMWX3KZ
ØMWX4ØZ
ØMWX47Z
ØMWX4JZ
ØMWX4KZ
ØMWYØØZ
ØMWYØ7Z
ØMWYØJZ
ØMWYØKZ
ØMWYØYZ
ØMWY3ØZ
ØMWY37Z
ØMWY3JZ
ØMWY3KZ
ØMWY4ØZ
ØMWY47Z
ØMWY4JZ
ØMWY4KZ
ØN5*
ØN8P*
ØN8Q*
ØN9PØØZ
ØN9PØZZ
ØN9P4ØZ
ØN9P4ZZ
ØN9QØØZ
ØN9QØZZ
ØN9Q4ØZ
ØN9Q4ZZ
ØNBØØZZ
ØNBØ3ZZ
ØNBØ4ZZ
ØNB1ØZZ
ØNB13ZZ
ØNB14ZZ
ØNB3ØZZ
ØNB33ZZ
ØNB34ZZ
ØNB4ØZZ
ØNB43ZZ
ØNB44ZZ
ØNB5ØZZ
ØNB53ZZ
ØNB54ZZ
ØNB6ØZZ
ØNB63ZZ
ØNB64ZZ
ØNB7ØZZ
ØNB73ZZ
ØNB74ZZ
ØNBBØZZ
ØNBB3ZZ
ØNBB4ZZ
ØNBCØZZ
ØNBC3ZZ
ØNBC4ZZ
ØNBFØZZ
ØNBF3ZZ
ØNBF4ZZ
ØNBGØZZ
ØNBG3ZZ
ØNBG4ZZ
ØNBHØZZ
ØNBH3ZZ
ØNBH4ZZ
ØNBJØZZ
ØNBJ3ZZ
ØNBJ4ZZ
ØNBKØZZ
ØNBK3ZZ
ØNBK4ZZ
ØNBLØZZ
ØNBL3ZZ
ØNBL4ZZ
ØNBMØZZ
ØNBM3ZZ
ØNBM4ZZ
ØNBNØZZ
ØNBN3ZZ
ØNBN4ZZ
ØNBPØZZ
ØNBP3ZZ
ØNBP4ZZ
ØNBQØZZ
ØNBQ3ZZ
ØNBQ4ZZ
ØNBRØZZ
ØNBR3ZZ
ØNBR4ZZ
ØNBTØZZ
ØNBT3ZZ
ØNBT4ZZ
ØNBVØZZ
ØNBV3ZZ
ØNBV4ZZ
ØNBXØZZ
ØNBX3ZZ
ØNBX4ZZ
ØNC1*
ØNC3*
ØNC4*
ØNC5*
ØNC6*
ØNC7*
ØNDØØZZ
ØND1ØZZ
ØND3ØZZ
ØND4ØZZ
ØND5ØZZ
ØND6ØZZ
ØND7ØZZ
ØNDBØZZ
ØNDCØZZ
ØNDFØZZ
ØNDGØZZ
ØNDHØZZ
ØNDJØZZ
ØNDKØZZ
ØNDLØZZ
ØNDMØZZ
ØNDNØZZ
ØNDPØZZ
ØNDQØZZ
ØNDRØZZ
ØNDTØZZ
ØNDVØZZ
ØNDXØZZ
ØNHØØ3Z
ØNHØØ4Z
ØNHØ33Z
ØNHØ34Z
ØNHØ43Z
ØNHØ44Z
ØNH1*
ØNH3*
ØNH4*
ØNH5Ø4Z
ØNH534Z
ØNH544Z
ØNH6Ø4Z
ØNH634Z
ØNH644Z
ØNH7*
ØNJØØZZ
ØNJØ4ZZ
ØNJBØZZ
ØNJB4ZZ
ØNJWØZZ
ØNJW4ZZ
ØNN1*
ØNN3*
ØNN4*
ØNN5*
ØNN6*
ØNN7*
ØNNC*
ØNNF*
ØNNG*
ØNNH*
ØNNJ*
ØNNK*
ØNNL*
ØNNM*
ØNNN*
ØNNP*
ØNNQ*
ØNNR*
ØNNT*
ØNNV*
ØNNX*
ØNPØØJZ
ØNPØ3JZ
ØNPØ4JZ
ØNPWØ4Z
ØNPWØJZ
ØNPW34Z
ØNPW3JZ
ØNPW44Z
ØNPW4JZ
ØNPWX4Z
ØNQØØZZ
ØNQØ3ZZ
ØNQØ4ZZ
ØNQ1ØZZ
ØNQ13ZZ
ØNQ14ZZ
ØNQ3ØZZ
ØNQ33ZZ
ØNQ34ZZ
ØNQ4ØZZ
ØNQ43ZZ
ØNQ44ZZ
ØNQ5ØZZ
ØNQ53ZZ
ØNQ54ZZ
ØNQ6ØZZ
ØNQ63ZZ
ØNQ64ZZ
ØNQ7ØZZ
ØNQ73ZZ
ØNQ74ZZ
ØNQBØZZ
ØNQB3ZZ
ØNQB4ZZ
ØNQCØZZ
ØNQC3ZZ
ØNQC4ZZ
ØNQFØZZ
ØNQF3ZZ
ØNQF4ZZ
ØNQGØZZ
ØNQG3ZZ
ØNQG4ZZ
ØNQHØZZ
ØNQH3ZZ
ØNQH4ZZ
ØNQJØZZ
ØNQJ3ZZ
ØNQJ4ZZ
ØNQKØZZ
ØNQK3ZZ
ØNQK4ZZ
ØNQLØZZ
ØNQL3ZZ
ØNQL4ZZ
ØNQMØZZ
ØNQM3ZZ
ØNQM4ZZ
ØNQNØZZ
ØNQN3ZZ
ØNQN4ZZ
ØNQPØZZ
ØNQP3ZZ
ØNQP4ZZ
ØNQQØZZ
ØNQQ3ZZ
ØNQQ4ZZ
ØNQRØZZ
ØNQR3ZZ
ØNQR4ZZ
ØNQTØZZ
ØNQT3ZZ
ØNQT4ZZ
ØNQVØZZ
ØNQV3ZZ
ØNQV4ZZ
ØNQXØZZ
ØNQX3ZZ
ØNQX4ZZ
ØNRØ*
ØNR1ØJZ
ØNR13JZ
ØNR14JZ
ØNR3ØJZ
ØNR33JZ
ØNR34JZ
ØNR4ØJZ
ØNR43JZ
ØNR44JZ
ØNR5ØJZ
ØNR53JZ
ØNR54JZ
ØNR6ØJZ
ØNR63JZ
ØNR64JZ
ØNR7ØJZ
ØNR73JZ
ØNR74JZ
ØNRB*
ØNRCØJZ
ØNRC3JZ
ØNRC4JZ
ØNRFØJZ
ØNRF3JZ
ØNRF4JZ
ØNRGØJZ
ØNRG3JZ
ØNRG4JZ
ØNRHØJZ
ØNRH3JZ
ØNRH4JZ
ØNRJØJZ
ØNRJ3JZ
ØNRJ4JZ
ØNRKØJZ
ØNRK3JZ
ØNRK4JZ
ØNRLØJZ
ØNRL3JZ
ØNRL4JZ
ØNRMØJZ
ØNRM3JZ
ØNRM4JZ
ØNRNØJZ
ØNRN3JZ
ØNRN4JZ
ØNRPØ7Z
ØNRPØJZ
ØNRP37Z
ØNRP3JZ
ØNRP47Z
ØNRP4JZ
ØNRQØ7Z
ØNRQØJZ
ØNRQ37Z
ØNRQ3JZ
ØNRQ47Z
ØNRQ4JZ
ØNRR*
ØNRT*
ØNRV*
ØNRXØJZ
ØNRX3JZ
ØNRX4JZ
ØNSØØ4Z
ØNSØØ5Z
ØNSØØZZ
ØNSØ34Z
ØNSØ35Z
ØNSØ3ZZ
ØNSØ44Z
ØNSØ45Z
ØNSØ4ZZ
ØNS1Ø4Z
ØNS1ØZZ
ØNS134Z
ØNS13ZZ
ØNS144Z
ØNS14ZZ
ØNS3Ø4Z
ØNS3ØZZ
ØNS334Z
ØNS33ZZ
ØNS344Z
ØNS34ZZ
ØNS4Ø4Z
ØNS4ØZZ
ØNS434Z
ØNS43ZZ
ØNS444Z
ØNS44ZZ
ØNS5Ø4Z
ØNS5ØZZ
ØNS534Z
ØNS53ZZ
ØNS544Z
ØNS54ZZ
ØNS6Ø4Z
ØNS6ØZZ
ØNS634Z
ØNS63ZZ
ØNS644Z
ØNS64ZZ
ØNS7Ø4Z
ØNS7ØZZ
ØNS734Z
ØNS73ZZ
ØNS744Z
ØNS74ZZ
ØNSBØ4Z
ØNSBØZZ
ØNSCØ4Z
ØNSCØZZ
ØNSFØ4Z
ØNSFØZZ
ØNSGØ4Z
ØNSGØZZ
ØNSHØ4Z
ØNSHØZZ
ØNSJØ4Z
ØNSJØZZ
ØNSKØ4Z
ØNSKØZZ
ØNSLØ4Z
ØNSLØZZ
ØNSMØ4Z
ØNSMØZZ
ØNSNØ4Z
ØNSNØZZ
ØNSPØ4Z
ØNSPØZZ
ØNSQØ4Z
ØNSQØZZ
ØNSRØ4Z
ØNSRØ5Z
ØNSRØZZ
ØNSTØ4Z
ØNSTØ5Z
ØNSTØZZ
ØNSVØ4Z
ØNSVØ5Z
ØNSVØZZ
ØNSXØ4Z
ØNSXØZZ
ØNT*
ØNUØØJZ
ØNUØ3JZ
ØNUØ4JZ
ØNU1ØJZ
ØNU13JZ
ØNU14JZ
ØNU3ØJZ
ØNU33JZ
ØNU34JZ
ØNU4ØJZ
ØNU43JZ
ØNU44JZ
ØNU5ØJZ
ØNU53JZ
ØNU54JZ
ØNU6ØJZ
ØNU63JZ
ØNU64JZ
ØNU7ØJZ
ØNU73JZ
ØNU74JZ
ØNUB*
ØNUCØJZ
ØNUC3JZ
ØNUC4JZ
ØNUFØJZ
ØNUF3JZ
ØNUF4JZ
ØNUGØJZ
ØNUG3JZ
ØNUG4JZ
ØNUHØJZ
ØNUH3JZ
ØNUH4JZ
ØNUJØJZ
ØNUJ3JZ
ØNUJ4JZ
ØNUKØJZ
ØNUK3JZ
ØNUK4JZ
ØNULØJZ
ØNUL3JZ
ØNUL4JZ
ØNUMØJZ
ØNUM3JZ
ØNUM4JZ
ØNUNØJZ
ØNUN3JZ
ØNUN4JZ
ØNUPØJZ
ØNUP3JZ
ØNUP4JZ
ØNUQØJZ
ØNUQ3JZ
ØNUQ4JZ
ØNUR*
ØNUT*
ØNUV*
ØNUXØJZ
ØNUX3JZ
ØNUX4JZ
ØP5Ø*
ØP51*
ØP52*
ØP53*
ØP54*
ØP55*
ØP56*
ØP57*
ØP58*
ØP59*
ØP5B*
ØP5C*
ØP5D*
ØP5F*
ØP5G*
ØP5H*
ØP5J*
ØP5K*
ØP5L*
ØP5R*
ØP5S*
ØP5T*
ØP5V*
ØP8Ø*
ØP81*
ØP82*
ØP83*
ØP84*
ØP85*
ØP86*
ØP87*
ØP88*
ØP89*
ØP8B*
ØP8C*
ØP8D*
ØP8F*
ØP8G*
ØP8H*
ØP8J*
ØP8K*
ØP8L*
ØP8R*
ØP8S*
ØP8T*
ØP8V*
ØPBØØZZ
ØPBØ3ZZ
ØPBØ4ZZ
ØPB1ØZZ
ØPB13ZZ
ØPB14ZZ
ØPB2ØZZ
ØPB23ZZ
ØPB24ZZ
ØPB3ØZZ
ØPB33ZZ
ØPB34ZZ
ØPB4ØZZ
ØPB43ZZ
ØPB44ZZ
ØPB5ØZZ
ØPB53ZZ
ØPB54ZZ
ØPB6ØZZ
ØPB63ZZ
ØPB64ZZ
ØPB7ØZZ
ØPB73ZZ
ØPB74ZZ
ØPB8ØZZ
ØPB83ZZ
ØPB84ZZ
ØPB9ØZZ
ØPB93ZZ
ØPB94ZZ
ØPBBØZZ
ØPBB3ZZ
ØPBB4ZZ
ØPBCØZZ
ØPBC3ZZ
ØPBC4ZZ
ØPBDØZZ
ØPBD3ZZ
ØPBD4ZZ
ØPBFØZZ
ØPBF3ZZ
ØPBF4ZZ
ØPBGØZZ
ØPBG3ZZ
ØPBG4ZZ
ØPBHØZZ
ØPBH3ZZ
ØPBH4ZZ
ØPBJØZZ
ØPBJ3ZZ
ØPBJ4ZZ
ØPBKØZZ
ØPBK3ZZ
ØPBK4ZZ
ØPBLØZZ
ØPBL3ZZ
ØPBL4ZZ
ØPBRØZZ
ØPBR3ZZ
ØPBR4ZZ
ØPBSØZZ
ØPBS3ZZ
ØPBS4ZZ
ØPBTØZZ
ØPBT3ZZ
ØPBT4ZZ
ØPBVØZZ
ØPBV3ZZ
ØPBV4ZZ
ØPCØ*
ØPC1*
ØPC2*
ØPC3*
ØPC4*
ØPC5*
ØPC6*
ØPC7*
ØPC8*
ØPC9*
ØPCB*
ØPCC*
ØPCD*
ØPCF*
ØPCG*
ØPCH*
ØPCJ*
ØPCK*
ØPCL*
ØPCR*
ØPCS*
ØPCT*
ØPCV*
ØPDØØZZ
ØPD1ØZZ
ØPD2ØZZ
ØPD3ØZZ
ØPD4ØZZ
ØPD5ØZZ
ØPD6ØZZ
ØPD7ØZZ
ØPD8ØZZ
ØPD9ØZZ
ØPDBØZZ
ØPDCØZZ
ØPDDØZZ
ØPDFØZZ
ØPDGØZZ
ØPDHØZZ
ØPDJØZZ
ØPDKØZZ
ØPDLØZZ
ØPHØ*
ØPH1*
ØPH2*
ØPH3*
ØPH4*
ØPH5*
ØPH6*
ØPH7*
ØPH8*
ØPH9*
ØPHB*
ØPHCØ4Z
ØPHCØ5Z
ØPHCØ6Z
ØPHCØBZ
ØPHCØCZ
ØPHCØDZ
ØPHC34Z
ØPHC35Z
ØPHC36Z
ØPHC3BZ
ØPHC3CZ
ØPHC3DZ
ØPHC44Z
ØPHC45Z
ØPHC46Z
ØPHC4BZ
ØPHC4CZ
ØPHC4DZ
ØPHDØ4Z
ØPHDØ5Z
ØPHDØ6Z
ØPHDØBZ
ØPHDØCZ
ØPHDØDZ
ØPHD34Z
ØPHD35Z
ØPHD36Z
ØPHD3BZ
ØPHD3CZ
ØPHD3DZ
ØPHD44Z
ØPHD45Z
ØPHD46Z
ØPHD4BZ
ØPHD4CZ
ØPHD4DZ
ØPHFØ4Z
ØPHFØ5Z
ØPHFØ6Z
ØPHFØ7Z
ØPHFØBZ
ØPHFØCZ
ØPHFØDZ
ØPHF34Z
ØPHF35Z
ØPHF36Z
ØPHF37Z
ØPHF3BZ
ØPHF3CZ
ØPHF3DZ
ØPHF44Z
ØPHF45Z
ØPHF46Z
ØPHF47Z
ØPHF4BZ
ØPHF4CZ
ØPHF4DZ
ØPHGØ4Z

ØPHGØ5Z
ØPHGØ6Z
ØPHGØ7Z
ØPHGØBZ
ØPHGØCZ
ØPHGØDZ
ØPHG34Z
ØPHG35Z
ØPHG36Z
ØPHG37Z
ØPHG3BZ
ØPHG3CZ
ØPHG3DZ
ØPHG44Z
ØPHG45Z
ØPHG46Z
ØPHG47Z
ØPHG4BZ
ØPHG4CZ
ØPHG4DZ
ØPHHØ4Z
ØPHHØ5Z
ØPHHØ6Z
ØPHHØBZ
ØPHHØCZ
ØPHHØDZ
ØPHH34Z
ØPHH35Z
ØPHH36Z
ØPHH3BZ
ØPHH3CZ
ØPHH3DZ
ØPHH44Z
ØPHH45Z
ØPHH46Z
ØPHH4BZ
ØPHH4CZ
ØPHH4DZ
ØPHJØ4Z
ØPHJØ5Z
ØPHJØ6Z
ØPHJØBZ
ØPHJØCZ
ØPHJØDZ
ØPHJ34Z
ØPHJ35Z
ØPHJ36Z
ØPHJ3BZ
ØPHJ3CZ
ØPHJ3DZ
ØPHJ44Z
ØPHJ45Z
ØPHJ46Z
ØPHJ4BZ
ØPHJ4CZ
ØPHJ4DZ
ØPHKØ4Z
ØPHKØ5Z
ØPHKØ6Z
ØPHKØBZ
ØPHKØCZ
ØPHKØDZ
ØPHK34Z
ØPHK35Z
ØPHK36Z
ØPHK3BZ
ØPHK3CZ
ØPHK3DZ
ØPHK44Z
ØPHK45Z
ØPHK46Z
ØPHK4BZ
ØPHK4CZ
ØPHK4DZ
ØPHLØ4Z
ØPHLØ5Z
ØPHLØ6Z
ØPHLØBZ
ØPHLØCZ
ØPHLØDZ
ØPHL34Z
ØPHL35Z
ØPHL36Z
ØPHL3BZ
ØPHL3CZ
ØPHL3DZ
ØPHL44Z
ØPHL45Z
ØPHL46Z
ØPHL4BZ
ØPHL4CZ
ØPHL4DZ
ØPHR*
ØPHS*
ØPHT*
ØPHV*
ØPHY*
ØPNØ*
ØPN1*
ØPN2*
ØPN5*
ØPN6*
ØPN7*
ØPN8*
ØPN9*
ØPNB*
ØPNC*
ØPND*
ØPNF*
ØPNG*
ØPNH*
ØPNJ*
ØPNK*
ØPNL*
ØPPØØ4Z
ØPPØØ7Z
ØPPØØJZ
ØPPØØKZ
ØPPØ34Z
ØPPØ37Z
ØPPØ3JZ
ØPPØ3KZ
ØPPØ44Z
ØPPØ47Z
ØPPØ4JZ
ØPPØ4KZ
ØPP1Ø4Z
ØPP1Ø7Z
ØPP1ØJZ
ØPP1ØKZ
ØPP134Z
ØPP137Z
ØPP13JZ
ØPP13KZ
ØPP144Z
ØPP147Z
ØPP14JZ
ØPP14KZ
ØPP2Ø4Z
ØPP2Ø7Z
ØPP2ØJZ
ØPP2ØKZ
ØPP234Z
ØPP237Z
ØPP23JZ
ØPP23KZ
ØPP244Z
ØPP247Z
ØPP24JZ
ØPP24KZ
ØPP3Ø4Z
ØPP3Ø7Z
ØPP3ØJZ
ØPP3ØKZ
ØPP334Z
ØPP337Z
ØPP33JZ
ØPP33KZ
ØPP344Z
ØPP347Z
ØPP34JZ
ØPP34KZ
ØPP4Ø4Z
ØPP4Ø7Z
ØPP4ØJZ
ØPP4ØKZ
ØPP434Z
ØPP437Z
ØPP43JZ
ØPP43KZ
ØPP444Z
ØPP447Z
ØPP44JZ
ØPP44KZ
ØPP5Ø4Z
ØPP5Ø7Z
ØPP5ØJZ
ØPP5ØKZ
ØPP534Z
ØPP537Z
ØPP53JZ
ØPP53KZ
ØPP544Z
ØPP547Z
ØPP54JZ
ØPP54KZ
ØPP6Ø4Z
ØPP6Ø7Z
ØPP6ØJZ
ØPP6ØKZ
ØPP634Z
ØPP637Z
ØPP63JZ
ØPP63KZ
ØPP644Z
ØPP647Z
ØPP64JZ
ØPP64KZ
ØPP7Ø4Z
ØPP7Ø7Z
ØPP7ØJZ
ØPP7ØKZ
ØPP734Z
ØPP737Z
ØPP73JZ
ØPP73KZ
ØPP744Z
ØPP747Z
ØPP74JZ
ØPP74KZ
ØPP8Ø4Z
ØPP8Ø7Z
ØPP8ØJZ
ØPP8ØKZ
ØPP834Z
ØPP837Z
ØPP83JZ
ØPP83KZ
ØPP844Z
ØPP847Z
ØPP84JZ
ØPP84KZ
ØPP9Ø4Z
ØPP9Ø7Z
ØPP9ØJZ
ØPP9ØKZ
ØPP934Z
ØPP937Z
ØPP93JZ
ØPP93KZ
ØPP944Z
ØPP947Z
ØPP94JZ
ØPP94KZ
ØPPBØ4Z
ØPPBØ7Z
ØPPBØJZ
ØPPBØKZ
ØPPB34Z
ØPPB37Z
ØPPB3JZ
ØPPB3KZ
ØPPB44Z
ØPPB47Z
ØPPB4JZ
ØPPB4KZ
ØPPCØ4Z
ØPPCØ5Z
ØPPCØ7Z
ØPPCØJZ
ØPPCØKZ
ØPPC34Z
ØPPC35Z
ØPPC37Z
ØPPC3JZ
ØPPC3KZ
ØPPC44Z
ØPPC45Z
ØPPC47Z
ØPPC4JZ
ØPPC4KZ
ØPPDØ4Z
ØPPDØ5Z
ØPPDØ7Z
ØPPDØJZ
ØPPDØKZ
ØPPD34Z
ØPPD35Z
ØPPD37Z
ØPPD3JZ
ØPPD3KZ
ØPPD44Z
ØPPD45Z
ØPPD47Z
ØPPD4JZ
ØPPD4KZ
ØPPFØ4Z
ØPPFØ5Z
ØPPFØ7Z
ØPPFØJZ
ØPPFØKZ
ØPPF34Z
ØPPF35Z
ØPPF37Z
ØPPF3JZ
ØPPF3KZ
ØPPF44Z
ØPPF45Z
ØPPF47Z
ØPPF4JZ
ØPPF4KZ
ØPPGØ4Z
ØPPGØ5Z
ØPPGØ7Z
ØPPGØJZ
ØPPGØKZ
ØPPG34Z
ØPPG35Z
ØPPG37Z
ØPPG3JZ
ØPPG3KZ
ØPPG44Z
ØPPG45Z
ØPPG47Z
ØPPG4JZ
ØPPG4KZ
ØPPHØ4Z
ØPPHØ5Z
ØPPHØ7Z
ØPPHØJZ
ØPPHØKZ
ØPPH34Z
ØPPH35Z
ØPPH37Z
ØPPH3JZ
ØPPH3KZ
ØPPH44Z
ØPPH45Z
ØPPH47Z
ØPPH4JZ
ØPPH4KZ
ØPPJØ4Z
ØPPJØ5Z
ØPPJØ7Z
ØPPJØJZ
ØPPJØKZ
ØPPJ34Z
ØPPJ35Z
ØPPJ37Z
ØPPJ3JZ
ØPPJ3KZ
ØPPJ44Z
ØPPJ45Z
ØPPJ47Z
ØPPJ4JZ
ØPPJ4KZ
ØPPKØ4Z
ØPPKØ5Z
ØPPKØ7Z
ØPPKØJZ
ØPPKØKZ
ØPPK34Z
ØPPK35Z
ØPPK37Z
ØPPK3JZ
ØPPK3KZ
ØPPK44Z
ØPPK45Z
ØPPK47Z
ØPPK4JZ
ØPPK4KZ
ØPPLØ4Z
ØPPLØ5Z
ØPPLØ7Z
ØPPLØJZ
ØPPLØKZ
ØPPL34Z
ØPPL35Z
ØPPL37Z
ØPPL3JZ
ØPPL3KZ
ØPPL44Z
ØPPL45Z
ØPPL47Z
ØPPL4JZ
ØPPL4KZ
ØPPRØ4Z
ØPPRØ5Z
ØPPRØ7Z
ØPPRØJZ
ØPPRØKZ
ØPPR34Z
ØPPR35Z
ØPPR37Z
ØPPR3JZ
ØPPR3KZ
ØPPR44Z
ØPPR45Z
ØPPR47Z
ØPPR4JZ
ØPPR4KZ
ØPPSØ4Z
ØPPSØ5Z
ØPPSØ7Z
ØPPSØJZ
ØPPSØKZ
ØPPS34Z
ØPPS35Z
ØPPS37Z
ØPPS3JZ
ØPPS3KZ
ØPPS44Z
ØPPS45Z
ØPPS47Z
ØPPS4JZ
ØPPS4KZ
ØPPTØ4Z
ØPPTØ5Z
ØPPTØ7Z
ØPPTØJZ
ØPPTØKZ
ØPPT34Z
ØPPT35Z
ØPPT37Z
ØPPT3JZ
ØPPT3KZ
ØPPT44Z
ØPPT45Z
ØPPT47Z
ØPPT4JZ
ØPPT4KZ
ØPPVØ4Z
ØPPVØ5Z
ØPPVØ7Z
ØPPVØJZ
ØPPVØKZ
ØPPV34Z
ØPPV35Z
ØPPV37Z
ØPPV3JZ
ØPPV3KZ
ØPPV44Z
ØPPV45Z
ØPPV47Z
ØPPV4JZ
ØPPV4KZ
ØPPYØMZ
ØPPY3MZ
ØPPY4MZ
ØPQØØZZ
ØPQØ3ZZ
ØPQØ4ZZ
ØPQ1ØZZ
ØPQ13ZZ
ØPQ14ZZ
ØPQ2ØZZ
ØPQ23ZZ
ØPQ24ZZ
ØPQ5ØZZ
ØPQ53ZZ
ØPQ54ZZ
ØPQ6ØZZ
ØPQ63ZZ
ØPQ64ZZ
ØPQ7ØZZ
ØPQ73ZZ
ØPQ74ZZ
ØPQ8ØZZ
ØPQ83ZZ
ØPQ84ZZ
ØPQ9ØZZ
ØPQ93ZZ
ØPQ94ZZ
ØPQBØZZ
ØPQB3ZZ
ØPQB4ZZ
ØPQCØZZ
ØPQC3ZZ
ØPQC4ZZ
ØPQDØZZ
ØPQD3ZZ
ØPQD4ZZ
ØPQFØZZ
ØPQF3ZZ
ØPQF4ZZ
ØPQGØZZ
ØPQG3ZZ
ØPQG4ZZ
ØPQHØZZ
ØPQH3ZZ
ØPQH4ZZ
ØPQJØZZ
ØPQJ3ZZ
ØPQJ4ZZ
ØPQKØZZ
ØPQK3ZZ
ØPQK4ZZ
ØPQLØZZ
ØPQL3ZZ
ØPQL4ZZ
ØPRØØJZ
ØPRØ3JZ
ØPRØ4JZ
ØPR1ØJZ
ØPR13JZ
ØPR14JZ
ØPR2ØJZ
ØPR23JZ
ØPR24JZ
ØPR5ØJZ
ØPR53JZ
ØPR54JZ
ØPR6ØJZ
ØPR63JZ
ØPR64JZ
ØPR7ØJZ
ØPR73JZ
ØPR74JZ
ØPR8ØJZ
ØPR83JZ
ØPR84JZ
ØPR9ØJZ
ØPR93JZ
ØPR94JZ
ØPRBØJZ
ØPRB3JZ
ØPRB4JZ
ØPRCØ7Z
ØPRCØKZ
ØPRC37Z
ØPRC3JZ
ØPRC3KZ
ØPRC47Z
ØPRC4JZ
ØPRC4KZ
ØPRDØ7Z
ØPRDØKZ
ØPRD37Z
ØPRD3JZ
ØPRD3KZ
ØPRD47Z
ØPRD4JZ
ØPRD4KZ
ØPRF*
ØPRG*
ØPRH*
ØPRJ*
ØPRK*
ØPRL*
ØPSØØØZ
ØPSØØ4Z
ØPSØØZZ
ØPSØ3ØZ
ØPSØ34Z
ØPSØ4ØZ
ØPSØ44Z
ØPS1Ø4Z
ØPS1ØZZ
ØPS134Z
ØPS144Z
ØPS2Ø4Z
ØPS2ØZZ
ØPS234Z
ØPS244Z
ØPS3Ø4Z
ØPS3ØZZ
ØPS334Z
ØPS344Z
ØPS34ZZ
ØPS4Ø3Z
ØPS4Ø4Z
ØPS4ØZZ
ØPS434Z
ØPS443Z
ØPS444Z
ØPS44ZZ
ØPS5Ø4Z
ØPS5ØZZ
ØPS534Z
ØPS544Z
ØPS6Ø4Z
ØPS6ØZZ
ØPS634Z
ØPS644Z
ØPS7Ø4Z
ØPS7ØZZ
ØPS734Z
ØPS744Z
ØPS8Ø4Z
ØPS8ØZZ
ØPS834Z
ØPS844Z
ØPS9Ø4Z
ØPS9ØZZ
ØPS934Z
ØPS944Z
ØPSBØ4Z
ØPSBØZZ
ØPSB34Z
ØPSB44Z
ØPSCØ4Z
ØPSCØ5Z
ØPSCØ6Z
ØPSCØBZ
ØPSCØCZ
ØPSCØDZ
ØPSCØZZ
ØPSC34Z
ØPSC35Z
ØPSC36Z
ØPSC3BZ
ØPSC3CZ
ØPSC3DZ
ØPSC44Z
ØPSC45Z
ØPSC46Z
ØPSC4BZ
ØPSC4CZ
ØPSC4DZ
ØPSDØ4Z
ØPSDØ5Z
ØPSDØ6Z
ØPSDØBZ
ØPSDØCZ
ØPSDØDZ
ØPSDØZZ
ØPSD34Z
ØPSD35Z
ØPSD36Z
ØPSD3BZ
ØPSD3CZ
ØPSD3DZ
ØPSD44Z
ØPSD45Z
ØPSD46Z
ØPSD4BZ
ØPSD4CZ
ØPSD4DZ
ØPSFØ4Z
ØPSFØ5Z
ØPSFØ6Z
ØPSFØBZ
ØPSFØCZ
ØPSFØDZ
ØPSFØZZ
ØPSF34Z
ØPSF35Z
ØPSF36Z
ØPSF3BZ
ØPSF3CZ
ØPSF3DZ
ØPSF44Z
ØPSF45Z
ØPSF46Z
ØPSF4BZ
ØPSF4CZ
ØPSF4DZ
ØPSGØ4Z
ØPSGØ5Z
ØPSGØ6Z
ØPSGØBZ
ØPSGØCZ
ØPSGØDZ
ØPSGØZZ
ØPSG34Z
ØPSG35Z
ØPSG36Z
ØPSG3BZ
ØPSG3CZ
ØPSG3DZ
ØPSG44Z
ØPSG45Z
ØPSG46Z
ØPSG4BZ
ØPSG4CZ
ØPSG4DZ
ØPSHØ4Z
ØPSHØ5Z
ØPSHØ6Z
ØPSHØBZ
ØPSHØCZ
ØPSHØDZ
ØPSHØZZ
ØPSH34Z
ØPSH35Z
ØPSH36Z
ØPSH3BZ
ØPSH3CZ
ØPSH3DZ
ØPSH44Z
ØPSH45Z
ØPSH46Z
ØPSH4BZ
ØPSH4CZ
ØPSH4DZ
ØPSJØ4Z
ØPSJØ5Z
ØPSJØ6Z
ØPSJØBZ
ØPSJØCZ
ØPSJØDZ
ØPSJØZZ
ØPSJ34Z
ØPSJ35Z
ØPSJ36Z
ØPSJ3BZ
ØPSJ3CZ
ØPSJ3DZ
ØPSJ44Z
ØPSJ45Z
ØPSJ46Z
ØPSJ4BZ
ØPSJ4CZ
ØPSJ4DZ
ØPSKØ4Z
ØPSKØ5Z
ØPSKØ6Z
ØPSKØBZ
ØPSKØCZ
ØPSKØDZ
ØPSKØZZ
ØPSK34Z
ØPSK35Z
ØPSK36Z
ØPSK3BZ
ØPSK3CZ
ØPSK3DZ
ØPSK44Z
ØPSK45Z
ØPSK46Z
ØPSK4BZ
ØPSK4CZ
ØPSK4DZ
ØPSLØ4Z
ØPSLØ5Z
ØPSLØ6Z
ØPSLØBZ
ØPSLØCZ
ØPSLØDZ
ØPSLØZZ
ØPSL34Z
ØPSL35Z
ØPSL36Z
ØPSL3BZ
ØPSL3CZ
ØPSL3DZ
ØPSL44Z
ØPSL45Z
ØPSL46Z
ØPSL4BZ
ØPSL4CZ
ØPSL4DZ
ØPSRØ5Z
ØPSR35Z
ØPSR45Z
ØPSSØ5Z
ØPSS35Z
ØPSS45Z
ØPSTØ5Z
ØPST35Z
ØPST45Z
ØPSVØ5Z
ØPSV35Z
ØPSV45Z
ØPTØØZZ
ØPT1ØZZ
ØPT2ØZZ
ØPT5ØZZ
ØPT6ØZZ
ØPT7ØZZ
ØPT8ØZZ
ØPT9ØZZ
ØPTBØZZ
ØPTCØZZ
ØPTDØZZ
ØPTFØZZ
ØPTGØZZ
ØPTHØZZ
ØPTJØZZ
ØPTKØZZ
ØPTLØZZ
ØPTRØZZ
ØPTSØZZ
ØPTTØZZ
ØPTVØZZ
ØPUØØJZ
ØPUØ3JZ
ØPUØ4JZ
ØPU1ØJZ
ØPU13JZ
ØPU14JZ
ØPU2ØJZ
ØPU23JZ
ØPU24JZ
ØPU3ØJZ
ØPU33JZ
ØPU34JZ
ØPU4ØJZ
ØPU43JZ
ØPU44JZ
ØPU5ØJZ
ØPU53JZ
ØPU54JZ
ØPU6ØJZ
ØPU63JZ
ØPU64JZ
ØPU7ØJZ
ØPU73JZ
ØPU74JZ
ØPU8ØJZ
ØPU83JZ
ØPU84JZ
ØPU9ØJZ
ØPU93JZ
ØPU94JZ
ØPUBØJZ
ØPUB3JZ
ØPUB4JZ
ØPUC*
ØPUD*
ØPUF*
ØPUG*
ØPUH*
ØPUJ*
ØPUK*
ØPUL*
ØQ5*
ØQ8*
ØQ9DØØZ
ØQ9DØZZ
ØQ9D4ØZ
ØQ9D4ZZ
ØQ9FØØZ
ØQ9FØZZ
ØQ9F4ØZ
ØQ9F4ZZ
ØQBØØZZ
ØQBØ3ZZ
ØQBØ4ZZ
ØQB1ØZZ
ØQB13ZZ
ØQB14ZZ
ØQB2ØZZ
ØQB23ZZ
ØQB24ZZ
ØQB3ØZZ
ØQB33ZZ
ØQB34ZZ
ØQB4ØZZ
ØQB43ZZ
ØQB44ZZ
ØQB5ØZZ
ØQB53ZZ
ØQB54ZZ
ØQB6ØZZ
ØQB63ZZ
ØQB64ZZ
ØQB7ØZZ
ØQB73ZZ
ØQB74ZZ
ØQB8ØZZ
ØQB83ZZ
ØQB84ZZ
ØQB9ØZZ
ØQB93ZZ
ØQB94ZZ
ØQBBØZZ
ØQBB3ZZ
ØQBB4ZZ
ØQBCØZZ
ØQBC3ZZ
ØQBC4ZZ
ØQBDØZZ
ØQBD3ZZ
ØQBD4ZZ

ØQBFØZZ
ØQBF3ZZ
ØQBF4ZZ
ØQBGØZZ
ØQBG3ZZ
ØQBG4ZZ
ØQBHØZZ
ØQBH3ZZ
ØQBH4ZZ
ØQBJØZZ
ØQBJ3ZZ
ØQBJ4ZZ
ØQBKØZZ
ØQBK3ZZ
ØQBK4ZZ
ØQBLØZZ
ØQBL3ZZ
ØQBL4ZZ
ØQBMØZZ
ØQBM3ZZ
ØQBM4ZZ
ØQBNØZ2
ØQBNØZZ
ØQBN3Z2
ØQBN3ZZ
ØQBN4Z2
ØQBN4ZZ
ØQBPØZ2
ØQBPØZZ
ØQBP3Z2
ØQBP3ZZ
ØQBP4Z2
ØQBP4ZZ
ØQBQØZZ
ØQBQ3ZZ
ØQBQ4ZZ
ØQBRØZZ
ØQBR3ZZ
ØQBR4ZZ
ØQBSØZZ
ØQBS3ZZ
ØQBS4ZZ
ØQC*
ØQDØØZZ
ØQD1ØZZ
ØQD2ØZZ
ØQD3ØZZ
ØQD4ØZZ
ØQD5ØZZ
ØQD6ØZZ
ØQD7ØZZ
ØQD8ØZZ
ØQD9ØZZ
ØQDBØZZ
ØQDCØZZ
ØQDDØZZ
ØQDFØZZ
ØQDGØZZ
ØQDHØZZ
ØQDJØZZ
ØQDKØZZ
ØQDLØZZ
ØQDMØZZ
ØQDNØZZ
ØQDPØZZ
ØQDQØZZ
ØQDRØZZ
ØQDSØZZ
ØQHØ*
ØQH1*
ØQH2*
ØQH3*
ØQH4*
ØQH5*
ØQH6Ø4Z
ØQH6Ø5Z
ØQH6Ø6Z
ØQH6ØBZ
ØQH6ØCZ
ØQH6ØDZ
ØQH634Z
ØQH635Z
ØQH636Z
ØQH63BZ
ØQH63CZ
ØQH63DZ
ØQH644Z
ØQH645Z
ØQH646Z
ØQH64BZ
ØQH64CZ
ØQH64DZ
ØQH7Ø4Z
ØQH7Ø5Z
ØQH7Ø6Z
ØQH7ØBZ
ØQH7ØCZ
ØQH7ØDZ
ØQH734Z
ØQH735Z
ØQH736Z
ØQH73BZ
ØQH73CZ
ØQH73DZ
ØQH744Z
ØQH745Z
ØQH746Z
ØQH74BZ
ØQH74CZ
ØQH74DZ
ØQH8Ø4Z
ØQH8Ø5Z
ØQH8Ø6Z
ØQH8Ø7Z
ØQH8ØBZ
ØQH8ØCZ
ØQH8ØDZ
ØQH834Z
ØQH835Z
ØQH836Z
ØQH837Z
ØQH83BZ
ØQH83CZ
ØQH83DZ
ØQH844Z
ØQH845Z
ØQH846Z
ØQH847Z
ØQH84BZ
ØQH84CZ
ØQH84DZ
ØQH9Ø4Z
ØQH9Ø5Z
ØQH9Ø6Z
ØQH9Ø7Z
ØQH9ØBZ
ØQH9ØCZ
ØQH9ØDZ
ØQH934Z
ØQH935Z
ØQH936Z
ØQH937Z
ØQH93BZ
ØQH93CZ
ØQH93DZ
ØQH944Z
ØQH945Z
ØQH946Z
ØQH947Z
ØQH94BZ
ØQH94CZ
ØQH94DZ
ØQHBØ4Z
ØQHBØ5Z
ØQHBØ6Z
ØQHBØBZ
ØQHBØCZ
ØQHBØDZ
ØQHB34Z
ØQHB35Z
ØQHB36Z
ØQHB3BZ
ØQHB3CZ
ØQHB3DZ
ØQHB44Z
ØQHB45Z
ØQHB46Z
ØQHB4BZ
ØQHB4CZ
ØQHB4DZ
ØQHCØ4Z
ØQHCØ5Z
ØQHCØ6Z
ØQHCØBZ
ØQHCØCZ
ØQHCØDZ
ØQHC34Z
ØQHC35Z
ØQHC36Z
ØQHC3BZ
ØQHC3CZ
ØQHC3DZ
ØQHC44Z
ØQHC45Z
ØQHC46Z
ØQHC4BZ
ØQHC4CZ
ØQHC4DZ
ØQHD*
ØQHF*
ØQHGØ4Z
ØQHGØ5Z
ØQHGØ6Z
ØQHGØ7Z
ØQHGØBZ
ØQHGØCZ
ØQHGØDZ
ØQHG34Z
ØQHG35Z
ØQHG36Z
ØQHG37Z
ØQHG3BZ
ØQHG3CZ
ØQHG3DZ
ØQHG44Z
ØQHG45Z
ØQHG46Z
ØQHG47Z
ØQHG4BZ
ØQHG4CZ
ØQHG4DZ
ØQHHØ4Z
ØQHHØ5Z
ØQHHØ6Z
ØQHHØ7Z
ØQHHØBZ
ØQHHØCZ
ØQHHØDZ
ØQHH34Z
ØQHH35Z
ØQHH36Z
ØQHH37Z
ØQHH3BZ
ØQHH3CZ
ØQHH3DZ
ØQHH44Z
ØQHH45Z
ØQHH46Z
ØQHH47Z
ØQHH4BZ
ØQHH4CZ
ØQHH4DZ
ØQHJØ4Z
ØQHJØ5Z
ØQHJØ6Z
ØQHJØBZ
ØQHJØCZ
ØQHJØDZ
ØQHJ34Z
ØQHJ35Z
ØQHJ36Z
ØQHJ3BZ
ØQHJ3CZ
ØQHJ3DZ
ØQHJ44Z
ØQHJ45Z
ØQHJ46Z
ØQHJ4BZ
ØQHJ4CZ
ØQHJ4DZ
ØQHKØ4Z
ØQHKØ5Z
ØQHKØ6Z
ØQHKØBZ
ØQHKØCZ
ØQHKØDZ
ØQHK34Z
ØQHK35Z
ØQHK36Z
ØQHK3BZ
ØQHK3CZ
ØQHK3DZ
ØQHK44Z
ØQHK45Z
ØQHK46Z
ØQHK4BZ
ØQHK4CZ
ØQHK4DZ
ØQHL*
ØQHM*
ØQHN*
ØQHP*
ØQHQ*
ØQHR*
ØQHS*
ØQHY*
ØQN6*
ØQN7*
ØQN8*
ØQN9*
ØQNB*
ØQNC*
ØQND*
ØQNF*
ØQNG*
ØQNH*
ØQNJ*
ØQNK*
ØQNL*
ØQNM*
ØQNN*
ØQNP*
ØQPØØ4Z
ØQPØØ5Z
ØQPØØ7Z
ØQPØØJZ
ØQPØØKZ
ØQPØ34Z
ØQPØ35Z
ØQPØ37Z
ØQPØ3JZ
ØQPØ3KZ
ØQPØ44Z
ØQPØ45Z
ØQPØ47Z
ØQPØ4JZ
ØQPØ4KZ
ØQP1Ø4Z
ØQP1Ø5Z
ØQP1Ø7Z
ØQP1ØJZ
ØQP1ØKZ
ØQP134Z
ØQP135Z
ØQP137Z
ØQP13JZ
ØQP13KZ
ØQP144Z
ØQP145Z
ØQP147Z
ØQP14JZ
ØQP14KZ
ØQP2Ø4Z
ØQP2Ø5Z
ØQP2Ø7Z
ØQP2ØJZ
ØQP2ØKZ
ØQP234Z
ØQP235Z
ØQP237Z
ØQP23JZ
ØQP23KZ
ØQP244Z
ØQP245Z
ØQP247Z
ØQP24JZ
ØQP24KZ
ØQP3Ø4Z
ØQP3Ø5Z
ØQP3Ø7Z
ØQP3ØJZ
ØQP3ØKZ
ØQP334Z
ØQP335Z
ØQP337Z
ØQP33JZ
ØQP33KZ
ØQP344Z
ØQP345Z
ØQP347Z
ØQP34JZ
ØQP34KZ
ØQP4Ø4Z
ØQP4Ø5Z
ØQP4Ø7Z
ØQP4ØJZ
ØQP4ØKZ
ØQP434Z
ØQP435Z
ØQP437Z
ØQP43JZ
ØQP43KZ
ØQP444Z
ØQP445Z
ØQP447Z
ØQP44JZ
ØQP44KZ
ØQP5Ø4Z
ØQP5Ø5Z
ØQP5Ø7Z
ØQP5ØJZ
ØQP5ØKZ
ØQP534Z
ØQP535Z
ØQP537Z
ØQP53JZ
ØQP53KZ
ØQP544Z
ØQP545Z
ØQP547Z
ØQP54JZ
ØQP54KZ
ØQP6Ø4Z
ØQP6Ø5Z
ØQP6Ø7Z
ØQP6ØJZ
ØQP6ØKZ
ØQP634Z
ØQP635Z
ØQP637Z
ØQP63JZ
ØQP63KZ
ØQP644Z
ØQP645Z
ØQP647Z
ØQP64JZ
ØQP64KZ
ØQP7Ø4Z
ØQP7Ø5Z
ØQP7Ø7Z
ØQP7ØJZ
ØQP7ØKZ
ØQP734Z
ØQP735Z
ØQP737Z
ØQP73JZ
ØQP73KZ
ØQP744Z
ØQP745Z
ØQP747Z
ØQP74JZ
ØQP74KZ
ØQP8Ø4Z
ØQP8Ø5Z
ØQP8Ø7Z
ØQP8ØJZ
ØQP8ØKZ
ØQP834Z
ØQP835Z
ØQP837Z
ØQP83JZ
ØQP83KZ
ØQP844Z
ØQP845Z
ØQP847Z
ØQP84JZ
ØQP84KZ
ØQP9Ø4Z
ØQP9Ø5Z
ØQP9Ø7Z
ØQP9ØJZ
ØQP9ØKZ
ØQP934Z
ØQP935Z
ØQP937Z
ØQP93JZ
ØQP93KZ
ØQP944Z
ØQP945Z
ØQP947Z
ØQP94JZ
ØQP94KZ
ØQPBØ4Z
ØQPBØ5Z
ØQPBØ7Z
ØQPBØJZ
ØQPBØKZ
ØQPB34Z
ØQPB35Z
ØQPB37Z
ØQPB3JZ
ØQPB3KZ
ØQPB44Z
ØQPB45Z
ØQPB47Z
ØQPB4JZ
ØQPB4KZ
ØQPCØ4Z
ØQPCØ5Z
ØQPCØ7Z
ØQPCØJZ
ØQPCØKZ
ØQPC34Z
ØQPC35Z
ØQPC37Z
ØQPC3JZ
ØQPC3KZ
ØQPC44Z
ØQPC45Z
ØQPC47Z
ØQPC4JZ
ØQPC4KZ
ØQPDØ4Z
ØQPDØ5Z
ØQPDØ7Z
ØQPDØJZ
ØQPDØKZ
ØQPD34Z
ØQPD35Z
ØQPD37Z
ØQPD3JZ
ØQPD3KZ
ØQPD44Z
ØQPD45Z
ØQPD47Z
ØQPD4JZ
ØQPD4KZ
ØQPFØ4Z
ØQPFØ5Z
ØQPFØ7Z
ØQPFØJZ
ØQPFØKZ
ØQPF34Z
ØQPF35Z
ØQPF37Z
ØQPF3JZ
ØQPF3KZ
ØQPF44Z
ØQPF45Z
ØQPF47Z
ØQPF4JZ
ØQPF4KZ
ØQPGØ4Z
ØQPGØ5Z
ØQPGØ7Z
ØQPGØJZ
ØQPGØKZ
ØQPG34Z
ØQPG35Z
ØQPG37Z
ØQPG3JZ
ØQPG3KZ
ØQPG44Z
ØQPG45Z
ØQPG47Z
ØQPG4JZ
ØQPG4KZ
ØQPHØ4Z
ØQPHØ5Z
ØQPHØ7Z
ØQPHØJZ
ØQPHØKZ
ØQPH34Z
ØQPH35Z
ØQPH37Z
ØQPH3JZ
ØQPH3KZ
ØQPH44Z
ØQPH45Z
ØQPH47Z
ØQPH4JZ
ØQPH4KZ
ØQPJØ4Z
ØQPJØ5Z
ØQPJØ7Z
ØQPJØJZ
ØQPJØKZ
ØQPJ34Z
ØQPJ35Z
ØQPJ37Z
ØQPJ3JZ
ØQPJ3KZ
ØQPJ44Z
ØQPJ45Z
ØQPJ47Z
ØQPJ4JZ
ØQPJ4KZ
ØQPKØ4Z
ØQPKØ5Z
ØQPKØ7Z
ØQPKØJZ
ØQPKØKZ
ØQPK34Z
ØQPK35Z
ØQPK37Z
ØQPK3JZ
ØQPK3KZ
ØQPK44Z
ØQPK45Z
ØQPK47Z
ØQPK4JZ
ØQPK4KZ
ØQPLØ4Z
ØQPLØ5Z
ØQPLØ7Z
ØQPLØJZ
ØQPLØKZ
ØQPL34Z
ØQPL35Z
ØQPL37Z
ØQPL3JZ
ØQPL3KZ
ØQPL44Z
ØQPL45Z
ØQPL47Z
ØQPL4JZ
ØQPL4KZ
ØQPMØ4Z
ØQPMØ5Z
ØQPMØ7Z
ØQPMØJZ
ØQPMØKZ
ØQPM34Z
ØQPM35Z
ØQPM37Z
ØQPM3JZ
ØQPM3KZ
ØQPM44Z
ØQPM45Z
ØQPM47Z
ØQPM4JZ
ØQPM4KZ
ØQPNØ4Z
ØQPNØ5Z
ØQPNØ7Z
ØQPNØJZ
ØQPNØKZ
ØQPN34Z
ØQPN35Z
ØQPN37Z
ØQPN3JZ
ØQPN3KZ
ØQPN44Z
ØQPN45Z
ØQPN47Z
ØQPN4JZ
ØQPN4KZ
ØQPPØ4Z
ØQPPØ5Z
ØQPPØ7Z
ØQPPØJZ
ØQPPØKZ
ØQPP34Z
ØQPP35Z
ØQPP37Z
ØQPP3JZ
ØQPP3KZ
ØQPP44Z
ØQPP45Z
ØQPP47Z
ØQPP4JZ
ØQPP4KZ
ØQPQØ4Z
ØQPQØ5Z
ØQPQØ7Z
ØQPQØJZ
ØQPQØKZ
ØQPQ34Z
ØQPQ35Z
ØQPQ37Z
ØQPQ3JZ
ØQPQ3KZ
ØQPQ44Z
ØQPQ45Z
ØQPQ47Z
ØQPQ4JZ
ØQPQ4KZ
ØQPRØ4Z
ØQPRØ5Z
ØQPRØ7Z
ØQPRØJZ
ØQPRØKZ
ØQPR34Z
ØQPR35Z
ØQPR37Z
ØQPR3JZ
ØQPR3KZ
ØQPR44Z
ØQPR45Z
ØQPR47Z
ØQPR4JZ
ØQPR4KZ
ØQPSØ4Z
ØQPSØ5Z
ØQPSØ7Z
ØQPSØJZ
ØQPSØKZ
ØQPS34Z
ØQPS35Z
ØQPS37Z
ØQPS3JZ
ØQPS3KZ
ØQPS44Z
ØQPS45Z
ØQPS47Z
ØQPS4JZ
ØQPS4KZ
ØQPYØMZ
ØQPY3MZ
ØQPY4MZ
ØQQ6ØZZ
ØQQ63ZZ
ØQQ64ZZ
ØQQ7ØZZ
ØQQ73ZZ
ØQQ74ZZ
ØQQ8ØZZ
ØQQ83ZZ
ØQQ84ZZ
ØQQ9ØZZ
ØQQ93ZZ
ØQQ94ZZ
ØQQBØZZ
ØQQB3ZZ
ØQQB4ZZ
ØQQCØZZ
ØQQC3ZZ
ØQQC4ZZ
ØQQDØZZ
ØQQD4ZZ
ØQQFØZZ
ØQQF4ZZ
ØQQGØZZ
ØQQG3ZZ
ØQQG4ZZ
ØQQHØZZ
ØQQH3ZZ
ØQQH4ZZ
ØQQJØZZ
ØQQJ3ZZ
ØQQJ4ZZ
ØQQKØZZ
ØQQK3ZZ
ØQQK4ZZ
ØQQLØZZ
ØQQL3ZZ
ØQQL4ZZ
ØQQMØZZ
ØQQM3ZZ
ØQQM4ZZ
ØQQNØZZ
ØQQN3ZZ
ØQQN4ZZ
ØQQPØZZ
ØQQP3ZZ
ØQQP4ZZ
ØQQQØZZ
ØQQQ3ZZ
ØQQQ4ZZ
ØQQRØZZ
ØQQR3ZZ
ØQQR4ZZ
ØQR4ØJZ
ØQR43JZ
ØQR44JZ
ØQR5ØJZ
ØQR53JZ
ØQR54JZ
ØQR6*
ØQR7*
ØQR8*
ØQR9*
ØQRB*
ØQRC*
ØQRD*
ØQRF*
ØQRG*
ØQRH*
ØQRJ*
ØQRK*
ØQRL*
ØQRM*
ØQRN*
ØQRP*
ØQSØØ3Z
ØQSØØ4Z
ØQSØØZZ
ØQSØ34Z
ØQSØ43Z
ØQSØ44Z
ØQSØ4ZZ
ØQS1Ø4Z
ØQS1ØZZ
ØQS134Z
ØQS144Z
ØQS14ZZ
ØQS2Ø4Z
ØQS2Ø5Z
ØQS2ØZZ
ØQS234Z
ØQS235Z
ØQS244Z
ØQS245Z
ØQS3Ø4Z
ØQS3Ø5Z
ØQS3ØZZ
ØQS334Z
ØQS335Z
ØQS344Z
ØQS345Z
ØQS4Ø4Z
ØQS4ØZZ
ØQS434Z
ØQS444Z
ØQS5Ø4Z
ØQS5ØZZ
ØQS534Z
ØQS544Z
ØQS6Ø4Z
ØQS6Ø5Z
ØQS6Ø6Z
ØQS6ØBZ
ØQS6ØCZ
ØQS6ØDZ
ØQS6ØZZ
ØQS634Z
ØQS635Z
ØQS636Z
ØQS63BZ
ØQS63CZ
ØQS63DZ
ØQS644Z
ØQS645Z
ØQS646Z
ØQS64BZ
ØQS64CZ
ØQS64DZ
ØQS7Ø4Z
ØQS7Ø5Z
ØQS7Ø6Z
ØQS7ØBZ
ØQS7ØCZ
ØQS7ØDZ
ØQS7ØZZ
ØQS734Z
ØQS735Z
ØQS736Z
ØQS73BZ
ØQS73CZ
ØQS73DZ
ØQS744Z
ØQS745Z
ØQS746Z
ØQS74BZ
ØQS74CZ
ØQS74DZ
ØQS8Ø4Z
ØQS8Ø5Z
ØQS8Ø6Z
ØQS8ØBZ
ØQS8ØCZ
ØQS8ØDZ
ØQS8ØZZ
ØQS834Z
ØQS835Z
ØQS836Z
ØQS83BZ
ØQS83CZ
ØQS83DZ
ØQS844Z
ØQS845Z
ØQS846Z
ØQS84BZ
ØQS84CZ
ØQS84DZ
ØQS9Ø4Z
ØQS9Ø5Z
ØQS9Ø6Z
ØQS9ØBZ
ØQS9ØCZ
ØQS9ØDZ
ØQS9ØZZ
ØQS934Z
ØQS935Z
ØQS936Z
ØQS93BZ
ØQS93CZ
ØQS93DZ
ØQS944Z
ØQS945Z
ØQS946Z
ØQS94BZ
ØQS94CZ
ØQS94DZ
ØQSBØ4Z

ØQSBØ5Z
ØQSBØ6Z
ØQSBØBZ
ØQSBØCZ
ØQSBØDZ
ØQSBØZZ
ØQSB34Z
ØQSB35Z
ØQSB36Z
ØQSB3BZ
ØQSB3CZ
ØQSB3DZ
ØQSB44Z
ØQSB45Z
ØQSB46Z
ØQSB4BZ
ØQSB4CZ
ØQSB4DZ
ØQSCØ4Z
ØQSCØ5Z
ØQSCØ6Z
ØQSCØBZ
ØQSCØCZ
ØQSCØDZ
ØQSCØZZ
ØQSC34Z
ØQSC35Z
ØQSC36Z
ØQSC3BZ
ØQSC3CZ
ØQSC3DZ
ØQSC44Z
ØQSC45Z
ØQSC46Z
ØQSC4BZ
ØQSC4CZ
ØQSC4DZ
ØQSDØ4Z
ØQSDØ5Z
ØQSDØZZ
ØQSD34Z
ØQSD35Z
ØQSD44Z
ØQSD45Z
ØQSFØ4Z
ØQSFØ5Z
ØQSFØZZ
ØQSF34Z
ØQSF35Z
ØQSF44Z
ØQSF45Z
ØQSGØ4Z
ØQSGØ5Z
ØQSGØ6Z
ØQSGØBZ
ØQSGØCZ
ØQSGØDZ
ØQSGØZZ
ØQSG34Z
ØQSG35Z
ØQSG36Z
ØQSG3BZ
ØQSG3CZ
ØQSG3DZ
ØQSG44Z
ØQSG45Z
ØQSG46Z
ØQSG4BZ
ØQSG4CZ
ØQSG4DZ
ØQSHØ4Z
ØQSHØ5Z
ØQSHØ6Z
ØQSHØBZ
ØQSHØCZ
ØQSHØDZ
ØQSHØZZ
ØQSH34Z
ØQSH35Z
ØQSH36Z
ØQSH3BZ
ØQSH3CZ
ØQSH3DZ
ØQSH44Z
ØQSH45Z
ØQSH46Z
ØQSH4BZ
ØQSH4CZ
ØQSH4DZ
ØQSJØ4Z
ØQSJØ5Z
ØQSJØ6Z
ØQSJØBZ
ØQSJØCZ
ØQSJØDZ
ØQSJØZZ
ØQSJ34Z
ØQSJ35Z
ØQSJ36Z
ØQSJ3BZ
ØQSJ3CZ
ØQSJ3DZ
ØQSJ44Z
ØQSJ45Z
ØQSJ46Z
ØQSJ4BZ
ØQSJ4CZ
ØQSJ4DZ
ØQSKØ4Z
ØQSKØ5Z
ØQSKØ6Z
ØQSKØBZ
ØQSKØCZ
ØQSKØDZ
ØQSKØZZ
ØQSK34Z
ØQSK35Z
ØQSK36Z
ØQSK3BZ
ØQSK3CZ
ØQSK3DZ
ØQSK44Z
ØQSK45Z
ØQSK46Z
ØQSK4BZ
ØQSK4CZ
ØQSK4DZ
ØQSLØ4Z
ØQSLØ5Z
ØQSLØZZ
ØQSL34Z
ØQSL35Z
ØQSL44Z
ØQSL45Z
ØQSMØ4Z
ØQSMØ5Z
ØQSMØZZ
ØQSM34Z
ØQSM35Z
ØQSM44Z
ØQSM45Z
ØQSNØ42
ØQSNØ4Z
ØQSNØ52
ØQSNØ5Z
ØQSNØZ2
ØQSNØZZ
ØQSN342
ØQSN34Z
ØQSN352
ØQSN35Z
ØQSN442
ØQSN44Z
ØQSN452
ØQSN45Z
ØQSPØ42
ØQSPØ4Z
ØQSPØ52
ØQSPØ5Z
ØQSPØZ2
ØQSPØZZ
ØQSP342
ØQSP34Z
ØQSP352
ØQSP35Z
ØQSP442
ØQSP44Z
ØQSP452
ØQSP45Z
ØQSQØ4Z
ØQSQØ5Z
ØQSQØZZ
ØQSQ34Z
ØQSQ35Z
ØQSQ44Z
ØQSQ45Z
ØQSRØ4Z
ØQSRØ5Z
ØQSRØZZ
ØQSR34Z
ØQSR35Z
ØQSR44Z
ØQSR45Z
ØQSSØ4Z
ØQSSØZZ
ØQSS34Z
ØQSS3ZZ
ØQSS44Z
ØQSS4ZZ
ØQT*
ØQUØØJZ
ØQUØ3JZ
ØQUØ4JZ
ØQU1ØJZ
ØQU13JZ
ØQU14JZ
ØQU4ØJZ
ØQU43JZ
ØQU44JZ
ØQU5ØJZ
ØQU53JZ
ØQU54JZ
ØQU6*
ØQU7*
ØQU8*
ØQU9*
ØQUB*
ØQUC*
ØQUD*
ØQUF*
ØQUG*
ØQUH*
ØQUJ*
ØQUK*
ØQUL*
ØQUM*
ØQUN*
ØQUP*
ØQWDØ4Z
ØQWDØ5Z
ØQWDØ7Z
ØQWDØJZ
ØQWDØKZ
ØQWD34Z
ØQWD35Z
ØQWD37Z
ØQWD3JZ
ØQWD3KZ
ØQWD44Z
ØQWD45Z
ØQWD47Z
ØQWD4JZ
ØQWD4KZ
ØQWFØ4Z
ØQWFØ5Z
ØQWFØ7Z
ØQWFØJZ
ØQWFØKZ
ØQWF34Z
ØQWF35Z
ØQWF37Z
ØQWF3JZ
ØQWF3KZ
ØQWF44Z
ØQWF45Z
ØQWF47Z
ØQWF4JZ
ØQWF4KZ
ØR5Ø*
ØR51*
ØR53ØZZ
ØR54*
ØR55ØZZ
ØR56*
ØR59ØZZ
ØR5A*
ØR5BØZZ
ØR5C*
ØR5D*
ØR5E*
ØR5F*
ØR5G*
ØR5H*
ØR5J*
ØR5K*
ØR5L*
ØR5M*
ØR9EØØZ
ØR9EØZZ
ØR9FØØZ
ØR9FØZZ
ØR9GØØZ
ØR9GØZZ
ØR9HØØZ
ØR9HØZZ
ØR9JØØZ
ØR9JØZZ
ØR9KØØZ
ØR9KØZZ
ØR9LØØZ
ØR9LØZZ
ØR9MØØZ
ØR9MØZZ
ØRBØØZZ
ØRBØ3ZZ
ØRBØ4ZZ
ØRB1ØZZ
ØRB13ZZ
ØRB14ZZ
ØRB3ØZZ
ØRB33ZZ
ØRB34ZZ
ØRB4ØZZ
ØRB43ZZ
ØRB44ZZ
ØRB5ØZZ
ØRB53ZZ
ØRB54ZZ
ØRB6ØZZ
ØRB63ZZ
ØRB64ZZ
ØRB9ØZZ
ØRB93ZZ
ØRB94ZZ
ØRBAØZZ
ØRBA3ZZ
ØRBA4ZZ
ØRBBØZZ
ØRBB3ZZ
ØRBB4ZZ
ØRBCØZZ
ØRBC3ZZ
ØRBC4ZZ
ØRBDØZZ
ØRBD3ZZ
ØRBD4ZZ
ØRBEØZZ
ØRBE3ZZ
ØRBE4ZZ
ØRBFØZZ
ØRBF3ZZ
ØRBF4ZZ
ØRBGØZZ
ØRBG3ZZ
ØRBG4ZZ
ØRBHØZZ
ØRBH3ZZ
ØRBH4ZZ
ØRBJØZZ
ØRBJ3ZZ
ØRBJ4ZZ
ØRBKØZZ
ØRBK3ZZ
ØRBK4ZZ
ØRBLØZZ
ØRBL3ZZ
ØRBL4ZZ
ØRBMØZZ
ØRBM3ZZ
ØRBM4ZZ
ØRCC*
ØRCD*
ØRCE*
ØRCF*
ØRCG*
ØRCH*
ØRCJ*
ØRCK*
ØRCL*
ØRCM*
ØRGØØ7Ø
ØRGØØ71
ØRGØØ7J
ØRGØØAØ
ØRGØØAJ
ØRGØØJØ
ØRGØØJ1
ØRGØØJJ
ØRGØØKØ
ØRGØØK1
ØRGØØKJ
ØRGØ37Ø
ØRGØ371
ØRGØ37J
ØRGØ3AØ
ØRGØ3AJ
ØRGØ3JØ
ØRGØ3J1
ØRGØ3JJ
ØRGØ3KØ
ØRGØ3K1
ØRGØ3KJ
ØRGØ47Ø
ØRGØ471
ØRGØ47J
ØRGØ4AØ
ØRGØ4AJ
ØRGØ4JØ
ØRGØ4J1
ØRGØ4JJ
ØRGØ4KØ
ØRGØ4K1
ØRGØ4KJ
ØRG1Ø7Ø
ØRG1Ø71
ØRG1Ø7J
ØRG1ØAØ
ØRG1ØAJ
ØRG1ØJØ
ØRG1ØJ1
ØRG1ØJJ
ØRG1ØKØ
ØRG1ØK1
ØRG1ØKJ
ØRG137Ø
ØRG1371
ØRG137J
ØRG13AØ
ØRG13AJ
ØRG13JØ
ØRG13J1
ØRG13JJ
ØRG13KØ
ØRG13K1
ØRG13KJ
ØRG147Ø
ØRG1471
ØRG147J
ØRG14AØ
ØRG14AJ
ØRG14JØ
ØRG14J1
ØRG14JJ
ØRG14KØ
ØRG14K1
ØRG14KJ
ØRG2Ø7Ø
ØRG2Ø71
ØRG2Ø7J
ØRG2ØAØ
ØRG2ØAJ
ØRG2ØJØ
ØRG2ØJ1
ØRG2ØJJ
ØRG2ØKØ
ØRG2ØK1
ØRG2ØKJ
ØRG237Ø
ØRG2371
ØRG237J
ØRG23AØ
ØRG23AJ
ØRG23JØ
ØRG23J1
ØRG23JJ
ØRG23KØ
ØRG23K1
ØRG23KJ
ØRG247Ø
ØRG2471
ØRG247J
ØRG24AØ
ØRG24AJ
ØRG24JØ
ØRG24J1
ØRG24JJ
ØRG24KØ
ØRG24K1
ØRG24KJ
ØRG4Ø7Ø
ØRG4Ø71
ØRG4Ø7J
ØRG4ØAØ
ØRG4ØAJ
ØRG4ØJØ
ØRG4ØJ1
ØRG4ØJJ
ØRG4ØKØ
ØRG4ØK1
ØRG4ØKJ
ØRG437Ø
ØRG4371
ØRG437J
ØRG43AØ
ØRG43AJ
ØRG43JØ
ØRG43J1
ØRG43JJ
ØRG43KØ
ØRG43K1
ØRG43KJ
ØRG447Ø
ØRG4471
ØRG447J
ØRG44AØ
ØRG44AJ
ØRG44JØ
ØRG44J1
ØRG44JJ
ØRG44KØ
ØRG44K1
ØRG44KJ
ØRG6Ø7Ø
ØRG6Ø71
ØRG6Ø7J
ØRG6ØAØ
ØRG6ØAJ
ØRG6ØJØ
ØRG6ØJ1
ØRG6ØJJ
ØRG6ØKØ
ØRG6ØK1
ØRG6ØKJ
ØRG637Ø
ØRG6371
ØRG637J
ØRG63AØ
ØRG63AJ
ØRG63JØ
ØRG63J1
ØRG63JJ
ØRG63KØ
ØRG63K1
ØRG63KJ
ØRG647Ø
ØRG6471
ØRG647J
ØRG64AØ
ØRG64AJ
ØRG64JØ
ØRG64J1
ØRG64JJ
ØRG64KØ
ØRG64K1
ØRG64KJ
ØRG7Ø7Ø
ØRG7Ø71
ØRG7Ø7J
ØRG7ØAØ
ØRG7ØAJ
ØRG7ØJØ
ØRG7ØJ1
ØRG7ØJJ
ØRG7ØKØ
ØRG7ØK1
ØRG7ØKJ
ØRG737Ø
ØRG7371
ØRG737J
ØRG73AØ
ØRG73AJ
ØRG73JØ
ØRG73J1
ØRG73JJ
ØRG73KØ
ØRG73K1
ØRG73KJ
ØRG747Ø
ØRG7471
ØRG747J
ØRG74AØ
ØRG74AJ
ØRG74JØ
ØRG74J1
ØRG74JJ
ØRG74KØ
ØRG74K1
ØRG74KJ
ØRG8Ø7Ø
ØRG8Ø71
ØRG8Ø7J
ØRG8ØAØ
ØRG8ØAJ
ØRG8ØJØ
ØRG8ØJ1
ØRG8ØJJ
ØRG8ØKØ
ØRG8ØK1
ØRG8ØKJ
ØRG837Ø
ØRG8371
ØRG837J
ØRG83AØ
ØRG83AJ
ØRG83JØ
ØRG83J1
ØRG83JJ
ØRG83KØ
ØRG83K1
ØRG83KJ
ØRG847Ø
ØRG8471
ØRG847J
ØRG84AØ
ØRG84AJ
ØRG84JØ
ØRG84J1
ØRG84JJ
ØRG84KØ
ØRG84K1
ØRG84KJ
ØRGAØ7Ø
ØRGAØ71
ØRGAØ7J
ØRGAØAØ
ØRGAØAJ
ØRGAØJØ
ØRGAØJ1
ØRGAØJJ
ØRGAØKØ
ØRGAØK1
ØRGAØKJ
ØRGA37Ø
ØRGA371
ØRGA37J
ØRGA3AØ
ØRGA3AJ
ØRGA3JØ
ØRGA3J1
ØRGA3JJ
ØRGA3KØ
ØRGA3K1
ØRGA3KJ
ØRGA47Ø
ØRGA471
ØRGA47J
ØRGA4AØ
ØRGA4AJ
ØRGA4JØ
ØRGA4J1
ØRGA4JJ
ØRGA4KØ
ØRGA4K1
ØRGA4KJ
ØRGCØ4Z
ØRGCØ7Z
ØRGCØJZ
ØRGCØKZ
ØRGC34Z
ØRGC37Z
ØRGC3JZ
ØRGC3KZ
ØRGC44Z
ØRGC47Z
ØRGC4JZ
ØRGC4KZ
ØRGDØ4Z
ØRGDØ7Z
ØRGDØJZ
ØRGDØKZ
ØRGD34Z
ØRGD37Z
ØRGD3JZ
ØRGD3KZ
ØRGD44Z
ØRGD47Z
ØRGD4JZ
ØRGD4KZ
ØRGLØ3Z
ØRGLØ4Z
ØRGLØ5Z
ØRGLØ7Z
ØRGLØJZ
ØRGLØKZ
ØRGL33Z
ØRGL34Z
ØRGL35Z
ØRGL37Z
ØRGL3JZ
ØRGL3KZ
ØRGL43Z
ØRGL44Z
ØRGL45Z
ØRGL47Z
ØRGL4JZ
ØRGL4KZ
ØRGMØ3Z
ØRGMØ4Z
ØRGMØ5Z
ØRGMØ7Z
ØRGMØJZ
ØRGMØKZ
ØRGM33Z
ØRGM34Z
ØRGM35Z
ØRGM37Z
ØRGM3JZ
ØRGM3KZ
ØRGM43Z
ØRGM44Z
ØRGM45Z
ØRGM47Z
ØRGM4JZ
ØRGM4KZ
ØRHØØBZ
ØRHØØCZ
ØRHØØDZ
ØRHØ3BZ
ØRHØ3CZ
ØRHØ3DZ
ØRHØ4BZ
ØRHØ4CZ
ØRHØ4DZ
ØRH1ØBZ
ØRH1ØCZ
ØRH1ØDZ
ØRH13BZ
ØRH13CZ
ØRH13DZ
ØRH14BZ
ØRH14CZ
ØRH14DZ
ØRH4ØBZ
ØRH4ØCZ
ØRH4ØDZ
ØRH43BZ
ØRH43CZ
ØRH43DZ
ØRH44BZ
ØRH44CZ
ØRH44DZ
ØRH6ØBZ
ØRH6ØCZ
ØRH6ØDZ
ØRH63BZ
ØRH63CZ
ØRH63DZ
ØRH64BZ
ØRH64CZ
ØRH64DZ
ØRHAØBZ
ØRHAØCZ
ØRHAØDZ
ØRHA3BZ
ØRHA3CZ
ØRHA3DZ
ØRHA4BZ
ØRHA4CZ
ØRHA4DZ
ØRHEØ4Z
ØRHE34Z
ØRHE44Z
ØRHFØ4Z
ØRHF34Z
ØRHF44Z
ØRHGØ4Z
ØRHG34Z
ØRHG44Z
ØRHHØ4Z
ØRHH34Z
ØRHH44Z
ØRHJØ4Z
ØRHJ34Z
ØRHJ44Z
ØRHKØ4Z
ØRHK34Z
ØRHK44Z
ØRHLØ4Z
ØRHLØ5Z
ØRHL34Z
ØRHL35Z
ØRHL44Z
ØRHL45Z
ØRHMØ4Z
ØRHMØ5Z
ØRHM34Z
ØRHM35Z
ØRHM44Z
ØRHM45Z
ØRJØ4ZZ
ØRJ14ZZ
ØRJ34ZZ
ØRJ44ZZ
ØRJ54ZZ
ØRJ64ZZ
ØRJ94ZZ
ØRJA4ZZ
ØRJB4ZZ
ØRJCØZZ
ØRJC4ZZ
ØRJDØZZ
ØRJD4ZZ
ØRJEØZZ
ØRJE4ZZ
ØRJFØZZ
ØRJF4ZZ
ØRJGØZZ
ØRJG4ZZ
ØRJHØZZ
ØRJH4ZZ
ØRJJØZZ
ØRJJ4ZZ
ØRJKØZZ
ØRJK4ZZ
ØRJLØZZ
ØRJL4ZZ
ØRJMØZZ
ØRJM4ZZ
ØRJN4ZZ
ØRJP4ZZ
ØRJQ4ZZ
ØRJR4ZZ
ØRJS4ZZ
ØRJT4ZZ
ØRJU4ZZ
ØRJV4ZZ
ØRJW4ZZ
ØRJX4ZZ
ØRNØØZZ
ØRNØ3ZZ
ØRNØ4ZZ
ØRN1ØZZ
ØRN13ZZ
ØRN14ZZ
ØRN3ØZZ
ØRN33ZZ
ØRN34ZZ
ØRN4ØZZ
ØRN43ZZ
ØRN44ZZ
ØRN5ØZZ
ØRN53ZZ
ØRN54ZZ
ØRN6ØZZ
ØRN63ZZ
ØRN64ZZ
ØRN9ØZZ
ØRN93ZZ
ØRN94ZZ
ØRNAØZZ
ØRNA3ZZ
ØRNA4ZZ
ØRNBØZZ
ØRNB3ZZ
ØRNB4ZZ
ØRNCØZZ
ØRNC3ZZ
ØRNC4ZZ
ØRNDØZZ
ØRND3ZZ
ØRND4ZZ
ØRNEØZZ
ØRNE3ZZ
ØRNE4ZZ
ØRNFØZZ
ØRNF3ZZ
ØRNF4ZZ
ØRNGØZZ
ØRNG3ZZ
ØRNG4ZZ
ØRNHØZZ
ØRNH3ZZ
ØRNH4ZZ
ØRNJØZZ
ØRNJ3ZZ
ØRNJ4ZZ
ØRNKØZZ
ØRNK3ZZ
ØRNK4ZZ
ØRNLØZZ
ØRNL3ZZ
ØRNL4ZZ
ØRNMØZZ
ØRNM3ZZ
ØRNM4ZZ
ØRPØØJZ
ØRPØ3JZ
ØRPØ4JZ
ØRP1ØJZ
ØRP13JZ
ØRP14JZ
ØRP3ØJZ
ØRP33JZ
ØRP34JZ
ØRP4ØJZ

ØRP43JZ
ØRP44JZ
ØRP5ØJZ
ØRP53JZ
ØRP54JZ
ØRP6ØJZ
ØRP63JZ
ØRP64JZ
ØRP9ØJZ
ØRP93JZ
ØRP94JZ
ØRPAØJZ
ØRPA3JZ
ØRPA4JZ
ØRPBØJZ
ØRPB3JZ
ØRPB4JZ
ØRPCØ4Z
ØRPC34Z
ØRPC44Z
ØRPCX4Z
ØRPDØ4Z
ØRPD34Z
ØRPD44Z
ØRPDX4Z
ØRPEØØZ
ØRPEØ3Z
ØRPEØ4Z
ØRPEØ7Z
ØRPEØJZ
ØRPEØKZ
ØRPE34Z
ØRPE37Z
ØRPE3JZ
ØRPE3KZ
ØRPE4ØZ
ØRPE43Z
ØRPE44Z
ØRPE47Z
ØRPE4JZ
ØRPE4KZ
ØRPFØØZ
ØRPFØ3Z
ØRPFØ4Z
ØRPFØ7Z
ØRPFØJZ
ØRPFØKZ
ØRPF34Z
ØRPF37Z
ØRPF3JZ
ØRPF3KZ
ØRPF4ØZ
ØRPF43Z
ØRPF44Z
ØRPF47Z
ØRPF4JZ
ØRPF4KZ
ØRPGØØZ
ØRPGØ3Z
ØRPGØ4Z
ØRPGØ7Z
ØRPGØJZ
ØRPGØKZ
ØRPG34Z
ØRPG37Z
ØRPG3JZ
ØRPG3KZ
ØRPG4ØZ
ØRPG43Z
ØRPG44Z
ØRPG47Z
ØRPG4JZ
ØRPG4KZ
ØRPHØØZ
ØRPHØ3Z
ØRPHØ4Z
ØRPHØ7Z
ØRPHØJZ
ØRPHØKZ
ØRPH34Z
ØRPH37Z
ØRPH3JZ
ØRPH3KZ
ØRPH4ØZ
ØRPH43Z
ØRPH44Z
ØRPH47Z
ØRPH4JZ
ØRPH4KZ
ØRPJØØZ
ØRPJØ3Z
ØRPJØ4Z
ØRPJØ7Z
ØRPJØJ6
ØRPJØJ7
ØRPJØJZ
ØRPJØKZ
ØRPJ34Z
ØRPJ37Z
ØRPJ3J6
ØRPJ3J7
ØRPJ3JZ
ØRPJ3KZ
ØRPJ4ØZ
ØRPJ43Z
ØRPJ44Z
ØRPJ47Z
ØRPJ4J6
ØRPJ4J7
ØRPJ4JZ
ØRPJ4KZ
ØRPKØØZ
ØRPKØ3Z
ØRPKØ4Z
ØRPKØ7Z
ØRPKØJ6
ØRPKØJ7
ØRPKØJZ
ØRPKØKZ
ØRPK34Z
ØRPK37Z
ØRPK3J6
ØRPK3J7
ØRPK3JZ
ØRPK3KZ
ØRPK4ØZ
ØRPK43Z
ØRPK44Z
ØRPK47Z
ØRPK4J6
ØRPK4J7
ØRPK4JZ
ØRPK4KZ
ØRPLØØZ
ØRPLØ3Z
ØRPLØ4Z
ØRPLØ5Z
ØRPLØ7Z
ØRPLØJZ
ØRPLØKZ
ØRPL34Z
ØRPL35Z
ØRPL37Z
ØRPL3JZ
ØRPL3KZ
ØRPL4ØZ
ØRPL43Z
ØRPL44Z
ØRPL45Z
ØRPL47Z
ØRPL4JZ
ØRPL4KZ
ØRPMØØZ
ØRPMØ3Z
ØRPMØ4Z
ØRPMØ5Z
ØRPMØ7Z
ØRPMØJZ
ØRPMØKZ
ØRPM34Z
ØRPM35Z
ØRPM37Z
ØRPM3JZ
ØRPM3KZ
ØRPM4ØZ
ØRPM43Z
ØRPM44Z
ØRPM45Z
ØRPM47Z
ØRPM4JZ
ØRPM4KZ
ØRQ3ØZZ
ØRQ9ØZZ
ØRQBØZZ
ØRQCØZZ
ØRQC3ZZ
ØRQC4ZZ
ØRQDØZZ
ØRQD3ZZ
ØRQD4ZZ
ØRQEØZZ
ØRQE3ZZ
ØRQE4ZZ
ØRQFØZZ
ØRQF3ZZ
ØRQF4ZZ
ØRQGØZZ
ØRQG3ZZ
ØRQG4ZZ
ØRQHØZZ
ØRQH3ZZ
ØRQH4ZZ
ØRQJØZZ
ØRQJ3ZZ
ØRQJ4ZZ
ØRQKØZZ
ØRQK3ZZ
ØRQK4ZZ
ØRQLØZZ
ØRQL3ZZ
ØRQL4ZZ
ØRQMØZZ
ØRQM3ZZ
ØRQM4ZZ
ØRR3ØJZ
ØRR5ØJZ
ØRR9ØJZ
ØRRBØJZ
ØRRC*
ØRRD*
ØRRE*
ØRRF*
ØRRG*
ØRRH*
ØRRJ*
ØRRK*
ØRRL*
ØRRM*
ØRRN*
ØRRP*
ØRSØØ4Z
ØRSØØZZ
ØRS1Ø4Z
ØRS1ØZZ
ØRS4Ø4Z
ØRS4ØZZ
ØRS6Ø4Z
ØRS6ØZZ
ØRSAØ4Z
ØRSAØZZ
ØRSCØ4Z
ØRSCØZZ
ØRSDØ4Z
ØRSDØZZ
ØRSEØ4Z
ØRSEØZZ
ØRSFØ4Z
ØRSFØZZ
ØRSGØ4Z
ØRSGØZZ
ØRSHØ4Z
ØRSHØZZ
ØRSJØ4Z
ØRSJØZZ
ØRSKØ4Z
ØRSKØZZ
ØRSLØ4Z
ØRSLØ5Z
ØRSLØZZ
ØRSMØ4Z
ØRSMØ5Z
ØRSMØZZ
ØRT3ØZZ
ØRT4ØZZ
ØRT5ØZZ
ØRT9ØZZ
ØRTBØZZ
ØRTCØZZ
ØRTDØZZ
ØRTEØZZ
ØRTFØZZ
ØRTGØZZ
ØRTHØZZ
ØRTJØZZ
ØRTKØZZ
ØRTLØZZ
ØRTMØZZ
ØRUØØJZ
ØRUØ3JZ
ØRUØ4JZ
ØRU1ØJZ
ØRU13JZ
ØRU14JZ
ØRU3*
ØRU4ØJZ
ØRU43JZ
ØRU44JZ
ØRU5ØJZ
ØRU53JZ
ØRU54JZ
ØRU6ØJZ
ØRU63JZ
ØRU64JZ
ØRU9*
ØRUAØJZ
ØRUA3JZ
ØRUA4JZ
ØRUB*
ØRUC*
ØRUD*
ØRUE*
ØRUF*
ØRUG*
ØRUH*
ØRUJ*
ØRUK*
ØRUL*
ØRUM*
ØRWØØ4Z
ØRWØØJZ
ØRWØ34Z
ØRWØ3JZ
ØRWØ44Z
ØRWØ4JZ
ØRW1Ø4Z
ØRW1ØJZ
ØRW134Z
ØRW13JZ
ØRW144Z
ØRW14JZ
ØRW3ØJZ
ØRW33JZ
ØRW34JZ
ØRW4Ø4Z
ØRW4ØJZ
ØRW434Z
ØRW43JZ
ØRW444Z
ØRW44JZ
ØRW5ØJZ
ØRW53JZ
ØRW54JZ
ØRW6Ø4Z
ØRW6ØJZ
ØRW634Z
ØRW63JZ
ØRW644Z
ØRW64JZ
ØRW9ØJZ
ØRW93JZ
ØRW94JZ
ØRWAØ4Z
ØRWAØJZ
ØRWA34Z
ØRWA3JZ
ØRWA44Z
ØRWA4JZ
ØRWBØJZ
ØRWB3JZ
ØRWB4JZ
ØRWEØØZ
ØRWEØ3Z
ØRWEØ4Z
ØRWEØ7Z
ØRWEØ8Z
ØRWEØJZ
ØRWEØKZ
ØRWE3ØZ
ØRWE33Z
ØRWE34Z
ØRWE37Z
ØRWE38Z
ØRWE3JZ
ØRWE3KZ
ØRWE4ØZ
ØRWE43Z
ØRWE44Z
ØRWE47Z
ØRWE48Z
ØRWE4JZ
ØRWE4KZ
ØRWFØØZ
ØRWFØ3Z
ØRWFØ4Z
ØRWFØ7Z
ØRWFØ8Z
ØRWFØJZ
ØRWFØKZ
ØRWF3ØZ
ØRWF33Z
ØRWF34Z
ØRWF37Z
ØRWF38Z
ØRWF3JZ
ØRWF3KZ
ØRWF4ØZ
ØRWF43Z
ØRWF44Z
ØRWF47Z
ØRWF48Z
ØRWF4JZ
ØRWF4KZ
ØRWGØØZ
ØRWGØ3Z
ØRWGØ4Z
ØRWGØ7Z
ØRWGØ8Z
ØRWGØJZ
ØRWGØKZ
ØRWG3ØZ
ØRWG33Z
ØRWG34Z
ØRWG37Z
ØRWG38Z
ØRWG3JZ
ØRWG3KZ
ØRWG4ØZ
ØRWG43Z
ØRWG44Z
ØRWG47Z
ØRWG48Z
ØRWG4JZ
ØRWG4KZ
ØRWHØØZ
ØRWHØ3Z
ØRWHØ4Z
ØRWHØ7Z
ØRWHØ8Z
ØRWHØJZ
ØRWHØKZ
ØRWH3ØZ
ØRWH33Z
ØRWH34Z
ØRWH37Z
ØRWH38Z
ØRWH3JZ
ØRWH3KZ
ØRWH4ØZ
ØRWH43Z
ØRWH44Z
ØRWH47Z
ØRWH48Z
ØRWH4JZ
ØRWH4KZ
ØRWJØØZ
ØRWJØ3Z
ØRWJØ4Z
ØRWJØ7Z
ØRWJØ8Z
ØRWJØJ6
ØRWJØJ7
ØRWJØJZ
ØRWJØKZ
ØRWJ3ØZ
ØRWJ33Z
ØRWJ34Z
ØRWJ37Z
ØRWJ38Z
ØRWJ3J6
ØRWJ3J7
ØRWJ3JZ
ØRWJ3KZ
ØRWJ4ØZ
ØRWJ43Z
ØRWJ44Z
ØRWJ47Z
ØRWJ48Z
ØRWJ4J6
ØRWJ4J7
ØRWJ4JZ
ØRWJ4KZ
ØRWKØØZ
ØRWKØ3Z
ØRWKØ4Z
ØRWKØ7Z
ØRWKØ8Z
ØRWKØJ6
ØRWKØJ7
ØRWKØJZ
ØRWKØKZ
ØRWK3ØZ
ØRWK33Z
ØRWK34Z
ØRWK37Z
ØRWK38Z
ØRWK3J6
ØRWK3J7
ØRWK3JZ
ØRWK3KZ
ØRWK4ØZ
ØRWK43Z
ØRWK44Z
ØRWK47Z
ØRWK48Z
ØRWK4J6
ØRWK4J7
ØRWK4JZ
ØRWK4KZ
ØRWLØØZ
ØRWLØ3Z
ØRWLØ4Z
ØRWLØ5Z
ØRWLØ7Z
ØRWLØ8Z
ØRWLØJZ
ØRWLØKZ
ØRWL3ØZ
ØRWL33Z
ØRWL34Z
ØRWL35Z
ØRWL37Z
ØRWL38Z
ØRWL3JZ
ØRWL3KZ
ØRWL4ØZ
ØRWL43Z
ØRWL44Z
ØRWL45Z
ØRWL47Z
ØRWL48Z
ØRWL4JZ
ØRWL4KZ
ØRWMØØZ
ØRWMØ3Z
ØRWMØ4Z
ØRWMØ5Z
ØRWMØ7Z
ØRWMØ8Z
ØRWMØJZ
ØRWMØKZ
ØRWM3ØZ
ØRWM33Z
ØRWM34Z
ØRWM35Z
ØRWM37Z
ØRWM38Z
ØRWM3JZ
ØRWM3KZ
ØRWM4ØZ
ØRWM43Z
ØRWM44Z
ØRWM45Z
ØRWM47Z
ØRWM48Z
ØRWM4JZ
ØRWM4KZ
ØRWNØJZ
ØRWN3JZ
ØRWN4JZ
ØRWPØJZ
ØRWP3JZ
ØRWP4JZ
ØRWQØJZ
ØRWQ3JZ
ØRWQ4JZ
ØRWRØJZ
ØRWR3JZ
ØRWR4JZ
ØRWSØJZ
ØRWS3JZ
ØRWS4JZ
ØRWTØJZ
ØRWT3JZ
ØRWT4JZ
ØRWUØJZ
ØRWU3JZ
ØRWU4JZ
ØRWVØJZ
ØRWV3JZ
ØRWV4JZ
ØRWWØJZ
ØRWW3JZ
ØRWW4JZ
ØRWXØJZ
ØRWX3JZ
ØRWX4JZ
ØS5*
ØS99ØØZ
ØS99ØZZ
ØS9BØØZ
ØS9BØZZ
ØS9CØØZ
ØS9CØZZ
ØS9DØØZ
ØS9DØZZ
ØS9FØØZ
ØS9FØZZ
ØS9GØØZ
ØS9GØZZ
ØS9HØØZ
ØS9HØZZ
ØS9JØØZ
ØS9JØZZ
ØS9KØØZ
ØS9KØZZ
ØS9LØØZ
ØS9LØZZ
ØS9MØØZ
ØS9MØZZ
ØS9NØØZ
ØS9NØZZ
ØS9PØØZ
ØS9PØZZ
ØS9QØØZ
ØS9QØZZ
ØSBØØZZ
ØSBØ3ZZ
ØSBØ4ZZ
ØSB2ØZZ
ØSB23ZZ
ØSB24ZZ
ØSB3ØZZ
ØSB33ZZ
ØSB34ZZ
ØSB4ØZZ
ØSB43ZZ
ØSB44ZZ
ØSB5ØZZ
ØSB53ZZ
ØSB54ZZ
ØSB6ØZZ
ØSB63ZZ
ØSB64ZZ
ØSB7ØZZ
ØSB73ZZ
ØSB74ZZ
ØSB8ØZZ
ØSB83ZZ
ØSB84ZZ
ØSB9ØZZ
ØSB93ZZ
ØSB94ZZ
ØSBBØZZ
ØSBB3ZZ
ØSBB4ZZ
ØSBCØZZ
ØSBC3ZZ
ØSBC4ZZ
ØSBDØZZ
ØSBD3ZZ
ØSBD4ZZ
ØSBFØZZ
ØSBF3ZZ
ØSBF4ZZ
ØSBGØZZ
ØSBG3ZZ
ØSBG4ZZ
ØSBHØZZ
ØSBH3ZZ
ØSBH4ZZ
ØSBJØZZ
ØSBJ3ZZ
ØSBJ4ZZ
ØSBKØZZ
ØSBK3ZZ
ØSBK4ZZ
ØSBLØZZ
ØSBL3ZZ
ØSBL4ZZ
ØSBMØZZ
ØSBM3ZZ
ØSBM4ZZ
ØSBNØZZ
ØSBN3ZZ
ØSBN4ZZ
ØSBPØZZ
ØSBP3ZZ
ØSBP4ZZ
ØSBQØZZ
ØSBQ3ZZ
ØSBQ4ZZ
ØSC9*
ØSCB*
ØSCC*
ØSCD*
ØSCF*
ØSCG*
ØSCH*
ØSCJ*
ØSCK*
ØSCL*
ØSCM*
ØSCN*
ØSCP*
ØSCQ*
ØSGØ*
ØSG1*
ØSG3*
ØSG5*
ØSG6*
ØSG7*
ØSG8*
ØSG9*
ØSGB*
ØSGC*
ØSGD*
ØSGF*
ØSGG*
ØSGH*
ØSGJ*
ØSGK*
ØSGL*
ØSGM*
ØSGN*
ØSHØØBZ
ØSHØØCZ
ØSHØØDZ
ØSHØ3BZ
ØSHØ3CZ
ØSHØ3DZ
ØSHØ4BZ
ØSHØ4CZ
ØSHØ4DZ
ØSH3ØBZ
ØSH3ØCZ
ØSH3ØDZ
ØSH33BZ
ØSH33CZ
ØSH33DZ
ØSH34BZ
ØSH34CZ
ØSH34DZ
ØSH9Ø4Z
ØSH9Ø5Z
ØSH934Z
ØSH935Z
ØSH944Z
ØSH945Z
ØSHBØ4Z
ØSHBØ5Z
ØSHB34Z
ØSHB35Z
ØSHB44Z
ØSHB45Z
ØSHCØ4Z
ØSHCØ5Z
ØSHC34Z
ØSHC35Z
ØSHC44Z
ØSHC45Z
ØSHDØ4Z
ØSHDØ5Z
ØSHD34Z
ØSHD35Z
ØSHD44Z
ØSHD45Z
ØSHFØ4Z
ØSHFØ5Z
ØSHF34Z
ØSHF35Z
ØSHF44Z
ØSHF45Z
ØSHGØ4Z
ØSHGØ5Z
ØSHG34Z
ØSHG35Z
ØSHG44Z
ØSHG45Z
ØSHHØ4Z
ØSHHØ5Z
ØSHH34Z
ØSHH35Z
ØSHH44Z
ØSHH45Z
ØSHJØ4Z
ØSHJØ5Z
ØSHJ34Z
ØSHJ35Z
ØSHJ44Z
ØSHJ45Z
ØSHKØ4Z
ØSHKØ5Z
ØSHK34Z
ØSHK35Z
ØSHK44Z
ØSHK45Z
ØSHLØ4Z
ØSHLØ5Z
ØSHL34Z
ØSHL35Z
ØSHL44Z
ØSHL45Z
ØSHMØ4Z
ØSHMØ5Z
ØSHM34Z
ØSHM35Z
ØSHM44Z
ØSHM45Z
ØSHNØ4Z
ØSHNØ5Z
ØSHN34Z
ØSHN35Z
ØSHN44Z
ØSHN45Z
ØSHPØ4Z
ØSHPØ5Z
ØSHP34Z
ØSHP35Z
ØSHP44Z
ØSHP45Z
ØSHQØ4Z
ØSHQØ5Z
ØSHQ34Z
ØSHQ35Z
ØSHQ44Z
ØSHQ45Z
ØSJØ4ZZ
ØSJ34ZZ
ØSJ54ZZ
ØSJ64ZZ
ØSJ74ZZ
ØSJ84ZZ
ØSJ9ØZZ
ØSJ94ZZ
ØSJBØZZ
ØSJB4ZZ
ØSJCØZZ
ØSJC4ZZ
ØSJDØZZ
ØSJD4ZZ
ØSJFØZZ
ØSJF4ZZ
ØSJGØZZ
ØSJG4ZZ
ØSJHØZZ
ØSJH4ZZ
ØSJJØZZ
ØSJJ4ZZ
ØSJKØZZ
ØSJK4ZZ
ØSJLØZZ
ØSJL4ZZ
ØSJMØZZ
ØSJM4ZZ
ØSJNØZZ
ØSJN4ZZ
ØSJPØZZ
ØSJP4ZZ
ØSJQØZZ
ØSJQ4ZZ
ØSNØØZZ
ØSNØ3ZZ
ØSNØ4ZZ
ØSN2ØZZ
ØSN23ZZ
ØSN24ZZ
ØSN3ØZZ
ØSN33ZZ
ØSN34ZZ
ØSN4ØZZ
ØSN43ZZ
ØSN44ZZ
ØSN5ØZZ
ØSN53ZZ
ØSN54ZZ
ØSN6ØZZ
ØSN63ZZ
ØSN64ZZ
ØSN7ØZZ
ØSN73ZZ
ØSN74ZZ
ØSN8ØZZ
ØSN83ZZ
ØSN84ZZ
ØSN9ØZZ
ØSN93ZZ
ØSN94ZZ
ØSNBØZZ
ØSNB3ZZ
ØSNB4ZZ
ØSNCØZZ
ØSNC3ZZ
ØSNC4ZZ
ØSNDØZZ
ØSND3ZZ

ØSND4ZZ
ØSNFØZZ
ØSNF3ZZ
ØSNF4ZZ
ØSNGØZZ
ØSNG3ZZ
ØSNG4ZZ
ØSNHØZZ
ØSNH3ZZ
ØSNH4ZZ
ØSNJØZZ
ØSNJ3ZZ
ØSNJ4ZZ
ØSNKØZZ
ØSNK3ZZ
ØSNK4ZZ
ØSNLØZZ
ØSNL3ZZ
ØSNL4ZZ
ØSNMØZZ
ØSNM3ZZ
ØSNM4ZZ
ØSNNØZZ
ØSNN3ZZ
ØSNN4ZZ
ØSNPØZZ
ØSNP3ZZ
ØSNP4ZZ
ØSNQØZZ
ØSNQ3ZZ
ØSNQ4ZZ
ØSPØØJZ
ØSPØ3JZ
ØSPØ4JZ
ØSP2ØJZ
ØSP23JZ
ØSP24JZ
ØSP3ØJZ
ØSP33JZ
ØSP34JZ
ØSP4ØJZ
ØSP43JZ
ØSP44JZ
ØSP5ØJZ
ØSP53JZ
ØSP54JZ
ØSP6ØJZ
ØSP63JZ
ØSP64JZ
ØSP7ØJZ
ØSP73JZ
ØSP74JZ
ØSP8ØJZ
ØSP83JZ
ØSP84JZ
ØSP9ØØZ
ØSP9Ø3Z
ØSP9Ø4Z
ØSP9Ø5Z
ØSP9Ø7Z
ØSP9Ø9Z
ØSP9ØBZ
ØSP9ØJZ
ØSP9ØKZ
ØSP934Z
ØSP935Z
ØSP937Z
ØSP93JZ
ØSP93KZ
ØSP94ØZ
ØSP943Z
ØSP944Z
ØSP945Z
ØSP947Z
ØSP94JZ
ØSP94KZ
ØSPAØJZ
ØSPA3JZ
ØSPA4JZ
ØSPBØØZ
ØSPBØ3Z
ØSPBØ4Z
ØSPBØ5Z
ØSPBØ7Z
ØSPBØ9Z
ØSPBØBZ
ØSPBØJZ
ØSPBØKZ
ØSPB34Z
ØSPB35Z
ØSPB37Z
ØSPB3JZ
ØSPB3KZ
ØSPB4ØZ
ØSPB43Z
ØSPB44Z
ØSPB45Z
ØSPB47Z
ØSPB4JZ
ØSPB4KZ
ØSPCØØZ
ØSPCØ3Z
ØSPCØ4Z
ØSPCØ5Z
ØSPCØ7Z
ØSPCØ9Z
ØSPCØJC
ØSPCØJZ
ØSPCØKZ
ØSPCØLZ
ØSPCØMZ
ØSPCØNZ
ØSPC34Z
ØSPC35Z
ØSPC37Z
ØSPC3JC
ØSPC3JZ
ØSPC3KZ
ØSPC3LZ
ØSPC3MZ
ØSPC3NZ
ØSPC4ØZ
ØSPC43Z
ØSPC44Z
ØSPC45Z
ØSPC47Z
ØSPC4JC
ØSPC4JZ
ØSPC4KZ
ØSPC4LZ
ØSPC4MZ
ØSPC4NZ
ØSPDØØZ
ØSPDØ3Z
ØSPDØ4Z
ØSPDØ5Z
ØSPDØ7Z
ØSPDØ9Z
ØSPDØJC
ØSPDØJZ
ØSPDØKZ
ØSPDØLZ
ØSPDØMZ
ØSPDØNZ
ØSPD34Z
ØSPD35Z
ØSPD37Z
ØSPD3JC
ØSPD3JZ
ØSPD3KZ
ØSPD3LZ
ØSPD3MZ
ØSPD3NZ
ØSPD4ØZ
ØSPD43Z
ØSPD44Z
ØSPD45Z
ØSPD47Z
ØSPD4JC
ØSPD4JZ
ØSPD4KZ
ØSPD4LZ
ØSPD4MZ
ØSPD4NZ
ØSPEØJZ
ØSPE3JZ
ØSPE4JZ
ØSPFØØZ
ØSPFØ3Z
ØSPFØ4Z
ØSPFØ5Z
ØSPFØ7Z
ØSPFØJZ
ØSPFØKZ
ØSPF34Z
ØSPF35Z
ØSPF37Z
ØSPF3JZ
ØSPF3KZ
ØSPF4ØZ
ØSPF43Z
ØSPF44Z
ØSPF45Z
ØSPF47Z
ØSPF4JZ
ØSPF4KZ
ØSPGØØZ
ØSPGØ3Z
ØSPGØ4Z
ØSPGØ5Z
ØSPGØ7Z
ØSPGØJZ
ØSPGØKZ
ØSPG34Z
ØSPG35Z
ØSPG37Z
ØSPG3JZ
ØSPG3KZ
ØSPG4ØZ
ØSPG43Z
ØSPG44Z
ØSPG45Z
ØSPG47Z
ØSPG4JZ
ØSPG4KZ
ØSPHØØZ
ØSPHØ3Z
ØSPHØ4Z
ØSPHØ5Z
ØSPHØ7Z
ØSPHØJZ
ØSPHØKZ
ØSPH34Z
ØSPH35Z
ØSPH37Z
ØSPH3JZ
ØSPH3KZ
ØSPH4ØZ
ØSPH43Z
ØSPH44Z
ØSPH45Z
ØSPH47Z
ØSPH4JZ
ØSPH4KZ
ØSPJØØZ
ØSPJØ3Z
ØSPJØ4Z
ØSPJØ5Z
ØSPJØ7Z
ØSPJØJZ
ØSPJØKZ
ØSPJ34Z
ØSPJ35Z
ØSPJ37Z
ØSPJ3JZ
ØSPJ3KZ
ØSPJ4ØZ
ØSPJ43Z
ØSPJ44Z
ØSPJ45Z
ØSPJ47Z
ØSPJ4JZ
ØSPJ4KZ
ØSPKØØZ
ØSPKØ3Z
ØSPKØ4Z
ØSPKØ5Z
ØSPKØ7Z
ØSPKØJZ
ØSPKØKZ
ØSPK34Z
ØSPK35Z
ØSPK37Z
ØSPK3JZ
ØSPK3KZ
ØSPK4ØZ
ØSPK43Z
ØSPK44Z
ØSPK45Z
ØSPK47Z
ØSPK4JZ
ØSPK4KZ
ØSPLØØZ
ØSPLØ3Z
ØSPLØ4Z
ØSPLØ5Z
ØSPLØ7Z
ØSPLØJZ
ØSPLØKZ
ØSPL34Z
ØSPL35Z
ØSPL37Z
ØSPL3JZ
ØSPL3KZ
ØSPL4ØZ
ØSPL43Z
ØSPL44Z
ØSPL45Z
ØSPL47Z
ØSPL4JZ
ØSPL4KZ
ØSPMØØZ
ØSPMØ3Z
ØSPMØ4Z
ØSPMØ5Z
ØSPMØ7Z
ØSPMØJZ
ØSPMØKZ
ØSPM34Z
ØSPM35Z
ØSPM37Z
ØSPM3JZ
ØSPM3KZ
ØSPM4ØZ
ØSPM43Z
ØSPM44Z
ØSPM45Z
ØSPM47Z
ØSPM4JZ
ØSPM4KZ
ØSPNØØZ
ØSPNØ3Z
ØSPNØ4Z
ØSPNØ5Z
ØSPNØ7Z
ØSPNØJZ
ØSPNØKZ
ØSPN34Z
ØSPN35Z
ØSPN37Z
ØSPN3JZ
ØSPN3KZ
ØSPN4ØZ
ØSPN43Z
ØSPN44Z
ØSPN45Z
ØSPN47Z
ØSPN4JZ
ØSPN4KZ
ØSPPØØZ
ØSPPØ3Z
ØSPPØ4Z
ØSPPØ5Z
ØSPPØ7Z
ØSPPØJZ
ØSPPØKZ
ØSPP34Z
ØSPP35Z
ØSPP37Z
ØSPP3JZ
ØSPP3KZ
ØSPP4ØZ
ØSPP43Z
ØSPP44Z
ØSPP45Z
ØSPP47Z
ØSPP4JZ
ØSPP4KZ
ØSPQØØZ
ØSPQØ3Z
ØSPQØ4Z
ØSPQØ5Z
ØSPQØ7Z
ØSPQØJZ
ØSPQØKZ
ØSPQ34Z
ØSPQ35Z
ØSPQ37Z
ØSPQ3JZ
ØSPQ3KZ
ØSPQ4ØZ
ØSPQ43Z
ØSPQ44Z
ØSPQ45Z
ØSPQ47Z
ØSPQ4JZ
ØSPQ4KZ
ØSPRØJZ
ØSPR3JZ
ØSPR4JZ
ØSPSØJZ
ØSPS3JZ
ØSPS4JZ
ØSPTØJZ
ØSPT3JZ
ØSPT4JZ
ØSPUØJZ
ØSPU3JZ
ØSPU4JZ
ØSPVØJZ
ØSPV3JZ
ØSPV4JZ
ØSPWØJZ
ØSPW3JZ
ØSPW4JZ
ØSQ2ØZZ
ØSQ4ØZZ
ØSQ9ØZZ
ØSQ93ZZ
ØSQ94ZZ
ØSQBØZZ
ØSQB3ZZ
ØSQB4ZZ
ØSQCØZZ
ØSQC3ZZ
ØSQC4ZZ
ØSQDØZZ
ØSQD3ZZ
ØSQD4ZZ
ØSQFØZZ
ØSQF3ZZ
ØSQF4ZZ
ØSQGØZZ
ØSQG3ZZ
ØSQG4ZZ
ØSR2ØJZ
ØSR4ØJZ
ØSR9Ø19
ØSR9Ø1A
ØSR9Ø1Z
ØSR9Ø29
ØSR9Ø2A
ØSR9Ø2Z
ØSR9Ø39
ØSR9Ø3A
ØSR9Ø3Z
ØSR9Ø49
ØSR9Ø4A
ØSR9Ø4Z
ØSR9Ø69
ØSR9Ø6A
ØSR9Ø6Z
ØSR9Ø7Z
ØSR9ØEZ
ØSR9ØJ9
ØSR9ØJA
ØSR9ØJZ
ØSR9ØKZ
ØSRA*
ØSRBØ19
ØSRBØ1A
ØSRBØ1Z
ØSRBØ29
ØSRBØ2A
ØSRBØ2Z
ØSRBØ39
ØSRBØ3A
ØSRBØ3Z
ØSRBØ49
ØSRBØ4A
ØSRBØ4Z
ØSRBØ69
ØSRBØ6A
ØSRBØ6Z
ØSRBØ7Z
ØSRBØEZ
ØSRBØJ9
ØSRBØJA
ØSRBØJZ
ØSRBØKZ
ØSRCØ69
ØSRCØ6A
ØSRCØ6Z
ØSRCØ7Z
ØSRCØEZ
ØSRCØJ9
ØSRCØJA
ØSRCØJZ
ØSRCØKZ
ØSRCØL9
ØSRCØLA
ØSRCØLZ
ØSRCØM9
ØSRCØMA
ØSRCØMZ
ØSRCØN9
ØSRCØNA
ØSRCØNZ
ØSRDØ69
ØSRDØ6A
ØSRDØ6Z
ØSRDØ7Z
ØSRDØEZ
ØSRDØJ9
ØSRDØJA
ØSRDØJZ
ØSRDØKZ
ØSRDØL9
ØSRDØLA
ØSRDØLZ
ØSRDØM9
ØSRDØMA
ØSRDØMZ
ØSRDØN9
ØSRDØNA
ØSRDØNZ
ØSRE*
ØSRF*
ØSRG*
ØSRH*
ØSRJ*
ØSRK*
ØSRL*
ØSRM*
ØSRN*
ØSRP*
ØSRQ*
ØSRR*
ØSRS*
ØSRT*
ØSRU*
ØSRV*
ØSRW*
ØSSØØ4Z
ØSSØØZZ
ØSS3Ø4Z
ØSS3ØZZ
ØSS5Ø4Z
ØSS5ØZZ
ØSS6Ø4Z
ØSS6ØZZ
ØSS7Ø4Z
ØSS7ØZZ
ØSS8Ø4Z
ØSS8ØZZ
ØSS9Ø4Z
ØSS9Ø5Z
ØSS9ØZZ
ØSSBØ4Z
ØSSBØ5Z
ØSSBØZZ
ØSSCØ4Z
ØSSCØ5Z
ØSSCØZZ
ØSSDØ4Z
ØSSDØ5Z
ØSSDØZZ
ØSSFØ4Z
ØSSFØ5Z
ØSSFØZZ
ØSSGØ4Z
ØSSGØ5Z
ØSSGØZZ
ØSSHØ4Z
ØSSHØ5Z
ØSSHØZZ
ØSSJØ4Z
ØSSJØ5Z
ØSSJØZZ
ØSSKØ4Z
ØSSKØ5Z
ØSSKØZZ
ØSSLØ4Z
ØSSLØ5Z
ØSSLØZZ
ØSSMØ4Z
ØSSMØ5Z
ØSSMØZZ
ØSSNØ4Z
ØSSNØ5Z
ØSSNØZZ
ØSSPØ4Z
ØSSPØ5Z
ØSSPØZZ
ØSSQØ4Z
ØSSQØ5Z
ØSSQØZZ
ØST*
ØSUØØJZ
ØSUØ3JZ
ØSUØ4JZ
ØSU2*
ØSU3ØJZ
ØSU33JZ
ØSU34JZ
ØSU4*
ØSU5ØJZ
ØSU53JZ
ØSU54JZ
ØSU6ØJZ
ØSU63JZ
ØSU64JZ
ØSU9ØBZ
ØSUAØBZ
ØSUBØBZ
ØSUEØBZ
ØSUHØJZ
ØSUH3JZ
ØSUH4JZ
ØSUJØJZ
ØSUJ3JZ
ØSUJ4JZ
ØSUR*
ØSUS*
ØSUVØ9Z
ØSUWØ9Z
ØSWØØ4Z
ØSWØØJZ
ØSWØ34Z
ØSWØ3JZ
ØSWØ44Z
ØSWØ4JZ
ØSW2ØJZ
ØSW23JZ
ØSW24JZ
ØSW3Ø4Z
ØSW3ØJZ
ØSW334Z
ØSW33JZ
ØSW344Z
ØSW34JZ
ØSW4ØJZ
ØSW43JZ
ØSW44JZ
ØSW9ØØZ
ØSW9Ø3Z
ØSW9Ø4Z
ØSW9Ø5Z
ØSW9Ø7Z
ØSW9Ø8Z
ØSW9Ø9Z
ØSW9ØBZ
ØSW9ØJZ
ØSW9ØKZ
ØSW93ØZ
ØSW933Z
ØSW934Z
ØSW935Z
ØSW937Z
ØSW938Z
ØSW93JZ
ØSW93KZ
ØSW94ØZ
ØSW943Z
ØSW944Z
ØSW945Z
ØSW947Z
ØSW948Z
ØSW94JZ
ØSW94KZ
ØSWAØJZ
ØSWA3JZ
ØSWA4JZ
ØSWBØØZ
ØSWBØ3Z
ØSWBØ4Z
ØSWBØ5Z
ØSWBØ7Z
ØSWBØ8Z
ØSWBØ9Z
ØSWBØBZ
ØSWBØJZ
ØSWBØKZ
ØSWB3ØZ
ØSWB33Z
ØSWB34Z
ØSWB35Z
ØSWB37Z
ØSWB38Z
ØSWB3JZ
ØSWB3KZ
ØSWB4ØZ
ØSWB43Z
ØSWB44Z
ØSWB45Z
ØSWB47Z
ØSWB48Z
ØSWB4JZ
ØSWB4KZ
ØSWCØØZ
ØSWCØ3Z
ØSWCØ4Z
ØSWCØ5Z
ØSWCØ7Z
ØSWCØ8Z
ØSWCØ9Z
ØSWCØJC
ØSWCØJZ
ØSWCØKZ
ØSWC3ØZ
ØSWC33Z
ØSWC34Z
ØSWC35Z
ØSWC37Z
ØSWC38Z
ØSWC3JC
ØSWC3JZ
ØSWC3KZ
ØSWC4ØZ
ØSWC43Z
ØSWC44Z
ØSWC45Z
ØSWC47Z
ØSWC48Z
ØSWC4JC
ØSWC4JZ
ØSWC4KZ
ØSWDØØZ
ØSWDØ3Z
ØSWDØ4Z
ØSWDØ5Z
ØSWDØ7Z
ØSWDØ8Z
ØSWDØ9Z
ØSWDØJC
ØSWDØJZ
ØSWDØKZ
ØSWD3ØZ
ØSWD33Z
ØSWD34Z
ØSWD35Z
ØSWD37Z
ØSWD38Z
ØSWD3JC
ØSWD3JZ
ØSWD3KZ
ØSWD4ØZ
ØSWD43Z
ØSWD44Z
ØSWD45Z
ØSWD47Z
ØSWD48Z
ØSWD4JC
ØSWD4JZ
ØSWD4KZ
ØSWEØJZ
ØSWE3JZ
ØSWE4JZ
ØSWFØØZ
ØSWFØ3Z
ØSWFØ4Z
ØSWFØ5Z
ØSWFØ7Z
ØSWFØ8Z
ØSWFØJZ
ØSWFØKZ
ØSWF3ØZ
ØSWF33Z
ØSWF34Z
ØSWF35Z
ØSWF37Z
ØSWF38Z
ØSWF3JZ
ØSWF3KZ
ØSWF4ØZ
ØSWF43Z
ØSWF44Z
ØSWF45Z
ØSWF47Z
ØSWF48Z
ØSWF4JZ
ØSWF4KZ
ØSWGØØZ
ØSWGØ3Z
ØSWGØ4Z
ØSWGØ5Z
ØSWGØ7Z
ØSWGØ8Z
ØSWGØJZ
ØSWGØKZ
ØSWG3ØZ
ØSWG33Z
ØSWG34Z
ØSWG35Z
ØSWG37Z
ØSWG38Z
ØSWG3JZ
ØSWG3KZ
ØSWG4ØZ
ØSWG43Z
ØSWG44Z
ØSWG45Z
ØSWG47Z
ØSWG48Z
ØSWG4JZ
ØSWG4KZ
ØSWHØØZ
ØSWHØ3Z
ØSWHØ4Z
ØSWHØ5Z
ØSWHØ7Z
ØSWHØ8Z
ØSWHØJZ
ØSWHØKZ
ØSWH3ØZ
ØSWH33Z
ØSWH34Z
ØSWH35Z
ØSWH37Z
ØSWH38Z
ØSWH3JZ
ØSWH3KZ
ØSWH4ØZ
ØSWH43Z
ØSWH44Z
ØSWH45Z
ØSWH47Z
ØSWH48Z
ØSWH4JZ
ØSWH4KZ
ØSWJØØZ
ØSWJØ3Z
ØSWJØ4Z
ØSWJØ5Z
ØSWJØ7Z
ØSWJØ8Z
ØSWJØJZ
ØSWJØKZ
ØSWJ3ØZ
ØSWJ33Z
ØSWJ34Z
ØSWJ35Z
ØSWJ37Z
ØSWJ38Z
ØSWJ3JZ
ØSWJ3KZ
ØSWJ4ØZ
ØSWJ43Z
ØSWJ44Z
ØSWJ45Z
ØSWJ47Z
ØSWJ48Z
ØSWJ4JZ
ØSWJ4KZ
ØSWKØØZ
ØSWKØ3Z
ØSWKØ4Z
ØSWKØ5Z
ØSWKØ7Z
ØSWKØ8Z
ØSWKØJZ
ØSWKØKZ
ØSWK3ØZ
ØSWK33Z
ØSWK34Z
ØSWK35Z
ØSWK37Z
ØSWK38Z
ØSWK3JZ
ØSWK3KZ
ØSWK4ØZ
ØSWK43Z
ØSWK44Z
ØSWK45Z
ØSWK47Z
ØSWK48Z
ØSWK4JZ
ØSWK4KZ
ØSWLØØZ
ØSWLØ3Z
ØSWLØ4Z
ØSWLØ5Z
ØSWLØ7Z
ØSWLØ8Z
ØSWLØJZ
ØSWLØKZ
ØSWL3ØZ
ØSWL33Z
ØSWL34Z
ØSWL35Z
ØSWL37Z
ØSWL38Z
ØSWL3JZ
ØSWL3KZ
ØSWL4ØZ
ØSWL43Z
ØSWL44Z
ØSWL45Z
ØSWL47Z
ØSWL48Z
ØSWL4JZ
ØSWL4KZ
ØSWMØØZ
ØSWMØ3Z
ØSWMØ4Z

ØSWMØ5Z
ØSWMØ7Z
ØSWMØ8Z
ØSWMØJZ
ØSWMØKZ
ØSWM3ØZ
ØSWM33Z
ØSWM34Z
ØSWM35Z
ØSWM37Z
ØSWM38Z
ØSWM3JZ
ØSWM3KZ
ØSWM4ØZ
ØSWM43Z
ØSWM44Z
ØSWM45Z
ØSWM47Z
ØSWM48Z
ØSWM4JZ
ØSWM4KZ
ØSWNØØZ
ØSWNØ3Z
ØSWNØ4Z
ØSWNØ5Z
ØSWNØ7Z
ØSWNØ8Z
ØSWNØJZ
ØSWNØKZ
ØSWN3ØZ
ØSWN33Z
ØSWN34Z
ØSWN35Z
ØSWN37Z
ØSWN38Z
ØSWN3JZ
ØSWN3KZ
ØSWN4ØZ
ØSWN43Z
ØSWN44Z
ØSWN45Z
ØSWN47Z
ØSWN48Z
ØSWN4JZ
ØSWN4KZ
ØSWPØØZ
ØSWPØ3Z
ØSWPØ4Z
ØSWPØ5Z
ØSWPØ7Z
ØSWPØ8Z
ØSWPØJZ
ØSWPØKZ
ØSWP3ØZ
ØSWP33Z
ØSWP34Z
ØSWP35Z
ØSWP37Z
ØSWP38Z
ØSWP3JZ
ØSWP3KZ
ØSWP4ØZ
ØSWP43Z
ØSWP44Z
ØSWP45Z
ØSWP47Z
ØSWP48Z
ØSWP4JZ
ØSWP4KZ
ØSWQØØZ
ØSWQØ3Z
ØSWQØ4Z
ØSWQØ5Z
ØSWQØ7Z
ØSWQØ8Z
ØSWQØJZ
ØSWQØKZ
ØSWQ3ØZ
ØSWQ33Z
ØSWQ34Z
ØSWQ35Z
ØSWQ37Z
ØSWQ38Z
ØSWQ3JZ
ØSWQ3KZ
ØSWQ4ØZ
ØSWQ43Z
ØSWQ44Z
ØSWQ45Z
ØSWQ47Z
ØSWQ48Z
ØSWQ4JZ
ØSWQ4KZ
ØSWRØJZ
ØSWR3JZ
ØSWR4JZ
ØSWSØJZ
ØSWS3JZ
ØSWS4JZ
ØSWTØJZ
ØSWT3JZ
ØSWT4JZ
ØSWUØJZ
ØSWU3JZ
ØSWU4JZ
ØSWVØJZ
ØSWV3JZ
ØSWV4JZ
ØSWWØJZ
ØSWW3JZ
ØSWW4JZ
ØT13Ø7B
ØT13ØJB
ØT13ØKB
ØT13ØZB
ØT1347B
ØT134JB
ØT134KB
ØT134ZB
ØT14Ø7B
ØT14ØJB
ØT14ØKB
ØT14ØZB
ØT1447B
ØT144JB
ØT144KB
ØT144ZB
ØT16*
ØT17*
ØT18*
ØT1BØZD
ØT1B4ZD
ØT56*
ØT57*
ØT76ØZZ
ØT763ZZ
ØT764ZZ
ØT768DZ
ØT768ZZ
ØT77ØZZ
ØT773ZZ
ØT774ZZ
ØT778DZ
ØT778ZZ
ØT78ØZZ
ØT783ZZ
ØT784ZZ
ØT788DZ
ØT7BØDZ
ØT7BØZZ
ØT7B3DZ
ØT7B3ZZ
ØT7B4DZ
ØT7B4ZZ
ØT7B8DZ
ØT7B8ZZ
ØT7DØZZ
ØT7D3ZZ
ØT7D4ZZ
ØT9ØØØZ
ØT9ØØZX
ØT9ØØZZ
ØT9Ø4ØZ
ØT9Ø7ØZ
ØT9Ø7ZZ
ØT9Ø8ØZ
ØT9Ø8ZZ
ØT91ØØZ
ØT91ØZX
ØT91ØZZ
ØT914ØZ
ØT917ØZ
ØT917ZZ
ØT918ØZ
ØT918ZZ
ØT93ØØZ
ØT93ØZX
ØT93ØZZ
ØT934ØZ
ØT937ØZ
ØT937ZZ
ØT938ØZ
ØT938ZZ
ØT94ØØZ
ØT94ØZX
ØT94ØZZ
ØT944ØZ
ØT947ØZ
ØT947ZZ
ØT948ØZ
ØT948ZZ
ØT9BØØZ
ØT9BØZZ
ØT9CØØZ
ØT9CØZZ
ØT9DØØZ
ØT9D4ØZ
ØTBØØZX
ØTBØØZZ
ØTBØ3ZZ
ØTBØ4ZZ
ØTBØ7ZZ
ØTBØ8ZZ
ØTB1ØZX
ØTB1ØZZ
ØTB13ZZ
ØTB14ZZ
ØTB17ZZ
ØTB18ZZ
ØTB3ØZX
ØTB3ØZZ
ØTB33ZZ
ØTB34ZZ
ØTB37ZZ
ØTB38ZZ
ØTB4ØZX
ØTB4ØZZ
ØTB43ZZ
ØTB44ZZ
ØTB47ZZ
ØTB48ZZ
ØTB6ØZZ
ØTB63ZZ
ØTB64ZZ
ØTB67ZZ
ØTB68ZZ
ØTB7ØZZ
ØTB73ZZ
ØTB74ZZ
ØTB77ZZ
ØTB78ZZ
ØTBBØZZ
ØTBB3ZZ
ØTBB4ZZ
ØTBCØZZ
ØTBC3ZZ
ØTBC4ZZ
ØTCØØZZ
ØTCØ3ZZ
ØTCØ4ZZ
ØTCØ7ZZ
ØTC1ØZZ
ØTC13ZZ
ØTC14ZZ
ØTC17ZZ
ØTC3ØZZ
ØTC33ZZ
ØTC34ZZ
ØTC37ZZ
ØTC4ØZZ
ØTC43ZZ
ØTC44ZZ
ØTC47ZZ
ØTC67ZZ
ØTC77ZZ
ØTCBØZZ
ØTCB3ZZ
ØTCB4ZZ
ØTCCØZZ
ØTCC3ZZ
ØTCC4ZZ
ØTCDØZZ
ØTCD3ZZ
ØTCD4ZZ
ØTF33ZZ
ØTF34ZZ
ØTF43ZZ
ØTF44ZZ
ØTH5Ø1Z
ØTH5Ø2Z
ØTH5ØYZ
ØTH532Z
ØTH541Z
ØTH542Z
ØTH581Z
ØTH58YZ
ØTHBØ1Z
ØTHBØ2Z
ØTHBØLZ
ØTHBØYZ
ØTHB32Z
ØTHB3LZ
ØTHB41Z
ØTHB42Z
ØTHB4LZ
ØTHB7LZ
ØTHB81Z
ØTHB8LZ
ØTHB8YZ
ØTHC*
ØTHDØ1Z
ØTHDØ2Z
ØTHDØLZ
ØTHDØYZ
ØTHD32Z
ØTHD3LZ
ØTHD41Z
ØTHD42Z
ØTHD4LZ
ØTHD7LZ
ØTHD81Z
ØTHD8LZ
ØTHDX2Z
ØTHDXLZ
ØTJ5ØZZ
ØTJBØZZ
ØTJB4ZZ
ØTJDØZZ
ØTL3*
ØTL4*
ØTL6*
ØTL7*
ØTLB*
ØTLC*
ØTM6*
ØTM7*
ØTM8*
ØTMB*
ØTMC*
ØTMD*
ØTNØ*
ØTN1*
ØTN3*
ØTN4*
ØTN6*
ØTN7*
ØTNBØZZ
ØTNB3ZZ
ØTNB4ZZ
ØTNCØZZ
ØTNC3ZZ
ØTNC4ZZ
ØTND*
ØTP5ØØZ
ØTP5Ø2Z
ØTP5Ø3Z
ØTP5Ø7Z
ØTP5ØCZ
ØTP5ØDZ
ØTP5ØJZ
ØTP5ØKZ
ØTP5ØYZ
ØTP53ØZ
ØTP532Z
ØTP533Z
ØTP537Z
ØTP53CZ
ØTP53DZ
ØTP53JZ
ØTP53KZ
ØTP54ØZ
ØTP542Z
ØTP543Z
ØTP547Z
ØTP54CZ
ØTP54DZ
ØTP54JZ
ØTP54KZ
ØTP577Z
ØTP57CZ
ØTP57JZ
ØTP57KZ
ØTP587Z
ØTP58CZ
ØTP58JZ
ØTP58KZ
ØTP58YZ
ØTPBØØZ
ØTPBØ2Z
ØTPBØ3Z
ØTPBØ7Z
ØTPBØCZ
ØTPBØDZ
ØTPBØJZ
ØTPBØKZ
ØTPBØLZ
ØTPBØYZ
ØTPB3ØZ
ØTPB32Z
ØTPB33Z
ØTPB37Z
ØTPB3CZ
ØTPB3DZ
ØTPB3JZ
ØTPB3KZ
ØTPB3LZ
ØTPB4ØZ
ØTPB42Z
ØTPB43Z
ØTPB47Z
ØTPB4CZ
ØTPB4DZ
ØTPB4JZ
ØTPB4KZ
ØTPB4LZ
ØTPB77Z
ØTPB7CZ
ØTPB7JZ
ØTPB7KZ
ØTPB7LZ
ØTPB87Z
ØTPB8CZ
ØTPB8JZ
ØTPB8KZ
ØTPB8LZ
ØTPB8YZ
ØTPDØØZ
ØTPDØ2Z
ØTPDØ3Z
ØTPDØ7Z
ØTPDØCZ
ØTPDØDZ
ØTPDØJZ
ØTPDØKZ
ØTPDØYZ
ØTPD3ØZ
ØTPD32Z
ØTPD33Z
ØTPD37Z
ØTPD3CZ
ØTPD3DZ
ØTPD3JZ
ØTPD3KZ
ØTPD4ØZ
ØTPD42Z
ØTPD43Z
ØTPD47Z
ØTPD4CZ
ØTPD4DZ
ØTPD4JZ
ØTPD4KZ
ØTPD77Z
ØTPD7CZ
ØTPD7JZ
ØTPD7KZ
ØTPD87Z
ØTPD8CZ
ØTPD8JZ
ØTPD8KZ
ØTQ3*
ØTQ4*
ØTQ6*
ØTQ7*
ØTQB*
ØTQD*
ØTR6*
ØTR7*
ØTRB*
ØTRC*
ØTRD*
ØTSØ*
ØTS1*
ØTS2*
ØTTØ*
ØTT1*
ØTT2*
ØTT3*
ØTT4*
ØTT6*
ØTT7*
ØTTB*
ØTTC*
ØTU6*
ØTU7*
ØTUB*
ØTUD*
ØTV6*
ØTV7*
ØTVB*
ØTVD*
ØTW5ØØZ
ØTW5Ø2Z
ØTW5Ø3Z
ØTW5Ø7Z
ØTW5ØCZ
ØTW5ØDZ
ØTW5ØJZ
ØTW5ØKZ
ØTW5ØYZ
ØTW53ØZ
ØTW532Z
ØTW533Z
ØTW537Z
ØTW53CZ
ØTW53DZ
ØTW53JZ
ØTW53KZ
ØTW54ØZ
ØTW542Z
ØTW543Z
ØTW547Z
ØTW54CZ
ØTW54DZ
ØTW54JZ
ØTW54KZ
ØTW57ØZ
ØTW572Z
ØTW573Z
ØTW577Z
ØTW57CZ
ØTW57DZ
ØTW57JZ
ØTW57KZ
ØTW58ØZ
ØTW582Z
ØTW583Z
ØTW587Z
ØTW58CZ
ØTW58DZ
ØTW58JZ
ØTW58KZ
ØTW58YZ
ØTWBØØZ
ØTWBØ2Z
ØTWBØ3Z
ØTWBØ7Z
ØTWBØCZ
ØTWBØDZ
ØTWBØJZ
ØTWBØKZ
ØTWBØLZ
ØTWBØMZ
ØTWBØYZ
ØTWB3ØZ
ØTWB32Z
ØTWB33Z
ØTWB37Z
ØTWB3CZ
ØTWB3DZ
ØTWB3JZ
ØTWB3KZ
ØTWB3LZ
ØTWB3MZ
ØTWB4ØZ
ØTWB42Z
ØTWB43Z
ØTWB47Z
ØTWB4CZ
ØTWB4DZ
ØTWB4JZ
ØTWB4KZ
ØTWB4LZ
ØTWB4MZ
ØTWB7ØZ
ØTWB72Z
ØTWB73Z
ØTWB77Z
ØTWB7CZ
ØTWB7DZ
ØTWB7JZ
ØTWB7KZ
ØTWB7LZ
ØTWB7MZ
ØTWB8ØZ
ØTWB82Z
ØTWB83Z
ØTWB87Z
ØTWB8CZ
ØTWB8DZ
ØTWB8JZ
ØTWB8KZ
ØTWB8LZ
ØTWB8MZ
ØTWB8YZ
ØTWDØØZ
ØTWDØ2Z
ØTWDØ3Z
ØTWDØ7Z
ØTWDØCZ
ØTWDØDZ
ØTWDØJZ
ØTWDØKZ
ØTWDØYZ
ØTWD3ØZ
ØTWD32Z
ØTWD33Z
ØTWD37Z
ØTWD3CZ
ØTWD3DZ
ØTWD3JZ
ØTWD3KZ
ØTWD4ØZ
ØTWD42Z
ØTWD43Z
ØTWD47Z
ØTWD4CZ
ØTWD4DZ
ØTWD4JZ
ØTWD4KZ
ØTWD7ØZ
ØTWD72Z
ØTWD73Z
ØTWD77Z
ØTWD7CZ
ØTWD7DZ
ØTWD7JZ
ØTWD7KZ
ØTWD8ØZ
ØTWD82Z
ØTWD83Z
ØTWD87Z
ØTWD8CZ
ØTWD8DZ
ØTWD8JZ
ØTWD8KZ
ØU79*
ØU7GØDZ
ØU7GØZZ
ØU7G3DZ
ØU7G3ZZ
ØU7G4DZ
ØU7G4ZZ
ØU7K*
ØU99ØØZ
ØU99ØZZ
ØU994ØZ
ØU994ZZ
ØU997ØZ
ØU997ZZ
ØU998ØZ
ØU998ZZ
ØUC9ØZZ
ØUC93ZZ
ØUC94ZZ
ØUCC*
ØUF5ØZZ
ØUF53ZZ
ØUF54ZZ
ØUF57ZZ
ØUF58ZZ
ØUF6ØZZ
ØUF63ZZ
ØUF64ZZ
ØUF67ZZ
ØUF68ZZ
ØUF7ØZZ
ØUF73ZZ
ØUF74ZZ
ØUF77ZZ
ØUF78ZZ
ØUHCØ1Z
ØUHC31Z
ØUHC41Z
ØUHC71Z
ØUHC81Z
ØUHGØ1Z
ØUHG31Z
ØUHG41Z
ØUHG71Z
ØUHG81Z
ØUHGX1Z
ØUMØ*
ØUM1*
ØUM2*
ØUM4*
ØUM5*
ØUM6*
ØUM7*
ØUMG*
ØUMMXZZ
ØUNØ*
ØUN1*
ØUN2*
ØUN4*
ØUN5*
ØUN6*
ØUN7*
ØUNG*
ØUNM*
ØUPDØØZ
ØUPDØ1Z
ØUPDØ3Z
ØUPDØ7Z
ØUPDØDZ
ØUPDØHZ
ØUPDØJZ
ØUPDØKZ
ØUPDØYZ
ØUPD3ØZ
ØUPD31Z
ØUPD33Z
ØUPD37Z
ØUPD3DZ
ØUPD3HZ
ØUPD3JZ
ØUPD3KZ
ØUPD4ØZ
ØUPD41Z
ØUPD43Z
ØUPD47Z
ØUPD4DZ
ØUPD4HZ
ØUPD4JZ
ØUPD4KZ
ØUPD71Z
ØUPD77Z
ØUPD7JZ
ØUPD7KZ
ØUPD81Z
ØUPD87Z
ØUPD8JZ
ØUPD8KZ
ØUQØ*
ØUQ1*
ØUQ2*
ØUQ4*
ØUQ5*
ØUQ6*
ØUQ7*
ØUQ9*
ØUQC*
ØUQGØZZ
ØUQG3ZZ
ØUQG4ZZ
ØUQG8ZZ
ØUQMØZZ
ØUSØ*
ØUS1*
ØUS2*
ØUS4*
ØUS5*
ØUS6*
ØUS7*
ØUSC*
ØUU4*
ØUU5Ø7Z
ØUU5ØKZ
ØUU547Z
ØUU54KZ
ØUU577Z
ØUU57KZ
ØUU587Z
ØUU58KZ
ØUU6Ø7Z
ØUU6ØKZ
ØUU647Z
ØUU64KZ
ØUU677Z
ØUU67KZ
ØUU687Z
ØUU68KZ
ØUU7Ø7Z
ØUU7ØKZ
ØUU747Z
ØUU74KZ
ØUU777Z
ØUU77KZ
ØUU787Z
ØUU78KZ
ØUUG*
ØUUM*
ØUV*
ØUWDØØZ
ØUWDØ1Z
ØUWDØ3Z
ØUWDØ7Z
ØUWDØDZ
ØUWDØHZ
ØUWDØJZ
ØUWDØKZ
ØUWDØYZ
ØUWD3ØZ
ØUWD31Z
ØUWD33Z
ØUWD37Z
ØUWD3DZ
ØUWD3HZ
ØUWD3JZ
ØUWD3KZ
ØUWD4ØZ
ØUWD41Z
ØUWD43Z
ØUWD47Z
ØUWD4DZ
ØUWD4HZ
ØUWD4JZ
ØUWD4KZ
ØUWD7ØZ
ØUWD71Z
ØUWD73Z
ØUWD77Z
ØUWD7DZ
ØUWD7HZ
ØUWD7JZ
ØUWD7KZ
ØUWD8ØZ
ØUWD81Z
ØUWD83Z
ØUWD87Z
ØUWD8DZ
ØUWD8HZ
ØUWD8JZ
ØUWD8KZ
ØV7*
ØV99ØØZ
ØV99ØZZ
ØV9BØØZ
ØV9BØZZ
ØV9CØØZ
ØV9CØZZ
ØVC9*
ØVCB*
ØVCC*
ØVHØ*
ØVLNØDZ
ØVLN3DZ
ØVLN4DZ
ØVLN8DZ
ØVLPØDZ
ØVLP3DZ
ØVLP4DZ
ØVLP8DZ
ØVLQØDZ
ØVLQ3DZ
ØVLQ4DZ
ØVLQ8DZ
ØVM*
ØVNØ*
ØVN5*
ØVN6*
ØVN7*
ØVNF*
ØVNG*
ØVNH*
ØVNJ*
ØVNK*
ØVNL*
ØVNN*
ØVNP*
ØVNQ*
ØVPDØØZ
ØVPDØ3Z
ØVPDØ7Z
ØVPDØJZ
ØVPDØKZ
ØVPDØYZ
ØVPD3ØZ
ØVPD33Z
ØVPD37Z
ØVPD3JZ
ØVPD3KZ
ØVPD4ØZ
ØVPD43Z
ØVPD47Z
ØVPD4JZ
ØVPD4KZ
ØVPD77Z
ØVPD7JZ
ØVPD7KZ
ØVPD87Z
ØVPD8JZ
ØVPD8KZ
ØVQØ*
ØVQ9*
ØVQB*

ØVQC*
ØVQF*
ØVQG*
ØVQH*
ØVQJ*
ØVQK*
ØVQL*
ØVQN*
ØVQP*
ØVQQ*
ØVQS*
ØVQT*
ØVSF*
ØVSG*
ØVSH*
ØVT9*
ØVTB*
ØVTC*
ØVU5*
ØVU6*
ØVU7*
ØVU9*
ØVUB*
ØVUC*
ØVUF*
ØVUG*
ØVUH*
ØVUJ*
ØVUK*
ØVUL*
ØVUN*
ØVUP*
ØVUQ*
ØVUSØ7Z
ØVUSØKZ
ØVUS47Z
ØVUS4KZ
ØVUT*
ØVWDØØZ
ØVWDØ3Z
ØVWDØ7Z
ØVWDØJZ
ØVWDØKZ
ØVWDØYZ
ØVWD3ØZ
ØVWD33Z
ØVWD37Z
ØVWD3JZ
ØVWD3KZ
ØVWD4ØZ
ØVWD43Z
ØVWD47Z
ØVWD4JZ
ØVWD4KZ
ØVWD7ØZ
ØVWD73Z
ØVWD77Z
ØVWD7JZ
ØVWD7KZ
ØVWD8ØZ
ØVWD83Z
ØVWD87Z
ØVWD8JZ
ØVWD8KZ
ØVXTØZD
ØVXTØZS
ØVXTXZD
ØVXTXZS
ØVY5ØZØ
ØVY5ØZ1
ØVY5ØZ2
ØVYSØZØ
ØVYSØZ1
ØVYSØZ2
ØWØ*
ØW11*
ØW19ØJ9
ØW19ØJB
ØW19ØJJ
ØW193J9
ØW193JB
ØW193JJ
ØW194J9
ØW194JB
ØW194JJ
ØW1BØJ9
ØW1BØJB
ØW1BØJJ
ØW1B3J9
ØW1B3JB
ØW1B3JJ
ØW1B4J9
ØW1B4JB
ØW1B4JJ
ØW1GØJ4
ØW1G3J4
ØW1G4J4
ØW3Ø*
ØW31*
ØW32*
ØW33*
ØW34*
ØW35*
ØW36*
ØW38*
ØW39*
ØW3B*
ØW3C*
ØW3D*
ØW3F*
ØW3GØZZ
ØW3G3ZZ
ØW3G4ZZ
ØW3H*
ØW3J*
ØW3K*
ØW3L*
ØW3M*
ØW3N*
ØW3PØZZ
ØW3P3ZZ
ØW3P4ZZ
ØW3P7ZZ
ØW3Q*
ØW3R*
ØW91ØØZ
ØW91ØZZ
ØW92ØØZ
ØW92ØZZ
ØW924ØZ
ØW924ZZ
ØW93ØØZ
ØW93ØZZ
ØW934ØZ
ØW934ZZ
ØW94ØØZ
ØW94ØZZ
ØW944ØZ
ØW944ZZ
ØW95ØØZ
ØW95ØZZ
ØW954ØZ
ØW954ZZ
ØW96ØØZ
ØW96ØZZ
ØW964ØZ
ØW964ZZ
ØW9CØØZ
ØW9CØZZ
ØW9C4ØZ
ØW9C4ZZ
ØW9DØØZ
ØW9DØZX
ØW9DØZZ
ØW9D4ØZ
ØW9D4ZX
ØW9D4ZZ
ØW9FØØZ
ØW9FØZX
ØW9FØZZ
ØW9F3ZX
ØW9F4ZX
ØW9GØØZ
ØW9GØZX
ØW9GØZZ
ØW9G4ØZ
ØW9G4ZX
ØW9G4ZZ
ØW9HØØZ
ØW9HØZX
ØW9HØZZ
ØW9H3ZX
ØW9H4ØZ
ØW9H4ZX
ØW9H4ZZ
ØW9JØØZ
ØW9JØZX
ØW9JØZZ
ØW9J4ØZ
ØW9J4ZX
ØW9J4ZZ
ØWBØØZZ
ØWBØ3ZZ
ØWBØ4ZZ
ØWBØXZZ
ØWB2ØZZ
ØWB23ZZ
ØWB24ZZ
ØWB2XZZ
ØWB4ØZZ
ØWB43ZZ
ØWB44ZZ
ØWB4XZZ
ØWB5ØZZ
ØWB53ZZ
ØWB54ZZ
ØWB5XZZ
ØWB6ØZZ
ØWB63ZZ
ØWB64ZZ
ØWB6XZ2
ØWB6XZZ
ØWBFØZX
ØWBF3ZX
ØWBF4ZX
ØWBFXZX
ØWBKØZZ
ØWBK3ZZ
ØWBK4ZZ
ØWBKXZZ
ØWBLØZZ
ØWBL3ZZ
ØWBL4ZZ
ØWBLXZZ
ØWBMØZZ
ØWBM3ZZ
ØWBM4ZZ
ØWBMXZZ
ØWC1ØZZ
ØWC13ZZ
ØWC14ZZ
ØWC3ØZZ
ØWC33ZZ
ØWC34ZZ
ØWCCØZZ
ØWCC3ZZ
ØWCC4ZZ
ØWCDØZZ
ØWCD3ZZ
ØWCD4ZZ
ØWCGØZZ
ØWCG3ZZ
ØWCG4ZZ
ØWCHØZZ
ØWCH3ZZ
ØWCH4ZZ
ØWCJØZZ
ØWCJ3ZZ
ØWCJ4ZZ
ØWCPØZZ
ØWCP3ZZ
ØWCP4ZZ
ØWCQ7ZZ
ØWCQ8ZZ
ØWCRØZZ
ØWCR3ZZ
ØWCR4ZZ
ØWF1ØZZ
ØWF13ZZ
ØWF14ZZ
ØWF3ØZZ
ØWF33ZZ
ØWF34ZZ
ØWF9ØZZ
ØWF93ZZ
ØWF94ZZ
ØWFBØZZ
ØWFB3ZZ
ØWFB4ZZ
ØWFCØZZ
ØWFC3ZZ
ØWFC4ZZ
ØWFD*
ØWFGØZZ
ØWFG3ZZ
ØWFG4ZZ
ØWFQØZZ
ØWFQ3ZZ
ØWFQ4ZZ
ØWFQ7ZZ
ØWFQ8ZZ
ØWHØØ1Z
ØWHØ31Z
ØWHØ41Z
ØWH1Ø1Z
ØWH131Z
ØWH141Z
ØWH2Ø1Z
ØWH231Z
ØWH241Z
ØWH3*
ØWH4Ø1Z
ØWH431Z
ØWH441Z
ØWH5Ø1Z
ØWH531Z
ØWH541Z
ØWH6Ø1Z
ØWH631Z
ØWH641Z
ØWH8Ø1Z
ØWH831Z
ØWH841Z
ØWH9Ø1Z
ØWH931Z
ØWH941Z
ØWHBØ1Z
ØWHB31Z
ØWHB41Z
ØWHCØ1Z
ØWHCØ3Z
ØWHCØYZ
ØWHC31Z
ØWHC33Z
ØWHC3YZ
ØWHC41Z
ØWHC43Z
ØWHC4YZ
ØWHD*
ØWHF*
ØWHGØ1Z
ØWHGØ3Z
ØWHG31Z
ØWHG41Z
ØWHG43Z
ØWHHØ1Z
ØWHH31Z
ØWHH41Z
ØWHJØ1Z
ØWHJ31Z
ØWHJ41Z
ØWHKØ1Z
ØWHK31Z
ØWHK41Z
ØWHLØ1Z
ØWHL31Z
ØWHL41Z
ØWHMØ1Z
ØWHM31Z
ØWHM41Z
ØWHNØ1Z
ØWHN31Z
ØWHN41Z
ØWHPØ1Z
ØWHP31Z
ØWHP41Z
ØWHP71Z
ØWHP81Z
ØWHQØ1Z
ØWHQ31Z
ØWHQ33Z
ØWHQ3YZ
ØWHQ41Z
ØWHQ43Z
ØWHQ4YZ
ØWHQ71Z
ØWHQ81Z
ØWHRØ1Z
ØWHR31Z
ØWHR41Z
ØWHR71Z
ØWHR81Z
ØWJ1ØZZ
ØWJ14ZZ
ØWJ6ØZZ
ØWJ64ZZ
ØWJ9ØZZ
ØWJ94ZZ
ØWJBØZZ
ØWJB4ZZ
ØWJCØZZ
ØWJFØZZ
ØWJF4ZZ
ØWJGØZZ
ØWJG4ZZ
ØWJHØZZ
ØWJH4ZZ
ØWJJØZZ
ØWJJ4ZZ
ØWJPØZZ
ØWJP4ZZ
ØWJQØZZ
ØWJQ4ZZ
ØWJRØZZ
ØWJR4ZZ
ØWM*
ØWPCØØZ
ØWPCØ1Z
ØWPCØ3Z
ØWPCØ7Z
ØWPCØGZ
ØWPCØJZ
ØWPCØKZ
ØWPCØYZ
ØWPC3ØZ
ØWPC31Z
ØWPC33Z
ØWPC37Z
ØWPC3GZ
ØWPC3JZ
ØWPC3KZ
ØWPC3YZ
ØWPC4ØZ
ØWPC41Z
ØWPC43Z
ØWPC47Z
ØWPC4GZ
ØWPC4JZ
ØWPC4KZ
ØWPC4YZ
ØWPDØØZ
ØWPDØ1Z
ØWPDØ3Z
ØWPDØYZ
ØWPD3ØZ
ØWPD31Z
ØWPD33Z
ØWPD3YZ
ØWPD4ØZ
ØWPD41Z
ØWPD43Z
ØWPD4YZ
ØWPFØØZ
ØWPFØ1Z
ØWPFØ3Z
ØWPFØ7Z
ØWPFØJZ
ØWPFØKZ
ØWPFØYZ
ØWPF3ØZ
ØWPF31Z
ØWPF33Z
ØWPF37Z
ØWPF3JZ
ØWPF3KZ
ØWPF3YZ
ØWPF4ØZ
ØWPF41Z
ØWPF43Z
ØWPF47Z
ØWPF4JZ
ØWPF4KZ
ØWPF4YZ
ØWPGØ3Z
ØWPG43Z
ØWPQ31Z
ØWPQ33Z
ØWPQ3YZ
ØWPQ41Z
ØWPQ43Z
ØWPQ4YZ
ØWPQ71Z
ØWPQ7YZ
ØWPQ81Z
ØWQØ*
ØWQ2*
ØWQ3ØZZ
ØWQ33ZZ
ØWQ34ZZ
ØWQ3XZZ
ØWQ4*
ØWQ5*
ØWQ6*
ØWQ8*
ØWQC*
ØWQF*
ØWQK*
ØWQL*
ØWQM*
ØWQNØZZ
ØWQN3ZZ
ØWQN4ZZ
ØWUØØJZ
ØWUØØKZ
ØWUØ4JZ
ØWUØ4KZ
ØWU2*
ØWU4*
ØWU5*
ØWU6ØJZ
ØWU6ØKZ
ØWU64JZ
ØWU64KZ
ØWUC*
ØWUF*
ØWUKØJZ
ØWUKØKZ
ØWUK4JZ
ØWUK4KZ
ØWULØJZ
ØWULØKZ
ØWUL4JZ
ØWUL4KZ
ØWUMØJZ
ØWUMØKZ
ØWUM4JZ
ØWUM4KZ
ØWUN*
ØWWCØØZ
ØWWCØ1Z
ØWWCØ3Z
ØWWCØ7Z
ØWWCØGZ
ØWWCØJZ
ØWWCØKZ
ØWWCØYZ
ØWWC3ØZ
ØWWC31Z
ØWWC33Z
ØWWC37Z
ØWWC3GZ
ØWWC3JZ
ØWWC3KZ
ØWWC3YZ
ØWWC4ØZ
ØWWC41Z
ØWWC43Z
ØWWC47Z
ØWWC4GZ
ØWWC4JZ
ØWWC4KZ
ØWWC4YZ
ØWWDØØZ
ØWWDØ1Z
ØWWDØ3Z
ØWWDØYZ
ØWWD3ØZ
ØWWD31Z
ØWWD33Z
ØWWD3YZ
ØWWD4ØZ
ØWWD41Z
ØWWD43Z
ØWWD4YZ
ØWWFØØZ
ØWWFØ1Z
ØWWFØ3Z
ØWWFØ7Z
ØWWFØJZ
ØWWFØKZ
ØWWFØYZ
ØWWF3ØZ
ØWWF31Z
ØWWF33Z
ØWWF37Z
ØWWF3JZ
ØWWF3KZ
ØWWF3YZ
ØWWF4ØZ
ØWWF41Z
ØWWF43Z
ØWWF47Z
ØWWF4JZ
ØWWF4KZ
ØWWF4YZ
ØWWGØ3Z
ØWWGØJZ
ØWWG43Z
ØWWG4JZ
ØWWQ31Z
ØWWQ33Z
ØWWQ3YZ
ØWWQ41Z
ØWWQ43Z
ØWWQ4YZ
ØWWQ71Z
ØWWQ73Z
ØWWQ7YZ
ØWWQ81Z
ØWWQ83Z
ØWWQ8YZ
ØWY2ØZØ
ØWY2ØZ1
ØXØ*
ØX3*
ØX6ØØZZ
ØX61ØZZ
ØX62ØZZ
ØX63ØZZ
ØX68*
ØX69*
ØX6BØZZ
ØX6CØZZ
ØX6D*
ØX6F*
ØX6J*
ØX6K*
ØXB2ØZZ
ØXB23ZZ
ØXB24ZZ
ØXB3ØZZ
ØXB33ZZ
ØXB34ZZ
ØXB4ØZZ
ØXB43ZZ
ØXB44ZZ
ØXB5ØZZ
ØXB53ZZ
ØXB54ZZ
ØXB6ØZZ
ØXB63ZZ
ØXB64ZZ
ØXB7ØZZ
ØXB73ZZ
ØXB74ZZ
ØXB8ØZZ
ØXB83ZZ
ØXB84ZZ
ØXB9ØZZ
ØXB93ZZ
ØXB94ZZ
ØXBBØZZ
ØXBB3ZZ
ØXBB4ZZ
ØXBCØZZ
ØXBC3ZZ
ØXBC4ZZ
ØXBDØZZ
ØXBD3ZZ
ØXBD4ZZ
ØXBFØZZ
ØXBF3ZZ
ØXBF4ZZ
ØXBGØZZ
ØXBG3ZZ
ØXBG4ZZ
ØXBHØZZ
ØXBH3ZZ
ØXBH4ZZ
ØXBJØZZ
ØXBJ3ZZ
ØXBJ4ZZ
ØXBKØZZ
ØXBK3ZZ
ØXBK4ZZ
ØXH2Ø1Z
ØXH231Z
ØXH241Z
ØXH3Ø1Z
ØXH331Z
ØXH341Z
ØXH4Ø1Z
ØXH431Z
ØXH441Z
ØXH5Ø1Z
ØXH531Z
ØXH541Z
ØXH6Ø1Z
ØXH631Z
ØXH641Z
ØXH7Ø1Z
ØXH731Z
ØXH741Z
ØXH8Ø1Z
ØXH831Z
ØXH841Z
ØXH9Ø1Z
ØXH931Z
ØXH941Z
ØXHBØ1Z
ØXHB31Z
ØXHB41Z
ØXHCØ1Z
ØXHC31Z
ØXHC41Z
ØXHDØ1Z
ØXHD31Z
ØXHD41Z
ØXHFØ1Z
ØXHF31Z
ØXHF41Z
ØXHGØ1Z
ØXHG31Z
ØXHG41Z
ØXHHØ1Z
ØXHH31Z
ØXHH41Z
ØXHJØ1Z
ØXHJ31Z
ØXHJ41Z
ØXHKØ1Z
ØXHK31Z
ØXHK41Z
ØXMØØZZ
ØXM1ØZZ
ØXM2ØZZ
ØXM3ØZZ
ØXM4ØZZ
ØXM5ØZZ
ØXM6ØZZ
ØXM7ØZZ
ØXM8ØZZ
ØXM9ØZZ
ØXMBØZZ
ØXMCØZZ
ØXMDØZZ
ØXMFØZZ
ØXMGØZZ
ØXMHØZZ
ØXMJØZZ
ØXMKØZZ
ØXQ*
ØXU2ØJZ
ØXU2ØKZ
ØXU24JZ
ØXU24KZ
ØXU3ØJZ
ØXU3ØKZ
ØXU34JZ
ØXU34KZ
ØXU4ØJZ
ØXU4ØKZ
ØXU44JZ
ØXU44KZ
ØXU5ØJZ
ØXU5ØKZ
ØXU54JZ
ØXU54KZ
ØXU6ØJZ
ØXU6ØKZ
ØXU64JZ
ØXU64KZ
ØXU7ØJZ
ØXU7ØKZ
ØXU74JZ
ØXU74KZ
ØXU8ØJZ
ØXU8ØKZ
ØXU84JZ
ØXU84KZ
ØXU9ØJZ
ØXU9ØKZ
ØXU94JZ
ØXU94KZ
ØXUBØJZ
ØXUBØKZ
ØXUB4JZ
ØXUB4KZ
ØXUCØJZ
ØXUCØKZ
ØXUC4JZ
ØXUC4KZ
ØXUDØJZ
ØXUDØKZ
ØXUD4JZ
ØXUD4KZ
ØXUFØJZ
ØXUFØKZ
ØXUF4JZ
ØXUF4KZ
ØXUGØJZ
ØXUGØKZ
ØXUG4JZ
ØXUG4KZ
ØXUHØJZ
ØXUHØKZ
ØXUH4JZ
ØXUH4KZ
ØXUJØJZ
ØXUJØKZ
ØXUJ4JZ
ØXUJ4KZ
ØXUKØJZ
ØXUKØKZ
ØXUK4JZ
ØXUK4KZ
ØXULØJZ
ØXULØKZ
ØXUL4JZ
ØXUL4KZ
ØXUMØJZ
ØXUMØKZ
ØXUM4JZ
ØXUM4KZ
ØXUNØJZ
ØXUNØKZ
ØXUN4JZ
ØXUN4KZ
ØXUPØJZ
ØXUPØKZ
ØXUP4JZ
ØXUP4KZ
ØXUQØJZ
ØXUQØKZ
ØXUQ4JZ
ØXUQ4KZ
ØXURØJZ
ØXURØKZ
ØXUR4JZ
ØXUR4KZ
ØXUSØJZ
ØXUSØKZ
ØXUS4JZ
ØXUS4KZ
ØXUTØJZ
ØXUTØKZ
ØXUT4JZ
ØXUT4KZ
ØXUVØJZ
ØXUVØKZ
ØXUV4JZ
ØXUV4KZ
ØXUWØJZ
ØXUWØKZ
ØXUW4JZ
ØXUW4KZ
ØXYJØZØ
ØXYJØZ1
ØXYKØZØ
ØXYKØZ1
ØYØ*
ØY3*
ØY6*
ØY95ØØZ
ØY95ØZX
ØY95ØZZ
ØY953ZX
ØY954ØZ
ØY954ZX
ØY954ZZ
ØY96ØØZ
ØY96ØZX
ØY96ØZZ
ØY963ZX
ØY964ØZ
ØY964ZX
ØY964ZZ
ØYBØØZZ
ØYBØ3ZZ
ØYBØ4ZZ
ØYB1ØZZ
ØYB13ZZ
ØYB14ZZ
ØYB5ØZX
ØYB53ZX
ØYB54ZX
ØYB6ØZX
ØYB63ZX
ØYB64ZX
ØYB7ØZX
ØYB73ZX
ØYB74ZX
ØYB8ØZX
ØYB83ZX
ØYB84ZX
ØYB9ØZZ
ØYB93ZZ
ØYB94ZZ
ØYBBØZZ
ØYBB3ZZ
ØYBB4ZZ
ØYBCØZZ
ØYBC3ZZ
ØYBC4ZZ
ØYBDØZZ
ØYBD3ZZ
ØYBD4ZZ
ØYBFØZZ
ØYBF3ZZ
ØYBF4ZZ
ØYBGØZZ
ØYBG3ZZ
ØYBG4ZZ
ØYBHØZZ
ØYBH3ZZ

ØYBH4ZZ
ØYBJØZZ
ØYBJ3ZZ
ØYBJ4ZZ
ØYBKØZZ
ØYBK3ZZ
ØYBK4ZZ
ØYBLØZZ
ØYBL3ZZ
ØYBL4ZZ
ØYBMØZZ
ØYBM3ZZ
ØYBM4ZZ
ØYBNØZZ
ØYBN3ZZ
ØYBN4ZZ
ØYHØØ1Z
ØYHØ31Z
ØYHØ41Z
ØYH1Ø1Z
ØYH131Z
ØYH141Z
ØYH5Ø1Z
ØYH531Z
ØYH541Z
ØYH6Ø1Z
ØYH631Z
ØYH641Z
ØYH7Ø1Z
ØYH731Z
ØYH741Z
ØYH8Ø1Z
ØYH831Z
ØYH841Z
ØYH9Ø1Z
ØYH931Z
ØYH941Z
ØYHBØ1Z
ØYHB31Z
ØYHB41Z
ØYHCØ1Z
ØYHC31Z
ØYHC41Z
ØYHDØ1Z
ØYHD31Z
ØYHD41Z
ØYHFØ1Z
ØYHF31Z
ØYHF41Z
ØYHGØ1Z
ØYHG31Z
ØYHG41Z
ØYHHØ1Z
ØYHH31Z
ØYHH41Z
ØYHJØ1Z
ØYHJ31Z
ØYHJ41Z
ØYHKØ1Z
ØYHK31Z
ØYHK41Z
ØYHLØ1Z
ØYHL31Z
ØYHL41Z
ØYHMØ1Z
ØYHM31Z
ØYHM41Z
ØYHNØ1Z
ØYHN31Z
ØYHN41Z
ØYJ5ØZZ
ØYJ54ZZ
ØYJ6ØZZ
ØYJ64ZZ
ØYJ7ØZZ
ØYJ74ZZ
ØYJ84ZZ
ØYJAØZZ
ØYJA4ZZ
ØYJE4ZZ
ØYM*
ØYQØ*
ØYQ1*
ØYQ9*
ØYQB*
ØYQC*
ØYQD*
ØYQF*
ØYQG*
ØYQH*
ØYQJ*
ØYQK*
ØYQL*
ØYQM*
ØYQN*
ØYQP*
ØYQQ*
ØYQR*
ØYQS*
ØYQT*
ØYQU*
ØYQV*
ØYQW*
ØYQX*
ØYQY*
ØYUØ*
ØYU1*
ØYU9*
ØYUB*
ØYUC*
ØYUD*
ØYUF*
ØYUG*
ØYUH*
ØYUJ*
ØYUK*
ØYUL*
ØYUM*
ØYUN*
ØYUP*
ØYUQ*
ØYUR*
ØYUS*
ØYUT*
ØYUU*
ØYUV*
ØYUW*
ØYUX*
ØYUY*
XØHK3Q8
XØHQ3R8
X27H385
X27H395
X27H3B5
X27H3C5
X27J385
X27J395
X27J3B5
X27J3C5
X2CP3T7
X2CS3T7
X2CT3T7
X2CY3T7
X2H13R9
X2H2ØR9
X2H3ØR9
X2KB317
X2KC317
X2RXØN7
X2U4Ø79
X2UQØP9
X2URØP9
X2VWØN7
XNH6Ø58
XNH6358
XNH7Ø58
XNH7358
XNR8ØD9
XNRLØ99
XNRMØ99
XNSØØ32
XNSØØC7
XNSØ332
XNSØ3C7
XNS3Ø32
XNS3332
XNS4Ø32
XNS4ØC7
XNS4332
XNS43C7
XNUØ356
XNU4356
XRGAØR7
XRGA3R7
XRGA4R7
XRGBØR7
XRGB3R7
XRGB4R7
XRGCØR7
XRGC3R7
XRGC4R7
XRGDØR7
XRGD3R7
XRGD4R7
XRGEØ58
XRGE358
XRGFØ58
XRGF358
XRGJØB9
XRGKØB9
XRGLØB9
XRGMØB9
XRHBØ18
XRHDØ18
XRRGØL8
XRRGØM8
XRRHØL8
XRRHØM8

OR

Nonoperating Room Procedures

Ø2H63JZ
Ø2H73JZ
Ø2HK3JZ
Ø2HL3JZ

DRG 908

Select operating room procedure OR nonoperating room procedure listed under DRG 907

DRG 909

Select operating room procedure OR nonoperating room procedure listed under DRG 907

DRG 913

Principal Diagnosis

SØ5.7ØXS
SØ5.71XS
SØ5.72XS
SØ5.8X1S
SØ5.8X2S
SØ5.8X9S
SØ5.9ØXS
SØ5.91XS
SØ5.92XS
SØ6.AØXS
SØ6.A1XS
SØ7.ØXXA
SØ7.1XXA
SØ7.8XXA
SØ7.9XXA
SØ9.ØXXA
SØ9.1ØXA
SØ9.1ØXS
SØ9.11XA
SØ9.19XA
SØ9.19XS
SØ9.2ØXS
SØ9.3Ø1S
SØ9.3Ø2S
SØ9.3Ø9S
SØ9.391S
SØ9.392S
SØ9.399S
SØ9.8XXA
SØ9.8XXS
SØ9.9ØXA
SØ9.9ØXS
SØ9.91XS
SØ9.92XA
SØ9.92XS
SØ9.93XA
SØ9.93XS
S15.ØØ1A
S15.ØØ2A
S15.ØØ9A
S15.Ø11A
S15.Ø12A
S15.Ø19A
S15.Ø21A
S15.Ø22A
S15.Ø29A
S15.Ø91A
S15.Ø92A
S15.Ø99A
S15.1Ø1A
S15.1Ø2A
S15.1Ø9A
S15.111A
S15.112A
S15.119A
S15.121A
S15.122A
S15.129A
S15.191A
S15.192A
S15.199A
S15.2Ø1A
S15.2Ø2A
S15.2Ø9A
S15.211A
S15.212A
S15.219A
S15.221A
S15.222A
S15.229A
S15.291A
S15.292A
S15.299A
S15.3Ø1A
S15.3Ø2A
S15.3Ø9A
S15.311A
S15.312A
S15.319A
S15.321A
S15.322A
S15.329A
S15.391A
S15.392A
S15.399A
S15.8XXA
S15.9XXA
S16.8XXA
S16.8XXS
S16.9XXA
S16.9XXS
S17.ØXXA
S17.8XXA
S17.9XXA
S19.8ØXA
S19.8ØXS
S19.81XA
S19.81XS
S19.82XA
S19.82XS
S19.83XA
S19.83XS
S19.84XA
S19.84XS
S19.85XA
S19.85XS
S19.89XA
S19.89XS
S19.9XXA
S19.9XXS
S21.121A
S21.122A
S21.129A
S21.141A
S21.142A
S21.149A
S21.3Ø1A
S21.3Ø2A
S21.3Ø9A
S21.311A
S21.312A
S21.319A
S21.321A
S21.322A
S21.329A
S21.331A
S21.332A
S21.339A
S21.341A
S21.342A
S21.349A
S21.351A
S21.352A
S21.359A
S21.4Ø1A
S21.4Ø2A
S21.4Ø9A
S21.411A
S21.412A
S21.419A
S21.421A
S21.422A
S21.429A
S21.431A
S21.432A
S21.439A
S21.441A
S21.442A
S21.449A
S21.451A
S21.452A
S21.459A
S21.92XA
S21.94XA
S25.ØØXA
S25.Ø1XA
S25.Ø2XA
S25.Ø9XA
S25.1Ø1A
S25.1Ø2A
S25.1Ø9A
S25.111A
S25.112A
S25.119A
S25.121A
S25.122A
S25.129A
S25.191A
S25.192A
S25.199A
S25.2ØXA
S25.21XA
S25.22XA
S25.29XA
S25.3Ø1A
S25.3Ø2A
S25.3Ø9A
S25.311A
S25.312A
S25.319A
S25.321A
S25.322A
S25.329A
S25.391A
S25.392A
S25.399A
S25.4Ø1A
S25.4Ø2A
S25.4Ø9A
S25.411A
S25.412A
S25.419A
S25.421A
S25.422A
S25.429A
S25.491A
S25.492A
S25.499A
S25.5Ø1A
S25.5Ø2A
S25.5Ø9A
S25.511A
S25.512A
S25.519A
S25.591A
S25.592A
S25.599A
S25.8Ø1A
S25.8Ø2A
S25.8Ø9A
S25.811A
S25.812A
S25.819A
S25.891A
S25.892A
S25.899A
S25.9ØXA
S25.91XA
S25.99XA
S27.9XXA
S28.ØXXA
S29.ØØ1A
S29.ØØ1S
S29.ØØ2A
S29.ØØ2S
S29.ØØ9A
S29.ØØ9S
S29.Ø91A
S29.Ø91S
S29.Ø92A
S29.Ø92S
S29.Ø99A
S29.Ø99S
S29.8XXA
S29.8XXS
S29.9XXA
S29.9XXS
S31.12ØA
S31.121A
S31.122A
S31.123A
S31.124A
S31.125A
S31.129A
S31.14ØA
S31.141A
S31.142A
S31.143A
S31.144A
S31.145A
S31.149A
S31.832A
S31.834A
S35.ØØXA
S35.Ø1XA
S35.Ø2XA
S35.Ø9XA
S35.1ØXA
S35.11XA
S35.12XA
S35.19XA
S35.211A
S35.212A
S35.218A
S35.219A
S35.221A
S35.222A
S35.228A
S35.229A
S35.231A
S35.232A
S35.238A
S35.239A
S35.291A
S35.292A
S35.298A
S35.299A
S35.311A
S35.318A
S35.319A
S35.321A
S35.328A
S35.329A
S35.331A
S35.338A
S35.339A
S35.341A
S35.348A
S35.349A
S35.4Ø1A
S35.4Ø2A
S35.4Ø3A
S35.4Ø4A
S35.4Ø5A
S35.4Ø6A
S35.411A
S35.412A
S35.413A
S35.414A
S35.415A
S35.416A
S35.491A
S35.492A
S35.493A
S35.494A
S35.495A
S35.496A
S35.5ØXA
S35.511A
S35.512A
S35.513A
S35.514A
S35.515A
S35.516A
S35.531A
S35.532A
S35.533A
S35.534A
S35.535A
S35.536A
S35.59XA
S35.8X1A
S35.8X8A
S35.8X9A
S35.9ØXA
S35.91XA
S35.99XA
S36.892A
S36.893A
S36.898A
S36.899A
S38.1XXA
S39.ØØ1A
S39.ØØ1S
S39.ØØ2A
S39.ØØ2S
S39.ØØ3A
S39.ØØ3S
S39.Ø91A
S39.Ø91S
S39.Ø92A
S39.Ø92S
S39.Ø93A
S39.Ø93S
S39.81XA
S39.81XS
S39.82XA
S39.82XS
S39.83XA
S39.83XS
S39.84ØA
S39.84ØS
S39.848A
S39.848S
S39.91XA
S39.91XS
S39.92XA
S39.92XS
S39.93XA
S39.93XS
S39.94XA
S39.94XS
S41.Ø21A
S41.Ø22A
S41.Ø29A
S41.Ø41A
S41.Ø42A
S41.Ø49A
S41.121A
S41.122A
S41.129A
S41.141A
S41.142A
S41.149A
S45.ØØ1A
S45.ØØ2A
S45.ØØ9A
S45.Ø11A
S45.Ø12A
S45.Ø19A
S45.Ø91A
S45.Ø92A
S45.Ø99A
S45.1Ø1A
S45.1Ø2A
S45.1Ø9A
S45.111A
S45.112A
S45.119A
S45.191A
S45.192A
S45.199A
S45.2Ø1A
S45.2Ø2A
S45.2Ø9A
S45.211A
S45.212A
S45.219A
S45.291A
S45.292A
S45.299A
S45.3Ø1A
S45.3Ø2A
S45.3Ø9A
S45.311A
S45.312A
S45.319A
S45.391A
S45.392A
S45.399A
S45.8Ø1A
S45.8Ø2A
S45.8Ø9A
S45.811A
S45.812A
S45.819A
S45.891A
S45.892A
S45.899A
S45.9Ø1A
S45.9Ø2A
S45.9Ø9A
S45.911A
S45.912A
S45.919A
S45.991A
S45.992A
S45.999A
S46.ØØ1A
S46.ØØ1S
S46.ØØ2A
S46.ØØ2S
S46.ØØ9A
S46.ØØ9S
S46.Ø91A
S46.Ø91S
S46.Ø92A
S46.Ø92S
S46.Ø99A
S46.Ø99S
S46.1Ø1A
S46.1Ø1S
S46.1Ø2A
S46.1Ø2S
S46.1Ø9A
S46.1Ø9S
S46.191A
S46.191S
S46.192A
S46.192S
S46.199A
S46.199S
S46.2Ø1A
S46.2Ø1S
S46.2Ø2A
S46.2Ø2S
S46.2Ø9A
S46.2Ø9S
S46.291A
S46.291S
S46.292A
S46.292S
S46.299A
S46.299S
S46.3Ø1A
S46.3Ø1S
S46.3Ø2A
S46.3Ø2S
S46.3Ø9A
S46.3Ø9S
S46.391A
S46.391S
S46.392A
S46.392S
S46.399A
S46.399S
S46.8Ø1A
S46.8Ø1S
S46.8Ø2A
S46.8Ø2S
S46.8Ø9A
S46.8Ø9S
S46.891A
S46.891S
S46.892A
S46.892S
S46.899A
S46.899S
S46.9Ø1A
S46.9Ø1S
S46.9Ø2A
S46.9Ø2S
S46.9Ø9A
S46.9Ø9S
S46.991A
S46.991S
S46.992A
S46.992S
S46.999A
S46.999S
S47.1XXA
S47.2XXA
S47.9XXA
S48.Ø11A
S48.Ø12A
S48.Ø19A
S48.Ø21A
S48.Ø22A
S48.Ø29A
S48.111A
S48.112A
S48.119A
S48.121A
S48.122A
S48.129A
S48.911A
S48.912A
S48.919A
S48.921A
S48.922A
S48.929A
S49.8ØXA
S49.8ØXS
S49.81XA
S49.81XS
S49.82XA
S49.82XS
S49.9ØXA
S49.9ØXS
S49.91XA
S49.91XS
S49.92XA
S49.92XS
S51.Ø21A
S51.Ø22A
S51.Ø29A
S51.Ø41A
S51.Ø42A
S51.Ø49A
S51.821A
S51.822A
S51.829A
S51.841A
S51.842A
S51.849A
S55.ØØ1A
S55.ØØ2A
S55.ØØ9A
S55.Ø11A
S55.Ø12A
S55.Ø19A
S55.Ø91A
S55.Ø92A
S55.Ø99A
S55.1Ø1A
S55.1Ø2A
S55.1Ø9A
S55.111A
S55.112A
S55.119A
S55.191A
S55.192A
S55.199A
S55.2Ø1A
S55.2Ø2A
S55.2Ø9A
S55.211A
S55.212A
S55.219A
S55.291A
S55.292A
S55.299A
S55.8Ø1A
S55.8Ø2A
S55.8Ø9A
S55.811A
S55.812A
S55.819A
S55.891A
S55.892A
S55.899A
S55.9Ø1A
S55.9Ø2A
S55.9Ø9A
S55.911A
S55.912A
S55.919A
S55.991A
S55.992A
S55.999A
S56.ØØ1A
S56.ØØ1S
S56.ØØ2A
S56.ØØ2S
S56.ØØ9A
S56.ØØ9S
S56.Ø91A
S56.Ø91S
S56.Ø92A
S56.Ø92S
S56.Ø99A
S56.Ø99S
S56.1Ø1A
S56.1Ø1S
S56.1Ø2A
S56.1Ø2S
S56.1Ø3A
S56.1Ø3S
S56.1Ø4A
S56.1Ø4S
S56.1Ø5A
S56.1Ø5S
S56.1Ø6A
S56.1Ø6S
S56.1Ø7A
S56.1Ø7S
S56.1Ø8A
S56.1Ø8S
S56.1Ø9A
S56.1Ø9S
S56.191A
S56.191S
S56.192A
S56.192S
S56.193A
S56.193S
S56.194A
S56.194S
S56.195A
S56.195S
S56.196A
S56.196S
S56.197A

S56.197S
S56.198A
S56.198S
S56.199A
S56.199S
S56.201A
S56.201S
S56.202A
S56.202S
S56.209A
S56.209S
S56.291A
S56.291S
S56.292A
S56.292S
S56.299A
S56.299S
S56.301A
S56.301S
S56.302A
S56.302S
S56.309A
S56.309S
S56.391A
S56.391S
S56.392A
S56.392S
S56.399A
S56.399S
S56.401A
S56.401S
S56.402A
S56.402S
S56.403A
S56.403S
S56.404A
S56.404S
S56.405A
S56.405S
S56.406A
S56.406S
S56.407A
S56.407S
S56.408A
S56.408S
S56.409A
S56.409S
S56.491A
S56.491S
S56.492A
S56.492S
S56.493A
S56.493S
S56.494A
S56.494S
S56.495A
S56.495S
S56.496A
S56.496S
S56.497A
S56.497S
S56.498A
S56.498S
S56.499A
S56.499S
S56.501A
S56.501S
S56.502A
S56.502S
S56.509A
S56.509S
S56.591A
S56.591S
S56.592A
S56.592S
S56.599A
S56.599S
S56.801A
S56.801S
S56.802A
S56.802S
S56.809A
S56.809S
S56.891A
S56.891S
S56.892A
S56.892S
S56.899A
S56.899S
S56.901A
S56.901S
S56.902A
S56.902S
S56.909A
S56.909S
S56.991A
S56.991S
S56.992A
S56.992S
S56.999A
S56.999S
S57.00XA
S57.01XA
S57.02XA
S57.80XA
S57.81XA
S57.82XA
S58.011A
S58.012A
S58.019A
S58.021A
S58.022A
S58.029A
S58.111A
S58.112A
S58.119A
S58.121A
S58.122A
S58.129A
S58.911A
S58.912A
S58.919A
S58.921A
S58.922A
S58.929A
S59.801A
S59.801S
S59.802A
S59.802S
S59.809A
S59.809S
S59.811A
S59.811S
S59.812A
S59.812S
S59.819A
S59.819S
S59.901A
S59.901S
S59.902A
S59.902S
S59.909A
S59.909S
S59.911A
S59.911S
S59.912A
S59.912S
S59.919A
S59.919S
S61.021A
S61.022A
S61.029A
S61.041A
S61.042A
S61.049A
S61.121A
S61.122A
S61.129A
S61.141A
S61.142A
S61.149A
S61.220A
S61.221A
S61.222A
S61.223A
S61.224A
S61.225A
S61.226A
S61.227A
S61.228A
S61.229A
S61.240A
S61.241A
S61.242A
S61.243A
S61.244A
S61.245A
S61.246A
S61.247A
S61.248A
S61.249A
S61.320A
S61.321A
S61.322A
S61.323A
S61.324A
S61.325A
S61.326A
S61.327A
S61.328A
S61.329A
S61.340A
S61.341A
S61.342A
S61.343A
S61.344A
S61.345A
S61.346A
S61.347A
S61.348A
S61.349A
S61.421A
S61.422A
S61.429A
S61.441A
S61.442A
S61.449A
S61.521A
S61.522A
S61.529A
S61.541A
S61.542A
S61.549A
S65.001A
S65.002A
S65.009A
S65.011A
S65.012A
S65.019A
S65.091A
S65.092A
S65.099A
S65.101A
S65.102A
S65.109A
S65.111A
S65.112A
S65.119A
S65.191A
S65.192A
S65.199A
S65.201A
S65.202A
S65.209A
S65.211A
S65.212A
S65.219A
S65.291A
S65.292A
S65.299A
S65.301A
S65.302A
S65.309A
S65.311A
S65.312A
S65.319A
S65.391A
S65.392A
S65.399A
S65.401A
S65.402A
S65.409A
S65.411A
S65.412A
S65.419A
S65.491A
S65.492A
S65.499A
S65.500A
S65.501A
S65.502A
S65.503A
S65.504A
S65.505A
S65.506A
S65.507A
S65.508A
S65.509A
S65.510A
S65.511A
S65.512A
S65.513A
S65.514A
S65.515A
S65.516A
S65.517A
S65.518A
S65.519A
S65.590A
S65.591A
S65.592A
S65.593A
S65.594A
S65.595A
S65.596A
S65.597A
S65.598A
S65.599A
S65.801A
S65.802A
S65.809A
S65.811A
S65.812A
S65.819A
S65.891A
S65.892A
S65.899A
S65.901A
S65.902A
S65.909A
S65.911A
S65.912A
S65.919A
S65.991A
S65.992A
S65.999A
S66.001A
S66.001S
S66.002A
S66.002S
S66.009A
S66.009S
S66.091A
S66.091S
S66.092A
S66.092S
S66.099A
S66.099S
S66.100A
S66.100S
S66.101A
S66.101S
S66.102A
S66.102S
S66.103A
S66.103S
S66.104A
S66.104S
S66.105A
S66.105S
S66.106A
S66.106S
S66.107A
S66.107S
S66.108A
S66.108S
S66.109A
S66.109S
S66.190A
S66.190S
S66.191A
S66.191S
S66.192A
S66.192S
S66.193A
S66.193S
S66.194A
S66.194S
S66.195A
S66.195S
S66.196A
S66.196S
S66.197A
S66.197S
S66.198A
S66.198S
S66.199A
S66.199S
S66.201A
S66.201S
S66.202A
S66.202S
S66.209A
S66.209S
S66.291A
S66.291S
S66.292A
S66.292S
S66.299A
S66.299S
S66.300A
S66.300S
S66.301A
S66.301S
S66.302A
S66.302S
S66.303A
S66.303S
S66.304A
S66.304S
S66.305A
S66.305S
S66.306A
S66.306S
S66.307A
S66.307S
S66.308A
S66.308S
S66.309A
S66.309S
S66.390A
S66.390S
S66.391A
S66.391S
S66.392A
S66.392S
S66.393A
S66.393S
S66.394A
S66.394S
S66.395A
S66.395S
S66.396A
S66.396S
S66.397A
S66.397S
S66.398A
S66.398S
S66.399A
S66.399S
S66.401A
S66.401S
S66.402A
S66.402S
S66.409A
S66.409S
S66.491A
S66.491S
S66.492A
S66.492S
S66.499A
S66.499S
S66.500A
S66.500S
S66.501A
S66.501S
S66.502A
S66.502S
S66.503A
S66.503S
S66.504A
S66.504S
S66.505A
S66.505S
S66.506A
S66.506S
S66.507A
S66.507S
S66.508A
S66.508S
S66.509A
S66.509S
S66.590A
S66.590S
S66.591A
S66.591S
S66.592A
S66.592S
S66.593A
S66.593S
S66.594A
S66.594S
S66.595A
S66.595S
S66.596A
S66.596S
S66.597A
S66.597S
S66.598A
S66.598S
S66.599A
S66.599S
S66.801A
S66.801S
S66.802A
S66.802S
S66.809A
S66.809S
S66.891A
S66.891S
S66.892A
S66.892S
S66.899A
S66.899S
S66.901A
S66.901S
S66.902A
S66.902S
S66.909A
S66.909S
S66.991A
S66.991S
S66.992A
S66.992S
S66.999A
S66.999S
S67.00XA
S67.01XA
S67.02XA
S67.10XA
S67.190A
S67.191A
S67.192A
S67.193A
S67.194A
S67.195A
S67.196A
S67.197A
S67.198A
S67.20XA
S67.21XA
S67.22XA
S67.30XA
S67.31XA
S67.32XA
S67.40XA
S67.41XA
S67.42XA
S67.90XA
S67.91XA
S67.92XA
S68.011A
S68.012A
S68.019A
S68.021A
S68.022A
S68.029A
S68.110A
S68.111A
S68.112A
S68.113A
S68.114A
S68.115A
S68.116A
S68.117A
S68.118A
S68.119A
S68.120A
S68.121A
S68.122A
S68.123A
S68.124A
S68.125A
S68.126A
S68.127A
S68.128A
S68.129A
S68.411A
S68.412A
S68.419A
S68.421A
S68.422A
S68.429A
S68.511A
S68.512A
S68.519A
S68.521A
S68.522A
S68.529A
S68.610A
S68.611A
S68.612A
S68.613A
S68.614A
S68.615A
S68.616A
S68.617A
S68.618A
S68.619A
S68.620A
S68.621A
S68.622A
S68.623A
S68.624A
S68.625A
S68.626A
S68.627A
S68.628A
S68.629A
S68.711A
S68.712A
S68.719A
S68.721A
S68.722A
S68.729A
S69.80XA
S69.80XS
S69.81XA
S69.81XS
S69.82XA
S69.82XS
S69.90XA
S69.90XS
S69.91XA
S69.91XS
S69.92XA
S69.92XS
S71.021A
S71.022A
S71.029A
S71.041A
S71.042A
S71.049A
S71.121A
S71.122A
S71.129A
S71.141A
S71.142A
S71.149A
S75.001A
S75.002A
S75.009A
S75.011A
S75.012A
S75.019A
S75.021A
S75.022A
S75.029A
S75.091A
S75.092A
S75.099A
S75.101A
S75.102A
S75.109A
S75.111A
S75.112A
S75.119A
S75.121A
S75.122A
S75.129A
S75.191A
S75.192A
S75.199A
S75.201A
S75.202A
S75.209A
S75.211A
S75.212A
S75.219A
S75.221A
S75.222A
S75.229A
S75.291A
S75.292A
S75.299A
S75.801A
S75.802A
S75.809A
S75.811A
S75.812A
S75.819A
S75.891A
S75.892A
S75.899A
S75.901A
S75.902A
S75.909A
S75.911A
S75.912A
S75.919A
S75.991A
S75.992A
S75.999A
S76.001A
S76.001S
S76.002A
S76.002S
S76.009A
S76.009S
S76.091A
S76.091S
S76.092A
S76.092S
S76.099A
S76.099S
S76.101A
S76.101S
S76.102A
S76.102S
S76.109A
S76.109S
S76.191A
S76.191S
S76.192A
S76.192S
S76.199A
S76.199S
S76.201A
S76.201S
S76.202A
S76.202S
S76.209A
S76.209S
S76.291A
S76.291S
S76.292A
S76.292S
S76.299A
S76.299S
S76.301A
S76.301S
S76.302A
S76.302S
S76.309A
S76.309S
S76.391A
S76.391S
S76.392A
S76.392S
S76.399A
S76.399S
S76.801A
S76.801S
S76.802A
S76.802S
S76.809A
S76.809S
S76.891A
S76.891S
S76.892A
S76.892S
S76.899A
S76.899S
S76.901A
S76.901S
S76.902A
S76.902S
S76.909A
S76.909S
S76.991A
S76.991S
S76.992A
S76.992S
S76.999A
S76.999S
S77.00XA
S77.01XA
S77.02XA
S77.10XA
S77.11XA
S77.12XA
S77.20XA
S77.21XA
S77.22XA
S78.011A
S78.012A
S78.019A
S78.021A
S78.022A
S78.029A
S78.111A
S78.112A
S78.119A
S78.121A
S78.122A
S78.129A
S78.911A
S78.912A
S78.919A
S78.921A
S78.922A
S78.929A
S79.811A
S79.811S
S79.812A
S79.812S
S79.819A
S79.819S
S79.821A
S79.821S
S79.822A
S79.822S
S79.829A
S79.829S
S79.911A
S79.911S
S79.912A
S79.912S
S79.919A
S79.919S
S79.921A
S79.921S
S79.922A
S79.922S
S79.929A
S79.929S
S81.021A
S81.022A
S81.029A
S81.041A
S81.042A
S81.049A
S81.821A
S81.822A
S81.829A
S81.841A
S81.842A
S81.849A
S85.001A
S85.002A
S85.009A
S85.011A
S85.012A
S85.019A
S85.091A
S85.092A
S85.099A
S85.101A
S85.102A
S85.109A
S85.111A
S85.112A
S85.119A
S85.121A
S85.122A
S85.129A
S85.131A
S85.132A
S85.139A
S85.141A
S85.142A
S85.149A
S85.151A
S85.152A
S85.159A
S85.161A
S85.162A
S85.169A
S85.171A
S85.172A
S85.179A
S85.181A
S85.182A
S85.189A
S85.201A
S85.202A
S85.209A
S85.211A
S85.212A
S85.219A
S85.291A
S85.292A
S85.299A
S85.301A
S85.302A
S85.309A
S85.311A
S85.312A
S85.319A
S85.391A
S85.392A
S85.399A
S85.401A
S85.402A
S85.409A
S85.411A
S85.412A
S85.419A
S85.491A
S85.492A
S85.499A
S85.501A
S85.502A
S85.509A
S85.511A

S85.512A
S85.519A
S85.591A
S85.592A
S85.599A
S85.8Ø1A
S85.8Ø2A
S85.8Ø9A
S85.811A
S85.812A
S85.819A
S85.891A
S85.892A
S85.899A
S85.9Ø1A
S85.9Ø2A
S85.9Ø9A
S85.911A
S85.912A
S85.919A
S85.991A
S85.992A
S85.999A
S86.ØØ1A
S86.ØØ1S
S86.ØØ2A
S86.ØØ2S
S86.ØØ9A
S86.ØØ9S
S86.Ø91A
S86.Ø91S
S86.Ø92A
S86.Ø92S
S86.Ø99A
S86.Ø99S
S86.1Ø1A
S86.1Ø1S
S86.1Ø2A
S86.1Ø2S
S86.1Ø9A
S86.1Ø9S
S86.191A
S86.191S
S86.192A
S86.192S
S86.199A
S86.199S
S86.2Ø1A
S86.2Ø1S
S86.2Ø2A
S86.2Ø2S
S86.2Ø9A
S86.2Ø9S
S86.291A
S86.291S
S86.292A
S86.292S
S86.299A
S86.299S
S86.3Ø1A
S86.3Ø1S
S86.3Ø2A
S86.3Ø2S
S86.3Ø9A
S86.3Ø9S
S86.391A
S86.391S
S86.392A
S86.392S
S86.399A
S86.399S
S86.8Ø1A
S86.8Ø1S
S86.8Ø2A
S86.8Ø2S
S86.8Ø9A
S86.8Ø9S
S86.891A
S86.891S
S86.892A
S86.892S
S86.899A
S86.899S
S86.9Ø1A
S86.9Ø1S
S86.9Ø2A
S86.9Ø2S
S86.9Ø9A
S86.9Ø9S
S86.991A
S86.991S
S86.992A
S86.992S
S86.999A
S86.999S
S87.ØØXA
S87.Ø1XA
S87.Ø2XA
S87.8ØXA
S87.81XA
S87.82XA
S88.Ø11A
S88.Ø12A
S88.Ø19A
S88.Ø21A
S88.Ø22A
S88.Ø29A
S88.111A
S88.112A
S88.119A
S88.121A
S88.122A
S88.129A
S88.911A
S88.912A
S88.919A
S88.921A
S88.922A
S88.929A
S89.8ØXA
S89.8ØXS
S89.81XA
S89.81XS
S89.82XA
S89.82XS
S89.9ØXA
S89.9ØXS
S89.91XA
S89.91XS
S89.92XA
S89.92XS
S91.Ø21A
S91.Ø22A
S91.Ø29A
S91.Ø41A
S91.Ø42A
S91.Ø49A
S91.121A
S91.122A
S91.123A
S91.124A
S91.125A
S91.126A
S91.129A
S91.141A
S91.142A
S91.143A
S91.144A
S91.145A
S91.146A
S91.149A
S91.221A
S91.222A
S91.223A
S91.224A
S91.225A
S91.226A
S91.229A
S91.241A
S91.242A
S91.243A
S91.244A
S91.245A
S91.246A
S91.249A
S91.321A
S91.322A
S91.329A
S91.341A
S91.342A
S91.349A
S95.ØØ1A
S95.ØØ2A
S95.ØØ9A
S95.Ø11A
S95.Ø12A
S95.Ø19A
S95.Ø91A
S95.Ø92A
S95.Ø99A
S95.1Ø1A
S95.1Ø2A
S95.1Ø9A
S95.111A
S95.112A
S95.119A
S95.191A
S95.192A
S95.199A
S95.2Ø1A
S95.2Ø2A
S95.2Ø9A
S95.211A
S95.212A
S95.219A
S95.291A
S95.292A
S95.299A
S95.8Ø1A
S95.8Ø2A
S95.8Ø9A
S95.811A
S95.812A
S95.819A
S95.891A
S95.892A
S95.899A
S95.9Ø1A
S95.9Ø2A
S95.9Ø9A
S95.911A
S95.912A
S95.919A
S95.991A
S95.992A
S95.999A
S96.ØØ1A
S96.ØØ1S
S96.ØØ2A
S96.ØØ2S
S96.ØØ9A
S96.ØØ9S
S96.Ø91A
S96.Ø91S
S96.Ø92A
S96.Ø92S
S96.Ø99A
S96.Ø99S
S96.1Ø1A
S96.1Ø1S
S96.1Ø2A
S96.1Ø2S
S96.1Ø9A
S96.1Ø9S
S96.191A
S96.191S
S96.192A
S96.192S
S96.199A
S96.199S
S96.2Ø1A
S96.2Ø1S
S96.2Ø2A
S96.2Ø2S
S96.2Ø9A
S96.2Ø9S
S96.291A
S96.291S
S96.292A
S96.292S
S96.299A
S96.299S
S96.8Ø1A
S96.8Ø1S
S96.8Ø2A
S96.8Ø2S
S96.8Ø9A
S96.8Ø9S
S96.891A
S96.891S
S96.892A
S96.892S
S96.899A
S96.899S
S96.9Ø1A
S96.9Ø1S
S96.9Ø2A
S96.9Ø2S
S96.9Ø9A
S96.9Ø9S
S96.991A
S96.991S
S96.992A
S96.992S
S96.999A
S96.999S
S97.ØØXA
S97.Ø1XA
S97.Ø2XA
S97.1Ø1A
S97.1Ø2A
S97.1Ø9A
S97.111A
S97.112A
S97.119A
S97.121A
S97.122A
S97.129A
S97.8ØXA
S97.81XA
S97.82XA
S98.Ø11A
S98.Ø12A
S98.Ø19A
S98.Ø21A
S98.Ø22A
S98.Ø29A
S98.111A
S98.112A
S98.119A
S98.121A
S98.122A
S98.129A
S98.131A
S98.132A
S98.139A
S98.141A
S98.142A
S98.149A
S98.211A
S98.212A
S98.219A
S98.221A
S98.222A
S98.229A
S98.311A
S98.312A
S98.319A
S98.321A
S98.322A
S98.329A
S98.911A
S98.912A
S98.919A
S98.921A
S98.922A
S98.929A
S99.ØØ1A
S99.ØØ1B
S99.ØØ1S
S99.ØØ2A
S99.ØØ2B
S99.ØØ2S
S99.ØØ9A
S99.ØØ9B
S99.ØØ9S
S99.Ø11A
S99.Ø11B
S99.Ø11S
S99.Ø12A
S99.Ø12B
S99.Ø12S
S99.Ø19A
S99.Ø19B
S99.Ø19S
S99.Ø21A
S99.Ø21B
S99.Ø21S
S99.Ø22A
S99.Ø22B
S99.Ø22S
S99.Ø29A
S99.Ø29B
S99.Ø29S
S99.Ø31A
S99.Ø31B
S99.Ø31S
S99.Ø32A
S99.Ø32B
S99.Ø32S
S99.Ø39A
S99.Ø39B
S99.Ø39S
S99.Ø41A
S99.Ø41B
S99.Ø41S
S99.Ø42A
S99.Ø42B
S99.Ø42S
S99.Ø49A
S99.Ø49B
S99.Ø49S
S99.Ø91A
S99.Ø91B
S99.Ø91S
S99.Ø92A
S99.Ø92B
S99.Ø92S
S99.Ø99A
S99.Ø99B
S99.Ø99S
S99.1Ø1A
S99.1Ø1B
S99.1Ø1S
S99.1Ø2A
S99.1Ø2B
S99.1Ø2S
S99.1Ø9A
S99.1Ø9B
S99.1Ø9S
S99.111A
S99.111B
S99.111S
S99.112A
S99.112B
S99.112S
S99.119A
S99.119B
S99.119S
S99.121A
S99.121B
S99.121S
S99.122A
S99.122B
S99.122S
S99.129A
S99.129B
S99.129S
S99.131A
S99.131B
S99.131S
S99.132A
S99.132B
S99.132S
S99.139A
S99.139B
S99.139S
S99.141A
S99.141B
S99.141S
S99.142A
S99.142B
S99.142S
S99.149A
S99.149B
S99.149S
S99.191A
S99.191B
S99.191S
S99.192A
S99.192B
S99.192S
S99.199A
S99.199B
S99.199S
S99.2Ø1A
S99.2Ø1B
S99.2Ø1S
S99.2Ø2A
S99.2Ø2B
S99.2Ø2S
S99.2Ø9A
S99.2Ø9B
S99.2Ø9S
S99.211A
S99.211B
S99.211S
S99.212A
S99.212B
S99.212S
S99.219A
S99.219B
S99.219S
S99.221A
S99.221B
S99.221S
S99.222A
S99.222B
S99.222S
S99.229A
S99.229B
S99.229S
S99.231A
S99.231B
S99.231S
S99.232A
S99.232B
S99.232S
S99.239A
S99.239B
S99.239S
S99.241A
S99.241B
S99.241S
S99.242A
S99.242B
S99.242S
S99.249A
S99.249B
S99.249S
S99.291A
S99.291B
S99.291S
S99.292A
S99.292B
S99.292S
S99.299A
S99.299B
S99.299S
S99.811A
S99.811S
S99.812A
S99.812S
S99.819A
S99.819S
S99.821A
S99.821S
S99.822A
S99.822S
S99.829A
S99.829S
S99.911A
S99.911S
S99.912A
S99.912S
S99.919A
S99.919S
S99.921A
S99.921S
S99.922A
S99.922S
S99.929A
S99.929S
TØ7.XXXA
TØ7.XXXS
T14.8XXA
T14.8XXS
T14.9ØXA
T14.9ØXS
T14.91XA
T14.91XS
T15.ØØXS
T15.Ø1XS
T15.Ø2XS
T15.1ØXS
T15.11XS
T15.12XS
T15.8ØXS
T15.81XS
T15.82XS
T15.9ØXS
T15.91XS
T15.92XS
T16.1XXS
T16.2XXS
T16.9XXS
T17.ØXXS
T17.1XXS
T17.2ØØS
T17.2Ø8S
T17.21ØS
T17.218S
T17.22ØS
T17.228S
T17.29ØS
T17.298S
T17.3ØØS
T17.3Ø8S
T17.31ØS
T17.318S
T17.32ØS
T17.328S
T17.39ØS
T17.398S
T17.4ØØS
T17.4Ø8S
T17.41ØS
T17.418S
T17.42ØS
T17.428S
T17.49ØS
T17.498S
T17.5ØØS
T17.5Ø8S
T17.51ØS
T17.518S
T17.52ØS
T17.528S
T17.59ØS
T17.598S
T17.8ØØS
T17.8Ø8S
T17.81ØS
T17.818S
T17.82ØS
T17.828S
T17.89ØS
T17.898S
T17.9ØØS
T17.9Ø8S
T17.91ØS
T17.918S
T17.92ØS
T17.928S
T17.99ØS
T17.998S
T18.ØXXS
T18.1ØØS
T18.1Ø8S
T18.11ØS
T18.118S
T18.12ØS
T18.128S
T18.19ØS
T18.198S
T18.2XXS
T18.3XXS
T18.4XXS
T18.5XXS
T18.8XXS
T18.9XXS
T19.ØXXS
T19.1XXS
T19.2XXS
T19.3XXS
T19.4XXS
T19.8XXS
T19.9XXS
T79.ØXXS
T79.1XXS
T79.2XXS
T79.4XXS
T79.5XXS
T79.6XXS
T79.7XXS
T79.8XXS
T79.9XXS
T79.AØXS
T79.A11S
T79.A12S
T79.A19S
T79.A21S
T79.A22S
T79.A29S
T79.A3XS
T79.A9XS

DRG 914

Select principal diagnosis listed under DRG 913

DRG 915

Principal Diagnosis

T78.ØØXA
T78.Ø1XA
T78.Ø2XA
T78.Ø3XA
T78.Ø4XA
T78.Ø5XA
T78.Ø6XA
T78.Ø7XA
T78.Ø8XA
T78.Ø9XA
T78.2XXA
T78.3XXA
T78.4ØXA
T78.49XA
T8Ø.51XA
T8Ø.52XA
T8Ø.59XA
T8Ø.61XA
T8Ø.62XA
T8Ø.69XA
T88.6XXA

DRG 916

Select principal diagnosis listed under DRG 915

DRG 917

Principal Diagnosis

M1A.1*
T36.ØX1A
T36.ØX2A
T36.ØX3A
T36.ØX4A
T36.ØX5A
T36.1X1A
T36.1X2A
T36.1X3A
T36.1X4A
T36.1X5A
T36.2X1A
T36.2X2A
T36.2X3A
T36.2X4A
T36.2X5A
T36.3X1A
T36.3X2A
T36.3X3A
T36.3X4A
T36.3X5A
T36.4X1A
T36.4X2A
T36.4X3A
T36.4X4A
T36.4X5A
T36.5X1A
T36.5X2A
T36.5X3A
T36.5X4A
T36.5X5A
T36.6X1A
T36.6X2A
T36.6X3A
T36.6X4A
T36.6X5A
T36.7X1A
T36.7X2A
T36.7X3A
T36.7X4A
T36.7X5A
T36.8X1A
T36.8X2A
T36.8X3A
T36.8X4A
T36.8X5A
T36.91XA
T36.92XA
T36.93XA
T36.94XA
T36.95XA
T37.ØX1A
T37.ØX2A
T37.ØX3A
T37.ØX4A
T37.ØX5A
T37.1X1A
T37.1X2A
T37.1X3A
T37.1X4A
T37.1X5A
T37.2X1A
T37.2X2A
T37.2X3A
T37.2X4A
T37.2X5A
T37.3X1A
T37.3X2A
T37.3X3A
T37.3X4A
T37.3X5A
T37.4X1A
T37.4X2A
T37.4X3A
T37.4X4A
T37.4X5A
T37.5X1A
T37.5X2A
T37.5X3A
T37.5X4A
T37.5X5A
T37.8X1A
T37.8X2A
T37.8X3A
T37.8X4A
T37.8X5A
T37.91XA
T37.92XA
T37.93XA
T37.94XA
T37.95XA
T38.ØX1A
T38.ØX2A
T38.ØX3A
T38.ØX4A
T38.ØX5A
T38.1X1A
T38.1X2A
T38.1X3A
T38.1X4A
T38.1X5A
T38.2X1A
T38.2X2A
T38.2X3A
T38.2X4A
T38.2X5A
T38.3X1A
T38.3X2A
T38.3X3A
T38.3X4A
T38.3X5A
T38.4X1A
T38.4X2A
T38.4X3A
T38.4X4A
T38.4X5A
T38.5X1A
T38.5X2A
T38.5X3A
T38.5X4A
T38.5X5A
T38.6X1A
T38.6X2A
T38.6X3A
T38.6X4A
T38.6X5A
T38.7X1A
T38.7X2A
T38.7X3A
T38.7X4A
T38.7X5A
T38.8Ø1A
T38.8Ø2A
T38.8Ø3A
T38.8Ø4A
T38.8Ø5A
T38.811A
T38.812A
T38.813A
T38.814A
T38.815A
T38.891A
T38.892A
T38.893A
T38.894A
T38.895A
T38.9Ø1A
T38.9Ø2A
T38.9Ø3A
T38.9Ø4A
T38.9Ø5A
T38.991A
T38.992A
T38.993A
T38.994A
T38.995A
T39.Ø11A
T39.Ø12A
T39.Ø13A
T39.Ø14A
T39.Ø15A
T39.Ø91A
T39.Ø92A
T39.Ø93A
T39.Ø94A
T39.Ø95A
T39.1X1A
T39.1X2A
T39.1X3A
T39.1X4A
T39.1X5A
T39.2X1A
T39.2X2A
T39.2X3A
T39.2X4A
T39.2X5A
T39.311A
T39.312A
T39.313A
T39.314A
T39.315A
T39.391A
T39.392A
T39.393A
T39.394A
T39.395A
T39.4X1A
T39.4X2A
T39.4X3A
T39.4X4A
T39.4X5A
T39.8X1A

T39.8X2A
T39.8X3A
T39.8X4A
T39.8X5A
T39.91XA
T39.92XA
T39.93XA
T39.94XA
T39.95XA
T4Ø.ØX1A
T4Ø.ØX2A
T4Ø.ØX3A
T4Ø.ØX4A
T4Ø.ØX5A
T4Ø.1X1A
T4Ø.1X2A
T4Ø.1X3A
T4Ø.1X4A
T4Ø.2X1A
T4Ø.2X2A
T4Ø.2X3A
T4Ø.2X4A
T4Ø.2X5A
T4Ø.3X1A
T4Ø.3X2A
T4Ø.3X3A
T4Ø.3X4A
T4Ø.3X5A
T4Ø.411A
T4Ø.412A
T4Ø.413A
T4Ø.414A
T4Ø.415A
T4Ø.421A
T4Ø.422A
T4Ø.423A
T4Ø.424A
T4Ø.425A
T4Ø.491A
T4Ø.492A
T4Ø.493A
T4Ø.494A
T4Ø.495A
T4Ø.5X1A
T4Ø.5X2A
T4Ø.5X3A
T4Ø.5X4A
T4Ø.5X5A
T4Ø.6Ø1A
T4Ø.6Ø2A
T4Ø.6Ø3A
T4Ø.6Ø4A
T4Ø.6Ø5A
T4Ø.691A
T4Ø.692A
T4Ø.693A
T4Ø.694A
T4Ø.695A
T4Ø.711A
T4Ø.712A
T4Ø.713A
T4Ø.714A
T4Ø.715A
T4Ø.721A
T4Ø.722A
T4Ø.723A
T4Ø.724A
T4Ø.725A
T4Ø.8X1A
T4Ø.8X2A
T4Ø.8X3A
T4Ø.8X4A
T4Ø.9Ø1A
T4Ø.9Ø2A
T4Ø.9Ø3A
T4Ø.9Ø4A
T4Ø.9Ø5A
T4Ø.991A
T4Ø.992A
T4Ø.993A
T4Ø.994A
T4Ø.995A
T41.ØX1A
T41.ØX2A
T41.ØX3A
T41.ØX4A
T41.ØX5A
T41.1X1A
T41.1X2A
T41.1X3A
T41.1X4A
T41.1X5A
T41.2Ø1A
T41.2Ø2A
T41.2Ø3A
T41.2Ø4A
T41.2Ø5A
T41.291A
T41.292A
T41.293A
T41.294A
T41.295A
T41.3X1A
T41.3X2A
T41.3X3A
T41.3X4A
T41.3X5A
T41.41XA
T41.42XA
T41.43XA
T41.44XA
T41.45XA
T41.5X1A
T41.5X2A
T41.5X3A
T41.5X4A
T41.5X5A
T42.ØX1A
T42.ØX2A
T42.ØX3A
T42.ØX4A
T42.ØX5A
T42.1X1A
T42.1X2A
T42.1X3A
T42.1X4A
T42.1X5A
T42.2X1A
T42.2X2A
T42.2X3A
T42.2X4A
T42.2X5A
T42.3X1A
T42.3X2A
T42.3X3A
T42.3X4A
T42.3X5A
T42.4X1A
T42.4X2A
T42.4X3A
T42.4X4A
T42.4X5A
T42.5X1A
T42.5X2A
T42.5X3A
T42.5X4A
T42.5X5A
T42.6X1A
T42.6X2A
T42.6X3A
T42.6X4A
T42.6X5A
T42.71XA
T42.72XA
T42.73XA
T42.74XA
T42.75XA
T42.8X1A
T42.8X2A
T42.8X3A
T42.8X4A
T42.8X5A
T43.Ø11A
T43.Ø12A
T43.Ø13A
T43.Ø14A
T43.Ø15A
T43.Ø21A
T43.Ø22A
T43.Ø23A
T43.Ø24A
T43.Ø25A
T43.1X1A
T43.1X2A
T43.1X3A
T43.1X4A
T43.1X5A
T43.2Ø1A
T43.2Ø2A
T43.2Ø3A
T43.2Ø4A
T43.2Ø5A
T43.211A
T43.212A
T43.213A
T43.214A
T43.215A
T43.221A
T43.222A
T43.223A
T43.224A
T43.225A
T43.291A
T43.292A
T43.293A
T43.294A
T43.295A
T43.3X1A
T43.3X2A
T43.3X3A
T43.3X4A
T43.3X5A
T43.4X1A
T43.4X2A
T43.4X3A
T43.4X4A
T43.4X5A
T43.5Ø1A
T43.5Ø2A
T43.5Ø3A
T43.5Ø4A
T43.5Ø5A
T43.591A
T43.592A
T43.593A
T43.594A
T43.595A
T43.6Ø1A
T43.6Ø2A
T43.6Ø3A
T43.6Ø4A
T43.6Ø5A
T43.611A
T43.612A
T43.613A
T43.614A
T43.615A
T43.621A
T43.622A
T43.623A
T43.624A
T43.625A
T43.631A
T43.632A
T43.633A
T43.634A
T43.635A
T43.641A
T43.642A
T43.643A
T43.644A
T43.651A
T43.652A
T43.653A
T43.654A
T43.655A
T43.691A
T43.692A
T43.693A
T43.694A
T43.695A
T43.8X1A
T43.8X2A
T43.8X3A
T43.8X4A
T43.8X5A
T43.91XA
T43.92XA
T43.93XA
T43.94XA
T43.95XA
T44.ØX1A
T44.ØX2A
T44.ØX3A
T44.ØX4A
T44.ØX5A
T44.1X1A
T44.1X2A
T44.1X3A
T44.1X4A
T44.1X5A
T44.2X1A
T44.2X2A
T44.2X3A
T44.2X4A
T44.2X5A
T44.3X1A
T44.3X2A
T44.3X3A
T44.3X4A
T44.3X5A
T44.4X1A
T44.4X2A
T44.4X3A
T44.4X4A
T44.4X5A
T44.5X1A
T44.5X2A
T44.5X3A
T44.5X4A
T44.5X5A
T44.6X1A
T44.6X2A
T44.6X3A
T44.6X4A
T44.6X5A
T44.7X1A
T44.7X2A
T44.7X3A
T44.7X4A
T44.7X5A
T44.8X1A
T44.8X2A
T44.8X3A
T44.8X4A
T44.8X5A
T44.9Ø1A
T44.9Ø2A
T44.9Ø3A
T44.9Ø4A
T44.9Ø5A
T44.991A
T44.992A
T44.993A
T44.994A
T44.995A
T45.ØX1A
T45.ØX2A
T45.ØX3A
T45.ØX4A
T45.ØX5A
T45.1X1A
T45.1X2A
T45.1X3A
T45.1X4A
T45.1X5A
T45.2X1A
T45.2X2A
T45.2X3A
T45.2X4A
T45.2X5A
T45.3X1A
T45.3X2A
T45.3X3A
T45.3X4A
T45.3X5A
T45.4X1A
T45.4X2A
T45.4X3A
T45.4X4A
T45.4X5A
T45.511A
T45.512A
T45.513A
T45.514A
T45.515A
T45.521A
T45.522A
T45.523A
T45.524A
T45.525A
T45.6Ø1A
T45.6Ø2A
T45.6Ø3A
T45.6Ø4A
T45.6Ø5A
T45.611A
T45.612A
T45.613A
T45.614A
T45.615A
T45.621A
T45.622A
T45.623A
T45.624A
T45.625A
T45.691A
T45.692A
T45.693A
T45.694A
T45.695A
T45.7X1A
T45.7X2A
T45.7X3A
T45.7X4A
T45.7X5A
T45.8X1A
T45.8X2A
T45.8X3A
T45.8X4A
T45.8X5A
T45.91XA
T45.92XA
T45.93XA
T45.94XA
T45.95XA
T46.ØX1A
T46.ØX2A
T46.ØX3A
T46.ØX4A
T46.ØX5A
T46.1X1A
T46.1X2A
T46.1X3A
T46.1X4A
T46.1X5A
T46.2X1A
T46.2X2A
T46.2X3A
T46.2X4A
T46.2X5A
T46.3X1A
T46.3X2A
T46.3X3A
T46.3X4A
T46.3X5A
T46.4X1A
T46.4X2A
T46.4X3A
T46.4X4A
T46.4X5A
T46.5X1A
T46.5X2A
T46.5X3A
T46.5X4A
T46.5X5A
T46.6X1A
T46.6X2A
T46.6X3A
T46.6X4A
T46.6X5A
T46.7X1A
T46.7X2A
T46.7X3A
T46.7X4A
T46.7X5A
T46.8X1A
T46.8X2A
T46.8X3A
T46.8X4A
T46.8X5A
T46.9Ø1A
T46.9Ø2A
T46.9Ø3A
T46.9Ø4A
T46.9Ø5A
T46.991A
T46.992A
T46.993A
T46.994A
T46.995A
T47.ØX1A
T47.ØX2A
T47.ØX3A
T47.ØX4A
T47.ØX5A
T47.1X1A
T47.1X2A
T47.1X3A
T47.1X4A
T47.1X5A
T47.2X1A
T47.2X2A
T47.2X3A
T47.2X4A
T47.2X5A
T47.3X1A
T47.3X2A
T47.3X3A
T47.3X4A
T47.3X5A
T47.4X1A
T47.4X2A
T47.4X3A
T47.4X4A
T47.4X5A
T47.5X1A
T47.5X2A
T47.5X3A
T47.5X4A
T47.5X5A
T47.6X1A
T47.6X2A
T47.6X3A
T47.6X4A
T47.6X5A
T47.7X1A
T47.7X2A
T47.7X3A
T47.7X4A
T47.7X5A
T47.8X1A
T47.8X2A
T47.8X3A
T47.8X4A
T47.8X5A
T47.91XA
T47.92XA
T47.93XA
T47.94XA
T47.95XA
T48.ØX1A
T48.ØX2A
T48.ØX3A
T48.ØX4A
T48.ØX5A
T48.1X1A
T48.1X2A
T48.1X3A
T48.1X4A
T48.1X5A
T48.2Ø1A
T48.2Ø2A
T48.2Ø3A
T48.2Ø4A
T48.2Ø5A
T48.291A
T48.292A
T48.293A
T48.294A
T48.295A
T48.3X1A
T48.3X2A
T48.3X3A
T48.3X4A
T48.3X5A
T48.4X1A
T48.4X2A
T48.4X3A
T48.4X4A
T48.4X5A
T48.5X1A
T48.5X2A
T48.5X3A
T48.5X4A
T48.5X5A
T48.6X1A
T48.6X2A
T48.6X3A
T48.6X4A
T48.6X5A
T48.9Ø1A
T48.9Ø2A
T48.9Ø3A
T48.9Ø4A
T48.9Ø5A
T48.991A
T48.992A
T48.993A
T48.994A
T48.995A
T49.ØX1A
T49.ØX2A
T49.ØX3A
T49.ØX4A
T49.ØX5A
T49.1X1A
T49.1X2A
T49.1X3A
T49.1X4A
T49.1X5A
T49.2X1A
T49.2X2A
T49.2X3A
T49.2X4A
T49.2X5A
T49.3X1A
T49.3X2A
T49.3X3A
T49.3X4A
T49.3X5A
T49.4X1A
T49.4X2A
T49.4X3A
T49.4X4A
T49.4X5A
T49.5X1A
T49.5X2A
T49.5X3A
T49.5X4A
T49.5X5A
T49.6X1A
T49.6X2A
T49.6X3A
T49.6X4A
T49.6X5A
T49.7X1A
T49.7X2A
T49.7X3A
T49.7X4A
T49.7X5A
T49.8X1A
T49.8X2A
T49.8X3A
T49.8X4A
T49.8X5A
T49.91XA
T49.92XA
T49.93XA
T49.94XA
T49.95XA
T5Ø.ØX1A
T5Ø.ØX2A
T5Ø.ØX3A
T5Ø.ØX4A
T5Ø.ØX5A
T5Ø.1X1A
T5Ø.1X2A
T5Ø.1X3A
T5Ø.1X4A
T5Ø.1X5A
T5Ø.2X1A
T5Ø.2X2A
T5Ø.2X3A
T5Ø.2X4A
T5Ø.2X5A
T5Ø.3X1A
T5Ø.3X2A
T5Ø.3X3A
T5Ø.3X4A
T5Ø.3X5A
T5Ø.4X1A
T5Ø.4X2A
T5Ø.4X3A
T5Ø.4X4A
T5Ø.4X5A
T5Ø.5X1A
T5Ø.5X2A
T5Ø.5X3A
T5Ø.5X4A
T5Ø.5X5A
T5Ø.6X1A
T5Ø.6X2A
T5Ø.6X3A
T5Ø.6X4A
T5Ø.6X5A
T5Ø.7X1A
T5Ø.7X2A
T5Ø.7X3A
T5Ø.7X4A
T5Ø.7X5A
T5Ø.8X1A
T5Ø.8X2A
T5Ø.8X3A
T5Ø.8X4A
T5Ø.8X5A
T5Ø.9Ø1A
T5Ø.9Ø2A
T5Ø.9Ø3A
T5Ø.9Ø4A
T5Ø.9Ø5A
T5Ø.911A
T5Ø.912A
T5Ø.913A
T5Ø.914A
T5Ø.915A
T5Ø.991A
T5Ø.992A
T5Ø.993A
T5Ø.994A
T5Ø.995A
T5Ø.A11A
T5Ø.A12A
T5Ø.A13A
T5Ø.A14A
T5Ø.A15A
T5Ø.A21A
T5Ø.A22A
T5Ø.A23A
T5Ø.A24A
T5Ø.A25A
T5Ø.A91A
T5Ø.A92A
T5Ø.A93A
T5Ø.A94A
T5Ø.A95A
T5Ø.B11A
T5Ø.B12A
T5Ø.B13A
T5Ø.B14A
T5Ø.B15A
T5Ø.B91A
T5Ø.B92A
T5Ø.B93A
T5Ø.B94A
T5Ø.B95A
T5Ø.Z11A
T5Ø.Z12A
T5Ø.Z13A
T5Ø.Z14A
T5Ø.Z15A
T5Ø.Z91A
T5Ø.Z92A
T5Ø.Z93A
T5Ø.Z94A
T5Ø.Z95A
T51.ØX1A
T51.ØX2A
T51.ØX3A
T51.ØX4A
T51.1X1A
T51.1X2A
T51.1X3A
T51.1X4A
T51.2X1A
T51.2X2A
T51.2X3A
T51.2X4A
T51.3X1A
T51.3X2A
T51.3X3A
T51.3X4A
T51.8X1A
T51.8X2A
T51.8X3A
T51.8X4A
T51.91XA
T51.92XA
T51.93XA
T51.94XA
T52.ØX1A
T52.ØX2A
T52.ØX3A
T52.ØX4A
T52.1X1A
T52.1X2A
T52.1X3A
T52.1X4A
T52.2X1A
T52.2X2A
T52.2X3A
T52.2X4A
T52.3X1A
T52.3X2A
T52.3X3A
T52.3X4A
T52.4X1A
T52.4X2A
T52.4X3A
T52.4X4A
T52.8X1A
T52.8X2A
T52.8X3A
T52.8X4A
T52.91XA
T52.92XA
T52.93XA
T52.94XA
T53.ØX1A
T53.ØX2A
T53.ØX3A
T53.ØX4A
T53.1X1A
T53.1X2A
T53.1X3A
T53.1X4A
T53.2X1A
T53.2X2A
T53.2X3A
T53.2X4A
T53.3X1A
T53.3X2A
T53.3X3A
T53.3X4A
T53.4X1A
T53.4X2A
T53.4X3A
T53.4X4A
T53.5X1A
T53.5X2A
T53.5X3A
T53.5X4A
T53.6X1A
T53.6X2A
T53.6X3A
T53.6X4A
T53.7X1A
T53.7X2A
T53.7X3A
T53.7X4A
T53.91XA
T53.92XA
T53.93XA
T53.94XA
T54.ØX1A
T54.ØX2A
T54.ØX3A
T54.ØX4A
T54.1X1A
T54.1X2A
T54.1X3A
T54.1X4A
T54.2X1A
T54.2X2A
T54.2X3A
T54.2X4A
T54.3X1A
T54.3X2A
T54.3X3A
T54.3X4A
T54.91XA
T54.92XA
T54.93XA
T54.94XA
T55.ØX1A
T55.ØX2A
T55.ØX3A
T55.ØX4A
T55.1X1A
T55.1X2A
T55.1X3A
T55.1X4A
T56.ØX1A
T56.ØX2A
T56.ØX3A
T56.ØX4A
T56.1X1A
T56.1X2A
T56.1X3A
T56.1X4A
T56.2X1A
T56.2X2A
T56.2X3A
T56.2X4A
T56.3X1A
T56.3X2A
T56.3X3A
T56.3X4A
T56.4X1A
T56.4X2A
T56.4X3A
T56.4X4A
T56.5X1A
T56.5X2A
T56.5X3A
T56.5X4A
T56.6X1A
T56.6X2A
T56.6X3A
T56.6X4A
T56.7X1A
T56.7X2A
T56.7X3A
T56.7X4A
T56.811A
T56.812A
T56.813A
T56.814A
T56.821A
T56.822A
T56.823A
T56.824A
T56.891A
T56.892A
T56.893A
T56.894A
T56.91XA
T56.92XA
T56.93XA
T56.94XA
T57.ØX1A
T57.ØX2A
T57.ØX3A
T57.ØX4A
T57.1X1A

T57.1X2A
T57.1X3A
T57.1X4A
T57.2X1A
T57.2X2A
T57.2X3A
T57.2X4A
T57.3X1A
T57.3X2A
T57.3X3A
T57.3X4A
T57.8X1A
T57.8X2A
T57.8X3A
T57.8X4A
T57.91XA
T57.92XA
T57.93XA
T57.94XA
T58.Ø1XA
T58.Ø2XA
T58.Ø3XA
T58.Ø4XA
T58.11XA
T58.12XA
T58.13XA
T58.14XA
T58.2X1A
T58.2X2A
T58.2X3A
T58.2X4A
T58.8X1A
T58.8X2A
T58.8X3A
T58.8X4A
T58.91XA
T58.92XA
T58.93XA
T58.94XA
T59.ØX1A
T59.ØX2A
T59.ØX3A
T59.ØX4A
T59.1X1A
T59.1X2A
T59.1X3A
T59.1X4A
T59.2X1A
T59.2X2A
T59.2X3A
T59.2X4A
T59.3X1A
T59.3X2A
T59.3X3A
T59.3X4A
T59.4X1A
T59.4X2A
T59.4X3A
T59.4X4A
T59.5X1A
T59.5X2A
T59.5X3A
T59.5X4A
T59.6X1A
T59.6X2A
T59.6X3A
T59.6X4A
T59.7X1A
T59.7X2A
T59.7X3A
T59.7X4A
T59.811A
T59.812A
T59.813A
T59.814A
T59.891A
T59.892A
T59.893A
T59.894A
T59.91XA
T59.92XA
T59.93XA
T59.94XA
T6Ø.ØX1A
T6Ø.ØX2A
T6Ø.ØX3A
T6Ø.ØX4A
T6Ø.1X1A
T6Ø.1X2A
T6Ø.1X3A
T6Ø.1X4A
T6Ø.2X1A
T6Ø.2X2A
T6Ø.2X3A
T6Ø.2X4A
T6Ø.3X1A
T6Ø.3X2A
T6Ø.3X3A
T6Ø.3X4A
T6Ø.4X1A
T6Ø.4X2A
T6Ø.4X3A
T6Ø.4X4A
T6Ø.8X1A
T6Ø.8X2A
T6Ø.8X3A
T6Ø.8X4A
T6Ø.91XA
T6Ø.92XA
T6Ø.93XA
T6Ø.94XA
T61.Ø1XA
T61.Ø2XA
T61.Ø3XA
T61.Ø4XA
T61.11XA
T61.12XA
T61.13XA
T61.14XA
T61.771A
T61.772A
T61.773A
T61.774A
T61.781A
T61.782A
T61.783A
T61.784A
T61.8X1A
T61.8X2A
T61.8X3A
T61.8X4A
T61.91XA
T61.92XA
T61.93XA
T61.94XA
T62.ØX1A
T62.ØX2A
T62.ØX3A
T62.ØX4A
T62.1X1A
T62.1X2A
T62.1X3A
T62.1X4A
T62.2X1A
T62.2X2A
T62.2X3A
T62.2X4A
T62.8X1A
T62.8X2A
T62.8X3A
T62.8X4A
T62.91XA
T62.92XA
T62.93XA
T62.94XA
T63.ØØ1A
T63.ØØ2A
T63.ØØ3A
T63.ØØ4A
T63.Ø11A
T63.Ø12A
T63.Ø13A
T63.Ø14A
T63.Ø21A
T63.Ø22A
T63.Ø23A
T63.Ø24A
T63.Ø31A
T63.Ø32A
T63.Ø33A
T63.Ø34A
T63.Ø41A
T63.Ø42A
T63.Ø43A
T63.Ø44A
T63.Ø61A
T63.Ø62A
T63.Ø63A
T63.Ø64A
T63.Ø71A
T63.Ø72A
T63.Ø73A
T63.Ø74A
T63.Ø81A
T63.Ø82A
T63.Ø83A
T63.Ø84A
T63.Ø91A
T63.Ø92A
T63.Ø93A
T63.Ø94A
T63.111A
T63.112A
T63.113A
T63.114A
T63.121A
T63.122A
T63.123A
T63.124A
T63.191A
T63.192A
T63.193A
T63.194A
T63.2X1A
T63.2X2A
T63.2X3A
T63.2X4A
T63.3Ø1A
T63.3Ø2A
T63.3Ø3A
T63.3Ø4A
T63.311A
T63.312A
T63.313A
T63.314A
T63.321A
T63.322A
T63.323A
T63.324A
T63.331A
T63.332A
T63.333A
T63.334A
T63.391A
T63.392A
T63.393A
T63.394A
T63.411A
T63.412A
T63.413A
T63.414A
T63.421A
T63.422A
T63.423A
T63.424A
T63.431A
T63.432A
T63.433A
T63.434A
T63.441A
T63.442A
T63.443A
T63.444A
T63.451A
T63.452A
T63.453A
T63.454A
T63.461A
T63.462A
T63.463A
T63.464A
T63.481A
T63.482A
T63.483A
T63.484A
T63.511A
T63.512A
T63.513A
T63.514A
T63.591A
T63.592A
T63.593A
T63.594A
T63.611A
T63.612A
T63.613A
T63.614A
T63.621A
T63.622A
T63.623A
T63.624A
T63.631A
T63.632A
T63.633A
T63.634A
T63.691A
T63.692A
T63.693A
T63.694A
T63.711A
T63.712A
T63.713A
T63.714A
T63.791A
T63.792A
T63.793A
T63.794A
T63.811A
T63.812A
T63.813A
T63.814A
T63.821A
T63.822A
T63.823A
T63.824A
T63.831A
T63.832A
T63.833A
T63.834A
T63.891A
T63.892A
T63.893A
T63.894A
T63.91XA
T63.92XA
T63.93XA
T63.94XA
T64.Ø1XA
T64.Ø2XA
T64.Ø3XA
T64.Ø4XA
T64.81XA
T64.82XA
T64.83XA
T64.84XA
T65.ØX1A
T65.ØX2A
T65.ØX3A
T65.ØX4A
T65.1X1A
T65.1X2A
T65.1X3A
T65.1X4A
T65.211A
T65.212A
T65.213A
T65.214A
T65.221A
T65.222A
T65.223A
T65.224A
T65.291A
T65.292A
T65.293A
T65.294A
T65.3X1A
T65.3X2A
T65.3X3A
T65.3X4A
T65.4X1A
T65.4X2A
T65.4X3A
T65.4X4A
T65.5X1A
T65.5X2A
T65.5X3A
T65.5X4A
T65.6X1A
T65.6X2A
T65.6X3A
T65.6X4A
T65.811A
T65.812A
T65.813A
T65.814A
T65.821A
T65.822A
T65.823A
T65.824A
T65.831A
T65.832A
T65.833A
T65.834A
T65.891A
T65.892A
T65.893A
T65.894A
T65.91XA
T65.92XA
T65.93XA
T65.94XA
T78.41XA
T88.52XA
T88.53XA
T88.59XA

DRG 918

Select principal diagnosis listed under DRG 917

DRG 919

Principal Diagnosis

D47.Z1
D78*
E36*
E89.8*
G96.11
G97.4*
G97.5*
G97.61
G97.62
G97.63
G97.64
H59.Ø1*
H59.Ø3*
H59.Ø9*
H59.1*
H59.2*
H59.3*
H59.8*
H95.2*
H95.3*
H95.4*
H95.51
H95.52
H95.53
H95.54
H95.8*
I97.3
I97.4*
I97.5*
I97.6*
J95.6*
J95.7*
J95.83Ø
J95.831
J95.86Ø
J95.861
J95.862
J95.863
K91.6*
K91.7*
K91.84Ø
K91.841
K91.87Ø
K91.871
K91.872
K91.873
L76*
M96.8*
N98.1
N98.2
N98.3
N98.8
N98.9
N99.6*
N99.7*
N99.82Ø
N99.821
N99.84Ø
N99.841
N99.842
N99.843
T81.1ØXA
T81.11XA
T81.12XA
T81.19XA
T81.3ØXA
T81.31XA
T81.32XA
T81.33XA
T81.5ØØA
T81.5Ø1A
T81.5Ø2A
T81.5Ø3A
T81.5Ø4A
T81.5Ø5A
T81.5Ø6A
T81.5Ø7A
T81.5Ø8A
T81.5Ø9A
T81.51ØA
T81.511A
T81.512A
T81.513A
T81.514A
T81.515A
T81.516A
T81.517A
T81.518A
T81.519A
T81.52ØA
T81.521A
T81.522A
T81.523A
T81.524A
T81.525A
T81.526A
T81.527A
T81.528A
T81.529A
T81.53ØA
T81.531A
T81.532A
T81.533A
T81.534A
T81.535A
T81.536A
T81.537A
T81.538A
T81.539A
T81.59ØA
T81.591A
T81.592A
T81.593A
T81.594A
T81.595A
T81.596A
T81.597A
T81.598A
T81.599A
T81.6ØXA
T81.61XA
T81.69XA
T81.81XA
T81.82XA
T81.83XA
T81.89XA
T81.9XXA
T85.31ØA
T85.311A
T85.32ØA
T85.321A
T85.39ØA
T85.391A
T85.51ØA
T85.511A
T85.518A
T85.52ØA
T85.521A
T85.528A
T85.59ØA
T85.591A
T85.598A
T85.611A
T85.612A
T85.613A
T85.614A
T85.618A
T85.621A
T85.622A
T85.623A
T85.624A
T85.628A
T85.631A
T85.633A
T85.638A
T85.691A
T85.692A
T85.693A
T85.694A
T85.698A
T85.71XA
T85.72XA
T85.79XA
T85.818A
T85.828A
T85.838A
T85.848A
T85.858A
T85.868A
T85.898A
T85.9XXA
T86.5
T86.82*
T86.83*
T86.842*
T86.848*
T86.849*
T86.85*
T86.9*
T88.4XXA
T88.7XXA
T88.8XXA
T88.9XXA

DRG 920

Select principal diagnosis listed under DRG 919

DRG 921

Select principal diagnosis listed under DRG 919

DRG 922

Principal Diagnosis

M97.Ø1XS
M97.Ø2XS
M97.11XS
M97.12XS
M97.21XS
M97.22XS
M97.31XS
M97.32XS
M97.41XS
M97.42XS
M97.8XXS
M97.9XXS
SØ2.121S
SØ2.122S
SØ2.129S
SØ2.831S
SØ2.832S
SØ2.839S
SØ2.841S
SØ2.842S
SØ2.849S
SØ2.85XS
T33.Ø11A
T33.Ø11S
T33.Ø12A
T33.Ø12S
T33.Ø19A
T33.Ø19S
T33.Ø2XA
T33.Ø2XS
T33.Ø9XA
T33.Ø9XS
T33.1XXA
T33.1XXS
T33.2XXA
T33.2XXS
T33.3XXA
T33.3XXS
T33.4ØXA
T33.4ØXS
T33.41XA
T33.41XS
T33.42XA
T33.42XS
T33.511A
T33.511S
T33.512A
T33.512S
T33.519A
T33.519S
T33.521A
T33.521S
T33.522A
T33.522S
T33.529A
T33.529S
T33.531A
T33.531S
T33.532A
T33.532S
T33.539A
T33.539S
T33.6ØXA
T33.6ØXS
T33.61XA
T33.61XS
T33.62XA
T33.62XS
T33.7ØXA
T33.7ØXS
T33.71XA
T33.71XS
T33.72XA
T33.72XS
T33.811A
T33.811S
T33.812A
T33.812S
T33.819A
T33.819S
T33.821A
T33.821S
T33.822A
T33.822S
T33.829A
T33.829S
T33.831A
T33.831S
T33.832A
T33.832S
T33.839A
T33.839S
T33.9ØXA
T33.9ØXS
T33.99XA
T33.99XS
T34.Ø11A
T34.Ø11S
T34.Ø12A
T34.Ø12S
T34.Ø19A
T34.Ø19S
T34.Ø2XA
T34.Ø2XS
T34.Ø9XA
T34.Ø9XS
T34.1XXA
T34.1XXS
T34.2XXA
T34.2XXS
T34.3XXA
T34.3XXS
T34.4ØXA
T34.4ØXS
T34.41XA
T34.41XS
T34.42XA
T34.42XS
T34.511A
T34.511S
T34.512A
T34.512S
T34.519A
T34.519S
T34.521A
T34.521S
T34.522A
T34.522S
T34.529A
T34.529S
T34.531A
T34.531S
T34.532A
T34.532S
T34.539A
T34.539S
T34.6ØXA
T34.6ØXS
T34.61XA
T34.61XS
T34.62XA
T34.62XS
T34.7ØXA
T34.7ØXS
T34.71XA
T34.71XS
T34.72XA
T34.72XS
T34.811A
T34.811S
T34.812A
T34.812S
T34.819A
T34.819S
T34.821A
T34.821S
T34.822A
T34.822S
T34.829A
T34.829S
T34.831A
T34.831S
T34.832A
T34.832S
T34.839A
T34.839S
T34.9ØXA
T34.9ØXS
T34.99XA
T34.99XS
T36.ØX1S
T36.ØX2S
T36.ØX3S
T36.ØX4S
T36.ØX5S
T36.1X1S
T36.1X2S
T36.1X3S
T36.1X4S
T36.1X5S
T36.2X1S
T36.2X2S
T36.2X3S
T36.2X4S
T36.2X5S
T36.3X1S
T36.3X2S
T36.3X3S
T36.3X4S
T36.3X5S
T36.4X1S
T36.4X2S
T36.4X3S
T36.4X4S
T36.4X5S
T36.5X1S
T36.5X2S
T36.5X3S
T36.5X4S
T36.5X5S
T36.6X1S
T36.6X2S
T36.6X3S
T36.6X4S
T36.6X5S
T36.7X1S
T36.7X2S
T36.7X3S
T36.7X4S
T36.7X5S
T36.8X1S
T36.8X2S
T36.8X3S
T36.8X4S
T36.8X5S
T36.91XS
T36.92XS
T36.93XS
T36.94XS
T36.95XS
T37.ØX1S
T37.ØX2S
T37.ØX3S
T37.ØX4S
T37.ØX5S
T37.1X1S
T37.1X2S
T37.1X3S
T37.1X4S
T37.1X5S
T37.2X1S
T37.2X2S
T37.2X3S
T37.2X4S
T37.2X5S
T37.3X1S
T37.3X2S
T37.3X3S
T37.3X4S
T37.3X5S
T37.4X1S
T37.4X2S
T37.4X3S
T37.4X4S
T37.4X5S
T37.5X1S
T37.5X2S
T37.5X3S
T37.5X4S
T37.5X5S
T37.8X1S
T37.8X2S
T37.8X3S
T37.8X4S
T37.8X5S
T37.91XS
T37.92XS
T37.93XS
T37.94XS
T37.95XS
T38.ØX1S
T38.ØX2S
T38.ØX3S
T38.ØX4S
T38.ØX5S
T38.1X1S
T38.1X2S
T38.1X3S
T38.1X4S
T38.1X5S
T38.2X1S
T38.2X2S

T38.2X3S
T38.2X4S
T38.2X5S
T38.3X1S
T38.3X2S
T38.3X3S
T38.3X4S
T38.3X5S
T38.4X1S
T38.4X2S
T38.4X3S
T38.4X4S
T38.4X5S
T38.5X1S
T38.5X2S
T38.5X3S
T38.5X4S
T38.5X5S
T38.6X1S
T38.6X2S
T38.6X3S
T38.6X4S
T38.6X5S
T38.7X1S
T38.7X2S
T38.7X3S
T38.7X4S
T38.7X5S
T38.801S
T38.802S
T38.803S
T38.804S
T38.805S
T38.811S
T38.812S
T38.813S
T38.814S
T38.815S
T38.891S
T38.892S
T38.893S
T38.894S
T38.895S
T38.901S
T38.902S
T38.903S
T38.904S
T38.905S
T38.991S
T38.992S
T38.993S
T38.994S
T38.995S
T39.011S
T39.012S
T39.013S
T39.014S
T39.015S
T39.091S
T39.092S
T39.093S
T39.094S
T39.095S
T39.1X1S
T39.1X2S
T39.1X3S
T39.1X4S
T39.1X5S
T39.2X1S
T39.2X2S
T39.2X3S
T39.2X4S
T39.2X5S
T39.311S
T39.312S
T39.313S
T39.314S
T39.315S
T39.391S
T39.392S
T39.393S
T39.394S
T39.395S
T39.4X1S
T39.4X2S
T39.4X3S
T39.4X4S
T39.4X5S
T39.8X1S
T39.8X2S
T39.8X3S
T39.8X4S
T39.8X5S
T39.91XS
T39.92XS
T39.93XS
T39.94XS
T39.95XS
T40.0X1S
T40.0X2S
T40.0X3S
T40.0X4S
T40.0X5S
T40.1X1S
T40.1X2S
T40.1X3S
T40.1X4S
T40.2X1S
T40.2X2S
T40.2X3S
T40.2X4S
T40.2X5S
T40.3X1S
T40.3X2S
T40.3X3S
T40.3X4S
T40.3X5S
T40.411S
T40.412S
T40.413S
T40.414S
T40.415S
T40.421S
T40.422S
T40.423S
T40.424S
T40.425S
T40.491S
T40.492S
T40.493S
T40.494S
T40.495S
T40.5X1S
T40.5X2S
T40.5X3S
T40.5X4S
T40.5X5S
T40.601S
T40.602S
T40.603S
T40.604S
T40.605S
T40.691S
T40.692S
T40.693S
T40.694S
T40.695S
T40.711S
T40.712S
T40.713S
T40.714S
T40.715S
T40.721S
T40.722S
T40.723S
T40.724S
T40.725S
T40.8X1S
T40.8X2S
T40.8X3S
T40.8X4S
T40.901S
T40.902S
T40.903S
T40.904S
T40.905S
T40.991S
T40.992S
T40.993S
T40.994S
T40.995S
T41.0X1S
T41.0X2S
T41.0X3S
T41.0X4S
T41.0X5S
T41.1X1S
T41.1X2S
T41.1X3S
T41.1X4S
T41.1X5S
T41.201S
T41.202S
T41.203S
T41.204S
T41.205S
T41.291S
T41.292S
T41.293S
T41.294S
T41.295S
T41.3X1S
T41.3X2S
T41.3X3S
T41.3X4S
T41.3X5S
T41.41XS
T41.42XS
T41.43XS
T41.44XS
T41.45XS
T41.5X1S
T41.5X2S
T41.5X3S
T41.5X4S
T41.5X5S
T42.0X1S
T42.0X2S
T42.0X3S
T42.0X4S
T42.0X5S
T42.1X1S
T42.1X2S
T42.1X3S
T42.1X4S
T42.1X5S
T42.2X1S
T42.2X2S
T42.2X3S
T42.2X4S
T42.2X5S
T42.3X1S
T42.3X2S
T42.3X3S
T42.3X4S
T42.3X5S
T42.4X1S
T42.4X2S
T42.4X3S
T42.4X4S
T42.4X5S
T42.5X1S
T42.5X2S
T42.5X3S
T42.5X4S
T42.5X5S
T42.6X1S
T42.6X2S
T42.6X3S
T42.6X4S
T42.6X5S
T42.71XS
T42.72XS
T42.73XS
T42.74XS
T42.75XS
T42.8X1S
T42.8X2S
T42.8X3S
T42.8X4S
T42.8X5S
T43.011S
T43.012S
T43.013S
T43.014S
T43.015S
T43.021S
T43.022S
T43.023S
T43.024S
T43.025S
T43.1X1S
T43.1X2S
T43.1X3S
T43.1X4S
T43.1X5S
T43.201S
T43.202S
T43.203S
T43.204S
T43.205S
T43.211S
T43.212S
T43.213S
T43.214S
T43.215S
T43.221S
T43.222S
T43.223S
T43.224S
T43.225S
T43.291S
T43.292S
T43.293S
T43.294S
T43.295S
T43.3X1S
T43.3X2S
T43.3X3S
T43.3X4S
T43.3X5S
T43.4X1S
T43.4X2S
T43.4X3S
T43.4X4S
T43.4X5S
T43.501S
T43.502S
T43.503S
T43.504S
T43.505S
T43.591S
T43.592S
T43.593S
T43.594S
T43.595S
T43.601S
T43.602S
T43.603S
T43.604S
T43.605S
T43.611S
T43.612S
T43.613S
T43.614S
T43.615S
T43.621S
T43.622S
T43.623S
T43.624S
T43.625S
T43.631S
T43.632S
T43.633S
T43.634S
T43.635S
T43.641S
T43.642S
T43.643S
T43.644S
T43.651S
T43.652S
T43.653S
T43.654S
T43.655S
T43.691S
T43.692S
T43.693S
T43.694S
T43.695S
T43.8X1S
T43.8X2S
T43.8X3S
T43.8X4S
T43.8X5S
T43.91XS
T43.92XS
T43.93XS
T43.94XS
T43.95XS
T44.0X1S
T44.0X2S
T44.0X3S
T44.0X4S
T44.0X5S
T44.1X1S
T44.1X2S
T44.1X3S
T44.1X4S
T44.1X5S
T44.2X1S
T44.2X2S
T44.2X3S
T44.2X4S
T44.2X5S
T44.3X1S
T44.3X2S
T44.3X3S
T44.3X4S
T44.3X5S
T44.4X1S
T44.4X2S
T44.4X3S
T44.4X4S
T44.4X5S
T44.5X1S
T44.5X2S
T44.5X3S
T44.5X4S
T44.5X5S
T44.6X1S
T44.6X2S
T44.6X3S
T44.6X4S
T44.6X5S
T44.7X1S
T44.7X2S
T44.7X3S
T44.7X4S
T44.7X5S
T44.8X1S
T44.8X2S
T44.8X3S
T44.8X4S
T44.8X5S
T44.901S
T44.902S
T44.903S
T44.904S
T44.905S
T44.991S
T44.992S
T44.993S
T44.994S
T44.995S
T45.0X1S
T45.0X2S
T45.0X3S
T45.0X4S
T45.0X5S
T45.1X1S
T45.1X2S
T45.1X3S
T45.1X4S
T45.1X5S
T45.2X1S
T45.2X2S
T45.2X3S
T45.2X4S
T45.2X5S
T45.3X1S
T45.3X2S
T45.3X3S
T45.3X4S
T45.3X5S
T45.4X1S
T45.4X2S
T45.4X3S
T45.4X4S
T45.4X5S
T45.511S
T45.512S
T45.513S
T45.514S
T45.515S
T45.521S
T45.522S
T45.523S
T45.524S
T45.525S
T45.601S
T45.602S
T45.603S
T45.604S
T45.605S
T45.611S
T45.612S
T45.613S
T45.614S
T45.615S
T45.621S
T45.622S
T45.623S
T45.624S
T45.625S
T45.691S
T45.692S
T45.693S
T45.694S
T45.695S
T45.7X1S
T45.7X2S
T45.7X3S
T45.7X4S
T45.7X5S
T45.8X1S
T45.8X2S
T45.8X3S
T45.8X4S
T45.8X5S
T45.91XS
T45.92XS
T45.93XS
T45.94XS
T45.95XS
T46.0X1S
T46.0X2S
T46.0X3S
T46.0X4S
T46.0X5S
T46.1X1S
T46.1X2S
T46.1X3S
T46.1X4S
T46.1X5S
T46.2X1S
T46.2X2S
T46.2X3S
T46.2X4S
T46.2X5S
T46.3X1S
T46.3X2S
T46.3X3S
T46.3X4S
T46.3X5S
T46.4X1S
T46.4X2S
T46.4X3S
T46.4X4S
T46.4X5S
T46.5X1S
T46.5X2S
T46.5X3S
T46.5X4S
T46.5X5S
T46.6X1S
T46.6X2S
T46.6X3S
T46.6X4S
T46.6X5S
T46.7X1S
T46.7X2S
T46.7X3S
T46.7X4S
T46.7X5S
T46.8X1S
T46.8X2S
T46.8X3S
T46.8X4S
T46.8X5S
T46.901S
T46.902S
T46.903S
T46.904S
T46.905S
T46.991S
T46.992S
T46.993S
T46.994S
T46.995S
T47.0X1S
T47.0X2S
T47.0X3S
T47.0X4S
T47.0X5S
T47.1X1S
T47.1X2S
T47.1X3S
T47.1X4S
T47.1X5S
T47.2X1S
T47.2X2S
T47.2X3S
T47.2X4S
T47.2X5S
T47.3X1S
T47.3X2S
T47.3X3S
T47.3X4S
T47.3X5S
T47.4X1S
T47.4X2S
T47.4X3S
T47.4X4S
T47.4X5S
T47.5X1S
T47.5X2S
T47.5X3S
T47.5X4S
T47.5X5S
T47.6X1S
T47.6X2S
T47.6X3S
T47.6X4S
T47.6X5S
T47.7X1S
T47.7X2S
T47.7X3S
T47.7X4S
T47.7X5S
T47.8X1S
T47.8X2S
T47.8X3S
T47.8X4S
T47.8X5S
T47.91XS
T47.92XS
T47.93XS
T47.94XS
T47.95XS
T48.0X1S
T48.0X2S
T48.0X3S
T48.0X4S
T48.0X5S
T48.1X1S
T48.1X2S
T48.1X3S
T48.1X4S
T48.1X5S
T48.201S
T48.202S
T48.203S
T48.204S
T48.205S
T48.291S
T48.292S
T48.293S
T48.294S
T48.295S
T48.3X1S
T48.3X2S
T48.3X3S
T48.3X4S
T48.3X5S
T48.4X1S
T48.4X2S
T48.4X3S
T48.4X4S
T48.4X5S
T48.5X1S
T48.5X2S
T48.5X3S
T48.5X4S
T48.5X5S
T48.6X1S
T48.6X2S
T48.6X3S
T48.6X4S
T48.6X5S
T48.901S
T48.902S
T48.903S
T48.904S
T48.905S
T48.991S
T48.992S
T48.993S
T48.994S
T48.995S
T49.0X1S
T49.0X2S
T49.0X3S
T49.0X4S
T49.0X5S
T49.1X1S
T49.1X2S
T49.1X3S
T49.1X4S
T49.1X5S
T49.2X1S
T49.2X2S
T49.2X3S
T49.2X4S
T49.2X5S
T49.3X1S
T49.3X2S
T49.3X3S
T49.3X4S
T49.3X5S
T49.4X1S
T49.4X2S
T49.4X3S
T49.4X4S
T49.4X5S
T49.5X1S
T49.5X2S
T49.5X3S
T49.5X4S
T49.5X5S
T49.6X1S
T49.6X2S
T49.6X3S
T49.6X4S
T49.6X5S
T49.7X1S
T49.7X2S
T49.7X3S
T49.7X4S
T49.7X5S
T49.8X1S
T49.8X2S
T49.8X3S
T49.8X4S
T49.8X5S
T49.91XS
T49.92XS
T49.93XS
T49.94XS
T49.95XS
T50.0X1S
T50.0X2S
T50.0X3S
T50.0X4S
T50.0X5S
T50.1X1S
T50.1X2S
T50.1X3S
T50.1X4S
T50.1X5S
T50.2X1S
T50.2X2S
T50.2X3S
T50.2X4S
T50.2X5S
T50.3X1S
T50.3X2S
T50.3X3S
T50.3X4S
T50.3X5S
T50.4X1S
T50.4X2S
T50.4X3S
T50.4X4S
T50.4X5S
T50.5X1S
T50.5X2S
T50.5X3S
T50.5X4S
T50.5X5S
T50.6X1S
T50.6X2S
T50.6X3S
T50.6X4S
T50.6X5S
T50.7X1S
T50.7X2S
T50.7X3S
T50.7X4S
T50.7X5S
T50.8X1S
T50.8X2S
T50.8X3S
T50.8X4S
T50.8X5S
T50.901S
T50.902S
T50.903S
T50.904S
T50.905S
T50.911S
T50.912S
T50.913S
T50.914S
T50.915S
T50.916S
T50.991S
T50.992S
T50.993S
T50.994S
T50.995S
T50.A11S
T50.A12S
T50.A13S
T50.A14S
T50.A15S
T50.A21S
T50.A22S
T50.A23S
T50.A24S
T50.A25S
T50.A91S
T50.A92S
T50.A93S
T50.A94S
T50.A95S
T50.B11S
T50.B12S
T50.B13S
T50.B14S
T50.B15S
T50.B91S
T50.B92S
T50.B93S
T50.B94S
T50.B95S
T50.Z11S
T50.Z12S
T50.Z13S
T50.Z14S
T50.Z15S
T50.Z91S
T50.Z92S
T50.Z93S
T50.Z94S
T50.Z95S
T51.0X1S
T51.0X2S
T51.0X3S
T51.0X4S
T51.1X1S
T51.1X2S
T51.1X3S
T51.1X4S
T51.2X1S
T51.2X2S
T51.2X3S
T51.2X4S
T51.3X1S
T51.3X2S
T51.3X3S
T51.3X4S
T51.8X1S
T51.8X2S
T51.8X3S
T51.8X4S
T51.91XS
T51.92XS
T51.93XS
T51.94XS
T52.0X1S
T52.0X2S
T52.0X3S
T52.0X4S
T52.1X1S
T52.1X2S
T52.1X3S
T52.1X4S
T52.2X1S
T52.2X2S
T52.2X3S
T52.2X4S
T52.3X1S
T52.3X2S
T52.3X3S
T52.3X4S
T52.4X1S
T52.4X2S
T52.4X3S
T52.4X4S
T52.8X1S
T52.8X2S
T52.8X3S
T52.8X4S
T52.91XS
T52.92XS
T52.93XS
T52.94XS
T53.0X1S
T53.0X2S
T53.0X3S
T53.0X4S
T53.1X1S
T53.1X2S
T53.1X3S
T53.1X4S
T53.2X1S
T53.2X2S
T53.2X3S
T53.2X4S
T53.3X1S
T53.3X2S
T53.3X3S
T53.3X4S
T53.4X1S
T53.4X2S
T53.4X3S
T53.4X4S
T53.5X1S
T53.5X2S
T53.5X3S
T53.5X4S
T53.6X1S
T53.6X2S
T53.6X3S

T53.6X4S
T53.7X1S
T53.7X2S
T53.7X3S
T53.7X4S
T53.91XS
T53.92XS
T53.93XS
T53.94XS
T54.ØX1S
T54.ØX2S
T54.ØX3S
T54.ØX4S
T54.1X1S
T54.1X2S
T54.1X3S
T54.1X4S
T54.2X1S
T54.2X2S
T54.2X3S
T54.2X4S
T54.3X1S
T54.3X2S
T54.3X3S
T54.3X4S
T54.91XS
T54.92XS
T54.93XS
T54.94XS
T55.ØX1S
T55.ØX2S
T55.ØX3S
T55.ØX4S
T55.1X1S
T55.1X2S
T55.1X3S
T55.1X4S
T56.ØX1S
T56.ØX2S
T56.ØX3S
T56.ØX4S
T56.1X1S
T56.1X2S
T56.1X3S
T56.1X4S
T56.2X1S
T56.2X2S
T56.2X3S
T56.2X4S
T56.3X1S
T56.3X2S
T56.3X3S
T56.3X4S
T56.4X1S
T56.4X2S
T56.4X3S
T56.4X4S
T56.5X1S
T56.5X2S
T56.5X3S
T56.5X4S
T56.6X1S
T56.6X2S
T56.6X3S
T56.6X4S
T56.7X1S
T56.7X2S
T56.7X3S
T56.7X4S
T56.811S
T56.812S
T56.813S
T56.814S
T56.821S
T56.822S
T56.823S
T56.824S
T56.891S
T56.892S
T56.893S
T56.894S
T56.91XS
T56.92XS
T56.93XS
T56.94XS
T57.ØX1S
T57.ØX2S
T57.ØX3S
T57.ØX4S
T57.1X1S
T57.1X2S
T57.1X3S
T57.1X4S
T57.2X1S
T57.2X2S
T57.2X3S
T57.2X4S
T57.3X1S
T57.3X2S
T57.3X3S
T57.3X4S
T57.8X1S
T57.8X2S
T57.8X3S
T57.8X4S
T57.91XS
T57.92XS
T57.93XS
T57.94XS
T58.Ø1XS
T58.Ø2XS
T58.Ø3XS
T58.Ø4XS
T58.11XS
T58.12XS
T58.13XS
T58.14XS
T58.2X1S
T58.2X2S
T58.2X3S
T58.2X4S
T58.8X1S
T58.8X2S
T58.8X3S
T58.8X4S
T58.91XS
T58.92XS
T58.93XS
T58.94XS
T59.ØX1S
T59.ØX2S
T59.ØX3S
T59.ØX4S
T59.1X1S
T59.1X2S
T59.1X3S
T59.1X4S
T59.2X1S
T59.2X2S
T59.2X3S
T59.2X4S
T59.3X1S
T59.3X2S
T59.3X3S
T59.3X4S
T59.4X1S
T59.4X2S
T59.4X3S
T59.4X4S
T59.5X1S
T59.5X2S
T59.5X3S
T59.5X4S
T59.6X1S
T59.6X2S
T59.6X3S
T59.6X4S
T59.7X1S
T59.7X2S
T59.7X3S
T59.7X4S
T59.811S
T59.812S
T59.813S
T59.814S
T59.891S
T59.892S
T59.893S
T59.894S
T59.91XS
T59.92XS
T59.93XS
T59.94XS
T6Ø.ØX1S
T6Ø.ØX2S
T6Ø.ØX3S
T6Ø.ØX4S
T6Ø.1X1S
T6Ø.1X2S
T6Ø.1X3S
T6Ø.1X4S
T6Ø.2X1S
T6Ø.2X2S
T6Ø.2X3S
T6Ø.2X4S
T6Ø.3X1S
T6Ø.3X2S
T6Ø.3X3S
T6Ø.3X4S
T6Ø.4X1S
T6Ø.4X2S
T6Ø.4X3S
T6Ø.4X4S
T6Ø.8X1S
T6Ø.8X2S
T6Ø.8X3S
T6Ø.8X4S
T6Ø.91XS
T6Ø.92XS
T6Ø.93XS
T6Ø.94XS
T61.Ø1XS
T61.Ø2XS
T61.Ø3XS
T61.Ø4XS
T61.11XS
T61.12XS
T61.13XS
T61.14XS
T61.771S
T61.772S
T61.773S
T61.774S
T61.781S
T61.782S
T61.783S
T61.784S
T61.8X1S
T61.8X2S
T61.8X3S
T61.8X4S
T61.91XS
T61.92XS
T61.93XS
T61.94XS
T62.ØX1S
T62.ØX2S
T62.ØX3S
T62.ØX4S
T62.1X1S
T62.1X2S
T62.1X3S
T62.1X4S
T62.2X1S
T62.2X2S
T62.2X3S
T62.2X4S
T62.8X1S
T62.8X2S
T62.8X3S
T62.8X4S
T62.91XS
T62.92XS
T62.93XS
T62.94XS
T63.ØØ1S
T63.ØØ2S
T63.ØØ3S
T63.ØØ4S
T63.Ø11S
T63.Ø12S
T63.Ø13S
T63.Ø14S
T63.Ø21S
T63.Ø22S
T63.Ø23S
T63.Ø24S
T63.Ø31S
T63.Ø32S
T63.Ø33S
T63.Ø34S
T63.Ø41S
T63.Ø42S
T63.Ø43S
T63.Ø44S
T63.Ø61S
T63.Ø62S
T63.Ø63S
T63.Ø64S
T63.Ø71S
T63.Ø72S
T63.Ø73S
T63.Ø74S
T63.Ø81S
T63.Ø82S
T63.Ø83S
T63.Ø84S
T63.Ø91S
T63.Ø92S
T63.Ø93S
T63.Ø94S
T63.111S
T63.112S
T63.113S
T63.114S
T63.121S
T63.122S
T63.123S
T63.124S
T63.191S
T63.192S
T63.193S
T63.194S
T63.2X1S
T63.2X2S
T63.2X3S
T63.2X4S
T63.3Ø1S
T63.3Ø2S
T63.3Ø3S
T63.3Ø4S
T63.311S
T63.312S
T63.313S
T63.314S
T63.321S
T63.322S
T63.323S
T63.324S
T63.331S
T63.332S
T63.333S
T63.334S
T63.391S
T63.392S
T63.393S
T63.394S
T63.411S
T63.412S
T63.413S
T63.414S
T63.421S
T63.422S
T63.423S
T63.424S
T63.431S
T63.432S
T63.433S
T63.434S
T63.441S
T63.442S
T63.443S
T63.444S
T63.451S
T63.452S
T63.453S
T63.454S
T63.461S
T63.462S
T63.463S
T63.464S
T63.481S
T63.482S
T63.483S
T63.484S
T63.511S
T63.512S
T63.513S
T63.514S
T63.591S
T63.592S
T63.593S
T63.594S
T63.611S
T63.612S
T63.613S
T63.614S
T63.621S
T63.622S
T63.623S
T63.624S
T63.631S
T63.632S
T63.633S
T63.634S
T63.691S
T63.692S
T63.693S
T63.694S
T63.711S
T63.712S
T63.713S
T63.714S
T63.791S
T63.792S
T63.793S
T63.794S
T63.811S
T63.812S
T63.813S
T63.814S
T63.821S
T63.822S
T63.823S
T63.824S
T63.831S
T63.832S
T63.833S
T63.834S
T63.891S
T63.892S
T63.893S
T63.894S
T63.91XS
T63.92XS
T63.93XS
T63.94XS
T64.Ø1XS
T64.Ø2XS
T64.Ø3XS
T64.Ø4XS
T64.81XS
T64.82XS
T64.83XS
T64.84XS
T65.ØX1S
T65.ØX2S
T65.ØX3S
T65.ØX4S
T65.1X1S
T65.1X2S
T65.1X3S
T65.1X4S
T65.211S
T65.212S
T65.213S
T65.214S
T65.221S
T65.222S
T65.223S
T65.224S
T65.291S
T65.292S
T65.293S
T65.294S
T65.3X1S
T65.3X2S
T65.3X3S
T65.3X4S
T65.4X1S
T65.4X2S
T65.4X3S
T65.4X4S
T65.5X1S
T65.5X2S
T65.5X3S
T65.5X4S
T65.6X1S
T65.6X2S
T65.6X3S
T65.6X4S
T65.811S
T65.812S
T65.813S
T65.814S
T65.821S
T65.822S
T65.823S
T65.824S
T65.831S
T65.832S
T65.833S
T65.834S
T65.891S
T65.892S
T65.893S
T65.894S
T65.91XS
T65.92XS
T65.93XS
T65.94XS
T66.XXXA
T66.XXXS
T67.Ø1XA
T67.Ø1XS
T67.Ø2XA
T67.Ø2XS
T67.Ø9XA
T67.Ø9XS
T67.1XXA
T67.1XXS
T67.2XXA
T67.2XXS
T67.3XXA
T67.3XXS
T67.4XXA
T67.4XXS
T67.5XXA
T67.5XXS
T67.6XXA
T67.6XXS
T67.7XXA
T67.7XXS
T67.8XXA
T67.8XXS
T67.9XXA
T67.9XXS
T68.XXXA
T68.XXXS
T69.Ø11A
T69.Ø11S
T69.Ø12A
T69.Ø12S
T69.Ø19A
T69.Ø19S
T69.Ø21A
T69.Ø21S
T69.Ø22A
T69.Ø22S
T69.Ø29A
T69.Ø29S
T69.1XXA
T69.1XXS
T69.8XXA
T69.8XXS
T69.9XXA
T69.9XXS
T7Ø.ØXXS
T7Ø.1XXS
T7Ø.2ØXA
T7Ø.2ØXS
T7Ø.29XA
T7Ø.29XS
T7Ø.3XXA
T7Ø.3XXS
T7Ø.4XXA
T7Ø.4XXS
T7Ø.8XXA
T7Ø.8XXS
T7Ø.9XXA
T7Ø.9XXS
T71.111A
T71.111S
T71.112A
T71.112S
T71.113A
T71.113S
T71.114A
T71.114S
T71.121A
T71.121S
T71.122A
T71.122S
T71.123A
T71.123S
T71.124A
T71.124S
T71.131A
T71.131S
T71.132A
T71.132S
T71.133A
T71.133S
T71.134A
T71.134S
T71.141A
T71.141S
T71.143A
T71.143S
T71.144A
T71.144S
T71.151A
T71.151S
T71.152A
T71.152S
T71.153A
T71.153S
T71.154A
T71.154S
T71.161A
T71.161S
T71.162A
T71.162S
T71.163A
T71.163S
T71.164A
T71.164S
T71.191A
T71.191S
T71.192A
T71.192S
T71.193A
T71.193S
T71.194A
T71.194S
T71.2ØXA
T71.2ØXS
T71.21XA
T71.21XS
T71.221A
T71.221S
T71.222A
T71.222S
T71.223A
T71.223S
T71.224A
T71.224S
T71.231A
T71.231S
T71.232A
T71.232S
T71.233A
T71.233S
T71.234A
T71.234S
T71.29XA
T71.29XS
T71.9XXA
T71.9XXS
T73.ØXXA
T73.ØXXS
T73.1XXA
T73.1XXS
T73.2XXA
T73.2XXS
T73.3XXA
T73.3XXS
T73.8XXA
T73.8XXS
T73.9XXA
T73.9XXS
T74.Ø1XA
T74.Ø1XS
T74.Ø2XA
T74.Ø2XS
T74.11XA
T74.11XS
T74.12XA
T74.12XS
T74.21XA
T74.21XS
T74.22XA
T74.22XS
T74.31XA
T74.31XS
T74.32XA
T74.32XS
T74.4XXA
T74.4XXS
T74.51XA
T74.51XS
T74.52XA
T74.52XS
T74.61XA
T74.61XS
T74.62XA
T74.62XS
T74.91XA
T74.91XS
T74.92XA
T74.92XS
T74.A1XA
T74.A1XS
T74.A2XA
T74.A2XS
T75.ØØXA
T75.ØØXS
T75.Ø1XA
T75.Ø1XS
T75.Ø9XA
T75.Ø9XS
T75.1XXA
T75.1XXS
T75.2ØXA
T75.2ØXS
T75.21XA
T75.21XS
T75.22XA
T75.22XS
T75.23XA
T75.23XS
T75.29XA
T75.29XS
T75.3XXS
T75.4XXA
T75.4XXS
T75.81XA
T75.81XS
T75.82XA
T75.82XS
T75.89XA
T75.89XS
T76.Ø1XA
T76.Ø1XS
T76.Ø2XA
T76.Ø2XS
T76.11XA
T76.11XS
T76.12XA
T76.12XS
T76.21XA
T76.21XS
T76.22XA
T76.22XS
T76.31XA
T76.31XS
T76.32XA
T76.32XS
T76.51XA
T76.51XS
T76.52XA
T76.52XS
T76.61XA
T76.61XS
T76.62XA
T76.62XS
T76.91XA
T76.91XS
T76.92XA
T76.92XS
T76.A1XA
T76.A1XS
T76.A2XA
T76.A2XS
T78.ØØXS
T78.Ø1XS
T78.Ø2XS
T78.Ø3XS
T78.Ø4XS
T78.Ø5XS
T78.Ø6XS
T78.Ø7XS
T78.Ø8XS
T78.Ø9XS
T78.1XXA
T78.1XXS
T78.2XXS
T78.3XXS
T78.4ØXS
T78.41XS
T78.49XS
T78.8XXA
T78.8XXS
T79.2XXA
T79.4XXA
T79.8XXA
T79.9XXA
T79.AØXA
T79.A11A
T79.A12A
T79.A19A
T79.A21A
T79.A22A
T79.A29A
T79.A3XA
T79.A9XA
T8Ø.ØXXS
T8Ø.1XXS
T8Ø.211S
T8Ø.212S
T8Ø.218S
T8Ø.219S
T8Ø.22XS
T8Ø.29XS
T8Ø.3ØXS
T8Ø.31ØS
T8Ø.311S
T8Ø.319S
T8Ø.39XS
T8Ø.4ØXS
T8Ø.41ØS
T8Ø.411S
T8Ø.419S
T8Ø.49XS
T8Ø.51XS
T8Ø.52XS
T8Ø.59XS
T8Ø.61XS
T8Ø.62XS
T8Ø.69XS
T8Ø.81ØS
T8Ø.818S
T8Ø.82XS
T8Ø.89XS
T8Ø.9ØXS
T8Ø.91ØS
T8Ø.911S
T8Ø.919S
T8Ø.92XS
T8Ø.AØXS
T8Ø.A1ØS
T8Ø.A11S
T8Ø.A19S
T8Ø.A9XS
T81.1ØXS
T81.11XS
T81.12XS
T81.19XS
T81.3ØXS
T81.31XS
T81.32XS
T81.33XS
T81.4ØXS
T81.41XS
T81.42XS
T81.43XS
T81.44XS
T81.49XS
T81.5ØØS
T81.5Ø1S
T81.5Ø2S
T81.5Ø3S
T81.5Ø4S
T81.5Ø5S
T81.5Ø6S
T81.5Ø7S
T81.5Ø8S
T81.5Ø9S
T81.51ØS
T81.511S
T81.512S
T81.513S
T81.514S
T81.515S
T81.516S
T81.517S
T81.518S
T81.519S
T81.52ØS
T81.521S
T81.522S
T81.523S
T81.524S
T81.525S
T81.526S
T81.527S
T81.528S
T81.529S
T81.53ØS
T81.531S
T81.532S
T81.533S
T81.534S
T81.535S
T81.536S
T81.537S
T81.538S
T81.539S
T81.59ØS
T81.591S
T81.592S
T81.593S
T81.594S
T81.595S
T81.596S
T81.597S
T81.598S
T81.599S
T81.6ØXS
T81.61XS
T81.69XS
T81.71ØS
T81.711S
T81.718S
T81.719S
T81.72XS
T81.81XS
T81.82XS
T81.83XS
T81.89XS
T81.9XXS
T82.Ø1XS
T82.Ø2XS
T82.Ø3XS
T82.Ø9XS

T82.11ØS
T82.111S
T82.118S
T82.119S
T82.12ØS
T82.121S
T82.128S
T82.129S
T82.19ØS
T82.191S
T82.198S
T82.199S
T82.211S
T82.212S
T82.213S
T82.218S
T82.221S
T82.222S
T82.223S
T82.228S
T82.31ØS
T82.311S
T82.312S
T82.318S
T82.319S
T82.32ØS
T82.321S
T82.322S
T82.328S
T82.329S
T82.33ØS
T82.331S
T82.332S
T82.338S
T82.339S
T82.39ØS
T82.391S
T82.392S
T82.398S
T82.399S
T82.41XS
T82.42XS
T82.43XS
T82.49XS
T82.51ØS
T82.511S
T82.512S
T82.513S
T82.514S
T82.515S
T82.518S
T82.519S
T82.52ØS
T82.521S
T82.522S
T82.523S
T82.524S
T82.525S
T82.528S
T82.529S
T82.53ØS
T82.531S
T82.532S
T82.533S
T82.534S
T82.535S
T82.538S
T82.539S
T82.59ØS
T82.591S
T82.592S
T82.593S
T82.594S
T82.595S
T82.598S
T82.599S
T82.6XXS
T82.7XXS
T82.817S
T82.818S
T82.827S
T82.828S
T82.837S
T82.838S
T82.847S
T82.848S
T82.855S
T82.856S
T82.857S
T82.858S
T82.867S
T82.868S
T82.897S
T82.898S
T82.9XXS
T83.Ø1ØS
T83.Ø11S
T83.Ø12S
T83.Ø18S
T83.Ø2ØS
T83.Ø21S
T83.Ø22S
T83.Ø28S
T83.Ø3ØS
T83.Ø31S
T83.Ø32S
T83.Ø38S
T83.Ø9ØS
T83.Ø91S
T83.Ø92S
T83.Ø98S
T83.11ØS
T83.111S
T83.112S
T83.113S
T83.118S
T83.12ØS
T83.121S
T83.122S
T83.123S
T83.128S
T83.19ØS
T83.191S
T83.192S
T83.193S
T83.198S
T83.21XS
T83.22XS
T83.23XS
T83.24XS
T83.25XS
T83.29XS
T83.31XS
T83.32XS
T83.39XS
T83.41ØS
T83.411S
T83.418S
T83.42ØS
T83.421S
T83.428S
T83.49ØS
T83.491S
T83.498S
T83.51ØS
T83.511S
T83.512S
T83.518S
T83.59ØS
T83.591S
T83.592S
T83.593S
T83.598S
T83.61XS
T83.62XS
T83.69XS
T83.711S
T83.712S
T83.713S
T83.714S
T83.718S
T83.719S
T83.721S
T83.722S
T83.723S
T83.724S
T83.728S
T83.729S
T83.79XS
T83.81XS
T83.82XS
T83.83XS
T83.84XS
T83.85XS
T83.86XS
T83.89XS
T83.9XXS
T84.Ø1ØS
T84.Ø11S
T84.Ø12S
T84.Ø13S
T84.Ø18S
T84.Ø19S
T84.Ø2ØS
T84.Ø21S
T84.Ø22S
T84.Ø23S
T84.Ø28S
T84.Ø29S
T84.Ø3ØS
T84.Ø31S
T84.Ø32S
T84.Ø33S
T84.Ø38S
T84.Ø39S
T84.Ø5ØS
T84.Ø51S
T84.Ø52S
T84.Ø53S
T84.Ø58S
T84.Ø59S
T84.Ø6ØS
T84.Ø61S
T84.Ø62S
T84.Ø63S
T84.Ø68S
T84.Ø69S
T84.Ø9ØS
T84.Ø91S
T84.Ø92S
T84.Ø93S
T84.Ø98S
T84.Ø99S
T84.11ØS
T84.111S
T84.112S
T84.113S
T84.114S
T84.115S
T84.116S
T84.117S
T84.119S
T84.12ØS
T84.121S
T84.122S
T84.123S
T84.124S
T84.125S
T84.126S
T84.127S
T84.129S
T84.19ØS
T84.191S
T84.192S
T84.193S
T84.194S
T84.195S
T84.196S
T84.197S
T84.199S
T84.21ØS
T84.213S
T84.216S
T84.218S
T84.22ØS
T84.223S
T84.226S
T84.228S
T84.29ØS
T84.293S
T84.296S
T84.298S
T84.31ØS
T84.318S
T84.32ØS
T84.328S
T84.39ØS
T84.398S
T84.41ØS
T84.418S
T84.42ØS
T84.428S
T84.49ØS
T84.498S
T84.5ØXS
T84.51XS
T84.52XS
T84.53XS
T84.54XS
T84.59XS
T84.6ØXS
T84.61ØS
T84.611S
T84.612S
T84.613S
T84.614S
T84.615S
T84.619S
T84.62ØS
T84.621S
T84.622S
T84.623S
T84.624S
T84.625S
T84.629S
T84.63XS
T84.69XS
T84.7XXS
T84.81XS
T84.82XS
T84.83XS
T84.84XS
T84.85XS
T84.86XS
T84.89XS
T84.9XXS
T85.Ø1XS
T85.Ø2XS
T85.Ø3XS
T85.Ø9XS
T85.11ØS
T85.111S
T85.112S
T85.113S
T85.118S
T85.12ØS
T85.121S
T85.122S
T85.123S
T85.128S
T85.19ØS
T85.191S
T85.192S
T85.193S
T85.199S
T85.21XS
T85.22XS
T85.29XS
T85.31ØS
T85.311S
T85.318S
T85.32ØS
T85.321S
T85.328S
T85.39ØS
T85.391S
T85.398S
T85.41XS
T85.42XS
T85.43XS
T85.44XS
T85.49XS
T85.51ØS
T85.511S
T85.518S
T85.52ØS
T85.521S
T85.528S
T85.59ØS
T85.591S
T85.598S
T85.61ØS
T85.611S
T85.612S
T85.613S
T85.614S
T85.615S
T85.618S
T85.62ØS
T85.621S
T85.622S
T85.623S
T85.624S
T85.625S
T85.628S
T85.63ØS
T85.631S
T85.633S
T85.635S
T85.638S
T85.69ØS
T85.691S
T85.692S
T85.693S
T85.694S
T85.695S
T85.698S
T85.71XS
T85.72XS
T85.73ØS
T85.731S
T85.732S
T85.733S
T85.734S
T85.735S
T85.738S
T85.79XS
T85.81ØS
T85.818S
T85.82ØS
T85.828S
T85.83ØS
T85.838S
T85.84ØS
T85.848S
T85.85ØS
T85.858S
T85.86ØS
T85.868S
T85.89ØS
T85.898S
T85.9XXS
T88.ØXXS
T88.1XXS
T88.2XXA
T88.2XXS
T88.3XXA
T88.3XXS
T88.4XXS
T88.51XA
T88.51XS
T88.52XS
T88.53XS
T88.59XS
T88.6XXS
T88.7XXS
T88.8XXS
T88.9XXS
ZØ4.1
ZØ4.2
ZØ4.3

DRG 923

Select principal diagnosis listed under DRG 922

MDC 22

DRG 927

Full Thickness Burns Principal or Secondary Diagnosis

T2Ø.3ØXA
T2Ø.311A
T2Ø.312A
T2Ø.319A
T2Ø.32XA
T2Ø.33XA
T2Ø.34XA
T2Ø.35XA
T2Ø.36XA
T2Ø.37XA
T2Ø.39XA
T2Ø.7ØXA
T2Ø.711A
T2Ø.712A
T2Ø.719A
T2Ø.72XA
T2Ø.73XA
T2Ø.74XA
T2Ø.75XA
T2Ø.76XA
T2Ø.77XA
T2Ø.79XA
T21.3ØXA
T21.31XA
T21.32XA
T21.33XA
T21.34XA
T21.35XA
T21.36XA
T21.37XA
T21.39XA
T21.7ØXA
T21.71XA
T21.72XA
T21.73XA
T21.74XA
T21.75XA
T21.76XA
T21.77XA
T21.79XA
T22.3ØXA
T22.311A
T22.312A
T22.319A
T22.321A
T22.322A
T22.329A
T22.331A
T22.332A
T22.339A
T22.341A
T22.342A
T22.349A
T22.351A
T22.352A
T22.359A
T22.361A
T22.362A
T22.369A
T22.391A
T22.392A
T22.399A
T22.7ØXA
T22.711A
T22.712A
T22.719A
T22.721A
T22.722A
T22.729A
T22.731A
T22.732A
T22.739A
T22.741A
T22.742A
T22.749A
T22.751A
T22.752A
T22.759A
T22.761A
T22.762A
T22.769A
T22.791A
T22.792A
T22.799A
T23.3Ø1A
T23.3Ø2A
T23.3Ø9A
T23.311A
T23.312A
T23.319A
T23.321A
T23.322A
T23.329A
T23.331A
T23.332A
T23.339A
T23.341A
T23.342A
T23.349A
T23.351A
T23.352A
T23.359A
T23.361A
T23.362A
T23.369A
T23.371A
T23.372A
T23.379A
T23.391A
T23.392A
T23.399A
T23.7Ø1A
T23.7Ø2A
T23.7Ø9A
T23.711A
T23.712A
T23.719A
T23.721A
T23.722A
T23.729A
T23.731A
T23.732A
T23.739A
T23.741A
T23.742A
T23.749A
T23.751A
T23.752A
T23.759A
T23.761A
T23.762A
T23.769A
T23.771A
T23.772A
T23.779A
T23.791A
T23.792A
T23.799A
T24.3Ø1A
T24.3Ø2A
T24.3Ø9A
T24.311A
T24.312A
T24.319A
T24.321A
T24.322A
T24.329A
T24.331A
T24.332A
T24.339A
T24.391A
T24.392A
T24.399A
T24.7Ø1A
T24.7Ø2A
T24.7Ø9A
T24.711A
T24.712A
T24.719A
T24.721A
T24.722A
T24.729A
T24.731A
T24.732A
T24.739A
T24.791A
T24.792A
T24.799A
T25.311A
T25.312A
T25.319A
T25.321A
T25.322A
T25.329A
T25.331A
T25.332A
T25.339A
T25.391A
T25.392A
T25.399A
T25.711A
T25.712A
T25.719A
T25.721A
T25.722A
T25.729A
T25.731A
T25.732A
T25.739A
T25.791A
T25.792A
T25.799A
T31.11
T32.11

AND

Nonoperating Room Procedures

5A1955Z

AND

Operating Room Procedures

ØHRØX72
ØHRØX73
ØHRØX74
ØHRØXJ3
ØHRØXJ4
ØHRØXJZ
ØHRØXK3
ØHRØXK4
ØHR1X72
ØHR1X73
ØHR1X74
ØHR1XJ3
ØHR1XJ4
ØHR1XJZ
ØHR1XK3
ØHR1XK4
ØHR4X72
ØHR4X73
ØHR4X74
ØHR4XJ3
ØHR4XJ4
ØHR4XJZ
ØHR4XK3
ØHR4XK4
ØHR5X72
ØHR5X73
ØHR5X74
ØHR5XJ3
ØHR5XJ4
ØHR5XJZ
ØHR5XK3
ØHR5XK4
ØHR6X72
ØHR6X73
ØHR6X74
ØHR6XJ3
ØHR6XJ4
ØHR6XJZ
ØHR6XK3
ØHR6XK4
ØHR7X72
ØHR7X73
ØHR7X74
ØHR7XJ3
ØHR7XJ4
ØHR7XJZ
ØHR7XK3
ØHR7XK4
ØHR8X72
ØHR8X73
ØHR8X74
ØHR8XJ3
ØHR8XJ4
ØHR8XJZ
ØHR8XK3
ØHR8XK4
ØHRAX72
ØHRAX73
ØHRAX74
ØHRAXJ3
ØHRAXJ4
ØHRAXJZ
ØHRAXK3
ØHRAXK4
ØHRBX72
ØHRBX73
ØHRBX74
ØHRBXJ3
ØHRBXJ4
ØHRBXJZ
ØHRBXK3
ØHRBXK4
ØHRCX72
ØHRCX73
ØHRCX74
ØHRCXJ3
ØHRCXJ4
ØHRCXJZ
ØHRCXK3
ØHRCXK4
ØHRDX72
ØHRDX73
ØHRDX74
ØHRDXJ3
ØHRDXJ4
ØHRDXJZ
ØHRDXK3
ØHRDXK4
ØHREX72
ØHREX73
ØHREX74
ØHREXJ3
ØHREXJ4
ØHREXJZ
ØHREXK3
ØHREXK4
ØHRFX72
ØHRFX73
ØHRFX74
ØHRFXJ3
ØHRFXJ4
ØHRFXJZ
ØHRFXK3
ØHRFXK4
ØHRGX72
ØHRGX73
ØHRGX74
ØHRGXJ3
ØHRGXJ4
ØHRGXJZ
ØHRGXK3
ØHRGXK4
ØHRHX72
ØHRHX73
ØHRHX74
ØHRHXJ3
ØHRHXJ4
ØHRHXJZ
ØHRHXK3
ØHRHXK4
ØHRJX72
ØHRJX73
ØHRJX74
ØHRJXJ3
ØHRJXJ4
ØHRJXJZ
ØHRJXK3
ØHRJXK4
ØHRKX72
ØHRKX73
ØHRKX74
ØHRKXJ3
ØHRKXJ4
ØHRKXJZ
ØHRKXK3
ØHRKXK4
ØHRLX72
ØHRLX73
ØHRLX74
ØHRLXJ3
ØHRLXJ4
ØHRLXJZ
ØHRLXK3
ØHRLXK4
ØHRMX72
ØHRMX73
ØHRMX74
ØHRMXJ3
ØHRMXJ4
ØHRMXJZ
ØHRMXK3
ØHRMXK4
ØHRNX72
ØHRNX73
ØHRNX74
ØHRNXJ3
ØHRNXJ4
ØHRNXJZ
ØHRNXK3
ØHRNXK4
ØHXØXZZ
ØHX1XZZ
ØHX4XZZ
ØHX5XZZ
ØHX6XZZ
ØHX7XZZ
ØHX8XZZ
ØHX9XZZ
ØHXAXZZ
ØHXBXZZ
ØHXCXZZ
ØHXDXZZ
ØHXEXZZ
ØHXFXZZ
ØHXGXZZ
ØHXHXZZ
ØHXJXZZ
ØHXKXZZ
ØHXLXZZ
ØHXMXZZ
ØHXNXZZ
ØJHØØNZ
ØJHØ3NZ
ØJH1ØNZ
ØJH13NZ
ØJH4ØNZ
ØJH43NZ
ØJH5ØNZ
ØJH53NZ
ØJH6ØNZ

ØJH63NZ
ØJH7ØNZ
ØJH73NZ
ØJH8ØNZ
ØJH83NZ
ØJH9ØNZ
ØJH93NZ
ØJHBØNZ
ØJHB3NZ
ØJHCØNZ
ØJHC3NZ
ØJHDØNZ
ØJHD3NZ
ØJHFØNZ
ØJHF3NZ
ØJHGØNZ
ØJHG3NZ
ØJHHØNZ
ØJHH3NZ
ØJHJØNZ
ØJHJ3NZ
ØJHKØNZ
ØJHK3NZ
ØJHLØNZ
ØJHL3NZ
ØJHMØNZ
ØJHM3NZ
ØJHNØNZ
ØJHN3NZ
ØJHPØNZ
ØJHP3NZ
ØJHQØNZ
ØJHQ3NZ
ØJHRØNZ
ØJHR3NZ
ØJXØØZB
ØJXØØZC
ØJXØ3ZB
ØJXØ3ZC
ØJX1ØZB
ØJX1ØZC
ØJX13ZB
ØJX13ZC
ØJX4ØZB
ØJX4ØZC
ØJX43ZB
ØJX43ZC
ØJX5ØZB
ØJX5ØZC
ØJX53ZB
ØJX53ZC
ØJX6ØZB
ØJX6ØZC
ØJX63ZB
ØJX63ZC
ØJX7ØZB
ØJX7ØZC
ØJX73ZB
ØJX73ZC
ØJX8ØZB
ØJX8ØZC
ØJX83ZB
ØJX83ZC
ØJX9ØZB
ØJX9ØZC
ØJX93ZB
ØJX93ZC
ØJXBØZB
ØJXBØZC
ØJXB3ZB
ØJXB3ZC
ØJXCØZB
ØJXCØZC
ØJXC3ZB
ØJXC3ZC
ØJXDØZB
ØJXDØZC
ØJXD3ZB
ØJXD3ZC
ØJXFØZB
ØJXFØZC
ØJXF3ZB
ØJXF3ZC
ØJXGØZB
ØJXGØZC
ØJXG3ZB
ØJXG3ZC
ØJXHØZB
ØJXHØZC
ØJXH3ZB
ØJXH3ZC
ØJXJØZB
ØJXJØZC
ØJXJ3ZB
ØJXJ3ZC
ØJXKØZB
ØJXKØZC
ØJXK3ZB
ØJXK3ZC
ØJXLØZB
ØJXLØZC
ØJXL3ZB
ØJXL3ZC
ØJXMØZB
ØJXMØZC
ØJXM3ZB
ØJXM3ZC
ØJXNØZB
ØJXNØZC
ØJXN3ZB
ØJXN3ZC
ØJXPØZB
ØJXPØZC
ØJXP3ZB
ØJXP3ZC
ØJXQØZB
ØJXQØZC
ØJXQ3ZB
ØJXQ3ZC
ØJXRØZB
ØJXRØZC
ØJXR3ZB
ØJXR3ZC
ØWUØØ7Z
ØWUØ47Z
ØWU2Ø7Z
ØWU247Z
ØWU6Ø7Z
ØWU647Z
ØWUKØ7Z
ØWUK47Z
ØWULØ7Z
ØWUL47Z
ØXU2Ø7Z
ØXU247Z
ØXU3Ø7Z
ØXU347Z
ØXU4Ø7Z
ØXU447Z
ØXU5Ø7Z
ØXU547Z
ØXU6Ø7Z
ØXU647Z
ØXU7Ø7Z
ØXU747Z
ØXU8Ø7Z
ØXU847Z
ØXU9Ø7Z
ØXU947Z
ØXUBØ7Z
ØXUB47Z
ØXUCØ7Z
ØXUC47Z
ØXUDØ7Z
ØXUD47Z
ØXUFØ7Z
ØXUF47Z
ØXUGØ7Z
ØXUG47Z
ØXUHØ7Z
ØXUH47Z
ØXUJØ7Z
ØXUJ47Z
ØXUKØ7Z
ØXUK47Z
ØXULØ7Z
ØXUL47Z
ØXUMØ7Z
ØXUM47Z
ØXUNØ7Z
ØXUN47Z
ØXUPØ7Z
ØXUP47Z
ØXUQØ7Z
ØXUQ47Z
ØXURØ7Z
ØXUR47Z
ØXUSØ7Z
ØXUS47Z
ØXUTØ7Z
ØXUT47Z
ØXUVØ7Z
ØXUV47Z
ØXUWØ7Z
ØXUW47Z
XHRPXF7

OR

Extensive Burns Principal or Secondary Diagnosis

T31.21
T31.22
T31.31
T31.32
T31.33
T31.41
T31.42
T31.43
T31.44
T31.51
T31.52
T31.53
T31.54
T31.55
T31.61
T31.62
T31.63
T31.64
T31.65
T31.66
T31.71
T31.72
T31.73
T31.74
T31.75
T31.76
T31.77
T31.81
T31.82
T31.83
T31.84
T31.85
T31.86
T31.87
T31.88
T31.91
T31.92
T31.93
T31.94
T31.95
T31.96
T31.97
T31.98
T31.99
T32.21
T32.22
T32.31
T32.32
T32.33
T32.41
T32.42
T32.43
T32.44
T32.51
T32.52
T32.53
T32.54
T32.55
T32.61
T32.62
T32.63
T32.64
T32.65
T32.66
T32.71
T32.72
T32.73
T32.74
T32.75
T32.76
T32.77
T32.81
T32.82
T32.83
T32.84
T32.85
T32.86
T32.87
T32.88
T32.91
T32.92
T32.93
T32.94
T32.95
T32.96
T32.97
T32.98
T32.99

DRG 928

Principal or Secondary Diagnosis

T2Ø.3ØXA
T2Ø.311A
T2Ø.312A
T2Ø.319A
T2Ø.32XA
T2Ø.33XA
T2Ø.34XA
T2Ø.35XA
T2Ø.36XA
T2Ø.37XA
T2Ø.39XA
T2Ø.7ØXA
T2Ø.711A
T2Ø.712A
T2Ø.719A
T2Ø.72XA
T2Ø.73XA
T2Ø.74XA
T2Ø.75XA
T2Ø.76XA
T2Ø.77XA
T2Ø.79XA
T21.3ØXA
T21.31XA
T21.32XA
T21.33XA
T21.34XA
T21.35XA
T21.36XA
T21.37XA
T21.39XA
T21.7ØXA
T21.71XA
T21.72XA
T21.73XA
T21.74XA
T21.75XA
T21.76XA
T21.77XA
T21.79XA
T22.3ØXA
T22.311A
T22.312A
T22.319A
T22.321A
T22.322A
T22.329A
T22.331A
T22.332A
T22.339A
T22.341A
T22.342A
T22.349A
T22.351A
T22.352A
T22.359A
T22.361A
T22.362A
T22.369A
T22.391A
T22.392A
T22.399A
T22.7ØXA
T22.711A
T22.712A
T22.719A
T22.721A
T22.722A
T22.729A
T22.731A
T22.732A
T22.739A
T22.741A
T22.742A
T22.749A
T22.751A
T22.752A
T22.759A
T22.761A
T22.762A
T22.769A
T22.791A
T22.792A
T22.799A
T23.3Ø1A
T23.3Ø2A
T23.3Ø9A
T23.311A
T23.312A
T23.319A
T23.321A
T23.322A
T23.329A
T23.331A
T23.332A
T23.339A
T23.341A
T23.342A
T23.349A
T23.351A
T23.352A
T23.359A
T23.361A
T23.362A
T23.369A
T23.371A
T23.372A
T23.379A
T23.391A
T23.392A
T23.399A
T23.7Ø1A
T23.7Ø2A
T23.7Ø9A
T23.711A
T23.712A
T23.719A
T23.721A
T23.722A
T23.729A
T23.731A
T23.732A
T23.739A
T23.741A
T23.742A
T23.749A
T23.751A
T23.752A
T23.759A
T23.761A
T23.762A
T23.769A
T23.771A
T23.772A
T23.779A
T23.791A
T23.792A
T23.799A
T24.3Ø1A
T24.3Ø2A
T24.3Ø9A
T24.311A
T24.312A
T24.319A
T24.321A
T24.322A
T24.329A
T24.331A
T24.332A
T24.339A
T24.391A
T24.392A
T24.399A
T24.7Ø1A
T24.7Ø2A
T24.7Ø9A
T24.711A
T24.712A
T24.719A
T24.721A
T24.722A
T24.729A
T24.731A
T24.732A
T24.739A
T24.791A
T24.792A
T24.799A
T25.311A
T25.312A
T25.319A
T25.321A
T25.322A
T25.329A
T25.331A
T25.332A
T25.339A
T25.391A
T25.392A
T25.399A
T25.711A
T25.712A
T25.719A
T25.721A
T25.722A
T25.729A
T25.731A
T25.732A
T25.739A
T25.791A
T25.792A
T25.799A
T31.11
T32.11

AND

Operating Room Procedures

ØHRØ*
ØHR1*
ØHR4*
ØHR5*
ØHR6*
ØHR7*
ØHR8*
ØHRA*
ØHRB*
ØHRC*
ØHRD*
ØHRE*
ØHRF*
ØHRG*
ØHRH*
ØHRJ*
ØHRK*
ØHRL*
ØHRM*
ØHRN*
ØHXØXZZ
ØHX1XZZ
ØHX4XZZ
ØHX5XZZ
ØHX6XZZ
ØHX7XZZ
ØHX8XZZ
ØHX9XZZ
ØHXAXZZ
ØHXBXZZ
ØHXCXZZ
ØHXDXZZ
ØHXEXZZ
ØHXFXZZ
ØHXGXZZ
ØHXHXZZ
ØHXJXZZ
ØHXKXZZ
ØHXLXZZ
ØHXMXZZ
ØHXNXZZ
ØJHØ*
ØJH1*
ØJH4*
ØJH5*
ØJH6ØNZ
ØJH63NZ
ØJH7ØNZ
ØJH73NZ
ØJH8ØNZ
ØJH83NZ
ØJH9*
ØJHB*
ØJHC*
ØJHDØNZ
ØJHD3NZ
ØJHFØNZ
ØJHF3NZ
ØJHGØNZ
ØJHG3NZ
ØJHHØNZ
ØJHH3NZ
ØJHJ*
ØJHK*
ØJHLØNZ
ØJHL3NZ
ØJHMØNZ
ØJHM3NZ
ØJHNØNZ
ØJHN3NZ
ØJHPØNZ
ØJHP3NZ
ØJHQ*
ØJHR*
ØJXØØZB
ØJXØØZC
ØJXØ3ZB
ØJXØ3ZC
ØJX1ØZB
ØJX1ØZC
ØJX13ZB
ØJX13ZC
ØJX4ØZB
ØJX4ØZC
ØJX43ZB
ØJX43ZC
ØJX5ØZB
ØJX5ØZC
ØJX53ZB
ØJX53ZC
ØJX6ØZB
ØJX6ØZC
ØJX63ZB
ØJX63ZC
ØJX7ØZB
ØJX7ØZC
ØJX73ZB
ØJX73ZC
ØJX8ØZB
ØJX8ØZC
ØJX83ZB
ØJX83ZC
ØJX9ØZB
ØJX9ØZC
ØJX93ZB
ØJX93ZC
ØJXBØZB
ØJXBØZC
ØJXB3ZB
ØJXB3ZC
ØJXCØZB
ØJXCØZC
ØJXC3ZB
ØJXC3ZC
ØJXDØZB
ØJXDØZC
ØJXD3ZB
ØJXD3ZC
ØJXFØZB
ØJXFØZC
ØJXF3ZB
ØJXF3ZC
ØJXGØZB
ØJXGØZC
ØJXG3ZB
ØJXG3ZC
ØJXHØZB
ØJXHØZC
ØJXH3ZB
ØJXH3ZC
ØJXJØZB
ØJXJØZC
ØJXJ3ZB
ØJXJ3ZC
ØJXKØZB
ØJXKØZC
ØJXK3ZB
ØJXK3ZC
ØJXLØZB
ØJXLØZC
ØJXL3ZB
ØJXL3ZC
ØJXMØZB
ØJXMØZC
ØJXM3ZB
ØJXM3ZC
ØJXNØZB
ØJXNØZC
ØJXN3ZB
ØJXN3ZC
ØJXPØZB
ØJXPØZC
ØJXP3ZB
ØJXP3ZC
ØJXQØZB
ØJXQØZC
ØJXQ3ZB
ØJXQ3ZC
ØJXRØZB
ØJXRØZC
ØJXR3ZB
ØJXR3ZC
ØWUØØ7Z
ØWUØ47Z
ØWU2Ø7Z
ØWU247Z
ØWU6Ø7Z
ØWU647Z
ØWUKØ7Z
ØWUK47Z
ØWULØ7Z
ØWUL47Z
ØXU2Ø7Z
ØXU247Z
ØXU3Ø7Z
ØXU347Z
ØXU4Ø7Z
ØXU447Z
ØXU5Ø7Z
ØXU547Z
ØXU6Ø7Z
ØXU647Z
ØXU7Ø7Z
ØXU747Z
ØXU8Ø7Z
ØXU847Z
ØXU9Ø7Z
ØXU947Z
ØXUBØ7Z
ØXUB47Z
ØXUCØ7Z
ØXUC47Z
ØXUDØ7Z
ØXUD47Z
ØXUFØ7Z
ØXUF47Z
ØXUGØ7Z
ØXUG47Z
ØXUHØ7Z
ØXUH47Z
ØXUJØ7Z
ØXUJ47Z
ØXUKØ7Z
ØXUK47Z
ØXULØ7Z
ØXUL47Z
ØXUMØ7Z
ØXUM47Z
ØXUNØ7Z
ØXUN47Z
ØXUPØ7Z
ØXUP47Z
ØXUQØ7Z
ØXUQ47Z
ØXURØ7Z
ØXUR47Z
ØXUSØ7Z
ØXUS47Z
ØXUTØ7Z
ØXUT47Z
ØXUVØ7Z
ØXUV47Z
ØXUWØ7Z
ØXUW47Z
XHRPXF7

OR

Secondary Diagnosis

J7Ø.5
J95.1
J95.2
J95.3
J95.82*
J96.Ø*
J96.2*
J96.9*
T27.ØXXA
T27.1XXA
T27.2XXA
T27.3XXA
T27.4XXA
T27.5XXA
T27.6XXA
T27.7XXA
T59.811A
T59.812A
T59.813A
T59.814A
T59.891A
T59.892A
T59.893A
T59.894A
T59.91XA
T59.92XA
T59.93XA
T59.94XA

DRG 929

Select principal or secondary diagnosis AND EITHER operating room procedure OR secondary diagnosis of inhalation injury listed under DRG 928

DRG 933

Full Thickness Burns Principal or Secondary Diagnosis

T2Ø.3ØXA
T2Ø.311A
T2Ø.312A
T2Ø.319A
T2Ø.32XA
T2Ø.33XA
T2Ø.34XA
T2Ø.35XA
T2Ø.36XA
T2Ø.37XA
T2Ø.39XA
T2Ø.7ØXA
T2Ø.711A
T2Ø.712A
T2Ø.719A
T2Ø.72XA
T2Ø.73XA
T2Ø.74XA
T2Ø.75XA
T2Ø.76XA
T2Ø.77XA
T2Ø.79XA
T21.3ØXA
T21.31XA
T21.32XA
T21.33XA
T21.34XA
T21.35XA
T21.36XA
T21.37XA
T21.39XA
T21.7ØXA
T21.71XA
T21.72XA
T21.73XA
T21.74XA
T21.75XA
T21.76XA
T21.77XA
T21.79XA
T22.3ØXA
T22.311A
T22.312A
T22.319A
T22.321A
T22.322A
T22.329A
T22.331A
T22.332A
T22.339A
T22.341A
T22.342A
T22.349A
T22.351A
T22.352A
T22.359A
T22.361A
T22.362A
T22.369A
T22.391A
T22.392A
T22.399A
T22.7ØXA
T22.711A
T22.712A
T22.719A
T22.721A
T22.722A
T22.729A
T22.731A
T22.732A
T22.739A
T22.741A
T22.742A
T22.749A
T22.751A
T22.752A
T22.759A
T22.761A
T22.762A
T22.769A
T22.791A
T22.792A
T22.799A
T23.3Ø1A
T23.3Ø2A
T23.3Ø9A
T23.311A
T23.312A
T23.319A
T23.321A
T23.322A
T23.329A
T23.331A
T23.332A
T23.339A
T23.341A
T23.342A
T23.349A
T23.351A
T23.352A
T23.359A
T23.361A

ICD-10-CM/PCS Codes by MS-DRG

T23.362A
T23.369A
T23.371A
T23.372A
T23.379A
T23.391A
T23.392A
T23.399A
T23.701A
T23.702A
T23.709A
T23.711A
T23.712A
T23.719A
T23.721A
T23.722A
T23.729A
T23.731A
T23.732A
T23.739A
T23.741A
T23.742A
T23.749A
T23.751A
T23.752A
T23.759A
T23.761A
T23.762A
T23.769A
T23.771A
T23.772A
T23.779A
T23.791A
T23.792A
T23.799A
T24.301A
T24.302A
T24.309A
T24.311A
T24.312A
T24.319A
T24.321A
T24.322A
T24.329A
T24.331A
T24.332A
T24.339A
T24.391A
T24.392A
T24.399A
T24.701A
T24.702A
T24.709A
T24.711A
T24.712A
T24.719A
T24.721A
T24.722A
T24.729A
T24.731A
T24.732A
T24.739A
T24.791A
T24.792A
T24.799A
T25.311A
T25.312A
T25.319A
T25.321A
T25.322A
T25.329A
T25.331A
T25.332A
T25.339A
T25.391A
T25.392A
T25.399A
T25.711A
T25.712A
T25.719A
T25.721A
T25.722A
T25.729A
T25.731A
T25.732A
T25.739A
T25.791A
T25.792A
T25.799A
T31.11
T32.11

AND

Nonoperating Room Procedure

5A1955Z

OR

Extensive Burns Principal or Secondary Diagnosis

T31.21
T31.22
T31.31
T31.32
T31.33
T31.41
T31.42
T31.43
T31.44
T31.51
T31.52
T31.53
T31.54
T31.55
T31.61
T31.62
T31.63
T31.64
T31.65
T31.66
T31.71
T31.72
T31.73
T31.74
T31.75
T31.76
T31.77
T31.81
T31.82
T31.83
T31.84
T31.85
T31.86
T31.87
T31.88
T31.91
T31.92
T31.93
T31.94
T31.95
T31.96
T31.97
T31.98
T31.99
T32.21
T32.22
T32.31
T32.32
T32.33
T32.41
T32.42
T32.43
T32.44
T32.51
T32.52
T32.53
T32.54
T32.55
T32.61
T32.62
T32.63
T32.64
T32.65
T32.66
T32.71
T32.72
T32.73
T32.74
T32.75
T32.76
T32.77
T32.81
T32.82
T32.83
T32.84
T32.85
T32.86
T32.87
T32.88
T32.91
T32.92
T32.93
T32.94
T32.95
T32.96
T32.97
T32.98
T32.99

DRG 934

Principal or Secondary Diagnosis

T20.30XA
T20.311A
T20.312A
T20.319A
T20.32XA
T20.33XA
T20.34XA
T20.35XA
T20.36XA
T20.37XA
T20.39XA
T20.70XA
T20.711A
T20.712A
T20.719A
T20.72XA
T20.73XA
T20.74XA
T20.75XA
T20.76XA
T20.77XA
T20.79XA
T21.30XA
T21.31XA
T21.32XA
T21.33XA
T21.34XA
T21.35XA
T21.36XA
T21.37XA
T21.39XA
T21.70XA
T21.71XA
T21.72XA
T21.73XA
T21.74XA
T21.75XA
T21.76XA
T21.77XA
T21.79XA
T22.30XA
T22.311A
T22.312A
T22.319A
T22.321A
T22.322A
T22.329A
T22.331A
T22.332A
T22.339A
T22.341A
T22.342A
T22.349A
T22.351A
T22.352A
T22.359A
T22.361A
T22.362A
T22.369A
T22.391A
T22.392A
T22.399A
T22.70XA
T22.711A
T22.712A
T22.719A
T22.721A
T22.722A
T22.729A
T22.731A
T22.732A
T22.739A
T22.741A
T22.742A
T22.749A
T22.751A
T22.752A
T22.759A
T22.761A
T22.762A
T22.769A
T22.791A
T22.792A
T22.799A
T23.301A
T23.302A
T23.309A
T23.311A
T23.312A
T23.319A
T23.321A
T23.322A
T23.329A
T23.331A
T23.332A
T23.339A
T23.341A
T23.342A
T23.349A
T23.351A
T23.352A
T23.359A
T23.361A
T23.362A
T23.369A
T23.371A
T23.372A
T23.379A
T23.391A
T23.392A
T23.399A
T23.701A
T23.702A
T23.709A
T23.711A
T23.712A
T23.719A
T23.721A
T23.722A
T23.729A
T23.731A
T23.732A
T23.739A
T23.741A
T23.742A
T23.749A
T23.751A
T23.752A
T23.759A
T23.761A
T23.762A
T23.769A
T23.771A
T23.772A
T23.779A
T23.791A
T23.792A
T23.799A
T24.301A
T24.302A
T24.309A
T24.311A
T24.312A
T24.319A
T24.321A
T24.322A
T24.329A
T24.331A
T24.332A
T24.339A
T24.391A
T24.392A
T24.399A
T24.701A
T24.702A
T24.709A
T24.711A
T24.712A
T24.719A
T24.721A
T24.722A
T24.729A
T24.731A
T24.732A
T24.739A
T24.791A
T24.792A
T24.799A
T25.311A
T25.312A
T25.319A
T25.321A
T25.322A
T25.329A
T25.331A
T25.332A
T25.339A
T25.391A
T25.392A
T25.399A
T25.711A
T25.712A
T25.719A
T25.721A
T25.722A
T25.729A
T25.731A
T25.732A
T25.739A
T25.791A
T25.792A
T25.799A
T31.11
T32.11

DRG 935

Principal or Secondary Diagnosis

T20.00XA
T20.011A
T20.012A
T20.019A
T20.02XA
T20.03XA
T20.04XA
T20.05XA
T20.06XA
T20.07XA
T20.09XA
T20.10XA
T20.111A
T20.112A
T20.119A
T20.12XA
T20.13XA
T20.14XA
T20.15XA
T20.16XA
T20.17XA
T20.19XA
T20.20XA
T20.211A
T20.212A
T20.219A
T20.22XA
T20.23XA
T20.24XA
T20.25XA
T20.26XA
T20.27XA
T20.29XA
T20.40XA
T20.411A
T20.412A
T20.419A
T20.42XA
T20.43XA
T20.44XA
T20.45XA
T20.46XA
T20.47XA
T20.49XA
T20.50XA
T20.511A
T20.512A
T20.519A
T20.52XA
T20.53XA
T20.54XA
T20.55XA
T20.56XA
T20.57XA
T20.59XA
T20.60XA
T20.611A
T20.612A
T20.619A
T20.62XA
T20.63XA
T20.64XA
T20.65XA
T20.66XA
T20.67XA
T20.69XA
T21.00XA
T21.01XA
T21.02XA
T21.03XA
T21.04XA
T21.05XA
T21.06XA
T21.07XA
T21.09XA
T21.10XA
T21.11XA
T21.12XA
T21.13XA
T21.14XA
T21.15XA
T21.16XA
T21.17XA
T21.19XA
T21.20XA
T21.21XA
T21.22XA
T21.23XA
T21.24XA
T21.25XA
T21.26XA
T21.27XA
T21.29XA
T21.40XA
T21.41XA
T21.42XA
T21.43XA
T21.44XA
T21.45XA
T21.46XA
T21.47XA
T21.49XA
T21.50XA
T21.51XA
T21.52XA
T21.53XA
T21.54XA
T21.55XA
T21.56XA
T21.57XA
T21.59XA
T21.60XA
T21.61XA
T21.62XA
T21.63XA
T21.64XA
T21.65XA
T21.66XA
T21.67XA
T21.69XA
T22.00XA
T22.011A
T22.012A
T22.019A
T22.021A
T22.022A
T22.029A
T22.031A
T22.032A
T22.039A
T22.041A
T22.042A
T22.049A
T22.051A
T22.052A
T22.059A
T22.061A
T22.062A
T22.069A
T22.091A
T22.092A
T22.099A
T22.10XA
T22.111A
T22.112A
T22.119A
T22.121A
T22.122A
T22.129A
T22.131A
T22.132A
T22.139A
T22.141A
T22.142A
T22.149A
T22.151A
T22.152A
T22.159A
T22.161A
T22.162A
T22.169A
T22.191A
T22.192A
T22.199A
T22.20XA
T22.211A
T22.212A
T22.219A
T22.221A
T22.222A
T22.229A
T22.231A
T22.232A
T22.239A
T22.241A
T22.242A
T22.249A
T22.251A
T22.252A
T22.259A
T22.261A
T22.262A
T22.269A
T22.291A
T22.292A
T22.299A
T22.40XA
T22.411A
T22.412A
T22.419A
T22.421A
T22.422A
T22.429A
T22.431A
T22.432A
T22.439A
T22.441A
T22.442A
T22.449A
T22.451A
T22.452A
T22.459A
T22.461A
T22.462A
T22.469A
T22.491A
T22.492A
T22.499A
T22.50XA
T22.511A
T22.512A
T22.519A
T22.521A
T22.522A
T22.529A
T22.531A
T22.532A
T22.539A
T22.541A
T22.542A
T22.549A
T22.551A
T22.552A
T22.559A
T22.561A
T22.562A
T22.569A
T22.591A
T22.592A
T22.599A
T22.60XA
T22.611A
T22.612A
T22.619A
T22.621A
T22.622A
T22.629A
T22.631A
T22.632A
T22.639A
T22.641A
T22.642A
T22.649A
T22.651A
T22.652A
T22.659A
T22.661A
T22.662A
T22.669A
T22.691A
T22.692A
T22.699A
T23.001A
T23.002A
T23.009A
T23.011A
T23.012A
T23.019A
T23.021A
T23.022A
T23.029A
T23.031A
T23.032A
T23.039A
T23.041A
T23.042A
T23.049A
T23.051A
T23.052A
T23.059A
T23.061A
T23.062A
T23.069A
T23.071A
T23.072A
T23.079A
T23.091A
T23.092A
T23.099A
T23.101A
T23.102A
T23.109A
T23.111A
T23.112A
T23.119A
T23.121A
T23.122A
T23.129A
T23.131A
T23.132A
T23.139A
T23.141A
T23.142A
T23.149A
T23.151A
T23.152A
T23.159A
T23.161A
T23.162A
T23.169A
T23.171A
T23.172A
T23.179A
T23.191A
T23.192A
T23.199A
T23.201A
T23.202A
T23.209A
T23.211A
T23.212A
T23.219A
T23.221A
T23.222A
T23.229A
T23.231A
T23.232A
T23.239A
T23.241A
T23.242A
T23.249A
T23.251A
T23.252A
T23.259A
T23.261A
T23.262A
T23.269A
T23.271A
T23.272A
T23.279A
T23.291A
T23.292A
T23.299A
T23.401A
T23.402A
T23.409A
T23.411A
T23.412A
T23.419A
T23.421A
T23.422A
T23.429A
T23.431A
T23.432A
T23.439A
T23.441A
T23.442A
T23.449A
T23.451A
T23.452A
T23.459A
T23.461A
T23.462A
T23.469A
T23.471A
T23.472A
T23.479A
T23.491A
T23.492A
T23.499A
T23.501A
T23.502A
T23.509A
T23.511A
T23.512A
T23.519A
T23.521A
T23.522A
T23.529A
T23.531A
T23.532A
T23.539A
T23.541A
T23.542A
T23.549A
T23.551A
T23.552A
T23.559A
T23.561A
T23.562A
T23.569A
T23.571A
T23.572A
T23.579A
T23.591A
T23.592A
T23.599A
T23.601A
T23.602A
T23.609A
T23.611A
T23.612A
T23.619A
T23.621A
T23.622A
T23.629A
T23.631A
T23.632A
T23.639A
T23.641A
T23.642A
T23.649A
T23.651A
T23.652A
T23.659A
T23.661A
T23.662A
T23.669A
T23.671A
T23.672A
T23.679A
T23.691A
T23.692A
T23.699A
T24.001A
T24.002A
T24.009A
T24.011A
T24.012A
T24.019A
T24.021A
T24.022A
T24.029A
T24.031A
T24.032A
T24.039A
T24.091A
T24.092A
T24.099A
T24.101A
T24.102A
T24.109A
T24.111A
T24.112A
T24.119A
T24.121A
T24.122A
T24.129A
T24.131A
T24.132A
T24.139A
T24.191A
T24.192A
T24.199A
T24.201A
T24.202A
T24.209A
T24.211A
T24.212A
T24.219A
T24.221A
T24.222A
T24.229A
T24.231A
T24.232A
T24.239A
T24.291A
T24.292A
T24.299A
T24.401A
T24.402A
T24.409A
T24.411A

T24.412A
T24.419A
T24.421A
T24.422A
T24.429A
T24.431A
T24.432A
T24.439A
T24.491A
T24.492A
T24.499A
T24.5Ø1A
T24.5Ø2A
T24.5Ø9A
T24.511A
T24.512A
T24.519A
T24.521A
T24.522A
T24.529A
T24.531A
T24.532A
T24.539A
T24.591A
T24.592A
T24.599A
T24.6Ø1A
T24.6Ø2A
T24.6Ø9A
T24.611A
T24.612A
T24.619A
T24.621A
T24.622A
T24.629A
T24.631A
T24.632A
T24.639A
T24.691A
T24.692A
T24.699A
T25.Ø11A
T25.Ø12A
T25.Ø19A
T25.Ø21A
T25.Ø22A
T25.Ø29A
T25.Ø31A
T25.Ø32A
T25.Ø39A
T25.Ø91A
T25.Ø92A
T25.Ø99A
T25.111A
T25.112A
T25.119A
T25.121A
T25.122A
T25.129A
T25.131A
T25.132A
T25.139A
T25.191A
T25.192A
T25.199A
T25.211A
T25.212A
T25.219A
T25.221A
T25.222A
T25.229A
T25.231A
T25.232A
T25.239A
T25.291A
T25.292A
T25.299A
T25.411A
T25.412A
T25.419A
T25.421A
T25.422A
T25.429A
T25.431A
T25.432A
T25.439A
T25.491A
T25.492A
T25.499A
T25.511A
T25.512A
T25.519A
T25.521A
T25.522A
T25.529A
T25.531A
T25.532A
T25.539A
T25.591A
T25.592A
T25.599A
T25.611A
T25.612A
T25.619A
T25.621A
T25.622A
T25.629A
T25.631A
T25.632A
T25.639A
T25.691A
T25.692A
T25.699A
T28.3XXA
T28.4ØXA
T28.411A
T28.412A
T28.419A
T28.49XA
T28.8XXA
T28.9ØXA
T28.911A
T28.912A
T28.919A
T28.99XA
T3Ø.Ø
T3Ø.4
T31.Ø
T31.1Ø
T31.2Ø
T31.3Ø
T31.4Ø
T31.5Ø
T31.6Ø
T31.7Ø
T31.8Ø
T31.9Ø
T32.Ø
T32.1Ø
T32.2Ø
T32.3Ø
T32.4Ø
T32.5Ø
T32.6Ø
T32.7Ø
T32.8Ø
T32.9Ø

MDC 23

DRG 939
Select any operating room procedure

DRG 940
Select any operating room procedure

DRG 941
Select any operating room procedure

DRG 945
Principal Diagnosis
Z44.8
Z44.9
OR
Rehabilitation Procedures
FØØ*
FØ1*
FØ2*
FØ6*
FØ7*
FØ8*
FØ9*
FØB*
FØC*
FØDZØ5Z
FØDZØZZ
FØDZ11Z
FØDZ12Z
FØDZ15Z
FØDZ1KZ
FØDZ1LZ
FØDZ1ZZ
FØDZ21Z
FØDZ22Z
FØDZ25Z
FØDZ2KZ
FØDZ2LZ
FØDZ2ZZ
FØDZ3MZ
FØDZ4SZ
FØDZ4VZ
FØDZ51Z
FØDZ52Z
FØDZ55Z
FØDZ5KZ
FØDZ5LZ
FØDZ5ZZ
FØDZ6EZ
FØDZ6FZ
FØDZ6UZ
FØDZ6ZZ
FØDZ7EZ
FØDZ7FZ
FØDZ7UZ
FØDZ7ZZ
FØDZ8EZ
FØDZ8FZ
FØDZ8UZ
FØF*
AND
Any principal diagnosis from MDC 23 except the following
Z45.1
Z45.2
Z46.82
Z48.Ø3
Z48.1
Z48.21
Z48.22
Z48.23
Z48.24
Z48.28Ø
Z48.288
Z48.29Ø
Z48.298
Z48.3
Z48.81Ø
Z48.811
Z48.812
Z48.813
Z48.814
Z48.815
Z48.816
Z48.817
Z48.89
Z51.81

DRG 946
Select principal diagnosis OR rehabilitation procedures AND principal diagnosis listed under DRG 945

DRG 947
Principal Diagnosis
EØ7.81
E79.Ø
G89.1*
G89.3
G93.3*
PØ9*
R18*
R23.Ø
R23.1
R23.2
R41.Ø
R41.1
R41.2
R41.3
R41.82
R41.9
R45.83
R45.84
R52
R53.Ø
R53.1
R53.2
R53.8*
R6Ø*
R64
R68.Ø
R68.11
R68.12
R68.81
R68.83
R68.89
R7Ø*
R74*
R77*
R78.1
R78.2
R78.3
R78.4
R78.5
R78.6
R78.7*
R78.89
R78.9
R79*
R82.1
R84*
R85.Ø
R85.1
R85.2
R85.3
R85.4
R85.5
R85.69
R85.7
R85.89
R85.9
R87.Ø
R87.1
R87.2
R87.3
R87.4
R87.5
R87.618
R87.619
R87.629
R87.69
R87.7
R87.89
R87.9
R88*
R89.Ø
R89.1
R89.2
R89.3
R89.4
R89.5
R89.6
R89.7
R89.8
R9Ø.89
R93.89
R93.9
R97.Ø
R97.1
R97.2Ø
R97.21
R97.8

DRG 948
Select principal diagnosis listed under DRG 947

DRG 949
Principal Diagnosis
SØØ.ØØXD
SØØ.Ø1XD
SØØ.Ø2XD
SØØ.Ø3XD
SØØ.Ø4XD
SØØ.Ø5XD
SØØ.Ø6XD
SØØ.Ø7XD
SØØ.1ØXD
SØØ.11XD
SØØ.12XD
SØØ.2Ø1D
SØØ.2Ø2D
SØØ.2Ø9D
SØØ.211D
SØØ.212D
SØØ.219D
SØØ.221D
SØØ.222D
SØØ.229D
SØØ.241D
SØØ.242D
SØØ.249D
SØØ.251D
SØØ.252D
SØØ.259D
SØØ.261D
SØØ.262D
SØØ.269D
SØØ.271D
SØØ.272D
SØØ.279D
SØØ.3ØXD
SØØ.31XD
SØØ.32XD
SØØ.33XD
SØØ.34XD
SØØ.35XD
SØØ.36XD
SØØ.37XD
SØØ.4Ø1D
SØØ.4Ø2D
SØØ.4Ø9D
SØØ.411D
SØØ.412D
SØØ.419D
SØØ.421D
SØØ.422D
SØØ.429D
SØØ.431D
SØØ.432D
SØØ.439D
SØØ.441D
SØØ.442D
SØØ.449D
SØØ.451D
SØØ.452D
SØØ.459D
SØØ.461D
SØØ.462D
SØØ.469D
SØØ.471D
SØØ.472D
SØØ.479D
SØØ.5Ø1D
SØØ.5Ø2D
SØØ.511D
SØØ.512D
SØØ.521D
SØØ.522D
SØØ.531D
SØØ.532D
SØØ.541D
SØØ.542D
SØØ.551D
SØØ.552D
SØØ.561D
SØØ.562D
SØØ.571D
SØØ.572D
SØØ.8ØXD
SØØ.81XD
SØØ.82XD
SØØ.83XD
SØØ.84XD
SØØ.85XD
SØØ.86XD
SØØ.87XD
SØØ.9ØXD
SØØ.91XD
SØØ.92XD
SØØ.93XD
SØØ.94XD
SØØ.95XD
SØØ.96XD
SØØ.97XD
SØ1.ØØXD
SØ1.Ø1XD
SØ1.Ø2XD
SØ1.Ø3XD
SØ1.Ø4XD
SØ1.Ø5XD
SØ1.1Ø1D
SØ1.1Ø2D
SØ1.1Ø9D
SØ1.111D
SØ1.112D
SØ1.119D
SØ1.121D
SØ1.122D
SØ1.129D
SØ1.131D
SØ1.132D
SØ1.139D
SØ1.141D
SØ1.142D
SØ1.149D
SØ1.151D
SØ1.152D
SØ1.159D
SØ1.2ØXD
SØ1.21XD
SØ1.22XD
SØ1.23XD
SØ1.24XD
SØ1.25XD
SØ1.3Ø1D
SØ1.3Ø2D
SØ1.3Ø9D
SØ1.311D
SØ1.312D
SØ1.319D
SØ1.321D
SØ1.322D
SØ1.329D
SØ1.331D
SØ1.332D
SØ1.339D
SØ1.341D
SØ1.342D
SØ1.349D
SØ1.351D
SØ1.352D
SØ1.359D
SØ1.4Ø1D
SØ1.4Ø2D
SØ1.4Ø9D
SØ1.411D
SØ1.412D
SØ1.419D
SØ1.421D
SØ1.422D
SØ1.429D
SØ1.431D
SØ1.432D
SØ1.439D
SØ1.441D
SØ1.442D
SØ1.449D
SØ1.451D
SØ1.452D
SØ1.459D
SØ1.5Ø1D
SØ1.5Ø2D
SØ1.511D
SØ1.512D
SØ1.521D
SØ1.522D
SØ1.531D
SØ1.532D
SØ1.541D
SØ1.542D
SØ1.551D
SØ1.552D
SØ1.8ØXD
SØ1.81XD
SØ1.82XD
SØ1.83XD
SØ1.84XD
SØ1.85XD
SØ1.9ØXD
SØ1.91XD
SØ1.92XD
SØ1.93XD
SØ1.94XD
SØ1.95XD
SØ2.121D
SØ2.121G
SØ2.121K
SØ2.122D
SØ2.122G
SØ2.122K
SØ2.129D
SØ2.129G
SØ2.129K
SØ2.831D
SØ2.831G
SØ2.831K
SØ2.832D
SØ2.832G
SØ2.832K
SØ2.839D
SØ2.839G
SØ2.839K
SØ2.841D
SØ2.841G
SØ2.841K
SØ2.842D
SØ2.842G
SØ2.842K
SØ2.849D
SØ2.849G
SØ2.849K
SØ2.85XD
SØ2.85XG
SØ2.85XK
SØ3.ØØXD
SØ3.Ø1XD
SØ3.Ø2XD
SØ3.Ø3XD
SØ3.1XXD
SØ3.2XXD
SØ3.4ØXD
SØ3.41XD
SØ3.42XD
SØ3.43XD
SØ3.8XXD
SØ3.9XXD
SØ4.Ø11D
SØ4.Ø12D
SØ4.Ø19D
SØ4.Ø2XD
SØ4.Ø31D
SØ4.Ø32D
SØ4.Ø39D
SØ4.Ø41D
SØ4.Ø42D
SØ4.Ø49D
SØ4.1ØXD
SØ4.11XD
SØ4.12XD
SØ4.2ØXD
SØ4.21XD
SØ4.22XD
SØ4.3ØXD
SØ4.31XD
SØ4.32XD
SØ4.4ØXD
SØ4.41XD
SØ4.42XD
SØ4.5ØXD
SØ4.51XD
SØ4.52XD
SØ4.6ØXD
SØ4.61XD
SØ4.62XD
SØ4.7ØXD
SØ4.71XD
SØ4.72XD
SØ4.811D
SØ4.812D
SØ4.819D
SØ4.891D
SØ4.892D
SØ4.899D
SØ4.9XXD
SØ5.ØØXD
SØ5.Ø1XD
SØ5.Ø2XD
SØ5.1ØXD
SØ5.11XD
SØ5.12XD
SØ5.2ØXD
SØ5.21XD
SØ5.22XD
SØ5.3ØXD
SØ5.31XD
SØ5.32XD
SØ5.4ØXD
SØ5.41XD
SØ5.42XD
SØ5.5ØXD
SØ5.51XD
SØ5.52XD
SØ5.6ØXD
SØ5.61XD
SØ5.62XD
SØ5.7ØXD
SØ5.71XD
SØ5.72XD
SØ5.8X1D
SØ5.8X2D
SØ5.8X9D
SØ5.9ØXD
SØ5.91XD
SØ5.92XD
SØ6.ØXØD
SØ6.ØX1D
SØ6.ØX9D
SØ6.ØXAD
SØ6.1XØD
SØ6.1X1D
SØ6.1X2D
SØ6.1X3D
SØ6.1X4D
SØ6.1X5D
SØ6.1X6D
SØ6.1X9D
SØ6.1XAD
SØ6.2XØD
SØ6.2X1D
SØ6.2X2D
SØ6.2X3D
SØ6.2X4D
SØ6.2X5D
SØ6.2X6D
SØ6.2X9D
SØ6.2XAD
SØ6.3ØØD
SØ6.3Ø1D
SØ6.3Ø2D
SØ6.3Ø3D
SØ6.3Ø4D
SØ6.3Ø5D
SØ6.3Ø6D
SØ6.3Ø9D
SØ6.3ØAD
SØ6.31ØD
SØ6.311D
SØ6.312D
SØ6.313D
SØ6.314D
SØ6.315D
SØ6.316D
SØ6.319D
SØ6.31AD
SØ6.32ØD
SØ6.321D
SØ6.322D
SØ6.323D
SØ6.324D
SØ6.325D
SØ6.326D
SØ6.329D
SØ6.32AD
SØ6.33ØD
SØ6.331D
SØ6.332D
SØ6.333D
SØ6.334D
SØ6.335D
SØ6.336D
SØ6.339D
SØ6.33AD
SØ6.34ØD
SØ6.341D
SØ6.342D
SØ6.343D
SØ6.344D
SØ6.345D
SØ6.346D
SØ6.349D
SØ6.34AD
SØ6.35ØD
SØ6.351D
SØ6.352D
SØ6.353D
SØ6.354D
SØ6.355D
SØ6.356D
SØ6.359D
SØ6.35AD
SØ6.36ØD
SØ6.361D
SØ6.362D
SØ6.363D
SØ6.364D
SØ6.365D
SØ6.366D
SØ6.369D
SØ6.36AD
SØ6.37ØD
SØ6.371D
SØ6.372D
SØ6.373D
SØ6.374D
SØ6.375D
SØ6.376D
SØ6.379D
SØ6.37AD
SØ6.38ØD
SØ6.381D
SØ6.382D
SØ6.383D
SØ6.384D
SØ6.385D
SØ6.386D
SØ6.389D
SØ6.38AD
SØ6.4XØD
SØ6.4X1D
SØ6.4X2D
SØ6.4X3D
SØ6.4X4D
SØ6.4X5D
SØ6.4X6D
SØ6.4X9D
SØ6.4XAD
SØ6.5XØD
SØ6.5X1D
SØ6.5X2D
SØ6.5X3D
SØ6.5X4D
SØ6.5X5D
SØ6.5X6D
SØ6.5X9D
SØ6.5XAD
SØ6.6XØD
SØ6.6X1D
SØ6.6X2D
SØ6.6X3D
SØ6.6X4D
SØ6.6X5D
SØ6.6X6D
SØ6.6X9D
SØ6.6XAD
SØ6.81ØD
SØ6.811D
SØ6.812D
SØ6.813D
SØ6.814D
SØ6.815D
SØ6.816D
SØ6.819D
SØ6.81AD
SØ6.82ØD
SØ6.821D
SØ6.822D
SØ6.823D
SØ6.824D
SØ6.825D
SØ6.826D
SØ6.829D
SØ6.82AD
SØ6.89ØD
SØ6.891D
SØ6.892D
SØ6.893D
SØ6.894D
SØ6.895D
SØ6.896D
SØ6.899D
SØ6.89AD
SØ6.8AØD
SØ6.8A1D
SØ6.8A2D
SØ6.8A3D
SØ6.8A4D
SØ6.8A5D
SØ6.8A6D
SØ6.8A9D
SØ6.8AAD
SØ6.9XØD
SØ6.9X1D
SØ6.9X2D
SØ6.9X3D
SØ6.9X4D
SØ6.9X5D

S06.9X6D
S06.9X9D
S06.9XAD
S06.A0XD
S06.A1XD
S07.0XXD
S07.1XXD
S07.8XXD
S07.9XXD
S08.0XXD
S08.111D
S08.112D
S08.119D
S08.121D
S08.122D
S08.129D
S08.811D
S08.812D
S08.89XD
S09.0XXD
S09.10XD
S09.11XD
S09.12XD
S09.19XD
S09.20XD
S09.21XD
S09.22XD
S09.301D
S09.302D
S09.309D
S09.311D
S09.312D
S09.313D
S09.319D
S09.391D
S09.392D
S09.399D
S09.8XXD
S09.90XD
S09.91XD
S09.92XD
S09.93XD
S10.0XXD
S10.10XD
S10.11XD
S10.12XD
S10.14XD
S10.15XD
S10.16XD
S10.17XD
S10.80XD
S10.81XD
S10.82XD
S10.83XD
S10.84XD
S10.85XD
S10.86XD
S10.87XD
S10.90XD
S10.91XD
S10.92XD
S10.93XD
S10.94XD
S10.95XD
S10.96XD
S10.97XD
S11.011D
S11.012D
S11.013D
S11.014D
S11.015D
S11.019D
S11.021D
S11.022D
S11.023D
S11.024D
S11.025D
S11.029D
S11.031D
S11.032D
S11.033D
S11.034D
S11.035D
S11.039D
S11.10XD
S11.11XD
S11.12XD
S11.13XD
S11.14XD
S11.15XD
S11.20XD
S11.21XD
S11.22XD
S11.23XD
S11.24XD
S11.25XD
S11.80XD
S11.81XD
S11.82XD
S11.83XD
S11.84XD
S11.85XD
S11.89XD
S11.90XD
S11.91XD
S11.92XD
S11.93XD
S11.94XD
S11.95XD
S13.0XXD
S13.100D
S13.101D
S13.110D
S13.111D
S13.120D
S13.121D
S13.130D
S13.131D
S13.140D
S13.141D
S13.150D
S13.151D
S13.160D
S13.161D
S13.170D
S13.171D
S13.180D
S13.181D
S13.20XD
S13.29XD
S13.4XXD
S13.5XXD
S13.8XXD
S13.9XXD
S14.0XXD
S14.101D
S14.102D
S14.103D
S14.104D
S14.105D
S14.106D
S14.107D
S14.108D
S14.109D
S14.111D
S14.112D
S14.113D
S14.114D
S14.115D
S14.116D
S14.117D
S14.118D
S14.119D
S14.121D
S14.122D
S14.123D
S14.124D
S14.125D
S14.126D
S14.127D
S14.128D
S14.129D
S14.131D
S14.132D
S14.133D
S14.134D
S14.135D
S14.136D
S14.137D
S14.138D
S14.139D
S14.141D
S14.142D
S14.143D
S14.144D
S14.145D
S14.146D
S14.147D
S14.148D
S14.149D
S14.151D
S14.152D
S14.153D
S14.154D
S14.155D
S14.156D
S14.157D
S14.158D
S14.159D
S14.2XXD
S14.3XXD
S14.4XXD
S14.5XXD
S14.8XXD
S14.9XXD
S15.001D
S15.002D
S15.009D
S15.011D
S15.012D
S15.019D
S15.021D
S15.022D
S15.029D
S15.091D
S15.092D
S15.099D
S15.101D
S15.102D
S15.109D
S15.111D
S15.112D
S15.119D
S15.121D
S15.122D
S15.129D
S15.191D
S15.192D
S15.199D
S15.201D
S15.202D
S15.209D
S15.211D
S15.212D
S15.219D
S15.221D
S15.222D
S15.229D
S15.291D
S15.292D
S15.299D
S15.301D
S15.302D
S15.309D
S15.311D
S15.312D
S15.319D
S15.321D
S15.322D
S15.329D
S15.391D
S15.392D
S15.399D
S15.8XXD
S15.9XXD
S16.1XXD
S16.2XXD
S16.8XXD
S16.9XXD
S17.0XXD
S17.8XXD
S17.9XXD
S19.80XD
S19.81XD
S19.82XD
S19.83XD
S19.84XD
S19.85XD
S19.89XD
S19.9XXD
S20.00XD
S20.01XD
S20.02XD
S20.101D
S20.102D
S20.109D
S20.111D
S20.112D
S20.119D
S20.121D
S20.122D
S20.129D
S20.141D
S20.142D
S20.149D
S20.151D
S20.152D
S20.159D
S20.161D
S20.162D
S20.169D
S20.171D
S20.172D
S20.179D
S20.20XD
S20.211D
S20.212D
S20.213D
S20.214D
S20.219D
S20.221D
S20.222D
S20.223D
S20.224D
S20.229D
S20.301D
S20.302D
S20.303D
S20.304D
S20.309D
S20.311D
S20.312D
S20.313D
S20.314D
S20.319D
S20.321D
S20.322D
S20.323D
S20.324D
S20.329D
S20.341D
S20.342D
S20.343D
S20.344D
S20.349D
S20.351D
S20.352D
S20.353D
S20.354D
S20.359D
S20.361D
S20.362D
S20.363D
S20.364D
S20.369D
S20.371D
S20.372D
S20.373D
S20.374D
S20.379D
S20.401D
S20.402D
S20.409D
S20.411D
S20.412D
S20.419D
S20.421D
S20.422D
S20.429D
S20.441D
S20.442D
S20.449D
S20.451D
S20.452D
S20.459D
S20.461D
S20.462D
S20.469D
S20.471D
S20.472D
S20.479D
S20.90XD
S20.91XD
S20.92XD
S20.94XD
S20.95XD
S20.96XD
S20.97XD
S21.001D
S21.002D
S21.009D
S21.011D
S21.012D
S21.019D
S21.021D
S21.022D
S21.029D
S21.031D
S21.032D
S21.039D
S21.041D
S21.042D
S21.049D
S21.051D
S21.052D
S21.059D
S21.101D
S21.102D
S21.109D
S21.111D
S21.112D
S21.119D
S21.121D
S21.122D
S21.129D
S21.131D
S21.132D
S21.139D
S21.141D
S21.142D
S21.149D
S21.151D
S21.152D
S21.159D
S21.201D
S21.202D
S21.209D
S21.211D
S21.212D
S21.219D
S21.221D
S21.222D
S21.229D
S21.231D
S21.232D
S21.239D
S21.241D
S21.242D
S21.249D
S21.251D
S21.252D
S21.259D
S21.301D
S21.302D
S21.309D
S21.311D
S21.312D
S21.319D
S21.321D
S21.322D
S21.329D
S21.331D
S21.332D
S21.339D
S21.341D
S21.342D
S21.349D
S21.351D
S21.352D
S21.359D
S21.401D
S21.402D
S21.409D
S21.411D
S21.412D
S21.419D
S21.421D
S21.422D
S21.429D
S21.431D
S21.432D
S21.439D
S21.441D
S21.442D
S21.449D
S21.451D
S21.452D
S21.459D
S21.90XD
S21.91XD
S21.92XD
S21.93XD
S21.94XD
S21.95XD
S23.0XXD
S23.100D
S23.101D
S23.110D
S23.111D
S23.120D
S23.121D
S23.122D
S23.123D
S23.130D
S23.131D
S23.132D
S23.133D
S23.140D
S23.141D
S23.142D
S23.143D
S23.150D
S23.151D
S23.152D
S23.153D
S23.160D
S23.161D
S23.162D
S23.163D
S23.170D
S23.171D
S23.20XD
S23.29XD
S23.3XXD
S23.41XD
S23.420D
S23.421D
S23.428D
S23.429D
S23.8XXD
S23.9XXD
S24.0XXD
S24.101D
S24.102D
S24.103D
S24.104D
S24.109D
S24.111D
S24.112D
S24.113D
S24.114D
S24.119D
S24.131D
S24.132D
S24.133D
S24.134D
S24.139D
S24.141D
S24.142D
S24.143D
S24.144D
S24.149D
S24.151D
S24.152D
S24.153D
S24.154D
S24.159D
S24.2XXD
S24.3XXD
S24.4XXD
S24.8XXD
S24.9XXD
S25.00XD
S25.01XD
S25.02XD
S25.09XD
S25.101D
S25.102D
S25.109D
S25.111D
S25.112D
S25.119D
S25.121D
S25.122D
S25.129D
S25.191D
S25.192D
S25.199D
S25.20XD
S25.21XD
S25.22XD
S25.29XD
S25.301D
S25.302D
S25.309D
S25.311D
S25.312D
S25.319D
S25.321D
S25.322D
S25.329D
S25.391D
S25.392D
S25.399D
S25.401D
S25.402D
S25.409D
S25.411D
S25.412D
S25.419D
S25.421D
S25.422D
S25.429D
S25.491D
S25.492D
S25.499D
S25.501D
S25.502D
S25.509D
S25.511D
S25.512D
S25.519D
S25.591D
S25.592D
S25.599D
S25.801D
S25.802D
S25.809D
S25.811D
S25.812D
S25.819D
S25.891D
S25.892D
S25.899D
S25.90XD
S25.91XD
S25.99XD
S26.00XD
S26.01XD
S26.020D
S26.021D
S26.022D
S26.09XD
S26.10XD
S26.11XD
S26.12XD
S26.19XD
S26.90XD
S26.91XD
S26.92XD
S26.99XD
S27.0XXD
S27.1XXD
S27.2XXD
S27.301D
S27.302D
S27.309D
S27.311D
S27.312D
S27.319D
S27.321D
S27.322D
S27.329D
S27.331D
S27.332D
S27.339D
S27.391D
S27.392D
S27.399D
S27.401D
S27.402D
S27.409D
S27.411D
S27.412D
S27.419D
S27.421D
S27.422D
S27.429D
S27.431D
S27.432D
S27.439D
S27.491D
S27.492D
S27.499D
S27.50XD
S27.51XD
S27.52XD
S27.53XD
S27.59XD
S27.60XD
S27.63XD
S27.69XD
S27.802D
S27.803D
S27.808D
S27.809D
S27.812D
S27.813D
S27.818D
S27.819D
S27.892D
S27.893D
S27.898D
S27.899D
S27.9XXD
S28.0XXD
S28.1XXD
S28.211D
S28.212D
S28.219D
S28.221D
S28.222D
S28.229D
S29.001D
S29.002D
S29.009D
S29.011D
S29.012D
S29.019D
S29.021D
S29.022D
S29.029D
S29.091D
S29.092D
S29.099D
S29.8XXD
S29.9XXD
S30.0XXD
S30.1XXD
S30.201D
S30.202D
S30.21XD
S30.22XD
S30.23XD
S30.3XXD
S30.810D
S30.811D
S30.812D
S30.813D
S30.814D
S30.815D
S30.816D
S30.817D
S30.820D
S30.821D
S30.822D
S30.823D
S30.824D
S30.825D
S30.826D
S30.827D
S30.840D
S30.841D
S30.842D
S30.843D
S30.844D
S30.845D
S30.846D
S30.850D
S30.851D
S30.852D
S30.853D
S30.854D
S30.855D
S30.856D
S30.857D
S30.860D
S30.861D
S30.862D
S30.863D
S30.864D
S30.865D
S30.866D
S30.867D
S30.870D
S30.871D
S30.872D
S30.873D
S30.874D
S30.875D
S30.876D
S30.877D
S30.91XD
S30.92XD
S30.93XD
S30.94XD
S30.95XD
S30.96XD
S30.97XD
S30.98XD
S31.000D
S31.001D
S31.010D
S31.011D
S31.020D
S31.021D
S31.030D
S31.031D
S31.040D
S31.041D
S31.050D
S31.051D
S31.100D
S31.101D
S31.102D
S31.103D
S31.104D
S31.105D
S31.109D
S31.110D
S31.111D
S31.112D
S31.113D
S31.114D
S31.115D
S31.119D
S31.120D
S31.121D
S31.122D
S31.123D
S31.124D
S31.125D
S31.129D
S31.130D
S31.131D
S31.132D
S31.133D
S31.134D
S31.135D
S31.139D
S31.140D
S31.141D
S31.142D
S31.143D
S31.144D
S31.145D
S31.149D
S31.150D
S31.151D
S31.152D
S31.153D
S31.154D
S31.155D
S31.159D
S31.20XD
S31.21XD
S31.22XD
S31.23XD
S31.24XD
S31.25XD
S31.30XD
S31.31XD
S31.32XD
S31.33XD
S31.34XD
S31.35XD
S31.40XD
S31.41XD
S31.42XD
S31.43XD
S31.44XD
S31.45XD
S31.501D
S31.502D
S31.511D
S31.512D
S31.521D
S31.522D
S31.531D
S31.532D
S31.541D
S31.542D
S31.551D
S31.552D
S31.600D
S31.601D
S31.602D
S31.603D
S31.604D
S31.605D
S31.609D
S31.610D
S31.611D
S31.612D
S31.613D
S31.614D
S31.615D
S31.619D
S31.620D
S31.621D
S31.622D
S31.623D
S31.624D
S31.625D
S31.629D
S31.630D
S31.631D
S31.632D
S31.633D
S31.634D
S31.635D
S31.639D
S31.640D
S31.641D
S31.642D

S31.643D
S31.644D
S31.645D
S31.649D
S31.650D
S31.651D
S31.652D
S31.653D
S31.654D
S31.655D
S31.659D
S31.801D
S31.802D
S31.803D
S31.804D
S31.805D
S31.809D
S31.811D
S31.812D
S31.813D
S31.814D
S31.815D
S31.819D
S31.821D
S31.822D
S31.823D
S31.824D
S31.825D
S31.829D
S31.831D
S31.832D
S31.833D
S31.834D
S31.835D
S31.839D
S33.0XXD
S33.100D
S33.101D
S33.110D
S33.111D
S33.120D
S33.121D
S33.130D
S33.131D
S33.140D
S33.141D
S33.2XXD
S33.30XD
S33.39XD
S33.4XXD
S33.5XXD
S33.6XXD
S33.8XXD
S33.9XXD
S34.01XD
S34.02XD
S34.101D
S34.102D
S34.103D
S34.104D
S34.105D
S34.109D
S34.111D
S34.112D
S34.113D
S34.114D
S34.115D
S34.119D
S34.121D
S34.122D
S34.123D
S34.124D
S34.125D
S34.129D
S34.131D
S34.132D
S34.139D
S34.21XD
S34.22XD
S34.3XXD
S34.4XXD
S34.5XXD
S34.6XXD
S34.8XXD
S34.9XXD
S35.00XD
S35.01XD
S35.02XD
S35.09XD
S35.10XD
S35.11XD
S35.12XD
S35.19XD
S35.211D
S35.212D
S35.218D
S35.219D
S35.221D
S35.222D
S35.228D
S35.229D
S35.231D
S35.232D
S35.238D
S35.239D
S35.291D
S35.292D
S35.298D
S35.299D
S35.311D
S35.318D
S35.319D
S35.321D
S35.328D
S35.329D
S35.331D
S35.338D
S35.339D
S35.341D
S35.348D
S35.349D
S35.401D
S35.402D
S35.403D
S35.404D
S35.405D
S35.406D
S35.411D
S35.412D
S35.413D
S35.414D
S35.415D
S35.416D
S35.491D
S35.492D
S35.493D
S35.494D
S35.495D
S35.496D
S35.50XD
S35.511D
S35.512D
S35.513D
S35.514D
S35.515D
S35.516D
S35.531D
S35.532D
S35.533D
S35.534D
S35.535D
S35.536D
S35.59XD
S35.8X1D
S35.8X8D
S35.8X9D
S35.90XD
S35.91XD
S35.99XD
S36.00XD
S36.020D
S36.021D
S36.029D
S36.030D
S36.031D
S36.032D
S36.039D
S36.09XD
S36.112D
S36.113D
S36.114D
S36.115D
S36.116D
S36.118D
S36.119D
S36.122D
S36.123D
S36.128D
S36.129D
S36.13XD
S36.200D
S36.201D
S36.202D
S36.209D
S36.220D
S36.221D
S36.222D
S36.229D
S36.230D
S36.231D
S36.232D
S36.239D
S36.240D
S36.241D
S36.242D
S36.249D
S36.250D
S36.251D
S36.252D
S36.259D
S36.260D
S36.261D
S36.262D
S36.269D
S36.290D
S36.291D
S36.292D
S36.299D
S36.30XD
S36.32XD
S36.33XD
S36.39XD
S36.400D
S36.408D
S36.409D
S36.410D
S36.418D
S36.419D
S36.420D
S36.428D
S36.429D
S36.430D
S36.438D
S36.439D
S36.490D
S36.498D
S36.499D
S36.500D
S36.501D
S36.502D
S36.503D
S36.508D
S36.509D
S36.510D
S36.511D
S36.512D
S36.513D
S36.518D
S36.519D
S36.520D
S36.521D
S36.522D
S36.523D
S36.528D
S36.529D
S36.530D
S36.531D
S36.532D
S36.533D
S36.538D
S36.539D
S36.590D
S36.591D
S36.592D
S36.593D
S36.598D
S36.599D
S36.60XD
S36.61XD
S36.62XD
S36.63XD
S36.69XD
S36.81XD
S36.892D
S36.893D
S36.898D
S36.899D
S36.90XD
S36.92XD
S36.93XD
S36.99XD
S37.001D
S37.002D
S37.009D
S37.011D
S37.012D
S37.019D
S37.021D
S37.022D
S37.029D
S37.031D
S37.032D
S37.039D
S37.041D
S37.042D
S37.049D
S37.051D
S37.052D
S37.059D
S37.061D
S37.062D
S37.069D
S37.091D
S37.092D
S37.099D
S37.10XD
S37.12XD
S37.13XD
S37.19XD
S37.20XD
S37.22XD
S37.23XD
S37.29XD
S37.30XD
S37.32XD
S37.33XD
S37.39XD
S37.401D
S37.402D
S37.409D
S37.421D
S37.422D
S37.429D
S37.431D
S37.432D
S37.439D
S37.491D
S37.492D
S37.499D
S37.501D
S37.502D
S37.509D
S37.511D
S37.512D
S37.519D
S37.521D
S37.522D
S37.529D
S37.531D
S37.532D
S37.539D
S37.591D
S37.592D
S37.599D
S37.60XD
S37.62XD
S37.63XD
S37.69XD
S37.812D
S37.813D
S37.818D
S37.819D
S37.822D
S37.823D
S37.828D
S37.829D
S37.892D
S37.893D
S37.898D
S37.899D
S37.90XD
S37.92XD
S37.93XD
S37.99XD
S38.001D
S38.002D
S38.01XD
S38.02XD
S38.03XD
S38.1XXD
S38.211D
S38.212D
S38.221D
S38.222D
S38.231D
S38.232D
S38.3XXD
S39.001D
S39.002D
S39.003D
S39.011D
S39.012D
S39.013D
S39.021D
S39.022D
S39.023D
S39.091D
S39.092D
S39.093D
S39.81XD
S39.82XD
S39.83XD
S39.840D
S39.848D
S39.91XD
S39.92XD
S39.93XD
S39.94XD
S40.011D
S40.012D
S40.019D
S40.021D
S40.022D
S40.029D
S40.211D
S40.212D
S40.219D
S40.221D
S40.222D
S40.229D
S40.241D
S40.242D
S40.249D
S40.251D
S40.252D
S40.259D
S40.261D
S40.262D
S40.269D
S40.271D
S40.272D
S40.279D
S40.811D
S40.812D
S40.819D
S40.821D
S40.822D
S40.829D
S40.841D
S40.842D
S40.849D
S40.851D
S40.852D
S40.859D
S40.861D
S40.862D
S40.869D
S40.871D
S40.872D
S40.879D
S40.911D
S40.912D
S40.919D
S40.921D
S40.922D
S40.929D
S41.001D
S41.002D
S41.009D
S41.011D
S41.012D
S41.019D
S41.021D
S41.022D
S41.029D
S41.031D
S41.032D
S41.039D
S41.041D
S41.042D
S41.049D
S41.051D
S41.052D
S41.059D
S41.101D
S41.102D
S41.109D
S41.111D
S41.112D
S41.119D
S41.121D
S41.122D
S41.129D
S41.131D
S41.132D
S41.139D
S41.141D
S41.142D
S41.149D
S41.151D
S41.152D
S41.159D
S43.001D
S43.002D
S43.003D
S43.004D
S43.005D
S43.006D
S43.011D
S43.012D
S43.013D
S43.014D
S43.015D
S43.016D
S43.021D
S43.022D
S43.023D
S43.024D
S43.025D
S43.026D
S43.031D
S43.032D
S43.033D
S43.034D
S43.035D
S43.036D
S43.081D
S43.082D
S43.083D
S43.084D
S43.085D
S43.086D
S43.101D
S43.102D
S43.109D
S43.111D
S43.112D
S43.119D
S43.121D
S43.122D
S43.129D
S43.131D
S43.132D
S43.139D
S43.141D
S43.142D
S43.149D
S43.151D
S43.152D
S43.159D
S43.201D
S43.202D
S43.203D
S43.204D
S43.205D
S43.206D
S43.211D
S43.212D
S43.213D
S43.214D
S43.215D
S43.216D
S43.221D
S43.222D
S43.223D
S43.224D
S43.225D
S43.226D
S43.301D
S43.302D
S43.303D
S43.304D
S43.305D
S43.306D
S43.311D
S43.312D
S43.313D
S43.314D
S43.315D
S43.316D
S43.391D
S43.392D
S43.393D
S43.394D
S43.395D
S43.396D
S43.401D
S43.402D
S43.409D
S43.411D
S43.412D
S43.419D
S43.421D
S43.422D
S43.429D
S43.431D
S43.432D
S43.439D
S43.491D
S43.492D
S43.499D
S43.50XD
S43.51XD
S43.52XD
S43.60XD
S43.61XD
S43.62XD
S43.80XD
S43.81XD
S43.82XD
S43.90XD
S43.91XD
S43.92XD
S44.00XD
S44.01XD
S44.02XD
S44.10XD
S44.11XD
S44.12XD
S44.20XD
S44.21XD
S44.22XD
S44.30XD
S44.31XD
S44.32XD
S44.40XD
S44.41XD
S44.42XD
S44.50XD
S44.51XD
S44.52XD
S44.8X1D
S44.8X2D
S44.8X9D
S44.90XD
S44.91XD
S44.92XD
S45.001D
S45.002D
S45.009D
S45.011D
S45.012D
S45.019D
S45.091D
S45.092D
S45.099D
S45.101D
S45.102D
S45.109D
S45.111D
S45.112D
S45.119D
S45.191D
S45.192D
S45.199D
S45.201D
S45.202D
S45.209D
S45.211D
S45.212D
S45.219D
S45.291D
S45.292D
S45.299D
S45.301D
S45.302D
S45.309D
S45.311D
S45.312D
S45.319D
S45.391D
S45.392D
S45.399D
S45.801D
S45.802D
S45.809D
S45.811D
S45.812D
S45.819D
S45.891D
S45.892D
S45.899D
S45.901D
S45.902D
S45.909D
S45.911D
S45.912D
S45.919D
S45.991D
S45.992D
S45.999D
S46.001D
S46.002D
S46.009D
S46.011D
S46.012D
S46.019D
S46.021D
S46.022D
S46.029D
S46.091D
S46.092D
S46.099D
S46.101D
S46.102D
S46.109D
S46.111D
S46.112D
S46.119D
S46.121D
S46.122D
S46.129D
S46.191D
S46.192D
S46.199D
S46.201D
S46.202D
S46.209D
S46.211D
S46.212D
S46.219D
S46.221D
S46.222D
S46.229D
S46.291D
S46.292D
S46.299D
S46.301D
S46.302D
S46.309D
S46.311D
S46.312D
S46.319D
S46.321D
S46.322D
S46.329D
S46.391D
S46.392D
S46.399D
S46.801D
S46.802D
S46.809D
S46.811D
S46.812D
S46.819D
S46.821D
S46.822D
S46.829D
S46.891D
S46.892D
S46.899D
S46.901D
S46.902D
S46.909D
S46.911D
S46.912D
S46.919D
S46.921D
S46.922D
S46.929D
S46.991D
S46.992D
S46.999D
S47.1XXD
S47.2XXD
S47.9XXD
S48.011D
S48.012D
S48.019D
S48.021D
S48.022D
S48.029D
S48.111D
S48.112D
S48.119D
S48.121D
S48.122D
S48.129D
S48.911D
S48.912D
S48.919D
S48.921D
S48.922D
S48.929D
S49.80XD
S49.81XD
S49.82XD
S49.90XD
S49.91XD
S49.92XD
S50.00XD
S50.01XD
S50.02XD
S50.10XD
S50.11XD
S50.12XD
S50.311D
S50.312D
S50.319D
S50.321D
S50.322D
S50.329D
S50.341D
S50.342D
S50.349D
S50.351D
S50.352D
S50.359D
S50.361D
S50.362D
S50.369D
S50.371D
S50.372D
S50.379D
S50.811D
S50.812D
S50.819D
S50.821D
S50.822D
S50.829D
S50.841D
S50.842D
S50.849D
S50.851D
S50.852D
S50.859D
S50.861D
S50.862D
S50.869D
S50.871D
S50.872D
S50.879D
S50.901D
S50.902D
S50.909D
S50.911D
S50.912D
S50.919D
S51.001D
S51.002D
S51.009D
S51.011D
S51.012D
S51.019D
S51.021D
S51.022D
S51.029D
S51.031D
S51.032D
S51.039D
S51.041D
S51.042D
S51.049D
S51.051D
S51.052D
S51.059D
S51.801D
S51.802D
S51.809D
S51.811D
S51.812D
S51.819D
S51.821D
S51.822D
S51.829D
S51.831D
S51.832D
S51.839D
S51.841D
S51.842D
S51.849D
S51.851D
S51.852D
S51.859D
S53.001D
S53.002D
S53.003D
S53.004D
S53.005D
S53.006D
S53.011D
S53.012D
S53.013D
S53.014D
S53.015D

S53.016D
S53.021D
S53.022D
S53.023D
S53.024D
S53.025D
S53.026D
S53.031D
S53.032D
S53.033D
S53.091D
S53.092D
S53.093D
S53.094D
S53.095D
S53.096D
S53.101D
S53.102D
S53.103D
S53.104D
S53.105D
S53.106D
S53.111D
S53.112D
S53.113D
S53.114D
S53.115D
S53.116D
S53.121D
S53.122D
S53.123D
S53.124D
S53.125D
S53.126D
S53.131D
S53.132D
S53.133D
S53.134D
S53.135D
S53.136D
S53.141D
S53.142D
S53.143D
S53.144D
S53.145D
S53.146D
S53.191D
S53.192D
S53.193D
S53.194D
S53.195D
S53.196D
S53.20XD
S53.21XD
S53.22XD
S53.30XD
S53.31XD
S53.32XD
S53.401D
S53.402D
S53.409D
S53.411D
S53.412D
S53.419D
S53.421D
S53.422D
S53.429D
S53.431D
S53.432D
S53.439D
S53.441D
S53.442D
S53.449D
S53.491D
S53.492D
S53.499D
S54.00XD
S54.01XD
S54.02XD
S54.10XD
S54.11XD
S54.12XD
S54.20XD
S54.21XD
S54.22XD
S54.30XD
S54.31XD
S54.32XD
S54.8X1D
S54.8X2D
S54.8X9D
S54.90XD
S54.91XD
S54.92XD
S55.001D
S55.002D
S55.009D
S55.011D
S55.012D
S55.019D
S55.091D
S55.092D
S55.099D
S55.101D
S55.102D
S55.109D
S55.111D
S55.112D
S55.119D
S55.191D
S55.192D
S55.199D
S55.201D
S55.202D
S55.209D
S55.211D
S55.212D
S55.219D
S55.291D
S55.292D
S55.299D
S55.801D
S55.802D
S55.809D
S55.811D
S55.812D
S55.819D
S55.891D
S55.892D
S55.899D
S55.901D
S55.902D
S55.909D
S55.911D
S55.912D
S55.919D
S55.991D
S55.992D
S55.999D
S56.001D
S56.002D
S56.009D
S56.011D
S56.012D
S56.019D
S56.021D
S56.022D
S56.029D
S56.091D
S56.092D
S56.099D
S56.101D
S56.102D
S56.103D
S56.104D
S56.105D
S56.106D
S56.107D
S56.108D
S56.109D
S56.111D
S56.112D
S56.113D
S56.114D
S56.115D
S56.116D
S56.117D
S56.118D
S56.119D
S56.121D
S56.122D
S56.123D
S56.124D
S56.125D
S56.126D
S56.127D
S56.128D
S56.129D
S56.191D
S56.192D
S56.193D
S56.194D
S56.195D
S56.196D
S56.197D
S56.198D
S56.199D
S56.201D
S56.202D
S56.209D
S56.211D
S56.212D
S56.219D
S56.221D
S56.222D
S56.229D
S56.291D
S56.292D
S56.299D
S56.301D
S56.302D
S56.309D
S56.311D
S56.312D
S56.319D
S56.321D
S56.322D
S56.329D
S56.391D
S56.392D
S56.399D
S56.401D
S56.402D
S56.403D
S56.404D
S56.405D
S56.406D
S56.407D
S56.408D
S56.409D
S56.411D
S56.412D
S56.413D
S56.414D
S56.415D
S56.416D
S56.417D
S56.418D
S56.419D
S56.421D
S56.422D
S56.423D
S56.424D
S56.425D
S56.426D
S56.427D
S56.428D
S56.429D
S56.491D
S56.492D
S56.493D
S56.494D
S56.495D
S56.496D
S56.497D
S56.498D
S56.499D
S56.501D
S56.502D
S56.509D
S56.511D
S56.512D
S56.519D
S56.521D
S56.522D
S56.529D
S56.591D
S56.592D
S56.599D
S56.801D
S56.802D
S56.809D
S56.811D
S56.812D
S56.819D
S56.821D
S56.822D
S56.829D
S56.891D
S56.892D
S56.899D
S56.901D
S56.902D
S56.909D
S56.911D
S56.912D
S56.919D
S56.921D
S56.922D
S56.929D
S56.991D
S56.992D
S56.999D
S57.00XD
S57.01XD
S57.02XD
S57.80XD
S57.81XD
S57.82XD
S58.011D
S58.012D
S58.019D
S58.021D
S58.022D
S58.029D
S58.111D
S58.112D
S58.119D
S58.121D
S58.122D
S58.129D
S58.911D
S58.912D
S58.919D
S58.921D
S58.922D
S58.929D
S59.801D
S59.802D
S59.809D
S59.811D
S59.812D
S59.819D
S59.901D
S59.902D
S59.909D
S59.911D
S59.912D
S59.919D
S60.00XD
S60.011D
S60.012D
S60.019D
S60.021D
S60.022D
S60.029D
S60.031D
S60.032D
S60.039D
S60.041D
S60.042D
S60.049D
S60.051D
S60.052D
S60.059D
S60.10XD
S60.111D
S60.112D
S60.119D
S60.121D
S60.122D
S60.129D
S60.131D
S60.132D
S60.139D
S60.141D
S60.142D
S60.149D
S60.151D
S60.152D
S60.159D
S60.211D
S60.212D
S60.219D
S60.221D
S60.222D
S60.229D
S60.311D
S60.312D
S60.319D
S60.321D
S60.322D
S60.329D
S60.341D
S60.342D
S60.349D
S60.351D
S60.352D
S60.359D
S60.361D
S60.362D
S60.369D
S60.371D
S60.372D
S60.379D
S60.391D
S60.392D
S60.399D
S60.410D
S60.411D
S60.412D
S60.413D
S60.414D
S60.415D
S60.416D
S60.417D
S60.418D
S60.419D
S60.420D
S60.421D
S60.422D
S60.423D
S60.424D
S60.425D
S60.426D
S60.427D
S60.428D
S60.429D
S60.440D
S60.441D
S60.442D
S60.443D
S60.444D
S60.445D
S60.446D
S60.447D
S60.448D
S60.449D
S60.450D
S60.451D
S60.452D
S60.453D
S60.454D
S60.455D
S60.456D
S60.457D
S60.458D
S60.459D
S60.460D
S60.461D
S60.462D
S60.463D
S60.464D
S60.465D
S60.466D
S60.467D
S60.468D
S60.469D
S60.470D
S60.471D
S60.472D
S60.473D
S60.474D
S60.475D
S60.476D
S60.477D
S60.478D
S60.479D
S60.511D
S60.512D
S60.519D
S60.521D
S60.522D
S60.529D
S60.541D
S60.542D
S60.549D
S60.551D
S60.552D
S60.559D
S60.561D
S60.562D
S60.569D
S60.571D
S60.572D
S60.579D
S60.811D
S60.812D
S60.819D
S60.821D
S60.822D
S60.829D
S60.841D
S60.842D
S60.849D
S60.851D
S60.852D
S60.859D
S60.861D
S60.862D
S60.869D
S60.871D
S60.872D
S60.879D
S60.911D
S60.912D
S60.919D
S60.921D
S60.922D
S60.929D
S60.931D
S60.932D
S60.939D
S60.940D
S60.941D
S60.942D
S60.943D
S60.944D
S60.945D
S60.946D
S60.947D
S60.948D
S60.949D
S61.001D
S61.002D
S61.009D
S61.011D
S61.012D
S61.019D
S61.021D
S61.022D
S61.029D
S61.031D
S61.032D
S61.039D
S61.041D
S61.042D
S61.049D
S61.051D
S61.052D
S61.059D
S61.101D
S61.102D
S61.109D
S61.111D
S61.112D
S61.119D
S61.121D
S61.122D
S61.129D
S61.131D
S61.132D
S61.139D
S61.141D
S61.142D
S61.149D
S61.151D
S61.152D
S61.159D
S61.200D
S61.201D
S61.202D
S61.203D
S61.204D
S61.205D
S61.206D
S61.207D
S61.208D
S61.209D
S61.210D
S61.211D
S61.212D
S61.213D
S61.214D
S61.215D
S61.216D
S61.217D
S61.218D
S61.219D
S61.220D
S61.221D
S61.222D
S61.223D
S61.224D
S61.225D
S61.226D
S61.227D
S61.228D
S61.229D
S61.230D
S61.231D
S61.232D
S61.233D
S61.234D
S61.235D
S61.236D
S61.237D
S61.238D
S61.239D
S61.240D
S61.241D
S61.242D
S61.243D
S61.244D
S61.245D
S61.246D
S61.247D
S61.248D
S61.249D
S61.250D
S61.251D
S61.252D
S61.253D
S61.254D
S61.255D
S61.256D
S61.257D
S61.258D
S61.259D
S61.300D
S61.301D
S61.302D
S61.303D
S61.304D
S61.305D
S61.306D
S61.307D
S61.308D
S61.309D
S61.310D
S61.311D
S61.312D
S61.313D
S61.314D
S61.315D
S61.316D
S61.317D
S61.318D
S61.319D
S61.320D
S61.321D
S61.322D
S61.323D
S61.324D
S61.325D
S61.326D
S61.327D
S61.328D
S61.329D
S61.330D
S61.331D
S61.332D
S61.333D
S61.334D
S61.335D
S61.336D
S61.337D
S61.338D
S61.339D
S61.340D
S61.341D
S61.342D
S61.343D
S61.344D
S61.345D
S61.346D
S61.347D
S61.348D
S61.349D
S61.350D
S61.351D
S61.352D
S61.353D
S61.354D
S61.355D
S61.356D
S61.357D
S61.358D
S61.359D
S61.401D
S61.402D
S61.409D
S61.411D
S61.412D
S61.419D
S61.421D
S61.422D
S61.429D
S61.431D
S61.432D
S61.439D
S61.441D
S61.442D
S61.449D
S61.451D
S61.452D
S61.459D
S61.501D
S61.502D
S61.509D
S61.511D
S61.512D
S61.519D
S61.521D
S61.522D
S61.529D
S61.531D
S61.532D
S61.539D
S61.541D
S61.542D
S61.549D
S61.551D
S61.552D
S61.559D
S63.001D
S63.002D
S63.003D
S63.004D
S63.005D
S63.006D
S63.011D
S63.012D
S63.013D
S63.014D
S63.015D
S63.016D
S63.021D
S63.022D
S63.023D
S63.024D
S63.025D
S63.026D
S63.031D
S63.032D
S63.033D
S63.034D
S63.035D
S63.036D
S63.041D
S63.042D
S63.043D
S63.044D
S63.045D
S63.046D
S63.051D
S63.052D
S63.053D
S63.054D
S63.055D
S63.056D
S63.061D
S63.062D
S63.063D
S63.064D
S63.065D
S63.066D
S63.071D
S63.072D
S63.073D
S63.074D
S63.075D
S63.076D
S63.091D
S63.092D
S63.093D
S63.094D
S63.095D
S63.096D
S63.101D
S63.102D
S63.103D
S63.104D
S63.105D
S63.106D
S63.111D
S63.112D
S63.113D
S63.114D
S63.115D
S63.116D
S63.121D
S63.122D
S63.123D
S63.124D
S63.125D
S63.126D
S63.200D
S63.201D
S63.202D
S63.203D
S63.204D
S63.205D
S63.206D
S63.207D
S63.208D
S63.209D
S63.210D
S63.211D
S63.212D
S63.213D
S63.214D
S63.215D
S63.216D
S63.217D
S63.218D
S63.219D
S63.220D
S63.221D
S63.222D
S63.223D
S63.224D
S63.225D
S63.226D
S63.227D
S63.228D
S63.229D
S63.230D
S63.231D
S63.232D
S63.233D
S63.234D
S63.235D
S63.236D
S63.237D
S63.238D
S63.239D
S63.240D
S63.241D
S63.242D
S63.243D
S63.244D
S63.245D
S63.246D
S63.247D
S63.248D
S63.249D
S63.250D
S63.251D
S63.252D
S63.253D
S63.254D
S63.255D
S63.256D
S63.257D
S63.258D
S63.259D
S63.260D
S63.261D
S63.262D
S63.263D
S63.264D
S63.265D
S63.266D
S63.267D
S63.268D
S63.269D
S63.270D
S63.271D
S63.272D
S63.273D
S63.274D
S63.275D
S63.276D
S63.277D
S63.278D
S63.279D
S63.280D
S63.281D
S63.282D
S63.283D
S63.284D
S63.285D
S63.286D
S63.287D
S63.288D
S63.289D
S63.290D
S63.291D
S63.292D
S63.293D
S63.294D
S63.295D
S63.296D
S63.297D

S63.298D
S63.299D
S63.301D
S63.302D
S63.309D
S63.311D
S63.312D
S63.319D
S63.321D
S63.322D
S63.329D
S63.331D
S63.332D
S63.339D
S63.391D
S63.392D
S63.399D
S63.400D
S63.401D
S63.402D
S63.403D
S63.404D
S63.405D
S63.406D
S63.407D
S63.408D
S63.409D
S63.410D
S63.411D
S63.412D
S63.413D
S63.414D
S63.415D
S63.416D
S63.417D
S63.418D
S63.419D
S63.420D
S63.421D
S63.422D
S63.423D
S63.424D
S63.425D
S63.426D
S63.427D
S63.428D
S63.429D
S63.430D
S63.431D
S63.432D
S63.433D
S63.434D
S63.435D
S63.436D
S63.437D
S63.438D
S63.439D
S63.490D
S63.491D
S63.492D
S63.493D
S63.494D
S63.495D
S63.496D
S63.497D
S63.498D
S63.499D
S63.501D
S63.502D
S63.509D
S63.511D
S63.512D
S63.519D
S63.521D
S63.522D
S63.529D
S63.591D
S63.592D
S63.599D
S63.601D
S63.602D
S63.609D
S63.610D
S63.611D
S63.612D
S63.613D
S63.614D
S63.615D
S63.616D
S63.617D
S63.618D
S63.619D
S63.621D
S63.622D
S63.629D
S63.630D
S63.631D
S63.632D
S63.633D
S63.634D
S63.635D
S63.636D
S63.637D
S63.638D
S63.639D
S63.641D
S63.642D
S63.649D
S63.650D
S63.651D
S63.652D
S63.653D
S63.654D
S63.655D
S63.656D
S63.657D
S63.658D
S63.659D
S63.681D
S63.682D
S63.689D
S63.690D
S63.691D
S63.692D
S63.693D
S63.694D
S63.695D
S63.696D
S63.697D
S63.698D
S63.699D
S63.8X1D
S63.8X2D
S63.8X9D
S63.90XD
S63.91XD
S63.92XD
S64.00XD
S64.01XD
S64.02XD
S64.10XD
S64.11XD
S64.12XD
S64.20XD
S64.21XD
S64.22XD
S64.30XD
S64.31XD
S64.32XD
S64.40XD
S64.490D
S64.491D
S64.492D
S64.493D
S64.494D
S64.495D
S64.496D
S64.497D
S64.498D
S64.8X1D
S64.8X2D
S64.8X9D
S64.90XD
S64.91XD
S64.92XD
S65.001D
S65.002D
S65.009D
S65.011D
S65.012D
S65.019D
S65.091D
S65.092D
S65.099D
S65.101D
S65.102D
S65.109D
S65.111D
S65.112D
S65.119D
S65.191D
S65.192D
S65.199D
S65.201D
S65.202D
S65.209D
S65.211D
S65.212D
S65.219D
S65.291D
S65.292D
S65.299D
S65.301D
S65.302D
S65.309D
S65.311D
S65.312D
S65.319D
S65.391D
S65.392D
S65.399D
S65.401D
S65.402D
S65.409D
S65.411D
S65.412D
S65.419D
S65.491D
S65.492D
S65.499D
S65.500D
S65.501D
S65.502D
S65.503D
S65.504D
S65.505D
S65.506D
S65.507D
S65.508D
S65.509D
S65.510D
S65.511D
S65.512D
S65.513D
S65.514D
S65.515D
S65.516D
S65.517D
S65.518D
S65.519D
S65.590D
S65.591D
S65.592D
S65.593D
S65.594D
S65.595D
S65.596D
S65.597D
S65.598D
S65.599D
S65.801D
S65.802D
S65.809D
S65.811D
S65.812D
S65.819D
S65.891D
S65.892D
S65.899D
S65.901D
S65.902D
S65.909D
S65.911D
S65.912D
S65.919D
S65.991D
S65.992D
S65.999D
S66.001D
S66.002D
S66.009D
S66.011D
S66.012D
S66.019D
S66.021D
S66.022D
S66.029D
S66.091D
S66.092D
S66.099D
S66.100D
S66.101D
S66.102D
S66.103D
S66.104D
S66.105D
S66.106D
S66.107D
S66.108D
S66.109D
S66.110D
S66.111D
S66.112D
S66.113D
S66.114D
S66.115D
S66.116D
S66.117D
S66.118D
S66.119D
S66.120D
S66.121D
S66.122D
S66.123D
S66.124D
S66.125D
S66.126D
S66.127D
S66.128D
S66.129D
S66.190D
S66.191D
S66.192D
S66.193D
S66.194D
S66.195D
S66.196D
S66.197D
S66.198D
S66.199D
S66.201D
S66.202D
S66.209D
S66.211D
S66.212D
S66.219D
S66.221D
S66.222D
S66.229D
S66.291D
S66.292D
S66.299D
S66.300D
S66.301D
S66.302D
S66.303D
S66.304D
S66.305D
S66.306D
S66.307D
S66.308D
S66.309D
S66.310D
S66.311D
S66.312D
S66.313D
S66.314D
S66.315D
S66.316D
S66.317D
S66.318D
S66.319D
S66.320D
S66.321D
S66.322D
S66.323D
S66.324D
S66.325D
S66.326D
S66.327D
S66.328D
S66.329D
S66.390D
S66.391D
S66.392D
S66.393D
S66.394D
S66.395D
S66.396D
S66.397D
S66.398D
S66.399D
S66.401D
S66.402D
S66.409D
S66.411D
S66.412D
S66.419D
S66.421D
S66.422D
S66.429D
S66.491D
S66.492D
S66.499D
S66.500D
S66.501D
S66.502D
S66.503D
S66.504D
S66.505D
S66.506D
S66.507D
S66.508D
S66.509D
S66.510D
S66.511D
S66.512D
S66.513D
S66.514D
S66.515D
S66.516D
S66.517D
S66.518D
S66.519D
S66.520D
S66.521D
S66.522D
S66.523D
S66.524D
S66.525D
S66.526D
S66.527D
S66.528D
S66.529D
S66.590D
S66.591D
S66.592D
S66.593D
S66.594D
S66.595D
S66.596D
S66.597D
S66.598D
S66.599D
S66.801D
S66.802D
S66.809D
S66.811D
S66.812D
S66.819D
S66.821D
S66.822D
S66.829D
S66.891D
S66.892D
S66.899D
S66.901D
S66.902D
S66.909D
S66.911D
S66.912D
S66.919D
S66.921D
S66.922D
S66.929D
S66.991D
S66.992D
S66.999D
S67.00XD
S67.01XD
S67.02XD
S67.10XD
S67.190D
S67.191D
S67.192D
S67.193D
S67.194D
S67.195D
S67.196D
S67.197D
S67.198D
S67.20XD
S67.21XD
S67.22XD
S67.30XD
S67.31XD
S67.32XD
S67.40XD
S67.41XD
S67.42XD
S67.90XD
S67.91XD
S67.92XD
S68.011D
S68.012D
S68.019D
S68.021D
S68.022D
S68.029D
S68.110D
S68.111D
S68.112D
S68.113D
S68.114D
S68.115D
S68.116D
S68.117D
S68.118D
S68.119D
S68.120D
S68.121D
S68.122D
S68.123D
S68.124D
S68.125D
S68.126D
S68.127D
S68.128D
S68.129D
S68.411D
S68.412D
S68.419D
S68.421D
S68.422D
S68.429D
S68.511D
S68.512D
S68.519D
S68.521D
S68.522D
S68.529D
S68.610D
S68.611D
S68.612D
S68.613D
S68.614D
S68.615D
S68.616D
S68.617D
S68.618D
S68.619D
S68.620D
S68.621D
S68.622D
S68.623D
S68.624D
S68.625D
S68.626D
S68.627D
S68.628D
S68.629D
S68.711D
S68.712D
S68.719D
S68.721D
S68.722D
S68.729D
S69.80XD
S69.81XD
S69.82XD
S69.90XD
S69.91XD
S69.92XD
S70.00XD
S70.01XD
S70.02XD
S70.10XD
S70.11XD
S70.12XD
S70.211D
S70.212D
S70.219D
S70.221D
S70.222D
S70.229D
S70.241D
S70.242D
S70.249D
S70.251D
S70.252D
S70.259D
S70.261D
S70.262D
S70.269D
S70.271D
S70.272D
S70.279D
S70.311D
S70.312D
S70.319D
S70.321D
S70.322D
S70.329D
S70.341D
S70.342D
S70.349D
S70.351D
S70.352D
S70.359D
S70.361D
S70.362D
S70.369D
S70.371D
S70.372D
S70.379D
S70.911D
S70.912D
S70.919D
S70.921D
S70.922D
S70.929D
S71.001D
S71.002D
S71.009D
S71.011D
S71.012D
S71.019D
S71.021D
S71.022D
S71.029D
S71.031D
S71.032D
S71.039D
S71.041D
S71.042D
S71.049D
S71.051D
S71.052D
S71.059D
S71.101D
S71.102D
S71.109D
S71.111D
S71.112D
S71.119D
S71.121D
S71.122D
S71.129D
S71.131D
S71.132D
S71.139D
S71.141D
S71.142D
S71.149D
S71.151D
S71.152D
S71.159D
S73.001D
S73.002D
S73.003D
S73.004D
S73.005D
S73.006D
S73.011D
S73.012D
S73.013D
S73.014D
S73.015D
S73.016D
S73.021D
S73.022D
S73.023D
S73.024D
S73.025D
S73.026D
S73.031D
S73.032D
S73.033D
S73.034D
S73.035D
S73.036D
S73.041D
S73.042D
S73.043D
S73.044D
S73.045D
S73.046D
S73.101D
S73.102D
S73.109D
S73.111D
S73.112D
S73.119D
S73.121D
S73.122D
S73.129D
S73.191D
S73.192D
S73.199D
S74.00XD
S74.01XD
S74.02XD
S74.10XD
S74.11XD
S74.12XD
S74.20XD
S74.21XD
S74.22XD
S74.8X1D
S74.8X2D
S74.8X9D
S74.90XD
S74.91XD
S74.92XD
S75.001D
S75.002D
S75.009D
S75.011D
S75.012D
S75.019D
S75.021D
S75.022D
S75.029D
S75.091D
S75.092D
S75.099D
S75.101D
S75.102D
S75.109D
S75.111D
S75.112D
S75.119D
S75.121D
S75.122D
S75.129D
S75.191D
S75.192D
S75.199D
S75.201D
S75.202D
S75.209D
S75.211D
S75.212D
S75.219D
S75.221D
S75.222D
S75.229D
S75.291D
S75.292D
S75.299D
S75.801D
S75.802D
S75.809D
S75.811D
S75.812D
S75.819D
S75.891D
S75.892D
S75.899D
S75.901D
S75.902D
S75.909D
S75.911D
S75.912D
S75.919D
S75.991D
S75.992D
S75.999D
S76.001D
S76.002D
S76.009D
S76.011D
S76.012D
S76.019D
S76.021D
S76.022D
S76.029D
S76.091D
S76.092D
S76.099D
S76.101D
S76.102D
S76.109D
S76.111D
S76.112D
S76.119D
S76.121D
S76.122D
S76.129D
S76.191D
S76.192D
S76.199D
S76.201D
S76.202D
S76.209D
S76.211D
S76.212D
S76.219D
S76.221D
S76.222D
S76.229D
S76.291D
S76.292D
S76.299D
S76.301D
S76.302D
S76.309D
S76.311D
S76.312D
S76.319D
S76.321D
S76.322D
S76.329D
S76.391D
S76.392D
S76.399D
S76.801D
S76.802D
S76.809D
S76.811D
S76.812D
S76.819D
S76.821D
S76.822D
S76.829D
S76.891D
S76.892D
S76.899D
S76.901D
S76.902D
S76.909D
S76.911D
S76.912D
S76.919D
S76.921D
S76.922D
S76.929D
S76.991D
S76.992D
S76.999D
S77.00XD
S77.01XD
S77.02XD
S77.10XD
S77.11XD
S77.12XD
S77.20XD
S77.21XD
S77.22XD
S78.011D
S78.012D
S78.019D
S78.021D
S78.022D
S78.029D
S78.111D
S78.112D
S78.119D
S78.121D
S78.122D
S78.129D
S78.911D
S78.912D
S78.919D
S78.921D
S78.922D
S78.929D
S79.811D
S79.812D
S79.819D
S79.821D
S79.822D
S79.829D
S79.911D
S79.912D
S79.919D
S79.921D
S79.922D
S79.929D
S80.00XD
S80.01XD
S80.02XD
S80.10XD
S80.11XD
S80.12XD
S80.211D
S80.212D
S80.219D
S80.221D
S80.222D
S80.229D
S80.241D
S80.242D
S80.249D
S80.251D

ICD-10-CM/PCS Codes by MS-DRG

S80.252D
S80.259D
S80.261D
S80.262D
S80.269D
S80.271D
S80.272D
S80.279D
S80.811D
S80.812D
S80.819D
S80.821D
S80.822D
S80.829D
S80.841D
S80.842D
S80.849D
S80.851D
S80.852D
S80.859D
S80.861D
S80.862D
S80.869D
S80.871D
S80.872D
S80.879D
S80.911D
S80.912D
S80.919D
S80.921D
S80.922D
S80.929D
S81.001D
S81.002D
S81.009D
S81.011D
S81.012D
S81.019D
S81.021D
S81.022D
S81.029D
S81.031D
S81.032D
S81.039D
S81.041D
S81.042D
S81.049D
S81.051D
S81.052D
S81.059D
S81.801D
S81.802D
S81.809D
S81.811D
S81.812D
S81.819D
S81.821D
S81.822D
S81.829D
S81.831D
S81.832D
S81.839D
S81.841D
S81.842D
S81.849D
S81.851D
S81.852D
S81.859D
S83.001D
S83.002D
S83.003D
S83.004D
S83.005D
S83.006D
S83.011D
S83.012D
S83.013D
S83.014D
S83.015D
S83.016D
S83.091D
S83.092D
S83.093D
S83.094D
S83.095D
S83.096D
S83.101D
S83.102D
S83.103D
S83.104D
S83.105D
S83.106D
S83.111D
S83.112D
S83.113D
S83.114D
S83.115D
S83.116D
S83.121D
S83.122D
S83.123D
S83.124D
S83.125D
S83.126D
S83.131D
S83.132D
S83.133D
S83.134D
S83.135D
S83.136D
S83.141D
S83.142D
S83.143D
S83.144D
S83.145D
S83.146D
S83.191D
S83.192D
S83.193D
S83.194D
S83.195D
S83.196D
S83.200D
S83.201D
S83.202D
S83.203D
S83.204D
S83.205D
S83.206D
S83.207D
S83.209D
S83.211D
S83.212D
S83.219D
S83.221D
S83.222D
S83.229D
S83.231D
S83.232D
S83.239D
S83.241D
S83.242D
S83.249D
S83.251D
S83.252D
S83.259D
S83.261D
S83.262D
S83.269D
S83.271D
S83.272D
S83.279D
S83.281D
S83.282D
S83.289D
S83.30XD
S83.31XD
S83.32XD
S83.401D
S83.402D
S83.409D
S83.411D
S83.412D
S83.419D
S83.421D
S83.422D
S83.429D
S83.501D
S83.502D
S83.509D
S83.511D
S83.512D
S83.519D
S83.521D
S83.522D
S83.529D
S83.60XD
S83.61XD
S83.62XD
S83.8X1D
S83.8X2D
S83.8X9D
S83.90XD
S83.91XD
S83.92XD
S84.00XD
S84.01XD
S84.02XD
S84.10XD
S84.11XD
S84.12XD
S84.20XD
S84.21XD
S84.22XD
S84.801D
S84.802D
S84.809D
S84.90XD
S84.91XD
S84.92XD
S85.001D
S85.002D
S85.009D
S85.011D
S85.012D
S85.019D
S85.091D
S85.092D
S85.099D
S85.101D
S85.102D
S85.109D
S85.111D
S85.112D
S85.119D
S85.121D
S85.122D
S85.129D
S85.131D
S85.132D
S85.139D
S85.141D
S85.142D
S85.149D
S85.151D
S85.152D
S85.159D
S85.161D
S85.162D
S85.169D
S85.171D
S85.172D
S85.179D
S85.181D
S85.182D
S85.189D
S85.201D
S85.202D
S85.209D
S85.211D
S85.212D
S85.219D
S85.291D
S85.292D
S85.299D
S85.301D
S85.302D
S85.309D
S85.311D
S85.312D
S85.319D
S85.391D
S85.392D
S85.399D
S85.401D
S85.402D
S85.409D
S85.411D
S85.412D
S85.419D
S85.491D
S85.492D
S85.499D
S85.501D
S85.502D
S85.509D
S85.511D
S85.512D
S85.519D
S85.591D
S85.592D
S85.599D
S85.801D
S85.802D
S85.809D
S85.811D
S85.812D
S85.819D
S85.891D
S85.892D
S85.899D
S85.901D
S85.902D
S85.909D
S85.911D
S85.912D
S85.919D
S85.991D
S85.992D
S85.999D
S86.001D
S86.002D
S86.009D
S86.011D
S86.012D
S86.019D
S86.021D
S86.022D
S86.029D
S86.091D
S86.092D
S86.099D
S86.101D
S86.102D
S86.109D
S86.111D
S86.112D
S86.119D
S86.121D
S86.122D
S86.129D
S86.191D
S86.192D
S86.199D
S86.201D
S86.202D
S86.209D
S86.211D
S86.212D
S86.219D
S86.221D
S86.222D
S86.229D
S86.291D
S86.292D
S86.299D
S86.301D
S86.302D
S86.309D
S86.311D
S86.312D
S86.319D
S86.321D
S86.322D
S86.329D
S86.391D
S86.392D
S86.399D
S86.801D
S86.802D
S86.809D
S86.811D
S86.812D
S86.819D
S86.821D
S86.822D
S86.829D
S86.891D
S86.892D
S86.899D
S86.901D
S86.902D
S86.909D
S86.911D
S86.912D
S86.919D
S86.921D
S86.922D
S86.929D
S86.991D
S86.992D
S86.999D
S87.00XD
S87.01XD
S87.02XD
S87.80XD
S87.81XD
S87.82XD
S88.011D
S88.012D
S88.019D
S88.021D
S88.022D
S88.029D
S88.111D
S88.112D
S88.119D
S88.121D
S88.122D
S88.129D
S88.911D
S88.912D
S88.919D
S88.921D
S88.922D
S88.929D
S89.80XD
S89.81XD
S89.82XD
S89.90XD
S89.91XD
S89.92XD
S90.00XD
S90.01XD
S90.02XD
S90.111D
S90.112D
S90.119D
S90.121D
S90.122D
S90.129D
S90.211D
S90.212D
S90.219D
S90.221D
S90.222D
S90.229D
S90.30XD
S90.31XD
S90.32XD
S90.411D
S90.412D
S90.413D
S90.414D
S90.415D
S90.416D
S90.421D
S90.422D
S90.423D
S90.424D
S90.425D
S90.426D
S90.441D
S90.442D
S90.443D
S90.444D
S90.445D
S90.446D
S90.451D
S90.452D
S90.453D
S90.454D
S90.455D
S90.456D
S90.461D
S90.462D
S90.463D
S90.464D
S90.465D
S90.466D
S90.471D
S90.472D
S90.473D
S90.474D
S90.475D
S90.476D
S90.511D
S90.512D
S90.519D
S90.521D
S90.522D
S90.529D
S90.541D
S90.542D
S90.549D
S90.551D
S90.552D
S90.559D
S90.561D
S90.562D
S90.569D
S90.571D
S90.572D
S90.579D
S90.811D
S90.812D
S90.819D
S90.821D
S90.822D
S90.829D
S90.841D
S90.842D
S90.849D
S90.851D
S90.852D
S90.859D
S90.861D
S90.862D
S90.869D
S90.871D
S90.872D
S90.879D
S90.911D
S90.912D
S90.919D
S90.921D
S90.922D
S90.929D
S90.931D
S90.932D
S90.933D
S90.934D
S90.935D
S90.936D
S91.001D
S91.002D
S91.009D
S91.011D
S91.012D
S91.019D
S91.021D
S91.022D
S91.029D
S91.031D
S91.032D
S91.039D
S91.041D
S91.042D
S91.049D
S91.051D
S91.052D
S91.059D
S91.101D
S91.102D
S91.103D
S91.104D
S91.105D
S91.106D
S91.109D
S91.111D
S91.112D
S91.113D
S91.114D
S91.115D
S91.116D
S91.119D
S91.121D
S91.122D
S91.123D
S91.124D
S91.125D
S91.126D
S91.129D
S91.131D
S91.132D
S91.133D
S91.134D
S91.135D
S91.136D
S91.139D
S91.141D
S91.142D
S91.143D
S91.144D
S91.145D
S91.146D
S91.149D
S91.151D
S91.152D
S91.153D
S91.154D
S91.155D
S91.156D
S91.159D
S91.201D
S91.202D
S91.203D
S91.204D
S91.205D
S91.206D
S91.209D
S91.211D
S91.212D
S91.213D
S91.214D
S91.215D
S91.216D
S91.219D
S91.221D
S91.222D
S91.223D
S91.224D
S91.225D
S91.226D
S91.229D
S91.231D
S91.232D
S91.233D
S91.234D
S91.235D
S91.236D
S91.239D
S91.241D
S91.242D
S91.243D
S91.244D
S91.245D
S91.246D
S91.249D
S91.251D
S91.252D
S91.253D
S91.254D
S91.255D
S91.256D
S91.259D
S91.301D
S91.302D
S91.309D
S91.311D
S91.312D
S91.319D
S91.321D
S91.322D
S91.329D
S91.331D
S91.332D
S91.339D
S91.341D
S91.342D
S91.349D
S91.351D
S91.352D
S91.359D
S93.01XD
S93.02XD
S93.03XD
S93.04XD
S93.05XD
S93.06XD
S93.101D
S93.102D
S93.103D
S93.104D
S93.105D
S93.106D
S93.111D
S93.112D
S93.113D
S93.114D
S93.115D
S93.116D
S93.119D
S93.121D
S93.122D
S93.123D
S93.124D
S93.125D
S93.126D
S93.129D
S93.131D
S93.132D
S93.133D
S93.134D
S93.135D
S93.136D
S93.139D
S93.141D
S93.142D
S93.143D
S93.144D
S93.145D
S93.146D
S93.149D
S93.301D
S93.302D
S93.303D
S93.304D
S93.305D
S93.306D
S93.311D
S93.312D
S93.313D
S93.314D
S93.315D
S93.316D
S93.321D
S93.322D
S93.323D
S93.324D
S93.325D
S93.326D
S93.331D
S93.332D
S93.333D
S93.334D
S93.335D
S93.336D
S93.401D
S93.402D
S93.409D
S93.411D
S93.412D
S93.419D
S93.421D
S93.422D
S93.429D
S93.431D
S93.432D
S93.439D
S93.491D
S93.492D
S93.499D
S93.501D
S93.502D
S93.503D
S93.504D
S93.505D
S93.506D
S93.509D
S93.511D
S93.512D
S93.513D
S93.514D
S93.515D
S93.516D
S93.519D
S93.521D
S93.522D
S93.523D
S93.524D
S93.525D
S93.526D
S93.529D
S93.601D
S93.602D
S93.609D
S93.611D
S93.612D
S93.619D
S93.621D
S93.622D
S93.629D
S93.691D
S93.692D
S93.699D
S94.00XD
S94.01XD
S94.02XD
S94.10XD
S94.11XD
S94.12XD
S94.20XD
S94.21XD
S94.22XD
S94.30XD
S94.31XD
S94.32XD
S94.8X1D
S94.8X2D
S94.8X9D
S94.90XD
S94.91XD
S94.92XD
S95.001D
S95.002D
S95.009D
S95.011D
S95.012D
S95.019D
S95.091D
S95.092D
S95.099D
S95.101D
S95.102D
S95.109D
S95.111D
S95.112D
S95.119D
S95.191D
S95.192D
S95.199D
S95.201D
S95.202D
S95.209D
S95.211D
S95.212D
S95.219D
S95.291D
S95.292D
S95.299D
S95.801D
S95.802D
S95.809D
S95.811D
S95.812D
S95.819D
S95.891D
S95.892D
S95.899D
S95.901D
S95.902D
S95.909D
S95.911D
S95.912D
S95.919D
S95.991D
S95.992D
S95.999D
S96.001D
S96.002D
S96.009D
S96.011D
S96.012D
S96.019D
S96.021D
S96.022D
S96.029D
S96.091D
S96.092D
S96.099D
S96.101D
S96.102D
S96.109D
S96.111D
S96.112D
S96.119D
S96.121D
S96.122D
S96.129D
S96.191D
S96.192D
S96.199D
S96.201D
S96.202D
S96.209D
S96.211D
S96.212D
S96.219D
S96.221D
S96.222D
S96.229D
S96.291D
S96.292D
S96.299D
S96.801D
S96.802D
S96.809D
S96.811D
S96.812D
S96.819D
S96.821D
S96.822D
S96.829D
S96.891D
S96.892D
S96.899D
S96.901D
S96.902D
S96.909D
S96.911D
S96.912D
S96.919D
S96.921D
S96.922D
S96.929D
S96.991D
S96.992D
S96.999D
S97.00XD
S97.01XD
S97.02XD
S97.101D
S97.102D
S97.109D

S97.111D
S97.112D
S97.119D
S97.121D
S97.122D
S97.129D
S97.80XD
S97.81XD
S97.82XD
S98.011D
S98.012D
S98.019D
S98.021D
S98.022D
S98.029D
S98.111D
S98.112D
S98.119D
S98.121D
S98.122D
S98.129D
S98.131D
S98.132D
S98.139D
S98.141D
S98.142D
S98.149D
S98.211D
S98.212D
S98.219D
S98.221D
S98.222D
S98.229D
S98.311D
S98.312D
S98.319D
S98.321D
S98.322D
S98.329D
S98.911D
S98.912D
S98.919D
S98.921D
S98.922D
S98.929D
S99.001D
S99.001G
S99.001K
S99.001P
S99.002D
S99.002G
S99.002K
S99.002P
S99.009D
S99.009G
S99.009K
S99.009P
S99.011D
S99.011G
S99.011K
S99.011P
S99.012D
S99.012G
S99.012K
S99.012P
S99.019D
S99.019G
S99.019K
S99.019P
S99.021D
S99.021G
S99.021K
S99.021P
S99.022D
S99.022G
S99.022K
S99.022P
S99.029D
S99.029G
S99.029K
S99.029P
S99.031D
S99.031G
S99.031K
S99.031P
S99.032D
S99.032G
S99.032K
S99.032P
S99.039D
S99.039G
S99.039K
S99.039P
S99.041D
S99.041G
S99.041K
S99.041P
S99.042D
S99.042G
S99.042K
S99.042P
S99.049D
S99.049G
S99.049K
S99.049P
S99.091D
S99.091G
S99.091K
S99.091P
S99.092D
S99.092G
S99.092K
S99.092P
S99.099D
S99.099G
S99.099K
S99.099P
S99.101D
S99.101G
S99.101K
S99.101P
S99.102D
S99.102G
S99.102K
S99.102P
S99.109D
S99.109G
S99.109K
S99.109P
S99.111D
S99.111G
S99.111K
S99.111P
S99.112D
S99.112G
S99.112K
S99.112P
S99.119D
S99.119G
S99.119K
S99.119P
S99.121D
S99.121G
S99.121K
S99.121P
S99.122D
S99.122G
S99.122K
S99.122P
S99.129D
S99.129G
S99.129K
S99.129P
S99.131D
S99.131G
S99.131K
S99.131P
S99.132D
S99.132G
S99.132K
S99.132P
S99.139D
S99.139G
S99.139K
S99.139P
S99.141D
S99.141G
S99.141K
S99.141P
S99.142D
S99.142G
S99.142K
S99.142P
S99.149D
S99.149G
S99.149K
S99.149P
S99.191D
S99.191G
S99.191K
S99.191P
S99.192D
S99.192G
S99.192K
S99.192P
S99.199D
S99.199G
S99.199K
S99.199P
S99.201D
S99.201G
S99.201K
S99.201P
S99.202D
S99.202G
S99.202K
S99.202P
S99.209D
S99.209G
S99.209K
S99.209P
S99.211D
S99.211G
S99.211K
S99.211P
S99.212D
S99.212G
S99.212K
S99.212P
S99.219D
S99.219G
S99.219K
S99.219P
S99.221D
S99.221G
S99.221K
S99.221P
S99.222D
S99.222G
S99.222K
S99.222P
S99.229D
S99.229G
S99.229K
S99.229P
S99.231D
S99.231G
S99.231K
S99.231P
S99.232D
S99.232G
S99.232K
S99.232P
S99.239D
S99.239G
S99.239K
S99.239P
S99.241D
S99.241G
S99.241K
S99.241P
S99.242D
S99.242G
S99.242K
S99.242P
S99.249D
S99.249G
S99.249K
S99.249P
S99.291D
S99.291G
S99.291K
S99.291P
S99.292D
S99.292G
S99.292K
S99.292P
S99.299D
S99.299G
S99.299K
S99.299P
S99.811D
S99.812D
S99.819D
S99.821D
S99.822D
S99.829D
S99.911D
S99.912D
S99.919D
S99.921D
S99.922D
S99.929D
T07.XXXD
T14.8XXD
T14.90XD
T14.91XD
T15.00XD
T15.01XD
T15.02XD
T15.10XD
T15.11XD
T15.12XD
T15.80XD
T15.81XD
T15.82XD
T15.90XD
T15.91XD
T15.92XD
T16.1XXD
T16.2XXD
T16.9XXD
T17.0XXD
T17.1XXD
T17.200D
T17.208D
T17.210D
T17.218D
T17.220D
T17.228D
T17.290D
T17.298D
T17.300D
T17.308D
T17.310D
T17.318D
T17.320D
T17.328D
T17.390D
T17.398D
T17.400D
T17.408D
T17.410D
T17.418D
T17.420D
T17.428D
T17.490D
T17.498D
T17.500D
T17.508D
T17.510D
T17.518D
T17.520D
T17.528D
T17.590D
T17.598D
T17.800D
T17.808D
T17.810D
T17.818D
T17.820D
T17.828D
T17.890D
T17.898D
T17.900D
T17.908D
T17.910D
T17.918D
T17.920D
T17.928D
T17.990D
T17.998D
T18.0XXD
T18.100D
T18.108D
T18.110D
T18.118D
T18.120D
T18.128D
T18.190D
T18.198D
T18.2XXD
T18.3XXD
T18.4XXD
T18.5XXD
T18.8XXD
T18.9XXD
T19.0XXD
T19.1XXD
T19.2XXD
T19.3XXD
T19.4XXD
T19.8XXD
T19.9XXD
T20.00XD
T20.011D
T20.012D
T20.019D
T20.02XD
T20.03XD
T20.04XD
T20.05XD
T20.06XD
T20.07XD
T20.09XD
T20.10XD
T20.111D
T20.112D
T20.119D
T20.12XD
T20.13XD
T20.14XD
T20.15XD
T20.16XD
T20.17XD
T20.19XD
T20.20XD
T20.211D
T20.212D
T20.219D
T20.22XD
T20.23XD
T20.24XD
T20.25XD
T20.26XD
T20.27XD
T20.29XD
T20.30XD
T20.311D
T20.312D
T20.319D
T20.32XD
T20.33XD
T20.34XD
T20.35XD
T20.36XD
T20.37XD
T20.39XD
T20.40XD
T20.411D
T20.412D
T20.419D
T20.42XD
T20.43XD
T20.44XD
T20.45XD
T20.46XD
T20.47XD
T20.49XD
T20.50XD
T20.511D
T20.512D
T20.519D
T20.52XD
T20.53XD
T20.54XD
T20.55XD
T20.56XD
T20.57XD
T20.59XD
T20.60XD
T20.611D
T20.612D
T20.619D
T20.62XD
T20.63XD
T20.64XD
T20.65XD
T20.66XD
T20.67XD
T20.69XD
T20.70XD
T20.711D
T20.712D
T20.719D
T20.72XD
T20.73XD
T20.74XD
T20.75XD
T20.76XD
T20.77XD
T20.79XD
T21.00XD
T21.01XD
T21.02XD
T21.03XD
T21.04XD
T21.05XD
T21.06XD
T21.07XD
T21.09XD
T21.10XD
T21.11XD
T21.12XD
T21.13XD
T21.14XD
T21.15XD
T21.16XD
T21.17XD
T21.19XD
T21.20XD
T21.21XD
T21.22XD
T21.23XD
T21.24XD
T21.25XD
T21.26XD
T21.27XD
T21.29XD
T21.30XD
T21.31XD
T21.32XD
T21.33XD
T21.34XD
T21.35XD
T21.36XD
T21.37XD
T21.39XD
T21.40XD
T21.41XD
T21.42XD
T21.43XD
T21.44XD
T21.45XD
T21.46XD
T21.47XD
T21.49XD
T21.50XD
T21.51XD
T21.52XD
T21.53XD
T21.54XD
T21.55XD
T21.56XD
T21.57XD
T21.59XD
T21.60XD
T21.61XD
T21.62XD
T21.63XD
T21.64XD
T21.65XD
T21.66XD
T21.67XD
T21.69XD
T21.70XD
T21.71XD
T21.72XD
T21.73XD
T21.74XD
T21.75XD
T21.76XD
T21.77XD
T21.79XD
T22.00XD
T22.011D
T22.012D
T22.019D
T22.021D
T22.022D
T22.029D
T22.031D
T22.032D
T22.039D
T22.041D
T22.042D
T22.049D
T22.051D
T22.052D
T22.059D
T22.061D
T22.062D
T22.069D
T22.091D
T22.092D
T22.099D
T22.10XD
T22.111D
T22.112D
T22.119D
T22.121D
T22.122D
T22.129D
T22.131D
T22.132D
T22.139D
T22.141D
T22.142D
T22.149D
T22.151D
T22.152D
T22.159D
T22.161D
T22.162D
T22.169D
T22.191D
T22.192D
T22.199D
T22.20XD
T22.211D
T22.212D
T22.219D
T22.221D
T22.222D
T22.229D
T22.231D
T22.232D
T22.239D
T22.241D
T22.242D
T22.249D
T22.251D
T22.252D
T22.259D
T22.261D
T22.262D
T22.269D
T22.291D
T22.292D
T22.299D
T22.30XD
T22.311D
T22.312D
T22.319D
T22.321D
T22.322D
T22.329D
T22.331D
T22.332D
T22.339D
T22.341D
T22.342D
T22.349D
T22.351D
T22.352D
T22.359D
T22.361D
T22.362D
T22.369D
T22.391D
T22.392D
T22.399D
T22.40XD
T22.411D
T22.412D
T22.419D
T22.421D
T22.422D
T22.429D
T22.431D
T22.432D
T22.439D
T22.441D
T22.442D
T22.449D
T22.451D
T22.452D
T22.459D
T22.461D
T22.462D
T22.469D
T22.491D
T22.492D
T22.499D
T22.50XD
T22.511D
T22.512D
T22.519D
T22.521D
T22.522D
T22.529D
T22.531D
T22.532D
T22.539D
T22.541D
T22.542D
T22.549D
T22.551D
T22.552D
T22.559D
T22.561D
T22.562D
T22.569D
T22.591D
T22.592D
T22.599D
T22.60XD
T22.611D
T22.612D
T22.619D
T22.621D
T22.622D
T22.629D
T22.631D
T22.632D
T22.639D
T22.641D
T22.642D
T22.649D
T22.651D
T22.652D
T22.659D
T22.661D
T22.662D
T22.669D
T22.691D
T22.692D
T22.699D
T22.70XD
T22.711D
T22.712D
T22.719D
T22.721D
T22.722D
T22.729D
T22.731D
T22.732D
T22.739D
T22.741D
T22.742D
T22.749D
T22.751D
T22.752D
T22.759D
T22.761D
T22.762D
T22.769D
T22.791D
T22.792D
T22.799D
T23.001D
T23.002D
T23.009D
T23.011D
T23.012D
T23.019D
T23.021D
T23.022D
T23.029D
T23.031D
T23.032D
T23.039D
T23.041D
T23.042D
T23.049D
T23.051D
T23.052D
T23.059D
T23.061D
T23.062D
T23.069D
T23.071D
T23.072D
T23.079D
T23.091D
T23.092D
T23.099D
T23.101D
T23.102D
T23.109D
T23.111D
T23.112D
T23.119D
T23.121D
T23.122D
T23.129D
T23.131D
T23.132D
T23.139D
T23.141D
T23.142D
T23.149D
T23.151D
T23.152D
T23.159D
T23.161D
T23.162D
T23.169D
T23.171D
T23.172D
T23.179D
T23.191D
T23.192D
T23.199D
T23.201D
T23.202D
T23.209D
T23.211D
T23.212D
T23.219D
T23.221D
T23.222D
T23.229D
T23.231D
T23.232D
T23.239D
T23.241D
T23.242D
T23.249D
T23.251D
T23.252D
T23.259D
T23.261D
T23.262D
T23.269D
T23.271D
T23.272D
T23.279D
T23.291D
T23.292D
T23.299D
T23.301D
T23.302D
T23.309D
T23.311D
T23.312D
T23.319D
T23.321D
T23.322D
T23.329D
T23.331D
T23.332D
T23.339D
T23.341D
T23.342D
T23.349D
T23.351D
T23.352D
T23.359D
T23.361D
T23.362D
T23.369D
T23.371D
T23.372D
T23.379D
T23.391D
T23.392D
T23.399D
T23.401D
T23.402D
T23.409D
T23.411D
T23.412D
T23.419D
T23.421D
T23.422D
T23.429D
T23.431D
T23.432D
T23.439D
T23.441D
T23.442D
T23.449D
T23.451D
T23.452D
T23.459D
T23.461D
T23.462D
T23.469D
T23.471D
T23.472D
T23.479D
T23.491D
T23.492D
T23.499D
T23.501D
T23.502D
T23.509D
T23.511D
T23.512D
T23.519D
T23.521D
T23.522D
T23.529D
T23.531D
T23.532D
T23.539D
T23.541D
T23.542D
T23.549D
T23.551D
T23.552D
T23.559D
T23.561D
T23.562D

T23.569D
T23.571D
T23.572D
T23.579D
T23.591D
T23.592D
T23.599D
T23.6Ø1D
T23.6Ø2D
T23.6Ø9D
T23.611D
T23.612D
T23.619D
T23.621D
T23.622D
T23.629D
T23.631D
T23.632D
T23.639D
T23.641D
T23.642D
T23.649D
T23.651D
T23.652D
T23.659D
T23.661D
T23.662D
T23.669D
T23.671D
T23.672D
T23.679D
T23.691D
T23.692D
T23.699D
T23.7Ø1D
T23.7Ø2D
T23.7Ø9D
T23.711D
T23.712D
T23.719D
T23.721D
T23.722D
T23.729D
T23.731D
T23.732D
T23.739D
T23.741D
T23.742D
T23.749D
T23.751D
T23.752D
T23.759D
T23.761D
T23.762D
T23.769D
T23.771D
T23.772D
T23.779D
T23.791D
T23.792D
T23.799D
T24.ØØ1D
T24.ØØ2D
T24.ØØ9D
T24.Ø11D
T24.Ø12D
T24.Ø19D
T24.Ø21D
T24.Ø22D
T24.Ø29D
T24.Ø31D
T24.Ø32D
T24.Ø39D
T24.Ø91D
T24.Ø92D
T24.Ø99D
T24.1Ø1D
T24.1Ø2D
T24.1Ø9D
T24.111D
T24.112D
T24.119D
T24.121D
T24.122D
T24.129D
T24.131D
T24.132D
T24.139D
T24.191D
T24.192D
T24.199D
T24.2Ø1D
T24.2Ø2D
T24.2Ø9D
T24.211D
T24.212D
T24.219D
T24.221D
T24.222D
T24.229D
T24.231D
T24.232D
T24.239D
T24.291D
T24.292D
T24.299D
T24.3Ø1D
T24.3Ø2D
T24.3Ø9D
T24.311D
T24.312D
T24.319D
T24.321D
T24.322D
T24.329D
T24.331D
T24.332D
T24.339D
T24.391D
T24.392D
T24.399D
T24.4Ø1D
T24.4Ø2D
T24.4Ø9D
T24.411D
T24.412D
T24.419D
T24.421D
T24.422D
T24.429D
T24.431D
T24.432D
T24.439D
T24.491D
T24.492D
T24.499D
T24.5Ø1D
T24.5Ø2D
T24.5Ø9D
T24.511D
T24.512D
T24.519D
T24.521D
T24.522D
T24.529D
T24.531D
T24.532D
T24.539D
T24.591D
T24.592D
T24.599D
T24.6Ø1D
T24.6Ø2D
T24.6Ø9D
T24.611D
T24.612D
T24.619D
T24.621D
T24.622D
T24.629D
T24.631D
T24.632D
T24.639D
T24.691D
T24.692D
T24.699D
T24.7Ø1D
T24.7Ø2D
T24.7Ø9D
T24.711D
T24.712D
T24.719D
T24.721D
T24.722D
T24.729D
T24.731D
T24.732D
T24.739D
T24.791D
T24.792D
T24.799D
T25.Ø11D
T25.Ø12D
T25.Ø19D
T25.Ø21D
T25.Ø22D
T25.Ø29D
T25.Ø31D
T25.Ø32D
T25.Ø39D
T25.Ø91D
T25.Ø92D
T25.Ø99D
T25.111D
T25.112D
T25.119D
T25.121D
T25.122D
T25.129D
T25.131D
T25.132D
T25.139D
T25.191D
T25.192D
T25.199D
T25.211D
T25.212D
T25.219D
T25.221D
T25.222D
T25.229D
T25.231D
T25.232D
T25.239D
T25.291D
T25.292D
T25.299D
T25.311D
T25.312D
T25.319D
T25.321D
T25.322D
T25.329D
T25.331D
T25.332D
T25.339D
T25.391D
T25.392D
T25.399D
T25.411D
T25.412D
T25.419D
T25.421D
T25.422D
T25.429D
T25.431D
T25.432D
T25.439D
T25.491D
T25.492D
T25.499D
T25.511D
T25.512D
T25.519D
T25.521D
T25.522D
T25.529D
T25.531D
T25.532D
T25.539D
T25.591D
T25.592D
T25.599D
T25.611D
T25.612D
T25.619D
T25.621D
T25.622D
T25.629D
T25.631D
T25.632D
T25.639D
T25.691D
T25.692D
T25.699D
T25.711D
T25.712D
T25.719D
T25.721D
T25.722D
T25.729D
T25.731D
T25.732D
T25.739D
T25.791D
T25.792D
T25.799D
T26.ØØXD
T26.Ø1XD
T26.Ø2XD
T26.1ØXD
T26.11XD
T26.12XD
T26.2ØXD
T26.21XD
T26.22XD
T26.3ØXD
T26.31XD
T26.32XD
T26.4ØXD
T26.41XD
T26.42XD
T26.5ØXD
T26.51XD
T26.52XD
T26.6ØXD
T26.61XD
T26.62XD
T26.7ØXD
T26.71XD
T26.72XD
T26.8ØXD
T26.81XD
T26.82XD
T26.9ØXD
T26.91XD
T26.92XD
T27.ØXXD
T27.1XXD
T27.2XXD
T27.3XXD
T27.4XXD
T27.5XXD
T27.6XXD
T27.7XXD
T28.ØXXD
T28.1XXD
T28.2XXD
T28.3XXD
T28.4ØXD
T28.411D
T28.412D
T28.419D
T28.49XD
T28.5XXD
T28.6XXD
T28.7XXD
T28.8XXD
T28.9ØXD
T28.911D
T28.912D
T28.919D
T28.99XD
T33.Ø11D
T33.Ø12D
T33.Ø19D
T33.Ø2XD
T33.Ø9XD
T33.1XXD
T33.2XXD
T33.3XXD
T33.4ØXD
T33.41XD
T33.42XD
T33.511D
T33.512D
T33.519D
T33.521D
T33.522D
T33.529D
T33.531D
T33.532D
T33.539D
T33.6ØXD
T33.61XD
T33.62XD
T33.7ØXD
T33.71XD
T33.72XD
T33.811D
T33.812D
T33.819D
T33.821D
T33.822D
T33.829D
T33.831D
T33.832D
T33.839D
T33.9ØXD
T33.99XD
T34.Ø11D
T34.Ø12D
T34.Ø19D
T34.Ø2XD
T34.Ø9XD
T34.1XXD
T34.2XXD
T34.3XXD
T34.4ØXD
T34.41XD
T34.42XD
T34.511D
T34.512D
T34.519D
T34.521D
T34.522D
T34.529D
T34.531D
T34.532D
T34.539D
T34.6ØXD
T34.61XD
T34.62XD
T34.7ØXD
T34.71XD
T34.72XD
T34.811D
T34.812D
T34.819D
T34.821D
T34.822D
T34.829D
T34.831D
T34.832D
T34.839D
T34.9ØXD
T34.99XD
T36.ØX1D
T36.ØX2D
T36.ØX3D
T36.ØX4D
T36.ØX5D
T36.ØX6D
T36.ØX6S
T36.1X1D
T36.1X2D
T36.1X3D
T36.1X4D
T36.1X5D
T36.1X6D
T36.1X6S
T36.2X1D
T36.2X2D
T36.2X3D
T36.2X4D
T36.2X5D
T36.2X6D
T36.2X6S
T36.3X1D
T36.3X2D
T36.3X3D
T36.3X4D
T36.3X5D
T36.3X6D
T36.3X6S
T36.4X1D
T36.4X2D
T36.4X3D
T36.4X4D
T36.4X5D
T36.4X6D
T36.4X6S
T36.5X1D
T36.5X2D
T36.5X3D
T36.5X4D
T36.5X5D
T36.5X6D
T36.5X6S
T36.6X1D
T36.6X2D
T36.6X3D
T36.6X4D
T36.6X5D
T36.6X6D
T36.6X6S
T36.7X1D
T36.7X2D
T36.7X3D
T36.7X4D
T36.7X5D
T36.7X6D
T36.7X6S
T36.8X1D
T36.8X2D
T36.8X3D
T36.8X4D
T36.8X5D
T36.8X6D
T36.8X6S
T36.91XD
T36.92XD
T36.93XD
T36.94XD
T36.95XD
T36.96XD
T36.96XS
T37.ØX1D
T37.ØX2D
T37.ØX3D
T37.ØX4D
T37.ØX5D
T37.ØX6D
T37.ØX6S
T37.1X1D
T37.1X2D
T37.1X3D
T37.1X4D
T37.1X5D
T37.1X6D
T37.1X6S
T37.2X1D
T37.2X2D
T37.2X3D
T37.2X4D
T37.2X5D
T37.2X6D
T37.2X6S
T37.3X1D
T37.3X2D
T37.3X3D
T37.3X4D
T37.3X5D
T37.3X6D
T37.3X6S
T37.4X1D
T37.4X2D
T37.4X3D
T37.4X4D
T37.4X5D
T37.4X6D
T37.4X6S
T37.5X1D
T37.5X2D
T37.5X3D
T37.5X4D
T37.5X5D
T37.5X6D
T37.5X6S
T37.8X1D
T37.8X2D
T37.8X3D
T37.8X4D
T37.8X5D
T37.8X6D
T37.8X6S
T37.91XD
T37.92XD
T37.93XD
T37.94XD
T37.95XD
T37.96XD
T37.96XS
T38.ØX1D
T38.ØX2D
T38.ØX3D
T38.ØX4D
T38.ØX5D
T38.ØX6D
T38.ØX6S
T38.1X1D
T38.1X2D
T38.1X3D
T38.1X4D
T38.1X5D
T38.1X6D
T38.1X6S
T38.2X1D
T38.2X2D
T38.2X3D
T38.2X4D
T38.2X5D
T38.2X6D
T38.2X6S
T38.3X1D
T38.3X2D
T38.3X3D
T38.3X4D
T38.3X5D
T38.3X6D
T38.3X6S
T38.4X1D
T38.4X2D
T38.4X3D
T38.4X4D
T38.4X5D
T38.4X6D
T38.4X6S
T38.5X1D
T38.5X2D
T38.5X3D
T38.5X4D
T38.5X5D
T38.5X6D
T38.5X6S
T38.6X1D
T38.6X2D
T38.6X3D
T38.6X4D
T38.6X5D
T38.6X6D
T38.6X6S
T38.7X1D
T38.7X2D
T38.7X3D
T38.7X4D
T38.7X5D
T38.7X6D
T38.7X6S
T38.8Ø1D
T38.8Ø2D
T38.8Ø3D
T38.8Ø4D
T38.8Ø5D
T38.8Ø6D
T38.8Ø6S
T38.811D
T38.812D
T38.813D
T38.814D
T38.815D
T38.816D
T38.816S
T38.891D
T38.892D
T38.893D
T38.894D
T38.895D
T38.896D
T38.896S
T38.9Ø1D
T38.9Ø2D
T38.9Ø3D
T38.9Ø4D
T38.9Ø5D
T38.9Ø6D
T38.9Ø6S
T38.991D
T38.992D
T38.993D
T38.994D
T38.995D
T38.996D
T38.996S
T39.Ø11D
T39.Ø12D
T39.Ø13D
T39.Ø14D
T39.Ø15D
T39.Ø16D
T39.Ø16S
T39.Ø91D
T39.Ø92D
T39.Ø93D
T39.Ø94D
T39.Ø95D
T39.Ø96D
T39.Ø96S
T39.1X1D
T39.1X2D
T39.1X3D
T39.1X4D
T39.1X5D
T39.1X6D
T39.1X6S
T39.2X1D
T39.2X2D
T39.2X3D
T39.2X4D
T39.2X5D
T39.2X6D
T39.2X6S
T39.311D
T39.312D
T39.313D
T39.314D
T39.315D
T39.316D
T39.316S
T39.391D
T39.392D
T39.393D
T39.394D
T39.395D
T39.396D
T39.396S
T39.4X1D
T39.4X2D
T39.4X3D
T39.4X4D
T39.4X5D
T39.4X6D
T39.4X6S
T39.8X1D
T39.8X2D
T39.8X3D
T39.8X4D
T39.8X5D
T39.8X6D
T39.8X6S
T39.91XD
T39.92XD
T39.93XD
T39.94XD
T39.95XD
T39.96XD
T39.96XS
T4Ø.ØX1D
T4Ø.ØX2D
T4Ø.ØX3D
T4Ø.ØX4D
T4Ø.ØX5D
T4Ø.ØX6D
T4Ø.ØX6S
T4Ø.1X1D
T4Ø.1X2D
T4Ø.1X3D
T4Ø.1X4D
T4Ø.2X1D
T4Ø.2X2D
T4Ø.2X3D
T4Ø.2X4D
T4Ø.2X5D
T4Ø.2X6D
T4Ø.2X6S
T4Ø.3X1D
T4Ø.3X2D
T4Ø.3X3D
T4Ø.3X4D
T4Ø.3X5D
T4Ø.3X6D
T4Ø.3X6S
T4Ø.411D
T4Ø.412D
T4Ø.413D
T4Ø.414D
T4Ø.415D
T4Ø.416D
T4Ø.416S
T4Ø.421D
T4Ø.422D
T4Ø.423D
T4Ø.424D
T4Ø.425D
T4Ø.426D
T4Ø.426S
T4Ø.491D
T4Ø.492D
T4Ø.493D
T4Ø.494D
T4Ø.495D
T4Ø.496D
T4Ø.496S
T4Ø.5X1D
T4Ø.5X2D
T4Ø.5X3D
T4Ø.5X4D
T4Ø.5X5D
T4Ø.5X6D
T4Ø.5X6S
T4Ø.6Ø1D
T4Ø.6Ø2D
T4Ø.6Ø3D
T4Ø.6Ø4D
T4Ø.6Ø5D
T4Ø.6Ø6D
T4Ø.6Ø6S
T4Ø.691D
T4Ø.692D
T4Ø.693D
T4Ø.694D
T4Ø.695D
T4Ø.696D
T4Ø.696S
T4Ø.711D
T4Ø.712D
T4Ø.713D
T4Ø.714D
T4Ø.715D
T4Ø.716D
T4Ø.716S
T4Ø.721D
T4Ø.722D
T4Ø.723D
T4Ø.724D
T4Ø.725D
T4Ø.726D
T4Ø.726S
T4Ø.8X1D
T4Ø.8X2D
T4Ø.8X3D
T4Ø.8X4D
T4Ø.9Ø1D
T4Ø.9Ø2D
T4Ø.9Ø3D
T4Ø.9Ø4D
T4Ø.9Ø5D
T4Ø.9Ø6D
T4Ø.9Ø6S
T4Ø.991D
T4Ø.992D
T4Ø.993D
T4Ø.994D
T4Ø.995D
T4Ø.996D
T4Ø.996S
T41.ØX1D
T41.ØX2D
T41.ØX3D
T41.ØX4D
T41.ØX5D
T41.ØX6D
T41.ØX6S
T41.1X1D
T41.1X2D
T41.1X3D
T41.1X4D
T41.1X5D
T41.1X6D
T41.1X6S
T41.2Ø1D
T41.2Ø2D
T41.2Ø3D
T41.2Ø4D
T41.2Ø5D
T41.2Ø6D
T41.2Ø6S
T41.291D
T41.292D
T41.293D
T41.294D
T41.295D
T41.296D
T41.296S
T41.3X1D
T41.3X2D
T41.3X3D
T41.3X4D
T41.3X5D
T41.3X6D
T41.3X6S
T41.41XD
T41.42XD
T41.43XD
T41.44XD
T41.45XD
T41.46XD
T41.46XS
T41.5X1D
T41.5X2D
T41.5X3D
T41.5X4D
T41.5X5D
T41.5X6D
T41.5X6S
T42.ØX1D
T42.ØX2D
T42.ØX3D
T42.ØX4D
T42.ØX5D
T42.ØX6D
T42.ØX6S
T42.1X1D
T42.1X2D
T42.1X3D
T42.1X4D
T42.1X5D
T42.1X6D
T42.1X6S
T42.2X1D
T42.2X2D
T42.2X3D
T42.2X4D
T42.2X5D
T42.2X6D

T42.2X6S
T42.3X1D
T42.3X2D
T42.3X3D
T42.3X4D
T42.3X5D
T42.3X6D
T42.3X6S
T42.4X1D
T42.4X2D
T42.4X3D
T42.4X4D
T42.4X5D
T42.4X6D
T42.4X6S
T42.5X1D
T42.5X2D
T42.5X3D
T42.5X4D
T42.5X5D
T42.5X6D
T42.5X6S
T42.6X1D
T42.6X2D
T42.6X3D
T42.6X4D
T42.6X5D
T42.6X6D
T42.6X6S
T42.71XD
T42.72XD
T42.73XD
T42.74XD
T42.75XD
T42.76XD
T42.76XS
T42.8X1D
T42.8X2D
T42.8X3D
T42.8X4D
T42.8X5D
T42.8X6D
T42.8X6S
T43.011D
T43.012D
T43.013D
T43.014D
T43.015D
T43.016D
T43.016S
T43.021D
T43.022D
T43.023D
T43.024D
T43.025D
T43.026D
T43.026S
T43.1X1D
T43.1X2D
T43.1X3D
T43.1X4D
T43.1X5D
T43.1X6D
T43.1X6S
T43.201D
T43.202D
T43.203D
T43.204D
T43.205D
T43.206D
T43.206S
T43.211D
T43.212D
T43.213D
T43.214D
T43.215D
T43.216D
T43.216S
T43.221D
T43.222D
T43.223D
T43.224D
T43.225D
T43.226D
T43.226S
T43.291D
T43.292D
T43.293D
T43.294D
T43.295D
T43.296D
T43.296S
T43.3X1D
T43.3X2D
T43.3X3D
T43.3X4D
T43.3X5D
T43.3X6D
T43.3X6S
T43.4X1D
T43.4X2D
T43.4X3D
T43.4X4D
T43.4X5D
T43.4X6D
T43.4X6S
T43.501D
T43.502D
T43.503D
T43.504D
T43.505D
T43.506D
T43.506S
T43.591D
T43.592D
T43.593D
T43.594D
T43.595D
T43.596D
T43.596S
T43.601D
T43.602D
T43.603D
T43.604D
T43.605D
T43.606D
T43.606S
T43.611D
T43.612D
T43.613D
T43.614D
T43.615D
T43.616D
T43.616S
T43.621D
T43.622D
T43.623D
T43.624D
T43.625D
T43.626D
T43.626S
T43.631D
T43.632D
T43.633D
T43.634D
T43.635D
T43.636D
T43.636S
T43.641D
T43.642D
T43.643D
T43.644D
T43.651D
T43.652D
T43.653D
T43.654D
T43.655D
T43.656D
T43.656S
T43.691D
T43.692D
T43.693D
T43.694D
T43.695D
T43.696D
T43.696S
T43.8X1D
T43.8X2D
T43.8X3D
T43.8X4D
T43.8X5D
T43.8X6D
T43.8X6S
T43.91XD
T43.92XD
T43.93XD
T43.94XD
T43.95XD
T43.96XD
T43.96XS
T44.0X1D
T44.0X2D
T44.0X3D
T44.0X4D
T44.0X5D
T44.0X6D
T44.0X6S
T44.1X1D
T44.1X2D
T44.1X3D
T44.1X4D
T44.1X5D
T44.1X6D
T44.1X6S
T44.2X1D
T44.2X2D
T44.2X3D
T44.2X4D
T44.2X5D
T44.2X6D
T44.2X6S
T44.3X1D
T44.3X2D
T44.3X3D
T44.3X4D
T44.3X5D
T44.3X6D
T44.3X6S
T44.4X1D
T44.4X2D
T44.4X3D
T44.4X4D
T44.4X5D
T44.4X6D
T44.4X6S
T44.5X1D
T44.5X2D
T44.5X3D
T44.5X4D
T44.5X5D
T44.5X6D
T44.5X6S
T44.6X1D
T44.6X2D
T44.6X3D
T44.6X4D
T44.6X5D
T44.6X6D
T44.6X6S
T44.7X1D
T44.7X2D
T44.7X3D
T44.7X4D
T44.7X5D
T44.7X6D
T44.7X6S
T44.8X1D
T44.8X2D
T44.8X3D
T44.8X4D
T44.8X5D
T44.8X6D
T44.8X6S
T44.901D
T44.902D
T44.903D
T44.904D
T44.905D
T44.906D
T44.906S
T44.991D
T44.992D
T44.993D
T44.994D
T44.995D
T44.996D
T44.996S
T45.0X1D
T45.0X2D
T45.0X3D
T45.0X4D
T45.0X5D
T45.0X6D
T45.0X6S
T45.1X1D
T45.1X2D
T45.1X3D
T45.1X4D
T45.1X5D
T45.1X6D
T45.1X6S
T45.2X1D
T45.2X2D
T45.2X3D
T45.2X4D
T45.2X5D
T45.2X6D
T45.2X6S
T45.3X1D
T45.3X2D
T45.3X3D
T45.3X4D
T45.3X5D
T45.3X6D
T45.3X6S
T45.4X1D
T45.4X2D
T45.4X3D
T45.4X4D
T45.4X5D
T45.4X6D
T45.4X6S
T45.511D
T45.512D
T45.513D
T45.514D
T45.515D
T45.516D
T45.516S
T45.521D
T45.522D
T45.523D
T45.524D
T45.525D
T45.526D
T45.526S
T45.601D
T45.602D
T45.603D
T45.604D
T45.605D
T45.606D
T45.606S
T45.611D
T45.612D
T45.613D
T45.614D
T45.615D
T45.616D
T45.616S
T45.621D
T45.622D
T45.623D
T45.624D
T45.625D
T45.626D
T45.626S
T45.691D
T45.692D
T45.693D
T45.694D
T45.695D
T45.696D
T45.696S
T45.7X1D
T45.7X2D
T45.7X3D
T45.7X4D
T45.7X5D
T45.7X6D
T45.7X6S
T45.8X1D
T45.8X2D
T45.8X3D
T45.8X4D
T45.8X5D
T45.8X6D
T45.8X6S
T45.91XD
T45.92XD
T45.93XD
T45.94XD
T45.95XD
T45.96XD
T45.96XS
T46.0X1D
T46.0X2D
T46.0X3D
T46.0X4D
T46.0X5D
T46.0X6D
T46.0X6S
T46.1X1D
T46.1X2D
T46.1X3D
T46.1X4D
T46.1X5D
T46.1X6D
T46.1X6S
T46.2X1D
T46.2X2D
T46.2X3D
T46.2X4D
T46.2X5D
T46.2X6D
T46.2X6S
T46.3X1D
T46.3X2D
T46.3X3D
T46.3X4D
T46.3X5D
T46.3X6D
T46.3X6S
T46.4X1D
T46.4X2D
T46.4X3D
T46.4X4D
T46.4X5D
T46.4X6D
T46.4X6S
T46.5X1D
T46.5X2D
T46.5X3D
T46.5X4D
T46.5X5D
T46.5X6D
T46.5X6S
T46.6X1D
T46.6X2D
T46.6X3D
T46.6X4D
T46.6X5D
T46.6X6D
T46.6X6S
T46.7X1D
T46.7X2D
T46.7X3D
T46.7X4D
T46.7X5D
T46.7X6D
T46.7X6S
T46.8X1D
T46.8X2D
T46.8X3D
T46.8X4D
T46.8X5D
T46.8X6D
T46.8X6S
T46.901D
T46.902D
T46.903D
T46.904D
T46.905D
T46.906D
T46.906S
T46.991D
T46.992D
T46.993D
T46.994D
T46.995D
T46.996D
T46.996S
T47.0X1D
T47.0X2D
T47.0X3D
T47.0X4D
T47.0X5D
T47.0X6D
T47.0X6S
T47.1X1D
T47.1X2D
T47.1X3D
T47.1X4D
T47.1X5D
T47.1X6D
T47.1X6S
T47.2X1D
T47.2X2D
T47.2X3D
T47.2X4D
T47.2X5D
T47.2X6D
T47.2X6S
T47.3X1D
T47.3X2D
T47.3X3D
T47.3X4D
T47.3X5D
T47.3X6D
T47.3X6S
T47.4X1D
T47.4X2D
T47.4X3D
T47.4X4D
T47.4X5D
T47.4X6D
T47.4X6S
T47.5X1D
T47.5X2D
T47.5X3D
T47.5X4D
T47.5X5D
T47.5X6D
T47.5X6S
T47.6X1D
T47.6X2D
T47.6X3D
T47.6X4D
T47.6X5D
T47.6X6D
T47.6X6S
T47.7X1D
T47.7X2D
T47.7X3D
T47.7X4D
T47.7X5D
T47.7X6D
T47.7X6S
T47.8X1D
T47.8X2D
T47.8X3D
T47.8X4D
T47.8X5D
T47.8X6D
T47.8X6S
T47.91XD
T47.92XD
T47.93XD
T47.94XD
T47.95XD
T47.96XD
T47.96XS
T48.0X1D
T48.0X2D
T48.0X3D
T48.0X4D
T48.0X5D
T48.0X6D
T48.0X6S
T48.1X1D
T48.1X2D
T48.1X3D
T48.1X4D
T48.1X5D
T48.1X6D
T48.1X6S
T48.201D
T48.202D
T48.203D
T48.204D
T48.205D
T48.206D
T48.206S
T48.291D
T48.292D
T48.293D
T48.294D
T48.295D
T48.296D
T48.296S
T48.3X1D
T48.3X2D
T48.3X3D
T48.3X4D
T48.3X5D
T48.3X6D
T48.3X6S
T48.4X1D
T48.4X2D
T48.4X3D
T48.4X4D
T48.4X5D
T48.4X6D
T48.4X6S
T48.5X1D
T48.5X2D
T48.5X3D
T48.5X4D
T48.5X5D
T48.5X6D
T48.5X6S
T48.6X1D
T48.6X2D
T48.6X3D
T48.6X4D
T48.6X5D
T48.6X6D
T48.6X6S
T48.901D
T48.902D
T48.903D
T48.904D
T48.905D
T48.906D
T48.906S
T48.991D
T48.992D
T48.993D
T48.994D
T48.995D
T48.996D
T48.996S
T49.0X1D
T49.0X2D
T49.0X3D
T49.0X4D
T49.0X5D
T49.0X6D
T49.0X6S
T49.1X1D
T49.1X2D
T49.1X3D
T49.1X4D
T49.1X5D
T49.1X6D
T49.1X6S
T49.2X1D
T49.2X2D
T49.2X3D
T49.2X4D
T49.2X5D
T49.2X6D
T49.2X6S
T49.3X1D
T49.3X2D
T49.3X3D
T49.3X4D
T49.3X5D
T49.3X6D
T49.3X6S
T49.4X1D
T49.4X2D
T49.4X3D
T49.4X4D
T49.4X5D
T49.4X6D
T49.4X6S
T49.5X1D
T49.5X2D
T49.5X3D
T49.5X4D
T49.5X5D
T49.5X6D
T49.5X6S
T49.6X1D
T49.6X2D
T49.6X3D
T49.6X4D
T49.6X5D
T49.6X6D
T49.6X6S
T49.7X1D
T49.7X2D
T49.7X3D
T49.7X4D
T49.7X5D
T49.7X6D
T49.7X6S
T49.8X1D
T49.8X2D
T49.8X3D
T49.8X4D
T49.8X5D
T49.8X6D
T49.8X6S
T49.91XD
T49.92XD
T49.93XD
T49.94XD
T49.95XD
T49.96XD
T49.96XS
T50.0X1D
T50.0X2D
T50.0X3D
T50.0X4D
T50.0X5D
T50.0X6D
T50.0X6S
T50.1X1D
T50.1X2D
T50.1X3D
T50.1X4D
T50.1X5D
T50.1X6D
T50.1X6S
T50.2X1D
T50.2X2D
T50.2X3D
T50.2X4D
T50.2X5D
T50.2X6D
T50.2X6S
T50.3X1D
T50.3X2D
T50.3X3D
T50.3X4D
T50.3X5D
T50.3X6D
T50.3X6S
T50.4X1D
T50.4X2D
T50.4X3D
T50.4X4D
T50.4X5D
T50.4X6D
T50.4X6S
T50.5X1D
T50.5X2D
T50.5X3D
T50.5X4D
T50.5X5D
T50.5X6D
T50.5X6S
T50.6X1D
T50.6X2D
T50.6X3D
T50.6X4D
T50.6X5D
T50.6X6D
T50.6X6S
T50.7X1D
T50.7X2D
T50.7X3D
T50.7X4D
T50.7X5D
T50.7X6D
T50.7X6S
T50.8X1D
T50.8X2D
T50.8X3D
T50.8X4D
T50.8X5D
T50.8X6D
T50.8X6S
T50.901D
T50.902D
T50.903D
T50.904D
T50.905D
T50.906D
T50.906S
T50.911D
T50.912D
T50.913D
T50.914D
T50.915D
T50.916D
T50.991D
T50.992D
T50.993D
T50.994D
T50.995D
T50.996D
T50.996S
T50.A11D
T50.A12D
T50.A13D
T50.A14D
T50.A15D
T50.A16D
T50.A16S
T50.A21D
T50.A22D
T50.A23D
T50.A24D
T50.A25D
T50.A26D
T50.A26S
T50.A91D
T50.A92D
T50.A93D
T50.A94D
T50.A95D
T50.A96D
T50.A96S
T50.B11D
T50.B12D
T50.B13D
T50.B14D
T50.B15D
T50.B16D
T50.B16S
T50.B91D
T50.B92D
T50.B93D
T50.B94D
T50.B95D
T50.B96D
T50.B96S
T50.Z11D
T50.Z12D
T50.Z13D
T50.Z14D
T50.Z15D
T50.Z16D
T50.Z16S
T50.Z91D
T50.Z92D
T50.Z93D
T50.Z94D
T50.Z95D
T50.Z96D
T50.Z96S
T51.0X1D
T51.0X2D
T51.0X3D
T51.0X4D
T51.1X1D
T51.1X2D
T51.1X3D
T51.1X4D
T51.2X1D
T51.2X2D
T51.2X3D
T51.2X4D
T51.3X1D
T51.3X2D
T51.3X3D
T51.3X4D
T51.8X1D
T51.8X2D
T51.8X3D
T51.8X4D
T51.91XD
T51.92XD
T51.93XD
T51.94XD
T52.0X1D
T52.0X2D
T52.0X3D
T52.0X4D
T52.1X1D
T52.1X2D
T52.1X3D
T52.1X4D
T52.2X1D
T52.2X2D
T52.2X3D
T52.2X4D
T52.3X1D
T52.3X2D
T52.3X3D
T52.3X4D
T52.4X1D
T52.4X2D
T52.4X3D
T52.4X4D
T52.8X1D
T52.8X2D
T52.8X3D
T52.8X4D
T52.91XD
T52.92XD
T52.93XD
T52.94XD
T53.0X1D
T53.0X2D
T53.0X3D
T53.0X4D
T53.1X1D
T53.1X2D
T53.1X3D
T53.1X4D
T53.2X1D
T53.2X2D
T53.2X3D
T53.2X4D
T53.3X1D
T53.3X2D
T53.3X3D
T53.3X4D
T53.4X1D
T53.4X2D
T53.4X3D
T53.4X4D
T53.5X1D
T53.5X2D
T53.5X3D
T53.5X4D
T53.6X1D
T53.6X2D
T53.6X3D
T53.6X4D
T53.7X1D

ICD-10-CM/PCS Codes by MS-DRG

T53.7X2D
T53.7X3D
T53.7X4D
T53.91XD
T53.92XD
T53.93XD
T53.94XD
T54.0X1D
T54.0X2D
T54.0X3D
T54.0X4D
T54.1X1D
T54.1X2D
T54.1X3D
T54.1X4D
T54.2X1D
T54.2X2D
T54.2X3D
T54.2X4D
T54.3X1D
T54.3X2D
T54.3X3D
T54.3X4D
T54.91XD
T54.92XD
T54.93XD
T54.94XD
T55.0X1D
T55.0X2D
T55.0X3D
T55.0X4D
T55.1X1D
T55.1X2D
T55.1X3D
T55.1X4D
T56.0X1D
T56.0X2D
T56.0X3D
T56.0X4D
T56.1X1D
T56.1X2D
T56.1X3D
T56.1X4D
T56.2X1D
T56.2X2D
T56.2X3D
T56.2X4D
T56.3X1D
T56.3X2D
T56.3X3D
T56.3X4D
T56.4X1D
T56.4X2D
T56.4X3D
T56.4X4D
T56.5X1D
T56.5X2D
T56.5X3D
T56.5X4D
T56.6X1D
T56.6X2D
T56.6X3D
T56.6X4D
T56.7X1D
T56.7X2D
T56.7X3D
T56.7X4D
T56.811D
T56.812D
T56.813D
T56.814D
T56.821D
T56.822D
T56.823D
T56.824D
T56.891D
T56.892D
T56.893D
T56.894D
T56.91XD
T56.92XD
T56.93XD
T56.94XD
T57.0X1D
T57.0X2D
T57.0X3D
T57.0X4D
T57.1X1D
T57.1X2D
T57.1X3D
T57.1X4D
T57.2X1D
T57.2X2D
T57.2X3D
T57.2X4D
T57.3X1D
T57.3X2D
T57.3X3D
T57.3X4D
T57.8X1D
T57.8X2D
T57.8X3D
T57.8X4D
T57.91XD
T57.92XD
T57.93XD
T57.94XD
T58.01XD
T58.02XD
T58.03XD
T58.04XD
T58.11XD
T58.12XD
T58.13XD
T58.14XD
T58.2X1D
T58.2X2D
T58.2X3D
T58.2X4D
T58.8X1D
T58.8X2D
T58.8X3D
T58.8X4D
T58.91XD
T58.92XD
T58.93XD
T58.94XD
T59.0X1D
T59.0X2D
T59.0X3D
T59.0X4D
T59.1X1D
T59.1X2D
T59.1X3D
T59.1X4D
T59.2X1D
T59.2X2D
T59.2X3D
T59.2X4D
T59.3X1D
T59.3X2D
T59.3X3D
T59.3X4D
T59.4X1D
T59.4X2D
T59.4X3D
T59.4X4D
T59.5X1D
T59.5X2D
T59.5X3D
T59.5X4D
T59.6X1D
T59.6X2D
T59.6X3D
T59.6X4D
T59.7X1D
T59.7X2D
T59.7X3D
T59.7X4D
T59.811D
T59.812D
T59.813D
T59.814D
T59.891D
T59.892D
T59.893D
T59.894D
T59.91XD
T59.92XD
T59.93XD
T59.94XD
T60.0X1D
T60.0X2D
T60.0X3D
T60.0X4D
T60.1X1D
T60.1X2D
T60.1X3D
T60.1X4D
T60.2X1D
T60.2X2D
T60.2X3D
T60.2X4D
T60.3X1D
T60.3X2D
T60.3X3D
T60.3X4D
T60.4X1D
T60.4X2D
T60.4X3D
T60.4X4D
T60.8X1D
T60.8X2D
T60.8X3D
T60.8X4D
T60.91XD
T60.92XD
T60.93XD
T60.94XD
T61.01XD
T61.02XD
T61.03XD
T61.04XD
T61.11XD
T61.12XD
T61.13XD
T61.14XD
T61.771D
T61.772D
T61.773D
T61.774D
T61.781D
T61.782D
T61.783D
T61.784D
T61.8X1D
T61.8X2D
T61.8X3D
T61.8X4D
T61.91XD
T61.92XD
T61.93XD
T61.94XD
T62.0X1D
T62.0X2D
T62.0X3D
T62.0X4D
T62.1X1D
T62.1X2D
T62.1X3D
T62.1X4D
T62.2X1D
T62.2X2D
T62.2X3D
T62.2X4D
T62.8X1D
T62.8X2D
T62.8X3D
T62.8X4D
T62.91XD
T62.92XD
T62.93XD
T62.94XD
T63.001D
T63.002D
T63.003D
T63.004D
T63.011D
T63.012D
T63.013D
T63.014D
T63.021D
T63.022D
T63.023D
T63.024D
T63.031D
T63.032D
T63.033D
T63.034D
T63.041D
T63.042D
T63.043D
T63.044D
T63.061D
T63.062D
T63.063D
T63.064D
T63.071D
T63.072D
T63.073D
T63.074D
T63.081D
T63.082D
T63.083D
T63.084D
T63.091D
T63.092D
T63.093D
T63.094D
T63.111D
T63.112D
T63.113D
T63.114D
T63.121D
T63.122D
T63.123D
T63.124D
T63.191D
T63.192D
T63.193D
T63.194D
T63.2X1D
T63.2X2D
T63.2X3D
T63.2X4D
T63.301D
T63.302D
T63.303D
T63.304D
T63.311D
T63.312D
T63.313D
T63.314D
T63.321D
T63.322D
T63.323D
T63.324D
T63.331D
T63.332D
T63.333D
T63.334D
T63.391D
T63.392D
T63.393D
T63.394D
T63.411D
T63.412D
T63.413D
T63.414D
T63.421D
T63.422D
T63.423D
T63.424D
T63.431D
T63.432D
T63.433D
T63.434D
T63.441D
T63.442D
T63.443D
T63.444D
T63.451D
T63.452D
T63.453D
T63.454D
T63.461D
T63.462D
T63.463D
T63.464D
T63.481D
T63.482D
T63.483D
T63.484D
T63.511D
T63.512D
T63.513D
T63.514D
T63.591D
T63.592D
T63.593D
T63.594D
T63.611D
T63.612D
T63.613D
T63.614D
T63.621D
T63.622D
T63.623D
T63.624D
T63.631D
T63.632D
T63.633D
T63.634D
T63.691D
T63.692D
T63.693D
T63.694D
T63.711D
T63.712D
T63.713D
T63.714D
T63.791D
T63.792D
T63.793D
T63.794D
T63.811D
T63.812D
T63.813D
T63.814D
T63.821D
T63.822D
T63.823D
T63.824D
T63.831D
T63.832D
T63.833D
T63.834D
T63.891D
T63.892D
T63.893D
T63.894D
T63.91XD
T63.92XD
T63.93XD
T63.94XD
T64.01XD
T64.02XD
T64.03XD
T64.04XD
T64.81XD
T64.82XD
T64.83XD
T64.84XD
T65.0X1D
T65.0X2D
T65.0X3D
T65.0X4D
T65.1X1D
T65.1X2D
T65.1X3D
T65.1X4D
T65.211D
T65.212D
T65.213D
T65.214D
T65.221D
T65.222D
T65.223D
T65.224D
T65.291D
T65.292D
T65.293D
T65.294D
T65.3X1D
T65.3X2D
T65.3X3D
T65.3X4D
T65.4X1D
T65.4X2D
T65.4X3D
T65.4X4D
T65.5X1D
T65.5X2D
T65.5X3D
T65.5X4D
T65.6X1D
T65.6X2D
T65.6X3D
T65.6X4D
T65.811D
T65.812D
T65.813D
T65.814D
T65.821D
T65.822D
T65.823D
T65.824D
T65.831D
T65.832D
T65.833D
T65.834D
T65.891D
T65.892D
T65.893D
T65.894D
T65.91XD
T65.92XD
T65.93XD
T65.94XD
T66.XXXD
T67.01XD
T67.02XD
T67.09XD
T67.1XXD
T67.2XXD
T67.3XXD
T67.4XXD
T67.5XXD
T67.6XXD
T67.7XXD
T67.8XXD
T67.9XXD
T68.XXXD
T69.011D
T69.012D
T69.019D
T69.021D
T69.022D
T69.029D
T69.1XXD
T69.8XXD
T69.9XXD
T70.0XXD
T70.1XXD
T70.20XD
T70.29XD
T70.3XXD
T70.4XXD
T70.8XXD
T70.9XXD
T71.111D
T71.112D
T71.113D
T71.114D
T71.121D
T71.122D
T71.123D
T71.124D
T71.131D
T71.132D
T71.133D
T71.134D
T71.141D
T71.143D
T71.144D
T71.151D
T71.152D
T71.153D
T71.154D
T71.161D
T71.162D
T71.163D
T71.164D
T71.191D
T71.192D
T71.193D
T71.194D
T71.20XD
T71.21XD
T71.221D
T71.222D
T71.223D
T71.224D
T71.231D
T71.232D
T71.233D
T71.234D
T71.29XD
T71.9XXD
T73.0XXD
T73.1XXD
T73.2XXD
T73.3XXD
T73.8XXD
T73.9XXD
T74.01XD
T74.02XD
T74.11XD
T74.12XD
T74.21XD
T74.22XD
T74.31XD
T74.32XD
T74.4XXD
T74.51XD
T74.52XD
T74.61XD
T74.62XD
T74.91XD
T74.92XD
T74.A1XD
T74.A2XD
T75.00XD
T75.01XD
T75.09XD
T75.1XXD
T75.20XD
T75.21XD
T75.22XD
T75.23XD
T75.29XD
T75.3XXD
T75.4XXD
T75.81XD
T75.82XD
T75.89XD
T76.01XD
T76.02XD
T76.11XD
T76.12XD
T76.21XD
T76.22XD
T76.31XD
T76.32XD
T76.51XD
T76.52XD
T76.61XD
T76.62XD
T76.91XD
T76.92XD
T76.A1XD
T76.A2XD
T78.00XD
T78.01XD
T78.02XD
T78.03XD
T78.04XD
T78.05XD
T78.06XD
T78.07XD
T78.08XD
T78.09XD
T78.1XXD
T78.2XXD
T78.3XXD
T78.40XD
T78.41XD
T78.49XD
T78.8XXD
T79.0XXD
T79.1XXD
T79.2XXD
T79.4XXD
T79.5XXD
T79.6XXD
T79.7XXD
T79.8XXD
T79.9XXD
T79.A0XD
T79.A11D
T79.A12D
T79.A19D
T79.A21D
T79.A22D
T79.A29D
T79.A3XD
T79.A9XD
T80.0XXD
T80.1XXD
T80.211D
T80.212D
T80.218D
T80.219D
T80.22XD
T80.29XD
T80.30XD
T80.310D
T80.311D
T80.319D
T80.39XD
T80.40XD
T80.410D
T80.411D
T80.419D
T80.49XD
T80.51XD
T80.52XD
T80.59XD
T80.61XD
T80.62XD
T80.69XD
T80.810D
T80.818D
T80.82XD
T80.89XD
T80.90XD
T80.910D
T80.911D
T80.919D
T80.92XD
T80.A0XD
T80.A10D
T80.A11D
T80.A19D
T80.A9XD
T81.10XD
T81.11XD
T81.12XD
T81.19XD
T81.30XD
T81.31XD
T81.32XD
T81.33XD
T81.40XD
T81.41XD
T81.42XD
T81.43XD
T81.44XD
T81.49XD
T81.500D
T81.501D
T81.502D
T81.503D
T81.504D
T81.505D
T81.506D
T81.507D
T81.508D
T81.509D
T81.510D
T81.511D
T81.512D
T81.513D
T81.514D
T81.515D
T81.516D
T81.517D
T81.518D
T81.519D
T81.520D
T81.521D
T81.522D
T81.523D
T81.524D
T81.525D
T81.526D
T81.527D
T81.528D
T81.529D
T81.530D
T81.531D
T81.532D
T81.533D
T81.534D
T81.535D
T81.536D
T81.537D
T81.538D
T81.539D
T81.590D
T81.591D
T81.592D
T81.593D
T81.594D
T81.595D
T81.596D
T81.597D
T81.598D
T81.599D
T81.60XD
T81.61XD
T81.69XD
T81.710D
T81.711D
T81.718D
T81.719D
T81.72XD
T81.81XD
T81.82XD
T81.83XD
T81.89XD
T81.9XXD
T82.01XD
T82.02XD
T82.03XD
T82.09XD
T82.110D
T82.111D
T82.118D
T82.119D
T82.120D
T82.121D
T82.128D
T82.129D
T82.190D
T82.191D
T82.198D
T82.199D
T82.211D
T82.212D
T82.213D
T82.218D
T82.221D
T82.222D
T82.223D
T82.228D
T82.310D
T82.311D
T82.312D
T82.318D
T82.319D
T82.320D
T82.321D
T82.322D
T82.328D
T82.329D
T82.330D
T82.331D
T82.332D
T82.338D
T82.339D
T82.390D
T82.391D
T82.392D
T82.398D
T82.399D
T82.41XD
T82.42XD
T82.43XD
T82.49XD
T82.510D
T82.511D
T82.512D
T82.513D
T82.514D
T82.515D
T82.518D
T82.519D
T82.520D
T82.521D
T82.522D
T82.523D
T82.524D
T82.525D
T82.528D
T82.529D
T82.530D
T82.531D
T82.532D
T82.533D
T82.534D
T82.535D
T82.538D
T82.539D
T82.590D
T82.591D
T82.592D
T82.593D
T82.594D
T82.595D
T82.598D
T82.599D
T82.6XXD
T82.7XXD
T82.817D
T82.818D
T82.827D
T82.828D
T82.837D
T82.838D
T82.847D
T82.848D
T82.855D
T82.856D
T82.857D
T82.858D
T82.867D
T82.868D
T82.897D
T82.898D
T82.9XXD
T83.010D
T83.011D
T83.012D
T83.018D
T83.020D
T83.021D
T83.022D
T83.028D
T83.030D
T83.031D
T83.032D
T83.038D
T83.090D
T83.091D
T83.092D
T83.098D
T83.110D
T83.111D
T83.112D
T83.113D
T83.118D
T83.120D
T83.121D
T83.122D

T83.123D
T83.128D
T83.19ØD
T83.191D
T83.192D
T83.193D
T83.198D
T83.21XD
T83.22XD
T83.23XD
T83.24XD
T83.25XD
T83.29XD
T83.31XD
T83.32XD
T83.39XD
T83.41ØD
T83.411D
T83.418D
T83.42ØD
T83.421D
T83.428D
T83.49ØD
T83.491D
T83.498D
T83.51ØD
T83.511D
T83.512D
T83.518D
T83.59ØD
T83.591D
T83.592D
T83.593D
T83.598D
T83.61XD
T83.62XD
T83.69XD
T83.711D
T83.712D
T83.713D
T83.714D
T83.718D
T83.719D
T83.721D
T83.722D
T83.723D
T83.724D
T83.728D
T83.729D
T83.79XD
T83.81XD
T83.82XD
T83.83XD
T83.84XD
T83.85XD
T83.86XD
T83.89XD
T83.9XXD
T84.Ø1ØD
T84.Ø11D
T84.Ø12D
T84.Ø13D
T84.Ø18D
T84.Ø19D
T84.Ø2ØD
T84.Ø21D
T84.Ø22D
T84.Ø23D
T84.Ø28D
T84.Ø29D
T84.Ø3ØD
T84.Ø31D
T84.Ø32D
T84.Ø33D
T84.Ø38D
T84.Ø39D
T84.Ø5ØD
T84.Ø51D
T84.Ø52D
T84.Ø53D
T84.Ø58D
T84.Ø59D
T84.Ø6ØD
T84.Ø61D
T84.Ø62D
T84.Ø63D
T84.Ø68D
T84.Ø69D
T84.Ø9ØD
T84.Ø91D
T84.Ø92D
T84.Ø93D
T84.Ø98D
T84.Ø99D
T84.11ØD
T84.111D
T84.112D
T84.113D
T84.114D
T84.115D
T84.116D
T84.117D
T84.119D
T84.12ØD
T84.121D
T84.122D
T84.123D
T84.124D
T84.125D
T84.126D
T84.127D
T84.129D
T84.19ØD
T84.191D
T84.192D
T84.193D
T84.194D
T84.195D
T84.196D
T84.197D
T84.199D
T84.21ØD
T84.213D
T84.216D
T84.218D
T84.22ØD
T84.223D
T84.226D
T84.228D
T84.29ØD
T84.293D
T84.296D
T84.298D
T84.31ØD
T84.318D
T84.32ØD
T84.328D
T84.39ØD
T84.398D
T84.41ØD
T84.418D
T84.42ØD
T84.428D
T84.49ØD
T84.498D
T84.5ØXD
T84.51XD
T84.52XD
T84.53XD
T84.54XD
T84.59XD
T84.6ØXD
T84.61ØD
T84.611D
T84.612D
T84.613D
T84.614D
T84.615D
T84.619D
T84.62ØD
T84.621D
T84.622D
T84.623D
T84.624D
T84.625D
T84.629D
T84.63XD
T84.69XD
T84.7XXD
T84.81XD
T84.82XD
T84.83XD
T84.84XD
T84.85XD
T84.86XD
T84.89XD
T84.9XXD
T85.Ø1XD
T85.Ø2XD
T85.Ø3XD
T85.Ø9XD
T85.11ØD
T85.111D
T85.112D
T85.113D
T85.118D
T85.12ØD
T85.121D
T85.122D
T85.123D
T85.128D
T85.19ØD
T85.191D
T85.192D
T85.193D
T85.199D
T85.21XD
T85.22XD
T85.29XD
T85.31ØD
T85.311D
T85.318D
T85.32ØD
T85.321D
T85.328D
T85.39ØD
T85.391D
T85.398D
T85.41XD
T85.42XD
T85.43XD
T85.44XD
T85.49XD
T85.51ØD
T85.511D
T85.518D
T85.52ØD
T85.521D
T85.528D
T85.59ØD
T85.591D
T85.598D
T85.61ØD
T85.611D
T85.612D
T85.613D
T85.614D
T85.615D
T85.618D
T85.62ØD
T85.621D
T85.622D
T85.623D
T85.624D
T85.625D
T85.628D
T85.63ØD
T85.631D
T85.633D
T85.635D
T85.638D
T85.69ØD
T85.691D
T85.692D
T85.693D
T85.694D
T85.695D
T85.698D
T85.71XD
T85.72XD
T85.73ØD
T85.731D
T85.732D
T85.733D
T85.734D
T85.735D
T85.738D
T85.79XD
T85.81ØD
T85.818D
T85.82ØD
T85.828D
T85.83ØD
T85.838D
T85.84ØD
T85.848D
T85.85ØD
T85.858D
T85.86ØD
T85.868D
T85.89ØD
T85.898D
T85.9XXD
T88.ØXXD
T88.1XXD
T88.2XXD
T88.3XXD
T88.4XXD
T88.51XD
T88.52XD
T88.53XD
T88.59XD
T88.6XXD
T88.7XXD
T88.8XXD
T88.9XXD
Z45.1
Z45.2
Z46.82
Z48.Ø3
Z48.1
Z48.2*
Z48.3
Z48.8*
Z51.8*
Z79.Ø*
Z79.1
Z79.2
Z79.3
Z79.4
Z79.5*
Z79.6Ø
Z79.61
Z79.62Ø
Z79.621
Z79.622
Z79.623
Z79.624
Z79.63Ø
Z79.631
Z79.632
Z79.633
Z79.634
Z79.64
Z79.69
Z79.82
Z79.83
Z79.84
Z79.85
Z79.891
Z79.899
Z92.2*

DRG 950

Select any principal diagnosis listed under DRG 949

DRG 951

Principal Diagnosis

F17.2ØØ
F17.2Ø1
F17.21Ø
F17.211
F17.22Ø
F17.221
F17.29Ø
F17.291
J95.85Ø
PØØ.2
PØØ.82
PØØ.89
Q89.9
Q92*
Q93.Ø
Q93.1
Q93.2
Q95*
Q99.9
R29.7*
R4Ø.213Ø
R4Ø.2131
R4Ø.2132
R4Ø.2133
R4Ø.2134
R4Ø.214Ø
R4Ø.2141
R4Ø.2142
R4Ø.2143
R4Ø.2144
R4Ø.223Ø
R4Ø.2231
R4Ø.2232
R4Ø.2233
R4Ø.2234
R4Ø.224Ø
R4Ø.2241
R4Ø.2242
R4Ø.2243
R4Ø.2244
R4Ø.225Ø
R4Ø.2251
R4Ø.2252
R4Ø.2253
R4Ø.2254
R4Ø.233Ø
R4Ø.2331
R4Ø.2332
R4Ø.2333
R4Ø.2334
R4Ø.235Ø
R4Ø.2351
R4Ø.2352
R4Ø.2353
R4Ø.2354
R4Ø.236Ø
R4Ø.2361
R4Ø.2362
R4Ø.2363
R4Ø.2364
R4Ø.241Ø
R4Ø.2411
R4Ø.2412
R4Ø.2413
R4Ø.2414
R4Ø.242Ø
R4Ø.2421
R4Ø.2422
R4Ø.2423
R4Ø.2424
R4Ø.243Ø
R4Ø.2431
R4Ø.2432
R4Ø.2433
R4Ø.2434
R4Ø.244*
R41.83
R44.8
R44.9
R45.85Ø
R46*
R68.13
R68.19
R68.82
R69
R99
T36.ØX6A
T36.1X6A
T36.2X6A
T36.3X6A
T36.4X6A
T36.5X6A
T36.6X6A
T36.7X6A
T36.8X6A
T36.96XA
T37.ØX6A
T37.1X6A
T37.2X6A
T37.3X6A
T37.4X6A
T37.5X6A
T37.8X6A
T37.96XA
T38.ØX6A
T38.1X6A
T38.2X6A
T38.3X6A
T38.4X6A
T38.5X6A
T38.6X6A
T38.7X6A
T38.8Ø6A
T38.816A
T38.896A
T38.9Ø6A
T38.996A
T39.Ø16A
T39.Ø96A
T39.1X6A
T39.2X6A
T39.316A
T39.396A
T39.4X6A
T39.8X6A
T39.96XA
T4Ø.ØX6A
T4Ø.2X6A
T4Ø.3X6A
T4Ø.416A
T4Ø.426A
T4Ø.496A
T4Ø.5X6A
T4Ø.6Ø6A
T4Ø.696A
T4Ø.716A
T4Ø.726A
T4Ø.9Ø6A
T4Ø.996A
T41.ØX6A
T41.1X6A
T41.2Ø6A
T41.296A
T41.3X6A
T41.46XA
T41.5X6A
T42.ØX6A
T42.1X6A
T42.2X6A
T42.3X6A
T42.4X6A
T42.5X6A
T42.6X6A
T42.76XA
T42.8X6A
T43.Ø16A
T43.Ø26A
T43.1X6A
T43.2Ø6A
T43.216A
T43.226A
T43.296A
T43.3X6A
T43.4X6A
T43.5Ø6A
T43.596A
T43.6Ø6A
T43.616A
T43.626A
T43.636A
T43.656A
T43.696A
T43.8X6A
T43.96XA
T44.ØX6A
T44.1X6A
T44.2X6A
T44.3X6A
T44.4X6A
T44.5X6A
T44.6X6A
T44.7X6A
T44.8X6A
T44.9Ø6A
T44.996A
T45.ØX6A
T45.1X6A
T45.2X6A
T45.3X6A
T45.4X6A
T45.516A
T45.526A
T45.6Ø6A
T45.616A
T45.626A
T45.696A
T45.7X6A
T45.8X6A
T45.96XA
T46.ØX6A
T46.1X6A
T46.2X6A
T46.3X6A
T46.4X6A
T46.5X6A
T46.6X6A
T46.7X6A
T46.8X6A
T46.9Ø6A
T46.996A
T47.ØX6A
T47.1X6A
T47.2X6A
T47.3X6A
T47.4X6A
T47.5X6A
T47.6X6A
T47.7X6A
T47.8X6A
T47.96XA
T48.ØX6A
T48.1X6A
T48.2Ø6A
T48.296A
T48.3X6A
T48.4X6A
T48.5X6A
T48.6X6A
T48.9Ø6A
T48.996A
T49.ØX6A
T49.1X6A
T49.2X6A
T49.3X6A
T49.4X6A
T49.5X6A
T49.6X6A
T49.7X6A
T49.8X6A
T49.96XA
T5Ø.ØX6A
T5Ø.1X6A
T5Ø.2X6A
T5Ø.3X6A
T5Ø.4X6A
T5Ø.5X6A
T5Ø.6X6A
T5Ø.7X6A
T5Ø.8X6A
T5Ø.9Ø6A
T5Ø.916A
T5Ø.996A
T5Ø.A16A
T5Ø.A26A
T5Ø.A96A
T5Ø.B16A
T5Ø.B96A
T5Ø.Z16A
T5Ø.Z96A
UØ9.9
ZØØ*
ZØ1*
ZØ2*
ZØ3*
ZØ4.4*
ZØ4.6
ZØ4.7*
ZØ4.81
ZØ4.82
ZØ4.89
ZØ4.9
ZØ5.Ø
ZØ5.1
ZØ5.2
ZØ5.3
ZØ5.41
ZØ5.42
ZØ5.43
ZØ5.5
ZØ5.6
ZØ5.71
ZØ5.72
ZØ5.73
ZØ5.8*
ZØ5.9
ZØ9
Z11*
Z12*
Z13.Ø
Z13.1
Z13.21
Z13.22Ø
Z13.228
Z13.29
Z13.3Ø
Z13.31
Z13.32
Z13.39
Z13.4Ø
Z13.41
Z13.42
Z13.49
Z13.5
Z13.6
Z13.71
Z13.79
Z13.81Ø
Z13.811
Z13.818
Z13.82Ø
Z13.828
Z13.83
Z13.84
Z13.85Ø
Z13.858
Z13.88
Z13.89
Z13.9
Z14*
Z15*
Z17*
Z18*
Z19.1
Z19.2
Z2Ø.Ø1
Z2Ø.Ø9
Z2Ø.1
Z2Ø.2
Z2Ø.3
Z2Ø.4
Z2Ø.5
Z2Ø.6
Z2Ø.7
Z2Ø.81Ø
Z2Ø.811
Z2Ø.818
Z2Ø.82Ø
Z2Ø.821
Z2Ø.822
Z2Ø.828
Z2Ø.89
Z2Ø.9
Z22.Ø
Z22.1
Z22.2
Z22.3*
Z22.4
Z22.6
Z22.7
Z22.8
Z22.9
Z23
Z28.Ø1
Z28.Ø2
Z28.Ø3
Z28.Ø4
Z28.Ø9
Z28.1
Z28.2Ø
Z28.21
Z28.29
Z28.3*
Z28.81
Z28.82
Z28.83
Z28.89
Z28.9
Z29.11
Z29.12
Z29.13
Z29.14
Z29.3
Z29.8*
Z29.9
Z3Ø.Ø*
Z3Ø.4*
Z3Ø.8
Z3Ø.9
Z31.4*
Z31.5
Z31.6*
Z31.7
Z31.8*
Z31.9
Z32*
Z33.1
Z33.3
Z34*
Z36*
Z37*
Z39.1
Z39.2
Z3A*
Z4Ø.ØØ
Z4Ø.Ø9
Z4Ø.8
Z4Ø.9
Z41.3
Z41.8
Z41.9
Z43.8
Z43.9
Z44.2*
Z44.3*
Z45.8*
Z45.9
Z46.Ø
Z46.1
Z46.3
Z46.4
Z46.81
Z46.89
Z46.9
Z48.ØØ
Z48.Ø1
Z48.Ø2
Z51.5
Z51.6
Z52.Ø*
Z52.3
Z52.5
Z52.8*
Z52.9
Z53*
Z55*
Z56*
Z57*
Z58.6
Z58.81
Z58.89
Z59*
Z6Ø*
Z62.Ø
Z62.1
Z62.21
Z62.22
Z62.23
Z62.24
Z62.29
Z62.3
Z62.6
Z62.81Ø
Z62.811
Z62.812
Z62.813
Z62.814
Z62.815
Z62.819
Z62.82Ø
Z62.821
Z62.822
Z62.823
Z62.831
Z62.832
Z62.833
Z62.89Ø
Z62.891
Z62.892
Z62.898
Z62.9
Z63*
Z64.4
Z65*
Z66
Z67*
Z68.1
Z68.2*
Z68.3*
Z68.5*
Z69*
Z7Ø*
Z71*
Z72.Ø
Z72.3
Z72.4
Z72.5*
Z72.6
Z72.82Ø
Z72.821
Z72.823
Z72.89
Z72.9
Z73*
Z74*
Z75*
Z76*
Z77*
Z78*
Z79.81Ø
Z79.811
Z79.818
Z79.89Ø
Z8Ø*
Z81*
Z82*
Z83.Ø
Z83.1
Z83.2
Z83.3
Z83.41
Z83.42
Z83.43Ø
Z83.438
Z83.49
Z83.511
Z83.518
Z83.52
Z83.6
Z83.71*
Z83.79
Z84*
Z86*
Z87.Ø*
Z87.1*
Z87.2
Z87.3*
Z87.411
Z87.412
Z87.42
Z87.43Ø
Z87.438
Z87.44Ø
Z87.441
Z87.442
Z87.448

Z87.5*
Z87.61
Z87.68
Z87.7*
Z87.81
Z87.820
Z87.821
Z87.828
Z87.891
Z87.892
Z87.898
Z88*
Z89*
Z90.02
Z90.09
Z90.1*
Z90.3
Z90.4*
Z90.5
Z90.8*
Z91.010
Z91.011
Z91.012
Z91.013
Z91.014
Z91.018
Z91.02
Z91.030
Z91.038
Z91.040
Z91.041
Z91.048
Z91.09
Z91.11*
Z91.120
Z91.128
Z91.130
Z91.138
Z91.14*
Z91.15*
Z91.19*
Z91.410
Z91.411
Z91.412
Z91.413
Z91.414
Z91.419
Z91.42
Z91.49
Z91.5*
Z91.81
Z91.82
Z91.83
Z91.841
Z91.842
Z91.843
Z91.849
Z91.85
Z91.89
Z91.A10
Z91.A18
Z91.A20
Z91.A28
Z91.A3
Z91.A4*
Z91.A5*
Z91.A9*
Z92.0
Z92.3
Z92.8*
Z93*
Z94.82
Z94.89
Z94.9
Z95.0
Z95.1
Z95.5
Z95.810
Z95.818
Z95.9
Z96.2*
Z96.3
Z96.4*
Z96.5
Z96.8*
Z96.9
Z97.2
Z97.3
Z97.4
Z97.5
Z97.8
Z98*
Z99*

MDC 24

DRG 955

Select combinations of MDC 24 diagnoses of significant trauma listed under DRG 963
AND
Operating Room Procedures

001607A
001607B
00160JA
00160JB
00160KA
00160KB
00160ZB
001637A
001637B
00163JA
00163JB
00163KA
00163KB
00163ZB
001647A
001647B
00164JA
00164JB
00164KA
00164KB
00164ZB
0050*
0051*
0052*
0056*
0057*
0058*
0059*
005A*
005B*
005C*
005D*
00760ZZ
00763ZZ
00764ZZ
0080*
0087*
0088*
009000Z
00900ZZ
009030Z
00903ZZ
009040Z
00904ZZ
009100Z
00910ZZ
009200Z
00920ZZ
009300Z
00930ZZ
009330Z
00933ZZ
009340Z
00934ZZ
009400Z
00940ZZ
009500Z
00950ZZ
009600Z
00960ZZ
009630Z
009640Z
009700Z
00970ZZ
009730Z
00973ZZ
009740Z
00974ZZ
009800Z
00980ZZ
009830Z
00983ZZ
009840Z
00984ZZ
009900Z
00990ZZ
009930Z
00993ZZ
009940Z
00994ZZ
009A00Z
009A0ZZ
009A30Z
009A3ZZ
009A40Z
009A4ZZ
009B00Z
009B0ZZ
009B30Z
009B3ZZ
009B40Z
009B4ZZ
009C00Z
009C0ZZ
009C30Z
009C3ZZ
009C40Z
009C4ZZ
009D00Z
009D0ZZ
009D30Z
009D3ZZ
009D40Z
009D4ZZ
00B00ZZ
00B03ZZ
00B04ZZ
00B10ZZ
00B13ZZ
00B14ZZ
00B20ZZ
00B23ZZ
00B24ZZ
00B60ZZ
00B63ZZ
00B64ZZ
00B70ZZ
00B73ZZ
00B74ZZ
00B80ZZ
00B83ZZ
00B84ZZ
00B90ZZ
00B93ZZ
00B94ZZ
00BA0ZZ
00BA3ZZ
00BA4ZZ
00BB0ZZ
00BB3ZZ
00BB4ZZ
00BC0ZZ
00BC3ZZ
00BC4ZZ
00BD0ZZ
00BD3ZZ
00BD4ZZ
00C0*
00C1*
00C2*
00C4*
00C5*
00C6*
00C7*
00C8*
00C9*
00CA*
00CB*
00CC*
00CD*
00D00ZZ
00D03ZZ
00D04ZZ
00D1*
00D2*
00D70ZZ
00D73ZZ
00D74ZZ
00DC0ZZ
00DC3ZZ
00DC4ZZ
00F30ZZ
00F33ZZ
00F34ZZ
00F40ZZ
00F43ZZ
00F44ZZ
00F50ZZ
00F53ZZ
00F54ZZ
00F60ZZ
00F63ZZ
00F64ZZ
00H001Z
00H002Z
00H003Z
00H00YZ
00H031Z
00H032Z
00H033Z
00H03YZ
00H041Z
00H042Z
00H043Z
00H04YZ
00H601Z
00H602Z
00H603Z
00H60YZ
00H631Z
00H632Z
00H633Z
00H63YZ
00H641Z
00H642Z
00H643Z
00H64YZ
00J00ZZ
00N6*
00N8*
00N9*
00NA*
00NB*
00NC*
00ND*
00NK*
00P000Z
00P002Z
00P003Z
00P007Z
00P00JZ
00P00KZ
00P00YZ
00P037Z
00P03JZ
00P03KZ
00P040Z
00P042Z
00P043Z
00P047Z
00P04JZ
00P04KZ
00P600Z
00P602Z
00P603Z
00P60YZ
00P640Z
00P642Z
00P643Z
00Q0*
00Q1*
00Q2*
00Q6*
00Q7*
00Q8*
00Q9*
00QA*
00QB*
00QC*
00QD*
00R107Z
00R10JZ
00R10KZ
00R147Z
00R14JZ
00R14KZ
00R207Z
00R20JZ
00R20KZ
00R247Z
00R24JZ
00R24KZ
00R607Z
00R60JZ
00R60KZ
00R647Z
00R64JZ
00R64KZ
00T*
00U1*
00U2*
00U607Z
00U60JZ
00U60KZ
00U637Z
00U63JZ
00U63KZ
00U647Z
00U64JZ
00U64KZ
00W000Z
00W002Z
00W003Z
00W007Z
00W00MZ
00W00YZ
00W030Z
00W032Z
00W033Z
00W037Z
00W03JZ
00W03KZ
00W03MZ
00W040Z
00W042Z
00W043Z
00W047Z
00W04JZ
00W04KZ
00W04MZ
00W600Z
00W602Z
00W603Z
00W60MZ
00W60YZ
00W630Z
00W632Z
00W633Z
00W63MZ
00W640Z
00W642Z
00W643Z
00W64MZ
03LG0CZ
03LG0ZZ
03LG3CZ
03LG3ZZ
03LG4CZ
03LG4ZZ
05LL*
0N50*
0N51*
0N53*
0N54*
0N55*
0N56*
0N57*
0N9000Z
0N900ZZ
0N9040Z
0N904ZZ
0N9100Z
0N910ZZ
0N9140Z
0N914ZZ
0N9300Z
0N930ZZ
0N9340Z
0N934ZZ
0N9400Z
0N940ZZ
0N9440Z
0N944ZZ
0N9500Z
0N950ZZ
0N9540Z
0N954ZZ
0N9600Z
0N960ZZ
0N9640Z
0N964ZZ
0N9700Z
0N970ZZ
0N9740Z
0N974ZZ
0NB00ZZ
0NB03ZZ
0NB04ZZ
0NB10ZZ
0NB13ZZ
0NB14ZZ
0NB30ZZ
0NB33ZZ
0NB34ZZ
0NB40ZZ
0NB43ZZ
0NB44ZZ
0NB50ZZ
0NB53ZZ
0NB54ZZ
0NB60ZZ
0NB63ZZ
0NB64ZZ
0NB70ZZ
0NB73ZZ
0NB74ZZ
0NC1*
0NC3*
0NC4*
0NC5*
0NC6*
0NC7*
0NH003Z
0NH004Z
0NH033Z
0NH034Z
0NH043Z
0NH044Z
0NH1*
0NH3*
0NH4*
0NH504Z
0NH534Z
0NH544Z
0NH604Z
0NH634Z
0NH644Z
0NH7*
0NN1*
0NN3*
0NN4*
0NN5*
0NN6*
0NN7*
0NQ00ZZ
0NQ03ZZ
0NQ04ZZ
0NQ10ZZ
0NQ13ZZ
0NQ14ZZ
0NQ30ZZ
0NQ33ZZ
0NQ34ZZ
0NQ40ZZ
0NQ43ZZ
0NQ44ZZ
0NQ50ZZ
0NQ53ZZ
0NQ54ZZ
0NQ60ZZ
0NQ63ZZ
0NQ64ZZ
0NQ70ZZ
0NQ73ZZ
0NQ74ZZ
0NR0*
0NR10JZ
0NR13JZ
0NR14JZ
0NR30JZ
0NR33JZ
0NR34JZ
0NR40JZ
0NR43JZ
0NR44JZ
0NR50JZ
0NR53JZ
0NR54JZ
0NR60JZ
0NR63JZ
0NR64JZ
0NR70JZ
0NR73JZ
0NR74JZ
0NS004Z
0NS005Z
0NS00ZZ
0NS034Z
0NS035Z
0NS03ZZ
0NS044Z
0NS045Z
0NS04ZZ
0NS104Z
0NS10ZZ
0NS134Z
0NS13ZZ
0NS144Z
0NS14ZZ
0NS304Z
0NS30ZZ
0NS334Z
0NS33ZZ
0NS344Z
0NS34ZZ
0NS404Z
0NS40ZZ
0NS434Z
0NS43ZZ
0NS444Z
0NS44ZZ
0NS504Z
0NS50ZZ
0NS534Z
0NS53ZZ
0NS544Z
0NS54ZZ
0NS604Z
0NS60ZZ
0NS634Z
0NS63ZZ
0NS644Z
0NS64ZZ
0NS704Z
0NS70ZZ
0NS734Z
0NS73ZZ
0NS744Z
0NS74ZZ
0NT10ZZ
0NT30ZZ
0NT40ZZ
0NT50ZZ
0NT60ZZ
0NT70ZZ
0NU00JZ
0NU03JZ
0NU04JZ
0NU10JZ
0NU13JZ
0NU14JZ
0NU30JZ
0NU33JZ
0NU34JZ
0NU40JZ
0NU43JZ
0NU44JZ
0NU50JZ
0NU53JZ
0NU54JZ
0NU60JZ
0NU63JZ
0NU64JZ
0NU70JZ
0NU73JZ
0NU74JZ
0W9100Z
0W910ZZ
0WC10ZZ
0WC13ZZ
0WC14ZZ
0WF10ZZ
0WF13ZZ
0WF14ZZ
0WJ10ZZ
XNR80D9

DRG 956

Select combinations of MDC 24 diagnoses of significant trauma listed under DRG 963
AND
Operating Room Procedures

0L8J*
0L8K*
0Q86*
0Q87*
0Q88*
0Q89*
0Q8B*
0Q8C*
0QC6*
0QC7*
0QC8*
0QC9*
0QCB*
0QCC*
0QH604Z
0QH605Z
0QH606Z
0QH60BZ
0QH60CZ
0QH60DZ
0QH634Z
0QH635Z
0QH636Z
0QH63BZ
0QH63CZ
0QH63DZ
0QH644Z
0QH645Z
0QH646Z
0QH64BZ
0QH64CZ
0QH64DZ
0QH704Z
0QH705Z
0QH706Z
0QH70BZ
0QH70CZ
0QH70DZ
0QH734Z
0QH735Z
0QH736Z
0QH73BZ
0QH73CZ
0QH73DZ
0QH744Z
0QH745Z
0QH746Z
0QH74BZ
0QH74CZ
0QH74DZ
0QH804Z
0QH805Z
0QH806Z
0QH807Z
0QH80BZ
0QH80CZ
0QH80DZ
0QH834Z
0QH835Z
0QH836Z
0QH837Z
0QH83BZ
0QH83CZ
0QH83DZ
0QH844Z
0QH845Z
0QH846Z
0QH847Z
0QH84BZ
0QH84CZ
0QH84DZ
0QH904Z
0QH905Z
0QH906Z
0QH907Z
0QH90BZ
0QH90CZ
0QH90DZ
0QH934Z
0QH935Z
0QH936Z
0QH937Z
0QH93BZ
0QH93CZ
0QH93DZ
0QH944Z
0QH945Z
0QH946Z
0QH947Z
0QH94BZ
0QH94CZ
0QH94DZ
0QHB04Z
0QHB05Z
0QHB06Z
0QHB0BZ
0QHB0CZ
0QHB0DZ
0QHB34Z
0QHB35Z
0QHB36Z
0QHB3BZ
0QHB3CZ
0QHB3DZ
0QHB44Z
0QHB45Z
0QHB46Z
0QHB4BZ
0QHB4CZ
0QHB4DZ
0QHC04Z
0QHC05Z
0QHC06Z
0QHC0BZ
0QHC0CZ
0QHC0DZ
0QHC34Z
0QHC35Z
0QHC36Z
0QHC3BZ
0QHC3CZ
0QHC3DZ
0QHC44Z
0QHC45Z
0QHC46Z
0QHC4BZ
0QHC4CZ
0QHC4DZ
0QN6*
0QN7*
0QN8*
0QN9*
0QNB*
0QNC*
0QQ60ZZ
0QQ63ZZ
0QQ64ZZ
0QQ70ZZ
0QQ73ZZ
0QQ74ZZ
0QQ80ZZ
0QQ83ZZ
0QQ84ZZ
0QQ90ZZ
0QQ93ZZ
0QQ94ZZ
0QQB0ZZ
0QQB3ZZ
0QQB4ZZ
0QQC0ZZ
0QQC3ZZ
0QQC4ZZ
0QR6*
0QR7*
0QR8*
0QR9*
0QRB*
0QRC*
0QS604Z
0QS605Z
0QS606Z
0QS60BZ
0QS60CZ
0QS60DZ
0QS60ZZ
0QS634Z
0QS635Z
0QS636Z
0QS63BZ
0QS63CZ
0QS63DZ
0QS644Z
0QS645Z
0QS646Z
0QS64BZ
0QS64CZ
0QS64DZ
0QS704Z
0QS705Z
0QS706Z
0QS70BZ
0QS70CZ
0QS70DZ
0QS70ZZ

ØQS734Z
ØQS735Z
ØQS736Z
ØQS73BZ
ØQS73CZ
ØQS73DZ
ØQS744Z
ØQS745Z
ØQS746Z
ØQS74BZ
ØQS74CZ
ØQS74DZ
ØQS8Ø4Z
ØQS8Ø5Z
ØQS8Ø6Z
ØQS8ØBZ
ØQS8ØCZ
ØQS8ØDZ
ØQS8ØZZ
ØQS834Z
ØQS835Z
ØQS836Z
ØQS83BZ
ØQS83CZ
ØQS83DZ
ØQS844Z
ØQS845Z
ØQS846Z
ØQS84BZ
ØQS84CZ
ØQS84DZ
ØQS9Ø4Z
ØQS9Ø5Z
ØQS9Ø6Z
ØQS9ØBZ
ØQS9ØCZ
ØQS9ØDZ
ØQS9ØZZ
ØQS934Z
ØQS935Z
ØQS936Z
ØQS93BZ
ØQS93CZ
ØQS93DZ
ØQS944Z
ØQS945Z
ØQS946Z
ØQS94BZ
ØQS94CZ
ØQS94DZ
ØQSBØ4Z
ØQSBØ5Z
ØQSBØ6Z
ØQSBØBZ
ØQSBØCZ
ØQSBØDZ
ØQSBØZZ
ØQSB34Z
ØQSB35Z
ØQSB36Z
ØQSB3BZ
ØQSB3CZ
ØQSB3DZ
ØQSB44Z
ØQSB45Z
ØQSB46Z
ØQSB4BZ
ØQSB4CZ
ØQSB4DZ
ØQSCØ4Z
ØQSCØ5Z
ØQSCØ6Z
ØQSCØBZ
ØQSCØCZ
ØQSCØDZ
ØQSCØZZ
ØQSC34Z
ØQSC35Z
ØQSC36Z
ØQSC3BZ
ØQSC3CZ
ØQSC3DZ
ØQSC44Z
ØQSC45Z
ØQSC46Z
ØQSC4BZ
ØQSC4CZ
ØQSC4DZ
ØQT6ØZZ
ØQT7ØZZ
ØQT8ØZZ
ØQT9ØZZ
ØQTBØZZ
ØQTCØZZ
ØQU6*
ØQU7*
ØQU8*
ØQU9*
ØQUB*
ØQUC*
ØSB9ØZZ
ØSB93ZZ
ØSB94ZZ
ØSBBØZZ
ØSBB3ZZ
ØSBB4ZZ
ØSG9*
ØSGB*
ØSH9Ø4Z
ØSH9Ø5Z
ØSH934Z
ØSH935Z
ØSH944Z
ØSH945Z
ØSHBØ4Z
ØSHBØ5Z
ØSHB34Z
ØSHB35Z
ØSHB44Z
ØSHB45Z
ØSN9ØZZ
ØSN93ZZ
ØSN94ZZ
ØSNBØZZ
ØSNB3ZZ
ØSNB4ZZ
ØSP9Ø9Z
ØSP9ØJZ
ØSP93JZ
ØSP94JZ
ØSPAØJZ
ØSPA3JZ
ØSPA4JZ
ØSPBØ9Z
ØSPBØJZ
ØSPB3JZ
ØSPB4JZ
ØSPEØJZ
ØSPE3JZ
ØSPE4JZ
ØSPRØJZ
ØSPR3JZ
ØSPR4JZ
ØSPSØJZ
ØSPS3JZ
ØSPS4JZ
ØSQ9ØZZ
ØSQ93ZZ
ØSQ94ZZ
ØSQBØZZ
ØSQB3ZZ
ØSQB4ZZ
ØSR9Ø19
ØSR9Ø1A
ØSR9Ø1Z
ØSR9Ø29
ØSR9Ø2A
ØSR9Ø2Z
ØSR9Ø39
ØSR9Ø3A
ØSR9Ø3Z
ØSR9Ø49
ØSR9Ø4A
ØSR9Ø4Z
ØSR9Ø69
ØSR9Ø6A
ØSR9Ø6Z
ØSR9Ø7Z
ØSR9ØEZ
ØSR9ØJ9
ØSR9ØJA
ØSR9ØJZ
ØSR9ØKZ
ØSRA*
ØSRBØ19
ØSRBØ1A
ØSRBØ1Z
ØSRBØ29
ØSRBØ2A
ØSRBØ2Z
ØSRBØ39
ØSRBØ3A
ØSRBØ3Z
ØSRBØ49
ØSRBØ4A
ØSRBØ4Z
ØSRBØ69
ØSRBØ6A
ØSRBØ6Z
ØSRBØ7Z
ØSRBØEZ
ØSRBØJ9
ØSRBØJA
ØSRBØJZ
ØSRBØKZ
ØSRE*
ØSRR*
ØSRS*
ØSS9Ø4Z
ØSS9Ø5Z
ØSS9ØZZ
ØSSBØ4Z
ØSSBØ5Z
ØSSBØZZ
ØST9ØZZ
ØSTBØZZ
ØSU9ØBZ
ØSUAØBZ
ØSUBØBZ
ØSUEØBZ
ØSURØBZ
ØSUSØBZ
ØSW9ØJZ
ØSW93JZ
ØSW94JZ
ØSWAØJZ
ØSWA3JZ
ØSWA4JZ
ØSWBØJZ
ØSWB3JZ
ØSWB4JZ
ØSWEØJZ
ØSWE3JZ
ØSWE4JZ
ØSWRØJZ
ØSWR3JZ
ØSWR4JZ
ØSWSØJZ
ØSWS3JZ
ØSWS4JZ
ØXMØØZZ
ØXM1ØZZ
ØXM2ØZZ
ØXM3ØZZ
ØXM4ØZZ
ØXM5ØZZ
ØXM6ØZZ
ØXM7ØZZ
ØXM8ØZZ
ØXM9ØZZ
ØXMBØZZ
ØXMCØZZ
ØXMDØZZ
ØXMFØZZ
ØXMGØZZ
ØXMHØZZ
ØXMJØZZ
ØXMKØZZ
ØYM7ØZZ
ØYM8ØZZ
ØYMCØZZ
ØYMDØZZ
ØYMFØZZ
ØYMGØZZ
ØYMHØZZ
ØYMJØZZ
ØYMKØZZ
ØYMLØZZ
ØYMMØZZ
ØYMNØZZ

DRG 957

Select combinations of MDC 24 diagnoses of significant trauma listed under DRG 963
AND
Operating Room Procedures

16Ø7Ø
16Ø71
16Ø72
16Ø73
16Ø74
16Ø75
16Ø76
16Ø77
16Ø78
ØØ16ØJØ
ØØ16ØJ1
ØØ16ØJ2
ØØ16ØJ3
ØØ16ØJ4
ØØ16ØJ5
ØØ16ØJ6
ØØ16ØJ7
ØØ16ØJ8
ØØ16ØKØ
ØØ16ØK1
ØØ16ØK2
ØØ16ØK3
ØØ16ØK4
ØØ16ØK5
ØØ16ØK6
ØØ16ØK7
ØØ16ØK8
1637Ø
16371
16372
16373
16374
16375
16376
16377
16378
ØØ163JØ
ØØ163J1
ØØ163J2
ØØ163J3
ØØ163J4
ØØ163J5
ØØ163J6
ØØ163J7
ØØ163J8
ØØ163KØ
ØØ163K1
ØØ163K2
ØØ163K3
ØØ163K4
ØØ163K5
ØØ163K6
ØØ163K7
ØØ163K8
1647Ø
16471
16472
16473
16474
16475
16476
16477
16478
ØØ164JØ
ØØ164J1
ØØ164J2
ØØ164J3
ØØ164J4
ØØ164J5
ØØ164J6
ØØ164J7
ØØ164J8
ØØ164KØ
ØØ164K1
ØØ164K2
ØØ164K3
ØØ164K4
ØØ164K5
ØØ164K6
ØØ164K7
ØØ164K8
ØØ8FØZZ
ØØ8F3ZZ
ØØ8F4ZZ
ØØ8GØZZ
ØØ8G3ZZ
ØØ8G4ZZ
ØØ8HØZZ
ØØ8H3ZZ
ØØ8H4ZZ
ØØ8JØZZ
ØØ8J3ZZ
ØØ8J4ZZ
ØØ8KØZZ
ØØ8K3ZZ
ØØ8K4ZZ
ØØ8LØZZ
ØØ8L3ZZ
ØØ8L4ZZ
ØØ8MØZZ
ØØ8M3ZZ
ØØ8M4ZZ
ØØ8NØZZ
ØØ8N3ZZ
ØØ8N4ZZ
ØØ8RØZZ
ØØ8R3ZZ
ØØ8R4ZZ
ØØ8SØZZ
ØØ8S3ZZ
ØØ8S4ZZ
ØØ8WØZZ
ØØ8W3ZZ
ØØ8W4ZZ
ØØ8XØZZ
ØØ8X3ZZ
ØØ8X4ZZ
ØØ8YØZZ
ØØ8Y3ZZ
ØØ8Y4ZZ
ØØ9FØZX
ØØ9GØZX
ØØ9HØZX
ØØ9JØZX
ØØ9KØZX
ØØ9LØZX
ØØ9MØZX
ØØ9NØZX
ØØ9PØZX
ØØ9QØZX
ØØ9RØZX
ØØ9SØZX
ØØ9TØØZ
ØØ9TØZZ
ØØ9T4ØZ
ØØ9T4ZZ
ØØ9UØØZ
ØØ9UØZZ
ØØ9WØØZ
ØØ9WØZZ
ØØ9W4ØZ
ØØ9W4ZZ
ØØ9XØØZ
ØØ9XØZZ
ØØ9X4ØZ
ØØ9X4ZZ
ØØ9YØØZ
ØØ9YØZZ
ØØ9Y4ØZ
ØØ9Y4ZZ
ØØBFØZX
ØØBGØZX
ØØBHØZX
ØØBJØZX
ØØBKØZX
ØØBKØZZ
ØØBK3ZZ
ØØBK4ZZ
ØØBLØZX
ØØBMØZX
ØØBNØZX
ØØBPØZX
ØØBQØZX
ØØBRØZX
ØØBSØZX
ØØC3ØZZ
ØØC33ZZ
ØØC34ZZ
ØØCTØZZ
ØØCT3ZZ
ØØCT4ZZ
ØØCUØZZ
ØØCU3ZZ
ØØCU4ZZ
ØØCWØZZ
ØØCW3ZZ
ØØCW4ZZ
ØØCXØZZ
ØØCX3ZZ
ØØCX4ZZ
ØØCYØZZ
ØØCY3ZZ
ØØCY4ZZ
ØØDTØZZ
ØØDT3ZZ
ØØDT4ZZ
ØØFUØZZ
ØØFU3ZZ
ØØFU4ZZ
ØØFUXZZ
ØØHØØMZ
ØØHØ3MZ
ØØHØ4MZ
ØØH6ØMZ
ØØH63MZ
ØØH64MZ
ØØHEØMZ
ØØHE3MZ
ØØHE4MZ
ØØHUØ1Z
ØØHUØ2Z
ØØHUØMZ
ØØHUØYZ
ØØHU31Z
ØØHU3MZ
ØØHU41Z
ØØHU42Z
ØØHU4MZ
ØØHVØ1Z
ØØHVØ2Z
ØØHVØMZ
ØØHVØYZ
ØØHV31Z
ØØHV3MZ
ØØHV3YZ
ØØHV41Z
ØØHV42Z
ØØHV4MZ
ØØHV4YZ
ØØJØ4ZZ
ØØJUØZZ
ØØJVØZZ
ØØKØØZZ
ØØKØ3ZZ
ØØKØ4ZZ
ØØK7ØZZ
ØØK73ZZ
ØØK74ZZ
ØØK8ØZZ
ØØK83ZZ
ØØK84ZZ
ØØK9ØZZ
ØØK93ZZ
ØØK94ZZ
ØØKAØZZ
ØØKA3ZZ
ØØKA4ZZ
ØØKBØZZ
ØØKB3ZZ
ØØKB4ZZ
ØØKCØZZ
ØØKC3ZZ
ØØKC4ZZ
ØØKDØZZ
ØØKD3ZZ
ØØKD4ZZ
ØØNØØZZ
ØØNØ3ZZ
ØØNØ4ZZ
ØØN1ØZZ
ØØN13ZZ
ØØN14ZZ
ØØN2ØZZ
ØØN23ZZ
ØØN24ZZ
ØØN7ØZZ
ØØN73ZZ
ØØN74ZZ
ØØNFØZZ
ØØNF3ZZ
ØØNF4ZZ
ØØNGØZZ
ØØNG3ZZ
ØØNG4ZZ
ØØNHØZZ
ØØNH3ZZ
ØØNH4ZZ
ØØNJØZZ
ØØNJ3ZZ
ØØNJ4ZZ
ØØNLØZZ
ØØNL3ZZ
ØØNL4ZZ
ØØNMØZZ
ØØNM3ZZ
ØØNM4ZZ
ØØNNØZZ
ØØNN3ZZ
ØØNN4ZZ
ØØNPØZZ
ØØNP3ZZ
ØØNP4ZZ
ØØNQØZZ
ØØNQ3ZZ
ØØNQ4ZZ
ØØNRØZZ
ØØNR3ZZ
ØØNR4ZZ
ØØNSØZZ
ØØNS3ZZ
ØØNS4ZZ
ØØNTØZZ
ØØNT3ZZ
ØØNT4ZZ
ØØNWØZZ
ØØNW3ZZ
ØØNW4ZZ
ØØNXØZZ
ØØNX3ZZ
ØØNX4ZZ
ØØNYØZZ
ØØNY3ZZ
ØØNY4ZZ
ØØP6ØJZ
ØØP63JZ
ØØP64JZ
ØØPEØMZ
ØØPE3MZ
ØØPE4MZ
ØØPUØØZ
ØØPUØ2Z
ØØPUØ3Z
ØØPUØJZ
ØØPUØMZ
ØØPUØYZ
ØØPU3JZ
ØØPU3MZ
ØØPU4ØZ
ØØPU42Z
ØØPU43Z
ØØPU4JZ
ØØPU4MZ
ØØPVØØZ
ØØPVØ2Z
ØØPVØ3Z
ØØPVØ7Z
ØØPVØJZ
ØØPVØKZ
ØØPVØMZ
ØØPVØYZ
ØØPV37Z
ØØPV3JZ
ØØPV3KZ
ØØPV3MZ
ØØPV4ØZ
ØØPV42Z
ØØPV43Z
ØØPV47Z
ØØPV4JZ
ØØPV4KZ
ØØPV4MZ
ØØQFØZZ
ØØQF3ZZ
ØØQF4ZZ
ØØQGØZZ
ØØQG3ZZ
ØØQG4ZZ
ØØQHØZZ
ØØQH3ZZ
ØØQH4ZZ
ØØQJØZZ
ØØQJ3ZZ
ØØQJ4ZZ
ØØQKØZZ
ØØQK3ZZ
ØØQK4ZZ
ØØQLØZZ
ØØQL3ZZ
ØØQL4ZZ
ØØQMØZZ
ØØQM3ZZ
ØØQM4ZZ
ØØQNØZZ
ØØQN3ZZ
ØØQN4ZZ
ØØQPØZZ
ØØQP3ZZ
ØØQP4ZZ
ØØQQØZZ
ØØQQ3ZZ
ØØQQ4ZZ
ØØQRØZZ
ØØQR3ZZ
ØØQR4ZZ
ØØQSØZZ
ØØQS3ZZ
ØØQS4ZZ
ØØQTØZZ
ØØQT3ZZ
ØØQT4ZZ
ØØQWØZZ
ØØQW3ZZ
ØØQW4ZZ
ØØQXØZZ
ØØQX3ZZ
ØØQX4ZZ
ØØQYØZZ
ØØQY3ZZ
ØØQY4ZZ
ØØRFØ7Z
ØØRFØJZ
ØØRFØKZ
ØØRF47Z
ØØRF4JZ
ØØRF4KZ
ØØRGØ7Z
ØØRGØJZ
ØØRGØKZ
ØØRG47Z
ØØRG4JZ
ØØRG4KZ
ØØRHØ7Z
ØØRHØJZ
ØØRHØKZ
ØØRH47Z
ØØRH4JZ
ØØRH4KZ
ØØRJØ7Z
ØØRJØJZ
ØØRJØKZ
ØØRJ47Z
ØØRJ4JZ
ØØRJ4KZ
ØØRKØ7Z
ØØRKØJZ
ØØRKØKZ
ØØRK47Z
ØØRK4JZ
ØØRK4KZ
ØØRLØ7Z
ØØRLØJZ
ØØRLØKZ
ØØRL47Z
ØØRL4JZ
ØØRL4KZ
ØØRMØ7Z
ØØRMØJZ
ØØRMØKZ
ØØRM47Z
ØØRM4JZ
ØØRM4KZ
ØØRNØ7Z
ØØRNØJZ
ØØRNØKZ
ØØRN47Z
ØØRN4JZ
ØØRN4KZ
ØØRPØ7Z
ØØRPØJZ
ØØRPØKZ
ØØRP47Z
ØØRP4JZ
ØØRP4KZ
ØØRQØ7Z
ØØRQØJZ
ØØRQØKZ
ØØRQ47Z
ØØRQ4JZ
ØØRQ4KZ
ØØRRØ7Z
ØØRRØJZ
ØØRRØKZ
ØØRR47Z
ØØRR4JZ
ØØRR4KZ
ØØRSØ7Z
ØØRSØJZ
ØØRSØKZ
ØØRS47Z
ØØRS4JZ
ØØRS4KZ
ØØRTØ7Z
ØØRTØJZ
ØØRTØKZ
ØØRT47Z
ØØRT4JZ
ØØRT4KZ
ØØSFØZZ
ØØSF3ZZ
ØØSF4ZZ
ØØSGØZZ
ØØSG3ZZ
ØØSG4ZZ
ØØSHØZZ
ØØSH3ZZ
ØØSH4ZZ
ØØSJØZZ
ØØSJ3ZZ
ØØSJ4ZZ
ØØSKØZZ
ØØSK3ZZ
ØØSK4ZZ
ØØSLØZZ
ØØSL3ZZ
ØØSL4ZZ
ØØSMØZZ
ØØSM3ZZ
ØØSM4ZZ
ØØSNØZZ
ØØSN3ZZ
ØØSN4ZZ
ØØSPØZZ
ØØSP3ZZ
ØØSP4ZZ
ØØSQØZZ
ØØSQ3ZZ
ØØSQ4ZZ
ØØSRØZZ
ØØSR3ZZ
ØØSR4ZZ
ØØSSØZZ
ØØSS3ZZ
ØØSS4ZZ
ØØSWØZZ
ØØSW3ZZ
ØØSW4ZZ
ØØSXØZZ
ØØSX3ZZ
ØØSX4ZZ
ØØSYØZZ
ØØSY3ZZ
ØØSY4ZZ
ØØUFØ7Z
ØØUFØJZ
ØØUFØKZ
ØØUF37Z
ØØUF3JZ
ØØUF3KZ
ØØUF47Z
ØØUF4JZ
ØØUF4KZ
ØØUGØ7Z
ØØUGØJZ
ØØUGØKZ
ØØUG37Z
ØØUG3JZ
ØØUG3KZ
ØØUG47Z
ØØUG4JZ
ØØUG4KZ
ØØUHØ7Z
ØØUHØJZ
ØØUHØKZ
ØØUH37Z
ØØUH3JZ
ØØUH3KZ
ØØUH47Z
ØØUH4JZ
ØØUH4KZ
ØØUJØ7Z
ØØUJØJZ
ØØUJØKZ
ØØUJ37Z
ØØUJ3JZ
ØØUJ3KZ
ØØUJ47Z
ØØUJ4JZ
ØØUJ4KZ
ØØUKØ7Z
ØØUKØJZ
ØØUKØKZ
ØØUK37Z
ØØUK3JZ
ØØUK3KZ
ØØUK47Z
ØØUK4JZ
ØØUK4KZ
ØØULØ7Z
ØØULØJZ
ØØULØKZ
ØØUL37Z
ØØUL3JZ
ØØUL3KZ
ØØUL47Z
ØØUL4JZ
ØØUL4KZ
ØØUMØ7Z
ØØUMØJZ
ØØUMØKZ
ØØUM37Z
ØØUM3JZ
ØØUM3KZ
ØØUM47Z
ØØUM4JZ
ØØUM4KZ
ØØUNØ7Z
ØØUNØJZ
ØØUNØKZ
ØØUN37Z
ØØUN3JZ
ØØUN3KZ
ØØUN47Z
ØØUN4JZ
ØØUN4KZ
ØØUPØ7Z

ØØUPØJZ
ØØUPØKZ
ØØUP37Z
ØØUP3JZ
ØØUP3KZ
ØØUP47Z
ØØUP4JZ
ØØUP4KZ
ØØUQØ7Z
ØØUQØJZ
ØØUQØKZ
ØØUQ37Z
ØØUQ3JZ
ØØUQ3KZ
ØØUQ47Z
ØØUQ4JZ
ØØUQ4KZ
ØØURØ7Z
ØØURØJZ
ØØURØKZ
ØØUR37Z
ØØUR3JZ
ØØUR3KZ
ØØUR47Z
ØØUR4JZ
ØØUR4KZ
ØØUSØ7Z
ØØUSØJZ
ØØUSØKZ
ØØUS37Z
ØØUS3JZ
ØØUS3KZ
ØØUS47Z
ØØUS4JZ
ØØUS4KZ
ØØUTØ7Z
ØØUTØJZ
ØØUTØKZ
ØØUT37Z
ØØUT3JZ
ØØUT3KZ
ØØUT47Z
ØØUT4JZ
ØØUT4KZ
ØØW6ØJZ
ØØW63JZ
ØØW64JZ
ØØWUØØZ
ØØWUØ2Z
ØØWUØ3Z
ØØWUØJZ
ØØWUØMZ
ØØWUØYZ
ØØWU3ØZ
ØØWU32Z
ØØWU33Z
ØØWU3JZ
ØØWU3MZ
ØØWU4ØZ
ØØWU42Z
ØØWU43Z
ØØWU4JZ
ØØWU4MZ
ØØWVØØZ
ØØWVØ2Z
ØØWVØ3Z
ØØWVØ7Z
ØØWVØJZ
ØØWVØKZ
ØØWVØMZ
ØØWVØYZ
ØØWV3ØZ
ØØWV32Z
ØØWV33Z
ØØWV37Z
ØØWV3JZ
ØØWV3KZ
ØØWV3MZ
ØØWV4ØZ
ØØWV42Z
ØØWV43Z
ØØWV47Z
ØØWV4JZ
ØØWV4KZ
ØØWV4MZ
ØØXFØZF
ØØXFØZG
ØØXFØZH
ØØXFØZJ
ØØXFØZK
ØØXFØZL
ØØXFØZM
ØØXFØZN
ØØXFØZP
ØØXFØZQ
ØØXFØZR
ØØXFØZS
ØØXF4ZF
ØØXF4ZG
ØØXF4ZH
ØØXF4ZJ
ØØXF4ZK
ØØXF4ZL
ØØXF4ZM
ØØXF4ZN
ØØXF4ZP
ØØXF4ZQ
ØØXF4ZR
ØØXF4ZS
ØØXGØZF
ØØXGØZG
ØØXGØZH
ØØXGØZJ
ØØXGØZK
ØØXGØZL
ØØXGØZM
ØØXGØZN
ØØXGØZP
ØØXGØZQ
ØØXGØZR
ØØXGØZS
ØØXG4ZF
ØØXG4ZG
ØØXG4ZH
ØØXG4ZJ
ØØXG4ZK
ØØXG4ZL
ØØXG4ZM
ØØXG4ZN
ØØXG4ZP
ØØXG4ZQ
ØØXG4ZR
ØØXG4ZS
ØØXHØZF
ØØXHØZG
ØØXHØZH
ØØXHØZJ
ØØXHØZK
ØØXHØZL
ØØXHØZM
ØØXHØZN
ØØXHØZP
ØØXHØZQ
ØØXHØZR
ØØXHØZS
ØØXH4ZF
ØØXH4ZG
ØØXH4ZH
ØØXH4ZJ
ØØXH4ZK
ØØXH4ZL
ØØXH4ZM
ØØXH4ZN
ØØXH4ZP
ØØXH4ZQ
ØØXH4ZR
ØØXH4ZS
ØØXJØZF
ØØXJØZG
ØØXJØZH
ØØXJØZJ
ØØXJØZK
ØØXJØZL
ØØXJØZM
ØØXJØZN
ØØXJØZP
ØØXJØZQ
ØØXJØZR
ØØXJØZS
ØØXJ4ZF
ØØXJ4ZG
ØØXJ4ZH
ØØXJ4ZJ
ØØXJ4ZK
ØØXJ4ZL
ØØXJ4ZM
ØØXJ4ZN
ØØXJ4ZP
ØØXJ4ZQ
ØØXJ4ZR
ØØXJ4ZS
ØØXKØZF
ØØXKØZG
ØØXKØZH
ØØXKØZJ
ØØXKØZK
ØØXKØZL
ØØXKØZM
ØØXKØZN
ØØXKØZP
ØØXKØZQ
ØØXKØZR
ØØXKØZS
ØØXK4ZF
ØØXK4ZG
ØØXK4ZH
ØØXK4ZJ
ØØXK4ZK
ØØXK4ZL
ØØXK4ZM
ØØXK4ZN
ØØXK4ZP
ØØXK4ZQ
ØØXK4ZR
ØØXK4ZS
ØØXLØZF
ØØXLØZG
ØØXLØZH
ØØXLØZJ
ØØXLØZK
ØØXLØZL
ØØXLØZM
ØØXLØZN
ØØXLØZP
ØØXLØZQ
ØØXLØZR
ØØXLØZS
ØØXL4ZF
ØØXL4ZG
ØØXL4ZH
ØØXL4ZJ
ØØXL4ZK
ØØXL4ZL
ØØXL4ZM
ØØXL4ZN
ØØXL4ZP
ØØXL4ZQ
ØØXL4ZR
ØØXL4ZS
ØØXMØZF
ØØXMØZG
ØØXMØZH
ØØXMØZJ
ØØXMØZK
ØØXMØZL
ØØXMØZM
ØØXMØZN
ØØXMØZP
ØØXMØZQ
ØØXMØZR
ØØXMØZS
ØØXM4ZF
ØØXM4ZG
ØØXM4ZH
ØØXM4ZJ
ØØXM4ZK
ØØXM4ZL
ØØXM4ZM
ØØXM4ZN
ØØXM4ZP
ØØXM4ZQ
ØØXM4ZR
ØØXM4ZS
ØØXNØZF
ØØXNØZG
ØØXNØZH
ØØXNØZJ
ØØXNØZK
ØØXNØZL
ØØXNØZM
ØØXNØZN
ØØXNØZP
ØØXNØZQ
ØØXNØZR
ØØXNØZS
ØØXN4ZF
ØØXN4ZG
ØØXN4ZH
ØØXN4ZJ
ØØXN4ZK
ØØXN4ZL
ØØXN4ZM
ØØXN4ZN
ØØXN4ZP
ØØXN4ZQ
ØØXN4ZR
ØØXN4ZS
ØØXPØZF
ØØXPØZG
ØØXPØZH
ØØXPØZJ
ØØXPØZK
ØØXPØZL
ØØXPØZM
ØØXPØZN
ØØXPØZP
ØØXPØZQ
ØØXPØZR
ØØXPØZS
ØØXP4ZF
ØØXP4ZG
ØØXP4ZH
ØØXP4ZJ
ØØXP4ZK
ØØXP4ZL
ØØXP4ZM
ØØXP4ZN
ØØXP4ZP
ØØXP4ZQ
ØØXP4ZR
ØØXP4ZS
ØØXQØZF
ØØXQØZG
ØØXQØZH
ØØXQØZJ
ØØXQØZK
ØØXQØZL
ØØXQØZM
ØØXQØZN
ØØXQØZP
ØØXQØZQ
ØØXQØZR
ØØXQØZS
ØØXQ4ZF
ØØXQ4ZG
ØØXQ4ZH
ØØXQ4ZJ
ØØXQ4ZK
ØØXQ4ZL
ØØXQ4ZM
ØØXQ4ZN
ØØXQ4ZP
ØØXQ4ZQ
ØØXQ4ZR
ØØXQ4ZS
ØØXRØZF
ØØXRØZG
ØØXRØZH
ØØXRØZJ
ØØXRØZK
ØØXRØZL
ØØXRØZM
ØØXRØZN
ØØXRØZP
ØØXRØZQ
ØØXRØZR
ØØXRØZS
ØØXR4ZF
ØØXR4ZG
ØØXR4ZH
ØØXR4ZJ
ØØXR4ZK
ØØXR4ZL
ØØXR4ZM
ØØXR4ZN
ØØXR4ZP
ØØXR4ZQ
ØØXR4ZR
ØØXR4ZS
ØØXSØZF
ØØXSØZG
ØØXSØZH
ØØXSØZJ
ØØXSØZK
ØØXSØZL
ØØXSØZM
ØØXSØZN
ØØXSØZP
ØØXSØZQ
ØØXSØZR
ØØXSØZS
ØØXS4ZF
ØØXS4ZG
ØØXS4ZH
ØØXS4ZJ
ØØXS4ZK
ØØXS4ZL
ØØXS4ZM
ØØXS4ZN
ØØXS4ZP
ØØXS4ZQ
ØØXS4ZR
ØØXS4ZS
Ø151ØZZ
Ø1514ZZ
Ø158ØZZ
Ø1584ZZ
Ø15BØZZ
Ø15B4ZZ
Ø15RØZZ
Ø15R4ZZ
Ø18ØØZZ
Ø18Ø3ZZ
Ø18Ø4ZZ
Ø181ØZZ
Ø1813ZZ
Ø1814ZZ
Ø182ØZZ
Ø1823ZZ
Ø1824ZZ
Ø183ØZZ
Ø1833ZZ
Ø1834ZZ
Ø184ØZZ
Ø1843ZZ
Ø1844ZZ
Ø185ØZZ
Ø1853ZZ
Ø1854ZZ
Ø186ØZZ
Ø1863ZZ
Ø1864ZZ
Ø188ØZZ
Ø1883ZZ
Ø1884ZZ
Ø189ØZZ
Ø1893ZZ
Ø1894ZZ
Ø18AØZZ
Ø18A3ZZ
Ø18A4ZZ
Ø18BØZZ
Ø18B3ZZ
Ø18B4ZZ
Ø18CØZZ
Ø18C3ZZ
Ø18C4ZZ
Ø18DØZZ
Ø18D3ZZ
Ø18D4ZZ
Ø18FØZZ
Ø18F3ZZ
Ø18F4ZZ
Ø18GØZZ
Ø18G3ZZ
Ø18G4ZZ
Ø18HØZZ
Ø18H3ZZ
Ø18H4ZZ
Ø18QØZZ
Ø18Q3ZZ
Ø18Q4ZZ
Ø18RØZZ
Ø18R3ZZ
Ø18R4ZZ
Ø19ØØZX
Ø191ØZX
Ø192ØZX
Ø193ØZX
Ø194ØZX
Ø195ØZX
Ø196ØZX
Ø198ØZX
Ø199ØZX
Ø19AØZX
Ø19BØZX
Ø19CØZX
Ø19DØZX
Ø19FØZX
Ø19GØZX
Ø19HØZX
Ø19QØZX
Ø19RØZX
Ø1BØØZX
Ø1B1ØZX
Ø1B2ØZX
Ø1B3ØZX
Ø1B4ØZX
Ø1B5ØZX
Ø1B6ØZX
Ø1B8ØZX
Ø1B9ØZX
Ø1BAØZX
Ø1BBØZX
Ø1BCØZX
Ø1BDØZX
Ø1BFØZX
Ø1BGØZX
Ø1BHØZX
Ø1BQØZX
Ø1BRØZX
Ø1HYØMZ
Ø1HY3MZ
Ø1HY4MZ
Ø1NØØZZ
Ø1NØ3ZZ
Ø1NØ4ZZ
Ø1N1ØZZ
Ø1N13ZZ
Ø1N14ZZ
Ø1N2ØZZ
Ø1N23ZZ
Ø1N24ZZ
Ø1N3ØZZ
Ø1N33ZZ
Ø1N34ZZ
Ø1N4ØZZ
Ø1N43ZZ
Ø1N44ZZ
Ø1N5ØZZ
Ø1N53ZZ
Ø1N54ZZ
Ø1N6ØZZ
Ø1N63ZZ
Ø1N64ZZ
Ø1N8ØZZ
Ø1N83ZZ
Ø1N84ZZ
Ø1N9ØZZ
Ø1N93ZZ
Ø1N94ZZ
Ø1NAØZZ
Ø1NA3ZZ
Ø1NA4ZZ
Ø1NBØZZ
Ø1NB3ZZ
Ø1NB4ZZ
Ø1NCØZZ
Ø1NC3ZZ
Ø1NC4ZZ
Ø1NDØZZ
Ø1ND3ZZ
Ø1ND4ZZ
Ø1NFØZZ
Ø1NF3ZZ
Ø1NF4ZZ
Ø1NGØZZ
Ø1NG3ZZ
Ø1NG4ZZ
Ø1NHØZZ
Ø1NH3ZZ
Ø1NH4ZZ
Ø1NQØZZ
Ø1NQ3ZZ
Ø1NQ4ZZ
Ø1NRØZZ
Ø1NR3ZZ
Ø1NR4ZZ
Ø1PYØMZ
Ø1PY3MZ
Ø1PY4MZ
Ø1QØØZZ
Ø1QØ3ZZ
Ø1QØ4ZZ
Ø1Q1ØZZ
Ø1Q13ZZ
Ø1Q14ZZ
Ø1Q2ØZZ
Ø1Q23ZZ
Ø1Q24ZZ
Ø1Q3ØZZ
Ø1Q33ZZ
Ø1Q34ZZ
Ø1Q4ØZZ
Ø1Q43ZZ
Ø1Q44ZZ
Ø1Q5ØZZ
Ø1Q53ZZ
Ø1Q54ZZ
Ø1Q6ØZZ
Ø1Q63ZZ
Ø1Q64ZZ
Ø1Q8ØZZ
Ø1Q83ZZ
Ø1Q84ZZ
Ø1Q9ØZZ
Ø1Q93ZZ
Ø1Q94ZZ
Ø1QAØZZ
Ø1QA3ZZ
Ø1QA4ZZ
Ø1QBØZZ
Ø1QB3ZZ
Ø1QB4ZZ
Ø1QCØZZ
Ø1QC3ZZ
Ø1QC4ZZ
Ø1QDØZZ
Ø1QD3ZZ
Ø1QD4ZZ
Ø1QFØZZ
Ø1QF3ZZ
Ø1QF4ZZ
Ø1QGØZZ
Ø1QG3ZZ
Ø1QG4ZZ
Ø1QHØZZ
Ø1QH3ZZ
Ø1QH4ZZ
Ø1QQØZZ
Ø1QQ3ZZ
Ø1QQ4ZZ
Ø1QRØZZ
Ø1QR3ZZ
Ø1QR4ZZ
Ø1R1Ø7Z
Ø1R1ØJZ
Ø1R1ØKZ
Ø1R147Z
Ø1R14JZ
Ø1R14KZ
Ø1R2Ø7Z
Ø1R2ØJZ
Ø1R2ØKZ
Ø1R247Z
Ø1R24JZ
Ø1R24KZ
Ø1R4Ø7Z
Ø1R4ØJZ
Ø1R4ØKZ
Ø1R447Z
Ø1R44JZ
Ø1R44KZ
Ø1R5Ø7Z
Ø1R5ØJZ
Ø1R5ØKZ
Ø1R547Z
Ø1R54JZ
Ø1R54KZ
Ø1R6Ø7Z
Ø1R6ØJZ
Ø1R6ØKZ
Ø1R647Z
Ø1R64JZ
Ø1R64KZ
Ø1R8Ø7Z
Ø1R8ØJZ
Ø1R8ØKZ
Ø1R847Z
Ø1R84JZ
Ø1R84KZ
Ø1RBØ7Z
Ø1RBØJZ
Ø1RBØKZ
Ø1RB47Z
Ø1RB4JZ
Ø1RB4KZ
Ø1RCØ7Z
Ø1RCØJZ
Ø1RCØKZ
Ø1RC47Z
Ø1RC4JZ
Ø1RC4KZ
Ø1RDØ7Z
Ø1RDØJZ
Ø1RDØKZ
Ø1RD47Z
Ø1RD4JZ
Ø1RD4KZ
Ø1RFØ7Z
Ø1RFØJZ
Ø1RFØKZ
Ø1RF47Z
Ø1RF4JZ
Ø1RF4KZ
Ø1RGØ7Z
Ø1RGØJZ
Ø1RGØKZ
Ø1RG47Z
Ø1RG4JZ
Ø1RG4KZ
Ø1RHØ7Z
Ø1RHØJZ
Ø1RHØKZ
Ø1RH47Z
Ø1RH4JZ
Ø1RH4KZ
Ø1RRØ7Z
Ø1RRØJZ
Ø1RRØKZ
Ø1RR47Z
Ø1RR4JZ
Ø1RR4KZ
Ø1SØØZZ
Ø1SØ3ZZ
Ø1SØ4ZZ
Ø1S1ØZZ
Ø1S13ZZ
Ø1S14ZZ
Ø1S2ØZZ
Ø1S23ZZ
Ø1S24ZZ
Ø1S3ØZZ
Ø1S33ZZ
Ø1S34ZZ
Ø1S4ØZZ
Ø1S43ZZ
Ø1S44ZZ
Ø1S5ØZZ
Ø1S53ZZ
Ø1S54ZZ
Ø1S6ØZZ
Ø1S63ZZ
Ø1S64ZZ
Ø1S8ØZZ
Ø1S83ZZ
Ø1S84ZZ
Ø1S9ØZZ
Ø1S93ZZ
Ø1S94ZZ
Ø1SAØZZ
Ø1SA3ZZ
Ø1SA4ZZ
Ø1SBØZZ
Ø1SB3ZZ
Ø1SB4ZZ
Ø1SCØZZ
Ø1SC3ZZ
Ø1SC4ZZ
Ø1SDØZZ
Ø1SD3ZZ
Ø1SD4ZZ
Ø1SFØZZ
Ø1SF3ZZ
Ø1SF4ZZ
Ø1SGØZZ
Ø1SG3ZZ
Ø1SG4ZZ
Ø1SHØZZ
Ø1SH3ZZ
Ø1SH4ZZ
Ø1SQØZZ
Ø1SQ3ZZ
Ø1SQ4ZZ
Ø1SRØZZ
Ø1SR3ZZ
Ø1SR4ZZ
Ø1U1Ø7Z
Ø1U1ØJZ
Ø1U1ØKZ
Ø1U137Z
Ø1U13JZ
Ø1U13KZ
Ø1U147Z
Ø1U14JZ
Ø1U14KZ
Ø1U2Ø7Z
Ø1U2ØJZ
Ø1U2ØKZ
Ø1U237Z
Ø1U23JZ
Ø1U23KZ
Ø1U247Z
Ø1U24JZ
Ø1U24KZ
Ø1U4Ø7Z
Ø1U4ØJZ
Ø1U4ØKZ
Ø1U437Z
Ø1U43JZ
Ø1U43KZ
Ø1U447Z
Ø1U44JZ
Ø1U44KZ
Ø1U5Ø7Z
Ø1U5ØJZ
Ø1U5ØKZ
Ø1U537Z
Ø1U53JZ
Ø1U53KZ
Ø1U547Z
Ø1U54JZ
Ø1U54KZ
Ø1U6Ø7Z
Ø1U6ØJZ
Ø1U6ØKZ
Ø1U637Z
Ø1U63JZ
Ø1U63KZ
Ø1U647Z
Ø1U64JZ
Ø1U64KZ
Ø1U8Ø7Z
Ø1U8ØJZ
Ø1U8ØKZ
Ø1U837Z
Ø1U83JZ
Ø1U83KZ
Ø1U847Z
Ø1U84JZ
Ø1U84KZ
Ø1UBØ7Z
Ø1UBØJZ
Ø1UBØKZ
Ø1UB37Z
Ø1UB3JZ
Ø1UB3KZ
Ø1UB47Z
Ø1UB4JZ
Ø1UB4KZ
Ø1UCØ7Z
Ø1UCØJZ
Ø1UCØKZ
Ø1UC37Z
Ø1UC3JZ
Ø1UC3KZ
Ø1UC47Z
Ø1UC4JZ
Ø1UC4KZ
Ø1UDØ7Z
Ø1UDØJZ
Ø1UDØKZ
Ø1UD37Z
Ø1UD3JZ
Ø1UD3KZ
Ø1UD47Z
Ø1UD4JZ
Ø1UD4KZ
Ø1UFØ7Z
Ø1UFØJZ
Ø1UFØKZ
Ø1UF37Z
Ø1UF3JZ
Ø1UF3KZ
Ø1UF47Z
Ø1UF4JZ
Ø1UF4KZ
Ø1UGØ7Z
Ø1UGØJZ
Ø1UGØKZ
Ø1UG37Z
Ø1UG3JZ
Ø1UG3KZ
Ø1UG47Z
Ø1UG4JZ
Ø1UG4KZ
Ø1UHØ7Z
Ø1UHØJZ
Ø1UHØKZ
Ø1UH37Z
Ø1UH3JZ
Ø1UH3KZ
Ø1UH47Z
Ø1UH4JZ
Ø1UH4KZ
Ø1URØ7Z
Ø1URØJZ
Ø1URØKZ
Ø1UR37Z
Ø1UR3JZ
Ø1UR3KZ
Ø1UR47Z
Ø1UR4JZ
Ø1UR4KZ
Ø217Ø8S
Ø217Ø8T
Ø217Ø8U
Ø217Ø9S
Ø217Ø9T
Ø217Ø9U
Ø217ØAS
Ø217ØAT
Ø217ØAU
Ø217ØJS
Ø217ØJT
Ø217ØJU
Ø217ØKS
Ø217ØKT
Ø217ØKU
Ø217ØZS
Ø217ØZT
Ø217ØZU
Ø21748S
Ø21748T
Ø21748U

Ø21749S
Ø21749T
Ø21749U
Ø2174AS
Ø2174AT
Ø2174AU
Ø2174JS
Ø2174JT
Ø2174JU
Ø2174KS
Ø2174KT
Ø2174KU
Ø2174ZS
Ø2174ZT
Ø2174ZU
Ø21PØ8A
Ø21PØ8B
Ø21PØ8D
Ø21PØ9A
Ø21PØ9B
Ø21PØ9D
Ø21PØAA
Ø21PØAB
Ø21PØAD
Ø21PØJA
Ø21PØJB
Ø21PØJD
Ø21PØKA
Ø21PØKB
Ø21PØKD
Ø21PØZA
Ø21PØZB
Ø21PØZD
Ø21P48A
Ø21P48B
Ø21P48D
Ø21P49A
Ø21P49B
Ø21P49D
Ø21P4AA
Ø21P4AB
Ø21P4AD
Ø21P4JA
Ø21P4JB
Ø21P4JD
Ø21P4KA
Ø21P4KB
Ø21P4KD
Ø21P4ZA
Ø21P4ZB
Ø21P4ZD
Ø21QØ8A
Ø21QØ8B
Ø21QØ8D
Ø21QØ9A
Ø21QØ9B
Ø21QØ9D
Ø21QØAA
Ø21QØAB
Ø21QØAD
Ø21QØJA
Ø21QØJB
Ø21QØJD
Ø21QØKA
Ø21QØKB
Ø21QØKD
Ø21QØZA
Ø21QØZB
Ø21QØZD
Ø21Q48A
Ø21Q48B
Ø21Q48D
Ø21Q49A
Ø21Q49B
Ø21Q49D
Ø21Q4AA
Ø21Q4AB
Ø21Q4AD
Ø21Q4JA
Ø21Q4JB
Ø21Q4JD
Ø21Q4KA
Ø21Q4KB
Ø21Q4KD
Ø21Q4ZA
Ø21Q4ZB
Ø21Q4ZD
Ø21RØ8A
Ø21RØ8B
Ø21RØ8D
Ø21RØ9A
Ø21RØ9B
Ø21RØ9D
Ø21RØAA
Ø21RØAB
Ø21RØAD
Ø21RØJA
Ø21RØJB
Ø21RØJD
Ø21RØKA
Ø21RØKB
Ø21RØKD
Ø21RØZA
Ø21RØZB
Ø21RØZD
Ø21R48A
Ø21R48B
Ø21R48D
Ø21R49A
Ø21R49B
Ø21R49D
Ø21R4AA
Ø21R4AB
Ø21R4AD
Ø21R4JA
Ø21R4JB
Ø21R4JD
Ø21R4KA
Ø21R4KB
Ø21R4KD
Ø21R4ZA
Ø21R4ZB
Ø21R4ZD
Ø21VØ8S
Ø21VØ8T
Ø21VØ8U
Ø21VØ9S
Ø21VØ9T
Ø21VØ9U
Ø21VØAS
Ø21VØAT
Ø21VØAU
Ø21VØJS
Ø21VØJT
Ø21VØJU
Ø21VØKS
Ø21VØKT
Ø21VØKU
Ø21VØZS
Ø21VØZT
Ø21VØZU
Ø21V48S
Ø21V48T
Ø21V48U
Ø21V49S
Ø21V49T
Ø21V49U
Ø21V4AS
Ø21V4AT
Ø21V4AU
Ø21V4JS
Ø21V4JT
Ø21V4JU
Ø21V4KS
Ø21V4KT
Ø21V4KU
Ø21V4ZS
Ø21V4ZT
Ø21V4ZU
Ø21WØ8A
Ø21WØ8B
Ø21WØ8D
Ø21WØ8G
Ø21WØ8H
Ø21WØ9A
Ø21WØ9B
Ø21WØ9D
Ø21WØ9G
Ø21WØ9H
Ø21WØAA
Ø21WØAB
Ø21WØAD
Ø21WØAG
Ø21WØAH
Ø21WØJA
Ø21WØJB
Ø21WØJD
Ø21WØJG
Ø21WØJH
Ø21WØKA
Ø21WØKB
Ø21WØKD
Ø21WØKG
Ø21WØKH
Ø21WØZA
Ø21WØZB
Ø21WØZD
Ø21W48A
Ø21W48B
Ø21W48D
Ø21W49A
Ø21W49B
Ø21W49D
Ø21W4AA
Ø21W4AB
Ø21W4AD
Ø21W4JA
Ø21W4JB
Ø21W4JD
Ø21W4KA
Ø21W4KB
Ø21W4KD
Ø21W4ZA
Ø21W4ZB
Ø21W4ZD
Ø21XØ8A
Ø21XØ8B
Ø21XØ8D
Ø21XØ9A
Ø21XØ9B
Ø21XØ9D
Ø21XØAA
Ø21XØAB
Ø21XØAD
Ø21XØJA
Ø21XØJB
Ø21XØJD
Ø21XØKA
Ø21XØKB
Ø21XØKD
Ø21XØZA
Ø21XØZB
Ø21XØZD
Ø21X48A
Ø21X48B
Ø21X48D
Ø21X49A
Ø21X49B
Ø21X49D
Ø21X4AA
Ø21X4AB
Ø21X4AD
Ø21X4JA
Ø21X4JB
Ø21X4JD
Ø21X4KA
Ø21X4KB
Ø21X4KD
Ø21X4ZA
Ø21X4ZB
Ø21X4ZD
Ø25NØZZ
Ø25N3ZZ
Ø25N4ZZ
Ø2BNØZZ
Ø2BN3ZZ
Ø2BN4ZZ
Ø2BP3ZZ
Ø2BQ3ZZ
Ø2BR3ZZ
Ø2BS3ZZ
Ø2BT3ZZ
Ø2BV3ZZ
Ø2BWØZZ
Ø2BW3ZZ
Ø2BW4ZZ
Ø2BXØZZ
Ø2BX3ZZ
Ø2BX4ZZ
Ø2CNØZZ
Ø2CN3ZZ
Ø2CN4ZZ
Ø2CPØZZ
Ø2CP3ZZ
Ø2CP4ZZ
Ø2CQØZZ
Ø2CQ3ZZ
Ø2CQ4ZZ
Ø2CRØZZ
Ø2CR3ZZ
Ø2CR4ZZ
Ø2CSØZZ
Ø2CS3ZZ
Ø2CS4ZZ
Ø2CTØZZ
Ø2CT3ZZ
Ø2CT4ZZ
Ø2CVØZZ
Ø2CV3ZZ
Ø2CV4ZZ
Ø2CWØZZ
Ø2CW3ZZ
Ø2CW4ZZ
Ø2CXØZZ
Ø2CX3ZZ
Ø2CX4ZZ
Ø2H6Ø2Z
Ø2H642Z
Ø2H7Ø2Z
Ø2H742Z
Ø2HLØ2Z
Ø2HL42Z
Ø2HNØØZ
Ø2HNØ2Z
Ø2HNØYZ
Ø2HN3ØZ
Ø2HN3YZ
Ø2HN4ØZ
Ø2HN42Z
Ø2HN4YZ
Ø2HVØ2Z
Ø2HVØDZ
Ø2HV3DZ
Ø2HV42Z
Ø2HV4DZ
Ø2JAØZZ
Ø2JYØZZ
Ø2LPØCZ
Ø2LPØDZ
Ø2LPØZZ
Ø2LP3CZ
Ø2LP3DZ
Ø2LP3ZZ
Ø2LP4CZ
Ø2LP4DZ
Ø2LP4ZZ
Ø2LQØCZ
Ø2LQØDZ
Ø2LQØZZ
Ø2LQ3CZ
Ø2LQ3DZ
Ø2LQ3ZZ
Ø2LQ4CZ
Ø2LQ4DZ
Ø2LQ4ZZ
Ø2LRØCZ
Ø2LRØDZ
Ø2LRØZZ
Ø2LR3CZ
Ø2LR3DZ
Ø2LR3ZZ
Ø2LR4CZ
Ø2LR4DZ
Ø2LR4ZZ
Ø2LVØCZ
Ø2LVØDZ
Ø2LVØZZ
Ø2LV3CZ
Ø2LV3DZ
Ø2LV3ZZ
Ø2LV4CZ
Ø2LV4DZ
Ø2LV4ZZ
Ø2NNØZZ
Ø2NN3ZZ
Ø2NN4ZZ
Ø2PAØMZ
Ø2PA3MZ
Ø2PA4MZ
Ø2QAØZZ
Ø2QPØZZ
Ø2QP3ZZ
Ø2QP4ZZ
Ø2QQØZZ
Ø2QQ3ZZ
Ø2QQ4ZZ
Ø2QRØZZ
Ø2QR3ZZ
Ø2QR4ZZ
Ø2QSØZZ
Ø2QS3ZZ
Ø2QS4ZZ
Ø2QTØZZ
Ø2QT3ZZ
Ø2QT4ZZ
Ø2QVØZZ
Ø2QV3ZZ
Ø2QV4ZZ
Ø2QWØZZ
Ø2QW3ZZ
Ø2QW4ZZ
Ø2QXØZZ
Ø2QX3ZZ
Ø2QX4ZZ
Ø2RPØ7Z
Ø2RPØ8Z
Ø2RPØJZ
Ø2RPØKZ
Ø2RP47Z
Ø2RP48Z
Ø2RP4JZ
Ø2RP4KZ
Ø2RQØ7Z
Ø2RQØ8Z
Ø2RQØJZ
Ø2RQØKZ
Ø2RQ47Z
Ø2RQ48Z
Ø2RQ4JZ
Ø2RQ4KZ
Ø2RRØ7Z
Ø2RRØ8Z
Ø2RRØJZ
Ø2RRØKZ
Ø2RR47Z
Ø2RR48Z
Ø2RR4JZ
Ø2RR4KZ
Ø2RSØ7Z
Ø2RSØ8Z
Ø2RSØJZ
Ø2RSØKZ
Ø2RS47Z
Ø2RS48Z
Ø2RS4JZ
Ø2RS4KZ
Ø2RTØ7Z
Ø2RTØ8Z
Ø2RTØJZ
Ø2RTØKZ
Ø2RT47Z
Ø2RT48Z
Ø2RT4JZ
Ø2RT4KZ
Ø2RVØ7Z
Ø2RVØ8Z
Ø2RVØJZ
Ø2RVØKZ
Ø2RV47Z
Ø2RV48Z
Ø2RV4JZ
Ø2RV4KZ
Ø2RWØ7Z
Ø2RWØ8Z
Ø2RWØJZ
Ø2RWØKZ
Ø2RW47Z
Ø2RW48Z
Ø2RW4JZ
Ø2RW4KZ
Ø2RXØ7Z
Ø2RXØ8Z
Ø2RXØJZ
Ø2RXØKZ
Ø2RX47Z
Ø2RX48Z
Ø2RX4JZ
Ø2RX4KZ
Ø2SØØZZ
Ø2S1ØZZ
Ø2SPØZZ
Ø2SQØZZ
Ø2SRØZZ
Ø2SSØZZ
Ø2STØZZ
Ø2SVØZZ
Ø2SWØZZ
Ø2SXØZZ
Ø2TNØZZ
Ø2TN3ZZ
Ø2TN4ZZ
Ø2UPØ7Z
Ø2UPØ8Z
Ø2UPØKZ
Ø2UP37Z
Ø2UP38Z
Ø2UP3KZ
Ø2UP47Z
Ø2UP48Z
Ø2UP4KZ
Ø2UQØ7Z
Ø2UQØ8Z
Ø2UQØKZ
Ø2UQ37Z
Ø2UQ38Z
Ø2UQ3KZ
Ø2UQ47Z
Ø2UQ48Z
Ø2UQ4KZ
Ø2URØ7Z
Ø2URØ8Z
Ø2URØKZ
Ø2UR37Z
Ø2UR38Z
Ø2UR3KZ
Ø2UR47Z
Ø2UR48Z
Ø2UR4KZ
Ø2USØ7Z
Ø2USØ8Z
Ø2USØKZ
Ø2US37Z
Ø2US38Z
Ø2US3KZ
Ø2US47Z
Ø2US48Z
Ø2US4KZ
Ø2UTØ7Z
Ø2UTØ8Z
Ø2UTØKZ
Ø2UT37Z
Ø2UT38Z
Ø2UT3KZ
Ø2UT47Z
Ø2UT48Z
Ø2UT4KZ
Ø2UVØ7Z
Ø2UVØ8Z
Ø2UVØKZ
Ø2UV37Z
Ø2UV38Z
Ø2UV3KZ
Ø2UV47Z
Ø2UV48Z
Ø2UV4KZ
Ø2UWØ7Z
Ø2UWØ8Z
Ø2UWØKZ
Ø2UW37Z
Ø2UW38Z
Ø2UW3JZ
Ø2UW3KZ
Ø2UW47Z
Ø2UW48Z
Ø2UW4JZ
Ø2UW4KZ
Ø2UXØ7Z
Ø2UXØ8Z
Ø2UXØKZ
Ø2UX37Z
Ø2UX38Z
Ø2UX3JZ
Ø2UX3KZ
Ø2UX47Z
Ø2UX48Z
Ø2UX4JZ
Ø2UX4KZ
Ø2VVØCZ
Ø2VVØDZ
Ø2VVØZZ
Ø2VV3CZ
Ø2VV3DZ
Ø2VV3ZZ
Ø2VV4CZ
Ø2VV4DZ
Ø2VV4ZZ
Ø2VWØDZ
Ø2VWØEZ
Ø2VWØFZ
Ø2VW3DZ
Ø2VW3EZ
Ø2VW3FZ
Ø2VW4DZ
Ø2VW4EZ
Ø2VW4FZ
Ø2VXØDZ
Ø2VXØEZ
Ø2VXØFZ
Ø2VX3DZ
Ø2VX3EZ
Ø2VX3FZ
Ø2VX4DZ
Ø2VX4EZ
Ø2VX4FZ
Ø2WAØKZ
Ø2WAØMZ
Ø2WA3JZ
Ø2WA3KZ
Ø2WA3MZ
Ø2WA4JZ
Ø2WA4KZ
Ø2WA4MZ
Ø312Ø9W
Ø312ØAW
Ø312ØJW
Ø312ØKW
Ø312ØZW
Ø313Ø9W
Ø313ØAW
Ø313ØJW
Ø313ØKW
Ø313ØZD
Ø313ØZW
Ø314Ø9W
Ø314ØAW
Ø314ØJW
Ø314ØKW
Ø314ØZD
Ø314ØZW
Ø315Ø9W
Ø315ØAW
Ø315ØJW
Ø315ØKW
Ø315ØZD
Ø315ØZT
Ø315ØZV
Ø315ØZW
Ø316Ø9W
Ø316ØAW
Ø316ØJW
Ø316ØKW
Ø316ØZD
Ø316ØZT
Ø316ØZV
Ø316ØZW
Ø317Ø9D
Ø317Ø9F
Ø317Ø9V
Ø317Ø9W
Ø317ØAD
Ø317ØAF
Ø317ØAV
Ø317ØAW
Ø317ØJD
Ø317ØJF
Ø317ØJV
Ø317ØJW
Ø317ØKD
Ø317ØKF
Ø317ØKV
Ø317ØKW
Ø317ØZD
Ø317ØZF
Ø317ØZV
Ø317ØZW
Ø3173ZF
Ø318Ø9D
Ø318Ø9F
Ø318Ø9V
Ø318Ø9W
Ø318ØAD
Ø318ØAF
Ø318ØAV
Ø318ØAW
Ø318ØJD
Ø318ØJF
Ø318ØJV
Ø318ØJW
Ø318ØKD
Ø318ØKF
Ø318ØKV
Ø318ØKW
Ø318ØZD
Ø318ØZF
Ø318ØZV
Ø318ØZW
Ø3183ZF
Ø319Ø9F
Ø319ØAF
Ø319ØJF
Ø319ØKF
Ø319ØZF
Ø3193ZF
Ø31AØ9F
Ø31AØAF
Ø31AØJF
Ø31AØKF
Ø31AØZF
Ø31A3ZF
Ø31BØ9F
Ø31BØAF
Ø31BØJF
Ø31BØKF
Ø31BØZF
Ø31B3ZF
Ø31CØ9F
Ø31CØAF
Ø31CØJF
Ø31CØKF
Ø31CØZF
Ø31C3ZF
Ø31HØ9G
Ø31HØ9J
Ø31HØ9K
Ø31HØ9Y
Ø31HØAG
Ø31HØAJ
Ø31HØAK
Ø31HØAY
Ø31HØJG
Ø31HØJJ
Ø31HØJK
Ø31HØJY
Ø31HØKG
Ø31HØKJ
Ø31HØKK
Ø31HØKY
Ø31HØZG
Ø31HØZJ
Ø31HØZK
Ø31HØZY
Ø31JØ9G
Ø31JØ9J
Ø31JØ9K
Ø31JØ9Y
Ø31JØAG
Ø31JØAJ
Ø31JØAK
Ø31JØAY
Ø31JØJG
Ø31JØJJ
Ø31JØJK
Ø31JØJY
Ø31JØKG
Ø31JØKJ
Ø31JØKK
Ø31JØKY
Ø31JØZG
Ø31JØZJ
Ø31JØZK
Ø31JØZY
Ø31KØ9J
Ø31KØ9K
Ø31KØAJ
Ø31KØAK
Ø31KØJJ
Ø31KØJK
Ø31KØKJ
Ø31KØKK
Ø31KØZJ
Ø31KØZK
Ø31LØ9J
Ø31LØ9K
Ø31LØAJ
Ø31LØAK
Ø31LØJJ
Ø31LØJK
Ø31LØKJ
Ø31LØKK
Ø31LØZJ
Ø31LØZK
Ø31MØ9J
Ø31MØ9K
Ø31MØAJ
Ø31MØAK
Ø31MØJJ
Ø31MØJK
Ø31MØKJ
Ø31MØKK
Ø31MØZJ
Ø31MØZK
Ø31NØ9J
Ø31NØ9K
Ø31NØAJ
Ø31NØAK
Ø31NØJJ
Ø31NØJK
Ø31NØKJ
Ø31NØKK
Ø31NØZJ
Ø31NØZK
Ø31SØ9G
Ø31SØAG
Ø31SØJG
Ø31SØKG
Ø31SØZG
Ø31TØ9G
Ø31TØAG
Ø31TØJG
Ø31TØKG
Ø31TØZG
Ø35GØZZ
Ø35G3ZZ
Ø35G4ZZ
Ø37334Z
Ø37335Z
Ø37336Z
Ø37337Z
Ø3733D1
Ø3733DZ
Ø3733EZ
Ø3733FZ
Ø3733GZ
Ø3733Z1
Ø3733ZZ
Ø37434Z
Ø37435Z
Ø37436Z
Ø37437Z
Ø3743D1
Ø3743DZ
Ø3743EZ
Ø3743FZ
Ø3743GZ
Ø3743Z1
Ø3743ZZ
Ø37734Z
Ø37735Z
Ø37736Z
Ø37737Z
Ø3773D1
Ø3773DZ
Ø3773EZ
Ø3773FZ
Ø3773GZ
Ø3773Z1
Ø3773ZZ
Ø37834Z
Ø37835Z
Ø37836Z
Ø37837Z
Ø3783D1
Ø3783DZ
Ø3783EZ
Ø3783FZ
Ø3783GZ
Ø3783Z1
Ø3783ZZ
Ø37934Z
Ø37935Z
Ø37936Z
Ø37937Z
Ø3793D1
Ø3793DZ
Ø3793EZ
Ø3793FZ
Ø3793GZ
Ø3793Z1
Ø3793ZZ
Ø37A34Z
Ø37A35Z
Ø37A36Z
Ø37A37Z
Ø37A3D1
Ø37A3DZ
Ø37A3EZ
Ø37A3FZ
Ø37A3GZ
Ø37A3Z1
Ø37A3ZZ
Ø37G34Z
Ø37G35Z
Ø37G36Z
Ø37G37Z
Ø37G3DZ
Ø37G3EZ
Ø37G3FZ
Ø37G3GZ
Ø37G3ZZ
Ø37G44Z
Ø37G45Z
Ø37G46Z
Ø37G47Z
Ø37G4DZ
Ø37G4EZ
Ø37G4FZ
Ø37G4GZ
Ø37G4ZZ
Ø37H34Z
Ø37H35Z
Ø37H36Z
Ø37H37Z
Ø37H3DZ
Ø37H3EZ
Ø37H3FZ
Ø37H3GZ
Ø37H3ZZ
Ø37H44Z
Ø37H45Z
Ø37H46Z
Ø37H47Z
Ø37H4DZ
Ø37H4EZ
Ø37H4FZ
Ø37H4GZ

Ø37H4ZZ
Ø37J34Z
Ø37J35Z
Ø37J36Z
Ø37J37Z
Ø37J3DZ
Ø37J3EZ
Ø37J3FZ
Ø37J3GZ
Ø37J3ZZ
Ø37J44Z
Ø37J45Z
Ø37J46Z
Ø37J47Z
Ø37J4DZ
Ø37J4EZ
Ø37J4FZ
Ø37J4GZ
Ø37J4ZZ
Ø37K34Z
Ø37K35Z
Ø37K36Z
Ø37K37Z
Ø37K3DZ
Ø37K3EZ
Ø37K3FZ
Ø37K3GZ
Ø37K3ZZ
Ø37K44Z
Ø37K45Z
Ø37K46Z
Ø37K47Z
Ø37K4DZ
Ø37K4EZ
Ø37K4FZ
Ø37K4GZ
Ø37K4ZZ
Ø37L34Z
Ø37L35Z
Ø37L36Z
Ø37L37Z
Ø37L3DZ
Ø37L3EZ
Ø37L3FZ
Ø37L3GZ
Ø37L3ZZ
Ø37L44Z
Ø37L45Z
Ø37L46Z
Ø37L47Z
Ø37L4DZ
Ø37L4EZ
Ø37L4FZ
Ø37L4GZ
Ø37L4ZZ
Ø37M34Z
Ø37M35Z
Ø37M36Z
Ø37M37Z
Ø37M3DZ
Ø37M3EZ
Ø37M3FZ
Ø37M3GZ
Ø37M3ZZ
Ø37M44Z
Ø37M45Z
Ø37M46Z
Ø37M47Z
Ø37M4DZ
Ø37M4EZ
Ø37M4FZ
Ø37M4GZ
Ø37M4ZZ
Ø37N34Z
Ø37N35Z
Ø37N36Z
Ø37N37Z
Ø37N3DZ
Ø37N3EZ
Ø37N3FZ
Ø37N3GZ
Ø37N3ZZ
Ø37N44Z
Ø37N45Z
Ø37N46Z
Ø37N47Z
Ø37N4DZ
Ø37N4EZ
Ø37N4FZ
Ø37N4GZ
Ø37N4ZZ
Ø37P34Z
Ø37P35Z
Ø37P36Z
Ø37P37Z
Ø37P3DZ
Ø37P3EZ
Ø37P3FZ
Ø37P3GZ
Ø37P3ZZ
Ø37P44Z
Ø37P45Z
Ø37P46Z
Ø37P47Z
Ø37P4DZ
Ø37P4EZ
Ø37P4FZ
Ø37P4GZ
Ø37P4ZZ
Ø37Q34Z
Ø37Q35Z
Ø37Q36Z
Ø37Q37Z
Ø37Q3DZ
Ø37Q3EZ
Ø37Q3FZ
Ø37Q3GZ
Ø37Q3ZZ
Ø37Q44Z
Ø37Q45Z
Ø37Q46Z
Ø37Q47Z
Ø37Q4DZ
Ø37Q4EZ
Ø37Q4FZ
Ø37Q4GZ
Ø37Q4ZZ
Ø37Y34Z
Ø37Y35Z
Ø37Y36Z
Ø37Y37Z
Ø37Y3DZ
Ø37Y3EZ
Ø37Y3FZ
Ø37Y3GZ
Ø37Y3ZZ
Ø3BØ3ZZ
Ø3B13ZZ
Ø3B23ZZ
Ø3B33ZZ
Ø3B43ZZ
Ø3B5ØZZ
Ø3B53ZZ
Ø3B54ZZ
Ø3B6ØZZ
Ø3B63ZZ
Ø3B64ZZ
Ø3B7ØZZ
Ø3B73ZZ
Ø3B74ZZ
Ø3B8ØZZ
Ø3B83ZZ
Ø3B84ZZ
Ø3B9ØZZ
Ø3B93ZZ
Ø3B94ZZ
Ø3BAØZZ
Ø3BA3ZZ
Ø3BA4ZZ
Ø3BBØZZ
Ø3BB3ZZ
Ø3BB4ZZ
Ø3BCØZZ
Ø3BC3ZZ
Ø3BC4ZZ
Ø3BDØZZ
Ø3BD3ZZ
Ø3BD4ZZ
Ø3BFØZZ
Ø3BF3ZZ
Ø3BF4ZZ
Ø3BGØZZ
Ø3BG3ZZ
Ø3BG4ZZ
Ø3BHØZZ
Ø3BH3ZZ
Ø3BH4ZZ
Ø3BJØZZ
Ø3BJ3ZZ
Ø3BJ4ZZ
Ø3BKØZZ
Ø3BK3ZZ
Ø3BK4ZZ
Ø3BLØZZ
Ø3BL3ZZ
Ø3BL4ZZ
Ø3BMØZZ
Ø3BM3ZZ
Ø3BM4ZZ
Ø3BNØZZ
Ø3BN3ZZ
Ø3BN4ZZ
Ø3BPØZZ
Ø3BP3ZZ
Ø3BP4ZZ
Ø3BQØZZ
Ø3BQ3ZZ
Ø3BQ4ZZ
Ø3BRØZZ
Ø3BR3ZZ
Ø3BR4ZZ
Ø3BSØZZ
Ø3BS3ZZ
Ø3BS4ZZ
Ø3BTØZZ
Ø3BT3ZZ
Ø3BT4ZZ
Ø3BUØZZ
Ø3BU3ZZ
Ø3BU4ZZ
Ø3BVØZZ
Ø3BV3ZZ
Ø3BV4ZZ
Ø3BYØZZ
Ø3BY3ZZ
Ø3BY4ZZ
Ø3CØØZZ
Ø3CØ3ZZ
Ø3CØ4ZZ
Ø3C1ØZZ
Ø3C13ZZ
Ø3C14ZZ
Ø3C2ØZZ
Ø3C23ZZ
Ø3C24ZZ
Ø3C3ØZZ
Ø3C33ZZ
Ø3C34ZZ
Ø3C4ØZZ
Ø3C43ZZ
Ø3C44ZZ
Ø3C5ØZZ
Ø3C53ZZ
Ø3C54ZZ
Ø3C6ØZZ
Ø3C63ZZ
Ø3C64ZZ
Ø3C7ØZZ
Ø3C73ZZ
Ø3C74ZZ
Ø3C8ØZZ
Ø3C83ZZ
Ø3C84ZZ
Ø3C9ØZZ
Ø3C93ZZ
Ø3C94ZZ
Ø3CAØZZ
Ø3CA3ZZ
Ø3CA4ZZ
Ø3CBØZZ
Ø3CB3ZZ
Ø3CB4ZZ
Ø3CCØZZ
Ø3CC3ZZ
Ø3CC4ZZ
Ø3CDØZZ
Ø3CD3ZZ
Ø3CD4ZZ
Ø3CFØZZ
Ø3CF3ZZ
Ø3CF4ZZ
Ø3CGØZZ
Ø3CG3Z7
Ø3CG3ZZ
Ø3CG4ZZ
Ø3CHØZZ
Ø3CH3Z7
Ø3CH3ZZ
Ø3CH4ZZ
Ø3CJØZZ
Ø3CJ3Z7
Ø3CJ3ZZ
Ø3CJ4ZZ
Ø3CKØZZ
Ø3CK3Z7
Ø3CK3ZZ
Ø3CK4ZZ
Ø3CLØZZ
Ø3CL3Z7
Ø3CL3ZZ
Ø3CL4ZZ
Ø3CMØZZ
Ø3CM3Z7
Ø3CM3ZZ
Ø3CM4ZZ
Ø3CNØZZ
Ø3CN3Z7
Ø3CN3ZZ
Ø3CN4ZZ
Ø3CPØZZ
Ø3CP3Z7
Ø3CP3ZZ
Ø3CP4ZZ
Ø3CQØZZ
Ø3CQ3Z7
Ø3CQ3ZZ
Ø3CQ4ZZ
Ø3CRØZZ
Ø3CR3ZZ
Ø3CR4ZZ
Ø3CSØZZ
Ø3CS3ZZ
Ø3CS4ZZ
Ø3CTØZZ
Ø3CT3ZZ
Ø3CT4ZZ
Ø3CUØZZ
Ø3CU3ZZ
Ø3CU4ZZ
Ø3CVØZZ
Ø3CV3ZZ
Ø3CV4ZZ
Ø3CYØZZ
Ø3CY3ZZ
Ø3CY4ZZ
Ø3HØØDZ
Ø3HØ3DZ
Ø3HØ4DZ
Ø3H1ØDZ
Ø3H13DZ
Ø3H14DZ
Ø3H2ØDZ
Ø3H23DZ
Ø3H24DZ
Ø3H3ØDZ
Ø3H33DZ
Ø3H34DZ
Ø3H4ØDZ
Ø3H43DZ
Ø3H44DZ
Ø3H5ØDZ
Ø3H53DZ
Ø3H54DZ
Ø3H6ØDZ
Ø3H63DZ
Ø3H64DZ
Ø3H7ØDZ
Ø3H73DZ
Ø3H74DZ
Ø3H8ØDZ
Ø3H83DZ
Ø3H84DZ
Ø3H9ØDZ
Ø3H93DZ
Ø3H94DZ
Ø3HAØDZ
Ø3HA3DZ
Ø3HA4DZ
Ø3HBØDZ
Ø3HB3DZ
Ø3HB4DZ
Ø3HCØDZ
Ø3HC3DZ
Ø3HC4DZ
Ø3HDØDZ
Ø3HD3DZ
Ø3HD4DZ
Ø3HFØDZ
Ø3HF3DZ
Ø3HF4DZ
Ø3HGØDZ
Ø3HG3DZ
Ø3HG4DZ
Ø3HHØDZ
Ø3HH3DZ
Ø3HH4DZ
Ø3HJØDZ
Ø3HJ3DZ
Ø3HJ4DZ
Ø3HKØDZ
Ø3HK3DZ
Ø3HK4DZ
Ø3HLØDZ
Ø3HL3DZ
Ø3HL4DZ
Ø3HMØDZ
Ø3HM3DZ
Ø3HM4DZ
Ø3HNØDZ
Ø3HN3DZ
Ø3HN4DZ
Ø3HPØDZ
Ø3HP3DZ
Ø3HP4DZ
Ø3HQØDZ
Ø3HQ3DZ
Ø3HQ4DZ
Ø3HRØDZ
Ø3HR3DZ
Ø3HR4DZ
Ø3HSØDZ
Ø3HS3DZ
Ø3HS4DZ
Ø3HTØDZ
Ø3HT3DZ
Ø3HT4DZ
Ø3HUØDZ
Ø3HU3DZ
Ø3HU4DZ
Ø3HVØDZ
Ø3HV3DZ
Ø3HV4DZ
Ø3HYØDZ
Ø3HY3DZ
Ø3HY4DZ
Ø3L5ØCZ
Ø3L5ØDZ
Ø3L5ØZZ
Ø3L53CZ
Ø3L53DZ
Ø3L53ZZ
Ø3L54CZ
Ø3L54DZ
Ø3L54ZZ
Ø3L6ØCZ
Ø3L6ØDZ
Ø3L6ØZZ
Ø3L63CZ
Ø3L63DZ
Ø3L63ZZ
Ø3L64CZ
Ø3L64DZ
Ø3L64ZZ
Ø3L7ØCZ
Ø3L7ØDZ
Ø3L7ØZZ
Ø3L73CZ
Ø3L73DZ
Ø3L73ZZ
Ø3L74CZ
Ø3L74DZ
Ø3L74ZZ
Ø3L8ØCZ
Ø3L8ØDZ
Ø3L8ØZZ
Ø3L83CZ
Ø3L83DZ
Ø3L83ZZ
Ø3L84CZ
Ø3L84DZ
Ø3L84ZZ
Ø3L9ØCZ
Ø3L9ØDZ
Ø3L9ØZZ
Ø3L93CZ
Ø3L93DZ
Ø3L93ZZ
Ø3L94CZ
Ø3L94DZ
Ø3L94ZZ
Ø3LAØCZ
Ø3LAØDZ
Ø3LAØZZ
Ø3LA3CZ
Ø3LA3DZ
Ø3LA3ZZ
Ø3LA4CZ
Ø3LA4DZ
Ø3LA4ZZ
Ø3LBØCZ
Ø3LBØDZ
Ø3LBØZZ
Ø3LB3CZ
Ø3LB3DZ
Ø3LB3ZZ
Ø3LB4CZ
Ø3LB4DZ
Ø3LB4ZZ
Ø3LCØCZ
Ø3LCØDZ
Ø3LCØZZ
Ø3LC3CZ
Ø3LC3DZ
Ø3LC3ZZ
Ø3LC4CZ
Ø3LC4DZ
Ø3LC4ZZ
Ø3LDØCZ
Ø3LDØDZ
Ø3LDØZZ
Ø3LD3CZ
Ø3LD3DZ
Ø3LD3ZZ
Ø3LD4CZ
Ø3LD4DZ
Ø3LD4ZZ
Ø3LFØCZ
Ø3LFØDZ
Ø3LFØZZ
Ø3LF3CZ
Ø3LF3DZ
Ø3LF3ZZ
Ø3LF4CZ
Ø3LF4DZ
Ø3LF4ZZ
Ø3LGØBZ
Ø3LGØDZ
Ø3LG3BZ
Ø3LG3DZ
Ø3LG4BZ
Ø3LG4DZ
Ø3LHØBZ
Ø3LHØCZ
Ø3LHØDZ
Ø3LHØZZ
Ø3LH3BZ
Ø3LH3CZ
Ø3LH3DZ
Ø3LH3ZZ
Ø3LH4BZ
Ø3LH4CZ
Ø3LH4DZ
Ø3LH4ZZ
Ø3LJØBZ
Ø3LJØCZ
Ø3LJØDZ
Ø3LJØZZ
Ø3LJ3BZ
Ø3LJ3CZ
Ø3LJ3DZ
Ø3LJ3ZZ
Ø3LJ4BZ
Ø3LJ4CZ
Ø3LJ4DZ
Ø3LJ4ZZ
Ø3LKØBZ
Ø3LKØDZ
Ø3LK3BZ
Ø3LK3DZ
Ø3LK4BZ
Ø3LK4DZ
Ø3LLØBZ
Ø3LLØDZ
Ø3LL3BZ
Ø3LL3DZ
Ø3LL4BZ
Ø3LL4DZ
Ø3LMØBZ
Ø3LMØCZ
Ø3LMØDZ
Ø3LMØZZ
Ø3LM3BZ
Ø3LM3CZ
Ø3LM3DZ
Ø3LM3ZZ
Ø3LM4BZ
Ø3LM4CZ
Ø3LM4DZ
Ø3LM4ZZ
Ø3LNØBZ
Ø3LNØCZ
Ø3LNØDZ
Ø3LNØZZ
Ø3LN3BZ
Ø3LN3CZ
Ø3LN3DZ
Ø3LN3ZZ
Ø3LN4BZ
Ø3LN4CZ
Ø3LN4DZ
Ø3LN4ZZ
Ø3LPØBZ
Ø3LPØCZ
Ø3LPØDZ
Ø3LPØZZ
Ø3LP3BZ
Ø3LP3CZ
Ø3LP3DZ
Ø3LP3ZZ
Ø3LP4BZ
Ø3LP4CZ
Ø3LP4DZ
Ø3LP4ZZ
Ø3LQØBZ
Ø3LQØCZ
Ø3LQØDZ
Ø3LQØZZ
Ø3LQ3BZ
Ø3LQ3CZ
Ø3LQ3DZ
Ø3LQ3ZZ
Ø3LQ4BZ
Ø3LQ4CZ
Ø3LQ4DZ
Ø3LQ4ZZ
Ø3LRØCZ
Ø3LRØDZ
Ø3LRØZZ
Ø3LR3CZ
Ø3LR3DZ
Ø3LR3ZZ
Ø3LR4CZ
Ø3LR4DZ
Ø3LR4ZZ
Ø3LSØCZ
Ø3LSØDZ
Ø3LSØZZ
Ø3LS3CZ
Ø3LS3DZ
Ø3LS3ZZ
Ø3LS4CZ
Ø3LS4DZ
Ø3LS4ZZ
Ø3LTØCZ
Ø3LTØDZ
Ø3LTØZZ
Ø3LT3CZ
Ø3LT3DZ
Ø3LT3ZZ
Ø3LT4CZ
Ø3LT4DZ
Ø3LT4ZZ
Ø3LUØCZ
Ø3LUØDZ
Ø3LUØZZ
Ø3LU3CZ
Ø3LU3DZ
Ø3LU3ZZ
Ø3LU4CZ
Ø3LU4DZ
Ø3LU4ZZ
Ø3LVØCZ
Ø3LVØDZ
Ø3LVØZZ
Ø3LV3CZ
Ø3LV3DZ
Ø3LV3ZZ
Ø3LV4CZ
Ø3LV4DZ
Ø3LV4ZZ
Ø3LYØCZ
Ø3LYØDZ
Ø3LYØZZ
Ø3LY3CZ
Ø3LY3DZ
Ø3LY3ZZ
Ø3LY4CZ
Ø3LY4DZ
Ø3LY4ZZ
Ø3PYØ7Z
Ø3PYØJZ
Ø3PYØKZ
Ø3PY37Z
Ø3PY3JZ
Ø3PY3KZ
Ø3PY47Z
Ø3PY4JZ
Ø3PY4KZ
Ø3QØØZZ
Ø3QØ3ZZ
Ø3QØ4ZZ
Ø3Q1ØZZ
Ø3Q13ZZ
Ø3Q14ZZ
Ø3Q2ØZZ
Ø3Q23ZZ
Ø3Q24ZZ
Ø3Q3ØZZ
Ø3Q33ZZ
Ø3Q34ZZ
Ø3Q4ØZZ
Ø3Q43ZZ
Ø3Q44ZZ
Ø3Q5ØZZ
Ø3Q53ZZ
Ø3Q54ZZ
Ø3Q6ØZZ
Ø3Q63ZZ
Ø3Q64ZZ
Ø3Q7ØZZ
Ø3Q73ZZ
Ø3Q74ZZ
Ø3Q8ØZZ
Ø3Q83ZZ
Ø3Q84ZZ
Ø3Q9ØZZ
Ø3Q93ZZ
Ø3Q94ZZ
Ø3QAØZZ
Ø3QA3ZZ
Ø3QA4ZZ
Ø3QBØZZ
Ø3QB3ZZ
Ø3QB4ZZ
Ø3QCØZZ
Ø3QC3ZZ
Ø3QC4ZZ
Ø3QDØZZ
Ø3QD3ZZ
Ø3QD4ZZ
Ø3QFØZZ
Ø3QF3ZZ
Ø3QF4ZZ
Ø3QGØZZ
Ø3QG3ZZ
Ø3QG4ZZ
Ø3QHØZZ
Ø3QH3ZZ
Ø3QH4ZZ
Ø3QJØZZ
Ø3QJ3ZZ
Ø3QJ4ZZ
Ø3QKØZZ
Ø3QK3ZZ
Ø3QK4ZZ
Ø3QLØZZ
Ø3QL3ZZ
Ø3QL4ZZ
Ø3QMØZZ
Ø3QM3ZZ
Ø3QM4ZZ
Ø3QNØZZ
Ø3QN3ZZ
Ø3QN4ZZ
Ø3QPØZZ
Ø3QP3ZZ
Ø3QP4ZZ
Ø3QQØZZ
Ø3QQ3ZZ
Ø3QQ4ZZ
Ø3QRØZZ
Ø3QR3ZZ
Ø3QR4ZZ
Ø3QSØZZ
Ø3QS3ZZ
Ø3QS4ZZ
Ø3QTØZZ
Ø3QT3ZZ
Ø3QT4ZZ
Ø3QUØZZ
Ø3QU3ZZ
Ø3QU4ZZ
Ø3QVØZZ
Ø3QV3ZZ
Ø3QV4ZZ
Ø3QYØZZ
Ø3QY3ZZ
Ø3QY4ZZ
Ø3RØØ7Z
Ø3RØØJZ
Ø3RØØKZ
Ø3RØ47Z
Ø3RØ4JZ
Ø3RØ4KZ
Ø3R1Ø7Z
Ø3R1ØJZ
Ø3R1ØKZ
Ø3R147Z
Ø3R14JZ
Ø3R14KZ
Ø3R2Ø7Z
Ø3R2ØJZ
Ø3R2ØKZ
Ø3R247Z
Ø3R24JZ
Ø3R24KZ
Ø3R3Ø7Z
Ø3R3ØJZ
Ø3R3ØKZ
Ø3R347Z
Ø3R34JZ
Ø3R34KZ
Ø3R4Ø7Z
Ø3R4ØJZ
Ø3R4ØKZ
Ø3R447Z
Ø3R44JZ
Ø3R44KZ
Ø3RGØ7Z
Ø3RGØJZ
Ø3RGØKZ
Ø3RG47Z
Ø3RG4JZ
Ø3RG4KZ
Ø3SØØZZ
Ø3SØ3ZZ
Ø3SØ4ZZ
Ø3S1ØZZ
Ø3S13ZZ
Ø3S14ZZ
Ø3S2ØZZ
Ø3S23ZZ
Ø3S24ZZ
Ø3S3ØZZ
Ø3S33ZZ
Ø3S34ZZ
Ø3S4ØZZ
Ø3S43ZZ
Ø3S44ZZ
Ø3S5ØZZ
Ø3S53ZZ
Ø3S54ZZ
Ø3S6ØZZ
Ø3S63ZZ
Ø3S64ZZ
Ø3S7ØZZ
Ø3S73ZZ
Ø3S74ZZ
Ø3S8ØZZ
Ø3S83ZZ
Ø3S84ZZ
Ø3S9ØZZ
Ø3S93ZZ
Ø3S94ZZ
Ø3SAØZZ
Ø3SA3ZZ
Ø3SA4ZZ
Ø3SBØZZ
Ø3SB3ZZ
Ø3SB4ZZ
Ø3SCØZZ
Ø3SC3ZZ
Ø3SC4ZZ
Ø3SDØZZ
Ø3SD3ZZ
Ø3SD4ZZ
Ø3SFØZZ
Ø3SF3ZZ
Ø3SF4ZZ
Ø3SGØZZ
Ø3SG3ZZ
Ø3SG4ZZ
Ø3SHØZZ
Ø3SH3ZZ
Ø3SH4ZZ
Ø3SJØZZ
Ø3SJ3ZZ
Ø3SJ4ZZ
Ø3SKØZZ
Ø3SK3ZZ
Ø3SK4ZZ
Ø3SLØZZ
Ø3SL3ZZ
Ø3SL4ZZ
Ø3SMØZZ
Ø3SM3ZZ
Ø3SM4ZZ
Ø3SNØZZ
Ø3SN3ZZ
Ø3SN4ZZ
Ø3SPØZZ
Ø3SP3ZZ
Ø3SP4ZZ
Ø3SQØZZ
Ø3SQ3ZZ
Ø3SQ4ZZ
Ø3SRØZZ
Ø3SR3ZZ
Ø3SR4ZZ
Ø3SSØZZ
Ø3SS3ZZ
Ø3SS4ZZ
Ø3STØZZ
Ø3ST3ZZ
Ø3ST4ZZ

03SU0ZZ
03SU3ZZ
03SU4ZZ
03SV0ZZ
03SV3ZZ
03SV4ZZ
03SY0ZZ
03SY3ZZ
03SY4ZZ
03U007Z
03U037Z
03U047Z
03U107Z
03U137Z
03U147Z
03U207Z
03U237Z
03U247Z
03U307Z
03U337Z
03U347Z
03U407Z
03U437Z
03U447Z
03U507Z
03U537Z
03U547Z
03U607Z
03U637Z
03U647Z
03U707Z
03U737Z
03U747Z
03U807Z
03U837Z
03U847Z
03U907Z
03U937Z
03U947Z
03UA07Z
03UA37Z
03UA47Z
03UB07Z
03UB37Z
03UB47Z
03UC07Z
03UC37Z
03UC47Z
03UD07Z
03UD37Z
03UD47Z
03UF07Z
03UF37Z
03UF47Z
03UG07Z
03UG37Z
03UG47Z
03UH07Z
03UH37Z
03UH47Z
03UJ07Z
03UJ37Z
03UJ47Z
03UK07Z
03UK37Z
03UK47Z
03UL07Z
03UL37Z
03UL47Z
03UM07Z
03UM37Z
03UM47Z
03UN07Z
03UN37Z
03UN47Z
03UP07Z
03UP37Z
03UP47Z
03UQ07Z
03UQ37Z
03UQ47Z
03UR07Z
03UR37Z
03UR47Z
03US07Z
03US37Z
03US47Z
03UT07Z
03UT37Z
03UT47Z
03UU07Z
03UU37Z
03UU47Z
03UV07Z
03UV37Z
03UV47Z
03UY07Z
03UY37Z
03UY47Z
03V00DZ
03V03DZ
03V04DZ
03V10DZ
03V13DZ
03V14DZ
03V20DZ
03V23DZ
03V24DZ
03V30DZ
03V33DZ
03V34DZ
03V40DZ
03V43DZ
03V44DZ
03V50DZ
03V53DZ
03V54DZ
03V60DZ
03V63DZ
03V64DZ
03V70DZ
03V73DZ
03V74DZ
03V80DZ
03V83DZ
03V84DZ
03V90DZ
03V93DZ
03V94DZ
03VA0DZ
03VA3DZ
03VA4DZ
03VB0DZ
03VB3DZ
03VB4DZ
03VC0DZ
03VC3DZ
03VC4DZ
03VD0DZ
03VD3DZ
03VD4DZ
03VF0DZ
03VF3DZ
03VF4DZ
03VG0BZ
03VG0DZ
03VG0HZ
03VG3BZ
03VG3DZ
03VG3HZ
03VG4BZ
03VG4DZ
03VG4HZ
03VH0BZ
03VH0DZ
03VH0HZ
03VH3BZ
03VH3DZ
03VH3HZ
03VH4BZ
03VH4DZ
03VH4HZ
03VJ0BZ
03VJ0DZ
03VJ0HZ
03VJ3BZ
03VJ3DZ
03VJ3HZ
03VJ4BZ
03VJ4DZ
03VJ4HZ
03VK0BZ
03VK0DZ
03VK0HZ
03VK3BZ
03VK3DZ
03VK3HZ
03VK4BZ
03VK4DZ
03VK4HZ
03VL0BZ
03VL0DZ
03VL0HZ
03VL3BZ
03VL3DZ
03VL3HZ
03VL4BZ
03VL4DZ
03VL4HZ
03VM0BZ
03VM0DZ
03VM0HZ
03VM3BZ
03VM3DZ
03VM3HZ
03VM4BZ
03VM4DZ
03VM4HZ
03VN0BZ
03VN0DZ
03VN0HZ
03VN3BZ
03VN3DZ
03VN3HZ
03VN4BZ
03VN4DZ
03VN4HZ
03VP0BZ
03VP0DZ
03VP0HZ
03VP3BZ
03VP3DZ
03VP3HZ
03VP4BZ
03VP4DZ
03VP4HZ
03VQ0BZ
03VQ0DZ
03VQ0HZ
03VQ3BZ
03VQ3DZ
03VQ3HZ
03VQ4BZ
03VQ4DZ
03VQ4HZ
03VR0DZ
03VR3DZ
03VR4DZ
03VS0DZ
03VS3DZ
03VS4DZ
03VT0DZ
03VT3DZ
03VT4DZ
03VU0DZ
03VU3DZ
03VU4DZ
03VV0DZ
03VV3DZ
03VV4DZ
03VY0DZ
03VY3DZ
03VY4DZ
410093
410094
410095
04100A3
04100A4
04100A5
04100J3
04100J4
04100J5
04100K3
04100K4
04100K5
04100Z3
04100Z4
04100Z5
410493
410494
410495
04104A3
04104A4
04104A5
04104J3
04104J4
04104J5
04104K3
04104K4
04104K5
04104Z3
04104Z4
04104Z5
413093
413094
413095
04130A3
04130A4
04130A5
04130J3
04130J4
04130J5
04130K3
04130K4
04130K5
04130Z3
04130Z4
04130Z5
413493
413494
413495
04134A3
04134A4
04134A5
04134J3
04134J4
04134J5
04134K3
04134K4
04134K5
04134Z3
04134Z4
04134Z5
04500ZZ
04503ZZ
04504ZZ
045K0ZZ
045K3ZZ
045K4ZZ
045L0ZZ
045L3ZZ
045L4ZZ
045M0ZZ
045M3ZZ
045M4ZZ
045N0ZZ
045N3ZZ
045N4ZZ
045P0ZZ
045P3ZZ
045P4ZZ
045Q0ZZ
045Q3ZZ
045Q4ZZ
045R0ZZ
045R3ZZ
045R4ZZ
045S0ZZ
045S3ZZ
045S4ZZ
045T0ZZ
045T3ZZ
045T4ZZ
045U0ZZ
045U3ZZ
045U4ZZ
045V0ZZ
045V3ZZ
045V4ZZ
045W0ZZ
045W3ZZ
045W4ZZ
045Y0ZZ
045Y3ZZ
045Y4ZZ
470341
047034Z
047035Z
047036Z
047037Z
04703D1
04703DZ
04703EZ
04703FZ
04703GZ
04703Z1
04703ZZ
471341
047134Z
047135Z
047136Z
047137Z
04713D1
04713DZ
04713EZ
04713FZ
04713GZ
04713Z1
04713ZZ
472341
047234Z
047235Z
047236Z
047237Z
04723D1
04723DZ
04723EZ
04723FZ
04723GZ
04723Z1
04723ZZ
473341
047334Z
047335Z
047336Z
047337Z
04733D1
04733DZ
04733EZ
04733FZ
04733GZ
04733Z1
04733ZZ
474341
047434Z
047435Z
047436Z
047437Z
04743D1
04743DZ
04743EZ
04743FZ
04743GZ
04743Z1
04743ZZ
475341
047534Z
047535Z
047536Z
047537Z
04753D1
04753DZ
04753EZ
04753FZ
04753GZ
04753Z1
04753ZZ
476341
047634Z
047635Z
047636Z
047637Z
04763D1
04763DZ
04763EZ
04763FZ
04763GZ
04763Z1
04763ZZ
477341
047734Z
047735Z
047736Z
047737Z
04773D1
04773DZ
04773EZ
04773FZ
04773GZ
04773Z1
04773ZZ
478341
047834Z
047835Z
047836Z
047837Z
04783D1
04783DZ
04783EZ
04783FZ
04783GZ
04783Z1
04783ZZ
479341
047934Z
047935Z
047936Z
047937Z
04793D1
04793DZ
04793EZ
04793FZ
04793GZ
04793Z1
04793ZZ
047A341
047A34Z
047A35Z
047A36Z
047A37Z
047A3D1
047A3DZ
047A3EZ
047A3FZ
047A3GZ
047A3Z1
047A3ZZ
047B341
047B34Z
047B35Z
047B36Z
047B37Z
047B3D1
047B3DZ
047B3EZ
047B3FZ
047B3GZ
047B3Z1
047B3ZZ
047C341
047C34Z
047C35Z
047C36Z
047C37Z
047C3D1
047C3DZ
047C3EZ
047C3FZ
047C3GZ
047C3Z1
047C3ZZ
047D341
047D34Z
047D35Z
047D36Z
047D37Z
047D3D1
047D3DZ
047D3EZ
047D3FZ
047D3GZ
047D3Z1
047D3ZZ
047E341
047E34Z
047E35Z
047E36Z
047E37Z
047E3D1
047E3DZ
047E3EZ
047E3FZ
047E3GZ
047E3Z1
047E3ZZ
047F341
047F34Z
047F35Z
047F36Z
047F37Z
047F3D1
047F3DZ
047F3EZ
047F3FZ
047F3GZ
047F3Z1
047F3ZZ
047H341
047H34Z
047H35Z
047H36Z
047H37Z
047H3D1
047H3DZ
047H3EZ
047H3FZ
047H3GZ
047H3Z1
047H3ZZ
047J341
047J34Z
047J35Z
047J36Z
047J37Z
047J3D1
047J3DZ
047J3EZ
047J3FZ
047J3GZ
047J3Z1
047J3ZZ
047K041
047K0D1
047K0Z1
047K341
047K34Z
047K35Z
047K36Z
047K37Z
047K3D1
047K3DZ
047K3EZ
047K3FZ
047K3GZ
047K3Z1
047K3ZZ
047K441
047K4D1
047K4Z1
047L041
047L0D1
047L0Z1
047L341
047L34Z
047L35Z
047L36Z
047L37Z
047L3D1
047L3DZ
047L3EZ
047L3FZ
047L3GZ
047L3Z1
047L3ZZ
047L441
047L4D1
047L4Z1
047M041
047M0D1
047M0Z1
047M341
047M3D1
047M3Z1
047M441
047M4D1
047M4Z1
047N041
047N0D1
047N0Z1
047N341
047N3D1
047N3Z1
047N441
047N4D1
047N4Z1
047Y341
047Y34Z
047Y35Z
047Y36Z
047Y37Z
047Y3D1
047Y3DZ
047Y3EZ
047Y3FZ
047Y3GZ
047Y3Z1
047Y3ZZ
04B00ZZ
04B03ZZ
04B04ZZ
04B10ZZ
04B14ZZ
04B20ZZ
04B24ZZ
04B30ZZ
04B34ZZ
04B40ZZ
04B44ZZ
04B50ZZ
04B54ZZ
04B60ZZ
04B64ZZ
04B70ZZ
04B74ZZ
04B80ZZ
04B84ZZ
04B90ZZ
04B94ZZ
04BA0ZZ
04BA4ZZ
04BB0ZZ
04BB4ZZ
04BC0ZZ
04BC4ZZ
04BD0ZZ
04BD4ZZ
04BE0ZZ
04BE4ZZ
04BF0ZZ
04BF4ZZ
04BH0ZZ
04BH4ZZ
04BJ0ZZ
04BJ4ZZ
04BK0ZZ
04BK3ZZ
04BK4ZZ
04BL0ZZ
04BL3ZZ
04BL4ZZ
04BM0ZZ
04BM3ZZ
04BM4ZZ
04BN0ZZ
04BN3ZZ
04BN4ZZ
04BP0ZZ
04BP3ZZ
04BP4ZZ
04BQ0ZZ
04BQ3ZZ
04BQ4ZZ
04BR0ZZ
04BR3ZZ
04BR4ZZ
04BS0ZZ
04BS3ZZ
04BS4ZZ
04BT0ZZ
04BT3ZZ
04BT4ZZ
04BU0ZZ
04BU3ZZ
04BU4ZZ
04BV0ZZ
04BV3ZZ
04BV4ZZ
04BW0ZZ
04BW3ZZ
04BW4ZZ
04BY0ZZ
04BY3ZZ
04BY4ZZ
04C00ZZ
04C03ZZ
04C04ZZ
04C10ZZ
04C13ZZ
04C14ZZ
04C20ZZ
04C23ZZ
04C24ZZ
04C30ZZ
04C33ZZ
04C34ZZ
04C40ZZ
04C43ZZ
04C44ZZ
04C50ZZ
04C53ZZ
04C54ZZ
04C60ZZ
04C63ZZ
04C64ZZ
04C70ZZ
04C73ZZ
04C74ZZ
04C80ZZ
04C83ZZ
04C84ZZ
04C90ZZ
04C93ZZ
04C94ZZ
04CA0ZZ
04CA3ZZ
04CA4ZZ
04CB0ZZ
04CB3ZZ
04CB4ZZ
04CC0ZZ
04CC3ZZ
04CC4ZZ
04CD0ZZ
04CD3ZZ
04CD4ZZ
04CE0ZZ
04CE3ZZ
04CE4ZZ
04CF0ZZ
04CF3ZZ
04CF4ZZ
04CH0ZZ
04CH3ZZ
04CH4ZZ
04CJ0ZZ
04CJ3ZZ
04CJ4ZZ
04CK0ZZ
04CK3ZZ
04CK4ZZ
04CL0ZZ
04CL3ZZ
04CL4ZZ
04CM0ZZ
04CM3ZZ
04CM4ZZ
04CN0ZZ
04CN3ZZ
04CN4ZZ
04CP0ZZ
04CP3ZZ
04CP4ZZ
04CQ0ZZ
04CQ3ZZ
04CQ4ZZ
04CR0ZZ
04CR3ZZ
04CR4ZZ
04CS0ZZ
04CS3ZZ
04CS4ZZ
04CT0ZZ
04CT3ZZ
04CT4ZZ
04CU0ZZ
04CU3ZZ
04CU4ZZ
04CV0ZZ
04CV3ZZ
04CV4ZZ
04CW0ZZ
04CW3ZZ
04CW4ZZ
04CY0ZZ
04CY3ZZ
04CY4ZZ
04H00DZ
04H03DZ
04H04DZ
04H10DZ
04H13DZ
04H14DZ
04H20DZ
04H23DZ
04H24DZ
04H30DZ
04H33DZ
04H34DZ
04H40DZ
04H43DZ
04H44DZ
04H50DZ
04H53DZ
04H54DZ
04H60DZ
04H63DZ
04H64DZ
04H70DZ
04H73DZ
04H74DZ
04H80DZ
04H83DZ
04H84DZ
04H90DZ
04H93DZ
04H94DZ
04HA0DZ
04HA3DZ
04HA4DZ
04HB0DZ
04HB3DZ
04HB4DZ
04HC0DZ
04HC3DZ
04HC4DZ
04HD0DZ
04HD3DZ
04HD4DZ
04HE0DZ
04HE3DZ
04HE4DZ
04HF0DZ
04HF3DZ
04HF4DZ
04HH0DZ
04HH3DZ
04HH4DZ
04HJ0DZ
04HJ3DZ
04HJ4DZ
04HK0DZ
04HK3DZ
04HK4DZ
04HL0DZ
04HL3DZ

04HL4DZ
04HM0DZ
04HM3DZ
04HM4DZ
04HN0DZ
04HN3DZ
04HN4DZ
04HP0DZ
04HP3DZ
04HP4DZ
04HQ0DZ
04HQ3DZ
04HQ4DZ
04HR0DZ
04HR3DZ
04HR4DZ
04HS0DZ
04HS3DZ
04HS4DZ
04HT0DZ
04HT3DZ
04HT4DZ
04HU0DZ
04HU3DZ
04HU4DZ
04HV0DZ
04HV3DZ
04HV4DZ
04HW0DZ
04HW3DZ
04HW4DZ
04HY02Z
04HY0DZ
04HY0YZ
04HY3DZ
04HY42Z
04HY4DZ
04L00CZ
04L00DJ
04L00DZ
04L00ZZ
04L03CZ
04L03DJ
04L03DZ
04L03ZZ
04L04CZ
04L04DZ
04L04ZZ
04L10CZ
04L10DZ
04L10ZZ
04L13CZ
04L13DZ
04L13ZZ
04L14CZ
04L14DZ
04L14ZZ
04L20CZ
04L20DZ
04L20ZZ
04L23CZ
04L23DZ
04L23ZZ
04L24CZ
04L24DZ
04L24ZZ
04L30CZ
04L30DZ
04L30ZZ
04L33CZ
04L33DZ
04L33ZZ
04L34CZ
04L34DZ
04L34ZZ
04L40CZ
04L40DZ
04L40ZZ
04L43CZ
04L43DZ
04L43ZZ
04L44CZ
04L44DZ
04L44ZZ
04L50CZ
04L50DZ
04L50ZZ
04L53CZ
04L53DZ
04L53ZZ
04L54CZ
04L54DZ
04L54ZZ
04L60CZ
04L60DZ
04L60ZZ
04L63CZ
04L63DZ
04L63ZZ
04L64CZ
04L64DZ
04L64ZZ
04L70CZ
04L70DZ
04L70ZZ
04L73CZ
04L73DZ
04L73ZZ
04L74CZ
04L74DZ
04L74ZZ
04L80CZ
04L80DZ
04L80ZZ
04L83CZ
04L83DZ
04L83ZZ
04L84CZ
04L84DZ
04L84ZZ
04L90CZ
04L90DZ
04L90ZZ
04L93CZ
04L93DZ
04L93ZZ
04L94CZ
04L94DZ
04L94ZZ
04LA0CZ
04LA0DZ
04LA0ZZ
04LA3CZ
04LA3DZ
04LA3ZZ
04LA4CZ
04LA4DZ
04LA4ZZ
04LB0CZ
04LB0DZ
04LB0ZZ
04LB3CZ
04LB3DZ
04LB3ZZ
04LB4CZ
04LB4DZ
04LB4ZZ
04LC0CZ
04LC0DZ
04LC0ZZ
04LC3CZ
04LC3DZ
04LC3ZZ
04LC4CZ
04LC4DZ
04LC4ZZ
04LD0CZ
04LD0DZ
04LD0ZZ
04LD3CZ
04LD3DZ
04LD3ZZ
04LD4CZ
04LD4DZ
04LD4ZZ
04LE0CV
04LE0CZ
04LE0DV
04LE0DZ
04LE0ZV
04LE0ZZ
04LE3CV
04LE3CZ
04LE3DV
04LE3DZ
04LE3ZV
04LE3ZZ
04LE4CV
04LE4CZ
04LE4DV
04LE4DZ
04LE4ZV
04LE4ZZ
04LF0CW
04LF0CZ
04LF0DW
04LF0DZ
04LF0ZW
04LF0ZZ
04LF3CW
04LF3CZ
04LF3DW
04LF3DZ
04LF3ZW
04LF3ZZ
04LF4CW
04LF4CZ
04LF4DW
04LF4DZ
04LF4ZW
04LF4ZZ
04LH0CZ
04LH0DZ
04LH0ZZ
04LH3CZ
04LH3DZ
04LH3ZZ
04LH4CZ
04LH4DZ
04LH4ZZ
04LJ0CZ
04LJ0DZ
04LJ0ZZ
04LJ3CZ
04LJ3DZ
04LJ3ZZ
04LJ4CZ
04LJ4DZ
04LJ4ZZ
04LK0CZ
04LK0DZ
04LK0ZZ
04LK3CZ
04LK3DZ
04LK3ZZ
04LK4CZ
04LK4DZ
04LK4ZZ
04LL0CZ
04LL0DZ
04LL0ZZ
04LL3CZ
04LL3DZ
04LL3ZZ
04LL4CZ
04LL4DZ
04LL4ZZ
04LM0CZ
04LM0DZ
04LM0ZZ
04LM3CZ
04LM3DZ
04LM3ZZ
04LM4CZ
04LM4DZ
04LM4ZZ
04LN0CZ
04LN0DZ
04LN0ZZ
04LN3CZ
04LN3DZ
04LN3ZZ
04LN4CZ
04LN4DZ
04LN4ZZ
04LP0CZ
04LP0DZ
04LP0ZZ
04LP3CZ
04LP3DZ
04LP3ZZ
04LP4CZ
04LP4DZ
04LP4ZZ
04LQ0CZ
04LQ0DZ
04LQ0ZZ
04LQ3CZ
04LQ3DZ
04LQ3ZZ
04LQ4CZ
04LQ4DZ
04LQ4ZZ
04LR0CZ
04LR0DZ
04LR0ZZ
04LR3CZ
04LR3DZ
04LR3ZZ
04LR4CZ
04LR4DZ
04LR4ZZ
04LS0CZ
04LS0DZ
04LS0ZZ
04LS3CZ
04LS3DZ
04LS3ZZ
04LS4CZ
04LS4DZ
04LS4ZZ
04LT0CZ
04LT0DZ
04LT0ZZ
04LT3CZ
04LT3DZ
04LT3ZZ
04LT4CZ
04LT4DZ
04LT4ZZ
04LU0CZ
04LU0DZ
04LU0ZZ
04LU3CZ
04LU3DZ
04LU3ZZ
04LU4CZ
04LU4DZ
04LU4ZZ
04LV0CZ
04LV0DZ
04LV0ZZ
04LV3CZ
04LV3DZ
04LV3ZZ
04LV4CZ
04LV4DZ
04LV4ZZ
04LW0CZ
04LW0DZ
04LW0ZZ
04LW3CZ
04LW3DZ
04LW3ZZ
04LW4CZ
04LW4DZ
04LW4ZZ
04LY0CZ
04LY0DZ
04LY0ZZ
04LY3CZ
04LY3DZ
04LY3ZZ
04LY4CZ
04LY4DZ
04LY4ZZ
04PY00Z
04PY02Z
04PY03Z
04PY0CZ
04PY0DZ
04PY0YZ
04PY3CZ
04PY40Z
04PY42Z
04PY43Z
04PY4CZ
04PY4DZ
04Q00ZZ
04Q03ZZ
04Q04ZZ
04Q10ZZ
04Q13ZZ
04Q14ZZ
04Q20ZZ
04Q23ZZ
04Q24ZZ
04Q30ZZ
04Q33ZZ
04Q34ZZ
04Q40ZZ
04Q43ZZ
04Q44ZZ
04Q50ZZ
04Q53ZZ
04Q54ZZ
04Q60ZZ
04Q63ZZ
04Q64ZZ
04Q70ZZ
04Q73ZZ
04Q74ZZ
04Q80ZZ
04Q83ZZ
04Q84ZZ
04Q90ZZ
04Q93ZZ
04Q94ZZ
04QA0ZZ
04QA3ZZ
04QA4ZZ
04QB0ZZ
04QB3ZZ
04QB4ZZ
04QC0ZZ
04QC3ZZ
04QC4ZZ
04QD0ZZ
04QD3ZZ
04QD4ZZ
04QE0ZZ
04QE3ZZ
04QE4ZZ
04QF0ZZ
04QF3ZZ
04QF4ZZ
04QH0ZZ
04QH3ZZ
04QH4ZZ
04QJ0ZZ
04QJ3ZZ
04QJ4ZZ
04QK0ZZ
04QK3ZZ
04QK4ZZ
04QL0ZZ
04QL3ZZ
04QL4ZZ
04QM0ZZ
04QM3ZZ
04QM4ZZ
04QN0ZZ
04QN3ZZ
04QN4ZZ
04QP0ZZ
04QP3ZZ
04QP4ZZ
04QQ0ZZ
04QQ3ZZ
04QQ4ZZ
04QR0ZZ
04QR3ZZ
04QR4ZZ
04QS0ZZ
04QS3ZZ
04QS4ZZ
04QT0ZZ
04QT3ZZ
04QT4ZZ
04QU0ZZ
04QU3ZZ
04QU4ZZ
04QV0ZZ
04QV3ZZ
04QV4ZZ
04QW0ZZ
04QW3ZZ
04QW4ZZ
04QY0ZZ
04QY3ZZ
04QY4ZZ
04R007Z
04R00JZ
04R00KZ
04R047Z
04R04JZ
04R04KZ
04R107Z
04R10JZ
04R10KZ
04R147Z
04R14JZ
04R14KZ
04R207Z
04R20JZ
04R20KZ
04R247Z
04R24JZ
04R24KZ
04R307Z
04R30JZ
04R30KZ
04R347Z
04R34JZ
04R34KZ
04R407Z
04R40JZ
04R40KZ
04R447Z
04R44JZ
04R44KZ
04R507Z
04R50JZ
04R50KZ
04R547Z
04R54JZ
04R54KZ
04R607Z
04R60JZ
04R60KZ
04R647Z
04R64JZ
04R64KZ
04R707Z
04R70JZ
04R70KZ
04R747Z
04R74JZ
04R74KZ
04R807Z
04R80JZ
04R80KZ
04R847Z
04R84JZ
04R84KZ
04RB07Z
04RB0JZ
04RB0KZ
04RB47Z
04RB4JZ
04RB4KZ
04RC07Z
04RC0JZ
04RC0KZ
04RC47Z
04RC4JZ
04RC4KZ
04RD07Z
04RD0JZ
04RD0KZ
04RD47Z
04RD4JZ
04RD4KZ
04RE07Z
04RE0JZ
04RE0KZ
04RE47Z
04RE4JZ
04RE4KZ
04RF07Z
04RF0JZ
04RF0KZ
04RF47Z
04RF4JZ
04RF4KZ
04RH07Z
04RH0JZ
04RH0KZ
04RH47Z
04RH4JZ
04RH4KZ
04RJ07Z
04RJ0JZ
04RJ0KZ
04RJ47Z
04RJ4JZ
04RJ4KZ
04RK07Z
04RK0JZ
04RK0KZ
04RK47Z
04RK4JZ
04RK4KZ
04RL07Z
04RL0JZ
04RL0KZ
04RL47Z
04RL4JZ
04RL4KZ
04RM07Z
04RM0JZ
04RM0KZ
04RM47Z
04RM4JZ
04RM4KZ
04RN07Z
04RN0JZ
04RN0KZ
04RN47Z
04RN4JZ
04RN4KZ
04RP07Z
04RP0JZ
04RP0KZ
04RP47Z
04RP4JZ
04RP4KZ
04RQ07Z
04RQ0JZ
04RQ0KZ
04RQ47Z
04RQ4JZ
04RQ4KZ
04RR07Z
04RR0JZ
04RR0KZ
04RR47Z
04RR4JZ
04RR4KZ
04RS07Z
04RS0JZ
04RS0KZ
04RS47Z
04RS4JZ
04RS4KZ
04RT07Z
04RT0JZ
04RT0KZ
04RT47Z
04RT4JZ
04RT4KZ
04RU07Z
04RU0JZ
04RU0KZ
04RU47Z
04RU4JZ
04RU4KZ
04RV07Z
04RV0JZ
04RV0KZ
04RV47Z
04RV4JZ
04RV4KZ
04RW07Z
04RW0JZ
04RW0KZ
04RW47Z
04RW4JZ
04RW4KZ
04RY07Z
04RY0JZ
04RY0KZ
04RY47Z
04RY4JZ
04RY4KZ
04S00ZZ
04S03ZZ
04S04ZZ
04S10ZZ
04S13ZZ
04S14ZZ
04S20ZZ
04S23ZZ
04S24ZZ
04S30ZZ
04S33ZZ
04S34ZZ
04S40ZZ
04S43ZZ
04S44ZZ
04S50ZZ
04S53ZZ
04S54ZZ
04S60ZZ
04S63ZZ
04S64ZZ
04S70ZZ
04S73ZZ
04S74ZZ
04S80ZZ
04S83ZZ
04S84ZZ
04SB0ZZ
04SB3ZZ
04SB4ZZ
04SC0ZZ
04SC3ZZ
04SC4ZZ
04SD0ZZ
04SD3ZZ
04SD4ZZ
04SE0ZZ
04SE3ZZ
04SE4ZZ
04SF0ZZ
04SF3ZZ
04SF4ZZ
04SH0ZZ
04SH3ZZ
04SH4ZZ
04SJ0ZZ
04SJ3ZZ
04SJ4ZZ
04SK0ZZ
04SK3ZZ
04SK4ZZ
04SL0ZZ
04SL3ZZ
04SL4ZZ
04SM0ZZ
04SM3ZZ
04SM4ZZ
04SN0ZZ
04SN3ZZ
04SN4ZZ
04SP0ZZ
04SP3ZZ
04SP4ZZ
04SQ0ZZ
04SQ3ZZ
04SQ4ZZ
04SR0ZZ
04SR3ZZ
04SR4ZZ
04SS0ZZ
04SS3ZZ
04SS4ZZ
04ST0ZZ
04ST3ZZ
04ST4ZZ
04SU0ZZ
04SU3ZZ
04SU4ZZ
04SV0ZZ
04SV3ZZ
04SV4ZZ
04SW0ZZ
04SW3ZZ
04SW4ZZ
04SY0ZZ
04SY3ZZ
04SY4ZZ
04U007Z
04U037Z
04U03JZ
04U047Z
04U04JZ
04U107Z
04U137Z
04U147Z
04U207Z
04U237Z
04U247Z
04U307Z
04U337Z
04U347Z
04U407Z
04U437Z
04U447Z
04U507Z
04U537Z
04U547Z
04U607Z
04U637Z
04U647Z
04U707Z
04U737Z
04U747Z
04U807Z
04U837Z
04U847Z
04U907Z
04U937Z
04U947Z
04UA07Z
04UA37Z
04UA47Z
04UB07Z
04UB37Z
04UB47Z
04UC07Z
04UC37Z
04UC47Z
04UD07Z
04UD37Z
04UD47Z
04UE07Z
04UE37Z
04UE47Z
04UF07Z
04UF37Z
04UF47Z
04UH07Z
04UH37Z
04UH47Z
04UJ07Z
04UJ37Z
04UJ47Z
04UK07Z
04UK37Z
04UK47Z
04UL07Z
04UL37Z
04UL47Z
04UM07Z
04UM37Z
04UM47Z
04UN07Z
04UN37Z
04UN47Z
04UP07Z
04UP37Z
04UP47Z
04UQ07Z
04UQ37Z
04UQ47Z
04UR07Z
04UR37Z
04UR47Z
04US07Z
04US37Z
04US47Z
04UT07Z
04UT37Z
04UT47Z
04UU07Z
04UU37Z
04UU47Z
04UV07Z
04UV37Z
04UV47Z
04UW07Z
04UW37Z
04UW47Z
04UY07Z
04UY37Z
04UY47Z
04V00DJ
04V00DZ
04V00EZ
04V00FZ
04V03DJ
04V03DZ
04V03EZ
04V03FZ
04V04DJ
04V04DZ
04V04EZ
04V04FZ
04V10DZ
04V13DZ
04V14DZ
04V20DZ
04V23DZ
04V24DZ
04V30DZ
04V33DZ
04V34DZ
04V40DZ
04V43DZ
04V44DZ
04V50DZ
04V53DZ
04V54DZ
04V60DZ
04V63DZ
04V64DZ
04V70DZ
04V73DZ
04V74DZ
04V80DZ
04V83DZ
04V84DZ
04V90DZ
04V93DZ
04V94DZ
04VA0DZ
04VA3DZ
04VA4DZ
04VB0DZ
04VB3DZ
04VB4DZ
04VC0DZ
04VC0EZ
04VC3DZ
04VC3EZ
04VC4DZ
04VC4EZ
04VD0DZ
04VD0EZ
04VD3DZ
04VD3EZ
04VD4DZ
04VD4EZ
04VE0DZ

Ø4VE3DZ
Ø4VE4DZ
Ø4VFØDZ
Ø4VF3DZ
Ø4VF4DZ
Ø4VHØDZ
Ø4VH3DZ
Ø4VH4DZ
Ø4VJØDZ
Ø4VJ3DZ
Ø4VJ4DZ
Ø4VKØDZ
Ø4VK3DZ
Ø4VK4DZ
Ø4VLØDZ
Ø4VL3DZ
Ø4VL4DZ
Ø4VMØDZ
Ø4VM3DZ
Ø4VM4DZ
Ø4VNØDZ
Ø4VN3DZ
Ø4VN4DZ
Ø4VPØDZ
Ø4VP3DZ
Ø4VP4DZ
Ø4VQØDZ
Ø4VQ3DZ
Ø4VQ4DZ
Ø4VRØDZ
Ø4VR3DZ
Ø4VR4DZ
Ø4VSØDZ
Ø4VS3DZ
Ø4VS4DZ
Ø4VTØDZ
Ø4VT3DZ
Ø4VT4DZ
Ø4VUØDZ
Ø4VU3DZ
Ø4VU4DZ
Ø4VVØDZ
Ø4VV3DZ
Ø4VV4DZ
Ø4VWØDZ
Ø4VW3DZ
Ø4VW4DZ
Ø4VYØDZ
Ø4VY3DZ
Ø4VY4DZ
Ø4WYØØZ
Ø4WYØ2Z
Ø4WYØ3Z
Ø4WYØCZ
Ø4WYØDZ
Ø4WYØYZ
Ø4WY3CZ
Ø4WY4ØZ
Ø4WY42Z
Ø4WY43Z
Ø4WY4CZ
Ø4WY4DZ
Ø51ØØ7Y
Ø51ØØ9Y
Ø51ØØAY
Ø51ØØJY
Ø51ØØKY
Ø51ØØZY
Ø51Ø47Y
Ø51Ø49Y
Ø51Ø4AY
Ø51Ø4JY
Ø51Ø4KY
Ø51Ø4ZY
Ø511Ø7Y
Ø511Ø9Y
Ø511ØAY
Ø511ØJY
Ø511ØKY
Ø511ØZY
Ø51147Y
Ø51149Y
Ø5114AY
Ø5114JY
Ø5114KY
Ø5114ZY
Ø513Ø7Y
Ø513Ø9Y
Ø513ØAY
Ø513ØJY
Ø513ØKY
Ø513ØZY
Ø51347Y
Ø51349Y
Ø5134AY
Ø5134JY
Ø5134KY
Ø5134ZY
Ø514Ø7Y
Ø514Ø9Y
Ø514ØAY
Ø514ØJY
Ø514ØKY
Ø514ØZY
Ø51447Y
Ø51449Y
Ø5144AY
Ø5144JY
Ø5144KY
Ø5144ZY
Ø515Ø7Y
Ø515Ø9Y
Ø515ØAY
Ø515ØJY
Ø515ØKY
Ø515ØZY
Ø51547Y
Ø51549Y
Ø5154AY
Ø5154JY
Ø5154KY
Ø5154ZY
Ø516Ø7Y
Ø516Ø9Y
Ø516ØAY
Ø516ØJY
Ø516ØKY
Ø516ØZY
Ø51647Y
Ø51649Y
Ø5164AY
Ø5164JY
Ø5164KY
Ø5164ZY
Ø55LØZZ
Ø55L3ZZ
Ø55L4ZZ
Ø5793D1
Ø5793DZ
Ø5793Z1
Ø5793ZZ
Ø57A3D1
Ø57A3DZ
Ø57A3Z1
Ø57A3ZZ
Ø57B3D1
Ø57B3DZ
Ø57B3Z1
Ø57B3ZZ
Ø57C3D1
Ø57C3DZ
Ø57C3Z1
Ø57C3ZZ
Ø57D3D1
Ø57D3DZ
Ø57D3Z1
Ø57D3ZZ
Ø57F3D1
Ø57F3DZ
Ø57F3Z1
Ø57F3ZZ
Ø57L3DZ
Ø57L4DZ
Ø57M3DZ
Ø57M4DZ
Ø57N3DZ
Ø57N4DZ
Ø57P3DZ
Ø57P4DZ
Ø57Q3DZ
Ø57Q4DZ
Ø57R3DZ
Ø57R4DZ
Ø57S3DZ
Ø57S4DZ
Ø57T3DZ
Ø57T4DZ
Ø5B7ØZZ
Ø5B74ZZ
Ø5B8ØZZ
Ø5B84ZZ
Ø5B9ØZZ
Ø5B94ZZ
Ø5BAØZZ
Ø5BA4ZZ
Ø5BBØZZ
Ø5BB4ZZ
Ø5BCØZZ
Ø5BC4ZZ
Ø5BDØZZ
Ø5BD4ZZ
Ø5BFØZZ
Ø5BF4ZZ
Ø5BGØZZ
Ø5BG4ZZ
Ø5BHØZZ
Ø5BH4ZZ
Ø5BLØZZ
Ø5BL3ZZ
Ø5BL4ZZ
Ø5BMØZZ
Ø5BM4ZZ
Ø5BNØZZ
Ø5BN4ZZ
Ø5BPØZZ
Ø5BP4ZZ
Ø5BQØZZ
Ø5BQ4ZZ
Ø5BRØZZ
Ø5BR4ZZ
Ø5BSØZZ
Ø5BS4ZZ
Ø5BTØZZ
Ø5BT4ZZ
Ø5BVØZZ
Ø5BV4ZZ
Ø5BYØZZ
Ø5BY3ZZ
Ø5BY4ZZ
Ø5CLØZZ
Ø5CL3ZZ
Ø5CL4ZZ
Ø5CMØZZ
Ø5CM3ZZ
Ø5CM4ZZ
Ø5CNØZZ
Ø5CN3ZZ
Ø5CN4ZZ
Ø5CPØZZ
Ø5CP3ZZ
Ø5CP4ZZ
Ø5CQØZZ
Ø5CQ3ZZ
Ø5CQ4ZZ
Ø5CRØZZ
Ø5CR3ZZ
Ø5CR4ZZ
Ø5CSØZZ
Ø5CS3ZZ
Ø5CS4ZZ
Ø5CTØZZ
Ø5CT3ZZ
Ø5CT4ZZ
Ø5CVØZZ
Ø5CV3ZZ
Ø5CV4ZZ
Ø5CYØZZ
Ø5CY3ZZ
Ø5CY4ZZ
Ø5HØØDZ
Ø5HØØMZ
Ø5HØ3DZ
Ø5HØ3MZ
Ø5HØ4DZ
Ø5HØ4MZ
Ø5H1ØDZ
Ø5H13DZ
Ø5H14DZ
Ø5H3ØDZ
Ø5H3ØMZ
Ø5H33DZ
Ø5H33MZ
Ø5H34DZ
Ø5H34MZ
Ø5H4ØDZ
Ø5H4ØMZ
Ø5H43DZ
Ø5H43MZ
Ø5H44DZ
Ø5H44MZ
Ø5H5ØDZ
Ø5H53DZ
Ø5H54DZ
Ø5H6ØDZ
Ø5H63DZ
Ø5H64DZ
Ø5H7ØDZ
Ø5H73DZ
Ø5H74DZ
Ø5H8ØDZ
Ø5H83DZ
Ø5H84DZ
Ø5H9ØDZ
Ø5H93DZ
Ø5H94DZ
Ø5HAØDZ
Ø5HA3DZ
Ø5HA4DZ
Ø5HBØDZ
Ø5HB3DZ
Ø5HB4DZ
Ø5HCØDZ
Ø5HC3DZ
Ø5HC4DZ
Ø5HDØDZ
Ø5HD3DZ
Ø5HD4DZ
Ø5HFØDZ
Ø5HF3DZ
Ø5HF4DZ
Ø5HGØDZ
Ø5HG3DZ
Ø5HG4DZ
Ø5HHØDZ
Ø5HH3DZ
Ø5HH4DZ
Ø5HLØDZ
Ø5HL3DZ
Ø5HL4DZ
Ø5HMØDZ
Ø5HM3DZ
Ø5HM4DZ
Ø5HNØDZ
Ø5HN3DZ
Ø5HN4DZ
Ø5HPØDZ
Ø5HP3DZ
Ø5HP4DZ
Ø5HQØDZ
Ø5HQ3DZ
Ø5HQ4DZ
Ø5HRØDZ
Ø5HR3DZ
Ø5HR4DZ
Ø5HSØDZ
Ø5HS3DZ
Ø5HS4DZ
Ø5HTØDZ
Ø5HT3DZ
Ø5HT4DZ
Ø5HVØDZ
Ø5HV3DZ
Ø5HV4DZ
Ø5HYØ2Z
Ø5HYØDZ
Ø5HYØYZ
Ø5HY3DZ
Ø5HY42Z
Ø5HY4DZ
Ø5L7ØCZ
Ø5L7ØDZ
Ø5L7ØZZ
Ø5L73CZ
Ø5L73DZ
Ø5L73ZZ
Ø5L74CZ
Ø5L74DZ
Ø5L74ZZ
Ø5L8ØCZ
Ø5L8ØDZ
Ø5L8ØZZ
Ø5L83CZ
Ø5L83DZ
Ø5L83ZZ
Ø5L84CZ
Ø5L84DZ
Ø5L84ZZ
Ø5L9ØCZ
Ø5L9ØDZ
Ø5L9ØZZ
Ø5L93CZ
Ø5L93DZ
Ø5L93ZZ
Ø5L94CZ
Ø5L94DZ
Ø5L94ZZ
Ø5LAØCZ
Ø5LAØDZ
Ø5LAØZZ
Ø5LA3CZ
Ø5LA3DZ
Ø5LA3ZZ
Ø5LA4CZ
Ø5LA4DZ
Ø5LA4ZZ
Ø5LBØCZ
Ø5LBØDZ
Ø5LBØZZ
Ø5LB3CZ
Ø5LB3DZ
Ø5LB3ZZ
Ø5LB4CZ
Ø5LB4DZ
Ø5LB4ZZ
Ø5LCØCZ
Ø5LCØDZ
Ø5LCØZZ
Ø5LC3CZ
Ø5LC3DZ
Ø5LC3ZZ
Ø5LC4CZ
Ø5LC4DZ
Ø5LC4ZZ
Ø5LDØCZ
Ø5LDØDZ
Ø5LDØZZ
Ø5LD3CZ
Ø5LD3DZ
Ø5LD3ZZ
Ø5LD4CZ
Ø5LD4DZ
Ø5LD4ZZ
Ø5LFØCZ
Ø5LFØDZ
Ø5LFØZZ
Ø5LF3CZ
Ø5LF3DZ
Ø5LF3ZZ
Ø5LF4CZ
Ø5LF4DZ
Ø5LF4ZZ
Ø5LGØCZ
Ø5LGØDZ
Ø5LGØZZ
Ø5LG3CZ
Ø5LG3DZ
Ø5LG3ZZ
Ø5LG4CZ
Ø5LG4DZ
Ø5LG4ZZ
Ø5LHØCZ
Ø5LHØDZ
Ø5LHØZZ
Ø5LH3CZ
Ø5LH3DZ
Ø5LH3ZZ
Ø5LH4CZ
Ø5LH4DZ
Ø5LH4ZZ
Ø5LMØCZ
Ø5LMØDZ
Ø5LMØZZ
Ø5LM3CZ
Ø5LM3DZ
Ø5LM3ZZ
Ø5LM4CZ
Ø5LM4DZ
Ø5LM4ZZ
Ø5LNØCZ
Ø5LNØDZ
Ø5LNØZZ
Ø5LN3CZ
Ø5LN3DZ
Ø5LN3ZZ
Ø5LN4CZ
Ø5LN4DZ
Ø5LN4ZZ
Ø5LPØCZ
Ø5LPØDZ
Ø5LPØZZ
Ø5LP3CZ
Ø5LP3DZ
Ø5LP3ZZ
Ø5LP4CZ
Ø5LP4DZ
Ø5LP4ZZ
Ø5LQØCZ
Ø5LQØDZ
Ø5LQØZZ
Ø5LQ3CZ
Ø5LQ3DZ
Ø5LQ3ZZ
Ø5LQ4CZ
Ø5LQ4DZ
Ø5LQ4ZZ
Ø5LRØCZ
Ø5LRØDZ
Ø5LRØZZ
Ø5LR3CZ
Ø5LR3DZ
Ø5LR3ZZ
Ø5LR4CZ
Ø5LR4DZ
Ø5LR4ZZ
Ø5LSØCZ
Ø5LSØDZ
Ø5LSØZZ
Ø5LS3CZ
Ø5LS3DZ
Ø5LS3ZZ
Ø5LS4CZ
Ø5LS4DZ
Ø5LS4ZZ
Ø5LTØCZ
Ø5LTØDZ
Ø5LTØZZ
Ø5LT3CZ
Ø5LT3DZ
Ø5LT3ZZ
Ø5LT4CZ
Ø5LT4DZ
Ø5LT4ZZ
Ø5LVØCZ
Ø5LVØDZ
Ø5LVØZZ
Ø5LV3CZ
Ø5LV3DZ
Ø5LV3ZZ
Ø5LV4CZ
Ø5LV4DZ
Ø5LV4ZZ
Ø5LYØCZ
Ø5LYØZZ
Ø5LY3CZ
Ø5LY3DZ
Ø5LY3ZZ
Ø5LY4CZ
Ø5LY4DZ
Ø5LY4ZZ
Ø5PØØMZ
Ø5PØ3MZ
Ø5PØ4MZ
Ø5PØXMZ
Ø5P3ØMZ
Ø5P33MZ
Ø5P34MZ
Ø5P3XMZ
Ø5P4ØMZ
Ø5P43MZ
Ø5P44MZ
Ø5P4XMZ
Ø5QØØZZ
Ø5QØ3ZZ
Ø5QØ4ZZ
Ø5Q1ØZZ
Ø5Q13ZZ
Ø5Q14ZZ
Ø5Q3ØZZ
Ø5Q33ZZ
Ø5Q34ZZ
Ø5Q4ØZZ
Ø5Q43ZZ
Ø5Q44ZZ
Ø5Q5ØZZ
Ø5Q53ZZ
Ø5Q54ZZ
Ø5Q6ØZZ
Ø5Q63ZZ
Ø5Q64ZZ
Ø5Q7ØZZ
Ø5Q73ZZ
Ø5Q74ZZ
Ø5Q8ØZZ
Ø5Q83ZZ
Ø5Q84ZZ
Ø5Q9ØZZ
Ø5Q93ZZ
Ø5Q94ZZ
Ø5QAØZZ
Ø5QA3ZZ
Ø5QA4ZZ
Ø5QBØZZ
Ø5QB3ZZ
Ø5QB4ZZ
Ø5QCØZZ
Ø5QC3ZZ
Ø5QC4ZZ
Ø5QDØZZ
Ø5QD3ZZ
Ø5QD4ZZ
Ø5QFØZZ
Ø5QF3ZZ
Ø5QF4ZZ
Ø5QGØZZ
Ø5QG3ZZ
Ø5QG4ZZ
Ø5QHØZZ
Ø5QH3ZZ
Ø5QH4ZZ
Ø5QLØZZ
Ø5QL3ZZ
Ø5QL4ZZ
Ø5QMØZZ
Ø5QM3ZZ
Ø5QM4ZZ
Ø5QNØZZ
Ø5QN3ZZ
Ø5QN4ZZ
Ø5QPØZZ
Ø5QP3ZZ
Ø5QP4ZZ
Ø5QQØZZ
Ø5QQ3ZZ
Ø5QQ4ZZ
Ø5QRØZZ
Ø5QR3ZZ
Ø5QR4ZZ
Ø5QSØZZ
Ø5QS3ZZ
Ø5QS4ZZ
Ø5QTØZZ
Ø5QT3ZZ
Ø5QT4ZZ
Ø5QVØZZ
Ø5QV3ZZ
Ø5QV4ZZ
Ø5QYØZZ
Ø5QY3ZZ
Ø5QY4ZZ
Ø5RØØ7Z
Ø5RØØJZ
Ø5RØØKZ
Ø5RØ47Z
Ø5RØ4JZ
Ø5RØ4KZ
Ø5R1Ø7Z
Ø5R1ØJZ
Ø5R1ØKZ
Ø5R147Z
Ø5R14JZ
Ø5R14KZ
Ø5R3Ø7Z
Ø5R3ØJZ
Ø5R3ØKZ
Ø5R347Z
Ø5R34JZ
Ø5R34KZ
Ø5R4Ø7Z
Ø5R4ØJZ
Ø5R4ØKZ
Ø5R447Z
Ø5R44JZ
Ø5R44KZ
Ø5R5Ø7Z
Ø5R5ØJZ
Ø5R5ØKZ
Ø5R547Z
Ø5R54JZ
Ø5R54KZ
Ø5R6Ø7Z
Ø5R6ØJZ
Ø5R6ØKZ
Ø5R647Z
Ø5R64JZ
Ø5R64KZ
Ø5RLØ7Z
Ø5RLØJZ
Ø5RLØKZ
Ø5RL47Z
Ø5RL4JZ
Ø5RL4KZ
Ø5SØØZZ
Ø5SØ3ZZ
Ø5SØ4ZZ
Ø5S1ØZZ
Ø5S13ZZ
Ø5S14ZZ
Ø5S3ØZZ
Ø5S33ZZ
Ø5S34ZZ
Ø5S4ØZZ
Ø5S43ZZ
Ø5S44ZZ
Ø5S5ØZZ
Ø5S53ZZ
Ø5S54ZZ
Ø5S6ØZZ
Ø5S63ZZ
Ø5S64ZZ
Ø5S7ØZZ
Ø5S73ZZ
Ø5S74ZZ
Ø5S8ØZZ
Ø5S83ZZ
Ø5S84ZZ
Ø5S9ØZZ
Ø5S93ZZ
Ø5S94ZZ
Ø5SAØZZ
Ø5SA3ZZ
Ø5SA4ZZ
Ø5SBØZZ
Ø5SB3ZZ
Ø5SB4ZZ
Ø5SCØZZ
Ø5SC3ZZ
Ø5SC4ZZ
Ø5SDØZZ
Ø5SD3ZZ
Ø5SD4ZZ
Ø5SFØZZ
Ø5SF3ZZ
Ø5SF4ZZ
Ø5SGØZZ
Ø5SG3ZZ
Ø5SG4ZZ
Ø5SHØZZ
Ø5SH3ZZ
Ø5SH4ZZ
Ø5SLØZZ
Ø5SL3ZZ
Ø5SL4ZZ
Ø5SMØZZ
Ø5SM3ZZ
Ø5SM4ZZ
Ø5SNØZZ
Ø5SN3ZZ
Ø5SN4ZZ
Ø5SPØZZ
Ø5SP3ZZ
Ø5SP4ZZ
Ø5SQØZZ
Ø5SQ3ZZ
Ø5SQ4ZZ
Ø5SRØZZ
Ø5SR3ZZ
Ø5SR4ZZ
Ø5SSØZZ
Ø5SS3ZZ
Ø5SS4ZZ
Ø5STØZZ
Ø5ST3ZZ
Ø5ST4ZZ
Ø5SVØZZ
Ø5SV3ZZ
Ø5SV4ZZ
Ø5SYØZZ
Ø5SY3ZZ
Ø5SY4ZZ
Ø5UØØ7Z
Ø5UØ37Z
Ø5UØ47Z
Ø5U1Ø7Z
Ø5U137Z
Ø5U147Z
Ø5U3Ø7Z
Ø5U337Z
Ø5U347Z
Ø5U4Ø7Z
Ø5U437Z
Ø5U447Z
Ø5U5Ø7Z
Ø5U537Z
Ø5U547Z
Ø5U6Ø7Z
Ø5U637Z
Ø5U647Z
Ø5U7Ø7Z
Ø5U737Z
Ø5U747Z
Ø5U8Ø7Z
Ø5U837Z
Ø5U847Z
Ø5U9Ø7Z
Ø5U937Z
Ø5U947Z
Ø5UAØ7Z
Ø5UA37Z
Ø5UA47Z
Ø5UBØ7Z
Ø5UB37Z
Ø5UB47Z
Ø5UCØ7Z
Ø5UC37Z
Ø5UC47Z
Ø5UDØ7Z
Ø5UD37Z
Ø5UD47Z
Ø5UFØ7Z
Ø5UF37Z
Ø5UF47Z
Ø5UGØ7Z
Ø5UG37Z
Ø5UG47Z
Ø5UHØ7Z
Ø5UH37Z
Ø5UH47Z
Ø5ULØ7Z
Ø5UL37Z
Ø5UL47Z
Ø5UMØ7Z
Ø5UM37Z
Ø5UM47Z
Ø5UNØ7Z
Ø5UN37Z
Ø5UN47Z
Ø5UPØ7Z
Ø5UP37Z
Ø5UP47Z
Ø5UQØ7Z
Ø5UQ37Z
Ø5UQ47Z
Ø5URØ7Z
Ø5UR37Z
Ø5UR47Z
Ø5USØ7Z
Ø5US37Z
Ø5US47Z
Ø5UTØ7Z
Ø5UT37Z
Ø5UT47Z
Ø5UVØ7Z
Ø5UV37Z
Ø5UV47Z
Ø5UYØ7Z
Ø5UY37Z
Ø5UY47Z
Ø5VØØDZ
Ø5VØ3DZ
Ø5VØ4DZ
Ø5V1ØDZ
Ø5V13DZ
Ø5V14DZ
Ø5V3ØDZ
Ø5V33DZ
Ø5V34DZ
Ø5V4ØDZ
Ø5V43DZ
Ø5V44DZ
Ø5V5ØDZ
Ø5V53DZ
Ø5V54DZ
Ø5V6ØDZ
Ø5V63DZ
Ø5V64DZ
Ø5V7ØDZ
Ø5V73DZ
Ø5V74DZ
Ø5V8ØDZ
Ø5V83DZ
Ø5V84DZ
Ø5V9ØDZ
Ø5V93DZ
Ø5V94DZ
Ø5VAØDZ
Ø5VA3DZ
Ø5VA4DZ
Ø5VBØDZ
Ø5VB3DZ
Ø5VB4DZ
Ø5VCØDZ
Ø5VC3DZ
Ø5VC4DZ
Ø5VDØDZ
Ø5VD3DZ
Ø5VD4DZ
Ø5VFØDZ
Ø5VF3DZ
Ø5VF4DZ
Ø5VGØDZ
Ø5VG3DZ
Ø5VG4DZ
Ø5VHØDZ
Ø5VH3DZ
Ø5VH4DZ
Ø5VLØDZ
Ø5VL3DZ
Ø5VL4DZ
Ø5VMØDZ
Ø5VM3DZ
Ø5VM4DZ
Ø5VNØDZ
Ø5VN3DZ
Ø5VN4DZ
Ø5VPØDZ

Ø5VP3DZ
Ø5VP4DZ
Ø5VQØDZ
Ø5VQ3DZ
Ø5VQ4DZ
Ø5VRØDZ
Ø5VR3DZ
Ø5VR4DZ
Ø5VSØDZ
Ø5VS3DZ
Ø5VS4DZ
Ø5VTØDZ
Ø5VT3DZ
Ø5VT4DZ
Ø5VVØDZ
Ø5VV3DZ
Ø5VV4DZ
Ø65MØZZ
Ø65M3ZZ
Ø65M4ZZ
Ø65NØZZ
Ø65N3ZZ
Ø65N4ZZ
Ø65PØZZ
Ø65P3ZZ
Ø65P4ZZ
Ø65QØZZ
Ø65Q3ZZ
Ø65Q4ZZ
Ø65TØZZ
Ø65T3ZZ
Ø65T4ZZ
Ø65VØZZ
Ø65V3ZZ
Ø65V4ZZ
Ø65YØZZ
Ø65Y3ZZ
Ø65Y4ZZ
Ø67Ø3DZ
Ø67Ø3ZZ
Ø693ØØZ
Ø693ØZZ
Ø6934ØZ
Ø6934ZZ
Ø6BMØZZ
Ø6BM3ZZ
Ø6BM4ZZ
Ø6BNØZZ
Ø6BN3ZZ
Ø6BN4ZZ
Ø6BPØZZ
Ø6BP3ZZ
Ø6BP4ZZ
Ø6BQØZZ
Ø6BQ3ZZ
Ø6BQ4ZZ
Ø6BTØZZ
Ø6BT3ZZ
Ø6BT4ZZ
Ø6BVØZZ
Ø6BV3ZZ
Ø6BV4ZZ
Ø6BYØZZ
Ø6BY3ZZ
Ø6BY4ZZ
Ø6C3ØZZ
Ø6C33ZZ
Ø6C34ZZ
Ø6CMØZZ
Ø6CM3ZZ
Ø6CM4ZZ
Ø6CNØZZ
Ø6CN3ZZ
Ø6CN4ZZ
Ø6CPØZZ
Ø6CP3ZZ
Ø6CP4ZZ
Ø6CQØZZ
Ø6CQ3ZZ
Ø6CQ4ZZ
Ø6CTØZZ
Ø6CT3ZZ
Ø6CT4ZZ
Ø6CVØZZ
Ø6CV3ZZ
Ø6CV4ZZ
Ø6CYØZZ
Ø6CY3ZZ
Ø6CY4ZZ
Ø6HØØDZ
Ø6HØ4DZ
Ø6H1ØDZ
Ø6H13DZ
Ø6H14DZ
Ø6H2ØDZ
Ø6H23DZ
Ø6H24DZ
Ø6H3ØDZ
Ø6H33DZ
Ø6H34DZ
Ø6H4ØDZ
Ø6H43DZ
Ø6H44DZ
Ø6H5ØDZ
Ø6H53DZ
Ø6H54DZ
Ø6H6ØDZ
Ø6H63DZ
Ø6H64DZ
Ø6H7ØDZ
Ø6H73DZ
Ø6H74DZ
Ø6H8ØDZ
Ø6H83DZ
Ø6H84DZ
Ø6H9ØDZ
Ø6H93DZ
Ø6H94DZ
Ø6HBØDZ
Ø6HB3DZ
Ø6HB4DZ
Ø6HCØDZ
Ø6HC3DZ
Ø6HC4DZ
Ø6HDØDZ
Ø6HD3DZ
Ø6HD4DZ
Ø6HFØDZ
Ø6HF3DZ
Ø6HF4DZ
Ø6HGØDZ
Ø6HG3DZ
Ø6HG4DZ
Ø6HHØDZ
Ø6HH3DZ
Ø6HH4DZ
Ø6HJØDZ
Ø6HJ3DZ
Ø6HJ4DZ
Ø6HMØDZ
Ø6HM3DZ
Ø6HM4DZ
Ø6HNØDZ
Ø6HN3DZ
Ø6HN4DZ
Ø6HPØDZ
Ø6HP3DZ
Ø6HP4DZ
Ø6HQØDZ
Ø6HQ3DZ
Ø6HQ4DZ
Ø6HTØDZ
Ø6HT3DZ
Ø6HT4DZ
Ø6HVØDZ
Ø6HV3DZ
Ø6HV4DZ
Ø6HYØ2Z
Ø6HYØDZ
Ø6HYØYZ
Ø6HY3DZ
Ø6HY42Z
Ø6HY4DZ
Ø6LØØCZ
Ø6LØØDZ
Ø6LØØZZ
Ø6LØ3CZ
Ø6LØ3DZ
Ø6LØ3ZZ
Ø6LØ4CZ
Ø6LØ4DZ
Ø6LØ4ZZ
Ø6L1ØCZ
Ø6L1ØDZ
Ø6L1ØZZ
Ø6L13CZ
Ø6L13DZ
Ø6L13ZZ
Ø6L14CZ
Ø6L14DZ
Ø6L14ZZ
Ø6L2ØCZ
Ø6L2ØDZ
Ø6L2ØZZ
Ø6L23CZ
Ø6L23DZ
Ø6L23ZZ
Ø6L24CZ
Ø6L24DZ
Ø6L24ZZ
Ø6L3ØCZ
Ø6L3ØDZ
Ø6L3ØZZ
Ø6L4ØCZ
Ø6L4ØDZ
Ø6L4ØZZ
Ø6L43CZ
Ø6L43DZ
Ø6L43ZZ
Ø6L44CZ
Ø6L44DZ
Ø6L44ZZ
Ø6L5ØCZ
Ø6L5ØDZ
Ø6L5ØZZ
Ø6L53CZ
Ø6L53DZ
Ø6L53ZZ
Ø6L54CZ
Ø6L54DZ
Ø6L54ZZ
Ø6L6ØCZ
Ø6L6ØDZ
Ø6L6ØZZ
Ø6L63CZ
Ø6L63DZ
Ø6L63ZZ
Ø6L64CZ
Ø6L64DZ
Ø6L64ZZ
Ø6L7ØCZ
Ø6L7ØDZ
Ø6L7ØZZ
Ø6L73CZ
Ø6L73DZ
Ø6L73ZZ
Ø6L74CZ
Ø6L74DZ
Ø6L74ZZ
Ø6L8ØCZ
Ø6L8ØDZ
Ø6L8ØZZ
Ø6L83CZ
Ø6L83DZ
Ø6L83ZZ
Ø6L84CZ
Ø6L84DZ
Ø6L84ZZ
Ø6L9ØCZ
Ø6L9ØDZ
Ø6L9ØZZ
Ø6L93CZ
Ø6L93DZ
Ø6L93ZZ
Ø6L94CZ
Ø6L94DZ
Ø6L94ZZ
Ø6LBØCZ
Ø6LBØDZ
Ø6LBØZZ
Ø6LB3CZ
Ø6LB3DZ
Ø6LB3ZZ
Ø6LB4CZ
Ø6LB4DZ
Ø6LB4ZZ
Ø6LCØCZ
Ø6LCØDZ
Ø6LCØZZ
Ø6LC3CZ
Ø6LC3DZ
Ø6LC3ZZ
Ø6LC4CZ
Ø6LC4DZ
Ø6LC4ZZ
Ø6LDØCZ
Ø6LDØDZ
Ø6LDØZZ
Ø6LD3CZ
Ø6LD3DZ
Ø6LD3ZZ
Ø6LD4CZ
Ø6LD4DZ
Ø6LD4ZZ
Ø6LFØCZ
Ø6LFØDZ
Ø6LFØZZ
Ø6LF3CZ
Ø6LF3DZ
Ø6LF3ZZ
Ø6LF4CZ
Ø6LF4DZ
Ø6LF4ZZ
Ø6LGØCZ
Ø6LGØDZ
Ø6LGØZZ
Ø6LG3CZ
Ø6LG3DZ
Ø6LG3ZZ
Ø6LG4CZ
Ø6LG4DZ
Ø6LG4ZZ
Ø6LHØCZ
Ø6LHØDZ
Ø6LHØZZ
Ø6LH3CZ
Ø6LH3DZ
Ø6LH3ZZ
Ø6LH4CZ
Ø6LH4DZ
Ø6LH4ZZ
Ø6LJØCZ
Ø6LJØDZ
Ø6LJØZZ
Ø6LJ3CZ
Ø6LJ3DZ
Ø6LJ3ZZ
Ø6LJ4CZ
Ø6LJ4DZ
Ø6LJ4ZZ
Ø6LMØCZ
Ø6LMØDZ
Ø6LMØZZ
Ø6LM3CZ
Ø6LM3DZ
Ø6LM3ZZ
Ø6LM4CZ
Ø6LM4DZ
Ø6LM4ZZ
Ø6LNØCZ
Ø6LNØDZ
Ø6LNØZZ
Ø6LN3CZ
Ø6LN3DZ
Ø6LN3ZZ
Ø6LN4CZ
Ø6LN4DZ
Ø6LN4ZZ
Ø6LPØCZ
Ø6LPØDZ
Ø6LPØZZ
Ø6LP3CZ
Ø6LP3DZ
Ø6LP3ZZ
Ø6LP4CZ
Ø6LP4DZ
Ø6LP4ZZ
Ø6LQØCZ
Ø6LQØDZ
Ø6LQØZZ
Ø6LQ3CZ
Ø6LQ3DZ
Ø6LQ3ZZ
Ø6LQ4CZ
Ø6LQ4DZ
Ø6LQ4ZZ
Ø6LTØCZ
Ø6LTØDZ
Ø6LTØZZ
Ø6LT3CZ
Ø6LT3DZ
Ø6LT3ZZ
Ø6LT4CZ
Ø6LT4DZ
Ø6LT4ZZ
Ø6LVØCZ
Ø6LVØDZ
Ø6LVØZZ
Ø6LV3CZ
Ø6LV3DZ
Ø6LV3ZZ
Ø6LV4CZ
Ø6LV4DZ
Ø6LV4ZZ
Ø6LYØCZ
Ø6LYØDZ
Ø6LYØZZ
Ø6LY3CZ
Ø6LY3DZ
Ø6LY3ZZ
Ø6LY4CZ
Ø6LY4DZ
Ø6LY4ZZ
Ø6LY7CZ
Ø6LY7DZ
Ø6LY7ZZ
Ø6LY8CZ
Ø6LY8DZ
Ø6LY8ZZ
Ø6PYØØZ
Ø6PYØ2Z
Ø6PYØ3Z
Ø6PYØCZ
Ø6PYØDZ
Ø6PYØYZ
Ø6PY3CZ
Ø6PY4ØZ
Ø6PY42Z
Ø6PY43Z
Ø6PY4CZ
Ø6PY4DZ
Ø6QØØZZ
Ø6QØ3ZZ
Ø6QØ4ZZ
Ø6Q1ØZZ
Ø6Q13ZZ
Ø6Q14ZZ
Ø6Q2ØZZ
Ø6Q23ZZ
Ø6Q24ZZ
Ø6Q3ØZZ
Ø6Q33ZZ
Ø6Q34ZZ
Ø6Q4ØZZ
Ø6Q43ZZ
Ø6Q44ZZ
Ø6Q5ØZZ
Ø6Q53ZZ
Ø6Q54ZZ
Ø6Q6ØZZ
Ø6Q63ZZ
Ø6Q64ZZ
Ø6Q7ØZZ
Ø6Q73ZZ
Ø6Q74ZZ
Ø6Q8ØZZ
Ø6Q83ZZ
Ø6Q84ZZ
Ø6Q9ØZZ
Ø6Q93ZZ
Ø6Q94ZZ
Ø6QBØZZ
Ø6QB3ZZ
Ø6QB4ZZ
Ø6QCØZZ
Ø6QC3ZZ
Ø6QC4ZZ
Ø6QDØZZ
Ø6QD3ZZ
Ø6QD4ZZ
Ø6QFØZZ
Ø6QF3ZZ
Ø6QF4ZZ
Ø6QGØZZ
Ø6QG3ZZ
Ø6QG4ZZ
Ø6QHØZZ
Ø6QH3ZZ
Ø6QH4ZZ
Ø6QJØZZ
Ø6QJ3ZZ
Ø6QJ4ZZ
Ø6QMØZZ
Ø6QM3ZZ
Ø6QM4ZZ
Ø6QNØZZ
Ø6QN3ZZ
Ø6QN4ZZ
Ø6QPØZZ
Ø6QP3ZZ
Ø6QP4ZZ
Ø6QQØZZ
Ø6QQ3ZZ
Ø6QQ4ZZ
Ø6QTØZZ
Ø6QT3ZZ
Ø6QT4ZZ
Ø6QVØZZ
Ø6QV3ZZ
Ø6QV4ZZ
Ø6QYØZZ
Ø6QY3ZZ
Ø6QY4ZZ
Ø6RMØ7Z
Ø6RMØJZ
Ø6RMØKZ
Ø6RM47Z
Ø6RM4JZ
Ø6RM4KZ
Ø6RNØ7Z
Ø6RNØJZ
Ø6RNØKZ
Ø6RN47Z
Ø6RN4JZ
Ø6RN4KZ
Ø6RPØ7Z
Ø6RPØJZ
Ø6RPØKZ
Ø6RP47Z
Ø6RP4JZ
Ø6RP4KZ
Ø6RQØ7Z
Ø6RQØJZ
Ø6RQØKZ
Ø6RQ47Z
Ø6RQ4JZ
Ø6RQ4KZ
Ø6RTØ7Z
Ø6RTØJZ
Ø6RTØKZ
Ø6RT47Z
Ø6RT4JZ
Ø6RT4KZ
Ø6RVØ7Z
Ø6RVØJZ
Ø6RVØKZ
Ø6RV47Z
Ø6RV4JZ
Ø6RV4KZ
Ø6RYØ7Z
Ø6RYØJZ
Ø6RYØKZ
Ø6RY47Z
Ø6RY4JZ
Ø6RY4KZ
Ø6SØØZZ
Ø6SØ3ZZ
Ø6SØ4ZZ
Ø6S1ØZZ
Ø6S13ZZ
Ø6S14ZZ
Ø6S2ØZZ
Ø6S23ZZ
Ø6S24ZZ
Ø6S3ØZZ
Ø6S33ZZ
Ø6S34ZZ
Ø6S4ØZZ
Ø6S43ZZ
Ø6S44ZZ
Ø6S5ØZZ
Ø6S53ZZ
Ø6S54ZZ
Ø6S6ØZZ
Ø6S63ZZ
Ø6S64ZZ
Ø6S7ØZZ
Ø6S73ZZ
Ø6S74ZZ
Ø6S8ØZZ
Ø6S83ZZ
Ø6S84ZZ
Ø6SCØZZ
Ø6SC3ZZ
Ø6SC4ZZ
Ø6SDØZZ
Ø6SD3ZZ
Ø6SD4ZZ
Ø6SFØZZ
Ø6SF3ZZ
Ø6SF4ZZ
Ø6SGØZZ
Ø6SG3ZZ
Ø6SG4ZZ
Ø6SHØZZ
Ø6SH3ZZ
Ø6SH4ZZ
Ø6SJØZZ
Ø6SJ3ZZ
Ø6SJ4ZZ
Ø6SMØZZ
Ø6SM3ZZ
Ø6SM4ZZ
Ø6SNØZZ
Ø6SN3ZZ
Ø6SN4ZZ
Ø6SPØZZ
Ø6SP3ZZ
Ø6SP4ZZ
Ø6SQØZZ
Ø6SQ3ZZ
Ø6SQ4ZZ
Ø6STØZZ
Ø6ST3ZZ
Ø6ST4ZZ
Ø6SVØZZ
Ø6SV3ZZ
Ø6SV4ZZ
Ø6SYØZZ
Ø6SY3ZZ
Ø6SY4ZZ
Ø6UØØ7Z
Ø6UØ37Z
Ø6UØ47Z
Ø6U1Ø7Z
Ø6U137Z
Ø6U147Z
Ø6U2Ø7Z
Ø6U237Z
Ø6U247Z
Ø6U3Ø7Z
Ø6U337Z
Ø6U347Z
Ø6U4Ø7Z
Ø6U437Z
Ø6U447Z
Ø6U5Ø7Z
Ø6U537Z
Ø6U547Z
Ø6U6Ø7Z
Ø6U637Z
Ø6U647Z
Ø6U7Ø7Z
Ø6U737Z
Ø6U747Z
Ø6U8Ø7Z
Ø6U837Z
Ø6U847Z
Ø6U9Ø7Z
Ø6U937Z
Ø6U947Z
Ø6UBØ7Z
Ø6UB37Z
Ø6UB47Z
Ø6UCØ7Z
Ø6UC37Z
Ø6UC47Z
Ø6UDØ7Z
Ø6UD37Z
Ø6UD47Z
Ø6UFØ7Z
Ø6UF37Z
Ø6UF47Z
Ø6UGØ7Z
Ø6UG37Z
Ø6UG47Z
Ø6UHØ7Z
Ø6UH37Z
Ø6UH47Z
Ø6UJØ7Z
Ø6UJ37Z
Ø6UJ47Z
Ø6UMØ7Z
Ø6UM37Z
Ø6UM47Z
Ø6UNØ7Z
Ø6UN37Z
Ø6UN47Z
Ø6UPØ7Z
Ø6UP37Z
Ø6UP47Z
Ø6UQØ7Z
Ø6UQ37Z
Ø6UQ47Z
Ø6UTØ7Z
Ø6UT37Z
Ø6UT47Z
Ø6UVØ7Z
Ø6UV37Z
Ø6UV47Z
Ø6UYØ7Z
Ø6UY37Z
Ø6UY47Z
Ø6VØØCZ
Ø6VØØDZ
Ø6VØØZZ
Ø6VØ3CZ
Ø6VØ3DZ
Ø6VØ3ZZ
Ø6VØ4CZ
Ø6VØ4DZ
Ø6VØ4ZZ
Ø6V1ØDZ
Ø6V13DZ
Ø6V14DZ
Ø6V2ØDZ
Ø6V23DZ
Ø6V24DZ
Ø6V3ØDZ
Ø6V33DZ
Ø6V34DZ
Ø6V4ØDZ
Ø6V43DZ
Ø6V44DZ
Ø6V5ØDZ
Ø6V53DZ
Ø6V54DZ
Ø6V6ØDZ
Ø6V63DZ
Ø6V64DZ
Ø6V7ØDZ
Ø6V73DZ
Ø6V74DZ
Ø6V8ØDZ
Ø6V83DZ
Ø6V84DZ
Ø6V9ØDZ
Ø6V93DZ
Ø6V94DZ
Ø6VBØDZ
Ø6VB3DZ
Ø6VB4DZ
Ø6VCØDZ
Ø6VC3DZ
Ø6VC4DZ
Ø6VDØDZ
Ø6VD3DZ
Ø6VD4DZ
Ø6VFØDZ
Ø6VF3DZ
Ø6VF4DZ
Ø6VGØDZ
Ø6VG3DZ
Ø6VG4DZ
Ø6VHØDZ
Ø6VH3DZ
Ø6VH4DZ
Ø6VJØDZ
Ø6VJ3DZ
Ø6VJ4DZ
Ø6VMØDZ
Ø6VM3DZ
Ø6VM4DZ
Ø6VNØDZ
Ø6VN3DZ
Ø6VN4DZ
Ø6VPØDZ
Ø6VP3DZ
Ø6VP4DZ
Ø6VQØDZ
Ø6VQ3DZ
Ø6VQ4DZ
Ø6VTØDZ
Ø6VT3DZ
Ø6VT4DZ
Ø6VVØDZ
Ø6VV3DZ
Ø6VV4DZ
Ø6WYØØZ
Ø6WYØ2Z
Ø6WYØ3Z
Ø6WYØCZ
Ø6WYØDZ
Ø6WYØYZ
Ø6WY3CZ
Ø6WY4ØZ
Ø6WY42Z
Ø6WY43Z
Ø6WY4CZ
Ø6WY4DZ
Ø75MØZZ
Ø75M3ZZ
Ø75M4ZZ
Ø75PØZZ
Ø75P3ZZ
Ø75P4ZZ
Ø79KØØZ
Ø79KØZZ
Ø79K4ØZ
Ø79K4ZZ
Ø79LØØZ
Ø79LØZZ
Ø79L4ØZ
Ø79L4ZZ
Ø79MØØZ
Ø79MØZZ
Ø79M4ØZ
Ø79M4ZZ
Ø79PØØZ
Ø79PØZZ
Ø7BMØZZ
Ø7BM3ZZ
Ø7BM4ZZ
Ø7BPØZZ
Ø7BP3ZZ
Ø7BP4ZZ
Ø7CMØZZ
Ø7CM3ZZ
Ø7CM4ZZ
Ø7CPØZZ
Ø7HKØ1Z
Ø7HKØYZ
Ø7HK41Z
Ø7HK4YZ
Ø7HLØ1Z
Ø7HLØYZ
Ø7HL41Z
Ø7HL4YZ
Ø7HMØ1Z
Ø7HMØYZ
Ø7HM41Z
Ø7HM4YZ
Ø7HPØ1Z
Ø7HPØYZ
Ø7HP41Z
Ø7JMØZZ
Ø7JM4ZZ
Ø7JPØZZ
Ø7LKØCZ
Ø7LKØDZ
Ø7LKØZZ
Ø7LK3CZ
Ø7LK3DZ
Ø7LK3ZZ
Ø7LK4CZ
Ø7LK4DZ
Ø7LK4ZZ
Ø7LLØCZ
Ø7LLØDZ
Ø7LLØZZ
Ø7LL3CZ
Ø7LL3DZ
Ø7LL3ZZ
Ø7LL4CZ
Ø7LL4DZ
Ø7LL4ZZ
Ø7NMØZZ
Ø7NM3ZZ
Ø7NM4ZZ
Ø7NPØZZ
Ø7NP3ZZ
Ø7NP4ZZ
Ø7PMØØZ
Ø7PMØ3Z
Ø7PMØYZ
Ø7PM3ØZ
Ø7PM33Z
Ø7PM4ØZ
Ø7PM43Z
Ø7PPØØZ
Ø7PPØ3Z
Ø7PPØYZ
Ø7PP3ØZ
Ø7PP33Z
Ø7PP4ØZ
Ø7PP43Z
Ø7QKØZZ
Ø7QK3ZZ
Ø7QK4ZZ
Ø7QK8ZZ
Ø7QMØZZ
Ø7QM3ZZ
Ø7QM4ZZ
Ø7QPØZZ
Ø7QP3ZZ
Ø7QP4ZZ
Ø7SMØZZ
Ø7SPØZZ
Ø7TMØZZ
Ø7TM4ZZ
Ø7TPØZZ
Ø7TP4ZZ
Ø7WMØØZ
Ø7WMØ3Z
Ø7WMØYZ
Ø7WM3ØZ
Ø7WM33Z
Ø7WM4ØZ
Ø7WM43Z
Ø7WPØØZ
Ø7WPØ3Z
Ø7WPØYZ
Ø7WP3ØZ
Ø7WP33Z
Ø7WP4ØZ
Ø7WP43Z
Ø8123J4
Ø8123K4
Ø8123Z4
Ø8133J4
Ø8133K4
Ø8133Z4
Ø81XØJ3
Ø81XØK3
Ø81XØZ3

ICD-10-CM/PCS Codes by MS-DRG

Ø81X3J3
Ø81X3K3
Ø81X3Z3
Ø81YØJ3
Ø81YØK3
Ø81YØZ3
Ø81Y3J3
Ø81Y3K3
Ø81Y3Z3
Ø8523ZZ
Ø8533ZZ
Ø8543ZZ
Ø8553ZZ
Ø856XZZ
Ø857XZZ
Ø858XZZ
Ø859XZZ
Ø85AØZZ
Ø85A3ZZ
Ø85BØZZ
Ø85B3ZZ
Ø85C3ZZ
Ø85D3ZZ
Ø85G3ZZ
Ø85H3ZZ
Ø85LØZZ
Ø85L3ZZ
Ø85MØZZ
Ø85M3ZZ
Ø85NØZZ
Ø85N3ZZ
Ø85NXZZ
Ø85PØZZ
Ø85P3ZZ
Ø85PXZZ
Ø85QØZZ
Ø85Q3ZZ
Ø85QXZZ
Ø85RØZZ
Ø85R3ZZ
Ø85RXZZ
Ø85SXZZ
Ø85TXZZ
Ø85VØZZ
Ø85V3ZZ
Ø85WØZZ
Ø85W3ZZ
Ø85XØZZ
Ø85X3ZZ
Ø85X7ZZ
Ø85X8ZZ
Ø85YØZZ
Ø85Y3ZZ
Ø85Y7ZZ
Ø85Y8ZZ
Ø87XØDZ
Ø87X3DZ
Ø87X7DZ
Ø87X8DZ
Ø87YØDZ
Ø87Y3DZ
Ø87Y7DZ
Ø87Y8DZ
Ø8923ØZ
Ø8923ZX
Ø8923ZZ
Ø8933ØZ
Ø8933ZX
Ø8933ZZ
Ø8943ØZ
Ø8943ZZ
Ø8953ØZ
Ø8953ZZ
Ø896XØZ
Ø897XØZ
Ø898XØZ
Ø899XØZ
Ø89AØØZ
Ø89AØZZ
Ø89A3ØZ
Ø89A3ZZ
Ø89BØØZ
Ø89BØZZ
Ø89B3ØZ
Ø89B3ZZ
Ø89C3ØZ
Ø89C3ZX
Ø89C3ZZ
Ø89D3ØZ
Ø89D3ZX
Ø89D3ZZ
Ø89E3ØZ
Ø89E3ZZ
Ø89F3ØZ
Ø89F3ZZ
Ø89G3ØZ
Ø89G3ZZ
Ø89H3ØZ
Ø89H3ZZ
Ø89J3ØZ
Ø89J3ZX
Ø89J3ZZ
Ø89K3ØZ
Ø89K3ZX
Ø89K3ZZ
Ø89LØØZ
Ø89LØZZ
Ø89L3ØZ
Ø89L3ZZ
Ø89MØØZ
Ø89MØZZ
Ø89M3ØZ
Ø89M3ZZ
Ø89NØZX
Ø89PØZX
Ø89QØZX
Ø89RØZX
Ø89VØZX
Ø89V3ZX
Ø89WØZX
Ø89W3ZX
Ø89X7ØZ
Ø89X7ZZ
Ø89X8ØZ
Ø89X8ZZ
Ø89Y7ØZ
Ø89Y7ZZ
Ø89Y8ØZ
Ø89Y8ZZ
Ø8BØØZZ
Ø8BØ3ZZ
Ø8BØXZZ
Ø8B1ØZZ
Ø8B13ZZ
Ø8B1XZZ
Ø8B43ZZ
Ø8B53ZZ
Ø8B6XZX
Ø8B6XZZ
Ø8B7XZX
Ø8B7XZZ
Ø8B8XZX
Ø8B8XZZ
Ø8B9XZX
Ø8B9XZZ
Ø8BAØZZ
Ø8BA3ZZ
Ø8BBØZZ
Ø8BB3ZZ
Ø8BC3ZX
Ø8BC3ZZ
Ø8BD3ZX
Ø8BD3ZZ
Ø8BJ3ZX
Ø8BK3ZX
Ø8BNØZX
Ø8BNØZZ
Ø8BN3ZX
Ø8BN3ZZ
Ø8BNXZX
Ø8BNXZZ
Ø8BPØZX
Ø8BPØZZ
Ø8BP3ZX
Ø8BP3ZZ
Ø8BPXZX
Ø8BPXZZ
Ø8BQØZX
Ø8BQØZZ
Ø8BQ3ZX
Ø8BQ3ZZ
Ø8BQXZX
Ø8BQXZZ
Ø8BRØZX
Ø8BRØZZ
Ø8BR3ZX
Ø8BR3ZZ
Ø8BRXZX
Ø8BRXZZ
Ø8BSXZZ
Ø8BTXZZ
Ø8BVØZX
Ø8BVØZZ
Ø8BV3ZX
Ø8BV3ZZ
Ø8BWØZX
Ø8BWØZZ
Ø8BW3ZX
Ø8BW3ZZ
Ø8BXØZZ
Ø8BX3ZZ
Ø8BX7ZZ
Ø8BX8ZZ
Ø8BYØZZ
Ø8BY3ZZ
Ø8BY7ZZ
Ø8BY8ZZ
Ø8C23ZZ
Ø8C33ZZ
Ø8C43ZZ
Ø8C4XZZ
Ø8C53ZZ
Ø8C5XZZ
Ø8C8XZZ
Ø8C9XZZ
Ø8CAØZZ
Ø8CA3ZZ
Ø8CAXZZ
Ø8CBØZZ
Ø8CB3ZZ
Ø8CBXZZ
Ø8CC3ZZ
Ø8CCXZZ
Ø8CD3ZZ
Ø8CDXZZ
Ø8CE3ZZ
Ø8CEXZZ
Ø8CF3ZZ
Ø8CFXZZ
Ø8CG3ZZ
Ø8CGXZZ
Ø8CH3ZZ
Ø8CHXZZ
Ø8CJ3ZZ
Ø8CJXZZ
Ø8CK3ZZ
Ø8CKXZZ
Ø8CLØZZ
Ø8CL3ZZ
Ø8CLXZZ
Ø8CMØZZ
Ø8CM3ZZ
Ø8CMXZZ
Ø8CV3ZZ
Ø8CVXZZ
Ø8CW3ZZ
Ø8CWXZZ
Ø8F43ZZ
Ø8F53ZZ
Ø8HØØ5Z
Ø8HØØYZ
Ø8H1Ø5Z
Ø8H1ØYZ
Ø8LXØCZ
Ø8LXØDZ
Ø8LXØZZ
Ø8LX3CZ
Ø8LX3DZ
Ø8LX3ZZ
Ø8LX7DZ
Ø8LX7ZZ
Ø8LX8DZ
Ø8LX8ZZ
Ø8LYØCZ
Ø8LYØDZ
Ø8LYØZZ
Ø8LY3CZ
Ø8LY3DZ
Ø8LY3ZZ
Ø8LY7DZ
Ø8LY7ZZ
Ø8LY8DZ
Ø8LY8ZZ
Ø8MNXZZ
Ø8MPXZZ
Ø8MQXZZ
Ø8MRXZZ
Ø8N23ZZ
Ø8N33ZZ
Ø8N43ZZ
Ø8N53ZZ
Ø8N6XZZ
Ø8N7XZZ
Ø8N8XZZ
Ø8N9XZZ
Ø8NAØZZ
Ø8NA3ZZ
Ø8NBØZZ
Ø8NB3ZZ
Ø8NC3ZZ
Ø8ND3ZZ
Ø8NE3ZZ
Ø8NF3ZZ
Ø8NG3ZZ
Ø8NH3ZZ
Ø8NJ3ZZ
Ø8NK3ZZ
Ø8NLØZZ
Ø8NL3ZZ
Ø8NMØZZ
Ø8NM3ZZ
Ø8NNØZZ
Ø8NN3ZZ
Ø8NNXZZ
Ø8NPØZZ
Ø8NP3ZZ
Ø8NPXZZ
Ø8NQØZZ
Ø8NQ3ZZ
Ø8NQXZZ
Ø8NRØZZ
Ø8NR3ZZ
Ø8NRXZZ
Ø8NVØZZ
Ø8NV3ZZ
Ø8NWØZZ
Ø8NW3ZZ
Ø8NXØZZ
Ø8NX3ZZ
Ø8NX7ZZ
Ø8NX8ZZ
Ø8NYØZZ
Ø8NY3ZZ
Ø8NY7ZZ
Ø8NY8ZZ
Ø8PØØ3Z
Ø8PØØJZ
Ø8PØ3JZ
Ø8P1Ø3Z
Ø8P1ØJZ
Ø8P13JZ
Ø8PJ3JZ
Ø8PK3JZ
Ø8PLØØZ
Ø8PLØYZ
Ø8PL3ØZ
Ø8PMØØZ
Ø8PMØYZ
Ø8PM3ØZ
Ø8QØXZZ
Ø8Q1XZZ
Ø8Q23ZZ
Ø8Q33ZZ
Ø8Q43ZZ
Ø8Q53ZZ
Ø8Q6XZZ
Ø8Q7XZZ
Ø8Q8XZZ
Ø8Q9XZZ
Ø8QAØZZ
Ø8QA3ZZ
Ø8QBØZZ
Ø8QB3ZZ
Ø8QC3ZZ
Ø8QD3ZZ
Ø8QE3ZZ
Ø8QF3ZZ
Ø8QG3ZZ
Ø8QH3ZZ
Ø8QJ3ZZ
Ø8QK3ZZ
Ø8QLØZZ
Ø8QL3ZZ
Ø8QMØZZ
Ø8QM3ZZ
Ø8QSXZZ
Ø8QTXZZ
Ø8QVØZZ
Ø8QV3ZZ
Ø8QWØZZ
Ø8QW3ZZ
Ø8QXØZZ
Ø8QX3ZZ
Ø8QX7ZZ
Ø8QX8ZZ
Ø8QYØZZ
Ø8QY3ZZ
Ø8QY7ZZ
Ø8QY8ZZ
Ø8RØØ7Z
Ø8RØØJZ
Ø8RØØKZ
Ø8RØ37Z
Ø8RØ3JZ
Ø8RØ3KZ
Ø8R1Ø7Z
Ø8R1ØJZ
Ø8R1ØKZ
Ø8R137Z
Ø8R13JZ
Ø8R13KZ
Ø8R437Z
Ø8R43JZ
Ø8R43KZ
Ø8R537Z
Ø8R53JZ
Ø8R53KZ
Ø8R6X7Z
Ø8R6XJZ
Ø8R6XKZ
Ø8R7X7Z
Ø8R7XJZ
Ø8R7XKZ
Ø8R837Z
Ø8R83JZ
Ø8R83KZ
Ø8R8X7Z
Ø8R8XJZ
Ø8R8XKZ
Ø8R937Z
Ø8R93JZ
Ø8R93KZ
Ø8R9X7Z
Ø8R9XJZ
Ø8R9XKZ
Ø8RAØ7Z
Ø8RAØJZ
Ø8RAØKZ
Ø8RA37Z
Ø8RA3JZ
Ø8RA3KZ
Ø8RBØ7Z
Ø8RBØJZ
Ø8RBØKZ
Ø8RB37Z
Ø8RB3JZ
Ø8RB3KZ
Ø8RC37Z
Ø8RC3JZ
Ø8RC3KZ
Ø8RD37Z
Ø8RD3JZ
Ø8RD3KZ
Ø8RG37Z
Ø8RG3JZ
Ø8RG3KZ
Ø8RH37Z
Ø8RH3JZ
Ø8RH3KZ
Ø8RJ3ØZ
Ø8RJ37Z
Ø8RJ3JZ
Ø8RJ3KZ
Ø8RK3ØZ
Ø8RK37Z
Ø8RK3JZ
Ø8RK3KZ
Ø8RNØ7Z
Ø8RNØJZ
Ø8RNØKZ
Ø8RN37Z
Ø8RN3JZ
Ø8RN3KZ
Ø8RNX7Z
Ø8RNXJZ
Ø8RNXKZ
Ø8RPØ7Z
Ø8RPØJZ
Ø8RPØKZ
Ø8RP37Z
Ø8RP3JZ
Ø8RP3KZ
Ø8RPX7Z
Ø8RPXJZ
Ø8RPXKZ
Ø8RQØ7Z
Ø8RQØJZ
Ø8RQØKZ
Ø8RQ37Z
Ø8RQ3JZ
Ø8RQ3KZ
Ø8RQX7Z
Ø8RQXJZ
Ø8RQXKZ
Ø8RRØ7Z
Ø8RRØJZ
Ø8RRØKZ
Ø8RR37Z
Ø8RR3JZ
Ø8RR3KZ
Ø8RRX7Z
Ø8RRXJZ
Ø8RRXKZ
Ø8RSX7Z
Ø8RSXJZ
Ø8RSXKZ
Ø8RTX7Z
Ø8RTXJZ
Ø8RTXKZ
Ø8RXØ7Z
Ø8RXØJZ
Ø8RXØKZ
Ø8RX37Z
Ø8RX3JZ
Ø8RX3KZ
Ø8RX77Z
Ø8RX7JZ
Ø8RX7KZ
Ø8RX87Z
Ø8RX8JZ
Ø8RX8KZ
Ø8RYØ7Z
Ø8RYØJZ
Ø8RYØKZ
Ø8RY37Z
Ø8RY3JZ
Ø8RY3KZ
Ø8RY77Z
Ø8RY7JZ
Ø8RY7KZ
Ø8RY87Z
Ø8RY8JZ
Ø8RY8KZ
Ø8SC3ZZ
Ø8SD3ZZ
Ø8SG3ZZ
Ø8SH3ZZ
Ø8SJ3ZZ
Ø8SK3ZZ
Ø8SNØZZ
Ø8SN3ZZ
Ø8SNXZZ
Ø8SPØZZ
Ø8SP3ZZ
Ø8SPXZZ
Ø8SQØZZ
Ø8SQ3ZZ
Ø8SQXZZ
Ø8SRØZZ
Ø8SR3ZZ
Ø8SRXZZ
Ø8SVØZZ
Ø8SV3ZZ
Ø8SWØZZ
Ø8SW3ZZ
Ø8SXØZZ
Ø8SX3ZZ
Ø8SX7ZZ
Ø8SX8ZZ
Ø8SYØZZ
Ø8SY3ZZ
Ø8SY7ZZ
Ø8SY8ZZ
Ø8TØXZZ
Ø8T1XZZ
Ø8T43ZZ
Ø8T53ZZ
Ø8T8XZZ
Ø8T9XZZ
Ø8TC3ZZ
Ø8TD3ZZ
Ø8TJ3ZZ
Ø8TK3ZZ
Ø8TNØZZ
Ø8TNXZZ
Ø8TPØZZ
Ø8TPXZZ
Ø8TQØZZ
Ø8TQXZZ
Ø8TRØZZ
Ø8TRXZZ
Ø8TVØZZ
Ø8TV3ZZ
Ø8TWØZZ
Ø8TW3ZZ
Ø8TXØZZ
Ø8TX3ZZ
Ø8TX7ZZ
Ø8TX8ZZ
Ø8TYØZZ
Ø8TY3ZZ
Ø8TY7ZZ
Ø8TY8ZZ
Ø8UØØ7Z
Ø8UØØJZ
Ø8UØØKZ
Ø8UØ37Z
Ø8UØ3JZ
Ø8UØ3KZ
Ø8U1Ø7Z
Ø8U1ØJZ
Ø8U1ØKZ
Ø8U137Z
Ø8U13JZ
Ø8U13KZ
Ø8U8Ø7Z
Ø8U8ØJZ
Ø8U8ØKZ
Ø8U837Z
Ø8U83JZ
Ø8U83KZ
Ø8U8X7Z
Ø8U8XJZ
Ø8U8XKZ
Ø8U9Ø7Z
Ø8U9ØJZ
Ø8U9ØKZ
Ø8U937Z
Ø8U93JZ
Ø8U93KZ
Ø8U9X7Z
Ø8U9XJZ
Ø8U9XKZ
Ø8UCØ7Z
Ø8UCØJZ
Ø8UCØKZ
Ø8UC37Z
Ø8UC3JZ
Ø8UC3KZ
Ø8UDØ7Z
Ø8UDØJZ
Ø8UDØKZ
Ø8UD37Z
Ø8UD3JZ
Ø8UD3KZ
Ø8UEØJZ
Ø8UE3JZ
Ø8UFØJZ
Ø8UF3JZ
Ø8UGØ7Z
Ø8UGØJZ
Ø8UGØKZ
Ø8UG37Z
Ø8UG3JZ
Ø8UG3KZ
Ø8UHØ7Z
Ø8UHØJZ
Ø8UHØKZ
Ø8UH37Z
Ø8UH3JZ
Ø8UH3KZ
Ø8ULØ7Z
Ø8ULØJZ
Ø8ULØKZ
Ø8UL37Z
Ø8UL3JZ
Ø8UL3KZ
Ø8UMØ7Z
Ø8UMØJZ
Ø8UMØKZ
Ø8UM37Z
Ø8UM3JZ
Ø8UM3KZ
Ø8UNØ7Z
Ø8UNØJZ
Ø8UNØKZ
Ø8UN37Z
Ø8UN3JZ
Ø8UN3KZ
Ø8UNX7Z
Ø8UNXJZ
Ø8UNXKZ
Ø8UPØ7Z
Ø8UPØJZ
Ø8UPØKZ
Ø8UP37Z
Ø8UP3JZ
Ø8UP3KZ
Ø8UPX7Z
Ø8UPXJZ
Ø8UPXKZ
Ø8UQØ7Z
Ø8UQØJZ
Ø8UQØKZ
Ø8UQ37Z
Ø8UQ3JZ
Ø8UQ3KZ
Ø8UQX7Z
Ø8UQXJZ
Ø8UQXKZ
Ø8URØ7Z
Ø8URØJZ
Ø8URØKZ
Ø8UR37Z
Ø8UR3JZ
Ø8UR3KZ
Ø8URX7Z
Ø8URXJZ
Ø8URXKZ
Ø8UXØ7Z
Ø8UXØJZ
Ø8UXØKZ
Ø8UX37Z
Ø8UX3JZ
Ø8UX3KZ
Ø8UX77Z
Ø8UX7JZ
Ø8UX7KZ
Ø8UX87Z
Ø8UX8JZ
Ø8UX8KZ
Ø8UYØ7Z
Ø8UYØJZ
Ø8UYØKZ
Ø8UY37Z
Ø8UY3JZ
Ø8UY3KZ
Ø8UY77Z
Ø8UY7JZ
Ø8UY7KZ
Ø8UY87Z
Ø8UY8JZ
Ø8UY8KZ
Ø8VXØCZ
Ø8VXØDZ
Ø8VXØZZ
Ø8VX3CZ
Ø8VX3DZ
Ø8VX3ZZ
Ø8VX7DZ
Ø8VX7ZZ
Ø8VX8DZ
Ø8VX8ZZ
Ø8VYØCZ
Ø8VYØDZ
Ø8VYØZZ
Ø8VY3CZ
Ø8VY3DZ
Ø8VY3ZZ
Ø8VY7DZ
Ø8VY7ZZ
Ø8VY8DZ
Ø8VY8ZZ
Ø8WØØJZ
Ø8WØ3JZ
Ø8W1ØJZ
Ø8W13JZ
Ø8WJ3JZ
Ø8WK3JZ
Ø8WLØØZ
Ø8WLØYZ
Ø8WL3ØZ
Ø8WMØØZ
Ø8WMØYZ
Ø8WM3ØZ
Ø9ØØØ7Z
Ø9ØØØJZ
Ø9ØØØKZ
Ø9ØØØZZ
Ø9ØØ37Z
Ø9ØØ3JZ
Ø9ØØ3KZ
Ø9ØØ3ZZ
Ø9ØØ47Z
Ø9ØØ4JZ
Ø9ØØ4KZ
Ø9ØØ4ZZ
Ø9ØØX7Z
Ø9ØØXJZ
Ø9ØØXKZ
Ø9ØØXZZ
Ø9Ø1Ø7Z
Ø9Ø1ØJZ
Ø9Ø1ØKZ
Ø9Ø1ØZZ
Ø9Ø137Z
Ø9Ø13JZ
Ø9Ø13KZ
Ø9Ø13ZZ
Ø9Ø147Z
Ø9Ø14JZ
Ø9Ø14KZ
Ø9Ø14ZZ
Ø9Ø1X7Z
Ø9Ø1XJZ
Ø9Ø1XKZ
Ø9Ø1XZZ
Ø9Ø2Ø7Z
Ø9Ø2ØJZ
Ø9Ø2ØKZ
Ø9Ø2ØZZ
Ø9Ø237Z
Ø9Ø23JZ
Ø9Ø23KZ
Ø9Ø23ZZ
Ø9Ø247Z
Ø9Ø24JZ
Ø9Ø24KZ
Ø9Ø24ZZ
Ø9Ø2X7Z
Ø9Ø2XJZ
Ø9Ø2XKZ
Ø9Ø2XZZ
Ø9ØKØ7Z
Ø9ØKØJZ
Ø9ØKØKZ
Ø9ØKØZZ
Ø9ØK37Z
Ø9ØK3JZ
Ø9ØK3KZ
Ø9ØK3ZZ
Ø9ØK47Z
Ø9ØK4JZ
Ø9ØK4KZ
Ø9ØK4ZZ
Ø9ØKX7Z
Ø9ØKXJZ
Ø9ØKXKZ
Ø9ØKXZZ
Ø98LØZZ
Ø98L3ZZ
Ø98L4ZZ
Ø98L7ZZ
Ø98L8ZZ
Ø99NØØZ
Ø99NØZZ
Ø99N4ØZ
Ø99N4ZZ
Ø99N7ØZ
Ø99N7ZZ
Ø99N8ØZ
Ø99N8ZZ
Ø9BLØZZ
Ø9BL3ZZ
Ø9BL4ZZ
Ø9BL7ZZ
Ø9BL8ZZ
Ø9BMØZZ
Ø9BM3ZZ
Ø9BM4ZZ
Ø9BM8ZZ
Ø9CNØZZ
Ø9CN3ZZ
Ø9CN4ZZ
Ø9CN7ZZ
Ø9CN8ZZ
Ø9DLØZZ
Ø9DL3ZZ
Ø9DL4ZZ
Ø9DL7ZZ
Ø9DL8ZZ
Ø9DMØZZ
Ø9DM3ZZ
Ø9DM4ZZ
Ø9MØXZZ
Ø9M1XZZ
Ø9MKXZZ
Ø9NØØZZ
Ø9NØ3ZZ
Ø9NØ4ZZ
Ø9N1ØZZ
Ø9N13ZZ
Ø9N14ZZ
Ø9N3ØZZ
Ø9N33ZZ
Ø9N34ZZ
Ø9N37ZZ
Ø9N38ZZ
Ø9N4ØZZ
Ø9N43ZZ
Ø9N44ZZ
Ø9N47ZZ
Ø9N48ZZ
Ø9QØØZZ
Ø9QØ3ZZ
Ø9QØ4ZZ
Ø9Q1ØZZ
Ø9Q13ZZ
Ø9Q14ZZ
Ø9Q2ØZZ
Ø9Q23ZZ
Ø9Q24ZZ
Ø9Q3ØZZ
Ø9Q33ZZ
Ø9Q34ZZ

Ø9Q37ZZ
Ø9Q38ZZ
Ø9Q4ØZZ
Ø9Q43ZZ
Ø9Q44ZZ
Ø9Q47ZZ
Ø9Q48ZZ
Ø9QKØZZ
Ø9QK3ZZ
Ø9QK4ZZ
Ø9QK8ZZ
Ø9QLØZZ
Ø9QL3ZZ
Ø9QL4ZZ
Ø9QL7ZZ
Ø9QL8ZZ
Ø9QMØZZ
Ø9QM3ZZ
Ø9QM4ZZ
Ø9QM8ZZ
Ø9QNØZZ
Ø9QN3ZZ
Ø9QN4ZZ
Ø9QN7ZZ
Ø9QN8ZZ
Ø9RØØ7Z
Ø9RØØJZ
Ø9RØØKZ
Ø9RØX7Z
Ø9RØXJZ
Ø9RØXKZ
Ø9R1Ø7Z
Ø9R1ØJZ
Ø9R1ØKZ
Ø9R1X7Z
Ø9R1XJZ
Ø9R1XKZ
Ø9R2Ø7Z
Ø9R2ØJZ
Ø9R2ØKZ
Ø9R2X7Z
Ø9R2XJZ
Ø9R2XKZ
Ø9RKØ7Z
Ø9RKØJZ
Ø9RKØKZ
Ø9RKX7Z
Ø9RKXJZ
Ø9RKXKZ
Ø9RLØ7Z
Ø9RLØJZ
Ø9RLØKZ
Ø9RL37Z
Ø9RL3JZ
Ø9RL3KZ
Ø9RL47Z
Ø9RL4JZ
Ø9RL4KZ
Ø9RL77Z
Ø9RL7JZ
Ø9RL7KZ
Ø9RL87Z
Ø9RL8JZ
Ø9RL8KZ
Ø9RMØ7Z
Ø9RMØJZ
Ø9RMØKZ
Ø9RM37Z
Ø9RM3JZ
Ø9RM3KZ
Ø9RM47Z
Ø9RM4JZ
Ø9RM4KZ
Ø9RNØ7Z
Ø9RNØJZ
Ø9RNØKZ
Ø9RN77Z
Ø9RN7JZ
Ø9RN7KZ
Ø9RN87Z
Ø9RN8JZ
Ø9RN8KZ
Ø9SØØZZ
Ø9SØ4ZZ
Ø9SØXZZ
Ø9S1ØZZ
Ø9S14ZZ
Ø9S1XZZ
Ø9S2ØZZ
Ø9S24ZZ
Ø9S2XZZ
Ø9SKØZZ
Ø9SK4ZZ
Ø9SKXZZ
Ø9SLØZZ
Ø9SL4ZZ
Ø9SL7ZZ
Ø9SL8ZZ
Ø9SMØZZ
Ø9SM4ZZ
Ø9TØØZZ
Ø9TØ4ZZ
Ø9TØXZZ
Ø9T1ØZZ
Ø9T14ZZ
Ø9T1XZZ
Ø9TKØZZ
Ø9TK4ZZ
Ø9TK8ZZ
Ø9TKXZZ
Ø9TLØZZ
Ø9TL4ZZ
Ø9TL7ZZ
Ø9TL8ZZ
Ø9TMØZZ
Ø9TM4ZZ
Ø9TM8ZZ
Ø9UØØ7Z
Ø9UØØJZ
Ø9UØØKZ
Ø9UØX7Z
Ø9UØXJZ
Ø9UØXKZ
Ø9U1Ø7Z
Ø9U1ØJZ
Ø9U1ØKZ
Ø9U1X7Z
Ø9U1XJZ
Ø9U1XKZ
Ø9U2Ø7Z
Ø9U2ØJZ
Ø9U2ØKZ
Ø9U2X7Z
Ø9U2XJZ
Ø9U2XKZ
Ø9UKØ7Z
Ø9UKØJZ
Ø9UKØKZ
Ø9UK87Z
Ø9UK8JZ
Ø9UK8KZ
Ø9UKX7Z
Ø9UKXJZ
Ø9UKXKZ
Ø9ULØ7Z
Ø9ULØJZ
Ø9ULØKZ
Ø9UL37Z
Ø9UL3JZ
Ø9UL3KZ
Ø9UL47Z
Ø9UL4JZ
Ø9UL4KZ
Ø9UL77Z
Ø9UL7JZ
Ø9UL7KZ
Ø9UL87Z
Ø9UL8JZ
Ø9UL8KZ
Ø9UMØ7Z
Ø9UMØJZ
Ø9UMØKZ
Ø9UM37Z
Ø9UM3JZ
Ø9UM3KZ
Ø9UM47Z
Ø9UM4JZ
Ø9UM4KZ
Ø9UM87Z
Ø9UM8JZ
Ø9UM8KZ
Ø9UNØ7Z
Ø9UNØJZ
Ø9UNØKZ
Ø9UN77Z
Ø9UN7JZ
Ø9UN7KZ
Ø9UN87Z
Ø9UN8JZ
Ø9UN8KZ
ØB5KØZ3
ØB5KØZZ
ØB5K4Z3
ØB5K7ZZ
ØB5LØZ3
ØB5LØZZ
ØB5L4Z3
ØB5L7ZZ
ØB5MØZ3
ØB5MØZZ
ØB5M4Z3
ØB5M7ZZ
ØB5NØZZ
ØB5N3ZZ
ØB5N4ZZ
ØB5PØZZ
ØB5P3ZZ
ØB5P4ZZ
ØB71ØDZ
ØB71ØZZ
ØB713DZ
ØB713ZZ
ØB714DZ
ØB714ZZ
ØB717DZ
ØB717ZZ
ØB718DZ
ØB718ZZ
ØB72ØDZ
ØB72ØZZ
ØB723DZ
ØB723ZZ
ØB724DZ
ØB724ZZ
ØB727DZ
ØB727ZZ
ØB728DZ
ØB728ZZ
ØBBC4ZZ
ØBBD4ZZ
ØBBF4ZZ
ØBBG4ZZ
ØBBH4ZZ
ØBBJ4ZZ
ØBBK4ZZ
ØBBL4ZZ
ØBBMØZZ
ØBBM3ZZ
ØBBM7ZZ
ØBBNØZZ
ØBBN3ZZ
ØBBN4ZZ
ØBBN8ZZ
ØBBPØZZ
ØBBP3ZZ
ØBBP4ZZ
ØBBP8ZZ
ØBDNØZX
ØBDNØZZ
ØBDN3ZX
ØBDN3ZZ
ØBDN4ZX
ØBDN4ZZ
ØBDPØZX
ØBDPØZZ
ØBDP3ZX
ØBDP3ZZ
ØBDP4ZX
ØBDP4ZZ
ØBF1ØZZ
ØBF13ZZ
ØBF14ZZ
ØBF17ZZ
ØBF18ZZ
ØBF2ØZZ
ØBF23ZZ
ØBF24ZZ
ØBF27ZZ
ØBF28ZZ
ØBHTØMZ
ØBHT3MZ
ØBHT4MZ
ØBHT4YZ
ØBJØ4ZZ
ØBJK4ZZ
ØBJL4ZZ
ØBL1ØCZ
ØBL1ØDZ
ØBL1ØZZ
ØBL13CZ
ØBL13DZ
ØBL13ZZ
ØBL14CZ
ØBL14DZ
ØBL14ZZ
ØBL17DZ
ØBL17ZZ
ØBL18DZ
ØBL18ZZ
ØBL2ØCZ
ØBL2ØDZ
ØBL2ØZZ
ØBL23CZ
ØBL23DZ
ØBL23ZZ
ØBL24CZ
ØBL24DZ
ØBL24ZZ
ØBL27DZ
ØBL27ZZ
ØBL28DZ
ØBL28ZZ
ØBM1ØZZ
ØBM2ØZZ
ØBN1ØZZ
ØBN13ZZ
ØBN14ZZ
ØBN17ZZ
ØBN18ZZ
ØBN2ØZZ
ØBN23ZZ
ØBN24ZZ
ØBN27ZZ
ØBN28ZZ
ØBNNØZZ
ØBNN3ZZ
ØBNN4ZZ
ØBNPØZZ
ØBNP3ZZ
ØBNP4ZZ
ØBPQØYZ
ØBQ1ØZZ
ØBQ13ZZ
ØBQ14ZZ
ØBQ17ZZ
ØBQ18ZZ
ØBQ2ØZZ
ØBQ23ZZ
ØBQ24ZZ
ØBQ27ZZ
ØBQ28ZZ
ØBQ3ØZZ
ØBQ33ZZ
ØBQ34ZZ
ØBQ37ZZ
ØBQ38ZZ
ØBQ4ØZZ
ØBQ43ZZ
ØBQ44ZZ
ØBQ47ZZ
ØBQ48ZZ
ØBQ5ØZZ
ØBQ53ZZ
ØBQ54ZZ
ØBQ57ZZ
ØBQ58ZZ
ØBQ6ØZZ
ØBQ63ZZ
ØBQ64ZZ
ØBQ67ZZ
ØBQ68ZZ
ØBQ7ØZZ
ØBQ73ZZ
ØBQ74ZZ
ØBQ77ZZ
ØBQ78ZZ
ØBQ8ØZZ
ØBQ83ZZ
ØBQ84ZZ
ØBQ87ZZ
ØBQ88ZZ
ØBQ9ØZZ
ØBQ93ZZ
ØBQ94ZZ
ØBQ97ZZ
ØBQ98ZZ
ØBQBØZZ
ØBQB3ZZ
ØBQB4ZZ
ØBQB7ZZ
ØBQB8ZZ
ØBQKØZZ
ØBQK3ZZ
ØBQK4ZZ
ØBQK7ZZ
ØBQK8ZZ
ØBQLØZZ
ØBQL3ZZ
ØBQL4ZZ
ØBQL7ZZ
ØBQL8ZZ
ØBQMØZZ
ØBQM3ZZ
ØBQM4ZZ
ØBQM7ZZ
ØBQM8ZZ
ØBQNØZZ
ØBQN3ZZ
ØBQN4ZZ
ØBQPØZZ
ØBQP3ZZ
ØBQP4ZZ
ØBQTØZZ
ØBQT3ZZ
ØBQT4ZZ
ØBR1Ø7Z
ØBR1ØJZ
ØBR1ØKZ
ØBR147Z
ØBR14JZ
ØBR14KZ
ØBR2Ø7Z
ØBR2ØJZ
ØBR2ØKZ
ØBR247Z
ØBR24JZ
ØBR24KZ
ØBR3Ø7Z
ØBR3ØJZ
ØBR3ØKZ
ØBR347Z
ØBR34JZ
ØBR34KZ
ØBR4Ø7Z
ØBR4ØJZ
ØBR4ØKZ
ØBR447Z
ØBR44JZ
ØBR44KZ
ØBR5Ø7Z
ØBR5ØJZ
ØBR5ØKZ
ØBR547Z
ØBR54JZ
ØBR54KZ
ØBR6Ø7Z
ØBR6ØJZ
ØBR6ØKZ
ØBR647Z
ØBR64JZ
ØBR64KZ
ØBR7Ø7Z
ØBR7ØJZ
ØBR7ØKZ
ØBR747Z
ØBR74JZ
ØBR74KZ
ØBR8Ø7Z
ØBR8ØJZ
ØBR8ØKZ
ØBR847Z
ØBR84JZ
ØBR84KZ
ØBR9Ø7Z
ØBR9ØJZ
ØBR9ØKZ
ØBR947Z
ØBR94JZ
ØBR94KZ
ØBRBØ7Z
ØBRBØJZ
ØBRBØKZ
ØBRB47Z
ØBRB4JZ
ØBRB4KZ
ØBRTØ7Z
ØBRTØJZ
ØBRTØKZ
ØBRT47Z
ØBRT4JZ
ØBRT4KZ
ØBS1ØZZ
ØBS2ØZZ
ØBT1ØZZ
ØBT14ZZ
ØBT2ØZZ
ØBT24ZZ
ØBT3ØZZ
ØBT34ZZ
ØBT4ØZZ
ØBT44ZZ
ØBT5ØZZ
ØBT54ZZ
ØBT6ØZZ
ØBT64ZZ
ØBT7ØZZ
ØBT74ZZ
ØBT8ØZZ
ØBT84ZZ
ØBT9ØZZ
ØBT94ZZ
ØBTBØZZ
ØBTB4ZZ
ØBTCØZZ
ØBTC4ZZ
ØBTDØZZ
ØBTD4ZZ
ØBTFØZZ
ØBTF4ZZ
ØBTGØZZ
ØBTG4ZZ
ØBTHØZZ
ØBTH4ZZ
ØBTJØZZ
ØBTJ4ZZ
ØBTKØZZ
ØBTK4ZZ
ØBTLØZZ
ØBTL4ZZ
ØBTMØZZ
ØBTM4ZZ
ØBTTØZZ
ØBTT4ZZ
ØBU1Ø7Z
ØBU1ØJZ
ØBU1ØKZ
ØBU147Z
ØBU14JZ
ØBU14KZ
ØBU187Z
ØBU18JZ
ØBU18KZ
ØBU2Ø7Z
ØBU2ØJZ
ØBU2ØKZ
ØBU247Z
ØBU24JZ
ØBU24KZ
ØBU287Z
ØBU28JZ
ØBU28KZ
ØBUTØ7Z
ØBUTØJZ
ØBUTØKZ
ØBUT47Z
ØBUT4JZ
ØBUT4KZ
ØBV1ØCZ
ØBV1ØDZ
ØBV1ØZZ
ØBV13CZ
ØBV13DZ
ØBV13ZZ
ØBV14CZ
ØBV14DZ
ØBV14ZZ
ØBV17DZ
ØBV17ZZ
ØBV18DZ
ØBV18ZZ
ØBV2ØCZ
ØBV2ØDZ
ØBV2ØZZ
ØBV23CZ
ØBV23DZ
ØBV23ZZ
ØBV24CZ
ØBV24DZ
ØBV24ZZ
ØBV27DZ
ØBV27ZZ
ØBV28DZ
ØBV28ZZ
ØBW1ØFZ
ØBW13FZ
ØBW14FZ
ØCØØX7Z
ØCØØXJZ
ØCØØXKZ
ØCØØXZZ
ØCØ1X7Z
ØCØ1XJZ
ØCØ1XKZ
ØCØ1XZZ
ØC53ØZZ
ØC533ZZ
ØC53XZZ
ØC54ØZZ
ØC543ZZ
ØC54XZZ
ØC5RØZZ
ØC5R3ZZ
ØC5R4ZZ
ØC5R7ZZ
ØC5R8ZZ
ØC9ØØØZ
ØC9ØØZZ
ØC9ØXØZ
ØC9ØXZZ
ØC91ØØZ
ØC91ØZZ
ØC91XØZ
ØC91XZZ
ØC94ØØZ
ØC94ØZZ
ØC94XØZ
ØC94XZZ
ØC9MØØZ
ØC9MØZZ
ØC9M4ØZ
ØC9M4ZZ
ØC9M7ØZ
ØC9M7ZZ
ØC9M8ØZ
ØC9M8ZZ
ØCB3ØZZ
ØCB33ZZ
ØCB3XZZ
ØCB4ØZZ
ØCB43ZZ
ØCB4XZZ
ØCBRØZZ
ØCBR3ZZ
ØCBR4ZZ
ØCBR7ZZ
ØCBR8ZZ
ØCBSØZZ
ØCBS3ZZ
ØCBS4ZZ
ØCBS7ZZ
ØCBS8ZZ
ØCBTØZZ
ØCBT3ZZ
ØCBT4ZZ
ØCBT7ZZ
ØCBT8ZZ
ØCBVØZZ
ØCBV3ZZ
ØCBV4ZZ
ØCBV7ZZ
ØCBV8ZZ
ØCCØØZZ
ØCCØ3ZZ
ØCC1ØZZ
ØCC13ZZ
ØCC4ØZZ
ØCC43ZZ
ØCCMØZZ
ØCCM3ZZ
ØCCM4ZZ
ØCCPØZZ
ØCCP3ZZ
ØCCQØZZ
ØCCQ3ZZ
ØCMØØZZ
ØCM1ØZZ
ØCM3ØZZ
ØCM7ØZZ
ØCN2ØZZ
ØCN23ZZ
ØCN2XZZ
ØCN3ØZZ
ØCN33ZZ
ØCN3XZZ
ØCN4ØZZ
ØCN43ZZ
ØCN8ØZZ
ØCN83ZZ
ØCN9ØZZ
ØCN93ZZ
ØCNBØZZ
ØCNB3ZZ
ØCNCØZZ
ØCNC3ZZ
ØCNDØZZ
ØCND3ZZ
ØCNFØZZ
ØCNF3ZZ
ØCNGØZZ
ØCNG3ZZ
ØCNHØZZ
ØCNH3ZZ
ØCNJØZZ
ØCNJ3ZZ
ØCNRØZZ
ØCNR3ZZ
ØCNR4ZZ
ØCNR7ZZ
ØCNR8ZZ
ØCNSØZZ
ØCNS3ZZ
ØCNS4ZZ
ØCNS7ZZ
ØCNS8ZZ
ØCNTØZZ
ØCNT3ZZ
ØCNT4ZZ
ØCNT7ZZ
ØCNT8ZZ
ØCNVØZZ
ØCNV3ZZ
ØCNV4ZZ
ØCNV7ZZ
ØCNV8ZZ
ØCPYØØZ
ØCPYØ1Z
ØCPYØ7Z
ØCPYØDZ
ØCPYØJZ
ØCPYØKZ
ØCPYØYZ
ØCPY3ØZ
ØCPY31Z
ØCPY37Z
ØCPY3DZ
ØCPY3JZ
ØCPY3KZ
ØCPY71Z
ØCPY77Z
ØCPY7JZ
ØCPY7KZ
ØCPY81Z
ØCPY87Z
ØCPY8JZ
ØCPY8KZ
ØCQØØZZ
ØCQØ3ZZ
ØCQ1ØZZ
ØCQ13ZZ
ØCQ2ØZZ
ØCQ23ZZ
ØCQ2XZZ
ØCQ3ØZZ
ØCQ33ZZ
ØCQ3XZZ
ØCQ4ØZZ
ØCQ43ZZ
ØCQ8ØZZ
ØCQ83ZZ
ØCQ9ØZZ
ØCQ93ZZ
ØCQBØZZ
ØCQB3ZZ
ØCQCØZZ
ØCQC3ZZ
ØCQDØZZ
ØCQD3ZZ
ØCQFØZZ
ØCQF3ZZ
ØCQGØZZ
ØCQG3ZZ
ØCQHØZZ
ØCQH3ZZ
ØCQJØZZ
ØCQJ3ZZ
ØCQMØZZ
ØCQM3ZZ
ØCQM4ZZ
ØCQM7ZZ
ØCQM8ZZ
ØCQSØZZ
ØCQS3ZZ
ØCQS4ZZ
ØCQS7ZZ
ØCQS8ZZ
ØCRØØ7Z
ØCRØØJZ
ØCRØØKZ
ØCRØ37Z
ØCRØ3JZ
ØCRØ3KZ
ØCRØX7Z
ØCRØXJZ
ØCRØXKZ
ØCR1Ø7Z
ØCR1ØJZ
ØCR1ØKZ
ØCR137Z
ØCR13JZ
ØCR13KZ
ØCR1X7Z
ØCR1XJZ
ØCR1XKZ
ØCR4Ø7Z
ØCR4ØJZ
ØCR4ØKZ
ØCR437Z
ØCR43JZ
ØCR43KZ
ØCR4X7Z
ØCR4XJZ
ØCR4XKZ
ØCR5Ø7Z
ØCR5ØJZ
ØCR5ØKZ
ØCR537Z
ØCR53JZ
ØCR53KZ
ØCR5X7Z
ØCR5XJZ
ØCR5XKZ
ØCR6Ø7Z
ØCR6ØJZ
ØCR6ØKZ
ØCR637Z
ØCR63JZ
ØCR63KZ
ØCR6X7Z
ØCR6XJZ
ØCR6XKZ
ØCR7Ø7Z
ØCR7ØJZ
ØCR7ØKZ
ØCR737Z
ØCR73JZ
ØCR73KZ
ØCR7X7Z
ØCR7XJZ
ØCR7XKZ
ØCRBØ7Z
ØCRBØJZ
ØCRBØKZ
ØCRB37Z
ØCRB3JZ
ØCRB3KZ
ØCRCØ7Z
ØCRCØJZ
ØCRCØKZ
ØCRC37Z
ØCRC3JZ
ØCRC3KZ
ØCRMØ7Z
ØCRMØJZ
ØCRMØKZ
ØCRM77Z
ØCRM7JZ
ØCRM7KZ
ØCRM87Z
ØCRM8JZ
ØCRM8KZ
ØCSØØZZ
ØCSØXZZ
ØCS1ØZZ
ØCS1XZZ
ØCS7ØZZ
ØCS7XZZ
ØCSBØZZ
ØCSB3ZZ
ØCSCØZZ
ØCSC3ZZ
ØCSSØZZ
ØCSS7ZZ
ØCSS8ZZ
ØCTØØZZ
ØCTØXZZ
ØCT1ØZZ
ØCT1XZZ
ØCT3ØZZ
ØCT3XZZ
ØCTRØZZ
ØCTR4ZZ
ØCTR7ZZ
ØCTR8ZZ
ØCTTØZZ
ØCTT4ZZ
ØCTT7ZZ
ØCTT8ZZ
ØCTVØZZ
ØCTV4ZZ
ØCTV7ZZ
ØCTV8ZZ
ØCUØØ7Z
ØCUØØJZ
ØCUØØKZ
ØCUØ37Z
ØCUØ3JZ
ØCUØ3KZ
ØCUØX7Z
ØCUØXJZ
ØCUØXKZ
ØCU1Ø7Z
ØCU1ØJZ
ØCU1ØKZ
ØCU137Z
ØCU13JZ

ØCU13KZ
ØCU1X7Z
ØCU1XJZ
ØCU1XKZ
ØCU4Ø7Z
ØCU4ØJZ
ØCU4ØKZ
ØCU437Z
ØCU43JZ
ØCU43KZ
ØCU4X7Z
ØCU4XJZ
ØCU4XKZ
ØCU5Ø7Z
ØCU5ØJZ
ØCU5ØKZ
ØCU537Z
ØCU53JZ
ØCU53KZ
ØCU5X7Z
ØCU5XJZ
ØCU5XKZ
ØCU6Ø7Z
ØCU6ØJZ
ØCU6ØKZ
ØCU637Z
ØCU63JZ
ØCU63KZ
ØCU6X7Z
ØCU6XJZ
ØCU6XKZ
ØCU7Ø7Z
ØCU7ØJZ
ØCU7ØKZ
ØCU737Z
ØCU73JZ
ØCU73KZ
ØCU7X7Z
ØCU7XJZ
ØCU7XKZ
ØCUMØ7Z
ØCUMØJZ
ØCUMØKZ
ØCUM77Z
ØCUM7JZ
ØCUM7KZ
ØCUM87Z
ØCUM8JZ
ØCUM8KZ
ØCVB7DZ
ØCVB7ZZ
ØCVB8DZ
ØCVB8ZZ
ØCVC7DZ
ØCVC7ZZ
ØCVC8DZ
ØCVC8ZZ
ØCWYØØZ
ØCWYØ1Z
ØCWYØDZ
ØCWYØJZ
ØCWYØKZ
ØCWYØYZ
ØCWY3ØZ
ØCWY31Z
ØCWY37Z
ØCWY3DZ
ØCWY3JZ
ØCWY3KZ
ØCWY7ØZ
ØCWY71Z
ØCWY77Z
ØCWY7DZ
ØCWY7JZ
ØCWY7KZ
ØCWY8ØZ
ØCWY81Z
ØCWY87Z
ØCWY8DZ
ØCWY8JZ
ØCWY8KZ
ØCXØØZZ
ØCXØXZZ
ØCX1ØZZ
ØCX1XZZ
ØCX3ØZZ
ØCX3XZZ
ØCX4ØZZ
ØCX4XZZ
ØCX5ØZZ
ØCX5XZZ
ØCX6ØZZ
ØCX6XZZ
ØCX7ØZZ
ØCX7XZZ
ØD11Ø74
ØD11Ø76
ØD11ØJ4
ØD11ØJ6
ØD11ØK4
ØD11ØK6
ØD11ØZ4
ØD11ØZ6
ØD113J4
ØD11474
ØD11476
ØD114J4
ØD114J6
ØD114K4
ØD114K6
ØD114Z4
ØD114Z6
ØD11874
ØD11876
ØD118J4
ØD118J6
ØD118K4
ØD118K6
ØD118Z4
ØD118Z6
ØD12Ø74
ØD12Ø76
ØD12ØJ4
ØD12ØJ6
ØD12ØK4
ØD12ØK6
ØD12ØZ4
ØD12ØZ6
ØD123J4
ØD12474
ØD12476
ØD124J4
ØD124J6
ØD124K4
ØD124K6
ØD124Z4
ØD124Z6
ØD12874
ØD12876
ØD128J4
ØD128J6
ØD128K4
ØD128K6
ØD128Z4
ØD128Z6
ØD13Ø74
ØD13Ø76
ØD13ØJ4
ØD13ØJ6
ØD13ØK4
ØD13ØK6
ØD13ØZ4
ØD13ØZ6
ØD133J4
ØD13474
ØD13476
ØD134J4
ØD134J6
ØD134K4
ØD134K6
ØD134Z4
ØD134Z6
ØD13874
ØD13876
ØD138J4
ØD138J6
ØD138K4
ØD138K6
ØD138Z4
ØD138Z6
ØD15Ø74
ØD15Ø76
ØD15Ø79
ØD15Ø7A
ØD15Ø7B
ØD15ØJ4
ØD15ØJ6
ØD15ØJ9
ØD15ØJA
ØD15ØJB
ØD15ØK4
ØD15ØK6
ØD15ØK9
ØD15ØKA
ØD15ØKB
ØD15ØZ4
ØD15ØZ6
ØD15ØZ9
ØD15ØZA
ØD15ØZB
ØD153J4
ØD15474
ØD15476
ØD15479
ØD1547A
ØD1547B
ØD154J4
ØD154J6
ØD154J9
ØD154JA
ØD154JB
ØD154K4
ØD154K6
ØD154K9
ØD154KA
ØD154KB
ØD154Z4
ØD154Z6
ØD154Z9
ØD154ZA
ØD154ZB
ØD15874
ØD15876
ØD15879
ØD1587A
ØD1587B
ØD158J4
ØD158J6
ØD158J9
ØD158JA
ØD158JB
ØD158K4
ØD158K6
ØD158K9
ØD158KA
ØD158KB
ØD158Z4
ØD158Z6
ØD158Z9
ØD158ZA
ØD158ZB
ØD18Ø74
ØD18Ø78
ØD18Ø7H
ØD18Ø7K
ØD18Ø7L
ØD18Ø7M
ØD18Ø7N
ØD18Ø7P
ØD18Ø7Q
ØD18ØJ4
ØD18ØJ8
ØD18ØJH
ØD18ØJK
ØD18ØJL
ØD18ØJM
ØD18ØJN
ØD18ØJP
ØD18ØJQ
ØD18ØK4
ØD18ØK8
ØD18ØKH
ØD18ØKK
ØD18ØKL
ØD18ØKM
ØD18ØKN
ØD18ØKP
ØD18ØKQ
ØD18ØZ4
ØD18ØZ8
ØD18ØZH
ØD18ØZK
ØD18ØZL
ØD18ØZM
ØD18ØZN
ØD18ØZP
ØD18ØZQ
ØD18474
ØD18478
ØD1847H
ØD1847K
ØD1847L
ØD1847M
ØD1847N
ØD1847P
ØD1847Q
ØD184J4
ØD184J8
ØD184JH
ØD184JK
ØD184JL
ØD184JM
ØD184JN
ØD184JP
ØD184JQ
ØD184K4
ØD184K8
ØD184KH
ØD184KK
ØD184KL
ØD184KM
ØD184KN
ØD184KP
ØD184KQ
ØD184Z4
ØD184Z8
ØD184ZH
ØD184ZK
ØD184ZL
ØD184ZM
ØD184ZN
ØD184ZP
ØD184ZQ
ØD18874
ØD18878
ØD1887H
ØD1887K
ØD1887L
ØD1887M
ØD1887N
ØD1887P
ØD1887Q
ØD188J4
ØD188J8
ØD188JH
ØD188JK
ØD188JL
ØD188JM
ØD188JN
ØD188JP
ØD188JQ
ØD188K4
ØD188K8
ØD188KH
ØD188KK
ØD188KL
ØD188KM
ØD188KN
ØD188KP
ØD188KQ
ØD188Z4
ØD188Z8
ØD188ZH
ØD188ZK
ØD188ZL
ØD188ZM
ØD188ZN
ØD188ZP
ØD188ZQ
ØD19Ø74
ØD19Ø79
ØD19Ø7A
ØD19Ø7B
ØD19ØJ4
ØD19ØJ9
ØD19ØJA
ØD19ØJB
ØD19ØK4
ØD19ØK9
ØD19ØKA
ØD19ØKB
ØD19ØZ4
ØD19ØZ9
ØD19ØZA
ØD19ØZB
ØD193J4
ØD19474
ØD19479
ØD1947A
ØD1947B
ØD194J4
ØD194J9
ØD194JA
ØD194JB
ØD194K4
ØD194K9
ØD194KA
ØD194KB
ØD194Z4
ØD194Z9
ØD194ZA
ØD194ZB
ØD19874
ØD19879
ØD1987A
ØD1987B
ØD198J4
ØD198J9
ØD198JA
ØD198JB
ØD198K4
ØD198K9
ØD198KA
ØD198KB
ØD198Z4
ØD198Z9
ØD198ZA
ØD198ZB
ØD1AØ74
ØD1AØ7A
ØD1AØ7B
ØD1AØ7P
ØD1AØ7Q
ØD1AØJ4
ØD1AØJA
ØD1AØJB
ØD1AØJP
ØD1AØJQ
ØD1AØK4
ØD1AØKA
ØD1AØKB
ØD1AØKP
ØD1AØKQ
ØD1AØZ4
ØD1AØZA
ØD1AØZB
ØD1AØZP
ØD1AØZQ
ØD1A3J4
ØD1A474
ØD1A47A
ØD1A47B
ØD1A47P
ØD1A47Q
ØD1A4J4
ØD1A4JA
ØD1A4JB
ØD1A4JP
ØD1A4JQ
ØD1A4K4
ØD1A4KA
ØD1A4KB
ØD1A4KP
ØD1A4KQ
ØD1A4Z4
ØD1A4ZA
ØD1A4ZB
ØD1A4ZP
ØD1A4ZQ
ØD1A874
ØD1A87A
ØD1A87B
ØD1A87H
ØD1A87P
ØD1A87Q
ØD1A8J4
ØD1A8JA
ØD1A8JB
ØD1A8JH
ØD1A8JP
ØD1A8JQ
ØD1A8K4
ØD1A8KA
ØD1A8KB
ØD1A8KH
ØD1A8KP
ØD1A8KQ
ØD1A8Z4
ØD1A8ZA
ØD1A8ZB
ØD1A8ZH
ØD1A8ZP
ØD1A8ZQ
ØD1BØ74
ØD1BØ7B
ØD1BØ7P
ØD1BØ7Q
ØD1BØJ4
ØD1BØJB
ØD1BØJP
ØD1BØJQ
ØD1BØK4
ØD1BØKB
ØD1BØKP
ØD1BØKQ
ØD1BØZ4
ØD1BØZB
ØD1BØZP
ØD1BØZQ
ØD1B3J4
ØD1B474
ØD1B47B
ØD1B47P
ØD1B47Q
ØD1B4J4
ØD1B4JB
ØD1B4JP
ØD1B4JQ
ØD1B4K4
ØD1B4KB
ØD1B4KP
ØD1B4KQ
ØD1B4Z4
ØD1B4ZB
ØD1B4ZP
ØD1B4ZQ
ØD1B874
ØD1B87B
ØD1B87H
ØD1B87P
ØD1B87Q
ØD1B8J4
ØD1B8JB
ØD1B8JH
ØD1B8JP
ØD1B8JQ
ØD1B8K4
ØD1B8KB
ØD1B8KH
ØD1B8KP
ØD1B8KQ
ØD1B8Z4
ØD1B8ZB
ØD1B8ZH
ØD1B8ZP
ØD1B8ZQ
ØD1EØ74
ØD1EØ7E
ØD1EØ7P
ØD1EØJ4
ØD1EØJE
ØD1EØJP
ØD1EØK4
ØD1EØKE
ØD1EØKP
ØD1EØZ4
ØD1EØZE
ØD1EØZP
ØD1E474
ØD1E47E
ØD1E47P
ØD1E4J4
ØD1E4JE
ØD1E4JP
ØD1E4K4
ØD1E4KE
ØD1E4KP
ØD1E4Z4
ØD1E4ZE
ØD1E4ZP
ØD1E874
ØD1E87E
ØD1E87P
ØD1E8J4
ØD1E8JE
ØD1E8JP
ØD1E8K4
ØD1E8KE
ØD1E8KP
ØD1E8Z4
ØD1E8ZE
ØD1E8ZP
ØD1HØ74
ØD1HØJ4
ØD1HØK4
ØD1HØZ4
ØD1H3J4
ØD1H474
ØD1H4J4
ØD1H4K4
ØD1H4Z4
ØD1H874
ØD1H87P
ØD1H8J4
ØD1H8JP
ØD1H8K4
ØD1H8KP
ØD1H8Z4
ØD1H8ZP
ØD1KØ74
ØD1KØJ4
ØD1KØK4
ØD1KØZ4
ØD1K3J4
ØD1K474
ØD1K4J4
ØD1K4K4
ØD1K4Z4
ØD1K874
ØD1K8J4
ØD1K8K4
ØD1K8Z4
ØD1LØ74
ØD1LØJ4
ØD1LØK4
ØD1LØZ4
ØD1L3J4
ØD1L474
ØD1L4J4
ØD1L4K4
ØD1L4Z4
ØD1L874
ØD1L8J4
ØD1L8K4
ØD1L8Z4
ØD1MØ74
ØD1MØJ4
ØD1MØK4
ØD1MØZ4
ØD1M3J4
ØD1M474
ØD1M4J4
ØD1M4K4
ØD1M4Z4
ØD1M874
ØD1M8J4
ØD1M8K4
ØD1M8Z4
ØD1NØ74
ØD1NØJ4
ØD1NØK4
ØD1N3J4
ØD1N474
ØD1N4J4
ØD1N4K4
ØD1N4Z4
ØD1N874
ØD1N8J4
ØD1N8K4
ØD1N8Z4
ØD71ØDZ
ØD71ØZZ
ØD713DZ
ØD713ZZ
ØD714DZ
ØD714ZZ
ØD72ØDZ
ØD72ØZZ
ØD723DZ
ØD723ZZ
ØD724DZ
ØD724ZZ
ØD73ØDZ
ØD73ØZZ
ØD733DZ
ØD733ZZ
ØD734DZ
ØD734ZZ
ØD74ØDZ
ØD74ØZZ
ØD743DZ
ØD743ZZ
ØD744DZ
ØD744ZZ
ØD75ØDZ
ØD75ØZZ
ØD753DZ
ØD753ZZ
ØD754DZ
ØD754ZZ
ØD76ØDZ
ØD76ØZZ
ØD763DZ
ØD763ZZ
ØD764DZ
ØD764ZZ
ØD7QØDZ
ØD7QØZZ
ØD7Q3DZ
ØD7Q3ZZ
ØD7Q4DZ
ØD7Q4ZZ
ØD84ØZZ
ØD843ZZ
ØD844ZZ
ØD847ZZ
ØD848ZZ
ØD99ØØZ
ØD99ØZZ
ØD994ØZ
ØD994ZZ
ØD997ZZ
ØD998ZZ
ØD9PØØZ
ØD9PØZZ
ØD9P4ØZ
ØD9P4ZZ
ØD9P7ZZ
ØD9P8ZZ
ØDB1ØZZ
ØDB13ZZ
ØDB17ZZ
ØDB2ØZZ
ØDB23ZZ
ØDB27ZZ
ØDB3ØZZ
ØDB33ZZ
ØDB37ZZ
ØDB4ØZZ
ØDB43ZZ
ØDB44ZZ
ØDB47ZZ
ØDB5ØZZ
ØDB53ZZ
ØDB57ZZ
ØDB6ØZ3
ØDB6ØZZ
ØDB63Z3
ØDB63ZZ
ØDB67Z3
ØDB67ZZ
ØDB68Z3
ØDB8ØZZ
ØDB84ZZ
ØDB87ZZ
ØDB97ZZ
ØDBA7ZZ
ØDBB7ZZ
ØDBEØZZ
ØDBE3ZZ
ØDBE4ZZ
ØDBFØZZ
ØDBF3ZZ
ØDBF4ZZ
ØDBGØZZ
ØDBG3ZZ
ØDBG4ZZ
ØDBHØZZ
ØDBH3ZZ
ØDBH4ZZ
ØDBKØZZ
ØDBK3ZZ
ØDBK4ZZ
ØDBLØZZ
ØDBL3ZZ
ØDBL4ZZ
ØDBMØZZ
ØDBM3ZZ
ØDBM4ZZ
ØDBNØZZ
ØDBN3ZZ
ØDBN4ZZ
ØDBPØZZ
ØDBP3ZZ
ØDBP4ZZ
ØDBP7ZZ
ØDBQØZZ
ØDBQ3ZZ
ØDBQ4ZZ
ØDC9ØZZ
ØDC93ZZ
ØDC94ZZ
ØDCPØZZ
ØDCP3ZZ
ØDCP4ZZ
ØDCUØZZ
ØDCU3ZZ
ØDCU4ZZ
ØDCVØZZ
ØDCV3ZZ
ØDCV4ZZ
ØDCWØZZ
ØDCW3ZZ
ØDCW4ZZ
ØDF6ØZZ
ØDF63ZZ
ØDF64ZZ
ØDF67ZZ
ØDF68ZZ
ØDFPØZZ
ØDFP3ZZ
ØDFP4ZZ
ØDFP7ZZ
ØDFP8ZZ
ØDFQØZZ
ØDFQ3ZZ
ØDFQ4ZZ
ØDFQ7ZZ
ØDFQ8ZZ
ØDH6ØDZ
ØDH6ØMZ
ØDH63DZ
ØDH63MZ
ØDH64DZ
ØDH64MZ
ØDH9Ø2Z
ØDH9Ø3Z
ØDH932Z
ØDH933Z
ØDH942Z
ØDH943Z
ØDHQØDZ
ØDHQØLZ
ØDHQ3DZ
ØDHQ3LZ
ØDHQ4DZ
ØDHQ4LZ
ØDHQ7DZ
ØDHQ8DZ
ØDJØØZZ
ØDJØ4ZZ
ØDJ6ØZZ
ØDJ64ZZ
ØDJDØZZ
ØDJD4ZZ
ØDJUØZZ
ØDJU4ZZ
ØDJVØZZ
ØDJV4ZZ
ØDJWØZZ
ØDJW4ZZ
ØDL6ØCZ
ØDL6ØDZ
ØDL6ØZZ
ØDL63CZ
ØDL63DZ
ØDL63ZZ
ØDL64CZ
ØDL64DZ
ØDL64ZZ
ØDL67DZ
ØDL67ZZ
ØDL68DZ
ØDL68ZZ
ØDL7ØCZ
ØDL7ØDZ
ØDL7ØZZ
ØDL73CZ
ØDL73DZ
ØDL73ZZ
ØDL74CZ
ØDL74DZ
ØDL74ZZ
ØDL77DZ
ØDL77ZZ
ØDL78DZ
ØDL78ZZ
ØDLQØCZ
ØDLQØDZ
ØDLQØZZ
ØDLQ3CZ
ØDLQ3DZ
ØDLQ3ZZ
ØDLQ4CZ
ØDLQ4DZ
ØDLQ4ZZ
ØDLQ7DZ
ØDLQ7ZZ
ØDLQ8DZ
ØDLQ8ZZ
ØDLQXCZ
ØDLQXDZ
ØDLQXZZ
ØDM6ØZZ
ØDM64ZZ
ØDN6ØZZ
ØDN63ZZ
ØDN64ZZ
ØDN67ZZ
ØDN68ZZ
ØDN8ØZZ
ØDN83ZZ
ØDN84ZZ
ØDN9ØZZ
ØDN93ZZ
ØDN94ZZ
ØDNAØZZ
ØDNA3ZZ
ØDNA4ZZ
ØDNBØZZ
ØDNB3ZZ
ØDNB4ZZ
ØDNCØZZ
ØDNC3ZZ
ØDNC4ZZ

ØDNEØZZ
ØDNE3ZZ
ØDNE4ZZ
ØDNFØZZ
ØDNF3ZZ
ØDNF4ZZ
ØDNGØZZ
ØDNG3ZZ
ØDNG4ZZ
ØDNHØZZ
ØDNH3ZZ
ØDNH4ZZ
ØDNJØZZ
ØDNJ3ZZ
ØDNJ4ZZ
ØDNKØZZ
ØDNK3ZZ
ØDNK4ZZ
ØDNLØZZ
ØDNL3ZZ
ØDNL4ZZ
ØDNMØZZ
ØDNM3ZZ
ØDNM4ZZ
ØDNNØZZ
ØDNN3ZZ
ØDNN4ZZ
ØDNPØZZ
ØDNP3ZZ
ØDNP4ZZ
ØDNP7ZZ
ØDNP8ZZ
ØDNRØZZ
ØDNR3ZZ
ØDNR4ZZ
ØDNUØZZ
ØDNU3ZZ
ØDNU4ZZ
ØDNVØZZ
ØDNV3ZZ
ØDNV4ZZ
ØDNWØZZ
ØDNW3ZZ
ØDNW4ZZ
ØDP6ØMZ
ØDP63MZ
ØDP64MZ
ØDPPØ1Z
ØDPP31Z
ØDPP41Z
ØDPQØLZ
ØDPQ3LZ
ØDPQ4LZ
ØDPQ7LZ
ØDPQ8LZ
ØDPRØMZ
ØDPR3MZ
ØDPR4MZ
ØDQ4ØZZ
ØDQ43ZZ
ØDQ44ZZ
ØDQ47ZZ
ØDQ48ZZ
ØDQ5ØZZ
ØDQ53ZZ
ØDQ54ZZ
ØDQ57ZZ
ØDQ58ZZ
ØDQ6ØZZ
ØDQ63ZZ
ØDQ64ZZ
ØDQ67ZZ
ØDQ68ZZ
ØDQ8ØZZ
ØDQ83ZZ
ØDQ84ZZ
ØDQ87ZZ
ØDQ88ZZ
ØDQ9ØZZ
ØDQ93ZZ
ØDQ94ZZ
ØDQ97ZZ
ØDQ98ZZ
ØDQAØZZ
ØDQA3ZZ
ØDQA4ZZ
ØDQA7ZZ
ØDQA8ZZ
ØDQBØZZ
ØDQB3ZZ
ØDQB4ZZ
ØDQB7ZZ
ØDQB8ZZ
ØDQEØZZ
ØDQE3ZZ
ØDQE4ZZ
ØDQE7ZZ
ØDQE8ZZ
ØDQHØZZ
ØDQH3ZZ
ØDQH4ZZ
ØDQH7ZZ
ØDQH8ZZ
ØDQJØZZ
ØDQJ3ZZ
ØDQJ4ZZ
ØDQJ7ZZ
ØDQJ8ZZ
ØDQKØZZ
ØDQK3ZZ
ØDQK4ZZ
ØDQK7ZZ
ØDQK8ZZ
ØDQNØZZ
ØDQN3ZZ
ØDQN4ZZ
ØDQN7ZZ
ØDQN8ZZ
ØDQPØZZ
ØDQP3ZZ
ØDQP4ZZ
ØDQP7ZZ
ØDQP8ZZ
ØDQQØZZ
ØDQQ3ZZ
ØDQQ4ZZ
ØDQQ7ZZ
ØDQQ8ZZ
ØDQQXZZ
ØDQRØZZ
ØDQR3ZZ
ØDQR4ZZ
ØDQVØZZ
ØDQV3ZZ
ØDQV4ZZ
ØDQWØZZ
ØDQW3ZZ
ØDQW4ZZ
ØDR5Ø7Z
ØDR5ØJZ
ØDR5ØKZ
ØDR547Z
ØDR54JZ
ØDR54KZ
ØDR577Z
ØDR57JZ
ØDR57KZ
ØDR587Z
ØDR58JZ
ØDR58KZ
ØDRRØ7Z
ØDRRØJZ
ØDRRØKZ
ØDRR47Z
ØDRR4JZ
ØDRR4KZ
ØDRUØ7Z
ØDRUØJZ
ØDRUØKZ
ØDRU47Z
ØDRU4JZ
ØDRU4KZ
ØDRVØ7Z
ØDRVØJZ
ØDRVØKZ
ØDRV47Z
ØDRV4JZ
ØDRV4KZ
ØDRWØ7Z
ØDRWØJZ
ØDRWØKZ
ØDRW47Z
ØDRW4JZ
ØDRW4KZ
ØDS6ØZZ
ØDS64ZZ
ØDS67ZZ
ØDS68ZZ
ØDS8ØZZ
ØDS84ZZ
ØDS87ZZ
ØDS88ZZ
ØDSBØZZ
ØDSB4ZZ
ØDSB7ZZ
ØDSB8ZZ
ØDSEØZZ
ØDSE4ZZ
ØDSE7ZZ
ØDSE8ZZ
ØDSHØZZ
ØDSH4ZZ
ØDSH7ZZ
ØDSH8ZZ
ØDSPØZZ
ØDSP4ZZ
ØDSP7ZZ
ØDSP8ZZ
ØDT1ØZZ
ØDT14ZZ
ØDT17ZZ
ØDT18ZZ
ØDT2ØZZ
ØDT24ZZ
ØDT27ZZ
ØDT28ZZ
ØDT3ØZZ
ØDT34ZZ
ØDT37ZZ
ØDT38ZZ
ØDT4ØZZ
ØDT44ZZ
ØDT47ZZ
ØDT48ZZ
ØDT5ØZZ
ØDT54ZZ
ØDT57ZZ
ØDT58ZZ
ØDT6ØZZ
ØDT64ZZ
ØDT67ZZ
ØDT68ZZ
ØDT7ØZZ
ØDT74ZZ
ØDT77ZZ
ØDT78ZZ
ØDT8ØZZ
ØDT84ZZ
ØDT87ZZ
ØDT88ZZ
ØDT9ØZZ
ØDT94ZZ
ØDT97ZZ
ØDT98ZZ
ØDTAØZZ
ØDTA4ZZ
ØDTA7ZZ
ØDTA8ZZ
ØDTBØZZ
ØDTB4ZZ
ØDTB7ZZ
ØDTB8ZZ
ØDTCØZZ
ØDTC4ZZ
ØDTC7ZZ
ØDTC8ZZ
ØDTEØZZ
ØDTE4ZZ
ØDTE7ZZ
ØDTE8ZZ
ØDTFØZZ
ØDTF4ZZ
ØDTF7ZZ
ØDTF8ZZ
ØDTGØZZ
ØDTG4ZZ
ØDTG7ZZ
ØDTG8ZZ
ØDTGFZZ
ØDTHØZZ
ØDTH4ZZ
ØDTH7ZZ
ØDTH8ZZ
ØDTJØZZ
ØDTJ4ZZ
ØDTJ7ZZ
ØDTJ8ZZ
ØDTKØZZ
ØDTK4ZZ
ØDTK7ZZ
ØDTK8ZZ
ØDTLØZZ
ØDTL4ZZ
ØDTL7ZZ
ØDTL8ZZ
ØDTLFZZ
ØDTMØZZ
ØDTM4ZZ
ØDTM7ZZ
ØDTM8ZZ
ØDTMFZZ
ØDTNØZZ
ØDTN4ZZ
ØDTN7ZZ
ØDTN8ZZ
ØDTNFZZ
ØDTPØZZ
ØDTP4ZZ
ØDU1Ø7Z
ØDU1ØJZ
ØDU1ØKZ
ØDU147Z
ØDU14JZ
ØDU14KZ
ØDU177Z
ØDU17JZ
ØDU17KZ
ØDU187Z
ØDU18JZ
ØDU18KZ
ØDU2Ø7Z
ØDU2ØJZ
ØDU2ØKZ
ØDU247Z
ØDU24JZ
ØDU24KZ
ØDU277Z
ØDU27JZ
ØDU27KZ
ØDU287Z
ØDU28JZ
ØDU28KZ
ØDU3Ø7Z
ØDU3ØJZ
ØDU3ØKZ
ØDU347Z
ØDU34JZ
ØDU34KZ
ØDU377Z
ØDU37JZ
ØDU37KZ
ØDU387Z
ØDU38JZ
ØDU38KZ
ØDU4Ø7Z
ØDU4ØJZ
ØDU4ØKZ
ØDU447Z
ØDU44JZ
ØDU44KZ
ØDU477Z
ØDU47JZ
ØDU47KZ
ØDU487Z
ØDU48JZ
ØDU48KZ
ØDU5Ø7Z
ØDU5ØJZ
ØDU5ØKZ
ØDU547Z
ØDU54JZ
ØDU54KZ
ØDU577Z
ØDU57JZ
ØDU57KZ
ØDU587Z
ØDU58JZ
ØDU58KZ
ØDU6Ø7Z
ØDU6ØJZ
ØDU6ØKZ
ØDU647Z
ØDU64JZ
ØDU64KZ
ØDU677Z
ØDU67JZ
ØDU67KZ
ØDU687Z
ØDU68JZ
ØDU68KZ
ØDUPØ7Z
ØDUPØJZ
ØDUPØKZ
ØDUP47Z
ØDUP4JZ
ØDUP4KZ
ØDUP77Z
ØDUP7JZ
ØDUP7KZ
ØDUP87Z
ØDUP8JZ
ØDUP8KZ
ØDUQØ7Z
ØDUQØJZ
ØDUQØKZ
ØDUQ47Z
ØDUQ4JZ
ØDUQ4KZ
ØDUQ77Z
ØDUQ7JZ
ØDUQ7KZ
ØDUQ87Z
ØDUQ8JZ
ØDUQ8KZ
ØDUQX7Z
ØDUQXJZ
ØDUQXKZ
ØDURØ7Z
ØDURØJZ
ØDURØKZ
ØDUR47Z
ØDUR4JZ
ØDUR4KZ
ØDUUØ7Z
ØDUUØJZ
ØDUUØKZ
ØDUU47Z
ØDUU4JZ
ØDUU4KZ
ØDUVØ7Z
ØDUVØJZ
ØDUVØKZ
ØDUV47Z
ØDUV4JZ
ØDUV4KZ
ØDUWØ7Z
ØDUWØJZ
ØDUWØKZ
ØDUW47Z
ØDUW4JZ
ØDUW4KZ
ØDV4ØCZ
ØDV4ØDZ
ØDV4ØZZ
ØDV43CZ
ØDV43DZ
ØDV43ZZ
ØDV44CZ
ØDV44DZ
ØDV44ZZ
ØDV47DZ
ØDV47ZZ
ØDV48DZ
ØDV48ZZ
ØDV6ØCZ
ØDV6ØDZ
ØDV6ØZZ
ØDV63CZ
ØDV63DZ
ØDV63ZZ
ØDV64CZ
ØDV64DZ
ØDV64ZZ
ØDV67ZZ
ØDV68ZZ
ØDVPØCZ
ØDVPØDZ
ØDVPØZZ
ØDVP3CZ
ØDVP3DZ
ØDVP3ZZ
ØDVP4CZ
ØDVP4DZ
ØDVP4ZZ
ØDVP7DZ
ØDVP7ZZ
ØDVP8DZ
ØDVP8ZZ
ØDW8Ø7Z
ØDW8ØJZ
ØDW8ØKZ
ØDW847Z
ØDW84JZ
ØDW84KZ
ØDW877Z
ØDW87JZ
ØDW87KZ
ØDW887Z
ØDW88JZ
ØDW88KZ
ØDWEØ7Z
ØDWEØJZ
ØDWEØKZ
ØDWE47Z
ØDWE4JZ
ØDWE4KZ
ØDWE77Z
ØDWE7JZ
ØDWE7KZ
ØDWE87Z
ØDWE8JZ
ØDWE8KZ
ØDWQØLZ
ØDWQ3LZ
ØDWQ4LZ
ØDWQ7LZ
ØDWQ8LZ
ØDX6ØZ5
ØDX64Z5
ØDX8ØZ5
ØDX8ØZB
ØDX8ØZC
ØDX8ØZD
ØDX8ØZF
ØDX84Z5
ØDX84ZB
ØDX84ZC
ØDX84ZD
ØDX84ZF
ØDXEØZ5
ØDXEØZ7
ØDXEØZB
ØDXE4Z5
ØDXE4Z7
ØDXE4ZB
ØDY6ØZØ
ØDY6ØZ1
ØDY6ØZ2
ØF14ØD3
ØF14ØD4
ØF14ØD5
ØF14ØD6
ØF14ØD7
ØF14ØD8
ØF14ØD9
ØF14ØDB
ØF14ØZ3
ØF14ØZ4
ØF14ØZ5
ØF14ØZ6
ØF14ØZ7
ØF14ØZ8
ØF14ØZ9
ØF14ØZB
ØF144D3
ØF144D4
ØF144D5
ØF144D6
ØF144D7
ØF144D8
ØF144D9
ØF144DB
ØF144Z3
ØF144Z4
ØF144Z5
ØF144Z6
ØF144Z7
ØF144Z8
ØF144Z9
ØF144ZB
ØF15ØD3
ØF15ØD4
ØF15ØD5
ØF15ØD6
ØF15ØD7
ØF15ØD8
ØF15ØD9
ØF15ØDB
ØF15ØZ3
ØF15ØZ4
ØF15ØZ5
ØF15ØZ6
ØF15ØZ7
ØF15ØZ8
ØF15ØZ9
ØF15ØZB
ØF154D3
ØF154D4
ØF154D5
ØF154D6
ØF154D7
ØF154D8
ØF154D9
ØF154DB
ØF154Z3
ØF154Z4
ØF154Z5
ØF154Z6
ØF154Z7
ØF154Z8
ØF154Z9
ØF154ZB
ØF16ØD3
ØF16ØD4
ØF16ØD5
ØF16ØD6
ØF16ØD7
ØF16ØD8
ØF16ØD9
ØF16ØDB
ØF16ØZ3
ØF16ØZ4
ØF16ØZ5
ØF16ØZ6
ØF16ØZ7
ØF16ØZ8
ØF16ØZ9
ØF16ØZB
ØF164D3
ØF164D4
ØF164D5
ØF164D6
ØF164D7
ØF164D8
ØF164D9
ØF164DB
ØF164Z3
ØF164Z4
ØF164Z5
ØF164Z6
ØF164Z7
ØF164Z8
ØF164Z9
ØF164ZB
ØF17ØD3
ØF17ØD4
ØF17ØD5
ØF17ØD6
ØF17ØD7
ØF17ØD8
ØF17ØD9
ØF17ØDB
ØF17ØZ3
ØF17ØZ4
ØF17ØZ5
ØF17ØZ6
ØF17ØZ7
ØF17ØZ8
ØF17ØZ9
ØF17ØZB
ØF174D3
ØF174D4
ØF174D5
ØF174D6
ØF174D7
ØF174D8
ØF174D9
ØF174DB
ØF174Z3
ØF174Z4
ØF174Z5
ØF174Z6
ØF174Z7
ØF174Z8
ØF174Z9
ØF174ZB
ØF18ØD3
ØF18ØD4
ØF18ØD5
ØF18ØD6
ØF18ØD7
ØF18ØD8
ØF18ØD9
ØF18ØDB
ØF18ØZ3
ØF18ØZ4
ØF18ØZ5
ØF18ØZ6
ØF18ØZ7
ØF18ØZ8
ØF18ØZ9
ØF18ØZB
ØF184D3
ØF184D4
ØF184D5
ØF184D6
ØF184D7
ØF184D8
ØF184D9
ØF184DB
ØF184Z3
ØF184Z4
ØF184Z5
ØF184Z6
ØF184Z7
ØF184Z8
ØF184Z9
ØF184ZB
ØF19ØD3
ØF19ØD4
ØF19ØD5
ØF19ØD6
ØF19ØD7
ØF19ØD8
ØF19ØD9
ØF19ØDB
ØF19ØZ3
ØF19ØZ4
ØF19ØZ5
ØF19ØZ6
ØF19ØZ7
ØF19ØZ8
ØF19ØZ9
ØF19ØZB
ØF194D3
ØF194D4
ØF194D5
ØF194D6
ØF194D7
ØF194D8
ØF194D9
ØF194DB
ØF194Z3
ØF194Z4
ØF194Z5
ØF194Z6
ØF194Z7
ØF194Z8
ØF194Z9
ØF194ZB
ØF1DØD3
ØF1DØD4
ØF1DØDB
ØF1DØDC
ØF1DØZ3
ØF1DØZ4
ØF1DØZB
ØF1DØZC
ØF1D4D3
ØF1D4D4
ØF1D4DB
ØF1D4DC
ØF1D4Z3
ØF1D4Z4
ØF1D4ZB
ØF1D4ZC
ØF1FØD3
ØF1FØDB
ØF1FØDC
ØF1FØZ3
ØF1FØZB
ØF1FØZC
ØF1F4D3
ØF1F4DB
ØF1F4DC
ØF1F4Z3
ØF1F4ZB
ØF1F4ZC
ØF1GØD3
ØF1GØDB
ØF1GØDC
ØF1GØZ3
ØF1GØZB
ØF1GØZC
ØF1G4D3
ØF1G4DB
ØF1G4DC
ØF1G4Z3
ØF1G4ZB
ØF1G4ZC
ØF54ØZ3
ØF54ØZZ
ØF543Z3
ØF543ZZ
ØF544Z3
ØF544ZZ
ØF548ZZ
ØF75ØDZ
ØF75ØZZ
ØF757ZZ
ØF76ØDZ
ØF76ØZZ
ØF767ZZ
ØF77ØDZ
ØF77ØZZ
ØF777ZZ
ØF78ØDZ
ØF78ØZZ
ØF787ZZ
ØF79ØDZ
ØF79ØZZ
ØF797ZZ
ØF7CØDZ
ØF7CØZZ
ØF7C3DZ
ØF7C3ZZ
ØF7C4DZ
ØF7C4ZZ
ØF7C7DZ
ØF7C7ZZ
ØF7DØDZ
ØF7DØZZ
ØF7D3DZ
ØF7D3ZZ
ØF7D7ZZ
ØF7FØDZ
ØF7FØZZ
ØF7F3DZ
ØF7F3ZZ
ØF7F7DZ
ØF7F7ZZ
ØF8ØØZZ
ØF8Ø4ZZ
ØF81ØZZ
ØF814ZZ
ØF82ØZZ
ØF824ZZ
ØF8GØZZ
ØF8G3ZZ
ØF9ØØØZ
ØF9ØØZX
ØF9ØØZZ
ØF91ØØZ
ØF91ØZX
ØF91ØZZ
ØF92ØØZ
ØF92ØZX
ØF92ØZZ
ØF997ØZ
ØF9CØØZ
ØF9CØZZ
ØF9C7ØZ
ØF9C7ZZ
ØF9FØZX
ØF9GØZX
ØFBØØZX
ØFBØØZZ
ØFBØ3ZZ
ØFBØ4ZX
ØFBØ4ZZ
ØFB1ØZX
ØFB1ØZZ
ØFB13ZZ
ØFB14ZX
ØFB14ZZ
ØFB2ØZX
ØFB2ØZZ
ØFB23ZZ
ØFB24ZX
ØFB24ZZ
ØFB4ØZZ
ØFB43ZZ
ØFB44ZZ
ØFB48ZZ
ØFB8ØZZ
ØFB83ZZ
ØFB87ZZ
ØFBDØZX
ØFBFØZX
ØFBGØZX
ØFBGØZZ
ØFBG3ZZ
ØFBG4ZZ
ØFBG8ZZ
ØFCØØZZ
ØFCØ3ZZ
ØFCØ4ZZ
ØFC1ØZZ
ØFC13ZZ
ØFC14ZZ
ØFC2ØZZ
ØFC23ZZ
ØFC24ZZ
ØFC9ØZZ
ØFCCØZZ
ØFCC3ZZ
ØFCC7ZZ
ØFDØ4ZX
ØFD14ZX
ØFD24ZX
ØFHØØ1Z
ØFHØØ2Z
ØFHØØYZ
ØFHØ32Z
ØFHØ41Z
ØFHØ42Z
ØFH1Ø2Z
ØFH132Z
ØFH142Z
ØFH2Ø2Z
ØFH232Z
ØFH242Z
ØFHBØDZ
ØFHB3DZ
ØFHB7DZ

ØFHDØDZ
ØFHD3DZ
ØFHD7DZ
ØFJØØZZ
ØFJØ4ZZ
ØFJ44ZZ
ØFJDØZZ
ØFJD4ZZ
ØFJGØZZ
ØFJG4ZZ
ØFL5ØCZ
ØFL5ØDZ
ØFL5ØZZ
ØFL6ØCZ
ØFL6ØDZ
ØFL6ØZZ
ØFL7ØCZ
ØFL7ØDZ
ØFL7ØZZ
ØFL8ØCZ
ØFL8ØDZ
ØFL8ØZZ
ØFL9ØCZ
ØFL9ØDZ
ØFL9ØZZ
ØFLCØCZ
ØFLCØDZ
ØFLCØZZ
ØFLC3CZ
ØFLC3DZ
ØFLC3ZZ
ØFLC4CZ
ØFLC4DZ
ØFLC4ZZ
ØFLC7DZ
ØFLC7ZZ
ØFLC8DZ
ØFLC8ZZ
ØFLDØCZ
ØFLDØDZ
ØFLDØZZ
ØFLD3CZ
ØFLD3DZ
ØFLD3ZZ
ØFLD4CZ
ØFLD4DZ
ØFLD4ZZ
ØFLD7DZ
ØFLD7ZZ
ØFLD8DZ
ØFLD8ZZ
ØFLFØCZ
ØFLFØDZ
ØFLFØZZ
ØFLF3CZ
ØFLF3DZ
ØFLF3ZZ
ØFLF4CZ
ØFLF4DZ
ØFLF4ZZ
ØFLF7DZ
ØFLF7ZZ
ØFLF8DZ
ØFLF8ZZ
ØFMØØZZ
ØFMØ4ZZ
ØFM1ØZZ
ØFM14ZZ
ØFM2ØZZ
ØFM24ZZ
ØFM4ØZZ
ØFM5ØZZ
ØFM6ØZZ
ØFM7ØZZ
ØFM8ØZZ
ØFM9ØZZ
ØFMCØZZ
ØFMC4ZZ
ØFMDØZZ
ØFMD4ZZ
ØFMFØZZ
ØFMF4ZZ
ØFMGØZZ
ØFMG4ZZ
ØFNØØZZ
ØFNØ3ZZ
ØFNØ4ZZ
ØFN1ØZZ
ØFN13ZZ
ØFN14ZZ
ØFN2ØZZ
ØFN23ZZ
ØFN24ZZ
ØFN4ØZZ
ØFN43ZZ
ØFN44ZZ
ØFN48ZZ
ØFN5ØZZ
ØFN53ZZ
ØFN54ZZ
ØFN57ZZ
ØFN58ZZ
ØFN6ØZZ
ØFN63ZZ
ØFN64ZZ
ØFN67ZZ
ØFN68ZZ
ØFN7ØZZ
ØFN73ZZ
ØFN74ZZ
ØFN77ZZ
ØFN78ZZ
ØFN8ØZZ
ØFN83ZZ
ØFN84ZZ
ØFN87ZZ
ØFN88ZZ
ØFN9ØZZ
ØFN93ZZ
ØFN94ZZ
ØFN97ZZ
ØFN98ZZ
ØFNCØZZ
ØFNC3ZZ
ØFNC4ZZ
ØFNC7ZZ
ØFNC8ZZ
ØFNDØZZ
ØFND3ZZ
ØFND4ZZ
ØFND7ZZ
ØFND8ZZ
ØFNFØZZ
ØFNF3ZZ
ØFNF4ZZ
ØFNF7ZZ
ØFNF8ZZ
ØFNGØZZ
ØFNG3ZZ
ØFNG4ZZ
ØFNG8ZZ
ØFPØØØZ
ØFPØØ2Z
ØFPØØ3Z
ØFPØØYZ
ØFPØ3ØZ
ØFPØ32Z
ØFPØ33Z
ØFPØ4ØZ
ØFPØ42Z
ØFPØ43Z
ØFP4ØDZ
ØFP43DZ
ØFP44DZ
ØFQØØZZ
ØFQØ3ZZ
ØFQØ4ZZ
ØFQ1ØZZ
ØFQ13ZZ
ØFQ14ZZ
ØFQ2ØZZ
ØFQ23ZZ
ØFQ24ZZ
ØFQ4ØZZ
ØFQ43ZZ
ØFQ44ZZ
ØFQ48ZZ
ØFQ5ØZZ
ØFQ53ZZ
ØFQ54ZZ
ØFQ57ZZ
ØFQ58ZZ
ØFQ6ØZZ
ØFQ63ZZ
ØFQ64ZZ
ØFQ67ZZ
ØFQ68ZZ
ØFQ7ØZZ
ØFQ73ZZ
ØFQ74ZZ
ØFQ77ZZ
ØFQ78ZZ
ØFQ8ØZZ
ØFQ83ZZ
ØFQ84ZZ
ØFQ87ZZ
ØFQ88ZZ
ØFQ9ØZZ
ØFQ93ZZ
ØFQ94ZZ
ØFQ97ZZ
ØFQ98ZZ
ØFQCØZZ
ØFQC3ZZ
ØFQC4ZZ
ØFQC7ZZ
ØFQC8ZZ
ØFQDØZZ
ØFQD3ZZ
ØFQD4ZZ
ØFQD7ZZ
ØFQD8ZZ
ØFQFØZZ
ØFQF3ZZ
ØFQF4ZZ
ØFQF7ZZ
ØFQF8ZZ
ØFQGØZZ
ØFQG3ZZ
ØFQG4ZZ
ØFQG8ZZ
ØFR5Ø7Z
ØFR5ØJZ
ØFR5ØKZ
ØFR547Z
ØFR54JZ
ØFR54KZ
ØFR587Z
ØFR58JZ
ØFR58KZ
ØFR6Ø7Z
ØFR6ØJZ
ØFR6ØKZ
ØFR647Z
ØFR64JZ
ØFR64KZ
ØFR687Z
ØFR68JZ
ØFR68KZ
ØFR7Ø7Z
ØFR7ØJZ
ØFR7ØKZ
ØFR747Z
ØFR74JZ
ØFR74KZ
ØFR787Z
ØFR78JZ
ØFR78KZ
ØFR8Ø7Z
ØFR8ØJZ
ØFR8ØKZ
ØFR847Z
ØFR84JZ
ØFR84KZ
ØFR887Z
ØFR88JZ
ØFR88KZ
ØFR9Ø7Z
ØFR9ØJZ
ØFR9ØKZ
ØFR947Z
ØFR94JZ
ØFR94KZ
ØFR987Z
ØFR98JZ
ØFR98KZ
ØFRCØ7Z
ØFRCØJZ
ØFRCØKZ
ØFRC47Z
ØFRC4JZ
ØFRC4KZ
ØFRC87Z
ØFRC8JZ
ØFRC8KZ
ØFRDØ7Z
ØFRDØJZ
ØFRDØKZ
ØFRD47Z
ØFRD4JZ
ØFRD4KZ
ØFRD87Z
ØFRD8JZ
ØFRD8KZ
ØFRFØ7Z
ØFRFØJZ
ØFRFØKZ
ØFRF47Z
ØFRF4JZ
ØFRF4KZ
ØFRF87Z
ØFRF8JZ
ØFRF8KZ
ØFSØØZZ
ØFSØ4ZZ
ØFS4ØZZ
ØFS44ZZ
ØFS5ØZZ
ØFS54ZZ
ØFS6ØZZ
ØFS64ZZ
ØFS7ØZZ
ØFS74ZZ
ØFS8ØZZ
ØFS84ZZ
ØFS9ØZZ
ØFS94ZZ
ØFSCØZZ
ØFSC4ZZ
ØFSDØZZ
ØFSD4ZZ
ØFSFØZZ
ØFSF4ZZ
ØFTØØZZ
ØFTØ4ZZ
ØFT1ØZZ
ØFT14ZZ
ØFT2ØZZ
ØFT24ZZ
ØFT4ØZZ
ØFT44ZZ
ØFTGØZZ
ØFTG4ZZ
ØFU5Ø7Z
ØFU5ØJZ
ØFU5ØKZ
ØFU537Z
ØFU53JZ
ØFU53KZ
ØFU547Z
ØFU54JZ
ØFU54KZ
ØFU587Z
ØFU58JZ
ØFU58KZ
ØFU6Ø7Z
ØFU6ØJZ
ØFU6ØKZ
ØFU637Z
ØFU63JZ
ØFU63KZ
ØFU647Z
ØFU64JZ
ØFU64KZ
ØFU687Z
ØFU68JZ
ØFU68KZ
ØFU7Ø7Z
ØFU7ØJZ
ØFU7ØKZ
ØFU737Z
ØFU73JZ
ØFU73KZ
ØFU747Z
ØFU74JZ
ØFU74KZ
ØFU787Z
ØFU78JZ
ØFU78KZ
ØFU8Ø7Z
ØFU8ØJZ
ØFU8ØKZ
ØFU837Z
ØFU83JZ
ØFU83KZ
ØFU847Z
ØFU84JZ
ØFU84KZ
ØFU887Z
ØFU88JZ
ØFU88KZ
ØFU9Ø7Z
ØFU9ØJZ
ØFU9ØKZ
ØFU937Z
ØFU93JZ
ØFU93KZ
ØFU947Z
ØFU94JZ
ØFU94KZ
ØFU987Z
ØFU98JZ
ØFU98KZ
ØFUCØ7Z
ØFUCØJZ
ØFUCØKZ
ØFUC37Z
ØFUC3JZ
ØFUC3KZ
ØFUC47Z
ØFUC4JZ
ØFUC4KZ
ØFUC87Z
ØFUC8JZ
ØFUC8KZ
ØFUDØ7Z
ØFUDØJZ
ØFUDØKZ
ØFUD37Z
ØFUD3JZ
ØFUD3KZ
ØFUD47Z
ØFUD4JZ
ØFUD4KZ
ØFUD87Z
ØFUD8JZ
ØFUD8KZ
ØFUFØ7Z
ØFUFØJZ
ØFUFØKZ
ØFUF37Z
ØFUF3JZ
ØFUF3KZ
ØFUF47Z
ØFUF4JZ
ØFUF4KZ
ØFUF87Z
ØFUF8JZ
ØFUF8KZ
ØFV5ØCZ
ØFV5ØDZ
ØFV5ØZZ
ØFV6ØCZ
ØFV6ØDZ
ØFV6ØZZ
ØFV7ØCZ
ØFV7ØDZ
ØFV7ØZZ
ØFV8ØCZ
ØFV8ØDZ
ØFV8ØZZ
ØFV9ØCZ
ØFV9ØDZ
ØFV9ØZZ
ØFVCØCZ
ØFVCØDZ
ØFVCØZZ
ØFVC3CZ
ØFVC3DZ
ØFVC3ZZ
ØFVC4CZ
ØFVC4DZ
ØFVC4ZZ
ØFVC7DZ
ØFVC7ZZ
ØFVC8DZ
ØFVC8ZZ
ØFVDØCZ
ØFVDØDZ
ØFVDØZZ
ØFVD3CZ
ØFVD3DZ
ØFVD3ZZ
ØFVD4CZ
ØFVD4DZ
ØFVD4ZZ
ØFVD7DZ
ØFVD7ZZ
ØFVD8DZ
ØFVD8ZZ
ØFVFØCZ
ØFVFØDZ
ØFVFØZZ
ØFVF3CZ
ØFVF3DZ
ØFVF3ZZ
ØFVF4CZ
ØFVF4DZ
ØFVF4ZZ
ØFVF7DZ
ØFVF7ZZ
ØFVF8DZ
ØFVF8ZZ
ØFWØØØZ
ØFWØØ2Z
ØFWØØ3Z
ØFWØØYZ
ØFWØ3ØZ
ØFWØ32Z
ØFWØ33Z
ØFWØ4ØZ
ØFWØ42Z
ØFWØ43Z
ØG9GØØZ
ØG9GØZZ
ØG9HØØZ
ØG9HØZZ
ØG9KØØZ
ØG9KØZZ
ØG9LØØZ
ØG9LØZZ
ØG9MØØZ
ØG9MØZZ
ØG9NØØZ
ØG9NØZZ
ØG9PØØZ
ØG9PØZZ
ØG9QØØZ
ØG9QØZZ
ØG9RØØZ
ØG9RØZZ
ØGCGØZZ
ØGCG3ZZ
ØGCG4ZZ
ØGCHØZZ
ØGCH3ZZ
ØGCH4ZZ
ØGCKØZZ
ØGCK3ZZ
ØGCK4ZZ
ØGCLØZZ
ØGCL3ZZ
ØGCL4ZZ
ØGCMØZZ
ØGCM3ZZ
ØGCM4ZZ
ØGCNØZZ
ØGCN3ZZ
ØGCN4ZZ
ØGCPØZZ
ØGCP3ZZ
ØGCP4ZZ
ØGCQØZZ
ØGCQ3ZZ
ØGCQ4ZZ
ØGCRØZZ
ØGCR3ZZ
ØGCR4ZZ
ØGHSØ1Z
ØGHSØ2Z
ØGHSØ3Z
ØGHSØYZ
ØGHS32Z
ØGHS33Z
ØGHS41Z
ØGHS42Z
ØGHS43Z
ØGJKØZZ
ØGJRØZZ
ØGJSØZZ
ØGM2ØZZ
ØGM24ZZ
ØGM3ØZZ
ØGM34ZZ
ØGN2ØZZ
ØGN23ZZ
ØGN24ZZ
ØGN3ØZZ
ØGN33ZZ
ØGN34ZZ
ØGN4ØZZ
ØGN43ZZ
ØGN44ZZ
ØGPKØØZ
ØGPK3ØZ
ØGPK4ØZ
ØGPRØØZ
ØGPR3ØZ
ØGPR4ØZ
ØGQ2ØZZ
ØGQ23ZZ
ØGQ24ZZ
ØGQ3ØZZ
ØGQ33ZZ
ØGQ34ZZ
ØGQ4ØZZ
ØGQ43ZZ
ØGQ44ZZ
ØGQGØZZ
ØGQG3ZZ
ØGQG4ZZ
ØGQHØZZ
ØGQH3ZZ
ØGQH4ZZ
ØGQJØZZ
ØGQJ3ZZ
ØGQJ4ZZ
ØGQKØZZ
ØGQK3ZZ
ØGQK4ZZ
ØGS2ØZZ
ØGS24ZZ
ØGS3ØZZ
ØGS34ZZ
ØGWKØØZ
ØGWK3ØZ
ØGWK4ØZ
ØGWRØØZ
ØGWR3ØZ
ØGWR4ØZ
ØHØTØ7Z
ØHØT37Z
ØHØUØ7Z
ØHØU37Z
ØHØVØ7Z
ØHØVØJZ
ØHØVØKZ
ØHØV37Z
ØHØV3KZ
ØH5TØZ3
ØH5TØZZ
ØH5T3Z3
ØH5T3ZZ
ØH5T7ZZ
ØH5T8ZZ
ØH5UØZ3
ØH5UØZZ
ØH5U3Z3
ØH5U3ZZ
ØH5U7ZZ
ØH5U8ZZ
ØH5VØZ3
ØH5VØZZ
ØH5V3Z3
ØH5V3ZZ
ØH5V7ZZ
ØH5V8ZZ
ØH5WØZZ
ØH5W3ZZ
ØH5W7ZZ
ØH5W8ZZ
ØH5WXZZ
ØH5XØZZ
ØH5X3ZZ
ØH5X7ZZ
ØH5X8ZZ
ØH5XXZZ
ØH9TØZX
ØH9TØZZ
ØH9UØZX
ØH9UØZZ
ØH9VØZX
ØH9VØZZ
ØH9WØZX
ØH9WØZZ
ØH9XØZX
ØH9XØZZ
ØHBTØZX
ØHBTØZZ
ØHBT3ZZ
ØHBT7ZZ
ØHBT8ZZ
ØHBUØZX
ØHBUØZZ
ØHBU3ZZ
ØHBU7ZZ
ØHBU8ZZ
ØHBVØZX
ØHBVØZZ
ØHBV3ZZ
ØHBV7ZZ
ØHBV8ZZ
ØHBWØZX
ØHBWØZZ
ØHBW3ZZ
ØHBW7ZZ
ØHBW8ZZ
ØHBWXZZ
ØHBXØZX
ØHBXØZZ
ØHBX3ZZ
ØHBX7ZZ
ØHBX8ZZ
ØHBXXZZ
ØHBYØZX
ØHBYØZZ
ØHBY3ZZ
ØHBY7ZZ
ØHBY8ZZ
ØHCTØZZ
ØHCUØZZ
ØHCVØZZ
ØHCWØZZ
ØHCXØZZ
ØHDTØZZ
ØHDUØZZ
ØHDVØZZ
ØHDYØZZ
ØHHTØNZ
ØHHTØYZ
ØHHT3NZ
ØHHT7NZ
ØHHT8NZ
ØHHUØNZ
ØHHUØYZ
ØHHU3NZ
ØHHU7NZ
ØHHU8NZ
ØHHVØNZ
ØHHV3NZ
ØHHV7NZ
ØHHV8NZ
ØHHWØNZ
ØHHW3NZ
ØHHW7NZ
ØHHW8NZ
ØHHXØNZ
ØHHX3NZ
ØHHX7NZ
ØHHX8NZ
ØHM2XZZ
ØHM3XZZ
ØHM9XZZ
ØHMWXZZ
ØHMXXZZ
ØHNØXZZ
ØHN1XZZ
ØHN2XZZ
ØHN3XZZ
ØHN4XZZ
ØHN5XZZ
ØHN6XZZ
ØHN7XZZ
ØHN8XZZ
ØHN9XZZ
ØHNAXZZ
ØHNBXZZ
ØHNCXZZ
ØHNDXZZ
ØHNEXZZ
ØHNFXZZ
ØHNGXZZ
ØHNHXZZ
ØHNJXZZ
ØHNKXZZ
ØHNLXZZ
ØHNMXZZ
ØHNNXZZ
ØHPTØJZ
ØHPTØNZ
ØHPTØYZ
ØHPT3JZ
ØHPT3NZ
ØHPUØJZ
ØHPUØNZ
ØHPUØYZ
ØHPU3JZ
ØHPU3NZ
ØHQQXZZ
ØHQRXZZ
ØHQTØZZ
ØHQT3ZZ
ØHQT7ZZ
ØHQT8ZZ
ØHQUØZZ
ØHQU3ZZ
ØHQU7ZZ
ØHQU8ZZ
ØHQWØZZ
ØHQW3ZZ
ØHQW7ZZ
ØHQW8ZZ
ØHQWXZZ
ØHQXØZZ
ØHQX3ZZ
ØHQX7ZZ
ØHQX8ZZ
ØHQXXZZ
ØHRØX72
ØHRØX73
ØHRØX74
ØHRØXJ3
ØHRØXJ4
ØHRØXJZ
ØHRØXK3
ØHRØXK4
ØHR1X72
ØHR1X73
ØHR1X74
ØHR1XJ3
ØHR1XJ4
ØHR1XJZ
ØHR1XK3
ØHR1XK4
ØHR2X72
ØHR2X73
ØHR2X74
ØHR2XJ3
ØHR2XJ4
ØHR2XJZ
ØHR2XK3
ØHR2XK4
ØHR3X72
ØHR3X73
ØHR3X74
ØHR3XJ3
ØHR3XJ4
ØHR3XJZ
ØHR3XK3
ØHR3XK4
ØHR4X72
ØHR4X73
ØHR4X74
ØHR4XJ3
ØHR4XJ4
ØHR4XJZ
ØHR4XK3
ØHR4XK4
ØHR5X72
ØHR5X73
ØHR5X74
ØHR5XJ3
ØHR5XJ4
ØHR5XJZ
ØHR5XK3
ØHR5XK4
ØHR6X72
ØHR6X73
ØHR6X74
ØHR6XJ3
ØHR6XJ4
ØHR6XJZ
ØHR6XK3
ØHR6XK4
ØHR7X72
ØHR7X73
ØHR7X74
ØHR7XJ3
ØHR7XJ4
ØHR7XJZ
ØHR7XK3
ØHR7XK4
ØHR8X72
ØHR8X73
ØHR8X74
ØHR8XJ3
ØHR8XJ4
ØHR8XJZ
ØHR8XK3
ØHR8XK4
ØHR9X72
ØHR9X73
ØHR9X74
ØHR9XJ3
ØHR9XJ4
ØHR9XJZ
ØHR9XK3
ØHR9XK4
ØHRAX72
ØHRAX73
ØHRAX74
ØHRAXJ3
ØHRAXJ4
ØHRAXJZ
ØHRAXK3
ØHRAXK4
ØHRBX72
ØHRBX73
ØHRBX74
ØHRBXJ3
ØHRBXJ4
ØHRBXJZ
ØHRBXK3
ØHRBXK4
ØHRCX72
ØHRCX73
ØHRCX74
ØHRCXJ3
ØHRCXJ4
ØHRCXJZ
ØHRCXK3
ØHRCXK4
ØHRDX72
ØHRDX73
ØHRDX74

ØHRDXJ3
ØHRDXJ4
ØHRDXJZ
ØHRDXK3
ØHRDXK4
ØHREX72
ØHREX73
ØHREX74
ØHREXJ3
ØHREXJ4
ØHREXJZ
ØHREXK3
ØHREXK4
ØHRFX72
ØHRFX73
ØHRFX74
ØHRFXJ3
ØHRFXJ4
ØHRFXJZ
ØHRFXK3
ØHRFXK4
ØHRGX72
ØHRGX73
ØHRGX74
ØHRGXJ3
ØHRGXJ4
ØHRGXJZ
ØHRGXK3
ØHRGXK4
ØHRHX72
ØHRHX73
ØHRHX74
ØHRHXJ3
ØHRHXJ4
ØHRHXJZ
ØHRHXK3
ØHRHXK4
ØHRJX72
ØHRJX73
ØHRJX74
ØHRJXJ3
ØHRJXJ4
ØHRJXJZ
ØHRJXK3
ØHRJXK4
ØHRKX72
ØHRKX73
ØHRKX74
ØHRKXJ3
ØHRKXJ4
ØHRKXJZ
ØHRKXK3
ØHRKXK4
ØHRLX72
ØHRLX73
ØHRLX74
ØHRLXJ3
ØHRLXJ4
ØHRLXJZ
ØHRLXK3
ØHRLXK4
ØHRMX72
ØHRMX73
ØHRMX74
ØHRMXJ3
ØHRMXJ4
ØHRMXJZ
ØHRMXK3
ØHRMXK4
ØHRNX72
ØHRNX73
ØHRNX74
ØHRNXJ3
ØHRNXJ4
ØHRNXJZ
ØHRNXK3
ØHRNXK4
ØHRQX7Z
ØHRQXJZ
ØHRQXKZ
ØHRRX7Z
ØHRRXJZ
ØHRRXKZ
ØHRTØ75
ØHRTØ76
ØHRTØ77
ØHRTØ78
ØHRTØ79
ØHRTØ7Z
ØHRTØJZ
ØHRTØKZ
ØHRT3JZ
ØHRUØ75
ØHRUØ76
ØHRUØ77
ØHRUØ78
ØHRUØ79
ØHRUØ7Z
ØHRUØJZ
ØHRUØKZ
ØHRU3JZ
ØHRVØ75
ØHRVØ76
ØHRVØ77
ØHRVØ78
ØHRVØ79
ØHRVØJZ
ØHRV3JZ
ØHRWØ7Z
ØHRWØJZ
ØHRWØKZ
ØHRW37Z
ØHRW3JZ
ØHRW3KZ
ØHRWX7Z
ØHRWXJZ
ØHRWXKZ
ØHRXØ7Z
ØHRXØJZ
ØHRXØKZ
ØHRX37Z
ØHRX3JZ
ØHRX3KZ
ØHRXX7Z
ØHRXXJZ
ØHRXXKZ
ØHSTØZZ
ØHSUØZZ
ØHSVØZZ
ØHSWXZZ
ØHSXXZZ
ØHTTØZZ
ØHTUØZZ
ØHTVØZZ
ØHTWXZZ
ØHTXXZZ
ØHTYØZZ
ØHUWØ7Z
ØHUWØJZ
ØHUWØKZ
ØHUW37Z
ØHUW3JZ
ØHUW3KZ
ØHUW77Z
ØHUW7JZ
ØHUW7KZ
ØHUW87Z
ØHUW8JZ
ØHUW8KZ
ØHUWX7Z
ØHUWXJZ
ØHUWXKZ
ØHUXØ7Z
ØHUXØJZ
ØHUXØKZ
ØHUX37Z
ØHUX3JZ
ØHUX3KZ
ØHUX77Z
ØHUX7JZ
ØHUX7KZ
ØHUX87Z
ØHUX8JZ
ØHUX8KZ
ØHUXX7Z
ØHUXXJZ
ØHUXXKZ
ØHWTØJZ
ØHWTØYZ
ØHWT3JZ
ØHWUØJZ
ØHWUØYZ
ØHWU3JZ
ØHXØXZZ
ØHX1XZZ
ØHX2XZZ
ØHX3XZZ
ØHX4XZZ
ØHX5XZZ
ØHX6XZZ
ØHX7XZZ
ØHX8XZZ
ØHX9XZZ
ØHXAXZZ
ØHXBXZZ
ØHXCXZZ
ØHXDXZZ
ØHXEXZZ
ØHXFXZZ
ØHXGXZZ
ØHXHXZZ
ØHXJXZZ
ØHXKXZZ
ØHXLXZZ
ØHXMXZZ
ØHXNXZZ
ØJØ1ØZZ
ØJØ13ZZ
ØJ8ØØZZ
ØJ8Ø3ZZ
ØJ81ØZZ
ØJ813ZZ
ØJ84ØZZ
ØJ843ZZ
ØJ85ØZZ
ØJ853ZZ
ØJ86ØZZ
ØJ863ZZ
ØJ87ØZZ
ØJ873ZZ
ØJ88ØZZ
ØJ883ZZ
ØJ89ØZZ
ØJ893ZZ
ØJ8BØZZ
ØJ8B3ZZ
ØJ8CØZZ
ØJ8C3ZZ
ØJ8DØZZ
ØJ8D3ZZ
ØJ8FØZZ
ØJ8F3ZZ
ØJ8GØZZ
ØJ8G3ZZ
ØJ8HØZZ
ØJ8H3ZZ
ØJ8JØZZ
ØJ8J3ZZ
ØJ8KØZZ
ØJ8K3ZZ
ØJ8LØZZ
ØJ8L3ZZ
ØJ8MØZZ
ØJ8M3ZZ
ØJ8NØZZ
ØJ8N3ZZ
ØJ8PØZZ
ØJ8P3ZZ
ØJ8QØZZ
ØJ8Q3ZZ
ØJ8RØZZ
ØJ8R3ZZ
ØJ8SØZZ
ØJ8S3ZZ
ØJ8TØZZ
ØJ8T3ZZ
ØJ8VØZZ
ØJ8V3ZZ
ØJ8WØZZ
ØJ8W3ZZ
ØJBØØZZ
ØJB1ØZZ
ØJB4ØZZ
ØJB5ØZZ
ØJB6ØZZ
ØJB7ØZZ
ØJB8ØZZ
ØJB9ØZZ
ØJBBØZZ
ØJBCØZZ
ØJBDØZZ
ØJBFØZZ
ØJBGØZZ
ØJBHØZZ
ØJBJØZZ
ØJBJ3ZZ
ØJBKØZZ
ØJBK3ZZ
ØJBLØZZ
ØJBMØZZ
ØJBNØZZ
ØJBPØZZ
ØJBQØZZ
ØJBRØZZ
ØJDØØZZ
ØJD1ØZZ
ØJD4ØZZ
ØJD5ØZZ
ØJD6ØZZ
ØJD7ØZZ
ØJD8ØZZ
ØJD9ØZZ
ØJDBØZZ
ØJDCØZZ
ØJDDØZZ
ØJDFØZZ
ØJDGØZZ
ØJDHØZZ
ØJDJØZZ
ØJDKØZZ
ØJDLØZZ
ØJDMØZZ
ØJDNØZZ
ØJDPØZZ
ØJDQØZZ
ØJDRØZZ
ØJHØØNZ
ØJHØ3NZ
ØJH1ØNZ
ØJH13NZ
ØJH4ØNZ
ØJH43NZ
ØJH5ØNZ
ØJH53NZ
ØJH6Ø2Z
ØJH6ØNZ
ØJH6ØVZ
ØJH6ØYZ
ØJH632Z
ØJH63NZ
ØJH63VZ
ØJH7ØNZ
ØJH7ØVZ
ØJH7ØYZ
ØJH73NZ
ØJH73VZ
ØJH8ØNZ
ØJH8ØVZ
ØJH8ØYZ
ØJH83NZ
ØJH83VZ
ØJH9ØNZ
ØJH93NZ
ØJHBØNZ
ØJHB3NZ
ØJHCØNZ
ØJHC3NZ
ØJHDØNZ
ØJHDØVZ
ØJHD3NZ
ØJHD3VZ
ØJHFØNZ
ØJHFØVZ
ØJHF3NZ
ØJHF3VZ
ØJHGØNZ
ØJHGØVZ
ØJHG3NZ
ØJHG3VZ
ØJHHØNZ
ØJHHØVZ
ØJHH3NZ
ØJHH3VZ
ØJHJØNZ
ØJHJ3NZ
ØJHKØNZ
ØJHK3NZ
ØJHLØNZ
ØJHLØVZ
ØJHL3NZ
ØJHL3VZ
ØJHMØNZ
ØJHMØVZ
ØJHM3NZ
ØJHM3VZ
ØJHNØNZ
ØJHNØVZ
ØJHN3NZ
ØJHN3VZ
ØJHPØNZ
ØJHPØVZ
ØJHP3NZ
ØJHP3VZ
ØJHQØNZ
ØJHQ3NZ
ØJHRØNZ
ØJHR3NZ
ØJHTØVZ
ØJHTØYZ
ØJHT3VZ
ØJNJØZZ
ØJNJ3ZZ
ØJNKØZZ
ØJNK3ZZ
ØJPTØFZ
ØJPTØPZ
ØJPT3FZ
ØJPT3PZ
ØJQØØZZ
ØJQBØZZ
ØJQJØZZ
ØJQKØZZ
ØJRØ37Z
ØJR1Ø7Z
ØJR1ØKZ
ØJR137Z
ØJR13KZ
ØJR437Z
ØJR537Z
ØJR637Z
ØJR737Z
ØJR837Z
ØJR937Z
ØJRB37Z
ØJRC37Z
ØJRD37Z
ØJRF37Z
ØJRG37Z
ØJRH37Z
ØJRJØ7Z
ØJRJØJZ
ØJRJØKZ
ØJRJ37Z
ØJRJ3JZ
ØJRJ3KZ
ØJRKØ7Z
ØJRKØJZ
ØJRKØKZ
ØJRK37Z
ØJRK3JZ
ØJRK3KZ
ØJRL37Z
ØJRM37Z
ØJRN37Z
ØJRP37Z
ØJRQ37Z
ØJRR37Z
ØJUJØ7Z
ØJUJØJZ
ØJUJØKZ
ØJUJ37Z
ØJUJ3JZ
ØJUJ3KZ
ØJUKØ7Z
ØJUKØJZ
ØJUKØKZ
ØJUK37Z
ØJUK3JZ
ØJUK3KZ
ØJWTØ2Z
ØJWTØFZ
ØJWTØPZ
ØJWTØYZ
ØJWT32Z
ØJWT3FZ
ØJWT3PZ
ØJXØØZB
ØJXØØZC
ØJXØ3ZB
ØJXØ3ZC
ØJX1ØZB
ØJX1ØZC
ØJX13ZB
ØJX13ZC
ØJX4ØZB
ØJX4ØZC
ØJX43ZB
ØJX43ZC
ØJX5ØZB
ØJX5ØZC
ØJX53ZB
ØJX53ZC
ØJX6ØZB
ØJX6ØZC
ØJX63ZB
ØJX63ZC
ØJX7ØZB
ØJX7ØZC
ØJX73ZB
ØJX73ZC
ØJX8ØZB
ØJX8ØZC
ØJX83ZB
ØJX83ZC
ØJX9ØZB
ØJX9ØZC
ØJX93ZB
ØJX93ZC
ØJXBØZB
ØJXBØZC
ØJXB3ZB
ØJXB3ZC
ØJXCØZB
ØJXCØZC
ØJXC3ZB
ØJXC3ZC
ØJXDØZB
ØJXDØZC
ØJXD3ZB
ØJXD3ZC
ØJXFØZB
ØJXFØZC
ØJXF3ZB
ØJXF3ZC
ØJXGØZB
ØJXGØZC
ØJXG3ZB
ØJXG3ZC
ØJXHØZB
ØJXHØZC
ØJXH3ZB
ØJXH3ZC
ØJXJØZB
ØJXJØZC
ØJXJ3ZB
ØJXJ3ZC
ØJXKØZB
ØJXKØZC
ØJXK3ZB
ØJXK3ZC
ØJXLØZB
ØJXLØZC
ØJXL3ZB
ØJXL3ZC
ØJXMØZB
ØJXMØZC
ØJXM3ZB
ØJXM3ZC
ØJXNØZB
ØJXNØZC
ØJXN3ZB
ØJXN3ZC
ØJXPØZB
ØJXPØZC
ØJXP3ZB
ØJXP3ZC
ØJXQØZB
ØJXQØZC
ØJXQ3ZB
ØJXQ3ZC
ØJXRØZB
ØJXRØZC
ØJXR3ZB
ØJXR3ZC
ØK5ØØZZ
ØK5Ø3ZZ
ØK5Ø4ZZ
ØK51ØZZ
ØK513ZZ
ØK514ZZ
ØK52ØZZ
ØK523ZZ
ØK524ZZ
ØK53ØZZ
ØK533ZZ
ØK534ZZ
ØK54ØZZ
ØK543ZZ
ØK544ZZ
ØK55ØZZ
ØK553ZZ
ØK554ZZ
ØK56ØZZ
ØK563ZZ
ØK564ZZ
ØK57ØZZ
ØK573ZZ
ØK574ZZ
ØK58ØZZ
ØK583ZZ
ØK584ZZ
ØK59ØZZ
ØK593ZZ
ØK594ZZ
ØK5BØZZ
ØK5B3ZZ
ØK5B4ZZ
ØK5CØZZ
ØK5C3ZZ
ØK5C4ZZ
ØK5DØZZ
ØK5D3ZZ
ØK5D4ZZ
ØK5FØZZ
ØK5F3ZZ
ØK5F4ZZ
ØK5GØZZ
ØK5G3ZZ
ØK5G4ZZ
ØK5HØZZ
ØK5H3ZZ
ØK5H4ZZ
ØK5JØZZ
ØK5J3ZZ
ØK5J4ZZ
ØK5KØZZ
ØK5K3ZZ
ØK5K4ZZ
ØK5LØZZ
ØK5L3ZZ
ØK5L4ZZ
ØK5MØZZ
ØK5M3ZZ
ØK5M4ZZ
ØK5NØZZ
ØK5N3ZZ
ØK5N4ZZ
ØK5PØZZ
ØK5P3ZZ
ØK5P4ZZ
ØK5QØZZ
ØK5Q3ZZ
ØK5Q4ZZ
ØK5RØZZ
ØK5R3ZZ
ØK5R4ZZ
ØK5SØZZ
ØK5S3ZZ
ØK5S4ZZ
ØK5TØZZ
ØK5T3ZZ
ØK5T4ZZ
ØK5VØZZ
ØK5V3ZZ
ØK5V4ZZ
ØK5WØZZ
ØK5W3ZZ
ØK5W4ZZ
ØK8ØØZZ
ØK8Ø3ZZ
ØK8Ø4ZZ
ØK81ØZZ
ØK813ZZ
ØK814ZZ
ØK82ØZZ
ØK823ZZ
ØK824ZZ
ØK83ØZZ
ØK833ZZ
ØK834ZZ
ØK85ØZZ
ØK853ZZ
ØK854ZZ
ØK86ØZZ
ØK863ZZ
ØK864ZZ
ØK87ØZZ
ØK873ZZ
ØK874ZZ
ØK88ØZZ
ØK883ZZ
ØK884ZZ
ØK89ØZZ
ØK893ZZ
ØK894ZZ
ØK8BØZZ
ØK8B3ZZ
ØK8B4ZZ
ØK8CØZZ
ØK8C3ZZ
ØK8C4ZZ
ØK8DØZZ
ØK8D3ZZ
ØK8D4ZZ
ØK8FØZZ
ØK8F3ZZ
ØK8F4ZZ
ØK8GØZZ
ØK8G3ZZ
ØK8G4ZZ
ØK8HØZZ
ØK8H3ZZ
ØK8H4ZZ
ØK8JØZZ
ØK8J3ZZ
ØK8J4ZZ
ØK8KØZZ
ØK8K3ZZ
ØK8K4ZZ
ØK8LØZZ
ØK8L3ZZ
ØK8L4ZZ
ØK8MØZZ
ØK8M3ZZ
ØK8M4ZZ
ØK8NØZZ
ØK8N3ZZ
ØK8N4ZZ
ØK8PØZZ
ØK8P3ZZ
ØK8P4ZZ
ØK8QØZZ
ØK8Q3ZZ
ØK8Q4ZZ
ØK8RØZZ
ØK8R3ZZ
ØK8R4ZZ
ØK8SØZZ
ØK8S3ZZ
ØK8S4ZZ
ØK8TØZZ
ØK8T3ZZ
ØK8T4ZZ
ØK8VØZZ
ØK8V3ZZ
ØK8V4ZZ
ØK8WØZZ
ØK8W3ZZ
ØK8W4ZZ
ØK9CØØZ
ØK9CØZZ
ØK9C4ØZ
ØK9DØØZ
ØK9DØZZ
ØK9D4ØZ
ØKBØØZZ
ØKBØ3ZZ
ØKBØ4ZZ
ØKB1ØZZ
ØKB13ZZ
ØKB14ZZ
ØKB2ØZZ
ØKB23ZZ
ØKB24ZZ
ØKB3ØZZ
ØKB33ZZ
ØKB34ZZ
ØKB4ØZZ
ØKB43ZZ
ØKB44ZZ
ØKB5ØZZ
ØKB53ZZ
ØKB54ZZ
ØKB6ØZZ
ØKB63ZZ
ØKB64ZZ
ØKB7ØZZ
ØKB73ZZ
ØKB74ZZ
ØKB8ØZZ
ØKB83ZZ
ØKB84ZZ
ØKB9ØZZ
ØKB93ZZ
ØKB94ZZ
ØKBBØZZ
ØKBB3ZZ
ØKBB4ZZ
ØKBCØZZ
ØKBC3ZZ
ØKBC4ZZ
ØKBDØZZ
ØKBD3ZZ
ØKBD4ZZ
ØKBFØZZ
ØKBF3ZZ
ØKBF4ZZ
ØKBGØZZ
ØKBG3ZZ
ØKBG4ZZ
ØKBHØZZ
ØKBH3ZZ
ØKBH4ZZ
ØKBJØZZ
ØKBJ3ZZ
ØKBJ4ZZ
ØKBKØZZ
ØKBK3ZZ
ØKBK4ZZ
ØKBLØZZ
ØKBL3ZZ
ØKBL4ZZ
ØKBMØZZ
ØKBM3ZZ
ØKBM4ZZ
ØKBNØZZ
ØKBN4ZZ
ØKBPØZZ
ØKBP4ZZ
ØKBQØZZ
ØKBQ3ZZ
ØKBQ4ZZ
ØKBRØZZ
ØKBR3ZZ
ØKBR4ZZ
ØKBSØZZ
ØKBS3ZZ
ØKBS4ZZ
ØKBTØZZ
ØKBT3ZZ
ØKBT4ZZ
ØKBVØZZ
ØKBV3ZZ
ØKBV4ZZ
ØKBWØZZ
ØKBW3ZZ
ØKBW4ZZ
ØKCCØZZ
ØKCC3ZZ
ØKCC4ZZ
ØKCDØZZ
ØKCD3ZZ
ØKCD4ZZ
ØKDØØZZ
ØKD1ØZZ
ØKD2ØZZ
ØKD3ØZZ
ØKD4ØZZ
ØKD5ØZZ
ØKD6ØZZ
ØKD7ØZZ
ØKD8ØZZ
ØKD9ØZZ
ØKDBØZZ
ØKDCØZZ
ØKDDØZZ
ØKDFØZZ
ØKDGØZZ
ØKDHØZZ
ØKDJØZZ
ØKDKØZZ
ØKDLØZZ
ØKDMØZZ
ØKDNØZZ
ØKDPØZZ
ØKDQØZZ
ØKDRØZZ
ØKDSØZZ
ØKDTØZZ
ØKDVØZZ
ØKDWØZZ
ØKHXØMZ
ØKHXØYZ
ØKHX3MZ
ØKHX4MZ
ØKHYØMZ
ØKHYØYZ
ØKHY3MZ
ØKHY4MZ
ØKMØØZZ
ØKMØ4ZZ
ØKM1ØZZ
ØKM14ZZ
ØKM2ØZZ
ØKM24ZZ
ØKM3ØZZ
ØKM34ZZ
ØKM4ØZZ
ØKM44ZZ
ØKM5ØZZ
ØKM54ZZ
ØKM6ØZZ
ØKM64ZZ
ØKM7ØZZ
ØKM74ZZ
ØKM8ØZZ
ØKM84ZZ
ØKM9ØZZ
ØKM94ZZ
ØKMBØZZ
ØKMB4ZZ
ØKMCØZZ
ØKMC4ZZ
ØKMDØZZ
ØKMD4ZZ
ØKMFØZZ
ØKMF4ZZ
ØKMGØZZ
ØKMG4ZZ
ØKMHØZZ
ØKMH4ZZ
ØKMJØZZ
ØKMJ4ZZ
ØKMKØZZ
ØKMK4ZZ

ØKMLØZZ
ØKML4ZZ
ØKMMØZZ
ØKMM4ZZ
ØKMNØZZ
ØKMN4ZZ
ØKMPØZZ
ØKMP4ZZ
ØKMQØZZ
ØKMQ4ZZ
ØKMRØZZ
ØKMR4ZZ
ØKMSØZZ
ØKMS4ZZ
ØKMTØZZ
ØKMT4ZZ
ØKMVØZZ
ØKMV4ZZ
ØKMWØZZ
ØKMW4ZZ
ØKNCØZZ
ØKNC3ZZ
ØKNC4ZZ
ØKNDØZZ
ØKND3ZZ
ØKND4ZZ
ØKPXØMZ
ØKPX3MZ
ØKPX4MZ
ØKPYØØZ
ØKPYØJZ
ØKPYØMZ
ØKPYØYZ
ØKPY3ØZ
ØKPY3JZ
ØKPY3MZ
ØKPY4ØZ
ØKPY4JZ
ØKPY4MZ
ØKQØØZZ
ØKQØ3ZZ
ØKQØ4ZZ
ØKQ1ØZZ
ØKQ13ZZ
ØKQ14ZZ
ØKQ2ØZZ
ØKQ23ZZ
ØKQ24ZZ
ØKQ3ØZZ
ØKQ33ZZ
ØKQ34ZZ
ØKQ4ØZZ
ØKQ43ZZ
ØKQ44ZZ
ØKQ5ØZZ
ØKQ53ZZ
ØKQ54ZZ
ØKQ6ØZZ
ØKQ63ZZ
ØKQ64ZZ
ØKQ7ØZZ
ØKQ73ZZ
ØKQ74ZZ
ØKQ8ØZZ
ØKQ83ZZ
ØKQ84ZZ
ØKQ9ØZZ
ØKQ93ZZ
ØKQ94ZZ
ØKQBØZZ
ØKQB3ZZ
ØKQB4ZZ
ØKQCØZZ
ØKQC3ZZ
ØKQC4ZZ
ØKQDØZZ
ØKQD3ZZ
ØKQD4ZZ
ØKQFØZZ
ØKQF3ZZ
ØKQF4ZZ
ØKQGØZZ
ØKQG3ZZ
ØKQG4ZZ
ØKQHØZZ
ØKQH3ZZ
ØKQH4ZZ
ØKQJØZZ
ØKQJ3ZZ
ØKQJ4ZZ
ØKQKØZZ
ØKQK3ZZ
ØKQK4ZZ
ØKQLØZZ
ØKQL3ZZ
ØKQL4ZZ
ØKQMØZZ
ØKQM3ZZ
ØKQM4ZZ
ØKQNØZZ
ØKQN3ZZ
ØKQN4ZZ
ØKQPØZZ
ØKQP3ZZ
ØKQP4ZZ
ØKQQØZZ
ØKQQ3ZZ
ØKQQ4ZZ
ØKQRØZZ
ØKQR3ZZ
ØKQR4ZZ
ØKQSØZZ
ØKQS3ZZ
ØKQS4ZZ
ØKQTØZZ
ØKQT3ZZ
ØKQT4ZZ
ØKQVØZZ
ØKQV3ZZ
ØKQV4ZZ
ØKQWØZZ
ØKQW3ZZ
ØKQW4ZZ
ØKRØØ7Z
ØKRØØJZ
ØKRØØKZ
ØKRØ47Z
ØKRØ4JZ
ØKRØ4KZ
ØKR1Ø7Z
ØKR1ØJZ
ØKR1ØKZ
ØKR147Z
ØKR14JZ
ØKR14KZ
ØKR2Ø7Z
ØKR2ØJZ
ØKR2ØKZ
ØKR247Z
ØKR24JZ
ØKR24KZ
ØKR3Ø7Z
ØKR3ØJZ
ØKR3ØKZ
ØKR347Z
ØKR34JZ
ØKR34KZ
ØKR4Ø7Z
ØKR4ØJZ
ØKR4ØKZ
ØKR447Z
ØKR44JZ
ØKR44KZ
ØKR5Ø7Z
ØKR5ØJZ
ØKR5ØKZ
ØKR547Z
ØKR54JZ
ØKR54KZ
ØKR6Ø7Z
ØKR6ØJZ
ØKR6ØKZ
ØKR647Z
ØKR64JZ
ØKR64KZ
ØKR7Ø7Z
ØKR7ØJZ
ØKR7ØKZ
ØKR747Z
ØKR74JZ
ØKR74KZ
ØKR8Ø7Z
ØKR8ØJZ
ØKR8ØKZ
ØKR847Z
ØKR84JZ
ØKR84KZ
ØKR9Ø7Z
ØKR9ØJZ
ØKR9ØKZ
ØKR947Z
ØKR94JZ
ØKR94KZ
ØKRBØ7Z
ØKRBØJZ
ØKRBØKZ
ØKRB47Z
ØKRB4JZ
ØKRB4KZ
ØKRCØ7Z
ØKRCØJZ
ØKRCØKZ
ØKRC47Z
ØKRC4JZ
ØKRC4KZ
ØKRDØ7Z
ØKRDØJZ
ØKRDØKZ
ØKRD47Z
ØKRD4JZ
ØKRD4KZ
ØKRFØ7Z
ØKRFØJZ
ØKRFØKZ
ØKRF47Z
ØKRF4JZ
ØKRF4KZ
ØKRGØ7Z
ØKRGØJZ
ØKRGØKZ
ØKRG47Z
ØKRG4JZ
ØKRG4KZ
ØKRHØ7Z
ØKRHØJZ
ØKRHØKZ
ØKRH47Z
ØKRH4JZ
ØKRH4KZ
ØKRJØ7Z
ØKRJØJZ
ØKRJØKZ
ØKRJ47Z
ØKRJ4JZ
ØKRJ4KZ
ØKRKØ7Z
ØKRKØJZ
ØKRKØKZ
ØKRK47Z
ØKRK4JZ
ØKRK4KZ
ØKRLØ7Z
ØKRLØJZ
ØKRLØKZ
ØKRL47Z
ØKRL4JZ
ØKRL4KZ
ØKRMØ7Z
ØKRMØJZ
ØKRMØKZ
ØKRM47Z
ØKRM4JZ
ØKRM4KZ
ØKRNØ7Z
ØKRNØJZ
ØKRNØKZ
ØKRN47Z
ØKRN4JZ
ØKRN4KZ
ØKRPØ7Z
ØKRPØJZ
ØKRPØKZ
ØKRP47Z
ØKRP4JZ
ØKRP4KZ
ØKRQØ7Z
ØKRQØJZ
ØKRQØKZ
ØKRQ47Z
ØKRQ4JZ
ØKRQ4KZ
ØKRRØ7Z
ØKRRØJZ
ØKRRØKZ
ØKRR47Z
ØKRR4JZ
ØKRR4KZ
ØKRSØ7Z
ØKRSØJZ
ØKRSØKZ
ØKRS47Z
ØKRS4JZ
ØKRS4KZ
ØKRTØ7Z
ØKRTØJZ
ØKRTØKZ
ØKRT47Z
ØKRT4JZ
ØKRT4KZ
ØKRVØ7Z
ØKRVØJZ
ØKRVØKZ
ØKRV47Z
ØKRV4JZ
ØKRV4KZ
ØKRWØ7Z
ØKRWØJZ
ØKRWØKZ
ØKRW47Z
ØKRW4JZ
ØKRW4KZ
ØKSØØZZ
ØKSØ4ZZ
ØKS1ØZZ
ØKS14ZZ
ØKS2ØZZ
ØKS24ZZ
ØKS3ØZZ
ØKS34ZZ
ØKS4ØZZ
ØKS44ZZ
ØKS5ØZZ
ØKS54ZZ
ØKS6ØZZ
ØKS64ZZ
ØKS7ØZZ
ØKS74ZZ
ØKS8ØZZ
ØKS84ZZ
ØKS9ØZZ
ØKS94ZZ
ØKSBØZZ
ØKSB4ZZ
ØKSCØZZ
ØKSC4ZZ
ØKSDØZZ
ØKSD4ZZ
ØKSFØZZ
ØKSF4ZZ
ØKSGØZZ
ØKSG4ZZ
ØKSHØZZ
ØKSH4ZZ
ØKSJØZZ
ØKSJ4ZZ
ØKSKØZZ
ØKSK4ZZ
ØKSLØZZ
ØKSL4ZZ
ØKSMØZZ
ØKSM4ZZ
ØKSNØZZ
ØKSN4ZZ
ØKSPØZZ
ØKSP4ZZ
ØKSQØZZ
ØKSQ4ZZ
ØKSRØZZ
ØKSR4ZZ
ØKSSØZZ
ØKSS4ZZ
ØKSTØZZ
ØKST4ZZ
ØKSVØZZ
ØKSV4ZZ
ØKSWØZZ
ØKSW4ZZ
ØKTCØZZ
ØKTC4ZZ
ØKTDØZZ
ØKTD4ZZ
ØKUCØ7Z
ØKUCØJZ
ØKUCØKZ
ØKUC47Z
ØKUC4JZ
ØKUC4KZ
ØKUDØ7Z
ØKUDØJZ
ØKUDØKZ
ØKUD47Z
ØKUD4JZ
ØKUD4KZ
ØKWYØØZ
ØKWYØJZ
ØKWYØMZ
ØKWYØYZ
ØKWY3ØZ
ØKWY3JZ
ØKWY3MZ
ØKWY4ØZ
ØKWY4JZ
ØKWY4MZ
ØKXCØZØ
ØKXCØZ1
ØKXCØZ2
ØKXCØZZ
ØKXC4ZØ
ØKXC4Z1
ØKXC4Z2
ØKXC4ZZ
ØKXDØZØ
ØKXDØZ1
ØKXDØZ2
ØKXDØZZ
ØKXD4ZØ
ØKXD4Z1
ØKXD4Z2
ØKXD4ZZ
ØKXFØZ5
ØKXFØZ7
ØKXFØZ8
ØKXFØZ9
ØKXF4Z5
ØKXF4Z7
ØKXF4Z8
ØKXF4Z9
ØKXGØZ5
ØKXGØZ7
ØKXGØZ8
ØKXGØZ9
ØKXG4Z5
ØKXG4Z7
ØKXG4Z8
ØKXG4Z9
ØKXHØZZ
ØKXH4ZZ
ØKXJØZZ
ØKXJ4ZZ
ØKXKØZ6
ØKXK4Z6
ØKXLØZ6
ØKXL4Z6
ØL5ØØZZ
ØL5Ø3ZZ
ØL5Ø4ZZ
ØL51ØZZ
ØL513ZZ
ØL514ZZ
ØL52ØZZ
ØL523ZZ
ØL524ZZ
ØL53ØZZ
ØL533ZZ
ØL534ZZ
ØL54ØZZ
ØL543ZZ
ØL544ZZ
ØL55ØZZ
ØL553ZZ
ØL554ZZ
ØL56ØZZ
ØL563ZZ
ØL564ZZ
ØL57ØZZ
ØL573ZZ
ØL574ZZ
ØL58ØZZ
ØL583ZZ
ØL584ZZ
ØL59ØZZ
ØL593ZZ
ØL594ZZ
ØL5BØZZ
ØL5B3ZZ
ØL5B4ZZ
ØL5CØZZ
ØL5C3ZZ
ØL5C4ZZ
ØL5DØZZ
ØL5D3ZZ
ØL5D4ZZ
ØL5FØZZ
ØL5F3ZZ
ØL5F4ZZ
ØL5GØZZ
ØL5G3ZZ
ØL5G4ZZ
ØL5HØZZ
ØL5H3ZZ
ØL5H4ZZ
ØL5JØZZ
ØL5J3ZZ
ØL5J4ZZ
ØL5KØZZ
ØL5K3ZZ
ØL5K4ZZ
ØL5LØZZ
ØL5L3ZZ
ØL5L4ZZ
ØL5MØZZ
ØL5M3ZZ
ØL5M4ZZ
ØL5NØZZ
ØL5N3ZZ
ØL5N4ZZ
ØL5PØZZ
ØL5P3ZZ
ØL5P4ZZ
ØL5QØZZ
ØL5Q3ZZ
ØL5Q4ZZ
ØL5RØZZ
ØL5R3ZZ
ØL5R4ZZ
ØL5SØZZ
ØL5S3ZZ
ØL5S4ZZ
ØL5TØZZ
ØL5T3ZZ
ØL5T4ZZ
ØL5VØZZ
ØL5V3ZZ
ØL5V4ZZ
ØL5WØZZ
ØL5W3ZZ
ØL5W4ZZ
ØL87ØZZ
ØL873ZZ
ØL874ZZ
ØL88ØZZ
ØL883ZZ
ØL884ZZ
ØL8NØZZ
ØL8N3ZZ
ØL8N4ZZ
ØL8PØZZ
ØL8P3ZZ
ØL8P4ZZ
ØL97ØØZ
ØL97ØZZ
ØL974ØZ
ØL98ØØZ
ØL98ØZZ
ØL984ØZ
ØLBØØZZ
ØLBØ3ZZ
ØLBØ4ZZ
ØLB1ØZZ
ØLB13ZZ
ØLB14ZZ
ØLB2ØZZ
ØLB23ZZ
ØLB24ZZ
ØLB3ØZZ
ØLB33ZZ
ØLB34ZZ
ØLB4ØZZ
ØLB43ZZ
ØLB44ZZ
ØLB5ØZZ
ØLB53ZZ
ØLB54ZZ
ØLB6ØZZ
ØLB63ZZ
ØLB64ZZ
ØLB7ØZZ
ØLB73ZZ
ØLB74ZZ
ØLB8ØZZ
ØLB83ZZ
ØLB84ZZ
ØLB9ØZZ
ØLB93ZZ
ØLB94ZZ
ØLBBØZZ
ØLBB3ZZ
ØLBB4ZZ
ØLBCØZZ
ØLBC3ZZ
ØLBC4ZZ
ØLBDØZZ
ØLBD3ZZ
ØLBD4ZZ
ØLBFØZZ
ØLBF3ZZ
ØLBF4ZZ
ØLBGØZZ
ØLBG3ZZ
ØLBG4ZZ
ØLBHØZZ
ØLBH3ZZ
ØLBH4ZZ
ØLBJØZZ
ØLBJ3ZZ
ØLBJ4ZZ
ØLBKØZZ
ØLBK3ZZ
ØLBK4ZZ
ØLBLØZZ
ØLBL3ZZ
ØLBL4ZZ
ØLBMØZZ
ØLBM3ZZ
ØLBM4ZZ
ØLBNØZZ
ØLBN3ZZ
ØLBN4ZZ
ØLBPØZZ
ØLBP3ZZ
ØLBP4ZZ
ØLBQØZZ
ØLBQ3ZZ
ØLBQ4ZZ
ØLBRØZZ
ØLBR3ZZ
ØLBR4ZZ
ØLBSØZZ
ØLBS3ZZ
ØLBS4ZZ
ØLBTØZZ
ØLBT3ZZ
ØLBT4ZZ
ØLBVØZZ
ØLBV3ZZ
ØLBV4ZZ
ØLBWØZZ
ØLBW3ZZ
ØLBW4ZZ
ØLC7ØZZ
ØLC73ZZ
ØLC74ZZ
ØLC8ØZZ
ØLC83ZZ
ØLC84ZZ
ØLDØØZZ
ØLD1ØZZ
ØLD2ØZZ
ØLD3ØZZ
ØLD4ØZZ
ØLD5ØZZ
ØLD6ØZZ
ØLD7ØZZ
ØLD8ØZZ
ØLD9ØZZ
ØLDBØZZ
ØLDCØZZ
ØLDDØZZ
ØLDFØZZ
ØLDGØZZ
ØLDHØZZ
ØLDJØZZ
ØLDKØZZ
ØLDLØZZ
ØLDMØZZ
ØLDNØZZ
ØLDPØZZ
ØLDQØZZ
ØLDRØZZ
ØLDSØZZ
ØLDTØZZ
ØLDVØZZ
ØLDWØZZ
ØLHXØYZ
ØLHYØYZ
ØLJXØZZ
ØLJX4ZZ
ØLMØØZZ
ØLMØ4ZZ
ØLM1ØZZ
ØLM14ZZ
ØLM2ØZZ
ØLM24ZZ
ØLM3ØZZ
ØLM34ZZ
ØLM4ØZZ
ØLM44ZZ
ØLM5ØZZ
ØLM54ZZ
ØLM6ØZZ
ØLM64ZZ
ØLM7ØZZ
ØLM74ZZ
ØLM8ØZZ
ØLM84ZZ
ØLM9ØZZ
ØLM94ZZ
ØLMBØZZ
ØLMB4ZZ
ØLMCØZZ
ØLMC4ZZ
ØLMDØZZ
ØLMD4ZZ
ØLMFØZZ
ØLMF4ZZ
ØLMGØZZ
ØLMG4ZZ
ØLMHØZZ
ØLMH4ZZ
ØLMJØZZ
ØLMJ4ZZ
ØLMKØZZ
ØLMK4ZZ
ØLMLØZZ
ØLML4ZZ
ØLMMØZZ
ØLMM4ZZ
ØLMNØZZ
ØLMN4ZZ
ØLMPØZZ
ØLMP4ZZ
ØLMQØZZ
ØLMQ4ZZ
ØLMRØZZ
ØLMR4ZZ
ØLMSØZZ
ØLMS4ZZ
ØLMTØZZ
ØLMT4ZZ
ØLMVØZZ
ØLMV4ZZ
ØLMWØZZ
ØLMW4ZZ
ØLN7ØZZ
ØLN73ZZ
ØLN74ZZ
ØLN8ØZZ
ØLN83ZZ
ØLN84ZZ
ØLQØØZZ
ØLQØ3ZZ
ØLQØ4ZZ
ØLQ1ØZZ
ØLQ13ZZ
ØLQ14ZZ
ØLQ2ØZZ
ØLQ23ZZ
ØLQ24ZZ
ØLQ3ØZZ
ØLQ33ZZ
ØLQ34ZZ
ØLQ4ØZZ
ØLQ43ZZ
ØLQ44ZZ
ØLQ5ØZZ
ØLQ53ZZ
ØLQ54ZZ
ØLQ6ØZZ
ØLQ63ZZ
ØLQ64ZZ
ØLQ7ØZZ
ØLQ73ZZ
ØLQ74ZZ
ØLQ8ØZZ
ØLQ83ZZ
ØLQ84ZZ
ØLQ9ØZZ
ØLQ93ZZ
ØLQ94ZZ
ØLQBØZZ
ØLQB3ZZ
ØLQB4ZZ
ØLQCØZZ
ØLQC3ZZ
ØLQC4ZZ
ØLQDØZZ
ØLQD3ZZ
ØLQD4ZZ
ØLQFØZZ
ØLQF3ZZ
ØLQF4ZZ
ØLQGØZZ
ØLQG3ZZ
ØLQG4ZZ
ØLQHØZZ
ØLQH3ZZ
ØLQH4ZZ
ØLQJØZZ
ØLQJ3ZZ
ØLQJ4ZZ
ØLQKØZZ
ØLQK3ZZ
ØLQK4ZZ
ØLQLØZZ
ØLQL3ZZ
ØLQL4ZZ
ØLQMØZZ
ØLQM3ZZ
ØLQM4ZZ
ØLQNØZZ
ØLQN3ZZ
ØLQN4ZZ
ØLQPØZZ
ØLQP3ZZ
ØLQP4ZZ
ØLQQØZZ
ØLQQ3ZZ
ØLQQ4ZZ
ØLQRØZZ
ØLQR3ZZ
ØLQR4ZZ
ØLQSØZZ
ØLQS3ZZ
ØLQS4ZZ
ØLQTØZZ
ØLQT3ZZ
ØLQT4ZZ
ØLQVØZZ
ØLQV3ZZ
ØLQV4ZZ
ØLQWØZZ
ØLQW3ZZ
ØLQW4ZZ
ØLR7Ø7Z
ØLR7ØJZ
ØLR7ØKZ
ØLR747Z
ØLR74JZ
ØLR74KZ
ØLR8Ø7Z
ØLR8ØJZ
ØLR8ØKZ
ØLR847Z
ØLR84JZ
ØLR84KZ
ØLSØØZZ
ØLSØ4ZZ
ØLS1ØZZ
ØLS14ZZ
ØLS2ØZZ
ØLS24ZZ
ØLS3ØZZ
ØLS34ZZ
ØLS4ØZZ
ØLS44ZZ
ØLS5ØZZ
ØLS54ZZ
ØLS6ØZZ
ØLS64ZZ
ØLS7ØZZ
ØLS74ZZ
ØLS8ØZZ
ØLS84ZZ
ØLS9ØZZ
ØLS94ZZ
ØLSBØZZ
ØLSB4ZZ
ØLSCØZZ
ØLSC4ZZ
ØLSDØZZ
ØLSD4ZZ
ØLSFØZZ
ØLSF4ZZ
ØLSGØZZ
ØLSG4ZZ
ØLSHØZZ
ØLSH4ZZ
ØLSJØZZ
ØLSJ4ZZ
ØLSKØZZ
ØLSK4ZZ
ØLSLØZZ
ØLSL4ZZ
ØLSMØZZ
ØLSM4ZZ
ØLSNØZZ
ØLSN4ZZ
ØLSPØZZ
ØLSP4ZZ
ØLSQØZZ
ØLSQ4ZZ
ØLSRØZZ
ØLSR4ZZ
ØLSSØZZ
ØLSS4ZZ
ØLSTØZZ
ØLST4ZZ
ØLSVØZZ
ØLSV4ZZ
ØLSWØZZ
ØLSW4ZZ
ØLT7ØZZ
ØLT74ZZ
ØLT8ØZZ
ØLT84ZZ

0LU707Z
0LU70JZ
0LU70KZ
0LU747Z
0LU74JZ
0LU74KZ
0LU807Z
0LU80JZ
0LU80KZ
0LU847Z
0LU84JZ
0LU84KZ
0LX00ZZ
0LX04ZZ
0LX10ZZ
0LX14ZZ
0LX20ZZ
0LX24ZZ
0LX30ZZ
0LX34ZZ
0LX40ZZ
0LX44ZZ
0LX50ZZ
0LX54ZZ
0LX60ZZ
0LX64ZZ
0LX70ZZ
0LX74ZZ
0LX80ZZ
0LX84ZZ
0LX90ZZ
0LX94ZZ
0LXB0ZZ
0LXB4ZZ
0LXC0ZZ
0LXC4ZZ
0LXD0ZZ
0LXD4ZZ
0LXF0ZZ
0LXF4ZZ
0LXG0ZZ
0LXG4ZZ
0LXH0ZZ
0LXH4ZZ
0LXJ0ZZ
0LXJ4ZZ
0LXK0ZZ
0LXK4ZZ
0LXL0ZZ
0LXL4ZZ
0LXM0ZZ
0LXM4ZZ
0LXN0ZZ
0LXN4ZZ
0LXP0ZZ
0LXP4ZZ
0LXQ0ZZ
0LXQ4ZZ
0LXR0ZZ
0LXR4ZZ
0LXS0ZZ
0LXS4ZZ
0LXT0ZZ
0LXT4ZZ
0LXV0ZZ
0LXV4ZZ
0LXW0ZZ
0LXW4ZZ
0M500ZZ
0M503ZZ
0M504ZZ
0M510ZZ
0M513ZZ
0M514ZZ
0M520ZZ
0M523ZZ
0M524ZZ
0M530ZZ
0M533ZZ
0M534ZZ
0M540ZZ
0M543ZZ
0M544ZZ
0M550ZZ
0M553ZZ
0M554ZZ
0M560ZZ
0M563ZZ
0M564ZZ
0M570ZZ
0M573ZZ
0M574ZZ
0M580ZZ
0M583ZZ
0M584ZZ
0M590ZZ
0M593ZZ
0M594ZZ
0M5B0ZZ
0M5B3ZZ
0M5B4ZZ
0M5C0ZZ
0M5C3ZZ
0M5C4ZZ
0M5D0ZZ
0M5D3ZZ
0M5D4ZZ
0M5F0ZZ
0M5F3ZZ
0M5F4ZZ
0M5G0ZZ
0M5G3ZZ
0M5G4ZZ
0M5H0ZZ
0M5H3ZZ
0M5H4ZZ
0M5J0ZZ
0M5J3ZZ
0M5J4ZZ
0M5K0ZZ
0M5K3ZZ
0M5K4ZZ
0M5L0ZZ
0M5L3ZZ
0M5L4ZZ
0M5M0ZZ
0M5M3ZZ
0M5M4ZZ
0M5N0ZZ
0M5N3ZZ
0M5N4ZZ
0M5P0ZZ
0M5P3ZZ
0M5P4ZZ
0M5Q0ZZ
0M5Q3ZZ
0M5Q4ZZ
0M5R0ZZ
0M5R3ZZ
0M5R4ZZ
0M5S0ZZ
0M5S3ZZ
0M5S4ZZ
0M5T0ZZ
0M5T3ZZ
0M5T4ZZ
0M800ZZ
0M803ZZ
0M804ZZ
0M810ZZ
0M813ZZ
0M814ZZ
0M820ZZ
0M823ZZ
0M824ZZ
0M830ZZ
0M833ZZ
0M834ZZ
0M840ZZ
0M843ZZ
0M844ZZ
0M870ZZ
0M873ZZ
0M874ZZ
0M880ZZ
0M883ZZ
0M884ZZ
0M890ZZ
0M893ZZ
0M894ZZ
0M8B0ZZ
0M8B3ZZ
0M8B4ZZ
0M8C0ZZ
0M8C3ZZ
0M8C4ZZ
0M8D0ZZ
0M8D3ZZ
0M8D4ZZ
0M8F0ZZ
0M8F3ZZ
0M8F4ZZ
0M8G0ZZ
0M8G3ZZ
0M8G4ZZ
0M8H0ZZ
0M8H3ZZ
0M8H4ZZ
0M8J0ZZ
0M8J3ZZ
0M8J4ZZ
0M8K0ZZ
0M8K3ZZ
0M8K4ZZ
0M8L0ZZ
0M8L3ZZ
0M8L4ZZ
0M8M0ZZ
0M8M3ZZ
0M8M4ZZ
0M8N0ZZ
0M8N3ZZ
0M8N4ZZ
0M8P0ZZ
0M8P3ZZ
0M8P4ZZ
0M8Q0ZZ
0M8Q3ZZ
0M8Q4ZZ
0M8R0ZZ
0M8R3ZZ
0M8R4ZZ
0M8S0ZZ
0M8S3ZZ
0M8S4ZZ
0M8T0ZZ
0M8T3ZZ
0M8T4ZZ
0M8V0ZZ
0M8V3ZZ
0M8V4ZZ
0M8W0ZZ
0M8W3ZZ
0M8W4ZZ
0M9000Z
0M900ZZ
0M9100Z
0M910ZZ
0M9200Z
0M920ZZ
0M9300Z
0M930ZZ
0M9400Z
0M940ZZ
0M9700Z
0M970ZZ
0M9800Z
0M980ZZ
0M9900Z
0M990ZZ
0M9B00Z
0M9B0ZZ
0M9C00Z
0M9C0ZZ
0M9D00Z
0M9D0ZZ
0M9F00Z
0M9F0ZZ
0M9G00Z
0M9G0ZZ
0M9H00Z
0M9H0ZZ
0M9J00Z
0M9J0ZZ
0M9K00Z
0M9K0ZZ
0M9L00Z
0M9L0ZZ
0M9M00Z
0M9M0ZZ
0M9N00Z
0M9N0ZZ
0M9P00Z
0M9P0ZZ
0M9Q00Z
0M9Q0ZZ
0M9R00Z
0M9R0ZZ
0M9S00Z
0M9S0ZZ
0M9T00Z
0M9T0ZZ
0M9V00Z
0M9V0ZZ
0M9W00Z
0M9W0ZZ
0MB00ZZ
0MB03ZZ
0MB04ZZ
0MB70ZZ
0MB73ZZ
0MB74ZZ
0MB80ZZ
0MB83ZZ
0MB84ZZ
0MB90ZZ
0MB93ZZ
0MB94ZZ
0MBB0ZZ
0MBB3ZZ
0MBB4ZZ
0MBC0ZZ
0MBC3ZZ
0MBC4ZZ
0MBD0ZZ
0MBD3ZZ
0MBD4ZZ
0MBF0ZZ
0MBF3ZZ
0MBF4ZZ
0MBG0ZZ
0MBG3ZZ
0MBG4ZZ
0MBV0ZZ
0MBV3ZZ
0MBV4ZZ
0MBW0ZZ
0MBW3ZZ
0MBW4ZZ
0MC00ZZ
0MC03ZZ
0MC04ZZ
0MC10ZZ
0MC13ZZ
0MC14ZZ
0MC20ZZ
0MC23ZZ
0MC24ZZ
0MC30ZZ
0MC33ZZ
0MC34ZZ
0MC40ZZ
0MC43ZZ
0MC44ZZ
0MC70ZZ
0MC73ZZ
0MC74ZZ
0MC80ZZ
0MC83ZZ
0MC84ZZ
0MC90ZZ
0MC93ZZ
0MC94ZZ
0MCB0ZZ
0MCB3ZZ
0MCB4ZZ
0MCC0ZZ
0MCC3ZZ
0MCC4ZZ
0MCD0ZZ
0MCD3ZZ
0MCD4ZZ
0MCF0ZZ
0MCF3ZZ
0MCF4ZZ
0MCG0ZZ
0MCG3ZZ
0MCG4ZZ
0MCH0ZZ
0MCH3ZZ
0MCH4ZZ
0MCJ0ZZ
0MCJ3ZZ
0MCJ4ZZ
0MCK0ZZ
0MCK3ZZ
0MCK4ZZ
0MCL0ZZ
0MCL3ZZ
0MCL4ZZ
0MCM0ZZ
0MCM3ZZ
0MCM4ZZ
0MCN0ZZ
0MCN3ZZ
0MCN4ZZ
0MCP0ZZ
0MCP3ZZ
0MCP4ZZ
0MCQ0ZZ
0MCQ3ZZ
0MCQ4ZZ
0MCR0ZZ
0MCR3ZZ
0MCR4ZZ
0MCS0ZZ
0MCS3ZZ
0MCS4ZZ
0MCT0ZZ
0MCT3ZZ
0MCT4ZZ
0MCV0ZZ
0MCV3ZZ
0MCV4ZZ
0MCW0ZZ
0MCW3ZZ
0MCW4ZZ
0MD70ZZ
0MD73ZZ
0MD74ZZ
0MD80ZZ
0MD83ZZ
0MD84ZZ
0MHX0YZ
0MHY0YZ
0MN70ZZ
0MN73ZZ
0MN74ZZ
0MN80ZZ
0MN83ZZ
0MN84ZZ
0MPX07Z
0MPX0KZ
0MPX37Z
0MPX3KZ
0MPX47Z
0MPX4KZ
0MPY07Z
0MPY0KZ
0MPY37Z
0MPY3KZ
0MPY47Z
0MPY4KZ
0MQ10ZZ
0MQ13ZZ
0MQ14ZZ
0MQ20ZZ
0MQ23ZZ
0MQ24ZZ
0MQ30ZZ
0MQ33ZZ
0MQ34ZZ
0MQ40ZZ
0MQ43ZZ
0MQ44ZZ
0MQ50ZZ
0MQ53ZZ
0MQ54ZZ
0MQ60ZZ
0MQ63ZZ
0MQ64ZZ
0MQ70ZZ
0MQ73ZZ
0MQ74ZZ
0MQ80ZZ
0MQ83ZZ
0MQ84ZZ
0MQN0ZZ
0MQN3ZZ
0MQN4ZZ
0MQP0ZZ
0MQP3ZZ
0MQP4ZZ
0MQQ0ZZ
0MQQ3ZZ
0MQQ4ZZ
0MQR0ZZ
0MQR3ZZ
0MQR4ZZ
0MQS0ZZ
0MQS3ZZ
0MQS4ZZ
0MQT0ZZ
0MQT3ZZ
0MQT4ZZ
0MR107Z
0MR10JZ
0MR10KZ
0MR147Z
0MR14JZ
0MR14KZ
0MR207Z
0MR20JZ
0MR20KZ
0MR247Z
0MR24JZ
0MR24KZ
0MR307Z
0MR30JZ
0MR30KZ
0MR347Z
0MR34JZ
0MR34KZ
0MR407Z
0MR40JZ
0MR40KZ
0MR447Z
0MR44JZ
0MR44KZ
0MR507Z
0MR50JZ
0MR50KZ
0MR547Z
0MR54JZ
0MR54KZ
0MR607Z
0MR60JZ
0MR60KZ
0MR647Z
0MR64JZ
0MR64KZ
0MR707Z
0MR70JZ
0MR70KZ
0MR747Z
0MR74JZ
0MR74KZ
0MR807Z
0MR80JZ
0MR80KZ
0MR847Z
0MR84JZ
0MR84KZ
0MRN07Z
0MRN0JZ
0MRN0KZ
0MRN47Z
0MRN4JZ
0MRN4KZ
0MRP07Z
0MRP0JZ
0MRP0KZ
0MRP47Z
0MRP4JZ
0MRP4KZ
0MRQ07Z
0MRQ0JZ
0MRQ0KZ
0MRQ47Z
0MRQ4JZ
0MRQ4KZ
0MRR07Z
0MRR0JZ
0MRR0KZ
0MRR47Z
0MRR4JZ
0MRR4KZ
0MRS07Z
0MRS0JZ
0MRS0KZ
0MRS47Z
0MRS4JZ
0MRS4KZ
0MRT07Z
0MRT0JZ
0MRT0KZ
0MRT47Z
0MRT4JZ
0MRT4KZ
0MT00ZZ
0MT04ZZ
0MT70ZZ
0MT74ZZ
0MT80ZZ
0MT84ZZ
0MT90ZZ
0MT94ZZ
0MTB0ZZ
0MTB4ZZ
0MTC0ZZ
0MTC4ZZ
0MTD0ZZ
0MTD4ZZ
0MTF0ZZ
0MTF4ZZ
0MTG0ZZ
0MTG4ZZ
0MTV0ZZ
0MTV4ZZ
0MTW0ZZ
0MTW4ZZ
0MWX00Z
0MWX07Z
0MWX0JZ
0MWX0KZ
0MWX0YZ
0MWX30Z
0MWX37Z
0MWX3JZ
0MWX3KZ
0MWX40Z
0MWX47Z
0MWX4JZ
0MWX4KZ
0MWY00Z
0MWY07Z
0MWY0JZ
0MWY0KZ
0MWY0YZ
0MWY30Z
0MWY37Z
0MWY3JZ
0MWY3KZ
0MWY40Z
0MWY47Z
0MWY4JZ
0MWY4KZ
0N5B0ZZ
0N5B3ZZ
0N5B4ZZ
0N5C0ZZ
0N5C3ZZ
0N5C4ZZ
0N5F0ZZ
0N5F3ZZ
0N5F4ZZ
0N5G0ZZ
0N5G3ZZ
0N5G4ZZ
0N5H0ZZ
0N5H3ZZ
0N5H4ZZ
0N5J0ZZ
0N5J3ZZ
0N5J4ZZ
0N5K0ZZ
0N5K3ZZ
0N5K4ZZ
0N5L0ZZ
0N5L3ZZ
0N5L4ZZ
0N5M0ZZ
0N5M3ZZ
0N5M4ZZ
0N5N0ZZ
0N5N3ZZ
0N5N4ZZ
0N5P0ZZ
0N5P3ZZ
0N5P4ZZ
0N5Q0ZZ
0N5Q3ZZ
0N5Q4ZZ
0N5R0ZZ
0N5R3ZZ
0N5R4ZZ
0N5T0ZZ
0N5T3ZZ
0N5T4ZZ
0N5V0ZZ
0N5V3ZZ
0N5V4ZZ
0N5X0ZZ
0N5X3ZZ
0N5X4ZZ
0N8P0ZZ
0N8P3ZZ
0N8P4ZZ
0N8Q0ZZ
0N8Q3ZZ
0N8Q4ZZ
0N9P00Z
0N9P0ZZ
0N9P40Z
0N9P4ZZ
0N9Q00Z
0N9Q0ZZ
0N9Q40Z
0N9Q4ZZ
0NBB0ZZ
0NBB3ZZ
0NBB4ZZ
0NBC0ZZ
0NBC3ZZ
0NBC4ZZ
0NBF0ZZ
0NBF3ZZ
0NBF4ZZ
0NBG0ZZ
0NBG3ZZ
0NBG4ZZ
0NBH0ZZ
0NBH3ZZ
0NBH4ZZ
0NBJ0ZZ
0NBJ3ZZ
0NBJ4ZZ
0NBK0ZZ
0NBK3ZZ
0NBK4ZZ
0NBL0ZZ
0NBL3ZZ
0NBL4ZZ
0NBM0ZZ
0NBM3ZZ
0NBM4ZZ
0NBN0ZZ
0NBN3ZZ
0NBN4ZZ
0NBP0ZZ
0NBP3ZZ
0NBP4ZZ
0NBQ0ZZ
0NBQ3ZZ
0NBQ4ZZ
0NBR0ZZ
0NBR3ZZ
0NBR4ZZ
0NBT0ZZ
0NBT3ZZ
0NBT4ZZ
0NBV0ZZ
0NBV3ZZ
0NBV4ZZ
0NBX0ZZ
0NBX3ZZ
0NBX4ZZ
0ND00ZZ
0ND10ZZ
0ND30ZZ
0ND40ZZ
0ND50ZZ
0ND60ZZ
0ND70ZZ
0NDB0ZZ
0NDC0ZZ
0NDF0ZZ
0NDG0ZZ
0NDH0ZZ
0NDJ0ZZ
0NDK0ZZ
0NDL0ZZ
0NDM0ZZ
0NDN0ZZ
0NDP0ZZ
0NDQ0ZZ
0NDR0ZZ
0NDT0ZZ
0NDV0ZZ
0NDX0ZZ
0NJ00ZZ
0NJ04ZZ
0NJB0ZZ
0NJB4ZZ
0NJW0ZZ
0NJW4ZZ
0NNC0ZZ
0NNC3ZZ
0NNC4ZZ
0NNF0ZZ
0NNF3ZZ
0NNF4ZZ
0NNG0ZZ
0NNG3ZZ
0NNG4ZZ
0NNH0ZZ
0NNH3ZZ
0NNH4ZZ
0NNJ0ZZ
0NNJ3ZZ
0NNJ4ZZ
0NNK0ZZ
0NNK3ZZ
0NNK4ZZ
0NNL0ZZ
0NNL3ZZ
0NNL4ZZ
0NNM0ZZ
0NNM3ZZ
0NNM4ZZ
0NNN0ZZ
0NNN3ZZ
0NNN4ZZ
0NNP0ZZ
0NNP3ZZ
0NNP4ZZ
0NNQ0ZZ
0NNQ3ZZ
0NNQ4ZZ
0NNR0ZZ
0NNR3ZZ
0NNR4ZZ
0NNT0ZZ
0NNT3ZZ
0NNT4ZZ
0NNV0ZZ
0NNV3ZZ
0NNV4ZZ
0NNX0ZZ
0NNX3ZZ
0NNX4ZZ
0NP00JZ
0NP03JZ
0NP04JZ
0NPW04Z
0NPW0JZ
0NPW34Z
0NPW3JZ
0NPW44Z
0NPW4JZ
0NPWX4Z
0NQB0ZZ
0NQB3ZZ
0NQB4ZZ
0NQC0ZZ
0NQC3ZZ
0NQC4ZZ
0NQF0ZZ
0NQF3ZZ
0NQF4ZZ
0NQG0ZZ
0NQG3ZZ
0NQG4ZZ
0NQH0ZZ
0NQH3ZZ
0NQH4ZZ
0NQJ0ZZ
0NQJ3ZZ
0NQJ4ZZ
0NQK0ZZ
0NQK3ZZ
0NQK4ZZ
0NQL0ZZ
0NQL3ZZ
0NQL4ZZ
0NQM0ZZ
0NQM3ZZ
0NQM4ZZ
0NQN0ZZ
0NQN3ZZ
0NQN4ZZ
0NQP0ZZ
0NQP3ZZ
0NQP4ZZ
0NQQ0ZZ
0NQQ3ZZ
0NQQ4ZZ
0NQR0ZZ
0NQR3ZZ
0NQR4ZZ
0NQT0ZZ
0NQT3ZZ
0NQT4ZZ
0NQV0ZZ
0NQV3ZZ
0NQV4ZZ
0NQX0ZZ
0NQX3ZZ
0NQX4ZZ
0NRB07Z
0NRB0JZ
0NRB0KZ
0NRB37Z
0NRB3JZ
0NRB3KZ
0NRB47Z
0NRB4JZ
0NRB4KZ
0NRC0JZ
0NRC3JZ
0NRC4JZ
0NRF0JZ
0NRF3JZ
0NRF4JZ
0NRG0JZ
0NRG3JZ
0NRG4JZ
0NRH0JZ
0NRH3JZ
0NRH4JZ
0NRJ0JZ
0NRJ3JZ
0NRJ4JZ
0NRK0JZ
0NRK3JZ

ØNRK4JZ
ØNRLØJZ
ØNRL3JZ
ØNRL4JZ
ØNRMØJZ
ØNRM3JZ
ØNRM4JZ
ØNRNØJZ
ØNRN3JZ
ØNRN4JZ
ØNRPØ7Z
ØNRPØJZ
ØNRP37Z
ØNRP3JZ
ØNRP47Z
ØNRP4JZ
ØNRQØ7Z
ØNRQØJZ
ØNRQ37Z
ØNRQ3JZ
ØNRQ47Z
ØNRQ4JZ
ØNRRØ7Z
ØNRRØJZ
ØNRRØKZ
ØNRR37Z
ØNRR3JZ
ØNRR3KZ
ØNRR47Z
ØNRR4JZ
ØNRR4KZ
ØNRTØ7Z
ØNRTØJZ
ØNRTØKZ
ØNRT37Z
ØNRT3JZ
ØNRT3KZ
ØNRT47Z
ØNRT4JZ
ØNRT4KZ
ØNRVØ7Z
ØNRVØJZ
ØNRVØKZ
ØNRV37Z
ØNRV3JZ
ØNRV3KZ
ØNRV47Z
ØNRV4JZ
ØNRV4KZ
ØNRXØJZ
ØNRX3JZ
ØNRX4JZ
ØNSBØ4Z
ØNSBØZZ
ØNSCØ4Z
ØNSCØZZ
ØNSFØ4Z
ØNSFØZZ
ØNSGØ4Z
ØNSGØZZ
ØNSHØ4Z
ØNSHØZZ
ØNSJØ4Z
ØNSJØZZ
ØNSKØ4Z
ØNSKØZZ
ØNSLØ4Z
ØNSLØZZ
ØNSMØ4Z
ØNSMØZZ
ØNSNØ4Z
ØNSNØZZ
ØNSPØ4Z
ØNSPØZZ
ØNSQØ4Z
ØNSQØZZ
ØNSRØ4Z
ØNSRØ5Z
ØNSRØZZ
ØNSTØ4Z
ØNSTØ5Z
ØNSTØZZ
ØNSVØ4Z
ØNSVØ5Z
ØNSVØZZ
ØNSXØ4Z
ØNSXØZZ
ØNTBØZZ
ØNTCØZZ
ØNTFØZZ
ØNTGØZZ
ØNTHØZZ
ØNTJØZZ
ØNTKØZZ
ØNTLØZZ
ØNTMØZZ
ØNTNØZZ
ØNTPØZZ
ØNTQØZZ
ØNTRØZZ
ØNTTØZZ
ØNTVØZZ
ØNTXØZZ
ØNUBØ7Z
ØNUBØJZ
ØNUBØKZ
ØNUB37Z
ØNUB3JZ
ØNUB3KZ
ØNUB47Z
ØNUB4JZ
ØNUB4KZ
ØNUCØJZ
ØNUC3JZ
ØNUC4JZ
ØNUFØJZ
ØNUF3JZ
ØNUF4JZ
ØNUGØJZ
ØNUG3JZ
ØNUG4JZ
ØNUHØJZ
ØNUH3JZ
ØNUH4JZ
ØNUJØJZ
ØNUJ3JZ
ØNUJ4JZ
ØNUKØJZ
ØNUK3JZ
ØNUK4JZ
ØNULØJZ
ØNUL3JZ
ØNUL4JZ
ØNUMØJZ
ØNUM3JZ
ØNUM4JZ
ØNUNØJZ
ØNUN3JZ
ØNUN4JZ
ØNUPØJZ
ØNUP3JZ
ØNUP4JZ
ØNUQØJZ
ØNUQ3JZ
ØNUQ4JZ
ØNURØ7Z
ØNURØJZ
ØNURØKZ
ØNUR37Z
ØNUR3JZ
ØNUR3KZ
ØNUR47Z
ØNUR4JZ
ØNUR4KZ
ØNUTØ7Z
ØNUTØJZ
ØNUTØKZ
ØNUT37Z
ØNUT3JZ
ØNUT3KZ
ØNUT47Z
ØNUT4JZ
ØNUT4KZ
ØNUVØ7Z
ØNUVØJZ
ØNUVØKZ
ØNUV37Z
ØNUV3JZ
ØNUV3KZ
ØNUV47Z
ØNUV4JZ
ØNUV4KZ
ØNUXØJZ
ØNUX3JZ
ØNUX4JZ
ØP5ØØZZ
ØP5Ø3ZZ
ØP5Ø4ZZ
ØP51ØZZ
ØP513ZZ
ØP514ZZ
ØP52ØZZ
ØP523ZZ
ØP524ZZ
ØP53ØZ3
ØP53ØZZ
ØP533Z3
ØP533ZZ
ØP534Z3
ØP534ZZ
ØP54ØZ3
ØP54ØZZ
ØP543Z3
ØP543ZZ
ØP544Z3
ØP544ZZ
ØP55ØZZ
ØP553ZZ
ØP554ZZ
ØP56ØZZ
ØP563ZZ
ØP564ZZ
ØP57ØZZ
ØP573ZZ
ØP574ZZ
ØP58ØZZ
ØP583ZZ
ØP584ZZ
ØP59ØZZ
ØP593ZZ
ØP594ZZ
ØP5BØZZ
ØP5B3ZZ
ØP5B4ZZ
ØP5CØZZ
ØP5C3ZZ
ØP5C4ZZ
ØP5DØZZ
ØP5D3ZZ
ØP5D4ZZ
ØP5FØZZ
ØP5F3ZZ
ØP5F4ZZ
ØP5GØZZ
ØP5G3ZZ
ØP5G4ZZ
ØP5HØZZ
ØP5H3ZZ
ØP5H4ZZ
ØP5JØZZ
ØP5J3ZZ
ØP5J4ZZ
ØP5KØZZ
ØP5K3ZZ
ØP5K4ZZ
ØP5LØZZ
ØP5L3ZZ
ØP5L4ZZ
ØP5MØZZ
ØP5M3ZZ
ØP5M4ZZ
ØP5NØZZ
ØP5N3ZZ
ØP5N4ZZ
ØP5PØZZ
ØP5P3ZZ
ØP5P4ZZ
ØP5QØZZ
ØP5Q3ZZ
ØP5Q4ZZ
ØP5RØZZ
ØP5R3ZZ
ØP5R4ZZ
ØP5SØZZ
ØP5S3ZZ
ØP5S4ZZ
ØP5TØZZ
ØP5T3ZZ
ØP5T4ZZ
ØP5VØZZ
ØP5V3ZZ
ØP5V4ZZ
ØP8ØØZZ
ØP8Ø3ZZ
ØP8Ø4ZZ
ØP81ØZZ
ØP813ZZ
ØP814ZZ
ØP82ØZZ
ØP823ZZ
ØP824ZZ
ØP83ØZZ
ØP833ZZ
ØP834ZZ
ØP84ØZZ
ØP843ZZ
ØP844ZZ
ØP85ØZZ
ØP853ZZ
ØP854ZZ
ØP86ØZZ
ØP863ZZ
ØP864ZZ
ØP87ØZZ
ØP873ZZ
ØP874ZZ
ØP88ØZZ
ØP883ZZ
ØP884ZZ
ØP89ØZZ
ØP893ZZ
ØP894ZZ
ØP8BØZZ
ØP8B3ZZ
ØP8B4ZZ
ØP8CØZZ
ØP8C3ZZ
ØP8C4ZZ
ØP8DØZZ
ØP8D3ZZ
ØP8D4ZZ
ØP8FØZZ
ØP8F3ZZ
ØP8F4ZZ
ØP8GØZZ
ØP8G3ZZ
ØP8G4ZZ
ØP8HØZZ
ØP8H3ZZ
ØP8H4ZZ
ØP8JØZZ
ØP8J3ZZ
ØP8J4ZZ
ØP8KØZZ
ØP8K3ZZ
ØP8K4ZZ
ØP8LØZZ
ØP8L3ZZ
ØP8L4ZZ
ØP8MØZZ
ØP8M3ZZ
ØP8M4ZZ
ØP8NØZZ
ØP8N3ZZ
ØP8N4ZZ
ØP8PØZZ
ØP8P3ZZ
ØP8P4ZZ
ØP8QØZZ
ØP8Q3ZZ
ØP8Q4ZZ
ØP8RØZZ
ØP8R3ZZ
ØP8R4ZZ
ØP8SØZZ
ØP8S3ZZ
ØP8S4ZZ
ØP8TØZZ
ØP8T3ZZ
ØP8T4ZZ
ØP8VØZZ
ØP8V3ZZ
ØP8V4ZZ
ØP9MØZX
ØP9M3ZX
ØP9M4ZX
ØP9NØZX
ØP9N3ZX
ØP9N4ZX
ØP9PØZX
ØP9P3ZX
ØP9P4ZX
ØP9QØZX
ØP9Q3ZX
ØP9Q4ZX
ØPBØØZZ
ØPBØ3ZZ
ØPBØ4ZZ
ØPB1ØZZ
ØPB13ZZ
ØPB14ZZ
ØPB2ØZZ
ØPB23ZZ
ØPB24ZZ
ØPB3ØZZ
ØPB33ZZ
ØPB34ZZ
ØPB4ØZZ
ØPB43ZZ
ØPB44ZZ
ØPB5ØZZ
ØPB53ZZ
ØPB54ZZ
ØPB6ØZZ
ØPB63ZZ
ØPB64ZZ
ØPB7ØZZ
ØPB73ZZ
ØPB74ZZ
ØPB8ØZZ
ØPB83ZZ
ØPB84ZZ
ØPB9ØZZ
ØPB93ZZ
ØPB94ZZ
ØPBBØZZ
ØPBB3ZZ
ØPBB4ZZ
ØPBCØZZ
ØPBC3ZZ
ØPBC4ZZ
ØPBDØZZ
ØPBD3ZZ
ØPBD4ZZ
ØPBFØZZ
ØPBF3ZZ
ØPBF4ZZ
ØPBGØZZ
ØPBG3ZZ
ØPBG4ZZ
ØPBHØZZ
ØPBH3ZZ
ØPBH4ZZ
ØPBJØZZ
ØPBJ3ZZ
ØPBJ4ZZ
ØPBKØZZ
ØPBK3ZZ
ØPBK4ZZ
ØPBLØZZ
ØPBL3ZZ
ØPBL4ZZ
ØPBMØZX
ØPBMØZZ
ØPBM3ZX
ØPBM3ZZ
ØPBM4ZX
ØPBM4ZZ
ØPBNØZX
ØPBNØZZ
ØPBN3ZX
ØPBN3ZZ
ØPBN4ZX
ØPBN4ZZ
ØPBPØZX
ØPBPØZZ
ØPBP3ZX
ØPBP3ZZ
ØPBP4ZX
ØPBP4ZZ
ØPBQØZX
ØPBQØZZ
ØPBQ3ZX
ØPBQ3ZZ
ØPBQ4ZX
ØPBQ4ZZ
ØPBRØZZ
ØPBR3ZZ
ØPBR4ZZ
ØPBSØZZ
ØPBS3ZZ
ØPBS4ZZ
ØPBTØZZ
ØPBT3ZZ
ØPBT4ZZ
ØPBVØZZ
ØPBV3ZZ
ØPBV4ZZ
ØPCØØZZ
ØPCØ3ZZ
ØPCØ4ZZ
ØPC1ØZZ
ØPC13ZZ
ØPC14ZZ
ØPC2ØZZ
ØPC23ZZ
ØPC24ZZ
ØPC3ØZZ
ØPC33ZZ
ØPC34ZZ
ØPC4ØZZ
ØPC43ZZ
ØPC44ZZ
ØPC5ØZZ
ØPC53ZZ
ØPC54ZZ
ØPC6ØZZ
ØPC63ZZ
ØPC64ZZ
ØPC7ØZZ
ØPC73ZZ
ØPC74ZZ
ØPC8ØZZ
ØPC83ZZ
ØPC84ZZ
ØPC9ØZZ
ØPC93ZZ
ØPC94ZZ
ØPCBØZZ
ØPCB3ZZ
ØPCB4ZZ
ØPCCØZZ
ØPCC3ZZ
ØPCC4ZZ
ØPCDØZZ
ØPCD3ZZ
ØPCD4ZZ
ØPCFØZZ
ØPCF3ZZ
ØPCF4ZZ
ØPCGØZZ
ØPCG3ZZ
ØPCG4ZZ
ØPCHØZZ
ØPCH3ZZ
ØPCH4ZZ
ØPCJØZZ
ØPCJ3ZZ
ØPCJ4ZZ
ØPCKØZZ
ØPCK3ZZ
ØPCK4ZZ
ØPCLØZZ
ØPCL3ZZ
ØPCL4ZZ
ØPCMØZZ
ØPCM3ZZ
ØPCM4ZZ
ØPCNØZZ
ØPCN3ZZ
ØPCN4ZZ
ØPCPØZZ
ØPCP3ZZ
ØPCP4ZZ
ØPCQØZZ
ØPCQ3ZZ
ØPCQ4ZZ
ØPCRØZZ
ØPCR3ZZ
ØPCR4ZZ
ØPCSØZZ
ØPCS3ZZ
ØPCS4ZZ
ØPCTØZZ
ØPCT3ZZ
ØPCT4ZZ
ØPCVØZZ
ØPCV3ZZ
ØPCV4ZZ
ØPDØØZZ
ØPD1ØZZ
ØPD2ØZZ
ØPD3ØZZ
ØPD4ØZZ
ØPD5ØZZ
ØPD6ØZZ
ØPD7ØZZ
ØPD8ØZZ
ØPD9ØZZ
ØPDBØZZ
ØPDCØZZ
ØPDDØZZ
ØPDFØZZ
ØPDGØZZ
ØPDHØZZ
ØPDJØZZ
ØPDKØZZ
ØPDLØZZ
ØPDMØZZ
ØPDNØZZ
ØPDPØZZ
ØPDQØZZ
ØPDRØZZ
ØPDSØZZ
ØPDTØZZ
ØPDVØZZ
ØPHØØØZ
ØPHØØ4Z
ØPHØ3ØZ
ØPHØ34Z
ØPHØ4ØZ
ØPHØ44Z
ØPH1Ø4Z
ØPH134Z
ØPH144Z
ØPH2Ø4Z
ØPH234Z
ØPH244Z
ØPH3Ø4Z
ØPH334Z
ØPH344Z
ØPH4Ø4Z
ØPH434Z
ØPH444Z
ØPH5Ø4Z
ØPH534Z
ØPH544Z
ØPH6Ø4Z
ØPH634Z
ØPH644Z
ØPH7Ø4Z
ØPH734Z
ØPH744Z
ØPH8Ø4Z
ØPH834Z
ØPH844Z
ØPH9Ø4Z
ØPH934Z
ØPH944Z
ØPHBØ4Z
ØPHB34Z
ØPHB44Z
ØPHCØ4Z
ØPHCØ5Z
ØPHCØ6Z
ØPHCØBZ
ØPHCØCZ
ØPHCØDZ
ØPHC34Z
ØPHC35Z
ØPHC36Z
ØPHC3BZ
ØPHC3CZ
ØPHC3DZ
ØPHC44Z
ØPHC45Z
ØPHC46Z
ØPHC4BZ
ØPHC4CZ
ØPHC4DZ
ØPHDØ4Z
ØPHDØ5Z
ØPHDØ6Z
ØPHDØBZ
ØPHDØCZ
ØPHDØDZ
ØPHD34Z
ØPHD35Z
ØPHD36Z
ØPHD3BZ
ØPHD3CZ
ØPHD3DZ
ØPHD44Z
ØPHD45Z
ØPHD46Z
ØPHD4BZ
ØPHD4CZ
ØPHD4DZ
ØPHFØ4Z
ØPHFØ5Z
ØPHFØ6Z
ØPHFØ7Z
ØPHFØBZ
ØPHFØCZ
ØPHFØDZ
ØPHF34Z
ØPHF35Z
ØPHF36Z
ØPHF37Z
ØPHF3BZ
ØPHF3CZ
ØPHF3DZ
ØPHF44Z
ØPHF45Z
ØPHF46Z
ØPHF47Z
ØPHF4BZ
ØPHF4CZ
ØPHF4DZ
ØPHGØ4Z
ØPHGØ5Z
ØPHGØ6Z
ØPHGØ7Z
ØPHGØBZ
ØPHGØCZ
ØPHGØDZ
ØPHG34Z
ØPHG35Z
ØPHG36Z
ØPHG37Z
ØPHG3BZ
ØPHG3CZ
ØPHG3DZ
ØPHG44Z
ØPHG45Z
ØPHG46Z
ØPHG47Z
ØPHG4BZ
ØPHG4CZ
ØPHG4DZ
ØPHHØ4Z
ØPHHØ5Z
ØPHHØ6Z
ØPHHØBZ
ØPHHØCZ
ØPHHØDZ
ØPHH34Z
ØPHH35Z
ØPHH36Z
ØPHH3BZ
ØPHH3CZ
ØPHH3DZ
ØPHH44Z
ØPHH45Z
ØPHH46Z
ØPHH4BZ
ØPHH4CZ
ØPHH4DZ
ØPHJØ4Z
ØPHJØ5Z
ØPHJØ6Z
ØPHJØBZ
ØPHJØCZ
ØPHJØDZ
ØPHJ34Z
ØPHJ35Z
ØPHJ36Z
ØPHJ3BZ
ØPHJ3CZ
ØPHJ3DZ
ØPHJ44Z
ØPHJ45Z
ØPHJ46Z
ØPHJ4BZ
ØPHJ4CZ
ØPHJ4DZ
ØPHKØ4Z
ØPHKØ5Z
ØPHKØ6Z
ØPHKØBZ
ØPHKØCZ
ØPHKØDZ
ØPHK34Z
ØPHK35Z
ØPHK36Z
ØPHK3BZ
ØPHK3CZ
ØPHK3DZ
ØPHK44Z
ØPHK45Z
ØPHK46Z
ØPHK4BZ
ØPHK4CZ
ØPHK4DZ
ØPHLØ4Z
ØPHLØ5Z
ØPHLØ6Z
ØPHLØBZ
ØPHLØCZ
ØPHLØDZ
ØPHL34Z
ØPHL35Z
ØPHL36Z
ØPHL3BZ
ØPHL3CZ
ØPHL3DZ
ØPHL44Z
ØPHL45Z
ØPHL46Z
ØPHL4BZ
ØPHL4CZ
ØPHL4DZ
ØPHMØ4Z
ØPHMØ5Z
ØPHM34Z
ØPHM35Z
ØPHM44Z
ØPHM45Z
ØPHNØ4Z
ØPHNØ5Z
ØPHN34Z
ØPHN35Z
ØPHN44Z
ØPHN45Z
ØPHPØ4Z
ØPHPØ5Z
ØPHP34Z
ØPHP35Z
ØPHP44Z
ØPHP45Z
ØPHQØ4Z
ØPHQØ5Z
ØPHQ34Z
ØPHQ35Z
ØPHQ44Z
ØPHQ45Z
ØPHRØ4Z
ØPHRØ5Z
ØPHR34Z
ØPHR35Z
ØPHR44Z
ØPHR45Z
ØPHSØ4Z
ØPHSØ5Z
ØPHS34Z
ØPHS35Z
ØPHS44Z
ØPHS45Z
ØPHTØ4Z
ØPHTØ5Z
ØPHT34Z
ØPHT35Z
ØPHT44Z
ØPHT45Z
ØPHVØ4Z
ØPHVØ5Z
ØPHV34Z
ØPHV35Z
ØPHV44Z
ØPHV45Z
ØPHYØMZ
ØPHY3MZ
ØPHY4MZ
ØPNCØZZ
ØPNC3ZZ
ØPNC4ZZ
ØPNDØZZ
ØPND3ZZ
ØPND4ZZ
ØPNFØZZ
ØPNF3ZZ
ØPNF4ZZ
ØPNGØZZ
ØPNG3ZZ
ØPNG4ZZ
ØPNHØZZ
ØPNH3ZZ
ØPNH4ZZ
ØPNJØZZ
ØPNJ3ZZ
ØPNJ4ZZ
ØPNKØZZ
ØPNK3ZZ
ØPNK4ZZ
ØPNLØZZ
ØPNL3ZZ
ØPNL4ZZ
ØPNMØZZ
ØPNM3ZZ
ØPNM4ZZ
ØPNNØZZ
ØPNN3ZZ
ØPNN4ZZ
ØPNPØZZ
ØPNP3ZZ
ØPNP4ZZ
ØPNQØZZ
ØPNQ3ZZ
ØPNQ4ZZ
ØPPCØ4Z
ØPPCØ5Z
ØPPCØ7Z
ØPPCØJZ
ØPPCØKZ
ØPPC34Z
ØPPC35Z
ØPPC37Z
ØPPC3JZ
ØPPC3KZ
ØPPC44Z
ØPPC45Z
ØPPC47Z
ØPPC4JZ
ØPPC4KZ
ØPPDØ4Z
ØPPDØ5Z
ØPPDØ7Z
ØPPDØJZ
ØPPDØKZ
ØPPD34Z
ØPPD35Z
ØPPD37Z
ØPPD3JZ
ØPPD3KZ
ØPPD44Z

ØPPD45Z
ØPPD47Z
ØPPD4JZ
ØPPD4KZ
ØPPFØ4Z
ØPPFØ5Z
ØPPFØ7Z
ØPPFØJZ
ØPPFØKZ
ØPPF34Z
ØPPF35Z
ØPPF37Z
ØPPF3JZ
ØPPF3KZ
ØPPF44Z
ØPPF45Z
ØPPF47Z
ØPPF4JZ
ØPPF4KZ
ØPPGØ4Z
ØPPGØ5Z
ØPPGØ7Z
ØPPGØJZ
ØPPGØKZ
ØPPG34Z
ØPPG35Z
ØPPG37Z
ØPPG3JZ
ØPPG3KZ
ØPPG44Z
ØPPG45Z
ØPPG47Z
ØPPG4JZ
ØPPG4KZ
ØPPHØ4Z
ØPPHØ5Z
ØPPHØ7Z
ØPPHØJZ
ØPPHØKZ
ØPPH34Z
ØPPH35Z
ØPPH37Z
ØPPH3JZ
ØPPH3KZ
ØPPH44Z
ØPPH45Z
ØPPH47Z
ØPPH4JZ
ØPPH4KZ
ØPPJØ4Z
ØPPJØ5Z
ØPPJØ7Z
ØPPJØJZ
ØPPJØKZ
ØPPJ34Z
ØPPJ35Z
ØPPJ37Z
ØPPJ3JZ
ØPPJ3KZ
ØPPJ44Z
ØPPJ45Z
ØPPJ47Z
ØPPJ4JZ
ØPPJ4KZ
ØPPKØ4Z
ØPPKØ5Z
ØPPKØ7Z
ØPPKØJZ
ØPPKØKZ
ØPPK34Z
ØPPK35Z
ØPPK37Z
ØPPK3JZ
ØPPK3KZ
ØPPK44Z
ØPPK45Z
ØPPK47Z
ØPPK4JZ
ØPPK4KZ
ØPPLØ4Z
ØPPLØ5Z
ØPPLØ7Z
ØPPLØJZ
ØPPLØKZ
ØPPL34Z
ØPPL35Z
ØPPL37Z
ØPPL3JZ
ØPPL3KZ
ØPPL44Z
ØPPL45Z
ØPPL47Z
ØPPL4JZ
ØPPL4KZ
ØPPMØ4Z
ØPPMØ5Z
ØPPMØ7Z
ØPPMØJZ
ØPPMØKZ
ØPPM34Z
ØPPM35Z
ØPPM37Z
ØPPM3JZ
ØPPM3KZ
ØPPM44Z
ØPPM45Z
ØPPM47Z
ØPPM4JZ
ØPPM4KZ
ØPPNØ4Z
ØPPNØ5Z
ØPPNØ7Z
ØPPNØJZ
ØPPNØKZ
ØPPN34Z
ØPPN35Z
ØPPN37Z
ØPPN3JZ
ØPPN3KZ
ØPPN44Z
ØPPN45Z
ØPPN47Z
ØPPN4JZ
ØPPN4KZ
ØPPPØ4Z
ØPPPØ5Z
ØPPPØ7Z
ØPPPØJZ
ØPPPØKZ
ØPPP34Z
ØPPP35Z
ØPPP37Z
ØPPP3JZ
ØPPP3KZ
ØPPP44Z
ØPPP45Z
ØPPP47Z
ØPPP4JZ
ØPPP4KZ
ØPPQØ4Z
ØPPQØ5Z
ØPPQØ7Z
ØPPQØJZ
ØPPQØKZ
ØPPQ34Z
ØPPQ35Z
ØPPQ37Z
ØPPQ3JZ
ØPPQ3KZ
ØPPQ44Z
ØPPQ45Z
ØPPQ47Z
ØPPQ4JZ
ØPPQ4KZ
ØPQCØZZ
ØPQC3ZZ
ØPQC4ZZ
ØPQDØZZ
ØPQD3ZZ
ØPQD4ZZ
ØPQFØZZ
ØPQF3ZZ
ØPQF4ZZ
ØPQGØZZ
ØPQG3ZZ
ØPQG4ZZ
ØPQHØZZ
ØPQH3ZZ
ØPQH4ZZ
ØPQJØZZ
ØPQJ3ZZ
ØPQJ4ZZ
ØPQKØZZ
ØPQK3ZZ
ØPQK4ZZ
ØPQLØZZ
ØPQL3ZZ
ØPQL4ZZ
ØPQMØZZ
ØPQM3ZZ
ØPQM4ZZ
ØPQNØZZ
ØPQN3ZZ
ØPQN4ZZ
ØPQPØZZ
ØPQP3ZZ
ØPQP4ZZ
ØPQQØZZ
ØPQQ3ZZ
ØPQQ4ZZ
ØPR3Ø7Z
ØPR3ØKZ
ØPR337Z
ØPR33KZ
ØPR347Z
ØPR34KZ
ØPR4Ø7Z
ØPR4ØKZ
ØPR437Z
ØPR43KZ
ØPR447Z
ØPR44KZ
ØPRCØ7Z
ØPRCØKZ
ØPRC37Z
ØPRC3JZ
ØPRC3KZ
ØPRC47Z
ØPRC4JZ
ØPRC4KZ
ØPRDØ7Z
ØPRDØKZ
ØPRD37Z
ØPRD3JZ
ØPRD3KZ
ØPRD47Z
ØPRD4JZ
ØPRD4KZ
ØPRFØ7Z
ØPRFØJZ
ØPRFØKZ
ØPRF37Z
ØPRF3JZ
ØPRF3KZ
ØPRF47Z
ØPRF4JZ
ØPRF4KZ
ØPRGØ7Z
ØPRGØJZ
ØPRGØKZ
ØPRG37Z
ØPRG3JZ
ØPRG3KZ
ØPRG47Z
ØPRG4JZ
ØPRG4KZ
ØPRHØ7Z
ØPRHØJZ
ØPRHØKZ
ØPRH37Z
ØPRH3JZ
ØPRH3KZ
ØPRH47Z
ØPRH4JZ
ØPRH4KZ
ØPRJØ7Z
ØPRJØJZ
ØPRJØKZ
ØPRJ37Z
ØPRJ3JZ
ØPRJ3KZ
ØPRJ47Z
ØPRJ4JZ
ØPRJ4KZ
ØPRKØ7Z
ØPRKØJZ
ØPRKØKZ
ØPRK37Z
ØPRK3JZ
ØPRK3KZ
ØPRK47Z
ØPRK4JZ
ØPRK4KZ
ØPRLØ7Z
ØPRLØJZ
ØPRLØKZ
ØPRL37Z
ØPRL3JZ
ØPRL3KZ
ØPRL47Z
ØPRL4JZ
ØPRL4KZ
ØPRMØ7Z
ØPRMØJZ
ØPRMØKZ
ØPRM37Z
ØPRM3JZ
ØPRM3KZ
ØPRM47Z
ØPRM4JZ
ØPRM4KZ
ØPRNØ7Z
ØPRNØJZ
ØPRNØKZ
ØPRN37Z
ØPRN3JZ
ØPRN3KZ
ØPRN47Z
ØPRN4JZ
ØPRN4KZ
ØPRPØ7Z
ØPRPØJZ
ØPRPØKZ
ØPRP37Z
ØPRP3JZ
ØPRP3KZ
ØPRP47Z
ØPRP4JZ
ØPRP4KZ
ØPRQØ7Z
ØPRQØJZ
ØPRQØKZ
ØPRQ37Z
ØPRQ3JZ
ØPRQ3KZ
ØPRQ47Z
ØPRQ4JZ
ØPRQ4KZ
ØPRRØ7Z
ØPRRØKZ
ØPRR37Z
ØPRR3KZ
ØPRR47Z
ØPRR4KZ
ØPRSØ7Z
ØPRSØKZ
ØPRS37Z
ØPRS3KZ
ØPRS47Z
ØPRS4KZ
ØPRTØ7Z
ØPRTØKZ
ØPRT37Z
ØPRT3KZ
ØPRT47Z
ØPRT4KZ
ØPRVØ7Z
ØPRVØKZ
ØPRV37Z
ØPRV3KZ
ØPRV47Z
ØPRV4KZ
ØPSØØØZ
ØPSØØ4Z
ØPSØØZZ
ØPSØ3ØZ
ØPSØ34Z
ØPSØ4ØZ
ØPSØ44Z
ØPS1Ø4Z
ØPS1ØZZ
ØPS134Z
ØPS144Z
ØPS2Ø4Z
ØPS2ØZZ
ØPS234Z
ØPS244Z
ØPS3Ø4Z
ØPS3ØZZ
ØPS334Z
ØPS344Z
ØPS34ZZ
ØPS4Ø3Z
ØPS4Ø4Z
ØPS4ØZZ
ØPS434Z
ØPS443Z
ØPS444Z
ØPS44ZZ
ØPS5Ø4Z
ØPS5ØZZ
ØPS534Z
ØPS544Z
ØPS6Ø4Z
ØPS6ØZZ
ØPS634Z
ØPS644Z
ØPS7Ø4Z
ØPS7ØZZ
ØPS734Z
ØPS744Z
ØPS8Ø4Z
ØPS8ØZZ
ØPS834Z
ØPS844Z
ØPS9Ø4Z
ØPS9ØZZ
ØPS934Z
ØPS944Z
ØPSBØ4Z
ØPSBØZZ
ØPSB34Z
ØPSB44Z
ØPSCØ4Z
ØPSCØ5Z
ØPSCØ6Z
ØPSCØBZ
ØPSCØCZ
ØPSCØDZ
ØPSCØZZ
ØPSC34Z
ØPSC35Z
ØPSC36Z
ØPSC3BZ
ØPSC3CZ
ØPSC3DZ
ØPSC44Z
ØPSC45Z
ØPSC46Z
ØPSC4BZ
ØPSC4CZ
ØPSC4DZ
ØPSDØ4Z
ØPSDØ5Z
ØPSDØ6Z
ØPSDØBZ
ØPSDØCZ
ØPSDØDZ
ØPSDØZZ
ØPSD34Z
ØPSD35Z
ØPSD36Z
ØPSD3BZ
ØPSD3CZ
ØPSD3DZ
ØPSD44Z
ØPSD45Z
ØPSD46Z
ØPSD4BZ
ØPSD4CZ
ØPSD4DZ
ØPSFØ4Z
ØPSFØ5Z
ØPSFØ6Z
ØPSFØBZ
ØPSFØCZ
ØPSFØDZ
ØPSFØZZ
ØPSF34Z
ØPSF35Z
ØPSF36Z
ØPSF3BZ
ØPSF3CZ
ØPSF3DZ
ØPSF44Z
ØPSF45Z
ØPSF46Z
ØPSF4BZ
ØPSF4CZ
ØPSF4DZ
ØPSGØ4Z
ØPSGØ5Z
ØPSGØ6Z
ØPSGØBZ
ØPSGØCZ
ØPSGØDZ
ØPSGØZZ
ØPSG34Z
ØPSG35Z
ØPSG36Z
ØPSG3BZ
ØPSG3CZ
ØPSG3DZ
ØPSG44Z
ØPSG45Z
ØPSG46Z
ØPSG4BZ
ØPSG4CZ
ØPSG4DZ
ØPSHØ4Z
ØPSHØ5Z
ØPSHØ6Z
ØPSHØBZ
ØPSHØCZ
ØPSHØDZ
ØPSHØZZ
ØPSH34Z
ØPSH35Z
ØPSH36Z
ØPSH3BZ
ØPSH3CZ
ØPSH3DZ
ØPSH44Z
ØPSH45Z
ØPSH46Z
ØPSH4BZ
ØPSH4CZ
ØPSH4DZ
ØPSJØ4Z
ØPSJØ5Z
ØPSJØ6Z
ØPSJØBZ
ØPSJØCZ
ØPSJØDZ
ØPSJØZZ
ØPSJ34Z
ØPSJ35Z
ØPSJ36Z
ØPSJ3BZ
ØPSJ3CZ
ØPSJ3DZ
ØPSJ44Z
ØPSJ45Z
ØPSJ46Z
ØPSJ4BZ
ØPSJ4CZ
ØPSJ4DZ
ØPSKØ4Z
ØPSKØ5Z
ØPSKØ6Z
ØPSKØBZ
ØPSKØCZ
ØPSKØDZ
ØPSKØZZ
ØPSK34Z
ØPSK35Z
ØPSK36Z
ØPSK3BZ
ØPSK3CZ
ØPSK3DZ
ØPSK44Z
ØPSK45Z
ØPSK46Z
ØPSK4BZ
ØPSK4CZ
ØPSK4DZ
ØPSLØ4Z
ØPSLØ5Z
ØPSLØ6Z
ØPSLØBZ
ØPSLØCZ
ØPSLØDZ
ØPSLØZZ
ØPSL34Z
ØPSL35Z
ØPSL36Z
ØPSL3BZ
ØPSL3CZ
ØPSL3DZ
ØPSL44Z
ØPSL45Z
ØPSL46Z
ØPSL4BZ
ØPSL4CZ
ØPSL4DZ
ØPSMØ4Z
ØPSMØ5Z
ØPSMØZZ
ØPSM34Z
ØPSM35Z
ØPSM44Z
ØPSM45Z
ØPSNØ4Z
ØPSNØ5Z
ØPSNØZZ
ØPSN34Z
ØPSN35Z
ØPSN44Z
ØPSN45Z
ØPSPØ4Z
ØPSPØ5Z
ØPSPØZZ
ØPSP34Z
ØPSP35Z
ØPSP44Z
ØPSP45Z
ØPSQØ4Z
ØPSQØ5Z
ØPSQØZZ
ØPSQ34Z
ØPSQ35Z
ØPSQ44Z
ØPSQ45Z
ØPSRØ4Z
ØPSRØ5Z
ØPSRØZZ
ØPSR34Z
ØPSR35Z
ØPSR44Z
ØPSR45Z
ØPSSØ4Z
ØPSSØ5Z
ØPSSØZZ
ØPSS34Z
ØPSS35Z
ØPSS44Z
ØPSS45Z
ØPSTØ4Z
ØPSTØ5Z
ØPSTØZZ
ØPST34Z
ØPST35Z
ØPST44Z
ØPST45Z
ØPSVØ4Z
ØPSVØ5Z
ØPSVØZZ
ØPSV34Z
ØPSV35Z
ØPSV44Z
ØPSV45Z
ØPTØØZZ
ØPT1ØZZ
ØPT2ØZZ
ØPT5ØZZ
ØPT6ØZZ
ØPT7ØZZ
ØPT8ØZZ
ØPT9ØZZ
ØPTBØZZ
ØPTCØZZ
ØPTDØZZ
ØPTFØZZ
ØPTGØZZ
ØPTHØZZ
ØPTJØZZ
ØPTKØZZ
ØPTLØZZ
ØPTMØZZ
ØPTNØZZ
ØPTPØZZ
ØPTQØZZ
ØPTRØZZ
ØPTSØZZ
ØPTTØZZ
ØPTVØZZ
ØPU3Ø7Z
ØPU3ØJZ
ØPU3ØKZ
ØPU337Z
ØPU33JZ
ØPU33KZ
ØPU347Z
ØPU34JZ
ØPU34KZ
ØPU4Ø7Z
ØPU4ØJZ
ØPU4ØKZ
ØPU437Z
ØPU43JZ
ØPU43KZ
ØPU447Z
ØPU44JZ
ØPU44KZ
ØPUCØ7Z
ØPUCØJZ
ØPUCØKZ
ØPUC37Z
ØPUC3JZ
ØPUC3KZ
ØPUC47Z
ØPUC4JZ
ØPUC4KZ
ØPUDØ7Z
ØPUDØJZ
ØPUDØKZ
ØPUD37Z
ØPUD3JZ
ØPUD3KZ
ØPUD47Z
ØPUD4JZ
ØPUD4KZ
ØPUFØ7Z
ØPUFØJZ
ØPUFØKZ
ØPUF37Z
ØPUF3JZ
ØPUF3KZ
ØPUF47Z
ØPUF4JZ
ØPUF4KZ
ØPUGØ7Z
ØPUGØJZ
ØPUGØKZ
ØPUG37Z
ØPUG3JZ
ØPUG3KZ
ØPUG47Z
ØPUG4JZ
ØPUG4KZ
ØPUHØ7Z
ØPUHØJZ
ØPUHØKZ
ØPUH37Z
ØPUH3JZ
ØPUH3KZ
ØPUH47Z
ØPUH4JZ
ØPUH4KZ
ØPUJØ7Z
ØPUJØJZ
ØPUJØKZ
ØPUJ37Z
ØPUJ3JZ
ØPUJ3KZ
ØPUJ47Z
ØPUJ4JZ
ØPUJ4KZ
ØPUKØ7Z
ØPUKØJZ
ØPUKØKZ
ØPUK37Z
ØPUK3JZ
ØPUK3KZ
ØPUK47Z
ØPUK4JZ
ØPUK4KZ
ØPULØ7Z
ØPULØJZ
ØPULØKZ
ØPUL37Z
ØPUL3JZ
ØPUL3KZ
ØPUL47Z
ØPUL4JZ
ØPUL4KZ
ØPUMØ7Z
ØPUMØJZ
ØPUMØKZ
ØPUM37Z
ØPUM3JZ
ØPUM3KZ
ØPUM47Z
ØPUM4JZ
ØPUM4KZ
ØPUNØ7Z
ØPUNØJZ
ØPUNØKZ
ØPUN37Z
ØPUN3JZ
ØPUN3KZ
ØPUN47Z
ØPUN4JZ
ØPUN4KZ
ØPUPØ7Z
ØPUPØJZ
ØPUPØKZ
ØPUP37Z
ØPUP3JZ
ØPUP3KZ
ØPUP47Z
ØPUP4JZ
ØPUP4KZ
ØPUQØ7Z
ØPUQØJZ
ØPUQØKZ
ØPUQ37Z
ØPUQ3JZ
ØPUQ3KZ
ØPUQ47Z
ØPUQ4JZ
ØPUQ4KZ
ØPURØ7Z
ØPURØKZ
ØPUR37Z
ØPUR3KZ
ØPUR47Z
ØPUR4KZ
ØPUSØ7Z
ØPUSØKZ
ØPUS37Z
ØPUS3KZ
ØPUS47Z
ØPUS4KZ
ØPUTØ7Z
ØPUTØKZ
ØPUT37Z
ØPUT3KZ
ØPUT47Z
ØPUT4KZ
ØPUVØ7Z
ØPUVØKZ
ØPUV37Z
ØPUV3KZ
ØPUV47Z
ØPUV4KZ
ØQ5ØØZ3
ØQ5ØØZZ
ØQ5Ø3Z3
ØQ5Ø3ZZ
ØQ5Ø4Z3
ØQ5Ø4ZZ
ØQ51ØZ3
ØQ51ØZZ
ØQ513Z3
ØQ513ZZ
ØQ514Z3
ØQ514ZZ
ØQ52ØZZ
ØQ523ZZ
ØQ524ZZ
ØQ53ØZZ
ØQ533ZZ
ØQ534ZZ
ØQ54ØZZ
ØQ543ZZ
ØQ544ZZ
ØQ55ØZZ
ØQ553ZZ
ØQ554ZZ
ØQ56ØZZ
ØQ563ZZ
ØQ564ZZ
ØQ57ØZZ
ØQ573ZZ
ØQ574ZZ
ØQ58ØZZ
ØQ583ZZ
ØQ584ZZ
ØQ59ØZZ
ØQ593ZZ
ØQ594ZZ
ØQ5BØZZ
ØQ5B3ZZ
ØQ5B4ZZ
ØQ5CØZZ
ØQ5C3ZZ
ØQ5C4ZZ
ØQ5DØZZ
ØQ5D3ZZ
ØQ5D4ZZ
ØQ5FØZZ
ØQ5F3ZZ
ØQ5F4ZZ
ØQ5GØZZ
ØQ5G3ZZ
ØQ5G4ZZ
ØQ5HØZZ
ØQ5H3ZZ
ØQ5H4ZZ
ØQ5JØZZ
ØQ5J3ZZ
ØQ5J4ZZ
ØQ5KØZZ
ØQ5K3ZZ
ØQ5K4ZZ
ØQ5LØZZ
ØQ5L3ZZ
ØQ5L4ZZ
ØQ5MØZZ
ØQ5M3ZZ
ØQ5M4ZZ
ØQ5NØZZ
ØQ5N3ZZ
ØQ5N4ZZ
ØQ5PØZZ
ØQ5P3ZZ
ØQ5P4ZZ
ØQ5QØZZ
ØQ5Q3ZZ
ØQ5Q4ZZ
ØQ5RØZZ
ØQ5R3ZZ
ØQ5R4ZZ
ØQ5SØZZ
ØQ5S3ZZ
ØQ5S4ZZ
ØQ8ØØZZ
ØQ8Ø3ZZ
ØQ8Ø4ZZ
ØQ81ØZZ
ØQ813ZZ
ØQ814ZZ
ØQ82ØZZ
ØQ823ZZ

ØQ824ZZ
ØQ83ØZZ
ØQ833ZZ
ØQ834ZZ
ØQ84ØZZ
ØQ843ZZ
ØQ844ZZ
ØQ85ØZZ
ØQ853ZZ
ØQ854ZZ
ØQ8DØZZ
ØQ8D3ZZ
ØQ8D4ZZ
ØQ8FØZZ
ØQ8F3ZZ
ØQ8F4ZZ
ØQ8GØZZ
ØQ8G3ZZ
ØQ8G4ZZ
ØQ8HØZZ
ØQ8H3ZZ
ØQ8H4ZZ
ØQ8JØZZ
ØQ8J3ZZ
ØQ8J4ZZ
ØQ8KØZZ
ØQ8K3ZZ
ØQ8K4ZZ
ØQ8LØZZ
ØQ8L3ZZ
ØQ8L4ZZ
ØQ8MØZZ
ØQ8M3ZZ
ØQ8M4ZZ
ØQ8NØZZ
ØQ8N3ZZ
ØQ8N4ZZ
ØQ8PØZZ
ØQ8P3ZZ
ØQ8P4ZZ
ØQ8QØZZ
ØQ8Q3ZZ
ØQ8Q4ZZ
ØQ8RØZZ
ØQ8R3ZZ
ØQ8R4ZZ
ØQ8SØZZ
ØQ8S3ZZ
ØQ8S4ZZ
ØQ9DØØZ
ØQ9DØZZ
ØQ9D4ØZ
ØQ9D4ZZ
ØQ9FØØZ
ØQ9FØZZ
ØQ9F4ØZ
ØQ9F4ZZ
ØQBØØZZ
ØQBØ3ZZ
ØQBØ4ZZ
ØQB1ØZZ
ØQB13ZZ
ØQB14ZZ
ØQB2ØZZ
ØQB23ZZ
ØQB24ZZ
ØQB3ØZZ
ØQB33ZZ
ØQB34ZZ
ØQB4ØZZ
ØQB43ZZ
ØQB44ZZ
ØQB5ØZZ
ØQB53ZZ
ØQB54ZZ
ØQB6ØZZ
ØQB63ZZ
ØQB64ZZ
ØQB7ØZZ
ØQB73ZZ
ØQB74ZZ
ØQB8ØZZ
ØQB83ZZ
ØQB84ZZ
ØQB9ØZZ
ØQB93ZZ
ØQB94ZZ
ØQBBØZZ
ØQBB3ZZ
ØQBB4ZZ
ØQBCØZZ
ØQBC3ZZ
ØQBC4ZZ
ØQBDØZZ
ØQBD3ZZ
ØQBD4ZZ
ØQBFØZZ
ØQBF3ZZ
ØQBF4ZZ
ØQBGØZZ
ØQBG3ZZ
ØQBG4ZZ
ØQBHØZZ
ØQBH3ZZ
ØQBH4ZZ
ØQBJØZZ
ØQBJ3ZZ
ØQBJ4ZZ
ØQBKØZZ
ØQBK3ZZ
ØQBK4ZZ
ØQBLØZZ
ØQBL3ZZ
ØQBL4ZZ
ØQBMØZZ
ØQBM3ZZ
ØQBM4ZZ
ØQBNØZ2
ØQBNØZZ
ØQBN3Z2
ØQBN3ZZ
ØQBN4Z2
ØQBN4ZZ
ØQBPØZ2
ØQBPØZZ
ØQBP3Z2
ØQBP3ZZ
ØQBP4Z2
ØQBP4ZZ
ØQBQØZZ
ØQBQ3ZZ
ØQBQ4ZZ
ØQBRØZZ
ØQBR3ZZ
ØQBR4ZZ
ØQBSØZZ
ØQBS3ZZ
ØQBS4ZZ
ØQCØØZZ
ØQCØ3ZZ
ØQCØ4ZZ
ØQC1ØZZ
ØQC13ZZ
ØQC14ZZ
ØQC2ØZZ
ØQC23ZZ
ØQC24ZZ
ØQC3ØZZ
ØQC33ZZ
ØQC34ZZ
ØQC4ØZZ
ØQC43ZZ
ØQC44ZZ
ØQC5ØZZ
ØQC53ZZ
ØQC54ZZ
ØQCDØZZ
ØQCD3ZZ
ØQCD4ZZ
ØQCFØZZ
ØQCF3ZZ
ØQCF4ZZ
ØQCGØZZ
ØQCG3ZZ
ØQCG4ZZ
ØQCHØZZ
ØQCH3ZZ
ØQCH4ZZ
ØQCJØZZ
ØQCJ3ZZ
ØQCJ4ZZ
ØQCKØZZ
ØQCK3ZZ
ØQCK4ZZ
ØQCLØZZ
ØQCL3ZZ
ØQCL4ZZ
ØQCMØZZ
ØQCM3ZZ
ØQCM4ZZ
ØQCNØZZ
ØQCN3ZZ
ØQCN4ZZ
ØQCPØZZ
ØQCP3ZZ
ØQCP4ZZ
ØQCQØZZ
ØQCQ3ZZ
ØQCQ4ZZ
ØQCRØZZ
ØQCR3ZZ
ØQCR4ZZ
ØQCSØZZ
ØQCS3ZZ
ØQCS4ZZ
ØQDØØZZ
ØQD1ØZZ
ØQD2ØZZ
ØQD3ØZZ
ØQD4ØZZ
ØQD5ØZZ
ØQD6ØZZ
ØQD7ØZZ
ØQD8ØZZ
ØQD9ØZZ
ØQDBØZZ
ØQDCØZZ
ØQDDØZZ
ØQDFØZZ
ØQDGØZZ
ØQDHØZZ
ØQDJØZZ
ØQDKØZZ
ØQDLØZZ
ØQDMØZZ
ØQDNØZZ
ØQDPØZZ
ØQDQØZZ
ØQDRØZZ
ØQDSØZZ
ØQHØØ4Z
ØQHØØ5Z
ØQHØ34Z
ØQHØ35Z
ØQHØ44Z
ØQHØ45Z
ØQH1Ø4Z
ØQH1Ø5Z
ØQH134Z
ØQH135Z
ØQH144Z
ØQH145Z
ØQH2Ø4Z
ØQH2Ø5Z
ØQH234Z
ØQH235Z
ØQH244Z
ØQH245Z
ØQH3Ø4Z
ØQH3Ø5Z
ØQH334Z
ØQH335Z
ØQH344Z
ØQH345Z
ØQH4Ø4Z
ØQH4Ø5Z
ØQH434Z
ØQH435Z
ØQH444Z
ØQH445Z
ØQH5Ø4Z
ØQH5Ø5Z
ØQH534Z
ØQH535Z
ØQH544Z
ØQH545Z
ØQHDØ4Z
ØQHDØ5Z
ØQHD34Z
ØQHD35Z
ØQHD44Z
ØQHD45Z
ØQHFØ4Z
ØQHFØ5Z
ØQHF34Z
ØQHF35Z
ØQHF44Z
ØQHF45Z
ØQHGØ4Z
ØQHGØ5Z
ØQHGØ6Z
ØQHGØ7Z
ØQHGØBZ
ØQHGØCZ
ØQHGØDZ
ØQHG34Z
ØQHG35Z
ØQHG36Z
ØQHG37Z
ØQHG3BZ
ØQHG3CZ
ØQHG3DZ
ØQHG44Z
ØQHG45Z
ØQHG46Z
ØQHG47Z
ØQHG4BZ
ØQHG4CZ
ØQHG4DZ
ØQHHØ4Z
ØQHHØ5Z
ØQHHØ6Z
ØQHHØ7Z
ØQHHØBZ
ØQHHØCZ
ØQHHØDZ
ØQHH34Z
ØQHH35Z
ØQHH36Z
ØQHH37Z
ØQHH3BZ
ØQHH3CZ
ØQHH3DZ
ØQHH44Z
ØQHH45Z
ØQHH46Z
ØQHH47Z
ØQHH4BZ
ØQHH4CZ
ØQHH4DZ
ØQHJØ4Z
ØQHJØ5Z
ØQHJØ6Z
ØQHJØBZ
ØQHJØCZ
ØQHJØDZ
ØQHJ34Z
ØQHJ35Z
ØQHJ36Z
ØQHJ3BZ
ØQHJ3CZ
ØQHJ3DZ
ØQHJ44Z
ØQHJ45Z
ØQHJ46Z
ØQHJ4BZ
ØQHJ4CZ
ØQHJ4DZ
ØQHKØ4Z
ØQHKØ5Z
ØQHKØ6Z
ØQHKØBZ
ØQHKØCZ
ØQHKØDZ
ØQHK34Z
ØQHK35Z
ØQHK36Z
ØQHK3BZ
ØQHK3CZ
ØQHK3DZ
ØQHK44Z
ØQHK45Z
ØQHK46Z
ØQHK4BZ
ØQHK4CZ
ØQHK4DZ
ØQHLØ4Z
ØQHLØ5Z
ØQHL34Z
ØQHL35Z
ØQHL44Z
ØQHL45Z
ØQHMØ4Z
ØQHMØ5Z
ØQHM34Z
ØQHM35Z
ØQHM44Z
ØQHM45Z
ØQHNØ4Z
ØQHNØ5Z
ØQHN34Z
ØQHN35Z
ØQHN44Z
ØQHN45Z
ØQHPØ4Z
ØQHPØ5Z
ØQHP34Z
ØQHP35Z
ØQHP44Z
ØQHP45Z
ØQHQØ4Z
ØQHQØ5Z
ØQHQ34Z
ØQHQ35Z
ØQHQ44Z
ØQHQ45Z
ØQHRØ4Z
ØQHRØ5Z
ØQHR34Z
ØQHR35Z
ØQHR44Z
ØQHR45Z
ØQHSØ4Z
ØQHSØ5Z
ØQHS34Z
ØQHS35Z
ØQHS44Z
ØQHS45Z
ØQHYØMZ
ØQHY3MZ
ØQHY4MZ
ØQNDØZZ
ØQND3ZZ
ØQND4ZZ
ØQNFØZZ
ØQNF3ZZ
ØQNF4ZZ
ØQNGØZZ
ØQNG3ZZ
ØQNG4ZZ
ØQNHØZZ
ØQNH3ZZ
ØQNH4ZZ
ØQNJØZZ
ØQNJ3ZZ
ØQNJ4ZZ
ØQNKØZZ
ØQNK3ZZ
ØQNK4ZZ
ØQNLØZZ
ØQNL3ZZ
ØQNL4ZZ
ØQNMØZZ
ØQNM3ZZ
ØQNM4ZZ
ØQNNØZZ
ØQNN3ZZ
ØQNN4ZZ
ØQNPØZZ
ØQNP3ZZ
ØQNP4ZZ
ØQPDØ4Z
ØQPDØ5Z
ØQPDØ7Z
ØQPDØJZ
ØQPDØKZ
ØQPD34Z
ØQPD35Z
ØQPD37Z
ØQPD3JZ
ØQPD3KZ
ØQPD44Z
ØQPD45Z
ØQPD47Z
ØQPD4JZ
ØQPD4KZ
ØQPFØ4Z
ØQPFØ5Z
ØQPFØ7Z
ØQPFØJZ
ØQPFØKZ
ØQPF34Z
ØQPF35Z
ØQPF37Z
ØQPF3JZ
ØQPF3KZ
ØQPF44Z
ØQPF45Z
ØQPF47Z
ØQPF4JZ
ØQPF4KZ
ØQPGØ4Z
ØQPGØ5Z
ØQPGØ7Z
ØQPGØJZ
ØQPGØKZ
ØQPG34Z
ØQPG35Z
ØQPG37Z
ØQPG3JZ
ØQPG3KZ
ØQPG44Z
ØQPG45Z
ØQPG47Z
ØQPG4JZ
ØQPG4KZ
ØQPHØ4Z
ØQPHØ5Z
ØQPHØ7Z
ØQPHØJZ
ØQPHØKZ
ØQPH34Z
ØQPH35Z
ØQPH37Z
ØQPH3JZ
ØQPH3KZ
ØQPH44Z
ØQPH45Z
ØQPH47Z
ØQPH4JZ
ØQPH4KZ
ØQPJØ4Z
ØQPJØ5Z
ØQPJØ7Z
ØQPJØJZ
ØQPJØKZ
ØQPJ34Z
ØQPJ35Z
ØQPJ37Z
ØQPJ3JZ
ØQPJ3KZ
ØQPJ44Z
ØQPJ45Z
ØQPJ47Z
ØQPJ4JZ
ØQPJ4KZ
ØQPKØ4Z
ØQPKØ5Z
ØQPKØ7Z
ØQPKØJZ
ØQPKØKZ
ØQPK34Z
ØQPK35Z
ØQPK37Z
ØQPK3JZ
ØQPK3KZ
ØQPK44Z
ØQPK45Z
ØQPK47Z
ØQPK4JZ
ØQPK4KZ
ØQPLØ4Z
ØQPLØ5Z
ØQPLØ7Z
ØQPLØJZ
ØQPLØKZ
ØQPL34Z
ØQPL35Z
ØQPL37Z
ØQPL3JZ
ØQPL3KZ
ØQPL44Z
ØQPL45Z
ØQPL47Z
ØQPL4JZ
ØQPL4KZ
ØQPMØ4Z
ØQPMØ5Z
ØQPMØ7Z
ØQPMØJZ
ØQPMØKZ
ØQPM34Z
ØQPM35Z
ØQPM37Z
ØQPM3JZ
ØQPM3KZ
ØQPM44Z
ØQPM45Z
ØQPM47Z
ØQPM4JZ
ØQPM4KZ
ØQPNØ4Z
ØQPNØ5Z
ØQPNØ7Z
ØQPNØJZ
ØQPNØKZ
ØQPN34Z
ØQPN35Z
ØQPN37Z
ØQPN3JZ
ØQPN3KZ
ØQPN44Z
ØQPN45Z
ØQPN47Z
ØQPN4JZ
ØQPN4KZ
ØQPPØ4Z
ØQPPØ5Z
ØQPPØ7Z
ØQPPØJZ
ØQPPØKZ
ØQPP34Z
ØQPP35Z
ØQPP37Z
ØQPP3JZ
ØQPP3KZ
ØQPP44Z
ØQPP45Z
ØQPP47Z
ØQPP4JZ
ØQPP4KZ
ØQQDØZZ
ØQQD4ZZ
ØQQFØZZ
ØQQF4ZZ
ØQQGØZZ
ØQQG3ZZ
ØQQG4ZZ
ØQQHØZZ
ØQQH3ZZ
ØQQH4ZZ
ØQQJØZZ
ØQQJ3ZZ
ØQQJ4ZZ
ØQQKØZZ
ØQQK3ZZ
ØQQK4ZZ
ØQQLØZZ
ØQQL3ZZ
ØQQL4ZZ
ØQQMØZZ
ØQQM3ZZ
ØQQM4ZZ
ØQQNØZZ
ØQQN3ZZ
ØQQN4ZZ
ØQQPØZZ
ØQQP3ZZ
ØQQP4ZZ
ØQQQØZZ
ØQQQ3ZZ
ØQQQ4ZZ
ØQQRØZZ
ØQQR3ZZ
ØQQR4ZZ
ØQRØØ7Z
ØQRØØKZ
ØQRØ37Z
ØQRØ3KZ
ØQRØ47Z
ØQRØ4KZ
ØQR1Ø7Z
ØQR1ØKZ
ØQR137Z
ØQR13KZ
ØQR147Z
ØQR14KZ
ØQR2Ø7Z
ØQR2ØKZ
ØQR237Z
ØQR23KZ
ØQR247Z
ØQR24KZ
ØQR3Ø7Z
ØQR3ØKZ
ØQR337Z
ØQR33KZ
ØQR347Z
ØQR34KZ
ØQR4Ø7Z
ØQR4ØJZ
ØQR4ØKZ
ØQR437Z
ØQR43JZ
ØQR43KZ
ØQR447Z
ØQR44JZ
ØQR44KZ
ØQR5Ø7Z
ØQR5ØJZ
ØQR5ØKZ
ØQR537Z
ØQR53JZ
ØQR53KZ
ØQR547Z
ØQR54JZ
ØQR54KZ
ØQRDØ7Z
ØQRDØJZ
ØQRDØKZ
ØQRD37Z
ØQRD3JZ
ØQRD3KZ
ØQRD47Z
ØQRD4JZ
ØQRD4KZ
ØQRFØ7Z
ØQRFØJZ
ØQRFØKZ
ØQRF37Z
ØQRF3JZ
ØQRF3KZ
ØQRF47Z
ØQRF4JZ
ØQRF4KZ
ØQRGØ7Z
ØQRGØJZ
ØQRGØKZ
ØQRG37Z
ØQRG3JZ
ØQRG3KZ
ØQRG47Z
ØQRG4JZ
ØQRG4KZ
ØQRHØ7Z
ØQRHØJZ
ØQRHØKZ
ØQRH37Z
ØQRH3JZ
ØQRH3KZ
ØQRH47Z
ØQRH4JZ
ØQRH4KZ
ØQRJØ7Z
ØQRJØJZ
ØQRJØKZ
ØQRJ37Z
ØQRJ3JZ
ØQRJ3KZ
ØQRJ47Z
ØQRJ4JZ
ØQRJ4KZ
ØQRKØ7Z
ØQRKØJZ
ØQRKØKZ
ØQRK37Z
ØQRK3JZ
ØQRK3KZ
ØQRK47Z
ØQRK4JZ
ØQRK4KZ
ØQRLØ7Z
ØQRLØJZ
ØQRLØKZ
ØQRL37Z
ØQRL3JZ
ØQRL3KZ
ØQRL47Z
ØQRL4JZ
ØQRL4KZ
ØQRMØ7Z
ØQRMØJZ
ØQRMØKZ
ØQRM37Z
ØQRM3JZ
ØQRM3KZ
ØQRM47Z
ØQRM4JZ
ØQRM4KZ
ØQRNØ7Z
ØQRNØJZ
ØQRNØKZ
ØQRN37Z
ØQRN3JZ
ØQRN3KZ
ØQRN47Z
ØQRN4JZ
ØQRN4KZ
ØQRPØ7Z
ØQRPØJZ
ØQRPØKZ
ØQRP37Z
ØQRP3JZ
ØQRP3KZ
ØQRP47Z
ØQRP4JZ
ØQRP4KZ
ØQRQØ7Z
ØQRQØKZ
ØQRQ37Z
ØQRQ3KZ
ØQRQ47Z
ØQRQ4KZ
ØQRRØ7Z
ØQRRØKZ
ØQRR37Z
ØQRR3KZ
ØQRR47Z
ØQRR4KZ
ØQRSØ7Z
ØQRSØKZ
ØQRS37Z
ØQRS3KZ
ØQRS47Z
ØQRS4KZ
ØQSØØ3Z
ØQSØØ4Z
ØQSØØZZ
ØQSØ34Z
ØQSØ43Z
ØQSØ44Z
ØQSØ4ZZ
ØQS1Ø4Z
ØQS1ØZZ
ØQS134Z
ØQS144Z
ØQS14ZZ
ØQS2Ø4Z
ØQS2Ø5Z
ØQS2ØZZ
ØQS234Z
ØQS235Z
ØQS244Z
ØQS245Z
ØQS3Ø4Z
ØQS3Ø5Z
ØQS3ØZZ
ØQS334Z
ØQS335Z
ØQS344Z
ØQS345Z
ØQS4Ø4Z
ØQS4ØZZ
ØQS434Z
ØQS444Z
ØQS5Ø4Z
ØQS5ØZZ
ØQS534Z
ØQS544Z
ØQSDØ4Z
ØQSDØ5Z
ØQSDØZZ
ØQSD34Z
ØQSD35Z
ØQSD44Z
ØQSD45Z
ØQSFØ4Z
ØQSFØ5Z
ØQSFØZZ
ØQSF34Z
ØQSF35Z
ØQSF44Z
ØQSF45Z
ØQSGØ4Z
ØQSGØ5Z
ØQSGØ6Z
ØQSGØBZ
ØQSGØCZ
ØQSGØDZ
ØQSGØZZ
ØQSG34Z
ØQSG35Z
ØQSG36Z
ØQSG3BZ
ØQSG3CZ
ØQSG3DZ
ØQSG44Z
ØQSG45Z
ØQSG46Z
ØQSG4BZ
ØQSG4CZ
ØQSG4DZ
ØQSHØ4Z
ØQSHØ5Z
ØQSHØ6Z
ØQSHØBZ
ØQSHØCZ
ØQSHØDZ
ØQSHØZZ
ØQSH34Z
ØQSH35Z
ØQSH36Z
ØQSH3BZ
ØQSH3CZ
ØQSH3DZ
ØQSH44Z
ØQSH45Z
ØQSH46Z
ØQSH4BZ
ØQSH4CZ
ØQSH4DZ
ØQSJØ4Z
ØQSJØ5Z
ØQSJØ6Z
ØQSJØBZ
ØQSJØCZ
ØQSJØDZ
ØQSJØZZ
ØQSJ34Z
ØQSJ35Z
ØQSJ36Z
ØQSJ3BZ
ØQSJ3CZ
ØQSJ3DZ
ØQSJ44Z

ØQSJ45Z
ØQSJ46Z
ØQSJ4BZ
ØQSJ4CZ
ØQSJ4DZ
ØQSKØ4Z
ØQSKØ5Z
ØQSKØ6Z
ØQSKØBZ
ØQSKØCZ
ØQSKØDZ
ØQSKØZZ
ØQSK34Z
ØQSK35Z
ØQSK36Z
ØQSK3BZ
ØQSK3CZ
ØQSK3DZ
ØQSK44Z
ØQSK45Z
ØQSK46Z
ØQSK4BZ
ØQSK4CZ
ØQSK4DZ
ØQSLØ4Z
ØQSLØ5Z
ØQSLØZZ
ØQSL34Z
ØQSL35Z
ØQSL44Z
ØQSL45Z
ØQSMØ4Z
ØQSMØ5Z
ØQSMØZZ
ØQSM34Z
ØQSM35Z
ØQSM44Z
ØQSM45Z
ØQSNØ42
ØQSNØ4Z
ØQSNØ52
ØQSNØ5Z
ØQSNØZ2
ØQSNØZZ
ØQSN342
ØQSN34Z
ØQSN352
ØQSN35Z
ØQSN442
ØQSN44Z
ØQSN452
ØQSN45Z
ØQSPØ42
ØQSPØ4Z
ØQSPØ52
ØQSPØ5Z
ØQSPØZ2
ØQSPØZZ
ØQSP342
ØQSP34Z
ØQSP352
ØQSP35Z
ØQSP442
ØQSP44Z
ØQSP452
ØQSP45Z
ØQSQØ4Z
ØQSQØ5Z
ØQSQØZZ
ØQSQ34Z
ØQSQ35Z
ØQSQ44Z
ØQSQ45Z
ØQSRØ4Z
ØQSRØ5Z
ØQSRØZZ
ØQSR34Z
ØQSR35Z
ØQSR44Z
ØQSR45Z
ØQSSØ4Z
ØQSSØZZ
ØQSS34Z
ØQSS3ZZ
ØQSS44Z
ØQSS4ZZ
ØQT2ØZZ
ØQT3ØZZ
ØQT4ØZZ
ØQT5ØZZ
ØQTDØZZ
ØQTFØZZ
ØQTGØZZ
ØQTHØZZ
ØQTJØZZ
ØQTKØZZ
ØQTLØZZ
ØQTMØZZ
ØQTNØZZ
ØQTPØZZ
ØQTQØZZ
ØQTRØZZ
ØQTSØZZ
ØQUØØ7Z
ØQUØØJZ
ØQUØØKZ
ØQUØ37Z
ØQUØ3JZ
ØQUØ3KZ
ØQUØ47Z
ØQUØ4JZ
ØQUØ4KZ
ØQU1Ø7Z
ØQU1ØJZ
ØQU1ØKZ
ØQU137Z
ØQU13JZ
ØQU13KZ
ØQU147Z
ØQU14JZ
ØQU14KZ
ØQU2Ø7Z
ØQU2ØKZ
ØQU237Z
ØQU23KZ
ØQU247Z
ØQU24KZ
ØQU3Ø7Z
ØQU3ØKZ
ØQU337Z
ØQU33KZ
ØQU347Z
ØQU34KZ
ØQU4Ø7Z
ØQU4ØJZ
ØQU4ØKZ
ØQU437Z
ØQU43JZ
ØQU43KZ
ØQU447Z
ØQU44JZ
ØQU44KZ
ØQU5Ø7Z
ØQU5ØJZ
ØQU5ØKZ
ØQU537Z
ØQU53JZ
ØQU53KZ
ØQU547Z
ØQU54JZ
ØQU54KZ
ØQUDØ7Z
ØQUDØJZ
ØQUDØKZ
ØQUD37Z
ØQUD3JZ
ØQUD3KZ
ØQUD47Z
ØQUD4JZ
ØQUD4KZ
ØQUFØ7Z
ØQUFØJZ
ØQUFØKZ
ØQUF37Z
ØQUF3JZ
ØQUF3KZ
ØQUF47Z
ØQUF4JZ
ØQUF4KZ
ØQUGØ7Z
ØQUGØJZ
ØQUGØKZ
ØQUG37Z
ØQUG3JZ
ØQUG3KZ
ØQUG47Z
ØQUG4JZ
ØQUG4KZ
ØQUHØ7Z
ØQUHØJZ
ØQUHØKZ
ØQUH37Z
ØQUH3JZ
ØQUH3KZ
ØQUH47Z
ØQUH4JZ
ØQUH4KZ
ØQUJØ7Z
ØQUJØJZ
ØQUJØKZ
ØQUJ37Z
ØQUJ3JZ
ØQUJ3KZ
ØQUJ47Z
ØQUJ4JZ
ØQUJ4KZ
ØQUKØ7Z
ØQUKØJZ
ØQUKØKZ
ØQUK37Z
ØQUK3JZ
ØQUK3KZ
ØQUK47Z
ØQUK4JZ
ØQUK4KZ
ØQULØ7Z
ØQULØJZ
ØQULØKZ
ØQUL37Z
ØQUL3JZ
ØQUL3KZ
ØQUL47Z
ØQUL4JZ
ØQUL4KZ
ØQUMØ7Z
ØQUMØJZ
ØQUMØKZ
ØQUM37Z
ØQUM3JZ
ØQUM3KZ
ØQUM47Z
ØQUM4JZ
ØQUM4KZ
ØQUNØ7Z
ØQUNØJZ
ØQUNØKZ
ØQUN37Z
ØQUN3JZ
ØQUN3KZ
ØQUN47Z
ØQUN4JZ
ØQUN4KZ
ØQUPØ7Z
ØQUPØJZ
ØQUPØKZ
ØQUP37Z
ØQUP3JZ
ØQUP3KZ
ØQUP47Z
ØQUP4JZ
ØQUP4KZ
ØQUQØ7Z
ØQUQØKZ
ØQUQ37Z
ØQUQ3KZ
ØQUQ47Z
ØQUQ4KZ
ØQURØ7Z
ØQURØKZ
ØQUR37Z
ØQUR3KZ
ØQUR47Z
ØQUR4KZ
ØQUSØ7Z
ØQUSØKZ
ØQUS37Z
ØQUS3KZ
ØQUS47Z
ØQUS4KZ
ØQWDØ4Z
ØQWDØ5Z
ØQWDØ7Z
ØQWDØJZ
ØQWDØKZ
ØQWD34Z
ØQWD35Z
ØQWD37Z
ØQWD3JZ
ØQWD3KZ
ØQWD44Z
ØQWD45Z
ØQWD47Z
ØQWD4JZ
ØQWD4KZ
ØQWFØ4Z
ØQWFØ5Z
ØQWFØ7Z
ØQWFØJZ
ØQWFØKZ
ØQWF34Z
ØQWF35Z
ØQWF37Z
ØQWF3JZ
ØQWF3KZ
ØQWF44Z
ØQWF45Z
ØQWF47Z
ØQWF4JZ
ØQWF4KZ
ØR5ØØZZ
ØR5Ø3ZZ
ØR5Ø4ZZ
ØR51ØZZ
ØR513ZZ
ØR514ZZ
ØR53ØZZ
ØR54ØZZ
ØR543ZZ
ØR544ZZ
ØR55ØZZ
ØR56ØZZ
ØR563ZZ
ØR564ZZ
ØR59ØZZ
ØR5AØZZ
ØR5A3ZZ
ØR5A4ZZ
ØR5BØZZ
ØR5CØZZ
ØR5C3ZZ
ØR5C4ZZ
ØR5DØZZ
ØR5D3ZZ
ØR5D4ZZ
ØR5EØZZ
ØR5E3ZZ
ØR5E4ZZ
ØR5FØZZ
ØR5F3ZZ
ØR5F4ZZ
ØR5GØZZ
ØR5G3ZZ
ØR5G4ZZ
ØR5HØZZ
ØR5H3ZZ
ØR5H4ZZ
ØR5JØZZ
ØR5J3ZZ
ØR5J4ZZ
ØR5KØZZ
ØR5K3ZZ
ØR5K4ZZ
ØR5LØZZ
ØR5L3ZZ
ØR5L4ZZ
ØR5MØZZ
ØR5M3ZZ
ØR5M4ZZ
ØR5NØZZ
ØR5N3ZZ
ØR5N4ZZ
ØR5PØZZ
ØR5P3ZZ
ØR5P4ZZ
ØR5QØZZ
ØR5Q3ZZ
ØR5Q4ZZ
ØR5RØZZ
ØR5R3ZZ
ØR5R4ZZ
ØR5SØZZ
ØR5S3ZZ
ØR5S4ZZ
ØR5TØZZ
ØR5T3ZZ
ØR5T4ZZ
ØR5UØZZ
ØR5U3ZZ
ØR5U4ZZ
ØR5VØZZ
ØR5V3ZZ
ØR5V4ZZ
ØR5WØZZ
ØR5W3ZZ
ØR5W4ZZ
ØR5XØZZ
ØR5X3ZZ
ØR5X4ZZ
ØRBØØZZ
ØRBØ3ZZ
ØRBØ4ZZ
ØRB1ØZZ
ØRB13ZZ
ØRB14ZZ
ØRB3ØZZ
ØRB33ZZ
ØRB34ZZ
ØRB4ØZZ
ØRB43ZZ
ØRB44ZZ
ØRB5ØZZ
ØRB53ZZ
ØRB54ZZ
ØRB6ØZZ
ØRB63ZZ
ØRB64ZZ
ØRB9ØZZ
ØRB93ZZ
ØRB94ZZ
ØRBAØZZ
ØRBA3ZZ
ØRBA4ZZ
ØRBBØZZ
ØRBB3ZZ
ØRBB4ZZ
ØRBCØZZ
ØRBC3ZZ
ØRBC4ZZ
ØRBDØZZ
ØRBD3ZZ
ØRBD4ZZ
ØRBEØZZ
ØRBE3ZZ
ØRBE4ZZ
ØRBFØZZ
ØRBF3ZZ
ØRBF4ZZ
ØRBGØZZ
ØRBG3ZZ
ØRBG4ZZ
ØRBHØZZ
ØRBH3ZZ
ØRBH4ZZ
ØRBJØZZ
ØRBJ3ZZ
ØRBJ4ZZ
ØRBKØZZ
ØRBK3ZZ
ØRBK4ZZ
ØRBLØZZ
ØRBL3ZZ
ØRBL4ZZ
ØRBMØZZ
ØRBM3ZZ
ØRBM4ZZ
ØRBNØZZ
ØRBN3ZZ
ØRBN4ZZ
ØRBPØZZ
ØRBP3ZZ
ØRBP4ZZ
ØRBQØZZ
ØRBQ3ZZ
ØRBQ4ZZ
ØRBRØZZ
ØRBR3ZZ
ØRBR4ZZ
ØRBSØZZ
ØRBS3ZZ
ØRBS4ZZ
ØRBTØZZ
ØRBT3ZZ
ØRBT4ZZ
ØRBUØZZ
ØRBU3ZZ
ØRBU4ZZ
ØRBVØZZ
ØRBV3ZZ
ØRBV4ZZ
ØRBWØZZ
ØRBW3ZZ
ØRBW4ZZ
ØRBXØZZ
ØRBX3ZZ
ØRBX4ZZ
ØRCCØZZ
ØRCC3ZZ
ØRCC4ZZ
ØRCDØZZ
ØRCD3ZZ
ØRCD4ZZ
ØRGØØ7Ø
ØRGØØ71
ØRGØØ7J
ØRGØØAØ
ØRGØØAJ
ØRGØØJØ
ØRGØØJ1
ØRGØØJJ
ØRGØØKØ
ØRGØØK1
ØRGØØKJ
ØRGØ37Ø
ØRGØ371
ØRGØ37J
ØRGØ3AØ
ØRGØ3AJ
ØRGØ3JØ
ØRGØ3J1
ØRGØ3JJ
ØRGØ3KØ
ØRGØ3K1
ØRGØ3KJ
ØRGØ47Ø
ØRGØ471
ØRGØ47J
ØRGØ4AØ
ØRGØ4AJ
ØRGØ4JØ
ØRGØ4J1
ØRGØ4JJ
ØRGØ4KØ
ØRGØ4K1
ØRGØ4KJ
ØRG1Ø7Ø
ØRG1Ø71
ØRG1Ø7J
ØRG1ØAØ
ØRG1ØAJ
ØRG1ØJØ
ØRG1ØJ1
ØRG1ØJJ
ØRG1ØKØ
ØRG1ØK1
ØRG1ØKJ
ØRG137Ø
ØRG1371
ØRG137J
ØRG13AØ
ØRG13AJ
ØRG13JØ
ØRG13J1
ØRG13JJ
ØRG13KØ
ØRG13K1
ØRG13KJ
ØRG147Ø
ØRG1471
ØRG147J
ØRG14AØ
ØRG14AJ
ØRG14JØ
ØRG14J1
ØRG14JJ
ØRG14KØ
ØRG14K1
ØRG14KJ
ØRG2Ø7Ø
ØRG2Ø71
ØRG2Ø7J
ØRG2ØAØ
ØRG2ØAJ
ØRG2ØJØ
ØRG2ØJ1
ØRG2ØJJ
ØRG2ØKØ
ØRG2ØK1
ØRG2ØKJ
ØRG237Ø
ØRG2371
ØRG237J
ØRG23AØ
ØRG23AJ
ØRG23JØ
ØRG23J1
ØRG23JJ
ØRG23KØ
ØRG23K1
ØRG23KJ
ØRG247Ø
ØRG2471
ØRG247J
ØRG24AØ
ØRG24AJ
ØRG24JØ
ØRG24J1
ØRG24JJ
ØRG24KØ
ØRG24K1
ØRG24KJ
ØRG4Ø7Ø
ØRG4Ø71
ØRG4Ø7J
ØRG4ØAØ
ØRG4ØAJ
ØRG4ØJØ
ØRG4ØJ1
ØRG4ØJJ
ØRG4ØKØ
ØRG4ØK1
ØRG4ØKJ
ØRG437Ø
ØRG4371
ØRG437J
ØRG43AØ
ØRG43AJ
ØRG43JØ
ØRG43J1
ØRG43JJ
ØRG43KØ
ØRG43K1
ØRG43KJ
ØRG447Ø
ØRG4471
ØRG447J
ØRG44AØ
ØRG44AJ
ØRG44JØ
ØRG44J1
ØRG44JJ
ØRG44KØ
ØRG44K1
ØRG44KJ
ØRG6Ø7Ø
ØRG6Ø71
ØRG6Ø7J
ØRG6ØAØ
ØRG6ØAJ
ØRG6ØJØ
ØRG6ØJ1
ØRG6ØJJ
ØRG6ØKØ
ØRG6ØK1
ØRG6ØKJ
ØRG637Ø
ØRG6371
ØRG637J
ØRG63AØ
ØRG63AJ
ØRG63JØ
ØRG63J1
ØRG63JJ
ØRG63KØ
ØRG63K1
ØRG63KJ
ØRG647Ø
ØRG6471
ØRG647J
ØRG64AØ
ØRG64AJ
ØRG64JØ
ØRG64J1
ØRG64JJ
ØRG64KØ
ØRG64K1
ØRG64KJ
ØRG7Ø7Ø
ØRG7Ø71
ØRG7Ø7J
ØRG7ØAØ
ØRG7ØAJ
ØRG7ØJØ
ØRG7ØJ1
ØRG7ØJJ
ØRG7ØKØ
ØRG7ØK1
ØRG7ØKJ
ØRG737Ø
ØRG7371
ØRG737J
ØRG73AØ
ØRG73AJ
ØRG73JØ
ØRG73J1
ØRG73JJ
ØRG73KØ
ØRG73K1
ØRG73KJ
ØRG747Ø
ØRG7471
ØRG747J
ØRG74AØ
ØRG74AJ
ØRG74JØ
ØRG74J1
ØRG74JJ
ØRG74KØ
ØRG74K1
ØRG74KJ
ØRG8Ø7Ø
ØRG8Ø71
ØRG8Ø7J
ØRG8ØAØ
ØRG8ØAJ
ØRG8ØJØ
ØRG8ØJ1
ØRG8ØJJ
ØRG8ØKØ
ØRG8ØK1
ØRG8ØKJ
ØRG837Ø
ØRG8371
ØRG837J
ØRG83AØ
ØRG83AJ
ØRG83JØ
ØRG83J1
ØRG83JJ
ØRG83KØ
ØRG83K1
ØRG83KJ
ØRG847Ø
ØRG8471
ØRG847J
ØRG84AØ
ØRG84AJ
ØRG84JØ
ØRG84J1
ØRG84JJ
ØRG84KØ
ØRG84K1
ØRG84KJ
ØRGAØ7Ø
ØRGAØ71
ØRGAØ7J
ØRGAØAØ
ØRGAØAJ
ØRGAØJØ
ØRGAØJ1
ØRGAØJJ
ØRGAØKØ
ØRGAØK1
ØRGAØKJ
ØRGA37Ø
ØRGA371
ØRGA37J
ØRGA3AØ
ØRGA3AJ
ØRGA3JØ
ØRGA3J1
ØRGA3JJ
ØRGA3KØ
ØRGA3K1
ØRGA3KJ
ØRGA47Ø
ØRGA471
ØRGA47J
ØRGA4AØ
ØRGA4AJ
ØRGA4JØ
ØRGA4J1
ØRGA4JJ
ØRGA4KØ
ØRGA4K1
ØRGA4KJ
ØRGCØ4Z
ØRGCØ7Z
ØRGCØJZ
ØRGCØKZ
ØRGC34Z
ØRGC37Z
ØRGC3JZ
ØRGC3KZ
ØRGC44Z
ØRGC47Z
ØRGC4JZ
ØRGC4KZ
ØRGDØ4Z
ØRGDØ7Z
ØRGDØJZ
ØRGDØKZ
ØRGD34Z
ØRGD37Z
ØRGD3JZ
ØRGD3KZ
ØRGD44Z
ØRGD47Z
ØRGD4JZ
ØRGD4KZ
ØRGLØ3Z
ØRGLØ4Z
ØRGLØ5Z
ØRGLØ7Z
ØRGLØJZ
ØRGLØKZ
ØRGL33Z
ØRGL34Z
ØRGL35Z
ØRGL37Z
ØRGL3JZ
ØRGL3KZ
ØRGL43Z
ØRGL44Z
ØRGL45Z
ØRGL47Z
ØRGL4JZ
ØRGL4KZ
ØRGMØ3Z
ØRGMØ4Z
ØRGMØ5Z
ØRGMØ7Z
ØRGMØJZ
ØRGMØKZ
ØRGM33Z
ØRGM34Z
ØRGM35Z
ØRGM37Z
ØRGM3JZ
ØRGM3KZ
ØRGM43Z
ØRGM44Z
ØRGM45Z
ØRGM47Z
ØRGM4JZ
ØRGM4KZ
ØRGNØ3Z
ØRGNØ4Z
ØRGNØ5Z
ØRGNØ7Z
ØRGNØJZ
ØRGNØKZ
ØRGN33Z
ØRGN34Z
ØRGN35Z
ØRGN37Z
ØRGN3JZ
ØRGN3KZ
ØRGN43Z
ØRGN44Z
ØRGN45Z
ØRGN47Z
ØRGN4JZ
ØRGN4KZ
ØRGPØ3Z
ØRGPØ4Z
ØRGPØ5Z
ØRGPØ7Z
ØRGPØJZ
ØRGPØKZ
ØRGP33Z
ØRGP34Z
ØRGP35Z
ØRGP37Z
ØRGP3JZ
ØRGP3KZ
ØRGP43Z
ØRGP44Z
ØRGP45Z
ØRGP47Z
ØRGP4JZ
ØRGP4KZ
ØRGQØ3Z
ØRGQØ4Z
ØRGQØ5Z
ØRGQØ7Z
ØRGQØJZ
ØRGQØKZ
ØRGQ33Z
ØRGQ34Z
ØRGQ35Z
ØRGQ37Z
ØRGQ3JZ
ØRGQ3KZ
ØRGQ43Z
ØRGQ44Z
ØRGQ45Z
ØRGQ47Z
ØRGQ4JZ
ØRGQ4KZ
ØRGRØ3Z
ØRGRØ4Z
ØRGRØ5Z
ØRGRØ7Z
ØRGRØJZ
ØRGRØKZ
ØRGR33Z
ØRGR34Z
ØRGR35Z
ØRGR37Z
ØRGR3JZ
ØRGR3KZ
ØRGR43Z
ØRGR44Z
ØRGR45Z
ØRGR47Z

ØRGR4JZ
ØRGR4KZ
ØRGSØ3Z
ØRGSØ4Z
ØRGSØ5Z
ØRGSØ7Z
ØRGSØJZ
ØRGSØKZ
ØRGS33Z
ØRGS34Z
ØRGS35Z
ØRGS37Z
ØRGS3JZ
ØRGS3KZ
ØRGS43Z
ØRGS44Z
ØRGS45Z
ØRGS47Z
ØRGS4JZ
ØRGS4KZ
ØRGTØ3Z
ØRGTØ4Z
ØRGTØ5Z
ØRGTØ7Z
ØRGTØJZ
ØRGTØKZ
ØRGT33Z
ØRGT34Z
ØRGT35Z
ØRGT37Z
ØRGT3JZ
ØRGT3KZ
ØRGT43Z
ØRGT44Z
ØRGT45Z
ØRGT47Z
ØRGT4JZ
ØRGT4KZ
ØRGUØ3Z
ØRGUØ4Z
ØRGUØ5Z
ØRGUØ7Z
ØRGUØJZ
ØRGUØKZ
ØRGU33Z
ØRGU34Z
ØRGU35Z
ØRGU37Z
ØRGU3JZ
ØRGU3KZ
ØRGU43Z
ØRGU44Z
ØRGU45Z
ØRGU47Z
ØRGU4JZ
ØRGU4KZ
ØRGVØ3Z
ØRGVØ4Z
ØRGVØ5Z
ØRGVØ7Z
ØRGVØJZ
ØRGVØKZ
ØRGV33Z
ØRGV34Z
ØRGV35Z
ØRGV37Z
ØRGV3JZ
ØRGV3KZ
ØRGV43Z
ØRGV44Z
ØRGV45Z
ØRGV47Z
ØRGV4JZ
ØRGV4KZ
ØRGWØ3Z
ØRGWØ4Z
ØRGWØ5Z
ØRGWØ7Z
ØRGWØJZ
ØRGWØKZ
ØRGW33Z
ØRGW34Z
ØRGW35Z
ØRGW37Z
ØRGW3JZ
ØRGW3KZ
ØRGW43Z
ØRGW44Z
ØRGW45Z
ØRGW47Z
ØRGW4JZ
ØRGW4KZ
ØRGXØ3Z
ØRGXØ4Z
ØRGXØ5Z
ØRGXØ7Z
ØRGXØJZ
ØRGXØKZ
ØRGX33Z
ØRGX34Z
ØRGX35Z
ØRGX37Z
ØRGX3JZ
ØRGX3KZ
ØRGX43Z
ØRGX44Z
ØRGX45Z
ØRGX47Z
ØRGX4JZ
ØRGX4KZ
ØRHØØ4Z
ØRHØØBZ
ØRHØØCZ
ØRHØØDZ
ØRHØ34Z
ØRHØ3BZ
ØRHØ3CZ
ØRHØ3DZ
ØRHØ44Z
ØRHØ4BZ
ØRHØ4CZ
ØRHØ4DZ
ØRH1Ø4Z
ØRH1ØBZ
ØRH1ØCZ
ØRH1ØDZ
ØRH134Z
ØRH13BZ
ØRH13CZ
ØRH13DZ
ØRH144Z
ØRH14BZ
ØRH14CZ
ØRH14DZ
ØRH4Ø4Z
ØRH4ØBZ
ØRH4ØCZ
ØRH4ØDZ
ØRH434Z
ØRH43BZ
ØRH43CZ
ØRH43DZ
ØRH444Z
ØRH44BZ
ØRH44CZ
ØRH44DZ
ØRH6Ø4Z
ØRH6ØBZ
ØRH6ØCZ
ØRH6ØDZ
ØRH634Z
ØRH63BZ
ØRH63CZ
ØRH63DZ
ØRH644Z
ØRH64BZ
ØRH64CZ
ØRH64DZ
ØRHAØ4Z
ØRHAØBZ
ØRHAØCZ
ØRHAØDZ
ØRHA34Z
ØRHA3BZ
ØRHA3CZ
ØRHA3DZ
ØRHA44Z
ØRHA4BZ
ØRHA4CZ
ØRHA4DZ
ØRHEØ4Z
ØRHE34Z
ØRHE44Z
ØRHFØ4Z
ØRHF34Z
ØRHF44Z
ØRHGØ4Z
ØRHG34Z
ØRHG44Z
ØRHHØ4Z
ØRHH34Z
ØRHH44Z
ØRHJØ4Z
ØRHJ34Z
ØRHJ44Z
ØRHKØ4Z
ØRHK34Z
ØRHK44Z
ØRHLØ4Z
ØRHLØ5Z
ØRHL34Z
ØRHL35Z
ØRHL44Z
ØRHL45Z
ØRHMØ4Z
ØRHMØ5Z
ØRHM34Z
ØRHM35Z
ØRHM44Z
ØRJØ4ZZ
ØRJ14ZZ
ØRJ34ZZ
ØRJ44ZZ
ØRJ54ZZ
ØRJ64ZZ
ØRJ94ZZ
ØRJA4ZZ
ØRJB4ZZ
ØRJCØZZ
ØRJC4ZZ
ØRJDØZZ
ØRJD4ZZ
ØRJE4ZZ
ØRJF4ZZ
ØRJG4ZZ
ØRJH4ZZ
ØRJJ4ZZ
ØRJK4ZZ
ØRJL4ZZ
ØRJM4ZZ
ØRJN4ZZ
ØRJP4ZZ
ØRJQ4ZZ
ØRJR4ZZ
ØRJS4ZZ
ØRJT4ZZ
ØRJU4ZZ
ØRJV4ZZ
ØRJW4ZZ
ØRJX4ZZ
ØRNØØZZ
ØRNØ3ZZ
ØRNØ4ZZ
ØRN1ØZZ
ØRN13ZZ
ØRN14ZZ
ØRN3ØZZ
ØRN33ZZ
ØRN34ZZ
ØRN4ØZZ
ØRN43ZZ
ØRN44ZZ
ØRN5ØZZ
ØRN53ZZ
ØRN54ZZ
ØRN6ØZZ
ØRN63ZZ
ØRN64ZZ
ØRN9ØZZ
ØRN93ZZ
ØRN94ZZ
ØRNAØZZ
ØRNA3ZZ
ØRNA4ZZ
ØRNBØZZ
ØRNB3ZZ
ØRNB4ZZ
ØRNCØZZ
ØRNC3ZZ
ØRNC4ZZ
ØRNDØZZ
ØRND3ZZ
ØRND4ZZ
ØRNEØZZ
ØRNE3ZZ
ØRNE4ZZ
ØRNFØZZ
ØRNF3ZZ
ØRNF4ZZ
ØRNGØZZ
ØRNG3ZZ
ØRNG4ZZ
ØRNHØZZ
ØRNH3ZZ
ØRNH4ZZ
ØRNJØZZ
ØRNJ3ZZ
ØRNJ4ZZ
ØRNKØZZ
ØRNK3ZZ
ØRNK4ZZ
ØRNLØZZ
ØRNL3ZZ
ØRNL4ZZ
ØRNMØZZ
ØRNM3ZZ
ØRNM4ZZ
ØRNNØZZ
ØRNN3ZZ
ØRNN4ZZ
ØRNPØZZ
ØRNP3ZZ
ØRNP4ZZ
ØRNQØZZ
ØRNQ3ZZ
ØRNQ4ZZ
ØRNRØZZ
ØRNR3ZZ
ØRNR4ZZ
ØRNSØZZ
ØRNS3ZZ
ØRNS4ZZ
ØRNTØZZ
ØRNT3ZZ
ØRNT4ZZ
ØRNUØZZ
ØRNU3ZZ
ØRNU4ZZ
ØRNVØZZ
ØRNV3ZZ
ØRNV4ZZ
ØRNWØZZ
ØRNW3ZZ
ØRNW4ZZ
ØRNXØZZ
ØRNX3ZZ
ØRNX4ZZ
ØRPØØJZ
ØRPØ3JZ
ØRPØ4JZ
ØRP1ØJZ
ØRP13JZ
ØRP14JZ
ØRP3ØJZ
ØRP33JZ
ØRP34JZ
ØRP4ØJZ
ØRP43JZ
ØRP44JZ
ØRP5ØJZ
ØRP53JZ
ØRP54JZ
ØRP6ØJZ
ØRP63JZ
ØRP64JZ
ØRP9ØJZ
ØRP93JZ
ØRP94JZ
ØRPAØJZ
ØRPA3JZ
ØRPA4JZ
ØRPBØJZ
ØRPB3JZ
ØRPB4JZ
ØRPCØ4Z
ØRPC34Z
ØRPC44Z
ØRPCX4Z
ØRPDØ4Z
ØRPD34Z
ØRPD44Z
ØRPDX4Z
ØRPEØJZ
ØRPE3JZ
ØRPE4JZ
ØRPFØJZ
ØRPF3JZ
ØRPF4JZ
ØRPGØJZ
ØRPG3JZ
ØRPG4JZ
ØRPHØJZ
ØRPH3JZ
ØRPH4JZ
ØRPJØJ6
ØRPJØJ7
ØRPJØJZ
ØRPJ3J6
ØRPJ3J7
ØRPJ3JZ
ØRPJ4J6
ØRPJ4J7
ØRPJ4JZ
ØRPKØJ6
ØRPKØJ7
ØRPKØJZ
ØRPK3J6
ØRPK3J7
ØRPK3JZ
ØRPK4J6
ØRPK4J7
ØRPK4JZ
ØRPLØJZ
ØRPL3JZ
ØRPL4JZ
ØRPMØJZ
ØRPM3JZ
ØRPM4JZ
ØRPNØJZ
ØRPN3JZ
ØRPN4JZ
ØRPPØJZ
ØRPP3JZ
ØRPP4JZ
ØRPQØJZ
ØRPQ3JZ
ØRPQ4JZ
ØRPRØJZ
ØRPR3JZ
ØRPR4JZ
ØRPSØJZ
ØRPS3JZ
ØRPS4JZ
ØRPTØJZ
ØRPT3JZ
ØRPT4JZ
ØRPUØJZ
ØRPU3JZ
ØRPU4JZ
ØRPVØJZ
ØRPV3JZ
ØRPV4JZ
ØRPWØJZ
ØRPW3JZ
ØRPW4JZ
ØRPXØJZ
ØRPX3JZ
ØRPX4JZ
ØRQ3ØZZ
ØRQ9ØZZ
ØRQBØZZ
ØRQCØZZ
ØRQC3ZZ
ØRQC4ZZ
ØRQDØZZ
ØRQD3ZZ
ØRQD4ZZ
ØRQEØZZ
ØRQE3ZZ
ØRQE4ZZ
ØRQFØZZ
ØRQF3ZZ
ØRQF4ZZ
ØRQGØZZ
ØRQG3ZZ
ØRQG4ZZ
ØRQHØZZ
ØRQH3ZZ
ØRQH4ZZ
ØRQJØZZ
ØRQJ3ZZ
ØRQJ4ZZ
ØRQKØZZ
ØRQK3ZZ
ØRQK4ZZ
ØRQLØZZ
ØRQL3ZZ
ØRQL4ZZ
ØRQMØZZ
ØRQM3ZZ
ØRQM4ZZ
ØRQNØZZ
ØRQN3ZZ
ØRQN4ZZ
ØRQPØZZ
ØRQP3ZZ
ØRQP4ZZ
ØRQQØZZ
ØRQQ3ZZ
ØRQQ4ZZ
ØRQRØZZ
ØRQR3ZZ
ØRQR4ZZ
ØRQSØZZ
ØRQS3ZZ
ØRQS4ZZ
ØRQTØZZ
ØRQT3ZZ
ØRQT4ZZ
ØRQUØZZ
ØRQU3ZZ
ØRQU4ZZ
ØRQVØZZ
ØRQV3ZZ
ØRQV4ZZ
ØRQWØZZ
ØRQW3ZZ
ØRQW4ZZ
ØRQXØZZ
ØRQX3ZZ
ØRQX4ZZ
ØRR3ØJZ
ØRR5ØJZ
ØRR9ØJZ
ØRRBØJZ
ØRRCØ7Z
ØRRCØJZ
ØRRCØKZ
ØRRDØ7Z
ØRRDØJZ
ØRRDØKZ
ØRREØ7Z
ØRREØJZ
ØRREØKZ
ØRRFØ7Z
ØRRFØJZ
ØRRFØKZ
ØRRGØ7Z
ØRRGØJZ
ØRRGØKZ
ØRRHØ7Z
ØRRHØJZ
ØRRHØKZ
ØRRJØØZ
ØRRJØ7Z
ØRRJØJ6
ØRRJØJ7
ØRRJØJZ
ØRRJØKZ
ØRRKØØZ
ØRRKØ7Z
ØRRKØJ6
ØRRKØJ7
ØRRKØJZ
ØRRKØKZ
ØRRLØ7Z
ØRRLØJZ
ØRRLØKZ
ØRRMØ7Z
ØRRMØJZ
ØRRMØKZ
ØRRNØ7Z
ØRRNØJZ
ØRRNØKZ
ØRRPØ7Z
ØRRPØJZ
ØRRPØKZ
ØRRQØ7Z
ØRRQØJZ
ØRRQØKZ
ØRRRØ7Z
ØRRRØJZ
ØRRRØKZ
ØRRSØ7Z
ØRRSØJZ
ØRRSØKZ
ØRRTØ7Z
ØRRTØJZ
ØRRTØKZ
ØRRUØ7Z
ØRRUØJZ
ØRRUØKZ
ØRRVØ7Z
ØRRVØJZ
ØRRVØKZ
ØRRWØ7Z
ØRRWØJZ
ØRRWØKZ
ØRRXØ7Z
ØRRXØJZ
ØRRXØKZ
ØRSØØ4Z
ØRSØØZZ
ØRS1Ø4Z
ØRS1ØZZ
ØRS4Ø4Z
ØRS4ØZZ
ØRS6Ø4Z
ØRS6ØZZ
ØRSAØ4Z
ØRSAØZZ
ØRSCØ4Z
ØRSCØZZ
ØRSDØ4Z
ØRSDØZZ
ØRSEØ4Z
ØRSEØZZ
ØRSFØ4Z
ØRSFØZZ
ØRSGØ4Z
ØRSGØZZ
ØRSHØ4Z
ØRSHØZZ
ØRSJØ4Z
ØRSJØZZ
ØRSKØ4Z
ØRSKØZZ
ØRSLØ4Z
ØRSLØ5Z
ØRSLØZZ
ØRSMØ4Z
ØRSMØ5Z
ØRSMØZZ
ØRSNØ4Z
ØRSNØ5Z
ØRSNØZZ
ØRSPØ4Z
ØRSPØ5Z
ØRSPØZZ
ØRSQØ4Z
ØRSQØ5Z
ØRSQØZZ
ØRSRØ4Z
ØRSRØ5Z
ØRSRØZZ
ØRSSØ4Z
ØRSSØ5Z
ØRSSØZZ
ØRSTØ4Z
ØRSTØ5Z
ØRSTØZZ
ØRSUØ4Z
ØRSUØ5Z
ØRSUØZZ
ØRSVØ4Z
ØRSVØ5Z
ØRSVØZZ
ØRSWØ4Z
ØRSWØ5Z
ØRSWØZZ
ØRSXØ4Z
ØRSXØ5Z
ØRSXØZZ
ØRT3ØZZ
ØRT4ØZZ
ØRT5ØZZ
ØRT9ØZZ
ØRTBØZZ
ØRTCØZZ
ØRTDØZZ
ØRTEØZZ
ØRTFØZZ
ØRTGØZZ
ØRTHØZZ
ØRTJØZZ
ØRTKØZZ
ØRTLØZZ
ØRTMØZZ
ØRTNØZZ
ØRTPØZZ
ØRTQØZZ
ØRTRØZZ
ØRTSØZZ
ØRTTØZZ
ØRTUØZZ
ØRTVØZZ
ØRTWØZZ
ØRTXØZZ
ØRUØØJZ
ØRUØ3JZ
ØRUØ4JZ
ØRU1ØJZ
ØRU13JZ
ØRU14JZ
ØRU3Ø7Z
ØRU3ØJZ
ØRU3ØKZ
ØRU337Z
ØRU33JZ
ØRU33KZ
ØRU347Z
ØRU34JZ
ØRU34KZ
ØRU4ØJZ
ØRU43JZ
ØRU44JZ
ØRU5ØJZ
ØRU53JZ
ØRU54JZ
ØRU6ØJZ
ØRU63JZ
ØRU64JZ
ØRU9Ø7Z
ØRU9ØJZ
ØRU9ØKZ
ØRU937Z
ØRU93JZ
ØRU93KZ
ØRU947Z
ØRU94JZ
ØRU94KZ
ØRUAØJZ
ØRUA3JZ
ØRUA4JZ
ØRUBØ7Z
ØRUBØJZ
ØRUBØKZ
ØRUB37Z
ØRUB3JZ
ØRUB3KZ
ØRUB47Z
ØRUB4JZ
ØRUB4KZ
ØRUCØ7Z
ØRUCØJZ
ØRUCØKZ
ØRUC37Z
ØRUC3JZ
ØRUC3KZ
ØRUC47Z
ØRUC4JZ
ØRUC4KZ
ØRUDØ7Z
ØRUDØJZ
ØRUDØKZ
ØRUD37Z
ØRUD3JZ
ØRUD3KZ
ØRUD47Z
ØRUD4JZ
ØRUD4KZ
ØRUEØ7Z
ØRUEØJZ
ØRUEØKZ
ØRUE37Z
ØRUE3JZ
ØRUE3KZ
ØRUE47Z
ØRUE4JZ
ØRUE4KZ
ØRUFØ7Z
ØRUFØJZ
ØRUFØKZ
ØRUF37Z
ØRUF3JZ
ØRUF3KZ
ØRUF47Z
ØRUF4JZ
ØRUF4KZ
ØRUGØ7Z
ØRUGØJZ
ØRUGØKZ
ØRUG37Z
ØRUG3JZ
ØRUG3KZ
ØRUG47Z
ØRUG4JZ
ØRUG4KZ
ØRUHØ7Z
ØRUHØJZ
ØRUHØKZ
ØRUH37Z
ØRUH3JZ
ØRUH3KZ
ØRUH47Z
ØRUH4JZ
ØRUH4KZ
ØRUJØ7Z
ØRUJØJZ
ØRUJØKZ
ØRUJ37Z
ØRUJ3JZ
ØRUJ3KZ
ØRUJ47Z
ØRUJ4JZ
ØRUJ4KZ
ØRUKØ7Z
ØRUKØJZ
ØRUKØKZ
ØRUK37Z
ØRUK3JZ
ØRUK3KZ
ØRUK47Z
ØRUK4JZ
ØRUK4KZ
ØRULØ7Z
ØRULØJZ
ØRULØKZ
ØRUL37Z
ØRUL3JZ
ØRUL3KZ
ØRUL47Z
ØRUL4JZ
ØRUL4KZ
ØRUMØ7Z
ØRUMØJZ
ØRUMØKZ
ØRUM37Z
ØRUM3JZ
ØRUM3KZ
ØRUM47Z
ØRUM4JZ
ØRUM4KZ
ØRUNØ7Z
ØRUNØJZ
ØRUNØKZ
ØRUN37Z
ØRUN3JZ
ØRUN3KZ
ØRUN47Z
ØRUN4JZ
ØRUN4KZ
ØRUPØ7Z
ØRUPØJZ
ØRUPØKZ
ØRUP37Z
ØRUP3JZ
ØRUP3KZ
ØRUP47Z
ØRUP4JZ
ØRUP4KZ
ØRUQØ7Z
ØRUQØJZ
ØRUQØKZ
ØRUQ37Z
ØRUQ3JZ
ØRUQ3KZ
ØRUQ47Z
ØRUQ4JZ
ØRUQ4KZ
ØRURØ7Z
ØRURØJZ
ØRURØKZ
ØRUR37Z
ØRUR3JZ
ØRUR3KZ
ØRUR47Z
ØRUR4JZ
ØRUR4KZ
ØRUSØ7Z
ØRUSØJZ
ØRUSØKZ
ØRUS37Z
ØRUS3JZ
ØRUS3KZ
ØRUS47Z
ØRUS4JZ
ØRUS4KZ
ØRUTØ7Z
ØRUTØJZ
ØRUTØKZ
ØRUT37Z
ØRUT3JZ
ØRUT3KZ
ØRUT47Z
ØRUT4JZ
ØRUT4KZ
ØRUUØ7Z
ØRUUØJZ
ØRUUØKZ
ØRUU37Z
ØRUU3JZ
ØRUU3KZ
ØRUU47Z
ØRUU4JZ
ØRUU4KZ
ØRUVØ7Z
ØRUVØJZ
ØRUVØKZ
ØRUV37Z
ØRUV3JZ
ØRUV3KZ
ØRUV47Z
ØRUV4JZ
ØRUV4KZ
ØRUWØ7Z
ØRUWØJZ
ØRUWØKZ
ØRUW37Z
ØRUW3JZ
ØRUW3KZ
ØRUW47Z
ØRUW4JZ
ØRUW4KZ
ØRUXØ7Z

0RUX0JZ
0RUX0KZ
0RUX37Z
0RUX3JZ
0RUX3KZ
0RUX47Z
0RUX4JZ
0RUX4KZ
0RW004Z
0RW00JZ
0RW034Z
0RW03JZ
0RW044Z
0RW04JZ
0RW104Z
0RW10JZ
0RW134Z
0RW13JZ
0RW144Z
0RW14JZ
0RW30JZ
0RW33JZ
0RW34JZ
0RW404Z
0RW40JZ
0RW434Z
0RW43JZ
0RW444Z
0RW44JZ
0RW50JZ
0RW53JZ
0RW54JZ
0RW604Z
0RW60JZ
0RW634Z
0RW63JZ
0RW644Z
0RW64JZ
0RW90JZ
0RW93JZ
0RW94JZ
0RWA04Z
0RWA0JZ
0RWA34Z
0RWA3JZ
0RWA44Z
0RWA4JZ
0RWB0JZ
0RWB3JZ
0RWB4JZ
0RWG0JZ
0RWG3JZ
0RWG4JZ
0RWH0JZ
0RWH3JZ
0RWH4JZ
0RWJ0J6
0RWJ0J7
0RWJ0JZ
0RWJ3J6
0RWJ3J7
0RWJ3JZ
0RWJ4J6
0RWJ4J7
0RWJ4JZ
0RWK0J6
0RWK0J7
0RWK0JZ
0RWK3J6
0RWK3J7
0RWK3JZ
0RWK4J6
0RWK4J7
0RWK4JZ
0RWL0JZ
0RWL3JZ
0RWL4JZ
0RWM0JZ
0RWM3JZ
0RWM4JZ
0RWN0JZ
0RWN3JZ
0RWN4JZ
0RWP0JZ
0RWP3JZ
0RWP4JZ
0RWQ0JZ
0RWQ3JZ
0RWQ4JZ
0RWR0JZ
0RWR3JZ
0RWR4JZ
0RWS0JZ
0RWS3JZ
0RWS4JZ
0RWT0JZ
0RWT3JZ
0RWT4JZ
0RWU0JZ
0RWU3JZ
0RWU4JZ
0RWV0JZ
0RWV3JZ
0RWV4JZ
0RWW0JZ
0RWW3JZ
0RWW4JZ
0RWX0JZ
0RWX3JZ
0RWX4JZ
0S500ZZ
0S503ZZ
0S504ZZ
0S520ZZ
0S523ZZ
0S524ZZ
0S530ZZ
0S533ZZ
0S534ZZ
0S540ZZ
0S543ZZ
0S544ZZ
0S550ZZ
0S553ZZ
0S554ZZ
0S560ZZ
0S563ZZ
0S564ZZ
0S570ZZ
0S573ZZ
0S574ZZ
0S580ZZ
0S583ZZ
0S584ZZ
0S590ZZ
0S593ZZ
0S594ZZ
0S5B0ZZ
0S5B3ZZ
0S5B4ZZ
0S5C0ZZ
0S5C3ZZ
0S5C4ZZ
0S5D0ZZ
0S5D3ZZ
0S5D4ZZ
0S5F0ZZ
0S5F3ZZ
0S5F4ZZ
0S5G0ZZ
0S5G3ZZ
0S5G4ZZ
0S5H0ZZ
0S5H3ZZ
0S5H4ZZ
0S5J0ZZ
0S5J3ZZ
0S5J4ZZ
0S5K0ZZ
0S5K3ZZ
0S5K4ZZ
0S5L0ZZ
0S5L3ZZ
0S5L4ZZ
0S5M0ZZ
0S5M3ZZ
0S5M4ZZ
0S5N0ZZ
0S5N3ZZ
0S5N4ZZ
0S5P0ZZ
0S5P3ZZ
0S5P4ZZ
0S5Q0ZZ
0S5Q3ZZ
0S5Q4ZZ
0SB00ZZ
0SB03ZZ
0SB04ZZ
0SB20ZZ
0SB23ZZ
0SB24ZZ
0SB30ZZ
0SB33ZZ
0SB34ZZ
0SB40ZZ
0SB43ZZ
0SB44ZZ
0SB50ZZ
0SB53ZZ
0SB54ZZ
0SB60ZZ
0SB63ZZ
0SB64ZZ
0SB70ZZ
0SB73ZZ
0SB74ZZ
0SB80ZZ
0SB83ZZ
0SB84ZZ
0SBC0ZZ
0SBC3ZZ
0SBC4ZZ
0SBD0ZZ
0SBD3ZZ
0SBD4ZZ
0SBF0ZZ
0SBF3ZZ
0SBF4ZZ
0SBG0ZZ
0SBG3ZZ
0SBG4ZZ
0SBH0ZZ
0SBH3ZZ
0SBH4ZZ
0SBJ0ZZ
0SBJ3ZZ
0SBJ4ZZ
0SBK0ZZ
0SBK3ZZ
0SBK4ZZ
0SBL0ZZ
0SBL3ZZ
0SBL4ZZ
0SBM0ZZ
0SBM3ZZ
0SBM4ZZ
0SBN0ZZ
0SBN3ZZ
0SBN4ZZ
0SBP0ZZ
0SBP3ZZ
0SBP4ZZ
0SBQ0ZZ
0SBQ3ZZ
0SBQ4ZZ
0SG0070
0SG0071
0SG007J
0SG00A0
0SG00AJ
0SG00J0
0SG00J1
0SG00JJ
0SG00K0
0SG00K1
0SG00KJ
0SG0370
0SG0371
0SG037J
0SG03A0
0SG03AJ
0SG03J0
0SG03J1
0SG03JJ
0SG03K0
0SG03K1
0SG03KJ
0SG0470
0SG0471
0SG047J
0SG04A0
0SG04AJ
0SG04J0
0SG04J1
0SG04JJ
0SG04K0
0SG04K1
0SG04KJ
0SG1070
0SG1071
0SG107J
0SG10A0
0SG10AJ
0SG10J0
0SG10J1
0SG10JJ
0SG10K0
0SG10K1
0SG10KJ
0SG1370
0SG1371
0SG137J
0SG13A0
0SG13AJ
0SG13J0
0SG13J1
0SG13JJ
0SG13K0
0SG13K1
0SG13KJ
0SG1470
0SG1471
0SG147J
0SG14A0
0SG14AJ
0SG14J0
0SG14J1
0SG14JJ
0SG14K0
0SG14K1
0SG14KJ
0SG3070
0SG3071
0SG307J
0SG30A0
0SG30AJ
0SG30J0
0SG30J1
0SG30JJ
0SG30K0
0SG30K1
0SG30KJ
0SG3370
0SG3371
0SG337J
0SG33A0
0SG33AJ
0SG33J0
0SG33J1
0SG33JJ
0SG33K0
0SG33K1
0SG33KJ
0SG3470
0SG3471
0SG347J
0SG34A0
0SG34AJ
0SG34J0
0SG34J1
0SG34JJ
0SG34K0
0SG34K1
0SG34KJ
0SG504Z
0SG507Z
0SG50JZ
0SG50KZ
0SG534Z
0SG537Z
0SG53JZ
0SG53KZ
0SG544Z
0SG547Z
0SG54JZ
0SG54KZ
0SG604Z
0SG607Z
0SG60JZ
0SG60KZ
0SG634Z
0SG637Z
0SG63JZ
0SG63KZ
0SG644Z
0SG647Z
0SG64JZ
0SG64KZ
0SG704Z
0SG707Z
0SG70JZ
0SG70KZ
0SG734Z
0SG737Z
0SG73JZ
0SG73KZ
0SG744Z
0SG747Z
0SG74JZ
0SG74KZ
0SG804Z
0SG807Z
0SG80JZ
0SG80KZ
0SG834Z
0SG837Z
0SG83JZ
0SG83KZ
0SG844Z
0SG847Z
0SG84JZ
0SG84KZ
0SGC03Z
0SGC04Z
0SGC05Z
0SGC07Z
0SGC0JZ
0SGC0KZ
0SGC33Z
0SGC34Z
0SGC35Z
0SGC37Z
0SGC3JZ
0SGC3KZ
0SGC43Z
0SGC44Z
0SGC45Z
0SGC47Z
0SGC4JZ
0SGC4KZ
0SGD03Z
0SGD04Z
0SGD05Z
0SGD07Z
0SGD0JZ
0SGD0KZ
0SGD33Z
0SGD34Z
0SGD35Z
0SGD37Z
0SGD3JZ
0SGD3KZ
0SGD43Z
0SGD44Z
0SGD45Z
0SGD47Z
0SGD4JZ
0SGD4KZ
0SGF03Z
0SGF04Z
0SGF05Z
0SGF07Z
0SGF0JZ
0SGF0KZ
0SGF33Z
0SGF34Z
0SGF35Z
0SGF37Z
0SGF3JZ
0SGF3KZ
0SGF43Z
0SGF44Z
0SGF45Z
0SGF47Z
0SGF4JZ
0SGF4KZ
0SGG03Z
0SGG04Z
0SGG05Z
0SGG07Z
0SGG0JZ
0SGG0KZ
0SGG33Z
0SGG34Z
0SGG35Z
0SGG37Z
0SGG3JZ
0SGG3KZ
0SGG43Z
0SGG44Z
0SGG45Z
0SGG47Z
0SGG4JZ
0SGG4KZ
0SGH03Z
0SGH04Z
0SGH05Z
0SGH07Z
0SGH0JZ
0SGH0KZ
0SGH33Z
0SGH34Z
0SGH35Z
0SGH37Z
0SGH3JZ
0SGH3KZ
0SGH43Z
0SGH44Z
0SGH45Z
0SGH47Z
0SGH4JZ
0SGH4KZ
0SGJ03Z
0SGJ04Z
0SGJ05Z
0SGJ07Z
0SGJ0JZ
0SGJ0KZ
0SGJ33Z
0SGJ34Z
0SGJ35Z
0SGJ37Z
0SGJ3JZ
0SGJ3KZ
0SGJ43Z
0SGJ44Z
0SGJ45Z
0SGJ47Z
0SGJ4JZ
0SGJ4KZ
0SGK03Z
0SGK04Z
0SGK05Z
0SGK07Z
0SGK0JZ
0SGK0KZ
0SGK33Z
0SGK34Z
0SGK35Z
0SGK37Z
0SGK3JZ
0SGK3KZ
0SGK43Z
0SGK44Z
0SGK45Z
0SGK47Z
0SGK4JZ
0SGK4KZ
0SGL03Z
0SGL04Z
0SGL05Z
0SGL07Z
0SGL0JZ
0SGL0KZ
0SGL33Z
0SGL34Z
0SGL35Z
0SGL37Z
0SGL3JZ
0SGL3KZ
0SGL43Z
0SGL44Z
0SGL45Z
0SGL47Z
0SGL4JZ
0SGL4KZ
0SGM03Z
0SGM04Z
0SGM05Z
0SGM07Z
0SGM0JZ
0SGM0KZ
0SGM33Z
0SGM34Z
0SGM35Z
0SGM37Z
0SGM3JZ
0SGM3KZ
0SGM43Z
0SGM44Z
0SGM45Z
0SGM47Z
0SGM4JZ
0SGM4KZ
0SGN03Z
0SGN04Z
0SGN05Z
0SGN07Z
0SGN0JZ
0SGN0KZ
0SGN33Z
0SGN34Z
0SGN35Z
0SGN37Z
0SGN3JZ
0SGN3KZ
0SGN43Z
0SGN44Z
0SGN45Z
0SGN47Z
0SGN4JZ
0SGN4KZ
0SH004Z
0SH00BZ
0SH00CZ
0SH00DZ
0SH034Z
0SH03BZ
0SH03CZ
0SH03DZ
0SH044Z
0SH04BZ
0SH04CZ
0SH04DZ
0SH304Z
0SH30BZ
0SH30CZ
0SH30DZ
0SH334Z
0SH33BZ
0SH33CZ
0SH33DZ
0SH344Z
0SH34BZ
0SH34CZ
0SH34DZ
0SH504Z
0SH534Z
0SH544Z
0SH604Z
0SH634Z
0SH644Z
0SH704Z
0SH734Z
0SH744Z
0SH804Z
0SH834Z
0SH844Z
0SHC04Z
0SHC05Z
0SHC34Z
0SHC35Z
0SHC44Z
0SHC45Z
0SHD04Z
0SHD05Z
0SHD34Z
0SHD35Z
0SHD44Z
0SHD45Z
0SHF04Z
0SHF05Z
0SHF34Z
0SHF35Z
0SHF44Z
0SHF45Z
0SHG04Z
0SHG05Z
0SHG34Z
0SHG35Z
0SHG44Z
0SHG45Z
0SJ04ZZ
0SJ34ZZ
0SJ54ZZ
0SJ64ZZ
0SJ74ZZ
0SJ84ZZ
0SJ94ZZ
0SJB4ZZ
0SJC4ZZ
0SJD4ZZ
0SJF4ZZ
0SJG4ZZ
0SJH4ZZ
0SJJ4ZZ
0SJK4ZZ
0SJL4ZZ
0SJM4ZZ
0SJN4ZZ
0SJP4ZZ
0SJQ4ZZ
0SN00ZZ
0SN03ZZ
0SN04ZZ
0SN20ZZ
0SN23ZZ
0SN24ZZ
0SN30ZZ
0SN33ZZ
0SN34ZZ
0SN40ZZ
0SN43ZZ
0SN44ZZ
0SN50ZZ
0SN53ZZ
0SN54ZZ
0SN60ZZ
0SN63ZZ
0SN64ZZ
0SN70ZZ
0SN73ZZ
0SN74ZZ
0SN80ZZ
0SN83ZZ
0SN84ZZ
0SNC0ZZ
0SNC3ZZ
0SNC4ZZ
0SND0ZZ
0SND3ZZ
0SND4ZZ
0SNF0ZZ
0SNF3ZZ
0SNF4ZZ
0SNG0ZZ
0SNG3ZZ
0SNG4ZZ
0SNH0ZZ
0SNH3ZZ
0SNH4ZZ
0SNJ0ZZ
0SNJ3ZZ
0SNJ4ZZ
0SNK0ZZ
0SNK3ZZ
0SNK4ZZ
0SNL0ZZ
0SNL3ZZ
0SNL4ZZ
0SNM0ZZ
0SNM3ZZ
0SNM4ZZ
0SNN0ZZ
0SNN3ZZ
0SNN4ZZ
0SNP0ZZ
0SNP3ZZ
0SNP4ZZ
0SNQ0ZZ
0SNQ3ZZ
0SNQ4ZZ
0SP00JZ
0SP03JZ
0SP04JZ
0SP20JZ
0SP23JZ
0SP24JZ
0SP30JZ
0SP33JZ
0SP34JZ
0SP40JZ
0SP43JZ
0SP44JZ
0SP50JZ
0SP53JZ
0SP54JZ
0SP60JZ
0SP63JZ
0SP64JZ
0SP70JZ
0SP73JZ
0SP74JZ
0SP80JZ
0SP83JZ
0SP84JZ
0SPC09Z
0SPC0JC
0SPC0JZ
0SPC0LZ
0SPC0MZ
0SPC0NZ
0SPC3JC
0SPC3JZ
0SPC3LZ
0SPC3MZ
0SPC3NZ
0SPC4JC
0SPC4JZ
0SPC4LZ
0SPC4MZ
0SPC4NZ
0SPD09Z
0SPD0JC
0SPD0JZ
0SPD0LZ
0SPD0MZ
0SPD0NZ
0SPD3JC
0SPD3JZ
0SPD3LZ
0SPD3MZ
0SPD3NZ
0SPD4JC
0SPD4JZ
0SPD4LZ
0SPD4MZ
0SPD4NZ
0SPF0JZ
0SPF3JZ
0SPF4JZ
0SPG0JZ
0SPG3JZ
0SPG4JZ
0SPH0JZ
0SPH3JZ
0SPH4JZ
0SPJ0JZ
0SPJ3JZ
0SPJ4JZ
0SPK0JZ
0SPK3JZ
0SPK4JZ
0SPL0JZ
0SPL3JZ
0SPL4JZ
0SPM0JZ
0SPM3JZ
0SPM4JZ
0SPN0JZ
0SPN3JZ
0SPN4JZ
0SPP0JZ
0SPP3JZ
0SPP4JZ
0SPQ0JZ
0SPQ3JZ
0SPQ4JZ
0SPT0JZ
0SPT3JZ
0SPT4JZ
0SPU0JZ
0SPU3JZ
0SPU4JZ
0SPV0JZ
0SPV3JZ
0SPV4JZ
0SPW0JZ
0SPW3JZ
0SPW4JZ
0SQ20ZZ
0SQ40ZZ
0SQC0ZZ
0SQC3ZZ
0SQC4ZZ
0SQD0ZZ
0SQD3ZZ
0SQD4ZZ
0SQF0ZZ
0SQF3ZZ
0SQF4ZZ
0SQG0ZZ
0SQG3ZZ
0SQG4ZZ
0SR20JZ
0SR40JZ
0SRC069
0SRC06A
0SRC06Z
0SRC07Z
0SRC0EZ
0SRC0J9
0SRC0JA
0SRC0JZ
0SRC0KZ
0SRC0L9
0SRC0LA
0SRC0LZ
0SRC0M9
0SRC0MA
0SRC0MZ
0SRC0N9
0SRC0NA
0SRC0NZ
0SRD069
0SRD06A
0SRD06Z
0SRD07Z
0SRD0EZ
0SRD0J9
0SRD0JA
0SRD0JZ
0SRD0KZ
0SRD0L9
0SRD0LA
0SRD0LZ
0SRD0M9
0SRD0MA
0SRD0MZ
0SRD0N9
0SRD0NA
0SRD0NZ
0SRF07Z
0SRF0J9

ØSRFØJA
ØSRFØJZ
ØSRFØKZ
ØSRGØ7Z
ØSRGØJ9
ØSRGØJA
ØSRGØJZ
ØSRGØKZ
ØSRHØ7Z
ØSRHØJZ
ØSRHØKZ
ØSRJØ7Z
ØSRJØJZ
ØSRJØKZ
ØSRKØ7Z
ØSRKØJZ
ØSRKØKZ
ØSRLØ7Z
ØSRLØJZ
ØSRLØKZ
ØSRMØ7Z
ØSRMØJZ
ØSRMØKZ
ØSRNØ7Z
ØSRNØJZ
ØSRNØKZ
ØSRPØ7Z
ØSRPØJZ
ØSRPØKZ
ØSRQØ7Z
ØSRQØJZ
ØSRQØKZ
ØSRTØ7Z
ØSRTØJ9
ØSRTØJA
ØSRTØJZ
ØSRTØKZ
ØSRUØ7Z
ØSRUØJ9
ØSRUØJA
ØSRUØJZ
ØSRUØKZ
ØSRVØ7Z
ØSRVØJ9
ØSRVØJA
ØSRVØJZ
ØSRVØKZ
ØSRWØ7Z
ØSRWØJ9
ØSRWØJA
ØSRWØJZ
ØSRWØKZ
ØSSØØ4Z
ØSSØØZZ
ØSS3Ø4Z
ØSS3ØZZ
ØSS5Ø4Z
ØSS5ØZZ
ØSS6Ø4Z
ØSS6ØZZ
ØSS7Ø4Z
ØSS7ØZZ
ØSS8Ø4Z
ØSS8ØZZ
ØSSCØ4Z
ØSSCØ5Z
ØSSCØZZ
ØSSDØ4Z
ØSSDØ5Z
ØSSDØZZ
ØSSFØ4Z
ØSSFØ5Z
ØSSFØZZ
ØSSGØ4Z
ØSSGØ5Z
ØSSGØZZ
ØSSHØ4Z
ØSSHØ5Z
ØSSHØZZ
ØSSJØ4Z
ØSSJØ5Z
ØSSJØZZ
ØSSKØ4Z
ØSSKØ5Z
ØSSKØZZ
ØSSLØ4Z
ØSSLØ5Z
ØSSLØZZ
ØSSMØ4Z
ØSSMØ5Z
ØSSMØZZ
ØSSNØ4Z
ØSSNØ5Z
ØSSNØZZ
ØSSPØ4Z
ØSSPØ5Z
ØSSPØZZ
ØSSQØ4Z
ØSSQØ5Z
ØSSQØZZ
ØST2ØZZ
ØST4ØZZ
ØST5ØZZ
ØST6ØZZ
ØST7ØZZ
ØST8ØZZ
ØSTCØZZ
ØSTDØZZ
ØSTFØZZ
ØSTGØZZ
ØSTHØZZ
ØSTJØZZ
ØSTKØZZ
ØSTLØZZ
ØSTMØZZ
ØSTNØZZ
ØSTPØZZ
ØSTQØZZ
ØSUØØJZ
ØSUØ3JZ
ØSUØ4JZ
ØSU2Ø7Z
ØSU2ØJZ
ØSU2ØKZ
ØSU237Z
ØSU23JZ
ØSU23KZ
ØSU247Z
ØSU24JZ
ØSU24KZ
ØSU3ØJZ
ØSU33JZ
ØSU34JZ
ØSU4Ø7Z
ØSU4ØJZ
ØSU4ØKZ
ØSU437Z
ØSU43JZ
ØSU43KZ
ØSU447Z
ØSU44JZ
ØSU44KZ
ØSU5ØJZ
ØSU53JZ
ØSU54JZ
ØSU6ØJZ
ØSU63JZ
ØSU64JZ
ØSUHØJZ
ØSUH3JZ
ØSUH4JZ
ØSUJØJZ
ØSUJ3JZ
ØSUJ4JZ
ØSURØ9Z
ØSUSØ9Z
ØSUVØ9Z
ØSUWØ9Z
ØSWØØ4Z
ØSWØØJZ
ØSWØ34Z
ØSWØ3JZ
ØSWØ44Z
ØSWØ4JZ
ØSW2ØJZ
ØSW23JZ
ØSW24JZ
ØSW3Ø4Z
ØSW3ØJZ
ØSW334Z
ØSW33JZ
ØSW344Z
ØSW34JZ
ØSW4ØJZ
ØSW43JZ
ØSW44JZ
ØSWCØJC
ØSWCØJZ
ØSWC3JC
ØSWC3JZ
ØSWC4JC
ØSWC4JZ
ØSWDØJC
ØSWDØJZ
ØSWD3JC
ØSWD3JZ
ØSWD4JC
ØSWD4JZ
ØSWFØJZ
ØSWF3JZ
ØSWF4JZ
ØSWGØJZ
ØSWG3JZ
ØSWG4JZ
ØSWHØJZ
ØSWH3JZ
ØSWH4JZ
ØSWJØJZ
ØSWJ3JZ
ØSWJ4JZ
ØSWKØJZ
ØSWK3JZ
ØSWK4JZ
ØSWLØJZ
ØSWL3JZ
ØSWL4JZ
ØSWMØJZ
ØSWM3JZ
ØSWM4JZ
ØSWNØJZ
ØSWN3JZ
ØSWN4JZ
ØSWPØJZ
ØSWP3JZ
ØSWP4JZ
ØSWQØJZ
ØSWQ3JZ
ØSWQ4JZ
ØSWTØJZ
ØSWT3JZ
ØSWT4JZ
ØSWUØJZ
ØSWU3JZ
ØSWU4JZ
ØSWVØJZ
ØSWV3JZ
ØSWV4JZ
ØSWWØJZ
ØSWW3JZ
ØSWW4JZ
ØT13Ø7B
ØT13ØJB
ØT13ØKB
ØT13ØZB
ØT1347B
ØT134JB
ØT134KB
ØT134ZB
ØT14Ø7B
ØT14ØJB
ØT14ØKB
ØT14ØZB
ØT1447B
ØT144JB
ØT144KB
ØT144ZB
ØT16Ø76
ØT16Ø77
ØT16Ø78
ØT16Ø79
ØT16Ø7A
ØT16Ø7B
ØT16Ø7C
ØT16Ø7D
ØT16ØJ6
ØT16ØJ7
ØT16ØJ8
ØT16ØJ9
ØT16ØJA
ØT16ØJB
ØT16ØJC
ØT16ØJD
ØT16ØK6
ØT16ØK7
ØT16ØK8
ØT16ØK9
ØT16ØKA
ØT16ØKB
ØT16ØKC
ØT16ØKD
ØT16ØZ6
ØT16ØZ7
ØT16ØZ8
ØT16ØZ9
ØT16ØZA
ØT16ØZB
ØT16ØZC
ØT16ØZD
ØT163JD
ØT16476
ØT16477
ØT16478
ØT16479
ØT1647A
ØT1647B
ØT1647C
ØT1647D
ØT164J6
ØT164J7
ØT164J8
ØT164J9
ØT164JA
ØT164JB
ØT164JC
ØT164JD
ØT164K6
ØT164K7
ØT164K8
ØT164K9
ØT164KA
ØT164KB
ØT164KC
ØT164KD
ØT164Z6
ØT164Z7
ØT164Z8
ØT164Z9
ØT164ZA
ØT164ZB
ØT164ZC
ØT164ZD
ØT17Ø76
ØT17Ø77
ØT17Ø78
ØT17Ø79
ØT17Ø7A
ØT17Ø7B
ØT17Ø7C
ØT17Ø7D
ØT17ØJ6
ØT17ØJ7
ØT17ØJ8
ØT17ØJ9
ØT17ØJA
ØT17ØJB
ØT17ØJC
ØT17ØJD
ØT17ØK6
ØT17ØK7
ØT17ØK8
ØT17ØK9
ØT17ØKA
ØT17ØKB
ØT17ØKC
ØT17ØKD
ØT17ØZ6
ØT17ØZ7
ØT17ØZ8
ØT17ØZ9
ØT17ØZA
ØT17ØZB
ØT17ØZC
ØT17ØZD
ØT173JD
ØT17476
ØT17477
ØT17478
ØT17479
ØT1747A
ØT1747B
ØT1747C
ØT1747D
ØT174J6
ØT174J7
ØT174J8
ØT174J9
ØT174JA
ØT174JB
ØT174JC
ØT174JD
ØT174K6
ØT174K7
ØT174K8
ØT174K9
ØT174KA
ØT174KB
ØT174KC
ØT174KD
ØT174Z6
ØT174Z7
ØT174Z8
ØT174Z9
ØT174ZA
ØT174ZB
ØT174ZC
ØT174ZD
ØT18Ø76
ØT18Ø77
ØT18Ø78
ØT18Ø79
ØT18Ø7A
ØT18Ø7B
ØT18Ø7C
ØT18Ø7D
ØT18ØJ6
ØT18ØJ7
ØT18ØJ8
ØT18ØJ9
ØT18ØJA
ØT18ØJB
ØT18ØJC
ØT18ØJD
ØT18ØK6
ØT18ØK7
ØT18ØK8
ØT18ØK9
ØT18ØKA
ØT18ØKB
ØT18ØKC
ØT18ØKD
ØT18ØZ6
ØT18ØZ7
ØT18ØZ8
ØT18ØZ9
ØT18ØZA
ØT18ØZB
ØT18ØZC
ØT18ØZD
ØT183JD
ØT18476
ØT18477
ØT18478
ØT18479
ØT1847A
ØT1847B
ØT1847C
ØT1847D
ØT184J6
ØT184J7
ØT184J8
ØT184J9
ØT184JA
ØT184JB
ØT184JC
ØT184JD
ØT184K6
ØT184K7
ØT184K8
ØT184K9
ØT184KA
ØT184KB
ØT184KC
ØT184KD
ØT184Z6
ØT184Z7
ØT184Z8
ØT184Z9
ØT184ZA
ØT184ZB
ØT184ZC
ØT184ZD
ØT1BØZD
ØT1B4ZD
ØT56ØZZ
ØT563ZZ
ØT564ZZ
ØT567ZZ
ØT568ZZ
ØT57ØZZ
ØT573ZZ
ØT574ZZ
ØT577ZZ
ØT578ZZ
ØT76ØZZ
ØT763ZZ
ØT764ZZ
ØT768DZ
ØT768ZZ
ØT77ØZZ
ØT773ZZ
ØT774ZZ
ØT778DZ
ØT778ZZ
ØT78ØZZ
ØT783ZZ
ØT784ZZ
ØT788DZ
ØT7BØDZ
ØT7BØZZ
ØT7B3DZ
ØT7B3ZZ
ØT7B4DZ
ØT7B4ZZ
ØT7B8DZ
ØT7B8ZZ
ØT7DØZZ
ØT7D3ZZ
ØT7D4ZZ
ØT9ØØØZ
ØT9ØØZX
ØT9Ø4ØZ
ØT9Ø7ØZ
ØT9Ø8ØZ
ØT91ØØZ
ØT91ØZX
ØT914ØZ
ØT917ØZ
ØT918ØZ
ØT93ØØZ
ØT93ØZX
ØT93ØZZ
ØT934ØZ
ØT937ØZ
ØT937ZZ
ØT938ØZ
ØT938ZZ
ØT94ØØZ
ØT94ØZX
ØT94ØZZ
ØT944ØZ
ØT947ØZ
ØT947ZZ
ØT948ØZ
ØT948ZZ
ØT9BØØZ
ØTBØØZX
ØTBØØZZ
ØTBØ3ZZ
ØTBØ4ZZ
ØTBØ7ZZ
ØTBØ8ZZ
ØTB1ØZX
ØTB1ØZZ
ØTB13ZZ
ØTB14ZZ
ØTB17ZZ
ØTB18ZZ
ØTB3ØZX
ØTB3ØZZ
ØTB33ZZ
ØTB34ZZ
ØTB37ZZ
ØTB38ZZ
ØTB4ØZX
ØTB4ØZZ
ØTB43ZZ
ØTB44ZZ
ØTB47ZZ
ØTB48ZZ
ØTB6ØZZ
ØTB63ZZ
ØTB64ZZ
ØTB67ZZ
ØTB68ZZ
ØTB7ØZZ
ØTB73ZZ
ØTB74ZZ
ØTB77ZZ
ØTB78ZZ
ØTBBØZZ
ØTBB3ZZ
ØTBB4ZZ
ØTBCØZZ
ØTBC3ZZ
ØTBC4ZZ
ØTCØ3ZZ
ØTCØ4ZZ
ØTC13ZZ
ØTC14ZZ
ØTC3ØZZ
ØTC33ZZ
ØTC34ZZ
ØTC37ZZ
ØTC4ØZZ
ØTC43ZZ
ØTC44ZZ
ØTC47ZZ
ØTC67ZZ
ØTC77ZZ
ØTF33ZZ
ØTF34ZZ
ØTF43ZZ
ØTF44ZZ
ØTHBØLZ
ØTHB3LZ
ØTHB4LZ
ØTHB7LZ
ØTHB8LZ
ØTHCØLZ
ØTHC3LZ
ØTHC4LZ
ØTHC7LZ
ØTHC8LZ
ØTHDØLZ
ØTHD3LZ
ØTHD4LZ
ØTHD7LZ
ØTHD8LZ
ØTHDXLZ
ØTJBØZZ
ØTJB4ZZ
ØTJDØZZ
ØTL3ØCZ
ØTL3ØDZ
ØTL3ØZZ
ØTL33CZ
ØTL33DZ
ØTL33ZZ
ØTL34CZ
ØTL34DZ
ØTL34ZZ
ØTL37DZ
ØTL37ZZ
ØTL38DZ
ØTL38ZZ
ØTL4ØCZ
ØTL4ØDZ
ØTL4ØZZ
ØTL43CZ
ØTL43DZ
ØTL43ZZ
ØTL44CZ
ØTL44DZ
ØTL44ZZ
ØTL47DZ
ØTL47ZZ
ØTL48DZ
ØTL48ZZ
ØTL6ØCZ
ØTL6ØDZ
ØTL6ØZZ
ØTL63CZ
ØTL63DZ
ØTL63ZZ
ØTL64CZ
ØTL64DZ
ØTL64ZZ
ØTL67DZ
ØTL67ZZ
ØTL68DZ
ØTL68ZZ
ØTL7ØCZ
ØTL7ØDZ
ØTL7ØZZ
ØTL73CZ
ØTL73DZ
ØTL73ZZ
ØTL74CZ
ØTL74DZ
ØTL74ZZ
ØTL77DZ
ØTL77ZZ
ØTL78DZ
ØTL78ZZ
ØTLBØCZ
ØTLBØDZ
ØTLBØZZ
ØTLB3CZ
ØTLB3DZ
ØTLB3ZZ
ØTLB4CZ
ØTLB4DZ
ØTLB4ZZ
ØTLB7DZ
ØTLB7ZZ
ØTLB8DZ
ØTLB8ZZ
ØTLCØCZ
ØTLCØDZ
ØTLCØZZ
ØTLC3CZ
ØTLC3DZ
ØTLC3ZZ
ØTLC4CZ
ØTLC4DZ
ØTLC4ZZ
ØTLC7DZ
ØTLC7ZZ
ØTLC8DZ
ØTLC8ZZ
ØTM6ØZZ
ØTM64ZZ
ØTM7ØZZ
ØTM74ZZ
ØTM8ØZZ
ØTM84ZZ
ØTMBØZZ
ØTMB4ZZ
ØTMCØZZ
ØTMC4ZZ
ØTMDØZZ
ØTMD4ZZ
ØTNØØZZ
ØTNØ3ZZ
ØTNØ4ZZ
ØTNØ7ZZ
ØTNØ8ZZ
ØTN1ØZZ
ØTN13ZZ
ØTN14ZZ
ØTN17ZZ
ØTN18ZZ
ØTN3ØZZ
ØTN33ZZ
ØTN34ZZ
ØTN37ZZ
ØTN38ZZ
ØTN4ØZZ
ØTN43ZZ
ØTN44ZZ
ØTN47ZZ
ØTN48ZZ
ØTN6ØZZ
ØTN63ZZ
ØTN64ZZ
ØTN67ZZ
ØTN68ZZ
ØTN7ØZZ
ØTN73ZZ
ØTN74ZZ
ØTN77ZZ
ØTN78ZZ
ØTNBØZZ
ØTNB3ZZ
ØTNB4ZZ
ØTNCØZZ
ØTNC3ZZ
ØTNC4ZZ
ØTNDØZZ
ØTND3ZZ
ØTND4ZZ
ØTND7ZZ
ØTND8ZZ
ØTNDXZZ
ØTQ3ØZZ
ØTQ33ZZ
ØTQ34ZZ
ØTQ37ZZ
ØTQ38ZZ
ØTQ4ØZZ
ØTQ43ZZ
ØTQ44ZZ
ØTQ47ZZ
ØTQ48ZZ
ØTQ6ØZZ
ØTQ63ZZ
ØTQ64ZZ
ØTQ67ZZ
ØTQ68ZZ
ØTQ7ØZZ
ØTQ73ZZ
ØTQ74ZZ
ØTQ77ZZ
ØTQ78ZZ
ØTQBØZZ
ØTQB3ZZ
ØTQB4ZZ
ØTQB7ZZ
ØTQB8ZZ
ØTQDØZZ
ØTQD3ZZ
ØTQD4ZZ
ØTQD7ZZ
ØTQD8ZZ
ØTQDXZZ
ØTR6Ø7Z
ØTR6ØJZ
ØTR6ØKZ
ØTR647Z
ØTR64JZ
ØTR64KZ
ØTR677Z
ØTR67JZ
ØTR67KZ
ØTR687Z
ØTR68JZ
ØTR68KZ
ØTR7Ø7Z
ØTR7ØJZ
ØTR7ØKZ
ØTR747Z
ØTR74JZ
ØTR74KZ
ØTR777Z
ØTR77JZ
ØTR77KZ
ØTR787Z
ØTR78JZ
ØTR78KZ
ØTRBØ7Z
ØTRBØJZ
ØTRBØKZ
ØTRB47Z
ØTRB4JZ
ØTRB4KZ
ØTRB77Z
ØTRB7JZ
ØTRB7KZ
ØTRB87Z
ØTRB8JZ
ØTRB8KZ
ØTRCØ7Z
ØTRCØJZ
ØTRCØKZ
ØTRC47Z
ØTRC4JZ
ØTRC4KZ
ØTRC77Z
ØTRC7JZ
ØTRC7KZ
ØTRC87Z
ØTRC8JZ
ØTRC8KZ
ØTRDØ7Z
ØTRDØJZ
ØTRDØKZ
ØTRD47Z
ØTRD4JZ
ØTRD4KZ
ØTRD77Z
ØTRD7JZ
ØTRD7KZ
ØTRD87Z
ØTRD8JZ
ØTRD8KZ
ØTRDX7Z
ØTRDXJZ
ØTRDXKZ
ØTSØØZZ
ØTSØ4ZZ
ØTS1ØZZ
ØTS14ZZ
ØTS2ØZZ
ØTS24ZZ
ØTTØØZZ
ØTTØ4ZZ
ØTT1ØZZ
ØTT14ZZ
ØTT2ØZZ
ØTT24ZZ
ØTT3ØZZ
ØTT34ZZ
ØTT37ZZ
ØTT38ZZ
ØTT4ØZZ
ØTT44ZZ
ØTT47ZZ
ØTT48ZZ
ØTT6ØZZ
ØTT64ZZ
ØTT67ZZ
ØTT68ZZ
ØTT7ØZZ
ØTT74ZZ
ØTT77ZZ
ØTT78ZZ
ØTTBØZZ
ØTTB4ZZ
ØTTB7ZZ
ØTTB8ZZ
ØTTCØZZ
ØTTC4ZZ
ØTTC7ZZ
ØTTC8ZZ
ØTU6Ø7Z
ØTU6ØJZ
ØTU6ØKZ
ØTU647Z
ØTU64JZ
ØTU64KZ
ØTU677Z
ØTU67JZ
ØTU67KZ
ØTU687Z
ØTU68JZ

ØTU68KZ
ØTU7Ø7Z
ØTU7ØJZ
ØTU7ØKZ
ØTU747Z
ØTU74JZ
ØTU74KZ
ØTU777Z
ØTU77JZ
ØTU77KZ
ØTU787Z
ØTU78JZ
ØTU78KZ
ØTUBØ7Z
ØTUBØJZ
ØTUBØKZ
ØTUB47Z
ØTUB4JZ
ØTUB4KZ
ØTUB77Z
ØTUB7JZ
ØTUB7KZ
ØTUB87Z
ØTUB8JZ
ØTUB8KZ
ØTUDØ7Z
ØTUDØJZ
ØTUDØKZ
ØTUD47Z
ØTUD4JZ
ØTUD4KZ
ØTUD77Z
ØTUD7JZ
ØTUD7KZ
ØTUD87Z
ØTUD8JZ
ØTUD8KZ
ØTUDX7Z
ØTUDXJZ
ØTUDXKZ
ØTV6ØCZ
ØTV6ØDZ
ØTV6ØZZ
ØTV63CZ
ØTV63DZ
ØTV63ZZ
ØTV64CZ
ØTV64DZ
ØTV64ZZ
ØTV67DZ
ØTV67ZZ
ØTV68DZ
ØTV68ZZ
ØTV7ØCZ
ØTV7ØDZ
ØTV7ØZZ
ØTV73CZ
ØTV73DZ
ØTV73ZZ
ØTV74CZ
ØTV74DZ
ØTV74ZZ
ØTV77DZ
ØTV77ZZ
ØTV78DZ
ØTV78ZZ
ØTVBØCZ
ØTVBØDZ
ØTVBØZZ
ØTVB3CZ
ØTVB3DZ
ØTVB3ZZ
ØTVB4CZ
ØTVB4DZ
ØTVB4ZZ
ØTVB7DZ
ØTVB7ZZ
ØTVB8DZ
ØTVB8ZZ
ØTVDØCZ
ØTVDØDZ
ØTVDØZZ
ØTVD3CZ
ØTVD3DZ
ØTVD3ZZ
ØTVD4CZ
ØTVD4DZ
ØTVD4ZZ
ØTVD7DZ
ØTVD7ZZ
ØTVD8DZ
ØTVD8ZZ
ØTVDXZZ
ØU79ØDZ
ØU79ØZZ

ØU793DZ
ØU793ZZ
ØU794DZ
ØU794ZZ
ØU797DZ
ØU797ZZ
ØU798DZ
ØU798ZZ
ØU7GØDZ
ØU7GØZZ
ØU7G3DZ
ØU7G3ZZ
ØU7G4DZ
ØU7G4ZZ
ØU7KØDZ
ØU7KØZZ
ØU7K3DZ
ØU7K3ZZ
ØU7K4DZ
ØU7K4ZZ
ØU7K7DZ
ØU7K7ZZ
ØU7K8DZ
ØU7K8ZZ
ØU7KXDZ
ØU7KXZZ
ØU99ØØZ
ØU99ØZZ
ØU994ØZ
ØU994ZZ
ØU997ØZ
ØU997ZZ
ØU998ØZ
ØU998ZZ
ØUC9ØZZ
ØUC93ZZ
ØUC94ZZ
ØUCCØZZ
ØUCC3ZZ
ØUCC4ZZ
ØUCC7ZZ
ØUCC8ZZ
ØUF5ØZZ
ØUF53ZZ
ØUF54ZZ
ØUF57ZZ
ØUF58ZZ
ØUF6ØZZ
ØUF63ZZ
ØUF64ZZ
ØUF67ZZ
ØUF68ZZ
ØUF7ØZZ
ØUF73ZZ
ØUF74ZZ
ØUF77ZZ
ØUF78ZZ
ØUMØØZZ
ØUMØ4ZZ
ØUM1ØZZ
ØUM14ZZ
ØUM2ØZZ
ØUM24ZZ
ØUM4ØZZ
ØUM44ZZ
ØUM5ØZZ
ØUM54ZZ
ØUM6ØZZ
ØUM64ZZ
ØUM7ØZZ
ØUM74ZZ
ØUMGØZZ
ØUMG4ZZ
ØUMMXZZ
ØUNØØZZ
ØUNØ3ZZ
ØUNØ4ZZ
ØUNØ8ZZ
ØUN1ØZZ
ØUN13ZZ
ØUN14ZZ
ØUN18ZZ
ØUN2ØZZ
ØUN23ZZ
ØUN24ZZ
ØUN28ZZ
ØUN4ØZZ
ØUN43ZZ
ØUN44ZZ
ØUN48ZZ
ØUN5ØZZ
ØUN53ZZ
ØUN54ZZ
ØUN57ZZ
ØUN58ZZ

ØUN6ØZZ
ØUN63ZZ
ØUN64ZZ
ØUN67ZZ
ØUN68ZZ
ØUN7ØZZ
ØUN73ZZ
ØUN74ZZ
ØUN77ZZ
ØUN78ZZ
ØUNGØZZ
ØUNG3ZZ
ØUNG4ZZ
ØUNG7ZZ
ØUNG8ZZ
ØUNGXZZ
ØUNMØZZ
ØUNMXZZ
ØUPDØØZ
ØUPDØ1Z
ØUPDØ3Z
ØUPDØ7Z
ØUPDØDZ
ØUPDØHZ
ØUPDØJZ
ØUPDØKZ
ØUPDØYZ
ØUPD3ØZ
ØUPD31Z
ØUPD33Z
ØUPD37Z
ØUPD3DZ
ØUPD3HZ
ØUPD3JZ
ØUPD3KZ
ØUPD4ØZ
ØUPD41Z
ØUPD43Z
ØUPD47Z
ØUPD4DZ
ØUPD4HZ
ØUPD4JZ
ØUPD4KZ
ØUPD71Z
ØUPD77Z
ØUPD7JZ
ØUPD7KZ
ØUPD81Z
ØUPD87Z
ØUPD8JZ
ØUPD8KZ
ØUQØØZZ
ØUQØ3ZZ
ØUQØ4ZZ
ØUQØ8ZZ
ØUQ1ØZZ
ØUQ13ZZ
ØUQ14ZZ
ØUQ18ZZ
ØUQ2ØZZ
ØUQ23ZZ
ØUQ24ZZ
ØUQ28ZZ
ØUQ4ØZZ
ØUQ43ZZ
ØUQ44ZZ
ØUQ48ZZ
ØUQ5ØZZ
ØUQ53ZZ
ØUQ54ZZ
ØUQ57ZZ
ØUQ58ZZ
ØUQ6ØZZ
ØUQ63ZZ
ØUQ64ZZ
ØUQ67ZZ
ØUQ68ZZ
ØUQ7ØZZ
ØUQ73ZZ
ØUQ74ZZ
ØUQ77ZZ
ØUQ78ZZ
ØUQ9ØZZ
ØUQ93ZZ
ØUQ94ZZ
ØUQ97ZZ
ØUQ98ZZ
ØUQCØZZ
ØUQC3ZZ
ØUQC4ZZ
ØUQC7ZZ
ØUQC8ZZ
ØUQGØZZ
ØUQG3ZZ
ØUQG4ZZ

ØUQG8ZZ
ØUQMØZZ
ØUSØØZZ
ØUSØ4ZZ
ØUSØ8ZZ
ØUS1ØZZ
ØUS14ZZ
ØUS18ZZ
ØUS2ØZZ
ØUS24ZZ
ØUS28ZZ
ØUS4ØZZ
ØUS44ZZ
ØUS48ZZ
ØUS5ØZZ
ØUS54ZZ
ØUS58ZZ
ØUS6ØZZ
ØUS64ZZ
ØUS68ZZ
ØUS7ØZZ
ØUS74ZZ
ØUS78ZZ
ØUSCØZZ
ØUSC4ZZ
ØUSC8ZZ
ØUU4Ø7Z
ØUU4ØJZ
ØUU4ØKZ
ØUU447Z
ØUU44JZ
ØUU44KZ
ØUU5Ø7Z
ØUU5ØKZ
ØUU547Z
ØUU54KZ
ØUU577Z
ØUU57KZ
ØUU587Z
ØUU58KZ
ØUU6Ø7Z
ØUU6ØKZ
ØUU647Z
ØUU64KZ
ØUU677Z
ØUU67KZ
ØUU687Z
ØUU68KZ
ØUU7Ø7Z
ØUU7ØKZ
ØUU747Z
ØUU74KZ
ØUU777Z
ØUU77KZ
ØUU787Z
ØUU78KZ
ØUUGØ7Z
ØUUGØJZ
ØUUGØKZ
ØUUG47Z
ØUUG4JZ
ØUUG4KZ
ØUUG77Z
ØUUG7JZ
ØUUG7KZ
ØUUG87Z
ØUUG8JZ
ØUUG8KZ
ØUUGX7Z
ØUUGXJZ
ØUUGXKZ
ØUUMØ7Z
ØUUMØJZ
ØUUMØKZ
ØUUMX7Z
ØUUMXJZ
ØUUMXKZ
ØUVCØCZ
ØUVCØDZ
ØUVCØZZ
ØUVC3CZ
ØUVC3DZ
ØUVC3ZZ
ØUVC4CZ
ØUVC4DZ
ØUVC4ZZ
ØUVC7DZ
ØUVC7ZZ
ØUVC8DZ
ØUVC8ZZ
ØUWDØØZ
ØUWDØ1Z
ØUWDØ3Z
ØUWDØ7Z
ØUWDØDZ

ØUWDØHZ
ØUWDØJZ
ØUWDØKZ
ØUWDØYZ
ØUWD3ØZ
ØUWD31Z
ØUWD33Z
ØUWD37Z
ØUWD3DZ
ØUWD3HZ
ØUWD3JZ
ØUWD3KZ
ØUWD4ØZ
ØUWD41Z
ØUWD43Z
ØUWD47Z
ØUWD4DZ
ØUWD4HZ
ØUWD4JZ
ØUWD4KZ
ØUWD7ØZ
ØUWD71Z
ØUWD73Z
ØUWD77Z
ØUWD7DZ
ØUWD7HZ
ØUWD7JZ
ØUWD7KZ
ØUWD8ØZ
ØUWD81Z
ØUWD83Z
ØUWD87Z
ØUWD8DZ
ØUWD8HZ
ØUWD8JZ
ØUWD8KZ
ØV7NØDZ
ØV7NØZZ
ØV7N3DZ
ØV7N3ZZ
ØV7N4DZ
ØV7N4ZZ
ØV7PØDZ
ØV7PØZZ
ØV7P3DZ
ØV7P3ZZ
ØV7P4DZ
ØV7P4ZZ
ØV7QØDZ
ØV7QØZZ
ØV7Q3DZ
ØV7Q3ZZ
ØV7Q4DZ
ØV7Q4ZZ
ØV99ØØZ
ØV99ØZZ
ØV9BØØZ
ØV9BØZZ
ØV9CØØZ
ØV9CØZZ
ØVC9ØZZ
ØVC93ZZ
ØVC94ZZ
ØVCBØZZ
ØVCB3ZZ
ØVCB4ZZ
ØVCCØZZ
ØVCC3ZZ
ØVCC4ZZ
ØVLNØDZ
ØVLN3DZ
ØVLN4DZ
ØVLN8DZ
ØVLPØDZ
ØVLP3DZ
ØVLP4DZ
ØVLP8DZ
ØVLQØDZ
ØVLQ3DZ
ØVLQ4DZ
ØVLQ8DZ
ØVM5XZZ
ØVM6ØZZ
ØVM64ZZ
ØVM7ØZZ
ØVM74ZZ
ØVM9ØZZ
ØVM94ZZ
ØVMBØZZ
ØVMB4ZZ
ØVMCØZZ
ØVMC4ZZ
ØVMFØZZ
ØVMF4ZZ
ØVMGØZZ

ØVMG4ZZ
ØVMHØZZ
ØVMH4ZZ
ØVMSXZZ
ØVNØØZZ
ØVNØ3ZZ
ØVNØ4ZZ
ØVNØ7ZZ
ØVNØ8ZZ
ØVN5ØZZ
ØVN53ZZ
ØVN54ZZ
ØVN5XZZ
ØVN6ØZZ
ØVN63ZZ
ØVN64ZZ
ØVN7ØZZ
ØVN73ZZ
ØVN74ZZ
ØVNFØZZ
ØVNF3ZZ
ØVNF4ZZ
ØVNF8ZZ
ØVNGØZZ
ØVNG3ZZ
ØVNG4ZZ
ØVNG8ZZ
ØVNHØZZ
ØVNH3ZZ
ØVNH4ZZ
ØVNH8ZZ
ØVNJØZZ
ØVNJ3ZZ
ØVNJ4ZZ
ØVNJ8ZZ
ØVNKØZZ
ØVNK3ZZ
ØVNK4ZZ
ØVNK8ZZ
ØVNLØZZ
ØVNL3ZZ
ØVNL4ZZ
ØVNL8ZZ
ØVNNØZZ
ØVNN3ZZ
ØVNN4ZZ
ØVNN8ZZ
ØVNPØZZ
ØVNP3ZZ
ØVNP4ZZ
ØVNP8ZZ
ØVNQØZZ
ØVNQ3ZZ
ØVNQ4ZZ
ØVNQ8ZZ
ØVPDØØZ
ØVPDØ3Z
ØVPDØ7Z
ØVPDØJZ
ØVPDØKZ
ØVPDØYZ
ØVPD3ØZ
ØVPD33Z
ØVPD37Z
ØVPD3JZ
ØVPD3KZ
ØVPD4ØZ
ØVPD43Z
ØVPD47Z
ØVPD4JZ
ØVPD4KZ
ØVPD77Z
ØVPD7JZ
ØVPD7KZ
ØVPD87Z
ØVPD8JZ
ØVPD8KZ
ØVQØØZZ
ØVQØ3ZZ
ØVQØ4ZZ
ØVQØ7ZZ
ØVQØ8ZZ
ØVQ9ØZZ
ØVQ93ZZ
ØVQ94ZZ
ØVQBØZZ
ØVQB3ZZ
ØVQB4ZZ
ØVQCØZZ
ØVQC3ZZ
ØVQC4ZZ
ØVQFØZZ
ØVQF3ZZ
ØVQF4ZZ
ØVQF8ZZ

ØVQGØZZ
ØVQG3ZZ
ØVQG4ZZ
ØVQG8ZZ
ØVQHØZZ
ØVQH3ZZ
ØVQH4ZZ
ØVQH8ZZ
ØVQJØZZ
ØVQJ3ZZ
ØVQJ4ZZ
ØVQJ8ZZ
ØVQKØZZ
ØVQK3ZZ
ØVQK4ZZ
ØVQK8ZZ
ØVQLØZZ
ØVQL3ZZ
ØVQL4ZZ
ØVQL8ZZ
ØVQNØZZ
ØVQN3ZZ
ØVQN4ZZ
ØVQN8ZZ
ØVQPØZZ
ØVQP3ZZ
ØVQP4ZZ
ØVQP8ZZ
ØVQQØZZ
ØVQQ3ZZ
ØVQQ4ZZ
ØVQQ8ZZ
ØVQSØZZ
ØVQS3ZZ
ØVQS4ZZ
ØVQSXZZ
ØVQTØZZ
ØVQT3ZZ
ØVQT4ZZ
ØVQTXZZ
ØVSFØZZ
ØVSF3ZZ
ØVSF4ZZ
ØVSF8ZZ
ØVSGØZZ
ØVSG3ZZ
ØVSG4ZZ
ØVSG8ZZ
ØVSHØZZ
ØVSH3ZZ
ØVSH4ZZ
ØVSH8ZZ
ØVT9ØZZ
ØVT94ZZ
ØVTBØZZ
ØVTB4ZZ
ØVTCØZZ
ØVTC4ZZ
ØVU5Ø7Z
ØVU5ØJZ
ØVU5ØKZ
ØVU547Z
ØVU54JZ
ØVU54KZ
ØVU5X7Z
ØVU5XJZ
ØVU5XKZ
ØVU6Ø7Z
ØVU6ØJZ
ØVU6ØKZ
ØVU647Z
ØVU64JZ
ØVU64KZ
ØVU687Z
ØVU68JZ
ØVU68KZ
ØVU7Ø7Z
ØVU7ØJZ
ØVU7ØKZ
ØVU747Z
ØVU74JZ
ØVU74KZ
ØVU787Z
ØVU78JZ
ØVU78KZ
ØVU9Ø7Z
ØVU9ØJZ
ØVU9ØKZ
ØVUBØ7Z
ØVUBØJZ
ØVUBØKZ
ØVUCØ7Z
ØVUCØJZ
ØVUCØKZ
ØVUFØ7Z

ØVUFØJZ
ØVUFØKZ
ØVUF47Z
ØVUF4JZ
ØVUF4KZ
ØVUF87Z
ØVUF8JZ
ØVUF8KZ
ØVUGØ7Z
ØVUGØJZ
ØVUGØKZ
ØVUG47Z
ØVUG4JZ
ØVUG4KZ
ØVUG87Z
ØVUG8JZ
ØVUG8KZ
ØVUHØ7Z
ØVUHØJZ
ØVUHØKZ
ØVUH47Z
ØVUH4JZ
ØVUH4KZ
ØVUH87Z
ØVUH8JZ
ØVUH8KZ
ØVUJØ7Z
ØVUJØJZ
ØVUJØKZ
ØVUJ47Z
ØVUJ4JZ
ØVUJ4KZ
ØVUJ87Z
ØVUJ8JZ
ØVUJ8KZ
ØVUKØ7Z
ØVUKØJZ
ØVUKØKZ
ØVUK47Z
ØVUK4JZ
ØVUK4KZ
ØVUK87Z
ØVUK8JZ
ØVUK8KZ
ØVULØ7Z
ØVULØJZ
ØVULØKZ
ØVUL47Z
ØVUL4JZ
ØVUL4KZ
ØVUL87Z
ØVUL8JZ
ØVUL8KZ
ØVUNØ7Z
ØVUNØJZ
ØVUNØKZ
ØVUN47Z
ØVUN4JZ
ØVUN4KZ
ØVUN87Z
ØVUN8JZ
ØVUN8KZ
ØVUPØ7Z
ØVUPØJZ
ØVUPØKZ
ØVUP47Z
ØVUP4JZ
ØVUP4KZ
ØVUP87Z
ØVUP8JZ
ØVUP8KZ
ØVUQØ7Z
ØVUQØJZ
ØVUQØKZ
ØVUQ47Z
ØVUQ4JZ
ØVUQ4KZ
ØVUQ87Z
ØVUQ8JZ
ØVUQ8KZ
ØVUSØ7Z
ØVUSØKZ
ØVUS47Z
ØVUS4KZ
ØVUTØ7Z
ØVUTØJZ
ØVUTØKZ
ØVUT47Z
ØVUT4JZ
ØVUT4KZ
ØVUTX7Z
ØVUTXJZ
ØVUTXKZ
ØVWDØØZ
ØVWDØ3Z

ØVWDØ7Z
ØVWDØJZ
ØVWDØKZ
ØVWDØYZ
ØVWD3ØZ
ØVWD33Z
ØVWD37Z
ØVWD3JZ
ØVWD3KZ
ØVWD4ØZ
ØVWD43Z
ØVWD47Z
ØVWD4JZ
ØVWD4KZ
ØVWD7ØZ
ØVWD73Z
ØVWD77Z
ØVWD7JZ
ØVWD7KZ
ØVWD8ØZ
ØVWD83Z
ØVWD87Z
ØVWD8JZ
ØVWD8KZ
ØVXTØZD
ØVXTØZS
ØVXTXZD
ØVXTXZS
ØVY5ØZØ
ØVY5ØZ1
ØVY5ØZ2
ØVYSØZØ
ØVYSØZ1
ØVYSØZ2
ØWØ2Ø7Z
ØWØ2ØJZ
ØWØ2ØKZ
ØWØ2ØZZ
ØWØ237Z
ØWØ23JZ
ØWØ23KZ
ØWØ23ZZ
ØWØ247Z
ØWØ24JZ
ØWØ24KZ
ØWØ24ZZ
ØWØ4Ø7Z
ØWØ4ØJZ
ØWØ4ØKZ
ØWØ4ØZZ
ØWØ437Z
ØWØ43JZ
ØWØ43KZ
ØWØ43ZZ
ØWØ447Z
ØWØ44JZ
ØWØ44KZ
ØWØ44ZZ
ØWØ5Ø7Z
ØWØ5ØJZ
ØWØ5ØKZ
ØWØ5ØZZ
ØWØ537Z
ØWØ53JZ
ØWØ53KZ
ØWØ53ZZ
ØWØ547Z
ØWØ54JZ
ØWØ54KZ
ØWØ54ZZ
ØWØ6Ø7Z
ØWØ6ØJZ
ØWØ6ØKZ
ØWØ6ØZZ
ØWØ637Z
ØWØ63JZ
ØWØ63KZ
ØWØ63ZZ
ØWØ647Z
ØWØ64JZ
ØWØ64KZ
ØWØ64ZZ
ØWØNØ7Z
ØWØNØJZ
ØWØNØKZ
ØWØNØZZ
ØWØN37Z
ØWØN3JZ
ØWØN3KZ
ØWØN3ZZ
ØWØN47Z
ØWØN4JZ
ØWØN4KZ
ØWØN4ZZ
ØW11ØJ9

ØW11ØJB
ØW11ØJG
ØW11ØJJ
ØW19ØJ9
ØW19ØJB
ØW19ØJJ
ØW193J9
ØW193JB
ØW193JJ
ØW194J9
ØW194JB
ØW194JJ
ØW1BØJ9
ØW1BØJB
ØW1BØJJ
ØW1B3J9
ØW1B3JB
ØW1B3JJ
ØW1B4J9
ØW1B4JB
ØW1B4JJ
ØW1GØJ4
ØW1G3J4
ØW1G4J4
ØW3ØØZZ
ØW3Ø3ZZ
ØW3Ø4ZZ
ØW31ØZZ
ØW313ZZ
ØW314ZZ
ØW32ØZZ
ØW323ZZ
ØW324ZZ
ØW33ØZZ
ØW333ZZ
ØW334ZZ
ØW337ZZ
ØW338ZZ
ØW33XZZ
ØW34ØZZ
ØW343ZZ
ØW344ZZ
ØW35ØZZ
ØW353ZZ
ØW354ZZ
ØW36ØZZ
ØW363ZZ
ØW364ZZ
ØW38ØZZ
ØW383ZZ
ØW384ZZ
ØW39ØZZ
ØW393ZZ
ØW394ZZ
ØW3BØZZ
ØW3B3ZZ
ØW3B4ZZ
ØW3CØZZ
ØW3C3ZZ
ØW3C4ZZ
ØW3DØZZ
ØW3D3ZZ
ØW3D4ZZ
ØW3FØZZ
ØW3F3ZZ
ØW3F4ZZ
ØW3GØZZ
ØW3G3ZZ
ØW3G4ZZ
ØW3HØZZ
ØW3H3ZZ
ØW3H4ZZ
ØW3JØZZ
ØW3J3ZZ
ØW3J4ZZ
ØW3KØZZ
ØW3K3ZZ
ØW3K4ZZ
ØW3LØZZ
ØW3L3ZZ
ØW3L4ZZ
ØW3MØZZ
ØW3M3ZZ
ØW3M4ZZ
ØW3NØZZ
ØW3N3ZZ
ØW3N4ZZ
ØW3PØZZ
ØW3P3ZZ
ØW3P4ZZ
ØW3P7ZZ
ØW3QØZZ
ØW3Q3ZZ
ØW3Q4ZZ
ØW3Q7ZZ
ØW3Q8ZZ
ØW3RØZZ
ØW3R3ZZ
ØW3R4ZZ
ØW3R7ZZ
ØW3R8ZZ
ØW92ØØZ
ØW92ØZZ
ØW924ØZ
ØW924ZZ
ØW93ØØZ
ØW93ØZZ
ØW934ØZ
ØW934ZZ
ØW94ØØZ
ØW94ØZZ
ØW944ØZ
ØW944ZZ
ØW95ØØZ
ØW95ØZZ
ØW954ØZ
ØW954ZZ
ØW96ØØZ
ØW96ØZZ
ØW964ØZ
ØW964ZZ
ØW9CØØZ
ØW9CØZZ
ØW9C4ØZ
ØW9C4ZZ
ØW9DØØZ
ØW9DØZX
ØW9DØZZ
ØW9D4ØZ
ØW9D4ZX
ØW9D4ZZ
ØW9FØZX
ØW9F3ZX
ØW9F4ZX
ØW9GØØZ
ØW9GØZX
ØW9GØZZ
ØW9G4ZX
ØW9HØZX
ØW9H3ZX
ØW9H4ZX
ØW9JØZX
ØW9J4ZX
ØWBØØZZ
ØWBØ3ZZ
ØWBØ4ZZ
ØWBØXZZ
ØWB2ØZZ
ØWB23ZZ
ØWB24ZZ
ØWB2XZZ
ØWB4ØZZ
ØWB43ZZ
ØWB44ZZ
ØWB4XZZ
ØWB5ØZZ
ØWB53ZZ
ØWB54ZZ
ØWB5XZZ
ØWB6ØZZ
ØWB63ZZ
ØWB64ZZ
ØWB6XZ2
ØWB6XZZ
ØWBFØZX
ØWBF3ZX
ØWBF4ZX
ØWBFXZX
ØWBKØZZ
ØWBK3ZZ
ØWBK4ZZ
ØWBKXZZ
ØWBLØZZ
ØWBL3ZZ
ØWBL4ZZ
ØWBLXZZ
ØWBMØZZ
ØWBM3ZZ
ØWBM4ZZ
ØWBMXZZ
ØWC3ØZZ
ØWC33ZZ
ØWC34ZZ
ØWCCØZZ
ØWCC3ZZ
ØWCC4ZZ
ØWCDØZZ
ØWCD3ZZ
ØWCD4ZZ
ØWCGØZZ
ØWCG3ZZ
ØWCG4ZZ
ØWCHØZZ
ØWCH3ZZ
ØWCH4ZZ
ØWCQ7ZZ
ØWCQ8ZZ
ØWF3ØZZ
ØWF33ZZ
ØWF34ZZ
ØWF9ØZZ
ØWF93ZZ
ØWF94ZZ
ØWFBØZZ
ØWFB3ZZ
ØWFB4ZZ
ØWFCØZZ
ØWFC3ZZ
ØWFC4ZZ
ØWFGØZZ
ØWFG3ZZ
ØWFG4ZZ
ØWFQØZZ
ØWFQ3ZZ
ØWFQ4ZZ
ØWFQ7ZZ
ØWFQ8ZZ
ØWH3Ø3Z
ØWH3ØYZ
ØWH333Z
ØWH33YZ
ØWH343Z
ØWH34YZ
ØWHCØ3Z
ØWHCØYZ
ØWHC33Z
ØWHC3YZ
ØWHC43Z
ØWHC4YZ
ØWHDØ3Z
ØWHDØYZ
ØWHD33Z
ØWHD3YZ
ØWHD43Z
ØWHD4YZ
ØWHQ33Z
ØWHQ3YZ
ØWHQ43Z
ØWHQ4YZ
ØWJ14ZZ
ØWJ6ØZZ
ØWJ64ZZ
ØWJ9ØZZ
ØWJ94ZZ
ØWJBØZZ
ØWJB4ZZ
ØWJCØZZ
ØWJF4ZZ
ØWJGØZZ
ØWJG4ZZ
ØWJH4ZZ
ØWJJØZZ
ØWJJ4ZZ
ØWJPØZZ
ØWJP4ZZ
ØWJQØZZ
ØWJQ4ZZ
ØWJRØZZ
ØWJR4ZZ
ØWM8ØZZ
ØWMFØZZ
ØWMNØZZ
ØWPCØØZ
ØWPCØ1Z
ØWPCØ3Z
ØWPCØ7Z
ØWPCØGZ
ØWPCØJZ
ØWPCØKZ
ØWPCØYZ
ØWPC3ØZ
ØWPC31Z
ØWPC33Z
ØWPC37Z
ØWPC3GZ
ØWPC3JZ
ØWPC3KZ
ØWPC3YZ
ØWPC4ØZ
ØWPC41Z
ØWPC43Z
ØWPC47Z
ØWPC4GZ
ØWPC4JZ
ØWPC4KZ
ØWPC4YZ
ØWPDØØZ
ØWPDØ1Z
ØWPDØ3Z
ØWPDØYZ
ØWPD3ØZ
ØWPD31Z
ØWPD33Z
ØWPD3YZ
ØWPD4ØZ
ØWPD41Z
ØWPD43Z
ØWPD4YZ
ØWPQ31Z
ØWPQ33Z
ØWPQ3YZ
ØWPQ41Z
ØWPQ43Z
ØWPQ4YZ
ØWPQ71Z
ØWPQ7YZ
ØWPQ81Z
ØWQ2XZZ
ØWQ3ØZZ
ØWQ33ZZ
ØWQ34ZZ
ØWQ3XZZ
ØWQ6XZ2
ØWQ8ØZZ
ØWQ83ZZ
ØWQ84ZZ
ØWQ8XZZ
ØWQCØZZ
ØWQC3ZZ
ØWQC4ZZ
ØWQFØZZ
ØWQF3ZZ
ØWQF4ZZ
ØWQFXZ2
ØWQFXZZ
ØWQNØZZ
ØWQN3ZZ
ØWQN4ZZ
ØWU2Ø7Z
ØWU247Z
ØWU4Ø7Z
ØWU4ØJZ
ØWU4ØKZ
ØWU447Z
ØWU44JZ
ØWU44KZ
ØWU5Ø7Z
ØWU5ØJZ
ØWU5ØKZ
ØWU547Z
ØWU54JZ
ØWU54KZ
ØWUCØ7Z
ØWUCØJZ
ØWUCØKZ
ØWUC47Z
ØWUC4JZ
ØWUC4KZ
ØWUFØ7Z
ØWUFØJZ
ØWUFØKZ
ØWUF47Z
ØWUF4JZ
ØWUF4KZ
ØWUNØ7Z
ØWUNØJZ
ØWUNØKZ
ØWUN47Z
ØWUN4JZ
ØWUN4KZ
ØWWCØØZ
ØWWCØ1Z
ØWWCØ3Z
ØWWCØ7Z
ØWWCØGZ
ØWWCØJZ
ØWWCØKZ
ØWWCØYZ
ØWWC3ØZ
ØWWC31Z
ØWWC33Z
ØWWC37Z
ØWWC3GZ
ØWWC3JZ
ØWWC3KZ
ØWWC3YZ
ØWWC4ØZ
ØWWC41Z
ØWWC43Z
ØWWC47Z
ØWWC4GZ
ØWWC4JZ
ØWWC4KZ
ØWWC4YZ
ØWWDØØZ
ØWWDØ1Z
ØWWDØ3Z
ØWWDØYZ
ØWWD3ØZ
ØWWD31Z
ØWWD33Z
ØWWD3YZ
ØWWD4ØZ
ØWWD41Z
ØWWD43Z
ØWWD4YZ
ØWWQ31Z
ØWWQ33Z
ØWWQ3YZ
ØWWQ41Z
ØWWQ43Z
ØWWQ4YZ
ØWWQ71Z
ØWWQ73Z
ØWWQ7YZ
ØWWQ81Z
ØWWQ83Z
ØWWQ8YZ
ØX32ØZZ
ØX323ZZ
ØX324ZZ
ØX33ØZZ
ØX333ZZ
ØX334ZZ
ØX34ØZZ
ØX343ZZ
ØX344ZZ
ØX35ØZZ
ØX353ZZ
ØX354ZZ
ØX36ØZZ
ØX363ZZ
ØX364ZZ
ØX37ØZZ
ØX373ZZ
ØX374ZZ
ØX38ØZZ
ØX383ZZ
ØX384ZZ
ØX39ØZZ
ØX393ZZ
ØX394ZZ
ØX3BØZZ
ØX3B3ZZ
ØX3B4ZZ
ØX3CØZZ
ØX3C3ZZ
ØX3C4ZZ
ØX3DØZZ
ØX3D3ZZ
ØX3D4ZZ
ØX3FØZZ
ØX3F3ZZ
ØX3F4ZZ
ØX3GØZZ
ØX3G3ZZ
ØX3G4ZZ
ØX3HØZZ
ØX3H3ZZ
ØX3H4ZZ
ØX3JØZZ
ØX3J3ZZ
ØX3J4ZZ
ØX3KØZZ
ØX3K3ZZ
ØX3K4ZZ
ØX6ØØZZ
ØX61ØZZ
ØX62ØZZ
ØX63ØZZ
ØX68ØZ1
ØX68ØZ2
ØX68ØZ3
ØX69ØZ1
ØX69ØZ2
ØX69ØZ3
ØX6BØZZ
ØX6CØZZ
ØX6DØZ1
ØX6DØZ2
ØX6DØZ3
ØX6FØZ1
ØX6FØZ2
ØX6FØZ3
ØX6JØZØ
ØX6JØZ4
ØX6JØZ5
ØX6JØZ6
ØX6JØZ7
ØX6JØZ8
ØX6JØZ9
ØX6JØZB
ØX6JØZC
ØX6JØZD
ØX6JØZF
ØX6KØZØ
ØX6KØZ4
ØX6KØZ5
ØX6KØZ6
ØX6KØZ7
ØX6KØZ8
ØX6KØZ9
ØX6KØZB
ØX6KØZC
ØX6KØZD
ØX6KØZF
ØX6LØZØ
ØX6LØZ1
ØX6LØZ2
ØX6LØZ3
ØX6MØZØ
ØX6MØZ1
ØX6MØZ2
ØX6MØZ3
ØX6NØZØ
ØX6NØZ1
ØX6NØZ2
ØX6NØZ3
ØX6PØZØ
ØX6PØZ1
ØX6PØZ2
ØX6PØZ3
ØX6QØZØ
ØX6QØZ1
ØX6QØZ2
ØX6QØZ3
ØX6RØZØ
ØX6RØZ1
ØX6RØZ2
ØX6RØZ3
ØX6SØZØ
ØX6SØZ1
ØX6SØZ2
ØX6SØZ3
ØX6TØZØ
ØX6TØZ1
ØX6TØZ2
ØX6TØZ3
ØX6VØZØ
ØX6VØZ1
ØX6VØZ2
ØX6VØZ3
ØX6WØZØ
ØX6WØZ1
ØX6WØZ2
ØX6WØZ3
ØXB2ØZZ
ØXB23ZZ
ØXB24ZZ
ØXB3ØZZ
ØXB33ZZ
ØXB34ZZ
ØXB4ØZZ
ØXB43ZZ
ØXB44ZZ
ØXB5ØZZ
ØXB53ZZ
ØXB54ZZ
ØXB6ØZZ
ØXB63ZZ
ØXB64ZZ
ØXB7ØZZ
ØXB73ZZ
ØXB74ZZ
ØXB8ØZZ
ØXB83ZZ
ØXB84ZZ
ØXB9ØZZ
ØXB93ZZ
ØXB94ZZ
ØXBBØZZ
ØXBB3ZZ
ØXBB4ZZ
ØXBCØZZ
ØXBC3ZZ
ØXBC4ZZ
ØXBDØZZ
ØXBD3ZZ
ØXBD4ZZ
ØXBFØZZ
ØXBF3ZZ
ØXBF4ZZ
ØXBGØZZ
ØXBG3ZZ
ØXBG4ZZ
ØXBHØZZ
ØXBH3ZZ
ØXBH4ZZ
ØXBJØZZ
ØXBJ3ZZ
ØXBJ4ZZ
ØXBKØZZ
ØXBK3ZZ
ØXBK4ZZ
ØXMLØZZ
ØXMMØZZ
ØXMNØZZ
ØXMPØZZ
ØXMQØZZ
ØXMRØZZ
ØXMSØZZ
ØXMTØZZ
ØXMVØZZ
ØXMWØZZ
ØXQ2ØZZ
ØXQ23ZZ
ØXQ24ZZ
ØXQ2XZZ
ØXQ3ØZZ
ØXQ33ZZ
ØXQ34ZZ
ØXQ3XZZ
ØXQ4ØZZ
ØXQ43ZZ
ØXQ44ZZ
ØXQ4XZZ
ØXQ5ØZZ
ØXQ53ZZ
ØXQ54ZZ
ØXQ5XZZ
ØXQ6ØZZ
ØXQ63ZZ
ØXQ64ZZ
ØXQ6XZZ
ØXQ7ØZZ
ØXQ73ZZ
ØXQ74ZZ
ØXQ7XZZ
ØXQ8ØZZ
ØXQ83ZZ
ØXQ84ZZ
ØXQ8XZZ
ØXQ9ØZZ
ØXQ93ZZ
ØXQ94ZZ
ØXQ9XZZ
ØXQBØZZ
ØXQB3ZZ
ØXQB4ZZ
ØXQBXZZ
ØXQCØZZ
ØXQC3ZZ
ØXQC4ZZ
ØXQCXZZ
ØXQDØZZ
ØXQD3ZZ
ØXQD4ZZ
ØXQDXZZ
ØXQFØZZ
ØXQF3ZZ
ØXQF4ZZ
ØXQFXZZ
ØXQGØZZ
ØXQG3ZZ
ØXQG4ZZ
ØXQGXZZ
ØXQHØZZ
ØXQH3ZZ
ØXQH4ZZ
ØXQHXZZ
ØXQJØZZ
ØXQJ3ZZ
ØXQJ4ZZ
ØXQJXZZ
ØXQKØZZ
ØXQK3ZZ
ØXQK4ZZ
ØXQKXZZ
ØXQLØZZ
ØXQL3ZZ
ØXQL4ZZ
ØXQLXZZ
ØXQMØZZ
ØXQM3ZZ
ØXQM4ZZ
ØXQMXZZ
ØXQNØZZ
ØXQN3ZZ
ØXQN4ZZ
ØXQNXZZ
ØXQPØZZ
ØXQP3ZZ
ØXQP4ZZ
ØXQPXZZ
ØXQQØZZ
ØXQQ3ZZ
ØXQQ4ZZ
ØXQQXZZ
ØXQRØZZ
ØXQR3ZZ
ØXQR4ZZ
ØXQRXZZ
ØXQSØZZ
ØXQS3ZZ
ØXQS4ZZ
ØXQSXZZ
ØXQTØZZ
ØXQT3ZZ
ØXQT4ZZ
ØXQTXZZ
ØXQVØZZ
ØXQV3ZZ
ØXQV4ZZ
ØXQVXZZ
ØXQWØZZ
ØXQW3ZZ
ØXQW4ZZ
ØXQWXZZ
ØXRLØ7N
ØXRLØ7P
ØXRL47N
ØXRL47P
ØXRMØ7N
ØXRMØ7P
ØXRM47N
ØXRM47P
ØXUJØ7Z
ØXUJ47Z
ØXUKØ7Z
ØXUK47Z
ØXULØ7Z
ØXUL47Z
ØXUMØ7Z
ØXUM47Z
ØXUNØ7Z
ØXUN47Z
ØXUPØ7Z
ØXUP47Z
ØXUQØ7Z
ØXUQ47Z
ØXURØ7Z
ØXUR47Z
ØXUSØ7Z
ØXUS47Z
ØXUTØ7Z
ØXUT47Z
ØXUVØ7Z
ØXUV47Z
ØXUWØ7Z
ØXUW47Z
ØXXNØZL
ØXXPØZM
ØXYJØZØ
ØXYJØZ1
ØXYKØZØ
ØXYKØZ1
ØY3ØØZZ
ØY3Ø3ZZ
ØY3Ø4ZZ
ØY31ØZZ
ØY313ZZ
ØY314ZZ
ØY35ØZZ
ØY353ZZ
ØY354ZZ
ØY36ØZZ
ØY363ZZ
ØY364ZZ
ØY37ØZZ
ØY373ZZ
ØY374ZZ
ØY38ØZZ
ØY383ZZ
ØY384ZZ
ØY39ØZZ
ØY393ZZ
ØY394ZZ
ØY3BØZZ
ØY3B3ZZ
ØY3B4ZZ
ØY3CØZZ
ØY3C3ZZ
ØY3C4ZZ
ØY3DØZZ
ØY3D3ZZ
ØY3D4ZZ
ØY3FØZZ
ØY3F3ZZ
ØY3F4ZZ
ØY3GØZZ
ØY3G3ZZ
ØY3G4ZZ
ØY3HØZZ
ØY3H3ZZ
ØY3H4ZZ
ØY3JØZZ
ØY3J3ZZ
ØY3J4ZZ
ØY3KØZZ
ØY3K3ZZ
ØY3K4ZZ
ØY3LØZZ
ØY3L3ZZ
ØY3L4ZZ
ØY3MØZZ
ØY3M3ZZ
ØY3M4ZZ
ØY3NØZZ
ØY3N3ZZ
ØY3N4ZZ
ØY62ØZZ
ØY63ØZZ
ØY64ØZZ
ØY67ØZZ
ØY68ØZZ
ØY6CØZ1
ØY6CØZ2
ØY6CØZ3
ØY6DØZ1
ØY6DØZ2
ØY6DØZ3
ØY6FØZZ
ØY6GØZZ
ØY6HØZ1
ØY6HØZ2
ØY6HØZ3
ØY6JØZ1
ØY6JØZ2
ØY6JØZ3
ØY6MØZØ
ØY6MØZ4
ØY6MØZ5
ØY6MØZ6
ØY6MØZ7
ØY6MØZ8
ØY6MØZ9
ØY6MØZB
ØY6MØZC
ØY6MØZD
ØY6MØZF
ØY6NØZØ
ØY6NØZ4
ØY6NØZ5
ØY6NØZ6
ØY6NØZ7
ØY6NØZ8
ØY6NØZ9
ØY6NØZB
ØY6NØZC
ØY6NØZD
ØY6NØZF
ØY6PØZØ
ØY6PØZ1
ØY6PØZ2
ØY6PØZ3
ØY6QØZØ
ØY6QØZ1
ØY6QØZ2
ØY6QØZ3
ØY6RØZØ
ØY6RØZ1
ØY6RØZ2
ØY6RØZ3
ØY6SØZØ
ØY6SØZ1
ØY6SØZ2
ØY6SØZ3
ØY6TØZØ
ØY6TØZ1
ØY6TØZ2
ØY6TØZ3
ØY6UØZØ
ØY6UØZ1
ØY6UØZ2
ØY6UØZ3

ØY6VØZØ
ØY6VØZ1
ØY6VØZ2
ØY6VØZ3
ØY6WØZØ
ØY6WØZ1
ØY6WØZ2
ØY6WØZ3
ØY6XØZØ
ØY6XØZ1
ØY6XØZ2
ØY6XØZ3
ØY6YØZØ
ØY6YØZ1
ØY6YØZ2
ØY6YØZ3
ØY95ØZX
ØY953ZX
ØY954ZX
ØY96ØZX
ØY963ZX
ØY964ZX
ØYBØØZZ
ØYBØ3ZZ
ØYBØ4ZZ
ØYB1ØZZ
ØYB13ZZ
ØYB14ZZ
ØYB5ØZX
ØYB53ZX
ØYB54ZX
ØYB6ØZX
ØYB63ZX
ØYB64ZX
ØYB7ØZX
ØYB73ZX
ØYB74ZX
ØYB8ØZX
ØYB83ZX
ØYB84ZX
ØYB9ØZZ
ØYB93ZZ
ØYB94ZZ
ØYBBØZZ
ØYBB3ZZ
ØYBB4ZZ
ØYBCØZZ
ØYBC3ZZ
ØYBC4ZZ
ØYBDØZZ
ØYBD3ZZ
ØYBD4ZZ
ØYBFØZZ
ØYBF3ZZ
ØYBF4ZZ
ØYBGØZZ
ØYBG3ZZ
ØYBG4ZZ
ØYBHØZZ
ØYBH3ZZ
ØYBH4ZZ
ØYBJØZZ
ØYBJ3ZZ
ØYBJ4ZZ
ØYBKØZZ
ØYBK3ZZ
ØYBK4ZZ
ØYBLØZZ
ØYBL3ZZ
ØYBL4ZZ
ØYBMØZZ
ØYBM3ZZ
ØYBM4ZZ
ØYBNØZZ
ØYBN3ZZ
ØYBN4ZZ
ØYJ5ØZZ
ØYJ54ZZ
ØYJ6ØZZ
ØYJ64ZZ
ØYJ7ØZZ
ØYJ74ZZ
ØYJ84ZZ
ØYJAØZZ
ØYJA4ZZ
ØYJE4ZZ
ØYM2ØZZ
ØYM3ØZZ
ØYM4ØZZ
ØYM5ØZZ
ØYM6ØZZ
ØYM9ØZZ
ØYMBØZZ
ØYMPØZZ
ØYMQØZZ
ØYMRØZZ
ØYMSØZZ
ØYMTØZZ
ØYMUØZZ
ØYMVØZZ
ØYMWØZZ
ØYMXØZZ
ØYMYØZZ
ØYQØØZZ
ØYQØ3ZZ
ØYQØ4ZZ
ØYQØXZZ
ØYQ1ØZZ
ØYQ13ZZ
ØYQ14ZZ
ØYQ1XZZ
ØYQ9ØZZ
ØYQ93ZZ
ØYQ94ZZ
ØYQ9XZZ
ØYQBØZZ
ØYQB3ZZ
ØYQB4ZZ
ØYQBXZZ
ØYQCØZZ
ØYQC3ZZ
ØYQC4ZZ
ØYQCXZZ
ØYQDØZZ
ØYQD3ZZ
ØYQD4ZZ
ØYQDXZZ
ØYQFØZZ
ØYQF3ZZ
ØYQF4ZZ
ØYQFXZZ
ØYQGØZZ
ØYQG3ZZ
ØYQG4ZZ
ØYQGXZZ
ØYQHØZZ
ØYQH3ZZ
ØYQH4ZZ
ØYQHXZZ
ØYQJØZZ
ØYQJ3ZZ
ØYQJ4ZZ
ØYQJXZZ
ØYQKØZZ
ØYQK3ZZ
ØYQK4ZZ
ØYQKXZZ
ØYQLØZZ
ØYQL3ZZ
ØYQL4ZZ
ØYQLXZZ
ØYQMØZZ
ØYQM3ZZ
ØYQM4ZZ
ØYQMXZZ
ØYQNØZZ
ØYQN3ZZ
ØYQN4ZZ
ØYQNXZZ
ØYQPØZZ
ØYQP3ZZ
ØYQP4ZZ
ØYQPXZZ
ØYQQØZZ
ØYQQ3ZZ
ØYQQ4ZZ
ØYQQXZZ
ØYQRØZZ
ØYQR3ZZ
ØYQR4ZZ
ØYQRXZZ
ØYQSØZZ
ØYQS3ZZ
ØYQS4ZZ
ØYQSXZZ
ØYQTØZZ
ØYQT3ZZ
ØYQT4ZZ
ØYQTXZZ
ØYQUØZZ
ØYQU3ZZ
ØYQU4ZZ
ØYQUXZZ
ØYQVØZZ
ØYQV3ZZ
ØYQV4ZZ
ØYQVXZZ
ØYQWØZZ
ØYQW3ZZ
ØYQW4ZZ
ØYQWXZZ
ØYQXØZZ
ØYQX3ZZ
ØYQX4ZZ
ØYQXXZZ
ØYQYØZZ
ØYQY3ZZ
ØYQY4ZZ
ØYQYXZZ
XØHK3Q8
XØHQ3R8
X27H385
X27H395
X27H3B5
X27H3C5
X27J385
X27J395
X27J3B5
X27J3C5
X2CP3T7
X2CS3T7
X2CT3T7
X2CY3T7
X2H13R9
X2H2ØR9
X2H3ØR9
X2KB317
X2KC317
X2RXØN7
X2VWØN7
XHRPXF7
XNH6Ø58
XNH6358
XNH7Ø58
XNH7358
XNRLØ99
XNRMØ99
XNSØØ32
XNSØØC7
XNSØ332
XNSØ3C7
XNS3Ø32
XNS3332
XNS4Ø32
XNS4ØC7
XNS4332
XNS43C7
XNUØ356
XNU4356
XRGAØR7
XRGA3R7
XRGA4R7
XRGBØR7
XRGB3R7
XRGB4R7
XRGCØR7
XRGC3R7
XRGC4R7
XRGDØR7
XRGD3R7
XRGD4R7
XRGEØ58
XRGE358
XRGFØ58
XRGF358
XRGJØB9
XRGKØB9
XRGLØB9
XRGMØB9
XRHBØ18
XRHDØ18
XRRGØL8
XRRGØM8
XRRHØL8
XRRHØM8

OR

Nonoperating Room Procedures

Ø2H63JZ
Ø2H73JZ
Ø2HK3JZ
Ø2HL3JZ

DRG 958

Select combinations of MDC 24 diagnoses of significant trauma listed under DRG 963

AND

Select operating room or nonoperating room procedures listed under DRG 957

DRG 959

Select combinations of MDC 24 diagnoses of significant trauma listed under DRG 963

AND

Select operating room or nonoperating room procedures listed under DRG 957

DRG 963

Select principal diagnosis from the Trauma Diagnosis List located below

AND

At least two different diagnoses from two different Significant Trauma Body Site Categories located below

OR

Select a principal diagnosis from one Significant Trauma Body Site Category located below

AND

Two or more significant trauma diagnoses from different Significant Trauma Body Site Categories located below

Trauma Diagnosis

M96.A1
M96.A2
M96.A3
M96.A4
M96.A9
M99.1Ø
M99.11
M99.12
M99.13
M99.14
M99.15
M99.16
M99.17
M99.18
M99.19
SØØ.ØØXA
SØØ.Ø1XA
SØØ.Ø2XA
SØØ.Ø3XA
SØØ.Ø4XA
SØØ.Ø5XA
SØØ.Ø6XA
SØØ.Ø7XA
SØØ.1ØXA
SØØ.11XA
SØØ.12XA
SØØ.2Ø1A
SØØ.2Ø2A
SØØ.2Ø9A
SØØ.211A
SØØ.212A
SØØ.219A
SØØ.221A
SØØ.222A
SØØ.229A
SØØ.241A
SØØ.242A
SØØ.249A
SØØ.251A
SØØ.252A
SØØ.259A
SØØ.261A
SØØ.262A
SØØ.269A
SØØ.271A
SØØ.272A
SØØ.279A
SØØ.3ØXA
SØØ.31XA
SØØ.32XA
SØØ.33XA
SØØ.34XA
SØØ.35XA
SØØ.36XA
SØØ.37XA
SØØ.4Ø1A
SØØ.4Ø2A
SØØ.4Ø9A
SØØ.411A
SØØ.412A
SØØ.419A
SØØ.421A
SØØ.422A
SØØ.429A
SØØ.431A
SØØ.432A
SØØ.439A
SØØ.441A
SØØ.442A
SØØ.449A
SØØ.451A
SØØ.452A
SØØ.459A
SØØ.461A
SØØ.462A
SØØ.469A
SØØ.471A
SØØ.472A
SØØ.479A
SØØ.5Ø1A
SØØ.5Ø2A
SØØ.511A
SØØ.512A
SØØ.521A
SØØ.522A
SØØ.531A
SØØ.532A
SØØ.541A
SØØ.542A
SØØ.551A
SØØ.552A
SØØ.561A
SØØ.562A
SØØ.571A
SØØ.572A
SØØ.8ØXA
SØØ.81XA
SØØ.82XA
SØØ.83XA
SØØ.84XA
SØØ.85XA
SØØ.86XA
SØØ.87XA
SØØ.9ØXA
SØØ.91XA
SØØ.92XA
SØØ.93XA
SØØ.94XA
SØØ.95XA
SØØ.96XA
SØØ.97XA
SØ1.ØØXA
SØ1.Ø1XA
SØ1.Ø2XA
SØ1.Ø3XA
SØ1.Ø4XA
SØ1.Ø5XA
SØ1.1Ø1A
SØ1.1Ø2A
SØ1.1Ø9A
SØ1.111A
SØ1.112A
SØ1.119A
SØ1.121A
SØ1.122A
SØ1.129A
SØ1.131A
SØ1.132A
SØ1.139A
SØ1.141A
SØ1.142A
SØ1.149A
SØ1.151A
SØ1.152A
SØ1.159A
SØ1.2ØXA
SØ1.21XA
SØ1.22XA
SØ1.23XA
SØ1.24XA
SØ1.25XA
SØ1.3Ø1A
SØ1.3Ø2A
SØ1.3Ø9A
SØ1.311A
SØ1.312A
SØ1.319A
SØ1.321A
SØ1.322A
SØ1.329A
SØ1.331A
SØ1.332A
SØ1.339A
SØ1.341A
SØ1.342A
SØ1.349A
SØ1.351A
SØ1.352A
SØ1.359A
SØ1.4Ø1A
SØ1.4Ø2A
SØ1.4Ø9A
SØ1.411A
SØ1.412A
SØ1.419A
SØ1.421A
SØ1.422A
SØ1.429A
SØ1.431A
SØ1.432A
SØ1.439A
SØ1.441A
SØ1.442A
SØ1.449A
SØ1.451A
SØ1.452A
SØ1.459A
SØ1.5Ø1A
SØ1.5Ø2A
SØ1.511A
SØ1.512A
SØ1.521A
SØ1.522A
SØ1.531A
SØ1.532A
SØ1.541A
SØ1.542A
SØ1.551A
SØ1.552A
SØ1.8ØXA
SØ1.81XA
SØ1.82XA
SØ1.83XA
SØ1.84XA
SØ1.85XA
SØ1.9ØXA
SØ1.91XA
SØ1.92XA
SØ1.93XA
SØ1.94XA
SØ1.95XA
SØ2.ØXXA
SØ2.ØXXB
SØ2.1Ø1A
SØ2.1Ø1B
SØ2.1Ø2A
SØ2.1Ø2B
SØ2.1Ø9A
SØ2.1Ø9B
SØ2.11ØA
SØ2.11ØB
SØ2.111A
SØ2.111B
SØ2.112A
SØ2.112B
SØ2.113A
SØ2.113B
SØ2.118A
SØ2.118B
SØ2.119A
SØ2.119B
SØ2.11AA
SØ2.11AB
SØ2.11BA
SØ2.11BB
SØ2.11CA
SØ2.11CB
SØ2.11DA
SØ2.11DB
SØ2.11EA
SØ2.11EB
SØ2.11FA
SØ2.11FB
SØ2.11GA
SØ2.11GB
SØ2.11HA
SØ2.11HB
SØ2.121A
SØ2.121B
SØ2.122A
SØ2.122B
SØ2.129A
SØ2.129B
SØ2.19XA
SØ2.19XB
SØ2.2XXA
SØ2.2XXB
SØ2.3ØXA
SØ2.3ØXB
SØ2.31XA
SØ2.31XB
SØ2.32XA
SØ2.32XB
SØ2.4ØØA
SØ2.4ØØB
SØ2.4Ø1A
SØ2.4Ø1B
SØ2.4Ø2A
SØ2.4Ø2B
SØ2.4ØAA
SØ2.4ØAB
SØ2.4ØBA
SØ2.4ØBB
SØ2.4ØCA
SØ2.4ØCB
SØ2.4ØDA
SØ2.4ØDB
SØ2.4ØEA
SØ2.4ØEB
SØ2.4ØFA
SØ2.4ØFB
SØ2.411A
SØ2.411B
SØ2.412A
SØ2.412B
SØ2.413A
SØ2.413B
SØ2.42XA
SØ2.42XB
SØ2.5XXA
SØ2.5XXB
SØ2.6ØØA
SØ2.6ØØB
SØ2.6Ø1A
SØ2.6Ø1B
SØ2.6Ø2A
SØ2.6Ø2B
SØ2.6Ø9A
SØ2.6Ø9B
SØ2.61ØA
SØ2.61ØB
SØ2.611A
SØ2.611B
SØ2.612A
SØ2.612B
SØ2.62ØA
SØ2.62ØB
SØ2.621A
SØ2.621B
SØ2.622A
SØ2.622B
SØ2.63ØA
SØ2.63ØB
SØ2.631A
SØ2.631B
SØ2.632A
SØ2.632B
SØ2.64ØA
SØ2.64ØB
SØ2.641A
SØ2.641B
SØ2.642A
SØ2.642B
SØ2.65ØA
SØ2.65ØB
SØ2.651A
SØ2.651B
SØ2.652A
SØ2.652B
SØ2.66XA
SØ2.66XB
SØ2.67ØA
SØ2.67ØB
SØ2.671A
SØ2.671B
SØ2.672A
SØ2.672B
SØ2.69XA
SØ2.69XB
SØ2.8ØXA
SØ2.8ØXB
SØ2.81XA
SØ2.81XB
SØ2.82XA
SØ2.82XB
SØ2.831A
SØ2.831B
SØ2.832A
SØ2.832B
SØ2.839A
SØ2.839B
SØ2.841A
SØ2.841B
SØ2.842A
SØ2.842B
SØ2.849A
SØ2.849B
SØ2.85XA
SØ2.85XB
SØ2.91XA
SØ2.91XB
SØ2.92XA
SØ2.92XB
SØ3.ØØXA
SØ3.Ø1XA
SØ3.Ø2XA
SØ3.Ø3XA
SØ3.1XXA
SØ3.2XXA
SØ3.4ØXA
SØ3.41XA
SØ3.42XA
SØ3.43XA
SØ3.8XXA
SØ3.9XXA
SØ4.Ø11A
SØ4.Ø12A
SØ4.Ø19A
SØ4.Ø2XA
SØ4.Ø31A
SØ4.Ø32A
SØ4.Ø39A
SØ4.Ø41A
SØ4.Ø42A
SØ4.Ø49A
SØ4.1ØXA
SØ4.11XA
SØ4.12XA
SØ4.2ØXA
SØ4.21XA
SØ4.22XA
SØ4.3ØXA
SØ4.31XA
SØ4.32XA
SØ4.4ØXA
SØ4.41XA
SØ4.42XA
SØ4.5ØXA
SØ4.51XA
SØ4.52XA
SØ4.6ØXA
SØ4.61XA
SØ4.62XA
SØ4.7ØXA
SØ4.71XA
SØ4.72XA
SØ4.811A
SØ4.812A
SØ4.819A
SØ4.891A
SØ4.892A
SØ4.899A
SØ4.9XXA
SØ5.ØØXA
SØ5.Ø1XA
SØ5.Ø2XA
SØ5.1ØXA
SØ5.11XA
SØ5.12XA
SØ5.2ØXA
SØ5.21XA
SØ5.22XA
SØ5.3ØXA
SØ5.31XA
SØ5.32XA
SØ5.4ØXA
SØ5.41XA
SØ5.42XA
SØ5.5ØXA
SØ5.51XA
SØ5.52XA
SØ5.6ØXA
SØ5.61XA
SØ5.62XA
SØ5.7ØXA
SØ5.71XA
SØ5.72XA
SØ5.8X1A
SØ5.8X2A
SØ5.8X9A
SØ5.9ØXA
SØ5.91XA
SØ5.92XA
SØ6.ØXØA
SØ6.ØX1A
SØ6.ØX9A
SØ6.ØXAA
SØ6.1XØA
SØ6.1X1A
SØ6.1X2A
SØ6.1X3A
SØ6.1X4A
SØ6.1X5A
SØ6.1X6A
SØ6.1X7A
SØ6.1X8A
SØ6.1X9A
SØ6.1XAA
SØ6.2XØA
SØ6.2X1A
SØ6.2X2A
SØ6.2X3A
SØ6.2X4A
SØ6.2X5A
SØ6.2X6A
SØ6.2X7A
SØ6.2X8A
SØ6.2X9A
SØ6.2XAA
SØ6.3ØØA
SØ6.3Ø1A
SØ6.3Ø2A
SØ6.3Ø3A
SØ6.3Ø4A
SØ6.3Ø5A
SØ6.3Ø6A
SØ6.3Ø7A
SØ6.3Ø8A
SØ6.3Ø9A
SØ6.3ØAA
SØ6.31ØA
SØ6.311A
SØ6.312A
SØ6.313A
SØ6.314A
SØ6.315A
SØ6.316A
SØ6.317A
SØ6.318A
SØ6.319A
SØ6.31AA
SØ6.32ØA
SØ6.321A
SØ6.322A
SØ6.323A
SØ6.324A
SØ6.325A
SØ6.326A
SØ6.327A
SØ6.328A
SØ6.329A
SØ6.32AA
SØ6.33ØA
SØ6.331A
SØ6.332A
SØ6.333A
SØ6.334A
SØ6.335A
SØ6.336A
SØ6.337A
SØ6.338A
SØ6.339A
SØ6.33AA
SØ6.34ØA
SØ6.341A
SØ6.342A
SØ6.343A
SØ6.344A
SØ6.345A
SØ6.346A
SØ6.347A
SØ6.348A
SØ6.349A
SØ6.34AA
SØ6.35ØA
SØ6.351A
SØ6.352A
SØ6.353A
SØ6.354A
SØ6.355A
SØ6.356A
SØ6.357A
SØ6.358A

S06.359A
S06.35AA
S06.360A
S06.361A
S06.362A
S06.363A
S06.364A
S06.365A
S06.366A
S06.367A
S06.368A
S06.369A
S06.36AA
S06.370A
S06.371A
S06.372A
S06.373A
S06.374A
S06.375A
S06.376A
S06.377A
S06.378A
S06.379A
S06.37AA
S06.380A
S06.381A
S06.382A
S06.383A
S06.384A
S06.385A
S06.386A
S06.387A
S06.388A
S06.389A
S06.38AA
S06.4X0A
S06.4X1A
S06.4X2A
S06.4X3A
S06.4X4A
S06.4X5A
S06.4X6A
S06.4X7A
S06.4X8A
S06.4X9A
S06.4XAA
S06.5X0A
S06.5X1A
S06.5X2A
S06.5X3A
S06.5X4A
S06.5X5A
S06.5X6A
S06.5X7A
S06.5X8A
S06.5X9A
S06.5XAA
S06.6X0A
S06.6X1A
S06.6X2A
S06.6X3A
S06.6X4A
S06.6X5A
S06.6X6A
S06.6X7A
S06.6X8A
S06.6X9A
S06.6XAA
S06.810A
S06.811A
S06.812A
S06.813A
S06.814A
S06.815A
S06.816A
S06.817A
S06.818A
S06.819A
S06.81AA
S06.820A
S06.821A
S06.822A
S06.823A
S06.824A
S06.825A
S06.826A
S06.827A
S06.828A
S06.829A
S06.82AA
S06.890A
S06.891A
S06.892A
S06.893A
S06.894A
S06.895A
S06.896A
S06.897A
S06.898A
S06.899A
S06.89AA
S06.8A0A
S06.8A1A
S06.8A2A
S06.8A3A
S06.8A4A
S06.8A5A
S06.8A6A
S06.8A7A
S06.8A8A
S06.8A9A
S06.8AAA
S06.9X0A
S06.9X1A
S06.9X2A
S06.9X3A
S06.9X4A
S06.9X5A
S06.9X6A
S06.9X7A
S06.9X8A
S06.9X9A
S06.9XAA
S06.A0XA
S06.A1XA
S07.0XXA
S07.1XXA
S07.8XXA
S07.9XXA
S08.0XXA
S08.111A
S08.112A
S08.119A
S08.121A
S08.122A
S08.129A
S08.811A
S08.812A
S08.89XA
S09.0XXA
S09.10XA
S09.11XA
S09.12XA
S09.19XA
S09.20XA
S09.21XA
S09.22XA
S09.301A
S09.302A
S09.309A
S09.311A
S09.312A
S09.313A
S09.319A
S09.391A
S09.392A
S09.399A
S09.8XXA
S09.90XA
S09.91XA
S09.92XA
S09.93XA
S10.0XXA
S10.10XA
S10.11XA
S10.12XA
S10.14XA
S10.15XA
S10.16XA
S10.17XA
S10.80XA
S10.81XA
S10.82XA
S10.83XA
S10.84XA
S10.85XA
S10.86XA
S10.87XA
S10.90XA
S10.91XA
S10.92XA
S10.93XA
S10.94XA
S10.95XA
S10.96XA
S10.97XA
S11.011A
S11.012A
S11.013A
S11.014A
S11.015A
S11.019A
S11.021A
S11.022A
S11.023A
S11.024A
S11.025A
S11.029A
S11.031A
S11.032A
S11.033A
S11.034A
S11.035A
S11.039A
S11.10XA
S11.11XA
S11.12XA
S11.13XA
S11.14XA
S11.15XA
S11.20XA
S11.21XA
S11.22XA
S11.23XA
S11.24XA
S11.25XA
S11.80XA
S11.81XA
S11.82XA
S11.83XA
S11.84XA
S11.85XA
S11.89XA
S11.90XA
S11.91XA
S11.92XA
S11.93XA
S11.94XA
S11.95XA
S12.000A
S12.000B
S12.001A
S12.001B
S12.01XA
S12.01XB
S12.02XA
S12.02XB
S12.030A
S12.030B
S12.031A
S12.031B
S12.040A
S12.040B
S12.041A
S12.041B
S12.090A
S12.090B
S12.091A
S12.091B
S12.100A
S12.100B
S12.101A
S12.101B
S12.110A
S12.110B
S12.111A
S12.111B
S12.112A
S12.112B
S12.120A
S12.120B
S12.121A
S12.121B
S12.130A
S12.130B
S12.131A
S12.131B
S12.14XA
S12.14XB
S12.150A
S12.150B
S12.151A
S12.151B
S12.190A
S12.190B
S12.191A
S12.191B
S12.200A
S12.200B
S12.201A
S12.201B
S12.230A
S12.230B
S12.231A
S12.231B
S12.24XA
S12.24XB
S12.250A
S12.250B
S12.251A
S12.251B
S12.290A
S12.290B
S12.291A
S12.291B
S12.300A
S12.300B
S12.301A
S12.301B
S12.330A
S12.330B
S12.331A
S12.331B
S12.34XA
S12.34XB
S12.350A
S12.350B
S12.351A
S12.351B
S12.390A
S12.390B
S12.391A
S12.391B
S12.400A
S12.400B
S12.401A
S12.401B
S12.430A
S12.430B
S12.431A
S12.431B
S12.44XA
S12.44XB
S12.450A
S12.450B
S12.451A
S12.451B
S12.490A
S12.490B
S12.491A
S12.491B
S12.500A
S12.500B
S12.501A
S12.501B
S12.530A
S12.530B
S12.531A
S12.531B
S12.54XA
S12.54XB
S12.550A
S12.550B
S12.551A
S12.551B
S12.590A
S12.590B
S12.591A
S12.591B
S12.600A
S12.600B
S12.601A
S12.601B
S12.630A
S12.630B
S12.631A
S12.631B
S12.64XA
S12.64XB
S12.650A
S12.650B
S12.651A
S12.651B
S12.690A
S12.690B
S12.691A
S12.691B
S12.8XXA
S12.9XXA
S13.0XXA
S13.100A
S13.101A
S13.110A
S13.111A
S13.120A
S13.121A
S13.130A
S13.131A
S13.140A
S13.141A
S13.150A
S13.151A
S13.160A
S13.161A
S13.170A
S13.171A
S13.180A
S13.181A
S13.20XA
S13.29XA
S13.4XXA
S13.5XXA
S13.8XXA
S13.9XXA
S14.0XXA
S14.101A
S14.102A
S14.103A
S14.104A
S14.105A
S14.106A
S14.107A
S14.108A
S14.109A
S14.111A
S14.112A
S14.113A
S14.114A
S14.115A
S14.116A
S14.117A
S14.118A
S14.119A
S14.121A
S14.122A
S14.123A
S14.124A
S14.125A
S14.126A
S14.127A
S14.128A
S14.129A
S14.131A
S14.132A
S14.133A
S14.134A
S14.135A
S14.136A
S14.137A
S14.138A
S14.139A
S14.141A
S14.142A
S14.143A
S14.144A
S14.145A
S14.146A
S14.147A
S14.148A
S14.149A
S14.151A
S14.152A
S14.153A
S14.154A
S14.155A
S14.156A
S14.157A
S14.158A
S14.159A
S14.2XXA
S14.3XXA
S14.4XXA
S14.5XXA
S14.8XXA
S14.9XXA
S15.001A
S15.002A
S15.009A
S15.011A
S15.012A
S15.019A
S15.021A
S15.022A
S15.029A
S15.091A
S15.092A
S15.099A
S15.101A
S15.102A
S15.109A
S15.111A
S15.112A
S15.119A
S15.121A
S15.122A
S15.129A
S15.191A
S15.192A
S15.199A
S15.201A
S15.202A
S15.209A
S15.211A
S15.212A
S15.219A
S15.221A
S15.222A
S15.229A
S15.291A
S15.292A
S15.299A
S15.301A
S15.302A
S15.309A
S15.311A
S15.312A
S15.319A
S15.321A
S15.322A
S15.329A
S15.391A
S15.392A
S15.399A
S15.8XXA
S15.9XXA
S16.1XXA
S16.2XXA
S16.8XXA
S16.9XXA
S17.0XXA
S17.8XXA
S17.9XXA
S19.80XA
S19.81XA
S19.82XA
S19.83XA
S19.84XA
S19.85XA
S19.89XA
S19.9XXA
S20.00XA
S20.01XA
S20.02XA
S20.101A
S20.102A
S20.109A
S20.111A
S20.112A
S20.119A
S20.121A
S20.122A
S20.129A
S20.141A
S20.142A
S20.149A
S20.151A
S20.152A
S20.159A
S20.161A
S20.162A
S20.169A
S20.171A
S20.172A
S20.179A
S20.20XA
S20.211A
S20.212A
S20.213A
S20.214A
S20.219A
S20.221A
S20.222A
S20.223A
S20.224A
S20.229A
S20.301A
S20.302A
S20.303A
S20.304A
S20.309A
S20.311A
S20.312A
S20.313A
S20.314A
S20.319A
S20.321A
S20.322A
S20.323A
S20.324A
S20.329A
S20.341A
S20.342A
S20.343A
S20.344A
S20.349A
S20.351A
S20.352A
S20.353A
S20.354A
S20.359A
S20.361A
S20.362A
S20.363A
S20.364A
S20.369A
S20.371A
S20.372A
S20.373A
S20.374A
S20.379A
S20.401A
S20.402A
S20.409A
S20.411A
S20.412A
S20.419A
S20.421A
S20.422A
S20.429A
S20.441A
S20.442A
S20.449A
S20.451A
S20.452A
S20.459A
S20.461A
S20.462A
S20.469A
S20.471A
S20.472A
S20.479A
S20.90XA
S20.91XA
S20.92XA
S20.94XA
S20.95XA
S20.96XA
S20.97XA
S21.001A
S21.002A
S21.009A
S21.011A
S21.012A
S21.019A
S21.021A
S21.022A
S21.029A
S21.031A
S21.032A
S21.039A
S21.041A
S21.042A
S21.049A
S21.051A
S21.052A
S21.059A
S21.101A
S21.102A
S21.109A
S21.111A
S21.112A
S21.119A
S21.121A
S21.122A
S21.129A
S21.131A
S21.132A
S21.139A
S21.141A
S21.142A
S21.149A
S21.151A
S21.152A
S21.159A
S21.201A
S21.202A
S21.209A
S21.211A
S21.212A
S21.219A
S21.221A
S21.222A
S21.229A
S21.231A
S21.232A
S21.239A
S21.241A
S21.242A
S21.249A
S21.251A
S21.252A
S21.259A
S21.301A
S21.302A
S21.309A
S21.311A
S21.312A
S21.319A
S21.321A
S21.322A
S21.329A
S21.331A
S21.332A
S21.339A
S21.341A
S21.342A
S21.349A
S21.351A
S21.352A
S21.359A
S21.401A
S21.402A
S21.409A
S21.411A
S21.412A
S21.419A
S21.421A
S21.422A
S21.429A
S21.431A
S21.432A
S21.439A
S21.441A
S21.442A
S21.449A
S21.451A
S21.452A
S21.459A
S21.90XA
S21.91XA
S21.92XA
S21.93XA
S21.94XA
S21.95XA
S22.000A
S22.000B
S22.001A
S22.001B
S22.002A
S22.002B
S22.008A
S22.008B
S22.009A
S22.009B
S22.010A
S22.010B
S22.011A
S22.011B
S22.012A
S22.012B
S22.018A
S22.018B
S22.019A
S22.019B
S22.020A
S22.020B
S22.021A
S22.021B
S22.022A
S22.022B
S22.028A
S22.028B
S22.029A
S22.029B
S22.030A
S22.030B
S22.031A
S22.031B
S22.032A
S22.032B
S22.038A
S22.038B
S22.039A
S22.039B
S22.040A
S22.040B
S22.041A
S22.041B
S22.042A
S22.042B
S22.048A
S22.048B
S22.049A
S22.049B
S22.050A
S22.050B
S22.051A
S22.051B
S22.052A
S22.052B
S22.058A
S22.058B
S22.059A
S22.059B
S22.060A
S22.060B
S22.061A
S22.061B
S22.062A
S22.062B
S22.068A
S22.068B
S22.069A
S22.069B
S22.070A
S22.070B
S22.071A
S22.071B
S22.072A
S22.072B
S22.078A
S22.078B
S22.079A
S22.079B
S22.080A
S22.080B
S22.081A
S22.081B
S22.082A
S22.082B
S22.088A
S22.088B
S22.089A
S22.089B
S22.20XA
S22.20XB
S22.21XA
S22.21XB
S22.22XA
S22.22XB
S22.23XA
S22.23XB
S22.24XA
S22.24XB
S22.31XA
S22.31XB
S22.32XA
S22.32XB
S22.39XA
S22.39XB
S22.41XA
S22.41XB
S22.42XA
S22.42XB
S22.43XA
S22.43XB
S22.49XA
S22.49XB
S22.5XXA
S22.5XXB
S22.9XXA
S22.9XXB
S23.0XXA
S23.100A
S23.101A
S23.110A
S23.111A
S23.120A
S23.121A
S23.122A
S23.123A
S23.130A
S23.131A
S23.132A
S23.133A
S23.140A
S23.141A
S23.142A
S23.143A
S23.150A
S23.151A
S23.152A
S23.153A
S23.160A
S23.161A

S23.162A
S23.163A
S23.170A
S23.171A
S23.20XA
S23.29XA
S23.3XXA
S23.41XA
S23.420A
S23.421A
S23.428A
S23.429A
S23.8XXA
S23.9XXA
S24.0XXA
S24.101A
S24.102A
S24.103A
S24.104A
S24.109A
S24.111A
S24.112A
S24.113A
S24.114A
S24.119A
S24.131A
S24.132A
S24.133A
S24.134A
S24.139A
S24.141A
S24.142A
S24.143A
S24.144A
S24.149A
S24.151A
S24.152A
S24.153A
S24.154A
S24.159A
S24.2XXA
S24.3XXA
S24.4XXA
S24.8XXA
S24.9XXA
S25.00XA
S25.01XA
S25.02XA
S25.09XA
S25.101A
S25.102A
S25.109A
S25.111A
S25.112A
S25.119A
S25.121A
S25.122A
S25.129A
S25.191A
S25.192A
S25.199A
S25.20XA
S25.21XA
S25.22XA
S25.29XA
S25.301A
S25.302A
S25.309A
S25.311A
S25.312A
S25.319A
S25.321A
S25.322A
S25.329A
S25.391A
S25.392A
S25.399A
S25.401A
S25.402A
S25.409A
S25.411A
S25.412A
S25.419A
S25.421A
S25.422A
S25.429A
S25.491A
S25.492A
S25.499A
S25.501A
S25.502A
S25.509A
S25.511A
S25.512A
S25.519A
S25.591A
S25.592A
S25.599A
S25.801A
S25.802A
S25.809A
S25.811A
S25.812A
S25.819A
S25.891A
S25.892A
S25.899A
S25.90XA
S25.91XA
S25.99XA
S26.00XA
S26.01XA
S26.020A
S26.021A
S26.022A
S26.09XA
S26.10XA
S26.11XA
S26.12XA
S26.19XA
S26.90XA
S26.91XA
S26.92XA
S26.99XA
S27.0XXA
S27.1XXA
S27.2XXA
S27.301A
S27.302A
S27.309A
S27.311A
S27.312A
S27.319A
S27.321A
S27.322A
S27.329A
S27.331A
S27.332A
S27.339A
S27.391A
S27.392A
S27.399A
S27.401A
S27.402A
S27.409A
S27.411A
S27.412A
S27.419A
S27.421A
S27.422A
S27.429A
S27.431A
S27.432A
S27.439A
S27.491A
S27.492A
S27.499A
S27.50XA
S27.51XA
S27.52XA
S27.53XA
S27.59XA
S27.60XA
S27.63XA
S27.69XA
S27.802A
S27.803A
S27.808A
S27.809A
S27.812A
S27.813A
S27.818A
S27.819A
S27.892A
S27.893A
S27.898A
S27.899A
S27.9XXA
S28.0XXA
S28.1XXA
S28.211A
S28.212A
S28.219A
S28.221A
S28.222A
S28.229A
S29.001A
S29.002A
S29.009A
S29.011A
S29.012A
S29.019A
S29.021A
S29.022A
S29.029A
S29.091A
S29.092A
S29.099A
S29.8XXA
S29.9XXA
S30.0XXA
S30.1XXA
S30.201A
S30.202A
S30.21XA
S30.22XA
S30.23XA
S30.3XXA
S30.810A
S30.811A
S30.812A
S30.813A
S30.814A
S30.815A
S30.816A
S30.817A
S30.820A
S30.821A
S30.822A
S30.823A
S30.824A
S30.825A
S30.826A
S30.827A
S30.840A
S30.841A
S30.842A
S30.843A
S30.844A
S30.845A
S30.846A
S30.850A
S30.851A
S30.852A
S30.853A
S30.854A
S30.855A
S30.856A
S30.857A
S30.860A
S30.861A
S30.862A
S30.863A
S30.864A
S30.865A
S30.866A
S30.867A
S30.870A
S30.871A
S30.872A
S30.873A
S30.874A
S30.875A
S30.876A
S30.877A
S30.91XA
S30.92XA
S30.93XA
S30.94XA
S30.95XA
S30.96XA
S30.97XA
S30.98XA
S31.000A
S31.001A
S31.010A
S31.011A
S31.020A
S31.021A
S31.030A
S31.031A
S31.040A
S31.041A
S31.050A
S31.051A
S31.100A
S31.101A
S31.102A
S31.103A
S31.104A
S31.105A
S31.109A
S31.110A
S31.111A
S31.112A
S31.113A
S31.114A
S31.115A
S31.119A
S31.120A
S31.121A
S31.122A
S31.123A
S31.124A
S31.125A
S31.129A
S31.130A
S31.131A
S31.132A
S31.133A
S31.134A
S31.135A
S31.139A
S31.140A
S31.141A
S31.142A
S31.143A
S31.144A
S31.145A
S31.149A
S31.150A
S31.151A
S31.152A
S31.153A
S31.154A
S31.155A
S31.159A
S31.20XA
S31.21XA
S31.22XA
S31.23XA
S31.24XA
S31.25XA
S31.30XA
S31.31XA
S31.32XA
S31.33XA
S31.34XA
S31.35XA
S31.40XA
S31.41XA
S31.42XA
S31.43XA
S31.44XA
S31.45XA
S31.501A
S31.502A
S31.511A
S31.512A
S31.521A
S31.522A
S31.531A
S31.532A
S31.541A
S31.542A
S31.551A
S31.552A
S31.600A
S31.601A
S31.602A
S31.603A
S31.604A
S31.605A
S31.609A
S31.610A
S31.611A
S31.612A
S31.613A
S31.614A
S31.615A
S31.619A
S31.620A
S31.621A
S31.622A
S31.623A
S31.624A
S31.625A
S31.629A
S31.630A
S31.631A
S31.632A
S31.633A
S31.634A
S31.635A
S31.639A
S31.640A
S31.641A
S31.642A
S31.643A
S31.644A
S31.645A
S31.649A
S31.650A
S31.651A
S31.652A
S31.653A
S31.654A
S31.655A
S31.659A
S31.801A
S31.802A
S31.803A
S31.804A
S31.805A
S31.809A
S31.811A
S31.812A
S31.813A
S31.814A
S31.815A
S31.819A
S31.821A
S31.822A
S31.823A
S31.824A
S31.825A
S31.829A
S31.831A
S31.832A
S31.833A
S31.834A
S31.835A
S31.839A
S32.000A
S32.000B
S32.001A
S32.001B
S32.002A
S32.002B
S32.008A
S32.008B
S32.009A
S32.009B
S32.010A
S32.010B
S32.011A
S32.011B
S32.012A
S32.012B
S32.018A
S32.018B
S32.019A
S32.019B
S32.020A
S32.020B
S32.021A
S32.021B
S32.022A
S32.022B
S32.028A
S32.028B
S32.029A
S32.029B
S32.030A
S32.030B
S32.031A
S32.031B
S32.032A
S32.032B
S32.038A
S32.038B
S32.039A
S32.039B
S32.040A
S32.040B
S32.041A
S32.041B
S32.042A
S32.042B
S32.048A
S32.048B
S32.049A
S32.049B
S32.050A
S32.050B
S32.051A
S32.051B
S32.052A
S32.052B
S32.058A
S32.058B
S32.059A
S32.059B
S32.10XA
S32.10XB
S32.110A
S32.110B
S32.111A
S32.111B
S32.112A
S32.112B
S32.119A
S32.119B
S32.120A
S32.120B
S32.121A
S32.121B
S32.122A
S32.122B
S32.129A
S32.129B
S32.130A
S32.130B
S32.131A
S32.131B
S32.132A
S32.132B
S32.139A
S32.139B
S32.14XA
S32.14XB
S32.15XA
S32.15XB
S32.16XA
S32.16XB
S32.17XA
S32.17XB
S32.19XA
S32.19XB
S32.2XXA
S32.2XXB
S32.301A
S32.301B
S32.302A
S32.302B
S32.309A
S32.309B
S32.311A
S32.311B
S32.312A
S32.312B
S32.313A
S32.313B
S32.314A
S32.314B
S32.315A
S32.315B
S32.316A
S32.316B
S32.391A
S32.391B
S32.392A
S32.392B
S32.399A
S32.399B
S32.401A
S32.401B
S32.402A
S32.402B
S32.409A
S32.409B
S32.411A
S32.411B
S32.412A
S32.412B
S32.413A
S32.413B
S32.414A
S32.414B
S32.415A
S32.415B
S32.416A
S32.416B
S32.421A
S32.421B
S32.422A
S32.422B
S32.423A
S32.423B
S32.424A
S32.424B
S32.425A
S32.425B
S32.426A
S32.426B
S32.431A
S32.431B
S32.432A
S32.432B
S32.433A
S32.433B
S32.434A
S32.434B
S32.435A
S32.435B
S32.436A
S32.436B
S32.441A
S32.441B
S32.442A
S32.442B
S32.443A
S32.443B
S32.444A
S32.444B
S32.445A
S32.445B
S32.446A
S32.446B
S32.451A
S32.451B
S32.452A
S32.452B
S32.453A
S32.453B
S32.454A
S32.454B
S32.455A
S32.455B
S32.456A
S32.456B
S32.461A
S32.461B
S32.462A
S32.462B
S32.463A
S32.463B
S32.464A
S32.464B
S32.465A
S32.465B
S32.466A
S32.466B
S32.471A
S32.471B
S32.472A
S32.472B
S32.473A
S32.473B
S32.474A
S32.474B
S32.475A
S32.475B
S32.476A
S32.476B
S32.481A
S32.481B
S32.482A
S32.482B
S32.483A
S32.483B
S32.484A
S32.484B
S32.485A
S32.485B
S32.486A
S32.486B
S32.491A
S32.491B
S32.492A
S32.492B
S32.499A
S32.499B
S32.501A
S32.501B
S32.502A
S32.502B
S32.509A
S32.509B
S32.511A
S32.511B
S32.512A
S32.512B
S32.519A
S32.519B
S32.591A
S32.591B
S32.592A
S32.592B
S32.599A
S32.599B
S32.601A
S32.601B
S32.602A
S32.602B
S32.609A
S32.609B
S32.611A
S32.611B
S32.612A
S32.612B
S32.613A
S32.613B
S32.614A
S32.614B
S32.615A
S32.615B
S32.616A
S32.616B
S32.691A
S32.691B
S32.692A
S32.692B
S32.699A
S32.699B
S32.810A
S32.810B
S32.811A
S32.811B
S32.82XA
S32.82XB
S32.89XA
S32.89XB
S32.9XXA
S32.9XXB
S33.0XXA
S33.100A
S33.101A
S33.110A
S33.111A
S33.120A
S33.121A
S33.130A
S33.131A
S33.140A
S33.141A
S33.2XXA
S33.30XA
S33.39XA
S33.4XXA
S33.5XXA
S33.6XXA
S33.8XXA
S33.9XXA
S34.01XA
S34.02XA
S34.101A
S34.102A
S34.103A
S34.104A
S34.105A
S34.109A
S34.111A
S34.112A
S34.113A
S34.114A
S34.115A
S34.119A
S34.121A
S34.122A
S34.123A
S34.124A
S34.125A
S34.129A
S34.131A
S34.132A
S34.139A
S34.21XA
S34.22XA
S34.3XXA
S34.4XXA
S34.5XXA
S34.6XXA
S34.8XXA
S34.9XXA
S35.00XA
S35.01XA
S35.02XA
S35.09XA
S35.10XA
S35.11XA
S35.12XA
S35.19XA
S35.211A
S35.212A
S35.218A
S35.219A
S35.221A
S35.222A
S35.228A
S35.229A
S35.231A
S35.232A
S35.238A
S35.239A
S35.291A
S35.292A
S35.298A
S35.299A
S35.311A
S35.318A
S35.319A
S35.321A
S35.328A
S35.329A
S35.331A
S35.338A
S35.339A
S35.341A
S35.348A
S35.349A
S35.401A
S35.402A
S35.403A
S35.404A
S35.405A
S35.406A
S35.411A
S35.412A
S35.413A
S35.414A
S35.415A
S35.416A
S35.491A
S35.492A
S35.493A
S35.494A
S35.495A
S35.496A
S35.50XA
S35.511A
S35.512A
S35.513A
S35.514A
S35.515A
S35.516A
S35.531A
S35.532A
S35.533A
S35.534A
S35.535A
S35.536A
S35.59XA
S35.8X1A
S35.8X8A
S35.8X9A
S35.90XA
S35.91XA
S35.99XA
S36.00XA
S36.020A
S36.021A
S36.029A
S36.030A
S36.031A
S36.032A
S36.039A
S36.09XA
S36.112A
S36.113A
S36.114A
S36.115A
S36.116A
S36.118A
S36.119A
S36.122A
S36.123A
S36.128A
S36.129A
S36.13XA
S36.200A
S36.201A
S36.202A
S36.209A
S36.220A
S36.221A
S36.222A
S36.229A
S36.230A
S36.231A
S36.232A
S36.239A
S36.240A
S36.241A
S36.242A

S36.249A
S36.250A
S36.251A
S36.252A
S36.259A
S36.260A
S36.261A
S36.262A
S36.269A
S36.290A
S36.291A
S36.292A
S36.299A
S36.30XA
S36.32XA
S36.33XA
S36.39XA
S36.400A
S36.408A
S36.409A
S36.410A
S36.418A
S36.419A
S36.420A
S36.428A
S36.429A
S36.430A
S36.438A
S36.439A
S36.490A
S36.498A
S36.499A
S36.500A
S36.501A
S36.502A
S36.503A
S36.508A
S36.509A
S36.510A
S36.511A
S36.512A
S36.513A
S36.518A
S36.519A
S36.520A
S36.521A
S36.522A
S36.523A
S36.528A
S36.529A
S36.530A
S36.531A
S36.532A
S36.533A
S36.538A
S36.539A
S36.590A
S36.591A
S36.592A
S36.593A
S36.598A
S36.599A
S36.60XA
S36.61XA
S36.62XA
S36.63XA
S36.69XA
S36.81XA
S36.892A
S36.893A
S36.898A
S36.899A
S36.90XA
S36.92XA
S36.93XA
S36.99XA
S37.001A
S37.002A
S37.009A
S37.011A
S37.012A
S37.019A
S37.021A
S37.022A
S37.029A
S37.031A
S37.032A
S37.039A
S37.041A
S37.042A
S37.049A
S37.051A
S37.052A
S37.059A
S37.061A
S37.062A
S37.069A
S37.091A
S37.092A
S37.099A
S37.10XA
S37.12XA
S37.13XA
S37.19XA
S37.20XA
S37.22XA
S37.23XA
S37.29XA
S37.30XA
S37.32XA
S37.33XA
S37.39XA
S37.60XA
S37.62XA
S37.63XA
S37.69XA
S37.812A
S37.813A
S37.818A
S37.819A
S37.892A
S37.893A
S37.898A
S37.899A
S37.90XA
S37.92XA
S37.93XA
S37.99XA
S38.001A
S38.002A
S38.01XA
S38.02XA
S38.03XA
S38.1XXA
S38.211A
S38.212A
S38.221A
S38.222A
S38.231A
S38.232A
S38.3XXA
S39.001A
S39.002A
S39.003A
S39.011A
S39.012A
S39.013A
S39.021A
S39.022A
S39.023A
S39.091A
S39.092A
S39.093A
S39.81XA
S39.82XA
S39.83XA
S39.840A
S39.848A
S39.91XA
S39.92XA
S39.93XA
S39.94XA
S40.011A
S40.012A
S40.019A
S40.021A
S40.022A
S40.029A
S40.211A
S40.212A
S40.219A
S40.221A
S40.222A
S40.229A
S40.241A
S40.242A
S40.249A
S40.251A
S40.252A
S40.259A
S40.261A
S40.262A
S40.269A
S40.271A
S40.272A
S40.279A
S40.811A
S40.812A
S40.819A
S40.821A
S40.822A
S40.829A
S40.841A
S40.842A
S40.849A
S40.851A
S40.852A
S40.859A
S40.861A
S40.862A
S40.869A
S40.871A
S40.872A
S40.879A
S40.911A
S40.912A
S40.919A
S40.921A
S40.922A
S40.929A
S41.001A
S41.002A
S41.009A
S41.011A
S41.012A
S41.019A
S41.021A
S41.022A
S41.029A
S41.031A
S41.032A
S41.039A
S41.041A
S41.042A
S41.049A
S41.051A
S41.052A
S41.059A
S41.101A
S41.102A
S41.109A
S41.111A
S41.112A
S41.119A
S41.121A
S41.122A
S41.129A
S41.131A
S41.132A
S41.139A
S41.141A
S41.142A
S41.149A
S41.151A
S41.152A
S41.159A
S42.001A
S42.001B
S42.002A
S42.002B
S42.009A
S42.009B
S42.011A
S42.011B
S42.012A
S42.012B
S42.013A
S42.013B
S42.014A
S42.014B
S42.015A
S42.015B
S42.016A
S42.016B
S42.017A
S42.017B
S42.018A
S42.018B
S42.019A
S42.019B
S42.021A
S42.021B
S42.022A
S42.022B
S42.023A
S42.023B
S42.024A
S42.024B
S42.025A
S42.025B
S42.026A
S42.026B
S42.031A
S42.031B
S42.032A
S42.032B
S42.033A
S42.033B
S42.034A
S42.034B
S42.035A
S42.035B
S42.036A
S42.036B
S42.101A
S42.101B
S42.102A
S42.102B
S42.109A
S42.109B
S42.111A
S42.111B
S42.112A
S42.112B
S42.113A
S42.113B
S42.114A
S42.114B
S42.115A
S42.115B
S42.116A
S42.116B
S42.121A
S42.121B
S42.122A
S42.122B
S42.123A
S42.123B
S42.124A
S42.124B
S42.125A
S42.125B
S42.126A
S42.126B
S42.131A
S42.131B
S42.132A
S42.132B
S42.133A
S42.133B
S42.134A
S42.134B
S42.135A
S42.135B
S42.136A
S42.136B
S42.141A
S42.141B
S42.142A
S42.142B
S42.143A
S42.143B
S42.144A
S42.144B
S42.145A
S42.145B
S42.146A
S42.146B
S42.151A
S42.151B
S42.152A
S42.152B
S42.153A
S42.153B
S42.154A
S42.154B
S42.155A
S42.155B
S42.156A
S42.156B
S42.191A
S42.191B
S42.192A
S42.192B
S42.199A
S42.199B
S42.201A
S42.201B
S42.202A
S42.202B
S42.209A
S42.209B
S42.211A
S42.211B
S42.212A
S42.212B
S42.213A
S42.213B
S42.214A
S42.214B
S42.215A
S42.215B
S42.216A
S42.216B
S42.221A
S42.221B
S42.222A
S42.222B
S42.223A
S42.223B
S42.224A
S42.224B
S42.225A
S42.225B
S42.226A
S42.226B
S42.231A
S42.231B
S42.232A
S42.232B
S42.239A
S42.239B
S42.241A
S42.241B
S42.242A
S42.242B
S42.249A
S42.249B
S42.251A
S42.251B
S42.252A
S42.252B
S42.253A
S42.253B
S42.254A
S42.254B
S42.255A
S42.255B
S42.256A
S42.256B
S42.261A
S42.261B
S42.262A
S42.262B
S42.263A
S42.263B
S42.264A
S42.264B
S42.265A
S42.265B
S42.266A
S42.266B
S42.271A
S42.272A
S42.279A
S42.291A
S42.291B
S42.292A
S42.292B
S42.293A
S42.293B
S42.294A
S42.294B
S42.295A
S42.295B
S42.296A
S42.296B
S42.301A
S42.301B
S42.302A
S42.302B
S42.309A
S42.309B
S42.311A
S42.312A
S42.319A
S42.321A
S42.321B
S42.322A
S42.322B
S42.323A
S42.323B
S42.324A
S42.324B
S42.325A
S42.325B
S42.326A
S42.326B
S42.331A
S42.331B
S42.332A
S42.332B
S42.333A
S42.333B
S42.334A
S42.334B
S42.335A
S42.335B
S42.336A
S42.336B
S42.341A
S42.341B
S42.342A
S42.342B
S42.343A
S42.343B
S42.344A
S42.344B
S42.345A
S42.345B
S42.346A
S42.346B
S42.351A
S42.351B
S42.352A
S42.352B
S42.353A
S42.353B
S42.354A
S42.354B
S42.355A
S42.355B
S42.356A
S42.356B
S42.361A
S42.361B
S42.362A
S42.362B
S42.363A
S42.363B
S42.364A
S42.364B
S42.365A
S42.365B
S42.366A
S42.366B
S42.391A
S42.391B
S42.392A
S42.392B
S42.399A
S42.399B
S42.401A
S42.401B
S42.402A
S42.402B
S42.409A
S42.409B
S42.411A
S42.411B
S42.412A
S42.412B
S42.413A
S42.413B
S42.414A
S42.414B
S42.415A
S42.415B
S42.416A
S42.416B
S42.421A
S42.421B
S42.422A
S42.422B
S42.423A
S42.423B
S42.424A
S42.424B
S42.425A
S42.425B
S42.426A
S42.426B
S42.431A
S42.431B
S42.432A
S42.432B
S42.433A
S42.433B
S42.434A
S42.434B
S42.435A
S42.435B
S42.436A
S42.436B
S42.441A
S42.441B
S42.442A
S42.442B
S42.443A
S42.443B
S42.444A
S42.444B
S42.445A
S42.445B
S42.446A
S42.446B
S42.447A
S42.447B
S42.448A
S42.448B
S42.449A
S42.449B
S42.451A
S42.451B
S42.452A
S42.452B
S42.453A
S42.453B
S42.454A
S42.454B
S42.455A
S42.455B
S42.456A
S42.456B
S42.461A
S42.461B
S42.462A
S42.462B
S42.463A
S42.463B
S42.464A
S42.464B
S42.465A
S42.465B
S42.466A
S42.466B
S42.471A
S42.471B
S42.472A
S42.472B
S42.473A
S42.473B
S42.474A
S42.474B
S42.475A
S42.475B
S42.476A
S42.476B
S42.481A
S42.482A
S42.489A
S42.491A
S42.491B
S42.492A
S42.492B
S42.493A
S42.493B
S42.494A
S42.494B
S42.495A
S42.495B
S42.496A
S42.496B
S42.90XA
S42.90XB
S42.91XA
S42.91XB
S42.92XA
S42.92XB
S43.001A
S43.002A
S43.003A
S43.004A
S43.005A
S43.006A
S43.011A
S43.012A
S43.013A
S43.014A
S43.015A
S43.016A
S43.021A
S43.022A
S43.023A
S43.024A
S43.025A
S43.026A
S43.031A
S43.032A
S43.033A
S43.034A
S43.035A
S43.036A
S43.081A
S43.082A
S43.083A
S43.084A
S43.085A
S43.086A
S43.101A
S43.102A
S43.109A
S43.111A
S43.112A
S43.119A
S43.121A
S43.122A
S43.129A
S43.131A
S43.132A
S43.139A
S43.141A
S43.142A
S43.149A
S43.151A
S43.152A
S43.159A
S43.201A
S43.202A
S43.203A
S43.204A
S43.205A
S43.206A
S43.211A
S43.212A
S43.213A
S43.214A
S43.215A
S43.216A
S43.221A
S43.222A
S43.223A
S43.224A
S43.225A
S43.226A
S43.301A
S43.302A
S43.303A
S43.304A
S43.305A
S43.306A
S43.311A
S43.312A
S43.313A
S43.314A
S43.315A
S43.316A
S43.391A
S43.392A
S43.393A
S43.394A
S43.395A
S43.396A
S43.401A
S43.402A
S43.409A
S43.411A
S43.412A
S43.419A
S43.421A
S43.422A
S43.429A
S43.431A
S43.432A
S43.439A
S43.491A
S43.492A
S43.499A
S43.50XA
S43.51XA
S43.52XA
S43.60XA
S43.61XA
S43.62XA
S43.80XA
S43.81XA
S43.82XA
S43.90XA
S43.91XA
S43.92XA
S44.00XA
S44.01XA
S44.02XA
S44.10XA
S44.11XA
S44.12XA
S44.20XA
S44.21XA
S44.22XA
S44.30XA
S44.31XA
S44.32XA
S44.40XA
S44.41XA
S44.42XA
S44.50XA
S44.51XA
S44.52XA
S44.8X1A
S44.8X2A
S44.8X9A
S44.90XA
S44.91XA
S44.92XA
S45.001A
S45.002A
S45.009A
S45.011A
S45.012A
S45.019A
S45.091A
S45.092A
S45.099A
S45.101A
S45.102A
S45.109A
S45.111A
S45.112A
S45.119A
S45.191A
S45.192A
S45.199A
S45.201A
S45.202A
S45.209A
S45.211A
S45.212A
S45.219A
S45.291A
S45.292A
S45.299A
S45.301A
S45.302A
S45.309A
S45.311A
S45.312A
S45.319A
S45.391A
S45.392A
S45.399A
S45.801A
S45.802A
S45.809A
S45.811A
S45.812A
S45.819A
S45.891A
S45.892A
S45.899A
S45.901A
S45.902A
S45.909A
S45.911A
S45.912A
S45.919A
S45.991A
S45.992A
S45.999A
S46.001A
S46.002A
S46.009A
S46.011A
S46.012A
S46.019A
S46.021A
S46.022A
S46.029A
S46.091A
S46.092A
S46.099A
S46.101A
S46.102A
S46.109A
S46.111A
S46.112A
S46.119A
S46.121A
S46.122A
S46.129A
S46.191A
S46.192A
S46.199A
S46.201A
S46.202A
S46.209A

S46.211A
S46.212A
S46.219A
S46.221A
S46.222A
S46.229A
S46.291A
S46.292A
S46.299A
S46.301A
S46.302A
S46.309A
S46.311A
S46.312A
S46.319A
S46.321A
S46.322A
S46.329A
S46.391A
S46.392A
S46.399A
S46.801A
S46.802A
S46.809A
S46.811A
S46.812A
S46.819A
S46.821A
S46.822A
S46.829A
S46.891A
S46.892A
S46.899A
S46.901A
S46.902A
S46.909A
S46.911A
S46.912A
S46.919A
S46.921A
S46.922A
S46.929A
S46.991A
S46.992A
S46.999A
S47.1XXA
S47.2XXA
S47.9XXA
S48.011A
S48.012A
S48.019A
S48.021A
S48.022A
S48.029A
S48.111A
S48.112A
S48.119A
S48.121A
S48.122A
S48.129A
S48.911A
S48.912A
S48.919A
S48.921A
S48.922A
S48.929A
S49.001A
S49.002A
S49.009A
S49.011A
S49.012A
S49.019A
S49.021A
S49.022A
S49.029A
S49.031A
S49.032A
S49.039A
S49.041A
S49.042A
S49.049A
S49.091A
S49.092A
S49.099A
S49.101A
S49.102A
S49.109A
S49.111A
S49.112A
S49.119A
S49.121A
S49.122A
S49.129A
S49.131A
S49.132A
S49.139A
S49.141A
S49.142A
S49.149A
S49.191A
S49.192A
S49.199A
S49.80XA
S49.81XA
S49.82XA
S49.90XA
S49.91XA
S49.92XA
S50.00XA
S50.01XA
S50.02XA
S50.10XA
S50.11XA
S50.12XA
S50.311A
S50.312A
S50.319A
S50.321A
S50.322A
S50.329A
S50.341A
S50.342A
S50.349A
S50.351A
S50.352A
S50.359A
S50.361A
S50.362A
S50.369A
S50.371A
S50.372A
S50.379A
S50.811A
S50.812A
S50.819A
S50.821A
S50.822A
S50.829A
S50.841A
S50.842A
S50.849A
S50.851A
S50.852A
S50.859A
S50.861A
S50.862A
S50.869A
S50.871A
S50.872A
S50.879A
S50.901A
S50.902A
S50.909A
S50.911A
S50.912A
S50.919A
S51.001A
S51.002A
S51.009A
S51.011A
S51.012A
S51.019A
S51.021A
S51.022A
S51.029A
S51.031A
S51.032A
S51.039A
S51.041A
S51.042A
S51.049A
S51.051A
S51.052A
S51.059A
S51.801A
S51.802A
S51.809A
S51.811A
S51.812A
S51.819A
S51.821A
S51.822A
S51.829A
S51.831A
S51.832A
S51.839A
S51.841A
S51.842A
S51.849A
S51.851A
S51.852A
S51.859A
S52.001A
S52.001B
S52.001C
S52.002A
S52.002B
S52.002C
S52.009A
S52.009B
S52.009C
S52.011A
S52.012A
S52.019A
S52.021A
S52.021B
S52.021C
S52.022A
S52.022B
S52.022C
S52.023A
S52.023B
S52.023C
S52.024A
S52.024B
S52.024C
S52.025A
S52.025B
S52.025C
S52.026A
S52.026B
S52.026C
S52.031A
S52.031B
S52.031C
S52.032A
S52.032B
S52.032C
S52.033A
S52.033B
S52.033C
S52.034A
S52.034B
S52.034C
S52.035A
S52.035B
S52.035C
S52.036A
S52.036B
S52.036C
S52.041A
S52.041B
S52.041C
S52.042A
S52.042B
S52.042C
S52.043A
S52.043B
S52.043C
S52.044A
S52.044B
S52.044C
S52.045A
S52.045B
S52.045C
S52.046A
S52.046B
S52.046C
S52.091A
S52.091B
S52.091C
S52.092A
S52.092B
S52.092C
S52.099A
S52.099B
S52.099C
S52.101A
S52.101B
S52.101C
S52.102A
S52.102B
S52.102C
S52.109A
S52.109B
S52.109C
S52.111A
S52.112A
S52.119A
S52.121A
S52.121B
S52.121C
S52.122A
S52.122B
S52.122C
S52.123A
S52.123B
S52.123C
S52.124A
S52.124B
S52.124C
S52.125A
S52.125B
S52.125C
S52.126A
S52.126B
S52.126C
S52.131A
S52.131B
S52.131C
S52.132A
S52.132B
S52.132C
S52.133A
S52.133B
S52.133C
S52.134A
S52.134B
S52.134C
S52.135A
S52.135B
S52.135C
S52.136A
S52.136B
S52.136C
S52.181A
S52.181B
S52.181C
S52.182A
S52.182B
S52.182C
S52.189A
S52.189B
S52.189C
S52.201A
S52.201B
S52.201C
S52.202A
S52.202B
S52.202C
S52.209A
S52.209B
S52.209C
S52.211A
S52.212A
S52.219A
S52.221A
S52.221B
S52.221C
S52.222A
S52.222B
S52.222C
S52.223A
S52.223B
S52.223C
S52.224A
S52.224B
S52.224C
S52.225A
S52.225B
S52.225C
S52.226A
S52.226B
S52.226C
S52.231A
S52.231B
S52.231C
S52.232A
S52.232B
S52.232C
S52.233A
S52.233B
S52.233C
S52.234A
S52.234B
S52.234C
S52.235A
S52.235B
S52.235C
S52.236A
S52.236B
S52.236C
S52.241A
S52.241B
S52.241C
S52.242A
S52.242B
S52.242C
S52.243A
S52.243B
S52.243C
S52.244A
S52.244B
S52.244C
S52.245A
S52.245B
S52.245C
S52.246A
S52.246B
S52.246C
S52.251A
S52.251B
S52.251C
S52.252A
S52.252B
S52.252C
S52.253A
S52.253B
S52.253C
S52.254A
S52.254B
S52.254C
S52.255A
S52.255B
S52.255C
S52.256A
S52.256B
S52.256C
S52.261A
S52.261B
S52.261C
S52.262A
S52.262B
S52.262C
S52.263A
S52.263B
S52.263C
S52.264A
S52.264B
S52.264C
S52.265A
S52.265B
S52.265C
S52.266A
S52.266B
S52.266C
S52.271A
S52.271B
S52.271C
S52.272A
S52.272B
S52.272C
S52.279A
S52.279B
S52.279C
S52.281A
S52.281B
S52.281C
S52.282A
S52.282B
S52.282C
S52.283A
S52.283B
S52.283C
S52.291A
S52.291B
S52.291C
S52.292A
S52.292B
S52.292C
S52.299A
S52.299B
S52.299C
S52.301A
S52.301B
S52.301C
S52.302A
S52.302B
S52.302C
S52.309A
S52.309B
S52.309C
S52.311A
S52.312A
S52.319A
S52.321A
S52.321B
S52.321C
S52.322A
S52.322B
S52.322C
S52.323A
S52.323B
S52.323C
S52.324A
S52.324B
S52.324C
S52.325A
S52.325B
S52.325C
S52.326A
S52.326B
S52.326C
S52.331A
S52.331B
S52.331C
S52.332A
S52.332B
S52.332C
S52.333A
S52.333B
S52.333C
S52.334A
S52.334B
S52.334C
S52.335A
S52.335B
S52.335C
S52.336A
S52.336B
S52.336C
S52.341A
S52.341B
S52.341C
S52.342A
S52.342B
S52.342C
S52.343A
S52.343B
S52.343C
S52.344A
S52.344B
S52.344C
S52.345A
S52.345B
S52.345C
S52.346A
S52.346B
S52.346C
S52.351A
S52.351B
S52.351C
S52.352A
S52.352B
S52.352C
S52.353A
S52.353B
S52.353C
S52.354A
S52.354B
S52.354C
S52.355A
S52.355B
S52.355C
S52.356A
S52.356B
S52.356C
S52.361A
S52.361B
S52.361C
S52.362A
S52.362B
S52.362C
S52.363A
S52.363B
S52.363C
S52.364A
S52.364B
S52.364C
S52.365A
S52.365B
S52.365C
S52.366A
S52.366B
S52.366C
S52.371A
S52.371B
S52.371C
S52.372A
S52.372B
S52.372C
S52.379A
S52.379B
S52.379C
S52.381A
S52.381B
S52.381C
S52.382A
S52.382B
S52.382C
S52.389A
S52.389B
S52.389C
S52.391A
S52.391B
S52.391C
S52.392A
S52.392B
S52.392C
S52.399A
S52.399B
S52.399C
S52.501A
S52.501B
S52.501C
S52.502A
S52.502B
S52.502C
S52.509A
S52.509B
S52.509C
S52.511A
S52.511B
S52.511C
S52.512A
S52.512B
S52.512C
S52.513A
S52.513B
S52.513C
S52.514A
S52.514B
S52.514C
S52.515A
S52.515B
S52.515C
S52.516A
S52.516B
S52.516C
S52.521A
S52.522A
S52.529A
S52.531A
S52.531B
S52.531C
S52.532A
S52.532B
S52.532C
S52.539A
S52.539B
S52.539C
S52.541A
S52.541B
S52.541C
S52.542A
S52.542B
S52.542C
S52.549A
S52.549B
S52.549C
S52.551A
S52.551B
S52.551C
S52.552A
S52.552B
S52.552C
S52.559A
S52.559B
S52.559C
S52.561A
S52.561B
S52.561C
S52.562A
S52.562B
S52.562C
S52.569A
S52.569B
S52.569C
S52.571A
S52.571B
S52.571C
S52.572A
S52.572B
S52.572C
S52.579A
S52.579B
S52.579C
S52.591A
S52.591B
S52.591C
S52.592A
S52.592B
S52.592C
S52.599A
S52.599B
S52.599C
S52.601A
S52.601B
S52.601C
S52.602A
S52.602B
S52.602C
S52.609A
S52.609B
S52.609C
S52.611A
S52.611B
S52.611C
S52.612A
S52.612B
S52.612C
S52.613A
S52.613B
S52.613C
S52.614A
S52.614B
S52.614C
S52.615A
S52.615B
S52.615C
S52.616A
S52.616B
S52.616C
S52.621A
S52.622A
S52.629A
S52.691A
S52.691B
S52.691C
S52.692A
S52.692B
S52.692C
S52.699A
S52.699B
S52.699C
S52.90XA
S52.90XB
S52.90XC
S52.91XA
S52.91XB
S52.91XC
S52.92XA
S52.92XB
S52.92XC
S53.001A
S53.002A
S53.003A
S53.004A
S53.005A
S53.006A
S53.011A
S53.012A
S53.013A
S53.014A
S53.015A
S53.016A
S53.021A
S53.022A
S53.023A
S53.024A
S53.025A
S53.026A
S53.031A
S53.032A
S53.033A
S53.091A
S53.092A
S53.093A
S53.094A
S53.095A
S53.096A
S53.101A
S53.102A
S53.103A
S53.104A
S53.105A
S53.106A
S53.111A
S53.112A
S53.113A
S53.114A
S53.115A
S53.116A
S53.121A
S53.122A
S53.123A
S53.124A
S53.125A
S53.126A
S53.131A
S53.132A
S53.133A
S53.134A
S53.135A
S53.136A
S53.141A
S53.142A
S53.143A
S53.144A
S53.145A
S53.146A
S53.191A
S53.192A
S53.193A
S53.194A
S53.195A
S53.196A
S53.20XA
S53.21XA
S53.22XA
S53.30XA
S53.31XA
S53.32XA
S53.401A
S53.402A
S53.409A
S53.411A
S53.412A
S53.419A
S53.421A
S53.422A
S53.429A
S53.431A
S53.432A
S53.439A
S53.441A
S53.442A
S53.449A
S53.491A
S53.492A
S53.499A
S54.00XA
S54.01XA
S54.02XA
S54.10XA
S54.11XA
S54.12XA
S54.20XA
S54.21XA
S54.22XA
S54.30XA
S54.31XA
S54.32XA
S54.8X1A
S54.8X2A
S54.8X9A
S54.90XA
S54.91XA
S54.92XA
S55.001A
S55.002A
S55.009A
S55.011A
S55.012A
S55.019A
S55.091A
S55.092A
S55.099A
S55.101A
S55.102A
S55.109A
S55.111A
S55.112A
S55.119A
S55.191A
S55.192A
S55.199A
S55.201A
S55.202A
S55.209A
S55.211A
S55.212A
S55.219A
S55.291A
S55.292A
S55.299A
S55.801A
S55.802A
S55.809A
S55.811A
S55.812A
S55.819A
S55.891A
S55.892A
S55.899A

S55.901A
S55.902A
S55.909A
S55.911A
S55.912A
S55.919A
S55.991A
S55.992A
S55.999A
S56.001A
S56.002A
S56.009A
S56.011A
S56.012A
S56.019A
S56.021A
S56.022A
S56.029A
S56.091A
S56.092A
S56.099A
S56.101A
S56.102A
S56.103A
S56.104A
S56.105A
S56.106A
S56.107A
S56.108A
S56.109A
S56.111A
S56.112A
S56.113A
S56.114A
S56.115A
S56.116A
S56.117A
S56.118A
S56.119A
S56.121A
S56.122A
S56.123A
S56.124A
S56.125A
S56.126A
S56.127A
S56.128A
S56.129A
S56.191A
S56.192A
S56.193A
S56.194A
S56.195A
S56.196A
S56.197A
S56.198A
S56.199A
S56.201A
S56.202A
S56.209A
S56.211A
S56.212A
S56.219A
S56.221A
S56.222A
S56.229A
S56.291A
S56.292A
S56.299A
S56.301A
S56.302A
S56.309A
S56.311A
S56.312A
S56.319A
S56.321A
S56.322A
S56.329A
S56.391A
S56.392A
S56.399A
S56.401A
S56.402A
S56.403A
S56.404A
S56.405A
S56.406A
S56.407A
S56.408A
S56.409A
S56.411A
S56.412A
S56.413A
S56.414A
S56.415A
S56.416A
S56.417A
S56.418A
S56.419A
S56.421A
S56.422A
S56.423A
S56.424A
S56.425A
S56.426A
S56.427A
S56.428A
S56.429A
S56.491A
S56.492A
S56.493A
S56.494A
S56.495A
S56.496A
S56.497A
S56.498A
S56.499A
S56.501A
S56.502A
S56.509A
S56.511A
S56.512A
S56.519A
S56.521A
S56.522A
S56.529A
S56.591A
S56.592A
S56.599A
S56.801A
S56.802A
S56.809A
S56.811A
S56.812A
S56.819A
S56.821A
S56.822A
S56.829A
S56.891A
S56.892A
S56.899A
S56.901A
S56.902A
S56.909A
S56.911A
S56.912A
S56.919A
S56.921A
S56.922A
S56.929A
S56.991A
S56.992A
S56.999A
S57.00XA
S57.01XA
S57.02XA
S57.80XA
S57.81XA
S57.82XA
S58.011A
S58.012A
S58.019A
S58.021A
S58.022A
S58.029A
S58.111A
S58.112A
S58.119A
S58.121A
S58.122A
S58.129A
S58.911A
S58.912A
S58.919A
S58.921A
S58.922A
S58.929A
S59.001A
S59.002A
S59.009A
S59.011A
S59.012A
S59.019A
S59.021A
S59.022A
S59.029A
S59.031A
S59.032A
S59.039A
S59.041A
S59.042A
S59.049A
S59.091A
S59.092A
S59.099A
S59.101A
S59.102A
S59.109A
S59.111A
S59.112A
S59.119A
S59.121A
S59.122A
S59.129A
S59.131A
S59.132A
S59.139A
S59.141A
S59.142A
S59.149A
S59.191A
S59.192A
S59.199A
S59.201A
S59.202A
S59.209A
S59.211A
S59.212A
S59.219A
S59.221A
S59.222A
S59.229A
S59.231A
S59.232A
S59.239A
S59.241A
S59.242A
S59.249A
S59.291A
S59.292A
S59.299A
S59.801A
S59.802A
S59.809A
S59.811A
S59.812A
S59.819A
S59.901A
S59.902A
S59.909A
S59.911A
S59.912A
S59.919A
S60.00XA
S60.011A
S60.012A
S60.019A
S60.021A
S60.022A
S60.029A
S60.031A
S60.032A
S60.039A
S60.041A
S60.042A
S60.049A
S60.051A
S60.052A
S60.059A
S60.10XA
S60.111A
S60.112A
S60.119A
S60.121A
S60.122A
S60.129A
S60.131A
S60.132A
S60.139A
S60.141A
S60.142A
S60.149A
S60.151A
S60.152A
S60.159A
S60.211A
S60.212A
S60.219A
S60.221A
S60.222A
S60.229A
S60.311A
S60.312A
S60.319A
S60.321A
S60.322A
S60.329A
S60.341A
S60.342A
S60.349A
S60.351A
S60.352A
S60.359A
S60.361A
S60.362A
S60.369A
S60.371A
S60.372A
S60.379A
S60.391A
S60.392A
S60.399A
S60.410A
S60.411A
S60.412A
S60.413A
S60.414A
S60.415A
S60.416A
S60.417A
S60.418A
S60.419A
S60.420A
S60.421A
S60.422A
S60.423A
S60.424A
S60.425A
S60.426A
S60.427A
S60.428A
S60.429A
S60.440A
S60.441A
S60.442A
S60.443A
S60.444A
S60.445A
S60.446A
S60.447A
S60.448A
S60.449A
S60.450A
S60.451A
S60.452A
S60.453A
S60.454A
S60.455A
S60.456A
S60.457A
S60.458A
S60.459A
S60.460A
S60.461A
S60.462A
S60.463A
S60.464A
S60.465A
S60.466A
S60.467A
S60.468A
S60.469A
S60.470A
S60.471A
S60.472A
S60.473A
S60.474A
S60.475A
S60.476A
S60.477A
S60.478A
S60.479A
S60.511A
S60.512A
S60.519A
S60.521A
S60.522A
S60.529A
S60.541A
S60.542A
S60.549A
S60.551A
S60.552A
S60.559A
S60.561A
S60.562A
S60.569A
S60.571A
S60.572A
S60.579A
S60.811A
S60.812A
S60.819A
S60.821A
S60.822A
S60.829A
S60.841A
S60.842A
S60.849A
S60.851A
S60.852A
S60.859A
S60.861A
S60.862A
S60.869A
S60.871A
S60.872A
S60.879A
S60.911A
S60.912A
S60.919A
S60.921A
S60.922A
S60.929A
S60.931A
S60.932A
S60.939A
S60.940A
S60.941A
S60.942A
S60.943A
S60.944A
S60.945A
S60.946A
S60.947A
S60.948A
S60.949A
S61.001A
S61.002A
S61.009A
S61.011A
S61.012A
S61.019A
S61.021A
S61.022A
S61.029A
S61.031A
S61.032A
S61.039A
S61.041A
S61.042A
S61.049A
S61.051A
S61.052A
S61.059A
S61.101A
S61.102A
S61.109A
S61.111A
S61.112A
S61.119A
S61.121A
S61.122A
S61.129A
S61.131A
S61.132A
S61.139A
S61.141A
S61.142A
S61.149A
S61.151A
S61.152A
S61.159A
S61.200A
S61.201A
S61.202A
S61.203A
S61.204A
S61.205A
S61.206A
S61.207A
S61.208A
S61.209A
S61.210A
S61.211A
S61.212A
S61.213A
S61.214A
S61.215A
S61.216A
S61.217A
S61.218A
S61.219A
S61.220A
S61.221A
S61.222A
S61.223A
S61.224A
S61.225A
S61.226A
S61.227A
S61.228A
S61.229A
S61.230A
S61.231A
S61.232A
S61.233A
S61.234A
S61.235A
S61.236A
S61.237A
S61.238A
S61.239A
S61.240A
S61.241A
S61.242A
S61.243A
S61.244A
S61.245A
S61.246A
S61.247A
S61.248A
S61.249A
S61.250A
S61.251A
S61.252A
S61.253A
S61.254A
S61.255A
S61.256A
S61.257A
S61.258A
S61.259A
S61.300A
S61.301A
S61.302A
S61.303A
S61.304A
S61.305A
S61.306A
S61.307A
S61.308A
S61.309A
S61.310A
S61.311A
S61.312A
S61.313A
S61.314A
S61.315A
S61.316A
S61.317A
S61.318A
S61.319A
S61.320A
S61.321A
S61.322A
S61.323A
S61.324A
S61.325A
S61.326A
S61.327A
S61.328A
S61.329A
S61.330A
S61.331A
S61.332A
S61.333A
S61.334A
S61.335A
S61.336A
S61.337A
S61.338A
S61.339A
S61.340A
S61.341A
S61.342A
S61.343A
S61.344A
S61.345A
S61.346A
S61.347A
S61.348A
S61.349A
S61.350A
S61.351A
S61.352A
S61.353A
S61.354A
S61.355A
S61.356A
S61.357A
S61.358A
S61.359A
S61.401A
S61.402A
S61.409A
S61.411A
S61.412A
S61.419A
S61.421A
S61.422A
S61.429A
S61.431A
S61.432A
S61.439A
S61.441A
S61.442A
S61.449A
S61.451A
S61.452A
S61.459A
S61.501A
S61.502A
S61.509A
S61.511A
S61.512A
S61.519A
S61.521A
S61.522A
S61.529A
S61.531A
S61.532A
S61.539A
S61.541A
S61.542A
S61.549A
S61.551A
S61.552A
S61.559A
S62.001A
S62.001B
S62.002A
S62.002B
S62.009A
S62.009B
S62.011A
S62.011B
S62.012A
S62.012B
S62.013A
S62.013B
S62.014A
S62.014B
S62.015A
S62.015B
S62.016A
S62.016B
S62.021A
S62.021B
S62.022A
S62.022B
S62.023A
S62.023B
S62.024A
S62.024B
S62.025A
S62.025B
S62.026A
S62.026B
S62.031A
S62.031B
S62.032A
S62.032B
S62.033A
S62.033B
S62.034A
S62.034B
S62.035A
S62.035B
S62.036A
S62.036B
S62.101A
S62.101B
S62.102A
S62.102B
S62.109A
S62.109B
S62.111A
S62.111B
S62.112A
S62.112B
S62.113A
S62.113B
S62.114A
S62.114B
S62.115A
S62.115B
S62.116A
S62.116B
S62.121A
S62.121B
S62.122A
S62.122B
S62.123A
S62.123B
S62.124A
S62.124B
S62.125A
S62.125B
S62.126A
S62.126B
S62.131A
S62.131B
S62.132A
S62.132B
S62.133A
S62.133B
S62.134A
S62.134B
S62.135A
S62.135B
S62.136A
S62.136B
S62.141A
S62.141B
S62.142A
S62.142B
S62.143A
S62.143B
S62.144A
S62.144B
S62.145A
S62.145B
S62.146A
S62.146B
S62.151A
S62.151B
S62.152A
S62.152B
S62.153A
S62.153B
S62.154A
S62.154B
S62.155A
S62.155B
S62.156A
S62.156B
S62.161A
S62.161B
S62.162A
S62.162B
S62.163A
S62.163B
S62.164A
S62.164B
S62.165A
S62.165B
S62.166A
S62.166B
S62.171A
S62.171B
S62.172A
S62.172B
S62.173A
S62.173B
S62.174A
S62.174B
S62.175A
S62.175B
S62.176A
S62.176B
S62.181A
S62.181B
S62.182A
S62.182B
S62.183A
S62.183B
S62.184A
S62.184B
S62.185A
S62.185B
S62.186A
S62.186B
S62.201A
S62.201B
S62.202A
S62.202B
S62.209A
S62.209B
S62.211A
S62.211B
S62.212A
S62.212B
S62.213A
S62.213B
S62.221A
S62.221B
S62.222A
S62.222B
S62.223A
S62.223B
S62.224A
S62.224B
S62.225A
S62.225B
S62.226A
S62.226B
S62.231A
S62.231B
S62.232A
S62.232B
S62.233A
S62.233B
S62.234A
S62.234B
S62.235A
S62.235B
S62.236A
S62.236B
S62.241A
S62.241B
S62.242A
S62.242B
S62.243A
S62.243B
S62.244A
S62.244B
S62.245A
S62.245B
S62.246A
S62.246B
S62.251A
S62.251B
S62.252A
S62.252B
S62.253A
S62.253B
S62.254A
S62.254B
S62.255A
S62.255B
S62.256A
S62.256B
S62.291A
S62.291B
S62.292A
S62.292B
S62.299A
S62.299B
S62.300A
S62.300B
S62.301A
S62.301B
S62.302A
S62.302B
S62.303A
S62.303B
S62.304A
S62.304B
S62.305A
S62.305B
S62.306A
S62.306B
S62.307A
S62.307B
S62.308A
S62.308B
S62.309A
S62.309B
S62.310A
S62.310B
S62.311A
S62.311B
S62.312A
S62.312B
S62.313A
S62.313B
S62.314A
S62.314B
S62.315A
S62.315B
S62.316A
S62.316B
S62.317A
S62.317B

S62.318A
S62.318B
S62.319A
S62.319B
S62.320A
S62.320B
S62.321A
S62.321B
S62.322A
S62.322B
S62.323A
S62.323B
S62.324A
S62.324B
S62.325A
S62.325B
S62.326A
S62.326B
S62.327A
S62.327B
S62.328A
S62.328B
S62.329A
S62.329B
S62.330A
S62.330B
S62.331A
S62.331B
S62.332A
S62.332B
S62.333A
S62.333B
S62.334A
S62.334B
S62.335A
S62.335B
S62.336A
S62.336B
S62.337A
S62.337B
S62.338A
S62.338B
S62.339A
S62.339B
S62.340A
S62.340B
S62.341A
S62.341B
S62.342A
S62.342B
S62.343A
S62.343B
S62.344A
S62.344B
S62.345A
S62.345B
S62.346A
S62.346B
S62.347A
S62.347B
S62.348A
S62.348B
S62.349A
S62.349B
S62.350A
S62.350B
S62.351A
S62.351B
S62.352A
S62.352B
S62.353A
S62.353B
S62.354A
S62.354B
S62.355A
S62.355B
S62.356A
S62.356B
S62.357A
S62.357B
S62.358A
S62.358B
S62.359A
S62.359B
S62.360A
S62.360B
S62.361A
S62.361B
S62.362A
S62.362B
S62.363A
S62.363B
S62.364A
S62.364B
S62.365A
S62.365B
S62.366A
S62.366B
S62.367A
S62.367B
S62.368A
S62.368B
S62.369A
S62.369B
S62.390A
S62.390B
S62.391A
S62.391B
S62.392A
S62.392B
S62.393A
S62.393B
S62.394A
S62.394B
S62.395A
S62.395B
S62.396A
S62.396B
S62.397A
S62.397B
S62.398A
S62.398B
S62.399A
S62.399B
S62.501A
S62.501B
S62.502A
S62.502B
S62.509A
S62.509B
S62.511A
S62.511B
S62.512A
S62.512B
S62.513A
S62.513B
S62.514A
S62.514B
S62.515A
S62.515B
S62.516A
S62.516B
S62.521A
S62.521B
S62.522A
S62.522B
S62.523A
S62.523B
S62.524A
S62.524B
S62.525A
S62.525B
S62.526A
S62.526B
S62.600A
S62.600B
S62.601A
S62.601B
S62.602A
S62.602B
S62.603A
S62.603B
S62.604A
S62.604B
S62.605A
S62.605B
S62.606A
S62.606B
S62.607A
S62.607B
S62.608A
S62.608B
S62.609A
S62.609B
S62.610A
S62.610B
S62.611A
S62.611B
S62.612A
S62.612B
S62.613A
S62.613B
S62.614A
S62.614B
S62.615A
S62.615B
S62.616A
S62.616B
S62.617A
S62.617B
S62.618A
S62.618B
S62.619A
S62.619B
S62.620A
S62.620B
S62.621A
S62.621B
S62.622A
S62.622B
S62.623A
S62.623B
S62.624A
S62.624B
S62.625A
S62.625B
S62.626A
S62.626B
S62.627A
S62.627B
S62.628A
S62.628B
S62.629A
S62.629B
S62.630A
S62.630B
S62.631A
S62.631B
S62.632A
S62.632B
S62.633A
S62.633B
S62.634A
S62.634B
S62.635A
S62.635B
S62.636A
S62.636B
S62.637A
S62.637B
S62.638A
S62.638B
S62.639A
S62.639B
S62.640A
S62.640B
S62.641A
S62.641B
S62.642A
S62.642B
S62.643A
S62.643B
S62.644A
S62.644B
S62.645A
S62.645B
S62.646A
S62.646B
S62.647A
S62.647B
S62.648A
S62.648B
S62.649A
S62.649B
S62.650A
S62.650B
S62.651A
S62.651B
S62.652A
S62.652B
S62.653A
S62.653B
S62.654A
S62.654B
S62.655A
S62.655B
S62.656A
S62.656B
S62.657A
S62.657B
S62.658A
S62.658B
S62.659A
S62.659B
S62.660A
S62.660B
S62.661A
S62.661B
S62.662A
S62.662B
S62.663A
S62.663B
S62.664A
S62.664B
S62.665A
S62.665B
S62.666A
S62.666B
S62.667A
S62.667B
S62.668A
S62.668B
S62.669A
S62.669B
S62.90XA
S62.90XB
S62.91XA
S62.91XB
S62.92XA
S62.92XB
S63.001A
S63.002A
S63.003A
S63.004A
S63.005A
S63.006A
S63.011A
S63.012A
S63.013A
S63.014A
S63.015A
S63.016A
S63.021A
S63.022A
S63.023A
S63.024A
S63.025A
S63.026A
S63.031A
S63.032A
S63.033A
S63.034A
S63.035A
S63.036A
S63.041A
S63.042A
S63.043A
S63.044A
S63.045A
S63.046A
S63.051A
S63.052A
S63.053A
S63.054A
S63.055A
S63.056A
S63.061A
S63.062A
S63.063A
S63.064A
S63.065A
S63.066A
S63.071A
S63.072A
S63.073A
S63.074A
S63.075A
S63.076A
S63.091A
S63.092A
S63.093A
S63.094A
S63.095A
S63.096A
S63.101A
S63.102A
S63.103A
S63.104A
S63.105A
S63.106A
S63.111A
S63.112A
S63.113A
S63.114A
S63.115A
S63.116A
S63.121A
S63.122A
S63.123A
S63.124A
S63.125A
S63.126A
S63.200A
S63.201A
S63.202A
S63.203A
S63.204A
S63.205A
S63.206A
S63.207A
S63.208A
S63.209A
S63.210A
S63.211A
S63.212A
S63.213A
S63.214A
S63.215A
S63.216A
S63.217A
S63.218A
S63.219A
S63.220A
S63.221A
S63.222A
S63.223A
S63.224A
S63.225A
S63.226A
S63.227A
S63.228A
S63.229A
S63.230A
S63.231A
S63.232A
S63.233A
S63.234A
S63.235A
S63.236A
S63.237A
S63.238A
S63.239A
S63.240A
S63.241A
S63.242A
S63.243A
S63.244A
S63.245A
S63.246A
S63.247A
S63.248A
S63.249A
S63.250A
S63.251A
S63.252A
S63.253A
S63.254A
S63.255A
S63.256A
S63.257A
S63.258A
S63.259A
S63.260A
S63.261A
S63.262A
S63.263A
S63.264A
S63.265A
S63.266A
S63.267A
S63.268A
S63.269A
S63.270A
S63.271A
S63.272A
S63.273A
S63.274A
S63.275A
S63.276A
S63.277A
S63.278A
S63.279A
S63.280A
S63.281A
S63.282A
S63.283A
S63.284A
S63.285A
S63.286A
S63.287A
S63.288A
S63.289A
S63.290A
S63.291A
S63.292A
S63.293A
S63.294A
S63.295A
S63.296A
S63.297A
S63.298A
S63.299A
S63.301A
S63.302A
S63.309A
S63.311A
S63.312A
S63.319A
S63.321A
S63.322A
S63.329A
S63.331A
S63.332A
S63.339A
S63.391A
S63.392A
S63.399A
S63.400A
S63.401A
S63.402A
S63.403A
S63.404A
S63.405A
S63.406A
S63.407A
S63.408A
S63.409A
S63.410A
S63.411A
S63.412A
S63.413A
S63.414A
S63.415A
S63.416A
S63.417A
S63.418A
S63.419A
S63.420A
S63.421A
S63.422A
S63.423A
S63.424A
S63.425A
S63.426A
S63.427A
S63.428A
S63.429A
S63.430A
S63.431A
S63.432A
S63.433A
S63.434A
S63.435A
S63.436A
S63.437A
S63.438A
S63.439A
S63.490A
S63.491A
S63.492A
S63.493A
S63.494A
S63.495A
S63.496A
S63.497A
S63.498A
S63.499A
S63.501A
S63.502A
S63.509A
S63.511A
S63.512A
S63.519A
S63.521A
S63.522A
S63.529A
S63.591A
S63.592A
S63.599A
S63.601A
S63.602A
S63.609A
S63.610A
S63.611A
S63.612A
S63.613A
S63.614A
S63.615A
S63.616A
S63.617A
S63.618A
S63.619A
S63.621A
S63.622A
S63.629A
S63.630A
S63.631A
S63.632A
S63.633A
S63.634A
S63.635A
S63.636A
S63.637A
S63.638A
S63.639A
S63.641A
S63.642A
S63.649A
S63.650A
S63.651A
S63.652A
S63.653A
S63.654A
S63.655A
S63.656A
S63.657A
S63.658A
S63.659A
S63.681A
S63.682A
S63.689A
S63.690A
S63.691A
S63.692A
S63.693A
S63.694A
S63.695A
S63.696A
S63.697A
S63.698A
S63.699A
S63.8X1A
S63.8X2A
S63.8X9A
S63.90XA
S63.91XA
S63.92XA
S64.00XA
S64.01XA
S64.02XA
S64.10XA
S64.11XA
S64.12XA
S64.20XA
S64.21XA
S64.22XA
S64.30XA
S64.31XA
S64.32XA
S64.40XA
S64.490A
S64.491A
S64.492A
S64.493A
S64.494A
S64.495A
S64.496A
S64.497A
S64.498A
S64.8X1A
S64.8X2A
S64.8X9A
S64.90XA
S64.91XA
S64.92XA
S65.001A
S65.002A
S65.009A
S65.011A
S65.012A
S65.019A
S65.091A
S65.092A
S65.099A
S65.101A
S65.102A
S65.109A
S65.111A
S65.112A
S65.119A
S65.191A
S65.192A
S65.199A
S65.201A
S65.202A
S65.209A
S65.211A
S65.212A
S65.219A
S65.291A
S65.292A
S65.299A
S65.301A
S65.302A
S65.309A
S65.311A
S65.312A
S65.319A
S65.391A
S65.392A
S65.399A
S65.401A
S65.402A
S65.409A
S65.411A
S65.412A
S65.419A
S65.491A
S65.492A
S65.499A
S65.500A
S65.501A
S65.502A
S65.503A
S65.504A
S65.505A
S65.506A
S65.507A
S65.508A
S65.509A
S65.510A
S65.511A
S65.512A
S65.513A
S65.514A
S65.515A
S65.516A
S65.517A
S65.518A
S65.519A
S65.590A
S65.591A
S65.592A
S65.593A
S65.594A
S65.595A
S65.596A
S65.597A
S65.598A
S65.599A
S65.801A
S65.802A
S65.809A
S65.811A
S65.812A
S65.819A
S65.891A
S65.892A
S65.899A
S65.901A
S65.902A
S65.909A
S65.911A
S65.912A
S65.919A
S65.991A
S65.992A
S65.999A
S66.001A
S66.002A
S66.009A
S66.011A
S66.012A
S66.019A
S66.021A
S66.022A
S66.029A
S66.091A
S66.092A
S66.099A
S66.100A
S66.101A
S66.102A
S66.103A
S66.104A
S66.105A
S66.106A
S66.107A
S66.108A
S66.109A
S66.110A
S66.111A
S66.112A
S66.113A
S66.114A
S66.115A
S66.116A
S66.117A
S66.118A
S66.119A
S66.120A
S66.121A
S66.122A
S66.123A
S66.124A
S66.125A
S66.126A
S66.127A
S66.128A
S66.129A
S66.190A
S66.191A
S66.192A
S66.193A
S66.194A
S66.195A
S66.196A
S66.197A
S66.198A
S66.199A
S66.201A
S66.202A
S66.209A
S66.211A
S66.212A
S66.219A
S66.221A
S66.222A
S66.229A
S66.291A
S66.292A
S66.299A
S66.300A
S66.301A
S66.302A
S66.303A
S66.304A
S66.305A
S66.306A
S66.307A
S66.308A
S66.309A
S66.310A
S66.311A
S66.312A
S66.313A
S66.314A
S66.315A
S66.316A
S66.317A
S66.318A
S66.319A
S66.320A
S66.321A
S66.322A
S66.323A
S66.324A
S66.325A
S66.326A
S66.327A
S66.328A
S66.329A
S66.390A
S66.391A
S66.392A
S66.393A
S66.394A
S66.395A
S66.396A
S66.397A
S66.398A
S66.399A
S66.401A
S66.402A
S66.409A
S66.411A
S66.412A
S66.419A
S66.421A
S66.422A
S66.429A
S66.491A
S66.492A
S66.499A
S66.500A
S66.501A
S66.502A
S66.503A
S66.504A
S66.505A
S66.506A
S66.507A
S66.508A
S66.509A
S66.510A

S66.511A
S66.512A
S66.513A
S66.514A
S66.515A
S66.516A
S66.517A
S66.518A
S66.519A
S66.520A
S66.521A
S66.522A
S66.523A
S66.524A
S66.525A
S66.526A
S66.527A
S66.528A
S66.529A
S66.590A
S66.591A
S66.592A
S66.593A
S66.594A
S66.595A
S66.596A
S66.597A
S66.598A
S66.599A
S66.801A
S66.802A
S66.809A
S66.811A
S66.812A
S66.819A
S66.821A
S66.822A
S66.829A
S66.891A
S66.892A
S66.899A
S66.901A
S66.902A
S66.909A
S66.911A
S66.912A
S66.919A
S66.921A
S66.922A
S66.929A
S66.991A
S66.992A
S66.999A
S67.00XA
S67.01XA
S67.02XA
S67.10XA
S67.190A
S67.191A
S67.192A
S67.193A
S67.194A
S67.195A
S67.196A
S67.197A
S67.198A
S67.20XA
S67.21XA
S67.22XA
S67.30XA
S67.31XA
S67.32XA
S67.40XA
S67.41XA
S67.42XA
S67.90XA
S67.91XA
S67.92XA
S68.011A
S68.012A
S68.019A
S68.021A
S68.022A
S68.029A
S68.110A
S68.111A
S68.112A
S68.113A
S68.114A
S68.115A
S68.116A
S68.117A
S68.118A
S68.119A
S68.120A
S68.121A
S68.122A
S68.123A
S68.124A
S68.125A
S68.126A
S68.127A
S68.128A
S68.129A
S68.411A
S68.412A
S68.419A
S68.421A
S68.422A
S68.429A
S68.511A
S68.512A
S68.519A
S68.521A
S68.522A
S68.529A
S68.610A
S68.611A
S68.612A
S68.613A
S68.614A
S68.615A
S68.616A
S68.617A
S68.618A
S68.619A
S68.620A
S68.621A
S68.622A
S68.623A
S68.624A
S68.625A
S68.626A
S68.627A
S68.628A
S68.629A
S68.711A
S68.712A
S68.719A
S68.721A
S68.722A
S68.729A
S69.80XA
S69.81XA
S69.82XA
S69.90XA
S69.91XA
S69.92XA
S70.00XA
S70.01XA
S70.02XA
S70.10XA
S70.11XA
S70.12XA
S70.211A
S70.212A
S70.219A
S70.221A
S70.222A
S70.229A
S70.241A
S70.242A
S70.249A
S70.251A
S70.252A
S70.259A
S70.261A
S70.262A
S70.269A
S70.271A
S70.272A
S70.279A
S70.311A
S70.312A
S70.319A
S70.321A
S70.322A
S70.329A
S70.341A
S70.342A
S70.349A
S70.351A
S70.352A
S70.359A
S70.361A
S70.362A
S70.369A
S70.371A
S70.372A
S70.379A
S70.911A
S70.912A
S70.919A
S70.921A
S70.922A
S70.929A
S71.001A
S71.002A
S71.009A
S71.011A
S71.012A
S71.019A
S71.021A
S71.022A
S71.029A
S71.031A
S71.032A
S71.039A
S71.041A
S71.042A
S71.049A
S71.051A
S71.052A
S71.059A
S71.101A
S71.102A
S71.109A
S71.111A
S71.112A
S71.119A
S71.121A
S71.122A
S71.129A
S71.131A
S71.132A
S71.139A
S71.141A
S71.142A
S71.149A
S71.151A
S71.152A
S71.159A
S72.001A
S72.001B
S72.001C
S72.002A
S72.002B
S72.002C
S72.009A
S72.009B
S72.009C
S72.011A
S72.011B
S72.011C
S72.012A
S72.012B
S72.012C
S72.019A
S72.019B
S72.019C
S72.021A
S72.021B
S72.021C
S72.022A
S72.022B
S72.022C
S72.023A
S72.023B
S72.023C
S72.024A
S72.024B
S72.024C
S72.025A
S72.025B
S72.025C
S72.026A
S72.026B
S72.026C
S72.031A
S72.031B
S72.031C
S72.032A
S72.032B
S72.032C
S72.033A
S72.033B
S72.033C
S72.034A
S72.034B
S72.034C
S72.035A
S72.035B
S72.035C
S72.036A
S72.036B
S72.036C
S72.041A
S72.041B
S72.041C
S72.042A
S72.042B
S72.042C
S72.043A
S72.043B
S72.043C
S72.044A
S72.044B
S72.044C
S72.045A
S72.045B
S72.045C
S72.046A
S72.046B
S72.046C
S72.051A
S72.051B
S72.051C
S72.052A
S72.052B
S72.052C
S72.059A
S72.059B
S72.059C
S72.061A
S72.061B
S72.061C
S72.062A
S72.062B
S72.062C
S72.063A
S72.063B
S72.063C
S72.064A
S72.064B
S72.064C
S72.065A
S72.065B
S72.065C
S72.066A
S72.066B
S72.066C
S72.091A
S72.091B
S72.091C
S72.092A
S72.092B
S72.092C
S72.099A
S72.099B
S72.099C
S72.101A
S72.101B
S72.101C
S72.102A
S72.102B
S72.102C
S72.109A
S72.109B
S72.109C
S72.111A
S72.111B
S72.111C
S72.112A
S72.112B
S72.112C
S72.113A
S72.113B
S72.113C
S72.114A
S72.114B
S72.114C
S72.115A
S72.115B
S72.115C
S72.116A
S72.116B
S72.116C
S72.121A
S72.121B
S72.121C
S72.122A
S72.122B
S72.122C
S72.123A
S72.123B
S72.123C
S72.124A
S72.124B
S72.124C
S72.125A
S72.125B
S72.125C
S72.126A
S72.126B
S72.126C
S72.131A
S72.131B
S72.131C
S72.132A
S72.132B
S72.132C
S72.133A
S72.133B
S72.133C
S72.134A
S72.134B
S72.134C
S72.135A
S72.135B
S72.135C
S72.136A
S72.136B
S72.136C
S72.141A
S72.141B
S72.141C
S72.142A
S72.142B
S72.142C
S72.143A
S72.143B
S72.143C
S72.144A
S72.144B
S72.144C
S72.145A
S72.145B
S72.145C
S72.146A
S72.146B
S72.146C
S72.21XA
S72.21XB
S72.21XC
S72.22XA
S72.22XB
S72.22XC
S72.23XA
S72.23XB
S72.23XC
S72.24XA
S72.24XB
S72.24XC
S72.25XA
S72.25XB
S72.25XC
S72.26XA
S72.26XB
S72.26XC
S72.301A
S72.301B
S72.301C
S72.302A
S72.302B
S72.302C
S72.309A
S72.309B
S72.309C
S72.321A
S72.321B
S72.321C
S72.322A
S72.322B
S72.322C
S72.323A
S72.323B
S72.323C
S72.324A
S72.324B
S72.324C
S72.325A
S72.325B
S72.325C
S72.326A
S72.326B
S72.326C
S72.331A
S72.331B
S72.331C
S72.332A
S72.332B
S72.332C
S72.333A
S72.333B
S72.333C
S72.334A
S72.334B
S72.334C
S72.335A
S72.335B
S72.335C
S72.336A
S72.336B
S72.336C
S72.341A
S72.341B
S72.341C
S72.342A
S72.342B
S72.342C
S72.343A
S72.343B
S72.343C
S72.344A
S72.344B
S72.344C
S72.345A
S72.345B
S72.345C
S72.346A
S72.346B
S72.346C
S72.351A
S72.351B
S72.351C
S72.352A
S72.352B
S72.352C
S72.353A
S72.353B
S72.353C
S72.354A
S72.354B
S72.354C
S72.355A
S72.355B
S72.355C
S72.356A
S72.356B
S72.356C
S72.361A
S72.361B
S72.361C
S72.362A
S72.362B
S72.362C
S72.363A
S72.363B
S72.363C
S72.364A
S72.364B
S72.364C
S72.365A
S72.365B
S72.365C
S72.366A
S72.366B
S72.366C
S72.391A
S72.391B
S72.391C
S72.392A
S72.392B
S72.392C
S72.399A
S72.399B
S72.399C
S72.401A
S72.401B
S72.401C
S72.402A
S72.402B
S72.402C
S72.409A
S72.409B
S72.409C
S72.411A
S72.411B
S72.411C
S72.412A
S72.412B
S72.412C
S72.413A
S72.413B
S72.413C
S72.414A
S72.414B
S72.414C
S72.415A
S72.415B
S72.415C
S72.416A
S72.416B
S72.416C
S72.421A
S72.421B
S72.421C
S72.422A
S72.422B
S72.422C
S72.423A
S72.423B
S72.423C
S72.424A
S72.424B
S72.424C
S72.425A
S72.425B
S72.425C
S72.426A
S72.426B
S72.426C
S72.431A
S72.431B
S72.431C
S72.432A
S72.432B
S72.432C
S72.433A
S72.433B
S72.433C
S72.434A
S72.434B
S72.434C
S72.435A
S72.435B
S72.435C
S72.436A
S72.436B
S72.436C
S72.441A
S72.441B
S72.441C
S72.442A
S72.442B
S72.442C
S72.443A
S72.443B
S72.443C
S72.444A
S72.444B
S72.444C
S72.445A
S72.445B
S72.445C
S72.446A
S72.446B
S72.446C
S72.451A
S72.451B
S72.451C
S72.452A
S72.452B
S72.452C
S72.453A
S72.453B
S72.453C
S72.454A
S72.454B
S72.454C
S72.455A
S72.455B
S72.455C
S72.456A
S72.456B
S72.456C
S72.461A
S72.461B
S72.461C
S72.462A
S72.462B
S72.462C
S72.463A
S72.463B
S72.463C
S72.464A
S72.464B
S72.464C
S72.465A
S72.465B
S72.465C
S72.466A
S72.466B
S72.466C
S72.471A
S72.472A
S72.479A
S72.491A
S72.491B
S72.491C
S72.492A
S72.492B
S72.492C
S72.499A
S72.499B
S72.499C
S72.8X1A
S72.8X1B
S72.8X1C
S72.8X2A
S72.8X2B
S72.8X2C
S72.8X9A
S72.8X9B
S72.8X9C
S72.90XA
S72.90XB
S72.90XC
S72.91XA
S72.91XB
S72.91XC
S72.92XA
S72.92XB
S72.92XC
S73.001A
S73.002A
S73.003A
S73.004A
S73.005A
S73.006A
S73.011A
S73.012A
S73.013A
S73.014A
S73.015A
S73.016A
S73.021A
S73.022A
S73.023A
S73.024A
S73.025A
S73.026A
S73.031A
S73.032A
S73.033A
S73.034A
S73.035A
S73.036A
S73.041A
S73.042A
S73.043A
S73.044A
S73.045A
S73.046A
S73.101A
S73.102A
S73.109A
S73.111A
S73.112A
S73.119A
S73.121A
S73.122A
S73.129A
S73.191A
S73.192A
S73.199A
S74.00XA
S74.01XA
S74.02XA
S74.10XA
S74.11XA
S74.12XA
S74.20XA
S74.21XA
S74.22XA
S74.8X1A
S74.8X2A
S74.8X9A
S74.90XA
S74.91XA
S74.92XA
S75.001A
S75.002A
S75.009A
S75.011A
S75.012A
S75.019A
S75.021A
S75.022A
S75.029A
S75.091A
S75.092A
S75.099A
S75.101A
S75.102A
S75.109A
S75.111A
S75.112A
S75.119A
S75.121A
S75.122A
S75.129A
S75.191A
S75.192A
S75.199A
S75.201A
S75.202A
S75.209A
S75.211A
S75.212A
S75.219A
S75.221A
S75.222A
S75.229A
S75.291A
S75.292A
S75.299A
S75.801A
S75.802A
S75.809A
S75.811A
S75.812A
S75.819A
S75.891A
S75.892A
S75.899A
S75.901A
S75.902A
S75.909A
S75.911A
S75.912A
S75.919A
S75.991A
S75.992A
S75.999A
S76.001A
S76.002A
S76.009A
S76.011A
S76.012A
S76.019A
S76.021A
S76.022A
S76.029A
S76.091A
S76.092A
S76.099A
S76.101A
S76.102A
S76.109A
S76.111A
S76.112A
S76.119A
S76.121A
S76.122A
S76.129A
S76.191A
S76.192A
S76.199A
S76.201A
S76.202A
S76.209A
S76.211A
S76.212A
S76.219A
S76.221A
S76.222A
S76.229A
S76.291A
S76.292A
S76.299A
S76.301A
S76.302A
S76.309A
S76.311A
S76.312A
S76.319A
S76.321A
S76.322A
S76.329A
S76.391A
S76.392A
S76.399A
S76.801A
S76.802A

S76.809A
S76.811A
S76.812A
S76.819A
S76.821A
S76.822A
S76.829A
S76.891A
S76.892A
S76.899A
S76.901A
S76.902A
S76.909A
S76.911A
S76.912A
S76.919A
S76.921A
S76.922A
S76.929A
S76.991A
S76.992A
S76.999A
S77.00XA
S77.01XA
S77.02XA
S77.10XA
S77.11XA
S77.12XA
S77.20XA
S77.21XA
S77.22XA
S78.011A
S78.012A
S78.019A
S78.021A
S78.022A
S78.029A
S78.111A
S78.112A
S78.119A
S78.121A
S78.122A
S78.129A
S78.911A
S78.912A
S78.919A
S78.921A
S78.922A
S78.929A
S79.001A
S79.002A
S79.009A
S79.011A
S79.012A
S79.019A
S79.091A
S79.092A
S79.099A
S79.101A
S79.102A
S79.109A
S79.111A
S79.112A
S79.119A
S79.121A
S79.122A
S79.129A
S79.131A
S79.132A
S79.139A
S79.141A
S79.142A
S79.149A
S79.191A
S79.192A
S79.199A
S79.811A
S79.812A
S79.819A
S79.821A
S79.822A
S79.829A
S79.911A
S79.912A
S79.919A
S79.921A
S79.922A
S79.929A
S80.00XA
S80.01XA
S80.02XA
S80.10XA
S80.11XA
S80.12XA
S80.211A
S80.212A
S80.219A
S80.221A
S80.222A
S80.229A
S80.241A
S80.242A
S80.249A
S80.251A
S80.252A
S80.259A
S80.261A
S80.262A
S80.269A
S80.271A
S80.272A
S80.279A
S80.811A
S80.812A
S80.819A
S80.821A
S80.822A
S80.829A
S80.841A
S80.842A
S80.849A
S80.851A
S80.852A
S80.859A
S80.861A
S80.862A
S80.869A
S80.871A
S80.872A
S80.879A
S80.911A
S80.912A
S80.919A
S80.921A
S80.922A
S80.929A
S81.001A
S81.002A
S81.009A
S81.011A
S81.012A
S81.019A
S81.021A
S81.022A
S81.029A
S81.031A
S81.032A
S81.039A
S81.041A
S81.042A
S81.049A
S81.051A
S81.052A
S81.059A
S81.801A
S81.802A
S81.809A
S81.811A
S81.812A
S81.819A
S81.821A
S81.822A
S81.829A
S81.831A
S81.832A
S81.839A
S81.841A
S81.842A
S81.849A
S81.851A
S81.852A
S81.859A
S82.001A
S82.001B
S82.001C
S82.002A
S82.002B
S82.002C
S82.009A
S82.009B
S82.009C
S82.011A
S82.011B
S82.011C
S82.012A
S82.012B
S82.012C
S82.013A
S82.013B
S82.013C
S82.014A
S82.014B
S82.014C
S82.015A
S82.015B
S82.015C
S82.016A
S82.016B
S82.016C
S82.021A
S82.021B
S82.021C
S82.022A
S82.022B
S82.022C
S82.023A
S82.023B
S82.023C
S82.024A
S82.024B
S82.024C
S82.025A
S82.025B
S82.025C
S82.026A
S82.026B
S82.026C
S82.031A
S82.031B
S82.031C
S82.032A
S82.032B
S82.032C
S82.033A
S82.033B
S82.033C
S82.034A
S82.034B
S82.034C
S82.035A
S82.035B
S82.035C
S82.036A
S82.036B
S82.036C
S82.041A
S82.041B
S82.041C
S82.042A
S82.042B
S82.042C
S82.043A
S82.043B
S82.043C
S82.044A
S82.044B
S82.044C
S82.045A
S82.045B
S82.045C
S82.046A
S82.046B
S82.046C
S82.091A
S82.091B
S82.091C
S82.092A
S82.092B
S82.092C
S82.099A
S82.099B
S82.099C
S82.101A
S82.101B
S82.101C
S82.102A
S82.102B
S82.102C
S82.109A
S82.109B
S82.109C
S82.111A
S82.111B
S82.111C
S82.112A
S82.112B
S82.112C
S82.113A
S82.113B
S82.113C
S82.114A
S82.114B
S82.114C
S82.115A
S82.115B
S82.115C
S82.116A
S82.116B
S82.116C
S82.121A
S82.121B
S82.121C
S82.122A
S82.122B
S82.122C
S82.123A
S82.123B
S82.123C
S82.124A
S82.124B
S82.124C
S82.125A
S82.125B
S82.125C
S82.126A
S82.126B
S82.126C
S82.131A
S82.131B
S82.131C
S82.132A
S82.132B
S82.132C
S82.133A
S82.133B
S82.133C
S82.134A
S82.134B
S82.134C
S82.135A
S82.135B
S82.135C
S82.136A
S82.136B
S82.136C
S82.141A
S82.141B
S82.141C
S82.142A
S82.142B
S82.142C
S82.143A
S82.143B
S82.143C
S82.144A
S82.144B
S82.144C
S82.145A
S82.145B
S82.145C
S82.146A
S82.146B
S82.146C
S82.151A
S82.151B
S82.151C
S82.152A
S82.152B
S82.152C
S82.153A
S82.153B
S82.153C
S82.154A
S82.154B
S82.154C
S82.155A
S82.155B
S82.155C
S82.156A
S82.156B
S82.156C
S82.161A
S82.162A
S82.169A
S82.191A
S82.191B
S82.191C
S82.192A
S82.192B
S82.192C
S82.199A
S82.199B
S82.199C
S82.201A
S82.201B
S82.201C
S82.202A
S82.202B
S82.202C
S82.209A
S82.209B
S82.209C
S82.221A
S82.221B
S82.221C
S82.222A
S82.222B
S82.222C
S82.223A
S82.223B
S82.223C
S82.224A
S82.224B
S82.224C
S82.225A
S82.225B
S82.225C
S82.226A
S82.226B
S82.226C
S82.231A
S82.231B
S82.231C
S82.232A
S82.232B
S82.232C
S82.233A
S82.233B
S82.233C
S82.234A
S82.234B
S82.234C
S82.235A
S82.235B
S82.235C
S82.236A
S82.236B
S82.236C
S82.241A
S82.241B
S82.241C
S82.242A
S82.242B
S82.242C
S82.243A
S82.243B
S82.243C
S82.244A
S82.244B
S82.244C
S82.245A
S82.245B
S82.245C
S82.246A
S82.246B
S82.246C
S82.251A
S82.251B
S82.251C
S82.252A
S82.252B
S82.252C
S82.253A
S82.253B
S82.253C
S82.254A
S82.254B
S82.254C
S82.255A
S82.255B
S82.255C
S82.256A
S82.256B
S82.256C
S82.261A
S82.261B
S82.261C
S82.262A
S82.262B
S82.262C
S82.263A
S82.263B
S82.263C
S82.264A
S82.264B
S82.264C
S82.265A
S82.265B
S82.265C
S82.266A
S82.266B
S82.266C
S82.291A
S82.291B
S82.291C
S82.292A
S82.292B
S82.292C
S82.299A
S82.299B
S82.299C
S82.301A
S82.301B
S82.301C
S82.302A
S82.302B
S82.302C
S82.309A
S82.309B
S82.309C
S82.311A
S82.312A
S82.319A
S82.391A
S82.391B
S82.391C
S82.392A
S82.392B
S82.392C
S82.399A
S82.399B
S82.399C
S82.401A
S82.401B
S82.401C
S82.402A
S82.402B
S82.402C
S82.409A
S82.409B
S82.409C
S82.421A
S82.421B
S82.421C
S82.422A
S82.422B
S82.422C
S82.423A
S82.423B
S82.423C
S82.424A
S82.424B
S82.424C
S82.425A
S82.425B
S82.425C
S82.426A
S82.426B
S82.426C
S82.431A
S82.431B
S82.431C
S82.432A
S82.432B
S82.432C
S82.433A
S82.433B
S82.433C
S82.434A
S82.434B
S82.434C
S82.435A
S82.435B
S82.435C
S82.436A
S82.436B
S82.436C
S82.441A
S82.441B
S82.441C
S82.442A
S82.442B
S82.442C
S82.443A
S82.443B
S82.443C
S82.444A
S82.444B
S82.444C
S82.445A
S82.445B
S82.445C
S82.446A
S82.446B
S82.446C
S82.451A
S82.451B
S82.451C
S82.452A
S82.452B
S82.452C
S82.453A
S82.453B
S82.453C
S82.454A
S82.454B
S82.454C
S82.455A
S82.455B
S82.455C
S82.456A
S82.456B
S82.456C
S82.461A
S82.461B
S82.461C
S82.462A
S82.462B
S82.462C
S82.463A
S82.463B
S82.463C
S82.464A
S82.464B
S82.464C
S82.465A
S82.465B
S82.465C
S82.466A
S82.466B
S82.466C
S82.491A
S82.491B
S82.491C
S82.492A
S82.492B
S82.492C
S82.499A
S82.499B
S82.499C
S82.51XA
S82.51XB
S82.51XC
S82.52XA
S82.52XB
S82.52XC
S82.53XA
S82.53XB
S82.53XC
S82.54XA
S82.54XB
S82.54XC
S82.55XA
S82.55XB
S82.55XC
S82.56XA
S82.56XB
S82.56XC
S82.61XA
S82.61XB
S82.61XC
S82.62XA
S82.62XB
S82.62XC
S82.63XA
S82.63XB
S82.63XC
S82.64XA
S82.64XB
S82.64XC
S82.65XA
S82.65XB
S82.65XC
S82.66XA
S82.66XB
S82.66XC
S82.811A
S82.812A
S82.819A
S82.821A
S82.822A
S82.829A
S82.831A
S82.831B
S82.831C
S82.832A
S82.832B
S82.832C
S82.839A
S82.839B
S82.839C
S82.841A
S82.841B
S82.841C
S82.842A
S82.842B
S82.842C
S82.843A
S82.843B
S82.843C
S82.844A
S82.844B
S82.844C
S82.845A
S82.845B
S82.845C
S82.846A
S82.846B
S82.846C
S82.851A
S82.851B
S82.851C
S82.852A
S82.852B
S82.852C
S82.853A
S82.853B
S82.853C
S82.854A
S82.854B
S82.854C
S82.855A
S82.855B
S82.855C
S82.856A
S82.856B
S82.856C
S82.861A
S82.861B
S82.861C
S82.862A
S82.862B
S82.862C
S82.863A
S82.863B
S82.863C
S82.864A
S82.864B
S82.864C
S82.865A
S82.865B
S82.865C
S82.866A
S82.866B
S82.866C
S82.871A
S82.871B
S82.871C
S82.872A
S82.872B
S82.872C
S82.873A
S82.873B
S82.873C
S82.874A
S82.874B
S82.874C
S82.875A
S82.875B
S82.875C
S82.876A
S82.876B
S82.876C
S82.891A
S82.891B
S82.891C
S82.892A
S82.892B
S82.892C
S82.899A
S82.899B
S82.899C
S82.90XA
S82.90XB
S82.90XC
S82.91XA
S82.91XB
S82.91XC
S82.92XA
S82.92XB
S82.92XC
S83.001A
S83.002A
S83.003A
S83.004A
S83.005A
S83.006A
S83.011A
S83.012A
S83.013A
S83.014A
S83.015A
S83.016A
S83.091A
S83.092A
S83.093A
S83.094A
S83.095A
S83.096A
S83.101A
S83.102A
S83.103A
S83.104A
S83.105A
S83.106A
S83.111A
S83.112A
S83.113A
S83.114A
S83.115A
S83.116A
S83.121A
S83.122A
S83.123A
S83.124A
S83.125A
S83.126A
S83.131A
S83.132A
S83.133A
S83.134A
S83.135A
S83.136A
S83.141A
S83.142A
S83.143A
S83.144A
S83.145A
S83.146A
S83.191A
S83.192A
S83.193A
S83.194A
S83.195A
S83.196A
S83.200A
S83.201A
S83.202A
S83.203A
S83.204A
S83.205A
S83.206A
S83.207A
S83.209A
S83.211A
S83.212A
S83.219A
S83.221A
S83.222A
S83.229A
S83.231A
S83.232A
S83.239A
S83.241A
S83.242A
S83.249A
S83.251A
S83.252A
S83.259A
S83.261A
S83.262A
S83.269A
S83.271A
S83.272A
S83.279A
S83.281A
S83.282A
S83.289A
S83.30XA
S83.31XA
S83.32XA
S83.401A
S83.402A
S83.409A
S83.411A
S83.412A
S83.419A
S83.421A
S83.422A
S83.429A
S83.501A
S83.502A
S83.509A
S83.511A
S83.512A

S83.519A
S83.521A
S83.522A
S83.529A
S83.60XA
S83.61XA
S83.62XA
S83.8X1A
S83.8X2A
S83.8X9A
S83.90XA
S83.91XA
S83.92XA
S84.00XA
S84.01XA
S84.02XA
S84.10XA
S84.11XA
S84.12XA
S84.20XA
S84.21XA
S84.22XA
S84.801A
S84.802A
S84.809A
S84.90XA
S84.91XA
S84.92XA
S85.001A
S85.002A
S85.009A
S85.011A
S85.012A
S85.019A
S85.091A
S85.092A
S85.099A
S85.101A
S85.102A
S85.109A
S85.111A
S85.112A
S85.119A
S85.121A
S85.122A
S85.129A
S85.131A
S85.132A
S85.139A
S85.141A
S85.142A
S85.149A
S85.151A
S85.152A
S85.159A
S85.161A
S85.162A
S85.169A
S85.171A
S85.172A
S85.179A
S85.181A
S85.182A
S85.189A
S85.201A
S85.202A
S85.209A
S85.211A
S85.212A
S85.219A
S85.291A
S85.292A
S85.299A
S85.301A
S85.302A
S85.309A
S85.311A
S85.312A
S85.319A
S85.391A
S85.392A
S85.399A
S85.401A
S85.402A
S85.409A
S85.411A
S85.412A
S85.419A
S85.491A
S85.492A
S85.499A
S85.501A
S85.502A
S85.509A
S85.511A
S85.512A
S85.519A
S85.591A
S85.592A
S85.599A
S85.801A
S85.802A
S85.809A
S85.811A
S85.812A
S85.819A
S85.891A
S85.892A
S85.899A
S85.901A
S85.902A
S85.909A
S85.911A
S85.912A
S85.919A
S85.991A
S85.992A
S85.999A
S86.001A
S86.002A
S86.009A
S86.011A
S86.012A
S86.019A
S86.021A
S86.022A
S86.029A
S86.091A
S86.092A
S86.099A
S86.101A
S86.102A
S86.109A
S86.111A
S86.112A
S86.119A
S86.121A
S86.122A
S86.129A
S86.191A
S86.192A
S86.199A
S86.201A
S86.202A
S86.209A
S86.211A
S86.212A
S86.219A
S86.221A
S86.222A
S86.229A
S86.291A
S86.292A
S86.299A
S86.301A
S86.302A
S86.309A
S86.311A
S86.312A
S86.319A
S86.321A
S86.322A
S86.329A
S86.391A
S86.392A
S86.399A
S86.801A
S86.802A
S86.809A
S86.811A
S86.812A
S86.819A
S86.821A
S86.822A
S86.829A
S86.891A
S86.892A
S86.899A
S86.901A
S86.902A
S86.909A
S86.911A
S86.912A
S86.919A
S86.921A
S86.922A
S86.929A
S86.991A
S86.992A
S86.999A
S87.00XA
S87.01XA
S87.02XA
S87.80XA
S87.81XA
S87.82XA
S88.011A
S88.012A
S88.019A
S88.021A
S88.022A
S88.029A
S88.111A
S88.112A
S88.119A
S88.121A
S88.122A
S88.129A
S88.911A
S88.912A
S88.919A
S88.921A
S88.922A
S88.929A
S89.001A
S89.002A
S89.009A
S89.011A
S89.012A
S89.019A
S89.021A
S89.022A
S89.029A
S89.031A
S89.032A
S89.039A
S89.041A
S89.042A
S89.049A
S89.091A
S89.092A
S89.099A
S89.101A
S89.102A
S89.109A
S89.111A
S89.112A
S89.119A
S89.121A
S89.122A
S89.129A
S89.131A
S89.132A
S89.139A
S89.141A
S89.142A
S89.149A
S89.191A
S89.192A
S89.199A
S89.201A
S89.202A
S89.209A
S89.211A
S89.212A
S89.219A
S89.221A
S89.222A
S89.229A
S89.291A
S89.292A
S89.299A
S89.301A
S89.302A
S89.309A
S89.311A
S89.312A
S89.319A
S89.321A
S89.322A
S89.329A
S89.391A
S89.392A
S89.399A
S89.80XA
S89.81XA
S89.82XA
S89.90XA
S89.91XA
S89.92XA
S90.00XA
S90.01XA
S90.02XA
S90.111A
S90.112A
S90.119A
S90.121A
S90.122A
S90.129A
S90.211A
S90.212A
S90.219A
S90.221A
S90.222A
S90.229A
S90.30XA
S90.31XA
S90.32XA
S90.411A
S90.412A
S90.413A
S90.414A
S90.415A
S90.416A
S90.421A
S90.422A
S90.423A
S90.424A
S90.425A
S90.426A
S90.441A
S90.442A
S90.443A
S90.444A
S90.445A
S90.446A
S90.451A
S90.452A
S90.453A
S90.454A
S90.455A
S90.456A
S90.461A
S90.462A
S90.463A
S90.464A
S90.465A
S90.466A
S90.471A
S90.472A
S90.473A
S90.474A
S90.475A
S90.476A
S90.511A
S90.512A
S90.519A
S90.521A
S90.522A
S90.529A
S90.541A
S90.542A
S90.549A
S90.551A
S90.552A
S90.559A
S90.561A
S90.562A
S90.569A
S90.571A
S90.572A
S90.579A
S90.811A
S90.812A
S90.819A
S90.821A
S90.822A
S90.829A
S90.841A
S90.842A
S90.849A
S90.851A
S90.852A
S90.859A
S90.861A
S90.862A
S90.869A
S90.871A
S90.872A
S90.879A
S90.911A
S90.912A
S90.919A
S90.921A
S90.922A
S90.929A
S90.931A
S90.932A
S90.933A
S90.934A
S90.935A
S90.936A
S91.001A
S91.002A
S91.009A
S91.011A
S91.012A
S91.019A
S91.021A
S91.022A
S91.029A
S91.031A
S91.032A
S91.039A
S91.041A
S91.042A
S91.049A
S91.051A
S91.052A
S91.059A
S91.101A
S91.102A
S91.103A
S91.104A
S91.105A
S91.106A
S91.109A
S91.111A
S91.112A
S91.113A
S91.114A
S91.115A
S91.116A
S91.119A
S91.121A
S91.122A
S91.123A
S91.124A
S91.125A
S91.126A
S91.129A
S91.131A
S91.132A
S91.133A
S91.134A
S91.135A
S91.136A
S91.139A
S91.141A
S91.142A
S91.143A
S91.144A
S91.145A
S91.146A
S91.149A
S91.151A
S91.152A
S91.153A
S91.154A
S91.155A
S91.156A
S91.159A
S91.201A
S91.202A
S91.203A
S91.204A
S91.205A
S91.206A
S91.209A
S91.211A
S91.212A
S91.213A
S91.214A
S91.215A
S91.216A
S91.219A
S91.221A
S91.222A
S91.223A
S91.224A
S91.225A
S91.226A
S91.229A
S91.231A
S91.232A
S91.233A
S91.234A
S91.235A
S91.236A
S91.239A
S91.241A
S91.242A
S91.243A
S91.244A
S91.245A
S91.246A
S91.249A
S91.251A
S91.252A
S91.253A
S91.254A
S91.255A
S91.256A
S91.259A
S91.301A
S91.302A
S91.309A
S91.311A
S91.312A
S91.319A
S91.321A
S91.322A
S91.329A
S91.331A
S91.332A
S91.339A
S91.341A
S91.342A
S91.349A
S91.351A
S91.352A
S91.359A
S92.001A
S92.001B
S92.002A
S92.002B
S92.009A
S92.009B
S92.011A
S92.011B
S92.012A
S92.012B
S92.013A
S92.013B
S92.014A
S92.014B
S92.015A
S92.015B
S92.016A
S92.016B
S92.021A
S92.021B
S92.022A
S92.022B
S92.023A
S92.023B
S92.024A
S92.024B
S92.025A
S92.025B
S92.026A
S92.026B
S92.031A
S92.031B
S92.032A
S92.032B
S92.033A
S92.033B
S92.034A
S92.034B
S92.035A
S92.035B
S92.036A
S92.036B
S92.041A
S92.041B
S92.042A
S92.042B
S92.043A
S92.043B
S92.044A
S92.044B
S92.045A
S92.045B
S92.046A
S92.046B
S92.051A
S92.051B
S92.052A
S92.052B
S92.053A
S92.053B
S92.054A
S92.054B
S92.055A
S92.055B
S92.056A
S92.056B
S92.061A
S92.061B
S92.062A
S92.062B
S92.063A
S92.063B
S92.064A
S92.064B
S92.065A
S92.065B
S92.066A
S92.066B
S92.101A
S92.101B
S92.102A
S92.102B
S92.109A
S92.109B
S92.111A
S92.111B
S92.112A
S92.112B
S92.113A
S92.113B
S92.114A
S92.114B
S92.115A
S92.115B
S92.116A
S92.116B
S92.121A
S92.121B
S92.122A
S92.122B
S92.123A
S92.123B
S92.124A
S92.124B
S92.125A
S92.125B
S92.126A
S92.126B
S92.131A
S92.131B
S92.132A
S92.132B
S92.133A
S92.133B
S92.134A
S92.134B
S92.135A
S92.135B
S92.136A
S92.136B
S92.141A
S92.141B
S92.142A
S92.142B
S92.143A
S92.143B
S92.144A
S92.144B
S92.145A
S92.145B
S92.146A
S92.146B
S92.151A
S92.151B
S92.152A
S92.152B
S92.153A
S92.153B
S92.154A
S92.154B
S92.155A
S92.155B
S92.156A
S92.156B
S92.191A
S92.191B
S92.192A
S92.192B
S92.199A
S92.199B
S92.201A
S92.201B
S92.202A
S92.202B
S92.209A
S92.209B
S92.211A
S92.211B
S92.212A
S92.212B
S92.213A
S92.213B
S92.214A
S92.214B
S92.215A
S92.215B
S92.216A
S92.216B
S92.221A
S92.221B
S92.222A
S92.222B
S92.223A
S92.223B
S92.224A
S92.224B
S92.225A
S92.225B
S92.226A
S92.226B
S92.231A
S92.231B
S92.232A
S92.232B
S92.233A
S92.233B
S92.234A
S92.234B
S92.235A
S92.235B
S92.236A
S92.236B
S92.241A
S92.241B
S92.242A
S92.242B
S92.243A
S92.243B
S92.244A
S92.244B
S92.245A
S92.245B
S92.246A
S92.246B
S92.251A
S92.251B
S92.252A
S92.252B
S92.253A
S92.253B
S92.254A
S92.254B
S92.255A
S92.255B
S92.256A
S92.256B
S92.301A
S92.301B
S92.302A
S92.302B
S92.309A
S92.309B
S92.311A
S92.311B
S92.312A
S92.312B
S92.313A
S92.313B
S92.314A
S92.314B
S92.315A
S92.315B
S92.316A
S92.316B
S92.321A
S92.321B
S92.322A
S92.322B
S92.323A
S92.323B
S92.324A
S92.324B
S92.325A
S92.325B
S92.326A
S92.326B
S92.331A
S92.331B
S92.332A
S92.332B
S92.333A
S92.333B
S92.334A
S92.334B
S92.335A
S92.335B
S92.336A
S92.336B
S92.341A
S92.341B
S92.342A
S92.342B
S92.343A
S92.343B
S92.344A
S92.344B
S92.345A
S92.345B
S92.346A
S92.346B
S92.351A
S92.351B
S92.352A
S92.352B
S92.353A
S92.353B
S92.354A
S92.354B
S92.355A
S92.355B
S92.356A
S92.356B
S92.401A
S92.401B
S92.402A
S92.402B
S92.403A
S92.403B
S92.404A
S92.404B
S92.405A
S92.405B
S92.406A
S92.406B
S92.411A
S92.411B
S92.412A
S92.412B
S92.413A
S92.413B
S92.414A
S92.414B
S92.415A
S92.415B
S92.416A
S92.416B
S92.421A
S92.421B
S92.422A
S92.422B
S92.423A
S92.423B
S92.424A
S92.424B
S92.425A
S92.425B
S92.426A
S92.426B
S92.491A
S92.491B
S92.492A
S92.492B
S92.499A
S92.499B
S92.501A
S92.501B
S92.502A
S92.502B
S92.503A
S92.503B
S92.504A
S92.504B
S92.505A
S92.505B
S92.506A
S92.506B
S92.511A
S92.511B
S92.512A
S92.512B
S92.513A
S92.513B
S92.514A
S92.514B
S92.515A
S92.515B
S92.516A
S92.516B
S92.521A
S92.521B
S92.522A
S92.522B
S92.523A

S92.523B
S92.524A
S92.524B
S92.525A
S92.525B
S92.526A
S92.526B
S92.531A
S92.531B
S92.532A
S92.532B
S92.533A
S92.533B
S92.534A
S92.534B
S92.535A
S92.535B
S92.536A
S92.536B
S92.591A
S92.591B
S92.592A
S92.592B
S92.599A
S92.599B
S92.811A
S92.811B
S92.812A
S92.812B
S92.819A
S92.819B
S92.901A
S92.901B
S92.902A
S92.902B
S92.909A
S92.909B
S92.911A
S92.911B
S92.912A
S92.912B
S92.919A
S92.919B
S93.01XA
S93.02XA
S93.03XA
S93.04XA
S93.05XA
S93.06XA
S93.101A
S93.102A
S93.103A
S93.104A
S93.105A
S93.106A
S93.111A
S93.112A
S93.113A
S93.114A
S93.115A
S93.116A
S93.119A
S93.121A
S93.122A
S93.123A
S93.124A
S93.125A
S93.126A
S93.129A
S93.131A
S93.132A
S93.133A
S93.134A
S93.135A
S93.136A
S93.139A
S93.141A
S93.142A
S93.143A
S93.144A
S93.145A
S93.146A
S93.149A
S93.301A
S93.302A
S93.303A
S93.304A
S93.305A
S93.306A
S93.311A
S93.312A
S93.313A
S93.314A
S93.315A
S93.316A
S93.321A
S93.322A
S93.323A
S93.324A
S93.325A
S93.326A
S93.331A
S93.332A
S93.333A
S93.334A
S93.335A
S93.336A
S93.401A
S93.402A
S93.409A
S93.411A
S93.412A
S93.419A
S93.421A
S93.422A
S93.429A
S93.431A
S93.432A
S93.439A
S93.491A
S93.492A
S93.499A
S93.501A
S93.502A
S93.503A
S93.504A
S93.505A
S93.506A
S93.509A
S93.511A
S93.512A
S93.513A
S93.514A
S93.515A
S93.516A
S93.519A
S93.521A
S93.522A
S93.523A
S93.524A
S93.525A
S93.526A
S93.529A
S93.601A
S93.602A
S93.609A
S93.611A
S93.612A
S93.619A
S93.621A
S93.622A
S93.629A
S93.691A
S93.692A
S93.699A
S94.00XA
S94.01XA
S94.02XA
S94.10XA
S94.11XA
S94.12XA
S94.20XA
S94.21XA
S94.22XA
S94.30XA
S94.31XA
S94.32XA
S94.8X1A
S94.8X2A
S94.8X9A
S94.90XA
S94.91XA
S94.92XA
S95.001A
S95.002A
S95.009A
S95.011A
S95.012A
S95.019A
S95.091A
S95.092A
S95.099A
S95.101A
S95.102A
S95.109A
S95.111A
S95.112A
S95.119A
S95.191A
S95.192A
S95.199A
S95.201A
S95.202A
S95.209A
S95.211A
S95.212A
S95.219A
S95.291A
S95.292A
S95.299A
S95.801A
S95.802A
S95.809A
S95.811A
S95.812A
S95.819A
S95.891A
S95.892A
S95.899A
S95.901A
S95.902A
S95.909A
S95.911A
S95.912A
S95.919A
S95.991A
S95.992A
S95.999A
S96.001A
S96.002A
S96.009A
S96.011A
S96.012A
S96.019A
S96.021A
S96.022A
S96.029A
S96.091A
S96.092A
S96.099A
S96.101A
S96.102A
S96.109A
S96.111A
S96.112A
S96.119A
S96.121A
S96.122A
S96.129A
S96.191A
S96.192A
S96.199A
S96.201A
S96.202A
S96.209A
S96.211A
S96.212A
S96.219A
S96.221A
S96.222A
S96.229A
S96.291A
S96.292A
S96.299A
S96.801A
S96.802A
S96.809A
S96.811A
S96.812A
S96.819A
S96.821A
S96.822A
S96.829A
S96.891A
S96.892A
S96.899A
S96.901A
S96.902A
S96.909A
S96.911A
S96.912A
S96.919A
S96.921A
S96.922A
S96.929A
S96.991A
S96.992A
S96.999A
S97.00XA
S97.01XA
S97.02XA
S97.101A
S97.102A
S97.109A
S97.111A
S97.112A
S97.119A
S97.121A
S97.122A
S97.129A
S97.80XA
S97.81XA
S97.82XA
S98.011A
S98.012A
S98.019A
S98.021A
S98.022A
S98.029A
S98.111A
S98.112A
S98.119A
S98.121A
S98.122A
S98.129A
S98.131A
S98.132A
S98.139A
S98.141A
S98.142A
S98.149A
S98.211A
S98.212A
S98.219A
S98.221A
S98.222A
S98.229A
S98.311A
S98.312A
S98.319A
S98.321A
S98.322A
S98.329A
S98.911A
S98.912A
S98.919A
S98.921A
S98.922A
S98.929A
S99.001A
S99.001B
S99.002A
S99.002B
S99.009A
S99.009B
S99.011A
S99.011B
S99.012A
S99.012B
S99.019A
S99.019B
S99.021A
S99.021B
S99.022A
S99.022B
S99.029A
S99.029B
S99.031A
S99.031B
S99.032A
S99.032B
S99.039A
S99.039B
S99.041A
S99.041B
S99.042A
S99.042B
S99.049A
S99.049B
S99.091A
S99.091B
S99.092A
S99.092B
S99.099A
S99.099B
S99.101A
S99.101B
S99.102A
S99.102B
S99.109A
S99.109B
S99.111A
S99.111B
S99.112A
S99.112B
S99.119A
S99.119B
S99.121A
S99.121B
S99.122A
S99.122B
S99.129A
S99.129B
S99.131A
S99.131B
S99.132A
S99.132B
S99.139A
S99.139B
S99.141A
S99.141B
S99.142A
S99.142B
S99.149A
S99.149B
S99.191A
S99.191B
S99.192A
S99.192B
S99.199A
S99.199B
S99.201A
S99.201B
S99.202A
S99.202B
S99.209A
S99.209B
S99.211A
S99.211B
S99.212A
S99.212B
S99.219A
S99.219B
S99.221A
S99.221B
S99.222A
S99.222B
S99.229A
S99.229B
S99.231A
S99.231B
S99.232A
S99.232B
S99.239A
S99.239B
S99.241A
S99.241B
S99.242A
S99.242B
S99.249A
S99.249B
S99.291A
S99.291B
S99.292A
S99.292B
S99.299A
S99.299B
S99.811A
S99.812A
S99.819A
S99.821A
S99.822A
S99.829A
S99.911A
S99.912A
S99.919A
S99.921A
S99.922A
S99.929A
T07.XXXA
T14.8XXA
T14.90XA
T14.91XA
T79.0XXA
T79.1XXA
T79.2XXA
T79.4XXA
T79.5XXA
T79.6XXA
T79.7XXA
T79.8XXA
T79.9XXA
T79.A0XA
T79.A11A
T79.A12A
T79.A19A
T79.A21A
T79.A22A
T79.A29A
T79.A3XA
T79.A9XA

Significant Trauma Body Site Category 1 - Head

S02.101B
S02.102B
S02.109B
S02.91XA
S02.91XB
S06.1X0A
S06.1X1A
S06.1X2A
S06.1X3A
S06.1X4A
S06.1X5A
S06.1X6A
S06.1X7A
S06.1X8A
S06.1X9A
S06.1XAA
S06.2X0A
S06.2X1A
S06.2X2A
S06.2X3A
S06.2X4A
S06.2X5A
S06.2X6A
S06.2X7A
S06.2X8A
S06.2X9A
S06.2XAA
S06.300A
S06.301A
S06.302A
S06.303A
S06.304A
S06.305A
S06.306A
S06.307A
S06.308A
S06.309A
S06.30AA
S06.310A
S06.311A
S06.312A
S06.313A
S06.314A
S06.315A
S06.316A
S06.317A
S06.318A
S06.319A
S06.31AA
S06.320A
S06.321A
S06.322A
S06.323A
S06.324A
S06.325A
S06.326A
S06.327A
S06.328A
S06.329A
S06.32AA
S06.330A
S06.331A
S06.332A
S06.333A
S06.334A
S06.335A
S06.336A
S06.337A
S06.338A
S06.339A
S06.33AA
S06.340A
S06.341A
S06.342A
S06.343A
S06.344A
S06.345A
S06.346A
S06.347A
S06.348A
S06.349A
S06.34AA
S06.350A
S06.351A
S06.352A
S06.353A
S06.354A
S06.355A
S06.356A
S06.357A
S06.358A
S06.359A
S06.35AA
S06.360A
S06.361A
S06.362A
S06.363A
S06.364A
S06.365A
S06.366A
S06.367A
S06.368A
S06.369A
S06.36AA
S06.370A
S06.371A
S06.372A
S06.373A
S06.374A
S06.375A
S06.376A
S06.377A
S06.378A
S06.379A
S06.37AA
S06.380A
S06.381A
S06.382A
S06.383A
S06.384A
S06.385A
S06.386A
S06.387A
S06.388A
S06.389A
S06.38AA
S06.4X0A
S06.4X1A
S06.4X2A
S06.4X3A
S06.4X4A
S06.4X5A
S06.4X6A
S06.4X7A
S06.4X8A
S06.4X9A
S06.4XAA
S06.5X0A
S06.5X1A
S06.5X2A
S06.5X3A
S06.5X4A
S06.5X5A
S06.5X6A
S06.5X7A
S06.5X8A
S06.5X9A
S06.5XAA
S06.6X0A
S06.6X1A
S06.6X2A
S06.6X3A
S06.6X4A
S06.6X5A
S06.6X6A
S06.6X7A
S06.6X8A
S06.6X9A
S06.6XAA
S06.810A
S06.811A
S06.812A
S06.813A
S06.814A
S06.815A
S06.816A
S06.817A
S06.818A
S06.819A
S06.81AA
S06.820A
S06.821A
S06.822A
S06.823A
S06.824A
S06.825A
S06.826A
S06.827A
S06.828A
S06.829A
S06.82AA
S06.890A
S06.891A
S06.892A
S06.893A
S06.894A
S06.895A
S06.896A
S06.897A
S06.898A
S06.899A
S06.89AA
S06.8A0A
S06.8A1A
S06.8A2A
S06.8A3A
S06.8A4A
S06.8A5A
S06.8A6A
S06.8A7A
S06.8A8A
S06.8A9A
S06.8AAA
S06.9X0A
S06.9X1A
S06.9X2A
S06.9X3A
S06.9X4A
S06.9X5A
S06.9X6A
S06.9X7A
S06.9X8A
S06.9X9A
S06.9XAA
S06.A0XA
S06.A1XA
S07.0XXA
S07.1XXA
S07.8XXA
S07.9XXA
S15.001A
S15.002A
S15.011A
S15.012A
S15.019A
S15.021A
S15.022A
S15.029A
S15.091A
S15.092A
S15.099A
S15.201A
S15.202A
S15.209A
S15.211A
S15.212A
S15.219A
S15.221A
S15.222A
S15.229A
S15.291A
S15.292A
S15.299A
S15.301A
S15.302A
S15.309A
S15.311A
S15.312A
S15.319A
S15.321A
S15.322A
S15.329A
S15.391A
S15.392A
S15.399A
S15.8XXA
S17.0XXA
S17.8XXA
S17.9XXA

Significant Trauma Body Site Category 2 - Chest

M96.A4
S11.012A
S11.014A
S11.022A
S11.024A
S11.032A
S11.034A
S12.8XXA
S21.301A
S21.302A
S21.309A
S21.311A
S21.312A
S21.319A
S21.321A
S21.322A
S21.329A
S21.331A
S21.332A
S21.339A
S21.341A
S21.342A
S21.349A
S21.351A
S21.352A
S21.359A
S21.401A
S21.402A
S21.409A
S21.411A
S21.412A
S21.419A
S21.421A
S21.422A
S21.429A
S21.431A
S21.432A
S21.439A
S21.441A
S21.442A
S21.449A
S21.451A
S21.452A
S21.459A
S22.20XB
S22.21XB
S22.22XB
S22.23XB
S22.24XB
S22.41XB
S22.42XB
S22.43XB
S22.5XXA
S22.5XXB
S25.00XA
S25.01XA
S25.02XA
S25.09XA
S25.101A
S25.102A
S25.109A
S25.111A
S25.112A
S25.119A
S25.121A
S25.122A
S25.129A
S25.191A
S25.192A
S25.199A
S25.20XA
S25.21XA
S25.22XA
S25.29XA
S25.301A
S25.302A
S25.309A
S25.311A
S25.312A
S25.319A
S25.321A
S25.322A
S25.329A
S25.391A
S25.392A
S25.399A
S25.401A
S25.402A
S25.409A
S25.411A
S25.412A
S25.419A
S25.421A
S25.422A
S25.429A
S25.491A
S25.492A
S25.499A
S25.801A
S25.802A
S25.809A
S25.811A
S25.812A
S25.819A
S25.891A
S25.892A
S25.899A
S25.90XA
S25.91XA
S25.99XA
S26.00XA
S26.01XA
S26.020A
S26.021A
S26.022A
S26.09XA
S26.10XA
S26.11XA
S26.12XA

S26.19XA
S26.9ØXA
S26.91XA
S26.92XA
S26.99XA
S27.ØXXA
S27.1XXA
S27.2XXA
S27.3Ø1A
S27.3Ø2A
S27.3Ø9A
S27.311A
S27.312A
S27.319A
S27.321A
S27.322A
S27.329A
S27.331A
S27.332A
S27.339A
S27.391A
S27.392A
S27.399A
S27.4Ø1A
S27.4Ø2A
S27.4Ø9A
S27.411A
S27.412A
S27.419A
S27.421A
S27.422A
S27.429A
S27.431A
S27.432A
S27.439A
S27.491A
S27.492A
S27.499A
S27.5ØXA
S27.51XA
S27.52XA
S27.53XA
S27.59XA
S27.6ØXA
S27.63XA
S27.69XA
S27.8Ø2A
S27.8Ø3A
S27.8Ø8A
S27.8Ø9A
S27.812A
S27.813A
S27.818A
S27.819A
S27.892A
S27.893A
S27.898A
S27.899A
S27.9XXA
T79.ØXXA
T79.1XXA

Significant Trauma Body Site Category 3 - Abdomen

S31.ØØ1A
S31.Ø11A
S31.Ø21A
S31.Ø31A
S31.Ø41A
S31.Ø51A
S31.6ØØA
S31.6Ø1A
S31.6Ø2A
S31.6Ø3A
S31.6Ø4A
S31.6Ø5A
S31.6Ø9A
S31.61ØA
S31.611A
S31.612A
S31.613A
S31.614A
S31.615A
S31.619A
S31.62ØA
S31.621A
S31.622A
S31.623A
S31.624A
S31.625A
S31.629A
S31.63ØA
S31.631A
S31.632A
S31.633A
S31.634A
S31.635A
S31.639A
S31.64ØA
S31.641A
S31.642A
S31.643A
S31.644A
S31.645A
S31.649A
S31.65ØA
S31.651A
S31.652A
S31.653A
S31.654A
S31.655A
S31.659A
S35.ØØXA
S35.Ø1XA
S35.Ø2XA
S35.Ø9XA
S35.1ØXA
S35.11XA
S35.12XA
S35.19XA
S35.211A
S35.212A
S35.218A
S35.219A
S35.221A
S35.222A
S35.228A
S35.229A
S35.231A
S35.232A
S35.238A
S35.239A
S35.291A
S35.292A
S35.298A
S35.299A
S35.311A
S35.318A
S35.319A
S35.321A
S35.328A
S35.329A
S35.331A
S35.338A
S35.339A
S35.341A
S35.348A
S35.349A
S35.4Ø1A
S35.4Ø2A
S35.4Ø3A
S35.4Ø4A
S35.4Ø5A
S35.4Ø6A
S35.411A
S35.412A
S35.413A
S35.414A
S35.415A
S35.416A
S35.491A
S35.492A
S35.493A
S35.494A
S35.495A
S35.496A
S35.5ØXA
S35.511A
S35.512A
S35.513A
S35.514A
S35.515A
S35.516A
S35.531A
S35.532A
S35.533A
S35.534A
S35.535A
S35.536A
S35.59XA
S35.8X1A
S35.8X8A
S35.8X9A
S35.9ØXA
S35.91XA
S35.99XA
S36.ØØXA
S36.Ø2ØA
S36.Ø21A
S36.Ø29A
S36.Ø3ØA
S36.Ø31A
S36.Ø32A
S36.Ø39A
S36.Ø9XA
S36.112A
S36.113A
S36.114A
S36.115A
S36.116A
S36.118A
S36.119A
S36.122A
S36.123A
S36.128A
S36.129A
S36.13XA
S36.2ØØA
S36.2Ø1A
S36.2Ø2A
S36.2Ø9A
S36.22ØA
S36.221A
S36.222A
S36.229A
S36.23ØA
S36.231A
S36.232A
S36.239A
S36.24ØA
S36.241A
S36.242A
S36.249A
S36.25ØA
S36.251A
S36.252A
S36.259A
S36.26ØA
S36.261A
S36.262A
S36.269A
S36.29ØA
S36.291A
S36.292A
S36.299A
S36.3ØXA
S36.32XA
S36.33XA
S36.39XA
S36.4ØØA
S36.4Ø8A
S36.4Ø9A
S36.41ØA
S36.418A
S36.419A
S36.42ØA
S36.428A
S36.429A
S36.43ØA
S36.438A
S36.439A
S36.49ØA
S36.498A
S36.499A
S36.5ØØA
S36.5Ø1A
S36.5Ø2A
S36.5Ø3A
S36.5Ø8A
S36.5Ø9A
S36.51ØA
S36.511A
S36.512A
S36.513A
S36.518A
S36.519A
S36.52ØA
S36.521A
S36.522A
S36.523A
S36.528A
S36.529A
S36.53ØA
S36.531A
S36.532A
S36.533A
S36.538A
S36.539A
S36.59ØA
S36.591A
S36.592A
S36.593A
S36.598A
S36.599A
S36.6ØXA
S36.61XA
S36.62XA
S36.63XA
S36.69XA
S36.892A
S36.893A
S36.898A
S36.899A
T79.A3XA

Significant Trauma Body Site Category 4 - Kidney

S37.ØØ1A
S37.ØØ2A
S37.ØØ9A
S37.Ø11A
S37.Ø12A
S37.Ø19A
S37.Ø21A
S37.Ø22A
S37.Ø29A
S37.Ø31A
S37.Ø32A
S37.Ø39A
S37.Ø41A
S37.Ø42A
S37.Ø49A
S37.Ø51A
S37.Ø52A
S37.Ø59A
S37.Ø61A
S37.Ø62A
S37.Ø69A
S37.Ø91A
S37.Ø92A
S37.Ø99A
S37.812A
S37.813A
S37.818A
S37.819A

Significant Trauma Body Site Category 5 - Urinary

S37.1ØXA
S37.12XA
S37.13XA
S37.19XA
S37.2ØXA
S37.22XA
S37.23XA
S37.29XA
S37.3ØXA
S37.32XA
S37.33XA
S37.39XA
S37.6ØXA
S37.62XA
S37.63XA
S37.69XA
S37.892A
S37.893A
S37.898A
S37.899A
S37.9ØXA
S37.92XA
S37.93XA
S37.99XA

Significant Trauma Body Site Category 6 - Pelvis or Spine

M99.1Ø
M99.11
S13.ØXXA
S13.1ØØA
S13.1Ø1A
S13.11ØA
S13.111A
S13.12ØA
S13.121A
S13.13ØA
S13.131A
S13.14ØA
S13.141A
S13.15ØA
S13.151A
S13.16ØA
S13.161A
S13.17ØA
S13.171A
S13.18ØA
S13.181A
S13.2ØXA
S13.29XA
S14.ØXXA
S14.1Ø1A
S14.1Ø2A
S14.1Ø3A
S14.1Ø4A
S14.1Ø5A
S14.1Ø6A
S14.1Ø7A
S14.1Ø8A
S14.1Ø9A
S14.111A
S14.112A
S14.113A
S14.114A
S14.115A
S14.116A
S14.117A
S14.118A
S14.119A
S14.121A
S14.122A
S14.123A
S14.124A
S14.125A
S14.126A
S14.127A
S14.128A
S14.129A
S14.131A
S14.132A
S14.133A
S14.134A
S14.135A
S14.136A
S14.137A
S14.138A
S14.139A
S14.141A
S14.142A
S14.143A
S14.144A
S14.145A
S14.146A
S14.147A
S14.148A
S14.149A
S14.151A
S14.152A
S14.153A
S14.154A
S14.155A
S14.156A
S14.157A
S14.158A
S14.159A
S22.9XXB
S24.ØXXA
S24.1Ø1A
S24.1Ø2A
S24.1Ø3A
S24.1Ø4A
S24.1Ø9A
S24.111A
S24.112A
S24.113A
S24.114A
S24.119A
S24.131A
S24.132A
S24.133A
S24.134A
S24.139A
S24.141A
S24.142A
S24.143A
S24.144A
S24.149A
S24.151A
S24.152A
S24.153A
S24.154A
S24.159A
S24.3XXA
S24.8XXA
S24.9XXA
S28.ØXXA
S32.1ØXA
S32.1ØXB
S32.11ØA
S32.11ØB
S32.111A
S32.111B
S32.112A
S32.112B
S32.119A
S32.119B
S32.12ØA
S32.12ØB
S32.121A
S32.121B
S32.122A
S32.122B
S32.129A
S32.129B
S32.13ØA
S32.13ØB
S32.131A
S32.131B
S32.132A
S32.132B
S32.139A
S32.139B
S32.14XA
S32.14XB
S32.15XA
S32.15XB
S32.16XA
S32.16XB
S32.17XA
S32.17XB
S32.19XA
S32.19XB
S32.2XXA
S32.2XXB
S32.3Ø1A
S32.3Ø1B
S32.3Ø2A
S32.3Ø2B
S32.3Ø9A
S32.3Ø9B
S32.311A
S32.311B
S32.312A
S32.312B
S32.313A
S32.313B
S32.314A
S32.314B
S32.315A
S32.315B
S32.316A
S32.316B
S32.391A
S32.391B
S32.392A
S32.392B
S32.399A
S32.399B
S32.4Ø1A
S32.4Ø1B
S32.4Ø2A
S32.4Ø2B
S32.4Ø9A
S32.4Ø9B
S32.411A
S32.411B
S32.412A
S32.412B
S32.413A
S32.413B
S32.414A
S32.414B
S32.415A
S32.415B
S32.416A
S32.416B
S32.421A
S32.421B
S32.422A
S32.422B
S32.423A
S32.423B
S32.424A
S32.424B
S32.425A
S32.425B
S32.426A
S32.426B
S32.431A
S32.431B
S32.432A
S32.432B
S32.433A
S32.433B
S32.434A
S32.434B
S32.435A
S32.435B
S32.436A
S32.436B
S32.441A
S32.441B
S32.442A
S32.442B
S32.443A
S32.443B
S32.444A
S32.444B
S32.445A
S32.445B
S32.446A
S32.446B
S32.451A
S32.451B
S32.452A
S32.452B
S32.453A
S32.453B
S32.454A
S32.454B
S32.455A
S32.455B
S32.456A
S32.456B
S32.461A
S32.461B
S32.462A
S32.462B
S32.463A
S32.463B
S32.464A
S32.464B
S32.465A
S32.465B
S32.466A
S32.466B
S32.471A
S32.471B
S32.472A
S32.472B
S32.473A
S32.473B
S32.474A
S32.474B
S32.475A
S32.475B
S32.476A
S32.476B
S32.481A
S32.481B
S32.482A
S32.482B
S32.483A
S32.483B
S32.484A
S32.484B
S32.485A
S32.485B
S32.486A
S32.486B
S32.491A
S32.491B
S32.492A
S32.492B
S32.499A
S32.499B
S32.5Ø1A
S32.5Ø1B
S32.5Ø2A
S32.5Ø2B
S32.5Ø9A
S32.5Ø9B
S32.511A
S32.511B
S32.512A
S32.512B
S32.519A
S32.519B
S32.591A
S32.591B
S32.592A
S32.592B
S32.599A
S32.599B
S32.6Ø1A
S32.6Ø1B
S32.6Ø2A
S32.6Ø2B
S32.6Ø9A
S32.6Ø9B
S32.611A
S32.611B
S32.612A
S32.612B
S32.613A
S32.613B
S32.614A
S32.614B
S32.615A
S32.615B
S32.616A
S32.616B
S32.691A
S32.691B
S32.692A
S32.692B
S32.699A
S32.699B
S32.81ØA
S32.81ØB
S32.811A
S32.811B
S32.82XA
S32.82XB
S32.89XA
S32.89XB
S32.9XXA
S32.9XXB
S34.Ø1XA
S34.Ø2XA
S34.1Ø1A
S34.1Ø2A
S34.1Ø3A
S34.1Ø4A
S34.1Ø5A
S34.1Ø9A
S34.111A
S34.112A
S34.113A
S34.114A
S34.115A
S34.119A
S34.121A
S34.122A
S34.123A
S34.124A
S34.125A
S34.129A
S34.131A
S34.132A
S34.139A
S34.3XXA
S34.4XXA
S34.6XXA
S34.8XXA
S34.9XXA
S36.81XA
S38.1XXA

Significant Trauma Body Site Category 7 - Upper Limb

S14.3XXA
S42.2Ø1B
S42.2Ø2B
S42.2Ø9B
S42.211B
S42.212B
S42.213B
S42.214B
S42.215B
S42.216B
S42.221B
S42.222B
S42.223B
S42.224B
S42.225B
S42.226B
S42.231B
S42.232B
S42.239B
S42.241B
S42.242B
S42.249B
S42.251B
S42.252B
S42.253B
S42.254B
S42.255B
S42.256B
S42.261B
S42.262B
S42.263B
S42.264B
S42.265B
S42.266B
S42.291B
S42.292B
S42.293B
S42.294B
S42.295B
S42.296B
S42.3Ø1B
S42.3Ø2B
S42.3Ø9B
S42.321B
S42.322B
S42.323B
S42.324B
S42.325B
S42.326B
S42.331B
S42.332B
S42.333B
S42.334B
S42.335B
S42.336B
S42.341B
S42.342B
S42.343B
S42.344B
S42.345B
S42.346B
S42.351B
S42.352B
S42.353B
S42.354B
S42.355B
S42.356B
S42.361B
S42.362B
S42.363B
S42.364B
S42.365B
S42.366B
S42.391B
S42.392B
S42.399B
S42.4Ø1B
S42.4Ø2B
S42.4Ø9B
S42.411B
S42.412B
S42.413B
S42.414B
S42.415B
S42.416B
S42.421B
S42.422B
S42.423B
S42.424B
S42.425B
S42.426B
S42.431B
S42.432B
S42.433B
S42.434B
S42.435B
S42.436B
S42.441B
S42.442B
S42.443B
S42.444B
S42.445B
S42.446B
S42.447B
S42.448B
S42.449B
S42.451B
S42.452B
S42.453B
S42.454B
S42.455B
S42.456B
S42.461B
S42.462B
S42.463B
S42.464B
S42.465B
S42.466B
S42.471B
S42.472B
S42.473B
S42.474B
S42.475B
S42.476B
S42.491B
S42.492B
S42.493B
S42.494B
S42.495B
S42.496B
S42.9ØXB
S42.91XB
S42.92XB
S44.ØØXA
S44.Ø1XA

ICD-10-CM/PCS Codes by MS-DRG

S44.Ø2XA
S44.1ØXA
S44.11XA
S44.12XA
S44.2ØXA
S44.21XA
S44.22XA
S44.3ØXA
S44.31XA
S44.32XA
S44.8X1A
S44.8X2A
S45.ØØ1A
S45.ØØ2A
S45.ØØ9A
S45.Ø11A
S45.Ø12A
S45.Ø19A
S45.Ø91A
S45.Ø92A
S45.Ø99A
S45.1Ø1A
S45.1Ø2A
S45.1Ø9A
S45.111A
S45.112A
S45.119A
S45.191A
S45.192A
S45.199A
S45.2Ø1A
S45.2Ø2A
S45.2Ø9A
S45.211A
S45.212A
S45.219A
S45.291A
S45.292A
S45.299A
S45.3Ø1A
S45.3Ø2A
S45.3Ø9A
S45.311A
S45.312A
S45.319A
S45.391A
S45.392A
S45.399A
S45.8Ø1A
S45.8Ø2A
S45.8Ø9A
S45.811A
S45.812A
S45.819A
S45.891A
S45.892A
S45.899A
S45.9Ø1A
S45.9Ø2A
S45.9Ø9A
S45.911A
S45.912A
S45.919A
S45.991A
S45.992A
S45.999A
S47.1XXA
S47.2XXA
S47.9XXA
S48.Ø11A
S48.Ø12A
S48.Ø19A
S48.Ø21A
S48.Ø22A
S48.Ø29A
S48.111A
S48.112A
S48.119A
S48.121A
S48.122A
S48.129A
S48.911A
S48.912A
S48.919A
S48.921A
S48.922A
S48.929A
S52.ØØ1B
S52.ØØ1C
S52.ØØ2B
S52.ØØ2C
S52.ØØ9B
S52.ØØ9C
S52.Ø21B
S52.Ø21C
S52.Ø22B
S52.Ø22C
S52.Ø23B
S52.Ø23C
S52.Ø24B
S52.Ø24C
S52.Ø25B
S52.Ø25C
S52.Ø26B
S52.Ø26C
S52.Ø31B
S52.Ø31C
S52.Ø32B
S52.Ø32C
S52.Ø33B
S52.Ø33C
S52.Ø34B
S52.Ø34C
S52.Ø35B
S52.Ø35C
S52.Ø36B
S52.Ø36C
S52.Ø41B
S52.Ø41C
S52.Ø42B
S52.Ø42C
S52.Ø43B
S52.Ø43C
S52.Ø44B
S52.Ø44C
S52.Ø45B
S52.Ø45C
S52.Ø46B
S52.Ø46C
S52.Ø91B
S52.Ø91C
S52.Ø92B
S52.Ø92C
S52.Ø99B
S52.Ø99C
S52.1Ø1B
S52.1Ø1C
S52.1Ø2B
S52.1Ø2C
S52.1Ø9B
S52.1Ø9C
S52.121B
S52.121C
S52.122B
S52.122C
S52.123B
S52.123C
S52.124B
S52.124C
S52.125B
S52.125C
S52.126B
S52.126C
S52.131B
S52.131C
S52.132B
S52.132C
S52.133B
S52.133C
S52.134B
S52.134C
S52.135B
S52.135C
S52.136B
S52.136C
S52.181B
S52.181C
S52.182B
S52.182C
S52.189B
S52.189C
S52.2Ø1B
S52.2Ø1C
S52.2Ø2B
S52.2Ø2C
S52.2Ø9B
S52.2Ø9C
S52.221B
S52.221C
S52.222B
S52.222C
S52.223B
S52.223C
S52.224B
S52.224C
S52.225B
S52.225C
S52.226B
S52.226C
S52.231B
S52.231C
S52.232B
S52.232C
S52.233B
S52.233C
S52.234B
S52.234C
S52.235B
S52.235C
S52.236B
S52.236C
S52.241B
S52.241C
S52.242B
S52.242C
S52.243B
S52.243C
S52.244B
S52.244C
S52.245B
S52.245C
S52.246B
S52.246C
S52.251B
S52.251C
S52.252B
S52.252C
S52.253B
S52.253C
S52.254B
S52.254C
S52.255B
S52.255C
S52.256B
S52.256C
S52.261B
S52.261C
S52.262B
S52.262C
S52.263B
S52.263C
S52.264B
S52.264C
S52.265B
S52.265C
S52.266B
S52.266C
S52.271B
S52.271C
S52.272B
S52.272C
S52.279B
S52.279C
S52.281B
S52.281C
S52.282B
S52.282C
S52.283B
S52.283C
S52.291B
S52.291C
S52.292B
S52.292C
S52.299B
S52.299C
S52.3Ø1B
S52.3Ø1C
S52.3Ø2B
S52.3Ø2C
S52.3Ø9B
S52.3Ø9C
S52.321B
S52.321C
S52.322B
S52.322C
S52.323B
S52.323C
S52.324B
S52.324C
S52.325B
S52.325C
S52.326B
S52.326C
S52.331B
S52.331C
S52.332B
S52.332C
S52.333B
S52.333C
S52.334B
S52.334C
S52.335B
S52.335C
S52.336B
S52.336C
S52.341B
S52.341C
S52.342B
S52.342C
S52.343B
S52.343C
S52.344B
S52.344C
S52.345B
S52.345C
S52.346B
S52.346C
S52.351B
S52.351C
S52.352B
S52.352C
S52.353B
S52.353C
S52.354B
S52.354C
S52.355B
S52.355C
S52.356B
S52.356C
S52.361B
S52.361C
S52.362B
S52.362C
S52.363B
S52.363C
S52.364B
S52.364C
S52.365B
S52.365C
S52.366B
S52.366C
S52.371B
S52.371C
S52.372B
S52.372C
S52.379B
S52.379C
S52.381B
S52.381C
S52.382B
S52.382C
S52.389B
S52.389C
S52.391B
S52.391C
S52.392B
S52.392C
S52.399B
S52.399C
S52.5Ø1B
S52.5Ø1C
S52.5Ø2B
S52.5Ø2C
S52.5Ø9B
S52.5Ø9C
S52.511B
S52.511C
S52.512B
S52.512C
S52.513B
S52.513C
S52.514B
S52.514C
S52.515B
S52.515C
S52.516B
S52.516C
S52.531B
S52.531C
S52.532B
S52.532C
S52.539B
S52.539C
S52.541B
S52.541C
S52.542B
S52.542C
S52.549B
S52.549C
S52.551B
S52.551C
S52.552B
S52.552C
S52.559B
S52.559C
S52.561B
S52.561C
S52.562B
S52.562C
S52.569B
S52.569C
S52.571B
S52.571C
S52.572B
S52.572C
S52.579B
S52.579C
S52.591B
S52.591C
S52.592B
S52.592C
S52.599B
S52.599C
S52.6Ø1B
S52.6Ø1C
S52.6Ø2B
S52.6Ø2C
S52.6Ø9B
S52.6Ø9C
S52.611B
S52.611C
S52.612B
S52.612C
S52.613B
S52.613C
S52.614B
S52.614C
S52.615B
S52.615C
S52.616B
S52.616C
S52.691B
S52.691C
S52.692B
S52.692C
S52.699B
S52.699C
S52.9ØXB
S52.9ØXC
S52.91XB
S52.91XC
S52.92XB
S52.92XC
S54.ØØXA
S54.Ø1XA
S54.Ø2XA
S54.1ØXA
S54.11XA
S54.12XA
S54.2ØXA
S54.21XA
S54.22XA
S54.8X1A
S54.8X2A
S54.8X9A
S55.ØØ1A
S55.ØØ2A
S55.ØØ9A
S55.Ø11A
S55.Ø12A
S55.Ø19A
S55.Ø91A
S55.Ø92A
S55.Ø99A
S55.1Ø1A
S55.1Ø2A
S55.1Ø9A
S55.111A
S55.112A
S55.119A
S55.191A
S55.192A
S55.199A
S55.2Ø1A
S55.2Ø2A
S55.2Ø9A
S55.211A
S55.212A
S55.219A
S55.291A
S55.292A
S55.299A
S55.8Ø1A
S55.8Ø2A
S55.8Ø9A
S55.811A
S55.812A
S55.819A
S55.891A
S55.892A
S55.899A
S55.9Ø1A
S55.9Ø2A
S55.9Ø9A
S55.911A
S55.912A
S55.919A
S55.991A
S55.992A
S55.999A
S57.ØØXA
S57.Ø1XA
S57.Ø2XA
S57.8ØXA
S57.81XA
S57.82XA
S58.Ø11A
S58.Ø12A
S58.Ø19A
S58.Ø21A
S58.Ø22A
S58.Ø29A
S58.111A
S58.112A
S58.119A
S58.121A
S58.122A
S58.129A
S58.911A
S58.912A
S58.919A
S58.921A
S58.922A
S58.929A
S62.9ØXB
S64.ØØXA
S64.Ø1XA
S64.Ø2XA
S64.1ØXA
S64.11XA
S64.12XA
S64.2ØXA
S64.21XA
S64.22XA
S64.8X1A
S64.8X2A
S64.8X9A
S65.ØØ1A
S65.ØØ2A
S65.ØØ9A
S65.Ø11A
S65.Ø12A
S65.Ø19A
S65.Ø91A
S65.Ø92A
S65.Ø99A
S65.1Ø1A
S65.1Ø2A
S65.1Ø9A
S65.111A
S65.112A
S65.119A
S65.191A
S65.192A
S65.199A
S65.8Ø1A
S65.8Ø2A
S65.8Ø9A
S65.811A
S65.812A
S65.819A
S65.891A
S65.892A
S65.899A
S65.9Ø1A
S65.9Ø2A
S65.9Ø9A
S65.911A
S65.912A
S65.919A
S65.991A
S65.992A
S65.999A
S68.411A
S68.412A
S68.419A
S68.421A
S68.422A
S68.429A
S68.711A
S68.712A
S68.719A
S68.721A
S68.722A
S68.729A
T79.6XXA
T79.A11A
T79.A12A
T79.A19A

Significant Trauma Body Site Category 8 - Lower Limb

S72.ØØ1A
S72.ØØ1B
S72.ØØ1C
S72.ØØ2A
S72.ØØ2B
S72.ØØ2C
S72.ØØ9A
S72.ØØ9B
S72.ØØ9C
S72.Ø11A
S72.Ø11B
S72.Ø11C
S72.Ø12A
S72.Ø12B
S72.Ø12C
S72.Ø19A
S72.Ø19B
S72.Ø19C
S72.Ø21A
S72.Ø21B
S72.Ø21C
S72.Ø22A
S72.Ø22B
S72.Ø22C
S72.Ø23A
S72.Ø23B
S72.Ø23C
S72.Ø24A
S72.Ø24B
S72.Ø24C
S72.Ø25A
S72.Ø25B
S72.Ø25C
S72.Ø26A
S72.Ø26B
S72.Ø26C
S72.Ø31A
S72.Ø31B
S72.Ø31C
S72.Ø32A
S72.Ø32B
S72.Ø32C
S72.Ø33A
S72.Ø33B
S72.Ø33C
S72.Ø34A
S72.Ø34B
S72.Ø34C
S72.Ø35A
S72.Ø35B
S72.Ø35C
S72.Ø36A
S72.Ø36B
S72.Ø36C
S72.Ø41A
S72.Ø41B
S72.Ø41C
S72.Ø42A
S72.Ø42B
S72.Ø42C
S72.Ø43A
S72.Ø43B
S72.Ø43C
S72.Ø44A
S72.Ø44B
S72.Ø44C
S72.Ø45A
S72.Ø45B
S72.Ø45C
S72.Ø46A
S72.Ø46B
S72.Ø46C
S72.Ø51A
S72.Ø51B
S72.Ø51C
S72.Ø52A
S72.Ø52B
S72.Ø52C
S72.Ø59A
S72.Ø59B
S72.Ø59C
S72.Ø61A
S72.Ø61B
S72.Ø61C
S72.Ø62A
S72.Ø62B
S72.Ø62C
S72.Ø63A
S72.Ø63B
S72.Ø63C
S72.Ø64A
S72.Ø64B
S72.Ø64C
S72.Ø65A
S72.Ø65B
S72.Ø65C
S72.Ø66A
S72.Ø66B
S72.Ø66C
S72.Ø91A
S72.Ø91B
S72.Ø91C
S72.Ø92A
S72.Ø92B
S72.Ø92C
S72.Ø99A
S72.Ø99B
S72.Ø99C
S72.1Ø1A
S72.1Ø1B
S72.1Ø1C
S72.1Ø2A
S72.1Ø2B
S72.1Ø2C
S72.1Ø9A
S72.1Ø9B
S72.1Ø9C
S72.111A
S72.111B
S72.111C
S72.112A
S72.112B
S72.112C
S72.113A
S72.113B
S72.113C
S72.114A
S72.114B
S72.114C
S72.115A
S72.115B
S72.115C
S72.116A
S72.116B
S72.116C
S72.121A
S72.121B
S72.121C
S72.122A
S72.122B
S72.122C
S72.123A
S72.123B
S72.123C
S72.124A
S72.124B
S72.124C
S72.125A
S72.125B
S72.125C
S72.126A
S72.126B
S72.126C
S72.131A
S72.131B
S72.131C
S72.132A
S72.132B
S72.132C
S72.133A
S72.133B
S72.133C
S72.134A
S72.134B
S72.134C
S72.135A
S72.135B
S72.135C
S72.136A
S72.136B
S72.136C
S72.141A
S72.141B
S72.141C
S72.142A
S72.142B
S72.142C
S72.143A
S72.143B
S72.143C
S72.144A
S72.144B
S72.144C
S72.145A
S72.145B
S72.145C
S72.146A
S72.146B
S72.146C
S72.21XA
S72.21XB
S72.21XC
S72.22XA
S72.22XB
S72.22XC
S72.23XA
S72.23XB
S72.23XC
S72.24XA
S72.24XB
S72.24XC
S72.25XA
S72.25XB
S72.25XC
S72.26XA
S72.26XB
S72.26XC
S72.3Ø1A
S72.3Ø1B
S72.3Ø1C
S72.3Ø2A
S72.3Ø2B
S72.3Ø2C
S72.3Ø9A
S72.3Ø9B
S72.3Ø9C
S72.321A
S72.321B
S72.321C
S72.322A
S72.322B
S72.322C
S72.323A
S72.323B
S72.323C
S72.324A
S72.324B
S72.324C
S72.325A
S72.325B
S72.325C
S72.326A
S72.326B
S72.326C
S72.331A
S72.331B
S72.331C
S72.332A
S72.332B
S72.332C
S72.333A
S72.333B
S72.333C
S72.334A
S72.334B
S72.334C
S72.335A
S72.335B
S72.335C
S72.336A
S72.336B
S72.336C
S72.341A
S72.341B
S72.341C
S72.342A
S72.342B
S72.342C
S72.343A
S72.343B
S72.343C
S72.344A
S72.344B
S72.344C
S72.345A
S72.345B
S72.345C
S72.346A
S72.346B
S72.346C
S72.351A
S72.351B
S72.351C
S72.352A
S72.352B
S72.352C
S72.353A
S72.353B
S72.353C
S72.354A
S72.354B
S72.354C

S72.355A
S72.355B
S72.355C
S72.356A
S72.356B
S72.356C
S72.361A
S72.361B
S72.361C
S72.362A
S72.362B
S72.362C
S72.363A
S72.363B
S72.363C
S72.364A
S72.364B
S72.364C
S72.365A
S72.365B
S72.365C
S72.366A
S72.366B
S72.366C
S72.391A
S72.391B
S72.391C
S72.392A
S72.392B
S72.392C
S72.399A
S72.399B
S72.399C
S72.4Ø1A
S72.4Ø1B
S72.4Ø1C
S72.4Ø2A
S72.4Ø2B
S72.4Ø2C
S72.4Ø9A
S72.4Ø9B
S72.4Ø9C
S72.411A
S72.411B
S72.411C
S72.412A
S72.412B
S72.412C
S72.413A
S72.413B
S72.413C
S72.414A
S72.414B
S72.414C
S72.415A
S72.415B
S72.415C
S72.416A
S72.416B
S72.416C
S72.421A
S72.421B
S72.421C
S72.422A
S72.422B
S72.422C
S72.423A
S72.423B
S72.423C
S72.424A
S72.424B
S72.424C
S72.425A
S72.425B
S72.425C
S72.426A
S72.426B
S72.426C
S72.431A
S72.431B
S72.431C
S72.432A
S72.432B
S72.432C
S72.433A
S72.433B
S72.433C
S72.434A
S72.434B
S72.434C
S72.435A
S72.435B
S72.435C
S72.436A
S72.436B
S72.436C
S72.441A
S72.441B
S72.441C
S72.442A
S72.442B
S72.442C
S72.443A
S72.443B
S72.443C
S72.444A
S72.444B
S72.444C
S72.445A
S72.445B
S72.445C
S72.446A
S72.446B
S72.446C
S72.451A
S72.451B
S72.451C
S72.452A
S72.452B
S72.452C
S72.453A
S72.453B
S72.453C
S72.454A
S72.454B
S72.454C
S72.455A
S72.455B
S72.455C
S72.456A
S72.456B
S72.456C
S72.461A
S72.461B
S72.461C
S72.462A
S72.462B
S72.462C
S72.463A
S72.463B
S72.463C
S72.464A
S72.464B
S72.464C
S72.465A
S72.465B
S72.465C
S72.466A
S72.466B
S72.466C
S72.471A
S72.472A
S72.479A
S72.491A
S72.491B
S72.491C
S72.492A
S72.492B
S72.492C
S72.499A
S72.499B
S72.499C
S72.8X1A
S72.8X1B
S72.8X1C
S72.8X2A
S72.8X2B
S72.8X2C
S72.8X9A
S72.8X9B
S72.8X9C
S72.9ØXA
S72.9ØXB
S72.9ØXC
S72.91XA
S72.91XB
S72.91XC
S72.92XA
S72.92XB
S72.92XC
S74.ØØXA
S74.Ø1XA
S74.Ø2XA
S74.1ØXA
S74.11XA
S74.12XA
S74.8X1A
S74.8X2A
S74.8X9A
S74.9ØXA
S74.91XA
S74.92XA
S75.ØØ1A
S75.ØØ2A
S75.ØØ9A
S75.Ø11A
S75.Ø12A
S75.Ø19A
S75.Ø21A
S75.Ø22A
S75.Ø29A
S75.Ø91A
S75.Ø92A
S75.Ø99A
S75.1Ø1A
S75.1Ø2A
S75.1Ø9A
S75.111A
S75.112A
S75.119A
S75.121A
S75.122A
S75.129A
S75.191A
S75.192A
S75.199A
S75.8Ø1A
S75.8Ø2A
S75.8Ø9A
S75.811A
S75.812A
S75.819A
S75.891A
S75.892A
S75.899A
S77.ØØXA
S77.Ø1XA
S77.Ø2XA
S77.1ØXA
S77.11XA
S77.12XA
S77.2ØXA
S77.21XA
S77.22XA
S78.Ø11A
S78.Ø12A
S78.Ø19A
S78.Ø21A
S78.Ø22A
S78.Ø29A
S78.111A
S78.112A
S78.119A
S78.121A
S78.122A
S78.129A
S78.911A
S78.912A
S78.919A
S78.921A
S78.922A
S78.929A
S79.ØØ1A
S79.ØØ2A
S79.ØØ9A
S79.Ø11A
S79.Ø12A
S79.Ø19A
S79.Ø91A
S79.Ø92A
S79.Ø99A
S79.1Ø1A
S79.1Ø2A
S79.1Ø9A
S79.111A
S79.112A
S79.119A
S79.121A
S79.122A
S79.129A
S79.131A
S79.132A
S79.139A
S79.141A
S79.142A
S79.149A
S79.191A
S79.192A
S79.199A
S82.1Ø1B
S82.1Ø1C
S82.1Ø2B
S82.1Ø2C
S82.1Ø9B
S82.1Ø9C
S82.111B
S82.111C
S82.112B
S82.112C
S82.113B
S82.113C
S82.114B
S82.114C
S82.115B
S82.115C
S82.116B
S82.116C
S82.121B
S82.121C
S82.122B
S82.122C
S82.123B
S82.123C
S82.124B
S82.124C
S82.125B
S82.125C
S82.126B
S82.126C
S82.131B
S82.131C
S82.132B
S82.132C
S82.133B
S82.133C
S82.134B
S82.134C
S82.135B
S82.135C
S82.136B
S82.136C
S82.141B
S82.141C
S82.142B
S82.142C
S82.143B
S82.143C
S82.144B
S82.144C
S82.145B
S82.145C
S82.146B
S82.146C
S82.151B
S82.151C
S82.152B
S82.152C
S82.153B
S82.153C
S82.154B
S82.154C
S82.155B
S82.155C
S82.156B
S82.156C
S82.161A
S82.162A
S82.169A
S82.191B
S82.191C
S82.192B
S82.192C
S82.199B
S82.199C
S82.2Ø1B
S82.2Ø1C
S82.2Ø2B
S82.2Ø2C
S82.2Ø9B
S82.2Ø9C
S82.221B
S82.221C
S82.222B
S82.222C
S82.223B
S82.223C
S82.224B
S82.224C
S82.225B
S82.225C
S82.226B
S82.226C
S82.231B
S82.231C
S82.232B
S82.232C
S82.233B
S82.233C
S82.234B
S82.234C
S82.235B
S82.235C
S82.236B
S82.236C
S82.241B
S82.241C
S82.242B
S82.242C
S82.243B
S82.243C
S82.244B
S82.244C
S82.245B
S82.245C
S82.246B
S82.246C
S82.251B
S82.251C
S82.252B
S82.252C
S82.253B
S82.253C
S82.254B
S82.254C
S82.255B
S82.255C
S82.256B
S82.256C
S82.261B
S82.261C
S82.262B
S82.262C
S82.263B
S82.263C
S82.264B
S82.264C
S82.265B
S82.265C
S82.266B
S82.266C
S82.291B
S82.291C
S82.292B
S82.292C
S82.299B
S82.299C
S82.311A
S82.312A
S82.319A
S82.4Ø1B
S82.4Ø1C
S82.4Ø2B
S82.4Ø2C
S82.4Ø9B
S82.4Ø9C
S82.421B
S82.421C
S82.422B
S82.422C
S82.423B
S82.423C
S82.424B
S82.424C
S82.425B
S82.425C
S82.426B
S82.426C
S82.431B
S82.431C
S82.432B
S82.432C
S82.433B
S82.433C
S82.434B
S82.434C
S82.435B
S82.435C
S82.436B
S82.436C
S82.441B
S82.441C
S82.442B
S82.442C
S82.443B
S82.443C
S82.444B
S82.444C
S82.445B
S82.445C
S82.446B
S82.446C
S82.451B
S82.451C
S82.452B
S82.452C
S82.453B
S82.453C
S82.454B
S82.454C
S82.455B
S82.455C
S82.456B
S82.456C
S82.461B
S82.461C
S82.462B
S82.462C
S82.463B
S82.463C
S82.464B
S82.464C
S82.465B
S82.465C
S82.466B
S82.466C
S82.491B
S82.491C
S82.492B
S82.492C
S82.499B
S82.499C
S82.811A
S82.812A
S82.819A
S82.821A
S82.822A
S82.829A
S82.831B
S82.831C
S82.832B
S82.832C
S82.839B
S82.839C
S82.861B
S82.861C
S82.862B
S82.862C
S82.863B
S82.863C
S82.864B
S82.864C
S82.865B
S82.865C
S82.866B
S82.866C
S84.ØØXA
S84.Ø1XA
S84.Ø2XA
S84.1ØXA
S84.11XA
S84.12XA
S84.8Ø1A
S84.8Ø2A
S84.8Ø9A
S84.9ØXA
S84.91XA
S84.92XA
S85.ØØ1A
S85.ØØ2A
S85.ØØ9A
S85.Ø11A
S85.Ø12A
S85.Ø19A
S85.Ø91A
S85.Ø92A
S85.Ø99A
S85.1Ø1A
S85.1Ø2A
S85.1Ø9A
S85.111A
S85.112A
S85.119A
S85.121A
S85.122A
S85.129A
S85.131A
S85.132A
S85.139A
S85.141A
S85.142A
S85.149A
S85.151A
S85.152A
S85.159A
S85.161A
S85.162A
S85.169A
S85.171A
S85.172A
S85.179A
S85.181A
S85.182A
S85.189A
S85.2Ø1A
S85.2Ø2A
S85.2Ø9A
S85.211A
S85.212A
S85.219A
S85.291A
S85.292A
S85.299A
S85.5Ø1A
S85.5Ø2A
S85.5Ø9A
S85.511A
S85.512A
S85.519A
S85.591A
S85.592A
S85.599A
S85.8Ø1A
S85.8Ø2A
S85.8Ø9A
S85.811A
S85.812A
S85.819A
S85.891A
S85.892A
S85.899A
S87.ØØXA
S87.Ø1XA
S87.Ø2XA
S87.8ØXA
S87.81XA
S87.82XA
S88.Ø11A
S88.Ø12A
S88.Ø19A
S88.Ø21A
S88.Ø22A
S88.Ø29A
S88.111A
S88.112A
S88.119A
S88.121A
S88.122A
S88.129A
S88.911A
S88.912A
S88.919A
S88.921A
S88.922A
S88.929A
S94.2ØXA
S94.21XA
S94.22XA
S94.8X1A
S94.8X2A
S94.8X9A
S94.9ØXA
S94.91XA
S94.92XA
S95.ØØ1A
S95.ØØ2A
S95.ØØ9A
S95.Ø11A
S95.Ø12A
S95.Ø19A
S95.Ø91A
S95.Ø92A
S95.Ø99A
S95.2Ø1A
S95.2Ø2A
S95.2Ø9A
S95.211A
S95.212A
S95.219A
S95.291A
S95.292A
S95.299A
S95.8Ø1A
S95.8Ø2A
S95.8Ø9A
S95.811A
S95.812A
S95.819A
S95.891A
S95.892A
S95.899A
S98.Ø11A
S98.Ø12A
S98.Ø19A
S98.Ø21A
S98.Ø22A
S98.Ø29A
S98.311A
S98.312A
S98.319A
S98.321A
S98.322A
S98.329A
S98.911A
S98.912A
S98.919A
S98.921A
S98.922A
S98.929A
T79.A21A
T79.A22A
T79.A29A

DRG 964

Select principal diagnosis from Trauma Diagnosis List located in DRG 963

AND

At least two different diagnoses from two different Significant Trauma Body Site Categories located in DRG 963

OR

Select a principal diagnosis from one Significant Trauma Body Site Category located in DRG 963

AND

Two or more significant trauma diagnoses from different Significant Trauma Body Site Categories located in DRG 963

DRG 965

Select principal diagnosis from Trauma Diagnosis List located in DRG 963

AND

At least two different diagnoses from two different Significant Trauma Body Site Categories located in DRG 963

OR

Select a principal diagnosis from one Significant Trauma Body Site Category located in DRG 963

AND

Two or more significant trauma diagnoses from different Significant Trauma Body Site Categories located in DRG 963

MDC 25

DRG 969

Principal or Secondary Diagnosis
B2Ø
AND
Any operating procedures excluding nonextensive operating room procedures (those procedures assigned to DRGs 987 - 989)

DRG 970

Principal or Secondary Diagnosis
B2Ø
AND
Any operating procedures excluding nonextensive operating room procedures (those procedures assigned to DRGs 987 - 989)

DRG 974

Principal or Secondary Diagnosis
B2Ø
AND
Major HIV-related Diagnosis

AØ2.1
AØ2.2*
AØ2.8
AØ2.9
AØ7.3
A15*
A17*
A18*
A19*
A31.2
A31.8
A31.9
A4Ø.9
A41*
A42*
A43*
A48.1
A6Ø.ØØ
A6Ø.Ø1
A6Ø.Ø4
A6Ø.Ø9
A6Ø.1
A6Ø.9
A81.2
A81.82
A81.83
A81.89
A81.9
A85.Ø
A85.1
A85.8
A86
A88.8
A89
BØØ.Ø
BØØ.1
BØØ.2
BØØ.3
BØØ.4
BØØ.5*
BØØ.7
BØØ.81
BØØ.89
BØØ.9
BØ2.Ø
BØ2.1
BØ2.21
BØ2.22
BØ2.23
BØ2.29
BØ2.3*
BØ2.7
BØ2.8
BØ2.9
B1Ø.Ø*
B25.8
B25.9
B37.Ø
B37.1
B37.2
B37.5
B37.6
B37.8*
B37.9
B38*
B39*
B45.Ø
B45.2
B45.3
B45.7
B45.8
B45.9
B47.1
B47.9
B48.8
B58*
B59
B6Ø.8
B78.Ø
B78.7
B78.9
B99.8
C46*
C82.5*
C83.Ø*
C83.1*
C83.3*
C83.7*
C83.8*
C83.9*
C84.4*
C84.6*
C84.7*
C84.9*
C84.A*
C84.Z*
C85*
C86*
C88.4
FØ3.9Ø
FØ6.7Ø
FØ6.71
FØ6.8
FØ7.9
FØ9
F28
F29
GØ4.81
GØ4.89
GØ4.9*
G36.9
G37.4
G37.9
G93.4*
G93.9
G95.2*
G95.9
G96.9
G98.8
I33*
I4Ø*
I67.3
I67.83
JØ9.X1
J1Ø.Ø8
J12.3
J12.8*
J12.9
J13
J14
J15.Ø
J15.1
J15.2*
J15.3
J15.4
J15.5
J15.6*
J15.8
J15.9
J18.1
J18.8
J18.9
LØ8.1
UØ7.1

DRG 975

Select principal AND secondary diagnoses listed under DRG 974

DRG 976

Select principal AND secondary diagnoses listed under DRG 974

DRG 977

Any combination of principal or secondary diagnoses including
B2Ø

MDC ALL

DRG 981

Discharges with any operating room procedures not listed for DRGs 987 through 989 that are unrelated to principal diagnosis

DRG 982

Discharges with any operating room procedures not listed for DRG 987 through 989 that are unrelated to principal diagnosis

DRG 983

Discharges with any operating room procedures not listed for DRG 987 through 989 that are unrelated to principal diagnosis

DRG 987

Operating Room Procedures

ØØ5Ø3Z3
ØØ5W3Z3
ØØ5X3Z3
ØØ5Y3Z3
ØØBFØZZ
ØØBF3ZZ
ØØBF4ZZ
ØØBGØZZ
ØØBG3ZZ
ØØBG4ZZ
ØØBHØZZ
ØØBH3ZZ
ØØBH4ZZ
ØØBJØZZ
ØØBJ3ZZ
ØØBJ4ZZ
ØØBKØZZ
ØØBK3ZZ
ØØBK4ZZ
ØØBLØZZ
ØØBL3ZZ
ØØBL4ZZ
ØØBMØZZ
ØØBM3ZZ
ØØBM4ZZ
ØØBN3ZZ
ØØBN4ZZ
ØØBPØZZ
ØØBP3ZZ
ØØBP4ZZ
ØØBQØZZ
ØØBQ3ZZ
ØØBQ4ZZ
ØØBRØZZ
ØØBR3ZZ
ØØBR4ZZ
ØØBSØZZ
ØØBS3ZZ
ØØBS4ZZ
ØØDC3ZZ
ØØDFØZZ
ØØDF3ZZ
ØØDF4ZZ
ØØDGØZZ
ØØDG3ZZ
ØØDG4ZZ
ØØDHØZZ
ØØDH3ZZ
ØØDH4ZZ
ØØDJØZZ
ØØDJ3ZZ
ØØDJ4ZZ
ØØDKØZZ
ØØDK3ZZ
ØØDK4ZZ
ØØDLØZZ
ØØDL3ZZ
ØØDL4ZZ
ØØDMØZZ
ØØDM3ZZ
ØØDM4ZZ
ØØDNØZZ
ØØDN3ZZ
ØØDN4ZZ
ØØDPØZZ
ØØDP3ZZ
ØØDP4ZZ
ØØDQØZZ
ØØDQ3ZZ
ØØDQ4ZZ
ØØDRØZZ
ØØDR3ZZ
ØØDR4ZZ
ØØDSØZZ
ØØDS3ZZ
ØØDS4ZZ
ØØHØ31Z
ØØH631Z
ØØHE31Z
ØØHU31Z
ØØHV31Z
ØØNFØZZ
ØØNF3ZZ
ØØNF4ZZ
ØØNGØZZ
ØØNG3ZZ
ØØNG4ZZ
ØØNHØZZ
ØØNH3ZZ
ØØNH4ZZ
ØØNJØZZ
ØØNJ3ZZ
ØØNJ4ZZ
ØØNKØZZ
ØØNK3ZZ
ØØNK4ZZ
ØØNLØZZ
ØØNL3ZZ
ØØNL4ZZ
ØØNMØZZ
ØØNM3ZZ
ØØNM4ZZ
ØØNNØZZ
ØØNN3ZZ
ØØNN4ZZ
ØØNPØZZ
ØØNP3ZZ
ØØNP4ZZ
ØØNQØZZ
ØØNQ3ZZ
ØØNQ4ZZ
ØØNRØZZ
ØØNR3ZZ
ØØNR4ZZ
ØØNSØZZ
ØØNS3ZZ
ØØNS4ZZ
Ø15NØZZ
Ø15N3ZZ
Ø15N4ZZ
Ø1BØØZZ
Ø1BØ3ZZ
Ø1BØ4ZZ
Ø1B1ØZZ
Ø1B13ZZ
Ø1B14ZZ
Ø1B2ØZZ
Ø1B23ZZ
Ø1B24ZZ
Ø1B3ØZZ
Ø1B33ZZ
Ø1B34ZZ
Ø1B4ØZZ
Ø1B43ZZ
Ø1B44ZZ
Ø1B5ØZZ
Ø1B53ZZ
Ø1B54ZZ
Ø1B6ØZZ
Ø1B63ZZ
Ø1B64ZZ
Ø1B8ØZZ
Ø1B83ZZ
Ø1B84ZZ
Ø1B9ØZZ
Ø1B93ZZ
Ø1B94ZZ
Ø1BAØZZ
Ø1BA3ZZ
Ø1BA4ZZ
Ø1BBØZZ
Ø1BB3ZZ
Ø1BB4ZZ
Ø1BCØZZ
Ø1BC3ZZ
Ø1BC4ZZ
Ø1BDØZZ
Ø1BD3ZZ
Ø1BD4ZZ
Ø1BFØZZ
Ø1BF3ZZ
Ø1BF4ZZ
Ø1BGØZZ
Ø1BG3ZZ
Ø1BG4ZZ
Ø1BHØZZ
Ø1BH3ZZ
Ø1BH4ZZ
Ø1BNØZZ
Ø1BN3ZZ
Ø1BN4ZZ
Ø1BQØZZ
Ø1BQ3ZZ
Ø1BQ4ZZ
Ø1BRØZZ
Ø1BR3ZZ
Ø1BR4ZZ
Ø1DØØZZ
Ø1DØ3ZZ
Ø1DØ4ZZ
Ø1D1ØZZ
Ø1D13ZZ
Ø1D14ZZ
Ø1D2ØZZ
Ø1D23ZZ
Ø1D24ZZ
Ø1D3ØZZ
Ø1D33ZZ
Ø1D34ZZ
Ø1D4ØZZ
Ø1D43ZZ
Ø1D44ZZ
Ø1D5ØZZ
Ø1D53ZZ
Ø1D54ZZ
Ø1D6ØZZ
Ø1D63ZZ
Ø1D64ZZ
Ø1D8ØZZ
Ø1D83ZZ
Ø1D84ZZ
Ø1D9ØZZ
Ø1D93ZZ
Ø1D94ZZ
Ø1DAØZZ
Ø1DA3ZZ
Ø1DA4ZZ
Ø1DBØZZ
Ø1DB3ZZ
Ø1DB4ZZ
Ø1DCØZZ
Ø1DC3ZZ
Ø1DC4ZZ
Ø1DDØZZ
Ø1DD3ZZ
Ø1DD4ZZ
Ø1DFØZZ
Ø1DF3ZZ
Ø1DF4ZZ
Ø1DGØZZ
Ø1DG3ZZ
Ø1DG4ZZ
Ø1DHØZZ
Ø1DH3ZZ
Ø1DH4ZZ
Ø1DNØZZ
Ø1DN3ZZ
Ø1DN4ZZ
Ø1DQØZZ
Ø1DQ3ZZ
Ø1DQ4ZZ
Ø1DRØZZ
Ø1DR3ZZ
Ø1DR4ZZ
Ø1HYØ1Z
Ø1HY41Z
Ø1NØØZZ
Ø1NØ3ZZ
Ø1NØ4ZZ
Ø1N1ØZZ
Ø1N13ZZ
Ø1N14ZZ
Ø1N2ØZZ
Ø1N23ZZ
Ø1N24ZZ
Ø1N3ØZZ
Ø1N33ZZ
Ø1N34ZZ
Ø1N4ØZZ
Ø1N43ZZ
Ø1N44ZZ
Ø1N5ØZZ
Ø1N53ZZ
Ø1N54ZZ
Ø1N6ØZZ
Ø1N63ZZ
Ø1N64ZZ
Ø1N8ØZZ
Ø1N83ZZ
Ø1N84ZZ
Ø1N9ØZZ
Ø1N93ZZ
Ø1N94ZZ
Ø1NAØZZ
Ø1NA3ZZ
Ø1NA4ZZ
Ø1NBØZZ
Ø1NB3ZZ
Ø1NB4ZZ
Ø1NCØZZ
Ø1NC3ZZ
Ø1NC4ZZ
Ø1NDØZZ
Ø1ND3ZZ
Ø1ND4ZZ
Ø1NFØZZ
Ø1NF3ZZ
Ø1NF4ZZ
Ø1NGØZZ
Ø1NG3ZZ
Ø1NG4ZZ
Ø1NHØZZ
Ø1NH3ZZ
Ø1NH4ZZ
Ø1NQØZZ
Ø1NQ3ZZ
Ø1NQ4ZZ
Ø1NRØZZ
Ø1NR3ZZ
Ø1NR4ZZ
Ø2BPØZX
Ø2BP3ZX
Ø2BP4ZX
Ø2BQØZX
Ø2BQ3ZX
Ø2BQ4ZX
Ø2BRØZX
Ø2BR3ZX
Ø2BR4ZX
Ø2BSØZX
Ø2BS3ZX
Ø2BS4ZX
Ø2BTØZX
Ø2BT3ZX
Ø2BT4ZX
Ø2BVØZX
Ø2BV3ZX
Ø2BV4ZX
Ø2BWØZX
Ø2BW3ZX
Ø2BW4ZX
Ø2BXØZX
Ø2BX3ZX
Ø2BX4ZX
Ø2FP3ZØ
Ø2FP3ZZ
Ø2FQ3ZØ
Ø2FQ3ZZ
Ø2FR3ZØ
Ø2FR3ZZ
Ø2FS3ZØ
Ø2FS3ZZ
Ø2FT3ZØ
Ø2FT3ZZ
Ø2RF38N
Ø2WY3DZ
Ø39ØØZX
Ø39Ø4ZX
Ø391ØZX
Ø3914ZX
Ø392ØZX
Ø3924ZX
Ø393ØZX
Ø3934ZX
Ø394ØZX
Ø3944ZX
Ø395ØZX
Ø3954ZX
Ø396ØZX
Ø3964ZX
Ø397ØZX
Ø3974ZX
Ø398ØZX
Ø3984ZX
Ø399ØZX
Ø3994ZX
Ø39AØZX
Ø39A4ZX
Ø39BØZX
Ø39B4ZX
Ø39CØZX
Ø39C4ZX
Ø39DØZX
Ø39D4ZX
Ø39FØZX
Ø39F4ZX
Ø39GØZX
Ø39G4ZX
Ø39HØZX
Ø39H4ZX
Ø39JØZX
Ø39J4ZX
Ø39KØZX
Ø39K4ZX
Ø39LØZX
Ø39L4ZX
Ø39MØZX
Ø39M4ZX
Ø39NØZX
Ø39N4ZX
Ø39PØZX
Ø39P4ZX
Ø39QØZX
Ø39Q4ZX
Ø39RØZX
Ø39R4ZX
Ø39SØZX
Ø39S4ZX
Ø39TØZX
Ø39T4ZX
Ø39UØZX
Ø39U4ZX
Ø39VØZX
Ø39V4ZX
Ø39YØZX
Ø39Y4ZX
Ø3BØØZX
Ø3BØ3ZX
Ø3BØ4ZX
Ø3B1ØZX
Ø3B13ZX
Ø3B14ZX
Ø3B2ØZX
Ø3B23ZX
Ø3B24ZX
Ø3B3ØZX
Ø3B33ZX
Ø3B34ZX
Ø3B4ØZX
Ø3B43ZX
Ø3B44ZX
Ø3B5ØZX
Ø3B53ZX
Ø3B54ZX
Ø3B6ØZX
Ø3B63ZX
Ø3B64ZX
Ø3B7ØZX
Ø3B73ZX
Ø3B74ZX
Ø3B8ØZX
Ø3B83ZX
Ø3B84ZX
Ø3B9ØZX
Ø3B93ZX
Ø3B94ZX
Ø3BAØZX
Ø3BA3ZX
Ø3BA4ZX
Ø3BBØZX
Ø3BB3ZX
Ø3BB4ZX
Ø3BCØZX
Ø3BC3ZX
Ø3BC4ZX
Ø3BDØZX
Ø3BD3ZX
Ø3BD4ZX
Ø3BFØZX
Ø3BF3ZX
Ø3BF4ZX
Ø3BGØZX
Ø3BG3ZX
Ø3BG4ZX
Ø3BHØZX
Ø3BH3ZX
Ø3BH4ZX
Ø3BJØZX
Ø3BJ3ZX
Ø3BJ4ZX
Ø3BKØZX
Ø3BK3ZX
Ø3BK4ZX
Ø3BLØZX
Ø3BL3ZX
Ø3BL4ZX
Ø3BMØZX
Ø3BM3ZX
Ø3BM4ZX
Ø3BNØZX
Ø3BN3ZX
Ø3BN4ZX
Ø3BPØZX
Ø3BP3ZX
Ø3BP4ZX
Ø3BQØZX
Ø3BQ3ZX
Ø3BQ4ZX
Ø3BRØZX
Ø3BR3ZX
Ø3BR4ZX
Ø3BSØZX
Ø3BS3ZX
Ø3BS4ZX
Ø3BTØZX
Ø3BT3ZX
Ø3BT4ZX
Ø3BUØZX
Ø3BU3ZX
Ø3BU4ZX
Ø3BVØZX
Ø3BV3ZX
Ø3BV4ZX
Ø3BYØZX
Ø3BY3ZX
Ø3BY4ZX
Ø3F23ZØ
Ø3F23ZZ
Ø3F33ZØ
Ø3F33ZZ
Ø3F43ZØ
Ø3F43ZZ
Ø3F53ZØ
Ø3F53ZZ
Ø3F63ZØ
Ø3F63ZZ
Ø3F73ZØ
Ø3F73ZZ
Ø3F83ZØ
Ø3F83ZZ
Ø3F93ZØ
Ø3F93ZZ
Ø3FA3ZØ
Ø3FA3ZZ
Ø3FB3ZØ
Ø3FB3ZZ
Ø3FC3ZØ
Ø3FC3ZZ
Ø3FG3ZØ
Ø3FG3ZZ
Ø3FY3ZØ
Ø3FY3ZZ
Ø3WYØ7Z
Ø3WYØKZ
Ø3WY37Z
Ø3WY3DZ
Ø3WY3KZ
Ø3WY47Z
Ø3WY4KZ
Ø49ØØZX
Ø49Ø4ZX
Ø491ØZX
Ø4914ZX
Ø492ØZX
Ø4924ZX
Ø493ØZX
Ø4934ZX
Ø494ØZX
Ø4944ZX
Ø495ØZX
Ø4954ZX
Ø496ØZX
Ø4964ZX
Ø497ØZX
Ø4974ZX
Ø498ØZX
Ø4984ZX
Ø499ØZX
Ø4994ZX
Ø49AØZX
Ø49A4ZX
Ø49BØZX
Ø49B4ZX
Ø49CØZX
Ø49C4ZX
Ø49DØZX
Ø49D4ZX
Ø49EØZX
Ø49E4ZX
Ø49FØZX
Ø49F4ZX
Ø49HØZX
Ø49H4ZX
Ø49JØZX
Ø49J4ZX
Ø49KØZX
Ø49K4ZX
Ø49LØZX
Ø49L4ZX
Ø49MØZX
Ø49M4ZX
Ø49NØZX
Ø49N4ZX
Ø49PØZX

Ø49P4ZX
Ø49QØZX
Ø49Q4ZX
Ø49RØZX
Ø49R4ZX
Ø49SØZX
Ø49S4ZX
Ø49TØZX
Ø49T4ZX
Ø49UØZX
Ø49U4ZX
Ø49VØZX
Ø49V4ZX
Ø49WØZX
Ø49W4ZX
Ø49YØZX
Ø49Y4ZX
Ø4BØØZX
Ø4BØ3ZX
Ø4BØ4ZX
Ø4B1ØZX
Ø4B13ZX
Ø4B14ZX
Ø4B2ØZX
Ø4B23ZX
Ø4B24ZX
Ø4B3ØZX
Ø4B33ZX
Ø4B34ZX
Ø4B4ØZX
Ø4B43ZX
Ø4B44ZX
Ø4B5ØZX
Ø4B53ZX
Ø4B54ZX
Ø4B6ØZX
Ø4B63ZX
Ø4B64ZX
Ø4B7ØZX
Ø4B73ZX
Ø4B74ZX
Ø4B8ØZX
Ø4B83ZX
Ø4B84ZX
Ø4B9ØZX
Ø4B93ZX
Ø4B94ZX
Ø4BAØZX
Ø4BA3ZX
Ø4BA4ZX
Ø4BBØZX
Ø4BB3ZX
Ø4BB4ZX
Ø4BCØZX
Ø4BC3ZX
Ø4BC4ZX
Ø4BDØZX
Ø4BD3ZX
Ø4BD4ZX
Ø4BEØZX
Ø4BE3ZX
Ø4BE4ZX
Ø4BFØZX
Ø4BF3ZX
Ø4BF4ZX
Ø4BHØZX
Ø4BH3ZX
Ø4BH4ZX
Ø4BJØZX
Ø4BJ3ZX
Ø4BJ4ZX
Ø4BKØZX
Ø4BK3ZX
Ø4BK4ZX
Ø4BLØZX
Ø4BL3ZX
Ø4BL4ZX
Ø4BMØZX
Ø4BM3ZX
Ø4BM4ZX
Ø4BNØZX
Ø4BN3ZX
Ø4BN4ZX
Ø4BPØZX
Ø4BP3ZX
Ø4BP4ZX
Ø4BQØZX
Ø4BQ3ZX
Ø4BQ4ZX
Ø4BRØZX
Ø4BR3ZX
Ø4BR4ZX
Ø4BSØZX
Ø4BS3ZX
Ø4BS4ZX
Ø4BTØZX
Ø4BT3ZX
Ø4BT4ZX
Ø4BUØZX
Ø4BU3ZX
Ø4BU4ZX
Ø4BVØZX
Ø4BV3ZX
Ø4BV4ZX
Ø4BWØZX
Ø4BW3ZX
Ø4BW4ZX
Ø4BYØZX
Ø4BY3ZX
Ø4BY4ZX
Ø4FC3ZØ
Ø4FC3ZZ
Ø4FD3ZØ
Ø4FD3ZZ
Ø4FE3ZØ
Ø4FE3ZZ
Ø4FF3ZØ
Ø4FF3ZZ
Ø4FH3ZØ
Ø4FH3ZZ
Ø4FJ3ZØ
Ø4FJ3ZZ
Ø4FK3ZØ
Ø4FK3ZZ
Ø4FL3ZØ
Ø4FL3ZZ
Ø4FM3ZØ
Ø4FM3ZZ
Ø4FN3ZØ
Ø4FN3ZZ
Ø4FP3ZØ
Ø4FP3ZZ
Ø4FQ3ZØ
Ø4FQ3ZZ
Ø4FR3ZØ
Ø4FR3ZZ
Ø4FS3ZØ
Ø4FS3ZZ
Ø4FT3ZØ
Ø4FT3ZZ
Ø4FU3ZØ
Ø4FU3ZZ
Ø4FY3ZØ
Ø4FY3ZZ
Ø4L1ØCZ
Ø4L1ØDZ
Ø4L1ØZZ
Ø4L13CZ
Ø4L13DZ
Ø4L13ZZ
Ø4L14CZ
Ø4L14DZ
Ø4L14ZZ
Ø4L2ØCZ
Ø4L2ØDZ
Ø4L2ØZZ
Ø4L23CZ
Ø4L23DZ
Ø4L23ZZ
Ø4L24CZ
Ø4L24DZ
Ø4L24ZZ
Ø4L3ØCZ
Ø4L3ØDZ
Ø4L3ØZZ
Ø4L33CZ
Ø4L33DZ
Ø4L33ZZ
Ø4L34CZ
Ø4L34DZ
Ø4L34ZZ
Ø4L4ØCZ
Ø4L4ØDZ
Ø4L4ØZZ
Ø4L43CZ
Ø4L43DZ
Ø4L43ZZ
Ø4L44CZ
Ø4L44DZ
Ø4L44ZZ
Ø4L5ØCZ
Ø4L5ØDZ
Ø4L5ØZZ
Ø4L53CZ
Ø4L53DZ
Ø4L53ZZ
Ø4L54CZ
Ø4L54DZ
Ø4L54ZZ
Ø4L6ØCZ
Ø4L6ØDZ
Ø4L6ØZZ
Ø4L63CZ
Ø4L63DZ
Ø4L63ZZ
Ø4L64CZ
Ø4L64DZ
Ø4L64ZZ
Ø4L7ØCZ
Ø4L7ØDZ
Ø4L7ØZZ
Ø4L73CZ
Ø4L73DZ
Ø4L73ZZ
Ø4L74CZ
Ø4L74DZ
Ø4L74ZZ
Ø4L8ØCZ
Ø4L8ØDZ
Ø4L8ØZZ
Ø4L83CZ
Ø4L83DZ
Ø4L83ZZ
Ø4L84CZ
Ø4L84DZ
Ø4L84ZZ
Ø4L9ØCZ
Ø4L9ØDZ
Ø4L9ØZZ
Ø4L93CZ
Ø4L93DZ
Ø4L93ZZ
Ø4L94CZ
Ø4L94DZ
Ø4L94ZZ
Ø4LAØCZ
Ø4LAØDZ
Ø4LAØZZ
Ø4LA3CZ
Ø4LA3DZ
Ø4LA3ZZ
Ø4LA4CZ
Ø4LA4DZ
Ø4LA4ZZ
Ø4LBØCZ
Ø4LBØDZ
Ø4LBØZZ
Ø4LB3CZ
Ø4LB3DZ
Ø4LB3ZZ
Ø4LB4CZ
Ø4LB4DZ
Ø4LB4ZZ
Ø4LCØCZ
Ø4LCØZZ
Ø4LC3CZ
Ø4LC3ZZ
Ø4LC4CZ
Ø4LC4ZZ
Ø4LDØCZ
Ø4LDØZZ
Ø4LD3CZ
Ø4LD3ZZ
Ø4LD4CZ
Ø4LD4ZZ
Ø4LEØCV
Ø4LEØCZ
Ø4LEØDV
Ø4LEØZV
Ø4LEØZZ
Ø4LE3CV
Ø4LE3CZ
Ø4LE3DV
Ø4LE3ZV
Ø4LE3ZZ
Ø4LE4CV
Ø4LE4CZ
Ø4LE4DV
Ø4LE4ZV
Ø4LE4ZZ
Ø4LFØCW
Ø4LFØCZ
Ø4LFØDW
Ø4LFØZW
Ø4LFØZZ
Ø4LF3CW
Ø4LF3CZ
Ø4LF3DW
Ø4LF3ZW
Ø4LF3ZZ
Ø4LF4CW
Ø4LF4CZ
Ø4LF4DW
Ø4LF4ZW
Ø4LF4ZZ
Ø4LHØCZ
Ø4LHØZZ
Ø4LH3CZ
Ø4LH3ZZ
Ø4LH4CZ
Ø4LH4ZZ
Ø4LJØCZ
Ø4LJØZZ
Ø4LJ3CZ
Ø4LJ3ZZ
Ø4LJ4CZ
Ø4LJ4ZZ
Ø4PYØ7Z
Ø4PYØJZ
Ø4PYØKZ
Ø4PY37Z
Ø4PY3JZ
Ø4PY3KZ
Ø4PY47Z
Ø4PY4JZ
Ø4PY4KZ
Ø4WYØ7Z
Ø4WYØJZ
Ø4WYØKZ
Ø4WY37Z
Ø4WY3DZ
Ø4WY3JZ
Ø4WY3KZ
Ø4WY47Z
Ø4WY4JZ
Ø4WY4KZ
Ø59ØØZX
Ø59Ø4ZX
Ø591ØZX
Ø5914ZX
Ø593ØZX
Ø5934ZX
Ø594ØZX
Ø5944ZX
Ø595ØZX
Ø5954ZX
Ø596ØZX
Ø5964ZX
Ø597ØZX
Ø5974ZX
Ø598ØZX
Ø5984ZX
Ø599ØZX
Ø5994ZX
Ø59AØZX
Ø59A4ZX
Ø59BØZX
Ø59B4ZX
Ø59CØZX
Ø59C4ZX
Ø59DØZX
Ø59D4ZX
Ø59FØZX
Ø59F4ZX
Ø59GØZX
Ø59G4ZX
Ø59HØZX
Ø59H4ZX
Ø59LØZX
Ø59L4ZX
Ø59MØZX
Ø59M4ZX
Ø59NØZX
Ø59N4ZX
Ø59PØZX
Ø59P4ZX
Ø59QØZX
Ø59Q4ZX
Ø59RØZX
Ø59R4ZX
Ø59SØZX
Ø59S4ZX
Ø59TØZX
Ø59T4ZX
Ø59VØZX
Ø59V4ZX
Ø59YØZX
Ø59Y4ZX
Ø5BØØZX
Ø5BØ3ZX
Ø5BØ4ZX
Ø5B1ØZX
Ø5B13ZX
Ø5B14ZX
Ø5B3ØZX
Ø5B33ZX
Ø5B34ZX
Ø5B4ØZX
Ø5B43ZX
Ø5B44ZX
Ø5B5ØZX
Ø5B53ZX
Ø5B54ZX
Ø5B6ØZX
Ø5B63ZX
Ø5B64ZX
Ø5B7ØZX
Ø5B73ZX
Ø5B74ZX
Ø5B8ØZX
Ø5B83ZX
Ø5B84ZX
Ø5B9ØZX
Ø5B93ZX
Ø5B94ZX
Ø5BAØZX
Ø5BA3ZX
Ø5BA4ZX
Ø5BBØZX
Ø5BB3ZX
Ø5BB4ZX
Ø5BCØZX
Ø5BC3ZX
Ø5BC4ZX
Ø5BDØZX
Ø5BD3ZX
Ø5BD4ZX
Ø5BFØZX
Ø5BF3ZX
Ø5BF4ZX
Ø5BGØZX
Ø5BG3ZX
Ø5BG4ZX
Ø5BHØZX
Ø5BH3ZX
Ø5BH4ZX
Ø5BLØZX
Ø5BL3ZX
Ø5BL4ZX
Ø5BMØZX
Ø5BM3ZX
Ø5BM4ZX
Ø5BNØZX
Ø5BN3ZX
Ø5BN4ZX
Ø5BPØZX
Ø5BP3ZX
Ø5BP4ZX
Ø5BQØZX
Ø5BQ3ZX
Ø5BQ4ZX
Ø5BRØZX
Ø5BR3ZX
Ø5BR4ZX
Ø5BSØZX
Ø5BS3ZX
Ø5BS4ZX
Ø5BTØZX
Ø5BT3ZX
Ø5BT4ZX
Ø5BVØZX
Ø5BV3ZX
Ø5BV4ZX
Ø5BYØZX
Ø5BY3ZX
Ø5BY4ZX
Ø5F33ZØ
Ø5F33ZZ
Ø5F43ZØ
Ø5F43ZZ
Ø5F53ZØ
Ø5F53ZZ
Ø5F63ZØ
Ø5F63ZZ
Ø5F73ZØ
Ø5F73ZZ
Ø5F83ZØ
Ø5F83ZZ
Ø5F93ZØ
Ø5F93ZZ
Ø5FA3ZØ
Ø5FA3ZZ
Ø5FB3ZØ
Ø5FB3ZZ
Ø5FC3ZØ
Ø5FC3ZZ
Ø5FD3ZØ
Ø5FD3ZZ
Ø5FF3ZØ
Ø5FF3ZZ
Ø5FY3ZØ
Ø5FY3ZZ
Ø5PYØ7Z
Ø5PYØJZ
Ø5PYØKZ
Ø5PY37Z
Ø5PY3JZ
Ø5PY3KZ
Ø5PY47Z
Ø5PY4JZ
Ø5PY4KZ
Ø5WYØ7Z
Ø5WYØJZ
Ø5WYØKZ
Ø5WY37Z
Ø5WY3DZ
Ø5WY3JZ
Ø5WY3KZ
Ø5WY47Z
Ø5WY4JZ
Ø5WY4KZ
Ø65YØZC
Ø65Y3ZC
Ø65Y4ZC
Ø69ØØZX
Ø69Ø4ZX
Ø691ØZX
Ø6914ZX
Ø692ØZX
Ø6924ZX
Ø693ØZX
Ø6934ZX
Ø694ØZX
Ø6944ZX
Ø695ØZX
Ø6954ZX
Ø696ØZX
Ø6964ZX
Ø697ØZX
Ø6974ZX
Ø698ØZX
Ø6984ZX
Ø699ØZX
Ø6994ZX
Ø69BØZX
Ø69B4ZX
Ø69CØZX
Ø69C4ZX
Ø69DØZX
Ø69D4ZX
Ø69FØZX
Ø69F4ZX
Ø69GØZX
Ø69G4ZX
Ø69HØZX
Ø69H4ZX
Ø69JØZX
Ø69J4ZX
Ø69MØZX
Ø69M4ZX
Ø69NØZX
Ø69N4ZX
Ø69PØZX
Ø69P4ZX
Ø69QØZX
Ø69Q4ZX
Ø69TØZX
Ø69T4ZX
Ø69VØZX
Ø69V4ZX
Ø69YØZX
Ø69Y4ZX
Ø6BØØZX
Ø6BØ3ZX
Ø6BØ4ZX
Ø6B1ØZX
Ø6B13ZX
Ø6B14ZX
Ø6B2ØZX
Ø6B23ZX
Ø6B24ZX
Ø6B3ØZX
Ø6B33ZX
Ø6B34ZX
Ø6B4ØZX
Ø6B43ZX
Ø6B44ZX
Ø6B5ØZX
Ø6B53ZX
Ø6B54ZX
Ø6B6ØZX
Ø6B63ZX
Ø6B64ZX
Ø6B7ØZX
Ø6B73ZX
Ø6B74ZX
Ø6B8ØZX
Ø6B83ZX
Ø6B84ZX
Ø6B9ØZX
Ø6B93ZX
Ø6B94ZX
Ø6BBØZX
Ø6BB3ZX
Ø6BB4ZX
Ø6BCØZX
Ø6BC3ZX
Ø6BC4ZX
Ø6BDØZX
Ø6BD3ZX
Ø6BD4ZX
Ø6BFØZX
Ø6BF3ZX
Ø6BF4ZX
Ø6BGØZX
Ø6BG3ZX
Ø6BG4ZX
Ø6BHØZX
Ø6BH3ZX
Ø6BH4ZX
Ø6BJØZX
Ø6BJ3ZX
Ø6BJ4ZX
Ø6BMØZX
Ø6BM3ZX
Ø6BM4ZX
Ø6BNØZX
Ø6BN3ZX
Ø6BN4ZX
Ø6BPØZX
Ø6BP3ZX
Ø6BP4ZX
Ø6BQØZX
Ø6BQ3ZX
Ø6BQ4ZX
Ø6BTØZX
Ø6BT3ZX
Ø6BT4ZX
Ø6BVØZX
Ø6BV3ZX
Ø6BV4ZX
Ø6BYØZC
Ø6BYØZX
Ø6BY3ZC
Ø6BY3ZX
Ø6BY4ZC
Ø6BY4ZX
Ø6CMØZZ
Ø6CM3ZZ
Ø6CM4ZZ
Ø6CNØZZ
Ø6CN3ZZ
Ø6CN4ZZ
Ø6CPØZZ
Ø6CP3ZZ
Ø6CP4ZZ
Ø6CQØZZ
Ø6CQ3ZZ
Ø6CQ4ZZ
Ø6CTØZZ
Ø6CT3ZZ
Ø6CT4ZZ
Ø6CVØZZ
Ø6CV3ZZ
Ø6CV4ZZ
Ø6DMØZZ
Ø6DM3ZZ
Ø6DM4ZZ
Ø6DNØZZ
Ø6DN3ZZ
Ø6DN4ZZ
Ø6DPØZZ
Ø6DP3ZZ
Ø6DP4ZZ
Ø6DQØZZ
Ø6DQ3ZZ
Ø6DQ4ZZ
Ø6DTØZZ
Ø6DT3ZZ
Ø6DT4ZZ
Ø6DVØZZ
Ø6DV3ZZ
Ø6DV4ZZ
Ø6DYØZZ
Ø6DY3ZZ
Ø6DY4ZZ
Ø6FC3ZØ
Ø6FC3ZZ
Ø6FD3ZØ
Ø6FD3ZZ
Ø6FF3ZØ
Ø6FF3ZZ
Ø6FG3ZØ
Ø6FG3ZZ
Ø6FH3ZØ
Ø6FH3ZZ
Ø6FJ3ZØ
Ø6FJ3ZZ
Ø6FM3ZØ
Ø6FM3ZZ
Ø6FN3ZØ
Ø6FN3ZZ
Ø6FP3ZØ
Ø6FP3ZZ
Ø6FQ3ZØ
Ø6FQ3ZZ
Ø6FY3ZØ
Ø6FY3ZZ
Ø6HYØ2Z
Ø6HYØYZ
Ø6HY42Z
Ø6LYØCC
Ø6LYØDC
Ø6LYØZC
Ø6LY3CC
Ø6LY3DC
Ø6LY3ZC
Ø6LY4CC
Ø6LY4DC
Ø6LY4ZC
Ø6LY7CC
Ø6LY7CZ
Ø6LY7DC
Ø6LY7DZ
Ø6LY7ZC
Ø6LY7ZZ
Ø6LY8CC
Ø6LY8CZ
Ø6LY8DC
Ø6LY8DZ
Ø6LY8ZC
Ø6LY8ZZ
Ø6PYØØZ
Ø6PYØ2Z
Ø6PYØ3Z
Ø6PYØ7Z
Ø6PYØCZ
Ø6PYØDZ
Ø6PYØJZ
Ø6PYØKZ
Ø6PYØYZ
Ø6PY37Z
Ø6PY3CZ
Ø6PY3JZ
Ø6PY3KZ
Ø6PY4ØZ
Ø6PY42Z
Ø6PY43Z
Ø6PY47Z
Ø6PY4CZ
Ø6PY4DZ
Ø6PY4JZ
Ø6PY4KZ
Ø6WYØØZ
Ø6WYØ2Z
Ø6WYØ3Z
Ø6WYØ7Z
Ø6WYØCZ
Ø6WYØDZ
Ø6WYØJZ
Ø6WYØKZ
Ø6WYØYZ
Ø6WY37Z
Ø6WY3CZ
Ø6WY3DZ
Ø6WY3JZ
Ø6WY3KZ
Ø6WY4ØZ
Ø6WY42Z
Ø6WY43Z
Ø6WY47Z
Ø6WY4CZ
Ø6WY4DZ
Ø6WY4JZ
Ø6WY4KZ
Ø79ØØØZ
Ø79ØØZX
Ø79ØØZZ
Ø79Ø3ZX
Ø79Ø4ØZ
Ø79Ø4ZX
Ø79Ø4ZZ
Ø791ØØZ
Ø791ØZX
Ø791ØZZ
Ø7913ZX
Ø7914ØZ
Ø7914ZX
Ø7914ZZ
Ø792ØØZ
Ø792ØZX
Ø792ØZZ
Ø7923ZX
Ø7924ØZ
Ø7924ZX
Ø7924ZZ
Ø793ØØZ
Ø793ØZX
Ø793ØZZ
Ø7933ZX
Ø7934ØZ
Ø7934ZX
Ø7934ZZ
Ø794ØØZ
Ø794ØZX
Ø794ØZZ
Ø7943ZX
Ø7944ØZ
Ø7944ZX
Ø7944ZZ
Ø795ØØZ
Ø795ØZX
Ø795ØZZ
Ø7953ZX
Ø7954ØZ
Ø7954ZX
Ø7954ZZ
Ø796ØØZ
Ø796ØZX
Ø796ØZZ
Ø7963ZX
Ø7964ØZ
Ø7964ZX
Ø7964ZZ
Ø797ØØZ
Ø797ØZX
Ø797ØZZ
Ø7973ZX
Ø7974ØZ
Ø7974ZX
Ø7974ZZ
Ø798ØØZ
Ø798ØZX
Ø798ØZZ
Ø7983ZX
Ø7984ØZ
Ø7984ZX
Ø7984ZZ
Ø799ØØZ
Ø799ØZX
Ø799ØZZ
Ø7993ZX
Ø7994ØZ
Ø7994ZX
Ø7994ZZ
Ø79BØØZ
Ø79BØZX
Ø79BØZZ
Ø79B3ZX
Ø79B4ØZ
Ø79B4ZX
Ø79B4ZZ
Ø79CØØZ
Ø79CØZX
Ø79CØZZ
Ø79C3ZX
Ø79C4ØZ
Ø79C4ZX
Ø79C4ZZ
Ø79DØØZ
Ø79DØZX
Ø79DØZZ
Ø79D3ZX
Ø79D4ØZ
Ø79D4ZX
Ø79D4ZZ
Ø79FØØZ
Ø79FØZX
Ø79FØZZ
Ø79F3ZX
Ø79F4ØZ
Ø79F4ZX
Ø79F4ZZ
Ø79GØØZ
Ø79GØZX
Ø79GØZZ
Ø79G3ZX
Ø79G4ØZ
Ø79G4ZX
Ø79G4ZZ
Ø79HØØZ
Ø79HØZX
Ø79HØZZ
Ø79H3ZX
Ø79H4ØZ

Ø79H4ZX
Ø79H4ZZ
Ø79JØØZ
Ø79JØZX
Ø79JØZZ
Ø79J3ZX
Ø79J4ØZ
Ø79J4ZX
Ø79J4ZZ
Ø79KØZX
Ø79K3ZX
Ø79K4ZX
Ø79LØZX
Ø79L3ZX
Ø79L4ZX
Ø7BØØZX
Ø7BØØZZ
Ø7BØ3ZX
Ø7BØ3ZZ
Ø7BØ4ZX
Ø7BØ4ZZ
Ø7B1ØZX
Ø7B1ØZZ
Ø7B13ZX
Ø7B13ZZ
Ø7B14ZX
Ø7B14ZZ
Ø7B2ØZX
Ø7B2ØZZ
Ø7B23ZX
Ø7B23ZZ
Ø7B24ZX
Ø7B24ZZ
Ø7B3ØZX
Ø7B3ØZZ
Ø7B33ZX
Ø7B33ZZ
Ø7B34ZX
Ø7B34ZZ
Ø7B4ØZX
Ø7B4ØZZ
Ø7B43ZX
Ø7B43ZZ
Ø7B44ZX
Ø7B44ZZ
Ø7B5ØZX
Ø7B5ØZZ
Ø7B53ZX
Ø7B53ZZ
Ø7B54ZX
Ø7B54ZZ
Ø7B6ØZX
Ø7B6ØZZ
Ø7B63ZX
Ø7B63ZZ
Ø7B64ZX
Ø7B64ZZ
Ø7B7ØZX
Ø7B7ØZZ
Ø7B73ZX
Ø7B73ZZ
Ø7B74ZX
Ø7B74ZZ
Ø7B8ØZX
Ø7B83ZX
Ø7B84ZX
Ø7B9ØZX
Ø7B93ZX
Ø7B94ZX
Ø7BBØZX
Ø7BBØZZ
Ø7BB3ZX
Ø7BB3ZZ
Ø7BB4ZX
Ø7BB4ZZ
Ø7BCØZX
Ø7BCØZZ
Ø7BC3ZX
Ø7BC3ZZ
Ø7BC4ZX
Ø7BC4ZZ
Ø7BDØZX
Ø7BDØZZ
Ø7BD3ZX
Ø7BD3ZZ
Ø7BD4ZX
Ø7BD4ZZ
Ø7BFØZX
Ø7BFØZZ
Ø7BF3ZX
Ø7BF3ZZ
Ø7BF4ZX
Ø7BF4ZZ
Ø7BGØZX
Ø7BGØZZ
Ø7BG3ZX
Ø7BG3ZZ
Ø7BG4ZX
Ø7BG4ZZ
Ø7BHØZX
Ø7BHØZZ
Ø7BH3ZX
Ø7BH3ZZ
Ø7BH4ZX
Ø7BH4ZZ
Ø7BJØZX
Ø7BJØZZ
Ø7BJ3ZX
Ø7BJ3ZZ
Ø7BJ4ZX
Ø7BJ4ZZ
Ø7BKØZX
Ø7BK3ZX
Ø7BK4ZX
Ø7BLØZX
Ø7BL3ZX
Ø7BL4ZX
Ø7CØØZZ
Ø7CØ3ZZ
Ø7CØ4ZZ
Ø7C1ØZZ
Ø7C13ZZ
Ø7C14ZZ
Ø7C2ØZZ
Ø7C23ZZ
Ø7C24ZZ
Ø7C3ØZZ
Ø7C33ZZ
Ø7C34ZZ
Ø7C4ØZZ
Ø7C43ZZ
Ø7C44ZZ
Ø7C5ØZZ
Ø7C53ZZ
Ø7C54ZZ
Ø7C6ØZZ
Ø7C63ZZ
Ø7C64ZZ
Ø7C7ØZZ
Ø7C73ZZ
Ø7C74ZZ
Ø7C8ØZZ
Ø7C83ZZ
Ø7C84ZZ
Ø7C9ØZZ
Ø7C93ZZ
Ø7C94ZZ
Ø7CBØZZ
Ø7CB3ZZ
Ø7CB4ZZ
Ø7CCØZZ
Ø7CC3ZZ
Ø7CC4ZZ
Ø7CDØZZ
Ø7CD3ZZ
Ø7CD4ZZ
Ø7CFØZZ
Ø7CF3ZZ
Ø7CF4ZZ
Ø7CGØZZ
Ø7CG3ZZ
Ø7CG4ZZ
Ø7CHØZZ
Ø7CH3ZZ
Ø7CH4ZZ
Ø7CJØZZ
Ø7CJ3ZZ
Ø7CJ4ZZ
Ø7CKØZZ
Ø7CK3ZZ
Ø7CK4ZZ
Ø7CLØZZ
Ø7CL3ZZ
Ø7CL4ZZ
Ø7HNØ1Z
Ø7HNØYZ
Ø7HN41Z
Ø7JKØZZ
Ø7JK4ZZ
Ø7JLØZZ
Ø7JL4ZZ
Ø7JNØZZ
Ø7JN4ZZ
Ø7PNØØZ
Ø7PNØ3Z
Ø7PNØCZ
Ø7PNØDZ
Ø7PNØYZ
Ø7PN3ØZ
Ø7PN33Z
Ø7PN3CZ
Ø7PN3DZ
Ø7PN4ØZ
Ø7PN43Z
Ø7PN4CZ
Ø7PN4DZ
Ø7WNØØZ
Ø7WNØ3Z
Ø7WNØCZ
Ø7WNØDZ
Ø7WNØYZ
Ø7WN3ØZ
Ø7WN33Z
Ø7WN3CZ
Ø7WN3DZ
Ø7WN4ØZ
Ø7WN43Z
Ø7WN4CZ
Ø7WN4DZ
Ø8123K4
Ø8123Z4
Ø8133K4
Ø8133Z4
Ø81XØJ3
Ø81XØK3
Ø81XØZ3
Ø81X3J3
Ø81X3K3
Ø81X3Z3
Ø81YØJ3
Ø81YØK3
Ø81YØZ3
Ø81Y3J3
Ø81Y3K3
Ø81Y3Z3
Ø85ØXZZ
Ø851XZZ
Ø8523ZZ
Ø8533ZZ
Ø8543ZZ
Ø8553ZZ
Ø856XZZ
Ø857XZZ
Ø858XZZ
Ø859XZZ
Ø85AØZZ
Ø85A3ZZ
Ø85BØZZ
Ø85B3ZZ
Ø85C3ZZ
Ø85D3ZZ
Ø85G3ZZ
Ø85H3ZZ
Ø85J3ZZ
Ø85K3ZZ
Ø85LØZZ
Ø85L3ZZ
Ø85MØZZ
Ø85M3ZZ
Ø85NØZZ
Ø85N3ZZ
Ø85NXZZ
Ø85PØZZ
Ø85P3ZZ
Ø85PXZZ
Ø85QØZZ
Ø85Q3ZZ
Ø85QXZZ
Ø85RØZZ
Ø85R3ZZ
Ø85RXZZ
Ø85SXZZ
Ø85TXZZ
Ø85VØZZ
Ø85V3ZZ
Ø85WØZZ
Ø85W3ZZ
Ø85XØZZ
Ø85X3ZZ
Ø85X7ZZ
Ø85X8ZZ
Ø85YØZZ
Ø85Y3ZZ
Ø85Y7ZZ
Ø85Y8ZZ
Ø87XØDZ
Ø87XØZZ
Ø87X3DZ
Ø87X3ZZ
Ø87X7DZ
Ø87X7ZZ
Ø87X8DZ
Ø87X8ZZ
Ø87YØDZ
Ø87YØZZ
Ø87Y3DZ
Ø87Y3ZZ
Ø87Y7DZ
Ø87Y7ZZ
Ø87Y8DZ
Ø87Y8ZZ
Ø89ØXØZ
Ø891XØZ
Ø8923ØZ
Ø8923ZX
Ø8923ZZ
Ø8933ØZ
Ø8933ZX
Ø8933ZZ
Ø8943ØZ
Ø8943ZX
Ø8943ZZ
Ø8953ØZ
Ø8953ZX
Ø8953ZZ
Ø896XØZ
Ø897XØZ
Ø898XØZ
Ø899XØZ
Ø89AØØZ
Ø89AØZX
Ø89AØZZ
Ø89A3ØZ
Ø89A3ZX
Ø89A3ZZ
Ø89BØØZ
Ø89BØZX
Ø89BØZZ
Ø89B3ØZ
Ø89B3ZX
Ø89B3ZZ
Ø89C3ØZ
Ø89C3ZX
Ø89C3ZZ
Ø89D3ØZ
Ø89D3ZX
Ø89D3ZZ
Ø89E3ØZ
Ø89E3ZX
Ø89E3ZZ
Ø89F3ØZ
Ø89F3ZX
Ø89F3ZZ
Ø89G3ØZ
Ø89G3ZX
Ø89G3ZZ
Ø89H3ØZ
Ø89H3ZX
Ø89H3ZZ
Ø89J3ØZ
Ø89J3ZX
Ø89J3ZZ
Ø89K3ØZ
Ø89K3ZX
Ø89K3ZZ
Ø89LØØZ
Ø89LØZX
Ø89LØZZ
Ø89L3ØZ
Ø89L3ZX
Ø89L3ZZ
Ø89MØØZ
Ø89MØZX
Ø89MØZZ
Ø89M3ØZ
Ø89M3ZX
Ø89M3ZZ
Ø89NØZX
Ø89PØZX
Ø89QØZX
Ø89RØZX
Ø89SXØZ
Ø89TXØZ
Ø89VØØZ
Ø89VØZX
Ø89VØZZ
Ø89V3ØZ
Ø89V3ZX
Ø89V3ZZ
Ø89WØØZ
Ø89WØZX
Ø89WØZZ
Ø89W3ØZ
Ø89W3ZX
Ø89W3ZZ
Ø89XØØZ
Ø89XØZX
Ø89XØZZ
Ø89X3ØZ
Ø89X3ZX
Ø89X3ZZ
Ø89X7ØZ
Ø89X7ZX
Ø89X7ZZ
Ø89X8ØZ
Ø89X8ZX
Ø89X8ZZ
Ø89YØØZ
Ø89YØZX
Ø89YØZZ
Ø89Y3ØZ
Ø89Y3ZX
Ø89Y3ZZ
Ø89Y7ØZ
Ø89Y7ZX
Ø89Y7ZZ
Ø89Y8ØZ
Ø89Y8ZX
Ø89Y8ZZ
Ø8BØØZX
Ø8BØØZZ
Ø8BØ3ZX
Ø8BØ3ZZ
Ø8BØXZX
Ø8BØXZZ
Ø8B1ØZX
Ø8B1ØZZ
Ø8B13ZX
Ø8B13ZZ
Ø8B1XZX
Ø8B1XZZ
Ø8B43ZX
Ø8B43ZZ
Ø8B53ZX
Ø8B53ZZ
Ø8B6XZX
Ø8B6XZZ
Ø8B7XZX
Ø8B7XZZ
Ø8B8XZX
Ø8B8XZZ
Ø8B9XZX
Ø8B9XZZ
Ø8BAØZX
Ø8BAØZZ
Ø8BA3ZX
Ø8BA3ZZ
Ø8BBØZX
Ø8BBØZZ
Ø8BB3ZX
Ø8BB3ZZ
Ø8BC3ZX
Ø8BC3ZZ
Ø8BD3ZX
Ø8BD3ZZ
Ø8BE3ZX
Ø8BE3ZZ
Ø8BF3ZX
Ø8BF3ZZ
Ø8BJ3ZX
Ø8BJ3ZZ
Ø8BK3ZX
Ø8BK3ZZ
Ø8BLØZX
Ø8BLØZZ
Ø8BL3ZX
Ø8BL3ZZ
Ø8BMØZX
Ø8BMØZZ
Ø8BM3ZX
Ø8BM3ZZ
Ø8BNØZX
Ø8BNØZZ
Ø8BN3ZX
Ø8BN3ZZ
Ø8BNXZX
Ø8BNXZZ
Ø8BPØZX
Ø8BPØZZ
Ø8BP3ZX
Ø8BP3ZZ
Ø8BPXZX
Ø8BPXZZ
Ø8BQØZX
Ø8BQØZZ
Ø8BQ3ZX
Ø8BQ3ZZ
Ø8BQXZX
Ø8BQXZZ
Ø8BRØZX
Ø8BRØZZ
Ø8BR3ZX
Ø8BR3ZZ
Ø8BRXZX
Ø8BRXZZ
Ø8BSXZX
Ø8BSXZZ
Ø8BTXZX
Ø8BTXZZ
Ø8BVØZX
Ø8BVØZZ
Ø8BV3ZX
Ø8BV3ZZ
Ø8BWØZX
Ø8BWØZZ
Ø8BW3ZX
Ø8BW3ZZ
Ø8BXØZX
Ø8BXØZZ
Ø8BX3ZX
Ø8BX3ZZ
Ø8BX7ZX
Ø8BX7ZZ
Ø8BX8ZX
Ø8BX8ZZ
Ø8BYØZX
Ø8BYØZZ
Ø8BY3ZX
Ø8BY3ZZ
Ø8BY7ZX
Ø8BY7ZZ
Ø8BY8ZX
Ø8BY8ZZ
Ø8C23ZZ
Ø8C33ZZ
Ø8C43ZZ
Ø8C4XZZ
Ø8C53ZZ
Ø8C5XZZ
Ø8C8XZZ
Ø8C9XZZ
Ø8CAØZZ
Ø8CA3ZZ
Ø8CAXZZ
Ø8CBØZZ
Ø8CB3ZZ
Ø8CBXZZ
Ø8CC3ZZ
Ø8CCXZZ
Ø8CD3ZZ
Ø8CDXZZ
Ø8CE3ZZ
Ø8CEXZZ
Ø8CF3ZZ
Ø8CFXZZ
Ø8CG3ZZ
Ø8CGXZZ
Ø8CH3ZZ
Ø8CHXZZ
Ø8CJ3ZZ
Ø8CJXZZ
Ø8CK3ZZ
Ø8CKXZZ
Ø8CLØZZ
Ø8CL3ZZ
Ø8CLXZZ
Ø8CMØZZ
Ø8CM3ZZ
Ø8CMXZZ
Ø8CVØZZ
Ø8CV3ZZ
Ø8CVXZZ
Ø8CWØZZ
Ø8CW3ZZ
Ø8CWXZZ
Ø8CXØZZ
Ø8CX3ZZ
Ø8CX7ZZ
Ø8CX8ZZ
Ø8CYØZZ
Ø8CY3ZZ
Ø8CY7ZZ
Ø8CY8ZZ
Ø8D8XZX
Ø8D8XZZ
Ø8D9XZX
Ø8D9XZZ
Ø8DJ3ZZ
Ø8DK3ZZ
Ø8F43ZZ
Ø8F53ZZ
Ø8HØ31Z
Ø8HØ33Z
Ø8HØX1Z
Ø8HØX3Z
Ø8H131Z
Ø8H133Z
Ø8H1X1Z
Ø8H1X3Z
Ø8JLØZZ
Ø8JMØZZ
Ø8LXØCZ
Ø8LXØDZ
Ø8LXØZZ
Ø8LX3CZ
Ø8LX3DZ
Ø8LX3ZZ
Ø8LX7DZ
Ø8LX7ZZ
Ø8LX8DZ
Ø8LX8ZZ
Ø8LYØCZ
Ø8LYØDZ
Ø8LYØZZ
Ø8LY3CZ
Ø8LY3DZ
Ø8LY3ZZ
Ø8LY7DZ
Ø8LY7ZZ
Ø8LY8DZ
Ø8LY8ZZ
Ø8MNXZZ
Ø8MPXZZ
Ø8MQXZZ
Ø8MRXZZ
Ø8NØXZZ
Ø8N1XZZ
Ø8N23ZZ
Ø8N33ZZ
Ø8N43ZZ
Ø8N53ZZ
Ø8N6XZZ
Ø8N7XZZ
Ø8N8XZZ
Ø8N9XZZ
Ø8NAØZZ
Ø8NA3ZZ
Ø8NBØZZ
Ø8NB3ZZ
Ø8NC3ZZ
Ø8ND3ZZ
Ø8NE3ZZ
Ø8NF3ZZ
Ø8NG3ZZ
Ø8NH3ZZ
Ø8NJ3ZZ
Ø8NK3ZZ
Ø8NLØZZ
Ø8NL3ZZ
Ø8NMØZZ
Ø8NM3ZZ
Ø8NNØZZ
Ø8NN3ZZ
Ø8NNXZZ
Ø8NPØZZ
Ø8NP3ZZ
Ø8NPXZZ
Ø8NQØZZ
Ø8NQ3ZZ
Ø8NQXZZ
Ø8NRØZZ
Ø8NR3ZZ
Ø8NRXZZ
Ø8NSXZZ
Ø8NTXZZ
Ø8NVØZZ
Ø8NV3ZZ
Ø8NWØZZ
Ø8NW3ZZ
Ø8NXØZZ
Ø8NX3ZZ
Ø8NX7ZZ
Ø8NX8ZZ
Ø8NYØZZ
Ø8NY3ZZ
Ø8NY7ZZ
Ø8NY8ZZ
Ø8PØØØZ
Ø8PØØ1Z
Ø8PØØ3Z
Ø8PØØ7Z
Ø8PØØCZ
Ø8PØØDZ
Ø8PØØJZ
Ø8PØØKZ
Ø8PØØYZ
Ø8PØ3ØZ
Ø8PØ31Z
Ø8PØ33Z
Ø8PØ37Z
Ø8PØ3CZ
Ø8PØ3DZ
Ø8PØ3JZ
Ø8PØ3KZ
Ø8PØ71Z
Ø8PØ77Z
Ø8PØ7CZ
Ø8PØ7JZ
Ø8PØ7KZ
Ø8PØ81Z
Ø8PØ87Z
Ø8PØ8CZ
Ø8PØ8JZ
Ø8PØ8KZ
Ø8PØX7Z
Ø8PØXKZ
Ø8P1ØØZ
Ø8P1Ø1Z
Ø8P1Ø3Z
Ø8P1Ø7Z
Ø8P1ØCZ
Ø8P1ØDZ
Ø8P1ØJZ
Ø8P1ØKZ
Ø8P1ØYZ
Ø8P13ØZ
Ø8P131Z
Ø8P133Z
Ø8P137Z
Ø8P13CZ
Ø8P13DZ
Ø8P13JZ
Ø8P13KZ
Ø8P171Z
Ø8P177Z
Ø8P17CZ
Ø8P17JZ
Ø8P17KZ
Ø8P181Z
Ø8P187Z
Ø8P18CZ
Ø8P18JZ
Ø8P18KZ
Ø8P1X7Z
Ø8P1XKZ
Ø8PJ3JZ
Ø8PK3JZ
Ø8PLØØZ
Ø8PLØ7Z
Ø8PLØJZ
Ø8PLØKZ
Ø8PLØYZ
Ø8PL3ØZ
Ø8PL37Z
Ø8PL3JZ
Ø8PL3KZ
Ø8PMØØZ
Ø8PMØ7Z
Ø8PMØJZ
Ø8PMØKZ
Ø8PMØYZ
Ø8PM3ØZ
Ø8PM37Z
Ø8PM3JZ
Ø8PM3KZ
Ø8QØXZZ
Ø8Q1XZZ
Ø8Q23ZZ
Ø8Q33ZZ
Ø8Q43ZZ
Ø8Q53ZZ
Ø8Q6XZZ
Ø8Q7XZZ
Ø8Q8XZZ
Ø8Q9XZZ
Ø8QAØZZ
Ø8QA3ZZ
Ø8QBØZZ
Ø8QB3ZZ
Ø8QC3ZZ
Ø8QD3ZZ
Ø8QE3ZZ
Ø8QF3ZZ
Ø8QG3ZZ
Ø8QH3ZZ
Ø8QJ3ZZ
Ø8QK3ZZ
Ø8QLØZZ
Ø8QL3ZZ
Ø8QMØZZ
Ø8QM3ZZ
Ø8QSXZZ
Ø8QTXZZ
Ø8QVØZZ
Ø8QV3ZZ
Ø8QWØZZ
Ø8QW3ZZ
Ø8QXØZZ
Ø8QX3ZZ
Ø8QX7ZZ
Ø8QX8ZZ
Ø8QYØZZ
Ø8QY3ZZ
Ø8QY7ZZ
Ø8QY8ZZ
Ø8RØØ7Z
Ø8RØØJZ
Ø8RØØKZ
Ø8RØ37Z
Ø8RØ3JZ
Ø8RØ3KZ
Ø8R1Ø7Z
Ø8R1ØJZ
Ø8R1ØKZ
Ø8R137Z
Ø8R13JZ
Ø8R13KZ
Ø8R437Z
Ø8R43JZ
Ø8R43KZ
Ø8R537Z
Ø8R53JZ
Ø8R53KZ
Ø8R6X7Z
Ø8R6XJZ
Ø8R6XKZ
Ø8R7X7Z
Ø8R7XJZ
Ø8R7XKZ
Ø8R837Z
Ø8R83JZ
Ø8R83KZ
Ø8R8X7Z
Ø8R8XJZ
Ø8R8XKZ
Ø8R937Z
Ø8R93JZ
Ø8R93KZ
Ø8R9X7Z
Ø8R9XJZ
Ø8R9XKZ
Ø8RAØ7Z
Ø8RAØJZ
Ø8RAØKZ
Ø8RA37Z
Ø8RA3JZ
Ø8RA3KZ
Ø8RBØ7Z
Ø8RBØJZ
Ø8RBØKZ
Ø8RB37Z
Ø8RB3JZ
Ø8RB3KZ
Ø8RC37Z
Ø8RC3JZ
Ø8RC3KZ
Ø8RD37Z
Ø8RD3JZ
Ø8RD3KZ
Ø8RG37Z
Ø8RG3JZ
Ø8RG3KZ
Ø8RH37Z
Ø8RH3JZ
Ø8RH3KZ
Ø8RJ3ØZ
Ø8RJ37Z
Ø8RJ3JZ
Ø8RJ3KZ
Ø8RK3ØZ
Ø8RK37Z
Ø8RK3JZ
Ø8RK3KZ
Ø8RNØ7Z
Ø8RNØJZ
Ø8RNØKZ
Ø8RN37Z
Ø8RN3JZ
Ø8RN3KZ
Ø8RNX7Z
Ø8RNXJZ
Ø8RNXKZ
Ø8RPØ7Z
Ø8RPØJZ
Ø8RPØKZ
Ø8RP37Z
Ø8RP3JZ
Ø8RP3KZ
Ø8RPX7Z
Ø8RPXJZ
Ø8RPXKZ
Ø8RQØ7Z
Ø8RQØJZ
Ø8RQØKZ
Ø8RQ37Z

Ø8RQ3JZ
Ø8RQ3KZ
Ø8RQX7Z
Ø8RQXJZ
Ø8RQXKZ
Ø8RRØ7Z
Ø8RRØJZ
Ø8RRØKZ
Ø8RR37Z
Ø8RR3JZ
Ø8RR3KZ
Ø8RRX7Z
Ø8RRXJZ
Ø8RRXKZ
Ø8RSX7Z
Ø8RSXJZ
Ø8RSXKZ
Ø8RTX7Z
Ø8RTXJZ
Ø8RTXKZ
Ø8RXØ7Z
Ø8RXØJZ
Ø8RXØKZ
Ø8RX37Z
Ø8RX3JZ
Ø8RX3KZ
Ø8RX77Z
Ø8RX7JZ
Ø8RX7KZ
Ø8RX87Z
Ø8RX8JZ
Ø8RX8KZ
Ø8RYØ7Z
Ø8RYØJZ
Ø8RYØKZ
Ø8RY37Z
Ø8RY3JZ
Ø8RY3KZ
Ø8RY77Z
Ø8RY7JZ
Ø8RY7KZ
Ø8RY87Z
Ø8RY8JZ
Ø8RY8KZ
Ø8SC3ZZ
Ø8SD3ZZ
Ø8SG3ZZ
Ø8SH3ZZ
Ø8SJ3ZZ
Ø8SK3ZZ
Ø8SLØZZ
Ø8SL3ZZ
Ø8SMØZZ
Ø8SM3ZZ
Ø8SNØZZ
Ø8SN3ZZ
Ø8SNXZZ
Ø8SPØZZ
Ø8SP3ZZ
Ø8SPXZZ
Ø8SQØZZ
Ø8SQ3ZZ
Ø8SQXZZ
Ø8SRØZZ
Ø8SR3ZZ
Ø8SRXZZ
Ø8SVØZZ
Ø8SV3ZZ
Ø8SWØZZ
Ø8SW3ZZ
Ø8SXØZZ
Ø8SX3ZZ
Ø8SX7ZZ
Ø8SX8ZZ
Ø8SYØZZ
Ø8SY3ZZ
Ø8SY7ZZ
Ø8SY8ZZ
Ø8TØXZZ
Ø8T1XZZ
Ø8T43ZZ
Ø8T53ZZ
Ø8T8XZZ
Ø8T9XZZ
Ø8TC3ZZ
Ø8TD3ZZ
Ø8TJ3ZZ
Ø8TK3ZZ
Ø8TLØZZ
Ø8TL3ZZ
Ø8TMØZZ
Ø8TM3ZZ
Ø8TNØZZ
Ø8TNXZZ
Ø8TPØZZ
Ø8TPXZZ
Ø8TQØZZ
Ø8TQXZZ
Ø8TRØZZ
Ø8TRXZZ
Ø8TVØZZ
Ø8TV3ZZ
Ø8TWØZZ
Ø8TW3ZZ
Ø8TXØZZ
Ø8TX3ZZ
Ø8TX7ZZ
Ø8TX8ZZ
Ø8TYØZZ
Ø8TY3ZZ
Ø8TY7ZZ
Ø8TY8ZZ
Ø8UØØ7Z
Ø8UØØJZ
Ø8UØØKZ
Ø8UØ37Z
Ø8UØ3JZ
Ø8UØ3KZ
Ø8U1Ø7Z
Ø8U1ØJZ
Ø8U1ØKZ
Ø8U137Z
Ø8U13JZ
Ø8U13KZ
Ø8U8Ø7Z
Ø8U8ØJZ
Ø8U8ØKZ
Ø8U837Z
Ø8U83JZ
Ø8U83KZ
Ø8U8X7Z
Ø8U8XJZ
Ø8U8XKZ
Ø8U9Ø7Z
Ø8U9ØJZ
Ø8U9ØKZ
Ø8U937Z
Ø8U93JZ
Ø8U93KZ
Ø8U9X7Z
Ø8U9XJZ
Ø8U9XKZ
Ø8UCØ7Z
Ø8UCØJZ
Ø8UCØKZ
Ø8UC37Z
Ø8UC3JZ
Ø8UC3KZ
Ø8UDØ7Z
Ø8UDØJZ
Ø8UDØKZ
Ø8UD37Z
Ø8UD3JZ
Ø8UD3KZ
Ø8UEØ7Z
Ø8UEØJZ
Ø8UEØKZ
Ø8UE37Z
Ø8UE3JZ
Ø8UE3KZ
Ø8UFØ7Z
Ø8UFØJZ
Ø8UFØKZ
Ø8UF37Z
Ø8UF3JZ
Ø8UF3KZ
Ø8UGØ7Z
Ø8UGØJZ
Ø8UGØKZ
Ø8UG37Z
Ø8UG3JZ
Ø8UG3KZ
Ø8UHØ7Z
Ø8UHØJZ
Ø8UHØKZ
Ø8UH37Z
Ø8UH3JZ
Ø8UH3KZ
Ø8ULØ7Z
Ø8ULØJZ
Ø8ULØKZ
Ø8UL37Z
Ø8UL3JZ
Ø8UL3KZ
Ø8UMØ7Z
Ø8UMØJZ
Ø8UMØKZ
Ø8UM37Z
Ø8UM3JZ
Ø8UM3KZ
Ø8UNØ7Z
Ø8UNØJZ
Ø8UNØKZ
Ø8UN37Z
Ø8UN3JZ
Ø8UN3KZ
Ø8UNX7Z
Ø8UNXJZ
Ø8UNXKZ
Ø8UPØ7Z
Ø8UPØJZ
Ø8UPØKZ
Ø8UP37Z
Ø8UP3JZ
Ø8UP3KZ
Ø8UPX7Z
Ø8UPXJZ
Ø8UPXKZ
Ø8UQØ7Z
Ø8UQØJZ
Ø8UQØKZ
Ø8UQ37Z
Ø8UQ3JZ
Ø8UQ3KZ
Ø8UQX7Z
Ø8UQXJZ
Ø8UQXKZ
Ø8URØ7Z
Ø8URØJZ
Ø8URØKZ
Ø8UR37Z
Ø8UR3JZ
Ø8UR3KZ
Ø8URX7Z
Ø8URXJZ
Ø8URXKZ
Ø8UXØ7Z
Ø8UXØJZ
Ø8UXØKZ
Ø8UX37Z
Ø8UX3JZ
Ø8UX3KZ
Ø8UX77Z
Ø8UX7JZ
Ø8UX7KZ
Ø8UX87Z
Ø8UX8JZ
Ø8UX8KZ
Ø8UYØ7Z
Ø8UYØJZ
Ø8UYØKZ
Ø8UY37Z
Ø8UY3JZ
Ø8UY3KZ
Ø8UY77Z
Ø8UY7JZ
Ø8UY7KZ
Ø8UY87Z
Ø8UY8JZ
Ø8UY8KZ
Ø8VXØCZ
Ø8VXØDZ
Ø8VXØZZ
Ø8VX3CZ
Ø8VX3DZ
Ø8VX3ZZ
Ø8VX7DZ
Ø8VX7ZZ
Ø8VX8DZ
Ø8VX8ZZ
Ø8VYØCZ
Ø8VYØDZ
Ø8VYØZZ
Ø8VY3CZ
Ø8VY3DZ
Ø8VY3ZZ
Ø8VY7DZ
Ø8VY7ZZ
Ø8VY8DZ
Ø8VY8ZZ
Ø8WØØØZ
Ø8WØØ3Z
Ø8WØØ7Z
Ø8WØØCZ
Ø8WØØDZ
Ø8WØØJZ
Ø8WØØKZ
Ø8WØØYZ
Ø8WØ3ØZ
Ø8WØ33Z
Ø8WØ37Z
Ø8WØ3CZ
Ø8WØ3DZ
Ø8WØ3JZ
Ø8WØ3KZ
Ø8WØ7ØZ
Ø8WØ73Z
Ø8WØ77Z
Ø8WØ7CZ
Ø8WØ7DZ
Ø8WØ7JZ
Ø8WØ7KZ
Ø8WØ8ØZ
Ø8WØ83Z
Ø8WØ87Z
Ø8WØ8CZ
Ø8WØ8DZ
Ø8WØ8JZ
Ø8WØ8KZ
Ø8W1ØØZ
Ø8W1Ø3Z
Ø8W1Ø7Z
Ø8W1ØCZ
Ø8W1ØDZ
Ø8W1ØJZ
Ø8W1ØKZ
Ø8W1ØYZ
Ø8W13ØZ
Ø8W133Z
Ø8W137Z
Ø8W13CZ
Ø8W13DZ
Ø8W13JZ
Ø8W13KZ
Ø8W17ØZ
Ø8W173Z
Ø8W177Z
Ø8W17CZ
Ø8W17DZ
Ø8W17JZ
Ø8W17KZ
Ø8W18ØZ
Ø8W183Z
Ø8W187Z
Ø8W18CZ
Ø8W18DZ
Ø8W18JZ
Ø8W18KZ
Ø8WJ3JZ
Ø8WK3JZ
Ø8WLØØZ
Ø8WLØ7Z
Ø8WLØJZ
Ø8WLØKZ
Ø8WLØYZ
Ø8WL3ØZ
Ø8WL37Z
Ø8WL3JZ
Ø8WL3KZ
Ø8WMØØZ
Ø8WMØ7Z
Ø8WMØJZ
Ø8WMØKZ
Ø8WMØYZ
Ø8WM3ØZ
Ø8WM37Z
Ø8WM3JZ
Ø8WM3KZ
Ø8XLØZZ
Ø8XL3ZZ
Ø8XMØZZ
Ø8XM3ZZ
ø9ØØØ7Z
Ø9ØØØJZ
Ø9ØØØKZ
Ø9ØØØZZ
Ø9ØØ37Z
Ø9ØØ3JZ
Ø9ØØ3KZ
Ø9ØØ3ZZ
Ø9ØØ47Z
Ø9ØØ4JZ
Ø9ØØ4KZ
Ø9ØØ4ZZ
Ø9ØØX7Z
Ø9ØØXJZ
Ø9ØØXKZ
Ø9ØØXZZ
Ø9Ø1Ø7Z
Ø9Ø1ØJZ
Ø9Ø1ØKZ
Ø9Ø1ØZZ
Ø9Ø137Z
Ø9Ø13JZ
Ø9Ø13KZ
Ø9Ø13ZZ
Ø9Ø147Z
Ø9Ø14JZ
Ø9Ø14KZ
Ø9Ø14ZZ
Ø9Ø1X7Z
Ø9Ø1XJZ
Ø9Ø1XKZ
Ø9Ø1XZZ
Ø9Ø2Ø7Z
Ø9Ø2ØJZ
Ø9Ø2ØKZ
Ø9Ø2ØZZ
Ø9Ø237Z
Ø9Ø23JZ
Ø9Ø23KZ
Ø9Ø23ZZ
Ø9Ø247Z
Ø9Ø24JZ
Ø9Ø24KZ
Ø9Ø24ZZ
Ø9Ø2X7Z
Ø9Ø2XJZ
Ø9Ø2XKZ
Ø9Ø2XZZ
Ø9ØKØ7Z
Ø9ØKØJZ
Ø9ØKØKZ
Ø9ØKØZZ
Ø9ØK37Z
Ø9ØK3JZ
Ø9ØK3KZ
Ø9ØK3ZZ
Ø9ØK47Z
Ø9ØK4JZ
Ø9ØK4KZ
Ø9ØK4ZZ
Ø9ØKX7Z
Ø9ØKXJZ
Ø9ØKXKZ
Ø9ØKXZZ
Ø959ØZZ
Ø9598ZZ
Ø95AØZZ
Ø95A8ZZ
Ø95UØZZ
Ø95U3ZZ
Ø95U4ZZ
Ø95U8ZZ
Ø95VØZZ
Ø95V3ZZ
Ø95V4ZZ
Ø95V8ZZ
Ø98LØZZ
Ø98L3ZZ
Ø98L4ZZ
Ø98L7ZZ
Ø98L8ZZ
Ø995ØØZ
Ø995ØZX
Ø9957ØZ
Ø996ØØZ
Ø996ØZX
Ø9967ØZ
Ø997ØØZ
Ø997ØZX
Ø9973ØZ
Ø9973ZX
Ø9974ØZ
Ø9974ZX
Ø9977ØZ
Ø9978ØZ
Ø998ØØZ
Ø998ØZX
Ø9983ØZ
Ø9983ZX
Ø9984ØZ
Ø9984ZX
Ø9987ØZ
Ø9988ØZ
Ø999ØZX
Ø99AØZX
Ø99BØØZ
Ø99BØZX
Ø99BØZZ
Ø99B3ZX
Ø99B4ØZ
Ø99B4ZX
Ø99B4ZZ
Ø99CØØZ
Ø99CØZX
Ø99CØZZ
Ø99C3ZX
Ø99C4ØZ
Ø99C4ZX
Ø99C4ZZ
Ø99DØZX
Ø99EØZX
Ø99FØZX
Ø99F3ZX
Ø99F4ZX
Ø99GØZX
Ø99G3ZX
Ø99G4ZX
Ø9B5ØZX
Ø9B5ØZZ
Ø9B58ZX
Ø9B58ZZ
Ø9B6ØZX
Ø9B6ØZZ
Ø9B68ZX
Ø9B68ZZ
Ø9B7ØZX
Ø9B7ØZZ
Ø9B73ZX
Ø9B73ZZ
Ø9B74ZX
Ø9B74ZZ
Ø9B77ZX
Ø9B77ZZ
Ø9B78ZX
Ø9B78ZZ
Ø9B8ØZX
Ø9B8ØZZ
Ø9B83ZX
Ø9B83ZZ
Ø9B84ZX
Ø9B84ZZ
Ø9B87ZX
Ø9B87ZZ
Ø9B88ZX
Ø9B88ZZ
Ø9B9ØZX
Ø9B9ØZZ
Ø9B98ZX
Ø9B98ZZ
Ø9BAØZX
Ø9BAØZZ
Ø9BA8ZX
Ø9BA8ZZ
Ø9BBØZX
Ø9BB3ZX
Ø9BB4ZX
Ø9BB8ZX
Ø9BCØZX
Ø9BC3ZX
Ø9BC4ZX
Ø9BC8ZX
Ø9BDØZX
Ø9BD8ZX
Ø9BEØZX
Ø9BE8ZX
Ø9BLØZZ
Ø9BL3ZZ
Ø9BL4ZZ
Ø9BL7ZZ
Ø9BL8ZZ
Ø9BMØZZ
Ø9BM3ZZ
Ø9BM4ZZ
Ø9BM8ZZ
Ø9BUØZZ
Ø9BU3ZZ
Ø9BU4ZZ
Ø9BU8ZZ
Ø9BVØZZ
Ø9BV3ZZ
Ø9BV4ZZ
Ø9BV8ZZ
Ø9C5ØZZ
Ø9C58ZZ
Ø9C6ØZZ
Ø9C68ZZ
Ø9CBØZZ
Ø9CB3ZZ
Ø9CB4ZZ
Ø9CB8ZZ
Ø9CCØZZ
Ø9CC3ZZ
Ø9CC4ZZ
Ø9CC8ZZ
Ø9D9ØZZ
Ø9DAØZZ
Ø9DLØZZ
Ø9DL3ZZ
Ø9DL4ZZ
Ø9DL7ZZ
Ø9DL8ZZ
Ø9DMØZZ
Ø9DM3ZZ
Ø9DM4ZZ
Ø9DUØZZ
Ø9DU3ZZ
Ø9DU4ZZ
Ø9DVØZZ
Ø9DV3ZZ
Ø9DV4ZZ
Ø9HYØ1Z
Ø9J7ØZZ
Ø9J74ZZ
Ø9J8ØZZ
Ø9J84ZZ
Ø9JDØZZ
Ø9JD4ZZ
Ø9JEØZZ
Ø9JE4ZZ
Ø9MØXZZ
Ø9M1XZZ
Ø9MKXZZ
Ø9NØØZZ
Ø9NØ3ZZ
Ø9NØ4ZZ
Ø9N1ØZZ
Ø9N13ZZ
Ø9N14ZZ
Ø9N3ØZZ
Ø9N33ZZ
Ø9N34ZZ
Ø9N37ZZ
Ø9N38ZZ
Ø9N4ØZZ
Ø9N43ZZ
Ø9N44ZZ
Ø9N47ZZ
Ø9N48ZZ
Ø9N5ØZZ
Ø9N58ZZ
Ø9N6ØZZ
Ø9N68ZZ
Ø9QØØZZ
Ø9QØ3ZZ
Ø9QØ4ZZ
Ø9Q1ØZZ
Ø9Q13ZZ
Ø9Q14ZZ
Ø9Q2ØZZ
Ø9Q23ZZ
Ø9Q24ZZ
Ø9Q3ØZZ
Ø9Q33ZZ
Ø9Q34ZZ
Ø9Q37ZZ
Ø9Q38ZZ
Ø9Q4ØZZ
Ø9Q43ZZ
Ø9Q44ZZ
Ø9Q47ZZ
Ø9Q48ZZ
Ø9Q5ØZZ
Ø9Q58ZZ
Ø9Q6ØZZ
Ø9Q68ZZ
Ø9Q7ØZZ
Ø9Q73ZZ
Ø9Q74ZZ
Ø9Q77ZZ
Ø9Q78ZZ
Ø9Q8ØZZ
Ø9Q83ZZ
Ø9Q84ZZ
Ø9Q87ZZ
Ø9Q88ZZ
Ø9QKØZZ
Ø9QK3ZZ
Ø9QK4ZZ
Ø9QK8ZZ
Ø9QLØZZ
Ø9QL3ZZ
Ø9QL4ZZ
Ø9QL7ZZ
Ø9QL8ZZ
Ø9QMØZZ
Ø9QM3ZZ
Ø9QM4ZZ
Ø9QM8ZZ
Ø9RØØ7Z
Ø9RØØJZ
Ø9RØØKZ
Ø9RØX7Z
Ø9RØXJZ
Ø9RØXKZ
Ø9R1Ø7Z
Ø9R1ØJZ
Ø9R1ØKZ
Ø9R1X7Z
Ø9R1XJZ
Ø9R1XKZ
Ø9R2Ø7Z
Ø9R2ØJZ
Ø9R2ØKZ
Ø9R2X7Z
Ø9R2XJZ
Ø9R2XKZ
Ø9R5Ø7Z
Ø9R5ØJZ
Ø9R5ØKZ
Ø9R6Ø7Z
Ø9R6ØJZ
Ø9R6ØKZ
Ø9R9Ø7Z
Ø9R9ØJZ
Ø9R9ØKZ
Ø9RAØ7Z
Ø9RAØJZ
Ø9RAØKZ
Ø9RKØ7Z
Ø9RKØJZ
Ø9RKØKZ
Ø9RKX7Z
Ø9RKXJZ
Ø9RKXKZ
Ø9RLØ7Z
Ø9RLØJZ
Ø9RLØKZ
Ø9RL37Z
Ø9RL3JZ
Ø9RL3KZ
Ø9RL47Z
Ø9RL4JZ
Ø9RL4KZ
Ø9RL77Z
Ø9RL7JZ
Ø9RL7KZ
Ø9RL87Z
Ø9RL8JZ
Ø9RL8KZ
Ø9RMØ7Z
Ø9RMØJZ
Ø9RMØKZ
Ø9RM37Z
Ø9RM3JZ
Ø9RM3KZ
Ø9RM47Z
Ø9RM4JZ
Ø9RM4KZ
Ø9RNØ7Z
Ø9RNØJZ
Ø9RNØKZ
Ø9RN77Z
Ø9RN7JZ
Ø9RN7KZ
Ø9RN87Z
Ø9RN8JZ
Ø9RN8KZ
Ø9SØØZZ
Ø9SØ4ZZ
Ø9SØXZZ
Ø9S1ØZZ
Ø9S14ZZ
Ø9S1XZZ
Ø9S2ØZZ
Ø9S24ZZ
Ø9S2XZZ
Ø9S7ØZZ
Ø9S74ZZ
Ø9S77ZZ
Ø9S78ZZ
Ø9S8ØZZ
Ø9S84ZZ
Ø9S87ZZ
Ø9S88ZZ
Ø9SKØZZ
Ø9SK4ZZ
Ø9SKXZZ
Ø9SLØZZ
Ø9SL4ZZ
Ø9SL7ZZ
Ø9SL8ZZ
Ø9SMØZZ
Ø9SM4ZZ
Ø9TØØZZ
Ø9TØ4ZZ
Ø9TØXZZ
Ø9T1ØZZ
Ø9T14ZZ
Ø9T1XZZ
Ø9T9ØZZ
Ø9T98ZZ
Ø9TAØZZ
Ø9TA8ZZ
Ø9TLØZZ
Ø9TL4ZZ
Ø9TL7ZZ
Ø9TL8ZZ
Ø9TMØZZ
Ø9TM4ZZ
Ø9TM8ZZ
Ø9TUØZZ
Ø9TU4ZZ
Ø9TU8ZZ
Ø9TVØZZ
Ø9TV4ZZ
Ø9TV8ZZ
Ø9UØØ7Z
Ø9UØØJZ
Ø9UØØKZ
Ø9UØX7Z
Ø9UØXJZ
Ø9UØXKZ
Ø9U1Ø7Z
Ø9U1ØJZ
Ø9U1ØKZ
Ø9U1X7Z
Ø9U1XJZ
Ø9U1XKZ
Ø9U2Ø7Z
Ø9U2ØJZ
Ø9U2ØKZ
Ø9U2X7Z
Ø9U2XJZ
Ø9U2XKZ
Ø9U5Ø7Z
Ø9U5ØJZ
Ø9U5ØKZ
Ø9U587Z
Ø9U58JZ
Ø9U58KZ
Ø9U6Ø7Z
Ø9U6ØJZ
Ø9U6ØKZ
Ø9U687Z
Ø9U68JZ
Ø9U68KZ
Ø9U7Ø7Z
Ø9U7ØJZ
Ø9U7ØKZ
Ø9U777Z
Ø9U77JZ
Ø9U77KZ
Ø9U787Z
Ø9U78JZ
Ø9U78KZ
Ø9U8Ø7Z
Ø9U8ØJZ
Ø9U8ØKZ
Ø9U877Z
Ø9U87JZ
Ø9U87KZ
Ø9U887Z
Ø9U88JZ
Ø9U88KZ
Ø9U9Ø7Z
Ø9U9ØJZ
Ø9U9ØKZ
Ø9U987Z
Ø9U98JZ
Ø9U98KZ
Ø9UAØ7Z
Ø9UAØJZ
Ø9UAØKZ
Ø9UA87Z
Ø9UA8JZ
Ø9UA8KZ
Ø9UKØ7Z
Ø9UKØJZ
Ø9UKØKZ
Ø9UK87Z
Ø9UK8JZ
Ø9UK8KZ
Ø9UKX7Z
Ø9UKXJZ
Ø9UKXKZ
Ø9ULØ7Z
Ø9ULØJZ
Ø9ULØKZ
Ø9UL37Z
Ø9UL3JZ
Ø9UL3KZ
Ø9UL47Z
Ø9UL4JZ
Ø9UL4KZ
Ø9UL77Z
Ø9UL7JZ
Ø9UL7KZ
Ø9UL87Z
Ø9UL8JZ
Ø9UL8KZ
Ø9UMØ7Z
Ø9UMØJZ
Ø9UMØKZ

Ø9UM37Z
Ø9UM3JZ
Ø9UM3KZ
Ø9UM47Z
Ø9UM4JZ
Ø9UM4KZ
Ø9UM87Z
Ø9UM8JZ
Ø9UM8KZ
Ø9UNØ7Z
Ø9UNØJZ
Ø9UNØKZ
Ø9UN77Z
Ø9UN7JZ
Ø9UN7KZ
Ø9UN87Z
Ø9UN8JZ
Ø9UN8KZ
ØB5C3Z3
ØB5D3Z3
ØB5F3Z3
ØB5G3Z3
ØB5H3Z3
ØB5J3Z3
ØB5K3Z3
ØB5L3Z3
ØB5M3Z3
ØBBC7ZX
ØBBC8ZX
ØBBD7ZX
ØBBD8ZX
ØBBF7ZX
ØBBF8ZX
ØBBG7ZX
ØBBG8ZX
ØBBH7ZX
ØBBH8ZX
ØBBJ7ZX
ØBBJ8ZX
ØBBK7ZX
ØBBK8ZX
ØBBL7ZX
ØBBL8ZX
ØBBM4ZX
ØBBM7ZX
ØBBM8ZX
ØBHØØ1Z
ØBHØ31Z
ØBHØ41Z
ØBHØ71Z
ØBHØ81Z
ØBHKØ1Z
ØBHK31Z
ØBHK41Z
ØBHK71Z
ØBHK81Z
ØBHLØ1Z
ØBHL31Z
ØBHL41Z
ØBHL71Z
ØBHL81Z
ØCØØX7Z
ØCØØXJZ
ØCØØXKZ
ØCØØXZZ
ØCØ1X7Z
ØCØ1XJZ
ØCØ1XKZ
ØCØ1XZZ
ØC5ØØZZ
ØC5Ø3ZZ
ØC5ØXZZ
ØC51ØZZ
ØC513ZZ
ØC51XZZ
ØC52ØZZ
ØC523ZZ
ØC52XZZ
ØC53ØZZ
ØC533ZZ
ØC53XZZ
ØC54ØZZ
ØC543ZZ
ØC54XZZ
ØC57ØZZ
ØC573ZZ
ØC57XZZ
ØC58ØZZ
ØC583ZZ
ØC59ØZZ
ØC593ZZ
ØC5BØZZ
ØC5B3ZZ
ØC5CØZZ
ØC5C3ZZ
ØC5DØZZ
ØC5D3ZZ
ØC5FØZZ
ØC5F3ZZ
ØC5GØZZ
ØC5G3ZZ
ØC5HØZZ
ØC5H3ZZ
ØC5JØZZ
ØC5J3ZZ
ØC5NØZZ
ØC5N3ZZ
ØC5NXZZ
ØC5SØZZ
ØC5S3ZZ
ØC5S4ZZ
ØC5S7ZZ
ØC5S8ZZ
ØC5TØZZ
ØC5T3ZZ
ØC5T4ZZ
ØC5T7ZZ
ØC5T8ZZ
ØC5VØZZ
ØC5V3ZZ
ØC5V4ZZ
ØC5V7ZZ
ØC5V8ZZ
ØC7SØDZ
ØC7SØZZ
ØC7S3DZ
ØC7S3ZZ
ØC7S4DZ
ØC7S4ZZ
ØC7S7DZ
ØC7S7ZZ
ØC7S8DZ
ØC7S8ZZ
ØC92ØZX
ØC923ZX
ØC92XZX
ØC93ØZX
ØC933ZX
ØC93XZX
ØC98ØZX
ØC98ØZZ
ØC99ØZX
ØC99ØZZ
ØC9BØZX
ØC9CØZX
ØC9DØZX
ØC9FØZX
ØC9GØZX
ØC9GØZZ
ØC9HØZX
ØC9HØZZ
ØC9JØZX
ØC9NØØZ
ØC9NØZX
ØC9NØZZ
ØC9N3ZX
ØC9NXØZ
ØC9NXZX
ØC9NXZZ
ØC9PØZX
ØC9P3ZX
ØC9PXZX
ØC9QØZX
ØC9Q3ZX
ØC9QXZX
ØCBØØZZ
ØCBØ3ZZ
ØCBØXZZ
ØCB1ØZZ
ØCB13ZZ
ØCB1XZZ
ØCB2ØZX
ØCB2ØZZ
ØCB23ZX
ØCB23ZZ
ØCB2XZX
ØCB2XZZ
ØCB3ØZX
ØCB3ØZZ
ØCB33ZX
ØCB33ZZ
ØCB3XZX
ØCB3XZZ
ØCB4ØZZ
ØCB43ZZ
ØCB4XZZ
ØCB8ØZX
ØCB8ØZZ
ØCB83ZZ
ØCB9ØZX
ØCB9ØZZ
ØCB93ZZ
ØCBBØZX
ØCBBØZZ
ØCBB3ZZ
ØCBCØZX
ØCBCØZZ
ØCBC3ZZ
ØCBDØZX
ØCBDØZZ
ØCBD3ZZ
ØCBFØZX
ØCBFØZZ
ØCBF3ZZ
ØCBGØZX
ØCBGØZZ
ØCBG3ZZ
ØCBHØZX
ØCBHØZZ
ØCBH3ZZ
ØCBJØZX
ØCBJØZZ
ØCBJ3ZZ
ØCBNØZX
ØCBNØZZ
ØCBN3ZX
ØCBN3ZZ
ØCBNXZX
ØCBNXZZ
ØCBPØZX
ØCBP3ZX
ØCBPXZX
ØCBQØZX
ØCBQ3ZX
ØCBQXZX
ØCCØØZZ
ØCCØ3ZZ
ØCC1ØZZ
ØCC13ZZ
ØCC4ØZZ
ØCC43ZZ
ØCC8ØZZ
ØCC9ØZZ
ØCCGØZZ
ØCCHØZZ
ØCCNØZZ
ØCCN3ZZ
ØCDTØZZ
ØCDT3ZZ
ØCDT4ZZ
ØCDT7ZZ
ØCDT8ZZ
ØCDVØZZ
ØCDV3ZZ
ØCDV4ZZ
ØCDV7ZZ
ØCDV8ZZ
ØCH7Ø1Z
ØCH731Z
ØCH7X1Z
ØCHAØYZ
ØCMØØZZ
ØCM1ØZZ
ØCM3ØZZ
ØCMNØZZ
ØCN2ØZZ
ØCN23ZZ
ØCN2XZZ
ØCN3ØZZ
ØCN33ZZ
ØCN3XZZ
ØCN4ØZZ
ØCN43ZZ
ØCNNØZZ
ØCNN3ZZ
ØCNNXZZ
ØCPSØJZ
ØCPS3JZ
ØCPS7JZ
ØCPS8JZ
ØCPYØØZ
ØCPYØ1Z
ØCPYØ7Z
ØCPYØDZ
ØCPYØJZ
ØCPYØKZ
ØCPYØYZ
ØCPY3ØZ
ØCPY31Z
ØCPY37Z
ØCPY3DZ
ØCPY3JZ
ØCPY3KZ
ØCQØØZZ
ØCQØ3ZZ
ØCQ1ØZZ
ØCQ13ZZ
ØCQ4ØZZ
ØCQ43ZZ
ØCQNØZZ
ØCQN3ZZ
ØCQNXZZ
ØCRØØ7Z
ØCRØØJZ
ØCRØØKZ
ØCRØ37Z
ØCRØ3JZ
ØCRØ3KZ
ØCRØX7Z
ØCRØXJZ
ØCRØXKZ
ØCR1Ø7Z
ØCR1ØJZ
ØCR1ØKZ
ØCR137Z
ØCR13JZ
ØCR13KZ
ØCR1X7Z
ØCR1XJZ
ØCR1XKZ
ØCR4Ø7Z
ØCR4ØJZ
ØCR4ØKZ
ØCR437Z
ØCR43JZ
ØCR43KZ
ØCR4X7Z
ØCR4XJZ
ØCR4XKZ
ØCRMØ7Z
ØCRMØJZ
ØCRMØKZ
ØCRM77Z
ØCRM7JZ
ØCRM7KZ
ØCRM87Z
ØCRM8JZ
ØCRM8KZ
ØCRNØ7Z
ØCRNØJZ
ØCRNØKZ
ØCRN37Z
ØCRN3JZ
ØCRN3KZ
ØCRNX7Z
ØCRNXJZ
ØCRNXKZ
ØCRTØJZ
ØCRT7JZ
ØCRT8JZ
ØCRVØJZ
ØCRV7JZ
ØCRV87Z
ØCSØØZZ
ØCSØXZZ
ØCS1ØZZ
ØCS1XZZ
ØCSNØZZ
ØCSNXZZ
ØCTØØZZ
ØCTØXZZ
ØCT1ØZZ
ØCT1XZZ
ØCT2ØZZ
ØCT2XZZ
ØCT3ØZZ
ØCT3XZZ
ØCT8ØZZ
ØCT9ØZZ
ØCTBØZZ
ØCTCØZZ
ØCTDØZZ
ØCTFØZZ
ØCTGØZZ
ØCTHØZZ
ØCTJØZZ
ØCTNØZZ
ØCTNXZZ
ØCTPØZZ
ØCTPXZZ
ØCUØØ7Z
ØCUØØJZ
ØCUØØKZ
ØCUØ37Z
ØCUØ3JZ
ØCUØ3KZ
ØCUØX7Z
ØCUØXJZ
ØCUØXKZ
ØCU1Ø7Z
ØCU1ØJZ
ØCU1ØKZ
ØCU137Z
ØCU13JZ
ØCU13KZ
ØCU1X7Z
ØCU1XJZ
ØCU1XKZ
ØCU4Ø7Z
ØCU4ØJZ
ØCU4ØKZ
ØCU437Z
ØCU43JZ
ØCU43KZ
ØCU4X7Z
ØCU4XJZ
ØCU4XKZ
ØCUMØ7Z
ØCUMØJZ
ØCUMØKZ
ØCUM77Z
ØCUM7JZ
ØCUM7KZ
ØCUM87Z
ØCUM8JZ
ØCUM8KZ
ØCUNØ7Z
ØCUNØJZ
ØCUNØKZ
ØCUN37Z
ØCUN3JZ
ØCUN3KZ
ØCUNX7Z
ØCUNXJZ
ØCUNXKZ
ØCWYØØZ
ØCWYØ1Z
ØCWYØDZ
ØCWYØJZ
ØCWYØKZ
ØCWYØYZ
ØCWY3ØZ
ØCWY31Z
ØCWY37Z
ØCWY3DZ
ØCWY3JZ
ØCWY3KZ
ØCXØØZZ
ØCXØXZZ
ØCX1ØZZ
ØCX1XZZ
ØCX3ØZZ
ØCX3XZZ
ØCX4ØZZ
ØCX4XZZ
ØCX5ØZZ
ØCX5XZZ
ØCX6ØZZ
ØCX6XZZ
ØD513Z3
ØD523Z3
ØD533Z3
ØD543Z3
ØD553Z3
ØD56ØZ3
ØD56ØZZ
ØD563Z3
ØD563ZZ
ØD567ZZ
ØD57ØZ3
ØD57ØZZ
ØD573Z3
ØD573ZZ
ØD577ZZ
ØD58ØZ3
ØD58ØZZ
ØD583Z3
ØD583ZZ
ØD584Z3
ØD584ZZ
ØD587ZZ
ØD59ØZ3
ØD59ØZZ
ØD593Z3
ØD593ZZ
ØD597ZZ
ØD5AØZ3
ØD5AØZZ
ØD5A3Z3
ØD5A3ZZ
ØD5A4Z3
ØD5A4ZZ
ØD5A7ZZ
ØD5BØZ3
ØD5BØZZ
ØD5B3Z3
ØD5B3ZZ
ØD5B4Z3
ØD5B4ZZ
ØD5B7ZZ
ØD5CØZ3
ØD5CØZZ
ØD5C3Z3
ØD5C3ZZ
ØD5C4Z3
ØD5C4ZZ
ØD5C7ZZ
ØD5EØZ3
ØD5EØZZ
ØD5E3Z3
ØD5E3ZZ
ØD5E7ZZ
ØD5FØZ3
ØD5FØZZ
ØD5F3Z3
ØD5F3ZZ
ØD5F7ZZ
ØD5GØZ3
ØD5GØZZ
ØD5G3Z3
ØD5G3ZZ
ØD5G7ZZ
ØD5HØZ3
ØD5HØZZ
ØD5H3Z3
ØD5H3ZZ
ØD5H7ZZ
ØD5J3Z3
ØD5KØZ3
ØD5KØZZ
ØD5K3Z3
ØD5K3ZZ
ØD5K7ZZ
ØD5LØZ3
ØD5LØZZ
ØD5L3Z3
ØD5L3ZZ
ØD5L7ZZ
ØD5MØZ3
ØD5MØZZ
ØD5M3Z3
ØD5M3ZZ
ØD5M7ZZ
ØD5NØZ3
ØD5NØZZ
ØD5N3Z3
ØD5N3ZZ
ØD5N7ZZ
ØD5QØZ3
ØD5QØZZ
ØD5Q3Z3
ØD5Q3ZZ
ØD5Q7ZZ
ØD5QXZZ
ØD5RØZZ
ØD5R3ZZ
ØD5UØZZ
ØD5U3ZZ
ØD5U4ZZ
ØD5VØZZ
ØD5V3ZZ
ØD5V4ZZ
ØD5WØZZ
ØD5W3ZZ
ØD5W4ZZ
ØD8RØZZ
ØD8R3ZZ
ØD96ØZX
ØD97ØZX
ØD9EØZX
ØD9FØZX
ØD9GØZX
ØD9HØZX
ØD9KØZX
ØD9LØZX
ØD9MØZX
ØD9NØZX
ØD9PØZX
ØD9RØØZ
ØD9RØZZ
ØD9R4ØZ
ØD9R4ZZ
ØD9WØØZ
ØD9WØZX
ØD9WØZZ
ØD9W4ØZ
ØD9W4ZX
ØD9W4ZZ
ØDB6ØZX
ØDB64Z3
ØDB64ZX
ØDB64ZZ
ØDB7ØZX
ØDB83ZZ
ØDB87ZZ
ØDB88ZZ
ØDB93ZZ
ØDBA3ZZ
ØDBA4ZZ
ØDBA7ZZ
ØDBA8ZZ
ØDBB3ZZ
ØDBB4ZZ
ØDBB7ZZ
ØDBB8ZZ
ØDBCØZZ
ØDBC3ZZ
ØDBC4ZZ
ØDBC7ZZ
ØDBC8ZZ
ØDBEØZX
ØDBE7ZZ
ØDBFØZX
ØDBF7ZZ
ØDBGØZX
ØDBG7ZZ
ØDBGFZZ
ØDBHØZX
ØDBH7ZZ
ØDBKØZX
ØDBK7ZZ
ØDBLØZX
ØDBL7ZZ
ØDBLFZZ
ØDBMØZX
ØDBM7ZZ
ØDBMFZZ
ØDBNØZX
ØDBN7ZZ
ØDBNFZZ
ØDBPØZX
ØDBP3ZZ
ØDBP7ZZ
ØDBQØZZ
ØDBQ3ZZ
ØDBQ4ZZ
ØDBQ7ZZ
ØDBQXZZ
ØDBRØZZ
ØDBR3ZZ
ØDBR4ZZ
ØDBUØZZ
ØDBU3ZZ
ØDBU4ZZ
ØDBVØZZ
ØDBV3ZZ
ØDBV4ZZ
ØDBWØZZ
ØDBW3ZZ
ØDBW4ZZ
ØDCRØZZ
ØDCR3ZZ
ØDCR4ZZ
ØDH5Ø1Z
ØDH531Z
ØDH541Z
ØDH571Z
ØDH581Z
ØDH6Ø1Z
ØDH641Z
ØDHPØ1Z
ØDHP31Z
ØDHP41Z
ØDHP71Z
ØDHP81Z
ØDJD4ZZ
ØDJU4ZZ
ØDJV4ZZ
ØDJW4ZZ
ØDNPØZZ
ØDNP3ZZ
ØDNP4ZZ
ØDNP7ZZ
ØDNP8ZZ
ØDNRØZZ
ØDNR3ZZ
ØDNR4ZZ
ØDP643Z
ØDP64CZ
ØDQ53ZZ
ØDQ57ZZ
ØDQ58ZZ
ØDQ64ZZ
ØDQRØZZ
ØDQR3ZZ
ØDQR4ZZ
ØDQWØZZ
ØDQW3ZZ
ØDQW4ZZ
ØDRRØ7Z
ØDRRØJZ
ØDRRØKZ
ØDRR47Z
ØDRR4JZ
ØDRR4KZ
ØDTQØZZ
ØDTQ4ZZ
ØDTQ7ZZ
ØDTQ8ZZ
ØDTRØZZ
ØDTR4ZZ
ØDTUØZZ
ØDTU4ZZ
ØDURØ7Z
ØDURØJZ
ØDURØKZ
ØDUR47Z
ØDUR4JZ
ØDUR4KZ
ØDV44CZ
ØDV44DZ
ØDV44ZZ
ØDV64CZ
ØDW643Z
ØDW64CZ
ØF5Ø3Z3
ØF513Z3
ØF523Z3
ØF543Z3
ØF553Z3
ØF563Z3
ØF573Z3
ØF583Z3
ØF593Z3
ØF5C3Z3
ØF5D3Z3
ØF5F3Z3
ØF5G3Z3
ØF94ØØZ
ØF94ØZX
ØF94ØZZ
ØF944ØZ
ØF944ZX
ØF944ZZ
ØFHBØ1Z
ØFHB31Z
ØFHB41Z
ØFHB71Z
ØFHB81Z
ØFHDØ1Z
ØFHD31Z
ØFHD41Z
ØFHD71Z
ØFHD81Z
ØFJØ4ZZ
ØFJ44ZZ
ØFJD4ZZ
ØFJG4ZZ
ØFL5ØCZ
ØFL5ØDZ
ØFL5ØZZ
ØFL6ØCZ
ØFL6ØDZ
ØFL6ØZZ
ØFL7ØCZ
ØFL7ØDZ
ØFL7ØZZ
ØFL8ØCZ
ØFL8ØDZ
ØFL8ØZZ
ØFL9ØCZ
ØFL9ØDZ
ØFL9ØZZ
ØFM4ØZZ
ØFR5ØJZ
ØFR54JZ
ØFR58JZ
ØFR6ØJZ
ØFR64JZ
ØFR68JZ
ØFR7ØJZ
ØFR74JZ
ØFR78JZ
ØFR8ØJZ
ØFR84JZ
ØFR88JZ
ØFR9ØJZ
ØFR94JZ
ØFR98JZ
ØFS4ØZZ
ØFS44ZZ
ØFT44ZZ
ØFV5ØCZ
ØFV5ØDZ
ØFV5ØZZ
ØFV6ØCZ
ØFV6ØDZ
ØFV6ØZZ
ØFV7ØCZ
ØFV7ØDZ
ØFV7ØZZ
ØFV8ØCZ
ØFV8ØDZ
ØFV8ØZZ
ØFV9ØCZ
ØFV9ØDZ
ØFV9ØZZ
ØG5Ø3Z3
ØG513Z3
ØG523Z3
ØG533Z3
ØG543Z3
ØG563Z3
ØG573Z3
ØG583Z3
ØG593Z3
ØG5B3Z3
ØG5C3Z3
ØG5D3Z3
ØG5F3Z3
ØG5G3Z3
ØG5H3Z3
ØG5K3Z3
ØG5L3Z3
ØG5M3Z3
ØG5N3Z3
ØG5P3Z3
ØG5Q3Z3
ØG5R3Z3
ØHØTØ7Z
ØHØTØJZ
ØHØTØKZ
ØHØT37Z
ØHØT3KZ
ØHØUØ7Z
ØHØUØJZ
ØHØUØKZ
ØHØU37Z
ØHØU3KZ
ØHØVØ7Z
ØHØVØJZ
ØHØVØKZ
ØHØV37Z
ØHØV3KZ
ØH5TØZ3
ØH5TØZZ
ØH5T3Z3
ØH5T3ZZ
ØH5T7ZZ
ØH5T8ZZ
ØH5UØZ3
ØH5UØZZ
ØH5U3Z3
ØH5U3ZZ
ØH5U7ZZ
ØH5U8ZZ
ØH5VØZ3
ØH5VØZZ
ØH5V3Z3
ØH5V3ZZ
ØH5V7ZZ
ØH5V8ZZ
ØH99XØZ
ØH99XZZ
ØH9TØZX
ØH9TØZZ
ØH9UØZX
ØH9UØZZ
ØH9VØZX
ØH9VØZZ
ØH9WØZX
ØH9WØZZ
ØH9XØZX
ØH9XØZZ
ØHBTØZX
ØHBTØZZ
ØHBT3ZZ
ØHBT7ZZ
ØHBT8ZZ
ØHBUØZX
ØHBUØZZ
ØHBU3ZZ
ØHBU7ZZ
ØHBU8ZZ
ØHBVØZX

ØHBVØZZ
ØHBV3ZZ
ØHBV7ZZ
ØHBV8ZZ
ØHBWØZX
ØHBXØZX
ØHBYØZX
ØHCTØZZ
ØHCUØZZ
ØHCVØZZ
ØHCWØZZ
ØHCXØZZ
ØHHTØ1Z
ØHHTØNZ
ØHHTØYZ
ØHHT31Z
ØHHT3NZ
ØHHT71Z
ØHHT7NZ
ØHHT81Z
ØHHT8NZ
ØHHUØ1Z
ØHHUØNZ
ØHHUØYZ
ØHHU31Z
ØHHU3NZ
ØHHU71Z
ØHHU7NZ
ØHHU81Z
ØHHU8NZ
ØHHVØ1Z
ØHHVØNZ
ØHHV31Z
ØHHV3NZ
ØHHV71Z
ØHHV7NZ
ØHHV81Z
ØHHV8NZ
ØHHWØ1Z
ØHHWØNZ
ØHHW31Z
ØHHW3NZ
ØHHW71Z
ØHHW7NZ
ØHHW81Z
ØHHW8NZ
ØHHWX1Z
ØHHXØ1Z
ØHHXØNZ
ØHHX31Z
ØHHX3NZ
ØHHX71Z
ØHHX7NZ
ØHHX81Z
ØHHX8NZ
ØHHXX1Z
ØHM1XZZ
ØHM2XZZ
ØHM3XZZ
ØHM4XZZ
ØHM5XZZ
ØHM6XZZ
ØHM7XZZ
ØHM8XZZ
ØHM9XZZ
ØHMAXZZ
ØHMBXZZ
ØHMCXZZ
ØHMDXZZ
ØHMEXZZ
ØHMFXZZ
ØHMGXZZ
ØHMHXZZ
ØHMJXZZ
ØHMKXZZ
ØHMLXZZ
ØHMMXZZ
ØHMNXZZ
ØHNØXZZ
ØHN1XZZ
ØHN2XZZ
ØHN3XZZ
ØHN4XZZ
ØHN5XZZ
ØHN6XZZ
ØHN7XZZ
ØHN8XZZ
ØHN9XZZ
ØHNAXZZ
ØHNBXZZ
ØHNCXZZ
ØHNDXZZ
ØHNEXZZ
ØHNFXZZ
ØHNGXZZ
ØHNHXZZ
ØHNJXZZ
ØHNKXZZ
ØHNLXZZ
ØHNMXZZ
ØHNNXZZ
ØHNQXZZ
ØHNRXZZ
ØHPTØJZ
ØHPTØNZ
ØHPTØYZ
ØHPT3JZ
ØHPT3NZ
ØHPUØJZ
ØHPUØNZ
ØHPUØYZ
ØHPU3JZ
ØHPU3NZ
ØHR2X72
ØHR2X73
ØHR2X74
ØHR2XJ3
ØHR2XJ4
ØHR2XJZ
ØHR2XK3
ØHR2XK4
ØHR3X72
ØHR3X73
ØHR3X74
ØHR3XJ3
ØHR3XJ4
ØHR3XJZ
ØHR3XK3
ØHR3XK4
ØHR9X72
ØHR9X73
ØHR9X74
ØHR9XJ3
ØHR9XJ4
ØHR9XJZ
ØHR9XK3
ØHR9XK4
ØHRFX72
ØHRFX74
ØHRGX72
ØHRGX74
ØHRSXJZ
ØHRSXKZ
ØHWTØJZ
ØHWTØYZ
ØHWT3JZ
ØHWUØJZ
ØHWUØYZ
ØHWU3JZ
ØHX2XZZ
ØHX3XZZ
ØJØ1ØZZ
ØJØ13ZZ
ØJØ4ØZZ
ØJØ43ZZ
ØJØ5ØZZ
ØJØ53ZZ
ØJØ6ØZZ
ØJØ63ZZ
ØJØ7ØZZ
ØJØ73ZZ
ØJØ8ØZZ
ØJØ83ZZ
ØJØ9ØZZ
ØJØ93ZZ
ØJØDØZZ
ØJØD3ZZ
ØJØFØZZ
ØJØF3ZZ
ØJØGØZZ
ØJØG3ZZ
ØJØHØZZ
ØJØH3ZZ
ØJØLØZZ
ØJØL3ZZ
ØJØMØZZ
ØJØM3ZZ
ØJØNØZZ
ØJØN3ZZ
ØJØPØZZ
ØJØP3ZZ
ØJ81ØZZ
ØJ813ZZ
ØJ8JØZZ
ØJ8J3ZZ
ØJ8KØZZ
ØJ8K3ZZ
ØJB13ZZ
ØJB6ØZZ
ØJB7ØZZ
ØJB8ØZZ
ØJBJØZZ
ØJBJ3ZZ
ØJBKØZZ
ØJBK3ZZ
ØJCØØZZ
ØJC1ØZZ
ØJC4ØZZ
ØJC5ØZZ
ØJC6ØZZ
ØJC7ØZZ
ØJC8ØZZ
ØJC9ØZZ
ØJCBØZZ
ØJCCØZZ
ØJCDØZZ
ØJCFØZZ
ØJCGØZZ
ØJCHØZZ
ØJCJØZZ
ØJCKØZZ
ØJCLØZZ
ØJCMØZZ
ØJCNØZZ
ØJCPØZZ
ØJCQØZZ
ØJCRØZZ
ØJH6ØYZ
ØJHSØ1Z
ØJHSØYZ
ØJHS31Z
ØJHTØ1Z
ØJHT31Z
ØJHVØ1Z
ØJHVØYZ
ØJHV31Z
ØJHWØ1Z
ØJHWØYZ
ØJHW31Z
ØJPTØFZ
ØJPTØPZ
ØJPT3FZ
ØJPT3PZ
ØJQ1ØZZ
ØJQ4ØZZ
ØJQ5ØZZ
ØJQ6ØZZ
ØJQ7ØZZ
ØJQ8ØZZ
ØJQ9ØZZ
ØJQBØZZ
ØJQDØZZ
ØJQFØZZ
ØJQGØZZ
ØJQHØZZ
ØJQJØZZ
ØJQKØZZ
ØJQLØZZ
ØJQMØZZ
ØJQNØZZ
ØJQPØZZ
ØJQQØZZ
ØJQRØZZ
ØK5ØØZZ
ØK5Ø3ZZ
ØK5Ø4ZZ
ØK51ØZZ
ØK513ZZ
ØK514ZZ
ØK52ØZZ
ØK523ZZ
ØK524ZZ
ØK53ØZZ
ØK533ZZ
ØK534ZZ
ØK54ØZZ
ØK543ZZ
ØK544ZZ
ØK55ØZZ
ØK553ZZ
ØK554ZZ
ØK56ØZZ
ØK563ZZ
ØK564ZZ
ØK57ØZZ
ØK573ZZ
ØK574ZZ
ØK58ØZZ
ØK583ZZ
ØK584ZZ
ØK59ØZZ
ØK593ZZ
ØK594ZZ
ØK5BØZZ
ØK5B3ZZ
ØK5B4ZZ
ØK5FØZZ
ØK5F3ZZ
ØK5F4ZZ
ØK5GØZZ
ØK5G3ZZ
ØK5G4ZZ
ØK5HØZZ
ØK5H3ZZ
ØK5H4ZZ
ØK5JØZZ
ØK5J3ZZ
ØK5J4ZZ
ØK5KØZZ
ØK5K3ZZ
ØK5K4ZZ
ØK5LØZZ
ØK5L3ZZ
ØK5L4ZZ
ØK5MØZZ
ØK5M3ZZ
ØK5M4ZZ
ØK5NØZZ
ØK5N3ZZ
ØK5N4ZZ
ØK5PØZZ
ØK5P3ZZ
ØK5P4ZZ
ØK5QØZZ
ØK5Q3ZZ
ØK5Q4ZZ
ØK5RØZZ
ØK5R3ZZ
ØK5R4ZZ
ØK5SØZZ
ØK5S3ZZ
ØK5S4ZZ
ØK5TØZZ
ØK5T3ZZ
ØK5T4ZZ
ØK5VØZZ
ØK5V3ZZ
ØK5V4ZZ
ØK5WØZZ
ØK5W3ZZ
ØK5W4ZZ
ØK847ZZ
ØK848ZZ
ØK9ØØØZ
ØK9ØØZX
ØK9ØØZZ
ØK9Ø4ØZ
ØK9Ø4ZZ
ØK91ØØZ
ØK91ØZX
ØK91ØZZ
ØK914ØZ
ØK914ZZ
ØK92ØØZ
ØK92ØZX
ØK92ØZZ
ØK924ØZ
ØK924ZZ
ØK93ØØZ
ØK93ØZX
ØK93ØZZ
ØK934ØZ
ØK934ZZ
ØK94ØØZ
ØK94ØZX
ØK94ØZZ
ØK944ØZ
ØK944ZZ
ØK95ØØZ
ØK95ØZX
ØK95ØZZ
ØK954ØZ
ØK954ZZ
ØK96ØØZ
ØK96ØZX
ØK96ØZZ
ØK964ØZ
ØK964ZZ
ØK97ØØZ
ØK97ØZX
ØK97ØZZ
ØK974ØZ
ØK974ZZ
ØK98ØØZ
ØK98ØZX
ØK98ØZZ
ØK984ØZ
ØK984ZZ
ØK99ØØZ
ØK99ØZX
ØK99ØZZ
ØK994ØZ
ØK994ZZ
ØK9BØØZ
ØK9BØZX
ØK9BØZZ
ØK9B4ØZ
ØK9B4ZZ
ØK9CØZX
ØK9DØZX
ØK9FØØZ
ØK9FØZX
ØK9FØZZ
ØK9F4ØZ
ØK9F4ZZ
ØK9GØØZ
ØK9GØZX
ØK9GØZZ
ØK9G4ØZ
ØK9G4ZZ
ØK9HØØZ
ØK9HØZX
ØK9HØZZ
ØK9H4ØZ
ØK9H4ZZ
ØK9JØØZ
ØK9JØZX
ØK9JØZZ
ØK9J4ØZ
ØK9J4ZZ
ØK9KØØZ
ØK9KØZX
ØK9KØZZ
ØK9K4ØZ
ØK9K4ZZ
ØK9LØØZ
ØK9LØZX
ØK9LØZZ
ØK9L4ØZ
ØK9L4ZZ
ØK9MØØZ
ØK9MØZX
ØK9MØZZ
ØK9M4ØZ
ØK9M4ZZ
ØK9NØØZ
ØK9NØZX
ØK9NØZZ
ØK9N4ØZ
ØK9N4ZZ
ØK9PØØZ
ØK9PØZX
ØK9PØZZ
ØK9P4ØZ
ØK9P4ZZ
ØK9QØØZ
ØK9QØZX
ØK9QØZZ
ØK9Q4ØZ
ØK9Q4ZZ
ØK9RØØZ
ØK9RØZX
ØK9RØZZ
ØK9R4ØZ
ØK9R4ZZ
ØK9SØØZ
ØK9SØZX
ØK9SØZZ
ØK9S4ØZ
ØK9S4ZZ
ØK9TØØZ
ØK9TØZX
ØK9TØZZ
ØK9T4ØZ
ØK9T4ZZ
ØK9VØØZ
ØK9VØZX
ØK9VØZZ
ØK9V4ØZ
ØK9V4ZZ
ØK9WØØZ
ØK9WØZX
ØK9WØZZ
ØK9W4ØZ
ØK9W4ZZ
ØKBØØZX
ØKB1ØZX
ØKB2ØZX
ØKB3ØZX
ØKB4ØZX
ØKB5ØZX
ØKB6ØZX
ØKB7ØZX
ØKB8ØZX
ØKB9ØZX
ØKBBØZX
ØKBCØZX
ØKBDØZX
ØKBFØZX
ØKBGØZX
ØKBHØZX
ØKBJØZX
ØKBKØZX
ØKBLØZX
ØKBMØZX
ØKBNØZX
ØKBPØZX
ØKBQØZX
ØKBRØZX
ØKBSØZX
ØKBTØZX
ØKBVØZX
ØKBWØZX
ØKCØØZZ
ØKCØ3ZZ
ØKCØ4ZZ
ØKC1ØZZ
ØKC13ZZ
ØKC14ZZ
ØKC2ØZZ
ØKC23ZZ
ØKC24ZZ
ØKC3ØZZ
ØKC33ZZ
ØKC34ZZ
ØKC4ØZZ
ØKC43ZZ
ØKC44ZZ
ØKC5ØZZ
ØKC53ZZ
ØKC54ZZ
ØKC6ØZZ
ØKC63ZZ
ØKC64ZZ
ØKC7ØZZ
ØKC73ZZ
ØKC74ZZ
ØKC8ØZZ
ØKC83ZZ
ØKC84ZZ
ØKC9ØZZ
ØKC93ZZ
ØKC94ZZ
ØKCBØZZ
ØKCB3ZZ
ØKCB4ZZ
ØKCFØZZ
ØKCF3ZZ
ØKCF4ZZ
ØKCGØZZ
ØKCG3ZZ
ØKCG4ZZ
ØKCHØZZ
ØKCH3ZZ
ØKCH4ZZ
ØKCJØZZ
ØKCJ3ZZ
ØKCJ4ZZ
ØKCKØZZ
ØKCK3ZZ
ØKCK4ZZ
ØKCLØZZ
ØKCL3ZZ
ØKCL4ZZ
ØKCMØZZ
ØKCM3ZZ
ØKCM4ZZ
ØKCNØZZ
ØKCN3ZZ
ØKCN4ZZ
ØKCPØZZ
ØKCP3ZZ
ØKCP4ZZ
ØKCQØZZ
ØKCQ3ZZ
ØKCQ4ZZ
ØKCRØZZ
ØKCR3ZZ
ØKCR4ZZ
ØKCSØZZ
ØKCS3ZZ
ØKCS4ZZ
ØKCTØZZ
ØKCT3ZZ
ØKCT4ZZ
ØKCVØZZ
ØKCV3ZZ
ØKCV4ZZ
ØKCWØZZ
ØKCW3ZZ
ØKCW4ZZ
ØKPXØØZ
ØKPXØ7Z
ØKPXØJZ
ØKPXØKZ
ØKPXØYZ
ØKPX3ØZ
ØKPX37Z
ØKPX3JZ
ØKPX3KZ
ØKPX4ØZ
ØKPX47Z
ØKPX4JZ
ØKPX4KZ
ØKPYØØZ
ØKPYØ7Z
ØKPYØJZ
ØKPYØKZ
ØKPYØYZ
ØKPY3ØZ
ØKPY37Z
ØKPY3JZ
ØKPY3KZ
ØKPY4ØZ
ØKPY47Z
ØKPY4JZ
ØKPY4KZ
ØKQØØZZ
ØKQØ3ZZ
ØKQØ4ZZ
ØKQ1ØZZ
ØKQ13ZZ
ØKQ14ZZ
ØKQ2ØZZ
ØKQ23ZZ
ØKQ24ZZ
ØKQ3ØZZ
ØKQ33ZZ
ØKQ34ZZ
ØKQ4ØZZ
ØKQ43ZZ
ØKQ44ZZ
ØKQ5ØZZ
ØKQ53ZZ
ØKQ54ZZ
ØKQ6ØZZ
ØKQ63ZZ
ØKQ64ZZ
ØKQ7ØZZ
ØKQ73ZZ
ØKQ74ZZ
ØKQ8ØZZ
ØKQ83ZZ
ØKQ84ZZ
ØKQ9ØZZ
ØKQ93ZZ
ØKQ94ZZ
ØKQBØZZ
ØKQB3ZZ
ØKQB4ZZ
ØKQCØZZ
ØKQC3ZZ
ØKQC4ZZ
ØKQDØZZ
ØKQD3ZZ
ØKQD4ZZ
ØKQFØZZ
ØKQF3ZZ
ØKQF4ZZ
ØKQGØZZ
ØKQG3ZZ
ØKQG4ZZ
ØKQHØZZ
ØKQH3ZZ
ØKQH4ZZ
ØKQJØZZ
ØKQJ3ZZ
ØKQJ4ZZ
ØKQKØZZ
ØKQK3ZZ
ØKQK4ZZ
ØKQLØZZ
ØKQL3ZZ
ØKQL4ZZ
ØKQMØZZ
ØKQM3ZZ
ØKQM4ZZ
ØKQNØZZ
ØKQN3ZZ
ØKQN4ZZ
ØKQPØZZ
ØKQP3ZZ
ØKQP4ZZ
ØKQSØZZ
ØKQS3ZZ
ØKQS4ZZ
ØKQTØZZ
ØKQT3ZZ
ØKQT4ZZ
ØKQVØZZ
ØKQV3ZZ
ØKQV4ZZ
ØKQWØZZ
ØKQW3ZZ
ØKQW4ZZ
ØKRØØ7Z
ØKRØØJZ
ØKRØØKZ
ØKRØ47Z
ØKRØ4JZ
ØKRØ4KZ
ØKR1Ø7Z
ØKR1ØJZ
ØKR1ØKZ
ØKR147Z
ØKR14JZ
ØKR14KZ
ØKR2Ø7Z
ØKR2ØJZ
ØKR2ØKZ
ØKR247Z
ØKR24JZ
ØKR24KZ
ØKR3Ø7Z
ØKR3ØJZ
ØKR3ØKZ
ØKR347Z
ØKR34JZ
ØKR34KZ
ØKR4Ø7Z
ØKR4ØJZ
ØKR4ØKZ
ØKR447Z
ØKR44JZ
ØKR44KZ
ØKR5Ø7Z
ØKR5ØJZ
ØKR5ØKZ
ØKR547Z
ØKR54JZ
ØKR54KZ
ØKR6Ø7Z
ØKR6ØJZ
ØKR6ØKZ
ØKR647Z
ØKR64JZ
ØKR64KZ
ØKR7Ø7Z
ØKR7ØJZ
ØKR7ØKZ
ØKR747Z
ØKR74JZ
ØKR74KZ
ØKR8Ø7Z
ØKR8ØJZ
ØKR8ØKZ
ØKR847Z
ØKR84JZ
ØKR84KZ
ØKR9Ø7Z
ØKR9ØJZ
ØKR9ØKZ
ØKR947Z
ØKR94JZ
ØKR94KZ
ØKRBØ7Z
ØKRBØJZ
ØKRBØKZ
ØKRB47Z
ØKRB4JZ
ØKRB4KZ
ØKRCØ7Z
ØKRCØJZ
ØKRCØKZ
ØKRC47Z
ØKRC4JZ
ØKRC4KZ
ØKRDØ7Z
ØKRDØJZ
ØKRDØKZ
ØKRD47Z
ØKRD4JZ
ØKRD4KZ
ØKRFØ7Z
ØKRFØJZ
ØKRFØKZ
ØKRF47Z
ØKRF4JZ
ØKRF4KZ
ØKRGØ7Z
ØKRGØJZ
ØKRGØKZ
ØKRG47Z
ØKRG4JZ
ØKRG4KZ
ØKRHØ7Z
ØKRHØJZ
ØKRHØKZ
ØKRH47Z
ØKRH4JZ
ØKRH4KZ
ØKRJØ7Z
ØKRJØJZ
ØKRJØKZ
ØKRJ47Z
ØKRJ4JZ
ØKRJ4KZ
ØKRKØ7Z
ØKRKØJZ
ØKRKØKZ
ØKRK47Z
ØKRK4JZ
ØKRK4KZ
ØKRLØ7Z
ØKRLØJZ
ØKRLØKZ
ØKRL47Z
ØKRL4JZ
ØKRL4KZ
ØKRMØ7Z
ØKRMØJZ
ØKRMØKZ
ØKRM47Z
ØKRM4JZ
ØKRM4KZ
ØKRNØ7Z
ØKRNØJZ
ØKRNØKZ
ØKRN47Z
ØKRN4JZ
ØKRN4KZ
ØKRPØ7Z
ØKRPØJZ
ØKRPØKZ
ØKRP47Z
ØKRP4JZ
ØKRP4KZ
ØKRSØ7Z
ØKRSØJZ
ØKRSØKZ
ØKRS47Z
ØKRS4JZ
ØKRS4KZ
ØKRTØ7Z
ØKRTØJZ
ØKRTØKZ
ØKRT47Z
ØKRT4JZ
ØKRT4KZ
ØKRVØ7Z
ØKRVØJZ
ØKRVØKZ
ØKRV47Z
ØKRV4JZ
ØKRV4KZ
ØKRWØ7Z
ØKRWØJZ
ØKRWØKZ
ØKRW47Z
ØKRW4JZ
ØKRW4KZ
ØKWXØØZ
ØKWXØ7Z
ØKWXØJZ
ØKWXØKZ
ØKWXØMZ
ØKWXØYZ
ØKWX3ØZ
ØKWX37Z
ØKWX3JZ
ØKWX3KZ
ØKWX3MZ
ØKWX4ØZ
ØKWX47Z
ØKWX4JZ
ØKWX4KZ
ØKWX4MZ
ØKWYØØZ
ØKWYØ7Z
ØKWYØJZ
ØKWYØKZ
ØKWYØMZ
ØKWYØYZ
ØKWY3ØZ
ØKWY37Z

ØKWY3JZ
ØKWY3KZ
ØKWY3MZ
ØKWY4ØZ
ØKWY47Z
ØKWY4JZ
ØKWY4KZ
ØKWY4MZ
ØL57ØZZ
ØL573ZZ
ØL574ZZ
ØL58ØZZ
ØL583ZZ
ØL584ZZ
ØL8ØØZZ
ØL8Ø3ZZ
ØL8Ø4ZZ
ØL81ØZZ
ØL813ZZ
ØL814ZZ
ØL82ØZZ
ØL823ZZ
ØL824ZZ
ØL83ØZZ
ØL833ZZ
ØL834ZZ
ØL84ØZZ
ØL843ZZ
ØL844ZZ
ØL85ØZZ
ØL853ZZ
ØL854ZZ
ØL86ØZZ
ØL863ZZ
ØL864ZZ
ØL87ØZZ
ØL873ZZ
ØL874ZZ
ØL88ØZZ
ØL883ZZ
ØL884ZZ
ØL89ØZZ
ØL893ZZ
ØL894ZZ
ØL8BØZZ
ØL8B3ZZ
ØL8B4ZZ
ØL8CØZZ
ØL8C3ZZ
ØL8C4ZZ
ØL8DØZZ
ØL8D3ZZ
ØL8D4ZZ
ØL8FØZZ
ØL8F3ZZ
ØL8F4ZZ
ØL8GØZZ
ØL8G3ZZ
ØL8G4ZZ
ØL8HØZZ
ØL8H3ZZ
ØL8H4ZZ
ØL8LØZZ
ØL8L3ZZ
ØL8L4ZZ
ØL8MØZZ
ØL8M3ZZ
ØL8M4ZZ
ØL8QØZZ
ØL8Q3ZZ
ØL8Q4ZZ
ØL8RØZZ
ØL8R3ZZ
ØL8R4ZZ
ØL8SØZZ
ØL8S3ZZ
ØL8S4ZZ
ØL8TØZZ
ØL8T3ZZ
ØL8T4ZZ
ØL8VØZZ
ØL8V3ZZ
ØL8V4ZZ
ØL8WØZZ
ØL8W3ZZ
ØL8W4ZZ
ØL9ØØØZ
ØL9ØØZX
ØL9ØØZZ
ØL9Ø4ØZ
ØL9Ø4ZZ
ØL91ØØZ
ØL91ØZX
ØL91ØZZ
ØL914ØZ
ØL914ZZ
ØL92ØØZ
ØL92ØZX
ØL92ØZZ
ØL924ØZ
ØL924ZZ
ØL93ØØZ
ØL93ØZX
ØL93ØZZ
ØL934ØZ
ØL934ZZ
ØL94ØØZ
ØL94ØZX
ØL94ØZZ
ØL944ØZ
ØL944ZZ
ØL95ØØZ
ØL95ØZX
ØL95ØZZ
ØL954ØZ
ØL954ZZ
ØL96ØØZ
ØL96ØZX
ØL96ØZZ
ØL964ØZ
ØL964ZZ
ØL97ØØZ
ØL97ØZX
ØL97ØZZ
ØL974ØZ
ØL98ØØZ
ØL98ØZX
ØL98ØZZ
ØL984ØZ
ØL99ØØZ
ØL99ØZX
ØL99ØZZ
ØL994ØZ
ØL994ZZ
ØL9BØØZ
ØL9BØZX
ØL9BØZZ
ØL9B4ØZ
ØL9B4ZZ
ØL9CØØZ
ØL9CØZX
ØL9CØZZ
ØL9C4ØZ
ØL9C4ZZ
ØL9DØØZ
ØL9DØZX
ØL9DØZZ
ØL9D4ØZ
ØL9D4ZZ
ØL9FØØZ
ØL9FØZX
ØL9FØZZ
ØL9F4ØZ
ØL9F4ZZ
ØL9GØØZ
ØL9GØZX
ØL9GØZZ
ØL9G4ØZ
ØL9G4ZZ
ØL9HØØZ
ØL9HØZX
ØL9HØZZ
ØL9H4ØZ
ØL9H4ZZ
ØL9JØØZ
ØL9JØZX
ØL9JØZZ
ØL9J4ØZ
ØL9J4ZZ
ØL9KØØZ
ØL9KØZX
ØL9KØZZ
ØL9K4ØZ
ØL9K4ZZ
ØL9LØØZ
ØL9LØZX
ØL9LØZZ
ØL9L4ØZ
ØL9L4ZZ
ØL9MØØZ
ØL9MØZX
ØL9MØZZ
ØL9M4ØZ
ØL9M4ZZ
ØL9NØØZ
ØL9NØZX
ØL9NØZZ
ØL9N4ØZ
ØL9N4ZZ
ØL9PØØZ
ØL9PØZX
ØL9PØZZ
ØL9P4ØZ
ØL9P4ZZ
ØL9QØØZ
ØL9QØZX
ØL9QØZZ
ØL9Q4ØZ
ØL9Q4ZZ
ØL9RØØZ
ØL9RØZX
ØL9RØZZ
ØL9R4ØZ
ØL9R4ZZ
ØL9SØØZ
ØL9SØZX
ØL9SØZZ
ØL9S4ØZ
ØL9S4ZZ
ØL9TØØZ
ØL9TØZX
ØL9TØZZ
ØL9T4ØZ
ØL9T4ZZ
ØL9VØØZ
ØL9VØZX
ØL9VØZZ
ØL9V4ØZ
ØL9V4ZZ
ØL9WØØZ
ØL9WØZX
ØL9WØZZ
ØL9W4ØZ
ØL9W4ZZ
ØLBØØZX
ØLB1ØZX
ØLB2ØZX
ØLB3ØZX
ØLB4ØZX
ØLB5ØZX
ØLB6ØZX
ØLB7ØZX
ØLB8ØZX
ØLB9ØZX
ØLBBØZX
ØLBCØZX
ØLBDØZX
ØLBFØZX
ØLBGØZX
ØLBHØZX
ØLBJØZX
ØLBKØZX
ØLBLØZX
ØLBMØZX
ØLBNØZX
ØLBPØZX
ØLBQØZX
ØLBRØZX
ØLBSØZX
ØLBTØZX
ØLBVØZX
ØLBWØZX
ØLCØØZZ
ØLCØ3ZZ
ØLCØ4ZZ
ØLC1ØZZ
ØLC13ZZ
ØLC14ZZ
ØLC2ØZZ
ØLC23ZZ
ØLC24ZZ
ØLC3ØZZ
ØLC33ZZ
ØLC34ZZ
ØLC4ØZZ
ØLC43ZZ
ØLC44ZZ
ØLC5ØZZ
ØLC53ZZ
ØLC54ZZ
ØLC6ØZZ
ØLC63ZZ
ØLC64ZZ
ØLC7ØZZ
ØLC73ZZ
ØLC74ZZ
ØLC8ØZZ
ØLC83ZZ
ØLC84ZZ
ØLC9ØZZ
ØLC93ZZ
ØLC94ZZ
ØLCBØZZ
ØLCB3ZZ
ØLCB4ZZ
ØLCCØZZ
ØLCC3ZZ
ØLCC4ZZ
ØLCDØZZ
ØLCD3ZZ
ØLCD4ZZ
ØLCFØZZ
ØLCF3ZZ
ØLCF4ZZ
ØLCGØZZ
ØLCG3ZZ
ØLCG4ZZ
ØLCHØZZ
ØLCH3ZZ
ØLCH4ZZ
ØLCJØZZ
ØLCJ3ZZ
ØLCJ4ZZ
ØLCKØZZ
ØLCK3ZZ
ØLCK4ZZ
ØLCLØZZ
ØLCL3ZZ
ØLCL4ZZ
ØLCMØZZ
ØLCM3ZZ
ØLCM4ZZ
ØLCNØZZ
ØLCN3ZZ
ØLCN4ZZ
ØLCPØZZ
ØLCP3ZZ
ØLCP4ZZ
ØLCQØZZ
ØLCQ3ZZ
ØLCQ4ZZ
ØLCRØZZ
ØLCR3ZZ
ØLCR4ZZ
ØLCSØZZ
ØLCS3ZZ
ØLCS4ZZ
ØLCTØZZ
ØLCT3ZZ
ØLCT4ZZ
ØLCVØZZ
ØLCV3ZZ
ØLCV4ZZ
ØLCWØZZ
ØLCW3ZZ
ØLCW4ZZ
ØLJXØZZ
ØLJX4ZZ
ØLPXØØZ
ØLPXØ7Z
ØLPXØJZ
ØLPXØKZ
ØLPXØYZ
ØLPX37Z
ØLPX3JZ
ØLPX3KZ
ØLPX4ØZ
ØLPX47Z
ØLPX4JZ
ØLPX4KZ
ØLPYØØZ
ØLPYØ7Z
ØLPYØJZ
ØLPYØKZ
ØLPYØYZ
ØLPY37Z
ØLPY3JZ
ØLPY3KZ
ØLPY4ØZ
ØLPY47Z
ØLPY4JZ
ØLPY4KZ
ØLQ1ØZZ
ØLQ13ZZ
ØLQ14ZZ
ØLQ2ØZZ
ØLQ23ZZ
ØLQ24ZZ
ØLQ7ØZZ
ØLQ73ZZ
ØLQ74ZZ
ØLQ8ØZZ
ØLQ83ZZ
ØLQ84ZZ
ØLQQØZZ
ØLQQ3ZZ
ØLQQ4ZZ
ØLQRØZZ
ØLQR3ZZ
ØLQR4ZZ
ØLQSØZZ
ØLQS3ZZ
ØLQS4ZZ
ØLQTØZZ
ØLQT3ZZ
ØLQT4ZZ
ØLWXØØZ
ØLWXØ7Z
ØLWXØJZ
ØLWXØKZ
ØLWXØYZ
ØLWX3ØZ
ØLWX37Z
ØLWX3JZ
ØLWX3KZ
ØLWX4ØZ
ØLWX47Z
ØLWX4JZ
ØLWX4KZ
ØLWYØØZ
ØLWYØ7Z
ØLWYØJZ
ØLWYØKZ
ØLWYØYZ
ØLWY3ØZ
ØLWY37Z
ØLWY3JZ
ØLWY3KZ
ØLWY4ØZ
ØLWY47Z
ØLWY4JZ
ØLWY4KZ
ØM5NØZZ
ØM5N3ZZ
ØM5N4ZZ
ØM5PØZZ
ØM5P3ZZ
ØM5P4ZZ
ØM5SØZZ
ØM5S3ZZ
ØM5S4ZZ
ØM5TØZZ
ØM5T3ZZ
ØM5T4ZZ
ØM8ØØZZ
ØM8Ø3ZZ
ØM8Ø4ZZ
ØM81ØZZ
ØM813ZZ
ØM814ZZ
ØM82ØZZ
ØM823ZZ
ØM824ZZ
ØM83ØZZ
ØM833ZZ
ØM834ZZ
ØM84ØZZ
ØM843ZZ
ØM844ZZ
ØM89ØZZ
ØM893ZZ
ØM894ZZ
ØM8BØZZ
ØM8B3ZZ
ØM8B4ZZ
ØM8CØZZ
ØM8C3ZZ
ØM8C4ZZ
ØM8DØZZ
ØM8D3ZZ
ØM8D4ZZ
ØM8FØZZ
ØM8F3ZZ
ØM8F4ZZ
ØM8GØZZ
ØM8G3ZZ
ØM8G4ZZ
ØM8HØZZ
ØM8H3ZZ
ØM8H4ZZ
ØM8JØZZ
ØM8J3ZZ
ØM8J4ZZ
ØM8KØZZ
ØM8K3ZZ
ØM8K4ZZ
ØM8LØZZ
ØM8L3ZZ
ØM8L4ZZ
ØM8MØZZ
ØM8M3ZZ
ØM8M4ZZ
ØM8NØZZ
ØM8N3ZZ
ØM8N4ZZ
ØM8PØZZ
ØM8P3ZZ
ØM8P4ZZ
ØM8QØZZ
ØM8Q3ZZ
ØM8Q4ZZ
ØM8RØZZ
ØM8R3ZZ
ØM8R4ZZ
ØM8SØZZ
ØM8S3ZZ
ØM8S4ZZ
ØM8TØZZ
ØM8T3ZZ
ØM8T4ZZ
ØM8VØZZ
ØM8V3ZZ
ØM8V4ZZ
ØM8WØZZ
ØM8W3ZZ
ØM8W4ZZ
ØM9ØØØZ
ØM9ØØZZ
ØM91ØØZ
ØM91ØZZ
ØM92ØØZ
ØM92ØZZ
ØM93ØØZ
ØM93ØZZ
ØM94ØØZ
ØM94ØZZ
ØM99ØØZ
ØM99ØZX
ØM99ØZZ
ØM9BØØZ
ØM9BØZX
ØM9BØZZ
ØM9CØØZ
ØM9CØZZ
ØM9DØØZ
ØM9DØZZ
ØM9FØØZ
ØM9FØZZ
ØM9GØØZ
ØM9GØZZ
ØM9HØØZ
ØM9HØZX
ØM9HØZZ
ØM9JØØZ
ØM9JØZX
ØM9JØZZ
ØM9KØØZ
ØM9KØZX
ØM9KØZZ
ØM9LØØZ
ØM9LØZZ
ØM9MØØZ
ØM9MØZZ
ØM9NØØZ
ØM9NØZZ
ØM9N4ØZ
ØM9PØØZ
ØM9PØZZ
ØM9P4ØZ
ØM9QØØZ
ØM9QØZZ
ØM9RØØZ
ØM9RØZZ
ØM9SØØZ
ØM9SØZZ
ØM9S4ØZ
ØM9TØØZ
ØM9TØZZ
ØM9T4ØZ
ØM9VØØZ
ØM9VØZX
ØM9VØZZ
ØM9WØØZ
ØM9WØZX
ØM9WØZZ
ØMBØØZZ
ØMBØ3ZZ
ØMBØ4ZZ
ØMB1ØZZ
ØMB13ZZ
ØMB14ZZ
ØMB2ØZZ
ØMB23ZZ
ØMB24ZZ
ØMB3ØZZ
ØMB33ZZ
ØMB34ZZ
ØMB4ØZZ
ØMB43ZZ
ØMB44ZZ
ØMB5ØZZ
ØMB53ZZ
ØMB54ZZ
ØMB6ØZZ
ØMB63ZZ
ØMB64ZZ
ØMB9ØZX
ØMB9ØZZ
ØMB93ZZ
ØMB94ZZ
ØMBBØZZ
ØMBB3ZZ
ØMBB4ZZ
ØMBCØZZ
ØMBC3ZZ
ØMBC4ZZ
ØMBDØZZ
ØMBD3ZZ
ØMBD4ZZ
ØMBFØZZ
ØMBF3ZZ
ØMBF4ZZ
ØMBGØZZ
ØMBG3ZZ
ØMBG4ZZ
ØMBHØZX
ØMBHØZZ
ØMBH3ZZ
ØMBH4ZZ
ØMBJØZX
ØMBJØZZ
ØMBJ3ZZ
ØMBJ4ZZ
ØMBKØZX
ØMBKØZZ
ØMBK3ZZ
ØMBK4ZZ
ØMBLØZZ
ØMBL3ZZ
ØMBL4ZZ
ØMBMØZZ
ØMBM3ZZ
ØMBM4ZZ
ØMBNØZZ
ØMBN3ZZ
ØMBN4ZZ
ØMBPØZZ
ØMBP3ZZ
ØMBP4ZZ
ØMBQØZZ
ØMBQ3ZZ
ØMBQ4ZZ
ØMBRØZZ
ØMBR3ZZ
ØMBR4ZZ
ØMBSØZZ
ØMBS3ZZ
ØMBS4ZZ
ØMBTØZZ
ØMBT3ZZ
ØMBT4ZZ
ØMBVØZX
ØMBVØZZ
ØMBV3ZZ
ØMBV4ZZ
ØMBWØZX
ØMBWØZZ
ØMBW3ZZ
ØMBW4ZZ
ØMCØØZZ
ØMCØ3ZZ
ØMCØ4ZZ
ØMC1ØZZ
ØMC13ZZ
ØMC14ZZ
ØMC2ØZZ
ØMC23ZZ
ØMC24ZZ
ØMC3ØZZ
ØMC33ZZ
ØMC34ZZ
ØMC4ØZZ
ØMC43ZZ
ØMC44ZZ
ØMC9ØZZ
ØMC93ZZ
ØMC94ZZ
ØMCBØZZ
ØMCB3ZZ
ØMCB4ZZ
ØMCCØZZ
ØMCC3ZZ
ØMCC4ZZ
ØMCDØZZ
ØMCD3ZZ
ØMCD4ZZ
ØMCFØZZ
ØMCF3ZZ
ØMCF4ZZ
ØMCGØZZ
ØMCG3ZZ
ØMCG4ZZ
ØMCHØZZ
ØMCH3ZZ
ØMCH4ZZ
ØMCJØZZ
ØMCJ3ZZ
ØMCJ4ZZ
ØMCKØZZ
ØMCK3ZZ
ØMCK4ZZ
ØMCLØZZ
ØMCL3ZZ
ØMCL4ZZ
ØMCMØZZ
ØMCM3ZZ
ØMCM4ZZ
ØMCNØZZ
ØMCN3ZZ
ØMCN4ZZ
ØMCPØZZ
ØMCP3ZZ
ØMCP4ZZ
ØMCQØZZ
ØMCQ3ZZ
ØMCQ4ZZ
ØMCRØZZ
ØMCR3ZZ
ØMCR4ZZ
ØMCSØZZ
ØMCS3ZZ
ØMCS4ZZ
ØMCTØZZ
ØMCT3ZZ
ØMCT4ZZ
ØMCVØZZ
ØMCV3ZZ
ØMCV4ZZ
ØMCWØZZ
ØMCW3ZZ
ØMCW4ZZ
ØMDØØZZ
ØMDØ3ZZ
ØMDØ4ZZ
ØMD1ØZZ
ØMD13ZZ
ØMD14ZZ
ØMD2ØZZ
ØMD23ZZ
ØMD24ZZ
ØMD3ØZZ
ØMD33ZZ
ØMD34ZZ
ØMD4ØZZ
ØMD43ZZ
ØMD44ZZ
ØMD5ØZZ
ØMD53ZZ
ØMD54ZZ
ØMD6ØZZ
ØMD63ZZ
ØMD64ZZ
ØMD9ØZZ
ØMD93ZZ
ØMD94ZZ
ØMDBØZZ
ØMDB3ZZ
ØMDB4ZZ
ØMDCØZZ
ØMDC3ZZ
ØMDC4ZZ
ØMDDØZZ
ØMDD3ZZ
ØMDD4ZZ
ØMDFØZZ
ØMDF3ZZ
ØMDF4ZZ
ØMDGØZZ
ØMDG3ZZ
ØMDG4ZZ
ØMDHØZZ
ØMDH3ZZ
ØMDH4ZZ
ØMDJØZZ
ØMDJ3ZZ
ØMDJ4ZZ
ØMDKØZZ
ØMDK3ZZ
ØMDK4ZZ
ØMDLØZZ
ØMDL3ZZ
ØMDL4ZZ
ØMDMØZZ
ØMDM3ZZ
ØMDM4ZZ
ØMDNØZZ
ØMDN3ZZ
ØMDN4ZZ
ØMDPØZZ
ØMDP3ZZ
ØMDP4ZZ
ØMDQØZZ
ØMDQ3ZZ
ØMDQ4ZZ
ØMDRØZZ
ØMDR3ZZ
ØMDR4ZZ
ØMDSØZZ
ØMDS3ZZ
ØMDS4ZZ
ØMDTØZZ
ØMDT3ZZ
ØMDT4ZZ
ØMDVØZZ
ØMDV3ZZ
ØMDV4ZZ
ØMDWØZZ
ØMDW3ZZ
ØMDW4ZZ
ØMPXØ7Z
ØMPXØKZ
ØMPX37Z
ØMPX3KZ
ØMPX47Z
ØMPX4KZ
ØMPYØ7Z
ØMPYØKZ
ØMPY37Z
ØMPY3KZ
ØMPY47Z
ØMPY4KZ
ØMTØØZZ
ØMTØ4ZZ
ØMT1ØZZ
ØMT14ZZ
ØMT2ØZZ
ØMT24ZZ
ØMT3ØZZ
ØMT34ZZ
ØMT4ØZZ
ØMT44ZZ
ØMT5ØZZ
ØMT54ZZ
ØMT6ØZZ
ØMT64ZZ
ØMT9ØZZ
ØMT94ZZ
ØMTBØZZ
ØMTB4ZZ
ØMTCØZZ
ØMTC4ZZ
ØMTDØZZ
ØMTD4ZZ
ØMTFØZZ
ØMTF4ZZ
ØMTGØZZ
ØMTG4ZZ
ØMTHØZZ
ØMTH4ZZ
ØMTJØZZ
ØMTJ4ZZ
ØMTKØZZ
ØMTK4ZZ
ØMTLØZZ
ØMTL4ZZ
ØMTMØZZ
ØMTM4ZZ
ØMTNØZZ
ØMTN4ZZ
ØMTPØZZ
ØMTP4ZZ
ØMTQØZZ
ØMTQ4ZZ
ØMTRØZZ
ØMTR4ZZ
ØMTSØZZ
ØMTS4ZZ
ØMTTØZZ
ØMTT4ZZ
ØMTVØZZ
ØMTV4ZZ
ØMTWØZZ
ØMTW4ZZ
ØMWXØØZ
ØMWXØ7Z

ØMWXØJZ
ØMWXØKZ
ØMWXØYZ
ØMWX3ØZ
ØMWX37Z
ØMWX3JZ
ØMWX3KZ
ØMWX4ØZ
ØMWX47Z
ØMWX4JZ
ØMWX4KZ
ØMWYØØZ
ØMWYØ7Z
ØMWYØJZ
ØMWYØKZ
ØMWYØYZ
ØMWY3ØZ
ØMWY37Z
ØMWY3JZ
ØMWY3KZ
ØMWY4ØZ
ØMWY47Z
ØMWY4JZ
ØMWY4KZ
ØN5BØZZ
ØN5B3ZZ
ØN5B4ZZ
ØN5CØZZ
ØN5C3ZZ
ØN5C4ZZ
ØN5FØZZ
ØN5F3ZZ
ØN5F4ZZ
ØN5GØZZ
ØN5G3ZZ
ØN5G4ZZ
ØN5HØZZ
ØN5H3ZZ
ØN5H4ZZ
ØN5JØZZ
ØN5J3ZZ
ØN5J4ZZ
ØN5KØZZ
ØN5K3ZZ
ØN5K4ZZ
ØN5LØZZ
ØN5L3ZZ
ØN5L4ZZ
ØN5MØZZ
ØN5M3ZZ
ØN5M4ZZ
ØN5NØZZ
ØN5N3ZZ
ØN5N4ZZ
ØN5PØZZ
ØN5P3ZZ
ØN5P4ZZ
ØN5QØZZ
ØN5Q3ZZ
ØN5Q4ZZ
ØN5RØZZ
ØN5R3ZZ
ØN5R4ZZ
ØN5TØZZ
ØN5T3ZZ
ØN5T4ZZ
ØN5VØZZ
ØN5V3ZZ
ØN5V4ZZ
ØN5XØZZ
ØN5X3ZZ
ØN5X4ZZ
ØN8PØZZ
ØN8P3ZZ
ØN8P4ZZ
ØN8QØZZ
ØN8Q3ZZ
ØN8Q4ZZ
ØN9CØZX
ØN9C3ZX
ØN9C4ZX
ØN9FØZX
ØN9F3ZX
ØN9F4ZX
ØN9GØZX
ØN9G3ZX
ØN9G4ZX
ØN9HØZX
ØN9H3ZX
ØN9H4ZX
ØN9JØZX
ØN9J3ZX
ØN9J4ZX
ØN9KØZX
ØN9K3ZX
ØN9K4ZX
ØN9LØZX
ØN9L3ZX
ØN9L4ZX
ØN9MØZX
ØN9M3ZX
ØN9M4ZX
ØN9NØZX
ØN9N3ZX
ØN9N4ZX
ØN9PØØZ
ØN9PØZX
ØN9PØZZ
ØN9P3ZX
ØN9P4ØZ
ØN9P4ZX
ØN9P4ZZ
ØN9QØØZ
ØN9QØZX
ØN9QØZZ
ØN9Q3ZX
ØN9Q4ØZ
ØN9Q4ZX
ØN9Q4ZZ
ØN9RØZX
ØN9R3ZX
ØN9R4ZX
ØN9TØZX
ØN9T3ZX
ØN9T4ZX
ØN9VØZX
ØN9V3ZX
ØN9V4ZX
ØN9XØZX
ØN9X3ZX
ØN9X4ZX
ØNBCØZX
ØNBC3ZX
ØNBC4ZX
ØNBFØZX
ØNBF3ZX
ØNBF4ZX
ØNBGØZX
ØNBG3ZX
ØNBG4ZX
ØNBHØZX
ØNBH3ZX
ØNBH4ZX
ØNBJØZX
ØNBJ3ZX
ØNBJ4ZX
ØNBKØZX
ØNBK3ZX
ØNBK4ZX
ØNBLØZX
ØNBL3ZX
ØNBL4ZX
ØNBMØZX
ØNBM3ZX
ØNBM4ZX
ØNBNØZX
ØNBN3ZX
ØNBN4ZX
ØNBPØZX
ØNBPØZZ
ØNBP3ZX
ØNBP3ZZ
ØNBP4ZX
ØNBP4ZZ
ØNBQØZX
ØNBQØZZ
ØNBQ3ZX
ØNBQ3ZZ
ØNBQ4ZX
ØNBQ4ZZ
ØNBXØZX
ØNBX3ZX
ØNBX4ZX
ØNNXØZZ
ØNNX3ZZ
ØNNX4ZZ
ØNPØØ3Z
ØNPØ33Z
ØNPØ43Z
ØNPWØJZ
ØNPW3JZ
ØNPW4JZ
ØNQBØZZ
ØNQB3ZZ
ØNQB4ZZ
ØNQPØZZ
ØNQP3ZZ
ØNQP4ZZ
ØNQQØZZ
ØNQQ3ZZ
ØNQQ4ZZ
ØNRBØ7Z
ØNRBØJZ
ØNRBØKZ
ØNRB37Z
ØNRB3JZ
ØNRB3KZ
ØNRB47Z
ØNRB4JZ
ØNRB4KZ
ØNRPØ7Z
ØNRPØJZ
ØNRP37Z
ØNRP3JZ
ØNRP47Z
ØNRP4JZ
ØNRQØ7Z
ØNRQØJZ
ØNRQ37Z
ØNRQ3JZ
ØNRQ47Z
ØNRQ4JZ
ØNSBØ4Z
ØNSBØZZ
ØNUBØ7Z
ØNUBØJZ
ØNUBØKZ
ØNUB37Z
ØNUB3JZ
ØNUB3KZ
ØNUB47Z
ØNUB4JZ
ØNUB4KZ
ØNUPØJZ
ØNUP3JZ
ØNUP4JZ
ØNUQØJZ
ØNUQ3JZ
ØNUQ4JZ
ØNWØØ3Z
ØNWØ33Z
ØNWØ43Z
ØP5ØØZZ
ØP5Ø3ZZ
ØP5Ø4ZZ
ØP51ØZZ
ØP513ZZ
ØP514ZZ
ØP52ØZZ
ØP523ZZ
ØP524ZZ
ØP53ØZ3
ØP53ØZZ
ØP533Z3
ØP533ZZ
ØP534Z3
ØP534ZZ
ØP54ØZ3
ØP54ØZZ
ØP543Z3
ØP543ZZ
ØP544Z3
ØP544ZZ
ØP55ØZZ
ØP553ZZ
ØP554ZZ
ØP56ØZZ
ØP563ZZ
ØP564ZZ
ØP57ØZZ
ØP573ZZ
ØP574ZZ
ØP58ØZZ
ØP583ZZ
ØP584ZZ
ØP59ØZZ
ØP593ZZ
ØP594ZZ
ØP5BØZZ
ØP5B3ZZ
ØP5B4ZZ
ØP5CØZZ
ØP5C3ZZ
ØP5C4ZZ
ØP5DØZZ
ØP5D3ZZ
ØP5D4ZZ
ØP5FØZZ
ØP5F3ZZ
ØP5F4ZZ
ØP5GØZZ
ØP5G3ZZ
ØP5G4ZZ
ØP5HØZZ
ØP5H3ZZ
ØP5H4ZZ
ØP5JØZZ
ØP5J3ZZ
ØP5J4ZZ
ØP5KØZZ
ØP5K3ZZ
ØP5K4ZZ
ØP5LØZZ
ØP5L3ZZ
ØP5L4ZZ
ØP5MØZZ
ØP5M3ZZ
ØP5M4ZZ
ØP5NØZZ
ØP5N3ZZ
ØP5N4ZZ
ØP5PØZZ
ØP5P3ZZ
ØP5P4ZZ
ØP5QØZZ
ØP5Q3ZZ
ØP5Q4ZZ
ØP5RØZZ
ØP5R3ZZ
ØP5R4ZZ
ØP5SØZZ
ØP5S3ZZ
ØP5S4ZZ
ØP5TØZZ
ØP5T3ZZ
ØP5T4ZZ
ØP5VØZZ
ØP5V3ZZ
ØP5V4ZZ
ØP9ØØZX
ØP9Ø3ZX
ØP9Ø4ZX
ØP91ØZX
ØP913ZX
ØP914ZX
ØP92ØZX
ØP923ZX
ØP924ZX
ØP93ØZX
ØP933ZX
ØP934ZX
ØP94ØZX
ØP943ZX
ØP944ZX
ØP95ØZX
ØP953ZX
ØP954ZX
ØP96ØZX
ØP963ZX
ØP964ZX
ØP97ØZX
ØP973ZX
ØP974ZX
ØP98ØZX
ØP983ZX
ØP984ZX
ØP99ØZX
ØP993ZX
ØP994ZX
ØP9BØZX
ØP9B3ZX
ØP9B4ZX
ØP9CØZX
ØP9C3ZX
ØP9C4ZX
ØP9DØZX
ØP9D3ZX
ØP9D4ZX
ØP9FØZX
ØP9F3ZX
ØP9F4ZX
ØP9GØZX
ØP9G3ZX
ØP9G4ZX
ØP9HØZX
ØP9H3ZX
ØP9H4ZX
ØP9JØZX
ØP9J3ZX
ØP9J4ZX
ØP9KØZX
ØP9K3ZX
ØP9K4ZX
ØP9LØZX
ØP9L3ZX
ØP9L4ZX
ØP9MØZX
ØP9M3ZX
ØP9M4ZX
ØP9NØZX
ØP9N3ZX
ØP9N4ZX
ØP9PØZX
ØP9P3ZX
ØP9P4ZX
ØP9QØZX
ØP9Q3ZX
ØP9Q4ZX
ØP9RØZX
ØP9R3ZX
ØP9R4ZX
ØP9SØZX
ØP9S3ZX
ØP9S4ZX
ØP9TØZX
ØP9T3ZX
ØP9T4ZX
ØP9VØZX
ØP9V3ZX
ØP9V4ZX
ØPBØØZX
ØPBØ3ZX
ØPBØ4ZX
ØPB1ØZX
ØPB13ZX
ØPB14ZX
ØPB2ØZX
ØPB23ZX
ØPB24ZX
ØPB3ØZX
ØPB33ZX
ØPB34ZX
ØPB4ØZX
ØPB43ZX
ØPB44ZX
ØPB5ØZX
ØPB53ZX
ØPB54ZX
ØPB6ØZX
ØPB63ZX
ØPB64ZX
ØPB7ØZX
ØPB73ZX
ØPB74ZX
ØPB8ØZX
ØPB83ZX
ØPB84ZX
ØPB9ØZX
ØPB93ZX
ØPB94ZX
ØPBBØZX
ØPBB3ZX
ØPBB4ZX
ØPBCØZX
ØPBC3ZX
ØPBC4ZX
ØPBDØZX
ØPBD3ZX
ØPBD4ZX
ØPBFØZX
ØPBF3ZX
ØPBF4ZX
ØPBGØZX
ØPBG3ZX
ØPBG4ZX
ØPBHØZX
ØPBH3ZX
ØPBH4ZX
ØPBJØZX
ØPBJ3ZX
ØPBJ4ZX
ØPBKØZX
ØPBK3ZX
ØPBK4ZX
ØPBLØZX
ØPBL3ZX
ØPBL4ZX
ØPBMØZX
ØPBM3ZX
ØPBM4ZX
ØPBNØZX
ØPBN3ZX
ØPBN4ZX
ØPBPØZX
ØPBP3ZX
ØPBP4ZX
ØPBQØZX
ØPBQ3ZX
ØPBQ4ZX
ØPBRØZX
ØPBR3ZX
ØPBR4ZX
ØPBSØZX
ØPBS3ZX
ØPBS4ZX
ØPBTØZX
ØPBT3ZX
ØPBT4ZX
ØPBVØZX
ØPBV3ZX
ØPBV4ZX
ØPPØØ4Z
ØPPØØ7Z
ØPPØØJZ
ØPPØØKZ
ØPPØ34Z
ØPPØ37Z
ØPPØ3JZ
ØPPØ3KZ
ØPPØ44Z
ØPPØ47Z
ØPPØ4JZ
ØPPØ4KZ
ØPP1Ø4Z
ØPP1Ø7Z
ØPP1ØJZ
ØPP1ØKZ
ØPP134Z
ØPP137Z
ØPP13JZ
ØPP13KZ
ØPP144Z
ØPP147Z
ØPP14JZ
ØPP14KZ
ØPP2Ø4Z
ØPP2Ø7Z
ØPP2ØJZ
ØPP2ØKZ
ØPP234Z
ØPP237Z
ØPP23JZ
ØPP23KZ
ØPP244Z
ØPP247Z
ØPP24JZ
ØPP24KZ
ØPP3Ø4Z
ØPP3Ø7Z
ØPP3ØJZ
ØPP3ØKZ
ØPP334Z
ØPP337Z
ØPP33JZ
ØPP33KZ
ØPP344Z
ØPP347Z
ØPP34JZ
ØPP34KZ
ØPP4Ø4Z
ØPP4Ø7Z
ØPP4ØJZ
ØPP4ØKZ
ØPP434Z
ØPP437Z
ØPP43JZ
ØPP43KZ
ØPP444Z
ØPP447Z
ØPP44JZ
ØPP44KZ
ØPP5Ø4Z
ØPP5Ø7Z
ØPP5ØJZ
ØPP5ØKZ
ØPP534Z
ØPP537Z
ØPP53JZ
ØPP53KZ
ØPP544Z
ØPP547Z
ØPP54JZ
ØPP54KZ
ØPP6Ø4Z
ØPP6Ø7Z
ØPP6ØJZ
ØPP6ØKZ
ØPP634Z
ØPP637Z
ØPP63JZ
ØPP63KZ
ØPP644Z
ØPP647Z
ØPP64JZ
ØPP64KZ
ØPP7Ø4Z
ØPP7Ø7Z
ØPP7ØJZ
ØPP7ØKZ
ØPP734Z
ØPP737Z
ØPP73JZ
ØPP73KZ
ØPP744Z
ØPP747Z
ØPP74JZ
ØPP74KZ
ØPP8Ø4Z
ØPP8Ø7Z
ØPP8ØJZ
ØPP8ØKZ
ØPP834Z
ØPP837Z
ØPP83JZ
ØPP83KZ
ØPP844Z
ØPP847Z
ØPP84JZ
ØPP84KZ
ØPP9Ø4Z
ØPP9Ø7Z
ØPP9ØJZ
ØPP9ØKZ
ØPP934Z
ØPP937Z
ØPP93JZ
ØPP93KZ
ØPP944Z
ØPP947Z
ØPP94JZ
ØPP94KZ
ØPPBØ4Z
ØPPBØ7Z
ØPPBØJZ
ØPPBØKZ
ØPPB34Z
ØPPB37Z
ØPPB3JZ
ØPPB3KZ
ØPPB44Z
ØPPB47Z
ØPPB4JZ
ØPPB4KZ
ØPPCØ4Z
ØPPCØ5Z
ØPPCØ7Z
ØPPCØJZ
ØPPCØKZ
ØPPC34Z
ØPPC35Z
ØPPC37Z
ØPPC3JZ
ØPPC3KZ
ØPPC44Z
ØPPC45Z
ØPPC47Z
ØPPC4JZ
ØPPC4KZ
ØPPDØ4Z
ØPPDØ5Z
ØPPDØ7Z
ØPPDØJZ
ØPPDØKZ
ØPPD34Z
ØPPD35Z
ØPPD37Z
ØPPD3JZ
ØPPD3KZ
ØPPD44Z
ØPPD45Z
ØPPD47Z
ØPPD4JZ
ØPPD4KZ
ØPPFØ4Z
ØPPFØ5Z
ØPPFØ7Z
ØPPFØJZ
ØPPFØKZ
ØPPF34Z
ØPPF35Z
ØPPF37Z
ØPPF3JZ
ØPPF3KZ
ØPPF44Z
ØPPF45Z
ØPPF47Z
ØPPF4JZ
ØPPF4KZ
ØPPGØ4Z
ØPPGØ5Z
ØPPGØ7Z
ØPPGØJZ
ØPPGØKZ
ØPPG34Z
ØPPG35Z
ØPPG37Z
ØPPG3JZ
ØPPG3KZ
ØPPG44Z
ØPPG45Z
ØPPG47Z
ØPPG4JZ
ØPPG4KZ
ØPPHØ4Z
ØPPHØ5Z
ØPPHØ7Z
ØPPHØJZ
ØPPHØKZ
ØPPH34Z
ØPPH35Z
ØPPH37Z
ØPPH3JZ
ØPPH3KZ
ØPPH44Z
ØPPH45Z
ØPPH47Z
ØPPH4JZ
ØPPH4KZ
ØPPJØ4Z
ØPPJØ5Z
ØPPJØ7Z
ØPPJØJZ
ØPPJØKZ
ØPPJ34Z
ØPPJ35Z
ØPPJ37Z
ØPPJ3JZ
ØPPJ3KZ
ØPPJ44Z
ØPPJ45Z
ØPPJ47Z
ØPPJ4JZ
ØPPJ4KZ
ØPPKØ4Z
ØPPKØ5Z
ØPPKØ7Z
ØPPKØJZ
ØPPKØKZ
ØPPK34Z
ØPPK35Z
ØPPK37Z
ØPPK3JZ
ØPPK3KZ
ØPPK44Z
ØPPK45Z
ØPPK47Z
ØPPK4JZ
ØPPK4KZ
ØPPLØ4Z
ØPPLØ5Z
ØPPLØ7Z
ØPPLØJZ
ØPPLØKZ
ØPPL34Z
ØPPL35Z
ØPPL37Z
ØPPL3JZ
ØPPL3KZ
ØPPL44Z
ØPPL45Z
ØPPL47Z
ØPPL4JZ
ØPPL4KZ
ØPPMØ4Z
ØPPMØ5Z
ØPPMØ7Z
ØPPMØJZ
ØPPMØKZ
ØPPM34Z
ØPPM35Z
ØPPM37Z
ØPPM3JZ
ØPPM3KZ
ØPPM44Z
ØPPM45Z
ØPPM47Z
ØPPM4JZ
ØPPM4KZ
ØPPNØ4Z
ØPPNØ5Z
ØPPNØ7Z
ØPPNØJZ
ØPPNØKZ
ØPPN34Z
ØPPN35Z
ØPPN37Z
ØPPN3JZ
ØPPN3KZ
ØPPN44Z
ØPPN45Z
ØPPN47Z
ØPPN4JZ
ØPPN4KZ
ØPPPØ4Z
ØPPPØ5Z
ØPPPØ7Z
ØPPPØJZ
ØPPPØKZ
ØPPP34Z
ØPPP35Z
ØPPP37Z
ØPPP3JZ
ØPPP3KZ
ØPPP44Z
ØPPP45Z
ØPPP47Z
ØPPP4JZ
ØPPP4KZ
ØPPQØ4Z
ØPPQØ5Z
ØPPQØ7Z
ØPPQØJZ
ØPPQØKZ
ØPPQ34Z
ØPPQ35Z
ØPPQ37Z
ØPPQ3JZ
ØPPQ3KZ
ØPPQ44Z
ØPPQ45Z
ØPPQ47Z
ØPPQ4JZ
ØPPQ4KZ
ØPPRØ4Z
ØPPRØ5Z
ØPPRØ7Z
ØPPRØJZ
ØPPRØKZ
ØPPR34Z
ØPPR35Z
ØPPR37Z
ØPPR3JZ
ØPPR3KZ
ØPPR44Z
ØPPR45Z
ØPPR47Z
ØPPR4JZ
ØPPR4KZ
ØPPSØ4Z
ØPPSØ5Z
ØPPSØ7Z
ØPPSØJZ
ØPPSØKZ
ØPPS34Z
ØPPS35Z
ØPPS37Z
ØPPS3JZ
ØPPS3KZ
ØPPS44Z
ØPPS45Z
ØPPS47Z
ØPPS4JZ
ØPPS4KZ
ØPPTØ4Z
ØPPTØ5Z
ØPPTØ7Z
ØPPTØJZ
ØPPTØKZ
ØPPT34Z
ØPPT35Z
ØPPT37Z
ØPPT3JZ
ØPPT3KZ
ØPPT44Z
ØPPT45Z
ØPPT47Z
ØPPT4JZ
ØPPT4KZ
ØPPVØ4Z
ØPPVØ5Z
ØPPVØ7Z
ØPPVØJZ
ØPPVØKZ
ØPPV34Z
ØPPV35Z
ØPPV37Z
ØPPV3JZ
ØPPV3KZ
ØPPV44Z
ØPPV45Z
ØPPV47Z
ØPPV4JZ
ØPPV4KZ
ØPPYØØZ
ØPPYØMZ

ØPPY3MZ
ØPPY4ØZ
ØPPY4MZ
ØPRHØ7Z
ØPRHØKZ
ØPRH37Z
ØPRH3KZ
ØPRH47Z
ØPRH4KZ
ØPRJØ7Z
ØPRJØKZ
ØPRJ37Z
ØPRJ3KZ
ØPRJ47Z
ØPRJ4KZ
ØPRKØ7Z
ØPRKØKZ
ØPRK37Z
ØPRK3KZ
ØPRK47Z
ØPRK4KZ
ØPRLØ7Z
ØPRLØKZ
ØPRL37Z
ØPRL3KZ
ØPRL47Z
ØPRL4KZ
ØPSH34Z
ØPSH36Z
ØPSH44Z
ØPSH46Z
ØPSJ34Z
ØPSJ36Z
ØPSJ44Z
ØPSJ46Z
ØPSK34Z
ØPSK36Z
ØPSK44Z
ØPSK46Z
ØPSL34Z
ØPSL36Z
ØPSL44Z
ØPSL46Z
ØPUHØ7Z
ØPUHØKZ
ØPUH37Z
ØPUH3KZ
ØPUH47Z
ØPUH4KZ
ØPUJØ7Z
ØPUJØKZ
ØPUJ37Z
ØPUJ3KZ
ØPUJ47Z
ØPUJ4KZ
ØPUKØ7Z
ØPUKØKZ
ØPUK37Z
ØPUK3KZ
ØPUK47Z
ØPUK4KZ
ØPULØ7Z
ØPULØKZ
ØPUL37Z
ØPUL3KZ
ØPUL47Z
ØPUL4KZ
ØQ5ØØZ3
ØQ5ØØZZ
ØQ5Ø3Z3
ØQ5Ø3ZZ
ØQ5Ø4Z3
ØQ5Ø4ZZ
ØQ51ØZ3
ØQ51ØZZ
ØQ513Z3
ØQ513ZZ
ØQ514Z3
ØQ514ZZ
ØQ52ØZZ
ØQ523ZZ
ØQ524ZZ
ØQ53ØZZ
ØQ533ZZ
ØQ534ZZ
ØQ54ØZZ
ØQ543ZZ
ØQ544ZZ
ØQ55ØZZ
ØQ553ZZ
ØQ554ZZ
ØQ56ØZZ
ØQ563ZZ
ØQ564ZZ
ØQ57ØZZ
ØQ573ZZ
ØQ574ZZ
ØQ58ØZZ
ØQ583ZZ
ØQ584ZZ
ØQ59ØZZ
ØQ593ZZ
ØQ594ZZ
ØQ5BØZZ
ØQ5B3ZZ
ØQ5B4ZZ
ØQ5CØZZ
ØQ5C3ZZ
ØQ5C4ZZ
ØQ5DØZZ
ØQ5D3ZZ
ØQ5D4ZZ
ØQ5FØZZ
ØQ5F3ZZ
ØQ5F4ZZ
ØQ5GØZZ
ØQ5G3ZZ
ØQ5G4ZZ
ØQ5HØZZ
ØQ5H3ZZ
ØQ5H4ZZ
ØQ5JØZZ
ØQ5J3ZZ
ØQ5J4ZZ
ØQ5KØZZ
ØQ5K3ZZ
ØQ5K4ZZ
ØQ5LØZZ
ØQ5L3ZZ
ØQ5L4ZZ
ØQ5MØZZ
ØQ5M3ZZ
ØQ5M4ZZ
ØQ5NØZZ
ØQ5N3ZZ
ØQ5N4ZZ
ØQ5PØZZ
ØQ5P3ZZ
ØQ5P4ZZ
ØQ5QØZZ
ØQ5Q3ZZ
ØQ5Q4ZZ
ØQ5RØZZ
ØQ5R3ZZ
ØQ5R4ZZ
ØQ5SØZZ
ØQ5S3ZZ
ØQ5S4ZZ
ØQ8LØZZ
ØQ8L3ZZ
ØQ8L4ZZ
ØQ8MØZZ
ØQ8M3ZZ
ØQ8M4ZZ
ØQ8NØZZ
ØQ8N3ZZ
ØQ8N4ZZ
ØQ8PØZZ
ØQ8P3ZZ
ØQ8P4ZZ
ØQ9ØØZX
ØQ9Ø3ZX
ØQ9Ø4ZX
ØQ91ØZX
ØQ913ZX
ØQ914ZX
ØQ92ØZX
ØQ923ZX
ØQ924ZX
ØQ93ØZX
ØQ933ZX
ØQ934ZX
ØQ94ØZX
ØQ943ZX
ØQ944ZX
ØQ95ØZX
ØQ953ZX
ØQ954ZX
ØQ96ØZX
ØQ963ZX
ØQ964ZX
ØQ97ØZX
ØQ973ZX
ØQ974ZX
ØQ98ØZX
ØQ983ZX
ØQ984ZX
ØQ99ØZX
ØQ993ZX
ØQ994ZX
ØQ9BØZX
ØQ9B3ZX
ØQ9B4ZX
ØQ9CØZX
ØQ9C3ZX
ØQ9C4ZX
ØQ9DØZX
ØQ9D3ZX
ØQ9D4ZX
ØQ9FØZX
ØQ9F3ZX
ØQ9F4ZX
ØQ9GØZX
ØQ9G3ZX
ØQ9G4ZX
ØQ9HØZX
ØQ9H3ZX
ØQ9H4ZX
ØQ9JØZX
ØQ9J3ZX
ØQ9J4ZX
ØQ9KØZX
ØQ9K3ZX
ØQ9K4ZX
ØQ9LØZX
ØQ9L3ZX
ØQ9L4ZX
ØQ9MØZX
ØQ9M3ZX
ØQ9M4ZX
ØQ9NØZX
ØQ9N3ZX
ØQ9N4ZX
ØQ9PØZX
ØQ9P3ZX
ØQ9P4ZX
ØQ9QØZX
ØQ9Q3ZX
ØQ9Q4ZX
ØQ9RØZX
ØQ9R3ZX
ØQ9R4ZX
ØQ9SØZX
ØQ9S3ZX
ØQ9S4ZX
ØQBØØZX
ØQBØ3ZX
ØQBØ4ZX
ØQB1ØZX
ØQB13ZX
ØQB14ZX
ØQB2ØZX
ØQB23ZX
ØQB24ZX
ØQB3ØZX
ØQB33ZX
ØQB34ZX
ØQB4ØZX
ØQB43ZX
ØQB44ZX
ØQB5ØZX
ØQB53ZX
ØQB54ZX
ØQB6ØZX
ØQB63ZX
ØQB64ZX
ØQB7ØZX
ØQB73ZX
ØQB74ZX
ØQB8ØZX
ØQB83ZX
ØQB84ZX
ØQB9ØZX
ØQB93ZX
ØQB94ZX
ØQBBØZX
ØQBB3ZX
ØQBB4ZX
ØQBCØZX
ØQBC3ZX
ØQBC4ZX
ØQBDØZX
ØQBD3ZX
ØQBD4ZX
ØQBFØZX
ØQBF3ZX
ØQBF4ZX
ØQBGØZX
ØQBG3ZX
ØQBG4ZX
ØQBHØZX
ØQBH3ZX
ØQBH4ZX
ØQBJØZX
ØQBJ3ZX
ØQBJ4ZX
ØQBKØZX
ØQBK3ZX
ØQBK4ZX
ØQBLØZX
ØQBLØZZ
ØQBL3ZX
ØQBL3ZZ
ØQBL4ZX
ØQBL4ZZ
ØQBMØZX
ØQBMØZZ
ØQBM3ZX
ØQBM3ZZ
ØQBM4ZX
ØQBM4ZZ
ØQBNØZ2
ØQBNØZX
ØQBNØZZ
ØQBN3Z2
ØQBN3ZX
ØQBN3ZZ
ØQBN4Z2
ØQBN4ZX
ØQBN4ZZ
ØQBPØZ2
ØQBPØZX
ØQBPØZZ
ØQBP3Z2
ØQBP3ZX
ØQBP3ZZ
ØQBP4Z2
ØQBP4ZX
ØQBP4ZZ
ØQBQØZX
ØQBQ3ZX
ØQBQ4ZX
ØQBRØZX
ØQBR3ZX
ØQBR4ZX
ØQBSØZX
ØQBS3ZX
ØQBS4ZX
ØQPØØ4Z
ØQPØØ5Z
ØQPØØ7Z
ØQPØØJZ
ØQPØØKZ
ØQPØ34Z
ØQPØ35Z
ØQPØ37Z
ØQPØ3JZ
ØQPØ3KZ
ØQPØ44Z
ØQPØ45Z
ØQPØ47Z
ØQPØ4JZ
ØQPØ4KZ
ØQP1Ø4Z
ØQP1Ø5Z
ØQP1Ø7Z
ØQP1ØJZ
ØQP1ØKZ
ØQP134Z
ØQP135Z
ØQP137Z
ØQP13JZ
ØQP13KZ
ØQP144Z
ØQP145Z
ØQP147Z
ØQP14JZ
ØQP14KZ
ØQP2Ø4Z
ØQP2Ø5Z
ØQP2Ø7Z
ØQP2ØJZ
ØQP2ØKZ
ØQP234Z
ØQP235Z
ØQP237Z
ØQP23JZ
ØQP23KZ
ØQP244Z
ØQP245Z
ØQP247Z
ØQP24JZ
ØQP24KZ
ØQP3Ø4Z
ØQP3Ø5Z
ØQP3Ø7Z
ØQP3ØJZ
ØQP3ØKZ
ØQP334Z
ØQP335Z
ØQP337Z
ØQP33JZ
ØQP33KZ
ØQP344Z
ØQP345Z
ØQP347Z
ØQP34JZ
ØQP34KZ
ØQP4Ø4Z
ØQP4Ø5Z
ØQP4Ø7Z
ØQP4ØJZ
ØQP4ØKZ
ØQP434Z
ØQP435Z
ØQP437Z
ØQP43JZ
ØQP43KZ
ØQP444Z
ØQP445Z
ØQP447Z
ØQP44JZ
ØQP44KZ
ØQP5Ø4Z
ØQP5Ø5Z
ØQP5Ø7Z
ØQP5ØJZ
ØQP5ØKZ
ØQP534Z
ØQP535Z
ØQP537Z
ØQP53JZ
ØQP53KZ
ØQP544Z
ØQP545Z
ØQP547Z
ØQP54JZ
ØQP54KZ
ØQP6Ø4Z
ØQP6Ø5Z
ØQP6Ø7Z
ØQP6ØJZ
ØQP6ØKZ
ØQP634Z
ØQP635Z
ØQP637Z
ØQP63JZ
ØQP63KZ
ØQP644Z
ØQP645Z
ØQP647Z
ØQP64JZ
ØQP64KZ
ØQP7Ø4Z
ØQP7Ø5Z
ØQP7Ø7Z
ØQP7ØJZ
ØQP7ØKZ
ØQP734Z
ØQP735Z
ØQP737Z
ØQP73JZ
ØQP73KZ
ØQP744Z
ØQP745Z
ØQP747Z
ØQP74JZ
ØQP74KZ
ØQP8Ø4Z
ØQP8Ø5Z
ØQP8Ø7Z
ØQP8ØJZ
ØQP8ØKZ
ØQP834Z
ØQP835Z
ØQP837Z
ØQP83JZ
ØQP83KZ
ØQP844Z
ØQP845Z
ØQP847Z
ØQP84JZ
ØQP84KZ
ØQP9Ø4Z
ØQP9Ø5Z
ØQP9Ø7Z
ØQP9ØJZ
ØQP9ØKZ
ØQP934Z
ØQP935Z
ØQP937Z
ØQP93JZ
ØQP93KZ
ØQP944Z
ØQP945Z
ØQP947Z
ØQP94JZ
ØQP94KZ
ØQPBØ4Z
ØQPBØ5Z
ØQPBØ7Z
ØQPBØJZ
ØQPBØKZ
ØQPB34Z
ØQPB35Z
ØQPB37Z
ØQPB3JZ
ØQPB3KZ
ØQPB44Z
ØQPB45Z
ØQPB47Z
ØQPB4JZ
ØQPB4KZ
ØQPCØ4Z
ØQPCØ5Z
ØQPCØ7Z
ØQPCØJZ
ØQPCØKZ
ØQPC34Z
ØQPC35Z
ØQPC37Z
ØQPC3JZ
ØQPC3KZ
ØQPC44Z
ØQPC45Z
ØQPC47Z
ØQPC4JZ
ØQPC4KZ
ØQPDØ4Z
ØQPDØ5Z
ØQPDØ7Z
ØQPDØJZ
ØQPDØKZ
ØQPD34Z
ØQPD35Z
ØQPD37Z
ØQPD3JZ
ØQPD3KZ
ØQPD44Z
ØQPD45Z
ØQPD47Z
ØQPD4JZ
ØQPD4KZ
ØQPFØ4Z
ØQPFØ5Z
ØQPFØ7Z
ØQPFØJZ
ØQPFØKZ
ØQPF34Z
ØQPF35Z
ØQPF37Z
ØQPF3JZ
ØQPF3KZ
ØQPF44Z
ØQPF45Z
ØQPF47Z
ØQPF4JZ
ØQPF4KZ
ØQPGØ4Z
ØQPGØ5Z
ØQPGØ7Z
ØQPGØJZ
ØQPGØKZ
ØQPG34Z
ØQPG35Z
ØQPG37Z
ØQPG3JZ
ØQPG3KZ
ØQPG44Z
ØQPG45Z
ØQPG47Z
ØQPG4JZ
ØQPG4KZ
ØQPHØ4Z
ØQPHØ5Z
ØQPHØ7Z
ØQPHØJZ
ØQPHØKZ
ØQPH34Z
ØQPH35Z
ØQPH37Z
ØQPH3JZ
ØQPH3KZ
ØQPH44Z
ØQPH45Z
ØQPH47Z
ØQPH4JZ
ØQPH4KZ
ØQPJØ4Z
ØQPJØ5Z
ØQPJØ7Z
ØQPJØJZ
ØQPJØKZ
ØQPJ34Z
ØQPJ35Z
ØQPJ37Z
ØQPJ3JZ
ØQPJ3KZ
ØQPJ44Z
ØQPJ45Z
ØQPJ47Z
ØQPJ4JZ
ØQPJ4KZ
ØQPKØ4Z
ØQPKØ5Z
ØQPKØ7Z
ØQPKØJZ
ØQPKØKZ
ØQPK34Z
ØQPK35Z
ØQPK37Z
ØQPK3JZ
ØQPK3KZ
ØQPK44Z
ØQPK45Z
ØQPK47Z
ØQPK4JZ
ØQPK4KZ
ØQPLØ4Z
ØQPLØ5Z
ØQPLØ7Z
ØQPLØJZ
ØQPLØKZ
ØQPL34Z
ØQPL35Z
ØQPL37Z
ØQPL3JZ
ØQPL3KZ
ØQPL44Z
ØQPL45Z
ØQPL47Z
ØQPL4JZ
ØQPL4KZ
ØQPMØ4Z
ØQPMØ5Z
ØQPMØ7Z
ØQPMØJZ
ØQPMØKZ
ØQPM34Z
ØQPM35Z
ØQPM37Z
ØQPM3JZ
ØQPM3KZ
ØQPM44Z
ØQPM45Z
ØQPM47Z
ØQPM4JZ
ØQPM4KZ
ØQPNØ4Z
ØQPNØ5Z
ØQPNØ7Z
ØQPNØJZ
ØQPNØKZ
ØQPN34Z
ØQPN35Z
ØQPN37Z
ØQPN3JZ
ØQPN3KZ
ØQPN44Z
ØQPN45Z
ØQPN47Z
ØQPN4JZ
ØQPN4KZ
ØQPPØ4Z
ØQPPØ5Z
ØQPPØ7Z
ØQPPØJZ
ØQPPØKZ
ØQPP34Z
ØQPP35Z
ØQPP37Z
ØQPP3JZ
ØQPP3KZ
ØQPP44Z
ØQPP45Z
ØQPP47Z
ØQPP4JZ
ØQPP4KZ
ØQPQØ4Z
ØQPQØ5Z
ØQPQØ7Z
ØQPQØJZ
ØQPQØKZ
ØQPQ34Z
ØQPQ35Z
ØQPQ37Z
ØQPQ3JZ
ØQPQ3KZ
ØQPQ44Z
ØQPQ45Z
ØQPQ47Z
ØQPQ4JZ
ØQPQ4KZ
ØQPRØ4Z
ØQPRØ5Z
ØQPRØ7Z
ØQPRØJZ
ØQPRØKZ
ØQPR34Z
ØQPR35Z
ØQPR37Z
ØQPR3JZ
ØQPR3KZ
ØQPR44Z
ØQPR45Z
ØQPR47Z
ØQPR4JZ
ØQPR4KZ
ØQPSØ4Z
ØQPSØ5Z
ØQPSØ7Z
ØQPSØJZ
ØQPSØKZ
ØQPS34Z
ØQPS35Z
ØQPS37Z
ØQPS3JZ
ØQPS3KZ
ØQPS44Z
ØQPS45Z
ØQPS47Z
ØQPS4JZ
ØQPS4KZ
ØQPYØØZ
ØQPYØMZ
ØQPY3MZ
ØQPY4ØZ
ØQPY4MZ
ØQTLØZZ
ØQTMØZZ
ØQTNØZZ
ØQTPØZZ
ØR5CØZZ
ØR5C3ZZ
ØR5C4ZZ
ØR5DØZZ
ØR5D3ZZ
ØR5D4ZZ
ØR9CØZX
ØR9C3ZX
ØR9C4ZX
ØR9DØZX
ØR9D3ZX
ØR9D4ZX
ØRBCØZX
ØRBCØZZ
ØRBC3ZX
ØRBC3ZZ
ØRBC4ZX
ØRBC4ZZ
ØRBDØZX
ØRBDØZZ
ØRBD3ZX
ØRBD3ZZ
ØRBD4ZX
ØRBD4ZZ
ØRBEØZZ
ØRBE3ZZ
ØRBE4ZZ
ØRBFØZZ
ØRBF3ZZ
ØRBF4ZZ
ØRBGØZZ
ØRBG3ZZ
ØRBG4ZZ
ØRBHØZZ
ØRBH3ZZ
ØRBH4ZZ
ØRBJØZZ
ØRBJ3ZZ
ØRBJ4ZZ
ØRBKØZZ
ØRBK3ZZ
ØRBK4ZZ
ØRBLØZZ
ØRBL3ZZ
ØRBL4ZZ
ØRBMØZZ
ØRBM3ZZ
ØRBM4ZZ
ØRBNØZZ
ØRBN3ZZ
ØRBN4ZZ
ØRBPØZZ
ØRBP3ZZ
ØRBP4ZZ
ØRBQØZZ
ØRBQ3ZZ
ØRBQ4ZZ
ØRBRØZZ
ØRBR3ZZ
ØRBR4ZZ
ØRBSØZZ
ØRBS3ZZ
ØRBS4ZZ
ØRBTØZZ
ØRBT3ZZ
ØRBT4ZZ
ØRBUØZZ
ØRBU3ZZ
ØRBU4ZZ
ØRBVØZZ
ØRBV3ZZ
ØRBV4ZZ
ØRBWØZZ
ØRBW3ZZ
ØRBW4ZZ
ØRBXØZZ
ØRBX3ZZ
ØRBX4ZZ
ØRGNØ3Z
ØRGN33Z
ØRGN43Z
ØRGPØ3Z
ØRGP33Z
ØRGP43Z
ØRGQØ3Z
ØRGQ33Z
ØRGQ43Z
ØRGRØ3Z
ØRGR33Z
ØRGR43Z
ØRGSØ3Z
ØRGS33Z
ØRGS43Z
ØRGTØ3Z
ØRGT33Z
ØRGT43Z
ØRGUØ3Z
ØRGU33Z
ØRGU43Z
ØRGVØ3Z
ØRGV33Z
ØRGV43Z
ØRGWØ3Z
ØRGW33Z
ØRGW43Z
ØRGXØ3Z
ØRGX33Z
ØRGX43Z
ØRHJØ8Z
ØRHJ48Z
ØRHKØ8Z
ØRHK48Z
ØRPJØ8Z
ØRPJØJ6
ØRPJØJ7
ØRPJ3J6
ØRPJ3J7
ØRPJ48Z
ØRPJ4J6
ØRPJ4J7
ØRPKØ8Z
ØRPKØJ6
ØRPKØJ7
ØRPK3J6
ØRPK3J7
ØRPK48Z
ØRPK4J6
ØRPK4J7
ØRQEØZZ
ØRQE3ZZ
ØRQE4ZZ
ØRQFØZZ
ØRQF3ZZ
ØRQF4ZZ
ØRQGØZZ
ØRQG3ZZ
ØRQG4ZZ
ØRQHØZZ
ØRQH3ZZ
ØRQH4ZZ
ØRQJØZZ
ØRQJ3ZZ
ØRQJ4ZZ

ICD-10-CM/PCS Codes by MS-DRG

ØRQKØZZ
ØRQK3ZZ
ØRQK4ZZ
ØRUEØ7Z
ØRUEØJZ
ØRUEØKZ
ØRUE37Z
ØRUE3JZ
ØRUE3KZ
ØRUE47Z
ØRUE4JZ
ØRUE4KZ
ØRUFØ7Z
ØRUFØJZ
ØRUFØKZ
ØRUF37Z
ØRUF3JZ
ØRUF3KZ
ØRUF47Z
ØRUF4JZ
ØRUF4KZ
ØRUGØ7Z
ØRUGØJZ
ØRUGØKZ
ØRUG37Z
ØRUG3JZ
ØRUG3KZ
ØRUG47Z
ØRUG4JZ
ØRUG4KZ
ØRUHØ7Z
ØRUHØJZ
ØRUHØKZ
ØRUH37Z
ØRUH3JZ
ØRUH3KZ
ØRUH47Z
ØRUH4JZ
ØRUH4KZ
ØRUJØ7Z
ØRUJØJZ
ØRUJØKZ
ØRUJ37Z
ØRUJ3JZ
ØRUJ3KZ
ØRUJ47Z
ØRUJ4JZ
ØRUJ4KZ
ØRUKØ7Z
ØRUKØJZ
ØRUKØKZ
ØRUK37Z
ØRUK3JZ
ØRUK3KZ
ØRUK47Z
ØRUK4JZ
ØRUK4KZ
ØRWJØJ6
ØRWJØJ7
ØRWJ3J6
ØRWJ3J7
ØRWJ4J6
ØRWJ4J7
ØRWKØJ6
ØRWKØJ7
ØRWK3J6
ØRWK3J7
ØRWK4J6
ØRWK4J7
ØS5CØZZ
ØS5C3ZZ
ØS5C4ZZ
ØS5DØZZ
ØS5D3ZZ
ØS5D4ZZ
ØS5HØZZ
ØS5H3ZZ
ØS5H4ZZ
ØS5JØZZ
ØS5J3ZZ
ØS5J4ZZ
ØS5KØZZ
ØS5K3ZZ
ØS5K4ZZ
ØS5LØZZ
ØS5L3ZZ
ØS5L4ZZ
ØS5MØZZ
ØS5M3ZZ
ØS5M4ZZ
ØS5NØZZ
ØS5N3ZZ
ØS5N4ZZ
ØS5PØZZ
ØS5P3ZZ
ØS5P4ZZ
ØS5QØZZ
ØS5Q3ZZ
ØS5Q4ZZ
ØS9CØØZ
ØS9CØZZ
ØS9DØØZ
ØS9DØZZ
ØS9HØØZ
ØS9HØZZ
ØS9JØØZ
ØS9JØZZ
ØS9KØØZ
ØS9KØZZ
ØS9LØØZ
ØS9LØZZ
ØS9MØØZ
ØS9MØZZ
ØS9NØØZ
ØS9NØZZ
ØS9PØØZ
ØS9PØZZ
ØS9QØØZ
ØS9QØZZ
ØSBCØZZ
ØSBC3ZZ
ØSBC4ZZ
ØSBDØZZ
ØSBD3ZZ
ØSBD4ZZ
ØSBFØZZ
ØSBF3ZZ
ØSBF4ZZ
ØSBGØZZ
ØSBG3ZZ
ØSBG4ZZ
ØSBHØZZ
ØSBH3ZZ
ØSBH4ZZ
ØSBJØZZ
ØSBJ3ZZ
ØSBJ4ZZ
ØSBKØZZ
ØSBK3ZZ
ØSBK4ZZ
ØSBLØZZ
ØSBL3ZZ
ØSBL4ZZ
ØSBMØZZ
ØSBM3ZZ
ØSBM4ZZ
ØSBNØZZ
ØSBN3ZZ
ØSBN4ZZ
ØSBPØZZ
ØSBP3ZZ
ØSBP4ZZ
ØSBQØZZ
ØSBQ3ZZ
ØSBQ4ZZ
ØSCCØZZ
ØSCC3ZZ
ØSCC4ZZ
ØSCDØZZ
ØSCD3ZZ
ØSCD4ZZ
ØSCHØZZ
ØSCH3ZZ
ØSCH4ZZ
ØSCJØZZ
ØSCJ3ZZ
ØSCJ4ZZ
ØSCKØZZ
ØSCK3ZZ
ØSCK4ZZ
ØSCLØZZ
ØSCL3ZZ
ØSCL4ZZ
ØSCMØZZ
ØSCM3ZZ
ØSCM4ZZ
ØSCNØZZ
ØSCN3ZZ
ØSCN4ZZ
ØSCPØZZ
ØSCP3ZZ
ØSCP4ZZ
ØSCQØZZ
ØSCQ3ZZ
ØSCQ4ZZ
ØSGFØ3Z
ØSGF33Z
ØSGF43Z
ØSGGØ3Z
ØSGG33Z
ØSGG43Z
ØSGHØ3Z
ØSGH33Z
ØSGH43Z
ØSGJØ3Z
ØSGJ33Z
ØSGJ43Z
ØSGKØ3Z
ØSGK33Z
ØSGK43Z
ØSGLØ3Z
ØSGL33Z
ØSGL43Z
ØSGMØ3Z
ØSGM33Z
ØSGM43Z
ØSGNØ3Z
ØSGN33Z
ØSGN43Z
ØSGPØ3Z
ØSGPØ4Z
ØSGPØ5Z
ØSGPØ7Z
ØSGPØJZ
ØSGPØKZ
ØSGP33Z
ØSGP34Z
ØSGP35Z
ØSGP37Z
ØSGP3JZ
ØSGP3KZ
ØSGP43Z
ØSGP44Z
ØSGP45Z
ØSGP47Z
ØSGP4JZ
ØSGP4KZ
ØSGQØ3Z
ØSGQØ4Z
ØSGQØ5Z
ØSGQØ7Z
ØSGQØJZ
ØSGQØKZ
ØSGQ33Z
ØSGQ34Z
ØSGQ35Z
ØSGQ37Z
ØSGQ3JZ
ØSGQ3KZ
ØSGQ43Z
ØSGQ44Z
ØSGQ45Z
ØSGQ47Z
ØSGQ4JZ
ØSGQ4KZ
ØSH9Ø8Z
ØSHBØ8Z
ØSHCØ4Z
ØSHCØ5Z
ØSHCØ8Z
ØSHC34Z
ØSHC35Z
ØSHC44Z
ØSHC45Z
ØSHDØ4Z
ØSHDØ5Z
ØSHDØ8Z
ØSHD34Z
ØSHD35Z
ØSHD44Z
ØSHD45Z
ØSHHØ4Z
ØSHHØ5Z
ØSHH34Z
ØSHH35Z
ØSHH44Z
ØSHH45Z
ØSHJØ4Z
ØSHJØ5Z
ØSHJ34Z
ØSHJ35Z
ØSHJ44Z
ØSHJ45Z
ØSHKØ4Z
ØSHKØ5Z
ØSHK34Z
ØSHK35Z
ØSHK44Z
ØSHK45Z
ØSHLØ4Z
ØSHLØ5Z
ØSHL34Z
ØSHL35Z
ØSHL44Z
ØSHL45Z
ØSHMØ4Z
ØSHMØ5Z
ØSHM34Z
ØSHM35Z
ØSHM44Z
ØSHM45Z
ØSHNØ4Z
ØSHNØ5Z
ØSHN34Z
ØSHN35Z
ØSHN44Z
ØSHN45Z
ØSHPØ4Z
ØSHPØ5Z
ØSHP34Z
ØSHP35Z
ØSHP44Z
ØSHP45Z
ØSHQØ4Z
ØSHQØ5Z
ØSHQ34Z
ØSHQ35Z
ØSHQ44Z
ØSHQ45Z
ØSJCØZZ
ØSJC4ZZ
ØSJDØZZ
ØSJD4ZZ
ØSJHØZZ
ØSJJØZZ
ØSJKØZZ
ØSJLØZZ
ØSJMØZZ
ØSJNØZZ
ØSJPØZZ
ØSJQØZZ
ØSNCØZZ
ØSNC3ZZ
ØSNC4ZZ
ØSNDØZZ
ØSND3ZZ
ØSND4ZZ
ØSP9Ø8Z
ØSP9ØEZ
ØSPBØ8Z
ØSPBØEZ
ØSPCØØZ
ØSPCØ3Z
ØSPCØ4Z
ØSPCØ5Z
ØSPCØ7Z
ØSPCØ8Z
ØSPCØEZ
ØSPCØKZ
ØSPC34Z
ØSPC35Z
ØSPC37Z
ØSPC3KZ
ØSPC4ØZ
ØSPC43Z
ØSPC44Z
ØSPC45Z
ØSPC47Z
ØSPC4KZ
ØSPDØØZ
ØSPDØ3Z
ØSPDØ4Z
ØSPDØ5Z
ØSPDØ7Z
ØSPDØ8Z
ØSPDØEZ
ØSPDØKZ
ØSPD34Z
ØSPD35Z
ØSPD37Z
ØSPD3KZ
ØSPD4ØZ
ØSPD43Z
ØSPD44Z
ØSPD45Z
ØSPD47Z
ØSPD4KZ
ØSPHØØZ
ØSPHØ3Z
ØSPHØ4Z
ØSPHØ5Z
ØSPHØ7Z
ØSPHØKZ
ØSPH34Z
ØSPH35Z
ØSPH37Z
ØSPH3KZ
ØSPH4ØZ
ØSPH43Z
ØSPH44Z
ØSPH45Z
ØSPH47Z
ØSPH4KZ
ØSPJØØZ
ØSPJØ3Z
ØSPJØ4Z
ØSPJØ5Z
ØSPJØ7Z
ØSPJØKZ
ØSPJ34Z
ØSPJ35Z
ØSPJ37Z
ØSPJ3KZ
ØSPJ4ØZ
ØSPJ43Z
ØSPJ44Z
ØSPJ45Z
ØSPJ47Z
ØSPJ4KZ
ØSPKØØZ
ØSPKØ3Z
ØSPKØ4Z
ØSPKØ5Z
ØSPKØ7Z
ØSPKØKZ
ØSPK34Z
ØSPK35Z
ØSPK37Z
ØSPK3KZ
ØSPK4ØZ
ØSPK43Z
ØSPK44Z
ØSPK45Z
ØSPK47Z
ØSPK4KZ
ØSPLØØZ
ØSPLØ3Z
ØSPLØ4Z
ØSPLØ5Z
ØSPLØ7Z
ØSPLØKZ
ØSPL34Z
ØSPL35Z
ØSPL37Z
ØSPL3KZ
ØSPL4ØZ
ØSPL43Z
ØSPL44Z
ØSPL45Z
ØSPL47Z
ØSPL4KZ
ØSPMØØZ
ØSPMØ3Z
ØSPMØ4Z
ØSPMØ5Z
ØSPMØ7Z
ØSPMØKZ
ØSPM34Z
ØSPM35Z
ØSPM37Z
ØSPM3KZ
ØSPM4ØZ
ØSPM43Z
ØSPM44Z
ØSPM45Z
ØSPM47Z
ØSPM4KZ
ØSPNØØZ
ØSPNØ3Z
ØSPNØ4Z
ØSPNØ5Z
ØSPNØ7Z
ØSPNØKZ
ØSPN34Z
ØSPN35Z
ØSPN37Z
ØSPN3KZ
ØSPN4ØZ
ØSPN43Z
ØSPN44Z
ØSPN45Z
ØSPN47Z
ØSPN4KZ
ØSPPØØZ
ØSPPØ3Z
ØSPPØ4Z
ØSPPØ5Z
ØSPPØ7Z
ØSPPØKZ
ØSPP34Z
ØSPP35Z
ØSPP37Z
ØSPP3KZ
ØSPP4ØZ
ØSPP43Z
ØSPP44Z
ØSPP45Z
ØSPP47Z
ØSPP4KZ
ØSPQØØZ
ØSPQØ3Z
ØSPQØ4Z
ØSPQØ5Z
ØSPQØ7Z
ØSPQØKZ
ØSPQ34Z
ØSPQ35Z
ØSPQ37Z
ØSPQ3KZ
ØSPQ4ØZ
ØSPQ43Z
ØSPQ44Z
ØSPQ45Z
ØSPQ47Z
ØSPQ4KZ
ØSRHØ7Z
ØSRHØJZ
ØSRHØKZ
ØSRJØ7Z
ØSRJØJZ
ØSRJØKZ
ØSRKØ7Z
ØSRKØJZ
ØSRKØKZ
ØSRLØ7Z
ØSRLØJZ
ØSRLØKZ
ØSRMØ7Z
ØSRMØJZ
ØSRMØKZ
ØSRNØ7Z
ØSRNØJZ
ØSRNØKZ
ØSRPØ7Z
ØSRPØJZ
ØSRPØKZ
ØSRQØ7Z
ØSRQØJZ
ØSRQØKZ
ØSS734Z
ØSS834Z
ØSS934Z
ØSSB34Z
ØSTHØZZ
ØSTJØZZ
ØSTKØZZ
ØSTLØZZ
ØSTMØZZ
ØSTNØZZ
ØSTPØZZ
ØSTQØZZ
ØSWCØØZ
ØSWCØ3Z
ØSWCØ4Z
ØSWCØ5Z
ØSWCØ7Z
ØSWCØ8Z
ØSWCØ9Z
ØSWCØKZ
ØSWC3ØZ
ØSWC33Z
ØSWC34Z
ØSWC35Z
ØSWC37Z
ØSWC38Z
ØSWC3KZ
ØSWC4ØZ
ØSWC43Z
ØSWC44Z
ØSWC45Z
ØSWC47Z
ØSWC48Z
ØSWC4KZ
ØSWDØØZ
ØSWDØ3Z
ØSWDØ4Z
ØSWDØ5Z
ØSWDØ7Z
ØSWDØ8Z
ØSWDØ9Z
ØSWDØKZ
ØSWD3ØZ
ØSWD33Z
ØSWD34Z
ØSWD35Z
ØSWD37Z
ØSWD38Z
ØSWD3KZ
ØSWD4ØZ
ØSWD43Z
ØSWD44Z
ØSWD45Z
ØSWD47Z
ØSWD48Z
ØSWD4KZ
ØSWHØØZ
ØSWHØ3Z
ØSWHØ4Z
ØSWHØ5Z
ØSWHØ7Z
ØSWHØ8Z
ØSWHØKZ
ØSWH3ØZ
ØSWH33Z
ØSWH34Z
ØSWH35Z
ØSWH37Z
ØSWH38Z
ØSWH3KZ
ØSWH4ØZ
ØSWH43Z
ØSWH44Z
ØSWH45Z
ØSWH47Z
ØSWH48Z
ØSWH4KZ
ØSWJØØZ
ØSWJØ3Z
ØSWJØ4Z
ØSWJØ5Z
ØSWJØ7Z
ØSWJØ8Z
ØSWJØKZ
ØSWJ3ØZ
ØSWJ33Z
ØSWJ34Z
ØSWJ35Z
ØSWJ37Z
ØSWJ38Z
ØSWJ3KZ
ØSWJ4ØZ
ØSWJ43Z
ØSWJ44Z
ØSWJ45Z
ØSWJ47Z
ØSWJ48Z
ØSWJ4KZ
ØSWKØØZ
ØSWKØ3Z
ØSWKØ4Z
ØSWKØ5Z
ØSWKØ7Z
ØSWKØ8Z
ØSWKØKZ
ØSWK3ØZ
ØSWK33Z
ØSWK34Z
ØSWK35Z
ØSWK37Z
ØSWK38Z
ØSWK3KZ
ØSWK4ØZ
ØSWK43Z
ØSWK44Z
ØSWK45Z
ØSWK47Z
ØSWK48Z
ØSWK4KZ
ØSWLØØZ
ØSWLØ3Z
ØSWLØ4Z
ØSWLØ5Z
ØSWLØ7Z
ØSWLØ8Z
ØSWLØKZ
ØSWL3ØZ
ØSWL33Z
ØSWL34Z
ØSWL35Z
ØSWL37Z
ØSWL38Z
ØSWL3KZ
ØSWL4ØZ
ØSWL43Z
ØSWL44Z
ØSWL45Z
ØSWL47Z
ØSWL48Z
ØSWL4KZ
ØSWMØØZ
ØSWMØ3Z
ØSWMØ4Z
ØSWMØ5Z
ØSWMØ7Z
ØSWMØ8Z
ØSWMØKZ
ØSWM3ØZ
ØSWM33Z
ØSWM34Z
ØSWM35Z
ØSWM37Z
ØSWM38Z
ØSWM3KZ
ØSWM4ØZ
ØSWM43Z
ØSWM44Z
ØSWM45Z
ØSWM47Z
ØSWM48Z
ØSWM4KZ
ØSWNØØZ
ØSWNØ3Z
ØSWNØ4Z
ØSWNØ5Z
ØSWNØ7Z
ØSWNØ8Z
ØSWNØKZ
ØSWN3ØZ
ØSWN33Z
ØSWN34Z
ØSWN35Z
ØSWN37Z
ØSWN38Z
ØSWN3KZ
ØSWN4ØZ
ØSWN43Z
ØSWN44Z
ØSWN45Z
ØSWN47Z
ØSWN48Z
ØSWN4KZ
ØSWPØØZ
ØSWPØ3Z
ØSWPØ4Z
ØSWPØ5Z
ØSWPØ7Z
ØSWPØ8Z
ØSWPØKZ
ØSWP3ØZ
ØSWP33Z
ØSWP34Z
ØSWP35Z
ØSWP37Z
ØSWP38Z
ØSWP3KZ
ØSWP4ØZ
ØSWP43Z
ØSWP44Z
ØSWP45Z
ØSWP47Z
ØSWP48Z
ØSWP4KZ
ØSWQØØZ
ØSWQØ3Z
ØSWQØ4Z
ØSWQØ5Z
ØSWQØ7Z
ØSWQØ8Z
ØSWQØKZ
ØSWQ3ØZ
ØSWQ33Z
ØSWQ34Z
ØSWQ35Z
ØSWQ37Z
ØSWQ38Z
ØSWQ3KZ
ØSWQ4ØZ
ØSWQ43Z
ØSWQ44Z
ØSWQ45Z
ØSWQ47Z
ØSWQ48Z
ØSWQ4KZ
ØT5BØZZ
ØT5B3ZZ
ØT5B4ZZ
ØT5B7ZZ
ØT5B8ZZ
ØT5CØZZ
ØT5C3ZZ
ØT5C4ZZ
ØT5C7ZZ
ØT5C8ZZ
ØT76ØZZ
ØT763ZZ
ØT764ZZ
ØT768DZ
ØT768ZZ
ØT77ØZZ
ØT773ZZ
ØT774ZZ
ØT778DZ
ØT778ZZ
ØT788DZ
ØT7DØZZ
ØT7D3ZZ
ØT7D4ZZ
ØT8CØZZ
ØT8C3ZZ
ØT8C4ZZ
ØT937ØZ
ØT938ØZ
ØT947ØZ
ØT948ØZ
ØT96ØZZ
ØT964ZZ
ØT967ZZ
ØT968ZZ
ØT97ØZZ
ØT974ZZ
ØT977ZZ
ØT978ZZ
ØT98ØZZ
ØT984ZZ
ØT987ZZ
ØT988ZZ
ØT9B3ZX
ØT9B4ZX
ØT9B7ZX
ØT9B8ZX
ØT9C3ZX
ØT9C4ZX
ØT9C7ZX
ØT9C8ZX
ØT9DØØZ
ØT9DØZZ
ØT9D4ØZ
ØTBB3ZX
ØTBB4ZX
ØTBB7ZX
ØTBB7ZZ
ØTBB8ZX
ØTBB8ZZ
ØTBC3ZX
ØTBC4ZX
ØTBC7ZX
ØTBC7ZZ
ØTBC8ZX
ØTBC8ZZ
ØTC37ZZ
ØTC47ZZ
ØTC6ØZZ
ØTC63ZZ
ØTC64ZZ
ØTC67ZZ
ØTC7ØZZ
ØTC73ZZ
ØTC74ZZ
ØTC77ZZ
ØTCDØZZ
ØTCD3ZZ
ØTCD4ZZ
ØTH5Ø1Z
ØTH541Z
ØTH581Z
ØTH9Ø1Z
ØTH9Ø2Z
ØTH9ØYZ
ØTH932Z
ØTH941Z
ØTH942Z
ØTH981Z
ØTH98YZ
ØTHBØ1Z
ØTHB41Z
ØTHB81Z
ØTHDØ1Z
ØTHDØ2Z
ØTHDØYZ
ØTHD32Z
ØTHD41Z
ØTHD42Z
ØTHD81Z
ØTHDX2Z
ØTJ9ØZZ
ØTJB4ZZ
ØTJDØZZ
ØTLDØCZ
ØTLDØDZ
ØTLDØZZ
ØTLD3CZ
ØTLD3DZ
ØTLD3ZZ
ØTLD4CZ
ØTLD4DZ

ØTLD4ZZ
ØTLD7DZ
ØTLD7ZZ
ØTLD8DZ
ØTLD8ZZ
ØTLDXCZ
ØTLDXDZ
ØTLDXZZ
ØTNDØZZ
ØTND3ZZ
ØTND4ZZ
ØTND7ZZ
ØTND8ZZ
ØTNDXZZ
ØTP9ØØZ
ØTP9Ø2Z
ØTP9Ø3Z
ØTP9Ø7Z
ØTP9ØCZ
ØTP9ØDZ
ØTP9ØJZ
ØTP9ØKZ
ØTP9ØYZ
ØTP93ØZ
ØTP932Z
ØTP933Z
ØTP937Z
ØTP93CZ
ØTP93DZ
ØTP93JZ
ØTP93KZ
ØTP94ØZ
ØTP942Z
ØTP943Z
ØTP947Z
ØTP94CZ
ØTP94DZ
ØTP94JZ
ØTP94KZ
ØTP977Z
ØTP97CZ
ØTP97JZ
ØTP97KZ
ØTP987Z
ØTP98CZ
ØTP98JZ
ØTP98KZ
ØTP98YZ
ØTPBØMZ
ØTPB3MZ
ØTPB4MZ
ØTPB7MZ
ØTPB8MZ
ØTPBXMZ
ØTPDØØZ
ØTPDØ2Z
ØTPDØ3Z
ØTPDØ7Z
ØTPDØCZ
ØTPDØDZ
ØTPDØJZ
ØTPDØKZ
ØTPDØLZ
ØTPDØYZ
ØTPD3ØZ
ØTPD32Z
ØTPD33Z
ØTPD37Z
ØTPD3CZ
ØTPD3DZ
ØTPD3JZ
ØTPD3KZ
ØTPD3LZ
ØTPD4ØZ
ØTPD42Z
ØTPD43Z
ØTPD47Z
ØTPD4CZ
ØTPD4DZ
ØTPD4JZ
ØTPD4KZ
ØTPD4LZ
ØTPD77Z
ØTPD7CZ
ØTPD7JZ
ØTPD7KZ
ØTPD7LZ
ØTPD87Z
ØTPD8CZ
ØTPD8JZ
ØTPD8KZ
ØTPD8LZ
ØTPDXLZ
ØTUCØJZ
ØTUC4JZ
ØTUC7JZ
ØTUC8JZ
ØTW9ØØZ
ØTW9Ø2Z
ØTW9Ø3Z
ØTW9Ø7Z
ØTW9ØCZ
ØTW9ØDZ
ØTW9ØJZ
ØTW9ØKZ
ØTW9ØMZ
ØTW9ØYZ
ØTW93ØZ
ØTW932Z
ØTW933Z
ØTW937Z
ØTW93CZ
ØTW93DZ
ØTW93JZ
ØTW93KZ
ØTW93MZ
ØTW94ØZ
ØTW942Z
ØTW943Z
ØTW947Z
ØTW94CZ
ØTW94DZ
ØTW94JZ
ØTW94KZ
ØTW94MZ
ØTW97ØZ
ØTW972Z
ØTW973Z
ØTW977Z
ØTW97CZ
ØTW97DZ
ØTW97JZ
ØTW97KZ
ØTW97MZ
ØTW98ØZ
ØTW982Z
ØTW983Z
ØTW987Z
ØTW98CZ
ØTW98DZ
ØTW98JZ
ØTW98KZ
ØTW98MZ
ØTW98YZ
ØTWDØØZ
ØTWDØ2Z
ØTWDØ3Z
ØTWDØ7Z
ØTWDØCZ
ØTWDØDZ
ØTWDØJZ
ØTWDØKZ
ØTWDØLZ
ØTWDØYZ
ØTWD3ØZ
ØTWD32Z
ØTWD33Z
ØTWD37Z
ØTWD3CZ
ØTWD3DZ
ØTWD3JZ
ØTWD3KZ
ØTWD3LZ
ØTWD4ØZ
ØTWD42Z
ØTWD43Z
ØTWD47Z
ØTWD4CZ
ØTWD4DZ
ØTWD4JZ
ØTWD4KZ
ØTWD4LZ
ØTWD7ØZ
ØTWD72Z
ØTWD73Z
ØTWD77Z
ØTWD7CZ
ØTWD7DZ
ØTWD7JZ
ØTWD7KZ
ØTWD7LZ
ØTWD8ØZ
ØTWD82Z
ØTWD83Z
ØTWD87Z
ØTWD8CZ
ØTWD8DZ
ØTWD8JZ
ØTWD8KZ
ØTWD8LZ
ØU57ØZZ
ØU573ZZ
ØU574ZZ
ØU577ZZ
ØU578ZZ
ØU59ØZZ
ØU593ZZ
ØU594ZZ
ØU597ZZ
ØU598ZZ
ØU5CØZZ
ØU5C3ZZ
ØU5C4ZZ
ØU5C7ZZ
ØU5C8ZZ
ØU5FØZZ
ØU5F3ZZ
ØU5F4ZZ
ØU5F7ZZ
ØU5F8ZZ
ØU5GØZZ
ØU5G3ZZ
ØU5G4ZZ
ØU5G7ZZ
ØU5G8ZZ
ØU5GXZZ
ØU5JØZZ
ØU5JXZZ
ØU5KØZZ
ØU5K3ZZ
ØU5K4ZZ
ØU5K7ZZ
ØU5K8ZZ
ØU5KXZZ
ØU5LØZZ
ØU5LXZZ
ØU5MØZZ
ØU5MXZZ
ØU943ZX
ØU944ZX
ØU993ZX
ØU994ZX
ØU997ZX
ØU998ZX
ØU9CØØZ
ØU9CØZX
ØU9CØZZ
ØU9C3ZX
ØU9C4ØZ
ØU9C4ZX
ØU9C4ZZ
ØU9C7ØZ
ØU9C7ZX
ØU9C7ZZ
ØU9C8ØZ
ØU9C8ZX
ØU9C8ZZ
ØU9FØZX
ØU9F3ZX
ØU9F4ZX
ØU9F7ZX
ØU9F8ZX
ØU9GØØZ
ØU9GØZX
ØU9GØZZ
ØU9G3ZX
ØU9G4ØZ
ØU9G4ZX
ØU9G4ZZ
ØU9G7ØZ
ØU9G7ZX
ØU9G7ZZ
ØU9G8ØZ
ØU9G8ZX
ØU9G8ZZ
ØU9GXØZ
ØU9GXZX
ØU9GXZZ
ØU9JØØZ
ØU9JØZX
ØU9JØZZ
ØU9JXØZ
ØU9JXZX
ØU9JXZZ
ØU9KØZX
ØU9K3ZX
ØU9K4ZX
ØU9K7ZX
ØU9K8ZX
ØU9KXZX
ØU9MØØZ
ØU9MØZX
ØU9MØZZ
ØU9MXØZ
ØU9MXZX
ØU9MXZZ
ØUB43ZX
ØUB44ZX
ØUB47ZX
ØUB48ZX
ØUB9ØZZ
ØUB93ZX
ØUB93ZZ
ØUB94ZX
ØUB94ZZ
ØUB97ZX
ØUB97ZZ
ØUB98ZX
ØUB98ZZ
ØUBCØZX
ØUBCØZZ
ØUBC3ZX
ØUBC3ZZ
ØUBC4ZX
ØUBC4ZZ
ØUBC7ZX
ØUBC7ZZ
ØUBC8ZX
ØUBC8ZZ
ØUBFØZX
ØUBFØZZ
ØUBF3ZX
ØUBF3ZZ
ØUBF4ZX
ØUBF4ZZ
ØUBF7ZX
ØUBF7ZZ
ØUBF8ZX
ØUBF8ZZ
ØUBGØZX
ØUBGØZZ
ØUBG3ZX
ØUBG3ZZ
ØUBG4ZX
ØUBG4ZZ
ØUBG7ZX
ØUBG7ZZ
ØUBG8ZX
ØUBG8ZZ
ØUBGXZX
ØUBGXZZ
ØUBJØZX
ØUBJØZZ
ØUBJXZX
ØUBJXZZ
ØUBKØZX
ØUBKØZZ
ØUBK3ZX
ØUBK3ZZ
ØUBK4ZX
ØUBK4ZZ
ØUBK7ZX
ØUBK7ZZ
ØUBK8ZX
ØUBK8ZZ
ØUBKXZX
ØUBKXZZ
ØUBLØZX
ØUBLØZZ
ØUBLXZX
ØUBLXZZ
ØUBMØZX
ØUBMXZX
ØUCGØZZ
ØUCG3ZZ
ØUCG4ZZ
ØUCJØZZ
ØUCJXZZ
ØUCLØZZ
ØUCLXZZ
ØUCMØZZ
ØUDB7ZX
ØUDB7ZZ
ØUDB8ZX
ØUDB8ZZ
ØUH3Ø1Z
ØUH341Z
ØUHCØ1Z
ØUHC31Z
ØUHC41Z
ØUHC71Z
ØUHC81Z
ØUHGØ1Z
ØUHG31Z
ØUHG41Z
ØUHG71Z
ØUHG81Z
ØUHGX1Z
ØUHHØ3Z
ØUHHØYZ
ØUHH33Z
ØUHH43Z
ØUJHØZZ
ØUJH4ZZ
ØUJMØZZ
ØUL5ØCZ
ØUL5ØDZ
ØUL5ØZZ
ØUL53CZ
ØUL53DZ
ØUL53ZZ
ØUL54CZ
ØUL54DZ
ØUL54ZZ
ØUL57DZ
ØUL57ZZ
ØUL58DZ
ØUL58ZZ
ØUL6ØCZ
ØUL6ØDZ
ØUL6ØZZ
ØUL63CZ
ØUL63DZ
ØUL63ZZ
ØUL64CZ
ØUL64DZ
ØUL64ZZ
ØUL67DZ
ØUL67ZZ
ØUL68DZ
ØUL68ZZ
ØUL7ØCZ
ØUL7ØDZ
ØUL7ØZZ
ØUL73CZ
ØUL73DZ
ØUL73ZZ
ØUL74CZ
ØUL74DZ
ØUL74ZZ
ØUL77DZ
ØUL77ZZ
ØUL78DZ
ØUL78ZZ
ØUMJXZZ
ØUMKØZZ
ØUMK4ZZ
ØUMKXZZ
ØUMMXZZ
ØUNJØZZ
ØUNJXZZ
ØUNKØZZ
ØUNK3ZZ
ØUNK4ZZ
ØUNK7ZZ
ØUNK8ZZ
ØUNKXZZ
ØUNLØZZ
ØUNLXZZ
ØUPDØCZ
ØUPHØØZ
ØUPHØ1Z
ØUPHØ3Z
ØUPHØ7Z
ØUPHØDZ
ØUPHØJZ
ØUPHØKZ
ØUPHØYZ
ØUPH3ØZ
ØUPH31Z
ØUPH33Z
ØUPH37Z
ØUPH3DZ
ØUPH3JZ
ØUPH3KZ
ØUPH4ØZ
ØUPH41Z
ØUPH43Z
ØUPH47Z
ØUPH4DZ
ØUPH4JZ
ØUPH4KZ
ØUPH71Z
ØUPH77Z
ØUPH7JZ
ØUPH7KZ
ØUPH81Z
ØUPH87Z
ØUPH8JZ
ØUPH8KZ
ØUPMØØZ
ØUPMØ7Z
ØUPMØJZ
ØUPMØKZ
ØUQJØZZ
ØUQJXZZ
ØUQKØZZ
ØUQK3ZZ
ØUQK4ZZ
ØUQK7ZZ
ØUQK8ZZ
ØUQLØZZ
ØUQLXZZ
ØUT9ØZL
ØUT94ZL
ØUT97ZL
ØUT97ZZ
ØUT98ZL
ØUT98ZZ
ØUT9FZL
ØUT9FZZ
ØUTJØZZ
ØUTJXZZ
ØUTKØZZ
ØUTK4ZZ
ØUTK7ZZ
ØUTK8ZZ
ØUTKXZZ
ØUTLØZZ
ØUTLXZZ
ØUUJØ7Z
ØUUJØJZ
ØUUJØKZ
ØUUJX7Z
ØUUJXJZ
ØUUJXKZ
ØUUMØ7Z
ØUUMØJZ
ØUUMØKZ
ØUUMX7Z
ØUUMXJZ
ØUUMXKZ
ØUWDØCZ
ØUWD3CZ
ØUWD4CZ
ØUWD7CZ
ØUWD8CZ
ØUWHØØZ
ØUWHØ1Z
ØUWHØ3Z
ØUWHØ7Z
ØUWHØDZ
ØUWHØJZ
ØUWHØKZ
ØUWHØYZ
ØUWH3ØZ
ØUWH31Z
ØUWH33Z
ØUWH37Z
ØUWH3DZ
ØUWH3JZ
ØUWH3KZ
ØUWH4ØZ
ØUWH41Z
ØUWH43Z
ØUWH47Z
ØUWH4DZ
ØUWH4JZ
ØUWH4KZ
ØUWH7ØZ
ØUWH71Z
ØUWH73Z
ØUWH77Z
ØUWH7DZ
ØUWH7JZ
ØUWH7KZ
ØUWH8ØZ
ØUWH81Z
ØUWH83Z
ØUWH87Z
ØUWH8DZ
ØUWH8JZ
ØUWH8KZ
ØUWMØØZ
ØUWMØ7Z
ØUWMØJZ
ØUWMØKZ
ØV5Ø3Z3
ØV5Ø7ZZ
ØV5Ø8ZZ
ØV5FØZZ
ØV5F3ZZ
ØV5F4ZZ
ØV5F8ZZ
ØV5GØZZ
ØV5G3ZZ
ØV5G4ZZ
ØV5G8ZZ
ØV5HØZZ
ØV5H3ZZ
ØV5H4ZZ
ØV5H8ZZ
ØV5JØZZ
ØV5J3ZZ
ØV5J4ZZ
ØV5J8ZZ
ØV5KØZZ
ØV5K3ZZ
ØV5K4ZZ
ØV5K8ZZ
ØV5LØZZ
ØV5L3ZZ
ØV5L4ZZ
ØV5L8ZZ
ØV5SØZZ
ØV5S3ZZ
ØV5S4ZZ
ØV5SXZZ
ØV5TØZZ
ØV5T3ZZ
ØV5T4ZZ
ØV5TXZZ
ØV9ØØØZ
ØV9ØØZX
ØV9ØØZZ
ØV9Ø7ØZ
ØV9Ø7ZZ
ØV9Ø8ØZ
ØV9Ø8ZZ
ØV95ØZZ
ØV9SØØZ
ØV9SØZX
ØV9SØZZ
ØV9S3ZX
ØV9S4ØZ
ØV9S4ZX
ØV9S4ZZ
ØV9SXØZ
ØV9SXZX
ØV9SXZZ
ØV9TØØZ
ØV9TØZX
ØV9TØZZ
ØV9T3ZX
ØV9T4ØZ
ØV9T4ZX
ØV9T4ZZ
ØV9TXØZ
ØV9TXZX
ØV9TXZZ
ØVBØØZX
ØVBØØZZ
ØVBØ3ZZ
ØVBØ4ZZ
ØVBØ7ZZ
ØVBØ8ZZ
ØVB5ØZZ
ØVB6ØZZ
ØVB7ØZZ
ØVBFØZZ
ØVBF3ZZ
ØVBF4ZZ
ØVBF8ZZ
ØVBGØZZ
ØVBG3ZZ
ØVBG4ZZ
ØVBG8ZZ
ØVBHØZZ
ØVBH3ZZ
ØVBH4ZZ
ØVBH8ZZ
ØVBJØZZ
ØVBJ3ZZ
ØVBJ4ZZ
ØVBJ8ZZ
ØVBKØZZ
ØVBK3ZZ
ØVBK4ZZ
ØVBK8ZZ
ØVBLØZZ
ØVBL3ZZ
ØVBL4ZZ
ØVBL8ZZ
ØVBSØZX
ØVBSØZZ
ØVBS3ZX
ØVBS3ZZ
ØVBS4ZX
ØVBS4ZZ
ØVBSXZX
ØVBSXZZ
ØVBTØZX
ØVBTØZZ
ØVBT3ZX
ØVBT3ZZ
ØVBT4ZX
ØVBT4ZZ
ØVBTXZX
ØVBTXZZ
ØVCØØZZ
ØVCØ3ZZ
ØVCØ4ZZ
ØVCØ7ZZ
ØVCØ8ZZ
ØVC5ØZZ
ØVCSØZZ
ØVCS3ZZ
ØVCS4ZZ
ØVCTØZZ
ØVCT3ZZ
ØVCT4ZZ
ØVCTXZZ
ØVHØØ1Z
ØVHØ31Z
ØVHØ41Z
ØVHØ71Z
ØVHØ81Z
ØVJ4ØZZ
ØVJ44ZZ
ØVJMØZZ
ØVJM4ZZ
ØVJRØZZ
ØVJR4ZZ
ØVJSØZZ
ØVNØØZZ
ØVNØ3ZZ
ØVNØ4ZZ
ØVNØ7ZZ
ØVNØ8ZZ
ØVNSØZZ
ØVNS3ZZ
ØVNS4ZZ
ØVP4ØØZ
ØVP4Ø1Z
ØVP4Ø3Z
ØVP4Ø7Z
ØVP4ØJZ
ØVP4ØKZ
ØVP4ØYZ
ØVP43ØZ
ØVP431Z
ØVP433Z
ØVP437Z
ØVP43JZ
ØVP43KZ
ØVP44ØZ
ØVP441Z
ØVP443Z
ØVP447Z
ØVP44JZ
ØVP44KZ
ØVP471Z
ØVP477Z
ØVP47JZ
ØVP47KZ
ØVP481Z
ØVP487Z
ØVP48JZ
ØVP48KZ
ØVPSØØZ
ØVPSØ3Z
ØVPSØ7Z
ØVPSØJZ
ØVPSØKZ
ØVPSØYZ
ØVPS3ØZ
ØVPS33Z
ØVPS37Z
ØVPS3JZ
ØVPS3KZ
ØVPS4ØZ
ØVPS43Z
ØVPS47Z
ØVPS4JZ
ØVPS4KZ
ØVPS77Z
ØVPS7JZ
ØVPS7KZ
ØVPS87Z
ØVPS8JZ
ØVPS8KZ
ØVQØØZZ
ØVQØ3ZZ
ØVQØ4ZZ
ØVQØ7ZZ
ØVQØ8ZZ
ØVQSØZZ
ØVQS3ZZ
ØVQS4ZZ
ØVQTØZZ
ØVQT3ZZ
ØVQT4ZZ
ØVQTXZZ
ØVTØ4ZZ
ØVTØ7ZZ
ØVTØ8ZZ
ØVTFØZZ
ØVTF4ZZ
ØVTGØZZ
ØVTG4ZZ
ØVTHØZZ
ØVTH4ZZ
ØVUSØJZ
ØVUS4JZ
ØVUTØ7Z
ØVUTØJZ
ØVUTØKZ
ØVUT47Z
ØVUT4JZ
ØVUT4KZ
ØVUTX7Z
ØVUTXJZ
ØVUTXKZ
ØVW4ØØZ
ØVW4Ø3Z
ØVW4Ø7Z
ØVW4ØJZ
ØVW4ØKZ
ØVW4ØYZ
ØVW43ØZ
ØVW433Z
ØVW437Z
ØVW43JZ
ØVW43KZ
ØVW44ØZ
ØVW443Z
ØVW447Z
ØVW44JZ
ØVW44KZ
ØVW47ØZ
ØVW473Z
ØVW477Z
ØVW47JZ
ØVW47KZ
ØVW48ØZ
ØVW483Z
ØVW487Z
ØVW48JZ
ØVW48KZ
ØVWSØØZ
ØVWSØ3Z
ØVWSØ7Z
ØVWSØJZ
ØVWSØKZ
ØVWSØYZ
ØVWS3ØZ
ØVWS33Z
ØVWS37Z
ØVWS3JZ
ØVWS3KZ
ØVWS4ØZ
ØVWS43Z
ØVWS47Z
ØVWS4JZ
ØVWS4KZ
ØVWS7ØZ
ØVWS73Z
ØVWS77Z
ØVWS7JZ
ØVWS7KZ
ØVWS8ØZ
ØVWS83Z
ØVWS87Z
ØVWS8JZ
ØVWS8KZ
ØVXTØZS
ØWØØØ7Z
ØWØØØJZ
ØWØØØKZ
ØWØØØZZ
ØWØØ37Z
ØWØØ3JZ
ØWØØ3KZ
ØWØØ3ZZ
ØWØØ47Z
ØWØØ4JZ
ØWØØ4KZ
ØWØØ4ZZ
ØWØ2Ø7Z
ØWØ2ØJZ
ØWØ2ØKZ
ØWØ2ØZZ
ØWØ237Z
ØWØ23JZ
ØWØ23KZ

ØWØ23ZZ
ØWØ247Z
ØWØ24JZ
ØWØ24KZ
ØWØ24ZZ
ØWØ6Ø7Z
ØWØ6ØJZ
ØWØ6ØKZ
ØWØ6ØZZ
ØWØ637Z
ØWØ63JZ
ØWØ63KZ
ØWØ63ZZ
ØWØ647Z
ØWØ64JZ
ØWØ64KZ
ØWØ64ZZ
ØWØ8Ø7Z
ØWØ8ØJZ
ØWØ8ØKZ
ØWØ8ØZZ
ØWØ837Z
ØWØ83JZ
ØWØ83KZ
ØWØ83ZZ
ØWØ847Z
ØWØ84JZ
ØWØ84KZ
ØWØ84ZZ
ØWØFØ7Z
ØWØFØJZ
ØWØFØKZ
ØWØFØZZ
ØWØF37Z
ØWØF3JZ
ØWØF3KZ
ØWØF3ZZ
ØWØF47Z
ØWØF4JZ
ØWØF4KZ
ØWØF4ZZ
ØWØKØ7Z
ØWØKØJZ
ØWØKØKZ
ØWØKØZZ
ØWØK37Z
ØWØK3JZ
ØWØK3KZ
ØWØK3ZZ
ØWØK47Z
ØWØK4JZ
ØWØK4KZ
ØWØK4ZZ
ØWØLØ7Z
ØWØLØJZ
ØWØLØKZ
ØWØLØZZ
ØWØL37Z
ØWØL3JZ
ØWØL3KZ
ØWØL3ZZ
ØWØL47Z
ØWØL4JZ
ØWØL4KZ
ØWØL4ZZ
ØWØMØ7Z
ØWØMØJZ
ØWØMØKZ
ØWØMØZZ
ØWØM37Z
ØWØM3JZ
ØWØM3KZ
ØWØM3ZZ
ØWØM47Z
ØWØM4JZ
ØWØM4KZ
ØWØM4ZZ
ØWØNØ7Z
ØWØNØJZ
ØWØNØKZ
ØWØNØZZ
ØWØN37Z
ØWØN3JZ
ØWØN3KZ
ØWØN3ZZ
ØWØN47Z
ØWØN4JZ
ØWØN4KZ
ØWØN4ZZ
ØW1GØJ6
ØW1G3J6
ØW1G4J6
ØW3G3ZZ
ØW3G4ZZ
ØW9FØZX
ØW9F3ZX
ØW9F4ZX
ØW9GØØZ
ØW9GØZX
ØW9GØZZ
ØW9G4ØZ
ØW9G4ZX
ØW9G4ZZ
ØW9HØZX
ØW9H3ZX
ØW9H4ZX
ØW9JØZX
ØW9J4ZX
ØW9NØØZ
ØW9NØZZ
ØW9N4ØZ
ØW9N4ZZ
ØWBØØZZ
ØWBØ3ZZ
ØWBØ4ZZ
ØWBØXZZ
ØWB2ØZZ
ØWB23ZZ
ØWB24ZZ
ØWB2XZZ
ØWB3ØZX
ØWB3ØZZ
ØWB33ZX
ØWB33ZZ
ØWB34ZX
ØWB34ZZ
ØWB3XZX
ØWB3XZZ
ØWB4ØZZ
ØWB43ZZ
ØWB44ZZ
ØWB4XZZ
ØWB5ØZZ
ØWB53ZZ
ØWB54ZZ
ØWB5XZZ
ØWB6ØZZ
ØWB63ZZ
ØWB64ZZ
ØWB6XZZ
ØWB8ØZZ
ØWB83ZZ
ØWB84ZZ
ØWB8XZZ
ØWBCØZX
ØWBCØZZ
ØWBC3ZX
ØWBC3ZZ
ØWBC4ZX
ØWBC4ZZ
ØWBFØZX
ØWBFØZZ
ØWBF3ZX
ØWBF3ZZ
ØWBF4ZX
ØWBF4ZZ
ØWBFXZ2
ØWBFXZX
ØWBFXZZ
ØWBKØZZ
ØWBK3ZZ
ØWBK4ZZ
ØWBKXZZ
ØWBLØZZ
ØWBL3ZZ
ØWBL4ZZ
ØWBLXZZ
ØWBMØZZ
ØWBM3ZZ
ØWBM4ZZ
ØWBMXZZ
ØWBNØZX
ØWBNØZZ
ØWBN3ZX
ØWBN3ZZ
ØWBN4ZX
ØWBN4ZZ
ØWBNXZX
ØWBNXZZ
ØWC3ØZZ
ØWC33ZZ
ØWC34ZZ
ØWC4ØZZ
ØWC44ZZ
ØWC5ØZZ
ØWC54ZZ
ØWF3ØZZ
ØWF33ZZ
ØWF34ZZ
ØWHØØ1Z
ØWHØ31Z
ØWHØ41Z
ØWH1Ø1Z
ØWH131Z
ØWH141Z
ØWH2Ø1Z
ØWH231Z
ØWH241Z
ØWH3Ø1Z
ØWH3Ø3Z
ØWH3ØYZ
ØWH331Z
ØWH333Z
ØWH33YZ
ØWH341Z
ØWH343Z
ØWH34YZ
ØWH4Ø1Z
ØWH431Z
ØWH441Z
ØWH5Ø1Z
ØWH531Z
ØWH541Z
ØWH6Ø1Z
ØWH631Z
ØWH641Z
ØWH8Ø1Z
ØWH831Z
ØWH841Z
ØWH9Ø1Z
ØWH931Z
ØWH941Z
ØWHBØ1Z
ØWHB31Z
ØWHB41Z
ØWHCØ1Z
ØWHC31Z
ØWHC41Z
ØWHDØ1Z
ØWHD31Z
ØWHD41Z
ØWHFØ1Z
ØWHF31Z
ØWHF41Z
ØWHGØ1Z
ØWHG31Z
ØWHG41Z
ØWHHØ1Z
ØWHH31Z
ØWHH41Z
ØWHJØ1Z
ØWHJ31Z
ØWHJ41Z
ØWHKØ1Z
ØWHK31Z
ØWHK41Z
ØWHLØ1Z
ØWHL31Z
ØWHL41Z
ØWHMØ1Z
ØWHM31Z
ØWHM41Z
ØWHNØ1Z
ØWHNØ3Z
ØWHNØYZ
ØWHN31Z
ØWHN33Z
ØWHN3YZ
ØWHN41Z
ØWHN43Z
ØWHN4YZ
ØWHPØ1Z
ØWHP31Z
ØWHP41Z
ØWHP71Z
ØWHP81Z
ØWHQØ1Z
ØWHQ31Z
ØWHQ41Z
ØWHQ71Z
ØWHQ81Z
ØWHRØ1Z
ØWHR31Z
ØWHR41Z
ØWHR71Z
ØWHR81Z
ØWJF4ZZ
ØWJG4ZZ
ØWJH4ZZ
ØWJJ4ZZ
ØWJP4ZZ
ØWJR4ZZ
ØWM2ØZZ
ØWM4ØZZ
ØWM5ØZZ
ØWM6ØZZ
ØWMKØZZ
ØWMLØZZ
ØWMMØZZ
ØWMNØZZ
ØWPMØ7Z
ØWPMØKZ
ØWPM37Z
ØWPM3KZ
ØWPM47Z
ØWPM4KZ
ØWPMX7Z
ØWPMXJZ
ØWPMXKZ
ØWPNØØZ
ØWPNØ1Z
ØWPNØ3Z
ØWPNØ7Z
ØWPNØJZ
ØWPNØKZ
ØWPNØYZ
ØWPN3ØZ
ØWPN31Z
ØWPN33Z
ØWPN37Z
ØWPN3JZ
ØWPN3KZ
ØWPN3YZ
ØWPN4ØZ
ØWPN41Z
ØWPN43Z
ØWPN47Z
ØWPN4JZ
ØWPN4KZ
ØWPN4YZ
ØWQØØZZ
ØWQØ3ZZ
ØWQØ4ZZ
ØWQØXZZ
ØWQ2ØZZ
ØWQ23ZZ
ØWQ24ZZ
ØWQ2XZZ
ØWQ4ØZZ
ØWQ43ZZ
ØWQ44ZZ
ØWQ4XZZ
ØWQ5ØZZ
ØWQ53ZZ
ØWQ54ZZ
ØWQ5XZZ
ØWQ6ØZZ
ØWQ63ZZ
ØWQ64ZZ
ØWQ6XZZ
ØWQFØZZ
ØWQFXZ2
ØWQFXZZ
ØWQKØZZ
ØWQK3ZZ
ØWQK4ZZ
ØWQKXZZ
ØWQLØZZ
ØWQL3ZZ
ØWQL4ZZ
ØWQLXZZ
ØWQMØZZ
ØWQM3ZZ
ØWQM4ZZ
ØWQMXZZ
ØWQNØZZ
ØWQN3ZZ
ØWQN4ZZ
ØWUØØ7Z
ØWUØØJZ
ØWUØØKZ
ØWUØ47Z
ØWUØ4JZ
ØWUØ4KZ
ØWU2ØJZ
ØWU2ØKZ
ØWU24JZ
ØWU24KZ
ØWU6Ø7Z
ØWU6ØJZ
ØWU6ØKZ
ØWU647Z
ØWU64JZ
ØWU64KZ
ØWUFØ7Z
ØWUFØJZ
ØWUFØKZ
ØWUKØ7Z
ØWUKØJZ
ØWUKØKZ
ØWUK47Z
ØWUK4JZ
ØWUK4KZ
ØWULØ7Z
ØWULØJZ
ØWULØKZ
ØWUL47Z
ØWUL4JZ
ØWUL4KZ
ØWUMØ7Z
ØWUMØJZ
ØWUMØKZ
ØWUM47Z
ØWUM4JZ
ØWUM4KZ
ØWUNØ7Z
ØWUNØJZ
ØWUNØKZ
ØWUN47Z
ØWUN4JZ
ØWUN4KZ
ØWWMØ7Z
ØWWMØKZ
ØWWM37Z
ØWWM3KZ
ØWWM47Z
ØWWM4KZ
ØWWNØØZ
ØWWNØ1Z
ØWWNØ3Z
ØWWNØ7Z
ØWWNØJZ
ØWWNØKZ
ØWWNØYZ
ØWWN3ØZ
ØWWN31Z
ØWWN33Z
ØWWN37Z
ØWWN3JZ
ØWWN3KZ
ØWWN3YZ
ØWWN4ØZ
ØWWN41Z
ØWWN43Z
ØWWN47Z
ØWWN4JZ
ØWWN4KZ
ØWWN4YZ
ØWY2ØZØ
ØWY2ØZ1
ØXØ2Ø7Z
ØXØ2ØJZ
ØXØ2ØKZ
ØXØ2ØZZ
ØXØ237Z
ØXØ23JZ
ØXØ23KZ
ØXØ23ZZ
ØXØ247Z
ØXØ24JZ
ØXØ24KZ
ØXØ24ZZ
ØXØ3Ø7Z
ØXØ3ØJZ
ØXØ3ØKZ
ØXØ3ØZZ
ØXØ337Z
ØXØ33JZ
ØXØ33KZ
ØXØ33ZZ
ØXØ347Z
ØXØ34JZ
ØXØ34KZ
ØXØ34ZZ
ØXØ4Ø7Z
ØXØ4ØJZ
ØXØ4ØKZ
ØXØ4ØZZ
ØXØ437Z
ØXØ43JZ
ØXØ43KZ
ØXØ43ZZ
ØXØ447Z
ØXØ44JZ
ØXØ44KZ
ØXØ44ZZ
ØXØ5Ø7Z
ØXØ5ØJZ
ØXØ5ØKZ
ØXØ5ØZZ
ØXØ537Z
ØXØ53JZ
ØXØ53KZ
ØXØ53ZZ
ØXØ547Z
ØXØ54JZ
ØXØ54KZ
ØXØ54ZZ
ØXØ6Ø7Z
ØXØ6ØJZ
ØXØ6ØKZ
ØXØ6ØZZ
ØXØ637Z
ØXØ63JZ
ØXØ63KZ
ØXØ63ZZ
ØXØ647Z
ØXØ64JZ
ØXØ64KZ
ØXØ64ZZ
ØXØ7Ø7Z
ØXØ7ØJZ
ØXØ7ØKZ
ØXØ7ØZZ
ØXØ737Z
ØXØ73JZ
ØXØ73KZ
ØXØ73ZZ
ØXØ747Z
ØXØ74JZ
ØXØ74KZ
ØXØ74ZZ
ØXØ8Ø7Z
ØXØ8ØJZ
ØXØ8ØKZ
ØXØ8ØZZ
ØXØ837Z
ØXØ83JZ
ØXØ83KZ
ØXØ83ZZ
ØXØ847Z
ØXØ84JZ
ØXØ84KZ
ØXØ84ZZ
ØXØ9Ø7Z
ØXØ9ØJZ
ØXØ9ØKZ
ØXØ9ØZZ
ØXØ937Z
ØXØ93JZ
ØXØ93KZ
ØXØ93ZZ
ØXØ947Z
ØXØ94JZ
ØXØ94KZ
ØXØ94ZZ
ØXØBØ7Z
ØXØBØJZ
ØXØBØKZ
ØXØBØZZ
ØXØB37Z
ØXØB3JZ
ØXØB3KZ
ØXØB3ZZ
ØXØB47Z
ØXØB4JZ
ØXØB4KZ
ØXØB4ZZ
ØXØCØ7Z
ØXØCØJZ
ØXØCØKZ
ØXØCØZZ
ØXØC37Z
ØXØC3JZ
ØXØC3KZ
ØXØC3ZZ
ØXØC47Z
ØXØC4JZ
ØXØC4KZ
ØXØC4ZZ
ØXØDØ7Z
ØXØDØJZ
ØXØDØKZ
ØXØDØZZ
ØXØD37Z
ØXØD3JZ
ØXØD3KZ
ØXØD3ZZ
ØXØD47Z
ØXØD4JZ
ØXØD4KZ
ØXØD4ZZ
ØXØFØ7Z
ØXØFØJZ
ØXØFØKZ
ØXØFØZZ
ØXØF37Z
ØXØF3JZ
ØXØF3KZ
ØXØF3ZZ
ØXØF47Z
ØXØF4JZ
ØXØF4KZ
ØXØF4ZZ
ØXØGØ7Z
ØXØGØJZ
ØXØGØKZ
ØXØGØZZ
ØXØG37Z
ØXØG3JZ
ØXØG3KZ
ØXØG3ZZ
ØXØG47Z
ØXØG4JZ
ØXØG4KZ
ØXØG4ZZ
ØXØHØ7Z
ØXØHØJZ
ØXØHØKZ
ØXØHØZZ
ØXØH37Z
ØXØH3JZ
ØXØH3KZ
ØXØH3ZZ
ØXØH47Z
ØXØH4JZ
ØXØH4KZ
ØXØH4ZZ
ØX6NØZØ
ØX6NØZ1
ØX6NØZ2
ØX6NØZ3
ØX6PØZØ
ØX6PØZ1
ØX6PØZ2
ØX6PØZ3
ØX6QØZØ
ØX6QØZ1
ØX6QØZ2
ØX6QØZ3
ØX6RØZØ
ØX6RØZ1
ØX6RØZ2
ØX6RØZ3
ØX6SØZØ
ØX6SØZ1
ØX6SØZ2
ØX6SØZ3
ØX6TØZØ
ØX6TØZ1
ØX6TØZ2
ØX6TØZ3
ØX6VØZØ
ØX6VØZ1
ØX6VØZ2
ØX6VØZ3
ØX6WØZØ
ØX6WØZ1
ØX6WØZ2
ØX6WØZ3
ØXB2ØZZ
ØXB23ZZ
ØXB24ZZ
ØXB3ØZZ
ØXB33ZZ
ØXB34ZZ
ØXB4ØZZ
ØXB43ZZ
ØXB44ZZ
ØXB5ØZZ
ØXB53ZZ
ØXB54ZZ
ØXB6ØZZ
ØXB63ZZ
ØXB64ZZ
ØXB7ØZZ
ØXB73ZZ
ØXB74ZZ
ØXB8ØZZ
ØXB83ZZ
ØXB84ZZ
ØXB9ØZZ
ØXB93ZZ
ØXB94ZZ
ØXBBØZZ
ØXBB3ZZ
ØXBB4ZZ
ØXBCØZZ
ØXBC3ZZ
ØXBC4ZZ
ØXBDØZZ
ØXBD3ZZ
ØXBD4ZZ
ØXBFØZZ
ØXBF3ZZ
ØXBF4ZZ
ØXBGØZZ
ØXBG3ZZ
ØXBG4ZZ
ØXBHØZZ
ØXBH3ZZ
ØXBH4ZZ
ØXBJØZZ
ØXBJ3ZZ
ØXBJ4ZZ
ØXBKØZZ
ØXBK3ZZ
ØXBK4ZZ
ØXH2Ø1Z
ØXH231Z
ØXH241Z
ØXH3Ø1Z
ØXH331Z
ØXH341Z
ØXH4Ø1Z
ØXH431Z
ØXH441Z
ØXH5Ø1Z
ØXH531Z
ØXH541Z
ØXH6Ø1Z
ØXH631Z
ØXH641Z
ØXH7Ø1Z
ØXH731Z
ØXH741Z
ØXH8Ø1Z
ØXH831Z
ØXH841Z
ØXH9Ø1Z
ØXH931Z
ØXH941Z
ØXHBØ1Z
ØXHB31Z
ØXHB41Z
ØXHCØ1Z
ØXHC31Z
ØXHC41Z
ØXHDØ1Z
ØXHD31Z
ØXHD41Z
ØXHFØ1Z
ØXHF31Z
ØXHF41Z
ØXHGØ1Z
ØXHG31Z
ØXHG41Z
ØXHHØ1Z
ØXHH31Z
ØXHH41Z
ØXHJØ1Z
ØXHJ31Z
ØXHJ41Z
ØXHKØ1Z
ØXHK31Z
ØXHK41Z
ØXU2Ø7Z
ØXU2ØJZ
ØXU2ØKZ
ØXU247Z
ØXU24JZ
ØXU24KZ
ØXU3Ø7Z
ØXU3ØJZ
ØXU3ØKZ
ØXU347Z
ØXU34JZ
ØXU34KZ
ØXU4Ø7Z
ØXU4ØJZ
ØXU4ØKZ
ØXU447Z
ØXU44JZ
ØXU44KZ
ØXU5Ø7Z
ØXU5ØJZ
ØXU5ØKZ
ØXU547Z
ØXU54JZ
ØXU54KZ
ØXU6Ø7Z
ØXU6ØJZ
ØXU6ØKZ
ØXU647Z
ØXU64JZ
ØXU64KZ
ØXU7Ø7Z
ØXU7ØJZ
ØXU7ØKZ
ØXU747Z
ØXU74JZ
ØXU74KZ
ØXU8Ø7Z
ØXU8ØJZ
ØXU8ØKZ
ØXU847Z
ØXU84JZ
ØXU84KZ
ØXU9Ø7Z
ØXU9ØJZ
ØXU9ØKZ
ØXU947Z
ØXU94JZ
ØXU94KZ
ØXUBØ7Z
ØXUBØJZ
ØXUBØKZ
ØXUB47Z
ØXUB4JZ
ØXUB4KZ
ØXUCØ7Z
ØXUCØJZ
ØXUCØKZ
ØXUC47Z
ØXUC4JZ
ØXUC4KZ
ØXUDØ7Z
ØXUDØJZ
ØXUDØKZ
ØXUD47Z
ØXUD4JZ
ØXUD4KZ
ØXUFØ7Z
ØXUFØJZ
ØXUFØKZ
ØXUF47Z
ØXUF4JZ
ØXUF4KZ
ØXUGØ7Z
ØXUGØJZ
ØXUGØKZ
ØXUG47Z
ØXUG4JZ
ØXUG4KZ
ØXUHØ7Z
ØXUHØJZ
ØXUHØKZ
ØXUH47Z
ØXUH4JZ
ØXUH4KZ
ØXUJØ7Z
ØXUJØJZ
ØXUJØKZ
ØXUJ47Z
ØXUJ4JZ
ØXUJ4KZ
ØXUKØ7Z
ØXUKØJZ
ØXUKØKZ
ØXUK47Z
ØXUK4JZ
ØXUK4KZ
ØXULØ7Z
ØXULØJZ
ØXULØKZ
ØXUL47Z
ØXUL4JZ
ØXUL4KZ
ØXUMØ7Z
ØXUMØJZ
ØXUMØKZ
ØXUM47Z
ØXUM4JZ
ØXUM4KZ
ØXUNØ7Z
ØXUNØJZ
ØXUNØKZ
ØXUN47Z
ØXUN4JZ
ØXUN4KZ
ØXUPØ7Z
ØXUPØJZ
ØXUPØKZ
ØXUP47Z
ØXUP4JZ
ØXUP4KZ
ØXUQØ7Z
ØXUQØJZ
ØXUQØKZ
ØXUQ47Z
ØXUQ4JZ
ØXUQ4KZ
ØXURØ7Z
ØXURØJZ
ØXURØKZ
ØXUR47Z

ØXUR4JZ
ØXUR4KZ
ØXUSØ7Z
ØXUSØJZ
ØXUSØKZ
ØXUS47Z
ØXUS4JZ
ØXUS4KZ
ØXUTØ7Z
ØXUTØJZ
ØXUTØKZ
ØXUT47Z
ØXUT4JZ
ØXUT4KZ
ØXUVØ7Z
ØXUVØJZ
ØXUVØKZ
ØXUV47Z
ØXUV4JZ
ØXUV4KZ
ØXUWØ7Z
ØXUWØJZ
ØXUWØKZ
ØXUW47Z
ØXUW4JZ
ØXUW4KZ
ØYØØØ7Z
ØYØØØJZ
ØYØØØKZ
ØYØØØZZ
ØYØØ37Z
ØYØØ3JZ
ØYØØ3KZ
ØYØØ3ZZ
ØYØØ47Z
ØYØØ4JZ
ØYØØ4KZ
ØYØØ4ZZ
ØYØ1Ø7Z
ØYØ1ØJZ
ØYØ1ØKZ
ØYØ1ØZZ
ØYØ137Z
ØYØ13JZ
ØYØ13KZ
ØYØ13ZZ
ØYØ147Z
ØYØ14JZ
ØYØ14KZ
ØYØ14ZZ
ØYØ9Ø7Z
ØYØ9ØJZ
ØYØ9ØKZ
ØYØ9ØZZ
ØYØ937Z
ØYØ93JZ
ØYØ93KZ
ØYØ93ZZ
ØYØ947Z
ØYØ94JZ
ØYØ94KZ
ØYØ94ZZ
ØYØBØ7Z
ØYØBØJZ
ØYØBØKZ
ØYØBØZZ
ØYØB37Z
ØYØB3JZ
ØYØB3KZ
ØYØB3ZZ
ØYØB47Z
ØYØB4JZ
ØYØB4KZ
ØYØB4ZZ
ØYØCØ7Z
ØYØCØJZ
ØYØCØKZ
ØYØCØZZ
ØYØC37Z
ØYØC3JZ
ØYØC3KZ
ØYØC3ZZ
ØYØC47Z
ØYØC4JZ
ØYØC4KZ
ØYØC4ZZ
ØYØDØ7Z
ØYØDØJZ
ØYØDØKZ
ØYØDØZZ
ØYØD37Z
ØYØD3JZ
ØYØD3KZ
ØYØD3ZZ
ØYØD47Z
ØYØD4JZ
ØYØD4KZ
ØYØD4ZZ
ØYØFØ7Z
ØYØFØJZ
ØYØFØKZ
ØYØFØZZ
ØYØF37Z
ØYØF3JZ
ØYØF3KZ
ØYØF3ZZ
ØYØF47Z
ØYØF4JZ
ØYØF4KZ
ØYØF4ZZ
ØYØGØ7Z
ØYØGØJZ
ØYØGØKZ
ØYØGØZZ
ØYØG37Z
ØYØG3JZ
ØYØG3KZ
ØYØG3ZZ
ØYØG47Z
ØYØG4JZ
ØYØG4KZ
ØYØG4ZZ
ØYØHØ7Z
ØYØHØJZ
ØYØHØKZ
ØYØHØZZ
ØYØH37Z
ØYØH3JZ
ØYØH3KZ
ØYØH3ZZ
ØYØH47Z
ØYØH4JZ
ØYØH4KZ
ØYØH4ZZ
ØYØJØ7Z
ØYØJØJZ
ØYØJØKZ
ØYØJØZZ
ØYØJ37Z
ØYØJ3JZ
ØYØJ3KZ
ØYØJ3ZZ
ØYØJ47Z
ØYØJ4JZ
ØYØJ4KZ
ØYØJ4ZZ
ØYØKØ7Z
ØYØKØJZ
ØYØKØKZ
ØYØKØZZ
ØYØK37Z
ØYØK3JZ
ØYØK3KZ
ØYØK3ZZ
ØYØK47Z
ØYØK4JZ
ØYØK4KZ
ØYØK4ZZ
ØYØLØ7Z
ØYØLØJZ
ØYØLØKZ
ØYØLØZZ
ØYØL37Z
ØYØL3JZ
ØYØL3KZ
ØYØL3ZZ
ØYØL47Z
ØYØL4JZ
ØYØL4KZ
ØYØL4ZZ
ØY95ØZX
ØY953ZX
ØY954ZX
ØY96ØZX
ØY963ZX
ØY964ZX
ØYBØØZZ
ØYBØ3ZZ
ØYBØ4ZZ
ØYB1ØZZ
ØYB13ZZ
ØYB14ZZ
ØYB5ØZX
ØYB5ØZZ
ØYB53ZX
ØYB53ZZ
ØYB54ZX
ØYB54ZZ
ØYB6ØZX
ØYB6ØZZ
ØYB63ZX
ØYB63ZZ
ØYB64ZX
ØYB64ZZ
ØYB7ØZX
ØYB7ØZZ
ØYB73ZX
ØYB73ZZ
ØYB74ZX
ØYB74ZZ
ØYB8ØZX
ØYB8ØZZ
ØYB83ZX
ØYB83ZZ
ØYB84ZX
ØYB84ZZ
ØYB9ØZZ
ØYB93ZZ
ØYB94ZZ
ØYBBØZZ
ØYBB3ZZ
ØYBB4ZZ
ØYBCØZZ
ØYBC3ZZ
ØYBC4ZZ
ØYBDØZZ
ØYBD3ZZ
ØYBD4ZZ
ØYBFØZZ
ØYBF3ZZ
ØYBF4ZZ
ØYBGØZZ
ØYBG3ZZ
ØYBG4ZZ
ØYBHØZZ
ØYBH3ZZ
ØYBH4ZZ
ØYBJØZZ
ØYBJ3ZZ
ØYBJ4ZZ
ØYBKØZZ
ØYBK3ZZ
ØYBK4ZZ
ØYBLØZZ
ØYBL3ZZ
ØYBL4ZZ
ØYBMØZZ
ØYBM3ZZ
ØYBM4ZZ
ØYBNØZZ
ØYBN3ZZ
ØYBN4ZZ
ØYHØØ1Z
ØYHØ31Z
ØYHØ41Z
ØYH1Ø1Z
ØYH131Z
ØYH141Z
ØYH5Ø1Z
ØYH531Z
ØYH541Z
ØYH6Ø1Z
ØYH631Z
ØYH641Z
ØYH7Ø1Z
ØYH731Z
ØYH741Z
ØYH8Ø1Z
ØYH831Z
ØYH841Z
ØYH9Ø1Z
ØYH931Z
ØYH941Z
ØYHBØ1Z
ØYHB31Z
ØYHB41Z
ØYHCØ1Z
ØYHC31Z
ØYHC41Z
ØYHDØ1Z
ØYHD31Z
ØYHD41Z
ØYHFØ1Z
ØYHF31Z
ØYHF41Z
ØYHGØ1Z
ØYHG31Z
ØYHG41Z
ØYHHØ1Z
ØYHH31Z
ØYHH41Z
ØYHJØ1Z
ØYHJ31Z
ØYHJ41Z
ØYHKØ1Z
ØYHK31Z
ØYHK41Z
ØYHLØ1Z
ØYHL31Z
ØYHL41Z
ØYHMØ1Z
ØYHM31Z
ØYHM41Z
ØYHNØ1Z
ØYHN31Z
ØYHN41Z
ØYJ54ZZ
ØYJ64ZZ
ØYJ74ZZ
ØYJ84ZZ
ØYJA4ZZ
ØYJE4ZZ
ØYMØØZZ
ØYM1ØZZ
ØYQ5ØZZ
ØYQ53ZZ
ØYQ54ZZ
ØYQ6ØZZ
ØYQ63ZZ
ØYQ64ZZ
ØYQ7ØZZ
ØYQ73ZZ
ØYQ74ZZ
ØYQ8ØZZ
ØYQ83ZZ
ØYQ84ZZ
ØYQAØZZ
ØYQA3ZZ
ØYQA4ZZ
ØYQEØZZ
ØYQE3ZZ
ØYQE4ZZ
ØYUØØ7Z
ØYUØØJZ
ØYUØØKZ
ØYUØ47Z
ØYUØ4JZ
ØYUØ4KZ
ØYU1Ø7Z
ØYU1ØJZ
ØYU1ØKZ
ØYU147Z
ØYU14JZ
ØYU14KZ
ØYU5Ø7Z
ØYU5ØJZ
ØYU5ØKZ
ØYU6Ø7Z
ØYU6ØJZ
ØYU6ØKZ
ØYU7Ø7Z
ØYU7ØJZ
ØYU7ØKZ
ØYU747Z
ØYU74JZ
ØYU74KZ
ØYU8Ø7Z
ØYU8ØJZ
ØYU8ØKZ
ØYU847Z
ØYU84JZ
ØYU84KZ
ØYU9Ø7Z
ØYU9ØJZ
ØYU9ØKZ
ØYU947Z
ØYU94JZ
ØYU94KZ
ØYUAØ7Z
ØYUAØJZ
ØYUAØKZ
ØYUBØ7Z
ØYUBØJZ
ØYUBØKZ
ØYUB47Z
ØYUB4JZ
ØYUB4KZ
ØYUCØ7Z
ØYUCØJZ
ØYUCØKZ
ØYUC47Z
ØYUC4JZ
ØYUC4KZ
ØYUDØ7Z
ØYUDØJZ
ØYUDØKZ
ØYUD47Z
ØYUD4JZ
ØYUD4KZ
ØYUEØ7Z
ØYUEØJZ
ØYUEØKZ
ØYUE47Z
ØYUE4JZ
ØYUE4KZ
ØYUFØ7Z
ØYUFØJZ
ØYUFØKZ
ØYUF47Z
ØYUF4JZ
ØYUF4KZ
ØYUGØ7Z
ØYUGØJZ
ØYUGØKZ
ØYUG47Z
ØYUG4JZ
ØYUG4KZ
ØYUHØ7Z
ØYUHØJZ
ØYUHØKZ
ØYUH47Z
ØYUH4JZ
ØYUH4KZ
ØYUJØ7Z
ØYUJØJZ
ØYUJØKZ
ØYUJ47Z
ØYUJ4JZ
ØYUJ4KZ
ØYUKØ7Z
ØYUKØJZ
ØYUKØKZ
ØYUK47Z
ØYUK4JZ
ØYUK4KZ
ØYULØ7Z
ØYULØJZ
ØYULØKZ
ØYUL47Z
ØYUL4JZ
ØYUL4KZ
ØYUMØ7Z
ØYUMØJZ
ØYUMØKZ
ØYUM47Z
ØYUM4JZ
ØYUM4KZ
ØYUNØ7Z
ØYUNØJZ
ØYUNØKZ
ØYUN47Z
ØYUN4JZ
ØYUN4KZ
ØYUPØ7Z
ØYUPØJZ
ØYUPØKZ
ØYUP47Z
ØYUP4JZ
ØYUP4KZ
ØYUQØ7Z
ØYUQØJZ
ØYUQØKZ
ØYUQ47Z
ØYUQ4JZ
ØYUQ4KZ
ØYURØ7Z
ØYURØJZ
ØYURØKZ
ØYUR47Z
ØYUR4JZ
ØYUR4KZ
ØYUSØ7Z
ØYUSØJZ
ØYUSØKZ
ØYUS47Z
ØYUS4JZ
ØYUS4KZ
ØYUTØ7Z
ØYUTØJZ
ØYUTØKZ
ØYUT47Z
ØYUT4JZ
ØYUT4KZ
ØYUUØ7Z
ØYUUØJZ
ØYUUØKZ
ØYUU47Z
ØYUU4JZ
ØYUU4KZ
ØYUVØ7Z
ØYUVØJZ
ØYUVØKZ
ØYUV47Z
ØYUV4JZ
ØYUV4KZ
ØYUWØ7Z
ØYUWØJZ
ØYUWØKZ
ØYUW47Z
ØYUW4JZ
ØYUW4KZ
ØYUXØ7Z
ØYUXØJZ
ØYUXØKZ
ØYUX47Z
ØYUX4JZ
ØYUX4KZ
ØYUYØ7Z
ØYUYØJZ
ØYUYØKZ
ØYUY47Z
ØYUY4JZ
ØYUY4KZ
1ØAØ7ZZ
1ØAØ8ZZ
1ØD2ØZZ
1ØD24ZZ
3EØL4GC
4AØ6Ø5Z
4AØ6ØBZ
4A16Ø5Z
4A16ØBZ
XNUØ356
XNU4356
XWØ2ØD8
XWØQ316

DRG 988

Select operating room procedures listed under DRG 987

DRG 989

Select operating room procedures listed under DRG 987

DRG 999

Discharges with invalid ICD-10-CM principal diagnosis, sex, or discharge status field (s) missing or invalid and necessary for DRG assignment.

Appendix A: DRG List

MS-DRG	Post-Acute DRG	Special Pay DRG	MDC	TYPE	MS-DRG TITLE	RW	GMLOS	AMLOS
001	No	No	PRE	SURG	HEART TRANSPLANT OR IMPLANT OF HEART ASSIST SYSTEM WITH MCC	27.0986	30.3	40.1
002	No	No	PRE	SURG	HEART TRANSPLANT OR IMPLANT OF HEART ASSIST SYSTEM WITHOUT MCC	12.2441	9.6	14.7
003	Yes	No	PRE	SURG	ECMO OR TRACHEOSTOMY WITH MV >96 HOURS OR PRINCIPAL DIAGNOSIS EXCEPT FACE, MOUTH AND NECK WITH MAJOR O.R. PROCEDURES	21.3203	26.7	36.5
004	Yes	No	PRE	SURG	TRACHEOSTOMY WITH MV >96 HOURS OR PRINCIPAL DIAGNOSIS EXCEPT FACE, MOUTH AND NECK WITHOUT MAJOR O.R. PROCEDURES	14.7000	26.1	32.0
005	No	No	PRE	SURG	LIVER TRANSPLANT WITH MCC OR INTESTINAL TRANSPLANT	10.3500	14.8	20.0
006	No	No	PRE	SURG	LIVER TRANSPLANT WITHOUT MCC	4.8369	7.8	8.8
007	No	No	PRE	SURG	LUNG TRANSPLANT	12.2664	18.5	22.2
008	No	No	PRE	SURG	SIMULTANEOUS PANCREAS AND KIDNEY TRANSPLANT	5.2617	8.7	9.8
010	No	No	PRE	SURG	PANCREAS TRANSPLANT	4.8136	9.5	10.4
011	No	No	PRE	SURG	TRACHEOSTOMY FOR FACE, MOUTH AND NECK DIAGNOSES OR LARYNGECTOMY WITH MCC	5.1563	11.5	14.8
012	No	No	PRE	SURG	TRACHEOSTOMY FOR FACE, MOUTH AND NECK DIAGNOSES OR LARYNGECTOMY WITH CC	4.0049	8.5	9.8
013	No	No	PRE	SURG	TRACHEOSTOMY FOR FACE, MOUTH AND NECK DIAGNOSES OR LARYNGECTOMY WITHOUT CC/MCC	2.6857	6.3	7.0
014	No	No	PRE	MED	ALLOGENEIC BONE MARROW TRANSPLANT	11.4609	25.6	28.7
016	No	No	PRE	MED	AUTOLOGOUS BONE MARROW TRANSPLANT WITH CC/MCC	6.1770	16.6	17.8
017	No	No	PRE	MED	AUTOLOGOUS BONE MARROW TRANSPLANT WITHOUT CC/MCC	6.1770	16.6	17.8
018	No	No	PRE	MED	CHIMERIC ANTIGEN RECEPTOR (CAR) T-CELL AND OTHER IMMUNOTHERAPIES	36.8427	12.9	15.1
019	No	No	PRE	SURG	SIMULTANEOUS PANCREAS AND KIDNEY TRANSPLANT WITH HEMODIALYSIS	7.9935	11.6	14.0
020	No	No	01	SURG	INTRACRANIAL VASCULAR PROCEDURES WITH PRINCIPAL DIAGNOSIS HEMORRHAGE WITH MCC	8.4524	10.2	14.1
021	No	No	01	SURG	INTRACRANIAL VASCULAR PROCEDURES WITH PRINCIPAL DIAGNOSIS HEMORRHAGE WITH CC	6.1414	6.3	9.0
022	No	No	01	SURG	INTRACRANIAL VASCULAR PROCEDURES WITH PRINCIPAL DIAGNOSIS HEMORRHAGE WITHOUT CC/MCC	3.4767	2.5	3.9
023	Yes	Yes	01	SURG	CRANIOTOMY WITH MAJOR DEVICE IMPLANT OR ACUTE COMPLEX CNS PRINCIPAL DIAGNOSIS WITH MCC OR CHEMOTHERAPY IMPLANT OR EPILEPSY WITH NEUROSTIMULATOR	5.6688	7.5	10.5
024	Yes	Yes	01	SURG	CRANIOTOMY WITH MAJOR DEVICE IMPLANT OR ACUTE COMPLEX CNS PRINCIPAL DIAGNOSIS WITHOUT MCC	3.7888	4.0	5.2
025	Yes	No	01	SURG	CRANIOTOMY AND ENDOVASCULAR INTRACRANIAL PROCEDURES WITH MCC	4.4160	6.6	9.1
026	Yes	No	01	SURG	CRANIOTOMY AND ENDOVASCULAR INTRACRANIAL PROCEDURES WITH CC	2.9531	3.1	4.7
027	Yes	No	01	SURG	CRANIOTOMY AND ENDOVASCULAR INTRACRANIAL PROCEDURES WITHOUT CC/MCC	2.4329	1.6	2.1
028	Yes	Yes	01	SURG	SPINAL PROCEDURES WITH MCC	6.0261	10.2	13.2
029	Yes	Yes	01	SURG	SPINAL PROCEDURES WITH CC OR SPINAL NEUROSTIMULATORS	3.4282	4.9	6.5
030	Yes	Yes	01	SURG	SPINAL PROCEDURES WITHOUT CC/MCC	2.3190	2.7	3.6
031	Yes	No	01	SURG	VENTRICULAR SHUNT PROCEDURES WITH MCC	4.1166	7.0	10.4
032	Yes	No	01	SURG	VENTRICULAR SHUNT PROCEDURES WITH CC	2.1538	2.7	4.1
033	Yes	No	01	SURG	VENTRICULAR SHUNT PROCEDURES WITHOUT CC/MCC	1.6229	1.6	2.0
034	No	No	01	SURG	CAROTID ARTERY STENT PROCEDURES WITH MCC	3.9014	4.9	7.4
035	No	No	01	SURG	CAROTID ARTERY STENT PROCEDURES WITH CC	2.2995	2.0	2.9
036	No	No	01	SURG	CAROTID ARTERY STENT PROCEDURES WITHOUT CC/MCC	1.8082	1.2	1.4
037	No	No	01	SURG	EXTRACRANIAL PROCEDURES WITH MCC	3.3756	5.1	8.1
038	No	No	01	SURG	EXTRACRANIAL PROCEDURES WITH CC	1.5999	1.9	2.8
039	No	No	01	SURG	EXTRACRANIAL PROCEDURES WITHOUT CC/MCC	1.1410	1.2	1.4
040	Yes	Yes	01	SURG	PERIPHERAL, CRANIAL NERVE AND OTHER NERVOUS SYSTEM PROCEDURES WITH MCC	3.8505	7.4	10.8
041	Yes	Yes	01	SURG	PERIPHERAL, CRANIAL NERVE AND OTHER NERVOUS SYSTEM PROCEDURES WITH CC OR PERIPHERAL NEUROSTIMULATOR	2.2307	3.9	5.0
042	Yes	Yes	01	SURG	PERIPHERAL, CRANIAL NERVE AND OTHER NERVOUS SYSTEM PROCEDURES WITHOUT CC/MCC	1.7398	2.4	3.0
052	No	No	01	MED	SPINAL DISORDERS AND INJURIES WITH CC/MCC	1.9445	4.6	6.6
053	No	No	01	MED	SPINAL DISORDERS AND INJURIES WITHOUT CC/MCC	0.9838	2.8	3.7
054	Yes	No	01	MED	NERVOUS SYSTEM NEOPLASMS WITH MCC	1.4735	4.0	5.8
055	Yes	No	01	MED	NERVOUS SYSTEM NEOPLASMS WITHOUT MCC	1.0732	3.0	4.3

MS-DRG	Post-Acute DRG	Special Pay DRG	MDC	TYPE	MS-DRG TITLE	RW	GMLOS	AMLOS
056	Yes	No	01	MED	DEGENERATIVE NERVOUS SYSTEM DISORDERS WITH MCC	2.3940	6.1	9.7
057	Yes	No	01	MED	DEGENERATIVE NERVOUS SYSTEM DISORDERS WITHOUT MCC	1.3632	4.0	6.4
058	No	No	01	MED	MULTIPLE SCLEROSIS AND CEREBELLAR ATAXIA WITH MCC	1.7279	4.7	7.1
059	No	No	01	MED	MULTIPLE SCLEROSIS AND CEREBELLAR ATAXIA WITH CC	1.1872	3.7	5.0
060	No	No	01	MED	MULTIPLE SCLEROSIS AND CEREBELLAR ATAXIA WITHOUT CC/MCC	0.8974	2.9	3.6
061	No	No	01	MED	ISCHEMIC STROKE, PRECEREBRAL OCCLUSION OR TRANSIENT ISCHEMIA WITH THROMBOLYTIC AGENT WITH MCC	2.8028	5.0	6.7
062	No	No	01	MED	ISCHEMIC STROKE, PRECEREBRAL OCCLUSION OR TRANSIENT ISCHEMIA WITH THROMBOLYTIC AGENT WITH CC	1.8717	3.2	3.8
063	No	No	01	MED	ISCHEMIC STROKE, PRECEREBRAL OCCLUSION OR TRANSIENT ISCHEMIA WITH THROMBOLYTIC AGENT WITHOUT CC/MCC	1.4868	2.2	2.5
064	Yes	No	01	MED	INTRACRANIAL HEMORRHAGE OR CEREBRAL INFARCTION WITH MCC	2.0030	4.6	6.7
065	Yes	No	01	MED	INTRACRANIAL HEMORRHAGE OR CEREBRAL INFARCTION WITH CC OR TPA IN 24 HOURS	1.0164	2.9	3.7
066	Yes	No	01	MED	INTRACRANIAL HEMORRHAGE OR CEREBRAL INFARCTION WITHOUT CC/MCC	0.6875	1.9	2.4
067	No	No	01	MED	NONSPECIFIC CVA AND PRECEREBRAL OCCLUSION WITHOUT INFARCTION WITH MCC	1.4169	3.3	4.7
068	No	No	01	MED	NONSPECIFIC CVA AND PRECEREBRAL OCCLUSION WITHOUT INFARCTION WITHOUT MCC	0.8710	2.1	2.6
069	No	No	01	MED	TRANSIENT ISCHEMIA WITHOUT THROMBOLYTIC	0.7987	2.1	2.6
070	Yes	No	01	MED	NONSPECIFIC CEREBROVASCULAR DISORDERS WITH MCC	1.7895	4.9	7.1
071	Yes	No	01	MED	NONSPECIFIC CEREBROVASCULAR DISORDERS WITH CC	1.0618	3.4	4.7
072	Yes	No	01	MED	NONSPECIFIC CEREBROVASCULAR DISORDERS WITHOUT CC/MCC	0.7830	2.4	3.1
073	No	No	01	MED	CRANIAL AND PERIPHERAL NERVE DISORDERS WITH MCC	1.5130	3.9	5.8
074	No	No	01	MED	CRANIAL AND PERIPHERAL NERVE DISORDERS WITHOUT MCC	1.0262	2.9	3.8
075	No	No	01	MED	VIRAL MENINGITIS WITH CC/MCC	1.9138	6.0	7.7
076	No	No	01	MED	VIRAL MENINGITIS WITHOUT CC/MCC	0.9225	3.2	3.9
077	No	No	01	MED	HYPERTENSIVE ENCEPHALOPATHY WITH MCC	1.5109	4.1	5.6
078	No	No	01	MED	HYPERTENSIVE ENCEPHALOPATHY WITH CC	1.0169	2.9	3.8
079	No	No	01	MED	HYPERTENSIVE ENCEPHALOPATHY WITHOUT CC/MCC	0.7408	2.2	2.6
080	No	No	01	MED	NONTRAUMATIC STUPOR AND COMA WITH MCC	2.2087	5.4	8.5
081	No	No	01	MED	NONTRAUMATIC STUPOR AND COMA WITHOUT MCC	0.9095	2.7	3.7
082	No	No	01	MED	TRAUMATIC STUPOR AND COMA >1 HOUR WITH MCC	2.2783	4.5	7.1
083	No	No	01	MED	TRAUMATIC STUPOR AND COMA >1 HOUR WITH CC	1.3564	3.3	4.4
084	No	No	01	MED	TRAUMATIC STUPOR AND COMA >1 HOUR WITHOUT CC/MCC	0.9197	2.1	2.6
085	Yes	No	01	MED	TRAUMATIC STUPOR AND COMA <1 HOUR WITH MCC	2.2728	4.7	6.7
086	Yes	No	01	MED	TRAUMATIC STUPOR AND COMA <1 HOUR WITH CC	1.3171	3.0	3.9
087	Yes	No	01	MED	TRAUMATIC STUPOR AND COMA <1 HOUR WITHOUT CC/MCC	0.8862	2.0	2.4
088	No	No	01	MED	CONCUSSION WITH MCC	1.5338	3.9	5.4
089	No	No	01	MED	CONCUSSION WITH CC	1.1499	2.5	3.4
090	No	No	01	MED	CONCUSSION WITHOUT CC/MCC	0.9348	1.9	2.4
091	Yes	No	01	MED	OTHER DISORDERS OF NERVOUS SYSTEM WITH MCC	1.7892	4.5	6.8
092	Yes	No	01	MED	OTHER DISORDERS OF NERVOUS SYSTEM WITH CC	1.0261	3.1	4.2
093	Yes	No	01	MED	OTHER DISORDERS OF NERVOUS SYSTEM WITHOUT CC/MCC	0.7744	2.2	2.8
094	No	No	01	MED	BACTERIAL AND TUBERCULOUS INFECTIONS OF NERVOUS SYSTEM WITH MCC	3.6227	8.6	11.5
095	No	No	01	MED	BACTERIAL AND TUBERCULOUS INFECTIONS OF NERVOUS SYSTEM WITH CC	2.3842	5.9	7.3
096	No	No	01	MED	BACTERIAL AND TUBERCULOUS INFECTIONS OF NERVOUS SYSTEM WITHOUT CC/MCC	2.1797	4.5	5.3
097	No	No	01	MED	NON-BACTERIAL INFECTION OF NERVOUS SYSTEM EXCEPT VIRAL MENINGITIS WITH MCC	3.6369	9.1	12.5
098	No	No	01	MED	NON-BACTERIAL INFECTION OF NERVOUS SYSTEM EXCEPT VIRAL MENINGITIS WITH CC	2.1545	6.1	8.2
099	No	No	01	MED	NON-BACTERIAL INFECTION OF NERVOUS SYSTEM EXCEPT VIRAL MENINGITIS WITHOUT CC/MCC	1.3202	3.9	4.8
100	Yes	No	01	MED	SEIZURES WITH MCC	1.9825	4.5	6.7
101	Yes	No	01	MED	SEIZURES WITHOUT MCC	0.9096	2.7	3.5
102	No	No	01	MED	HEADACHES WITH MCC	1.2066	3.1	4.5
103	No	No	01	MED	HEADACHES WITHOUT MCC	0.8424	2.3	3.1
113	No	No	02	SURG	ORBITAL PROCEDURES WITH CC/MCC	2.5073	4.9	7.9

MS-DRG	Post-Acute DRG	Special Pay DRG	MDC	TYPE	MS-DRG TITLE	RW	GMLOS	AMLOS
114	No	No	02	SURG	ORBITAL PROCEDURES WITHOUT CC/MCC	1.2318	2.1	2.5
115	No	No	02	SURG	EXTRAOCULAR PROCEDURES EXCEPT ORBIT	1.5644	3.6	4.9
116	No	No	02	SURG	INTRAOCULAR PROCEDURES WITH CC/MCC	1.8308	4.2	6.2
117	No	No	02	SURG	INTRAOCULAR PROCEDURES WITHOUT CC/MCC	1.1984	2.0	2.6
121	No	No	02	MED	ACUTE MAJOR EYE INFECTIONS WITH CC/MCC	1.2812	4.4	6.2
122	No	No	02	MED	ACUTE MAJOR EYE INFECTIONS WITHOUT CC/MCC	0.7445	3.0	3.7
123	No	No	02	MED	NEUROLOGICAL EYE DISORDERS	0.8040	2.1	2.7
124	No	No	02	MED	OTHER DISORDERS OF THE EYE WITH MCC OR THROMBOLYTIC AGENT	1.3219	3.4	5.0
125	No	No	02	MED	OTHER DISORDERS OF THE EYE WITHOUT MCC	0.7975	2.3	3.0
135	No	No	03	SURG	SINUS AND MASTOID PROCEDURES WITH CC/MCC	2.6521	4.2	6.7
136	No	No	03	SURG	SINUS AND MASTOID PROCEDURES WITHOUT CC/MCC	0.9391	1.3	1.5
137	No	No	03	SURG	MOUTH PROCEDURES WITH CC/MCC	1.5047	3.7	5.2
138	No	No	03	SURG	MOUTH PROCEDURES WITHOUT CC/MCC	0.8657	1.6	2.0
139	No	No	03	SURG	SALIVARY GLAND PROCEDURES	1.1877	2.2	3.3
140	No	No	03	SURG	MAJOR HEAD AND NECK PROCEDURES WITH MCC	3.7781	7.0	9.6
141	No	No	03	SURG	MAJOR HEAD AND NECK PROCEDURES WITH CC	2.0717	3.1	4.3
142	No	No	03	SURG	MAJOR HEAD AND NECK PROCEDURES WITHOUT CC/MCC	1.5450	2.0	2.5
143	No	No	03	SURG	OTHER EAR, NOSE, MOUTH AND THROAT O.R. PROCEDURES WITH MCC	3.3256	6.3	9.1
144	No	No	03	SURG	OTHER EAR, NOSE, MOUTH AND THROAT O.R. PROCEDURES WITH CC	1.7305	3.0	4.1
145	No	No	03	SURG	OTHER EAR, NOSE, MOUTH AND THROAT O.R. PROCEDURES WITHOUT CC/MCC	1.2211	1.7	2.1
146	No	No	03	MED	EAR, NOSE, MOUTH AND THROAT MALIGNANCY WITH MCC	2.1110	5.5	8.4
147	No	No	03	MED	EAR, NOSE, MOUTH AND THROAT MALIGNANCY WITH CC	1.2358	3.6	5.1
148	No	No	03	MED	EAR, NOSE, MOUTH AND THROAT MALIGNANCY WITHOUT CC/MCC	0.8897	2.2	2.8
149	No	No	03	MED	DYSEQUILIBRIUM	0.7447	1.9	2.4
150	No	No	03	MED	EPISTAXIS WITH MCC	1.3145	3.4	4.5
151	No	No	03	MED	EPISTAXIS WITHOUT MCC	0.7707	2.2	2.7
152	No	No	03	MED	OTITIS MEDIA AND URI WITH MCC	1.1882	3.2	4.4
153	No	No	03	MED	OTITIS MEDIA AND URI WITHOUT MCC	0.7348	2.3	2.9
154	No	No	03	MED	OTHER EAR, NOSE, MOUTH AND THROAT DIAGNOSES WITH MCC	1.5382	4.2	5.8
155	No	No	03	MED	OTHER EAR, NOSE, MOUTH AND THROAT DIAGNOSES WITH CC	0.9466	2.9	3.7
156	No	No	03	MED	OTHER EAR, NOSE, MOUTH AND THROAT DIAGNOSES WITHOUT CC/MCC	0.6555	2.1	2.6
157	No	No	03	MED	DENTAL AND ORAL DISEASES WITH MCC	1.7070	4.7	6.7
158	No	No	03	MED	DENTAL AND ORAL DISEASES WITH CC	0.9385	2.9	3.6
159	No	No	03	MED	DENTAL AND ORAL DISEASES WITHOUT CC/MCC	0.6752	2.0	2.5
163	Yes	No	04	SURG	MAJOR CHEST PROCEDURES WITH MCC	4.7136	7.5	10.3
164	Yes	No	04	SURG	MAJOR CHEST PROCEDURES WITH CC	2.5504	3.7	4.7
165	Yes	No	04	SURG	MAJOR CHEST PROCEDURES WITHOUT CC/MCC	1.8764	2.2	2.7
166	Yes	No	04	SURG	OTHER RESPIRATORY SYSTEM O.R. PROCEDURES WITH MCC	4.0578	8.4	11.9
167	Yes	No	04	SURG	OTHER RESPIRATORY SYSTEM O.R. PROCEDURES WITH CC	1.8198	3.5	4.8
168	Yes	No	04	SURG	OTHER RESPIRATORY SYSTEM O.R. PROCEDURES WITHOUT CC/MCC	1.3557	1.8	2.3
173	No	No	04	SURG	ULTRASOUND ACCELERATED AND OTHER THROMBOLYSIS WITH PRINCIPAL DIAGNOSIS PULMONARY EMBOLISM	3.0750	4.0	4.8
175	Yes	No	04	MED	PULMONARY EMBOLISM WITH MCC OR ACUTE COR PULMONALE	1.4030	4.0	5.2
176	Yes	No	04	MED	PULMONARY EMBOLISM WITHOUT MCC	0.8156	2.5	3.1
177	Yes	No	04	MED	RESPIRATORY INFECTIONS AND INFLAMMATIONS WITH MCC	1.6964	5.0	6.8
178	Yes	No	04	MED	RESPIRATORY INFECTIONS AND INFLAMMATIONS WITH CC	0.9867	3.3	4.3
179	Yes	No	04	MED	RESPIRATORY INFECTIONS AND INFLAMMATIONS WITHOUT CC/MCC	0.7633	2.5	3.3
180	No	No	04	MED	RESPIRATORY NEOPLASMS WITH MCC	1.7382	4.9	6.6
181	No	No	04	MED	RESPIRATORY NEOPLASMS WITH CC	1.1011	3.2	4.2
182	No	No	04	MED	RESPIRATORY NEOPLASMS WITHOUT CC/MCC	0.7590	2.2	2.8
183	No	No	04	MED	MAJOR CHEST TRAUMA WITH MCC	1.5745	4.5	6.0
184	No	No	04	MED	MAJOR CHEST TRAUMA WITH CC	1.0519	3.1	3.8

MS-DRG	Post-Acute DRG	Special Pay DRG	MDC	TYPE	MS-DRG TITLE	RW	GMLOS	AMLOS
185	No	No	04	MED	MAJOR CHEST TRAUMA WITHOUT CC/MCC	0.7557	2.2	2.6
186	Yes	No	04	MED	PLEURAL EFFUSION WITH MCC	1.5521	4.4	5.9
187	Yes	No	04	MED	PLEURAL EFFUSION WITH CC	0.9963	3.1	3.9
188	Yes	No	04	MED	PLEURAL EFFUSION WITHOUT CC/MCC	0.7465	2.3	2.9
189	No	No	04	MED	PULMONARY EDEMA AND RESPIRATORY FAILURE	1.2320	3.6	4.9
190	Yes	No	04	MED	CHRONIC OBSTRUCTIVE PULMONARY DISEASE WITH MCC	1.1020	3.5	4.4
191	Yes	No	04	MED	CHRONIC OBSTRUCTIVE PULMONARY DISEASE WITH CC	0.8490	2.7	3.4
192	Yes	No	04	MED	CHRONIC OBSTRUCTIVE PULMONARY DISEASE WITHOUT CC/MCC	0.6418	2.2	2.7
193	Yes	No	04	MED	SIMPLE PNEUMONIA AND PLEURISY WITH MCC	1.3266	4.1	5.2
194	Yes	No	04	MED	SIMPLE PNEUMONIA AND PLEURISY WITH CC	0.8222	2.9	3.6
195	Yes	No	04	MED	SIMPLE PNEUMONIA AND PLEURISY WITHOUT CC/MCC	0.6256	2.4	2.8
196	Yes	No	04	MED	INTERSTITIAL LUNG DISEASE WITH MCC	1.8954	5.2	7.0
197	Yes	No	04	MED	INTERSTITIAL LUNG DISEASE WITH CC	0.9975	3.0	3.9
198	Yes	No	04	MED	INTERSTITIAL LUNG DISEASE WITHOUT CC/MCC	0.7782	2.3	2.8
199	No	No	04	MED	PNEUMOTHORAX WITH MCC	1.7741	5.1	6.7
200	No	No	04	MED	PNEUMOTHORAX WITH CC	1.0770	3.2	4.1
201	No	No	04	MED	PNEUMOTHORAX WITHOUT CC/MCC	0.7061	2.4	2.9
202	No	No	04	MED	BRONCHITIS AND ASTHMA WITH CC/MCC	0.9575	2.9	3.7
203	No	No	04	MED	BRONCHITIS AND ASTHMA WITHOUT CC/MCC	0.6949	2.2	2.7
204	No	No	04	MED	RESPIRATORY SIGNS AND SYMPTOMS	0.8229	2.1	2.8
205	Yes	No	04	MED	OTHER RESPIRATORY SYSTEM DIAGNOSES WITH MCC	1.8103	4.5	6.4
206	Yes	No	04	MED	OTHER RESPIRATORY SYSTEM DIAGNOSES WITHOUT MCC	0.9135	2.5	3.2
207	Yes	No	04	MED	RESPIRATORY SYSTEM DIAGNOSIS WITH VENTILATOR SUPPORT >96 HOURS	6.9080	14.8	17.4
208	No	No	04	MED	RESPIRATORY SYSTEM DIAGNOSIS WITH VENTILATOR SUPPORT <=96 HOURS	2.7038	5.2	7.7
212	No	No	05	SURG	CONCOMITANT AORTIC AND MITRAL VALVE PROCEDURES	10.7707	12.6	15.7
215	No	No	05	SURG	OTHER HEART ASSIST SYSTEM IMPLANT	10.2148	5.0	9.0
216	Yes	Yes	05	SURG	CARDIAC VALVE AND OTHER MAJOR CARDIOTHORACIC PROCEDURES WITH CARDIAC CATHETERIZATION WITH MCC	9.7053	11.2	14.5
217	Yes	Yes	05	SURG	CARDIAC VALVE AND OTHER MAJOR CARDIOTHORACIC PROCEDURES WITH CARDIAC CATHETERIZATION WITH CC	6.3653	5.2	7.1
218	Yes	Yes	05	SURG	CARDIAC VALVE AND OTHER MAJOR CARDIOTHORACIC PROCEDURES WITH CARDIAC CATHETERIZATION WITHOUT CC/MCC	5.6967	2.2	3.1
219	Yes	Yes	05	SURG	CARDIAC VALVE AND OTHER MAJOR CARDIOTHORACIC PROCEDURES WITHOUT CARDIAC CATHETERIZATION WITH MCC	7.7112	8.7	10.7
220	Yes	Yes	05	SURG	CARDIAC VALVE AND OTHER MAJOR CARDIOTHORACIC PROCEDURES WITHOUT CARDIAC CATHETERIZATION WITH CC	5.2446	5.7	6.3
221	Yes	Yes	05	SURG	CARDIAC VALVE AND OTHER MAJOR CARDIOTHORACIC PROCEDURES WITHOUT CARDIAC CATHETERIZATION WITHOUT CC/MCC	4.6486	3.3	4.0
228	No	No	05	SURG	OTHER CARDIOTHORACIC PROCEDURES WITH MCC	5.0387	6.5	9.1
229	No	No	05	SURG	OTHER CARDIOTHORACIC PROCEDURES WITHOUT MCC	3.1796	2.6	3.4
231	No	No	05	SURG	CORONARY BYPASS WITH PTCA WITH MCC	8.1152	10.3	12.0
232	No	No	05	SURG	CORONARY BYPASS WITH PTCA WITHOUT MCC	5.9486	7.5	8.3
233	Yes	No	05	SURG	CORONARY BYPASS WITH CARDIAC CATHETERIZATION OR OPEN ABLATION WITH MCC	7.7996	11.4	12.8
234	Yes	No	05	SURG	CORONARY BYPASS WITH CARDIAC CATHETERIZATION OR OPEN ABLATION WITHOUT MCC	5.1979	8.1	8.6
235	Yes	No	05	SURG	CORONARY BYPASS WITHOUT CARDIAC CATHETERIZATION WITH MCC	5.8806	8.2	9.5
236	Yes	No	05	SURG	CORONARY BYPASS WITHOUT CARDIAC CATHETERIZATION WITHOUT MCC	4.0412	5.8	6.3
239	Yes	No	05	SURG	AMPUTATION FOR CIRCULATORY SYSTEM DISORDERS EXCEPT UPPER LIMB AND TOE WITH MCC	4.8068	11.1	14.2
240	Yes	No	05	SURG	AMPUTATION FOR CIRCULATORY SYSTEM DISORDERS EXCEPT UPPER LIMB AND TOE WITH CC	2.8092	7.1	8.7
241	Yes	No	05	SURG	AMPUTATION FOR CIRCULATORY SYSTEM DISORDERS EXCEPT UPPER LIMB AND TOE WITHOUT CC/MCC	1.3898	4.2	5.1
242	Yes	No	05	SURG	PERMANENT CARDIAC PACEMAKER IMPLANT WITH MCC	3.4551	5.1	6.7
243	Yes	No	05	SURG	PERMANENT CARDIAC PACEMAKER IMPLANT WITH CC	2.2776	2.9	3.6
244	Yes	No	05	SURG	PERMANENT CARDIAC PACEMAKER IMPLANT WITHOUT CC/MCC	1.8295	2.1	2.4
245	No	No	05	SURG	AICD GENERATOR PROCEDURES	4.5314	4.1	5.8

MS-DRG	Post-Acute DRG	Special Pay DRG	MDC	TYPE	MS-DRG TITLE	RW	GMLOS	AMLOS
250	No	No	05	SURG	PERCUTANEOUS CARDIOVASCULAR PROCEDURES WITHOUT INTRALUMINAL DEVICE WITH MCC	2.3508	3.4	4.8
251	No	No	05	SURG	PERCUTANEOUS CARDIOVASCULAR PROCEDURES WITHOUT INTRALUMINAL DEVICE WITHOUT MCC	1.5869	2.0	2.5
252	No	No	05	SURG	OTHER VASCULAR PROCEDURES WITH MCC	3.3538	5.4	8.0
253	No	No	05	SURG	OTHER VASCULAR PROCEDURES WITH CC	2.5511	3.8	5.2
254	No	No	05	SURG	OTHER VASCULAR PROCEDURES WITHOUT CC/MCC	1.7351	1.9	2.4
255	Yes	No	05	SURG	UPPER LIMB AND TOE AMPUTATION FOR CIRCULATORY SYSTEM DISORDERS WITH MCC	2.7474	7.0	9.1
256	Yes	No	05	SURG	UPPER LIMB AND TOE AMPUTATION FOR CIRCULATORY SYSTEM DISORDERS WITH CC	1.6397	5.0	6.0
257	Yes	No	05	SURG	UPPER LIMB AND TOE AMPUTATION FOR CIRCULATORY SYSTEM DISORDERS WITHOUT CC/MCC	0.9910	3.4	4.0
258	No	No	05	SURG	CARDIAC PACEMAKER DEVICE REPLACEMENT WITH MCC	2.7086	4.7	6.3
259	No	No	05	SURG	CARDIAC PACEMAKER DEVICE REPLACEMENT WITHOUT MCC	1.8666	2.4	3.0
260	No	No	05	SURG	CARDIAC PACEMAKER REVISION EXCEPT DEVICE REPLACEMENT WITH MCC	3.3152	5.7	8.4
261	No	No	05	SURG	CARDIAC PACEMAKER REVISION EXCEPT DEVICE REPLACEMENT WITH CC	1.8818	2.9	3.8
262	No	No	05	SURG	CARDIAC PACEMAKER REVISION EXCEPT DEVICE REPLACEMENT WITHOUT CC/MCC	1.6453	2.3	2.7
263	No	No	05	SURG	VEIN LIGATION AND STRIPPING	2.8252	4.6	6.8
264	Yes	No	05	SURG	OTHER CIRCULATORY SYSTEM O.R. PROCEDURES	3.2660	6.9	9.9
265	No	No	05	SURG	AICD LEAD PROCEDURES	3.5341	4.0	5.6
266	Yes	Yes	05	SURG	ENDOVASCULAR CARDIAC VALVE REPLACEMENT AND SUPPLEMENT PROCEDURES WITH MCC	6.2461	2.7	4.9
267	Yes	Yes	05	SURG	ENDOVASCULAR CARDIAC VALVE REPLACEMENT AND SUPPLEMENT PROCEDURES WITHOUT MCC	4.8802	1.3	1.6
268	No	No	05	SURG	AORTIC AND HEART ASSIST PROCEDURES EXCEPT PULSATION BALLOON WITH MCC	6.8547	6.1	9.5
269	No	No	05	SURG	AORTIC AND HEART ASSIST PROCEDURES EXCEPT PULSATION BALLOON WITHOUT MCC	4.1586	1.5	2.1
270	No	No	05	SURG	OTHER MAJOR CARDIOVASCULAR PROCEDURES WITH MCC	5.0569	6.5	9.5
271	No	No	05	SURG	OTHER MAJOR CARDIOVASCULAR PROCEDURES WITH CC	3.4562	4.0	5.4
272	No	No	05	SURG	OTHER MAJOR CARDIOVASCULAR PROCEDURES WITHOUT CC/MCC	2.4395	1.9	2.4
273	No	No	05	SURG	PERCUTANEOUS AND OTHER INTRACARDIAC PROCEDURES WITH MCC	3.8970	3.6	5.5
274	No	No	05	SURG	PERCUTANEOUS AND OTHER INTRACARDIAC PROCEDURES WITHOUT MCC	3.2408	1.2	1.5
275	No	No	05	SURG	CARDIAC DEFIBRILLATOR IMPLANT WITH CARDIAC CATHETERIZATION AND MCC	7.0358	8.0	9.9
276	Yes	Yes	05	SURG	CARDIAC DEFIBRILLATOR IMPLANT WITH MCC	6.2102	6.3	8.3
277	Yes	Yes	05	SURG	CARDIAC DEFIBRILLATOR IMPLANT WITHOUT MCC	4.7824	3.3	4.2
278	No	No	05	SURG	ULTRASOUND ACCELERATED AND OTHER THROMBOLYSIS OF PERIPHERAL VASCULAR STRUCTURES WITH MCC	4.4604	6.3	8.5
279	No	No	05	SURG	ULTRASOUND ACCELERATED AND OTHER THROMBOLYSIS OF PERIPHERAL VASCULAR STRUCTURES WITHOUT MCC	3.2006	3.1	4.3
280	Yes	No	05	MED	ACUTE MYOCARDIAL INFARCTION, DISCHARGED ALIVE WITH MCC	1.5865	4.2	5.5
281	Yes	No	05	MED	ACUTE MYOCARDIAL INFARCTION, DISCHARGED ALIVE WITH CC	0.9130	2.4	3.0
282	Yes	No	05	MED	ACUTE MYOCARDIAL INFARCTION, DISCHARGED ALIVE WITHOUT CC/MCC	0.7181	1.8	2.1
283	No	No	05	MED	ACUTE MYOCARDIAL INFARCTION, EXPIRED WITH MCC	1.9714	3.2	5.4
284	No	No	05	MED	ACUTE MYOCARDIAL INFARCTION, EXPIRED WITH CC	0.7397	1.7	2.4
285	No	No	05	MED	ACUTE MYOCARDIAL INFARCTION, EXPIRED WITHOUT CC/MCC	0.4887	1.2	1.4
286	No	No	05	MED	CIRCULATORY DISORDERS EXCEPT AMI, WITH CARDIAC CATHETERIZATION WITH MCC	2.1556	5.4	7.2
287	No	No	05	MED	CIRCULATORY DISORDERS EXCEPT AMI, WITH CARDIAC CATHETERIZATION WITHOUT MCC	1.0816	2.2	2.7
288	Yes	No	05	MED	ACUTE AND SUBACUTE ENDOCARDITIS WITH MCC	2.5930	7.7	9.9
289	Yes	No	05	MED	ACUTE AND SUBACUTE ENDOCARDITIS WITH CC	1.4777	5.1	6.2
290	Yes	No	05	MED	ACUTE AND SUBACUTE ENDOCARDITIS WITHOUT CC/MCC	1.0252	3.4	4.3
291	Yes	No	05	MED	HEART FAILURE AND SHOCK WITH MCC	1.2839	3.9	5.1
292	Yes	No	05	MED	HEART FAILURE AND SHOCK WITH CC	0.8565	3.0	3.9
293	Yes	No	05	MED	HEART FAILURE AND SHOCK WITHOUT CC/MCC	0.5615	2.1	2.6
294	No	No	05	MED	DEEP VEIN THROMBOPHLEBITIS WITH CC/MCC	1.0937	3.5	4.7
295	No	No	05	MED	DEEP VEIN THROMBOPHLEBITIS WITHOUT CC/MCC	0.6315	2.4	2.8
296	No	No	05	MED	CARDIAC ARREST, UNEXPLAINED WITH MCC	1.6032	2.0	3.3
297	No	No	05	MED	CARDIAC ARREST, UNEXPLAINED WITH CC	0.7286	1.3	1.6
298	No	No	05	MED	CARDIAC ARREST, UNEXPLAINED WITHOUT CC/MCC	0.4389	1.1	1.1

MS-DRG	Post-Acute DRG	Special Pay DRG	MDC	TYPE	MS-DRG TITLE	RW	GMLOS	AMLOS
299	Yes	No	05	MED	PERIPHERAL VASCULAR DISORDERS WITH MCC	1.5762	4.0	5.6
300	Yes	No	05	MED	PERIPHERAL VASCULAR DISORDERS WITH CC	1.0670	3.1	4.0
301	Yes	No	05	MED	PERIPHERAL VASCULAR DISORDERS WITHOUT CC/MCC	0.7098	2.1	2.6
302	No	No	05	MED	ATHEROSCLEROSIS WITH MCC	1.1211	2.8	3.9
303	No	No	05	MED	ATHEROSCLEROSIS WITHOUT MCC	0.6581	1.8	2.2
304	No	No	05	MED	HYPERTENSION WITH MCC	1.1490	3.0	4.2
305	No	No	05	MED	HYPERTENSION WITHOUT MCC	0.7535	2.1	2.7
306	No	No	05	MED	CARDIAC CONGENITAL AND VALVULAR DISORDERS WITH MCC	1.5368	3.8	5.3
307	No	No	05	MED	CARDIAC CONGENITAL AND VALVULAR DISORDERS WITHOUT MCC	0.9426	2.2	3.0
308	No	No	05	MED	CARDIAC ARRHYTHMIA AND CONDUCTION DISORDERS WITH MCC	1.2022	3.5	4.7
309	No	No	05	MED	CARDIAC ARRHYTHMIA AND CONDUCTION DISORDERS WITH CC	0.7447	2.3	2.9
310	No	No	05	MED	CARDIAC ARRHYTHMIA AND CONDUCTION DISORDERS WITHOUT CC/MCC	0.5530	1.8	2.1
311	No	No	05	MED	ANGINA PECTORIS	0.6981	2.0	2.5
312	No	No	05	MED	SYNCOPE AND COLLAPSE	0.8635	2.4	3.1
313	No	No	05	MED	CHEST PAIN	0.7236	1.7	2.2
314	Yes	No	05	MED	OTHER CIRCULATORY SYSTEM DIAGNOSES WITH MCC	2.0935	5.1	7.1
315	Yes	No	05	MED	OTHER CIRCULATORY SYSTEM DIAGNOSES WITH CC	0.9673	2.7	3.5
316	Yes	No	05	MED	OTHER CIRCULATORY SYSTEM DIAGNOSES WITHOUT CC/MCC	0.6927	1.8	2.2
319	No	No	05	SURG	OTHER ENDOVASCULAR CARDIAC VALVE PROCEDURES WITH MCC	4.3619	7.8	10.4
320	No	No	05	SURG	OTHER ENDOVASCULAR CARDIAC VALVE PROCEDURES WITHOUT MCC	2.2260	2.2	3.1
321	No	No	05	SURG	PERCUTANEOUS CARDIOVASCULAR PROCEDURES WITH INTRALUMINAL DEVICE WITH MCC OR 4+ ARTERIES/INTRALUMINAL DEVICES	2.8747	3.8	5.2
322	No	No	05	SURG	PERCUTANEOUS CARDIOVASCULAR PROCEDURES WITH INTRALUMINAL DEVICE WITHOUT MCC	1.8234	2.0	2.4
323	No	No	05	SURG	CORONARY INTRAVASCULAR LITHOTRIPSY WITH INTRALUMINAL DEVICE WITH MCC	4.1400	4.6	6.3
324	No	No	05	SURG	CORONARY INTRAVASCULAR LITHOTRIPSY WITH INTRALUMINAL DEVICE WITHOUT MCC	2.9686	2.3	2.9
325	No	No	05	SURG	CORONARY INTRAVASCULAR LITHOTRIPSY WITHOUT INTRALUMINAL DEVICE	2.6443	2.6	3.4
326	Yes	No	06	SURG	STOMACH, ESOPHAGEAL AND DUODENAL PROCEDURES WITH MCC	5.0790	9.4	13.0
327	Yes	No	06	SURG	STOMACH, ESOPHAGEAL AND DUODENAL PROCEDURES WITH CC	2.4974	4.3	6.0
328	Yes	No	06	SURG	STOMACH, ESOPHAGEAL AND DUODENAL PROCEDURES WITHOUT CC/MCC	1.5973	2.1	2.7
329	Yes	No	06	SURG	MAJOR SMALL AND LARGE BOWEL PROCEDURES WITH MCC	4.5168	9.8	12.7
330	Yes	No	06	SURG	MAJOR SMALL AND LARGE BOWEL PROCEDURES WITH CC	2.3721	5.1	6.4
331	Yes	No	06	SURG	MAJOR SMALL AND LARGE BOWEL PROCEDURES WITHOUT CC/MCC	1.6720	2.9	3.4
332	Yes	No	06	SURG	RECTAL RESECTION WITH MCC	3.6276	6.7	9.0
333	Yes	No	06	SURG	RECTAL RESECTION WITH CC	2.0795	3.4	4.4
334	Yes	No	06	SURG	RECTAL RESECTION WITHOUT CC/MCC	1.6051	2.3	2.7
335	Yes	No	06	SURG	PERITONEAL ADHESIOLYSIS WITH MCC	3.5750	8.9	11.2
336	Yes	No	06	SURG	PERITONEAL ADHESIOLYSIS WITH CC	2.1053	5.5	6.8
337	Yes	No	06	SURG	PERITONEAL ADHESIOLYSIS WITHOUT CC/MCC	1.4964	3.4	4.2
344	No	No	06	SURG	MINOR SMALL AND LARGE BOWEL PROCEDURES WITH MCC	2.7404	7.1	9.8
345	No	No	06	SURG	MINOR SMALL AND LARGE BOWEL PROCEDURES WITH CC	1.5406	4.2	5.3
346	No	No	06	SURG	MINOR SMALL AND LARGE BOWEL PROCEDURES WITHOUT CC/MCC	1.2878	2.9	3.4
347	No	No	06	SURG	ANAL AND STOMAL PROCEDURES WITH MCC	2.5491	5.6	7.8
348	No	No	06	SURG	ANAL AND STOMAL PROCEDURES WITH CC	1.3014	3.1	4.1
349	No	No	06	SURG	ANAL AND STOMAL PROCEDURES WITHOUT CC/MCC	0.9758	1.8	2.2
350	No	No	06	SURG	INGUINAL AND FEMORAL HERNIA PROCEDURES WITH MCC	2.4000	4.8	6.5
351	No	No	06	SURG	INGUINAL AND FEMORAL HERNIA PROCEDURES WITH CC	1.4556	3.0	3.8
352	No	No	06	SURG	INGUINAL AND FEMORAL HERNIA PROCEDURES WITHOUT CC/MCC	1.1090	2.0	2.4
353	No	No	06	SURG	HERNIA PROCEDURES EXCEPT INGUINAL AND FEMORAL WITH MCC	2.9243	6.0	8.1
354	No	No	06	SURG	HERNIA PROCEDURES EXCEPT INGUINAL AND FEMORAL WITH CC	1.7178	3.5	4.4
355	No	No	06	SURG	HERNIA PROCEDURES EXCEPT INGUINAL AND FEMORAL WITHOUT CC/MCC	1.3626	2.3	2.7
356	Yes	No	06	SURG	OTHER DIGESTIVE SYSTEM O.R. PROCEDURES WITH MCC	4.2787	8.0	11.0
357	Yes	No	06	SURG	OTHER DIGESTIVE SYSTEM O.R. PROCEDURES WITH CC	2.1968	4.4	5.7

MS-DRG	Post-Acute DRG	Special Pay DRG	MDC	TYPE	MS-DRG TITLE	RW	GMLOS	AMLOS
358	Yes	No	06	SURG	OTHER DIGESTIVE SYSTEM O.R. PROCEDURES WITHOUT CC/MCC	1.2811	2.5	3.2
368	No	No	06	MED	MAJOR ESOPHAGEAL DISORDERS WITH MCC	1.6520	4.2	5.6
369	No	No	06	MED	MAJOR ESOPHAGEAL DISORDERS WITH CC	0.9883	3.0	3.7
370	No	No	06	MED	MAJOR ESOPHAGEAL DISORDERS WITHOUT CC/MCC	0.7437	2.2	2.6
371	Yes	No	06	MED	MAJOR GASTROINTESTINAL DISORDERS AND PERITONEAL INFECTIONS WITH MCC	1.7477	5.4	7.2
372	Yes	No	06	MED	MAJOR GASTROINTESTINAL DISORDERS AND PERITONEAL INFECTIONS WITH CC	1.0423	3.8	4.7
373	Yes	No	06	MED	MAJOR GASTROINTESTINAL DISORDERS AND PERITONEAL INFECTIONS WITHOUT CC/MCC	0.7165	2.8	3.4
374	Yes	No	06	MED	DIGESTIVE MALIGNANCY WITH MCC	2.0990	5.6	7.7
375	Yes	No	06	MED	DIGESTIVE MALIGNANCY WITH CC	1.1983	3.6	4.7
376	Yes	No	06	MED	DIGESTIVE MALIGNANCY WITHOUT CC/MCC	0.8914	2.4	3.0
377	Yes	No	06	MED	GASTROINTESTINAL HEMORRHAGE WITH MCC	1.7903	4.6	6.0
378	Yes	No	06	MED	GASTROINTESTINAL HEMORRHAGE WITH CC	0.9838	3.0	3.6
379	Yes	No	06	MED	GASTROINTESTINAL HEMORRHAGE WITHOUT CC/MCC	0.6332	2.1	2.4
380	Yes	No	06	MED	COMPLICATED PEPTIC ULCER WITH MCC	1.9485	5.1	6.7
381	Yes	No	06	MED	COMPLICATED PEPTIC ULCER WITH CC	1.0730	3.2	3.9
382	Yes	No	06	MED	COMPLICATED PEPTIC ULCER WITHOUT CC/MCC	0.7571	2.4	2.9
383	No	No	06	MED	UNCOMPLICATED PEPTIC ULCER WITH MCC	1.3982	3.8	4.9
384	No	No	06	MED	UNCOMPLICATED PEPTIC ULCER WITHOUT MCC	0.8757	2.6	3.2
385	No	No	06	MED	INFLAMMATORY BOWEL DISEASE WITH MCC	1.5669	5.0	6.7
386	No	No	06	MED	INFLAMMATORY BOWEL DISEASE WITH CC	0.9716	3.4	4.3
387	No	No	06	MED	INFLAMMATORY BOWEL DISEASE WITHOUT CC/MCC	0.6841	2.6	3.2
388	Yes	No	06	MED	GASTROINTESTINAL OBSTRUCTION WITH MCC	1.4535	4.6	6.1
389	Yes	No	06	MED	GASTROINTESTINAL OBSTRUCTION WITH CC	0.7964	3.1	3.8
390	Yes	No	06	MED	GASTROINTESTINAL OBSTRUCTION WITHOUT CC/MCC	0.5590	2.3	2.7
391	No	No	06	MED	ESOPHAGITIS, GASTROENTERITIS AND MISCELLANEOUS DIGESTIVE DISORDERS WITH MCC	1.2757	3.9	5.3
392	No	No	06	MED	ESOPHAGITIS, GASTROENTERITIS AND MISCELLANEOUS DIGESTIVE DISORDERS WITHOUT MCC	0.7856	2.6	3.3
393	No	No	06	MED	OTHER DIGESTIVE SYSTEM DIAGNOSES WITH MCC	1.6196	4.4	6.2
394	No	No	06	MED	OTHER DIGESTIVE SYSTEM DIAGNOSES WITH CC	0.9369	3.0	3.8
395	No	No	06	MED	OTHER DIGESTIVE SYSTEM DIAGNOSES WITHOUT CC/MCC	0.6475	2.1	2.6
397	No	No	06	SURG	APPENDIX PROCEDURES WITH MCC	2.2466	4.7	6.4
398	No	No	06	SURG	APPENDIX PROCEDURES WITH CC	1.5133	3.1	4.0
399	No	No	06	SURG	APPENDIX PROCEDURES WITHOUT CC/MCC	1.1131	1.9	2.3
405	Yes	No	07	SURG	PANCREAS, LIVER AND SHUNT PROCEDURES WITH MCC	5.5052	9.0	12.6
406	Yes	No	07	SURG	PANCREAS, LIVER AND SHUNT PROCEDURES WITH CC	2.8874	5.0	6.2
407	Yes	No	07	SURG	PANCREAS, LIVER AND SHUNT PROCEDURES WITHOUT CC/MCC	2.1510	3.5	4.2
408	No	No	07	SURG	BILIARY TRACT PROCEDURES EXCEPT ONLY CHOLECYSTECTOMY WITH OR WITHOUT C.D.E. WITH MCC	3.7222	8.1	10.9
409	No	No	07	SURG	BILIARY TRACT PROCEDURES EXCEPT ONLY CHOLECYSTECTOMY WITH OR WITHOUT C.D.E. WITH CC	1.9573	4.6	5.7
410	No	No	07	SURG	BILIARY TRACT PROCEDURES EXCEPT ONLY CHOLECYSTECTOMY WITH OR WITHOUT C.D.E. WITHOUT CC/MCC	1.5652	3.1	3.6
411	No	No	07	SURG	CHOLECYSTECTOMY WITH C.D.E. WITH MCC	2.8805	6.2	8.1
412	No	No	07	SURG	CHOLECYSTECTOMY WITH C.D.E. WITH CC	2.0455	4.1	5.0
413	No	No	07	SURG	CHOLECYSTECTOMY WITH C.D.E. WITHOUT CC/MCC	1.5096	2.5	2.9
414	Yes	No	07	SURG	CHOLECYSTECTOMY EXCEPT BY LAPAROSCOPE WITHOUT C.D.E. WITH MCC	3.5252	7.6	9.9
415	Yes	No	07	SURG	CHOLECYSTECTOMY EXCEPT BY LAPAROSCOPE WITHOUT C.D.E. WITH CC	1.9758	4.7	5.7
416	Yes	No	07	SURG	CHOLECYSTECTOMY EXCEPT BY LAPAROSCOPE WITHOUT C.D.E. WITHOUT CC/MCC	1.3392	2.8	3.4
417	No	No	07	SURG	LAPAROSCOPIC CHOLECYSTECTOMY WITHOUT C.D.E. WITH MCC	2.3178	4.9	6.3
418	No	No	07	SURG	LAPAROSCOPIC CHOLECYSTECTOMY WITHOUT C.D.E. WITH CC	1.6347	3.4	4.1
419	No	No	07	SURG	LAPAROSCOPIC CHOLECYSTECTOMY WITHOUT C.D.E. WITHOUT CC/MCC	1.3132	2.3	2.7
420	No	No	07	SURG	HEPATOBILIARY DIAGNOSTIC PROCEDURES WITH MCC	3.2008	7.1	9.9
421	No	No	07	SURG	HEPATOBILIARY DIAGNOSTIC PROCEDURES WITH CC	1.7096	3.7	4.8
422	No	No	07	SURG	HEPATOBILIARY DIAGNOSTIC PROCEDURES WITHOUT CC/MCC	1.4110	2.4	3.1

MS-DRG	Post-Acute DRG	Special Pay DRG	MDC	TYPE	MS-DRG TITLE	RW	GMLOS	AMLOS
423	No	No	07	SURG	OTHER HEPATOBILIARY OR PANCREAS O.R. PROCEDURES WITH MCC	3.9109	8.0	11.0
424	No	No	07	SURG	OTHER HEPATOBILIARY OR PANCREAS O.R. PROCEDURES WITH CC	2.0873	4.5	6.0
425	No	No	07	SURG	OTHER HEPATOBILIARY OR PANCREAS O.R. PROCEDURES WITHOUT CC/MCC	1.6019	2.4	3.3
432	No	No	07	MED	CIRRHOSIS AND ALCOHOLIC HEPATITIS WITH MCC	1.9160	4.9	6.8
433	No	No	07	MED	CIRRHOSIS AND ALCOHOLIC HEPATITIS WITH CC	1.0310	3.3	4.3
434	No	No	07	MED	CIRRHOSIS AND ALCOHOLIC HEPATITIS WITHOUT CC/MCC	0.6695	2.3	2.8
435	No	No	07	MED	MALIGNANCY OF HEPATOBILIARY SYSTEM OR PANCREAS WITH MCC	1.7599	4.8	6.4
436	No	No	07	MED	MALIGNANCY OF HEPATOBILIARY SYSTEM OR PANCREAS WITH CC	1.1007	3.4	4.4
437	No	No	07	MED	MALIGNANCY OF HEPATOBILIARY SYSTEM OR PANCREAS WITHOUT CC/MCC	0.8311	2.4	2.9
438	No	No	07	MED	DISORDERS OF PANCREAS EXCEPT MALIGNANCY WITH MCC	1.6688	4.7	6.6
439	No	No	07	MED	DISORDERS OF PANCREAS EXCEPT MALIGNANCY WITH CC	0.8552	3.1	3.8
440	No	No	07	MED	DISORDERS OF PANCREAS EXCEPT MALIGNANCY WITHOUT CC/MCC	0.6156	2.4	2.8
441	Yes	No	07	MED	DISORDERS OF LIVER EXCEPT MALIGNANCY, CIRRHOSIS OR ALCOHOLIC HEPATITIS WITH MCC	1.8282	4.8	6.7
442	Yes	No	07	MED	DISORDERS OF LIVER EXCEPT MALIGNANCY, CIRRHOSIS OR ALCOHOLIC HEPATITIS WITH CC	0.9515	3.2	4.1
443	Yes	No	07	MED	DISORDERS OF LIVER EXCEPT MALIGNANCY, CIRRHOSIS OR ALCOHOLIC HEPATITIS WITHOUT CC/MCC	0.7147	2.5	3.1
444	No	No	07	MED	DISORDERS OF THE BILIARY TRACT WITH MCC	1.6332	4.4	5.9
445	No	No	07	MED	DISORDERS OF THE BILIARY TRACT WITH CC	1.0868	3.1	3.8
446	No	No	07	MED	DISORDERS OF THE BILIARY TRACT WITHOUT CC/MCC	0.8015	2.2	2.6
453	No	No	08	SURG	COMBINED ANTERIOR AND POSTERIOR SPINAL FUSION WITH MCC	8.8614	7.3	9.4
454	No	No	08	SURG	COMBINED ANTERIOR AND POSTERIOR SPINAL FUSION WITH CC	6.1163	3.7	4.4
455	No	No	08	SURG	COMBINED ANTERIOR AND POSTERIOR SPINAL FUSION WITHOUT CC/MCC	4.6056	2.3	2.7
456	No	No	08	SURG	SPINAL FUSION EXCEPT CERVICAL WITH SPINAL CURVATURE, MALIGNANCY, INFECTION OR EXTENSIVE FUSIONS WITH MCC	8.4294	10.6	13.3
457	No	No	08	SURG	SPINAL FUSION EXCEPT CERVICAL WITH SPINAL CURVATURE, MALIGNANCY, INFECTION OR EXTENSIVE FUSIONS WITH CC	6.0753	5.3	6.4
458	No	No	08	SURG	SPINAL FUSION EXCEPT CERVICAL WITH SPINAL CURVATURE, MALIGNANCY, INFECTION OR EXTENSIVE FUSIONS WITHOUT CC/MCC	4.5310	3.0	3.5
459	Yes	No	08	SURG	SPINAL FUSION EXCEPT CERVICAL WITH MCC	6.6323	7.6	9.8
460	Yes	No	08	SURG	SPINAL FUSION EXCEPT CERVICAL WITHOUT MCC	3.6579	2.8	3.5
461	No	No	08	SURG	BILATERAL OR MULTIPLE MAJOR JOINT PROCEDURES OF LOWER EXTREMITY WITH MCC	6.8185	7.4	10.6
462	No	No	08	SURG	BILATERAL OR MULTIPLE MAJOR JOINT PROCEDURES OF LOWER EXTREMITY WITHOUT MCC	2.8463	2.3	2.9
463	Yes	No	08	SURG	WOUND DEBRIDEMENT AND SKIN GRAFT EXCEPT HAND FOR MUSCULOSKELETAL AND CONNECTIVE TISSUE DISORDERS WITH MCC	5.6637	11.1	15.4
464	Yes	No	08	SURG	WOUND DEBRIDEMENT AND SKIN GRAFT EXCEPT HAND FOR MUSCULOSKELETAL AND CONNECTIVE TISSUE DISORDERS WITH CC	3.0014	5.6	7.4
465	Yes	No	08	SURG	WOUND DEBRIDEMENT AND SKIN GRAFT EXCEPT HAND FOR MUSCULOSKELETAL AND CONNECTIVE TISSUE DISORDERS WITHOUT CC/MCC	1.8708	2.4	3.3
466	Yes	No	08	SURG	REVISION OF HIP OR KNEE REPLACEMENT WITH MCC	5.1866	7.2	9.4
467	Yes	No	08	SURG	REVISION OF HIP OR KNEE REPLACEMENT WITH CC	3.4863	3.2	4.3
468	Yes	No	08	SURG	REVISION OF HIP OR KNEE REPLACEMENT WITHOUT CC/MCC	2.6696	1.6	2.0
469	Yes	No	08	SURG	MAJOR HIP AND KNEE JOINT REPLACEMENT OR REATTACHMENT OF LOWER EXTREMITY WITH MCC OR TOTAL ANKLE REPLACEMENT	3.3298	3.5	5.0
470	Yes	No	08	SURG	MAJOR HIP AND KNEE JOINT REPLACEMENT OR REATTACHMENT OF LOWER EXTREMITY WITHOUT MCC	1.8817	1.7	2.0
471	No	No	08	SURG	CERVICAL SPINAL FUSION WITH MCC	4.9190	7.1	9.7
472	No	No	08	SURG	CERVICAL SPINAL FUSION WITH CC	2.9554	2.6	3.6
473	No	No	08	SURG	CERVICAL SPINAL FUSION WITHOUT CC/MCC	2.4606	1.7	2.0
474	Yes	No	08	SURG	AMPUTATION FOR MUSCULOSKELETAL SYSTEM AND CONNECTIVE TISSUE DISORDERS WITH MCC	4.3028	10.1	13.1
475	Yes	No	08	SURG	AMPUTATION FOR MUSCULOSKELETAL SYSTEM AND CONNECTIVE TISSUE DISORDERS WITH CC	2.1447	5.9	7.3
476	Yes	No	08	SURG	AMPUTATION FOR MUSCULOSKELETAL SYSTEM AND CONNECTIVE TISSUE DISORDERS WITHOUT CC/MCC	1.1769	2.7	3.4
477	Yes	Yes	08	SURG	BIOPSIES OF MUSCULOSKELETAL SYSTEM AND CONNECTIVE TISSUE WITH MCC	3.3690	8.8	11.0
478	Yes	Yes	08	SURG	BIOPSIES OF MUSCULOSKELETAL SYSTEM AND CONNECTIVE TISSUE WITH CC	2.3837	5.4	6.8

MS-DRG	Post-Acute DRG	Special Pay DRG	MDC	TYPE	MS-DRG TITLE	RW	GMLOS	AMLOS
479	Yes	Yes	08	SURG	BIOPSIES OF MUSCULOSKELETAL SYSTEM AND CONNECTIVE TISSUE WITHOUT CC/MCC	1.8640	3.3	4.2
480	Yes	Yes	08	SURG	HIP AND FEMUR PROCEDURES EXCEPT MAJOR JOINT WITH MCC	2.9489	6.5	7.9
481	Yes	Yes	08	SURG	HIP AND FEMUR PROCEDURES EXCEPT MAJOR JOINT WITH CC	2.0749	4.5	5.0
482	Yes	Yes	08	SURG	HIP AND FEMUR PROCEDURES EXCEPT MAJOR JOINT WITHOUT CC/MCC	1.5884	3.2	3.6
483	No	No	08	SURG	MAJOR JOINT OR LIMB REATTACHMENT PROCEDURES OF UPPER EXTREMITIES	2.4842	1.7	2.3
485	No	No	08	SURG	KNEE PROCEDURES WITH PRINCIPAL DIAGNOSIS OF INFECTION WITH MCC	3.2940	8.3	10.1
486	No	No	08	SURG	KNEE PROCEDURES WITH PRINCIPAL DIAGNOSIS OF INFECTION WITH CC	2.0083	5.0	5.9
487	No	No	08	SURG	KNEE PROCEDURES WITH PRINCIPAL DIAGNOSIS OF INFECTION WITHOUT CC/MCC	1.5449	3.5	4.1
488	Yes	No	08	SURG	KNEE PROCEDURES WITHOUT PRINCIPAL DIAGNOSIS OF INFECTION WITH CC/MCC	2.1066	3.1	4.5
489	Yes	No	08	SURG	KNEE PROCEDURES WITHOUT PRINCIPAL DIAGNOSIS OF INFECTION WITHOUT CC/MCC	1.2377	1.5	1.9
492	Yes	Yes	08	SURG	LOWER EXTREMITY AND HUMERUS PROCEDURES EXCEPT HIP, FOOT AND FEMUR WITH MCC	3.4621	6.7	8.6
493	Yes	Yes	08	SURG	LOWER EXTREMITY AND HUMERUS PROCEDURES EXCEPT HIP, FOOT AND FEMUR WITH CC	2.4017	4.2	5.2
494	Yes	Yes	08	SURG	LOWER EXTREMITY AND HUMERUS PROCEDURES EXCEPT HIP, FOOT AND FEMUR WITHOUT CC/MCC	1.8692	2.8	3.4
495	Yes	Yes	08	SURG	LOCAL EXCISION AND REMOVAL OF INTERNAL FIXATION DEVICES EXCEPT HIP AND FEMUR WITH MCC	3.5812	7.7	10.5
496	Yes	Yes	08	SURG	LOCAL EXCISION AND REMOVAL OF INTERNAL FIXATION DEVICES EXCEPT HIP AND FEMUR WITH CC	1.9875	3.4	4.6
497	Yes	Yes	08	SURG	LOCAL EXCISION AND REMOVAL OF INTERNAL FIXATION DEVICES EXCEPT HIP AND FEMUR WITHOUT CC/MCC	1.4274	1.8	2.3
498	No	No	08	SURG	LOCAL EXCISION AND REMOVAL OF INTERNAL FIXATION DEVICES OF HIP AND FEMUR WITH CC/MCC	2.6110	5.9	8.4
499	No	No	08	SURG	LOCAL EXCISION AND REMOVAL OF INTERNAL FIXATION DEVICES OF HIP AND FEMUR WITHOUT CC/MCC	1.2898	1.9	2.6
500	Yes	Yes	08	SURG	SOFT TISSUE PROCEDURES WITH MCC	3.2428	7.8	10.6
501	Yes	Yes	08	SURG	SOFT TISSUE PROCEDURES WITH CC	1.7357	4.1	5.3
502	Yes	Yes	08	SURG	SOFT TISSUE PROCEDURES WITHOUT CC/MCC	1.3827	2.3	2.9
503	No	No	08	SURG	FOOT PROCEDURES WITH MCC	2.6819	7.3	9.1
504	No	No	08	SURG	FOOT PROCEDURES WITH CC	1.7271	4.5	5.6
505	No	No	08	SURG	FOOT PROCEDURES WITHOUT CC/MCC	1.7057	2.6	3.2
506	No	No	08	SURG	MAJOR THUMB OR JOINT PROCEDURES	1.4626	4.0	5.1
507	No	No	08	SURG	MAJOR SHOULDER OR ELBOW JOINT PROCEDURES WITH CC/MCC	2.1317	5.5	7.1
508	No	No	08	SURG	MAJOR SHOULDER OR ELBOW JOINT PROCEDURES WITHOUT CC/MCC	1.4340	2.3	2.9
509	No	No	08	SURG	ARTHROSCOPY	1.3262	3.3	4.2
510	Yes	No	08	SURG	SHOULDER, ELBOW OR FOREARM PROCEDURES, EXCEPT MAJOR JOINT PROCEDURES WITH MCC	2.7206	5.0	6.4
511	Yes	No	08	SURG	SHOULDER, ELBOW OR FOREARM PROCEDURES, EXCEPT MAJOR JOINT PROCEDURES WITH CC	1.9938	3.4	4.2
512	Yes	No	08	SURG	SHOULDER, ELBOW OR FOREARM PROCEDURES, EXCEPT MAJOR JOINT PROCEDURES WITHOUT CC/MCC	1.6138	2.2	2.6
513	No	No	08	SURG	HAND OR WRIST PROCEDURES, EXCEPT MAJOR THUMB OR JOINT PROCEDURES WITH CC/MCC	1.6210	3.9	5.5
514	No	No	08	SURG	HAND OR WRIST PROCEDURES, EXCEPT MAJOR THUMB OR JOINT PROCEDURES WITHOUT CC/MCC	1.0415	2.2	2.8
515	Yes	Yes	08	SURG	OTHER MUSCULOSKELETAL SYSTEM AND CONNECTIVE TISSUE O.R. PROCEDURES WITH MCC	3.1615	7.0	9.0
516	Yes	Yes	08	SURG	OTHER MUSCULOSKELETAL SYSTEM AND CONNECTIVE TISSUE O.R. PROCEDURES WITH CC	2.0408	3.9	5.0
517	Yes	Yes	08	SURG	OTHER MUSCULOSKELETAL SYSTEM AND CONNECTIVE TISSUE O.R. PROCEDURES WITHOUT CC/MCC	1.4944	2.3	2.9
518	Yes	Yes	08	SURG	BACK AND NECK PROCEDURES EXCEPT SPINAL FUSION WITH MCC OR DISC DEVICE OR NEUROSTIMULATOR	3.6518	5.5	8.0
519	Yes	Yes	08	SURG	BACK AND NECK PROCEDURES EXCEPT SPINAL FUSION WITH CC	1.9686	3.2	4.2
520	Yes	Yes	08	SURG	BACK AND NECK PROCEDURES EXCEPT SPINAL FUSION WITHOUT CC/MCC	1.4315	2.0	2.5
521	Yes	Yes	08	SURG	HIP REPLACEMENT WITH PRINCIPAL DIAGNOSIS OF HIP FRACTURE WITH MCC	2.9942	6.4	7.7
522	Yes	Yes	08	SURG	HIP REPLACEMENT WITH PRINCIPAL DIAGNOSIS OF HIP FRACTURE WITHOUT MCC	2.1122	4.1	4.6
533	Yes	No	08	MED	FRACTURES OF FEMUR WITH MCC	1.6314	4.6	6.5
534	Yes	No	08	MED	FRACTURES OF FEMUR WITHOUT MCC	0.8100	2.8	3.7
535	Yes	No	08	MED	FRACTURES OF HIP AND PELVIS WITH MCC	1.2967	3.9	5.2

MS-DRG	Post-Acute DRG	Special Pay DRG	MDC	TYPE	MS-DRG TITLE	RW	GMLOS	AMLOS
536	Yes	No	08	MED	FRACTURES OF HIP AND PELVIS WITHOUT MCC	0.7871	2.8	3.4
537	No	No	08	MED	SPRAINS, STRAINS, AND DISLOCATIONS OF HIP, PELVIS AND THIGH WITH CC/MCC	0.9670	3.1	4.0
538	No	No	08	MED	SPRAINS, STRAINS, AND DISLOCATIONS OF HIP, PELVIS AND THIGH WITHOUT CC/MCC	0.7091	2.2	2.7
539	Yes	No	08	MED	OSTEOMYELITIS WITH MCC	1.9844	6.4	8.6
540	Yes	No	08	MED	OSTEOMYELITIS WITH CC	1.2982	4.4	5.7
541	Yes	No	08	MED	OSTEOMYELITIS WITHOUT CC/MCC	0.8579	3.0	3.9
542	Yes	No	08	MED	PATHOLOGICAL FRACTURES AND MUSCULOSKELETAL AND CONNECTIVE TISSUE MALIGNANCY WITH MCC	1.8237	5.2	7.1
543	Yes	No	08	MED	PATHOLOGICAL FRACTURES AND MUSCULOSKELETAL AND CONNECTIVE TISSUE MALIGNANCY WITH CC	1.0907	3.5	4.5
544	Yes	No	08	MED	PATHOLOGICAL FRACTURES AND MUSCULOSKELETAL AND CONNECTIVE TISSUE MALIGNANCY WITHOUT CC/MCC	0.7675	2.6	3.2
545	Yes	No	08	MED	CONNECTIVE TISSUE DISORDERS WITH MCC	2.4932	5.8	8.6
546	Yes	No	08	MED	CONNECTIVE TISSUE DISORDERS WITH CC	1.1993	3.5	4.6
547	Yes	No	08	MED	CONNECTIVE TISSUE DISORDERS WITHOUT CC/MCC	0.8134	2.4	3.0
548	No	No	08	MED	SEPTIC ARTHRITIS WITH MCC	1.9498	6.1	8.4
549	No	No	08	MED	SEPTIC ARTHRITIS WITH CC	1.2062	4.1	5.3
550	No	No	08	MED	SEPTIC ARTHRITIS WITHOUT CC/MCC	0.9208	3.1	3.7
551	Yes	No	08	MED	MEDICAL BACK PROBLEMS WITH MCC	1.7019	4.6	6.2
552	Yes	No	08	MED	MEDICAL BACK PROBLEMS WITHOUT MCC	0.9663	2.9	3.7
553	No	No	08	MED	BONE DISEASES AND ARTHROPATHIES WITH MCC	1.3515	4.2	5.7
554	No	No	08	MED	BONE DISEASES AND ARTHROPATHIES WITHOUT MCC	0.8218	2.8	3.5
555	No	No	08	MED	SIGNS AND SYMPTOMS OF MUSCULOSKELETAL SYSTEM AND CONNECTIVE TISSUE WITH MCC	1.3990	3.9	5.6
556	No	No	08	MED	SIGNS AND SYMPTOMS OF MUSCULOSKELETAL SYSTEM AND CONNECTIVE TISSUE WITHOUT MCC	0.8244	2.6	3.3
557	Yes	No	08	MED	TENDONITIS, MYOSITIS AND BURSITIS WITH MCC	1.5568	5.1	7.0
558	Yes	No	08	MED	TENDONITIS, MYOSITIS AND BURSITIS WITHOUT MCC	0.8784	3.1	3.9
559	Yes	No	08	MED	AFTERCARE, MUSCULOSKELETAL SYSTEM AND CONNECTIVE TISSUE WITH MCC	1.8505	5.1	7.3
560	Yes	No	08	MED	AFTERCARE, MUSCULOSKELETAL SYSTEM AND CONNECTIVE TISSUE WITH CC	1.1321	3.9	5.3
561	Yes	No	08	MED	AFTERCARE, MUSCULOSKELETAL SYSTEM AND CONNECTIVE TISSUE WITHOUT CC/MCC	0.7802	2.7	3.9
562	Yes	No	08	MED	FRACTURE, SPRAIN, STRAIN AND DISLOCATION EXCEPT FEMUR, HIP, PELVIS AND THIGH WITH MCC	1.5207	4.3	5.8
563	Yes	No	08	MED	FRACTURE, SPRAIN, STRAIN AND DISLOCATION EXCEPT FEMUR, HIP, PELVIS AND THIGH WITHOUT MCC	0.8956	2.8	3.5
564	No	No	08	MED	OTHER MUSCULOSKELETAL SYSTEM AND CONNECTIVE TISSUE DIAGNOSES WITH MCC	1.5619	5.0	6.5
565	No	No	08	MED	OTHER MUSCULOSKELETAL SYSTEM AND CONNECTIVE TISSUE DIAGNOSES WITH CC	0.9994	3.3	4.2
566	No	No	08	MED	OTHER MUSCULOSKELETAL SYSTEM AND CONNECTIVE TISSUE DIAGNOSES WITHOUT CC/MCC	0.7505	2.4	3.0
570	Yes	No	09	SURG	SKIN DEBRIDEMENT WITH MCC	2.9222	7.9	10.7
571	Yes	No	09	SURG	SKIN DEBRIDEMENT WITH CC	1.6919	5.1	6.5
572	Yes	No	09	SURG	SKIN DEBRIDEMENT WITHOUT CC/MCC	1.1396	3.0	3.8
573	Yes	No	09	SURG	SKIN GRAFT FOR SKIN ULCER OR CELLULITIS WITH MCC	6.2181	12.2	17.6
574	Yes	No	09	SURG	SKIN GRAFT FOR SKIN ULCER OR CELLULITIS WITH CC	3.4058	8.0	11.3
575	Yes	No	09	SURG	SKIN GRAFT FOR SKIN ULCER OR CELLULITIS WITHOUT CC/MCC	2.0460	4.4	5.7
576	No	No	09	SURG	SKIN GRAFT EXCEPT FOR SKIN ULCER OR CELLULITIS WITH MCC	5.6831	9.3	14.7
577	No	No	09	SURG	SKIN GRAFT EXCEPT FOR SKIN ULCER OR CELLULITIS WITH CC	2.6491	4.6	6.9
578	No	No	09	SURG	SKIN GRAFT EXCEPT FOR SKIN ULCER OR CELLULITIS WITHOUT CC/MCC	1.6105	2.6	3.6
579	Yes	No	09	SURG	OTHER SKIN, SUBCUTANEOUS TISSUE AND BREAST PROCEDURES WITH MCC	3.3422	8.0	11.1
580	Yes	No	09	SURG	OTHER SKIN, SUBCUTANEOUS TISSUE AND BREAST PROCEDURES WITH CC	1.7466	4.1	5.6
581	Yes	No	09	SURG	OTHER SKIN, SUBCUTANEOUS TISSUE AND BREAST PROCEDURES WITHOUT CC/MCC	1.3467	2.1	2.6
582	No	No	09	SURG	MASTECTOMY FOR MALIGNANCY WITH CC/MCC	1.6671	2.4	3.5
583	No	No	09	SURG	MASTECTOMY FOR MALIGNANCY WITHOUT CC/MCC	1.5219	1.7	2.0
584	No	No	09	SURG	BREAST BIOPSY, LOCAL EXCISION AND OTHER BREAST PROCEDURES WITH CC/MCC	1.9586	3.5	4.5
585	No	No	09	SURG	BREAST BIOPSY, LOCAL EXCISION AND OTHER BREAST PROCEDURES WITHOUT CC/MCC	1.6840	2.1	2.4
592	Yes	No	09	MED	SKIN ULCERS WITH MCC	2.0901	5.9	8.7

MS-DRG	Post-Acute DRG	Special Pay DRG	MDC	TYPE	MS-DRG TITLE	RW	GMLOS	AMLOS
593	Yes	No	09	MED	SKIN ULCERS WITH CC	1.2099	4.3	5.7
594	Yes	No	09	MED	SKIN ULCERS WITHOUT CC/MCC	0.7874	3.1	3.9
595	No	No	09	MED	MAJOR SKIN DISORDERS WITH MCC	2.1750	5.7	8.0
596	No	No	09	MED	MAJOR SKIN DISORDERS WITHOUT MCC	1.0090	3.5	4.6
597	No	No	09	MED	MALIGNANT BREAST DISORDERS WITH MCC	1.6005	4.7	6.4
598	No	No	09	MED	MALIGNANT BREAST DISORDERS WITH CC	1.1988	3.4	4.9
599	No	No	09	MED	MALIGNANT BREAST DISORDERS WITHOUT CC/MCC	0.6214	1.9	2.2
600	No	No	09	MED	NON-MALIGNANT BREAST DISORDERS WITH CC/MCC	1.0255	3.4	4.4
601	No	No	09	MED	NON-MALIGNANT BREAST DISORDERS WITHOUT CC/MCC	0.6226	2.5	2.8
602	Yes	No	09	MED	CELLULITIS WITH MCC	1.4875	4.8	6.2
603	Yes	No	09	MED	CELLULITIS WITHOUT MCC	0.8847	3.2	3.9
604	No	No	09	MED	TRAUMA TO THE SKIN, SUBCUTANEOUS TISSUE AND BREAST WITH MCC	1.5062	3.9	5.5
605	No	No	09	MED	TRAUMA TO THE SKIN, SUBCUTANEOUS TISSUE AND BREAST WITHOUT MCC	0.9088	2.6	3.4
606	No	No	09	MED	MINOR SKIN DISORDERS WITH MCC	1.5858	4.7	6.8
607	No	No	09	MED	MINOR SKIN DISORDERS WITHOUT MCC	0.8935	3.0	3.9
614	No	No	10	SURG	ADRENAL AND PITUITARY PROCEDURES WITH CC/MCC	2.2524	2.8	4.1
615	No	No	10	SURG	ADRENAL AND PITUITARY PROCEDURES WITHOUT CC/MCC	1.4711	1.6	1.8
616	Yes	No	10	SURG	AMPUTATION OF LOWER LIMB FOR ENDOCRINE, NUTRITIONAL AND METABOLIC DISORDERS WITH MCC	3.9577	10.1	13.0
617	Yes	No	10	SURG	AMPUTATION OF LOWER LIMB FOR ENDOCRINE, NUTRITIONAL AND METABOLIC DISORDERS WITH CC	1.9845	5.8	7.0
618	Yes	No	10	SURG	AMPUTATION OF LOWER LIMB FOR ENDOCRINE, NUTRITIONAL AND METABOLIC DISORDERS WITHOUT CC/MCC	1.1615	3.4	3.9
619	No	No	10	SURG	O.R. PROCEDURES FOR OBESITY WITH MCC	2.5885	2.6	4.2
620	No	No	10	SURG	O.R. PROCEDURES FOR OBESITY WITH CC	1.6222	1.6	1.9
621	No	No	10	SURG	O.R. PROCEDURES FOR OBESITY WITHOUT CC/MCC	1.5173	1.3	1.4
622	Yes	No	10	SURG	SKIN GRAFTS AND WOUND DEBRIDEMENT FOR ENDOCRINE, NUTRITIONAL AND METABOLIC DISORDERS WITH MCC	3.8256	9.3	12.8
623	Yes	No	10	SURG	SKIN GRAFTS AND WOUND DEBRIDEMENT FOR ENDOCRINE, NUTRITIONAL AND METABOLIC DISORDERS WITH CC	1.8614	5.4	6.7
624	Yes	No	10	SURG	SKIN GRAFTS AND WOUND DEBRIDEMENT FOR ENDOCRINE, NUTRITIONAL AND METABOLIC DISORDERS WITHOUT CC/MCC	1.1145	2.9	3.7
625	No	No	10	SURG	THYROID, PARATHYROID AND THYROGLOSSAL PROCEDURES WITH MCC	2.9212	5.1	8.1
626	No	No	10	SURG	THYROID, PARATHYROID AND THYROGLOSSAL PROCEDURES WITH CC	1.4919	2.0	2.8
627	No	No	10	SURG	THYROID, PARATHYROID AND THYROGLOSSAL PROCEDURES WITHOUT CC/MCC	1.2360	1.3	1.5
628	Yes	No	10	SURG	OTHER ENDOCRINE, NUTRITIONAL AND METABOLIC O.R. PROCEDURES WITH MCC	4.0145	8.4	12.1
629	Yes	No	10	SURG	OTHER ENDOCRINE, NUTRITIONAL AND METABOLIC O.R. PROCEDURES WITH CC	2.2628	6.2	7.4
630	Yes	No	10	SURG	OTHER ENDOCRINE, NUTRITIONAL AND METABOLIC O.R. PROCEDURES WITHOUT CC/MCC	1.3963	2.1	2.8
637	Yes	No	10	MED	DIABETES WITH MCC	1.4493	4.1	5.6
638	Yes	No	10	MED	DIABETES WITH CC	0.8994	3.0	3.8
639	Yes	No	10	MED	DIABETES WITHOUT CC/MCC	0.6225	2.1	2.5
640	Yes	No	10	MED	MISCELLANEOUS DISORDERS OF NUTRITION, METABOLISM, FLUIDS AND ELECTROLYTES WITH MCC	1.3152	3.6	5.2
641	Yes	No	10	MED	MISCELLANEOUS DISORDERS OF NUTRITION, METABOLISM, FLUIDS AND ELECTROLYTES WITHOUT MCC	0.7814	2.6	3.4
642	No	No	10	MED	INBORN AND OTHER DISORDERS OF METABOLISM	1.3033	3.4	4.7
643	Yes	No	10	MED	ENDOCRINE DISORDERS WITH MCC	1.6451	5.1	6.6
644	Yes	No	10	MED	ENDOCRINE DISORDERS WITH CC	1.0617	3.6	4.5
645	Yes	No	10	MED	ENDOCRINE DISORDERS WITHOUT CC/MCC	0.7609	2.7	3.2
650	No	No	11	SURG	KIDNEY TRANSPLANT WITH HEMODIALYSIS WITH MCC	4.4975	6.4	7.9
651	No	No	11	SURG	KIDNEY TRANSPLANT WITH HEMODIALYSIS WITHOUT MCC	3.4584	5.4	6.1
652	No	No	11	SURG	KIDNEY TRANSPLANT	3.0044	4.4	4.9
653	Yes	No	11	SURG	MAJOR BLADDER PROCEDURES WITH MCC	5.4136	10.1	13.3
654	Yes	No	11	SURG	MAJOR BLADDER PROCEDURES WITH CC	2.7375	5.3	6.4

MS-DRG	Post-Acute DRG	Special Pay DRG	MDC	TYPE	MS-DRG TITLE	RW	GMLOS	AMLOS
655	Yes	No	11	SURG	MAJOR BLADDER PROCEDURES WITHOUT CC/MCC	2.1078	3.3	4.0
656	No	No	11	SURG	KIDNEY AND URETER PROCEDURES FOR NEOPLASM WITH MCC	3.1376	5.2	7.4
657	No	No	11	SURG	KIDNEY AND URETER PROCEDURES FOR NEOPLASM WITH CC	1.8442	2.8	3.5
658	No	No	11	SURG	KIDNEY AND URETER PROCEDURES FOR NEOPLASM WITHOUT CC/MCC	1.4804	1.7	2.0
659	Yes	No	11	SURG	KIDNEY AND URETER PROCEDURES FOR NON-NEOPLASM WITH MCC	2.5889	5.9	8.2
660	Yes	No	11	SURG	KIDNEY AND URETER PROCEDURES FOR NON-NEOPLASM WITH CC	1.3459	2.9	3.8
661	Yes	No	11	SURG	KIDNEY AND URETER PROCEDURES FOR NON-NEOPLASM WITHOUT CC/MCC	1.0484	1.8	2.2
662	No	No	11	SURG	MINOR BLADDER PROCEDURES WITH MCC	2.9967	7.1	10.0
663	No	No	11	SURG	MINOR BLADDER PROCEDURES WITH CC	1.4590	3.5	4.7
664	No	No	11	SURG	MINOR BLADDER PROCEDURES WITHOUT CC/MCC	1.0616	1.8	2.2
665	No	No	11	SURG	PROSTATECTOMY WITH MCC	3.0891	7.9	10.6
666	No	No	11	SURG	PROSTATECTOMY WITH CC	1.7174	3.8	5.0
667	No	No	11	SURG	PROSTATECTOMY WITHOUT CC/MCC	1.0496	2.0	2.6
668	No	No	11	SURG	TRANSURETHRAL PROCEDURES WITH MCC	2.8180	7.2	9.8
669	No	No	11	SURG	TRANSURETHRAL PROCEDURES WITH CC	1.5346	3.8	5.0
670	No	No	11	SURG	TRANSURETHRAL PROCEDURES WITHOUT CC/MCC	0.9626	2.0	2.5
671	No	No	11	SURG	URETHRAL PROCEDURES WITH CC/MCC	1.7119	3.9	5.6
672	No	No	11	SURG	URETHRAL PROCEDURES WITHOUT CC/MCC	0.9227	1.5	1.8
673	No	No	11	SURG	OTHER KIDNEY AND URINARY TRACT PROCEDURES WITH MCC	3.6980	8.8	12.2
674	No	No	11	SURG	OTHER KIDNEY AND URINARY TRACT PROCEDURES WITH CC	2.3822	6.1	7.8
675	No	No	11	SURG	OTHER KIDNEY AND URINARY TRACT PROCEDURES WITHOUT CC/MCC	1.5865	2.7	3.6
682	Yes	No	11	MED	RENAL FAILURE WITH MCC	1.5008	4.4	6.0
683	Yes	No	11	MED	RENAL FAILURE WITH CC	0.9008	3.1	3.9
684	Yes	No	11	MED	RENAL FAILURE WITHOUT CC/MCC	0.6085	2.2	2.7
686	No	No	11	MED	KIDNEY AND URINARY TRACT NEOPLASMS WITH MCC	1.8394	5.3	7.3
687	No	No	11	MED	KIDNEY AND URINARY TRACT NEOPLASMS WITH CC	1.0453	3.3	4.3
688	No	No	11	MED	KIDNEY AND URINARY TRACT NEOPLASMS WITHOUT CC/MCC	0.7809	1.9	2.4
689	Yes	No	11	MED	KIDNEY AND URINARY TRACT INFECTIONS WITH MCC	1.1744	3.9	5.2
690	Yes	No	11	MED	KIDNEY AND URINARY TRACT INFECTIONS WITHOUT MCC	0.8069	2.9	3.6
693	No	No	11	MED	URINARY STONES WITH MCC	1.4163	3.8	5.4
694	No	No	11	MED	URINARY STONES WITHOUT MCC	0.7827	2.1	2.7
695	No	No	11	MED	KIDNEY AND URINARY TRACT SIGNS AND SYMPTOMS WITH MCC	1.1960	3.7	4.9
696	No	No	11	MED	KIDNEY AND URINARY TRACT SIGNS AND SYMPTOMS WITHOUT MCC	0.6921	2.3	2.9
697	No	No	11	MED	URETHRAL STRICTURE	1.1131	2.7	3.7
698	Yes	No	11	MED	OTHER KIDNEY AND URINARY TRACT DIAGNOSES WITH MCC	1.6544	4.9	6.4
699	Yes	No	11	MED	OTHER KIDNEY AND URINARY TRACT DIAGNOSES WITH CC	1.0208	3.3	4.2
700	Yes	No	11	MED	OTHER KIDNEY AND URINARY TRACT DIAGNOSES WITHOUT CC/MCC	0.7083	2.3	2.8
707	No	No	12	SURG	MAJOR MALE PELVIC PROCEDURES WITH CC/MCC	1.9619	2.2	3.2
708	No	No	12	SURG	MAJOR MALE PELVIC PROCEDURES WITHOUT CC/MCC	1.4585	1.4	1.6
709	No	No	12	SURG	PENIS PROCEDURES WITH CC/MCC	2.1200	4.3	6.8
710	No	No	12	SURG	PENIS PROCEDURES WITHOUT CC/MCC	1.2343	1.7	2.3
711	No	No	12	SURG	TESTES PROCEDURES WITH CC/MCC	2.1229	5.1	7.1
712	No	No	12	SURG	TESTES PROCEDURES WITHOUT CC/MCC	1.1884	2.6	3.6
713	No	No	12	SURG	TRANSURETHRAL PROSTATECTOMY WITH CC/MCC	1.4507	2.6	3.9
714	No	No	12	SURG	TRANSURETHRAL PROSTATECTOMY WITHOUT CC/MCC	0.9585	1.5	1.7
715	No	No	12	SURG	OTHER MALE REPRODUCTIVE SYSTEM O.R. PROCEDURES FOR MALIGNANCY WITH CC/MCC	2.2075	5.4	7.7
716	No	No	12	SURG	OTHER MALE REPRODUCTIVE SYSTEM O.R. PROCEDURES FOR MALIGNANCY WITHOUT CC/MCC	1.4222	1.5	1.9
717	No	No	12	SURG	OTHER MALE REPRODUCTIVE SYSTEM O.R. PROCEDURES EXCEPT MALIGNANCY WITH CC/MCC	1.8137	3.5	5.3
718	No	No	12	SURG	OTHER MALE REPRODUCTIVE SYSTEM O.R. PROCEDURES EXCEPT MALIGNANCY WITHOUT CC/MCC	1.1758	1.8	2.3
722	No	No	12	MED	MALIGNANCY, MALE REPRODUCTIVE SYSTEM WITH MCC	1.8748	5.5	7.8
723	No	No	12	MED	MALIGNANCY, MALE REPRODUCTIVE SYSTEM WITH CC	1.1143	3.5	4.7

MS-DRG	Post-Acute DRG	Special Pay DRG	MDC	TYPE	MS-DRG TITLE	RW	GMLOS	AMLOS
724	No	No	12	MED	MALIGNANCY, MALE REPRODUCTIVE SYSTEM WITHOUT CC/MCC	0.8095	2.0	3.4
725	No	No	12	MED	BENIGN PROSTATIC HYPERTROPHY WITH MCC	1.2409	4.1	5.6
726	No	No	12	MED	BENIGN PROSTATIC HYPERTROPHY WITHOUT MCC	0.7309	2.4	3.1
727	No	No	12	MED	INFLAMMATION OF THE MALE REPRODUCTIVE SYSTEM WITH MCC	1.6210	4.9	6.8
728	No	No	12	MED	INFLAMMATION OF THE MALE REPRODUCTIVE SYSTEM WITHOUT MCC	0.8001	2.9	3.6
729	No	No	12	MED	OTHER MALE REPRODUCTIVE SYSTEM DIAGNOSES WITH CC/MCC	1.0039	3.0	3.9
730	No	No	12	MED	OTHER MALE REPRODUCTIVE SYSTEM DIAGNOSES WITHOUT CC/MCC	0.6216	1.9	2.3
734	No	No	13	SURG	PELVIC EVISCERATION, RADICAL HYSTERECTOMY AND RADICAL VULVECTOMY WITH CC/MCC	2.1736	3.4	4.8
735	No	No	13	SURG	PELVIC EVISCERATION, RADICAL HYSTERECTOMY AND RADICAL VULVECTOMY WITHOUT CC/MCC	1.2602	1.6	1.9
736	No	No	13	SURG	UTERINE AND ADNEXA PROCEDURES FOR OVARIAN OR ADNEXAL MALIGNANCY WITH MCC	3.8872	7.9	10.3
737	No	No	13	SURG	UTERINE AND ADNEXA PROCEDURES FOR OVARIAN OR ADNEXAL MALIGNANCY WITH CC	1.9738	3.9	4.7
738	No	No	13	SURG	UTERINE AND ADNEXA PROCEDURES FOR OVARIAN OR ADNEXAL MALIGNANCY WITHOUT CC/MCC	1.3646	2.3	2.6
739	No	No	13	SURG	UTERINE AND ADNEXA PROCEDURES FOR NON-OVARIAN AND NON-ADNEXAL MALIGNANCY WITH MCC	3.6163	6.3	9.0
740	No	No	13	SURG	UTERINE AND ADNEXA PROCEDURES FOR NON-OVARIAN AND NON-ADNEXAL MALIGNANCY WITH CC	1.7870	2.7	3.6
741	No	No	13	SURG	UTERINE AND ADNEXA PROCEDURES FOR NON-OVARIAN AND NON-ADNEXAL MALIGNANCY WITHOUT CC/MCC	1.2993	1.6	1.9
742	No	No	13	SURG	UTERINE AND ADNEXA PROCEDURES FOR NON-MALIGNANCY WITH CC/MCC	1.7819	2.7	3.8
743	No	No	13	SURG	UTERINE AND ADNEXA PROCEDURES FOR NON-MALIGNANCY WITHOUT CC/MCC	1.1620	1.6	1.8
744	No	No	13	SURG	D&C, CONIZATION, LAPAROSCOPY AND TUBAL INTERRUPTION WITH CC/MCC	1.8824	4.6	6.4
745	No	No	13	SURG	D&C, CONIZATION, LAPAROSCOPY AND TUBAL INTERRUPTION WITHOUT CC/MCC	1.0359	1.9	2.3
746	No	No	13	SURG	VAGINA, CERVIX AND VULVA PROCEDURES WITH CC/MCC	1.6761	3.3	5.5
747	No	No	13	SURG	VAGINA, CERVIX AND VULVA PROCEDURES WITHOUT CC/MCC	0.8872	1.4	1.6
748	No	No	13	SURG	FEMALE REPRODUCTIVE SYSTEM RECONSTRUCTIVE PROCEDURES	1.4049	1.4	1.8
749	No	No	13	SURG	OTHER FEMALE REPRODUCTIVE SYSTEM O.R. PROCEDURES WITH CC/MCC	2.5172	5.5	7.6
750	No	No	13	SURG	OTHER FEMALE REPRODUCTIVE SYSTEM O.R. PROCEDURES WITHOUT CC/MCC	1.3600	2.0	2.5
754	No	No	13	MED	MALIGNANCY, FEMALE REPRODUCTIVE SYSTEM WITH MCC	1.8525	5.1	7.4
755	No	No	13	MED	MALIGNANCY, FEMALE REPRODUCTIVE SYSTEM WITH CC	1.0847	3.3	4.4
756	No	No	13	MED	MALIGNANCY, FEMALE REPRODUCTIVE SYSTEM WITHOUT CC/MCC	0.9897	2.2	2.5
757	No	No	13	MED	INFECTIONS, FEMALE REPRODUCTIVE SYSTEM WITH MCC	1.4916	5.0	6.6
758	No	No	13	MED	INFECTIONS, FEMALE REPRODUCTIVE SYSTEM WITH CC	0.9926	3.7	4.6
759	No	No	13	MED	INFECTIONS, FEMALE REPRODUCTIVE SYSTEM WITHOUT CC/MCC	0.6462	2.6	3.2
760	No	No	13	MED	MENSTRUAL AND OTHER FEMALE REPRODUCTIVE SYSTEM DISORDERS WITH CC/MCC	0.9954	2.8	3.9
761	No	No	13	MED	MENSTRUAL AND OTHER FEMALE REPRODUCTIVE SYSTEM DISORDERS WITHOUT CC/MCC	0.6056	1.8	2.1
768	No	No	14	SURG	VAGINAL DELIVERY WITH O.R. PROCEDURES EXCEPT STERILIZATION AND/OR D&C	1.2181	3.2	4.0
769	No	No	14	SURG	POSTPARTUM AND POST ABORTION DIAGNOSES WITH O.R. PROCEDURES	1.5439	3.3	5.0
770	No	No	14	SURG	ABORTION WITH D&C, ASPIRATION CURETTAGE OR HYSTEROTOMY	0.7987	1.7	2.0
776	No	No	14	MED	POSTPARTUM AND POST ABORTION DIAGNOSES WITHOUT O.R. PROCEDURES	0.7167	2.4	3.2
779	No	No	14	MED	ABORTION WITHOUT D&C	0.9892	1.8	2.8
783	No	No	14	SURG	CESAREAN SECTION WITH STERILIZATION WITH MCC	1.7718	4.5	6.9
784	No	No	14	SURG	CESAREAN SECTION WITH STERILIZATION WITH CC	1.0241	3.1	3.8
785	No	No	14	SURG	CESAREAN SECTION WITH STERILIZATION WITHOUT CC/MCC	0.8663	2.5	2.8
786	No	No	14	SURG	CESAREAN SECTION WITHOUT STERILIZATION WITH MCC	1.7495	4.3	6.7
787	No	No	14	SURG	CESAREAN SECTION WITHOUT STERILIZATION WITH CC	1.0511	3.3	4.1
788	No	No	14	SURG	CESAREAN SECTION WITHOUT STERILIZATION WITHOUT CC/MCC	0.8550	2.7	3.1
789	No	No	15	MED	NEONATES, DIED OR TRANSFERRED TO ANOTHER ACUTE CARE FACILITY	1.8194	1.8	1.8
790	No	No	15	MED	EXTREME IMMATURITY OR RESPIRATORY DISTRESS SYNDROME, NEONATE	6.0001	17.9	17.9
791	No	No	15	MED	PREMATURITY WITH MAJOR PROBLEMS	4.0977	13.3	13.3
792	No	No	15	MED	PREMATURITY WITHOUT MAJOR PROBLEMS	2.4725	8.6	8.6
793	No	No	15	MED	FULL TERM NEONATE WITH MAJOR PROBLEMS	4.2093	4.7	4.7

MS-DRG	Post-Acute DRG	Special Pay DRG	MDC	TYPE	MS-DRG TITLE	RW	GMLOS	AMLOS
794	No	No	15	MED	NEONATE WITH OTHER SIGNIFICANT PROBLEMS	1.4899	3.4	3.4
795	No	No	15	MED	NORMAL NEWBORN	0.2017	3.1	3.1
796	No	No	14	SURG	VAGINAL DELIVERY WITH STERILIZATION AND/OR D&C WITH MCC	1.4184	2.5	4.5
797	No	No	14	SURG	VAGINAL DELIVERY WITH STERILIZATION AND/OR D&C WITH CC	0.9959	2.4	2.7
798	No	No	14	SURG	VAGINAL DELIVERY WITH STERILIZATION AND/OR D&C WITHOUT CC/MCC	0.8112	2.0	2.2
799	No	No	16	SURG	SPLENIC PROCEDURES WITH MCC	4.9546	7.7	10.2
800	No	No	16	SURG	SPLENIC PROCEDURES WITH CC	2.8177	4.2	5.7
801	No	No	16	SURG	SPLENIC PROCEDURES WITHOUT CC/MCC	1.7897	2.3	2.7
802	No	No	16	SURG	OTHER O.R. PROCEDURES OF THE BLOOD AND BLOOD FORMING ORGANS WITH MCC	3.3903	7.7	10.8
803	No	No	16	SURG	OTHER O.R. PROCEDURES OF THE BLOOD AND BLOOD FORMING ORGANS WITH CC	1.8582	3.8	5.3
804	No	No	16	SURG	OTHER O.R. PROCEDURES OF THE BLOOD AND BLOOD FORMING ORGANS WITHOUT CC/MCC	1.2104	1.7	2.3
805	No	No	14	MED	VAGINAL DELIVERY WITHOUT STERILIZATION OR D&C WITH MCC	1.0082	2.8	3.8
806	No	No	14	MED	VAGINAL DELIVERY WITHOUT STERILIZATION OR D&C WITH CC	0.7467	2.3	2.7
807	No	No	14	MED	VAGINAL DELIVERY WITHOUT STERILIZATION OR D&C WITHOUT CC/MCC	0.6543	2.0	2.2
808	No	No	16	MED	MAJOR HEMATOLOGICAL AND IMMUNOLOGICAL DIAGNOSES EXCEPT SICKLE CELL CRISIS AND COAGULATION DISORDERS WITH MCC	2.1901	5.3	7.4
809	No	No	16	MED	MAJOR HEMATOLOGICAL AND IMMUNOLOGICAL DIAGNOSES EXCEPT SICKLE CELL CRISIS AND COAGULATION DISORDERS WITH CC	1.2044	3.4	4.4
810	No	No	16	MED	MAJOR HEMATOLOGICAL AND IMMUNOLOGICAL DIAGNOSES EXCEPT SICKLE CELL CRISIS AND COAGULATION DISORDERS WITHOUT CC/MCC	1.0045	2.5	3.2
811	No	No	16	MED	RED BLOOD CELL DISORDERS WITH MCC	1.4036	3.8	5.1
812	No	No	16	MED	RED BLOOD CELL DISORDERS WITHOUT MCC	0.9007	2.8	3.6
813	No	No	16	MED	COAGULATION DISORDERS	1.5600	3.7	4.9
814	No	No	16	MED	RETICULOENDOTHELIAL AND IMMUNITY DISORDERS WITH MCC	2.1281	4.8	7.2
815	No	No	16	MED	RETICULOENDOTHELIAL AND IMMUNITY DISORDERS WITH CC	0.9942	3.0	3.9
816	No	No	16	MED	RETICULOENDOTHELIAL AND IMMUNITY DISORDERS WITHOUT CC/MCC	0.7102	2.3	2.9
817	No	No	14	SURG	OTHER ANTEPARTUM DIAGNOSES WITH O.R. PROCEDURES WITH MCC	2.2550	4.3	6.8
818	No	No	14	SURG	OTHER ANTEPARTUM DIAGNOSES WITH O.R. PROCEDURES WITH CC	1.1731	2.4	3.0
819	No	No	14	SURG	OTHER ANTEPARTUM DIAGNOSES WITH O.R. PROCEDURES WITHOUT CC/MCC	0.9072	1.9	2.4
820	No	No	17	SURG	LYMPHOMA AND LEUKEMIA WITH MAJOR O.R. PROCEDURES WITH MCC	6.0467	11.9	17.2
821	No	No	17	SURG	LYMPHOMA AND LEUKEMIA WITH MAJOR O.R. PROCEDURES WITH CC	2.2321	3.6	5.5
822	No	No	17	SURG	LYMPHOMA AND LEUKEMIA WITH MAJOR O.R. PROCEDURES WITHOUT CC/MCC	1.2388	1.6	2.0
823	No	No	17	SURG	LYMPHOMA AND NON-ACUTE LEUKEMIA WITH OTHER PROCEDURES WITH MCC	4.5019	10.5	14.0
824	No	No	17	SURG	LYMPHOMA AND NON-ACUTE LEUKEMIA WITH OTHER PROCEDURES WITH CC	2.2329	5.1	7.0
825	No	No	17	SURG	LYMPHOMA AND NON-ACUTE LEUKEMIA WITH OTHER PROCEDURES WITHOUT CC/MCC	1.2914	2.2	3.1
826	No	No	17	SURG	MYELOPROLIFERATIVE DISORDERS OR POORLY DIFFERENTIATED NEOPLASMS WITH MAJOR O.R. PROCEDURES WITH MCC	4.3888	8.7	11.8
827	No	No	17	SURG	MYELOPROLIFERATIVE DISORDERS OR POORLY DIFFERENTIATED NEOPLASMS WITH MAJOR O.R. PROCEDURES WITH CC	2.3172	4.2	5.5
828	No	No	17	SURG	MYELOPROLIFERATIVE DISORDERS OR POORLY DIFFERENTIATED NEOPLASMS WITH MAJOR O.R. PROCEDURES WITHOUT CC/MCC	1.6404	2.5	3.1
829	No	No	17	SURG	MYELOPROLIFERATIVE DISORDERS OR POORLY DIFFERENTIATED NEOPLASMS WITH OTHER PROCEDURES WITH CC/MCC	3.1538	6.1	9.2
830	No	No	17	SURG	MYELOPROLIFERATIVE DISORDERS OR POORLY DIFFERENTIATED NEOPLASMS WITH OTHER PROCEDURES WITHOUT CC/MCC	1.5812	2.4	3.1
831	No	No	14	MED	OTHER ANTEPARTUM DIAGNOSES WITHOUT O.R. PROCEDURES WITH MCC	1.0098	3.3	4.7
832	No	No	14	MED	OTHER ANTEPARTUM DIAGNOSES WITHOUT O.R. PROCEDURES WITH CC	0.7377	2.5	3.9
833	No	No	14	MED	OTHER ANTEPARTUM DIAGNOSES WITHOUT O.R. PROCEDURES WITHOUT CC/MCC	0.5118	1.9	2.7
834	No	No	17	MED	ACUTE LEUKEMIA WITHOUT MAJOR O.R. PROCEDURES WITH MCC	5.5990	9.9	16.3
835	No	No	17	MED	ACUTE LEUKEMIA WITHOUT MAJOR O.R. PROCEDURES WITH CC	2.2355	4.6	7.2
836	No	No	17	MED	ACUTE LEUKEMIA WITHOUT MAJOR O.R. PROCEDURES WITHOUT CC/MCC	1.1973	2.7	3.9
837	No	No	17	MED	CHEMOTHERAPY WITH ACUTE LEUKEMIA AS SECONDARY DIAGNOSIS OR WITH HIGH DOSE CHEMOTHERAPY AGENT WITH MCC	4.7566	10.9	16.0
838	No	No	17	MED	CHEMOTHERAPY WITH ACUTE LEUKEMIA AS SECONDARY DIAGNOSIS WITH CC OR HIGH DOSE CHEMOTHERAPY AGENT	1.9524	5.1	6.6

MS-DRG	Post-Acute DRG	Special Pay DRG	MDC	TYPE	MS-DRG TITLE	RW	GMLOS	AMLOS
839	No	No	17	MED	CHEMOTHERAPY WITH ACUTE LEUKEMIA AS SECONDARY DIAGNOSIS WITHOUT CC/MCC	1.3031	4.2	4.5
840	Yes	No	17	MED	LYMPHOMA AND NON-ACUTE LEUKEMIA WITH MCC	3.1252	6.8	9.9
841	Yes	No	17	MED	LYMPHOMA AND NON-ACUTE LEUKEMIA WITH CC	1.5735	4.0	5.5
842	Yes	No	17	MED	LYMPHOMA AND NON-ACUTE LEUKEMIA WITHOUT CC/MCC	1.0664	2.7	3.5
843	No	No	17	MED	OTHER MYELOPROLIFERATIVE DISORDERS OR POORLY DIFFERENTIATED NEOPLASTIC DIAGNOSES WITH MCC	1.8606	5.4	7.4
844	No	No	17	MED	OTHER MYELOPROLIFERATIVE DISORDERS OR POORLY DIFFERENTIATED NEOPLASTIC DIAGNOSES WITH CC	1.1572	3.7	5.0
845	No	No	17	MED	OTHER MYELOPROLIFERATIVE DISORDERS OR POORLY DIFFERENTIATED NEOPLASTIC DIAGNOSES WITHOUT CC/MCC	0.8649	2.7	3.6
846	No	No	17	MED	CHEMOTHERAPY WITHOUT ACUTE LEUKEMIA AS SECONDARY DIAGNOSIS WITH MCC	2.4440	5.8	7.9
847	No	No	17	MED	CHEMOTHERAPY WITHOUT ACUTE LEUKEMIA AS SECONDARY DIAGNOSIS WITH CC	1.2126	3.7	4.2
848	No	No	17	MED	CHEMOTHERAPY WITHOUT ACUTE LEUKEMIA AS SECONDARY DIAGNOSIS WITHOUT CC/MCC	0.7595	2.7	3.2
849	No	No	17	MED	RADIOTHERAPY	2.6914	6.9	10.4
853	Yes	No	18	SURG	INFECTIOUS AND PARASITIC DISEASES WITH O.R. PROCEDURES WITH MCC	4.9993	9.9	13.3
854	Yes	No	18	SURG	INFECTIOUS AND PARASITIC DISEASES WITH O.R. PROCEDURES WITH CC	2.0382	5.2	6.6
855	Yes	No	18	SURG	INFECTIOUS AND PARASITIC DISEASES WITH O.R. PROCEDURES WITHOUT CC/MCC	1.7018	3.7	4.5
856	Yes	No	18	SURG	POSTOPERATIVE OR POST-TRAUMATIC INFECTIONS WITH O.R. PROCEDURES WITH MCC	4.4284	9.4	12.5
857	Yes	No	18	SURG	POSTOPERATIVE OR POST-TRAUMATIC INFECTIONS WITH O.R. PROCEDURES WITH CC	2.1357	5.4	6.9
858	Yes	No	18	SURG	POSTOPERATIVE OR POST-TRAUMATIC INFECTIONS WITH O.R. PROCEDURES WITHOUT CC/MCC	1.2834	3.4	4.1
862	Yes	No	18	MED	POSTOPERATIVE AND POST-TRAUMATIC INFECTIONS WITH MCC	1.8420	5.1	6.8
863	Yes	No	18	MED	POSTOPERATIVE AND POST-TRAUMATIC INFECTIONS WITHOUT MCC	1.0055	3.5	4.3
864	No	No	18	MED	FEVER AND INFLAMMATORY CONDITIONS	0.8828	2.7	3.4
865	No	No	18	MED	VIRAL ILLNESS WITH MCC	1.6399	4.3	6.3
866	No	No	18	MED	VIRAL ILLNESS WITHOUT MCC	0.9177	2.8	3.8
867	Yes	No	18	MED	OTHER INFECTIOUS AND PARASITIC DISEASES DIAGNOSES WITH MCC	2.0923	5.5	7.8
868	Yes	No	18	MED	OTHER INFECTIOUS AND PARASITIC DISEASES DIAGNOSES WITH CC	1.0855	3.7	4.8
869	Yes	No	18	MED	OTHER INFECTIOUS AND PARASITIC DISEASES DIAGNOSES WITHOUT CC/MCC	0.6907	2.5	3.1
870	Yes	No	18	MED	SEPTICEMIA OR SEVERE SEPSIS WITH MV >96 HOURS	6.9649	13.5	16.1
871	Yes	No	18	MED	SEPTICEMIA OR SEVERE SEPSIS WITHOUT MV >96 HOURS WITH MCC	1.9826	5.1	6.9
872	Yes	No	18	MED	SEPTICEMIA OR SEVERE SEPSIS WITHOUT MV >96 HOURS WITHOUT MCC	1.0299	3.6	4.3
876	No	No	19	SURG	O.R. PROCEDURES WITH PRINCIPAL DIAGNOSIS OF MENTAL ILLNESS	3.7315	7.2	17.7
880	No	No	19	MED	ACUTE ADJUSTMENT REACTION AND PSYCHOSOCIAL DYSFUNCTION	0.9546	2.9	4.4
881	No	No	19	MED	DEPRESSIVE NEUROSES	0.9065	4.0	5.9
882	No	No	19	MED	NEUROSES EXCEPT DEPRESSIVE	0.9393	3.5	5.7
883	No	No	19	MED	DISORDERS OF PERSONALITY AND IMPULSE CONTROL	1.8754	5.4	11.4
884	Yes	No	19	MED	ORGANIC DISTURBANCES AND INTELLECTUAL DISABILITY	1.7569	5.0	9.2
885	No	No	19	MED	PSYCHOSES	1.3664	6.4	9.7
886	No	No	19	MED	BEHAVIORAL AND DEVELOPMENTAL DISORDERS	1.6817	5.4	10.3
887	No	No	19	MED	OTHER MENTAL DISORDER DIAGNOSES	1.2956	3.3	6.5
894	No	No	20	MED	ALCOHOL, DRUG ABUSE OR DEPENDENCE, LEFT AMA	0.5745	2.1	2.9
895	No	No	20	MED	ALCOHOL, DRUG ABUSE OR DEPENDENCE WITH REHABILITATION THERAPY	1.6088	8.3	11.6
896	Yes	No	20	MED	ALCOHOL, DRUG ABUSE OR DEPENDENCE WITHOUT REHABILITATION THERAPY WITH MCC	1.7781	5.0	7.4
897	Yes	No	20	MED	ALCOHOL, DRUG ABUSE OR DEPENDENCE WITHOUT REHABILITATION THERAPY WITHOUT MCC	0.8556	3.4	4.4
901	No	No	21	SURG	WOUND DEBRIDEMENTS FOR INJURIES WITH MCC	4.3278	9.1	14.7
902	No	No	21	SURG	WOUND DEBRIDEMENTS FOR INJURIES WITH CC	1.8847	4.6	6.6
903	No	No	21	SURG	WOUND DEBRIDEMENTS FOR INJURIES WITHOUT CC/MCC	1.2415	2.7	3.5
904	No	No	21	SURG	SKIN GRAFTS FOR INJURIES WITH CC/MCC	3.2562	6.9	10.0
905	No	No	21	SURG	SKIN GRAFTS FOR INJURIES WITHOUT CC/MCC	1.5837	3.2	4.7
906	No	No	21	SURG	HAND PROCEDURES FOR INJURIES	1.8816	2.9	5.1
907	Yes	No	21	SURG	OTHER O.R. PROCEDURES FOR INJURIES WITH MCC	3.7195	6.9	9.7
908	Yes	No	21	SURG	OTHER O.R. PROCEDURES FOR INJURIES WITH CC	2.0041	3.8	5.1
909	Yes	No	21	SURG	OTHER O.R. PROCEDURES FOR INJURIES WITHOUT CC/MCC	1.3563	2.3	2.8

MS-DRG	Post-Acute DRG	Special Pay DRG	MDC	TYPE	MS-DRG TITLE	RW	GMLOS	AMLOS
913	No	No	21	MED	TRAUMATIC INJURY WITH MCC	1.4945	3.9	5.7
914	No	No	21	MED	TRAUMATIC INJURY WITHOUT MCC	0.9077	2.5	3.2
915	No	No	21	MED	ALLERGIC REACTIONS WITH MCC	1.7740	3.8	5.4
916	No	No	21	MED	ALLERGIC REACTIONS WITHOUT MCC	0.6588	1.8	2.3
917	Yes	No	21	MED	POISONING AND TOXIC EFFECTS OF DRUGS WITH MCC	1.5959	3.9	5.7
918	Yes	No	21	MED	POISONING AND TOXIC EFFECTS OF DRUGS WITHOUT MCC	0.8609	2.5	3.5
919	No	No	21	MED	COMPLICATIONS OF TREATMENT WITH MCC	1.8247	4.4	6.2
920	No	No	21	MED	COMPLICATIONS OF TREATMENT WITH CC	1.0338	2.9	3.9
921	No	No	21	MED	COMPLICATIONS OF TREATMENT WITHOUT CC/MCC	0.6978	2.1	2.7
922	No	No	21	MED	OTHER INJURY, POISONING AND TOXIC EFFECT DIAGNOSES WITH MCC	1.7449	4.5	7.7
923	No	No	21	MED	OTHER INJURY, POISONING AND TOXIC EFFECT DIAGNOSES WITHOUT MCC	1.0114	2.9	4.8
927	No	No	22	SURG	EXTENSIVE BURNS OR FULL THICKNESS BURNS WITH MV >96 HOURS WITH SKIN GRAFT	26.3587	26.4	36.0
928	No	No	22	SURG	FULL THICKNESS BURN WITH SKIN GRAFT OR INHALATION INJURY WITH CC/MCC	6.9197	12.6	17.1
929	No	No	22	SURG	FULL THICKNESS BURN WITH SKIN GRAFT OR INHALATION INJURY WITHOUT CC/MCC	3.2155	6.0	8.3
933	No	No	22	MED	EXTENSIVE BURNS OR FULL THICKNESS BURNS WITH MV >96 HOURS WITHOUT SKIN GRAFT	3.0320	2.5	5.0
934	No	No	22	MED	FULL THICKNESS BURN WITHOUT SKIN GRAFT OR INHALATION INJURY	2.0925	4.9	7.3
935	No	No	22	MED	NON-EXTENSIVE BURNS	2.0411	3.7	5.5
939	No	No	23	SURG	O.R. PROCEDURES WITH DIAGNOSES OF OTHER CONTACT WITH HEALTH SERVICES WITH MCC	3.2153	6.3	9.4
940	No	No	23	SURG	O.R. PROCEDURES WITH DIAGNOSES OF OTHER CONTACT WITH HEALTH SERVICES WITH CC	2.1666	3.2	4.6
941	No	No	23	SURG	O.R. PROCEDURES WITH DIAGNOSES OF OTHER CONTACT WITH HEALTH SERVICES WITHOUT CC/MCC	1.8560	1.8	2.3
945	Yes	No	23	MED	REHABILITATION WITH CC/MCC	1.5095	4.8	6.7
946	Yes	No	23	MED	REHABILITATION WITHOUT CC/MCC	1.0127	3.2	4.5
947	Yes	No	23	MED	SIGNS AND SYMPTOMS WITH MCC	1.2516	3.7	5.3
948	Yes	No	23	MED	SIGNS AND SYMPTOMS WITHOUT MCC	0.8010	2.6	3.5
949	No	No	23	MED	AFTERCARE WITH CC/MCC	1.0361	4.4	6.4
950	No	No	23	MED	AFTERCARE WITHOUT CC/MCC	0.6282	2.9	4.0
951	No	No	23	MED	OTHER FACTORS INFLUENCING HEALTH STATUS	0.5900	1.8	2.8
955	No	No	24	SURG	CRANIOTOMY FOR MULTIPLE SIGNIFICANT TRAUMA	6.0902	8.3	12.2
956	Yes	No	24	SURG	LIMB REATTACHMENT, HIP AND FEMUR PROCEDURES FOR MULTIPLE SIGNIFICANT TRAUMA	3.8782	6.3	8.0
957	No	No	24	SURG	OTHER O.R. PROCEDURES FOR MULTIPLE SIGNIFICANT TRAUMA WITH MCC	7.2325	10.0	14.5
958	No	No	24	SURG	OTHER O.R. PROCEDURES FOR MULTIPLE SIGNIFICANT TRAUMA WITH CC	4.0448	6.7	8.2
959	No	No	24	SURG	OTHER O.R. PROCEDURES FOR MULTIPLE SIGNIFICANT TRAUMA WITHOUT CC/MCC	2.5324	4.0	5.0
963	No	No	24	MED	OTHER MULTIPLE SIGNIFICANT TRAUMA WITH MCC	2.7343	5.6	8.2
964	No	No	24	MED	OTHER MULTIPLE SIGNIFICANT TRAUMA WITH CC	1.5010	3.9	5.0
965	No	No	24	MED	OTHER MULTIPLE SIGNIFICANT TRAUMA WITHOUT CC/MCC	0.9559	2.7	3.2
969	No	No	25	SURG	HIV WITH EXTENSIVE O.R. PROCEDURES WITH MCC	6.8726	13.4	20.2
970	No	No	25	SURG	HIV WITH EXTENSIVE O.R. PROCEDURES WITHOUT MCC	2.4044	5.8	8.1
974	No	No	25	MED	HIV WITH MAJOR RELATED CONDITION WITH MCC	2.9165	7.0	10.5
975	No	No	25	MED	HIV WITH MAJOR RELATED CONDITION WITH CC	1.3633	4.1	5.9
976	No	No	25	MED	HIV WITH MAJOR RELATED CONDITION WITHOUT CC/MCC	0.8453	2.8	3.6
977	No	No	25	MED	HIV WITH OR WITHOUT OTHER RELATED CONDITION	1.4161	3.9	6.2
981	Yes	No		SURG	EXTENSIVE O.R. PROCEDURES UNRELATED TO PRINCIPAL DIAGNOSIS WITH MCC	4.7404	9.0	12.8
982	Yes	No		SURG	EXTENSIVE O.R. PROCEDURES UNRELATED TO PRINCIPAL DIAGNOSIS WITH CC	2.4860	4.3	5.9
983	Yes	No		SURG	EXTENSIVE O.R. PROCEDURES UNRELATED TO PRINCIPAL DIAGNOSIS WITHOUT CC/MCC	1.6352	1.9	2.5
987	Yes	Yes		SURG	NON-EXTENSIVE O.R. PROCEDURES UNRELATED TO PRINCIPAL DIAGNOSIS WITH MCC	3.3767	8.2	11.4
988	Yes	Yes		SURG	NON-EXTENSIVE O.R. PROCEDURES UNRELATED TO PRINCIPAL DIAGNOSIS WITH CC	1.6970	4.3	5.9
989	Yes	Yes		SURG	NON-EXTENSIVE O.R. PROCEDURES UNRELATED TO PRINCIPAL DIAGNOSIS WITHOUT CC/MCC	1.0803	2.3	3
998	No	No		**	PRINCIPAL DIAGNOSIS INVALID AS DISCHARGE DIAGNOSIS	.		
999	No	No		**	UNGROUPABLE	.		

**MS-DRGs 998 and 999 contain cases that could not be assigned to valid DRGs.

Appendix B: Numeric Lists of CCs and MCCs

Numeric CC List

AØØ.Ø
AØØ.1
AØØ.9
AØ1.ØØ
AØ1.Ø1
AØ1.Ø2
AØ1.Ø3
AØ1.Ø4
AØ1.Ø5
AØ1.Ø9
AØ1.1
AØ1.2
AØ1.3
AØ1.4
AØ2.Ø
AØ2.23
AØ2.24
AØ2.25
AØ2.29
AØ2.8
AØ2.9
AØ3.Ø
AØ4.Ø
AØ4.1
AØ4.2
AØ4.3
AØ4.4
AØ4.5
AØ4.6
AØ4.71
AØ4.72
AØ4.8
AØ4.9
AØ5.Ø
AØ5.1
AØ5.2
AØ5.3
AØ5.4
AØ5.5
AØ5.8
AØ6.Ø
AØ6.1
AØ6.2
AØ6.3
AØ6.81
AØ6.82
AØ6.89
AØ7.1
AØ7.2
AØ7.3
AØ7.4
AØ7.8
AØ7.9
AØ8.Ø
AØ8.11
AØ8.19
AØ8.2
AØ8.31
AØ8.32
AØ8.39
AØ9
A15.Ø
A15.4
A15.5
A15.6
A15.7
A15.8
A15.9
A17.9
A18.Ø1
A18.Ø2
A18.Ø3
A18.Ø9
A18.1Ø
A18.11
A18.12
A18.13
A18.14
A18.15
A18.16
A18.17
A18.18
A18.2
A18.32
A18.39
A18.4
A18.5Ø
A18.51
A18.52
A18.53
A18.54
A18.59
A18.6
A18.7
A18.81
A18.82
A18.83
A18.84
A18.85
A18.89
A21.Ø
A21.1
A21.2
A21.3
A21.7
A21.8
A21.9
A22.Ø
A22.2
A22.8
A22.9
A23.8
A23.9
A24.Ø
A24.1
A24.2
A24.3
A24.9
A25.Ø
A25.1
A25.9
A27.Ø
A27.89
A27.9
A28.Ø
A28.1
A28.2
A28.8
A28.9
A3Ø.Ø
A3Ø.1
A3Ø.2
A3Ø.3
A3Ø.4
A3Ø.5
A3Ø.8
A3Ø.9
A31.Ø
A31.1
A31.2
A31.8
A31.9
A32.Ø
A32.11
A32.12
A32.81
A32.82
A32.89
A32.9
A34
A36.Ø
A36.1
A36.2
A36.3
A36.81
A36.82
A36.83
A36.84
A36.85
A36.86
A36.89
A36.9
A37.ØØ
A37.1Ø
A37.8Ø
A37.9Ø
A38.Ø
A38.1
A38.8
A38.9
A39.82
A39.83
A39.84
A39.89
A39.9
A42.Ø
A42.1
A42.2
A42.81
A42.82
A42.89
A42.9
A43.Ø
A43.1
A43.8
A43.9
A44.Ø
A44.1
A44.8
A44.9
A48.51
A48.52
A5Ø.Ø1
A5Ø.Ø2
A5Ø.Ø3
A5Ø.Ø4
A5Ø.Ø5
A5Ø.Ø6
A5Ø.Ø7
A5Ø.Ø8
A5Ø.Ø9
A5Ø.2
A5Ø.3Ø
A5Ø.31
A5Ø.32
A5Ø.39
A5Ø.4Ø
A5Ø.43
A5Ø.44
A5Ø.45
A5Ø.49
A5Ø.51
A5Ø.52
A5Ø.53
A5Ø.54
A5Ø.55
A5Ø.56
A5Ø.57
A5Ø.59
A51.31
A51.32
A51.39
A51.42
A51.43
A51.44
A51.45
A51.46
A51.49
A52.ØØ
A52.Ø1
A52.Ø2
A52.Ø3
A52.Ø4
A52.Ø5
A52.Ø6
A52.Ø9
A52.1Ø
A52.11
A52.12
A52.15
A52.16
A52.17
A52.19
A52.2
A52.3
A52.71
A52.72
A52.73
A52.74
A52.75
A52.76
A52.77
A52.78
A52.79
A54.ØØ
A54.Ø1
A54.Ø2
A54.Ø3
A54.Ø9
A54.1
A54.21
A54.22
A54.23
A54.24
A54.29
A54.3Ø
A54.31
A54.32
A54.33
A54.39
A54.4Ø
A54.41
A54.42
A54.43
A54.49
A54.82
A54.83
A54.84
A54.85
A54.89
A54.9
A68.Ø
A68.1
A68.9
A69.1
A69.2Ø
A69.21
A69.22
A69.23
A69.29
A7Ø
A75.Ø
A75.1
A75.2
A75.3
A75.9
A77.Ø
A77.1
A77.2
A77.3
A77.4Ø
A77.41
A77.49
A77.8
A77.9
A78
A79.Ø
A79.1
A79.81
A79.82
A79.89
A79.9
A81.ØØ
A81.Ø1
A81.Ø9
A81.1
A81.2
A81.81
A81.82
A81.83
A81.89
A81.9
A82.Ø
A82.1
A82.9
A85.Ø
A85.1
A85.8
A86
A87.Ø
A87.1
A87.2
A87.8
A87.9
A88.Ø
A88.8
A89
A9Ø
A91
A92.Ø
A92.1
A92.2
A92.4
A92.5
A92.8
A92.9
A93.Ø
A93.1
A93.2
A93.8
A94
A95.Ø
A95.1
A95.9
A96.Ø
A96.1
A96.8
A96.9
A98.Ø
A98.1
A98.2
A98.5
A98.8
A99
BØØ.2
BØØ.5Ø
BØØ.51
BØØ.52
BØØ.53
BØØ.59
BØØ.81
BØØ.89
BØ1.Ø
BØ1.81
BØ1.89
BØ1.9
BØ2.Ø
BØ2.21
BØ2.22
BØ2.23
BØ2.29
BØ2.3Ø
BØ2.31
BØ2.32
BØ2.33
BØ2.34
BØ2.39
BØ2.7
BØ2.8
BØ3
BØ4
BØ5.1
BØ5.4
BØ5.81
BØ5.89
BØ6.ØØ
BØ6.Ø2
BØ6.Ø9
BØ6.81
BØ6.82
BØ6.89
BØ8.3
BØ8.71
B15.9
B16.1
B16.9
B17.Ø
B17.1Ø
B17.2
B17.8
B17.9
B18.Ø
B18.1
B18.8
B18.9
B19.1Ø
B19.9
B2Ø
B25.1
B25.8
B25.9
B26.Ø
B26.3
B26.81
B26.82
B26.83
B26.84
B26.85
B26.89
B33.1
B33.2Ø
B33.21
B33.22
B33.23
B33.4
B34.3
B37.Ø
B37.41
B37.49
B37.81
B37.82
B37.83
B37.84
B37.89
B38.Ø
B38.1
B38.2
B38.3
B38.7
B38.81
B38.89
B38.9
B39.3
B4Ø.Ø
B4Ø.1
B4Ø.2
B4Ø.3
B4Ø.7
B4Ø.81
B4Ø.89
B4Ø.9
B41.Ø
B41.7
B41.8
B41.9
B44.1
B44.2
B44.7
B44.81
B44.89
B44.9
B45.Ø
B45.2
B45.3
B45.7
B45.8
B45.9
B47.Ø
B47.1
B47.9
B48.2
B48.3
B48.4
B48.8
B49
B5Ø.Ø
B5Ø.8
B51.Ø
B51.8
B51.9
B52.Ø
B52.8
B52.9
B53.Ø
B53.1
B53.8
B54
B55.Ø
B55.1
B55.2
B55.9
B56.Ø
B56.1
B56.9
B57.Ø
B57.1
B57.2
B57.3Ø
B57.31
B57.32
B57.39
B57.4Ø
B57.41
B57.42
B57.49
B57.5
B58.ØØ
B58.Ø1
B58.Ø9
B58.1
B58.82
B58.83
B58.89
B58.9
B6Ø.ØØ
B6Ø.Ø1
B6Ø.Ø2
B6Ø.Ø3
B6Ø.Ø9
B6Ø.1Ø
B6Ø.19
B6Ø.2
B65.Ø
B65.1
B65.2
B65.3
B65.8
B65.9
B66.Ø
B66.1
B66.2
B66.3
B66.4
B66.5
B66.8
B67.Ø
B67.1
B67.2
B67.31
B67.32
B67.39
B67.4
B67.5
B67.61
B67.69
B67.7
B67.8
B67.9Ø
B67.99
B68.Ø
B68.1
B68.9
B69.Ø
B69.1
B69.81
B69.89
B69.9
B7Ø.Ø
B7Ø.1
B71.Ø
B71.1
B71.8
B72
B73.ØØ
B73.Ø1
B73.Ø2
B73.Ø9
B73.1
B74.Ø
B74.1
B74.2
B74.3
B74.4
B74.8
B74.9
B75
B76.Ø
B76.1
B76.8
B76.9
B77.Ø
B77.89
B77.9
B78.Ø
B78.7
B78.9
B79
B8Ø
B81.Ø
B81.1
B81.2
B81.3
B81.4
B81.8
B82.Ø
B97.21
B97.33
B97.34
B97.35
C15.3
C15.4
C15.5
C15.8
C15.9
C16.Ø
C16.1
C16.2
C16.3
C16.4
C16.5
C16.6
C16.8
C16.9
C17.Ø
C17.1
C17.2
C17.3
C17.8
C17.9
C18.Ø
C18.1
C18.2
C18.3
C18.4
C18.5
C18.6
C18.7
C18.8
C18.9
C19
C2Ø
C21.Ø
C21.1
C21.2
C21.8
C22.Ø
C22.1
C22.2
C22.3
C22.4
C22.7
C22.8
C22.9
C23
C24.Ø
C24.1
C24.8
C24.9
C25.Ø
C25.1
C25.2
C25.3
C25.4
C25.7
C25.8
C25.9
C33
C34.ØØ
C34.Ø1
C34.Ø2
C34.1Ø
C34.11
C34.12
C34.2
C34.3Ø
C34.31
C34.32
C34.8Ø
C34.81
C34.82
C34.9Ø
C34.91
C34.92
C37
C38.Ø
C38.1
C38.2
C38.3
C38.4
C38.8
C4Ø.ØØ
C4Ø.Ø1
C4Ø.Ø2
C4Ø.1Ø
C4Ø.11
C4Ø.12
C4Ø.2Ø
C4Ø.21
C4Ø.22
C4Ø.3Ø
C4Ø.31
C4Ø.32
C4Ø.8Ø
C4Ø.81
C4Ø.82
C4Ø.9Ø
C4Ø.91
C4Ø.92
C41.Ø
C41.1
C41.2
C41.3
C41.4
C41.9
C45.Ø
C45.1
C45.2
C46.Ø
C46.1
C46.2
C46.3
C46.4
C46.5Ø
C46.51
C46.52
C46.7
C46.9
C47.Ø
C47.1Ø
C47.11
C47.12
C47.2Ø
C47.21
C47.22
C47.3
C47.4
C47.5
C47.6
C47.8
C47.9
C48.Ø
C48.1
C48.2
C48.8
C49.Ø
C49.1Ø
C49.11
C49.12
C49.2Ø
C49.21
C49.22
C49.3
C49.4
C49.5
C49.6
C49.8
C49.9
C49.AØ
C49.A1
C49.A2
C49.A3
C49.A4
C49.A5
C49.A9
C56.1
C56.2
C56.3
C56.9
C64.1
C64.2
C64.9
C65.1
C65.2
C65.9
C66.1
C66.2
C66.9
C68.Ø
C68.1
C68.8
C68.9
C7Ø.Ø
C7Ø.1
C7Ø.9
C71.Ø
C71.1
C71.2
C71.3
C71.4
C71.5
C71.6
C71.7
C71.8
C71.9
C72.Ø
C72.1
C72.2Ø
C72.21
C72.22
C72.3Ø
C72.31
C72.32
C72.4Ø
C72.41
C72.42
C72.5Ø
C72.59
C72.9
C74.ØØ
C74.Ø1
C74.Ø2
C74.1Ø
C74.11
C74.12
C74.9Ø
C74.91
C74.92
C75.Ø
C75.1
C75.2
C75.3
C75.4
C75.5
C75.8
C75.9
C77.Ø
C77.1
C77.2
C77.3
C77.4
C77.5
C77.8
C77.9
C78.ØØ
C78.Ø1
C78.Ø2
C78.1
C78.2
C78.3Ø
C78.39
C78.4
C78.5
C78.6
C78.7
C78.8Ø
C78.89

C79.00
C79.01
C79.02
C79.10
C79.11
C79.19
C79.2
C79.31
C79.32
C79.40
C79.49
C79.51
C79.52
C79.60
C79.61
C79.62
C79.63
C79.70
C79.71
C79.72
C79.81
C79.82
C79.89
C79.9
C7A.00
C7A.010
C7A.011
C7A.012
C7A.019
C7A.020
C7A.021
C7A.022
C7A.023
C7A.024
C7A.025
C7A.026
C7A.029
C7A.090
C7A.091
C7A.092
C7A.093
C7A.094
C7A.095
C7A.096
C7A.098
C7A.1
C7A.8
C7B.01
C7B.02
C7B.03
C7B.04
C7B.09
C7B.8
C80.0
C80.2
C81.00
C81.01
C81.02
C81.03
C81.04
C81.05
C81.06
C81.07
C81.08
C81.09
C81.10
C81.11
C81.12
C81.13
C81.14
C81.15
C81.16
C81.17
C81.18
C81.19
C81.20
C81.21
C81.22
C81.23
C81.24
C81.25
C81.26
C81.27
C81.28
C81.29
C81.30
C81.31
C81.32
C81.33
C81.34
C81.35
C81.36
C81.37
C81.38
C81.39
C81.40
C81.41
C81.42
C81.43
C81.44
C81.45
C81.46
C81.47
C81.48
C81.49
C81.70
C81.71
C81.72
C81.73
C81.74
C81.75
C81.76
C81.77
C81.78
C81.79
C81.90
C81.91
C81.92
C81.93
C81.94
C81.95
C81.96
C81.97
C81.98
C81.99
C82.00
C82.01
C82.02
C82.03
C82.04
C82.05
C82.06
C82.07
C82.08
C82.09
C82.10
C82.11
C82.12
C82.13
C82.14
C82.15
C82.16
C82.17
C82.18
C82.19
C82.20
C82.21
C82.22
C82.23
C82.24
C82.25
C82.26
C82.27
C82.28
C82.29
C82.30
C82.31
C82.32
C82.33
C82.34
C82.35
C82.36
C82.37
C82.38
C82.39
C82.40
C82.41
C82.42
C82.43
C82.44
C82.45
C82.46
C82.47
C82.48
C82.49
C82.50
C82.51
C82.52
C82.53
C82.54
C82.55
C82.56
C82.57
C82.58
C82.59
C82.60
C82.61
C82.62
C82.63
C82.64
C82.65
C82.66
C82.67
C82.68
C82.69
C82.80
C82.81
C82.82
C82.83
C82.84
C82.85
C82.86
C82.87
C82.88
C82.89
C82.90
C82.91
C82.92
C82.93
C82.94
C82.95
C82.96
C82.97
C82.98
C82.99
C83.00
C83.01
C83.02
C83.03
C83.04
C83.05
C83.06
C83.07
C83.08
C83.09
C83.10
C83.11
C83.12
C83.13
C83.14
C83.15
C83.16
C83.17
C83.18
C83.19
C83.30
C83.31
C83.32
C83.33
C83.34
C83.35
C83.36
C83.37
C83.38
C83.39
C83.50
C83.51
C83.52
C83.53
C83.54
C83.55
C83.56
C83.57
C83.58
C83.59
C83.70
C83.71
C83.72
C83.73
C83.74
C83.75
C83.76
C83.77
C83.78
C83.79
C83.80
C83.81
C83.82
C83.83
C83.84
C83.85
C83.86
C83.87
C83.88
C83.89
C83.90
C83.91
C83.92
C83.93
C83.94
C83.95
C83.96
C83.97
C83.98
C83.99
C84.00
C84.01
C84.02
C84.03
C84.04
C84.05
C84.06
C84.07
C84.08
C84.09
C84.10
C84.11
C84.12
C84.13
C84.14
C84.15
C84.16
C84.17
C84.18
C84.19
C84.40
C84.41
C84.42
C84.43
C84.44
C84.45
C84.46
C84.47
C84.48
C84.49
C84.60
C84.61
C84.62
C84.63
C84.64
C84.65
C84.66
C84.67
C84.68
C84.69
C84.70
C84.71
C84.72
C84.73
C84.74
C84.75
C84.76
C84.77
C84.78
C84.79
C84.7A
C84.90
C84.91
C84.92
C84.93
C84.94
C84.95
C84.96
C84.97
C84.98
C84.99
C84.A0
C84.A1
C84.A2
C84.A3
C84.A4
C84.A5
C84.A6
C84.A7
C84.A8
C84.A9
C84.Z0
C84.Z1
C84.Z2
C84.Z3
C84.Z4
C84.Z5
C84.Z6
C84.Z7
C84.Z8
C84.Z9
C85.10
C85.11
C85.12
C85.13
C85.14
C85.15
C85.16
C85.17
C85.18
C85.19
C85.20
C85.21
C85.22
C85.23
C85.24
C85.25
C85.26
C85.27
C85.28
C85.29
C85.80
C85.81
C85.82
C85.83
C85.84
C85.85
C85.86
C85.87
C85.88
C85.89
C85.90
C85.91
C85.92
C85.93
C85.94
C85.95
C85.96
C85.97
C85.98
C85.99
C86.0
C86.1
C86.2
C86.3
C86.4
C86.5
C86.6
C88.2
C88.3
C88.4
C88.8
C88.9
C90.00
C90.01
C90.02
C90.10
C90.11
C90.12
C90.20
C90.21
C90.22
C90.30
C90.31
C90.32
C91.00
C91.01
C91.02
C91.10
C91.11
C91.12
C91.30
C91.31
C91.32
C91.40
C91.41
C91.42
C91.50
C91.51
C91.52
C91.60
C91.61
C91.62
C91.90
C91.91
C91.92
C91.A0
C91.A1
C91.A2
C91.Z0
C91.Z1
C91.Z2
C92.00
C92.01
C92.02
C92.10
C92.11
C92.12
C92.20
C92.21
C92.22
C92.30
C92.31
C92.32
C92.40
C92.41
C92.42
C92.50
C92.51
C92.52
C92.60
C92.61
C92.62
C92.90
C92.91
C92.92
C92.A0
C92.A1
C92.A2
C92.Z0
C92.Z1
C92.Z2
C93.00
C93.01
C93.02
C93.10
C93.11
C93.12
C93.30
C93.31
C93.32
C93.90
C93.91
C93.92
C93.Z0
C93.Z1
C93.Z2
C94.00
C94.01
C94.02
C94.20
C94.21
C94.22
C94.30
C94.31
C94.32
C94.40
C94.41
C94.42
C94.6
C94.80
C94.81
C94.82
C95.00
C95.01
C95.02
C95.10
C95.11
C95.12
C95.90
C95.91
C95.92
C96.0
C96.20
C96.21
C96.22
C96.29
C96.4
C96.5
C96.6
C96.9
C96.A
C96.Z
D46.22
D46.C
D47.01
D47.02
D47.09
D47.1
D47.9
D47.Z1
D47.Z2
D47.Z9
D58.8
D58.9
D59.0
D59.10
D59.11
D59.12
D59.13
D59.19
D59.2
D59.4
D59.9
D61.01
D61.02
D61.09
D61.818
D61.82
D61.9
D62
D68.00
D68.01
D68.020
D68.021
D68.022
D68.023
D68.029
D68.03
D68.04
D68.09
D68.1
D68.2
D68.311
D68.312
D68.318
D68.32
D68.4
D68.51
D68.52
D68.59
D68.61
D68.62
D68.69
D68.8
D68.9
D69.0
D69.3
D69.41
D69.42
D74.0
D74.8
D74.9
D75.81
D76.1
D76.2
D76.3
D78.01
D78.02
D78.11
D78.12
D78.21
D78.22
D78.31
D78.32
D78.33
D78.34
D78.81
D78.89
D80.0
D80.1
D80.2
D80.3
D80.4
D80.5
D80.6
D80.7
D80.8
D80.9
D81.0
D81.1
D81.2
D81.30
D81.31
D81.32
D81.39
D81.4
D81.5
D81.6
D81.7
D81.82
D81.89
D81.9
D82.0
D82.1
D83.0
D83.1
D83.2
D83.8
D83.9
D84.81
D84.821
D84.822
D84.89
D84.9
D89.810
D89.811
D89.812
D89.813
D89.833
D89.834
D89.835
E06.0
E08.52
E09.52
E10.52
E11.52
E13.52
E15
E22.1
E22.2
E22.8
E22.9
E23.0
E23.2
E24.0
E24.2
E24.3
E24.4
E24.8
E24.9
E27.0
E27.1
E27.2
E27.3
E27.40
E27.49
E27.5
E32.1
E34.0
E36.01
E36.02
E36.11
E36.12
E44.0
E44.1
E45
E46
E51.11
E51.12
E51.2
E51.8
E51.9
E53.0
E55.0
E64.0
E66.2
E70.0
E70.1
E70.20
E70.21
E70.29
E70.30
E70.310
E70.311
E70.318
E70.319
E70.320
E70.321
E70.328
E70.329
E70.330
E70.331
E70.338
E70.339
E70.39
E70.40
E70.41
E70.49
E70.5
E70.81
E70.89
E70.9
E71.0
E71.110
E71.111
E71.118
E71.120
E71.121
E71.128
E71.19
E71.2
E71.310
E71.311
E71.312
E71.313
E71.314
E71.318
E71.32
E71.39
E71.50
E71.510
E71.511
E71.518
E71.520
E71.521
E71.522
E71.528
E71.529
E71.53
E71.540
E71.541
E71.542
E71.548
E72.00
E72.01
E72.02
E72.03
E72.04
E72.09
E72.10
E72.11
E72.12
E72.19
E72.20
E72.21
E72.22
E72.23
E72.29
E72.3
E72.4
E72.50
E72.51
E72.52
E72.53
E72.59
E72.81
E72.89
E72.9
E74.00
E74.01
E74.02
E74.03
E74.04
E74.05
E74.09
E74.20
E74.21
E74.29
E74.4
E74.810
E74.818
E74.819
E74.89
E75.00
E75.01
E75.02
E75.09
E75.10
E75.11
E75.19
E75.23
E75.25
E75.26
E75.27
E75.28
E75.29
E75.4
E76.01
E76.02
E76.03
E76.1
E76.210
E76.211
E76.219
E76.22
E76.29
E76.3
E76.8
E76.9
E78.71
E78.72
E79.1
E79.2
E79.81
E79.82
E79.89
E79.9
E80.0
E80.1
E80.20
E80.21
E80.29
E80.3
E84.19
E84.8
E84.9
E85.0
E85.1
E85.2
E85.3
E85.4
E85.81
E85.82
E85.89
E85.9
E87.0
E87.1
E87.20
E87.21
E87.22
E87.29
E87.3
E87.4
E88.02
E88.40
E88.41
E88.42
E88.43
E88.49
E89.1
E89.6
E89.810
E89.811
E89.820
E89.821
E89.822
E89.823
E89.89
F01.511
F01.518
F01.52
F01.53
F01.54
F01.A11
F01.A18
F01.A2
F01.A3
F01.A4
F01.B11
F01.B18
F01.B2
F01.B3
F01.B4
F01.C11
F01.C18
F01.C2
F01.C3
F01.C4
F02.811
F02.818
F02.82
F02.83
F02.84
F02.A11
F02.A18
F02.A2
F02.A3
F02.A4
F02.B11
F02.B18
F02.B2
F02.B3
F02.B4
F02.C11
F02.C18
F02.C2
F02.C3

F02.C4
F03.911
F03.918
F03.92
F03.93
F03.94
F03.A11
F03.A18
F03.A2
F03.A3
F03.A4
F03.B11
F03.B18
F03.B2
F03.B3
F03.B4
F03.C11
F03.C18
F03.C2
F03.C3
F03.C4
F05
F06.0
F06.2
F06.71
F10.121
F10.130
F10.131
F10.132
F10.139
F10.14
F10.151
F10.159
F10.180
F10.181
F10.188
F10.19
F10.221
F10.230
F10.231
F10.232
F10.239
F10.24
F10.251
F10.259
F10.27
F10.280
F10.281
F10.288
F10.29
F10.921
F10.930
F10.931
F10.932
F10.939
F10.94
F10.951
F10.959
F10.980
F10.981
F10.988
F10.99
F11.121
F11.13
F11.150
F11.151
F11.20
F11.221
F11.222
F11.23
F11.250
F11.251
F11.259
F11.281
F11.282
F11.288
F11.921
F11.93
F11.950
F11.951
F12.121
F12.150
F12.151
F12.221
F12.250
F12.251
F12.921
F12.950
F12.951
F13.121
F13.130
F13.131
F13.132
F13.139
F13.150
F13.151
F13.20
F13.221
F13.230
F13.231
F13.232
F13.239
F13.250
F13.251
F13.259
F13.26
F13.27
F13.280
F13.281
F13.282
F13.288
F13.921
F13.930
F13.931
F13.932
F13.939
F13.950
F13.951
F13.97
F14.121
F14.13
F14.150
F14.151
F14.20
F14.221
F14.222
F14.229
F14.23
F14.250
F14.251
F14.259
F14.280
F14.281
F14.282
F14.288
F14.921
F14.93
F14.950
F14.951
F15.121
F15.13
F15.150
F15.151
F15.20
F15.221
F15.222
F15.23
F15.250
F15.251
F15.259
F15.280
F15.281
F15.282
F15.288
F15.921
F15.93
F15.950
F15.951
F16.121
F16.150
F16.151
F16.20
F16.221
F16.250
F16.251
F16.259
F16.280
F16.283
F16.288
F16.921
F16.950
F16.951
F17.203
F17.213
F17.223
F17.293
F18.121
F18.150
F18.151
F18.17
F18.20
F18.221
F18.250
F18.251
F18.259
F18.27
F18.280
F18.288
F18.921
F18.950
F18.951
F18.97
F19.121
F19.130
F19.131
F19.132
F19.139
F19.150
F19.151
F19.17
F19.20
F19.221
F19.222
F19.230
F19.231
F19.232
F19.239
F19.250
F19.251
F19.259
F19.26
F19.27
F19.280
F19.281
F19.282
F19.288
F19.921
F19.930
F19.931
F19.932
F19.939
F19.950
F19.951
F19.97
F20.0
F20.1
F20.2
F20.5
F20.81
F20.89
F23
F30.10
F30.11
F30.12
F30.13
F30.2
F30.9
F31.0
F31.10
F31.11
F31.12
F31.13
F31.2
F31.30
F31.31
F31.32
F31.4
F31.5
F31.60
F31.61
F31.62
F31.63
F31.64
F31.81
F31.89
F32.0
F32.1
F32.2
F32.3
F33.0
F33.1
F33.2
F33.3
F33.40
F33.8
F33.9
F34.81
F34.89
F34.9
F50.00
F50.01
F50.02
F50.2
F68.10
F68.12
F68.A
F72
F73
F84.0
F84.2
F84.3
F84.5
F84.8
F84.9
G03.1
G03.2
G04.1
G10
G11.0
G11.10
G11.11
G11.19
G11.2
G11.3
G11.4
G11.5
G11.6
G11.8
G11.9
G12.0
G12.1
G12.20
G12.21
G12.22
G12.23
G12.24
G12.25
G12.29
G12.8
G12.9
G21.11
G21.19
G21.2
G21.3
G21.8
G21.9
G23.0
G23.1
G23.2
G23.3
G23.8
G23.9
G24.02
G24.09
G24.2
G24.8
G25.82
G25.9
G31.81
G31.82
G32.0
G32.81
G36.0
G36.1
G36.8
G36.9
G37.0
G37.1
G37.2
G37.3
G37.5
G37.81
G37.89
G37.9
G40.001
G40.009
G40.011
G40.019
G40.101
G40.109
G40.111
G40.119
G40.201
G40.209
G40.211
G40.219
G40.411
G40.419
G40.501
G40.509
G40.801
G40.802
G40.803
G40.804
G40.811
G40.812
G40.813
G40.814
G40.821
G40.822
G40.823
G40.824
G40.833
G40.834
G40.89
G40.911
G40.919
G40.A11
G40.A19
G40.B01
G40.B09
G40.B11
G40.B19
G40.C01
G40.C09
G40.C11
G40.C19
G43.601
G43.609
G43.611
G43.619
G45.0
G45.1
G45.2
G45.3
G45.8
G45.9
G46.0
G46.1
G46.2
G60.1
G61.0
G61.81
G62.81
G70.80
G70.81
G71.20
G71.21
G71.220
G71.228
G71.29
G72.0
G72.1
G72.2
G72.81
G73.1
G73.3
G80.1
G80.2
G80.3
G81.00
G81.01
G81.02
G81.03
G81.04
G81.10
G81.11
G81.12
G81.13
G81.14
G81.90
G81.91
G81.92
G81.93
G81.94
G82.20
G82.21
G82.22
G83.0
G83.4
G90.3
G90.50
G90.511
G90.512
G90.513
G90.519
G90.521
G90.522
G90.523
G90.529
G90.59
G91.0
G91.1
G91.2
G91.3
G91.8
G91.9
G92.03
G92.04
G92.05
G93.1
G93.40
G93.42
G93.43
G93.44
G93.49
G95.0
G95.20
G95.29
G95.81
G95.89
G95.9
G96.00
G96.01
G96.02
G96.08
G96.09
G96.11
G97.0
G97.2
G97.31
G97.32
G97.41
G97.48
G97.49
G97.51
G97.52
G97.61
G97.62
G97.63
G97.64
G97.81
G97.82
G97.83
G97.84
G99.0
G99.2
H05.011
H05.012
H05.013
H05.019
H05.021
H05.022
H05.023
H05.029
H05.031
H05.032
H05.033
H05.039
H20.00
H20.011
H20.012
H20.013
H20.019
H20.021
H20.022
H20.023
H20.029
H20.031
H20.032
H20.033
H20.039
H20.9
H21.331
H21.332
H21.333
H21.339
H30.101
H30.102
H30.103
H30.109
H30.111
H30.112
H30.113
H30.119
H30.121
H30.122
H30.123
H30.129
H30.131
H30.132
H30.133
H30.139
H30.141
H30.142
H30.143
H30.149
H30.891
H30.892
H30.893
H30.899
H30.90
H30.91
H30.92
H30.93
H31.321
H31.322
H31.323
H31.329
H31.401
H31.402
H31.403
H31.409
H31.411
H31.412
H31.413
H31.419
H31.421
H31.422
H31.423
H31.429
H33.121
H33.122
H33.123
H33.129
H33.20
H33.21
H33.22
H33.23
H33.40
H33.41
H33.42
H33.43
H33.8
H34.00
H34.01
H34.02
H34.03
H34.10
H34.11
H34.12
H34.13
H34.211
H34.212
H34.213
H34.219
H34.231
H34.232
H34.233
H34.239
H34.8110
H34.8111
H34.8112
H34.8120
H34.8121
H34.8122
H34.8130
H34.8131
H34.8132
H34.8190
H34.8191
H34.8192
H34.9
H35.70
H35.721
H35.722
H35.723
H35.729
H35.731
H35.732
H35.733
H35.739
H35.82
H40.211
H40.212
H40.213
H40.219
H44.001
H44.002
H44.003
H44.009
H44.011
H44.012
H44.013
H44.019
H44.021
H44.022
H44.023
H44.029
H44.111
H44.112
H44.113
H44.119
H44.121
H44.122
H44.123
H44.129
H44.131
H44.132
H44.133
H44.139
H44.19
H46.00
H46.01
H46.02
H46.03
H46.10
H46.11
H46.12
H46.13
H46.8
H46.9
H47.10
H47.11
H47.41
H47.42
H47.43
H47.49
H47.511
H47.512
H47.519
H47.521
H47.522
H47.529
H47.531
H47.532
H47.539
H47.621
H47.622
H47.629
H47.631
H47.632
H47.639
H47.641
H47.642
H47.649
H49.811
H49.812
H49.813
H49.819
H53.121
H53.122
H53.123
H53.129
H53.131
H53.132
H53.133
H53.139
H59.011
H59.012
H59.013
H59.019
H59.031
H59.032
H59.033
H59.039
H59.091
H59.092
H59.093
H59.099
H59.111
H59.112
H59.113
H59.119
H59.121
H59.122
H59.123
H59.129
H59.211
H59.212
H59.213
H59.219
H59.221
H59.222
H59.223
H59.229
H59.311
H59.312
H59.313
H59.319
H59.321
H59.322
H59.323
H59.329
H59.331
H59.332
H59.333
H59.339
H59.341
H59.342
H59.343
H59.349
H59.351
H59.352
H59.353
H59.359
H59.361
H59.362
H59.363
H59.369
H59.811
H59.812
H59.813
H59.819
H59.88
H59.89
H60.20
H60.21
H60.22
H60.23
H70.001
H70.002
H70.003
H70.009
H70.011
H70.012
H70.013
H70.019
H70.091
H70.092
H70.093
H70.099
H95.21
H95.22
H95.31
H95.32
H95.41
H95.42
H95.51
H95.52
H95.53
H95.54
H95.811
H95.812
H95.813
H95.819
H95.88
H95.89
I01.0
I01.1
I01.2
I01.8
I01.9
I02.0
I02.9
I09.0
I09.2
I09.81
I12.0
I13.0
I13.11
I13.2
I16.1
I16.9
I20.0
I20.1
I20.2
I23.0
I23.1
I23.2
I23.3
I23.6
I23.7
I23.8
I24.0
I24.1
I24.81
I24.89
I24.9
I25.110
I25.112
I25.3
I25.700
I25.702
I25.710
I25.711
I25.712
I25.718
I25.719
I25.720
I25.721
I25.722
I25.728
I25.729
I25.730
I25.731
I25.732
I25.738
I25.739
I25.750
I25.751
I25.752
I25.758
I25.759
I25.760
I25.761
I25.762
I25.768
I25.769
I25.790
I25.791
I25.792
I25.798
I25.799
I25.810
I25.811
I25.812
I27.0
I27.1
I27.82
I28.0
I28.1
I30.0
I30.1
I30.8
I30.9
I31.0
I31.1
I31.2
I31.31
I31.39
I31.4
I31.8
I31.9
I32
I38
I39
I42.0
I42.1
I42.2
I42.3
I42.4
I42.5
I42.6
I42.7
I42.8
I42.9
I43
I44.2
I45.2
I45.3
I45.89
I47.0
I47.10
I47.11
I47.19
I47.20
I47.21
I47.29
I48.11
I48.19
I48.20
I48.21
I48.3
I48.4
I48.92
I49.2
I50.1
I50.20
I50.22
I50.30
I50.32
I50.40

I5Ø.42
I51.Ø
I51.81
I5A
I62.9
I67.3
I67.4
I67.5
I67.6
I67.7
I67.81
I67.82
I67.841
I67.848
I67.85Ø
I67.858
I67.89
I68.2
I69.Ø51
I69.Ø52
I69.Ø53
I69.Ø54
I69.Ø59
I69.151
I69.152
I69.153
I69.154
I69.159
I69.251
I69.252
I69.253
I69.254
I69.259
I69.351
I69.352
I69.353
I69.354
I69.359
I69.851
I69.852
I69.853
I69.854
I69.859
I69.951
I69.952
I69.953
I69.954
I69.959
I7Ø.261
I7Ø.262
I7Ø.263
I7Ø.268
I7Ø.269
I7Ø.331
I7Ø.332
I7Ø.333
I7Ø.334
I7Ø.338
I7Ø.339
I7Ø.341
I7Ø.342
I7Ø.343
I7Ø.344
I7Ø.348
I7Ø.349
I7Ø.361
I7Ø.362
I7Ø.363
I7Ø.368
I7Ø.369
I7Ø.431
I7Ø.432
I7Ø.433
I7Ø.434
I7Ø.438
I7Ø.439
I7Ø.441
I7Ø.442
I7Ø.443
I7Ø.444
I7Ø.448
I7Ø.449
I7Ø.461
I7Ø.462
I7Ø.463
I7Ø.468
I7Ø.469
I7Ø.531
I7Ø.532
I7Ø.533
I7Ø.534
I7Ø.538
I7Ø.539
I7Ø.541
I7Ø.542
I7Ø.543
I7Ø.544
I7Ø.548
I7Ø.549
I7Ø.561
I7Ø.562
I7Ø.563
I7Ø.568
I7Ø.569
I7Ø.631
I7Ø.632
I7Ø.633
I7Ø.634
I7Ø.638
I7Ø.639
I7Ø.641
I7Ø.642
I7Ø.643
I7Ø.644
I7Ø.648
I7Ø.649
I7Ø.661
I7Ø.662
I7Ø.663
I7Ø.668
I7Ø.669
I7Ø.731
I7Ø.732
I7Ø.733
I7Ø.734
I7Ø.738
I7Ø.739
I7Ø.741
I7Ø.742
I7Ø.743
I7Ø.744
I7Ø.748
I7Ø.749
I7Ø.761
I7Ø.762
I7Ø.763
I7Ø.768
I7Ø.769
I7Ø.92
I73.Ø1
I74.Ø9
I74.1Ø
I74.11
I74.19
I74.2
I74.3
I74.4
I74.5
I74.8
I74.9
I75.Ø11
I75.Ø12
I75.Ø13
I75.Ø19
I75.Ø21
I75.Ø22
I75.Ø23
I75.Ø29
I75.81
I75.89
I76
I77.2
I77.4
I77.5
I8Ø.1Ø
I8Ø.11
I8Ø.12
I8Ø.13
I8Ø.2Ø1
I8Ø.2Ø2
I8Ø.2Ø3
I8Ø.2Ø9
I8Ø.211
I8Ø.212
I8Ø.213
I8Ø.219
I8Ø.221
I8Ø.222
I8Ø.223
I8Ø.229
I8Ø.231
I8Ø.232
I8Ø.233
I8Ø.239
I8Ø.241
I8Ø.242
I8Ø.243
I8Ø.249
I8Ø.291
I8Ø.292
I8Ø.293
I8Ø.299
I82.1
I82.21Ø
I82.211
I82.29Ø
I82.291
I82.3
I82.4Ø1
I82.4Ø2
I82.4Ø3
I82.4Ø9
I82.411
I82.412
I82.413
I82.419
I82.421
I82.422
I82.423
I82.429
I82.431
I82.432
I82.433
I82.439
I82.441
I82.442
I82.443
I82.449
I82.451
I82.452
I82.453
I82.459
I82.491
I82.492
I82.493
I82.499
I82.4Y1
I82.4Y2
I82.4Y3
I82.4Y9
I82.4Z1
I82.4Z2
I82.4Z3
I82.4Z9
I82.5Ø1
I82.5Ø2
I82.5Ø3
I82.5Ø9
I82.511
I82.512
I82.513
I82.519
I82.521
I82.522
I82.523
I82.529
I82.531
I82.532
I82.533
I82.539
I82.541
I82.542
I82.543
I82.549
I82.551
I82.552
I82.553
I82.559
I82.591
I82.592
I82.593
I82.599
I82.5Y1
I82.5Y2
I82.5Y3
I82.5Y9
I82.5Z1
I82.5Z2
I82.5Z3
I82.5Z9
I82.6Ø1
I82.6Ø2
I82.6Ø3
I82.6Ø9
I82.611
I82.612
I82.613
I82.619
I82.621
I82.622
I82.623
I82.629
I82.7Ø1
I82.7Ø2
I82.7Ø3
I82.7Ø9
I82.711
I82.712
I82.713
I82.719
I82.721
I82.722
I82.723
I82.729
I82.811
I82.812
I82.813
I82.819
I82.89Ø
I82.891
I82.9Ø
I82.91
I82.A11
I82.A12
I82.A13
I82.A19
I82.A21
I82.A22
I82.A23
I82.A29
I82.B11
I82.B12
I82.B13
I82.B19
I82.B21
I82.B22
I82.B23
I82.B29
I82.C11
I82.C12
I82.C13
I82.C19
I82.C21
I82.C22
I82.C23
I82.C29
I83.2Ø1
I83.2Ø2
I83.2Ø3
I83.2Ø4
I83.2Ø5
I83.2Ø8
I83.2Ø9
I83.211
I83.212
I83.213
I83.214
I83.215
I83.218
I83.219
I83.221
I83.222
I83.223
I83.224
I83.225
I83.228
I83.229
I85.ØØ
I85.1Ø
I87.Ø11
I87.Ø12
I87.Ø13
I87.Ø19
I87.Ø31
I87.Ø32
I87.Ø33
I87.Ø39
I87.1
I87.311
I87.312
I87.313
I87.319
I87.331
I87.332
I87.333
I87.339
I96
I97.11Ø
I97.111
I97.12Ø
I97.121
I97.13Ø
I97.131
I97.19Ø
I97.191
I97.41Ø
I97.411
I97.418
I97.42
I97.51
I97.52
I97.61Ø
I97.611
I97.618
I97.62Ø
I97.621
I97.622
I97.63Ø
I97.631
I97.638
I97.64Ø
I97.641
I97.648
I97.71Ø
I97.711
I97.79Ø
I97.791
I97.81Ø
I97.811
I97.82Ø
I97.821
I97.88
I97.89
JØ5.1Ø
J18.2
J21.Ø
J21.1
J21.8
J21.9
J36
J39.Ø
J39.1
J44.Ø
J44.1
J45.21
J45.22
J45.31
J45.32
J45.41
J45.42
J45.51
J45.52
J45.9Ø1
J45.9Ø2
J47.Ø
J47.1
J67.7
J67.8
J67.9
J68.Ø
J7Ø.Ø
J7Ø.1
J81.1
J82.81
J82.82
J82.83
J82.89
J84.Ø1
J84.Ø2
J84.Ø3
J84.Ø9
J84.114
J84.116
J84.117
J84.2
J84.82
J84.9
J9Ø
J91.Ø
J91.8
J93.11
J93.12
J93.81
J93.82
J93.83
J93.9
J94.Ø
J94.2
J94.8
J95.ØØ
J95.Ø1
J95.Ø2
J95.Ø3
J95.Ø4
J95.Ø9
J95.4
J95.5
J95.61
J95.62
J95.71
J95.72
J95.811
J95.812
J95.83Ø
J95.831
J95.84
J95.85Ø
J95.851
J95.859
J95.86Ø
J95.861
J95.862
J95.863
J95.87
J95.88
J95.89
J96.1Ø
J96.11
J96.12
J98.11
J98.19
KØ4.Ø1
KØ4.Ø2
KØ4.4
K11.3
K11.4
K12.2
K22.1Ø
K25.3
K26.3
K27.3
K28.3
K31.Ø
K31.1
K31.5
K31.6
K35.2ØØ
K35.2Ø1
K35.2Ø9
K35.3Ø
K35.31
K35.8Ø
K35.89Ø
K35.891
K4Ø.ØØ
K4Ø.Ø1
K4Ø.3Ø
K4Ø.31
K41.ØØ
K41.Ø1
K41.3Ø
K41.31
K42.Ø
K43.Ø
K43.3
K43.6
K44.Ø
K45.Ø
K46.Ø
K5Ø.ØØ
K5Ø.Ø11
K5Ø.Ø12
K5Ø.Ø13
K5Ø.Ø14
K5Ø.Ø18
K5Ø.Ø19
K5Ø.1Ø
K5Ø.111
K5Ø.112
K5Ø.113
K5Ø.114
K5Ø.118
K5Ø.119
K5Ø.8Ø
K5Ø.811
K5Ø.812
K5Ø.813
K5Ø.814
K5Ø.818
K5Ø.819
K5Ø.9Ø
K5Ø.911
K5Ø.912
K5Ø.913
K5Ø.914
K5Ø.918
K5Ø.919
K51.ØØ
K51.Ø11
K51.Ø12
K51.Ø13
K51.Ø14
K51.Ø18
K51.Ø19
K51.2Ø
K51.211
K51.212
K51.213
K51.214
K51.218
K51.219
K51.3Ø
K51.311
K51.312
K51.313
K51.314
K51.318
K51.319
K51.4Ø
K51.411
K51.412
K51.413
K51.414
K51.418
K51.419
K51.5Ø
K51.511
K51.512
K51.513
K51.514
K51.518
K51.519
K51.8Ø
K51.811
K51.812
K51.813
K51.814
K51.818
K51.819
K51.9Ø
K51.911
K51.912
K51.913
K51.914
K51.918
K51.919
K52.Ø
K52.1
K55.1
K55.8
K55.9
K56.Ø
K56.1
K56.3
K56.49
K56.5Ø
K56.51
K56.52
K56.6ØØ
K56.6Ø1
K56.6Ø9
K56.69Ø
K56.691
K56.699
K56.7
K57.ØØ
K57.12
K57.2Ø
K57.32
K57.4Ø
K57.52
K57.8Ø
K57.92
K59.2
K59.31
K59.39
K61.Ø
K61.1
K61.2
K61.4
K62.5
K62.6
K63.Ø
K63.2
K63.3
K65.4
K68.11
K76.6
K77
K8Ø.ØØ
K8Ø.Ø1
K8Ø.1Ø
K8Ø.11
K8Ø.12
K8Ø.13
K8Ø.18
K8Ø.19
K8Ø.21
K8Ø.3Ø
K8Ø.31
K8Ø.32
K8Ø.33
K8Ø.34
K8Ø.35
K8Ø.36
K8Ø.37
K8Ø.4Ø
K8Ø.41
K8Ø.42
K8Ø.43
K8Ø.44
K8Ø.45
K8Ø.46
K8Ø.47
K8Ø.51
K8Ø.6Ø
K8Ø.61
K8Ø.62
K8Ø.63
K8Ø.64
K8Ø.65
K8Ø.66
K8Ø.71
K8Ø.81
K81.Ø
K81.2
K82.Ø
K82.1
K82.3
K82.A2
K83.Ø1
K83.Ø9
K83.3
K86.Ø
K86.1
K86.2
K86.3
K9Ø.1
K9Ø.2
K9Ø.3
K9Ø.41
K9Ø.49
K9Ø.81
K9Ø.821
K9Ø.822
K9Ø.829
K9Ø.83
K9Ø.89
K9Ø.9
K91.2
K91.3Ø
K91.31
K91.32
K91.61
K91.62
K91.71
K91.72
K91.81
K91.82
K91.83
K91.84Ø
K91.841
K91.85Ø
K91.858
K91.86
K91.87Ø
K91.871
K91.872
K91.873
K91.89
K92.Ø
K92.1
K92.2
K92.81
K94.Ø1
K94.Ø2
K94.Ø3
K94.Ø9
K94.11
K94.12
K94.13
K94.19
K94.22
K94.23
K94.3Ø
K94.31
K94.32
K94.33
K94.39
K95.Ø1
K95.Ø9
K95.81
K95.89
LØ2.Ø1
LØ2.11
LØ2.211
LØ2.212
LØ2.213
LØ2.214
LØ2.215
LØ2.216
LØ2.219
LØ2.31
LØ2.411
LØ2.412
LØ2.413
LØ2.414
LØ2.415
LØ2.416
LØ2.419
LØ2.511
LØ2.512
LØ2.519
LØ2.611
LØ2.612
LØ2.619
LØ2.811
LØ2.818
LØ2.91
LØ3.111
LØ3.112
LØ3.113
LØ3.114
LØ3.115
LØ3.116
LØ3.119
LØ3.121
LØ3.122
LØ3.123
LØ3.124
LØ3.125
LØ3.126
LØ3.129
LØ3.211
LØ3.212
LØ3.213
LØ3.221
LØ3.222
LØ3.311
LØ3.312
LØ3.313
LØ3.314
LØ3.315
LØ3.316
LØ3.317
LØ3.319
LØ3.321
LØ3.322
LØ3.323
LØ3.324
LØ3.325
LØ3.326
LØ3.327
LØ3.329
LØ3.811
LØ3.818
LØ3.891
LØ3.898
LØ3.9Ø
LØ3.91
LØ5.Ø1
LØ5.Ø2
LØ8.1
L1Ø.Ø
L1Ø.1
L1Ø.2
L1Ø.3
L1Ø.4
L1Ø.5
L1Ø.81
L1Ø.89
L1Ø.9
L12.Ø
L12.3Ø
L12.31
L12.35
L12.8
L12.9
L49.3
L49.4
L49.5
L49.6
L49.7
L49.8
L49.9
L51.1
L51.2
L51.3
L53.Ø
L53.1
L53.2
L53.3
L76.Ø1
L76.Ø2
L76.11
L76.12
L76.21
L76.22
L76.31
L76.32
L76.33
L76.34
L88
L97.1Ø1
L97.1Ø2
L97.1Ø3
L97.1Ø4
L97.1Ø5
L97.1Ø6
L97.1Ø8
L97.1Ø9
L97.111
L97.112
L97.113
L97.114
L97.115
L97.116
L97.118
L97.119
L97.121
L97.122
L97.123
L97.124
L97.125
L97.126
L97.128
L97.129
L97.2Ø1
L97.2Ø2
L97.2Ø3
L97.2Ø4
L97.2Ø5
L97.2Ø6
L97.2Ø8
L97.2Ø9
L97.211
L97.212
L97.213
L97.214
L97.215
L97.216
L97.218
L97.219
L97.221
L97.222
L97.223
L97.224
L97.225
L97.226
L97.228
L97.229
L97.3Ø1
L97.3Ø2

L97.303
L97.304
L97.305
L97.306
L97.308
L97.309
L97.311
L97.312
L97.313
L97.314
L97.315
L97.316
L97.318
L97.319
L97.321
L97.322
L97.323
L97.324
L97.325
L97.326
L97.328
L97.329
L97.401
L97.402
L97.403
L97.404
L97.405
L97.406
L97.408
L97.409
L97.411
L97.412
L97.413
L97.414
L97.415
L97.416
L97.418
L97.419
L97.421
L97.422
L97.423
L97.424
L97.425
L97.426
L97.428
L97.429
L97.505
L97.506
L97.508
L97.515
L97.516
L97.518
L97.525
L97.526
L97.528
L97.801
L97.802
L97.803
L97.804
L97.805
L97.806
L97.808
L97.809
L97.811
L97.812
L97.813
L97.814
L97.815
L97.816
L97.818
L97.819
L97.821
L97.822
L97.823
L97.824
L97.825
L97.826
L97.828
L97.829
L97.901
L97.902
L97.903
L97.904
L97.905
L97.906
L97.908
L97.909
L97.911
L97.912
L97.913
L97.914
L97.915
L97.916
L97.918
L97.919
L97.921
L97.922
L97.923
L97.924
L97.925
L97.926
L97.928
L97.929
L98.3
L98.415
L98.416
L98.418
L98.425
L98.426
L98.428
L98.495
L98.496
L98.498
M00.00
M00.011
M00.012
M00.019
M00.021
M00.022
M00.029
M00.031
M00.032
M00.039
M00.041
M00.042
M00.049
M00.051
M00.052
M00.059
M00.061
M00.062
M00.069
M00.071
M00.072
M00.079
M00.08
M00.09
M00.10
M00.111
M00.112
M00.119
M00.121
M00.122
M00.129
M00.131
M00.132
M00.139
M00.141
M00.142
M00.149
M00.151
M00.152
M00.159
M00.161
M00.162
M00.169
M00.171
M00.172
M00.179
M00.18
M00.19
M00.20
M00.211
M00.212
M00.219
M00.221
M00.222
M00.229
M00.231
M00.232
M00.239
M00.241
M00.242
M00.249
M00.251
M00.252
M00.259
M00.261
M00.262
M00.269
M00.271
M00.272
M00.279
M00.28
M00.29
M00.80
M00.811
M00.812
M00.819
M00.821
M00.822
M00.829
M00.831
M00.832
M00.839
M00.841
M00.842
M00.849
M00.851
M00.852
M00.859
M00.861
M00.862
M00.869
M00.871
M00.872
M00.879
M00.88
M00.89
M00.9
M01.X0
M01.X11
M01.X12
M01.X19
M01.X21
M01.X22
M01.X29
M01.X31
M01.X32
M01.X39
M01.X41
M01.X42
M01.X49
M01.X51
M01.X52
M01.X59
M01.X61
M01.X62
M01.X69
M01.X71
M01.X72
M01.X79
M01.X8
M01.X9
M02.10
M02.111
M02.112
M02.119
M02.121
M02.122
M02.129
M02.131
M02.132
M02.139
M02.141
M02.142
M02.149
M02.151
M02.152
M02.159
M02.161
M02.162
M02.169
M02.171
M02.172
M02.179
M02.18
M02.19
M02.30
M02.311
M02.312
M02.319
M02.321
M02.322
M02.329
M02.331
M02.332
M02.339
M02.341
M02.342
M02.349
M02.351
M02.352
M02.359
M02.361
M02.362
M02.369
M02.371
M02.372
M02.379
M02.38
M02.39
M02.80
M02.811
M02.812
M02.819
M02.821
M02.822
M02.829
M02.831
M02.832
M02.839
M02.841
M02.842
M02.849
M02.851
M02.852
M02.859
M02.861
M02.862
M02.869
M02.871
M02.872
M02.879
M02.88
M02.89
M05.40
M05.411
M05.412
M05.419
M05.421
M05.422
M05.429
M05.431
M05.432
M05.439
M05.441
M05.442
M05.449
M05.451
M05.452
M05.459
M05.461
M05.462
M05.469
M05.471
M05.472
M05.479
M05.49
M25.00
M25.011
M25.012
M25.019
M25.021
M25.022
M25.029
M25.031
M25.032
M25.039
M25.041
M25.042
M25.049
M25.051
M25.052
M25.059
M25.061
M25.062
M25.069
M25.071
M25.072
M25.073
M25.074
M25.075
M25.076
M25.08
M30.0
M30.1
M30.2
M30.3
M30.8
M31.0
M31.2
M31.30
M31.31
M31.4
M31.7
M31.8
M31.9
M32.11
M32.12
M33.00
M33.01
M33.02
M33.03
M33.09
M33.10
M33.11
M33.12
M33.13
M33.19
M33.20
M33.21
M33.22
M33.29
M33.90
M33.91
M33.92
M33.93
M33.99
M34.81
M34.82
M35.03
M35.07
M35.1
M35.2
M35.5
M35.81
M35.89
M36.0
M46.20
M46.21
M46.22
M46.23
M46.24
M46.25
M46.26
M46.27
M46.28
M46.30
M46.31
M46.32
M46.33
M46.34
M46.35
M46.36
M46.37
M46.38
M46.39
M47.011
M47.012
M47.013
M47.014
M47.015
M47.016
M47.019
M47.021
M47.022
M47.029
M47.10
M47.11
M47.12
M47.13
M47.14
M47.15
M47.16
M48.30
M48.31
M48.32
M48.33
M48.34
M48.35
M48.36
M48.37
M48.38
M48.50XA
M48.51XA
M48.52XA
M48.53XA
M48.54XA
M48.55XA
M48.56XA
M48.57XA
M48.58XA
M50.00
M50.01
M50.020
M50.021
M50.022
M50.023
M50.03
M51.04
M51.05
M51.06
M60.000
M60.001
M60.002
M60.003
M60.004
M60.005
M60.009
M60.011
M60.012
M60.019
M60.021
M60.022
M60.029
M60.031
M60.032
M60.039
M60.041
M60.042
M60.043
M60.044
M60.045
M60.046
M60.051
M60.052
M60.059
M60.061
M60.062
M60.069
M60.070
M60.071
M60.072
M60.073
M60.074
M60.075
M60.076
M60.077
M60.078
M60.08
M60.09
M62.82
M79.A11
M79.A12
M79.A19
M79.A21
M79.A22
M79.A29
M79.A3
M79.A9
M80.00XA
M80.00XK
M80.00XP
M80.011A
M80.011K
M80.011P
M80.012A
M80.012K
M80.012P
M80.019A
M80.019K
M80.019P
M80.021A
M80.021K
M80.021P
M80.022A
M80.022K
M80.022P
M80.029A
M80.029K
M80.029P
M80.031A
M80.031K
M80.031P
M80.032A
M80.032K
M80.032P
M80.039A
M80.039K
M80.039P
M80.041A
M80.041K
M80.041P
M80.042A
M80.042K
M80.042P
M80.049A
M80.049K
M80.049P
M80.051A
M80.051K
M80.051P
M80.052A
M80.052K
M80.052P
M80.059A
M80.059K
M80.059P
M80.061A
M80.061K
M80.061P
M80.062A
M80.062K
M80.062P
M80.069A
M80.069K
M80.069P
M80.071A
M80.071K
M80.071P
M80.072A
M80.072K
M80.072P
M80.079A
M80.079K
M80.079P
M80.08XA
M80.08XK
M80.08XP
M80.0AXA
M80.0AXK
M80.0AXP
M80.0B1A
M80.0B1K
M80.0B1P
M80.0B2A
M80.0B2K
M80.0B2P
M80.0B9A
M80.0B9K
M80.0B9P
M80.80XA
M80.80XK
M80.80XP
M80.811A
M80.811K
M80.811P
M80.812A
M80.812K
M80.812P
M80.819A
M80.819K
M80.819P
M80.821A
M80.821K
M80.821P
M80.822A
M80.822K
M80.822P
M80.829A
M80.829K
M80.829P
M80.831A
M80.831K
M80.831P
M80.832A
M80.832K
M80.832P
M80.839A
M80.839K
M80.839P
M80.841A
M80.841K
M80.841P
M80.842A
M80.842K
M80.842P
M80.849A
M80.849K
M80.849P
M80.851A
M80.851K
M80.851P
M80.852A
M80.852K
M80.852P
M80.859A
M80.859K
M80.859P
M80.861A
M80.861K
M80.861P
M80.862A
M80.862K
M80.862P
M80.869A
M80.869K
M80.869P
M80.871A
M80.871K
M80.871P
M80.872A
M80.872K
M80.872P
M80.879A
M80.879K
M80.879P
M80.88XA
M80.88XK
M80.88XP
M80.8AXA
M80.8AXK
M80.8AXP
M80.8B1A
M80.8B1K
M80.8B1P
M80.8B2A
M80.8B2K
M80.8B2P
M80.8B9A
M80.8B9K
M80.8B9P
M84.30XK
M84.30XP
M84.311K
M84.311P
M84.312K
M84.312P
M84.319K
M84.319P
M84.321K
M84.321P
M84.322K
M84.322P
M84.329K
M84.329P
M84.331K
M84.331P
M84.332K
M84.332P
M84.333K
M84.333P
M84.334K
M84.334P
M84.339K
M84.339P
M84.341K
M84.341P
M84.342K
M84.342P
M84.343K
M84.343P
M84.344K
M84.344P
M84.345K
M84.345P
M84.346K
M84.346P
M84.350K
M84.350P
M84.351K
M84.351P
M84.352K
M84.352P
M84.353K
M84.353P
M84.359K
M84.359P
M84.361K
M84.361P
M84.362K
M84.362P
M84.363K
M84.363P
M84.364K
M84.364P
M84.369K
M84.369P
M84.371K
M84.371P
M84.372K
M84.372P
M84.373K
M84.373P
M84.374K
M84.374P
M84.375K
M84.375P
M84.376K
M84.376P
M84.377K
M84.377P
M84.378K
M84.378P
M84.379K
M84.379P
M84.38XK
M84.38XP
M84.40XA
M84.40XK
M84.40XP
M84.411A
M84.411K
M84.411P
M84.412A
M84.412K
M84.412P
M84.419A
M84.419K
M84.419P
M84.421A
M84.421K
M84.421P
M84.422A
M84.422K
M84.422P
M84.429A
M84.429K
M84.429P
M84.431A
M84.431K
M84.431P
M84.432A
M84.432K
M84.432P
M84.433A
M84.433K
M84.433P
M84.434A
M84.434K
M84.434P
M84.439A
M84.439K
M84.439P
M84.441A
M84.441K
M84.441P
M84.442A
M84.442K
M84.442P
M84.443A
M84.443K
M84.443P
M84.444A
M84.444K
M84.444P
M84.445A
M84.445K
M84.445P
M84.446A
M84.446K
M84.446P
M84.451A
M84.451K
M84.451P
M84.452A
M84.452K
M84.452P
M84.453A
M84.453K
M84.453P
M84.454A
M84.454K
M84.454P
M84.459A
M84.459K
M84.459P
M84.461A
M84.461K
M84.461P
M84.462A
M84.462K
M84.462P
M84.463A
M84.463K
M84.463P
M84.464A
M84.464K
M84.464P
M84.469A
M84.469K
M84.469P
M84.471A
M84.471K
M84.471P
M84.472A
M84.472K
M84.472P
M84.473A
M84.473K
M84.473P
M84.474A
M84.474K
M84.474P
M84.475A
M84.475K
M84.475P
M84.476A
M84.476K
M84.476P
M84.477A
M84.477K
M84.477P
M84.478A
M84.478K
M84.478P
M84.479A
M84.479K
M84.479P
M84.48XA
M84.48XK
M84.48XP
M84.50XA
M84.50XK
M84.50XP
M84.511A
M84.511K
M84.511P
M84.512A
M84.512K
M84.512P
M84.519A
M84.519K
M84.519P
M84.521A
M84.521K
M84.521P
M84.522A
M84.522K
M84.522P
M84.529A
M84.529K
M84.529P
M84.531A
M84.531K
M84.531P
M84.532A
M84.532K
M84.532P
M84.533A
M84.533K
M84.533P
M84.534A
M84.534K
M84.534P
M84.539A
M84.539K
M84.539P
M84.541A
M84.541K
M84.541P
M84.542A
M84.542K
M84.542P
M84.549A
M84.549K
M84.549P
M84.550A
M84.550K
M84.550P
M84.551A
M84.551K

M84.551P
M84.552A
M84.552K
M84.552P
M84.553A
M84.553K
M84.553P
M84.559A
M84.559K
M84.559P
M84.561A
M84.561K
M84.561P
M84.562A
M84.562K
M84.562P
M84.563A
M84.563K
M84.563P
M84.564A
M84.564K
M84.564P
M84.569A
M84.569K
M84.569P
M84.571A
M84.571K
M84.571P
M84.572A
M84.572K
M84.572P
M84.573A
M84.573K
M84.573P
M84.574A
M84.574K
M84.574P
M84.575A
M84.575K
M84.575P
M84.576A
M84.576K
M84.576P
M84.58XA
M84.58XK
M84.58XP
M84.60XA
M84.60XK
M84.60XP
M84.611A
M84.611K
M84.611P
M84.612A
M84.612K
M84.612P
M84.619A
M84.619K
M84.619P
M84.621A
M84.621K
M84.621P
M84.622A
M84.622K
M84.622P
M84.629A
M84.629K
M84.629P
M84.631A
M84.631K
M84.631P
M84.632A
M84.632K
M84.632P
M84.633A
M84.633K
M84.633P
M84.634A
M84.634K
M84.634P
M84.639A
M84.639K
M84.639P
M84.641A
M84.641K
M84.641P
M84.642A
M84.642K
M84.642P
M84.649A
M84.649K
M84.649P
M84.650A
M84.650K
M84.650P
M84.651A
M84.651K
M84.651P
M84.652A
M84.652K
M84.652P
M84.653A
M84.653K
M84.653P
M84.659A
M84.659K
M84.659P
M84.661A
M84.661K
M84.661P
M84.662A
M84.662K
M84.662P
M84.663A
M84.663K
M84.663P
M84.664A
M84.664K
M84.664P
M84.669A
M84.669K
M84.669P
M84.671A
M84.671K
M84.671P
M84.672A
M84.672K
M84.672P
M84.673A
M84.673K
M84.673P
M84.674A
M84.674K
M84.674P
M84.675A
M84.675K
M84.675P
M84.676A
M84.676K
M84.676P
M84.68XA
M84.68XK
M84.68XP
M84.750A
M84.750K
M84.750P
M84.751A
M84.751K
M84.751P
M84.752A
M84.752K
M84.752P
M84.753A
M84.753K
M84.753P
M84.754A
M84.754K
M84.754P
M84.755A
M84.755K
M84.755P
M84.756A
M84.756K
M84.756P
M84.757A
M84.757K
M84.757P
M84.758A
M84.758K
M84.758P
M84.759A
M84.759K
M84.759P
M86.00
M86.011
M86.012
M86.019
M86.021
M86.022
M86.029
M86.031
M86.032
M86.039
M86.041
M86.042
M86.049
M86.051
M86.052
M86.059
M86.061
M86.062
M86.069
M86.071
M86.072
M86.079
M86.08
M86.09
M86.10
M86.111
M86.112
M86.119
M86.121
M86.122
M86.129
M86.131
M86.132
M86.139
M86.141
M86.142
M86.149
M86.151
M86.152
M86.159
M86.161
M86.162
M86.169
M86.171
M86.172
M86.179
M86.18
M86.19
M86.20
M86.211
M86.212
M86.219
M86.221
M86.222
M86.229
M86.231
M86.232
M86.239
M86.241
M86.242
M86.249
M86.251
M86.252
M86.259
M86.261
M86.262
M86.269
M86.271
M86.272
M86.279
M86.28
M86.29
M86.30
M86.311
M86.312
M86.319
M86.321
M86.322
M86.329
M86.331
M86.332
M86.339
M86.341
M86.342
M86.349
M86.351
M86.352
M86.359
M86.361
M86.362
M86.369
M86.371
M86.372
M86.379
M86.38
M86.39
M86.40
M86.411
M86.412
M86.419
M86.421
M86.422
M86.429
M86.431
M86.432
M86.439
M86.441
M86.442
M86.449
M86.451
M86.452
M86.459
M86.461
M86.462
M86.469
M86.471
M86.472
M86.479
M86.48
M86.49
M86.50
M86.511
M86.512
M86.519
M86.521
M86.522
M86.529
M86.531
M86.532
M86.539
M86.541
M86.542
M86.549
M86.551
M86.552
M86.559
M86.561
M86.562
M86.569
M86.571
M86.572
M86.579
M86.58
M86.59
M86.60
M86.611
M86.612
M86.619
M86.621
M86.622
M86.629
M86.631
M86.632
M86.639
M86.641
M86.642
M86.649
M86.651
M86.652
M86.659
M86.661
M86.662
M86.669
M86.671
M86.672
M86.679
M86.68
M86.69
M86.8X0
M86.8X1
M86.8X2
M86.8X3
M86.8X4
M86.8X5
M86.8X6
M86.8X7
M86.8X8
M86.8X9
M86.9
M87.00
M87.011
M87.012
M87.019
M87.021
M87.022
M87.029
M87.031
M87.032
M87.033
M87.034
M87.035
M87.036
M87.037
M87.038
M87.039
M87.041
M87.042
M87.043
M87.044
M87.045
M87.046
M87.050
M87.051
M87.052
M87.059
M87.061
M87.062
M87.063
M87.064
M87.065
M87.066
M87.071
M87.072
M87.073
M87.074
M87.075
M87.076
M87.077
M87.078
M87.079
M87.08
M87.09
M87.10
M87.111
M87.112
M87.119
M87.121
M87.122
M87.129
M87.131
M87.132
M87.133
M87.134
M87.135
M87.136
M87.137
M87.138
M87.139
M87.141
M87.142
M87.143
M87.144
M87.145
M87.146
M87.150
M87.151
M87.152
M87.159
M87.161
M87.162
M87.163
M87.164
M87.165
M87.166
M87.171
M87.172
M87.173
M87.174
M87.175
M87.176
M87.177
M87.178
M87.179
M87.180
M87.188
M87.19
M87.20
M87.211
M87.212
M87.219
M87.221
M87.222
M87.229
M87.231
M87.232
M87.233
M87.234
M87.235
M87.236
M87.237
M87.238
M87.239
M87.241
M87.242
M87.243
M87.244
M87.245
M87.246
M87.250
M87.251
M87.252
M87.256
M87.261
M87.262
M87.263
M87.264
M87.265
M87.266
M87.271
M87.272
M87.273
M87.274
M87.275
M87.276
M87.277
M87.278
M87.279
M87.28
M87.29
M87.30
M87.311
M87.312
M87.319
M87.321
M87.322
M87.329
M87.331
M87.332
M87.333
M87.334
M87.335
M87.336
M87.337
M87.338
M87.339
M87.341
M87.342
M87.343
M87.344
M87.345
M87.346
M87.350
M87.351
M87.352
M87.353
M87.361
M87.362
M87.363
M87.364
M87.365
M87.366
M87.371
M87.372
M87.373
M87.374
M87.375
M87.376
M87.377
M87.378
M87.379
M87.38
M87.39
M87.80
M87.811
M87.812
M87.819
M87.821
M87.822
M87.829
M87.831
M87.832
M87.833
M87.834
M87.835
M87.836
M87.837
M87.838
M87.839
M87.841
M87.842
M87.843
M87.844
M87.845
M87.849
M87.850
M87.851
M87.852
M87.859
M87.861
M87.862
M87.863
M87.864
M87.865
M87.869
M87.871
M87.872
M87.873
M87.874
M87.875
M87.876
M87.877
M87.878
M87.879
M87.88
M87.89
M87.9
M90.50
M90.511
M90.512
M90.519
M90.521
M90.522
M90.529
M90.531
M90.532
M90.539
M90.541
M90.542
M90.549
M90.551
M90.552
M90.559
M90.561
M90.562
M90.569
M90.571
M90.572
M90.579
M90.58
M90.59
M96.0
M96.621
M96.622
M96.629
M96.631
M96.632
M96.639
M96.65
M96.661
M96.662
M96.669
M96.671
M96.672
M96.679
M96.69
M96.810
M96.811
M96.820
M96.821
M96.830
M96.831
M96.840
M96.841
M96.842
M96.843
M96.89
M96.A1
M96.A2
M96.A3
M96.A9
M97.01XA
M97.02XA
M97.11XA
M97.12XA
M97.21XA
M97.22XA
M97.31XA
M97.32XA
M97.41XA
M97.42XA
M97.8XXA
M97.9XXA
M99.10
M99.11
M99.18
N02.0
N02.1
N02.2
N02.3
N02.4
N02.5
N02.6
N02.7
N02.8
N02.9
N02.A
N02.B1
N02.B2
N02.B3
N02.B4
N02.B5
N02.B6
N02.B9
N03.0
N03.1
N03.2
N03.3
N03.4
N03.5
N03.6
N03.7
N03.8
N03.9
N03.A
N04.0
N04.1
N04.20
N04.21
N04.22
N04.29
N04.3
N04.4
N04.5
N04.6
N04.7
N04.8
N04.9
N04.A
N05.2
N05.3
N05.4
N05.5
N05.A
N06.20
N06.21
N06.22
N06.29
N06.3
N06.4
N06.5
N06.A
N07.2
N07.3
N07.4
N07.5
N07.A
N10
N11.1
N11.8
N11.9
N12
N13.0
N13.1
N13.2
N13.30
N13.39
N13.4
N13.6
N13.8
N17.8
N17.9
N18.4
N18.5
N20.1
N20.2
N25.1
N25.81
N28.0
N28.84
N28.85
N28.86
N30.00
N30.01
N30.40
N30.41
N32.1
N32.2
N34.0
N36.0
N39.0
N41.0
N41.2
N43.1
N44.00
N44.01
N44.02
N44.03
N44.04
N45.4
N48.30
N48.31
N48.32
N48.33
N48.39
N70.01
N70.02
N70.03
N71.0
N73.0
N73.4
N75.1
N76.4
N76.81
N82.0
N82.1
N82.2
N82.3
N82.4
N82.5
N82.8
N82.9
N83.511
N83.512
N83.519
N83.521
N83.522
N83.529
N83.53
N98.0
N98.1
N98.2
N98.3
N98.8
N98.9
N99.510
N99.511
N99.512
N99.518
N99.61
N99.62
N99.71
N99.72
N99.820
N99.821
N99.840
N99.841
N99.842
N99.843
O00.00
O00.01
O00.101
O00.102
O00.109
O00.111
O00.112
O00.119
O00.201
O00.202
O00.209
O00.211
O00.212
O00.219
O00.80
O00.81
O00.90
O00.91
O03.0
O03.30
O03.33
O03.34
O03.35
O03.36
O03.37
O03.38
O03.39
O03.5
O03.7
O03.80
O03.83
O03.84
O03.85
O03.86
O03.87
O03.88
O03.89
O04.5
O04.80
O04.83
O04.84
O04.85
O04.86
O04.87
O04.88
O04.89
O07.0
O07.1
O07.30
O07.33
O07.34
O07.35
O07.36
O07.37
O07.38
O07.39
O08.0
O08.1
O08.5
O08.6
O08.7
O08.81
O08.82
O08.83
O08.89
O08.9
O10.011
O10.012
O10.013
O10.02
O10.411
O10.412
O10.413
O10.43
O10.911
O10.912
O10.913
O10.92
O12.11
O12.12
O12.13
O12.21
O12.22
O12.23
O14.02
O14.03
O14.92
O14.93
O16.1
O16.2
O16.3
O20.0
O20.9
O22.20
O22.21
O22.22
O22.23
O22.30
O22.40
O22.41
O22.42
O22.43
O22.50
O22.51
O22.52
O22.53
O22.8X1
O22.8X2
O22.8X3
O22.8X9
O22.90
O23.01
O23.02
O23.03
O23.11
O23.12
O23.13
O23.21
O23.22
O23.23
O23.31
O23.32
O23.33

O23.41
O23.42
O23.43
O23.511
O23.512
O23.513
O23.521
O23.522
O23.523
O23.591
O23.592
O23.593
O23.91
O23.92
O23.93
O24.011
O24.012
O24.013
O24.019
O24.03
O24.111
O24.112
O24.113
O24.119
O24.13
O24.311
O24.312
O24.313
O24.319
O24.33
O24.811
O24.812
O24.813
O24.819
O24.83
O24.911
O24.912
O24.913
O24.919
O24.93
O26.611
O26.612
O26.613
O26.62
O26.641
O26.642
O26.643
O26.831
O26.832
O26.833
O26.872
O26.873
O26.879
O30.101
O30.102
O30.103
O30.111
O30.112
O30.113
O30.121
O30.122
O30.123
O30.131
O30.132
O30.133
O30.191
O30.192
O30.193
O30.201
O30.202
O30.203
O30.211
O30.212
O30.213
O30.221
O30.222
O30.223
O30.231
O30.232
O30.233
O30.291
O30.292
O30.293
O30.801
O30.802
O30.803
O30.811
O30.812
O30.813
O30.821
O30.822
O30.823
O30.831
O30.832
O30.833
O30.891
O30.892
O30.893
O31.8X10
O31.8X11
O31.8X12
O31.8X13
O31.8X14
O31.8X15
O31.8X19
O31.8X20
O31.8X21
O31.8X22
O31.8X23
O31.8X24
O31.8X25
O31.8X29
O31.8X30
O31.8X31
O31.8X32
O31.8X33
O31.8X34
O31.8X35
O31.8X39
O33.0
O36.0110
O36.0111
O36.0112
O36.0113
O36.0114
O36.0115
O36.0119
O36.0120
O36.0121
O36.0122
O36.0123
O36.0124
O36.0125
O36.0129
O36.0130
O36.0131
O36.0132
O36.0133
O36.0134
O36.0135
O36.0139
O36.0910
O36.0911
O36.0912
O36.0913
O36.0914
O36.0915
O36.0919
O36.0920
O36.0921
O36.0922
O36.0923
O36.0924
O36.0925
O36.0929
O36.0930
O36.0931
O36.0932
O36.0933
O36.0934
O36.0935
O36.0939
O36.4XX0
O36.4XX1
O36.4XX2
O36.4XX3
O36.4XX4
O36.4XX5
O36.4XX9
O41.01X0
O41.01X1
O41.01X2
O41.01X3
O41.01X4
O41.01X5
O41.01X9
O41.02X0
O41.02X1
O41.02X2
O41.02X3
O41.02X4
O41.02X5
O41.02X9
O41.03X0
O41.03X1
O41.03X2
O41.03X3
O41.03X4
O41.03X5
O41.03X9
O44.01
O44.02
O44.03
O44.21
O44.22
O44.23
O44.41
O44.42
O44.43
O47.02
O47.03
O47.1
O60.10X0
O60.10X1
O60.10X2
O60.10X3
O60.10X4
O60.10X5
O60.10X9
O60.20X0
O60.20X1
O60.20X2
O60.20X3
O60.20X4
O60.20X5
O60.20X9
O63.9
O68
O70.20
O70.21
O70.22
O70.23
O70.3
O70.4
O71.2
O71.3
O71.4
O71.5
O71.6
O71.7
O72.0
O72.1
O72.2
O75.2
O86.11
O86.12
O86.13
O86.19
O86.20
O86.21
O86.22
O86.29
O86.4
O87.0
O87.2
O87.3
O87.8
O88.319
O98.011
O98.012
O98.013
O98.02
O98.03
O98.111
O98.112
O98.113
O98.12
O98.13
O98.211
O98.212
O98.213
O98.22
O98.23
O98.311
O98.312
O98.313
O98.32
O98.33
O98.411
O98.412
O98.413
O98.42
O98.43
O98.511
O98.512
O98.513
O98.52
O98.53
O98.611
O98.612
O98.613
O98.62
O98.63
O98.711
O98.712
O98.713
O98.72
O98.73
O98.811
O98.812
O98.813
O98.82
O98.83
O98.911
O98.912
O98.913
O98.92
O98.93
O99.111
O99.112
O99.113
O99.119
O99.12
O99.13
O99.321
O99.322
O99.323
O99.324
O99.325
O99.354
O99.355
O99.411
O99.412
O99.413
O99.43
O99.830
O99.834
O99.835
P10.2
P12.2
P28.0
P28.10
P28.11
P28.19
P28.2
P28.30
P28.31
P28.32
P28.33
P28.39
P28.40
P28.41
P28.42
P28.43
P28.49
P35.0
P38.1
P38.9
P39.0
P39.2
P39.3
P39.4
P39.8
P39.9
P52.0
P52.1
P52.3
P53
P54.4
P61.2
P61.3
P61.4
P61.6
P70.2
P70.8
P71.0
P71.1
P71.2
P71.3
P71.4
P71.8
P71.9
P72.0
P72.1
P72.2
P72.8
P74.41
P74.5
P74.6
P74.8
P76.1
P83.0
P83.30
P83.39
P91.60
P91.61
P91.62
P93.0
P93.8
P94.0
P96.1
P96.2
Q01.0
Q01.1
Q01.2
Q01.8
Q01.9
Q04.4
Q04.5
Q04.6
Q04.8
Q05.0
Q05.1
Q05.2
Q05.3
Q05.4
Q07.02
Q07.03
Q20.5
Q21.0
Q21.10
Q21.11
Q21.12
Q21.13
Q21.14
Q21.15
Q21.16
Q21.19
Q21.20
Q21.21
Q21.22
Q21.23
Q22.1
Q22.2
Q22.3
Q23.0
Q23.1
Q23.2
Q23.3
Q24.0
Q24.1
Q24.3
Q24.5
Q25.0
Q25.1
Q25.21
Q25.29
Q25.3
Q25.40
Q25.41
Q25.42
Q25.43
Q25.44
Q25.45
Q25.46
Q25.47
Q25.48
Q25.49
Q25.8
Q25.9
Q26.0
Q26.1
Q26.2
Q26.3
Q26.4
Q26.8
Q26.9
Q27.30
Q27.4
Q28.0
Q28.1
Q28.8
Q28.9
Q31.1
Q31.2
Q31.3
Q31.5
Q31.8
Q31.9
Q32.0
Q32.1
Q32.2
Q32.3
Q32.4
Q33.0
Q33.4
Q39.5
Q39.6
Q39.8
Q39.9
Q41.0
Q41.1
Q41.2
Q41.8
Q41.9
Q42.0
Q42.1
Q42.2
Q42.3
Q42.8
Q42.9
Q43.1
Q43.2
Q43.3
Q43.4
Q43.5
Q43.6
Q43.7
Q43.8
Q43.9
Q44.0
Q44.1
Q44.4
Q44.5
Q44.6
Q44.70
Q44.71
Q44.79
Q45.0
Q45.1
Q45.2
Q45.3
Q60.0
Q60.1
Q60.2
Q60.3
Q60.4
Q60.5
Q60.6
Q61.00
Q61.01
Q61.02
Q61.11
Q61.19
Q61.2
Q61.3
Q61.4
Q61.5
Q61.8
Q61.9
Q62.0
Q62.10
Q62.11
Q62.12
Q62.2
Q62.31
Q62.32
Q62.39
Q64.10
Q64.11
Q64.12
Q64.19
Q64.2
Q64.31
Q64.32
Q64.33
Q64.39
Q67.5
Q67.8
Q68.1
Q74.3
Q76.3
Q76.425
Q76.426
Q76.427
Q76.428
Q76.429
Q76.6
Q76.7
Q76.8
Q76.9
Q77.2
Q78.0
Q78.2
Q79.60
Q79.61
Q79.62
Q79.63
Q79.69
Q85.1
Q85.81
Q85.82
Q85.83
Q85.89
Q85.9
Q87.11
Q87.19
Q87.2
Q87.3
Q87.40
Q87.410
Q87.418
Q87.42
Q87.43
Q87.5
Q87.81
Q87.82
Q87.83
Q87.84
Q87.85
Q87.89
Q89.01
Q89.09
Q89.3
Q89.7
Q89.8
Q91.0
Q91.1
Q91.2
Q91.3
Q91.4
Q91.5
Q91.6
Q91.7
Q93.3
Q93.4
Q93.51
Q93.52
Q93.59
Q93.7
Q93.82
Q93.88
Q93.89
Q93.9
R04.2
R04.81
R04.89
R04.9
R06.3
R09.01
R17
R18.0
R18.8
R29.0
R29.1
R29.5
R39.0
R40.3
R41.4
R44.0
R44.2
R44.3
R45.851
R47.01
R56.00
R56.01
R56.1
R57.9
R64
R65.10
R71.0
R78.81
R82.0
R82.1
S01.101A
S01.102A
S01.109A
S02.0XXA
S02.0XXK
S02.101A
S02.101K
S02.102A
S02.102K
S02.109A
S02.109K
S02.110A
S02.110K
S02.111A
S02.111K
S02.112A
S02.112K
S02.113A
S02.113K
S02.118A
S02.118K
S02.119A
S02.119K
S02.11AA
S02.11AK
S02.11BA
S02.11BK
S02.11CA
S02.11CK
S02.11DA
S02.11DK
S02.11EA
S02.11EK
S02.11FA
S02.11FK
S02.11GA
S02.11GK
S02.11HA
S02.11HK
S02.121A
S02.121K
S02.122A
S02.122K
S02.129A
S02.129K
S02.19XA
S02.19XK
S02.2XXB
S02.2XXK
S02.30XA
S02.30XB
S02.30XK
S02.31XA
S02.31XB
S02.31XK
S02.32XA
S02.32XB
S02.32XK
S02.400A
S02.400B
S02.400K
S02.401A
S02.401B
S02.401K
S02.402A
S02.402B
S02.402K
S02.40AA
S02.40AB
S02.40AK
S02.40BA
S02.40BB
S02.40BK
S02.40CA
S02.40CB
S02.40CK
S02.40DA
S02.40DB
S02.40DK
S02.40EA
S02.40EB
S02.40EK
S02.40FA
S02.40FB
S02.40FK
S02.411A
S02.411B
S02.411K
S02.412A
S02.412B
S02.412K
S02.413A
S02.413B
S02.413K
S02.42XA
S02.42XB
S02.42XK
S02.5XXK
S02.600A
S02.600B
S02.600K
S02.601A
S02.601B
S02.601K
S02.602A
S02.602B
S02.602K
S02.609A
S02.609B
S02.609K
S02.610A
S02.610B
S02.610K
S02.611A
S02.611B
S02.611K
S02.612A
S02.612B
S02.612K
S02.620A
S02.620B
S02.620K
S02.621A
S02.621B
S02.621K
S02.622A
S02.622B
S02.622K
S02.630A
S02.630B
S02.630K
S02.631A
S02.631B
S02.631K
S02.632A
S02.632B
S02.632K
S02.640A
S02.640B
S02.640K
S02.641A
S02.641B
S02.641K
S02.642A
S02.642B
S02.642K
S02.650A
S02.650B
S02.650K
S02.651A
S02.651B
S02.651K
S02.652A
S02.652B
S02.652K
S02.66XA
S02.66XB
S02.66XK
S02.670A
S02.670B
S02.670K
S02.671A
S02.671B
S02.671K
S02.672A
S02.672B
S02.672K
S02.69XA
S02.69XB
S02.69XK
S02.80XA
S02.80XB
S02.80XK
S02.81XA
S02.81XB
S02.81XK
S02.82XA
S02.82XB
S02.82XK
S02.831A
S02.831B
S02.831K
S02.832A
S02.832B
S02.832K
S02.839A
S02.839B
S02.839K
S02.841A
S02.841B
S02.841K
S02.842A
S02.842B
S02.842K
S02.849A
S02.849B
S02.849K
S02.85XA
S02.85XB
S02.85XK
S02.91XA
S02.91XK
S02.92XA
S02.92XB
S02.92XK
S04.011A
S04.012A
S04.019A
S04.02XA
S04.031A
S04.032A
S04.039A
S04.041A
S04.042A
S04.049A
S04.10XA
S04.11XA
S04.12XA
S04.20XA
S04.21XA
S04.22XA
S04.30XA
S04.31XA
S04.32XA
S04.40XA
S04.41XA
S04.42XA
S04.50XA
S04.51XA
S04.52XA
S04.60XA
S04.61XA
S04.62XA
S04.70XA
S04.71XA
S04.72XA
S04.811A
S04.812A
S04.819A
S04.891A
S04.892A
S04.899A
S04.9XXA
S05.20XA
S05.21XA
S05.22XA
S05.30XA
S05.31XA
S05.32XA
S05.40XA
S05.41XA
S05.42XA
S05.50XA
S05.51XA
S05.52XA
S05.70XA
S05.71XA
S05.72XA
S05.8X1A
S05.8X2A
S05.8X9A
S05.91XA
S05.92XA
S06.0X1A
S06.0X9A
S06.0XAA
S06.2X1A
S06.2X2A
S06.2X3A
S06.2X4A
S06.2X5A
S06.2X9A
S06.2XAA
S06.301A
S06.302A
S06.303A
S06.304A
S06.305A
S06.309A

Appendix B: Numeric Lists of CCs and MCCs

S06.30AA
S06.371A
S06.372A
S06.373A
S06.374A
S06.375A
S06.379A
S06.381A
S06.382A
S06.383A
S06.384A
S06.385A
S06.389A
S06.811A
S06.812A
S06.813A
S06.814A
S06.815A
S06.819A
S06.81AA
S06.821A
S06.822A
S06.823A
S06.824A
S06.825A
S06.829A
S06.82AA
S06.891A
S06.892A
S06.893A
S06.894A
S06.895A
S06.899A
S06.89AA
S06.8A0A
S06.8A1A
S06.8A2A
S06.8A3A
S06.8A4A
S06.8A5A
S06.8A9A
S06.8AAA
S06.9X1A
S06.9X2A
S06.9X3A
S06.9X4A
S06.9X5A
S06.9X9A
S06.9XAA
S07.0XXA
S07.1XXA
S07.8XXA
S07.9XXA
S09.0XXA
S09.20XA
S09.21XA
S09.22XA
S09.301A
S09.302A
S09.309A
S09.311A
S09.312A
S09.313A
S09.319A
S09.391A
S09.392A
S09.399A
S11.10XA
S11.11XA
S11.12XA
S11.13XA
S11.14XA
S11.15XA
S11.20XA
S11.21XA
S11.22XA
S11.23XA
S11.24XA
S11.25XA
S12.000A
S12.000K
S12.001A
S12.001K
S12.01XA
S12.01XK
S12.02XA
S12.02XK
S12.030A
S12.030K
S12.031A
S12.031K
S12.040A
S12.040K
S12.041A
S12.041K
S12.090A
S12.090K
S12.091A
S12.091K
S12.100A
S12.100K
S12.101A
S12.101K
S12.110A
S12.110K
S12.111A
S12.111K
S12.112A
S12.112K
S12.120A
S12.120K
S12.121A
S12.121K
S12.130A
S12.130K
S12.131A
S12.131K
S12.14XA
S12.14XK
S12.150A
S12.150K
S12.151A
S12.151K
S12.190A
S12.190K
S12.191A
S12.191K
S12.200A
S12.200K
S12.201A
S12.201K
S12.230A
S12.230K
S12.231A
S12.231K
S12.24XA
S12.24XK
S12.250A
S12.250K
S12.251A
S12.251K
S12.290A
S12.290K
S12.291A
S12.291K
S12.300A
S12.300K
S12.301A
S12.301K
S12.330A
S12.330K
S12.331A
S12.331K
S12.34XA
S12.34XK
S12.350A
S12.350K
S12.351A
S12.351K
S12.390A
S12.390K
S12.391A
S12.391K
S12.400A
S12.400K
S12.401A
S12.401K
S12.430A
S12.430K
S12.431A
S12.431K
S12.44XA
S12.44XK
S12.450A
S12.450K
S12.451A
S12.451K
S12.490A
S12.490K
S12.491A
S12.491K
S12.500A
S12.500K
S12.501A
S12.501K
S12.530A
S12.530K
S12.531A
S12.531K
S12.54XA
S12.54XK
S12.550A
S12.550K
S12.551A
S12.551K
S12.590A
S12.590K
S12.591A
S12.591K
S12.600A
S12.600K
S12.601A
S12.601K
S12.630A
S12.630K
S12.631A
S12.631K
S12.64XA
S12.64XK
S12.650A
S12.650K
S12.651A
S12.651K
S12.690A
S12.690K
S12.691A
S12.691K
S12.9XXA
S13.0XXA
S13.100A
S13.101A
S13.110A
S13.111A
S13.120A
S13.121A
S13.130A
S13.131A
S13.140A
S13.141A
S13.150A
S13.151A
S13.160A
S13.161A
S13.170A
S13.171A
S13.180A
S13.181A
S13.20XA
S13.29XA
S15.001A
S15.002A
S15.009A
S15.011A
S15.012A
S15.019A
S15.021A
S15.022A
S15.029A
S15.091A
S15.092A
S15.099A
S15.101A
S15.102A
S15.109A
S15.111A
S15.112A
S15.119A
S15.121A
S15.122A
S15.129A
S15.191A
S15.192A
S15.199A
S15.201A
S15.202A
S15.209A
S15.211A
S15.212A
S15.219A
S15.221A
S15.222A
S15.229A
S15.291A
S15.292A
S15.299A
S15.301A
S15.302A
S15.309A
S15.311A
S15.312A
S15.319A
S15.321A
S15.322A
S15.329A
S15.391A
S15.392A
S15.399A
S15.8XXA
S15.9XXA
S17.0XXA
S17.8XXA
S17.9XXA
S21.101A
S21.102A
S21.109A
S21.111A
S21.112A
S21.119A
S21.121A
S21.122A
S21.129A
S21.131A
S21.132A
S21.139A
S21.141A
S21.142A
S21.149A
S21.151A
S21.152A
S21.159A
S21.90XA
S21.91XA
S21.92XA
S21.93XA
S21.94XA
S21.95XA
S22.000A
S22.000K
S22.001A
S22.001K
S22.002A
S22.002K
S22.008A
S22.008K
S22.009A
S22.009K
S22.010A
S22.010K
S22.011A
S22.011K
S22.012A
S22.012K
S22.018A
S22.018K
S22.019A
S22.019K
S22.020A
S22.020K
S22.021A
S22.021K
S22.022A
S22.022K
S22.028A
S22.028K
S22.029A
S22.029K
S22.030A
S22.030K
S22.031A
S22.031K
S22.032A
S22.032K
S22.038A
S22.038K
S22.039A
S22.039K
S22.040A
S22.040K
S22.041A
S22.041K
S22.042A
S22.042K
S22.048A
S22.048K
S22.049A
S22.049K
S22.050A
S22.050K
S22.051A
S22.051K
S22.052A
S22.052K
S22.058A
S22.058K
S22.059A
S22.059K
S22.060A
S22.060K
S22.061A
S22.061K
S22.062A
S22.062K
S22.068A
S22.068K
S22.069A
S22.069K
S22.070A
S22.070K
S22.071A
S22.071K
S22.072A
S22.072K
S22.078A
S22.078K
S22.079A
S22.079K
S22.080A
S22.080K
S22.081A
S22.081K
S22.082A
S22.082K
S22.088A
S22.088K
S22.089A
S22.089K
S22.20XA
S22.20XK
S22.21XA
S22.21XK
S22.22XA
S22.22XK
S22.23XA
S22.23XK
S22.24XA
S22.24XK
S22.31XA
S22.31XK
S22.32XA
S22.32XK
S22.39XA
S22.39XK
S22.41XA
S22.41XK
S22.42XA
S22.42XK
S22.43XA
S22.43XK
S22.49XA
S22.49XK
S22.5XXK
S22.9XXA
S22.9XXK
S25.501A
S25.502A
S25.509A
S25.511A
S25.512A
S25.519A
S25.591A
S25.592A
S25.599A
S25.801A
S25.802A
S25.809A
S25.811A
S25.812A
S25.819A
S25.891A
S25.892A
S25.899A
S25.90XA
S25.91XA
S25.99XA
S26.00XA
S26.01XA
S26.09XA
S26.10XA
S26.11XA
S26.19XA
S26.90XA
S26.91XA
S26.99XA
S27.0XXA
S27.301A
S27.302A
S27.309A
S27.311A
S27.312A
S27.319A
S27.321A
S27.322A
S27.329A
S27.391A
S27.392A
S27.399A
S27.50XA
S27.51XA
S27.52XA
S27.53XA
S27.59XA
S27.60XA
S27.63XA
S27.69XA
S27.802A
S27.803A
S27.808A
S27.809A
S27.892A
S27.893A
S27.898A
S27.899A
S27.9XXA
S28.1XXA
S29.021A
S29.029A
S32.000A
S32.000K
S32.001A
S32.001K
S32.002A
S32.002K
S32.008A
S32.008K
S32.009A
S32.009K
S32.010A
S32.010K
S32.011A
S32.011K
S32.012A
S32.012K
S32.018A
S32.018K
S32.019A
S32.019K
S32.020A
S32.020K
S32.021A
S32.021K
S32.022A
S32.022K
S32.028A
S32.028K
S32.029A
S32.029K
S32.030A
S32.030K
S32.031A
S32.031K
S32.032A
S32.032K
S32.038A
S32.038K
S32.039A
S32.039K
S32.040A
S32.040K
S32.041A
S32.041K
S32.042A
S32.042K
S32.048A
S32.048K
S32.049A
S32.049K
S32.050A
S32.050K
S32.051A
S32.051K
S32.052A
S32.052K
S32.058A
S32.058K
S32.059A
S32.059K
S32.10XA
S32.10XK
S32.110A
S32.110K
S32.111A
S32.111K
S32.112A
S32.112K
S32.119A
S32.119K
S32.120A
S32.120K
S32.121A
S32.121K
S32.122A
S32.122K
S32.129A
S32.129K
S32.130A
S32.130K
S32.131A
S32.131K
S32.132A
S32.132K
S32.139A
S32.139K
S32.14XA
S32.14XK
S32.15XA
S32.15XK
S32.16XA
S32.16XK
S32.17XA
S32.17XK
S32.19XA
S32.19XK
S32.2XXA
S32.2XXK
S32.301A
S32.301K
S32.302A
S32.302K
S32.309A
S32.309K
S32.311A
S32.311K
S32.312A
S32.312K
S32.313A
S32.313K
S32.314A
S32.314K
S32.315A
S32.315K
S32.316A
S32.316K
S32.391A
S32.391K
S32.392A
S32.392K
S32.399A
S32.399K
S32.401K
S32.402K
S32.409K
S32.411K
S32.412K
S32.413K
S32.414K
S32.415K
S32.416K
S32.421K
S32.422K
S32.423K
S32.424K
S32.425K
S32.426K
S32.431K
S32.432K
S32.433K
S32.434K
S32.435K
S32.436K
S32.441K
S32.442K
S32.443K
S32.444K
S32.445K
S32.446K
S32.451K
S32.452K
S32.453K
S32.454K
S32.455K
S32.456K
S32.461K
S32.462K
S32.463K
S32.464K
S32.465K
S32.466K
S32.471K
S32.472K
S32.473K
S32.474K
S32.475K
S32.476K
S32.481K
S32.482K
S32.483K
S32.484K
S32.485K
S32.486K
S32.491K
S32.492K
S32.499K
S32.501A
S32.501K
S32.502A
S32.502K
S32.509A
S32.509K
S32.511A
S32.511K
S32.512A
S32.512K
S32.519A
S32.519K
S32.591A
S32.591K
S32.592A
S32.592K
S32.599A
S32.599K
S32.601A
S32.601K
S32.602A
S32.602K
S32.609A
S32.609K
S32.611A
S32.611K
S32.612A
S32.612K
S32.613A
S32.613K
S32.614A
S32.614K
S32.615A
S32.615K
S32.616A
S32.616K
S32.691A
S32.691K
S32.692A
S32.692K
S32.699A
S32.699K
S32.810A
S32.810K
S32.811A
S32.811K
S32.82XA
S32.82XK
S32.89XA
S32.89XK
S32.9XXA
S32.9XXK
S35.531A
S35.532A
S35.533A
S35.534A
S35.535A
S35.536A
S35.8X1A
S35.8X8A
S35.8X9A
S35.90XA
S35.91XA
S35.99XA
S36.00XA
S36.020A
S36.021A
S36.029A
S36.030A
S36.039A
S36.09XA
S36.112A
S36.113A
S36.114A
S36.118A
S36.119A
S36.122A
S36.123A
S36.128A
S36.129A
S36.13XA
S36.200A
S36.201A
S36.202A
S36.209A
S36.220A
S36.221A
S36.222A
S36.229A
S36.230A
S36.231A
S36.232A
S36.239A
S36.240A
S36.241A
S36.242A
S36.249A
S36.250A
S36.251A
S36.252A
S36.259A
S36.260A
S36.261A
S36.262A
S36.269A
S36.290A
S36.291A
S36.292A
S36.299A
S36.30XA
S36.32XA
S36.33XA
S36.39XA
S36.400A
S36.408A
S36.409A
S36.410A
S36.418A
S36.419A
S36.420A
S36.428A
S36.429A
S36.430A
S36.438A
S36.439A
S36.490A
S36.498A
S36.499A
S36.500A
S36.501A
S36.502A
S36.503A
S36.508A
S36.509A
S36.510A
S36.511A
S36.512A
S36.513A
S36.518A
S36.519A
S36.520A
S36.521A
S36.522A
S36.523A
S36.528A
S36.529A
S36.530A
S36.531A
S36.532A
S36.533A
S36.538A
S36.539A
S36.590A
S36.591A
S36.592A
S36.593A
S36.598A
S36.599A
S36.60XA
S36.61XA
S36.62XA
S36.63XA
S36.69XA
S36.81XA
S36.892A
S36.893A
S36.898A
S36.899A
S36.90XA
S36.92XA
S36.93XA
S36.99XA
S37.001A
S37.002A
S37.009A
S37.011A
S37.012A
S37.019A
S37.021A
S37.022A
S37.029A
S37.031A
S37.032A
S37.039A
S37.041A
S37.042A
S37.049A
S37.051A
S37.052A
S37.059A
S37.10XA
S37.12XA
S37.13XA
S37.19XA
S37.20XA
S37.22XA
S37.23XA
S37.29XA
S37.30XA
S37.32XA
S37.33XA
S37.39XA
S37.60XA
S37.62XA
S37.63XA
S37.69XA
S37.812A
S37.813A
S37.818A
S37.819A
S37.892A
S37.893A
S37.898A
S37.899A
S37.90XA
S37.92XA
S37.93XA
S37.99XA
S42.001B
S42.001K
S42.001P
S42.002B
S42.002K
S42.002P
S42.009B
S42.009K
S42.009P
S42.011B
S42.011K
S42.011P
S42.012B
S42.012K
S42.012P
S42.013B
S42.013K
S42.013P
S42.014B
S42.014K
S42.014P
S42.015B
S42.015K

S42.015P
S42.016B
S42.016K
S42.016P
S42.017B
S42.017K
S42.017P
S42.018B
S42.018K
S42.018P
S42.019B
S42.019K
S42.019P
S42.021B
S42.021K
S42.021P
S42.022B
S42.022K
S42.022P
S42.023B
S42.023K
S42.023P
S42.024B
S42.024K
S42.024P
S42.025B
S42.025K
S42.025P
S42.026B
S42.026K
S42.026P
S42.031B
S42.031K
S42.031P
S42.032B
S42.032K
S42.032P
S42.033B
S42.033K
S42.033P
S42.034B
S42.034K
S42.034P
S42.035B
S42.035K
S42.035P
S42.036B
S42.036K
S42.036P
S42.101B
S42.101K
S42.101P
S42.102B
S42.102K
S42.102P
S42.109B
S42.109K
S42.109P
S42.111B
S42.111K
S42.111P
S42.112B
S42.112K
S42.112P
S42.113B
S42.113K
S42.113P
S42.114B
S42.114K
S42.114P
S42.115B
S42.115K
S42.115P
S42.116B
S42.116K
S42.116P
S42.121B
S42.121K
S42.121P
S42.122B
S42.122K
S42.122P
S42.123B
S42.123K
S42.123P
S42.124B
S42.124K
S42.124P
S42.125B
S42.125K
S42.125P
S42.126B
S42.126K
S42.126P
S42.131B
S42.131K
S42.131P
S42.132B
S42.132K
S42.132P
S42.133B
S42.133K
S42.133P
S42.134B
S42.134K
S42.134P
S42.135B
S42.135K
S42.135P
S42.136B
S42.136K
S42.136P
S42.141B
S42.141K
S42.141P
S42.142B
S42.142K
S42.142P
S42.143B
S42.143K
S42.143P
S42.144B
S42.144K
S42.144P
S42.145B
S42.145K
S42.145P
S42.146B
S42.146K
S42.146P
S42.151B
S42.151K
S42.151P
S42.152B
S42.152K
S42.152P
S42.153B
S42.153K
S42.153P
S42.154B
S42.154K
S42.154P
S42.155B
S42.155K
S42.155P
S42.156B
S42.156K
S42.156P
S42.191B
S42.191K
S42.191P
S42.192B
S42.192K
S42.192P
S42.199B
S42.199K
S42.199P
S42.201A
S42.201K
S42.201P
S42.202A
S42.202K
S42.202P
S42.209A
S42.209K
S42.209P
S42.211A
S42.211K
S42.211P
S42.212A
S42.212K
S42.212P
S42.213A
S42.213K
S42.213P
S42.214A
S42.214K
S42.214P
S42.215A
S42.215K
S42.215P
S42.216A
S42.216K
S42.216P
S42.221A
S42.221K
S42.221P
S42.222A
S42.222K
S42.222P
S42.223A
S42.223K
S42.223P
S42.224A
S42.224K
S42.224P
S42.225A
S42.225K
S42.225P
S42.226A
S42.226K
S42.226P
S42.231A
S42.231K
S42.231P
S42.232A
S42.232K
S42.232P
S42.239A
S42.239K
S42.239P
S42.241A
S42.241K
S42.241P
S42.242A
S42.242K
S42.242P
S42.249A
S42.249K
S42.249P
S42.251A
S42.251K
S42.251P
S42.252A
S42.252K
S42.252P
S42.253A
S42.253K
S42.253P
S42.254A
S42.254K
S42.254P
S42.255A
S42.255K
S42.255P
S42.256A
S42.256K
S42.256P
S42.261A
S42.261K
S42.261P
S42.262A
S42.262K
S42.262P
S42.263A
S42.263K
S42.263P
S42.264A
S42.264K
S42.264P
S42.265A
S42.265K
S42.265P
S42.266A
S42.266K
S42.266P
S42.271A
S42.271K
S42.271P
S42.272A
S42.272K
S42.272P
S42.279A
S42.279K
S42.279P
S42.291A
S42.291K
S42.291P
S42.292A
S42.292K
S42.292P
S42.293A
S42.293K
S42.293P
S42.294A
S42.294K
S42.294P
S42.295A
S42.295K
S42.295P
S42.296A
S42.296K
S42.296P
S42.301A
S42.301K
S42.301P
S42.302A
S42.302K
S42.302P
S42.309A
S42.309K
S42.309P
S42.311A
S42.311K
S42.311P
S42.312A
S42.312K
S42.312P
S42.319A
S42.319K
S42.319P
S42.321A
S42.321K
S42.321P
S42.322A
S42.322K
S42.322P
S42.323A
S42.323K
S42.323P
S42.324A
S42.324K
S42.324P
S42.325A
S42.325K
S42.325P
S42.326A
S42.326K
S42.326P
S42.331A
S42.331K
S42.331P
S42.332A
S42.332K
S42.332P
S42.333A
S42.333K
S42.333P
S42.334A
S42.334K
S42.334P
S42.335A
S42.335K
S42.335P
S42.336A
S42.336K
S42.336P
S42.341A
S42.341K
S42.341P
S42.342A
S42.342K
S42.342P
S42.343A
S42.343K
S42.343P
S42.344A
S42.344K
S42.344P
S42.345A
S42.345K
S42.345P
S42.346A
S42.346K
S42.346P
S42.351A
S42.351K
S42.351P
S42.352A
S42.352K
S42.352P
S42.353A
S42.353K
S42.353P
S42.354A
S42.354K
S42.354P
S42.355A
S42.355K
S42.355P
S42.356A
S42.356K
S42.356P
S42.361A
S42.361K
S42.361P
S42.362A
S42.362K
S42.362P
S42.363A
S42.363K
S42.363P
S42.364A
S42.364K
S42.364P
S42.365A
S42.365K
S42.365P
S42.366A
S42.366K
S42.366P
S42.391A
S42.391K
S42.391P
S42.392A
S42.392K
S42.392P
S42.399A
S42.399K
S42.399P
S42.401A
S42.401K
S42.401P
S42.402A
S42.402K
S42.402P
S42.409A
S42.409K
S42.409P
S42.411A
S42.411K
S42.411P
S42.412A
S42.412K
S42.412P
S42.413A
S42.413K
S42.413P
S42.414A
S42.414K
S42.414P
S42.415A
S42.415K
S42.415P
S42.416A
S42.416K
S42.416P
S42.421A
S42.421K
S42.421P
S42.422A
S42.422K
S42.422P
S42.423A
S42.423K
S42.423P
S42.424A
S42.424K
S42.424P
S42.425A
S42.425K
S42.425P
S42.426A
S42.426K
S42.426P
S42.431A
S42.431K
S42.431P
S42.432A
S42.432K
S42.432P
S42.433A
S42.433K
S42.433P
S42.434A
S42.434K
S42.434P
S42.435A
S42.435K
S42.435P
S42.436A
S42.436K
S42.436P
S42.441A
S42.441K
S42.441P
S42.442A
S42.442K
S42.442P
S42.443A
S42.443K
S42.443P
S42.444A
S42.444K
S42.444P
S42.445A
S42.445K
S42.445P
S42.446A
S42.446K
S42.446P
S42.447A
S42.447K
S42.447P
S42.448A
S42.448K
S42.448P
S42.449A
S42.449K
S42.449P
S42.451A
S42.451K
S42.451P
S42.452A
S42.452K
S42.452P
S42.453A
S42.453K
S42.453P
S42.454A
S42.454K
S42.454P
S42.455A
S42.455K
S42.455P
S42.456A
S42.456K
S42.456P
S42.461A
S42.461K
S42.461P
S42.462A
S42.462K
S42.462P
S42.463A
S42.463K
S42.463P
S42.464A
S42.464K
S42.464P
S42.465A
S42.465K
S42.465P
S42.466A
S42.466K
S42.466P
S42.471A
S42.471K
S42.471P
S42.472A
S42.472K
S42.472P
S42.473A
S42.473K
S42.473P
S42.474A
S42.474K
S42.474P
S42.475A
S42.475K
S42.475P
S42.476A
S42.476K
S42.476P
S42.481A
S42.481K
S42.481P
S42.482A
S42.482K
S42.482P
S42.489A
S42.489K
S42.489P
S42.491A
S42.491K
S42.491P
S42.492A
S42.492K
S42.492P
S42.493A
S42.493K
S42.493P
S42.494A
S42.494K
S42.494P
S42.495A
S42.495K
S42.495P
S42.496A
S42.496K
S42.496P
S42.90XA
S42.90XK
S42.90XP
S42.91XA
S42.91XK
S42.91XP
S42.92XA
S42.92XK
S42.92XP
S43.201A
S43.202A
S43.203A
S43.204A
S43.205A
S43.206A
S43.211A
S43.212A
S43.213A
S43.214A
S43.215A
S43.216A
S43.221A
S43.222A
S43.223A
S43.224A
S43.225A
S43.226A
S45.101A
S45.102A
S45.109A
S45.111A
S45.112A
S45.119A
S45.191A
S45.192A
S45.199A
S45.201A
S45.202A
S45.209A
S45.211A
S45.212A
S45.219A
S45.291A
S45.292A
S45.299A
S45.301A
S45.302A
S45.309A
S45.311A
S45.312A
S45.319A
S45.391A
S45.392A
S45.399A
S45.801A
S45.802A
S45.809A
S45.811A
S45.812A
S45.819A
S45.891A
S45.892A
S45.899A
S45.901A
S45.902A
S45.909A
S45.911A
S45.912A
S45.919A
S45.991A
S45.992A
S45.999A
S46.021A
S46.022A
S46.029A
S46.121A
S46.122A
S46.129A
S46.221A
S46.222A
S46.229A
S46.321A
S46.322A
S46.329A
S46.821A
S46.822A
S46.829A
S46.921A
S46.922A
S46.929A
S48.011A
S48.012A
S48.019A
S48.021A
S48.022A
S48.029A
S48.111A
S48.112A
S48.119A
S48.121A
S48.122A
S48.129A
S48.911A
S48.912A
S48.919A
S48.921A
S48.922A
S48.929A
S49.001A
S49.001K
S49.001P
S49.002A
S49.002K
S49.002P
S49.009A
S49.009K
S49.009P
S49.011A
S49.011K
S49.011P
S49.012A
S49.012K
S49.012P
S49.019A
S49.019K
S49.019P
S49.021A
S49.021K
S49.021P
S49.022A
S49.022K
S49.022P
S49.029A
S49.029K
S49.029P
S49.031A
S49.031K
S49.031P
S49.032A
S49.032K
S49.032P
S49.039A
S49.039K
S49.039P
S49.041A
S49.041K
S49.041P
S49.042A
S49.042K
S49.042P
S49.049A
S49.049K
S49.049P
S49.091A
S49.091K
S49.091P
S49.092A
S49.092K
S49.092P
S49.099A
S49.099K
S49.099P
S49.101A
S49.101K
S49.101P
S49.102A
S49.102K
S49.102P
S49.109A
S49.109K
S49.109P
S49.111A
S49.111K
S49.111P
S49.112A
S49.112K
S49.112P
S49.119A
S49.119K
S49.119P
S49.121A
S49.121K
S49.121P
S49.122A
S49.122K
S49.122P
S49.129A
S49.129K
S49.129P
S49.131A
S49.131K
S49.131P
S49.132A
S49.132K
S49.132P
S49.139A
S49.139K
S49.139P
S49.141A
S49.141K
S49.141P
S49.142A
S49.142K
S49.142P
S49.149A
S49.149K
S49.149P
S49.191A
S49.191K
S49.191P
S49.192A
S49.192K
S49.192P
S49.199A
S49.199K
S49.199P
S52.001K
S52.001M
S52.001N
S52.001P
S52.001Q
S52.001R
S52.002K
S52.002M
S52.002N
S52.002P
S52.002Q
S52.002R
S52.009K
S52.009M
S52.009N
S52.009P
S52.009Q
S52.009R
S52.011A
S52.011K
S52.011P
S52.012A
S52.012K
S52.012P
S52.019A
S52.019K
S52.019P
S52.021K
S52.021M
S52.021N
S52.021P
S52.021Q
S52.021R
S52.022K
S52.022M
S52.022N
S52.022P
S52.022Q
S52.022R
S52.023K
S52.023M
S52.023N
S52.023P
S52.023Q
S52.023R
S52.024K
S52.024M
S52.024N
S52.024P
S52.024Q
S52.024R
S52.025K
S52.025M
S52.025N
S52.025P
S52.025Q
S52.025R
S52.026K
S52.026M
S52.026N
S52.026P
S52.026Q
S52.026R
S52.031K
S52.031M
S52.031N
S52.031P
S52.031Q
S52.031R
S52.032K
S52.032M
S52.032N
S52.032P
S52.032Q
S52.032R
S52.033K
S52.033M
S52.033N
S52.033P
S52.033Q
S52.033R
S52.034K
S52.034M
S52.034N
S52.034P
S52.034Q
S52.034R
S52.035K
S52.035M
S52.035N
S52.035P
S52.035Q
S52.035R
S52.036K
S52.036M
S52.036N
S52.036P
S52.036Q
S52.036R
S52.041K
S52.041M
S52.041N
S52.041P
S52.041Q
S52.041R
S52.042K
S52.042M
S52.042N
S52.042P
S52.042Q
S52.042R
S52.043K
S52.043M
S52.043N
S52.043P
S52.043Q
S52.043R
S52.044K
S52.044M
S52.044N
S52.044P
S52.044Q
S52.044R
S52.045K
S52.045M
S52.045N

Appendix B: Numeric Lists of CCs and MCCs

S52.Ø45P
S52.Ø45Q
S52.Ø45R
S52.Ø46K
S52.Ø46M
S52.Ø46N
S52.Ø46P
S52.Ø46Q
S52.Ø46R
S52.Ø91K
S52.Ø91M
S52.Ø91N
S52.Ø91P
S52.Ø91Q
S52.Ø91R
S52.Ø92K
S52.Ø92M
S52.Ø92N
S52.Ø92P
S52.Ø92Q
S52.Ø92R
S52.Ø99K
S52.Ø99M
S52.Ø99N
S52.Ø99P
S52.Ø99Q
S52.Ø99R
S52.1Ø1K
S52.1Ø1M
S52.1Ø1N
S52.1Ø1P
S52.1Ø1Q
S52.1Ø1R
S52.1Ø2K
S52.1Ø2M
S52.1Ø2N
S52.1Ø2P
S52.1Ø2Q
S52.1Ø2R
S52.1Ø9K
S52.1Ø9M
S52.1Ø9N
S52.1Ø9P
S52.1Ø9Q
S52.1Ø9R
S52.111A
S52.111K
S52.111P
S52.112A
S52.112K
S52.112P
S52.119A
S52.119K
S52.119P
S52.121K
S52.121M
S52.121N
S52.121P
S52.121Q
S52.121R
S52.122K
S52.122M
S52.122N
S52.122P
S52.122Q
S52.122R
S52.123K
S52.123M
S52.123N
S52.123P
S52.123Q
S52.123R
S52.124K
S52.124M
S52.124N
S52.124P
S52.124Q
S52.124R
S52.125K
S52.125M
S52.125N
S52.125P
S52.125Q
S52.125R
S52.126K
S52.126M
S52.126N
S52.126P
S52.126Q
S52.126R
S52.131K
S52.131M
S52.131N
S52.131P
S52.131Q
S52.131R
S52.132K
S52.132M
S52.132N
S52.132P
S52.132Q
S52.132R
S52.133K
S52.133M
S52.133N
S52.133P
S52.133Q
S52.133R
S52.134K
S52.134M
S52.134N
S52.134P
S52.134Q
S52.134R
S52.135K
S52.135M
S52.135N
S52.135P
S52.135Q
S52.135R
S52.136K
S52.136M
S52.136N
S52.136P
S52.136Q
S52.136R
S52.181K
S52.181M
S52.181N
S52.181P
S52.181Q
S52.181R
S52.182K
S52.182M
S52.182N
S52.182P
S52.182Q
S52.182R
S52.189K
S52.189M
S52.189N
S52.189P
S52.189Q
S52.189R
S52.2Ø1A
S52.2Ø1K
S52.2Ø1M
S52.2Ø1N
S52.2Ø1P
S52.2Ø1Q
S52.2Ø1R
S52.2Ø2A
S52.2Ø2K
S52.2Ø2M
S52.2Ø2N
S52.2Ø2P
S52.2Ø2Q
S52.2Ø2R
S52.2Ø9A
S52.2Ø9K
S52.2Ø9M
S52.2Ø9N
S52.2Ø9P
S52.2Ø9Q
S52.2Ø9R
S52.211A
S52.211K
S52.211P
S52.212A
S52.212K
S52.212P
S52.219A
S52.219K
S52.219P
S52.221A
S52.221K
S52.221M
S52.221N
S52.221P
S52.221Q
S52.221R
S52.222A
S52.222K
S52.222M
S52.222N
S52.222P
S52.222Q
S52.222R
S52.223A
S52.223K
S52.223M
S52.223N
S52.223P
S52.223Q
S52.223R
S52.224A
S52.224K
S52.224M
S52.224N
S52.224P
S52.224Q
S52.224R
S52.225A
S52.225K
S52.225M
S52.225N
S52.225P
S52.225Q
S52.225R
S52.226A
S52.226K
S52.226M
S52.226N
S52.226P
S52.226Q
S52.226R
S52.231A
S52.231K
S52.231M
S52.231N
S52.231P
S52.231Q
S52.231R
S52.232A
S52.232K
S52.232M
S52.232N
S52.232P
S52.232Q
S52.232R
S52.233A
S52.233K
S52.233M
S52.233N
S52.233P
S52.233Q
S52.233R
S52.234A
S52.234K
S52.234M
S52.234N
S52.234P
S52.234Q
S52.234R
S52.235A
S52.235K
S52.235M
S52.235N
S52.235P
S52.235Q
S52.235R
S52.236A
S52.236K
S52.236M
S52.236N
S52.236P
S52.236Q
S52.236R
S52.241A
S52.241K
S52.241M
S52.241N
S52.241P
S52.241Q
S52.241R
S52.242A
S52.242K
S52.242M
S52.242N
S52.242P
S52.242Q
S52.242R
S52.243A
S52.243K
S52.243M
S52.243N
S52.243P
S52.243Q
S52.243R
S52.244A
S52.244K
S52.244M
S52.244N
S52.244P
S52.244Q
S52.244R
S52.245A
S52.245K
S52.245M
S52.245N
S52.245P
S52.245Q
S52.245R
S52.246A
S52.246K
S52.246M
S52.246N
S52.246P
S52.246Q
S52.246R
S52.251A
S52.251K
S52.251M
S52.251N
S52.251P
S52.251Q
S52.251R
S52.252A
S52.252K
S52.252M
S52.252N
S52.252P
S52.252Q
S52.252R
S52.253A
S52.253K
S52.253M
S52.253N
S52.253P
S52.253Q
S52.253R
S52.254A
S52.254K
S52.254M
S52.254N
S52.254P
S52.254Q
S52.254R
S52.255A
S52.255K
S52.255M
S52.255N
S52.255P
S52.255Q
S52.255R
S52.256A
S52.256K
S52.256M
S52.256N
S52.256P
S52.256Q
S52.256R
S52.261A
S52.261K
S52.261M
S52.261N
S52.261P
S52.261Q
S52.261R
S52.262A
S52.262K
S52.262M
S52.262N
S52.262P
S52.262Q
S52.262R
S52.263A
S52.263K
S52.263M
S52.263N
S52.263P
S52.263Q
S52.263R
S52.264A
S52.264K
S52.264M
S52.264N
S52.264P
S52.264Q
S52.264R
S52.265A
S52.265K
S52.265M
S52.265N
S52.265P
S52.265Q
S52.265R
S52.266A
S52.266K
S52.266M
S52.266N
S52.266P
S52.266Q
S52.266R
S52.271K
S52.271M
S52.271N
S52.271P
S52.271Q
S52.271R
S52.272K
S52.272M
S52.272N
S52.272P
S52.272Q
S52.272R
S52.279K
S52.279M
S52.279N
S52.279P
S52.279Q
S52.279R
S52.281A
S52.281K
S52.281M
S52.281N
S52.281P
S52.281Q
S52.281R
S52.282A
S52.282K
S52.282M
S52.282N
S52.282P
S52.282Q
S52.282R
S52.283A
S52.283K
S52.283M
S52.283N
S52.283P
S52.283Q
S52.283R
S52.291A
S52.291K
S52.291M
S52.291N
S52.291P
S52.291Q
S52.291R
S52.292A
S52.292K
S52.292M
S52.292N
S52.292P
S52.292Q
S52.292R
S52.299A
S52.299K
S52.299M
S52.299N
S52.299P
S52.299Q
S52.299R
S52.3Ø1A
S52.3Ø1K
S52.3Ø1M
S52.3Ø1N
S52.3Ø1P
S52.3Ø1Q
S52.3Ø1R
S52.3Ø2A
S52.3Ø2K
S52.3Ø2M
S52.3Ø2N
S52.3Ø2P
S52.3Ø2Q
S52.3Ø2R
S52.3Ø9A
S52.3Ø9K
S52.3Ø9M
S52.3Ø9N
S52.3Ø9P
S52.3Ø9Q
S52.3Ø9R
S52.311A
S52.311K
S52.311P
S52.312A
S52.312K
S52.312P
S52.319A
S52.319K
S52.319P
S52.321A
S52.321K
S52.321M
S52.321N
S52.321P
S52.321Q
S52.321R
S52.322A
S52.322K
S52.322M
S52.322N
S52.322P
S52.322Q
S52.322R
S52.323A
S52.323K
S52.323M
S52.323N
S52.323P
S52.323Q
S52.323R
S52.324A
S52.324K
S52.324M
S52.324N
S52.324P
S52.324Q
S52.324R
S52.325A
S52.325K
S52.325M
S52.325N
S52.325P
S52.325Q
S52.325R
S52.326A
S52.326K
S52.326M
S52.326N
S52.326P
S52.326Q
S52.326R
S52.331A
S52.331K
S52.331M
S52.331N
S52.331P
S52.331Q
S52.331R
S52.332A
S52.332K
S52.332M
S52.332N
S52.332P
S52.332Q
S52.332R
S52.333A
S52.333K
S52.333M
S52.333N
S52.333P
S52.333Q
S52.333R
S52.334A
S52.334K
S52.334M
S52.334N
S52.334P
S52.334Q
S52.334R
S52.335A
S52.335K
S52.335M
S52.335N
S52.335P
S52.335Q
S52.335R
S52.336A
S52.336K
S52.336M
S52.336N
S52.336P
S52.336Q
S52.336R
S52.341A
S52.341K
S52.341M
S52.341N
S52.341P
S52.341Q
S52.341R
S52.342A
S52.342K
S52.342M
S52.342N
S52.342P
S52.342Q
S52.342R
S52.343A
S52.343K
S52.343M
S52.343N
S52.343P
S52.343Q
S52.343R
S52.344A
S52.344K
S52.344M
S52.344N
S52.344P
S52.344Q
S52.344R
S52.345A
S52.345K
S52.345M
S52.345N
S52.345P
S52.345Q
S52.345R
S52.346A
S52.346K
S52.346M
S52.346N
S52.346P
S52.346Q
S52.346R
S52.351A
S52.351K
S52.351M
S52.351N
S52.351P
S52.351Q
S52.351R
S52.352A
S52.352K
S52.352M
S52.352N
S52.352P
S52.352Q
S52.352R
S52.353A
S52.353K
S52.353M
S52.353N
S52.353P
S52.353Q
S52.353R
S52.354A
S52.354K
S52.354M
S52.354N
S52.354P
S52.354Q
S52.354R
S52.355A
S52.355K
S52.355M
S52.355N
S52.355P
S52.355Q
S52.355R
S52.356A
S52.356K
S52.356M
S52.356N
S52.356P
S52.356Q
S52.356R
S52.361A
S52.361K
S52.361M
S52.361N
S52.361P
S52.361Q
S52.361R
S52.362A
S52.362K
S52.362M
S52.362N
S52.362P
S52.362Q
S52.362R
S52.363A
S52.363K
S52.363M
S52.363N
S52.363P
S52.363Q
S52.363R
S52.364A
S52.364K
S52.364M
S52.364N
S52.364P
S52.364Q
S52.364R
S52.365A
S52.365K
S52.365M
S52.365N
S52.365P
S52.365Q
S52.365R
S52.366A
S52.366K
S52.366M
S52.366N
S52.366P
S52.366Q
S52.366R
S52.371A
S52.371K
S52.371M
S52.371N
S52.371P
S52.371Q
S52.371R
S52.372A
S52.372K
S52.372M
S52.372N
S52.372P
S52.372Q
S52.372R
S52.379A
S52.379K
S52.379M
S52.379N
S52.379P
S52.379Q
S52.379R
S52.381A
S52.381K
S52.381M
S52.381N
S52.381P
S52.381Q
S52.381R
S52.382A
S52.382K
S52.382M
S52.382N
S52.382P
S52.382Q
S52.382R
S52.389A
S52.389K
S52.389M
S52.389N
S52.389P
S52.389Q
S52.389R
S52.391A
S52.391K
S52.391M
S52.391N
S52.391P
S52.391Q
S52.391R
S52.392A
S52.392K
S52.392M
S52.392N
S52.392P
S52.392Q
S52.392R
S52.399A
S52.399K
S52.399M
S52.399N
S52.399P
S52.399Q
S52.399R
S52.5Ø1A
S52.5Ø1K
S52.5Ø1M
S52.5Ø1N
S52.5Ø1P
S52.5Ø1Q
S52.5Ø1R
S52.5Ø2A
S52.5Ø2K
S52.5Ø2M
S52.5Ø2N
S52.5Ø2P
S52.5Ø2Q
S52.5Ø2R
S52.5Ø9A
S52.5Ø9K
S52.5Ø9M
S52.5Ø9N
S52.5Ø9P
S52.5Ø9Q
S52.5Ø9R
S52.511A
S52.511K
S52.511M
S52.511N
S52.511P
S52.511Q
S52.511R
S52.512A
S52.512K
S52.512M
S52.512N
S52.512P
S52.512Q
S52.512R
S52.513A
S52.513K
S52.513M
S52.513N
S52.513P
S52.513Q
S52.513R
S52.514A
S52.514K
S52.514M
S52.514N
S52.514P
S52.514Q
S52.514R
S52.515A
S52.515K
S52.515M
S52.515N
S52.515P
S52.515Q
S52.515R
S52.516A
S52.516K
S52.516M
S52.516N
S52.516P
S52.516Q
S52.516R
S52.521A
S52.521K
S52.521P
S52.522A
S52.522K
S52.522P
S52.529A
S52.529K
S52.529P
S52.531A
S52.531K
S52.531M
S52.531N
S52.531P
S52.531Q
S52.531R
S52.532A
S52.532K
S52.532M
S52.532N
S52.532P
S52.532Q
S52.532R
S52.539A
S52.539K
S52.539M
S52.539N
S52.539P
S52.539Q
S52.539R
S52.541A
S52.541K
S52.541M
S52.541N
S52.541P
S52.541Q
S52.541R
S52.542A
S52.542K
S52.542M
S52.542N
S52.542P
S52.542Q
S52.542R
S52.549A
S52.549K
S52.549M
S52.549N
S52.549P
S52.549Q
S52.549R
S52.551A
S52.551K
S52.551M
S52.551N
S52.551P
S52.551Q
S52.551R
S52.552A
S52.552K
S52.552M
S52.552N
S52.552P
S52.552Q
S52.552R
S52.559A
S52.559K
S52.559M
S52.559N
S52.559P
S52.559Q
S52.559R
S52.561A
S52.561K
S52.561M
S52.561N
S52.561P
S52.561Q
S52.561R
S52.562A
S52.562K
S52.562M
S52.562N
S52.562P
S52.562Q
S52.562R
S52.569A
S52.569K
S52.569M
S52.569N
S52.569P
S52.569Q
S52.569R
S52.571A
S52.571K
S52.571M
S52.571N
S52.571P
S52.571Q
S52.571R
S52.572A
S52.572K
S52.572M

S52.572N
S52.572P
S52.572Q
S52.572R
S52.579A
S52.579K
S52.579M
S52.579N
S52.579P
S52.579Q
S52.579R
S52.591A
S52.591K
S52.591M
S52.591N
S52.591P
S52.591Q
S52.591R
S52.592A
S52.592K
S52.592M
S52.592N
S52.592P
S52.592Q
S52.592R
S52.599A
S52.599K
S52.599M
S52.599N
S52.599P
S52.599Q
S52.599R
S52.601A
S52.601K
S52.601M
S52.601N
S52.601P
S52.601Q
S52.601R
S52.602A
S52.602K
S52.602M
S52.602N
S52.602P
S52.602Q
S52.602R
S52.609A
S52.609K
S52.609M
S52.609N
S52.609P
S52.609Q
S52.609R
S52.611A
S52.611K
S52.611M
S52.611N
S52.611P
S52.611Q
S52.611R
S52.612A
S52.612K
S52.612M
S52.612N
S52.612P
S52.612Q
S52.612R
S52.613A
S52.613K
S52.613M
S52.613N
S52.613P
S52.613Q
S52.613R
S52.614A
S52.614K
S52.614M
S52.614N
S52.614P
S52.614Q
S52.614R
S52.615A
S52.615K
S52.615M
S52.615N
S52.615P
S52.615Q
S52.615R
S52.616A
S52.616K
S52.616M
S52.616N
S52.616P
S52.616Q
S52.616R
S52.621A
S52.621K
S52.621P
S52.622A
S52.622K
S52.622P
S52.629A
S52.629K
S52.629P
S52.691A
S52.691K
S52.691M
S52.691N
S52.691P
S52.691Q
S52.691R
S52.692A
S52.692K
S52.692M
S52.692N
S52.692P
S52.692Q
S52.692R
S52.699A
S52.699K
S52.699M
S52.699N
S52.699P
S52.699Q
S52.699R
S52.90XA
S52.90XK
S52.90XM
S52.90XN
S52.90XP
S52.90XQ
S52.90XR
S52.91XA
S52.91XK
S52.91XM
S52.91XN
S52.91XP
S52.91XQ
S52.91XR
S52.92XA
S52.92XK
S52.92XM
S52.92XN
S52.92XP
S52.92XQ
S52.92XR
S55.001A
S55.002A
S55.009A
S55.011A
S55.012A
S55.019A
S55.091A
S55.092A
S55.099A
S55.101A
S55.102A
S55.109A
S55.111A
S55.112A
S55.119A
S55.191A
S55.192A
S55.199A
S55.201A
S55.202A
S55.209A
S55.211A
S55.212A
S55.219A
S55.291A
S55.292A
S55.299A
S55.801A
S55.802A
S55.809A
S55.811A
S55.812A
S55.819A
S55.891A
S55.892A
S55.899A
S55.901A
S55.902A
S55.909A
S55.911A
S55.912A
S55.919A
S55.991A
S55.992A
S55.999A
S56.021A
S56.022A
S56.029A
S56.121A
S56.122A
S56.123A
S56.124A
S56.125A
S56.126A
S56.127A
S56.128A
S56.129A
S56.221A
S56.222A
S56.229A
S56.321A
S56.322A
S56.329A
S56.421A
S56.422A
S56.423A
S56.424A
S56.425A
S56.426A
S56.427A
S56.428A
S56.429A
S56.521A
S56.522A
S56.529A
S56.821A
S56.822A
S56.829A
S56.921A
S56.922A
S56.929A
S58.011A
S58.012A
S58.019A
S58.021A
S58.022A
S58.029A
S58.111A
S58.112A
S58.119A
S58.121A
S58.122A
S58.129A
S58.911A
S58.912A
S58.919A
S58.921A
S58.922A
S58.929A
S59.001A
S59.001K
S59.001P
S59.002A
S59.002K
S59.002P
S59.009A
S59.009K
S59.009P
S59.011A
S59.011K
S59.011P
S59.012A
S59.012K
S59.012P
S59.019A
S59.019K
S59.019P
S59.021A
S59.021K
S59.021P
S59.022A
S59.022K
S59.022P
S59.029A
S59.029K
S59.029P
S59.031A
S59.031K
S59.031P
S59.032A
S59.032K
S59.032P
S59.039A
S59.039K
S59.039P
S59.041A
S59.041K
S59.041P
S59.042A
S59.042K
S59.042P
S59.049A
S59.049K
S59.049P
S59.091A
S59.091K
S59.091P
S59.092A
S59.092K
S59.092P
S59.099A
S59.099K
S59.099P
S59.101K
S59.101P
S59.102K
S59.102P
S59.109K
S59.109P
S59.111K
S59.111P
S59.112K
S59.112P
S59.119K
S59.119P
S59.121K
S59.121P
S59.122K
S59.122P
S59.129K
S59.129P
S59.131K
S59.131P
S59.132K
S59.132P
S59.139K
S59.139P
S59.141K
S59.141P
S59.142K
S59.142P
S59.149K
S59.149P
S59.191K
S59.191P
S59.192K
S59.192P
S59.199K
S59.199P
S59.201A
S59.201K
S59.201P
S59.202A
S59.202K
S59.202P
S59.209A
S59.209K
S59.209P
S59.211A
S59.211K
S59.211P
S59.212A
S59.212K
S59.212P
S59.219A
S59.219K
S59.219P
S59.221A
S59.221K
S59.221P
S59.222A
S59.222K
S59.222P
S59.229A
S59.229K
S59.229P
S59.231A
S59.231K
S59.231P
S59.232A
S59.232K
S59.232P
S59.239A
S59.239K
S59.239P
S59.241A
S59.241K
S59.241P
S59.242A
S59.242K
S59.242P
S59.249A
S59.249K
S59.249P
S59.291A
S59.291K
S59.291P
S59.292A
S59.292K
S59.292P
S59.299A
S59.299K
S59.299P
S62.001B
S62.001K
S62.001P
S62.002B
S62.002K
S62.002P
S62.009B
S62.009K
S62.009P
S62.011B
S62.011K
S62.011P
S62.012B
S62.012K
S62.012P
S62.013B
S62.013K
S62.013P
S62.014B
S62.014K
S62.014P
S62.015B
S62.015K
S62.015P
S62.016B
S62.016K
S62.016P
S62.021B
S62.021K
S62.021P
S62.022B
S62.022K
S62.022P
S62.023B
S62.023K
S62.023P
S62.024B
S62.024K
S62.024P
S62.025B
S62.025K
S62.025P
S62.026B
S62.026K
S62.026P
S62.031B
S62.031K
S62.031P
S62.032B
S62.032K
S62.032P
S62.033B
S62.033K
S62.033P
S62.034B
S62.034K
S62.034P
S62.035B
S62.035K
S62.035P
S62.036B
S62.036K
S62.036P
S62.101B
S62.101K
S62.101P
S62.102B
S62.102K
S62.102P
S62.109B
S62.109K
S62.109P
S62.111B
S62.111K
S62.111P
S62.112B
S62.112K
S62.112P
S62.113B
S62.113K
S62.113P
S62.114B
S62.114K
S62.114P
S62.115B
S62.115K
S62.115P
S62.116B
S62.116K
S62.116P
S62.121B
S62.121K
S62.121P
S62.122B
S62.122K
S62.122P
S62.123B
S62.123K
S62.123P
S62.124B
S62.124K
S62.124P
S62.125B
S62.125K
S62.125P
S62.126B
S62.126K
S62.126P
S62.131B
S62.131K
S62.131P
S62.132B
S62.132K
S62.132P
S62.133B
S62.133K
S62.133P
S62.134B
S62.134K
S62.134P
S62.135B
S62.135K
S62.135P
S62.136B
S62.136K
S62.136P
S62.141B
S62.141K
S62.141P
S62.142B
S62.142K
S62.142P
S62.143B
S62.143K
S62.143P
S62.144B
S62.144K
S62.144P
S62.145B
S62.145K
S62.145P
S62.146B
S62.146K
S62.146P
S62.151B
S62.151K
S62.151P
S62.152B
S62.152K
S62.152P
S62.153B
S62.153K
S62.153P
S62.154B
S62.154K
S62.154P
S62.155B
S62.155K
S62.155P
S62.156B
S62.156K
S62.156P
S62.161B
S62.161K
S62.161P
S62.162B
S62.162K
S62.162P
S62.163B
S62.163K
S62.163P
S62.164B
S62.164K
S62.164P
S62.165B
S62.165K
S62.165P
S62.166B
S62.166K
S62.166P
S62.171B
S62.171K
S62.171P
S62.172B
S62.172K
S62.172P
S62.173B
S62.173K
S62.173P
S62.174B
S62.174K
S62.174P
S62.175B
S62.175K
S62.175P
S62.176B
S62.176K
S62.176P
S62.181B
S62.181K
S62.181P
S62.182B
S62.182K
S62.182P
S62.183B
S62.183K
S62.183P
S62.184B
S62.184K
S62.184P
S62.185B
S62.185K
S62.185P
S62.186B
S62.186K
S62.186P
S62.201B
S62.201K
S62.201P
S62.202B
S62.202K
S62.202P
S62.209B
S62.209K
S62.209P
S62.211B
S62.211K
S62.211P
S62.212B
S62.212K
S62.212P
S62.213B
S62.213K
S62.213P
S62.221B
S62.221K
S62.221P
S62.222B
S62.222K
S62.222P
S62.223B
S62.223K
S62.223P
S62.224B
S62.224K
S62.224P
S62.225B
S62.225K
S62.225P
S62.226B
S62.226K
S62.226P
S62.231B
S62.231K
S62.231P
S62.232B
S62.232K
S62.232P
S62.233B
S62.233K
S62.233P
S62.234B
S62.234K
S62.234P
S62.235B
S62.235K
S62.235P
S62.236B
S62.236K
S62.236P
S62.241B
S62.241K
S62.241P
S62.242B
S62.242K
S62.242P
S62.243B
S62.243K
S62.243P
S62.244B
S62.244K
S62.244P
S62.245B
S62.245K
S62.245P
S62.246B
S62.246K
S62.246P
S62.251B
S62.251K
S62.251P
S62.252B
S62.252K
S62.252P
S62.253B
S62.253K
S62.253P
S62.254B
S62.254K
S62.254P
S62.255B
S62.255K
S62.255P
S62.256B
S62.256K
S62.256P
S62.291B
S62.291K
S62.291P
S62.292B
S62.292K
S62.292P
S62.299B
S62.299K
S62.299P
S62.300B
S62.300K
S62.300P
S62.301B
S62.301K
S62.301P
S62.302B
S62.302K
S62.302P
S62.303B
S62.303K
S62.303P
S62.304B
S62.304K
S62.304P
S62.305B
S62.305K
S62.305P
S62.306B
S62.306K
S62.306P
S62.307B
S62.307K
S62.307P
S62.308B
S62.308K
S62.308P
S62.309B
S62.309K
S62.309P
S62.310B
S62.310K
S62.310P
S62.311B
S62.311K
S62.311P
S62.312B
S62.312K
S62.312P
S62.313B
S62.313K
S62.313P
S62.314B
S62.314K
S62.314P
S62.315B
S62.315K
S62.315P
S62.316B
S62.316K
S62.316P
S62.317B
S62.317K
S62.317P
S62.318B
S62.318K
S62.318P
S62.319B
S62.319K
S62.319P
S62.320B
S62.320K
S62.320P
S62.321B
S62.321K
S62.321P
S62.322B
S62.322K
S62.322P
S62.323B
S62.323K
S62.323P
S62.324B
S62.324K
S62.324P
S62.325B
S62.325K
S62.325P
S62.326B
S62.326K
S62.326P
S62.327B
S62.327K
S62.327P
S62.328B
S62.328K
S62.328P
S62.329B
S62.329K
S62.329P
S62.330B
S62.330K
S62.330P
S62.331B
S62.331K
S62.331P
S62.332B
S62.332K
S62.332P
S62.333B
S62.333K
S62.333P
S62.334B
S62.334K
S62.334P
S62.335B
S62.335K
S62.335P
S62.336B
S62.336K
S62.336P
S62.337B
S62.337K
S62.337P
S62.338B
S62.338K
S62.338P
S62.339B
S62.339K
S62.339P
S62.340B
S62.340K
S62.340P
S62.341B
S62.341K
S62.341P
S62.342B
S62.342K
S62.342P
S62.343B
S62.343K
S62.343P
S62.344B
S62.344K
S62.344P
S62.345B
S62.345K
S62.345P
S62.346B
S62.346K
S62.346P
S62.347B
S62.347K
S62.347P
S62.348B
S62.348K
S62.348P
S62.349B
S62.349K
S62.349P
S62.350B
S62.350K
S62.350P
S62.351B
S62.351K
S62.351P
S62.352B
S62.352K
S62.352P
S62.353B
S62.353K
S62.353P
S62.354B
S62.354K
S62.354P
S62.355B
S62.355K
S62.355P
S62.356B
S62.356K
S62.356P
S62.357B
S62.357K
S62.357P
S62.358B
S62.358K
S62.358P
S62.359B
S62.359K
S62.359P
S62.360B
S62.360K
S62.360P
S62.361B
S62.361K
S62.361P
S62.362B
S62.362K
S62.362P
S62.363B
S62.363K
S62.363P
S62.364B
S62.364K
S62.364P
S62.365B
S62.365K
S62.365P
S62.366B
S62.366K
S62.366P
S62.367B
S62.367K
S62.367P
S62.368B
S62.368K
S62.368P
S62.369B
S62.369K

S62.369P
S62.390B
S62.390K
S62.390P
S62.391B
S62.391K
S62.391P
S62.392B
S62.392K
S62.392P
S62.393B
S62.393K
S62.393P
S62.394B
S62.394K
S62.394P
S62.395B
S62.395K
S62.395P
S62.396B
S62.396K
S62.396P
S62.397B
S62.397K
S62.397P
S62.398B
S62.398K
S62.398P
S62.399B
S62.399K
S62.399P
S62.501B
S62.501K
S62.501P
S62.502B
S62.502K
S62.502P
S62.509B
S62.509K
S62.509P
S62.511B
S62.511K
S62.511P
S62.512B
S62.512K
S62.512P
S62.513B
S62.513K
S62.513P
S62.514B
S62.514K
S62.514P
S62.515B
S62.515K
S62.515P
S62.516B
S62.516K
S62.516P
S62.521B
S62.521K
S62.521P
S62.522B
S62.522K
S62.522P
S62.523B
S62.523K
S62.523P
S62.524B
S62.524K
S62.524P
S62.525B
S62.525K
S62.525P
S62.526B
S62.526K
S62.526P
S62.600B
S62.600K
S62.600P
S62.601B
S62.601K
S62.601P
S62.602B
S62.602K
S62.602P
S62.603B
S62.603K
S62.603P
S62.604B
S62.604K
S62.604P
S62.605B
S62.605K
S62.605P
S62.606B
S62.606K
S62.606P
S62.607B
S62.607K
S62.607P
S62.608B
S62.608K
S62.608P
S62.609B
S62.609K
S62.609P
S62.610B
S62.610K
S62.610P
S62.611B
S62.611K
S62.611P
S62.612B
S62.612K
S62.612P
S62.613B
S62.613K
S62.613P
S62.614B
S62.614K
S62.614P
S62.615B
S62.615K
S62.615P
S62.616B
S62.616K
S62.616P
S62.617B
S62.617K
S62.617P
S62.618B
S62.618K
S62.618P
S62.619B
S62.619K
S62.619P
S62.620B
S62.620K
S62.620P
S62.621B
S62.621K
S62.621P
S62.622B
S62.622K
S62.622P
S62.623B
S62.623K
S62.623P
S62.624B
S62.624K
S62.624P
S62.625B
S62.625K
S62.625P
S62.626B
S62.626K
S62.626P
S62.627B
S62.627K
S62.627P
S62.628B
S62.628K
S62.628P
S62.629B
S62.629K
S62.629P
S62.630B
S62.630K
S62.630P
S62.631B
S62.631K
S62.631P
S62.632B
S62.632K
S62.632P
S62.633B
S62.633K
S62.633P
S62.634B
S62.634K
S62.634P
S62.635B
S62.635K
S62.635P
S62.636B
S62.636K
S62.636P
S62.637B
S62.637K
S62.637P
S62.638B
S62.638K
S62.638P
S62.639B
S62.639K
S62.639P
S62.640B
S62.640K
S62.640P
S62.641B
S62.641K
S62.641P
S62.642B
S62.642K
S62.642P
S62.643B
S62.643K
S62.643P
S62.644B
S62.644K
S62.644P
S62.645B
S62.645K
S62.645P
S62.646B
S62.646K
S62.646P
S62.647B
S62.647K
S62.647P
S62.648B
S62.648K
S62.648P
S62.649B
S62.649K
S62.649P
S62.650B
S62.650K
S62.650P
S62.651B
S62.651K
S62.651P
S62.652B
S62.652K
S62.652P
S62.653B
S62.653K
S62.653P
S62.654B
S62.654K
S62.654P
S62.655B
S62.655K
S62.655P
S62.656B
S62.656K
S62.656P
S62.657B
S62.657K
S62.657P
S62.658B
S62.658K
S62.658P
S62.659B
S62.659K
S62.659P
S62.660B
S62.660K
S62.660P
S62.661B
S62.661K
S62.661P
S62.662B
S62.662K
S62.662P
S62.663B
S62.663K
S62.663P
S62.664B
S62.664K
S62.664P
S62.665B
S62.665K
S62.665P
S62.666B
S62.666K
S62.666P
S62.667B
S62.667K
S62.667P
S62.668B
S62.668K
S62.668P
S62.669B
S62.669K
S62.669P
S62.90XB
S62.90XK
S62.90XP
S62.91XB
S62.91XK
S62.91XP
S62.92XB
S62.92XK
S62.92XP
S65.001A
S65.002A
S65.009A
S65.011A
S65.012A
S65.019A
S65.091A
S65.092A
S65.099A
S65.101A
S65.102A
S65.109A
S65.111A
S65.112A
S65.119A
S65.191A
S65.192A
S65.199A
S65.201A
S65.202A
S65.209A
S65.211A
S65.212A
S65.219A
S65.291A
S65.292A
S65.299A
S65.301A
S65.302A
S65.309A
S65.311A
S65.312A
S65.319A
S65.391A
S65.392A
S65.399A
S65.401A
S65.402A
S65.409A
S65.411A
S65.412A
S65.419A
S65.491A
S65.492A
S65.499A
S65.500A
S65.501A
S65.502A
S65.503A
S65.504A
S65.505A
S65.506A
S65.507A
S65.508A
S65.509A
S65.510A
S65.511A
S65.512A
S65.513A
S65.514A
S65.515A
S65.516A
S65.517A
S65.518A
S65.519A
S65.590A
S65.591A
S65.592A
S65.593A
S65.594A
S65.595A
S65.596A
S65.597A
S65.598A
S65.599A
S65.801A
S65.802A
S65.809A
S65.811A
S65.812A
S65.819A
S65.891A
S65.892A
S65.899A
S65.901A
S65.902A
S65.909A
S65.911A
S65.912A
S65.919A
S65.991A
S65.992A
S65.999A
S66.021A
S66.022A
S66.029A
S66.120A
S66.121A
S66.122A
S66.123A
S66.124A
S66.125A
S66.126A
S66.127A
S66.128A
S66.129A
S66.221A
S66.222A
S66.229A
S66.320A
S66.321A
S66.322A
S66.323A
S66.324A
S66.325A
S66.326A
S66.327A
S66.328A
S66.329A
S66.421A
S66.422A
S66.429A
S66.520A
S66.521A
S66.522A
S66.523A
S66.524A
S66.525A
S66.526A
S66.527A
S66.528A
S66.529A
S66.821A
S66.822A
S66.829A
S66.921A
S66.922A
S66.929A
S68.411A
S68.412A
S68.419A
S68.421A
S68.422A
S68.429A
S68.711A
S68.712A
S68.719A
S68.721A
S68.722A
S68.729A
S72.001K
S72.001M
S72.001N
S72.001P
S72.001Q
S72.001R
S72.002K
S72.002M
S72.002N
S72.002P
S72.002Q
S72.002R
S72.009K
S72.009M
S72.009N
S72.009P
S72.009Q
S72.009R
S72.011K
S72.011M
S72.011N
S72.011P
S72.011Q
S72.011R
S72.012K
S72.012M
S72.012N
S72.012P
S72.012Q
S72.012R
S72.019K
S72.019M
S72.019N
S72.019P
S72.019Q
S72.019R
S72.021K
S72.021M
S72.021N
S72.021P
S72.021Q
S72.021R
S72.022K
S72.022M
S72.022N
S72.022P
S72.022Q
S72.022R
S72.023K
S72.023M
S72.023N
S72.023P
S72.023Q
S72.023R
S72.024K
S72.024M
S72.024N
S72.024P
S72.024Q
S72.024R
S72.025K
S72.025M
S72.025N
S72.025P
S72.025Q
S72.025R
S72.026K
S72.026M
S72.026N
S72.026P
S72.026Q
S72.026R
S72.031K
S72.031M
S72.031N
S72.031P
S72.031Q
S72.031R
S72.032K
S72.032M
S72.032N
S72.032P
S72.032Q
S72.032R
S72.033K
S72.033M
S72.033N
S72.033P
S72.033Q
S72.033R
S72.034K
S72.034M
S72.034N
S72.034P
S72.034Q
S72.034R
S72.035K
S72.035M
S72.035N
S72.035P
S72.035Q
S72.035R
S72.036K
S72.036M
S72.036N
S72.036P
S72.036Q
S72.036R
S72.041K
S72.041M
S72.041N
S72.041P
S72.041Q
S72.041R
S72.042K
S72.042M
S72.042N
S72.042P
S72.042Q
S72.042R
S72.043K
S72.043M
S72.043N
S72.043P
S72.043Q
S72.043R
S72.044K
S72.044M
S72.044N
S72.044P
S72.044Q
S72.044R
S72.045K
S72.045M
S72.045N
S72.045P
S72.045Q
S72.045R
S72.046K
S72.046M
S72.046N
S72.046P
S72.046Q
S72.046R
S72.051K
S72.051M
S72.051N
S72.051P
S72.051Q
S72.051R
S72.052K
S72.052M
S72.052N
S72.052P
S72.052Q
S72.052R
S72.059K
S72.059M
S72.059N
S72.059P
S72.059Q
S72.059R
S72.061K
S72.061M
S72.061N
S72.061P
S72.061Q
S72.061R
S72.062K
S72.062M
S72.062N
S72.062P
S72.062Q
S72.062R
S72.063K
S72.063M
S72.063N
S72.063P
S72.063Q
S72.063R
S72.064K
S72.064M
S72.064N
S72.064P
S72.064Q
S72.064R
S72.065K
S72.065M
S72.065N
S72.065P
S72.065Q
S72.065R
S72.066K
S72.066M
S72.066N
S72.066P
S72.066Q
S72.066R
S72.091K
S72.091M
S72.091N
S72.091P
S72.091Q
S72.091R
S72.092K
S72.092M
S72.092N
S72.092P
S72.092Q
S72.092R
S72.099K
S72.099M
S72.099N
S72.099P
S72.099Q
S72.099R
S72.101K
S72.101M
S72.101N
S72.101P
S72.101Q
S72.101R
S72.102K
S72.102M
S72.102N
S72.102P
S72.102Q
S72.102R
S72.109K
S72.109M
S72.109N
S72.109P
S72.109Q
S72.109R
S72.111K
S72.111M
S72.111N
S72.111P
S72.111Q
S72.111R
S72.112K
S72.112M
S72.112N
S72.112P
S72.112Q
S72.112R
S72.113K
S72.113M
S72.113N
S72.113P
S72.113Q
S72.113R
S72.114K
S72.114M
S72.114N
S72.114P
S72.114Q
S72.114R
S72.115K
S72.115M
S72.115N
S72.115P
S72.115Q
S72.115R
S72.116K
S72.116M
S72.116N
S72.116P
S72.116Q
S72.116R
S72.121K
S72.121M
S72.121N
S72.121P
S72.121Q
S72.121R
S72.122K
S72.122M
S72.122N
S72.122P
S72.122Q
S72.122R
S72.123K
S72.123M
S72.123N
S72.123P
S72.123Q
S72.123R
S72.124K
S72.124M
S72.124N
S72.124P
S72.124Q
S72.124R
S72.125K
S72.125M
S72.125N
S72.125P
S72.125Q
S72.125R
S72.126K
S72.126M
S72.126N
S72.126P
S72.126Q
S72.126R
S72.131K
S72.131M
S72.131N
S72.131P
S72.131Q
S72.131R
S72.132K
S72.132M
S72.132N
S72.132P
S72.132Q
S72.132R
S72.133K
S72.133M
S72.133N
S72.133P
S72.133Q
S72.133R
S72.134K
S72.134M
S72.134N
S72.134P
S72.134Q
S72.134R
S72.135K
S72.135M
S72.135N
S72.135P
S72.135Q
S72.135R
S72.136K
S72.136M
S72.136N
S72.136P
S72.136Q
S72.136R
S72.141K
S72.141M
S72.141N
S72.141P
S72.141Q
S72.141R
S72.142K
S72.142M
S72.142N
S72.142P
S72.142Q
S72.142R
S72.143K
S72.143M
S72.143N
S72.143P
S72.143Q
S72.143R
S72.144K
S72.144M
S72.144N
S72.144P
S72.144Q
S72.144R
S72.145K
S72.145M
S72.145N
S72.145P
S72.145Q
S72.145R
S72.146K
S72.146M
S72.146N
S72.146P
S72.146Q
S72.146R
S72.21XK
S72.21XM
S72.21XN
S72.21XP
S72.21XQ
S72.21XR
S72.22XK
S72.22XM
S72.22XN
S72.22XP
S72.22XQ
S72.22XR
S72.23XK
S72.23XM
S72.23XN
S72.23XP
S72.23XQ
S72.23XR
S72.24XK
S72.24XM
S72.24XN
S72.24XP
S72.24XQ
S72.24XR
S72.25XK
S72.25XM
S72.25XN
S72.25XP
S72.25XQ
S72.25XR
S72.26XK
S72.26XM
S72.26XN
S72.26XP
S72.26XQ
S72.26XR
S72.301K
S72.301M
S72.301N
S72.301P
S72.301Q
S72.301R
S72.302K
S72.302M
S72.302N
S72.302P
S72.302Q
S72.302R
S72.309K
S72.309M
S72.309N
S72.309P
S72.309Q
S72.309R
S72.321K
S72.321M
S72.321N
S72.321P
S72.321Q
S72.321R
S72.322K
S72.322M
S72.322N
S72.322P
S72.322Q
S72.322R
S72.323K
S72.323M
S72.323N
S72.323P
S72.323Q
S72.323R
S72.324K
S72.324M
S72.324N
S72.324P
S72.324Q
S72.324R
S72.325K
S72.325M
S72.325N
S72.325P
S72.325Q
S72.325R
S72.326K
S72.326M
S72.326N
S72.326P
S72.326Q
S72.326R

S72.331K
S72.331M
S72.331N
S72.331P
S72.331Q
S72.331R
S72.332K
S72.332M
S72.332N
S72.332P
S72.332Q
S72.332R
S72.333K
S72.333M
S72.333N
S72.333P
S72.333Q
S72.333R
S72.334K
S72.334M
S72.334N
S72.334P
S72.334Q
S72.334R
S72.335K
S72.335M
S72.335N
S72.335P
S72.335Q
S72.335R
S72.336K
S72.336M
S72.336N
S72.336P
S72.336Q
S72.336R
S72.341K
S72.341M
S72.341N
S72.341P
S72.341Q
S72.341R
S72.342K
S72.342M
S72.342N
S72.342P
S72.342Q
S72.342R
S72.343K
S72.343M
S72.343N
S72.343P
S72.343Q
S72.343R
S72.344K
S72.344M
S72.344N
S72.344P
S72.344Q
S72.344R
S72.345K
S72.345M
S72.345N
S72.345P
S72.345Q
S72.345R
S72.346K
S72.346M
S72.346N
S72.346P
S72.346Q
S72.346R
S72.351K
S72.351M
S72.351N
S72.351P
S72.351Q
S72.351R
S72.352K
S72.352M
S72.352N
S72.352P
S72.352Q

S72.352R
S72.353K
S72.353M
S72.353N
S72.353P
S72.353Q
S72.353R
S72.354K
S72.354M
S72.354N
S72.354P
S72.354Q
S72.354R
S72.355K
S72.355M
S72.355N
S72.355P
S72.355Q
S72.355R
S72.356K
S72.356M
S72.356N
S72.356P
S72.356Q
S72.356R
S72.361K
S72.361M
S72.361N
S72.361P
S72.361Q
S72.361R
S72.362K
S72.362M
S72.362N
S72.362P
S72.362Q
S72.362R
S72.363K
S72.363M
S72.363N
S72.363P
S72.363Q
S72.363R
S72.364K
S72.364M
S72.364N
S72.364P
S72.364Q
S72.364R
S72.365K
S72.365M
S72.365N
S72.365P
S72.365Q
S72.365R
S72.366K
S72.366M
S72.366N
S72.366P
S72.366Q
S72.366R
S72.391K
S72.391M
S72.391N
S72.391P
S72.391Q
S72.391R
S72.392K
S72.392M
S72.392N
S72.392P
S72.392Q
S72.392R
S72.399K
S72.399M
S72.399N
S72.399P
S72.399Q
S72.399R
S72.401A
S72.401K
S72.401M
S72.401N

S72.401P
S72.401Q
S72.401R
S72.402A
S72.402K
S72.402M
S72.402N
S72.402P
S72.402Q
S72.402R
S72.409A
S72.409K
S72.409M
S72.409N
S72.409P
S72.409Q
S72.409R
S72.411A
S72.411K
S72.411M
S72.411N
S72.411P
S72.411Q
S72.411R
S72.412A
S72.412K
S72.412M
S72.412N
S72.412P
S72.412Q
S72.412R
S72.413A
S72.413K
S72.413M
S72.413N
S72.413P
S72.413Q
S72.413R
S72.414A
S72.414K
S72.414M
S72.414N
S72.414P
S72.414Q
S72.414R
S72.415A
S72.415K
S72.415M
S72.415N
S72.415P
S72.415Q
S72.415R
S72.416A
S72.416K
S72.416M
S72.416N
S72.416P
S72.416Q
S72.416R
S72.421A
S72.421K
S72.421M
S72.421N
S72.421P
S72.421Q
S72.421R
S72.422A
S72.422K
S72.422M
S72.422N
S72.422P
S72.422Q
S72.422R
S72.423A
S72.423K
S72.423M
S72.423N
S72.423P
S72.423Q
S72.423R
S72.424A
S72.424K
S72.424M

S72.424N
S72.424P
S72.424Q
S72.424R
S72.425A
S72.425K
S72.425M
S72.425N
S72.425P
S72.425Q
S72.425R
S72.426A
S72.426K
S72.426M
S72.426N
S72.426P
S72.426Q
S72.426R
S72.431A
S72.431K
S72.431M
S72.431N
S72.431P
S72.431Q
S72.431R
S72.432A
S72.432K
S72.432M
S72.432N
S72.432P
S72.432Q
S72.432R
S72.433A
S72.433K
S72.433M
S72.433N
S72.433P
S72.433Q
S72.433R
S72.434A
S72.434K
S72.434M
S72.434N
S72.434P
S72.434Q
S72.434R
S72.435A
S72.435K
S72.435M
S72.435N
S72.435P
S72.435Q
S72.435R
S72.436A
S72.436K
S72.436M
S72.436N
S72.436P
S72.436Q
S72.436R
S72.441A
S72.441K
S72.441M
S72.441N
S72.441P
S72.441Q
S72.441R
S72.442A
S72.442K
S72.442M
S72.442N
S72.442P
S72.442Q
S72.442R
S72.443A
S72.443K
S72.443M
S72.443N
S72.443P
S72.443Q
S72.443R
S72.444A
S72.444K

S72.444M
S72.444N
S72.444P
S72.444Q
S72.444R
S72.445A
S72.445K
S72.445M
S72.445N
S72.445P
S72.445Q
S72.445R
S72.446A
S72.446K
S72.446M
S72.446N
S72.446P
S72.446Q
S72.446R
S72.451A
S72.451K
S72.451M
S72.451N
S72.451P
S72.451Q
S72.451R
S72.452A
S72.452K
S72.452M
S72.452N
S72.452P
S72.452Q
S72.452R
S72.453A
S72.453K
S72.453M
S72.453N
S72.453P
S72.453Q
S72.453R
S72.454A
S72.454K
S72.454M
S72.454N
S72.454P
S72.454Q
S72.454R
S72.455A
S72.455K
S72.455M
S72.455N
S72.455P
S72.455Q
S72.455R
S72.456A
S72.456K
S72.456M
S72.456N
S72.456P
S72.456Q
S72.456R
S72.461A
S72.461K
S72.461M
S72.461N
S72.461P
S72.461Q
S72.461R
S72.462A
S72.462K
S72.462M
S72.462N
S72.462P
S72.462Q
S72.462R
S72.463A
S72.463K
S72.463M
S72.463N
S72.463P
S72.463Q
S72.463R
S72.464A

S72.464K
S72.464M
S72.464N
S72.464P
S72.464Q
S72.464R
S72.465A
S72.465K
S72.465M
S72.465N
S72.465P
S72.465Q
S72.465R
S72.466A
S72.466K
S72.466M
S72.466N
S72.466P
S72.466Q
S72.466R
S72.471A
S72.471K
S72.471P
S72.472A
S72.472K
S72.472P
S72.479A
S72.479K
S72.479P
S72.491A
S72.491K
S72.491M
S72.491N
S72.491P
S72.491Q
S72.491R
S72.492A
S72.492K
S72.492M
S72.492N
S72.492P
S72.492Q
S72.492R
S72.499A
S72.499K
S72.499M
S72.499N
S72.499P
S72.499Q
S72.499R
S72.8X1K
S72.8X1M
S72.8X1N
S72.8X1P
S72.8X1Q
S72.8X1R
S72.8X2K
S72.8X2M
S72.8X2N
S72.8X2P
S72.8X2Q
S72.8X2R
S72.8X9K
S72.8X9M
S72.8X9N
S72.8X9P
S72.8X9Q
S72.8X9R
S72.90XK
S72.90XM
S72.90XN
S72.90XP
S72.90XQ
S72.90XR
S72.91XK
S72.91XM
S72.91XN
S72.91XP
S72.91XQ
S72.91XR
S72.92XK
S72.92XM
S72.92XN

S72.92XP
S72.92XQ
S72.92XR
S73.001A
S73.002A
S73.003A
S73.004A
S73.005A
S73.006A
S73.011A
S73.012A
S73.013A
S73.014A
S73.015A
S73.016A
S73.021A
S73.022A
S73.023A
S73.024A
S73.025A
S73.026A
S73.031A
S73.032A
S73.033A
S73.034A
S73.035A
S73.036A
S73.041A
S73.042A
S73.043A
S73.044A
S73.045A
S73.046A
S75.201A
S75.202A
S75.209A
S75.211A
S75.212A
S75.219A
S75.221A
S75.222A
S75.229A
S75.291A
S75.292A
S75.299A
S75.801A
S75.802A
S75.809A
S75.811A
S75.812A
S75.819A
S75.891A
S75.892A
S75.899A
S75.901A
S75.902A
S75.909A
S75.911A
S75.912A
S75.919A
S75.991A
S75.992A
S75.999A
S76.021A
S76.022A
S76.029A
S76.121A
S76.122A
S76.129A
S76.221A
S76.222A
S76.229A
S76.321A
S76.322A
S76.329A
S76.821A
S76.822A
S76.829A
S76.921A
S76.922A
S76.929A
S77.00XA
S77.01XA

S77.02XA
S77.10XA
S77.11XA
S77.12XA
S78.011A
S78.012A
S78.019A
S78.021A
S78.022A
S78.029A
S78.111A
S78.112A
S78.119A
S78.121A
S78.122A
S78.129A
S78.911A
S78.912A
S78.919A
S78.921A
S78.922A
S78.929A
S79.001K
S79.001P
S79.002K
S79.002P
S79.009K
S79.009P
S79.011K
S79.011P
S79.012K
S79.012P
S79.019K
S79.019P
S79.091K
S79.091P
S79.092K
S79.092P
S79.099K
S79.099P
S79.101A
S79.101K
S79.101P
S79.102A
S79.102K
S79.102P
S79.109A
S79.109K
S79.109P
S79.111A
S79.111K
S79.111P
S79.112A
S79.112K
S79.112P
S79.119A
S79.119K
S79.119P
S79.121A
S79.121K
S79.121P
S79.122A
S79.122K
S79.122P
S79.129A
S79.129K
S79.129P
S79.131A
S79.131K
S79.131P
S79.132A
S79.132K
S79.132P
S79.139A
S79.139K
S79.139P
S79.141A
S79.141K
S79.141P
S79.142A
S79.142K
S79.142P
S79.149A

S79.149K
S79.149P
S79.191A
S79.191K
S79.191P
S79.192A
S79.192K
S79.192P
S79.199A
S79.199K
S79.199P
S82.001A
S82.001B
S82.001C
S82.001K
S82.001M
S82.001N
S82.001P
S82.001Q
S82.001R
S82.002A
S82.002B
S82.002C
S82.002K
S82.002M
S82.002N
S82.002P
S82.002Q
S82.002R
S82.009A
S82.009B
S82.009C
S82.009K
S82.009M
S82.009N
S82.009P
S82.009Q
S82.009R
S82.011A
S82.011B
S82.011C
S82.011K
S82.011M
S82.011N
S82.011P
S82.011Q
S82.011R
S82.012A
S82.012B
S82.012C
S82.012K
S82.012M
S82.012N
S82.012P
S82.012Q
S82.012R
S82.013A
S82.013B
S82.013C
S82.013K
S82.013M
S82.013N
S82.013P
S82.013Q
S82.013R
S82.014A
S82.014B
S82.014C
S82.014K
S82.014M
S82.014N
S82.014P
S82.014Q
S82.014R
S82.015A
S82.015B
S82.015C
S82.015K
S82.015M
S82.015N
S82.015P
S82.015Q
S82.015R

S82.016A
S82.016B
S82.016C
S82.016K
S82.016M
S82.016N
S82.016P
S82.016Q
S82.016R
S82.021A
S82.021B
S82.021C
S82.021K
S82.021M
S82.021N
S82.021P
S82.021Q
S82.021R
S82.022A
S82.022B
S82.022C
S82.022K
S82.022M
S82.022N
S82.022P
S82.022Q
S82.022R
S82.023A
S82.023B
S82.023C
S82.023K
S82.023M
S82.023N
S82.023P
S82.023Q
S82.023R
S82.024A
S82.024B
S82.024C
S82.024K
S82.024M
S82.024N
S82.024P
S82.024Q
S82.024R
S82.025A
S82.025B
S82.025C
S82.025K
S82.025M
S82.025N
S82.025P
S82.025Q
S82.025R
S82.026A
S82.026B
S82.026C
S82.026K
S82.026M
S82.026N
S82.026P
S82.026Q
S82.026R
S82.031A
S82.031B
S82.031C
S82.031K
S82.031M
S82.031N
S82.031P
S82.031Q
S82.031R
S82.032A
S82.032B
S82.032C
S82.032K
S82.032M
S82.032N
S82.032P
S82.032Q
S82.032R
S82.033A
S82.033B

S82.033C
S82.033K
S82.033M
S82.033N
S82.033P
S82.033Q
S82.033R
S82.034A
S82.034B
S82.034C
S82.034K
S82.034M
S82.034N
S82.034P
S82.034Q
S82.034R
S82.035A
S82.035B
S82.035C
S82.035K
S82.035M
S82.035N
S82.035P
S82.035Q
S82.035R
S82.036A
S82.036B
S82.036C
S82.036K
S82.036M
S82.036N
S82.036P
S82.036Q
S82.036R
S82.041A
S82.041B
S82.041C
S82.041K
S82.041M
S82.041N
S82.041P
S82.041Q
S82.041R
S82.042A
S82.042B
S82.042C
S82.042K
S82.042M
S82.042N
S82.042P
S82.042Q
S82.042R
S82.043A
S82.043B
S82.043C
S82.043K
S82.043M
S82.043N
S82.043P
S82.043Q
S82.043R
S82.044A
S82.044B
S82.044C
S82.044K
S82.044M
S82.044N
S82.044P
S82.044Q
S82.044R
S82.045A
S82.045B
S82.045C
S82.045K
S82.045M
S82.045N
S82.045P
S82.045Q
S82.045R
S82.046A
S82.046B
S82.046C
S82.046K

S82.Ø46M
S82.Ø46N
S82.Ø46P
S82.Ø46Q
S82.Ø46R
S82.Ø91A
S82.Ø91B
S82.Ø91C
S82.Ø91K
S82.Ø91M
S82.Ø91N
S82.Ø91P
S82.Ø91Q
S82.Ø91R
S82.Ø92A
S82.Ø92B
S82.Ø92C
S82.Ø92K
S82.Ø92M
S82.Ø92N
S82.Ø92P
S82.Ø92Q
S82.Ø92R
S82.Ø99A
S82.Ø99B
S82.Ø99C
S82.Ø99K
S82.Ø99M
S82.Ø99N
S82.Ø99P
S82.Ø99Q
S82.Ø99R
S82.1Ø1A
S82.1Ø1K
S82.1Ø1M
S82.1Ø1N
S82.1Ø1P
S82.1Ø1Q
S82.1Ø1R
S82.1Ø2A
S82.1Ø2K
S82.1Ø2M
S82.1Ø2N
S82.1Ø2P
S82.1Ø2Q
S82.1Ø2R
S82.1Ø9A
S82.1Ø9K
S82.1Ø9M
S82.1Ø9N
S82.1Ø9P
S82.1Ø9Q
S82.1Ø9R
S82.111A
S82.111K
S82.111M
S82.111N
S82.111P
S82.111Q
S82.111R
S82.112A
S82.112K
S82.112M
S82.112N
S82.112P
S82.112Q
S82.112R
S82.113A
S82.113K
S82.113M
S82.113N
S82.113P
S82.113Q
S82.113R
S82.114A
S82.114K
S82.114M
S82.114N
S82.114P
S82.114Q
S82.114R
S82.115A
S82.115K
S82.115M
S82.115N
S82.115P
S82.115Q
S82.115R
S82.116A
S82.116K
S82.116M
S82.116N
S82.116P
S82.116Q
S82.116R
S82.121A
S82.121K
S82.121M
S82.121N
S82.121P
S82.121Q
S82.121R
S82.122A
S82.122K
S82.122M
S82.122N
S82.122P
S82.122Q
S82.122R
S82.123A
S82.123K
S82.123M
S82.123N
S82.123P
S82.123Q
S82.123R
S82.124A
S82.124K
S82.124M
S82.124N
S82.124P
S82.124Q
S82.124R
S82.125A
S82.125K
S82.125M
S82.125N
S82.125P
S82.125Q
S82.125R
S82.126A
S82.126K
S82.126M
S82.126N
S82.126P
S82.126Q
S82.126R
S82.131A
S82.131K
S82.131M
S82.131N
S82.131P
S82.131Q
S82.131R
S82.132A
S82.132K
S82.132M
S82.132N
S82.132P
S82.132Q
S82.132R
S82.133A
S82.133K
S82.133M
S82.133N
S82.133P
S82.133Q
S82.133R
S82.134A
S82.134K
S82.134M
S82.134N
S82.134P
S82.134Q
S82.134R
S82.135A
S82.135K
S82.135M
S82.135N
S82.135P
S82.135Q
S82.135R
S82.136A
S82.136K
S82.136M
S82.136N
S82.136P
S82.136Q
S82.136R
S82.141A
S82.141K
S82.141M
S82.141N
S82.141P
S82.141Q
S82.141R
S82.142A
S82.142K
S82.142M
S82.142N
S82.142P
S82.142Q
S82.142R
S82.143A
S82.143K
S82.143M
S82.143N
S82.143P
S82.143Q
S82.143R
S82.144A
S82.144K
S82.144M
S82.144N
S82.144P
S82.144Q
S82.144R
S82.145A
S82.145K
S82.145M
S82.145N
S82.145P
S82.145Q
S82.145R
S82.146A
S82.146K
S82.146M
S82.146N
S82.146P
S82.146Q
S82.146R
S82.151A
S82.151K
S82.151M
S82.151N
S82.151P
S82.151Q
S82.151R
S82.152A
S82.152K
S82.152M
S82.152N
S82.152P
S82.152Q
S82.152R
S82.153A
S82.153K
S82.153M
S82.153N
S82.153P
S82.153Q
S82.153R
S82.154A
S82.154K
S82.154M
S82.154N
S82.154P
S82.154Q
S82.154R
S82.155A
S82.155K
S82.155M
S82.155N
S82.155P
S82.155Q
S82.155R
S82.156A
S82.156K
S82.156M
S82.156N
S82.156P
S82.156Q
S82.156R
S82.161A
S82.161K
S82.161P
S82.162A
S82.162K
S82.162P
S82.169A
S82.169K
S82.169P
S82.191A
S82.191K
S82.191M
S82.191N
S82.191P
S82.191Q
S82.191R
S82.192A
S82.192K
S82.192M
S82.192N
S82.192P
S82.192Q
S82.192R
S82.199A
S82.199K
S82.199M
S82.199N
S82.199P
S82.199Q
S82.199R
S82.2Ø1A
S82.2Ø1K
S82.2Ø1M
S82.2Ø1N
S82.2Ø1P
S82.2Ø1Q
S82.2Ø1R
S82.2Ø2A
S82.2Ø2K
S82.2Ø2M
S82.2Ø2N
S82.2Ø2P
S82.2Ø2Q
S82.2Ø2R
S82.2Ø9A
S82.2Ø9K
S82.2Ø9M
S82.2Ø9N
S82.2Ø9P
S82.2Ø9Q
S82.2Ø9R
S82.221A
S82.221K
S82.221M
S82.221N
S82.221P
S82.221Q
S82.221R
S82.222A
S82.222K
S82.222M
S82.222N
S82.222P
S82.222Q
S82.222R
S82.223A
S82.223K
S82.223M
S82.223N
S82.223P
S82.223Q
S82.223R
S82.224A
S82.224K
S82.224M
S82.224N
S82.224P
S82.224Q
S82.224R
S82.225A
S82.225K
S82.225M
S82.225N
S82.225P
S82.225Q
S82.225R
S82.226A
S82.226K
S82.226M
S82.226N
S82.226P
S82.226Q
S82.226R
S82.231A
S82.231K
S82.231M
S82.231N
S82.231P
S82.231Q
S82.231R
S82.232A
S82.232K
S82.232M
S82.232N
S82.232P
S82.232Q
S82.232R
S82.233A
S82.233K
S82.233M
S82.233N
S82.233P
S82.233Q
S82.233R
S82.234A
S82.234K
S82.234M
S82.234N
S82.234P
S82.234Q
S82.234R
S82.235A
S82.235K
S82.235M
S82.235N
S82.235P
S82.235Q
S82.235R
S82.236A
S82.236K
S82.236M
S82.236N
S82.236P
S82.236Q
S82.236R
S82.241A
S82.241K
S82.241M
S82.241N
S82.241P
S82.241Q
S82.241R
S82.242A
S82.242K
S82.242M
S82.242N
S82.242P
S82.242Q
S82.242R
S82.243A
S82.243K
S82.243M
S82.243N
S82.243P
S82.243Q
S82.243R
S82.244A
S82.244K
S82.244M
S82.244N
S82.244P
S82.244Q
S82.244R
S82.245A
S82.245K
S82.245M
S82.245N
S82.245P
S82.245Q
S82.245R
S82.246A
S82.246K
S82.246M
S82.246N
S82.246P
S82.246Q
S82.246R
S82.251A
S82.251K
S82.251M
S82.251N
S82.251P
S82.251Q
S82.251R
S82.252A
S82.252K
S82.252M
S82.252N
S82.252P
S82.252Q
S82.252R
S82.253A
S82.253K
S82.253M
S82.253N
S82.253P
S82.253Q
S82.253R
S82.254A
S82.254K
S82.254M
S82.254N
S82.254P
S82.254Q
S82.254R
S82.255A
S82.255K
S82.255M
S82.255N
S82.255P
S82.255Q
S82.255R
S82.256A
S82.256K
S82.256M
S82.256N
S82.256P
S82.256Q
S82.256R
S82.261A
S82.261K
S82.261M
S82.261N
S82.261P
S82.261Q
S82.261R
S82.262A
S82.262K
S82.262M
S82.262N
S82.262P
S82.262Q
S82.262R
S82.263A
S82.263K
S82.263M
S82.263N
S82.263P
S82.263Q
S82.263R
S82.264A
S82.264K
S82.264M
S82.264N
S82.264P
S82.264Q
S82.264R
S82.265A
S82.265K
S82.265M
S82.265N
S82.265P
S82.265Q
S82.265R
S82.266A
S82.266K
S82.266M
S82.266N
S82.266P
S82.266Q
S82.266R
S82.291A
S82.291K
S82.291M
S82.291N
S82.291P
S82.291Q
S82.291R
S82.292A
S82.292K
S82.292M
S82.292N
S82.292P
S82.292Q
S82.292R
S82.299A
S82.299K
S82.299M
S82.299N
S82.299P
S82.299Q
S82.299R
S82.3Ø1B
S82.3Ø1C
S82.3Ø1K
S82.3Ø1M
S82.3Ø1N
S82.3Ø1P
S82.3Ø1Q
S82.3Ø1R
S82.3Ø2B
S82.3Ø2C
S82.3Ø2K
S82.3Ø2M
S82.3Ø2N
S82.3Ø2P
S82.3Ø2Q
S82.3Ø2R
S82.3Ø9B
S82.3Ø9C
S82.3Ø9K
S82.3Ø9M
S82.3Ø9N
S82.3Ø9P
S82.3Ø9Q
S82.3Ø9R
S82.311A
S82.311K
S82.311P
S82.312A
S82.312K
S82.312P
S82.319A
S82.319K
S82.319P
S82.391B
S82.391C
S82.391K
S82.391M
S82.391N
S82.391P
S82.391Q
S82.391R
S82.392B
S82.392C
S82.392K
S82.392M
S82.392N
S82.392P
S82.392Q
S82.392R
S82.399B
S82.399C
S82.399K
S82.399M
S82.399N
S82.399P
S82.399Q
S82.399R
S82.4Ø1K
S82.4Ø1M
S82.4Ø1N
S82.4Ø1P
S82.4Ø1Q
S82.4Ø1R
S82.4Ø2K
S82.4Ø2M
S82.4Ø2N
S82.4Ø2P
S82.4Ø2Q
S82.4Ø2R
S82.4Ø9K
S82.4Ø9M
S82.4Ø9N
S82.4Ø9P
S82.4Ø9Q
S82.4Ø9R
S82.421K
S82.421M
S82.421N
S82.421P
S82.421Q
S82.421R
S82.422K
S82.422M
S82.422N
S82.422P
S82.422Q
S82.422R
S82.423K
S82.423M
S82.423N
S82.423P
S82.423Q
S82.423R
S82.424K
S82.424M
S82.424N
S82.424P
S82.424Q
S82.424R
S82.425K
S82.425M
S82.425N
S82.425P
S82.425Q
S82.425R
S82.426K
S82.426M
S82.426N
S82.426P
S82.426Q
S82.426R
S82.431K
S82.431M
S82.431N
S82.431P
S82.431Q
S82.431R
S82.432K
S82.432M
S82.432N
S82.432P
S82.432Q
S82.432R
S82.433K
S82.433M
S82.433N
S82.433P
S82.433Q
S82.433R
S82.434K
S82.434M
S82.434N
S82.434P
S82.434Q
S82.434R
S82.435K
S82.435M
S82.435N
S82.435P
S82.435Q
S82.435R
S82.436K
S82.436M
S82.436N
S82.436P
S82.436Q
S82.436R
S82.441K
S82.441M
S82.441N
S82.441P
S82.441Q
S82.441R
S82.442K
S82.442M
S82.442N
S82.442P
S82.442Q
S82.442R
S82.443K
S82.443M
S82.443N
S82.443P
S82.443Q
S82.443R
S82.444K
S82.444M
S82.444N
S82.444P
S82.444Q
S82.444R
S82.445K
S82.445M
S82.445N
S82.445P
S82.445Q
S82.445R
S82.446K
S82.446M
S82.446N
S82.446P
S82.446Q
S82.446R
S82.451K
S82.451M
S82.451N
S82.451P
S82.451Q
S82.451R
S82.452K
S82.452M
S82.452N
S82.452P
S82.452Q
S82.452R
S82.453K
S82.453M
S82.453N
S82.453P
S82.453Q
S82.453R
S82.454K
S82.454M
S82.454N
S82.454P
S82.454Q
S82.454R
S82.455K
S82.455M
S82.455N
S82.455P
S82.455Q
S82.455R
S82.456K
S82.456M
S82.456N
S82.456P
S82.456Q
S82.456R
S82.461K
S82.461M
S82.461N
S82.461P
S82.461Q
S82.461R
S82.462K
S82.462M
S82.462N
S82.462P
S82.462Q
S82.462R
S82.463K
S82.463M
S82.463N
S82.463P
S82.463Q
S82.463R
S82.464K
S82.464M
S82.464N
S82.464P
S82.464Q
S82.464R
S82.465K
S82.465M
S82.465N
S82.465P
S82.465Q
S82.465R
S82.466K
S82.466M
S82.466N
S82.466P
S82.466Q
S82.466R
S82.491K
S82.491M
S82.491N
S82.491P
S82.491Q
S82.491R
S82.492K
S82.492M
S82.492N
S82.492P
S82.492Q
S82.492R
S82.499K
S82.499M
S82.499N
S82.499P
S82.499Q
S82.499R
S82.51XB
S82.51XC
S82.51XK
S82.51XM
S82.51XN
S82.51XP
S82.51XQ
S82.51XR
S82.52XB
S82.52XC
S82.52XK
S82.52XM
S82.52XN
S82.52XP
S82.52XQ
S82.52XR
S82.53XB
S82.53XC
S82.53XK
S82.53XM
S82.53XN
S82.53XP
S82.53XQ
S82.53XR
S82.54XB
S82.54XC
S82.54XK
S82.54XM
S82.54XN
S82.54XP
S82.54XQ
S82.54XR
S82.55XB
S82.55XC
S82.55XK
S82.55XM
S82.55XN
S82.55XP
S82.55XQ
S82.55XR
S82.56XB
S82.56XC
S82.56XK
S82.56XM
S82.56XN
S82.56XP
S82.56XQ
S82.56XR
S82.61XB
S82.61XC
S82.61XK
S82.61XM
S82.61XN
S82.61XP
S82.61XQ
S82.61XR
S82.62XB
S82.62XC
S82.62XK
S82.62XM
S82.62XN
S82.62XP
S82.62XQ
S82.62XR
S82.63XB
S82.63XC
S82.63XK
S82.63XM
S82.63XN
S82.63XP
S82.63XQ
S82.63XR
S82.64XB
S82.64XC
S82.64XK
S82.64XM
S82.64XN
S82.64XP
S82.64XQ
S82.64XR
S82.65XB
S82.65XC
S82.65XK
S82.65XM
S82.65XN
S82.65XP
S82.65XQ
S82.65XR
S82.66XB
S82.66XC
S82.66XK
S82.66XM
S82.66XN
S82.66XP
S82.66XQ

S82.66XR
S82.811K
S82.811P
S82.812K
S82.812P
S82.819K
S82.819P
S82.821K
S82.821P
S82.822K
S82.822P
S82.829K
S82.829P
S82.831K
S82.831M
S82.831N
S82.831P
S82.831Q
S82.831R
S82.832K
S82.832M
S82.832N
S82.832P
S82.832Q
S82.832R
S82.839K
S82.839M
S82.839N
S82.839P
S82.839Q
S82.839R
S82.841B
S82.841C
S82.841K
S82.841M
S82.841N
S82.841P
S82.841Q
S82.841R
S82.842B
S82.842C
S82.842K
S82.842M
S82.842N
S82.842P
S82.842Q
S82.842R
S82.843B
S82.843C
S82.843K
S82.843M
S82.843N
S82.843P
S82.843Q
S82.843R
S82.844B
S82.844C
S82.844K
S82.844M
S82.844N
S82.844P
S82.844Q
S82.844R
S82.845B
S82.845C
S82.845K
S82.845M
S82.845N
S82.845P
S82.845Q
S82.845R
S82.846B
S82.846C
S82.846K
S82.846M
S82.846N
S82.846P
S82.846Q
S82.846R
S82.851B
S82.851C
S82.851K
S82.851M
S82.851N
S82.851P
S82.851Q
S82.851R
S82.852B
S82.852C
S82.852K
S82.852M
S82.852N
S82.852P
S82.852Q
S82.852R
S82.853B
S82.853C
S82.853K
S82.853M
S82.853N
S82.853P
S82.853Q
S82.853R
S82.854B
S82.854C
S82.854K
S82.854M
S82.854N
S82.854P
S82.854Q
S82.854R
S82.855B
S82.855C
S82.855K
S82.855M
S82.855N
S82.855P
S82.855Q
S82.855R
S82.856B
S82.856C
S82.856K
S82.856M
S82.856N
S82.856P
S82.856Q
S82.856R
S82.861K
S82.861M
S82.861N
S82.861P
S82.861Q
S82.861R
S82.862K
S82.862M
S82.862N
S82.862P
S82.862Q
S82.862R
S82.863K
S82.863M
S82.863N
S82.863P
S82.863Q
S82.863R
S82.864K
S82.864M
S82.864N
S82.864P
S82.864Q
S82.864R
S82.865K
S82.865M
S82.865N
S82.865P
S82.865Q
S82.865R
S82.866K
S82.866M
S82.866N
S82.866P
S82.866Q
S82.866R
S82.871B
S82.871C
S82.871K
S82.871M
S82.871N
S82.871P
S82.871Q
S82.871R
S82.872B
S82.872C
S82.872K
S82.872M
S82.872N
S82.872P
S82.872Q
S82.872R
S82.873B
S82.873C
S82.873K
S82.873M
S82.873N
S82.873P
S82.873Q
S82.873R
S82.874B
S82.874C
S82.874K
S82.874M
S82.874N
S82.874P
S82.874Q
S82.874R
S82.875B
S82.875C
S82.875K
S82.875M
S82.875N
S82.875P
S82.875Q
S82.875R
S82.876B
S82.876C
S82.876K
S82.876M
S82.876N
S82.876P
S82.876Q
S82.876R
S82.891B
S82.891C
S82.891K
S82.891M
S82.891N
S82.891P
S82.891Q
S82.891R
S82.892B
S82.892C
S82.892K
S82.892M
S82.892N
S82.892P
S82.892Q
S82.892R
S82.899B
S82.899C
S82.899K
S82.899M
S82.899N
S82.899P
S82.899Q
S82.899R
S82.90XB
S82.90XC
S82.90XK
S82.90XM
S82.90XN
S82.90XP
S82.90XQ
S82.90XR
S82.91XB
S82.91XC
S82.91XK
S82.91XM
S82.91XN
S82.91XP
S82.91XQ
S82.91XR
S82.92XB
S82.92XC
S82.92XK
S82.92XM
S82.92XN
S82.92XP
S82.92XQ
S82.92XR
S85.101A
S85.102A
S85.109A
S85.111A
S85.112A
S85.119A
S85.121A
S85.122A
S85.129A
S85.131A
S85.132A
S85.139A
S85.141A
S85.142A
S85.149A
S85.151A
S85.152A
S85.159A
S85.161A
S85.162A
S85.169A
S85.171A
S85.172A
S85.179A
S85.181A
S85.182A
S85.189A
S85.201A
S85.202A
S85.209A
S85.211A
S85.212A
S85.219A
S85.291A
S85.292A
S85.299A
S85.301A
S85.302A
S85.309A
S85.311A
S85.312A
S85.319A
S85.391A
S85.392A
S85.399A
S85.401A
S85.402A
S85.409A
S85.411A
S85.412A
S85.419A
S85.491A
S85.492A
S85.499A
S85.801A
S85.802A
S85.809A
S85.811A
S85.812A
S85.819A
S85.891A
S85.892A
S85.899A
S85.901A
S85.902A
S85.909A
S85.911A
S85.912A
S85.919A
S85.991A
S85.992A
S85.999A
S86.021A
S86.022A
S86.029A
S86.121A
S86.122A
S86.129A
S86.221A
S86.222A
S86.229A
S86.321A
S86.322A
S86.329A
S86.821A
S86.822A
S86.829A
S86.921A
S86.922A
S86.929A
S88.011A
S88.012A
S88.019A
S88.021A
S88.022A
S88.029A
S88.111A
S88.112A
S88.119A
S88.121A
S88.122A
S88.129A
S88.911A
S88.912A
S88.919A
S88.921A
S88.922A
S88.929A
S89.001A
S89.001K
S89.001P
S89.002A
S89.002K
S89.002P
S89.009A
S89.009K
S89.009P
S89.011A
S89.011K
S89.011P
S89.012A
S89.012K
S89.012P
S89.019A
S89.019K
S89.019P
S89.021A
S89.021K
S89.021P
S89.022A
S89.022K
S89.022P
S89.029A
S89.029K
S89.029P
S89.031A
S89.031K
S89.031P
S89.032A
S89.032K
S89.032P
S89.039A
S89.039K
S89.039P
S89.041A
S89.041K
S89.041P
S89.042A
S89.042K
S89.042P
S89.049A
S89.049K
S89.049P
S89.091A
S89.091K
S89.091P
S89.092A
S89.092K
S89.092P
S89.099A
S89.099K
S89.099P
S89.101K
S89.101P
S89.102K
S89.102P
S89.109K
S89.109P
S89.111K
S89.111P
S89.112K
S89.112P
S89.119K
S89.119P
S89.121K
S89.121P
S89.122K
S89.122P
S89.129K
S89.129P
S89.131K
S89.131P
S89.132K
S89.132P
S89.139K
S89.139P
S89.141K
S89.141P
S89.142K
S89.142P
S89.149K
S89.149P
S89.191K
S89.191P
S89.192K
S89.192P
S89.199K
S89.199P
S89.201K
S89.201P
S89.202K
S89.202P
S89.209K
S89.209P
S89.211K
S89.211P
S89.212K
S89.212P
S89.219K
S89.219P
S89.221K
S89.221P
S89.222K
S89.222P
S89.229K
S89.229P
S89.291K
S89.291P
S89.292K
S89.292P
S89.299K
S89.299P
S89.301K
S89.301P
S89.302K
S89.302P
S89.309K
S89.309P
S89.311K
S89.311P
S89.312K
S89.312P
S89.319K
S89.319P
S89.321K
S89.321P
S89.322K
S89.322P
S89.329K
S89.329P
S89.391K
S89.391P
S89.392K
S89.392P
S89.399K
S89.399P
S92.001B
S92.001K
S92.001P
S92.002B
S92.002K
S92.002P
S92.009B
S92.009K
S92.009P
S92.011B
S92.011K
S92.011P
S92.012B
S92.012K
S92.012P
S92.013B
S92.013K
S92.013P
S92.014B
S92.014K
S92.014P
S92.015B
S92.015K
S92.015P
S92.016B
S92.016K
S92.016P
S92.021B
S92.021K
S92.021P
S92.022B
S92.022K
S92.022P
S92.023B
S92.023K
S92.023P
S92.024B
S92.024K
S92.024P
S92.025B
S92.025K
S92.025P
S92.026B
S92.026K
S92.026P
S92.031B
S92.031K
S92.031P
S92.032B
S92.032K
S92.032P
S92.033B
S92.033K
S92.033P
S92.034B
S92.034K
S92.034P
S92.035B
S92.035K
S92.035P
S92.036B
S92.036K
S92.036P
S92.041B
S92.041K
S92.041P
S92.042B
S92.042K
S92.042P
S92.043B
S92.043K
S92.043P
S92.044B
S92.044K
S92.044P
S92.045B
S92.045K
S92.045P
S92.046B
S92.046K
S92.046P
S92.051B
S92.051K
S92.051P
S92.052B
S92.052K
S92.052P
S92.053B
S92.053K
S92.053P
S92.054B
S92.054K
S92.054P
S92.055B
S92.055K
S92.055P
S92.056B
S92.056K
S92.056P
S92.061B
S92.061K
S92.061P
S92.062B
S92.062K
S92.062P
S92.063B
S92.063K
S92.063P
S92.064B
S92.064K
S92.064P
S92.065B
S92.065K
S92.065P
S92.066B
S92.066K
S92.066P
S92.101B
S92.101K
S92.101P
S92.102B
S92.102K
S92.102P
S92.109B
S92.109K
S92.109P
S92.111B
S92.111K
S92.111P
S92.112B
S92.112K
S92.112P
S92.113B
S92.113K
S92.113P
S92.114B
S92.114K
S92.114P
S92.115B
S92.115K
S92.115P
S92.116B
S92.116K
S92.116P
S92.121B
S92.121K
S92.121P
S92.122B
S92.122K
S92.122P
S92.123B
S92.123K
S92.123P
S92.124B
S92.124K
S92.124P
S92.125B
S92.125K
S92.125P
S92.126B
S92.126K
S92.126P
S92.131B
S92.131K
S92.131P
S92.132B
S92.132K
S92.132P
S92.133B
S92.133K
S92.133P
S92.134B
S92.134K
S92.134P
S92.135B
S92.135K
S92.135P
S92.136B
S92.136K
S92.136P
S92.141B
S92.141K
S92.141P
S92.142B
S92.142K
S92.142P
S92.143B
S92.143K
S92.143P
S92.144B
S92.144K
S92.144P
S92.145B
S92.145K
S92.145P
S92.146B
S92.146K
S92.146P
S92.151B
S92.151K
S92.151P
S92.152B
S92.152K
S92.152P
S92.153B
S92.153K
S92.153P
S92.154B
S92.154K
S92.154P
S92.155B
S92.155K
S92.155P
S92.156B
S92.156K
S92.156P
S92.191B
S92.191K
S92.191P
S92.192B
S92.192K
S92.192P
S92.199B
S92.199K
S92.199P
S92.201B
S92.201K
S92.201P
S92.202B
S92.202K
S92.202P
S92.209B
S92.209K
S92.209P
S92.211B
S92.211K
S92.211P
S92.212B
S92.212K
S92.212P
S92.213B
S92.213K
S92.213P
S92.214B
S92.214K
S92.214P
S92.215B
S92.215K
S92.215P
S92.216B
S92.216K
S92.216P
S92.221B
S92.221K
S92.221P
S92.222B
S92.222K
S92.222P
S92.223B
S92.223K
S92.223P
S92.224B
S92.224K
S92.224P
S92.225B
S92.225K
S92.225P
S92.226B
S92.226K
S92.226P
S92.231B
S92.231K
S92.231P
S92.232B
S92.232K
S92.232P
S92.233B
S92.233K
S92.233P
S92.234B
S92.234K
S92.234P
S92.235B
S92.235K
S92.235P
S92.236B
S92.236K
S92.236P
S92.241B
S92.241K
S92.241P
S92.242B
S92.242K
S92.242P
S92.243B
S92.243K
S92.243P
S92.244B
S92.244K
S92.244P
S92.245B
S92.245K
S92.245P
S92.246B
S92.246K
S92.246P
S92.251B
S92.251K
S92.251P
S92.252B
S92.252K
S92.252P
S92.253B
S92.253K
S92.253P
S92.254B
S92.254K
S92.254P
S92.255B
S92.255K
S92.255P
S92.256B
S92.256K
S92.256P
S92.301B
S92.301K
S92.301P
S92.302B
S92.302K
S92.302P
S92.309B
S92.309K
S92.309P
S92.311B
S92.311K
S92.311P
S92.312B
S92.312K
S92.312P
S92.313B
S92.313K
S92.313P
S92.314B
S92.314K
S92.314P
S92.315B
S92.315K
S92.315P
S92.316B
S92.316K
S92.316P
S92.321B
S92.321K
S92.321P
S92.322B
S92.322K
S92.322P
S92.323B
S92.323K
S92.323P
S92.324B
S92.324K
S92.324P
S92.325B
S92.325K
S92.325P
S92.326B
S92.326K
S92.326P
S92.331B
S92.331K
S92.331P
S92.332B
S92.332K
S92.332P
S92.333B
S92.333K
S92.333P
S92.334B
S92.334K
S92.334P
S92.335B
S92.335K
S92.335P
S92.336B
S92.336K
S92.336P
S92.341B
S92.341K
S92.341P
S92.342B
S92.342K
S92.342P
S92.343B
S92.343K
S92.343P
S92.344B
S92.344K
S92.344P
S92.345B
S92.345K
S92.345P
S92.346B
S92.346K
S92.346P
S92.351B
S92.351K
S92.351P

S92.352B
S92.352K
S92.352P
S92.353B
S92.353K
S92.353P
S92.354B
S92.354K
S92.354P
S92.355B
S92.355K
S92.355P
S92.356B
S92.356K
S92.356P
S92.401K
S92.401P
S92.402K
S92.402P
S92.403K
S92.403P
S92.404K
S92.404P
S92.405K
S92.405P
S92.406K
S92.406P
S92.411K
S92.411P
S92.412K
S92.412P
S92.413K
S92.413P
S92.414K
S92.414P
S92.415K
S92.415P
S92.416K
S92.416P
S92.421K
S92.421P
S92.422K
S92.422P
S92.423K
S92.423P
S92.424K
S92.424P
S92.425K
S92.425P
S92.426K
S92.426P
S92.491K
S92.491P
S92.492K
S92.492P
S92.499K
S92.499P
S92.501K
S92.501P
S92.502K
S92.502P
S92.503K
S92.503P
S92.504K
S92.504P
S92.505K
S92.505P
S92.506K
S92.506P
S92.511K
S92.511P
S92.512K
S92.512P
S92.513K
S92.513P
S92.514K
S92.514P
S92.515K
S92.515P
S92.516K
S92.516P
S92.521K
S92.521P
S92.522K
S92.522P
S92.523K
S92.523P
S92.524K
S92.524P
S92.525K
S92.525P
S92.526K
S92.526P
S92.531K
S92.531P
S92.532K
S92.532P
S92.533K
S92.533P
S92.534K
S92.534P
S92.535K
S92.535P
S92.536K
S92.536P
S92.591K
S92.591P
S92.592K
S92.592P
S92.599K
S92.599P
S92.811B
S92.811K
S92.811P
S92.812B
S92.812K
S92.812P
S92.819B
S92.819K
S92.819P
S92.901B
S92.901K
S92.901P
S92.902B
S92.902K
S92.902P
S92.909B
S92.909K
S92.909P
S92.911K
S92.911P
S92.912K
S92.912P
S92.919K
S92.919P
S95.001A
S95.002A
S95.009A
S95.011A
S95.012A
S95.019A
S95.091A
S95.092A
S95.099A
S95.101A
S95.102A
S95.109A
S95.111A
S95.112A
S95.119A
S95.191A
S95.192A
S95.199A
S95.201A
S95.202A
S95.209A
S95.211A
S95.212A
S95.219A
S95.291A
S95.292A
S95.299A
S95.801A
S95.802A
S95.809A
S95.811A
S95.812A
S95.819A
S95.891A
S95.892A
S95.899A
S95.901A
S95.902A
S95.909A
S95.911A
S95.912A
S95.919A
S95.991A
S95.992A
S95.999A
S96.021A
S96.022A
S96.029A
S96.121A
S96.122A
S96.129A
S96.221A
S96.222A
S96.229A
S96.821A
S96.822A
S96.829A
S96.921A
S96.922A
S96.929A
S98.011A
S98.012A
S98.019A
S98.021A
S98.022A
S98.029A
S98.311A
S98.312A
S98.319A
S98.321A
S98.322A
S98.329A
S98.911A
S98.912A
S98.919A
S98.921A
S98.922A
S98.929A
T17.400A
T17.408A
T17.410A
T17.418A
T17.420A
T17.428A
T17.490A
T17.498A
T17.500A
T17.508A
T17.510A
T17.518A
T17.520A
T17.528A
T17.590A
T17.598A
T17.800A
T17.808A
T17.810A
T17.818A
T17.820A
T17.828A
T17.890A
T17.898A
T20.30XA
T20.311A
T20.312A
T20.319A
T20.32XA
T20.33XA
T20.34XA
T20.35XA
T20.36XA
T20.37XA
T20.39XA
T20.70XA
T20.711A
T20.712A
T20.719A
T20.72XA
T20.73XA
T20.74XA
T20.75XA
T20.76XA
T20.77XA
T20.79XA
T21.30XA
T21.31XA
T21.32XA
T21.33XA
T21.34XA
T21.35XA
T21.36XA
T21.37XA
T21.39XA
T21.70XA
T21.71XA
T21.72XA
T21.73XA
T21.74XA
T21.75XA
T21.76XA
T21.77XA
T21.79XA
T22.30XA
T22.311A
T22.312A
T22.319A
T22.321A
T22.322A
T22.329A
T22.331A
T22.332A
T22.339A
T22.341A
T22.342A
T22.349A
T22.351A
T22.352A
T22.359A
T22.361A
T22.362A
T22.369A
T22.391A
T22.392A
T22.399A
T22.70XA
T22.711A
T22.712A
T22.719A
T22.721A
T22.722A
T22.729A
T22.731A
T22.732A
T22.739A
T22.741A
T22.742A
T22.749A
T22.751A
T22.752A
T22.759A
T22.761A
T22.762A
T22.769A
T22.791A
T22.792A
T22.799A
T23.301A
T23.302A
T23.309A
T23.311A
T23.312A
T23.319A
T23.321A
T23.322A
T23.329A
T23.331A
T23.332A
T23.339A
T23.341A
T23.342A
T23.349A
T23.351A
T23.352A
T23.359A
T23.361A
T23.362A
T23.369A
T23.371A
T23.372A
T23.379A
T23.391A
T23.392A
T23.399A
T23.701A
T23.702A
T23.709A
T23.711A
T23.712A
T23.719A
T23.721A
T23.722A
T23.729A
T23.731A
T23.732A
T23.739A
T23.741A
T23.742A
T23.749A
T23.751A
T23.752A
T23.759A
T23.761A
T23.762A
T23.769A
T23.771A
T23.772A
T23.779A
T23.791A
T23.792A
T23.799A
T24.301A
T24.302A
T24.309A
T24.311A
T24.312A
T24.319A
T24.321A
T24.322A
T24.329A
T24.331A
T24.332A
T24.339A
T24.391A
T24.392A
T24.399A
T24.701A
T24.702A
T24.709A
T24.711A
T24.712A
T24.719A
T24.721A
T24.722A
T24.729A
T24.731A
T24.732A
T24.739A
T24.791A
T24.792A
T24.799A
T25.311A
T25.312A
T25.319A
T25.321A
T25.322A
T25.329A
T25.331A
T25.332A
T25.339A
T25.391A
T25.392A
T25.399A
T25.711A
T25.712A
T25.719A
T25.721A
T25.722A
T25.729A
T25.731A
T25.732A
T25.739A
T25.791A
T25.792A
T25.799A
T26.20XA
T26.21XA
T26.22XA
T26.70XA
T26.71XA
T26.72XA
T27.0XXA
T27.1XXA
T27.2XXA
T27.3XXA
T27.4XXA
T27.5XXA
T27.6XXA
T27.7XXA
T28.1XXA
T28.2XXA
T28.6XXA
T28.7XXA
T31.10
T31.11
T31.20
T31.30
T31.40
T31.50
T31.60
T31.70
T31.80
T31.90
T32.10
T32.11
T32.20
T32.30
T32.40
T32.50
T32.60
T32.70
T32.80
T32.90
T33.011A
T33.012A
T33.019A
T33.02XA
T33.09XA
T33.1XXA
T33.2XXA
T33.3XXA
T33.40XA
T33.41XA
T33.42XA
T33.511A
T33.512A
T33.519A
T33.521A
T33.522A
T33.529A
T33.531A
T33.532A
T33.539A
T33.60XA
T33.61XA
T33.62XA
T33.70XA
T33.71XA
T33.72XA
T33.811A
T33.812A
T33.819A
T33.821A
T33.822A
T33.829A
T33.831A
T33.832A
T33.839A
T33.90XA
T33.99XA
T34.011A
T34.012A
T34.019A
T34.02XA
T34.09XA
T34.1XXA
T34.2XXA
T34.3XXA
T34.40XA
T34.41XA
T34.42XA
T34.511A
T34.512A
T34.519A
T34.521A
T34.522A
T34.529A
T34.531A
T34.532A
T34.539A
T34.60XA
T34.61XA
T34.62XA
T34.70XA
T34.71XA
T34.72XA
T34.811A
T34.812A
T34.819A
T34.821A
T34.822A
T34.829A
T34.831A
T34.832A
T34.839A
T34.90XA
T34.99XA
T67.01XA
T67.02XA
T67.09XA
T69.021A
T69.022A
T69.029A
T70.3XXA
T71.111A
T71.112A
T71.113A
T71.114A
T71.121A
T71.122A
T71.123A
T71.124A
T71.131A
T71.132A
T71.133A
T71.134A
T71.141A
T71.143A
T71.144A
T71.151A
T71.152A
T71.153A
T71.154A
T71.161A
T71.162A
T71.163A
T71.164A
T71.191A
T71.192A
T71.193A
T71.194A
T71.20XA
T71.21XA
T71.221A
T71.222A
T71.223A
T71.224A
T71.231A
T71.232A
T71.233A
T71.234A
T71.29XA
T71.9XXA
T74.01XA
T74.02XA
T74.11XA
T74.12XA
T74.21XA
T74.22XA
T74.32XA
T74.4XXA
T74.51XA
T74.52XA
T74.61XA
T74.62XA
T74.91XA
T74.92XA
T75.1XXA
T76.01XA
T76.02XA
T76.11XA
T76.12XA
T76.21XA
T76.22XA
T76.32XA
T76.51XA
T76.52XA
T76.61XA
T76.62XA
T76.91XA
T76.92XA
T78.00XA
T78.01XA
T78.02XA
T78.03XA
T78.04XA
T78.05XA
T78.06XA
T78.07XA
T78.08XA
T78.09XA
T78.2XXA
T79.2XXA
T79.7XXA
T79.A0XA
T79.A11A
T79.A12A
T79.A19A
T79.A21A
T79.A22A
T79.A29A
T79.A3XA
T79.A9XA
T80.1XXA
T80.211A
T80.212A
T80.218A
T80.219A
T80.22XA
T80.29XA
T80.30XA
T80.310A
T80.311A
T80.319A
T80.39XA
T80.40XA
T80.410A
T80.411A
T80.419A
T80.49XA
T80.51XA
T80.52XA
T80.59XA
T80.61XA
T80.62XA
T80.69XA
T80.810A
T80.818A
T80.910A
T80.911A
T80.919A
T80.A0XA
T80.A10A
T80.A11A
T80.A19A
T80.A9XA
T81.10XA
T81.30XA
T81.31XA
T81.32XA
T81.33XA
T81.40XA
T81.41XA
T81.42XA
T81.43XA
T81.44XA
T81.49XA
T81.500A
T81.501A
T81.502A
T81.503A
T81.504A
T81.505A
T81.506A
T81.507A
T81.508A
T81.509A
T81.510A
T81.511A
T81.512A
T81.513A
T81.514A
T81.515A
T81.516A
T81.517A
T81.518A
T81.519A
T81.520A
T81.521A
T81.522A
T81.523A
T81.524A
T81.525A
T81.526A
T81.527A
T81.528A
T81.529A
T81.530A
T81.531A
T81.532A
T81.533A
T81.534A
T81.535A
T81.536A
T81.537A
T81.538A
T81.539A
T81.590A
T81.591A
T81.592A
T81.593A
T81.594A
T81.595A
T81.596A
T81.597A
T81.598A
T81.599A
T81.60XA
T81.61XA
T81.69XA
T81.710A
T81.711A
T81.718A
T81.719A
T81.72XA
T81.83XA
T82.01XA
T82.02XA
T82.03XA
T82.09XA
T82.110A
T82.111A
T82.118A
T82.119A
T82.120A
T82.121A
T82.128A
T82.129A
T82.190A
T82.191A
T82.198A
T82.199A
T82.211A
T82.212A
T82.213A
T82.218A
T82.221A
T82.222A
T82.223A
T82.228A
T82.310A
T82.311A
T82.312A
T82.318A
T82.319A
T82.320A
T82.321A
T82.322A
T82.328A
T82.329A
T82.330A
T82.331A
T82.332A
T82.338A
T82.339A
T82.390A
T82.391A
T82.392A
T82.398A
T82.399A
T82.41XA
T82.42XA
T82.43XA
T82.49XA
T82.510A
T82.511A
T82.512A
T82.513A
T82.514A
T82.515A
T82.518A
T82.519A
T82.520A
T82.521A
T82.522A
T82.523A
T82.524A
T82.525A
T82.528A
T82.529A
T82.530A
T82.531A
T82.532A
T82.533A
T82.534A
T82.535A
T82.538A
T82.539A
T82.590A
T82.591A
T82.592A
T82.593A
T82.594A
T82.595A
T82.598A
T82.599A
T82.6XXA
T82.7XXA
T82.817A
T82.818A
T82.827A
T82.828A
T82.837A
T82.838A
T82.847A
T82.848A
T82.855A
T82.856A
T82.857A
T82.858A
T82.867A
T82.868A
T82.897A
T82.898A
T82.9XXA
T83.010A
T83.020A
T83.030A
T83.090A
T83.110A
T83.111A
T83.112A
T83.113A
T83.118A
T83.120A
T83.121A
T83.122A
T83.123A
T83.128A
T83.190A
T83.191A
T83.192A
T83.193A
T83.198A
T83.21XA
T83.22XA
T83.23XA
T83.24XA
T83.25XA
T83.29XA
T83.410A
T83.411A
T83.418A
T83.420A
T83.421A
T83.428A
T83.490A
T83.491A
T83.498A
T83.510A
T83.511A
T83.512A
T83.518A
T83.590A
T83.591A
T83.592A
T83.593A
T83.598A
T83.61XA
T83.62XA
T83.69XA
T83.712A
T83.713A
T83.714A
T83.718A
T83.719A
T83.722A
T83.723A
T83.724A
T83.728A
T83.729A
T83.79XA
T83.81XA
T83.82XA
T83.83XA
T83.84XA
T83.85XA
T83.86XA
T83.89XA
T83.9XXA
T84.010A
T84.011A
T84.012A
T84.013A
T84.018A
T84.019A
T84.020A
T84.021A
T84.022A

T84.023A
T84.028A
T84.029A
T84.030A
T84.031A
T84.032A
T84.033A
T84.038A
T84.039A
T84.050A
T84.051A
T84.052A
T84.053A
T84.058A
T84.059A
T84.060A
T84.061A
T84.062A
T84.063A
T84.068A
T84.069A
T84.090A
T84.091A
T84.092A
T84.093A
T84.098A
T84.099A
T84.110A
T84.111A
T84.112A
T84.113A
T84.114A
T84.115A
T84.116A
T84.117A
T84.119A
T84.120A
T84.121A
T84.122A
T84.123A
T84.124A
T84.125A
T84.126A
T84.127A
T84.129A
T84.190A
T84.191A
T84.192A
T84.193A
T84.194A
T84.195A
T84.196A
T84.197A
T84.199A
T84.210A
T84.213A
T84.216A
T84.218A
T84.220A
T84.223A
T84.226A
T84.228A
T84.290A
T84.293A
T84.296A
T84.298A
T84.310A
T84.318A
T84.320A
T84.328A
T84.390A
T84.398A
T84.410A
T84.418A
T84.420A
T84.428A
T84.490A
T84.498A
T84.50XA
T84.51XA
T84.52XA
T84.53XA
T84.54XA
T84.59XA
T84.60XA
T84.610A
T84.611A
T84.612A
T84.613A
T84.614A
T84.615A
T84.619A
T84.620A
T84.621A
T84.622A
T84.623A
T84.624A
T84.625A
T84.629A
T84.63XA
T84.69XA
T84.7XXA
T84.81XA
T84.82XA
T84.83XA
T84.84XA
T84.85XA
T84.86XA
T84.89XA
T84.9XXA
T85.01XA
T85.02XA
T85.03XA
T85.09XA
T85.110A
T85.111A
T85.112A
T85.113A
T85.118A
T85.120A
T85.121A
T85.122A
T85.123A
T85.128A
T85.190A
T85.191A
T85.192A
T85.193A
T85.199A
T85.21XA
T85.22XA
T85.29XA
T85.310A
T85.311A
T85.320A
T85.321A
T85.390A
T85.391A
T85.41XA
T85.42XA
T85.43XA
T85.44XA
T85.49XA
T85.510A
T85.511A
T85.518A
T85.520A
T85.521A
T85.528A
T85.590A
T85.591A
T85.598A
T85.610A
T85.611A
T85.612A
T85.613A
T85.614A
T85.615A
T85.618A
T85.620A
T85.621A
T85.622A
T85.623A
T85.624A
T85.625A
T85.628A
T85.630A
T85.631A
T85.633A
T85.635A
T85.638A
T85.690A
T85.691A
T85.692A
T85.693A
T85.694A
T85.695A
T85.698A
T85.71XA
T85.72XA
T85.730A
T85.731A
T85.732A
T85.733A
T85.734A
T85.735A
T85.738A
T85.79XA
T85.810A
T85.810D
T85.820A
T85.820D
T85.830A
T85.830D
T85.840A
T85.840D
T85.850A
T85.850D
T85.860A
T85.860D
T85.890A
T85.890D
T86.00
T86.01
T86.02
T86.03
T86.09
T86.10
T86.11
T86.12
T86.13
T86.19
T86.20
T86.21
T86.22
T86.23
T86.290
T86.298
T86.30
T86.31
T86.32
T86.33
T86.39
T86.40
T86.41
T86.42
T86.43
T86.49
T86.5
T86.810
T86.811
T86.812
T86.818
T86.819
T86.820
T86.821
T86.822
T86.828
T86.829
T86.830
T86.831
T86.832
T86.838
T86.839
T86.8401
T86.8402
T86.8403
T86.8409
T86.8411
T86.8412
T86.8413
T86.8419
T86.8421
T86.8422
T86.8423
T86.8429
T86.8481
T86.8482
T86.8483
T86.8489
T86.8491
T86.8492
T86.8493
T86.8499
T86.850
T86.851
T86.852
T86.858
T86.859
T86.890
T86.891
T86.892
T86.898
T86.899
T86.90
T86.91
T86.92
T86.93
T86.99
T87.0X1
T87.0X2
T87.0X9
T87.1X1
T87.1X2
T87.1X9
T87.2
T87.40
T87.41
T87.42
T87.43
T87.44
T88.0XXA
T88.1XXA
T88.2XXA
T88.3XXA
T88.6XXA
Z16.10
Z16.11
Z16.12
Z16.13
Z16.19
Z16.20
Z16.21
Z16.22
Z16.23
Z16.24
Z16.29
Z16.30
Z16.31
Z16.32
Z16.33
Z16.341
Z16.342
Z16.35
Z16.39
Z43.1
Z48.21
Z48.22
Z48.23
Z48.24
Z48.280
Z48.290
Z59.00
Z59.01
Z59.02
Z68.1
Z68.41
Z68.42
Z68.43
Z68.44
Z68.45
Z94.0
Z94.1
Z94.2
Z94.3
Z94.4
Z94.81
Z94.82
Z94.83
Z94.84
Z95.811
Z95.812
Z99.11
Z99.12

Numeric MCC List

A02.1
A02.21
A02.22
A06.4
A06.5
A06.6
A17.0
A17.1
A17.81
A17.82
A17.83
A17.89
A18.31
A19.0
A19.1
A19.2
A19.8
A19.9
A20.0
A20.1
A20.2
A20.3
A20.7
A20.8
A20.9
A22.1
A22.7
A26.7
A27.81
A32.7
A33
A35
A37.01
A37.11
A37.81
A37.91
A39.0
A39.1
A39.2
A39.3
A39.4
A39.50
A39.51
A39.52
A39.53
A39.81
A40.0
A40.1
A40.3
A40.8
A40.9
A41.01
A41.02
A41.1
A41.2
A41.3
A41.4
A41.50
A41.51
A41.52
A41.53
A41.54
A41.59
A41.81
A41.89
A41.9
A42.7
A48.0
A48.1
A48.3
A50.41
A50.42
A51.41
A52.13
A52.14
A54.81
A54.86
A80.0
A80.1
A80.2
A80.30
A80.39
A83.0
A83.1
A83.2
A83.3
A83.4
A83.5
A83.6
A83.8
A83.9
A84.0
A84.1
A84.81
A84.89
A84.9
A85.2
A92.30
A92.31
A92.32
A92.39
B00.3
B00.4
B00.7
B00.82
B01.11
B01.12
B01.2
B02.1
B02.24
B05.0
B05.2
B06.01
B10.01
B10.09
B15.0
B16.0
B16.2
B17.11
B19.0
B19.11
B19.21
B25.0
B25.2
B26.1
B26.2
B37.1
B37.5
B37.6
B37.7
B38.4
B39.0
B39.1
B39.2
B44.0
B45.1
B46.0
B46.1
B46.2
B46.3
B46.4
B46.5
B46.8
B46.9
B50.9
B58.2
B58.3
B58.81
B59
B77.81
D57.00
D57.01
D57.02
D57.03
D57.04
D57.09
D57.211
D57.212
D57.213
D57.214
D57.218
D57.219
D57.411
D57.412
D57.413
D57.414
D57.418
D57.419
D57.431
D57.432
D57.433
D57.434
D57.438
D57.439
D57.451
D57.452
D57.453
D57.454
D57.458
D57.459
D57.811
D57.812
D57.813
D57.814
D57.818
D57.819
D59.30
D59.31
D59.32
D59.39
D60.0
D60.1
D60.8
D60.9
D61.1
D61.2
D61.3
D61.810
D61.811
D61.89
D65
D66
D67
E03.5
E05.01
E05.11
E05.21
E05.31
E05.41
E05.81
E05.91
E08.00
E08.01
E08.10
E08.11
E08.641
E09.00
E09.01
E09.10
E09.11
E09.641
E10.10
E10.11
E10.641
E11.00
E11.01
E11.10
E11.11
E11.641
E13.00
E13.01
E13.10
E13.11
E13.641
E40
E41
E42
E43
E84.0
E84.11
E88.3
G00.0
G00.1
G00.2
G00.3
G00.8
G00.9
G01
G02
G03.0
G03.8
G03.9
G04.00
G04.01
G04.02
G04.2
G04.30
G04.31
G04.32
G04.39
G04.81
G04.82
G04.89
G04.90
G04.91
G05.3
G05.4
G06.0
G06.1
G06.2
G07
G08
G21.0
G37.4
G40.301
G40.311
G40.319
G70.01
G80.0
G82.50
G82.51
G82.52
G82.53
G82.54
G83.5
G92.8
G92.9
G93.41
G93.5
G93.6
G93.7
G93.82
G95.11
G95.19
I21.01
I21.02
I21.09
I21.11
I21.19
I21.21
I21.29
I21.3
I21.4
I21.9
I21.A1
I21.A9
I21.B
I22.0
I22.1
I22.2
I22.8
I22.9
I23.4
I23.5
I25.42
I26.01
I26.02
I26.09
I26.90
I26.92
I26.93
I26.94
I26.99
I33.0
I33.9
I40.0
I40.1
I40.8
I40.9
I41
I46.2
I46.8
I46.9
I49.01
I49.02
I50.21
I50.23
I50.31
I50.33
I50.41
I50.43
I51.1
I51.2
I60.00
I60.01
I60.02
I60.10
I60.11
I60.12
I60.2
I60.30
I60.31
I60.32
I60.4
I60.50
I60.51
I60.52
I60.6
I60.7
I60.8
I60.9
I61.0
I61.1
I61.2
I61.3
I61.4
I61.5
I61.6
I61.8
I61.9
I62.00
I62.01
I62.02
I62.03
I62.1
I63.00
I63.011
I63.012
I63.013
I63.019
I63.02
I63.031
I63.032
I63.033
I63.039
I63.09
I63.10
I63.111
I63.112
I63.113
I63.119
I63.12
I63.131
I63.132
I63.133
I63.139
I63.19
I63.20
I63.211
I63.212
I63.213
I63.219
I63.22
I63.231
I63.232
I63.233
I63.239
I63.29
I63.30
I63.311
I63.312
I63.313
I63.319
I63.321
I63.322
I63.323
I63.329
I63.331
I63.332
I63.333
I63.339
I63.341
I63.342
I63.343
I63.349
I63.39
I63.40
I63.411
I63.412
I63.413
I63.419
I63.421
I63.422
I63.423
I63.429
I63.431
I63.432
I63.433
I63.439
I63.441
I63.442
I63.443
I63.449
I63.49
I63.50
I63.511
I63.512
I63.513
I63.519
I63.521
I63.522
I63.523
I63.529
I63.531
I63.532
I63.533
I63.539
I63.541
I63.542
I63.543
I63.549
I63.59
I63.6
I63.81
I63.89
I63.9
I67.0
I67.83
I71.00
I71.010
I71.011
I71.012
I71.019
I71.02
I71.03
I71.10
I71.11
I71.12
I71.13
I71.30
I71.31
I71.32
I71.33
I71.50
I71.51
I71.52
I71.8
I74.01
I77.70
I77.71
I77.72
I77.73
I77.74
I77.75
I77.76
I77.77
I77.79
I81
I82.0
I82.220
I82.221
I85.01
I85.11
J04.11
J04.31
J05.11
J09.X1
J10.00
J10.01
J10.08
J11.00
J11.08
J12.0
J12.1
J12.2
J12.3
J12.81
J12.82
J12.89
J12.9
J13
J14
J15.0
J15.1
J15.20
J15.211
J15.212
J15.29
J15.3
J15.4
J15.5
J15.61
J15.69
J15.7
J15.8
J15.9
J16.0
J16.8
J17
J18.0
J18.1
J18.8
J18.9
J68.1
J69.0
J69.1
J69.8
J80
J81.0
J84.81
J84.83
J84.841
J84.842
J84.843
J84.848
J85.0
J85.1
J85.2
J85.3
J86.0
J86.9
J93.0
J95.1
J95.2
J95.3
J95.821
J95.822
J96.00
J96.01
J96.02
J96.20
J96.21
J96.22
J96.90
J96.91
J96.92
J98.51
J98.59
K20.81
K20.91
K21.01
K22.11
K22.3
K22.6
K25.0
K25.1
K25.2
K25.4
K25.5
K25.6
K26.0
K26.1
K26.2
K26.4
K26.5
K26.6
K27.0
K27.1
K27.2
K27.4
K27.5
K27.6
K28.0
K28.1
K28.2
K28.4
K28.5
K28.6
K29.01
K29.21
K29.31
K29.41
K29.51
K29.61
K29.71
K29.81
K29.91
K31.811
K31.82
K35.210
K35.211
K35.219
K35.32
K35.33
K40.10
K40.11
K40.40
K40.41
K41.10
K41.11
K41.40
K41.41
K42.1
K43.1
K43.4
K43.7
K44.1
K45.1
K46.1
K55.011
K55.012
K55.019
K55.021
K55.022
K55.029
K55.031
K55.032
K55.039
K55.041
K55.042
K55.049
K55.051
K55.052
K55.059
K55.061
K55.062
K55.069
K55.21
K55.30
K55.31
K55.32
K55.33
K56.2
K57.01
K57.11
K57.13
K57.21
K57.31
K57.33
K57.41
K57.51
K57.53
K57.81
K57.91
K57.93
K63.1
K63.81
K65.0
K65.1
K65.2
K65.3
K65.8
K65.9
K66.1
K67
K68.12
K68.19
K68.2
K68.3
K68.9
K70.41
K71.11
K72.00
K72.01
K72.11
K72.91
K75.0
K75.1
K76.2
K76.3
K76.7
K80.67
K82.2
K83.1
K83.2
K85.00
K85.01
K85.02
K85.10
K85.11
K85.12
K85.20
K85.21
K85.22
K85.30
K85.31
K85.32
K85.80
K85.81
K85.82
K85.90
K85.91
K85.92
L89.003
L89.004
L89.013
L89.014
L89.023
L89.024
L89.103
L89.104
L89.113
L89.114
L89.123
L89.124
L89.133
L89.134
L89.143
L89.144
L89.153
L89.154
L89.203
L89.204
L89.213
L89.214
L89.223
L89.224
L89.303
L89.304
L89.313
L89.314
L89.323
L89.324
L89.43
L89.44
L89.503
L89.504
L89.513
L89.514
L89.523
L89.524
L89.603
L89.604
L89.613
L89.614
L89.623
L89.624
L89.813
L89.814
L89.893
L89.894
L89.93
L89.94
M31.10
M31.11
M31.19
M72.6
M96.A4
N00.0
N00.1
N00.2
N00.3
N00.4
N00.5
N00.6
N00.7
N00.8
N00.9
N00.A
N01.0
N01.1
N01.2
N01.3
N01.4
N01.5
N01.6
N01.7
N01.8
N01.9
N01.A
N15.1
N17.0
N17.1
N17.2
N18.6
N73.3
O03.2
O03.31
O03.32
O03.81
O03.82
O04.7
O04.81
O04.82
O07.2
O07.31
O07.32
O08.2
O08.3
O08.4
O10.42
O11.1
O11.2
O11.3
O14.12
O14.13
O14.22
O14.23
O15.02
O15.03
O15.1
O15.2
O22.31
O22.32
O22.33
O24.02
O24.12
O24.32
O24.82
O34.31
O34.32
O34.33
O41.1010
O41.1011
O41.1012
O41.1013
O41.1014
O41.1015
O41.1019
O41.1020
O41.1021
O41.1022
O41.1023
O41.1024
O41.1025
O41.1029
O41.1030
O41.1031
O41.1032
O41.1033
O41.1034
O41.1035
O41.1039
O41.1210
O41.1211
O41.1212
O41.1213
O41.1214
O41.1215
O41.1219
O41.1220
O41.1221
O41.1222
O41.1223
O41.1224
O41.1225
O41.1229
O41.1230
O41.1231
O41.1232

O41.1233
O41.1234
O41.1235
O41.1239
O41.1410
O41.1411
O41.1412
O41.1413
O41.1414
O41.1415
O41.1419
O41.1420
O41.1421
O41.1422
O41.1423
O41.1424
O41.1425
O41.1429
O41.1430
O41.1431
O41.1432
O41.1433
O41.1434
O41.1435
O41.1439
O44.11
O44.12
O44.13
O44.31
O44.32
O44.33
O44.51
O44.52
O44.53
O45.001
O45.002
O45.003
O45.011
O45.012
O45.013
O45.021
O45.022
O45.023
O45.091
O45.092
O45.093
O45.8X1
O45.8X2
O45.8X3
O45.91
O45.92
O45.93
O46.001
O46.002
O46.003
O46.011
O46.012
O46.013
O46.021
O46.022
O46.023
O46.091
O46.092
O46.093
O60.02
O60.03
O60.12X0
O60.12X1
O60.12X2
O60.12X3
O60.12X4
O60.12X5
O60.12X9
O60.13X0
O60.13X1
O60.13X2
O60.13X3
O60.13X4
O60.13X5
O60.13X9
O60.14X0
O60.14X1
O60.14X2
O60.14X3
O60.14X4
O60.14X5
O60.14X9
O60.22X0
O60.22X1
O60.22X2
O60.22X3
O60.22X4
O60.22X5
O60.22X9
O60.23X0
O60.23X1
O60.23X2
O60.23X3
O60.23X4
O60.23X5
O60.23X9
O67.0
O71.02
O71.03
O71.1
O75.1
O75.3
O85
O86.04
O86.81
O86.89
O87.1
O88.011
O88.012
O88.013
O88.02
O88.03
O88.111
O88.112
O88.113
O88.12
O88.13
O88.211
O88.212
O88.213
O88.22
O88.23
O88.311
O88.312
O88.313
O88.32
O88.33
O88.811
O88.812
O88.813
O88.82
O88.83
O90.3
O90.41
O90.49
O99.42
P10.0
P10.1
P10.3
P10.4
P10.8
P10.9
P11.0
P11.2
P11.9
P22.0
P23.0
P23.1
P23.2
P23.3
P23.4
P23.5
P23.6
P23.8
P23.9
P24.01
P24.11
P24.21
P24.31
P24.81
P25.0
P25.1
P25.2
P25.3
P25.8
P26.0
P26.1
P26.8
P26.9
P27.0
P27.1
P27.8
P27.9
P28.5
P28.81
P29.30
P29.38
P29.81
P35.1
P35.2
P35.3
P35.4
P35.8
P35.9
P36.0
P36.10
P36.19
P36.2
P36.30
P36.39
P36.4
P36.5
P36.8
P36.9
P37.0
P37.1
P37.2
P37.3
P37.4
P37.8
P37.9
P52.21
P52.22
P52.4
P52.5
P52.6
P52.8
P52.9
P54.1
P54.2
P54.3
P56.0
P56.90
P56.99
P57.0
P57.8
P57.9
P59.1
P59.20
P59.29
P60
P61.0
P61.5
P74.0
P77.1
P77.2
P77.3
P77.9
P78.0
P83.2
P90
P91.0
P91.1
P91.2
P91.3
P91.4
P91.5
P91.63
P91.821
P91.822
P91.823
P91.829
P92.01
Q00.0
Q00.1
Q00.2
Q04.0
Q04.1
Q04.2
Q04.3
Q20.0
Q20.1
Q20.2
Q20.3
Q20.4
Q21.3
Q22.0
Q22.4
Q22.5
Q22.6
Q22.8
Q22.9
Q23.4
Q24.2
Q24.4
Q24.6
Q25.5
Q25.6
Q25.71
Q25.72
Q25.79
Q28.2
Q28.3
Q33.2
Q33.3
Q33.6
Q39.0
Q39.1
Q39.2
Q39.3
Q39.4
Q44.2
Q44.3
Q79.0
Q79.1
Q79.2
Q79.3
Q79.4
Q79.51
Q79.59
Q89.4
Q93.81
R09.2
R40.20
R40.2110
R40.2111
R40.2112
R40.2113
R40.2114
R40.2120
R40.2121
R40.2122
R40.2123
R40.2124
R40.2210
R40.2211
R40.2212
R40.2213
R40.2214
R40.2220
R40.2221
R40.2222
R40.2223
R40.2224
R40.2310
R40.2311
R40.2312
R40.2313
R40.2314
R40.2320
R40.2321
R40.2322
R40.2323
R40.2324
R40.2340
R40.2341
R40.2342
R40.2343
R40.2344
R40.2A
R53.2
R57.0
R57.1
R57.8
R65.11
R65.20
R65.21
S02.0XXB
S02.101B
S02.102B
S02.109B
S02.110B
S02.111B
S02.112B
S02.113B
S02.118B
S02.119B
S02.11AB
S02.11BB
S02.11CB
S02.11DB
S02.11EB
S02.11FB
S02.11GB
S02.11HB
S02.121B
S02.122B
S02.129B
S02.19XB
S02.91XB
S06.1X0A
S06.1X1A
S06.1X2A
S06.1X3A
S06.1X4A
S06.1X5A
S06.1X6A
S06.1X7A
S06.1X8A
S06.1X9A
S06.1XAA
S06.2X6A
S06.2X7A
S06.2X8A
S06.306A
S06.307A
S06.308A
S06.310A
S06.311A
S06.312A
S06.313A
S06.314A
S06.315A
S06.316A
S06.317A
S06.318A
S06.319A
S06.31AA
S06.320A
S06.321A
S06.322A
S06.323A
S06.324A
S06.325A
S06.326A
S06.327A
S06.328A
S06.329A
S06.32AA
S06.330A
S06.331A
S06.332A
S06.333A
S06.334A
S06.335A
S06.336A
S06.337A
S06.338A
S06.339A
S06.33AA
S06.340A
S06.341A
S06.342A
S06.343A
S06.344A
S06.345A
S06.346A
S06.347A
S06.348A
S06.349A
S06.34AA
S06.350A
S06.351A
S06.352A
S06.353A
S06.354A
S06.355A
S06.356A
S06.357A
S06.358A
S06.359A
S06.35AA
S06.360A
S06.361A
S06.362A
S06.363A
S06.364A
S06.365A
S06.366A
S06.367A
S06.368A
S06.369A
S06.36AA
S06.370A
S06.376A
S06.377A
S06.378A
S06.37AA
S06.380A
S06.386A
S06.387A
S06.388A
S06.38AA
S06.4X0A
S06.4X1A
S06.4X2A
S06.4X3A
S06.4X4A
S06.4X5A
S06.4X6A
S06.4X7A
S06.4X8A
S06.4X9A
S06.4XAA
S06.5X0A
S06.5X1A
S06.5X2A
S06.5X3A
S06.5X4A
S06.5X5A
S06.5X6A
S06.5X7A
S06.5X8A
S06.5X9A
S06.5XAA
S06.6X0A
S06.6X1A
S06.6X2A
S06.6X3A
S06.6X4A
S06.6X5A
S06.6X6A
S06.6X7A
S06.6X8A
S06.6X9A
S06.6XAA
S06.816A
S06.817A
S06.818A
S06.826A
S06.827A
S06.828A
S06.896A
S06.897A
S06.898A
S06.8A6A
S06.8A7A
S06.8A8A
S06.9X6A
S06.9X7A
S06.9X8A
S06.A0XA
S06.A1XA
S11.011A
S11.012A
S11.013A
S11.014A
S11.015A
S11.019A
S11.021A
S11.022A
S11.023A
S11.024A
S11.025A
S11.029A
S11.031A
S11.032A
S11.033A
S11.034A
S11.035A
S11.039A
S12.000B
S12.001B
S12.01XB
S12.02XB
S12.030B
S12.031B
S12.040B
S12.041B
S12.090B
S12.091B
S12.100B
S12.101B
S12.110B
S12.111B
S12.112B
S12.120B
S12.121B
S12.130B
S12.131B
S12.14XB
S12.150B
S12.151B
S12.190B
S12.191B
S12.200B
S12.201B
S12.230B
S12.231B
S12.24XB
S12.250B
S12.251B
S12.290B
S12.291B
S12.300B
S12.301B
S12.330B
S12.331B
S12.34XB
S12.350B
S12.351B
S12.390B
S12.391B
S12.400B
S12.401B
S12.430B
S12.431B
S12.44XB
S12.450B
S12.451B
S12.490B
S12.491B
S12.500B
S12.501B
S12.530B
S12.531B
S12.54XB
S12.550B
S12.551B
S12.590B
S12.591B
S12.600B
S12.601B
S12.630B
S12.631B
S12.64XB
S12.650B
S12.651B
S12.690B
S12.691B
S12.8XXA
S14.0XXA
S14.101A
S14.102A
S14.103A
S14.104A
S14.105A
S14.106A
S14.107A
S14.108A
S14.111A
S14.112A
S14.113A
S14.114A
S14.115A
S14.116A
S14.117A
S14.118A
S14.121A
S14.122A
S14.123A
S14.124A
S14.125A
S14.126A
S14.127A
S14.128A
S14.131A
S14.132A
S14.133A
S14.134A
S14.135A
S14.136A
S14.137A
S14.138A
S14.141A
S14.142A
S14.143A
S14.144A
S14.145A
S14.146A
S14.147A
S14.148A
S14.151A
S14.152A
S14.153A
S14.154A
S14.155A
S14.156A
S14.157A
S14.158A
S21.301A
S21.302A
S21.309A
S21.311A
S21.312A
S21.319A
S21.321A
S21.322A
S21.329A
S21.331A
S21.332A
S21.339A
S21.341A
S21.342A
S21.349A
S21.351A
S21.352A
S21.359A
S21.401A
S21.402A
S21.409A
S21.411A
S21.412A
S21.419A
S21.421A
S21.422A
S21.429A
S21.431A
S21.432A
S21.439A
S21.441A
S21.442A
S21.449A
S21.451A
S21.452A
S21.459A
S22.000B
S22.001B
S22.002B
S22.008B
S22.009B
S22.010B
S22.011B
S22.012B
S22.018B
S22.019B
S22.020B
S22.021B
S22.022B
S22.028B
S22.029B
S22.030B
S22.031B
S22.032B
S22.038B
S22.039B
S22.040B
S22.041B
S22.042B
S22.048B
S22.049B
S22.050B
S22.051B
S22.052B
S22.058B
S22.059B
S22.060B
S22.061B
S22.062B
S22.068B
S22.069B
S22.070B
S22.071B
S22.072B
S22.078B
S22.079B
S22.080B
S22.081B
S22.082B
S22.088B
S22.089B
S22.20XB
S22.21XB
S22.22XB
S22.23XB
S22.24XB
S22.31XB
S22.32XB
S22.39XB
S22.41XB
S22.42XB
S22.43XB
S22.49XB
S22.5XXA
S22.5XXB
S22.9XXB
S24.0XXA
S24.101A
S24.102A
S24.103A
S24.104A
S24.111A
S24.112A
S24.113A
S24.114A
S24.131A
S24.132A
S24.133A
S24.134A
S24.141A
S24.142A
S24.143A
S24.144A
S24.151A
S24.152A
S24.153A
S24.154A
S25.00XA
S25.01XA
S25.02XA
S25.09XA
S25.101A
S25.102A
S25.109A
S25.111A
S25.112A
S25.119A
S25.121A
S25.122A
S25.129A
S25.191A
S25.192A
S25.199A
S25.20XA
S25.21XA
S25.22XA
S25.29XA
S25.301A
S25.302A
S25.309A
S25.311A
S25.312A
S25.319A
S25.321A
S25.322A
S25.329A
S25.391A
S25.392A
S25.399A
S25.401A
S25.402A
S25.409A
S25.411A
S25.412A
S25.419A
S25.421A
S25.422A
S25.429A
S25.491A
S25.492A
S25.499A
S26.020A
S26.021A
S26.022A
S26.12XA
S26.92XA
S27.1XXA
S27.2XXA
S27.331A
S27.332A
S27.339A
S27.401A
S27.402A
S27.409A
S27.411A
S27.412A
S27.419A
S27.421A
S27.422A
S27.429A
S27.431A
S27.432A
S27.439A
S27.491A
S27.492A
S27.499A
S27.812A
S27.813A
S27.818A
S27.819A
S31.001A
S31.011A
S31.021A
S31.031A
S31.041A
S31.051A
S31.600A
S31.601A
S31.602A
S31.603A
S31.604A
S31.605A
S31.609A
S31.610A
S31.611A
S31.612A
S31.613A
S31.614A
S31.615A
S31.619A
S31.620A
S31.621A
S31.622A
S31.623A
S31.624A
S31.625A
S31.629A
S31.630A
S31.631A
S31.632A
S31.633A
S31.634A
S31.635A
S31.639A
S31.640A
S31.641A
S31.642A
S31.643A
S31.644A
S31.645A
S31.649A
S31.650A
S31.651A
S31.652A
S31.653A
S31.654A
S31.655A
S31.659A
S32.000B
S32.001B
S32.002B
S32.008B
S32.009B
S32.010B
S32.011B
S32.012B
S32.018B
S32.019B
S32.020B
S32.021B
S32.022B
S32.028B
S32.029B
S32.030B
S32.031B
S32.032B
S32.038B
S32.039B
S32.040B
S32.041B
S32.042B
S32.048B
S32.049B
S32.050B
S32.051B
S32.052B
S32.058B
S32.059B

S32.10XB
S32.110B
S32.111B
S32.112B
S32.119B
S32.120B
S32.121B
S32.122B
S32.129B
S32.130B
S32.131B
S32.132B
S32.139B
S32.14XB
S32.15XB
S32.16XB
S32.17XB
S32.19XB
S32.2XXB
S32.301B
S32.302B
S32.309B
S32.311B
S32.312B
S32.313B
S32.314B
S32.315B
S32.316B
S32.391B
S32.392B
S32.399B
S32.401A
S32.401B
S32.402A
S32.402B
S32.409A
S32.409B
S32.411A
S32.411B
S32.412A
S32.412B
S32.413A
S32.413B
S32.414A
S32.414B
S32.415A
S32.415B
S32.416A
S32.416B
S32.421A
S32.421B
S32.422A
S32.422B
S32.423A
S32.423B
S32.424A
S32.424B
S32.425A
S32.425B
S32.426A
S32.426B
S32.431A
S32.431B
S32.432A
S32.432B
S32.433A
S32.433B
S32.434A
S32.434B
S32.435A
S32.435B
S32.436A
S32.436B
S32.441A
S32.441B
S32.442A
S32.442B
S32.443A
S32.443B
S32.444A
S32.444B
S32.445A
S32.445B
S32.446A
S32.446B
S32.451A
S32.451B
S32.452A
S32.452B
S32.453A
S32.453B
S32.454A
S32.454B
S32.455A
S32.455B
S32.456A
S32.456B
S32.461A
S32.461B
S32.462A
S32.462B
S32.463A
S32.463B
S32.464A
S32.464B
S32.465A
S32.465B
S32.466A
S32.466B
S32.471A
S32.471B
S32.472A
S32.472B
S32.473A
S32.473B
S32.474A
S32.474B
S32.475A
S32.475B
S32.476A
S32.476B
S32.481A
S32.481B
S32.482A
S32.482B
S32.483A
S32.483B
S32.484A
S32.484B
S32.485A
S32.485B
S32.486A
S32.486B
S32.491A
S32.491B
S32.492A
S32.492B
S32.499A
S32.499B
S32.501B
S32.502B
S32.509B
S32.511B
S32.512B
S32.519B
S32.591B
S32.592B
S32.599B
S32.601B
S32.602B
S32.609B
S32.611B
S32.612B
S32.613B
S32.614B
S32.615B
S32.616B
S32.691B
S32.692B
S32.699B
S32.810B
S32.811B
S32.82XB
S32.89XB
S32.9XXB
S34.01XA
S34.02XA
S34.101A
S34.102A
S34.103A
S34.104A
S34.105A
S34.109A
S34.111A
S34.112A
S34.113A
S34.114A
S34.115A
S34.119A
S34.121A
S34.122A
S34.123A
S34.124A
S34.125A
S34.129A
S34.131A
S34.132A
S34.139A
S34.3XXA
S35.00XA
S35.01XA
S35.02XA
S35.09XA
S35.10XA
S35.11XA
S35.12XA
S35.19XA
S35.211A
S35.212A
S35.218A
S35.219A
S35.221A
S35.222A
S35.228A
S35.229A
S35.231A
S35.232A
S35.238A
S35.239A
S35.291A
S35.292A
S35.298A
S35.299A
S35.311A
S35.318A
S35.319A
S35.321A
S35.328A
S35.329A
S35.331A
S35.338A
S35.339A
S35.341A
S35.348A
S35.349A
S35.401A
S35.402A
S35.403A
S35.404A
S35.405A
S35.406A
S35.411A
S35.412A
S35.413A
S35.414A
S35.415A
S35.416A
S35.491A
S35.492A
S35.493A
S35.494A
S35.495A
S35.496A
S35.50XA
S35.511A
S35.512A
S35.513A
S35.514A
S35.515A
S35.516A
S35.59XA
S36.031A
S36.032A
S36.115A
S36.116A
S37.061A
S37.062A
S37.069A
S37.091A
S37.092A
S37.099A
S42.201B
S42.202B
S42.209B
S42.211B
S42.212B
S42.213B
S42.214B
S42.215B
S42.216B
S42.221B
S42.222B
S42.223B
S42.224B
S42.225B
S42.226B
S42.231B
S42.232B
S42.239B
S42.241B
S42.242B
S42.249B
S42.251B
S42.252B
S42.253B
S42.254B
S42.255B
S42.256B
S42.261B
S42.262B
S42.263B
S42.264B
S42.265B
S42.266B
S42.291B
S42.292B
S42.293B
S42.294B
S42.295B
S42.296B
S42.301B
S42.302B
S42.309B
S42.321B
S42.322B
S42.323B
S42.324B
S42.325B
S42.326B
S42.331B
S42.332B
S42.333B
S42.334B
S42.335B
S42.336B
S42.341B
S42.342B
S42.343B
S42.344B
S42.345B
S42.346B
S42.351B
S42.352B
S42.353B
S42.354B
S42.355B
S42.356B
S42.361B
S42.362B
S42.363B
S42.364B
S42.365B
S42.366B
S42.391B
S42.392B
S42.399B
S42.401B
S42.402B
S42.409B
S42.411B
S42.412B
S42.413B
S42.414B
S42.415B
S42.416B
S42.421B
S42.422B
S42.423B
S42.424B
S42.425B
S42.426B
S42.431B
S42.432B
S42.433B
S42.434B
S42.435B
S42.436B
S42.441B
S42.442B
S42.443B
S42.444B
S42.445B
S42.446B
S42.447B
S42.448B
S42.449B
S42.451B
S42.452B
S42.453B
S42.454B
S42.455B
S42.456B
S42.461B
S42.462B
S42.463B
S42.464B
S42.465B
S42.466B
S42.471B
S42.472B
S42.473B
S42.474B
S42.475B
S42.476B
S42.491B
S42.492B
S42.493B
S42.494B
S42.495B
S42.496B
S42.90XB
S42.91XB
S42.92XB
S45.001A
S45.002A
S45.009A
S45.011A
S45.012A
S45.019A
S45.091A
S45.092A
S45.099A
S52.001B
S52.001C
S52.002B
S52.002C
S52.009B
S52.009C
S52.021B
S52.021C
S52.022B
S52.022C
S52.023B
S52.023C
S52.024B
S52.024C
S52.025B
S52.025C
S52.026B
S52.026C
S52.031B
S52.031C
S52.032B
S52.032C
S52.033B
S52.033C
S52.034B
S52.034C
S52.035B
S52.035C
S52.036B
S52.036C
S52.041B
S52.041C
S52.042B
S52.042C
S52.043B
S52.043C
S52.044B
S52.044C
S52.045B
S52.045C
S52.046B
S52.046C
S52.091B
S52.091C
S52.092B
S52.092C
S52.099B
S52.099C
S52.101B
S52.101C
S52.102B
S52.102C
S52.109B
S52.109C
S52.121B
S52.121C
S52.122B
S52.122C
S52.123B
S52.123C
S52.124B
S52.124C
S52.125B
S52.125C
S52.126B
S52.126C
S52.131B
S52.131C
S52.132B
S52.132C
S52.133B
S52.133C
S52.134B
S52.134C
S52.135B
S52.135C
S52.136B
S52.136C
S52.181B
S52.181C
S52.182B
S52.182C
S52.189B
S52.189C
S52.201B
S52.201C
S52.202B
S52.202C
S52.209B
S52.209C
S52.221B
S52.221C
S52.222B
S52.222C
S52.223B
S52.223C
S52.224B
S52.224C
S52.225B
S52.225C
S52.226B
S52.226C
S52.231B
S52.231C
S52.232B
S52.232C
S52.233B
S52.233C
S52.234B
S52.234C
S52.235B
S52.235C
S52.236B
S52.236C
S52.241B
S52.241C
S52.242B
S52.242C
S52.243B
S52.243C
S52.244B
S52.244C
S52.245B
S52.245C
S52.246B
S52.246C
S52.251B
S52.251C
S52.252B
S52.252C
S52.253B
S52.253C
S52.254B
S52.254C
S52.255B
S52.255C
S52.256B
S52.256C
S52.261B
S52.261C
S52.262B
S52.262C
S52.263B
S52.263C
S52.264B
S52.264C
S52.265B
S52.265C
S52.266B
S52.266C
S52.271B
S52.271C
S52.272B
S52.272C
S52.279B
S52.279C
S52.281B
S52.281C
S52.282B
S52.282C
S52.283B
S52.283C
S52.291B
S52.291C
S52.292B
S52.292C
S52.299B
S52.299C
S52.301B
S52.301C
S52.302B
S52.302C
S52.309B
S52.309C
S52.321B
S52.321C
S52.322B
S52.322C
S52.323B
S52.323C
S52.324B
S52.324C
S52.325B
S52.325C
S52.326B
S52.326C
S52.331B
S52.331C
S52.332B
S52.332C
S52.333B
S52.333C
S52.334B
S52.334C
S52.335B
S52.335C
S52.336B
S52.336C
S52.341B
S52.341C
S52.342B
S52.342C
S52.343B
S52.343C
S52.344B
S52.344C
S52.345B
S52.345C
S52.346B
S52.346C
S52.351B
S52.351C
S52.352B
S52.352C
S52.353B
S52.353C
S52.354B
S52.354C
S52.355B
S52.355C
S52.356B
S52.356C
S52.361B
S52.361C
S52.362B
S52.362C
S52.363B
S52.363C
S52.364B
S52.364C
S52.365B
S52.365C
S52.366B
S52.366C
S52.371B
S52.371C
S52.372B
S52.372C
S52.379B
S52.379C
S52.381B
S52.381C
S52.382B
S52.382C
S52.389B
S52.389C
S52.391B
S52.391C
S52.392B
S52.392C
S52.399B
S52.399C
S52.501B
S52.501C
S52.502B
S52.502C
S52.509B
S52.509C
S52.511B
S52.511C
S52.512B
S52.512C
S52.513B
S52.513C
S52.514B
S52.514C
S52.515B
S52.515C
S52.516B
S52.516C
S52.531B
S52.531C
S52.532B
S52.532C
S52.539B
S52.539C
S52.541B
S52.541C
S52.542B
S52.542C
S52.549B
S52.549C
S52.551B
S52.551C
S52.552B
S52.552C
S52.559B
S52.559C
S52.561B
S52.561C
S52.562B
S52.562C
S52.569B
S52.569C
S52.571B
S52.571C
S52.572B
S52.572C
S52.579B
S52.579C
S52.591B
S52.591C
S52.592B
S52.592C
S52.599B
S52.599C
S52.601B
S52.601C
S52.602B
S52.602C
S52.609B
S52.609C
S52.611B
S52.611C
S52.612B
S52.612C
S52.613B
S52.613C
S52.614B
S52.614C
S52.615B
S52.615C
S52.616B
S52.616C
S52.691B
S52.691C
S52.692B
S52.692C
S52.699B
S52.699C
S52.90XB
S52.90XC
S52.91XB
S52.91XC
S52.92XB
S52.92XC
S72.001A
S72.001B
S72.001C
S72.002A
S72.002B
S72.002C
S72.009A
S72.009B
S72.009C
S72.011A
S72.011B
S72.011C
S72.012A
S72.012B
S72.012C
S72.019A
S72.019B
S72.019C
S72.021A
S72.021B
S72.021C
S72.022A
S72.022B
S72.022C
S72.023A
S72.023B
S72.023C
S72.024A
S72.024B
S72.024C
S72.025A
S72.025B
S72.025C
S72.026A
S72.026B
S72.026C
S72.031A
S72.031B
S72.031C
S72.032A
S72.032B
S72.032C
S72.033A
S72.033B
S72.033C
S72.034A
S72.034B
S72.034C
S72.035A
S72.035B
S72.035C
S72.036A
S72.036B
S72.036C
S72.041A
S72.041B
S72.041C
S72.042A
S72.042B
S72.042C
S72.043A
S72.043B
S72.043C
S72.044A
S72.044B
S72.044C
S72.045A
S72.045B
S72.045C
S72.046A
S72.046B
S72.046C
S72.051A
S72.051B
S72.051C
S72.052A
S72.052B
S72.052C
S72.059A
S72.059B
S72.059C
S72.061A
S72.061B
S72.061C
S72.062A
S72.062B
S72.062C
S72.063A
S72.063B
S72.063C
S72.064A
S72.064B
S72.064C
S72.065A
S72.065B
S72.065C
S72.066A
S72.066B
S72.066C
S72.091A
S72.091B
S72.091C
S72.092A
S72.092B
S72.092C
S72.099A
S72.099B
S72.099C
S72.101A
S72.101B
S72.101C
S72.102A
S72.102B
S72.102C
S72.109A
S72.109B
S72.109C
S72.111A
S72.111B
S72.111C
S72.112A
S72.112B
S72.112C
S72.113A
S72.113B
S72.113C
S72.114A
S72.114B
S72.114C
S72.115A
S72.115B
S72.115C
S72.116A
S72.116B
S72.116C
S72.121A
S72.121B
S72.121C
S72.122A
S72.122B
S72.122C
S72.123A
S72.123B
S72.123C
S72.124A
S72.124B
S72.124C
S72.125A
S72.125B
S72.125C
S72.126A
S72.126B
S72.126C
S72.131A
S72.131B
S72.131C
S72.132A
S72.132B
S72.132C
S72.133A
S72.133B
S72.133C
S72.134A
S72.134B
S72.134C
S72.135A
S72.135B
S72.135C
S72.136A
S72.136B
S72.136C
S72.141A
S72.141B
S72.141C
S72.142A

S72.142B
S72.142C
S72.143A
S72.143B
S72.143C
S72.144A
S72.144B
S72.144C
S72.145A
S72.145B
S72.145C
S72.146A
S72.146B
S72.146C
S72.21XA
S72.21XB
S72.21XC
S72.22XA
S72.22XB
S72.22XC
S72.23XA
S72.23XB
S72.23XC
S72.24XA
S72.24XB
S72.24XC
S72.25XA
S72.25XB
S72.25XC
S72.26XA
S72.26XB
S72.26XC
S72.3Ø1A
S72.3Ø1B
S72.3Ø1C
S72.3Ø2A
S72.3Ø2B
S72.3Ø2C
S72.3Ø9A
S72.3Ø9B
S72.3Ø9C
S72.321A
S72.321B
S72.321C
S72.322A
S72.322B
S72.322C
S72.323A
S72.323B
S72.323C
S72.324A
S72.324B
S72.324C
S72.325A
S72.325B
S72.325C
S72.326A
S72.326B
S72.326C
S72.331A
S72.331B
S72.331C
S72.332A
S72.332B
S72.332C
S72.333A
S72.333B
S72.333C
S72.334A
S72.334B
S72.334C
S72.335A
S72.335B
S72.335C
S72.336A
S72.336B
S72.336C
S72.341A
S72.341B
S72.341C
S72.342A
S72.342B
S72.342C
S72.343A
S72.343B
S72.343C
S72.344A
S72.344B
S72.344C
S72.345A
S72.345B
S72.345C
S72.346A
S72.346B
S72.346C
S72.351A
S72.351B
S72.351C
S72.352A
S72.352B
S72.352C
S72.353A
S72.353B
S72.353C
S72.354A
S72.354B
S72.354C
S72.355A
S72.355B
S72.355C
S72.356A
S72.356B
S72.356C
S72.361A
S72.361B
S72.361C
S72.362A
S72.362B
S72.362C
S72.363A
S72.363B
S72.363C
S72.364A
S72.364B
S72.364C
S72.365A
S72.365B
S72.365C
S72.366A
S72.366B
S72.366C
S72.391A
S72.391B
S72.391C
S72.392A
S72.392B
S72.392C
S72.399A
S72.399B
S72.399C
S72.4Ø1B
S72.4Ø1C
S72.4Ø2B
S72.4Ø2C
S72.4Ø9B
S72.4Ø9C
S72.411B
S72.411C
S72.412B
S72.412C
S72.413B
S72.413C
S72.414B
S72.414C
S72.415B
S72.415C
S72.416B
S72.416C
S72.421B
S72.421C
S72.422B
S72.422C
S72.423B
S72.423C
S72.424B
S72.424C
S72.425B
S72.425C
S72.426B
S72.426C
S72.431B
S72.431C
S72.432B
S72.432C
S72.433B
S72.433C
S72.434B
S72.434C
S72.435B
S72.435C
S72.436B
S72.436C
S72.441B
S72.441C
S72.442B
S72.442C
S72.443B
S72.443C
S72.444B
S72.444C
S72.445B
S72.445C
S72.446B
S72.446C
S72.451B
S72.451C
S72.452B
S72.452C
S72.453B
S72.453C
S72.454B
S72.454C
S72.455B
S72.455C
S72.456B
S72.456C
S72.461B
S72.461C
S72.462B
S72.462C
S72.463B
S72.463C
S72.464B
S72.464C
S72.465B
S72.465C
S72.466B
S72.466C
S72.491B
S72.491C
S72.492B
S72.492C
S72.499B
S72.499C
S72.8X1A
S72.8X1B
S72.8X1C
S72.8X2A
S72.8X2B
S72.8X2C
S72.8X9A
S72.8X9B
S72.8X9C
S72.9ØXA
S72.9ØXB
S72.9ØXC
S72.91XA
S72.91XB
S72.91XC
S72.92XA
S72.92XB
S72.92XC
S75.ØØ1A
S75.ØØ2A
S75.ØØ9A
S75.Ø11A
S75.Ø12A
S75.Ø19A
S75.Ø21A
S75.Ø22A
S75.Ø29A
S75.Ø91A
S75.Ø92A
S75.Ø99A
S75.1Ø1A
S75.1Ø2A
S75.1Ø9A
S75.111A
S75.112A
S75.119A
S75.121A
S75.122A
S75.129A
S75.191A
S75.192A
S75.199A
S79.ØØ1A
S79.ØØ2A
S79.ØØ9A
S79.Ø11A
S79.Ø12A
S79.Ø19A
S79.Ø91A
S79.Ø92A
S79.Ø99A
S82.1Ø1B
S82.1Ø1C
S82.1Ø2B
S82.1Ø2C
S82.1Ø9B
S82.1Ø9C
S82.111B
S82.111C
S82.112B
S82.112C
S82.113B
S82.113C
S82.114B
S82.114C
S82.115B
S82.115C
S82.116B
S82.116C
S82.121B
S82.121C
S82.122B
S82.122C
S82.123B
S82.123C
S82.124B
S82.124C
S82.125B
S82.125C
S82.126B
S82.126C
S82.131B
S82.131C
S82.132B
S82.132C
S82.133B
S82.133C
S82.134B
S82.134C
S82.135B
S82.135C
S82.136B
S82.136C
S82.141B
S82.141C
S82.142B
S82.142C
S82.143B
S82.143C
S82.144B
S82.144C
S82.145B
S82.145C
S82.146B
S82.146C
S82.151B
S82.151C
S82.152B
S82.152C
S82.153B
S82.153C
S82.154B
S82.154C
S82.155B
S82.155C
S82.156B
S82.156C
S82.191B
S82.191C
S82.192B
S82.192C
S82.199B
S82.199C
S82.2Ø1B
S82.2Ø1C
S82.2Ø2B
S82.2Ø2C
S82.2Ø9B
S82.2Ø9C
S82.221B
S82.221C
S82.222B
S82.222C
S82.223B
S82.223C
S82.224B
S82.224C
S82.225B
S82.225C
S82.226B
S82.226C
S82.231B
S82.231C
S82.232B
S82.232C
S82.233B
S82.233C
S82.234B
S82.234C
S82.235B
S82.235C
S82.236B
S82.236C
S82.241B
S82.241C
S82.242B
S82.242C
S82.243B
S82.243C
S82.244B
S82.244C
S82.245B
S82.245C
S82.246B
S82.246C
S82.251B
S82.251C
S82.252B
S82.252C
S82.253B
S82.253C
S82.254B
S82.254C
S82.255B
S82.255C
S82.256B
S82.256C
S82.261B
S82.261C
S82.262B
S82.262C
S82.263B
S82.263C
S82.264B
S82.264C
S82.265B
S82.265C
S82.266B
S82.266C
S82.291B
S82.291C
S82.292B
S82.292C
S82.299B
S82.299C
S82.4Ø1B
S82.4Ø1C
S82.4Ø2B
S82.4Ø2C
S82.4Ø9B
S82.4Ø9C
S82.421B
S82.421C
S82.422B
S82.422C
S82.423B
S82.423C
S82.424B
S82.424C
S82.425B
S82.425C
S82.426B
S82.426C
S82.431B
S82.431C
S82.432B
S82.432C
S82.433B
S82.433C
S82.434B
S82.434C
S82.435B
S82.435C
S82.436B
S82.436C
S82.441B
S82.441C
S82.442B
S82.442C
S82.443B
S82.443C
S82.444B
S82.444C
S82.445B
S82.445C
S82.446B
S82.446C
S82.451B
S82.451C
S82.452B
S82.452C
S82.453B
S82.453C
S82.454B
S82.454C
S82.455B
S82.455C
S82.456B
S82.456C
S82.461B
S82.461C
S82.462B
S82.462C
S82.463B
S82.463C
S82.464B
S82.464C
S82.465B
S82.465C
S82.466B
S82.466C
S82.491B
S82.491C
S82.492B
S82.492C
S82.499B
S82.499C
S82.831B
S82.831C
S82.832B
S82.832C
S82.839B
S82.839C
S82.861B
S82.861C
S82.862B
S82.862C
S82.863B
S82.863C
S82.864B
S82.864C
S82.865B
S82.865C
S82.866B
S82.866C
S85.ØØ1A
S85.ØØ2A
S85.ØØ9A
S85.Ø11A
S85.Ø12A
S85.Ø19A
S85.Ø91A
S85.Ø92A
S85.Ø99A
S85.5Ø1A
S85.5Ø2A
S85.5Ø9A
S85.511A
S85.512A
S85.519A
S85.591A
S85.592A
S85.599A
T31.21
T31.22
T31.31
T31.32
T31.33
T31.41
T31.42
T31.43
T31.44
T31.51
T31.52
T31.53
T31.54
T31.55
T31.61
T31.62
T31.63
T31.64
T31.65
T31.66
T31.71
T31.72
T31.73
T31.74
T31.75
T31.76
T31.77
T31.81
T31.82
T31.83
T31.84
T31.85
T31.86
T31.87
T31.88
T31.91
T31.92
T31.93
T31.94
T31.95
T31.96
T31.97
T31.98
T31.99
T32.21
T32.22
T32.31
T32.32
T32.33
T32.41
T32.42
T32.43
T32.44
T32.51
T32.52
T32.53
T32.54
T32.55
T32.61
T32.62
T32.63
T32.64
T32.65
T32.66
T32.71
T32.72
T32.73
T32.74
T32.75
T32.76
T32.77
T32.81
T32.82
T32.83
T32.84
T32.85
T32.86
T32.87
T32.88
T32.91
T32.92
T32.93
T32.94
T32.95
T32.96
T32.97
T32.98
T32.99
T79.ØXXA
T79.1XXA
T79.4XXA
T79.5XXA
T8Ø.ØXXA
T81.11XA
T81.12XA
T81.19XA
UØ7.1

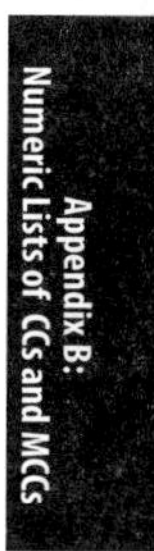

Appendix C: Major HIV-Related Conditions (Principal or Secondary Diagnosis)

AØ2.1	Salmonella sepsis
AØ2.2Ø	Localized salmonella infection, unspecified
AØ2.21	Salmonella meningitis
AØ2.22	Salmonella pneumonia
AØ2.23	Salmonella arthritis
AØ2.24	Salmonella osteomyelitis
AØ2.25	Salmonella pyelonephritis
AØ2.29	Salmonella with other localized infection
AØ2.8	Other specified salmonella infections
AØ2.9	Salmonella infection, unspecified
AØ7.3	Isosporiasis
A15.Ø	Tuberculosis of lung
A15.4	Tuberculosis of intrathoracic lymph nodes
A15.5	Tuberculosis of larynx, trachea and bronchus
A15.6	Tuberculous pleurisy
A15.7	Primary respiratory tuberculosis
A15.8	Other respiratory tuberculosis
A15.9	Respiratory tuberculosis unspecified
A17.Ø	Tuberculous meningitis
A17.1	Meningeal tuberculoma
A17.81	Tuberculoma of brain and spinal cord
A17.82	Tuberculous meningoencephalitis
A17.83	Tuberculous neuritis
A17.89	Other tuberculosis of nervous system
A17.9	Tuberculosis of nervous system, unspecified
A18.Ø1	Tuberculosis of spine
A18.Ø2	Tuberculous arthritis of other joints
A18.Ø3	Tuberculosis of other bones
A18.Ø9	Other musculoskeletal tuberculosis
A18.1Ø	Tuberculosis of genitourinary system, unspecified
A18.11	Tuberculosis of kidney and ureter
A18.12	Tuberculosis of bladder
A18.13	Tuberculosis of other urinary organs
A18.14	Tuberculosis of prostate
A18.15	Tuberculosis of other male genital organs
A18.16	Tuberculosis of cervix
A18.17	Tuberculous female pelvic inflammatory disease
A18.18	Tuberculosis of other female genital organs
A18.2	Tuberculous peripheral lymphadenopathy
A18.31	Tuberculous peritonitis
A18.32	Tuberculous enteritis
A18.39	Retroperitoneal tuberculosis
A18.4	Tuberculosis of skin and subcutaneous tissue
A18.5Ø	Tuberculosis of eye, unspecified
A18.51	Tuberculous episcleritis
A18.52	Tuberculous keratitis
A18.53	Tuberculous chorioretinitis
A18.54	Tuberculous iridocyclitis
A18.59	Other tuberculosis of eye
A18.6	Tuberculosis of (inner) (middle) ear
A18.7	Tuberculosis of adrenal glands
A18.81	Tuberculosis of thyroid gland
A18.82	Tuberculosis of other endocrine glands
A18.83	Tuberculosis of digestive tract organs, not elsewhere classified
A18.84	Tuberculosis of heart
A18.85	Tuberculosis of spleen
A18.89	Tuberculosis of other sites
A19.Ø	Acute miliary tuberculosis of a single specified site
A19.1	Acute miliary tuberculosis of multiple sites
A19.2	Acute miliary tuberculosis, unspecified
A19.8	Other miliary tuberculosis
A19.9	Miliary tuberculosis, unspecified
A31.2	Disseminated mycobacterium avium-intracellulare complex (DMAC)
A31.8	Other mycobacterial infections
A31.9	Mycobacterial infection, unspecified
A4Ø.9	Streptococcal sepsis, unspecified
A41.Ø1	Sepsis due to Methicillin susceptible Staphylococcus aureus
A41.Ø2	Sepsis due to Methicillin resistant Staphylococcus aureus
A41.1	Sepsis due to other specified staphylococcus
A41.2	Sepsis due to unspecified staphylococcus
A41.3	Sepsis due to Hemophilus influenzae
A41.4	Sepsis due to anaerobes
A41.5Ø	Gram-negative sepsis, unspecified
A41.51	Sepsis due to Escherichia coli [E. coli]
A41.52	Sepsis due to Pseudomonas
A41.53	Sepsis due to Serratia
A41.54	Sepsis due to Acinetobacter Baumannii
A41.59	Other Gram-negative sepsis
A41.81	Sepsis due to Enterococcus
A41.89	Other specified sepsis
A41.9	Sepsis, unspecified organism
A42.Ø	Pulmonary actinomycosis
A42.1	Abdominal actinomycosis
A42.2	Cervicofacial actinomycosis
A42.7	Actinomycotic sepsis
A42.81	Actinomycotic meningitis
A42.82	Actinomycotic encephalitis
A42.89	Other forms of actinomycosis
A42.9	Actinomycosis, unspecified
A43.Ø	Pulmonary nocardiosis
A43.1	Cutaneous nocardiosis
A43.8	Other forms of nocardiosis
A43.9	Nocardiosis, unspecified
A48.1	Legionnaires' disease
A6Ø.ØØ	Herpesviral infection of urogenital system, unspecified
A6Ø.Ø1	Herpesviral infection of penis
A6Ø.Ø4	Herpesviral vulvovaginitis
A6Ø.Ø9	Herpesviral infection of other urogenital tract
A6Ø.1	Herpesviral infection of perianal skin and rectum
A6Ø.9	Anogenital herpesviral infection, unspecified
A81.2	Progressive multifocal leukoencephalopathy
A81.82	Gerstmann-Straussler-Scheinker syndrome
A81.83	Fatal familial insomnia
A81.89	Other atypical virus infections of central nervous system
A81.9	Atypical virus infection of central nervous system, unspecified
A85.Ø	Enteroviral encephalitis
A85.1	Adenoviral encephalitis
A85.8	Other specified viral encephalitis
A86	Unspecified viral encephalitis
A88.8	Other specified viral infections of central nervous system
A89	Unspecified viral infection of central nervous system
BØØ.Ø	Eczema herpeticum
BØØ.1	Herpesviral vesicular dermatitis
BØØ.2	Herpesviral gingivostomatitis and pharyngotonsillitis
BØØ.3	Herpesviral meningitis
BØØ.4	Herpesviral encephalitis
BØØ.5Ø	Herpesviral ocular disease, unspecified
BØØ.51	Herpesviral iridocyclitis
BØØ.52	Herpesviral keratitis
BØØ.53	Herpesviral conjunctivitis
BØØ.59	Other herpesviral disease of eye
BØØ.7	Disseminated herpesviral disease

B00.81 Herpesviral hepatitis
B00.89 Other herpesviral infection
B00.9 Herpesviral infection, unspecified
B02.0 Zoster encephalitis
B02.1 Zoster meningitis
B02.21 Postherpetic geniculate ganglionitis
B02.22 Postherpetic trigeminal neuralgia
B02.23 Postherpetic polyneuropathy
B02.29 Other postherpetic nervous system involvement
B02.30 Zoster ocular disease, unspecified
B02.31 Zoster conjunctivitis
B02.32 Zoster iridocyclitis
B02.33 Zoster keratitis
B02.34 Zoster scleritis
B02.39 Other herpes zoster eye disease
B02.7 Disseminated zoster
B02.8 Zoster with other complications
B02.9 Zoster without complications
B10.01 Human herpesvirus 6 encephalitis
B10.09 Other human herpesvirus encephalitis
B25.8 Other cytomegaloviral diseases
B25.9 Cytomegaloviral disease, unspecified
B37.0 Candidal stomatitis
B37.1 Pulmonary candidiasis
B37.2 Candidiasis of skin and nail
B37.5 Candidal meningitis
B37.6 Candidal endocarditis
B37.81 Candidal esophagitis
B37.82 Candidal enteritis
B37.83 Candidal cheilitis
B37.84 Candidal otitis externa
B37.89 Other sites of candidiasis
B37.9 Candidiasis, unspecified
B38.0 Acute pulmonary coccidioidomycosis
B38.1 Chronic pulmonary coccidioidomycosis
B38.2 Pulmonary coccidioidomycosis, unspecified
B38.3 Cutaneous coccidioidomycosis
B38.4 Coccidioidomycosis meningitis
B38.7 Disseminated coccidioidomycosis
B38.81 Prostatic coccidioidomycosis
B38.89 Other forms of coccidioidomycosis
B38.9 Coccidioidomycosis, unspecified
B39.0 Acute pulmonary histoplasmosis capsulati
B39.1 Chronic pulmonary histoplasmosis capsulati
B39.2 Pulmonary histoplasmosis capsulati, unspecified
B39.3 Disseminated histoplasmosis capsulati
B39.4 Histoplasmosis capsulati, unspecified
B39.5 Histoplasmosis duboisii
B39.9 Histoplasmosis, unspecified
B45.0 Pulmonary cryptococcosis
B45.2 Cutaneous cryptococcosis
B45.3 Osseous cryptococcosis
B45.7 Disseminated cryptococcosis
B45.8 Other forms of cryptococcosis
B45.9 Cryptococcosis, unspecified
B47.1 Actinomycetoma
B47.9 Mycetoma, unspecified
B48.8 Other specified mycoses
B58.00 Toxoplasma oculopathy, unspecified
B58.01 Toxoplasma chorioretinitis
B58.09 Other toxoplasma oculopathy
B58.1 Toxoplasma hepatitis
B58.2 Toxoplasma meningoencephalitis
B58.3 Pulmonary toxoplasmosis
B58.81 Toxoplasma myocarditis
B58.82 Toxoplasma myositis
B58.83 Toxoplasma tubulo-interstitial nephropathy
B58.89 Toxoplasmosis with other organ involvement
B58.9 Toxoplasmosis, unspecified
B59 Pneumocystosis
B60.8 Other specified protozoal diseases
B78.0 Intestinal strongyloidiasis
B78.7 Disseminated strongyloidiasis
B78.9 Strongyloidiasis, unspecified
B99.8 Other infectious disease
C46.0 Kaposi's sarcoma of skin
C46.1 Kaposi's sarcoma of soft tissue
C46.2 Kaposi's sarcoma of palate
C46.3 Kaposi's sarcoma of lymph nodes
C46.4 Kaposi's sarcoma of gastrointestinal sites
C46.50 Kaposi's sarcoma of unspecified lung
C46.51 Kaposi's sarcoma of right lung
C46.52 Kaposi's sarcoma of left lung
C46.7 Kaposi's sarcoma of other sites
C46.9 Kaposi's sarcoma, unspecified
C82.50 Diffuse follicle center lymphoma, unspecified site
C82.51 Diffuse follicle center lymphoma, lymph nodes of head, face, and neck
C82.52 Diffuse follicle center lymphoma, intrathoracic lymph nodes
C82.53 Diffuse follicle center lymphoma, intra-abdominal lymph nodes
C82.54 Diffuse follicle center lymphoma, lymph nodes of axilla and upper limb
C82.55 Diffuse follicle center lymphoma, lymph nodes of inguinal region and lower limb
C82.56 Diffuse follicle center lymphoma, intrapelvic lymph nodes
C82.57 Diffuse follicle center lymphoma, spleen
C82.58 Diffuse follicle center lymphoma, lymph nodes of multiple sites
C82.59 Diffuse follicle center lymphoma, extranodal and solid organ sites
C83.00 Small cell B-cell lymphoma, unspecified site
C83.01 Small cell B-cell lymphoma, lymph nodes of head, face, and neck
C83.02 Small cell B-cell lymphoma, intrathoracic lymph nodes
C83.03 Small cell B-cell lymphoma, intra-abdominal lymph nodes
C83.04 Small cell B-cell lymphoma, lymph nodes of axilla and upper limb
C83.05 Small cell B-cell lymphoma, lymph nodes of inguinal region and lower limb
C83.06 Small cell B-cell lymphoma, intrapelvic lymph nodes
C83.07 Small cell B-cell lymphoma, spleen
C83.08 Small cell B-cell lymphoma, lymph nodes of multiple sites
C83.09 Small cell B-cell lymphoma, extranodal and solid organ sites
C83.10 Mantle cell lymphoma, unspecified site
C83.11 Mantle cell lymphoma, lymph nodes of head, face, and neck
C83.12 Mantle cell lymphoma, intrathoracic lymph nodes
C83.13 Mantle cell lymphoma, intra-abdominal lymph nodes
C83.14 Mantle cell lymphoma, lymph nodes of axilla and upper limb
C83.15 Mantle cell lymphoma, lymph nodes of inguinal region and lower limb
C83.16 Mantle cell lymphoma, intrapelvic lymph nodes
C83.17 Mantle cell lymphoma, spleen
C83.18 Mantle cell lymphoma, lymph nodes of multiple sites
C83.19 Mantle cell lymphoma, extranodal and solid organ sites
C83.30 Diffuse large B-cell lymphoma, unspecified site
C83.31 Diffuse large B-cell lymphoma, lymph nodes of head, face, and neck
C83.32 Diffuse large B-cell lymphoma, intrathoracic lymph nodes
C83.33 Diffuse large B-cell lymphoma, intra-abdominal lymph nodes
C83.34 Diffuse large B-cell lymphoma, lymph nodes of axilla and upper limb
C83.35 Diffuse large B-cell lymphoma, lymph nodes of inguinal region and lower limb
C83.36 Diffuse large B-cell lymphoma, intrapelvic lymph nodes
C83.37 Diffuse large B-cell lymphoma, spleen
C83.38 Diffuse large B-cell lymphoma, lymph nodes of multiple sites
C83.39 Diffuse large B-cell lymphoma, extranodal and solid organ sites
C83.70 Burkitt lymphoma, unspecified site
C83.71 Burkitt lymphoma, lymph nodes of head, face, and neck
C83.72 Burkitt lymphoma, intrathoracic lymph nodes
C83.73 Burkitt lymphoma, intra-abdominal lymph nodes
C83.74 Burkitt lymphoma, lymph nodes of axilla and upper limb

C83.75 Burkitt lymphoma, lymph nodes of inguinal region and lower limb
C83.76 Burkitt lymphoma, intrapelvic lymph nodes
C83.77 Burkitt lymphoma, spleen
C83.78 Burkitt lymphoma, lymph nodes of multiple sites
C83.79 Burkitt lymphoma, extranodal and solid organ sites
C83.8Ø Other non-follicular lymphoma, unspecified site
C83.81 Other non-follicular lymphoma, lymph nodes of head, face, and neck
C83.82 Other non-follicular lymphoma, intrathoracic lymph nodes
C83.83 Other non-follicular lymphoma, intra-abdominal lymph nodes
C83.84 Other non-follicular lymphoma, lymph nodes of axilla and upper limb
C83.85 Other non-follicular lymphoma, lymph nodes of inguinal region and lower limb
C83.86 Other non-follicular lymphoma, intrapelvic lymph nodes
C83.87 Other non-follicular lymphoma, spleen
C83.88 Other non-follicular lymphoma, lymph nodes of multiple sites
C83.89 Other non-follicular lymphoma, extranodal and solid organ sites
C83.9Ø Non-follicular (diffuse) lymphoma, unspecified, unspecified site
C83.91 Non-follicular (diffuse) lymphoma, unspecified, lymph nodes of head, face, and neck
C83.92 Non-follicular (diffuse) lymphoma, unspecified, intrathoracic lymph nodes
C83.93 Non-follicular (diffuse) lymphoma, unspecified, intra-abdominal lymph nodes
C83.94 Non-follicular (diffuse) lymphoma, unspecified, lymph nodes of axilla and upper limb
C83.95 Non-follicular (diffuse) lymphoma, unspecified, lymph nodes of inguinal region and lower limb
C83.96 Non-follicular (diffuse) lymphoma, unspecified, intrapelvic lymph nodes
C83.97 Non-follicular (diffuse) lymphoma, unspecified, spleen
C83.98 Non-follicular (diffuse) lymphoma, unspecified, lymph nodes of multiple sites
C83.99 Non-follicular (diffuse) lymphoma, unspecified, extranodal and solid organ sites
C84.4Ø Peripheral T-cell lymphoma, not elsewhere classified, unspecified site
C84.41 Peripheral T-cell lymphoma, not elsewhere classified, lymph nodes of head, face, and neck
C84.42 Peripheral T-cell lymphoma, not elsewhere classified, intrathoracic lymph nodes
C84.43 Peripheral T-cell lymphoma, not elsewhere classified, intra-abdominal lymph nodes
C84.44 Peripheral T-cell lymphoma, not elsewhere classified, lymph nodes of axilla and upper limb
C84.45 Peripheral T-cell lymphoma, not elsewhere classified, lymph nodes of inguinal region and lower limb
C84.46 Peripheral T-cell lymphoma, not elsewhere classified, intrapelvic lymph nodes
C84.47 Peripheral T-cell lymphoma, not elsewhere classified, spleen
C84.48 Peripheral T-cell lymphoma, not elsewhere classified, lymph nodes of multiple sites
C84.49 Peripheral T-cell lymphoma, not elsewhere classified, extranodal and solid organ sites
C84.6Ø Anaplastic large cell lymphoma, ALK-positive, unspecified site
C84.61 Anaplastic large cell lymphoma, ALK-positive, lymph nodes of head, face, and neck
C84.62 Anaplastic large cell lymphoma, ALK-positive, intrathoracic lymph nodes
C84.63 Anaplastic large cell lymphoma, ALK-positive, intra-abdominal lymph nodes
C84.64 Anaplastic large cell lymphoma, ALK-positive, lymph nodes of axilla and upper limb
C84.65 Anaplastic large cell lymphoma, ALK-positive, lymph nodes of inguinal region and lower limb
C84.66 Anaplastic large cell lymphoma, ALK-positive, intrapelvic lymph nodes
C84.67 Anaplastic large cell lymphoma, ALK-positive, spleen
C84.68 Anaplastic large cell lymphoma, ALK-positive, lymph nodes of multiple sites
C84.69 Anaplastic large cell lymphoma, ALK-positive, extranodal and solid organ sites
C84.7Ø Anaplastic large cell lymphoma, ALK-negative, unspecified site
C84.71 Anaplastic large cell lymphoma, ALK-negative, lymph nodes of head, face, and neck
C84.72 Anaplastic large cell lymphoma, ALK-negative, intrathoracic lymph nodes
C84.73 Anaplastic large cell lymphoma, ALK-negative, intra-abdominal lymph nodes
C84.74 Anaplastic large cell lymphoma, ALK-negative, lymph nodes of axilla and upper limb
C84.75 Anaplastic large cell lymphoma, ALK-negative, lymph nodes of inguinal region and lower limb
C84.76 Anaplastic large cell lymphoma, ALK-negative, intrapelvic lymph nodes
C84.77 Anaplastic large cell lymphoma, ALK-negative, spleen
C84.78 Anaplastic large cell lymphoma, ALK-negative, lymph nodes of multiple sites
C84.79 Anaplastic large cell lymphoma, ALK-negative, extranodal and solid organ sites
C84.7A Anaplastic large cell lymphoma, ALK-negative, breast
C84.9Ø Mature T/NK-cell lymphomas, unspecified, unspecified site
C84.91 Mature T/NK-cell lymphomas, unspecified, lymph nodes of head, face, and neck
C84.92 Mature T/NK-cell lymphomas, unspecified, intrathoracic lymph nodes
C84.93 Mature T/NK-cell lymphomas, unspecified, intra-abdominal lymph nodes
C84.94 Mature T/NK-cell lymphomas, unspecified, lymph nodes of axilla and upper limb
C84.95 Mature T/NK-cell lymphomas, unspecified, lymph nodes of inguinal region and lower limb
C84.96 Mature T/NK-cell lymphomas, unspecified, intrapelvic lymph nodes
C84.97 Mature T/NK-cell lymphomas, unspecified, spleen
C84.98 Mature T/NK-cell lymphomas, unspecified, lymph nodes of multiple sites
C84.99 Mature T/NK-cell lymphomas, unspecified, extranodal and solid organ sites
C84.AØ Cutaneous T-cell lymphoma, unspecified, unspecified site
C84.A1 Cutaneous T-cell lymphoma, unspecified lymph nodes of head, face, and neck
C84.A2 Cutaneous T-cell lymphoma, unspecified, intrathoracic lymph nodes
C84.A3 Cutaneous T-cell lymphoma, unspecified, intra-abdominal lymph nodes
C84.A4 Cutaneous T-cell lymphoma, unspecified, lymph nodes of axilla and upper limb
C84.A5 Cutaneous T-cell lymphoma, unspecified, lymph nodes of inguinal region and lower limb
C84.A6 Cutaneous T-cell lymphoma, unspecified, intrapelvic lymph nodes
C84.A7 Cutaneous T-cell lymphoma, unspecified, spleen
C84.A8 Cutaneous T-cell lymphoma, unspecified, lymph nodes of multiple sites
C84.A9 Cutaneous T-cell lymphoma, unspecified, extranodal and solid organ sites
C84.ZØ Other mature T/NK-cell lymphomas, unspecified site
C84.Z1 Other mature T/NK-cell lymphomas, lymph nodes of head, face, and neck
C84.Z2 Other mature T/NK-cell lymphomas, intrathoracic lymph nodes
C84.Z3 Other mature T/NK-cell lymphomas, intra-abdominal lymph nodes
C84.Z4 Other mature T/NK-cell lymphomas, lymph nodes of axilla and upper limb
C84.Z5 Other mature T/NK-cell lymphomas, lymph nodes of inguinal region and lower limb
C84.Z6 Other mature T/NK-cell lymphomas, intrapelvic lymph nodes
C84.Z7 Other mature T/NK-cell lymphomas, spleen
C84.Z8 Other mature T/NK-cell lymphomas, lymph nodes of multiple sites
C84.Z9 Other mature T/NK-cell lymphomas, extranodal and solid organ sites
C85.1Ø Unspecified B-cell lymphoma, unspecified site
C85.11 Unspecified B-cell lymphoma, lymph nodes of head, face, and neck
C85.12 Unspecified B-cell lymphoma, intrathoracic lymph nodes
C85.13 Unspecified B-cell lymphoma, intra-abdominal lymph nodes
C85.14 Unspecified B-cell lymphoma, lymph nodes of axilla and upper limb
C85.15 Unspecified B-cell lymphoma, lymph nodes of inguinal region and lower limb
C85.16 Unspecified B-cell lymphoma, intrapelvic lymph nodes

C85.17 Unspecified B-cell lymphoma, spleen
C85.18 Unspecified B-cell lymphoma, lymph nodes of multiple sites
C85.19 Unspecified B-cell lymphoma, extranodal and solid organ sites
C85.20 Mediastinal (thymic) large B-cell lymphoma, unspecified site
C85.21 Mediastinal (thymic) large B-cell lymphoma, lymph nodes of head, face, and neck
C85.22 Mediastinal (thymic) large B-cell lymphoma, intrathoracic lymph nodes
C85.23 Mediastinal (thymic) large B-cell lymphoma, intra-abdominal lymph nodes
C85.24 Mediastinal (thymic) large B-cell lymphoma, lymph nodes of axilla and upper limb
C85.25 Mediastinal (thymic) large B-cell lymphoma, lymph nodes of inguinal region and lower limb
C85.26 Mediastinal (thymic) large B-cell lymphoma, intrapelvic lymph nodes
C85.27 Mediastinal (thymic) large B-cell lymphoma, spleen
C85.28 Mediastinal (thymic) large B-cell lymphoma, lymph nodes of multiple sites
C85.29 Mediastinal (thymic) large B-cell lymphoma, extranodal and solid organ sites
C85.80 Other specified types of non-Hodgkin lymphoma, unspecified site
C85.81 Other specified types of non-Hodgkin lymphoma, lymph nodes of head, face, and neck
C85.82 Other specified types of non-Hodgkin lymphoma, intrathoracic lymph nodes
C85.83 Other specified types of non-Hodgkin lymphoma, intra-abdominal lymph nodes
C85.84 Other specified types of non-Hodgkin lymphoma, lymph nodes of axilla and upper limb
C85.85 Other specified types of non-Hodgkin lymphoma, lymph nodes of inguinal region and lower limb
C85.86 Other specified types of non-Hodgkin lymphoma, intrapelvic lymph nodes
C85.87 Other specified types of non-Hodgkin lymphoma, spleen
C85.88 Other specified types of non-Hodgkin lymphoma, lymph nodes of multiple sites
C85.89 Other specified types of non-Hodgkin lymphoma, extranodal and solid organ sites
C85.90 Non-Hodgkin lymphoma, unspecified, unspecified site
C85.91 Non-Hodgkin lymphoma, unspecified, lymph nodes of head, face, and neck
C85.92 Non-Hodgkin lymphoma, unspecified, intrathoracic lymph nodes
C85.93 Non-Hodgkin lymphoma, unspecified, intra-abdominal lymph nodes
C85.94 Non-Hodgkin lymphoma, unspecified, lymph nodes of axilla and upper limb
C85.95 Non-Hodgkin lymphoma, unspecified, lymph nodes of inguinal region and lower limb
C85.96 Non-Hodgkin lymphoma, unspecified, intrapelvic lymph nodes
C85.97 Non-Hodgkin lymphoma, unspecified, spleen
C85.98 Non-Hodgkin lymphoma, unspecified, lymph nodes of multiple sites
C85.99 Non-Hodgkin lymphoma, unspecified, extranodal and solid organ sites
C86.0 Extranodal NK/T-cell lymphoma, nasal type
C86.1 Hepatosplenic T-cell lymphoma
C86.2 Enteropathy-type (intestinal) T-cell lymphoma
C86.3 Subcutaneous panniculitis-like T-cell lymphoma
C86.4 Blastic NK-cell lymphoma
C86.5 Angioimmunoblastic T-cell lymphoma
C86.6 Primary cutaneous CD30-positive T-cell proliferations
C88.4 Extranodal marginal zone B-cell lymphoma of mucosa-associated lymphoid tissue [MALT lymphoma]
F03.90 Unspecified dementia, unspecified severity, without behavioral disturbance, psychotic disturbance, mood disturbance, and anxiety
F06.70 Mild neurocognitive disorder due to known physiological condition without behavioral disturbance
F06.71 Mild neurocognitive disorder due to known physiological condition with behavioral disturbance
F06.8 Other specified mental disorders due to known physiological condition
F07.9 Unspecified personality and behavioral disorder due to known physiological condition
F09 Unspecified mental disorder due to known physiological condition
F28 Other psychotic disorder not due to a substance or known physiological condition
F29 Unspecified psychosis not due to a substance or known physiological condition
G04.81 Other encephalitis and encephalomyelitis
G04.89 Other myelitis
G04.90 Encephalitis and encephalomyelitis, unspecified
G04.91 Myelitis, unspecified
G36.9 Acute disseminated demyelination, unspecified
G37.4 Subacute necrotizing myelitis of central nervous system
G37.9 Demyelinating disease of central nervous system, unspecified
G93.40 Encephalopathy, unspecified
G93.41 Metabolic encephalopathy
G93.42 Megaloencephalic leukoencephalopathy with subcortical cysts
G93.43 Leukoencephalopathy with calcifications and cysts
G93.44 Adult-onset leukodystrophy with axonal spheroids
G93.49 Other encephalopathy
G93.9 Disorder of brain, unspecified
G95.20 Unspecified cord compression
G95.29 Other cord compression
G95.9 Disease of spinal cord, unspecified
G96.9 Disorder of central nervous system, unspecified
G98.8 Other disorders of nervous system
I33.0 Acute and subacute infective endocarditis
I33.9 Acute and subacute endocarditis, unspecified
I40.0 Infective myocarditis
I40.1 Isolated myocarditis
I40.8 Other acute myocarditis
I40.9 Acute myocarditis, unspecified
I67.3 Progressive vascular leukoencephalopathy
I67.83 Posterior reversible encephalopathy syndrome
J09.X1 Influenza due to identified novel influenza A virus with pneumonia
J10.08 Influenza due to other identified influenza virus with other specified pneumonia
J12.3 Human metapneumovirus pneumonia
J12.81 Pneumonia due to SARS-associated coronavirus
J12.82 Pneumonia due to coronavirus disease 2019
J12.89 Other viral pneumonia
J12.9 Viral pneumonia, unspecified
J13 Pneumonia due to Streptococcus pneumoniae
J14 Pneumonia due to Hemophilus influenzae
J15.0 Pneumonia due to Klebsiella pneumoniae
J15.1 Pneumonia due to Pseudomonas
J15.20 Pneumonia due to staphylococcus, unspecified
J15.211 Pneumonia due to Methicillin susceptible Staphylococcus aureus
J15.212 Pneumonia due to Methicillin resistant Staphylococcus aureus
J15.29 Pneumonia due to other staphylococcus
J15.3 Pneumonia due to streptococcus, group B
J15.4 Pneumonia due to other streptococci
J15.5 Pneumonia due to Escherichia coli
J15.61 Pneumonia due to Acinetobacter baumannii
J15.69 Pneumonia du to other Gram-negative bacteria
J15.8 Pneumonia due to other specified bacteria
J15.9 Unspecified bacterial pneumonia
J18.1 Lobar pneumonia, unspecified organism
J18.8 Other pneumonia, unspecified organism
J18.9 Pneumonia, unspecified organism
L08.1 Erythrasma
U07.1 COVID-19

Appendix D: Neonate Major Problems (Principal or Secondary Diagnosis)

E84.11 Meconium ileus in cystic fibrosis

PØ3.4 Newborn affected by Cesarean delivery

PØ5.11 Newborn small for gestational age, less than 5ØØ grams

PØ5.12 Newborn small for gestational age, 5ØØ-749 grams

PØ5.13 Newborn small for gestational age, 75Ø-999 grams

PØ5.14 Newborn small for gestational age, 1ØØØ-1249 grams

PØ5.15 Newborn small for gestational age, 125Ø-1499 grams

PØ5.16 Newborn small for gestational age, 15ØØ-1749 grams

PØ5.17 Newborn small for gestational age, 175Ø-1999 grams

PØ5.2 Newborn affected by fetal (intrauterine) malnutrition not light or small for gestational age

P1Ø.Ø Subdural hemorrhage due to birth injury

P1Ø.1 Cerebral hemorrhage due to birth injury

P1Ø.2 Intraventricular hemorrhage due to birth injury

P1Ø.3 Subarachnoid hemorrhage due to birth injury

P1Ø.4 Tentorial tear due to birth injury

P1Ø.8 Other intracranial lacerations and hemorrhages due to birth injury

P1Ø.9 Unspecified intracranial laceration and hemorrhage due to birth injury

P11.Ø Cerebral edema due to birth injury

P11.2 Unspecified brain damage due to birth injury

P11.4 Birth injury to other cranial nerves

P11.5 Birth injury to spine and spinal cord

P11.9 Birth injury to central nervous system, unspecified

P12.2 Epicranial subaponeurotic hemorrhage due to birth injury

P14.2 Phrenic nerve paralysis due to birth injury

P14.8 Birth injuries to other parts of peripheral nervous system

P14.9 Birth injury to peripheral nervous system, unspecified

P23.Ø Congenital pneumonia due to viral agent

P23.1 Congenital pneumonia due to Chlamydia

P23.2 Congenital pneumonia due to staphylococcus

P23.3 Congenital pneumonia due to streptococcus, group B

P23.4 Congenital pneumonia due to Escherichia coli

P23.5 Congenital pneumonia due to Pseudomonas

P23.6 Congenital pneumonia due to other bacterial agents

P23.8 Congenital pneumonia due to other organisms

P23.9 Congenital pneumonia, unspecified

P24.ØØ Meconium aspiration without respiratory symptoms

P24.Ø1 Meconium aspiration with respiratory symptoms

P24.1Ø Neonatal aspiration of (clear) amniotic fluid and mucus without respiratory symptoms

P24.11 Neonatal aspiration of (clear) amniotic fluid and mucus with respiratory symptoms

P24.2Ø Neonatal aspiration of blood without respiratory symptoms

P24.21 Neonatal aspiration of blood with respiratory symptoms

P24.3Ø Neonatal aspiration of milk and regurgitated food without respiratory symptoms

P24.31 Neonatal aspiration of milk and regurgitated food with respiratory symptoms

P24.8Ø Other neonatal aspiration without respiratory symptoms

P24.81 Other neonatal aspiration with respiratory symptoms

P24.9 Neonatal aspiration, unspecified

P25.Ø Interstitial emphysema originating in the perinatal period

P25.1 Pneumothorax originating in the perinatal period

P25.2 Pneumomediastinum originating in the perinatal period

P25.3 Pneumopericardium originating in the perinatal period

P25.8 Other conditions related to interstitial emphysema originating in the perinatal period

P26.Ø Tracheobronchial hemorrhage originating in the perinatal period

P26.1 Massive pulmonary hemorrhage originating in the perinatal period

P26.8 Other pulmonary hemorrhages originating in the perinatal period

P26.9 Unspecified pulmonary hemorrhage originating in the perinatal period

P28.Ø Primary atelectasis of newborn

P28.5 Respiratory failure of newborn

P29.3Ø Pulmonary hypertension of newborn

P29.38 Other persistent fetal circulation

P29.81 Cardiac arrest of newborn

P35.Ø Congenital rubella syndrome

P35.1 Congenital cytomegalovirus infection

P35.2 Congenital herpesviral [herpes simplex] infection

P35.3 Congenital viral hepatitis

P35.4 Congenital Zika virus disease

P35.8 Other congenital viral diseases

P35.9 Congenital viral disease, unspecified

P36.Ø Sepsis of newborn due to streptococcus, group B

P36.1Ø Sepsis of newborn due to unspecified streptococci

P36.19 Sepsis of newborn due to other streptococci

P36.2 Sepsis of newborn due to Staphylococcus aureus

P36.3Ø Sepsis of newborn due to unspecified staphylococci

P36.39 Sepsis of newborn due to other staphylococci

P36.4 Sepsis of newborn due to Escherichia coli

P36.5 Sepsis of newborn due to anaerobes

P36.8 Other bacterial sepsis of newborn

P36.9 Bacterial sepsis of newborn, unspecified

P37.Ø Congenital tuberculosis

P37.1 Congenital toxoplasmosis

P37.2 Neonatal (disseminated) listeriosis

P37.3 Congenital falciparum malaria

P37.4 Other congenital malaria

P37.8 Other specified congenital infectious and parasitic diseases

P37.9 Congenital infectious or parasitic disease, unspecified

P38.1 Omphalitis with mild hemorrhage

P38.9 Omphalitis without hemorrhage

P39.Ø Neonatal infective mastitis

P39.2 Intra-amniotic infection affecting newborn, not elsewhere classified

P39.3 Neonatal urinary tract infection

P39.4 Neonatal skin infection

P39.8 Other specified infections specific to the perinatal period

P39.9 Infection specific to the perinatal period, unspecified

P5Ø.Ø Newborn affected by intrauterine (fetal) blood loss from vasa previa

P5Ø.1 Newborn affected by intrauterine (fetal) blood loss from ruptured cord

P5Ø.2 Newborn affected by intrauterine (fetal) blood loss from placenta

P5Ø.3 Newborn affected by hemorrhage into co-twin

P5Ø.4 Newborn affected by hemorrhage into maternal circulation

P5Ø.5 Newborn affected by intrauterine (fetal) blood loss from cut end of co-twin's cord

P5Ø.8 Newborn affected by other intrauterine (fetal) blood loss

P5Ø.9 Newborn affected by intrauterine (fetal) blood loss, unspecified

P52.Ø Intraventricular (nontraumatic) hemorrhage, grade 1, of newborn

P52.1 Intraventricular (nontraumatic) hemorrhage, grade 2, of newborn

P52.21 Intraventricular (nontraumatic) hemorrhage, grade 3, of newborn

P52.22 Intraventricular (nontraumatic) hemorrhage, grade 4, of newborn

P52.3 Unspecified intraventricular (nontraumatic) hemorrhage of newborn

P52.4 Intracerebral (nontraumatic) hemorrhage of newborn

P52.5 Subarachnoid (nontraumatic) hemorrhage of newborn

P52.6 Cerebellar (nontraumatic) and posterior fossa hemorrhage of newborn

P52.8 Other intracranial (nontraumatic) hemorrhages of newborn

P52.9 Intracranial (nontraumatic) hemorrhage of newborn, unspecified

P53 Hemorrhagic disease of newborn

P54.1 Neonatal melena

P54.2 Neonatal rectal hemorrhage
P54.3 Other neonatal gastrointestinal hemorrhage
P54.4 Neonatal adrenal hemorrhage
P55.8 Other hemolytic diseases of newborn
P55.9 Hemolytic disease of newborn, unspecified
P56.Ø Hydrops fetalis due to isoimmunization
P56.9Ø Hydrops fetalis due to unspecified hemolytic disease
P56.99 Hydrops fetalis due to other hemolytic disease
P57.Ø Kernicterus due to isoimmunization
P57.8 Other specified kernicterus
P57.9 Kernicterus, unspecified
P59.1 Inspissated bile syndrome
P59.2Ø Neonatal jaundice from unspecified hepatocellular damage
P59.29 Neonatal jaundice from other hepatocellular damage
P6Ø Disseminated intravascular coagulation of newborn
P61.Ø Transient neonatal thrombocytopenia
P61.2 Anemia of prematurity
P61.6 Other transient neonatal disorders of coagulation
P7Ø.2 Neonatal diabetes mellitus
P7Ø.3 Iatrogenic neonatal hypoglycemia
P7Ø.4 Other neonatal hypoglycemia
P71.Ø Cow's milk hypocalcemia in newborn
P71.1 Other neonatal hypocalcemia
P71.2 Neonatal hypomagnesemia
P71.3 Neonatal tetany without calcium or magnesium deficiency
P71.4 Transitory neonatal hypoparathyroidism
P71.8 Other transitory neonatal disorders of calcium and magnesium metabolism
P71.9 Transitory neonatal disorder of calcium and magnesium metabolism, unspecified
P72.1 Transitory neonatal hyperthyroidism
P74.Ø Late metabolic acidosis of newborn
P74.1 Dehydration of newborn
P74.21 Hypernatremia of newborn
P74.22 Hyponatremia of newborn
P74.31 Hyperkalemia of newborn
P74.32 Hypokalemia of newborn
P74.421 Hyperchloremia of newborn
P74.422 Hypochloremia of newborn
P74.49 Other transitory electrolyte disturbance of newborn
P76.Ø Meconium plug syndrome
P76.2 Intestinal obstruction due to inspissated milk
P77.1 Stage 1 necrotizing enterocolitis in newborn
P77.2 Stage 2 necrotizing enterocolitis in newborn
P77.3 Stage 3 necrotizing enterocolitis in newborn
P77.9 Necrotizing enterocolitis in newborn, unspecified
P78.Ø Perinatal intestinal perforation
P83.2 Hydrops fetalis not due to hemolytic disease
P9Ø Convulsions of newborn
P91.Ø Neonatal cerebral ischemia
P91.1 Acquired periventricular cysts of newborn
P91.3 Neonatal cerebral irritability
P91.4 Neonatal cerebral depression
P91.5 Neonatal coma
P91.62 Moderate hypoxic ischemic encephalopathy [HIE]
P91.63 Severe hypoxic ischemic encephalopathy [HIE]
P91.811 Neonatal encephalopathy in diseases classified elsewhere
P91.819 Neonatal encephalopathy, unspecified
P91.821 Neonatal cerebral infarction, right side of brain
P91.822 Neonatal cerebral infarction, left side of brain
P91.823 Neonatal cerebral infarction, bilateral
P91.829 Neonatal cerebral infarction, unspecified side
P91.88 Other specified disturbances of cerebral status of newborn
P91.9 Disturbance of cerebral status of newborn, unspecified
P92.Ø1 Bilious vomiting of newborn
P93.Ø Grey baby syndrome
P93.8 Other reactions and intoxications due to drugs administered to newborn
P94.Ø Transient neonatal myasthenia gravis
P96.1 Neonatal withdrawal symptoms from maternal use of drugs of addiction
P96.2 Withdrawal symptoms from therapeutic use of drugs in newborn

Appendix E: Neonate Other Significant Problems (Principal or Secondary Diagnosis)

A33 Tetanus neonatorum

PØØ.Ø Newborn affected by maternal hypertensive disorders

PØØ.1 Newborn affected by maternal renal and urinary tract diseases

PØØ.4 Newborn affected by maternal nutritional disorders

PØØ.5 Newborn affected by maternal injury

PØØ.6 Newborn affected by surgical procedure on mother

PØØ.7 Newborn affected by other medical procedures on mother, not elsewhere classified

PØØ.81 Newborn affected by periodontal disease in mother

PØ1.Ø Newborn affected by incompetent cervix

PØ1.1 Newborn affected by premature rupture of membranes

PØ1.2 Newborn affected by oligohydramnios

PØ1.3 Newborn affected by polyhydramnios

PØ1.4 Newborn affected by ectopic pregnancy

PØ1.5 Newborn affected by multiple pregnancy

PØ1.6 Newborn affected by maternal death

PØ1.7 Newborn affected by malpresentation before labor

PØ1.8 Newborn affected by other maternal complications of pregnancy

PØ1.9 Newborn affected by maternal complication of pregnancy, unspecified

PØ2.Ø Newborn affected by placenta previa

PØ2.1 Newborn affected by other forms of placental separation and hemorrhage

PØ2.2Ø Newborn affected by unspecified morphological and functional abnormalities of placenta

PØ2.29 Newborn affected by other morphological and functional abnormalities of placenta

PØ2.3 Newborn affected by placental transfusion syndromes

PØ2.7Ø Newborn affected by fetal inflammatory response syndrome

PØ2.78 Newborn affected by other conditions from chorioamnionitis

PØ2.8 Newborn affected by other abnormalities of membranes

PØ2.9 Newborn affected by abnormality of membranes, unspecified

PØ3.6 Newborn affected by abnormal uterine contractions

PØ3.81Ø Newborn affected by abnormality in fetal (intrauterine) heart rate or rhythm before the onset of labor

PØ3.811 Newborn affected by abnormality in fetal (intrauterine) heart rate or rhythm during labor

PØ3.819 Newborn affected by abnormality in fetal (intrauterine) heart rate or rhythm, unspecified as to time of onset

PØ3.82 Meconium passage during delivery

PØ3.89 Newborn affected by other specified complications of labor and delivery

PØ4.Ø Newborn affected by maternal anesthesia and analgesia in pregnancy, labor and delivery

PØ4.11 Newborn affected by maternal antineoplastic chemotherapy

PØ4.12 Newborn affected by maternal cytotoxic drugs

PØ4.13 Newborn affected by maternal use of anticonvulsants

PØ4.14 Newborn affected by maternal use of opiates

PØ4.15 Newborn affected by maternal use of antidepressants

PØ4.16 Newborn affected by maternal use of amphetamines

PØ4.17 Newborn affected by maternal use of sedative-hypnotics

PØ4.18 Newborn affected by other maternal medication

PØ4.19 Newborn affected by maternal use of unspecified medication

PØ4.1A Newborn affected by maternal use of anxiolytics

PØ4.2 Newborn affected by maternal use of tobacco

PØ4.3 Newborn affected by maternal use of alcohol

PØ4.4Ø Newborn affected by maternal use of unspecified drugs of addition

PØ4.41 Newborn affected by maternal use of cocaine

PØ4.42 Newborn affected by maternal use of hallucinogens

PØ4.49 Newborn affected by maternal use of other drugs of addiction

PØ4.5 Newborn affected by maternal use of nutritional chemical substances

PØ4.6 Newborn affected by maternal exposure to environmental chemical substances

PØ4.81 Newborn affected by maternal use of cannabis

PØ4.89 Newborn affected by other maternal noxious substances

PØ4.9 Newborn affected by maternal noxious substance, unspecified

PØ5.ØØ Newborn light for gestational age, unspecified weight

PØ5.Ø1 Newborn light for gestational age, less than 5ØØ grams

PØ5.Ø2 Newborn light for gestational age, 5ØØ-749 grams

PØ5.Ø3 Newborn light for gestational age, 75Ø-999 grams

PØ5.Ø4 Newborn light for gestational age, 1ØØØ-1249 grams

PØ5.Ø5 Newborn light for gestational age, 125Ø-1499 grams

PØ5.Ø6 Newborn light for gestational age, 15ØØ-1749 grams

PØ5.Ø7 Newborn light for gestational age, 175Ø-1999 grams

PØ5.Ø9 Newborn light for gestational age, 25ØØ grams and over

PØ5.1Ø Newborn small for gestational age, unspecified weight

PØ5.19 Newborn small for gestational age, other

PØ5.9 Newborn affected by slow intrauterine growth, unspecified

P11.1 Other specified brain damage due to birth injury

P11.3 Birth injury to facial nerve

P13.Ø Fracture of skull due to birth injury

P13.1 Other birth injuries to skull

P13.2 Birth injury to femur

P13.3 Birth injury to other long bones

P13.4 Fracture of clavicle due to birth injury

P13.8 Birth injuries to other parts of skeleton

P13.9 Birth injury to skeleton, unspecified

P14.Ø Erb's paralysis due to birth injury

P14.1 Klumpke's paralysis due to birth injury

P14.3 Other brachial plexus birth injuries

P15.Ø Birth injury to liver

P15.1 Birth injury to spleen

P15.2 Sternomastoid injury due to birth injury

P15.3 Birth injury to eye

P15.4 Birth injury to face

P15.5 Birth injury to external genitalia

P15.6 Subcutaneous fat necrosis due to birth injury

P15.8 Other specified birth injuries

P15.9 Birth injury, unspecified

P19.Ø Metabolic acidemia in newborn first noted before onset of labor

P19.1 Metabolic acidemia in newborn first noted during labor

P19.2 Metabolic acidemia noted at birth

P19.9 Metabolic acidemia in newborn, unspecified

P22.1 Transient tachypnea of newborn

P22.8 Other respiratory distress of newborn

P22.9 Respiratory distress of newborn, unspecified

P28.1Ø Unspecified atelectasis of newborn

P28.11 Resorption atelectasis without respiratory distress syndrome

P28.19 Other atelectasis of newborn

P28.2 Cyanotic attacks of newborn

P28.3Ø Primary sleep apnea of newborn, unspecified

P28.31 Primary central sleep apnea of newborn

P28.32 Primary obstructive sleep apnea of newborn

P28.33 Primary mixed sleep apnea of newborn

P28.39 Other primary sleep apnea of newborn

P28.4Ø Unspecified apnea of newborn

P28.41 Central neonatal apnea of newborn

P28.42 Obstructive apnea of newborn

P28.43 Mixed neonatal apnea of newborn

P28.49 Other apnea of newborn

P28.4 Other apnea of newborn
P28.81 Respiratory arrest of newborn
P28.89 Other specified respiratory conditions of newborn
P28.9 Respiratory condition of newborn, unspecified
P29.Ø Neonatal cardiac failure
P29.11 Neonatal tachycardia
P29.12 Neonatal bradycardia
P29.2 Neonatal hypertension
P29.4 Transient myocardial ischemia in newborn
P29.89 Other cardiovascular disorders originating in the perinatal period
P29.9 Cardiovascular disorder originating in the perinatal period, unspecified
P37.5 Neonatal candidiasis
P39.1 Neonatal conjunctivitis and dacryocystitis
P51.Ø Massive umbilical hemorrhage of newborn
P51.8 Other umbilical hemorrhages of newborn
P51.9 Umbilical hemorrhage of newborn, unspecified
P54.Ø Neonatal hematemesis
P54.6 Neonatal vaginal hemorrhage
P54.8 Other specified neonatal hemorrhages
P54.9 Neonatal hemorrhage, unspecified
P55.Ø Rh isoimmunization of newborn
P55.1 ABO isoimmunization of newborn
P58.Ø Neonatal jaundice due to bruising
P58.1 Neonatal jaundice due to bleeding
P58.2 Neonatal jaundice due to infection
P58.3 Neonatal jaundice due to polycythemia
P58.41 Neonatal jaundice due to drugs or toxins transmitted from mother
P58.42 Neonatal jaundice due to drugs or toxins given to newborn
P58.5 Neonatal jaundice due to swallowed maternal blood
P58.8 Neonatal jaundice due to other specified excessive hemolysis
P58.9 Neonatal jaundice due to excessive hemolysis, unspecified
P59.Ø Neonatal jaundice associated with preterm delivery
P61.1 Polycythemia neonatorum
P61.3 Congenital anemia from fetal blood loss
P61.4 Other congenital anemias, not elsewhere classified
P61.5 Transient neonatal neutropenia
P61.8 Other specified perinatal hematological disorders
P61.9 Perinatal hematological disorder, unspecified
P7Ø.Ø Syndrome of infant of mother with gestational diabetes
P7Ø.1 Syndrome of infant of a diabetic mother
P7Ø.8 Other transitory disorders of carbohydrate metabolism of newborn
P7Ø.9 Transitory disorder of carbohydrate metabolism of newborn, unspecified
P72.Ø Neonatal goiter, not elsewhere classified
P72.2 Other transitory neonatal disorders of thyroid function, not elsewhere classified
P72.8 Other specified transitory neonatal endocrine disorders
P72.9 Transitory neonatal endocrine disorder, unspecified
P74.41 Alkalosis of newborn
P74.5 Transitory tyrosinemia of newborn
P74.6 Transitory hyperammonemia of newborn
P74.8 Other transitory metabolic disturbances of newborn
P74.9 Transitory metabolic disturbance of newborn, unspecified
P76.1 Transitory ileus of newborn
P76.8 Other specified intestinal obstruction of newborn
P76.9 Intestinal obstruction of newborn, unspecified
P78.1 Other neonatal peritonitis
P78.2 Neonatal hematemesis and melena due to swallowed maternal blood
P78.3 Noninfective neonatal diarrhea
P78.81 Congenital cirrhosis (of liver)
P78.82 Peptic ulcer of newborn
P78.83 Newborn esophageal reflux
P78.84 Gestational alloimmune liver disease
P78.89 Other specified perinatal digestive system disorders
P78.9 Perinatal digestive system disorder, unspecified
P8Ø.Ø Cold injury syndrome
P8Ø.8 Other hypothermia of newborn
P8Ø.9 Hypothermia of newborn, unspecified
P81.Ø Environmental hyperthermia of newborn
P81.8 Other specified disturbances of temperature regulation of newborn
P81.9 Disturbance of temperature regulation of newborn, unspecified
P83.Ø Sclerema neonatorum
P83.3Ø Unspecified edema specific to newborn
P83.39 Other edema specific to newborn
P83.4 Breast engorgement of newborn
P83.5 Congenital hydrocele
P83.9 Condition of the integument specific to newborn, unspecified
P84 Other problems with newborn
P91.6Ø Hypoxic ischemic encephalopathy [HIE], unspecified
P91.61 Mild hypoxic ischemic encephalopathy [HIE]
P94.1 Congenital hypertonia
P94.2 Congenital hypotonia
P94.8 Other disorders of muscle tone of newborn
P94.9 Disorder of muscle tone of newborn, unspecified
P95 Stillbirth
P96.Ø Congenital renal failure
P96.3 Wide cranial sutures of newborn
P96.5 Complication to newborn due to (fetal) intrauterine procedure
P96.81 Exposure to (parental) (environmental) tobacco smoke in the perinatal period
P96.83 Meconium staining
P96.89 Other specified conditions originating in the perinatal period
P96.9 Condition originating in the perinatal period, unspecified
Q86.Ø Fetal alcohol syndrome (dysmorphic)
Q86.1 Fetal hydantoin syndrome
Q86.2 Dysmorphism due to warfarin
Q86.8 Other congenital malformation syndromes due to known exogenous causes

Appendix F: Root Operation Definitions

Ø Medical and Surgical

ICD-10-PCS Value		Definition	
Ø	Alteration	Definition:	Modifying the anatomic structure of a body part without affecting the function of the body part
		Explanation:	Principal purpose is to improve appearance
		Examples:	Face lift, breast augmentation
1	Bypass	Definition:	Altering the route of passage of the contents of a tubular body part
		Explanation:	Rerouting contents of a body part to a downstream area of the normal route, to a similar route and body part, or to an abnormal route and dissimilar body part. Includes one or more anastomoses, with or without the use of a device.
		Examples:	Coronary artery bypass, colostomy formation
2	Change	Definition:	Taking out or off a device from a body part and putting back an identical or similar device in or on the same body part without cutting or puncturing the skin or a mucous membrane
		Explanation:	All CHANGE procedures are coded using the approach EXTERNAL
		Examples:	Urinary catheter change, gastrostomy tube change
3	Control	Definition:	Stopping, or attempting to stop, postprocedural or other acute bleeding
		Explanation:	None
		Examples:	Control of post-prostatectomy hemorrhage, control of intracranial subdural hemorrhage, control of bleeding duodenal ulcer, control of retroperitoneal hemorrhage
4	Creation	Definition:	Putting in or on biological or synthetic material to form a new body part that to the extent possible replicates the anatomic structure or function of an absent body part
		Explanation:	Used for gender reassignment surgery and corrective procedures in individuals with congenital anomalies
		Examples:	Creation of vagina in a male, creation of right and left atrioventricular valve from common atrioventricular valve
5	Destruction	Definition:	Physical eradication of all or a portion of a body part by the direct use of energy, force, or a destructive agent
		Explanation:	None of the body part is physically taken out
		Examples:	Fulguration of rectal polyp, cautery of skin lesion
6	Detachment	Definition:	Cutting off all or a portion of the upper or lower extremities
		Explanation:	The body part value is the site of the detachment, with a qualifier if applicable to further specify the level where the extremity was detached
		Examples:	Below knee amputation, disarticulation of shoulder
7	Dilation	Definition:	Expanding an orifice or the lumen of a tubular body part
		Explanation:	The orifice can be a natural orifice or an artificially created orifice. Accomplished by stretching a tubular body part using intraluminal pressure or by cutting part of the orifice or wall of the tubular body part.
		Examples:	Percutaneous transluminal angioplasty, internal urethrotomy
8	Division	Definition:	Cutting into a body part, without draining fluids and/or gases from the body part, in order to separate or transect a body part
		Explanation:	All or a portion of the body part is separated into two or more portions
		Examples:	Spinal cordotomy, osteotomy
9	Drainage	Definition:	Taking or letting out fluids and/or gases from a body part
		Explanation:	The qualifier DIAGNOSTIC is used to identify drainage procedures that are biopsies
		Examples:	Thoracentesis, incision and drainage
B	Excision	Definition:	Cutting out or off, without replacement, a portion of a body part
		Explanation:	The qualifier DIAGNOSTIC is used to identify excision procedures that are biopsies
		Examples:	Partial nephrectomy, liver biopsy
C	Extirpation	Definition:	Taking or cutting out solid matter from a body part
		Explanation:	The solid matter may be an abnormal byproduct of a biological function or a foreign body; it may be imbedded in a body part or in the lumen of a tubular body part. The solid matter may or may not have been previously broken into pieces.
		Examples:	Thrombectomy, choledocholithotomy

Continued on next page

Ø	Medical and Surgical		(Continued)
ICD-10-PCS Value		**Definition**	
D	Extraction	Definition:	Pulling or stripping out or off all or a portion of a body part by the use of force
		Explanation:	The qualifier DIAGNOSTIC is used to identify extractions that are biopsies
		Examples:	Dilation and curettage, vein stripping
F	Fragmentation	Definition:	Breaking solid matter in a body part into pieces
		Explanation:	Physical force (e.g., manual, ultrasonic) applied directly or indirectly is used to break the solid matter into pieces. The solid matter may be an abnormal byproduct of a biological function or a foreign body. The pieces of solid matter are not taken out.
		Examples:	Extracorporeal shockwave lithotripsy, transurethral lithotripsy
G	Fusion	Definition:	Joining together portions of an articular body part rendering the articular body part immobile
		Explanation:	The body part is joined together by fixation device, bone graft, or other means
		Examples:	Spinal fusion, ankle arthrodesis
H	Insertion	Definition:	Putting in a nonbiological appliance that monitors, assists, performs, or prevents a physiological function but does not physically take the place of a body part
		Explanation:	None
		Examples:	Insertion of radioactive implant, insertion of central venous catheter
J	Inspection	Definition:	Visually and/or manually exploring a body part
		Explanation:	Visual exploration may be performed with or without optical instrumentation. Manual exploration may be performed directly or through intervening body layers.
		Examples:	Diagnostic arthroscopy, exploratory laparotomy
K	Map	Definition:	Locating the route of passage of electrical impulses and/or locating functional areas in a body part
		Explanation:	Applicable only to the cardiac conduction mechanism and the central nervous system
		Examples:	Cardiac mapping, cortical mapping
L	Occlusion	Definition:	Completely closing an orifice or lumen of a tubular body part
		Explanation:	The orifice can be a natural orifice or an artificially created orifice
		Examples:	Fallopian tube ligation, ligation of inferior vena cava
M	Reattachment	Definition:	Putting back in or on all or a portion of a separated body part to its normal location or other suitable location
		Explanation:	Vascular circulation and nervous pathways may or may not be reestablished
		Examples:	Reattachment of hand, reattachment of avulsed kidney
N	Release	Definition:	Freeing a body part from an abnormal physical constraint by cutting or by use of force
		Explanation:	Some of the restraining tissue may be taken out but none of the body part is taken out
		Examples:	Adhesiolysis, carpal tunnel release
P	Removal	Definition:	Taking out or off a device from a body part
		Explanation:	If a device is taken out and a similar device put in without cutting or puncturing the skin or mucous membrane, the procedure is coded to the root operation CHANGE. Otherwise, the procedure for taking out a device is coded to the root operation REMOVAL.
		Examples:	Drainage tube removal, cardiac pacemaker removal
Q	Repair	Definition:	Restoring, to the extent possible, a body part to its normal anatomic structure and function
		Explanation:	Used only when the method to accomplish the repair is not one of the other root operations
		Examples:	Colostomy takedown, suture of laceration
R	Replacement	Definition:	Putting in or on biological or synthetic material that physically takes the place and/or function of all or a portion of a body part
		Explanation:	The body part may have been taken out or replaced, or may be taken out, physically eradicated, or rendered nonfunctional during the REPLACEMENT procedure. A REMOVAL procedure is coded for taking out the device used in a previous replacement procedure.
		Examples:	Total hip replacement, bone graft, free skin graft
S	Reposition	Definition:	Moving to its normal location, or other suitable location, all or a portion of a body part
		Explanation:	The body part is moved to a new location from an abnormal location, or from a normal location where it is not functioning correctly. The body part may or may not be cut out or off to be moved to the new location.
		Examples:	Reposition of undescended testicle, fracture reduction

Continued on next page

Ø	Medical and Surgical		(Continued)
ICD-10-PCS Value		**Definition**	
T	Resection	Definition:	Cutting out or off, without replacement, all of a body part
		Explanation:	None
		Examples:	Total nephrectomy, total lobectomy of lung
V	Restriction	Definition:	Partially closing an orifice or the lumen of a tubular body part
		Explanation:	The orifice can be a natural orifice or an artificially created orifice
		Examples:	Esophagogastric fundoplication, cervical cerclage
W	Revision	Definition:	Correcting, to the extent possible, a portion of a malfunctioning device or the position of a displaced device
		Explanation:	Revision can include correcting a malfunctioning or displaced device by taking out or putting in components of the device such as a screw or pin
		Examples:	Adjustment of position of pacemaker lead, recementing of hip prosthesis
U	Supplement	Definition:	Putting in or on biological or synthetic material that physically reinforces and/or augments the function of a portion of a body part
		Explanation:	The biological material is non-living, or is living and from the same individual. The body part may have been previously replaced, and the SUPPLEMENT procedure is performed to physically reinforce and/or augment the function of the replaced body part.
		Examples:	Herniorrhaphy using mesh, mitral valve ring annuloplasty, put a new acetabular liner in a previous hip replacement
X	Transfer	Definition:	Moving, without taking out, all or a portion of a body part to another location to take over the function of all or a portion of a body part
		Explanation:	The body part transferred remains connected to its vascular and nervous supply
		Examples:	Tendon transfer, skin pedicle flap transfer
Y	Transplantation	Definition:	Putting in or on all or a portion of a living body part taken from another individual or animal to physically take the place and/or function of all or a portion of a similar body part
		Explanation:	The native body part may or may not be taken out, and the transplanted body part may take over all or a portion of its function
		Examples:	Kidney transplant, heart transplant

Root Operation Definitions for Other Sections

1	Obstetrics		
ICD-10-PCS Value		**Definition**	
2	Change	Definition:	Taking out or off a device from a body part and putting back an identical or similar device in or on the same body part without cutting or puncturing the skin or a mucous membrane
		Explanation:	None
		Example:	Replacement of fetal scalp electrode
9	Drainage	Definition:	Taking or letting out fluids and/or gases from a body part
		Explanation:	None
		Example:	Biopsy of amniotic fluid
A	Abortion	Definition:	Artificially terminating a pregnancy
		Explanation:	None
		Example:	Transvaginal abortion using vacuum aspiration technique
D	Extraction	Definition:	Pulling or stripping out or off all or a portion of a body part by the use of force
		Explanation:	None
		Example:	Low-transverse C-section
E	Delivery	Definition:	Assisting the passage of the products of conception from the genital canal
		Explanation:	None
		Example:	Manually-assisted delivery
H	Insertion	Definition:	Putting in a nonbiological appliance that monitors, assists, performs, or prevents a physiological function but does not physically take the place of a body part
		Explanation:	None
		Example:	Placement of fetal scalp electrode

Continued on next page

1 Obstetrics (Continued)

ICD-10-PCS Value		Definition	
J	Inspection	Definition:	Visually and/or manually exploring a body part
		Explanation:	Visual exploration may be performed with or without optical instrumentation. Manual exploration may be performed directly or through intervening body layers.
		Example:	Bimanual pregnancy exam
P	Removal	Definition:	Taking out or off a device from a body part, region or orifice
		Explanation:	If a device is taken out and a similar device put in without cutting or puncturing the skin or mucous membrane, the procedure is coded to the root operation CHANGE. Otherwise, the procedure for taking out a device is coded to the root operation REMOVAL.
		Example:	Removal of fetal monitoring electrode
Q	Repair	Definition:	Restoring, to the extent possible, a body part to its normal anatomic structure and function
		Explanation:	Used only when the method to accomplish the repair is not one of the other root operations
		Example:	In utero repair of congenital diaphragmatic hernia
S	Reposition	Definition:	Moving to its normal location, or other suitable location, all or a portion of a body part
		Explanation:	The body part is moved to a new location from an abnormal location, or from a normal location where it is not functioning correctly. The body part may or may not be cut out or off to be moved to the new location.
		Example:	External version of fetus
T	Resection	Definition:	Cutting out or off, without replacement, all of a body part
		Explanation:	None
		Example:	Total excision of tubal pregnancy
Y	Transplantation	Definition:	Putting in or on all or a portion of a living body part taken from another individual or animal to physically take the place and/or function of all or a portion of a similar body part
		Explanation:	The native body part may or may not be taken out, and the transplanted body part may take over all or a portion of its function
		Example:	In utero fetal kidney transplant

2 Placement

ICD-10-PCS Value		Definition	
Ø	Change	Definition:	Taking out or off a device from a body part and putting back an identical or similar device in or on the same body part without cutting or puncturing the skin or a mucous membrane
		Example:	Change of vaginal packing
1	Compression	Definition:	Putting pressure on a body region
		Example:	Placement of pressure dressing on abdominal wall
2	Dressing	Definition:	Putting material on a body region for protection
		Example:	Application of sterile dressing to head wound
3	Immobilization	Definition:	Limiting or preventing motion of a body region
		Example:	Placement of splint on left finger
4	Packing	Definition:	Putting material in a body region or orifice
		Example:	Placement of nasal packing
5	Removal	Definition:	Taking out or off a device from a body part
		Example:	Removal of stereotactic head frame
6	Traction	Definition:	Exerting a pulling force on a body region in a distal direction
		Example:	Lumbar traction using motorized split-traction table

3 Administration

ICD-10-PCS Value		Definition	
Ø	Introduction	Definition:	Putting in or on a therapeutic, diagnostic, nutritional, physiological, or prophylactic substance except blood or blood products
		Example:	Nerve block injection to median nerve
1	Irrigation	Definition:	Putting in or on a cleansing substance
		Example:	Flushing of eye
2	Transfusion	Definition:	Putting in blood or blood products
		Example:	Transfusion of cell saver red cells into central venous line

4 Measurement and Monitoring

ICD-10-PCS Value		Definition	
Ø	Measurement	Definition:	Determining the level of a physiological or physical function at a point in time
		Example:	External electrocardiogram(EKG), single reading
1	Monitoring	Definition:	Determining the level of a physiological or physical function repetitively over a period of time
		Example:	Urinary pressure monitoring

5 Extracorporeal or Systemic Assistance and Performance

ICD-10-PCS Value		Definition	
Ø	Assistance	Definition:	Taking over a portion of a physiological function by extracorporeal means
		Example:	Hyperbaric oxygenation of wound
1	Performance	Definition:	Completely taking over a physiological function by extracorporeal means
		Example:	Cardiopulmonary bypass in conjunction with CABG
2	Restoration	Definition:	Returning, or attempting to return, a physiological function to its original state by extracorporeal means
		Example:	Attempted cardiac defibrillation, unsuccessful

6 Extracorporeal or Systemic Therapies

ICD-10-PCS Value		Definition	
Ø	Atmospheric Control	Definition:	Extracorporeal control of atmospheric pressure and composition
		Example:	Antigen-free air conditioning, series treatment
1	Decompression	Definition:	Extracorporeal elimination of undissolved gas from body fluids
		Example:	Hyperbaric decompression treatment, single
2	Electromagnetic Therapy	Definition:	Extracorporeal treatment by electromagnetic rays
		Example:	TMS (transcranial magnetic stimulation), series treatment
3	Hyperthermia	Definition:	Extracorporeal raising of body temperature
		Example:	None
4	Hypothermia	Definition:	Extracorporeal lowering of body temperature
		Example:	Whole body hypothermia treatment for temperature imbalances, series
5	Pheresis	Definition:	Extracorporeal separation of blood products
		Example:	Therapeutic leukopheresis, single treatment
6	Phototherapy	Definition:	Extracorporeal treatment by light rays
		Example:	Phototherapy of circulatory system, series treatment
7	Ultrasound Therapy	Definition:	Extracorporeal treatment by ultrasound
		Example:	Therapeutic ultrasound of peripheral vessels, single treatment
8	Ultraviolet Light Therapy	Definition:	Extracorporeal treatment by ultraviolet light
		Example:	Ultraviolet light phototherapy, series treatment
9	Shock Wave Therapy	Definition:	Extracorporeal treatment by shock waves
		Example:	Shockwave therapy of plantar fascia, single treatment
B	Perfusion	Definition:	Extracorporeal treatment by diffusion of therapeutic fluid
		Example:	Perfusion of donor liver while preparing transplant patient

7 Osteopathic

ICD-10-PCS Value		Definition	
Ø	Treatment	Definition:	Manual treatment to eliminate or alleviate somatic dysfunction and related disorders
		Examples:	Fascial release of abdomen, osteopathic treatment

8 Other Procedures

ICD-10-PCS Value		Definition	
Ø	Other Procedures	Definition:	Methodologies which attempt to remediate or cure a disorder or disease
		Examples:	Acupuncture, yoga therapy

9 Chiropractic

ICD-10-PCS Value		Definition	
B	Manipulation	Definition:	Manual procedure that involves a directed thrust to move a joint past the physiological range of motion, without exceeding the anatomical limit
		Example:	Chiropractic treatment of cervical spine, short lever specific contact

Appendix G: Body Part Key

Term	ICD-10-PCS Value
Abdominal aortic plexus	Abdominal Sympathetic Nerve
Abdominal cavity	Peritoneal Cavity
Abdominal esophagus	Esophagus, Lower
Abductor hallucis muscle	Foot Muscle, Right
	Foot Muscle, Left
Accessory cephalic vein	Cephalic Vein, Right
	Cephalic Vein, Left
Accessory obturator nerve	Lumbar Plexus
Accessory phrenic nerve	Phrenic nerve
Accessory spleen	Spleen
Acetabulofemoral joint	Hip Joint, Right
	Hip Joint, Left
Achilles tendon	Lower Leg Tendon, Right
	Lower Leg Tendon, Left
Acromioclavicular ligament	Shoulder Bursa and Ligament, Right
	Shoulder Bursa and Ligament, Left
Acromion (process)	Scapula, Right
	Scapula, Left
Adductor brevis muscle	Upper Leg Muscle, Right
	Upper Leg Muscle, Left
Adductor hallucis muscle	Foot Muscle, Right
	Foot Muscle, Left
Adductor longus muscle	Upper Leg Muscle, Right
	Upper Leg Muscle, Left
Adductor magnus muscle	Upper Leg Muscle, Right
	Upper Leg Muscle, Left
Adenohypophysis	Pituitary Gland
Alar ligament of axis	Head and Neck Bursa and Ligament
Alveolar process of mandible	Mandible, Right
	Mandible, Left
Alveolar process of maxilla	Maxilla
Anal orifice	Anus
Anatomical snuffbox	Lower Arm and Wrist Muscle, Right
	Lower Arm and Wrist Muscle, Left
Angular artery	Face Artery
Angular vein	Face Vein, Right
	Face Vein, Left
Annular ligament	Elbow Bursa and Ligament, Right
	Elbow Bursa and Ligament, Left
Anorectal junction	Rectum
Ansa cervicalis	Cervical Plexus
Antebrachial fascia	Subcutaneous Tissue and Fascia, Right Lower Arm
	Subcutaneous Tissue and Fascia, Left Lower Arm
Anterior (pectoral) lymph node	Lymphatic, Right Axillary
	Lymphatic, Left Axillary
Anterior cerebral artery	Intracranial Artery
Anterior cerebral vein	Intracranial Vein
Anterior choroidal artery	Intracranial Artery
Anterior circumflex humeral artery	Axillary Artery, Right
	Axillary Artery, Left
Anterior communicating artery	Intracranial Artery

Term	ICD-10-PCS Value
Anterior cruciate ligament (ACL)	Knee Bursa and Ligament, Right
	Knee Bursa and Ligament, Left
Anterior crural nerve	Femoral Nerve
Anterior facial vein	Face Vein, Right
	Face Vein, Left
Anterior intercostal artery	Internal Mammary Artery, Right
	Internal Mammary Artery, Left
Anterior interosseous nerve	Median Nerve
Anterior lateral malleolar artery	Anterior Tibial Artery, Right
	Anterior Tibial Artery, Left
Anterior lingual gland	Minor Salivary Gland
Anterior medial malleolar artery	Anterior Tibial Artery, Right
	Anterior Tibial Artery, Left
Anterior spinal artery	Vertebral Artery, Right
	Vertebral Artery, Left
Anterior tibial recurrent artery	Anterior Tibial Artery, Right
	Anterior Tibial Artery, Left
Anterior ulnar recurrent artery	Ulnar Artery, Right
	Ulnar Artery, Left
Anterior vagal trunk	Vagus Nerve
Anterior vertebral muscle	Neck Muscle, Right
	Neck Muscle, Left
Antihelix	External Ear, Right
	External Ear, Left
	External Ear, Bilateral
Antitragus	External Ear, Right
	External Ear, Left
	External Ear, Bilateral
Antrum of Highmore	Maxillary Sinus, Right
	Maxillary Sinus, Left
Aortic annulus	Aortic Valve
Aortic arch	Thoracic Aorta, Ascending/Arch
Aortic intercostal artery	Upper Artery
Apical (subclavicular) lymph node	Lymphatic, Right Axillary
	Lymphatic, Left Axillary
Apneustic center	Pons
Appendiceal orifice	Appendix
Aqueduct of Sylvius	Cerebral Ventricle
Aqueous humour	Anterior Chamber, Right
	Anterior Chamber, Left
Arachnoid mater, intracranial	Cerebral Meninges
Arachnoid mater, spinal	Spinal Meninges
Arcuate artery	Foot Artery, Right
	Foot Artery, Left
Areola	Nipple, Right
	Nipple, Left
Arterial canal (duct)	Pulmonary Artery, Left
Aryepiglottic fold	Larynx
Arytenoid cartilage	Larynx
Arytenoid muscle	Neck Muscle, Right
	Neck Muscle, Left
Ascending aorta	Thoracic Aorta, Ascending/Arch
Ascending palatine artery	Face Artery

Term	ICD-10-PCS Value
Ascending pharyngeal artery	External Carotid Artery, Right
	External Carotid Artery, Left
Atlantoaxial joint	Cervical Vertebral Joint
Atrioventricular node	Conduction Mechanism
Atrium dextrum cordis	Atrium, Right
Atrium pulmonale	Atrium, Left
Auditory tube	Eustachian Tube, Right
	Eustachian Tube, Left
Auerbach's (myenteric) plexus	Abdominal Sympathetic Nerve
Auricle	External Ear, Right
	External Ear, Left
	External Ear, Bilateral
Auricularis muscle	Head Muscle
Axillary fascia	Subcutaneous Tissue and Fascia, Right Upper Arm
	Subcutaneous Tissue and Fascia, Left Upper Arm
Axillary nerve	Brachial Plexus
Bartholin's (greater vestibular) gland	Vestibular Gland
Basal (internal) cerebral vein	Intracranial Vein
Basal nuclei	Basal Ganglia
Base of tongue	Pharynx
Basilar artery	Intracranial Artery
Basis pontis	Pons
Biceps brachii muscle	Upper Arm Muscle, Right
	Upper Arm Muscle, Left
Biceps femoris muscle	Upper Leg Muscle, Right
	Upper Leg Muscle, Left
Bicipital aponeurosis	Subcutaneous Tissue and Fascia, Right Lower Arm
	Subcutaneous Tissue and Fascia, Left Lower Arm
Bicuspid valve	Mitral Valve
Body of femur	Femoral Shaft, Right
	Femoral Shaft, Left
Body of fibula	Fibula, Right
	Fibula, Left
Bony labyrinth	Inner Ear, Right
	Inner Ear, Left
Bony orbit	Orbit, Right
	Orbit, Left
Bony vestibule	Inner Ear, Right
	Inner Ear, Left
Botallo's duct	Pulmonary Artery, Left
Brachial (lateral) lymph node	Lymphatic, Right Axillary
	Lymphatic, Left Axillary
Brachialis muscle	Upper Arm Muscle, Right
	Upper Arm Muscle, Left
Brachiocephalic artery	Innominate Artery
Brachiocephalic trunk	Innominate Artery
Brachiocephalic vein	Innominate Vein, Right
	Innominate Vein, Left
Brachioradialis muscle	Lower Arm and Wrist Muscle, Right
	Lower Arm and Wrist Muscle, Left
Breast procedures, skin only	Skin, Chest
Broad ligament	Uterine Supporting Structure

Term	ICD-10-PCS Value
Bronchial artery	Upper Artery
Bronchus intermedius	Main Bronchus, Right
Buccal gland	Buccal Mucosa
Buccinator lymph node	Lymphatic, Head
Buccinator muscle	Facial Muscle
Bulbospongiosus muscle	Perineum Muscle
Bulbourethral (Cowper's) gland	Urethra
Bundle of His	Conduction Mechanism
Bundle of Kent	Conduction Mechanism
Calcaneocuboid joint	Tarsal Joint, Right
	Tarsal Joint, Left
Calcaneocuboid ligament	Foot Bursa and Ligament, Right
	Foot Bursa and Ligament, Left
Calcaneofibular ligament	Ankle Bursa and Ligament, Right
	Ankle Bursa and Ligament, Left
Calcaneus	Tarsal, Right
	Tarsal, Left
Capitate bone	Carpal, Right
	Carpal, Left
Cardia	Esophagogastric Junction
Cardiac plexus	Thoracic Sympathetic Nerve
Cardioesophageal junction	Esophagogastric Junction
Caroticotympanic artery	Internal Carotid Artery, Right
	Internal Carotid Artery, Left
Carotid glomus	Carotid Body, Right
	Carotid Body, Left
	Carotid Bodies, Bilateral
Carotid sinus	Internal Carotid Artery, Right
	Internal Carotid Artery, Left
Carotid sinus nerve	Glossopharyngeal Nerve
Carpometacarpal ligament	Hand Bursa and Ligament, Right
	Hand Bursa and Ligament, Left
Cauda equina	Lumbar Spinal Cord
Cavernous plexus	Head and Neck Sympathetic Nerve
Cavoatrial junction	Superior Vena Cava
Celiac ganglion	Abdominal Sympathetic Nerve
Celiac (solar) plexus	Abdominal Sympathetic Nerve
Celiac lymph node	Lymphatic, Aortic
Celiac trunk	Celiac Artery
Central axillary lymph node	Lymphatic, Right Axillary
	Lymphatic, Left Axillary
Cerebral aqueduct (Sylvius)	Cerebral Ventricle
Cerebrum	Brain
Cervical esophagus	Esophagus, Upper
Cervical facet joint	Cervical Vertebral Joint
	Cervical Vertebral Joints, 2 or more
Cervical ganglion	Head and Neck Sympathetic Nerve
Cervical interspinous ligament	Head and Neck Bursa and Ligament
Cervical intertransverse ligament	Head and Neck Bursa and Ligament
Cervical ligamentum flavum	Head and Neck Bursa and Ligament
Cervical lymph node	Lymphatic, Right Neck
	Lymphatic, Left Neck
Cervicothoracic facet joint	Cervicothoracic Vertebral Joint
Chin	Subcutaneous Tissue and Fascia, Face
Choana	Nasopharynx
Chondroglossus muscle	Tongue, Palate, Pharynx Muscle

Term	ICD-10-PCS Value
Chorda tympani	Facial Nerve
Choroid plexus	Cerebral Ventricle
Ciliary body	Eye, Right
	Eye, Left
Ciliary ganglion	Head and Neck Sympathetic Nerve
Circle of Willis	Intracranial Artery
Circumflex iliac artery	Femoral Artery, Right
	Femoral Artery, Left
Claustrum	Basal Ganglia
Coccygeal body	Coccygeal Glomus
Coccygeus muscle	Trunk Muscle, Right
	Trunk Muscle, Left
Cochlea	Inner Ear, Right
	Inner Ear, Left
Cochlear nerve	Acoustic Nerve
Columella	Nasal Mucosa and Soft Tissue
Common digital vein	Foot Vein, Right
	Foot Vein, Left
Common facial vein	Face Vein, Right
	Face Vein, Left
Common fibular nerve	Peroneal Nerve
Common hepatic artery	Hepatic Artery
Common iliac (subaortic) lymph node	Lymphatic, Pelvis
Common interosseous artery	Ulnar Artery, Right
	Ulnar Artery, Left
Common peroneal nerve	Peroneal Nerve
Condyloid process	Mandible, Right
	Mandible, Left
Conus arteriosus	Ventricle, Right
Conus medullaris	Lumbar Spinal Cord
Coracoacromial ligament	Shoulder Bursa and Ligament, Right
	Shoulder Bursa and Ligament, Left
Coracobrachialis muscle	Upper Arm Muscle, Right
	Upper Arm Muscle, Left
Coracoclavicular ligament	Shoulder Bursa and Ligament, Right
	Shoulder Bursa and Ligament, Left
Coracohumeral ligament	Shoulder Bursa and Ligament, Right
	Shoulder Bursa and Ligament, Left
Coracoid process	Scapula, Right
	Scapula, Left
Corniculate cartilage	Larynx
Corpus callosum	Brain
Corpus cavernosum	Penis
Corpus spongiosum	Penis
Corpus striatum	Basal Ganglia
Corrugator supercilii muscle	Facial Muscle
Costocervical trunk	Subclavian Artery, Right
	Subclavian Artery, Left
Costoclavicular ligament	Shoulder Bursa and Ligament, Right
	Shoulder Bursa and Ligament, Left
Costotransverse joint	Thoracic Vertebral Joint
Costotransverse ligament	Rib(s) Bursa and Ligament
Costovertebral joint	Thoracic Vertebral Joint
Costoxiphoid ligament	Sternum Bursa and Ligament
Cowper's (bulbourethral) gland	Urethra
Cremaster muscle	Perineum Muscle

Term	ICD-10-PCS Value
Cribriform plate	Ethmoid Bone, Right
	Ethmoid Bone, Left
Cricoid cartilage	Trachea
Cricothyroid artery	Thyroid Artery, Right
	Thyroid Artery, Left
Cricothyroid muscle	Neck Muscle, Right
	Neck Muscle, Left
Crural fascia	Subcutaneous Tissue and Fascia, Right Upper Leg
	Subcutaneous Tissue and Fascia, Left Upper Leg
Cubital lymph node	Lymphatic, Right Upper Extremity
	Lymphatic, Left Upper Extremity
Cubital nerve	Ulnar Nerve
Cuboid bone	Tarsal, Right
	Tarsal, Left
Cuboideonavicular joint	Tarsal Joint, Right
	Tarsal Joint, Left
Culmen	Cerebellum
Cuneiform cartilage	Larynx
Cuneonavicular joint	Tarsal Joint, Right
	Tarsal Joint, Left
Cuneonavicular ligament	Foot Bursa and Ligament, Right
	Foot Bursa and Ligament, Left
Cutaneous (transverse) cervical nerve	Cervical Plexus
Deep cervical fascia	Subcutaneous Tissue and Fascia, Right Neck
	Subcutaneous Tissue and Fascia, Left Neck
Deep cervical vein	Vertebral Vein, Right
	Vertebral Vein, Left
Deep circumflex iliac artery	External Iliac Artery, Right
	External Iliac Artery, Left
Deep facial vein	Face Vein, Right
	Face Vein, Left
Deep femoral artery	Femoral Artery, Right
	Femoral Artery, Left
Deep femoral (profunda femoris) vein	Femoral Vein, Right
	Femoral Vein, Left
Deep palmar arch	Hand Artery, Right
	Hand Artery, Left
Deep transverse perineal muscle	Perineum Muscle
Deferential artery	Internal Iliac Artery, Right
	Internal Iliac Artery, Left
Deltoid fascia	Subcutaneous Tissue and Fascia, Right Upper Arm
	Subcutaneous Tissue and Fascia, Left Upper Arm
Deltoid ligament	Ankle Bursa and Ligament, Right
	Ankle Bursa and Ligament, Left
Deltoid muscle	Shoulder Muscle, Right
	Shoulder Muscle, Left
Deltopectoral (infraclavicular) lymph node	Lymphatic, Right Upper Extremity
	Lymphatic, Left Upper Extremity
Dens	Cervical Vertebra
Denticulate (dentate) ligament	Spinal Meninges
Depressor anguli oris muscle	Facial Muscle

Term	ICD-10-PCS Value
Depressor labii inferioris muscle	Facial Muscle
Depressor septi nasi muscle	Facial Muscle
Depressor supercilii muscle	Facial Muscle
Dermis	Skin
Descending genicular artery	Femoral Artery, Right
	Femoral Artery, Left
Diaphragma sellae	Dura Mater
Distal humerus	Humeral Shaft, Right
	Humeral Shaft, Left
Distal humerus, involving joint	Elbow Joint, Right
	Elbow Joint, Left
Distal radioulnar joint	Wrist Joint, Right
	Wrist Joint, Left
Dorsal digital nerve	Radial Nerve
Dorsal metacarpal vein	Hand Vein, Right
	Hand Vein, Left
Dorsal metatarsal artery	Foot Artery, Right
	Foot Artery, Left
Dorsal metatarsal vein	Foot Vein, Right
	Foot Vein, Left
Dorsal root ganglion	Cervical Spinal Cord
	Lumbar Spinal Cord
	Spinal Cord
	Thoracic Spinal Cord
Dorsal scapular artery	Subclavian Artery, Right
	Subclavian Artery, Left
Dorsal scapular nerve	Brachial Plexus
Dorsal venous arch	Foot Vein, Right
	Foot Vein, Left
Dorsalis pedis artery	Anterior Tibial Artery, Right
	Anterior Tibial Artery, Left
Duct of Santorini	Pancreatic Duct, Accessory
Duct of Wirsung	Pancreatic Duct
Ductus deferens	Vas Deferens, Right
	Vas Deferens, Left
	Vas Deferens, Bilateral
	Vas Deferens
Duodenal ampulla	Ampulla of Vater
Duodenojejunal flexure	Jejunum
Dura mater, intracranial	Dura Mater
Dura mater, spinal	Spinal Meninges
Dural venous sinus	Intracranial Vein
Earlobe	External Ear, Right
	External Ear, Left
	External Ear, Bilateral
Eighth cranial nerve	Acoustic Nerve
Ejaculatory duct	Vas Deferens, Right
	Vas Deferens, Left
	Vas Deferens, Bilateral
	Vas Deferens
Eleventh cranial nerve	Accessory Nerve
Encephalon	Brain
Ependyma	Cerebral Ventricle
Epidermis	Skin
Epidural space, spinal	Spinal Canal
Epiploic foramen	Peritoneum

Term	ICD-10-PCS Value
Epithalamus	Thalamus
Epitrochlear lymph node	Lymphatic, Right Upper Extremity
	Lymphatic, Left Upper Extremity
Erector spinae muscle	Trunk Muscle, Right
	Trunk Muscle, Left
Esophageal artery	Upper Artery
Esophageal plexus	Thoracic Sympathetic Nerve
Ethmoidal air cell	Ethmoid Sinus, Right
	Ethmoid Sinus, Left
Extensor carpi radialis muscle	Lower Arm and Wrist Muscle, Right
	Lower Arm and Wrist Muscle, Left
Extensor carpi ulnaris muscle	Lower Arm and Wrist Muscle, Right
	Lower Arm and Wrist Muscle, Left
Extensor digitorum brevis muscle	Foot Muscle, Right
	Foot Muscle, Left
Extensor digitorum longus muscle	Lower Leg Muscle, Right
	Lower Leg Muscle, Left
Extensor hallucis brevis muscle	Foot Muscle, Right
	Foot Muscle, Left
Extensor hallucis longus muscle	Lower Leg Muscle, Right
	Lower Leg Muscle, Left
External anal sphincter	Anal Sphincter
External auditory meatus	External Auditory Canal, Right
	External Auditory Canal, Left
External maxillary artery	Face Artery
External naris	Nasal Mucosa and Soft Tissue
External oblique aponeurosis	Subcutaneous Tissue and Fascia, Trunk
External oblique muscle	Abdomen Muscle, Right
	Abdomen Muscle, Left
External popliteal nerve	Peroneal Nerve
External pudendal artery	Femoral Artery, Right
	Femoral Artery, Left
External pudendal vein	Saphenous Vein, Right
	Saphenous Vein, Left
External urethral sphincter	Urethra
Extradural space, intracranial	Epidural Space, Intracranial
Extradural space, spinal	Spinal Canal
Facial artery	Face Artery
False vocal cord	Larynx
Falx cerebri	Dura Mater
Fascia lata	Subcutaneous Tissue and Fascia, Right Upper Leg
	Subcutaneous Tissue and Fascia, Left Upper Leg
Femoral head	Upper Femur, Right
	Upper Femur, Left
Femoral lymph node	Lymphatic, Right Lower Extremity
	Lymphatic, Left Lower Extremity
Femoropatellar joint	Knee Joint, Right
	Knee Joint, Left
	Knee Joint, Femoral Surface, Right
	Knee Joint, Femoral Surface, Left
Femorotibial joint	Knee Joint, Right
	Knee Joint, Left
	Knee Joint, Tibial Surface, Right
	Knee Joint, Tibial Surface, Left

Term	ICD-10-PCS Value
Fibular artery	Peroneal Artery, Right
	Peroneal Artery, Left
Fibular sesamoid	Metatarsal, Right
	Metatarsal, Left
Fibularis brevis muscle	Lower Leg Muscle, Right
	Lower Leg Muscle, Left
Fibularis longus muscle	Lower Leg Muscle, Right
	Lower Leg Muscle, Left
Fifth cranial nerve	Trigeminal Nerve
Filum terminale	Spinal Meninges
First cranial nerve	Olfactory Nerve
First intercostal nerve	Brachial Plexus
Flexor carpi radialis muscle	Lower Arm and Wrist Muscle, Right
	Lower Arm and Wrist Muscle, Left
Flexor carpi ulnaris muscle	Lower Arm and Wrist Muscle, Right
	Lower Arm and Wrist Muscle, Left
Flexor digitorum brevis muscle	Foot Muscle, Right
	Foot Muscle, Left
Flexor digitorum longus muscle	Lower Leg Muscle, Right
	Lower Leg Muscle, Left
Flexor hallucis brevis muscle	Foot Muscle, Right
	Foot Muscle, Left
Flexor hallucis longus muscle	Lower Leg Muscle, Right
	Lower Leg Muscle, Left
Flexor pollicis longus muscle	Lower Arm and Wrist Muscle, Right
	Lower Arm and Wrist Muscle, Left
Foramen magnum	Occipital Bone
Foramen of Monro (intraventricular)	Cerebral Ventricle
Foreskin	Prepuce
Fossa of Rosenmuller	Nasopharynx
Fourth cranial nerve	Trochlear Nerve
Fourth ventricle	Cerebral Ventricle
Fovea	Retina, Right
	Retina, Left
Frenulum labii inferioris	Lower Lip
Frenulum labii superioris	Upper Lip
Frenulum linguae	Tongue
Frontal lobe	Cerebral Hemisphere
Frontal vein	Face Vein, Right
	Face Vein, Left
Fundus uteri	Uterus
Galea aponeurotica	Subcutaneous Tissue and Fascia, Scalp
Ganglion impar (ganglion of Walther)	Sacral Sympathetic Nerve
Gasserian ganglion	Trigeminal Nerve
Gastric lymph node	Lymphatic, Aortic
Gastric plexus	Abdominal Sympathetic Nerve
Gastrocnemius muscle	Lower Leg Muscle, Right
	Lower Leg Muscle, Left
Gastrocolic ligament	Omentum
Gastrocolic omentum	Omentum
Gastroduodenal artery	Hepatic Artery
Gastroesophageal (GE) junction	Esophagogastric Junction
Gastrohepatic omentum	Omentum
Gastrophrenic ligament	Omentum
Gastrosplenic ligament	Omentum

Term	ICD-10-PCS Value
Gemellus muscle	Hip Muscle, Right
	Hip Muscle, Left
Geniculate ganglion	Facial Nerve
Geniculate nucleus	Thalamus
Genioglossus muscle	Tongue, Palate, Pharynx Muscle
Genitofemoral nerve	Lumbar Plexus
Glans penis	Prepuce
Glenohumeral joint	Shoulder Joint, Right
	Shoulder Joint, Left
Glenohumeral ligament	Shoulder Bursa and Ligament, Right
	Shoulder Bursa and Ligament, Left
Glenoid fossa (of scapula)	Glenoid Cavity, Right
	Glenoid Cavity, Left
Glenoid ligament (labrum)	Shoulder Joint, Right
	Shoulder Joint, Left
Globus pallidus	Basal Ganglia
Glossoepiglottic fold	Epiglottis
Glottis	Larynx
Gluteal lymph node	Lymphatic, Pelvis
Gluteal vein	Hypogastric Vein, Right
	Hypogastric Vein, Left
Gluteus maximus muscle	Hip Muscle, Right
	Hip Muscle, Left
Gluteus medius muscle	Hip Muscle, Right
	Hip Muscle, Left
Gluteus minimus muscle	Hip Muscle, Right
	Hip Muscle, Left
Gracilis muscle	Upper Leg Muscle, Right
	Upper Leg Muscle, Left
Great auricular nerve	Cervical Plexus
Great cerebral vein	Intracranial Vein
Great(er) saphenous vein	Saphenous Vein, Right
	Saphenous Vein, Left
Greater alar cartilage	Nasal Mucosa and Soft Tissue
Greater occipital nerve	Cervical Nerve
Greater omentum	Omentum
Greater splanchnic nerve	Thoracic Sympathetic Nerve
Greater superficial petrosal nerve	Facial Nerve
Greater trochanter	Upper Femur, Right
	Upper Femur, Left
Greater tuberosity	Humeral Head, Right
	Humeral Head, Left
Greater vestibular (Bartholin's) gland	Vestibular Gland
Greater wing	Sphenoid Bone
Hallux	1st Toe, Right
	1st Toe, Left
Hamate bone	Carpal, Right
	Carpal, Left
Head of fibula	Fibula, Right
	Fibula, Left
Helix	External Ear, Right
	External Ear, Left
	External Ear, Bilateral
Hepatic artery proper	Hepatic Artery
Hepatic flexure	Transverse Colon

Term	ICD-10-PCS Value
Hepatic lymph node	Lymphatic, Aortic
Hepatic plexus	Abdominal Sympathetic Nerve
Hepatic portal vein	Portal Vein
Hepatogastric ligament	Omentum
Hepatopancreatic ampulla	Ampulla of Vater
Humeroradial joint	Elbow Joint, Right
	Elbow Joint, Left
Humeroulnar joint	Elbow Joint, Right
	Elbow Joint, Left
Humerus, distal	Humeral Shaft, Right
	Humeral Shaft, Left
Hyoglossus muscle	Tongue, Palate, Pharynx Muscle
Hyoid artery	Thyroid Artery, Right
	Thyroid Artery, Left
Hypogastric artery	Internal Iliac Artery, Right
	Internal Iliac Artery, Left
Hypopharynx	Pharynx
Hypophysis	Pituitary Gland
Hypothenar muscle	Hand Muscle, Right
	Hand Muscle, Left
Ileal artery	Superior Mesenteric Artery
Ileocolic artery	Superior Mesenteric Artery
Ileocolic vein	Colic Vein
Iliac crest	Pelvic Bone, Right
	Pelvic Bone, Left
Iliac fascia	Subcutaneous Tissue and Fascia, Right Upper Leg
	Subcutaneous Tissue and Fascia, Left Upper Leg
Iliac lymph node	Lymphatic, Pelvis
Iliacus muscle	Hip Muscle, Right
	Hip Muscle, Left
Iliofemoral ligament	Hip Bursa and Ligament, Right
	Hip Bursa and Ligament, Left
Iliohypogastric nerve	Lumbar Plexus
Ilioinguinal nerve	Lumbar Plexus
Iliolumbar artery	Internal Iliac Artery, Right
	Internal Iliac Artery, Left
Iliolumbar ligament	Lower Spine Bursa and Ligament
Iliotibial tract (band)	Subcutaneous Tissue and Fascia, Right Upper Leg
	Subcutaneous Tissue and Fascia, Left Upper Leg
Ilium	Pelvic Bone, Right
	Pelvic Bone, Left
Incus	Auditory Ossicle, Right
	Auditory Ossicle, Left
Inferior cardiac nerve	Thoracic Sympathetic Nerve
Inferior cerebellar vein	Intracranial Vein
Inferior cerebral vein	Intracranial Vein
Inferior epigastric artery	External Iliac Artery, Right
	External Iliac Artery, Left
Inferior epigastric lymph node	Lymphatic, Pelvis
Inferior genicular artery	Popliteal Artery, Right
	Popliteal Artery, Left
Inferior gluteal artery	Internal Iliac Artery, Right
	Internal Iliac Artery, Left

Term	ICD-10-PCS Value
Inferior gluteal nerve	Sacral Plexus
Inferior hypogastric plexus	Abdominal Sympathetic Nerve
Inferior labial artery	Face Artery
Inferior longitudinal muscle	Tongue, Palate, Pharynx Muscle
Inferior mesenteric ganglion	Abdominal Sympathetic Nerve
Inferior mesenteric lymph node	Lymphatic, Mesenteric
Inferior mesenteric plexus	Abdominal Sympathetic Nerve
Inferior oblique muscle	Extraocular Muscle, Right
	Extraocular Muscle, Left
Inferior pancreaticoduodenal artery	Superior Mesenteric Artery
Inferior phrenic artery	Abdominal Aorta
Inferior rectus muscle	Extraocular Muscle, Right
	Extraocular Muscle, Left
Inferior suprarenal artery	Renal Artery, Right
	Renal Artery, Left
Inferior tarsal plate	Lower Eyelid, Right
	Lower Eyelid, Left
Inferior thyroid vein	Innominate Vein, Right
	Innominate Vein, Left
Inferior tibiofibular joint	Ankle Joint, Right
	Ankle Joint, Left
Inferior turbinate	Nasal Turbinate
Inferior ulnar collateral artery	Brachial Artery, Right
	Brachial Artery, Left
Inferior vesical artery	Internal Iliac Artery, Right
	Internal Iliac Artery, Left
Infraauricular lymph node	Lymphatic, Head
Infraclavicular (deltopectoral) lymph node	Lymphatic, Right Upper Extremity
	Lymphatic, Left Upper Extremity
Infrahyoid muscle	Neck Muscle, Right
	Neck Muscle, Left
Infraparotid lymph node	Lymphatic, Head
Infraspinatus fascia	Subcutaneous Tissue and Fascia, Right Upper Arm
	Subcutaneous Tissue and Fascia, Left Upper Arm
Infraspinatus muscle	Shoulder Muscle, Right
	Shoulder Muscle, Left
Infundibulopelvic ligament	Uterine Supporting Structure
Inguinal canal	Inguinal Region, Right
	Inguinal Region, Left
	Inguinal Region, Bilateral
Inguinal triangle	Inguinal Region, Right
	Inguinal Region, Left
	Inguinal Region, Bilateral
Interatrial septum	Atrial Septum
Intercarpal joint	Carpal Joint, Right
	Carpal Joint, Left
Intercarpal ligament	Hand Bursa and Ligament, Right
	Hand Bursa and Ligament, Left
Interclavicular ligament	Shoulder Bursa and Ligament, Right
	Shoulder Bursa and Ligament, Left
Intercostal lymph node	Lymphatic, Thorax
Intercostal muscle	Thorax Muscle, Right
	Thorax Muscle, Left
Intercostal nerve	Thoracic Nerve

Term	ICD-10-PCS Value
Intercostobrachial nerve	Thoracic Nerve
Intercuneiform joint	Tarsal Joint, Right
	Tarsal Joint, Left
Intercuneiform ligament	Foot Bursa and Ligament, Right
	Foot Bursa and Ligament, Left
Intermediate bronchus	Main Bronchus, Right
Intermediate cuneiform bone	Tarsal, Right
	Tarsal, Left
Internal anal sphincter	Anal Sphincter
Internal (basal) cerebral vein	Intracranial Vein
Internal carotid artery, intracranial portion	Intracranial Artery
Internal carotid plexus	Head and Neck Sympathetic Nerve
Internal iliac vein	Hypogastric Vein, Right
	Hypogastric Vein, Left
Internal maxillary artery	External Carotid Artery, Right
	External Carotid Artery, Left
Internal naris	Nasal Mucosa and Soft Tissue
Internal oblique muscle	Abdomen Muscle, Right
	Abdomen Muscle, Left
Internal pudendal artery	Internal Iliac Artery, Right
	Internal Iliac Artery, Left
Internal pudendal vein	Hypogastric Vein, Right
	Hypogastric Vein, Left
Internal thoracic artery	Internal Mammary Artery, Right
	Internal Mammary Artery, Left
	Subclavian Artery, Right
	Subclavian Artery, Left
Internal urethral sphincter	Urethra
Interphalangeal (IP) joint	Finger Phalangeal Joint, Right
	Finger Phalangeal Joint, Left
	Toe Phalangeal Joint, Right
	Toe Phalangeal Joint, Left
Interphalangeal ligament	Foot Bursa and Ligament, Right
	Foot Bursa and Ligament, Left
	Hand Bursa and Ligament, Right
	Hand Bursa and Ligament, Left
Interspinalis muscle	Trunk Muscle, Right
	Trunk Muscle, Left
Interspinous ligament, cervical	Head and Neck Bursa and Ligament
Interspinous ligament, lumbar	Lower Spine Bursa and Ligament
Interspinous ligament, thoracic	Upper Spine Bursa and Ligament
Intertransversarius muscle	Trunk Muscle, Right
	Trunk Muscle, Left
Intertransverse ligament, cervical	Head and Neck Bursa and Ligament
Intertransverse ligament, lumbar	Lower Spine Bursa and Ligament
Intertransverse ligament, thoracic	Upper Spine Bursa and Ligament
Interventricular foramen (Monro)	Cerebral Ventricle
Interventricular septum	Ventricular Septum
Intestinal lymphatic trunk	Cisterna Chyli
Ischiatic nerve	Sciatic Nerve
Ischiocavernosus muscle	Perineum Muscle

Term	ICD-10-PCS Value
Ischiofemoral ligament	Hip Bursa and Ligament, Right
	Hip Bursa and Ligament, Left
Ischium	Pelvic Bone, Right
	Pelvic Bone, Left
Jejunal artery	Superior Mesenteric Artery
Jugular body	Glomus Jugulare
Jugular lymph node	Lymphatic, Right Neck
	Lymphatic, Left Neck
Labia majora	Vulva
Labia minora	Vulva
Labial gland	Upper Lip
	Lower Lip
Lacrimal canaliculus	Lacrimal Duct, Right
	Lacrimal Duct, Left
Lacrimal punctum	Lacrimal Duct, Right
	Lacrimal Duct, Left
Lacrimal sac	Lacrimal Duct, Right
	Lacrimal Duct, Left
Laryngopharynx	Pharynx
Lateral (brachial) lymph node	Lymphatic, Right Axillary
	Lymphatic, Left Axillary
Lateral canthus	Upper Eyelid, Right
	Upper Eyelid, Left
Lateral collateral ligament (LCL)	Knee Bursa and Ligament, Right
	Knee Bursa and Ligament, Left
Lateral condyle of femur	Lower Femur, Right
	Lower Femur, Left
Lateral condyle of tibia	Tibia, Right
	Tibia, Left
Lateral cuneiform bone	Tarsal, Right
	Tarsal, Left
Lateral epicondyle of femur	Lower Femur, Right
	Lower Femur, Left
Lateral epicondyle of humerus	Humeral Shaft, Right
	Humeral Shaft, Left
Lateral femoral cutaneous nerve	Lumbar Plexus
Lateral malleolus	Fibula, Right
	Fibula, Left
Lateral meniscus	Knee Joint, Right
	Knee Joint, Left
Lateral nasal cartilage	Nasal Mucosa and Soft Tissue
Lateral plantar artery	Foot Artery, Right
	Foot Artery, Left
Lateral plantar nerve	Tibial Nerve
Lateral rectus muscle	Extraocular Muscle, Right
	Extraocular Muscle, Left
Lateral sacral artery	Internal Iliac Artery, Right
	Internal Iliac Artery, Left
Lateral sacral vein	Hypogastric Vein, Right
	Hypogastric Vein, Left
Lateral sural cutaneous nerve	Peroneal Nerve
Lateral tarsal artery	Foot Artery, Right
	Foot Artery, Left
Lateral temporo- mandibular ligament	Head and Neck Bursa and Ligament
Lateral thoracic artery	Axillary Artery, Right
	Axillary Artery, Left

Term	ICD-10-PCS Value
Latissimus dorsi muscle	Trunk Muscle, Right
	Trunk Muscle, Left
Least splanchnic nerve	Thoracic Sympathetic Nerve
Left ascending lumbar vein	Hemiazygos Vein
Left atrioventricular valve	Mitral Valve
Left auricular appendix	Atrium, Left
Left colic vein	Colic Vein
Left coronary sulcus	Heart, Left
Left gastric artery	Gastric Artery
Left gastroepiploic artery	Splenic Artery
Left gastroepiploic vein	Splenic Vein
Left inferior phrenic vein	Renal Vein, Left
Left inferior pulmonary vein	Pulmonary Vein, Left
Left jugular trunk	Thoracic Duct
Left lateral ventricle	Cerebral Ventricle
Left ovarian vein	Renal Vein, Left
Left second lumbar vein	Renal Vein, Left
Left subclavian trunk	Thoracic Duct
Left subcostal vein	Hemiazygos Vein
Left superior pulmonary vein	Pulmonary Vein, Left
Left suprarenal vein	Renal Vein, Left
Left testicular vein	Renal Vein, Left
Leptomeninges, intracranial	Cerebral Meninges
Leptomeninges, spinal	Spinal Meninges
Lesser alar cartilage	Nasal Mucosa and Soft Tissue
Lesser occipital nerve	Cervical Plexus
Lesser omentum	Omentum
Lesser saphenous vein	Saphenous Vein, Right
	Saphenous Vein, Left
Lesser splanchnic nerve	Thoracic Sympathetic Nerve
Lesser trochanter	Upper Femur, Right
	Upper Femur, Left
Lesser tuberosity	Humeral Head, Right
	Humeral Head, Left
Lesser wing	Sphenoid Bone
Levator anguli oris muscle	Facial Muscle
Levator ani muscle	Perineum Muscle
Levator labii superioris alaeque nasi muscle	Facial Muscle
Levator labii superioris muscle	Facial Muscle
Levator palpebrae superioris muscle	Upper Eyelid, Right
	Upper Eyelid, Left
Levator scapulae muscle	Neck Muscle, Right
	Neck Muscle, Left
Levator veli palatini muscle	Tongue, Palate, Pharynx Muscle
Levatores costarum muscle	Thorax Muscle, Right
	Thorax Muscle, Left
Ligament of head of fibula	Knee Bursa and Ligament, Right
	Knee Bursa and Ligament, Left
Ligament of the lateral malleolus	Ankle Bursa and Ligament, Right
	Ankle Bursa and Ligament, Left
Ligamentum flavum, cervical	Head and Neck Bursa and Ligament
Ligamentum flavum, lumbar	Lower Spine Bursa and Ligament
Ligamentum flavum, thoracic	Upper Spine Bursa and Ligament
Lingual artery	External Carotid Artery, Right
	External Carotid Artery, Left
Lingual tonsil	Pharynx

Term	ICD-10-PCS Value
Locus ceruleus	Pons
Long thoracic nerve	Brachial Plexus
Lumbar artery	Abdominal Aorta
Lumbar facet joint	Lumbar Vertebral Joint
Lumbar ganglion	Lumbar Sympathetic Nerve
Lumbar lymph node	Lymphatic, Aortic
Lumbar lymphatic trunk	Cisterna Chyli
Lumbar splanchnic nerve	Lumbar Sympathetic Nerve
Lumbosacral facet joint	Lumbosacral Joint
Lumbosacral trunk	Lumbar Nerve
Lunate bone	Carpal, Right
	Carpal, Left
Lunotriquetral ligament	Hand Bursa and Ligament, Right
	Hand Bursa and Ligament, Left
Macula	Retina, Right
	Retina, Left
Malleus	Auditory Ossicle, Right
	Auditory Ossicle, Left
Mammary duct	Breast, Right
	Breast, Left
	Breast, Bilateral
Mammary gland	Breast, Right
	Breast, Left
	Breast, Bilateral
Mammillary body	Hypothalamus
Mandibular nerve	Trigeminal Nerve
Mandibular notch	Mandible, Right
	Mandible, Left
Manubrium	Sternum
Masseter muscle	Head Muscle
Masseteric fascia	Subcutaneous Tissue and Fascia, Face
Mastoid (postauricular) lymph node	Lymphatic, Right Neck
	Lymphatic, Left Neck
Mastoid air cells	Mastoid Sinus, Right
	Mastoid Sinus, Left
Mastoid process	Temporal Bone, Right
	Temporal Bone, Left
Maxillary artery	External Carotid Artery, Right
	External Carotid Artery, Left
Maxillary nerve	Trigeminal Nerve
Medial canthus	Lower Eyelid, Right
	Lower Eyelid, Left
Medial collateral ligament (MCL)	Knee Bursa and Ligament, Right
	Knee Bursa and Ligament, Left
Medial condyle of femur	Lower Femur, Right
	Lower Femur, Left
Medial condyle of tibia	Tibia, Right
	Tibia, Left
Medial cuneiform bone	Tarsal, Right
	Tarsal, Left
Medial epicondyle of femur	Lower Femur, Right
	Lower Femur, Left
Medial epicondyle of humerus	Humeral Shaft, Right
	Humeral Shaft, Left
Medial malleolus	Tibia, Right
	Tibia, Left

Term	ICD-10-PCS Value
Medial meniscus	Knee Joint, Right
	Knee Joint, Left
Medial plantar artery	Foot Artery, Right
	Foot Artery, Left
Medial plantar nerve	Tibial Nerve
Medial popliteal nerve	Tibial Nerve
Medial rectus muscle	Extraocular Muscle, Right
	Extraocular Muscle, Left
Medial sural cutaneous nerve	Tibial Nerve
Median antebrachial vein	Basilic Vein, Right
	Basilic Vein, Left
Median cubital vein	Basilic Vein, Right
	Basilic Vein, Left
Median sacral artery	Abdominal Aorta
Mediastinal cavity	Mediastinum
Mediastinal lymph node	Lymphatic, Thorax
Mediastinal space	Mediastinum
Meissner's (submucous) plexus	Abdominal Sympathetic Nerve
Membranous urethra	Urethra
Mental foramen	Mandible, Right
	Mandible, Left
Mentalis muscle	Facial Muscle
Mesoappendix	Mesentery
Mesocolon	Mesentery
Metacarpal ligament	Hand Bursa and Ligament, Right
	Hand Bursa and Ligament, Left
Metacarpophalangeal ligament	Hand Bursa and Ligament, Right
	Hand Bursa and Ligament, Left
Metatarsal ligament	Foot Bursa and Ligament, Right
	Foot Bursa and Ligament, Left
Metatarsophalangeal ligament	Foot Bursa and Ligament, Right
	Foot Bursa and Ligament, Left
Metatarsophalangeal (MTP) joint	Metatarsal-Phalangeal Joint, Right
	Metatarsal-Phalangeal Joint, Left
Metathalamus	Thalamus
Midcarpal joint	Carpal Joint, Right
	Carpal Joint, Left
Middle cardiac nerve	Thoracic Sympathetic Nerve
Middle cerebral artery	Intracranial Artery
Middle cerebral vein	Intracranial Vein
Middle colic vein	Colic Vein
Middle genicular artery	Popliteal Artery, Right
	Popliteal Artery, Left
Middle hemorrhoidal vein	Hypogastric Vein, Right
	Hypogastric Vein, Left
Middle meningeal artery, intracranial portion	Intracranial Artery
Middle rectal artery	Internal Iliac Artery, Right
	Internal Iliac Artery, Left
Middle suprarenal artery	Abdominal Aorta
Middle temporal artery	Temporal Artery, Right
	Temporal Artery, Left
Middle turbinate	Nasal Turbinate
Mitral annulus	Mitral Valve
Molar gland	Buccal Mucosa
Musculocutaneous nerve	Brachial Plexus

Term	ICD-10-PCS Value
Musculophrenic artery	Internal Mammary Artery, Right
	Internal Mammary Artery, Left
Musculospiral nerve	Radial Nerve
Myelencephalon	Medulla Oblongata
Myenteric (Auerbach's) plexus	Abdominal Sympathetic Nerve
Myometrium	Uterus
Nail bed	Finger Nail
	Toe Nail
Nail plate	Finger Nail
	Toe Nail
Nasal cavity	Nasal Mucosa and Soft Tissue
Nasal concha	Nasal Turbinate
Nasalis muscle	Facial Muscle
Nasolacrimal duct	Lacrimal Duct, Right
	Lacrimal Duct, Left
Navicular bone	Tarsal, Right
	Tarsal, Left
Neck of femur	Upper Femur, Right
	Upper Femur, Left
Neck of humerus (anatomical) (surgical)	Humeral Head, Right
	Humeral Head, Left
Nerve to the stapedius	Facial Nerve
Neurohypophysis	Pituitary Gland
Ninth cranial nerve	Glossopharyngeal Nerve
Nostril	Nasal Mucosa and Soft Tissue
Obturator artery	Internal Iliac Artery, Right
	Internal Iliac Artery, Left
Obturator lymph node	Lymphatic, Pelvis
Obturator muscle	Hip Muscle, Right
	Hip Muscle, Left
Obturator nerve	Lumbar Plexus
Obturator vein	Hypogastric Vein, Right
	Hypogastric Vein, Left
Obtuse margin	Heart, Left
Occipital artery	External Carotid Artery, Right
	External Carotid Artery, Left
Occipital lobe	Cerebral Hemisphere
Occipital lymph node	Lymphatic, Right Neck
	Lymphatic, Left Neck
Occipitofrontalis muscle	Facial Muscle
Odontoid process	Cervical Vertebra
Olecranon bursa	Elbow Bursa and Ligament, Right
	Elbow Bursa and Ligament, Left
Olecranon process	Ulna, Right
	Ulna, Left
Olfactory bulb	Olfactory Nerve
Ophthalmic artery	Intracranial Artery
Ophthalmic nerve	Trigeminal Nerve
Ophthalmic vein	Intracranial Vein
Optic chiasma	Optic Nerve
Optic disc	Retina, Right
	Retina, Left
Optic foramen	Sphenoid Bone
Orbicularis oculi muscle	Upper Eyelid, Right
	Upper Eyelid, Left
Orbicularis oris muscle	Facial Muscle

Term	ICD-10-PCS Value
Orbital fascia	Subcutaneous Tissue and Fascia, Face
Orbital portion of ethmoid bone	Orbit, Right
	Orbit, Left
Orbital portion of frontal bone	Orbit, Right
	Orbit, Left
Orbital portion of lacrimal bone	Orbit, Right
	Orbit, Left
Orbital portion of maxilla	Orbit, Right
	Orbit, Left
Orbital portion of palatine bone	Orbit, Right
	Orbit, Left
Orbital portion of sphenoid bone	Orbit, Right
	Orbit, Left
Orbital portion of zygomatic bone	Orbit, Right
	Orbit, Left
Oropharynx	Pharynx
Otic ganglion	Head and Neck Sympathetic Nerve
Oval window	Middle Ear, Right
	Middle Ear, Left
Ovarian artery	Abdominal Aorta
Ovarian ligament	Uterine Supporting Structure
Oviduct	Fallopian Tube, Right
	Fallopian Tube, Left
Palatine gland	Buccal Mucosa
Palatine tonsil	Tonsils
Palatine uvula	Uvula
Palatoglossal muscle	Tongue, Palate, Pharynx Muscle
Palatopharyngeal muscle	Tongue, Palate, Pharynx Muscle
Palmar (volar) digital vein	Hand Vein, Right
	Hand Vein, Left
Palmar (volar) metacarpal vein	Hand Vein, Right
	Hand Vein, Left
Palmar cutaneous nerve	Median Nerve
	Radial Nerve
Palmar fascia (aponeurosis)	Subcutaneous Tissue and Fascia, Right Hand
	Subcutaneous Tissue and Fascia, Left Hand
Palmar interosseous muscle	Hand Muscle, Right
	Hand Muscle, Left
Palmar ulnocarpal ligament	Wrist Bursa and Ligament, Right
	Wrist Bursa and Ligament, Left
Palmaris longus muscle	Lower Arm and Wrist Muscle, Right
	Lower Arm and Wrist Muscle, Left
Pancreatic artery	Splenic Artery
Pancreatic plexus	Abdominal Sympathetic Nerve
Pancreatic vein	Splenic Vein
Pancreaticosplenic lymph node	Lymphatic, Aortic
Paraaortic lymph node	Lymphatic, Aortic
Parapharyngeal space	Neck
Pararectal lymph node	Lymphatic, Mesenteric
Parasternal lymph node	Lymphatic, Thorax
Paratracheal lymph node	Lymphatic, Thorax
Paraurethral (Skene's) gland	Vestibular Gland
Parietal lobe	Cerebral Hemisphere
Parotid lymph node	Lymphatic, Head
Parotid plexus	Facial Nerve
Pars flaccida	Tympanic Membrane, Right
	Tympanic Membrane, Left
Patellar ligament	Knee Bursa and Ligament, Right
	Knee Bursa and Ligament, Left
Patellar tendon	Knee Tendon, Right
	Knee Tendon, Left
Patellofemoral joint	Knee Joint, Right
	Knee Joint, Left
	Knee Joint, Femoral Surface, Right
	Knee Joint, Femoral Surface, Left
Pectineus muscle	Upper Leg Muscle, Right
	Upper Leg Muscle, Left
Pectoral (anterior) lymph node	Lymphatic, Right Axillary
	Lymphatic, Left Axillary
Pectoral fascia	Subcutaneous Tissue and Fascia, Chest
Pectoralis major muscle	Thorax Muscle, Right
	Thorax Muscle, Left
Pectoralis minor muscle	Thorax Muscle, Right
	Thorax Muscle, Left
Pelvic splanchnic nerve	Abdominal Sympathetic Nerve
	Sacral Sympathetic Nerve
Penile urethra	Urethra
Perianal skin	Skin, Perineum
Pericardiophrenic artery	Internal Mammary Artery, Right
	Internal Mammary Artery, Left
Perimetrium	Uterus
Peroneus brevis muscle	Lower Leg Muscle, Right
	Lower Leg Muscle, Left
Peroneus longus muscle	Lower Leg Muscle, Right
	Lower Leg Muscle, Left
Petrous part of temporal bone	Temporal Bone, Right
	Temporal Bone, Left
Pharyngeal constrictor muscle	Tongue, Palate, Pharynx Muscle
Pharyngeal plexus	Vagus Nerve
Pharyngeal recess	Nasopharynx
Pharyngeal tonsil	Adenoids
Pharyngotympanic tube	Eustachian Tube, Right
	Eustachian Tube, Left
Pia mater, intracranial	Cerebral Meninges
Pia mater, spinal	Spinal Meninges
Pinna	External Ear, Right
	External Ear, Left
	External Ear, Bilateral
Piriform recess (sinus)	Pharynx
Piriformis muscle	Hip Muscle, Right
	Hip Muscle, Left
Pisiform bone	Carpal, Right
	Carpal, Left
Pisohamate ligament	Hand Bursa and Ligament, Right
	Hand Bursa and Ligament, Left
Pisometacarpal ligament	Hand Bursa and Ligament, Right
	Hand Bursa and Ligament, Left
Plantar digital vein	Foot Vein, Right
	Foot Vein, Left

Term	ICD-10-PCS Value
Plantar fascia (aponeurosis)	Subcutaneous Tissue and Fascia, Right Foot
	Subcutaneous Tissue and Fascia, Left Foot
Plantar metatarsal vein	Foot Vein, Right
	Foot Vein, Left
Plantar venous arch	Foot Vein, Right
	Foot Vein, Left
Platysma muscle	Neck Muscle, Right
	Neck Muscle, Left
Plica semilunaris	Conjunctiva, Right
	Conjunctiva, Left
Pneumogastric nerve	Vagus Nerve
Pneumotaxic center	Pons
Pontine tegmentum	Pons
Popliteal ligament	Knee Bursa and Ligament, Right
	Knee Bursa and Ligament, Left
Popliteal lymph node	Lymphatic, Left Lower Extremity
	Lymphatic, Right Lower Extremity
Popliteal vein	Femoral Vein, Right
	Femoral Vein, Left
Popliteus muscle	Lower Leg Muscle, Right
	Lower Leg Muscle, Left
Postauricular (mastoid) lymph node	Lymphatic, Right Neck
	Lymphatic, Left Neck
Postcava	Inferior Vena Cava
Posterior (subscapular) lymph node	Lymphatic, Right Axillary
	Lymphatic, Left Axillary
Posterior auricular artery	External Carotid Artery, Right
	External Carotid Artery, Left
Posterior auricular nerve	Facial Nerve
Posterior auricular vein	External Jugular Vein, Right
	External Jugular Vein, Left
Posterior cerebral artery	Intracranial Artery
Posterior chamber	Eye, Right
	Eye, Left
Posterior circumflex humeral artery	Axillary Artery, Right
	Axillary Artery, Left
Posterior communicating artery	Intracranial Artery
Posterior cruciate ligament (PCL)	Knee Bursa and Ligament, Right
	Knee Bursa and Ligament, Left
Posterior facial (retromandibular) vein	Face Vein, Right
	Face Vein, Left
Posterior femoral cutaneous nerve	Sacral Plexus
Posterior inferior cerebellar artery (PICA)	Intracranial Artery
Posterior interosseous nerve	Radial Nerve
Posterior labial nerve	Pudendal Nerve
Posterior scrotal nerve	Pudendal Nerve
Posterior spinal artery	Vertebral Artery, Right
	Vertebral Artery, Left
Posterior tibial recurrent artery	Anterior Tibial Artery, Right
	Anterior Tibial Artery, Left
Posterior ulnar recurrent artery	Ulnar Artery, Right
	Ulnar Artery, Left
Posterior vagal trunk	Vagus Nerve
Preauricular lymph node	Lymphatic, Head
Precava	Superior Vena Cava
Prepatellar bursa	Knee Bursa and Ligament, Right
	Knee Bursa and Ligament, Left
Pretracheal fascia	Subcutaneous Tissue and Fascia, Right Neck
	Subcutaneous Tissue and Fascia, Left Neck
Prevertebral fascia	Subcutaneous Tissue and Fascia, Right Neck
	Subcutaneous Tissue and Fascia, Left Neck
Princeps pollicis artery	Hand Artery, Right
	Hand Artery, Left
Procerus muscle	Facial Muscle
Profunda brachii	Brachial Artery, Right
	Brachial Artery, Left
Profunda femoris (deep femoral) vein	Femoral Vein, Right
	Femoral Vein, Left
Pronator quadratus muscle	Lower Arm and Wrist Muscle, Right
	Lower Arm and Wrist Muscle, Left
Pronator teres muscle	Lower Arm and Wrist Muscle, Right
	Lower Arm and Wrist Muscle, Left
Prostatic artery	Internal Iliac Artery, Right
	Internal Iliac Artery, Left
Prostatic urethra	Urethra
Proximal radioulnar joint	Elbow Joint, Right
	Elbow Joint, Left
Psoas muscle	Hip Muscle, Right
	Hip Muscle, Left
Pterygoid muscle	Head Muscle
Pterygoid process	Sphenoid Bone
Pterygopalatine (sphenopalatine) ganglion	Head and Neck Sympathetic Nerve
Pubis	Pelvic Bone, Right
	Pelvic Bone, Left
Pubofemoral ligament	Hip Bursa and Ligament, Right
	Hip Bursa and Ligament, Left
Pudendal nerve	Sacral Plexus
Pulmoaortic canal	Pulmonary Artery, Left
Pulmonary annulus	Pulmonary Valve
Pulmonary plexus	Thoracic Sympathetic Nerve
	Vagus Nerve
Pulmonic valve	Pulmonary Valve
Pulvinar	Thalamus
Pyloric antrum	Stomach, Pylorus
Pyloric canal	Stomach, Pylorus
Pyloric sphincter	Stomach, Pylorus
Pyramidalis muscle	Abdomen Muscle, Right
	Abdomen Muscle, Left
Quadrangular cartilage	Nasal Septum
Quadrate lobe	Liver
Quadratus femoris muscle	Hip Muscle, Right
	Hip Muscle, Left
Quadratus lumborum muscle	Trunk Muscle, Right
	Trunk Muscle, Left

Term	ICD-10-PCS Value
Quadratus plantae muscle	Foot Muscle, Right
	Foot Muscle, Left
Quadriceps (femoris)	Upper Leg Muscle, Right
	Upper Leg Muscle, Left
Radial collateral carpal ligament	Wrist Bursa and Ligament, Right
	Wrist Bursa and Ligament, Left
Radial collateral ligament	Elbow Bursa and Ligament, Right
	Elbow Bursa and Ligament, Left
Radial notch	Ulna, Right
	Ulna, Left
Radial recurrent artery	Radial Artery, Right
	Radial Artery, Left
Radial vein	Brachial Vein, Right
	Brachial Vein, Left
Radialis indicis	Hand Artery, Right
	Hand Artery, Left
Radiocarpal joint	Wrist Joint, Right
	Wrist Joint, Left
Radiocarpal ligament	Wrist Bursa and Ligament, Right
	Wrist Bursa and Ligament, Left
Radioulnar ligament	Wrist Bursa and Ligament, Right
	Wrist Bursa and Ligament, Left
Rectosigmoid junction	Sigmoid Colon
Rectus abdominis muscle	Abdomen Muscle, Right
	Abdomen Muscle, Left
Rectus femoris muscle	Upper Leg Muscle, Right
	Upper Leg Muscle, Left
Recurrent laryngeal nerve	Vagus Nerve
Renal calyx	Kidney, Right
	Kidney, Left
	Kidneys, Bilateral
	Kidney
Renal capsule	Kidney, Right
	Kidney, Left
	Kidneys, Bilateral
	Kidney
Renal cortex	Kidney, Right
	Kidney, Left
	Kidneys, Bilateral
	Kidney
Renal nerve	Abdominal sympathetic Nerve
Renal plexus	Abdominal Sympathetic Nerve
Renal segment	Kidney, Right
	Kidney, Left
	Kidneys, Bilateral
	Kidney
Renal segmental artery	Renal Artery, Right
	Renal Artery, Left
Retroperitoneal cavity	Retroperitoneum
Retroperitoneal lymph node	Lymphatic, Aortic
Retroperitoneal space	Retroperitoneum
Retropharyngeal lymph node	Lymphatic, Right Neck
	Lymphatic, Left Neck
Retropharyngeal space	Neck
Retropubic space	Pelvic Cavity
Rhinopharynx	Nasopharynx

Term	ICD-10-PCS Value
Rhomboid major muscle	Trunk Muscle, Right
	Trunk Muscle, Left
Rhomboid minor muscle	Trunk Muscle, Right
	Trunk Muscle, Left
Right ascending lumbar vein	Azygos Vein
Right atrioventricular valve	Tricuspid Valve
Right auricular appendix	Atrium, Right
Right colic vein	Colic Vein
Right coronary sulcus	Heart, Right
Right gastric artery	Gastric Artery
Right gastroepiploic vein	Superior Mesenteric Vein
Right inferior phrenic vein	Inferior Vena Cava
Right inferior pulmonary vein	Pulmonary Vein, Right
Right jugular trunk	Lymphatic, Right Neck
Right lateral ventricle	Cerebral Ventricle
Right lymphatic duct	Lymphatic, Right Neck
Right ovarian vein	Inferior Vena Cava
Right second lumbar vein	Inferior Vena Cava
Right subclavian trunk	Lymphatic, Right Neck
Right subcostal vein	Azygos Vein
Right superior pulmonary vein	Pulmonary Vein, Right
Right suprarenal vein	Inferior Vena Cava
Right testicular vein	Inferior Vena Cava
Rima glottidis	Larynx
Risorius muscle	Facial Muscle
Round ligament of uterus	Uterine Supporting Structure
Round window	Inner Ear, Right
	Inner Ear, Left
Sacral ganglion	Sacral Sympathetic Nerve
Sacral lymph node	Lymphatic, Pelvis
Sacral splanchnic nerve	Sacral Sympathetic Nerve
Sacrococcygeal ligament	Lower Spine Bursa and Ligament
Sacrococcygeal symphysis	Sacrococcygeal Joint
Sacroiliac ligament	Lower Spine Bursa and Ligament
Sacrospinous ligament	Lower Spine Bursa and Ligament
Sacrotuberous ligament	Lower Spine Bursa and Ligament
Salpingopharyngeus muscle	Tongue, Palate, Pharynx Muscle
Salpinx	Fallopian Tube, Right
	Fallopian Tube, Left
Saphenous nerve	Femoral Nerve
Sartorius muscle	Upper Leg Muscle, Right
	Upper Leg Muscle, Left
Scalene muscle	Neck Muscle, Right
	Neck Muscle, Left
Scaphoid bone	Carpal, Right
	Carpal, Left
Scapholunate ligament	Wrist Bursa and Ligament, Right
	Wrist Bursa and Ligament, Left
Scaphotrapezium ligament	Hand Bursa and Ligament, Right
	Hand Bursa and Ligament, Left
Scarpa's (vestibular) ganglion	Acoustic Nerve
Sebaceous gland	Skin
Second cranial nerve	Optic Nerve
Sella turcica	Sphenoid Bone
Semicircular canal	Inner Ear, Right
	Inner Ear, Left

Term	ICD-10-PCS Value
Semimembranosus muscle	Upper Leg Muscle, Right
	Upper Leg Muscle, Left
Semitendinosus muscle	Upper Leg Muscle, Right
	Upper Leg Muscle, Left
Septal cartilage	Nasal Septum
Serratus anterior muscle	Thorax Muscle, Right
	Thorax Muscle, Left
Serratus posterior muscle	Trunk Muscle, Right
	Trunk Muscle, Left
Seventh cranial nerve	Facial Nerve
Short gastric artery	Splenic Artery
Sigmoid artery	Inferior Mesenteric Artery
Sigmoid flexure	Sigmoid Colon
Sigmoid vein	Inferior Mesenteric Vein
Sinoatrial node	Conduction Mechanism
Sinus venosus	Atrium, Right
Sixth cranial nerve	Abducens Nerve
Skene's (paraurethral) gland	Vestibular Gland
Small saphenous vein	Saphenous Vein, Right
	Saphenous Vein, Left
Solar (celiac) plexus	Abdominal Sympathetic Nerve
Soleus muscle	Lower Leg Muscle, Right
	Lower Leg Muscle, Left
Space of Retzius	Pelvic Cavity
Sphenomandibular ligament	Head and Neck Bursa and Ligament
Sphenopalatine (pterygopalatine) ganglion	Head and Neck Sympathetic Nerve
Spinal nerve, cervical	Cervical Nerve
Spinal nerve, lumbar	Lumbar Nerve
Spinal nerve, sacral	Sacral Nerve
Spinal nerve, thoracic	Thoracic Nerve
Spinous process	Cervical Vertebra
	Lumbar Vertebra
	Thoracic Vertebra
Spiral ganglion	Acoustic Nerve
Splenic flexure	Transverse Colon
Splenic plexus	Abdominal Sympathetic Nerve
Splenius capitis muscle	Head Muscle
Splenius cervicis muscle	Neck Muscle, Right
	Neck Muscle, Left
Stapes	Auditory Ossicle, Right
	Auditory Ossicle, Left
Stellate ganglion	Head and Neck Sympathetic Nerve
Stensen's duct	Parotid Duct, Right
	Parotid Duct, Left
Sternoclavicular ligament	Shoulder Bursa and Ligament, Right
	Shoulder Bursa and Ligament, Left
Sternocleidomastoid artery	Thyroid Artery, Right
	Thyroid Artery, Left
Sternocleidomastoid muscle	Neck Muscle, Right
	Neck Muscle, Left
Sternocostal ligament	Sternum Bursa and Ligament
Styloglossus muscle	Tongue, Palate, Pharynx Muscle
Stylomandibular ligament	Head and Neck Bursa and Ligament
Stylopharyngeus muscle	Tongue, Palate, Pharynx Muscle
Subacromial bursa	Shoulder Bursa and Ligament, Right
	Shoulder Bursa and Ligament, Left

Term	ICD-10-PCS Value
Subaortic (common iliac) lymph node	Lymphatic, Pelvis
Subarachnoid space, spinal	Spinal Canal
Subclavicular (apical) lymph node	Lymphatic, Right Axillary
	Lymphatic, Left Axillary
Subclavius muscle	Thorax Muscle, Right
	Thorax Muscle, Left
Subclavius nerve	Brachial Plexus
Subcostal artery	Upper Artery
Subcostal muscle	Thorax Muscle, Right
	Thorax Muscle, Left
Subcostal nerve	Thoracic Nerve
Subdural space, spinal	Spinal Canal
Submandibular ganglion	Facial Nerve
	Head and Neck Sympathetic Nerve
Submandibular gland	Submaxillary Gland, Right
	Submaxillary Gland, Left
Submandibular lymph node	Lymphatic, Head
Submandibular space	Subcutaneous Tissue and Fascia, Face
Submaxillary ganglion	Head and Neck Sympathetic Nerve
Submaxillary lymph node	Lymphatic, Head
Submental artery	Face Artery
Submental lymph node	Lymphatic, Head
Submucous (Meissner's) plexus	Abdominal Sympathetic Nerve
Suboccipital nerve	Cervical Nerve
Suboccipital venous plexus	Vertebral Vein, Right
	Vertebral Vein, Left
Subparotid lymph node	Lymphatic, Head
Subscapular aponeurosis	Subcutaneous Tissue and Fascia, Right Upper Arm
	Subcutaneous Tissue and Fascia, Left Upper Arm
Subscapular artery	Axillary Artery, Right
	Axillary Artery, Left
Subscapular (posterior) lymph node	Lymphatic, Right Axillary
	Lymphatic, Left Axillary
Subscapularis muscle	Shoulder Muscle, Right
	Shoulder Muscle, Left
Substantia nigra	Basal Ganglia
Subtalar (talocalcaneal) joint	Tarsal Joint, Right
	Tarsal Joint, Left
Subtalar ligament	Foot Bursa and Ligament, Right
	Foot Bursa and Ligament, Left
Subthalamic nucleus	Basal Ganglia
Superficial circumflex iliac vein	Saphenous Vein, Right
	Saphenous Vein, Left
Superficial epigastric artery	Femoral Artery, Right
	Femoral Artery, Left
Superficial epigastric vein	Saphenous Vein, Right
	Saphenous Vein, Left
Superficial palmar arch	Hand Artery, Right
	Hand Artery, Left
Superficial palmar venous arch	Hand Vein, Right
	Hand Vein, Left
Superficial temporal artery	Temporal Artery, Right
	Temporal Artery, Left

Term	ICD-10-PCS Value
Superficial transverse perineal muscle	Perineum Muscle
Superior cardiac nerve	Thoracic Sympathetic Nerve
Superior cerebellar vein	Intracranial Vein
Superior cerebral vein	Intracranial Vein
Superior clunic (cluneal) nerve	Lumbar Nerve
Superior epigastric artery	Internal Mammary Artery, Right
	Internal Mammary Artery, Left
Superior genicular artery	Popliteal Artery, Right
	Popliteal Artery, Left
Superior gluteal artery	Internal Iliac Artery, Right
	Internal Iliac Artery, Left
Superior gluteal nerve	Lumbar Plexus
Superior hypogastric plexus	Abdominal Sympathetic Nerve
Superior labial artery	Face Artery
Superior laryngeal artery	Thyroid Artery, Right
	Thyroid Artery, Left
Superior laryngeal nerve	Vagus Nerve
Superior longitudinal muscle	Tongue, Palate, Pharynx Muscle
Superior mesenteric ganglion	Abdominal Sympathetic Nerve
Superior mesenteric lymph node	Lymphatic, Mesenteric
Superior mesenteric plexus	Abdominal Sympathetic Nerve
Superior oblique muscle	Extraocular Muscle, Right
	Extraocular Muscle, Left
Superior olivary nucleus	Pons
Superior rectal artery	Inferior Mesenteric Artery
Superior rectal vein	Inferior Mesenteric Vein
Superior rectus muscle	Extraocular Muscle, Right
	Extraocular Muscle, Left
Superior tarsal plate	Upper Eyelid, Right
	Upper Eyelid, Left
Superior thoracic artery	Axillary Artery, Right
	Axillary Artery, Left
Superior thyroid artery	External Carotid Artery, Right
	External Carotid Artery, Left
	Thyroid Artery, Right
	Thyroid Artery, Left
Superior turbinate	Nasal Turbinate
Superior ulnar collateral artery	Brachial Artery, Right
	Brachial Artery, Left
Superior vesical artery	Internal Iliac Artery, Right
	Internal Iliac Artery, Left
Supraclavicular nerve	Cervical Plexus
Supraclavicular (Virchow's) lymph node	Lymphatic, Right Neck
	Lymphatic, Left Neck
Suprahyoid lymph node	Lymphatic, Head
Suprahyoid muscle	Neck Muscle, Right
	Neck Muscle, Left
Suprainguinal lymph node	Lymphatic, Pelvis
Supraorbital vein	Face Vein, Right
	Face Vein, Left
Suprarenal gland	Adrenal Gland, Right
	Adrenal Gland, Left
	Adrenal Glands, Bilateral
	Adrenal Gland
Suprarenal plexus	Abdominal Sympathetic Nerve
Suprascapular nerve	Brachial Plexus

Term	ICD-10-PCS Value
Supraspinatus fascia	Subcutaneous Tissue and Fascia, Right Upper Arm
	Subcutaneous Tissue and Fascia, Left Upper Arm
Supraspinatus muscle	Shoulder Muscle, Right
	Shoulder Muscle, Left
Supraspinous ligament	Upper Spine Bursa and Ligament
	Lower Spine Bursa and Ligament
Suprasternal notch	Sternum
Supratrochlear lymph node	Lymphatic, Right Upper Extremity
	Lymphatic, Left Upper Extremity
Sural artery	Popliteal Artery, Right
	Popliteal Artery, Left
Sweat gland	Skin
Talocalcaneal ligament	Foot Bursa and Ligament, Right
	Foot Bursa and Ligament, Left
Talocalcaneal (subtalar) joint	Tarsal Joint, Right
	Tarsal Joint, Left
Talocalcaneonavicular joint	Tarsal Joint, Right
	Tarsal Joint, Left
Talocalcaneonavicular ligament	Foot Bursa and Ligament, Right
	Foot Bursa and Ligament, Left
Talocrural joint	Ankle Joint, Right
	Ankle Joint, Left
Talofibular ligament	Ankle Bursa and Ligament, Right
	Ankle Bursa and Ligament, Left
Talus bone	Tarsal, Right
	Tarsal, Left
Tarsometatarsal ligament	Foot Bursa and Ligament, Right
	Foot Bursa and Ligament, Left
Temporal lobe	Cerebral Hemisphere
Temporalis muscle	Head Muscle
Temporoparietalis muscle	Head Muscle
Tensor fasciae latae muscle	Hip Muscle, Right
	Hip Muscle, Left
Tensor veli palatini muscle	Tongue, Palate, Pharynx Muscle
Tenth cranial nerve	Vagus Nerve
Tentorium cerebelli	Dura Mater
Teres major muscle	Shoulder Muscle, Right
	Shoulder Muscle, Left
Teres minor muscle	Shoulder Muscle, Right
	Shoulder Muscle, Left
Testicular artery	Abdominal Aorta
Thenar muscle	Hand Muscle, Right
	Hand Muscle, Left
Third cranial nerve	Oculomotor Nerve
Third occipital nerve	Cervical Nerve
Third ventricle	Cerebral Ventricle
Thoracic aortic plexus	Thoracic Sympathetic Nerve
Thoracic esophagus	Esophagus, Middle
Thoracic facet joint	Thoracic Vertebral Joint
Thoracic ganglion	Thoracic Sympathetic Nerve
Thoracoacromial artery	Axillary Artery, Right
	Axillary Artery, Left
Thoracolumbar facet joint	Thoracolumbar Vertebral Joint
Thymus gland	Thymus

Term	ICD-10-PCS Value
Thyroarytenoid muscle	Neck Muscle, Right
	Neck Muscle, Left
Thyrocervical trunk	Thyroid Artery, Right
	Thyroid Artery, Left
Thyroid cartilage	Larynx
Tibial sesamoid	Metatarsal, Right
	Metatarsal, Left
Tibialis anterior muscle	Lower Leg Muscle, Right
	Lower Leg Muscle, Left
Tibialis posterior muscle	Lower Leg Muscle, Right
	Lower Leg Muscle, Left
Tibiofemoral joint	Knee Joint, Right
	Knee Joint, Left
	Knee Joint, Tibial Surface, Right
	Knee Joint, Tibial Surface, Left
Tibioperoneal trunk	Popliteal Artery, Right
	Popliteal Artery, Left
Tongue, base of	Pharynx
Tracheobronchial lymph node	Lymphatic, Thorax
Tragus	External Ear, Right
	External Ear, Left
	External Ear, Bilateral
Transversalis fascia	Subcutaneous Tissue and Fascia, Trunk
Transverse acetabular ligament	Hip Bursa and Ligament, Right
	Hip Bursa and Ligament, Left
Transverse (cutaneous) cervical nerve	Cervical Plexus
Transverse facial artery	Temporal Artery, Right
	Temporal Artery, Left
Transverse foramen	Cervical Vertebra
Transverse humeral ligament	Shoulder Bursa and Ligament, Right
	Shoulder Bursa and Ligament, Left
Transverse ligament of atlas	Head and Neck Bursa and Ligament
Transverse process	Cervical Vertebra
	Thoracic Vertebra
	Lumbar Vertebra
Transverse scapular ligament	Shoulder Bursa and Ligament, Right
	Shoulder Bursa and Ligament, Left
Transverse thoracis muscle	Thorax Muscle, Right
	Thorax Muscle, Left
Transversospinalis muscle	Trunk Muscle, Right
	Trunk Muscle, Left
Transversus abdominis muscle	Abdomen Muscle, Right
	Abdomen Muscle, Left
Trapezium bone	Carpal, Right
	Carpal, Left
Trapezius muscle	Trunk Muscle, Right
	Trunk Muscle, Left
Trapezoid bone	Carpal, Right
	Carpal, Left
Triceps brachii muscle	Upper Arm Muscle, Right
	Upper Arm Muscle, Left
Tricuspid annulus	Tricuspid Valve
Trifacial nerve	Trigeminal Nerve
Trigone of bladder	Bladder
Triquetral bone	Carpal, Right
	Carpal, Left

Term	ICD-10-PCS Value
Trochanteric bursa	Hip Bursa and Ligament, Right
	Hip Bursa and Ligament, Left
Twelfth cranial nerve	Hypoglossal Nerve
Tympanic cavity	Middle Ear, Right
	Middle Ear, Left
Tympanic nerve	Glossopharyngeal Nerve
Tympanic part of temoporal bone	Temporal Bone, Right
	Temporal Bone, Left
Ulnar collateral carpal ligament	Wrist Bursa and Ligament, Right
	Wrist Bursa and Ligament, Left
Ulnar collateral ligament	Elbow Bursa and Ligament, Right
	Elbow Bursa and Ligament, Left
Ulnar notch	Radius, Right
	Radius, Left
Ulnar vein	Brachial Vein, Right
	Brachial Vein, Left
Umbilical artery	Internal Iliac Artery, Right
	Internal Iliac Artery, Left
	Lower Artery
Ureteral orifice	Ureter, Right
	Ureter, Left
	Ureters, Bilateral
	Ureter
Ureteropelvic junction (UPJ)	Kidney Pelvis, Right
	Kidney Pelvis, Left
Ureterovesical orifice	Ureter, Right
	Ureter, Left
	Ureters, Bilateral
	Ureter
Uterine artery	Internal Iliac Artery, Right
	Internal Iliac Artery, Left
Uterine cornu	Uterus
Uterine tube	Fallopian Tube, Right
	Fallopian Tube, Left
Uterine vein	Hypogastric Vein, Right
	Hypogastric Vein, Left
Vaginal artery	Internal Iliac Artery, Right
	Internal Iliac Artery, Left
Vaginal vein	Hypogastric Vein, Right
	Hypogastric Vein, Left
Vastus intermedius muscle	Upper Leg Muscle, Right
	Upper Leg Muscle, Left
Vastus lateralis muscle	Upper Leg Muscle, Right
	Upper Leg Muscle, Left
Vastus medialis muscle	Upper Leg Muscle, Right
	Upper Leg Muscle, Left
Ventricular fold	Larynx
Vermiform appendix	Appendix
Vermilion border	Upper Lip
	Lower Lip
Vertebral arch	Cervical Vertebra
	Lumbar Vertebra
	Thoracic Vertebra
Vertebral artery, intracranial portion	Intracranial Artery

Term	ICD-10-PCS Value
Vertebral body	Cervical Vertebra
	Lumbar Vertebra
	Thoracic Vertebra
Vertebral canal	Spinal Canal
Vertebral foramen	Cervical Vertebra
	Lumbar Vertebra
	Thoracic Vertebra
Vertebral lamina	Cervical Vertebra
	Lumbar Vertebra
	Thoracic Vertebra
Vertebral pedicle	Cervical Vertebra
	Lumbar Vertebra
	Thoracic Vertebra
Vesical vein	Hypogastric Vein, Right
	Hypogastric Vein, Left
Vestibular (Scarpa's) ganglion	Acoustic Nerve
Vestibular nerve	Acoustic Nerve
Vestibulocochlear nerve	Acoustic Nerve
Virchow's (supraclavicular) lymph node	Lymphatic, Right Neck
	Lymphatic, Left Neck
Vitreous body	Vitreous, Right
	Vitreous, Left
Vocal fold	Vocal Cord, Right
	Vocal Cord, Left
Volar (palmar) digital vein	Hand Vein, Right
	Hand Vein, Left
Volar (palmar) metacarpal vein	Hand Vein, Right
	Hand Vein, Left
Vomer bone	Nasal Septum
Vomer of nasal septum	Nasal Bone
Xiphoid process	Sternum
Zonule of Zinn	Lens, Right
	Lens, Left
Zygomatic process of frontal bone	Frontal Bone
Zygomatic process of temporal bone	Temporal Bone, Right
	Temporal Bone, Left
Zygomaticus muscle	Facial Muscle

Appendix H: Device Key and Aggregation Table

Device Key

Term	ICD-10-PCS Value
3f (Aortic) Bioprosthesis valve	Zooplastic Tissue in Heart and Great Vessels
AbioCor® Total Replacement Heart	Synthetic Substitute
Absolute Pro Vascular (OTW) Self-Expanding Stent System	Intraluminal Device
Acculink (RX) Carotid Stent System	Intraluminal Device
Acellular Hydrated Dermis	Nonautologous Tissue Substitute
Acetabular cup	Liner in Lower Joints
Activa PC neurostimulator	Stimulator Generator, Multiple Array for Insertion in Subcutaneous Tissue and Fascia
Activa RC neurostimulator	Stimulator Generator, Multiple Array Rechargeable for Insertion in Subcutaneous Tissue and Fascia
Activa SC neurostimulator	Stimulator Generator, Single Array for Insertion in Subcutaneous Tissue and Fascia
ACUITY™ Steerable Lead	Cardiac Lead, Pacemaker for Insertion in Heart and Great Vessels Cardiac Lead, Defibrillator for Insertion in Heart and Great Vessels
Advisa (MRI)	Pacemaker, Dual Chamber for Insertion in Subcutaneous Tissue and Fascia
AFX® Endovascular AAA System	Intraluminal Device
Alfapump® system	Other Device
AMPLATZER® Muscular VSD Occluder	Synthetic Substitute
AMS 800® Urinary Control System	Artificial Sphincter in Urinary System
AneuRx® AAA Advantage®	Intraluminal Device
Ankle Truss System™ (ATS)	Internal Fixation Device, Open-truss Design in New Technology
Annuloplasty ring	Synthetic Substitute
Aortix™ System	Short-term External Heart Assist System in Heart and Great Vessels
ApiFix® Minimally Invasive Deformity Correction (MID-C) System (C)	Posterior (Dynamic) Distraction Device in New Technology
aprevo™	Interbody Fusion Device, Custom-made Anatomically Designed in New Technology
Articulating Spacer (Antibiotic)	Articulating Spacer in Lower Joints
Artificial anal sphincter (AAS)	Artificial Sphincter in Gastrointestinal System
Artificial bowel sphincter (neosphincter)	Artificial Sphincter in Gastrointestinal System
Artificial urinary sphincter (AUS)	Artificial Sphincter in Urinary System
Ascenda Intrathecal Catheter	Infusion Device
Assurant (Cobalt) stent	Intraluminal Device
AtriClip LAA Exclusion System	Extraluminal Device
Attain Ability® Lead	Cardiac Lead, Pacemaker for Insertion in Heart and Great Vessels Cardiac Lead, Defibrillator for Insertion in Heart and Great Vessels
Attain StarFix® (OTW) Lead	Cardiac Lead, Pacemaker for Insertion in Heart and Great Vessels Cardiac Lead, Defibrillator for Insertion in Heart and Great Vessels
Autograft	Autologous Tissue Substitute
Autologous artery graft	Autologous Arterial Tissue in Heart and Great Vessels Autologous Arterial Tissue in Upper Arteries Autologous Arterial Tissue in Lower Arteries Autologous Arterial Tissue in Upper Veins Autologous Arterial Tissue in Lower Veins
Autologous vein graft	Autologous Venous Tissue in Heart and Great Vessels Autologous Venous Tissue in Upper Arteries Autologous Venous Tissue in Lower Arteries Autologous Venous Tissue in Upper Veins Autologous Venous Tissue in Lower Veins
Aveir™ AR, as dual chamber	Intracardiac Pacemaker, Dual-Chamber in New Technology
Aveir™ DR, dual chamber	Intracardiac Pacemaker, Dual-Chamber in New Technology
Aveir™ VR, as single chamber	Intracardiac Pacemaker in the Heart and Great Vessels
Axial Lumbar Interbody Fusion System	Interbody Fusion Device in Lower Joints
AxiaLIF® System	Interbody Fusion Device in Lower Joints
BAK/C® Interbody Cervical Fusion System	Interbody Fusion Device in Upper Joints
Bard® Composix® (E/X)(LP) mesh	Synthetic Substitute
Bard® Composix® Kugel® patch	Synthetic Substitute
Bard® Dulex™ mesh	Synthetic Substitute
Bard® Ventralex™ hernia patch	Synthetic Substitute
Baroreflex Activation Therapy® (BAT®)	Stimulator Lead in Upper Arteries Stimulator Generator in Subcutaneous Tissue and Fascia
Barricaid® Annular Closure Device (ACD)	Synthetic Substitute
Berlin Heart Ventricular Assist Device	Implantable Heart Assist System in Heart and Great Vessels
Bioactive embolization coil(s)	Intraluminal Device, Bioactive in Upper Arteries
Biventricular external heart assist system	Short-term External Heart Assist System in Heart and Great Vessels
Blood glucose monitoring system	Monitoring Device
Bone anchored hearing device	Hearing Device, Bone Conduction for Insertion in Ear, Nose, Sinus Hearing Device, in Head and Facial Bones
Bone bank bone graft	Nonautologous Tissue Substitute
Bone screw (interlocking)(lag)(pedicle)(recessed)	Internal Fixation Device in Head and Facial Bones Internal Fixation Device in Upper Bones Internal Fixation Device in Lower Bones
Bovine pericardial valve	Zooplastic Tissue in Heart and Great Vessels
Bovine pericardium graft	Zooplastic Tissue in Heart and Great Vessels

Term	ICD-10-PCS Value
Brachytherapy seeds	Radioactive Element
BRYAN® Cervical Disc System	Synthetic Substitute
BVS 5000 Ventricular Assist Device	Short-term External Heart Assist System in Heart and Great Vessels
Canturio™ te (Tibial Extension)	Tibial Extension with Motion Sensors in New Technology
Cardiac contractility modulation lead	Cardiac Lead in Heart and Great Vessels
Cardiac event recorder	Monitoring Device
Cardiac resynchronization therapy (CRT) lead	Cardiac Lead, Pacemaker for Insertion in Heart and Great Vessels Cardiac Lead, Defibrillator for Insertion in Heart and Great Vessels
CardioMEMS® pressure sensor	Monitoring Device, Pressure Sensor for Insertion in Heart and Great Vessels
Carmat total artificial heart (TAH)	Biologic with Synthetic Substitute, Autoregulated Electrohydraulic for Replacement in Heart and Great Vessels
Carotid (artery) sinus (baroreceptor) lead	Stimulator Lead in Upper Arteries
Carotid WALLSTENT® Monorail® Endoprosthesis	Intraluminal Device
Centrimag® Blood Pump	Short-term External Heart Assist System in Heart and Great Vessels
Ceramic on ceramic bearing surface	Synthetic Substitute, Ceramic for Replacement in Lower Joints
Cesium-131 Collagen Implant	Radioactive Element, Cesium-131 Collagen Implant for Insertion in Central Nervous System and Cranial Nerves
CivaSheet®	Radioactive Element
Clamp and rod internal fixation system (CRIF)	Internal Fixation Device in Upper Bones Internal Fixation Device in Lower Bones
COALESCE® radiolucent interbody fusion device	Interbody Fusion Device in Upper Joints Interbody Fusion Device in Lower Joints
CoAxia NeuroFlo catheter	Intraluminal Device
Cobalt/chromium head and polyethylene socket	Synthetic Substitute, Metal on Polyethylene for Replacement in Lower Joints
Cobalt/chromium head and socket	Synthetic Substitute, Metal for Replacement in Lower Joints
Cochlear implant (CI), multiple channel (electrode)	Hearing Device, Multiple Channel Cochlear Prosthesis for Insertion in Ear, Nose, Sinus
Cochlear implant (CI), single channel (electrode)	Hearing Device, Single Channel Cochlear Prosthesis for Insertion in Ear, Nose, Sinus
COGNIS® CRT-D	Cardiac Resynchronization Defibrillator Pulse Generator for Insertion in Subcutaneous Tissue and Fascia
COHERE® radiolucent interbody fusion device	Interbody Fusion Device in Upper Joints Interbody Fusion Device in Lower Joints
Colonic Z-Stent®	Intraluminal Device
Complete (SE) stent	Intraluminal Device
Concerto II CRT-D	Cardiac Resynchronization Defibrillator Pulse Generator for Insertion in Subcutaneous Tissue and Fascia
CONSERVE® PLUS Total Resurfacing Hip System	Resurfacing Device in Lower Joints
Consulta CRT-D	Cardiac Resynchronization Defibrillator Pulse Generator for Insertion in Subcutaneous Tissue and Fascia
Consulta CRT-P	Cardiac Resynchronization Pacemaker Pulse Generator for Insertion in Subcutaneous Tissue and Fascia
CONTAK RENEWAL® 3 RF (HE) CRT-D	Cardiac Resynchronization Defibrillator Pulse Generator for Insertion in Subcutaneous Tissue and Fascia
Contegra Pulmonary Valved Conduit	Zooplastic Tissue in Heart and Great Vessels
Continuous Glucose Monitoring (CGM) device	Monitoring Device
Cook Biodesign® Fistula Plug(s)	Nonautologous Tissue Substitute
Cook Biodesign® Hernia Graft(s)	Nonautologous Tissue Substitute
Cook Biodesign® Layered Graft(s)	Nonautologous Tissue Substitute
Cook Zenapro™ Layered Graft(s)	Nonautologous Tissue Substitute
Cook Zenith AAA Endovascular Graft	Intraluminal Device
Cook Zenith® Fenestrated AAA Endovascular Graft	Intraluminal Device, Branched or Fenestrated, One or Two Arteries for Restriction in Lower Arteries Intraluminal Device, Branched or Fenestrated, Three or More Arteries for Restriction in Lower Arteries
CoreValve transcatheter aortic valve	Zooplastic Tissue in Heart and Great Vessels
Cormet Hip Resurfacing System	Resurfacing Device in Lower Joints
CoRoent® XL	Interbody Fusion Device in Lower Joints
Corox (OTW) Bipolar Lead	Cardiac Lead, Pacemaker for Insertion in Heart and Great Vessels Cardiac Lead, Defibrillator for Insertion in Heart and Great Vessels
Cortical strip neurostimulator lead	Neurostimulator Lead in Central Nervous System and Cranial Nerves
Corvia IASD®	Synthetic Substitute
Cultured epidermal cell autograft	Autologous Tissue Substitute
CYPHER® Stent	Intraluminal Device, Drug-eluting in Heart and Great Vessels
Cystostomy tube	Drainage Device
DBS lead	Neurostimulator Lead in Central Nervous System and Cranial Nerves
DeBakey Left Ventricular Assist Device	Implantable Heart Assist System in Heart and Great Vessels
Deep brain neurostimulator lead	Neurostimulator Lead in Central Nervous System and Cranial Nerves
Delta frame external fixator	External Fixation Device, Hybrid for Insertion in Upper Bones External Fixation Device, Hybrid for Reposition in Upper Bones External Fixation Device, Hybrid for Insertion in Lower Bones External Fixation Device, Hybrid for Reposition in Lower Bones
Delta III Reverse shoulder prosthesis	Synthetic Substitute, Reverse Ball and Socket for Replacement in Upper Joints
DETOUR® System	Conduit through Femoral Vein to Popliteal Artery in New Technology Conduit through Femoral Vein to Superficial Femoral Artery in New Technology
Diaphragmatic pacemaker generator	Stimulator Generator in Subcutaneous Tissue and Fascia
Direct Lateral Interbody Fusion (DLIF) device	Interbody Fusion Device in Lower Joints
Driver stent (RX) (OTW)	Intraluminal Device

Appendix H: Device Key and Aggregation Table

Term	ICD-10-PCS Value
DuraHeart Left Ventricular Assist System	Implantable Heart Assist System in Heart and Great Vessels
Durata® Defibrillation Lead	Cardiac Lead, Defibrillator for Insertion in Heart and Great Vessels
DynaClip® (Forte)	Internal Fixation Device, Sustained Compression for Fusion in Upper Joints Internal Fixation Device, Sustained Compression for Fusion in Lower Joints
DynaNail® (Helix) (Hybrid) (Mini)	Internal Fixation Device, Sustained Compression for Fusion in Upper Joints Internal Fixation Device, Sustained Compression for Fusion in Lower Joints
Dynesys® Dynamic Stabilization System	Spinal Stabilization Device, Pedicle-Based for Insertion in Upper Joints Spinal Stabilization Device, Pedicle-Based for Insertion in Lower Joints
E-Luminexx™ (Biliary) (Vascular) Stent	Intraluminal Device
Electrical bone growth stimulator (EBGS)	Bone Growth Stimulator in Head and Facial Bones Bone Growth Stimulator in Upper Bones Bone Growth Stimulator in Lower Bones
Electrical muscle stimulation (EMS) lead	Stimulator Lead in Muscles
Electronic muscle stimulator lead	Stimulator Lead in Muscles
Eluvia™ Drug-eluting Vascular Stent System	Intraluminal Device, Sustained Release Drug-eluting in New Technology Intraluminal Device, Sustained Release Drug-eluting, Two in New Technology Intraluminal Device, Sustained Release Drug-eluting, Three in New Technology Intraluminal Device, Sustained Release Drug-eluting, Four or More in New Technology
Embolization coil(s)	Intraluminal Device
Endeavor® (III) (IV) (Sprint) Zotarolimus-eluting Coronary Stent System	Intraluminal Device, Drug-eluting in Heart and Great Vessels
Endologix AFX® Endovascular AAA System	Intraluminal Device
EndoSure® sensor	Monitoring Device, Pressure Sensor for Insertion in Heart and Great Vessels
ENDOTAK RELIANCE® (G) Defibrillation Lead	Cardiac Lead, Defibrillator for Insertion in Heart and Great Vessels
Endotracheal tube (cuffed) (double-lumen)	Intraluminal Device, Endotracheal Airway in Respiratory System
Endurant® Endovascular Stent Graft	Intraluminal Device
Endurant® II AAA stent graft system	Intraluminal Device
EnRhythm	Pacemaker, Dual Chamber for Insertion in Subcutaneous Tissue and Fascia
Enterra gastric neurostimulator	Stimulator Generator, Multiple Array for Insertion in Subcutaneous Tissue and Fascia
Epic™ Stented Tissue Valve (aortic)	Zooplastic Tissue in Heart and Great Vessels
Epicel® cultured epidermal autograft	Autologous Tissue Substitute
Esophageal obturator airway (EOA)	Intraluminal Device, Airway in Gastrointestinal System
Esteem® implantable hearing system	Hearing Device in Ear, Nose, Sinus
EV ICD System (Extravascular implantable defibrillator lead)	Defibrillator Lead in Anatomical Regions, General

Term	ICD-10-PCS Value
Evera (XT)(S)(DR/VR)	Defibrillator Generator for Insertion in Subcutaneous Tissue and Fascia
Everolimus-eluting coronary stent	Intraluminal Device, Drug-eluting in Heart and Great Vessels
Ex-PRESS™ mini glaucoma shunt	Synthetic Substitute
EXCLUDER® AAA Endoprosthesis	Intraluminal Device Intraluminal Device, Branched or Fenestrated, One or Two Arteries for Restriction in Lower Arteries Intraluminal Device, Branched or Fenestrated, Three or More Arteries for Restriction in Lower Arteries
EXCLUDER® IBE Endoprosthesis	Intraluminal Device, Branched or Fenestrated, One or Two Arteries for Restriction in Lower Arteries
Express® (LD) Premounted Stent System	Intraluminal Device
Express® Biliary SD Monorail® Premounted Stent System	Intraluminal Device
Express® SD Renal Monorail® Premounted Stent System	Intraluminal Device
External fixator	External Fixation Device in Head and Facial Bones External Fixation Device in Upper Bones External Fixation Device in Lower Bones External Fixation Device in Upper Joints External Fixation Device in Lower Joints
EXtreme Lateral Interbody Fusion (XLIF) device	Interbody Fusion Device in Lower Joints
Facet replacement spinal stabilization device	Spinal Stabilization Device, Facet Replacement for Insertion in Upper Joints Spinal Stabilization Device, Facet Replacement for Insertion in Lower Joints
FLAIR® Endovascular Stent Graft	Intraluminal Device
Flexible Composite Mesh	Synthetic Substitute
Flourish® Pediatric Esophageal Atresia Device	Magnetic Lengthening Device in Gastrointestinal System
Flow Diverter embolization device	Intraluminal Device, Flow Diverter for Restriction in Upper Arteries
Foley catheter	Drainage Device
Formula™ Balloon-Expandable Renal Stent System	Intraluminal Device
Freestyle (Stentless) Aortic Root Bioprosthesis	Zooplastic Tissue in Heart and Great Vessels
Fusion screw (compression)(lag)(locking)	Internal Fixation Device in Upper Joints Internal Fixation Device in Lower Joints
GammaTile™	Radioactive Element, Cesium-131 Collagen Implant for Insertion in Central Nervous System and Cranial Nerves
Gastric electrical stimulation (GES) lead	Stimulator Lead in Gastrointestinal System
Gastric pacemaker lead	Stimulator Lead in Gastrointestinal System
GORE EXCLUDER® AAA Endoprosthesis	Intraluminal Device Intraluminal Device, Branched or Fenestrated, One or Two Arteries for Restriction in Lower Arteries Intraluminal Device, Branched or Fenestrated, Three or More Arteries for Restriction in Lower Arteries
GORE EXCLUDER® IBE Endoprosthesis	Intraluminal Device, Branched or Fenestrated, One or Two Arteries for Restriction in Lower Arteries

Term	ICD-10-PCS Value
GORE TAG® Thoracic Endoprosthesis	Intraluminal Device
GORE® DUALMESH®	Synthetic Substitute
Guedel airway	Intraluminal Device, Airway in Mouth and Throat
Hancock Bioprosthesis (aortic)(mitral) valve	Zooplastic Tissue in Heart and Great Vessels
Hancock Bioprosthetic Valved Conduit	Zooplastic Tissue in Heart and Great Vessels
HeartMate 3™ LVAS	Implantable Heart Assist System in Heart and Great Vessels
HeartMate II® Left Ventricular Assist Device (LVAD)	Implantable Heart Assist System in Heart and Great Vessels
HeartMate XVE® Left Ventricular Assist Device (LVAD)	Implantable Heart Assist System in Heart and Great Vessels
Herculink (RX) Elite Renal Stent System	Intraluminal Device
Hip (joint) liner	Liner in Lower Joints
Holter valve ventricular shunt	Synthetic Substitute
IASD® (InterAtrial Shunt Device), Corvia	Synthetic Substitute
iFuse Bedrock™ Granite Implant System	Internal Fixation Device with Tulip Connector in New Technology
Ilizarov external fixator	External Fixation Device, Ring for Insertion in Upper Bones External Fixation Device, Ring for Reposition in Upper Bones External Fixation Device, Ring for Insertion in Lower Bones External Fixation Device, Ring for Reposition in Lower Bones
Ilizarov-Vecklich device	External Fixation Device, Limb Lengthening for Insertion in Upper Bones External Fixation Device, Limb Lengthening for Insertion in Lower Bones
Impella® 5.5 with SmartAssist® System	Conduit To Short-term External Heart Assist System in New Technology
Impella® heart pump	Short-term External Heart Assist System in Heart and Great Vessels
Implantable cardioverter-defibrillator (ICD)	Defibrillator Generator for Insertion in Subcutaneous Tissue and Fascia
Implantable drug infusion pump (anti-spasmodic) (chemotherapy)(pain)	Infusion Device, Pump in Subcutaneous Tissue and Fascia
Implantable glucose monitoring device	Monitoring Device
Implantable hemodynamic monitor (IHM)	Monitoring Device, Hemodynamic for Insertion in Subcutaneous Tissue and Fascia
Implantable hemodynamic monitoring system (IHMS)	Monitoring Device, Hemodynamic for Insertion in Subcutaneous Tissue and Fascia
Implantable Miniature Telescope™ (IMT)	Synthetic Substitute, Intraocular Telescope for Replacement in Eye
Implanted (venous)(access) port	Vascular Access Device, Totally Implantable in Subcutaneous Tissue and Fascia
InDura, intrathecal catheter (1P) (spinal)	Infusion Device
Injection reservoir, port	Vascular Access Device, Totally Implantable in Subcutaneous Tissue and Fascia
Injection reservoir, pump	Infusion Device, Pump in Subcutaneous Tissue and Fascia
Intellis™ neurostimulator	Stimulator Generator, Multiple Array Rechargeable for Insertion in Subcutaneous Tissue and Fascia
InterAtrial Shunt Device IASD®, Corvia	Synthetic Substitute
Interbody fusion (spine) cage	Interbody Fusion Device in Upper Joints Interbody Fusion Device in Lower Joints
Interspinous process spinal stabilization device	Spinal Stabilization Device, Interspinous Process for Insertion in Upper Joints Spinal Stabilization Device, Interspinous Process for Insertion in Lower Joints
InterStim™ Micro Therapy neurostimulator	Stimulator Generator, Single Array Rechargeable for Insertion in Subcutaneous Tissue and Fascia
InterStim® Therapy lead	Neurostimulator Lead in Peripheral Nervous System
InterStim™ II Therapy neurostimulator	Stimulator Generator, Single Array for Insertion in Subcutaneous Tissue and Fascia
Intramedullary (IM) rod (nail)	Internal Fixation Device, Intramedullary in Upper Bones Internal Fixation Device, Intramedullary in Lower Bones
Intramedullary skeletal kinetic distractor (ISKD)	Internal Fixation Device, Intramedullary in Upper Bones Internal Fixation Device, Intramedullary in Lower Bones
Intrauterine Device (IUD)	Contraceptive Device in Female Reproductive System
Ischemic Stroke System (ISS500)	Neurostimulator Lead in New Technology
ISS500 (Ischemic Stroke System)	Neurostimulator Lead in New Technology
Itrel (3)(4) neurostimulator	Stimulator Generator, Single Array for Insertion in Subcutaneous Tissue and Fascia
Joint fixation plate	Internal Fixation Device in Upper Joints Internal Fixation Device in Lower Joints
Joint liner (insert)	Liner in Lower Joints
Joint spacer (antibiotic)	Spacer in Upper Joints Spacer in Lower Joints
Kappa	Pacemaker, Dual Chamber for Insertion in Subcutaneous Tissue and Fascia
Kirschner wire (K-wire)	Internal Fixation Device in Head and Facial Bones Internal Fixation Device in Upper Bones Internal Fixation Device in Lower Bones Internal Fixation Device in Upper Joints Internal Fixation Device in Lower Joints
Knee (implant) insert	Liner in Lower Joints
Kuntscher nail	Internal Fixation Device, Intramedullary in Upper Bones Internal Fixation Device, Intramedullary in Lower Bones
LAP-BAND® adjustable gastric banding system	Extraluminal Device
LifeStent® (Flexstar)(XL) Vascular Stent System	Intraluminal Device
LigaPASS 2.0™ PJK Prevention System	Posterior Vertebral Tether in New Technology
LIVIAN™ CRT-D	Cardiac Resynchronization Defibrillator Pulse Generator for Insertion in Subcutaneous Tissue and Fascia
Longeviti ClearFit® Cranial Implant	Synthetic Substitute, Ultrasound Penetrable in New Technology

Term	ICD-10-PCS Value
Longeviti ClearFit® OTS Cranial Implant	Synthetic Substitute, Ultrasound Penetrable in New Technology
Loop recorder, implantable	Monitoring Device
MAGEC® Spinal Bracing and Distraction System	Magnetically Controlled Growth Rod(s) in New Technology
Mark IV Breathing Pacemaker System	Stimulator Generator in Subcutaneous Tissue and Fascia
Maximo II DR (VR)	Defibrillator Generator for Insertion in Subcutaneous Tissue and Fascia
Maximo II DR CRT-D	Cardiac Resynchronization Defibrillator Pulse Generator for Insertion in Subcutaneous Tissue and Fascia
Medtronic Endurant® II AAA stent graft system	Intraluminal Device
Melody® transcatheter pulmonary valve	Zooplastic Tissue in Heart and Great Vessels
Metal on metal bearing surface	Synthetic Substitute, Metal for Replacement in Lower Joints
Micro-Driver stent (RX) (OTW)	Intraluminal Device
MicroMed HeartAssist	Implantable Heart Assist System in Heart and Great Vessels
Micrus CERECYTE microcoil	Intraluminal Device, Bioactive in Upper Arteries
MIRODERM™ Biologic Wound Matrix	Nonautologous Tissue Substitute
MitraClip valve repair system	Synthetic Substitute
Mitroflow® Aortic Pericardial Heart Valve	Zooplastic Tissue in Heart and Great Vessels
Mosaic Bioprosthesis (aortic) (mitral) valve	Zooplastic Tissue in Heart and Great Vessels
MULTI-LINK (VISION)(MINI-VISION)(ULTRA) Coronary Stent System	Intraluminal Device
nanoLOCK™ interbody fusion device	Interbody Fusion Device in Upper Joints Interbody Fusion Device in Lower Joints
Nasopharyngeal airway (NPA)	Intraluminal Device, Airway in Ear, Nose, Sinus
Neovasc Reducer™	Reduction Device in New Technology
Neuromuscular electrical stimulation (NEMS) lead	Stimulator Lead in Muscles
Neurostimulator generator, multiple channel	Stimulator Generator, Multiple Array for Insertion in Subcutaneous Tissue and Fascia
Neurostimulator generator, multiple channel rechargeable	Stimulator Generator, Multiple Array Rechargeable for Insertion in Subcutaneous Tissue and Fascia
Neurostimulator generator, single channel	Stimulator Generator, Single Array for Insertion in Subcutaneous Tissue and Fascia
Neurostimulator generator, single channel rechargeable	Stimulator Generator, Single Array Rechargeable for Insertion in Subcutaneous Tissue and Fascia
Neutralization plate	Internal Fixation Device in Head and Facial Bones Internal Fixation Device in Upper Bones Internal Fixation Device in Lower Bones
Nitinol framed polymer mesh	Synthetic Substitute
Non-tunneled central venous catheter	Infusion Device
Novacor Left Ventricular Assist Device	Implantable Heart Assist System in Heart and Great Vessels
Novation® Ceramic AHS® (Articulation Hip System)	Synthetic Substitute, Ceramic for Replacement in Lower Joints
NUsurface® Meniscus Implant	Synthetic Substitute, Lateral Meniscus in New Technology Synthetic Substitute, Medial Meniscus in New Technology
Omnilink Elite Vascular Balloon Expandable Stent System	Intraluminal Device
Open Pivot Aortic Valve Graft (AVG)	Synthetic Substitute
Open Pivot (mechanical) Valve	Synthetic Substitute
Optimizer™ III implantable pulse generator	Contractility Modulation Device for Insertion in Subcutaneous Tissue and Fascia
Oropharyngeal airway (OPA)	Intraluminal Device, Airway in Mouth and Throat
Ovatio™ CRT-D	Cardiac Resynchronization Defibrillator Pulse Generator for Insertion in Subcutaneous Tissue and Fascia
OXINIUM	Synthetic Substitute, Oxidized Zirconium on Polyethylene for Replacement in Lower Joints
Paclitaxel-eluting coronary stent	Intraluminal Device, Drug-eluting in Heart and Great Vessels
Paclitaxel-eluting peripheral stent	Intraluminal Device, Drug-eluting in Upper Arteries Intraluminal Device, Drug-eluting in Lower Arteries
Partially absorbable mesh	Synthetic Substitute
Pedicle-based dynamic stabilization device	Spinal Stabilization Device, Pedicle-Based for Insertion in Upper Joints Spinal Stabilization Device, Pedicle-Based for Insertion in Lower Joints
PERCEPT™ PC neurostimulator	Stimulator Generator, Multiple Array for Insertion in Subcutaneous Tissue and Fascia
Percutaneous endoscopic gastrojejunostomy (PEG/J) tube	Feeding Device in Gastrointestinal System
Percutaneous endoscopic gastrostomy (PEG) tube	Feeding Device in Gastrointestinal System
Percutaneous nephrostomy catheter	Drainage Device
Peripherally inserted central catheter (PICC)	Infusion Device
Pessary ring	Intraluminal Device, Pessary in Female Reproductive System
Phrenic nerve stimulator generator	Stimulator Generator in Subcutaneous Tissue and Fascia
Phrenic nerve stimulator lead	Diaphragmatic Pacemaker Lead in Respiratory System
PHYSIOMESH™ Flexible Composite Mesh	Synthetic Substitute
Pipeline™ (Flex) embolization device	Intraluminal Device, Flow Diverter for Restriction in Upper Arteries
Polyethylene socket	Synthetic Substitute, Polyethylene for Replacement in Lower Joints
Polymethylmethacrylate (PMMA)	Synthetic Substitute
Polypropylene mesh	Synthetic Substitute
Porcine (bioprosthetic) valve	Zooplastic Tissue in Heart and Great Vessels

Term	ICD-10-PCS Value
PRECICE intramedullary limb lengthening system	Internal Fixation Device, Intramedullary Limb Lengthening for Insertion in Upper Bones Internal Fixation Device, Intramedullary Limb Lengthening for Insertion in Lower Bones
PRESTIGE® Cervical Disc	Synthetic Substitute
PrimeAdvanced neurostimulator (SureScan)(MRI Safe)	Stimulator Generator, Multiple Array for Insertion in Subcutaneous Tissue and Fascia
PROCEED™ Ventral Patch	Synthetic Substitute
Prodisc-C	Synthetic Substitute
Prodisc-L	Synthetic Substitute
PROLENE Polypropylene Hernia System (PHS)	Synthetic Substitute
Protecta XT CRT-D	Cardiac Resynchronization Defibrillator Pulse Generator for Insertion in Subcutaneous Tissue and Fascia
Protecta XT DR (XT VR)	Defibrillator Generator for Insertion in Subcutaneous Tissue and Fascia
Protégé® RX Carotid Stent System	Intraluminal Device
Pump reservoir	Infusion Device, Pump in Subcutaneous Tissue and Fascia
REALIZE® Adjustable Gastric Band	Extraluminal Device
Rebound HRD® (Hernia Repair Device)	Synthetic Substitute
Reducer™ System	Reduction Device in New Technology
RestoreAdvanced neurostimulator (SureScan)(MRI Safe)	Stimulator Generator, Multiple Array Rechargeable for Insertion in Subcutaneous Tissue and Fascia
RestoreSensor neurostimulator (SureScan)(MRI Safe)	Stimulator Generator, Multiple Array Rechargeable for Insertion in Subcutaneous Tissue and Fascia
RestoreUltra neurostimulator (SureScan)(MRI Safe)	Stimulator Generator, Multiple Array Rechargeable for Insertion in Subcutaneous Tissue and Fascia
Reveal (LINQ)(DX)(XT)	Monitoring Device
Reverse® Shoulder Prosthesis	Synthetic Substitute, Reverse Ball and Socket for Replacement in Upper Joints
Revo MRI™ SureScan® pacemaker	Pacemaker, Dual Chamber for Insertion in Subcutaneous Tissue and Fascia
Rheos® System device	Stimulator Generator in Subcutaneous Tissue and Fascia
Rheos® System lead	Stimulator Lead in Upper Arteries
RNS System lead	Neurostimulator Lead in Central Nervous System and Cranial Nerves
RNS system neurostimulator generator	Neurostimulator Generator in Head and Facial Bones
S-ICD™ lead	Subcutaneous Defibrillator Lead in Subcutaneous Tissue and Fascia
Sacral nerve modulation (SNM) lead	Stimulator Lead in Urinary System
Sacral neuromodulation lead	Stimulator Lead in Urinary System
SAPIEN transcatheter aortic valve	Zooplastic Tissue in Heart and Great Vessels
SAVAL below-the-knee (BTK) drug-eluting stent system	Intraluminal Device, Sustained Release Drug-eluting in New Technology Intraluminal Device, Sustained Release Drug-eluting, Two in New Technology Intraluminal Device, Sustained Release Drug-eluting, Three in New Technology Intraluminal Device, Sustained Release Drug-eluting, Four or More in New Technology
Secura (DR) (VR)	Defibrillator Generator for Insertion in Subcutaneous Tissue and Fascia
Sheffield hybrid external fixator	External Fixation Device, Hybrid for Insertion in Upper Bones External Fixation Device, Hybrid for Reposition in Upper Bones External Fixation Device, Hybrid for Insertion in Lower Bones External Fixation Device, Hybrid for Reposition in Lower Bones
Sheffield ring external fixator	External Fixation Device, Ring for Insertion in Upper Bones External Fixation Device, Ring for Reposition in Upper Bones External Fixation Device, Ring for Insertion in Lower Bones External Fixation Device, Ring for Reposition in Lower Bones
Single lead pacemaker (atrium)(ventricle)	Pacemaker, Single Chamber for Insertion in Subcutaneous Tissue and Fascia
Single lead rate responsive pacemaker (atrium)(ventricle)	Pacemaker, Single Chamber Rate Responsive for Insertion in Subcutaneous Tissue and Fascia
Sirolimus-eluting coronary stent	Intraluminal Device, Drug-eluting in Heart and Great Vessels
SJM Biocor® Stented Valve System	Zooplastic Tissue in Heart and Great Vessels
Spacer, Articulating (Antibiotic)	Articulating Spacer in Lower Joints
Spacer, Static (Antibiotic)	Spacer in Lower Joints
Spinal cord neurostimulator lead	Neurostimulator Lead in Central Nervous System and Cranial Nerves
Spinal growth rods, magnetically controlled	Magnetically Controlled Growth Rod(s) in New Technology
SpineJack® system	Synthetic Substitute, Mechanically Expandable (Paired) in New Technology
Spiration IBV™ Valve System	Intraluminal Device, Endobronchial Valve in Respiratory System
Static Spacer (Antibiotic)	Spacer in Lower Joints
Stent, intraluminal (cardiovascular) (gastrointestinal) (hepatobiliary)(urinary)	Intraluminal Device
Stented tissue valve	Zooplastic Tissue in Heart and Great Vessels
Stratos LV	Cardiac Resynchronization Pacemaker Pulse Generator for Insertion in Subcutaneous Tissue and Fascia
Subcutaneous injection reservoir, port	Vascular Access Device, Totally Implantable in Subcutaneous Tissue and Fascia
Subcutaneous injection reservoir, pump	Infusion Device, Pump in Subcutaneous Tissue and Fascia
Subdermal progesterone implant	Contraceptive Device in Subcutaneous Tissue and Fascia
Surpass Streamline™ Flow Diverter	Intraluminal Device, Flow Diverter for Restriction in Upper Arteries

Term	ICD-10-PCS Value
SynCardia (temporary) Total Artificial Heart (TAH)	Synthetic Substitute, Pneumatic for Replacement in Heart and Great Vessels
SynCardia Total Artificial Heart	Synthetic Substitute
Synchra CRT-P	Cardiac Resynchronization Pacemaker Pulse Generator for Insertion in Subcutaneous Tissue and Fascia
SynchroMed Pump	Infusion Device, Pump in Subcutaneous Tissue and Fascia
Talent® Converter	Intraluminal Device
Talent® Occluder	Intraluminal Device
Talent® Stent Graft (abdominal)(thoracic)	Intraluminal Device
TandemHeart® System	Short-term External Heart Assist System in Heart and Great Vessels
TAXUS® Liberté® Paclitaxel-eluting Coronary Stent System	Intraluminal Device, Drug-eluting in Heart and Great Vessels
Therapeutic occlusion coil(s)	Intraluminal Device
Thoracostomy tube	Drainage Device
Thoraflex™ Hybrid device	Branched Synthetic Substitute with Intraluminal Device in New Technology
Thoratec IVAD (Implantable Ventricular Assist Device)	Implantable Heart Assist System in Heart and Great Vessels
Thoratec Paracorporeal Ventricular Assist Device	Short-term External Heart Assist System in Heart and Great Vessels
Tibial insert	Liner in Lower Joints
Tissue bank graft	Nonautologous Tissue Substitute
Tissue expander (inflatable)(injectable)	Tissue Expander in Skin and Breast Tissue Expander in Subcutaneous Tissue and Fascia
Titan Endoskeleton™	Interbody Fusion Device in Upper Joints Interbody Fusion Device in Lower Joints
Titanium Sternal Fixation System (TSFS)	Internal Fixation Device, Rigid Plate for Insertion in Upper Bones Internal Fixation Device, Rigid Plate for Reposition in Upper Bones
TOPS™ System	Posterior Spinal Motion Preservation Device in New Technology
Total Ankle Talar Replacement™ (TATR)	Synthetic Substitute, Talar Prosthesis in New Technology
Total artificial (replacement) heart	Synthetic Substitute
Tracheostomy tube	Tracheostomy Device in Respiratory System
TricValve® Transcatheter Bicaval Valve System	Intraluminal Device, Bioprosthetic Valve in New Technology
Trifecta™ Valve (aortic)	Zooplastic Tissue in Heart and Great Vessels
Tunneled central venous catheter	Vascular Access Device, Tunneled in Subcutaneous Tissue and Fascia
Tunneled spinal (intrathecal) catheter	Infusion Device
Two lead pacemaker	Pacemaker, Dual Chamber for Insertion in Subcutaneous Tissue and Fascia
Ultraflex™ Precision Colonic Stent System	Intraluminal Device
ULTRAPRO Hernia System (UHS)	Synthetic Substitute
ULTRAPRO Partially Absorbable Lightweight Mesh	Synthetic Substitute
ULTRAPRO Plug	Synthetic Substitute
Ultrasonic osteogenic stimulator	Bone Growth Stimulator in Head and Facial Bones Bone Growth Stimulator in Upper Bones Bone Growth Stimulator in Lower Bones
Ultrasound bone healing system	Bone Growth Stimulator in Head and Facial Bones Bone Growth Stimulator in Upper Bones Bone Growth Stimulator in Lower Bones
Uniplanar external fixator	External Fixation Device, Monoplanar for Insertion in Upper Bones External Fixation Device, Monoplanar for Reposition in Upper Bones External Fixation Device, Monoplanar for Insertion in Lower Bones External Fixation Device, Monoplanar for Reposition in Lower Bones
Urinary incontinence stimulator lead	Stimulator Lead in Urinary System
V-Wave Interatrial Shunt System	Synthetic Substitute
Vaginal pessary	Intraluminal Device, Pessary in Female Reproductive System
Valiant Thoracic Stent Graft	Intraluminal Device
Vanta™ PC neurostimulator	Stimulator Generator, Multiple Array for Insertion in Subcutaneous Tissue and Fascia
VasQ™ External Support device	Synthetic Substitute, Extraluminal Support Device in New Technology
Vectra® Vascular Access Graft	Vascular Access Device, Tunneled in Subcutaneous Tissue and Fascia
VenoValve®	Intraluminal Device, Bioprosthetic Valve in New Technology
Ventrio™ Hernia Patch	Synthetic Substitute
Versa	Pacemaker, Dual Chamber for Insertion in Subcutaneous Tissue and Fascia
VEST™ Venous External Support device	Vein Graft Extraluminal Support Device(s) in New Technology
Virtuoso (II) (DR) (VR)	Defibrillator Generator for Insertion in Subcutaneous Tissue and Fascia
Viva(XT)(S)	Cardiac Resynchronization Defibrillator Pulse Generator for Insertion in Subcutaneous Tissue and Fascia
Vivistim® Paired VNS System Lead	Neurostimulator Lead with Paired Stimulation System in New Technology
WALLSTENT® Endoprosthesis	Intraluminal Device
X-Spine Axle Cage	Spinal Stabilization Device, Interspinous Process for Insertion in Upper Joints Spinal Stabilization Device, Interspinous Process for Insertion in Lower Joints
X-STOP® Spacer	Spinal Stabilization Device, Interspinous Process for Insertion in Upper Joints Spinal Stabilization Device, Interspinous Process for Insertion in Lower Joints
Xact Carotid Stent System	Intraluminal Device
Xenograft	Zooplastic Tissue in Heart and Great Vessels
XIENCE Everolimus Eluting Coronary Stent System	Intraluminal Device, Drug-eluting in Heart and Great Vessels
XLIF® System	Interbody Fusion Device in Lower Joints
Zenith AAA Endovascular Graft	Intraluminal Device

Term	ICD-10-PCS Value
Zenith® Fenestrated AAA Endovascular Graft	Intraluminal Device, Branched or Fenestrated, One or Two Arteries for Restriction in Lower Arteries Intraluminal Device, Branched or Fenestrated, Three or More Arteries for Restriction in Lower Arteries
Zenith Flex® AAA Endovascular Graft	Intraluminal Device
Zenith® Renu™ AAA Ancillary Graft	Intraluminal Device
Zenith TX2® TAA Endovascular Graft	Intraluminal Device
Zilver® PTX® (paclitaxel) Drug-Eluting Peripheral Stent	Intraluminal Device, Drug-eluting in Upper Arteries Intraluminal Device, Drug-eluting in Lower Arteries
Zimmer® NexGen® LPS Mobile Bearing Knee	Synthetic Substitute
Zimmer® NexGen® LPS-Flex Mobile Knee	Synthetic Substitute
Zotarolimus-eluting coronary stent	Intraluminal Device, Drug-eluting in Heart and Great Vessels

Device Aggregation Table

This table crosswalks specific device character value definitions for specific root operations in a specific body system to the more general device character value to be used when the root operation covers a wide range of body parts and the device character represents an entire family of devices.

Specific Device	for Operation	in Body System	General Device
Autologous Arterial Tissue (A)	All applicable	Heart and Great Vessels Lower Arteries Lower Veins Upper Arteries Upper Veins	**7** Autologous Tissue Substitute
Autologous Venous Tissue (9)	All applicable	Heart and Great Vessels Lower Arteries Lower Veins Upper Arteries Upper Veins	**7** Autologous Tissue Substitute
Cardiac Lead, Defibrillator (K)	Insertion	Heart and Great Vessels	**M** Cardiac Lead
Cardiac Lead, Pacemaker (J)	Insertion	Heart and Great Vessels	**M** Cardiac Lead
Cardiac Resynchronization Defibrillator Pulse Generator (9)	Insertion	Subcutaneous Tissue and Fascia	**P** Cardiac Rhythm Related Device
Cardiac Resynchronization Pacemaker Pulse Generator (7)	Insertion	Subcutaneous Tissue and Fascia	**P** Cardiac Rhythm Related Device
Contractility Modulation Device (A)	Insertion	Subcutaneous Tissue and Fascia	**P** Cardiac Rhythm Related Device
Defibrillator Generator (8)	Insertion	Subcutaneous Tissue and Fascia	**P** Cardiac Rhythm Related Device
Epiretinal Visual Prosthesis (5)	All applicable	Eye	**J** Synthetic Substitute
External Fixation Device, Hybrid (D)	Insertion	Lower Bones Upper Bones	**5** External Fixation Device
External Fixation Device, Hybrid (D)	Reposition	Lower Bones Upper Bones	**5** External Fixation Device
External Fixation Device, Limb Lengthening (8)	Insertion	Lower Bones Upper Bones	**5** External Fixation Device
External Fixation Device, Monoplanar (B)	Insertion	Lower Bones Upper Bones	**5** External Fixation Device
External Fixation Device, Monoplanar (B)	Reposition	Lower Bones Upper Bones	**5** External Fixation Device
External Fixation Device, Ring (C)	Insertion	Lower Bones Upper Bones	**5** External Fixation Device
External Fixation Device, Ring (C)	Reposition	Lower Bones Upper Bones	**5** External Fixation Device
Hearing Device, Bone Conduction (4)	Insertion	Ear, Nose, Sinus	**S** Hearing Device
Hearing Device, Multiple Channel Cochlear Prosthesis (6)	Insertion	Ear, Nose, Sinus	**S** Hearing Device
Hearing Device, Single Channel Cochlear Prosthesis (5)	Insertion	Ear, Nose, Sinus	**S** Hearing Device
Internal Fixation Device, Intramedullary (6)	All applicable	Lower Bones Upper Bones	**4** Internal Fixation Device
Internal Fixation Device, Intramedullary Limb Lengthening (7)	Insertion	Lower Bones Upper Bones	**6** Internal Fixation Device, Intramedullary
Internal Fixation Device, Rigid Plate (Ø)	Insertion	Upper Bones	**4** Internal Fixation Device
Internal Fixation Device, Rigid Plate (Ø)	Reposition	Upper Bones	**4** Internal Fixation Device
Intraluminal Device, Airway (B)	All applicable	Ear, Nose, Sinus Gastrointestinal System Mouth and Throat	**D** Intraluminal Device
Intraluminal Device, Bioactive (B)	All applicable	Upper Arteries	**D** Intraluminal Device
Intraluminal Device, Branched or Fenestrated, One or Two Arteries (E)	Restriction	Heart and Great Vessels Lower Arteries	**D** Intraluminal Device
Intraluminal Device, Branched or Fenestrated, Three or More Arteries (F)	Restriction	Heart and Great Vessels Lower Arteries	**D** Intraluminal Device
Intraluminal Device, Drug-eluting (4)	All applicable	Heart and Great Vessels Lower Arteries Upper Arteries	**D** Intraluminal Device
Intraluminal Device, Drug-eluting, Four or More (7)	All applicable	Heart and Great Vessels Lower Arteries Upper Arteries	**D** Intraluminal Device

Specific Device	for Operation	in Body System	General Device
Intraluminal Device, Drug-eluting, Three (6)	All applicable	Heart and Great Vessels Lower Arteries Upper Arteries	**D** Intraluminal Device
Intraluminal Device, Drug-eluting, Two (5)	All applicable	Heart and Great Vessels Lower Arteries Upper Arteries	**D** Intraluminal Device
Intraluminal Device, Endobronchial Valve (G)	All applicable	Respiratory System	**D** Intraluminal Device
Intraluminal Device, Endotracheal Airway (E)	All applicable	Respiratory System	**D** Intraluminal Device
Intraluminal Device, Flow Diverter (H)	Restriction	Upper Arteries	**D** Intraluminal Device
Intraluminal Device, Four or More (G)	All applicable	Heart and Great Vessels Lower Arteries Upper Arteries	**D** Intraluminal Device
Intraluminal Device, Pessary (G)	All applicable	Female Reproductive System	**D** Intraluminal Device
Intraluminal Device, Radioactive (T)	All applicable	Heart and Great Vessels	**D** Intraluminal Device
Intraluminal Device, Three (F)	All applicable	Heart and Great Vessels Lower Arteries Upper Arteries	**D** Intraluminal Device
Intraluminal Device, Two (E)	All applicable	Heart and Great Vessels Lower Arteries Upper Arteries	**D** Intraluminal Device
Monitoring Device, Hemodynamic (Ø)	Insertion	Subcutaneous Tissue and Fascia	**2** Monitoring Device
Monitoring Device, Pressure Sensor (Ø)	Insertion	Heart and Great Vessels	**2** Monitoring Device
Pacemaker, Dual Chamber (6)	Insertion	Subcutaneous Tissue and Fascia	**P** Cardiac Rhythm Related Device
Pacemaker, Single Chamber (4)	Insertion	Subcutaneous Tissue and Fascia	**P** Cardiac Rhythm Related Device
Pacemaker, Single Chamber Rate Responsive (5)	Insertion	Subcutaneous Tissue and Fascia	**P** Cardiac Rhythm Related Device
Spinal Stabilization Device, Facet Replacement (D)	Insertion	Lower Joints Upper Joints	**4** Internal Fixation Device
Spinal Stabilization Device, Interspinous Process (B)	Insertion	Lower Joints Upper Joints	**4** Internal Fixation Device
Spinal Stabilization Device, Pedicle-Based (C)	Insertion	Lower Joints Upper Joints	**4** Internal Fixation Device
Spinal Stabilization Device, Vertebral Body Tether (3)	Reposition	Lower Bones Upper Bones	**4** Internal Fixation Device
Stimulator Generator, Multiple Array (D)	Insertion	Subcutaneous Tissue and Fascia	**M** Stimulator Generator
Stimulator Generator, Multiple Array Rechargeable (E)	Insertion	Subcutaneous Tissue and Fascia	**M** Stimulator Generator
Stimulator Generator, Single Array (B)	Insertion	Subcutaneous Tissue and Fascia	**M** Stimulator Generator
Stimulator Generator, Single Array Rechargeable (C)	Insertion	Subcutaneous Tissue and Fascia	**M** Stimulator Generator
Synthetic Substitute, Ceramic (3)	Replacement	Lower Joints	**J** Synthetic Substitute
Synthetic Substitute, Ceramic on Polyethylene (4)	Replacement	Lower Joints	**J** Synthetic Substitute
Synthetic Substitute, Intraocular Telescope (Ø)	Replacement	Eye	**J** Synthetic Substitute
Synthetic Substitute, Metal (1)	Replacement	Lower Joints	**J** Synthetic Substitute
Synthetic Substitute, Metal on Polyethylene (2)	Replacement	Lower Joints	**J** Synthetic Substitute
Synthetic Substitute, Oxidized Zirconium on Polyethylene (6)	Replacement	Lower Joints	**J** Synthetic Substitute
Synthetic Substitute, Polyethylene (Ø)	Replacement	Lower Joints	**J** Synthetic Substitute
Synthetic Substitute, Reverse Ball and Socket (Ø)	Replacement	Upper Joints	**J** Synthetic Substitute

Glossary

against medical advice. Discharge status of patients who leave the hospital after signing a form that releases the hospital from responsibility, or those who leave the hospital premises without notifying hospital personnel.

arithmetic mean length of stay. Average number of days within a given DRG-stay in the hospital, also referred to as the average length of stay. The AMLOS is used to determine payment for outlier cases.

base rate. Payment weight assigned to hospitals to calculate diagnosis-related group (DRG) reimbursement. The base payment rate is divided into labor-related and nonlabor shares. The labor-related share is adjusted by the wage index applicable to the area where the hospital is located, and if the hospital is located in Alaska or Hawaii, the nonlabor share is adjusted by a cost of living adjustment factor. This base payment rate is multiplied by the DRG relative weight to calculate DRG reimbursement.

case mix index. Sum of all DRG relative weights for cases over a given period of time, divided by the number of Medicare cases.

charges. Dollar amount assigned to a service or procedure by a provider and reported to a payer.

code cluster. Group of two or more ICD-10-CM or ICD-10-PCS codes that must be used together to replicate the meaning of one ICD-9-CM code.

complication/comorbidity (CC). Condition that, when present, leads to substantially increased hospital resource use, such as intensive monitoring, expensive and technically complex services, and extensive care requiring a greater number of caregivers. Significant acute disease, acute exacerbations of significant chronic diseases, advanced or end stage chronic diseases, and chronic diseases associated with extensive debility are representative of CC conditions.

complication or comorbidity(CC) exclusion. Diagnosis on the basic list of complications and comorbidities that is excluded as a CC or MCC because the diagnosis is too closely related to the principal diagnosis. Excluded secondary diagnoses were established using five principles, chronic and acute manifestations of the same condition should not be considered CC/MCCs for one another; specific and nonspecific (that is, not otherwise specified (NOS)) diagnosis codes for the same condition should not be considered CC/MCCs for one another; codes for the same condition that cannot coexist, such as partial/total, unilateral/bilateral, obstructed/unobstructed, and benign/malignant, should not be considered CC/MCCs for one another; codes for the same condition in anatomically proximal sites should not be considered CC/MCCs for one another; and closely related conditions should not be considered CC/MCCs for one another.

discharge. Situation in which the patient leaves an acute care (prospective payment) hospital after receiving complete acute care treatment.

discharge status. Disposition of the patient at discharge (e.g., left against medical advice, discharged home, transferred to an acute care hospital, expired).

geometric mean length of stay. Statistically adjusted value for all cases for a given diagnosis-related group, allowing for the outliers, transfer cases, and negative outlier cases that would normally skew the data. The GMLOS is used to determine payment only for transfer cases (i.e., the per diem rate).

grouper. Software program that assigns diagnosis-related groups (DRGs).

homogeneous. Group of patients consuming similar types and amounts of hospital resources.

hospital-acquired condition (HAC). A significant, reasonably preventable condition determined to have occurred during a hospital visit, identified via the assignment of certain present on admission (POA) indicators. The MCC or CC status for the code for the HAC condition is invalidated when the POA indicator is N or U, thus potentially affecting DRG reimbursement.

major complication/comorbidity (MCC). Diagnosis codes that reflect the highest level of severity and have the potential to increase DRG reimbursement. See also complication/comorbidity.

major diagnostic category (MDC). Broad classification of diagnoses typically grouped by body system.

Medicare severity-adjusted diagnosis-related group (MS-DRG). One of the 761 classifications of diagnoses in which patients demonstrate similar resource consumption and length-of-stay patterns. MS-DRGs are a modification of the prior system that more accurately reflect the severity of a patient's illness and resources used.

nonoperating room procedure. Procedure that does not normally require the use of the operating room and that can affect MS-DRG assignment.

operating room (OR) procedure. Defined group of procedures that normally require the use of an operating room.

other diagnosis. All conditions (secondary) that exist at the time of admission or that develop subsequently that affect the treatment received and/or the length of stay. Diagnoses that relate to an earlier episode and that have no bearing on the current hospital stay are not to be reported.

outliers. There are two types of outliers: cost and day outliers. A cost outlier is a case in which the costs for treating the patient are extraordinarily high compared with other cases classified to the same MS-DRG. A cost outlier is paid an amount in excess of the cut-off threshold for a given MS-DRG. Payment for day outliers was eliminated with discharges occurring on or after October 1, 1997.

per diem rate. Payment made to the hospital from which a patient is transferred for each day of stay. It is determined by dividing the full MS-DRG payment by the GMLOS for the MS-DRG. The payment rate for the first day of stay is twice the per diem rate, and subsequent days are paid at the per diem rate up to the full DRG amount.

PMDC (Pre-major diagnostic category). Fifteen MS-DRGs to which cases are directly assigned based upon procedure codes before classification to an MDC, including MS-DRGs for the heart, liver, bone marrow transplants, simultaneous pancreas/kidney transplant, pancreas transplant, lung transplant, and five MS-DRGs for tracheostomies.

present on admission (POA). CMS-mandated assignment of indicators Y (Yes), N (No), U (Unknown), W (Clinically undetermined), or 1 (Exempt) to identify each condition as present or not present at the time the order for inpatient admission occurs for Medicare patients. A POA indicator should be listed for the principal diagnosis as well as secondary diagnoses and external cause of injury codes.

principal diagnosis. Condition established after study to be chiefly responsible for occasioning the admission of the patient to the hospital for care.

principal procedure. Procedure performed for definitive treatment rather than for diagnostic or exploratory purposes, or that was necessary to treat a complication. Usually related to the principal diagnosis.

relative weight. Assigned weight that is intended to reflect the relative resource consumption associated with each MS-DRG. The higher the relative weight, the greater the payment to the hospital. The relative weights are calculated by CMS and published in the final prospective payment system rule.

surgical hierarchy. Ordering of surgical cases from most to least resource intensive. Application of this decision rule is necessary when patient stays involve multiple surgical procedures, each of which, occurring by itself, could result in assignment to a different MS-DRG. All patients must be assigned to only one MS-DRG per admission.

transfer. A situation in which the patient is transferred to another acute care hospital for related care.

DRG Decision Trees

MDC | Description

Pre-MDC
All Patients
1 | Diseases and Disorders of the Nervous System
2 | Diseases and Disorders of the Eye
3 | Diseases and Disorders of the Ear, Nose, Mouth and Throat
4 | Diseases and Disorders of the Respiratory System
5 | Diseases and Disorders of the Circulatory System
6 | Diseases and Disorders of the Digestive System
7 | Diseases and Disorders of the Hepatobiliary System and Pancreas
8 | Diseases and Disorders of the Musculoskeletal System and Connective Tissue
9 | Diseases and Disorders of the Skin, Subcutaneous Tissue and Breast
10 | Endocrine, Nutritional and Metabolic Diseases and Disorders
11 | Diseases and Disorders of the Kidney and Urinary Tract
12 | Diseases and Disorders of the Male Reproductive System
13 | Diseases and Disorders of the Female Reproductive System
14 | Pregnancy, Childbirth and the Puerperium
15 | Newborns and Other Neonates with Conditions Originating in Perinatal Period
16 | Diseases and Disorders of Blood, Blood Forming Organs and Immunological Disorders
17 | Myeloproliferative Diseases and Disorders, Poorly Differentiated Neoplasms
18 | Infectious and Parasitic Diseases, Systemic or Unspecified Sites
19 | Mental Diseases and Disorders
20 | Alcohol or Drug Use or Induced Organic Mental Disorders
21 | Injuries, Poisonings and Toxic Effects of Drugs
22 | Burns
23 | Factors Influencing Health Status and Other Contacts with Health Services
24 | Multiple Significant Trauma
25 | Human Immunodeficiency Virus Infections

Definitions

AICD	Automatic Implantation Cardioverter Defibrillator
AMI	Acute Myocardial Infarction
CC	Complication/Comorbidity
C.D.E	Common Duct Exploration
CNS	Central Nervous System
CV	Cardiovascular
CVA	Cerebrovascular Accident
DRG Non O.R	Non Operating Room Procedure that Affects the DRG
DX	Diagnosis
ECMO	Extracorporeal Membrane Oxygenation
ESWL	Extracorporeal Shock Wave Lithotripsy
GI	Gastrointestinal
MCC	Major Complication/Comorbidity
MV	Mechanical Ventilation
O.R.	Operating Room Procedure
PDX	Principal Diagnosis
PTCA	Percutaneous Coronary Angioplasty
SDX	Secondary Diagnosis

Symbols

= Procedure (and/or Diagnosis, when appropriate)

= Diagnosis

= MS-DRG

= Severity Split

= MDC Continued on Next Page

= Discharge Status

Pre-MDC

ALL PATIENTS
MS-DRG
Chimeric Antigen Receptor (CAR) T-cell and Other Immunotherapies
018
Heart Transplant or Implant of Heart Assist System
MCC
Yes
001
No
002
ECMO
003
Tracheostomy with MV > 96 Hours or PDX Except Face, Mouth and Neck
O.R. or DRG Non O.R. Procedure
Major O.R. Procedure
Yes
003
No
004
Intestinal Transplant
005
Liver Transplant
MCC
Yes
005
No
006
Allogeneic Bone Marrow Transplant
014
Lung Transplant
007
1

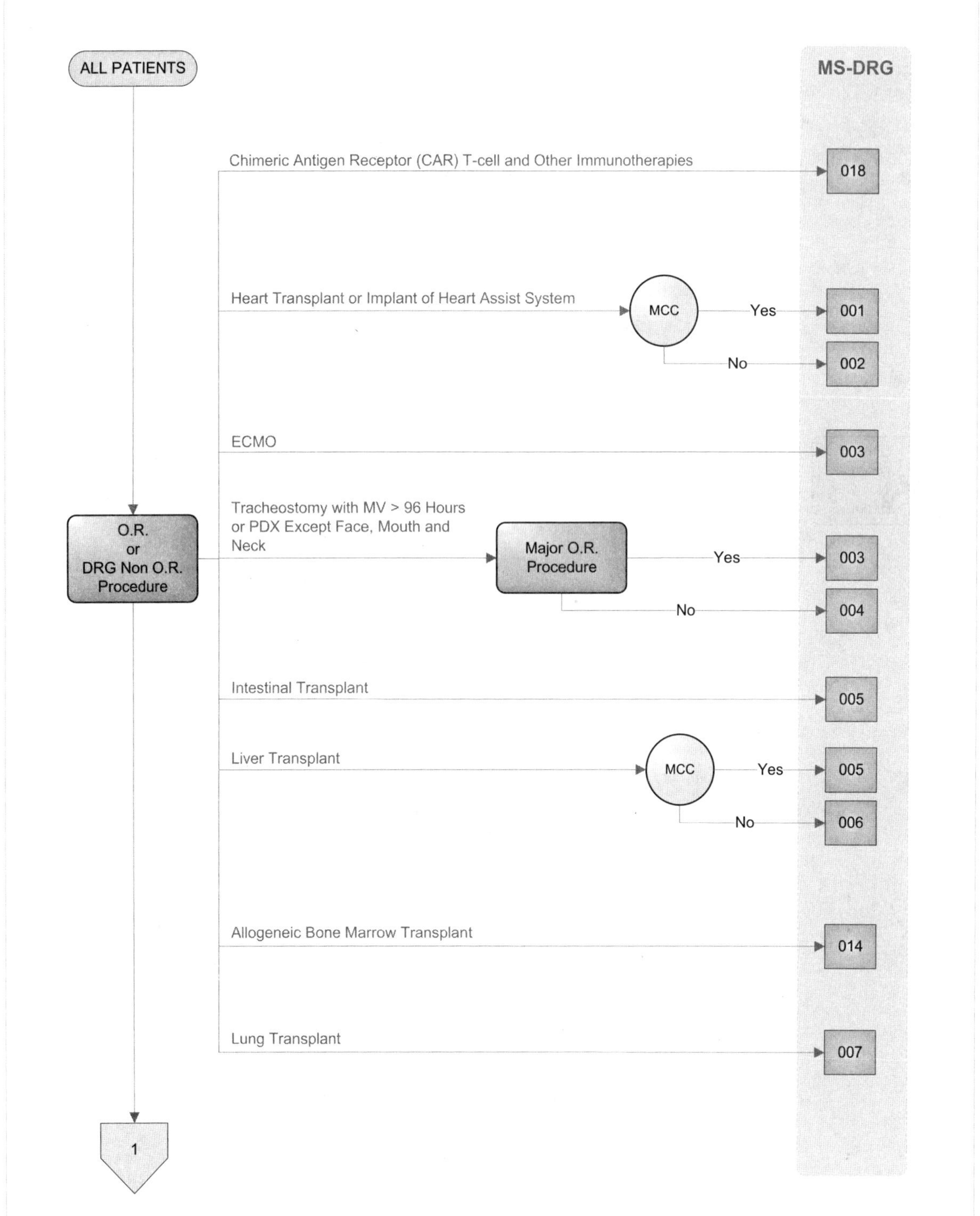

Pre-MDC

MS-DRG
1
Simultaneous Pancreas and Kidney Transplant
Hemodialysis
Yes
019
No
008
Autologous Bone Marrow Transplant
MCC or CC
Yes
016
No
017
O.R. or DRG Non O.R. Procedure
Pancreas Transplant
010
Yes, MCC
011
Tracheostomy for Face, Mouth and Neck Diagnoses or Laryngectomy
MCC/ CC
Yes, CC
012
No
013
1

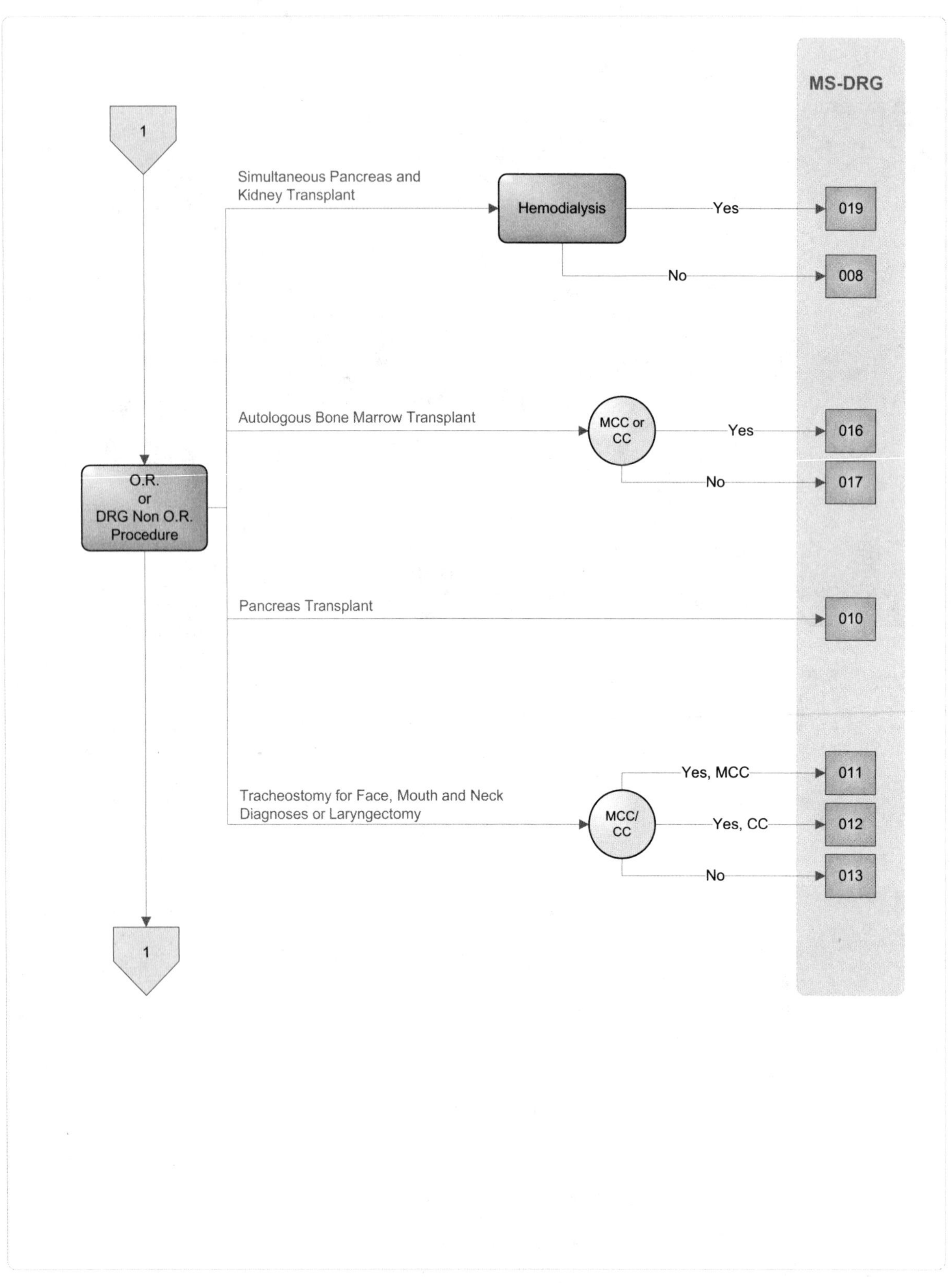

All Patients

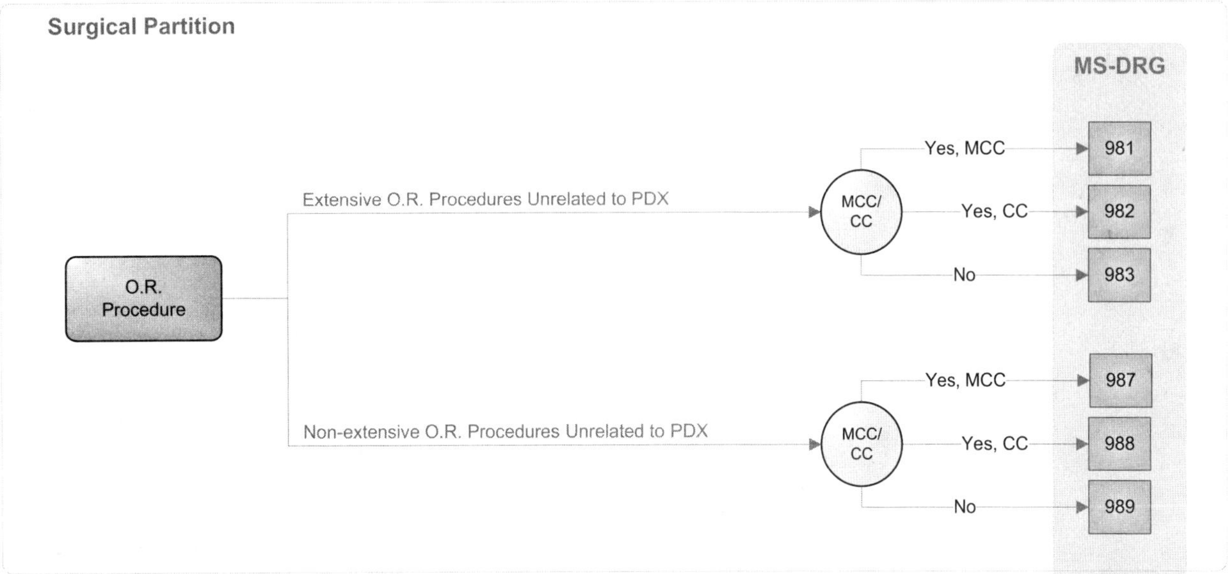

Surgical Partition

MS-DRG

O.R. Procedure

Extensive O.R. Procedures Unrelated to PDX → MCC/CC
- Yes, MCC → 981
- Yes, CC → 982
- No → 983

Non-extensive O.R. Procedures Unrelated to PDX → MCC/CC
- Yes, MCC → 987
- Yes, CC → 988
- No → 989

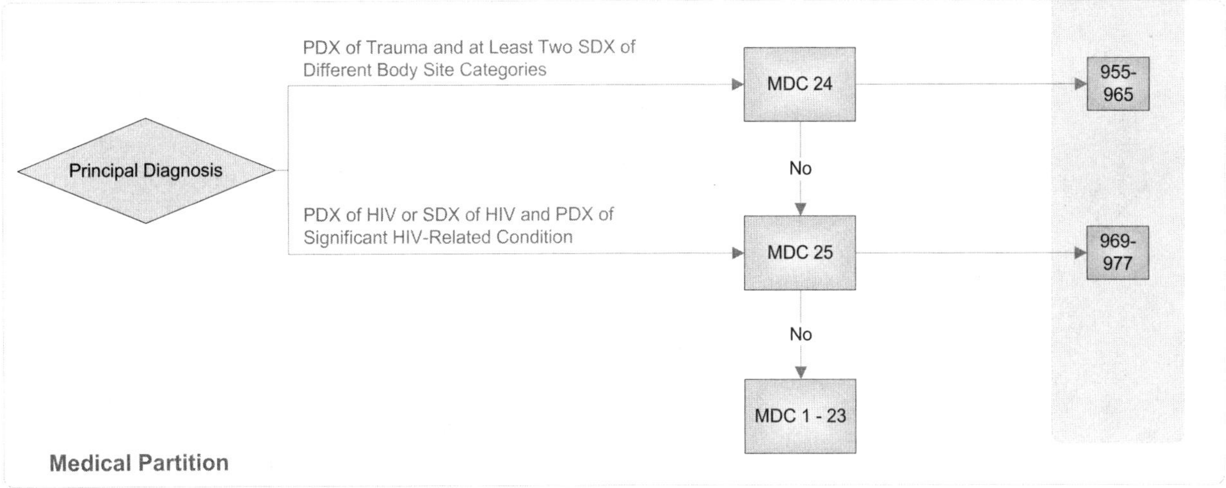

Medical Partition

Principal Diagnosis

PDX of Trauma and at Least Two SDX of Different Body Site Categories → MDC 24 → 955-965

No

PDX of HIV or SDX of HIV and PDX of Significant HIV-Related Condition → MDC 25 → 969-977

No

MDC 1 - 23

Major Diagnostic Category 1
Diseases and Disorders of the Nervous System

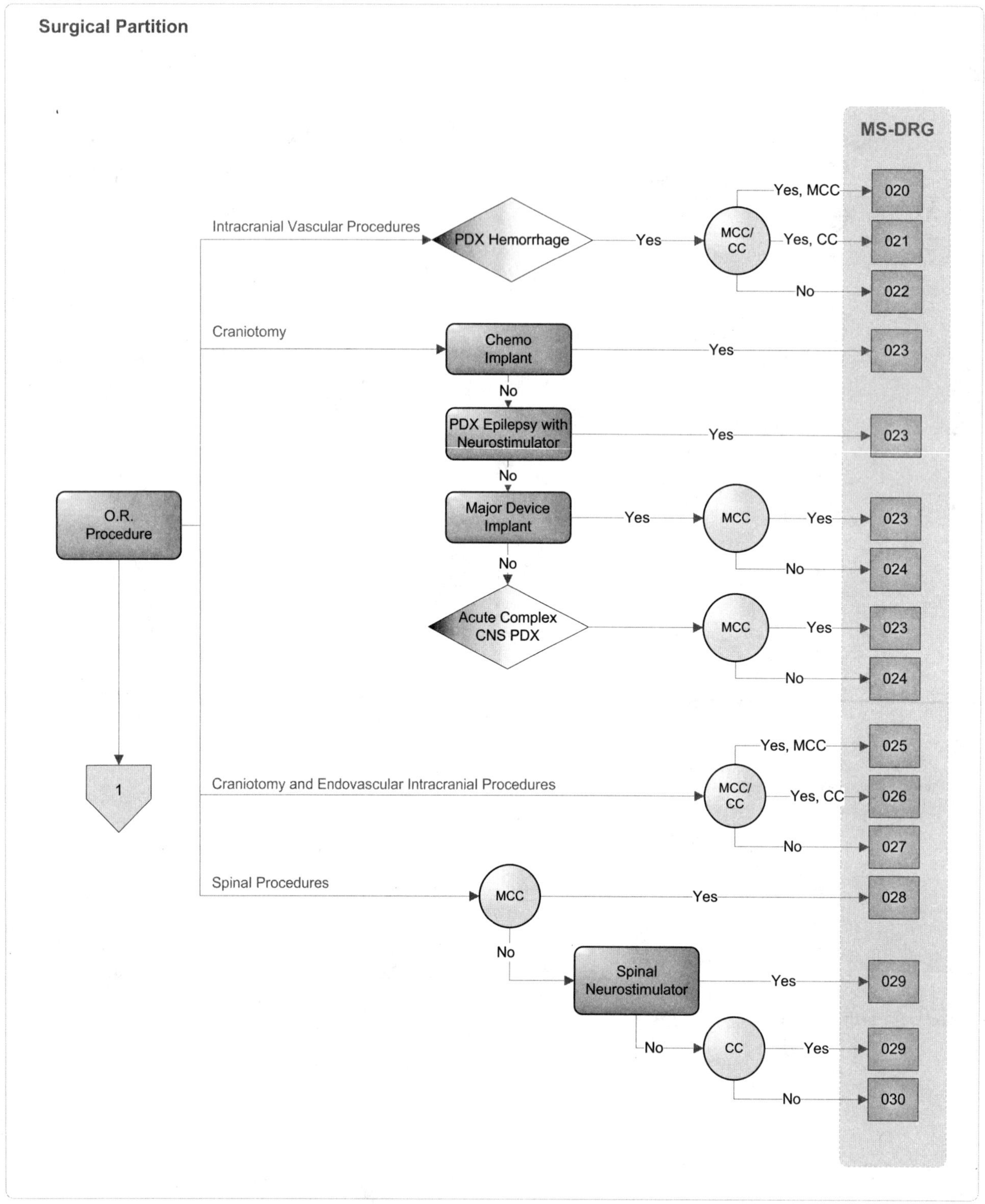

Major Diagnostic Category 1
Diseases and Disorders of the Nervous System

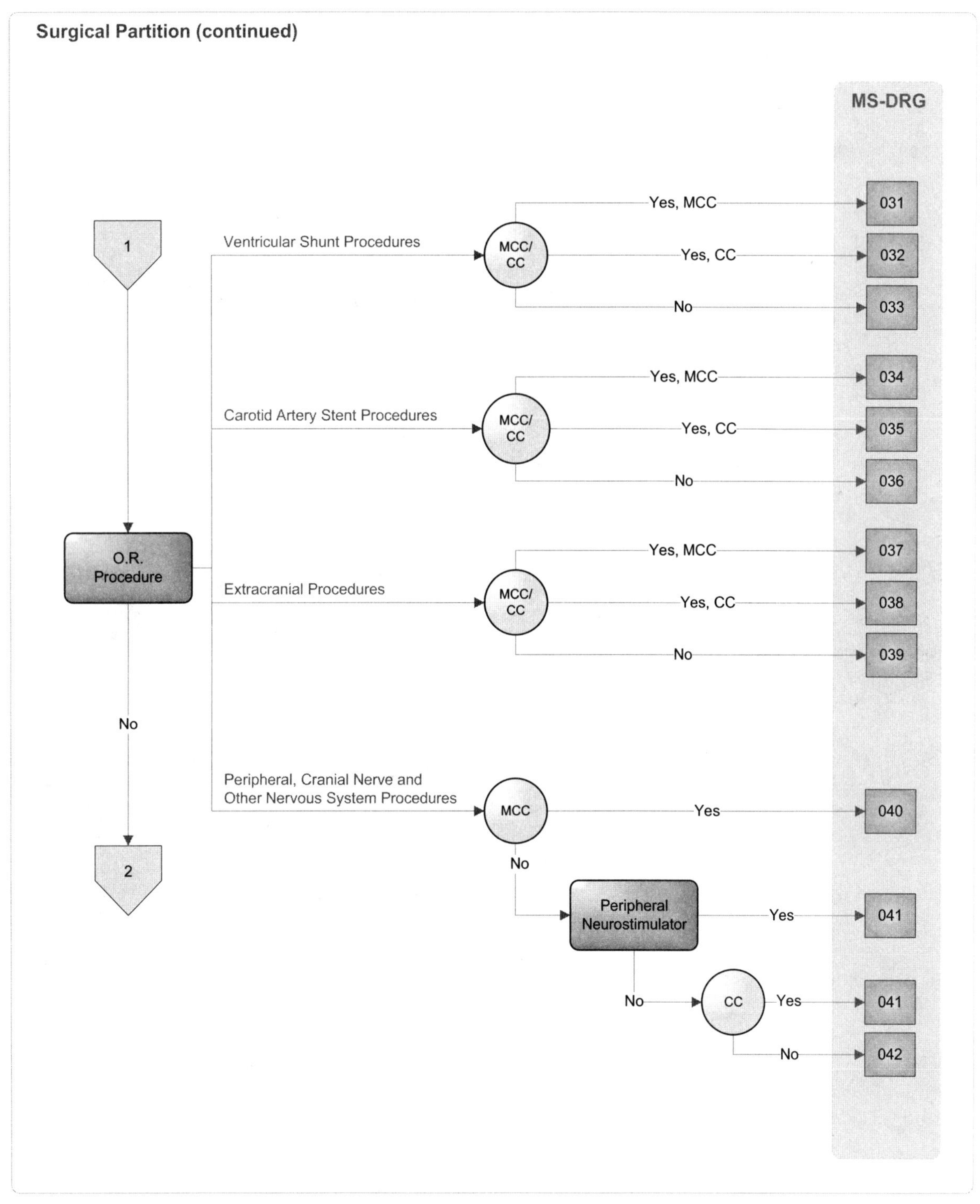

Major Diagnostic Category 1
Diseases and Disorders of the Nervous System

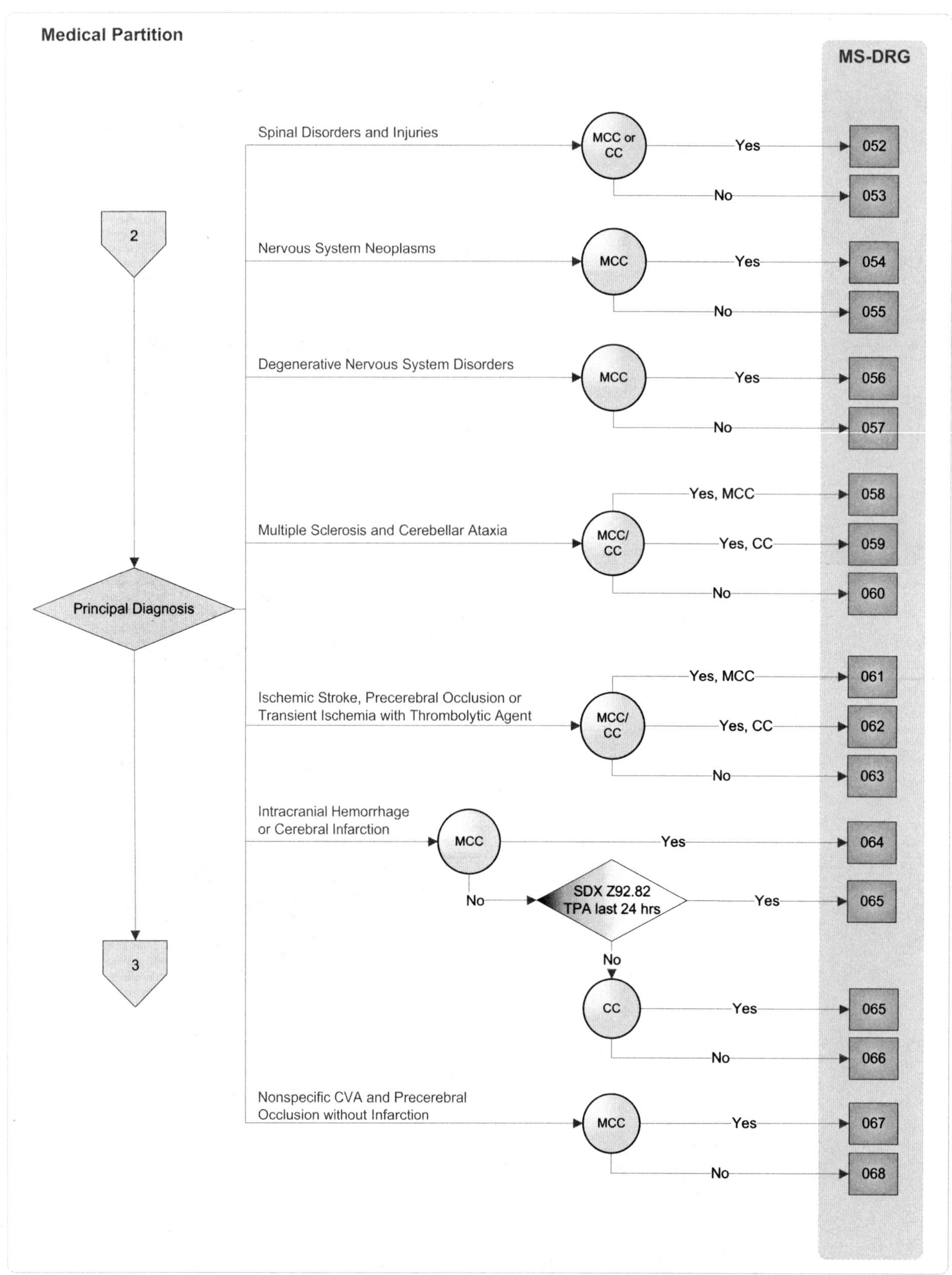

Major Diagnostic Category 1
Diseases and Disorders of the Nervous System

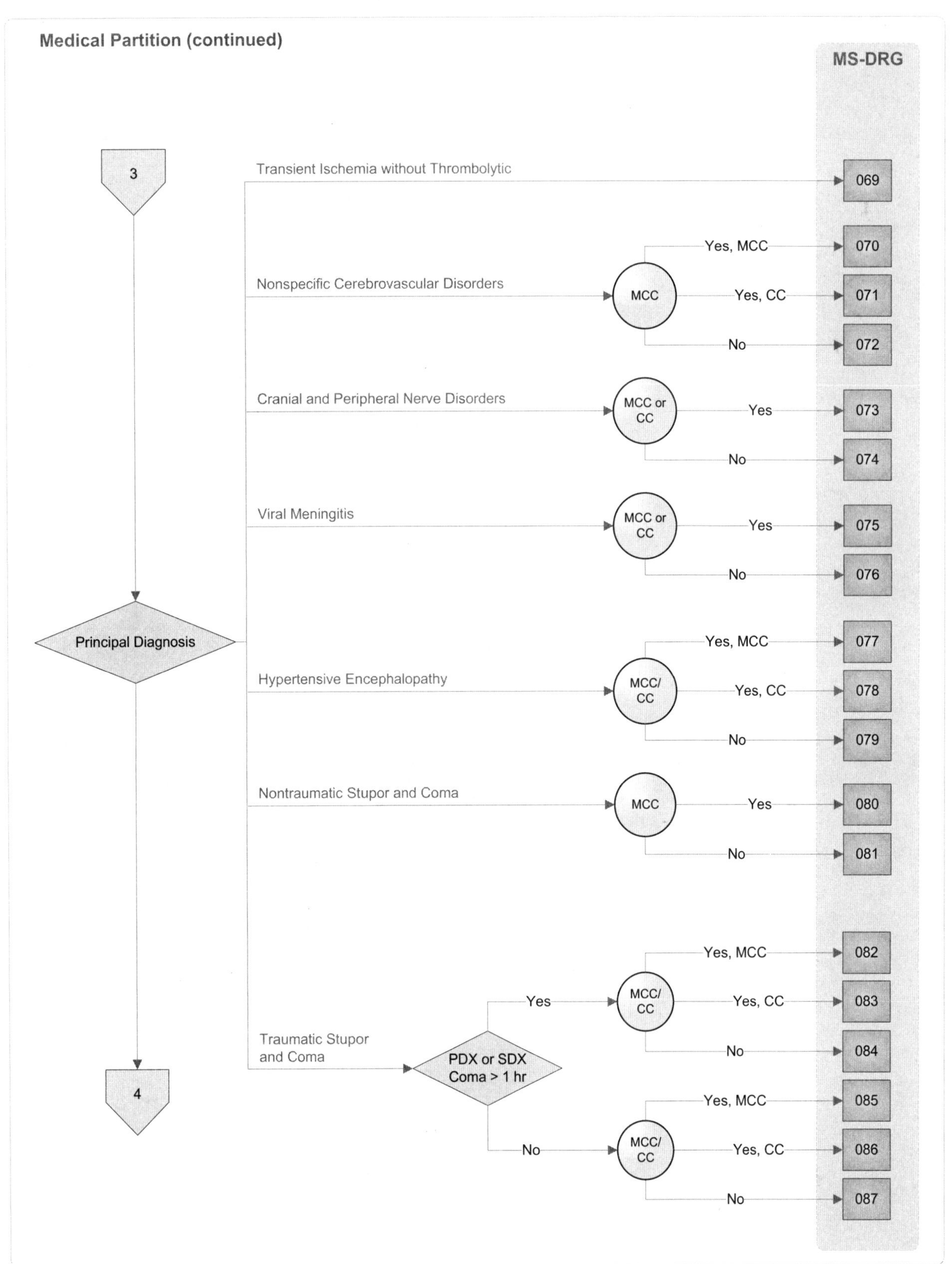

Major Diagnostic Category 1
Diseases and Disorders of the Nervous System

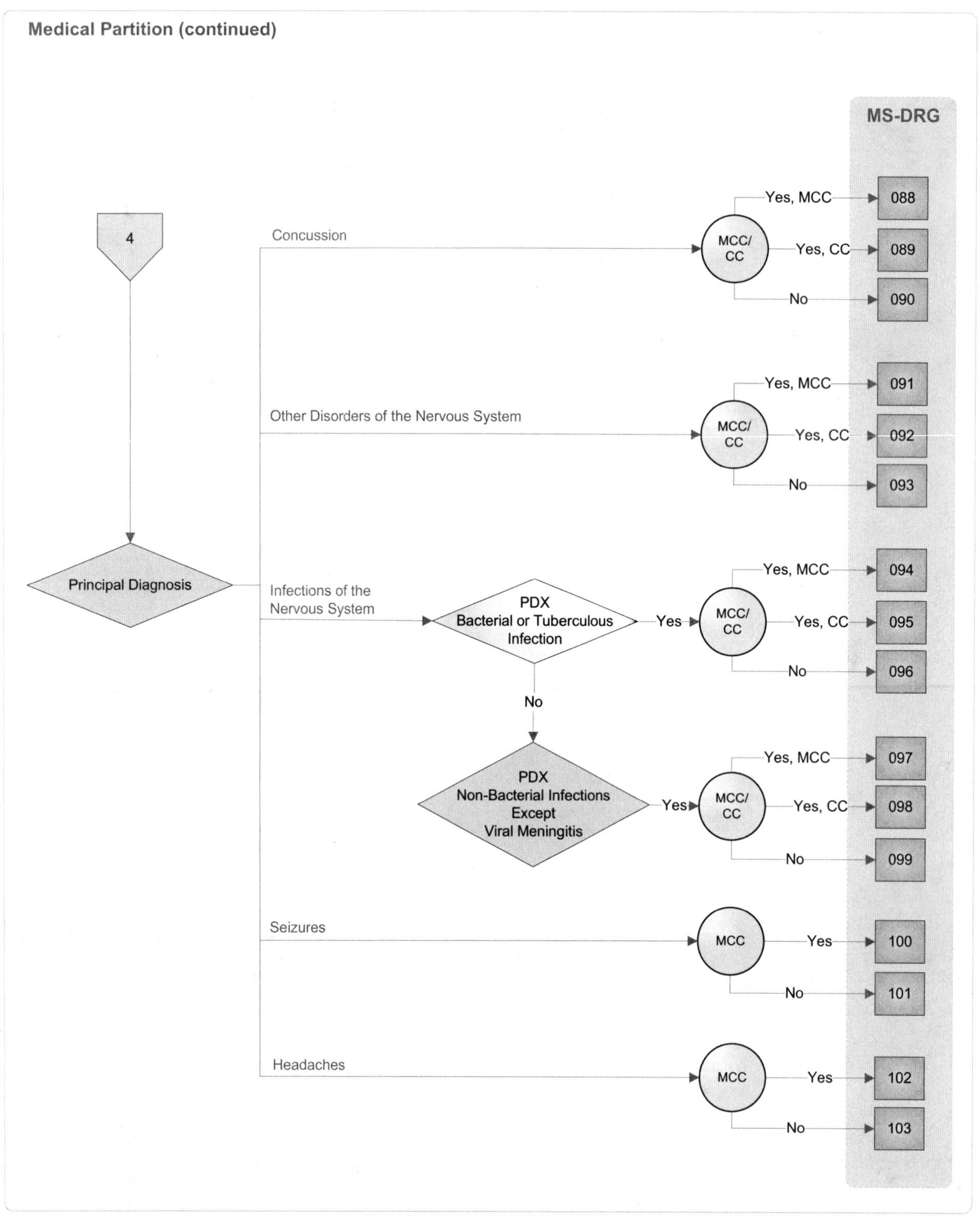

Major Diagnostic Category 2
Diseases and Disorders of the Eye

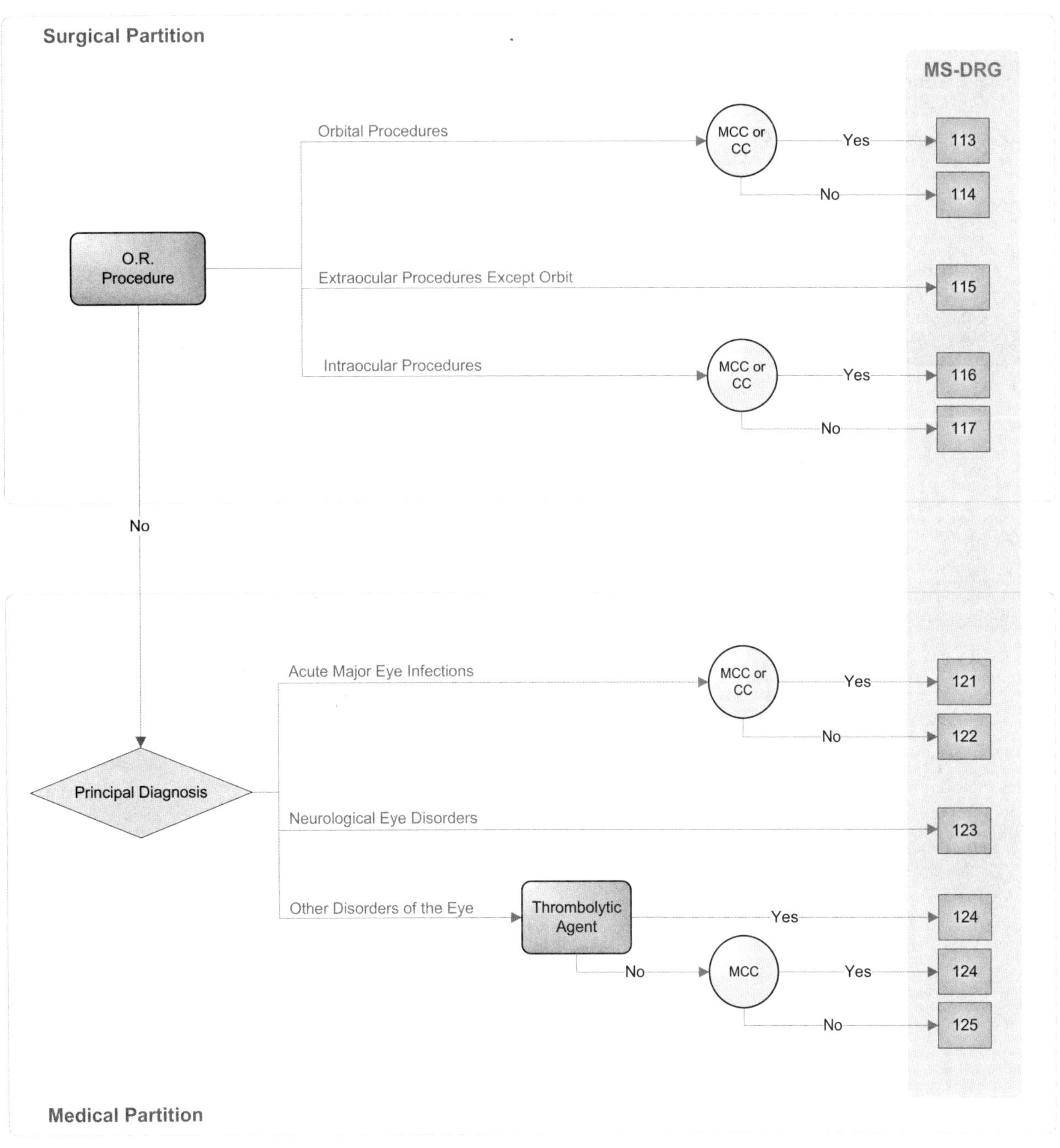

Major Diagnostic Category 3
Diseases and Disorders of the Ear, Nose, Mouth and Throat

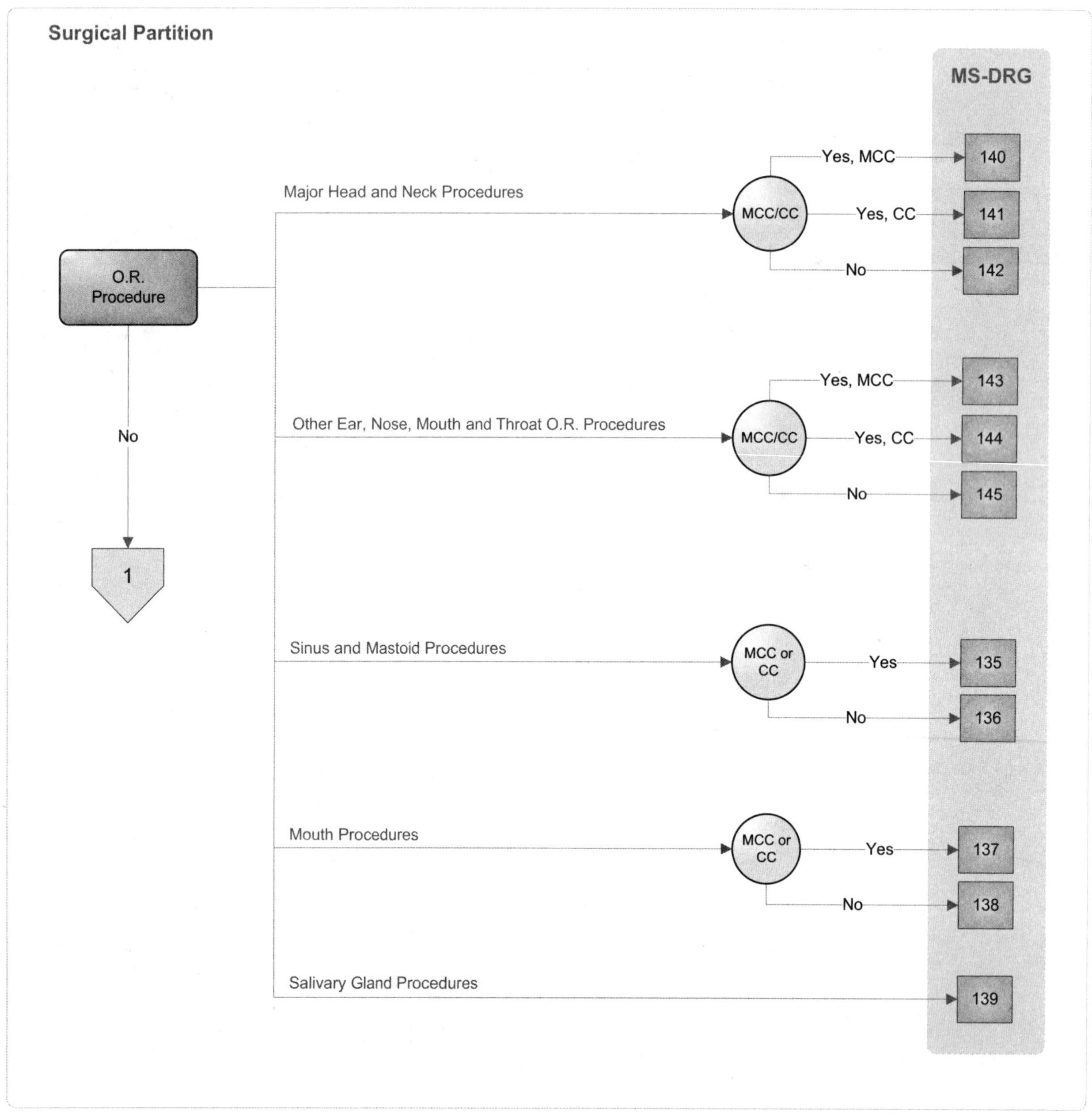

Major Diagnostic Category 3

Diseases and Disorders of the Ear, Nose, Mouth and Throat

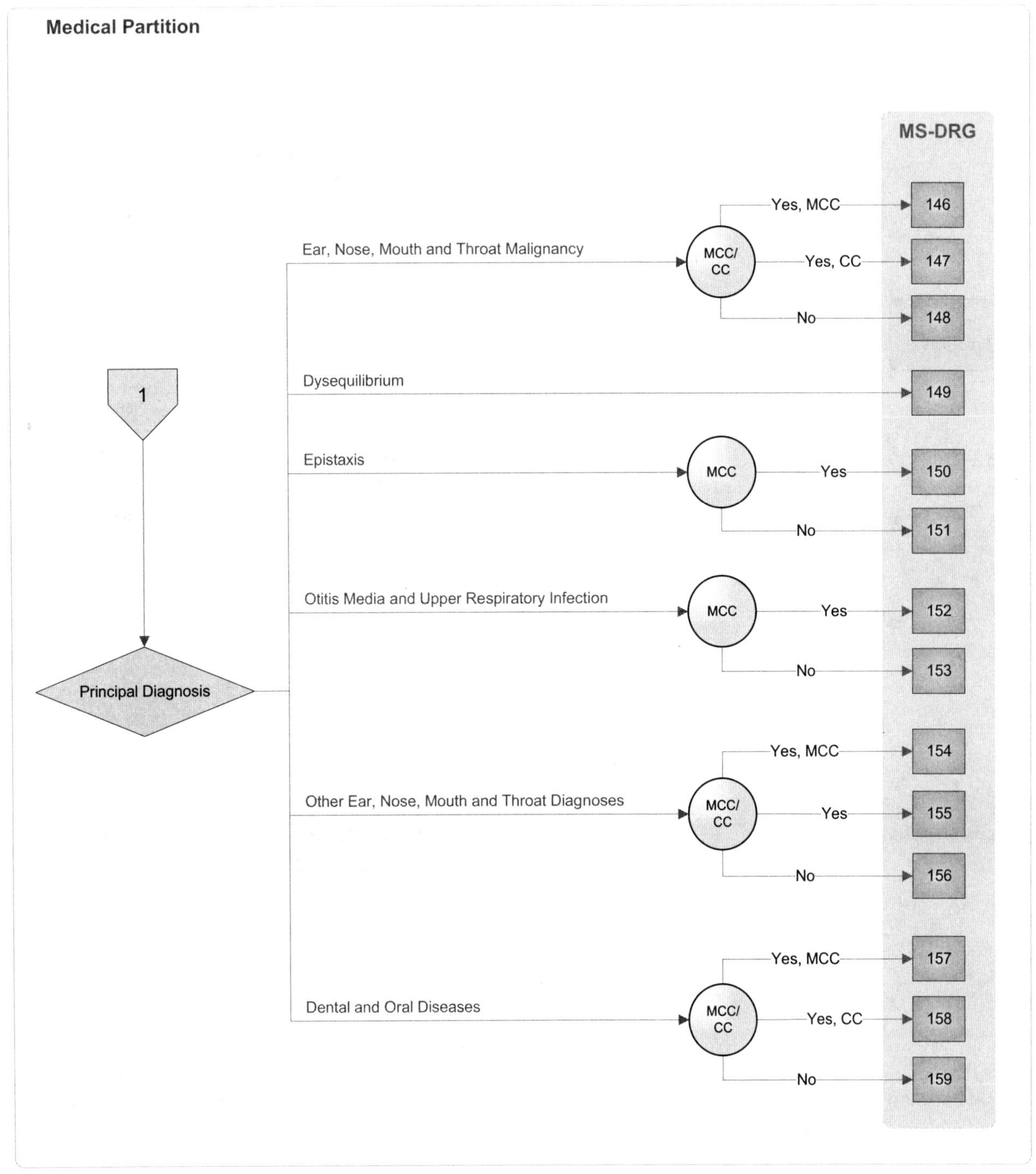

Major Diagnostic Category 4
Diseases and Disorders of the Respiratory System

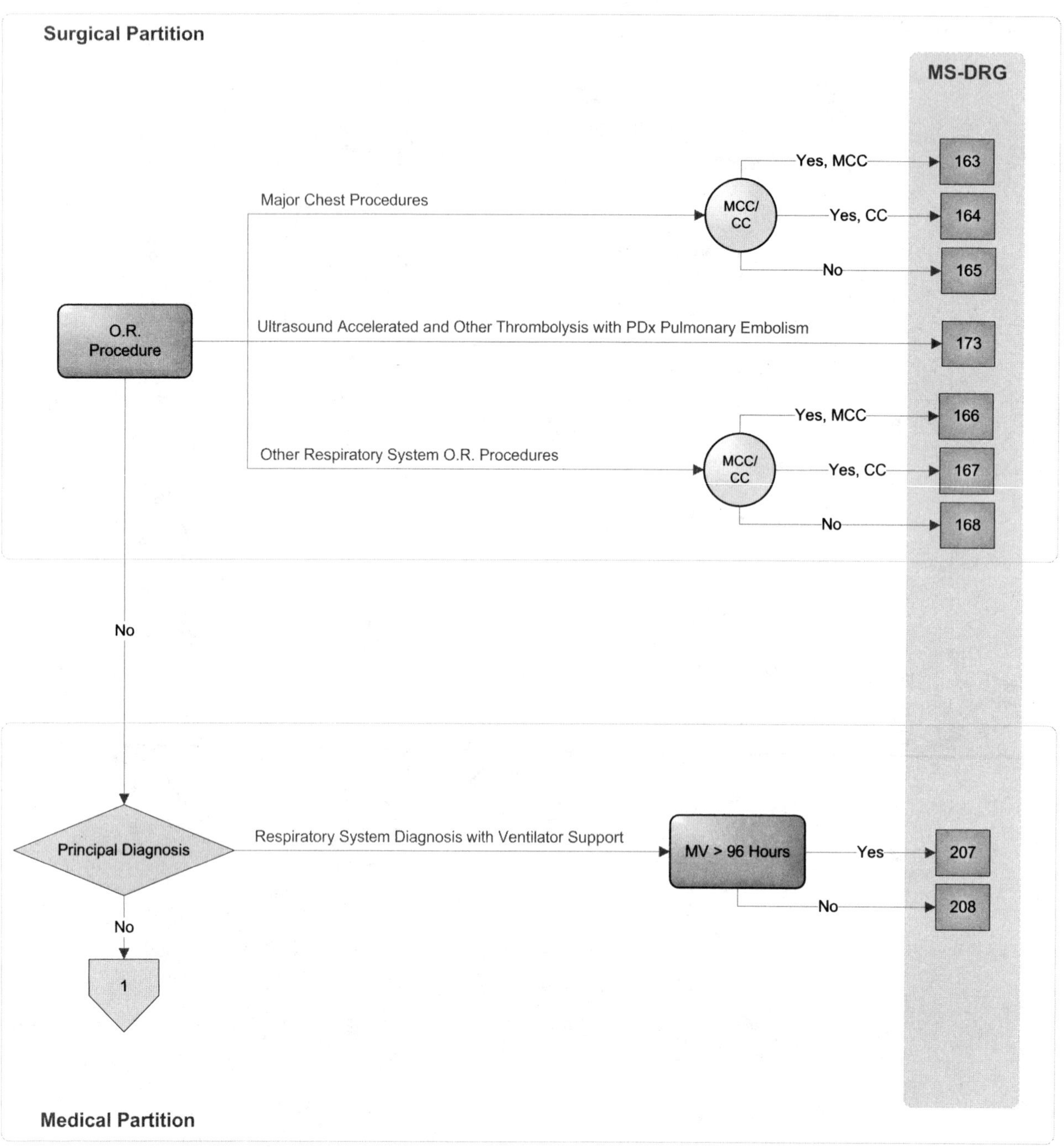

Major Diagnostic Category 4
Diseases and Disorders of the Respiratory System

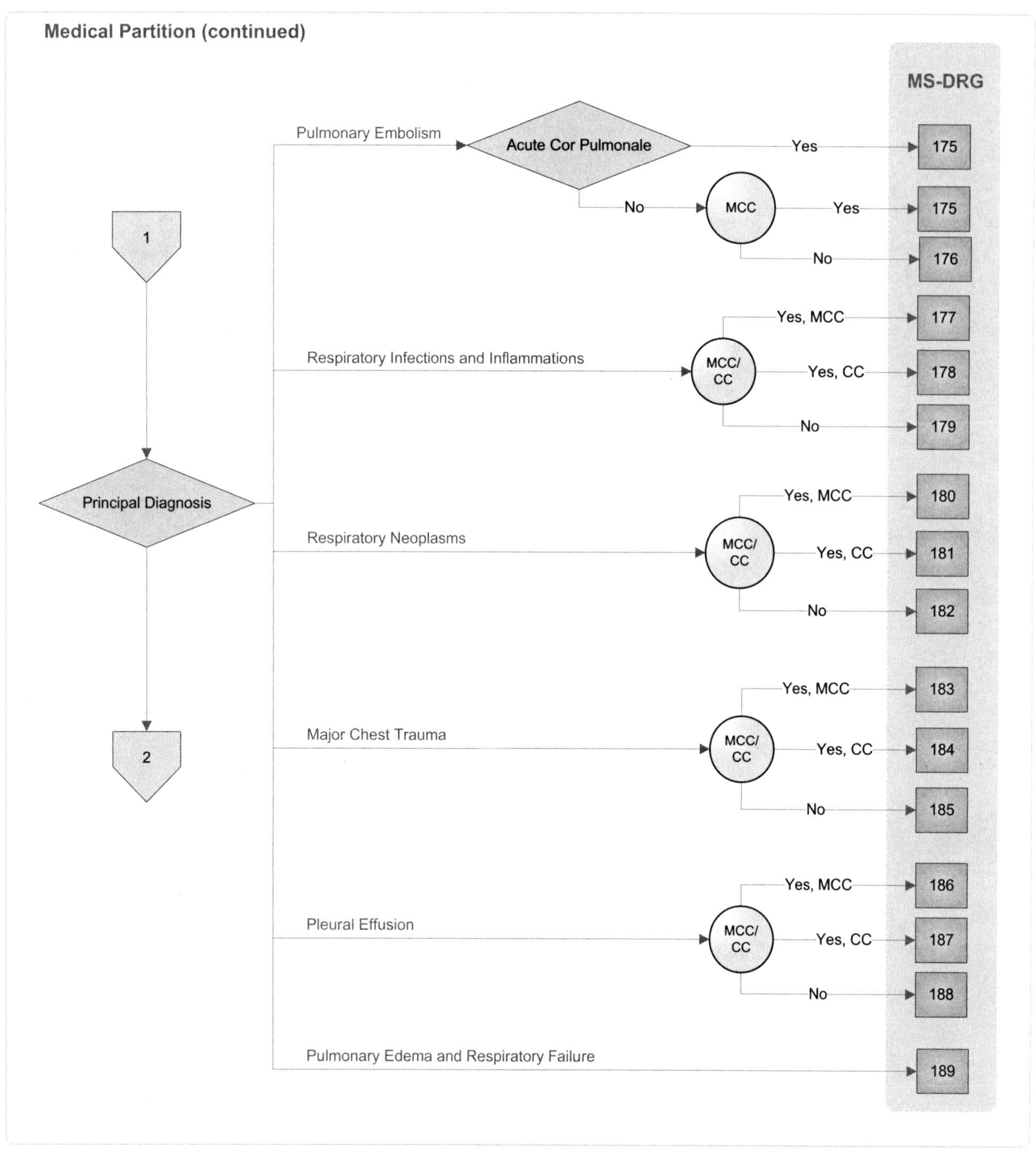

Major Diagnostic Category 4
Diseases and Disorders of the Respiratory System

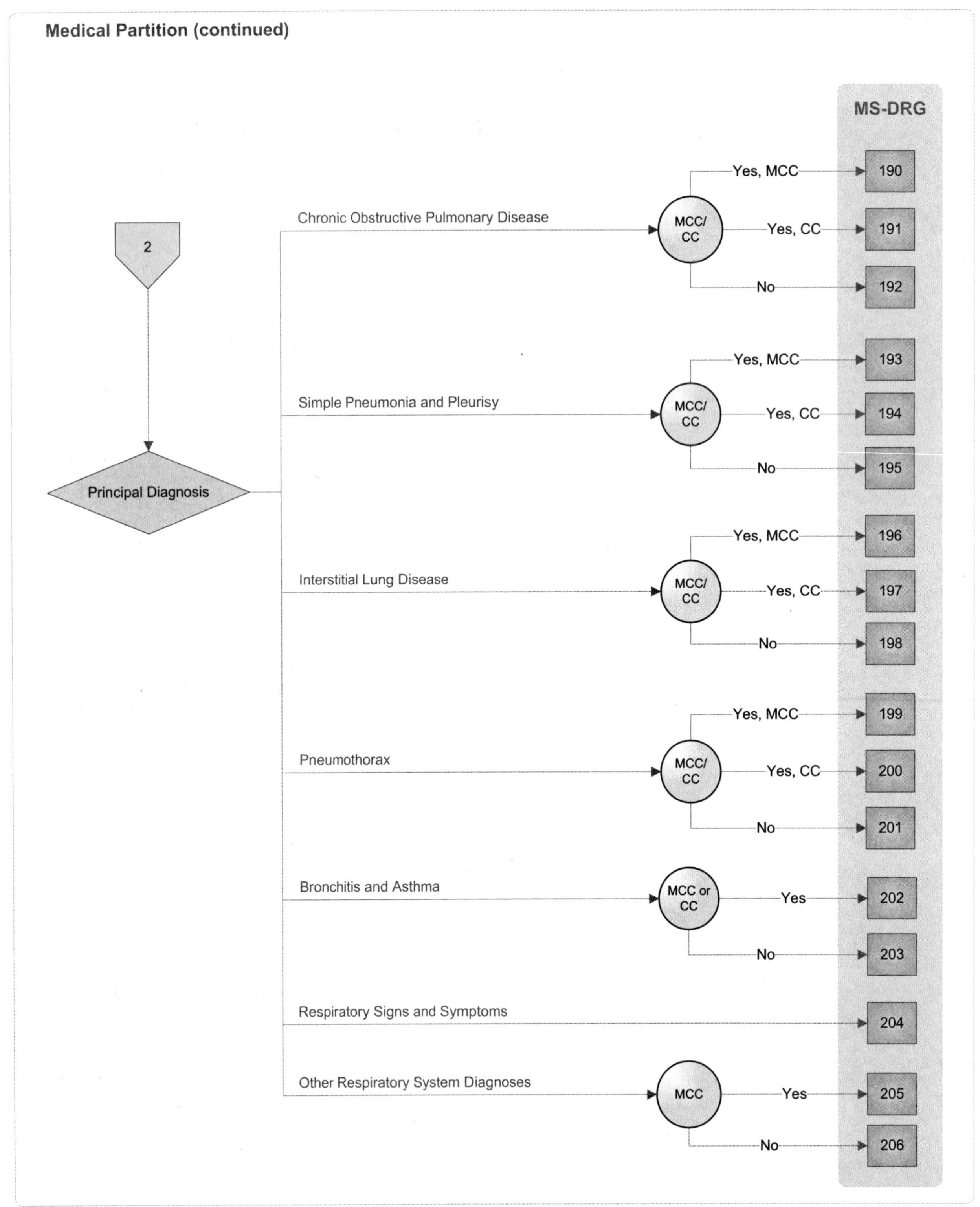

Major Diagnostic Category 5
Diseases and Disorders of the Circulatory System

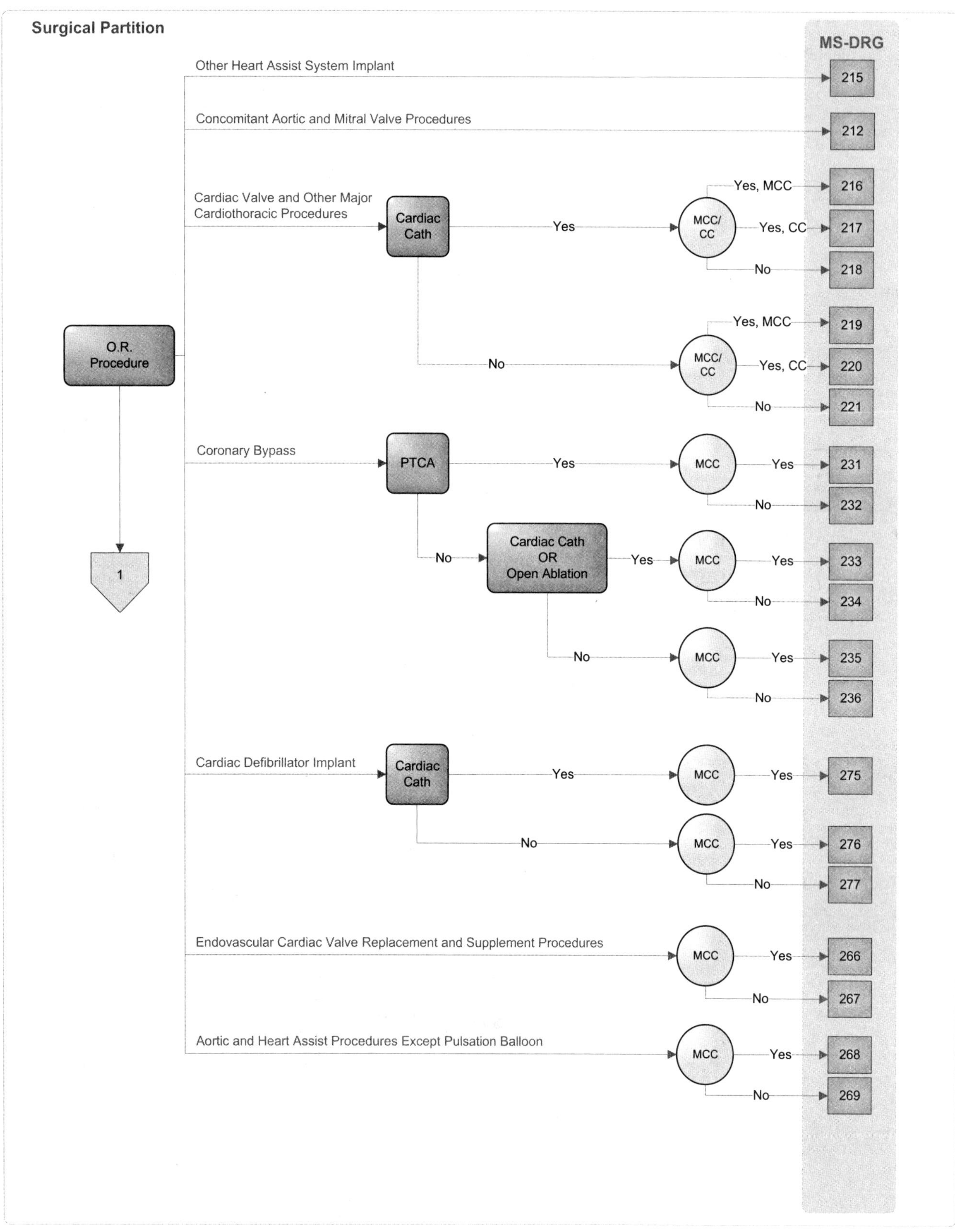

Major Diagnostic Category 5

Diseases and Disorders of the Circulatory System

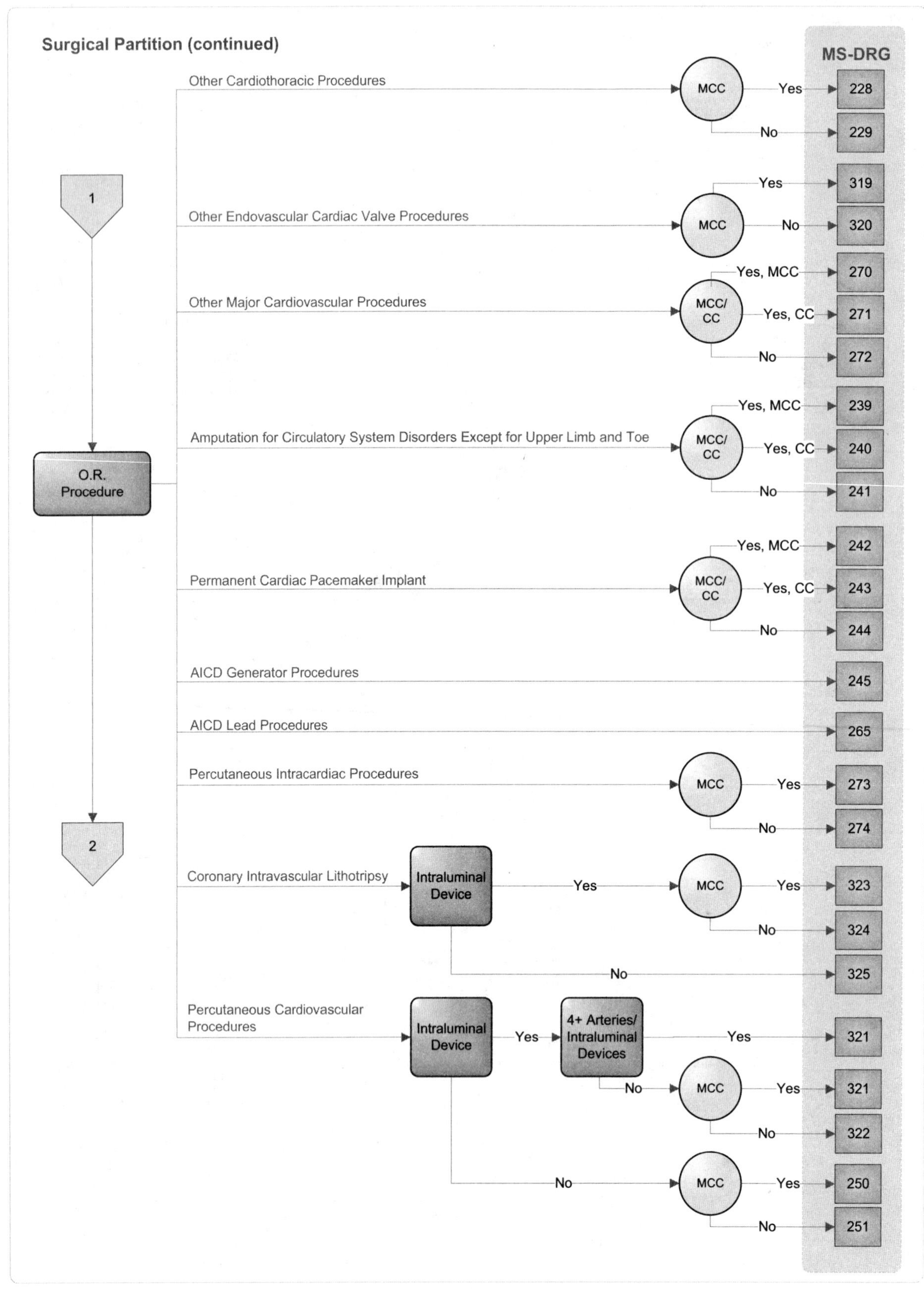

Major Diagnostic Category 5
Diseases and Disorders of the Circulatory System

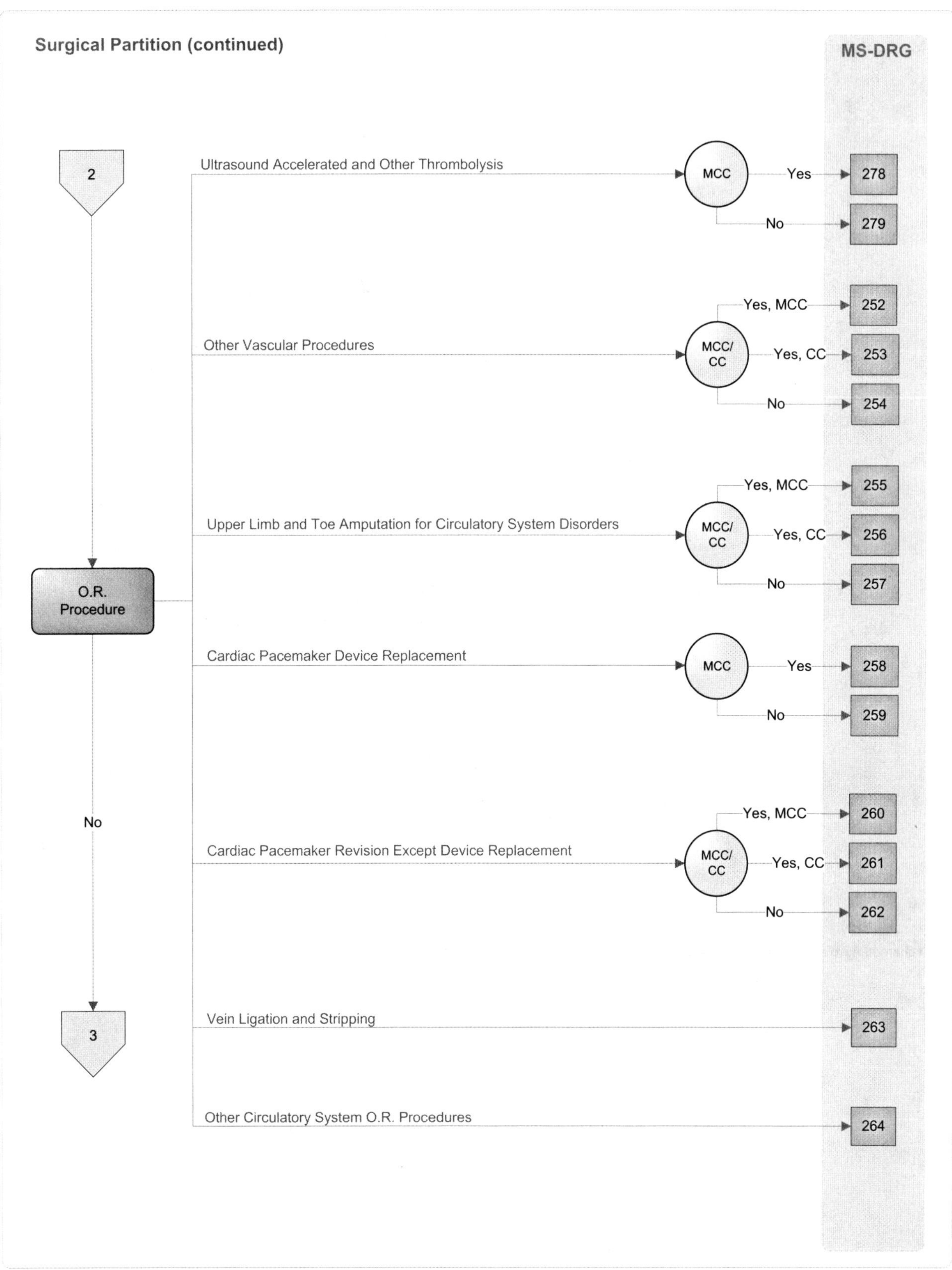

Major Diagnostic Category 5
Diseases and Disorders of the Circulatory System

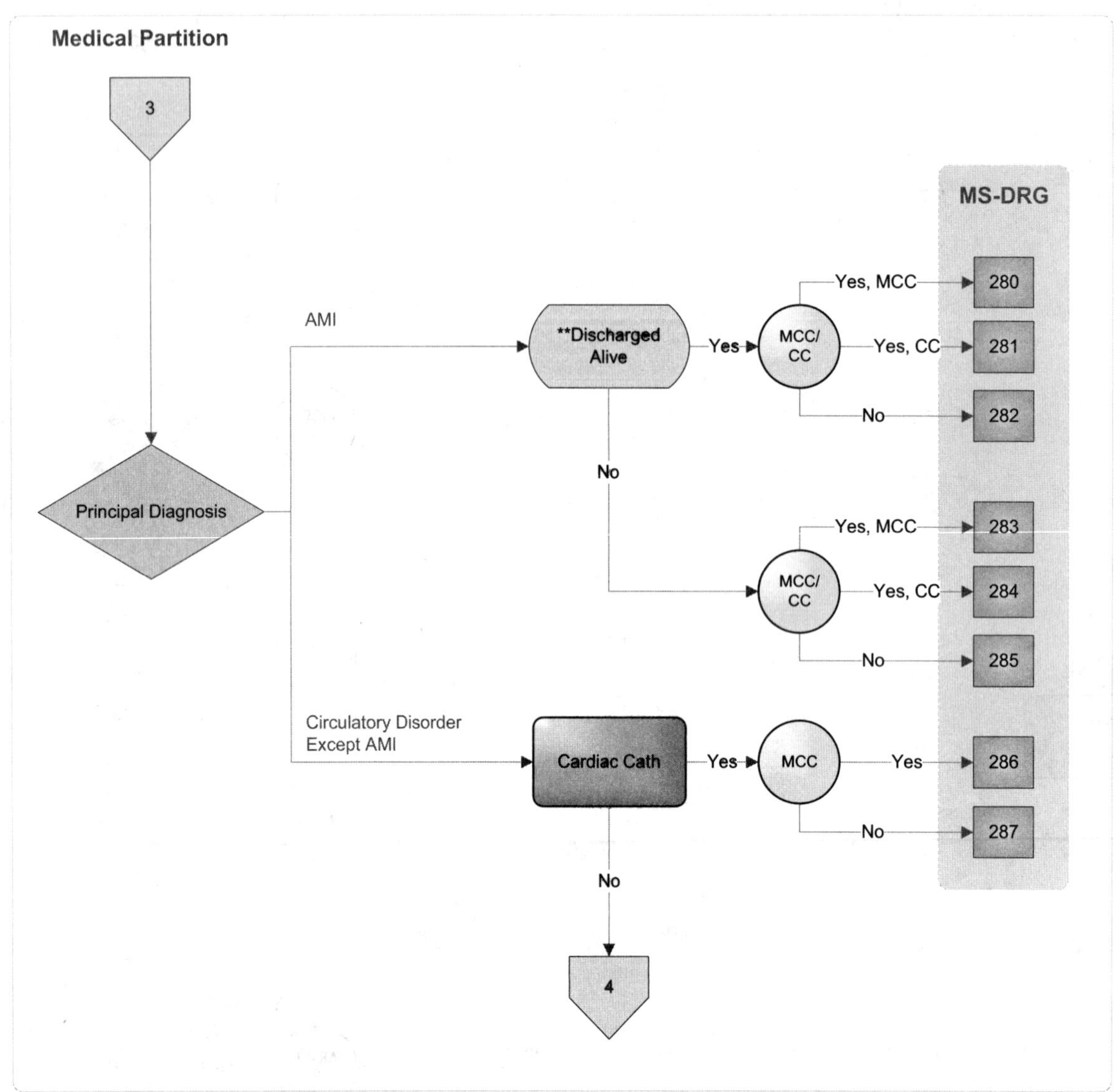

**Discharged Alive = Any discharge status except for Discharge Status of 20 (Died).

Major Diagnostic Category 5
Diseases and Disorders of the Circulatory System

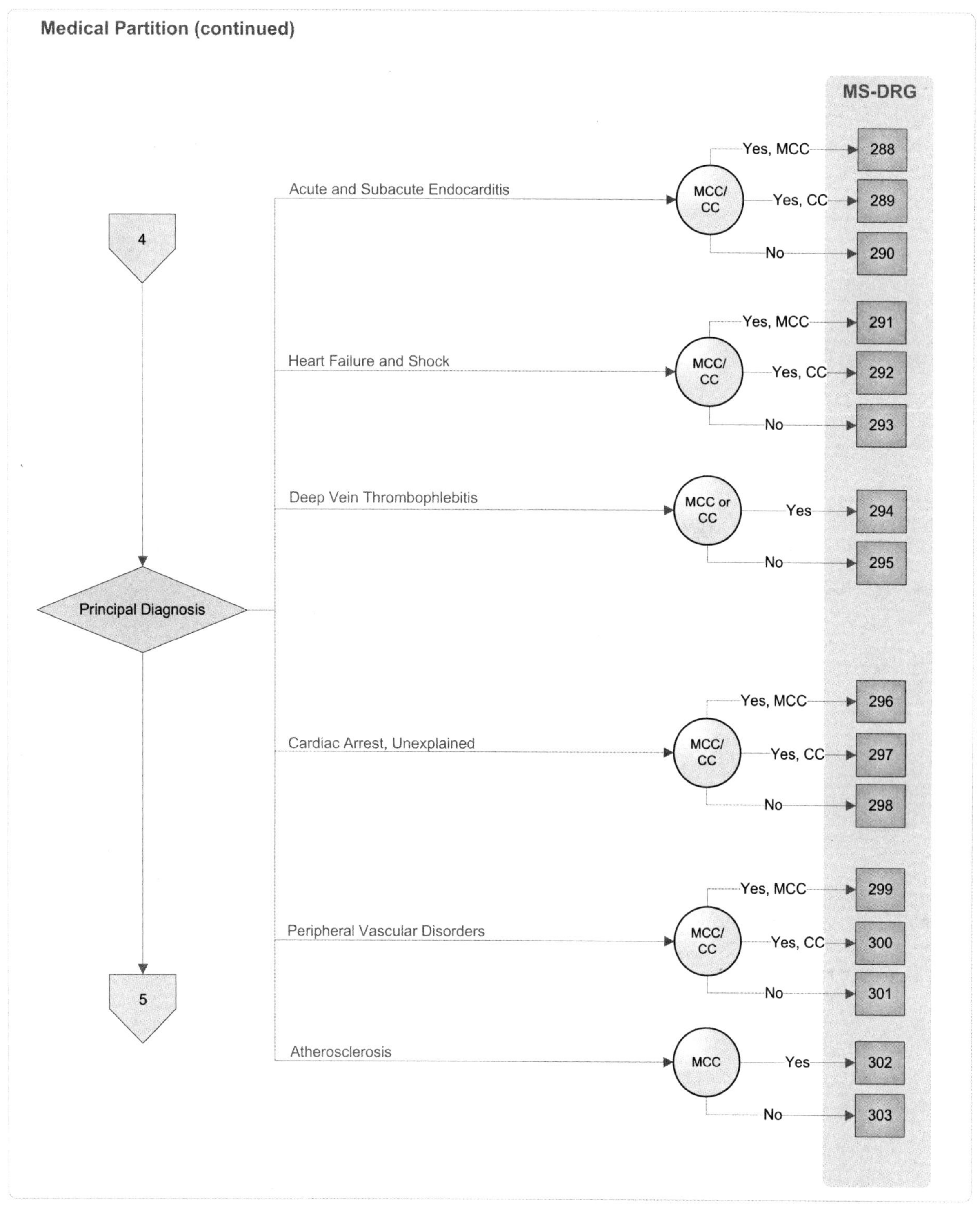

Major Diagnostic Category 5
Diseases and Disorders of the Circulatory System

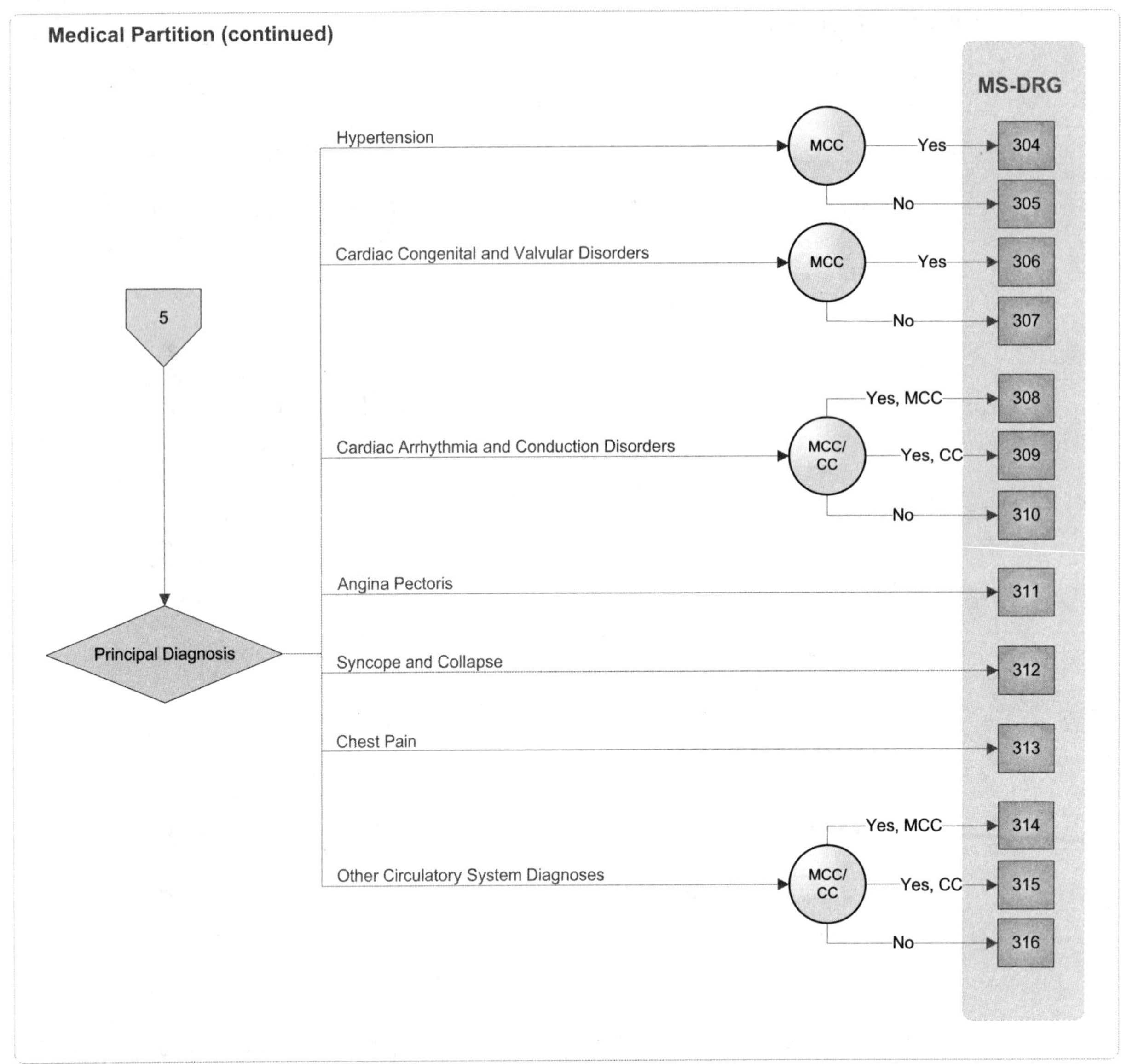

Major Diagnostic Category 6

Diseases and Disorders of the Digestive System

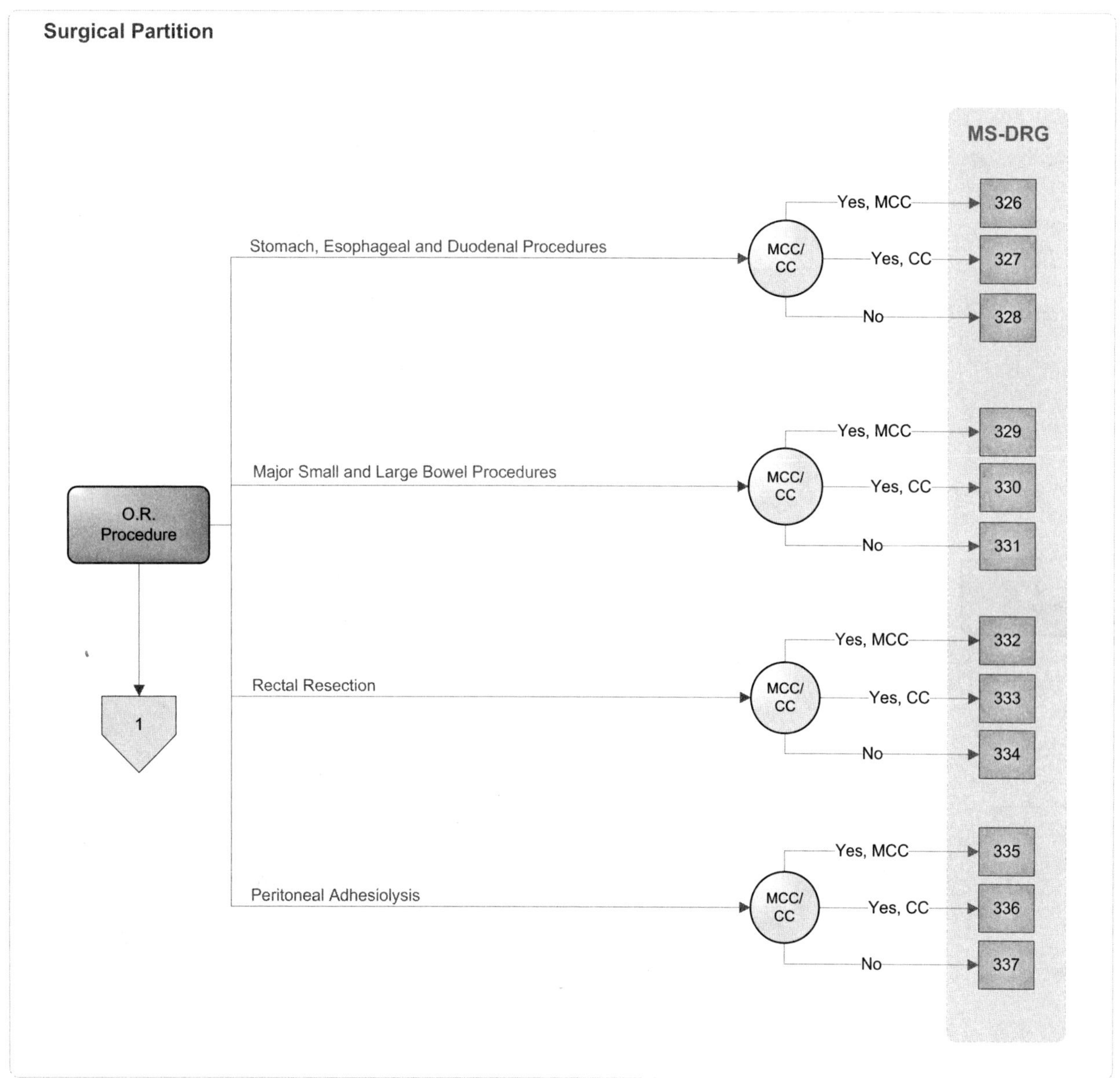

Major Diagnostic Category 6

Diseases and Disorders of the Digestive System

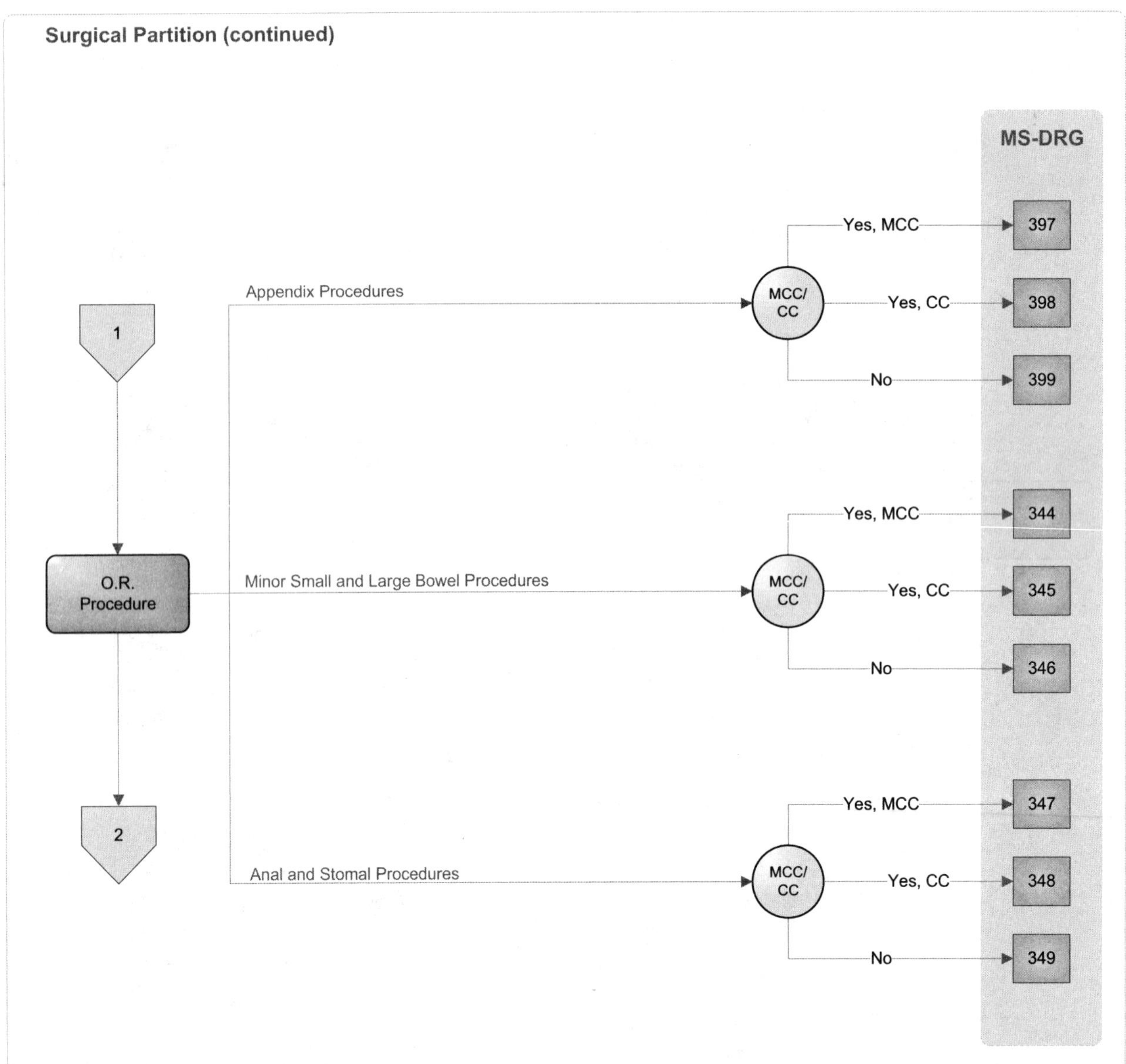

Major Diagnostic Category 6
Diseases and Disorders of the Digestive System

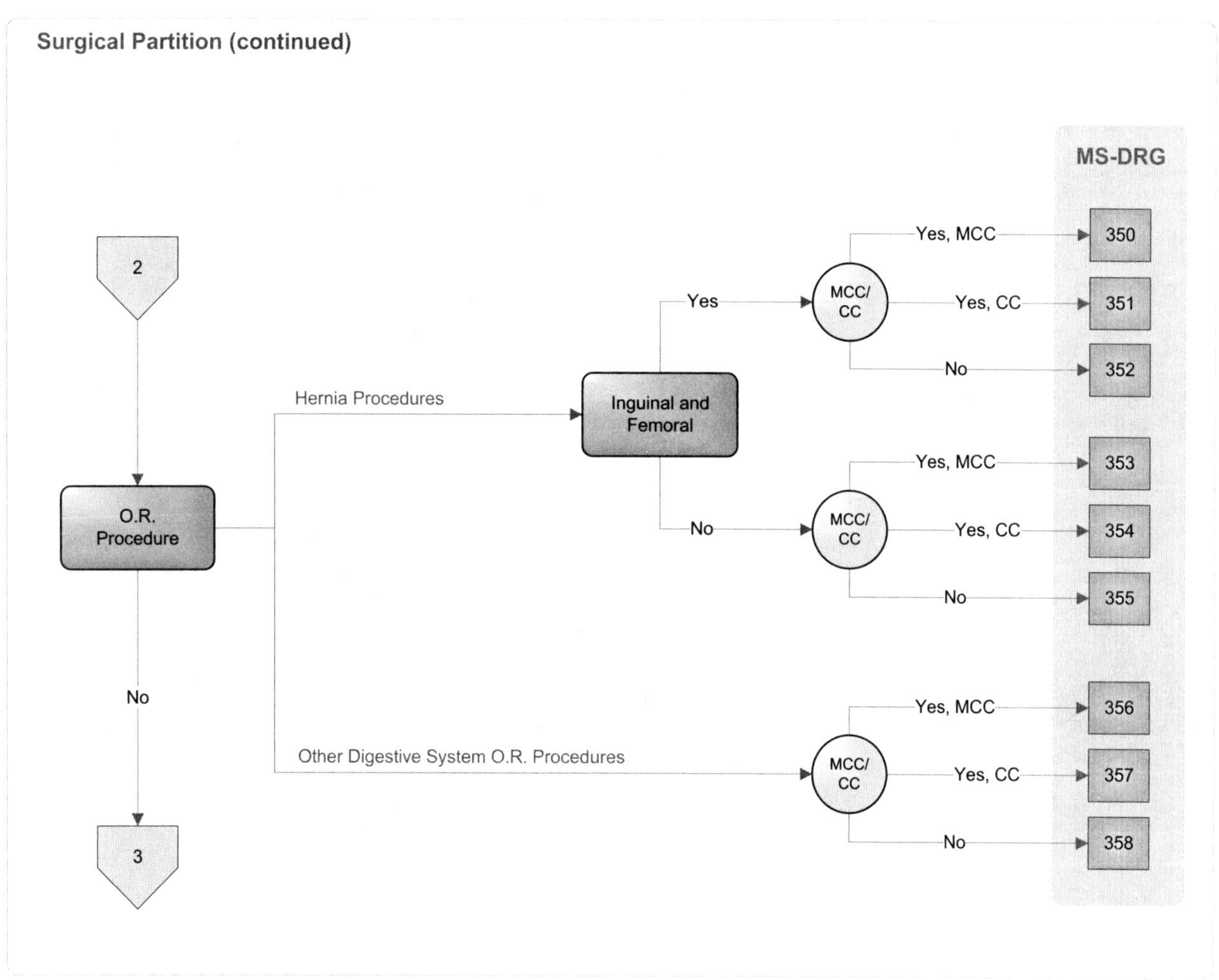

Major Diagnostic Category 6
Diseases and Disorders of the Digestive System

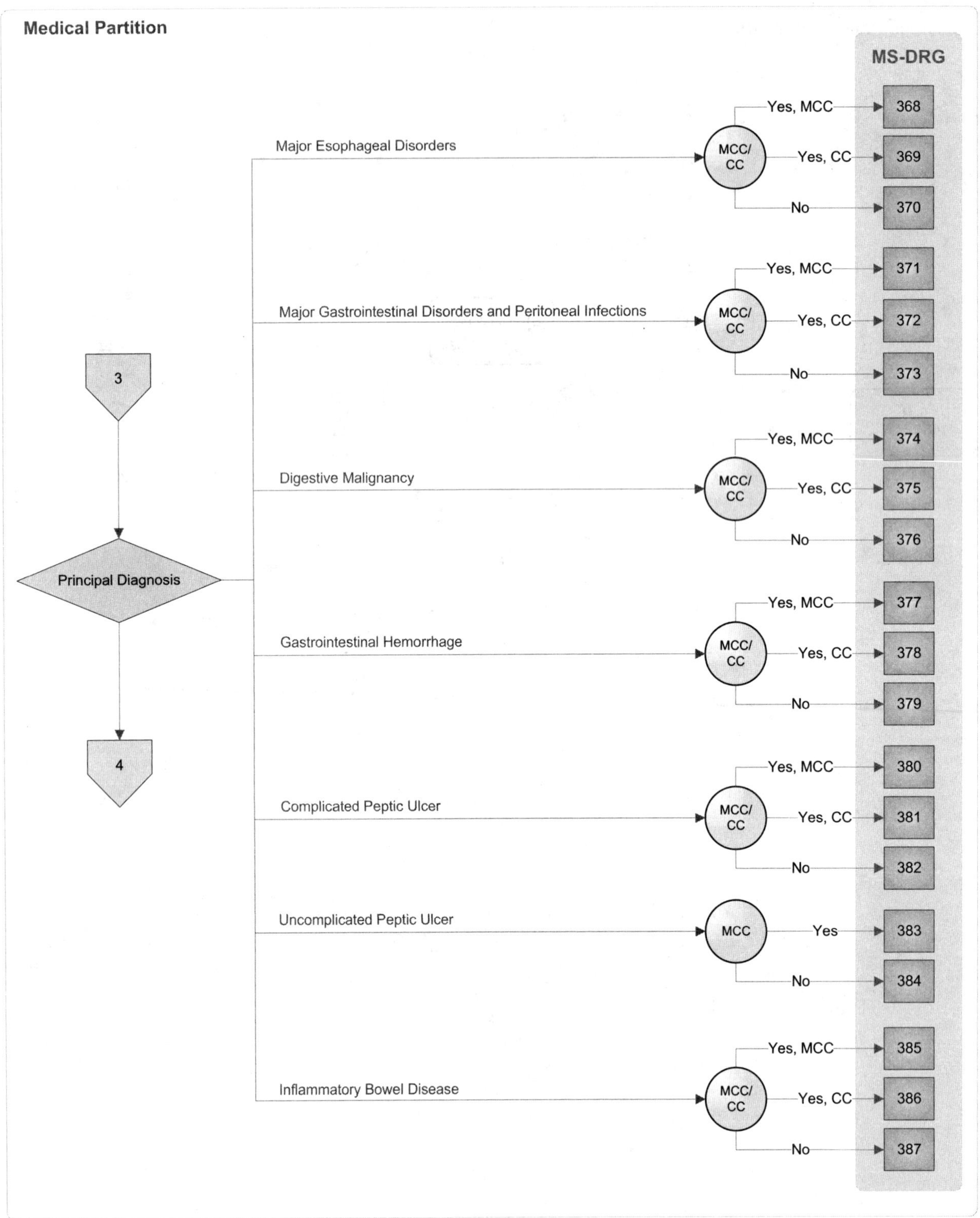

Major Diagnostic Category 6
Diseases and Disorders of the Digestive System

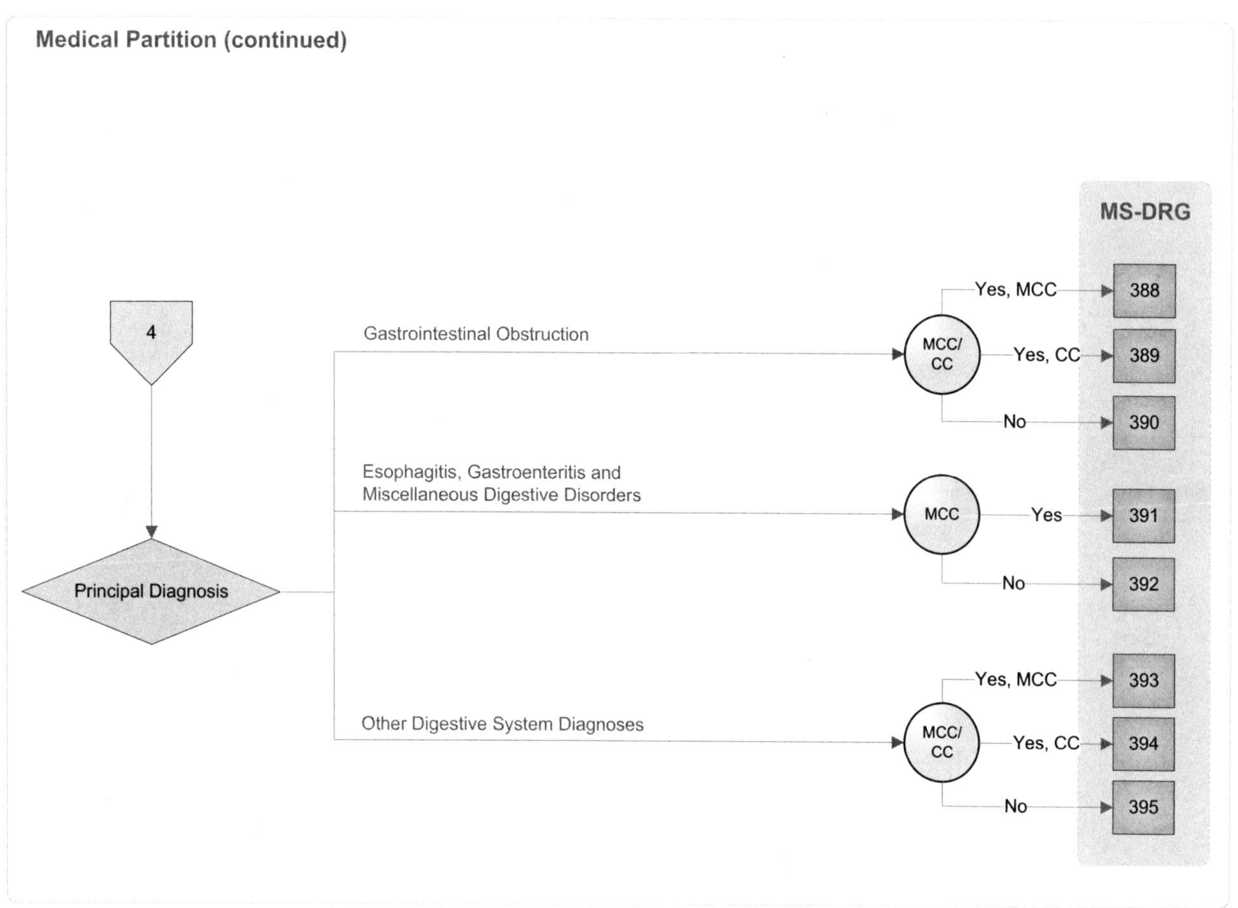

Major Diagnostic Category 7

Diseases and Disorders of the Hepatobiliary System and Pancreas

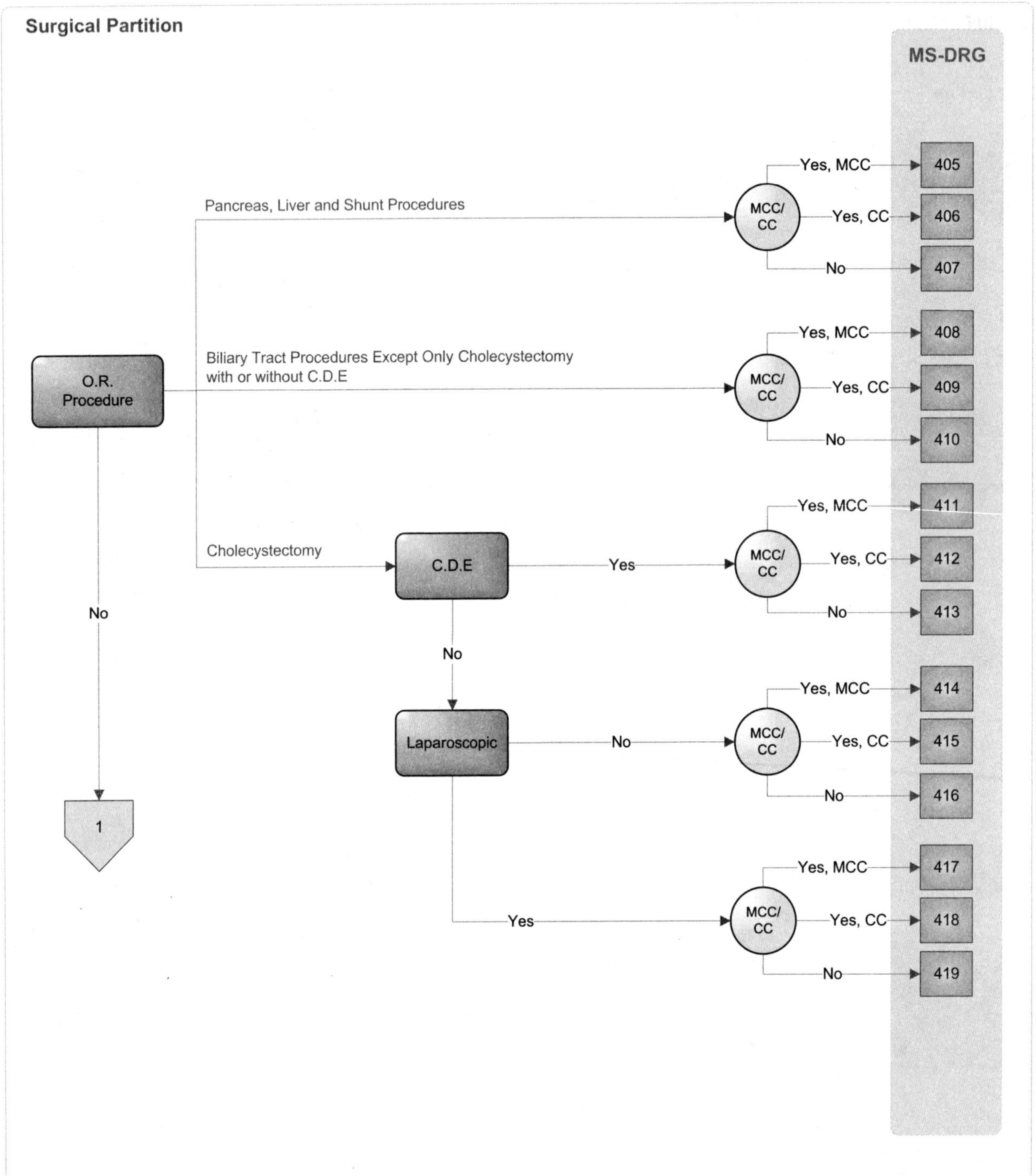

Major Diagnostic Category 7

Diseases and Disorders of the Hepatobiliary System and Pancreas

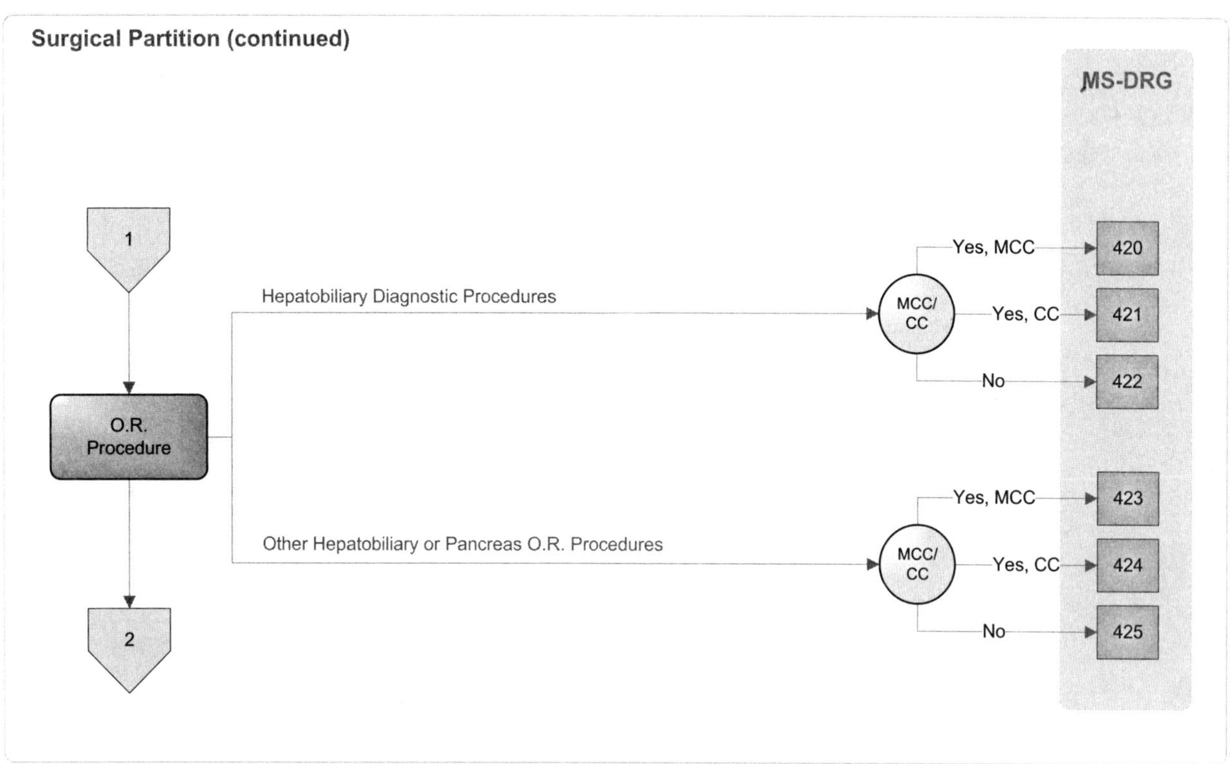

Major Diagnostic Category 7

Diseases and Disorders of the Hepatobiliary System and Pancreas

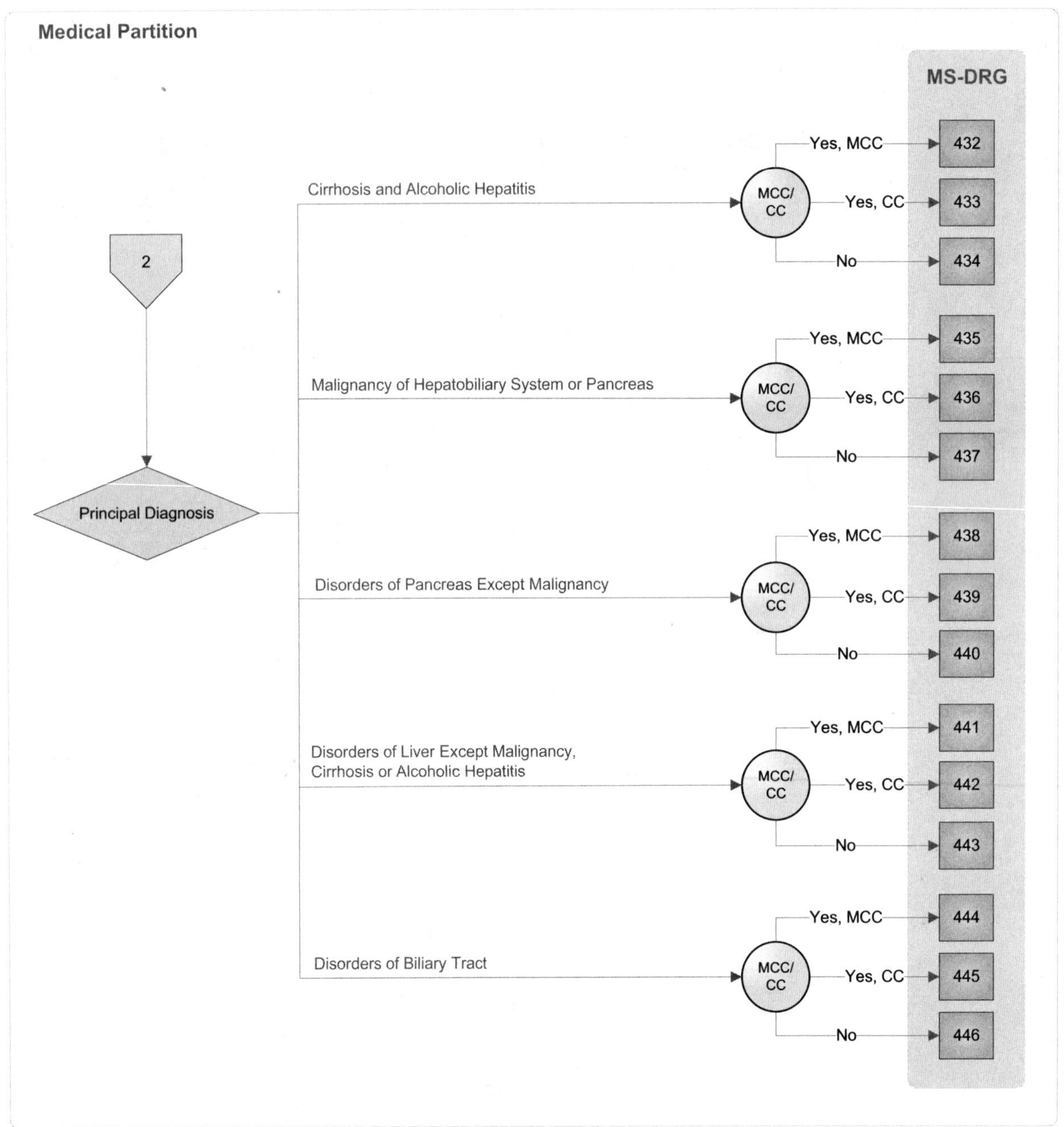

Major Diagnostic Category 8
Diseases and Disorders of the Musculoskeletal System and Connective Tissue

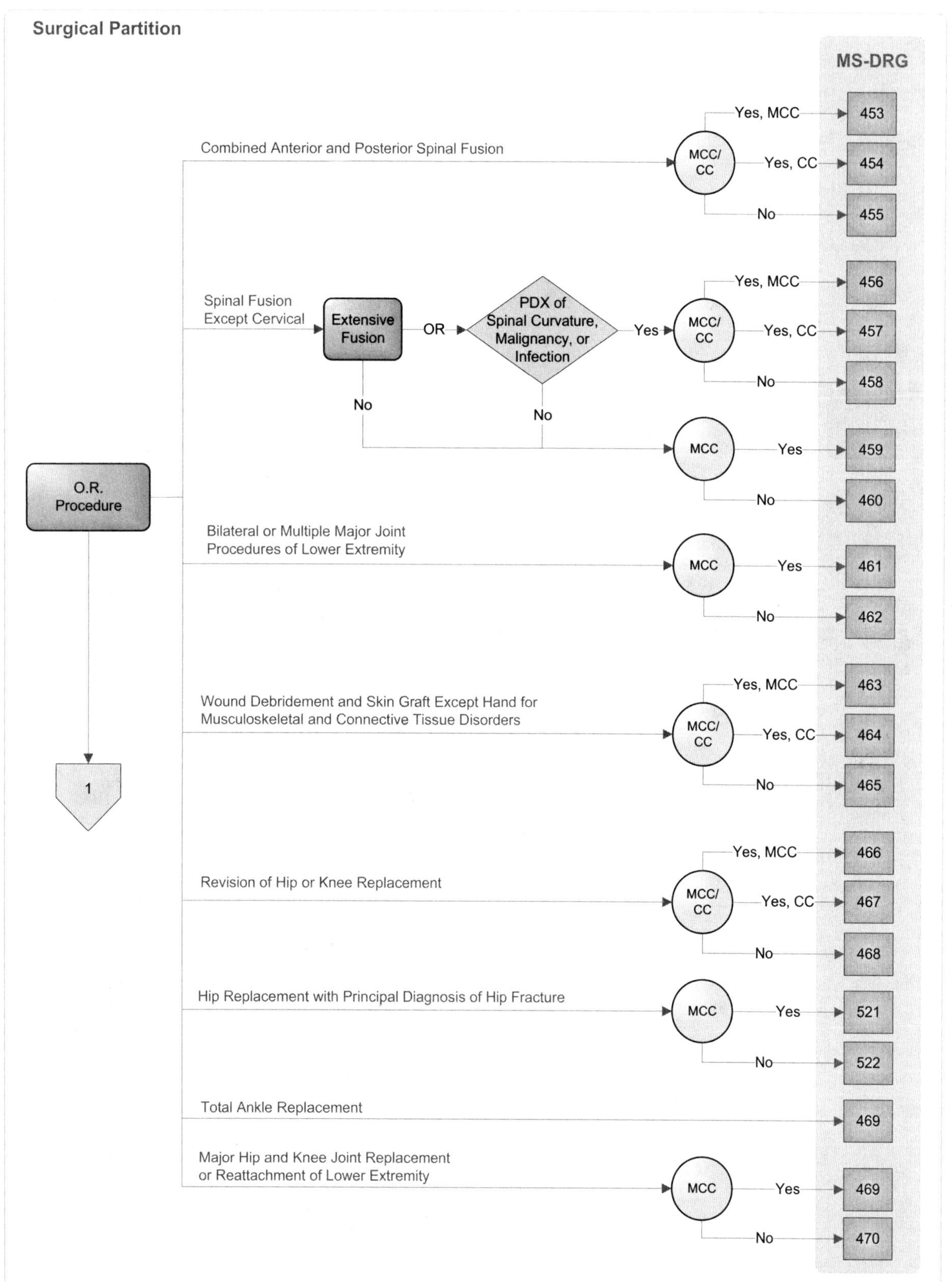

Major Diagnostic Category 8

Diseases and Disorders of the Musculoskeletal System and Connective Tissue

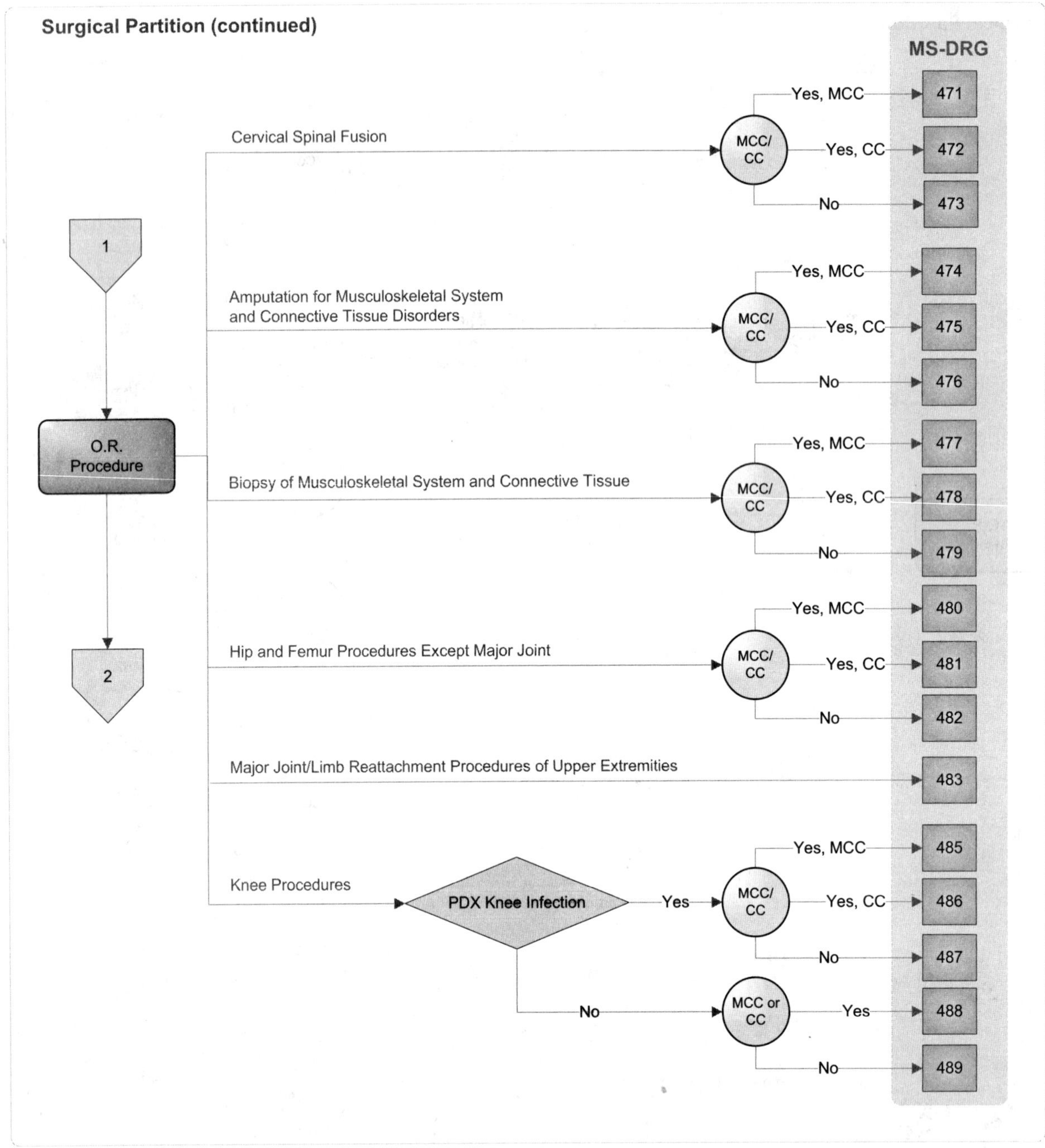

Major Diagnostic Category 8
Diseases and Disorders of the Musculoskeletal System and Connective Tissue

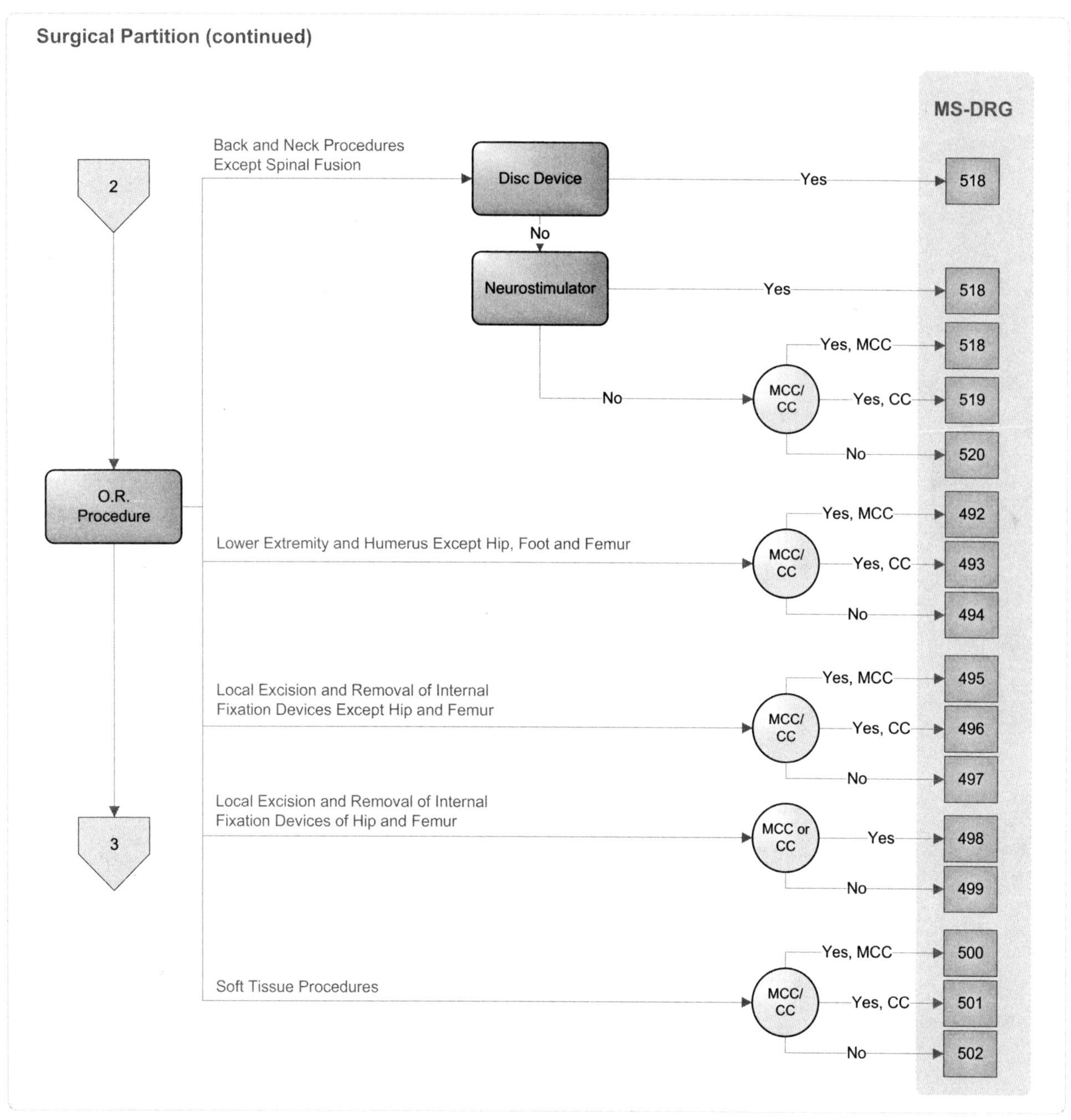

Major Diagnostic Category 8

Diseases and Disorders of the Musculoskeletal System and Connective Tissue

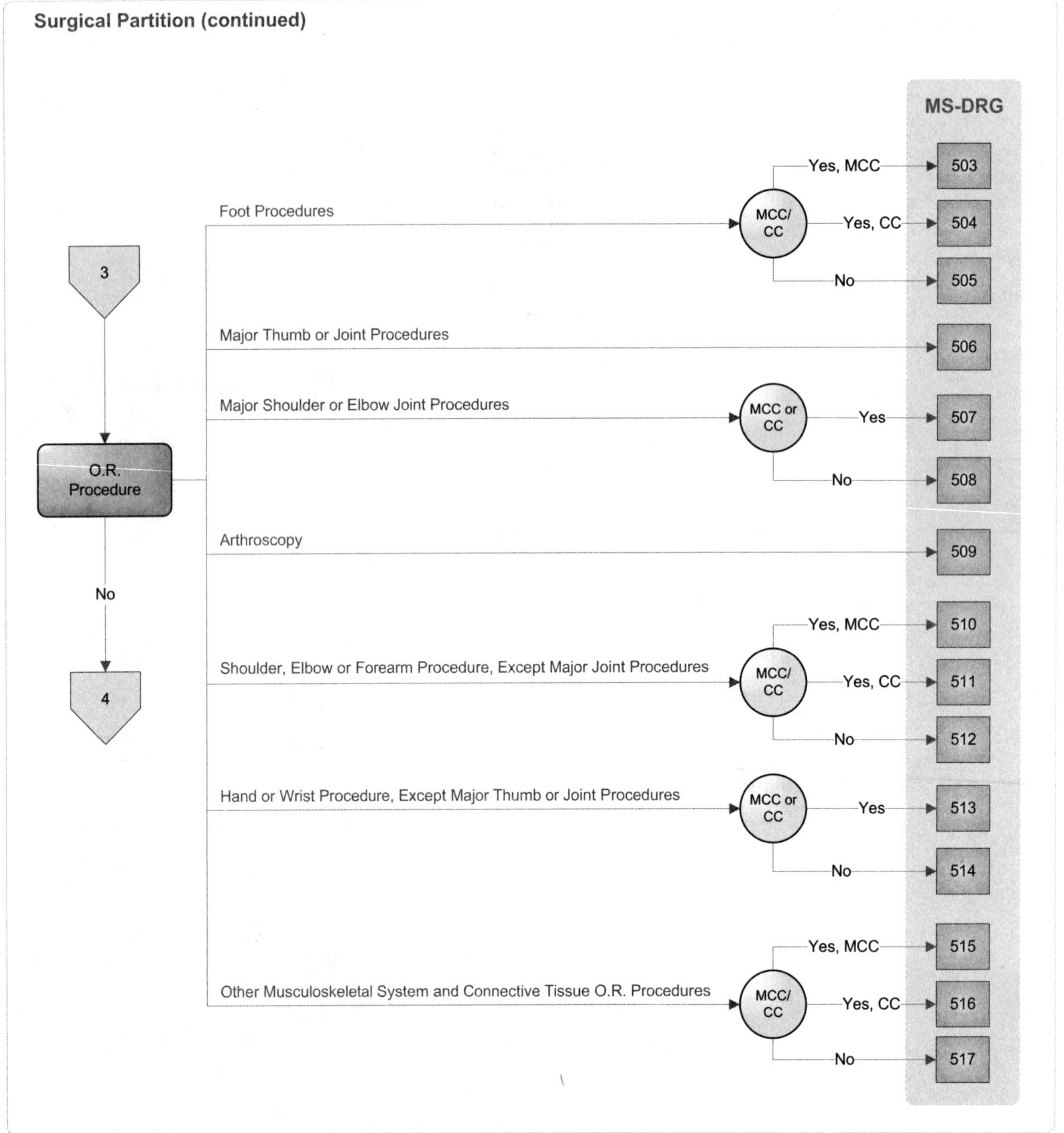

Major Diagnostic Category 8
Diseases and Disorders of the Musculoskeletal System and Connective Tissue

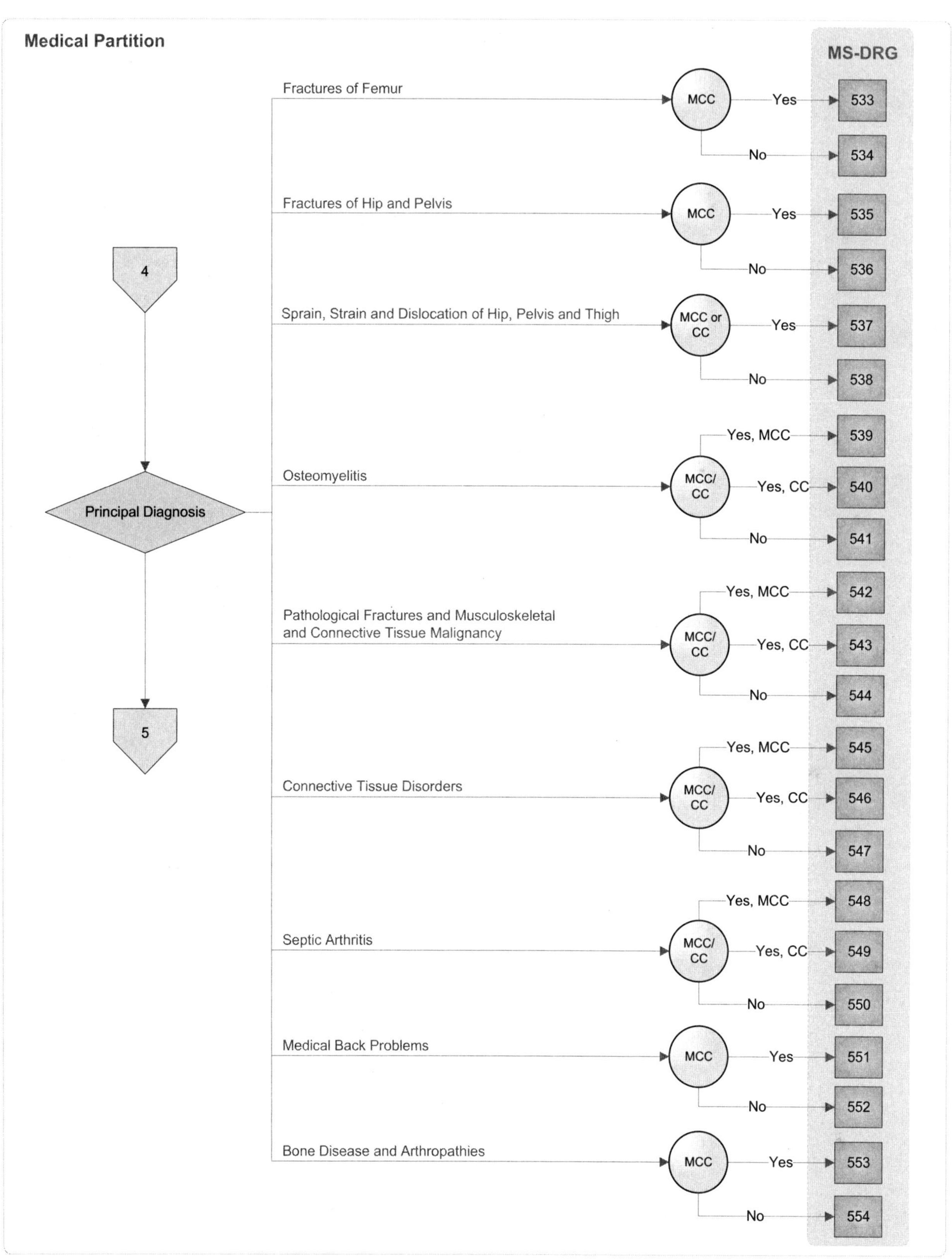

Major Diagnostic Category 8
Diseases and Disorders of the Musculoskeletal System and Connective Tissue

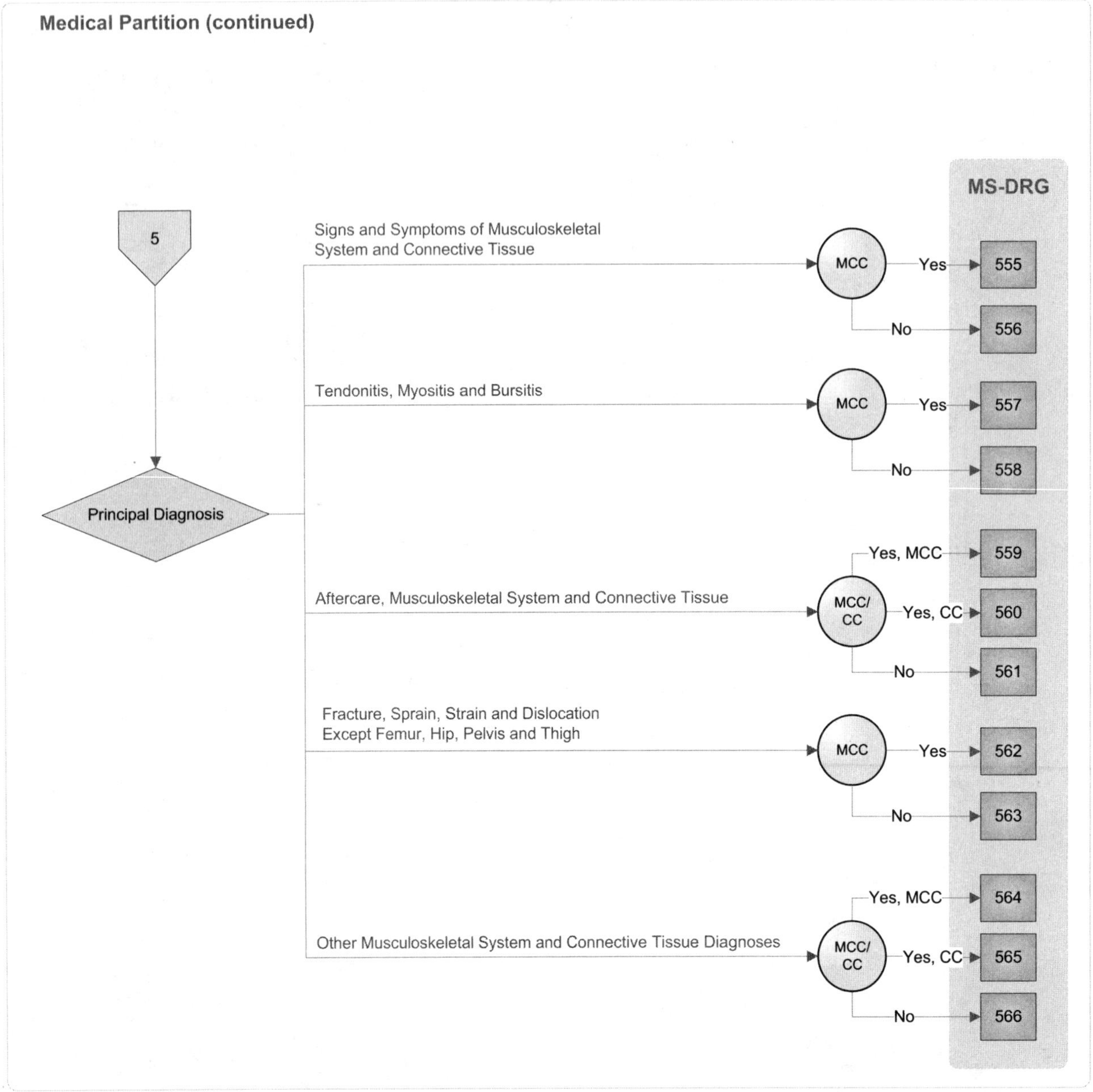

Major Diagnostic Category 9
Diseases and Disorders of the Skin, Subcutaneous Tissue and Breast

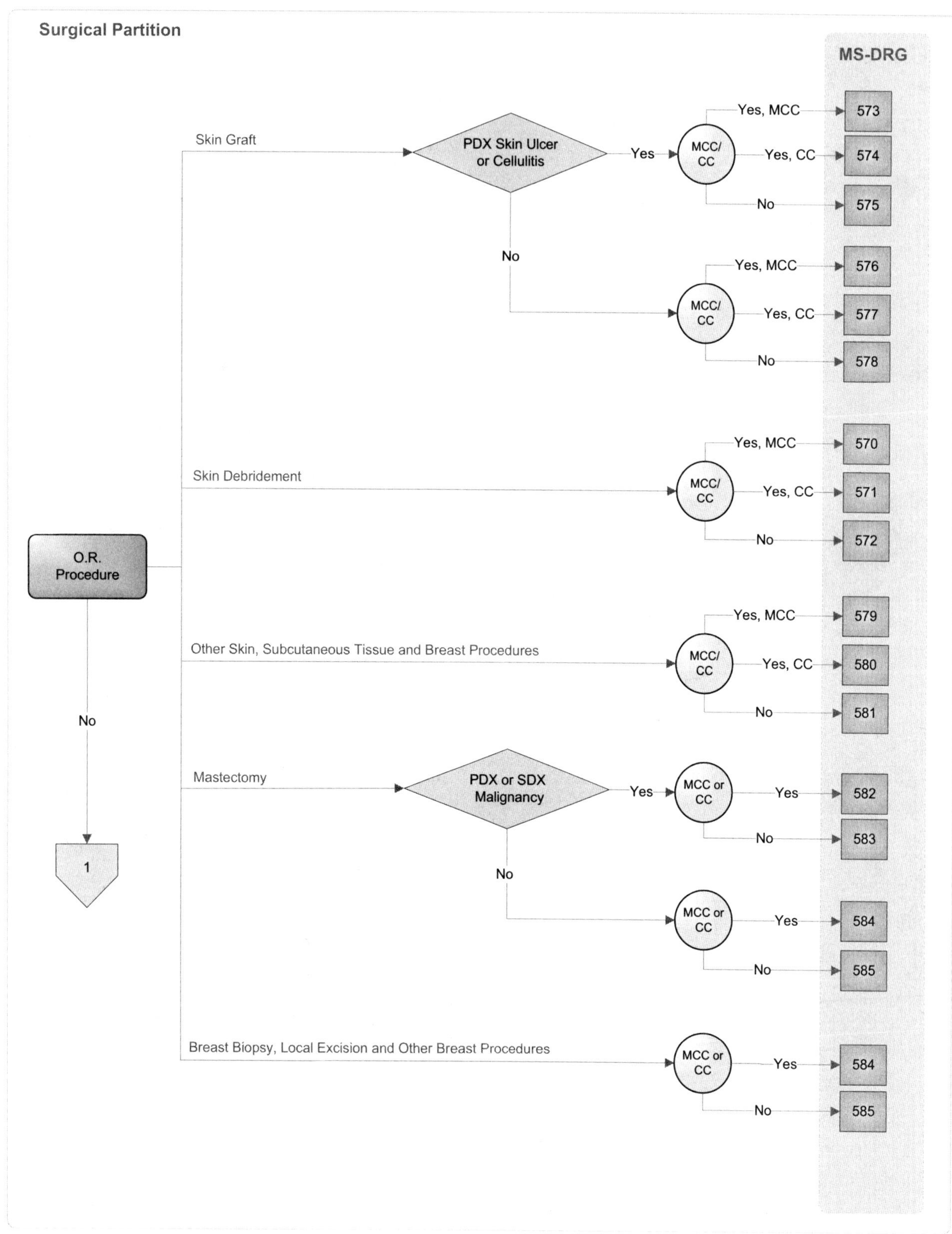

Major Diagnostic Category 9

Diseases and Disorders of the Skin, Subcutaneous Tissue and Breast

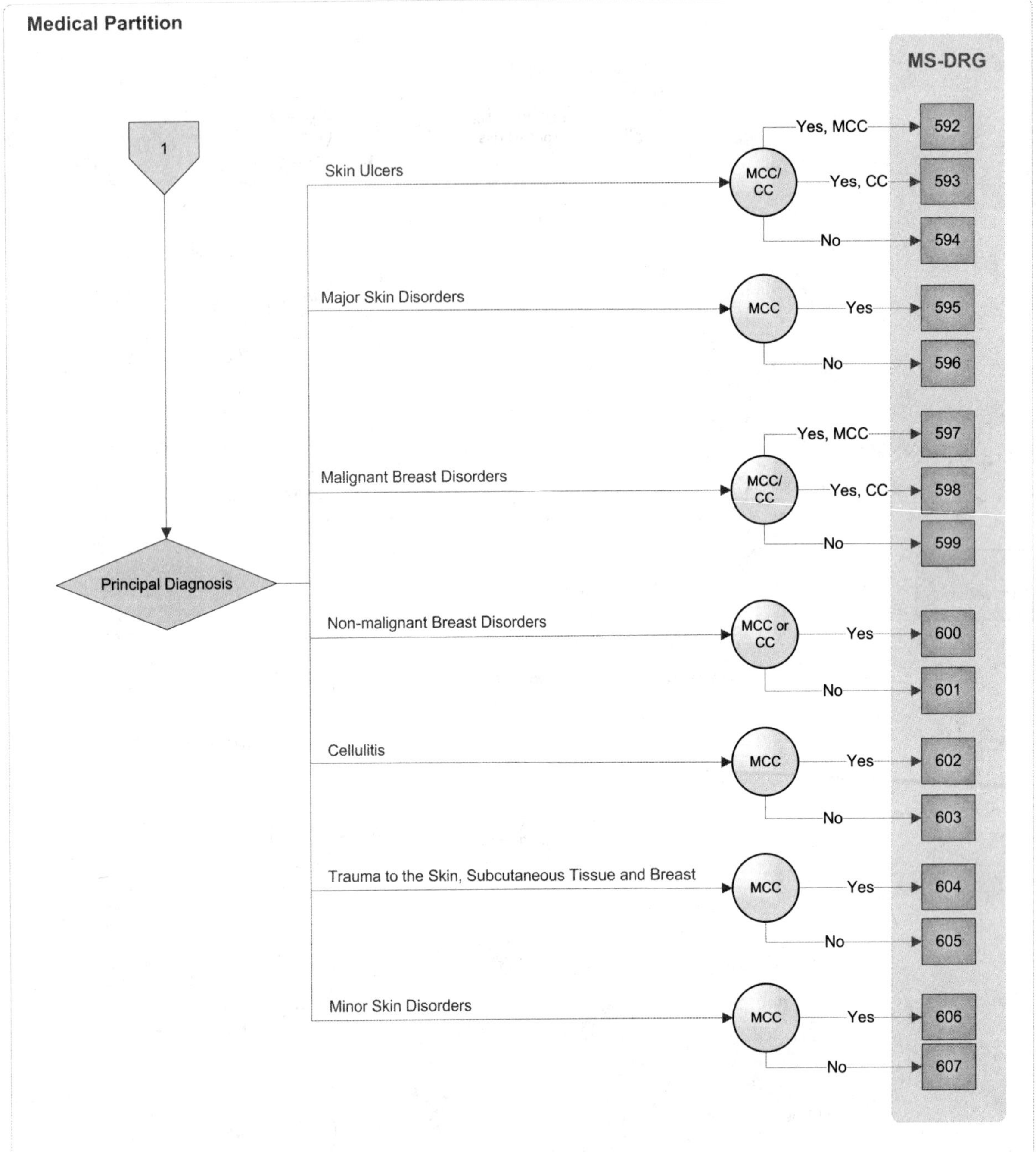

Major Diagnostic Category 10
Endocrine, Nutritional and Metabolic Diseases and Disorders

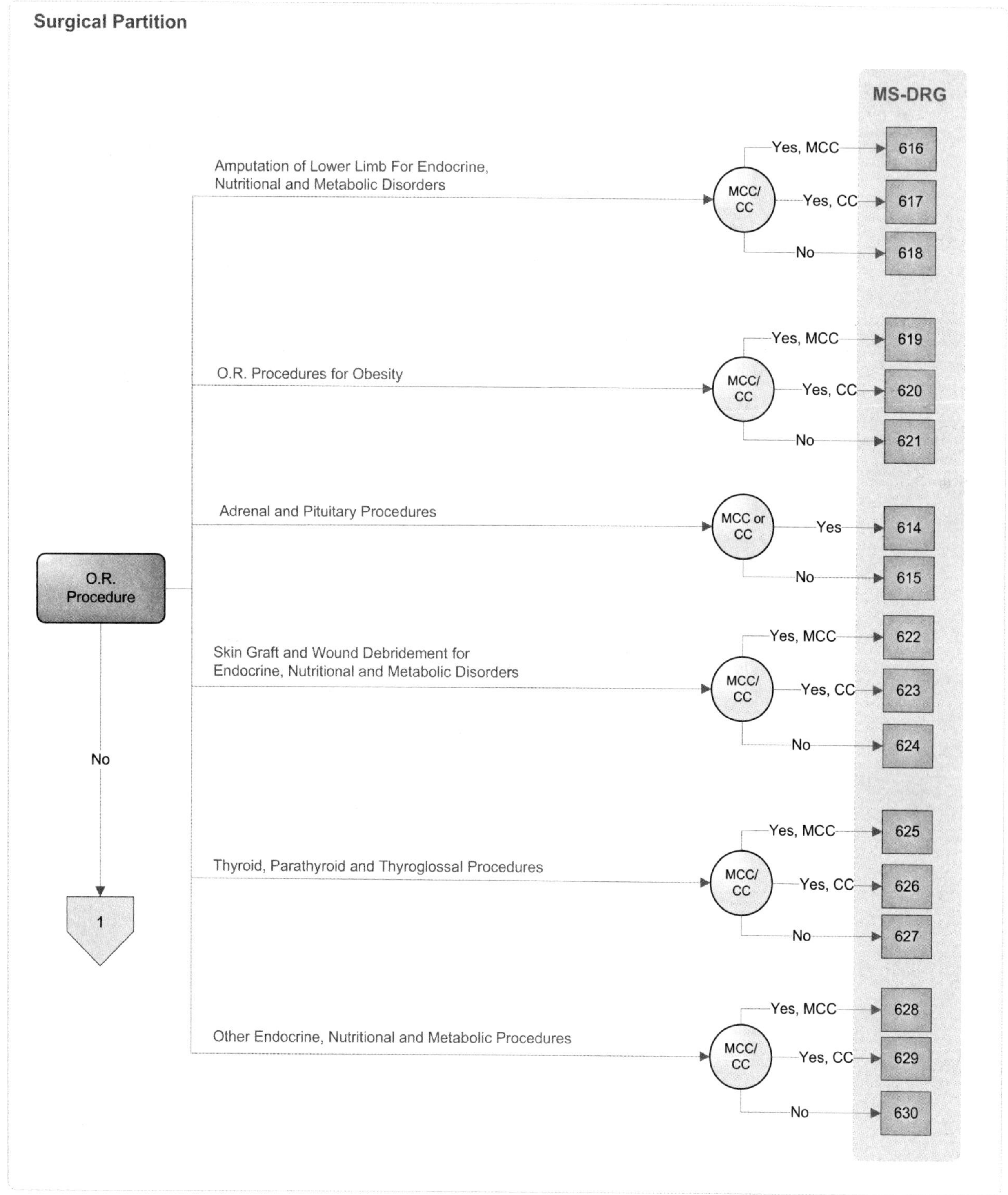

Major Diagnostic Category 10

Endocrine, Nutritional and Metabolic Diseases and Disorders

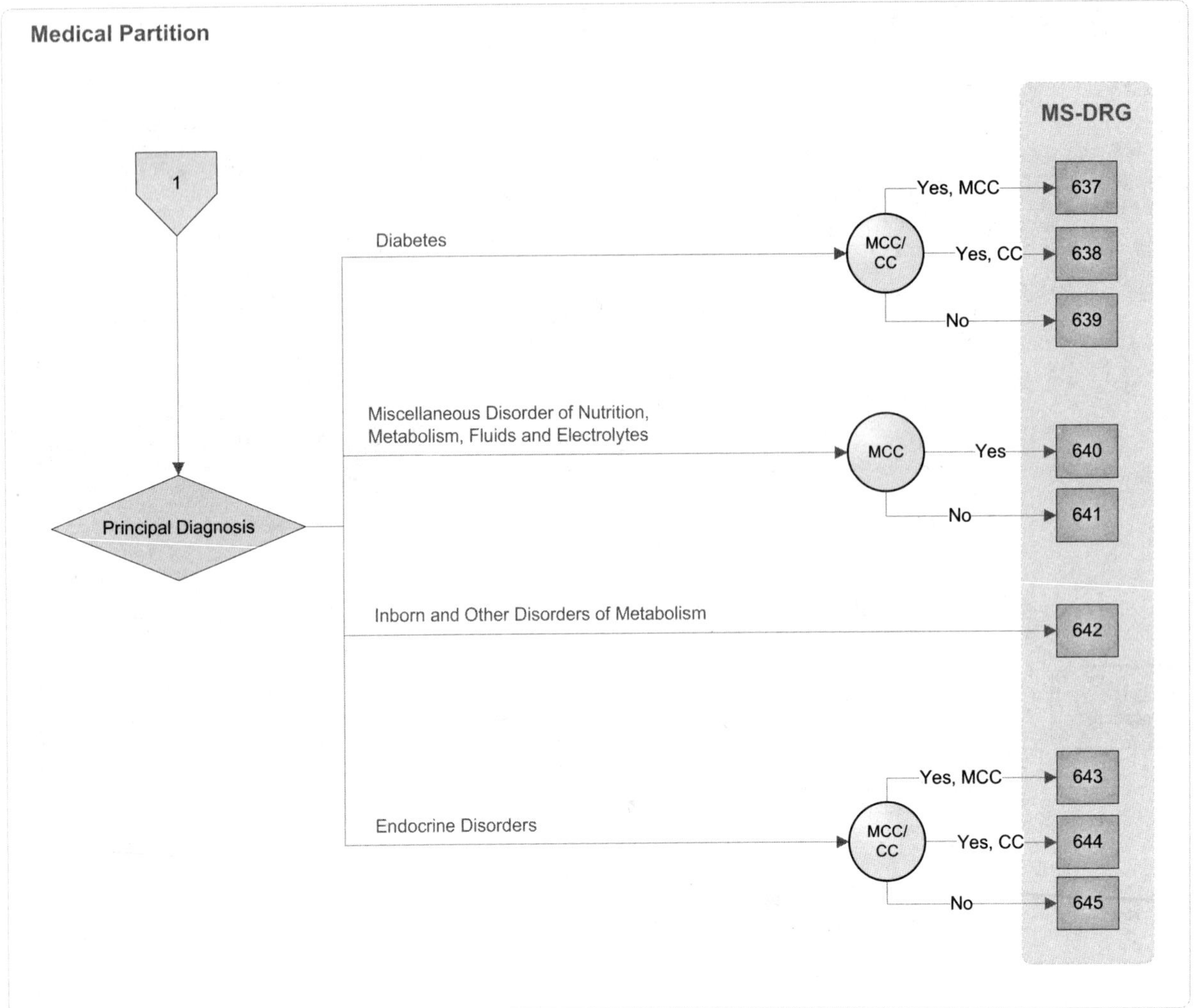

DRG Decision Trees

Major Diagnostic Category 11
Diseases and Disorders of the Kidney and Urinary Tract

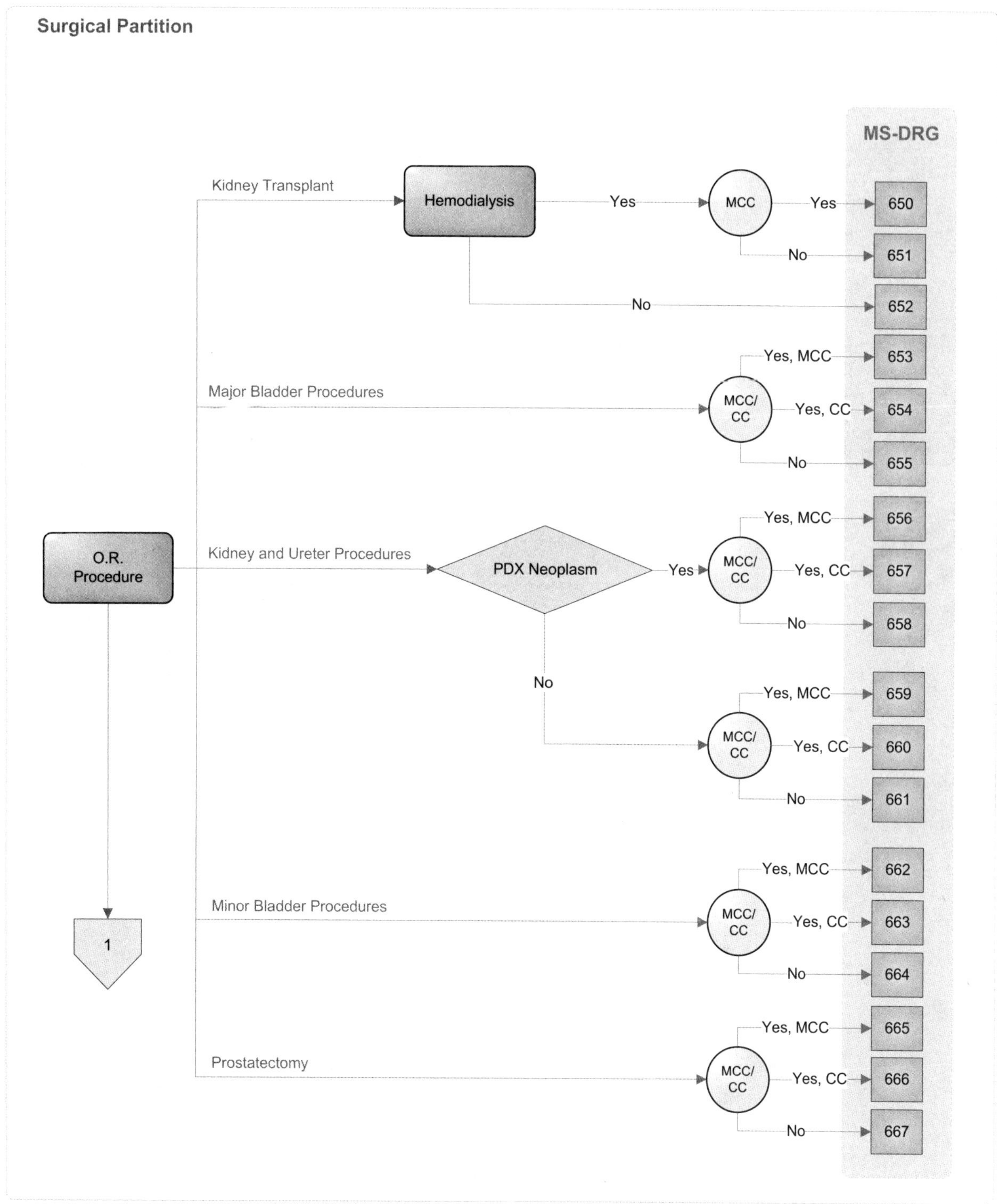

Major Diagnostic Category 11
Diseases and Disorders of the Kidney and Urinary Tract

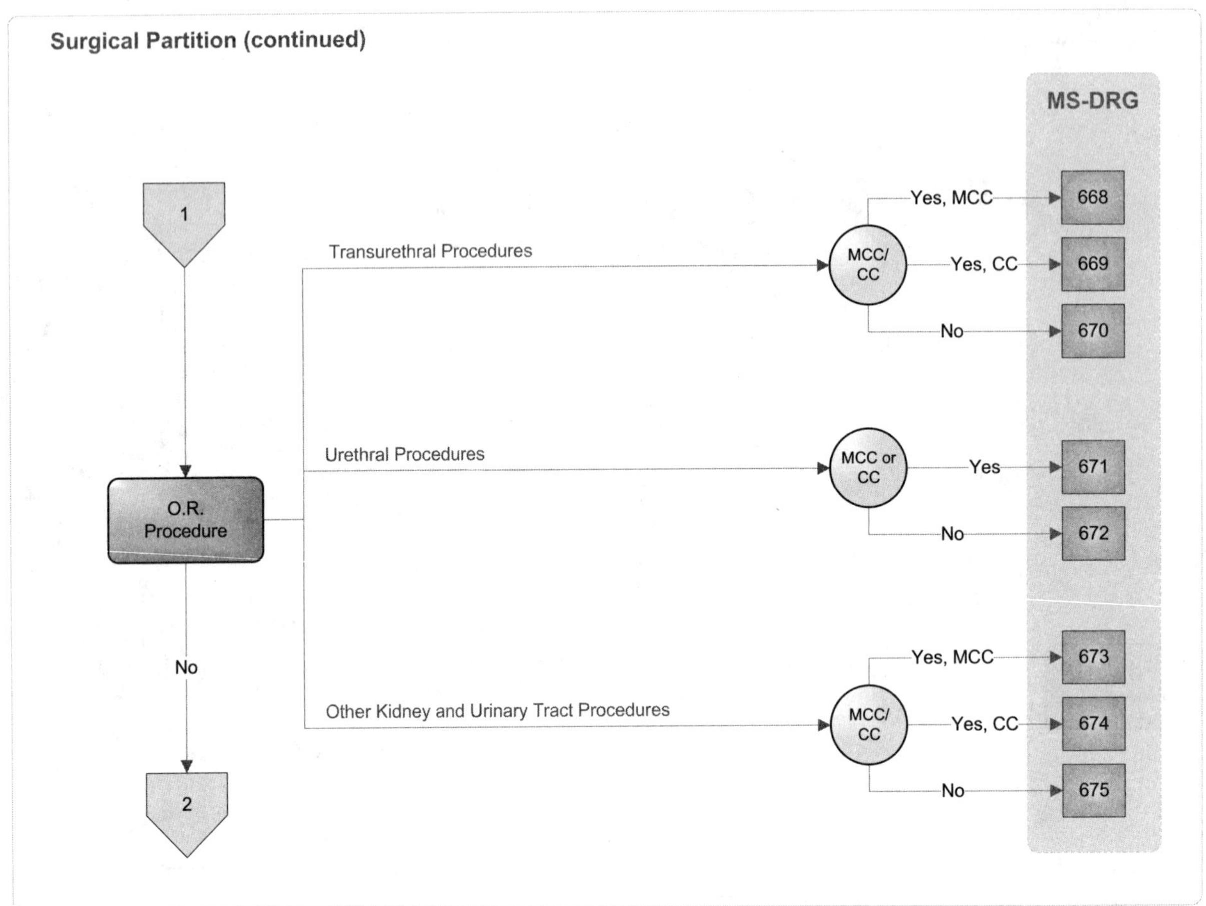

Major Diagnostic Category 11
Diseases and Disorders of the Kidney and Urinary Tract

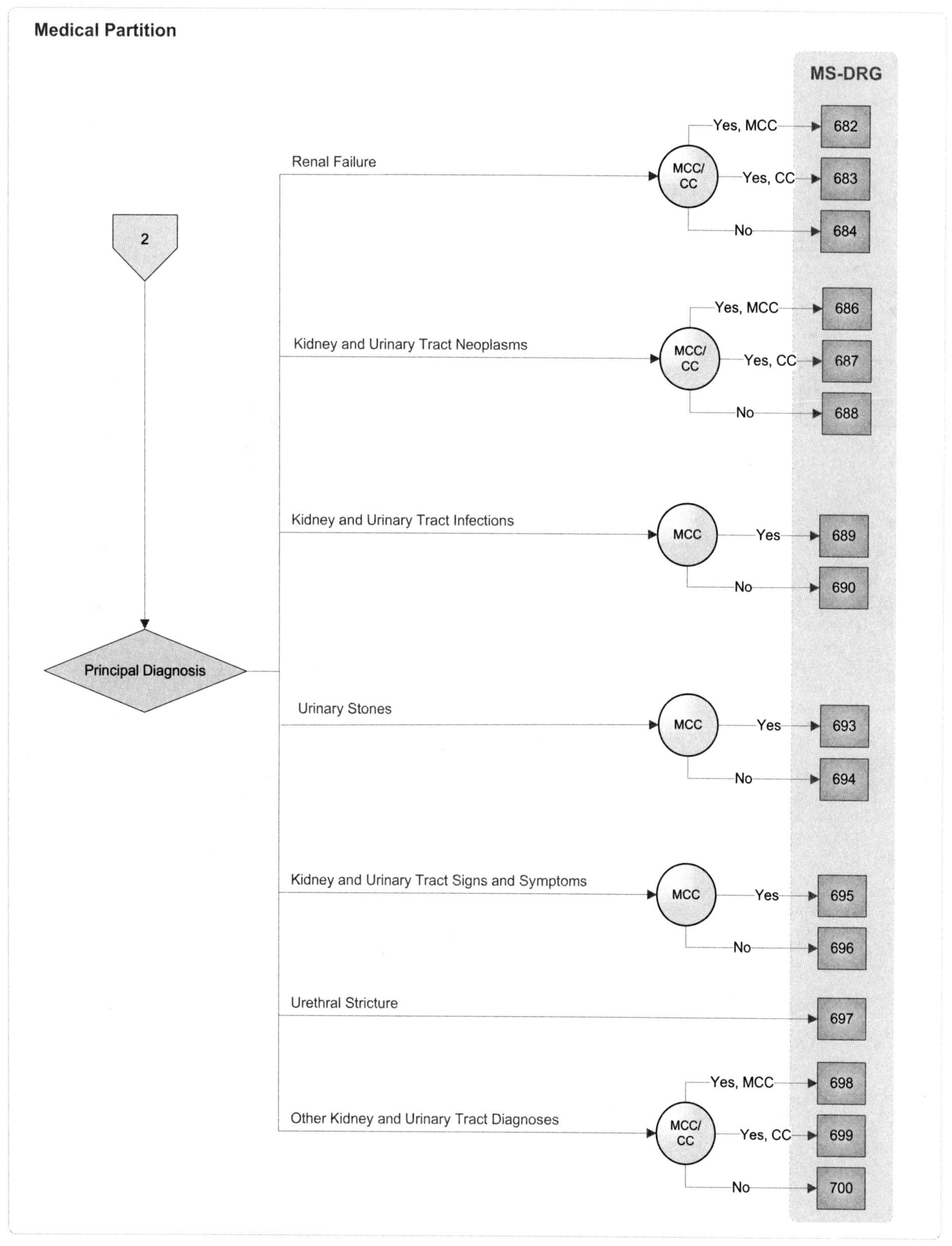

Major Diagnostic Category 12

Diseases and Disorders of the Male Reproductive System

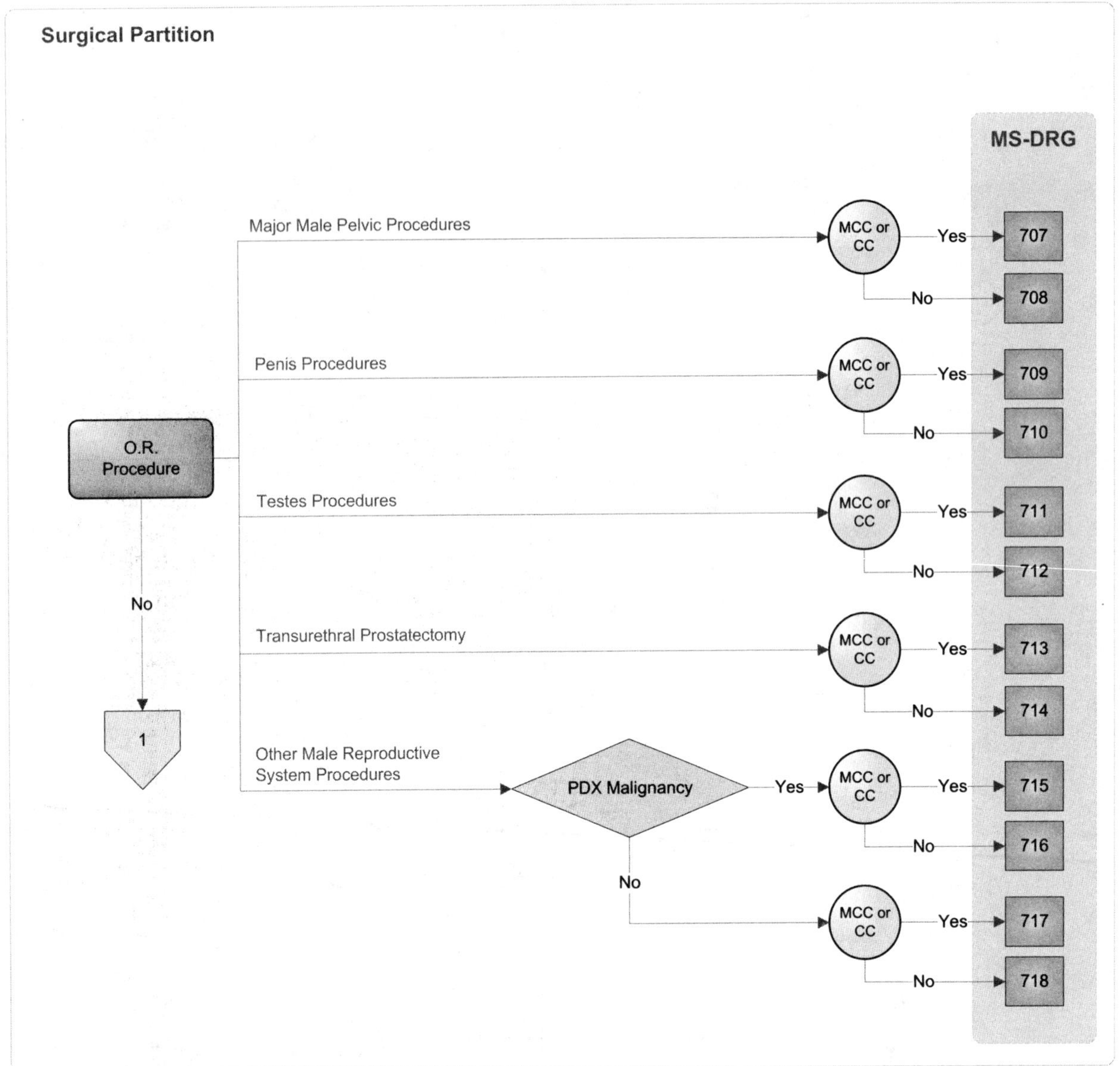

Major Diagnostic Category 12
Diseases and Disorders of the Male Reproductive System

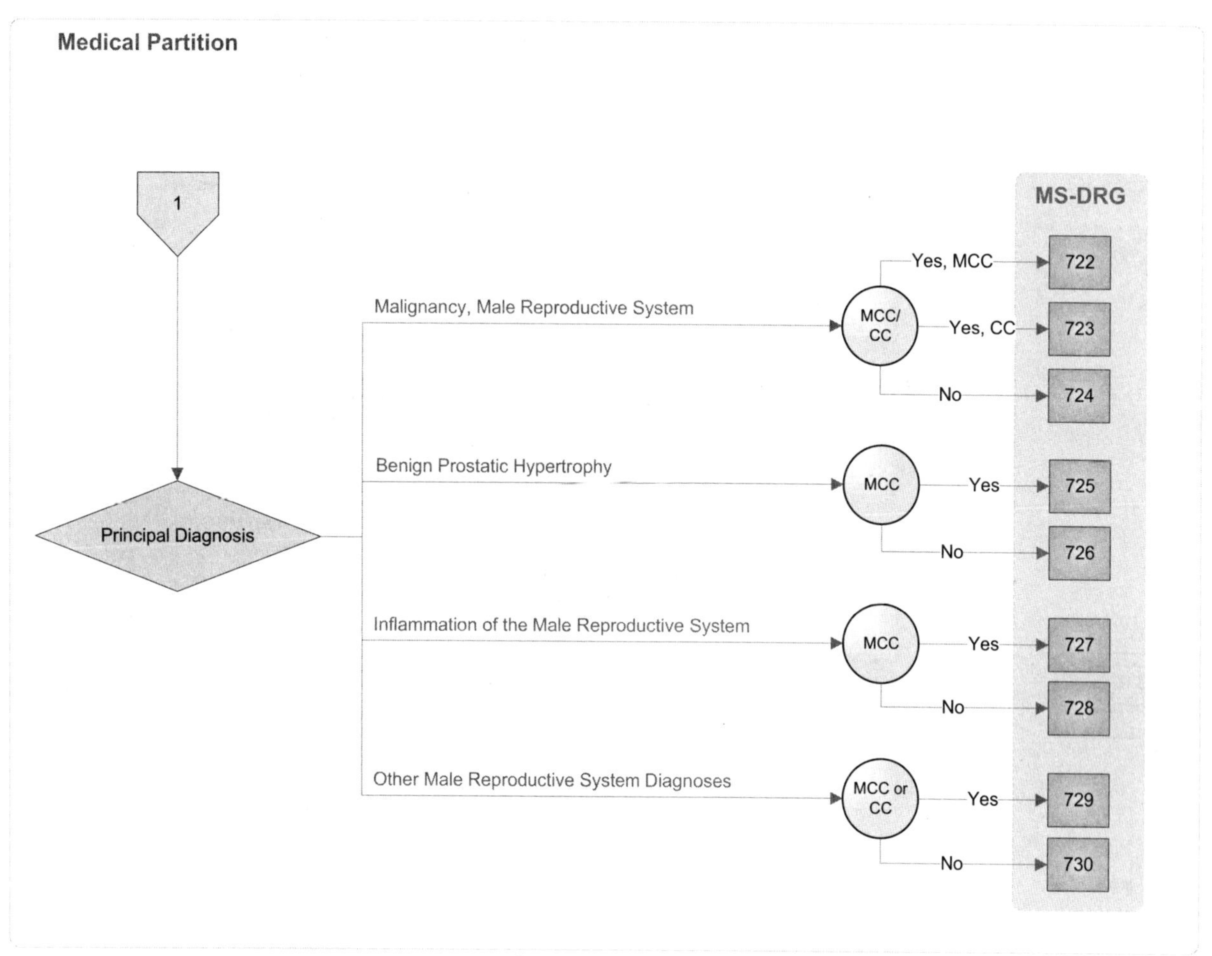

Major Diagnostic Category 13
Diseases and Disorders of the Female Reproductive System

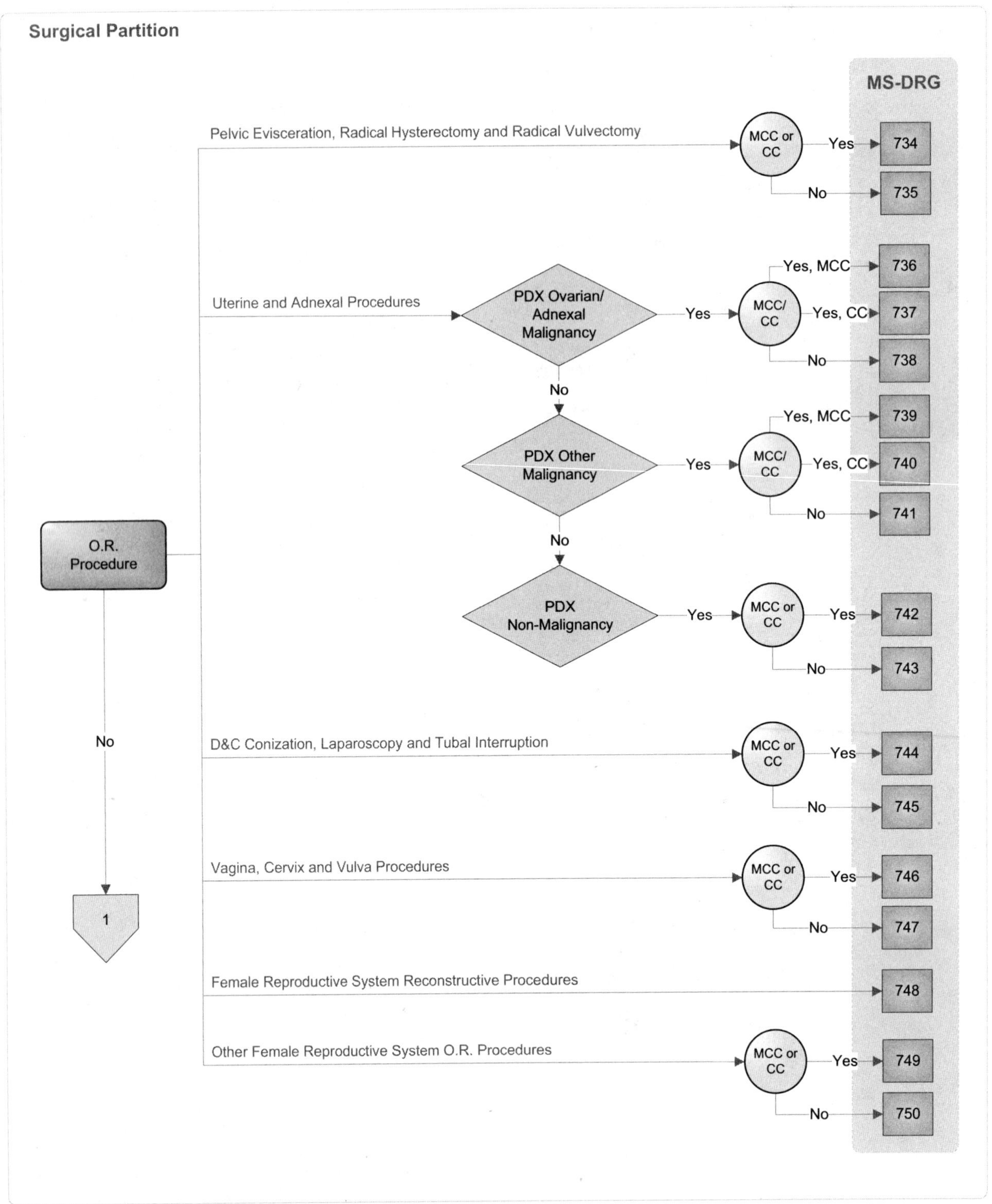

Major Diagnostic Category 13
Diseases and Disorders of the Female Reproductive System

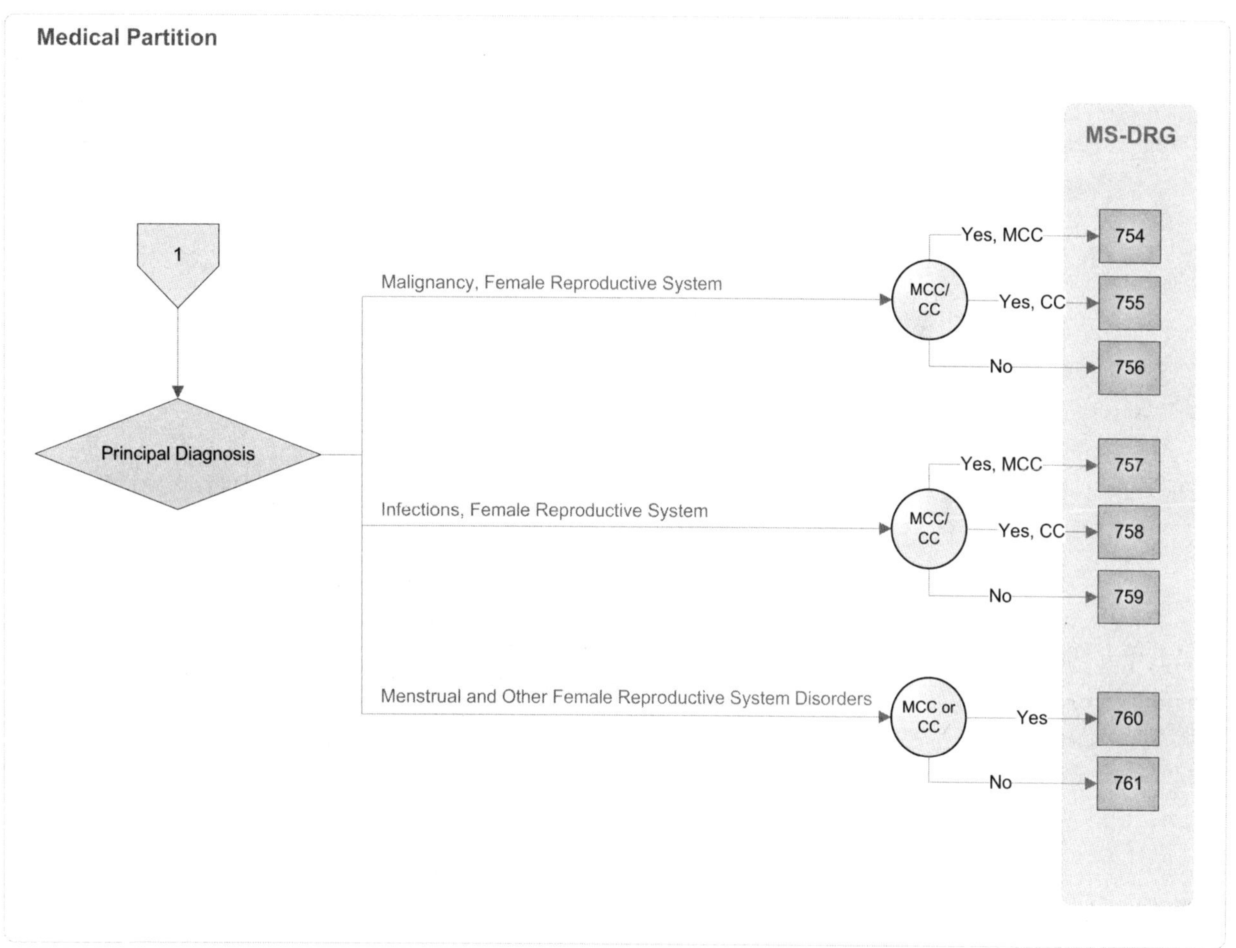

Major Diagnostic Category 14

Pregnancy, Childbirth and Puerperium

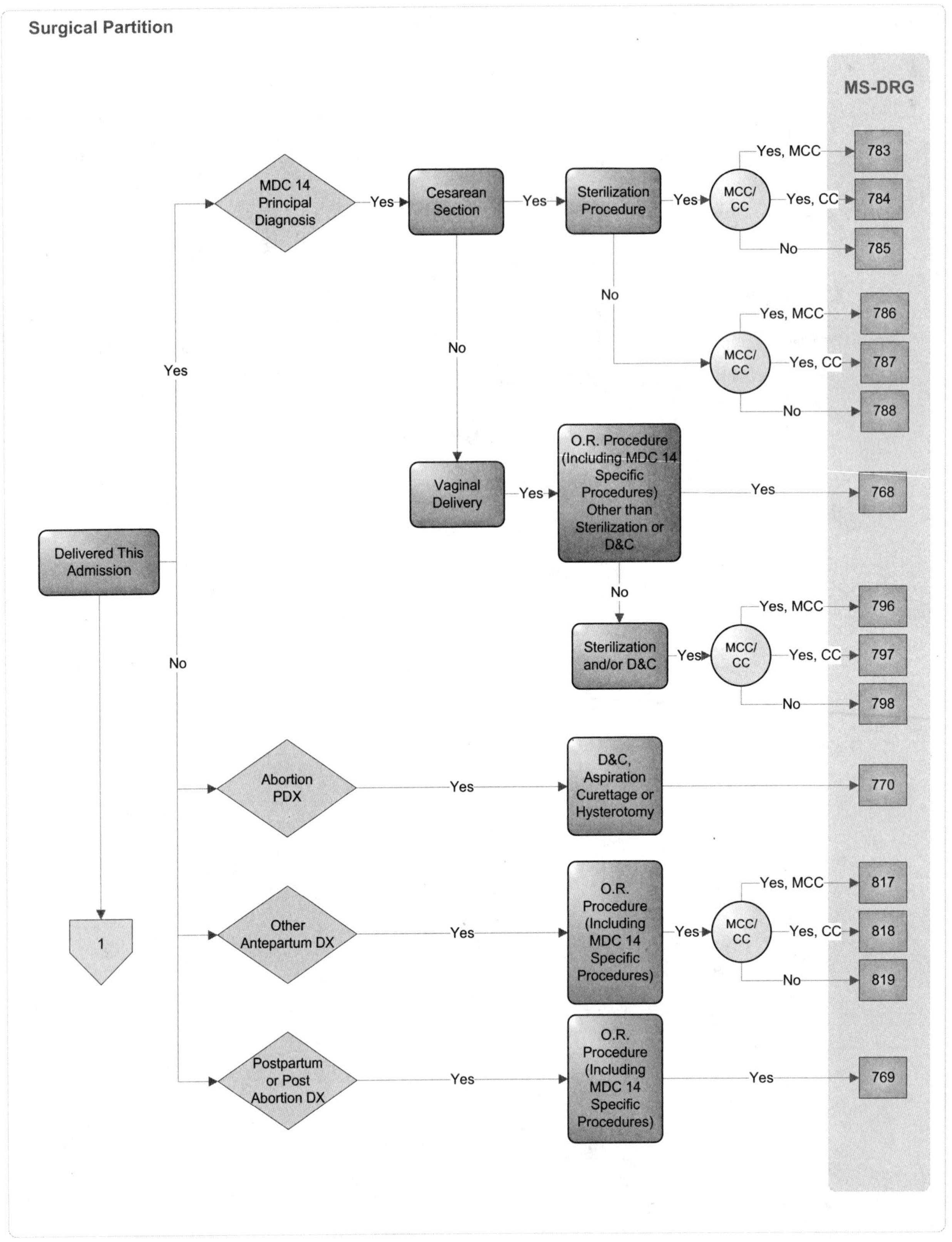

Major Diagnostic Category 14
Pregnancy, Childbirth and Puerperium

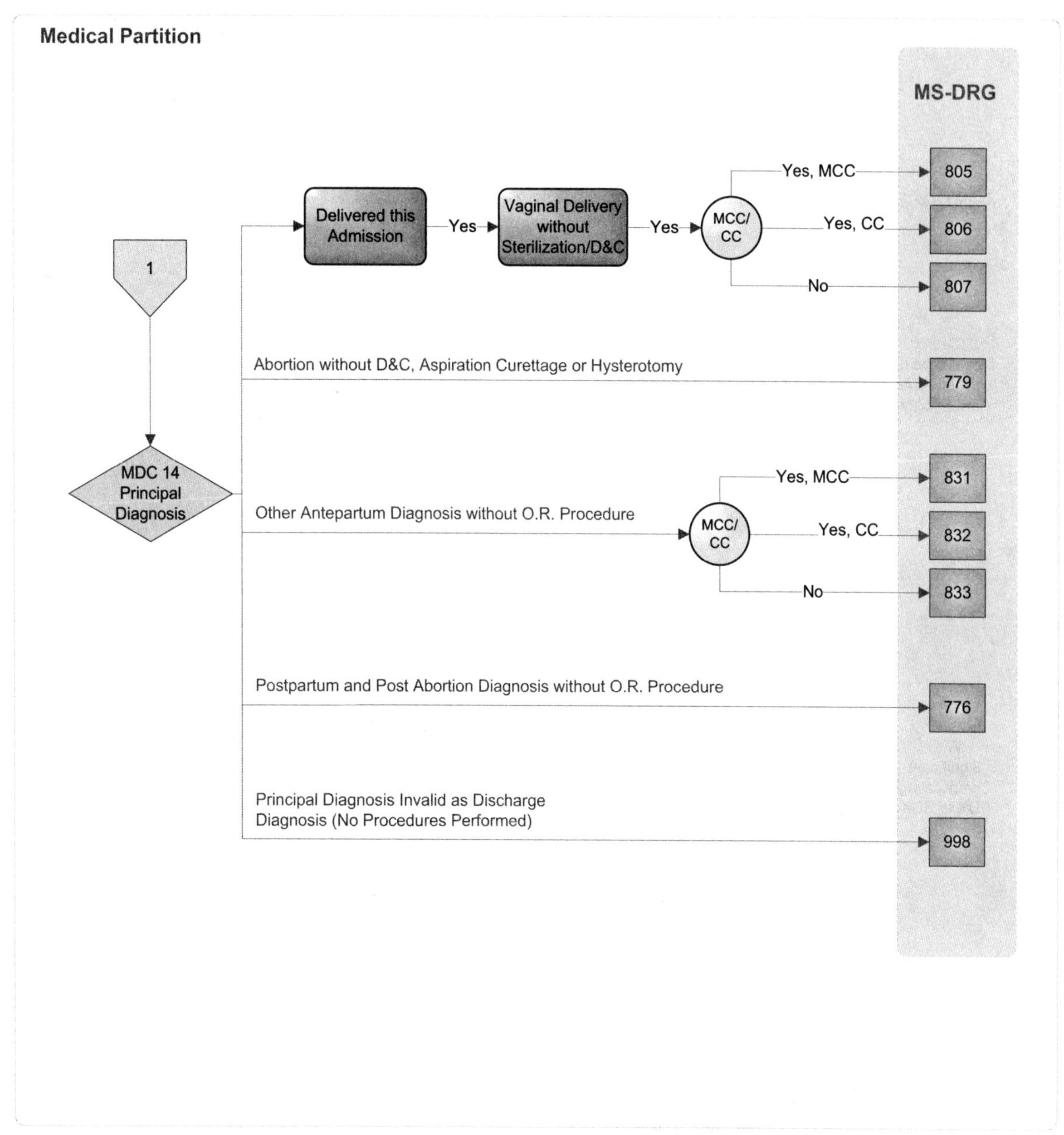

Major Diagnostic Category 15

Newborns and Other Neonates with Conditions Originating in Perinatal Period

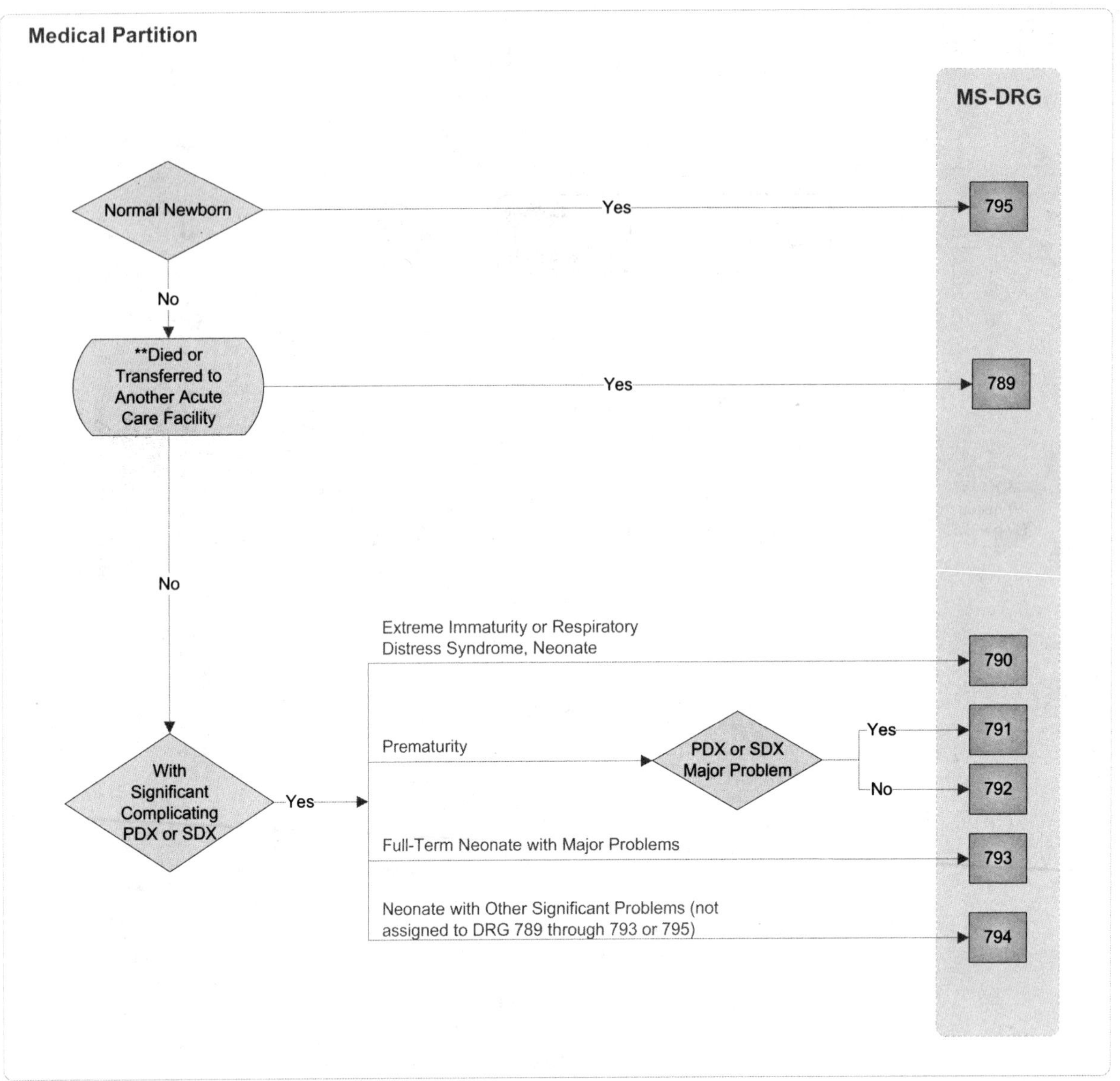

**Died = Discharge Status of 20

Acute Care Facilities:

Discharge Status of 02 = Short-Term General Hospital or;

Discharge Status of 05 = Designated Cancer Center or Children's Hospital or;

Discharge Status of 66 = Critical Access Hospital or;

Discharge Status of 82 = Discharged/Transferred to a Short Term General Hospital for Inpatient Care with a Planned Acute Care Hospital Inpatient Readmission or;

Discharge Status of 85 = Discharged/Transferred to a Designated Cancer Center or Children's Hospital with a Planned Acute Care Hospital Inpatient Readmission or;

Discharge Status of 94 = Discharged/Transferred to a Critical Access Hospital (CAH) with a Planned Acute Care Hospital Inpatient Readmission

Major Diagnostic Category 16
Diseases and Disorders of Blood, Blood Forming Organs and Immunological Disorders

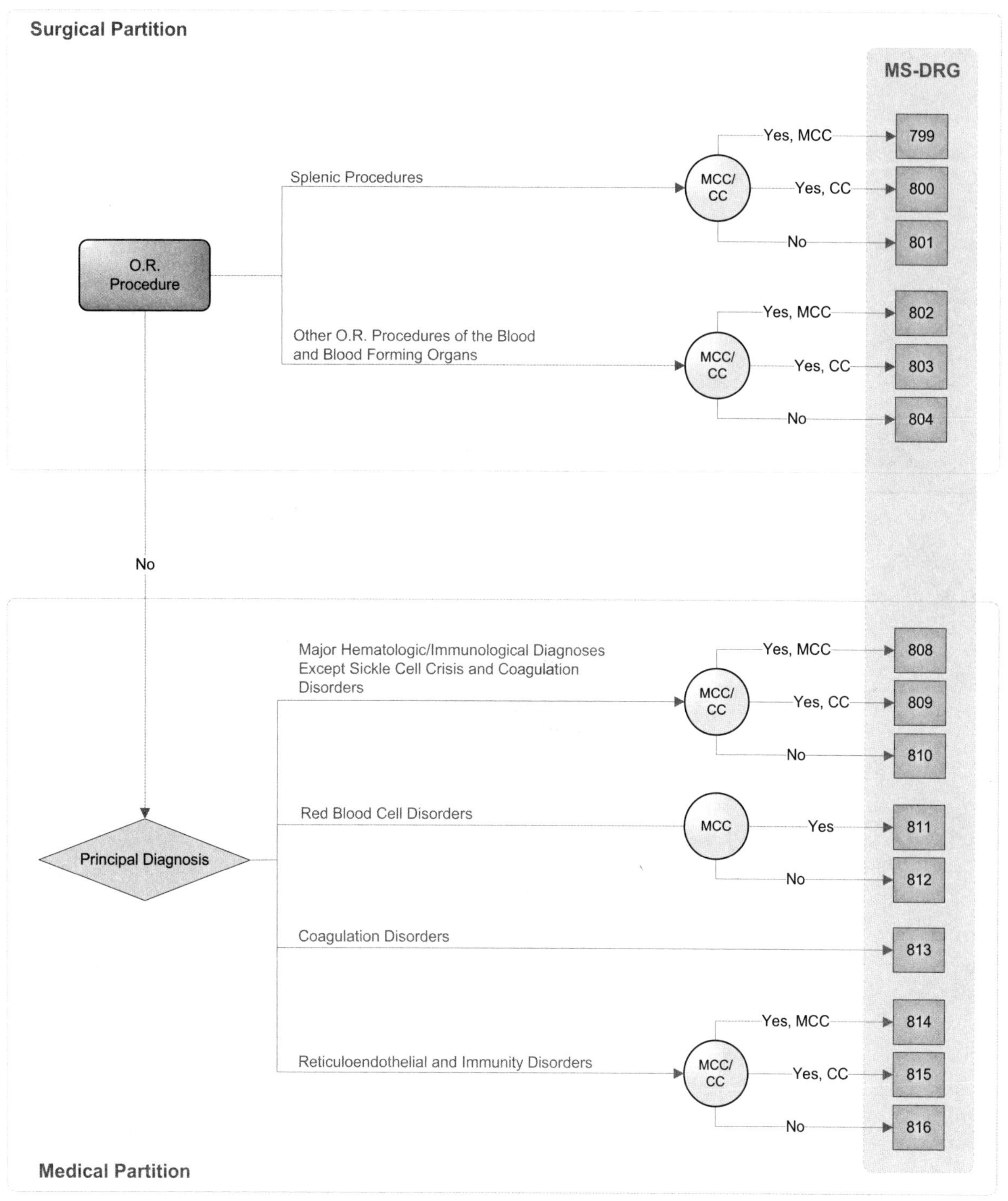

Major Diagnostic Category 17

Myeloproliferative Diseases and Disorders, Poorly Differentiated Neoplasm

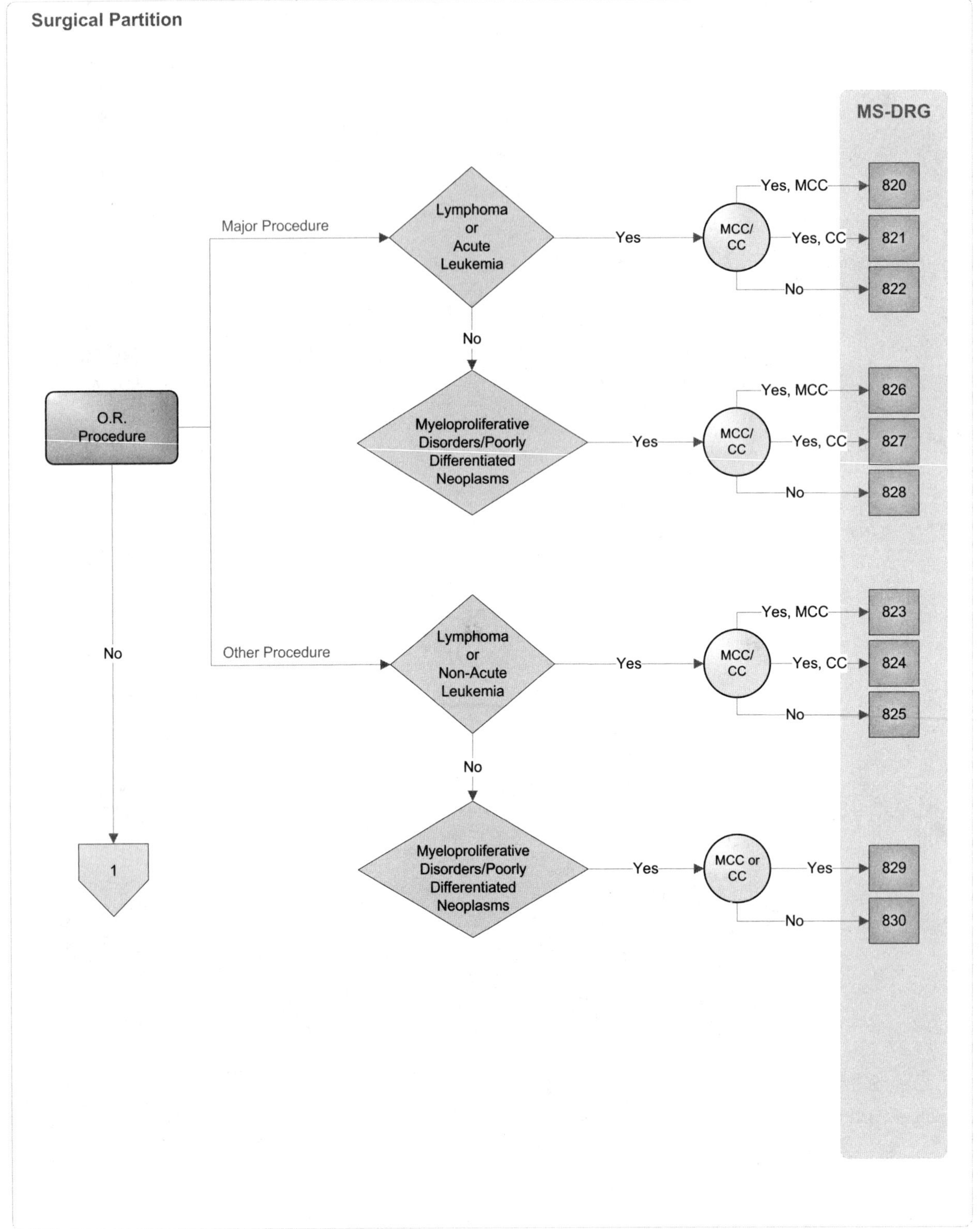

Major Diagnostic Category 17

Myeloproliferative Diseases and Disorders, Poorly Differentiated Neoplasm

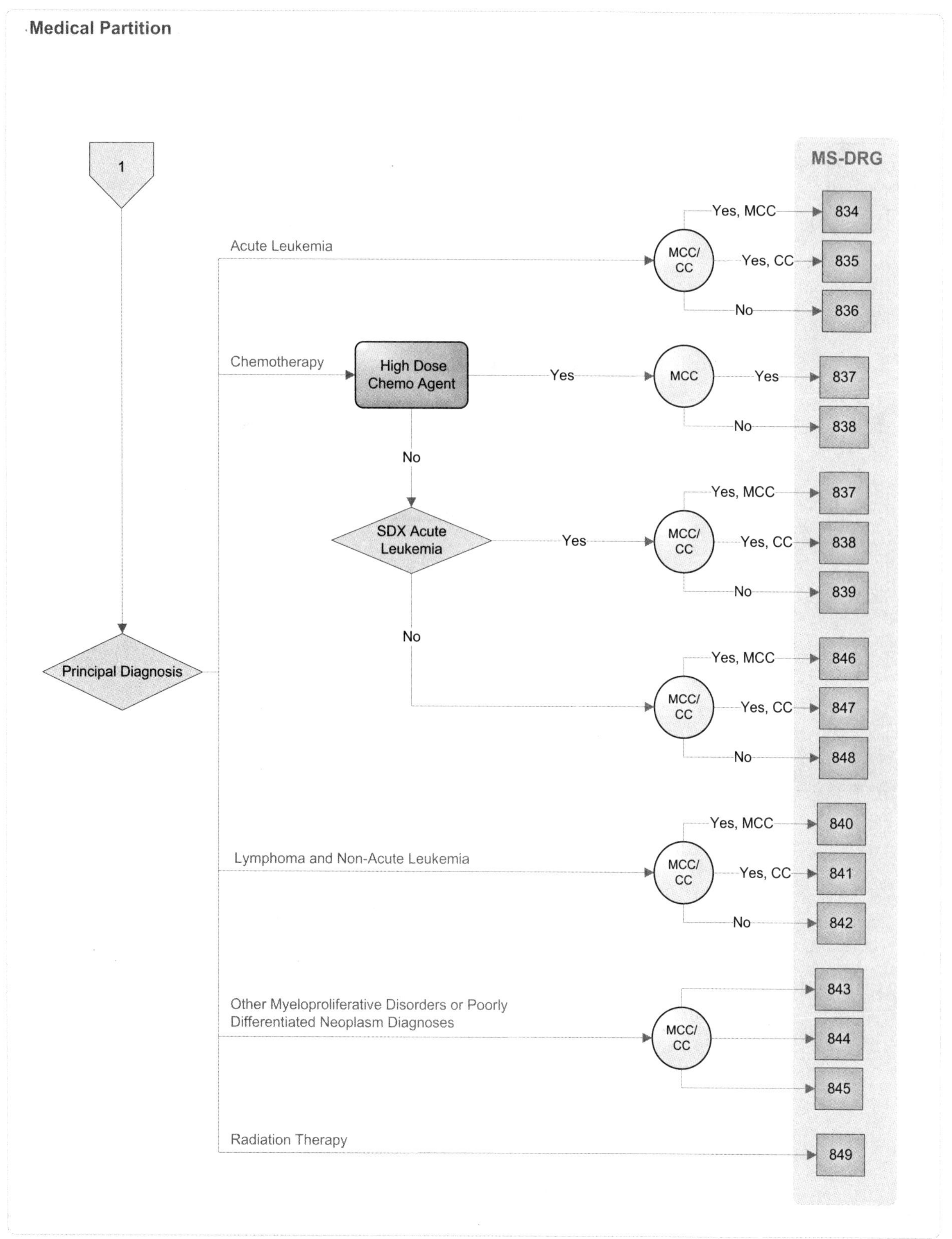

Major Diagnostic Category 18

Infections and Parasitic Diseases (Systemic or Unspecified Sites)

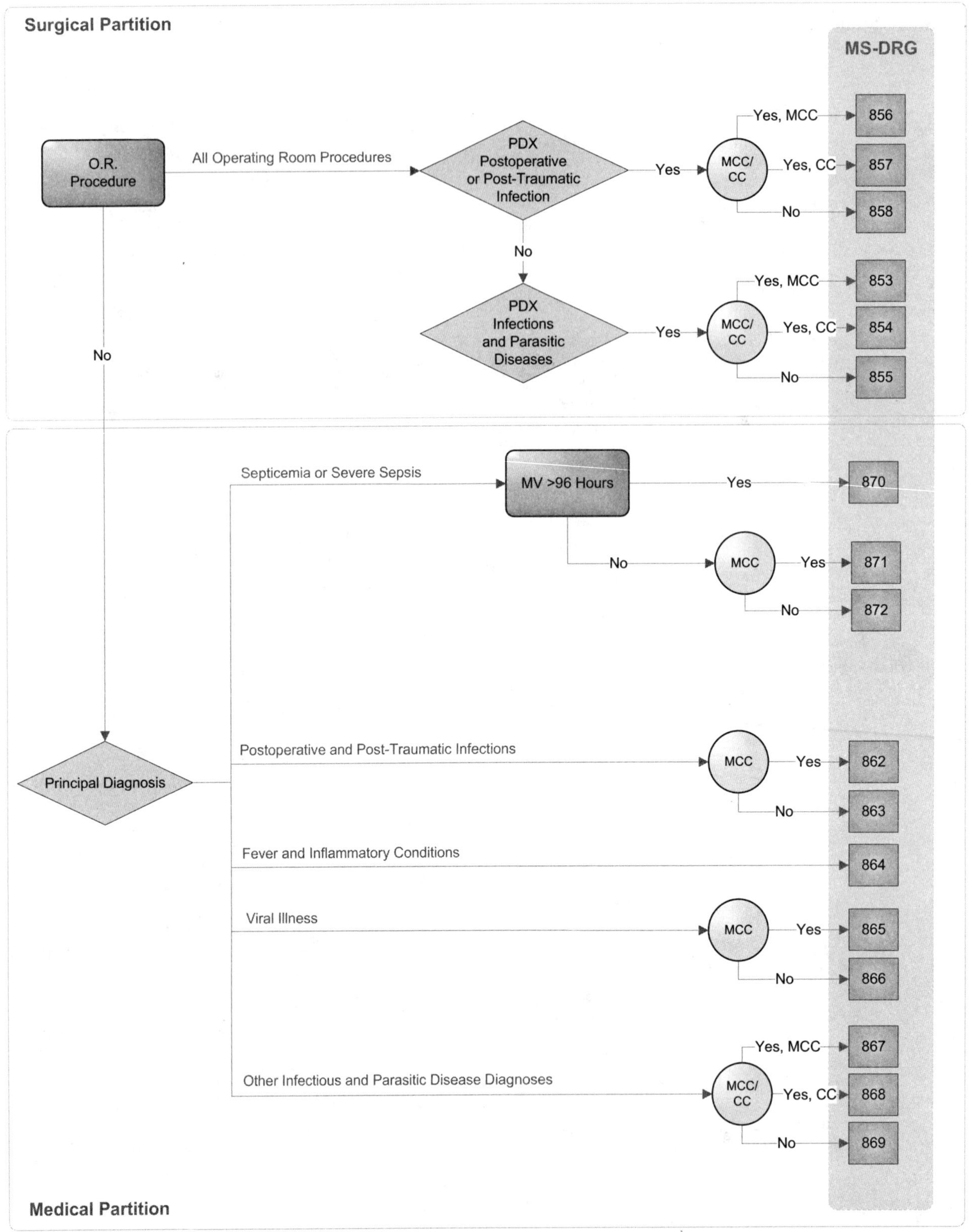

Major Diagnostic Category 19
Mental Diseases and Disorders

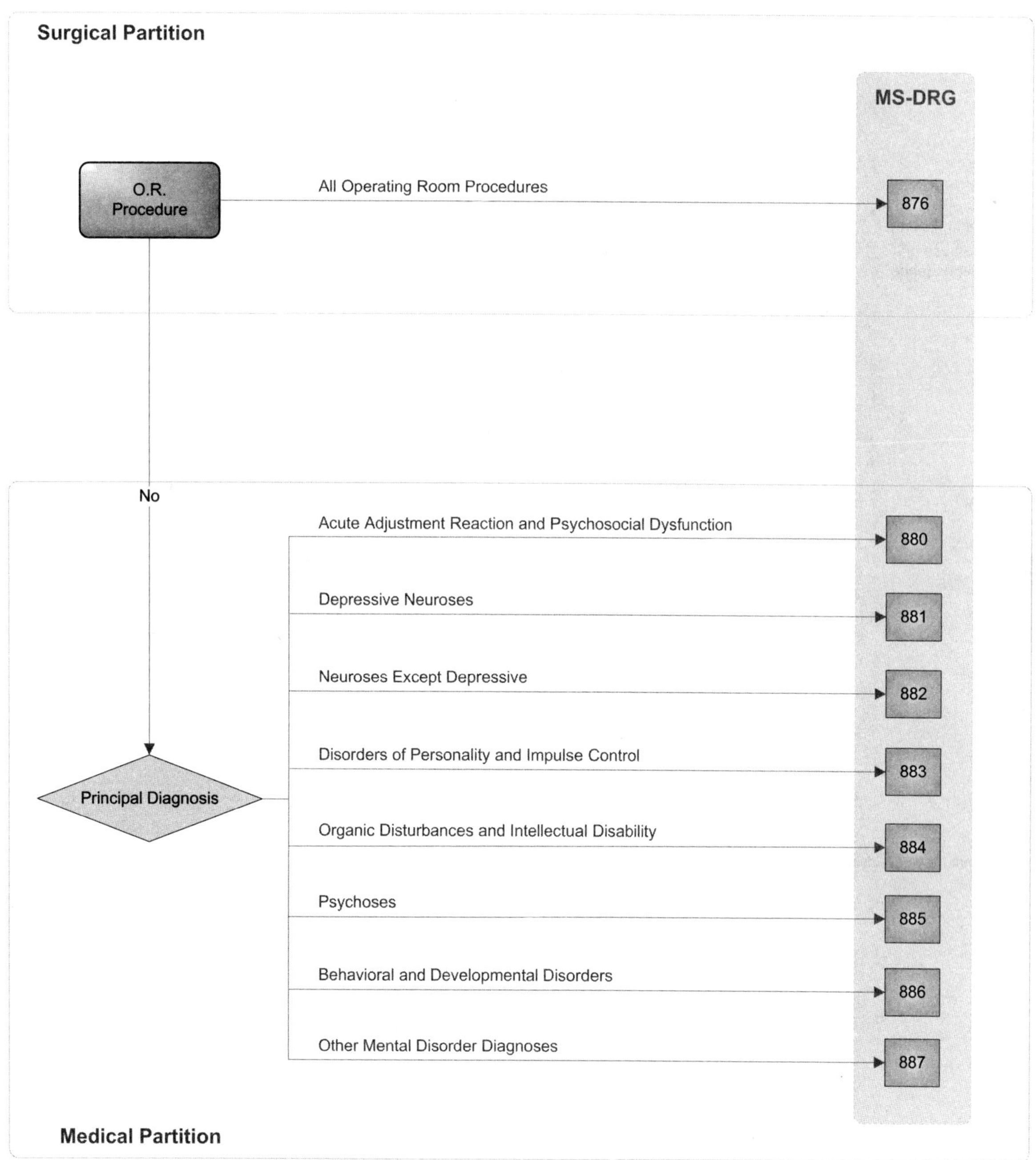

Major Diagnostic Category 20

Alcohol or Drug Use or Induced Organic Mental Disorders

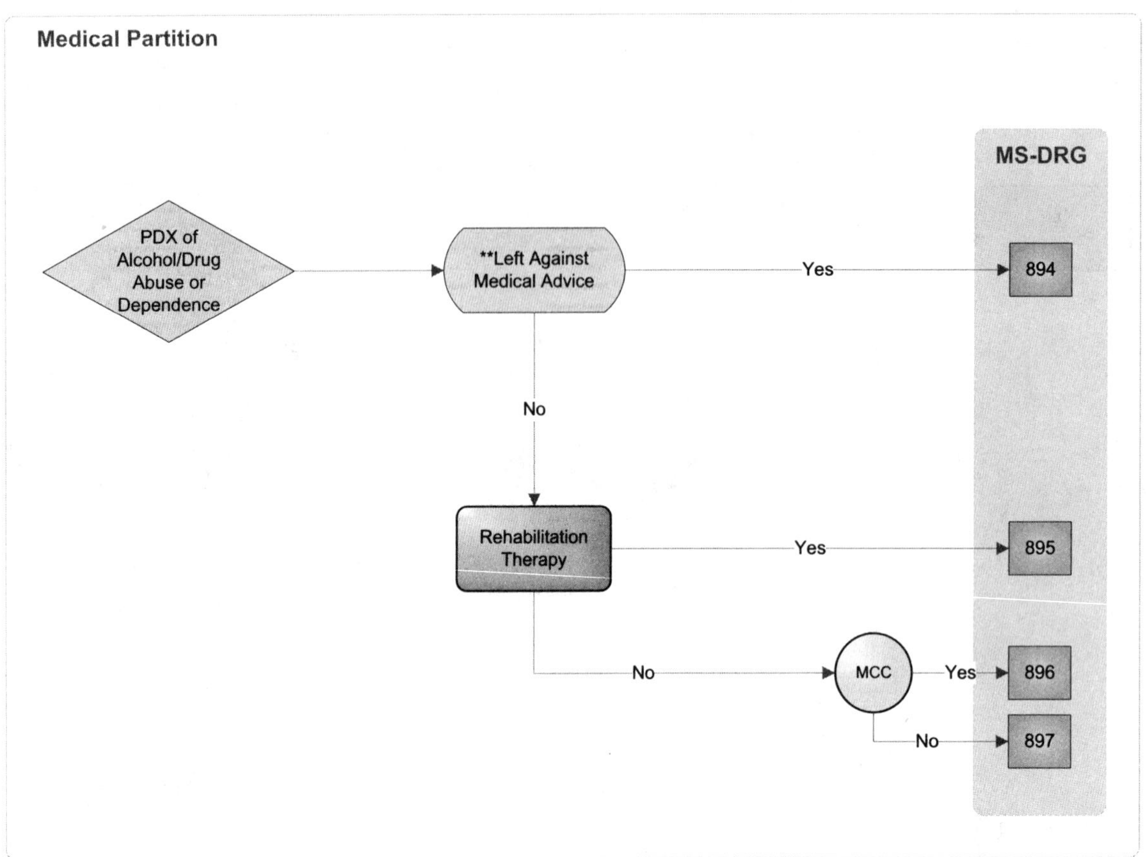

** Left Against Medical Advice = Discharge Status of 07

Major Diagnostic Category 21
Injuries, Poisonings and Toxic Effects of Drugs

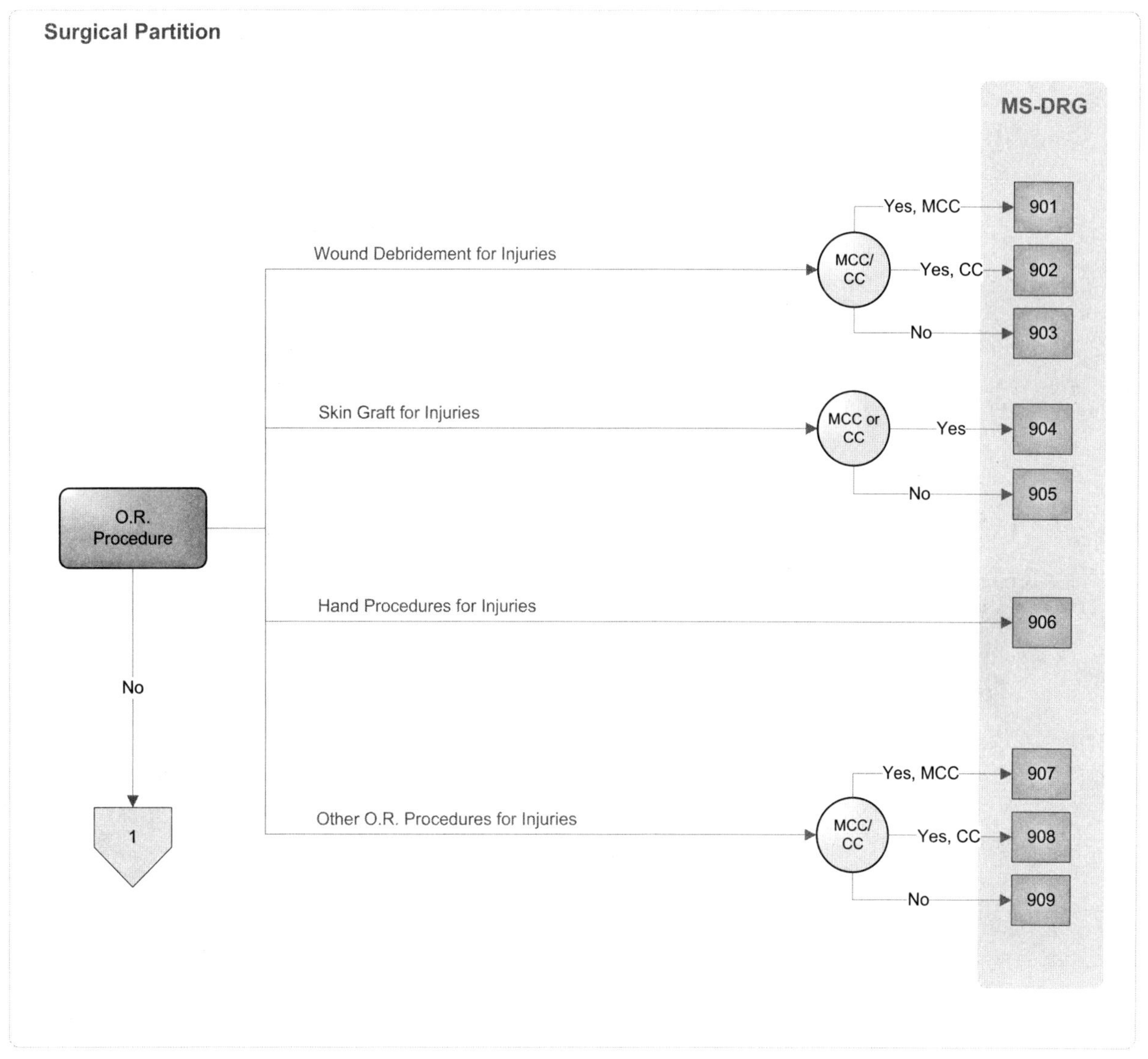

Major Diagnostic Category 21
Injuries, Poisonings and Toxic Effects of Drugs

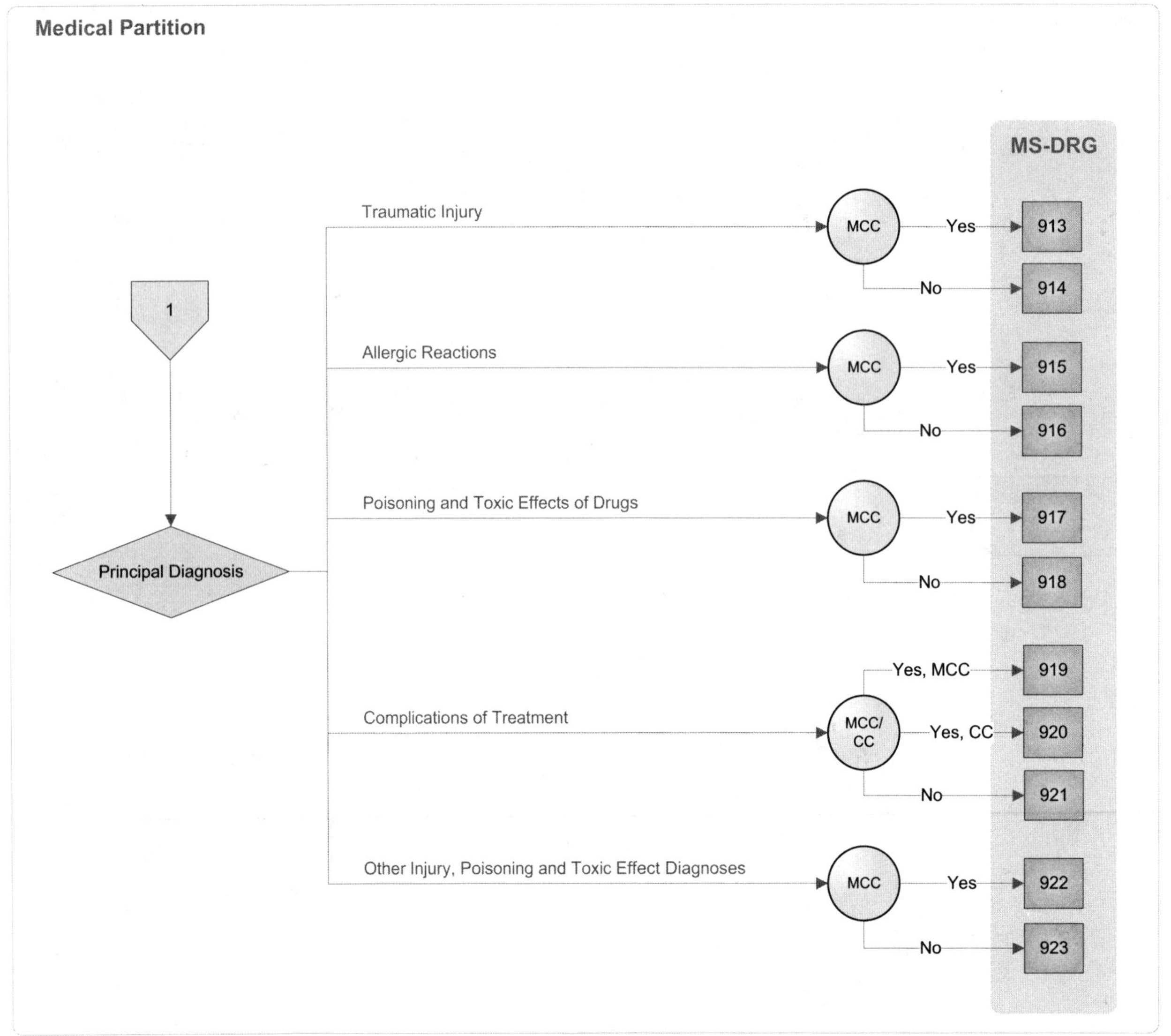

Major Diagnostic Category 22
Burns

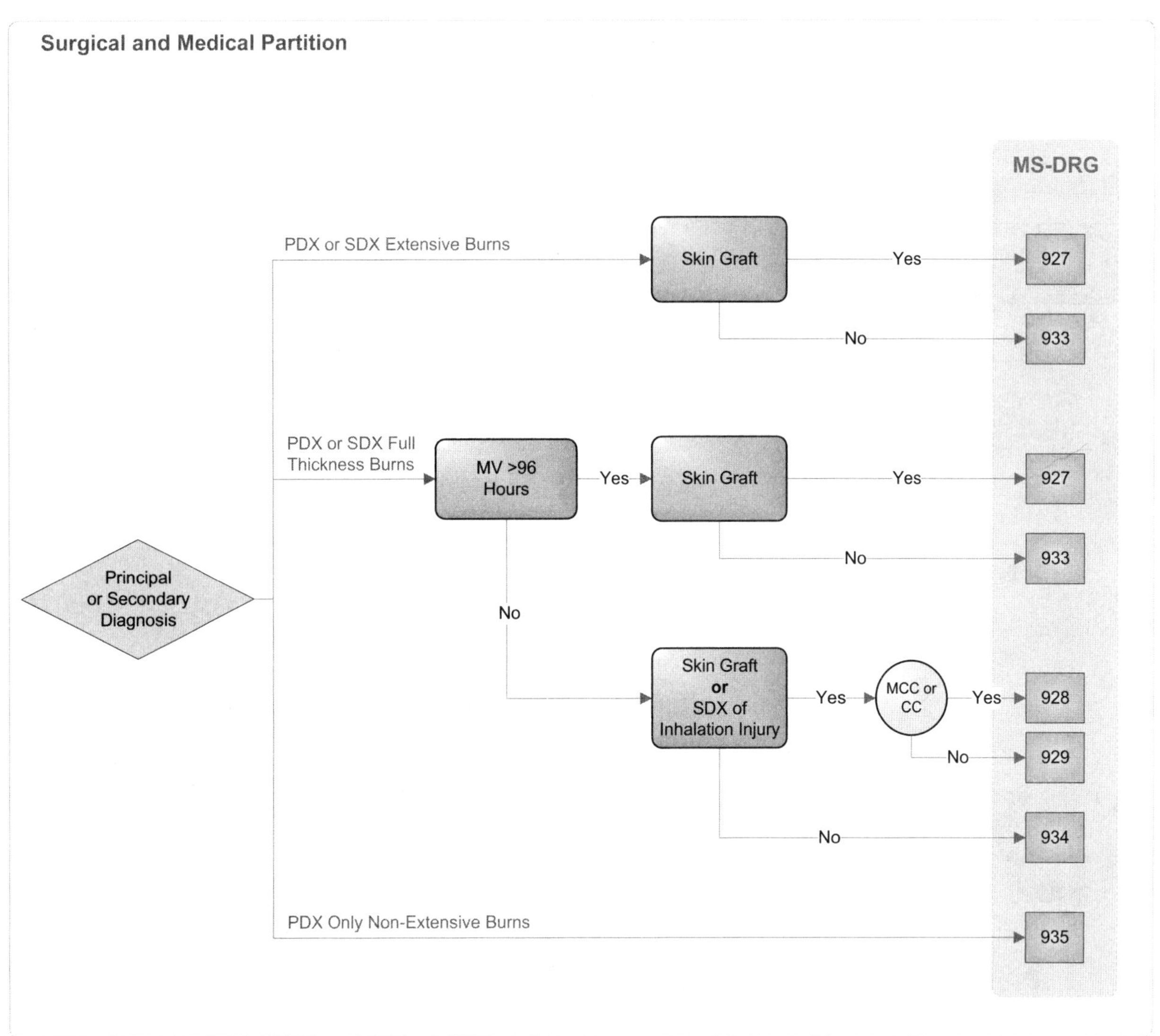

Major Diagnostic Category 23
Factors Influencing Health Status and Other Contacts with Health Services

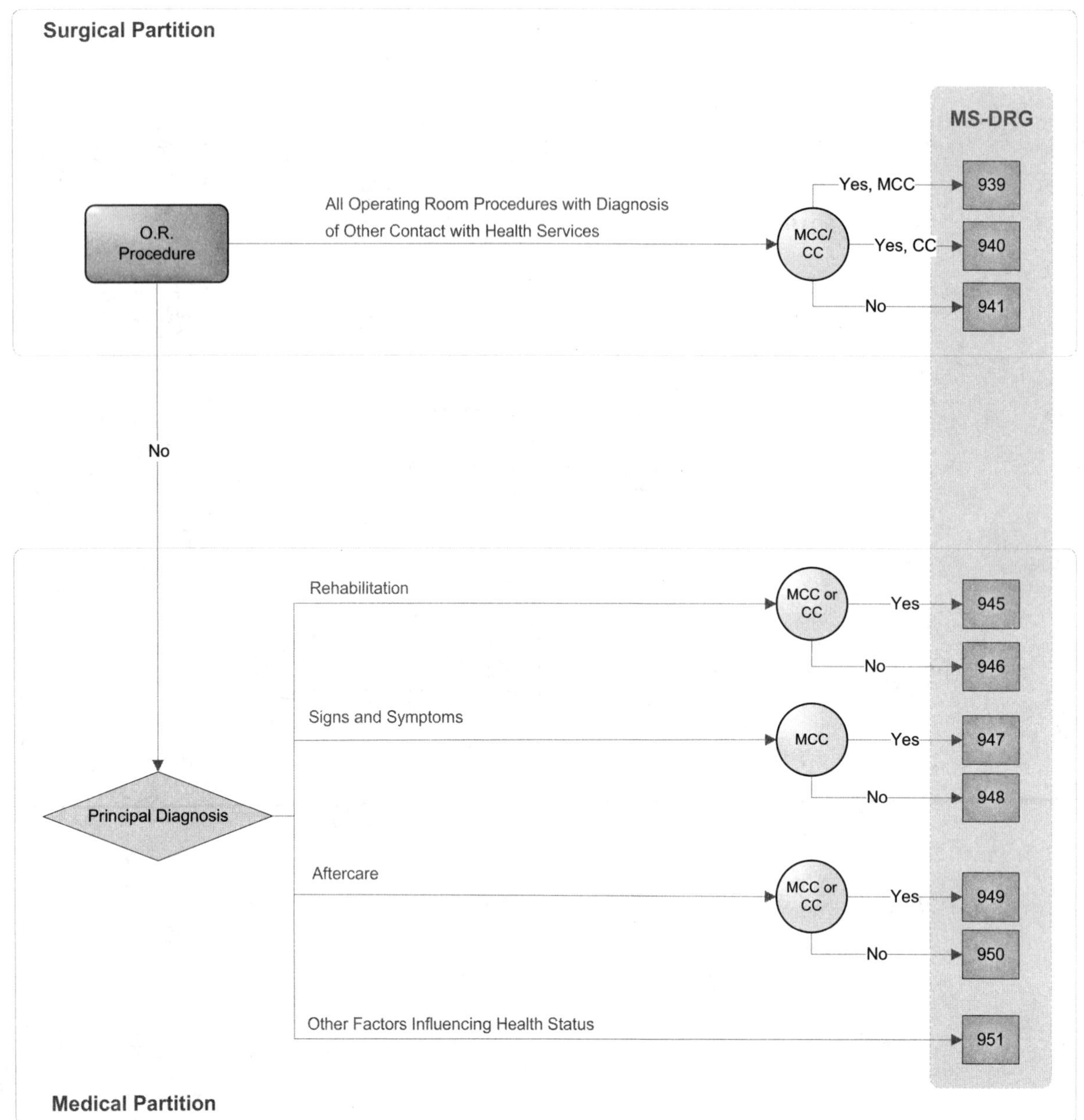

Major Diagnostic Category 24
Multiple Significant Trauma

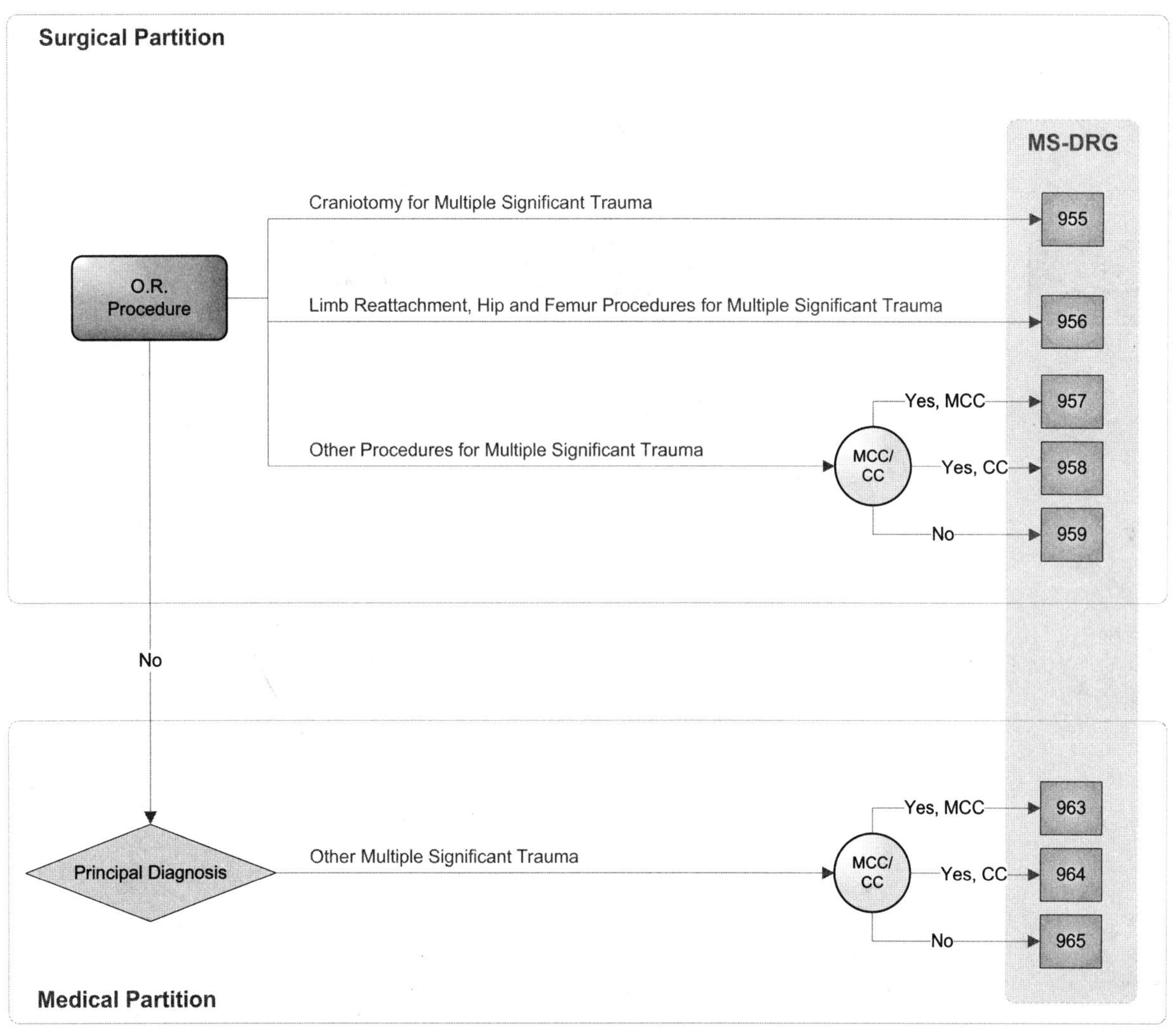

Major Diagnostic Category 25
Human Immunodeficiency Virus (HIV) Infections

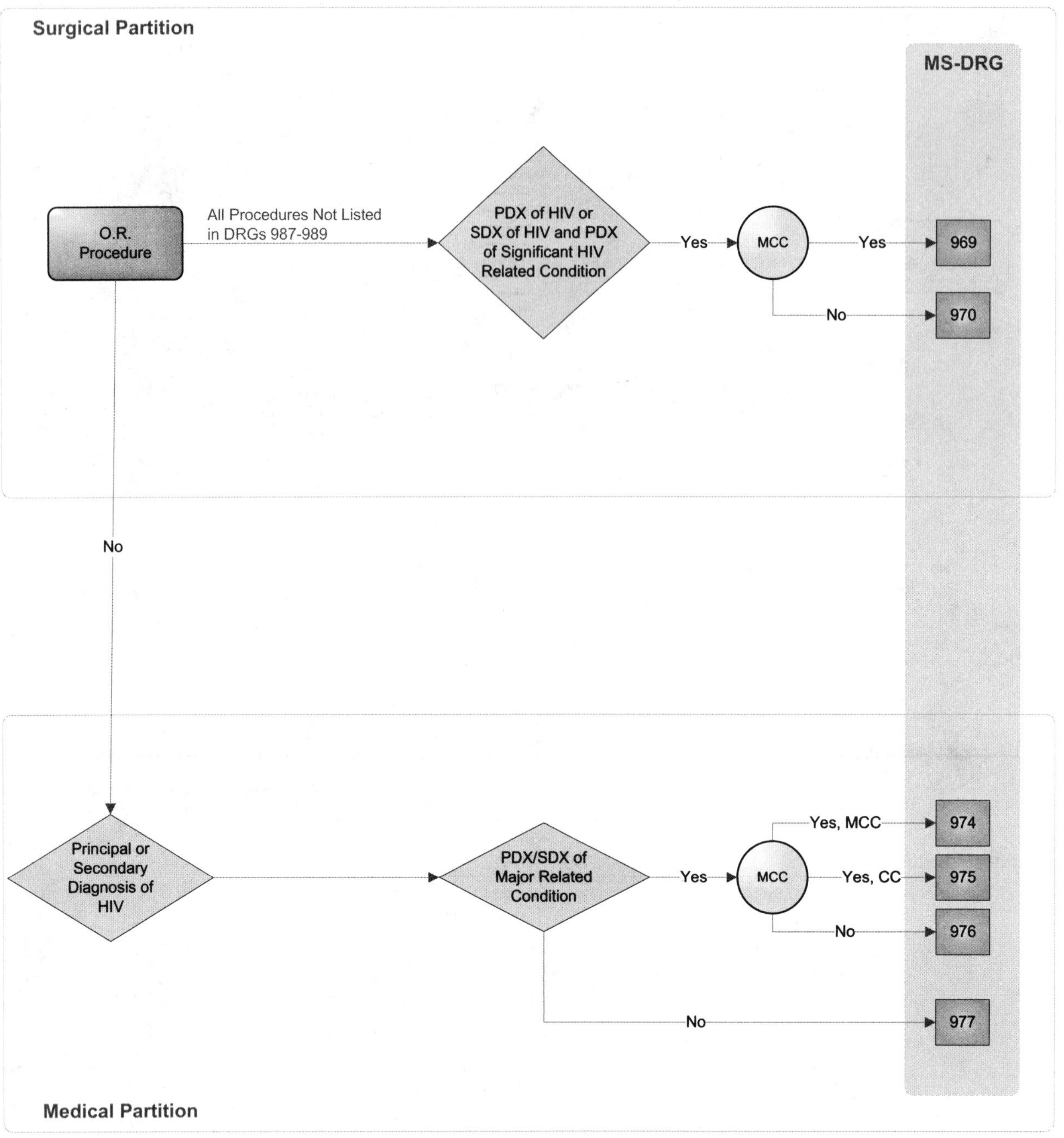

